Brief Table of Contents

Pharmacotherapeutics

Kathleen Gutierrez, PhD, RN, ANP, CNS

Associate Professor of Nursing

Department of Nursing

Regis University

Denver, Colorado

and

Adult Nurse Practitioner in Private Practice

Littleton, Colorado

Pharmacotherapeutics

Clinical Decision-Making in Nursing

W.B. SAUNDERS COMPANY

A Division of Harcourt Brace & Company

Philadelphia London Toronto Montreal Sydney Tokyo

W.B. SAUNDERS COMPANY
A Division of Harcourt Brace & Company

The Curtis Center
Independence Square West
Philadelphia, Pennsylvania 19106

Library of Congress Cataloging-in-Publication Data

Gutierrez, Kathleen.
Pharmacotherapeutics : clinical decision-making in nursing /
Kathleen Gutierrez.

p. cm.

ISBN 0–7216–5405–3

1. Chemotherapy. 2. Pharmacology. 3. Nursing. I. Title.
[DNLM: 1. Drug Therapy nurses' instruction. 2. Pharmaceutical Preparations nurses' instruction. 3. Decision-Making nurses' instruction. WB 330 G984p 1999]

RM262.G88 1999 615.5′8—dc21

DNLM/DLC 98–12900

PHARMACOTHERAPEUTICS: Clinical Decision-Making in Nursing ISBN 0–7216–5405–3

Printed in the United States of America

Last digit is the print number: 9 8 7 6 5 4 3 2 1

Dedication

Now that all is said and done, I wish to dedicate this book to my family, whose unwavering care, thoughtfulness, and guidance supported me through this lengthy endeavor.

To my husband and soul-mate Pat, who stands beside me through thick and thin, maintains our home, nourishes me, and helps me to keep my sanity—I don't know what I would do without you.

To my lovely daughter and friend Pam, whose ability to be forthright and honest with me helps keep my life in perspective especially through life's challenges.

And to my son Michael, who remains the most honest, compassionate, devoted, nonjudgmental individual I have ever known.

With all our love,
Michael Patrick Gutierrez
1970-1995

The Man in the Glass

When you get what you want in your struggle for self,
And the world makes you king for a day,
Just go to a mirror and look at yourself,
And see what that man has to say.

For it isn't your father or mother or wife,
Whose judgment upon you must pass,
The fellow whose verdict counts most in your life,
Is the one staring back from the glass.

Some people might think you're a straight-shootin' chum,
And call you a wonderful guy,
But the man in the glass says you're only a bum,
If you can't look him straight in the eye.

He's the fellow to please, never mind all the rest,
For he's with you clear up to the end.
And you've passed your most dangerous, difficult test,
If the guy in the glass is your friend.

You may fool the whole world down the pathway of years,
And get pats on the back as you pass,
But your final reward will be heartaches and tears,
If you've cheated the man in the glass.

NOTICE

Pharmacology is an ever-changing field. Standard safety precautions must be followed, but as new research and clinical experience broaden our knowledge, changes in treatment and drug therapy become necessary or appropriate. Readers are advised to check the product information currently provided by the manufacturer of each drug to be administered to verify the recommended dose, the method and duration of administration, and the contraindications. It is the responsibility of the treating physician, relying on experience and knowledge of the patient, to determine dosages and the best treatment for the patient. Neither the publisher nor the editor assumes any responsibility for any injury and/or damage to persons or property.

THE PUBLISHER

Contributors

Patricia S. Alfrey, RN, BSN, MSN
Discharge Coordinator, Home Dialysis Training, Department of Veterans Affairs Medical Center, Denver, Colorado
Drugs Used in Renal Dysfunction

Kristen Arney
Disaster Specialist, American Red Cross, Denver, Colorado
Spanish and English Phrases for Pharmacotherapeutic Assessment

Arlyne S. Barnett, MN, RN, BSPI
Senior Specialist in Poison Information, Massachusetts Poison Control Center, Boston, Massachusetts
Anticonvulsants

Marilyn Booker, RN, MS, CRNI
Consultant, Sunnybrook Services; Case Manager, Diversified Health Services, Baltimore, Maryland
Blood and Blood Products

Sheryl J. Bourque, RN, BSN, BBA/CIS, MAOM
Nursing Informatics Consultant, Self-employed; Q.A. Analyst, Surgical Services, Presbyterian Healthcare Systems, Albuquerque, New Mexico
Peptic Ulcer and Hyperacidity Drugs

Janice M. Brencick, RN, CS, PhD
Visiting Assistant Professor of Nursing, Bethel College of Nursing, University of Colorado, Colorado Springs, Colorado
Substance Abuse; Central Nervous System Stimulants

MaryAnne Bruno, BSN, MSN, PNNP
Perinatal Nurse Practitioner (PNNP), Columbia/Presbyterian St. Luke's Women's & Children's Hospital, Denver, Colorado
Fertility Drugs

Margaret Burns, RN, MSN
Travel Nurse, Medical Express
Antineoplastic Drugs

Tonya Schrader Buttry, MSN, RN-C
Chairperson, College of Nursing, Southeast Missouri Hospital, Cape Girardeau, Missouri
Anticoagulant and Antiplatelet Drugs

Judi R. Davis, MS, BS, RD
Chief HCS Dietitian Tarrant County Mental Health Mental Retardation; Nutrition Consultant, Day Care Association of Fort Worth and Tarrant County, Texas
Enteral Products Appendix G: Product Information for Selected Nutritional Supplements and Enteral Formulas

Anne Dill, MSN, RN, PNNP, CNM
Affiliate Faculty, Regis University; Perinatal Nurse Practitioner, Presbyterian/St. Luke's Medical Center, Denver, Colorado
Uterine Motility Drugs

Steven F. Finder, MD, MBA, MPH
Associate Professor, University of Texas College of Pharmacy, University of Texas, Austin, Texas; President, Med Analysis, Inc, San Antonio, Texas
Pharmacoeconomics

Sandra Franklin, RN, MS
Nursing Faculty, Arapahoe Community College, Littleton, Colorado
Antitubercular and Antileprotic Drugs; Controversy for Chapter 26

Leslie A. Gardner, MSN, RN, PNNP
Adjunct Faculty, Regis University; Perinatal Nurse Practitioner, Presbyterian/St. Luke's Medical Center, Denver, Colorado
Hormonal Contraceptives and Related Drugs

Kathleen Gutierrez, PhD, RN, ANP, CNS
Associate Professor of Nursing, Department of Nursing, Regis University, Denver, Colorado; Adult Nurse Practitioner, in Private Practice, Littleton, Colorado
The History of Pharmacology; Pharmacotherapeutics; Pharmaceutics and Pharmacokinetics; Pharmacodynamics; Geriatric Pharmacotherapeutics; Sympathetic Nervous System Drugs; Opioid Analgesics and Related Drugs; Nonsteroidal Anti-Inflammatory, Disease-Modifying Antirheumatic, and Related Drugs; Antianxiety and Sedative-Hypnotic Drugs; Biologic Response Modifiers; Inotropic Drugs; Antianginal Drugs; Antiarrhythmic Drugs; Antilipemic Drugs; Laxatives and Antidiarrheal Drugs; Antiemetic Drugs; Cation-Exchange Resins and Ammonia-Detoxifying Drugs; Antiasthmatic and Bronchodilator Drugs; Antihistamines and Related Drugs; Expectorants, Antitussives, Decongestants, and Mucolytics; Pancreatic Drugs; Alkalinizing and Acidifying Drugs; Ophthalmic Drugs; Appendix A: Resources in Supporting Orphan Drug Development; Appendix B: Selected Internet Accessible Information Databases; Appendix C: Dietary Considerations; Appendix D: Influence of Drugs on Laboratory Values; Appendix E: Selected Formulas Used in Pharmacotherapeutics

Kamal Hijjazi, PhD, RN
Assistant Professor, Department of Nursing, Simmons College; Research Analyst, US Department of Health and Human Services; Fellow, Gerontology Institute, University of Massachusetts, Boston, Massachusetts
Pituitary Drugs

Mary J. Hillyard, RN, MSN
Nurse Manager, Dialysis Unit, Veterans Affairs Medical Center, Denver, Colorado
Diuretic Drugs

Karen A. Karlowicz, MSN, RN, CURN
Lecturer—Adult Health, Gerontology and Rehabilitation Nursing, School of Nursing, College of Health Science, Old Dominion University, Norfolk, Virginia
Urinary Antimicrobial and Related Drugs

E. Jacquelyn Kirkis, BSN, BSc, MSc, RNP
Nursing Faculty, Pima Community College; CEO, Echoes and Associates, Inc, Tucson, Arizona
Anthelmintic, Antimalarial and Antiparasitic Drugs

Elizabeth W. Kissell, BSN, MSNE
Affiliate Faculty, Regis University, Denver, Colorado
Appendix F: Administration Techniques

Jane Koeckeritz, PhD, CANP, RN
Associate Professor, University of Northern Colorado, Greeley, Colorado; Staff Nurse, Emergency Department, Poudre Valley Hospital, Fort Collins, Colorado
Intravenous Therapy

Pamala D. Larsen, PhD
Director, Undergraduate Nursing Program, School of Nursing, Wichita State University, Wichita, Kansas
Androgens and Anabolic Steroids

Karen LeDuc, BSN, MSN
Affiliate Faculty, Clinical Instructor, Regis University, University of Colorado Health Science Center; Level V Staff Nurse, The Children's Hospital, Denver, Colorado
Pediatric Pharmacotherapeutics

Linda Eilee Schmidt McCuistion, RN, BSN, MN, PhD
Associate Professor, Our Lady of Holy Cross College, New Orleans, Louisiana
Antibiotic Drugs

Maureen McDonald, MS, RN, CS
Associate Professor, Massasait Community College, Brockton Hospital School of Nursing, Brockton, Massachusetts
Antiviral and Antifungal Drugs; Controversy for Chapter 25; Antihypertensive Drugs

Deborah Cooper McGee, BSN, MSN, PNNP
Clinical Liaison, Perinatal Nurse Practitioner Program, Adjunct Faculty, Regis University, Department of Nursing; Coordinator, Perinatal Nurse Practitioner Services, Columbia Presbyterian/St Luke's Medical Center, Denver, Colorado
Perinatal Pharmacotherapeutics; Appendix G: Effects of Selected Maternal Drug Ingestion on the Fetus or Neonate

Judy Malkiewicz, RN, PhD
Professor, University of Northern Colorado, School of Nursing, Greeley, Colorado
Adrenal Cortex Drugs and Inhibitors; Otic Drugs

Jan Hoot Martin, RN, PhD, GNP
Associate Professor, University of Northern Colorado, Greeley, Colorado
Adrenal Cortex Drugs and Inhibitors; Otic Drugs

Kimberly Mathai, MS, RD
Adjunct Professor, North Seattle Community College Nutritional Consultant, Nutrition by Design, Inc.; Corporate Wellness Presenter, Nutrition Concepts, Inc. Seattle, Washington
Complementary and Adjunctive Therapies

Phyllis S. Moore, DNSc, RN, CS
Professor, Department of Nursing, Simmons College, Boston, Massachusetts
Anticonvulsants

Sandra Maree Ouellette, CRNA, MEd, FAAN
Visiting Assistant Professor, The University of North Carolina, Greensboro, Greensboro, North Carolina; Program Director, Wake Forest University Baptist Medical Center, Winston-Salem, North Carolina
Anesthetic Drugs

Barbara A. Pedersen, MSN, RNC, ANP
Adult Nurse Practitioner, Rheumatology and Dermatology Departments; Department of Veterans Affairs Medical Center—Denver, Denver, Colorado
Community Pharmacotherapeutics

Phyllis G. Peterson, BA, RN, BSN, MN
Assistant Professor, Division of Nursing, Our Lady of Holy Cross College, New Orleans, Louisiana
Antineoplastic Drugs

Barbara Pfretzschner, RN, MSN, CNS
Staff Nurse, Emergency Department, Centura Health–St. Anthony Central Hospital, Denver, Colorado
Antiparkinsonian and Myasthenia Gravis Drugs

Keith A. Rains, BSN, RN
Infection Control Practitioner, Department of Veterans Affairs Medical Center, Denver, Colorado
Antianxiety and Sedative-Hypnotic Drugs

Elizabeth Anne DeSalvo Rankin, PhD, RNC, NBCCH, CHES
Professor, Department of Nursing, Henson School of Science and Technology, Salisbury State University, Salisbury, Maryland
Antipsychotic Drugs

Eve Romero, MSN, RN
Registered Nurse, Western Medical Services, Denver, Colorado
Dermatologic Drugs

Sally Schnell, RN, MSN, CNRN
Professional Education Coordinator, Regional Organ Bank of Illinois, Chicago, Illinois
Parasympathetic Nervous System Drugs; Controversy for Chapter 13

Elizabeth Lamb Shannon, MSN, BSN, CPNP
Assistant Professor, Simmons College, Boston, Massachusetts
Neuromuscular Blocking Drugs

Donna Shirrell, MSN
Assistant Professor, Coordinator—Medical Surgical Nursing, Southeast Missouri Hospital College of Nursing, Cape Girardeau, Missouri
Thrombolytic and Sclerosing Drugs

Golden M. Tradewell, MA, MSN
Assistant Professor, Adult Health Clinical Nurse Specialist, College of Nursing, McNeese State University, Lake Charles, Louisiana
Vitamins and Minerals

Glenn A. Webster, PhD
Associate Professor of Philosophy, University of Colorado, Denver, Colorado
Substance Abuse; Central Nervous System Stimulants

Carol M. Wester, RN, MSN, CS, CNA
Hopewell Associates, Inc., President; Consultant; Director of Continuing Education; Director of Psychopharmacology Services, Mattapoisette, Massachusetts
Antidepressant and Antimania Drugs

Sheila Winters, BS Ed, MEd
Adjunct Faculty, University of Colorado School of Nursing; Instructor, University of Phoenix; Nurse Practitioner, Veterans Affairs Medical Center, Denver, Colorado
Skeletal Muscle Relaxants; Thyroid and Parathyroid Drugs

Jonathan J. Wolfe, PhD, RPH
Associate Professor, University of Arkansas for Medical Sciences, Department of Pharmacy Practice, Little Rock, Arkansas
Controversies for Chapters 6, 8, 9, 14, 15, 16, 17, 18, 20, 21, 22, 24, 25, 28, 29, 31, 33, 34, 35, 36, 42, 43, 48, 49, 53, 54, 55, 56, 58, 59, 60, and 64

Deborah Wujcik, RN, MSN, AOCN
Adjunct Faculty, Vanderbilt School of Nursing, Nashville, Tennessee; Clinical Director, Vanderbilt Cancer Center, Nashville, Tennessee
Biologic Response Modifiers

Yvonne Yousey, BSN, MS, CPNP
Clinical Faculty, University of Colorado Health Sciences Center, School of Nursing, Denver, Colorado
Sera, Vaccines, and Immunizing Drugs

Preface

Most contacts between health care providers and their patients end with a prescription for drugs or other kinds of therapy. Today, health care providers and patients are influenced by advertising and promotion, managed health care and restricted formularies, and time limitations that complicate the decision-making process in the choice of one drug over another. New information floods the market daily, rendering previously memorized drug data useless.

This text was conceived and designed to help students understand the multidisciplinary science of pharmacology, which is based on physical and chemical principles applied to living systems. Learning pharmacology focuses on the unifying elements in specific groups of drugs that exhibit common effects and mechanisms of action. Students integrate knowledge of drugs, physiology, pathophysiology, and disease with patient profiles in order to make clinical decisions and apply the mechanisms of pharmacotherapeutics.

Drug regimens and patients are dynamic. Throughout this text, drugs are discussed with the disorders for which they are generally accepted to be the most appropriate treatment. Often, the clinical use of a drug changes over time, with previous indications being either deleted or new ones added. And as scientists explore better treatment options, improved drug therapies continually replace older agents. There are always areas in which treatment engenders substantial debate, and this may cause a drug regimen discussed here to seem inappropriate to some clinicians. In order to disseminate the most accurate and clinically appropriate information, contributors to this volume include practicing clinicians, academicians, and pharmacists. Professionals in relevant specialty areas extensively analyzed all details. Their joint efforts have produced a resource that is in accord with current clinical practice.

Philosophy

Pharmacotherapeutics must be based on factual information about chemical and functional drug classifications, indications, adverse effects and contraindications, age-related variables, dosages, and nursing implications. However, successful clinical practice is built on a decision-making process that identifies concepts and principles that illuminate the importance, meaning, and rationale for choosing one drug over another. This text moves beyond memorization in a ground-breaking approach that uses clinical application of all pertinent facts to promote the best patient care.

Organization

This text is organized around two distinct content areas. The 10 chapters in Unit I focus on the link between pharmacology and professional nursing practice. This unit grounds the student in the history of pharmacology and thoroughly explains the concepts of pharmacotherapeutics, pharmacoeconomics, pharmaceutics, pharmacokinetics, and pharmacodynamics. Age-related variables are explored in detail in the chapters on perinatal, pediatric, and geriatric pharmacotherapeutics. The chapter on community issues addresses over-the-counter medications, legislative concerns, drug compliance, patient education, and community resources. And the chapter on substance abuse discusses the use of both prescriptive and illicit drugs in a culture that sometimes promotes dependence.

The remaining units are organized around the influence of drugs on the various body systems and nutritional balance. Units II, III, and IV provide an introductory discussion of appropriate physiology: the autonomic and central nervous systems and the immune system. Chapters include discussions on diseases or disorders relevant to the particular system, beginning with an overview of the pathology involved. To correlate pathophysiology with pharmacology, these topics are followed by a discussion of treatment objectives that include pharmacotherapeutic options with listings of appropriate drugs including the generic name, brand name, and Canadian equivalents where applicable. Indications, adverse effects and contraindications, pharmacodynamics, pharmacokinetics, dosage regimen, and laboratory considerations are also discussed. Each discussion includes a clinical case study within a framework of patient assessment. Finally, the sections on analysis and management, intervention, and evaluation demonstrate the application of the decision-making process.

Special Features

Pharmacotherapeutic Decision-Making Process

Clinical chapters provide the expected requisite drug information and apply the knowledge, decision-making process, and case management techniques through the case studies. The basic purpose of this model is to focus on pharmacotherapeutics, ruling in some factors as germane to the drug decision and ruling out others because of their lesser importance to patient outcomes. The utility of the model comes from the systematic organization it provides for thinking, observing, and analyzing treatment regimens. In addition, it provides structure and rationale for specific nursing activities and a mechanism for professional accountability. The model also provides criteria for knowing when a patient problem has been solved.

Body System Organization

The body system approach helps the reader make logical connections between major drug groups and the conditions for which drugs are commonly used. Each of the clinical units represents major body systems. A chapter on complementary and adjunctive therapies is also included and addresses the roles of naturopathy, homeopathy, acupuncture, and herbs in pharmacotherapy.

Integration of Physiology, Pathophysiology, and Pharmacology

The integration of physiology and pathophysiology with the study of pharmacology provides students with an understanding of the physical and cellular causes of specific diseases and the advantage of specific drugs for therapy. Examples of physiologic and pathophysiologic processes discussed include pain and the use of opioid analgesics and nonsteroidal anti-inflammatory drugs, multiple sclerosis and the role of skeletal muscle relaxants, the antimicrobial therapy used for tuberculosis, and the role of antiarrhythmic drugs in treating arrhythmias.

Clinical Case Studies

Forty-six individual case studies present patient profiles and highlight the many variables that influence the clinical decision-making process in pharmacotherapeutics. Each case study explores how factors such as age, economic status, co-morbidity, and drug characteristics affect drug selection. Inclusion of average wholesale drug prices from the 1998 *Drug Topics Redbook* in each case study clearly demonstrates the importance that economic considerations play in pharmacotherapeutic decision-making.

Controversies

Throughout the text, readers will find controversy boxes, designed to increase awareness of the ethical, legal, and practical dilemmas associated with pharmacology. More than 30 controversies address issues such as why we question the use of generic drugs, the administration of opioids to chemically dependent patients, immunization policy issues, the use of the antidepressant fluoxetine for managing weight loss, and the wisdom of using directly observed therapy in the management of tuberculosis. Each controversy presents the pros and cons of the issue, and provides critical thinking questions for readers to ponder and formulate their own opinions on the topic.

Pharmacokinetic Tables

Pharmacokinetics describes what happens to a drug following administration—what the body does with the drug. These tables appear in each of the clinical chapters and provide an overview of drug absorption, distribution, biotransformation, elimination, protein binding, and half-life.

Drug-Drug Interaction Tables

Drug-drug interactions are often the by-product of concurrent administration of two or more drugs or of a food-drug combination. The results can be physical, chemical, or biologic effects. Although some drug-drug interactions are intentional and seen as beneficial, others may diminish a drug's therapeutic benefits or increase the risk of adverse effects. The number of potentially significant drug-drug interactions increases as pharmacotherapy becomes more complex and drugs more potent. Each of the clinical chapters contains Drug-Drug Interaction tables.

Dosage Regimen Tables

There are no common characteristics among dosage regimens, nor is there an overall pattern to their numeric figures or dosing frequency. Even the terms dose and dosage are used interchangeably. The Dosage Regimen tables in this book include the usual routes of drug administration, along with the adult and pediatric dosages and units of measurement commonly used in the management of disease.

Illustrations

The illustrations in this text begin with a timeline on drug development and progress through graphs, charts, algorithms, products, and human physiology at the system and cellular levels. All were carefully chosen and designed to maximize visual communication and enable students to understand better how drugs work. Whether the drawings show the pharmacokinetic phases, examine toxic range, outline the nervous system, describe antidepressants or antibiotics action, or follow the steps from an injured blood vessel to fibrin-platelet plug, all became integral to the written text and enhance the learning process.

Additional Resources

For Instructors

The teaching package includes an Instructor's Manual consisting of lecture outlines and learning activities. Also, on adoption, instructors will receive a complimentary printed test bank, a set of two-color transparencies, and test-generating software called ExaMaster.

For Students

Pharmacology is a demanding science. The companion Study Guide for *Pharmacotherapeutics: Clinical Decision-Making in Nursing* complements the text. It provides a wealth of learning opportunities that help reinforce pharmacology content and foster understanding of pharmacotherapeutic decision-making. The case studies help the student apply the pharmacotherapeutic decision-making process to various clinical scenarios. Review exercises expand the student's understanding of the importance of patient education. Puzzles are interjected for fun but are also designed to encourage critical thinking in a way that has previously been underused. Because suggested responses to exercises and case studies are provided in the back of this guide, students have a valuable opportunity to check learning effectiveness immediately.

Comments

Every effort has been made to ensure that this comprehensive text is accurate and user friendly. We hope that it will provide students, educators, and clinicians with a valuable frame of reference, as well as expand their understanding and practice of pharmacotherapeutics. We look forward to your comments and suggestions as you use this text and its companion resources.

Kathleen Gutierrez
kgutierr@usa.net

Acknowledgments

No author writes a book alone. A project of this size could not come to fruition without the collaboration of many people. First and foremost, my thanks and appreciation to Janet Velasquez, RN, MS, retired nursing educator from the Community College of Denver, who 29 years ago fostered an initial interest in pharmacology and nursing and facilitated my first opportunity to teach these subjects. My first group of students and I struggled with the abundance of pharmacology information and teaching strategies to enhance their learning. Over the years students have contributed valuable insight into sorting the information that is *need-to-know* from *nice-to-know* and *fluff*.

My thanks also go to the many nurse educators and clinicians for their collaboration over a number of years. Their patience and sharing of expertise have permitted the development of a text that will become a gold standard in nursing pharmacology education.

Most of the Controversies were written by Jonathan J. Wolfe, PhD, RPh, Associate Professor at the University of Arkansas for Medical Sciences Department of Pharmacy Practice, College of Pharmacy. Thank you Jonathan for your diligence, expertise, and understanding of deadlines. You have been a valuable asset and resource to this project.

The excellent illustrations are the work of Hans Neuhart of the Electronic Illustrators Group in Fountain Hills, Arizona, and Risa J. Clow, Matt Andrews, and Sharon Iwanczuk at W. B. Saunders.

There are many individuals at W. B. Saunders who have made this book a reality. Thank you, Thomas Eoyang, Vice-President and Editor-in-Chief of Nursing Books, for your willingness to take on a new author, ongoing support, and encouragement. Thank you, Maura Connor, Senior Editor, for continually sound advice, marketing savvy, friendship, and the gracious permission to use your photograph in a very pregnant state. Thank you Sue Bredensteiner, Developmental Editor, for your day-to-day accessibility, realistic perspective, help, guidance, and encouragement to complete the project. Thank you, Carol DiBerardino, Copy Editor, for your patience and understanding as this new author successfully waded through the copy editing process and for fielding the myriad changes, additions, and deletions with unwavering poise; to Pat Morrison, Art Director, for coordinating the artwork; to Jeff Gunning, Production Manager, for keeping the text on schedule despite overwhelming odds and delays. Thank you, Rachel Hubbs, former Assistant Developmental Editor, and Victoria Legnini, Editorial Assistant, for coordinating the peer reviews of the many chapters and handling numerous administrative tasks associated with publication of a book.

My thanks also to the many individuals who reviewed the initial manuscript drafts and provided valuable insight regarding content and structure. Although the reviews were not always pleasant to read, they helped keep my ego in check and fostered the quality of the final product.

Last, my thanks to you—nursing educators and students—for permitting me to join you in the teaching and learning of pharmacology. I trust that you will find this first edition of *Pharmacotherapeutics: Clinical Decision-Making in Nursing* a valuable addition to your repertoire of educational materials.

Kathleen Gutierrez, PhD, RN, ANP, CNS

Reviewer List

Jeanette Adams, DrPH, RN, ANP, AOCN
School of Nursing
University of Texas–Houston
Health Science Center
Houston, Texas

Donna Baker, MSN, RN
Central Missouri State University
Warrensburg, Missouri

Linda C. Baker, RN, C, MSN, FNP
Scottsdale Community College
Scottsdale, Arizona

Jean Krajicek Bartek, PhD, RN, ARNP, CARN
Associate Professor
Colleges of Nursing & Medicine
University of Nebraska Medical Center
Omaha, Nebraska

Linda J. Becker, MSN, RNC
St. Clair County Community College
Port Huron, Michigan

Carita A. Bird, MSN, RNC
Haywood Community College–Region A Nursing Consortium
Clyde, North Carolina

Ilene Borze, MS, RN, CEN
Gateway Community College
Phoenix, Arizona

Susanne Boustany, BSN, RN
State University of New York Health Science Center at Syracuse
Syracuse, New York

Angel A. Brown, MSN, RN, CNM, C-FNP
New River Birth Center
New River Family Health Center
Scarbo, West Virginia

Carol Cassini, MS, RN
Rush University
Chicago, Illinois

Anne O'Rourke Cloutier, MSN, RN, AOCN
Schering Oncology Biotech
Kenilworth, New Jersey

Deborah Padgett Coehlo, MN, RN, C-PNP
School of Nursing
Oregon Health Sciences University at Southern Oregon State College
Ashland, Oregon

JoAnn Coleman, MS, RN, CS, CANP, OCN
Johns Hopkins Hospital
Baltimore, Maryland

Sharon I. Decker, MSN, RN, CS, CCRN
Associate Professor of Clinical Nursing
Director, Clinical Simulation Center
Texas Tech University Health Sciences Center
Lubbock, Texas

Deborah Deierlein, MS, RN, ANP, CS
Stony Brook Medical Center
Stony Brook, New York

Janet Duffy Dionne, MS, RN
Community College of Denver
Denver, Colorado

Janet M. Farahmand, EdD, MSN
Associate Professor of Nursing
Division of Nursing
Neumann College
Aston, Pennsylvania

Mary Kay Flynn, DNSc, RN, CCRN
Samaritan College of Nursing
Grand Canyon University
Phoenix, Arizona

Edward M. Freeman, PhD, ARNP, CS
Associate Professor
College of Nursing
Florida Atlantic University
Boca Raton, Florida

Jacquelyn L. Gaddy, MS, RN, CDE
School of Nursing
Southern Illinois University at Edwardsville
Edwardsville, Illinois

Mary Jo Gerlach, MSNEd, RN
School of Nursing
Medical College of Georgia
Athens, Georgia

Margaret M. Gingrich, MSN, RN
Harrisburg Area Community College
Harrisburg, Pennsylvania

Judy L. Goodhart, MSN, RN
Associate Professor
Baccalaureate Nursing Program
Mesa State College
Grand Junction, Colorado

Karen E. Groth, MN, RN, CS
Doctoral Candidate
Department of Nursing
Gonzaga University
Spokane, Washington

Paul O. Gubbins, PharmD
Department of Pharmacy Practice
College of Pharmacy
University of Arkansas for Medical Sciences
Little Rock, Arkansas

Pamala K. Hays, MSN, RN
Nursing Instructor
John A. Logan College
Carterville, Illinois

Patricia C. Hermanson, MSN, FNP
Gerontological Nurse Practitioner
MedCenter One College of Nursing
Bismarck, North Dakota

Barbara D. Horton, MS, RN
Nursing Educator
School of Nursing
Arnot Ogden Medical Center
Elmira, New York

Paulette J. Perrone Hoyer, PhD, RNC
College of Nursing
Wayne State University
Detroit, Michigan

Brenda P. Johnson, MSN
Geriatric Nurse Practitioner
Southeast Missouri State University
Cape Girardeau, Missouri

Mary Jane Jones, MN, RN
Henderson Community College
Henderson, Kentucky; and
St. Mary's Hospital
Evansville, Indiana

Cara J. Krulewitch, PhD, MS, RN
Adjunct Instructor
Columbia Union College
Takoma Park, Maryland

Nita Liptak, MSEd, MSN, RN
School of Nursing
Shadyside Hospital
Pittsburgh, Pennsylvania

Anita Loos-Hannifan, MSN, RN, C-GNP
Department of Veterans Affairs
Long Beach, California

Catherine M. MacLeod, MD
Rush-Presbyterian-St. Luke's Medical Center
Chicago, Illinois

William James McIntyre, PharmD
Arkansas Cancer Research Center
College of Pharmacy
University of Arkansas for Medical Sciences
Little Rock, Arkansas

Sandra G. Mattox, BSN, RNP, OCN
Arkansas Cancer Research Center
University of Arkansas for Medical Sciences
Little Rock, Arkansas

Elaine Negley, MSN, RNC
Veterans Affairs Nursing Home Care Unit
Wilmington, Delaware

Sheila F. Norton, MSN, RN, CNM
Doctoral Student, Harvard Graduate School of Education
Clinical Practice
Harvard Community Health Plan
Boston, Massachusetts

Dorothy M. Obester, PhD, MSN, RN
St. Francis College
Loretto, Pennsylvania

Nancy O'Donnell, MSN, RN
J. Sargeant Reynolds Community College
Richmond, Virginia

Barbara L. Ogden, MSN, RNC
College of Nursing
University of Florida
Gainesville Veterans Affairs Medical Center
Gainesville, Florida

Barbara K. Polacsek, MA, RN
Norwalk Community-Technical College
Norwalk, Connecticut

Lois H. Rafenski, EdD, RN
State University of New York at Farmingdale
Farmingdale, New York

Margaret A. Reilly, PhD, MS
School of Nursing
Concordia College
Bronxville, New York; and
Phillips Beth Israel
New York, New York

Rob Rockhold, PhD
Professor of Pharmacology & Toxicology
Associate Professor of Research
Department of Emergency Medicine
University of Mississippi Medical Center
Jackson, Mississippi

Lynn M. Stover, MSN, RNC
University of Alabama
Capstone College of Nursing
Tuscaloosa, Alabama

Barbara Ann Stuart, MS, RN, FNP
Oregon Health Sciences University at Oregon Institute of Technology
Klamath Falls, Oregon

Gregory M. Susla, PharmD
National Institutes of Health
Bethesda, Maryland

Diane M. Tomasic, EdD, RN
Professor of Nursing
West Liberty State College
West Liberty, West Virginia

Constance R. Uphold, PhD, ARNP, RN, CNS
University of Florida
Gainesville, Florida

Karen Kay Vietz, MS, RN
Johns Hopkins Hospital
Baltimore, Maryland

M.J.A. Walker, PhD
Department of Pharmacology & Therapeutics
University of British Columbia
Vancouver, British Columbia

Kathleen S. Whalen, MN, RN, CCRN
Community College of Denver
Denver, Colorado

Jonathan J. Wolfe, PhD, RPh
Department of Pharmacy Practice
College of Pharmacy
University of Arkansas for Medical Sciences
Little Rock, Arkansas

Bruce H. Woolley, PharmD
Professor of Pharmacology & Nutrition
Brigham Young University
Provo, Utah

Contents

Unit I
Pharmacology and Professional Nursing Practice

Chapter 1
The History of Pharmacology 2
Kathleen Gutierrez

Chapter 2
Pharmacotherapeutics 19
Kathleen Gutierrez

Chapter 3
Pharmacoeconomics 30
Steven F. Finder

Chapter 4
Pharmaceutics and Pharmacokinetics 41
Kathleen Gutierrez

Chapter 9

Chapter 10

Unit II
Drugs Influencing the Autonomic Nervous System

Chapter 11

Chapter 12

Chapter 13

Parasympathetic Nervous System Drugs 201

Sally Schnell

Unit III

Drugs Influencing the Central Nervous System

Kathleen Gutierrez

Chapter 14

Opioid Analgesics and Related Drugs 226

Kathleen Gutierrez

Chapter 15

Nonsteroidal Anti-Inflammatory, Disease-Modifying Antirheumatic, and Related Drugs 248

Kathleen Gutierrez

Chapter 28

Sera, Vaccines, and Immunizing Drugs 582

Yvonne Yousey

Chapter 29

Biologic Response Modifiers 605

Deborah Wujcik and Kathleen Gutierrez

Chapter 30

Antineoplastic Drugs 627

Phyllis G. Peterson and Margaret Burns

Unit V
Drugs Influencing the Cardiovascular System

Chapter 31

Chapter 32

Chapter 33

Chapter 34

Chapter 35

Unit VI
Drugs Influencing the Hematologic System

Chapter 36
Anticoagulant and Antiplatelet Drugs 774
Tonya Schrader Buttry

Chapter 37
Thrombolytic and Sclerosing Drugs 791
Donna Shirrell

Chapter 38
Blood and Blood Products 806
Marilyn Booker

Unit VII
Drugs Influencing the Renal and Urinary Systems

Chapter 39
Diuretic Drugs 822
Mary J. Hillyard

Chapter 40

Chapter 41

Unit VIII
Drugs Influencing the Gastrointestinal Tract

Chapter 42

Chapter 43

Unit X
Drugs Influencing the Endocrine System

Chapter 49

Chapter 50

Chapter 51

Chapter 52

Adrenal Cortex Drugs and Inhibitors 1091

Jan Hoot Martin and Judy Malkiewicz

Chapter 53

Androgens and Anabolic Steroids 1114

Pamala D. Larsen

Chapter 54

Hormonal Contraceptives and Related Drugs 1129

Leslie A. Gardner

Chapter 55

Uterine Motility Drugs 1155

Anne Dill

Chapter 56

Fertility Drugs 1170

MaryAnne Bruno

Unit XI

Drugs Influencing Nutritional Balance

Chapter 57

Intravenous Therapy 1190

Jane Koeckeritz

Chapter 58

Vitamins and Minerals 1208

Golden M. Tradewell

Chapter 64

Unit XIII
Appendices

Appendix A

Appendix B

Appendix C

Appendix D

Appendix E

Selected Formulas Used in Pharmacotherapeutics 1362

Kathleen Gutierrez

Appendix F

Administration Techniques 1364

Elizabeth Kissell

Appendix G

Effects of Selected Maternal Drug Ingestion on the Fetus or Neonate 1371

Deborah Cooper McGee

Appendix H

Product Information for Selected Nutritional Supplements and Enteral Formulas 1375

Judi R. Davis

Index

Back Pages: Spanish and English Phrases for Pharmacotherapeutic Assessment

Kristen Arney

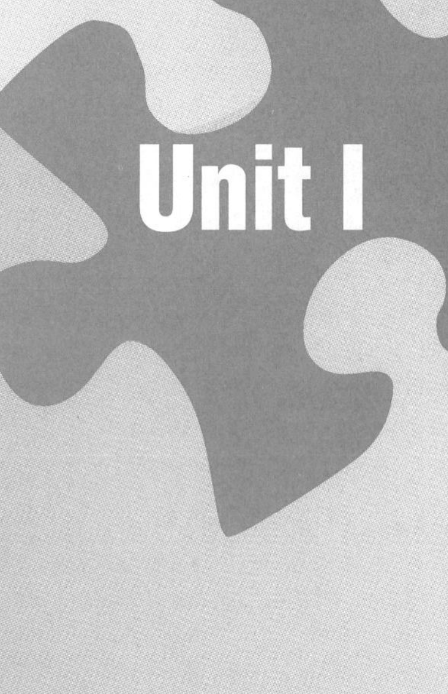

Pharmacology and Professional Nursing Practice

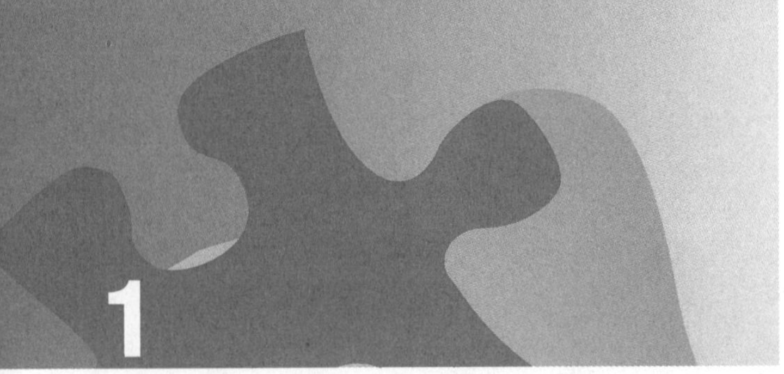

The History of Pharmacology

The history of pharmacology helps us understand the development and uses of drugs in religious, psychosocial, political, and economic frameworks. Since a *drug* is defined broadly as any chemical agent affecting living processes, the subject of pharmacotherapeutics is strikingly extensive. The health care provider essentially is interested in drugs useful in the prevention, diagnosis, and treatment of disease. Although a drug's societal impact may be far reaching, we are concerned here in providing a clear understanding and appreciation for the principles of *pharmacodynamics* (what the drug does to the body) and *pharmacokinetics* (what the body does to the drug). Understanding these principles allows us to practice pharmacotherapeutics safely and effectively because whether a drug is useful for therapy depends on its ability to produce desired effects with minimal adverse reactions. Thus, the standards required for preparation, identification of ingredients, efficacy, and government intervention, largely a result of innovations during the 20th century, are important components within the structure of pharmacology and professional nursing practice.

HISTORICAL PERSPECTIVE

Four distinct stages of pharmacotherapeutics evolved as humankind searched for substances to treat illness and cure disease. These stages chronicle the development of medicinal treatment by natural and derived substances. The mystical period of pharmacotherapeutics persisted in primitive and prehistoric cultures before 3000 BC and was followed by the empirical period, which lasted until approximately 200 BC. The medieval period began from 1200 to 1400 AD and extended through the 1800s. The early 1800s mark the advent of contemporary pharmacotherapeutics, which continues today.

Mystical Period

Primitive and prehistoric cultures believed in the supernatural and relied on these beliefs to explain disease and its cure. People thought illness was the result of malevolent external influences, such as evil spirits or hostile sorcerers. Treatments were magical and mystical, employing three primary modes of healing: prayer, crude surgeries, and potions.

Powerful medicine men formed a separate caste and surrounded themselves with mystery. Some among them became shrewd observers; thus, many cultural superstitions contain elements of empirical truth. The Incas knew the therapeutic value of maté, a tea made from the leaves of *Ilex paraguayensis*. This plant contains tannin and caffeine, and it was used in large quantities for its diaphoretic and diuretic effects. They also used *guarana,* a paste of seeds obtained from the *Paullinia cupana* tree to make an astringent drink that also contained tannin and caffeine. The Incas knew about the stimulating effects of coca, as well as the analgesic value found in a variety of other plants.

North American Indians used charms, spells, and other spiritual practices but also engaged in effective pharmacotherapeutic practices. Digestive disorders were treated with emetics, laxatives, carminatives, and enemas. Lobelia (Indian tobacco), flax, and cupping were used to treat respiratory diseases. Of the 144 drugs known to have been used by the Indians, 59 are still included in the modern pharmacopeia.

Religious mysticism is still practiced in some communities in the United States. In the Southwest, members of the Native American Church of North America use mescal (from the peyote cactus) in religious ceremonies, a practice upheld by the federal courts in 1962. The Supreme Court decision found peyote to be a sacramental symbol comparable to the bread and wine used in Christian churches. As such, it is the very heart of Indian religion.

Spiritual beliefs and practices governed the treatments of the mystical period, and substances used in healing were discovered by trial and error. Each generation orally passed the resulting knowledge on to the next. However, as knowledge about the effects of plant and animal compounds increased, their use moved from the supernatural to a more scientific base. Although this view implies a straight line of progress, history covers a broad spectrum of cultures moving forward at varying and overlapping rates across a lengthy period of development.

Empirical Period

During the empirical period, treatment began to be based on observations that a substance was effective even when the mechanism by which it acted remained unknown. The earliest records were preserved in cuneiform script on a clay tablet by a Sumerian physician nearly 5000 years ago in the Euphrates River Valley of what is now known as Iraq.

Although the Sumerians are credited with the first written prescriptions, the empirical stage is often associated with an inventory of mixtures that appeared in China about 2700 BC. One book from that period recommends ephedra, which is used today as a sympathomimetic drug. Rhubarb, important today for its mineral content, has astringent and cathartic properties; and senna, a cathartic, is also still used. In 1873, a German Egyptologist, George Maurice Ebers, edited *The Medical Papyrus of Egypt,* a collection of scrolls with drug information dating from about 1550 BC. The 22-foot manuscript contained 700 magical formulas and folk remedies meant to cure afflictions ranging from crocodile bites to toenail pain and to rid the house of such pests as scorpions. The manuscript also demonstrated Egyptian attempts to standardize drug preparations. In addition to prescriptions, the manuscript contains information about preventing decay of a body after death. The document also provides information about the drug formulations available at the time: tablets, powders, gargles, salves, and poultices.

The Greco-Roman people incorporated many substances in medicinal practices. Hippocrates (460 to 357 BC), commonly known as the Father of Medicine, practiced an early form of holistic medicine. Hippocratic medicine was based on cooperation with nature. Instead of reliance on dramatic measures, it emphasized the healing power of nature, which often led to what appeared to be a spontaneous recovery. Although Hippocrates mentioned many drugs in his writings, surviving evidence of clinical practice suggests that he used very few of today's so-called important drugs.

Hindu practices dating from about 200 BC recognized the usefulness of preparations such as colchicum, gentian, castor bean, and digitalis. Drugs derived from these products are still in current use. Colchicum is used in the treatment of gout, gentian may be used as a topical antimicrobial, the oil from castor beans may be used for its laxative effects, and digitalis is used in the treatment of heart failure and arrhythmias.

The empirical stage of pharmacotherapeutics was reached at different times in different cultures because it was dependent on the scientific and religious development of a particular region. In Europe, the empirical period lasted until the late Middle Ages, when the so-called period of specifics emerged and encouraged closer scrutiny of mysticism and superstitious practices.

Medieval Period

The Greeks introduced their practice of pharmacy throughout the Mediterranean world even before Rome came to dominate the region. Galen (131 to 201 AD), a Greek physician living in Rome, is recognized as the Father of Pharmacy. He prepared vegetables as medicinal aids, and his recipes became known as galenicals. Dioscorides, a Greek physician who later traveled to Rome, had written *De Materia Medica,* a text on drugs and their use.

After the fall of the Roman Empire, Muslims settled throughout Egypt, North Africa, Spain, and the Holy Land. They blended the mathematical and scientific knowledge of their culture with that of the Greek, Roman, and Jewish peoples. They introduced many new substances to the region including musk, myrrh, tamarind, and cloves. Syrups, juleps, and aromatic water preparations were created, adding significantly to the body of pharmaceutical knowledge. The new formularies represented the first sets of drug standards and, along with the southern European compilations, served as models for the first *London Pharmacopoeia,* published in 1618. This book contained 1028 simple drugs and 932 preparations and compounds. The most complex preparation combined 130 ingredients. Muslim apothecaries (pharmaceutical houses) were inspected on a regular basis. Those found selling deteriorated or adulterated drugs were punished.

The best-known pharmaceutical authority of the late Middle Ages was Nicholas of Salerno, director of the University of Salerno Medical School. The Salerno Medical School was one of the earliest organized medical schools in Europe. It flourished from 900 to 1200 AD. While at the university, Nicholas wrote a book entitled *The Antidotarium.* The standard for pharmaceutical preparations for centuries, it used the basic units of the apothecary system—the grain, the scruple (20 grains in apothecary weight), and the dram. According to laws drafted by Spanish Emperor Frederick II in 1240, ownership of an apothecary shop or any business relationship with an apothecary was limited to licensed pharmacists. In addition, the drug preparation was supervised by inspectors.

Pharmacy flourished in the Renaissance (1400 to 1500), and pharmaceutical advancements occurred on a regular basis. Paracelsus, the Swiss-born son of a German physician, advocated the use of simple preparations in the treatment of illness and disease. He introduced remedies such as sulfur and calomel (used today in powder form to treat ulcers and skin rashes), as well as other chemical compounds. In addition, he attempted to change the relatively common practice of overdosing the patient.

Two advances in the late 1700s were significant and remain so today. Digitalis, a cardiac glycoside derived from the foxglove plant, was introduced in 1785 by Englishman William Withering to treat heart disease. Edmund Jenner, also an Englishman, introduced smallpox immunization and began public inoculations in May 1796. The result was a dramatic reduction in the numbers of smallpox and confirmation that immunization could prevent disease.

Contemporary Period

Great advances were made in pharmacy, chemistry, and medicine during the 19th century. Pharmaceutical chemistry became a specialized science following the first significant discovery made by Frederick Serturner. He isolated the first active ingredient, opium, from the flowers of the poppy. The discovery led to further research and to the isolation of other active compounds in previously known drugs.

Research during this period focused on the effects of active compounds on organs and tissues. Pelletier and Caventou discovered quinine, strychnine, and veratrine; Brandes uncovered atropine; Magendie and Pelletier found emetine; and codeine was isolated by Robiquet. Dr. Crawford Long first reported using ether as general anesthesia in 1842. Later, Morton and Wells successfully demonstrated the use of ether in dentistry. In the 1850s, as Perkins searched for a synthetic quinine, he discovered coal tar products. Coal tar dye later became known as Perkins' purple.

Problems related to drug efficacy were recognized. Scientists examined (1) dosage, time, and effect; (2) processes involved in absorption, distribution, biotransformation, and elimination of drugs; (3) sites of drug action; (4) specific mechanisms of drug action; and (5) relationships between chemical composition and biologic activity of substances.

Early in the 1900s, two significant advances occurred: (1) an improved understanding of the relationship between the pancreas and diabetes mellitus and (2) the development of antimicrobial compounds. In 1899, Joseph von Mering and Oskar Minkowski conducted experiments that linked the pancreas to diabetes mellitus. Banting and Best formulated an early preparation of insulin in 1922. This outstanding achievement allowed control of alterations in carbohydrate metabolism. Four years later, John Abel became the first to crystallize insulin. His experiments revealed its molecular structure and hormonal action. Later, insulin was combined with protamine, a protein complex that delays and prolongs its activity. Development of other delayed-acting insulins soon followed.

German physician Paul Ehrlich introduced modern drug therapy in 1907 with the development of a specific drug against a specific microorganism. He experimented for years with chemical compounds while looking for a cure for syphilis. His 606th experiment was a success; arsphenamine was the chemical compound that could cure syphilis.

The discovery of penicillin by Alexander Fleming in 1928 dramatically changed the treatment of infectious diseases. He had observed that the *Penicillium notatum* mold secreted a substance that inhibited the growth of certain types of gram-positive organisms. The physicians Howard Florey, of Oxford University, and Ernest Chain went on to demonstrate the value of penicillin in the treatment of infectious diseases in 1941. Penicillin became the best drug at that time for the treatment of gonococcal infections and pneumococcal pneumonia.

Subsequent investigators developed other important therapeutic drugs. Antihistamines, other antibiotics, glucocorticoids, oral contraceptives, and antihypertensives, as well as parenteral poliomyelitis vaccine, were developed. Antiviral drugs and the oral form of polio vaccine were developed in the 1960s. During the 1970s, antineoplastic drugs such as doxorubicin and bleomycin and the histamine-2 antagonist cimetidine appeared. Calcium-channel blockers were introduced in the 1980s for the treatment of arrhythmias, angina pectoris, and hypertension. Drugs effective in the prevention and treatment of conditions associated with the human immunodeficiency virus have been developed throughout the 1990s. Today, virtually every body function can be enhanced, suppressed, or manipulated by pharmaceutical means.

In 1958, 1375 companies manufactured prescription drugs in the United States. Of this number, 187 companies provided close to 90 percent of the pharmaceuticals in the marketplace. Many major pharmaceutical firms were founded between 1850 and 1920. Survivors include Smith Kline Beecham; Wyeth Laboratories; Warner-Lambert Pharmaceutical Company; Eli Lilly and Company; Merck, Sharp and Dohme; Parke, Davis, and Company; Warner-Chilcott; Upjohn-Pharmacia; Abbott Laboratories; G.D. Searle and Company; Johnson and Johnson; Mead Johnson and Company; Miles Laboratories; Bristol-Myers Squibb; and Lederle Laboratories. European pharmaceutical companies with American branches include Merck and Company, Ciba, Geigy, Hoffman-La Roche, Sandoz, Charles Pfizer and Company, and Schering Corporation.

NEW DRUG DEVELOPMENT

New drug development has evolved significantly. Contemporary scientists still use natural materials in formulating some drugs; however, advanced technology has changed drug production, eliminating the process of trial and error. Although the importance and the variety of laboratory-synthesized drugs are expanding at a phenomenal rate, drugs obtained from plant and animal sources continue to play important roles in therapeutic practice.

Historically, drug preparations were derived from minerals, plants, and animals. The term *pharmacognosy* refers to the study of such natural drug sources. Plants were the earliest source of drugs, with their use dating back to the primitive-prehistoric period. Commonly used drugs derived from plant sources include digitalis (from the purple foxglove), vincristine (from the periwinkle plant), and morphine (from the opium poppy). Drugs derived from plant sources are organized by their physical and chemical characteristics. These include alkaloids, glycosides, oils, gums, and resins. Drugs derived from animal sources include insulin (from pork and beef pancreas) and pituitary hormones.

The majority of drugs today are either inorganic or organic compounds. Synthetic drugs are far more easily standardized and less often associated with allergic reactions than those made of natural ingredients. In fact, many drugs in use today are directly related to the increasing sophistication of chemical synthesis.

Phases of Clinical Development

It takes an average of about 12 years for an experimental drug to travel from laboratory to market. Only five of every 1000 compounds screened in preclinical drug trials make it to the phase of human testing. Furthermore, only one in five drugs tested in humans is approved for sale in the United States.

The Food and Drug Administration (FDA) monitors new drug development. The process of new drug development begins with preclinical studies (laboratory and animal studies), progresses through several phases of clinical testing, and ends with postmarketing surveillance studies (Fig. 1–1).

The effectiveness and safety of a drug are based on the uniformity of its strength, the purity of the preparation, and the consistency of drug action. Biochemical assay testing is performed to determine identity and potency. Biologic assays measure the amount of drug required to produce a predetermined biologic effect. Clinical studies determine toxicity and dosing.

Preclinical Testing

Preclinical testing can take about 3½ years. During preclinical studies, the FDA requires testing with both male and female animals of at least two different mammalian species. Special attention is given to toxicity and the reversal of toxic effects, carcinogenicity, and teratogenicity. The FDA approves an application for an investigational new drug (IND) only after reviewing extensive animal studies and data on the safety and effectiveness of the proposed new drug.

Clinical Trials

Clinical trials begin after approval of an IND application and require an additional 6 to 9 years for investigation. Clinical trials are designed to provide information about the drug's purity, bioavailability, potency, efficacy, safety, and toxicity through controlled experiments with volunteers. Studies can be stopped at any time, depending on the results. During Phases I, II, and III, the FDA may suspend or shorten the IND process. The FDA may also allow health care providers to treat selected patients with what are called treatment INDs, drugs that have not reached final approval. Emerging treatments for acquired immunodeficiency syndrome (AIDS) have used treatment INDs. Once approved as a treatment IND, the company supplies drugs to physicians treating patients who meet the required criteria.

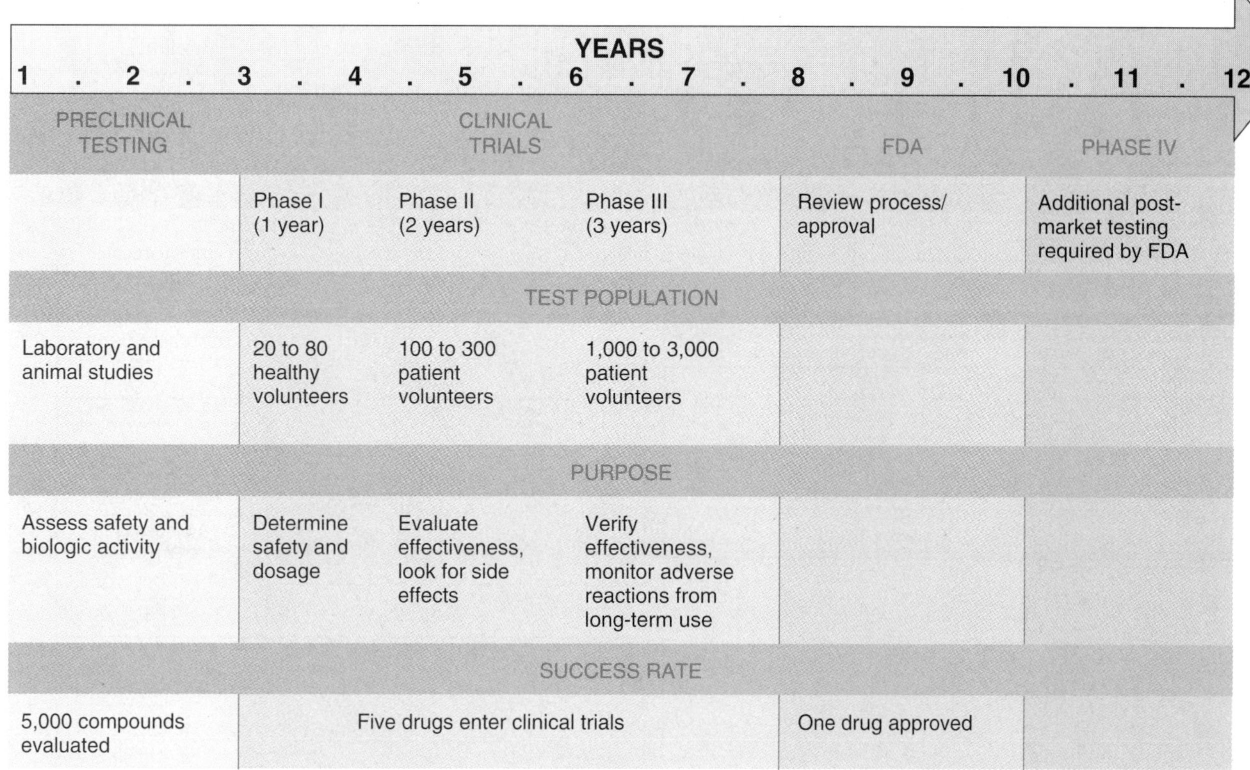

Figure 1–1 The drug development and approval process. (From Wierenga, D., and Eaton, C. [1993]. *The drug development and approval process.* Office of Research and Development, Washington, DC: Pharmaceutical Manufacturers Association. Used with permission.)

Phase I Phase I clinical trials involve the initial evaluation of a drug. A pharmacologist typically supervises studies involving 20 to 80 healthy people. During this phase, emphasis is placed on absorption, distribution, biotransformation, elimination, the preferred route of administration, and the establishment of a safe dosage range. The clinical data obtained determine the need for further testing.

Phase II During Phase II of clinical trials, the drug is tested on 100 to 300 diseased or ill volunteers. This phase evaluates the same aspects as those in Phase I, with the emphasis shifted to compare the effects of the drug in healthy people with those in diseased people. Therapeutic dosage levels are also refined during Phase II.

Phase III Once an effective dosage range has been established (and provided there have been no serious adverse effects), a more lengthy study of the drug's effects on diseased people is undertaken. The therapeutic effectiveness of the drug is verified because larger numbers of individuals (1000 to 3000) are included in this phase of the clinical trial. To remove bias from the study, double-blind research designs are used. In this process, neither the patient nor the health care provider knows who received the investigational drug and who received an alternative therapy. The new drug is usually compared with a known effective treatment. There were several ethical problems with the use of placebo, particularly when an accepted effective therapy exists. A cross-over research design may also be used in some clinical trials, in which the patients receive the drug for part of the time and an alternative for the remaining part of the study. Most risks associated with the new drug are determined during Phase III trials. However, there is always an aspect of the unknown.

FDA Reporting After the first three phases have been completed, a report is made to the FDA. The company developing the drug may submit a new drug application (NDA) after an evaluation of the report. Approval of the NDA means that the new drug has been accepted and therefore can be marketed exclusively by that company on a limited basis.

Phase IV Phase IV clinical trials involve monitoring all people taking the drug. This postmarketing surveillance period evolves over a period of 2 to 3 years. During early Phase IV testing, the new drug is released to the public on a limited basis. Early Phase IV testing is important because it permits observation and monitoring of the drug's effects in larger numbers of people. Later in Phase IV testing, the drug is released for general marketing.

PHARMACOVIGILANCE

Preclinical and clinical trials of new drugs cannot discern all adverse effects that a new drug may produce. Consequently, information about a drug's adverse effects is incomplete when it is released to the marketplace. Because newly released drugs may have as yet unreported adverse effects,

MEDWATCH

THE FDA MEDICAL PRODUCTS REPORTING PROGRAM

For VOLUNTARY reporting by health professionals of adverse events and product problems

Page ___ of ___

Form Approved: OMB No. 0910-0291 Expires:12/31/94
See OMB statement on reverse

FDA Use Only

Triage unit sequence #

A. Patient information

1. Patient identifier — In confidence
2. Age at time of event: ______ or Date of birth:
3. Sex ☐ female ☐ male
4. Weight ____ lbs or ____ kgs

B. Adverse event or product problem

1. ☐ Adverse event and/or ☐ Product problem (e.g., defects/malfunctions)
2. Outcomes attributed to adverse event (check all that apply)
   - ☐ death ________ (mo/day/yr)
   - ☐ life-threatening
   - ☐ hospitalization – initial or prolonged
   - ☐ disability
   - ☐ congenital anomaly
   - ☐ required intervention to prevent permanent impairment/damage
   - ☐ other: ________
3. Date of event (mo/day/yr)
4. Date of this report (mo/day/yr)
5. Describe event or problem
6. Relevant tests/laboratory data, including dates
7. Other relevant history, including preexisting medical conditions (e.g., allergies, race, pregnancy, smoking and alcohol use, hepatic/renal dysfunction, etc.)

C. Suspect medication(s)

1. Name (give labeled strength & mfr/labeler, if known)
   #1
   #2
2. Dose, frequency & route used
   #1
   #2
3. Therapy dates (if unknown, give duration) from/to (or best estimate)
   #1
   #2
4. Diagnosis for use (indication)
   #1
   #2
5. Event abated after use stopped or dose reduced
   #1 ☐ yes ☐ no ☐ doesn't apply
   #2 ☐ yes ☐ no ☐ doesn't apply
6. Lot # (if known)
   #1
   #2
7. Exp. date (if known)
   #1
   #2
8. Event reappeared after reintroduction
   #1 ☐ yes ☐ no ☐ doesn't apply
   #2 ☐ yes ☐ no ☐ doesn't apply
9. NDC # (for product problems only)
   – –
10. Concomitant medical products and therapy dates (exclude treatment of event)

D. Suspect medical device

1. Brand name
2. Type of device
3. Manufacturer name & address
4. Operator of device
   - ☐ health professional
   - ☐ lay user/patient
   - ☐ other: ________
5. Expiration date (mo/day/yr)
6. model # ________
   catalog # ________
   serial # ________
   lot # ________
   other #
7. If implanted, give date (mo/day/yr)
8. If explanted, give date (mo/day/yr)
9. Device available for evaluation? (Do not send to FDA)
   ☐ yes ☐ no ☐ returned to manufacturer on ________ (mo/day/yr)
10. Concomitant medical products and therapy dates (exclude treatment of event)

E. Reporter (see confidentiality section on back)

1. Name, address & phone #
2. Health professional? ☐ yes ☐ no
3. Occupation
4. Also reported to
   - ☐ manufacturer
   - ☐ user facility
   - ☐ distributor
5. If you do NOT want your identity disclosed to the manufacturer, place an " X " in this box. ☐

FDA

Mail to: MEDWATCH
5600 Fishers Lane
Rockville, MD 20852-9787

or FAX to:
1-800-FDA-0178

FDA Form 3500 (6/93)

Submission of a report does not constitute an admission that medical personnel or the product caused or contributed to the event.

Figure 1–2 The FDA MedWatch reporting form.

the health care provider should be alert for unusual responses, especially if the drug has been in the marketplace for less than 3 years. If the patient develops new signs or symptoms, it is wise to suspect that the new drug is responsible—even if those specific signs and symptoms are not described in the literature.

When a drug is suspected of producing a heretofore unknown adverse effect, that effect should be reported to the FDA. Even without equivocal proof of a drug's complicity, all suspected adverse effects should be reported. The purpose of the reporting system is to collect, sort, and scrutinize reports of clinically relevant adverse effects; evaluate the likelihood that the event was drug related; identify patterns that may help prevent further reactions; and provide guidelines for managing reactions. These reports may lead to withdrawal of the drug from the market or produce changes in product labeling. Prompt, voluntary reporting by alert health care providers affords a means whereby the drug's potential for harm can be made known. The MedWatch form shown in Figure 1–2 is used for reporting adverse effects and is available from the FDA at the address noted. The FDA also has a computerized reporting system that is available via the Internet and the World Wide Web.

In both the hospital and ambulatory settings, adverse drug effects are underreported. The Joint Commission on the Accreditation of Health Care Organizations (JCAHO) requires reporting of adverse effects that occur in hospitals. The JCAHO also requires that all significant reactions be reviewed to ensure quality care. According to the JCAHO, a significant event is one in which the drug must be discontinued, the patient requires treatment with another drug to diminish the drug's effects, or the length of the hospitalization is prolonged.

Pharmacovigilance is a branch of *pharmacoepidemiology* (the study of the use and effects of drugs in large numbers of people). Pharmacovigilance is the study of drug-related adverse effects. The field of pharmacovigilance uses epidemiologic methods to gather information about all aspects of the benefit-risk ratio of drugs.

ORPHAN DRUGS

Orphan drugs are a special category of drugs found to be useful in the treatment of certain rare diseases. However, because of patent laws or a limited market, these drugs often are not considered a good financial investment for pharmaceutical companies. Pharmaceutical companies most often choose to develop drugs that provide, with reasonable certainty, substantial returns on their research and development dollars. Congress passed the Orphan Drug Act (Public Law 97-414) in 1983 to motivate companies to develop orphan drugs. Revisions were made in 1984 (The Drug Price Competition and Patent Term Restoration Act), 1985, and 1988. The act, with its amendments, offers substantial tax incentives and longer patent protection to companies that develop such drugs. The 1984 act makes it possible for generic drug companies to market generic drugs by proving bioequiva-

TABLE 1–1 EXAMPLES OF ORPHAN DRUGS AND THEIR INDICATIONS

Drug/Biologic (Trade Name)	Proposed Use	Sponsor
AIDS and AIDS-related Disorders		
2′3′-Dideoxyadenosine (DDA)	AIDS	Bristol-Myers Squibb, National Cancer Institute
Ganciclovir (CYTOVENE)	Cytomegalovirus, severe retinitis	Syntex (USA), Inc.
Molgramostim (LEUKOMAX)	Neutropenia	Schering Corporation
Cancers		
Interferon alfa-2a (ROFERON-A)	Metastatic renal cell cancer	Hoffman-La Roche Inc.
Monoclonal antibody 17-1A (PANOREX)	Pancreatic cancer	Centocor, Inc.
Filgrastim (NEUPOGEN)	Neutropenia associated with bone marrow transplant	Amgen
Gastrointestinal Disorders		
Ethanolamine oleate (ETHAMOLIN)	Esophageal varices	Block Drug Company
Somatostatin (ZECNIL)	Secreting enterocutaneous fistulas	Ferring Laboratories, Inc.
Neurologic Disorders		
Mazindol (SANOREX)	Duchenne muscular dystrophy	Platon J. Collipp, MD; Sandoz
Baclofen (intrathecal) (LIORESAL)	Intractable spasticity related to multiple sclerosis or spinal cord injury	Medtronic, Inc.

AIDS, Acquired immunodeficiency syndrome.

lence rather than duplicating costly clinical trials that are performed when the drugs are first introduced.

The act defines an orphan drug as one used for the diagnosis, treatment, or prevention of diseases or conditions affecting less than 200,000 people in the United States. A drug also may have an orphan status when the cost of developing and marketing it to more than 200,000 affected people would not be covered by sales in the United States. Some companies receive federal research grants to help them develop orphan drugs. Application for an orphan designation must be made before filing a NDA. More than 400 products have been given orphan designations to date. Table 1–1 provides a brief overview of selected drugs with designated indications.

Programs Supporting Orphan Drug Development

In addition to the Orphan Drug Act, other programs support the development of orphan drugs. The Federal Technology Transfer Act of 1986 (Public Law 99-502) permits commercial development of products originating in U.S. government laboratories. The laboratories may enter into cooperative research and development agreements with state or local governments, business and industry, private profit and nonprofit foundations, and universities.

The Small Business Innovation Research (SBIR) program (Public Law 97-219) is designed to encourage for-profit small businesses to develop products with the help of various governmental agencies. Examples of orphan products supported by SBIR funds include vaccines, lung surfactant, and diagnostic drugs.

In 1981, the Pharmaceutical Research Manufacturers of America (PhRMA) established a Commission on Drugs for Rare Diseases. It invites proposals from scientific investigators, voluntary and governmental health agencies, research institutions, and other interested persons. Proposals are screened, and information on promising drugs or other research efforts is distributed to prospective sponsors. The PhRMA also provides grant support in 11 different research areas.

There are several sources of information on rare diseases and orphan drugs. The Office of Orphan Product Development of the FDA provides information and guidance in applying for sponsorship of an orphan product or grant support for research on orphan products. Questions regarding the Public Health Service's SBIR program are directed to the Program Coordinator. The National Organization for Rare Disorders (NORD) acts as a clearinghouse for current information on rare diseases. It is a nonprofit organization created by a group of voluntary agencies, medical researchers in both academia and the pharmaceutical industry, and concerned individuals. It provides patients and their families with accurate, comprehensive explanations of their condition and offers a network of programs that link together people with the same disorder for mutual support. Assistance in forming new support groups is also provided.

The National Information Center for Orphan Drugs and Rare Diseases (NICODARD) provides the names of orphan drug sponsors. Questions from the public are referred to the appropriate voluntary support group or, where none exists, to NORD (for additional resources, see Appendix A).

DRUG STANDARDS

Drug standards are developed by the United States Pharmacopeial Convention (USP) to ensure the uniform quality of drugs. Under federal food and drug law, the FDA enforces adherence to these standards for all drugs offered for sale in interstate commerce. The standards pertain to purity, bioavailability, potency, efficacy, safety, and toxicity. *Purity* refers to the uncontaminated state of a drug. Single-entity drugs are relatively uncommon. Additives are usually needed to facilitate formulation or to alter absorption. The type and concentration of such additives, termed excipient substances, permitted are also specified by USP standards of purity.

Bioavailability is the degree to which a drug can be absorbed by the body and transported to its site of action. Factors influencing bioavailability include solubility, polarity, crystalline structure, and particle size. Serum drug concentrations are commonly used to measure bioavailability.

Potency is generally dependent on the concentration of active drug in the preparation. Potency is determined through bioassay procedures when the active ingredient in a drug is unknown. If the active ingredient is known, potency is determined through chemical assay procedures.

Efficacy refers to the ability of a drug used in treatment of illness or disease to be effective. Objective measures are rarely available for determining efficacy; therefore, subjective data are cautiously interpreted. Double-blind studies are used to distinguish greatest efficacy among alternative drugs.

The incidence and severity of adverse reactions determine the safety of a drug. As a general rule, no active chemical agent is free of toxic effects. The therapeutic index (margin of safety) of a drug is the difference between the therapeutic and the toxic dosages. The risk-benefit ratio is examined when a particular drug is considered for use.

NAMING NEW DRUGS

The name given a new drug is almost as important as the drug itself. Systematic study of pharmacology requires the use of standardized nomenclature. A drug usually has three designations: a chemical name that is based on the drug's precise chemical structure and that conforms to a specific set of international rules; a generic name, or common name, that is simpler than the chemical name and identifies or classifies the drug in scientific literature; and a trade name, or brand name, that identifies the drug as the product of a specific manufacturer (Table 1–2). For example, 7-chloro-1,3-dihydro-1-methyl-5-phenyl-2H-1,4-benzodiazepin-2-1 is the chemical name for the drug generically known as diazepam. Trade names are important for distinguishing a company and its product from the competition. Diazepam was first produced by Roche Laboratories under the trade name VALIUM.

Chemical names are complex and therefore not practical for everyday use. The generic name is assigned to the compound by the United States Adopted Name (USAN) Council, with consultation with the pharmaceutical company developing the drug. The USAN Council is jointly sponsored

TABLE 1–2 SELECTED DRUGS—A COMPARISON OF CHEMICAL, GENERIC, AND TRADE NAMES

Chemical Name	Generic Name	Trade Name
N-Acetyl-para-aminophenol	Acetaminophen	TYLENOL
Acetylsalicylic acid	Aspirin	BUFFERIN
7-Chloro-1,3-dihydro-1-methyl-5-phenyl-2H-1,4-benzodiazepin-2-1	Diazepam	VALIUM
1-Methyl-4-phenylisonipecotate hydrochloride	Meperidine	DEMEROL
17, 21-Dihydroxypregna-1,4-diene-3,11,20-trione	Prednisone	DELTASONE

by the American Medical Association (AMA), the American Pharmaceutical Association (APA), and the United States Pharmacopeial Convention. As a general rule, the USAN Council accepts whatever name the company suggests. In clinical practice, using a drug's generic name facilitates communication and promotes safe, effective drug use.

Manufacturers assign a drug's trade name. Trade names are copyrighted by the company and are legally on record for 17 years. Pharmaceutical companies want names that are easily recognized by patients and health care providers. Unfortunately, having multiple trade names for a single generic drug can impair recognition of the drug and increase the possibility of drug errors.

As more and more drugs enter the marketplace, health care providers, pharmacists, and the public are often bewildered by subtle differences in spelling. Between 1977 and 1987, more than 50 new sound-alike drug names were introduced. Sometimes the similarities in name produced errors detrimental to some patients. Most drug errors occurred when the drug name was similar to that of a more frequently prescribed product, it could be misread, misheard, or miswritten (Table 1–3).

Because no organization is addressing the problem of sound-alike trade names, health care providers and their patients must become familiar with the name, appearance, and the disorder for which a drug is prescribed. When a new prescription is filled, the drug should be double checked and the pharmacist informed of the reason the drug was prescribed.

UNITED STATES DRUG LEGISLATION

A review of the history of drug legislation in the United States reflects the government's increased commitment to ensure safety and efficacy of marketed drugs (Table 1–4). Before 1906, there were no legal controls for the sale or use of any drug. Patented drugs and remedies were sold by traveling medicine men from the back of wagons, in drugstores, by mail order, and by real and self-professed physicians. In addition, drug manufacturers were not required to list ingredients on the container. As a result, many products contained alcohol, opium, or heroin. Illnesses and injuries were reported as a result of a tonic's ingredients as well as the quantities of ingredients.

Federal Food, Drug, and Cosmetic Act

Legislated drug controls in the United States began in 1906 with the passage of the Federal Food, Drug, and Cos-

TABLE 1–3 DRUG NAMES TOO SIMILAR FOR COMFORT

Instead of	For	The Patient Received	For
Acetazolamide (DIAMOX)	Glaucoma	Acetohexamide (DYMELOR)	Diabetes
ANTURANE (sulfinpyrazone)	Gout	ANTABUSE (disulfiram)	Alcoholism
Disopyramide (NORPACE)	Arrhythmias	Desipramine (PERTOFRANE)	Depression
ENDURON (methyclothiazide)	Thiazide diuretic	INDERAL (propranolol)	Arrhythmias
FELDENE (piroxicam)	Inflammation	SELDANE (terfenadine)	Allergies, hay fever
Hydroxyzine (VISTARIL)	Anxiety	Hydralazine (APRESOLINE)	Hypertension
ORINASE (tolbutamide)	Diabetes mellitus	ORNADE (phenylpropanolamine with orpheniramine)	Sinus congestion
Metolazone (ZAROXOLYN)	Thiazide diuretic	Metaxalone (SKELAXIN)	Skeletal muscle relaxant
Ritodrine (YUTOPAR)	Prevent uterine contractions	RITALIN (methylphenidate)	Attention deficit disorder
Selegiline (ELDEPRYL)	Parkinson's disease	STELAZINE (trifluoperazine)	Anxiety states

TABLE 1–4 SUMMARY OF UNITED STATES FEDERAL DRUG LEGISLATION

Year	Legislation	Significance of Legislation
1906	Federal Food, Drug and Cosmetic Act (FFDCA)	Restricted the manufacture and sale of drugs; established *The National Formulary* and *The U.S. Pharmacopeia* as official standards
1912	Sherley Amendment (to the FFDCA)	Prohibited fraudulent therapeutic claims by drug manufacturers
1914	Harrison Narcotic Act	Established word narcotic as legal term. Regulated the import, manufacture, sale, and use of habit-forming drugs
1938	Amendment to Sherley Amendment of 1912	Mandated that drug manufacturers test all drugs for harmful effects before they enter interstate commerce and all drug labels must be accurate and complete
1938	Wheeler-Lea Act	Defined criteria for nonfraudulent advertising
1952	Durham-Humphrey Amendments of 1945 and 1952	Distinguished between OTC and prescription drugs specifying procedures for distribution of prescription drugs
1962	Kefauver-Harris Amendment (to the FFDCA)	Tightened controls regarding safety and effectiveness of drugs; made statements about adverse reactions and contraindications; and introduced drug-testing methodologies
1970	Comprehensive Drug Abuse Prevention Act of 1970 (Controlled Substances Act)	Categorized controlled substances based on their abuse potential. Established governmental programs to prevent and treat drug abuse. Assigned drugs to schedules (see Table 1–6)
1978	Drug Regulation Reform Act	Established a more expedient process for release of new drugs to the public
1983	Orphan Drug Act	Offered drug manufacturers incentives to develop drugs for rare disorders or that have a limited market

OTC, Over the counter.

metic Act (FFDCA), but the act primarily addressed the issue of food purity. Drug manufacturers were not required to establish drug efficacy. The act also designated *The United States Pharmacopeia (USP)* and *The National Formulary (NF)* as official drug references.*

Sherley Amendment

The Sherley Amendment (1912) prohibited fraudulent claims by pharmaceutical companies. The Sherley Amendment was subsequently modified in 1938 after the deaths of 100 children from a solution of sulfanilamide in diethylene glycol, an excellent but highly toxic solvent.

The 1938 amendment deals primarily with truth in labeling and drug safety. According to the amendment, drug labels are to contain the following elements before products can enter the marketplace:

- A statement describing package contents
- Reference to the presence, quantity, and proportion of certain drugs such as alcohol, atropine, digitalis, and bromides
- A statement that the product contains habit-forming substances and a listing of their effects
- The name of the manufacturer, packager, and distributor
- Directions for safe use with recommendations for dosage and frequency
- A statement that the product has not yet been approved for interstate commerce, where appropriate
- The brand name and generic names must be included on the label and no false or misleading statements are to appear

Toxicity studies were required as well as NDA before a drug could be promoted and distributed. No proof of efficacy was required. As a result, extravagant claims for therapeutic uses were made. At the time, drugs went from the laboratory to the clinical arena without FDA approval.

Durham-Humphrey Amendment

The FFDCA was further amended in 1945 to provide for direct supervision and inspection of drugs during the production process. It was amended again in 1952 to distinguish between over-the-counter (OTC) and prescription drugs. The 1952 amendment also identified procedures required for distribution of prescription drugs.

Harris-Kefauver Amendment

The Harris-Kefauver Amendment to the FFDCA was an attempt to control untested drug use. The act requires sufficient pharmacologic and toxicologic research in animals before drugs can be tested in humans. As a result, research flourished during the 1940s and 1950s. A number of drugs used in the treatment of organic and infectious diseases flowed out of the academic and industrial laboratories. The risk-benefit ratio of the new drugs was seldom mentioned, and efficacy was not strictly defined. During this period of relaxed research, thalidomide was introduced into the European and United States marketplaces. The drug was used to treat nausea associated with pregnancy; however, in a short time, it became obvious that thalidomide was teratogenic.

***The National Formulary (NF)* was established by the American Pharmaceutical Association in 1888. It, too, was a privately issued compendium that was the project of pharmacists. In 1906, both *The United States Pharmacopeia* and *The National Formulary* were established as official standards by the U.S. government. In 1974, the United States Pharmacopeial Convention purchased *The National Formulary* from the American Pharmaceutical Association, merging the *USP* and the *NF*.

Harrison Narcotic Act

The Harrison Narcotic Act of 1914 followed the Sherley Amendment. It was the first significant piece of legislation classifying certain drugs (e.g., marijuana, opium, cocaine, and their derivatives) as habit forming. The act also placed regulations on the import, manufacture, sale, and use of habit-forming substances.

Controlled Substances Act

The most stringent regulation is the Controlled Substances Act (i.e., Title II of the Comprehensive Drug Abuse Prevention and Control Act). Passed by Congress in 1970, it was designed to contain the rapidly increasing problem of drug abuse. The act encourages research into the prevention and treatment of drug abuse and dependency and promotes drug education programs. In addition, it provides for the establishment of treatment and rehabilitation centers. Drug enforcement was further strengthened by the creation of drug schedules based on abuse potential. Table 1–5 provides an overview of the controlled drug schedules with defined prescriptive components.

Both health care provider and pharmacist are legally responsible for drugs covered by the Controlled Substances Act. In order to prescribe, dispense, or administer any controlled substance, the health care provider must be registered with the federal Drug Enforcement Administration (DEA). Once an application is approved, the certificate is valid for 3 years. Separate registrations are required if the health care provider practices in more than one location. An outline of the Controlled Substances Act of 1970, contained in *A Manual for the Medical Practitioner* may be obtained from the DEA.

Schedule I

Schedule I drugs have a high potential for abuse and have no accepted medical use. They may be available for research use or for chemical analysis by forwarding an application and supporting protocols to the DEA. Under normal circumstances, health care providers cannot write and pharmacists cannot fill prescriptions for Schedule I drugs.

TABLE 1–5 UNITED STATES SCHEDULES FOR CONTROLLED SUBSTANCES

Schedule	Selected Examples	Schedule Characteristics	Restrictions Required
C_I	Cannabis, heroin, LSD, mescaline, methaqualone, peyote, psilocybin, tetrahydrocannabinol	All nonresearch, analysis, or instructional use prohibited High potential for abuse May lead to severe dependence	Approved research protocol only
C_{II}	Amphetamine, cocaine, codeine, hydromorphone, morphine, opium, meperidine, methadone, methylphenidate, oxycodone, pentobarbital, phenmetrazine, secobarbital	Accepted medical uses. High abuse potential May lead to severe psychological or physiologic dependence, or both	Written prescription necessary No telephone renewals May prescribe over telephone if an emergency Container must have warning label*
C_{III}	Preparations containing limited amounts of, or which are combined with, one or more active ingredients considered to be noncontrolled substances: codeine, dihydrocodeine or ethylmorphine, hydrocodone, morphine, and non-narcotic agents such as derivatives of barbituric acid except those that are listed in another schedule, chlorphentermine, glutethimide, methyprylon, paregoric, and others	Accepted medical uses Potential for abuse lower than with drugs in Schedules I and II May lead to low to moderate physical dependence or high psychological dependence	Written or verbal prescription required Prescription expires in 6 months No more than five refills permitted within 6-month period Container must have warning label*
C_{IV}	Alprazolam, barbital, chloral hydrate, chlordiazepoxide, clorazepate, dextropropoxyphene diazepam, fenfluramine, flurazepam, lorazepam, phenobarbital, mazindol, meprobamate, oxazepam, pentazocine, and others	Accepted medical uses Potential for abuse lower than with Schedule III drugs May lead to limited physical or psychological dependence	Written or verbal prescription required Prescription expires in 6 months with no more than five refills permitted Container must have warning label*
C_V	Generally OTC drugs used for the relief of coughs or diarrhea. Contain limited amounts of select opioid controlled substances.	Accepted medical uses Potential for abuse lower than with Schedule IV drugs May lead to limited physical or psychological dependence	May require written prescription or may be sold without a prescription Check state law

*Caution: Federal law prohibits the transfer of this drug to any person other than the patient for whom it was prescribed.
Note: Some states may have their own schedules (e.g., pentazocine is a C_{II} drug in several states).
OTC, Over the counter; LSD, lysergic acid diethylamide.

Schedule II

Drugs in this schedule also have high abuse potential, but they have accepted medical uses. The inappropriate or indiscriminate use of Schedule II drugs may result in psychological or physiologic dependence. A written prescription is required; however, federal law permits emergency telephone orders for Schedule II controlled drugs under the following circumstances:

- Immediate administration of the drug is necessary for proper treatment
- There are no alternative treatments available
- It is not possible to provide a written prescription for the drug at that time

Under these circumstances, the amount of the drug prescribed is limited to that used to treat the patient during the emergency. A written, signed prescription must be provided to the pharmacy within 72 hours. In addition, "authorization for emergency dispensing" and the date of the verbal order must be written on the face of the prescription. The pharmacist is required to notify the DEA if the written prescription is not received within 72 hours.

Schedule III

Schedule III drugs have a lower potential for abuse than drugs in Schedules I and II. These drugs are accepted for medical use in the United States. Abuse of these drugs may lead to low to moderate physical dependency or to high psychological dependency. Schedule III drugs are those that often contain a noncontrolled substance along with a controlled substance (for example, acetaminophen with 30 mg of codeine). Preparations with less than 1.8 g of codeine per 100 mL, depressants such as butabarbital and glutethimide, and certain anabolic steroids fall into this schedule.

Prescriptions for Schedule III drugs may be presented in writing or given verbally to the pharmacist. If authorized on the prescription, the order may be refilled five times within 6 months of the date of issue. A new prescription is needed at the end of the 6-month period. Federal law permits verbal authorization for additional refills under the following circumstances:

- The total quantity of the drug does not exceed five refills or extend beyond 6 months from the date of issue of the original prescription (including the amount of the original prescription)
- The quantity of each additional refill is equal to or less than the quantity originally authorized
- A new prescription for any additional quantities beyond the five refills or 6-month limitation must be provided

For example, the health care provider who originally wrote for 60 tablets with three refills could provide a verbal order for two additional refills of no more than 60 tablets each.

Schedule IV

Schedule IV drugs have a low abuse potential. The potential is primarily for limited physical or psychological dependency relative to those drugs in Schedule III. Schedule IV drugs have acceptable medical uses in the United States. The primary difference between Schedule III and Schedule IV drugs is the penalty for unlawful possession. Prescription requirements for drugs in Schedule IV are similar to those of Schedule III.

Schedule V

Drugs in this schedule are thought to have less abuse potential than those of Schedule IV. This schedule includes drugs containing moderate quantities of opioids but that are generally used for their antitussive and antidiarrheal properties. They may be distributed without a prescription under the following conditions:

- The purchaser is at least 18 years of age and proper identification is obtained
- Distribution is made only by a pharmacist
- No more than 240 mL of any Schedule V substance containing opium, or more than 120 mL or more than 24 solid dosage units of any other controlled substance can be sold to the same person in any 48-hour period without a valid prescription
- Records are kept of the name and address of the person purchasing the drug, the name and quantity of the controlled substance, date of sale, and the name or initials of the pharmacist
- Other federal, state, and local laws do not require a prescription to obtain the drug

CANADIAN DRUG LEGISLATION

Canadian Food and Drugs Act

Canadian drug laws evolved in a manner analogous to those in the United States. The present Food and Drugs Act was passed in 1953 and has been amended almost every year since. The act states that no drug, food, cosmetic, or medical device can be fraudulently advertised or sold to the public for the treatment, prevention, or cure of certain diseases. In addition, the act prohibits sale of contaminated, adulterated, or unsafe drugs. In addition, the sale of certain drugs is forbidden unless the process and conditions of manufacture have been approved by the Minister of National Health and Welfare.

The drugs must comply with standards contained in recognized formularies and pharmacopeias. The legend CSD (Canadian Standard Drug) must appear on the inner and outer labels of drug packaging to indicate it meets standards contained in the following formularies and pharmacopeias:

- *The British Pharmaceutical Codex*
- *Pharmacopeia Française*
- *Pharmacopoeia Internationalis*
- *The British Pharmacopoeia*
- *The Canadian Formulary*
- *The United States Pharmacopeia/National Formulary*

The British Pharmacopoeia (BP) is similar in scope and purpose to *The United States Pharmacopeia. The* British Pharmaceutical Codex is published by the Pharmaceutical Society of Great Britain. It includes standards for new drugs prescribed in Canada but which are not included in *The BP. The*

United States Pharmacopeia is used a great deal in Canada. Some drugs used in Canada conform to *The United States Pharmacopeia* instead of *The BP* because, although they are used in Canada, they are manufactured in the United States.*

In Canada, the Drugs Directorate of the Health Protection Branch (HPB) of the Department of National Health and Welfare is responsible for the administration and enforcement of the Foods and Drugs Act. The Directorate is also responsible for the Proprietary or Patent Medicine Act and the Narcotic Control Act. These acts are designed to control and continuously monitor the research, development, advertising, and product information of all drug products.

Narcotic Control Act

The most recent Canadian legislation is the Narcotic Control Act of 1982. The act is similar in scope to the U.S. Controlled Substances Act (1970). It designates drug classifications with drug schedules based on abuse potential (Table 1–6). Although the administration of the Narcotic Control Act is legally the responsibility of the Department of National Health and Welfare, the enforcement of the law falls primarily to the Royal Canadian Mounted Police. Health care providers are advised to check with appropriate government officials regarding drug controls and standards if they will be working within Canadian boundaries.

The implications of the act cover several areas. Much as in the United States, a PRN order for narcotics must be rewritten every 72 hours. A standing order is not permitted for narcotics. In an emergency situation, a verbal order is permitted if the nature of the emergency is documented in the record and the order is validated within 24 hours. Diligent record keeping is mandated and must include the date, the administration time, and the names of the patient and health care providers and their signatures. When a narcotic previously prepared for administration is refused, contaminated, or wasted, it should be disposed of in the sewage system in the presence of a witness, and then proper documentation completed. All controlled substances stored on nursing units must be kept in locked cabinets with access available only to authorized personnel.

CONCEPTS AND PRINCIPLES OF PRESCRIBING

The prescription is a means of communicating therapeutic treatment plans between the health care provider and the pharmacist. The most carefully written prescription becomes useless if it does not clearly communicate the drug regimen.

*Canadian drugs within this book's drug lists are identified with a maple leaf icon (e.g., ampicillin (OMNIPEN; [🍁] APO-AMPI).

TABLE 1–6 OVERVIEW OF CANADIAN DRUG SCHEDULES

Sch	Selected Examples	Schedule Characteristics	Restrictions Required
Restricted Drugs			
H	*N,N*-Diethyltryptamine (DET), *N,N*-dimethyltryptamine (DMT), 4-methyl-2,5-dimethoxyamphetamine (STP, DOM), lysergic acid diethylamide (LSD), mescaline, peyote	No recognized medicinal uses Sale is prohibited Possess dangerous physiologic and psychological effects	Available for investigational use with authorization from Minister of National Health and Welfare
N	Anileride, cannabis, cocaine, codeine, morphine, opium, phencyclidine, and preparations containing controlled substances with noncontrolled substances (e.g., acetaminophen with codeine, diphenoxylate with atropine)	Stringently restricted High potential for abuse *Parenteral Forms:* All narcotics containing less than two other non-narcotic ingredients All narcotic compounds containing more than one narcotic drug	Letter N must appear on all labels and professional advertisements Refills not permitted Reorders require new written prescription Oral formulations require written or verbal order
Controlled Drugs			c symbol must appear on all labels and professional advertisements
G	Amphetamines, anabolic steroids, barbiturates	Potential for abuse All combinations containing more than one controlled drug All combinations with one controlled drug and one or more ingredients in recognized therapeutic dosage	Refills not permitted if original order was verbal Refills authorized if identified on original prescription Prescription required
F	Antipsychotics, benzodiazepines, oral antibiotics, oral contraceptives, steroids, hormones	Some have relatively low abuse potential Can be sold and refilled only on prescription (Pr) Pr symbol must appear on label	Orders may be written, verbal, or electronic Refills are permitted at specified intervals but cannot exceed 6 months
C and D	Anterior pituitary extracts, antibiotics, injectable liver extracts, low-dose codeine preparations, insulin, muscle relaxants, nitroglycerine, radioactive isotopes, parenteral serums, vaccines not of bacterial origin	Nonprescription drug schedule Limited public access	Drugs available only in pharmacy and used only on physician recommendation

Essential Components of Drug Orders

There are several essential components in a drug order (Fig. 1–3). The components are related to the five rights of drug administration: right patient, right drug, right dose, right route, and right time. All components of the order should be legible and clearly expressed. If there is doubt, the order must be clarified.

Federal law does not require that a particular form be used for prescription writing, nor does it identify what information should be included. Labeling requirements dictate the information that must be included; some states may require that a prescription be displayed graphically in a specific manner.

Regulations for prescription of controlled substances are stringent. There is additional information that must be included on the prescription blank. Some state laws require the patient's address, telephone number, and age, along with the health care provider's address and telephone number. Federal law also requires the health care provider's DEA registration number. Some states require use of a duplicate or triplicate prescription blank for some or all controlled substances.

Types of Drug Orders

Several different types of drug orders exist (see Types of Drug Orders with Examples). A routine order directs drug administration on a regular basis until formal instructions are provided to stop or until a specific termination date (stop policy) is reached. Automatic stop policies act as stimuli to re-evaluate the continued need for the drug. Automatic stop policies are usually explicit in agency policies. A pro re nata (PRN) order means that the drug is to be administered as necessary. Criteria that spell out how often a drug may be administered are specified within the drug order.

Although patients are free to treat themselves with any OTC drug available while at home, once they are admitted to a clinical institution, a written drug order is required. A prescription is written on an inpatient order sheet found in the patient's medical record in an institutional setting. It is

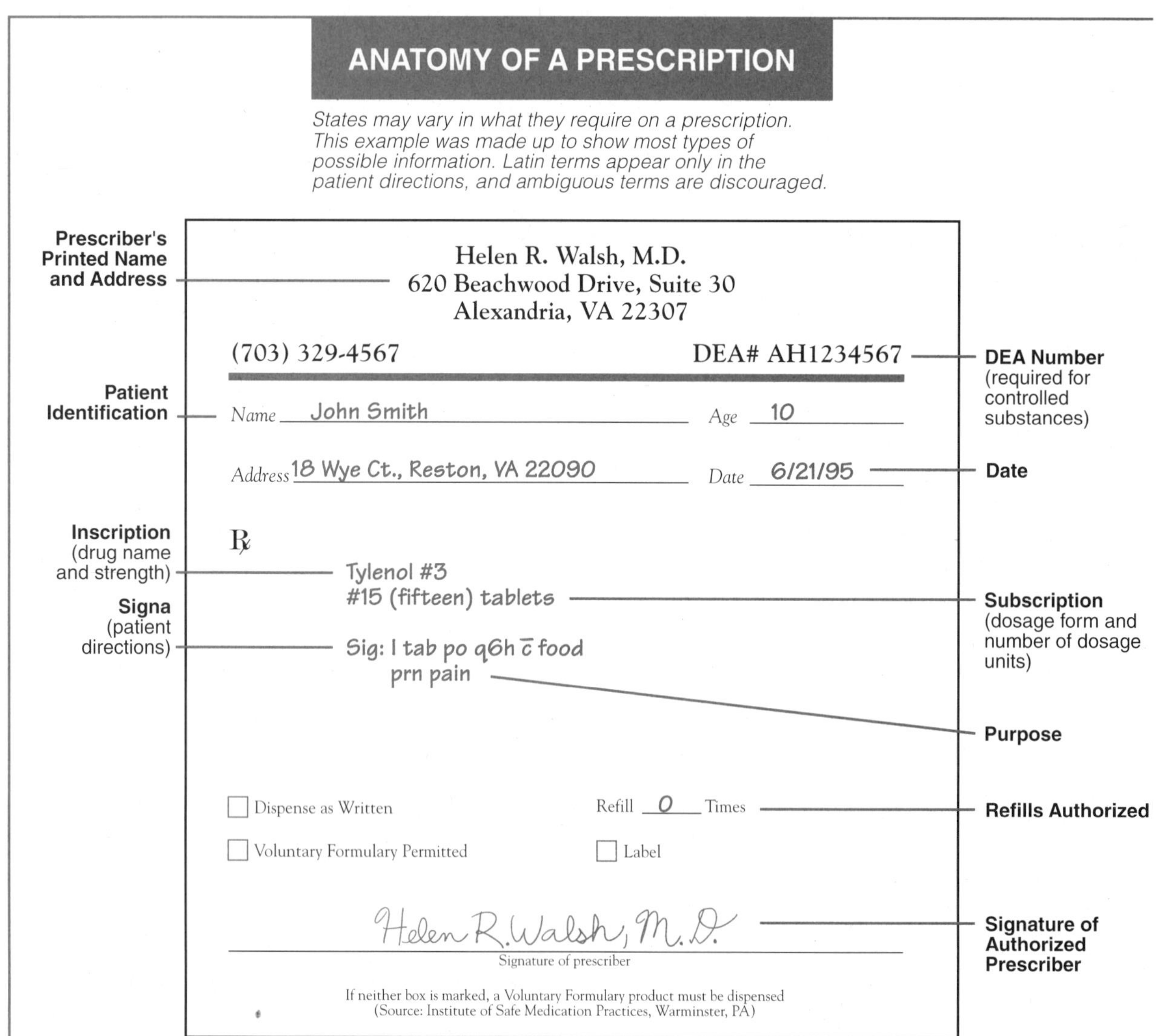
ANATOMY OF A PRESCRIPTION

States may vary in what they require on a prescription. This example was made up to show most types of possible information. Latin terms appear only in the patient directions, and ambiguous terms are discouraged.

Helen R. Walsh, M.D.
620 Beachwood Drive, Suite 30
Alexandria, VA 22307

(703) 329-4567 DEA# AH1234567

Name John Smith Age 10

Address 18 Wye Ct., Reston, VA 22090 Date 6/21/95

℞

Tylenol #3
#15 (fifteen) tablets

Sig: I tab po q6h c̄ food
prn pain

☐ Dispense as Written Refill 0 Times

☐ Voluntary Formulary Permitted ☐ Label

Helen R. Walsh, M.D.
Signature of prescriber

If neither box is marked, a Voluntary Formulary product must be dispensed
(Source: Institute of Safe Medication Practices, Warminster, PA)

Figure 1–3 Anatomy of a prescription. (From Farley, D. [1995]. Making it easier to read prescriptions. *FDA Consumer.* July-August.)

TYPES OF DRUG ORDERS WITH EXAMPLES

Routine order	Enalapril maleate 10 mg po each AM (#30 tablets)
PRN order	Ibuprofen 400 mg po q4–6 hr. PRN pain
Single order	Diazepam 10 mg po ×1 preoperatively at 9 AM
Stat order	Furosemide 40 mg IV push now
Protocol order	*Sliding scale insulin:* If fingerstick glucose is 120–160 mg/dL, give 2 units regular insulin 160–200 mg/dL, give 4 units regular insulin 200–220 mg/dL, give 6 units regular insulin over 220 mg/dL, call health care provider

filled by the institution's pharmacy or a contract pharmacy. A prescription blank is used when patients are discharged and in outpatient settings. Although the process of ordering drugs has been computerized in recent years, the principles remain the same.

Prescription Writing

Latin served a useful purpose when it was used in the 1400s to write entire prescriptions. Today, Latin may appear in the directions for taking the drug. On some prescriptions the abbreviation R_x is used; it is Latin for recipe. The cross at the end of the R has been explained as a substitute period. Although the terms *signa* (write) and *signetur* (let it be labeled) are still commonly used, health care providers have accepted recommendations that offer greater clarity.

At the 1994 annual meeting of the AMA, several recommendations were made that make prescription writing clearer. The recommendations include writing out directions rather than using ambiguous abbreviations. For example, write out the word daily rather than using QD, a Latin abbreviation meaning every day. This abbreviation can be misinterpreted as QID, meaning four times a day, or even OD, meaning right eye. Vague instructions, such as "take as directed," and the use of apothecary or chemical symbols such as K for potassium should be avoided.

Decimal figures should be avoided as much as possible. For example, it may be less problematic to prescribe 500 mg rather than 0.5 g. When a decimal is required, a zero should precede the decimal, denoting less than one (e.g., 0.5 mg rather than .5 mg). Additionally, the word *unit* should be used rather than its abbreviation, U. The metric system is preferred over the apothecary system.

It is good practice to use one prescription pad at a time, securing the remaining pads in a safe location to reduce the possibility of theft. Prescription blanks should never be signed in advance. Additionally, state laws and practical aspects of use should be considered before having prescription blanks printed. The dimensions of the prescription blank, the amount of space available to write directions, the location of refill instructions, purpose of the drug, and spaces for names, signature or signatures, and DEA number should be considered.

Prescriptions may be written in ink or typewritten, but they must be signed by the health care provider. Stamped signatures are not considered valid. Federal law mandates that erasable pens not be used to write or sign prescriptions for controlled substances. The ink in erasable pens does not become permanent for approximately 3 days. During this time, it is possible that prescription information could be altered without notice.

In some states, only one drug order may be written per prescription blank. Preprinted prescriptions may be forbidden. Preprinted blanks have the drug name, strength, amount, dosage, route, frequency, use, or some combination of the above information preprinted on the blank.

Federal law permits an authorized representative, usually a nurse or secretary, to prepare prescriptions (including those for controlled substances) for the signature of the health care provider. The patient is not an authorized representative. Ordering greater quantities of drug than required should be avoided. Representatives must make sure that the prescription conforms in all essential respects to the law and regulations. The pharmacist has an equal responsibility to make sure the prescription meets all federal as well as state requirements.

Record-Keeping Requirements

The Controlled Substances Act requires that records of drugs purchased, distributed, and dispensed be kept. The scope of the health care provider's activities determines what records must be kept.

Controlled drugs prescribed in the course of professional practice do not require specific record keeping of the transactions. However, they must be documented in patient records. When controlled substances are dispensed, a record of each transaction is required.

A health care provider who regularly administers controlled substances is required to keep records if patients are charged for the drugs either separately or with other patient services. Health care providers who dispense controlled substances and who administer the drug (from the same inventory) are required to keep a record of all transactions. All records, including those for controlled substances, are maintained as part of a patient's file. The records must be made available to a duly authorized DEA official on request.

Drug transaction records must document inventory of all stock on hand every 2 years. Specific requirements related to taking inventory are found in the *DEA Physician's Manual* that is available from a DEA field office.

Substitutions

Most states have regulations specifying circumstances under which a pharmacist may substitute a generic drug or a different brand for the prescribed drug. The substitution must be the same chemical entity and must be the same dosage form as in the original prescription. Many states use a formulary system to help in the selection process. Some formularies indicate which drug may be substituted, whereas other state formularies may indicate which drug may not be substituted. Individual state laws should be consulted. The substitution must be authorized by the health care provider through a variety of means. Authorization is usually noted through a specific statement or abbreviation.

Prescription Refills

The health care provider should always clearly indicate whether or not a prescription may be refilled. Prescriptions are refilled when authorized on the original prescription or through a verbal order. The most effective method for identifying refills is to indicate a specific number of times it may be refilled. It can be as simple as filling in a blank (e.g., Refill: two times), or a series of numbers that can be circled to indicate the refills (e.g., Refill: 0 1 2 3). The absence of refill instructions means that no refills are permitted.

The FDA discourages the use of the designation "refill PRN." It is not up to the pharmacist to determine the number of times a prescription should be refilled. A variation on the PRN theme (e.g., PRN—6 months) may be occasionally seen. In this case, a limit to the number of refills exists. Lifetime refills are unsafe and pointless. In addition, the FDA directs that a prescription is no longer valid when the relationship with the patient is severed, as in the death of the health care provider.

The Durham-Humphrey Amendment permits pharmacists to take refill orders by telephone for noncontrolled drugs, as well as for Schedule III and IV controlled substances. The order must be authorized by the health care provider or a legally authorized representative and must be recorded by the pharmacist. Furthermore, because the health care provider cannot delegate decision-making authority to others, the legally authorized representative may only relay the instructions to the pharmacist.

Expired Prescriptions

Federal law does not stipulate that a prescription be filled within a specified period after it is written. Some states, however, have established time limits, especially for controlled substances. For example, New York pharmacists will fill a prescription for controlled substances within 30 days of being written. The pharmacist should question the person, and the health care provider should be concerned about persons who present prescriptions an extended period of time after they were written. Patients should be encouraged to have all prescriptions filled within a reasonable time period.

Prescription Labeling

Explicit labeling requirements have been established by the FFDCA, the Controlled Substances Act, and various state acts. Prescription labels may also require the name and address of the pharmacy, prescription number, date the prescription was filled or refilled, and any caution or warning statements, in addition to essential drug components. Information such as the dispensing pharmacist's name or initials, lot numbers, expiration dates, the name of the manufacturer or distributor, and the telephone number of the pharmacy may be required. For controlled substances, caution and warning statements, and the federal warning statement for drugs in Schedules I to IV must be included:

> Caution: Federal law prohibits the transfer of this drug to any person other than the patient for whom it was prescribed.

Some states, such as New York, require a specific label color for controlled substances. Texas law requires that all prescriptions include the intended use of the drug (e.g., for pain), unless the health care provider decides this inclusion is not in the patient's best interest.

Prescription Copies

Patients have the right to request a copy of their prescription. However, copies have no legal status and cannot be filled or refilled. The copy should be marked with a statement such as "Copy—For Information Purposes Only" before being given to the patient. Without this statement on the prescription, there is no guarantee that the prescription is factual and genuine, and that the prescription has not been filled previously by other pharmacies. There is also no assurance that a copy of the prescription will not be recognized for the remaining refills. Pharmacists presented with a copy of a prescription should contact the health care provider for authorization to fill or refill the prescription.

Out-of-State Prescriptions

Health care providers may legally write prescriptions only in the states in which they are licensed to practice. A health care provider licensed in at least one state but employed in a federal institution may have prescriptive authority in any federal facility. Nevertheless, whether a pharmacist can fill a prescription written by a health care provider licensed in another state depends on state laws. There is no federal requirement that the prescription be filled in the state in which the health care provider is licensed. The prescription must have been valid in the location where it was written.

Drug Samples

A 1987 amendment to the FFDCA, the Prescription Drug Marketing Act, defines a sample as a drug unit that is not intended for sale, but which is distributed to promote drug sales. Health care providers who receive drug samples have provided a written request to the manufacturer or distributor. A written receipt of the samples must be returned to the manufacturer or distributor.

SOURCES OF DRUG INFORMATION

The need for objective, concise, well-organized information on drugs is obvious. However, there is no single source of drug information that covers all clinical situations. Resources include pharmacology and therapeutic textbooks, professional journals, drug compendia, continuing education seminars and meetings, advertising, drug information centers, and online computer databases.

Official Sources

The only official book of drug standards in the United States is *The United States Pharmacopeia/National Formulary*, a privately issued compendium. The first edition of *The United States Pharmacopeia* was published in 1820. It is revised every 5 years by a group of elected experts from a variety of fields, including nursing, pharmacy, pharmacology, and chemistry, and by consumers. Drugs included in the reference meet high standards of quality, purity, and strength and are identified by the letters *USP-NF* following the official name.

Clinical References

Numerous additional reference books and guides are available in the marketplace. Two valuable sources for drug information are the *USP Dispensing Information (USPDI)* and the *American Hospital Formulary Service (AHFS) Drug Information* book. These unbiased, relatively accessible sources of information provide data on the clinical uses of drugs. The *AHFS* is a collection of monographs published by the American Society of Health System Pharmacists (ASHP). The collection is kept current by annual republication. It frequently reviews the newer or investigational uses for drugs.

The *USPDI* is published annually, with regular updates issued during the year. It contains information for both the health care provider (Volumes I and III) and the patient (Volume II). The volumes for the health care provider offer information about approved drug products, drug indications, pharmacokinetics, dosing, warnings, adverse effects, and precautions.

Volume II, which is written for patients, is a valuable resource for patient teaching. Information contained in the patient volume may be used in patient counseling. It does not require that the user obtain permission from the publisher for its use. Automatic permission is granted to health care providers who copy a limited quantity of monographs to distribute free of charge to their patients.

Nonofficial Sources

Goodman and Gilman's The Pharmacological Basis of Therapeutics is the classic reference on pharmacology. As the name implies, the primary focus is on the basic science information that underlies drug use and not on individual drugs. New editions are published approximately every 5 years.

Drug Evaluations is a comprehensive reference compiled by the AMA. It discusses drugs from a therapeutic perspective and emphasizes clinical care rather than basic science information.

Drug Facts and Comparisons is another valuable resource. It is organized by drug classification and is updated monthly. It contains a comprehensive list of drugs with a cost index guide to the average wholesale price (AWP) for equivalent quantities of similar or identical drugs

The *Physicians' Desk Reference (PDR)* is another unofficial source of information that is commonly used by health care providers. The information contained in the *PDR* is identical to that found in drug package inserts and is submitted and paid for by drug companies. The information is largely based on the results of Phase III clinical trials. Its primary value is in identifying the clinical indications for an FDA-approved drug. It does not include care implications associated with a particular drug.

Objective journals not supported by drug manufacturers include *Clinical Pharmacology and Therapeutics* and *Drugs*. The first journal is devoted to original articles that evaluate actions and effects of drugs on humans. *Drugs* publishes timely reviews of individual drugs and drug classifications.

In addition, three publications effectively provide objective information in an easy-to-understand form. *The Medical Letter,* a biweekly publication of a nonprofit corporation, provides summaries of scientific reports and consultant evaluations as to the safety, efficacy, and rationale for using particular drugs. *Clin-Alert* consists chiefly of abstracts from the literature on drugs. *Rationale Drug Therapy* provides a monthly review article on drug groups or on the management of specific conditions.

Nurses' Drug Alert, a newsletter produced monthly, reviews other journal articles on the use of drugs for specific disorders. The *Nurse Practitioners' Prescribing Reference* is a quarterly publication produced in New York. It provides the advanced practice nurse with an up-to-date guide to commonly prescribed products available by prescription, as well as selected OTC drugs.

Textbooks

Depending on their purpose and scope, pharmacology textbooks offer basic pharmacologic principles, critical appraisal of useful categories of therapeutic drugs, and descriptions of individual prototype drugs. Prototypes serve as standards of reference for assessing new drugs. Pharmacodynamics and pharmacokinetics are also covered in textbooks. Administration techniques, patient assessment and monitoring, and patient teaching are included in most of the textbooks. However, most are somewhat out of date by the time of publication, so therefore they cannot contain information on recently introduced drugs.

Pocket reference books offer another resource. These references provide specific information regarding administration, assessment and evaluation of patient responses, and patient education considerations.

Health Care Providers

Inevitably, clinical situations occur in which needed information is not contained in presently available resources. The health care provider is then wise to consult with a pharmacist. A pharmacist may be able to provide a brochure or other reference material on the drug. As an expert in the field of drug therapy, the pharmacist is a valuable member of the health care team and should be actively involved in drug regimen decisions.

Each health care provider adopts sources found to be useful and convenient but should guard against undue reliance on one reference for drug information. Periodic use of other resources helps minimize systematic bias in the selection of drugs and drug information data that influence pharmacotherapeutic judgments.

Online Databases

A number of online computer databases have been developed in recent years that provide drug and treatment information to health care providers and the public alike. The most popular of these are accessed through the Internet. The Internet has its roots in the network designed to centralize military computing by the Department of Defense in the late 1960s. This network also linked researchers and defense contractors at colleges and universities across the country through a network of supercomputing centers accessible by personal computers for heavy-duty statistical analyses funded by the National Science Foundation (NSF). Today, the Internet is used by more than 63 million people.

Resources available through the Internet include medical subject directories, clinical resources, conditions and diseases, consumer and patient information, dictionaries and glossaries, online medical journals and news, statistics, and drug information (see Appendix B). A working knowledge of computer databases and resources will continue to be important to successful pharmacotherapeutics as more information becomes available online.

SUMMARY

- Historical writings show that early pharmacotherapeutic efforts were for the most part mystical, based on magic, prayers, and incantations.
- A period of empirical pharmacotherapeutics emerged as clinical evidence of the effectiveness of early drugs became known.
- New drug development during the contemporary period fostered an exponential growth of new drugs entering the marketplace.
- The process of new drug development begins with preclinical studies, progresses through several phases of clinical testing, and ends with postmarketing surveillance studies.
- A drug usually has three designations: a chemical name, a generic name or common name, and a trade name or brand name that identifies the drug as the product of a specific manufacturer.
- The FDA monitors new drug development, often over a period of 6 to 12 years before a drug reaches the marketplace.
- The Orphan Drug Act, private institutions, and other programs support the development of orphan drugs.
- Drug standards were developed as a means of establishing controls that regulate the manufacture, distribution, and use of drugs.
- Formal drug controls have been established through legislation and the policies and procedures of individual institutions.
- The Harrison Narcotic Act of 1914 was the first significant legislation that classified certain drugs as habit-forming.
- The Controlled Substances Act of 1970 classified habit-forming drugs into five schedules and established drug education programs, treatment programs, and rehabilitation centers.
- The only official book of drug standards in the United States is *The United States Pharmacopeia/National Formulary,* whereas Canada uses the *USP, The Canadian Formulary,* and *The British Pharmacopoeia.*
- A prescription order communicates the therapeutic treatment plan to the pharmacist and includes the patient name, date order was written, drug name, dosage, route, frequency, quantity to be dispensed, health care provider's signature, and DEA number (when appropriate).
- There are five different types of drug orders: routine, PRN, single, stat, and protocol orders.
- The AMA recommends that drug orders be written out rather than using unclear, sometimes ambiguous abbreviations.
- Generic drug substitutions for the prescribed drug are acceptable as long as it is the same chemical entity and dosage form as the original prescription.
- Health care providers must check state practice requirements for information regarding record-keeping requirements, prescription refills, expired prescriptions, prescription labeling, prescription copies, out-of-state prescriptions, and drug samples.
- Official sources that will assist the practitioner in making decisions regarding specific drug therapies include *The United States Pharmacopeia/National Formulary* and *The United States Pharmacopeia Dispensing Information (USPDI).*

BIBLIOGRAPHY

Code of Federal Regulations. Title 21, 1300. Washington, D.C.: Superintendent of Documents. Washington, D.C.: United States Government Printing Office.

Compendium of Pharmaceuticals and Specialties. (1990). (25th ed.) Ottawa, Ontario: Canadian Pharmaceutical Association.

Drug Enforcement Administration. (1983). *Physician's Manual.* Washington, D.C.: Drug Enforcement Administration.

Farley, D. (1987–1988). How FDA approves new drugs. *FDA Consumer,* 21(10):6–13.

Goodman, L., Rall, T., Nies, A., Taylor, P. (1990). *Goodman and Gilman's the pharmacologic basis of therapeutics* (8th ed.). New York: Pergamon Press.

Leake, C. (1975). *An historical account of pharmacology to the twentieth century.* Springfield: Charles C Thomas.

Navarra, T. (1990). The history of a love affair. *American Journal of Nursing,* 10, 91–97.

O'Donnell, J. (1992). Understanding adverse drug reactions. *Nursing '92,* 22(8), 34–40.

Rawlins, M. (1995). Pharmacovigilance: Paradise lost, regained or postponed? *Journal of the Royal College of Physicians of London,* 29, 41–49.

Segal, M. (1993). *Rx to OTC: The switch is on.* Rockville, MD: Department of Health and Human Services, Public Health Service, Food and Drug Administration, Office of Public Affairs (Pub. No. 92-3195).

Stehlin, D. (1995). *Getting information from FDA.* Rockville, MD: Department of Health and Human Services, Public Health Service, Food and Drug Administration (Pub. No. 95-1167).

The R_x legend—an FDA manual for pharmacists. Rockville, MD: U.S. Food and Drug Administration.

Thorwald, J. (1963). *Science and secrets of early medicine.* New York: Harcourt, Brace and World.

USPDI. (1991). *Drug Information for the Health Care Professional.* Rockville, MD: United States Pharmacopeial Convention, 1:11.

United States Pharmacopeial Convention. (1990). *The United States pharmacopeia* (22nd rev.). Easton, PA: Mack Printing Company.

United States Pharmacopeial Convention. (1990). *The National Formulary* (17th ed.). Easton, PA: Mack Printing Company.

York, J. (1993). *FDA ensures equivalence of generic drugs.* Rockville, MD: Department of Health and Human Services, Public Health Service, Food and Drug Administration, Office of Public Affairs (Pub. No. 93-3206).

Ziporyn, T. (1985). The Food and Drug Administration: How those regulations came to be. *Journal of the American Medical Association,* 254(15), 2037–2039, 2043–2046.

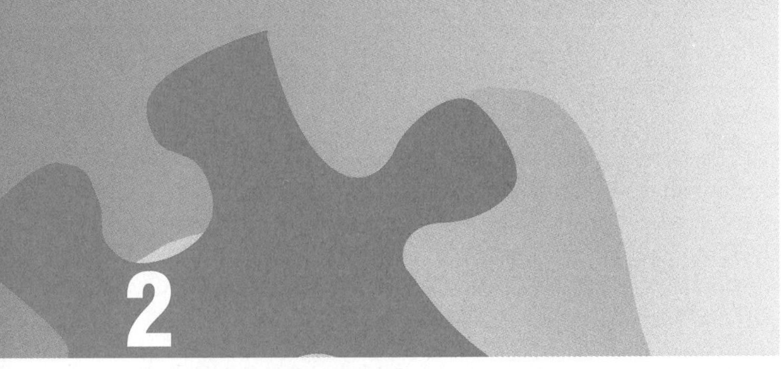

2 Pharmacotherapeutics

The relationship between professional nursing practice and pharmacology has unquestionably changed. Today, professional nurses and certified nurse practitioners need the knowledge and skill to apply advanced treatment technologies and drug therapy. This increased collaboration among health care providers demands in-depth understanding of drug actions and interactions, recognition of therapeutic and adverse effects, and the exercise of judgment in drug administration. Independent nursing practice brings with it increased responsibility for the appropriate use of drugs, identification of safe and appropriate dosages, and accurate monitoring and evaluation of drug effectiveness.

Pharmacotherapeutics is the study of drug use in the treatment of disease as associated with patient care. *Pharmaco-* relates to the science of drug therapy; *therapeutics* speaks to the art of application that results from educated practice. Pharmacotherapeutics is closely interrelated with the individual patient care that is basic to nursing practice.

COLLABORATIVE NATURE OF PHARMACOTHERAPEUTICS

Collaboration means to work together, cooperate, or unite, especially in a joint intellectual effort such as pharmacotherapy. The purpose of collaboration among health care providers is to enhance quality of care and improve patient outcomes. Although patient needs are the primary focus, collaboration also is a synergistic alliance that optimizes the contributions of each professional participant. Historically, prescribing drugs was exclusively a medical function. There was no delegation of the responsibility to others. However, times have changed and now there are a variety of health care providers involved in drug therapies. Further, much remains to be learned about the actual mechanism of drug action as well as the effects of prolonged use. There are also increasing concerns from the public and the health care community about drug-induced illness and disease. Therefore, an awareness of each health care provider's role in pharmacotherapy and the ability and willingness to interact with each other are vital to safe and effective drug management.

Physicians, Dentists, and Nurses

Traditionally, physicians and dentists are responsible for assessing the state of a patient's health, identifying disease, and determining appropriate treatment. When required, they write a prescription and the drug is dispensed by a pharmacist. The person prescribing the drug is accountable for monitoring therapeutic response, treating adverse reactions, and modifying the treatment regimen, if necessary. Increasingly however, the responsibility for assessment, diagnosis, and treatment has expanded to include nurse practitioners, clinical nurse specialists, nurse midwives, and nurse anesthetists.

As advanced practice nurses, these nurses engage in pharmacotherapy through the use of protocols or they have some level of legislated prescriptive authority. Protocols consist of written recommendations, rules, or standards to be followed for any medical situation in which rational procedures can be specified. They are guidelines that provide authorization for the medical aspects of advanced practice nursing. Protocols offer parameters outlining the scope of practice and responsibilities of the advanced practice nurse and the physician for the care of patients with specific diagnoses.

Independent prescriptive authority permits the advanced practice nurse to assess, plan, implement, and evaluate pharmacotherapeutic regimens. In most states, advanced practice nurses have the authority to prescribe by virtue of a Nurse Practice Act, a pharmacy law, a Medical Practice Act, or any combination of the three. Statutory authority indicates that an amendment to a Practice Act or a bill that specifically addresses prescriptive authority has passed the state legislature with the governor's signature. Because prescriptive authority is regulated by the state, the legislative process for obtaining prescriptive authority differs from state to state. In states without legislated prescriptive authority for advanced practice nurses, many nurses are nonetheless actively prescribing for patients through one or more activities. For example, a physician writes the prescription for the patient and the prescription is called into the pharmacy by a nurse under the physician's name. A nurse co-signs the physician's prescription pad, or a nurse carries out prescribing activities using collaboratively developed protocols. Formularies and chart audits have been used to review and monitor prescribing activities. Although there are questions and issues that remain to be addressed (see Questions and Issues to Be Addressed Regarding Prescriptive Authority), most states now have some degree of prescriptive authority for advanced practice nurses.

The issue of prescriptive authority for advanced practice nurses became important as education and expertise progressed to expanded nursing roles. Two early documents recognized the need for prescriptive authority: a 1970 report from the American Medical Association (AMA) and a 1971 report from the Department of Health, Education, and Welfare (HEW). Both documents clearly indicate that prescribing may be the practice of medicine when carried out by a physician, and it may be the practice of nursing when carried out by the nurse. As a result of the publication of these two documents, a number of states are amending nurse practice acts to accommodate this perspective and expansion of the nurse's role.

A 1983 study of nurse-prescribing activities demonstrated high levels of precision and accountability on the part of nurses. Of 1000 nurse-generated prescriptions, 25 percent were for pain relief, 25 percent were for birth control, 40 percent for antimicrobial drugs, and 6 percent were

QUESTIONS AND ISSUES TO BE ADDRESSED REGARDING PRESCRIPTIVE AUTHORITY

- What is the state's existing definition of prescription?
- What is the state's existing definition of dispensing?
- Who are the individuals licensed to prescribe in the state?
- What restrictions are placed on prescriptive authority in the state?
- Do advanced practice nurses see a need to prescribe?
- Is the quality of rural health care a problem without the advanced practice nurse's ability to prescribe?
- What other groups or organizations have an interest in prescriptive authority?
- Would interaction with regulatory boards help or hinder the nurses' cause toward prescriptive authority?
- How do we educate the state legislature and other special interest groups regarding the issue of prescriptive authority?
- What roles and responsibilities do paraprofessionals have or desire regarding prescriptive authority?
- Are advanced practice nurses who presently have prescriptive authority, providing cost-effective care?
- How many nurses are actively engaging in advanced practice roles that may require prescriptive authority?

for drugs used in the management of stable chronic illnesses. Only a handful were prescriptions for controlled substances. Ninety percent of the prescriptions were found to be appropriate in terms of therapeutic usefulness and safety considerations, and they were consistent with explicit protocols. Corresponding but more current research has similar findings. It should be noted that the ratio of nurse-generated prescriptions was lower than those generated by physicians. The functional effectiveness of advanced practice nurses may offer one solution to today's high costs, long waiting periods, and depersonalized health care.

Pharmacologists and Pharmacists

A *pharmacologist* is considered a specialist in pharmacology by virtue of education and experience. A *pharmacist* has the legal authority to compound and dispense drugs on written prescription from a licensed practitioner. The profession of pharmacy includes the provision of drug and therapeutic information to other members of the health care team and the public. The terms pharmacologist and pharmacist are often used interchangeably. Most pharmacists are baccalaureate graduates of a 5- or 6-year education program. The Pharm.D. degree is generally awarded after an additional 6 or 7 years of study. Their education includes advanced, more comprehensive coursework in pathophysiology, pharmacokinetics, and pharmacotherapeutics.

Contemporary pharmacists are employed in a wide variety of settings. Pharmacists can be found in community pharmacies (e.g., in retail or home health care pharmacies) or as consultants to extended care facilities. A clinical pharmacologist is often involved in the initial selection and monitoring of drug therapies. Industrial pharmacists who are employed in drug manufacturing transform raw materials into appropriate drug forms. In contrast, pharmacists in large medical care institutions are less likely to be involved in compounding. They prepare drugs to be dispensed to inpatient care units and, in many cases, to outpatients. In addition, they may be involved with persons who volunteer to be part of research protocols during new drug research, development, and testing. Some pharmacists work with the Food and Drug Administration, the Indian Health Service, or the Armed Forces. An important aspect of the pharmacist's role is to ensure the proper storage and security of drugs.

Associated Health Care Providers

Pharmacy technicians are trained to collect information about patient allergies, transcribe drug orders, prepare drug records or treatment sheets, and order drugs from the manufacturer or supplier. In some settings, they prepare simple prescriptions for dispensing. In some states, the institutionally employed pharmacy technician may be a licensed practical or vocational nurse (LPN/LVN) whose responsibility is to administer prescribed drugs. No formal license is required of pharmacy technicians in many instances. A licensed pharmacist remains responsible for delegated tasks. Evaluation of therapeutic response, however, still falls to the professional nurse.

Registered respiratory therapists (RRTs) may administer drugs (other than anesthetics) that are given by inhalation and are well informed about machines that deliver drugs to the lungs. The educational background of an RRT varies from a 2-year associate degree to more advanced degrees. Like many other health care providers, their scope of practice is dictated by health care agency policies and procedures, job descriptions, state licensure boards, and credentialing agencies. In tertiary care institutions, professional nurses still monitor patient response.

The legal status of the physician's assistant varies from state to state, but in many areas, this individual prescribes drugs following established protocols. Because the legal authority to diagnose and prescribe is limited to the physician, dentist, and select advanced practice nurses, the wisdom of delegating this responsibility has been challenged. In many cases, the physician's assistant has less professional education and experience than the nurse. The nurse may refuse to follow the orders of a physician's assistant in some agencies, and this is particularly true in institutional settings.

PHARMACOTHERAPEUTIC DECISION MAKING

The model of decision making used in this text provides a framework for understanding pharmacotherapeutic decision-making processes (Fig. 2–1). Clinical chapters delineate the expected requisite drug information but then apply the decision-making process through case studies. The model's basic purpose is to focus, factoring in some information as germane to the drug choice and ruling others out as less important to patient outcomes.

The utility of the model comes from the systematic organization it provides for thinking, observing, and analyzing treatment regimens. In addition, it gives structure and rationale for specific activities and a mechanism for professional accountability. The model also offers general criteria for knowing when a patient's problem has been solved. However, it is also important to note a few terms that are commonly misunderstood and misused but that are relevant in considering drug regimens (see Commonly Misused Word Pairs).

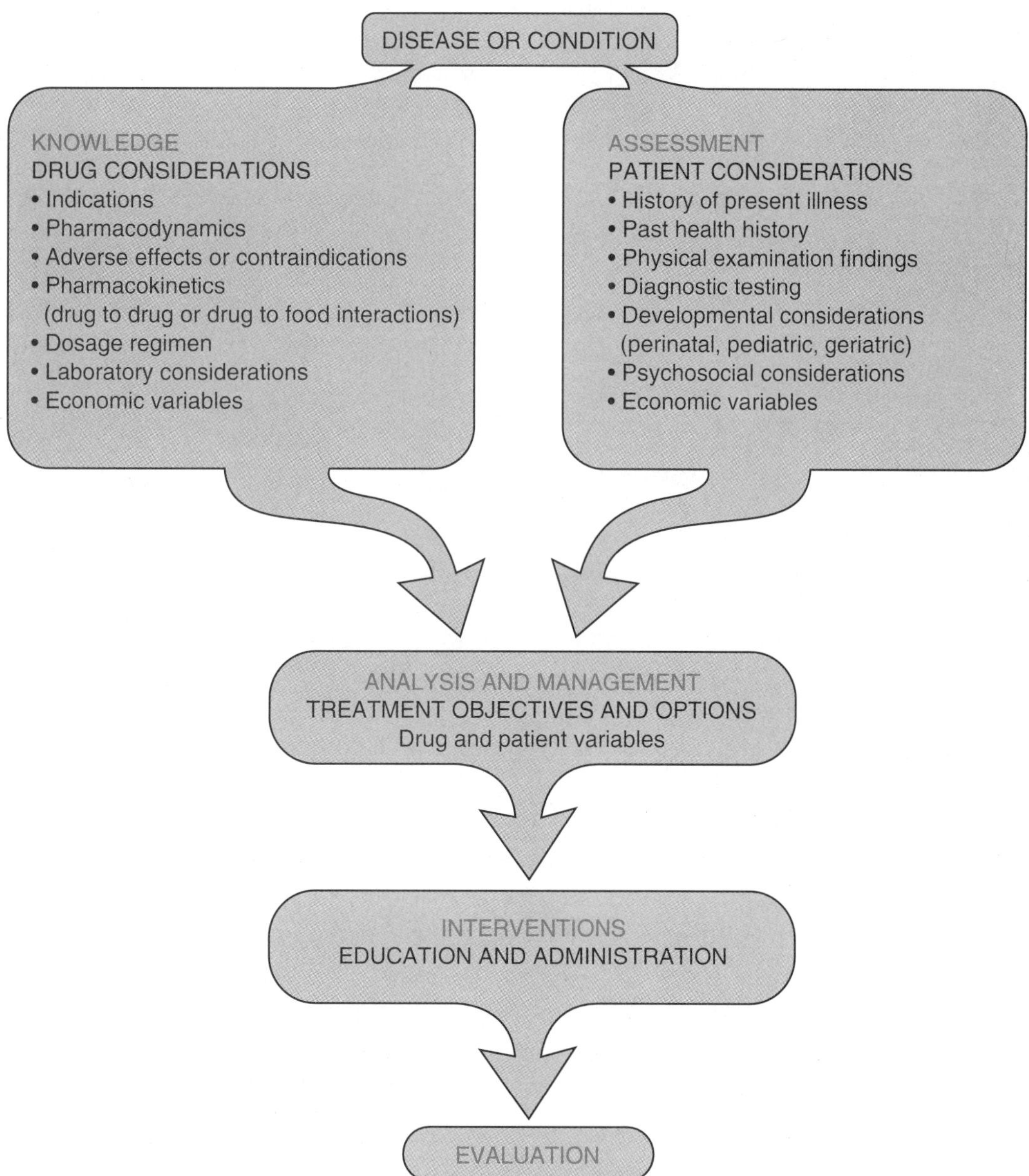

Figure 2–1 Visual representation of pharmacotherapeutic decision-making model.

Requisite Drug Knowledge

No single decision-making model is complete in itself; all components are interrelated and interdependent in some fashion. Drug knowledge begins to interplay with the assessment process as the health care provider works toward a pharmacotherapeutic decision. Because drug knowledge is requisite to drug decisions, in each chapter, attention is first directed at pharmacotherapeutic options.

Various strategies have been used over the years to organize the vast number and variety of drugs into classification schemes. The schemes functionally relate one drug to another in some fashion. For example, drug information has been organized according to body system, therapeutic uses, chemical characteristics, or by drug class. One of the more common ways is by drug class, usually through the use of a prototype drug. Using the drug classification scheme, rote memorization of multiple, isolated facts about individual drugs is minimized, and learning is enhanced.

A prototype drug represents all other drugs in a particular class, as the best example of a drug within the class. In many cases, the prototype was the first drug identified in that class.

At the beginning of each clinical unit, a classification scheme is provided as an overview of the drug class. However, baseline data are needed to determine appropriate drug therapies and to evaluate therapeutic as well as adverse drug effects. Accordingly, in order to make appropriate drug decisions, we must first know the information about the drugs.

The pharmacologic characteristics of a drug group are presented within each of the clinical chapters. The characteristics include indications for the drugs, pharmacodynamics, adverse effects and contraindications, pharmacokinetics,

COMMONLY MISUSED WORD PAIRS

- **Patient:** The person cared for by the physician, nurse, or other health care provider *versus* **Case:** not a patient but an episode or example of illness, injury, or asymptomatic disease
- **Effect:** The result of an action, or to bring about or to cause to come into being *versus* **Affect:** the sum of feelings that accompany a mental state, the appearance of emotion or mood
- **Incidence:** The number of cases developing in a specific unit of population in a specific time *versus* **Prevalence:** the number of cases existing in a specific unit of the population at a specific time.
- **Sign:** Any objective evidence of disease or dysfunction, an observable physical phenomenon frequently associated with a given condition *versus* **Symptom:** An indication of disease or illness perceived by the patient
- **Management:** The process of controlling how something is done or used, a more active process *versus* **Planning:** Consciously setting forth a scheme to achieve a desired end or goal; applies to overall management of a disorder for which a drug is used and much less to the drug itself
- **Dosage:** The amount of drug taken or given in a period, the total amount *versus* **Dose:** the amount of drug to be taken or given at one time; the sum of the doses may be dosage or total dose.

dosage regimens, laboratory considerations, and economic considerations.

Indications

Food and Drug Administration (FDA)–approved therapeutic uses for the drug or drug class are detailed in this section. Newer significant but unlabeled (non–FDA-approved) uses of specific drugs are also discussed here.

Pharmacodynamics

The mechanism of action does not always play a significant role in pharmacotherapeutic decision making. However, it is relevant for some drugs. For example, central nervous system (CNS) depressants indirectly produce respiratory depression. If the patient has a pre-existing respiratory disorder, the use of a CNS depressant may be inadvisable. The initial concepts and principles of pharmacodynamics are discussed in Chapter 5.

Adverse Effects and Contraindications

All drugs have the potential to produce undesirable *effects*. Common examples of undesirable effects include the gastrointestinal (GI) distress produced by aspirin, the sedation often caused by antihistamines, hypoglycemia caused by insulin, and excessive fluid loss caused by diuretics. Some effects can be extremely dangerous, whereas others are only bothersome. Irreversible injury or death may result if toxicity is not identified early and a response quickly generated.

When considering the use of a specific drug, the potential for predictable and unpredictable reactions is taken into account. An effort has been made to include major adverse effects and contraindications, because it is nearly impossible to include all reported reactions in this section. Information regarding cautious use of the drugs is also included. The types of adverse effects are discussed further in Chapter 5. The *incidence* of such effects can be reduced when drugs are used correctly.

Pharmacokinetics

Pharmacokinetics describes what happens to a drug following administration (i.e., what the body does with the drug). Discussions include analyses of absorption, distribution, biotransformation, elimination, protein binding, and half-life. Pharmacokinetic tables provide an overview of these variables. The basic concepts and principles of pharmacokinetics are discussed in Chapter 4, and pharmacokinetic tables are included in each clinical chapter.

Drug-Drug Interactions

Drug-drug interactions are the by-product of the concurrent administration of two or more drugs or of a combination of food and drugs. The resulting interaction can be physical, chemical, or biologic. The interactions that occur can diminish therapeutic effects or increase adverse effects. For example, oral contraceptives are designed to protect against pregnancy. However, their ability to do so can be decreased with concurrent administration of an anticonvulsant drug (e.g., phenobarbital) or certain antibiotics (e.g., tetracycline). Likewise, the risk of thromboembolism secondary to oral contraceptive use can be increased if the woman smokes. A table of drug-drug interactions is included in each clinical chapter.

The number of potentially significant drug-drug interactions increases as pharmacotherapy becomes more complex and drugs more potent. Some drug-drug interactions are intentional and are seen as beneficial. However, most others are unintentional and have potentially harmful effects. Drug-drug interactions often result in treatment delays and hospitalization or, in some cases, increase the length of a hospital stay.

Drug-Food Interactions

Drug-food interactions produce alterations in the therapeutic effects of a drug or in the use of nutrients. Foods interact in various ways to alter drug effectiveness (see Appendix C). They may bind with the drug, decreasing absorption; increase the chemical decomposition of the drug in the intestines; or increase the time it takes for the drug to reach therapeutic levels.

Dosage Regimen

The only common characteristic of dosage regimens is that they have nothing in common. There is no overall pattern to their numeric figures or dosing frequency. Even discussions of regimens sometimes use the term dose and at other times use dosage.

The usual routes of administration are identified together in tables that include adult and pediatric dosages (where appropriate). Drug regimens are provided in commonly used units of measurement. For example, penicillin G is given in units rather than milligrams (mg). Common dosing intervals are also identified. For example, every 4 hours. Situations in which the dosage or interval is different from those commonly encountered are discussed. Administration schedules for drugs to be given pro re nata (PRN) are not fixed. In order to rationally administer a drug PRN, the health care provider needs to know the reason for drug use and be able to assess patient needs.

Laboratory Considerations

Many drugs alter clinical laboratory test results (see Appendix D). Altered results are generally related to the pharmacologic properties of a drug or to interference with the testing procedure. The pharmacologic properties of a drug cause actual changes in the laboratory tests themselves. The changes frequently result from a drug's adverse effects, such as the elevated aspartate aminotransferase (AST, SGPT) level that results from isoniazid hepatotoxicity. Interference with the testing procedure is usually related to the drug itself or its metabolites. For example, the antimicrobial drug cephalothin produces a black-brown or green-brown color when Clinitest tablets are used to check for the presence of glucose in the urine. The results may be misinterpreted as a positive urine test for glucose. Many other cephalosporins, such as cefazolin and cefoxitin, contain noncreatinine chromogens that are not differentiated using the colorimetric method. An overestimation of serum creatinine levels may lead to inadequate drug dosage.

There are many situations that warrant therapeutic drug monitoring. Drug monitoring is warranted when there has been a change in a drug source, dose, or regimen; when noncompliance is suspected; and when patient motivation to maintain a drug regimen is in question. Monitoring may also be warranted when the physiologic status of the patient is altered by factors such as weight gain or loss, menstrual cycle abnormalities, changes in body water, stress, age, or alterations in thyroid function. In addition, concomitant drug therapies can cause synergistic or antagonistic drug interactions. Cardiovascular, renal, or hepatic disorders that influence drug absorption and elimination also provide valid reasons for testing. Monitoring is especially important when there is a narrow margin of safety between therapeutic and toxic drug levels. Drugs that typically have a narrow margin of safety include antiarrhythmics, antibiotics, anticonvulsants, bronchodilators, and cardiac glycosides.

Reliable assessment of a patient's condition and knowledge of drug interactions are used in interpreting laboratory test results. Furthermore, the importance of identifying the sampling time when obtaining specimens cannot be overstated. Whatever the sampling procedure used, it is important that the same time interval that occurred between sampling and drug administration be used in comparing results of serial testing. When interpreting serum drug levels, a current laboratory manual or reference should be consulted. To interpret drug levels accurately, the concepts of peak drug concentration (the time when drug absorption and drug elimination are equal) and the steady-state duration of action must be understood. Serum drug levels provide an easy and more rapid estimation of the patient's drug requirement than does observing for drug effects.

Requisite Patient Database

The nursing process provides a systematic method for gathering information to plan, provide, and evaluate pharmacotherapy. Knowledge and skill in this specific decision-making modality are as requisite for drug therapy as for other aspects of patient care. An assessment database involves collecting subjective and objective data about the patient. The data are used to identify actual and potential health needs. The information contained in the patient's database establishes a foundation for subsequent pharmacotherapeutic decision making. In its simplest form, nursing process, which is referred to as the critical thinking process in this text, has four basic components: assessment, analysis and management, intervention, and evaluation.

Critical Thinking Process

Assessment

History of Present Illness

Assessment begins by eliciting the patient's chief complaint or the reason for the visit to the health care provider. Principal *symptoms* are elicited as they relate to location, quality, quantity, or severity of symptoms. Onset, duration, frequency of occurrence, and the setting in which symptoms occur are noted. In addition, query is made regarding factors that aggravate or alleviate symptoms.

Past Health History

A past health history includes the patient's allergies, concomitant disease or illnesses, accidents, injuries, hospitalizations, and previous surgical procedures. A drug history is a significant component of the patient's past health history. The drug history includes information about a patient's experiences with drugs, although the scope of the drug history varies with the setting and patient situation (Table 2–1). Any drug history, however, should summon similar information

TABLE 2–1 INFORMATION RELEVANT TO DRUG HISTORY DATABASE

Assessment	***Prescription Drug Use*** • Prescription drugs used to treat illness/disease • Self-prescribed drugs (over-the-counter medications) • Street drug use, borrowed prescriptions, home/folk remedies, use of obsolete prescriptions • Caffeine use, smoking history • Drugs prescribed by other providers that may be unknown to current care health care provider ***Responses to Drug Use*** • Therapeutic responses to drugs used in the past • Side effects, adverse drug reactions • Idiosyncratic, paradoxical reactions • Allergic reactions • Tolerance and dependence ***Attitudes Toward Drug Use*** • Attitudes toward drugs and reasons for use and chosen route • Compliance with use or with any special monitoring required • Placebo effects that may have occurred • Knowledge of drug-drug and drug-food interactions • Educational level (impact on current health status and future planned drug regimens)
Analysis	• Identify contraindications to drug use or factors warranting cautious use of a drug • Determine the patient's risk for undesirable reactions • Determine physiologic and psychologic response to previous drug use • Use information in a database to identify potential problems with a planned drug regimen • Identify factors affecting administration or compliance, or both

each time the activity is undertaken. It should include the purpose for prescription, over-the-counter (OTC), street drugs, caffeine, alcohol, and herbal remedies and the dosages, frequency, and duration of use. Smoking history is important because tobacco contains pharmacologically active ingredients. In many cases, the patient may share information about alterations in dosage schedules, use of obsolete prescriptions, home remedies, "borrowed" prescriptions, or drugs prescribed by others. A drug history helps identify the potential for drug-drug and food-drug interactions, aids in accurate interpretation of laboratory test results, provides clues about unreported chronic illnesses and disorders, and even assists in explaining strange new symptoms.

Physical, psychosocial, cultural, and spiritual responses to drug use are ascertained, as well as perspectives the patient and family may have toward drug use in general. Additional information to be elicited includes therapeutic responses, adverse effects, idiosyncratic and paradoxic responses, tolerance, and drug dependency concerns. A family history of idiosyncrasy or other unusual reactions is also important to note.

Many patients are unaware of drug-drug interactions; therefore, it is appropriate to ask about the use of all types of drugs. Certain drugs interact with foods, so it is also important to assess dietary habits in some patients. Information about drug storage may not be an important consideration in a health care environment, but it is important in the home (see Chapter 9).

It is important to know whether or not the patient understands the reason for taking a particular drug, the reason for the route chosen, the adverse effects of the drug, and when it is appropriate to contact the health care provider. Compliance with special monitoring should also be noted (e.g., checking the pulse before taking digoxin, or using fingersticks to monitor blood glucose levels before taking insulin).

Physical Exam Findings

Physical exam findings help identify and verify health-related concerns and explain *signs* and symptoms. Findings help answer patient questions, provide an opportunity for patient teaching, supply a database for future evaluation, and increase both the credibility of and the patient's belief in the advice, recommendations, or reassurance that is provided.

Most patients view a physical exam with some degree of anxiety. They are physically exposed in many cases and feel vulnerable and apprehensive. Patients may be uneasy about what will be found in the exam. At the same time, however, patients often value the detailed attention to their health care concerns and may even enjoy the attention they receive. As the exam proceeds, the patient should be kept informed as to what is happening, especially if discomfort or embarrassment is anticipated.

Diagnostic Testing

Because the health care system involves many different personnel, a working knowledge of other systems and services including the role of diagnostic evaluation is needed. Laboratory and diagnostic tests are tools that, in and of themselves, are almost useless. When these tools are used in combination with a history and physical exam, they help confirm a diagnosis or provide information necessary to monitor the patient's response to therapy.

It is vital to know laboratory reference values. So-called normal reference values are often misleading because of variation in testing procedures from laboratory to laboratory. Theoretically, the term normal refers to the ideal or average value, or it could refer to types of distribution. The reported normal range differs with the methods used and the population tested. Each laboratory provides a normal range for the particular testing method it uses. A sampling of factors that affect or interfere with accurate test results is included in Chapter 9. Conscious attention to these factors improves the likelihood of accurately interpreting test results.

Developmental Considerations

Age is a significant variable that determines how a patient responds to a particular drug regimen. The very young, pregnant women, and older adults tend to respond differently to drugs. The immature liver and kidneys of the very young delay drug biotransformation and elimination. Normal changes of pregnancy influence drug response in the woman as well as the unborn child. The older adult is susceptible to adverse drug effects and toxicity because of age-related changes in liver and kidney functioning. Chapters 6, 7, and 8 discuss the impact that maturational and physiologic changes have on drug response in perinatal, pediatric, and geriatric patients.

Psychosocial Considerations

Health beliefs and practices are an integral feature of every known culture and society. The perspective of the individual is a major factor in how health and illness are defined in that community. Health is most often viewed as a continuum. Wellness is located on one end of the continuum, the optimal level of functioning, with illness at the other end, culminating in death. At any point along the continuum, a patient has both positive attributes of wellness and negative attributes of illness (Fig. 2–2). Health and illness are dynamic and vary as interactions between the patient and the internal and external environments change. Health beliefs reflect what is considered a healthy state, and what can be gained with intervention by the health care provider. For example, a patient who does not perceive dizziness and early morning occipital headaches as abnormal is unlikely to seek attention for hypertension.

Illness is culturally defined. What is diagnosed as illness in one society may be viewed as a normal phenomenon in another. Further, within a single society, there may be a lack of consensus as to what signs and symptoms indicate illness. For some persons, the term normal is not a statistical concept but a personal judgment. In other words, in a group of people with the same symptoms, some would seek medical care, whereas others would ignore the symptoms, failing to associate them with illness. Heavy reliance on signs and symptoms is one of the primary problems with the medical model of illness. Except for gross abnormalities, manifestations that differentiate normal from abnormal are vague. The challenge is to determine at what point a change in structure and function becomes a sign or a symptom of disease requiring drug therapy.

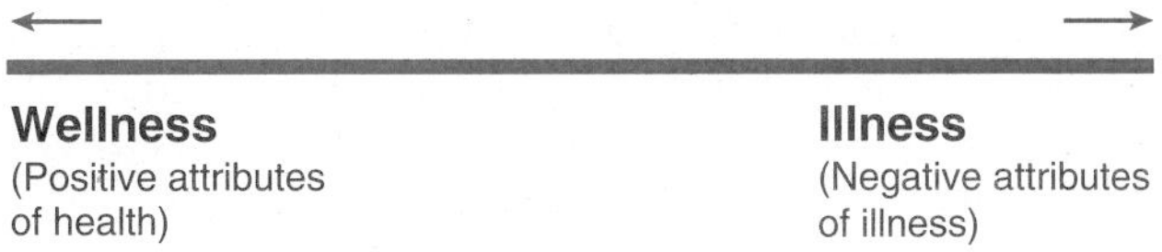

←   →

Wellness
(Positive attributes of health)

Illness
(Negative attributes of illness)

Figure 2–2 Health-illness continuum.

Cultural dimensions are a vital consideration in pharmacotherapeutics because the rich variety of patients' cultural and ethnic backgrounds has resulted in a wealth of folk practices. Each of the four major ethnic subgroups in American society (i.e., blacks, Hispanic, Asian, and Native Americans) have culturally diverse health beliefs and practices that influence health and illness. Further, the science of *ethnopharmacology* is attempting to bridge the gap between traditional use of medicinal plants and their role in health care today. The many factors that influence ethnopharmacologic practices are inherent in cultural beliefs about the causes of illness.

Ethnopharmacologic practices view the individual as a composite of psycho-socio-cultural-spiritual and physiologic forces that interact with the internal and external environments. This belief is in contrast to Western medicine, in which diagnosis of disease is made by categorizing pathophysiologic deviations in body systems. An exploration of folk beliefs and practices may reveal many cross-cultural similarities and, as such, help explain epidemiologic differences in morbidity. The differences may be an indication of the culture-specific significance placed on certain disease-related problems. What is commonplace and unavoidable may be considered insignificant, whereas unacceptable symptomatic behaviors, regardless of the cause, may be denied. Further, societal differences in health and illness-related practices influence both the degree to which a patient is aware of body symptoms and the decision to act on those symptoms. Relief of symptoms, or lack thereof, is not a reliable basis in determining whether symptoms are somatic or psychogenic in origin. In most cases, drugs are generally more effective when the patient has a positive outlook and anticipates a therapeutic response.

All things being equal, the cost of a drug regimen is important when evaluating treatment options. Consideration should be given to the impact a specific regimen will have on the financial resources of the patient, particularly the older adult, who is often a victim of polypharmacy. For example, 1 g of an antibiotic such as cefazolin given every 8 hours for 5 days costs between $42 and $110. On the other hand, ceftriaxone, a newer antibiotic, costs approximately $300 for a 2-g dose given every 12 hours for 7 days.

Analysis and Management

Treatment Objectives

The first step of management is to determine treatment objectives. Treatment objectives are developed based on all available patient and drug information. Goals, priorities, interventions, and evaluation criteria should be individualized and set. It is important to recognize that the locus of decision making includes both the patient and family. Management decisions should not be a unilateral process. Treatment objectives are influenced by the severity, urgency, and prognosis. Prevention, cure, alleviation, and palliation therapies are interrelated and interdependent in many instances. Therefore, drugs may be prescribed for any or all of these purposes.

Initial drug regimens are chosen from among a variety of reasonable alternatives. It should be noted that reasonable alternatives and adjuncts include nondrug therapies. Specific interventions are directed at resolving or preventing problems identified in the analysis.

Prevention Primary preventative health behaviors are most commonly viewed as voluntary actions taken to decrease the threat of illness. Actions taken with this objective in mind are not curative or restorative because they occur before symptoms appear. Identification and correction of precipitating factors constitute an important component of preventive regimens. Primary prevention measures such as proper diet, exercise, and immunizations may avert a specific disease or illness.

Immunizations are a deliberate attempt to protect the individual against disease. Active immunity is obtained by developing antibodies that render a person immune to a particular disease. Antigenic stimulation is produced either by having the disease or through inoculation with a vaccine. Passive immunity is acquired in utero from antibodies that pass from the mother through the placenta to the fetus or that are acquired by the newborn by breastfeeding. Passive immunity may also be produced by injecting antibodies. Drugs used to cause active and passive immunity are discussed further in Chapter 28.

Steps should be taken to ensure that the patient has the requisite knowledge with which to make an informed decision. Explaining the consequences of the disease for which a patient is at risk and providing information about how they can reduce vulnerability to the disease is a vital component. Societal group norms and peer pressure have been used in some situations to promote preventive health behaviors.

Cure Three sets of criteria are used in identifying a disease in the traditional biologic perspective of health and illness: the patient's subjective experience of illness, the finding that the patient has some disorder of body system or function, and symptoms forming an identifiable pattern that meets diagnostic criteria. In other words, the person is said to be ill or diseased when signs and symptoms or results of laboratory testing and physical exam fit a particular model or pattern of disease.

In one sense, illness is viewed as the body's attempt to adapt to internal and external stressors and noxious conditions. The signs and symptoms that result tend to draw attention to bodily functions when they are sufficiently disturbing or intense. There may be apprehension about minor alterations in body function that in health would go unnoticed. Unusual sensations act as stimuli to remind the patient of the illness or disease. Minor variations in temperature, pulse, digestion, or elimination take on an importance that would in other circumstances go unnoticed. Relief of the alterations begin to take precedence over other needs.

For an individual to function in the sick role, however, persons around them must perceive that the patient is ill. The classic components of the sick role were defined by Parsons in the early 1950s and include the right of the individual to be held blameless for the illness. Thus, the patient has a right to be released from routine responsibilities. Further, the patient has a duty to view illness and disease as undesirable and to try to get well, to seek competent assistance from a health care provider, and to cooperate with the plan of care.

Relief of signs and symptoms as well as the illness are usually a priority concern for patients. However, the extent to which signs and symptoms can be relieved is dependent on the extent and the severity of the illness or disease. Drugs used in the treatment of disease and illness may be organized into three major groups: replacement, supportive, and maintenance therapies, or a combination of all three. Replacement drug therapies are appropriate when there is an identifiable deficiency and may be short-term or long-term in nature. For example, a patient who has a deficiency of thyroid hormone requires life-long supplemental thyroid hormone replacement. Ferrous sulfate, for example, is an iron preparation used in the short-term treatment of iron deficiency anemia until the patient's own iron reserves are replenished.

Relieving signs and symptoms of illness or disease also includes psychological as well as physical interventions such as providing reassurance, limiting activity, or providing oxygen. Symptomatic illness management may require life-style redesign in some cases. For example, a patient with ulcerative colitis may elect to go only to events in locations where the restrooms are nearby.

Alleviation On the other hand, supportive therapy may be required when a certain illness threatens other body systems. Drugs may be used until the primary condition is alleviated or under control. For example, a patient with an acute myocardial infarction may require a histamine-2 antagonist such as famotidine to minimize the potential for stress-related duodenal ulcers.

Supportive therapies may be used for patients who have chronic long-term conditions. The objective of supportive therapy is to maintain a patient's level of wellness while halting further progression of the disease. For example, hypertension is not curable. However, it can be managed effectively by using a variety of drugs and through life-style modification. A postmenopausal woman uses calcium supplements and hormones to minimize the debilitating effects of osteoporosis.

Drugs that are used for a specific disease or condition are many and varied or limited. The most appropriate treatment regimen takes into account the specific characteristics of the drug and patient variables that relate to compliance, the benefits and risks of using a particular drug, serum drug levels desired, concerns related to toxicity, dosing frequency, and last but not least, the cost. At times, the identification and correction of precipitating factors may require drug therapy, surgery, or other interventions. For example, a patient with congestive heart failure may require antiarrhythmic drugs to treat cardiac irregularities, surgery to correct a preexisting valvular dysfunction, or thrombolytic drugs to treat an ischemic problem. In this example, the drugs are used as a secondary intervention because several other pathologic processes are present.

Palliation The term palliation means to alleviate without curing. As used in common practice, palliation therapy is typically used for patients with end-stage illness or disease. Interventions are used to make the patient as comfortable as possible. For example, home oxygen therapy (oxygen is considered a drug) may be used for someone with end-stage pulmonary disease. Pain management is accomplished with around-the-clock, reliable, high-dose intravenous infusions of opioid analgesics.

Treatment Options

Drug Variables

There are a multitude of factors influencing the decision to use a particular drug regimen. The therapeutic value of the drug (i.e., risk-benefit ratio) is weighed against its inherent risks. Historically, this risk-benefit ratio has been determined by the health care provider. With an increased understanding of health care needs and the health care system, patients take a more active role in pharmacotherapeutic regimens. The seriousness of the disease or illness and the availability of less toxic, more reliable drugs are still taken into consideration.

Whether a drug is useful depends on its ability to produce only the desired effects with tolerable undesired effects. Thus, from the viewpoint of therapeutic indications, the selectivity of effects is one of the most important characteristics. *Selectivity* is the ability of a drug to act at specific sites to produce an action, whereas the presence of the drug at other sites does not lead to any measurable response.

Patient Variables

In considering a particular drug regimen, it should be acknowledged that there are risks inherent in every beneficial therapy. Will possible adverse effects compromise an already stressed cardiovascular, respiratory, renal, or hepatic system? Will the drug alter the patient's mental status to such an extent that it increases the possibility of injury or dependence on others? Do adverse effects of a drug include the possibility of bladder or bowel incontinence, which, in turn, may cause a loss of dignity? The patient's unique set of circumstances should be taken into consideration when the benefits and risks of a particular drug regimen are weighed.

In making pharmacotherapeutic decisions, the likelihood of patient compliance and, at times, the cost of the therapy are also analyzed. Individual patient preferences impact specific drug regimens.

Intervention

Intervention involves carrying out therapeutic activities. Most interventions are independent nursing actions but some require collaboration with other health care providers. The two key interventions are drug administration and patient and family education.

Administration

Drugs can be of great value to the patient but only if they are taken correctly. Successful therapy requires informed and active patient participation. Therefore, knowledge of the degree to which a patient will follow through with a planned treatment regimen influences not only the drug that is ordered but also the dosing frequency and route of administration. For example, if there is a choice between prescribing oral cimetidine four times a day or ranitidine twice a day, the twice-daily regimen is more likely to promote compliance.

This is especially true if the patient does not like taking pills or cannot remember to take them at all.

Although drug administration can occur without a detailed understanding of pharmacology, having such knowledge helps reduce medication errors. Administration times are dictated in part by agency policy, patient preference, diagnostic testing, drug characteristics, and other treatment regimens currently in use. For example, some health care agencies routinely give drugs at 9 AM, 1 PM, 5 PM, and 9 PM when the drug is to be given four times a day. On the other hand, specialty areas, such as intensive care, maternal-infant, or pediatric units, may have other administration times to better coincide with patient needs. However, dosing intervals for a given drug are seldom changed. For example, dosages of anticoagulants are titrated based on the patient's partial thromboplastin time (PTT) or similar measure. In many cases, a drug is administered once daily in the afternoon to permit time for the test results to return. In another example, diuretics are usually taken early in the day to avoid interference with patient rest. Corticosteroids are frequently administered on a twice-daily schedule. Two-thirds of the daily dose is taken in the morning, with the remaining third taken in the late afternoon. The split-dose regimen closely matches most patients' normal secretion biorhythm of corticosteroids. Still another example is the dosing schedules for many antimicrobial drugs. They are most often administered around the clock in order to maintain a steady-state level of drug in the serum.

Drugs taken on a daily basis can usually be taken on a more flexible schedule; however, they should be taken as close to the same time each day as possible. Exempt from flexible schedules are one-time-only drug orders, such as those given before surgery or diagnostic procedures, and those that require more frequent administration schedules (e.g., every 2 hours, every 4 hours). Stat orders should be given when ordered.

The rationale for using a particular drug dose and frequency requires a basic understanding of the drug in question and the number of variables associated with dose-response and time-response relationships (see Chapter 5). Variables influencing dose–response time relationships include

- *Drug potency:* the absolute amount of drug required to produce a desired effect
- *Therapeutic index:* the ratio of effective dose to lethal dose
- *Maximum effect:* the greatest response possible regardless of the dose given

Time-response variables include

- *Latency:* the time necessary for a therapeutic effect to occur
- *Peak:* the time it takes for drug effects to reach maximum
- *Duration:* the length of time the drug is effective

The time-response variables are affected by a patient's biorhythms, how the body reacts to the drug, and the route of administration. Doses are given at appropriate intervals to avoid accumulation of the drug and toxicity. If the dosing interval is too short, drug accumulation occurs. Serum drug concentrations drop if the dosing interval is too long. The drop occurs because the drug continues to be excreted and not replaced. Orally administered drugs with short half-lives do not accumulate if they are taken frequently because a short dosing interval is necessary to maintain a steady state. In contrast, drugs with long half-lives are often taken only once daily.

Dosing relationships are interpreted on the basis of a normal curve (the average person in the population). The normal curve explains why certain drugs with relatively long half-lives can be taken once daily. Likewise, it explains why a drug scheduled to be given every 6 hours may not be as effective if it is given four times a day. That is, there are 6 hours between doses with a dosing frequency of every 6 hours (6–12–6–12) but only 4 hours between doses given 4 times daily (9–1–5–9). This means that there are 12 hours between the last dose on one day and the first dose of the next day. It is less likely that optimal serum or tissue levels will be maintained by the later schedule. It also explains why drug regimens must be continually reassessed. Increasing the dose or frequency of administration increases the pharmacologic effect, within limits. It can also increase the risk of adverse effects. Chapters 3 and 4 discuss the relationships and dose-response curve in more depth. On another note, to prevent errors related to drug orders, a few practical guidelines should be observed (Table 2–2).

Dosage calculations and drug administration skills are topics that are thoroughly addressed in the *Saunders Nursing Drug Handbook 1998* and *Clinical Calculations* (3rd edition) by Kee and Marshall. General supplemental material is included in Appendix E, Dosing Formulas, and Appendix F, Administration Techniques.

Education

The objective of patient education is to assist the individual to incorporate health-related behaviors into everyday life. The void between a patient's knowledge level and what information is needed for compliance is referred to as a learning deficit. In order to reduce adverse drug effects, knowledge of the major effects that taking the drug can produce, the time when these reactions are likely to occur, and the early signs that a reaction is developing must be known. Measures used to reduce adverse drug effects include identifying the high-risk patient through gathering the patient history, ensuring proper administration through patient education, and forewarning the patient about activities that might precipitate an adverse reaction. Patient education is seen as vital to the successful outcome of drug therapy (see Chapter 9). By educating the patient about the drugs being taken, the health care provider can elicit the required level of participation.

A great amount of time can be spent in pharmacotherapeutic teaching-learning activities. Yet poor understanding of verbal instructions and written materials remains a major factor in failure to achieve treatment objectives. Patients vary greatly in their ability to hear, read, and translate verbal language and written instructions into a meaningful whole. Close attention should be given to the patient's reading and comprehension abilities. Drug compliance is best achieved when both verbal and written information is presented at the appropriate level of understanding.

TABLE 2–2 SELECTED STRATEGIES FOR PREVENTING DRUG ERRORS

Potential Problem with Drug Orders	Recommended Action
Unusually large dosage or excessive increase in dosage ordered Drug form used in an unfamiliar fashion Single order contains more than one drug Ambiguous orders, drug names that include numerals	Check order with health care provider, pharmacist, or literature.
Multiple tablets or several vials are necessary to prepare single dose	Check all dosage calculations with a peer.
Illegible, incomplete orders	Obtain clear copy of order.
Nonstandard abbreviations or symbols Slang names, colloquialisms	Avoid use when transcribing drug orders, writing notes, or prescriptions.
Telephone and verbal orders	Do not take or give a telephone or verbal order except in an emergency.
First time patient has taken drug	Read package insert carefully. Double check for patient allergies.
New drug is added to drug regimen	Check for drug-drug interactions. Commit common interactions to memory.

Evaluation

Like assessment and intervention, evaluation of patient response is an important aspect of drug therapy. After all, evaluation is the process that tells us if the drug therapy worked. The evaluation of patient response is organized around four areas: therapeutic response, secondary or adverse effects, compliance and accurate self-administration, and the patient's satisfaction with prescribed therapy. Evaluating patient response to a drug that has more than one application requires that the health care provider know the specific indication for which the drug is used.

Evaluation of therapeutic response may be accomplished by monitoring physiologic parameters (e.g., vital signs, absence of infection, serum or urine drug levels, body weight, and serum and urine chemistry values). For example, in the patient receiving nifedipine to treat hypertension, his or her blood pressure should be monitored for reduction in systolic and diastolic pressures. In contrast, when the same drug is used to treat angina, the patient should be evaluated for decreased chest pain. Knowing the purpose of drug use helps guide the health care provider in the evaluation process. When beneficial responses develop as hoped, ignorance of expected adverse effects might not be so bad. However, when desired responses do not occur, it is essential to identify the situation early because intervention with an alternative therapy may be needed.

Evaluation of secondary or adverse effects is also conducted. The responses may be predictable (dose related) or unpredictable (patient sensitivity related). Dose-related responses result from unknown pharmacologic effects of a drug. Sensitivity-related responses cannot be predicted or foreseen. An allergic reaction is an example of a sensitivity-related response that is unrelated to dosage. Secondary or adverse effects are discussed in Chapter 5.

Methods available to assess the degree of patient compliance and self-satisfaction with the treatment regimen may include pill counts, the review of a drug diary, self-reports, direct observation, assessment of physiologic parameters, and input from other health care workers, family members, or friends. Combining several methods provides for a more accurate assessment. Other assessment and intervention strategies to promote compliance are discussed in Chapter 9.

Satisfaction with the treatment regimen is an important consideration that is often ignored or skimmed over when evaluating drug effectiveness. However, patient satisfaction is closely tied to compliance. Dissatisfaction may lead to noncompliance and failure of an otherwise adequate drug regimen. Dissatisfaction can be prevented if therapy is designed around the patient's life-style, resources and preferences, and health care needs. Hence, patient and family involvement is a necessity.

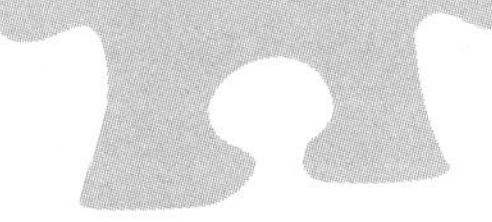

SUMMARY

- A variety of health care providers are included in pharmacotherapeutics: physicians and dentists, advanced practice nurses, pharmacologists and pharmacists, pharmacy technicians, RRTs, and physician assistants.
- Requisite drug knowledge includes indications, pharmacodynamics, adverse effects and contraindications, pharmacokinetics, dosage regimens, laboratory considerations, and economic variables.
- Requisite patient database includes a history of present illness, past health history, physical exam findings, diagnostic testing, developmental considerations (perinatal, pediatric, geriatric), psychosocial considerations, and economic variables.
- Management involves the development of treatment objectives and consideration of treatment options.

- Interventions include activities that surround drug administration, and patient and family education.
- Evaluation of patient response is ongoing. It is organized around therapeutic response, secondary or adverse effects, compliance and accurate self-administration, and the patient's satisfaction with prescribed therapy.
- Patient satisfaction with the prescribed drug regimen promotes compliance and increases quality of life in the long term.

BIBLIOGRAPHY

American Nurses Association. (1993). Advanced nursing practice: A new age in health care. In *Nursing facts*. Washington DC: Author.

American Nurses Association. (1993). Primary health care: The nurse solution. In *Nursing facts*. Washington DC: Author.

Babcock, D., and Miller, M. (1994). *Client education: Theory and practice*. St. Louis: C.V. Mosby.

Batey, M., and Holland, J. (1985). Prescribing practices among nurse practitioners in adult and family health. *American Journal of Public Health,* 75(3), 258–262.

Bigbee, J. (1984). Territoriality and prescriptive authority for nurse practitioners. *Nursing and Health Care,* 5(2), 106–110.

Bigbee, J., Lundin, S., Corbett, J., et al. (1984). Prescriptive authority for nurse practitioners: A comparative study of professional attitudes. *American Journal of Public Health,* 74(2), 162–163.

Bradford, R. (1989). Obstacles to collaborative practice. *Nursing Management,* 20(4), 72I–72P.

Bullough, B. (1992). Alternative models for specialty nursing practice. *Nursing and Health Care,* 13(5), 254–259.

Cohn, S. (1984). Prescriptive authority for nurses. *Law, Medicine and Health Care,* 4, 72–75.

Congress of the United States Office of Technology Assessment. (1986). *Nurse practitioners, physician assistants, and certified nurse-midwives: A policy analysis*. HCS 37. December.

Dukes, J., and Stewart, R. (1993). Be prepared. *Health Service Journal,* 103, 24–25.

Faucher, M. (1992). Prescriptive authority for advanced nurse practitioners: A blueprint for action. *Journal of Pediatric Health Care,* 6(1), 25–31.

Fennell, K. (1991). Prescriptive authority for nurse-midwives: A historical review. *Nursing Clinics of North America,* 26(2), 511–522.

Fondiller, S. (1991). How case management is changing the picture. *American Journal of Nursing,* 91(1), 64–80.

Fry, E. (1968). A readability formula that saves time. *Journal of Reading,* 11, 513–516, 575–577.

Hadley, E. (1989). Nurses and prescriptive authority: A legal and economic analysis. *American Journal of Law and Medicine,* 15(2/3), 245–299.

Holden, R. (1991). Responsibility and autonomous nursing practice. *Journal of Advanced Nursing,* 16, 398–403.

Kassirer, J. (1994). What role for nurse practitioners in primary care? *New England Journal of Medicine,* 330(3), 204–205.

Le Breck, D. (1989). Clinical judgement: A comparison of theoretical perspectives. In *Review of research in nursing education* (Vol. II). New York: National League for Nursing.

McLain, B. (1988). Collaborative practice: A critical theory perspective. *Research in Nursing and Health,* 11, 391–398.

National Council of State Boards for Nursing, Inc. (1991). *Advanced Practice Survey Results,* 12(2), 12–14.

Nunn, C. (1997). Pathways, guidelines, and cookbook medicine: Are we all becoming Betty Crocker? *Journal of Clinical Outcomes Management,* 4(1), 17–24.

Pauker, S., and Kassirer, J. (1980). The threshold approach to clinical decision-making. *New England Journal of Medicine,* 302(20), 1110–1116.

Pearson, L. (1997). Annual update on how each state stands on legislative issues affecting advanced nursing practice. *The Nurse Practitioner: The American Journal of Primary Health Care,* 22(1), 18–86.

Phelps, C., and Mushlin, A. (1988). Focusing medical technology assessment using medical decision theory. *Medical Decision Making,* 8, 279–289.

Safreit, B. (1992). Health care dollars and regulatory sense: The role of advanced practice nursing. *Yale Journal on Regulation,* 9(2), 417–487.

Sekscenski, E., Sansom, S., Bazell, C., et al. (1994). State practice environments and the supply of physician assistants, nurse practitioners, and certified nurse-midwives. *New England Journal of Medicine,* 331(19), 1266–1271.

Sellards, S., and Mills, M. (1995). Administrative issues for use of nurse practitioners. *Journal of Nursing Administration,* 25(5), 64–70.

Tanner, C. (1986). Research on clinical judgement. In W. Holzemer (Ed.), *Review of research in nursing education* (Vol I). New York: National League for Nursing.

Tanner, C. (1987). Teaching clinical judgement. In J. Fitzpatrick and R. Taunton (Eds.), *Annual review of nursing research* (Vol. V). New York: Springer Publishing Company.

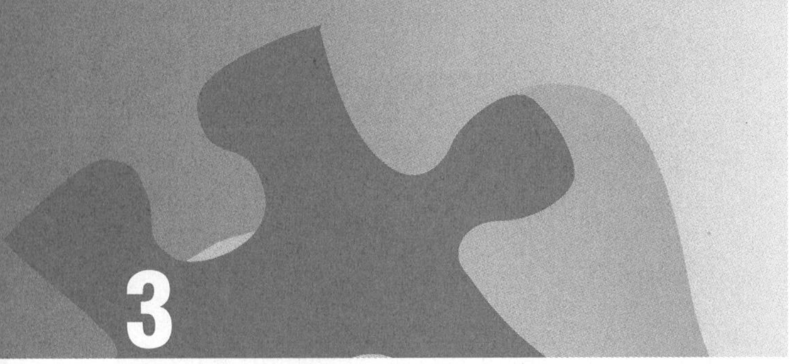

3 Pharmacoeconomics

In just a few years, pharmacoeconomics has grown from relative obscurity to having a prominent role in the development and application of clinical pharmacology. This is because the provision of health care has dramatically changed in recent years. Health care's guiding principle was once "the best that money could buy," with little consideration given to cost. When a health care provider believed a patient needed treatment, it was ordered and the responsible party, whether it was the patient, insurance company, Medicare, or Medicaid, paid the bill. Furthermore, pharmaceutical companies created new products in the belief that health care providers would use them even if the benefits were only marginal or the number of adverse effects decreased.

Increasingly, the operating principle is changing to "the best health care we can afford." Today's payors for health care services are demanding that new pharmaceuticals demonstrate benefits that are worth additional costs. At the same time, employers, insurance companies, and the government are firmly encouraging health care providers to consider the cost effectiveness as well as the safety and efficacy of their treatment options. In response, pharmacy programs are offering courses and fellowships in pharmacoeconomics and nursing programs are including health care economics in curricula. Indeed, it is estimated that 20 percent of the $300 to 400 million spent by the pharmaceutical industry to bring a new drug to market is directed toward its pharmacoeconomics.

Pharmacoeconomics is much like the story of the blind men and the elephant, in which each man had a different belief as to what an elephant was depending on the tactile sensations he felt. This chapter is an introduction to the subject and offers the reader an opportunity to sample the variety and depth of this discipline while beginning to appreciate claims made by researchers in the field. Additional information about pharmacoeconomics is available from resources in the bibliography and through the International Society of Pharmacoeconomics and Outcomes Research.*

PHARMACOECONOMICS DEFINED

Pharmacoeconomics is defined as an analysis that identifies, measures, and compares the costs and consequences of pharmaceutical products and services. This new emerging science is the means by which cost factors are incorporated into clinical decisions for pharmacotherapy. As cost limitations increase and cost effectiveness becomes more critical in the day-to-day treatment of patients, health care providers must have a basic understanding of pharmacoeconomics so as to grasp the rationale for choices made, make cost-effective treatment decisions themselves, and educate and advise patients better.

Pharmacoeconomics was initially concerned with only evaluating drug treatment. But as the field matures, it is becoming apparent that a complete evaluation of disease treatment must include consideration of nondrug treatments. For example, a thorough evaluation of treatment for depression must include consideration not only of the various antidepressant drugs but also of psychotherapy, a possible adjunct to drug treatment. In keeping with that philosophy, this chapter discusses the evaluation of treatment options, not just drug therapy, though the vast majority of treatment options are pharmaceuticals.

PHILOSOPHICAL BASIS OF PHARMACOECONOMICS

Pharmacoeconomic analyses encompass two related but separate philosophies—resource allocation and increased efficiency. The first is primarily concerned with allocating health care resources between broad treatment choices. The second is concerned with increasing the efficacy of medical care.

Resource Allocation

In a society with unlimited resources, it would be unnecessary to have methods that determine the best way to allocate resources among alternatives. However, in today's health care environment, resources are limited. In the mid-1990s, U.S. spending for health care exceeded one trillion dollars for the first time and spending is projected to grow 50 percent faster than the gross national product for the remainder of the decade. Throughout the world, there are pressures on public budgets as policymakers and the public begin to recognize that every dollar spent on health care is one dollar no longer available for education, crime prevention, or improvement in infrastructure. Further, much of what we now spend is used for care that does not improve our health and yields small improvements at an exorbitant cost. Even the Food and Drug Administration (FDA) and Medicare do not use cost effectiveness as a criterion for making what are, in essence, decisions about resource allocation. The use of criteria by the private sector, hospitals, health maintenance organizations, insurers, and other decision-makers is limited.

The basic question has been as follows: Given a variety of treatment choices and limited resources, which options should we choose? A common example is whether society is better off spending its limited resources on high-cost drugs that are marginally more effective or that have fewer adverse effects, or whether society would be better off spending its limited resources on older, less expensive drugs that allow us to treat a greater number of people. The field of pharmacoeconomics has traditionally focused on society and its choices to provide an optimal mix of services to all recipi-

* The International Society of Pharmacoeconomics and Outcomes Research. Five Independence way, Suite 300, Princeton, NJ 08540-6627. Tel: (609) 452-0209. Fax: (609) 452-7473.

ents. Its roots are in health care economics and public health, and has concentrated on the greater good.

Resource allocation has been the main concern of governmental agencies such as the Health Care Financing Agency when determining which treatments to fund under Medicare, or the Agency for Health Care Policy and Research when developing treatment guidelines. Pharmaceutical companies have generally used a policymaking approach when conducting studies that evaluate the cost effectiveness of products. Economic studies are conducted to meet the regulatory requirements of the FDA or to convince managed care providers that their product is more cost effective than a competitor's product.

Increased Efficiency

Although resource allocation is useful for a governmental agency trying to determine whether to fund an expensive new treatment, this philosophy provides little guidance to a health care provider or managed care organization trying to determine the most efficient means of treating a disease. Whereas general pharmacoeconomics helps determine the best allocation of resources across society, health care providers are concerned with how to treat a disease state most efficiently, given that the disease must be treated and that there are competing treatment options. This is the field of *applied pharmacoeconomics*. The field emerged as providers and managed care organizations looked for more efficient ways to provide quality health care.

An example might provide a clearer understanding of the distinction between the philosophies of resource allocation and increased efficiency. It is generally agreed that in treating depression, there is little difference in the efficacy of the various treatment options. The differences are in the level of adverse effects and adverse outcomes between the various treatments. One question facing an organization is whether it should pay the additional cost of newer antidepressants that appear to have fewer adverse effects or continue to pay for older drugs that are just as effective but that have potentially more adverse effects. One way to answer this question would be to conduct a pharmacoeconomic study to determine whether the marginal benefit to be gained by using a new drug was greater than the marginal cost of an older drug. This is the approach taken by *general pharmacoeconomics*. The answer suggests to the organization how to allocate its limited resources between the various antidepressant drugs.

At the same time, this information is of little benefit to the health care provider who must choose, from over 20 different drug treatment options and psychotherapy, the option that will best treat the patient for the least total cost. Instead, it is necessary to assess all reasonable treatment options and compare them among themselves to make the most efficient choice. Finally, it is possible that a new antidepressant can be cost effective from a resource allocation point of view and still not be the best choice for treating the patient.

MODELS FOR ECONOMIC ANALYSES

There are four basic pharmacoeconomic models—cost-benefit analysis (CBA), cost-effectiveness analysis (CEA), cost-utility analysis (CUA), and cost-minimization analysis (CMA). Each of these approaches measures costs in dollars but measures outcomes (consequences) differently. CBA measures outcomes in dollars, whereas CEA measures outcomes in terms of natural units (e.g., reduction in blood pressure in millimeters of mercury [mmHg]). CUA measures outcomes by incorporating preferences (utilities) with natural outcomes (e.g., quality-adjusted life-years [QALYs]). CMA assumes equal outcomes between treatment options (e.g., generic products). Each of these approaches has its own advantages and disadvantages, degrees of usefulness, and value. Table 3–1 compares the four approaches to economic analysis.

Cost-Benefit Analysis

CBA has traditionally been the choice of economists. In CBA, all costs and benefits are valued in monetary terms, generally dollars. If the value (in dollars) is more than the cost (in dollars), then the option is cost-beneficial and should be undertaken. Because CBA values everything in a common denominator (dollars), it allows comparisons to be made between unrelated options. One advantage of CBA compared with other types of analyses is that alternatives for different types of consequences can be compared. For example, a decision maker with limited resources could chose between building a new road or funding a new treatment for Medicaid patients.

TABLE 3–1 COMPARISON OF APPROACHES TO PHARMACOECONOMIC ANALYSIS

Approach	Costs (Input)	Outcomes (Consequences)	Formula
Cost-benefit (CB) analysis	Dollars	Dollars	CB ratio = \$ benefit − \$ cost
Cost-effectiveness (CE) analysis	Dollars	Natural units (e.g., blood pressure, lipid levels, lives saved, days of illness averted)	$\text{CE ratio} = \frac{\$\text{ cost}}{\text{unit of effectiveness}}$
Cost-utility (CU) analysis	Dollars	Quality adjusted life-years	$\text{CU ratio} = \frac{\$\text{ cost}}{(\text{X years})\ (\text{health state preference})}$
Cost-minimization analysis	Dollars	Equality of outcomes*	—

*Assumes a constant outcome (consequence).

It is generally possible to assign value to the costs of an intervention. However, trouble begins in attempts to value its benefit. The disadvantage of CBA is that it is difficult to place a monetary value on health benefits. How does one value the benefit of a few days of better health, much less the value of surviving an illness? Because answering this question is plagued with many problems, the CBA approach to pharmacoeconomic analysis is rarely used. There are occasional reports of research conducted using this approach, but those articles must be carefully scrutinized.

There are two methods that have been commonly used to estimate a value for these types of questions—the human capital approach and the willingness-to-pay approach. The human capital approach presumes that the value of health benefits is equal to the economic productivity that they permit. The cost of a disease is related to the cost of lost productivity due to the disease. A person's expected income (before taxes) or an imputed value for nonemployment activities (e.g., housework or child care) is used as an estimate of the value of any health benefits for that person. However, earnings may not reflect a person's true worth to society.

The willingness-to-pay method estimates the value of benefits by estimating how much people would pay to reduce their chance of an adverse health outcome. The difficulty with this approach is that what people say they are willing to pay may not correspond with what they would actually do. The willingness of third parties (i.e., insurers) to pay should also be taken into consideration.

Cost-Effectiveness Analysis

CEA measures the outcomes of intervention in terms of natural health units. In CEA, the costs of providing a treatment option are valued in dollars. The value of a CEA is the ratio between a dollar amount and the unit of effectiveness. The simplest form of CEA is based on objective, natural units, such as reduction in blood pressure or lipid levels, the probability of cure, or days of illness averted. The choice of units is determined by what is most relevant to the disease state or treatment in question. The benefit to this approach is that it is generally similar to the logic used by health care providers when they make clinical pharmacotherapeutic decisions.

The CEA ratio depends on the nonmonetary unit chosen, but the advantage is that the researcher is not responsible for assigning a monetary value to health. The disadvantage of CEA is that it becomes difficult to compare unrelated options. The alternatives compared must have similar outcomes that are measurable in the same units.

Cost-Utility Analysis

In CUA, the effectiveness unit is not a natural condition of the disease or treatment in question but rather an artificial measure designed to allow for comparisons between different diseases or populations. CUA can take patient preferences into account when measuring health outcomes. The most commonly used utility measures are life-years saved, the number of years that a treatment option saves compared with some other option, or QALYs, in which the LYs are adjusted to include a preference for the quality of life. The QALY is based on the notion that a year of being healthy is preferable to and worth more than a year of illness. For example, 1 year of life in perfect health has a score of 1.0 QALY. If the health-related quality of life is diminished by disease or treatment, that 1 year of life is worth less than 1.0 QALY. This method allows for comparisons of mortality and morbidity. In another example, a woman with hypertension dies at age 65 but otherwise would have been expected to live to age 85. Hypertension is associated with 20 lost life-years. If 100 women die at age 65 (women who also had a life expectancy of 85 years), 20 times 100, or 2000, life-years would be lost. However, death is not the only outcome of hypertension. The disease leaves many people disabled over long periods of time (e.g., due to stroke, myocardial infarction, or renal failure). Although the patient remains alert and active, the quality of life has decreased. QALYs take into account the quality of life consequences of illness. For example, a disease that reduces the quality of life by one-half will take away 0.5 QALY over the course of 1 year. If the disease affects five people, it will take away 5 times 0.5, or 2.5, QALYs over a period of 1 year. A drug that improves the quality of life by 0.2 for each of the five people will result in the equivalent of 1.0 QALY if the benefit is maintained over a period of 1 year.

Although there is considerable debate about which dimensions should be used as QALY units, the most common are physical functioning, the ability to carry out prescribed roles, and mental health status. A common strategy is to report outcomes along multiple dimensions, but it is unclear whether multiple dimensions are more likely to detect clinical differences than is use of a single measure. A number of other utility measures of varying complexity have been used. The benefit of CUA is that it allows comparison between unrelated treatment options. The problem is that health care providers or managed care organizations must carefully apply these utility measures in a meaningful way.

Cost-Minimization and Cost-of-Illness Analyses

Two other common economic analyses are often encountered—CMA and *cost-of-illness analysis.* CMA is a variation of CEA in which the outcomes are assumed to be equivalent among the possible options. Only the costs are evaluated. Although costs are explicitly measured, the consequences are not. One example of a CMA is the measurement and comparison of costs for two equivalent generic drugs. Another example is the measurement and comparison of total costs required for home intravenous antibiotic therapy with the total costs of providing this therapy in the hospital. The strength of CMA depends on the assumption that the outcomes are the same. This evidence can be based on previous studies, publications, FDA data, or expert opinion.

The second common analysis encountered is a cost-of-illness analysis. Cost-of-illness analysis attempts to measure the cost factors associated with a particular disease, including direct costs like medical services and indirect costs such as loss of productivity due to illness or premature death.

PERSPECTIVES

In attempting to understand pharmacoeconomic concepts and especially when evaluating pharmacoeconomic claims, the single most important issue is perspective. *Perspective* broadly relates to the focus and orientation of an analysis. Perspective has been previously mentioned but warrants a separate discussion because of its overriding importance in determining the direction and value of a specific analysis. The analysis, treatment options, costs, and values that are chosen depend on the perspective. For example, a societal perspective could use the average wholesale price of a drug in an analysis. On the other hand, a payor perspective could use the actual cost of that drug to that payor. This is important because a real difference between the two costs dramatically changes the results and, therefore, the choice of the most cost-effective treatment. It is not uncommon for two separate analyses to reach different conclusions because of perspective.

The following are four of the more common perspectives used in pharmacoeconomic analyses. As will become apparent, there is no correct perspective. Like the approaches to pharmacoeconomic analysis, each perspective has its own advantages and disadvantages. Thus, it is important that the user of a pharmacoeconomic evaluation explicitly consider the perspective of the analysis when evaluating the results.

Society

The societal perspective is the most commonly used type in pharmacoeconomics today. This is because of the early influence of health economic research, which usually focused on society, and the interest of governmental policy-making bodies to regulate and allocate resources across societal interests. It is also the most commonly used type because pharmaceutical firms try to satisfy the FDA, which as a governmental regulatory body, tends to favor a societal perspective.

From this perspective, the costs and values of treatment are based on the interest of society as a whole. A strong argument can be made that the societal perspective is the only one that should be used in pharmacoeconomic analyses because it considers the well-being of all members of society. On the other hand, society is made up of many different values and interests, and it is not always possible to determine which costs and values best reflect the interests of all members. In addition, the societal perspective does not take into account the particular interests and circumstances of individual organizations. In an effort to find a common denominator, the societal perspective can actually produce results that are not in the best interest of an organization or its patients.

Payor

From the payor's perspective, the costs and values chosen reflect those that apply to a specific payor or organization. Because this perspective begins with a specific organization and uses its costs, it can provide the most cost-effective and efficient treatment choice. But because the costs and values are specific to that organization, it is often difficult to generalize the results to other organizations unless the costs and values are similar, something that is not always true. For example, the cost to a payor (e.g., Blue Cross/Blue Shield or Medicare) equals the charges that are allowed by that payor. This perspective has historically not been used to any great extent, although it is gaining favor as payors demand pharmacoeconomic analyses relevant to their organizations.

Health Care Provider

From the health care provider's perspective, the values and costs of the health care provider (e.g., the hospital) are chosen for the analysis. This perspective is often closely aligned with the payor perspective, especially when the values of the providers coincide with the interests of managed care organizations. To determine the provider's cost, it is often necessary to carry out cost-finding exercises using techniques that have been developed by accountants and industrial engineers (e.g., time and motion studies). For example, the savings to a hospital can be calculated by changing from a drug that requires multiple daily doses to one that requires once-daily dosing. This perspective has traditionally focused less on the cost differences between treatment options and more on the differences in effectiveness. This perspective reflects the traditional role of the health care provider as patient advocate.

Patient

The patient's perspective has occasionally been used in pharmacoeconomic analyses, and a persuasive argument can be made that it should be used more often. Unfortunately, this argument suffers from three major faults. First, there may be significant differences in perspective between various individuals' or groups' interests. Should the interests of patients whose diseases are uncommon be valued less because their disorders are not as prevalent as others? Second, owing to insurance coverage, many patients are divorced from paying directly for the health care resources they consume. This distorts the true ratio of costs to benefits. And finally, by its very nature, pharmacoeconomics is population based rather than being based on the individual patient. Thus, there is an inherent conflict between what is in the best interest of individual patients and what is in the best interest of a population of patients. A patient-based perspective must chart this tricky ground very carefully.

TECHNIQUES FOR CONDUCTING PHARMACOECONOMIC ANALYSES

Independent of the perspective or approach chosen, there are several strategies that can be used to conduct pharmacoeconomic analyses. The choice of strategy depends to some extent on the purpose of the analysis and the expectations of the audience.

Clinical Trials

The majority of pharmacoeconomic analyses are evaluations that have been piggy-backed onto clinical trials that are evaluating the efficacy and safety of specific treatment or intervention. The FDA has requested that a pharmacoeconomic analysis be attached to clinical trials. This request stems from the FDA's past experience with clinical trials and it's lack of experience with other analytic strategies. Economic data are collected as part of the clinical trial and used to determine the cost effectiveness of the treatment under study.

As the field matures, pharmacoeconomists are realizing the inherent limitation of the clinical trial because of inclusion and exclusion criteria, observational effects, and strict assignment of patients to control and treatment groups. In other words, the results of experimental research do not accurately represent what occurs in the real world. Therefore, the results of clinical trials are difficult to generalize to clinical practice settings.

In an attempt to resolve these limitations, some researchers are using open-label clinical trials. Using this strategy, a clinical trial is conducted without control groups or the blinding of variables normally found in standard clinical trials. Patients and health care providers are allowed to participate in the treatment option of their choosing and even to change treatments if desired. Costs and effectiveness of the interventions are followed and the results evaluated to determine the most cost-effective treatment.

The assumption is that an open-label trial more closely mimics what happens in real life. Although there are fewer limitations than with normal clinical trials, it is still difficult to generalize results beyond the specifics of the open-label trial. In addition, many researchers and health care providers are suspicious of the results of open-label trials because they lack control groups and blinding, the components designed to produce unbiased results. Finally, open-label trials are expensive. The expense limits the number of treatment options that can be evaluated at any one time, making it difficult to evaluate more than just a few treatment options.

Retrospective Database Analysis

The retrospective database analysis is another approach to pharmacoeconomic analysis. In this approach, a database of clinical and economic information is evaluated using statistical and mathematical methods to determine the relationship between treatment options, outcomes, and costs. The advantage of this approach is that the data are usually readily available and reflect the historical experience of the particular organization.

This approach can provide significant results and information to an organization, especially when external factors are properly controlled; however, three limitations must be kept in mind. Data analysis can be technically challenging, especially when there are large unrelated data sets. Also, the data may not be accurate. For example, evaluation of current procedural terminology (CPT) coding can be useful, but one cannot forget that CPT codes are collected to support reimbursement rather than to measure accurately treatment choices. The more complicated and strict the reimbursement policies, the more likely CPT codes will not accurately reflect the real consumption of resources. This is especially true when significant cost shifting (shifting costs from low-reimbursing patients to higher reimbursing patients) occurs. Biases can and do distort the results of any analysis.

Finally, owing to policies, circumstances, or changes in treatments over time, the data may not truly reflect a fair comparison of all treatment options. For example, some data sets may not include certain drugs (i.e., those drugs not contained in the formulary), or there is a perception among health care providers that a particular drug should be reserved for sicker patients, thereby distorting the cost experience of that drug. The limitations to data sets can often be controlled by statistical means, but there is a limit to these types of corrections, especially when subtle biases are not recognized. The net result is that retrospective database analyses can provide information with which to make accurate cost-effective determinations, but the analysis must be carefully evaluated by the reader and user of the studies.

Mathematical Modeling

A third strategy to pharmacoeconomic analyses is mathematical modeling. Modeling has only recently gained wider acceptance, although it has a long and lustrous history in a wide range of fields from scientific research to meteorology and manufacturing. Mathematical modeling is based on the notion that although it may be impossible or difficult to measure specific phenomena, it is possible to describe the phenomena mathematically. Models can range from simple approximations of what is being measured to much more complex and accurate representations of reality. Modeling allows the researcher to predict a phenomenon that would be impossible to actually measure directly. In pharmacoeconomics, modeling permits an evaluation of the cost-effectiveness of a disease state that would otherwise be impossible to measure through a clinical trial. For example, there are dozens of drugs available for the treatment of primary hypertension, all of which could be used singly or in many different combinations. Only a model could evaluate these combinations of treatment.

A mathematical model begins with a framework that presumes to represent reality. The framework is developed based on assumptions about what really happens in a specific disease state or with a particular treatment. Further, all models contain assumptions about the reality that is portrayed. How well the reader or user of the analysis believes the model depends on the extent of agreement with the assumptions. Experimental or observational data such as cost, efficacy, and adverse effect profile are then used for the variables within the mathematical model, and results calculated. The results of mathematical modeling include predictions that can be tested. It is this testing of predictions that helps validate the model's reliability.

The advantage of using a mathematical model is the ability to evaluate questions that cannot be directly analyzed because of complexity or cost. The disadvantage of modeling, especially as the model becomes more complex, is its underlying mathematical nature. A certain degree of comfort and familiarity with mathematical concepts and techniques is required. In addition, developing accurate models is as much an art as a science. Traditionally, mathematical models have not been the preferred means of conducting pharmacoeconomic analyses. However, this attitude may change as more people become familiar with the necessary techniques, managed care organizations begin to demand more applied pharmacoeconomic analyses, and people realize that some pharmacoeconomic questions can be answered only by mathematical models.

METHODS FOR PHARMACOECONOMIC ANALYSES

A second way to understand pharmacoeconomic analyses is by the type of method or structure used. Ultimately, the data must be evaluated by using one of several methods. For example, during a clinical trial, economic data can be captured that could be used to determine the cost effectiveness of the treatment options. But a pharmacoeconomic method must then be chosen to analyze those data. The following discussion includes some of the more commonly used methods.

Proactive Methods

Decision Analysis

A decision analysis (decision analytic) is the most common method used. This method reduces the management of a disease into a series of treatment choices to be made by the health care provider. Using this method, a decision tree is created that includes options or decision points from which the health care provider or health care system must choose. Costs and outcomes are assigned to these decisions, and ultimately, the cost effectiveness for a particular decision is determined. This methodology can be used in conjunction with clinical trials, databases, or models.

Decision analysis is easy to use, and several computer programs are available to create the decision trees. Unfortunately, as the number of treatment options increases, the number of decision points grow exponentially. Very quickly, a decision tree becomes a decision forest. This growth limits the usefulness of this method when more than a few drug choices must be evaluated.

Decision trees are a simple way to structure problems of decision-making. Consider the management of a sore throat. The treatment options include giving antibiotics to all patients, culturing for strep throat and giving antibiotics to patients with positive cultures, or giving antibiotics to none of the patients (Fig. 3–1). The leftmost arm of the tree is connected to branches that specify alternative actions. Customarily, decision points are depicted as a rectangle. At a decision point, the health care provider chooses whichever branch is most appropriate. The upper branch represents the option of treating the patient empirically (i.e., giving an antibiotic without culturing for the streptococcus organism). The middle branch represents the option of culturing for the streptococcus organism but then waiting for the results before determining the need for an antibiotic. The lower branch, no treatment, represents the option of not giving antibiotics. In analyses comparing various antibiotics, there would be a branch for each drug.

Additionally, allergic reactions are a possible adverse effect of antibiotics. The uncertain possibility of an allergic reaction is represented by a chance node (●), leading to branches "reaction" and "no reaction." Under the reaction branch is the probability (p) with which a reaction may occur. The other branch indicates the much more likely situation that there is no reaction. The branches extending from a chance node partition the set of probabilities. That is, the probability of all possible occurrences should equal one.

Simulation Modeling

Simulation modeling is a mathematical method that simulates or mimics real world events from inputs and choices made by health care providers. In many ways, this is directly analogous to mathematical modeling, which was discussed earlier. When it is handled properly, this method can be easy to understand and provide tremendous insight into the choices and efficiencies of providers when making treatment decisions. At the same time, this approach can be difficult to implement. The results can also be difficult to understand and believe if the mathematics underlying the simulation are overly obtuse and complex. Despite this problem, simulation modeling remains the approach best able to answer complex questions of cost effectiveness when the decision involves multiple treatment options.

Reactive Methods

Statistical Analysis

Statistical analysis is best used with large data sets. It can also be applied in clinical trials and models when sufficient data are available. Descriptive statistics (i.e., means, medi-

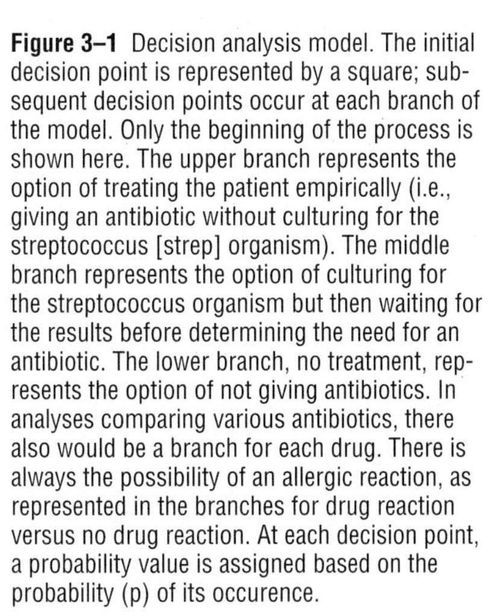

Figure 3–1 Decision analysis model. The initial decision point is represented by a square; subsequent decision points occur at each branch of the model. Only the beginning of the process is shown here. The upper branch represents the option of treating the patient empirically (i.e., giving an antibiotic without culturing for the streptococcus [strep] organism). The middle branch represents the option of culturing for the streptococcus organism but then waiting for the results before determining the need for an antibiotic. The lower branch, no treatment, represents the option of not giving antibiotics. In analyses comparing various antibiotics, there also would be a branch for each drug. There is always the possibility of an allergic reaction, as represented in the branches for drug reaction versus no drug reaction. At each decision point, a probability value is assigned based on the probability (p) of its occurence.

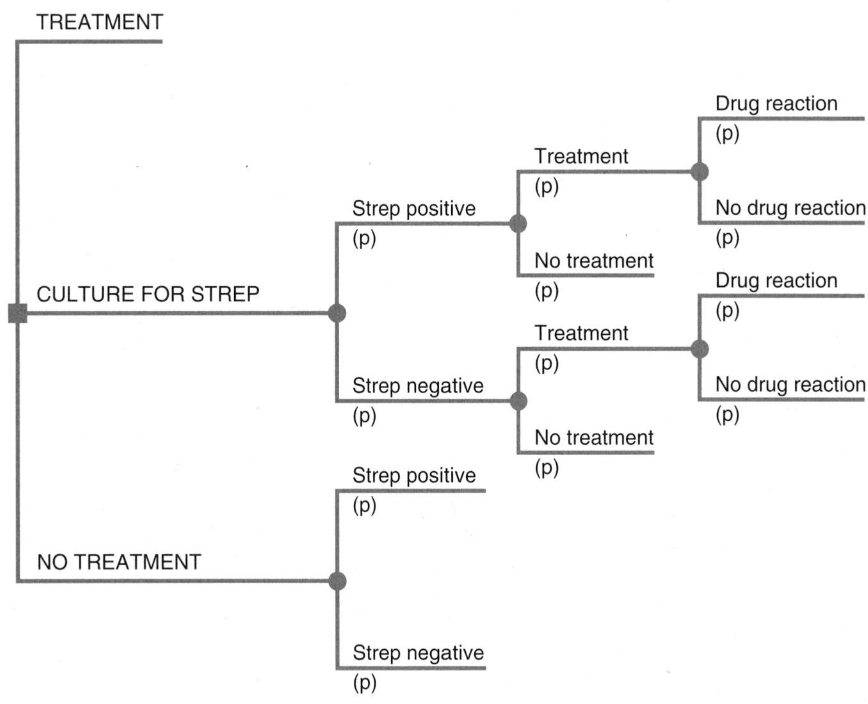

ums, standard deviations), inferential statistics (i.e., t-test, paired t-tests, chi-square analysis), and more advanced inferential techniques, such as regression analysis, factor analysis, and logistic regression, are used to evaluate both the costs and effectiveness of each treatment option.

Statistical analysis works best when the data already exist, either in a database or as the result of a clinical trial or mathematical model. Statistical evaluation of alternative treatment regimens requires a thorough understanding and modeling of the process that generated the health care provider's and the patient's behaviors as well as the data collection effort. It is important to go beyond simple univariate statistical analysis to understand how much confidence can be placed in the results (i.e., estimated cost-effectiveness ratio). Sensitivity analysis shows which parametric variables will have a dramatic effect on the conclusions, but it fails to capture all of the variability that results from estimating multiple parameter values.

Whereas other methods are predictive, statistical methods are descriptive, finding results already in the data. Such statistical analysis looks for relationships within a data set, whereas the other two methods begin with the data and predict (based on assumptions and an analytic framework) the cost effectiveness. This means that statistical analysis is preferred when the data are extensive and complete.

ADVANCED CONCEPTS IN PHARMACOECONOMICS

A brief discussion of advanced concepts within pharmacoeconomics analyses will focus on sensitivity analysis and discounting, Markov analysis, and incremental analysis. The intent is to provide an appreciation for the methods and issues addressed in the pharmacoeconomic literature.

Sensitivity Analysis

Few costs in a pharmacoeconomic evaluation are known with certainty. Therefore, one can ask whether the results would change if the researchers were incorrect in their estimate of variables. For example, would the results change if the cost of one drug was 10 percent higher or 10 percent lower? Would the results change if the effectiveness of the treatment options was better or worse than predicted? Would the results change if every patient complied with treatment or if none of the patients complied with treatment? These are extremely important questions. An analysis that fails to address these and similar questions is of limited usefulness. The method by which an analysis addresses these questions is called sensitivity analysis and is as critical to the final result as the analysis itself.

Sensitivity analysis is the process by which one measures how well the results withstand changes in assumptions or initial conditions. There are several different techniques for measuring sensitivity. The most common is to modify a few variables within the model or data set and evaluate the results. This is called univariate sensitivity analysis. A more advanced technique often encountered is called a Monte Carlo analysis, which before the advent of computers, involved rolling dice. Using a Monte Carlo analysis, the model is run multiple times (as many as a thousand times) and some or all of the variables are randomly changed for each run. The results of the trials are then statistically analyzed to determine the sensitivity of the results to changes in the variables.

A conclusion is called robust if the results change little, even with large changes in costs or other variables. This means that the result is consistent over a large range of variables. The more robust an analysis, the more one can believe the results. The more robust the conclusion, the easier it is to generalize the findings to conditions different from those of the original study.

Discounting: The Time Value of Money

An important issue in evaluating pharmacoeconomic claims concerns the time value of money. Most people and businesses prefer to receive money today rather than at a later date. Therefore, a dollar today is worth more than a dollar tomorrow, or next year. For example, assume you have $100. You can spend it or invest it. If you spend it, you enjoy $100 worth of value. If you invest it, you receive interest on that money. To the extent that the interest received is greater than the rate of inflation, you have received added value. The interest earned is the time value of money and includes both a component for inflation and a component for the real return money brings in investment. The actual rate of return is the value returned if the money is invested in a business or venture, even if inflation is nonexistent.

Discounting is the process by which future costs are standardized to present-day values by a particular interest rate. In discounting, the effect of inflation is usually canceled and the interest rate is the actual rate of return. If an evaluation covers less than 1 year, the time value of money can be ignored; otherwise, all costs must be discounted to reflect this difference in value. In many analyses, this actual interest rate has been assumed to be 5 percent, although this number has been questioned. There are various arguments concerning whether the interest rate should be higher or lower depending on the purpose of the study. Regardless, the analysis should include a discussion of the interest rate chosen and the rationale for its choice.

Table 3–2 demonstrates the time value of money and the need for discounting. Assume we have two choices, both which cost $1000 today, but option A (no discounting) will return $2000 next year, whereas option B (with discounting) will return $2000 in 5 years. If we ignore the time value of money (i.e., if we do not care when we get the money back), both choices are worth $1000 (the $2000 we receive in the future less the $1000 we pay today). But $2000 next year is worth more than $2000 in 5 years. Instead, if we discount the return at 5 percent, we realize that option A is really worth $905 (in present dollars), whereas option B is worth only $567. Without taking into account the time value of money, we could choose either option, but by discounting, we discover that option A is better (i.e., it is worth more to us). The final section of the table (option C) illustrates that if we invested the proceeds of option A ($2000) at 5 percent in the second year, it would be worth $2431 by the fifth year. This is more than option B returns in the fifth year and again demonstrates that option A is the better option. On the other hand, if option B were to pay out more than $2431 in the fifth year, then it would be the better choice.

TABLE 3–2 DISCOUNTING: THE TIME VALUE OF MONEY

Time Value of Money	Option	Today's Dollars	Next Year's Dollars	Fifth-Year Dollars	Total Value
No discounting	A	$1000	$2000	—	$1000
	B	$1000	—	$2000	$1000
With discounting at 5 percent	A	$1000	$1905	—	$ 905
	B	$1000	—	$1567	$ 567
Investing at 5 percent the proceeds of option A	C	—	$2000 invested	$2431	—

A more difficult question concerns whether the benefits should be discounted. Should the decrease in blood pressure, QALYs gained, or number of cases prevented be discounted when it is calculated over multiple years? This difficult question has yet to be resolved. One side argues that by not discounting the benefits, it is always more cost effective to put off a choice until the future (i.e., the most cost-effective choice is to do nothing). The other side argues that the benefits of health cannot be invested; therefore, health cannot be discounted. Until such time as consensus is found among researchers, the reasonable approach is to evaluate each situation on a case-by-case basis, and understand the rationale for discounting or not discounting the effectiveness measure.

Markov Analysis

One problem with decision analysis methods is that they reduce all decisions to a set of deterministic processes. In a decision tree, one would choose either option A or B. Option E or F would be available only if option B is chosen. However, this rarely happens in real life because there are usually interconnections between the options. *Markov analysis*, a methodology often encountered in economic literature, allows decision analysis methods to deal with the flexible choices of real life. The basic idea of a Markov model is that individuals at any time are in one of a finite set of states of health. Health status varies according to a set of transition probabilities. For example, in the most rudimentary form, transition probabilities are fixed.

The model could be used to analyze health changes of a patient with kidney failure who is on dialysis. Here, the two states are life on dialysis and death (for simplicity we will ignore the possibility of a transplant). Data are gathered for specific time periods. During each period examined, living people either make the transition to death or survive. Applying such simplistic focus allows clinical problems with continuous risk or in which events occur numerous times to be assessed for quality of life and cost effectiveness of treatment. The technique for conducting Markov analysis is complex; although it extends the power of decision analysis methodologies, it does not alleviate other problems associated with that approach.

Incremental Analysis

Many applications of cost-effectiveness analysis in health care involve comparisons among competing alternatives for the same condition. Examples include treatment options among drug treatment regimens for cholesterol reduction or hypertension, alternative drug doses for a given condition, and comparisons between drug treatment and nonpharmacologic treatment.

In *incremental analysis*, the incremental cost effectiveness that occurs as a result of changing one treatment option to another is analyzed. The idea is to determine whether the incremental improvement in benefit is worth the incremental cost. This incremental difference is then compared with a standard to determine whether the new treatment option should be undertaken. For example, a new drug might be shown to cost incrementally only $3000 more per QALY than the current standard of care. The argument could then be made that this cost compares favorably with other incremental costs for similar or reasonably different treatments, and therefore, the new drug should be funded. This method has gained much favor within pharmaceutical and academic communities. However, it has not proved as successful at answering the needs of managed care. When confronted with a patient, a disease, and a host of possible treatment options, what health care providers and managed care providers need to know is not whether one treatment is incrementally more cost effective than another but the rank-ordering of cost effectiveness among the various treatments. Generally, health care providers have the flexibility to use a stepwise approach to treatment (i.e., start with one treatment and switch to another if it does not work). By its nature, incremental analysis makes this approach to drug therapy difficult to evaluate.

THE FUTURE OF PHARMACOECONOMICS

The field of pharmacoeconomics and the data it evaluates will change rapidly as the field evolves. Increasingly, several themes will play a role in the field and will be reflected in the published literature. These themes include increased pressure on health care providers to consider the economic impact of their decisions on individual patients and on the populations they serve; demands by managed care organizations for pharmacoeconomic evaluations that meet their specific needs rather than the needs of policymakers; and a push toward standardization and guidelines in conducting and reporting pharmacoeconomic evaluations.

Mathematical modeling will become the dominant means of conducting pharmacoeconomic evaluation, with clinical trials and retrospective database analysis used to support and validate the clinical and economic models. Analysis techniques will improve, and new methodologies will be developed to help resolve many of the controversies currently debated within the field.

POINTS TO CONSIDER WHEN EVALUATING PHARMACOECONOMIC STUDIES

- Consider the question—Is it well defined? Can it be answered?
- Review the analysis used. Does it state its perspective clearly and consider all alternatives?
- Does the study describe the competing alternatives (i.e., Can you tell who? Did what? To whom? Where? How often?)?
- Does the study provide evidence that the treatment's or program's effectiveness has been established?
- Does the study identify important and relevant costs and outcomes for each alternative?
- Does the study measure important costs and outcomes accurately in appropriate physical units (e.g., hours of nursing time, number of visits to health care provider, lost work days, life-years gained)?
- Does the study credibly value costs and outcomes?
- Does the study adjust costs and consequences for differential timing?
- Does the study address incremental analysis of costs and consequences of alternatives performed?
- Does the study identify assumptions clearly?
- Does the study justify its choice and use of surveys or other instruments?
- Does the study apply discounting to multi-year research?
- Does the study use sensitivity analysis?
- Does the study present results that include all issues of concern to users?
- Does the study address its limitations and present information in an unbiased manner?

Data from Drummond, M., Stoddart, G., and Torrance, G. (1987). *Methods for the economic evaluation of healthcare programmes.* Oxford: Oxford University Press.

In order to understand and apply pharmacoeconomic research, health care professionals must be able to critique the quality of that research. Guidelines for research evaluation can help in this process (see Points to Consider when Evaluating Pharmacoeconomic Studies).

SUMMARY

- Pharmacoeconomics is defined as an analysis that identifies, measures, and compares the costs and consequences of pharmaceutical products and services.
- Pharmacoeconomic analyses encompass two related but separate philosophies: resource allocation and increased efficiency.
- The basic question has been: Given a variety of treatment choices and limited resources, which choices should we make?
- One question confronting health care providers and organizations is whether they should pay the additional cost for newer drugs that appear to have fewer adverse effects or continue to pay for older drugs that are just as effective but with potentially more adverse effects.
- There are many different approaches to pharmacoeconomic analysis: CBA, CEA, CUA, and CMA.
- Strategies for conducting pharmacoeconomic analyses include retrospective database analysis and mathematical modeling.
- Decision analysis, statistical analysis, simulation modeling, discounting/time value of money, sensitivity analysis, Markov analysis, and incremental analysis are advanced techniques of analysis.
- The choice of which analytic method, strategy, or structure to use depends on the purpose of the analysis and the expectations of the audience.
- CBAs measure outcomes in dollars, whereas CEA measures outcomes in terms of natural units (e.g., reduction in blood pressure in mmHg).
- CUA measures outcomes by incorporating preferences, or utilities, with natural outcomes (e.g., QALYs).
- CMA assumes equal outcomes between treatment options (e.g., generic products).
- Perspective relates to the focus and orientation of an analysis, and includes those of society, the payor, health care provider, and patient.
- The majority of pharmacoeconomic analyses are evaluations that have been piggy-backed onto clinical trials being done to evaluate efficacy and safety of an intervention.
- In retrospective database analysis, a database of clinical and economic information is evaluated using statistical and mathematical methods to determine the relationship between treatment options, outcomes, and costs.
- Mathematical modeling is based on the idea that although it may be impossible or difficult to measure a phenomenon, it is possible to describe the phenomenon mathematically.
- Decision analysis is based on the concept of reducing the management of a disease into a series of treatment choices to be made by the health care provider and the patient. This methodology can be used in conjunction with clinical trials, databases, or models.
- Statistical analysis is best used in combination with large data sets. It can also be applied in clinical trials and models when sufficient data are available.
- Simulation modeling is a mathematical method that simulates or mimics real-world events from inputs and choices made by health care providers.
- When a treatment continues for more than 1 year, dollars should be measured using their present value. This is referred to discounting and states that there is a time value associated with costs.
- Sensitivity analysis is the process by which one measures how well the results withstand changes in assumptions or initial conditions.
- A conclusion is called robust if the results change little, even with large changes in costs or other variables.
- Markov analysis allows decision analysis methods to deal with the flexible choices of real life.
- In incremental analysis, what is evaluated is the incremental cost effectiveness that occurs as a result of changing one treatment option to another.

BIBLIOGRAPHY

Bootman J., Townsend, R., and McGhan, W. (Eds.) (1996). *Principles of pharmacoeconomics* (2nd ed.). Cincinnati, OH: Harvey Whitney Books Company.

Department of Health and Human Services. Office of Disease Prevention and Promotion. (1992). *A framework for cost-utility analysis of government health care program.* Washington, DC: Government Printing Office.

Doubilet, P., Weinstein, M., and McNeil, B. (1986). Use and misuse of the term "cost-effective" in medicine. *New England Journal of Medicine,* 314, 253–256.

Drummond, M., Stoddart, G., and Torrance, G. (1987). *Methods for the economic evaluation of healthcare programmes.* Oxford: Oxford University Press.

Gold, M., Siegel, J., Russell, L., et al. (1996). *Cost-effectiveness in health and medicine.* New York: Oxford University Press.

Heller, B. (1996). Pharmacoeconomics guidelines galore coming. *Drug Topics,* 140(11), 106.

Kozma, C., Reeder, C., and Shultz, R. (1993). Economic, clinical, and humanistic outcomes: A planning model for pharmacoeconomic research. *Clinical Therapeutics,* 15, 1121–1132.

Muirhead, G. (1995). Batty up! Pharmacoeconomics, the rookie, enters game. *Drug Topics,* 139(8), 33–34.

Muirhead, G. (1994). Pharmacoeconomics: A still-fuzzy buzzword. *Drug Topics,* 138(9), 74–75.

Naimark, D., Krahn, M., Naglie, G., et al. (1997). Primer on medical decision analysis: Part 5—working with Markov processes. *Medical Decision Making,* 17, 151–159.

Riesenberg, D. (Ed.) (1989). Clinical economics: A guide to the economic analysis of clinical practices. *Clinical Economics,* 262(20), 2879–2886.

Revicki, D., and Kaplan, K. (1993). Relationship between psychometric and utility-based approaches to the measurement of health-related quality of life. *Quality of Life Research,* 2, 477–487.

Sloan, F. (1995). *Valuing health care: Cost, benefits, and effectiveness of pharmaceuticals and other medical technologies.* New York: Cambridge University Press.

Sonnenberg, F., and Beck, R. (1993). Markov models in medical decision making: A practical guide. *Medical Decision Making,* 13, 322–338.

Wilke, R. (1995). What's all this about pharmacoeconomics? *Business Economics,* 30(2), 26–31.

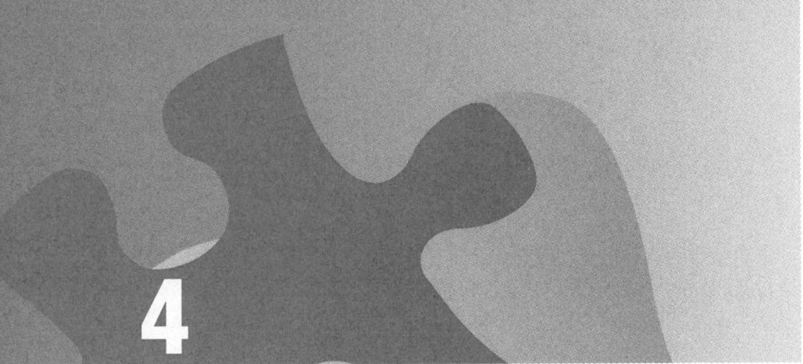

4

Pharmaceutics and Pharmacokinetics

Health care providers understand that drugs alter physiologic functions. There are, moreover, three basic principles of drug action that are crucial to a comprehensive understanding of pharmacokinetics (see General Principles of Drug Action). The first principle states that drugs modify existing functions within the body—they do not create function. Second, no drug has a single action. All drugs are capable of producing desirable as well as undesirable effects. The third principle states that drug response is determined by the drug's interaction within the body. Drugs act in specific as well as nonspecific ways with the body. For example, most drugs act on specific receptor sites to cause responses. Other drugs act in nonspecific ways by interacting with cell membranes. Still others alter the characteristics of body fluids.

PHASES OF DRUG ACTIVITY

Drug activity occurs in three phases: the pharmaceutic phase, pharmacokinetic phase, and the pharmacodynamic phase. These phases are interrelated and interdependent; thus, the phases are not as clearly delineated as they first appear to be. The *pharmaceutic phase* of drug activity begins with formulating drugs into dosage forms suited for delivery to the site of action (Fig. 4–1). The pharmaceutic phase also describes the stage during which the drug enters the body in one form and changes to another form in order to be used. *Pharmacokinetics* refers to the processes of absorption, distribution, biotransformation, and elimination (Fig. 4–2). The *pharmacodynamic* phase occurs when a drug reaches its site of action and produces an effect. Pharmacodynamics is discussed in Chapter 5.

GENERAL PRINCIPLES OF DRUG ACTION

Principle 1:
Drugs modify existing functions within the body; they do not create function

Principle 2:
No drug has a single action

Principle 3:
Drug effects are determined by the drug's interaction with the body

Pharmaceutic Phase

Once a solid dosage form is in solution in the gastrointestinal (GI) tract or body fluid, it is available for absorption and distribution. Formulations such as syrups and elixirs are already in a liquid state and are generally absorbed faster than tablets or capsules. When action is needed more quickly, drugs may be given parenterally. Solubility characteristics can be manipulated to delay disintegration and dissolution in the GI tract, or to alter the location where disintegration takes place. By altering solubility characteristics, drug action can be prolonged.

Particle size is an important determinant in solubility. When particle size is reduced, surface area is increased and dissolution is facilitated. On the other hand, large crystals delay dissolution and prolong drug absorption. The dissolution rate is usually slowest for drugs given as powders, or when disintegration of a tablet or capsule results in solid particles. Generally, salts of weak acids or bases are more rapidly dissolved than is the parent compound.

When two drug forms contain the same active ingredient, they are considered *chemically equivalent*. Chemical equivalence, however, does not guarantee that two drugs have identical pharmacologic activity. Most dosage forms contain additives such as starches or protamine that affect drug stability, size, shape, ease of manufacture, absorbability, and patient acceptance.

Drug Constituents

A drug is made up of one or more active ingredients and various additives. Active ingredients are responsible for producing desired effects and vary considerably in their chemical structure. The major classes of active ingredients include alkaloids, glycosides, polypeptides, salts, and steroids. They are categorized based on chemical and physical properties. Additives are used to alter certain properties of the final formulation (Table 4–1).

Active Ingredients

Alkaloids are organic compounds that contain nitrogen and have a basic pH. They are found in the seeds, roots, leaves, or bark of plants such as the opium poppy, tobacco, and cinchona bark. Most drugs whose names end in "ine" are alkaloid derivatives (e.g., atropine, nicotine).

Glycosides are secured from plants that, when hydrolyzed, produce a sugar and one or more other products. Sugars obtained from glycosides are usually glucose (from glucosides) and galactose (from galactosides). Digitalis is a cardiac glycoside derived from the foxglove plant.

Polypeptides are high-molecular-weight protein compounds. They are usually amphoteric (i.e., they exhibit electrical charges at two or more sites on the molecule), although their molecules do not ionize. Most polypeptides are administered parenterally because they are easily hydrolyzed by proteases in the digestive tract. Hormones such as insulin are polypeptides.

Salts are made up of a positive ion (other than hydrogen) and a negative ion (other than hydroxyl). Solid salts tend to form crystals. In solution, a certain percentage of their molecules separate, releasing electrically charged ions that are often chemically active. Drug activity is usually confined to either the negatively charged ion (anion) or the positively

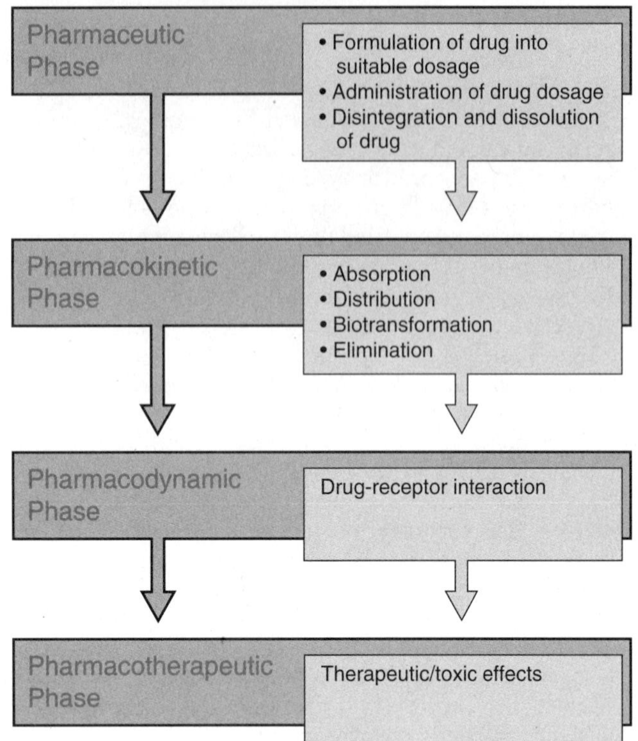

Figure 4–1 Phases of drug activity. The phases of drug activity between administration and effect include pharmaceutical, pharmacokinetic, pharmacodynamic, and pharmacotherapeutic. The pharmaceutic phase portrays the stage during which the drug enters the body in one form and changes to another in order to be used. In the pharmacokinetic phase, the drug is absorbed into the circulation, distributed to its site of action, biotransformed in the liver, and eliminated via the liver or kidneys. The pharmacodynamic phase is the phase of action of the drug on cellular receptors. The pharmacodynamic and pharmacotherapeutic phases assist in determining the proper dose and dosing schedule.

charged ion (cation). Compounds containing ions with like charges tend to be chemically compatible. Those ions with unlike charges tend to form inactive precipitates when joined.

Steroids contain a characteristic chemical structure made up of three hexagonal carbon rings and one pentagonal ring. Naturally occurring compounds containing a steroid nucleus include adrenocortical hormones and cholesterol. Steroids used as drugs include cortisone, estrogen, and testosterone. These drugs are ordinarily unaffected by digestive enzymes and can be taken orally.

Additives

Additives are used to impart a desired property to the drug formulation. They typically consist of binders, diluents, disintegrators, dyes, flavorings, fillers, and vehicles. They must be nontoxic and compatible with the active ingredient as well as with each of the other additives.

Binders are added to solid formulations to improve the cohesiveness of dry ingredients. They help shape the durable dosage forms. Dextrose and lactose are typical binders.

Diluents are used to increase the bulk of the formulation. By adding a diluent, such as water or petrolatum, the concentration of the active ingredients is reduced.

Disintegrators facilitate disaggregation and dissolution when the solid drug is placed in water. Starches are disintegrators.

Dyes are added to drug formulations to make them more eye appealing and to facilitate drug identification in case of overdose or poisoning. The dyes used are under scrutiny of the Food and Drug Administration (FDA). Some have been banned as carcinogenic (e.g., certain red dyes). Tartrazine (FDA yellow number 5) has been shown to cause allergic re-

TABLE 4–1 DRUG CONSTITUENTS

	Form	Example(s)
Active ingredients	Alkaloids	Atropine, nicotine
	Glycosides	Digitalis
	Polypeptides	Insulin
	Salts	Morphine sulfate, potassium chloride
	Steroids	Estrogen, testosterone, cortisone
Additives	Binders	Dextrose, lactose
	Diluents	Vehicles, fillers
	Disintegrators	Starch
	Dyes	Tartrazine (FDA yellow no. 5)
	Flavorings	Cherry, raspberry, licorice syrups
	Fillers	Dextrose, lactose, starch
	Lubricants	Hydrogenated vegetable oils, stearates, talc
	Vehicles	Cocoa butter, oils, petrolatum, syrups, water

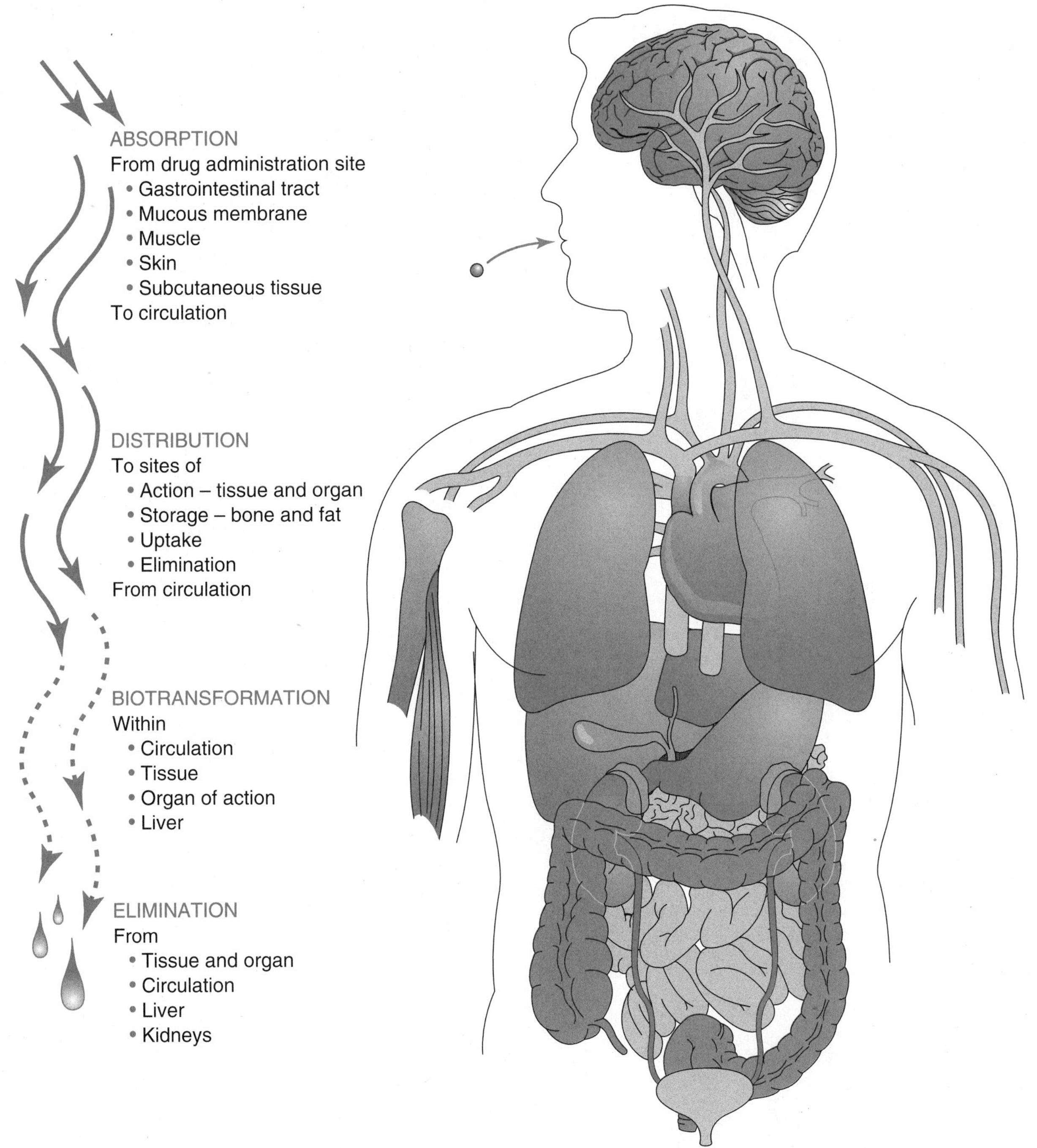

Figure 4–2 Pharmacokinetic phases of drug activity. Dispositional changes that drugs and chemicals undergo within the body during the pharmacokinetic phase of drug activity.

actions in susceptible individuals (i.e., asthmatics with aspirin allergy and persons who are prone to the development of nasal polyps).

Flavorings are usually added to liquids or chewable tablets to improve palatability. Cherry, raspberry, banana, and licorice syrups are examples of flavorings.

Fillers are usually relatively inert substances added to dry drugs to provide the bulk needed to produce a solid preparation of a uniform dose. Hydrophobic fillers (those that do not readily dissolve in water) are sometimes used to delay dissolution of the drug, thereby achieving a timed-release effect. Individuals with a lactose deficiency may be unable to tolerate a lactose filler in a drug and develop GI upset.

Lubricants prevent tablets and caplets from adhering to machinery during the compression of solid dosage forms. Examples of lubricants include hydrogenated vegetable oils, stearates, and talc.

Vehicles are substances added to active ingredients to give it substance and form. Common vehicles include cocoa butter, oils, petrolatum, syrups, and water. Other solvents and solids can also be used. Vehicles can have a significant effect on the chemical and physical properties of a drug.

Drug Formulations

Drugs are formulated and administered in such a way as to produce either local or systemic effects. Local effects are confined to one area of the body (e.g., antiseptics, anti-inflammatories, local anesthetics). Systemic effects occur when the drug is absorbed and delivered to body tissues by way of the circulatory system.

Drug formulations for local use come in many forms, including aerosols, ointments, creams, pastes, powders, tinctures, and lotions. They can also be obtained as gels, foams, and suppositories for rectal, vaginal, or urethral use. Drug formulations can be administered by douche (i.e., vaginal irrigation) or as an enema (i.e., rectal irrigation). Sprays, aerosols, gases, and nebulizers are methods of introducing local or systemic drugs, or both, to the respiratory system.

Local drug formulations can be water based (aqueous) or oil based. Water-based formulations are readily absorbed whereas oil-based formulations are absorbed more slowly. Oil-based drugs are not used in the respiratory tract since the oil may be carried to the alveoli, resulting in a lipoid pneumonia.

Systemic drug formulations are absorbed into the circulatory system to affect one or more tissue groups. They can be administered orally, topically, or parenterally, or applied to mucous membranes. Parenterally administered drugs are introduced into the body by any route other than enteral. For example, intradermal (ID), subcutaneous (SC or SQ), intramuscular (IM), and intravenous (IV) routes. An overview of formulations is seen in Drug Formulations, and Table 4–2 provides the absorption speeds of various drugs.

Solid Formulations

Tablets are the most complex common dosage forms. In addition to the active ingredient, an average tablet contains a filler, a binder, a disintegrator, and a lubricant. These additives influence the rate of disintegration. In addition, some tablets contain preservatives, pH stabilizers, coatings, flavorings, or coloring. Bioavailability may be compromised if the tablet is poorly compounded. For example, excessive compaction of the tablet during the manufacturing process may slow disintegration. Some tablets deteriorate (especially in humid conditions), whereas others harden enough to impair disintegration. Well-formulated tablets actually result in more complete absorption than capsules of the same drug.

There are various types of tablets. Buccal tablets are held in the mouth between the cheek and gum until they are dissolved and absorbed. Sublingual tablets are placed beneath the tongue until they are dissolved and absorbed. Coated tablets have an outside layer, usually of sugar or chocolate, to make them more palatable. Effervescent tablets contain a mixture of sodium bicarbonate and an acidulant, such as citric acid, that generates carbon dioxide when added to water.

Enteric-coated tablets are designed to prevent disintegration of the tablet in gastric juices. They are formulated to dissolve instead in the alkaline environment of the small intestine. Occasionally, enteric-coated drugs disintegrate in the stomach despite the coating, resulting in relatively poor absorption. In practice, enteric-coated drugs are less reliable with respect to their onset of action than uncoated dosage forms. If gastric emptying time is prolonged, enteric-coated drugs may remain inactive in the stomach for several hours. Even when enteric-coated drugs reach the small intestine, absorption can be delayed if the coating does not readily dissolve. In some cases, the enteric-coated drug passes right through the GI tract to be eliminated intact in the stool. For these reasons, enteric-coated drugs should not be used when immediate drug action is desired. It is also recommended that the patient avoid fatty meals just before taking an enteric-coated drug because fatty meals delay gastric emptying.

Sustained-release or timed-release dosage forms contain small particles of drug coated with substances that require varying amounts of time to dissolve. Sustained-release dosage forms are most useful for drugs that are rapidly biotransformed or excreted or that would otherwise need to be taken on a more frequent basis. Because sustained-release dosage forms contain more total drug than single dose tablets or capsules, irregular absorption can occur. These dosage forms are not used for drugs with a narrow margin of safety (i.e., therapeutic index).

TABLE 4–2 ABSORPTION SPEED OF VARIOUS DRUG FORMULATIONS

Absorption Speed of Various Oral Formulations	
Fastest	Liquids, syrups, elixirs
↓	Suspensions
	Powders
↓	Capsules
	Tablets
↓	Coated tablets
Slowest	Enteric-coated tablets
Absorption Speed of Various Parenteral Formulations	
Fastest	Intravenous
	Intramuscular
↓	Subcutaneous
	Intrathecal
Slowest	Epidural

DRUG FORMULATIONS

Solid Formulations	*Semisolid Formulations*	*Liquids*
Tablets	Ointments	Aromatic waters
Oral	Creams	Elixirs
Buccal	Pastes	Extracts
Sublingual	Suppositories	Emulsions
Coated	Foams	Liniments
Effervescent		Lotions
Sustained release		Solutions
Enteric coated		Suspensions
Caplets		Syrups
Capsules		Tinctures
Immediate release		
Sustained release		
Powders, dusts, granules		
Patches		
Pellets, needles		
Troches, lozenges		

Capsules are gelatin cases enclosing solid drugs. They melt quickly after being taken. Powders contained in capsules dissolve and are rapidly absorbed. Some capsules contain sustained-release beads designed for prolonged drug action. *Caplets* are tablets that resemble capsules in shape. Capsules are more easily tampered with after manufacturing than caplets but are still widely used.

Powders are measured doses of solid drug in powder form. They are ordinarily dissolved in water for administration. *Dusts* are very fine powders applied topically to the skin or mucous membranes. They can also be administered by inhalation (e.g., cromolyn is given prophylactically by inhalation to control asthma). *Granules* resemble powders in appearance, but the particles are larger. They are prepared in bulk or as single-dose packets.

Patches look like adhesive dressings in appearance. The drug is usually embedded in either the adhesive ring or a central area. Patches are designed so that the drug is gradually absorbed through the skin.

Pellets and *needles* are also solid drug forms. Pellets are small pills or spherical tablets. They are made of materials that are slowly absorbed from subcutaneous tissue or muscle after being surgically implanted. Needles are long, thin cylinders that are surgically implanted for sustained-release actions. Norplant, a systemically used contraceptive, is an example of a needle formulation.

Troches and *lozenges* are flat, round, or oval-shaped formulations made primarily of a drug powder, sugar, and mucilage. Lozenges are designed for oral use, whereas troches may be used either orally or vaginally.

Semisolid Formulations

Semisolid drug formulations include ointments, creams, pastes, suppositories, and foams. Their use in dermatologic disorders is discussed in Chapter 64.

Ointments are soft, fatty substances that are applied to the skin or eyes. They may be oil based or water based. Terms synonymous with ointment are salve, unction, and unguent.

Creams are topical preparations less viscous than ointments but more viscous than lotions. Creams spread easily but tend to hold their shape when left undisturbed.

Pastes are thick, gelatinous substances that are intended for topical use. Vehicles and fillers in pastes include oils, starches, and waxes.

Suppositories are cone-shaped or cylindrical drugs whose vehicles (e.g., cocoa butter) melt at body temperature. They are molded to conform to the contour of body cavities such as the vagina, rectum, or urethra.

Foams are combinations of finely dispersed gas bubbles interspersed in a liquid. Contraceptive vaginal foams are an example.

Liquid Formulations

Liquid drug formulations include solutions, aromatic waters, elixirs, extracts, tinctures, emulsions, liniments, lotions, suspensions, and syrups. They each have their own characteristics.

Solutions are mixtures of two or more substances dissolved in another substance. The molecules of each solute disperse homogeneously but do not change chemically. Drug solutions are primarily liquids, although they can be solid, liquid, or gas. Solutions can be administered orally, rectally, topically, by inhalation, or by parenteral routes. They can also be used as sprays or irrigations, or instilled in the nose, eye, or ear.

Aromatic waters are saturated aqueous solutions of volatile substances. Spearmint oil and peppermint oil are aromatic waters.

Elixirs are clear liquids containing alcohol, water, sweeteners, and flavoring. They are usually administered by mouth. Elixir of phenobarbital is an example. *Extracts,* on the other hand, are concentrated solutions of an active ingredient dissolved or diluted with an alcoholic solvent. The strength of an extract is usually several times stronger than the crude drug. Fluid extracts are alcoholic solutions of 100 percent concentration. That is, each milliliter of solution contains 1 g of pure drug. In contrast, *tinctures* are alcoholic extracts of vegetable or animal substances and are administered topically or by mouth. Tinctures often contain tannic acid. Examples of a tincture include tincture of belladonna and tincture of benzoin. The usual dose of an oral tincture is 5 mL. Potent drugs are dispensed as 10 percent concentrations, and less potent drugs are dispensed as 20 percent.

Emulsions are combinations of two liquids, usually oil and water. When the emulsion is thoroughly shaken, the oil divides into globules that disperse throughout the mixture. Emulsions tend to separate if they are left undisturbed but can be stabilized by the addition of an agent that reduces surface tension. Drugs formulated as emulsions may contain oils that are less than palatable. The emulsion tends to disguise the taste and alters the consistency of the substance.

Liniments are liquids containing an alcoholic, oily, or soapy vehicle. They act as counterirritants when rubbed on the skin.

Lotions are emollient liquids that may be clear solutions, suspensions, or emulsions. They are used on the skin.

Suspensions are combinations of a solid and liquid in which the solid particles do not dissolve. Gels and magmas are viscous suspensions of mineral precipitates in water. Examples of a magma and a gel are milk of magnesia and aluminum hydroxide gel, respectively.

Syrups are solutions of sugar and water to which a drug is added. Syrups are usually added to drug mixtures to increase palatability. They are especially useful in pediatric formulations (e.g., syrup of ipecac).

Oils are of two types, volatile and fixed. Volatile oils evaporate easily, leaving no greasy residue. Fixed oils do not readily evaporate. Oils can be used as vehicles to dissolve other drugs or as the drugs themselves (e.g., castor oil). The viscous, greasy liquids are insoluble in water.

Pharmacokinetic Phase

The term pharmacokinetics is derived from the Greek words *pharmacon,* meaning drug or poison, and *kinesis,* meaning motion. The four processes of absorption, distribution, biotransformation, and elimination, along with the dosage, determine drug concentration at the site of action, the intensity of effects, and the duration of drug action. There are several factors influencing each of the pharmacokinetic processes (see Factors Affecting Pharmacokinetic Phase).

FACTORS AFFECTING PHARMACOKINETIC PHASES

Absorption
Bioavailability
Solubility
Ionization
Absorbing surface
Presystemic biotransformation

Distribution
Blood flow
Protein binding
Tissue binding
Solubility

Biotransformation
Age
Pregnancy
Disease
Genetics

Elimination
Renal clearance
Half-life
Steady state

Absorption

For a drug to produce a pharmacologic effect, it must be absorbed, that is, transferred from its site of administration (e.g., skin, GI tract, muscle) into the blood stream. Absorption must occur before active ingredients can reach the central circulation, where the drug is distributed throughout the body. Exceptions are drugs administered IV, those injected into a body space for local effects, topically applied drugs, and drugs administered for their action within the GI tract.

Factors influencing the rate and extent of drug absorption into the circulation include dosage form, administration route, age, pregnancy, and disease states. The rate at which drugs are absorbed determines the onset of effects. In turn, the amount of drug absorbed determines the intensity of effects.

There are several physiologic variables affecting the transport of drugs across membranes. In general, the factors include absorptive surface area, contact time with the absorptive surface, concentration gradient, and the extent of presystemic biotransformation.

Mechanisms of Transport

In many cases, drug absorption obeys the same pathways as those of nutrients: passive mechanisms, pinocytosis, and active transport (Fig. 4–3). These mechanisms allow drugs to penetrate cell membranes to create physiologic effects.

Passive Mechanisms Passive mechanisms involve simple diffusion, filtration, and carrier-mediated diffusion. *Simple passive diffusion* moves drugs from higher to lower concentrations. Absorption occurs as drugs randomly move from high concentrations in the original compartment to areas of lower concentration in another. This mechanism accounts for the absorption of most drugs from the GI tract into the circulation and from the circulation to target cells.

During *filtration,* small drug molecules move along with fluid through the pores in cell walls. This is how water-soluble drugs and some electrolytes are absorbed through tissue pores (rather than through the lipid matrix of the cells) into systemic circulation. The capillary membrane pores act as barriers only to very large drug molecules.

Carrier-mediated diffusion (i.e., facilitated transport) occurs in harmony with concentration gradients. A carrier is needed to move the drug across membranes, but a driving force is not required. Carrier-mediated diffusion is used for physiologic substances such as glucose, certain vitamins, amino acids, and organic acids. Any drug that resembles these substances can be transported by carriers. The classic example of carrier-mediated diffusion is dietary vitamin B_{12}. Vitamin B_{12} binds with intrinsic factor in the GI tract to form a complex. The complex is then selectively but passively carried from areas of higher concentrations to areas of lower concentrations.

Pinocytosis *Pinocytosis* facilitates absorption of drug molecules by engulfing the particles and moving them across cell membranes. The term pinocytosis is derived from the Greek word *pino,* meaning I drink, *kytos* meaning hollow vessel (representing cells), and *osis,* meaning a process. The drug does not have to be dissolved because during pinocytosis, the cell wall invaginates, forms a vacuole for drug transport, breaks off, and moves into the cell. Fat-soluble vitamins such as vitamins A, D, E, and K are commonly transported by pinocytosis.

Active Transport *Active transport* moves drug molecules against a concentration gradient using metabolic energy, usually in the form of adenosine triphosphate (ATP). The ATP:drug complex forms on the surface of the cell membrane, carries the drug through the membrane, and then dissociates. The rate of active transport is proportional to drug concentration. When carrier mechanisms become saturated, the transfer rate cannot increase.

The size of drug molecules plays a part in drug transport. For example, urea molecules are small and pass easily across cell membranes. In contrast, glucose molecules are rather large and do not pass easily. Once the concentrations on both sides of the cell membrane are equal, drug movement stops. Thus, small, lipid-soluble, nonionized drugs readily diffuse across cell membranes, whereas larger, water-soluble, ionized drugs do not.

Factors Affecting Absorption

Bioavailability *Bioavailability,* as defined by the FDA, is the rate and extent to which an active drug, or its therapeutic metabolite, is absorbed and becomes available at the site of action. In other words, the percentage of drug available to produce a pharmacologic effect. Bioavailability is determined by measuring drug concentration in body fluids (serum levels) and by assessing the magnitude of response. The amount of bioavailable drug is dependent on its solubility, chemical structure, size, and polarity. Bioavailability is influenced by the presence of food within the GI tract. Food reduces the amount of fluid in the GI tract, slowing the dissolution of drugs and thus the absorption rate. In contrast, fasting for more than 18 to 20 hours causes vasoconstriction

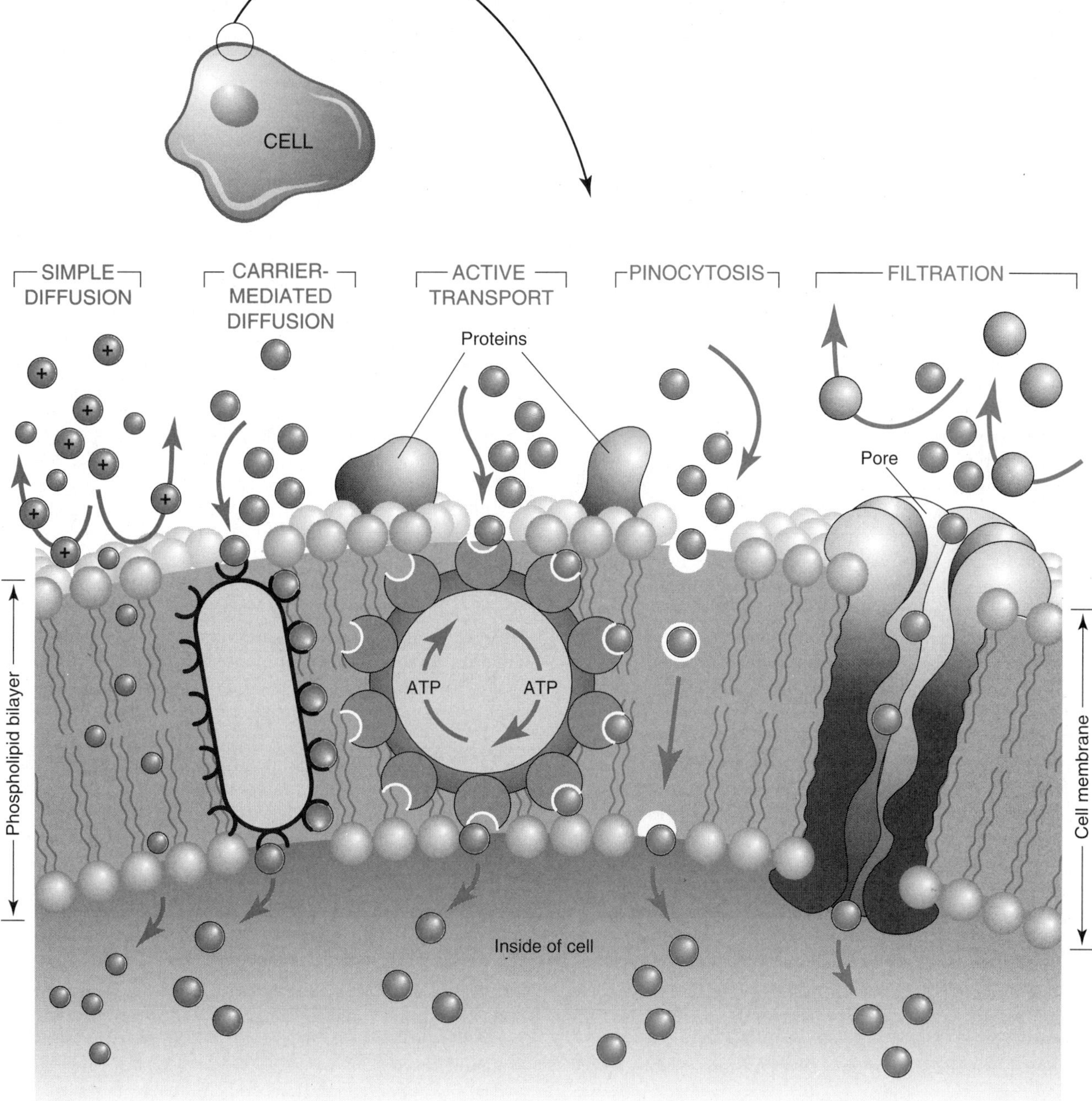

Figure 4–3 Mechanisms of transport. The majority of drugs cross cell membranes via simple passive diffusion. Only nonionized (uncharged), lipid molecules diffuse easily. Movement of drug molecules also occurs via carrier-mediated diffusion, active transport, pinocytosis, and filtration mechanisms.

of blood vessels supplying the GI tract and delays the absorption of any drugs that may be present.

The concept of bioavailability is important when one considers the large number of drugs in the marketplace. Different brands of drugs may contain the same active ingredient in the same unit dose, and yet the amount delivered to the tissues may vary greatly. Bioavailability becomes especially important when drugs with narrow therapeutic indices (i.e., margins of safety) are prescribed. In some cases, substitution of a generic drug for a brand name leads to toxicity because the amount of drug bioavailable in the generic form is greater. Substitution of one drug for another may also provide inadequate amounts of the drug to produce a therapeutic effect.

The increasing array of new and existing drug formulations led manufacturers and the FDA to set standards for bioavailability. In 1970, the FDA began requiring data on bioequivalence. When two drugs are chemically equivalent and the bioavailabilities are similar, they are said to be *bioequivalent*. Therapeutic equivalence is a separate matter, because even when two drugs are not bioequivalent, or even chemically equivalent, they may produce similar therapeutic effects in a particular group of people.

Manufacturers of solid oral dosage forms must demonstrate the rate and extent of absorption of a new drug compared with a standard preparation, usually an oral solution, or an IV dosage form. Once the drug is marketed, it becomes the standard for bioavailability. Other manufacturers must demonstrate bioequivalence to the established industry standard if they wish to market a generic equivalent.

Ionization The movement of a drug by one or more transport mechanisms is influenced by the electrical charge (polarity) of the cell membrane and by the charge on the drug molecule. In order to understand the effect *ionization* has on the absorption of drug molecules, the effect of ionization on solubility must first be understood.

There are two basic rules regarding ionization of drugs: substances of like electric charge repel each other, and unlike forms attract one another. Alkaloids, bases, and metallic radicals are positively charged. Acids and acid radicals are negatively charged. Nonionized (uncharged) drug molecules are usually lipid soluble and capable of crossing cell membranes. In contrast, ionized (charged) drug molecules are unable to penetrate lipoid cell membranes (see Interrelationship of Pharmacokinetic Variables). A charge on a drug molecule that is similar to that of the membrane will delay absorption. Both the dissolution and ionization of drugs are affected by the pH values of body solutions.

The ratio of a nonionized drug to an ionized drug is related to two factors: the pH of the aqueous medium in which it is dissolved, and its *pKa value.* The pH of an environment in which exactly half of the drug molecules are charged and the other half are not is called the pKa, or the ionization constant, of a drug. Each acid and base has a characteristic pKa. For example, aspirin (a weak acid) has a pKa value of 3.5. This means that if the pH of the solution in which the aspirin is dissolved is greater than 3.5, the drug will be ionized and relatively insoluble in lipid environments. At pH levels less than 3.5, aspirin will be almost entirely nonionized and lipid soluble. It will, therefore, readily cross cell membranes.

A phenomenon called *ion trapping* occurs when the pH is different on the two sides of a cell membrane. Because ionization of drugs is pH dependent, drug molecules tend to accumulate on the side of the cell membrane where the pH is most favorable. When an acid drug is in an environment more acidic than its pKa value, it has fewer ionized molecules and thus is more lipid soluble. For example, aspirin, nonionized in the stomach, crosses cell membranes into plasma. There, where the pH is about 7.4, it becomes ionized and lipid insoluble. Thus, it is trapped in the plasma. Ion trapping is used therapeutically in the treatment of drug overdose and poisoning. For example, alkalinization of the urine promotes ionization of an acid drug such as phenobarbital (pKa of 7.4) and facilitates its elimination by trapping it in the urine.

Basic drugs act in the opposite way. A weak organic base such as codeine will be almost completely ionized when placed in an acid environment. In this form, it is not lipid soluble and will not be absorbed. When there is a pH difference between two sides of a membrane, basic drugs tend to accumulate on the side that is more acidic. The plasma pH and the pH of the administration site are such that drug molecules have a greater tendency to be ionized in the plasma than at the administration site. Any drug can be absorbed to some extent in both the stomach and intestines.

Solubility *Solubility* refers to the ability of the drug to dissolve and form a solution. To facilitate absorption, the solubility of the drug must be similar to the polar characteristics (i.e., electrical charge) of the absorption site. The more lipid soluble a drug is, the faster it crosses lipoid cell membranes. Although a drug may be nonionized in one environment, when it moves to an environment with a different pH, it becomes ionized. The next section discusses these relationships.

Absorbing Surface Cell membranes determine the speed at which drugs reach systemic circulation. Drug molecules that pass through a single layer of cells, as in the case of intestinal epithelium, do so faster than when they must pass several layers of cells. A rich blood supply to the absorptive surface is a significant factor in the absorption of drugs because it allows drugs to enter the circulation, and then blood flow removes them from that area. In so doing, the body maintains a steady-state environment that encourages absorption and transport of the drug. Blood flow may be increased with local massage, local application of heat, certain metabolic diseases, or the concurrent administration of vasodilator drugs.

The rich blood supply of oral mucous membranes enhances absorption of drugs administered by the sublingual route. In contrast, absorption is delayed from subcutaneous tissues because of poor vascularity. Disease states such as peripheral vascular disease or shock, or the administration of vasoconstrictive drugs may delay absorption.

It is assumed that the gastric mucosa is a simple lipoid membrane permeable to nonionized, lipid-soluble forms of a drug. The stomach wall, however, limits absorption to some extent. The surface area of the stomach is relatively small and lacks mucosal villi, and most of its cells are primarily adapted for secretion. Lipid-soluble substances such as ethanol and acid drugs are relatively nonionized at low gastric pH and therefore are absorbed in the stomach owing to its rich blood supply. However, because the absorptive surface is small compared with that of the intestine, even acid drugs are significantly absorbed in the intestine.

INTERRELATIONSHIP OF PHARMACOKINETIC VARIABLES

Small, nonionized (uncharged) drug molecules are lipid-soluble and readily cross cell membranes

Large, ionized (charged) drug molecules are water-soluble and do not readily cross cell membranes

High water solubility + high serum protein binding = $\downarrow V_d$ & $\uparrow$ serum levels

High lipid solubility + high serum protein binding = $\uparrow V_d$ & $\downarrow$ serum levels

V_d, Volume of distribution.

Delayed gastric emptying slows the absorption of most drugs because it increases transit time to the intestine. High gastric acidity, hot meals, vigorous exercise, pain, and emotion all delay gastric emptying. Many drugs such as morphine, amphetamines, and anticholinergics slow gastric emptying. Gastric emptying time also may be increased by hunger, lying on the right side, the ingestion of dilute solutions, and mild exercise.

The larger the surface area, the more fully a drug is absorbed. For example, most absorption of orally administered drugs occurs in the small intestine, where many mucosal villi and microvilli provide an extensive surface area. The number of folds in the lining of the small intestine decreases from the proximal to the distal end. Therefore, drugs tend to be absorbed more in the duodenum, less in the jejunum, and least in the ileum. When large sections of the small intestine are diseased or surgically removed, drug absorption decreases. In select cases, a shortened small intestine also causes a decrease in the transit time of substances moving through the intestine.

The rectal route may be used when oral administration of a drug is not possible. The rectum, although it has a good blood supply, has a limited surface area. Dissolution of drugs occurs slowly, and absorption is irregular, unpredictable, and incomplete. In addition, many of the drugs formulated for a rectal route are irritating to the fragile, thin mucosa of the rectum. Approximately half of a rectally administered drug enters the enterohepatic circulation before entering the systemic circulation.

Drugs delivered to the lungs as gases or aerosols are rapidly absorbed because of the rich blood supply, large surface area, and high permeability of alveolar epithelium. Bronchodilator drugs, anesthetics, and the nicotine found in tobacco smoke are examples of substances that may be rapidly absorbed when inhaled.

Few drugs readily penetrate the skin. It is low in lipid and water content. Absorption of drugs can be facilitated by suspending the drug in an oily vehicle and rubbing it into the skin. Absorption of the drug is proportional to lipid solubility and the surface area over which it is applied. Because hydrated skin is more permeable than dry skin, dosage forms may be modified or an occlusive dressing used to facilitate absorption. Systemic absorption occurs more readily through abraded, burned, or denuded skin surfaces. Inflammation or other conditions that increase circulation to the skin surfaces also enhance absorption. Body surfaces containing scar tissue generally have poor absorptive surfaces and therefore are not recommended for topical administration of drugs.

Topically applied ophthalmic and otic drugs are used primarily for their local effects. To produce local effects, absorption of the drug through the cornea or the auditory canal is required. Systemic absorption is usually not desired. Ophthalmic and otic drugs are discussed in more depth in Chapters 62 and 63.

Presystemic Biotransformation Drugs may be biotransformed, usually to inactive metabolites, before reaching the systemic circulation. Orally administered drugs are transformed in the GI tract by acids, digestive enzymes, bacterial action, and enzymes in the cells of the intestinal walls. Venous blood from the GI tract (except the mouth and rectum) passes through the liver via the portal system prior to entering systemic circulation. Therefore, drugs that are highly cleared by the liver will undergo considerable biotransformation before entering systemic circulation. This phenomenon is known as the *first-pass effect.* Drugs highly cleared via the first-pass effect include certain tricyclic antidepressants (e.g., amitriptyline), analgesics (e.g., meperidine, morphine, propoxyphene), and antiarrhythmics (e.g., propranolol). Lidocaine, an anesthetic drug, when taken by mouth is almost completely biotransformed on the first pass through the liver and, therefore, has no pharmacologic effect.

As a general rule, drugs with significant first-pass effects require much larger oral than parenteral doses to achieve the same effects. Variable serum levels occur in the same individual as a result of a large variation in the metabolic activity in the liver. Dosage requirements for drugs that undergo a first-pass effect vary widely between individuals.

Distribution

Following absorption, drugs are distributed via the circulation to inert plasma and tissue-binding sites, to the site of action, and to the organs of elimination (Fig. 4–4). Several factors influence the distribution of an absorbed drug, including blood flow, protein binding, tissue-binding, and solubility.

Factors Affecting Distribution

Blood Flow Cardiac output and blood flow influence the time required for a drug to be distributed to body tissues. The uptake of a drug is faster in tissues that are well perfused, such as the kidneys, heart, liver, and brain. The uptake of a drug in poorly perfused tissues, such as muscle and adipose tissue, is slower. High-blood-flow areas receive the drug before other body tissues. Unless a drug is given for its effect on the blood itself, drug molecules in the circulation must leave that fluid compartment and cross capillary membranes to reach their site of action. Drug concentrations rapidly equalize between blood and organs with high blood flow and then equalize more slowly within other tissues. When an IV bolus is given, redistribution is responsible for termination of drug action. For example, a patient who received an IV barbiturate for anesthesia will awaken within a few minutes even though the half-life of the drug is several hours. The rapid response is due to the decline of drug levels in the brain as the drug is redistributed to adipose tissue. It is the redistribution rather than drug elimination that terminates the anesthetic effect.

Protein Binding Once they are absorbed, most drugs are bound, to a greater or lesser extent, to various tissues in the body. Storage reservoirs within the body permit the accumulation of a drug. Drugs with an affinity for lipoid tissues, for example, readily cross cell membranes. They take less time arriving at their site of action than lipid-soluble drugs.

Drugs bind to proteins throughout the body. In so doing, binding restrains the drug, decreasing plasma concentration of unbound drug. Because only free drug is available to cross cell membranes to sites of action, the bound drug is lost to pharmacologic action. The effect is only temporary, however, because as the unbound drug is eliminated, bound drug is released from the prote'n-binding site to exert pharmacologic action.

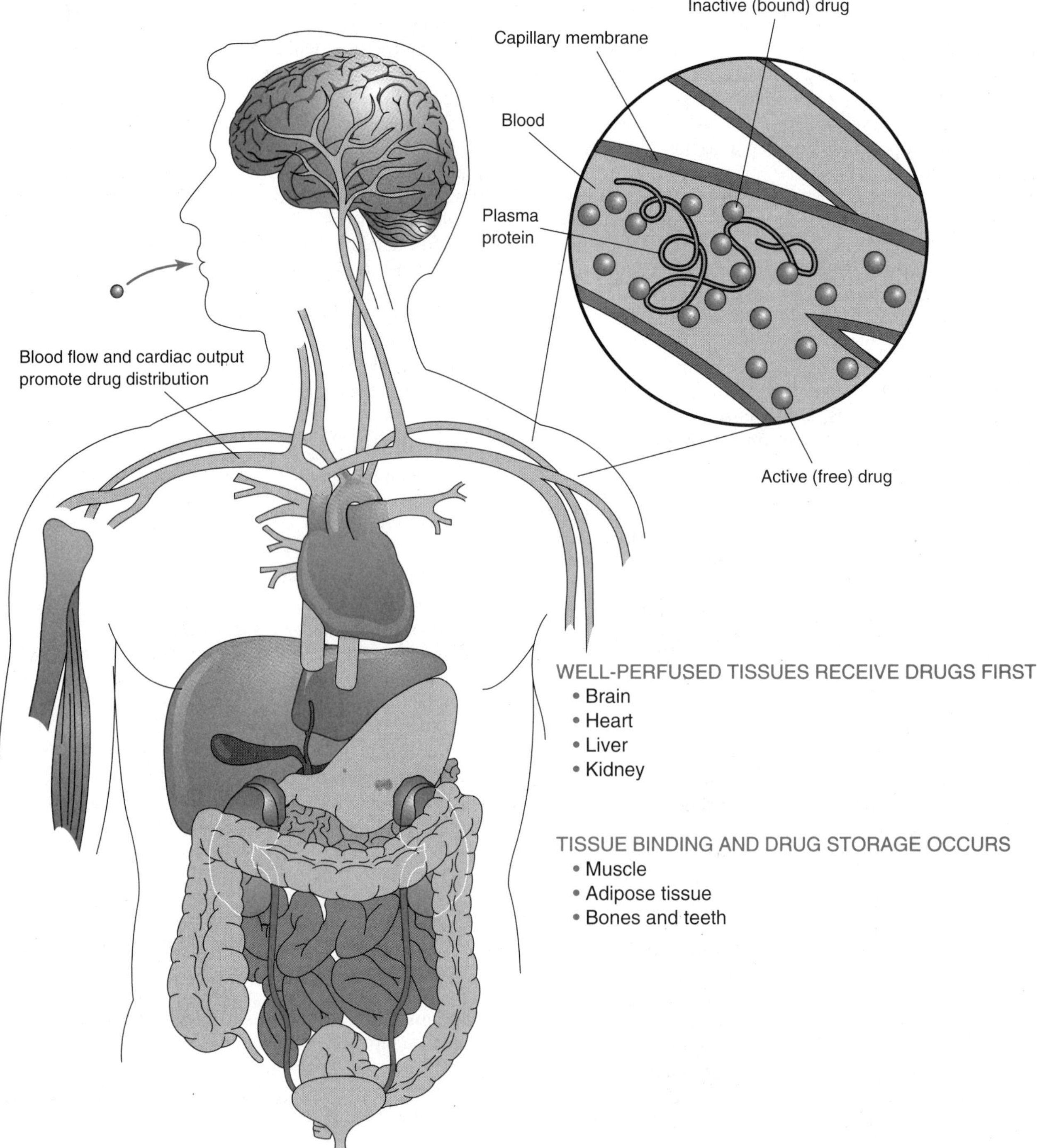

Figure 4–4 Drug distribution and the concept of bound versus free drug in the circulation. Once the drug is absorbed from the site of administration, tissues that are well perfused receive the drug molecules first. Some drug molecules are reversibly bound to plasma proteins, particularly albumin. Because the drug-protein complex is large, it is trapped in the circulation and serves as a storage site for the drug. The percentage of bound or free drug depends on the drug itself and the availability of protein-binding sites. Some drug molecules are also bound to tissues such as muscle, adipose tissue, bone, and teeth.

Two independent protein-binding sites have been identified: alpha-1-acid glycoproteins and albumin. Different drugs tend to bind at each site. Basic drugs such as quinidine, meperidine, imipramine, dipyridamole, and chlorpromazine tend to bind to alpha-1-acid glycoproteins for distribution. Acid drugs, on the other hand, bind to albumin, the most abundant plasma protein, to form a drug-protein carrier complex. Examples of such drugs include warfarin, penicillins, sulfonamides, tolbutamide, and phenylbutazone. Binding to other plasma proteins occurs to a much smaller extent. Various disease states can alter the plasma concentrations of albumin and alpha-1-acid glycoprotein and thus affect drug-protein binding (Table 4–3).

TABLE 4–3 CHANGES IN PLASMA PROTEIN CONCENTRATIONS IN VARIOUS DISEASE STATES

Disease States	Changes in Albumin Concentration	Changes in Alpha-1-Acid Glycoprotein Concentration
Arthritis	Slight decrease	Increase
Burns	Decrease	Increase
Cirrhosis	Decrease	Varies
Hepatitis	Slight decrease	Increase
Myocardial infarction	Decrease	Increase
Obesity	No change	Increase
Pregnancy	Decrease	Slight decrease
Renal failure	Decrease	Increase
Stress or trauma	Varies	Increase
Surgery	Varies	Increase

Bound drugs are considered pharmacologically inactive. The large molecular size prevents the carrier complex from reaching the site of action. Further, bound drugs cannot be biotransformed or excreted. The exceptions are high-hepatic-clearance drugs and those eliminated by renal tubular secretion. Binding of a drug to plasma proteins limits its concentration in tissues and at the site of action because only unbound drugs exert pharmacologic actions.

To some extent, plasma protein binding prolongs drug action. The stronger the drug-protein bond, the slower the release of the bonds and the longer the duration of drug action. As drug molecules are released from their bonds, they become free to create an effect. For example, sulfonamide drugs are highly bound to plasma proteins. To maintain drug equilibrium within the circulation, sulfonamide molecules are slowly released from the proteins and are then free to produce antimicrobial action.

The degree of drug-protein binding is expressed as a percentage. The percentage of protein binding in the circulation depends largely on the chemical nature of the drug. It may range from nearly zero to almost 100 percent. For example, warfarin, an anticoagulant, is 99 percent protein bound. The remaining 1 percent is free to create pharmacologic effects. As a result, it is necessary to administer the drug only once a day in most cases because of the long duration of action. In contrast, a therapeutic dose of the analgesic acetaminophen is virtually free from protein binding. This permits more drug molecules to reach the site of action.

It should be noted that an individual who has low serum protein levels (i.e., hypoalbuminemia) may have difficulty transporting some drugs. This patient has fewer proteins available to bind with the drug. The result of large amounts of unbound drug is an exaggerated drug effect that could prove hazardous to the patient.

Some proteins are nonspecific in that they are capable of binding with many different drugs at any given time. Several different drugs can compete with one another for the binding sites. For example, one drug that is poorly bound to albumin will not offer much competition to the molecules of another drug that possesses a strong bond to albumin. If two drug molecules are somewhat equivalent in terms of bonding ability, the one with the stronger protein binding or the one present in higher concentration will be more extensively bound.

Tissue Binding Body compartments in which a drug accumulates are also potential drug storage sites. Tissue mass determines the amount of drug that accumulates outside the vascular space. A stored drug in equilibrium with that found in the plasma is released as the plasma concentration diminishes. The plasma concentration of drug at its site of action is thus sustained, and the pharmacologic effects of the drug are prolonged.

Lipid-soluble drugs have a high affinity for adipose tissue. Even in starvation states, the percentage of body fat can constitute 10 percent or more of body mass. Moreover, the relatively low blood flow to adipose tissue makes this area a stable environment for drug storage. Barbiturates, antibiotics, anesthetics, and anticoagulants are commonly stored in body fat.

With obesity, the proportion of the body that is fat is greater and the proportion that is lean is less. Fat tissue contains less water than does lean body mass, so the amount of body water per kilogram of total body weight is less in the obese person than in the nonobese person. For some drugs, alterations in body makeup that accompany obesity require changes in drug dosages. Drugs that are lipophilic (e.g., thiopental) and distribute well into fat tissues must often be given in larger doses to achieve the desired results. Drugs that distribute primarily to extracellular fluids (e.g., aminoglycoside antibiotics) may be given in higher doses to the obese person, but the overall milligram per kilogram dose is lower.

Bones and teeth, structures primarily made up of calcium salts, can accumulate substances that bind to calcium ions. Tetracycline antibiotics, heavy metals such as lead, radioactive elements such as radium, and environmental pollutants such as fluoride are stored in the bone and may lead to toxicity.

Solubility The distribution of a drug depends on its solubility once it has been absorbed. Diffusion occurs rapidly because of the highly permeable nature of capillary endothelial membranes. Lipid-soluble drugs readily move across the membrane. Drugs that are insoluble in lipids are limited in their ability to pass capillary endothelial membranes and, therefore, have a restricted distribution.

Barriers to Distribution

The capillary networks of certain endothelial structures act as barriers to drug distribution. The two most significant of these structures are the placental membranes and blood-brain barrier.

Placental Membranes The layer of epithelial cells separating maternal from fetal circulation make up the placental membranes. The long-standing notion that the placenta is a barrier to drugs is inaccurate. The placental membranes may serve as a means to protect the fetus against potentially harmful drug effects. However, it is believed that the fetus is exposed to the same drug concentrations as those in the mother or to even higher drug levels. Teratogenic effects of drugs may develop. Nonionized, lipid-soluble drugs readily reach the fetus through maternal circulation. The same factors that affect drug movement across other membranes also determine drug movement across placental membranes. Chapter 6 discusses in more depth the physiologic changes of pregnancy and their influence on pharmacokinetics.

Blood-Brain Barrier The distribution of drugs from the circulation to the central nervous system (CNS) is limited by the blood-brain barrier. The capillary endothelial cells of the brain and its glial sheath effectively create a second membrane between the plasma and the brain interstitium. The membrane limits the ability of many drugs to diffuse across the membranes and reach effective concentrations in the brain. Highly ionized and protein-bound drugs cannot enter the CNS. The membrane between the plasma and brain cells is less permeable to water-soluble drugs.

The membrane becomes important in individuals with infection. Antimicrobial drugs may be ineffective for CNS infections if they are unable to cross the blood-brain barrier. Only drugs that are very lipid soluble and poorly bound to plasma proteins are capable of crossing the membrane to produce effects within the CNS. The active transport system of the blood-brain barrier pumps drug molecules out of the brain when diffusion has permitted them to enter. In select instances, such as with meningitis, the active transport system fails and large amounts of antibiotics such as penicillin are allowed to remain in the brain.

Volume of Distribution

The actual volume of fluid in which a drug is distributed within the body cannot be measured. However, an estimate, the *apparent volume of distribution* (V_d), can be obtained. V_d is an abstraction. It describes the volume of fluid necessary to contain all of the drug in the body in the same concentration as that in the blood. The V_d serves as a guide to determine whether a drug is bound primarily to plasma or tissue sites. One method for calculating the V_d is to divide the amount of drug administered IV by the drug concentration in the plasma 1 hour after the drug is given. Thus, the formula is as follows:

$$V_d = \frac{\text{total amount of drug administered}}{\text{concentration of drug in plasma}}$$

Many drugs exhibit V_d far in excess of known body fluid volumes. For drugs that are lipid soluble, the apparent V_d is greater than the entire fluid volume of the body (over 0.6 L/kg). Drugs with extensive tissue binding can have an apparent V_d greater than total body volume (over 1.0 L/kg). For example, when 500 mcg of digoxin is administered to a young, healthy 70-kg male, a plasma concentration of approximately 0.78 ng/mL results. Dividing the amount of drug in the body by the plasma concentration yields an apparent V_d for digoxin of 645 L, about nine times the total body volume of a 70-kg male. This example illustrates that V_d does not represent a real volume but must be thought of as the pool of body fluids that would be required if the drug were distributed equally throughout all portions of the body. In fact, digoxin is relatively hydrophobic, distributing to muscle and adipose tissue. Only a very small amount of drug is in the plasma.

The V_d and therefore drug concentration is influenced by age, body mass, gender, drug dosage, extent of protein binding, and solubility. Males and females have different percentages of body fat and body water, so drug distribution also differs. Differences in the V_d are also evident during pregnancy, when the fetal-placental unit provides additional tissue storage sites for certain drugs.

High water solubility and high plasma protein binding keep a drug in circulation. This results in a small V_d and high blood levels (see Interrelationship of Pharmacokinetic Variables). High lipid solubility and high tissue binding result in a large V_d and lower blood levels. Drugs with a large V_d are more spread out to plasma proteins and tissues and, therefore, are less frequently exposed to sites of elimination. Less frequent dosing may be required. A drug with a small apparent V_d is most likely contained only within the plasma.

Biotransformation

Characteristics of drug molecules such as size, lipid solubility, and polarity facilitate their passage across cell membranes during absorption and distribution. The same characteristics also impair elimination of the drug. Most lipid-soluble drugs are not eliminated from the body because they are readily reabsorbed from glomerular filtrate by the renal tubular cells. The biotransformation of lipid-soluble drugs to a more polar, less lipid-soluble metabolite enhances elimination and reduces the V_d. Chemical alterations required to accomplish the change are referred to as detoxification, metabolism, or biotransformation.

The term *detoxification* has historical significance in that the first foreign compounds chemically altered by the body were converted to less toxic substances. The term is used less often today because it has been shown that chemical reactions may produce a compound with toxicity greater than that of the parent drug.

The term *metabolism*, as originally used, referred to the process by which carbohydrates, proteins, fats, vitamins, and minerals were built into living matter, and by which the living matter is broken down to simpler compounds. Metabolism is the sum total of intracellular chemical changes relating to catabolism and anabolism. In contrast, chemical changes that drugs undergo do not ordinarily provide new materials or energy. Thus, the term *biotransformation* is preferable. It more accurately describes the physiochemical reactions that take place and that are not normally considered a part of carbohydrate, protein, fat, vitamin, or mineral metabolism.

Mechanisms of Biotransformation

Most drugs are chemically altered by many body tissues or organs. Reactions may take place in the intestines, for example, where drugs are biotransformed either by epithelial

TABLE 4–4 BIOTRANSFORMATION PROCESSES

Phase I (Nonsynthetic) Reactions	
Oxidation	The loss of electrons by an atom; molecular oxygen serves as the final electron acceptor; usually carried out by a family of isoenzymes called cytochrome P_{450}
Reduction	The gain of electrons by an atom
Hydrolysis	The combination of a water with a salt to produce an acid and a base
Phase II (Synthetic) Reactions	
Conjugation	An acid or base formed when an acid or base either accepts or gives up a proton to another molecule; a coupling together
Alkylation	A chemical process in which an alkyl radical replaces a hydrogen atom
Acetylation	The introduction of one or more acetyl groups into an organic compound
Methylation	The introduction of a methyl group into a compound

cells or by normal digestive enzymes. The reactions may also occur as a result of normal flora in the intestines. Biotransformation also occurs in the plasma, kidneys, and brain. By far, the greatest number of chemical transformation reactions occur in the liver.

Biotransformation reactions are many and varied but may be divided into two primary categories (Table 4–4). Phase I, or nonsynthetic, reactions include oxidation, reduction, and hydrolysis. Phase II, or synthetic, reactions include conjugation, alkylation, acetylation, and methylation. The resultant metabolites are usually more polar and less lipid soluble than the parent molecule. Oxidation and conjugation are most important and are discussed further.

Phase I Reactions In the process of *oxidation,* the parent drug is converted to one that is usually more water soluble than the parent drug. The metabolite may be pharmacologically inactive, less active, or occasionally more active than the parent drug. Some drugs are administered as inactive prodrugs, which then must be metabolized into the pharmacologically active form.

Although many older drugs such as castor oil or cascara and newer ones like primaquine, an antimalarial drug, are known to be inactive until biotransformed, their utility as prodrugs was incidental. Today, prodrugs are widely used to overcome problems of absorption, to improve the distribution of drugs with poor lipid solubility, to increase the duration of action for drugs that are rapidly eliminated, to suppress problems of patient noncompliance, and to promote delivery of the drug to a specific site.

Oxidation is one of the most general biochemical reactions because there are so many ways in which a compound can be oxidized. In quantitative terms, most oxidative reactions are carried out by a large family of isoenzymes called cytochromes P_{450}. At least 10 families of cytochrome P_{450} genes are known. The ancestral cytochrome was probably present more than one and one-half billion years ago. It is thought that some P_{450} gene families evolved and split as a result of exposure to plant metabolites and decayed plant products. The exposure led to a remarkable overlap of specific substrates of the P_{450} enzymes.

The microsomal P_{450} enzyme system is embedded in the lipid bilayer of the hepatic smooth endoplasmic reticulum, most often affecting the transformation of lipid-soluble, nonionized drugs. The enzyme system renders them more water soluble. Although the liver is the primary organ in which oxidation reactions occur, similar reactions are also catalyzed by microsomal fractions in the lung, kidneys, and small intestine.

Phase II Reactions Phase II reactions combine the drug with an endogenous substrate. The conjugating agent is ordinarily a carbohydrate, an amino acid, or a substance derived from these nutrients (e.g., glucuronic acid, sulfate, glycine, and acetate). The endogenous substances yield polar molecules that are usually inactive and readily excreted in the urine or bile. Some drug conjugates are thought to contribute to hepatotoxic reactions. Drugs that are considered to be major hepatotoxic agents are identified in Examples of Major Hepatotoxic Drugs and Drug Classes.

EXAMPLES OF MAJOR HEPATOTOXIC DRUGS

Antimicrobial Drugs
Chloramphenicol (Chloromycetin)
Isoniazid (INH)
Nitrofurantoin (Furadantin)
Penicillins
Sulfonamides
Tetracyclines

Analgesics
Acetaminophen (Tylenol)
Allopurinol (Zyloprim)
Indomethacin (Indocin)
Phenylbutazone (Butazolidin)

Antiemetics
Prochlorperazine (Compazine)

Anticonvulsants
Barbiturates
Phenytoin (Dilantin)

Antineoplastics
Chlorambucil (Leukeran)
Mercaptopurine (6-MP, Purinethol)
Methotrexate (Folex, Mexate, MTX)

Cardiovascular Drugs
Digoxin (Lanoxin)
Hydralazine
Methyldopa (Aldomet)
Nitroglycerine (Nitrostat)

Diuretics
Furosemide (Lasix)

Psychoactive Drugs
Chlorpromazine (Thorazine)
Isocarboxazide (Marplan)
Perphenazine (Trilafon)
Phenelzine (Nardil)
Prochlorperazine (Compazine)
Promazine (Sparine)
Thioridazine (Mellaril)
Trifluoperazine (Stelazine)
Diazepam (Valium)

Factors Influencing Biotransformation

Age Neonates and infants up to 1 year of age do not yet have fully developed and operational microsomal enzyme systems. The combination of poorly developed blood-brain barriers, weak drug-metabolizing activity, and immature elimination mechanisms combine to make the fetus, neonates, and very young children sensitive to toxic effects of drugs. They are unable to handle either the range or total quantity of chemicals that adult systems manage. See Chapter 7 for further discussion of pediatric pharmacotherapeutics.

Likewise, older adults also have a limited capacity to manage drugs. Their limited capacity is related to changes in GI absorption and in the V_d owing to changes in body composition, in metabolism, and in the elimination of drugs that decrease renal clearance. With declining functional capacity of body systems, the biotransformation of drugs is reduced. Chapter 8 discusses geriatric pharmacotherapeutics further.

Pregnancy

Chapter 6 discusses further the effect of pregnancy on liver blood flow and the intrinsic activity of biotransformation enzymes.

Disease

In persons with liver disease (e.g., hepatitis), drugs may circulate for longer periods of time because the enzymes responsible for the breakdown of certain drugs exist in lower than normal concentrations. As a result, plasma drug concentrations remain elevated and predispose the patient to toxicity. In patients with cirrhosis, circulation to the liver is reduced or altered to such an extent that drug exposure to the microsomal enzyme systems is decreased. In other circumstances, a particular enzyme may exist in larger concentrations, hastening transformation of a drug to an inactive metabolite. Its effectiveness is thereby decreased. Biotransformation rates are directly proportional to the concentration of enzymes. If a change occurs in the concentration of an enzyme, there is a proportionate change in the rate of biotransformation.

Hypothyroid states and acute hypoxemia are associated with decreased hepatic enzyme activity. In addition, because lipids, proteins, vitamins, and iron are required for the production and function of hepatic microsomal enzymes, malnutrition impairs enzyme activity. For example, the biotransformation of barbiturates is impaired with prolonged protein malnutrition. Conversely, a balanced diet fosters drug biotransformation. Dietary constituents such as caffeine, ethanol, cruciferous vegetables (e.g., cabbage, cauliflower, broccoli, Brussels sprouts), and charcoal-broiled meats stimulate enzyme induction. As an example of enzyme induction, persons taking the bronchodilating drug theophylline who consume large amounts of broccoli may experience an asthma attack. In this example, microsomal enzymes rapidly biotransformed the drug and serum levels dropped.

Air pollutants, insecticides, and food additives can increase or decrease the activity of microsomal enzyme systems. In addition, cigarette smoke contains compounds that promote enzyme induction. Therefore, smokers have considerably higher levels of hepatic and pulmonary drug–metabolizing enzymes.

Genetics Genetically determined differences also affect biotransformation. The differences may be evident in one group of individuals or marginally present to completely absent in another group. For example, identical twins metabolize drugs at the same rates, whereas fraternal twins do not. One of the most prevalent genetically determined alterations involves acetylation, a phase II reaction. About half of the population of the United States are *slow acetylators,* an autosomal recessive trait. These persons biotransform drugs more slowly than the rest of the population. As a result, they are more likely to develop toxicity and often require lower doses. A syndrome resembling lupus erythematosus (joint pain, arthritis, and pleuritic pain) is more likely to develop in patients who are slow acetylators and who are taking such drugs as hydralazine, procainamide, or isoniazid. In another example, a bimodal distribution of drug metabolism rates is evident in a population of individuals who are considered *rapid acetylators.* These individuals metabolize a drug more rapidly and consequently may develop reactions caused by the increased metabolites.

Another group of individuals have a genetic defect in the enzyme glucose-6-phosphate dehydrogenase (G6PD) and are more likely to develop more severe drug reactions. G6PD deficiency is more common in blacks and in certain Mediterranean and Asian populations (i.e., Sardinians, Sephardic Jews, Greeks, Iranians). With the sex-linked incomplete codominant pattern of inheritance, males are more frequently and severely affected. Heterozygous females can exhibit a milder form of the disease. After an initial episode, the disease is usually self-limiting.

Elimination

Drug elimination refers to the movement of a drug or its metabolites from the tissues back into the circulation and then to the organs of elimination. The primary organ system responsible for drug elimination is the kidneys, but to lesser degrees the GI tract, respiratory system, sweat, saliva, tears, and breast milk also are involved. Efficient elimination depends on proper functioning of the system involved. Lipid-soluble drugs are not eliminated until they have been biotransformed to a more polar compound.

Routes of Elimination

Renal Elimination Several factors affect the rate of drug elimination through the kidneys. The ability of the heart and blood vessels to deliver an adequate blood supply to the kidney, renal maturity, the presence or absence of renal disease, and urinary pH affect the rate of elimination. In addition, some drugs (e.g., nonsteroidal anti-inflammatory drugs) decrease renal blood flow and the glomerular filtration rate, thereby altering the elimination of many other drugs.

The kidneys, as primary organs of elimination, use glomerular filtration and active tubular secretion to rid the body of unchanged drug molecules and their metabolites. Only free, unbound drug molecules are filtered by the glomeruli. Most drugs passively filter into the tubules, but those bound to plasma proteins are poorly filtered and remain in the plasma. Ionized compounds become trapped in the urine because they do not readily diffuse back across lipid membranes of the tubules into the systemic circulation. Large protein-bound compounds do not pass through the glomeruli. Nonionized, lipid-soluble weak acids and bases, once filtered by the glomeruli, are passively reabsorbed from the proximal and distal tubules. With tubular cells less permeable to ionized drug forms, passive reabsorption of these substances is pH dependent.

Urinary pH affects the amount of the drug passively reabsorbed by renal tubules. When tubular urine is made more alkaline by consuming milk, vegetables, or most fruits, weak acids are excreted more rapidly. The rapid elimination rate occurs primarily because they are more ionized and passive reabsorption is decreased. When tubular urine is more acid (as after eating cranberries, plums, or prunes) the elimination of weak acids is reduced. The alkalinization and acidification of urine produce opposite effects on the elimination of weak bases.

By manipulating urinary pH, the passive reabsorption of a drug can be decreased and elimination enhanced. The effect is greatest for weak acids and bases with pKa values in the range of urinary pH (5 to 8). The administration of systemic alkalizers (e.g., sodium bicarbonate, tromethamine) causes tubular urine to become more alkaline. In contrast, high doses of ascorbic acid or ammonium chloride acidify the tubular urine and promote the elimination of basic drugs.

Biliary-Fecal Elimination Although the vast proportion of drugs are eliminated through the kidneys, there are some that are eliminated through the intestine via biliary elimination. The secretion and reabsorption process is called *enterohepatic recirculation.* Drugs present in bile enter the small intestine, where a portion may be reabsorbed, returned to the liver, and again secreted into the bile. Lipid-soluble drugs usually have prolonged effects because the enterohepatic recirculation cycle continues until the drug is eliminated.

Small doses of oral contraceptives produce therapeutic effects because of enterohepatic recirculation. However, if the woman concurrently takes an antibiotic, the bacteria that normally cleave chemical bonds of drugs found in the GI tract are killed. Oral contraceptive serum levels then drop. This mechanism explains some cases of contraceptive failure.

Elimination by Other Routes Other drug elimination routes include breast milk and the lungs. The lungs are the preferred route for elimination of gaseous and volatile compounds. Drugs that are administered by inhalation are generally eliminated in their original form (not metabolites) by this route. Inhaled drugs enter the systemic circulation after passing through alveolar membranes. The rate of drug elimination depends in part on the respiratory rate. For example, deep breathing or exercise increases cardiac output, with a subsequent increase in pulmonary blood flow. Drug elimination is thus fostered. The reverse is also true if the respiratory rate is impaired.

Drugs taken by women who are breast feeding cross epithelial membranes of the mammary glands to be excreted in breast milk. Breast milk is acidic in nature, and therefore, basic compounds such as morphine or codeine reach high concentrations in the milk. Weak acids such as barbiturates, sulfonamides, or diuretics are found in lower concentrations. Although relatively small quantities of any drug pass to the fetus, there is considerable concern about the cumulative effects of drugs on the infant. Because of the potential for a drug's reaching the infant, lactating women should check with their health care provider before taking any drug. When the mother's health requires her to take a drug, the risk to the infant can be diminished if the drug is given immediately after breast feeding.

Small amounts of drug also appear in the sweat, saliva, hair, and tears. However, these elimination routes have little therapeutic or toxicologic importance. Although the routes are insignificant in most cases, they may become important if the primary route of elimination is not functional. For lipid drugs to be eliminated in the sweat, they diffuse through the epithelial cells of the sweat glands to the skin surface. Drugs excreted in the saliva are usually swallowed and undergo the same fate as orally administered drugs. Although drug elimination into hair is quantitatively insignificant, it can aid in diagnosis. Some tests for drug abuse involve analysis of hair samples. Arsenic was detected in hair samples obtained during Napoleon's lifetime but that were examined 150 years after his death. Some now suggest that he was poisoned.

Factors Influencing Elimination

Relatively few unchanged drugs or active metabolites depend on renal clearance for elimination. A few drugs still produce toxic symptoms in the presence of renal impairment if the dosage is not adjusted. Drugs likely to produce toxicity include the cardiac glycoside digoxin, the histamine-2 antagonist cimetidine, aminoglycoside antibiotics such as gentamicin, and some antihypertensive drugs. The creatinine clearance test is a good indicator of renal function and is often used as the basis for dosage adjustment.

Renal Clearance Clearance reflects the integrity of glomerular filtration. *Creatinine clearance* describes the volume of plasma that needs to be cleared per unit of time (milliliters per minute) to account for the rate of drug removal taking place in the kidneys. Creatinine, a by-product of muscle metabolism, is produced at a constant rate in a healthy individual as long as muscle mass remains constant. Assuming 100 percent bioavailability and steady state, a therapeutic range is reached when the rate of drug elimination equals the rate of drug administration.

Clearance measured in terms of blood flow measurements may take on proportions that are not physiologic. A drug concentrated in red blood cells can display a plasma clearance of tens of liters per minute. However, if blood concentration is used to define clearance, the maximum possible clearance is equal to the sum of blood flow to the various organs of elimination. Because drug elimination takes place in the kidneys, lungs, liver, or other structures, it is important to remember the additive characteristic of clearance:

$$CL_{systemic} = CL_{kidneys} + CL_{liver} + CL_{other}$$

A drug that is slowly removed from the plasma and eliminated through the kidneys has a low clearance rate and requires less frequent dosing. A drug with a high renal clearance is rapidly removed from the plasma. The patient may thus require more frequent dosing and/or higher doses of the drug. Both clearance and half-life vary greatly from one drug to another.

Half-Life The term *half-life* ($t_{1/2}$) describes the relationship between drug volume (V_d) and clearance. It is the time required by the body to biotransform and decrease the original plasma concentration of a drug by half. It is a useful parameter in that it indicates the time required to attain 50 percent of steady state, or a 50-percent decay from steady-state conditions after stopping a drug. Half-life is an important factor in determining proper dosage and frequency of administration. However, as an indicator of either drug elimination or distribution, it has little value because disease states affect both physiology-related parameters, the V_d, and clearance. Thus, the derived parameters will not necessarily reflect the expected change in drug elimination.

$$t_{1/2} = \frac{0.693 \times V_d}{\text{clearance}}$$

The handling of a drug by the body can be very complex because several processes work to alter drug concentrations in tissues and fluids. Simplifications of body processes are necessary to predict a drug's behavior in the body. On a practical note, and most useful in designing dosage regimens, the body may be thought of as a single compartment equal to the size of the V_d. However, the organs of elimination can clear drug only from blood that is in direct contact with the organ. Thus, the time course of a drug in the body depends on both the V_d and the clearance. A single-compartment model portrays the body as a single, homogeneous unit. In other words, all body tissues and fluids are considered a part of this compartment. Furthermore, it is assumed that after a dose of drug is administered, it distributes instantaneously to all body areas, much like chemicals added to an aquarium. Figure 4–5 simplifies the difference between one- and two-compartment models.

But some drugs do not distribute instantly to all parts of the body (even after IV bolus administration). A common distribution pattern is for the drug to distribute rapidly in the blood stream and to the highly perfused organs such as the heart, liver, lungs, and kidneys. Then, at a slower rate, the drug is distributed to other body tissues such as fat, muscle, and cerebrospinal fluid. This pattern of drug distribution can be represented by a two-compartment model, much like a two-compartment aquarium. Chemicals placed in the first compartment equilibrate rapidly with those of the second compartment. Drugs transfer back and forth between these compartments to maintain equilibrium. The amount of drug in the first compartment declines logarithmically to a new steady state. When an avenue is created to drain the aquarium (i.e., an elimination route), a more realistic combination of elimination and equilibration results. A graph of this process would show an early distribution phase followed by a slower elimination phase, with curves made by plotting the logarithm of the amount of drug on one axis against time on the other axis (Fig. 4–6).

In a practical sense, the half-life of a drug determines the dosing frequency. Owing to long half-lives, certain drugs may accumulate, posing an increased risk of toxicity. For

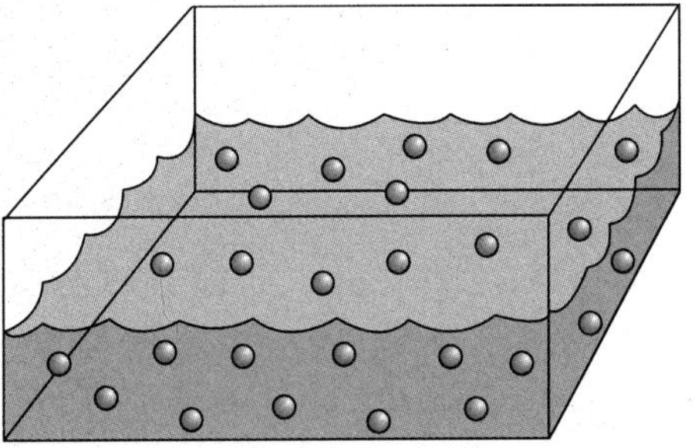

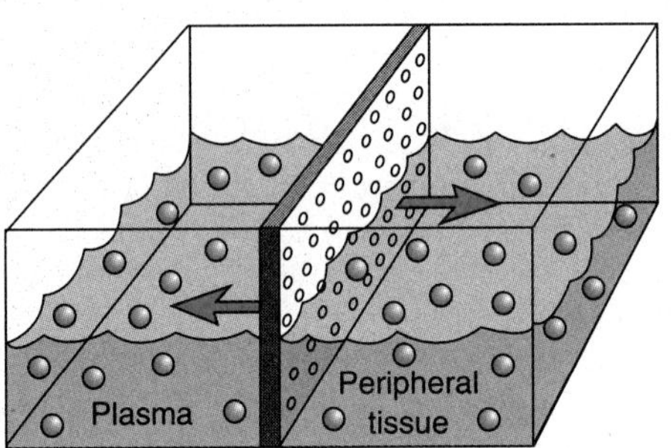

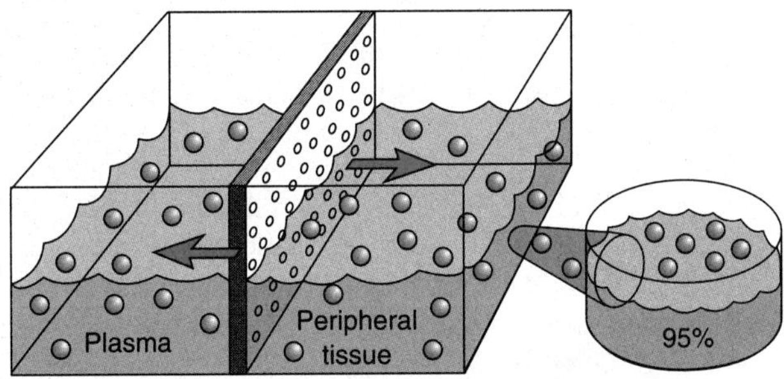

Figure 4–5 Compartment models. A one-compartment model portrays the body as a single, homogeneous unit. In other words, all body tissues and fluids are considered a part of this compartment. The assumption is that after a dose of drug is administered, it distributes instantaneously to all body areas, much like chemicals added to an aquarium. However, some drugs do not distribute instantaneously to all parts of the body (even after intravenous bolus administration). A common distribution pattern is for the drug to distribute rapidly in the blood stream and to the highly perfused organs such as the heart, liver, lungs, and kidneys. Then, at a slower rate, the drug is distributed to other body tissues such as fat, muscle, and cerebrospinal fluid. This pattern of drug distribution can be represented by a two-compartment model, much like a two-compartment aquarium. Chemicals placed in the first compartment equilibrate rapidly with those of the second compartment. Drugs transfer back and forth between these compartments to maintain equilibrium. The amount of drug in the first compartment declines logarithmically to a new steady state. When an avenue is created to drain the aquarium (i.e., an elimination route), a more realistic combination of elimination and equilibration results.

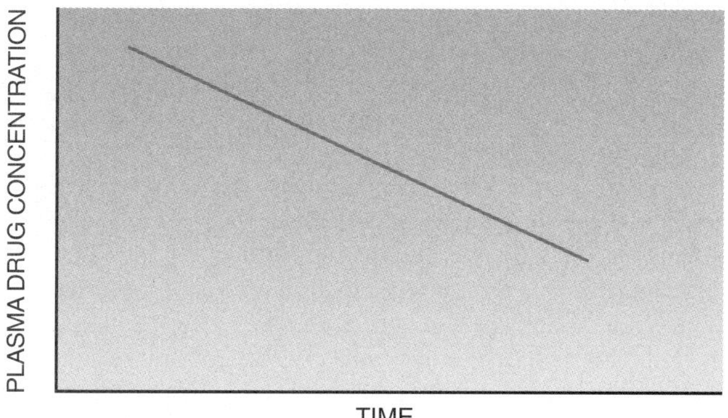

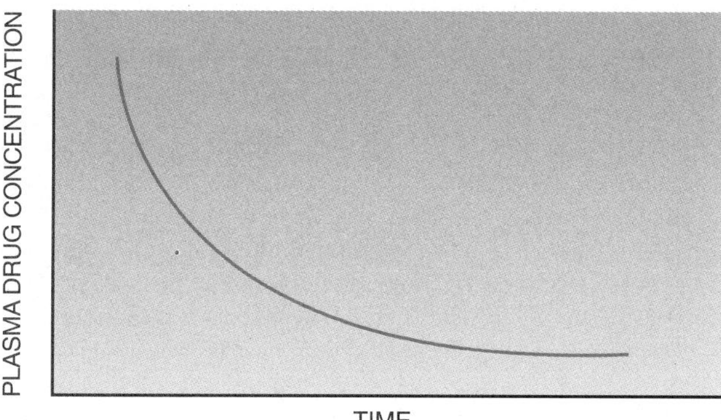

Figure 4–6 Drug elimination. Graphs of drug elimination using one- and two-compartment models. The top figure represents a one-compartment model and assumes instantaneous mixing of the drug. Drug concentration in plasma is plotted against the time course after a single intravenous bolus of the drug. In a two-compartment model, drug concentration in plasma is again plotted against time after a single intravenous dose and also assumes instantaneous mixing. In this model, the amount of drug in the compartment declines exponentially.

example, a single one gram (1000 mg) dose of a drug with a half-life of 4 hours is administered. The total amount of drug in the patient's body decreases by half to 500 mg after 4 hours, to 250 mg after 8 hours, and to 125 mg after 12 hours. The drug amount would continue to decrease accordingly with each subsequent half-life.

The half-life of a given drug usually remains the same within each person, assuming that all elimination systems are functioning normally. For example, a patient arrives at acute care facility with a diagnosis of drug overdose. Assuming that all elimination systems are functioning and the elimination rate of the drug is not compromised, approximately 97 percent of the original dose will be eliminated after five half-lives. For example:

- t_0 = time drug is administered
- t_1 = 50 percent of administered drug remains
- t_2 = 25 percent remains
- t_3 = 12.5 percent remains
- t_4 = 6.25 percent remains
- t_5 = 3.13 percent remains

Patients with renal or hepatic disease ordinarily have increased drug half-lives. By understanding the concept of half-life, the health care provider can appreciate why some drugs are administered daily, some twice a day, and others four times a day.

In the past decade, it has become apparent that early pharmacokinetic studies were compromised by reliance on half-life as the sole measure of alterations in drug disposition. It is now recognized that the half-life is a derived parameter that changes as a function of both renal clearance and V_d.

Steady State The route by which a drug is administered affects how quickly it reaches a steady state and therapeutic level. With repeated dosing, drugs accumulate in the body until they reach a plateau, or *steady state*. Drug absorption then equals drug elimination during the dosing interval. It takes approximately five half-lives for plasma drug levels to reach a steady state, with peak and valley (trough) levels remaining constant after each dosing. A practical guide to the time it takes for a drug concentration to reach steady state can be obtained by multiplying the half-life by five. This figure is very close to the time it will take to reach 90 percent of the steady-state value.

CHRONOTHERAPY

Many body functions such as hormone production, blood pressure, blood clotting, sleep-wake cycles, and response to drugs exhibit a certain rhythmicity. *Ultracadian rhythms* are shorter than a day. For example, a 90-minute sleep cycle or the millisecond it takes for a neuron to fire is reflective of ultracadian rhythms. *Circadian rhythms* last about 24 hours. For example, a circadian variation exists for susceptibility to noxious stimuli, endotoxins, and drugs. Sleep-wake cycles are directed by circadian rhythm. *Infracadian rhythms* are cycles that are longer than 24 hours. A woman's menses usually cycle anywhere from 21 days to 5 weeks. *Seasonal rhythms* influence our reactions and behaviors during particular seasons of the year (e.g., late spring, early fall). For example, seasonal affective disorder causes depression in susceptible individuals during the short days of winter.

Body functions take their cue from the environment and the rhythms of the solar system that change night to day and lead us from one season to another. Biologic rhythms are also dictated by our genetic makeup. Biologic rhythms influence drug behavior and subsequently patient response. The rate of drug absorption, hepatic clearance, half-life, duration of action, and the magnitude of drug effect have all been shown to differ depending on the time of day the drug is administered.

Coordinating these biologic rhythms with medical and pharmacotherapy is referred to as *chronotherapy*. Chronotherapy is being studied in relation to diseases such as asthma, arthritis, and cancer. Chronotherapy for asthma is directed at obtaining maximal effects from bronchodilator drugs during the early morning hours, when lung function normally undergoes circadian changes, reaching a low point. For example, a long-acting theophylline bronchodilator drug (UNIPHYL) is taken once daily in the evening. Theophylline blood levels reach their peak during the early morning hours to improve lung function. In general, health care providers believe that unless asthma treatment improves nighttime symptoms, it is difficult to improve its daytime manifestations. For patients with severe asthma who wake during the night gasping for breath, a good night's sleep can be a dream come true.

Chronobiologic patterns have also been noted in patients with pain from osteoarthritis. These patients tend to have less pain in the morning and more at night. For patients with rheumatoid arthritis, the pain is usually worse in the morning and decreases as the day goes on. Thus, it appears that joint inflammation fluctuates over a 24-hour period. In chronotherapy, drug dosing with corticosteroids and nonsteroidal anti-inflammatory drugs is timed to ensure that the highest blood levels of the drug coincide with peak pain periods. For patients with osteoarthritis, the optimal time for administration of a nonsteroidal drug such as ibuprofen would be at lunch time or mid-afternoon. For the patient with rheumatoid arthritis, the best administration time would be after the evening meal.

It is also becoming apparent that cancer therapy may be more effective and less toxic if antineoplastic drugs are administered at carefully selected times. It has been noted that there may be different chronobiologic cycles for normal cells and cancer cells. If this is indeed true, the treatment goal would be to time drug administration to coincide with the chronobiologic cycles of tumor cells, making them more effective against cancer and less toxic to normal tissues. Because some patients may be better served by receiving antineoplastic drugs in the late afternoon or even during the night, perhaps an implantable infusion pump might be more appealing. Chronotherapy means that not all patients can receive their antineoplastic drugs first thing in the morning, an otherwise common practice today.

Furthermore, it is believed that timing breast cancer surgery to coincide with the last half of the menstrual cycle can increase the number of patients who are tumor free after 5 years. In the first half of the menstrual cycle, estrogen levels are high and progesterone is not produced. However, in the last half of the cycle, progesterone levels rise and estrogen falls. It is thought that progesterone may inhibit the production of some enzymes that help cancer to metastasize.

In other examples, patients who received test doses of intradermal histamine experienced the mildest skin response at 11 AM. The most severe responses were noted to occur at 11 PM. Thus, administration of cyproheptadine, an antihistamine, provided 16 hours of relief when it was taken at 7 AM but only 7 hours of relief when it was taken at 7 PM.

The plasma cortisol rhythm for daytime-active persons is one in which cortisol levels begin to rise in the latter part of the usual sleep cycle. These peak shortly before or just after awakening, then irregularly decline throughout the day and evening until minimal levels are reached early in the next sleep cycle. Transplant recipients, for example, are placed on lifetime steroid therapy to augment their endogenous cortisol levels and to prevent rejection of the donor organ. Under these conditions, the goal of treatment is to reinforce intrinsic adrenocortical activity with minimal suppression. In order to achieve this goal, a synthetic glucocorticoid such as prednisone is given after the peak secretion of endogenous cortisol on a daily or alternate-day midmorning schedule.

On the other hand, when the treatment goal is replacement, such as in a person with adrenocortical insufficiency, it is recommended that the steroid be given at a time that mimics natural endogenous rhythm. That is, approximately two-thirds of the daily dose would be taken in the morning upon awakening, and the remaining one third prior to bedtime in the evening.

Patients are more likely to follow drug regimen schedules when the drugs are formulated for chronotherapy. That is, reformulating a drug so absorption into the blood stream is delayed, revising the dosing schedule, or using programmable pumps that deliver drugs to the patient at precise intervals optimizes a drug's desirable effects, minimizes undesirable effects, and promotes patient compliance. Although susceptible biologic rhythms are not as well documented in human beings as in animals, research in this area is rapidly growing. Drugs that are reformulated to be chronotherapeutic agents are regulated by the FDA.

SUMMARY

- The three phases of drug activity include the pharmaceutic phase, the pharmacokinetic phase, and the pharmacodynamic phase.
- The pharmaceutic phase begins with the formulation of a drug into a dosage form best suited for delivery to its site of action.
- Drug constituents include active ingredients and additives.
- Compounded drugs include solid, semisolid, and liquid formulations.
- The pharmacokinetic phase refers to the action of drugs as it relates to absorption by body tissues, distribution of the drug throughout the body, biotransformation, and elimination.
- Simple passive diffusion, filtration, carrier-mediated diffusion, pinocytosis, and active transport are responsible for the absorption of drugs into systemic circulation.
- Factors affecting absorption include bioavailability, solubility, ionization, absorbing surfaces, drug forms, and routes of administration.
- Distribution is influenced by blood flow, the degree of protein and tissue binding, and the affinity of the drug for lipoid or aqueous tissues.
- The volume of distribution (V_d) represents an abstraction describing the fluid volume necessary to contain all of the drug in the body at the same concentration as that of the blood. Thus, a large V_d represents a lower blood concentration level of a drug.
- The major barriers to drug distribution include the placental membranes and the blood-brain barrier.
- The biotransformation of drugs, most often by oxidation and conjugation, alters a drug in such a way that the renal and biliary systems can excrete them more readily.
- Age, various diseases and conditions, and genetic variations influence biotransformation, and therefore, undertreatment or toxicity is possible.
- Elimination of drugs is primarily through the kidneys and biliary-fecal route, but it may also occur through the respiratory system, breast milk, saliva, and tears.
- Factors influencing elimination include renal clearance, half-life, and steady state.
- Knowledge of a drug's half-life, renal clearance, and steady state can assist in predicting the frequency of administration and in assessing drug accumulation.

- Coordinating biologic rhythms with medical and pharmacotherapeutic regimens is called chronotherapy. This approach considers the patient's biologic rhythms in determining the timing (and sometimes the dosage) of drug to optimize desired effects and minimize adverse effects.

BIBLIOGRAPHY

Bakutis, A. (1983). The P_{450} enzyme system: A key to understanding the metabolism of drugs. *Journal of the American Association of Nurse Anesthetists,* 51, 272–274.

Bourne, D. (1986). *Pharmacokinetics for the non-mathematical.* Higham, MA: Kluwer Academic Publishers.

Dipiro, J. (1991). *Concepts in clinical pharmacokinetics: A self-instructional course.* Bethesda, MD: American Society of Hospital-System Pharmacists.

Evans, W. (1986). *Applied pharmacokinetics: Principles of therapeutic drug monitoring* (2nd ed.) Vancouver, WA: Applied Therapeutics.

Gilman, A., Rall, T., Nies, A., and Taylor, P. (1990). *Goodman and Gilman's the pharmacological basis of therapeutics* (8th ed.) New York: Pergamon Press.

Katzung, B. (1992). *Basic and clinical pharmacology* (5th ed.) Norwalk, CT: Appleton & Lange.

Moore-Ede, M., Sulzman, F., and Fuller, C. (1982). Circadian timing of physiologic systems. In M. Moore-Ede and C. Czeisler (Eds.), *The clocks that time us.* Cambridge: Harvard University Press.

Reinberg, A., Smolensky, M., and Labrecque, G. (1987). Aspects of chronopharmacology and chronotherapy in children. *Chronobiologia,* 14: 303–323.

Stehlin, I. (1997). A time to heal: Chronotherapy tunes in to body's rhythms. *FDA Consumer,* 31(3), 16–19.

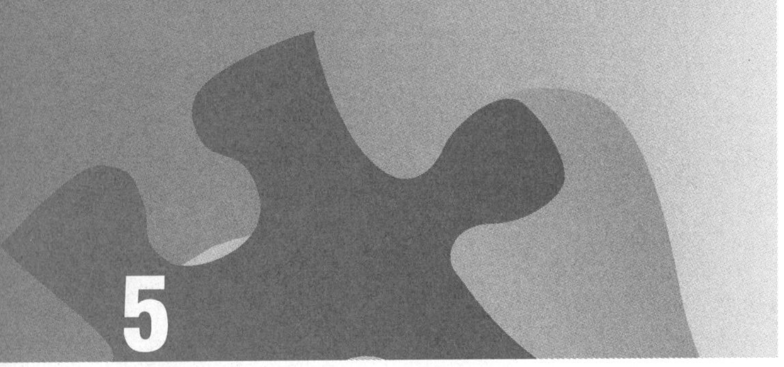

5 Pharmacodynamics

The pharmacodynamic phase of drug activity occurs when a drug reaches its site of action and produces an effect; in other words, how the drug acts in the body. Together, the pharmacokinetics and pharmacodynamics of a drug determine the route by which it will be administered, how often it will be given, and what the dosage will be. The following major factors influence the site of drug action: drug actions versus drug effects, receptors, dose-time-effect relationships, and a drug's therapeutic indices.

Adverse effects are possible when any patient receives a drug. Patient factors as well as drug-related factors contribute to adverse reactions. The effects can be classified as dose related or sensitivity related.

SITE OF ACTION

One of the fundamental concepts of pharmacodynamics relates to the site of drug action. The site of action is the specific cell, tissue, or organ where the drug works. Although the site of action for many drugs has been identified, there are many drugs for which a site of action has not been identified. The site of action and the effects produced are mutually dependent—one cannot be demonstrated in the absence of the other. Drug effects can be produced at nearby physiologic sites or by drug action at sites far away from the target organ. The more complex the physiologic processes, the more sites the drug may act on to produce an alteration in functioning.

Drug Action Versus Drug Effects

The difference between drug action and drug effect is important to the understanding of pharmacodynamics. The interaction between a drug and cellular components constitutes the *mechanism of action*—how the drug works. A patient's response to a drug's action represents the *effect.* Once a drug reaches the site of action, it produces effects through nonspecific modification of the cellular environment or through specific physical and chemical alterations in cell functioning, or both. The effects produced by a particular drug may be the consequence of a single mechanism of action, but they appear at a variety of sites.

In most cases, the effects are easily recognized and are expressed as changes in the patient's physiologic state. For example, morphine sulfate minimizes pain and suffering, acetaminophen or aspirin relieves fever, and digoxin slows the heart rate and strengthens its contractions. Figure 5–1 provides a visual representation of the relationships between the pharmacologic effects of a drug and the levels at which it produces therapeutic or toxic effects.

Nonspecific Changes of Cell Environment

Mechanisms that alter a cell's environment range from creating a physical barrier and altering surface tension to lubrication and ionizing radiation. The environment can also be modified by altering the osmolality, chemistry, or pH of the surrounding body fluids. Drugs that modify a cell's environment do so without physically attaching to cell membranes.

Specific Changes of Cell Function

In contrast, alterations in cell function occur when a drug structurally interacts with cell components or target tissue. Commonly, the interactions inhibit or support energy metabolism, foster drug transport across cell membranes, or depress membrane function. Specific effects are produced by drug-receptor interactions, drug-enzyme reactions, and nonspecific drug interactions. Regardless of the target cell, tissue, or process, drug actions accelerate or inhibit cell functioning.

DRUG ACTION AND INTERACTION

Drug-Receptor Interactions

The majority of drugs are thought to act by attaching to *receptors* on cell surfaces—the receptor being that portion of the cell whose site of action is occupied by a drug (Fig. 5–2). In general, the body uses a variety of receptors to regulate each of its physiologic activities (Table 5–1). The characteristics of drug receptors and of the drug-receptor complex are important to the subsequent understanding of pharmacotherapeutics.

Proteins of the cell membrane are the most important drug receptors. They are physiologic points of control. However, enzymes, carbohydrates, and lipids also act as receptor sites. On a day-to-day basis and under normal homeostatic conditions, receptors interact with cell membranes to serve normal physiologic functions. Theoretically, it should be possible to synthesize a drug that could alter any physiologic process for which receptors exist. As a general rule, though, if a physiologic process is not regulated through receptors, it is unlikely to be influenced by a drug.

A drug-receptor complex is similar to the relationship between a lock and key, or to the biochemical action of enzymes and substrates. Drugs and receptors combine in a reciprocal manner. Thus, when a drug attaches to a receptor, the resultant drug-receptor complex initiates reactions. It is known that a single receptor can react with a number of drugs, provided that each drug structurally conforms to the receptor site. In a sense, drugs that possess similar chemical or physiochemical properties and produce selective pharmacologic responses probably produce the responses by acting on the same population of receptors. Assumptions about drug-receptor interaction provide a theoretic basis for the

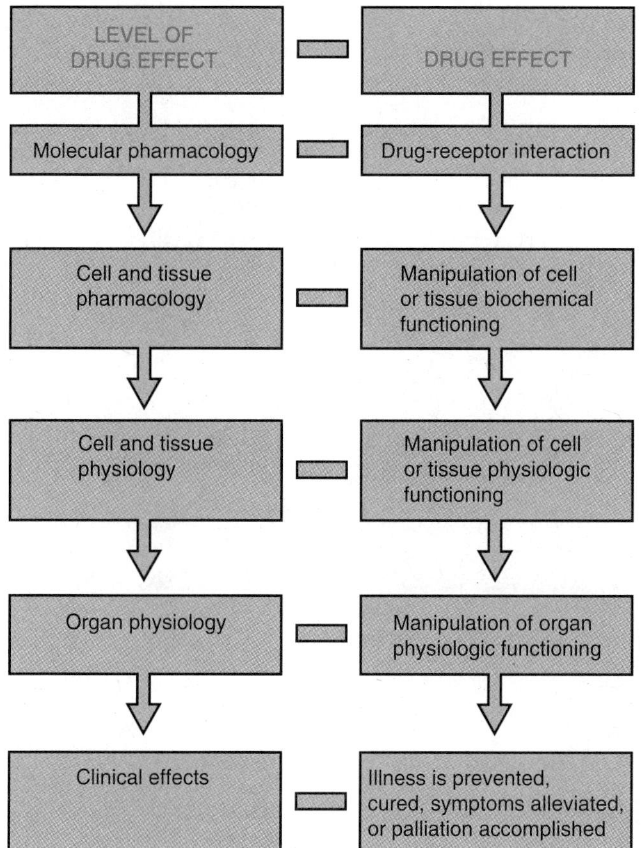

Figure 5–1 Comparison of drug effects with the level of effect. A visual representation of the relationships between the pharmacologic effects of a drug and the levels at which it produces therapeutic or toxic effects. (From Grahame-Smith, D.G., and Aronson, J.K. [1984]. *Oxford textbook of clinical pharmacology and drug therapy.* Oxford: Oxford University Press. Used by permission of Oxford University Press.)

ASSUMPTIONS APPLICABLE TO DRUG-RECEPTOR INTERACTIONS

- All receptors are identical in structure and equally accessible to drug agents.
- The intensity of the drug-mediated response is proportional to the number of receptors occupied by the drug agent.
- The amount of drug that combines with receptors is negligible compared with the amount of drug to which the receptors are exposed.

dose-time-effect phenomenon that follows (see Assumptions Applicable to Drug-Receptor Interactions). The attachment of drugs to receptors is the first step leading to a response. The terms agonist and antagonist describe drugs that enhance or diminish a physiologic response.

Agonists

Drugs that mimic the effects of an endogenous compound are referred to as *agonists.* To be termed an agonist, a drug must display two characteristics: it must have an affinity for a specific receptor and it must display some degree of intrinsic activity. Agonists produce actions through two different mechanisms. Agonist I drugs bind to the same site as an endogenous substance (e.g., neurotransmitter) to produce the similar type of response. The response usually equals or is greater than that of the endogenous substance. Agonist II drugs bind to different extracellular sites from those of agonist I drugs, with no response produced in the sole presence of the agonist. However, an enhanced response is generated when the endogenous substance also binds to its site.

The degree of intrinsic activity displayed by an agonist is referred to as *efficacy*—the ability to initiate physiologic re-

TABLE 5–1 EXAMPLES OF RECEPTORS

Receptor Type	Subtype*†	Endogenous Transmitter
Acetylcholine	Nicotinic	Acetylcholine
	Muscarinic (M_1, M_2, M_3, M_4, M_5)	Acetylcholine
ACTH	—	ACTH
Acidic amino acids	NMDA, kainate, quisqualate	Glutamate or aspartate
Adenosine	A_1, A_2	Adenosine
Adrenergic	α_1, α_2	Epinephrine and norepinephrine
	β_1, β_2, β_3	Epinephrine and norepinephrine
Dopamine	D_1, D_2, D_3, D_4, D_5	Dopamine
GABA	A	GABA
	B	GABA
Glucagon	—	Glucagon
Glycine	—	Glycine
Histamine	H_1, H_2, H_3	Histamine
Insulin	—	Insulin
Opioid	μ, μ_1, κ, δ, ϵ	Enkephalins
Serotonin	5-HT_1, 5-HT_2, 5-HT_3	5-HT
Steroids	—	Several

5-HT, 5-Hydroxytryptamine (serotonin); ACTH, adrenocorticotrophic hormone; GABA, gamma-aminobutyric acid; NMDA, *N*-methyl-D-aspartate.
* Receptor identification and classification are based in large part on ligand-binding specificity.
† Other receptor subtypes in various stages of documentation have been proposed, especially where no endogenous transmitter is yet defined.

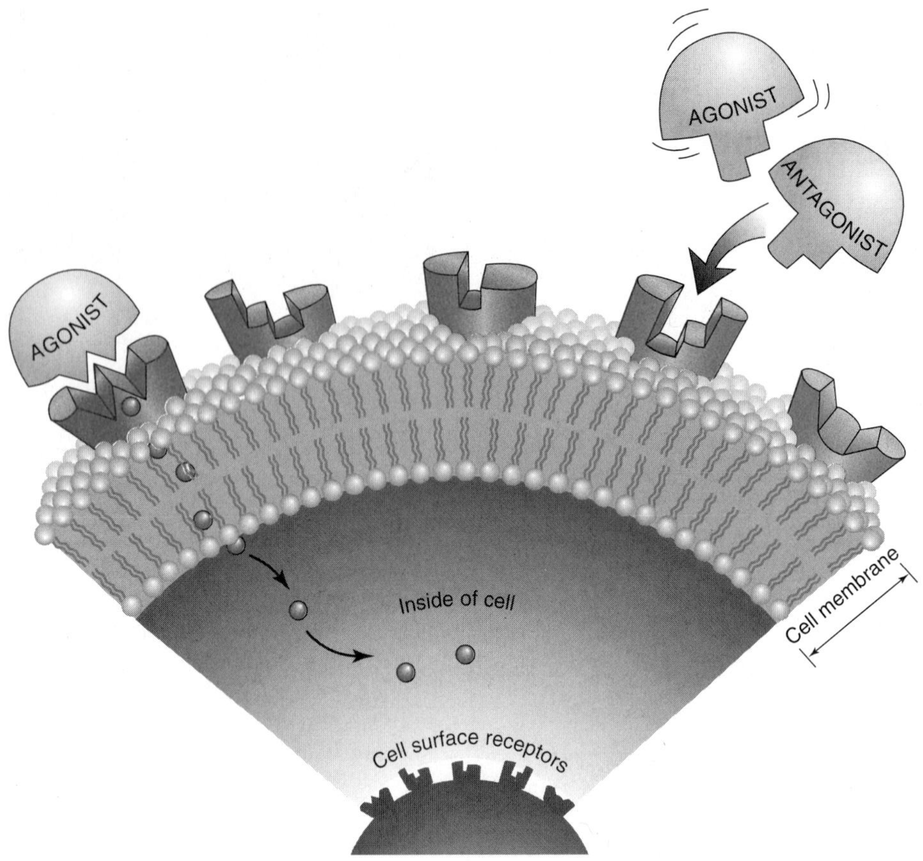

Figure 5–2 Drug-receptor interaction. *Agonists* interact with a receptor to form a drug-receptor complex. In so doing, cell function is altered, causing a response. Agonists with shapes that match an endogenous substance produce the same response as that of the endogenous substance. The response usually equals or is greater than that of the endogenous substance. Drugs with somewhat different shapes that do not allow a perfect fit at weaker agonists produce weaker effects. Antagonists inhibit or counteract receptor activity. They do so through competitive or noncompetitive inhibition, thereby preventing stimulation of receptors. *Competitive antagonists* have an affinity for the same receptor sites as that of an agonist. Inhibition occurs when the concentration of the antagonist increases without a change in the amount of available agonist. *Noncompetitive inhibitors* combine with different parts of the receptor to inactivate the receptor, or by binding in a covalent fashion to the same site as the agonist.

sponse as a result of binding with a receptor (regardless of how intense the response).

Affinity refers to the strength of the attraction between a drug and its receptor site. Affinity is reflected in the potency of the drug.

Potency, not to be confused with efficacy, refers to the dosage needed to produce a response. Potency is influenced by the drug's affinity for receptors and by the body's absorptive, distributive, biotransformational, and elimination capabilities.

Drugs with a high affinity are strongly attracted to receptors and are generally considered potent drugs. For example, a 10-mg dose of morphine sulfate is equivalent to a 1-mg dose of hydromorphone. Therefore, hydromorphone is the more potent drug. In other words, drugs with a great affinity for particular receptors are capable of eliciting a response at lower doses. The reverse is also true. Drugs with low affinity are less strongly attracted to receptors. They are generally weak drugs that require large dosages to elicit a response.

Antagonists

Antagonists inhibit or counteract receptor activity. They do so through competitive or noncompetitive inhibition, thereby preventing stimulation of receptors. Antagonist I drugs bind to the same sites used by endogenous substances, so diminishing or blocking the responses generated by the endogenous substances. Antagonist II drugs bind to extracellular sites, producing diminished responses. Antagonist III drugs are somewhat different, in that they dissolve in the cell membrane or cross the membrane to intercept the response generated by the endogenous substance. Thus, in and of themselves, antagonists have no intrinsic regulatory activity.

The potency of some antagonists, especially those that inhibit enzyme activity, are expressed as the *TI_{50} value.* This value is merely the concentration of antagonist needed to elicit 50 percent inhibition of enzyme activity (see later discussion of therapeutic indices).

Competitive Inhibitors

Antagonists with affinity for the same receptor sites as that of agonists are called *competitive inhibitors.* A competitive inhibitor prevents a response by interfering with the action of the agonist. Inhibition occurs when the concentration of the antagonist increases without a change in the amount of available agonist.

A common example of competitive inhibition is vitamin K, which acts on the same receptors as the oral anticoagulant warfarin. The interaction between the two compounds is usually reversible by the use of excess agonist.

Noncompetitive Inhibitors

Noncompetitive inhibitors either combine with different parts of the receptor to inactivate the receptor or bind in a covalent fashion to the same site as the agonist. The result is a decrease in the maximum effect originally created by the agonist. For example, certain toxins and drugs bind to the gamma-aminobutyric acid receptor, blocking the ion channel much like a cork plugs the opening of a bottle. Environmental pollutants, pesticides, nerve gas, and heavy metals such as lead, mercury, and arsenic are noncompetitive inhibitors. The inhibitory effects cannot be overcome by increasing the concentration of the agonist. The drug-receptor complex is altered to such an extent that it becomes inseparable.

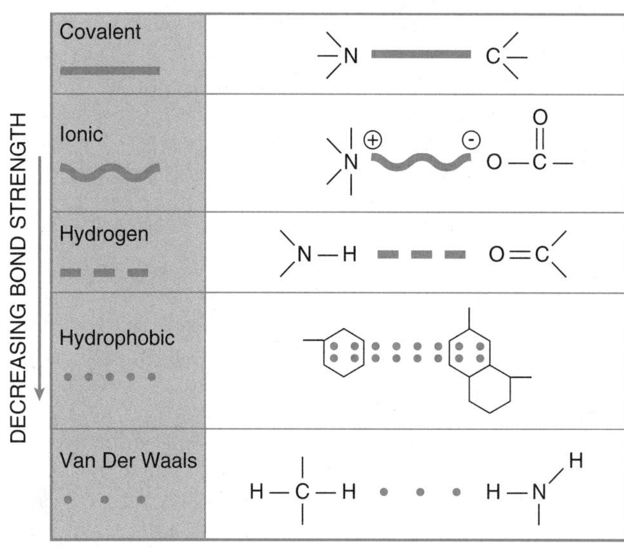

Figure 5–3 Drug-receptor bonding. The majority of drugs have a remarkable degree of selectivity and specificity for receptor sites. It has been postulated that specific forces attract a drug to a receptor, creating a complex and retaining it long enough to produce specific effects. It is likely that a variety of bonding forms are involved in drug-receptor interactions. Bonding may result from the formation of covalent, ionic, hydrogen, hydrophobic, or van der Waals bonding. The duration of drug action is prolonged when the binding is covalent. The other forms are more easily cleaved.

Selectivity and Specificity

A drug can produce more than one effect and still fit the picture of a lock-and-key mechanism. *Selectivity* occurs because a specific receptor is located at more than one site. The response triggered at each site by the drug-receptor complex produces an alteration in the physiologic functioning of that region of the body.

The majority of drugs have a remarkable level of selectivity and *specificity* for receptor sites. It has been postulated that specific forces attract a drug to a receptor, creating a complex and retaining it long enough to produce specific effects. It is likely that a variety of bonding forms are involved in drug-receptor interactions. Bonding may result from the formation of covalent, ionic, hydrogen, hydrophobic, or van der Waals bonding (Fig. 5–3). The duration of drug action is prolonged when the binding is covalent. The other forms are more easily cleaved.

It is generally considered good practice to prescribe drugs that are highly selective and specific, because the more selective the drug, the fewer the adverse effects. Likewise, a drug that interacts with many receptors is likely to elicit a wide range and variety of responses.

Receptor Numbers and Response

Receptor activation initiates or changes the rate of cell functioning. The drug occupying the most sites determines the predominant type of reaction. The number of receptor sites available to a drug and their affinity for binding determine the magnitude of drug action. It has been suggested that the number of receptor sites available at any given time for drug attachment ranges from 2000 to 200,000 per cell. Drug-receptor interactions throughout the body can produce widespread and unpredictable effects. If, however, a drug interacts only with specific receptors of highly differentiated cells, the response is much more predictable. To understand the variability in numbers, the concept of up-regulation and down-regulation is helpful.

Down-regulation is a state of receptor desensitization. It is seen as a decrease in the responsiveness of the receptors. Decreased responsiveness may be due to an actual reduction in the number of receptors, to changes in existing receptors, or both. For example, down-regulation occurs with repeated use of isoproterenol, a beta-adrenergic bronchodilator used in the treatment of asthma. Down-regulation reduces receptor sensitivity to the drug, thereby lowering its effectiveness. An increase in dosage or a change of drug may be required to achieve therapeutic effects.

In contrast, *up-regulation* is associated with an increase in the number of receptors triggered by hormones and neurotransmitters. Dose-dependent exaggerated responses may result.

A patient's response can vary considerably during the course of treatment. The patient can experience different responses to the same drug at different times. The responses may range from exaggerated to virtually no response. A state of up-regulation can occur when receptor activity is at an ongoing level. In other words, the patient's heightened response to the drug exceeds the response seen in most other persons. Up-regulation may occur, for example, with the long-term use of a beta-adrenergic blocking drug such as propranolol. If the drug is abruptly withdrawn, the patient may experience a hypertensive episode or an exacerbation of anginal attacks that had previously been controlled. In this example, the response is due to the increased sensitivity of beta-adrenergic receptors to norepinephrine.

Drug-Enzyme Interactions

Drug-enzyme interactions also result in a response. An enzyme is a protein that catalyzes a response without itself changing. Because enzymes determine the rate of biochemical reactions, their levels directly influence cellular activity. Drugs that combine with enzymes do so because of a structural similarity to the enzyme substrate. The drug, in some cases, may so closely resemble the substrate structure that the enzyme combines with the drug instead of its normal substrate.

Drugs closely resembling the chemical structure of enzymatic substrates are called antimetabolites and are commonly used in the treatment of cancer. Antimetabolites act to block normal enzyme activity or to produce other substances that have unique biochemical properties. The ability of antimetabolites to interact with nucleic acids or other cellular components slows or causes a regression of the cancerous processes (see Chapter 30).

Non-Receptor Interactions

Some drugs have little or no structural specificity with receptor sites and yet still elicit a response. Presumably, drugs enter the cell or accumulate in the membrane, where they influence chemical or physical functioning.

For example, vitamins and trace elements influence cell function and therefore are considered pharmacologically active. General anesthetics are also nonreceptor drugs. They are unrelated, lipid-soluble compounds with properties similar to those of cell membranes. Their effects are mediated through ionic interactions with cell membranes. The electrochemical gradient between the interior and exterior cell surfaces regulates the flow of ions in a highly discriminating fashion.

Another example of nonreceptor drug action is psyllium hydrophilic mucilloid, a bulk-producing laxative. Psyllium forms a nonabsorbable gel that absorbs water, keeping the stool hydrated and soft.

DRUG EFFECTS

To this point, the fundamental concepts and principles of pharmacology have been discussed. They provide the basis for understanding drug safety and effectiveness and for the rational association of drug effects with therapeutics. One of the most basic principles of pharmacology states that drug effects are a function of time and of the dose administered. The properties—dose, time, and effects—are interdependent and interrelated (Fig. 5–4).

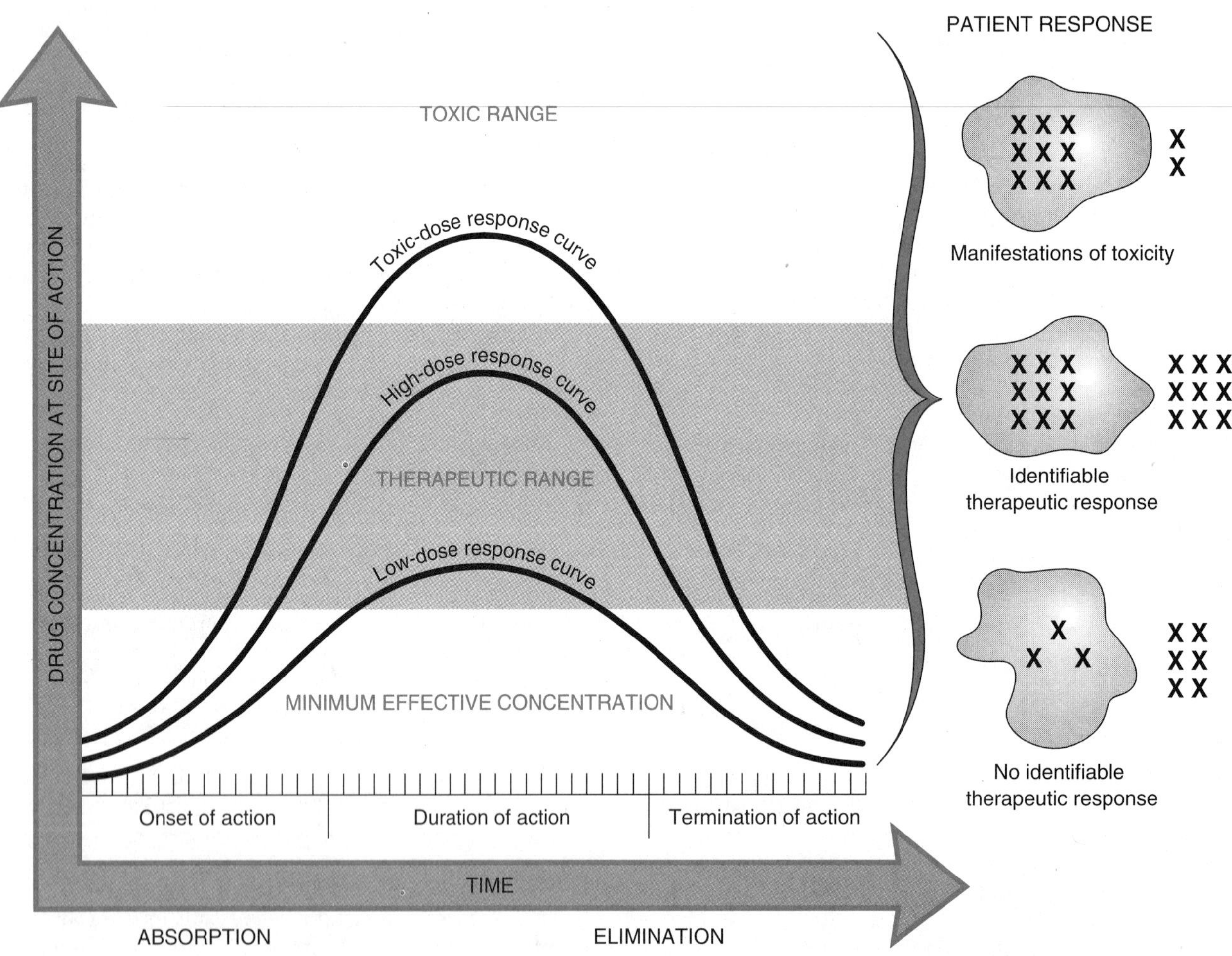

Figure 5–4 Interrelationship of dose-time-effect. Dose-time-effect relationships compare minimum amounts of drug given with the maximum response elicited in a given time. The curve reflects the onset, duration of drug action, and elimination time. Graded drug dosing usually results in a greater magnitude of response as dosage is increased. With routine dosing schedules, the serum level of a drug is prevented from dropping below the desired therapeutic range. A threshold dose is needed in order for a given response to be elicited. Using the dose-time-effect curve, an initial low dose usually corresponds with a low response, or none at all. In most cases, a drug-induced response reaches a plateau rather than increase indefinitely. Increasing the amount of drug administered often produces undesirable effects to a greater degree than it produces therapeutic effects. The ideal drug produces three separate curves that do not overlap: a low-dose response curve, a high-dose response curve, and an adverse/toxic effect curve. With adequate distance between the three curves, the possibility of an adverse drug reaction is minimized.

Dose-Time-Effect Relationships

Dose-time-effect relationships compare the minimum amounts of drug given with the maximum response elicited in a given time. They also illustrate the ease with which the dosage can be safely adjusted. The dose-time-effect curve (see Fig. 5–4) reflects the onset—the time when the drug is absorbed to enter the central circulation. It also reflects the duration of action and elimination time, thereby terminating drug action. It is during the last phase that the next dose of a drug is usually administered. Graded drug dosing usually results in a greater magnitude of response as dosage is increased. With routine dosing schedules, the serum level of a drug is prevented from dropping below the desired therapeutic range.

A threshold dose is needed for a given response to be elicited. According to the dose-time-effect curve, an initial low dose usually corresponds with a low response, or none at all. Likewise, in most cases, a drug-induced response will reach a plateau rather than indefinitely increase. Increasing the amount of drug administered often produces undesirable effects to a greater extent than it produces therapeutic effects.

The ideal drug produces three separate curves that do not overlap: a low-dose response curve, a high-dose response curve, and an adverse/toxic effect curve. With adequate distance between the three curves, the possibility of an adverse drug reaction is minimized.

Therapeutic Indices

The *therapeutic index* (TI) is the ratio relating the drug concentration needed to produce a therapeutic response to that producing a toxic response. It expresses the relative safety of a drug. Therapeutic indices are derived from animal studies during the developmental phase of new drug development. They are then redefined during clinical trials. Drugs with a high therapeutic index are said to be safe (i.e., to have a wide margin of safety). Those with a low therapeutic index are relatively unsafe. They have a narrow margin of safety.

The index is computed using the following formula, where TI equals the therapeutic index, TD_{50} equals the dose that would be toxic in 50 percent of patients, and ED_{50} equals the dose that produces the desired therapeutic effect in 50 percent of test animals:

$$\mathrm{TI} = \mathrm{TD}_{50}/\mathrm{ED}_{50}$$

The closer the ratio is to 1, the greater the possibility of toxicity. For example, digoxin is a cardiac glycoside used in the treatment of congestive heart failure and arrhythmias. In many cases, the TI value for digoxin approaches 1. This means there is an increased likelihood of digoxin toxicity compared with some other drugs. Digoxin may be difficult to use without encountering significant toxicity.

The TI of a drug is often less important than the dose that causes an adverse effect or an early sign of a toxic response. However, the TI is important in terms of dosage frequency and clinical monitoring.

There is no reliable method to guide therapeutic effectiveness when drugs are used prophylactically. Serum drug level monitoring is thus indicated. Drug level monitoring is warranted when there are concerns about patient compliance, when known or suspected pharmacokinetic factors complicate a treatment regimen, or when complications are anticipated. Unusual drug concentrations may be the result of variation in dosage, drug formulation, route or time of administration, concurrent hepatic, renal, gastrointestinal (GI), or cardiac disease, drug-food interactions, or patient weight, gender, or age.

DRUG RESPONSES

Drug responses are categorized as those that are predictable and those that are unpredictable. The incidence of drug-drug interactions and adverse effects has risen with the greater prevalence of drug use. A study by the Boston Collaborative Drug Surveillance Program (1992) found that the incidence of adverse drug reactions in hospitalized patients ranges from 10 to 30 percent. In addition, 2 to 3 percent of hospital admissions were the result of adverse reactions. Further, toxicities leading to death affected 0.2 to 0.5 percent of hospitalized patients. Digoxin and cytotoxic drugs were most often associated with adverse reactions. Antibiotics, anticoagulants, cardiac glycosides, diuretics, corticosteroids, and salicylates were implicated most commonly in patients who required hospitalization as the result of a drug reaction. Adverse reactions may occur in all persons, but females, the very young, the elderly, and persons with impaired renal functioning are most vulnerable.

In general, when drug use is warranted, the expected benefits should outweigh the potential risks. It should be noted, however, that no drug is totally safe and that all drugs produce a variety of effects. Drug responses may be desirable or undesirable. Desirable responses are anticipated and therapeutic. Clinically, an *adverse effect* is any unexpected or unintended response to a therapeutic dose of a drug. An adverse effect usually requires a change in dosage, cessation of the drug, or administration of an antidote for its termination.

Adverse drug responses, sometimes called side effects (see later), fall into two groups: predictable effects that occur as a result of dose-related known pharmacologic effects, and unpredictable effects that are unrelated to the drug's characteristics. Reactions in this second group are often the result of something distinctive to the affected individual, such as drug allergies, hypersensitivities, or idiosyncratic reactions. The adverse effects can range in severity from those that are merely annoying to those that are life-threatening. Although it is not always possible to predict who will experience adverse effects, knowledge of factors known to increase a patient's risk will help minimize their occurrence.

Predictable Adverse Effects

Side Effects

Most adverse responses resulting from the pharmacologic characteristics of a drug are predictable. They are typically dose related. To be precise, *side effects* are the aftermath of a drug that are not specifically desired in the treatment situation. Although the effects are generally undesirable, many drugs are chosen specifically for their side effects. The care provider may often regard these as additional therapeutic effects. Which effects are therapeutic and which are side effects depend on the situation. For example, the use of diphenhydramine produces side effects that are both desirable and undesirable. The drowsiness experienced with this antihistamine may be troublesome for some persons. On the other hand, diphenhydramine may be specifically prescribed in a short course of therapy for its sedative properties. The side effects of some drugs subside with continued therapy.

Common undesirable side effects include nausea, vomiting, skin rashes, electrolyte imbalances, and changes in the level of consciousness. These side effects can be mild or severe to life-threatening. Less serious side effects often go undiagnosed. However, with long-term therapy, such minor effects persist as troublesome, distressing symptoms that are unresponsive to treatment. Dermatologic reactions can be caused by almost any drug and, in many cases, manifest as highly pruritic macules (flat red spots) or papules (raised red spots). Patients with pre-existing pathologic skin conditions are often more prone to skin reactions.

Numerous drugs can produce undesirable effects on the hematologic system. These effects are reflected in blood cell destruction or the inhibition of cell development in the bone marrow. Because hematologic responses affect the formed elements of the blood (red blood cells, white blood cells, and platelets), the resulting reactions include aplastic anemia, leukopenia, and thrombocytopenia.

Complications can also occur following systemic and topical administration of ophthalmic drugs (see Chapter 62). A wide variety of drugs can adversely affect almost any portion of the eye. Patients may complain of blurring vision when taking anticholinergic drugs, or of disturbances of color vision when taking a cardiac glycoside. These symptoms are usually reversible with changes in drug dosage or upon withdrawal of the drug. Because it is not possible to predict when ophthalmic complications will occur, initial and follow-up exams should be performed.

The mechanisms by which drugs produce sexual dysfunction are poorly understood. The effects are usually drug specific but include decreased libido, erectile dysfunction, and impaired ejaculation. Drug categories that significantly interfere with sexual function include antihypertensives such as calcium channel blockers (e.g., diltiazem), psychoactive drugs such as fluoxetine, and dopaminergic drugs such as levodopa.

Toxic Effects

Toxic effects are associated with excessive drug levels in a given patient. In some cases, the effects are characterized by exaggeration of the usual pharmacologic effects. If drug concentration does not exceed a critical level, the effects are usually reversible. The risk of a toxic response is inversely related to the TI of the drug. For example, toxicity with water-soluble vitamins is rarely seen. However, when drugs such as digoxin or insulin—each has a narrow TI—are administered, therapy must be closely monitored and carefully managed to avoid toxicity. Many drugs are not toxic in and of themselves, but are activated into toxic metabolites through biotransformation. The toxic response then depends on the rate at which the toxic metabolite is produced and destroyed.

Most systemic toxic drugs predominantly affect few organs. The target organ of toxicity is not necessarily the site of drug accumulation. Adverse effects require varying amounts of time to develop. They can therefore be classified as short-term or delayed. Short-term effects are those that occur immediately after drug exposure (e.g., apnea related to use of central nervous system [CNS] depressants), within a few days (e.g., GI bleeding), or after several weeks (e.g., nephrotoxicity). Toxic effects, on the other hand, may be delayed; that is, the manifestations of toxicity do not appear until months or years after the drug was administered.

Adverse effects can mimic many naturally occurring diseases, making diagnosis difficult. Awareness and identification of potential causative drugs and modification of therapy are of prime importance. Drugs capable of affecting tissues, structures, and organs within the body do so either directly or indirectly. The organs most often affected are the liver, kidneys, ears, eyes, and sexual organs. *Teratogenesis*—abnormal development of the human embryo that leads to birth defects—can occur with a variety drugs if they are taken during pregnancy. Because many drugs have been implicated in causing drowsiness, nausea, vomiting, or diarrhea, GI and CNS toxicities are not included in this discussion.

Because the liver is the first organ to receive a drug once it is absorbed from the intestine, that organ is prone to both parenchymal (functional liver cells) and bile duct injury. Persons with liver dysfunction are more prone to drug-induced hepatic injury and necrosis. Liver function tests are commonly performed before the initiation of therapy with drugs known to cause liver injury, and they are then performed periodically to monitor hepatic status.

The kidneys can be injured by drugs that are eliminated through the kidneys or that are carried in the blood and therefore flow through the kidneys. The kidneys are at risk because they have the greatest blood supply per gram of any tissue in the body, second only to the CNS. Drug-induced kidney diseases such as interstitial nephritis and toxic nephropathy can occur secondary to various antibiotics, analgesics such as salicylates and nonsteroidal anti-inflammatory drugs (see Chapter 15), biologic response modifiers (see Chapter 29), antineoplastics (see Chapter 30), and heavy metals. Patients receiving potentially nephrotoxic drugs should have baseline determinations of blood urea nitrogen (BUN) and creatinine levels before the start of therapy and periodically thereafter. Any drug suspected of causing renal damage should be discontinued.

Ototoxic drugs cause detrimental effects on the eighth cranial nerve—vestibular and auditory branches—and the structures of hearing. Ototoxic effects range from dizziness and balance difficulties to an annoying ringing in the ear (*tinnitus*) and total, irreversible deafness. Ototoxicity and nephrotoxicity often occur concurrently, because drugs not eliminated accumulate in body tissues. Aminoglycoside antibiotics (see Chapter 24) are known to be ototoxic and nephrotoxic. Kanamycin and neomycin affect the cochlear portion of the labyrinth, whereas the effects of gentamicin and streptomycin occur mainly at the vestibular portion.

Toxicology is concerned with the detection and analysis of pharmaceutical and environmental chemicals. As a division of medicine and biologic science, toxicology has grown in popularity as our communities receive long-term environmental exposure to low levels of various natural and synthetic chemicals. Toxicologists establish antidotes and treatments for toxicity and work toward the prevention and control of environmental and occupational exposure to toxic drugs.

Cumulative Effects

Cumulative effects result when the effects of one drug dose have not dissipated before the administration of another dose. Although they are somewhat unpredictable, cumulative effects develop when the rate of administration exceeds the rate of biotransformation or elimination. Cumulative effects occur most often with drugs whose biologic half-lives are measured in days, weeks, or months, unlike those whose half-lives are measured in hours (whose concentrations fall to ineffective levels long before the drugs disappear from the body). However, as the drug concentration rises (often owing to reduced elimination but continued dosing), toxic symptoms may appear. Cumulative toxicity can rapidly progress, as in the case of ethyl alcohol intoxication, or slowly, as with the slow and insidious poisoning with heavy metals.

Unpredictable Adverse Effects

There are two unpredictable, sensitivity-related adverse effects: idiosyncratic reactions and allergic reactions.

Idiosyncratic Reactions

The term idiosyncratic reaction is a catchall for side effects that are inadequately understood. The term idiosyncrasy is derived from the Greek works *idios,* meaning "one's own," "peculiar," or "distinct," and *synkrasis,* meaning "mixing together." As defined here, *idiosyncrasy* is a genetically determined, unusual or abnormal response to a drug. Idiosyncratic reactions affect a small portion of the total population and tend not to be dose related.

Idiosyncratic reactions result from (1) extreme sensitivity to a low dose of a drug, (2) extreme insensitivity to high doses of a drug, indicating an abnormal tolerance, or (3) unpredictable and unexplainable symptoms. Sometimes an idiosyncratic reaction takes on a *paradoxical* response, an effect opposite to that desired.

Pharmacogenetic Reactions

Variations in drug response can also result from genetic differences in drug disposition. *Pharmacogenetics* is the study of genetic differences in biotransformation. The importance of pharmacogenetics is twofold: the investigation and identification of the genetic basis for unusual drug responses, and the development of methods for predicting who will react abnormally to drugs. The practical value of pharmacogenetic studies lies in their predictive ability, enabling potentially injurious responses to be avoided.

Genetic differences are inherited much like inborn errors of metabolism, but with two major differences. Patients with pharmacogenetic disorders lead normal lives and do not have difficulty unless they are challenged with a drug producing an aberrant response. Further, a nutrient or its metabolite is not involved. Rather, the problem substrate is the drug. Pharmacogenetic differences result in either increased or decreased response intensity to a drug with a longer or shorter duration of action.

Genetic changes in enzyme activity and biotransformation are major mechanisms encountered in pharmacogenetics. For example, about 10 percent of black males have a decreased production of erythrocytic glucose-6-phosphate dehydrogenase (G6PD). The lack of G6PD leads to the development of serious hemolytic anemia if the patient receives the antimalarial preparation primaquine phosphate. Further, it has been estimated that a G6PD variant is present in approximately 200 million persons worldwide.

Other persons may not hydrolyze a standard dose of succinylcholine, a skeletal muscle relaxant used during general anesthesia. The result is prolonged muscle relaxation and ensuing apnea. In these persons, atypical plasma cholinesterase is present. An abnormally long duration of action results from a reduced affinity of the aberrant enzyme for succinylcholine. This genetic difference has a worldwide distribution but is rare to undetectable among blacks, Filipinos, Eskimos, and the Japanese.

Malignant hyperthermia has developed in some persons receiving a general anesthetic such as halothane (Chapter 16). The disorder is associated with high fever and skeletal muscle rigidity. Affected patients can be tested for creatine phosphokinase, an enzyme found in high concentrations in the heart and skeletal muscles, and in much smaller concentrations in brain tissue. Isoenzyme studies help distinguish whether the creatine phosphokinase originated from the heart (isoenzyme MB) or the skeletal muscle (isoenzyme MM). The information obtained from these studies assists in the diagnosis and treatment of cardiac and skeletal muscle disorders.

Allergic Reactions

Allergic reactions are difficult both to predict and to prevent. A careful and complete drug history helps avoid allergic reactions caused by a drug to which a patient has reported a prior allergy. Although allergies generally can occur with any route of administration, the oral route is less likely to result in sensitization. Topical drug application presents the greatest risk. Some drug classifications are more likely to cause drug reactions than others, but there is no known way to estimate the allergic potential of any drug. As with most undesirable responses to drug therapy, the health care provider is well advised to limit the number of drugs prescribed.

All allergic drug reactions are the result of an immune system response. Contrary to popular belief, allergic reactions do not occur with the first exposure to an antigen. An allergic reaction is manifest only after a second or subsequent exposure, and then as a reaction different from the usual pharmacologic response. Because drugs are ordinarily not proteins, they do not, in and of themselves, act as antigens. However, following biotransformation, drugs or their metabolites can combine with endogenous proteins to form reactive compounds. Undesirable immunologic responses are often called "drug allergies." The broad term includes genetic variations and toxic effects of drugs that result from idiosyncratic reactions. Documented allergic reactions account for as few as 10 percent of all adverse effects of drugs.

Hypersensitivity is commonly used to describe an allergic reaction when a drug acts as the antigen. However, there is a lack of precision in defining hypersensitivity as an entity dis-

TABLE 5–2 CLASSIFICATION OF ALLERGIC REACTIONS*

Type	Synonyms	Antibody	Effector Cells	Mechanism	Example
I	Anaphylaxis	IgE	Mast cells	Antigen binds with basophils on surface of mast cells and basophils with release of histamine, leukotrienes, serotonin, and prostaglandins	Penicillin, pollens, insect bites, household cleaning agents
II	Cytotoxic	IgG, IgM	Polymorpho-nuclear leukocytes	Antigen binds to allergen on cell membranes; complement system activated with cell destruction	Penicillin, methyldopa, sulfonamides, hydralazine, procainamide, quinidine
III	Immune complex–mediated response	IgG, IgM	Polymorpho–nuclear leukocytes	Antigen binds to allergen in fluid phase and deposits in small blood vessels; complement system is activated with cell destruction	Penicillin, phenytoin, streptomycin, iodides, sulfonamides
IV	Cell-mediated response	Not involved	Not involved	Sensitized cells bind to allergen and release lymphokines	Tuberculosis skin tests, rabies vaccination, poison ivy, phenol, benzene products, halothane

* Type I, II, and III allergic responses are immediately produced. Type IV has a delayed rate of development.
Adapted with permission from McCance, K., and Huether, S. (1997). *Pathophysiology: The biologic basis for disease in adults and children* (3rd ed., p. 240). St. Louis: C.V. Mosby.

tinctly different from other unpredictable responses. Thus, it is generally wise to avoid using the term.

On the basis of the immunologic mechanism in operation, drug allergies may be classified as anaphylactoid or atopic reactions (Type I), cytotoxic reactions (Type II), autoimmune reactions (Type III), and cell-mediated hypersensitivities (Type IV) (Table 5–2).

Anaphylactoid Reactions

Immediate *anaphylactoid reactions* (Type I) are acute, life-threatening events. They are mediated through immunoglobulin (Ig) E antibodies produced by drugs binding to the surface of mast cells and basophils. The reaction results in a cross-linking of antibodies with subsequent degranulation and the release of chemical mediators. The released mediators—histamine, leukotrienes, serotonin, and prostaglandins—trigger a rapid immune response (usually within 5 to 20 minutes after exposure). Signs and symptoms of a Type I reaction include apprehension, itching of the palms, chin, or throat, tearing, laryngeal edema, wheezing, and dyspnea. When it is severe, the reaction progresses to shock, hypotension, and cardiovascular collapse. Anaphylaxis can occur with all routes of administration but is most often seen following use of parenteral formulations.

Type I reactions are also activated by environmental pollens, foods, insect bites, and certain household cleaning products. Penicillin is a particularly offensive drug. Treatment of a penicillin reaction usually requires the administration of subcutaneous epinephrine, intravenous or intramuscular diphenhydramine, and intravenous corticosteroids. Adequate fluid volume replacement precedes the administration of vasopressors used for the profound and persistent hypotension of shock.

Cytotoxic Responses

Cytotoxic or *autoimmune reactions* (Type II) involve drug-protein complexes that adhere to the surfaces of red or white blood cells or platelets and evoke an antibody response. Circulating IgG and IgM antibodies then activate complement, a series of enzymatic proteins present in normal serum. The result is cytolysis and cell death.

Cytotoxic responses can become apparent in a few minutes or a few days. The primary target is the circulatory system. Manifestations of cytotoxic responses include a penicillin-induced hemolytic anemia, methyldopa-induced autoimmune hemolytic anemia, sulfonamide-induced granulocytopenia, hydralazine-induced or procainamide-induced systemic lupus erythematosus, and quinidine-induced thrombocytopenia purpura. In most cases, the reactions subside a few months after the drug is discontinued.

Immune Complex–Mediated Reactions

Immune complex–mediated reactions (Type III) involve circulating antigen-antibody complexes with increased amounts of IgG. The antigen-antibody complexes are deposited in vascular endothelium, and a destructive inflammatory response takes place locally. The best known immune-complex mediated reaction is serum sickness, seen after exposure to penicillin, phenytoin, streptomycin, iodides, and sulfonamides. The signs and symptoms of serum sickness are urticarial skin eruptions, arthritis or arthralgia, lymphadenopathy, and fever. The symptoms usually resolve after the drug is discontinued. However, Stevens-Johnson syndrome is a severe form of sulfonamide-induced vasculitis. It manifests as erythema multiforme, arthritis, nephritis, CNS abnormalities, and myocarditis.

Cell-Mediated Responses

Cell-mediated responses (Type IV) are the result of interactions between T lymphocytes (T cells), macrophages, and neutrophils rather than antibodies. The T-cell/antigen complex most often combines with skin proteins, evoking an immune response. The sensitized T-cells release macrophage migration–inhibiting factor, macrophage-activating factor, chemotactic factors, and other substances that attract macrophages and neutrophils to the area. Infiltration by these substances contributes to a local inflammatory response. Examples of cell-mediated allergic responses are the reactions to tuberculin skin tests or rabies vaccination, contact dermatitis caused by poison ivy, and reaction to exposure to phenol and benzene products. Halothane-induced hepatitis is another example of a cell-mediated response.

Tolerance

Tolerance is a state of decreased drug responsiveness. It is acquired with repeated exposure to a drug. Tolerance develops to many drugs, especially opioids, various other CNS depressants, and organic nitrates. It can develop not only to the drug in use but also to drugs that are closely related to it in pharmacologic activity, particularly those acting at the same receptor sites. The level of tolerance varies from person to person, but drug dosage must be increased in order to maintain a given therapeutic effect. Tolerance usually disappears when the drug that produced the phenomenon is discontinued.

The mechanisms involved in the development of tolerance are only partially understood. It is thought that tolerance develops as the result of (1) a reduction in absorption, (2) a reduction in the rate of drug transfer across biologic membranes, (3) a drug-induced synthesis of hepatic microsomal enzymes, or (4) increased elimination. Because tolerance does not usually develop to all effects of a drug, the TI of the drug may decrease.

A drug-disposition (pharmacokinetic) tolerance is created by drugs such as phenobarbital, glutethimide, and meprobamate. These drugs increase their own rate of biotransformation by stimulating the hepatic microsomal enzyme system. Pharmacodynamic tolerance involves multiple mechanisms. It is often a slowly developing phenomenon rather than an acute tolerance. Pharmacodynamic tolerance occurs with drugs that act on the CNS to produce changes in mood or behavior. In general terms, this type of tolerance is related to a modification of target receptor sites within the brain. Thus, receptors are rendered insensitive to the action of the drugs.

Tolerance generally results from prolonged and repeated administration of a drug. Tolerance may also occur, however, after only one or two doses. In such a case, the term *tachyphylaxis* is used. Tachyphylaxis occurs quickly. Even with larger doses of the drug, the patient's initial response to the drug cannot be reproduced. Tachyphylaxis may occur as a result of a change in the sensitivity of the target cells.

Drug Dependence

The World Health Organization has suggested the use of the term *drug dependence* rather than *addiction* or *habituation.* The terms are synonymous, however. The reason for using the general term drug dependence is to avoid the connotations of serious harm to the drug user and to society and of the interventions needed to solve the problems associated with drug abuse (see Chapter 10).

Drug dependence has two distinct and interdependent components: physiologic and psychological. Psychological dependence is characterized by an emotional drive to continue taking a drug in order to maintain an optimal sense of well-being. Manifestations of psychological dependence range from a mild desire for the drug to craving and compulsive use. Craving and compulsivity represent a major problem to the drug abuser, because they suggest a loss of control over the drug and its effects.

Physical dependence describes an alteration in physiologic state produced by the repeated administration of a drug. The body adapts to the drug's effects until it can function only in the presence of the drug. Physical dependence and its concomitant changes in health status do not result from excessive use of all drugs but depend on each drug's properties. *Abstinence syndrome* is an intense physiologic disturbance that occurs when a drug is no longer available to the body. For drugs such as alcohol, barbiturates, and opioid analgesics, the physiologic effects of withdrawal are so unpleasant and threatening that they become important factors in continued use of the drug and in motivating drug-seeking behaviors.

DRUG INTERACTIONS

As pharmacotherapeutics become more complex and drugs more potent, beneficial as well as detrimental drug-drug interactions may occur. It has been estimated that the average patient receives as many as 6 to 10 different drugs during a hospital stay. Further, many outpatients are taking six to eight drugs on a somewhat regular basis. Geriatric patients may be taking as many as 15 to 20 drugs concurrently. These practices present many opportunities for drug-drug interactions to occur. Therefore, for the ultimate benefit of the patient, the health care provider must have a working knowledge of potential drug-drug interactions and must share that knowledge and experience.

Drug-drug interaction refers to a change in the magnitude or duration of a response to one drug in the presence of another drug. Interactions can be related to the pharmacokinetic or pharmacodynamic characteristics of the interacting drugs. Several mechanisms are involved with drug-drug interactions (see Mechanisms of Drug Interactions). The result is an increase or decrease in the concentration of the drug at the site of action. The most commonly encountered mechanisms involve displacement of the drug from plasma proteins, a very rapid or very slow biotransformation, and poor absorption from the GI tract. Interactions that increase therapeutic or adverse effects of drugs include additive effects, synergistic (e.g., potentiation) effects, interference, and displacement. Interactions in which decreased drug effects re-

MECHANISMS OF DRUG INTERACTIONS

- Acceleration or inhibition of drug biotransformation*
- Displacement of plasma protein–bound drug*
- Impaired uptake of drug from the gastrointestinal tract*
- Altered renal clearance of drug
- Modifications in receptors or blockade of receptor channels
- Changes in electrolyte balance or body fluid pH
- Changes in the rate of protein synthesis

* Most commonly encountered mechanisms by which drug interactions occur.

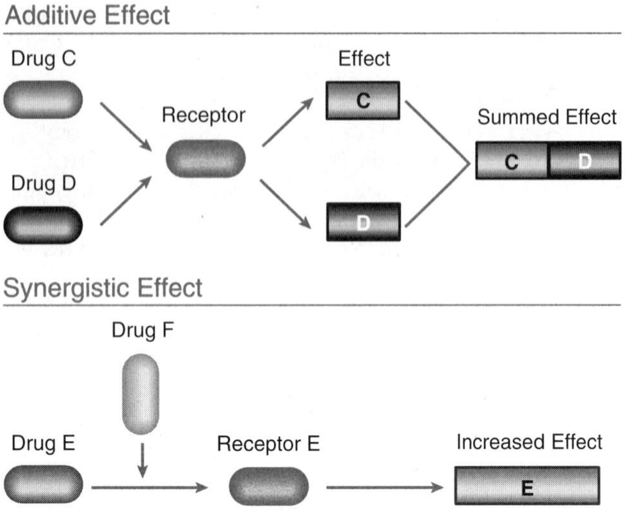

Additive Effect

Drug C

Receptor

Effect

C

Summed Effect

C D

Drug D

D

Synergistic Effect

Drug F

Drug E

Receptor E

Increased Effect

E

Figure 5–5 Additive and synergistic effects. *Additive effects* occur when two drugs with similar pharmacologic actions are taken. In some cases, combining two drugs at lower dosages produces increased therapeutic effects with a resultant decrease in adverse reactions. *Synergistic effects* are produced when two drugs whose combined effects are greater than the sum of each individual drug acting alone. The term is usually reserved for situations in which the two drugs act at different sites or have different mechanisms of action.

sult are generally grouped under the category *antagonism*. Antagonistic effects may be physiologic, biochemical, or chemical in nature.

Additive Effects

Additive effects occur when two drugs with similar pharmacologic actions are taken (Fig. 5–5). In some cases, combining two drugs at lower dosages produces increased therapeutic effects with a resultant decrease in adverse reactions.

Synergism

Synergism describes the results of two drugs whose combined effects are greater than the sum of each drug acting alone (see Fig. 5–5). The term is usually reserved for situations in which the two drugs act at different sites or have different mechanisms of action. One of the drugs, the synergist, increases the effect of the second drug by altering its absorption, biotransformation, distribution, or elimination. Thus, the intensity of effects is increased or the duration of action prolonged. An example of a common synergistic effect is that produced when penicillin is given concurrently with probenecid. Each drug alone produces its own effect. However, the combination provides penicillin with a longer duration of action than it would alone, because probenecid inhibits the elimination of penicillin.

Potentiation

Potentiation occurs when one drug increases the effect of a second drug. The term is often used interchangeably (although not necessarily accurately) with synergism. With potentiation, the first drug may be devoid of an observable effect when given alone but produces a measurable response when combined with a second drug.

For example, tyramine is an intermediate product in the conversion of tyrosine, an amino acid, to epinephrine and norepinephrine. In and of itself, tyramine has no pharmacologic effects. However, tyramine is commonly found in a variety of foods and is particularly plentiful in cheese (see Appendix D). Patients taking monoamine oxidase inhibitor drugs are unable to metabolize ingested tyramine. Thus, an ordinarily harmless food is turned into a toxic substance. A sharp rise in blood pressure and, in a few cases, cerebral hemorrhage, has occurred. This response is sometimes referred to as the "cheese response."

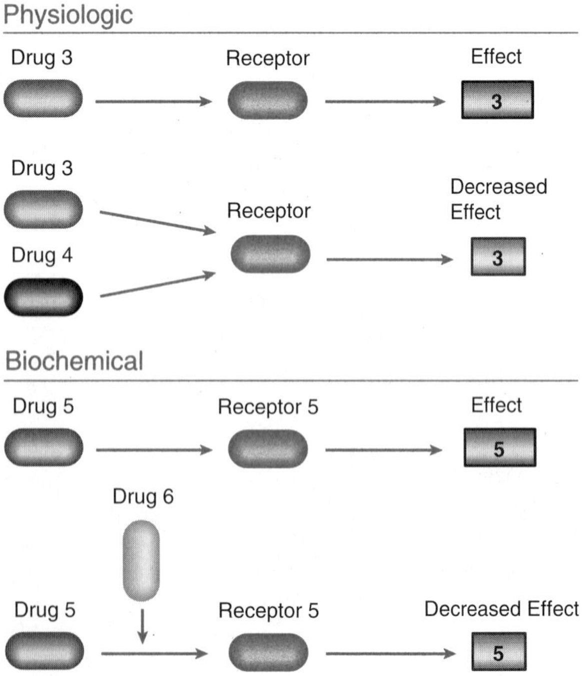

Physiologic

Drug 3

Receptor

Effect

3

Drug 3

Receptor

Decreased Effect

Drug 4

3

Biochemical

Drug 5

Receptor 5

Effect

5

Drug 6

Drug 5

Receptor 5

Decreased Effect

5

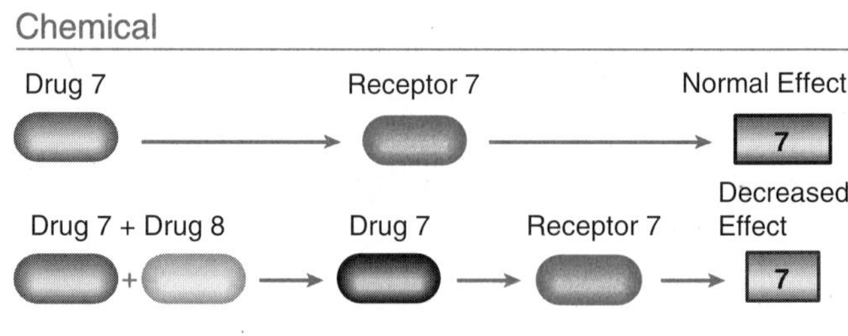

Figure 5–6 Physiologic, chemical, and biochemical antagonism. Antagonism occurs any time the effect of two drugs is less than the sum of the effects of the drugs acting separately. Drug antagonism causes a diminished therapeutic effect. With functional or *physiologic antagonism,* two agonists acting at different sites counterbalance each other by producing opposite effects on the same physiologic function. *Chemical antagonism* occurs when an agonist and an antagonist combine to form an inactive product. *Biochemical antagonism* is the opposite of synergism. It occurs whenever one drug indirectly decreases the amount of a second drug available at its site of action.

Antagonism

Antagonism occurs any time the effect of two drugs is less than the sum of the effects of the drugs acting separately (Fig. 5–6). In general, drug antagonism causes a diminished therapeutic effect.

With functional or *physiologic antagonism,* two agonists acting at different sites counterbalance each other by producing opposite effects on the same physiologic function. For example, the effects of histamine on the respiratory tract can be offset by epinephrine.

Chemical antagonism occurs when an agonist and an antagonist combine to form an inactive product. The effect of heparin on antithrombin II, prothrombin, and fibrinogen is reduced in the presence of protein protamine sulfate.

Biochemical antagonism is the opposite of synergism. It occurs whenever one drug indirectly decreases the amount of a second drug available at its site of action. For example, diphenhydramine prevents histamine from exerting effects without pharmacokinetic properties of the drug being affected.

VARIABLES AFFECTING DRUG ACTIONS, INTERACTIONS, AND REACTIONS

Numerous physiologic and environmental factors alter a patient's response to drugs and contribute to the possibility of adverse effects. Physiologic factors are age and body mass, gender, genetics, general state of health, maturity of body systems, biologic rhythms, and the developmental changes associated with pregnancy. Conditions related to drug administration and iatrogenic or exogenous factors also influence a patient's response to drugs.

Physiologic Factors

Age

Pharmacokinetic drug action in infants and elderly patients are different from those in the middle age group. Infants have a greater proportion of total body water than adults, resulting in expanded distribution and diminished blood levels of water-soluble drugs. Infants and young children also have a low percentage of body fat, thus contributing to increased blood levels of lipid-soluble drugs. A relative lack of gastric acid contributes to an exaggerated absorption of drugs that would normally be inactivated by gastric acid. An exaggerated absorption of drugs normally ionized at a low pH also occurs. Further, an infant's body system lacks the enzymes responsible for drug biotransformation. Most of the enzyme systems develop quickly, however, with levels reaching those of an adult 1 to 8 weeks after birth. By the first year of life, the enzyme systems are probably as active as they will ever be. Additionally, rapid dehydration caused by immature temperature regulation mechanisms can elevate serum drug levels. The renal elimination of drugs is also reduced in an infant as a result of decreased renal blood flow, and a greater volume of distribution. The breastfeeding infant can develop adverse reactions to drugs that pass from the mother into breast milk (see Chapter 6).

On the other end of the age spectrum, the elderly are prone to drug interactions as a result of the normal changes of aging and concomitant disease. Alterations in drug absorption, distribution, biotransformation, and elimination are common in the elderly. A high gastric pH decreases the absorption of drugs that are normally nonionized at a low pH. Proportional increases in body fat lead to less fat-soluble drug deposition. Reduced body water contributes to higher serum concentrations of water-soluble drugs. Lowered serum albumin levels result in increased amounts of unbound drug, leading to greater drug activity. Further, a reduction in cardiac output and renal blood flow affects the biotransformation and elimination of drugs. All of these changes result in higher drug concentration levels and a greater chance of toxicity.

Body Weight

Body weight is a significant determinant of drug effects. The magnitude of drug response is a function of drug concentration at the site of action. The concentration, in turn, is related to the volume of distribution (V_d) of the drug. As a general rule, a particular quantity of drug might be less effective in a heavier individual, provided that renal, hepatic, and cardiovascular functions are adequate. The average adult dose of a drug is calculated on the basis of the amount that will produce a particular effect in half of the population between the ages of 18 and 65 years who weigh approximately 154 pounds (70 kg). The dosage required to obtain a therapeutic effect is roughly proportional to body size. Any variation in effect is minimized when dosage is calculated using kilograms of body weight. The recommended dosages for many drugs are listed in terms of grams or milligrams per kilogram (g/kg or mg/kg) of body weight. Pediatric dosages are most often calculated on the basis of body weight.

Gender

Gender does not play a significant role in drug action. However, women generally require smaller doses of drugs than men to manifest the same magnitude of response, simply because of lower average weight. For women taking drugs that have a narrow TI, the differences in drug response may require a reduction in dosage. There can also be gender-related differences in drug response because of an unequal proportion of lean body mass to fat mass.

Genetics

An exaggerated response or lack of response to a drug can be the result of genetically determined susceptibility. Genetically determined drug responses require that the patient be closely assessed and monitored for abnormal susceptibility, especially at the start of therapy.

General State of Health

Almost all pharmacokinetic and pharmacodynamic principles have been formulated using data collected from healthy persons. Drugs, however, are administered to persons in whom a physiologic process is taking place at an abnormal level. The presence of disease contributes to variability in drug response, especially when organs responsible for the absorption, distribution, biotransformation, and elimination of drugs are affected. For example, drugs tend to accumulate in the presence of liver disease. As the liver ceases to function, the rate of biotransformation falls, and drug levels rise. Liver disease does not alter plasma levels of drugs that are primarily removed by renal or pulmonary elimination. As with liver disease, kidney disease interferes with the elimination of water-soluble drugs, causing the drugs to accumulate in the body. A decrease in dosage levels is required so that drug levels remain below toxic range.

Biologic Rhythms

Normal biologic rhythms influence drug action and can, in some cases, lead to adverse drug reactions. Circadian rhythms continue to operate even when external factors that influence behaviors, such as clocks and social and work routines, are removed. For example, cortisol levels normally rise between 8 and 10 AM, decline toward evening, and then rise again in the morning. Human growth hormone and prolactin secretions peak within the first 2 hours after sleep. Thyroid-stimulating hormone is also at maximum levels the first few hours after sleep begins. Thyroid-stimulating hormone levels ebb about 3 hours after awakening in the morning. Biologic rhythms must be considered in the interpretation of laboratory results related to drug and hormone levels.

Developmental Changes

Changes associated with pregnancy influence pharmacokinetics, pharmacodynamics, and patient response to drugs. Although the numerous physiologic changes that occur during pregnancy affect drug action, the pregnant patient is not necessarily at higher risk for adverse effects. Body water and plasma volume increase by as much as 50 percent in a normal pregnancy. Therefore, a drug dose is "diluted" compared with a nonpregnant state. As a result, dosage requirements may increase. This and other factors associated with drug therapy during pregnancy are discussed in depth in Chapter 6.

No woman of childbearing age should receive a drug before it is determined whether or not she is pregnant. A fundamental concept to remember when administering a drug to a pregnant patient is that the drug will be received by two persons, the mother and the fetus.

Psychosocial Factors

Psychosocial, cultural, religious, and personal belief systems influence patient drug regimens and can predispose a patient to adverse drug reactions. Even with our present-day knowledge of normal body functioning and the manner in which these functions are affected by disease, it is commonly difficult to separate the pharmacologic effects of drugs from their psychological effects. Certain symptoms of disease, such as headache, nausea, and even more serious signs, can be brought about by impulses that originate in the cerebral cortex.

Placebo effects are temporally correlated with administration and cannot be attributed to a drug's pharmacodynamic properties. Placebos are usually inert substances (e.g., lactose). The term placebo is derived from the Latin meaning "I shall please." An inactive substance is administered specifically for the purpose of satisfying an individual's need for drug dosing.

A positive health care provider–patient relationship influences the effectiveness of a placebo. The level of effectiveness is related to the patient's belief that the substance has desirable powers. Although the effects obtained from a placebo are determined by psychological factors rather than physiologic ones, the presence of a placebo response does not suggest that the patient's original problem was imaginary.

Several factors are known to influence both beneficial and adverse drug response. They are the patient's physical environment; bioavailability and drug additives; dosage; dietary considerations; compliance, noncompliance, and misuse; administration routes; and the number of drugs the patient is receiving. The concept referred to as "acquired resistance" is also a variable affecting drug action and effect.

Environment

Physical environment affects drug response. For example, environmental temperature affects the action and effects of nitrates and antihypertensives. These drugs, when used by an individual exposed to high temperatures, relax peripheral vessels to the extent that excessive vasodilation occurs. Pesticide exposure, smoking, and alcohol use alter the pharmacokinetics of certain drugs, thereby increasing the risk of adverse effects.

Bioavailability and Additives

Numerous brands of the same drug can vary in bioavailability because of differences in manufacturing. Variance in onset, peak concentration levels, and duration of action among the different drugs can lead to adverse effects. Therefore, caution must be used when substituting one brand of drug for another, or when changing from a brand name to a generic drug and vice versa.

Although they are relatively uncommon, adverse effects have occurred when a drug past its expiration date (an expired drug) is administered. Improper storage of drugs contributes to their degradation, rendering some more or less potent.

Drug additives such as buffers, stabilizing agents, or dyes can produce adverse responses in susceptible individuals. When adverse responses to an additive are numerous, the manufacturer may reformulate a drug to remove the offending additive.

Dosage and Number of Drugs Administered

The dosage a patient receives contributes to adverse effects. The probability of an adverse response increases for the patient who is on high doses for extended periods. For example, a patient on the antihypertensive drug hydralazine is more likely to develop drug-induced systemic lupus erythematosus with orally administered dosages greater than 200 mg/day and during therapy lasting longer than 6 months.

The dose administered, the formulation, and the route and frequency of administration all modify drug effects. However, the risk of adverse effects increases in direct proportion to the number of drugs the patient takes. These factors all have one thing in common: The effects produced depend on the previous administration of the same or a different drug.

The repeated administration of a single drug may create a state referred to as *acquired resistance.* Acquired resistance is most often associated with antimicrobial or antineoplastic drugs. It describes a state of decreased, or complete lack of, responsiveness to a particular drug. When the antimicrobial activity of a drug is first tested, a pattern of sensitivity and resistance is usually defined. Unfortunately, the spectrum of activity may subsequently change to a surprising degree. The spectrum changes because pathogens develop a variety of mechanisms that allow them to survive in the presence of antimicrobial drugs.

When a susceptible pathogen is exposed for the first time to an antimicrobial drug, the effect produced is anticipated: retarded growth rate or a reduction in the numbers of pathogens, or both. The susceptible organism is thus referred to as *sensitive* to the antimicrobial drug. However, as therapy continues, the growth of pathogens also continues, and resistant strains of organisms increase in number. When plasma and tissue concentrations of the drug rise above the accepted therapeutic range with no therapeutic response, the microorganism is considered to be *resistant* to the drug. Persistent subtherapeutic dosage levels increase the likelihood of resistance among pathogenic organisms.

The mechanism of drug resistance varies from organism to organism and from drug to drug. Although mutation is commonly the cause of acquired resistance, resistance to antimicrobial drugs may be acquired by transfer of genetic material from one organism to another. This occurs through the processes of transduction (transfer of a genetic fragment from one organism to another), transformation (exchange of genetic material between strains of bacteria), or conjugation (a form of sexual reproduction in which genetic material is transferred between organisms).

Dietary Considerations

The presence of food in the stomach impairs the absorption of certain drugs. For example, when antacids are taken concurrently with iron preparations, the antacid binds the iron, making it unavailable for absorption by the GI tract. Green leafy vegetables are high in vitamin K. Their excessive intake decreases the effectiveness of oral anticoagulants such as warfarin. Cabbage, broccoli, charcoal-broiled meats, and products containing caffeine stimulate liver enzymes, thereby increasing the rate of drug biotransformation. As previously discussed, a hypertensive crisis can be precipitated when monoamine oxidase–inhibiting drugs and tyramine-containing foods are consumed at the same time.

Compliance, Noncompliance, and Misuse

Compliance (some prefer the term adherence) is defined as the extent to which a prescribed care plan is followed. Drugs are not always taken or administered as prescribed. Doses may be omitted, extra doses taken, or the drug taken at a wrong time. Patients receiving higher than normal dosages for extended periods are at increased risk for adverse effects. On the other hand, in patients receiving less than the dose prescribed, serum drug levels may remain at or below minimal effective concentrations, and therapeutic drug levels are never reached.

Failure of the prescribed drug regimen is often a result of *noncompliance* with (or nonadherence to)• the prescribed plan of care. It should be noted, however, that noncompliance is a term generated by health care providers. It defines the problem only from the health care provider's viewpoint.

Drug misuse is a related consideration. *Misuse,* the administration of a drug for the wrong purpose, is often the result of inaccurate self-diagnosis. In addition, the administration of a drug in situations in which contraindications are misunderstood or not recognized contributes to drug misuse. The administration of drugs by more than one person, each unaware of the other's actions, and administration of excessive doses based on the false impression that "if a little is good, more is better" are of concern. Patients at greatest risk for adverse reactions related to compliance or misuse behaviors are those taking drugs with narrow TIs, those taking drugs for which the precise timing of the dosage is important, and those in whom underlying medical conditions are likely to be aggravated by a particular drug.

Noncompliance and misuse commonly generate referrals to community health agencies. Noncompliance with a prescribed drug regimen (or misuse) is viewed as deviant behavior by health care providers. In reality, the patient may not be aware of the proper dose and regimen or may have chosen not to take the drug as prescribed for a variety of reasons. One reason for noncompliance is a belief that the drug is no longer needed; this is common with antimicrobial drugs. A patient feels better after 3 to 4 days of therapy and stops taking the drug. The offending organism remains in the body to produce additional signs and symptoms later, perhaps in a newly resistant form. Fears about the drug's adverse effects and of addiction are also possible causes of premature discontinuation of therapy.

Suggestions for improving compliance with the drug regimen include establishing a collaborative relationship with the patient and other members of the health care team. A working relationship helps simplify drug regimens. Understanding of the regimen is fostered by effective patient teaching. Manufacturers can assist with compliance issues by reducing costs and generating more once-a-day drugs. The health care provider's advocacy role assumes increasing importance in light of the growing numbers of drugs on the market. Contact with interdisciplinary care teams and the advisory role of pharmacists become vital. Further discussions of compliance are found in Chapters 2 and 9.

Administration Routes and Techniques

Drugs are manufactured with specific routes of administration in mind. Administration by routes other than those recommended can cause adverse reactions. Even use of the recommended routes of drug administration can cause adverse reactions at times. A parenterally administered drug does not have to be absorbed through the GI tract before entering systemic circulation. For this reason, drugs administered by this route, especially those given intravenously, reach receptor sites quickly and are more likely to cause adverse responses. Administering an intravenous drug too rapidly may cause an adverse response, because the speed with which a drug is given alters its rate of distribution. Similarly, a drug designed to treat ear problems will cause pain and irritation if administered in the eye. The pain and irritation occur because the buffer system and the pH of the solution differ from those of ophthalmic drugs.

SUMMARY

- A fundamental principle of pharmacology states that the intensity of response elicited by a drug is a function of the dose administered.
- As the dosage of a drug is increased, the proportion of persons experiencing a particular, stated response is also increased.
- Drug action represents the interaction between the drug and the environment, and the interactions between drug and cellular components.
- A patient's response to drug action represents the effect.
- Drug action occurs at the cellular level; however, drug effects influence total body functioning.
- Receptors are specialized proteins, cell membranes, or enzymes to which drugs display a chemical or biophysical attraction. The stronger the affinity for the receptor, the longer the drug action.
- Drugs are agonists when they interact with a receptor to produce an effect of their own.
- Drugs are antagonists when they interact with a receptor to produce no response of their own. Instead, they impair the receptor's ability to combine with an effector molecule.
- An antagonist is said to be competitive when it combines reversibly with the same sites as the drug and can be displaced from those sites by an excess of the agonist.
- Noncompetitive inhibitor drug effects cannot be overcome by increasing the concentration of the agonist.
- The dose-time-effect curve represents the relationship between drug dose, the time or times administered, and the effect observed in the patient.
- Therapeutic index, selectivity, and margin of safety all refer to the relationship between a drug's therapeutic and adverse effects.
- Drug idiosyncrasy, toxicity, and allergies are adverse effects considered unusual, in that they occur infrequently. The differences among them influence the subsequent use of a drug.
- Adverse drug reactions may be categorized as dose related or sensitivity related.
- Variables predisposing the patient to adverse reactions include physiologic and psychosocial factors as well as conditions of administration.
- Conditions of administration that affect drug action and effects are route, bioavailability of the drug and its additives, dietary considerations, and the compliance/noncompliance/misuse of a drug.
- Drug interaction refers to a change in the magnitude or duration of a response of one drug because of the presence of another drug.
- Interactions can be related to the pharmacokinetic or pharmacodynamic characteristics of the interacting drugs.
- Physiologic factors such as age, body mass, gender, genetics, general state of health, maturity of body systems, circadian rhythms, and developmental changes associated with pregnancy influence drug actions, interactions, and reactions.
- Conditions related to drug administration and iatrogenic or exogenous factors also influence a patient's response to drugs.
- Psychosocial, cultural, religious, and personal belief systems influence patient drug regimens and can predispose a patient to adverse drug reactions.
- Placebo effects are temporally related to drug administration rather than to a drug's pharmacodynamic properties.
- Factors influencing beneficial and adverse drug responses are the patient's environment, drug bioavailability, dosage, dietary considerations, compliance/noncompliance/misuse, administration route, and the number of drugs the patient is receiving.

BIBLIOGRAPHY

Benjamin, D. (1994). Recognizing and preventing adverse drug reactions. *Drug Therapy,* 24(6), 52.

Boston Collaborative Drug Surveillance Program. (1992). 25 years of the Boston Collaborative Drug Surveillance Program: A compilation of abstracts published by the BCDSP 1966–1991. *Hospital Pharmacy,* 27(4), Supp.

Davis, L. (1987). Timing is everything. *Hippocrates,* 2(4), 22–25.

DiPiro, J., Blouin, R., and Pruemer, J. (1991). *Concepts in clinical pharmacokinetics: A self-instructional course.* Bethesda, MD: American Society of Hospital System Pharmacists.

Gilman, A., Rall, T., Nies, A., et al. (1990). *Goodman and Gilman's the pharmacologic basis of therapeutics* (8th ed.). New York: Pergamon Press.

Levine, R. (1990). *Pharmacology: Drug actions and reactions* (4th ed.). Boston: Little, Brown and Company.

Pratt, W., Taylor, P. (Eds.) (1990). *Principles of drug action: The basis of pharmacology.* New York: Churchill Livingstone.

Rizack, M. (Ed.) (1996). *The medical letter handbook of adverse drug interactions.* New Rochelle, NY: The Medical Letter.

Shaikh, A. (1985). Application of pharmacokinetic principles in therapeutic drug monitoring. *Journal of Medical Technology,* 2(9), 583–587.

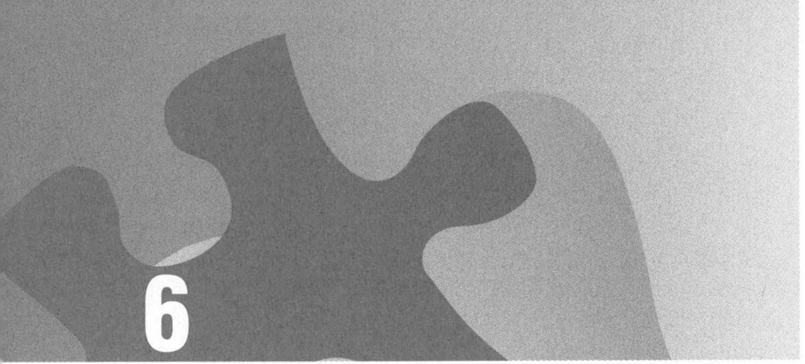

6

Perinatal Pharmacotherapeutics

The study of perinatal pharmacotherapeutics examines the complex interaction that exists between maternal physiologic changes, fetal development, and the placenta. In order to adequately grasp how pregnancy influences pharmacokinetics and pharmacodynamics, it is necessary to understand the physiologic changes that occur to both mother and fetus during its course. This chapter speaks to the physiologic changes of pregnancy that affect drugs administered during this developmental period.

ANATOMIC AND PHYSIOLOGIC VARIABLES

Pregnancy causes one of the most striking changes in physiology of any normal condition that appears in humans. From the moment conception occurs, changes begin in a woman's body (Fig. 6–1). The changes are related to several factors: hormonal influences, growth of the fetus inside the uterus, and the mother's physical adaptation to the changes that are occurring.

Reproductive System

The most obvious changes associated with pregnancy are those that occur in the reproductive system. The pear-shaped uterus normally weighs about 60 g, but it hypertrophies during pregnancy to become an organ weighing approximately 1000 g. To support the growing fetus, the blood flow increases dramatically from 30 to 40 mL/min to 500 mL/min. Uterine vascular resistance decreases, and blood flow to the uterus and placenta is maximized.

Fluid Balance

Pregnancy is characterized by water retention and an increase in extracellular volume. Total body water increases by 7 to 9 liters in the absence of edema. Extracellular fluid volume gain is 4 to 6 liters, including an increase in plasma volume of about 1200 mL. Sodium excretion during pregnancy is analogous to that of nonpregnant women, indicating that the body senses the "physiologic hypervolemia." Pregnancies failing to achieve the expanded plasma volume correlate with poor pregnancy outcomes.

A rise in plasma volume occurs despite reductions in plasma osmolarity and colloid osmotic pressure. Colloidal osmotic pressure drops during pregnancy because of decreased concentration of plasma proteins. Plasma osmolarity decreases 8 to 10 mOsm/kg below nonpregnant values as early as 10 weeks of gestation. This decrease is explained by the concomitant fall in plasma sodium and other associated anions. The fall in osmolarity from nonpregnant values to normal pregnancy levels can be equated to the drop in osmolarity that occurs in a nonpregnant person who quickly drinks a liter of water. The pregnant woman does not respond to the change in osmolarity by water diuresis, suggesting a resetting of the osmoreceptor system to a lower level. This theory is supported by the fact that plasma tonicity, urinary osmolality, and vasopressin levels normally increase after water deprivation and decrease after fluid loading. The osmotic threshold for thirst is also lower.

The normal kidney has an amazing ability to control water and electrolyte balance. Sodium is the major solute in the body's biochemical composition. Given the increase in extracellular fluid during pregnancy, it is not surprising that a considerable amount of sodium must be retained. Approximately 950 milliequivalents (mEq) of sodium is distributed between the products of conception and maternal extracellular fluid. The filtered load of sodium rises owing to the increase in glomerular filtration rate (GFR). This change must be accompanied by an increase in tubular reabsorption to prevent severe maternal sodium depletion. Serum sodium values drop from a nonpregnant value of approximately 139 mEq/L to around 136 mEq/L in pregnancy, in spite of the reabsorption efficiency of the tubules. Although their exact role in sodium conservation is unknown, increases in renin, aldosterone, deoxycorticosterone, human placental lactogen, and estrogen seem to enhance sodium levels.

Renin is a highly specific enzyme produced by the kidneys and found in the circulation. In nonpregnant women, renin acts on angiotensinogen, which is formed in the liver, to produce angiotensin I and subsequently angiotensin II, a powerful vasoconstrictor. Renin levels are elevated in some forms of hypertension. During a normal pregnancy, the circulating level of renin progressively increases until term, becoming five to 10 times greater than in the nonpregnant woman.

Angiotensinogen, a serum globulin fraction formed in the liver and converted to angiotensin, also increases from the mean nonpregnant value. The elevated levels of renin and angiotensinogen combine to form higher amounts of angiotensin I and II, but the vasoconstriction and associated rise in blood pressure that would be expected in the nonpregnant woman do not occur. Greater resistance to the pressor effects of angiotensin has been explained in several ways: elevated circulating levels of prostaglandins (which are vasodilatory), an increase in the level of the specific enzyme angiotensinase, and/or a decrease in smooth muscle responsiveness (due to activation of the renal kallikrein-kinin system).

Normally, increased levels of angiotensin II inhibit renin production, but in pregnancy, the levels of both angiotensin II and renin remain high. The normal physiologic stimuli that produce a renin response in the nonpregnant woman—for example, changes in posture or sodium restriction—also produce a response in the pregnant woman. The reduced vascular response seems to be specific to angiotensin II, since the response to exogenous norepinephrine remains unaltered.

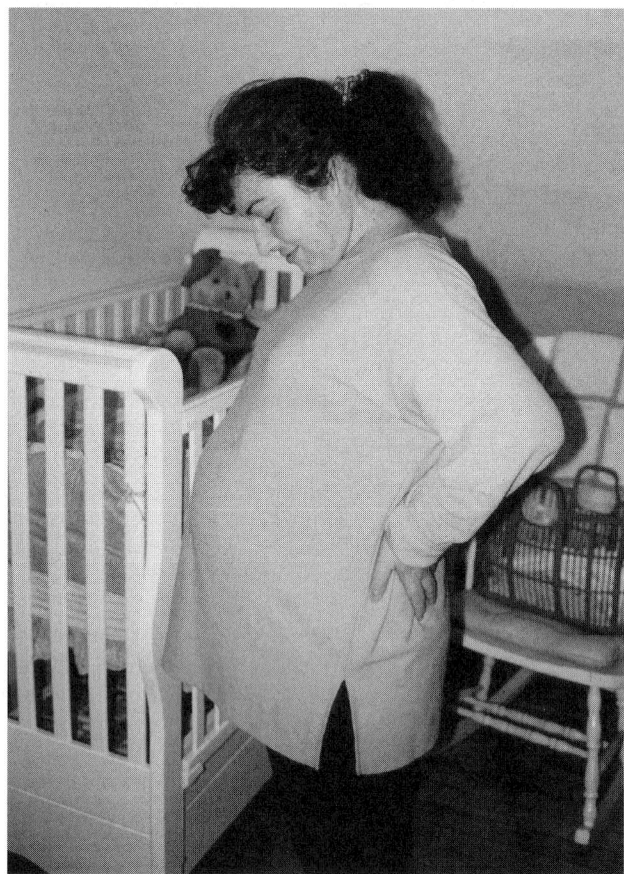

Figure 6–1 Changes during pregnancy that influence pharmacotherapy:
- Total body water increases by 40 to 50 percent at 6 weeks' gestation
- Cardiac output increases by 40 percent at 10 weeks' gestation
- Decreased peripheral vascular resistance
- Increased CO_2 gradient between mother and fetus, enabling the fetus to off-load its CO_2 to the maternal circulation
- High levels of progesterone result in decreased gastric emptying time
- Gastric acid secretion is decreased in the first and second trimesters then increases in third trimester
- Increased percentage of body fat and weight
- Gallbladder capacity expands, while emptying time slows
- Increased absorption of nutrients needed by the developing fetus
- Prolonged intestinal transit times
- Dilutional decrease in serum albumin levels
- Progesterone stimulates hepatic enzyme system
- Renal blood flow and glomerular filtration rate increased in early pregnancy decreasing in late pregnancy
- Circulating levels of renin progressively increase until term, becoming 5 to 10 times greater than in the nonpregnant woman
- Aldosterone levels significantly increase by about 15 weeks' gestation

(Courtesy of Dave Murcar.)

Gastrointestinal System

The most fundamental change in the gastrointestinal tract during pregnancy is the increased absorption of nutrients needed by the developing fetus. In the absence of morning sickness, most women experience an increase in their appetite that persists throughout pregnancy. Nausea and vomiting complicates 70 percent of all pregnancies. Typically, it begins at 4 to 6 weeks of gestation and continues until about 14 to 16 weeks. The cause is not well understood but has been associated with elevated levels of steroid hormones and human chorionic gonadotropin. There may also be a connection with higher levels of progesterone and the relaxation of smooth muscle of the stomach. Later in pregnancy, reflux esophagitis (heartburn) may also cause a reduction in appetite.

Gastric motility and tone are decreased during pregnancy, resulting in delayed gastric emptying. The delayed emptying prolongs the absorption phase and lowers peak drug concentrations. The decreased tone and motility are due to smooth muscle relaxation effects of progesterone. Gastric acid secretion is decreased in the first and second trimester but increases over nonpregnant levels in the third trimester. Decreased gastric acidity is thought to result from high levels of placental histaminase and other hormonal influences, especially estrogen.

Reduced gastrointestinal tone also leads to prolonged intestinal transit time, especially during the second and third trimesters. In addition, the height of intestinal villi increases, augmenting the absorption of calcium, glucose, sodium, chloride, amino acids, and water. Because of progesterone's influence on enzymatic transport mechanisms, absorption of niacin, riboflavin, and vitamin B_6 is decreased. Iron absorption rises in late pregnancy, possibly because of the depleted iron stores as pregnancy advances.

Progesterone's effect on smooth muscle relaxation is carried over to produce changes in the gallbladder. Gallbladder capacity is expanded but emptying time lengthens. Alterations in gallbladder tone lead to a tendency to retain bile salts and form gallstones, which may cause pruritus during pregnancy.

Drug absorption from the gastrointestinal tract is thought to be relatively unchanged in pregnancy. Slow gastric emptying and prolonged intestinal transit time probably have little effect on drugs. The decreased gastric tone and motility may enhance absorption of lipid-soluble drugs. In addition, the pH changes associated with heartburn and morning sickness, or the treatment of these symptoms with antacids, affects absorption of some orally administered drugs.

Several changes occur in the liver during pregnancy. Despite a 30 to 50 percent rise in cardiac output during pregnancy, liver size and hepatic blood flow do not change significantly. Proportionate to the increased cardiac output, the amount of blood arriving at the liver is decreased by about 28 to 35 percent. Estrogen enhances production of alpha- and beta-globulins, and liver production of albumin and total serum protein levels are reduced by 20 percent. In addition, the liver has greater fat and glycogen storage.

Adding to the lower concentration of serum albumin is the expansion of intravascular volume. These factors combine to create a progressive fall in serum albumin levels throughout pregnancy. At term, serum albumin levels are approximately 30 percent lower than nonpregnant values. The lowered concentration of serum albumin allows more free (unbound) drug to be available for placental transfer, with the transfer occurring at lower serum drug concentrations. Albumin binding capacity is also decreased, mainly because of competition with endogenous factors such as free fatty acids.

The liver is the primary site for drug biotransformation. The cytochrome P_{450} system is responsible for deactivation and detoxification of drugs. During pregnancy, biotransformation of drugs in the liver is influenced by elevated amounts of steroid hormones. The responsiveness of the hepatic microsomal enzyme system to induction or inhibition by certain drugs is not altered by pregnancy. Progesterone may be responsible for greater enzyme activity in the liver, leading to a measurable increase in liver clearance and the shortened half-life of a drug.

Cardiovascular System

When a woman becomes pregnant, her cardiovascular system has to adjust to meet not only physiologic demands but also the demands of her dynamically changing fetus. The mother's cardiovascular system supplies energy and growth substrates for the fetus while carrying away waste products and excess heat. To meet fetal requirements without unduly compromising maternal well-being, the system makes remarkable adjustments.

During pregnancy, the heart enlarges about 12 percent. The myocardium undergoes some hypertrophy, and the capacity of the heart for blood increases by about 10 percent. Electrocardiographic changes occur because of a positional shift in the heart but are usually of no clinical significance. The changes include transient ST segment and T wave changes and a left axis shift of the QRS complex. Heart rate progressively increases during pregnancy, averaging 15 to 20 beats per minute higher than in the nonpregnant state. The heart rate has the ability to fluctuate widely in order to contribute to the maintenance of cardiac output.

Early in pregnancy, cardiac output rises as a result of the increasing heart rate. Later in pregnancy, stroke volume rises by 40 mL above nonpregnant levels, reaching a peak at 20 to 24 weeks of gestation. Distribution of blood flow also changes as cardiac output increases. The mechanisms controlling these changes are not well understood. The most dramatic increase occurs in uterine blood flow, from 50 mL/min to 500 to 700 mL/min. This increase represents 10 to 20 percent of the cardiac output. The kidneys, skin, and breasts also receive higher blood flow. Cerebral and hepatic blood flow remain relatively unchanged.

Despite increases in both cardiac output and blood volume, there is no associated rise in blood pressure. Systolic pressures remain stable or fall slightly, whereas diastolic blood pressure drops more significantly. Blood pressure changes begin in the first trimester and continue until the middle of pregnancy. At that time, a gradual return to prepregnant blood pressure readings begins. The alterations in blood pressure are probably related to the hormone-mediated (i.e., by estrogen and progesterone) decreases in systemic vascular resistance.

As pregnancy progresses, the growing uterus can have a profound impact on maternal blood pressure. In the supine position, the uterus compresses the inferior vena cava. The compression decreases venous return to the heart, resulting in lowered cardiac output. If the compensatory rise in peripheral resistance is inadequate, "supine hypotension syndrome" ensues, accompanied by symptoms of dizziness and nausea. Symptoms can be relieved merely by changing to a lateral recumbent position.

Total blood volume, consisting of both red blood cell volume and plasma volume, increases beginning at 6 weeks of gestation. Plasma volume rises approximately 50 percent, but red blood cell volume only about 33 percent. This change leads to hemodilution and a fall in hematocrit. Iron supplementation during pregnancy cannot prevent the physiologic anemia, but women who have received iron supplementation demonstrate higher hematocrit levels in the third trimester than women who have not. These changes are amplified in multiple gestations.

The intravascular hemodynamic picture in pregnancy is complicated by lower serum protein levels. Decreased serum protein levels result in lowered colloid osmotic pressure and a tendency for fluid to shift from the intravascular to the interstitial space. The changes in colloidal osmotic pressure are reflected as dependent edema in the late second and third trimesters.

As previously mentioned, red blood cell volume rises during pregnancy, but not in as great a proportion as the rise in plasma volume. Mean red blood cell volume is virtually unchanged during pregnancy unless the woman has received regular iron supplementation. In this case, mean cell size increases progressively through term. This effect allows women who are given iron supplementation to maintain near-normal hemoglobin and hematocrit values in pregnancy despite the significant hemodilution.

Total leukocyte counts increase during normal pregnancy, ranging from 5000 to 12,000 cells/mL, with an average of 10,000 to 11,000 cells/mL. During labor and early puerperium, white blood cell counts may become markedly elevated, averaging 14,000 to 16,000 cells/mL. The elevation in white blood cell count is primarily related to an increase in the number of neutrophils. There is little change in other white blood cell components (i.e., monocytes, lymphocytes, eosinophils).

Although the mechanisms of hemostasis are unchanged during pregnancy, increases in production of certain clotting factors and venous stasis contribute to a hypercoagulable state. Fibrinogen concentrations increase 50 percent, from a nonpregnancy average of 250 to 400 mg/dL to as high as 600 mg/dL. Higher fibrinogen levels contribute to changes in the erythrocyte sedimentation rate, which is therefore an unreliable predictor of inflammatory activity. Levels of factors VII, VIII, IX, and X are also increased. Factor II (prothrombin) levels only slightly increase. In contrast, factors XI and XII decrease in pregnancy.

The levels of plasminogen (profibrinolysin) are considerably higher during pregnancy. This phenomenon is induced by estrogen treatment. In spite of higher levels of plasminogen, fibrinolytic activity is prolonged during normal pregnancy.

Renal System

The kidneys enlarge one to two centimeters owing to increases in renal blood flow and vascular volume. In the nonpregnant individual, the kidneys usually receive a total of 1000 to 1200 mL of blood per minute. The glomerular filtration rate—the amount of plasma filtered by the kidneys—rises 40 to 50 percent beginning soon after conception. GFR may reach 150 percent of normal; it peaks at 9 to 16 weeks, remaining relatively stable thereafter. The increase in glomerular filtration is due to the influences of higher glomerular blood flow. The rise in GFR results in greater elimination of urinary amino acids, glucose, protein, urea, uric acid, potassium, calcium, water-soluble vitamins, creatinine, and certain drugs.

The ability to concentrate and dilute urine remains unchanged in pregnancy. Interestingly enough, the volume of urine excreted in a 24-hour period remains stable and does not reflect the increase in GFR. Urea, uric acid, and creatinine clearance values are used to evaluate renal function. The creatinine clearance is markedly increased to 120 to 220 mL/min owing to the elevated GFR. Therefore, levels of 100 mL/min or lower indicate disease in a pregnant woman. Uric acid levels are used as a marker for preeclampsia.

Respiratory System

During pregnancy, a number of changes take place in the respiratory system, mediated by the mechanical effects of the enlarging uterus, higher oxygen demands, and the stimulant effect of progesterone. There is an estrogen-induced hyperemia of nasopharyngeal mucosa with concurrent edema and greater production of mucus. This leads to a feeling of stuffiness and greater tendency for epistaxis. Pregnant women should be warned of this normal change and advised against using over-the-counter drugs and nasal sprays in hopes of alleviating symptoms. A normal saline nasal spray may be helpful in reducing some of the discomfort and should be encouraged for women who find the stuffy feeling uncomfortable.

The most important biochemical influences on the respiratory system during pregnancy are elicited by progesterone and prostaglandins. Progesterone levels gradually rise, from 25 mcg/mL at 6 weeks to 150 mcg/mL at term. This hormone increases minute ventilation and thereby lowers the carbon dioxide threshold of the respiratory center. The greater minute ventilation creates a state of chronic hyperventilation, resulting in a fall in $PaCO_2$ (partial pressure of carbon dioxide, arterial). This important change increases the carbon dioxide gradient between mother and fetus, enabling the fetus to off-load its carbon dioxide to maternal circulation. The maternal response to the fall in $PaCO_2$ is greater renal elimination of bicarbonate, thus maintaining arterial pH within normal limits.

Dyspnea is a complaint in 60 to 70 percent of normal pregnant women. The fact that it generally begins in late first or early second trimester eliminates compression from a growing uterus as a likely cause. The sensation of dyspnea is probably related to reduced $PaCO_2$ levels and a greater sensitivity of the respiratory center to carbon dioxide.

The role of prostaglandins in influencing airway tone during pregnancy is unclear. Prostaglandins affect bronchial smooth muscle tissue. Prostaglandin F_2 has been identified as a smooth muscle constrictor, whereas prostaglandins E_1 and E_2 act as bronchial dilators. Although prostaglandin F_2 appears to be elevated throughout pregnancy, higher levels of prostaglandin E have been found only during the third trimester. Prostaglandin E may help counteract the structural effect of an elevated diaphragm. Administration of prostaglandin F_2, which has been used for termination of pregnancy or to control postpartum hemorrhage, is contraindicated in women with asthma, because of its potential constrictive effect on the bronchioles.

Endocrine System

Pituitary Gland

The pituitary gland enlarges in pregnancy because of the high circulating levels of estrogen. The higher number of prolactin-producing cells causes enlargement of the anterior pituitary. The pituitary gland has been called the "conductor of the hormone orchestra," but once a pregnancy is established, the pituitary gland is not necessary for the maintenance of pregnancy.

There is a marked increase in levels of circulating prolactin during pregnancy. The main function of prolactin is to ensure lactation. Prolactin initiates DNA synthesis and mitosis of glandular epithelial cells and presecretory alveolar cells in the breast.

Thyroid Gland

Maternal adaptations to pregnancy mimic hyperthyroidism, but thyroid function itself does not change. Pregnancy causes a slight enlargement of the thyroid gland, through an increase in vascularity and hyperplasia of the glandular tissue. The basal metabolic rate rises as much as 25 percent, with most of the increase attributed to the metabolic activity of the products of conception.

Marked enlargement of the thyroid gland is considered abnormal and requires further evaluation.

Changes in concentrations of thyroxine, triiodothyronine, and thyroxine-binding globulin occur during pregnancy. These changes are influenced by estrogen and human chorionic gonadotropin as well as by alterations in kidney and liver function. Increases in total thyroxine and triiodothyronine levels begin as early as the second month of pregnancy, but the concentrations of free thyroxine and triiodothyronine remain unchanged in the healthy pregnant woman. This situation is due to the influence of estrogen, which stimulates the liver to raise the synthesis of thyroxine-binding globulin by 50 to 100 percent. The additional thyroxine-binding globulin binds with thyroxine and triiodothyronine to increase total thyroxine and triiodothyronine. Concentrations of free thyroxine and triiodothyronine, however, remain within normal physiologic limits.

Thyroid hormones do not cross the placenta. Therefore, fetal thyroid function appears to be independent of maternal thyroid function. Thyrotropin-releasing hormone, a neurotransmitter found in the brain, stimulates the synthesis and release of thyroid-stimulating hormone. Thyrotropin-releasing hormone crosses the placenta, but the role of the endogenous part of this hormone in fetal homeostasis is not clear.

Thyroid-stimulating immunoglobulins may also cross the placenta and cause fetal and neonatal hyperthyroidism. The most common cause of hyperthyroidism in pregnancy is Graves' disease. Untreated hyperthyroidism has a very poor prognosis for the fetus. In addition, in a euthyroid woman with a history of Graves' disease, thyroid-stimulating immunoglobulins may continue to cross the placenta and leave the fetus at risk. Neonatal hyperthyroidism is usually temporary, since the half-life of thyroid-stimulating immunoglobulins is approximately 2 weeks.

Antithyroid drugs, such as propylthiouracil and methimazole (see Chapter 50), as well as iodine easily cross the placenta. Propylthiouracil is transported in smaller amounts than methimazole; therefore, propylthiouracil is the drug of choice during pregnancy in any attempt to avoid fetal hypothyroidism. Ablation of the thyroid by radioactive iodine is contraindicated in pregnancy because the agent is easily transported across the placenta.

Parathyroid Glands

The parathyroid hormone acts directly on bone and the kidneys and indirectly on the intestine to raise serum calcium levels. Parathyroid hormone does this by increasing bone resorption, decreasing renal elimination of calcium, and increasing calcium absorption from the intestines.

Parathyroid hormone levels are lowered in early pregnancy, then progressively rise until delivery. Ionized calcium is the major ion regulating the release of parathyroid hormone. The fact that ionized calcium levels are only slightly decreased in pregnancy suggests that a new setpoint for the stimulation of parathyroid hormone release exists in pregnancy. The ensuing physiologic hyperparathyroidism is probably the result of the body's attempt to supply the fetus with adequate calcium.

Calcitonin generally opposes parathyroid hormone and vitamin D. Elevated calcitonin inhibits calcium and phosphorus release from bone. This inhibition protects the maternal skeleton from decalcification during times of stress while allowing the renal and intestinal actions of parathyroid hormone to provide the additional calcium needed by the fetus. Pregnancy and lactation are causes of profound calcium stress, which can explain the elevated levels of calcitonin during these times.

Adrenal Glands

Hepatic synthesis of corticosteroid-binding globulin during pregnancy is enhanced by estrogen. The estrogen-mediated increase in this globulin results in higher levels of plasma cortisol. Only the fraction of cortisol that is unbound is metabolically active, but unlike with thyroid hormone, the concentration of free plasma cortisol is elevated in pregnancy. The higher free plasma cortisol levels may be the result of maternal feedback mechanisms' resetting themselves to higher levels. The resetting of cortisol levels is possibly due to tissue refractoriness to cortisol. In this case, higher levels of free plasma cortisol would be needed to maintain homeostasis.

Aldosterone levels are significantly increased at about 15 weeks of gestation. It has been suggested that higher aldosterone levels afford protection against the natriuretic effect of progesterone, which generally causes a loss of sodium. If sodium is restricted in pregnancy, there is a further rise in aldosterone secretion.

Pancreas

The placenta and the fetus depend on maternal glucose as their primary source of energy. Glucose crosses the placenta by facilitated diffusion, but insulin, owing to its large molecular size, does not cross the placenta. The fetal pancreas produces insulin by 10 to 12 weeks of gestation. Therefore, the fetus responds to maternal hyperglycemia by producing excessive amounts of insulin.

The insulin-producing beta cells of the pancreas demonstrate a characteristic hyperplasia during pregnancy. The first half of pregnancy is distinguished by elevated fasting concentrations of insulin despite increased insulin sensitivity. Blood glucose levels are therefore 15 to 20 mg/dL lower after a 12-hour fast than in the nonpregnant state. The lowered glucose levels can be attributed to fetal-placental utilization of glucose.

Insulin antagonism emerges during the second half of pregnancy, mediated by the rising levels of placental hormones—estrogen, progesterone, and human placental lactogen. The biphasic effect on glucose metabolism explains why glucose intolerance in pregnancy is often not evident until 24 to 30 weeks of gestation.

MATERNAL PHARMACOKINETIC CONSIDERATIONS

The pregnant woman manifests physiologic changes that impact pharmacokinetics and pharmacodynamics. The resulting pharmacokinetic changes may require adjustment of drug dosages. In addition, the hormones of pregnancy alter the effectiveness of some drugs. For example, human placental lactogen exerts antagonistic effects on insulin in patients with a healthy functioning placenta, thereby requiring larger insulin dosages. The role pregnancy plays in pharmacokinetics is explored in the following sections.

Absorption

Absorption of orally administered drugs is influenced by gastric acidity, the presence of bile acids, mucus, and intestinal transit time. Reduced acidity acts to slow the absorption of weakly acidic drugs (e.g., aspirin) and speed the absorption of weakly basic drugs (e.g., opioids).

Gastric motility is reduced in pregnancy. With gastric transit time prolonged under the influence of high levels of progesterone, the rate and completeness of drug absorption can be delayed. The bioavailability of slowly absorbed drugs (e.g., digoxin) may be increased because of the decreased motility. The absorption and peak plasma levels of readily absorbed drugs (e.g., acetaminophen) may be delayed.

Distribution

Weight gain in pregnancy results from increases in body fat, total body water, and the products of conception. Drug concentration in maternal circulation is diminished owing to increases in extracellular fluid. Water-soluble drugs may be diluted, whereas lipid-soluble drugs concentrate in adipose tissue of the mother and the membrane layers of the fetal-placental unit. Increased body water allows a greater volume in which drugs can be distributed. However, increased total body water has more profound effects on polar drugs, which are confined to extracellular spaces. The distribution of fat-soluble drugs is influenced by changes in protein and lipid binding. The higher body fat associated with pregnancy acts as a reservoir for fat-soluble drugs and free fatty acids. Free fatty acids compete with some drugs for albumin binding sites; therefore, the elevation in free fatty acids during pregnancy may alter drug distribution.

Drugs with low lipid solubility tend to be highly bound to plasma proteins, but drugs with high lipid solubility tend to concentrate in tissues. In pregnancy, the level of plasma albumin, to which most acidic drugs are bound, falls. Basic drugs (e.g., propranolol) tend to bind to alpha$_1$-acid glycoproteins. Endogenous ligands, such as free fatty acids, compete with drugs for binding sites on both albumin and alpha$_1$-acid glycoproteins. The implications of these changes, which influence the volume of distribution, are greatest for drugs with relatively low lipid solubility and high protein binding (e.g., benzodiazepines, anticonvulsants). Generally, the impact of an increased volume of distribution reduces peak plasma drug concentrations following a dose and decreases elimination, resulting in a prolonged half-life. This remains true unless there is a concurrent increase in clearance by biotransformation or elimination.

The higher GFR in pregnancy can lead to more rapid elimination of drugs, and at times, blood and tissue levels may be subtherapeutic. Serum levels and the half-life of many drugs, especially barbiturates and antibiotics, are decreased, primarily owing to greater elimination. Dosage and frequency of administration may need to be altered, and women need to be evaluated for signs of toxicity as well as for evidence of subtherapeutic drug levels.

The consequence of a reduction in plasma proteins is less binding of a given drug. The resultant larger fraction of unbound drug is free to be more widely distributed, to exert a pharmacologic effect, and to be eliminated through biotransformation or elimination. Greater elimination due to a rise in GFR means a decrease in tissue concentration. In pregnancy, the net result of the increase in unbound fraction is a lower total drug concentration in plasma. Plasma drug concentrations should be monitored closely during pregnancy to ensure therapeutic blood levels of important drugs.

Biotransformation

Drug biotransformation during pregnancy is heightened by the effects of progesterone. Accompanied by a rise in hepatic enzymes, liver clearance is increased, elimination accelerated, and drug half-life shortened. The microsomal enzyme system remains sensitive to inhibition as well as stimulation by certain drugs. Hepatic blood flow is not increased during pregnancy, although a small amount of biliary stasis may occur as pregnancy advances. If hepatic enzymatic processes slow, drug biotransformation and degradation may be delayed.

Other factors contributing to slowed drug biotransformation are the stable blood supply to the liver and lowered plasma concentration of the drug (from reduced serum protein levels). Drugs expected to have a shorter half-life in pregnancy (e.g., antibiotics, barbiturates) may have increased concentrations during labor, when the clearance of drugs is thought to decrease. Biotransformation during pregnancy also occurs in both the placenta and the fetal liver, although the contribution of the fetal-placental unit is thought to be very small.

Elimination

Increased renal blood flow and glomerular filtration result in an accelerated clearance of urea, uric acid, and creatinine. Along with those substances, drugs that are excreted unchanged (e.g., gentamycin, digoxin) are cleared in proportion to the creatinine clearance. Serum levels of these drugs need to be closely monitored to maintain therapeutic levels during pregnancy. Because blood flow through the liver is not appreciably changed in pregnancy, drugs that depend solely on hepatic blood flow for clearance are removed from the body at the same rate as in the nonpregnant woman.

Lipid-soluble, nonionized drugs are more likely to be reabsorbed. Drugs that are ionized at the pH of urine are more readily excreted. The higher the lipid solubility of a drug, the greater its half-life in pregnancy, and the more polar a drug, the shorter its half-life.

FETAL-PLACENTAL PHARMACOKINETIC CONSIDERATIONS

Absorption

The placenta allows transfer of substances between mother and fetus. It has a high basal metabolic rate, with energy needs supplied predominantly by oxygen and glucose. The placenta transports oxygen and nutrients to the fetus and clears urea, carbon dioxide, and other catabolites produced by the fetus. The placenta has five mechanisms of transfer: simple diffusion, facilitated diffusion, active transport, pinocytosis, and leakage (see also Chapter 4, Fig. 4–3).

Gases and some molecules cross the placenta by *simple diffusion*. Transport depends on the concentration gradient, the size of the molecule, and the surface area available for transfer.

Facilitated diffusion transports glucose, the major source of energy for the fetus. This transfer occurs more rapidly than simple diffusion, and it is accomplished by a carrier system in the direction of the concentration gradient. Normally, the fetal concentration of glucose is approximately 80 percent of the maternal value. The highest rate of diffusion across placental membranes occurs with substances of low molecular weight, minimal electrical charge, and high lipid solubility.

Essential amino acids and water-soluble vitamins are transferred by *active transport*. These substances are found in higher concentration in the fetus and are carried across the placenta against the concentration gradient.

Pinocytosis involves the ingestion of fluids and solute molecules through the formation of small vesicles. The particles are carried across the membrane virtually intact, to be released on the other side. Complex proteins, immune bodies, small amounts of fat, and viruses travel through the placenta in this manner.

Leakage of fetal cells into maternal circulation occurs when there are minute breaks in the placental membrane. This leakage is thought to be the mechanism by which Rh sensitization occurs between an Rh-negative mother and Rh-positive fetus.

Distribution

The effect of drugs on the fetus depends on whether the drug is distributed throughout the body or selectively. The distribution is significant in determining whether a drug can pass through the placental membranes. Many factors influence placental transfer of drugs, including physiochemical properties, molecular weight and configuration, ionization, lipid solubility, and protein binding.

Physiochemical Properties

The placenta is not an impermeable barrier (Fig. 6–2). It is living tissue that synthesizes a number of peptides, enzymes, and hormones. It actively transports molecules needed by the fetus and carries away wastes. The placenta usually provides an effective immunologic barrier between mother and fetus but does not act to protect the fetus in the same manner as the blood-brain barrier functions to protect the brain (Table 6–1).

Molecular Weight and Configuration

The placenta permits transfer of drugs with molecular weights of less than 600. Molecules of weights up to 1000, if unbound and nonionized, are usually lipid soluble and rapidly penetrate the tissues that separate the fetal and maternal circulation. The vast majority of drugs have molecular weights between 100 and 500.

Ionization

The distribution of weak acids and weak bases is somewhat complex. In the blood, a weak acid or weak base distributes to all compartments of the body differently, forming an equilibrium between charged and uncharged forms of the drug in each compartment. In addition, polar substances cross the placenta more slowly than drugs that are nonionized at a physiologic pH. For example, if a fetus becomes acidotic from prolonged cord compression, a weak base (e.g., amphetamine) that diffuses into the fetal compartment

TABLE 6–1 FACTORS AFFECTING PLACENTAL TRANSFER OF DRUGS

Drug Transfer Enhanced by	Drug Transfer Inhibited by
Lipid solubility	Increased diffusion distance
Nonionized substances	High molecular charge
Molecular weight less than 600	High molecular weight
Lack of significant albumin binding	Drug bound to maternal red blood cells and/or proteins
Higher maternal-to-fetal gradient	Drug altered or bound by placental enzymes
Increased placental blood flow	Decreased placental blood flow
Increased fetal acidity, which retains basic drugs	Drugs highly metabolized by mother
Larger surface area	

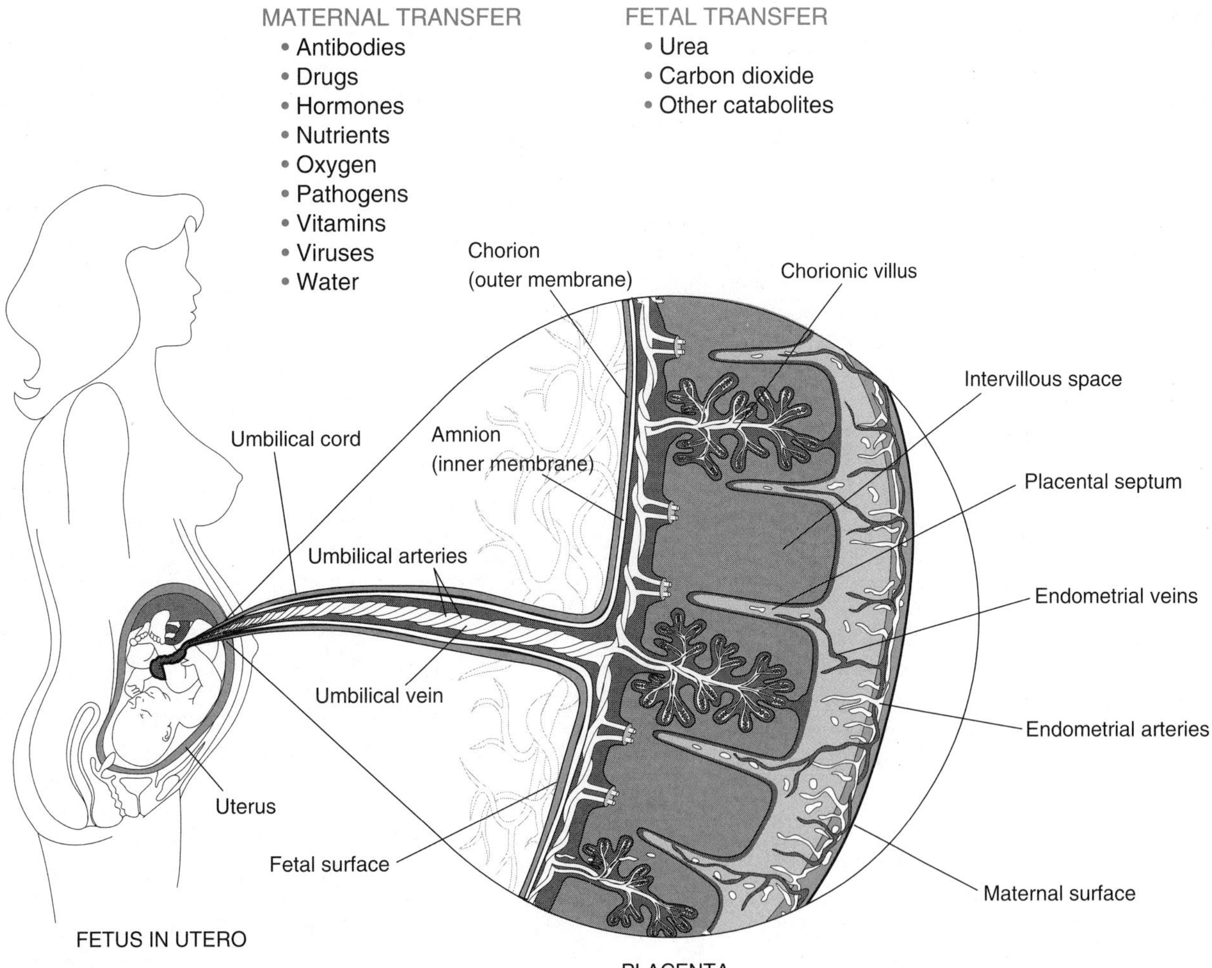

Figure 6–2 The maternal-fetal unit permits many substances to be transported from mother to fetus and back through the placenta. Maternal blood circulates through uterine arteries to intervillous spaces of the placenta and is returned to the maternal circulation through the uterine veins. Fetal blood flows through two umbilical arteries into the placenta and returns through the umbilical vein.

will become charged. The charged amphetamine does not diffuse passively back into the maternal circulation. The result is a higher amphetamine concentration in the acidotic fetus than if that fetus were more alkalotic.

Lipid Solubility

Lipid-soluble drugs passively diffuse across the placenta. Small molecules cross at rates dependent on their molecular weight, charge characteristics, and concentration in the maternal blood.

Tissue Binding

Just as drugs may bind to plasma proteins, they may also be removed from circulation and stored in tissue, such as bone, teeth, hair, and adipose tissue. Lipid-soluble drugs are stored in adipose tissue, which increases during pregnancy. This can lead to a slight decrease in the amount of free lipid-soluble drugs such as sedatives and hypnotics. When such a drug is discontinued, the tissue deposits of drugs may be slowly released, resulting in persistent drug effects.

Protein Binding

Circulating plasma proteins act either as a reservoir for drugs or as sites from which drugs are released. During pregnancy, plasma albumin levels are decreased, in part from dilutional effects of expanded plasma volumes. The decrease in albumin levels promotes an increase in free drug. It is important to remember that only free, unbound drug is able to exert a pharmacologic effect. In addition, only a free drug is able to cross the placenta into the fetal compartment.

A second important concept related to protein binding is that many drugs bind to the same protein sites. One drug therefore may displace another, resulting in a potentially dangerous increase in free drug concentration. During pregnancy, there is also an elevation in free fatty acids, which may contribute to further competition for albumin binding sites.

Maternal-Fetal Blood Flow

Several variables in blood flow affect the availability of drugs to the fetus. They are maternal blood pressure, maternal position, fetal cord compression, and uterine contractions.

Maternal blood pressure may increase or decrease the amount of unbound drug available to cross the placenta and ultimately reach the fetus. Maternal positions for optimal uterine-placental blood flow are right or left lateral recumbent and sitting positions. Uterine blood flow is impeded by the standing or supine position. Any maternal position that does not optimize uterine blood flow decreases the potential for fetal drug exposure.

Fetal Cord Compression and Uterine Contractions

Blood flow through the umbilical cord is probably an even more important factor in transfer of freely permeable drugs. Cord compression jeopardizes circulation and hence the delivery of oxygen to and removal of wastes from the fetus. Cord compression thus also affects the delivery of drugs to the fetus. Likewise, uterine contractions impair placental blood flow and reduce the transfer of intravenous drugs to the fetal compartment when bolus drug administration coincides with a uterine contraction.

Physiologic Properties of the Placenta

Drug transfer via the placenta is greatest late in gestation. As pregnancy progresses, chorionic villi become more numerous, providing a greater surface area across which diffusion between the two circulations can occur. Near term, the membrane separating maternal and fetal circulation thins considerably, so that fetal capillary endothelium is separated from maternal circulation by a single layer of fetal chorionic tissue. Inflammation, hypoxia, vascular degeneration, or partial separation of the placenta affects drug transfer just as it affects transfer of oxygen and nutrients to the fetus. For example, a woman with diabetes tends to have a larger, thicker placenta, creating a greater distance for molecules to travel before arriving in fetal circulation.

The placenta contains many of the drug-biotransforming enzymes that are present in the adult liver. This knowledge might lead one to assume that the placenta would act to protect the fetus from some maternal drugs. However, there is no evidence to suggest the placenta acts as a barrier to any significant degree.

Acid-Base Balance

Weak acids and weak bases create an equilibrium between charged and uncharged forms of a drug molecule, depending on the pH of the substance in which they are dissolved. At a low pH, there is a high concentration of hydrogen ions. In this situation, the nitrogen ion of many weak bases will accept a proton and become charged. Conversely, at a high pH, there is a low concentration of hydrogen ions. In this case, the nitrogen molecule will donate its proton to the solvent and become an uncharged molecule. This fact demonstrates how both maternal and fetal pH values affect the pH gradient. Transplacental distribution of a drug is based on the free nonionized component of that drug.

Biotransformation

Fetal biotransformation of drugs is believed to be minimal. Therefore, the fetus must rely on maternal plasma levels of a drug to clear that drug from fetal circulation. As maternal serum levels fall, drug diffuses from fetal circulation into the maternal blood stream. Different drugs take variable amounts of time to reach the fetus, on the basis of previously mentioned conditions. Highly lipid-soluble barbiturates equilibrate within a few minutes of maternal intravenous injection. On the other hand, dexamethasone takes several hours to equilibrate between maternal and fetal circulations. Consequently, a particular drug may have a profound or minimal effect on the fetus, as determined by its absorption, distribution, and elimination rates as well as by how long before birth it is administered.

The fetal liver contains the adult complement of enzymes, but the activities of these enzymes at term are only about half those in an adult. In addition, liver enzymes in the fetus are also poorly inducible compared with those in the adult.

Only drugs that are unbound in maternal circulation may cross the placenta to reach the fetus. Therefore, the protein-bound component of plasma drug concentration is often discounted. The fetus, however, also possesses the ability to store drugs through plasma protein binding. The protein content of fetal plasma increases with gestational age. Fetal albumin levels usually exceed maternal levels at time of delivery. A large bound component in the fetus promotes placental drug transfer by promoting the gradient for free drug. The bound component also increases the overall fetal dose after a brief administration of a drug, and thereby prolongs the fetal and, perhaps more important, the neonatal effects of a drug given to the mother. Following birth, the neonate is removed from the benefit of maternal metabolism and must rely on its own limited ability to biotransform and remove a drug from its circulation. Hence, drug action following birth may be prolonged and may have adverse neonatal consequences.

TABLE 6–2 DRUGS WITH AFFINITY FOR SPECIFIC FETAL TISSUE

Drug	Fetal Tissue
Tetracycline Warfarin	Teeth
Aminoglycosides	Middle ear
Quinine Chlorpromazine	Retina
Diethylstilbestrol	Mullerian duct Vagina
Corticosteroids Phenytoin	Adrenal gland
Iodides Propylthiouracil	Thyroid gland

Elimination

The presence of drug-biotransforming enzymes in the fetal liver supports the notion that the fetus is capable of eliminating drugs. Drug metabolites have been found in fetal serum, but because metabolites can freely cross the placenta in both directions, it has been difficult to prove that they are of fetal origin. Drug metabolites themselves may be pharmacologically active and able to cause adverse effects in the fetus.

A hydrophilic drug may cross the placenta slowly from mother to fetus, but once it reaches the fetus, it undergoes rapid elimination by the fetal kidneys. However, fetal urine voided into the amniotic cavity constitutes a substantial portion of the amniotic fluid. As the fetus goes through the normal process of swallowing amniotic fluid, it ingests the drug or its metabolites that have been excreted in fetal urine. The result is more prolonged fetal drug exposure. Appearance of a drug in amniotic fluid is usually delayed after a single dose is given to the mother. However, the concentration gradually increases. This delay suggests that the major portion of the drug enters the amniotic fluid via fetal urine.

Lipid-soluble drugs diffuse back across placental membranes to the mother, who provides the major route of elimination. Metabolites formed by the fetal liver are probably excreted in bile and deposited in meconium. Hair analysis can reflect drug exposure during the last 3 months of pregnancy.

PHARMACODYNAMICS

A drug demonstrates the same biochemical mechanism of action in all individuals. If a drug normally inhibits the transfer of a substance into a cell, it will do so in persons of any age group. The response to the drug, however, varies according to the physiologic changes associated with pregnancy. Consequently, a dosage adjustment may be necessary. The sensitivity of drug receptors is also variable.

Since the thalidomide crisis of the 1960s, health care providers and their patients have been concerned about the effects of drugs on the fetus. Prior to the crisis, the general rule of thumb was that a drug was safe until proven otherwise. Today, it is prudent for anyone who prescribes or administers drugs to a pregnant woman to function under the premise that few, if any drugs fail to cross the placenta. It is difficult to prove that any drug is safe for use during pregnancy, just as it is difficult to absolutely determine that a given drug is a teratogen. Drugs may have many teratogenic effects, such as spontaneous abortion, malformations, altered fetal growth, functional deficits, carcinogenesis, and mutagenesis.

The fetal central nervous system seems to be particularly susceptible to adverse effects of drug exposure. Permeability through the blood-brain barrier is greater in the fetus than in the adult; therefore, the developing brain is more susceptible to drug action. Drug elimination in the fetus is slower, owing to the immaturity of the fetal liver and kidneys. In addition, amniotic fluid, which is composed in part of fetal urine, is swallowed by the normal fetus and can recirculate the drug through the fetal enterohepatic circulation. The result of fetal immaturity is a greater total drug burden for the fetus. Immature fetal tissues also permit special tissue-specific accumulations of certain drugs (Table 6–2).

Certain factors influence whether or not a particular drug has an adverse effect on a fetus. The type and amount of drug, rate of elimination, distribution in fetal tissue, gestational age, and fetal receptor function affect drug action. The fetus is most vulnerable during the first trimester. During the pre-embryonic stage (conception to 14 days following conception), there is little morphologic differentiation. Exposure to teratogens at this time generally has an all-or-nothing effect on the zygote: either the zygote is damaged so severely that it is aborted or there are no apparent effects.

The greatest risk for malformations in the fetus is during the period of *organogenesis* (15 to 60 days after conception). After the first trimester, drugs do not cause gross structural abnormalities but can have toxic effects or can affect growth and developmental functioning. Drug exposure occurring at this time can lead to brain damage, deafness, growth retardation, stillbirth, infant death, or malignancy.

Teratogenicity

A *teratogen* is capable of causing abnormal development or function by interfering with embryonic and/or fetal development (see Appendix G). Because the use of prescription and over-the-counter drugs is common in women of childbearing age, the possibility of fetal abnormalities exists. It is difficult to establish the teratogenicity of individual drugs because of

FDA DRUG CATEGORIES

Category A

Controlled studies in women have failed to demonstrate fetal risk. The risk to the fetus throughout pregnancy appears to be remote.

Category B

Studies in animals have not demonstrated fetal risk. Risks demonstrated in animal studies have not been demonstrated in women in their first trimester.

Category C

Studies in women and animals are not available, or studies in animals have revealed adverse effects and no controlled studies are available in women.

Category D

There is positive evidence of human risk. The benefits of use in pregnancy may be acceptable in spite of this risk.

Category X

Studies or experience in humans and animals has demonstrated evidence of fetal risk. The risk of using this drug during pregnancy far outweighs any potential benefit. The drug is contraindicated in women who are pregnant or who may become pregnant.

the ethical implications of such studies. Therefore, drug use in pregnancy should be avoided as much as possible. When drugs are necessary, they should be taken at the lowest possible effective dose. Factors determining whether or not a drug will have an adverse effect include the type and amount of drug, rate of elimination, distribution in fetal tissue, gestational age, and specific fetal receptor function.

The Food and Drug Administration (FDA) classification system for systemic drug use in pregnancy is based on the level of known risk the drug presents to the fetus (see FDA Drug Categories). Category A and category B drugs are often used during pregnancy. Drugs in category C should be used only if the potential benefit outweighs the risks to the fetus. Category D contains drugs with documented evidence of risk to the human fetus; they should be used only in life-threatening situations or when maternal pathology is not treatable with a safer drug. Category X drugs should never be used in a woman who is or may become pregnant.

The FDA pregnancy categories are usually identified in drug reference books and materials. Drugs that were put on the market prior to the introduction of current FDA categories are generally not listed in patient package inserts, but this information may be found in textbooks on drug use in pregnancy.

The six variables associated with teratogenesis are susceptibility, timing, specific teratogen, mechanism of action, dosage, and manifestation.

Susceptibility

The biochemical and morphologic makeup of an individual embryo affects its particular sensitivity to a teratogenic drug. For example, the response of the human fetus to teratogens such as the rubella virus, thalidomide, and alcohol is variable.

Timing

The period of greatest susceptibility is during organogenesis, when cell differentiation is taking place. The timing of drug exposure determines which organ system is affected. After 12 weeks of gestation, drug exposure can result in decreased growth or function but generally not in a structural malformation.

Teratogen

Fetal exposure depends on the characteristics of the teratogen (e.g., lipid permeability, protein binding). Whether a teratogen reaches toxic or teratogenic concentrations depends on drug transmission across the placenta, maternal dosage, rate of absorption, maternal homeostatic capabilities, and the physical properties of the drug.

Mechanism

The mechanism of drug action can trigger changes in developing cells. Changes occurring at the molecular level early in pregnancy may not be discernible. Pathogenesis occurs when cellular damage is caused by secondary interference with cellular interactions or by cell necrosis.

Dosage

There appears to be a threshold above which embryotoxicity of a particular offending drug occurs. The same or similar teratogenic effects may result from a variety of drugs.

Manifestation

The result of early embryonic exposure is most likely death. Teratogenic events leading to malformation of organs or organ systems most often occur during organogenesis. Later exposures generally lead to functional deficit or growth retardation.

DRUGS AND LACTATION

Breastfeeding is the major form of neonatal nutrition. More than 60 percent of newborns are breastfed. Approximately 95 percent of breastfeeding women are taking at least one drug during the first week after delivery. The Committee on Drugs of the American Academy of Pediatrics (1994) has published a list of drugs and chemicals that transfer to breast milk. The list identifies drugs that are contraindicated during breastfeeding, drugs that require temporary cessation of breastfeeding, drugs that should be used with caution during breastfeeding, and drugs that are usually compatible with breastfeeding. Table 6–3 lists drugs that are contraindicated during breastfeeding, along with the reason for concern or the reported effect.

Drug Distribution

As a general rule, a breastfeeding infant ingests less than 1 to 2 percent of the total maternal drug dose. Several factors influence drug passage into breast milk. These factors are not unlike those determining the distribution of drugs in the mother. The pharmacologic factors should be considered when giving drugs to lactating women. Low-molecular-weight drugs penetrate more easily than high-molecular-

TABLE 6–3 DRUGS THAT ARE CONTRAINDICATED DURING BREASTFEEDING

Drug	Reason(s) for Concern or Reported Effect(s)
Amphetamine*†	Irritability, poor sleeping pattern
Bromocriptine	Suppresses lactation; may be hazardous to mother
Cocaine*	Cocaine intoxication
Cyclophosphamide	Possible immune suppression; unknown effect on growth or association with carcinogenesis; neutropenia
Cyclosporine	Possible immune suppression; unknown effect on growth or association with carcinogenesis
Doxorubicin†	Possible immune suppression; unknown effect on growth or association with carcinogenesis
Ergotamine	Vomiting, diarrhea, convulsions (doses used in migraine medication)
Heroin*	Tremors, restlessness, vomiting, poor feeding
Lithium	One-third to one-half therapeutic blood concentration in infants
Marijuana*	Only one report in literature; no effect mentioned
Methotrexate	Possible immune suppression; unknown effect on growth or association with carcinogenesis; neutropenia
Nicotine (smoking)*	Shock, vomiting, diarrhea, rapid heart rate, restlessness; decreased milk production
Phencyclidine (PCP)*	Potent hallucinogen
Phenindione	Anticoagulant; increased prothrombin and partial thromboplastin time in one infant; not used in United States

* The Committee on Drugs strongly believes that nursing mothers should not ingest any of these compounds. Not only are they hazardous to the nursing infant, but they are also detrimental to the physical and emotional health of the mother. This list is obviously not complete. No drug of abuse should be ingested by nursing mothers, even though adverse reports are not in the literature.

† Drug is concentrated in human milk.

Adapted from American Academy of Pediatrics Committee on Drugs (1994). The transfer of drugs and other chemicals into human milk. *Pediatrics*, 93 (1), 137–150. Used with permission of the American Academy of Pediatrics.

weight drugs. Only the unbound, free portion of drugs in maternal plasma diffuse into breast milk. Drugs that are widely distributed in the maternal body usually do not achieve high concentrations in breast milk. The pH of breast milk is lower pH than that of plasma (7.0 versus 7.4, respectively). The lower pH of breast milk may cause organic bases to ionize and become "trapped" in breast milk. Drugs that are highly fat soluble can concentrate in breast milk; however, milk fat represents only 3 to 5 percent of total milk volume. Highly protein-bound drugs enter breast milk poorly, because the concentration of protein in breast milk is only 10 percent of the concentration in plasma.

Drugs are transported to breast milk via simple diffusion, facilitated diffusion, or active transport. Mammary alveolar epithelium is a lipid barrier with water-filled pores. The pores are most permeable to drugs during the colostrum phase of milk secretion. Drugs enter into the breast in a nonionized, non–protein-bound form. Water-soluble drugs with a molecular weight of less than 200 pass through membrane pores. In addition, drugs can enter breast milk through spaces between mammary alveolar cells. Drugs leave the breast by diffusion or active transport. Drug-biotransforming capacity of the breast, if it even exists, is not understood.

Infant Factors Affecting Drug Exposure

An infant is immature and constantly changing. The concepts used to determine serum concentrations of a drug in an adult do not necessarily hold true for an infant. Compared with an adult, an infant's gastrointestinal tract has a high pH and changing microbial flora. The slow intestinal motility in an infant can prolong drug transit time. The infant's immature liver has a limited ability to detoxify a chemical and/or excrete it in the urine.

Because a newborn has lower serum protein levels than a nonpregnant adult, protein binding is less, contributing to higher levels of free drug in the infant. Some drugs (e.g., sulfadiazine, aspirin, furosemide, phenylbutazone) compete for binding sites with bilirubin. The competition for binding sites puts the newborn at risk for kernicterus because of a higher fraction of unbound bilirubin.

Clearly, the gestational age of an infant has an impact on how well a drug is tolerated. Not only are body systems less mature in a preterm infant, but also, body composition is different. The less mature an infant is, the higher the water content of the body and the greater the proportion of extracellular water. When body fat accounts for only a low percentage of body weight, highly lipid-soluble drugs are more likely to deposit in the brain. Compare the 1000-gram preterm infant, whose body fat is 3 percent, with a full-term, 3500-gram infant, whose body fat is 12 percent. Complications of birth such as acidosis and hypoxemia also contribute to the unavailability of albumin binding sites and result in higher levels of unbound drug.

The age of the infant not only influences its ability to metabolize a drug but also affects the total amount of breast milk consumed at a feeding. Drug exposure is intensified in an infant who is solely dependent on breast milk for nutrition. In general, healthy infants from birth to 5 months of age consume 150 to 225 mL/kg of breast milk per day. An older infant may also consume other food items, so that milk does not comprise the total nutritional intake.

Minimizing Infant Drug Exposure

The goal of the health care provider is to minimize the risk of potentially harmful drug exposure to the breastfed infant. Unfortunately, mothers are often discouraged from breastfeeding when they are taking a drug, because of a knowledge deficit about the impact of a specific drug or because of concern over the potential but undefined risk to the infant.

When a mother requires a drug that carries minimal hazards for the infant, the health care provider can make the following adjustments to diminish drug effects:

- Avoid sustained-release and long-acting drugs. They are difficult for an infant to excrete, and drug accumulation in the infant is a significant concern.
- Identify the usual rate of absorption and peak blood levels of the drug, and then schedule drug administration so the least amount possible gets into the milk. Having the mother take the drug immediately after breastfeeding is generally the safest for the infant.

- Short-acting drugs may never fully equilibrate with milk if the drug is rapidly cleared. In this case, expressing and discarding breast milk after drug administration may not be useful.
- When possible, an agent that produces the lowest levels of drug in the milk should be used.
- Use the American Academy of Pediatrics Committee on Drugs (1994) list of drugs and other chemicals transferred into milk to assist in selection of drugs compatible with breastfeeding.
- Watch the infant for signs of drug reaction (e.g., changes in sleep or feeding patterns, fussiness, rashes).

It is difficult to estimate the extent of infant drug exposure incurred with breastfeeding. Maternal plasma levels of a specific drug may not correlate with concentrations of that drug in breast milk. Steady-state drug concentrations are rarely achieved between serum and breast milk. A significant lag time may occur between peak levels in the blood and those in milk. Other factors interfering with prediction of infant drug exposure are problems identifying the bioavailability of a particular drug in a specific infant and the clearance rate for the substance.

The length of therapy influences the impact a drug might have on the infant. Single-dose or short-term therapy is less likely to achieve a steady state in milk or to produce metabolites that are excreted through the milk supply. In addition, the storage of milk in the breast permits drugs to accumulate even while maternal serum levels are declining.

A greater awareness of the benefits of breastfeeding in a more health-conscious society is evidenced by a dramatic increase in breastfeeding over the last decade. Organizations have been formed to support nursing mothers, and more health care providers are involved in parent education. Many institutions are offering prenatal breastfeeding classes, provide specially trained lactation consultants, and are developing policies that support family-centered care.

Accurate information must be available to evaluate the benefits and risks of breastfeeding while the mother is on drug therapy. The long-term consequences of infant exposure to drugs through breast milk is unknown. However, during the last 10 years, sound information about drugs and breastfeeding has become available. Members of the health care team may access literature on drugs and pregnancy or may use teratogen information resources or contact regional drug consultation centers.

The actual drug dose an infant consumes is determined by the volume of milk ingested. Depending on the drug involved, temporary interruption of breastfeeding combined with pumping and discarding the milk may be advisable. There is controversy, however, regarding the benefit of pumping to reduce drug levels in human milk. Drug concentrations in the milk decrease by retrograde diffusion; therefore, as maternal serum levels fall, levels of the drug in milk will follow the concentration gradient and also fall. Breast milk contains higher amounts of fat at midday, so the breastfed infant may be exposed to higher amounts of fat-soluble drugs at that feeding. Supplementing nursing with formula for the midday feedings may help reduce the amount of drug the infant receives.

Another strategy that may be used to reduce drug exposure is to instruct a mother to take the drugs immediately after breastfeeding so sufficient time elapses between the dose and the next feeding. This approach works well in the case of a single daily dose of a drug. It is more difficult when a drug must be taken four times a day. The strategy also provides marginal benefit for the young infant who feeds frequently, or with the use of specific drugs that have an extended half-life. Therefore, it is wise to know what type of drug the mother is taking. For example, a weak acid tends to produce lower milk concentrations, and a weak base ionizes at the lower pH of breast milk, resulting in higher maternal milk concentrations. Nonsteroidal anti-inflammatory drugs, barbiturates, sulfonamides, and penicillin are weakly acidic agents, whereas erythromycin, ephedrine, quinine, and trimethoprim are weakly basic drugs.

Using short-acting dosage forms reduces the risk of accumulation in both the mother and the breastfed infant. Using milk that has been expressed previous to the initiation of drug therapy, if there is a supply available, is a sure way to avoid drug exposure. A mother may also request a temporary supply of milk from a milk bank.

The last recommendation for nursing mothers is to take only the drug needed. Many over-the-counter drugs contain more than one compound (e.g., night-time cold remedies). If a decongestant is really all that is needed, the combination drug, which includes a cough suppressant, should be avoided, and a decongestant such as pseudoephedrine should be used.

FETAL DRUG THERAPIES

The ability to treat the unborn fetus with pharmacologic therapies is a relatively new and challenging area. The discovery that betamethasone augments fetal surfactant production ushered in the era of intentional maternal drug therapy directed at the fetus.

Fetal therapy requires drug administration to the mother with potentially higher doses used to obtain therapeutic levels in the fetus. However, higher dosages create a potential for maternal toxicity and subsequent fetal compromise. Because the fetus is more difficult to monitor than the newborn, inadvertent fetal toxicity or insufficient therapy may go unrecognized. Careful assessment of the risks and potential benefits to both mother and fetus must be considered before initiation of therapy.

Critical Thinking Process

Assessment

Although pregnancy is not considered an illness, it is important for the health care provider to gather a sufficient database with which to make safe pharmacotherapeutic decisions. Nurses are assuming a more important role in perinatal care, especially in the area of assessment. The progression of a pregnancy depends on a number of factors, including the presence of disease states, emotional status, and past health care. Diagnosis of pregnancy and accurate dating are essential to reduce maternal and fetal risk during the early weeks of gestation. All risk factors do not threaten the pregnancy to the same extent.

History of Present Illness

The database for a perinatal patient should include a menstrual, contraceptive, gynecologic, and obstetric history. Amenorrhea is often the first sign of conception. However, a lack of menses can be due to other factors, such as anovulation, chronic disease, lactation, and stress. Other presumptive signs of pregnancy are breast tenderness/fullness, skin changes, nausea, vomiting, urinary frequency, and fatigue.

A known menstrual history is usually the most reliable predictor of delivery date. The mean duration of pregnancy, as calculated from the last menstrual period, is 280 days or 40 weeks.

The health care provider should gather information related to the pregnancy, including the date of the last menstrual period and status of previous pregnancies as well as current problems. It is important to establish the patient's past and present use of drugs (e.g., tobacco, caffeine, alcohol, marijuana, cocaine, crack, crank). The patient should also be asked about current use of over-the-counter and prescription drugs.

The drug history can be obtained as part of the initial patient interview along with personal and family health data. It allows the health care provider to assess the patient's knowledge about drug use during pregnancy.

One area of public health concern is the substantial number of women of child-bearing age who have used illegal drugs or alcohol. Identification of these women and their fetuses may depend on successful interview techniques since the reliability of urinalysis depends on the pharmacokinetics of the abused substance and the time of the last exposure. The interview should begin with routine and non threatening open-ended questions. Something as easy as, "How is your life going?" may open the door for a woman to safely share important information with the health care provider.

A pregnant woman may present with a problem that requires the health care provider to assess the need for pharmacologic therapy. There are circumstances when an indicated drug therapy has a long history of use and can be given without excessive concern, for example, the use of magnesium sulfate for the treatment of pre-eclampsia or the use of heparin for thrombophlebitis. In other situations, the risks of therapy compared to the potential benefits must be weighed carefully. Consider the pregnant woman who has had a significant exposure to a disease with substantial risk of severe morbidity or mortality to herself or her fetus. Generally, immunization is discouraged in pregnancy. But in the case of certain diseases, such as varicella zoster, the risk of acquiring the disease is greater than the risk from passive immunization with varicella zoster immune globulin (VZIG).

Past Health History

Assessment of the pregnant woman's health concerns and concurrent medical condition is part of the data gathering. Questions regarding exposure to chemical substances shortly before the last menstrual period through the time of the interview are pertinent. Determining the woman's perception of her health and the effect of any drugs she is using will assist in gaining insights that may aid in effective intervention if necessary.

When a pregnant woman has a disease that predates her pregnancy, she may be taking medication for that condition when she begins perinatal care. If she is currently taking medication, the first step is to identify whether the drug is a potential hazard. If the drug is a human toxicant, the timing of exposure related to the pregnancy and its dose-response relationship becomes the next issue. For example, if a toxic drug is taken 1 week after the last menstrual period, one can feel relatively confident that the surviving embryo was not harmed. On the other hand, exposure during the period of organogenesis, which includes the first 2 to 3 weeks after conception through the first trimester, comes at a critical period for organ development and may cause malformation.

Physical Exam Findings

A complete physical exam begins with assessment of vital signs. A decrease in blood pressure from baseline during the second trimester is expected because of normal physiologic changes of pregnancy. The exam continues with evaluation of body weight, skin, head and neck, cardiovascular and respiratory systems, breasts, and musculoskeletal and neurologic systems. Abdominal and pelvic measurements are taken.

If it has been determined that a woman has not started perinatal counseling, this is the perfect time to introduce patient education regarding the use of drugs, alcohol, and environmental hazards. When a woman is required to take drugs during her pregnancy, the risks and benefits should be discussed, and the need to report adverse effects or lack of effectiveness of the drugs should be addressed.

Diagnostic Testing

Laboratory testing of the pregnant woman comprises a complete blood count, ABO and Rh blood typing, screening for sexually transmitted diseases (i.e., gonorrhea, *Chlamydia,* herpes, human immunodeficiency virus, syphilis), sickle cell disease, and rubella titer. A urinalysis and Papanicolaou smear are also included in diagnostic testing.

The health care provider also determines what risks a desired test might impose, what value the information gained would provide, and at what cost. In dealing with women of child-bearing age, one must always be open to the possibility of an unknown pre-existing pregnancy. If symptoms require a test that could adversely affect the outcome of a pregnancy, a pregnancy test should be performed to rule out the possibility of pregnancy. If the woman is indeed pregnant, she and her family or support person should be carefully counseled as to the potential impact of the testing.

Developmental Considerations

Pregnancy is a time of maternal psychological adjustment and concern. It is viewed as a period with distinctive developmental tasks. Family dynamics, social support, cultural influences, and whether or not the pregnancy was planned distinctly influence the mother's as well as the family's adjustment to pregnancy. Thus, the woman's personal situation and support systems must be explored as the family prepares for a new member.

During the first trimester, the woman normally feels some ambivalence about the pregnancy, even if it was planned. These feelings should be discussed with the patient, because she may feel the need to hide the negative feelings, believing that they are abnormal. Helping her to understand the feelings will benefit her, especially if the baby should subsequently be aborted or be born with a congenital defect. The ambivalence usually ends by the beginning of the second trimester.

When the pregnancy is well accepted, the woman will demonstrate feelings of happiness about it. On the other hand, failure to move toward maternal role attainment may be demonstrated through direct statements of dissatisfaction with being pregnant. Less directly, failure of role attainment may be demonstrated through excessive complaints of physical discomfort or illness, depression, expressions of feeling ugly, or failure to seek prenatal care and/or to comply with the plan of care. Other examples are missing appointments, refusal to take vitamins or other drugs that may be needed for concurrent medical conditions, and general noncompliance with recommended self-care activities such as diet, exercise, alcohol consumption, and drug use.

Other developmental considerations during pregnancy are related to cultural influences and beliefs. For example, awareness of a patient's use of indigenous healers or home remedies and adherence to folk beliefs are important for health professionals, because these factors influence health outcomes. Knowing the causes of noncompliance enables the health care provider to offer appropriate patient education or to incorporate the patient's cultural practices into her perinatal care.

Psychosocial Considerations

As part of the psychosocial assessment, information related to religious, cultural, and socioeconomic factors that influence the woman's expectations of the child-bearing experience should be noted. It is particularly helpful if the health care provider is familiar with common practices of various religious and cultural groups who reside in the community.

Birth, death, and marriage are generally considered the most important events in an individual's life. Rituals, customs, and practices connected with these events reflect value systems. Familiarity with these values aids the health care provider in understanding reactions and behaviors that may be different from expectations. Some examples of such cultural value systems follow.

Many Mexican American women believe that pregnancy is not an illness and that therefore prenatal care is unnecessary. Many Mexican American women prefer to receive their care from *parteras* (lay midwives) or *curanderas* (folk healers). Paradoxically, Mexican American women who receive prenatal care either late in pregnancy or not at all have surprisingly healthy birth outcomes. In their culture, walking is recommended to ensure quick birth. Motherhood is seen by many such women as the most important social role to be achieved. As a result, the times surrounding pregnancy and birth are especially rich in traditional beliefs and practices.

Women of Haitian background may believe that hot ginger tea should be taken during labor. During the postpartum period, such a woman may sit in a hot bath with added leaves, herbs, and roots. Some Haitian women believe that hot, spicy food should be avoided during pregnancy and that the diet should consist of okra and tisane, a tea made from lettuce. After the baby is born, a Haitian woman and her family may massage the baby's head with palm oil, pinch the nose to give it shape, or press the cheeks to give the child dimples. Castor oil or *lok* (castor oil with nutmeg powder and mashed garlic) is sometimes used to speed the passage of meconium stool.

Women of Southeast Asian background often deal with illness by self-medication. Herbal preparations are widely used in their communities, and facsimiles of Western prescription drugs are sold over the counter. A common belief in this culture is that if one pill is good, two are better. Traditional Southeast Asian healers will use herbal preparations, acupuncture, "coining" (rubbing the "sick" area with coins), or "cupping" (using small heated cups over the area). They believe that cutting into the body, such as occurs during episiotomies, cesarean section, and circumcision, makes an exit point for a person's spirit and should therefore be avoided. Many Southeast Asians may regard invasive treatments such as nasal oxygen or intravenous fluid administration as providing the means of exit for life's essence.

Southeast Asians believe in the balance between *yin* (hot) and *yang* (cold). Childbirth is a precarious time, when a woman is in a cold state that may lead to illness. In Thailand, women have been seen lying on cots placed over smoldering charcoal fires on days when the air temperature is 90 to 100°F. In Cambodia, the women usually lie next to the fire with their heads covered by blankets or towels. With antibiotics being unavailable, this process of raising the body temperature may provide a way to kill some infectious organisms.

An awareness of potential cultural differences and individual knowledge must be assessed by nurses providing patient care. Determining a patient's needs and expectations helps bridge the cultural gap. Individual beliefs and values that are beneficial or harmless must be supported in order to promote the use of health care systems. Practices that may be harmful can be modified through patient education. Flexibility, compromise, and respect for differences makes culturally appropriate nursing care an attainable goal.

Analysis and Management

Treatment Objectives

Pharmacotherapeutics involves assessing factors that may affect the administration, effectiveness, and safety of a given drug regimen. In pregnancy, drug use is avoided unless the benefits of such use outweigh the risks. The woman should received accurate information and teaching regarding any drugs to be used and, when appropriate, should be involved in the decision-making process.

Drug objectives are directed at prevention, cure, alleviation, or palliation. An example of a drug used for its preventive value is iron supplementation to avoid iron deficiency anemia. Anticonvulsants prevent maternal seizure, and phenobarbital may be used just before delivery in an attempt to prevent severe neonatal intraventricular hemorrhage.

Curative objectives are instituted during pregnancy in the treatment of infection. An antibiotic is chosen on the basis of its effectiveness against the offending organism. The antibiotic of choice would also be one that holds the lowest possible risk to the fetus. In the case of a urinary tract infection, for example, failure to treat and cure the infection could lead to preterm labor and subsequent delivery.

Objectives related to palliation are directed at preventing complications associated with pregnancy. Chronic hypertension requires treatment throughout pregnancy to reduce the risk of complications associated with an elevated blood pressure. Hypertension is one of the leading causes of maternal death and predisposes a pregnant woman to pregnancy-induced hypertension. In addition, chronic hypertension has been linked to intrauterine growth retardation and fetal death. Similarly, a woman with diabetes will require insulin to ensure optimum health for both her and the developing fetus.

Treatment Options

As a rule, some therapies are offered during pregnancy simply to promote maternal comfort and, therefore, caution is required. The objective is to select a drug that has been identified as safe for use in pregnancy or to substitute one drug for another that is suspected to be highly teratogenic. The gestational age of the fetus is taken into consideration. Further, well-chosen therapies that provide relief from discomforts can make a significant difference in how a woman views her pregnancy. The health care provider should consult the FDA pregnancy categories for a listing of drugs that are safe to administer (see Appendix G).

Analgesics Minor muscle aches and headaches are common during pregnancy. Acetaminophen is often used short term during pregnancy. High doses, on the other hand, especially during the first trimester, may result in severe fetal liver damage. Aspirin is commonly ingested by pregnant women. However, use of aspirin has been associated with maternal anemia, antepartal and postpartal hemorrhage, and prolonged gestation and labor. Aspirin's effects on the fetus and neonate include intrauterine growth retardation, congenital salicylate intoxication, depressed albumin binding capacity, and an increased perinatal mortality rate. Aspirin taken (even in low doses) during the week before delivery may affect the neonate's clotting abilities.

Opioids should be used cautiously, if at all, in a pregnant woman. When used on a regular basis, opiates induce an intense addiction in both mother and fetus. Pain relief during labor and delivery must be carefully coordinated with the time of delivery and the drug dose to protect the fetus from a potentially harmful drug effects. Chapters 14 and 15 discuss analgesia further.

Cardiovascular Drugs Cardiac glycosides are used extensively for the management of congestive heart failure and various supraventricular arrhythmias. Digoxin is the most commonly used cardiac glycoside. No evidence exists of any harmful fetal effects. Because of the expansion of maternal blood volume and the increased GFR, a higher dosage of digoxin is often necessary in order to maintain therapeutic serum levels as the pregnancy progresses. Chapter 31 discusses cardiac glycosides in more depth.

Secondary uterine effects should be considered in patients receiving cardiac drugs that result in either alpha (uterine contraction) or beta (uterine relaxation) effects. Likewise, women who are taking beta-adrenergic receptor agonists for complications of pregnancy may experience secondary but significant cardiac effects. There is controversy regarding the safety of beta-blocking drugs in pregnancy. No evidence exists to suggest that beta blockers are teratogenic, and they can be used for women with hypertension. Chapter 11 discusses sympathetic drugs in more depth.

Arrhythmias otherwise treated with atropine, quinidine, or procainamide can be so treated during pregnancy without adverse effects on the fetus or newborn. There is a paucity of studies on the use of calcium channel blockers in pregnancy. Antiarrhythmic drugs are discussed in Chapter 33.

Patients requiring anticoagulation during pregnancy because of underlying cardiovascular abnormalities pose a particular problem. A number of complications in both mother and fetus have been demonstrated with warfarin derivatives, particularly in the first and third trimesters of pregnancy. Heparin has been shown to be an effective prophylactic as well as therapeutic agent and is the drug of choice when anticoagulation is required. More information about anticoagulants can be found in Chapter 36.

Antibiotics Antibiotic choice should be guided by sensitivity testing and considerations of maternal and fetal toxicity. Penicillins are safe in pregnancy; they show no increase in maternal toxicity and no known fetal toxicity. Cephalosporins are safe and do not cause increased fetal toxicity. Tetracyclines are generally contraindicated in pregnancy.

Parenteral formulations can cause fulminant maternal hepatitis and pancreatitis when administered during the third trimester. Oral tetracycline causes staining and deformity of deciduous teeth and inhibition of fetal bone growth in the fetus. Sulfonamides should not be used within 4 weeks of delivery. Sulfonamides and nitrofurantoin can cause hemolysis in patients with glucose-6-phosphate dehydrogenase (G6PD) deficiency. Trimethoprim is contraindicated. The risk of ototoxicity and nephrotoxicity secondary to aminoglycoside use is the same in the pregnant and nonpregnant woman.

Antacids and Hyperacidity Drugs Antacids are used by approximately 50 percent of pregnant women for relief of heartburn. Most antacids that contain aluminum, magnesium, and calcium are safe in therapeutic dosages during the second and third trimesters. Sucralfate and histamine$_2$ antagonists are excellent therapeutic modalities among nonpregnant patients, but their safety during pregnancy is not yet well established. Although the histamine$_2$ antagonists, such as cimetidine and ranitidine, are FDA category B drugs, their extended use is not recommended. Antacids and hyperacidity drugs are discussed further in Chapter 42.

Laxatives Certain laxatives are not safe for use during pregnancy, when constipation and painful hemorrhoids may appear. Castor oil can initiate premature uterine contractions. Saline laxatives (e.g., magnesium hydroxide) can lead to sodium retention in the mother. Furthermore, frequent use of lubricants such as mineral oil can lead to reduced absorption of fat-soluble vitamins, resulting in neonatal hypoprothrombinemia and hemorrhage. Stimulant laxatives, such as bisacodyl and senna, and stool softeners, such as docusate, may be safe for use during pregnancy. Bulk-forming laxatives (e.g., psyllium hydrophilic mucilloid) may also be safe during pregnancy. As a component of patient teaching, the patient should be encouraged to use nondrug measures to alleviate constipation or hemorrhoidal discomfort, such as increasing fluid intake, dietary fiber, and activity, and avoiding straining as much as possible when defecating. Laxatives are discussed further in Chapter 43.

Antiemetics Many antiemetic drugs have been linked to an increased risk of fetal harm. Diphenhydramine may cause cleft palate. Trimethobenzamide may produce other congen-

Controversy

Perinatal Pharmacotherapeutics—What to Restrict?

JONATHAN J. WOLFE

Perinatal drug dosing places the health care provider in uncomfortable territory. It often involves a choice between the interests of the mother, who can express her needs, and the fetus or neonate, who cannot. Any use of drugs in the later stages of pregnancy and the birth process demands consideration of both parties. At this stage in development, the teratogenicity of drugs is not a significant issue. Developmental defects due to drugs are chiefly associated with administration in the second trimester of pregnancy. The uncertainty in perinatal drug use focuses rather on the passage of drugs across the placenta and their effect on an emerging child, whose systems for drug biotransformation and elimination are imperfectly developed.

The placenta does not function as an effective barrier to the transmission of pharmaceutical agents to the fetus. Lipid-soluble, nonionized drugs readily pass across the placenta from the maternal to the fetal circulation. Highly dissociated ionized drugs and those with low lipid solubility pass less easily. In either case, simple diffusion carries drugs across the placenta, and any drug administered to the mother will to some extent be presented to fetal circulation.

Drugs are also transferred from mother to the neonate through breast milk. Here again, the primary concern is that highly lipophilic drugs are carried in the fat content of the milk and are absorbed by the child. A countervailing concern may well be the value of the protective antibodies provided to the newborn through breast milk.

For these reasons, the therapeutic index relationship between blood level to achieve therapeutic effect and blood level associated with toxicity for both mother and fetus or neonate must be considered. Such evaluation lends itself to an interdisciplinary approach. The treatment choice must account for outcomes appropriate to the patient's choice for self and child, the best standard of current practice, and the most current available data about distribution and effects of each drug contemplated.

Critical Thinking Discussion

- A patient at 34 weeks of gestation develops a life-threatening gram-positive infection that is responsive to carbenicillin. What interests of mother and fetus are most important here? Are their interests compatible? Is this drug likely to cause significant harm to either party? May treatment reasonably be postponed?
- The same patient is diagnosed with a malignant breast tumor. The oncologist advises immediate excision, followed by combination antineoplastic therapy using 5-fluorouracil and cyclophosphamide. What interests of mother and fetus are most important here? Are their interests compatible? Is this drug likely to cause significant harm to either party? May treatment reasonably be postponed?
- Perinatal analgesia in the past involved use of "twilight sleep" with meperidine and scopolamine. The use of these drugs commonly resulted in neonates with low Apgar scores who required immediate resuscitation involving the use of naloxone. What circumstances might justify this approach to pain management during labor and delivery today? What precautions would you recommend to a mother in the first 24 hours postpartum who wants to breast-feed but has received significant doses of phenobarbital during labor for prophylaxis against a documented seizure disorder?

ital anomalies. Prochlorperazine has been linked to an increased risk of cardiovascular and other malformations. Phosphorated carbohydrate solution has not been linked to toxicity.

The best scheme for managing nausea and vomiting in pregnancy with antiemetics is to become familiar with two or three drugs. Many antiemetics have the potential for extrapyramidal (and other) adverse effects. With this potential in mind, nausea and vomiting can often be managed with nonpharmacologic practices (e.g., eating small, frequent meals; consuming liquid and dry foods separately; avoiding fried, odorous, spicy, greasy, or gas-forming foods; and keeping crackers or other dry food at the bedside to be eaten in the morning before rising). Antiemetics are discussed further in Chapter 44.

Lactation Treatment options should be discussed with the lactating patient as to whether or not she should continue breastfeeding while receiving drug therapy. Some drugs are contraindicated during breastfeeding. The health care provider should use the resource available from the American Academy of Pediatrics when determining which drugs are safe for use during lactation. Again, the timing of the drug dose in relation to breastfeeding should be carefully coordinated to minimize the infant's drug exposure.

Intervention

Administration

Collaboration among and between members of the health care team is the best insurance that appropriate identification and intervention for a woman and fetus or infant at risk will occur. To minimize the risk of drug exposure to mother and fetus, the following administration guidelines should be used:

- Clearly identify the need for any drug used.
- Choose the safest effective drug option available.
- Avoid use of the newest drugs on the market.
- Use the lowest effective dose for the shortest possible time.
- Use topical or local therapy whenever possible.
- Carefully schedule drug administration times so a breastfeeding mother does not receive the drug within a short time before nursing.
- Once-daily drug doses may be taken by a breastfeeding mother before the infant's longest sleep period (see Controversy—Perinatal Pharmacotherapeutics).

Education

Patient teaching should include the names of the drugs that have been ordered and why. Special instructions about the timing of drug doses and drug-food interactions should be clarified. Adverse effects that may occur should be reviewed. The patient should be told about adverse effects that should be reported as well as what to do if she forgets to take a dose. A patient should know the expected duration of the therapy and should be advised not to change the dosage or discontinue the drug without consulting the health care provider. The addition of any prescription or over-the-counter drugs should be approved before use. Written instructions are helpful as a reference after the patient leaves the office, clinic, or hospital.

Prenatal counseling is beneficial for women with underlying health problems. It provides the opportunity for the health care provider to counsel the woman regarding the potential risks of a drug and to offer an alternative therapy when available. For example, if a woman with chronic hypertension is considering pregnancy and has been taking an angiotensin-converting enzyme inhibitor in order to control blood pressure, she can be switched to a preferred drug, such as methyldopa.

Evaluation

Meticulous, ongoing assessment is essential to achieve optimal perinatal management outcomes. When drug exposure during pregnancy is inevitable, an awareness of the physiologic changes of pregnancy, attention to the pharmacokinetics and pharmacodynamics of the required drugs, and early recognition of potential complications are essential. Definitive management goals center, in most cases, on prevention and alleviation of potential problems.

Understanding the applications, benefits, and risks of drugs given during pregnancy and lactation assists the health care provider in safely using drugs and evaluating their effects. Drug therapy may be unavoidable during this period, and it becomes the responsibility of the health care professional to maintain a current knowledge base in order to best respond to the health needs of the pregnant or lactating woman and her infant.

SUMMARY

- Anatomic, physiologic, and psychological variables of pregnancy influence the pharmacokinetics and pharmacodynamics of drug therapy.
- Understanding the physical changes of pregnancy as well as the indications for and risk-benefit ratio of drugs used during pregnancy and lactation assists the health care provider in safely managing drug therapy.
- Maternal physiologic factors affecting drug response during pregnancy include reduced tone and motility of the gastrointestinal tract, altered secretion of hydrochloric acid, weight gain, rises in fluid volumes and blood pressure, higher production of plasma proteins, such as fibrinogen, and greater competition for plasma protein–binding sites.
- Fetal factors affecting drug response during pregnancy include the fetus's immature hepatic and renal systems, reduced plasma protein–binding sites, umbilical blood flow, immature blood-brain barrier, a high proportion of water to body mass, and placental metabolism.
- Only free, unbound drug exerts a pharmacologic effect. During pregnancy, the levels of serum albumin are reduced, promoting an increase in the amount of unbound drug.
- Unbound drugs in the maternal plasma are able to cross the placenta into the fetal compartment.
- Drug exposure may have therapeutic or teratogenic effects on the fetus. Teratogenicity is influenced by the susceptibility of the individual fetus, the timing of use of the offending drug, the characteristics of the teratogen, the mechanism of action that triggers changes in developing cells, the manifestation of the insult, and the dosage of the offending drug.
- The FDA pregnancy classification system for risk factors associated with systemic drug use is based on the level of known risk the drug presents to the fetus.
- When drug therapy is unavoidable, it becomes the responsibility of the health care provider to maintain a current knowledge base in order to best respond to the health needs of the pregnant or lactating woman and her baby.
- When possible, drug therapy for a breastfeeding woman should be delayed until her infant is weaned or is not totally dependent on breast milk for its nutrition.
- When exposure to drugs through breast milk is inevitable, the parents should be taught to monitor the infant and report any changes in levels of activity, changes in behavior or feeding patterns, or skin rashes.

BIBLIOGRAPHY

American Academy of Pediatrics Committee on Drugs. (1994). The transfer of drugs and other chemicals into human milk. *Pediatrics*, 93(1), 137–150.

Blackburn, S., and Loper, D. (1992). *Maternal, fetal and neonatal physiology: A clinical perspective.* Philadelphia: W. B. Saunders.

Brent, R., Beckkman, D., and Landel, C. (1993). Clinical teratology. *Current Opinions in Pediatrics*, 5(2), 201–211.

Callister, L. (1995). Beliefs and perceptions of childbearing women choosing different primary health care providers. *Clinical Nursing Research*, 4(2), 72–73.

Cunningham, F., MacDonald, P., and Gant, N. (1993). *Williams obstetrics* (19th ed.). Norwalk, CT: Appleton & Lange.

D'Avanzo, C. (1992). Bridging the cultural gap with Southeast Asians. *Maternal-Child Nursing*, 17, 204–208.

Dafnis, E., and Sabatini, S. (1992). The effects of pregnancy on renal function: Physiology and pathophysiology. *The American Journal of the Medical Sciences*, 303(3), 184–205.

Elkus, R., and Popovich, J. (1992). Respiratory physiology in pregnancy. *Clinics in Chest Medicine*, 13(4), 555–565.

Farrar, J., and Blumer, J. (1991). Fetal effects of maternal drug exposure. *Annual Review of Pharmacology and Toxicology*, 31, 525–547.

Gabbe, S., Niebyl, J., and Simpson, J. (Eds.). (1996). *Obstetrics: Normal and problem pregnancies.* New York: Churchill Livingstone.

Hou, S. (1991). Pregnancy in women with renal disease. *AKF Nephrology Letter*, 8(1), 1–11.

James, D., Steer, P., Weiner, P., et al. (Eds.). (1995). *High risk pregnancy: Management options.* London: W. B. Saunders, LTD.

Karboski, J. (1991). Medication selection for pregnant women. *The Female Patient*, 16(5), 15–23.

Knuppel, R., and Drukker, R. (Eds.). (1993). *High-risk pregnancy: A team approach.* Philadelphia: W. B. Saunders.

Lipson, J., Dibble, S., and Minarik, P. (1996). *Culture and nursing care: A pocket guide.* San Francisco: University of California San Francisco Nursing Press.

Mattson, S., and Lew, L. (1992). Culturally sensitive prenatal care for Southeast Asians. *Journal of Obstetric, Gynecologic, and Neonatal Nursing*, 21(1), 48–54.

McCance, K., and Huether, S. (Eds.). (1994). *Pathophysiology: The biologic basis for disease in adults and children.* St. Louis: C.V. Mosby.

Nicholes, F., and Zwelling, E. (1997). *Maternal-newborn nursing: Theory and practice.* Philadelphia: W. B. Saunders.

Niswander, K., and Evans, A. (Eds.). (1996). *Manual of obstetrics: Diagnosis and therapy.* Boston: Little, Brown & Co.

O'Dea, R. (1992). Medication use in the breastfeeding mother. *NAACOG's Clinical Issues in Perinatal and Women's Health Nursing,* 3(4), 598–604.

Olds, S., London, M., and Ladewig, P. (1996). Physical and psychological changes of pregnancy. In *Maternal newborn nursing.* Menlo Park, CA: Addison-Wesley Nursing.

Ornoy, A. (1993). Clinical teratology. In Fetal Medicine (Special Issue). *Western Journal of Medicine,* 159(3), 382–390.

Plessinger, M., and Woods, J. (1993). Maternal, placental and fetal pathophysiology of cocaine exposure during pregnancy. *Clinical Obstetrics and Gynecology,* 36(2), 267–278.

Porreco, R. (Ed.). (1991). *Contemporary obstetrics for medical students.* Ithaca, NY: Perinatology Press.

Queenan, J., and Hobbins, J. (Eds.). (1996). *Protocols for high risk pregnancy.* Cambridge, MA: Blackwell Scientific.

Rayburn, W., and Zuspan, F. (1992). *Drug therapy in obstetrics and gynecology.* St. Louis: Mosby-Year Book.

Reece, E., Hobbins, J., Mahoney, M., et al. (1995). *Handbook of medicine of the fetus & mother.* Philadelphia: J.B. Lippincott Co.

Rubin, P. (1990). Prescribing in pregnancy. *Practitioner,* 234(1489), 556–560.

Scott, J., DiSaia, P., Hammond, C., et al. (Eds.). (1994). *Danforth's obstetrics and gynecology.* Philadelphia: J.B. Lippincott Co.

Spector, R. (1991). *Cultural diversity in health and illness.* Norwalk, CT: Appleton & Lange.

Szeto, H. (1993). Kinetics of drug transfer to the fetus. *Clinical Obstetrics and Gynecology,* 36(2), 246–254.

Thorp, J., and Gaston, L. (1993). Antepartum prevention of intraventricular hemorrhage in the premature newborn. *Perinatal Hotline,* 7(1), 1–4.

Ward, R. (1992). Maternal drug therapy for fetal disorders. *Seminars in Perinatology,* 16(1), 12–20.

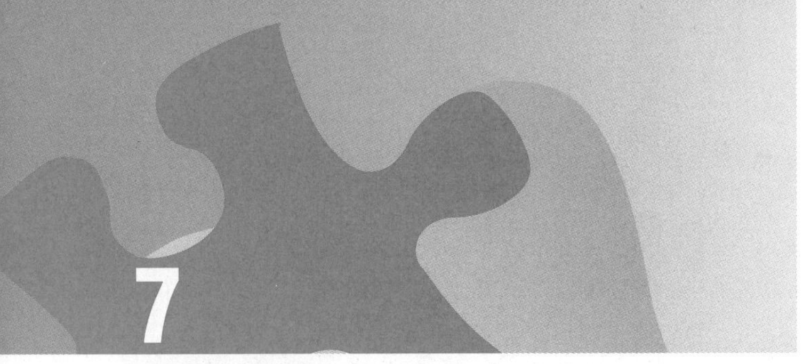

7 Pediatric Pharmacotherapeutics

In the last decade, an estimated 12 percent of all prescriptions written in the United States have been for children younger than 9 years of age. In spite of that fact, the term *therapeutic orphan* has been applied to pharmacotherapeutics in children because of the relative deficiency of information on drug safety and efficacy. The pharmaceutical industry has generated a wealth of data for adults, but similar studies in the pediatric population have not been done. Furthermore, only a quarter of the drugs approved by the Food and Drug Administration (FDA) have specific indications for use in the pediatric population. Children differ from adults and from one another in regard to drug absorption, distribution, biotransformation, and elimination. The pharmacokinetic and pharmacodynamic components of pediatric drug therapy become a unique challenge because of differences in body composition and in maturation of various organ systems (Fig. 7–1). There is every reason to believe that pharmacokinetic behavior during infancy and childhood, and even during adolescence, differs from that in adulthood. Application of the principles of pharmacodynamics to the pediatric patient has contributed to improved treatment regimens.

There are several reasons for the lack of extrinsic pharmacokinetic information in children. Pharmacokinetic studies require that multiple blood samples be taken to adequately define a dose-time-response curve; children and their parents are resistant to multiple venipunctures. There are also ethical constraints on clinical research in children. Important differences remain, however, in the way children of different ages absorb, distribute, biotransform, and eliminate drugs. These differences must be addressed as a foundation for understanding and managing pharmacotherapeutics in pediatric patients. Indeed, federal legislation enacted in 1997 calls for the FDA and the pharmaceutical industry to correct this deficiency.

ANATOMIC AND PHYSIOLOGIC VARIABLES

Drug therapy for children requires an understanding of the anatomic and physiologic differences between children and adults. Assessment of the pediatric patient is contingent upon the health care provider's understanding of these characteristics and their related clinical significance. Because children's body systems grow and develop at different rates, generalizations about the use of drugs in this population are not possible.

Body Composition and Size

Significant changes in body weight occur in infancy and childhood. The child is smaller in height and weight than an adult, and the proportions are different. A child's weight increases about 20 times between birth and adulthood, but height increases only three and one-half times. A child's weight in kilograms may be estimated using the following formula:

$$\text{Weight (kg)} = 8 + 2\ (\text{age in years})$$

Approximate weight may also be estimated according to age by using the following general rules:

- Two times the birth weight by 5 months
- Three times the birth weight by 12 months
- Seven times the birth weight by 7 years
- Fourteen times the birth weight by 14 years

Commercially available charts and devices have been developed to assist in the estimation of weight in infants and children in emergent situations. Accurate estimates of weight are essential for proper pharmacotherapy.

The concept of body surface area (BSA) is important in pediatrics, because many physiologic functions are proportional to body surface area (Fig. 7–2). The child's proportionally large head accounts for much of the exposed surface area. The BSA, estimated as the relationship between height and weight, is about seven times greater in adulthood than at birth. Physiologic parameters influenced by body surface area include the metabolic rate, extracellular fluid and plasma volumes, cardiac output, and glomerular filtration rate.

Infants are particularly susceptible to significant changes in total body water because of their high metabolic rates.

Fluid Balance

The amount and distribution of total body water change with age. Total body water comprises intracellular and extracellular fluids. Water is the major constituent of body tissues. Total body water generally ranges from 58 to 60 percent of total body weight (Table 7–1). The importance of body water to body function is related not only to its abundance but also to the medium in which solutes are dissolved and in which all metabolic reactions take place. Metabolism (all chemical and energy transformations in the body) is affected by an assortment of intrinsic and extrinsic factors. Therefore, metabolic needs vary among individuals and within each individual.

The basal metabolic rate changes distinctively throughout childhood. Highest in the infant, this rate closely relates to the proportion of surface area to body mass. In both sexes, the proportion decreases progressively to maturity. The rate of fluid intake and fluid elimination in the infant is seven times as great, in relation to body weight, as in the adult. In the premature infant, body water makes up approximately 86 percent of total body weight. In the immedi-

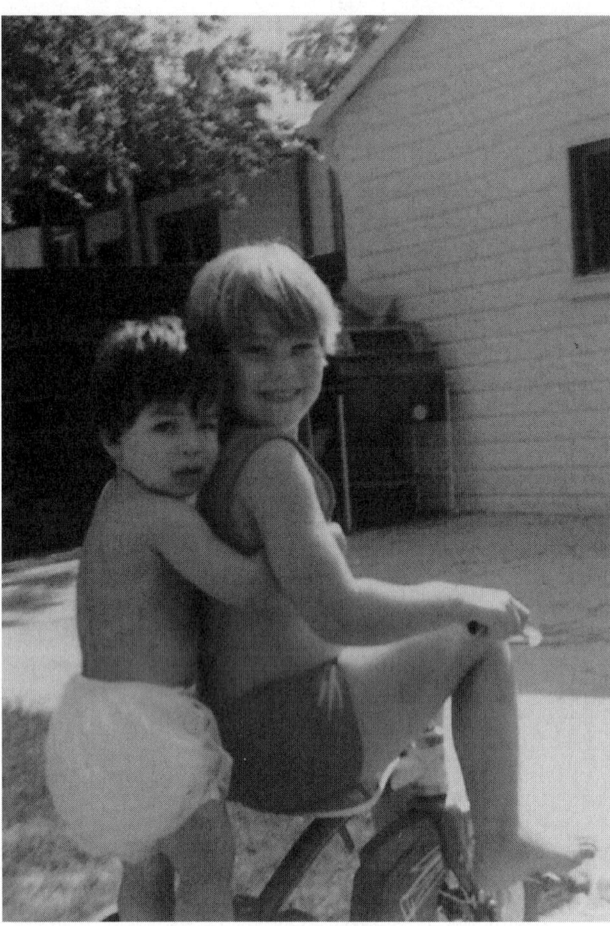

Figure 7–1 Developmental changes influencing pharmacotherapy:

- Cardiac output is rate dependent rather than stroke dependent until late school age and adolescence, which makes the heart rate more rapid
- Increased gastric pH; gastrointestinal motility is dependent on maturity of body systems
- Increased total body water in neonates and infants
- Proportion of body weight in water is greater before school age with more water in extracellular spaces
- Reduced albumin concentration and plasma protein binding
- Metabolic rates are two times higher than those of adults
- Unstable glucose concentrations, unable to concentrate bilirubin
- Twenty-five percent of an infant's weight is muscle; muscles lack tone, power, and coordination
- Ineffective renal concentration of urine before age 12 to 18 months
- Immature hepatic enzyme capacities and activity

ate postnatal period, as the infant adjusts to a new environment, there is a physiologic loss of body water amounting to 5 percent of body weight. Total body water, which in newborn infants is approximately 70 to 80 percent of body weight (50 percent contained in extracellular fluid), decreases to about 67 percent during the first year of life. It reaches adult levels of 60 percent by about the age of 2 years. The body weight of the infant is composed of 35 percent intracellular and 45 percent extracellular fluid.

Total body water throughout childhood is approximately 60 percent of body weight. During adolescence, the percentage of body water approaches that of an adult, but gender differences begin to appear. Males eventually have a greater percentage of body water because of increasing muscle mass. Proportionally, females have more body fat and less muscle mass as a function of estrogens. They therefore have comparatively less body water. Daily water turnover in children involves more than half of the extracellular fluid; in the adult, one-fifth of the extracellular fluid is exchanged daily. Because of a child's greater proportion of body fluid, especially in the extracellular compartment, larger milligram per kilogram doses of certain drugs are required in order to achieve therapeutic drug levels.

Tissue Mass

Skeletal growth and muscle development in healthy children consist of two concurrent processes: the creation of new cells and tissues (growth) and the consolidation of the new

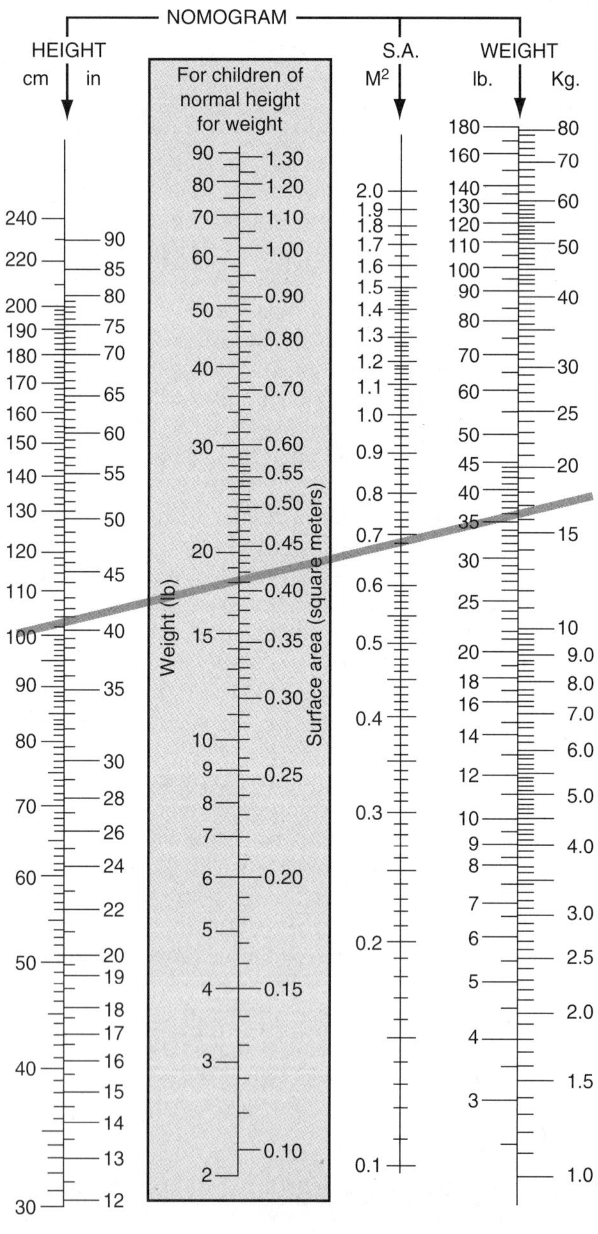

Figure 7–2 West Nomogram for estimating body surface area. Body surface area is indicated where the shaded line connecting height and weight intersect the surface area (SA) column or if the patient is of approximately normal proportion from weight alone (see highlighted central column). (Adapted from data of E. Boyd by C.D. West presented in Behrman, R.E., Kliegman, R.M., and Arvin, A.M. [1996]. *Nelson textbook of pediatrics* [15th ed., P. 670]. Philadelphia: W.B. Saunders. Used with permission.)

TABLE 7–1 BODY WEIGHT COMPOSITION IN PERCENTAGES

	Components (% of Body Weight)			
Age (Weight)	EXTRA-CELLULAR FLUID	INTRA-CELLULAR FLUID	TOTAL BODY WATER	FAT
Premature infant (1.5 kg)	60	40	83–86	1
Full-term infant (3.5 kg)	45–47	32–35	70–80	16
1 year old (10 kg)	40	60	60	22–24
4 year old	24	41	40	12
10 year old	15	40	60	18–20
Adult male	40	60	60	15

Adapted and used with permission from Howry, L., Bindler, R., and Tso, Y. (1981). *Pediatric medications.* Philadelphia: J.B. Lippincott.

tissues into a permanent form (maturation). In the infant, muscle mass accounts for approximately 25 percent of total body weight, compared with 40 percent in the adult. The composition and size of muscles vary with age. In the fetus, muscle tissue contains large amounts of water and intracellular matrix. After birth, both are considerably reduced as muscle fibers enlarge to accommodate additional cytoplasm.

Gender differences in muscle size and weight are minor during childhood but become considerable with the onset of puberty. Muscle growth during adolescence is a major factor in weight gain. Muscle fibers reach maximal size at about age 10 in females and age 14 in males. Therefore, the younger the child, the less muscle tissue is available for injections.

Body fat makes up approximately 16 percent of an infant's birth weight. Between the ages of 1 and 5 years, fat levels fall to between 8 and 12 percent. The levels increase again at about age 10, to 18 to 20 percent of body weight. Because drugs are water soluble or fat soluble, the percentage of body fat affects drug distribution. The relative mass of subcutaneous tissue in children also varies. Premature infants have very little fatty tissue. Fatty tissue development reaches a peak at 9 months and then decreases again until about 6 years. In adolescence, subcutaneous tissue once again increases.

Head and Neck

In children, the head is large in proportion to the rest of the body. The bones of the skull are softer and more pliable, and there is a greater percentage of blood in their heads. The cartilage of the larynx is softer. The larynx is positioned more anteriorly and cephaloid. The cricoid cartilage is the narrowest part of the larynx. Muscular support of the neck is weak in the young child, and the eustachian tube is shorter and straighter. Frequent ear infections occur owing to increased mucus in the eustachian tube during milk consumption, which creates a perfect medium for bacteria.

Respiratory System

The immature immune and respiratory systems of children allow for more respiratory disease than in the adult. Infants are obligate nose breathers for the first 2 to 4 months of life. Nasal passages must be kept clear of secretions to prevent respiratory distress. The child's tongue and epiglottis are larger than an adult's. The airways of a child are smaller and narrower from the trachea to the terminal bronchioles, so a relatively small amount of mucus or mucosal edema may cause obstruction. Any obstruction of the airway greatly lowers resistance to airflow and increases oxygen requirements as well as the work of breathing. The diameter of an infant's trachea approximates that of the infant's little finger. An infant relies primarily on the diaphragm for breathing. The thorax is pliable, the lungs have fewer alveoli than an adult's, and the intercostal muscles are poorly developed, leading to lower lung compliance.

The physiologic differences in the respiratory tracts of children and adults involve metabolic rates and immunocompetence. Because of higher metabolic rates and oxygen consumption, children rely on respiratory function to a greater extent than adults. The proportionately larger body surface area and respiratory rate of children lead to rapid heat and water loss during infection or fever. For example, dehydration and its resulting acidosis may occur rapidly during the times of decreased oral intake that frequently accompany acute infections in children.

Children are more vulnerable to infections of the respiratory tract than adults, have not had time to develop immunity to most organisms, and are commonly exposed to respiratory tract infections through contact with other children. They also have less compensatory reserve than adults, owing to the size and immaturity of the respiratory tract. Collateral pathways of ventilation are incompletely developed. Children have less elastic and collagen tissue in the lungs, and therefore greater susceptibility to edema. The metabolic rate in infants is approximately two times that in adults, thereby increasing the need for oxygen. Anything that raises the metabolic rate contributes to respiratory demands.

Cardiovascular System

Cardiovascular dynamics of the young child change during the transition from fetus to newborn, from newborn to young child, and from child to adult. These dynamics affect the uptake and distribution of drugs.

The heart rate and stroke volume are greater in a child than in an adult. Like respiration and body metabolism, the cardiac output of the newborn is about two times as much in relation to body weight as that of the adult, or approximately 550 mL/min. The child's circulating blood volume is less than that of the adult (infant, 90 mL/kg; child, 80 mL/kg; adult, 60 mL/kg). Further, peripheral circulation is poorly developed in the infant, so blood flow to various muscles changes a great deal during the first 2 weeks of life. The overall changes in cardiovascular dynamics ultimately affect the uptake and distribution of drugs.

Gastrointestinal System

Although most of the alterations in gastrointestinal (GI) functioning are caused by congenital obstructions, liver disease, and disorders of digestion and absorption, defects of nutrition also influence drug action. The characteristics of the GI system are a major influence on the speed and efficiency with which drugs are absorbed into the body. For example, the gastric emptying time in a newborn is 6 to 8 hours, compared with 2 hours in an adult. In addition, peristalsis may be irregular in young infants. Absorption of fats is somewhat lower than in the older child. Consequently, milk with a high fat content (e.g., cow's milk) commonly is inadequately utilized. The secretion of pancreatic amylase in the newborn infant is also deficient, so the infant utilizes starches less effectively.

The gastric pH in neonates ranges from 5 to 8. It drops to a more acidic pH of 1 to 3 within the first day of life, and then reaches adult levels at about 4 months of age. Mechanisms by which food interferes with drug therapy may also cause alterations in the amount, type, and osmolality of GI secretions, pH, transit time, and motility. The ionization, solubility, and stability of a drug may also be altered. As a result, a drug-food complex alters the drug's distribution, biotransformation, and elimination.

Liver function develops considerably during infancy, so the greatest risk for drug toxicity is to the newborn. The ability to produce biotransformational enzymes occurs at varying rates in the young child. The immature liver of the newborn is unable to form plasma proteins, so their concentrations are 15 to 20 percent less than those in older children. The lower plasma concentration of protein for binding with drugs makes children particularly vulnerable to the harmful effects of drugs. Idiosyncratic responses to various drugs may occur as a result of changes in protein binding at different stages of childhood.

Renal System

Most drugs are excreted in the urine through three mechanisms: glomerular filtration, tubular secretion, and tubular reabsorption. Glomerular filtration is the most common mechanism by which drugs are excreted. The glomerular filtration rate in infants is 30 to 50 percent that of an adult. Therefore, drugs excreted through the kidneys have a half-life approximately 50 percent longer in infants than in adults.

Tubular secretion employs carrier mechanisms to eliminate substances. The infant's secretory capacity is less than the adult's, because of fewer tubular cells, shorter tubule length, and smaller rates of tubular blood flow. Tubular secretion reaches adult levels by about 7 months of age.

Tubular reabsorption preserves substances coming through the renal tubule. The kidney of a newborn can concentrate urine to only one and one-half times the osmolality of plasma, instead of the three to four times normal found in the adult. When considering the immaturity of the kidneys and marked fluid turnover in the infant, one can readily understand that among the most important considerations in all drug, fluid, and electrolyte therapy for children are the ability to concentrate or dilute urine and the ability to excrete.

Neurologic System

The central nervous system of a young child is immature. Reflexes present in an adult may be absent in an infant. However, as an infant matures, neonatal reflexes disappear in a predictable sequence and are replaced by voluntary motor functions. During the first year of life, the presence or absence of the various reflexes is indicative of the extent of myelinization that has occurred.

All primary structures of the brain are present at birth but they grow over the first few years of life. The brain has 25 percent of its mature adult weight at birth, 75 percent by 2½ years, and 90 percent by 6 years. The mature brain is protected by a structure known as the blood-brain barrier, which prevents substances from diffusing freely out of the circulatory system into brain cells. The myelinization that produces the blood-brain barrier is not mature in children younger than 2 years, leading to unpredictable pharmacotherapeutic results. In certain pathologic conditions, such as hyperbilirubinemia, there is an increase in the permeability of the blood-brain barrier.

Immune System

An infant receives much of its passive immunity from its mother. Antibodies diffuse from the mother's blood through the placenta to the fetus. Infants less than 2 or 3 months old have immature immune systems and need this acquired immunity. Passively acquired antibodies are lost over the first 3 to 6 months of life. Although the immune mechanisms continue to mature during childhood, the immaturity of the young child's immune system increases the susceptibility to a number of childhood diseases. For example, the inherited antibodies against pertussis (whooping cough) are normally insufficient to protect the neonate. Therefore, the infant requires immunization against this disease by 2 months of age. Immunizations are discussed further in Chapter 28.

The immaturity of the immune system may also lead to altered or depressed allergic responses to foreign substances. It is not until the infant's own antibodies begin to form that allergic states can develop. Allergic responses include eczema, GI upset, drug rashes, scalded skin syndrome, and (rarely) anaphylaxis.

As the child grows older and establishes still higher levels of immunity, the allergic manifestations usually dissipate.

PHARMACOKINETIC CONSIDERATIONS

Data on the pharmacokinetics, pharmacodynamics, efficacy, and safety of drugs in infants and children are scarce. Thus, drug therapy in the pediatric patient presents a challenge to the health care provider. Maturational changes provide some guidance in understanding the complex nature of pharmacokinetic principles. A poorly developed blood-brain barrier, weak biotransformational activity, and immature mechanisms for elimination combine to make the fetus and neonate vulnerable to toxic drug effects.

Individualized pharmacokinetic evaluation allows optimization of drug therapy so that benefits may be maximized and risks minimized. The most pressing need in pediatric pharmacotherapy is the formulation of a distinct, rational therapeutic plan, with subsequent individualization of drug dosage based on careful assessment of the patient. There is little doubt that sound pharmacokinetic information can contribute to a more rapid achievement of optimal dosages. Table 7–2 summarizes age-related physiologic factors related to pharmacokinetic drug action.

TABLE 7–2 SUMMARY OF PHYSIOLOGIC FACTORS THAT ALTER PHARMACOKINETIC VARIABLES

Pharmacokinetic Component	Age Group	Physiologic Factor	Comment
Absorption	Neonates, infants, young children	Increased gastric pH	Increased bioavailability of basic drugs and reduced bioavailability of acidic drugs
	Neonates, infants	Reduced gastric and intestinal motility	
	Infants, children	Increased gastric and intestinal motility	Bioavailability unpredictable
	Neonates	Decreased bile acids	Bioavailability is reduced
Distribution	Neonates, infants	Increased total body water and extracellular fluid	Volume of distribution is increased
		Reduced albumin concentration and protein binding	Volume of distribution is increased. Concentration of free drug is increased
Biotransformation	Neonates, infants	Immature enzyme capacity	Half-life increases but clearance is reduced
Elimination	Neonates, infants	Immature glomerular and tubular function	Half-life increases
	Young children	Increased enzyme capacity	Clearance increases but half-life is reduced

Absorption

Drug absorption depends on the route of administration, disintegration, dissociation, drug concentration, blood flow to the site, and absorptive surface area. Two factors affecting the absorption of drugs from the GI tract are pH-dependent diffusion and gastric emptying time. Both processes are strikingly different in a premature infant compared with older children and adults. Age-related variables such as delayed gastric emptying time and irregular intestinal motility are examples of mechanisms that affect absorption. The rate of absorption also depends on the specific characteristics of the drug and the child.

Oral Route

Drug absorption *via* the oral route depends on a number of factors. Drug formulation, the degree of disintegration and dissociation, concentration, blood flow to the site and the absorptive surface area, pH-dependent diffusion, and gastric motility all influence the process.

Absorption of orally administered drugs is often delayed in neonates and young infants, owing primarily to differences in the pH of the GI tract and reduced gastric motility. Immediately after birth, gastric pH is high. By 4 months of age, gastric pH values have reached 50 percent of the adult value (pH 1 to 3.5), and by 3 years of age, they are thought to reach adult levels. Thus, the pH of gastric contents remains less acidic during infancy and early childhood. Acidic drugs, such as nalidixic acid, phenobarbital, and phenytoin, are less well absorbed. On the other hand, the absorption of acid-labile drugs (e.g., penicillin) may be enhanced.

Gastric emptying time is 6 to 8 hours in the neonate but reaches the adult time of 2 hours by 6 to 8 months of age. Prolonged exposure of certain drugs to gastric contents increases the disintegration of unstable drugs and also delays drug entry into the lower GI tract, so drug absorption and attainment of peak serum levels are delayed.

Parenteral Routes

Any condition that alters muscle growth decreases the number of muscle sites suitable for intramuscular injections. Intramuscular drug absorption may be uncertain because of unpredictable blood flow, decreased muscle tone, lower muscle oxygenation, and vasomotor instability. Repeated injections in the child's few available muscle sites may cause tissue breakdown and less absorption of the drug. The absorption of drugs administered by the percutaneous route, however, is increased because of an underdeveloped epidermal barrier and greater permeability of the skin.

The intravenous route of administration is commonly used in pediatric therapy. For some drugs, it is the only effective route. When a drug is administered intravenously, the effect is almost instantaneous, and further control is limited. Most drugs intended for intravenous administration require a specified minimum dilution and/or rate of infusion.

Intraosseous cannulation provides a reliable method for rapidly achieving venous access in emergent situations, particularly in children younger than 6 years. In general, any intravenous drug or fluid can be safely administered by the intraosseous route. Reports of successful administration of catecholamines, calcium, antibiotics, digitalis, heparin, lidocaine, atropine, phenytoin, sodium bicarbonate, neuromuscular blocking drugs, crystalloids, colloids, and blood can be found in the literature. This route is used temporarily, until other venous access sites become available. The flat, anteromedial surface of the tibia, approximately 1 to 3 cm below the tibial tuberosity, is the preferred site.

Topical Routes

The absorption rate of a topically administered drug is not different in a child. However, more of the drug is absorbed in a child because of greater body surface area and skin permeability in relation to total body mass. When occlusive dressings are used, absorption of a topically administered drug is enhanced, and the possibility of adverse reactions increased, particularly to steroid creams, salicylic acid, and silver sulfadiazine. Corticosteroids are purposefully applied sparingly in children to prevent absorption that may lead to adrenal suppression. Growth retardation may occur if the adrenal glands are suppressed before bone epiphyses mature.

A few drugs are known for their bioavailability when given rectally, and this avenue provides an alternative to oral or parenteral routes. Rectal administration is generally disliked but may be preferred over intramuscular injection. Furthermore, acceptance of rectal administration may be culturally influenced. Drugs available in suppository form include acetaminophen, sedatives, antiemetics, and analgesics such as morphine.

Distribution

Many age-related differences in drug distribution occur during the first 10 to 12 months of life. The distribution of a drug in children is affected by the changing percentage of body fat, total body water content, total blood volume, and blood flow to target tissues as well as by the ability of the drug to exit capillaries and move into cells.

Drug distribution and equilibration rates may be faster in children than in adults. Therefore, a larger average dose per kilogram of body weight is needed to reach desired serum concentration levels. The higher the percentage of body water, the greater the dilution of water-soluble drugs. The result is reduced serum concentration levels. As the percentage of body fat increases with age, so does the distribution of fat-soluble drugs. Therefore, the distribution of these drugs is more limited in children than in adults.

Decreased formation of plasma proteins in the immature liver of infants also affects drug distribution and results in higher serum drug levels. Factors influencing protein binding are the amount of albumin and/or alpha$_1$-acid glycoproteins available, the pH of the blood, the binding capacity of the albumin, and other substances in the child's system that compete for binding sites with the available albumin.

The albumin in neonates and infants has a lower binding capacity for certain drugs (e.g., phenytoin, penicillin) compared with the binding capacity of mature albumin. Therefore, more unbound drug is free to circulate and produce effects. Thus, it is possible that free drug levels will be high enough to produce adverse or toxic effects. To minimize the possibility of toxicity and to compensate for the shorter duration of drug action, it is often necessary to decrease the amount of the drug given and/or lengthen the time between doses.

In contrast, adverse effects may occur when drugs such as salicylates, penicillins, sulfonamides, phenytoin, phenobarbital, and imipramine compete with endogenous substances (e.g., free fatty acids, bilirubin) for the same protein binding sites. Competitive drug binding in the neonate increases the potential for adverse effects from increased concentrations of unbound, unconjugated bilirubin. *Kernicterus* (bilirubin encephalopathy) is a grave condition in which the basal ganglia and other areas of the brain and spinal cord are infiltrated with bilirubin. The higher permeability of the blood-brain barrier in children allows this to occur. Any drug that competes with bilirubin for protein binding sites or that inhibits the binding of bilirubin increases the risk. The signs of kernicterus are those of central nervous system depression or excitation, such as decreased activity, lethargy, irritability, and loss of interest in feeding, seizures, and gastric or pulmonary hemorrhage.

Biotransformation

Most biotransformation of drugs is performed in the liver by microsomal enzymes. The activities of the hepatic enzymes are low in the neonate and premature infants. The capacity of an infant's liver to biotransform drugs develops quickly during the first months after birth. The capacity to biotransform drugs varies with the enzymes involved. Phase I, nonsynthetic reaction of hydroxylation, is most affected. Depression of hydroxylation causes longer plasma half-lives in neonates, so the interval between doses should be increased and/or the daily dose decreased.

Phase II reactions, such as conjugation with glucuronic acid, are variably reduced. Lower conjugating activity contributes to *hyperbilirubinemia* and the risk of bilirubin-induced encephalopathy. Altered biotransformation processes persist for approximately the first month of life, undergoing a dramatic increase at about 6 months.

It is almost impossible to predict the effect of maturation on biotransformation solely on the basis of age. Metabolic rates and hepatic drug oxidation remain markedly elevated for the first 2 to 3 years of life. Rates gradually decrease until puberty, when adult levels are reached. The plasma half-lives of diazepam, digoxin, indomethacin, acetaminophen, and phenobarbital appear to be longer in infants.

The first pass effect has received little attention in pediatric populations but has been demonstrated with a number of drugs. For example, the mean plasma half-life for phenytoin and phenobarbital decreases from 80 hours between birth and 2 days of age to about 15 hours at age 3 to 14 days, and then declines to 6 hours (approximate adult level) between 14 and 150 days after birth.

Dosages and choice of drug may be altered for an infant with immature liver function or liver disease. For example, the antimicrobial drug chloramphenicol is not inadequately metabolized before toxic levels are reached. *Gray baby syndrome* results. This disorder is characterized by tachypnea, ashen-gray cyanosis, vomiting, loose green stools, progressive abdominal distention, vasomotor collapse, and perhaps death. Discontinuing the drug as soon as symptoms appear can reverse progression of symptoms.

Body temperature regulation is unstable in children, creating implications for drug action. When infants and toddlers develop an infection, the sudden high temperature increases basal metabolic rates. For each degree centigrade rise in body temperature, the metabolic rate increases by approximately 12 percent. The higher metabolic rate reduces drug half-lives and duration of therapeutic effects. Antipyretic effects of drugs are short-lived because of this phenomenon.

Elimination

Renal function is lower in infants and small children than in adults. Glomerular filtration rate, concentrating and acidifying functions, and tubular function, including secretion and reabsorption, all influence drug action. These factors are reflected in prolonged elimination, increasing the risk for toxicity. Each of the processes mature at a different rate, so the clearance of various drugs may be greater in infants than in older children or adults. There is a disproportionate development of renal filtration and secretion in relation to reabsorption. Full renal function develops in infants by 6 to 12 months of age.

The neonate has glomerular cells at birth, but they are functionally immature. Digoxin, for example, depends on the glomerular filtration rate for elimination. Because of the rapid increase in glomerular filtration rate during the first few weeks of life, the dosage of digoxin may have to be increased in order to maintain the desired serum drug level.

During the first 6 months of life, an infant has a small number of tubular cells, a shorter tubular length, and a lower tubular blood flow. Dosages of drugs that depend on the kidneys for elimination must be adjusted to avoid toxic responses. When renal blood flow increases in response to a rise in systemic arterial pressure, intrarenal vascular resistance decreases. This response permits the kidneys to receive a higher percentage of the cardiac output and the circulating drug. Therefore, drugs that depend on tubular secretion for elimination, such as the penicillins, have a longer half-life.

Drug elimination is also affected by the urinary pH, because some drugs are more readily eliminated in acid urine but others require a more basic urine in order to be excreted. An infant's kidneys are less able to excrete hydrogen ions and reabsorb bicarbonate. As a result, the infant's urine is slightly less acidic than an adult's.

The clearance of drugs is important to pharmacokinetics, mainly because there are no operative assumptions about drug distribution in pediatric patients. For example, clearance rates of theophylline are low in infancy but increase fivefold by 4 years of age and then slowly decline over the years. Theophylline is biotransformed to caffeine in the neonate, whereas adults rapidly biotransform theophylline to inactive metabolites. Both theophylline and caffeine are methylxanthines with similar drug actions. Toxicity can be produced in the neonate through additive mechanisms.

The net effect of organ immaturity is the potential for drugs to accumulate in the body. Drug dosages may need to be adjusted to maintain a desired serum level and to avoid toxicity.

PHARMACODYNAMIC CONSIDERATIONS

Drugs produce the same biochemical mechanism of action in all individuals, including children. If a drug normally inhibits the transfer of a substance into a cell, it does so in any age group. The response to the drug, however, varies according to the maturity of the target organ and the specific drug receptor's.

Critical Thinking Process

Assessment

History of Present Illness

Other than the obvious age-related differences between children and adults, assessment of the child resembles that of the adult, with certain additions. The patient's history should provide information pertinent to the course of the child's illness. Specific questions should address the onset, duration, and severity of signs and symptoms, and any treatment that was attempted. Children 5 years of age or older are usually able to add to the history. They often describe more accurately than parents the severity of symptoms and their own levels of concern. Sometimes the accuracy of the information can be improved by interviewing the child without the parent in attendance.

Further, it should be clearly determined whether the chief complaint is the problem of the patient, the parent(s), or both. It should be noted that the chief complaint may get the patient into the health care system, a sort of "admission ticket." However, once with the health care provider, the child or parent may bring up another problem that in and of itself was not viewed as a legitimate reason for seeking care. The provider should attempt to create an atmosphere that facilitates effective communication and allows the child or parent to express these concerns.

Past Health History

A pediatric past health history provides information about operations and injuries, hospitalizations, drug history, birth history (i.e., prenatal, natal, and neonatal history—particularly important during the first 2 years of life), feeding history, and childhood illnesses. Knowledge of the feeding history (i.e., breast, bottle, solid foods) helps the health care provider to identify problems of under- and over-nutrition. The use of vitamin and iron supplements and immunization history should also be noted.

Special attention should be paid to children who have immigrated, because they may have received immunizations that are not routinely administered in the United States. Specific dates of each vaccine should be noted so that an ongoing record can be maintained throughout childhood and adolescence. Any untoward reactions to specific vaccines should also be noted. For example, limited immunity can be produced by administration of bacille Calmette-Guérin vaccine, which produces definite but incomplete (about 50 percent) protection against tuberculosis. Bacille Calmette-Guérin vaccination is not generally recommended for use in the United States.

Particular attention should be paid to allergies prevalent during infancy and childhood. The allergies are often manifested as insect hypersensitivity, perennial allergic rhinitis, urticaria, and eczema.

Information on existing or past conditions that are familial or hereditary in parents, grandparents, aunts, uncles, and siblings should be obtained. Drug regimens can be affected in a patient with an existing history of, or potential for, glaucoma, cataracts, tuberculosis, asthma, heart disease, hypertension, kidney disease, arthritis, epilepsy, diabetes, and sickle cell disease.

Physical Exam

Emphasis during the pediatric physical exam should be placed on the anticipated findings and the signs and symptoms that accompany common pathologic conditions. The health care provider may anticipate a child's cooperative ability by merely asking the child where the physical exam should take place—in the parent's lap or on the exam table. A systematic approach to the exam minimizes the possibility of missing parts of it because of distraction by the child's behavior or the parent's questions.

Diagnostic Testing

Screening procedures, such as evaluations of vision and hearing, measurements of hemoglobin and hematocrit, and testing for phenylketonuria, galactosemia, sickle cell anemia, lead toxicity, and alpha$_1$-antitrypsin deficiency, may be indicated. Because pediatric patients have a limited ability to communicate when they are experiencing adverse drug effects, monitoring of therapeutic serum levels is especially useful. This is particularly true when the effects of a drug cannot be directly observed or when the drug has a narrow therapeutic index (e.g., anticonvulsants, antineoplastic drugs, theophylline, digoxin).

Developmental Considerations

The developmental status of a child places him or her at greater risk than an adult for physical and psychological trauma related to drug therapy. Taking the developmental aspects of a child into account can lead to a better understanding of the child's response to drug therapy. Considerations such as the developmental norms for fine motor skills, gross motor skills, feeding behavior, language, and social skills should be identified and used in the planning of appropriate medication administration techniques.

Psychosocial Considerations

Sensitivity to the issues of culture is essential in the care of children. The purpose of a cultural assessment is to identify health care patterns and beliefs that may be factors in treatment interventions. The detail and depth of the cultural assessment depend on the situation and the needs of the child and family. Cultural practices may involve the use of "protective devices" to keep the child from harm or illness or to help in the healing process (strings, cords, beads, amulets). These devices should be removed only by the patient or family and only when absolutely necessary. Cultural acceptance of clinical medicine may become a compliance issue as well.

Analysis and Management

As discussed in previous chapters, pharmacotherapeutics involves assessment of factors that affect administration, pharmacokinetics, effectiveness, and safety of a given drug regimen. The health care provider must be knowledgeable about common drug therapies and also about the biologic distinctions that affect pharmacokinetics in children.

Treatment Objectives

The primary treatment objective for the pediatric patient is to achieve appropriate outcomes while maintaining therapeutic drug levels and avoiding toxic effects. Treatment objectives include allaying fears and preventing injury associated with drug regimens. Principles relevant to pediatric pharmacotherapy are identified Pediatric Pharmacotherapeutic Principles.

Treatment Options

Treatment objectives may be accomplished by limiting the number of drugs prescribed (avoiding polypharmacy), avoiding inappropriate drug use (i.e., wanting to try out a new drug, or choosing a particular drug because samples are available), and ensuring that the drugs are taken as directed. Although some drugs pose a significant hazard to the pediatric patient, caution should be used until the health care provider has absolutely determined that a drug is indicated and appropriate for the child. Specific end points of therapy should be determined so that dosage can be optimized, irrational combinations avoided, and adverse effects minimized.

PEDIATRIC PHARMACOTHERAPEUTIC PRINCIPLES

- Provide explanations using language that is developmentally or age appropriate.
- Keep the time between explanation and administration to a minimum.
- Prepare drugs in advance, keeping needles and syringes out of sight.
- Expect success with positive approaches. Act smoothly and quickly.
- Be honest with the child, involving the child to gain cooperation (e.g., warning that a shot will hurt, emphasizing that drugs are not candy).
- Solicit the parent's help where appropriate.
- Provide distraction for a frightened or uncooperative child.
- Allow the child to express feelings; assure the child that crying is okay.
- Praise the child for doing his or her best.
- Spend time with the child after administering the medication.
- Let the child know he or she is accepted as a person of value.

In general, the least toxic, least expensive drug that treats the underlying cause of the child's illness (in preference to symptoms) should be chosen.

Intervention

Administration

Optimal tailoring of a drug dose to the neonate, infant, or child has long been a subject of discussion. Any method devised to calculate drug dosage for children (and adults) provides an estimate only, to be verified or corrected by clinical response and/or measurement of drug concentrations. No universal dosage rule can be recommended. Today, drug manufacturers usually recommend doses in milligrams per kilograms of body weight, which are generally expressed as ranges rather than fixed doses. There is ample evidence that dosage regimens cannot be based simply on data about body weight or surface area that has been extrapolated from adult data. Bioavailability, pharmacokinetics, efficacy, and adverse effects can differ markedly from patient to patient.

Pediatric pharmacotherapy requires that appropriate dosage regimens be designed to compensate for developmental changes and to optimize therapy at different stages of childhood. The fact that a pediatric dosage cannot be found in current publications and references should be evaluated carefully before any dose is calculated. If a pediatric dosage cannot be found in current drug references, the drug may not be suitable for pediatric use.

Table 7–3 is a summary of developmental considerations for each age group as they apply to drug administration. As is true for all procedures, parents and children require age-appropriate education about drug administration as well as information about the drug. Table 7–4 is a summary of nursing considerations for drug administration to infants and children. Further, an explanation of why the drug is given, what is expected of the child, and how the parent can participate and support the child should be given.

Infant. Oral drugs are delivered in liquid form by means of nipple, dropper, or syringe. The tongue move-

TABLE 7–3 DEVELOPMENTAL CONSIDERATIONS IN DRUG ADMINISTRATION

Developmental Age	Implications
Infancy (1 Month–1 Year)	
Period of most rapid growth	Poor head control requires support to minimize choking
Develops trust	Hands should be monitored to prevent interference
Limited to sensory and motor experiences	Drug agents require precise measurement
Enjoys sucking and eating	Physical comfort during administration calms the infant
Attends to environment	
Fears separation and strangers	
Toddler (1–2 Years)	
Growth rate decreases with a decrease in appetite	Allow child to choose a position to take the medication
Increased independence	Follow routine of home
Increased mobility	Taste of medication may be disguised
Enjoys exploration	Use single commands
Seeks parental reassurance	Allow child to familiarize self with dosing device
Fears loss of control, altered rituals	
Preschool (3–6 Years)	
Weight gain 2 kg/yr, height increases 6–8 cm/yr	Tablets and capsules should be crushed—most children this age are not capable of swallowing pills
Greater autonomy and initiative	Allow child to make decisions about dosage formulation and place of administration
Age of discovery, curiosity	More cooperative since understands relationships between illness and treatment
Sense of self vs. individual	
Increased muscle coordination	
Uses language as a tool to express self	
Trial-and-error learning	
Fears mutilation, loss of control, dark, ghosts	
School Age (6–12 Years)	
Growth relatively latent	Can usually swallow capsules or tablets
Develops logic	Praise child after drug administration
Develops skills and talents	Drug taking may have long-term benefits
Age of industry and increased competence	
Needs parental support	
Fears separation from friends, physical disability	
Adolescent (12–18 Years)	
Growth spurt begins at 9½ years for females and 10½ years for males	Include child in therapeutic decision-making to foster respect
Puberty between 8 and 13 years for females and 10 and 14 years for males	Incorporate group or peer activities as appropriate
Can project consequences	Able to appreciate causal relationships
Transition from childhood to adulthood	Minimize dependent drug regimens where possible
Quest for independence	
Risk-taking behaviors	
Fears change in appearance or functioning, dependency	

ments of sucking cause the infant to spit out materials other than the nipple. The infant should be positioned to avoid aspiration of a drug, which should be administered slowly to minimize choking, with the hands restrained if necessary. The infant younger than 3 to 4 months does not have a well-developed sense of taste. Medication administration requires feeding behavior that establishes an easy, comfortable situation to form a trusting relationship. A pacifier may be used to distract an infant before administration of an injection.

Toddler A toddler displays negativism and should be approached in a positive manner. The child's rituals should be followed to allow for a sense of control and decrease anxiety. Health care providers should make sure that the child is familiar with all equipment and use bandages decorated with drawings. Drugs should be administered promptly; the child should be restrained as necessary and rewarded for positive behavior. A favorite juice or other liquid should be given after an oral dose of drug. Caregivers should be taught proper storage and disposal of drugs and containers to avoid accidental ingestion and subsequent poisoning.

Toddlers have a limited concept of time and resistive behaviors are at a peak within this age group. Games may be used effectively to gain cooperation.

Preschooler A preschool child benefits from the opportunity to play with equipment and responds positively to explanations and comforting measures. A child of this age fears bodily intrusion and mutilation, so the use of suppositories can be especially upsetting. The health care provider should be truthful with the child about painful sensations, should address the child by name, and should be aware of the preschooler's well-developed coordination and sense of taste. The loss of deciduous teeth occurs in this age group and may need to be considered in the selection of drug formulation. The health care provider should involve the preschooler in choices, wherever possible, so that the patient feels some control over his or her treatment and environment.

School-Age Child The school-age child enjoys taking responsibility for himself or herself. A reward system is an effective feedback mechanism. Time limits should be enforced. The child should be given a means to express fears

TABLE 7–4 STRATEGIES FOR DRUG ADMINISTRATION

Administration Route	Nursing Implications
Ophthalmic	Apply finger pressure to lacrimal punctum aspect of inner lid for 1 minute to prevent drainage of the drug into nasopharynx and unpleasant tasting of drug.
Otic	For children less than 3 years of age, pull pinna down and back. For children more than 3 years of age, pull pinna up and back. Warm drops to avoid causing pain in the tympanic membrane.
Nasal	Hold the infant in the cradle position, stabilizing the head and tilting it back. Give nose drops 20 to 30 minutes before feeding, because infants are nose breathers and nasal congestion inhibits sucking.
Oral	Administer drug to infants using a syringe, nipple, or dropper. Do not add drugs to formulas or other essential foods. Crush chewable tablets and add them to a small amount of flavored syrup, jelly, or applesauce. Do not crush enteric-coated capsules. Do not open sustained-release capsules. In 1-month-old infants and in children with neurologic impairments, blow a small puff of air in the face to elicit a swallow reflex.
Subcutaneous	Make injections just below the skin at a 45-degree angle in the deltoid, anterior thigh, abdominal wall, or subscapular areas in volumes of 0.5 to 1.0 mL. Use 25- or 26-gauge, ⅜-inch needles for infants, and 25- or 26-gauge, ⅝-inch for older children.
Intramuscular	Consider placing a wrapped ice cube on the injection site for 1 minute before the injection to reduce discomfort. Select needle size appropriate to the volume to be administered, the drug viscosity, the muscle mass to be penetrated, and the child's age. Limit volume for injection to 0.5 mL for infants and 2.0 mL for older children. After drawing drug into syringe, change the needle before giving the injection. Insertion of the needle through a rubber stopper dulls the tip. After injection, comfort the child and give a reward. Use the following injection sites: vastus lateralis (largest muscle group in children younger than 3 years); ventrogluteal muscle (for a child older than 3 years; easily accessible; can tolerate large volumes); dorsogluteal (for children younger than 3 years; large mass in older children; danger of sciatic nerve injury), and deltoid (small muscle mass; rapid absorption rate).
Intravenous	Because desired effect is rapidly achieved, use volumetric device and/or infusion pump for infants and young children. Administer drugs according to guidelines for dilution and infusion time. Check drug-drug compatibilities.
Venous access device	Following required special procedures for access (i.e., Huber, Groshong, Broviac, Hickman catheters are above the skin; Mediport, Infus-a-port are below the skin). Clamp Broviac and Hickman devices; Groshong devices do not require clamping because they contain a two-way valve. Flush Broviac and Groshong devices daily or weekly to maintain patency. Flush implanted ports, such as the Mediport and Infus-a-port, monthly.
Rectal	Place the child in the side-lying position. Lubricate the suppository. Consult a pharmacist before cutting a suppository. If still appropriate, cut the suppository lengthwise, because the drugs are not distributed evenly throughout.

about injections. Play activities will assist with coping. Drawings can be used to explain the effects of drugs on the body. By age 9, the child can tell time and assume some responsibility for self-medication.

Adolescent The adolescent gains an identity through group membership. An adolescent patient should be allowed to manage his or her drug regimen when possible. It helps to foster identity formation. However, close monitoring is essential to ensure compliance. Disorders and drugs affecting body appearance may be particularly stressful for an adolescent. Preparation for drug administration is important. A confident, matter-of-fact approach should be used, and the adolescent should be given an opportunity to express feelings or concerns about the treatment regimen.

Education

Children's and adolescents' reactions to drug regimens are affected by physical and cognitive abilities, developmental characteristics, environmental influences, past experiences, current relationship with the health care provider, and perception of the present situation. Helpful approaches and explanations can increase the potential for compliance.

Management of pharmacotherapeutic regimens require of the caregiver or parent attention, coordination, and some understanding of the drug being given. Stress or fatigue from caring for a sick child may contribute to a drug administration error. In some cases, young or unseasoned parents do not have the experience to ask appropriate questions about a drug to clarify their understanding of the drug regimen. Drug misuse in pediatric patients has many common causes. The use of multiple medication dispensers (e.g., one each for father, mother, and day-care center personnel) may increase the risk of repeated or missed doses. Drugs prescribed for a previous illness or for a sibling with similar symptoms may be inappropriate for the present illness.

Considerable variation exists in the understanding of the term "teaspoon," causing errors in measurement. Misinterpretation of the route of administration may occur. For example, ear drops may be prescribed "for the ear" or prescribed to be placed "in the ear." The ability of the parent or caregiver to recognize side effects is complicated by the child's lack of language and inability to recognize, understand, and communicate symptoms. The belief that "if a little is good, more is better" can lead to accidental ingestion and possible overdose.

One solution to these potential problems is parent and caregiver education. Assessment of the parents' and caregivers' level of understanding is a must. Caregivers must know what the drug is. They must know the dosage, frequency, and route, the length of time the drug is to be administered, and the anticipated effects of the drug. Finally, they must be told whom to contact if they observe untoward signs and symptoms of the drug. A demonstration of administration techniques is appropriate to caregiver education, as well as the provision of written instructions. Following these general principles helps to ensure safe, accurate, and timely pharmacotherapeutic administration.

The issue of compliance with therapeutic regimens rests on the willingness of others to assist in the child's care. Follow-up by telephone or through a community health nurse may ensure that the pharmacotherapeutic regimen is accurately implemented.

Evaluation

Meticulous, ongoing assessment is essential to optimal pediatric pharmacotherapeutic regimens. When administration of a drug to a child is inevitable, an awareness of the physiologic and developmental changes, conscious attention paid to the pharmacokinetics and pharmacodynamics of the required drugs, and early recognition of potential complications are essential. Definitive management goals center, in most cases, on prevention and cure.

Children are not small adults. The physiology of their changing body systems affects pharmacotherapeutic regimens. Applied pediatric pharmacokinetics has not yet attained the clarity of modern adult drug therapy. Ethical and legal constraints on drug testing in the pediatric population have limited the health care provider's knowledge of drug action and response. There is little doubt that sound pharmacokinetic information can contribute to a more rapid achievement of optimal drug dosages for this population of patients. However, contemporary pediatric pharmacotherapeutics is based on cautious and conservative empiricism.

Application of the principles of normal growth and development and knowledge of what constitutes deviations from normal help individualize care. The approach chosen should facilitate a positive experience for the health care provider, the patient, and the family. Patient and family education should always be included in order to promote compliance with pharmacotherapeutic regimens, drug administration, and drug safety.

SUMMARY

- The anatomic and physiologic differences in body systems of a child have a clinical significance that affects pharmacotherapeutics.
- Children's body systems grow and develop at different rates; therefore, generalizations about the use of drugs in this population are not possible.
- The concept of body surface area is important in pediatrics, because many physiologic functions are proportional to body surface area.
- Because of a child's greater proportion of body fluid, higher milligram per kilogram doses of certain drugs may be needed in order to achieve therapeutic drug levels.
- The relative immaturity of a child's body systems contributes to differences in pharmacokinetics, drug efficacy, and drug effectiveness.
- Health care providers have a responsibility for knowing the biologic distinctions that affect pharmacokinetics in children.
- Physiologic differences in the pediatric patient influence drug absorption by oral, parenteral, and topical routes.
- Many age-related differences in drug distribution occur during the first 10 to 12 months of life. Distribution and equilibration rates may be faster in children than in adults.
- Immaturity of the liver in premature infants and neonates reduces the biotransformation of drugs.
- There are significant age-related changes in glomerular filtration rates, tubular secretion and reabsorption, and, thus, renal elimination of drugs and their metabolites.
- Drugs produce the same biochemical mechanism of action in all individuals, including children. The response to the drug, however, varies according to the maturity of the target organ, thereby necessitating a dosage adjustment.
- It should be clearly determined whether the chief complaint is the problem of the patient, the parent(s), or both.
- Particular attention should be paid to the allergies that are prevalent during infancy and childhood.
- Emphasis during the pediatric physical exam should be placed on the anticipated findings and the signs and symptoms that accompany common pathologic conditions of infancy, childhood, and adolescence.
- Considerations such as the developmental norms for fine motor skills, gross motor skills, feeding behavior, language, and social skills can be used in planning appropriate medication administration techniques.
- The developmental status of the child places him or her at greater risk for physical and psychological trauma related to drug therapy.
- Caution should be used until the health care provider has absolutely determined that a drug is indicated and appropriate for the child.
- In general, the least toxic, least expensive drug that treats the underlying cause of the child's illness (in preference to symptoms) should be chosen.
- Pharmacotherapeutics involves assessing factors that may affect administration, effectiveness, and safety of a given drug regimen. Specific pediatric disorders influence drug utilization in children as well as in adults.
- There are many common causes of drug misuse in the pediatric patient, related to multiple caregivers, misunderstanding of measurement parameters, and the inability of the caregiver to recognize adverse effects.

- Meticulous, ongoing assessment and evaluation are essential to optimize pediatric pharmacotherapeutic regimens.

BIBLIOGRAPHY

Bendayan, R., Pieper, T., Stewart, R., et al. (1984). Influence of age on serum protein binding. *European Journal of Clinical Pharmacology,* 26, 251–254.

Bernardo, L., and Bove, M. (1993). *Pediatric emergency nursing procedures.* Boston: Jones and Bartlett.

Byington, K. (1991). Your guide to pediatric nursing administration. *Nursing '91,* 21(8), 207–240.

Chameides, L., and Hazinski, M. (Eds.) (1994). *Textbook of advanced pediatric life support.* (2nd ed.). Dallas: American Heart Association.

Farrington, E. (1990). Pediatric drug information. *Pediatric Nursing,* 16, 64–65.

Geller, B. (1991). Psychopharmacology of children and pharmacokinetics and relationships of plasma/serum levels. *Psychopharmacology Bulletin,* 27(4), 401–409.

Goodman, A., Rall, T., Nies, A., et al. (1990). *The pharmacological basis of therapeutics.* (8th ed.). Elmsford, NY: Pergamon Press.

Haley, K., and Baker, P. (1993). *Emergency nursing pediatric course: Instructor manual.* Park Ridge, IL: Emergency Nurses Association.

Herfindal, J., Gourley, D., and Hart, L. (1992). *Clinical pharmacy and therapeutics.* (5th ed.). Baltimore: Williams & Wilkins.

Johnson, K. (1993). *The Harriet Lane handbook.* St. Louis: Mosby–Year Book.

Koda-Kimble, M., and Young, L. (1992). *Applied therapeutics: The clinical use of drugs.* Vancouver, WA: Applied Therapeutics, Inc.

Litteral, J. (1990). What are the clinically important drug-nutrient interactions? *Pediatric Nursing,* 16, 594–598.

Ludwig, S., Loiselle, J. (1993). Anatomy, growth, and development: Impact on injury. In Eichelberger, M. (Ed.), *Pediatric trauma; prevention, acute care, rehabilitation* (1st ed.). Chicago: Mosby.

Luwandowski, L. (1992). Psychosocial aspects of pediatric critical care. In Hazinski, M. (Ed.). *Nursing care of the critically ill child.* (2nd ed.). St. Louis: Mosby–Year Book.

MacLeod, H., and Evans, W. (1992). Pediatric pharmacokinetics and therapeutic drug monitoring. *Pediatric Review,* 13(11), 413–421.

Nahata, M. (1992). Advances in pediatric pharmacology. *Journal of Pharmacotherapy,* 17(3), 141–146.

Newton, M., Newton, D., and Fudin, J. (1992). Reviewing the big three injection routes. *Nursing '92,* 22(9), 34–42.

Phelps, S., and Hak, E. (1996). *Guidelines for administration of intravenous medications to pediatric patients.* (5th ed.). Bethesda, MD: American Society of Health-System Pharmacists, Inc.

Schwertz, D. (1991). Basic principles of pharmacologic action. *Nursing Clinics of North America,* 26(2), 245–262.

Skaer, T. (1991). Dosing considerations in the pediatric patient. *Clinical Therapeutics,* 13(5), 526–544.

Skale, N. (1992). *Manual of pediatric nursing procedures.* Philadelphia: J.B. Lippincott.

Thomas, D. (1991). Anatomical and physical variables. *Pediatric emergency nursing.* Gaithersburg, MD: Aspen Publishing.

Tripp-Reimer, R., and Afifi, L. (1989). Cross-cultural perspectives on patient teaching. *Nursing Clinics of North America,* 25, 613–619.

Wilson, J. (1993). Pediatric pharmacology: The path clears for a noble mission. *Journal of Clinical Pharmacology,* 33(3), 210–213.

Wink, D. (1991). Giving infants and children drugs. *American Journal of Maternal Child Nursing,* 16, 317–321.

Wong, E., and Whaley, L. (1995). *Nursing care of infants and children.* (5th ed.). St. Louis: Mosby–Year Book.

Yaffe, S., and Aranda, J. (1992). *Pediatric pharmacology: Therapeutic principles in practice.* (2nd ed.). Philadelphia: W.B. Saunders.

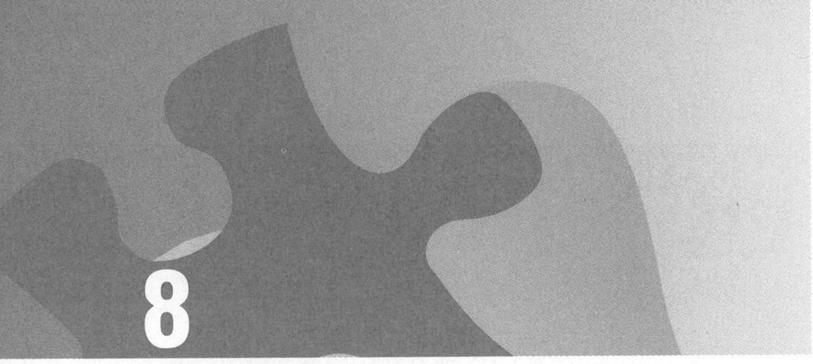

8 Geriatric Pharmacotherapeutics

Today, more people than ever are living into their senior years, and those older than 65 years represent more than 12 percent of the population in the United States. In 1930, slightly more than 6 million people were older than 65, and the average life expectancy was 59.7 years. In 1965, the numbers had grown to 20 million people older than 65 years with an average life expectancy of 70.2 years. Now, life expectancy has reached 74.9 years, and it is anticipated that 20 percent of the population will reach age 65 by the year 2020. Advances in disease control and health care technologies, reduced infant mortality rates, improved sanitation, and better living conditions have helped increase life expectancy for most Americans.

"Older" adults are now grouped into age categories for the purpose of epidemiologic studies. The "young-old" are between 55 and 65 years, the "old" between 65 and 75 years, and the "old-old" older than 75 years. The practicality of these categories in pharmacotherapy remains elusive. However, chronic illness represents a major obstacle for our older adult population. Most older adults have at least one chronic condition or disease, and many have several that must be concurrently managed (Table 8–1). Chronic illness contributes to self-care limitations in almost half of this population. Approximately one-fourth of older adults have difficulty with the activities of daily living. The older the individual is, the greater the prevalence of drug therapy and the need for assistance with the tasks of daily living becomes, while the likelihood of remaining totally independent declines.

Individuals older than 65 years purchase 35 percent of all prescription drugs and more than 40 percent of over-the-counter drugs sold in the United States at an annual cost of $3 billion. The average older American residing at home has 11 different prescriptions filled annually; residents of extended care facilities average 8 prescriptions a year. Ninety percent of all older adults take at least one drug daily. Drugs most commonly prescribed are diuretics, potassium salts, histamine-2 antagonists, nitroglycerin, insulin, cardiac glycosides, beta blockers, antianxiety drugs, and antihypertensives. The most common over-the-counter drugs purchased by older adults are analgesics, anti-inflammatory drugs, laxatives, and antacids (Table 8–2).

ANATOMIC AND PHYSIOLOGIC VARIABLES

As we age, a variety of physiologic changes increase the older adult's sensitivity to drugs and drug-induced disease. It should be noted that chronologic age is not necessarily related to physiologic age. With aging, however, there is a gradual decline in many body system functions, some systems being affected more than others (Fig. 8–1). There is a growing awareness that physiologic changes once considered to be inevitable are not evident in physically fit older adults. Indeed, the variations between people of the same age are so great that increased biologic variation is characteristic of this age group. This is particularly true of physiologic functions that affect drug disposition and response. Therefore, each person must be evaluated on his or her own merit.

The aging process is complex and varied, involving changes in cells, tissues, and organs. Tissue, organ, and system changes can be traced to alterations that occur at the cellular level. Ordinarily, there is a functional decline of all body systems beginning at the cellular level.

Body Composition

All body cells show age-related changes. Cell numbers gradually decline, leaving fewer functional body cells. The nucleus of each cell appears to enlarge, although there is no discernible increase in the amount of DNA present. The nucleoli increase in size and numbers, and there appears to be an increase in RNA. Protoplasmic changes include a rise in protein content but a fall in protein synthesis, an increase in lipids, accumulation of lipofuscin (especially in the fixed cells of nerve tissue and muscle), and glycogen depletion. Lysosomes needed for digestion and breakdown of cellular products accumulate because of either alterations in the rate of protein turnover or deficits in the catabolic process.

Age-related tissue changes are best seen in the extracellular matrix. Elastin, found in tissues associated with body movement (e.g., walls of major blood vessels, heart, lungs, and skin), is reduced and replaced with pseudoelastin. Tissues become less pliable and ultimately less efficient. Double chins, elongated ears, and baggy eyelids are obvious manifestations of the loss of elastin. Aortic stenosis may also develop as elastin is replaced with pseudoelastin.

Body fat increases until about age 85 and then decreases. In women, fat and lipids continue to accumulate. In men, there is a steady increase in lipids until age 60, after which there is a gradual decrease. As body fat atrophies, contours gain a bony appearance, with deepening of intercostal and supraclavicular spaces, orbits, and axillae. Skin-fold thickness is significantly reduced in the forearm and on the back of the hands. The loss of subcutaneous fat, responsible for the decrease in skin-fold thickness, is responsible for a decline in the body's natural insulation. This loss makes older adults sensitive to cold and puts them at risk for hypothermia. Many of the lipids are stored in endothelial tissues of arteries, contributing to atherosclerosis.

Bone mass decreases, resulting in a 2-inch loss of height by age 70. The loss in stature is due in part to loss of cartilage and thinning of vertebrae. This change causes long bones to seem disproportionately long. Loss of height is as

TABLE 8–1 RATES OF CHRONIC ILLNESS IN ADULTS BY AGE PER 1000 POPULATION

Illness/Condition	Age (yr) 18–44	45–64	65–74	>75
Arthritis	52.8	273.3	463.6	511.9
Hypertension	61.8	252.0	392.4	337.0
Hearing impairments	54.1	135.6	264.7	348.0
Heart conditions	40.7	126.1	284.7	322.2
Chronic sinusitis	149.5	192.1	154.0	131.4
Visual impairments	29.3	47.3	56.3	111.2
Orthopaedic problems	135.4	155.0	154.9	182.0
Diabetes mellitus	11.9	56.4	98.3	98.2
Varicose veins	26.8	54.1	82.5	64.8
Hemorrhoids	46.9	79.7	74.1	73.1

Adapted from U.S. Department of Commerce. (1990). Statistical Abstract of the US. (110th ed.). Washington, DC: Bureau of the Census.

much a result of dehydration of vertebral discs as a loss of bone mass or collapse of the vertebrae. Moreover, the loss of bone mass leaves the older adult susceptible to fractures of the wrist, hip, and vertebrae with all the known physical and psychological sequelae.

TABLE 8–2 DRUGS COMMONLY USED BY THE OLDER ADULT

Prescription Drugs	Over-the-Counter Drugs
Antianxiety drugs	Analgesics
Antihypertensives	Antacids
Beta blockers	Laxatives
Digitalis preparations	Nonsteroidal anti-inflammatory drugs
Diuretics	
Histamine-2 antagonists	
Insulin	
Nitroglycerin	
Potassium salts	

Although the quantity of extracellular fluids remains fairly constant, intracellular volume is decreased, resulting in less overall total body fluid. This change puts the older adult at risk for dehydration.

As with cells and tissues, there is a decrease in the functional capacity of body organs. Physiologic reserves display a linear decline beginning at age 30, especially in cardiac, respiratory, and renal function. As a result, maintenance of homeostasis becomes increasingly difficult. Although changes in these organ systems occur gradually over a long period and are generally insignificant, moderate or se-

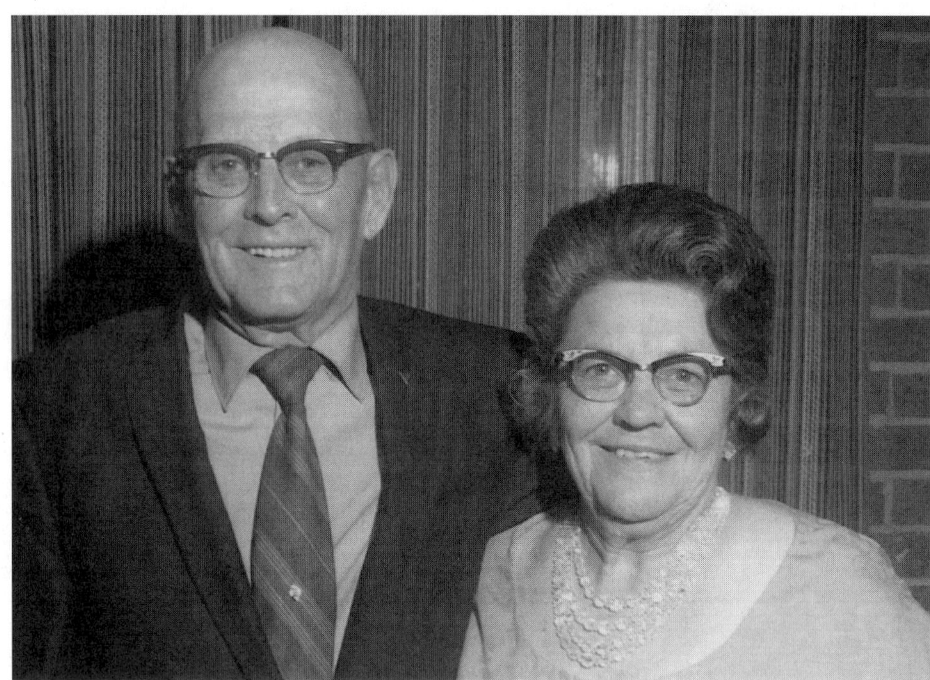

Figure 8–1 Developmental changes of aging that influence pharmacotherapy:
- Reduced long-term and short-term memory in some patients
- Reduced visual acuity
- Decreased cardiac output
- Decreased blood flow to organs and tissues
- Altered peripheral vascular tone and reduced baroreceptor activity
- Decreased enzymatic activity in the liver
- Decreased serum albumin levels
- Increased adipose tissue
- Decreased tissue elasticity and reduced muscle mass
- Increased gastric pH and reduced gastric acid
- Decreased body water
- Changes in sensitivity of receptor sites

vere stressors can precipitate unexpected problems or organ failure.

Cardiovascular System

Physiologic changes in the cardiovascular system manifest in a variety of ways. The efficiency and contractile strength of the myocardium decline, resulting in a 1 percent per year reduction in cardiac output. It is thought that stroke volume decreases by 0.7 percent yearly. The systolic and diastolic phases of the myocardial cycle are prolonged. Ordinarily, older adults adjust to these changes without much difficulty. However, when unusual demands are placed on the heart (e.g., shoveling snow, running to catch a bus), the changes become more evident. Pulse rates may not reach the levels in younger persons, and tachycardia lasts longer. There is some disagreement among health care providers as to when the normal elevation becomes hypertension. In some older adults, the blood pressure may remain stable but tachycardia progresses to heart failure. Furthermore, some health care providers suggest that only an elevated diastolic pressure should be treated.

Resistance to peripheral blood flow increases by 1 percent each year. Reduced elasticity of the arteries is responsible for vascular changes to the heart, kidneys, and pituitary gland. The rigidity of vessel walls and narrowing of lumens require more force to move blood through the vessels. These changes lead to a higher diastolic blood pressure. There is also a decrease in the ability of the aorta to distend, in turn causing a rise in systolic pressure. Vagal tone increases, and the heart becomes more sensitive to carotid sinus stimulation. Reduced sensitivity of the baroreceptors potentiates orthostatic hypotension. The normal changes of aging do not usually influence venous circulation.

Respiratory System

Various structural changes in the chest diminish respiratory functioning. In addition, there are reductions in the number of alveoli, diffusion capacity, and elastic recoil of the lungs during expiration. Vital capacity is decreased but residual volume increases approximately 40 percent by age 85; thus, more energy is required to achieve full respiratory capacity. A slight fall in arterial oxyhemoglobin saturation occurs, and cough efficiency is reduced. With less effective gas exchange and a lack of bibasilar inflation, the older adult is at risk for atelectasis and pulmonary infections.

Gastrointestinal System

Although gastrointestinal problems are not as life-threatening as some cardiovascular or respiratory problems, older adults are infamous for having gastrointestinal complaints. The gastrointestinal system is altered by the aging process at all points. Natural dentition is usually retained, primarily owing to an increased awareness of, and compliance with, recommended dental hygiene practices. Tooth loss is not a normal outcome of growing older, but results from poor dental care, diet, and environmental influences that contribute to tooth loss. Periodontal disease is the major cause of tooth loss after age 30. Decreased activity of the salivary gland and drier mucous membranes contribute to difficulty swallowing. Lowered esophageal motility and relaxation of the lower esophageal sphincter may occur. Aspiration becomes a risk when these factors combine with a weaker gag reflex and delayed esophageal emptying.

By age 70, gastric mucosa atrophies, increasing the risk of irritation and ulceration. Mucosal atrophy is thought to be due to changes in the ratio of gastrin-secreting and somatostatin-secreting cells. Somatostatin is a hormone that inhibits gastrin secretion. This change in ratio leads to a diminished ability to secrete hydrochloric acid (i.e., hypochlorhydria). The severity of hypochlorhydria is directly correlated with the extent of atrophy.

Many indigestion problems are related to an increased gastric pH and to reduced amounts of hydrochloric acid, pepsin, lipase, and pancreatic enzymes. The pancreas produces normal amounts of bicarbonate, amylase, and trypsin, but there is a decrease in lipase, resulting in subclinical abnormalities in fat absorption. Lowered fat absorption reduces the absorption of fat-soluble vitamins. There is also faulty absorption of vitamin B_1, vitamin B_{12}, calcium, and iron.

Liver cells change in size and character, and hepatic blood flow is altered. Hepatic protein synthesis is compromised, and there are changes in the microsomal enzyme systems involved in a variety of metabolic pathways.

Intestinal blood flow is decreased, so the absorption of substances actively transported from the intestinal lumen (e.g., some sugars, minerals, and vitamins) may be reduced. The intestinal mucosa atrophies, decreasing its surface area, and the intestinal musculature weakens. Peristalsis is slower, contributing to constipation.

Renal System

A 50 percent decrease in renal blood flow and glomerular filtration rate develops between the ages of 20 and 90 years. There is a possibility of protein loss because of decreased cardiac output, subsequently reduced renal blood flow, and lower glomerular filtration rates. Tubular reabsorption is decreased, and a lower threshold for glucose and creatinine clearance develops. As a result, the kidneys are less effective in concentrating urine. At younger ages, the urinary specific gravity is about 1.032, but at age 80, it may be 1.024. Blood urea nitrogen levels may reach a value of 21.2 mg/dL at age 70 (normal range for persons older than 60 years is 8 to 20 mg/dL).

Urinary frequency and urgency as well as nocturia result in smaller bladder capacities. Nocturia is a consequence of difficulty in concentrating urine. Although urine leakage is not a normal change of aging, some stress incontinence is common in women because of a weakening of pelvic musculature, particularly in multiparous women.

Prostatic enlargement occurs in many older men. Approximately 75 percent of men older than 65 years experience some degree of prostatism, which contributes to urinary frequency. Prostatic enlargement does not imply a cancerous or metastatic process.

Sensory-Perceptual Function

The eyes of an older adult reflect a variety of changes that affect functional capacity as well as the ability to protect the self from hazards and to enjoy a high quality of life. The aging eye loses the ability to accommodate and focus for near vision (*presbyopia*). As a result, many persons older than 40 years require corrective lenses. Lens opacity may develop and is accompanied by a decreased tolerance for glare. A gradual narrowing of the visual field occurs.

Yellowing of the lens and altered color perception make the older adult less able to differentiate the low tone colors of the blues, greens, and violets. Depth perception changes, causing problems in judging the height of steps or curbs. Bifocals compound this problem. Adaptation to light and dark takes longer. Sclerosis of the pupillary sphincter and a decrease in pupil size make the pupil less responsive to light. Further, reabsorption of intraocular fluid is less efficient, increasing the risk for glaucoma. Reduced tear production leads to less lustrous eyes and complaints of dry eyes.

Deterioration of the cochlea and neurons of the higher auditory pathways leads to sensorineural hearing loss (*presbycusis*). High-pitched sounds such as *s, sh, f, ch,* and *ph* are initially impaired, followed by the middle and low frequencies. The change is so gradual and subtle that affected persons may not realize the magnitude of the hearing loss. Stiffening of the cilia combined with the higher keratin content of cerumen causes ear wax to become easily impacted, further decreasing hearing.

There is some reduction in olfactory senses as sensory cells in the nasal lining decrease in number. The nasal mucosa becomes drier. A reduction in the number of taste buds alters taste sensations, especially to sweet and salty flavors.

Tactile sensation is reduced, evidenced in the older adult as diminished ability to sense pressure and pain and to differentiate temperatures. The sensory changes can cause faulty interpretation of the environment and increase the risk of harm.

Neuromuscular System

Over the years, the bulk, strength, and number of muscle fibers decline. Muscles become more rigid and easily fatigued. Resting tremors may be present in some people. Bone mass and strength are reduced. Bones fracture with less stress than in younger persons. Cartilage decreases, contributing to some discomfort with joint mobility and shortening of the vertebral column. Deep tendon reflexes are sluggish.

It is difficult to determine with accuracy the impact of aging on the nervous system, because of the system's interdependence with other body systems. Reductions in nerve cells, cerebral blood flow, and metabolism are seen. Nerve conduction velocity is slowed, leading to slower reflexes and delayed response to multiple stimuli. Kinesthetic sense lessens. Changes in the sleep pattern occur, with stages III and IV of sleep becoming less prominent. The average sleeping time shortens only a minimal amount, although frequent awakening during sleep is common.

Endocrine System

The pituitary gland shrinks by 20 percent. Human growth hormone remains present in usual amounts, although blood levels may be lower. Variable decreases in adrenocorticotropic hormone, thyroid-stimulating hormone, follicle-stimulating hormone, luteinizing hormone, and luteotrophic hormones are seen. Gonadal secretion declines with age, including gradual decreases in testosterone, estrogen, and progesterone. With the exception of changes in plasma calcium levels or dysfunction of other glands, the parathyroid glands maintain their function throughout life.

Thyroid function for the most part remains adequate for the reduced muscle mass of the older adult, because overall, the body is housing a "smaller engine." However, the thyroid gland becomes atrophic, fibrotic, and nodular. The secretion of thyroid-stimulating hormone and serum concentrations of thyroxin do not change. Any decrease in activity reduces the basal metabolic rate, with less thyrotropin secretion and release. Any loss of adrenal function further lowers thyroid activity.

Just as secretion of adrenocorticotropic hormone declines with age, secretory activity of adrenal glands also decreases. Although adrenocorticotropic hormone does not affect aldosterone secretion, less aldosterone is produced and excreted in the urine. The secretion of glucocorticoids, 17-ketosteroids, progesterone, androgens, and estrogen, also influenced by the adrenal gland, diminishes. There is delayed insufficient release of insulin by beta cells of the pancreas. The smaller quantities of insulin may make it difficult to maintain a euglycemic state for short or prolonged periods. In addition, a lesser sensitivity to circulating insulin is thought to exist. The older adult's ability to metabolize glucose is reduced, causing higher and more prolonged hyperglycemia. Therefore, it is not unusual to detect higher blood glucose levels in nondiabetic older adults.

Immune System

After midlife, there is a steady loss of thymic mass. Serum activity of thymic hormones is almost undetectable in the older adult. T-cell activity declines, with immature T cells present in the thymus. A significant decline in cell-mediated immunity occurs, with T cells less able to proliferate in response to antigens. Changes in T cells contribute to a reactivation of varicella-zoster virus (i.e., shingles) and *Mycobacterium tuberculosis* infections. Serum immunoglobulin concentrations remain essentially unchanged. Concentrations of immunoglobulin M (IgM) are lower, whereas those of immunoglobulins A and G (IgA, IgG) are higher. Responses to influenza, parainfluenza, pneumococcus, and tetanus vaccines are less pronounced. Inflammatory defenses decline, and often, inflammation is atypical. Older adults do not develop fevers in response to infection as readily as younger individuals.

Mental Status

A loss of mental function is not a normal change of aging, nor is a significant change in personality. Altered mental functioning must be evaluated in terms of the older adult's life-long behavioral patterns and potential health problems. Intelligence remains stable throughout the life-span, with the potential for learning unchanged. However, more time may be required for older adults to learn new and difficult tasks. Short-term memory becomes poorer, although there is some controversy as to the extent to which this is true. Long-term memory remains intact.

PHARMACOKINETIC CONSIDERATIONS

Drug effects are different in older adults from those in younger adults, owing to either pharmacokinetic or pharmacodynamic factors. Ordinarily, older adults have less difficulty with drug absorption than with distribution, biotransformation, or elimination. A summary of the physiologic changes of aging that result in pharmacokinetic alterations is found in Table 8–3.

Absorption

There is little evidence that passive absorption of drugs is diminished in older adults. However, conditions such as decreased gastric pH alter the absorption of weak acids and bases. Weak acids (e.g., barbiturates) are more ionized in the gastrointestinal tract and less well absorbed. Weak bases are less ionized and better absorbed. As a result, older adults may not respond as quickly as people in other age groups.

A number of variables affect drug absorption in the older adult. Decreases in gastric motility and in production of trypsin delay or impair drug absorption. Drugs affecting gastric acidity, motility, or trypsin production (e.g., laxatives, antacids, anticholinergics, levodopa) affect the absorption of other drugs. Pain, mucosal edema, diabetes mellitus, and hypokalemia have also been shown to decrease drug absorption.

In addition, the decrease in cardiac output results in a 40 to 50 percent reduction in perfusion of the gastrointestinal tract. This is because blood flow to the area must be sacrificed to maintain coronary and cerebral blood flow. The result is delayed, less thorough, and less reliable removal of drugs and other substances from the intestinal lumen.

To compensate for these changes, drug absorption can be enhanced. Exercise stimulates circulation and increases drug absorption. Prevention of dehydration, hypothermia, and hypotension promotes drug absorption. Drugs that neutralize gastric acid (e.g., antacids) should be avoided.

Distribution

It is more difficult to generalize the effect of advanced age on biotransformation. Because of wide differences in the decline of enzyme systems and organs of elimination, it is impossible to make blanket statements about drug distribution. Older adults are, in many ways, a more heterogeneous group than the very young. Although biotransformation of some drugs is decreased, there are no changes in the clearance of most drugs. However, because of the heterogeneity of older adults, a small subset of the more frail elderly does experience alterations in biotransformation. This population of older adults may not be identified in drug studies of healthy older adults.

Alterations in circulation and changes in body composition affect drug distribution and equilibration rates. The changes occur because aging alters many of the factors that influence protein binding, volume of distribution, the amount of body fat present, and regional perfusion patterns.

Total body mass decreases with age along with declines in body water. These two changes alter the distribution patterns of most drugs. Total body weight decreases, especially in the "old-old" (older than 75 years), but the ratio of fat to lean body mass is usually greater. Average adipose tissue levels increase, from 18 to 30 percent in men and from 35 to 48 percent in women. The enlarged fat compartment increases the volume of distribution of lipid-soluble drugs and reduces the volume of water-soluble drugs. In other words, changes in adipose tissue raise tissue drug concentrations and the duration of drug action while lowering plasma concentrations. For example, a highly fat-soluble drug (e.g., diazepam) has a greater volume of distribution and a prolonged distribution phase, leading to an extended half-life. On the other hand, highly water-soluble drugs (e.g., gentamicin) have a smaller volume of distribution. Lowered cardiac output leads to elevated plasma concentrations with less deposition in reservoirs. Older adults are therefore at higher risk of drug toxicity, so they should be given drugs with shorter half-lives.

TABLE 8–3 PHARMACOKINETIC CONSIDERATIONS RELATED TO CHANGES OF AGING

Normal Physiologic Changes	Pharmacokinetic Alterations
Reduced long- and short-term memory in some patients	Higher risk of unintentional noncompliance
Reduced visual acuity	Higher risk of drug errors due to poor vision
Diminished cardiac output	Decreased biotransformation and excretion of drugs, resulting in longer circulation time
Decreased blood flow to organs and tissues	Potentially decreased absorption of orally administered drugs Vaginal and rectal suppositories take longer to dissolve and may be prematurely expelled Decreased biotransformation or elimination of drugs.
Altered peripheral vascular tone and reduced baroreceptor activity	Exaggerated effects of antihypertensives and diuretic drugs
Decreased enzymatic activity in liver	Altered biotransformation and detoxification processes Biotransformation time is lengthened, and both parent drug and active metabolites exert effects for extended periods Drug toxicity may occur more readily
Reduced serum albumin	Less availability of albumin for binding, amounts of unbound drug and drug activity both increase
More adipose tissue	Altered distribution and higher concentration of fat-soluble drugs in adipose tissue Some drugs reach greater peak concentrations with longer half-lives
Decreases in tissue elasticity and muscle mass	Poor absorption of drugs with poor sealing of tissues after injection
Higher gastric pH and reduced gastric acid	Decreased absorption of drugs that are normally nonionized at low pH (weak acids and bases)
Decreased body water	Drier mucous membranes may cause drugs to stick to the oral cavity and cause irritation Higher water-soluble drug concentration in blood stream
Changes in sensitivity of receptor sites	Increase or decrease in drug activity

EXAMPLES OF HIGHLY PROTEIN-BOUND DRUGS

Acetazolamide	Nortriptyline
Amitriptyline	Phenylbutazone
Cefazolin	Phenytoin
Chlordiazepoxide	Propranolol
Chlorpromazine	Rifampin
Cloxacillin	Salicylates
Digitoxin	Spironolactone
Furosemide	Sulfisoxazole
Hydralazine	Warfarin

Depressed plasma albumin levels result in higher concentrations of unbound drug, especially when the drug competes with other protein-bound drugs. As a result, more unbound drug circulates, increasing the action of highly protein-bound drugs. This effect is not always predictable. Moreover, as the amount of unbound drug rises, so does the amount of drug available for biotransformation and elimination. For example, a highly protein-bound drug (e.g., phenytoin) undergoes greater biotransformation, decreasing the serum drug levels and the therapeutic effects. In contrast, another highly protein-bound drug such as warfarin, an anticoagulant, produces greater anticoagulation effects in persons with low serum albumin levels. The box entitled Examples of Highly Protein-Bound Drugs contains a partial listing of these compounds. States of dehydration and hypoalbuminemia require lower dosage levels.

Other factors altering drug distribution in the older adult are poor nutrition, extremes of body weight, electrolyte and mineral imbalances, inactivity, and prolonged bedrest. Perhaps the most significant factor is size: Older patients are typically smaller than younger patients. An older patient who receives the same dosage as a younger patient has a higher concentration of the drug in the blood because of the older patient's smaller volume.

Biotransformation

Although the liver remains functional, in the older adult the ability to biotransform drugs changes. A person who lives to be 100 has a 50 percent reduction in liver mass, with the greatest decrease occurring between the ages of 60 and 70 years.

Drug biotransformation in the liver depends primarily on two processes, hepatic blood flow and metabolic enzyme activity. With aging, blood flow to the liver is reduced, so less drug is delivered for biotransformation. The reduced blood flow and lower enzyme activity can be particularly significant with drugs for which metabolic rates depend on hepatic blood flow (e.g., propranolol).

The relationship between aging and hepatic enzyme function is complex, and depends on the type of metabolic reaction and the patient's gender. Biotransformation of drugs occurs in two phases (see Chapter 4). Oxidation, reduction, and hydrolysis make up phase I reactions. These processes lead to minor changes in drug molecules and typically produce active metabolites. Environmental factors such as cigarette smoking have a greater influence than age per se. Oxidative capacity declines with age, but the decline is thought to be greater in men than in women. The effect on oxidative metabolism is consistent for drugs with low hepatic extraction rates. The rate of hepatic conjugation is unaffected by age. Data are less clear about drugs with a high extraction ratios because their rate of biotransformation depends on hepatic blood flow in addition to hepatic enzyme activity. Liver size is a significant determinant in the elimination of drugs that have high extraction ratios, regardless of age.

Phase II reactions combine the drug or its metabolite with acetic, glucuronic, sulfuric, or amino acids, leading to the production of inactive compounds. Aging reduces the efficacy of both phases of biotransformation, but phase I reactions are more affected than phase II reactions. Although no significant effects have been reported, the smaller size and reduced function of the liver interfere with the formation of prothrombin, albumin, and vitamins A and D. Conditions such as dehydration, hyperthermia, immobility, and liver disease diminish the biotransformation of drugs. As a consequence, drugs can accumulate to toxic levels. Also, the extended biologic half-life of many drugs warrants close monitoring of drug clearance in older patients. Drugs such as morphine, meperidine, propoxyphene, propranolol, lidocaine, phenylbutazone, warfarin, amobarbital, and benzodiazepines have extended half-lives. Drugs that are normally subject to a considerable first-pass effect (e.g., propranolol) are especially likely to have exaggerated effects in older adults (see Chapter 5).

Elimination

The kidneys are primarily responsible for the body's excretory functions, including the elimination of most drugs. Drugs follow a path through the kidneys similar to that of most constituents of urine. After systemic circulation, the drug filters through the walls of the glomeruli into Bowman's capsule. It continues down the tubule, where substances beneficial to the body are reabsorbed into the blood stream. Waste products flow into the kidney pelvis for elimination through the urine.

With aging, however, the number of functional nephrons falls by as much as 64 percent, and the glomerular filtration rate by 46 percent. At age 30, the glomerular filtration rate is approximately 140 mL/min/1.73 m^2. The decline continues at an average rate of 8 mL/min/1.73 m^2 every decade. The normal decline in glomerular filtration rate related to aging is not reflected in the serum creatinine, because of the comparable loss in muscle mass, which lowers the production of creatinine. That means that an older patient may not demonstrate higher serum creatinine levels until the dysfunction is severe. The change is accompanied by a similar decrease in renal blood flow. Tubular secretory mechanisms and the ability to concentrate urine are diminished. In addition, cardiovascular disease, dehydration, and kidney disease commonly impair renal functioning. Thus, the half-life of a drug may be increased by as much as 40 percent. Because drugs remain in the body longer, they can have adverse effects. For these reasons, antibiotics such as penicillin, streptomycin, tetracycline, and kanamycin have prolonged half-lives and elevated peak plasma levels in older patients. Health care providers should be particularly alert to the toxic levels of drugs that may occur when kidney function is reduced.

PHARMACODYNAMIC CONSIDERATIONS

Systemic Effects

Many of the changes in patient responses do not result from pharmacokinetic factors. Instead, they can be caused by aging organ systems and their role in drug-receptor or drug-organ interactions. Aging reduces tissue responsiveness to drugs in a number of ways. Drug receptor response can be altered because the functional capacity of organs and thus the total number of receptors decline with age. Therefore, any adverse effects are more keenly felt. The effects of drugs that thwart liver, kidney, or cardiac function may go unnoticed in younger individuals but can be dangerous in the older adult. In addition, the vitality of control mechanisms is reduced, the maintenance of homeostasis is less dynamic, and compensatory responses to primary drug effects are less profound. For example, drugs that raise blood pressure often do so in a more profound manner, because the vagal reflex is less efficient in generating a compensatory reduction in cardiac output.

Drug response includes increased sensitivity of the myocardium to anesthetics. Cardiac glycosides (see Chapter 31) are well known for their narrow therapeutic index in all patients, but older adults are particularly prone to toxicities. Older adults also exhibit reduced pharmacodynamic responsiveness to quinidine but a greater sensitivity to lidocaine. Vascular responses to norepinephrine and cardiac response to isoproterenol and other catecholamines are somewhat diminished (see Chapter 11).

Orthostatic hypotension caused by antihypertensive drugs (see Chapter 34), antidepressants (see Chapter 18) and antipsychotic drugs (see Chapter 19) is more common in older adults who are volume depleted secondary to diuretic therapy (see Chapter 39). In addition, potassium-wasting diuretics such as furosemide can cause hypokalemia, which potentiates the effects of cardiac glycosides. The incidence of hyperkalemia in older patients taking potassium-sparing diuretics (e.g., spironolactone) is higher, possibly because renal function is impaired.

Older adults are more susceptible to the effects of neuromuscular blocking drugs (see Chapter 12). The blockade is more intense and prolonged with advanced age. In general, patients of advanced age are more sensitive to drugs acting within the central nervous system. Thus, barbiturates, benzodiazepines, lithium, opioid analgesics, tricyclic antidepressants, and phenothiazines demonstrate therapeutic and toxic effects at lower doses.

In the autonomic nervous system, beta-adrenergic receptor responses to both agonists and antagonists appear to be blunted. As a result, older adults show diminished response to drugs and increased toxicity to beta-adrenergic blocking drugs. Aging causes a decline in parasympathetic control, which enhances the effects of anticholinergic drugs (see Chapter 13). It also reduces the amounts of neurotransmitters, particularly dopamine and acetylcholine. Reduced dopamine in the brain increases the older adult's susceptibility to the extrapyramidal effects of neuroleptics, metoclopramide, and other drugs.

Central nervous system effects of sedative-hypnotics and antianxiety drugs include paradoxical responses, characterized by restlessness, disorientation, and confusion. Balance disturbances are also of concern, in that they often lead to falls and subsequent injury. In contrast, the effects of stimulants such as amphetamines on motor activity are less in the older adult, but their anorexic effects are enhanced (see the controversy entitled Dosing and Driving?).

Several endocrine changes influence drug response. For example, the age-related decline in glucose tolerance causes greater hyperglycemia than normal in response to a thiazide diuretic. Moreover, because the response to drug-induced

Controversy

Dosing and Driving?

JONATHAN J. WOLFE

Drug therapy of behavioral disorders opens many doors, particularly for the older adult. It is no longer necessary to accept endogenous depression, panic disorder, or phantom voices as necessary accompaniments to the aging process. The crude chemical straightjackets associated with the early psychotropic drugs are no longer satisfactory. The relative low cost of phenothiazines, for example, is not a proper argument against the use of more expensive drugs, which enhance the ability to live autonomously.

Operating a motor vehicle is a component of autonomy in most parts of America that reduces dependence on others. Driving, however, may well be considered separately from activities of daily living that relate to personal care.

Concerns about the older adult's driving may be grouped around two issues. The first, independent of issues of drug prescribing and administration, is a patient's maintenance of the skills and knowledge to safely operate an automobile. No one would argue that the patient whose vision is severely diminished or motor functions importantly impaired has a right to drive that outweighs the risk it may pose to others. The other focus of concern is impairment of driving ability when drugs are used that suppress central nervous system function.

In many cases involving drug therapy, restriction of driving is temporary. When a drug is first introduced into the treatment plan or doses are increased, the patient may experience somnolence, dizziness, or disorientation incompatible with safe driving. Once the sensorium adjusts to higher doses, driving may be appropriate. Permanent loss of driving privileges represents a graver choice. It is, however, necessary for the patient whose skills remain impaired or who requires indefinite use of a centrally acting drug.

Critical Thinking Discussion

- Think about your experience as a new driver. Having the car keys opened many opportunities. It also released you from direct parental scrutiny when you were driving alone. List three activities in your daily life that you would lose without access to a vehicle.
- Reflect privately on one activity in your adult life that you reluctantly would give up rather than explain or reveal to your family that you could no longer drive.
- What counseling is appropriate for a 72-year-old patient in otherwise good health who is to begin treatment of his anxiety disorder with a short-acting benzodiazepine?
- What is an appropriate response to a concerned adult child who reports that her 85-year-old mother experiences severe postural hypotension from her antihypertensive drug regimen, yet continues to drive on the interstate highway?
- You are asked to present a 30-minute educational program to your state's highway patrol officers. They want you to talk about prescription drugs and driving impairment. What three topics will you discuss?

hypoglycemia is reduced, older adults do not seek treatment as early as a younger adult would. In addition, diminished thyroid function decreases the metabolic rate, which in turn slows drug biotransformation.

Polypharmacy

Compounding the effect of physiologic aging on pharmacokinetics and pharmacodynamics is the presence of comorbid, chronic disease. The higher incidence of chronic diseases generally results in greater use of prescriptive and over-the-counter drugs. Specialty medical practice has to some extent added to the practice of *polypharmacy,* the prescription of many drugs given or taken at one time. Indeed, polypharmacy is the result of multiple disease processes, but also of the prescribing behaviors of multiple health care providers and of poorly coordinated patient management. Polypharmacy results in a higher risk of adverse effects, drug interactions, extended hospital stays, and reduced compliance. Ironically, drug reactions that mimic medical-physical complaints are often treated with yet another drug.

The rate of adverse effects is directly proportional to the number of drugs taken. Patients receiving two drugs have a 5.6 percent risk for a drug interaction, whereas those receiving five drugs have a 50 percent chance. Patients receiving eight different drugs have a 100 percent chance for drug interaction. Ninety-one percent of noninstitutionalized older adults experience adverse effects through taking an average of 11 different drugs. Drug reactions in older adults are responsible for more than 243,000 hospitalizations, 32,000 hip fractures, 160,000 changes in mental status, and 2 million cases of drug dependence. Although polypharmacy is significant in this population, it is commonly overlooked as a possible factor in patient symptoms.

The combination of an aging population and a proliferation of new drugs puts the frail old adult at even greater risk for polypharmacy. The most common intervention for managing aches, pains, and other complaints is drug therapy. For example, an agitated older adult can be treated with an antianxiety drug, which complicates arthritic mobility problems, which in turn leads to more complaints that are treated with additional drugs. In addition, excessive drug use by the older adult inadvertently creates an economically, psychologically, and physiologically costly cycle of events from which he or she may never recover.

Critical Thinking Process

Assessment

The examiner must first establish a climate of reassurance and trust with the older adult. A warm greeting with an extended hand and good eye contact almost always results in acceptance of the hand. The examiner should maintain the hand contact as long as the older adult shows an inclination to do so, but should be sensitive to painful, paralyzed, or traumatized hands.

Health care personnel should always address the older adult as "Mr.," "Mrs.," or "Miss" ("Ms."). Some older adults dislike being called by their first names by younger persons, and almost all take offense at being addressed as "Pop," "Grandma," "Sweetheart," or "Dear."

Physical limitations the patient may have should be considered in the planning of the interview and physical exam. Sensory-perceptual impairments are often present. The patient who is hearing impaired should be faced directly, so that the interviewer's mouth and face are fully visible. Contrary to popular practice, it does not help to shout. Shouting actually distorts speech.

In some cases, it may be necessary to break up the interview into more than one visit, collecting the most important historical data first. Certain portions of the data, such as past history or the review of systems, can be provided on a form that the patient fills out at home. However, using a form assumes that the older patient has the capacity to complete it. The completed form should then be reviewed with the patient during the interview.

It is important to pace the assessment of older adults, who often have a great deal of background material to sort through. Further, some older adults need more time to interpret questions and process answers. They should not be rushed. Any indication that he or she is being rushed may cause such a patient to retreat, so that valuable data are lost, and the patient's needs unmet.

Touch is a nonverbal skill that is significant to older adults. Their other senses may be impaired, so touch helps ground the interviewer in reality. A hand on the patient's arm or shoulder is an empathic message communicating interest.

Occasionally, an older adult asks personal questions about the interviewer's life or opinions. Such questions need not be answered. A brief response may be appropriate, but thought should be given to the motive behind the personal questions. Loneliness or anxiety may be directing the questions. Sexual innuendoes, flirtatious compliments, or advances occur on rare occasions. Some people perceive acute or chronic illness as threats to self-esteem and sexual adequacy. The interviewer should make sure to communicate acceptance of the older adult and understanding of the need to be self-assertive, but should make clear that sexual advances will not be tolerated.

History of Present Illness

The patient should be carefully questioned about the problems for which the patient is seeking care. History of the present illness should include the onset of the problem, the setting in which it occurred, manifestations, and any self-treatment attempted. Principal complaints should be described in terms of location, quality, quantity or severity, timing, the setting in which they occur, aggravating and alleviating factors, and any associated symptoms.

The history of present illness should also include the older adult's responses to symptoms and limitations. The interviewer should ask what the patient thinks caused the problem. What underlying worries might the patient have that led him or her to seek attention, and why it is a worry? Any effects the illness has had on the activities of daily living should be noted. An older adult may shrug off a symptom as evidence of growing older and may be unsure that it is worth mentioning. Furthermore, some older adults maintain a conservative philosophy that "if it ain't broken, don't fix it." These patients may present for care only when there is a blatant problem.

Past Health History

In addition to the history of the present illness, the general state of health as the patient perceives it over the past 5 years should be noted. The presence or occurrences of adult illnesses, accidents, injuries, operations, and hospitalizations should be elicited. It is usually not necessary to include obstetric history for a woman who has passed menopause and has no gynecologic symptoms. However, a perimenopausal history should be obtained, including any symptoms and whether or not estrogen replacement therapy is or was used.

Current use of prescribed and over-the-counter drugs, home remedies, herbals, and vitamins should be elicited. Drug allergies should be documented, including the description of an allergic response, when it occurred, interventions used, and any sequelae. A listing of the names, strength, and directions for use of each drug should be noted. As-needed drugs should be included, especially if the patient reports taking them one or more times weekly. The prescriber of the drug(s) should also be identified during the interview, and the elicited information checked against prescription labels.

Ideally, older adults should be encouraged to bring all drugs they are taking to their appointments. Prescription bottles provide additional information, such as the name of pharmacy that dispensed the drug. The reason for the use of more than one pharmacy should be elicited. Because the older adult tends to save leftover drugs, expiration dates should also be noted. Expired drugs should be destroyed because of the potential for ineffectiveness or toxicity; the patient's permission must be requested before disposal.

Additionally, older adults should be questioned about how they remember to take scheduled drugs, whether they ever forget to take a dose, and if so, what they do about it. Have they ever intentionally discontinued a drug, and if so, why? This information helps evaluate the patient's understanding of and compliance with the drug regimen, as well as its safety. The interviewer should explore the possibility of physical impairments, memory loss, health or cultural beliefs, financial constraints, or lack of support systems that impair safe self-administration of drugs.

Physical Exam Findings

When the history has been completed, the focus of the physical exam is established. The decision is made to perform either a baseline total exam or a limited, but detailed exam of body systems related to the patient's complaint.

The approach to assessment must be tailored to the older person's needs. The standard method for physical exams may be quite appropriate for the young person or an alert, oriented older adult who is not acutely ill and has no sensory deficits. However, the exam may need to be modified for the older person who is acutely ill and who may not be able to accomplish or tolerate the usual position for the exam. Rest periods may be required during the exam.

To organize the exam and to minimize omissions and patient fatigue, the examiner should follow three practices: minimize changes of patient position (where possible), organize the body into units for exam, and integrate the information sought according to body systems. The entire body can be examined by placing the patient in a sequence of positions: standing, sitting, supine, sitting again, and the lithotomy or side-lying position (when needed).

Because older adults are often cold and are at risk for hypothermia, it is necessary to limit exposure of body parts to a minimum. This is accomplished with the appropriate use of a patient gown and drapes, which also conveys to the patient the examiner's respect of concerns for privacy.

A major concern in working with the old-old is mobility and balance. The patient may need assistance getting into position for the exam because of limitations of sensory perception or physical mobility, confusion, agitation, or other problems. Assistance should be provided as indicated. Some physical exam techniques (e.g., deep knee bends) may not be appropriate. Other techniques need modification, such as testing the range of hip motion in a person who has had a total hip replacement or prosthesis. Care must be taken in performing any procedure that has the potential to result in injury or a fall.

Some patients have physical deformities that require modification in positioning. For example, the person with severe kyphosis may have difficulty maintaining a supine position. The person with hip contracture requires modifications in the lithotomy position. Patients who use wheelchairs or require walkers for balance cannot perform a Romberg test.

As the examination proceeds, each step should be prefaced with an explanation. Explanations help alleviate the fear, anger, and resistance that might appear if the patient were examined without explanation. For the hearing-impaired patient who can see, the demonstration of the instruments on the examiner before they are used on the elder improves understanding and increases cooperation.

For the patient who is both hearing and vision impaired, touch is the only means of communication. The examiner should gently guide the patient's hand to the examiner's face, shoulders, and hands. The patient should be allowed to feel the instruments before they are used in the exam. The investment of time and encouragement of touch communicates the examiner's good will and respect for the patient's identity.

Diagnostic Testing

Diagnostic testing of the older adult includes laboratory screening studies as well as hepatic and renal function testing to establish baselines and to monitor drug therapy. Because of the age-related decline in renal function and the use of potentially nephrotoxic drugs, monitoring of renal function is vital.

A variety of assessment instruments may also be used, such as the CADET, a self-care assessment tool. This tool addressed the patient's level of independence as it relates to Communication, Ambulation, activities of Daily living, Elimination, and Transfer abilities. The Comprehensive Older Person's Evaluation (COPE) instrument, similar to the CADET, uses cognition, social support, financial considerations, physical and psychological health, and activities of daily living categories. A number of other instruments are available to help assess the patient's functional status. These assessments are vital, particularly for older adults who are living alone or who have multiple limitations. Not all older adults are in need of supervision.

Developmental Considerations

The older adult has the potential for more personal losses than younger people. Losses o^r loved ones, of job status and prestige, of income, and of an energetic and resilient body occur with time. The grief and despair surrounding these losses can affect mental status, leading to disorientation, disability, or depression.

The interviewer should attempt to learn the priorities and goals of the older adult, as well as how he or she has handled crises in the past. Because the patient may pursue similar adaptive patterns in the present situation, this information can help with care planning. It is also helpful to determine the patient's perception of the situation. Such information can be elicited by asking questions such as, "Can you tell me how you feel about getting older?" "What kinds of things do you find most satisfying?" "What kinds of things worry you?" and "What would you like to change if you could?" It is normal for older adults to reminisce about the past and to reflect upon previous experiences, including joys, regrets, and conflicts. Listening to the life review process provides important insights into developmental conflicts.

Psychosocial Considerations

Although variations exist, the typical older adult has at least one serious illness or limiting condition and is aware of the increasing frequency of death among his or her peers. These issues, coupled with society's generally negative view of aging, lead to a fear that the person has lost all that remains of youth. The task, then, is not so much to look for new forms of youthfulness, but rather to seek forms of continued usefulness. The search may take the older adult toward new creative endeavors. The older adult has stepped off stage in both formal employment and the family circle. This change can be traumatic, because it means a loss of recognition and authority. However, there is now an attempt to direct energy inward. When financially and socially secure, the older adult can pursue whatever activity is important. Spending more time at home also affects the marriage relationship. Some couples find that having one or both at home means invasion of previously held "turf," such as the kitchen, garden, or workshop.

The older adult has the task of finding the meaning of life, the purpose for his or her own existence, and adjusting to the inevitability of death. The majority of older adults present with a calm demeanor and self-assurance, providing satisfying answers to questions. However, the interviewer must be alert for the occasional person who sounds hopeless and despairing about life at present and in the future. Requests for antianxiety drugs or sedative-hypnotics may help identify the person who has difficulty coping.

Analysis and Management

Treatment Objectives

The goal of drug therapy in the older adult is to maintain health status using the fewest drugs possible. Drug dosing should be individualized so as to decrease the likelihood of noncompliance, adverse drug reactions, or drug interactions. The purpose of and need for each drug should be weighed. The possibility of additive adverse effects from several drugs should be considered in the formulation of management objectives. Use of drugs that exacerbate the older adult's disease states should be questioned.

Treatment Options

Prescribing drugs for an older adult is complex, involving numerous considerations. Thus, there are six basic principles of prescribing for the older adult:

- Start low and go slow.
- Start one (drug), stop two.
- Do not use a drug if the adverse effects are worse than the disease.
- Use as few drugs as possible, choosing nondrug therapies when possible.
- Assess the patient's response frequently.
- Consider drug holidays from time to time.

Ideally, drug regimens are kept simple with the least frequent administration schedule used. Keeping the number of drugs to a minimum will reduce the potential for drug interactions and improve the patient's ability to comply with the drug regimen. Table 8–4 identifies selected reasons for noncompliance and possible solutions.

TABLE 8–4 REASONS FOR NONCOMPLIANCE WITH DRUG THERAPY AMONG OLDER ADULTS

Etiology	Possible Solution(s)
Inability to pay for prescribed drugs	Minimize number of drugs prescribed, and use therapeutic alternatives when possible Refer patient to appropriate agency for financial assistance
Forgetfulness	Use calendars, diaries
Knowledge deficit regarding drug or disease state	Educate patient
Confusion surrounding multiple drug regimen	Simplify drug regimen Make sure prescriptions are clearly labeled Provide written as well as verbal instructions
Misunderstandings of directions or instructions	Simplify directions and instructions Make sure directions are clear
Inability to tolerate adverse effects of drugs	Closely monitor patient condition Consider changing to another drug Consider reducing dosage or frequency of administration
Interference with prescribed drug regimen because of use of self-treatment strategies	Educate patient
Overdose or underdose based on patient's perception of need for the drug	Educate patient
Expiration of prescription supplies prior to follow-up appointment with health care provider	Closely monitor patient profile
Fatigue or illness that prevents drug ingestion	Educate patient Reevaluate patient condition

Although still somewhat controversial, "drug holidays" may also be considered from time to time. Drug holidays reduce the likelihood that drugs will accumulate to toxic levels in the blood stream, increase mental alertness (in some cases), and provide a cost savings. The use of drug holidays, however, requires interdisciplinary support, planning, and thorough assessment of the appropriateness of this strategy. Drugs that are usually not included in a drug holiday are antibiotics, anticoagulants, anticonvulsants, antidiabetic drugs, and ophthalmic drugs. The health care provider may have overlooked this option and may need to be reminded of the length of time the patient has been using the drug.

Intervention

Administration

Alterations in the dosage forms of some drugs may be required for the older adult. Dry mucous membranes can cause tablets and capsules to stick to the roof or sides of the mouth and not be swallowed. If tablets and capsules dissolve in the mouth, they can be irritating. If they are spit out, they are of no value. Water should be offered before and after administering oral drugs if the patient's condition permits. The patient should be positioned so that gravity assists passage of the drug through the esophagus and minimizes the risk of aspiration. Because of diminished sensation, the older adult may be unaware that a tablet or capsule is stuck between the lip and the gum. The patient should be asked to examine the mouth to ensure that the drug has been swallowed. Further, dentures can mask where the tablet is in the mouth. In some cases, a drug that is formulated as a liquid or suspension may be easier to take than tablets.

In some cases, capsules can be opened and the contents placed in applesauce, ice cream, or other soft food. The exceptions to this practice are with enteric-coated, slow-release, and extended-release drug formulations that are specifically designed to begin action in the small intestine. Furthermore, caution should be used when mixing drugs with food products, especially if the patient's appetite is already impaired.

Intramuscular and subcutaneous administration of drugs is necessary when immediate results are sought or when other routes are not available. Commonly, the older adult bleeds slightly or oozes after an injection because of decreased tissue elasticity or altered clotting mechanisms. Use of the Z-track technique facilitates sealing of the injection tract and reduces bleeding and leakage of drug. (Blood dyscrasias are also more common in the older adult.) A small bandage may be helpful. Injections should not be given in an immobile extremity, because inactivity reduces the rate of absorption. When frequent injections are required, the site of administration should be monitored for signs of irritation, inflammation, or infection. Reduction or absence of subcutaneous sensation in older persons may delay their awareness of a complication at the injection site.

At times, intravenous administration is necessary. In addition to monitoring for drug effects, attention should be paid to the amount of fluid in which the drug is administered. Declining cardiac and renal function make the older person more susceptible not only to dehydration but also to overhydration. Of course, the patient should also be monitored for complications such as infiltration, air embolism, thrombophlebitis, and pyrogenic reactions. As with injection sites, decreased sensation may mask these potential complications.

Suppositories can be expelled by the older adult, because circulation in the lower bowel and vagina is decreased and lower body temperature keeps the suppositories from melting. A special effort should be made to ensure that the suppository is not expelled. The suppository should be positioned above the rectal sphincter and away from any feces that may be present in the rectum. Having the patient remain in a supine or lateral recumbent position promotes retention of the suppository. Longer time should be permitted for the suppository to melt.

If the patient has a memory or sensory deficit, the use of prefilled syringes, prefilled envelopes, or containers labeled with the drug, day of the week, and time of administration may be helpful. Commercial medicine boxes are available that help organize the drugs and allow the patient and caregiver check how much drug has been taken (see Figure 9–1). A labeled egg carton can also serve the same compartmentalizing purpose at a much lower cost.

Education

The older adult's understanding of the prescribed therapy should be determined and the requisite teaching implemented. The aging process leaves mental status intact. There is no decrease in knowledge and little or no loss of vocabulary with aging, although response time is slower than in younger persons. Slower responses affect new learning. The Patient Teaching Guidelines, applicable to all people receiving drug therapy, are particularly useful with the aging population.

The health care provider should review all drugs with the patient or caregiver, clarifying information as needed. In some cases, complex drug regimens can be simplified by discussing the possible alterations with the health care provider. A homebound, confused, or isolated older adult is more likely to follow a drug regimen improperly. The functional assessment obtained during the history and physical exam helps determine whether the older adult needs a compliance aid or a memory cue to take the drugs. Additionally, the health care provider will need to determine whether a family member or a caregiver is available or required, if the older adult lives alone. Further, the ability of the patient to obtain necessary drugs should be facilitated when necessary. If the patient is essentially homebound, the use of a pharmacy that delivers can be helpful. Referral to a social worker may be necessary to obtain financial or other forms of assistance.

Evaluation

The overall purpose of evaluating drug therapy is to bring all parts of the regimen together. Evaluation involves looking at the overall drug regimen and answering the following questions:

- Were there any recent drug changes? Why were they made?
- Is cost or the patient's physical limitations a barrier to safe drug use?
- Are chronic symptoms improving, or are there new symptoms? Could the symptoms possibly be adverse drug effects?

PATIENT TEACHING GUIDELINES

The following information should be provided for each drug taken:

I. The name of the drug, both generic and brand name.
II. The purpose of the drug and what it does, and the disease or condition for which it is prescribed.
III. The color, size, and shape of the dosage form (e.g., tablet, capsule, liquid).
IV. The route of administration (by mouth, inhalation, topical, etc).
V. The dosing schedule. Consider these factors:
   A. The patient's activities of daily living schedule (e.g., eating, sleeping, activities).
      1. Work with the patient to develop a feasible schedule.
      2. Specify the times of day and associated meals or activities; for example: "Take one tablet at 7 am when you get up, one at noon with lunch, and one at 5 pm with your dinner."
      3. Do not assume the number of meals, time of meals, or hours of sleeping.
   B. Should the drug be taken on an empty stomach or with meals?
   C. Can the drug be taken at the same time as other drugs?
   D. Are there any restrictions on alcohol consumption while taking the drug?
   E. If the drug is prescribed on an as-needed basis, how often can it be taken? What signs or symptoms should the patient use to decide whether it can or should be taken?
   F. Indicate what to do if a dose is missed. Should the dose be skipped? Should two doses be taken at the same time?
   G. When the dosage is to be changed after a time, be specific about the instructions; for example: Rather than instructing the patient to "take one tablet each day for the next 3 days, then increase to two tablets per day," instruct them as follows: "Take one tablet in the morning each day for 3 days, starting tomorrow, Tuesday, January 15th. Then increase to one tablet in the morning and one tablet at night, starting Friday, January 18th."
VI. Indicate the length of time the drug should be taken, that is, a short time for an acute problem versus a prolonged time for a chronic one.
VII. Indicate whether the new drug is intended to replace or is to be added to current drug regimens.
VIII. Describe the adverse effects so that they are recognizable, and explain what action the patient should take. Point out what actions the patient should take if symptoms arise, and explain the degree of urgency in reporting them.
IX. Identify any special precautions; for example: "Do not take with drug at the same time as, or less than 2 hours after, you take your antacid."
X. Give special instructions regarding storage if this is an important consideration: Does the drug need to be refrigerated? Should it always be left in its original container? Does the drug have an especially short shelf-life? Is it wise for the patient to request a non-childproof cap for the drug container, or is a childproof cap warranted?
XI. Give instructions on how to refill the prescription: Are the number of refills indicated on the container, and if so, where? This is particularly important for hospitalized patients going home.
XII. Give instructions in writing, and review them orally with the patient; encourage the patient to call if he or she has any questions.
XIII. When and how should the patient follow up with the health care provider?
XIV. What is the procedure for disposing of noncurrent and expired drugs?

- Is the older adult concurrently using nonprescription drugs, home remedies, or street drugs?
- Could there be information that has not been reported to the health care provider?
- Have plans for follow-up care been outlined and follow-up done as necessary?

Further, older adults who are managing drug regimens at home may misuse drugs in more than one way. They may share drugs with friends or family or save the drugs for use in self-treatment in the future. Additionally, they may not understand the purpose of the drug and, as a result, may increase their risk of taking duplicate drugs; this situation is a consequence not so much of the aging process as of poor prescribing practices. With the growing availability of generic drugs, the prescriber can choose drugs that are different colors, sizes, and shapes, so as to help the patient differentiate them. This possibility exists whether the patient uses the same pharmacy each time or has prescriptions filled at multiple pharmacies.

The underlying reasons for sharing drugs is often the desire to help out a friend by providing something that has, after all, given oneself symptomatic relief. The recipient may not wish to refuse the friend, may believe that previous remedies did not work, or may not wish to consult a health care provider.

A similar problem is the use of drugs that have been prescribed for an earlier problem. Saving prescription drugs is common in the older adult. Cost and financial constraints often enter into the patient's desire to save or to be frugal. However, there are three risks associated with this practice: self-diagnosis, self-treatment, and the use of outdated drugs.

Self-treatment with drugs, vitamins, herbal remedies, or home remedies is not necessarily harmful but can become so if the practice keeps the older adult from seeking or receiving needed evaluation and treatment. Although vitamins, herbal remedies, or home remedies are not always viewed as drug therapy, such practices may aggravate underlying problems, affecting current disease or interacting with a prescribed drug regimen.

Some older adults maintain a such strong belief in the efficacy of drugs and the wisdom of the health care provider that they continue to take drugs even after significant adverse effects appear. Others are reluctant to bother the health care provider with "minor" complaints. Still others attribute their symptoms to normal aging or have a habit of disregarding signs and symptoms; these two factors may cause a delay in calling or even mentioning the onset of drug-related adverse effects. The health care provider should reinforce the notion that adverse effects sometimes do occur and that the patient is expected to contact the health care provider promptly if they do.

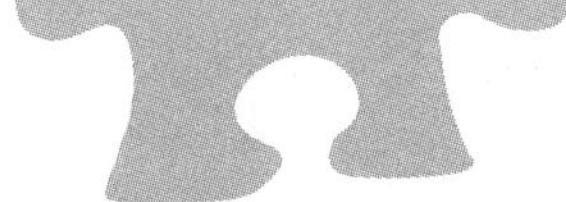

SUMMARY

- The cellular changes of aging are still not clearly understood. In general, changes of aging are related more to accumulation of pigments and metabolic processes and cell receptor unresponsiveness.
- The associated changes in the respiratory, cardiovascular, hepatic, and renal systems have significant implications for drug therapy.
- Signs and symptoms of adverse effects may manifest differently in the older adult and may not become apparent for extended periods.
- In most cases, older adults have less difficulty with absorption than with distribution, biotransformation, and elimination.
- Aging influences tissue responsiveness to drug concentrations in a number of ways.
- Polypharmacy is the result of the presence multiple disease processes, of the prescribing behaviors of the health care provider, and of poorly coordinated patient care management.
- Polypharmacy raises risk of adverse effects, drug interactions, and extended hospital stays and reduces the level of patient compliance.
- The rate of adverse effects is directly proportional to the number of drugs taken.
- Drug-related problems commonly affect the cardiovascular, central nervous, respiratory, renal, gastrointestinal, endocrine, and musculoskeletal systems.
- An invaluable tool for working with the older adult and effectively managing a drug regimen is the drug history.
- A drug history sets the background and provides data to begin evaluation of the patient in terms of drug therapy.
- A major cause of patient noncompliance is lack of understanding of the drug regimen. Frequent changing of the drugs prescribed is a common factor in misunderstanding of the drug regimen.
- Cost, memory deficits, physical limitations, and scheduling difficulties contribute to noncompliance.
- The goal of drug therapy is to maintain the patient on the fewest drugs possible and at optimal doses that will decrease the likelihood of noncompliance, adverse drug reactions, or drug interactions.
- Prescribing drugs for an older adult involves six basic principles: (1) start low and go slow; (2) start one (drug), stop two; (3) do not use a drug if the adverse effects are worse than the disease; (4) use as few drugs as possible using nondrug therapies when able; (5) assess response frequently; and (6) consider drug holidays from time to time.
- Many physiologic changes of aging affect the pharmacokinetic and pharmacodynamic characteristics of drugs. Knowledge of these changes helps minimize the potential for adverse effects and drug interactions.
- The objective of evaluating drug therapy is to bring all parts of the drug regimen together.
- Older adults managing their own drug regimens at home may misuse drugs by sharing them with friends or family, saving them to use for self-treatment in the future, or taking duplicate drugs.

BIBLIOGRAPHY

Abrams, W., and Berkow, R. (Eds.). (1990). *The Merck manual of geriatrics.* Rahway, NJ: Merck Sharp and Dohme Research Laboratories.

Alford, D. (1982). Bill of rights for elderly on drug therapy. *Nursing Clinics of North America,* 17(2), 282–302.

American Medical Association. (1995). *Drug evaluations annual 1995.* Washington, DC: American Medical Association.

Beers, M., and Ouslander, J. (1989). Risk factors in geriatric drug prescribing: A practical guide to avoiding problems. *Drugs,* 37, 105–112.

Bressler, R., and Katz, M. (1993). *Geriatric pharmacology.* New York: McGraw-Hill.

Cooper, J. (1989). The aging of America: How to deal with the geriatric patient in the community pharmacy. *Journal of Geriatric Drug Therapy,* 4(1), 33–49.

Fowles, D. (1990). *A profile of older Americans.* Washington, DC: American Association of Retired Persons.

Klein, R., Klein, B., Jensen, S., et al. (1994). The relation of socioeconomic factors to age-related cataract, maculopathy, and impaired vision: The Beaver Dam eye study. *Ophthalmology,* 101(12), 1969–1979.

Kroenke, L., and Pinholt, E. (1990). Reducing polypharmacy in the elderly: A controlled trial of physician feedback. *Journal of the American Geriatric Society,* 38(1), 31–36.

Lichtenstein, M. (1992). Hearing and visual impairments. *Clinics in Geriatric Medicine,* (8)1, 173–182.

Mahoney, C. (1991). Return to independence: Lessons from a hospital long-term care unit. *American Journal of Nursing,* March, 45–48.

McCue, J. (1993). *Geriatric drug handbook for long term care.* Baltimore: Williams & Wilkins.

Mead, G. (1934). *Mind, self, and society.* Chicago: University Press.

Miller, C. (1990). When medication harms as well as helps. *Geriatric Nursing,* 11(6), 301–302.

Moore, J., and Johnson, J. (1993). Over-the-counter drug use by the rural elderly. *Geriatric Nursing,* 14(4), 190–191.

Nielson, C. (1994). Pharmacologic considerations in critical care of the elderly. *Clinics in Geriatric Medicine,* 10(1), 71–89.

Pearlman, R. (1987). Development of a functional assessment questionnaire for geriatric patients: The comprehensive older persons' evaluation (COPE). *Journal of Chronic Disease,* 40, 85S–94S.

Pollow, R., Stoller, E., Forster, L., et al. (1994). Drug combinations and potential for risk of adverse drug reaction among community-dwelling elderly. *Nursing Research,* 43(1), 44–49.

Practice Trends. (1993). Geriatric assessment reduces mortality. *American Pharmacist,* NS33(7), 10.

Rameizl, P. (1983). CADET: A self-care assessment tool. *Geriatric Nursing,* 4(12), 377–378.

Stratton, M. (1991). Geriatric pharmacotherapy: Pharmaguide to hospital medicine. *Journal of Geriatric Drug Therapy,* 4(3), 1–5.
United States Department of Commerce. (1990). *Statistical abstract of the US.* (110th ed.). Washington, DC: Bureau of the Census.
Wade, B., and Bowling, A. (1986). Appropriate use of drugs by elderly people. *Journal of Advanced Nursing,* 11, 47–55.
Walker, J., and Wynne, H. (1994). Review: The frequency and severity of adverse drug reactions in elderly people. *Age and Aging,* 23(3), 255–259.
White, P. (1995). Pearls for practice: Polypharmacy and the older adult. *Journal of the American Academy of Nurse Practitioners,* 7(11), 545–548.

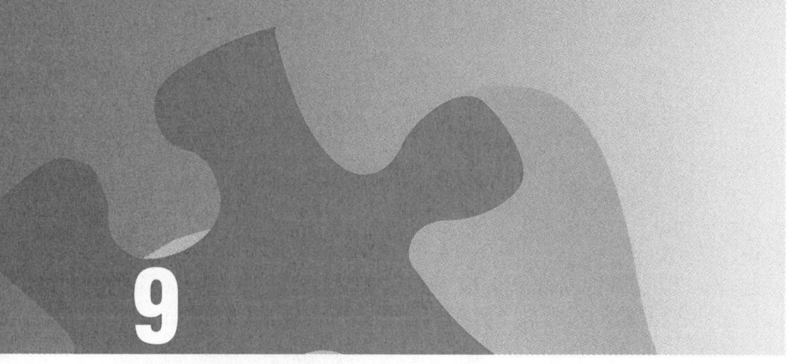

9 Community Pharmacotherapeutics

Knowledge of pharmacotherapeutics takes on growing importance as health care moves out of the institutional setting and into the community. Increasingly, the health care provider is managing the care of patients who are self-administering drugs while residing at home and in community settings. The purpose of the health care provider's involvement in community drug use is to promote health by facilitating safe, knowledgeable drug use. The patient at home is unsupervised, remaining independent within the confines of illness or disability.

The community provides a context in which the health care provider gains an understanding of the patient and family's past experience with the health care system. Knowledge of health-illness beliefs and practices, religious influences, educational level, sociocultural variables, level of compliance with treatment plans, and family and community support systems is vital to successful pharmacotherapy.

CONSUMER BUYING PRACTICES

The numbers of available over-the-counter (OTC) products are estimated to be from 300,000 to more than 600,000, and they are manufactured by some 12,000 companies. The number of OTC drugs used has increased exponentially, for a number of reasons. The gradual move of some prescription drugs to OTC status continues to gain momentum, making even more drugs and other products available. Drug companies continually introduce new products to the marketplace. Furthermore, OTC drugs are easily accessible in a free enterprise system. In addition, consumers in general are engaged in self-diagnosing and self-treatment as the cost of and accessibility to health care have changed. Health care providers promote this trend by encouraging consumers to make informed decisions about health care. Thus, nonprescription drugs and medical devices such as contraceptives, dental hygiene preparations, home diagnostic products (e.g., pregnancy testing, occult blood), and monitoring products (e.g., home glucose monitoring) continue to constitute a significant portion of OTC purchases.

Over $10 billion are spent on OTC drugs each year. Of the total sales, 45 percent of expenditures were made in pharmacies. The remaining expenditures were made in food stores and discount merchandising outlets. With the sales of OTC drugs increasing approximately 8 to 10 percent annually, the potential for adverse effects also rises. Like prescription drugs, over-the-counter drugs contain active and inactive ingredients. Active ingredients are those that produce therapeutic effects (e.g., reduce fever), whereas inactive ingredients have no therapeutic effects (e.g., flavorings, coloring, preservatives). As a general rule, the fewer active ingredients contained in an OTC drug, the fewer the potential problems.

Approximately 70 percent of consumers treat themselves on a regular basis. Approximately 40 percent of the U.S. population uses at least one OTC drug in any 48-hour period. Eighty percent of self-limiting illnesses and health problems can be treated with OTC drugs (see Problems Considered Amenable to Self-Treatment with OTC Drugs).

Self-care supports two important cultural values in U.S. society—independence and freedom of action. The accessibility of OTC products symbolizes the independence. The Nonprescription Drug Manufacturers Association emphasizes, however, that self-treatment decisions should include informed, appropriate, and responsible use of OTC products. In addition, the NDMA stresses that responsible self-treatment does not involve the use of prescription drugs without medical supervision.

Over-the-counter drugs and products are purchased most often without professional assistance. Consumers are more inclined to self-treat when they perceive their illnesses to be minor or not amenable to medical interventions, or the cost of medical care to be prohibitive. Consumers may also treat themselves because of distrust of the health care system or its providers.

OTC drugs have advantages and disadvantages (Table 9–1). In some cases, the consumer does not understand or cannot accurately determine the seriousness of signs and symptoms. Additionally, some OTC drugs can mask the actual problem and yet relieve the signs and symptoms. Further, many OTC drugs contain potentially harmful ingredients (e.g., caffeine, alcohol, phenylpropanolamine). If consumers do not, or cannot, read labels, they remain unaware of the potentially harmful ingredients until problems arise.

Use of OTC drugs appears to vary with gender and age. Women are more likely to use OTC drugs to treat anxiety, fatigue, headache, indigestion, obesity, and sleep and skin disorders. Men, on the other hand, self-treat muscle aches and pains, colds, cuts, and scratches. Persons younger than 55 years most often treat themselves for problems such as headaches, colds, sinus problems, cuts, and scratches. In contrast, persons older than 55 years typically treat themselves for age-related discomforts such as arthritis, constipation, and insomnia. Older persons also use more prescription drugs than younger adults. Thus, even though the use of OTC drugs tends to remain constant with age, the number of OTC products used by older adults continues to increase.

Self-care strategies are learned early and extend throughout life. Seventy percent of children younger than 2 years have been given OTC drugs at least once, and an average of 5.5 drugs are kept on hand by their caregivers. Some families keep as many as 16 different drugs on hand, and over 50 percent of ambulatory older adults have OTC drugs at home that are not being used.

PROBLEMS CONSIDERED AMENABLE TO SELF-TREATMENT WITH OTC DRUGS

Acne
Allergic rhinitis, nasal congestion
Athlete's foot
Bacterial infections (superficial, uncomplicated, topical)
Boils
Burns (minor thermal burns, sunburn)
Calluses, corns, and warts
Cold and canker sores
Constipation, flatulence
Contact dermatitis (e.g., poison ivy, poison oak)
Contraception
Coughs and colds, sore throat
Dandruff
Diabetes mellitus (insulin, supplies)
Diaper rash
Diarrhea (e.g., traveler's diarrhea)
Dry skin, dry mouth
Dysmenorrhea, premenstrual syndrome
Fever
Halitosis
Head lice
Heartburn, dyspepsia
Hemorrhoids
Insect bites, stings
Insomnia
"Jock itch," prickly heat
Mineral and vitamin deficiencies
Minor aches and pains, headache
Motion sickness
Nausea and vomiting
Pinworms
Sprains and strains
"Swimmer's ear"
Vaginal fungus infection

Data from Covington, T. (1992). Overview of nonprescription drug therapy and the self-care movement. Paper presented at the 139th annual meeting of the American Pharmaceutical Association in San Diego. March 14.

A number of factors influence consumer behaviors—social pressures that encourage self-reliance and self-responsibility for health, economy of time, and limited resources. Too many consumers are inclined to self-treat with prescription drugs already in the home. Cultural expectations, alternative health care options, education, sophistication, the wide range of OTC products, and the availability of pharmacists all contribute to the trend for self-treatment. In addition, when pharmacists are consulted, they often have recommendations for specific OTC drugs. These recommendations include drugs for sore throats, coughs, allergies, diarrhea, hemorrhoids, fungal vaginal tract infections, "jock itch," and athlete's foot.

Partly as a consequence of proliferation of OTC drugs and other health care products, a growing number of prescription drugs are going unclaimed. A patient visits the health care provider, obtains a prescription, and submits it to the pharmacy for processing. However, the prescription is never claimed. In many cases, the patient, once diagnosed, turns to OTC drugs and home remedies for symptom relief. Factors contributing to the number of unclaimed prescriptions are drug cost, forgetfulness, and improved condition. Some patients do not want the drug or believe that there was a lack of communication with the health care provider. Other patients disagree with the health care provider and choose not to pick up the prescription.

LEGISLATIVE CONTROL OF OTC DRUGS

Legislative control of OTC drugs is designed to protect consumers. In 1906, the initial focus of federal legislation on food and drug products was with adulterated products. A 1938 act mandated that all new drugs be proven safe for human use. Although there have been several amendments since, the 1952 Durham-Humphrey amendment was the first to address OTC drugs, thus distinguishing prescription from nonprescription drugs. The act was expanded in 1962 to provide assurance of a drug's safety and effectiveness for its intended use and to establish a means of improving communication about the drugs.

In 1970, the National Research Council of the National Academy of Sciences found that 75 percent of the OTC drugs reviewed were not effective for at least one or more of their intended uses. As a result, the Food and Drug Admin-

TABLE 9–1 ADVANTAGES AND DISADVANTAGES OF OTC DRUGS

Advantages	Disadvantages
Promotes consumer responsibility for health maintenance	Requires consumer self-diagnosis
Greater availability	Increased use of anecdotal and/or nonprofessional advice
Easily accessible and obtainable	Patient may not be able to read labels, may misread or misunderstand directions
Free professional advice (RPh) often available	Patient may not ask for or receive professional advice when uncertain about directions
Less costly to acquire, because visit to health care provider is not required	Increased susceptibility to incomplete or exaggerated advertising claims
Generally safe and effective for many conditions when used as directed	Greater potential for drug-drug and drug-food interactions
Lower cost	Higher risk of delay in seeking needed medical attention

OVER-THE-COUNTER DRUG CLASSIFICATIONS

Antacids
Antimicrobials I
Antimicrobials II
Antiperspirants
Bronchodilator and antiasthmatic drugs
Cold, cough, allergy drugs
Contraceptives and other vaginal drugs
Dentifrice and dental care drugs
Hemorrhoidal drugs
Internal analgesics, antipyretics, and antirheumatics
Laxatives, antidiarrheals, emetics, and antiemetics
Miscellaneous external drugs
Ophthalmics
Oral cavity drug preparations
Sedatives, tranquilizers, and sleeping aids
Vitamins, minerals, and hematinics

istration (FDA) established the OTC Drug Review panel in 1972, to ensure that OTC drugs were safe, effective, and not mislabeled. Prescription drugs are evaluated in their finished dosage forms, whereas only the active ingredients in OTC drugs are evaluated.

New OTC drugs are divided into two categories. Category I drugs are *recognized as safe and effective* (RASE). Category II drugs are *generally recognized as safe and effective* (GRASE). *Safe* refers to (1) the low potential for harm if the drug is misused and (2) the rarity of major adverse effects when the drug is used as directed. A drug is considered *effective* (used as directed) when it provides the relief intended for the majority of the population. A drug classified as GRASE has more relaxed requirements than one classified as RASE. No FDA preclearance is required for a GRASE drug. Approval is needed only for the active ingredient rather than for the entire formulation, and flexible labeling is permitted (although it must not be misleading and must meet the requirements of the 1938 act). All data about the drug are public information, and the marketing of the drug is not limited to the manufacturer. Classifications of OTC drugs have been established by the FDA (see OTC Drug Classifications).

Since the FDA's review of OTC products began in 1972, some ingredients have been removed from the market because they were not safe (e.g., phenacetin). Others have been reclassified as prescription drugs after clinical data revealed serious adverse effects (e.g., hexachlorophene). Conversely, FDA review has also led to the reclassification of some prescription drug ingredients as OTC drugs (e.g., ibuprofen and some hydrocortisone creams).

Drug Packaging

Drug packaging laws came into being in the early 1980s, after several reported episodes of cyanide poisoning in the U.S. via OTC analgesics. The cyanide was thought to have been added to the analgesic capsules once they reached store shelves. To prevent a recurrence of these problems, drug manufacturers developed sealed, tamper-resistant containers. The containers usually have an inner seal of aluminum foil, together with a plastic outer ring around the cap or a shrink-seal full-package plastic wrapper. Some drugs are packaged using a unit-dose system.

Drug packages should be carefully inspected before purchase and use. A discrepancy between the lot number on the container and that on the outer packaging many suggest tampering as well as breaks, cracks, or holes in the outer wrapping, or other indications that the outer packaging has been disturbed, unwrapped, or replaced. Distortion or stretching of the shrink-seal, a loose bottle cap, or traces of paper or glue around the outer rim of the container may indicate that the seal has been removed and replaced. Additionally, discoloration or disarray of the cotton plug, an overfilled or underfilled bottle, or an unusual appearance of the drug should also alert the consumer to possible tampering.

Tablets are suspect if they are not of the usual size, thickness, color, shine, smoothness, taste, odor, or manufacturer's insignia. Variations in color, size, length, odor, or manufacturer's insignia and the presence of fingerprints, cracks, dents, or surface dullness should be reported. Liquids should be checked for color, clarity, thickness, sediment, and odor. Ophthalmic solutions should have intact protective seals (manufacturers of such products are also required to ensure their sterility). Ointments, creams, and pastes contained in tubes should be properly sealed, and the bottom of the tube crimped and uniform in appearance. Ointments should have a smooth, uniform consistency.

If tampering is suspected, the package should be returned to the pharmacy from where it was dispensed. The pharmacy in turn will report suspected tampering to the Drug Product Problem Reporting Program. This program is coordinated by the FDA in collaboration with the United States Pharmacopeia and the American Society of Health System Pharmacists.

Drug Labeling

Labeling requirements for OTC drugs are strict and specific. Labels must be written so that the information is likely to be read and understood even by consumers whose intelligence, education levels, and reading skills are limited. Professional labeling in some drug monographs (the written mechanism by which drugs are evaluated by the FDA) provides more information than is otherwise required on an OTC label. Figure 9–1 illustrates a product label that meets FDA labeling requirements.

DRUG STORAGE, HANDLING, AND DISPOSAL

Storage

Variables affecting drug use in the home and community differ from those in the hospital. The United States Pharmacopeia establishes guidelines for drug storage. In an institutional setting, the nurse is most often the gatekeeper of the drug supply; in collaboration with colleagues, the nurse determines when and how drugs will be administered. In most cases, there is little input from the patient. Drugs are obtained from a stock supply or are accessible via unit-dose systems. The standard drug carts or cabinets are equipped with a drawer for each patient's drugs. Unused and discontinued drugs are returned to the pharmacy for proper disposal.

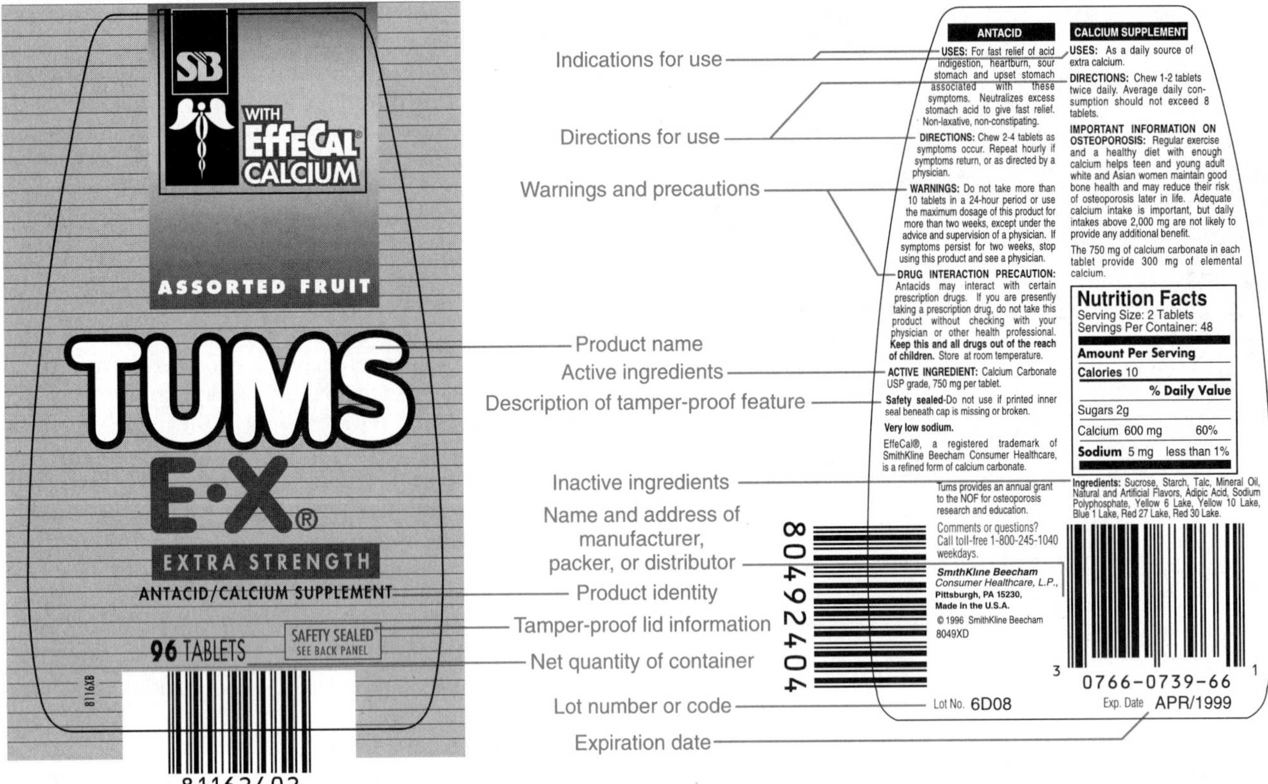

Figure 9–1 Labeling requirements for an OTC drug include statements that address several specific items including a description of the tamper-proof opener; product name; identity (type of drug); active ingredients; inactive ingredients; net quantity of the container (e.g., number of tablets); name and address of the manufacturer, packager, or distributor; indications for use; directions for administration; and warnings or precautions, expiration date, and the drug's lot number or code. (Label courtesy of Smith Kline Beecham, Pittsburgh, PA.)

In the home setting, however, the gatekeeper of the drug supply is the patient. Most drugs provided by community pharmacies are dispensed in a single container rather than a unit-dose container, posing a greater risk for misuse or overdosage. Further, any drug remaining after the condition for which it was purchased has improved is commonly saved rather than discarded, increasing the risk of later harm through misuse or reuse.

In the home, drugs should be kept in their original containers to ensure availability of correct directions and to avoid misidentification and unknown expiration dates. Storage in a secure, locked cabinet not located in the bathroom is recommended. Drug storage in the bathroom is not acceptable because bathroom cabinets rarely have a lock and are too easily accessible to children. These principles should be followed not only where children live but also where they may visit.

Further, chemical deterioration of drugs is hastened by heat, moisture, and, in some cases, light. Light-sensitive drugs should be stored in their original amber-colored containers and exposure to direct sunlight avoided. To prevent changes caused by moisture, silica gel inserts are packaged with some drugs. Moisture dissolves some solid dosage forms and heat melts the waxy base of suppositories and ointments.

Not all drugs should be stored at room temperature. Some drugs must be refrigerated at temperatures ranging from 35 to 60° F (2 to 15° C). Other drugs must be stored in a freezer, and still others must be stored where temperatures do not exceed 40° F. Multidose, injectable drugs and suppositories in airtight containers are refrigerated to protect them from humidity and food residues. Such a container is placed where it is least accessible to children but away from freezer coils. Accidental freezing may alter drug characteristics.

Insulin presents a special storage problem. Bacterial contamination is possible, owing to the multidose container in which insulin is manufactured and the prolonged time over which it is used. The potential for contamination of insulin is high even though a preservative is added. However, insulin should be administered at room temperature to reduce the risk of lipoatrophy and lipohypertrophy at injection sites. Insulin vials in current use are kept at room temperature, and additional vials are refrigerated.

Handling

Many drugs are dispensed in containers with childproof caps. Because the caps require complex manipulation, the time required for children to gain access to the drug is prolonged. The caps reduce the potential for accidental ingestion and have lowered the incidence of poisoning in children. Such caps are difficult for persons with impaired dexterity to use, however. Standard, easily opened containers are available and can be requested at the time a drug is dispensed. However, special safeguards must be taken to prevent access by children. Further, when drugs are handled, the container should be protected from soiling so that the label remains legible as long as possible.

Consumers should be discouraged from borrowing drugs from family members or others. The money saved by "borrowing" is likely to translate into a much greater expense in the form of ineffective treatment and higher risks of adverse effects and drug-drug interactions.

Disposal

Pharmaceutical manufacturers establish expiration dates and print them on the label or package insert of each drug. Expiration dates are only approximations and do not indicate that a drug is at once rendered useless or harmful on that date. However, most drugs lose potency over time, although some can become toxic (e.g., tetracycline, acetaminophen).

Consumers should be taught to discard drugs according to the following guidelines:

- Aspirin or acetaminophen (Tylenol) that smells like vinegar (has become toxic)
- Any drugs in solid dosage form (i.e., pills, tablets, capsules) that are damaged, discolored, softened, or stuck together
- Liquids that have lost their original color, smell, or taste or that have developed gas formations (indicate deterioration)
- Ointments or creams that have changed in odor, color, or consistency
- Any oral drug that is past its expiration date or is more than 2 years old
- Any drug that has not been stored as directed

Disposal of oral drugs is best accomplished by flushing down the toilet. In the absence of toilet facilities, tablets and capsules can be burned. Discarding drugs in a trash receptacle is asking for accidental poisoning of children or pets. The Centers for Disease Control and Prevention recommend disposing of needles, syringes, and vials by placing them in a sturdy (preferably metal) container with a tightly fitting lid. The container should be taped closed, double bagged, and placed with the regular household trash for disposal. Commercially available containers may also be used for disposal. However, some patients are not comfortable with disposal of needles, syringes, and vials at home. In that case, the container can be taken to a hospital or clinic, where it will be disposed of with other medical waste.

COMPLIANCE AND NONCOMPLIANCE

Compliance, how well the patient follows through with a drug regimen, has been a concern of health care providers for decades. Many assume that once a diagnosis is made and the prescription written, the patient will comply with the plan of care. Unfortunately, drug therapy of any kind is often compromised by lack of full compliance. In many cases, noncompliance is often the reason a patient reenters the health care system. One should note, however, that *noncompliance* is a term generated by health care providers and defines the problem from their viewpoint only. Not adhering to the drug regimen may be regarded as deviant behavior by the health care worker, but the patient may see the action as a cautious approach to self-administration of potentially harmful substances.

All health care providers have patients with the potential for noncompliance, whether through intentional or unintentional actions. The complex medical problems of many individuals and the varied drug regimens they are expected to follow lay the groundwork for noncompliance and drug interactions. One-third to one-half of prescription drugs are not taken as directed. In addition, some patients fail to have the prescription filled at all, or fail to pick up the filled prescription. Still others stop taking the drug too early in the treatment regimen, leading to treatment failure.

Noncompliance is the most common problem encountered in drug therapy administered at home. As many as 50 percent of patients engage in noncompliant behaviors, resulting in poor control of chronic illnesses and sometimes in extensive hospitalizations. Compliance by older adults, for example, is reduced when five or more drugs are prescribed, when drug labels cannot be read, or when containers are difficult to open.

The health care provider should consider noncompliance when inexplicable treatment failure occurs. Drugs that are not taken correctly when first prescribed may be used at a later date, when their chemical characteristics and potency have changed. Patients may discontinue a drug because of adverse effects, for a variety of reasons (e.g., failure to recognize them or to consider them important or relevant, health or cultural beliefs, life-style, confusion, or decreased memory). Sometimes, instead of investigating the cause of treatment failure, the health care provider simply increases the dosage of the same drug or changes to a new one. Table 9–2 provides examples of cues that may be predictive of noncompliance along with possible interventions.

COMMUNITY RESOURCES

Community Pharmacists

The role of the community pharmacist is growing as a result of the trend toward the use of OTC drugs. The expansion and greater availability of OTC drugs and the likelihood of more sophisticated and technical products provide the impetus for the consumer and health care provider alike to use the services and expertise of community pharmacists. Before 1972 and the FDA's review of OTC drugs, pharmacists avoided giving consumer advice or counseling about health care concerns. Now, this practice is encouraged, and pharmacists' expertise uniquely qualifies them to teach the patient as well as provide advice about OTC drugs. Many times, the community pharmacist is the first contact the consumer has with a health care provider.

Computer Information Systems

According to the American Society for Automation in Pharmacy, more than 90 percent of U.S. pharmacies use computers to process prescriptions. Within a computerized system, a patient's drug profile can be maintained for a de-

TABLE 9–2 ASSESSMENT AND INTERVENTIONS TO PROMOTE COMPLIANCE

Parameter	Factors Related to Noncompliance	Interview Questions	Possible Interventions
Personal health-illness beliefs and practices	Illness not as severe as perceived by health care provider Denial of problem results in patients' ignoring information Is susceptible to actual or potential illness	"How would you describe the severity of your illness?" "Would you describe yourself as healthy or unhealthy?"	Be sure questions asked and information provided are relevant from the patient's perspective
Beliefs regarding effectiveness of Western health care interventions	Patient does not believe Western health care is effective	"How would you describe the effectiveness of your care?"	Use nonjudgmental, active listening, e.g., ask, "Tell me about your beliefs."
Previous experience with health care system or health care provider	Patient expresses dissatisfaction with past or present interactions	"How do you feel about the care you received?"	Use non-judgmental, active listening Avoid false reassurance
Perception of complexity of management plan	Plan seems difficult to follow, vague, ambiguous, disruptive, or lengthy	"How does the plan of care affect your daily routine?"	Simplify regimen when possible Adapt it to patient's life-style
Level of trust	Patient lacks trust in health care provider or health care system Health care provider has failed to establish interest and trust	"To what degree do you trust your health care provider?" "What can we do that would foster your trust in us?"	Take a genuine interest in the patient. Follow up on patient responses, requests, and complaints
Compliance/ noncompliance	Patient never intends to comply Patient has history of noncompliance	"How do you plan to take your medications?" "How often did you take your medicine for your other illness?"	Acknowledge difficulty with compliance Explore strategies to improve it
Coping mechanisms	Patient uses denial, does not recognize need for treatment, exhibits repression, or is unable to mobilize energies to cope	Assess for cues such as, "I'm not so ill."	Educate patient about disease, drugs, etc., and effective coping mechanisms
Patient self-esteem	Negative self-image	Assess for verbal and/or nonverbal cues, such as, "Don't bother with me, I'm not worth the effort."	Provide resources for counseling relative to the patient's underlying problem
Economic status	Patient has lower socioeconomic status, is unemployed, lacks health insurance, or believes drugs are not worth the cost Patient believes self-care is a more efficient alternative to high-cost drugs.	"What resources do you have that help you with the cost of your treatment and medicines?"	Investigate situation and refer patient to appropriate resources for financial assistance Explore methods to alleviate environmental issues
Support systems	Patient lacks family or cultural support Patient lives alone	"When you want to talk about a problem, to whom do you go?"	Enlist family and friends to assist patient Refer to social services if appropriate
Reading and comprehension abilities	Inaccessible educational system Patient has limited reading and comprehension skills	Query patient about disease process, drug action, and adverse effects "Can you tell me what you see on this prescription bottle?" "What directions are on this container?"	Increase sensory exposure with pictures, charts, verbal reinforcement Assess baseline knowledge and build on that foundation Use nonjudgmental behaviors Refer to literacy hotline, local literacy council or other community service if appropriate
Physical capabilities to carry out plan of care	Patient physically unable to carry out plan of care Patient faces environmental obstacles	"What kind of problems do you have that make it difficult for you to take your medicine?" "Are you able to reach your medicines and open the containers?"	Assist patient to obtain non-childproof caps, if appropriate Explore alternative devices and methods of administration (e.g., automatic injection devices, magnifying glasses)

Adapted from Kuhn, M. (1991). *Pharmacotherapeutics: A nursing process approach.* (3rd ed.). Philadelphia: FA Davis. Used with permission.

fined number of years. Such systems are an avenue for checking food or drug allergies against each chemical contained in a drug and for compatibilities with other drugs the patient is taking. When incompatibility information is found, the pharmacy can notify the patient and health care provider before the drug is dispensed.

Tracking drug regimens through computerized information networks helps provide a safety net, but only to the extent that appropriate information has been provided by the patient. As more and more people engage in self-treatment, the importance of accurate, accessible information cannot be overestimated. It is imperative that the patient communicate information about food and drug allergies, the use of herbs and home remedies, prescription drugs that may have been dispensed by other health care providers, as well as OTC drugs that are used. Withholding such information places the patient at risk for harmful drug interactions and reactions and failure of the management plan.

Publications

Until the American Pharmaceutical Association published its first edition of the *Handbook of Nonprescription Drugs* in 1965, there was no information resource for nonprescription drugs. This handbook, the *United States Pharmacopeia Dispensing Information* (USPDI) compendia, and many lay publications and resource guides are now available to consumers (see Chapter 2). The *FDA Consumer* is a magazine that focuses on topics related to FDA-regulated products, including food safety, nutrition, prescription and OTC drugs, medical technology, cosmetics, and all of the other products and services under the FDA's jurisdiction. The magazine also provides a behindthe-scenes look at how the FDA uncovers fraudulent and illegal activities. The consumer also has easy access to professional resources, many of which are found in local bookstores. Health care providers can recommend publications and help patients evaluate such materials, which vary in accuracy, user friendliness, and completeness.

Critical Thinking Process

Assessment

Establishing a patient database at the patient's home is no different from performing the same activity in an office, clinic, or institutional setting. However, the health care provider must respect that the home is the patient's domain, where the provider is an invited guest. Obtaining information about where the health care provider should sit and other patient preferences is important. The provider should watch for nonverbal clues and respond accordingly.

History of Present Illness

The first step in assessing the patient at home is to identify the situation for which the patient seeks treatment. Patients may initially provide incomplete and vague information. The objective is to determine the patient's specific symptoms and whether they are amenable to self-treatment.

Past Health History

Pertinent past health information is important to effective drug management. Information to be elicited includes the patient's age, pre-existing medical problems or chronic disease, drug and food allergies, long-term (more than 2 weeks) use of prescription or OTC drugs and home remedies, and past use of vitamins, supplements, nicotine, alcohol, and illicit drugs.

Special monitoring is required for certain drug therapies. Therefore, the provider must assess the patient's understanding of current drug therapies, therapeutic and adverse effects, and motivation to learn and comply with the prescribed regimen. Attitudes influence compliance. For a patient with a newly diagnosed condition, the appropriateness of the drug regimen and factors that may necessitate a change in the management plan should be evaluated.

Several methods may be used to assess compliance with a drug regimen. Patient self-reporting may be inaccurate if the patient has memory problems or is reluctant to admit that the drug was not taken. When a drug history is obtained in the patient's home, the provider should request to see the drugs. It is not uncommon, especially with older adults, for the patient to forget about drugs used for self-medication or to store multiple drugs in a single, unlabeled container. The provider should note the drug storage site, which may be unsafe. Exposure to heat, light, and moisture adversely effects most drugs.

The patient's ability to read and understand drug labels and to locate expiration dates should also be evaluated, along with knowledge about proper disposal of drugs. Many persons cannot read, visualize, or understand information contained on packaging labels or inserts. The provider must also take into account factors that foster noncompliance.

Sleep patterns, exercise, and activity habits should be assessed in relation to drug therapy. Some drugs may alter sleep patterns and interfere with the rapid eye movement sleep cycle. Therefore, the total amount of sleep may be increased but rapid eye movement sleep time may be reduced (see Chapter 17). The patient may awake feeling more tired than before going to bed. Diuretics causing frequent urination are best taken when the patient will be awake and ambulatory (see Chapter 39). Drugs that alter the patient's level of consciousness should be taken at bedtime or when alertness is not required (e.g., not before driving a vehicle or operating machinery). The drug schedule or the activity pattern should be adjusted to minimize the risk of harm.

Physical Exam Findings

A physical exam in the home should be completed in a location where the patient's privacy is respected and the patient can be comfortable. The patient should choose where the exam is to be carried out. Only the body areas necessary for the exam should be exposed.

Physical assessments are directly related to and specific for the health problems being monitored. Physical findings often document specific responses to drug regimens. For example, serial blood pressure readings help monitor the use and effectiveness of antihypertensive drugs. Signs of dehydration or fluid overload (peripheral edema, weight gain or loss, and moist lung sounds) provide information about the therapeutic effectiveness of diuretics. A change in the mental status of an older adult may provide an early indication of drug toxicity. Whether the patient moves around easily in the home and can obtain drugs when needed provides further information about the patient's physical status and ability to comply with the management plan, as does appropriateness of the patient's dress and hygiene, posture, gait, and motor movements. The patient's physical ability to manage the route of drug administration (i.e., injections, rectal or vaginal suppositories) is also important to compliance. The ability to swallow is necessary for taking oral drugs.

Changes in sensory-perceptual abilities place patients at higher risk for accidents and injury. The patient must be able to read, hear, and comprehend for compliance with a drug regimen to be expected. In addition, alterations in taste and smell may affect ability and willingness to comply with drug or dietary regimens. Changes in tactile sensation may be evident with close observation, and touch may be used to compensate for losses of other senses. Decreases in fine motor function and sensation may create difficulty in moving small objects or in opening drug containers. Gross motor limitations may affect an individual's ability to obtain drugs in the home or may determine accessible storage sites.

Modifications in the management plan may be necessary if the physical exam findings suggest actual or potential problems. The nurse in the community setting is often the only health care provider regularly monitoring the patient; thus, attention to assessment findings and regular communication with other members of the health care team are vital to the patient's well-being.

Diagnostic Testing

Diagnostic tests may be safely performed in the home using standard precautions. Specimen collection in the home is similar to that in an institutional setting, except that the health care provider must physically transport the specimen to the laboratory. Laboratory protocols should be followed for storage of specimens that cannot be immediately transported to the designated laboratory. Some specimens, such as those for serum potassium, must be transported with minimum disturbance to ensure accurate test results. Required examination or interviewing activities should be completed before specimen collection. All specimens should be collected in appropriate containers to reduce errors and limit the need for repeated procedures.

Developmental Considerations

Three groups of individuals—pregnant women (see Chapter 6), pediatric patients (see Chapter 7), and older adults (see Chapter 8) often have higher incidences of adverse effects of drug therapy. Such high-risk patients require special consideration. Awareness of the patient's physiologic state, disease or illnesses, and special social context is necessary for the proper assessment and recommendations for treatment.

Furthermore, with earlier discharge from acute care institutions, many patients are returning home while still in early recovery and with limited self-care capabilities. Until a patient is able to manage his or her own care, drug administration is often the responsibility of a family member or other caregiver. Using commercial or homemade pill boxes may be helpful in organizing drugs and thus facilitate compliance.

For school-age children or patients living with limited supervision (e.g., group homes), drug administration may be the responsibility of supervisory personnel. In these situations, the health care provider may have primary care, delegatory, educational, and supervisory responsibilities. In some states, the health care provider has the legal power to delegate drug administration activities to nonprofessional staff. In many schools, however, permission must be obtained from the child's parent(s) and the prescribing health care provider for the drug to be administered on the premises.

Psychosocial Considerations

Psychosocial factors within the community provide valuable information to the health care provider. Because of the increasing interest in self-care and the trend toward nonprescription drug use, the health care provider must, more than ever, understand the factors influencing patients' treatment choices. Inherent in this understanding is knowledge of the patient's environment, dietary practices, sleeping patterns, and activity levels. Health-illness beliefs and practices, past experiences with the health care system, educational level, religious beliefs, language barriers, support system, and financial resources should also be considered.

Environment Home and environmental assessment is crucial in dealing with the patient in the home care setting. The health care provider should determine drug accessibility, storage areas, and temperature as well as check for disposal of expired prescription or OTC drugs.

Dietary Practices A working knowledge of the patient's dietary practices is essential to evaluating the therapeutic potential of drug regimens as well as the risk of drug-food interactions. The overall results of drug-food interactions are not well understood, but such interactions can have dramatic effects. For example, eating tyramine-containing foods while taking a monoamine oxidase inhibitor may precipitate a hypertensive crisis. Less dramatic reactions involve changes in the absorption of drugs related to the timing of food intake. Drugs may also alter nutrient absorption, which can lead over time to vitamin and mineral deficiencies. The health care provider should assess the patient's nutritional status before starting drug therapy and periodically throughout therapy to determine the need for dietary or vitamin supplementation.

Health-Illness Beliefs and Practices A patient's health-illness beliefs and practices and use of the health care system affect compliance with a drug regimen. When confronted with symptoms perceived to be minor or easily controlled, patients often seek self-care remedies or OTC drugs first. It is only when these attempts do not relieve symptoms, or the problem worsens, that patients seek advice. Consistent with the values of independence and freedom of action, American culture strongly supports the use of self-care products. With continued emphasis on individual responsibility for health, the importance of self-treatment may continue to increase.

Use of home remedies may be based on frustration with or distrust of the health care system or provider, or on a perception that the illness is not severe enough to need prescription drugs. In contrast, individuals who have the greatest trust in contemporary health care practices and technologies are least likely to purchase OTC drugs or to use questionably efficacious products on their own.

Self-treatment is not limited to OTC drugs. Non-Western traditional folk/cultural practices and beliefs are mysterious by Western standards. A patient's use of home remedies and other self-treatment strategies is important to note. As a constant presence in the community, the health care provider is in a unique position to acquire information about health and illness practices that may be unavailable to providers in clinics or institutional settings. Some of the most common practices are reviewed here.

Herbalism uses the flowers, stems, leaves, or roots of plants to treat illness. Not all herbal remedies are harmless, however. *Naturopathy* is based on the concept of using the healing force of nature. Naturopathic doctors avoid therapies that weaken the body's innate ability to heal itself or that take over a function of the body. *Homeopathy* uses drugs that produce, in healthy individuals, the same symptoms as the disease being treated. It is based on the principles of the law of similars, the minimum dose, and the single remedy. *Therapeutic touch* is a modern variation of the laying-on of hands. It involves touching with the intent to help or heal. This technique is used to assess and treat energy field imbalances by the movement of a practitioner's hands through a recipient's energy field. *Acupuncture* is the use of thin needles inserted into points on the body's meridians to stimulate the body's *chi* or vital energy. This therapy is used to treat disharmony in the body that leads to disease. *Phytotherapy* (*phyto* is the Greek word for plant) is the science of using plant-based medicines (phytomedicines) to treat illness. The effects of phytomedicines are the result of their pharmacologic actions.

Critics of these practices view them as trickery. Proponents often accept these practices without evaluation. (Chapter 60 discusses alternative and complementary therapies in more depth.) The values and beliefs held by groups within the community help determine health care practices.

Black Americans Many health care beliefs and practices of blacks arise from African and Caribbean ancestry. To many in this population, health denotes harmony of the body, mind, and spirit. Illness is viewed as a state of disharmony resulting from natural causes or divine punishment. Survival depends on restoring and maintaining a balance of harmony with nature.

The health care practices are derived from a fundamental belief in the power of the supernatural. They include the use of herbs, spices, and roots. Health care advice may come from a "granny," a voodoo practitioner. The first line of treatment is often prayer and the laying-on of hands, although there are no universally accepted practices. The concurrent use of a variety of practitioners and practices is not uncommon.

Black Americans may use diverse home remedies. For example, cooked cornmeal and peach leaves are wrapped in cloth and placed over an inflamed area or wound infection. It is thought that bactericidal enzymes are produced through the process of fermentation. A raw potato poultice may be used to treat inflammation and wound infections. For open wounds, salt pork may be secured in a cloth and placed over the affected area. Epsom salts are familiar ingredients in many folk remedies. The extent to which folk medicine is used in the Black American population is not well understood. Discriminatory practices, unfair treatment, and difficult access to the health care system has caused many Black Americans to distrust the establishment health care system and to seek other solutions.

Asian Americans Asian Americans have originated in China, Hawaii, the Philippines, Korea, Japan, Laos, Cambodia, and Vietnam. Their folk medicine practices evolved from China and the Far East and comprise complex and varying methodologies. Imbalance between *yin* (female, negative energy) and *yang* (male, positive energy) causes illness. Restoring the balance is the basis for most therapies, including acupuncture, herbal medicines, massage, skin scrapings, and cupping. Instead of destroying the "germs" that cause illness, much of folk medicine practice focuses on self-restraint, corrective diets, and herbs to restore balance. Rather than as an individual's property, the body is seen as a gift given by parents and forebears that must be cared for and maintained. The primary role of the physician in ancient China was to safeguard the body and to prevent illness. If a person became ill despite preventive measures, it was not necessary to pay for the treatment.

Traditional remedies used to prevent and treat ailments among Asian Americans include *jen shen lu jung wan*. This brown, thick liquid is used as a general tonic to support the body system and aid in digestion. *Tiger balm* is a salve used for temporary relief of minor aches and pains. *Huo li jian mei su* are small, brown, coated tablets taken twice a day to relieve fatigue, to counteract senility, and to maintain youth, health, and vigor. *White flower* is a liquid used to treat colds, influenza, headaches, and coughs. *Thousand-year eggs* are uncooked eggs that are covered with carbon and straw and stored in large vases for extended periods. They are eaten daily with rice for good health.

Ginseng root is the most widely known of the Chinese herbs. It has universal medicinal usage in "building the blood," especially after childbirth. Chinese legend has it that the more the root looks like a man, the more effective it is. Native to the United States, ginseng is used as a restorative tonic. It has scientifically proven antioxidant, antitumor, and antiviral effects.

Acupuncture, as already mentioned, is the practice of puncturing the skin at certain points on the body with metal needles. *Moxibustion* is the application of heat to the needles to increase the benefit.

Because of the focus on prevention in Asian medicine, many patients combine "Western" treatment with folk remedies. Such patients should be monitored for the development of toxicities. They may use folk remedies rather than seeking medical treatment, with sometimes serious consequences.

Hispanic Americans Hispanic cultural influences include European, Spanish, South American, and Indian folk beliefs. Eighty percent of the Hispanic American population consists of persons from Mexico, Cuba, and Puerto Rico. The remaining 20 percent are descendants of Central and South American peoples. The use of medicinal herbs and folk healers accompanied by religious rituals is representative of this group.

Many Hispanic Americans believe that health results from good luck, as a reward for good behavior, or as a reward from God. Health represents an equilibrium in a universe where the forces of "hot" and "cold" must be balanced. Body fluids reflect this perspective. Blood is hot and wet, phlegm is cold and wet, yellow bile is hot and dry, and black bile is cold and dry.

The concept of hot and cold forces originated with the early Hippocratic theory of health and the four humors. Health exists when the four humors are balanced and is maintained by diet and other practices. Examples of cold foods are chicken, honey, avocados, bananas, and lima beans. *Friadad del estomago,* a "cold stomach," is caused by eating too many cold foods. Cold foods are to be avoided during menstruation and after childbirth. In contrast, a pregnant woman avoids hot foods such as chocolate, coffee, cornmeal, garlic, kidney beans, onions, and peas. For restoration of health, hot diseases require cold treatments, and cold diseases need hot treatments.

Illness is also caused by "dislocation of body parts" and magic or supernatural forces outside the body such as *mal de ojo,* or "evil eye." *Envidia,* envy, causes illness and bad luck. Many people of Hispanic background believe that to succeed is to fail; that is, when a person's success provokes the envy of friends and neighbors, misfortune or illness may follow.

Hispanic Americans use a variety of remedies to prevent or treat illness. Novena candles may be burned to ward off evil. *Jabon de la mano milagrosa* (soap of the miraculous hand) cleanses and protects a person. Amulets such as *milagros* are worn to protect from evil. The *mano negro* (black hand) amulet of Puerto Rico may be placed on a baby at birth to protect it from the "evil eye." In addition, manzanilla, an herb made into tea, is used to treat abdominal pain, uterine cramps, anxiety, and insomnia. Anise is star-shaped seeds used to treat painful gases, upset stomach, colic, and anorexia and to increase breast milk. Several levels of practitioners, one of whom is the *curandero,* may carry out the folk system of medicine, incorporating herbs, spices, and the power of divine intervention.

Puerto Rican Americans' concepts of disease are similar to those of other Hispanic cultures. They view health as a state of equilibrium, with illness resulting from physical causes or conditions. The concepts of hot and cold are used. Conditions identified as "cold" (e.g., respiratory infections and menstruation) require hot remedies such as chocolate or alcohol. Conversely, "hot" conditions (e.g., ulcers or constipation) are treated with cool remedies like fruits.

Native Americans There are approximately 170 Native American tribes in the United States. They have varying health care beliefs and values. Consequently, it is difficult to generalize their cultural and health belief systems. Medicine, magic, and religion are closely bound beliefs for most Native American peoples. The concept of medicine extends beyond the treatment of illness to include life and death, and harmony with the universe. To stay healthy, one must maintain a positive, balanced, intimate spiritual relationship with nature and must treat the body and earth with respect.

Another interpretation of the Native American view of health is that the body is partitioned into halves, plus and minus. There are also positive and negative energy poles. Every person has the power to control the self, and with this energy, spiritual control (control of the body's energy) is derived. Health is then characterized as a harmony between the halves, or the energy poles. Illness is disharmony of the body, mind, and spirit.

The Navajo view illness as the result of displeasing holy people, annoying the elements, disturbing plant and animal life, neglecting the celestial bodies, misusing a sacred ceremony, or tampering with witches or witchcraft. Hopi associate illness with evil spirits and therefore strive to avoid or ward off these spirits. An eastern band Cherokee medicine man, Hawk Littlejohn, describes illness as the imbalance of the body, mind, or spirit caused by an excess in one domain and the neglect of the other. For example, a student who spends too much time studying (developing the mind) may neglect the body and spirit and is therefore susceptible to disharmony and illness.

To treat disharmony and illness, the Native American may wear a thunderbird amulet for protection and good luck. One may wear a mask to hide self from the devil or evil spirits. *Estafoate* are dried leaves made into a tea to treat stomach problems. A medicine man may burn sweet grass in a purification rite or create sand paintings in an elaborate diagnostic ceremony. The way the medicine man's hand moves while casting the sand indicates a specific illness. Correct treatment may then be prescribed. In some areas, the medicine men work in consultation with health care providers in contemporary health care systems.

White Americans Members of most White communities are of European descent and have been migrating to the United States since 1620. The 1980 census was the first attempt to break down the U.S. population by country of origin; the largest groups were found to be from England, Germany, Ireland, and France. White Americans define health and illness in many ways. Health is the ability to carry out activities of daily living, a state of physical and emotional well-being, and freedom from illness. Conversely, illness is often defined as the inability to carry out the activities of daily living, the presence of disease symptoms and pain, and the malfunction of body organs. Examples of etiologies of illness are breaking of religious rules, exposure to causative agents, punishment from God, drafts, climatic changes, and abuse of the body.

Whites reportedly have a wide variety of traditional and contemporary remedies. Father John's Medicine has been considered a wholesome, family medicine used for colds and coughs since 1855. Sloan's Liniment provides temporary relief of minor arthritic pain and other ailments. *Malocchio,* an Italian horn-shaped object, is worn as an amulet to prevent the "evil eye." Swamp root is an OTC liquid used as a diuretic. Syrup of Black Draught is an OTC laxative. Vicks VapoRub may be used in the treatment of head and chest congestion. *Olbas* and *magentropfen,* drugs sold in Germany, are used to treat sore throats and anorexia. Many of these remedies have withstood the test of time, having been transmitted from generation to generation.

Religious Beliefs Religious practices must be taken into account by the health care provider using or prescribing drugs and treatments in the home. The beliefs of some religious groups prohibit the use of blood and blood products and support other therapies such as faith healing and prayer. Health care providers must become familiar with the specific beliefs of each patient whose care they supervise. The legal implications of religious practices as they relate to health care must also be acknowledged.

Drug Use and Misuse The health care provider must always be aware of the possibility of drug misuse in any community setting. The drug history should include use of illicit drugs as well as the use and misuse of legal drugs such as alcohol and nicotine, all of which can significantly influence the effects of other pharmacologic agents. Because the patient may be hesitant to disclose such information, the health care provider may be the first to detect the use of substances of abuse. Chapter 10 further discusses substance abuse.

Language Barriers The health care provider should consider the ethnicity of the patient in the type of treatment prescribed, and the potential for compliance. As mentioned previously, ethnic groups often use folk remedies and folk healers because of distrust or dislike of the health care system. Language barriers impair access to health care and may further discourage use of the system. Language barriers also interfere with the health care provider's ability to accurately assess and to teach the patient. Interpreters may facilitate the process.

Family Support Network An assessment of family functioning is also an important component. Family living arrangements, the number, ages, and relationships of people in the home, communication patterns, the roles of family members, the power and authority structure of the family, and the presence of a caregiver all affect patient care. To effectively treat the patient, the health care provider must gain the cooperation of the family.

Support persons are important in caring for the patient at home. The patient who has cognitive difficulties and/or self-care deficits requires a caregiver with the ability to appropriately administer or monitor drug regimens as well as provide other care and services.

Education The patient's level of sophistication, education, and ability to use and interpret label information is important in determining the appropriateness of self-care and the use of OTC preparations. Consumer interpretation of drug instructions is culturally determined and relatively consistent, regardless of age, gender, or educational level.

Nearly 20 percent of the U.S. population is functionally illiterate. A subtle approach is necessary to assess a patient's ability to read and understand directions for prescribed and nonprescription drug therapy. Patients who are unable to read or comprehend are often ashamed of the deficit and try to compensate by indicating that they understand and will comply. The health care provider should have the patient read a drug instruction (label) and explain specifically how the product is to be taken (e.g., times, before or after meals, amount). The patient's vocabulary, knowledge, and intellectual level may be assessed through questioning about drug action, adverse effects, and the disease process. The discussion must involve not only the use of the drug but how and why to read a label.

Economic Factors The high cost of pharmaceuticals is a commonly acknowledged reason for noncompliance with drug regimens. Health care providers must evaluate the socioeconomic level, health insurance, and assistance program available to a patient for purchase of needed drugs. Assistance programs commonly require a needs assessment to determine eligibility. Interpretation of eligibility regulations often becomes the health care provider's responsibility. Many patients regard self-treatment as a more economical alternative, both in time and in money, and may try it before seeking professional advice. Astute pharmacists help patients save money by offering less expensive generic drug forms.

The availability of transportation and pharmacy delivery services may help patients obtain needed drugs. Health care providers should furnish information about delivery services to the patient, particularly when the cost of transportation may prevent access to a pharmacy. It is also possible to obtain pharmaceuticals by mail, through organizations such as the American Association of Retired Persons. And, many pharmacies are now commonly located in grocery stores, thus eliminating a special trip to the drug store.

Analysis and Management

Treatment Objectives

In general, drug therapy is directed at prevention, cure, alleviation, or palliation. Prevention of drug-related complications is a primary concern. Early detection may identify

Controversy

Why Do We Question the Use of Generic Drugs?
JONATHAN J. WOLFE

Generic drugs have engendered controversy since their introduction into the American marketplace in the 1960s. The advent of managed care and the use of drug formularies have brought new scrutiny to the growing use of generic drugs as opposed to brand-name products. The question revolved around more than price. Generic drugs initially offered lower price as a reason for their use. After a brand-name drug loses its patent protection, however, its price may be lowered below that of its generic counterpart as a strategy to guard market share.

Initially, concern focused on the efficacy and safety of generic drugs. Now, however, their worth is well established. The *Orange Book* provides documentation of the equivalence of generic drug products. Nonequivalent Drug Lists warn against substitution of generics whose equivalence to the standard brand name product is not established. Within this environment, the justice of substitution has emerged as a cogent concern.

Often, patients are the focus of the dilemma. Patients may refuse to accept a generic drug product after years of treatment with a brand-name drug. In other cases, patients who agree to a generic drug substitution may not receive the lower price. A prescription management company may keep part of the savings and pass on only a small percentage of the reduction to the patient. Additionally, the prescription plan manager may receive rebates from drug manufacturers in return for encouraging generic substitution.

Critical Thinking Discussion

- When a generic drug has been documented by reliable studies to be equivalent to a well-established brand-name product, what concerns do you have about administering the generic product when the prescriber has written for the brand name drug?
- There have been product quality problems with drugs from generic manufacturer X. Now your hospital has chosen X as its sole supplier of generic drugs. Under your formulary, you may administer a brand-name product in preference to the generic equivalent as long as the health care provider has ordered the brand-name drug. Are you justified in asking a physician to rewrite an order naming the more expensive brand-name product? Is it right for you to take a telephone order for the generic, but to enter the trade name into a patient's chart and the medication administration record?
- If you are the nursing department representative on the Pharmacy and Therapeutics Committee, what reservations may you properly express about awarding manufacturer X (see preceding question) a new 3-year contract as the hospital's sole supplier of generic drugs?

the onset of disease or complications and may allow for early intervention. *Cure* is the relief of the signs and symptoms as well as eradication or elimination of illness. *Supportive therapy* helps alleviate symptoms of certain illnesses, conditions, diseases that threaten other body systems. The objective of *palliation* is to relieve or alleviate a patient's symptoms without providing a cure.

Treatment Options

Effective health care, whether given inside or outside an institution, requires communication and collaboration among health care providers. Sharing patient histories with other providers is essential for appropriate follow-up care. Health care providers have a certain liberty in determining or recommending the most effective drug therapy. However, management strategies must recognize the patient's locus of control and must promote appropriate and accurate decision-making (see Controversy—Why Do We Question the Use of Generic Drugs?).

Intervention

Administration

The complexity of any patient's drug regimen should be constantly monitored. Health care providers should always consider the possibility of eliminating a drug from the regimen. Compliance is fostered when the patient feels in control of and knowledgeable about the management plan.

Tailoring the drug regimen to the patient's life-style helps him or her to remember to take the drugs. Often, it is helpful to schedule drug administration to coincide with mealtimes. Patients may also select other specific times during the day when an activity or routine can help "cue" them to take their drugs. The use of egg cartons, muffin tins, or commercially available drug boxes may help the patient organize the drug regimen. Drug boxes can be 7-day organizers but can also be subdivided into several daily-dose compartments (Fig. 9–2). The responsibility for filling the organizers may fall to the health care provider or a caregiver.

A drug diary can help the patient remember whether a particular dose was taken, thus eliminating missed or double doses. However, a diary is disadvantageous in that it requires concerted effort and consistency on the part of the patient or caregiver (see Improving Pharmacotherapeutic Compliance).

Pill counts are easy to perform and inexpensive. However, they provide no information about the timing of doses, misplaced bottles, dropped pills, or the addition of leftover doses from a previous prescription. A relatively new method used in the home today involves the placement of microprocessors in drug bottle caps. Each time the bottle is opened, the date and time are recorded. This system provides information about the timing of doses and does not rely on the patient's memory. The two disadvantages of the system are that it is based on the assumption that a dose of medicine is taken every time the bottle is opened and it is expensive.

Health care providers should address noncompliance as openly and as clearly as possible. Begin assessment of compliance by obtaining an accurate account of the drug regimen. The health care provider may also inquire, for example, how the patient remembers to take a prescribed drug four times a day, especially if the drug is stored out of sight and out of reach of children. Upon identification of a compliance problem due to poor memory or an inability to open containers, the health care provider may choose to initiate a

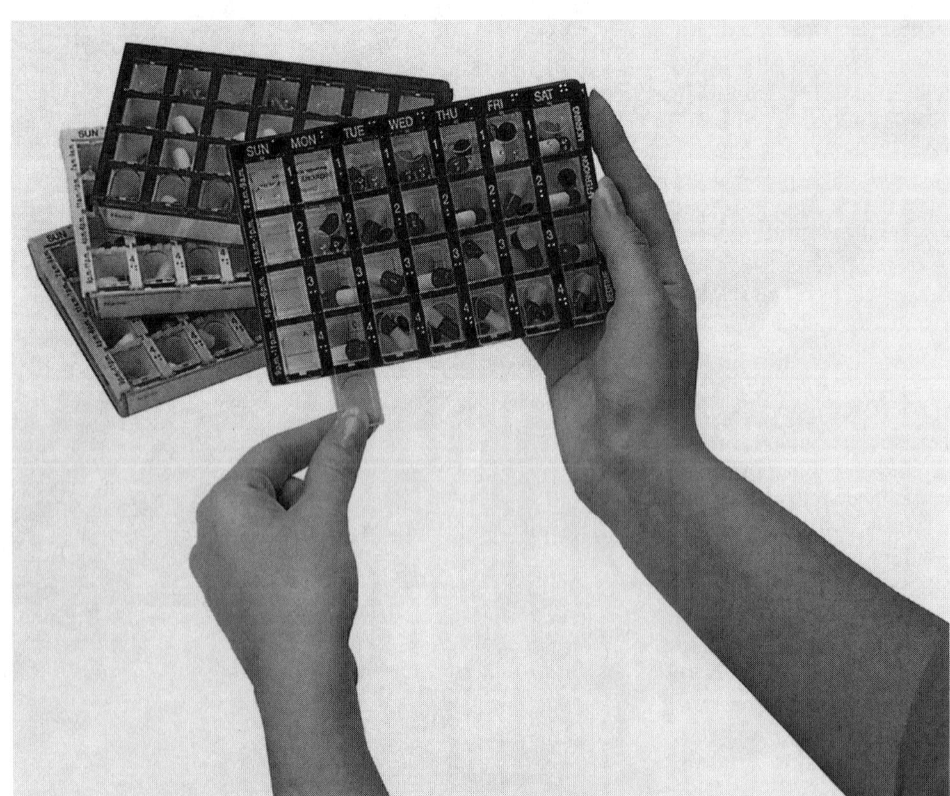

Figure 9–2 Commercially available drug boxes may contain a single compartment or multiple compartments. Some boxes contain just seven divisions, enough for a full week of medication. Others contain multiple compartments with space available for several doses throughout the day and the week. (Photo courtesy of Apothecary Products, Burnside, MN.)

IMPROVING PHARMACOTHERAPEUTIC COMPLIANCE

Relate
- Develop a therapeutic relationship with patients—they need to know that you care.

Communicate
- Communicate—be certain that patients understand what you are saying—ask them to repeat the message that you gave.

Motivate
- Set realistic short-term goals in order to gain long-term compliance.

Educate
- Educational materials will help patients keep track of medication regimen.

Collaborate
- Enlist family support and that of the neighborhood pharmacist. Refer patients when appropriate.

Facilitate
- Factor in the patient's daily routine, and interfere as little as possible. Keep medication regimens as simple as possible.

Innovate
- Institute a reward system for goals achieved.

Calculate
- Chart the patient's progress where it is available to patient and health care providers.

From United States Department of Health and Human Services. (1991. Eight moves to help your patients improve adherence. *Infomemo*, Spring, 9.

home drug-dispensing system (e.g., an egg carton, ice cube tray, or commercial device). Each compartment should be labeled with the time and day when that dose should be taken. Posting of reminders on the calendar, refrigerator door, bathroom medicine cabinet, and similar places in the home may help the patient remember to take the drug as prescribed. Enlisting the help of a family member is often beneficial. Caution must be used, however. In order for these strategies or others to be effective, the health care provider must have an understanding of the patient's life-style and health beliefs and practices.

Working from knowledge of the patient's ability to read, interpret, and understand directions on OTC labels, the health care provider has an important role in guiding, teaching, and supporting the patient in the appropriate administration of OTC drugs. Even though OTC drugs contain patient package inserts explaining drug actions, adverse effects, and how to take the drugs, the health care provider provides guidance in their selection and use.

Education

Patient education is an essential part of effective drug therapy. Most patients, upon receiving a prescription for a new drug or after purchase of an OTC drug, require a certain amount of information in order to effectively use it. The amount and type of information needed depends on the complexity of the health problem and the specific drug to be used. In some cases, teaching consists simply of a brief explanation of the therapy and instructions for taking the drug. This situation occurs most often in outpatient settings for patients with a simple health concern. In other cases, there is no teaching, because the patient has chosen to use an OTC product.

For complex situations, the health care provider should schedule a series of educational sessions to give the patient and/or family sufficient time to integrate detailed information and directions. This is more often necessary for patients with chronic conditions requiring the use of multiple drugs, patients for whom the acquisition of new psychomotor skills is necessary (e.g., insulin injections), or patients whose medical condition requires life-style alterations.

Teaching requires that the health care provider consider several factors (see Basic Principles of Teaching and Learning). However, there are specific issues to evaluate for each patient—demographic information such as age, gender, culture or ethnic background, and educational level—all of which influence the method and effectiveness of teaching and learning activities. Physiologic factors such as vision or hearing deficits may require alterations in teaching strategies. It is important also to tailor the amount and specific content to the patient's interest, knowledge base, motivational level, self-care requirements, literacy, and cognitive abilities. The health care provider must remember the key concept that learning and motivation are enhanced by positive reinforcement. Written materials may be helpful but should be appropriate for the patient's reading and comprehension abilities.

Assessing Patient Education Materials A number of criteria and methods can be used to assess the readability of

BASIC PRINCIPLES OF TEACHING AND LEARNING

Principles of Learning
- Determine patient's physical and emotional learning readiness.
- Encourage active participation throughout the learning activity.
- Base learning activities on patient's prior knowledge and experiences.
- Have patient apply learning immediately to increase effectiveness.
- Use repetition to reinforce learning.
- Enhance learning and motivation by rewarding positive behaviors.
- Present information that is congruent with the patient's expectations and goals.

Principles of Teaching
- Provide an atmosphere conducive to learning.
- Establish effective nurse-patient relationship.
- Consider psychosociocultural factors and spiritual beliefs when planning teaching-learning activities.
- Determine patient's present knowledge level.
- Use behavioral objectives to guide the teaching-learning activity and aid in evaluation.
- Present information at a level the patient can understand.
- Begin with simple information and build to the complex.
- Enhance learning and motivation by rewarding positive behaviors.
- Elicit feedback periodically to determine whether learning has taken place.

printed patient education materials. Qualitative criteria that help determine readability include how words and ideas are linked together, and what assumptions the patient must make to interpret the information. The number and complexity of required inferences should be noted. Does the patient need to combine experience with what is printed to formulate a conclusion, construct a new meaning, or both? When and how often are pronouns (e.g., he, she, it, we, they, you) used? Understanding pronouns requires a certain sophistication of language. How much and what kind of symbolic language is used? Are the meanings of terms and phrases commonly understood by the target population? What is the distance between the subject and predicate in a sentence? The greater the distance, the more difficult the message, because the reader must keep both parts of speech in mind throughout the entire sentence to discern its meaning.

Two methods may be used to evaluate the effectiveness of patient teaching. *Formative evaluation* (i.e., concurrent evaluation) takes place continuously throughout the teaching-learning process. The advantage of formative evaluation is that teaching strategies can be adjusted as necessary to enhance learning. The second method of evaluation is *summative* (i.e., retrospective evaluation). With this method, feedback is provided to the patient or family at the conclusion of the teaching-learning activity. The disadvantage to the second method is that it does not allow for adjustment of teaching strategies until the teaching-learning activity is completed.

Teaching in the home allows the health care provider to assess the impact of the environment on the patient's willingness and ability to learn. Such collaboration within the patient's environment places the locus of control firmly with the patient rather than with the health care provider. Because patients feel more comfortable at home, they may be more receptive and attentive to the information presented. On the other hand, distractions such as telephone interruptions and disruptions by family members may affect the length of teaching sessions in the home setting.

Evaluation

Treatment goals provide outcome criteria directed toward helping the patient make informed decisions. Evaluation of the patient using OTC drugs, for example, would include confirmation of the absence of adverse effects and the presence of therapeutic effects. Compliance with an agreed-upon regimen and improvement or maintenance of health status are long-term outcomes of drug regimens. Evaluation of patient teaching involves follow-up care at appropriate intervals.

There are several methods to assess compliance with a drug regimen. Patient self-reporting may be inaccurate if the patient has memory deficits or is reluctant to admit not taking the drugs as directed. Physical assessment of the patient will help determine whether the regimen was followed, but there is no guarantee that the presence of an improvement in the patient's health is a direct result of compliance with therapy. As mentioned earlier, pill counts are easy and inexpensive to perform, but they provide limited information. Use of containers that have microprocessors in the caps will provide information about when the bottle was entered but not whether the drug was taken; such a system does, however, avoid reliance on the patient's memory.

Drug therapy for any patient who is seen in the clinic, emergency room, or other outpatient facility should be followed as closely as that for a hospitalized patient. Regular assessment of physical findings and continued interim histories provide information needed to appropriately evaluate patient response.

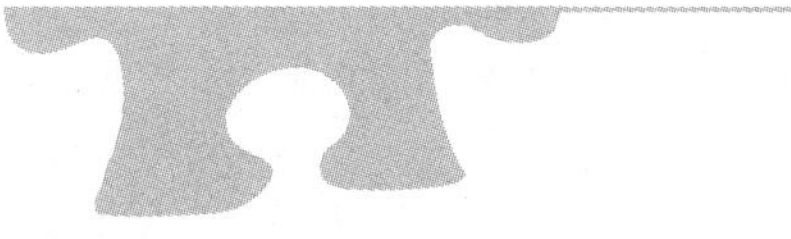

POISONINGS

Epidemiology and Etiology

Despite an extensive prevention campaign, poisoning remains a serious problem in the United States. According to the American Association of Poison Control Centers (AAPCC), although more than 1.8 million poison exposures are reported annually, an additional 2.1 million go unreported. Of the 1.8 million reported to the AAPCC, approximately 76 percent are intentional ingestions by adults that lead to death. Poisonings occur in people of all ages, and more than 92 percent in the home.

There are more than 300,000 different drug products on the market. Fewer than 20 drugs are responsible for 90 percent of the nonaccidental poisonings. Drugs most commonly associated with nonaccidental poisonings are amphetamines, antidepressants, barbiturates, benzodiazepines, cocaine, opioids, and analgesics.

The toxicity of a chemical substance is determined by the interactions of the specific substance with food and other drugs, the dose, susceptibility of the individual, biologic and genetic factors, and the route of contact. Poisons gain access to the body in a variety of ways, including gastrointestinal, inhalation, transcutaneous, and parenteral routes.

An unusual type of poisoning has surfaced with the proliferation of battery-operated watches, hearing aids, calculators, games, and cameras. An estimated 500 to 600 miniature, disk-shaped batteries are swallowed each year by persons of all ages. The batteries can lodge in the esophagus, cecum, or other areas of the gastrointestinal tract. Because the major component is potassium hydroxide, the batteries are corrosive to gastrointestinal tissues, causing ulceration or perforation in 1 to 2 hours. They can also cause mercury poisoning if the battery contents leak. A common inhalation poisoning results from inhalation of fumes produced by the interaction of bleach and ammonia in a diaper pail.

Critical Thinking Process

Assessment

History of Present Illness

When an ingestion occurs, the local poison control center should be contacted. Information that must be available for contacting the center is as follows:

- Generic, trade, or chemical name of the substance, if known
- Purpose, or how the substance was meant to be used

- The physical appearance of the substance
- Odor, color, texture, and any distinguishing characteristics of the substance
- Label statements related to "poison" content or flammability
- Quantity ingested
- The time of ingestion

The time of ingestion is important, because the elapsed time since ingestion helps determine the management strategies to be used. It should be noted, however, that approximately 50 percent of the data gathered during a poison crisis may be inaccurate.

The bottle from which an ingestion occurs should be kept, so that necessary information can be obtained. If the amount of an ingested liquid is not known, an assumption is made that the largest amount that could have been taken was consumed. As a general rule, a small child swallows approximately 5 mL at a time, a 10 year-old approximately 10 mL, and an adult approximately 15 mL. Saving the emesis or stool is often helpful in identifying the substance and may provide some clue to how much was ingested. Depending on the specific poisoning, assessment includes not only the patient but household members as well.

Past Health History

The health care provider elicits information about a history of suicidal thought or intent, cirrhosis, or thrombocytopenia. (Emesis induced with syrup of ipecac is contraindicated in patients with these last two disorders.) Information about prescription and OTC drugs used is also requested. Reports of previous poisonings or ingestion of foreign substances are important to note.

Physical Exam Findings

Toxidromes, the clinical manifestations of an ingestion, are helpful in determining the ingredients ingested (see Common Toxidromes). The health care provider should become familiar with the clinical manifestatious of specific drug ingestions and overdoses.

Other physical exam findings that may suggest poisoning are breath odor, respiratory rate, and the presence of dyspnea or cyanosis. Changes in pulse rate, the appearance and odor of any vomitus, and any abnormalities of stool and urine may also suggest the poison. Anything unusual about the patient, the clothing, or the surroundings should be noted; for example, evidence of burns around the lips and mouth, discolored gums, hypodermic pricks, pustules, or scars on the exposed and accessible surfaces of the body. Signs of nervous system involvement include excitement, muscular twitching, delirium, dysarthria, pupillary constriction or dilation, an elevated or subnormal temperature, stupor, and coma. Coma related to drug overdose is categorized as follows:

Grade I—Patient asleep but easily aroused, reacts to painful stimuli; deep tendon reflexes intact; pupils equal and react to light, ocular movements present; vital signs stable.

Grade II—Vital signs stable; pupils slightly dilated but reactive; pain response absent; deep tendon reflexes depressed.

Grade III—Vital signs stable; pupillary reflexes and deep tendon reflexes absent.

Grade IV—Respirations and circulation depressed.

COMMON TOXIDROMES

The common clinical manifestations of toxic ingestion are listed here according to the type of substance ingested.

Anticholinergics, Atropine, Scopolamine
Agitation
Coma
Delirium
Dilated pupils
Dry, beet-red skin
Hallucinations
Hyperthermia
Tachycardia

Barbiturates, Sedative-Hypnotics, Tranquilizers
Ataxia
Drowsiness
Hypotension
Slurred speech (without alcohol breath odor)

Organophosphates (Cholinergics), Mushrooms
Involuntary defecation, urination
Lacrimation
Miosis
Pulmonary congestion
Salivation
Seizures

Opioids
Coma
Hypotension
Miosis
Respiratory depression

Salicylates
Fever
Hyperglycemia
Hyperventilation
Mixed respiratory alkalosis and metabolic acidosis

Tricyclic Antidepressants
Anticholinergic signs & symptoms
Arrhythmias (prolonged QRS interval)
Coma
Seizures

Diagnostic Testing

Toxicology screens are used to diagnose, assess prognosis of, and manage acute poisoning, particularly in uncooperative or comatose patients. However, screening is time consuming, expensive, and often unreliable. Reliability of results depends on precise communication between the laboratory and the health care provider about the drugs under suspicion. Correct sampling of appropriate body fluids, prompt reporting of the results, and the number of substances listed on the analysis profile all contribute to effective diagnostic testing and subsequent management.

Toxicology screening is no substitute for assessment and critical judgments. The plasma levels of a few toxins may influence the plan of care (e.g., acetaminophen, carbon monoxide, ethylene glycol, iron, lithium, methanol, salicylates, theophylline). For others, however, there is a poor correlation between plasma drug levels and toxicity (e.g., tricyclic antidepressants). The interpretation of toxicology results should take into account the patient's clinical status, the time elapsed since exposure, and the potential for delayed toxic effects. For example, therapeutic levels of acetaminophen 4 to 8 hours after ingestion are associated with little risk of hepatotoxicity, but the same level obtained more than 16 hours after ingestion indicates a high risk of hepatotoxicity.

Developmental Considerations

Pediatric Drugs specifically packaged for children generally contain small quantities, so if the entire package were consumed it would be less likely to cause serious harm. For example, baby aspirin is packaged in containers of 36 or fewer tablets, to prevent a child who ingests the entire contents from receiving a lethal dose. Even with this safety factor, the majority of pediatric poisonings involve accidental ingestion by children younger than 5 years. Toddlers between the ages of 2 and 3 are the most common victims of accidental prescription drug poisoning, and 25 percent of all the solid prescription drugs involved in such poisonings are enclosed in child-resistant containers. Although the Poison Prevention Packaging Act (PPPA) of 1970 resulted in a 65 percent decrease in the ingestion of household products (e.g., antifreeze, lye), prescription drug ingestion by children has declined only 36 percent. In addition, most accidentally ingested drugs have been stored in ordinary containers or improperly used child-resistant containers; many in no containers at all.

Accidental ingestions of analgesics and antipyretics are the leading causes of pediatric poisoning emergencies. Other substances commonly ingested are flavored chewable vitamins, household cleaners and polishes, plants, cosmetics, pesticides, paints and solvents, and petroleum products.

Adolescent and Adult Though pediatric poisonings constitute the majority of calls to poison control centers, adolescent and adult poisonings more often result in serious morbidity and mortality. A high percentage of these poisonings are related to drug abuse or suicide attempts. Men 20 to 39 years old account for 70 percent of all drug abuse–related emergency room visits. Cocaine and heroin/morphine are involved in more than one-third of the deaths. Because of the growing prevalence of drug abuse, it may be difficult to distinguish a suicide attempt from a recreational overdose.

Geriatric Poisonings in older adults related to polypharmacy and suicide attempts are common. It is estimated that the average older adult has 11 prescriptions filled per year. An average of 8 drugs are administered to each nursing home resident. Although older adults constitute approximately 12 percent of the population, they consume 32 percent of all prescription drugs. Further, 25 percent of suicides reported each year in the United States involve older adults. The combination of increased drug use, declining organ function, and the potential for depression raises the risk of poisoning and drug toxicity in this population.

Analysis and Management

Treatment Objectives

Interventions for poisonings center on three major management objectives: supporting the patient's vital functions, preventing absorption of or eliminating the poison, and preventing or managing complications. The acronym SIRES is an aid to remembering the essentials of care, which are as follows:

- *Stabilize* the patient.
- *Identify* the toxic substance.
- *Reverse* its effects.
- *Eliminate* the substance from the body.
- *Support* the patient and significant others (physically and psychosocially).

Treatment Options

The key principle in the management of poisonings is, "Treat the patient, not the poison." This principle is important because treatment for most poisonings is symptomatic and supportive in nature. There is always time to stabilize the patient before treating the poisoning. Once the patient is stable, treatment options and interventions can be explored. Emotional support of the patient and others is crucial.

The most reliable information about poison emergencies is available through the network of regional poison control centers. These centers were established to provide current and comprehensive management guidelines to the general public and health care providers. Although several references on toxicity and the treatment of poisoning are available, the most up-to-date information on both human and animal poisonings is provided by *Poisondex*. Developed in conjunction with the Rocky Mountain Poison and Drug Centers in Denver, Colorado, *Poisondex* is reviewed and updated every 3 months. This detailed toxicology database is designed to identify and provide information on chemical composition, toxicity, and medical management of more than 750,000 drugs, household chemicals, industrial and environmental toxins, and biologics (including plant and animal toxins). *Poisondex* also provides a visual reference (e.g., drug color, shape, imprinted symbols) to facilitate identification of manufactured and street drugs. All regional poison control centers accept calls 24 hours a day, 7 days a week, 365 days a year. Many also have "800" numbers.

Antidotes or antagonists may be used in selected cases for management or diagnosis of the toxin (Table 9–3). However, one must remember that although an antidote may produce significant improvement initially, the half-life of the toxic substance may be longer than that of the antidote. For example, naloxone is a potent antagonist used in opiate overdose. The patient may initially respond rather quickly but, as the naloxone wears off, may become obtunded.

Interventions

Support Vital Functions

Treatment for most poisonings and complications is symptomatic and supportive. Basic and advanced life support should be implemented as patient condition dictates. Vital functions such as respirations, circulation, and acid-base and fluid-electrolyte balances should be supported. Supplemental oxygen and suction equipment should be readily available. A ventilator may be kept on hand in case the patient needs ventilatory assistance. Cardiac monitoring may be necessary, because many poisoning substances precipitate rhythm disturbances. A large-bore intravenous line should be established for all patients with actual or potentially unstable vital signs or a decreased level of conscious-

TABLE 9–3 ANTIDOTES COMMONLY USED IN MANAGING POISONED OR OVERDOSED PATIENTS

Poisonous Substance	Antidote(s)
Acetaminophen	Acetylcysteine (MUCOMYST)
Anticholinergics/antimuscarinics (atropine, scopolamine), tricyclic antidepressants	Physostigmine (ANTILIRIUM)
Anticoagulants (e.g., warfarin, salicylates)	Vitamin K
Benzodiazepines	Flumazenil (ROMAZICON)
Beta blockers	Isoproterenol (ISUPREL), glucagon
Calcium channel blockers	Calcium chloride
Carbon monoxide	Oxygen
Cholinergics and acetylcholinesterase inhibitors (e.g., organic phosphates, insecticides, nerve gases, carbamates)	Atropine Pralidoxime (2-PAM)
Cyanide, nitroprusside sodium	Amyl nitrate, then sodium nitrite, then sodium thiosulfate
Digoxin, digitoxin, oleander, foxglove	Digoxin immune FAB (DIGIBIND, DIGIDOTE)
Heparin	Protamine sulfate
Iron	Deferoxamine (DESFERAL)
Insulin	Dextrose 50%
Lead	Ethylenediaminetetraacetic acid (EDTA)
Mercury, arsenic, lead, other heavy metals	Dimercaprol (BAL), disodium edetate, penicillamine
Methanol, ethylene glycol	Ethanol
Opioids and opioid derivatives	Naloxone (NARCAN)

ness. Arterial blood gas specimens may be drawn for the patient who arrives in respiratory distress or who has ingested a poisoning substance that may alter acid-base balance.

Virtually every patient who arrives with a decreased level of consciousness will receive an intravenous dose of the opioid antagonist naloxone (see Chapter 14) and the benzodiazepine antagonist flumazenil (see Chapter 17). A positive response to the usual dose of naloxone or flumazenil indicates the presence of opioids or benzodiazepines, respectively. These two drugs serve not only as potential treatment for narcotic or benzodiazepine overdose but also as useful diagnostic aids.

It is important to monitor the patient's response after receiving these drugs. Both naloxone and flumazenil are short acting, so the patient's level of consciousness may fall once therapeutic effectiveness of the drug declines. Repeated administration of the antagonist may be necessary until the patient recovers sufficiently.

Prevent Absorption

Removal of the ingested substance may be accomplished by inducing emesis or through gastric aspiration and lavage. Vomiting should not be induced until recommended by a poison control center. The container label's antidote information should not be relied on because it may be out of date.

There are several treatment regimens for poisoning. The most effective method for removal of ingested toxins is usually the most natural one—inducing vomiting as soon as possible. The "universal antidote," a mixture of burnt toast, magnesium oxide (milk of magnesia), and tannic acid (tea), is ineffective and, in some instances, may even be harmful.

Syrup of Ipecac Syrup of ipecac (IPECAC), an emetic, is available without a prescription in 1-ounce bottles and is effective for inducing vomiting after ingestion of practically all poisons. It acts centrally to stimulate the chemoreceptor trigger zone in the medulla and by irritant action on the gastric mucosa.

Vomiting is contraindicated when corrosives (e.g., lye, acids, alkalis, petroleum products, hydrocarbons) have been ingested. Vomiting of such substances increases the risk of gastric perforation and esophageal necrosis. Syrup of ipecac is also contraindicated if the patient's gag or cough reflex is absent or if the patient is delirious, convulsing, or in a coma; inducing vomiting in these circumstances can result in aspiration of gastric contents. Other contraindications to induced emesis are ingestions of convulsants, of sharp objects (such as glass) along with the toxic substance and of central nervous system toxins (such as camphor or strychnine). These substances should be removed immediately by lavage. Vomiting should never be induced in children younger than 1 year. Instead, the poison should be diluted by having the child drink milk or water, and the poison control center should be contacted.

Only syrup of ipecac, not ipecac fluid extract, should be used. The usual dose for a child younger than 1 year is 5 to 10 mL; for a child between 1 and 12 years, 15 mL; and for an adolescent or adult, 15 to 30 mL. Consumption of 200 to 300 mL of water or fruit juice, or as much fluid as the patient can drink, should follow. Ipecac syrup is not effective on an empty stomach. Vomiting usually occurs 15 to 30 minutes after the ipecac syrup is given. The patient should be positioned so as to prevent aspiration of vomitus and to permit prompt attention to mouth care. The dose of ipecac may be repeated only once after 20 minutes if the first dose was not effective. If vomiting does not occur within 30 minutes, gastric lavage is indicated, because systemic absorption of ipecac may cause conduction disturbances, atrial fibrillation, and myocarditis.

Activated Charcoal Activated charcoal (SUPERCHAR, ACTIDOSE, LIQUI-CHAR) adsorbs (detoxifies) ingested toxic substances and irritants. Substances adsorbed by activated charcoal include alcohol, salicylates, opioids, barbiturates, benzodiazepines, phenothiazines, digitalis, atropine, and penicillin. The charcoal may also serve as a stool marker to indicate when gastrointestinal absorption of the ingested poison has ended. The occasional adverse effects are diarrhea, gastrointestinal discomfort, and intestinal gas.

The desired dose of activated charcoal in an adult is 30 to 100 g given as a slurry (30 g in at least 8 ounces of water) or 12.5 to 50 g in an aqueous or sorbitol suspension. If dosing is based on body weight, the dose is 1 g per kg, or approximately five to ten times the amount of poison ingested. Pediatric doses range from 25 to 50 g.

Activated charcoal is usually given as a single dose. For toxicants that are slowly absorbed or that undergo enterohepatic recirculation or secretion from the blood into the stomach, sequential doses can be beneficial. There is no upper limit to the amount that may be given. Further, the mixture need not be removed from the stomach after ingestion, because no known adverse effects have been identified. Because it inactivates syrup of ipecac, activated charcoal should be administered after emesis or lavage.

Saline Laxatives Saline laxatives (e.g., magnesium citrate, magnesium sulfate, sodium sulfate) foster the passage of toxicants through the intestine, thereby minimizing absorption. Saline laxatives do not reduce adsorption onto charcoal but do accelerate charcoal elimination. These drugs act quickly and have little toxicity. A commercial solution of magnesium citrate is available for adults (120 to 240 mL) and children (0.5 mL/kg). A 10 percent solution of magnesium sulfate (2.5 mL/kg for children; 150 to 200 mL for adults) is preferred to sodium sulfate for patients who are on low-sodium diets or have congestive heart failure or hypertension.

Eliminate Poison

Eliminating poisons usually consists of first aid for the system involved. Management of ocular exposure involves flushing the eye(s) with water or normal saline for up to 20 minutes. The eyelids should be held open to facilitate thorough washing of the eyes. Eye drops and other chemicals should be avoided after flushing. A follow-up ophthalmic exam should be scheduled.

Topical exposures should be managed by immediately flooding the body parts with water. A shower is the best strategy. Clothing should be removed while the patient is in the shower, to prevent exposure of the health care provider or others. The flooding should be followed by gentle washing of the area with soap and water, and thorough rinsing.

Inhaled poisons require immediate removal of the victim to fresh air. Patency of the airway and oxygen exchange should be evaluated. If necessary, mouth-to-mouth resuscitation should be instituted.

Other ways to block or eliminate toxins from the system are forced diuresis, cathartics and enemas, dialysis, hemoperfusion, and exchange transfusions. These methods are not universally effective and are used much less commonly than lavage. Altering urinary pH enhances elimination of certain drugs (see Chapters 41 and 61). The efficacy of dialysis in removing toxic substances has not been proven; thus, it is used primarily as an adjunct to other therapies. The usefulness of dialysis depends on the pharmacokinetics of the substance. It is often effective when the usual supportive or corrective measures do not suffice in preventing further organ damage, and when biotransformation or elimination routes are damaged, blocked, or otherwise dysfunctional. Drugs not amenable to dialysis are diazepam, digoxin, doxycycline, phenothiazines, propoxyphene, and zidovudine.

Education

It is often difficult for the general population to understand the dangers associated with various substances, including poisonous plants. Education about poison prevention is vital. Ideally, primary prevention activities occur before poison exposure; however, in many cases, the awareness of poison potential comes after an exposure. The combined efforts of poison control centers and health care providers have had a significant impact on the frequency of certain categories of drug poisonings, most notably aspirin poisoning.

Prevention of accidental drug ingestion involves teaching about the appropriate storage of drugs so that children do not gain access to them. Parents or guardians of small children must survey their homes for hazardous substances stored in unsafe locations. Even alcoholic beverages must be safely stored, because fatal poisonings have occurred in young children who ingested relatively small amounts.

Keeping all drugs in their original containers prevents confusion as to the contents. Furthermore, families should be cautioned that toxic substances must not be stored in food containers. Household cleaners and other toxic substances should be kept in original, well-marked containers and stored in a location inaccessible to children. Syrup of ipecac should be kept in the home and in the first aid kit for camping or traveling. The telephone numbers of the poison control center and the health care provider should be readily available.

Childproof caps delay, if not totally prevent, children's indiscriminate drug ingestion. Graphic symbols, such as "Mr. Yuk," an ugly, green-faced, scowling image, were placed on labels of poisoning substances in years past to alert adults and children to the potential hazards. It has been shown that such symbols did more to attract children to the poisonous substance than to keep them away. Poisonous plants should not be kept in homes where there are small children.

Evaluation

Treatment outcomes vary with the specific poison. In general, treatment outcomes are manifest as stable vital signs and the absorption, or elimation, of the poison.

Additionally, evaluation activities may include the use of epidemiologic methods that help identify drug-related problems. For example, poison prevention programs can be implemented at the primary prevention level, early diagnosis and screening for drug abuse at the secondary prevention level, and rehabilitation and restoration efforts at the tertiary prevention level.

SUMMARY

- The number and variety of OTC drugs have exponentially increased, but their use carries risks as well as benefits to the consumer.
- Noncompliance is the most common problem encountered with drug management in the home.
- The OTC drug resources available in the community include pharmacists, computer information systems, publications, poison control centers, and emergency alert systems.
- Assessment of the patient in the home is comparable to that performed in an institution, including history taking, physical exam, and diagnostic testing.
- Psychosocial and cultural influences in self-care behaviors and the use of OTC drugs are components vital to the patient database, as is information about dietary practices, health-illness beliefs, use of folk medicine, family support, language, financial status, and educational barriers.
- General objectives of OTC drug therapy are directed at cure, alleviation, or palliation of illness.
- Care plan strategies should recognize the patient's locus of control and promote appropriate and accurate decision-making.
- The use of pill boxes, calendars, diaries, etc., can help track patient compliance with the drug regimen.
- When necessary, noncompliance should be addressed as openly and directly as possible, with the intent being to understand the reasons behind the difficulty.
- There are more than 300,000 different OTC drug products on the market, but fewer than 20 are responsible for 90 percent of nonaccidental poisonings.
- Pediatric patients younger than 5 years are at highest risk for accidental drug poisonings.
- Adolescent and adult poisonings more often result in serious morbidity and mortality.
- It is sometimes difficult to distinguish between a suicidal drug overdose and recreational drug use.
- The local poison control center should be contacted when an accidental or nonaccidental ingestion of substances is suspected.
- A complete accounting of the suspected poison is needed, including the name of the substance (if known), quantity consumed, and time of ingestion.
- Toxidromes—the clinical manifestations of ingestion—and toxicology testing are helpful in determining the exposure.
- Treatment objectives center on supporting vital functions, preventing absorption of or eliminating the poison, and managing complications.
- The key principle in the treatment of poisonings is, "Treat the patient, not the poison." Treatment for most poisonings is symptomatic and supportive.
- Basic and advanced life support protocols should be used if the patient's condition warrants.
- Absorption of the poison may be prevented by inducing emesis, gastric aspiration, and lavage (ipecac syrup, activated charcoal).
- The poison is eliminated by removing the patient from the environment for inhaled poisons and flushing the skin or eyes for topical exposures.
- Forced diuresis, cathartics and enemas, dialysis, hemoperfusion, and exchange transfusions may also be used in some cases to eliminate the poison.
- Education emphasizes primary prevention; however, patient readiness to learn often peaks immediately after a poisoning has taken place.

BIBLIOGRAPHY

Aiken, L., and Fagin, C. (1991). *Charting nursing's future: Agenda for the 1990's*. Philadelphia: J.B. Lippincott.

American Society of Hospital Pharmacists. (1993). *PDR for nonprescription drugs*. Montvale, NJ: Medical Economics Company, Inc.

Bird, C. (1990). Drug administration: A prescription for self-help. *Nursing Times*, 86(43), 52–55.

Bruch, M., and Larson, E. (1989). An early historical perspective on the FDA's regulation of OTC drugs. *Infection Control & Hospital Epidemiology*, 10, 527–528.

Campbill, R., White, J., and Hansten, P. (1992). Prescription and over-the-counter drugs: The ins and outs. *Diabetes Forecast*, 45(2), 35–39.

Cargill, J. (1992). Medication compliance in elderly people: Influencing variables and interventions. *Journal of Advanced Nursing*, 17, 422–426.

Colucciello, M. (1993). Learning styles and instructional processes for home healthcare providers. *Home Healthcare Nurse*, 11(2), 43–50.

Conn, V. (1992). Self-management of over-the-counter medications in older adults. *Public Health Nursing*, 9(1), 29–36.

Conn, V. (1991). Older adults: Factors that predict the use of over-the-counter medication. *Journal of Advanced Nursing*, 16(10), 1190–1196.

Covington, T. (Ed.) (1993). *Handbook of Nonprescription Drugs*. (10th ed.). Washington, DC: American Pharmaceutical Association.

Covington, T. (1992). Overview of nonprescription drug therapy and the self-care movement. Paper presented at the 139th Annual Meeting of the American Pharmaceutical Association. San Diego, CA, March 14.

Emmett, A. (1994). Health care trends that will reshape nursing. *Nursing*, 9(4), 50–53.

Fielo, S., and Warren, S. (1993). Medication usage by the elderly. *Geriatric Nursing*, 14(1), 47–51.

Fineman, B., and DeFelice, C. (1992). A study of medication compliance. *Home Healthcare Nurse*, 10(5), 26–29.

Gannon, K. (1994). Hot, hot hot: New switches to brighten OTC market. *Drug Topics*, 135(15), 32.

Giger, J., and Davidhizar, R. (1991). *Transcultural Nursing*. St. Louis: Mosby–Yearbook.

Goldfrank, L. (1994). *Toxicologic Emergencies*. (5th ed.). New York: Appleton-Century-Crofts.

Hamilton, T. (1991). Appropriate use of the family medicine cabinet. *Vibrant Life*, 7(2), 5.

Holt, G., Dorcheus, L., and Hall, E. (1992). Patient interpretation of label instruction. *American Pharmacy*, 32(3), 58–62.

Holt, G., Hollon, J., and Hughes, S. (1990). OTC Labels: Can consumers read and understand them? *American Pharmacy*, NS30(11), 51–54.

Home health care update: Dealing with noncompliance. (1994). *Nursing*, 24(6), 53.

Jubeck, M. (1992). Are you sensitive to the cognitive needs of the elderly? *Home Healthcare Nurse*, 10(5), 20–25.

Kemper, D., Lorig, K., and Mettler, M. (1993). The effectiveness of medical self-care interventions: A focus on self-initiated responses to symptoms. *Patient Education and Counseling*, 21(1,2), 29–39.

Kluckowski, J. (1992). Solving medication noncompliance in home care. *Caring*, 11(11), 34–41.

Legislation and Regulation. (1995). FDA considers OTC drug labeling reform. *American Pharmacist*, 35(11), 5.

Lewin, N., Howland, M., and Goldfrank, L. (1994). *Goldfrank's toxicologic emergencies.* (5th ed.). Norwalk, CT: Appleton & Lange.

Lund, V., and Frank, D. (1991). Helping the medicine go down. *Journal of Psychosocial Nursing,* 29(7), 7–9.

McCaffrey, D., Smith, M., and Banahan, B. (1993). Why prescriptions go unclaimed. *U.S. Pharmacist,* 18(8), 58–65.

Nonprescription Drug Manufacturers Association. (1991, July). *Facts and figures.* Washington, DC.: Author.

O'Donnell, J. (1994). Drug therapy: Ways your role will change. Nursing, 4(3), 46–48.

Physicians desk reference for nonprescription drugs. (1995). Montvale, NJ: Medical Economics Data Production Company.

Salerno, E., Ries, D., Sank, J., et al. (1985). Self-medicating behaviors. *Florida Journal of Hospital Pharmacy,* 5(7), 13–21.

United States Department of Health and Human Services. (1991). Eight moves to help your patients improve adherence. *Infomemo,* Spring, 9.

United States Pharmacopeial Convention. (1994). USPDI: Drug information for the health care professional. (14th ed.). Rockville, MD: Author.

United States Pharmacopeial Convention. (1993). *Advice for the patient.* Rockville, MD: Mack Printing Company.

United States Pharmacopeial Convention. (1991). *Tips against tampering.* Rockville, MD: Author.

Wolfgang, A., Jankel, C., and McMillan, J. (1993). Drug information and educational needs. *Home Healthcare Nurse,* 11(3), 20–23.

Young, L., and Koda-Kimbel, M. (1995). *Applied therapeutics: The clinical use of drugs.* (6th ed.) Vancouver: Applied Therapeutics, Inc.

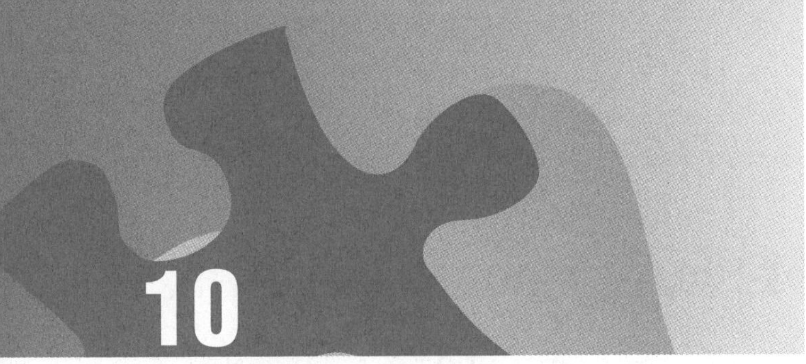

10 Substance Abuse

Psychostimulating plants have attracted humans and animals for thousands of years. Equally old is the controversy over the use of such plants and related substances. There is evidence that the Classical Greeks used psychedelics for mind-altering purposes, especially in connection with religious rituals, and that they employed other psychoactive substances for medical and recreational purposes. Hence, the use of psychoactive substances is as old as civilization.

The popularity of drugs of abuse tends to increase and decrease over time as each new generation learns the adverse effects and consequences of particular drugs or as new drug forms become available. Although the nation attempts to free its populace from the abuse of illegal substances, each generation has become known for its own prescription drug use and abuse (Fig. 10–1). Many terms are associated with substance abuse (see Terms Associated with Substance Abuse).

In the United States, there are four main categories of abused substances: sedatives, stimulants, hallucinogens, and anabolic steroids. Sedative-like substances include alcohol, opioids, barbiturates, and benzodiazepines. Stimulants comprise caffeine, nicotine, cannabis, amphetamines, and cocaine. Hallucinogens or psychedelics cover peyote, phencyclidine (PCP), and inhalants. Anabolic steroids have been abused by athletes in recent years in an attempt to build muscle mass and strength.

EPIDEMIOLOGY OF SUBSTANCE ABUSE

The prevalence of marijuana, alcohol, and cocaine use over the life-span is higher in men than in women. Men tend to obtain drugs illicitly, whereas women are more likely to abuse prescription drugs. Heroin use by blacks decreased in the 1970s, only to be replaced by cocaine and crack. Crack use among blacks peaked in 1988. Hispanics are less likely than whites or blacks to use stimulants or hallucinogens, but as a group, they have a longer history of abuse, arrests, and incarcerations and are slower seeking treatment.

There is a 20 to 30 percent incidence of alcohol abuse among the elderly, which frequently masks other health care problems. Also, there is a greater incidence of heavy drinking among blacks over the age of 20, whereas heavy drinking by whites tends to level off after the age of 20. Native Americans use alcohol in approximately the same proportion as the general population, although this group has a disproportional number of young people drinking. Young Native Americans also tend to use more marijuana and inhalants. The Jewish population has a low rate of alcohol abuse, most likely because they tolerate the drug poorly.

Thirty percent of the homeless—approximately two million people each year—have alcohol abuse problems. And 40 percent have abuse problems with other substances. Thus, the incidence and prevalence of substance use problems is significant. Further, prison populations have doubled since the 1970s as a result of substance abuse–related convictions. Additionally, two-thirds of the population who abuse alcohol have other psychiatric disorders. Over 50 percent of traffic fatalities involve alcohol, with 80 percent of the fatalities occurring between 8 PM and 4 AM, and alcohol has been linked to 40 percent of all reported assaults and 30 percent of forcible rapes and cases of child molestation.

The economic cost of substance abuse is significant. Accordingly, health insurance coverage for substance abuse has more limitations than for other illnesses or disorders. The use of alcohol by those responsible for operating automobiles, airplanes, or other high powered equipment, has resulted in loss of life and property, and has been blamed for disastrous effects on the environment (e.g., oil and chemical spills). Further, airline pilots, air traffic controllers, train engineers, ship pilots, truck drivers, and nuclear power plant operators who abuse drugs place the populace at risk for accidents and injury (see Controversy—Should Presently Controlled Substances Be Legalized?).

Populations at Risk

A number of populations are at risk for substance abuse. Adolescents tend to use alcohol as their primary substance of choice. Fifteen percent of adolescents have a definable problem with alcohol. However, less than 1 percent of adolescents who use alcohol or drugs are truly dependent on these substances.

Approximately 15 percent of community-based older adults are dependent on alcohol but as many as 44 percent of the older adults in inpatient medical and psychiatric facilities abuse alcohol. Individuals who have a dual diagnosis are more likely to become substance abusers than the rest of the population. A dual diagnosis is defined as a psychoactive substance use disorder and a co-existing psychological disorder that requires simultaneous treatment. A surprising discovery is that the highest rate of alcoholism for any professionally defined group is found among American Nobel laureates for literature. Of nine such individuals to date, four were alcoholic and a fifth was a very heavy drinker.

Health care providers are at risk for substance abuse. Health care providers older than 40 years of age typically abuse alcohol alone, whereas providers younger than 40 years of age tend to use other drugs, either alone, or in combination with alcohol. The most common substances abused by health care providers include opioids, benzodiazepines, alcohol, and tobacco. However, the incidence of substance abuse by health care providers is in line with that of the general population. Injectable drugs are more likely to be used by providers working in acute care settings. Pharmacists tend to abuse multiple orally administered drugs, with central nervous system (CNS) stimulants being most common.

SIGNE
PHILADELPHIA DAILY NEWS
Philadelphia
USA
DRUG-FREE AMERICA
HISTORY OF SOMEONE BORN BEFORE I WAS
12 MILLION LAYOFFS
GRIND
AGE 0-4
AMOXICILLIN
4-12
RITALIN
12-18
APPETITE SUPPRESSANTS
18-24
NO-DOZ
24-38
PROZAC
38-65
ZANTAC
65 —
EVERYTHING ELSE
Cartoonists & Writers Syndicate

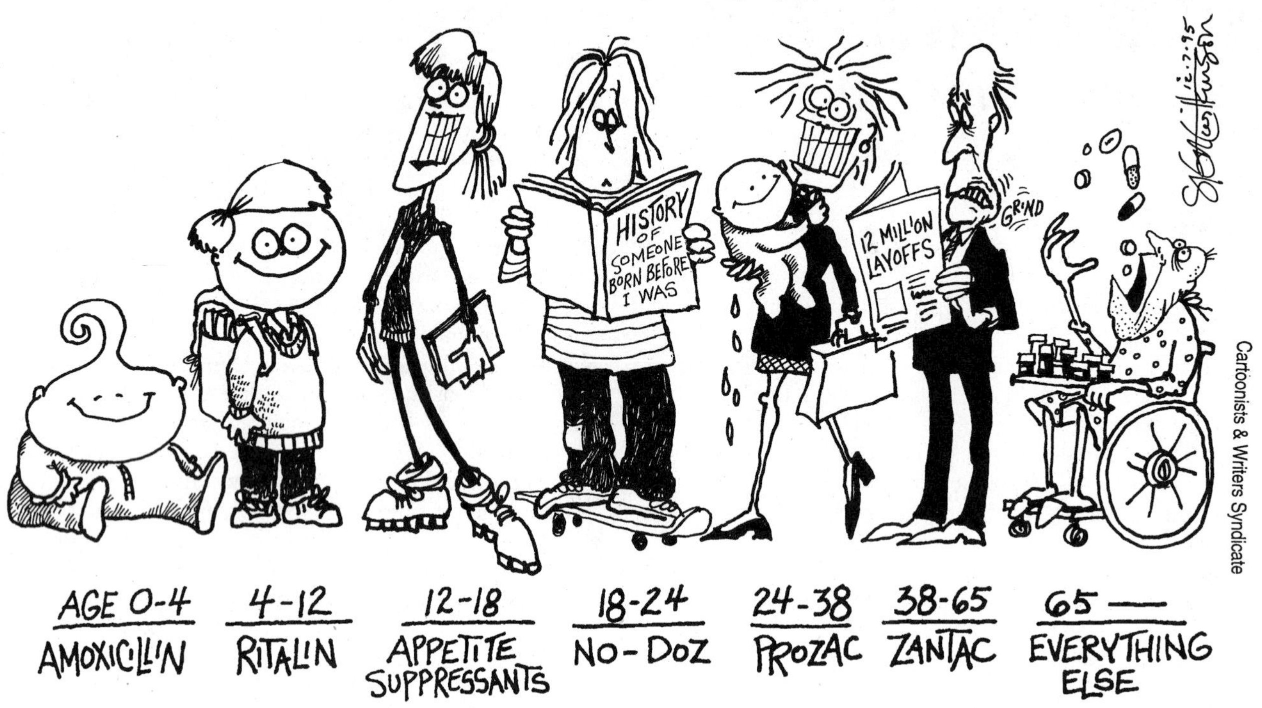

Figure 10–1 Drug use across American generations. How we view and use prescription and over-the-counter drugs as a society has an impact on the issue of all drug use and abuse. ("Drug-Free America" by Signe Wilkinson, published in the *Philadelphia Daily News,* 1997.)

Nitrous oxide use by dentists is not uncommon. Anesthesiologists and nurse anesthetists may use fentanyl or its analogs.

Vietnam veterans had a much larger problem with substance abuse than Gulf War veterans or veterans of World War I, World War II, or the Korean War. There are various reasons for this situation. Vietnam neighbored the so-called Golden Triangle for opiate production and use, which included Myanmar (formerly Burma), Laos, and Thailand. Thus, access to drugs of abuse was easy. Also, the Vietnam War was fought during a period when laws against these substances were not enforced as stringently as they are today. A legal substance, alcohol, remains at the heart of the greatest substance abuse problem for veterans. Over 100,000 alcoholic patients are treated yearly in veterans administration health care facilities.

Substance abuse is often associated with risky sexual behavior. Many substances break down inhibitions and increase desire so that the use of safe sex techniques and safe drug administration become secondary to immediate gratification. For example, homosexuals, particularly gay men, have been known to abuse nitrites, especially amyl nitrite, which is presumed to heighten orgasm. Drug abuse clinics are witnessing a larger number of substance abusers who are now positive for human immunodeficiency virus (HIV) as a result.

People with chronic pain are a diverse group, especially with respect to *drug abuse liability.* Few health care providers would deny appropriate analgesia to those suffering from terminal cancer. Yet neither would they freely give analgesics to people they suspect are drug seeking and using a physical condition as an excuse. Yet, there is a large middle ground that is difficult for the health care provider to assess. These are the individuals with chronic headaches, back or neck pains, fibromyalgia, and so forth. On the one hand, pain relief is important and humane. On the other hand, the health care provider does not want to be an unwitting enabler to a potential drug abuse problem. Because patients with chronic pain do not meet official diagnostic criteria for drug abuse or dependence, the diagnosis is often overlooked.

Since the time of the original Greek Olympiad, athletes have used substances to enhance their performance. Today's athletes are tempted to use anabolic steroids to enhance their muscle bulk and amphetamines to enhance confidence and performance. Athletes also perceive other substances, such as erythropoietin, and blood transfusions as giving them an edge in competition. Erythropoietin, a hormone produced by the kidney, increases red blood cell production. Blood transfusions (so-called blood doping) produce erythrocythemia. Both methods have been used to increase the oxygen-carrying capacity of the blood.

Other substances with abuse potential used by athletes for the purpose of increasing their prowess include CNS stimulants, such as strychnine and amiphenazole, and opioids, such as codeine, morphine, and heroin. Amphetamines and cocaine are used as psychomotor stimulants.

TERMS ASSOCIATED WITH SUBSTANCE ABUSE

Term	*Definition*
Abuse liability	Potential for causing addictive behavior.
Congeners	Substances with the same or similar functions.
Compulsive drug abuse	Irrational, irresistible, compelling abuse of substances.
Cross tolerance	A condition that exists between a drug and its congeners when a tolerance for one results in a corresponding tolerance for others. The need for an increased dosage of one carries over to its congeners.
Drug abuse	An evaluative phrase whose meaning differs from society to society. Drug abuse can be use of an illegal substance, use of a substance for other than the purpose or person for which it was prescribed, or in amounts larger than prescribed; use of a legal substance in excessive amounts (e.g., alcohol), or use of a substance despite known potentiality for harm (e.g., tobacco).
Drug addiction	Outdated term for drug dependence.
Drug dependence	A human or animal condition that manifests itself as either psychic or physical reliance on a drug. The drug comes to have higher value than other things formerly valued. (See psychic dependence and physical dependence.)
Drug misuse	Misuse is a term often used by the health care provider referring to the patient's use of the drug for other than the person or purpose for which it was prescribed or in an amount different than prescribed. But the term might also be applied to over prescribing and over reliance on medications by the health care provider rather than other therapies to resolve the patient's problem.
Experimental drug abuse	Exploratory use of a substance after which a decision is made to accept or reject continuing use.
Gateway drug	A substance more easily accessed by young people, experimentation with which can often lead to use of drugs which are illegal and addicting. The most often cited gateway drugs are alcohol, tobacco, marijuana, and inhalants.
Intensified drug	Abuse that is long term and patterned.abuse
Physical dependence	A condition in which a drug has altered neurons sufficiently so that there will be a physical withdrawal syndrome on diminishment or discontinuation of the drug.
Polydrug drug abuse	Use of multiple substances of abuse
Psychic dependence	A psychological craving for a drug.
Psychoactivity	The result of the stimulation of the neurons by natural or introduced substances.
Recreational/social drug abuse	Use of substances only in social contexts,most often alcohol, marijuana, cocaine and caffeine.
Situational drug abuse	The individual uses the drug to assist in task accomplishment.
Street drug	An illegal drug with no guarantee of purity; or a legally prescribed drug sold on the street illegally.
Tolerance	A condition in which it is necessary after repeated administration of a drug to increase the dose in order to achieve the same effect.

Patterns of Abuse

The choice of substances appears to follow a progressive pattern. The pattern of abuse usually begins early with the individual abusing wine or beer and, in most cases, nicotine in the form of cigarettes. This practice is followed by marijuana use and finally use of other illegal drugs (e.g., cocaine). Initially, the period of substance abuse is short term and without a defined pattern. During this *experimental phase,* the individual explores use of the substance, after which a decision is made to accept or reject continuing use of the drug. During the *recreational-social* phase, the individual begins using the substance in social contexts. A mood-altering experience is desired—no longer is experimentation the purpose for using the drug. *Situational drug abuse* follows, whereby the individual uses the drug in order to accomplish a specific task. In time, the substance abuse becomes patterned, long term, and intensive. *Compulsive* use ordinarily follows.

THEORIES OF SUBSTANCE ABUSE

One theory about the development of substance abuse posits that drugs are a panacea for life's problems. Drugs represent a quick fix for boredom and relief from pain and anxiety, and they promote self-confidence and a sense of well-being. Health care providers promote this philosophy when we attribute relief of many problems to the use of prescribed or over-the-counter (OTC) drugs. What we do not appreciate is the inconsistency between promoting legal drugs

Controversy

Should Presently Controlled Substances Be Legalized?

JANICE BRENCICK and GLENN WEBSTER

There is a parallel between the current use and abuse of controlled substances and that of alcohol during Prohibition. In both cases, legislated restriction resulted in increases in organized crime and black marketing, loss of tax revenues, difficulties in treatment and prevention, and violence. No reduction in dependency and other problems associated with the use of controlled substance has been evidenced.

On one hand, it is argued that abuse of controlled substances and attendant legal issues would disappear or be greatly diminished if controlled substances were legalized.

On the other hand, these substances are deemed so harmful and seductive that they must be outlawed and those who traffic in them punished if society is to be protected. The threat to society is related to the fear that many more people will use and grow to depend on these substances if they are legal and easily obtained. Additionally, there is concern that the use of drugs may increase violence that legalization was supposed to prevent.

Critical Thinking Discussion

- What are the potential health hazards that the use of controlled substances poses?
- What kinds of social problems are generated by the unregulated use of controlled substances?
- Is the threat to society related to the use of these substances sufficient to warrant government intervention in areas many would reserve to the individual?

while disparaging the use of illicit ones. On the one hand, we expect patients to "just say no" to street drugs, and on the other hand to "just say yes" to prescription drugs.

Another theory blames substance abuse on the patient or the patient's family. This viewpoint proposes that a patient's lack of will power or early environment produced conditions that promote the problem. Some theorists search for a biologic, chemical, or genetic tendency for substance abuse.

Freud's thesis is that there is a basic incompatibility between civilization and human nature. If we accept the thesis as stated, perhaps this is the reason substance use and abuse have been associated with every civilization since ancient times. Substance abuse is the result of internal tensions. The individual learns that substances reduce the tension to a tolerable level. This theory suggests that substance abuse is a learned response to tension.

The sociocultural theory suggests that substance abuse is communicated through the socialization process. Verbal and nonverbal behaviors convey the acceptability of substance use. Drug use by parents is often observed by children as a behavior to emulate. However, the acceptance or rejection of drug use by adolescents is often the result of pressure from peers.

The disease model was originally developed to describe alcoholism. According to this theory, substance abuse and dependency is a progressive disease that has both psychological and physiologic components. The psychological factors include an obsession with the substance, whereas physiologic factors include a genetic predisposition and altered brain function. Dependency occurs when the individual is physically and psychologically reliant on a substance.

COMMONLY ABUSED SUBSTANCES

Central Nervous System Depressants

ALCOHOL

Alcohol is the substance of choice for most of the population who are subject to substance abuse. Its only competitor in contemporary times is caffeine. Alcohol has been used at social events and in religious ceremonies from earliest recorded history. Most people do not view alcohol as a drug, and unless its use is excessive, most societies accept it as normal and unremarkable. Although there are many problems associated with alcohol abuse, there are positive benefits from low to moderate alcohol use.

Alcohol can be used as an astringent, antiseptic, and disinfectant. It is a solvent and a preservative in many drug formulations (e.g., spirits, elixirs, and fluid extracts). In some cases, 80 percent ethyl alcohol can be used to destroy sensory nerve fibers and relieve pain associated with severe, protracted neuralgias (e.g., tic douloureux). Similarly, patients with Buerger's disease (thromboangiitis obliterans) may profit from alcohol use because of its vasodilation effects. And many people with anorexia benefit from the appetite-stimulating feature of alcohol.

Pharmacodynamics

The exact mechanism of action of alcohol is unclear. It has been suggested that alcohol affects the brain by interacting with specific protein constituents of brain cell membranes. Gamma-aminobutyric acid (GABA), a major inhibitory neurotransmitter, has been implicated. The GABA receptor recognizes not only GABA but also barbiturates (see Fig.17–3) and benzodiazepines (see Fig.17–4), producing effects similar to those of alcohol. The glutamate system and its *N*-methyl-D-aspartate receptor, another neurotransmitter system, may mediate many of the acute effects of alcohol. The activity of amino acid glutamate appears to be the primary excitatory neurotransmitter and is stimulated by alcohol.

Effects and Adverse Effects

Alcohol has a very simple molecular structure. This makes it easy for it to cross almost every biologic membrane and affect almost every organ. The effects depend on the amount consumed, the number of years during which it has been consumed, and genetic factors.

Alcohol's most obvious effects are on the CNS. Many of the initial effects of alcohol affect the reticular activating system. This system extends upward through the middle portion of the brainstem to the thalamus to activate the cerebral cortex (see Fig. 17–1). The cortex is receptive to the depressant effects of alcohol. The effects include excitation, intoxication, ataxia, incoordination, sedation, and even anesthesia. Excessive use results in neurologic disorders such as Wernicke-Korsakoff syndrome (related to thiamine deficiency), stroke, cerebellar degeneration, a classic stocking-glove peripheral neuropathy, and peripheral nerve pressure palsies (so-called Saturday night paralysis).

Alcohol has a cross tolerance with other CNS depressant drugs because they share either similar metabolic pathways or receptor systems. This explains why other CNS-active drugs can be used to manage alcohol withdrawal. One theory about how drinkers build tolerance to alcohol itself is that the neuronal membranes (which must be penetrated for intoxication to occur) become resistant to penetration when they are repeatedly exposed to ethanol. One drink (i.e., 1 ounce of spirits or the equivalent) produces a slight mood elevation with a blood alcohol concentration of 0.02 to 0.03 percent. In most states, legal intoxication is defined as 0.1 percent. This level can be achieved by consuming about three drinks. Major impairment occurs by the fifth drink for most individuals. With additional alcohol intake, the effects increase from slight euphoria to sensory-motor disturbances, coma, and death. Twenty drinks produce a blood alcohol level of 0.6 percent, a level that can cause death from respiratory failure. Even so, there are tremendous individual variations.

Small amounts of alcohol increase salivary secretion and gastric acid production. However, large quantities of alcohol inhibit gastric acid secretion and prostaglandin activity, thus contributing to the risk of gastritis. Malnutrition, especially deficiencies of thiamine (B_1), pyridoxine (B_6), folic acid (B_9), cyanocobalamine (B_{12}), niacin (nicotinamide), iron, ascorbic acid (C), and vitamins A, D, and K, plays a major role in the problems associated with alcoholism. There is also likely to be a protein deficiency. The combination of protein deficiency and a zinc deficiency can result in night blindness, susceptibility to infection and injury, and slowness in wound healing. Large quantities of alcohol also suppress the appetite, complicating the nutritional problems.

Regular alcohol consumption irritates the gastrointestinal (GI) tract, precipitating inflammation of the esophagus, stomach, and duodenum. Heartburn is common. Severe vomiting may result in mucosal tears and bleeding at the junction between the esophagus and stomach (Mallory-Weiss syndrome.) Alcoholic patients who smoke increase the chance of esophageal cancer tenfold.

If given a choice, the liver prefers alcohol as a source of energy and stores fat instead of burning it for fuel. With alcoholism, storing of fat leads to steatosis (fatty liver), alcoholic hepatitis, and cirrhosis. The cirrhosis, in turn, can result portal hypertension and esophageal varices.

Acute and chronic pancreatitis are associated with heavy are alcohol consumption. Patients with this problem often have intractable abdominal pain. When opioids, in turn, are given for pain management, the potential for a secondary dependency is possible.

The hematopoietic and immunologic effects of alcoholism are also notable. Anemia results from nutritional deficits and bleeding. Bone marrow suppression by alcohol contributes to the problem. Splenomegaly produces pancytopenia. A decreased white blood cell count renders the individual immunocompromised and prone to infections, especially mycobacterial infections and pneumonia. The disinhibitory effects of alcohol increase the risk for sexually transmitted diseases, including HIV.

Excessive consumption of alcohol clearly results in an increased risk of cancer of the tongue, mouth, oropharynx, esophagus, and liver. Although it is not a true carcinogen, alcohol may act as a tumor promoter by chronically irritating mucous membranes. Alcohol may also dissolve tobacco carcinogens, thus increasing their concentration in these structures. This may explain the much higher incidence of these cancers in heavy drinkers who also smoke. Other evidence suggests that alcohol may act as an immunosuppressant, a co-factor in the development of cancer.

The endocrine system is also affected by alcohol. Of special interest is the effect of alcohol on antidiuretic hormone. Alcohol suppresses antidiuretic hormone. The net effect is an increased urinary output and the risk for dehydration. If excessive magnesium is also eliminated, muscular weakness and tetany can result. Pseudo-Cushing's syndrome is associated with an alcohol-induced stimulation of adrenocorticotropic hormone. Hypocalcemia is partly responsible for the osteoporosis and fractures in alcoholics. Transient hypoparathyroidism and suppression of human growth hormone can also occur with long-term use of alcohol. Alcohol causes a degree of hypoglycemia by interfering with gluconeogenesis. It also affects the production of sex hormones, resulting in reduced fertility, impotency, and amenorrhea.

Vasomotor center responses in the medulla are reduced, leading to peripheral vasodilation. The temperature-regulating mechanism is also affected. These two mechanisms reduce core body temperature and contribute to the risk of hypothermia. Small quantities of alcohol (25 to 30 mL) raise the pulse rate, although to a minor degree. Large quantities also increase the pulse rate but with greater effects on the vasomotor center. Hypotension is likely. Large quantities of alcohol significantly decrease cardiac output. Idiopathic cardiomyopathy and arrhythmias resulting in congestive heart failure refractory to cardiac glycoside therapy are possible.

Folate deficiency is the most common sign of malnutrition in chronic alcoholism. Thirty percent of patients with severe alcoholism develop megaloblastic anemia as a consequence of this deficiency. A number of factors contribute to folate deficiency. The factors include inadequate dietary intake of folate (i.e., green leafy vegetables and liver), impaired absorption, and a decreased retention and storage that accompanies severe liver disease. Other factors contributing to the deficiency include an alteration of the tissues to folate, modifications in enterohepatic cycling of folate, and elimination of greater amounts of folate secondary to hemolysis.

People who abuse alcohol have derangements of iron metabolism, which contribute to the risk of sideroblastic anemia and hemosiderosis. Iron deficiency anemia is common and due to inadequate dietary intake and an associated GI blood loss. Hemolytic anemia results from liver damage. Bleeding times are prolonged because alcohol interferes with platelet formation and function, and the production of vitamin K–dependent clotting factors by the liver.

Available evidence suggests that alcohol itself injures skeletal muscle. Alcoholic myopathy is a syndrome of muscle necrosis that varies greatly in severity. The initial presentation can range from asymptomatic, transient elevations of a specific fraction of creatine kinase to frank rhabdomyolysis (disintegration of striated muscles with elimination of myoglobin in the urine).

Pharmacokinetics

Alcohol does not require digestion for absorption to take place. Although small quantities of alcohol are absorbed in the stomach, most absorption takes place in the small intestine. The absorption rate of alcohol increases as the gastric alcohol concentration increases. As the alcohol begins to restrict blood supply to the stomach, the absorption rate decreases. The presence of food or milk also slows gastric absorption of alcohol. Alcohol is uniformly distributed to all body tissues in the same ratio as water.

Over 90 percent of the alcohol is biotransformed in the liver by alcohol dehydrogenase. Alcohol is oxidized to acetaldehyde and then to acetic acid. It is buffered to an acetate and then further oxidized to carbon dioxide and water. Although the rate of biotransformation differs with acute or chronic ingestion and other factors, it is generally about 10 mL/hour. This is the amount of alcohol contained in 3 to 4 ounces of wine or champagne (12 percent alcohol), 8 to 12 ounces of beer (4 percent alcohol), or 20 to 30 mL of 90 proof spirits (45 percent alcohol). Alcohol that is not oxidized is eliminated via the lungs and the kidneys. Large quantities of alcohol damage renal epithelium and alter urinary elimination.

The public and many health care providers alike are not entirely aware of the most significant alcohol-drug interactions. Table 10–1 provides an overview of the most important interactions. Understanding alcohol's interactions is important because these interactions increase the risk of CNS depression. The subsequent respiratory suppression can be fatal. For example, alcohol has an interaction with disulfiram that can be fatal.

TABLE 10–1 DRUG-DRUG INTERACTIONS OF SELECTED SUBSTANCES OF ABUSE

Drug	Interactive Drugs	Interaction
CNS Depressants		
Alcohol	Antianxiety drugs Antihistamines Antidepressants Antipsychotics Opioids Sedative-hypnotics	Additive CNS depression
	Salicylates	Additive GI irritation and bleeding
	Nitrates Nitroglycerine	Additive vasodilation leading to hypotension and syncope
	Phenytoin	May increase or decrease liver metabolism
	Chlorpropamide Disulfiram Metronidazole	Inhibits aldehyde dehydrogenase, leading to accumulation of acetaldehyde and a disulfiram reaction
CNS Stimulants		
Caffeine	CNS stimulants	Increased CNS stimulation
	MAO inhibitors	Increased risk of severe hypertension and arrhythmias
Nicotine	Acetaminophen Caffeine Oxazepam Pentazocine Propranolol Propoxyphene Theophylline	Increases biotransformation of interactive drug
	Adrenergic agonists Adrenergic blockers Catecholamines Cortisol	Increased plasma levels of interactive drug
	Furosemide	Reduced cardiac output and diuretic effects
	Insulin	Decreased effects of interactive drug

CNS, Central nervous system; GI, gastrointestinal; MAO, monoamine oxidase.

Alcohol Overdose and Withdrawal

Management of alcohol abuse can be divided into treatment of acute alcoholism, chronic alcoholism, and withdrawal syndromes. Acute intoxication does not usually require intervention. In most cases, the patient is simply allowed to sleep off the effects of the alcohol. If the patient is hyperactive or combative, a sedative may be administered. The problem with this intervention is that sedatives potentiate alcohol, and excessive CNS depression is possible. If the patient is comatose, supportive measures (e.g., artificial airway, mechanical ventilation) may be required.

Alcohol withdrawal of mild to moderate severity is characterized by tremors, restlessness, agitation, insomnia, and other signs and symptoms. Signs and symptoms of severe withdrawal involve those noted earlier but also include seizures, hallucinations, and delirium tremens. Intervention for withdrawal syndrome usually involves use of antianxiety drugs (i.e., benzodiazepines). These drugs provide sedation and possess a significant anticonvulsant property. The benzodiazepines are discussed further in Chapter 17. Other treatment measures for withdrawal include vitamins, nutritional therapy, and symptomatic measures. The primary purpose of short-term benzodiazepine therapy is to permit the patient to participate in a rehabilitation program. Long-term use of antianxiety drugs should be avoided because they, too, can be abused.

Long-term drug therapy for chronic alcoholism involves disulfiram (ANTABUSE). Disulfiram blocks the action of aldehyde dehydrogenase and allows acetaldehyde to accumulate. If alcohol is then ingested, flushing of the face, dyspnea, hypotension, tachycardia, nausea and vomiting, syncope, vertigo, blurred vision, headache, and confusion develop. Severe disulfiram reactions include respiratory depression, cardiovascular collapse, arrhythmias, myocardial infarction, congestive heart failure, unconsciousness, seizures, and death. The severity of the reaction is proportional to the amounts of alcohol and disulfiram taken. The reaction lasts as long as alcohol is present in the circulation, which may be a few minutes to several hours. Furthermore, use of prescription or OTC drugs containing alcohol can precipitate a disulfiram-like reaction. Table 10–2 provides a brief list of

TABLE 10–2 ALCOHOL CONCENTRATION OF COMMON OVER-THE-COUNTER PRODUCTS

Over-the-Counter Drug	Content (%)	Proof
CĒPACOL THROAT LOZENGES	15	28
COMTREX	20	40
FORMULA 44 MULTI-SYMPTOM COUGH & COLD	20	40
LISTERINE MOUTHWASH	26.9	53.8
NYQUIL LIQUICAPS	25	50
SCOPE MOUTHWASH	18.9	37.8
MULTI-SYMPTOM TYLENOL COUGH	10	20

the concentration of alcohol in some OTC drugs. Because drowsiness may occur with disulfiram therapy, it should be taken as a single bedtime dose.

OPIOIDS

Over 5 million people in the United States use opioid analgesics for nonmedical purposes. Approximately 3 million of these individuals report using heroin, with 500,000 being dependent on the drug. Approximately 80 percent of heroin abusers are in their mid-20s. The largest population of heroin abusers are located in New York, with Los Angeles holding second place.

Opioids and opioid-like drugs that cause dependence include opium alkaloids (heroin, morphine, codeine, and thebaine). Natural opioids come directly from the poppy. The semisynthetic group (e.g., hydromorphone, oxymorphone), and the synthetic group (e.g., meperidine, levorphanol, propoxyphene, and methadone) are manufactured. The opioids most often abused include heroin, propoxyphene, methadone, oxycodone, and morphine. Heroin is the most potent of this group. The opioids are discussed in greater depth in Chapter 14.

Opium has been used as a euphoric to combat anxiety, as an antidepressant, to relieve hunger and thirst, and to induce sleep. It has also been used to treat abdominal cramping and colic. Opium derivatives are CNS depressants that act on the thalamus, sensory cortex, and higher brain centers. Because opioids elevate mood; relieve tension, fear, and anxiety; and produce feelings of peace, euphoria, and tranquility, they are particularly likely to lead to physical and psychological dependence. The heroin user compares the ecstatic rush from intravenous (IV) injection of heroin with that of a sexual orgasm. Further, the high causes the individual to defer satisfying basic biologic needs (e.g., eating and drinking). The effects of IV opioids last about a minute. The high is followed by an interval of nodding, which is a pleasant drowsiness that alternates with sudden wakenings. If a person is smoking, nodding results in cigarette burns in the shape of a rosette on the chest. The nodding may be followed by periods of talkativeness called soap boxing. Opioids do not produce hallucinogenic effects.

Heroin is a derivative of morphine. It was initially introduced in Germany at the end of the 19th century as a stronger form of morphine. Heroin imported into the United States is about 95-percent pure. To increase profits to illegal drug dealers, heroin is reduced (cut) with other substances (e.g., lactose or quinine) to 3 to 5 percent purity and sold on the streets.

Heroin is a Schedule I drug in the United States and has no therapeutic use. In England, heroin is one of the constituents in Brompton's cocktail (a combination of drugs used to manage pain in terminally ill patients). Heroin produces psychological and physical dependence within a few weeks of continued use.

Methadone is used to alleviate opioid craving. It has been used since the 1960s in the rehabilitation of opioid-dependent patients. Methadone satisfies the craving but does not produce the euphoric effects of other opioids. Its use is not without controversy, however. Defenders assert that it is an effective adjunct for an individual determined to stay away from drugs. Detractors claim that its use simply substitutes one drug of abuse for another, that therapy often requires indefinite maintenance, and that detoxification is often accompanied by a return to heroin.

Opioid Overdose and Withdrawal

Opioid overdose can be managed with the administration of an opioid antagonist (see Chapter 14) and respiratory support. Naloxone (NARCAN) is a pure antagonist that reverses opioid toxicity and reverses the triad of miotic pupils, coma or stupor, and bradypnea (a respiratory rate of 4 to 6 breaths/minute). The usual adult dose of naloxone is 0.4 to 2 mg IV. The dose may be repeated at 2- to 3-minute intervals, if necessary. Larger doses may be required for the treatment of certain opioids. Failure to respond to naloxone may suggest a mixed substance overdose or involvement of a nonopioid substance. For example, the administration of naloxone can help differentiate opioid toxicity from benzodiazepine overdose.

Withdrawal from opioids without medical supervision is called going cold turkey because the skin is cold and the piloerection resembles a plucked turkey. There may be a crawling sensation of the skin. Histamine release is responsible for the sweating and itching and dilation of superficial blood vessels, especially of the face, neck, and upper thorax, The individual takes on a flushed appearance. Muscle spasms, especially of the back and limbs, result in kicking motions, and hence the phrase "kicking the habit." Yawning, sweating, rhinorrhea, hot flashes, nausea, vomiting, abdominal cramps, tachypnea, and tachycardia can also be present.

Clonidine (CATAPRES), a sympatholytic antihypertensive (see Chapter 34), is used in the management of opioid withdrawal. It stimulates alpha-2 receptors in the brain, resulting in reduction in sympathetic outflow and a decrease in peripheral vascular resistance, heart rate, and blood pressure. At present, it is under investigation for relieving symptoms of acute drug withdrawal. It takes 2 to 3 days to reach peak effect using clonidine patches, which is often too late to manage the worse effects of opioid withdrawal. The tablet formulation offers a rapid and more easily titrated treatment modality.

The dosage of clonidine required to prevent withdrawal symptoms is 5 mcg/kg/day, increasing to 17 mcg/kg/day, as necessary. The dosage is individualized based on patient tolerance, the quantity and type of opioid used, and patient response. It is administered daily in divided doses for a period of 10 days. The dosage is then reduced by 50 percent for the next 3 days and is discontinued on day 14.

The clinical efficacy of clonidine is limited by its sedative and hypotensive effects. Extremely close supervision is necessary to monitor for adverse effects and possible dosage manipulation by the patient.

BENZODIAZEPINES

The discovery of benzodiazepines in the 1950s was exciting because although they produced sedating and euphoric effects, they were thought to be less lethal than opioids or barbiturates. Moreover, these drugs did not appear to promote dependency in people who were not already predisposed. It takes ingestion of larger doses of benzodiazepines for longer periods of time to produce the life-threatening problems of the barbiturates. Today, benzodiazepines are rarely the primary drugs of abuse; however, they are commonly abused.

Use of benzodiazepine for other than sedative-hypnotic purposes is estimated to occur in 11 percent of the population each year. Approximately 37 percent of prescriptions for controlled substances are for benzodiazepines. This translates to about one prescription for every two adults. Of this figure, 80 percent report drug use for less than 4 months, 5 percent used the drug 4 to 11 months, and 15 percent used the drug 12 months or longer. Nearly two-thirds of benzodiazepine abusers are female. Older adults tend to be overrepresented in these figures, and they tend to use the drug on a chronic basis. Among alcohol or opioid abusers, the prevalence rates of benzodiazepine use is as high as 75 and 80 percent, respectively.

Benzodiazepines reduce fear and anxiety and produce euphoria, which explains their potential for abuse. But individuals who abuse benzodiazepines often combine them with alcohol or barbiturates because of the enhanced effects. The consequences, however, can be tragic.

The euphoric effect of benzodiazepines depends on the drug's onset of action. Although as a group benzodiazepines are slower to produce adverse effects than alcohol or the barbiturates, diazepam (VALIUM) is biotransformed the most quickly and, consequently, has the greatest potential for abuse. Lorazepam and alprazolam are the next most likely benzodiazepines to be abused. Oxazepam, prazepam, and clorazepate are the least likely to be abused. Chapter 17 discusses the benzodiazepines in more depth.

Persons on concurrent methadone maintenance may experience a boost with the simultaneous use of benzodiazepines. The theory is that both methadone and benzodiazepines compete for oxidation sites. Thus, there are higher levels of methadone in the blood and the brain.

BARBITURATES

The incidence and prevalence of nonmedical use of barbiturates exceeds that of the opioids. Opioid users frequently take barbiturates, benzodiazepines, and other sedative-hypnotics to augment the effects of weak illicit heroin or to produce psychological effects when they have become tolerant to prescribed opioids. The short-acting barbiturates such as pentobarbital (yellow-jackets) or secobarbital (reds) are preferred over long-acting drugs such as phenobarbital (purple hearts). Most users take the drugs by mouth, but a few individuals inject barbiturates IV or IM. Abusers who inject the tablet or capsule forms of barbiturates IV can develop serum hepatitis, septicemia, pulmonary emboli, papilloma, bacterial endocarditis, tetanus, and various skin rashes. Because of the highly alkaline sclerosing of veins, these individuals can be identified by the large abscesses that spread over the accessible areas of their bodies.

The amount of barbiturate used varies considerably, but an average dose of 1.5 g of a short-acting agent is not uncommon. Some individuals consume as much as 2.5 g daily over several months. Because tolerance develops to most of the actions of barbiturates, there may be no apparent signs of long-term use. For the patient taking barbiturates on a regular basis, the only manifestation of abuse may be rebound insomnia and some anxiety when the drug is stopped. For individuals attempting to maintain a state of intoxication, the acute and chronic effects resemble those of alcohol. This individual shows a general sluggishness, difficulty thinking, faulty judgment, poor comprehension and memory, has a narrow attention span, and is emotionally labile; also, there is an exaggeration of basic personality traits. Slurring and a slowness of speech is also noted. Quarrelsome behaviors and moroseness are common. The person may have an unkempt appearance, laugh or cry without provocation, and maintain hostile, paranoid, and suicidal ideations. Toxic doses of barbiturates lead to stupor and respiratory depression.

Long-term use of short-acting barbiturates results in both drug disposition and pharmacodynamic tolerance. Although there may be considerable tolerance to the sedative and intoxicant effects of barbiturates, the lethal dose is not much different than that in individuals who do not abuse the drugs. Consequently, acute barbiturate poisoning may be accidentally or deliberately superimposed on chronic intoxication. Cross tolerance to other barbiturates is common.

Barbiturates increase the biotransformation of other drugs by increasing microsomal enzyme activity. The combination of amphetamines and barbiturates produces greater euphoria than either drug alone. Hence, concurrent use of barbiturates with other drugs can be problematic. Specific and efficient antidotes to offset barbiturate overdoses are not available. Individuals who are dependent on barbiturates should never have them abruptly withdrawn because the withdrawal syndrome is one of the most dangerous in the field of drug abuse.

In its mildest form, the withdrawal syndrome from short-acting barbiturates may consist only of electroencephalographic changes, rebound increases in rapid-eye-movement sleep, insomnia, and anxiety. Somewhat greater degrees of dependency result in tremulousness, weakness, GI disturbances, and orthostatic hypotension that may last for 3 to 14 days. These signs may leave the patient unable to get out of bed. When the withdrawal syndrome is severe, there may be, in addition, symptoms of psychoses that progress to confusion, delirium, hallucinations, and tonic-clonic seizures. Seizure activity is more common in withdrawal from barbiturates than in alcohol withdrawal. The number of seizures varies from a single one to status epilepticus. Agitation and hyperthermia may lead to exhaustion, cardiovascular collapse, and death.

With the longer acting barbiturates, withdrawal symptoms may not begin until the second or third day and peak more slowly. Anxiety rises with time, and frightening dreams may be succeeded by refractory insomnia. Persecutory visual hallucinations generally start at the same time that clouding of the senses begins. Full blown delirium is manifested in disorientation to time and place. Once the delirium starts, even the administration of large doses of barbiturate may not suppress it immediately. This is true also of the delirium that develops during alcohol withdrawal. The reason for the irreversibility is unclear. The withdrawal syndrome, even if it is left untreated, usually clears by the eighth day.

Central Nervous System Stimulants

AMPHETAMINES

Amphetamines are a favorite drug of abuse across a wide range of age groups. Amphetamines were used by the military in World War II to heighten alertness, eliminate fatigue, strengthen endurance, and produce a heightened euphoria.

Benzedrine was a favorite drug for these purposes. Dexedrine was later used to decrease appetite for those who wanted to lose weight.

Methamphetamine has risen in popularity. Speed or meth is readily available and cheaper to produce than cocaine. Profit margins for the producer and for the dealer are thus greater and so is the desire for new recruits. Children as young as 11 years of age have become dependent on it. The price varies according to its purity. The purest form of methamphetamine is used for smoking. Other varieties are called glass, crystal, and crank, which is the cheapest. One analog of amphetamine is called methcatinone (cat), which can be produced from solvents purchased at almost any hardware store.

Pharmacodynamics

Amphetamines alter brain receptors for dopamine, norepinephrine, and serotonin. It also appears that the major mechanism by which amphetamines produce their reinforcing effects is their capacity to release newly synthesized dopamine and norepinephrine from intraneuronal stores. The release of other neurotransmitters along with inhibition of their uptake may also account for drug effects.

There are three types of amphetamines: salts of racemic amphetamines, dextroamphetamines, and methamphetamines. These types vary in potency and peripheral effects. Dextroamphetamine is said to have the fewest peripheral effects (i.e., hypertension and tachycardia).

Effects and Adverse Effects

The subjective effects of amphetamines, like those of all centrally active drugs, are dependent on the user, the environment, dose of the drug, and route of administration. Because drug action is associated with the sense of pleasure, amphetamines are very attractive to the user.

Amphetamines increase sociability in the early phases of use but tend to substitute for sociability in later phases. Moderate doses taken orally commonly produce an elevation in mood, a sense of increased energy and alertness, reduced need for sleep, a decreased appetite and improved task performance. They do not create extra physical or mental energy but rather promote expenditure of present resources, sometimes to the point of unsafe fatigue. The fatigue often goes unrecognized. The user feels little or no need for food, water, rest, or sleep. They may continually engage in vigorous activity that is perceived as exhilarating and creative. Amphetamines are sometimes called the trailer park drugs because of their use by truck drivers and others that need to stay awake.

The effects of amphetamines on the cardiovascular system can be profound. Tachycardia, chest pain, hypertension, and dyspnea may contribute to a panic state because these signs and symptoms are those of a myocardial infarction. To cope with these effects the individual is often also using depressants (downers). Some manufacturers combine a CNS stimulant such as dextroamphetamine with a CNS depressant such as amobarbital in an attempt to minimize overstimulation.

Amphetamines increase self-esteem to the point of grandiosity. Heavy users may develop amphetamine psychosis, which is characterized by aggression, delusions of persecution, depression, paranoia, euphoria, and fully formed visual and auditory hallucinations. Some users become loquacious. Some health care providers suggest that these symptoms are associated with sleep deprivation, which in and of itself leads to psychological disturbance. The paranoid rages of amphetamines have been associated with violent and unpredictable behavior. Grandiosity coupled with rage can be deadly. Amphetamines are responsible for some of the most audacious crimes. The saying speed kills is true in at least one context: Amphetamines trigger violent actions as well as pose a threat from toxic overdose.

Pharmacokinetics

Oral doses of amphetamines are absorbed from the GI tract to be concentrated in the brain, lungs, and kidneys. Amphetamines are biotransformed in the liver and eliminated via the kidneys. The half-life of metabolites varies with changes in urinary pH. A urine pH of 7 extends the half-life of amphetamines to 20 hours. In contrast, a pH of 5 reduces the half-life to 5 or 6 hours. Thus, the higher the urinary pH, the longer the half-life.

Overdose and Withdrawal

Acute intoxication from amphetamines and amphetamine-like drugs is more likely to occur in the neophyte user. Acute symptoms include dizziness, tremor, irritability, confusion, hallucinations, chest pain, palpitations, hypertension, sweating, and arrhythmias. Amphetamines can produce panic attacks, extreme paranoia, and death. Death is usually preceded by hyperpyrexia, seizures, and shock.

No specific antidote is available to manage amphetamine overdose. Treatment is primarily supportive and symptomatic. A conscious, nonconvulsant patient may be given an antiemetic, or gastric lavage can be used. An anticonvulsant may be used if seizures are present. Elimination of amphetamines can be enhanced with the administration of an osmotic diuretic (e.g., mannitol) along with a urinary acidifier (e.g., ammonium chloride).

Abrupt cessation of amphetamines after long-term use, or even after a binge of a few days, is commonly followed by depression, anxiety, and craving for the drug. These feelings are soon followed by general fatigue and a need for sleep (crash). On awaking, there is hyperphagia, continued sleepiness, depression, and anhedonia (lack of interest in usual activities). Mood returns to normal over a period of days, although the dysphoria and anhedonia may persist for weeks in some cases. Although these responses meet the criteria for a withdrawal syndrome, there are no obvious physiologic disruptions that require gradual withdrawal of the drug.

DESIGNER DRUGS

Designer drugs, mostly methylated amphetamines, are so called because they are manufactured in labs, although many of the substances can be found in more dilute form in nature. Here the distinction between artificial and natural is blurred and difficult. Of these drugs, methylenedioxymethamphetamine is a powerful stimulant as well as hallucinogen. Users say that it increases empathy as well as telepathic abilities. However, one also acquires knight's move thinking, which is a thought process involving logical hiatuses. Methylenedioxymethamphetamine heightens tactile sensations and the sense of well-being as well as the desire to be with others, and increases pleasures of sex and expressions of affection. When methylenedioxymethamphetamine is modified, it becomes monoethylmethylenedioxyamphetamine.

COCAINE

The early use of cocaine dates back to at least 500 AD. Spanish explorers noted that the people of Peru chewed the leaf of a certain plant because it seemed to give them energy and a sense of well-being. These explorers introduced the coca leaf to Europeans. Its popularity quickly spread. Before 1980, cocaine abuse was considered a minor drug abuse problem. However, in the 1980s, the use of cocaine increased dramatically.

Pharmacodynamics

Cocaine is ingested orally, chewed, snuffed, taken intravenously, administered topically, and smoked. It is an alkaloid found in the leaves of the plant *Erythroxylon coca*. Its effects have been linked directly to its action on cortical cells and to the alteration of central catecholamine levels. Cocaine is known to inhibit the reuptake of norepinephrine at adrenergic synapses, which may account for some of its central and peripheral effects. In the CNS, it potentiates neurotransmission of norepinephrine, dopamine, or serotonin. The reabsorption of the neurotransmitters is blocked, leaving circuits open that would otherwise close. The sequence of events associated with cocaine addiction is shown in Figure 10–2. A similar action occurs in the peripheral nervous system. The resulting effects depend on the dosage and the concentration in the blood.

Freebasing is the process for extracting cocaine from its hydrochloride salt. Freebase-cocaine (crack) contains impurities that were used to extract the cocaine base. Bicarbonate is one of these. When it is heated, the trapped bicarbonate is released, producing a crackling sound, hence the name crack. By concentrating the cocaine, stronger effects are produced.

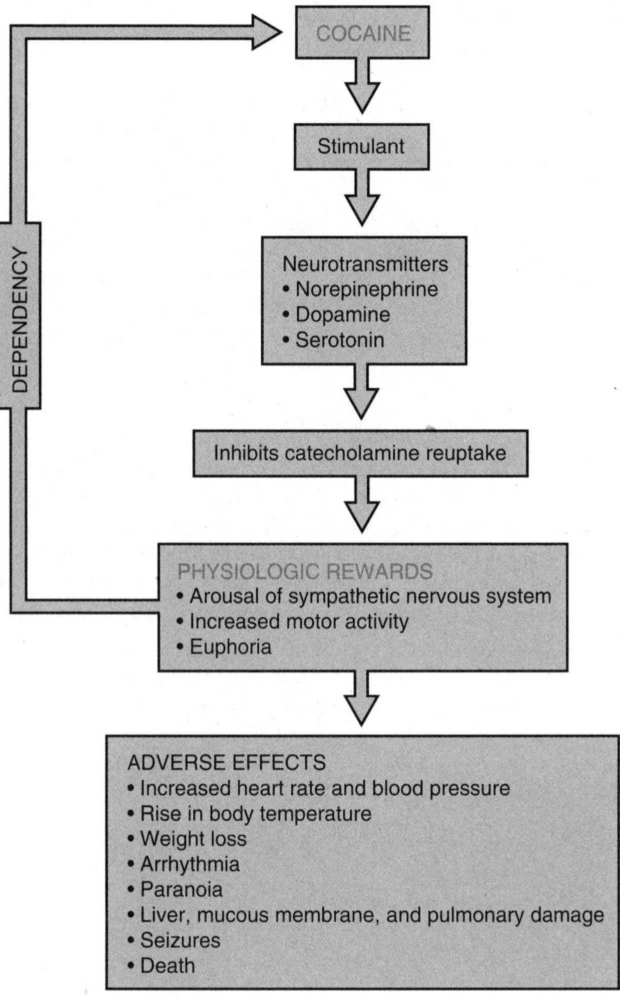

Figure 10–2 Addictive effects of cocaine. The algorithm follows the sequence of events leading to the physiologic rewards as well as adverse effects of cocaine addiction.

Effects and Adverse Effects

At low concentrations, there is a general arousal of the sympathetic nervous system and an increase in motor activity. It makes one more alert and active, which is the effect desired by many cocaine users. But at increased moderate concentrations, heart rate and blood pressure increase and body temperature rises, and there may be dilation of pupils. High concentrations can result in seizures. Cocaine can cause sudden death as a result of ventricular fibrillation, myocardial infarction, stroke, or respiratory arrest. When cocaine is snorted, perforation and bleeding of the nasal septum occurs. Pulmonary effects include wheezes and rhonchi.

Chronic cocaine abuse can result in arrhythmias, weight loss due to anorexia, paranoia, and liver and pulmonary damage. In addition, the user can experience unusual tactile sensations such as so-called cocaine bugs. This is the sensation of insects crawling all over the body. Lesions, scratches, and ulcerations of the skin occur when the user attempts to get rid of the "bugs."

Liver damage occurs, especially when the cocaine user also uses barbiturates. The combination of the metabolites of these two substances produces a liver toxin. However, cocaine use alone can produce liver damage, though the specific mechanism that produces the damage is unclear. When cocaine is inhaled chronically, it can produce pulmonary damage by constricting local blood vessels in the lung. In addition, impurities (e.g., kerosene) from solvents left behind in the freebasing procedure contribute to the damage.

The incidence of violence attributed to cocaine abusers is partially attributed to paranoia and increased motor activity. Part of cocaine psychosis consists of hallucinations and misperceptions, particularly, but not limited to, tactile misperceptions.

Abrupt withdrawal from cocaine use results in what many users call anguish, an extreme restless irritability. So intense is this feeling that the user attempts to ameliorate the effect by taking more cocaine in addition to opioids such as heroin. Speedballs are just such a combination of cocaine and heroin. Withdrawal from cocaine produces changes in electroencephalogram patterns and disruption of sleep cycles.

Pharmacokinetics

Cocaine is readily absorbed from its various routes of entry. It is biotransformed in the liver to benzoyl ecgonine. Cocaine has a very short half-life. After nasal or buccal absorption, the effects last 5 to 15 minutes. To maintain CNS stimulation over longer periods, cocaine must be inhaled or injected every 15 to 30 minutes. It is uncertain whether the liver damage reported from the use of cocaine is due to the cocaine itself or to the impurities associated with cocaine. Cocaine metabolites may be detected in the urine for 24 to 36 hours after use.

CAFFEINE

Caffeine is probably the world's most widely used psychoactive substance. It is found in many beverages, foods, and OTC and prescription drugs. It has been estimated that seven million kilograms of caffeine are consumed annually in the United States. The basis for the popularity of all caffeine-containing beverages has been the ancient belief that the beverages had stimulant and antisoporific actions that elevate mood, decrease fatigue, and increase the capacity for work.

Pharmacodynamics

The action of caffeine is similar to other stimulants such as the amphetamines and cocaine. Caffeine increases cyclic adenosine monophosphate (cAMP) levels by blocking phosphodiesterase, the enzyme responsible for degradation of cAMP. It also acts to antagonize the central neurotransmitter adenosine at the receptor site.

Effects and Adverse Effects

Although much of the populace does not consider caffeine a drug it does produce many long-term and short-term therapeutic and adverse effects on body systems. Although all levels of the CNS are affected by caffeine, regular doses (85 to 250 mg) of caffeine (the amount contained in three cups of coffee) produce increased capacity for intellectual activities and decreased motor reaction time to both visual and auditory events. However, tasks requiring delicate muscular coordination and accurate timing or arithmetic skills may be adversely affected. Drowsiness and fatigue generally disappear. However, in excess, caffeine causes nervousness or jittery feelings.

Large doses of caffeine produce a slowing of the heart rate, vasoconstriction, and increased respiratory rate. Caffeine stimulates the myocardium, increasing both heart rate and cardiac output. Because the effect is antagonistic to that produced on the vagus nerve, a slight slowing of the heart is noted in some individuals, whereas others note an increased rate.

Caffeine also dilates peripheral blood vessels, thereby decreasing peripheral vascular resistance. However, this effect is usually offset by the increased heart rate and cardiac output. Therefore, the effects on blood pressure depend on the dosage and individual effects.

Caffeine stimulates the respiratory center in the medulla, thus increasing the respiratory rate. Caffeine is sometimes used to treat apnea in preterm infants and Cheyne-Stokes respirations in adults.

The secretion of pepsin and hydrochloric acid is increased in the presence of caffeine. Thus, it should be avoided in patients who have history of peptic ulcer disease. Caffeine increases renal blood flow and the glomerular filtration rate by decreasing the reabsorption of sodium and water in the proximal tubules. A mild diuretic effect results.

Caffeine increases the contractual force and reduces voluntary muscle fatigue. It increases the metabolic rate, inhibits uterine contractions, transiently increases glucose levels by stimulating glycolysis, and increases plasma and urinary catecholamine levels. Caffeine has also been implicated in fibrocystic breast disease, birth defects, and cancer. It produces bladder irritation and frequent urination.

Caffeine constricts cerebral blood vessels, resulting in reduced cerebral blood flow and oxygen tension in the brain. When it is combined with ergotamine, caffeine may promote better absorption of ergotamine and enhances pain relief.

Signs of overdose include agitation, confusion, insomnia, irritability, nausea, vomiting, tinnitus, sensitivity to pain or touch, increased urination, abdominal pain, and muscle twitching. Seizures are possible.

A withdrawal syndrome including increased irritability, headache, and increased weakness has been reported when users who ingest more than 600 mg of caffeine per day decrease their consumption.

Pharmacokinetics

Caffeine is well absorbed from the GI tract and is distributed to all body compartments, including breast milk. Peak plasma levels are achieved 50 to 75 minutes after consumption. It is biotransformed in the adult liver to theophylline and theobromine. In the neonate, only a small portion is biotransformed to theophylline. The elimination half-life of caffeine is 6 hours in adults and 36 to 144 hours in the neonate. The adult half-life value is reached by age 4 to 6 months. In adults, caffeine's metabolites are eliminated by the kidneys, with only 1 to 2 percent eliminated unchanged. In neonates, caffeine is eliminated by the kidneys, with approximately 85 percent eliminated unchanged. A fatal dose of caffeine consists of between 50 and 100 cups of coffee.

TOBACCO AND NICOTINE

Nicotine is widely confirmed as the basis of the smoking habit. Nicotine has no therapeutic use but is of pharmacologic interest and toxicologic importance. Nicotine improves memory, especially long-term memory, and increases the accuracy and speed of information processing. Other benefits include an increase in pain threshold and a reduction of tension and anxiety. Perhaps it is the reduction of tension and anxiety that was responsible for its use in the peace pipe by some Native Americans.

In spite of the above-mentioned benefits, tobacco has been shown to cause heart disease, stroke, emphysema, and lung cancer. It can produce complications in pregnancy, including low birth weight, prematurity, and fetal injury. Some health care providers claim that any use of tobacco is substance abuse. Nicotine is the additive component of tobacco.

Pharmacodynamics

Nicotine is a liquid alkaloid that is freely soluble in water. It turns brown on exposure to air and is the chief alkaloid in tobacco. It both stimulates and then depresses the CNS, with the responses being dose related. In general, small doses stimulate whereas large doses depress. Stimulation occurs as a result of norepinephrine release from the sympathetic nervous system and acetylcholine from the parasympathetic nervous system. A period of depression follows that tends to last longer than the stimulant effects. The depressant effects of nicotine are due to curare-like action on skeletal muscle.

Effects and Adverse Effects

Nicotine stimulates the CNS, particularly the respiratory, emetic, and vasomotor centers in the medulla. Large doses of nicotine cause tremors and seizure activity. The curare-like effects of nicotine on nerve endings in the diaphragm contribute to the risk of respiratory failure and death.

The effects of nicotine on the cardiovascular system are multifarious. The heart rate is often slowed but later may increase above normal. Arrhythmias have been noted. Small peripheral blood vessels may first constrict, only to dilate with a fall in the blood pressure. Nicotine also has an antidiuretic effect. The adverse effects of smoking are reflected in Figure 10–3.

Pharmacokinetics

Nicotine can enter the system by inhaling tobacco smoke, by injection, by chewing tobacco, by snuffing tobacco, and by absorption through the skin by means of nicotine patches. It is readily absorbed from the GI tract, respiratory mucous membranes, and skin. The average cigarette provides between 0.05 and 2.5 mg of nicotine. Because it is most often inhaled, nicotine reaches the brain much more rapidly than if it had been injected (7 seconds). The nicotine is biotransformed in the liver. Its half-life is about 2 hours. The major metabolite, cotinine, is nonactive but has a half- life of 10 to 27 hours.

There are several drug-drug interactions with nicotine. Table 10–2 provides an overview of the interactive drugs. Smoking can increase the biotransformation of some drugs, resulting in reduced blood levels. Insulin doses may need to be increased in the smoking patient. Nicotine also decreases cardiac output and diuresis.

Overdose and Withdrawal

Acute signs and symptoms of nicotine toxicity most often involve the CNS, cardiovascular, and GI systems. There may be confusion or cold sweats. Fainting, hypotension, tachycardia, prostration, and collapse have been noted. Increased salivation, nausea, vomiting, diarrhea, and abdominal cramps may be apparent.

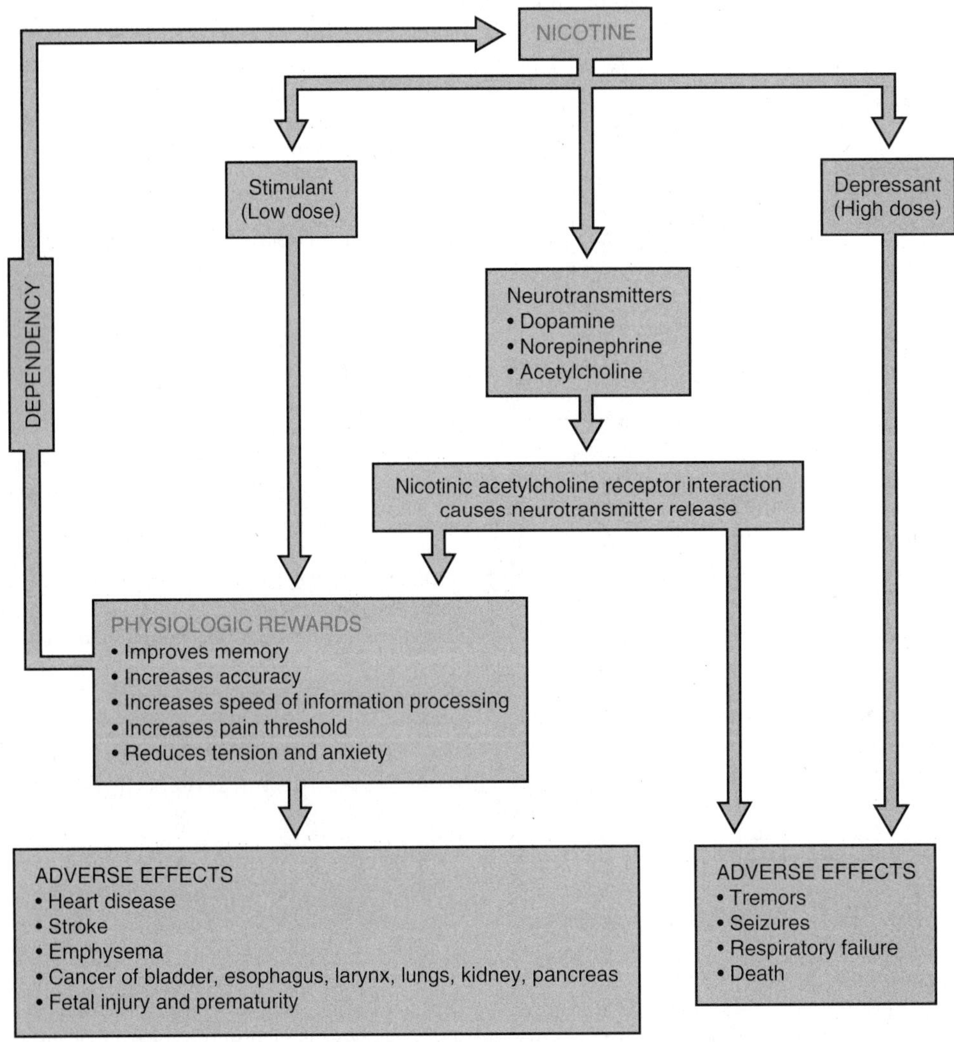

Figure 10–3 Addictive effects of nicotine. The algorithm follows the sequence of events leading to the physiologic rewards as well as adverse effects of nicotine addiction.

Smoking cessation produces withdrawal symptoms such as craving (which peaks at 24 to 48 hours), irritability, weight gain, restlessness, sleep disturbance, dullness, impaired judgment, lack of concentration, fatigue, depression, and GI upset. The lethal dosage of nicotine for an adult is 60 mg. If poisoning occurs, it is generally by accidental ingestion on the part of children.

Hallucinogens

Hallucinogens (psychedelics, psychotogens) are categorized according to their chemical composition. Group I substances contain an indole nucleus. This group of substances includes lysergic acid diethylamide (LSD), psilocybin, dimethyltryptamine (DMT), and diethyltriptyamine. Group II drugs include substances containing beta-phenethylamines or substituted phenyl alkylamines, such as mescaline and amphetamine-like drugs. Group III contains marijuana and PCP, which are not structurally related to one another or the other two groups (see Street Names of Commonly Abused Substances).

There are several factors influencing an individual's response to hallucinogens. Among these factors are dosage, the personality of the individual, the expectation the individual has in using the drug, and the immediate environment and social setting in which the drug was taken. Because many of the hallucinogens make an individual highly suggestible, this environment and the people in it, and especially the "guide" who is making the suggestions, are very important.

LYSERGIC ACID DIETHYLAMIDE

LSD is at the top of the list of popular hallucinogens. It is one of the most powerful psychoactive substances known. Because very small amounts are needed and because it is odorless and colorless, it is stored in an amazing variety of ways. It can be painted onto the fingernails, stored in blotters, or as dried droplets on paper.

Research has not been able to identify a common CNS receptor for LSD. The receptors seem to affect multiple transmitter systems. LSD produces increased empathy and euphoria, and decreased inhibitions, as well as kaleidoscopic hallucinations. Ten micrograms of LSD produce mild euphoria and increased empathy. Fifty to one hundred micro-

STREET NAMES OF COMMONLY ABUSED SUBSTANCES

Central Nervous System Depressants	
Amobarbital	Blue devils, blue angels, blue heavens, blues, bluebirds
Chlordiazepoxide	Green and whites, libs, roaches
Codeine	Schoolboy, robo, romo, syrup
Heroin	H, horse, junk, noise, pee, scag, shit, skid, smack, boy, doojee, hairy, Harry, TNT
Morphine	M, morph, morphie, morpho, white stuff, cube juice, emsel, hocus, Miss Emma, unkie, white merchandise
Opium	Black stuff, poppy, tar, hop, pin, yen, skee, wen shee, big O
Pentobarbital	Yellow jackets, yellowbirds, nembies, yellows
Phenobarbital	Purple hearts
Secobarbital	Seccy, red birds, red devils, reds
Tuinal	Tooeys, rainbows, double trouble
Cental Nervous System Stimulants	
Cocaine	Dope, coke, snow, lady, gold dust, rock, crack, Carrie, Cecil, dream, happy dust, heaven dust, joy powder, flake, girl, nose candy, crystal
Dextroamphetamine	Dexies, oranges, hearts, Christmas trees, wedges, spots
Amphetamine (racemic)	Uppers, bennies
Methamphetamine	Chris, Christine, speed, meth, crystal, whites, ice
Monoethymethylenedioxyamphetamine (MDEA)	Eve
Methylenedioxyamphetamine (MDA)	Love drug
Methylenedioxymethamphetamine (MDMA)	Ecstasy, XTC, Adam
Amphetamine complex	Black beauty, black Cadillacs
Hallucinogens	
Cannabis (marijuana)	Acapulco gold, ace, ashes, baby, broccoli, grass, hemp, jive, joint, Mary Jane, pot, THC, weed, Panama red, MJ, loco weed, Texas tea, Sweet Lucy, many others
Dimethyltryptamine (DMT)	Businessman's trip, mind blowing, DMT
Hash, hashish	Black hash (hashish containing opium), black Russian (potent, dark hashish)
Lysergic acid diethylamide (LSD)	Acid, cube, big D, California sunshine, blue dots, barrels, black magic, blue acid, blue heaven, chocolate chips, cupcakes, domes, Hawaiian sunshine, micro dots, peace tablets, squirrels, strawberry field, purple haze, purple ozone, battery acid, Berkeley blood, chief, HCP, sugar, window pane
Mescaline	Bad seed, big chief, cactus buttons, peyote, pink wedge, white light, mescal, half moon
Phencyclidine (PCP)	Angel dust, dummy dust, PCP, flying saucers, hair hog, mist, peace pill, tranq, whack, Shermans, rocket fuel, sheets
Psilocybin	God's flesh
Anabolic Steroids	
Anabolic steroids	Roids, juice

grams is a minimal psychedelic dose, whereas 400 to 500 mg produce maximal psychedelic effects. *Synesthesia* is common. It is a crossover phenomenon between the senses, such as seeing sounds or hearing colors. There is loss of identity and cosmic merging, which is self-reflection in which long repressed material comes to the surface. LSD is not physically addicting, nor is there evidence that it causes teratogenic problems, in spite of earlier speculation that this might be the case. But whether it produces a "good trip" or a "bad trip" is unpredictable and is seemingly dependent on personality traits of the user and variations in dosage and environment at the time of use.

The half-life of LSD is approximately 2 hours. Biotransformation is hepatoenteric, with elimination through the feces. There is cross tolerance of LSD with mescaline and psilocybin. A good indication of the potency of LSD can be obtained by noting that it takes 6000 times as much mescaline to produce a comparable psychedelic effect.

Magic mushrooms *(Psilocybe mexicana)* are a source of both psilocybin and psilocin. Timothy Leary, self-proclaimed guru of the drug culture, started with magic mushrooms, later adding LSD. However, most so-called magic mushrooms sold illegally are normal mushrooms laced with LSD.

The way LSD is administered, including whether the person is aware that the drug is being taken, is important. So little LSD is needed to produce strong effects that it is easy to ingest the substance without knowledge by the individual. Panic, paranoia, and terrifying visions are among the more frequently encountered symptoms or effects of LSD, especially when they produce a "bad trip."

With LSD and some other hallucinogens, intervention is based on the principle of keeping the patient calm and safe until the effects wear off. "Talking down" is important because of the high suggestibility of patients on LSD. Fears about long-term effects have not been justified.

DIMETHYLTRYPTAMINE

DMT is found in legumes in South America, but it is also manufactured. DMT is often called the "businessman's trip" or "mind blowing" because its effects last less than 1 hour, usually only 5 to 20 minutes. DMT does not cause physical dependence.

PEYOTE AND MESCALINE

Peyote, a substance present in the button of the peyote cactus *(Lophophora williamsii, L. diffusa)*, is the major source of mescaline. The only entity legally allowed to use peyote for any purpose is the Native American Church. Native Americans have used peyote and the mescal bean *(Sophora secundiflora)* in their religious services. Although peyote is still used in religious ceremonies, peyotism is controversial among the Native Americans.

Although mescaline comes from the peyote cactus, it was named in honor of the mescal bean, a red seed that comes from an evergreen shrub. The active substance in this seed, the alkaloid cytosine, is related to nicotine. Half a bean produces the desired hallucinations, whereas a whole bean might kill. More recently, wearing of a red bean is a symbol of loyalty to traditional Native American cultural values.

PHENYLETHYLAMINES

The phenylethylamine hallucinogens are chemically related to both hallucinogens and amphetamines because each contains varying amounts of serotonin and dopamine. Serotonin induces hallucinations, whereas dopamine stimulates the CNS. Dimethoxymethylamphetamine is nick-named STP after the oil additive said to increase the power of automobile engines. Dimethoxymethylamphetamine is associated with panic, violent behavior, seizures, death, vascular spasms, and limb ischemia. Limb ischemia has resulted in the need for bilateral above-the-knee amputations.

PHENCYCLIDINE

PCP is derived from a genus containing more than 30 similar chemical substances, all of them dissociative or cataleptoid anesthetics. PCP acts on the limbic cortex and the hippocampus, and the cholinergic and dopaminergic neurotransmitters. Classification of this substance is difficult because the effects range far beyond those of simple hallucinogens. These substances are cheap and are often used to adulterate or enhance other drugs. Hence, with the exception of marijuana, they are the most commonly abused drugs in the United States.

A helpful mnemonic device for remembering the eight cardinal signs of PCP intoxication is *red danes:* **r**ed skin, **e**nlarged pupils, **d**elusions, **d**issociations, **a**mnesia, **n**ystagmus, **e**xcitement, and dry **s**kin. PCP produces a subjective sense of intoxication, with staggering gait, slurred speech, nystagmus, and numbness of the extremities. Depending on the dose, users may not sweat, may display catatonic rigidity, and have a blank stare. They may also experience changes in body image, disorganized thought, drowsiness, and apathy. Hostile and bizarre behaviors may appear. PCP also gives the user the feeling of possessing abnormally great strength. Given the combination of these two features, special precautions must be taken for staff and patient safety when it becomes necessary to restrain the patient. Amnesia is possible. With increasing dosage, analgesia becomes more profound and anesthesia, stupor, or coma may occur, although the eyes may remain open. Heart rate and blood pressure are elevated, and there is hypersalivation, fever, and seizure activity.

Dosage is variable and is dependent on the user. Mild intoxication occurs with 0.5 mg, severe intoxication occurs with about 20 mg. Chronic users may ingest up to 1 g in 24 hours.

PCP is taken by almost every method: IV, IM, by smoking, ingestion, vaginal douching, and rectal enemas. The most rapid effects are obtained by smoking or IV injection. The half-life of PCP ranges from 10 hours to 4 days, but its effects can last for over a week. Biotransformation occurs primarily in the liver, and it is eliminated in the urine with nearly half of it unchanged.

Because PCP is a general psychoactive substance that affects many areas, there is no one antidote. Consequently, treatment should be focused on specific presenting symptoms. Haloperidol has been effective for PCP psychosis. Diazepam is used to help prevent seizures, but it is not useful for PCP psychosis. It merely delays its presentation by modulating downward the dopaminergic effects while blocking the breakdown of the PCP. The patient's psychosis may appear to be controlled well enough to allow the patient to be transferred from the emergency room to a general psychiatric unit, only to have the psychosis reappear after the breakdown of the diazepam. Atonic bladder and ileus that accompany PCP use can be treated with physostigmine. Because of the anesthetic effects of PCP and the paranoia and irritability it often precipitates, care should be taken to forestall the possibility of self-injury or injury to others. Because of the irritability that additional stimuli may elicit from the patient, "talking down" is contraindicated in favor of a quiet room that is free from provocation.

CANNABINOIDS

Marijuana, hashish, and hemp are the three better known cannabinoids. Of the three, marijuana is the most widely used in the United States and, in fact, is the most widely used illicit drug in the world. Approximately 20 million individuals in the United States are current users. Some estimate that one-third of all Americans have tried marijuana at least once.

Marijuana is obtained from the *Cannabis sativa* plant. This is the same plant that produces the fiber called *hemp,* which is used for rope, carpets, sails, linen, and clothes. The seed is used as bird seed. But the cannabinoids vary greatly from plant to plant and even in the same plant. No two plants are identical in chemical composition. Marijuana contains more than 400 different chemicals, 61 of them are cannabinoids. There are eleven tetrahydrocannabinoids (THC), of which D-9-THC is the most psychoactive.

Marijuana itself comes from the dried leaves and flowering tops of the plant. *Hashish* is a potent concentrate prepared from the resin secreted by the flowering tops of plants. *Hash oil* is a distillate of hashish made by boiling. Marijuana typically contains about 1 to 6 percent THC. Hashish contains 10 to 15 percent THC, and hash oil contains 15 to 30 percent THC. The variations in THC levels are partially responsible for the wide variety of reactions seen with its use. Marijuana may be laced with PCP or LSD, or it may be polluted with a weed killer such as paraquat. Jimsonweed may be an additive.

Part of the controversy over marijuana use concerns its therapeutic effects. It has been used as an antiemetic in cancer therapy. Marijuana reduces intraocular pressure in glaucoma. It has antidepressant effects and is used with some success for this purpose in Great Britain. Native South African women smoke it to reduce the pain of childbirth. Unlike the opioids, it does not suppress respiration. It is also a muscle relaxant that helps decrease the pain of muscle spasms. Marijuana has also been used as an antihistamine, as a bronchodilator, and as an antiseizure agent.

However, the nonspecificity of marijuana makes its use difficult and controversial. It can both stimulate and suppress such varied things as nausea and vomiting, seizure activity, and sexual interest. It can be helpful to asthma patients but, at the same time, cause other respiratory problems. Marijuana is also controversial because it is thought to be a so-called *gateway drug,* one that promotes the use of other drugs. However, many people never use any other drug beside marijuana.

Marijuana can be smoked, mixed with tobacco, used in a water pipe, or eaten alone or in foods, or it can be mixed with PCP. Inhalation of the smoke results in the absorption of the THC into the blood stream within seconds. Blood levels decline slowly over 2 to 3 hours. If it is ingested in food, effects occur 30 minutes to 2 hours later, with an average duration of action of about 6 hours. THC is rapidly absorbed and stored in body fat, which accounts for its detection in urine months after cessation of its use. Because it is stored in body fat, weight reduction results in its release back into the blood stream. Biotransformation takes place in 1 to 4 hours to the metabolites 8, 11-dihydroxy-THC and 11-hydroxy-delta-9-THC.

It is speculated that people enjoy smoking marijuana because of its effect on the limbic system in the brain. This is the system that is activated in sexual arousal and orgasm. But the after effects of this type of arousal seem to be indolence, a personality trait associated with marijuana use.

It is also speculated that marijuana alters the lipid membrane in all neurons, which may account for its wide range of effects and its nonspecificity and unpredictability. The responses can range from euphoria to paranoia, and from sedation to hallucinations. Time dilation, lack of motive to accomplish external tasks, an increased appetite, and dry mouth are commonly experienced.

Because marijuana users inhale more deeply than cigarette smokers, more tar builds up in the lungs from each cigarette. This is balanced by marijuana users smoking fewer cigarettes. However, when marijuana and tobacco are combined, the lung damage is greatly increased. Marijuana is thought to reduce the ability of the alveolar macrophages in the lungs to remove debris and combat bacteria. Hence, users have a higher incidence of respiratory problems. It also affects the immune system in a more general manner by reducing the T lymphocytes throughout the body.

Long-term use decreases libido and increases impotence. This may be due to chemicals that reduce the quantity of testosterone and lower the sperm count. Initially, it can be an aphrodisiac, perhaps because the slowing of time makes the pleasure of sex seem to last longer. The longer term effect is reduced interest in sex. In the cardiovascular system, marijuana use produces tachycardia. If marijuana is used during pregnancy, fetal toxicity and organ malformations may occur.

Marijuana use is detectable through a number of symptoms, among them reddening of the eyes. There is a sweet odor about the user, similar to the burning of rope. There may be the appearance of intoxication with no smell of alcohol and yellowish stains on the fingertips from smoking the joint closer to the fingers than is customary with cigarettes. Excessive laughter is not uncommon. The ability to engage in skilled tasks, such as driving, is reduced or not completed. Abusers drop out of school or are excessively absent.

OTHER HALLUCINOGENS

Nutmeg *(Myristica fragans)* and mace (the covering of nutmeg) also belong in this category. Nutmeg abuse is common among prison inmates in the United States. The oral ingestion of the equivalent of two nutmegs produces, after a latency of several hours, leaden feelings in the extremities and a sense of depersonalization and unreality. Agitation and apprehension are common. Dry mouth, thirst, rapid heart rate, and a red, flushed face are common and may mimic atropine poisoning (see Chapter 13). Both nutmeg and mace contain the hallucinogenic compound myristicin, which is structurally similar to mescaline.

Sassafras contains safrole, which is similar to myristicin. The harmala alkaloids are hallucinogens that produce a trance with intense imagery. These alkaloids are present in *Peganum harmala,* the seeds of which are chewed in India for their intoxicant effect. Catnip *(Nepeta cataria)* contains the hallucinogen nepetalactone, and the Mexican morning glory seed *(Rivea corymbosa)* and its American cousin, the morning glory seed *(Ipomoea),* are other examples of plants with natural hallucinogens. Panacea tea, available in health food stores, is made from morning glory seeds.

Inhalants

Inhalants present a major health problem, especially for children. These substances are called inhalants by some, solvents by others, and volatile substances by yet others. Inhalants include substances such as gasoline, spray paints, aerosol sprays, glue, lacquer thinners, amyl nitrite, ether, nitrous oxide, and correction fluids. In 1 year, 10 percent of 26- to 34-year-olds have abused inhalants and 20 percent of all American high school students were found to have abused inhalants. Ten percent of all children 12 to 17 years of age had done so, and a few children as young as 3 years of age were found to have used inhalants. Although amyl nitrite, nitrous oxide, and gasoline were the three most cited inhalants overall, those 12 to 17 years of age most often used, in decreasing order of frequency, gasoline, glue, spray paint, and correction fluids. The initial intoxicating effect of substances might be compared with the simple hypoxic effect of hyperventilation followed by breath-holding, a game played by young children.

The populations most involved are male (boys outnumber girls 10 to 1) Hispanics and Native Americans. In one Native American community, 50 percent of all children 4 to 18 years of age were chronic gasoline sniffers. The ages at which abuse of inhalants is found to begin varies from study to study, with very young children actively seeking substances in inner cities.

Most of the children who experiment with inhalants do so only once or for a short time, often at a social event. The more serious incidences occur when children are alone when they use the inhalant. This is not only more dangerous because no one is there to help, but it can indicate a tendency on the part of the child to continue substance abuse.

Many child and adolescent inhalant abusers either quit or turn to other substances for abuse as they become adults. The substances inhaled by adults are generally different than those used by children. Among those preferred by adults are amyl nitrite (to enhance orgasm in males), butyl nitrite, nitrous oxide, chloroform, and ether. Nitrite use by homosexual men to enhance orgasm has been found to decrease inhibitions and increase the risk of unsafe sexual practices.

For whatever reasons, certain activities produce higher numbers of inhalant abusers: shoe making, petroleum refining, service stations, bicycle repair shops, chemical plants, and the health care providers who have access to anesthetics. Inhalants are also used under circumstances in which other substances are unavailable, such as in the military and in prison.

Inhalation is the quickest way for a psychoactive substance to enter the CNS because it enters the blood stream directly through the large surface areas within the lungs, reaching the brain within seconds. The only competing administration route for rapid effects is IV injection. But given that the inhalants require no syringes and needles and given that the inhalants are inexpensive, it is not difficult to understand their widespread use.

The list of inhalants is surprisingly extensive (Table 10–3). Few of them are illegal, and most are products of our present civilization, unavailable in earlier times. The psychoactive properties of these substances are easily overlooked. Inhalants are commonly available and rather easily obtained from hardware and grocery stores. Items on the shelves are either bought, stolen, or used right in the store. For example, nitrous oxide can be extracted from whipped cream dispensers, resulting in an intoxicated child and a flat dispenser. Adults are often unaware that their children are experimenting with inhalants because the substances are everyday volatile materials that are found in or near the home. In addition, nondrug-using children may be unaware that their peers are using drugs because the users tend to form tight-knit secretive groups.

There are various methods for taking inhalants. Some are "huffed," that is, they are orally inhaled from a rag soaked in the desired liquid. Others are inhaled through the nose, called "sniffing," or are sprayed into a paper or plastic bag and then inhaled ("bagging"). Some are heated gently and the fumes inhaled. And still others (e.g., lighter fluid and nail polish) are ingested orally mixed in a soft drink or beer. Cleaning fluids are soaked on clothes and sniffed. A cloth over the head is effective for inhaling the fumes heated in a skillet.

One of the most dangerous methods of introducing inhalants is with the use of a plastic bag over the head. The sniffer may pass out from the substance and die of asphyxiation before help can be summoned. It is partially to protect the abuser from experiences of this kind that group activities are popular. Aerosols and butane lighter fluid are sprayed directly into the mouth. "Fire breathing," another dangerous route of entry, is used with propane or butane.

The effects of solvent abuse and inhalants vary with age and weight, personality characteristics, and environmental circumstances in which the substance is used. Users describe various pleasant effects within seconds or minutes after inhalation. These effects begin with intoxication, euphoria, sensation of flying, sensation of the ground moving, delusion of great strength, giddiness, depersonalization, loss of inhibitions, dream states, and auditory, tactile, olfactory, and visual hallucinations. Solvents can produce erotic visual hallucinations. Other effects include sensation of being touched by human hands or animals, numbness in face and extremities, sensation of crawling insects or being pricked with needles, dental pain, confusion, insomnia, muscular cramps in calves and sides, a buzzing noise and dizziness, anxiety, delusion of demonic possession, urge for self-mutilation, self-tattooing, visual distortions such as gory wounds or savage animals, paranoia, tremors, hypersensitivity to noise, chest pain, and dysuria. Hallucinations during intoxication differentiate inhalant intoxication from that of alcoholic and sedative intoxication.

The apparent lack of societal concern may be attributed to various factors, including underreporting due to reluctance to involve the children and the difficulty in detecting the substances used. It is often believed that because most of the children who experiment with inhalants do so only briefly, the time and energy would be better spent combating

TABLE 10–3 INHALANTS

Category	Active Chemical	Effects
Acrylic paint	Methylethyl ketone	Intoxicant
Adhesives	Hydrocarbons, aromatic hydrocarbons	Intoxicant
Aerosols	Fluorinated hydrocarbons, propane, isobutane, isopropanol, xylene, ethanol	Intoxicant
Amyl nitrite	Aliphatic nitrites	Intoxicant, enhanced orgasm
Anesthetics	Halothane, chloroform, ether	Intoxicant, euphoriant
Antifreeze	Ethyl glycol, methanol, isopropanol	Intoxicant
Butyl nitrite	Aliphatic nitrite	Intoxicant
Cement cleaners	Toluene and toluene mixtures	Intoxicant, narcotic
Degreasers	Isopropanol, benzene, ketones, *N*-butyl acetate, xylene, methylethyl ketone	Intoxicant
Dry cleaning solvents, spot removers	Trichloroethylene, trichloroethane petroleum distillates, perchloroethylene	Intoxicant
Fingernail polish remover	Acetone, alcohol, aliphatic acetates	Intoxicant
Fire extinguishers	Bromochlorodifluoromethane	Intoxicant
Foam dispensers	Nitrous oxide	Intoxicant, giddiness
Gasoline	Aliphatic and aromatic hydrocarbons	Intoxicant
Glue	Naphtha, petroleum distillates, acetone, polyvinyl chloride, benzene, hexane, heptanes	Intoxicant
Household cleaners	Chlorine, trichloroethane	Intoxicant
Lighter fluid	Butane, naphtha, aliphatic hydrocarbons	Intoxicant
Nitrous oxide	Nitrous oxide	Intoxicant, giddiness
Paint thinners, removers, lacquers	Benzene, naphthalene	Intoxicant hallucinogen
Printing ink	Ketones	Intoxicant
Refrigerant	Freon	Intoxicant
Room deodorizers	Amyl nitrite, butyl nitrite, isobutyl nitrite, isoamyl nitrite	Orgasm enhancers, giddiness
Shoe polish, spray	Isopropanol	Intoxicant
Spray paint (especially metallic gold or silver)	Ketones	Euphoriant
Correction fluid	Trichloroethylene, trichloroethane, chloroform, methylchloroform, amyl acetate	Euphoriant, intoxicant
Whipped cream dispensers	Nitrous oxide	Euphoriant, intoxicant

other more major drug problems. Yet it may not be well understood that experimentation is sometimes fatal, and children have been known to die after the first dose. Death can be attributed not only to the toxicity of the substances themselves but also to the methods of administration.

Another reason for the paucity of information about this problem is the possibility that a general alarm might result in an increase in experimentation rather than the intended opposite effect. Such was the case in the early 60s, when the national alarm sounded concerning the toxic effects of glue sniffing. The result was an increase of such activity, leading to experimentation with other substances in many instances.

Anabolic Steroids

The anabolic steroids are called anabolic because of their ability to convert nutrients into tissue mass, especially muscle tissue. They have an androgenic effect, that is, they accentuate the secondary male characteristics in both males and females. The desired effects are increased strength, lean body mass, aggressiveness, and enhanced athletic performance. It is still uncertain whether or not the increase in athletic ability is due to the steroid itself or the belief by the user that it is effective. Anabolic steroids are discussed further in Chapter 53.

Both sexes may show an increase in mood swings, aggressiveness (so called roid rages), depression, and psychosis. In addition, there are effects on the GI tract including arrest of bile secretion, cellular damage to the liver, and an increased risk of cancer. Endocrine system changes occur in the form of decreased glucose tolerance. The cardiovascular system may be affected by an overall increase in cholesterol, especially high-density lipoproteins, and an increase in blood pressure. There is some evidence that steroids may increase the incidence of Wilms' tumor in the urinary tract.

Steroids taken by children before growth is complete produce premature closure of the epiphyseal growth plates at the ends of the long bones, thus resulting in a short stature. There are some immunologic changes, including a decrease in immunoglobulin A (IgA).

Because lab tests are either too expensive or unreliable, the health care provider needs to rely on communication with the patient and the family about the use of androgenic steroids. But there are physical effects of steroid use that are sufficiently noticeable to justify further inquiry. The anabolic steroids can produce unusual growth in muscle mass in a short time, unusual secondary sex characteristics, acne, and so-called moon face. Unusual aggressiveness and mood swings are also associated with steroid use, although it may be difficult to decide what is unusual in the case of teenagers.

The health care provider might ask questions concerning whether the patient has experienced muscle tears or stress fractures that might open up the possibility of communication about steroid use, because steroid use is often associated with these conditions.

If the patient is taking steroids, he or she may also be taking human growth hormone, which is not detectable by current urine testing methods. Some of the desired effects include tissue building, faster repair of injured tissue, and the conversion of fats to lipids to increase energy. Undesirable effects include development of diabetes, muscle weakness, and cardiac muscle problems.

Erythropoietin and blood doping are methods used to increase energy by increasing the oxygen-carrying capacity of the blood to increase endurance. Erythropoietin, a hormone that stimulates red blood cell production, and blood transfusion (so-called doping) are used by some athletes to produce erythrocythemia. Both practices are unequivocally disapproved by sports officials and governing bodies like the International Olympics Committee. But their use is also not detectable by current testing methods. Increased blood pressure and cardiac workload could lead to heart failure or pulmonary edema.

Critical Thinking Process

Assessment

History of Present Illness

Assessing for substance abuse or misuse should be done, even though the patient presents to the health care provider with a different problem. Because these substances produce undesirable effects on the body in many ways, it is possible that the substances the patient is abusing or misusing could be the direct cause of the patient's complaint. Some patients cannot see a connection between misusing a prescribed medication and their present condition. This is especially important in assessing the older adult and those living at or below the poverty line.

A factual drug history may be difficult to obtain when polysubstance dependency exists. Nonetheless, elicit information about the initial use of substances, the drugs used, and the setting in which the drugs are used and how often. Inquire when the drugs were last taken and the route of administration. Explore how the patient feels when the drug is used and what behavior changes occur. Ask about withdrawal symptoms and if the patient has had contact with the legal system. Assume that the patient is a polysubstance abuser until you are convinced otherwise. Whenever possible, find an additional source of information to corroborate what the patient is saying. Often, the patient minimizes the amount of substances taken or may actually not know.

If there is a suspicion of alcohol abuse, sometimes it is useful to start by assessing the patient's attitudes about drinking. If the patient admits to drinking some alcohol regularly, then consider using a more specific assessment tool. One such strategy for alcohol abuse assessment employs a mnemonic device. *CAGE* is a metaphor for the manner in which the alcohol-abusing individual is imprisoned by both the self and the alcohol. "Have you felt you ought to **c**ut down on your drinking?" "Have people **a**nnoyed you by criticizing your drinking?" "Have you felt bad or **g**uilty about your drinking?" "Have you **e**ver had a drink first thing in the morning to steady your nerves or get rid of a hangover?" This last "e" is sometimes modified to "eye-opener." Two or more positive answers usually indicate the need for a much deeper assessment, including a history or presence of blackouts, legal problems involving alcohol, presence of alcohol related diseases, and possibly other substance abuse.

Past Health History

Ask about drug use in the home. What drugs are used? When was the last time the patient took an OTC drug? For what conditions? Has the patient ever borrowed his or her spouse's or friend's drugs?

Be alert for conditions that suggest substance abuse, remembering that these conditions are only suggestive because they can be caused by other things than substance abuse (see Characteristics That May Suggest Substance Abuse). Their presence does not prove substance abuse has occurred but may heighten suspicion of use. Determine whether or not there is a family history of substance abuse. Has the patient been treated for substance abuse in the past? If so, where, when, for what, and how long? Was the treatment successful for a period of time?

Physical Exam Findings

Physical manifestations of substance abuse depend on the type of substance, route of administration, frequency of use, and the individual's overall health status. The longer substance abuse persists, the more body systems that become involved. Some substances promote impulsive or unprovoked and unpredictable violent behavior.

During the exam, observe the general appearance of the patient. Is the patient well kept? Observe hygiene and dress. Patients may have concealed drugs and weapons in body cavities as well as in clothing or other personal items. Be sure to note the patient's affect or the presence of confusion or agitation. Does the patient appear to be underweight or overweight? Do you note any jaundice or skin discoloration. Does the patient have an unsteady gait? Is the speech slurred? Inspect the skin for needle tracks or lesions over veins. Tracks or lesions are commonly found on the forearms, in the antecubital fossa, on legs, or between the toes.

Examine the eyes, noting if they are red or glassy. Note pupil size and reaction. Are the pupils dilated or constricted? Check the patient's nose and throat. Is the nose red and bulbous with broken blood vessels? This finding is often associated with excessive alcohol intake over a long period of time. Is the nasal mucosa edematous, reddened, or necrotic? Is the septum intact, or is there evidence of perforation? Swelling, necrosis, bleeding, or perforation are usually associated with cocaine snorting, or inhalation of the powder through a straw or rolled currency.

Assess for the presence of tachycardia and arrhythmias. Measure the patient's blood pressure carefully because long-term substance abuse contributes to the development of hypertension. Observe for evidence of hyperventilation and cough, and auscultate for abnormal breath sounds. Test deep tendon reflexes. The physical exam should also include palpitation of the liver and spleen.

Diagnostic Testing

The choice of diagnostic tests depends on the particular circumstances of the patient. For example, if inhalant use is suspected, tests that indicate the condition of the respiratory tract would be important. If the patient uses mind-altering drugs, tests of higher cortical functions maybe warranted. If the patient shares needles, testing for HIV and sexually

CHARACTERISTICS THAT MAY SUGGEST SUBSTANCE ABUSE

Substance	*Characteristics*
Alcohol	Arrhythmias, idiopathic cardiomyopathy Behavioral problems in infants Cirrhosis, pancreatitis, splenomegaly Coma Conflicts with legal system (DUI, family violence, MVAs) Depression Eating disorders, malnutrition, gastritis Fetal alcohol syndrome Headaches, neurologic problems House fires Hypersexuality Hypertension Hypothermia Social isolation Unexplained accidents, changes in behavior, suicide attempt
Amphetamines	Anxiety, sleep disorders Conflicts with legal system (MVAs, violence) Hypersexuality Malnutrition Membership in high risk population group Mood swings Multiple skin disorders (infections, ulcerations) Needle marks and bruises on the arms Psychoses, unexplained changes in behavior
Barbiturates	Coma Depressed responses Endocrine imbalances Hypotension
Benzodiazepines	Anxiety Coma Suicide attempt
Caffeine	Arrhythmias Eating disorders Headaches Hyperactivity Hypertension Sleeping disorders
Cocaine	Behavior problems in infants (when consumed by the mother) Epistaxis Headaches Hypersexuality Impotence Masculinization Mood swings Nasal septal defects
Hallucinogens	Conflicts with legal system (MVAs, violence) Disorientation, fear of surroundings Unexplained accidents, changes in behavior, suicide attempt Psychosis, mood swings, unexplained changes in behavior
Inhalants	Burns around mouth, nose Epistaxis House fires Mood swings Respiratory difficulty, suffocation Social isolation
Opioids	Malnutrition Multiple skin disorders (infections, ulcerations)
Steroids	Conflicts with legal system (violence) Depression Hypertension Impotence Masculinization Mood swings Retarded growth in children

DUI, Driving under the influence, MVAs, motor vehicle accidents.

transmitted diseases may be warranted. Liver function tests can help establish the extent of alcohol or drug damage. Gamma-glutamyltransferase is the most common marker of alcohol use. It is often raised 75 to 80 percent above normal in alcoholics and heavy drinkers. Gamma-glutamyltransferase correlates with the total amount of alcohol consumed, but the results should be interpreted cautiously because it takes weeks to reflect alcohol use. Further, elevated levels may be caused by liver disease, gallbladder disorders, liver cancer, and metastasis. Other liver function tests indicative of impaired liver functioning include the alanine aminotransferase (ALT; serum glutamic-pyruvic transaminase [SGPT]) and aspartate aminotransferase (AST; serum glutamic-oxaloacetic transaminase [SGOT]), but they are also nonspecific for alcohol. However, there is greater specificity for alcohol if the AST:ALT ratio is greater than two. Albumin and total proteins are also important for determining liver damage.

A complete blood count, prothrombin time, partial thromboplastin time, and blood chemistry tests help evaluate the presence of blood dyscrasias as well as liver function. The mean corpuscular volume is an important and reliable but nonspecific indicator of hematology system damage. The mean corpuscular volume is elevated in many alcoholic patients. The mean corpuscular volume is slow to respond, so it is not a reliable indicator of abstinence and relapse.

Drug screens should be conducted on both blood and urine to determine what substances the patient has consumed and how much still remains in the body. In an acute care setting, drug screens should be conducted as soon as possible after admission. Many substances and their metabolites have very short half-lives and may be eliminated before they are detected. The health care provider cannot ensure the authenticity of the specimen unless the collection was witnessed. Here, the patient's right to privacy needs to be weighed against the need to ensure authenticity of the specimen. Patients have done many things in the past to foil the testing results, such as switching urine samples.

Sometimes a disparity is noted between the patient's clinical condition and the results of a drug screen. The patient appears to be under the influence of a substance or may even admit to being under its influence, but the lab results are inconclusive. The accuracy of test results depends not only on accurate specimen collection but the sophistication of the devices used to analyze it. Gas chromatography and mass spectrometry are often too expensive for smaller labs, yet some of the metabolites are not easily detected without it.

Developmental Considerations

Perinatal When considering the effects of substance abuse on the perinatal period, the primary concerns are the health of the mother and preventing or curtailing complications to the fetus. If the mother continues to abuse drugs throughout her pregnancy, neonatal complications and the potential to neglect or abuse her child are increased.

The effects of substance abuse on mothers and unborn infants have been studied intensely, although many questions remain unanswered. It is safe to say that the fetus is exposed to virtually all of the substances the mother consumes. Which effects are the direct result of the substances themselves and which are related to indirect consequences such as the mother's general health, prenatal nutrition status, or her general life-style and living conditions is unknown. Drugs with high lipid solubility are particularly dangerous to the fetus because they penetrate the fetal blood more easily through simple diffusion.

Although recent research has shown that heavy use of alcohol by pregnant women can have undesirable effects on unborn children, it is as yet uncertain what effects the moderate use of alcohol might have. There is a continuum of alcohol-related disorders, from fetal alcohol effects to fetal alcohol syndrome. Fetal alcohol syndrome effects range from indiscernible to severe. In extreme cases, there is growth deficiency, dysmorphology, and neurobehavioral effects. The dysmorphology is particularly noticeable in the face, and may include such features as epicanthal folds, ears rotated toward the back, a flattened midface, and other anomalies. There may be problems with hearing and the ears. The circumference of the skull is typically smaller. Neurobehavioral effects include reduced intellectual functioning, behavioral problems, attention deficits, and memory problems.

Cocaine readily passes through placental membranes and induces birth defects. The fetus can be affected either directly or indirectly by the mother's drug-induced vasoconstriction and lowered oxygen level. There is a high incidence of miscarriage and behavioral problems in infants whose mothers are chronic abusers. Further, skull defects and congenital heart defects in infants can result from cocaine use by the mother. Some babies experience strokes before birth or heart attacks after delivery.

Infants born to mothers using opioids show withdrawal symptoms. They are irritable, have tremors, hyperreflexia, restlessness, a high-pitched cry, and insomnia. These are all hallmarks of neonatal opioid withdrawal. The infant is less alert, less responsive to visual stimuli, and less cuddly. The onset of withdrawal symptoms in these infants occurs minutes to hours after birth. The average time is 72 hours, but symptoms may be delayed for as long as 2 weeks. Symptoms of delayed withdrawal include high-pitched crying, yawning, respiratory distress, mottling, sneezing, frantic sucking of fist or thumbs, and ineffective swallowing reflex. Fever, vomiting, and diarrhea are additional frequent symptoms. Acute heroin withdrawal symptoms usually last only a week, but protracted symptoms may last as long as 6 weeks. Dehydration and seizures are of major concern and can be fatal.

Pediatric In pediatric populations, substance abuse affects growth and development, contributes to school dropout rates and gang membership, can result in violence and death, and is a catalyst for sexual promiscuity, teen pregnancy, and transmission of sexually transmitted diseases. Adolescent males tend to abuse volatile substances and other inhalants. These, along with tobacco, marijuana, and alcohol, are called gateway drugs, because their use can be followed by the use of more serious substances later. One response to poverty in the inner cities is the formation of youth gangs. Dealing in abused substances is a source of finance for these gangs. Dealing in substances, the effects of substance abuse on mood or personality, and getting money to feed a habit are three causes of the violence that is associated with substance abuse.

Preadolescents and adolescents are at risk for abuse of different substances. Younger children tend to abuse inhalants, whereas alcohol is the substance of choice of older children. Dextromethorphan, the principal ingredient in many OTC cough syrups, produces mild hallucinations in high doses and stimulating effects similar to those of PCP.

Although there was a marked decrease in the use of many substances by high school and college students in the 1980s, PCP, marijuana, inhalants, and hallucinogens are still used by many young people. Consumption of alcohol in fraternities is sometimes used in initiation rites, occasionally with fatal results. Caffeine and other stimulants are used around exam times.

Geriatric The rates of alcohol and drug abuse in the elderly are low, but there is increasing worry that the actual rate may be higher and undetected. The expectation of a low abuse rate in this population results in the problem of health care providers not asking the appropriate questions during an assessment. Conventional wisdom holds that because alcoholism begins at younger ages and results in a reduced life expectancy, few alcoholics survive to become older adults. One theory holds that the reason that so few opioid-dependent individuals are reported between the ages of 35 and 45 is that there is "a maturing out," that is, they die, or become debilitated and are treated for something else, just get tired of their dependency and manage to stop using the substance, or know how to manage it well so that they do not come to the attention of the health care provider. If they are still abusing at middle age and beyond, they are probably obtaining the substances via OTC and prescription drugs. Loneliness, depression, and isolation that are seen in many older adults who have not abused drugs in the past can contribute to the potential for current substance abuse.

Psychosocial Considerations

Whatever the basis for substance abuse, the effect on those who are abusers and those who depend on them is re-

Case Study Hypertension Masking a Substance Abuse Problem

Patient History

History of Present Illness	CF is a 45-year-old white male successful businessman who is returning for a follow-up visit for hypertension of 10 years' duration. Despite aggressive treatment, CF's blood pressure has been increasing during the past few months. He complains of heartburn, headaches, irritability, intermittent recent memory loss, and occasional night sweats.
Past Health History	CF has had two hospitalizations in the past 10 years for a broken right femur, a result of what he reports as skiing accidents. Later he admitted that these were accidents in the lodge after skiing as a result of losing his balance. He has a 5-year history of gastric ulcer, for which he takes cimetidine daily. His blood pressure has been treated with a daily dose of 150 mg of atenolol. He admits to drinking on occasion and to relax his nerves when his office work becomes too hectic. He has no known allergies. He is a nonsmoker. CF has an adequate dietary intake.
Physical Exam	CFs blood pressure is 175/98. All other exam results are normal. He has full range of motion of his affected extremity. He is pleasant, cooperative, and articulate.
Diagnostic Testing	Upper GI series positive for healing ulcer. CBC, PT, and PTT results are all within normal limits. SMA-12 and GGT indicate slight liver involvement.
Developmental Considerations	Elevated liver function tests are not compatible with age. History of broken femur is not incompatible with skiing, but a repeat of the same accident is unusual.
Psychosocial Considerations	CF has been married to the same woman for 20 years. They have three children—a son, 19, who is in college; a 17-year-old daughter; and a 13-year-old-son. CF is the primary provider, but his wife teaches part time in elementary school while her children are in school. CF has been compliant with his medication and regularly exercises at a health club. He admits to experimentation at parties with some street drugs in the past, specifically marijuana and cocaine.
Economic Factors	CF is upper middle class in income. Although his salary is adequate for most of the family's needs, he worries about college expenses for his children. They do not qualify for public assistance progams.

Variables Influencing Decision

Treatment Objectives	• Patient will acknowledge that alcohol is his primary problem and will stop or greatly diminish his drinking.

Drug Variables	*Drug Summary*	*Patient Variables*
Indications	Disulfiram can help forestall the impulse to drink, because it takes 2 weeks for the medication to clear so that it is safe to consume alcohol.	CF may decide not to use disulfiram because he has not really tested his will power not to drink in excess or to abstain.
Pharmacodynamics	Disulfiram inhibits the enzyme aldehyde dehydrogenase, resulting in the blocking of the oxidation of alcohol at the acetaldehyde stage.The result is an accumulation of toxic concentrations of acetaldehyde following the ingestion of alcohol.	May be a decision point. This depends on CF's willingness to accept the benefits of disulfiram treatment. He may perceive his will power as too weak without the threat of harm from the disulfiram, or he may decide that his will power is sufficient, so that there is no need to run the risk of the disulfiram.

Case Study continued on following page

Drug Variables	Drug Summary	Patient Variables
Adverse Effects/ Contraindications	Acetaldehyde syndrome in the presence of alcohol. May be fatal. Disulfiram increases the absorption and toxicity of nickel and lead in the blood, leading to accumulation in the brain. Disulfiram may cause some blood dyscrasias. Contraindicated with other acetaldehyde agents such as metronidazole or hypoglycemic drugs.	May be a decision point. CF may decide the drug is too dangerous. Patient may not want to be bothered to screen out all alcohol from environment, such as mouth washes, fermented vinegar in sauces, cough medicines, inhalants, aerosols, aftershave lotion and cologne.
Pharmacokinetics	Onset of effects: 1 to 2 hrs after dose. Remains in system up to 14 days.	Should CF use alcohol in any amount in any way within 2 weeks of the last dose of disulfiram, the result may be a disulfiram reaction.
Laboratory Considerations	Liver function tests and cholesterol levels before treatment and periodically during disulfiram treatment. Complete blood count, transaminase and SMA-12 before treatment and periodically throughout treatment.	Liver function tests will indicate level of success in abstinence or moderation of drinking. If moderation does not improve liver function tests, abstinence may be necessary.
Dosage Regimen	Disulfiram may be continued indefinitely (if patient desires). Multivitamins may be recommended only initially. Disulfiram doses of 500 mg/day may increase cholesterol levels; this may be a decision point to stop the medication.	Disulfiram should not be given without CF's consent and full support. Disulfiram must not be given in the presence of any alcohol or alcohol containing substance. If CF's diet is good and there is no indication of neuropathy, multivitamins may be discontinued after the initial period.
Cost Index*	Disulfiram: 1 B-complex: 1 Multivitamins: 1	

Summary of Decision Points

- If CF decides to abstain, decision is made for disulfiram and/or group support meetings
- If patient chooses moderation, decision is made for other support groups or private therapy
- Disulfiram doses of 500 mg/day may increase cholesterol levels; this may be a decision point to stop the medication.

DRUG TO BE USED

- Disulfiram 500 mg po daily for 1–2 weeks, then 250 mg/day (range is 125 to 500 mg/day)
- B-complex vitamin daily
- Multivitamin daily

*Cost index
1 = $ < 30/mo.
2 = $ 30–40/mo.
3 = $ 40–50/mo.
4 = $ 50–60/mo.
5 = $ > 60/mo.

AWP of 100, 250-mg tablets of disulfiram is approximately $13.
AWP of 60 capsules of B-complex vitamins is approximately $8.
AWP of 100 tablets of multivitamin is approximately $3.

markable. When patients become dependent on or addicted to a drug, they are held hostage by the substance and their rational thinking functions are subverted to focus on obtaining and using the drug. Commitments to other people or to responsibilities are secondary. Cognitively, the abuser develops impaired judgment, recall, and problem-solving abilities. Psychosocial manifestations include anger, denial, withdrawal, and loss of self-control. Feelings of anxiety, paranoia, depression, apathy, shame, and failure arise. The individual may experience a sense of powerlessness and destructiveness toward the self and his or her family. The patient may realize that he needs to stop and often feels guilty about the effect of his substance abuse problem on his family and himself. People initially drink to feel good and then drink to stop feeling bad.

Interpersonal relationships, particularly those with the family, are impaired and disrupted. Communication, role performance, and sexual interactions become distorted. Concerned family or friends may show evidence of codependence or coping strategies that contribute to the progression of the illness. To protect the user, family and friends may act as if nothing is wrong or may terminate outside friendships and community involvement. Children's response to abuse may take the form of rigid, compulsive roles and emotional distancing. Children of dependent parents usually perform poorly in school and show withdrawal, anger, or aggressive behaviors.

The economic effects of substance abuse have many variations and a significant impact on worldwide economy. On an individual level, substance abuse has resulted in loss of income and dramatic changes in life-style. On a national level, billions of dollars have been spent on the war on drugs. On an international level, the revenues from illegal substances have supported criminal activities and have provided many developing countries with funding for weapons necessary to support international armed conflicts and uprisings (see Case Study—Hypertension Masking a Substance Abuse Problem).

Analysis and Management

Treatment Objectives

The primary treatment objective for patients with a substance abuse problem is to stop the abuse and to correct the physical conditions that were the result. Treatment objectives for the patient with an overdose is primarily symptomatic and supportive. The aim of treatment is usually to support vital functions until the drug is biotransformed and eliminated from the body.

Treatment Options

Treatment options vary depending upon the substance the patient is abusing, the extent of the dependence, the patient's incentive to stop the abuse, the depth of the commitment to stop, and the support structure available to the patient. Some patterns of substance abuse, such as weekly use of marijuana, do not require treatment any more than does the occasional smoking of tobacco or the social use of alcohol. Further, such patterns do not necessarily constitute a treatable disorder. Such casual use is not without hazard. Changing views of substance abuse will continue to create gray areas where the justification for drug testing and the necessity for treatment are unclear. There is a general agreement that treatment is warranted for the adverse consequences of drug use and for the compulsive user who voluntarily seeks help.

Overall interventions for the substance abuser should include maintenance of existing body system function along with adequate nutritional support. A multidisciplinary team approach can assist the patient to make the biologic and psychosocial adjustments necessary to successfully eliminate the substance abuse habit.

Drug Variables Drug therapy is relatively controversial for the management of patients with substance abuse for several reasons. First, specific antidotes are available only for benzodiazepines and opioids. Second, there is a high risk of substituting one abused substance for another. Third, there are significant drawbacks to giving CNS stimulants to reverse the effects of CNS depressants and vice versa. However, there are some clinical indications for pharmacotherapy. These indications include disulfiram as a deterrent for chronic alcohol abuse, methadone maintenance for opioid drug dependence, symptomatic treatment of acute drug toxicity or overdose, and treatment of withdrawal syndromes.

Benzodiazepines are the treatment of choice for many patients in need of assistance with substance abuse. Some controversy surrounds which benzodiazepine is most effective and yet carries the fewest adverse effects. Some are long acting (diazepam, lorazepam, and clorazepate), and others are short acting (oxazepam). The problem is that when the longer acting drugs are used in a patient with a compromised liver, the drug may remain in the system for extended periods and accumulate to excessive levels. Health care providers who prefer the longer acting benzodiazepines assert that the effects remain in the system long enough to prevent breakthrough gaps in sedation. Another positive effect of benzodiazepines is that they are known to increase the intake of food and water. However, benzodiazepines, if they are used long term, pose a problem for withdrawal themselves.

Another controversy is the use of barbiturates in acute withdrawal. Barbiturates have a potentiating effect with alcohol yet are beneficial for the management and prevention of seizures. Preferences are often area or health care–provider specific.

Patient Variables The patient bears the burden of stopping drug abuse. The health care provider must assume that the patient in treatment wants to stop and should proceed with this assumption. It is important that the health care provider convey the attitude that the patient will succeed. Many health care providers who have worked with patients who have tried to reform become cynical. The cynicism is a natural outcome of repeated disappointment when highly motivated patients are unable to remain drug free after completing drug treatment programs. In addition, patients who abuse drugs generally will do or say anything to obtain the drugs. This includes lying and manipulation of the health care team. Any health care provider who has ever been misled by a patient does not want to repeat the experience. It reveals a certain naiveté that fellow staff members are quick to point out.

Yet, if the health care provider presumes that the patient will fail, this expectation may be conveyed to the patient and unwittingly contribute to its fulfillment. The recovering patient needs all possible resources available to release assistance in stopping the abuse and an environment that has firm limits but one with a "can do" approach. Health care providers who work with patients who abuse substances walk a delicate line. It requires great skill and the willingness to appear foolish from time to time.

Although the approach is optimistic, the health care provider can look for some clues in the patient that would raise the possibility for success. The patient who accepts responsibility for choices made and does not blame external situations for the drug abuse has a better chance of success. The patient increases the likelihood for successful recovery if, after the acute withdrawal phase has passed, there is a willingness to accept the discomfort of the emotional withdrawal of the substances without seeking or demanding immediate relief. The chance of success is increased if the patient resists the temptation to think too soon that recovery has taken place. This means accepting the harsh reality that the substance has pervaded the person's life space, and as recovery evolves, the problems that were shielded by the substance abuse still remain. The process of confronting those problems extracts an emotional toll for which preparation is needed. If the patient substitutes a comfortable support system for the drugs, the chances for success are even greater.

Community Variables Measures that prevent development of alcohol and drug abuse should be explored. Although there are problems with trying to prevent a condition for which causes are essentially unknown, community-wide and individual measures may be helpful. Most efforts that are directed toward prevention of substance abuse are directed toward reducing the drug supply. Legislative intervention is often the outcome of such efforts—essentially, decrease the demand for drugs. Because these efforts involve changing attitudes, it is likely to be very difficult but more effective in the long run.

Encourage individuals to take personal responsibility for drinking alcohol and taking mind-altering drugs. When mind-altering drugs are prescribed for medical purposes, the patient must use them in the prescribed dose and preferably for a short time. Health care providers should prescribe drugs appropriately, using mild-altering drugs in limited amounts and for limited periods. Promoting nondrug measures when they are likely to be effective, educating patients about the drugs that are prescribed, participating in drug education programs, and recognizing as early as possible patients who are at risk for substance abuse all contribute to reducing the incidence and prevalence of this health care problem.

Parents can be encouraged to model appropriate behaviors by minimizing their own drug use and avoiding smoking. Children are apt to use a drug if their parents have a generally permissive attitude about drug use, if either parent uses mild-altering drugs, and if either parent is a heavy drinker or smoker.

Intervention

Administration

During the acute phase of withdrawal, it is important that the health care provider monitors the patient frequently for challenges to the patient's vital processes. Ensuring an adequate respiratory, cardiac, and circulatory function is a priority. It is important to know what substances the patient is withdrawing from to anticipate the characteristics of the withdrawal.

Maintain patient safety while the patient is in the acute withdrawal phase. Environmental stimuli should be reduced. Cardiovascular, respiratory, and neurologic functions; mental status; and behavior should be monitored regularly. Check laboratory reports, when available, for abnormal liver function tests, indications of anemia, and abnormal white blood cell or electrolyte counts. Hypocalcemia, hypomagnesemia, and acidosis are common in alcohol abusers. Also drug and alcohol blood levels should be monitored. Observe for use or avoidance of nonprescribed drugs.

Education

The best intervention for substance abuse is primary prevention. Educational programs are available in the elementary and secondary classrooms as well as public service announcements in the media. Public education about the deleterious effects of substance abuse is the best prevention.

Because substance abuse and child abuse and neglect are correlated, it is important to educate parents not only about the effects of the substance abuse but also about successful parenting techniques. Educating parents about the clues of substance abuse in their child is important, as well as enlightening parents about role-modeling behaviors that promote respect for moderation or abstinence and for healthy ways to resolve conflict.

Responsibility for recovery and optimal health is placed on the patient once physiologic and psychological stability has been established. This is often a long-term process and involves the attainment of patient self-awareness and acceptance. Education, along with support and encouragement regarding changes in life-style, plays a significant part in the patient's recovery. Self-help groups such as Alcoholics Anonymous, Synanon, Alateen, Alanon, and others educate the public about the dangers of substances.

When disulfiram therapy is chosen, the patient needs to be knowledgeable about the physiologic effects of this drug and its restrictions. The patient needs to be aware of the various OTC substances that contain alcohol and will elicit reactions. Some common substances such as mouthwash contain alcohol and must be avoided for safety. Foods containing alcohol are fermented vinegar and sauces. Some cough medicines also contain alcohol. Because alcohol can enter the body through inhalants and skin, the patient needs to know whether the common aerosol medications used in the treatment of asthma and respiratory problems contain alcohol and, if so, to find a substitute. The patient also needs to be alerted to alcohol wipes, backrub lotions, and skin bracers or aftershaves containing alcohol.

Question the patient about the work and home environment. Disulfiram should not be used by those who encounter lead in their environment, because disulfiram increases the absorption rate and the toxicity of lead and nickel in the blood and the accumulation of lead and nickel in the brain. The patient should be advised to avoid drugs such as metronidazole or oral hypoglycemic agents because these drugs may cause a disulfiram-like reaction. Warn the patient that it takes as long as 14 days to recover from the effects of disulfiram because of the slow rate of restoration of aldehyde dehydrogenase. Alcohol consumed within the 14-

day period can be dangerous. Once the patient has passed the acute stage of withdrawal, the patient should be advised that treatment is focused on prevention of relapse. The path to abstinence is divided into several options. Support networks such as Alcoholics Anonymous have been effective. Behavioral approaches, marital and family counseling, and hypnosis have been tried with varying degrees of success.

Many patients find smoking extremely difficult to stop, given the positive benefits of continuing and the very unpleasant withdrawal symptoms experienced on attempting withdrawal. Patients should be advised that nicotine patches; gum; aversion therapy; behavior modification; the substitution of other activities, especially physical activities; and avoidance of activities associated with smoking are all successful interventions.

Evaluation

Evaluating the effectiveness of interventions for substance abuse involves the patient's and family's response to the management plan. Some health care providers believe that management is considered successful when the patient is clean and sober. This means that the patient abstains from illegal drug use and abstains from alcohol completely or drinks alcohol in moderation. It also means that the patient uses prescription drugs according to directions and for the condition for which they were prescribed.

Success for some patients may be defined as diminishment of the undesirable adverse effects of the substance abused. If so, success might be defined in terms of the patient not engaging in high-risk behaviors.

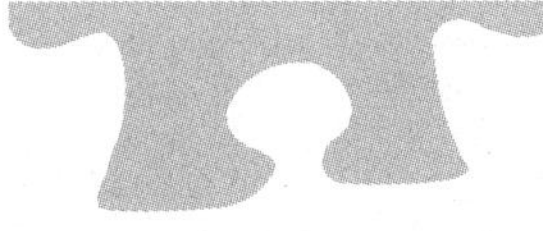

SUMMARY

- There are four main categories of abused substances in the United States: sedatives, stimulants, hallucinogens, and anabolic steroids.
- A number of populations are at risk for substance abuse: adolescents, older adults, health care providers, dual-diagnosis psychiatric patients, Vietnam veterans, individuals with chronic pain, and athletes.
- There are four primary patterns of substance abuse: experimental, recreational-social, situational, and compulsive.
- There are several theories about the cause of substance abuse: drugs as panacea for life's problems; biologic, chemical, or genetic predisposition; a basic incompatibility between civilization and human nature; acceptance communicated through the socialization process; and a progressive disease with psychological and physiologic components.
- Commonly abused CNS depressants include alcohol, opioids, benzodiazepines, and barbiturates.
- Commonly abused CNS stimulants include amphetamines, cocaine, caffeine, tobacco, and designer drugs.
- Other commonly abused drugs include hallucinogens, inhalants, and anabolic steroids.
- Assessment for substance abuse or misuse should be done even though the patient presents with a different problem. Health care providers should be alert for conditions that suggest substance abuse.
- Drug screens should be conducted on both blood and urine to determine what substances the patient has consumed and how much still remains in the body.
- Substance abuse affects growth and development, contributes to school dropout rates and gang membership, can result in violence and death, and is a catalyst for sexual promiscuity, teen pregnancy, and sexually transmitted disease.
- The primary treatment objective for patients with a substance abuse problem is to stop the abuse and correct the physical conditions that were the result.
- Treatment options vary depending on the substance abused, the extent of the dependence, the patient's incentive to stop the abuse, the depth of the commitment to stop, and the support available to the patient.
- Overall interventions for the substance abuser should include maintenance of existing body system function, along with adequate nutritional support.
- The patient bears the burden for stopping drug abuse. Health care providers must assume the patient in treatment wants to stop and proceed with this assumption.
- The best treatment for substance abuse is primary prevention.
- Responsibility for recovery and optimal health is placed on the patient once physiologic and psychological stability has been established.
- Evaluating the effectiveness of interventions for substance abuse involves the patient's and family's response to the management plan.

BIBLIOGRAPHY

American Psychological Association. (1994). *Diagnostic and statistical manual of mental disorders: DSM-IV* (4th ed.). Washington, DC: Author.

Baldwin, D., Hughes, P., Conard, S., et al. (1991). Substance use among senior medical students: A survey of 23 medical schools. *Journal of the American Medical Association,* 265(16), 2074–2078.

Balfour, D. (Ed.). (1990). Psychotropic drugs of abuse. In *International encyclopedia of pharmacology and therapeutics.* New York: Pergamon Press.

Brust, J. (1993). *Neurological aspects of substance abuse.* Boston: Butterworth-Heinemann.

Chalmers, E. (1991). Volatile substance abuse. *The Medical Journal of Australia,* 154(2), 269–274.

Chenitz, W., Salisbury, S., and Stone, J. (1990). Drug misuse and abuse in the elderly. *Issues in Mental Health Nursing,* 11, 1–16.

Denver General Hospital. (1994). *Nursing care plan for the patient experiencing alcohol withdrawal syndrome.* [Nursing care plan and protocols for the Denver General Hospital Alcohol Detoxification Program.]

Doherty, S., and Bennett, C. (Eds.). (1991). *Substance abuse in dentistry: a proviso for a drug-free profession.* Brentwood, TN: D. S. H. Publishing Company.

Esmail, A., Anderson, H., Ramsey, J., et al. (1992). Controlling deaths from volatile substance abuse in those under 18: The effects of legislation. *British Medical Journal,* 305(6858), 692.

Fleming, M., and Barry, K. (1992). *Addictive disorders.* St. Louis: Mosby–Year Book.

Frances, R., and Miller, S. (Eds.). (1991). *Clinical textbook of addictive disorders.* New York: The Guilford Press.

Gjerde, H., Smith-Kielland, A., Normann, P., et al. (1990). Driving under the influence of toluene. *Forensic Science International,* 44(1), 77–83.

Gold, M., and Slaby, A. (Eds.). (1991). *Dual diagnosis in substance abuse.* New York: Marcel Dekker.

Gossop, M., and Grant, M. (Eds.). (1990). *Preventing and controlling drug abuse.* Geneva: World Health Organization.

Gowett, G., Hanzlick, G., and Randy, L. (1992). Atypical autoerotic deaths. *American Journal of Forensic Medicine and Pathology,* 13(2), 115–119.

Hoffman, P., Rabe, C., Moses, F., et al. (1989). Ethanol and the GABA receptor complex: Studies with partial inverse benzodiazepine receptor agonist Ro 15-4513. *Pharmacological Biochemistry and Behavior,* 31, 767–772.

Hogstel, M. (Ed.). (1990). *Geropsychiatric nursing.* St. Louis: The C. V. Mosby Company.

Hughes, P., Conard, S., Baldwin, D., et al. (1991). Resident physician substance abuse in the United States. *Journal of the American Medical Association,* 265(16), 2069–2073.

Lovinger, D., White, G., and Weight, F. (1989). Ethanol inhibits NMDA-activated ion current in hippocampal neurons. *Science,* 243, 1721–1724.

Naegle, M. (Ed.). (1991). *Substance abuse education in nursing* (Vol. I). New York: National League for Nursing Press.

Naegle, M. (Ed.). (1992). *Substance abuse education in nursing* (Vol. II). New York: National League for Nursing Press.

Naegle, M. (Ed.). (1993). *Substance abuse education in nursing* (Vol. III). New York: National League for Nursing Press.

Nowinski, J. (1990). *Substance abuse in adolescents and young adults: a guide to treatment.* New York: W. W. Norton & Company.

Pernanen, K. (1991). *Alcohol in human violence.* New York: The Guilford Press.

Simpson, D., Knight, K., and Ray, S. (1993). Psychosocial correlates of AIDS: Risk drug use and sexual behaviors. *AIDS Education and Prevention,* 5(2), 121–130.

Sparks, S. (1993). *Children of prenatal substance abuse.* San Diego: Singular Publishing Group.

Substance Abuse and Mental Health Services Administration. (1993). *National household survey on drug abuse: Main findings 1991.* Rockville, MD: Department of Health and Human Services. DHHS Publication No. ADM 93–1980.

Swotinsky, R. (Ed.). (1992). *The medical review officer's guide to drug testing.* New York: Van Nostrand Reinhold.

Vega, W., Zimmerman, R., Warheit, G., et al. (1993). Risk factors for early adolescent drug use in four ethnic and racial groups. *American Journal of Public Health,* 83(2), 185–189.

Voth, E. (1992). The misprescribing physician. *Kansas Medicine,* 3, 82–83.

United States Pharmacopeial Convention. (1994). *The United States pharmacopeia dispensing information* (14th ed). Easton, PA: Mack Printing Co.

Vredevoe, D., Brecht, M., Schuler, P., et al. (1992). Risk factors for disease in a homeless population. *Public Health Nursing,* 2, 263–269.

Wagner, J., Melragon, B., and Menke, E. (1993). Homeless children: Interdisciplinary drug prevention intervention. *Journal of Child and Adolescent Psychiatric and Mental Health Nursing,* 1, 22–30.

Witters, W., Venturelli, P., and Hanson, G. (1992). *Drugs and Society* (3rd ed). Boston: Jones and Bartlett Publishers.

Wright, J., and Pearl, L. (1990). Knowledge and experience of young people regarding drug abuse, 1969–1989. *British Medical Journal,* 300(6717), 99–103.

Unit II

Drugs Influencing the Autonomic Nervous System

AUTONOMIC NERVOUS SYSTEM

This unit provides an overview of the peripheral nervous system, focusing primarily on those structures and functions affected by pharmacologic agents. Because the nervous system oversees the regulation of virtually all body processes, those same body processes can be influenced by drugs that alter neuronal regulation. Neuropharmacologic drugs that mimic or block neuronal regulation can modify such diverse processes as skeletal muscle contraction, cardiac output, vascular tone, respirations, gastrointestinal function, uterine motility, glandular secretion, and functions unique to the central nervous system (CNS), such as pain perception, cognition, sleep, and mood. Our understanding of peripheral nervous system pharmacology is much clearer than that of CNS pharmacology. This is so because the peripheral nervous system is much less complex than the CNS and also more accessible to experimentation.

FUNCTIONAL ORGANIZATION OF THE AUTONOMIC NERVOUS SYSTEM

The nervous system is made up of the central and peripheral nervous systems. The CNS is composed of the brain and spinal cord, whereas the peripheral nervous system includes the cranial nerves arising from the brain and the spinal nerves arising from the spinal cord. The CNS acts as a processing center, integrating and coordinating responses to both internal and external stimuli. Over 50 separate chemicals, including acetylcholine, norepinephrine, dopamine, serotonin, epinephrine, histamine, gamma-aminobutyric acid, glycine, and the enkephalins, act as excitatory or inhibitory neurotransmitters.

The peripheral nervous system is subdivided into the somatic and the autonomic nervous systems. The *somatic* or motor nervous system initiates voluntary skeletal muscle contraction in response to external sensory input. The *autonomic nervous system* (ANS) is further divided into the sympathetic and parasympathetic systems, which control internal body responses, particularly the involuntary actions of smooth muscles, cardiac muscles, and glands. These divisions are somewhat simplistic: Nervous system function depends on a delicate balance of complex interrelationships within the body. It is important to recognize the ANS as integral to the CNS (Fig. II–1). A continuous feedback circuit exists between the sensory gathering components of the ANS and the CNS command post (see Fig. 21–3).

Neurons are the basic unit in the nervous system. They respond to physical and chemical stimuli, conduct impulses, and release specific neurotransmitters, chemicals stored inside the synaptic vesicles. All neurons use neurotransmitters to communicate with other cells and neurons. Impulses that originate in the CNS are conducted via motor or efferent neurons to a muscle or gland. Impulses that originate at sensory receptors are conducted via afferent neurons back to the CNS. Somatic impulses travel directly from the brain or spinal cord to skeletal muscles via a preganglionic axon, whereas sympathetic and parasympathetic ganglia are composed of a two-neuron system of preganglionic and postganglionic axons.

When a nerve is stimulated, neurotransmitters are released at the axon; release of acetylcholine at the neuromuscular junction causes muscle cell contraction. The neurotransmitters move into the synapse where some are decomposed by the enzyme cholinesterase, whereas others cross the synapse to occupy specific receptors on the next neuron and continue stimulus transmission.

The effector junctions of the ANS allow pharmacologic manipulation of visceral function because transmission across the junctions is chemical. Neurotransmitters, such as norepinephrine, acetylcholine, and dopamine, are synthesized, stored in nerve endings, and released near the neurons and muscle or gland cells on which they act. Thus, the actions of ANS drugs can be understood and classified in terms of their ability to mimic or modify the actions of the neurotransmitters.

Sympathetic Division

The sympathetic nervous system includes two paravertebral ganglia that lie on each side of the spinal column, prevertebral ganglia, and nerves that extend from the ganglia to the various internal organs. Sympathetic nerves are innervated by cell bodies located in the thoracolumbar division of the spinal column between T_1 and L_2. The fibers then diverge with appropriate ganglions to synapse with postganglionic neurons; pass upward or downward in the paravertebral ganglia before synapse; or travel through the paravertebral ganglia without synapsing and terminate there. The postganglionic neurons originate in the paravertebral ganglia or one of the prevertebral ganglia. The fibers then travel to tissues and organs stimulated by sympathetic nerves (Fig. II–2).

The one exception to the two-neuron system in the ANS pathway is seen in the preganglionic axons that innervate the adrenal medulla. Here, no postganglionic neuron exists, and because the preganglionic fibers are myelinated, innervation causes rapid release of epinephrine and norepinephrine (see Fig. II–1).

Physical and emotional stress act to excite the sympathetic system. The body's response allows immediate action and elevated physical strength. Specific body responses include increased:

- Arterial blood pressure and cardiac output
- Blood flow to active muscles concurrent with decreased blood flow to organs not needed for flight or fight
- Rate and depth of respirations
- Rates of cellular metabolism (i.e., increased oxygen consumption and carbon dioxide production)
- Blood sugar levels through increased glycolysis in the liver and muscles
- Mental activity and ability to think clearly
- Rate of blood coagulation
- Pupil dilation to aid vision

Biosynthesis and Release of Catecholamines

The term catecholamine refers to a group of chemically related compounds: norepinephrine, epinephrine, and dopamine. The synthesis of epinephrine from tyrosine was

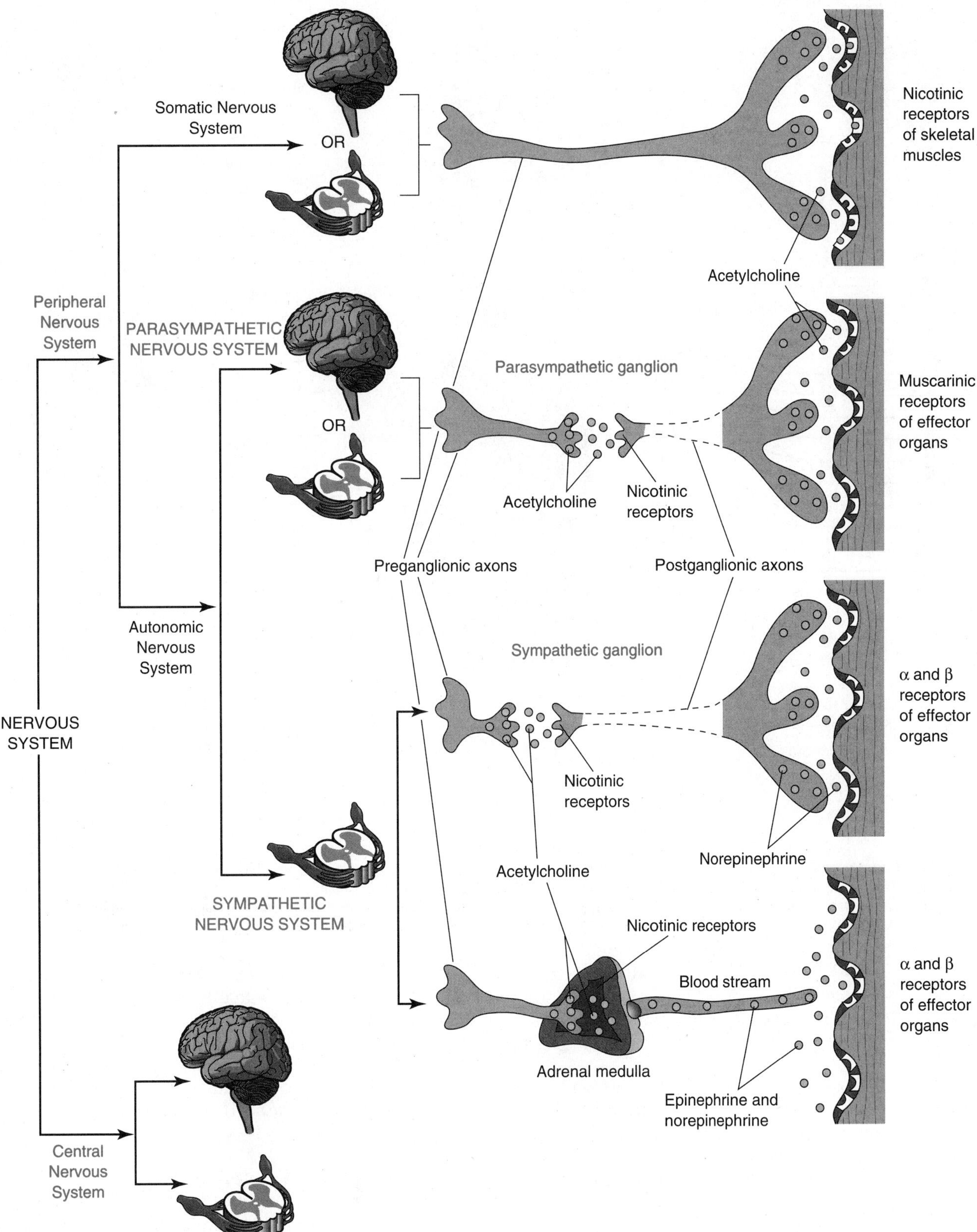

Figure II–1 Components of the autonomic and somatic nervous systems. All preganglionic nerves release acetylcholine. The acetylcholine interacts with nicotinic receptors of the postganglionic sympathetic and parasympathetic nerves, the adrenal medullae, or skeletal muscle within the somatic system. Norepinephrine is released from postganglionic sympathetic nerves. The norepinephrine acts on alpha or beta receptors on effector organs (smooth muscle, cardiac muscle, glands). Acetylcholine is released by postganglionic parasympathetic nerves to act on muscarinic receptors. The preganglionic fiber that innervates adrenal medullae without synapsing at a ganglion releases norepinephrine and epinephrine directly into the circulation to the effector organs.

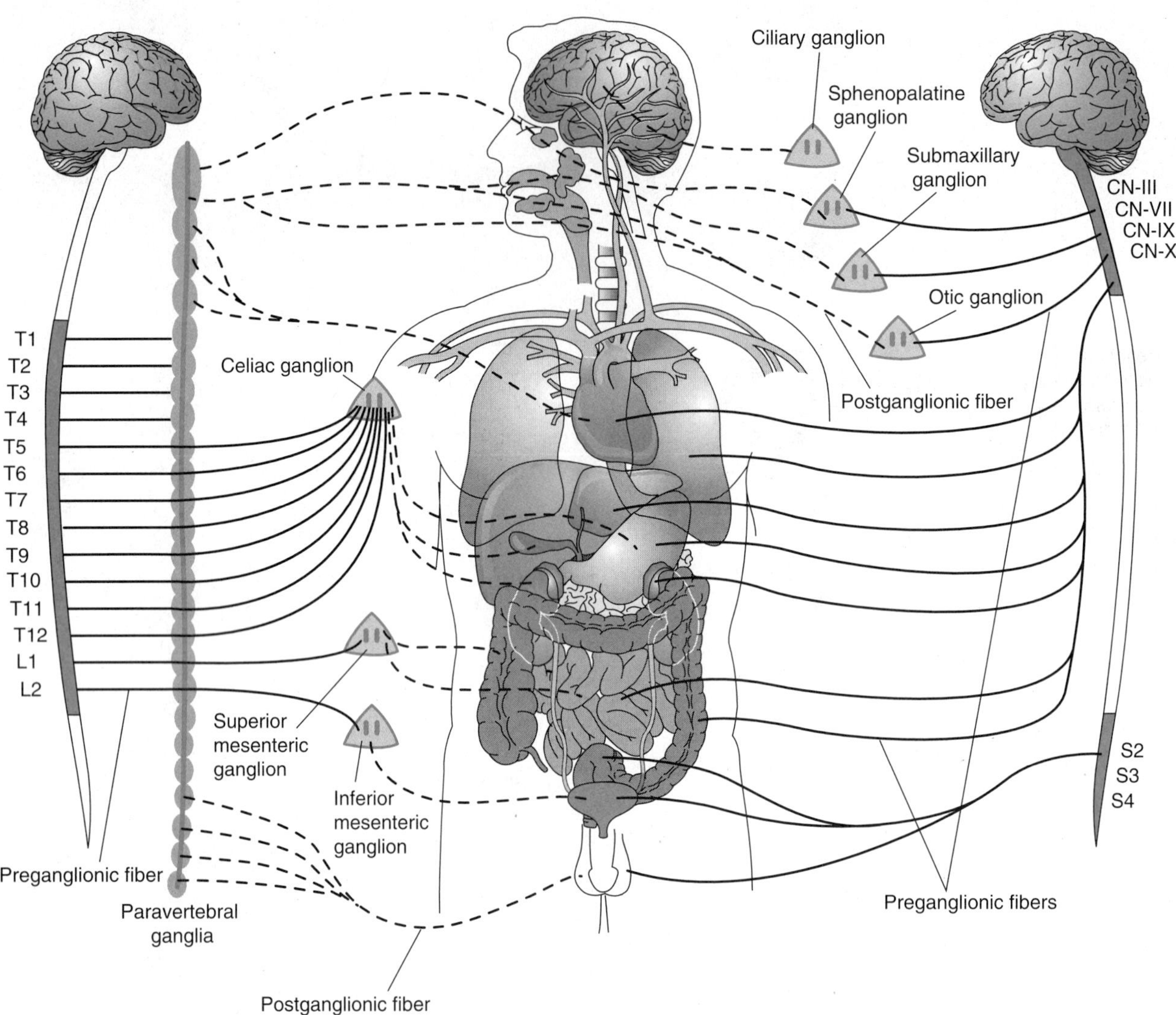

Figure II–2 The autonomic nervous system. Parasympathetic neurons originate in the craniosacral regions of the spinal cord. Preganglionic fibers are long and travel to ganglia located close to or in the walls of effector organs. Postganglionic fibers are short. Sympathetic neurons originate in the thoracolumbar region of the central nervous system. The preganglionic fibers are short, terminating in ganglia adjacent to the spinal cord. Postganglionic fibers are long, traveling some distance through effector cells to reach effector organs.

proposed in 1939 by Blaschko (see Fig. 11–1). The enzymes involved in the transition, however, exhibit broad substrate specificity. In other words, many endogenous substances, as well as certain drugs, are similarly acted on at the various steps.

Once norepinephrine is secreted by terminal nerve endings it is removed from the secretory site in three different ways. Reuptake of the neurotransmitter occurs through active transport by adrenergic nerve endings, which account for retrieval of 50 to 80 percent of the secreted norepinephrine. Movement away from the nerve endings into the surrounding body fluids with diffusion into the bloodstream accounts for removal of much of the remaining norepinephrine. And last, there is enzyme degradation of the neurotransmitter, especially by monoamine oxidase (MAO), an enzyme found in the nerve endings themselves.

Under normal circumstances, norepinephrine is secreted directly into tissues, remaining active for only a matter of seconds. The short activity time illustrates that uptake and diffusion away from tissues are rapid. However, norepinephrine and epinephrine secreted into the circulation by the adrenal medullae remain active until they diffuse back into tissue and are destroyed. Degradation occurs mainly in the liver by the enzyme catechol *O*-methyltransferase. Therefore, when they are secreted into the bloodstream, both norepinephrine and epinephrine remain active for 10 to 30 seconds.

Catecholamine Receptors

An understanding of the classification and properties of the different types of adrenergic receptors is critical to understanding the remarkably diverse effects of the catecholamines and related drugs. Although they are structurally related, different adrenergic receptors regulate distinct physiologic processes by controlling the synthesis or release of a variety of secondary messengers.

There are two major sympathetic receptors: alpha receptors and beta receptors. The alpha receptors are subdivided

TABLE II–1 CLASSIFICATION OF EFFECTOR ORGAN RESPONSES TO ANS IMPULSES

Effector Organs	Sympathetic Impulses RECEPTOR	Sympathetic Impulses RESPONSE	Parasympathetic Impulses RESPONSE
Cardiac			
SA Node	$Beta_1$	Increased heart rate ↑↑	Decreased heart rate ↓↓↓
AV Node	$Beta_1$	Increased automaticity ↑↑	Decreased conduction velocity ↓↓
Atria	$Beta_1$	Increase in contractility and conduction velocity ↑↑	Decrease in contractility and shortened AP duration ↓↓
Ventricles	$Beta_1$	Increased force of contraction and conduction velocity	Slight decrease in contractility
Purkinje fibers	$Beta_1$	Increased automaticity and propagation velocity ↑↑↑	Little effect
Vasculature			
Coronary arterioles	$Alpha_1$, $alpha_2$, $beta_2$	Constriction ↑ Dilation ↑↑	Constriction ↓
Pulmonary arterioles	$Alpha_1$, $beta_2$	Constriction ↑, Dilatation	Dilatation
Skeletal muscles	M,N	Constriction ↑↑ Dilatation ↑↑	Dilatation
Skin/mucosa	$Alpha_1$, $alpha_2$	Constriction ↑↑↑	Dilatation
Cerebral arterioles	$Alpha_1$	Slight Constriction	Dilatation
Abdominal viscera	$Alpha_1$, $beta_2$	Constriction ↑↑↑, Dilatation ↑	—
Adrenal medulla	—	—	Secretion EPI and NEPI (nicotinic effect)
Mesentery	$Alpha_1$, D_1	Constriction ↑↑	—
Renal arterioles	$Alpha_1$, $beta_1$, $beta_2$, D_1	Constriction ↑↑↑, Dilatation ↑	—
Systemic veins	$Alpha_1$, $beta_2$	Constriction ↑↑ Dilatation ↑	—
Respiratory Tract			
Tracheal/bronchial Smooth muscle	$Beta_2$	Relaxation ↑ (bronchodilation)	Contraction ↓↓
Bronchial glands	$Alpha_1$, $beta_2$	Decreased secretion Increased secretion	Stimulation ↓↓↓
GI Tract			
GI motility	$Alpha_1$, $beta_2$	Usually decreased ↓	Increased ↑↑↑
GI sphincters	$Alpha_1$	Usually contraction ↑	Usually relaxation ↓
Exocrine secretion	$Alpha_1$	Inhibition	Stimulation ↑↑
Salivary glands	$Alpha_1$, $alpha_2$	($Alpha_1$) Constriction ↑ K^+ and H_2O secretion ↑ ($Alpha_2$) Secretion amylase ↑	Dilation ↑ K^+ and H_2O secretion ↑↑↑
Gallbladder and ducts	$Beta_2$	Relaxation ↑	Contraction ↓
Liver	$Alpha_1$, $beta_2$	Glycogenolysis Gluconeogenesis	Glycogen synthesis
Pancreatic acini	Alpha	Decreased secretion ↓	Secretion ↑↑
Pancreatic islets	$Alpha_2$, $beta_2$	Decreased secretion ↓↓↓ Increased secretion ↑	—
Fat cells	$Alpha_2$, $beta_1$, $beta_2$	Inhibition lipolysis; stimulation lipolysis	—
Genitourinary Tract			
Kidneys	$Alpha_1$, $beta_2$	($Alpha_1$) ↑ Renin secretion ($Beta_2$) ↓ Renin secretion	—
Detrusor	$Beta_2$	Usually relaxation ↓	Contraction ↑↑↑
Trigone and sphincter	$Alpha_1$	Contraction ↓↓	Relaxation ↑↑
Ureter motility and tone	$Alpha_1$	Increased	Increased (?)
Uterus	$Alpha_1$, $beta_2$	Pregnant: contraction ($alpha_1$); relaxation ($beta_2$) Nonpregnant: relaxation ($beta_2$)	Variable
Male sex glands	$Alpha_1$	Ejaculation↑↑	Erection ↑↑↑
Eyes			
Radial muscle, iris	$Alpha_1$	Mydriasis ↓↓	—
Sphincter muscle, iris	$Alpha_1$	—	Miosis ↓↓↓
Lacrimal glands	—	—	Secretion
Ciliary muscle	$Beta_2$	Relaxation for distance vision ↑	Contraction for near vision ↓↓↓
Other			
Posterior pituitary	$Beta_1$	Antidiuretic hormone secretion	—
Sweat glands	$Alpha_1$	Localized secretion	Generalized secretion
Pineal gland	Beta	Melatonin synthesis	—
Piloerector cells	$Alpha_1$	Contract	—

D Dopaminergic receptors; M Muscarinic receptors; N Nicotinic receptors; ↑↓ The approximate strength of sympathetic and parasympathetic stimulation of the various organs and functions listed.

Adapted from Hardman, J. G., Limbird, L. E., Molinoff, P. B., et al. (1996). *Goodman and Gilman's The pharmacological basis of therapeutics* (9th ed., pp. 110–111). New York: McGraw-Hill.

into $alpha_1$ and $alpha_2$, which are identified by their location. The $alpha_1$ receptors are located on postsynaptic effector cells. The $alpha_2$ receptors are found on presynaptic nerve terminals. The beta receptors, in turn, are designated by organ location: $beta_1$ receptors are found primarily in the heart, and $beta_2$ receptors appear in the smooth muscle of the bronchioles, arterioles, and various other visceral organs. In addition, dopaminergic receptors are found in the brain and on coronary, renal, and mesenteric blood vessels.

Norepinephrine and epinephrine, both secreted by the adrenal medullae, have somewhat different effects on alpha and beta receptors. Norepinephrine primarily excites alpha receptors but stimulates beta receptors to a lesser degree. Epinephrine excites both types of receptors equally. The strength of sympathetic and parasympathetic activity in controlling organ function is shown in Table II–1.

Parasympathetic Division

The parasympathetic nervous system consists of preganglionic fibers originating in the midbrain, the medulla oblongata, and the sacral portion of the spinal cord. Neuronal fibers leave the CNS through cranial nerves III (oculomotor), VII (facial), IX (glossopharyngeal), and X (vagus); the second and third sacral spinal nerves and, occasionally, the first and fourth sacral nerves. Thus, the parasympathetic nervous system is often called the craniosacral division. Unlike the sympathetic system, the preganglionic fibers of the parasympathetic division travel to the organs they innervate before forming synapses with relatively short postganglionic neurons.

This division counterbalances the action of the sympathetic system. The parasympathetic nervous system conserves and restores energy, allowing rejuvenation of organ function, and is often described as resting in nature. Approximately ¾ of all parasympathetic fibers are in vagus nerves, passing to the thoracic and abdominal regions of the body. These nerves supply branches to the heart, lungs, esophagus, stomach and small intestine, the proximal half of the colon, liver, gallbladder and pancreas, and the upper portions of the ureters. Other parasympathetic fibers supply pupillary sphincters and ciliary muscles; lacrimal, nasal, submaxillary, and parotid glands; descending colon and rectum; lower portion of the ureters and bladder; and the genitalia.

Biosynthesis and Release of Acetylcholine

Synthesis of acetylcholine involves the interaction of choline and acetate with the active uptake of choline into cholinergic neurons. The interaction is catalyzed by the enzyme choline acetyltransferase (see Fig. 13–1). This enzyme is found in high concentrations in cholinergic nerve endings. The arrival of an impulse at a synapse increases the permeability of the membrane to calcium, which is necessary for an efficient release of acetylcholine. The resultant influx of calcium causes liberation of acetylcholine into the synapse for attachment to specialized receptors on the membrane of the next neuron. Binding of acetylcholine to the receptor increases the permeability of the membrane to sodium and potassium ions. Depolarization of nerve fibers results in excitation or inhibition of neural, muscular, or glandular activity.

Parasympathetic Receptors

Acetylcholine activates two different types of receptors—muscarinic and nicotinic. The reason for these names is that muscarine, the alkaloid responsible for the toxicity of toadstools, activates only the muscarinic receptors. Nicotine activates only nicotinic receptors. Acetylcholine activates both types of receptors.

Muscarinic receptors are found in the ganglia of both parasympathetic and sympathetic fibers of the heart, smooth muscle, adrenal medullae, and glands. Skeletal muscle is supplied by the somatic motor system. Nicotinic receptors are found in the synapses between the preganglionic and postganglionic neurons of both the sympathetic and parasympathetic nervous systems. They are also found in the membranes of skeletal muscle fibers at the neuromuscular junction.

CONFUSING TERMINOLOGY

A clear understanding of the terminology associated with the peripheral nervous system is essential to a study of ANS drugs. The actions of an ANS drug can often be predicted if the responses to nerve impulses that reach the organs are known and understood.

The terminology used to describe various ANS drugs is often confusing because assorted terms are used to refer to the same phenomenon (Table II–2). For example, the term *sympathomimetic* and *adrenergic* are both used to describe a drug that has the same effects on the body as that produced by stimulation of the sympathetic nervous system. They are considered sympathetic agonists. *Parasympathomimetic* and *cholinergic* are both used to describe a drug that has the same effects on the body as that produced by stimulation of the

TABLE II–2 TERMINOLOGY DESCRIBING AUTONOMIC NERVOUS SYSTEM DRUG ACTIVITY

	Sympathetic Nervous System	Parasympathetic Nervous System
Anatomic location	Thoracolumbar region	Craniosacral region
Primary neurotransmitters	Norepinephrine	Acetylcholine
Pharmacodynamic terms	Sympathomimetic	Parasympathomimetic
Functional agonist terms	Adrenergic	Anticholinergic
Functional antagonist terms	Antiadrenergic	Anticholinergic
	Alpha blocker	Antinicotinic
	Beta blocker	Antimuscarinic
		Anticholinesterase
		Cholinesterase inhibitor

parasympathetic nervous system. These are considered parasympathetic agonists.

Conversely, there are also drugs that oppose or block the stimulation of these systems. Terms associated with inhibition of parasympathetic stimulation include *parasympatholytic, anticholinergic,* and *cholinergic blocking* agents. The terms associated with inhibition of sympathetic stimulation include *sympatholytic, antiadrenergic,* or *alpha-blocking* and *beta-blocking* drugs.

PHARMACOLOGIC IMPLICATIONS

The point of transmission, which at most synapses is chemically mediated, is of great pharmacologic importance. The action of drugs affecting the ANS can be interpreted in terms of how they modify the synthesis, release, storage, or disposition of a neurotransmitter, or stimulate or inhibit interactions at receptor sites. Thus, the synapses are a logical point for drug manipulation of neural function. The biochemical phenomena that occur at a synapse are much more sensitive to drugs and hypoxia than events in the nerve fibers themselves. For example, anesthetic drugs produce a greater effect on neural pathways with multiple synapses than on neural pathways that have few synapses, which helps explain the mechanism operating in general anesthesia. Because transmission in the CNS and the peripheral nervous system is chemically mediated, pharmacologists should be able to develop drugs that regulate not only the somatic and visceral motor activities but also those of emotion, behavior, and other complex cerebral functions.

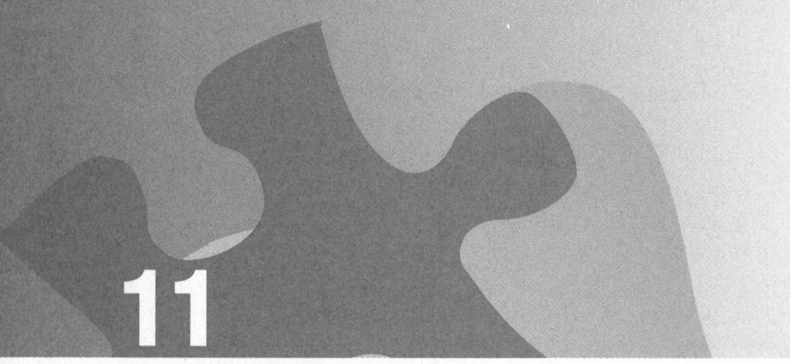

11 Sympathetic Nervous System Drugs

Adrenergics are chemical compounds that stimulate sympathetic nervous system activity. These drugs, also referred to as *sympathomimetic* or *adrenergic agonists,* are divided into three different groups: alpha and beta agonists, alpha agonists, and beta agonists. Adrenergics are chemically structured as catecholamines and noncatecholamines. Catecholamines are exogenous formulations of the naturally occurring neurotransmitters epinephrine and norepinephrine; noncatecholamines are chemical relatives. The first step in the synthesis of catecholamines from dietary phenylalanine (Fig. 11–1) takes place outside the nerve terminals. Subsequent steps take place within the cytoplasm of the nerve endings, with the final step occurring in the presynaptic vesicles. None of the enzymes involved in the sequence is specific for norepinephrine. The enzymes involved can catalyze similar reactions using other endogenous compounds and some drugs.

Catecholamines and noncatecholamines act on sympathetic nervous system receptors. Adrenergic compounds stimulate adrenergic receptors directly, thereby stimulating cells that respond to norepinephrine and epinephrine. The result is a sympathetic response that causes mydriasis, increased rate and force of myocardial contraction, vasoconstriction, bronchodilation, decreased gastric motility, pallor, perspiration, and sphincter constriction, as well as decreased motility, tone, and contractility of the urinary bladder. Additionally, there is a subjective increase in mental alertness. In general, the effects mimic the so-called fight or flight response. Indications for adrenergic agonists stem primarily from their effects on the heart, blood vessels, and bronchi. They are often used in the emergency management of acute shock, cardiovascular, respiratory, and allergic disorders.

Another group of sympathetic nervous system drugs are chemical compounds that inhibit sympathetic nervous system activity by interacting with the receptor site. These drugs are referred to as *sympatholytics* or *antiadrenergics.* There are two types of adrenergic blockers—*alpha blockers* and *beta blockers.* Alpha blockers block alpha receptors, and beta blockers block beta receptors. Antiadrenergic compounds inhibit sympathetic nervous system activity, dilate peripheral blood vessels, and reduce the heart rate. Additionally, the patient develops an increase in gastrointestinal (GI) and urinary activity. The effects are, in essence, vegetative in character. Indications for antiadrenergic drugs stem from their blockade effects on the heart and blood vessels.

PHYSIOLOGY AND PATHOPHYSIOLOGY

Circulatory Shock

The circulatory system supplies body tissues with oxygen. Adequate tissue perfusion relies on the pumping ability of the heart, the ability of blood vessels to expand and contract, sufficient blood to fill the circulatory system, and tissues capable of extracting oxygen and nutrients from the blood. *Circulatory shock* (i.e., failure of the vasculature) produces compensatory responses that result in decreased peripheral perfusion, inadequate oxygenation of vital organs, and eventually, decompensation to various shock states. Circulatory shock results in decreased peripheral perfusion and inadequate oxygenation of vital organs. Circulatory shock is not a specific disease but a cascade of events that occur in the course of trauma or disease states.

Types of Shock

There are three main categories of circulatory shock. Hypovolemic shock is a consequence of inadequate circulatory volume. Hypovolemic shock can be caused by hemorrhage, third-spacing (a shift of fluid from the intravascular space to potential spaces), loss of plasma from severe burns, or GI loss of fluids secondary to vomiting or diarrhea.

Obstructive shock is related to mechanical obstruction of arterial blood flow or of venous return. Obstructive shock can be caused by cardiac tamponade, pneumothorax, an aortic aneurysm, or evisceration of abdominal organs into the chest cavity.

Distributive shock is characterized by loss of blood vessel tone, enlargement of the vascular compartment, and displacement of vascular volume away from the heart and central circulation. Distributive shock occurs when the tissues are unable to use oxygen and nutrients to produce energy. The basic circulatory events are reflected in three subtypes of distributive shock—neurogenic shock, anaphylactic shock, and septic shock.

Neurogenic shock is correlated with reduced sympathetic control of vascular tone. It may be caused by a defect in the vasomotor center in the brain stem, or to sympathetic outflow to the vasculature. Neurogenic shock can be related to brain injury, the depressant action of drugs, general anesthesia, hypoxia, or hypoglycemia.

Anaphylactic shock is an immune-mediated reaction. Vasodilator chemicals that are released into the circulation bring about massive dilation of arterioles and venules, increased capillary permeability, and peripheral pooling of blood.

Septic shock may occur as the result of a systemic response to severe infection. It is most often caused by gram-negative or gram-positive bacteremia or systemic fungal infections. Unlike other types of shock, septic shock commonly results in pulmonary insufficiency, disseminated intravascular coagulation, and multiple organ dysfunction.

Mechanisms of Shock

In severe, prolonged shock, arterioles and venules relax, resulting in a drop of arterial pressure and venous pooling. Hypoxia at the capillary level and the products of cellular deterioration cause increased capillary permeability, stagnant blood flow, the formation of small blood clots, and

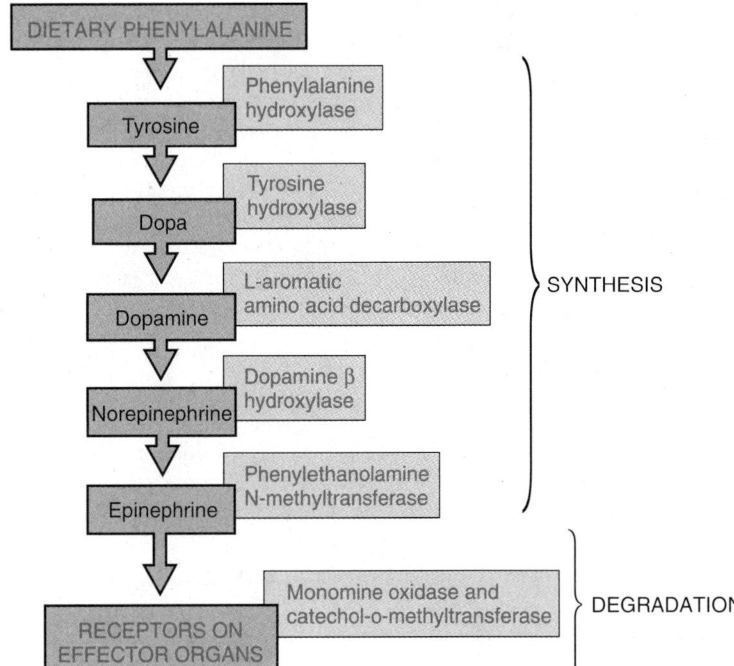

Figure 11–1 Synthesis and degradation of catecholamines. Dietary phenylalanine is converted to tyrosine with the aid of the enzyme phenylalanine hydroxylase, which, in turn, is converted to dopa with the aid of tyrosine hydroxylase. Additional enzymes continue the conversion to dopamine, norepinephrine, and finally, epinephrine. Monoamine oxidase (MAO) and catechol-*O*-methyltransferase (COMT) enzymes act to degrade the catecholamines in the synapse, while a portion of the catecholamines go on to interact with receptors on effector organs.

third-spacing. Without effective compensatory mechanisms, the loss of vascular volume results in rapid, progressive, irreversible shock.

The initial compensatory mechanism in shock is a sympathetic response designed to maintain cardiac output and blood pressure. Vasoconstriction reduces vessel size, increasing peripheral vascular resistance. Fluid is absorbed from interstitial spaces, the kidneys conserve sodium and water, and thirst develops in an effort to restore blood volume. Renal blood flow is reduced in shock due to sympathetic vasoconstriction. The reduced blood flow, in turn, causes a fall in the glomerular filtration rate and activation of the renal-angiotensin-aldosterone system. Further, antidiuretic hormone, also known as vasopressin, constricts peripheral arteries and veins and increases water retention. However, these compensatory mechanisms are not designed for long-term use and they begin to exert detrimental effects of their own. Vasoconstriction results in decreased tissue perfusion, impaired cellular metabolism, release of vasoactive inflammatory mediators (e.g., histamine), liberation of lactic acid, and cell death.

Within the cell, oxygen and nutrients are normally converted to adenosine triphosphate. The cell, in turn, uses adenosine triphosphate to operate the sodium-potassium pump to move sodium out and potassium back into the cells. Nutrients are converted to energy through the aerobic and anaerobic pathways. The aerobic pathway (i.e., Krebs' cycle) uses oxygen to move pyruvate, the end product of glycolysis, into mitochondria, where it is transformed to adenosine triphosphate, carbon dioxide, and water. When oxygen is lacking, pyruvate does not enter Krebs' cycle but is converted to lactic acid. The lactic acid builds up to accumulate in the cellular and extracellular compartments.

Normal cellular function cannot be sustained without adequate energy production. The sodium-potassium pump becomes impaired, sodium accumulates in the cells, and potassium moves outward. Cells swell as membranes become more permeable. Mitochondrial activity is severely depressed. Lysosomal membranes rupture, releasing the enzymes with further intracellular destruction taking place. Cell death follows as cellular contents are released into the extracellular spaces. Inflammatory mediators and intracellular enzymes (e.g., myocardial depressant factor) are released, and the adverse changes within the circulation become more evident. Regaining perfusion and cellular oxygenation abilities is critical to ensure cellular survival and, consequently, survival of the patient.

Complications of Shock

Many body systems are affected by shock. The five main complications include adult respiratory distress syndrome (ARDS), acute renal failure, GI ulceration, disseminated intravascular coagulation, and multiple organ dysfunction.

ARDS is thought to result from increased permeability of pulmonary capillaries to water and plasma proteins. Protein-rich fluids leak into alveolar and interstitial spaces, impairing gas exchange. The lungs become stiff and difficult to inflate. Despite high oxygen levels and the mechanical assistance of ventilators, most patients with ARDS remain hypoxic with deadly consequences.

The extent of acute renal failure is related to the severity and duration of shock. Compensatory mechanisms reduce renal blood as a means of diverting blood flow to the heart and brain. However, the normal kidney can withstand the severe ischemia associated with shock for only 15 to 20 minutes. Oliguria of less than 20 mL/hour indicates severe shock and inadequate renal perfusion. Sepsis and trauma are regarded as the primary causes of most cases of acute renal failure.

Gastrointestinal ulcerations are related to ischemic changes of its mucosal surface. In shock, there is widespread vasoconstriction, particularly of the splanchnic and mesenteric vascular beds. Further, these vascular beds have a proportionately greater vasoconstrictive response due to circulating catecholamines and angiotensin II than do other vascular beds. GI ulcerations of the stomach and duodenum can develop within hours of severe trauma, sepsis, or burns.

Disseminated intravascular coagulation is characterized by the formation of small clots in the microvasculature. This secondary disorder is a paradox in that the normal hemostatic sequence of blood coagulation, clot dissolution, and bleeding all take place at once. Consumption and depletion of fibrinogen, platelets, and other clotting factors lead to disruption of the normal clotting process. This disruption has been associated with certain obstetric conditions, metastatic cancer and leukemia, infections, shock, trauma, surgery, and blood transfusion reactions.

Multiple organ dysfunction results from severe, but selective, vasospasm of hepatic and mesenteric circulation. Endorphins potentiate the hypotensive effects of vasodilation, and free radicals and tumor necrosis factor (TNF) are released. Blood loss, impaired oxygen delivery due to hypotension, ARDS, sepsis, and anaphylaxis contribute to a deadly cycle of cellular necrosis.

Reactive Airway Disease

Reactive airway diseases are obstructive disorders characterized by limitation of expiratory air flow. These disorders can be caused by a variety of nonreversible airway diseases, including chronic bronchitis, emphysema, bronchiectasis, and cystic fibrosis. Asthma is a chronic, reversible airway disorder characterized by hypersensitivity of the airways and episodic attacks of bronchospasm. Acute asthma attacks can be triggered by an assortment of stimuli including allergens, respiratory tract infections, hyperventilation, cold air, exercise, drugs and chemicals, airborne pollutants, and emotional upset.

The early response results in immediate bronchoconstriction, which subsides in about 90 minutes. Although the early response is caused by inflammatory mediators, it tends to cause bronchospasm but not inflammation of the airways. The late response develops 3 to 5 hours after exposure and involves inflammation and increased airway responsiveness. Responsiveness to parasympathetic nervous system mediators is often heightened, suggesting changes in parasympathetic control of airway function. Reactive airway disease is discussed further in Chapter 46.

Benign Prostatic Hyperplasia

Benign prostatic hyperplasia (BPH) is an enlargement of the prostate. The disease is common in men over age 50; the incidence increases to almost 90 percent in men older than 80 years of age. It is more common in black men worldwide. With aging, the periurethral glands undergo hyperplasia (abnormal increase in the number of normal cells). The prostate enlarges, compressing surrounding normal prostatic tissue and pushing it toward the periphery, forming a capsule. Because of its position around the urethra, enlargement of the prostate gland quickly interferes with the normal outflow of urine from the bladder. Although the exact cause of BPH is unknown, urination becomes increasingly more difficult and the bladder never feels completely empty. The prostatic enlargement eventually obstructs urinary outflow completely. The usual remedy is prostatectomy. However, in some cases, alpha-blocking drugs can be used to relieve symptoms and improve urination. Autonomic innervation of the bladder neck and prostatic smooth muscle is abundant. Prostatic obstruction is caused in part by the neurogenic tone of the bladder neck and prostatic smooth muscle.

PHARMACOTHERAPEUTIC OPTIONS

Adrenergic Agonists

ALPHA AND BETA AGONISTS

- ❒ Dopamine (INTROPIN); (✱) REVIMINE
- ❒ Epinephrine (ASRELIN)
- ❒ Norepinephrine (levarterenol; LEVOPHED)

ALPHA AGONISTS

- ❒ Metaraminol (ARAMINE)
- ❒ Phenylephrine (NEO-SYNEPHRINE)

BETA AGONISTS

- ❒ Dobutamine (DOBUTREX)
- ❒ Isoetharine (BRONKOSOL)
- ❒ Isoproterenol (ISUPREL)

Indications

Adrenergic drugs are used to increase blood pressure in severe hypotension, to reverse anaphylactic shock, to reduce bleeding at the operative site in conjunction with local anesthetics, and to treat hypoglycemic episodes because epinephrine antagonizes the effects of insulin, causing blood sugar to rise.

In hypotension and shock, adrenergics (e.g., dopamine, epinephrine) are given to increase blood pressure. In hemorrhage or hypovolemic states, adrenergics are used as second-line drugs if adequate fluid volume replacement does not restore blood pressure and circulation sufficiently to maintain organ perfusion.

In reactive airway diseases and anaphylaxis, the drugs are used as bronchodilators to relieve bronchoconstriction and bronchospasm (e.g., epinephrine). In upper respiratory infections, including the common cold and sinusitis, they are used for their decongestant effects. The use of these drugs is discussed in more detail in Chapters 46, 47, and 48.

The drugs are used in allergic disorders because of their vasoconstricting effects and ability to relieve edema in the respiratory tract, skin, and other tissues. Thus, they are used in the management of allergic rhinitis, anaphylaxis to animal serums, insect stings and other allergens, serum sickness, urticaria, and angioedema.

Other clinical uses include relaxation of uterine musculature and to inhibit contractions in preterm labor (e.g., terbutaline) (see Chapter 55). Some of the drugs (e.g., epinephrine) can be added to local anesthetics to prolong anesthesia (see Chapter 16). Topical uses of adrenergic drugs for their vasoconstrictive and mydriatic effects are discussed in Chapter 62.

Pharmacodynamics

Adrenergics may act directly or indirectly to stimulate sympathetic nervous system receptors. Direct-acting drugs directly stimulate sympathetic nervous system receptors by combining with postsynaptic alpha or beta receptors (Fig. 11–2). The drugs alter permeability of cell membranes to

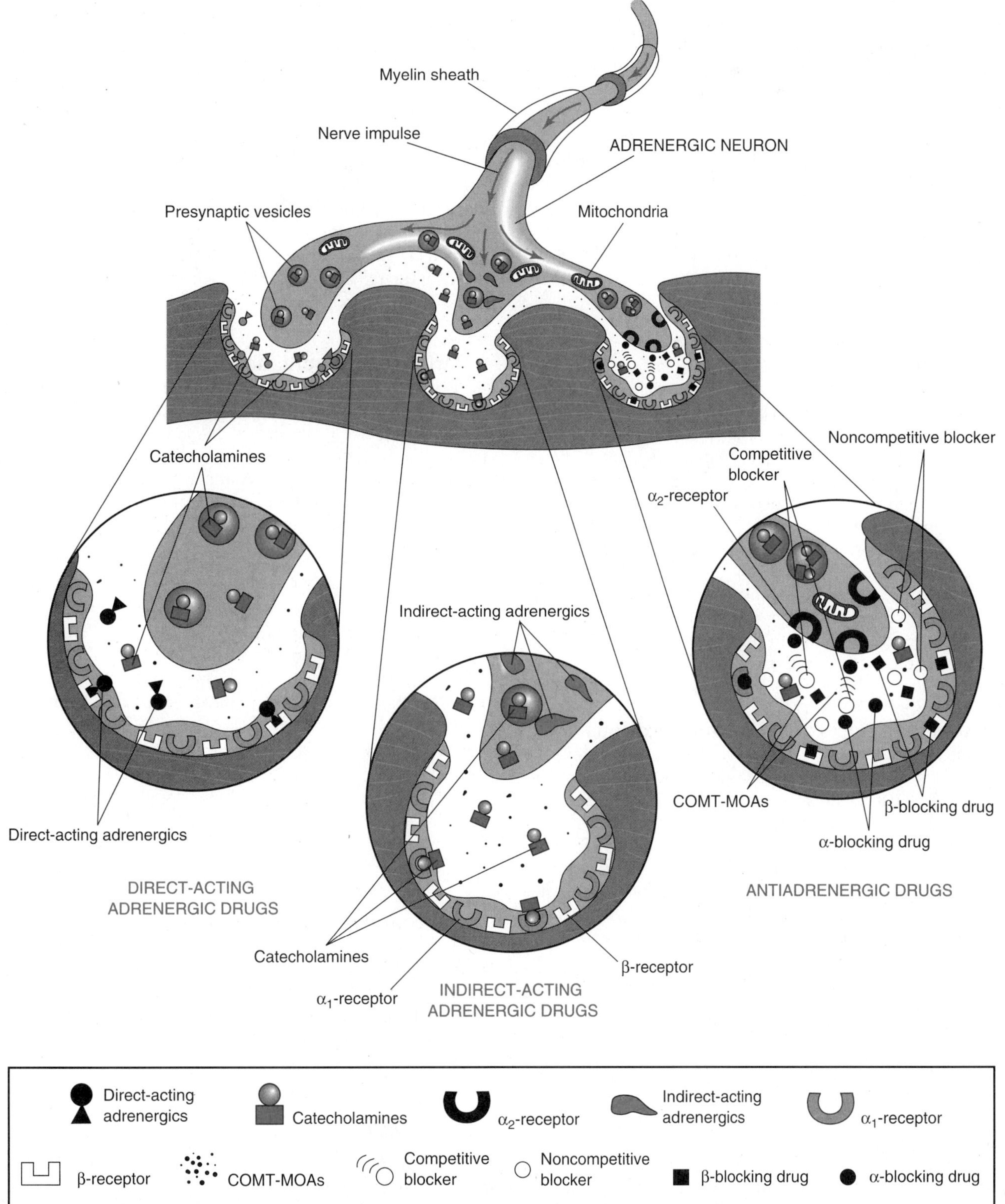

Figure 11–2 Sympathetic drug action. Catecholamines such as norepinephrine and epinephrine are normally released from storage sites within the adrenergic neuron with the arrival of a nerve impulse. Most adrenergic drugs directly mimic the action of these catecholamines on alpha or beta receptors. In contrast, indirect acting adrenergic drugs operate by first triggering the release of catecholamines from presynaptic vesicles. The neurotransmitters, in turn, activate alpha and beta receptors. Antiadrenergic drugs (i.e., alpha and beta blockers) are receptor specific or nonspecific and act by noncompetitive or competitive blocking activity of catecholamines at receptor sites. The catecholamines are degraded by monoamine oxidase (MAO) or by catechol-*O*-methyltransferase (COMT) in the synapse.

ions or intracellular enzymes. This, in turn, stimulates intracellular metabolism and production of other enzymes, structural proteins, and other products required for cell function and reproduction. The exception to this is activation of alpha$_2$ receptors on presynaptic membranes. Activation of alpha$_2$ receptors inhibits the release of additional norepinephrine.

Because most body tissues possess both alpha and beta receptors, drug effects depend largely on the drug's ability to activate specific receptors (see Table II–2) and the number of receptors available. Some drugs act on both alpha and beta receptors, whereas others are more discriminating, acting only on specific receptor subtypes. For example, alpha$_1$ activation of blood vessels results in vasoconstriction, blood pressure elevation, and a reduction in nasal congestion. Activation of beta$_1$ receptors in the heart results in an increased force of myocardial contraction (i.e., positive inotropic action) and an increased heart rate. Activation of beta$_2$ receptors in the lungs results in bronchodilation. Activation of beta$_2$ receptors in blood vessels results in vasodilation with increased blood flow to the heart, brain, and skeletal muscles, tissues essential for the fight or flight response. Other effects of adrenergic drugs include contraction of GI and urinary sphincters, decreased GI tone, lipolysis, changes in renin secretion, uterine relaxation, hepatic glycogenolysis and gluconeogenesis, and decreased insulin secretion.

In contrast, indirect-acting adrenergic drugs (e.g., phenylephrine, ephedrine) operate by first triggering the release of catecholamines from presynaptic vesicles. The neurotransmitters, in turn, activate alpha and beta receptors.

Adverse Effects and Contraindications

The adverse effects of adrenergic agonists are essentially extensions of their therapeutic effects. Adverse effects include nervousness, restlessness, insomnia, tremors, and headache. Tachycardia, arrhythmias, angina, and hypertension are present. A pink-red discoloration of saliva is noted with isoproterenol. A paradoxical bronchospasm has been noted with excessive use of adrenergic inhalers and pulmonary edema when terbutaline is used as a tocolytic agent.

Symptoms of drug overdose include persistent agitation, chest pain or discomfort, decreased blood pressure, dizziness, hyperglycemia, hypokalemia, seizures, tachyarrhythmias, persistent trembling, and vomiting.

Contraindications to the use of adrenergic agonists include cardiac arrhythmias, angina pectoris, hypertension, hyperthyroidism, cerebrovascular disease, narrow-angle glaucoma, and hypersensitivity to the drug or any component. Some of the drugs contain sulfites to which some persons are allergic. Adrenergic drugs are also contraindicated with local anesthesia of distal areas because of the potential for tissue damage and sloughing from vasoconstriction. The distal areas include the fingers, toes, ears, nose, and penis. Adrenergic drugs should also be avoided during the second stage of labor because they may delay progression. The drugs should be used with caution in patients with anxiety, insomnia, and psychiatric disorders because of their stimulant effects on the central nervous system (CNS) and in older adults because of their cardiac and CNS stimulating effects.

Pharmacokinetics

The pharmacokinetics of adrenergic drugs vary with the specific agent; however, because most of the drugs are given by the parenteral route, the time of drug onset ranges from immediate to 30 minutes. When given via the respiratory tract or any parenteral routes, effects occur almost immediately. Peak effects are noted immediately to 20 minutes. The duration of action for adrenergic agonists is short, often averaging minutes rather than hours (Table 11–1). The bioavailability of drugs given intravenously (IV) is 100 percent. Suspension formulations provide for a longer duration of drug action. Many adrenergic drugs are partially biotransformed by nerve endings through the monoamine oxidase system. The remaining circulating drug is biotransformed in the liver.

Drug-Drug Interactions

There is an increased risk of cardiac arrhythmias and pressor responses when adrenergic drugs are used in the presence of general anesthetics, digoxin, antihistamines, cocaine, monoamine oxidase inhibitors, thyroid hormones, and xanthines (Table 11–2). A number of other drugs cause increased bronchodilation. Because of the variety of drugs that interact with adrenergic agonists, the health care provider is advised to check for interactions before administering the drug.

Dosage Regimen

The dosage of adrenergic agonists depends on the specific drug and its use. For example, dopamine is used to maintain renal perfusion at a dosage range that is different from that used when dopamine is given to increase peripheral vascular resistance (Table 11–3) although the drug is given IV in both instances. Epinephrine on the other hand can be given subcutaneously, by the intramuscular route, as well as IV, with each route requiring different dosages. The dosage of many of these drugs is titrated based on the patient's response.

Laboratory Considerations

Adrenergic drugs may cause transient decreases in serum potassium concentrations when they are administered via nebulizer or in higher than recommended concentrations. Hypokalemia is rare at recommended dosages. Epinephrine may cause an increase in blood glucose and serum lactic acid concentrations.

Alpha Blockers

- ❐ Dihydroergotamine (DHE 45); (✱) DIHYDROERGOTAMINE-SANDOZ
- ❐ Doxazosin (CARDURA)
- ❐ Ergotamine; (✱) ERGOMAR
- ❐ Methysergide (SANSERT)
- ❐ Phenoxybenzamine (DIBENZYLINE)
- ❐ Phentolamine mesylate (REGITINE)
- ❐ Tamsulosin (FLOMAX)
- ❐ Terazosin (HYTRIN)
- ❐ Tolazoline (PRISCOLINE)

TABLE 11–1 PHARMACOKINETICS OF SELECTED SYMPATHETIC NERVOUS SYSTEM DRUGS

Drug	Route	Onset	Peak	Duration	PB (%)	$t_{1/2}$	BioA (%)
Alpha and Beta Agonists							
Dopamine	IV	1–2 min	10 min	Duration of infusion	UA	2 min	100
Epinephrine	IV	Immed	20 min	20–30 min	UA	UK	100
	SC	6–12 min	20 min	<1–4 hr			UA
	IM	6–12 min	20 min	<1–4 hr			
	INH	3–5 min	UK	1–3 hr			
Norepinephrine	IV	Rapid	Immed	1–2 min	UA	UK	100
Alpha Agonists							
Metaraminol	IV	1–2 min	UK	15–20 min	UA	UK	100
	SC	15–20 min		20–60 min			UA
	IM	10 min					
Phenylephrine	IV	Immed	UK	15–20 min	UA	UK	100
	SC	10–15 min	UK	1–2 hr			UA
	IM						
Beta Agonists							
Dobutamine	IV	1–2 min	10 min	Duration of infusion	UA	2 min	100
Isoetharine	INH	5 min	UA	1–3 hr	UA	UA	UA
Isoproterenol	IV	Immediate	UA	Duration of infusion	UA	1–2 min	100
Alpha Blockers							
Dihydroergotamine	IV	15–30 min	15 min–2hr	3–4 hr	UA	2.3–1.4 hr; 18–32 hr*	100
	SC						UA
	IM						
Doxazosin	po	1–2 hr	2–6 hr	24 hr	98	22 hr	UA
Ergotamine	SL	Rapid	½–3 hr	UA	UA	2.7 hr; 21 hr*	60
Phenoxybenzamine	po	2 hr	4–6 hr	3–4 days	UA	24 hr	20–30
Phentolamine	IV	Immed	2 min	15–30 min	UA	19 min	100
Tamsulosin	po	UA	5 days	UA	94–99	9–15 hr	>90
Terazosin	po	15 min; 2–6 wk†	6–8 wk; UK†	24 hr; UK	94	12 hr	UA
Tolazoline	IV	Varies	30–60 min	3–4 hr	UA	1.5–41 hr	100
Postganglionic Inhibitors							
Guanadrel	po	2 hr	4–6 hr	9 hr	UA	12 hr	UA
Guanethidine‡	po	1–3 wk	1–3 wk	1–3 wk	UA	5 days	UA
Reserpine	po	Days–3 wks	3–6 wk	1–6 wk	0	11 days	40–50
Miscellaneous							
Sumatriptan	po	<30 min	2–4 hr	24 hr	UA	2 hr	UA
	SC	30 min	To 2 hr				

*Dihydroergotamine and ergotamine have biphasic half-lives, phase one and phase two, respectively.
† Terazosin's onset time and peak effects after a single dose used for hypertension and prostatic hypertrophy, respectively.
‡Guanethidine's antihypertensive effects during chronic therapy. Effects are more rapidly achieved with loading doses. Maximum effects occur 8 hours after a single dose.
PB, Protein binding; $t_{1/2}$, elimination half-life; NA, not applicable; UA, unavailable; UK, unknown; INH, inhalation; BioA, bioavailability.

Indications

The alpha blockers are used to improve cerebral circulation. They may also be used in the management of pheochromocytoma and in select cases of hypertension, especially when the hypertension is associated with increased sympathetic nervous system activity.

Both phenoxybenzamine and phentolamine may be used by continuous IV infusion in a patient with pheochromocytoma crisis or in a patient with pressor crisis associated with clonidine or propranolol withdrawal, or use of MAO inhibitors. MAO inhibitors are still marketed as antihypertensives but more often as antidepressants. MAO inhibitors may be associated with a hypertensive crisis after the ingestion of certain foods containing tyramine such as Chianti wine, marinated foods, and certain cheeses.

The $alpha_1$ blockers (e.g., doxazosin, tamsulosin, terazosin) have been used for the treatment of obstructive uropathy resulting from benign prostatic hyperplasia. Phentolamine may be used intracavernosally with papaverine as adjunct therapy for impotence. Phentolamine is also used intracavernosally for the prevention and treatment of dermal necrosis and sloughing following IV administration or extravasation of norepinephrine and dopamine.

Unlabeled uses for alpha blockers include frostbite sequelae and Raynaud's acrocyanosis to improve circulation in peripheral vasospastic conditions. Phenoxybenzamine may also be used as an adjunct treatment of shock.

Ergotamine, dihydroergotamine, and methysergide are used in the management of vascular headaches (e.g., migraine, cluster).

Pharmacodynamics

Hemodynamically, the alpha blockers reduce arterial pressure by reducing total peripheral resistance. The reduc-

TABLE 11–2 DRUG-DRUG INTERACTIONS OF SELECTED SYMPATHETIC NERVOUS SYSTEM DRUGS

Drug	Interactive Drugs	Interaction
Alpha and beta agonists		
	General anesthetics	Increased risk of arrhythmias
	Digoxin	
	Anticholinergics	Increased bronchial relaxation and mydriasis
	Tricyclic antidepressants	Increased pressor response with IV epinephrine
	Antihistamines	May increase pressor effects
	Doxapram	
	Methylphenidate	
	Cocaine	Increases pressor and mydriatic effects, risk for arrhythmias, seizures, acute glaucoma
	Ergot alkaloids	Increased vasoconstriction and extremely high blood pressure
	Monoamine oxidase inhibitors	Increased risk of arrhythmias, respiratory depression, acute hypertensive crisis, seizures, coma, and death
	Thyroid hormones	Increased adrenergic effects and possible arrhythmias
	Xanthines	Enhanced bronchodilating effect, excessive CNS stimulation, arrhythmias, emotional disturbances, insomnia
	Beta blockers	May augment hypertensive response and decrease bronchodilating effect of adrenergic
	Anticholinesterase drugs	Decreased mydriatic effects of adrenergic
	Antihypertensives	Decreases pressor effects of adrenergics
	Phentolamine	
	Antipsychotic drugs	Block vasopressor effect of epinephrine
Alpha Blockers		
Dihydroergotamine	Antihypertensives	Additive effects of interactive drug
Ergotamine	CNS depressants	
Methysergide	Epinephrine	
Phentolamine	NSAIDs	
Phenoxybenzamine	Sumatriptan	Prolonged vasoconstriction
	Nitrates	Antagonizes effects of interactive drug
	Alpha-adrenergic agonists	Increased risk of peripheral vasoconstriction
	Beta blockers	
	Oral contraceptives	
	Vasoconstrictors	
	Macrolide antibiotics	
	Nicotine	
	Estrogens	Sodium and fluid retention, decreased antihypertensive effects of alpha blocker
	Oral contraceptives	
	NSAIDs	
Terazosin	Alcohol	Additive hypotension
	Antihypertensive drugs	
	Nitrates	
	Estrogens	May decrease the effects of antihypertensive therapy
	NSAIDs	
	Sympathomimetics	
Doxazosin	Alcohol	Additive hypotension
	Antihypertensive drugs	
	Nitrates	
	NSAIDs	May decrease antihypertensive effects
	Clonidin	May decrease antihypertensive effects of clonidine
Tamsulosin	Alpha blockers	Additive effects
	Cimetidine	Increased effects of tamulosin
	Warfarin	

CNS, Central nervous system; NSAIDs, nonsteroidal anti-inflammatory agents.

tion in pressure occurs without the associated baroreceptor reflex increase in heart rate, cardiac output, and contractility. Phentolamine and phenoxybenzamine block both presynaptic and postsynaptic alpha receptors to the action of norepinephrine.

Terazosin, tamsulosin, and doxazosin act by selectively blocking alpha$_1$ receptors. Blockade of these receptors causes smooth muscles in the bladder neck and prostate to relax, resulting in improvement in urine flow rate and a reduction in symptoms of BPH.

Ergotamine and similar drugs have agonist and antagonist actions with alpha adrenergic, serotonergic, and dopaminergic receptors. These drugs directly stimulate vascular smooth muscle, thus constricting arteries and veins. They may also inhibit the reuptake of norepinephrine.

Adverse Effects and Contraindications

The adverse effects of alpha blockers include tachycardia, arrhythmias, angina, abdominal pain, nausea, vomiting, and

TABLE 11–2 DRUG-DRUG INTERACTIONS OF SELECTED SYMPATHETIC NERVOUS SYSTEM DRUG *Continued*

Drug	Interactive Drugs	Interaction
Post Ganglionic Inhibitors		
Guanadrel	Beta blockers	Increases the risk of excessive orthostatic hypotension
	Vasodilators	
	NSAIDs	Decreased antihypertensive effects of guanadrel
	Phenothiazines	
	Sympathomimetics	
	Tricyclic antidepressants	
	Direct-acting sympathomimetics	May increase effects of interactive drugs
Guanethidine	Haloperidol	Hypotensive effects may be decreased by interactive drug
	Methylphenidate	
	MAO inhibitors	
	Nitrates	Decrease the antihypertensive effects of guanethidine
	NSAIDs	
	Oral contraceptives	
	Epinephrine	Increased pressor response and risk of arrhythmias
	Norepinephrine	
	Phenylephrine	
	Metaraminol	
	Methoxamine	
	Minoxidil	Profound hypotension
Reserpine	Alcohol	Additive hypotension
	Antihypertensives	
	Nitrates	
	Antiarrhythmic drugs	Increased risk of arrhythmias
	Cardiac glycosides	
	Procainamide	
	Quinidine	
	MAO inhibitors	Excitement and increased risk of hypertension
	Ephedrine	Decreased therapeutic response of interactive drug
	Levodopa	
	Dobutamine	Increased responsiveness to interactive drug
	Dopamine	
	Metaraminol	
	Phenylephrine	
	Alcohol	Additive CNS depression
	Antidepressants	
	Antihistamines	
	CNS depressants	
	Opioids	
	Sedative-hypnotics	
	NSAIDs	Decreased effectiveness of reserpine
Miscellaneous		
Sumatriptan	Ergotamine	Increased risk of vasospastic reactions
	Lithium	Combined effects of interactive drugs is unknown
	MAO inhibitors	
	SSRIs	

CNS, Central nervous system; MAO, monoamine oxidase; NSAIDs, nonsteroidal anti-inflammatory drugs; SSRIs, selective serotonin reuptake inhibitors.

diarrhea. Nasal stuffiness, weakness, and dizziness are also possible. The most life-threatening adverse effects include cerebrovascular spasm, hypotension, and myocardial infarction.

Alpha blockers are contraindicated in patients with hypersensitivity, peripheral vascular disease, severe hypertension, cardiovascular or renal disease, and atrioventricular (AV) block. Caution should be used when $alpha_1$ blocking drugs are used with patients who have chronic renal failure or hypertensive patients with cerebral thrombosis. Caution should also be used in men with sickle cell trait. CNS adverse effects include dizziness, headache, drowsiness, fatigue, weakness, and depression.

The common adverse effects of ergot preparations include numbness, tingling of fingers and toes, extremity muscle pain, nausea and vomiting (the drug stimulates the chemoreceptor trigger zone), precordial distress and pain, transient tachycardia, bradycardia, localized edema, and itching. Ergotism may occur with prolonged use. Symptoms of ergotism include nausea, vomiting, diarrhea, severe thirst, hypoperfusion, chest pain, blood pressure changes, and confusion. Drug dependence and abuse may occur with extended use. Neutropenia and eosinophilia are noted with methysergide but not with the other ergot preparations.

Pharmacokinetics

Phentolamine is well absorbed following intramuscular (IM) administration. Its distribution and half-life are un-

TABLE 11–3 DOSAGE REGIMEN FOR SELECTED SYMPATHETIC NERVOUS SYSTEM DRUGS

Drug	Use(s)	Dosage	Implications
Alpha and Beta Agonists			
Dopamine	Maintain renal perfusion	*Adults:* 0.5–3 mcg/kg/min IV *Child:* 5–20 mcg/kg/min IV based on desired response	Correct hypovolemia with volume expanders before initiating dopamine therapy. Give through large vein. Increase infusion rate as needed. Extravasation may cause severe irritation, Extravasation tissue necrosis and sloughing *Common dilution:* 250 mg/500 mL; 400 mg/500 mL; 800 mg/500 mL
	Improve cardiac output	*Adults:* 2–10 mcg/kg/min IV *Child:* 5–20 mcg/kg/min IV based on desired response	
	Increase peripheral vascular resistance	*Adults:* 10 mcg/kg/min IV *Child:* 5–20 mcg/kg/min IV based on desired response	
Epinephrine	Anaphylaxis	*Adults:* 0.1–0.5 mg SC/IM. Single dose not to exceed 1 mg. May repeat q10–15 min *or* 0.1–0.25 mg IV q5–15 min. May be followed by 1–4 mcg/min continuous infusion *Child:* 0.1 mg IV. May be followed by 0.1 mcg/kg/min continuous infusion	Assess breath sounds, respiratory pattern, and blood pressure before giving and during time of peak drug effects. Observe patient for tolerance and paradoxical or rebound bronchospasm *Common dilution:* 1 mg/250 mL = 4 mcg/mL 4.0 mcg/min = 60 mL/hr
	Cardiopulmonary resuscitation	*Adults:* 0.01 mg/kg IV. May repeat q3–5 min. May be followed by 1–4 mcg/min IV continuous infusion *or* 0.3–0.5 mg intracardiac *or* 1 mg endotracheal *or* for 1 mcg/min initially for bradycardia. Adjust as needed to range of 2–10 mcg/min *Child:* 0.01 mg/kg IV. May repeat q3–5 min. May be followed by 0.1 mcg/kg/min IV continuous infusion *or* 0.1–0.2 mg/kg endotracheal. May repeat q3–5 min	Monitor BP, pulse, ECG, and respiratory rate, hemodynamic parameters, and urinary output frequently during administration. Notify health care provider if chestpain, arrhythmias, heart rate over 100 bpm or hypertension develop
	Chronic airway limitation	*Adults:* 0.1–0.5 mg SC/IM. Repeat q20 min–4 hr single dose not to exceed 1 mg *or* 1 puff of MDI (200–275 mcg). May repeat after 1–2 min. Additional doses repeated q3hr *or* 1 INH of 1% solution. May repeat after 1–2 min. Additional doses given q3hr	Assess breath sounds, respiratory pattern, and blood pressure before administration and during time of peak drug effects. Observe patient for tolerance and paradoxical or rebound bronchospasm
Norepinephrine	Shock	*Adults:* 0.5–1 mcg/min initially. Range: 2–12 mcg/min depending on BP *Child:* 0.1 mcg/kg/min up to 1 mcg/kg/min depending on BP	Correct hypovolemia with volume expanders before initiating therapy
Alpha Agonists			
Metaraminol	Prevention and treatment of hypotension	*Adults:* 2–10 mg SC/IM *or* 15–100 mg in 250–500 mL sodium chloride or 5% dextrose solution IV. Adjust rate to maintain desired BP	At least 10 minutes should elapse between successive doses so that effects of previous dose are fully apparent. Adjust concentration based on patient's need for fluid.
Phenylephrine	Hypotension associated with shock	*Adult:* 100–180 mcg/min IV initally. Maintenance: 40–60 mcg/min *or* 2–5 mg SC/IM q10–15 min Initial dose not to exceed 5 mg	Monitor BP every 2–3 minutes until stabilized and every 5 minutes thereafter during IV administration. Monitor ECG continuously. Avoid extravasation *Common dilution:* 10 mg/500 mL = 20 mcg/mL 0.04 mg/min = 120 mL/hr
Beta Agonists			
Dobutamine	Short-term mangement of heart failure due to depressed contractility	*Adults:* 2.5–15 mcg/kg/min IV to increase cardiac output. Rates above 40 mcg/kg/min are rarely needed *Child:* 5–20 mcg/kg/min IV although safety and efficacy have not been established	Continuously monitor BP, heart rate, PCWP, cardiac output, CVP, and urinary output during therapy. Palpate peripheral pulses.Notify health care provider if arrhythmias occur, changes in VS, or if quality of pulse declines or extremities become cold or mottled *Common dilution:* 250 mg/1000 mL; 500 mg/1000 mL; 1000 mg/1000 mL

TABLE 11–3 DOSAGE REGIMEN FOR SELECTED SYMPATHETIC NERVOUS SYSTEM DRUGS *Continued*

Drug	Use(s)	Dosage	Implications
Beta Agonists *Continued*			
Isoetharine	Acute bronchospasm	*Adults:* 4 INH undiluted. May repeat up to 5 times/daily. Range: 3–7 INH *or* 1–2 INH by MDI q4hr *or* 0.5–1 mL of 0.5% *or* 0.5 mL of 1% solution diluted 1:3 by IPPB or nebulizer	Monitor rate, depth, rhythm of respirations, pulse quality, breath sounds, ABGs. Notify health care provider if changes in VS, hand tremors develop, quality of pulse declines or extremities become cold or mottled
Isoproterenol	Management heart block and shock	*Adults:* 10 mg SL initially with dose adjusted as needed. Range 5–50 mg *or* 0.5–5 mcg/min IV infusion *Child:* 5–10 mg SL. Not to exceed 30 mg/day, more than three doses/day, or more often than q3–4 hr *or* 0.1 mcg/kg/min IV initially. Adjust dose based on response. Range 0.1–1 mcg/kg/min	Frequently monitor BP, pulse, ECG, and respiratory rate, hemodynamic parameters, and urinary output during administration.Notify health care provider if chest pain, arrhythmias, heart rate over 100 bpm, or hypertension develop. Adjust dosage to keep heart rate under 110 bpm. *Common dilution:* 2 mg/500 mL 2 mcg/min = 30 mL/hr
	Reversible airway disease	*Adults:* 10–20 mg SL not to exceed 60 mg/day, more than three doses/day, or more often than q3–4 hr *or* 1–2 INH by MDI four to six times daily *or* 6–12 INH by nebulizer q15 min for three treatments up to eight times daily *or* 2 mL of 0.125% solution or 0.5 mL of 0.1% solution IPPB over 10–20 min *Child:* 5–10 mg SL not to exceed 30 mg/day, three doses/day, or more often than q3–4 hr *or* 1–2 INH by MDI four to six times daily *or* 6–12 INH by nebulizer q15 min for 3 treatments up to 8 times daily.	Assess breath sounds, respiratory pattern and blood pressure before giving and during time of peak drug effects. Observepatient for tolerance and paradoxical orrebound bronchospasm
	Cardiac standstill	*Adults:* 20–60 mcg IV initially followed with 10–200 mcg as bolus or 5 mcg/min continuous infusion	Monitor BP, pulse, ECG, and respiratory rate, hemodynamic parameters, and urinary output frequently during administration. Notify health care provider if chest pain, arrhythmias, heart rate over 100 bpm, or hypertension develop
Alpha Blockers			
Dihydroergotamine	Vascular headaches (migraine, cluster)	*Adults:* 1 mg SC/IM. May repeat in 1 hr to total of 3 mg. Not to exceed 3 mg/day or 6 mg/wk *or* 0.5 mg IV. May repeat in 1 hr. Not to exceed 2 mg/day or 6 mg/wk *or* 0.5–1 mg IV q8hr until relief. Not to exceed 6 mg/wk *Child age 12–16 yr:* 0.25–0.5 mg IV. One or two more doses may be given q20 min *Child age 9–12 yr:* 0.2 mg IV. 1–2 more doses may be given q20 min *Child age 6–9 yr:* 0.1–0.15 mg IV. One or two more doses may be given q20 min	Monitor BP and peripheral pulses during therapy. Inform health care provider if significant hypertension or signs of ergotism (cold, numb fingers, toes, nausea, vomiting, headache, muscle pain, weakness) develop
Doxazosin	Benign prostatic hypertrophy	Adults: 1 mg po initially once daily. May double the dose every 1–2 weeks. Maximum: 8 mg/day	Monitor BP and pulse 2–6 hr after first dose, with each increase in dose, and periodically throughout therapy
	Hypertension	Adults: 1 mg po once daily. May increase gradually at 2 week intervals to 2–16 mg/day	The incidence of postural hypotension is greatly increased at dosages greater than 4 mg/day.
Ergotamine	Vascular headaches (migraine, cluster)	*Adults:* 2 mg po/SL initially then 1–2 mg q30 min until attack subsides or a total of 6 mg has been given	Not to exceed two times weekly, with at least 5 days between courses
Methysergide	Prophylaxis of vascular headaches	*Adults:* 2–3 mg po BID with meals.	Titrate dose to patient response. Report dyspnea, paresthesias, urinary difficulty, pain in abdomen, chest, back, and legs. Observe for development of retroperitoneal fibrosis during long-term therapy

TABLE 11–3 DOSAGE REGIMEN FOR SELECTED SYMPATHETIC NERVOUS SYSTEM DRUGS *Continued*

Drug	Use(s)	Dosage	Implications
Phentolamine	Hypertension associated with pheochromocytoma, adrenergic excess, tyramine-containing foods in patients on MAO inhibitors or clonidine withdrawal	*Adults:* 5 mg IV given 1–2 hr preop. May repeat as necessary or be infused at a rate of 0.5–1 mg/min during surgery *Child:* 1 mg or 0.1 mg/kg (3 mg/m^2) IM/IV 1–2 hr preop. May repeat IV as necessary during surgery	Monitor BP, pulse, ECG every 2 minutes until stable during IV administration. Epinephrine is contraindicated if hypotensive crisis occurs and may cause paradoxical further decrease in blood pressure. Norepinephrine may be used to treat hypotensive crisis
Phenoxybenzamine	Hypertension associated with pheochromocytoma, partial prostatic obstruction, neurogenic bladder	*Adults:* 10 mg po initially BID. Increase dosage every other day until an optimal dosage is obtained. Range: 20–40 mg po BID–TID *Child:* 1–2 mg/kg/day po in divided doses q6–8 hr	Monitor BP and heart rate carefully. Do not ingest alcohol
Tamsulosin	Benign prostatic hypertrophy	*Adults:* 0.4 mg po once daily. May increase to 0.8 mg daily after 2–4 weeks if response is inadequate	Administer approximately 30 minutes following the same meal each day. If therapy is interrupted, resume at 0.4 mg po once daily and retitrate
Terazosin	Benign prostatic hypertrophy	*Adults:* 1 mg po initially at bedtime. Titrate upwards to 10 mg once daily. Maximum: 20 mg/day	Re-evaluate patient in 6 weeks if no response. Rule out prostate cancer and syncope before use
Tolazoline	Persistent pulmonary hypertension in newborns	*Infants:* 1–2 mg/kg IV initially, then 0.2 mg/kg/hr for each 1 mg/kg loading dose	Dosage reduction required for renal impairment
Postganglionic Blockers			
Guanadrel	Adjunct to moderate to severe hypertension	*Adults:* 5 mg po BID. Increase weekly or monthly as needed. Maintenance: 20–75 mg po in two to four divided doses *Child:* Safety and efficacy have not been established	Dosage adjustments should not be made unless there is no decrease in BP when taken supine and after standing for 10 minutes. Inform patient that severity of adverse effects usually lessens after the first 8 weeks of therapy. Usually given with diuretics to reduce tolerance and fluid retention
Guanethidine	Adjunct to moderate to severe hypertension	*Adults:* 10 mg po daily. May increase q5–7 days by 10–25 mg/day. Maintenance: single 25–50 mg dose. Hospitalized patients: 25–50 mg po initial dose. May increase by 25–50 mg/day or every other day as needed. *Child:* 0.2 mg/kg/day po as a single oral dose. Increase by 0.2 mg/kg/day every 7–10 days. Maximum: 3 mg/kg/day	For severely hypertensive adult patient a loading dose is given three times daily q6hr (no nighttime dose) for 1–3 days. Usually given with diuretics to reduce tolerance and fluid retention. Note prominently on patient chart that guanethidine is in use if emergency surgery is required
Reserpine	Adjunct to mild to moderate hypertension	*Adults:* 100–250 mcg/day po *Child:* 5–20 mcg/kg/day (150–600 mcg/m^2/day) in one to two divided doses	Monitor BP and pulse frequently during initial dosage adjustment and periodically thereafter
Miscellaneous			
Sumatriptan	Migraine headaches	*Adults:* 25 mg po initially. May increase to 100 mg as necessary *or* 6 mg SC. May repeat after 1 hour, not to exceed 12 mg in 24 hours	If headache recurs, doses may be repeated q2hr, not to exceed 300 mg/day. If potherapy is to follow SC injection, additional po drug may be taken q2hr, not to exceed 200 mg/day

known. The peak effects after IM administration are reached in 20 minutes, with a duration of drug action of 30 to 45 minutes. The onset of action when the drug is given IV is 10 minutes, with a duration of 4 hours.

Thirty percent of phenoxybenzamine is absorbed from the GI tract. Onset of action is 2 hours, with peak activity noted in 4 to 6 hours. Drug action lasts 3 to 4 days. Phenoxybenzamine has a cumulative effect. The onset of therapeutic effects may not occur until 2 weeks of therapy. Full therapeutic effects may not be apparent for several more weeks. Phenoxybenzamine accumulates in adipose tissue. The half-life is 24 hours; 80 percent is eliminated in urine and bile within 24 hours. Phenoxybenzamine is biotransformed in the liver.

Ergotamine is unpredictably absorbed from the GI tract. Oral absorption can be enhanced in the presence of caffeine. Sublingual absorption is poor. Dihydroergotamine is rapidly absorbed following SC or IM administration. Both ergotamine and dihydroergotamine are highly biotransformed (90 percent) in the liver, with elimination being a biphasic process.

Methysergide is rapidly absorbed from the GI tract and is widely distributed. Peak effects occur in 1 to 2 days. It is biotransformed in the liver to an active metabolite. The half-life of methysergide is approximately 10 hours.

Drug-Drug Interactions

Phentolamine use with other antihypertensives increases hypotensive effects. Epinephrine, guanethidine, and guanadrel increase hypotension and bradycardia. Dopamine decreases peripheral vasoconstriction.

Phenoxybenzamine interacts with compounds that stimulate both alpha- and beta-adrenergic receptors to produce an exaggerated hypotensive response and tachycardia. Tricyclic antidepressants, alcohol, and nitrates increase the hypotensive effect of phenoxybenzamine. MAO inhibitors block the antihypertensive effect of phenoxybenzamine.

Concurrent use of ergot preparations with beta blockers, oral contraceptives, vasoconstrictors, macrolide antibiotics, and nicotine (smoking) may increase the risk of peripheral vasoconstriction. Dihydroergotamine antagonizes the antianginal effects of nitrates. Concurrent use of sumatriptan (see later) may result in prolonged vasoconstriction.

Dosage Regimen

The dosage regimens of alpha blockers vary significantly depending on the use of the individual drugs (see Table 11–3). For example, phentolamine is administered 1 to 2 hours preoperatively for patients with hypertension related to pheochromocytoma. On the other hand, doxazosin is taken on a daily basis. Ergot preparations are taken by mouth prophylactically for migraine headaches; however, during an acute episode, the drugs may be given subcutaneously, IM or IV. Alpha blockers used in the management of prostatic hyperplasia are usually taken on a daily basis.

Laboratory Considerations

Phenoxybenzamine may increase urinary norepinephrine levels, but there are no significant laboratory considerations for phentolamine, ergotamine, and dihydroergotamine. Methysergide may increase blood urea nitrogen levels.

Beta Blockers

Although beta blockers are considered sympathetic nervous system drugs, they are most often used in the management of cardiovascular disorders such as hypertension, tachyarrhythmias, angina pectoris, hypertrophic subaortic stenosis, migraine prophylaxis, prevention of myocardial infarction, glaucoma (e.g., betaxolol, levobunolol, metipranolol, and timolol), pheochromocytoma, tremors (e.g. propranolol), and the symptoms of hyperthyroidism.

Beta blockers act by competing with the neurotransmitters epinephrine and norepinephrine for beta-receptor sites. Beta-receptor sites are primarily located in the heart, where blockade results in increased heart rate, contractility, and AV conduction. $Beta_2$ receptors are found primarily in bronchial and vascular smooth muscle. Stimulation of $beta_2$ receptors produces vasodilation and bronchodilation. Blockade of beta receptors antagonizes the effects of the neurotransmitters.

Nonselective beta blockers block both $beta_1$ and $beta_2$ receptors. Selective beta blockers block either $beta_1$ or $beta_2$ receptors. These nonselective and selective beta-blocking drugs are discussed further in Chapter 34 in relation to their use in hypertension, Chapter 35 in relation to their use as an antiarrhythmic drug, and in Chapters 46, 47, 48, and 62 in relation to their use in respiratory and ophthalmic disorders.

These drugs are contraindicated in patients with heart failure or obstructive airway disease, acute bronchospasm, some forms of valvular heart disease, bradyarrhythmias, and heart block. They should be used with caution in patients with any form of lung disease, or underlying compensated heart failure. They should also be used with caution in patients with diabetes or severe liver disease. Further, they should not be discontinued abruptly in patients with cardiovascular disease.

Beta blockers may cause additive myocardial depression and bradycardia when they are used with other drugs also having these effects (e.g., cardiac glycosides, certain antiarrhythmics). They can antagonize the therapeutic effects of bronchodilating drugs and alter insulin requirements in patients with diabetes. Cimetidine, a $histamine_2$ antagonist, may decrease biotransformation of the beta blocker and increase its effects.

Postganglionic Blockers

- ❐ Guanadrel (HYLOREL)
- ❐ Guanethidine (ISMELIN); (✱)
- ❐ Reserpine; (✱) NOVO-RESERPINE

Indications

Postganglionic blockers are alternative drugs for hypertension (see also Chapter 34). In recent years, as a result of the introduction of newer drugs having less bothersome adverse effects, postganglionic blockers are now used only in hypertensive emergencies.

The principal indication for reserpine is hypertension. Reserpine can also be used to treat agitated psychotic patients. An unlabeled use for reserpine is to reduce vasospastic attacks in patients with Raynaud's phenomenon. Reserpine has also been used for short-term symptomatic treatment of thyrotoxicosis.

The postganglionic blockers guanadrel, guanethidine, and reserpine as used in the treatment of hypertension are commonly administered with other drugs such as thiazide diuretics or hydralazine to increase their effectiveness and prevent resistance to their antihypertensive effects. Guanethidine has limited indications for hypertension because of the risk of profound orthostatic hypotension. Unlabeled uses for guanethidine include chronic open-angle glaucoma and endocrine ophthalmopathy.

Pharmacodynamics

These rauwolfia alkaloids have varying potencies and abilities to deplete neuronal tissue (brain, adrenal, and postganglionic sympathetic nerve endings) of the biogenic amines.

The long-term effects of rauwolfia alkaloids result from their ability to inhibit the storage of norepinephrine within the vesicles in adrenergic nerve endings. This leads to depletion of catecholamine stores.

Reserpine interferes with the binding of serotonin at receptor sites. Reserpine decreases the synthesis of norepinephrine by depleting dopamine, its precursor, and competitively inhibiting reuptake in storage granules.

There are two mechanisms by which reserpine depletes norepinephrine from postganglionic sympathetic neurons. First, reserpine acts on vesicles within the nerve terminal to cause displacement of stored norepinephrine. Reserpine suppresses norepinephrine synthesis.

Postganglionic blockers include guanethidine and guanadrel. Guanethidine has been used in the last 35 years in patients with more severe hypertension. Guanadrel has been introduced in recent years for patients with less severe hypertension. Both drugs demonstrate hemodynamic effects similar to those of other ganglion-blocking drugs without inhibition of parasympathetic effects. There is a slight fall in arteriolar resistance, peripheral venodilation, and decreased venous return to the heart with decreased cardiac output. Cardiovascular reflexive adjustments and reduced renal blood flow may impair renal excretory function.

By depleting sympathetic neurons of norepinephrine, reserpine decreases the activation of alpha and beta adrenergic receptors. Decreasing alpha activation promotes vasodilation. Decreasing activation of beta receptors slows heart rate and reduces cardiac output. The outcome is decreased blood pressure.

Adverse Effects and Contraindications

The most common adverse effects of guanadrel include fatigue, headache, fainting, drowsiness, visual disturbances, paresthesias, and confusion. Anorexia, glossitis, increased bowel movements, constipation, and gas pains and indigestion are also common. Nocturia, urinary urgency or frequency, peripheral edema, ejaculation disturbances, and impotence have been noted. Some patients also complain of excessive weight gain, weight loss, aching extremities, and leg cramps.

Guanadrel is contraindicated in patients with pheochromocytoma and heart failure (not due to hypertension), as well as in patients taking MAO inhibitors. Guanadrel is a pregnancy category B drug, although safe use in pregnant and nursing women has not been established. Guanadrel should be used cautiously in patients with asthma, coronary artery disease with insufficiency, or a recent myocardial infarction. These patients are at special risk of developing orthostatic hypotension. The drug should also be used with caution in patients who have an active peptic ulcer; ulcerative colitis (which may be aggravated by a relative increase in parasympathetic tone); peripheral vascular disease; and renal dysfunction. Caution should be employed when these drugs are used with the older adult patient.

Adverse effects of guanethidine include marked orthostatic and exertional hypotension with dizziness and lightheadedness. Cardiovascular effects include bradycardia, symptomatic sick sinus syndrome, angina, and edema with weight gain. Blurred vision and ptosis of the eyelids may occur, as well as nocturia, urinary retention, and incontinence. In men, impotence and inhibition of ejaculation may occur. Other adverse effects include dyspnea, fatigue, myalgia, asthma, and a rise in blood urea nitrogen levels.

Guanethidine is contraindicated in patients with pheochromocytoma or heart failure. It should be used cautiously in patients with diabetes mellitus, impaired renal or hepatic function, sinus bradycardia, limited cardiac reserve, coronary artery disease with insufficiency, or recent myocardial infarction. Guanethidine should also be used cautiously in older adults, patients with cerebrovascular insufficiency, and those with bronchial asthma.

The most common adverse effects of reserpine include drowsiness, lethargy, nasal stuffiness, dry mouth, nausea, abdominal cramps, and diarrhea. In addition, it can produce severe depression that persists months after the drug is withdrawn and can increase the risk of suicide. Reserpine can cause a parkinson-like syndrome with tremors and muscle rigidity. Respiratory depression, seizures, and hypothermia may also occur. The adverse effects of reserpine on the cardiovascular system include orthostatic hypotension, increased AV conduction time, angina, and arrhythmias. Impotence, impaired sexual function, breast engorgement, and menstrual irregularities may occur with reserpine.

Reserpine is contraindicated for patients with a history of depressive disorders, active peptic ulcer, ulcerative colitis, and gallstones, as well as for patients receiving electroconvulsive therapy. It should be used with caution in patients with cardiac, cerebrovascular, or renal insufficiency. Safe use during pregnancy and lactation or in children has not been established.

Pharmacokinetics

Guanadrel is rapidly absorbed following oral administration. Plasma concentrations peak in 1 to 2 hours. The half-life is about 10 hours, but there is great individual variability. Guanadrel is eliminated in the urine.

Guanethidine is completely absorbed by the GI tract. Guanethidine undergoes significant first-pass biotransformation by the liver. Three to fifty percent of the dose reaches systemic circulation. The peak effect occurs in 1 to 3 weeks.

The amount of guanethidine in plasma and urine is linearly related to dose. Large differences occur because of variation in absorption and biotransformation. It is incompletely absorbed (3 to 50 percent) from the GI tract following oral administration. Guanethidine is widely distributed to storage sites, including the adrenergic neurons. It does not appear to cross the blood-brain barrier. Adrenergic blockade occurs at a minimum concentration in plasma of 8 ng/mL; however, maximal effectiveness may take 1 to 3 weeks to become evident. Guanethidine is biotransformed in the liver but eliminated slowly because of extensive tissue binding. After chronic oral administration, the initial phase of elimination is 1 day, followed by a second phase of 4 to 8 days.

Forty to fifty percent of reserpine is absorbed following oral administration. It is widely distributed in tissues, especially adipose tissue. Reserpine crosses the blood-brain barrier and the placenta, and it is widely distributed in breast milk. It is not bound to plasma proteins. Reserpine is biotransformed in the liver, with at least 50 percent eliminated in feces as unabsorbed drug. Small amounts are eliminated unchanged by the kidneys. The half-life of reserpine is 11 days.

Drug-Drug Interactions

Guanadrel interacts with beta blockers or vasodilator drugs to increase the risk of excessive orthostatic hypotension. Thus, concurrent use of vasodilators is not recommended. The antihypertensive effects of guanadrel may be decreased with the concurrent use of phenothiazines, adrenergic agonists, nonsteroidal anti-inflammatory drugs, and tricyclic antidepressants. Abrupt withdrawal of tricyclic antidepressants may enhance guanadrel's effects.

The hypotensive effects of guanethidine are decreased by haloperidol, methylphenidate, MAO inhibitors, alcohol, levodopa, and nitrates may increase the hypotensive effects of guanethidine. Norepinephrine and phenylephrine increase the pressure and mydriatic effects of guanethidine. Oral contraceptives block the antihypertensive effect of guanethidine and increase hypertension.

Reserpine has additive hypotension when it is used with other antihypertensive drugs. Nitrates and alcohol ingestion potentiate hypotension. An increased risk of arrhythmias may occur with cardiac glycosides, quinidine, procainamide, and other antiarrhythmic drugs. Concurrent use of MAO inhibitors may cause excitement and hypertension. Reserpine may decrease the therapeutic response to ephedrine or levodopa. Patients receiving direct-acting sympathomimetic amines such as dopamine, dobutamine, metaraminol, and phenylephrine may demonstrate increased responses to those drugs.

Dosage Regimen

The dosage regimen of postganglionic blockers is individualized based on their use. The usual dose of guanadrel is 5 mg twice daily. Daily maintenance doses range from 20 to 75 mg in two to four divided doses. Three to four divided doses may be needed for larger dosages. The dosage is adjusted weekly or monthly until the blood pressure is controlled. The initial dosage should be reduced to 5 mg daily in older adults or those with renal disease for a creatinine clearance of 30 to 60 mL/min. Patients whose creatinine clearance values are less than 30 mL/min should receive 5 mg every 48 hours with the dosage cautiously adjusted at intervals of 7 to 14 days.

The initial doses of guanethidine should be small and the dosage increased slowly. It may take up to 2 weeks to evaluate the response to daily administration adequately. For ambulatory patients, the usual oral dose is 10 mg daily. The dosage should not be increased more often than every 5 to 7 days. The blood pressure should be taken in the supine position, after standing for 10 minutes and again immediately after exercise. Increase the dosage only if there has been no decrease in standing blood pressure from the previous levels. The dosage should be reduced if the patient develops a normal supine blood pressure, an excessive fall in orthostatic blood pressures, or severe diarrhea. The initial dose of guanethidine for hospitalized patients is 25 to 50 mg daily. The dosage is increased by 25 to 50 mg daily or every other day as indicated.

The usual adult dose of reserpine is 100 to 250 mg/day orally. For children whose dosage is based on mcg/kg, the usual oral dosage range is 5 to 20 mcg/kg/day.

Laboratory Considerations

Guanethidine interferes with blood urea nitrogen levels. Renal function of patients receiving guanethidine should be evaluated periodically. Decreases of urinary norepinephrine may occur with guanethidine. Blood glucose may also decrease with guanethidine.

Miscellaneous Drug

❐ Sumatriptan (IMITREX)

Sumatriptan is a vascular headache suppressant that is a selective agonist at specific vascular serotonin receptor sites. Its actions result in vasoconstriction of large intracranial arteries, resulting in relief of acute migraine headaches.

The mechanism causing vascular headaches is complex, although the early neurologic symptoms are caused by constriction of intracranial blood vessels. Later, dilation of extracranial and intracranial branches of the external carotid artery cause the throbbing headache typically associated with migraines. The underlying mechanism for the periodic spasm and dilation of cranial vessels is unknown.

The adverse effects of sumatriptan are less common following oral administration but include dizziness and vertigo, as well as a warm tingling sensation. For some patients, there is a feeling of chest heaviness or tightness, drowsiness, anxiety, malaise, fatigue, and weakness. There may be throat and sinus discomfort, as well as alterations in vision. Patients may note abdominal discomfort and dysphagia. The most life-threatening adverse effects include myocardial infarction in susceptible individuals.

Sumatriptan is contraindicated in patients with hypersensitivity, ischemic heart disease, or signs and symptoms of ischemic heart disease, Prinzmetal's angina, or uncontrolled hypertension. It should be used with caution in patients with any history of cardiovascular disease, patients of childbearing age, during pregnancy, and lactation, as well as in children younger than 18 years of age.

Sumatriptan is well absorbed (97 percent) when it is taken SC. Absorption following oral administration is incomplete, with significant amounts undergoing a first-pass effect. The substantial first-past effect results in 14 percent bioavailability. The distribution of sumatriptan is unknown but 80 percent of the drug is biotransformed in the liver.

Critical Thinking Process

Assessment

History of Present Illness

Inquire about the onset, intensity, and duration of the patient's symptoms. What has been done to relieve the symptoms? What activities or interventions make the symptoms worse? Determine whether the patient has had the symptoms previously and what treatment was rendered. Inquire about drugs the patient is currently taking, including over-the-counter and prescription drugs.

Past Health History

Because of the urgency with which many adrenergic drugs are used, there may be little time to obtain a thorough patient history. However, questions that should be asked include information about a past history of pheochromocytoma, tachyarrhythmias, ventricular fibrillation, hypovolemia, general anesthesia, and occlusive vascular disease. Determine whether the patient has sensitivities to specific drugs or components of the drug preparation. Elicit information regarding a past history of narrow-angle glaucoma, organic brain damage, cerebral arteriosclerosis, coronary insufficiency, and renal dysfunction. Information about diabetes, hyperthyroidism, prostatic hypertrophy, and seizure disorders should also be elicited.

Physical Exam Findings

Body weight and skin color should be noted. Temperature, pulse rate and rhythm, blood pressure, and respiratory rate and depth should also be noted. The chest should be auscultated for adventitious sounds. Urinary output should also be noted. In some patients, the prostate is palpated to note any enlargement.

Diagnostic Testing

Most patients require blood tests for serum electrolytes, hemoglobin and hematocrit, prothrombin time, partial thromboplastin time, thyroid function, glucose, blood urea nitrogen, and creatinine. An electrocardiographic tracing is also used to determine the heart's response. For patients with reactive airway disease, a chest radiograph and peak expiratory flow rate, or pulmonary function tests may be indicated as well as arterial blood gases.

Developmental Considerations

Perinatal Blood loss from vaginal delivery or cesarean section is notoriously underestimated. Compensatory mechanisms may provide a normal blood pressure until blood loss exceeds 1000 to 1500 mL. Blood loss can be concealed (e.g., abruptio placenta) and not appreciated until shock occurs. Patients who are at risk for obstetric hemorrhage are those of multiparity or those who have been diagnosed with placenta previa.

Because of the young age of most obstetric patients and their lack of underlying disease, mortality from septic shock is distinctly uncommon. This is true despite the frequent presence of infections in the upper and lower genital tracts. As in hemorrhage, compensatory mechanisms may mask the severity of sepsis, and shock may occur suddenly when they are overcome. ARDS and disseminated intravascular coagulation may accompany septic shock in the pregnant woman.

Pediatric The circulatory system of a healthy child is able to transport oxygen and nutrients to meet essential needs of the body tissues. The cardiac output and distribution of blood flow to various body tissues can change very rapidly in response to intrinsic (myocardial and intravascular) or extrinsic (neuronal) control mechanisms. In shock states, these mechanisms are altered or challenged. Septic shock is the most common form of shock seen in newborns.

Geriatric Physiologic changes in the cardiovascular system of an older adult manifest in a variety of ways. The efficiency and contractile strength of the myocardium declines, resulting in a 1-percent per year reduction in cardiac output. It is thought that stroke volume decreases by 0.7 percent yearly. The systolic and diastolic phases of the myocardial cycle are prolonged. Ordinarily, older adults adjust to these changes without much difficulty. However, when unusual demands are placed on the heart (e.g., shoveling snow, running to catch a bus), the changes become more evident. Pulse rates may not reach the levels of younger people, and tachycardia lasts longer.

Resistance to peripheral blood flow increases by 1 percent each year. Decreased elasticity of the arteries is responsible for vascular changes of the heart, kidneys, and pituitary gland. The rigidity of vessel walls and narrowing of lumens require more force to move blood through the vessels. These changes lead to a higher diastolic blood pressure. There is also a decrease in the ability of the aorta to distend, in turn causing an increase in systolic pressure. Vagal tone increases, and the heart becomes more sensitive to carotid sinus stimulation. Reduced sensitivity of the baroreceptors potentiates orthostatic hypotension. The normal changes of aging do not usually influence venous circulation.

Analysis and Management

Treatment Objectives

The treatment objectives for shock are determined by the type of shock but, in general, are threefold: (1) maintain mean arterial pressure above 60 mmHg (in a normal adult) to ensure adequate perfusion of vital organs, (2) maintain blood flow to those organs most often damaged by shock (i.e., kidneys, liver, CNS, lungs), and (3) maintain arterial blood lactate levels below 22 mmol/L. In hypovolemic shock, the objective is to restore vascular volume. In cardiogenic shock, treatment is directed toward reducing the workload of the heart while improving pumping efficacy. Treatment objectives for the patient with anaphylactic shock are directed toward maintaining adequate respiratory gas exchange, cardiac output, and tissue perfusion. Treatment objectives for the management of septic shock include maintenance of adequate organ system perfusion and function.

For patients with vascular headaches, the objective of treatment is to reduce the frequency and severity of the headache. Abortive therapy or symptomatic management may interrupt acute attacks in up to 70 to 80 percent of patients given sumatriptan and in 60 to 70 percent of patients given dihydroergotamine or ergots.

Treatment Options

Drug Variables

Shock and Reactive Airway Disease The choice of drug, dosage, and route of administration depend largely on the reason for its use (Table 11–4). As in any shock state, the airway is the first concern. The most important drug is epinephrine. It causes a beta$_2$-mediated bronchodilation and inhibition of mast cell degranulation. Further, epinephrine may immediately decrease angioedema in patients with anaphylaxis. Usually, a single dose is effective, but additional doses are given if needed. Dobutamine may be used to treat anaphylaxis if cardiac output remains decreased after other measures (e.g., nebulizer, corticosteroids) have been instituted.

Epinephrine is considered part of advanced cardiac life support protocol and can be used to manage asystole or ventricular fibrillation that is unresponsive to electrical cardioversion. It increases cardiac output but redistributes blood flow away from the kidney and splanchnic circulations toward skeletal muscle. At low doses, epinephrine primarily stimulates beta receptors to cause peripheral vasodilation and an increase in heart rate and contractility. As the infusion rate is increased, alpha vasoconstrictive effects become more prominent. Epinephrine is a potent renal artery vasoconstricting drug, even at low doses, and thus, its clinical utility is limited.

Subcutaneous epinephrine for the initial treatment of acute asthma has not been shown to be superior to inhaled beta$_2$ agonists. The inhaled form of epinephrine is not recommended for the initial treatment of acute asthma because

TABLE 11–4 SYMPATHETIC NERVOUS SYSTEM DRUGS BY RECEPTOR ACTIVITY AND INDICATIONS

Drug	Shock, Anaphylaxis	Respiratory Disorders	Hypertension	Headache	Ophthalmic Disorders	Angina, MI, Arrhythmias
Alpha and Beta Agonists						
Dipivefrin					√	√
Dopamine	√					
Ephedrine		√				
Epinephrine	√	√			√	
Norepinephrine	√					
Alpha Agonists						
Clonidine			√			
Guanabenz			√			
Guanfacine			√			
Metaraminol	√					
Methyldopa			√			
Naphazoline		√				
Oxymetazoline		√				
Phenylephrine	√	√			√	
Phenylpropanolamine		√				
Propylhexedrine		√				
Pseudoephedrine		√				
Tetrahydrozoline		√				
Xylometazoline		√				
Beta Agonists						
Dobutamine						√
Isoetharine		√				
Isoproterenol	√	√				
Alpha Blockers						
Dihydroergotamine				√		
Doxazosin			√			
Ergotamine				√		
Methysergide				√		
Phenoxybenzamine			√			
Phentolamine			√			
Prazosin			√			
Terazosin			√			
Postganglionic Blockers						
Guanadrel			√			
Guanethidine			√			
Reserpine			√			

it stimulates alpha and beta receptors and because there are selective $beta_2$ agonists available (e.g., terbutaline and salbutamol), which produce fewer adverse effects.

Isoproterenol administered by oral inhalation may be used to treat bronchoconstriction, although a selective $beta_2$ drug is preferred because it causes less cardiac stimulation. It also has a higher propensity to produce myocardial infarction and excessive tachycardia compared with the selective beta agonists. The magnitude of the vasodilator effect of isoproterenol varies in different vascular beds, depending on the density of $beta_2$ receptors and the affinity of the drug for them. The major vasodilator effect of isoproterenol is in vascular beds of skeletal muscle.

Dobutamine is the preferred drug for managing patients with low output states with heart failure in the setting of an acute myocardial infarction. In contrast to dopamine, dobutamine has much less alpha-vasoconstricting activity but equal positive inotropic effects. Thus, in equal doses, dobutamine tends to lower the pulmonary capillary wedge pressure, whereas dopamine tends to increase it. Dobutamine is also reported to have a lower incidence of arrhythmias.

Vascular Headaches Ergot-like drug therapy should be considered for the patient who has failed to respond to simple analgesics or who has moderate to severe symptoms. Dihydroergotamine is as effective and better tolerated (i.e., less nausea) and has only modest arterial effects compared with ergotamine, but it is only available parenterally. Ergotamine is advantageous compared with dihydroergotamine because it is available in oral, rectal, sublingual, and inhalation forms. Furthermore, ergotamine is most effective when it is used during the prodromal phase of the headache. Inhaled ergotamine is preferred because of its rapid onset of action.

Ergot preparations are not as effective when therapy has been delayed and the pain is well established. The use of ergotamine can be risky in patients with prolonged prodromal symptoms (i.e., complicated migraine) and may lead to irreversible sequelae in these circumstances. Ergotamine dosages should be titrated for each patient until the appropriate dose is determined for subsequent attacks. In some cases, prochlorperazine, an antiemetic drug, should be given before ergotamine is administered to reduce the occurrence of nausea associated with these drugs. Repeated dosing over an extended period may be less efficacious by allowing establishment of vasodilation. The bioavailability of oral and sublingual ergotamine is poor compared with that of inhalation formulations.

Dihydroergotamine is as effective as and better tolerated than ergotamine. The parenteral form is particularly helpful for patients with concomitant nausea and vomiting. Dihydroergotamine can be used at home for patients who find other drug therapy ineffective if the patient is taught how to administer the drug. A nasal spray formulation of dihydroergotamine has just become available and appears to offer some benefit in headache relief.

Sumatriptan is effective and well tolerated when given as a single SC or oral dose. Approximately 50 percent of patients respond within 2 hours of an oral dose of sumatriptan, and 70 percent of patients respond within 1 hour of SC administration. But sumatriptan does not work for all patients, and it is relatively expensive. It does appear to be more effective and safer than ergotamine, but further studies are needed. If headaches are persistent after 1 to 2 hours, alternative therapy should be instituted. However, allow an adequate trial of 4 to 6 weeks of prophylaxis at appropriate dosages before abandoning therapy.

Methysergide should be used only when other therapies have failed because of the risk of fibrosis.

Patient Variables

If blood pressure support is needed in the pregnant woman, dopamine is preferable because at low doses, it not only increases cardiac output and arterial blood pressure but also improves renal perfusion. Dopamine may decrease uterine blood flow and so should be used once it has been demonstrated that volume replacement is insufficient. Ephedrine is valuable to counteract hypotension from epidural or spinal anesthesia if fluids are ineffective.

The safety and efficacy of many of the adrenergic drugs has not been established for pediatric patients. Drug use in the older adult should be performed with caution because of the risk of reduced renal function secondary to the changes of aging and other co-morbid disorders.

Most drugs cause a reduction in the severity and number of vascular headaches; however, up to 25 percent of patients do not tolerate prophylactic drugs. Consider prophylaxis for patients with 2 headaches or more per month, who have significant impairment in quality of life, with regular and predictable attacks (e.g., menstrual migraine), and who require increased use of an opioid analgesic.

Intervention

Administration

Extreme caution should be used in calculating and preparing doses of adrenergic drugs. Some adrenergics are very potent; thus, small errors in dosage can cause serious adverse effects. Double check pediatric dosages. Hypovolemia should be corrected with volume expanders before initiating dopamine, epinephrine, or norepinephrine therapy. Use minimal doses for minimal periods of time because drug tolerance can occur with prolonged use of some drugs.

The drugs used in an emergency should be administered in large veins of the antecubital fossa in preference to veins of the hand or ankle. Phentolamine should be available in case of extravasation of alpha agonists. Five to ten milligrams of phentolamine is mixed with 10 to 15 mL of saline and the affected area infiltrated.

Monitor the cardiovascular effects of adrenergic drugs carefully, particularly in patients with a history of hypertension or other cardiovascular disorders. A rapid-acting alpha blocker such as phentolamine or a vasodilator (a nitrite) should be available in case of excessive hypertensive reaction.

Patients who have atrial fibrillation who are to be treated with dobutamine require digitalization before being given dobutamine. Dobutamine facilitates AV conduction.

Education

Because adrenergic drugs are most often used in emergency situations, patient teaching depends on the patient's awareness and medical status. Advise patients to notify the health care provider if they experience chest pain, dizziness, insomnia, weakness, tremor, or irregular heart beat while receiving sympathetic nervous system drugs.

Patients with recurrent vascular headaches should be taught the importance of the management of migraines. They should be taught to identify factors contributing to the headache (e.g., behaviors, food products, drugs, stress) to prevent or diminish precipitating factors. Instruction on the prodromal signs of an impending migraine and on prompt initiation of abortive therapy at the onset of attacks is needed in order for therapy to be most effective.

Evaluation

The desired outcome of drug therapy with adrenergic drugs is correction of hemodynamic imbalances and increase in cardiac output, blood pressure, peripheral circulation, and urinary output. The desired outcome of the patient with a vascular headache is relief from the signs and symptoms.

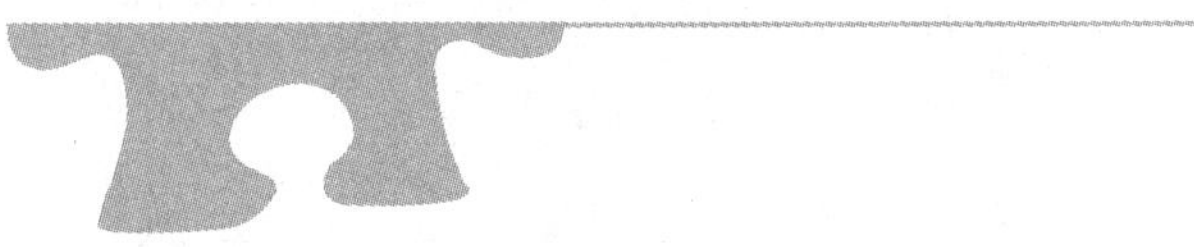

SUMMARY

- Adrenergics stimulate nervous system activity. These drugs are also referred to as sympathomimetic or adrenergic agonists and are divided into three different groups: alpha and beta agonists, alpha agonists, and beta agonists.
- Sympathetic responses include mydriasis, increased rate and force of myocardial contraction, vasoconstriction, bronchodilation, decreased gastric motility, pallor, perspiration, sphincter constriction, decreased motility, tone, and contractility of the urinary bladder.
- Chemical compounds that inhibit sympathetic nervous system activity by interacting with the receptor site are referred to as sympatholytics or antiadrenergics. There are two types of adrenergic blockers: alpha blockers and beta blockers.
- Antiadrenergic compounds inhibit sympathetic nervous system activity, dilate peripheral blood vessels, and reduce the heart rate. Additionally, the patient develops an increase in GI and urinary activity.
- Circulatory shock produces compensatory responses that result in decreased peripheral perfusion, inadequate oxygenation of vital organs, and eventually, decompensation to various shock states.

- Hypovolemic shock is a consequence of inadequate circulatory volume. Obstructive shock is related to mechanical obstruction of arterial blood flow or of venous return. Distributive shock occurs when the tissues are unable to use oxygen and nutrients to produce energy. The basic circulatory events are reflected in three subtypes of distributive shock: neurogenic shock, anaphylactic shock, and septic shock.
- In shock, arterioles and venules relax, resulting in a drop of arterial pressure and venous pooling. Hypoxia at the capillary level and the products of cellular deterioration cause increased capillary permeability, stagnant blood flow, the formation of small blood clots, and third-spacing.
- The five main complications of shock include ARDS, acute renal failure, GI ulceration, disseminated intravascular coagulation, and multiple system organ failure.
- Reactive airway diseases are obstructive disorders characterized by limitations of expiratory airflow.
- Adrenergic drugs are used to increase blood pressure in severe hypotension, reverse anaphylactic shock, reduce bleeding at the operative site in conjunction with local anesthetics, and treat hypoglycemic episodes.
- Alpha blockers are used to improve cerebral circulation and manage pheochromocytoma, and in selected cases of hypertension, especially when the hypertension is associated with increased sympathetic nervous system activity.
- Postganglionic blockers are alternative drugs for hypertension. Newer drugs have less bothersome adverse effects. The postganglionic blockers guanadrel, guanethidine, and reserpine are used in the treatment of hypertension in selected patients.
- The choice of drug, dosage, and route of administration depend largely on the reason for its use.

BIBLIOGRAPHY

Alpert, J., and Becker, P. (1993). Mechanisms and management of cardiogenic shock. *Critical Care Clinics,* 9(2), 205–218.

Bennett, J., and Plum, F. (Eds.). (1996). *Cecil textbook of medicine* (20th ed.). Philadelphia: W.B. Saunders.

Bochner, B., and Lichtenstein, L. (1991). Anaphylaxis. *New England Journal of Medicine,* 324, 1785–1790.

Brown, A. (1995). Anaphylactic shock: Mechanisms and treatment. *Journal of Accident and Emergency Medicine,* 12(2), 89–100.

Califf, R., and Bengton, J. (1994). Cardiogenic shock. *New England Journal of Medicine,* 330(24), 1724–1730.

Collins, A. (1990). Gastrointestinal complications in shock. *Critical Care Clinics of North America,* 2(2), 269–276.

Francis, G., and Chu, C. (1994). Compensatory and maladaptive responses to cardiac dysfunction. *Current Opinion in Cardiology,* 9(3), 280–288.

Gutierrez, G. (1991). Cellular energy metabolism during hypoxia. *Critical Care Medicine,* 19, 619–626.

Guyton, A., and Hall, J. (1996). *Textbook of medical physiology* (9th ed.). Philadelphia: W.B. Saunders.

Hachamovitch, R., Chang, J., Kuntz, R., et al. (1995). Recurrent reversible cardiogenic shock triggered by emotional distress with nonobstructive coronary disease. *American Heart Journal,* 129(5), 1026–1028.

Hardman, L., Limbird, L., Molinoff, P., et al. (1996). *Goodman and Gilman's The pharmacological basis of therapeutics* (9th ed.). New York: McGraw-Hill.

Hockman, J., Boland, J., Sleeper, L., et al. (1995). Current spectrum of cardiogenic shock and effect of early revascularization on mortality. *Circulation,* 91(3), 873–881.

Isselbacher, K., Braunwald, E., and Wilson, J. (Eds.). (1994). *Harrison's principles of internal medicine* (13th ed.). New York: McGraw-Hill, Inc.

Parillo, J. (1995). Pathogenetic mechanisms of septic shock. *New England Journal of Medicine,* 328(20), 1471–1477.

Shoemaker, W., Pietzman, A., Bellamy, R., et al. (1996). Resuscitation from severe hemorrhage. *Critical Care Medicine,* 24(2 Suppl), S12–S23.

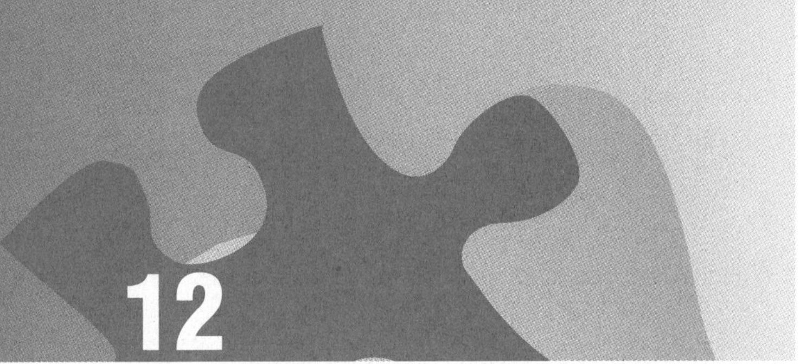

12 Neuromuscular Blocking Drugs

Neuromuscular blocking drugs are commonly referred to as muscle relaxants, although that term is a misnomer. Neuromuscular blockers work peripherally by blocking transmission of impulses at the neuromuscular junction. A true muscle relaxant works centrally to reduce transmission of impulses from spinal cord to skeletal muscle. Centrally acting skeletal muscle relaxants are discussed in detail in Chapter 21.

Neuromuscular blockers are one of the most frequently used classes of drugs in the operating room. They are used primarily as an adjunct to general anesthesia to facilitate endotracheal intubation and to relax skeletal muscle during surgery. More recently, health care providers in intensive care units and emergency rooms have found them useful in the management of respiratory problems. Neuromuscular blockers commonly are classified by type of block produced (depolarizing versus nondepolarizing), chemical structure (steroidal compound, acetylcholine derivative, isoquinoline derivative or benzylisoquinolinium ester), or duration of action (ultra short acting, short acting, intermediate acting, or long acting). In this chapter, the drugs are classified according to the type of blockade produced. However, to understand neuromuscular blockade, a brief review of physiology follows.

PHYSIOLOGY OF NEUROMUSCULAR TRANSMISSION

No muscle stays completely relaxed. So long as the patient is conscious, muscles remain slightly contracted. This condition is called *tonus*. It keeps the bones in place and enables posture to be maintained. When a muscle contracts, a nerve impulse is sent from the brain and spinal cord through a motor neuron to a muscle cell membrane at a communication point called the motor endplate. The space between the nerve and the muscle membrane is known as the neuromuscular junction. The neuromuscular junction is composed of the axon, presynaptic motor nerve terminals, synaptic cleft, and postsynaptic motor endplate membranes (Fig. 12–1). Nerve impulses arriving at the motor neuron evoke liberation of acetylcholine stored in presynaptic vesicles. Acetylcholine release occurs through the calcium-dependent process of exocytosis. Acetylcholine diffuses across the synapse to reversibly bind to cholinergic receptors located on the postsynaptic motor endplate. One molecule of acetylcholine binds to each of two sites on a single cholinergic receptor in order for the ion channel to open. Once the channel opens, sodium ions flow through, causing depolarization of the muscle cell. The degree of depolarization is proportional to the number of receptors occupied. After depolarization of the endplate, acetylcholine binds to acetylcholinesterase, where it is hydrolyzed to acetate and choline. Calcium released from the sarcoplasmic reticulum binds to troponin C (a complex of muscle proteins) uncovering myosin-binding sites on actin. Cross-linkages form between actin and myosin, resulting in contraction of skeletal muscle.

Sustained muscle contraction demands an endless series of action potentials. The generation of action potentials results in repeated release of acetylcholine. In turn, there is repeated stimulation of cholinergic receptors on the motor endplate. Repeating cycles of depolarization and repolarization result in sufficient release of calcium from the sarcoplasmic reticulum to sustain the contraction. If the motor endplate remains depolarized, as with the administration of a neuromuscular blocker, the stimulus for calcium release stops. There is an immediate reuptake of calcium by the sarcoplasmic reticulum, and muscle contraction ceases.

PHARMACOTHERAPEUTIC OPTIONS

Twelve neuromuscular blockers are approved for clinical use in the United States. They are classified according to their mechanism and duration of action. When these agents are organized by mechanism, they fall into two categories: nondepolarizing neuromuscular blockers and depolarizing neuromuscular blockers. When they are organized according to duration of action, they fall into four groups: long-acting (30 to 90 minutes), intermediate-acting (15 to 30 minutes), short-acting (10 to 15 minutes), and ultra short-acting (3 to 5 minutes) agents. Regardless of how they are categorized, the principal differences among the drugs relate to cardiovascular effects and duration of action.

Nondepolarizing Neuromuscular Blockers

- ❒ Atracurium (TRACRIUM)
- ❒ Cisatracurium (NIMBEX)
- ❒ Doxacurium (NUROMAX)
- ❒ Gallamine (FLAXEDIL)
- ❒ Metocurine (METUBINE IODIDE)
- ❒ Mivacurium (MIVACRON)
- ❒ Pancuronium (PAVULON)
- ❒ Pipecuronium (ARDUAN)
- ❒ Rocuronium (ZEMURON)
- ❒ Tubocurarine; (🍁) TUBARINE
- ❒ Vecuronium (NORCURON)

Indications

There are a limited number of uses for nondepolarizing neuromuscular blockers. They are used most often to produce muscle relaxation during endotracheal intubation and surgical procedures, and to facilitate mechanical ventilation. Some agents have been used as an adjunct during electroconvulsive therapy (ECT). The use of these drugs is also in-

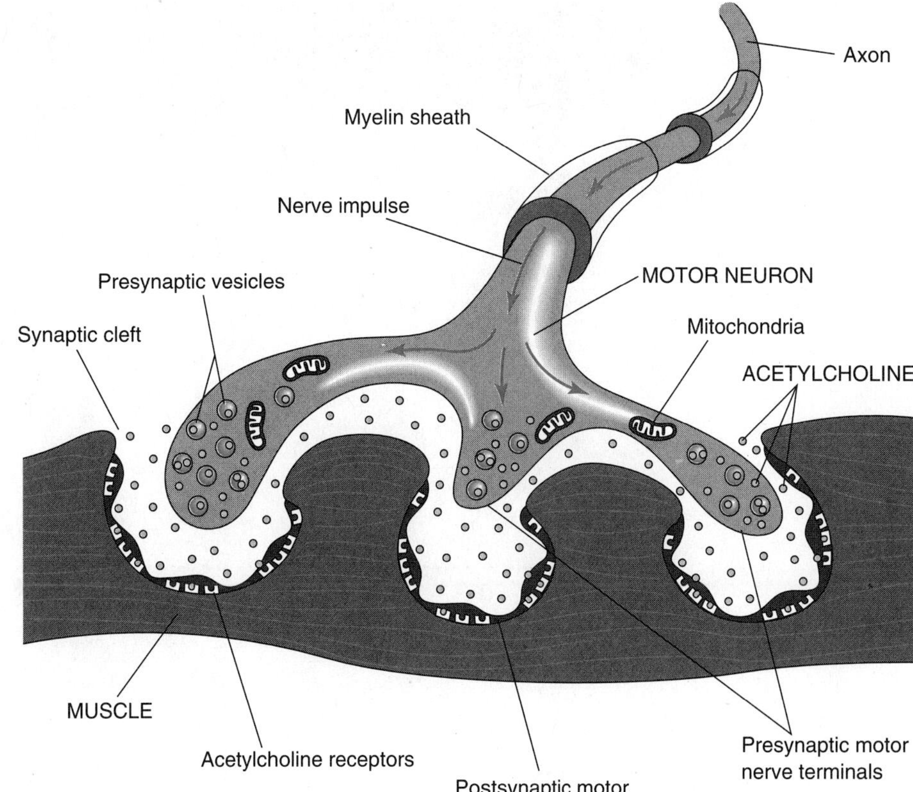

Figure 12–1 Schematic representation of neuromuscular junction. The term neuromuscular junction refers to the axon terminal of a motor neuron together with the motor endplate. The distal ends of the axon terminals expand into bulblike structures called presynaptic motor nerve terminals. The structures contain vesicles that store neurotransmitters (e.g., acetylcholine and norepinephrine). The presynaptic motor nerve terminals come into close approximation with the muscle fiber. The synaptic cleft is the region between the motor nerve terminals and postsynaptic membranes.

dicated for patients in status asthmaticus who need ventilatory assistance. Tubocurarine can be used to diagnose myasthenia gravis. Another use of nondepolarizing blockers is in the management of tetanus, a potentially fatal bacterial infection.

Intubation generally involves the use of neuromuscular blockers because laryngeal stimulation can be associated with reflex closure of the vocal cords and hypoxemia if intubation is unsuccessful. Neuromuscular blockers are used during intra-abdominal and intrathoracic procedures to prevent reflex muscle contraction and to permit surgical exposure and effective wound closure. Reflex muscle responses can be suppressed by high concentrations of a volatile anesthetic, but this practice results in circulatory depression.

Neuromuscular blockers are used in patients requiring mechanical ventilation for three primary reasons. First, they promote ventilation by reducing or eliminating spontaneous breathing efforts. Second, they reduce oxygen consumption in patients with severely compromised cardiopulmonary function. Third, neuromuscular blockers reduce motor activity that may disturb vascular catheters, access tubes, and surgical dressings.

ECT has been used for years as an effective treatment for severe depression. The benefit, however, is strictly related to the effects of electroshock on the brain. The convulsive movements that accompany ECT do not help relieve depression. Thus, neuromuscular blockers are used to prevent convulsive movements because such movements serve no useful purpose and can actually be harmful.

The blockers prevent the intense muscle contracture and rigidity associated with tetanus that can cause a host of serious systemic problems (e.g., electrolyte imbalances owing to muscle damage). They also aid in mechanical ventilation of the patient with tetanus.

Pharmacodynamics

Acetylcholine must bind to nicotinic cholinergic receptors for normal neuromuscular transmission to occur. Thus, nondepolarizing neuromuscular blockers compete with acetylcholine for binding to nicotinic cholinergic receptors on the motor endplate. Because the drug does not activate these receptors, binding does not result in muscle contraction. Muscle relaxation lasts as long as the quantity of drug at the neuromuscular junction is adequate to deter receptor occupation by acetylcholine. Muscle strength can be restored by increasing the amount of acetylcholine at the neuromuscular junction or by increasing elimination of the drug from the body.

Although nondepolarizing drugs paralyze all skeletal muscles, the paralysis affects muscles in a specific and predictable sequence. Small, rapidly moving muscles of the eyes, face, and neck are affected first. Muscles of the limbs, abdomen, and trunk are affected next, followed by the intercostal muscles and diaphragm. Muscle weakness rapidly progresses to *flaccid paralysis*. Typically, recovery from drug-induced paralysis occurs in reverse order from the induction sequence. Nondepolarizing drugs have no analgesic properties.

Adverse Effects and Contraindications

The principal adverse effects of nondepolarizing neuromuscular blockers are on the cardiovascular and respiratory systems. The underlying physiologic mechanisms for the car-

TABLE 12–1 PHYSIOLOGIC CAUSES OF CARDIOVASCULAR ADVERSE EFFECTS*

Drugs	Histamine Release	Ganglionic Blockade	Vagolytic Activity
Long-Acting Nondepolarizing Drugs			
Doxacurium	None	None	None
Metocurine	Slight	Weak	None
Pipecuronium	None	None	None
Tubocurarine	Moderate	Weak	Decreased
Intermediate-Acting Nondepolarizing Drugs			
Atracurium	Slight	None	Minimal effect
Cisatracurium	None	None	Minimal effect
Gallamine	High dose only	None	Increased
Pancuronium	Slight	None	Increased
Rocuronium	None	None	Increased
Vecuronium	None	None	None
Short-Acting Nondepolarizing Drug			
Mivacurium	Slight	None	Slight increase
Ultra Short-Acting Depolarizing Drug			
Succinylcholine	Slight	Stimulates	Increase or decrease

*Histamine release is related to the dose and speed of administration. Cardiovascular effects can be lessened by minimizing the dose and increasing the IV administration time. The histamine response can be minimized by pretreating the patient with histamine-1 and histamine-2 antagonists.

diovascular adverse effects are identified in Table 12–1. Neuromuscular blockers cause hypotension through two primary mechanisms: partial ganglionic blockade and histamine release. Ganglionic blockade decreases sympathetic tone of the arterioles and veins with subsequent vasodilation. Histamine release also promotes vasodilation. Ganglionic blockade is common with metocurine and tubocurarine. Metocurine, tubocurarine, and atracurium cause histamine release and thus a drop in blood pressure. Blockade of muscarinic receptors results in tachycardia. Bradycardia, arrhythmias, and cardiac arrest can also result. The mechanism that underlies these latter effects, however, is unclear.

Paralysis of intercostal muscles and the diaphragm can lead to respiratory arrest. Overadministration of drugs, an accumulation of active metabolites, and end-organ damage or dysfunction can result in short-term persistent paralysis that lasts from hours to days. The paralysis is clearly pharmacologically based. Long-term persistent paralysis lasts from days to weeks and is characterized by muscle and nerve degeneration.

Contraindications to nondepolarizing neuromuscular blockers include hypersensitivity this class of drugs and to bromides (pancuronium, vecuronium only) and iodides or iodine (gallamine, metocurine only). Products containing benzyl alcohol should be avoided in neonates.

There are many conditions that require cautious use of nondepolarizing drugs. Cautious use is warranted in patients with underlying cardiovascular disease (because of an increased risk of arrhythmias), dehydration, or electrolyte imbalance. Situations in which histamine release may occur (e.g., asthma, allergic conditions) could be problematic. Older adults and patients with impaired renal function (leading to decreased elimination of gallamine, metocurine, pancuronium, and tubocurarine) should be monitored closely. Hepatic disease reduces the biotransformation of vecuronium, and therefore, the drug should also be used with caution. Shock related to prolonged paralysis from gallamine, metocurine, and tubocurarine has been noted. Cautious use is also warranted in patients with low plasma pseudocholinesterase levels in association with anemia, dehydration, the use of cholinesterase inhibitors or insecticides, severe liver disease, or pregnancy. Safe use during pregnancy or lactation or in children has not been established for most agents. Extreme caution should be exercised when neuromuscular blockers are used for patients with myasthenia gravis or myasthenic syndromes. Patients with myasthenia gravis, an autoimmune disorder characterized by antibodies to the nicotinic acetylcholine receptor, are extremely sensitive to nondepolarizing neuromuscular blockers.

Pharmacokinetics

These drugs as a class are poorly absorbed from the gastrointestinal tract and therefore must be administered parenterally. Muscular paralysis develops in minutes following intravenous (IV) administration. Peak effects are reached in 2 to 10 minutes, with the duration of effective paralysis lasting from 45 minutes to hours (Table 12–2). Complete recovery may take several hours.

Pancuronium, vecuronium, and rocuronium are biotransformed in the liver. Atracurium and mivacurium are broken down in the plasma. The majority of the nondepolarizing neuromuscular blockers are eliminated primarily in an unchanged form in the urine. The half-life of nondepolarizing neuromuscular blockers ranges from 20 minutes to 4 hours.

Drug-Drug Interactions

Drug-drug interactions with nondepolarizing drugs are many. Drug interactions may occur at the nerve terminal, synapse, or motor endplate and sometimes at more than one site. Table 12–3 provides an overview of key interacting drugs. The intensity and duration of paralysis may be prolonged if the patient has been pretreated in some fashion

TABLE 12–2 PHARMACOKINETICS OF SELECTED NEUROMUSCULAR BLOCKERS

Drugs	Route	Onset	Time to Maximum Paralysis	Duration of Effective Paralysis*	Time to Spontaneous Recovery†	PB (%)	$t_{1/2}$
Long-Acting Nondepolarizing Drugs							
Doxacurium	IV	5 min	4–10 min	100 min	Hours	UA	99 min
Metocurine	IV	1–4 min	6 min	25–90 min	Hours	55	3.6 hr
Pipecuronium	IV	2.5–3 min	3–5 min	60–120 min	Hours	UA	1.7 hr
Tubocurarine	IV	1 min	2–5 min	35–60 min	Hours	40–45	2 hr
Intermediate-Acting Nondepolarizing Drugs							
Atracurium	IV	2–2.5 min	5 min	30–40 min	60–70 min	82	20 min
Cisatracurium	IV	1–2 min	5–7 min	22–63 min	60–70 min	UA‡	UA
Gallamine	IV	1–2 min	3–5 min	15–30 min	—	16	2.5 hr
Pancuronium	IV	30–45 sec	3–4.5 min	35–45 min	60–70 min	15	2 hr
Rocuronium	IV	1 min	1.8 min	31 min	13 min	30	1.4 hr
Vecuronium	IV	1 min	3–5 min	15–30 min	45–60 min	27	31–80 min
Short-Acting Nondepolarizing Drug							
Mivacurium	IV	2.5 min	3.3 min	26 min	6–8 min	UA	2 hr
Ultra Short-Acting Depolarizing Drug							
Succinylcholine	IV	0.5–1 min	1–2 min	4–10 min	—	UK	UK

* Duration of effective paralysis varies with dosage. Figures presented are for an average adult dose administered as a single IV injection.

† Spontaneous recovery from paralysis can take a long time. Recovery from nondepolarizing drugs may be accelerated by administering a cholinesterase inhibitor (see Chapter 13).

‡ Protein binding for cisatracurium has not been successfully studied owing to its rapid degradation at physiologic pH.

PB, Protein binding; UA, unavailable; UK, unknown.

TABLE 12–3 DRUG-DRUG INTERACTIONS OF SELECTED NEUROMUSCULAR BLOCKERS

Drug	Interactive Drugs	Interaction
Nondepolarizing Drugs		
Atracurium	Aminoglycoside antibiotics	Additive neuromuscular blockade, apnea, respiratory depression
Doxacurium chloride	Beta blockers	
Gallamine triethiodide	Clindamycin	
Metocurine iodide	Colistin	
Pancuronium bromide	Inhaled general anesthetics	
Pipecuronium bromide	Lidocaine	
Rocuronium bromide	Opioid analgesics	
Tubocurarine chloride	Magnesium	
Vecuronium bromide	MAO inhibitors	
	Polymyxin B	
	Potassium-losing diuretics	
	Procainimide	
	Quinidine	
	Succinylcholine	
	Anticholinesterase drugs	Reversal of effects of neuromuscular blocker
Depolarizing Drug		
Succinylcholine	Cimetidine	Prolonged apnea
	Local anesthetics	
	Anticholinesterase drugs	Reduce pseudocholinesterase activity and intensify paralysis
	Demecarium eye drops	
	Echothiophate	
	Isoflurophate	
	Cardiac glycosides	Increased risk of adverse cardiovascular effects
	Opioids	

MAO, monoamine oxidase.

TABLE 12–4 DOSAGE REGIMEN FOR SELECTED NEUROMUSCULAR BLOCKERS

Drug	Use(s)	Dosage	Implications
Long-Acting Nondepolarizing Drugs			
Doxacurium	Skeletal muscle paralysis and facilitation of intubation; facilitation of compliance during mechanical ventilation	*Adults:* 50 mcg/kg IV initially followed 60–100 minutes later by 5–10 mcg/kg repeated as necessary. May need up to 80 mcg/kg for prolonged effect, 25 mcg/kg for succinylcholine-assisted intubation *Children 2–12 yr:* 30–50 mcg/kg IV initially	Maintenance doses may be required more frequently in children than in adults
Metacurine	Adjunct to electroconvulsive therapy	*Adults:* 150–400 mcg/kg IV initially. May give additional doses of 0.5–1 mg q30–90 minutes. *Adjunct to electroconvulsive therapy:* 1.75–5.5 mg IV	Relaxation from initial dose usually averages 60 minutes. Administer supplemental doses as needed
Pipecuronium	Skeletal muscle paralysis and facilitation of intubation; facilitation of compliance during mechanical ventilation	*Adults:* 70–85 mcg/kg (if given following recovery from succinylcholine during intubation, decrease dose to 50 mcg/kg 70–85 mcg/kg if longer paralysis is desired). Additional doses of 10–15 mcg/kg may be required as maintenance *Children 1–14 yr:* 57 mcg/kg IV initial dose *Infants 3 mo–1 yr:* 40 mcg/kg IV initial dose	Dosage reduction is recommended if using concurrent inhalation anesthetics. Dose should be determined on the basis of ideal body weight in obese patients and may require adjustments in patients with renal impairment Recommended only for procedures lasting less than 90 minutes
Tubocurarine	Diagnosis of myasthenia gravis; adjunct to electroconvulsive therapy	*Adults:* 6–9 mg initially IV followed by 3–4.5 mg after 3–5 minutes, if needed. Additional doses of 0.165 mg/kg may be given as needed. *Infants and Children:* 500–600 mcg/kg IV *Neonates–4 weeks:* 250–500 mcg/kg initially; then additional increments that are 1/5th to 1/6th the initial dose may be given *Mechanical ventilation:* 16.5 mcg/kg with subsequent doses given as necessary *Adjunct to electroconvulsive therapy:* 165 mcg/kg IV. Initial doses should be 3 mg less than calculated dose *Diagnosis myasthenia gravis:* 4–33 mcg/kg IV	When drug is used for diagnosis of myasthenia gravis, profound myasthenic symptoms may occur. Do not use any solution that has developed a faint color
Intermediate-Acting Nondepolarizing Drugs			
Atracurium	Skeletal muscle paralysis and facilitation of intubation: facilitation of compliance during mechanical ventilation	*Adults and Children over 2 yr:* 0.4–0.5 mg/kg initially IV, followed by continuous infusion of 2–15 mcg/kg/minute. Dosage is 0.25–0.35 mg/kg if administered after steady-state anesthesia with enflurane or isoflurane or 0.3–0.4 mg/kg following succinylcholine *Children 1 mo–2 yr:* 0.3–0.4 mg/kg initially (while under halothane anesthesia)	Do not use before induction of unconsciousness. Bradycardia during anesthesia is common.
Cisatracurium		*Adults:* 0.15 mg/kg initially IV, followed by 0.03 mg/kg based on patient response to sustain neuromuscular blockade. 1–2 mcg/kg IV continuous infusion under nitrous oxide, oxygen, and opioid anesthesia. Maximum dose: 1.6 mg/kg *Children 2–12 yr:* 0.1 mg/kg IV during halothane or opioid anesthesia	Primarily used for short procedures. Relatively new drug.
Gallamine		*Adults and Children:* 1 mg/kg (not to exceed 100 mg/dose), then 0.5–1 mg/kg may be given 30–40 minutes later if needed during prolonged procedures	Dose cautiously in patients weighing less than 5 kg. Monitor patient for increased heart rate
Pancuronium		*Adults and Children older than 1 mo:* 40–100 mcg/kg initially. Incremental doses of 10 mcg/kg may be given q20–60 minutes to maintain paralysis.	Provision of relaxation to allow for mechanical ventilation—15 mcg/kg. Monitor patients for prolonged drug effects beyond the time needed or anticipated by drug use. Supportive care may be needed
Rocuronium		*Adults:* 0.6 mg/kg IV for rapid-sequence tracheal intubation. Maintenance dosing is 0.1–0.2 mg/kg. For continuous IV infusion, give 0.01–0.012 mg/kg/minute, with a range of 4–16 mcg/kg/minute *Children:* 0.6 mg/kg for intubation. Maintenance dose is 0.075–0.125 mg/kg IV. Continuous IV infusion dose is 0.012 mg/kg/minute	Dosages are not different in obese and nonobese patients when calculated on their actual body weight

TABLE 12–4 DOSAGE REGIMEN FOR SELECTED NEUROMUSCULAR BLOCKERS *Continued*

Drug	Use(s)	Dosage	Implications
Vecuronium		*Intubation of Adults and Children over 10 yr:* 80–100 mcg/kg (60–85 mcg/kg if given after steady-state anesthesia achieved or 40–60 mcg/kg after succinylcholine-assisted intubation and anesthesia. Wait for disappearance of succinylcholine effects or 50–60 mcg/kg during balanced anesthesia). Maintenance: 10–15 mcg/kg 25–40 minutes after initial dose, then q12–15 minutes as needed or as a continuous IV infusion at 0.8–1.2 mcg/kg/minute	Doses of 150–280 mcg/kg have been used in some patients for intubation. Prolongation of neuromuscular blockade has been reported. Monitor patient during recovery, and provide supportive care
Short-Acting Nondepolarizing Drug			
Mivacurium	Skeletal muscle paralysis and facilitation of intubation; facilitation of compliance during mechanical ventilation	*Adults:* 150–200 mcg/kg IV; initially, then 100 mcg/kg as bolus doses q15min or as a continuous infusion at 9–10 mcg/kg/minute. Start with rate of 4 mcg/kg/minute if infusion is begun at the same time as initial dose. Infusion rates may vary from 1–20 mcg/kg/minute *Children 2–12 yr:* 200 mcg/kg IV initially. May be repeated as needed or continued as an infusion at 14 mcg/kg/ minute. Average range 5–31 mcg/kg/minute	Do not use before unconsciousness has been induced
Ultra Short-Acting Depolarizing Drug			
Succinylcholine	Skeletal muscle paralysis; adjunct to electroconvulsive therapy	*Test dose in adults:* 0.1 mg/kg IV; then assess respiratory function *Short procedures in adults:* 0.3–1.1 mg/kg, with additional doses dependent on response *Short procedure in children:* 1–2 mg/kg, with additional doses dependent on response *Prolonged procedures in adults:* 0.6 mg/kg initially, then 0.04–0.07 mg/kg, as necessary *Electroshock therapy in adults:* 10–30 mg IV 1 minute before shock. Further individualization of dose may be required	Continuous IV infusion not recommended in children or neonates for short procedures. Continuous IV infusion is preferred in adults for prolonged procedures. Monitor patient for histamine release and resultant hypotension and flushing

with succinylcholine (see the discussion of depolarizing drugs), inhaled general anesthesia, aminoglycosides and certain other antibiotics, quinidine, procainamide, beta blockers, potassium-losing diuretics, and magnesium. Most neuromuscular blockers are incompatible with barbiturates and sodium bicarbonate. High-dose antibiotics may intensify or produce neuromuscular blockade on their own. They should not be admixed.

Dosage Regimen

The dosage regimen for nondepolarizing neuromuscular blockers depends on the purpose for their use (Table 12–4). The majority of these drugs are dosed based on micrograms per kilogram or milligram per kilogram of body weight. Standard dosing according to body weight alone often results in overadministration of neuromuscular blockers. Maintenance doses differ from those administered initially and are titrated to patient response. Many of the drugs can be administered by continuous IV infusion. The health care provider is cautioned to check dosage regimens closely before administering the drug. Although tubocurarine can be administered intramuscularly (IM), the preferred route is IV. The IM route can be used for infants and other patients who do not have venous access devices.

Depolarizing Neuromuscular Blocker

❒ Succinylcholine chloride (ANECTINE, QUELICIN, SUCOSTRIN)

Indications

Succinylcholine is the most commonly used depolarizing drug. It is used primarily to produce muscle relaxation during endotracheal intubation, ECT, endoscopy, and other short procedures.

Pharmacodynamics

Like acetylcholine, succinylcholine binds to cholinergic receptors at the motor endplate to produce depolarization. However, unlike acetylcholine, as a result of deactivation by acetylcholinesterase, succinylcholine remains receptor bound for several minutes, and muscles do not respond to the subsequent release of acetylcholine. After a few minutes, succinylcholine is biotransformed by plasma cholinesterase, and the postjunctional cholinergic membrane repolarizes. Repolarization and further muscle contractions are inhibited as long as an adequate concentration of drug remains at receptor sites. Histamine is released, which may contribute to hypotension. Like nondepolarizing drugs, depolarizing drugs have no analgesic properties.

Adverse Effects and Contraindications

Most adverse effects of succinylcholine are extension of pharmacologic effects. The adverse effects include bronchospasm and apnea, hypotension, arrhythmias, bradycardia, hyperkalemia, tachyphylaxis, and muscle fasciculations. The risk of myoglobinemia and myoglobinuria is increased in children. Malignant hyperthermia is the most life-threatening adverse effect of succinylcholine.

Muscle fasciculations that occur as a result of drug action often result in postoperative myalgia. Ten to seventy percent of patients complain of neck, shoulder, and back pain 12 to 24 hours after administration. The discomfort can persist for several hours or days. Succinylcholine is contraindicated in patients with hypersensitivity to the drug or hypersensitivity to parabens and in patients with pseudocholinesterase deficiency. A continuous infusion of succinylcholine is contraindicated in children and neonates. Succinylcholine raises intraocular pressure and thus is absolutely contraindicated in patients with glaucoma.

A history of malignant hyperthermia or pulmonary, renal, or liver impairment, or of myasthenia gravis or myasthenic syndromes, warrants cautious use of succinylcholine. It should also be used with caution in older adults or debilitated patients, patients with electrolyte disturbances, and patients receiving cardiac glycosides.

Pharmacokinetics

Succinylcholine is well absorbed with IV administration and is widely distributed into extracellular fluid. It crosses the placenta in small amounts. The onset of skeletal muscle relaxation occurs in 30 seconds to 1 minute, with peak paralysis noted in 1 to 2 minutes (see Table 12–2). Paralysis can last from 4 to 10 minutes. Ninety percent of the drug is biotransformed by pseudocholinesterase in the plasma. Ten percent is eliminated unchanged in the kidneys. The half-life of succinylcholine is unknown.

Drug-Drug Interactions

Concurrent administration of succinylcholine with cholinesterase inhibitors (i.e., echothiophate, isoflurophate, demecarium eye drops) reduces pseudocholinesterase activity and intensifies paralysis (see Table 12–3). The intensity and duration of paralysis may be prolonged by pretreatment with general anesthetics, aminoglycoside antibiotics, cimetidine, polymyxin B, colistin, clindamycin, lidocaine, quinidine, procainamide, beta blockers, lithium, cyclophosphamide, phenelzine, potassium-losing diuretics, and magnesium. There is an increased risk of adverse cardiovascular reactions with opioids or cardiac glycosides.

Dosage Regimen

Succinylcholine dosing hinges on the reason for its use. However, a test dose of 0.1 mg/kg, followed by assessment of respiratory function, is needed before administration. For short procedures in adults, the dosage of succinylcholine ranges from 0.3 to 1.1 mg/kg (see Table 12–4). In children, a dose of 1 to 2 mg/kg is used. Additional doses are dependent on response. Continuous IV infusion is not recommended for children or neonates.

For prolonged procedures in adults, the initial IV dose of succinylcholine ranges from 0.6 to 1.1 mg, followed by 0.04 to 0.07 mg/kg. Continuous IV infusion at a rate of 2.5 to 4.3 mg/minute is preferred over bolus doses. The dose is titrated to patient response and degree of paralysis required.

When succinylcholine is used as an adjunct to ECT, the dose is 10 to 30 mg given 1 minute before the treatment. Additional individualized doses may be required.

Laboratory Considerations

The sustained depolarization induced by succinylcholine is associated with potassium leakage from muscle. There is also a slight increase in serum potassium concentrations. In patients with recent burns, spinal cord injuries, and myopathies, however, succinylcholine can lead to sudden hyperkalemia and cardiac arrest.

Critical Thinking Process

Assessment

Assessment of the patient who is a candidate for neuromuscular blockade includes the history of present illness, past health history, physical exam, and diagnostic testing. There are a number of co-morbid conditions that place the patient at risk for complications. Patients with a history of myocardial infarction or deep vein thrombosis and those who have vasculopathy, hypertension, pulmonary disease, or a neuromuscular disease (e.g., myasthenia gravis) are at risk for complications. Patients with a history of chronic liver disease or kidney disease and those who are undergoing intraperitoneal or intrathoracic procedures need to be thoroughly screened before neuromuscular blockers are used. A personal or family history of malignant hyperthermia, myopathies, or acute narrow-angle glaucoma is significant to note. For female patients of child-bearing age, determine the date of their last menstrual period, because nondepolarizing neuromuscular blockers have not been approved for use during pregnancy. The depolarizing neuromuscular blocker drug succinylcholine is a Food and Drug Administration category C agent. Note the type of emotional support that is available to the patient. This is particularly important if it is known that the patient will be paralyzed for long periods.

A thorough drug history is important because of the potential for drug-drug interactions and adverse responses. Patients should be asked specifically if they have taken opioids, cardiac glycosides, monoamine oxidase (MAO) inhibitors, nonpenicillin antibiotics, quinidine, beta blockers, or diuretics in the previous 72 hours. The use of these drugs may influence the choice of anesthetic or preclude the use of certain other drugs.

Assess respiratory status before the use of neuromuscular blockers, including the rate, depth, and adequacy of breath sounds. Record vital signs. A basic neurologic assessment is performed with attention to vision, hearing, ability to swallow, facial expression, general movements, and the initiation of volitional movements. If deficits appear during this screening session, a more detailed neurologic assessment is performed.

Is the patient able to communicate verbally? Remember that once the patient is paralyzed, the ability to communicate is lost. Furthermore, symptoms of stroke, chest pain, and similar disorders will be extremely difficult to discern in the paralyzed patient. Furthermore, does the patient have pre-existing musculoskeletal disorders that will affect position changes required during paralysis?

Determine baseline laboratory values for factors that may alter the patient's response to neuromuscular blockade.

Baseline testing should include serum potassium, calcium, magnesium, blood urea nitrogen, and creatinine clearance. Serum levels of pseudocholinesterase may be needed for patients who are to receive succinylcholine.

Analysis and Management

Treatment Objectives

Neuromuscular blockers should be administered only by health care providers who are skilled in their use. There are three clinical outcomes related to muscular relaxation: no evidence of spontaneous patient movement, some patient movement but no spontaneous respirations, and movement and spontaneous respirations but without respiratory asynchrony. When the desired clinical outcome is no spontaneous movement, peripheral nerve stimulation is necessary to reduce the risk of excessive blockade.

Treatment Options

Drug Variables

The ideal neuromuscular blocker has five characteristics:

- It should be free of cardiovascular and autonomic adverse effects and should not increase intracranial pressure
- The onset and duration of neuromuscular blockade should be predictable
- Recovery of neuromuscular function after discontinuing the drug should occur quickly
- There should be no accumulation of parent drug or its metabolites with repetitive dosing
- There should be flexibility in administration to permit bolus injection or continuous IV infusion

Unfortunately, none of the currently available neuromuscular blockers meet all of these criteria.

The mode of administration influences the drug of choice. Long-acting neuromuscular blockers are usually given by intermittent injection. Short-acting or intermediate-acting drugs are suited for bolus injection or continuous infusion. Continuous infusion provides a stable degree of blockade for extended periods. Even though continuous infusions are more convenient, patients must be closely monitored to avoid excessive dosing. Intermittent doses of short-acting or intermediate-acting drugs may be used for short-term paralysis. However, with long-term use, this technique permits wide fluctuations in the degree of blockade and is inconvenient. On the other hand, this mode allows for assessment of patient movement before each dose is given, which minimizes the risk of unintentional overdose. If a drug or its metabolite begins to accumulate, the time between drug administration can be lengthened. The single disadvantage is simple. Dosing based on patient movement negates the original reason for the neuromuscular blockade.

In determining which nondepolarizing blocker to use, the health care provider takes into consideration the patient's history and physical exam results, as well as the drug's characteristics. Tubocurarine causes the greatest amount of histamine release and ganglionic blockade compared with other neuromuscular blockers. As a result, the risk of hypotension is relatively high. Doxacurium is essentially devoid of adverse cardiovascular effects. Pipecuronium does not cause histamine release and does not produce vagal blockade. It is relatively free of adverse cardiovascular effects. Age has no effect on pipecuronium's duration of paralysis.

Atracurium's organ-independent biotransformation makes it attractive for patients with multiple organ system failure. Gallamine causes histamine release in high doses. Other intermediate-acting neuromuscular blockers cause slight or no histamine release and no ganglionic blockade. Gallium, pancuronium, and rocuronium can cause tachycardia by blocking vagal input to the heart. Like gallamine, pancuronium can cause tachycardia via its vagolytic effects. Vecuronium does not produce ganglionic or vagal blockade and does not cause histamine release. Thus, cardiovascular effects are minimal.

Mivacurium causes cutaneous facial flushing secondary to histamine release. Other cardiovascular effects are minimal. Its duration of blockade at equipotent doses is two times greater than that of atracurium or vecuronium.

Succinylcholine causes large amounts of histamine to be released and stimulates ganglionic blockade. It may increase or decrease vagolytic activity.

Patient Variables

The preference for one neuromuscular blocker over another depends on the patient's end-organ dysfunction, route of drug biotransformation and elimination, and duration of therapy. The onset and duration of paralysis should be equivalent to that dictated by the procedure. Relatively short procedures (e.g., intubation) require a short-acting agent. Bolus administrations of intermediate-acting or long-acting drugs are used for longer procedures (e.g., radiologic scans or dressing changes). Lengthy procedures may require intermittent doses of long-acting agents or continuous infusions of short-acting or intermediate-acting drugs.

Because the health care provider loses the ability to interact with the paralyzed patient, physical examination of the patient cannot be accurately performed. Identification of changes in mental status and the presence of anginal pain, seizures, or peritonitis is difficult when the patient is paralyzed. Some health care providers advocate stopping neuromuscular blockade every 24 hours to reassess the patient and evaluate the need for continued paralysis. Reversing the paralysis, however, may result in deterioration of the condition that required the paralysis.

Patients on mechanical ventilation are at risk for respiratory distress syndrome. Signs of impending distress include desaturation with movement, rising peak inspiratory pressures, and difficulty maintaining adequate blood gas values despite sedation. Many times, pharmacologic paralysis helps prevent or minimize the risks of further complications in these patients.

Hyperkalemia may develop after a dose of succinylcholine in patients with burns, intra-abdominal abscess, or trauma, or in patients confined to bed. Atracurium should be used with caution in patients with asthma or allergies because of the likelihood of histamine-induced bronchospasm. Long-term administration of steroid-based neuromuscular blockers (e.g., pancuronium, pipecuronium, and vecuronium) should be avoided in patients with severe renal failure (owing to accumulation of active metabolites). Of the cur-

FACTORS ALTERING INDIVIDUAL RESPONSES TO NEUROMUSCULAR BLOCKING DRUGS

Potentiating Factors
Acidosis
Aminoglycosides
Benzodiazepines
Beta blockers
Calcium channel blockers
Corticosteroids
Droperidol
Hypocalcemia, hypokalemia
Hypothermia
Lincomycin
Lithium
Magnesium sulfate
Midazolam
Neomycin
Neuromuscular disease
Nitroglycerin
Phenytoin
Polymyxin A, B, E
Potassium-wasting diuretics
Procainamide
Tetracyclines
Vancomycin

Antagonizing Factors
Alkalosis
Aminophylline
Burns
Hypercalcemia, hyperkalemia
Pregnancy
Ranitidine

rently available neuromuscular blockers, doxacurium, pipecuronium, cisatracurium, and vecuronium are essentially devoid of clinically significant cardiovascular effects. These agents become the drugs of choice for patients with unstable cardiovascular profiles (see Factors Altering Individual Responses to Neuromuscular Blocking Drugs).

Children between the ages of 1 and 10 years may require higher doses and more frequent supplementation than adults receiving the same drug. Further, infants aged 7 weeks to 1 year are more sensitive to pancuronium and may require a longer recovery period from the drug owing to their immature hepatic and renal function.

Nondepolarizing drugs are safe to use in malignant hyperthermia–susceptible patients. The depolarizing drug succinylcholine can trigger malignant hyperthermia and is absolutely contraindicated in susceptible patients.

Many neuromuscular blockers contain iodides, bromides, parabens, or sulfites. The clinician should select drugs carefully in patients with known hypersensitivity.

Intervention

Administration

Neuromuscular blockers are not sedatives or analgesics. They do not affect consciousness or pain perception. Thus, sedatives (e.g., lorazapam and midazolam) or analgesics (e.g., morphine, alfentanil, fentanyl) should be administered concurrently when prolonged therapy is required. The benzodiazepine drug diazepam (see Chapter 17) should be avoided for sedation because significant accumulation of its metabolite can produce excessive sedation for days after stopping the drug. Propofol, an IV general anesthetic (see Chapter 16), has recently been approved for sedation of mechanically ventilated patients. Local or topical anesthetics should be used as appropriate for procedures such as wound débridement, dressing changes, or placement of IV catheters.

Increases in blood pressure and heart rate, diaphoresis, and tearing during a painful procedure (e.g., endotracheal tube suctioning) may indicate inadequate sedation and analgesia. The ability to assist or impede ventilator breaths or gagging or coughing during suctioning indicates that the patient is inadequately paralyzed or sedated. Conversely, failure to produce a physiologic response during stimulation may indicate that the level of sedation and analgesia is excessive.

Because the patient will be awake but will not appear to be, conversations taking place in the patient's presence should contain information suitable for the patient to hear. A sign should be placed on the patient's bed to alert visitors that the patient is in a drug-induced paralysis. Further, care should be taken to ensure the patient's comfort (e.g., frequent mouth care, frequent repositioning, and bathing) when neuromuscular blockers are used for prolonged periods. The patient's corneas should be protected with ocular lubricants (i.e., artificial tears) because the eyelids will remain open. If a patient will be paralyzed for extended periods, a special bed should be used to minimize pressure areas. Physical therapy and anticoagulation should be implemented to help maintain range of motion of joints and minimize the risk of deep vein thrombosis.

Vital signs and temperature should be checked every hour during neuromuscular blockade. Close monitoring of intake and output is necessary to predict drug excretion and end-organ function. In addition, neurologic signs (including pupillary reaction) must be monitored closely. Devastating neurologic events are often difficult to recognize because of the drug-induced muscular paralysis.

Respirations should be closely monitored during periods of peak drug activity. Because all neuromuscular blockers can cause respiratory arrest, intubation and ventilation equipment should be readily available. An Ambu bag and mask must always be kept at the patient's bedside. All ventilator alarms must be kept on. Patients also benefit from pulse oximetry and end-tidal carbon dioxide (CO_2) monitoring. Decreasing oxygen saturation or increasing CO_2 tension may indicate that the patient is not being effectively ventilated and oxygenated. Anticholinesterase drugs (see Chapter 13) should be readily available to reverse respiratory depression. Remember, reversal agents are not effective for succinylcholine-induced respiratory depression.

Malignant hyperthermia has been associated with the use of succinylcholine. Determine whether or not there is a patient or family history of this disorder before its use. Monitor the patient throughout administration for signs that malignant hyperthermia may be developing. Signs of malignant hyperthermia include development of tachycardia, tachypnea, hypercapnia, jaw muscle spasm, lack of laryngeal relaxation, and hyperthermia. The heart rate and rhythm and blood pressure should be monitored throughout the duration of the therapy.

Muscle fasciculations occurring during the initial phase of succinylcholine action account for patient complaints of muscle pain. A small dose of a nondepolarizing agent may be used before succinylcholine is administered to decrease the severity of muscle fasciculations and the resultant myalgia.

Monitoring Peripheral Nerve Stimulation The extent of neuromuscular blockade is objectively assessed using peripheral nerve stimulation. Peripheral nerve stimulation is performed before and throughout treatment with neuromuscular blockers. Peripheral nerve stimulation is extremely beneficial in patients who exhibit pharmacokinetic and pharmacodynamic characteristics predisposing them to prolonged paralysis. Failure to monitor blockade can result in an unintentional overdose.

Commonly employed tests performed with the peripheral nerve stimulator include train-of-four (TOF) stimulation, single-twitch stimulation, and tetanic stimulation. TOF is preferred because the degree of block can be read directly from the response, and because it is less painful than other forms of nerve stimulation. The ulnar nerve is used most often. The facial, common peroneal, or posterior tibial nerve can also be used. Electrocardiographic (ECG) electrodes are placed on the skin over the nerve. An electrical impulse is sent through to verify the ability of the nerve to prompt muscle movement.

TOF delivers four bursts of electricity over 2 seconds every 30 to 60 seconds. The desired response is one muscle twitch per four electrical impulses. This response indicates blockade of more than 90 percent of receptors. However, additional drug may be needed if two, three, or four twitches are elicited from one series. Clinical signs of movement that indicate additional drug is needed include the presence of reflexive and spontaneous movement, spontaneous respiratory efforts, and increasing levels of palpable muscle tone. Testing should be performed at least every four hours when neuromuscular blockers are administered by continuous IV infusion.

Reversal of Neuromuscular Blockade Muscle tone returns either spontaneously with the discontinuation of the drug or after administation of an anticholinesterase reversal drug. Spontaneous return of muscle tone is permitted when the drug was used to facilitate intubation and mechanical ventilation. Reversal drugs are used to return muscle tone and respirations after surgical procedures. Reversal drugs are also used when a patient is weaned from mechanical ventilation and immediate reversal of the neuromuscular blockade is unnecessary. Spontaneous patient movement usually begins within 1 hour of discontinuation or reversal of the drug activity.

Reversal of neuromuscular blockade is possible only with nondepolarizing drugs. The reversal drugs act at the neuromuscular junction to decrease the natural metabolism of acetylcholine and overcome the competitive block. The anticholinesterase drug (e.g., neostigmine, pyridostigmine, and edrophonium) is combined with a muscarinic receptor antagonist (e.g., atropine or glycopyrrolate) to prevent cardiac arrest and bronchospasm due to excess stimulation of muscarinic receptors.

Clinically adequate reversal is noted when the head can be lifted off the bed for at least 5 seconds. However, complete return of gross and fine motor movement depends on the duration of therapy, duration of immobility, muscle weakness, and the patient's nutritional status. Administration of reversal drugs to a patient in whom heavy neuromuscular blockade was used may not provide adequate clinical reversal, even though the drug had a pharmacologic effect. This results from oversaturation of drug receptors occupied by the neuromuscular blocker or its metabolites. Anticholinesterase drugs should be avoided in patients who have a significant past medical history of coronary artery disease, reactive airway disease, obstructive lung disease, or acute narrow-angle glaucoma.

Check the patient's gag reflex and ability to swallow before administering oral drugs or food to a patient recovering from neuromuscular blockade to reduce the possibility of aspiration. Monitor the respiratory rate, depth, and adequacy during the period of recovery. Note changes in heart rate and blood pressure as indications for supplemental drugs.

Education

Explain all procedures to the patient receiving neuromuscular blockers, particularly when they are used without general anesthesia. Remember, consciousness is not affected by these drugs alone. Patients should be routinely reminded why they are paralyzed and that the paralysis is only temporary. Reassure the patient that communication abilities and movement will return as drug effects wear off. The patient should also be reassured that they will be monitored closely during the period of paralysis. It is important to maintain the patient's dignity and comfort at all times.

Muscle fasciculations during the initial phase of succinylcholine action account for patient complaints of muscle pain. Reassure the patient that this response, although unpleasant, is not unusual. The discomfort can persist for several hours or days.

Evaluation

The effectiveness of therapy with neuromuscular blockers can be demonstrated by adequate suppression of the twitch response when it is tested with peripheral nerve stimulation and subsequent muscle paralysis.

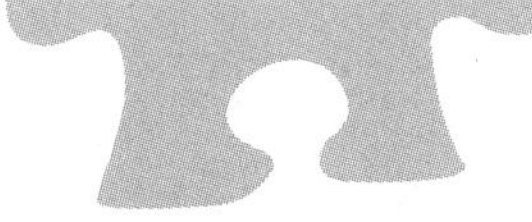

SUMMARY

- Indications for pharmacologic paralysis with neuromuscular blockers include endotracheal intubation and surgical procedures, and to facilitate mechanical ventilation. Some drugs have been used as adjunctive agents during electroconvulsive therapy. Tubocurarine can be used to diagnose myasthenia gravis.
- The specific drug to be administered, dose, route, adverse effect profile, underlying pathophysiologic process, and expected clinical outcomes should be determined.
- The primary differences in neuromuscular blockers are potency and duration of action. The degree of blockade required to facilitate patient management varies from patient to patient.
- There are three clinical outcomes related to muscular relaxation: no evidence of spontaneous patient movement, some pa-

tient movement but no spontaneous respirations, and movement and spontaneous respirations but without respiratory asynchrony.

- Peripheral nerve stimulation monitoring is necessary when the clinical objective is no patient movement. Monitoring is necessary to reduce the risk of excessive blockade that may result from overdose.
- Recovery from nondepolarizing neuromuscular blockade can be hastened by the administration of a anticholinesterase drug (e.g., neostigmine, pyridostigmine, and edrophonium). There is no reversal agent for succinylcholine.
- Clinically adequate reversal is noted when the patient can lift his or her head off the bed for at least 5 seconds.
- Anticipating, assessing, monitoring, treating, and evaluating the patient's pain and anxiety are paramount considerations for patients receiving neuromuscular blocking drugs.
- The health care provider has an essential role as patient advocate to ensure that every paralyzed patient, regardless of age, is adequately medicated with analgesics and sedatives. Neuromuscular blocking drugs should never be used as a substitute for analgesics and sedatives.
- The indications for neuromuscular blockade should be reviewed daily and the drug discontinued as soon as medically possible.
- Reassure the patient that myalgia associated with succinylcholine drug action, although unpleasant, is not unusual and will resolve.

BIBLIOGRAPHY

Collins, V. (1996). *Physiologic and pharmacologic bases of anesthesia.* Baltimore: Williams & Wilkins.

Cummins, R. (Ed.). (1994). *Textbook of advanced cardiac life support.* Dallas: American Heart Association.

Dulin, P., and Williams, C. (1994). Monitoring and preventative care of the paralyzed patient in respiratory failure. *Critical Care Clinics,* 10(4), 815–829.

Durbin, C. (1991). Neuromuscular blocking agents and sedative drugs: Clinical uses and toxic effects in the critical care unit. *Critical Care Clinician,* 7(3), 489–506.

Feldman, S., and Hood, J. (1996). Factors governing onset of neuromuscular block. *British Journal of Anesthesia,* 76(4), 596–598.

Jarpe, M. (1992). Nursing care of patients receiving long-term infusion of neuromuscular blocking agents. *Critical Care Nurse,* 12(7), 58–63.

Johnson, R. (1993). Reversal of neuromuscular blocking drugs. *Anesthesiology Clinics of North America,* 11(2), 391–407.

Mellinghoff, H., Radbruch, L., Diefenbach, C., et al. (1996). A comparison of cisatracurium and atracurium: Onset of neuromuscular block after bolus injection and recovery after subsequent infusion. *Anesthesia and Analgesia,* 83(5), 1072–1075.

Smith, S., Brown, H., Toman J., et al. (1947). The lack of cerebral effects of D-tubocurarine. *Anesthesiology,* 8, 1–14.

Susla, G. (1993). Neuromuscular blocking agents in critical care. *Critical Care Nursing Clinics of North America,* 5(2), 297–311.

Wild, L. (1991). Neuromuscular blocking agents in the critically ill patient: Neither sedating or pain relieving. *AACN Clinical Issues in Critical Care Nursing,* 2(4), 778–787.

Young, L., and Koda-Kimble, M. (1995). *Applied therapeutics: the clinical use of drugs.* Vancouver, WA: Applied Therapeutics, Inc.

13 Parasympathetic Nervous System Drugs

Most body organs are innervated by both the sympathetic and parasympathetic nervous systems. This allows each system to counterbalance individually the effects of the other on a particular organ or gland. The parasympathetic nervous system produces effects opposite those of the sympathetic nervous system. So when stress has passed, parasympathetic stimulation slows the heart rate and returns the body to physiologic stability.

The terms *parasympathomimetic* and *cholinergic* describe drugs that produce the same effects as those initiated by parasympathetic nerve stimulation. *Acetylcholine* (ACh), the primary parasympathetic nervous system neurotransmitter, is synthesized from choline and acetyl coenzyme A with the assistance of the enzyme choline acetyltransferase (Fig. 13–1). The large pyramidal cells of the motor cortex and the cells of the basal ganglia are major sources of ACh. Preganglionic neurons and motor neurons that innervate skeletal muscles are additional sources of ACh. ACh is also secreted by the postganglionic neurons of both the parasympathetic and sympathetic nervous systems.

ACh stimulates the ganglia, the adrenal medullae, the skeletal muscles, and the postganglionic nerve endings in cardiac muscle, smooth muscle, and glands. It binds to both the nicotinic and muscarinic receptors. *Nicotinic effects* include tachycardia, elevated blood pressure, and peripheral vasoconstriction. However, rapid biotransformation of ACh weakens these effects. *Muscarinic effects* include increased salivary secretion, gastric motility, and gastric acid secretion. As with other systems of the human body, there is a check and balance system in place that prevents normal functions from proceeding uncontrolled. In the case of ACh, the mechanism of balance is *acetylcholinesterase,* an enzyme that breaks down ACh.

A number of conditions, including urinary retention, dementia of the Alzheimer's type, nausea, peptic ulcer disease, irritable bowel syndrome, motion sickness, visual disorders, and Parkinson's disease, can be treated with parasympathetic nervous system drugs. To understand the use of parasympathetic nervous system drugs in the treatment of some of these disorders, a brief explanation of the disorders is appropriate.

URINARY RETENTION

Etiology and Epidemiology

Urinary retention is defined as a condition in which urine that is retained in the bladder. Urine production continues, but the accumulated urine is not released. The incidence of urinary retention varies with the etiology. It occurs in approximately 10 to 15 percent of patients who receive general anesthesia and 20 to 25 percent of patients following spinal anesthesia. More than half of men over the age of 50 have benign prostatic hyperplasia that contributes to urinary retention. Urinary retention can be serious because of the risk of urinary tract infection and stone formation. There is also a risk of direct damage to the bladder, ureters, or kidneys. Further, continued bladder distention leads to loss of bladder tone.

Patients who have received epidural anesthesia may experience urinary retention. Additionally, opioid analgesics are commonly used for pain management, and the level of voiding reflex inhibition is directly related to the level of analgesia. In other words, the more effective the pain control, the greater the risk of urinary retention. These effects are observed with both epidural and parenteral routes of drug administration. Depending on the dosage, opioid analgesics may impair bladder function for as long as 14 to 16 hours.

Preoperative drugs, anesthetics, and surgical manipulation, either alone or in combination, can also cause urinary retention. Because general anesthetics have an inhibitory effect on bladder function, the longer the patient is under general anesthesia, the greater the risk of urinary retention. Circumstances associated with surgery that may affect the patient's ability to void include the length of the procedure and the amount of intravenous fluids administered. The patient may have an overfull bladder on completion of the procedure or may not be alert enough to recognize the need to void. Thus, the bladder becomes distended, increasing the likelihood of retention.

Anorectal disorders such as hemorrhoids, abscess, or fecal impaction also contribute to urinary retention. The retention is caused by obstruction or spasms of perineal muscles, hampering the ability to relax. Anorectal surgery is associated with a particularly high incidence of postoperative urinary retention. Stimulation of the vesicoanal reflex inhibits contraction of the detrusor muscle, resulting in urinary retention. The reflex may be activated by physically stimulating the anus or rectum by the pres-ence of packing materials in the anus or rectal vault, or by pain associated with examination or procedures.

Autonomic dysfunction secondary to spinal cord injury initially results in an areflexive bladder that later leads to urinary retention and a neurogenic bladder. Immobility also contributes to urinary retention. Patients confined to bed, particularly those unable to sit upright, may find it difficult if not impossible to void using a bedpan. In an effort to avoid movement and the possibility of increased pain, patients may ignore the sensation of a full bladder. Or anxiety that someone will see or hear them using a bedpan or bedside commode may inhibit their ability to relax enough to void. Because privacy is an uncommon commodity in institutional settings, urinary retention may escalate.

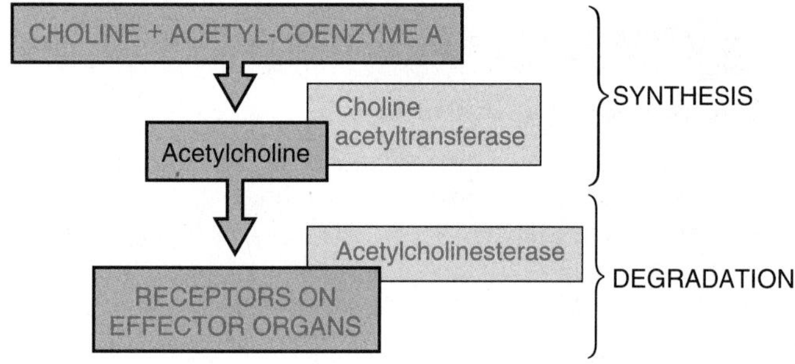

Figure 13–1 Acetylcholine is synthesized by combining choline with acetyl-coenzyme A and is degraded by the enzyme acetyl-cholinesterase.

Physiology and Pathophysiology

Bladder emptying requires contraction of the detrusor muscle and relaxation of urinary sphincters. Striated muscle of the external urinary sphincter is under voluntary control. The bladder has an amazing ability to stretch to accommodate urine, contract, empty, and return to its resting size. However, as the bladder becomes overstretched, its ability to contract rapidly diminishes.

Urinary retention produces a series of adverse consequences. As urine accumulates, hydrostatic pressure against the bladder wall increases. Hypertrophy of the detrusor muscle, development of connective tissue in the bladder wall, or development of diverticula may result. Ureteral peristalsis also increases as pressure against the accumulating urine rises. Ureters gradually distend and elongate, becoming fibrotic and tortuous. The pressure is transmitted through renal pelves and calices to the parenchyma. In turn, the resulting hydronephrosis exerts pressure on renal vasculature, causing ischemia and parenchymal damage. Without interruption, the process can progress to renal failure and death.

In addition, as pressure within the bladder continues to rise, the pressure overcomes the restraint of the sphincter and incontinence results. Urine is released until the intravesicular pressure is reduced but only to the extent that the external sphincter can regain control. The cycle is repeated as the bladder continues to overfill. Prolonged high intravesicular pressures predispose the patient to diverticula. A diverticulum is an outpocketing of the mucous membrane lining due to weakness in the bladder wall. Bladder diverticula contribute to the risk of urinary tract infections and malignancy. The infections are related to urinary stasis. The malignancy is thought to be related to chronic irritation.

Drug therapy can be used to treat urinary retention and thus reduce the likelihood of complications. Direct-acting and indirect-acting cholinergic drugs are used to facilitate voiding in some patients.

PHARMACOTHERAPEUTIC OPTIONS

Direct-Acting Cholinergics

❒ Bethanechol chloride (URECHOLINE, DUVOID, URABETH, UROCARB); (🍁) DUVOID, URECHOLINE

Indications

Bethanechol chloride is used for the short-term treatment of postoperative or postpartum urinary retention. The drug is also used on a long-term basis to treat patients who have urinary retention due to neurogenic atony of the bladder. Because bethanechol chloride also acts on the gastrointestinal (GI) tract, it may be used to treat gastroesophageal reflux disease and megacolon (dilation and hypertrophy of the colon).

Pharmacodynamics

Direct-acting cholinergics are structurally and pharmacologically similar to ACh. Drug effects are the result of direct stimulation of cholinergic receptors in postsynaptic membranes (Fig. 13–2). Bethanechol is a synthetic choline ester; however, unlike naturally occurring ACh, bethanechol is not destroyed in the synapse by acetylcholinesterase. Thus, the drug enhances the activity of naturally occurring ACh. The enhancement results in contraction of the detrusor muscle and emptying of the bladder. There is also stimulation of intestinal peristalsis, resulting in bowel elimination.

Adverse Effects and Contraindications

The most common adverse effects of bethanechol chloride are associated with the GI and urinary systems. Urinary urgency, nausea, vomiting, salivation, abdominal cramps, and diarrhea are frequent. Headache, malaise, increased lacrimation, increased bronchial secretions, miosis, flushing of the skin, and diaphoresis have also been reported. The adverse effects are more common when the drug is given subcutaneously (SC) rather than by mouth. The most life-threatening adverse effects include syncope, heart block, and cardiac arrest.

Bethanechol chloride should not be used in patients with urethral obstruction or if the urethral sphincter is unable to dilate. In these instances, intravesical pressure increases against an obstructed outlet, which, in turn, causes ureterovesical reflux and the risk of a ruptured bladder.

Bethanechol chloride is also contraindicated in patients in whom the strength or integrity of the bladder wall or GI tract is compromised. Patients with a mechanical obstruction or acute inflammatory lesions of the GI tract, a history of peptic ulcers, spastic disturbances, or peritonitis should not use bethanechol chloride because of the risk of damage to the GI tract.

Patients with latent or active asthma may experience life-threatening bronchial constriction in the presence of bethanechol chloride. The drug is also contraindicated for patients with pronounced bradycardia, hypotension, cardiac disease, vasomotor instability, hypertension, or marked vagotonia (irritability of the vagus nerve). The

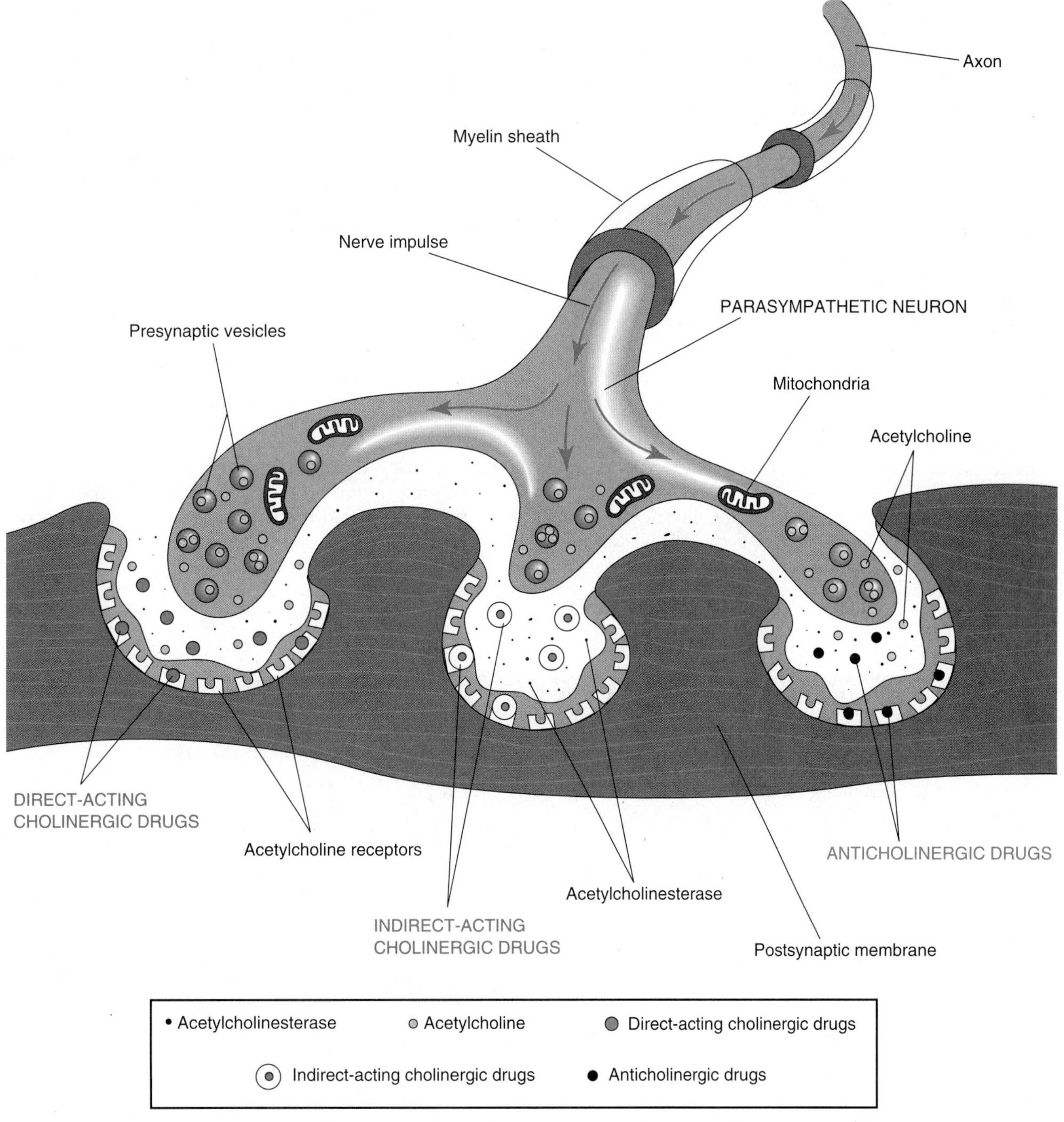

Figure 13–2 Parasympathetic drug action. Direct-acting cholinergics stimulate cholinergic receptors in postsynaptic membranes that are innervated by parasympathetic neurons. They mimic the action of acetylcholine. Indirect-acting cholinergics act primarily by shielding acetylcholine from the effects of acetylcholinesterase. The blocking effects result in accumulation of ACh at all sites where it is liberated. Anticholinergic drugs block the action of ACh at postganglionic sites.

drug causes significant changes in blood vessel diameter and resulting changes in cardiac function and blood pressure. Patients with hyperthyroidism or seizure disorders may have an exacerbation of their disease and are at increased risk for cardiac complications. Patients suffering from Parkinson's disease may notice an increase in tremors because of the cholinergic effect of bethanechol chloride.

Bethanechol chloride must never be given intravenously (IV) or intramuscularly (IM). The extreme stimulation of cholinergic receptors resulting from IV or IM administration can lead to circulatory collapse, profound hypotension, shock, and cardiac arrest. The symptoms of circulatory collapse are typically preceded by severe abdominal cramping and bloody diarrhea.

Bethanechol chloride is a pregnancy class C drug that should be used with caution. It is not known if the drug passes into breast milk, which is a concern because one of the prime indications of use for the drug is postpartum urinary retention.

Pharmacokinetics

Bethanechol chloride is poorly absorbed when it is administered by mouth, and thus, larger doses are needed when the drug is given orally. The onset of drug action occurs 30 to 90 minutes after oral administration (Table 13–1). The peak response by the detrusor muscle occurs in 1 hour, with drug effects lasting up to 6 hours. The onset of drug effects occurs 5 to 15 minutes after SC administration. Peak drug effects are reached in 15 to 30 minutes and last up to 2 hours.

Drug-Drug Interactions

Atropine, an anticholinergic drug, reverses the cholinergic effects of bethanechol chloride (Table 13–2). Although this phenomenon is useful in cases of toxicity, it can interfere with treatment if atropine or other anticholinergic drugs are used concurrently with bethanechol chloride. Procainamide and quinidine have similar effects. Cholinergic drugs and cholinesterase inhibitors produce synergistic effects and can result in toxicity if they are given concurrently. Concurrent use of ganglionic blocking drugs (e.g., mecamylamine) may result in severe hypotension. Patients typically complain of severe abdominal cramping and diarrhea before the hypotension becomes profound.

Dosage Regimen

The initial adult dose of bethanechol chloride is determined by orally administering 5 to 10 mg of the drug every 1 to 2 hours until the desired response is obtained or a total of 50 mg has been given (Table 13–3). Treatment can also be initiated by starting with 10 mg and giving 25 mg 6 hours later. If needed, a 50-mg dose may be given in another 6 hours. The usual maintenance dose of bethanechol chloride is 10 to 50 mg three times daily. Maintenance doses of 50 to 100 mg given four times daily have been used. It should be noted that this dosage is higher than that recommended by the FDA.

The SC dose of bethanechol chloride may be determined by administering 2.5 mg every 15 to 30 minutes until the desired response is obtained or a total of four doses has been administered. The maintenance dosage ranges from 2.5 to 5 mg three to four times daily. For children, the usual dose is 0.2 mg/kg/day in three to four divided doses.

Laboratory Considerations

Monitoring serum levels of bethanechol chloride is not ordinarily required. However, bethanechol chloride may increase serum aspartate aminotransferase (AST serum glutamic-oxaloacetic transaminase [SGOT]), serum amylase, and serum lipase concentrations.

TABLE 13–1 PHARMACOKINETICS OF SELECTED PARASYMPATHETIC NERVOUS SYSTEM DRUGS

Drug	Route	Onset	Peak	Duration	PB (%)	$t_{1/2}$
Direct-Acting Cholinergic						
Bethanechol	po	30–90 min	60 min	1–6 hr	UA	UA
	SC	5–15 min	15–30 min	2 hr	UA	UA
Indirect-Acting Cholinergic						
Tacrine	po	UK	1–2 hr	4–8 hr	55	2–4 hr
Cholinesterase Inhibitor						
Donepezil	po	Varies	2–4 hr	24 hr	UA	8–12 hr
Anticholinergics						
Atropine	po/SC	30–90 min	1–2 hr	4–6 hr	Mod	2.5 hr
	IM	30 min	1–1.6 hr	Brief	Mod	2.5 hr
Clidinium	po	60 min	UA	3 hr	UA	UA
Dicyclomine	po/IM	UK	60–90 min	UK	UA	1.8 hr
Glycopyrrolate	po	UK	UK	8–12 hr*	UA	0.6–4.6 hr
	IM	15–30 min	30–45 min	2–7 hr	UA	0.6–4.6 hr
	IV	1 min	UK	2–7 hr	UA	0.6–4.6 hr
Hyoscyamine	po/IM	5–30 min	30–60 min	4–12 hr	Mod	3.5 hr
	IV	2 min	15–30 min	4–12 hr	Mod	
Mepenzolate	po	60 min	UA	3–4 hr	UA	UA
Methscopolamine	po	60 min	UA	4–6 hr	UA	2–3 hr
Propantheline	po	30–60 min	2–6 hr	6 hr	UA	3–4 hr
Scopolamine	TD	UK	UK	3 days	UA	8 hr
	IM	30 min		4 hr	Low	UA
	IV	UK		UK	UA	
Autonomic Ganglionic Stimulants						
NICORETTE	Chew	Rapid	15–30 min	UK	UA	1–2 hr
NICODERM	TD	Slow	2–4 hr	UK	UA	1–2 hr
HABITROL	TD	Slow	6–12 hr	UK	UA	1–2 hr
PROSTEP	TD	Slow	9 hr	UK	UA	1–2 hr
Autonomic Ganglionic Blocker						
Mecamylamine	po	30 min–2 hr	3–5 hr	6–12 hr	UA	4–6 hr

*The antisecretory effects of glycopyrrolate last up to 7 hours. Vagal blockade lasts 2 to 3 hours.
PB, Protein binding; $t_{1/2}$, elimination half-life; TD, transdermal patch; UA, unavailable; UK, unknown.

TABLE 13–2 DRUG-DRUG INTERACTIONS OF SELECTED PARASYMPATHETIC NERVOUS SYSTEM DRUGS

Drug	Interactive Drugs	Interaction
Direct-Acting Cholinergic		
Bethanechol	Atropine	Reversal of cholinergic effects
	Anticholinergic drugs	
	Procainamide	
	Quinidine	
	Cholinergic drugs	Additive effects and increased risk of toxicity
	Cholinesterase inhibitors	
	Ganglionic blockers	Severe hypotension
	Anticholinergics	Decreased effectiveness of bethanechol chloride
Indirect-Acting Cholinergic		
Tacrine	Bethanechol chloride	Synergistic effects when used together, can cause bladder outlet obstruction if used together
	Theophylline	Decreased biotransformation of theophylline resulting in increased serum levels
	Cimetidine	Decreased biotransformation of tacrine resulting in increased serum levels
	Succinylcholine	Exaggerates neuromuscular blockade
	NSAIDs	Increased gastric irritation related to increased cholinergic activity
	Nicotine	Decreases blood levels of tacrine
Cholinesterase Inhibitor		
Donepezil	Theophylline	Increases drug effects and risk of toxicity
	Cholinesterase inhibitors	
	Anticholinergics	Decreases effects of interactive drug
	NSAIDs	Increases risk of GI bleeding
Anticholinergic Drugs		
Atropine	Antacids	Decreased absorption of anticholinergics
Dicyclomine	Amantadine	Synergistic action
Hyoscyamine	Antihistamines	
Scopolamine	Antiparkinsonian drugs	
	Disopyramide	
	Histamine-1 antagonists	
	Glutethimide	
	Meperidine	
	Monoamine oxidase inhibitors	
	Procainamide	
	Quinidine	
	Tricyclic antidepressants	
	Ketoconazole	Decreased absorption of interactive drug
	Levodopa	
	Phenothiazines	
	Methotrimeprazine	May cause extrapyramidal symptoms
	Wax matrix potassium chloride	Increased risk of mucosal lesions from atropine
	Digoxin	Increased levels of interactive drug
Scopolamine	Alcohol	Additive CNS depression
Methscopolamine	Haloperidol	Decreased antipsychotic effectiveness of interactive drug
Autonomic Ganglionic Stimulant		
Nicotine	Insulin	Insulin requirements may decrease during nicotine withdrawal
	Acetaminophen	Effects of interactive drug may be increased during nicotine withdrawal owing to reduced biotransformation
	Caffeine	
	Furosemide	
	Imipramine	
	Oxazepam	
	Pentazocine	
	Propranolol	
	Theophylline	
Autonomic Ganglionic Blocker		
Mecamylamine	Antihypertensive drugs	Enhanced antihypertensive effects

CNS, Central nervous system; GI, gastrointestinal; NSAIDs, nonsteroidal anti-inflammatory drugs.

TABLE 13–3 DOSAGE REGIMENS FOR SELECTED PARASYMPATHETIC NERVOUS SYSTEM DRUGS

Drug	Use(s)	Dosage	Implications
Direct-Acting Cholinergic			
Bethanechol	Nonobstructive urinary retention, postoperative or postpartum urinary retention, neurogenic atony of urinary bladder with retention	*Adult:* 10–50 mg po BID–QID *or* 2.5–5 mg SC TID–QID. *Child:* 0.6 mg/kg/day po in three to four divided doses *or* 0.2 mg/kg/day SC in three to four divided doses	Never give the injectable form IM or IV. Oral and SC formulations are not interchangeable. Administer oral formulation on empty stomach. Monitor for drug toxicity (sweating, abdominal cramps, nausea, salivation).
Indirect-Acting Cholinergic			
Tacrine	Mild to moderate cognitive deficits of dementia of the Alzheimer's type	*Adult:* Initial dose 10 mg po QID for 6 weeks, then 20 mg QID for 6 weeks if needed. Increase dosage to 30 mg QID for 6 weeks and then maintain at 40 mg QID if needed	Use and titration must be accompanied by evaluation of ALT (SGPT) levels. Teach caregivers the signs and symptoms of liver disease
Cholinesterase Inhibitor			
Donepezil	Mild to moderate dementia of the Alzheimer's type	*Adult:* 5 mg po daily at HS. Increase to 10 mg QD after first 4 to 6 weeks	Notify health care provider if surgery is required because exaggerated muscle relaxation may occur if succinylcholine-type drugs are used concurrently
Anticholinergic Drugs			
Atropine	Treatment of bradycardia and bradyarrhythmias	*Adult:* 0.5–1.0 mg IV push. Repeat every 3–5 min as needed to a maximum of 2 mg *Child:* 0.01 mg/kg IV push. Maximum: 0.4 mg	Doses less than 0.5 mg in adults can *cause* bradycardia. If overdose occurs, physostigmine is the antidote. Intense flushing of the face and trunk occurs 15–20 minutes after IM administration. In children, this response is called "atropine flush" and is not harmful. Instruct patient that oral rinses, sugarless gum or candy, and frequent oral hygiene may help relieve dry mouth. Caution patients that atropine impairs heat regulation. Strenuous activity in hot environment may cause heat stroke. Instruct patients with benign prostatic hyperplasia that drug may cause urinary hesitancy and retention.Changes in urinary stream should be reported to health care provider
	Preoperatively to decrease secretions and block cardiac vagal reflexes	*Adult and child over 20 kg:* 0.2–0.6 mg IM/IV/SC 30–60 minutes preoperatively *or* 2 mg po *Child 12–20 kg:* 0.3 mg IM/SC 30–60 minutes preoperatively *Child 7–9 kg:* 0.2 mg 30–60 mg IM/SC 30–60 minutes preoperatively *Child 3 kg:* 0.1 mg 30–60 mg IM/SC 30–60 minutes preoperatively	
	Adjunctive treatment of peptic ulcer disease or treatment of irritable bowel syndrome	*Adult:* 0.4–0.6 mg po every 4–6 hours *Child:* 0.01 mg/kg *or* 0.3 mg/m^2 to oral maximum dose of 0.4 mg	
	Reversal of cholinesterase inhibitor drug effects	*Adults:* 0.6–1.2 mg for each 0.5–2.5 mg of neostigmine methylsulfate or 10–20 mg of pyridostigmine currently with cholinesterase inhibitor	
Clidinium	Adjunct in peptic ulcer disease	*Adult:* 2.5–5 mg po TID–QID before meals and at HS *Older adult:* 2.5 mg po TID before meals	Administer 30 minutes to 1 hour before meals for better absorption
Dicyclomine	Irritable bowel syndrome	*Adult:* 10–20 mg po TID–QID to maximum of 160 mg/day *Child over 2 yr:* 10 mg po TID–QID. Adjust dose as tolerated *Child 6 mo–2 yr:* 5–10 mg po TID–QID. Adjust dose as tolerated	Do not use SC or IV. Separate administration of dicyclomine and antacids by 2–3 hours Administer 30–60 minutes before to meals. Bedtime dose should be administered at least 2 hours after last meal
Glycopyrrolate	Control of secretions during surgery	*Adult:* 4.4 mcg/kg 30–60 minutes preoperatively. Not to exceed 0.1 mg *Child:* 4.4–8.8 mcg/kg 30–60 minutes preoperatively	The antisecretory effects of glycopyrrolate last up to 7 hours. Vagal blockade lasts 2 to3 hours
	Peptic ulcer	*Adult:* 1–2 mg po BID–TID. An additional 2 mg may be given at HS. Not to exceed 8 mg po daily *or* 100–200 mcg q4hr IM/IV up to four times daily	Do not administer within 1 hour of antacids or antidiarrheal drugs to maximize absorption. Administer IV at rate of 0.2 mg over 1–2 minutes. If overdosage occurs, neostigmine is the antidote
	Antiarrhythmic	*Adult:* 100 mcg IV. May repeat q2–3 minutes. *Child:* 4.4 mcg/kg (up to 100 mcg). May repeat q2–3 minutes.	

TABLE 13–3 DOSAGE REGIMENS FOR SELECTED PARASYMPATHETIC NERVOUS SYSTEM DRUGS *Continued*

Drug	Use(s)	Dosage	Implications
Hyoscyamine	Management of irritable bowel syndrome, genitourinary tract spasm	*Adult and child over 12 yr:* 0.125–0.5 mg po TID–QID *or* 0.375 mg twice daily as extended-release capsule	Give before meals and HS. There are elixirs and oral solution, tablets, and extended-release formulations. The concentrations are not the same. Avoid mistakenly substituting one for the other. Administer 30–60 minutes before meals. Bedtime dose should be given at least 2 hours after last meal
Mepenzolate	Peptic ulcer disease, adjunct in irritable bowel syndrome	*Adult:* 25–50 mg po QID before meals and HS. Titrate based on patient response	Administer 30 minutes to 1 hour before meals for better absorption
Methscopolamine	Peptic ulcer disease	*Adult:* 2.5–5 mg po before meals and HS	Administer 30 minutes to 1 hour before meals for better absorption
Propantheline	Antisecretory or antispasmodic drug	*Adult:* 15 mg po TID with 30 mg at HS *Older adults:* 7.5 mg po TID–QID *Child:* 0.375 mg/kg (10 mg/m^2) QID	Administer 30 minutes before meals. Bedtime dose should be given at least 2 hours after last meal of the day
Scopolamine	Preoperatively to decrease secretions and block cardiac vagal reflexes	*Adult:* 0.2–0.6 mg IM/SC/IV 30–60 minutes before anesthesia *Child age 8–12 yr:* 0.3 mg IM 45 minutes before anesthesia *Child age 3–8 yr:* 0.2 mg IM 45 minutes before anesthesia *Child 7 mo-3 yr:* 0.15 mg IM 45 minutes before anesthesia *Infants 4–7 mo:* 0.1 mg IM or IV 45 minutes before anesthesia	Assess patient for signs of urinary retention periodically throughout therapy. May act as stimulant in presence of pain, producing delirium if used without morphine or meperidine
Autonomic Ganglionic Stimulants			
HABITROL NICODERM	Smoking cessation Smoking cessation	*Adult:* 21 mg/day patches for 4 to 8 weeks, followed by 14-mg/day patches for 2 to 4 weeks, and 7-mg/day patches for an additional 2- to 4-week period	Transdermal systems are worn 24 hours per day. Patients weighing less than 100 pounds, who smoke less than 10 cigarettes per day, or who have underlying cardiac disease should begin therapy at 14 mg/day. Total treatment period lasts 14–20 weeks
NICOTROL	Smoking cessation	*Adult:* 15-mg/day patches for 4 to 12 weeks, followed by 10 mg/day for 2 to 4 weeks, and 5 mg/day for the last 2 to 4 weeks	
PROSTEP	Smoking cessation	*Adult:* 22-mg/day patches for 4 to 8 weeks, then 11 mg/day for 2 to 4 weeks.	Total treatment period lasts 6–12 weeks. Patients weighing less than 100 pounds, who smoke less than 10 cigarettes per day, or who have underlying cardiac disease should begin therapy at 11 mg/day
NICORETTE	Smoking cessation	*Adult:* 2 or 4 mg (1 piece of gum) as needed. Initial requirement usually 20 mg of 2-mg strength pieces or 80 mg/day of the 4-mg strength	The amount needed is determined by smoking urge or rate of chewing, or on a fixed schedule every 1 to 2 hours. The gum should be chewed slowly until a tingling sensation is felt. Stop chewing and store gum between cheek and gums until tingling sensation disappears (about 1 minute). Resume the cycle for approximately 30 minutes
Autonomic Ganglionic Blocker			
Mecamylamine	Dissecting aortic aneurysm, uncomplicated malignant hypertension	*Adult:* 2.5 mg po BID initially. May increase by 2.5-mg increments every 2 days until desired BP response occurs. Average total daily dose is 25 mg in three divided doses	Give after meals for more gradual absorption and smoother control of BP. Discontinue drug gradually. Abrupt discontinuation may cause rebound hypertension and fatal cerebrovascular accident or acute heart failure

Critical Thinking Process

Assessment

History of Present Illness

Urinary retention typically develops while a patient is hospitalized rather than being an illness that brings the patient to the health care system. The patient may complain of bladder fullness or generalized pelvic discomfort. The patient reports the need to void but is unable to do so. The patient may also complain of overflow incontinence or a feeling that the bladder is not emptying with each voiding. Particular attention should be paid to patients who lack normal sensory function of the bladder and those who have received local or spinal anesthetics. Patients with neurogenic atony may not complain of urinary symptoms.

Past Health History

Recent childbirth and surgery are the two most relevant components of the past medical history. Also of importance is a history of stroke or diabetes. These two disorders can interfere with normal neurologic function of the bladder. The most common cause of neurogenic atony of the bladder is spinal cord injury.

Be sure to elicit information regarding a past history of peptic ulcer disease, asthma, cardiovascular disease, or hyperthyroidism. A previous history of mechanical obstruction of the GI or urinary tract may contraindicate use of cholinergic drugs. Patient allergies should also be noted.

Physical Exam Findings

The ability to palpate the bladder above the symphysis pubis indicates urinary retention. Depending on the patient's size and weight, palpation, even of a distended bladder, may be difficult. In very thin patients, it may be possible to visualize distention of the bladder. A dull sound is produced when a distended bladder is percussed. Patients voiding more than once per hour or in amounts smaller than 50 mL are probably experiencing urinary retention with overflow. Patients may become diaphoretic or restless owing to discomfort from the distended bladder. Furthermore, assess the patient for the presence of urinary incontinence, particularly if epidural analgesia has been administered. Urinary retention should always be considered when fluid intake is considerably greater than urinary output.

Diagnostic Testing

If urinary retention is suspected despite the patient's having voided, postvoiding catheterization is performed and the amount of urine voided measured. This allows comparison of the amount of urine voided and the amount of urine obtained through catheterization. Patients may think they are voiding adequately, when in reality only a small amount of urine is voided and the majority remains in the bladder. In some cases, it may be necessary to perform ultrasound examination of the bladder to estimate bladder size.

Developmental Considerations

Perinatal The normal physiologic changes accompanying pregnancy predispose women to postpartum urinary retention. During pregnancy and the weeks immediately following the delivery, smooth muscle tone is reduced owing to increased levels of progesterone. A dilated bladder with poor muscle tone is less likely to empty itself effectively. The pressure within the bladder nearly doubles during pregnancy and then rapidly returns to pre-pregnancy levels during the first postpartum week. This rapid change in pressure results in hypotonia of bladder muscles.

Bladder tone and sensation may be reduced as the result of operative vaginal procedures and the effects of analgesia and anesthesia. Epidural analgesia is frequently used for vaginal deliveries and cesarean sections. The duration of the voiding difficulty is also influenced by analgesic drugs. For example, long-acting bupivacaine can result in decreased detrusor strength for up to 8 hours after administration. Further, pain or fear of pain interferes with the woman's ability to relax. These factors in combination with postpartum diuresis frequently lead to bladder distention or to incomplete emptying of the bladder. Edema and increased blood flow to the bladder mucosa and urethra may interfere with free passage of urine.

Postpartum urinary retention is usually a short-lived complication. However, with recent decreases in the length of hospital stay following childbirth, patients not only need to be assessed for the problem but need to be taught about the possibility of urinary retention once they return home.

Pediatric The psychosocial impact of neurogenic atony once the patient has successfully attained bladder control can be significant. Children may feel ashamed if they can no longer control bladder function. This problem is compounded if the child's peers learn about the use of absorbent undergarments or episodes of incontinence.

Geriatric Urinary retention in the older adult is not uncommon. Causes include phimosis, meatal stenosis, urethral trauma or stricture, benign prostatic hyperplasia, cancer of the prostate, and bladder tumor. Bleeding with clot formation, uterine prolapse, fecal impaction, and neurologic impairment (diabetes mellitus, nerve damage related to neoplasms) may also contribute to urinary retention. Table 40–2 provides a listing of drug classifications that are commonly associated with urinary retention.

Psychosocial Considerations

Patients with chronic urinary retention may have life-style adjustments to make. Some adjustments are related to the underlying cause of the retention and some to the retention itself. Most patients with neurogenic atony have experienced overflow incontinence at some point. Fear of incontinence may keep these individuals from participating fully in school, vocational, and social activities. Some patients may choose to use external, indwelling, or intermittent catheterization rather than drugs to control the disorder. This is particularly true for patients unable to sense that they have been incontinent or who cannot perform personal hygiene tasks independently. Knowledge of the patient's current life-style, level of independence, and anticipated changes helps determine treatment goals and interventions.

Analysis and Management

Treatment Objectives

The treatment objective for the patient with urinary retention is to stimulate complete bladder emptying. Cholinergic drugs are used on a short-term basis until the effects of surgery, childbirth, or other drugs have diminished. Avoidance of urinary retention also minimizes the risk of damage to the urinary system and urinary tract infection. Establishing a routine schedule for voiding is a major factor in the patient's ability to be independent and function in the community.

Treatment Options

Drug Variables

Bethanechol is the only drug in this class that is prescribed for urinary retention. SC administration typically results in a more rapid and stronger response than that seen with oral administration does. However, oral administration results in longer duration of action.

Patient Variables

Not all cases of urinary retention require intervention. Using a drug that stimulates bladder contraction is generally not advised if swelling of perineal tissues is obstructing urine flow. If the patient is unable to void because of positioning or privacy concerns, stimulating bladder contractions probably will not help. However, for patients whose bladders are not contracting adequately, use of a cholinergic drug may be appropriate. Bethanechol is not suitable for use in patients who have questionable structural integrity of the urinary or GI tract. It should be used very cautiously in patients with a previous history of bronchial asthma or cardiac disease.

When bethanechol is used in the acute care setting, both the oral and SC forms are used. Bethanechol is rarely used in the ambulatory care environment. Use of the SC formulation in the home setting requires the patient or caregiver to have adequate vision to prepare the drug correctly for administration. This may be an issue for individuals with poor vision related to diabetes, stroke, or visual changes related to aging. Patients who have had a stroke or high-level spinal cord injury may not have the manual dexterity to prepare and administer the drug.

Intervention

Administration

Monitor blood pressure, pulse, and respirations before administering bethanechol chloride and for at least 1 hour following SC administration. A test dose is ordinarily given before maintenance therapy to determine the minimum effective dosage. Oral and SC dosage formulations are not interchangeable; thus, attention to the dosage is important. The parenteral formulation is designed only for SC administration. It should not be given IM or IV. Regardless of the formulation used, the health care provider should assure the patient that a bathroom, bedside commode, or bedpan is readily available

Equipment to support respiratory function and atropine, the cholinergic antagonist, should be readily available in the event of respiratory depression. The adult dose of atropine is 0.5 to 0.6 mg SC or slow IV. The dosage of atropine for a child 12 years of age or younger is 0.01 mg/kg to a maximum total single dose of 0.4 mg. These doses may be repeated every 2 hours, if needed.

Dizziness and orthostatic hypotension are common adverse effects; therefore, the patient should be instructed to call for help before getting up after the first dose of the drug. Intake and output should be carefully monitored to evaluate drug effectiveness.

Education

Instruct the patient to take the drug exactly as directed. Forgotten doses should be taken as soon as possible if it is within 2 hours of the scheduled administration time. If it is past the 2-hour limit, the regular administration schedule should be followed. Double dosing is not recommended. Teach the patient to take the drug during the day, when fluid intake is higher, so as to minimize nocturnal voiding patterns. However, advise the patient to report flushing, salivation, and abdominal cramping to the health care provider because these symptoms suggest overdose.

Caution the patient taking bethanechol chloride to change positions slowly, particularly when first starting the drug, to minimize orthostatic blood pressure changes. This measure is especially important for patients with spinal cord injuries, who are already at risk for orthostatic hypotension.

Evaluation

The expected outcome for patients using bethanechol chloride is regular, complete emptying of the bladder. For hospitalized patients, this would be observed as relative balance between fluid intake and urine output, no distention of the bladder, and no complaints of pelvic discomfort. The health care provider should expect that urinary output exceeds 50 mL per void. For patients using bethanechol chloride on a regular basis, the expectation is regular emptying of the bladder without incontinence.

DEMENTIA OF THE ALZHEIMER'S TYPE

Epidemiology and Etiology

There are approximately four million people in the United States living with Alzheimer's disease, a form of dementia. Dementia involves progressive deterioration in cognition (usually memory), language, calculation, visuospatial perception, judgment, the ability to abstract, and personality. Dementia of the Alzheimer's type (DAT) makes up at least 50 percent of all dementias. The prevalence of DAT doubles for every 5 years a person lives beyond the age of 65. DAT occurs in 10 to 15 percent of people older than 65 years of age, in 19 percent of people older than 75 years of age, and in 47 percent of people older than 85 years of age. The lifetime risk for the disease is approximately 25.5 percent for men and 32 percent for women. The differences in risk correlate with the longer life span of today's women.

The exact etiology of DAT has not been identified. At least four chromosomes are involved in some forms of familial DAT. The lack of 100 percent concordance in identical twins suggests that environmental, metabolic, and other factors may also play a role. It is believed that DAT may be associated with aluminum intoxication, disordered immune function, and viral infection; however, these factors have not been proved. Female gender, head trauma, lack of education, and myocardial infarction have been linked to DAT, but the associations are weak. Although the risk factors for DAT (age, family history) are not modifiable, efforts to reduce the incidence of head trauma and cardiovascular disease may reduce the incidence of DAT and other types of dementia. There is no cure for DAT.

Physiology and Pathophysiology

DAT is named after the German neurologist Galen, who described the autopsy findings in a 55-year-old woman who had symptoms of progressive dementia. The disease is invariably fatal. *Neurofibrillary tangles* and *neuritic plaques* characterize DAT. The remnants from disintegration of dendrite branches and axon terminals result in neuritic plaques. The orderly arrangement of neurons normally found in the brain is lost. The neurofibrillary tangles are composed of tubules and filaments within the brain. Although the structural changes begin in small areas of the brain, axonal spread allows transmission to other areas of the brain. The more areas of the brain that are affected, the more severe the symptoms.

The hippocampus is the fir t area of the brain to be affected by DAT. Short-term memory requires a functional hippocampus. Impairment of this structure is correlated with mild memory loss, one of the first signs of DAT. Neurofibrillary tangles and neuritic plaques are also seen in the raphe nuclei within the cerebellum. The raphe nuclei secrete serotonin, a neurotransmitter responsible for mood control. Lower than normal levels of serotonin can result in depression. Depression that is superimposed on top of DAT can make the patient's cognitive function even worse. Antidepressant drugs may improve the depression but will not change the course of the disease. In some cases, the adverse effects of the antidepressant drugs further compromise the patient's condition.

DAT is typically divided into three stages (see Table 13–4). From the time symptoms appear, the median survival time is a little over a decade. The patient and family may have trouble pinpointing when symptoms first appeared. Mild memory impairment, particularly short-term memory, and difficulty learning new information characterize the first stage. The patient may compensate by making lists and notes, by avoiding new situations and environments, and by blaming others for misplaced items or forgotten tasks. Job performance may suffer if the patient is still employed. The judgment of patients with DAT becomes impaired without the patient's realizing the extent of the deficit. This raises safety issues regarding driving and the ability to be alone and unsupervised. The patient's family and caregivers are faced with the problem of protecting the patient and others while helping the patient retain as much independence as possible.

Patients with stage two DAT experience profound loss of memory and judgment. They may not recognize friends or people who are not immediate members of the family. The skills needed to function in social situations are forgotten. Changes in personality occur, and the ability to perform skilled purposeful movements is lost. At this point, the patient's family and caregiver may become overwhelmed and consider institutionalizing the patient.

Stage three is characterized by a state of progressive helplessness. The patient can no longer express himself or herself, recognize family members, or carry out the activities of daily living. The patient needs constant care and supervision. Many of these patients are placed in skilled health care facilities.

PHARMACOTHERAPEUTIC OPTIONS

Indirect-Acting Cholinergics

- ❐ Ambenonium chloride (MYTELASE)
- ❐ Edrophonium chloride (TENSILON, ENLON, REVERSOL)
- ❐ Neostigmine (PROSTIGIMIN); (🍁) PROSTIGMIN
- ❐ Pyridostigmine (MESTINON, REGONOL); (🍁) MESTINON, MESTINON-SR, REGONOL
- ❐ Tacrine hydrochloride (COGNEX)

Indications

Tacrine is used to treat mild to moderate cognitive deficits associated with DAT. Use of tacrine does not cure the disease but is thought to slow cognitive deterioration. Uses of tacrine that have not been approved by the Food and Drug Administration (FDA) include treatment of tardive dyskinesia and dementias associated with acquired immune deficiency syndrome (AIDS). A noticeable increase in the $CD4^+$ lymphocyte count is noted when tacrine is used to treat AIDS dementia. Ambenonium, edrophonium, neostigmine, and pyridostigmine are used in the management of myasthenia gravis, a descending degenerative neuromuscular disorder. These drugs are discussed in Chapter 23. Neostigmine has also been used in some patients for the management of urinary retention.

Pharmacodynamics

In contrast to direct-acting cholinergics, indirect-acting cholinergics act primarily by shielding ACh from degradation by the enzyme acetylcholinesterase. This results in accumulation of ACh at all sites where ACh is liberated. By rendering enzymatic action ineffective, tacrine causes a prolonged and intensified cholinergic response. However, as DAT progresses, more and more ACh-producing cells are destroyed. The fewer of these cells that are available, the less ACh is produced. As the level of ACh drops, inhibiting cholinesterase activity does little to maintain adequate levels for functioning, and the patient's symptoms worsen. Slowing cognitive deterioration will not cure the disease, nor will it stop its progression.

Adverse Effects and Contraindications

Common adverse effects of tacrine include diarrhea, loss of appetite, clumsiness or unsteadiness, nausea, and vomiting. The cholinergic action of tacrine increases gastric secretions and can be problematic for patients with peptic ulcer disease. Agitation and hallucinations are seen in a small percentage of patients. These adverse effects may be particularly troublesome if the patient has a history of behavioral problems. The major adverse effect of tacrine is elevation of alanine aminotransferase (ALT; serum glutamic-pyruvic transaminase [SGPT]). The degree of elevation of this liver enzyme determines the ability to increase the dosage or continue the drug, or both.

Because of its cholinergic effects, tacrine should be used cautiously in patients with GI obstruction, urinary tract obstruction, asthma, or cardiac disease. Tacrine is a pregnancy category C drug.

Pharmacokinetics

Tacrine is rapidly absorbed from the GI tract following oral administration. However, the bioavailability of the drug is low (17 percent). Food decreases the absorption of tacrine 30 to 40 percent. Although the onset of drug action occurs within 6 weeks, improvement in cognitive function may take 18 to 24 weeks to become noticeable (see Table 13–1). Plasma concentrations of tacrine are approximately 50 percent higher in women than in men. Further, plasma drug concentrations are two thirds lower in patients who smoke. It is theorized that smoking increases the rate of drug biotransformation in the liver.

Drug-Drug Interactions

Because bethanechol chloride and tacrine are cholinergic drugs that act synergistically when taken together, concurrent use should be carefully undertaken (see Table 13–2). Like bethanechol chloride, tacrine can cause bladder outlet obstruction. Use of tacrine with theophylline or cholinesterase inhibitors increases the effects of these drugs and the risk of toxicity. Concurrent use of cimetidine increases the effects of tacrine. Anticholinergic drug effects are decreased in the presence of tacrine.

Dosage Regimen

Tacrine's dosage regimen depends on the patient's ability to take the drug without experiencing unacceptable adverse effects or increases in liver enzymes. Tacrine appears to be most effective when it is taken at regular intervals. The initial dosage is 10 mg four times per day for 6 weeks with regular monitoring of serum ALT (SGPT) levels. If the drug is tolerated and there are no elevations in liver function tests, the dosage is increased to 20 mg four times daily. The dosage is increased to 30 mg for 6 weeks and finally 40 mg four times daily. If the patient tolerates this dosage, it is continued until the patient demonstrates significant cognitive deterioration. It is theorized that at this point, tacrine-mediated inhibition of ACh breakdown is not therapeutic because not enough ACh is being produced. Continuation of tacrine beyond this stage is ordinarily not effective.

Tacrine therapy should not be discontinued abruptly in spite of adverse effects, lab results, or decreased efficacy. Lowering the dose by 80 mg/day or more may result in behavioral abnormalities and significant worsening of cognitive deficits. If a patient is taken off tacrine for 4 weeks or more and then therapy is subsequently restarted, the entire titration schedule must be resumed.

Laboratory Considerations

Approximately 50 percent of patients taking tacrine will have at least one episode of elevated ALT (SGPT) levels. Twenty-five percent of these patients have elevations that are three times the upper limits of normal. Approximately 7 percent of patients taking tacrine will have ALT (SGPT) levels ten times the upper limits of normal. The extreme elevations usually occur 6 weeks from the time of the first elevation. Bi-weekly monitoring should be resumed for at least 6 weeks after any dose increase. If the AST (SGPT) level is less than three times the upper limit of normal, dosage titration may be continued. If the levels are greater than three times but less than five times the upper limit of normal, decrease the dosage of tacrine by 40 mg per day, and resume dosage titration when ALT (SGPT) levels return to normal. Tacrine therapy should be discontinued if ALT (SGPT) levels are greater than five times the upper limit of normal. ALT (SGPT) levels ordinarily return to normal 4 to 6 weeks after therapy is discontinued. Patients with clinical jaundice and a total bilirubin level over 3 mg/dL should have therapy discontinued, and a new trial period should not be attempted.

Newer Cholinesterase Inhibitor

❒ Donepezil (ARICEPT)

Donepezil is the newest drug available for the management of DAT. It is a reversible cholinesterase inhibitor that permits elevated ACh levels in the cerebral cortex. Elevated levels of ACh slow the neuronal degradation that occurs with DAT. It improves or stabilizes symptoms of DAT in 50 to 80 percent of patients.

Common adverse effects of donepezil include insomnia, fatigue, dizziness, confusion, ataxia, somnolence, tremor, agitation, depression, and difficulty in problem solving. Adverse effects on the GI tract include anorexia, nausea, vomiting, dyspepsia, abdominal pain, and diarrhea. Donepezil-induced hepatotoxicity is possible, although the type of liver dysfunction is less severe than that seen with tacrine. Donepezil is contraindicated in patients with hypersensitivity to the drug, in pregnancy, and in women who are breastfeeding. It should be used with caution in patients who have sick sinus syndrome, GI bleeding, seizures, or asthma.

Donepezil is rapidly absorbed from the GI tract when it is taken by mouth. The time to onset of drug action varies, but peak drug effects are ordinarily reached in 2 to 4 hours. Its duration of action lasts for up to 24 hours. The half-life of donepezil is 8 to 12 hours.

Concurrent use of theophylline and cholinesterase inhibitors increases drug effects and increases the risk of toxicity. Donepezil decreases the effects of anticholinergics, and there is an increased risk of GI bleeding with concurrent use of nonsteroidal anti-inflammatory drugs.

Donepezil is administered orally in a dose of 5 mg daily at bedtime. The dosage may be increased to 10 mg daily after the first 4 to 6 weeks. Regularly scheduled blood tests should be performed before and periodically throughout therapy while the patient adjusts to this drug.

Critical Thinking Process

Assessment

History of Present Illness

Many older adults have relatives who have DAT. These individuals may be reluctant to consider the possibility that they are developing symptoms of DAT. Forgetfulness and difficulty learning new information may be attributed to aging. Contact with the health care system may be initiated by the patient or by significant others. If the memory deficits and judgment impairments are significant, it will probably be the significant others who schedule an evaluation. Ask specifically about difficulties with activities of daily living, judgment, increasing forgetfulness, and changes in personality. Family members or significant others may relate episodes of leaving a stove on, not shutting the front door, or blaming others when objects have been misplaced. They may note that the patient does not initiate activities that were previously enjoyable and does not socialize with friends. The common manifestations of DAT are identified in Table 13–4.

Past Health History

Patients and the family or significant others should be questioned closely about the patient's use of drugs, both prescription and over-the-counter forms. Particular attention should be paid to any recently added drugs. Older individuals are particularly prone to drug interactions, owing in part to slower biotransformation of drugs and in part to multidrug therapies for co-morbid conditions. If patients are receiving care and prescriptions from several health care providers, the possibility of drug-drug interactions increases.

TABLE 13–4 COMMON MANIFESTATIONS OF DEMENTIA OF THE ALZHEIMER'S TYPE

Characteristic	Stage I	Stage II	Stage III
Duration of symptoms	1–3 years	2–10 years	8–12 years
Cognition and memory	Difficulty learning Mild impairment of short-term memory	Profound impairment of short-term and long-term memory	
Visuospatial skills	Topographic disorientation Poor complex constructions	Poor spatial orientation and ability to perform purposeful skilled movement	
Language skills	Difficult to generate word list Word construction impaired	Aphasia	
Mental state	Indifference Occasional irritability Sorrowful Occasional delusions	Indifference Irritability Delusional Social skills lost	
Motor function	Within normal limits	Restless Paces	Limb rigidity and flexed posture
Diagnostic testing	*EEG, CT, MRI:* Essentially normal *PET scan:* Hypometabolism and hyperperfusion of bilateral parietal lobe	*EEG:* Slowing of background rhythm *CT and MRI:* Normal or ventricular dilation and enlargement of sulcus *PET scan:* Hypometabolism and hypoperfusion of parietal and frontal lobes	*EEG:* Diffusely slow *CT and MRI:* Ventricular dilation and enlargement of sulcus *PET scan:* Hypometabolism and hypoperfusion of parietal and frontal lobes

EEG, Electroencephalogram; CT, computed tomography; MRI, magnetic resonance imaging; PET, positron emission tomography.

Questions should be asked about the possible occurrence of head injury, recent falls, headache, transient ischemic attacks (TIAs), or stroke. Has the patient ever felt numbness or clumsiness in one arm or leg ? Has he or she ever been unable to speak for a brief period of time? Patients may have had episodes of ischemia to the brain without realizing what was happening. Multiple infarctions, whether symptomatic or not, may result in dementia. Also, ask about use of alcohol and illicit drugs. Do not assume that an individual is not a substance abuser based simply on age.

Patients and family members should be asked if anyone else in the family has or has had similar symptoms. Although DAT is not directly inherited, there is evidence to suggest a familial tendency. If the patient is unable to remember, it may be necessary to contact members of the extended family. This line of questioning should be approached with sensitivity. The possible diagnosis of DAT is frightening in itself. The possibility that it could affect several members of the family may be new information.

Physical Exam Findings

DAT does not typically manifest as changes in physical exam findings. In the early stages, the patient has relatively normal physiologic function. As the disease progresses, however, the ability to walk, talk, and care for oneself deteriorates. Most patients are diagnosed in the first stage of the disease. A Mini Mental State Exam may provide objective data for ongoing evaluation of the patient.

Diagnostic Testing

The definitive diagnosis of DAT can be made only by examining the brain following the patient's death for pathologic changes. However, most health care providers will diagnose the disease based on clinical exam and cognitive testing findings, and by ruling out other causes of symptoms. Neurofibrillary tangles and neuritic plaques can be identified on computed tomography and magnetic resonance imaging scans. A positron emission tomography scan may detect areas of the brain that have reduced metabolism. A recently developed test shows promise in confirming the diagnosis of DAT. The test is called AD7C and is performed on the cerebrospinal fluid of the patient. This neural thread protein is believed to function in the regeneration of brain tissue and repair of neurons. Because patients with DAT have degeneration of neurons, one would expect to find higher levels of neural thread protein in the cerebrospinal fluid. The AD7C test has detected elevations of the protein in 80 to 90 percent of patients. The presence of DAT in these patients was confirmed on autopsy. AD7C has a low incidence of false-positive results.

Developmental Considerations

Perinatal DAT is a disorder of late middle to old age. The gene associated with DAT is found on chromosome 21, the same chromosome responsible for Down syndrome. Most individuals with Down syndrome begin exhibiting changes in brain structure associated with DAT by 20 years of age. By the time these individuals reach 40 years of age, they may begin showing symptoms of DAT. Individuals with Down syndrome may be the only population to use tacrine during child-bearing years, with the likelihood of such use being very small. No studies of tacrine specifically targeting this population have been conducted.

Pediatric DAT does not affect children. Tacrine has not been widely studied as a treatment for childhood dementia.

Geriatric Tacrine is used primarily by the older adult population. Therefore, the recommendations for use are based on geriatric patients (see Controversy—Clinical Trials Involving Alzheimer's Disease Patients).

Psychosocial Considerations

DAT is a devastating disorder. The health care provider should inquire about the patient's reactions to changes in routine or in the environment. It is not uncommon for a pa-

Controversy

Clinical Trials Involving Alzheimer's Disease Patients

SALLY SCHNELL

During new product development, most drugs are initially tested on healthy volunteers to determine adverse effects and safe dosages. After safe dosages have been established, the drug is tested on individuals suffering from the targeted disease. It is at this point that the ethics surrounding the inclusion of patients with cognitive impairment comes into play.

One school of thought posits that a patient who is not cognitively competent to give consent to participate should not be included in such trial. This belief assumes that if the patient cannot express his wishes, no one else should presume to do so. Adherence to this perspective would effectively block the drug trials for the products designed to treat dementia of the Alzheimer's type.

The opposite perspective counters that if a competent significant other understands the risks and benefits of the trial and consents to enrollment, then the patient should be allowed to participate. This point of view assumes that the significant other knows the patient's wishes and will act in his best interest.

Critical Thinking Discussion

- Who should decide on participation in clinical trials if the patient is not competent to make the decision?
- How much risk is acceptable?
- Is it acceptable to force a confused patient to undergo the blood tests necessary for monitoring of the clinical trial?

tient with DAT to become extremely agitated over small changes. Similarly, apathy, social isolation, and irritability may be noted. As the brain atrophies, the patient exhibits paranoia, uses abusive language, and becomes suspicious of others. Be sure to assess for the impact of DAT on the family. Determine their strengths and weaknesses, their ability to provide care for the patient, and financial concerns (see Case Study—Dementia of the Alzheimer's Type).

Analysis and Management

Treatment Objectives

The goal of tacrine therapy is to slow the cognitive deterioration that inevitably occurs in patients with DAT. Use of the drug may allow the patient to maintain a more independent life-style and lessen the burden on family and significant others. The longer duration of independence has immense implications for family functioning, caregiver burnout, and the financial strain of placement in a skilled health care facility.

Treatment Options

Drug Variables

Tacrine and donepezil carry a significant risk of hepatotoxicity, thus requiring regular monitoring of liver function. Tacrine also has the potential to cause clumsiness and unsteadiness. This may be particularly problematic for older individuals, who are not as steady on their feet as younger individuals.

Patient Variables

Tacrine interacts with a variety of drugs commonly taken by older adults. Further, the ability of the patient, family, and significant others to comply with treatment regimens and lab work schedules is very important. Tacrine therapy may not be a safe therapy if the patient does not have the ability or the resources to comply. Donepezil does not require lab work, but the patient's ability to understand and comply with administration schedules is an important factor.

Intervention

Administration

Tacrine should be taken on an empty stomach unless gastric upset requires that it be administered with food. Concurrent use of tacrine with cimetidine or theophylline should be avoided without careful monitoring of serum concentrations and dosage. The dosage of tacrine should not be decreased abruptly or therapy discontinued suddenly to avoid a relapse in patient symptoms.

Education

Patients, family, and significant others should be advised to contact the health care provider who is prescribing tacrine before taking any new prescribed or over-the-counter medication. They should also be instructed to tell all of the health care providers, including dentists, about the use of tacrine. The medication should not be stored in a location that is accessible to the patient because of the possibility of overdose.

The patient, family, and significant others need to understand that tacrine does not cure DAT. They should also know that it is not effective for all patients. In addition, the risk of liver enzyme elevation should be explained and the necessity of stopping treatment if ALT (SGPT) reaches dangerous levels reinforced. Stopping treatment can be devastating to these individuals if the drug was noticeably effective. It is possible to retry the drug after liver function test values return to normal. As DAT worsens, the effectiveness of tacrine eventually declines. This fact should also be clearly explained.

Evaluation

The effectiveness of tacrine therapy is monitored by the patient's ability to perform activities of daily living. The degree of supervision needed and the relative safety in performing tasks are evaluated. Many health care providers use the Mini Mental State Exam as an objective measure of cognitive functioning. Although the family and significant others provide the most comprehensive information, the Mini Mental State Exam is subjective in nature. Functional assessment may be colored by the strong desire for tacrine therapy to be effective.

GASTROINTESTINAL DISORDERS

Peptic Ulcer Disease

Approximately 10 percent of the population will suffer from peptic ulcer disease in their lifetime. Gastric and duodenal ulcers occur more frequently in men than in women. Gastric ulcerations are more commonly found between the ages of 55 and 65 years, with the peak age for duodenal forms being 45 to 54 years. Males tend to develop peptic ul-

Case Study Dementia of the Alzheimer's Type

Patient History

History of Present Illness	HW is a 74-year-old Hispanic female who states that she has developed some memory difficulty over the last 6 months. She also reports pain in her hips and knees. She is accompanied by two of her daughters. Her daughters state that their mother is experiencing significant memory and judgment impairment. HW's daughters also state that she does not maintain her personal hygiene and diet as well as she used to.
Past Health History	HW gives no significant past medical history. She currently takes ibuprofen PRN for joint pain. She denies use of alcohol or tobacco, and her daughters concur.
Physical Exam	VSS. HWs daughters state she has lost 5 pounds in the last 6 months. HW ambulates independently but slowly. She is essentially expressionless.
Diagnostic Testing	MRI of the brain reveals neurofibrillary tangles and neuritic plaques. Mini-Mental State Exam score is 26.
Developmental Considerations	HW may have less effective hepatic function owing to the changes of aging.
Psychosocial Considerations	HW lives alone. Her two daughters live within 15 minutes of her. They will no longer allow her to supervise their children alone, a situation that causes HW a great deal of frustration. She has a group of close friends, all of whom are about her age. HW has three siblings. Her oldest sister died in a skilled nursing facility after spending 4 years there with a diagnosis of dementia of the Alzheimer's type. She still drives locally, but her daughters want her to stop driving.
Economic Factors	HW has Social Security as her main source of income and Medicare as her insurance provider.

Variables Influencing Decision

Treatment Objectives
- Slow the rate of cognitive deterioration as much as possible.
- Allow patient to function as independently as possible.

Drug Variables	*Drug Summary*	*Patient Variables*
Indications	Tacrine and donepezil both slow the cognitive deterioration associated with dementia of the Alzheimer's type.	HW has been diagnosed with dementia of the Alzheimer's type. This will be a decision point.
Pharmacodynamics	Both tacrine and donepezil are cholinesterase inhibitors.	There are no identifiable pharmacodynamic variables that will affect the decision for drug use at this time.
Adverse Effects/ Contraindications	Tacrine: hepatotoxicity, diarrhea, clumsiness, unsteadiness Donepezil: nausea and vomiting. HW uses an NSAID for joint pain.	HW is at risk for clumsiness and unsteadiness. Concurrent use with tacrine may place her at risk for increased gastric secretion and peptic ulcer disease. This will be a decision point.
Pharmacokinetics	Donepezil is estimated to have an effectiveness of up to 24 months. The length of effectiveness of tacrine has not been established.	There are no identifiable pharmacokinetic variables that will affect the decision for drug use at this time.
Dosage Regimen	Both agents are taken orally. Donepezil is taken once a day. Tacrine is taken four times a day.	HW wishes to remain living alone. Her memory impairment will make compliance with either drug regimen a problem. This will be a decision point.

Case Study Dementia of the Alzheimer's Type—cont'd

Drug Variables	Drug Summary	Patient Variables
Lab Considerations	Tacrine will require every other week ALT (SGPT) levels for 16 weeks, then every month, then every 3 months. Donepezil does not require lab work.	Will be a decision point based on the daughters' willingness to monitor HW for signs of liver dysfunction and compliance with medication regimen and lab work.
Cost Index*	Tacrine: 3 Donepezil: 2	HW has Medicare but no other pharmacy coverage. This will be a decision point because she lives on Social Security.

Summary of Decision Points

- HW has been diagnosed with dementia of the Alzheimer's type.
- Cognitive impairment may interfere with HW's ability to comply with the medication regimen for either drug.
- Concurrent use of NSAIDs with tacrine may place HW at risk for increased gastric secretion and peptic ulcer disease.
- The significant risk for hepatic dysfunction requires frequent lab work and may require discontinuation of tacrine.
- Donepezil has an easier dosage regimen and fewer adverse reactions than tacrine.
- HW has Medicare but no other pharmacy coverage. Donepezil is comparably cheaper than tacrine.

DRUG TO BE USED

- Donepezil 5 mg po daily at bedtime. May increase dose to 10 mg after the first 4 to 6 weeks of therapy.

*Cost Index:
1 \$ < 30/mo.
2 \$ 30–40.
3 \$ 40–50/mo.
4 \$ 50–60/mo.
5 \$ > 60/mo.

AWP of 100, 5-mg tablets of donepezil is approximately \$120.
AWP of 100, 10-mg capsules of tacrine is approximately \$137.

cer more often than women. There are a number of etiologic factors that are believed to be involved in the origin of peptic ulcer disease, including the presence of the organism *Helicobacter pylori,* reduced endogenous prostaglandins, alcohol, genetics, smoking, stress, gastroesophageal reflux disease, and nonsteroidal anti-inflammatory drugs.

Peptic ulcer disease is characterized by an imbalance between the corrosive action of hydrochloric acid and pepsin and the mucosal protective factor of prostaglandins. Hydrochloric acid and pepsin are the naturally occurring digestive juices. In some individuals, secretion of these juices is increased or the contents of the stomach rapidly emptied. In these situations, the natural buffering effect of food is lost and the mucosa of the duodenum is affected by the acidic gastric juices. Some individuals experience bile acid reflux into the stomach via an incompetent pylorus. These bile acids can break down the mucosa of the stomach, resulting in ulceration.

The principal manifestation of peptic ulcer disease is dyspepsia, an aching, burning, cramplike, gnawing pain. Hydrochloric acid secretion produces inflammation and edema with resultant pain and can activate motor changes with increased spasm, intragastric pressure, and motility, also with resultant pain. Severe retching and vomiting associated with an gastric ulcer or pyloric obstruction can lead to an esophageal tear.

Irritable Bowel Syndrome

Theoretical causes of irritable bowel syndrome (spastic colon, irritable colon, mucous colitis) range from fear and anxiety to depression, foods, drugs, toxins, and colonic distention. Contributing factors include diverticular disease, caffeine and other gastric stimulants, and lactose intolerance. Irritable bowel syndrome is a functional disorder whose exact cause is unknown. It is the most common digestive disorder in the United States, although reliable data are essentially unavailable. Irritable bowel disease affects 15 to 20 percent of the population, with two thirds of the cases involving women. Most patients who report symptoms are between the ages of 35 and 40 years. The symptoms include a changes in bowel habits with abdominal pain and distention. There may be alternating periods of constipation and diarrhea, with cramping and abdominal discomfort. Belching and increased flatus are also noted.

PHARMACOTHERAPEUTIC OPTIONS

Anticholinergics

- ❒ Atropine
- ❒ Benztropine (COGENTIN)
- ❒ Clidinium (QUARZAN)
- ❒ Dicyclomine (ANTISPAS, BENTYL, BYCLOMINE, DIBENT, DI-SPAZ, NEOQUESS, others); (🍁) BENTYLOL, FORMULEX
- ❒ Glycopyrrolate (ROBINUL)
- ❒ Hyoscyamine (ANASPAZ, CYSTOSPAZ, LEVSIN, LEVSINEX TIMECAPS); (🍁) LEVSIN
- ❒ Mepenzolate (CANTIL)
- ❒ Methscopolamine (PAMINE)
- ❒ Procyclidine (KEMADRIN); (🍁) PROCYCLID
- ❒ Propantheline (PRO-BANTHINE)
- ❒ Scopolamine (TRANSDERM SCOP); (🍁) BUSCOPAN, TRANSDERM-V
- ❒ Trihexyphenidyl (ARTANE, TRIHEXY); (🍁) PMS-TRIHEXYPHENIDYL

Indications

There are many uses for anticholinergic drugs. Atropine is the best known anticholinergic agent and has the most indications for use. Atropine, clidinium, dicyclomine, hyoscyamine, methscopolamine, mepenzolate, and propantheline are used in the treatment of peptic ulcer disease and irritable bowel syndrome. These drugs are discussed in more depth in Chapters 42 and 43. Hyoscyamine is also used to treat hypermobility of the bladder associated with cystitis.

Some of these anticholinergic drugs may be used to decrease secretions preoperatively. Glycopyrrolate is used as a preoperative agent to inhibit salivation and excessive respiratory secretions. Glycopyrrolate is also used as a adjunct to reverse the secretory and vagal actions of cholinesterase inhibitors used to treat nondepolarizing neuromuscular blockade. Atropine is also used to reverse toxicity associated with cholinesterase inhibitor drugs and to treat cardiac arrhythmias.

Benztropine, procyclidine, and trihexyphenidyl are used primarily in the management of Parkinson's disease and are discussed in Chapter 23. Scopolamine is used transdermally for the prophylactic treatment of motion sickness (see Chapter 44). Atropine, scopolamine, and cyclopentolate are also used as ophthalmic mydriatics (see Chapter 62).

Pharmacodynamics

Anticholinergic drugs block the action of ACh at postganglionic receptor sites located in smooth muscle, secretory glands, the central nervous system (CNS) (antimuscarinic activity), the sinoatria (SA) and atrioventricular (AV) nodes, and cardiac muscle. Drug actions and adverse effects of anticholinergic drugs are opposite those of cholinergic drugs. Low doses decrease sweating, salivation, and respiratory secretions. Intermediate doses cause *mydriasis* (pupillary dilation), *cycloplegia* (loss of visual accommodation), and increased heart rate. In larger doses, the motility of the GI and genitourinary tracts is decreased. The excessive hydrochloric acid secretion and gastric motility associated with peptic ulcer disease can be partially reduced by decreasing vagal stimulation. Anticholinergic drugs are occasionally used to accomplish this. Anticholinergics enhance pain relief by relieving gastric distress caused by gastric spasm and hyperperistalsis.

Adverse Effects and Contraindications

The adverse effects and contraindications associated with anticholinergic drugs are many. They produce a high incidence of adverse effects such as dilated pupils, dry mouth and skin, flushing, thirst, tachycardia, and urinary retention. Because of their tendency to decrease gastric motility, anticholinergic drugs should be avoided in cases in which delayed gastric emptying increases the patient's level of discomfort. All anticholinergic drugs suppress perspiration, thus contributing to the possibility of overheating.

Anticholinergics are contraindicated in patients with hypersensitivity, narrow-angle glaucoma, severe hemorrhage, tachycardia due to thyrotoxicosis, cardiac insufficiency, or myasthenia gravis. Pediatric patients and older adults are more susceptible to the adverse effects of these drugs than are younger individuals.

Anticholinergic drugs should be used with caution in patients with urinary tract pathology, those at risk for GI obstruction or GI atony, patients with toxic megacolon, and those with chronic renal, hepatic, pulmonary, or cardiac disease. These drugs are considered pregnancy category C.

Pharmacokinetics

The pharmacokinetics of selected anticholinergic drugs is identified in Table 13–1. The onset of drug action for most of the drugs identified ranges from 5 minutes for hyoscyamine to as long as 90 minutes for atropine. The duration of drug action ranges from 3 hours to 3 days, depending on the specific drug.

Drug-Drug Interactions

Concurrent use of antacids and anticholinergics may result in decreased absorption of the anticholinergics. Table 13–2 provides a listing of drug classes that act synergistically with anticholinergic drugs, thereby increasing their action. Among the more commonly used drugs that have anticholinergic effects are antihistamines, procainamide, meperidine, and tricyclic antidepressants. Use of methotrimeprazine with atropine, dicyclomine, or hyoscyamine may result in extrapyramidal symptoms. Concurrent use of anticholinergic drugs with ketoconazole or levodopa may cause decreased absorption and efficacy. Wax matrix formulations of potassium chloride should be used cautiously with atropine because of the risk of mucosal lesions.

Simultaneous use of ethanol or CNS depressants and scopolamine results in increased CNS depression. This interaction should be stressed to patients who use the scopolamine patch for motion sickness prophylaxis. Even moderate use of alcohol while using the patch may result in significant CNS depression.

Dosage Regimen

The dosages of anticholinergic drugs are identified in Table 13–3. Because of the many uses of anticholinergic drugs, the health care provider must carefully check drug references for appropriate dosages. When using atropine for treatment of bradycardia and bradyarrhythmias, remember that doses of less than 0.5 mg can actually cause bradycardia. The maximum cumulative adult dose of IV atropine is 2 mg. Children's dosages of atropine are calculated based on body weight or square meters of body surface.

Laboratory Considerations

Serum drug levels are not required with anticholinergic drugs. Some drugs may provide false values on certain laboratory tests. For example, dicyclomine and glycopyrrolate should not be used 24 hours before the pentagastrin and histamine gastric acid secretion tests. Dicyclomine acts as an antagonist to these other drugs. Glycopyrrolate may cause decreased uric acid levels in patients with gout or hyperuricemia. Propantheline may cause elevated antinuclear antibody titers, a condition that is usually asymptomatic and reversible.

Critical Thinking Process

Assessment

History of Present Illness

In the case of peptic ulcer disease, the patient may complain of pain and burning in the stomach and indigestion. Complaints of nausea and vomiting are rare, although epigastric pain is present when the stomach is empty, usually 2 to 3 hours after eating and on awakening.

Complaints associated with irritable bowel syndrome center on diarrhea that alternates with constipation, abdominal cramping, and in some cases, weight loss. For patients with any of the GI disorders, elicit information about factors that worsen symptoms and factors that relieve symptoms. Determine when the symptoms began, their severity, and what has been done to self-treat.

Past Health History

It is important to carefully question the patient about concurrent or previous illnesses. A past history of myasthenia gravis or glaucoma should be prominently noted on the patient's chart and communicated to all health care providers. A history of GI or urinary tract obstruction may influence the decision to use anticholinergics.

Physical Exam Findings

Patients may or may not demonstrate weight loss due to irritable bowel syndrome or peptic ulcer disease. There may be epigastric pain and palpable tenderness with peptic ulcer disease. Melena is more common than hematemesis in patients with duodenal disease, whereas hematemesis is more common in patients with gastric ulcerations. The patient with duodenal ulcers is usually well nourished, whereas with gastric ulcerations the patient is probably malnourished.

Diagnostic Testing

Radiographic studies of the upper and lower portions of the GI tract may be ordered. Patients with bradycardia or bradyarrhythmias should undergo an electrocardiogram.

Developmental Considerations

Perinatal Atropine, hyoscyamine, and the transdermal form of scopolamine can cross into the placenta. IV administration of atropine or hyoscyamine can result in tachycardia in the fetus. There have been isolated reports of fetal malformations associated with dicyclomine administration. Retrospective studies did not confirm the association. Parenteral administration of scopolamine hydrobromide during labor may cause CNS depression in the neonate. Owing to a reduction in clotting factors dependent on vitamin K, administration of parenteral scopolamine may contribute to neonatal hemorrhage. All of these factors make the use of these drugs in pregnant women a risk-versus-benefit decision. If the drugs are administered, both the mother and fetus or neonate should be closely monitored.

All of the anticholinergic drugs have the capacity to inhibit lactation. Atropine and hyoscyamine cross into breast milk. Infants are very sensitive to anticholinergics. Again, in the population of nursing mothers, the anticholinergics must be used very carefully. If long-term use is necessary, the mother must be counseled about the advisability of breast-feeding.

Pediatric In a hot environment, the decrease in perspiration caused by anticholinergics may result in the body temperature's reaching dangerous levels. Use of dicyclomine syrup in infants younger than 3 months old may result in respiratory distress. The parenteral form of hyoscyamine contains benzyl alcohol as a preservative. This form should not be used in neonates and very young infants.

Geriatric Any patient taking an anticholinergic may experience excitement, agitation, drowsiness, or confusion. In the older adult, these adverse effects occur more frequently and with a greater severity. Memory impairment associated with anticholinergic drug use is due to the inhibition of ACh action. If the patient has underlying cognitive dysfunction, the behavioral compromise may be severe. Anticholinergics should be used cautiously in this population because many may have undiagnosed glaucoma. Further, as a result of the changes of aging, these individuals are particularly prone to the constipation, dry mouth, and urinary retention that may accompany use of anticholinergics.

Psychosocial Considerations

Anticholinergic use does not typically affect an individual's psychosocial function or his or her ability to function in the community. If older adults are taking an anticholinergic over an extended period of time, they may experience disorientation or agitation, which would interfere with their interactions with others.

Analysis and Management

Treatment Objectives

The goal of treatment for the patient with irritable bowel syndrome is to diminish the motility of the GI tract. If peptic ulcer disease is the diagnosis, the goal is to decrease gastric secretions that are ulcerating the gastric lining and to slow gastric emptying. When atropine is administered as an antidote to acetylcholinesterase inhibitor toxicity, the objective is to re-establish the effect of the acetylcholinesterase. Use of atropine to treat bradycardia or bradyarrhythmia should result in a functional heart rhythm.

Treatment Options

Drug Variables

For treatment of irritable bowel syndrome or peptic ulcer disease, hyoscyamine is more potent than atropine. It also comes in a variety of formulations and strengths, which helps in individualizing therapy and promoting patient compliance. Scopolamine has the disadvantage of increased occurrence of CNS adverse effects compared with other anticholinergics. It is used primarily in the perioperative setting. Controversy exists as to whether or not transdermal scopolamine has the ability to decrease postoperative nausea and vomiting. Many anticholinergics are used on a short-term basis as adjunctive agents to treatment because newer drugs of different classes are used to treat GI disorders.

Patient Variables

Many patients find the adverse effects of anticholinergic drugs difficult to tolerate. These adverse effects are very similar among the different medications; therefore, switching to a different anticholinergic may not provide relief.

Intervention

Administration

Anticholinergics are best given to the patient with peptic ulcer disease approximately 1 hour after meals, when food-stimulated acid production is at its peak. Unfortunately, anticholinergics suppress basal acid secretion more effectively than they suppress secretion in response to food. In order to achieve sufficient suppression of secretion, the patient must receive a large dose of anticholinergic drug. Large doses cause intolerable adverse effects, such as dry mouth, blurred vision, constipation, and occasionally, urinary retention caused by bladder atony. Anticholinergic effects last 4 to 5 hours. Anticholinergics should not be administered to the patient who has GI bleeding because the stomach may become distended. Monitor vital signs and urinary output. The patient should maintain a good fluid intake.

Education

Instruct patients, family, and significant others that anticholinergics may have an undesirable effect on the CNS. Encourage the patient to refrain from driving or other potentially dangerous activity until the effect of the drug is known. Encourage him or her to report any occurrence of dizziness, agitation, or disorientation to the health care provider. Adjustments in dosage may be required.

Individuals who take anticholinergics should be warned about the risk of overheating in hot environments due to decreased perspiration. This is particularly true in children and older adults, who may experience significant increases in body temperature. Prolonged use of anticholinergics decreases salivary flow and contributes to dental disorders. Patients should be told to notify their dentist that they are taking anticholinergics. Decreased salivation makes patients more prone to periodontal disease, oral candidal infections, and dental caries.

Dry mouth is a common complaint among patients taking anticholinergics. Encourage the use of sugarless hard candy and regular consultation with a dentist. Constipation may be lessened by an increase in activity and in fluid and fiber intake. Encourage the patient to consult the health care provider before beginning to use laxatives.

Evaluation

Successful treatment is determined by relief or decrease of symptoms. Patients with peptic ulcer disease would expect a decrease in their gastric pain. Patients with irritable bowel syndrome would expect less muscle spasm and less abdominal cramping. The frequency or amount of diarrhea may not be greatly affected.

RELATED DRUGS

Autonomic Ganglionic Stimulants

❒ Nicotine (HABITROL, NICODERM, NICORETTE, NICOTROL, PROSTEP)

With the exception of nicotine gum and transdermal nicotine patches, there are no therapeutically useful ganglionic stimulant drugs. However, they must be understood because of their toxic effects. Nicotine is available for use in smoking cessation programs. The gum and transdermal formulations provide a source of nicotine for the nicotine-dependent patient who is attempting smoking cessation.

Nicotine improves memory, especially long-term memory, and increases the accuracy and speed of information processing. Other benefits include an increase in pain threshold and a reduction of tensions and anxiety. Despite the perceived benefits, nicotine has been shown to cause heart disease, stroke, emphysema, and lung cancer. It can cause problems in pregnancy, resulting in low birth weight, prematurity, and fetal injury. Some health care providers suggest that use of any nicotine formulation is potentially harmful to the fetus. Autonomic ganglionic stimulants activate nicotinic receptors at ganglionic sites rather than at effector organs such as muscle. Thus, stimulation occurs as a result of norepinephrine release from sympathetic fibers and ACh release from parasympathetic fibers. This action ultimately generates nerve impulses down the postganglionic fibers to produce specific effects on smooth muscle, cardiac muscle, and glands. Nicotine stimulates the CNS, particularly the respiratory, vomiting, and vasomotor centers in the medulla. Large doses of nicotine cause tremors and seizure activity. The curare-like effects of nicotine on diaphragmatic nerve endings contribute to the risk of respiratory failure and death. The effects of nicotine on the cardiovascular system are many. The heart rate slows but later may increase above normal, with arrhythmias noted. Small peripheral blood vessels may first constrict, only to dilate with a resultant fall in the blood pressure. Nicotine also has an antidiuretic effect. The adverse effects of nicotine are discussed in Chapter 10.

Nicotine is readily absorbed from the GI tract, respiratory mucous membranes, and skin. The average cigarette provides between 0.05 to 2.5 mg of nicotine. Because it is most often inhaled, nicotine reaches the brain very much more rapidly than if it had been injected (7 seconds). Nicotine is biotransformed in the liver. Its half-life is about 2 hours. The major metabolite cotinine is nonactive but has a half-life of 10 to 27 hours. There are several drug-drug interactions with nicotine. Table 10–2 provides an overview of the interactive drugs. The dosage of ganglionic stimulant drugs is found in Table 13–3.

Autonomic Ganglionic Blockers

❐ Mecamylamine (INVERSINE)

Ganglionic blockers were the mainstay of treatment for severe hypertension several years ago. They have since been replaced by superior agents for the treatment of chronic hypertension and hypertensive crisis (see Chapter 34). The only remaining use of ganglionic blockers in hypertension is for the initial control of blood pressure in patients with acute dissecting aortic aneurysm and for uncomplicated malignant hypertension. Ganglionic blockers are ideal for these purposes because they not only reduce blood pressure but also inhibit sympathetic reflexes. Thus, they reduce the rate of rise of pressure at the site of the aneurysm. By blocking all transmission in the autonomic nervous system, ganglionic blockers effectively prevent the autonomic nervous system from participating in body responses.

Mecamylamine reduces arterial blood pressure by diminishing autonomic outflow to the heart and vascular smooth muscle at the level of the thoracolumbar autonomic ganglia. Arteriolar and venous smooth muscle tone is thus reduced. Venous dilation promotes peripheral pooling of blood and diminishes venous return to the heart. Arteriolar dilation decreases total peripheral resistance and organ vascular resistance. Autonomic inhibition of the heart results in diminished cardiac reflexes.

The effects of mecamylamine interfere with parasympathetic as well as sympathetic function. The adverse effects include orthostatic hypotension; an inability to accommodate vision for near sight (accommodation); drying of secretions in the eyes, mouth, and stomach; paralytic ileus; retention of urine; and failure of erection and ejaculation. Mecamylamine readily penetrates into the brain and may produce CNS effects. Syncope, paresthesia, weakness, fatigue, sedation, tremor, choreiform movements, mental aberrations, and convulsions may occur. These effects occur when large doses of the drug are given and may be worsened in patients with renal insufficiency. Glossitis, anorexia, nausea, and vomiting are possible. Mecamylamine should not be used in patients with mild, moderate, or labile hypertension and may be unsuitable for uncooperative patients. The drug is contraindicated in patients with coronary insufficiency or recent myocardial infarction. Mecamylamine crosses the blood-brain and placental barriers and is distributed in breast milk (pregnancy category C).

Patients receiving antibiotics and sulfonamides should not be given ganglionic blockers. The action of mecamylamine may be potentiated by anesthesia, other antihypertensive drugs, and alcohol.

Mecamylamine is completely absorbed from the GI tract. It has a gradual onset of action of $^{1}/_{2}$ to 2 hours, and its effects last for 6 to 12 hours. Mecamylamine is slowly eliminated in the urine in its unchanged form. The rate of renal elimination is markedly influenced by the urinary pH. Alkaline urine reduces the elimination of the drug, whereas acidic urine promotes renal elimination. Patients taking mecamylamine should be monitored for elevated blood urea nitrogen and creatinine.

Mecamylamine therapy is usually started with one 2.5-mg tablet twice a day. This initial dose should be adjusted in increments of 2.5 mg at intervals of no less than 2 days until the desired blood pressure response occurs (i.e., dosage below that which causes signs of mild postural hypotension). The average total daily dose of mecamylamine is 25 mg, given in three divided doses. Patients may develop a partial tolerance, thus requiring increased dosage. Hypertensive levels return if ganglionic blockers or other potent antihypertensive drugs are suddenly discontinued. In patients with malignant hypertension, this return of hypertensive levels may occur abruptly and cause fatal cerebrovascular accidents or heart failure.

SUMMARY

- Urinary retention is a common occurrence following surgery or childbirth and in patients with neurogenic atony of the bladder.
- The objective of treatment is regular and complete emptying of the bladder.
- Unlike naturally occurring ACh, bethanechol is not destroyed in the synapse by acetylcholinesterase. Thus, the drug enhances the activity of naturally occurring ACh to cause bladder contraction.
- Pre-existing obstruction of the GI or urinary tract must be ruled out before administration of bethanechol chloride.
- Chronic administration requires patient education and individualization of the dose to fit the patient's life-style.
- Alzheimer's disease is a progressive fatal dementia affecting 47 percent of people over the age of 85.
- The treatment objective for Alzheimer's disease is to slow the progress of the dementia. The disease is not curable.
- Treatment options for Alzheimer's disease include tacrine, an indirect-acting cholinergic drug, and the cholinesterase inhibitor donepezil.
- Indirect-acting cholinergics act primarily by shielding ACh from degradation by the enzyme acetylcholinesterase. This results in accumulation of ACh at all sites where ACh is liberated. Donepezil is a reversible cholinesterase inhibitor that permits elevated ACh levels in the cerebral cortex.
- Although it is effective in reducing the cognitive dysfunction associated with Alzheimer's disease, tacrine carries a significant risk of liver dysfunction and requires frequent monitoring of AST (SGPT).
- Peptic ulcer disease and irritable bowel syndrome are common disorders that may be treated with anticholinergic drugs to reduce cramping.
- Anticholinergic drugs block the action of ACh at postganglionic receptor sites that are located in smooth muscle, secretory glands, the CNS (antimuscarinic activity), the SA and AV nodes, and cardiac muscle.
- Significant adverse effects of anticholinergics (e.g., dry mouth, blurred, vision, urinary retention) may decrease patient compliance.
- With the exception of nicotine gum and transdermal nicotine patches, there are no therapeutically useful ganglionic stimulant

drugs. This group of drugs must be understood because of their toxic effects.

- Autonomic ganglionic stimulants activate nicotinic receptors at ganglionic sites rather than at effector organs such as muscle. Thus, stimulation occurs as a result of norepinephrine release from sympathetic fibers and ACh release from parasympathetic fibers.
- Nicotine improves memory, especially long-term memory, and increases the accuracy and speed of information processing. Other benefits include an increase in pain threshold and a reduction of tension and anxiety.
- Nicotine use causes heart disease, stroke, emphysema, lung cancer, low birth weight, prematurity, and fetal injury.
- Ganglionic blockers effectively prevent the autonomic nervous system from participating in body responses by blocking all transmission in the autonomic nervous system.
- The only remaining use of ganglionic blockers in hypertension is for the initial control of blood pressure in patients with acute dissecting aortic aneurysm and in patients with uncomplicated malignant hypertension.
- The adverse effects of mecamylamine include orthostatic hypotension; an inability to accommodate vision for near sight (accommodation); drying of secretions in the eyes, mouth, and stomach; paralytic ileus; retention of urine; and failure of erection and ejaculation.

BIBLIOGRAPHY

Abramowicz, M. (1997). Donepezil (Aricept) for Alzheimer's disease. *The Medical Letter on Drugs and Therapeutics,* 39(1002), 53–54.

Andolf, E., Iosif, C., Jorgensen, C., et al. (1994). Insidious urinary retention after vaginal delivery: Prevalence and symptoms at follow-up in a population-based study. *Gynecologic and Obstetric Investigations,* 38(1), 51–53.

Black, J., and Matassarin-Jacobs, E. (1997). *Medical-surgical nursing: Clinical management for continuity of care* (5th ed). Philadelphia: W. B. Saunders.

Delieu, J., and Keady, J. (1996). The biology of Alzheimer's disease: Part 1. *British Journal of Nursing,* 5(3), 162–168.

Delieu, J., and Keady, J. (1996). The biology of Alzheimer's disease: Part 2. *British Journal of Nursing,* 5(4), 216–220.

Geldmacher, D. (1997). Donepezil (Aricept) therapy for Alzheimer's disease. *Comprehensive Therapy,* 23(7), 492–493.

Gilman, A., Rall, T., Nies, A., et al. (Eds.). (1990). *Goodman and Gilman's the pharmacologic basis of therapeutics.* (8th ed.). New York: Pergamon Press.

Henke, C., and Burchmore, M. (1997). The economic impact of tacrine in the treatment of Alzheimer's disease. *Clinical Therapeutics,* 19(2), 330–345.

Hickey, J. (1997). *The clinical practice of neurological and neurosurgical nursing* (4th ed). Philadelphia: J. B. Lippincott.

Long, J., and Rybacki, J. (1995). *The essential guide to prescription drugs.* New York: Harper Perennial.

Medical Economics Company, Inc. (1997). *Physicians' desk reference* (51st ed). Montvale, NJ: Author.

Medical Economics Company, Inc. (1996). *The PDR family guide to prescription drugs* (4th ed.) Montvale, NJ: Author.

Sohi, H., Heipel, J., Inman, K., et al. (1994). Preoperative transdermal scopolamine does not reduce the level of nausea and frequency of vomiting after laparoscopic cholecystectomy. *Canadian Journal of Surgery,* 37(4), 307–312.

Tammela, T. (1995). Postoperative urinary retention—why the patient cannot void. *Scandinavian Journal of Urology and Nephrology Supplement,* 175, 75–77.

U.S. Pharmacopeial Convention, Inc. (1997). *Drug Information for the Health Care Professional: USP DI.* (17th ed). Rockville, MD: Author.

Zurlinden, J. (1997). New hope for patients with Alzheimer's disease. *The Nursing Spectrum,* 10(22), 24.

Unit III

Drugs Influencing the Central Nervous System

THE CENTRAL NERVOUS SYSTEM

Despite the widespread use of central nervous system (CNS) drugs, our understanding of the anatomic and neurochemical complexity of the brain and spinal cord is limited. Given this deficit, it is important to have a basic understanding of CNS anatomy and physiology in order to appreciate the indications and implications of CNS drugs.

Billions of cells, each cell a functional unit in its own right, are interdependent and interrelated components of a single entity, a human being. Chemical mechanisms and the endocrine system play a major role in controlling and integrating body functions. But it is the CNS that is the information system of the body—processing, integrating, and coordinating all stimuli and activity. The CNS, enclosed and protected by the vertebrae and the skull, is composed of the brain, spinal cord, and nerve cells, and mediates overall adjustments and reactions within the body to changes in internal and external environments.

FUNCTIONAL ORGANIZATION OF THE CENTRAL NERVOUS SYSTEM

The brain is divided into major components: the cerebrum, parietal lobe, frontal lobe, occipital lobe, temporal lobe, thalamus, midbrain, cerebellum, pons, medulla oblongata, reticular activating system, limbic system, and blood-brain barrier. And it is the human brain's high degree of specialization that permits us to integrate information, reason, and be creative and sets us apart from other animals.

The spinal cord serves as a communication pathway between the brain and the peripheral nervous system. The gray matter of the brain functions as a center for spinal reflexes. The peripheral nervous system relays impulses to and from the CNS, thus alerting it to internal and external changes. The white matter on either side of the anterior and posterior gray horns contains distinct bundles of myelinated fibers than run within the spinal cord. These bundles are called tracts. The long ascending tracts contain sensory fibers that conduct impulses upward to the brain. The long descending tracts contain motor fibers that conduct impulses from the brain downward into the spinal cord. The fibers of descending tracts converge with other neurons whose axons pass out to muscles and glands. Thus, the ascending tracts are sensory tracts and the descending tracts are motor tracts (Fig. III–1).

Neurons characteristically consist of dendrites, a nucleated cell body, and an axon. Dendrites receive impulses from neurons or other cell types and conduct them to the cell body. Cell bodies transmit *afferent* (sensory) or *efferent* (motor) impulses. Afferent neurons conduct impulses toward the CNS from the sensory organs (e.g., the eye or ear) or from receptors in tissue that has adapted to respond to various stimuli. Efferent neurons transmit impulses from the CNS to muscles, glands, or other tissues and organs. The axon conducts impulses away from the cell body and stimulates other cells.

Impulse Transmission

Most information transmitted in the CNS results from alterations in electrical currents. Neurons are surrounded by a polarized membrane; the outer surface of the neuronal membrane is positively charged, whereas the inner surface is negatively charged. Polarization results from a disparate ion distribution on either side of the membrane. The three most notable ions are sodium, potassium, and chloride.

When neurons are left undisturbed (i.e., not conducting an impulse), the cell membranes remain quiescent and there is a greater concentration of sodium ions outside the neuronal cell and a greater concentration of potassium inside. This difference in electrical charge is referred to as the *resting potential*. However, when the resting neuron is stimulated, its membranes resting potential becomes less negative. And after repeated stimulation, a threshold potential is reached. When this threshold is reached, the membrane's permeability to sodium changes and sodium ions enter as potassium ions diffuse out of the cell. The neuron becomes depolarized by losing its electrical charge. This sequence of change is called *action potential,* and describes the depolarization and repolarization of the neurons. When an action potential occurs at one point in a nerve cell, it triggers other action potentials. The action potentials cause the nerve fiber to fire an impulse.

The junction between two neurons is called the *synapse,* the point at which impulses are transmitted from one neuron to another. Transmission at the synapse is unidirectional. The impulse is conveyed from the axon of one neuron (presynaptic cell) to another neuron (the postsynaptic cell). Because the terminal branches of a solitary axon may encroach on a number of different cells, one axon may transmit impulses to hundreds of other neurons. Likewise, any one neuron can receive impulses from many different axons. In the CNS, impulses from the presynaptic fibers may excite or inhibit postsynaptic neurons.

As discussed in Unit II, over 50 separate chemicals act as excitatory or inhibitory neurotransmitters. Small-molecule, rapid-acting transmitters produce most acute responses. Aspartic acid and glutamate are among the excitatory transmitters. Gamma-aminobutyric acid (GABA) and glycine are two of the inhibitory transmitters. Monoamine neurotransmitters (i.e., norepinephrine, epinephrine, dopamine, and serotonin) are excitatory at some synapses and inhibitory at others.

Neuropeptides are large-molecule, slow-acting transmitters whose effects last for days or even months in some cases. Some of the significant neuropeptides include endorphins, enkephalins, and substance P. Certain neuropeptides also function as hormones.

Cerebrum

The *cerebrum* is the largest and uppermost part of the brain. The cerebral cortex is its outer layer covering the two cerebral hemispheres; each hemisphere is divided into four lobes. The parietal lobe interprets sensations of heat, cold, touch, and pressure. The frontal lobe contains areas concerned with behavior, intellect, control of muscular movement, and speech as well as coordination of functional muscular activity within the vital organs. The occipital lobe is responsible for perception and interpretation of visual stimuli, while a large part of the temporal lobe is involved in the processes of hearing and memory.

Cortical activity may be slowed by CNS depressant drugs (e.g., alcohol, opioids, phenobarbital, and phenytoin) or

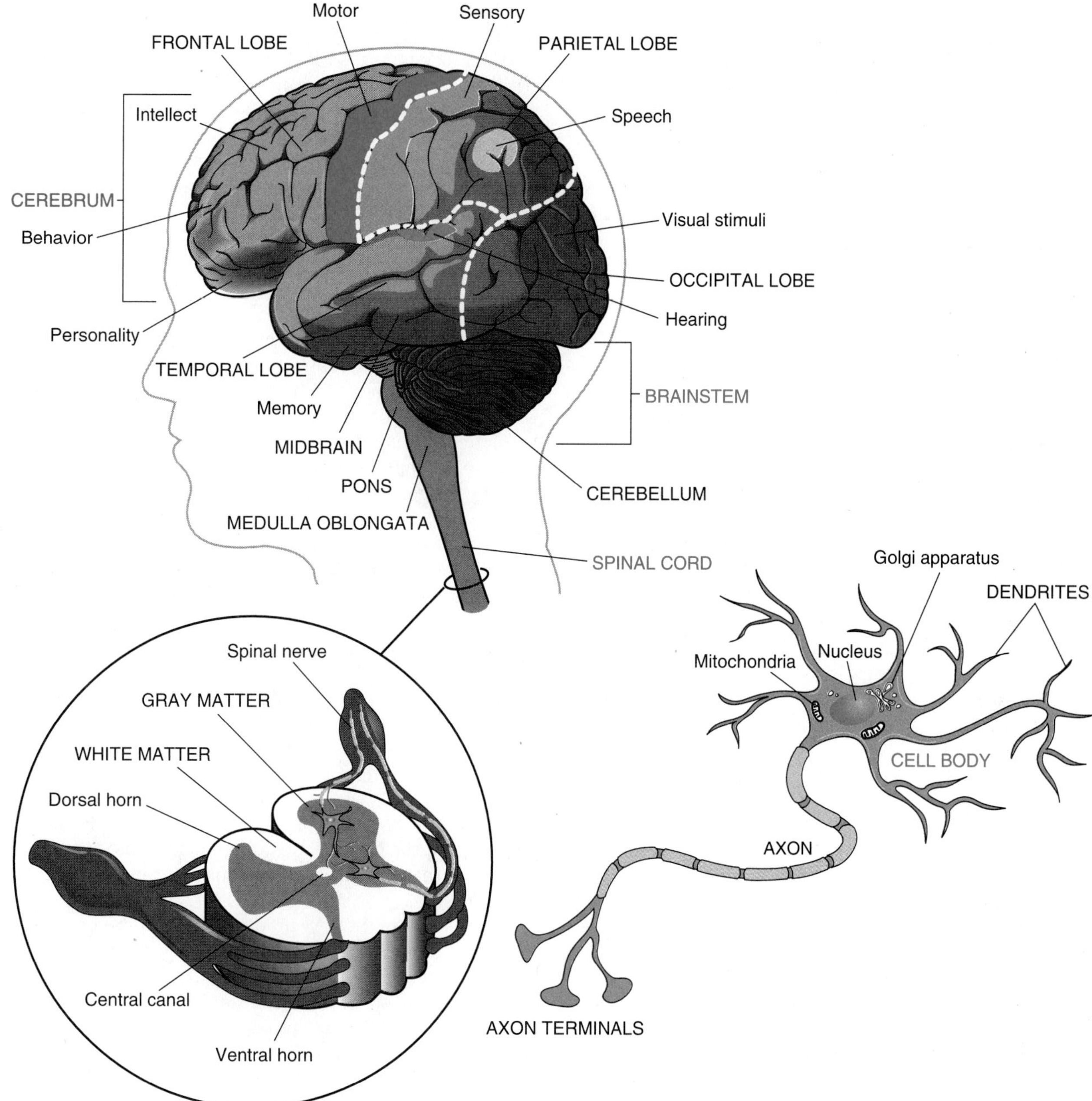

Figure III–1 Components of the central nervous system. The central nervous system is composed of the brain and spinal cord. The brain consists of the cerebrum, which includes the frontal, parietal, occipital, and temporal lobes, and a number of other structures, each with a specialized function. The spinal cord begins as a continuation of the medulla oblongata and is made up of both white and gray matter. The lipid substance myelin has a whitish color that gives white matter its name. The gray matter contains nerve cell bodies and dendrites, as well as bundles of unmyelinated axons; the absence of myelin in these components accounts for its gray color. A neuron may have many dendrites but has only one axon, which carries impulses away from the cell body. Nerve impulses from other cells are transmitted from knobs of incoming axons to dendrites or directly to the nerve cell body. A single neuron may receive impulses from many other neurons.

stimulated by drugs such as caffeine and amphetamines. Depressant activity is manifested as a decrease in muscular activity or the acuity of sensory perception. Conversely, CNS stimulation is seen as wakefulness, increased mental or muscular activity, reduced fatigue, or elation. However, drug actions that produce either depression or stimulation are exerted on portions of the brain not directly concerned with motor function.

The *extrapyramidal system* is a somatic pathway out of the cerebral cortex that affects skeletal muscles. The fibers of the extrapyramidal system originate mainly in the premotor area of the cerebral cortex and travel to the basal ganglia and brainstem. The structure of the extrapyramidal system is important to the control and coordination of motor activity. The complex adjustments needed to maintain balance, posture, and the proper degree of muscle contraction also are mediated here with assistance from the pyramidal system.

Drugs affecting the extrapyramidal network work by stimulating or depressing the system. Their effect is one of relaxation or rigidity of skeletal muscles.

The *pyramidal system* (corticospinal tract) nerve fibers originate in the cerebral cortex and extend down the brainstem to the medulla, where the fibers cross. The fibers continue down the spinal cord to specific levels of use. Impulses are then carried from the spinal cord to skeletal muscle. Because the fibers cross in the medulla, pulses originating in the right side of the cerebral cortex regulate muscle movement on the left side of the body. Impulses from the left side of the cortex regulate muscle movement on the right side of the body. Pyramidal and extrapyramidal systems intermingle in the spinal cord. Disease processes affecting higher levels of the CNS involve both nerve tracts.

Thalamus

The *thalamus* lies above and to the right and left of the midbrain, which is one of the three parts of the brainstem. It is concerned primarily with sensory transmission and perception. All sensory impulses entering the spinal cord or brainstem pass through a synapse at the thalamus. The impulses are then organized and interpreted before they are relayed to the cerebral cortex. However, thalamic perception and interpretation of heat, cold, pain, touch, or other sensory phenomena are rather crude and nondiscriminating. The cerebrum refines and carefully scrutinizes the sensations.

Drugs acting on the thalamus interfere with the orderly transmission of sensory impulses. This interference may be partially responsible for the action of some analgesic drugs. However, little is definitively known about the action of drugs on the thalamus.

Hypothalamus

The *hypothalamus* lies below the thalamus. It is a major link between the mind and the body, connecting the CNS with endocrine gland mechanisms. The major functions of the hypothalamus are fairly clear-cut visceral reflexes. Other functions include complex behavioral and emotional responses, but all involve distinctive responses to stimuli.

The hypothalamus regulates many body functions including the production of oxytocin and antidiuretic hormone, regulation of body temperature, assistance with regulation of arterial blood pressure through its effects on the vasomotor center in the medulla oblongata, and regulation of anterior pituitary hormone release through the secretion of releasing factors. The regulation of food and water intake by the hypothalamic thirst, appetite, hunger, and satiety centers is also mediated here. And there is evidence that a center for the sleep-wake cycle exists in the hypothalamus.

Some sedative-hypnotic drugs are thought to depress hypothalamic centers. Other drugs acting on the hypothalamus are helpful in treating the symptoms of weight loss, anorexia, decreased libido, and insomnia associated with depression. Selected drugs may also be used for a variety of conditions in which there is a hormonal deficit.

Cerebellum

The *cerebellum* is located somewhat above the medulla oblongata and is connected to the brainstem by large tracts of nerve fibers. It modulates and controls equilibrium, posture, and movement. The cerebellum coordinates and refines muscular activity and movement through feedback mechanisms to the periphery of the body and other parts of the brain.

The brainstem is made up of the *pons* and *midbrain* along with the medulla oblongata. Afferent and efferent fibers course through the pons; some of the descending fibers connect at synapses with neurons in the cerebellum. The midbrain serves as a relay station for impulses to and from the higher regions of the brain and for impulses related to vision and hearing.

Medulla Oblongata

The *medulla oblongata* is a direct extension of the spinal cord. It contains the vital centers that regulate blood pressure, heart rate and contractile force, and respirations. The synapses concerned with reflex control of swallowing, coughing, and vomiting also lie within the medulla.

Many drugs stimulate or depress one of the medullary centers. For example, barbiturates and opioids depress respirations by their action on receptors in the respiratory center. The therapeutic effectiveness of some drugs are related to their ability to affect specific medullary centers at doses below those that produce effects at other sites (e.g., cough suppression by codeine or the induction of vomiting by apomorphine).

Reticular Activating System

The *reticular activating system* (RAS) is a diffuse system of neurons that ascends from the spinal cord through the medulla and pons to the thalamus and hypothalamus (see Fig. 17–1). It permits two-way communication between the RAS and the cerebral cortex. It plays a significant role in the integration of both sensory and motor activity. Portions of the RAS appear to filter incoming sensory information and relay only that information requiring a response by the cerebral cortex.

Stimulation of the RAS produces wakefulness and mental alertness, whereas its depression causes sedation and loss of consciousness. For arousal to occur, the RAS must be stimulated by input signals. Almost any input can activate the RAS: pain; sensory, perceptual, or positional input; bright lights; or an alarm clock. Once the RAS is activated, the cerebral cortex is also activated and arousal is experienced. Following arousal, the RAS and cerebral cortex continue to activate one another through a feedback mechanism that is made up of many circuits. During the wakeful state, the RAS controls the general level of attentiveness to external surroundings. The RAS can excite or inhibit specific areas of the cortex through its links with the hypothalamus. Because humans experience different levels of wakefulness, it is assumed that the level of wakefulness is subject to the number of feedback currents operating at any given time.

It appears that the RAS plays a role in selecting appropriate responses to a given stimuli and, in general, provides for integration of the activity of the various parts of the CNS. Excitation or inhibition of the cortex may be one of the mechanisms whereby we can direct attention to certain aspects of the conscious mind while ignoring others.

Many CNS drugs act via the RAS. Psychomotor stimulants such as the amphetamines probably activate the RAS to produce a state of wakefulness and alertness. On the other hand, meditation or sedation caused by certain drugs produces a relaxed, focused state of consciousness. Anesthetics, the most potent of all CNS depressant drugs, produce a state of consciousness called anesthesia.

Limbic System

The *limbic system* anatomically involves several structures but is seen as a wishbone-shaped group of subcortical tissues (see Fig. 17–1). It forms a ring around the top of the brainstem and has little intrinsic activity of its own. This system is instantly responsive to emotions such as fear, anger, aggression, docility, sorrow, pleasure, affection, and sexual feelings. The limbic system also regulates behaviors such as laughing or crying. Although behavior is an outcome of the entire nervous system functioning, the limbic system controls most of the involuntary aspects. Additionally, learning and memory have been associated with the hippocampus portion of the limbic system. Further, because many nerve impulses from the limbic system are transmitted through the hypothalamus, changes in blood pressure, heart rate, respirations, and hormonal secretion occur in response to emotions.

Drugs affecting the limbic system work by first preventing the activation of the RAS. Subsequently, drowsiness and sleep or changes in the level of fear, anger, aggression, sorrow, pleasure, and sexual feelings are affected.

Basal Ganglia

Basal ganglia are concerned with skeletal muscle tone and orderly activity. Normal function is influenced by dopamine, a neurotransmitter produced in the midbrain by a specific group of cells called the substantia nigra (see Figs. 18–1 and 23–1). Degenerative changes in these cells cause dopamine to be released in reduced amounts.

Blood-Brain Barrier

The blood-brain barrier is composed of capillaries that serve the CNS. The barrier forms tight junctions between the cells of the capillary walls and separates the blood from the brain parenchyma everywhere except in the hypothalamus. The barrier is permeable to water, oxygen, carbon dioxide, and nonionic solutes (e.g., glucose, alcohol, and general anesthetics). The membrane is only slightly permeable to electrolytes and other ionic substances. However, lipid-soluble drugs or those compounds with an active transport system are capable of crossing the barrier to a significant degree.

The presence of the blood-brain barrier is a mixed blessing in that it protects the brain from injury by potentially toxic substances. In contrast, however, the barrier can be a significant obstacle to drug therapy of certain CNS disorders. In large dosages or in instances of meningeal inflammation, the permeation of substances across the blood-brain barrier increases. At present, research is being directed toward methods to increase the permeability of the barrier to specific therapeutic drugs, such as antineoplastics or antibiotics, which are needed to treat brain tumors or localized brain infections.

PHARMACOLOGIC IMPLICATIONS

Drugs affecting the CNS are broadly classified as depressants or stimulants according to their function. Such a simple classification is insufficient to describe the overall effect of a particular drug on CNS activity. Generally, opioids, general anesthetics, and sedative-hypnotics produce depression of the CNS when given in sufficient dosages. Lack of attention to surroundings and a short attention span are signs of mild CNS depression. As depression of the CNS deepens, muscle tone and the ability to move are reduced, and the perception of sensations such as pain, heat, and cold are decreased, followed by drowsiness and sleep. Unconsciousness or coma, loss of reflexes, respiratory failure, and death are outcomes of a severely depressed CNS.

CNS stimulants produce a variety of effects. Mild arousal is characterized by wakefulness, increased mental alertness, and decreased fatigue. Increased stimulation produces hyperactivity, excessive verbalizing, nervousness, and insomnia. Intense stimulation can lead to seizures, arrhythmias, and death. CNS stimulants are hard to regulate and thus have fewer therapeutic uses than CNS depressants.

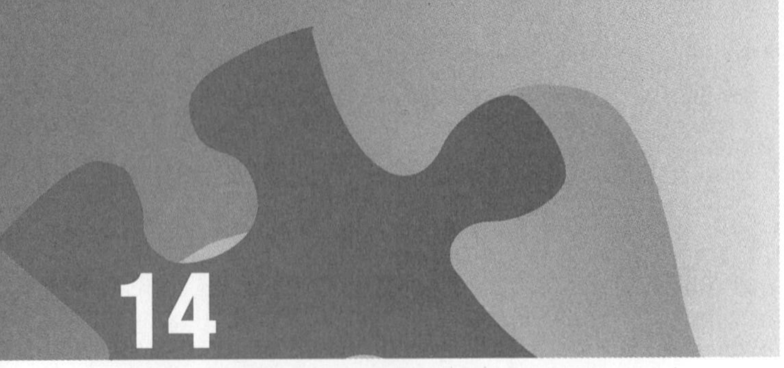

14

Opioid Analgesics and Related Drugs

Pain is a normal manifestation of everyday life and is an essential defense mechanism. *Pain* is defined as an unpleasant sensory and emotional experience that arises from actual or potential tissue damage. It is useful because it protects us from injury caused by extreme temperatures, mechanical pressure, or penetrating wounds. But beyond this capacity for warning, pain serves no beneficial purpose.

A person in pain usually takes action to eliminate the pain or its cause. Indeed, it is the main symptom that causes people to seek health care intervention. Further, unmanaged or undermanaged pain dramatically diminishes the quality of life more than any other single health-related problem. This is because pain is associated with psychological disturbances and profound changes in autonomic nervous system function.

One of the principal objectives of pain management is the alleviation of suffering. Opioids, which are derived from the opium poppy, accomplish this objective in many cases. The importance of effective pain management, however, goes beyond alleviating patient suffering. Additional benefits are gained for the patient when earlier mobilization, shortened hospital stays, reduced cost, and improved quality of life are realized.

PAIN

Epidemiology and Etiology

Pain has many definitions. It has been defined by the International Association for the Study of Pain as an unpleasant sensory and emotional experience arising from actual or potential tissue damage, or is described in terms of such damage. The most popular definition is put forth by Margo McCaffery, a registered nurse who is a recognized pain expert. According to McCaffery, *"pain is whatever the experiencing person says it is and exists whenever he says it does."* This definition requires that the patient be seen as the authority on his pain and the only person who can define the experience.

The events leading to pain begin when pain fibers are stimulated by a variety of stimuli. The stimuli can be mechanical (i.e., stretching of organs or pressure), temperature extremes (i.e., heat or cold), or chemical (e.g., ischemia or inflammation). There are many pathologic origins of pain. Pain can result from central or peripheral nervous system disorders, musculoskeletal damage, vascular disease, inflammation, or malignancy. Back pain is one of the most common pain complaints, second only to headache. Psychogenic pain, although not related to physiologic dysfunction, can nonetheless still result in pain.

Pain is a response to the trauma of surgery. Over 23 million operations were performed in the United States since 1989. In addition, pain related to malignancy occurs in 60 to 80 percent of patients with solid tumors.

Reports on the prevalence of pain in patients with human immunodeficiency virus infection range from 25 to 40 percent in early and ambulatory patients to 60 to 100 percent in patients with end-stage disease. The sources of pain in this population are many. Gastrointestinal pain can be related to oropharyngeal candidiasis or herpes, esophagitis, gastritis, or colitis. Herpes and cytomegalovirus infections, peripheral neuropathy, headache, pleuritic pain from pneumonia, and pain from Kaposi's sarcoma secondary to lymphatic obstruction are also causes of pain.

Pathogenesis

Regardless of the definition or the etiology, pain has both sensory (*perception*) and behavioral components (*interpretation*). An understanding of the elements that control pain perception from damaged tissues, the spinal cord, and higher brain centers is needed to provide effective pain management. However, pain interpretation varies among patients and health care providers alike, which, in turn, strongly influences pain management strategies.

Pain Perception

The first phase of the pain process involves chemical mediators such as bradykinin, serotonin, histamine, substance P, potassium ions, acids, proteolytic enzymes, prostaglandins, and acetylcholine. These mediators are released from damaged cells at the site of tissue injury, disease, or inflammation; magnify *nociceptor* (pain-specific receptors) input; and therefore increase pain.

Nociceptors are simply exposed nerve endings located in almost all types of tissue, including the skin, muscle, and deep viscera. Nociceptors require a relatively high level of stimulation to be activated but respond only to changes occurring in close proximity. The chemical mediators identified earlier increase the pain input to the nociceptors. Once they are stimulated, nociceptors actively communicate the presence of a painful stimulus. They can also become sensitized so that communication persists long after the stimulus has been removed. Much is known about pain originating from pain receptors in the skin. However, pain receptors located in deeper tissues may operate differently.

During the second stage of the pain process, impulses traverse myelinated A delta fibers in the periphery to reach the spinal cord. Acute pain (so-called fast pain) is usually elicited by A delta fibers. It is the pain felt when the skin is cut or burned, or when an electrical shock is felt. A delta fibers are provoked by superficial stimuli, so acute pain is uncommon in deep tissues. Acute pain is often described as sharp, pricking, acute, or electrical in nature. In contrast, nonmyelinated C fibers transmit impulses associated with chronic pain (so-called slow pain). C fibers are more primitive and transmit impulses slowly. Chronic pain is less well defined, localized, and described as a dull, burning, aching, or throbbing sensation.

The cell bodies of both A delta and C fibers lie within the dorsal root ganglion. Ganglionic filaments enter the substantia gelatinosa in the dorsal horns of the spinal cord. This area receives, transmits, and processes sensory input. The afferent nociceptors terminate at the level of the first, second, and fifth laminae. The substantia gelatinosa is found in the second lamina. This area is hypothesized to be the gating mechanism originally described by Melzack and Wall in their gate control theory of the mid 1960s (Fig. 14–1).

The third phase of the pain process is the transmission of impulses to higher brain centers. Distinct transmission pathways in the spinal cord contribute to the diverse qualities of pain. The major structure carrying impulses to higher brain centers is the ascending spinothalamic tract. Some fibers in this tract lead directly to the thalamus. The more direct pathway is along the neospinothalamic tract, which occupies the more lateral portion of the spinal cord. This pathway has few synapses and thus permits rapid impulse conduction. Its fibers project into the posterior nucleus of the thalamus to provide discriminatory functions such as the location, intensity, and duration of the painful stimulus.

A more diffuse pathway is the paleospinothalamic tract, which is located more medial within the spinal cord. This pathway leads to more diverse centers such as the medulla, hypothalamus, the reticular activating system, and limbic systems. Slower impulses are transmitted through this multisynaptic pathway. Impulse transmission through this structure is associated with autonomic nervous system responses and the unpleasant emotional aspect of pain.

There is a great deal of variation in pain perception and interpretation. Pain perception is modulated via the dorsal horn of the spinal cord, descending pathways, and endogenous chemicals. The dorsal horn of the spinal cord was once considered nothing more than a simple relay center for impulses. It is now thought to be a highly interpretative center for regulating sensory impulses.

The neurotransmitters serotonin and substance P are released into descending pathway fibers. The inhibitory fibers originate in the midbrain and descend downward into the dorsal horn at the level of the first and fifth laminae.

Pain perception and interpretation is also modulated via endogenous chemicals such as histamine, bradykinin, serotonin, substance P, and prostaglandin E. Substance P, a neuropeptide, appears to be a pain-specific transmitter that is present in the gate of the second lamina. Other peptides, such as *endorphins,* also inhibit pain. Endorphins, including alpha and beta endorphins, are a group of peptides with similar properties. Stimulation of the brainstem by endorphins provides profound analgesic effects. Endorphin effects are long lasting, whereas enkephalin action is much shorter. *Enkephalins* are smaller peptides found throughout the brain and dorsal horn of the spinal cord. They inhibit the release of substance P, thereby modulating pain. Serotonin facilitates pain transmission in peripheral nociceptors. It also acts as one of the neurotransmitters in the descending pain inhibition system.

Neurotransmitter levels vary throughout the day. The patient's pain threshold (i.e., pain sensitivity) is higher in the afternoon than in the morning. Further, the patient's analgesia requirement may differ at different times of the day. In addition, there is increasing evidence that patients with chronic pain may be lacking in some neurotransmitter. This evidence may help explain the relationship of certain antidepressant drugs to pain management (see Chapter 18).

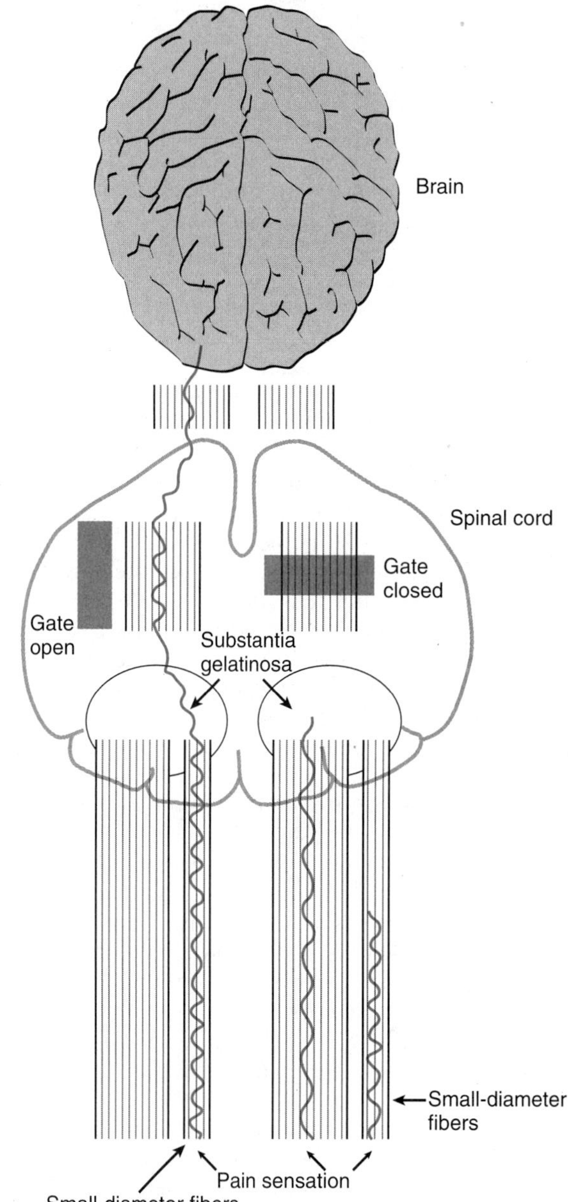

Figure 14–1 Gate control theory of pain. (From Ignatavicius D.D., Workman M.L., and Mishler M.A. [1995]. *Medical-surgical nursing: A nursing process approach* [2nd ed., p. 121]. Philadelphia: W.B. Saunders. Used with permission.)

Types of Pain

There are several ways to define types of pain including the onset of occurrence, duration, severity or intensity, mode of transmission, location or source, and causation. *Acute pain* is short term, generally lasting only for the duration of tissue damage. It has an identifiable etiology (e.g., inflammation, trauma, or surgery) and an immediate onset. Acute pain is relieved once the chemical mediators have been removed.

Acute pain can be classified further as somatic, visceral, or neuropathic. *Somatic pain* originates in cutaneous tissues such as skin and superficial tissues. Pain in these structures is well defined and localized. Although it is of low to moderate intensity, it stimulates the sympathetic nervous system to increase blood pressure, pulse rate, and respirations; dilates pupils; and increases the tension of skeletal muscles. In contrast, deep pain originates in bone, nerves, muscles, blood vessels, and other supporting tissues of the abdominal or thoracic cavities. It produces a dull, aching sensation that is hard to localize. Deep pain stimulates the parasympathetic nervous system, reducing blood pressure and pulse, but often causing nausea and vomiting, weakness, syncope, and possibly loss of consciousness.

Visceral pain arises from body organs. Because there are few nociceptors in body organs pain sensations are diffuse and poorly localized. Visceral nociceptors are insensitive to cuts and temperature extremes, but they are sensitive to ischemia, inflammation, and stretching. Nerve fibers innervating body organs follow sympathetic nerves to the spinal cord. This may explain why autonomic manifestations (i.e., diarrhea, cramps, sweating, and hypertension) frequently accompany visceral pain. Typical visceral pain includes that associated with acute appendicitis, cholecystitis, biliary and pancreatic tract inflammation, gastroduodenal disease, cardiovascular disease, pleurisy, and renal and ureteral colic.

Visceral nociceptors transmit referred pain. *Referred pain* occurs because visceral nerve fibers synapse at a level in the spinal cord close to fibers supplying certain subcutaneous tissues of the body. It is peculiar in that it is sometimes intense, although there is little or no pain at the point of the noxious stimulus. For example, pain associated with cholecystitis is referred to the back and the scapula. Pleural pain from the diaphragm is referred to the shoulder, and myocardial ischemia is often felt in the left arm, shoulder, or jaw.

In contrast to somatic and visceral pain, *neuropathic pain* is caused by injury or damage to nerve fibers in the periphery or damage to the CNS. With injury, there is interruption in the ability of nerve fibers to conduct sensory impulses. The brain interprets the painful stimuli even though no documented physiologic cause exists for the pain. Other names for neuropathic pain include deafferentation, hyperpathia, causalgia, or spontaneous pain. Neuropathic pain is often present in the absence of pathologic processes known to produce pain or in the absence of otherwise painful stimuli. The pain may seemingly arise from a body part whose pain pathway to the brain has been destroyed. *Phantom pain* is associated with the traumatic or surgical amputation of a body part. Patients describe the pain as residing in the missing body part, with the sensations described as itching, tingling, stabbing, or burning.

Vascular pain is believed to originate from some pathologic condition of vascular or perivascular tissues. Distention, displacement, or pulling on cranial vessels may account for a large portion of migraine headaches and headaches associated with arterial hypertension, brain tumors, and variations in the hydrodynamics of cerebrospinal fluid. Blood vessel responses are thought to be associated with pain induced by cold.

Cancer pain has multiple causes and can be composed of several types at any given time. Pain can be caused by pressure on or displacement of nerves, interference with blood supply, or blockage within hollow organs. Metastasis to the bone is a common cause of cancer pain. Metastatic pain occurs as a result of pathologic fracture, with resultant muscle spasms. Other causes are iatrogenic, such as surgery, radiation therapy, and antineoplastic therapy. Immobility and inflammation contribute to cancer pain.

Chronic pain is usually defined as pain of 6 months' duration. It may occur with or without evidence of tissue damage, and like other types of pain, it serves no useful purpose. When it is allowed to persist, chronic pain results in fatigue and irritability. Chronic pain is not characterized by physical signs but is often accompanied by depression and changes in personality, life-style, and reduced functional ability. Chronic pain is difficult to describe and difficult to manage because often it is not responsive to conventional management strategies.

Other types of pain, although they are not encountered as frequently, deserve a brief discussion. *Central pain* is associated with lesions, tumors, trauma, or inflammation in the brain. This pain manifests as high-frequency bursts of impulses that patients describe as severe, spontaneous, and often unyielding. Central pain can occur with any disorder that produces CNS damage, including cancer, diabetes, stroke, multiple sclerosis, or trauma. *Thalamic pain* is extremely rare. This pain occurs after a thalamic injury and is described by patients as hyperesthesia (i.e., abnormally increased sensitivity to stimuli) in one half of the body. Thalamic pain can range in intensity from paresthesias (i.e., numbness, tingling, or prickling) to agonizing, boring, burning pain. *Psychogenic pain* is distress primarily due to psychological factors rather than to physiologic dysfunction. It is very real to that patient. Patients with psychogenic pain undergo a genuine experience. The tension or stress the patient feels may lead to pronounced physiologic changes. Unfortunately, this type of pain is often thought to be "all in the head," and the diagnosis is assigned to the patient prematurely. However, careful assessment may uncover a treatable physiologic cause for the pain. Further, pain relief obtained with a placebo does not mean the patient does not have pain. When the psychogenic effect of stress, anxiety, fear, and anger produces painful physiologic responses, the pain is known as *psychophysiologic pain.*

Pain Interpretation

The *pain threshold,* which is the lowest intensity of stimulus that is perceived by the patient as pain, is essentially the same for all people as long as the central and peripheral nervous systems remain intact. However, the threshold may vary within each person based on a number of physiologic and psychosocial factors (e.g., age, gender, disease or condition, fatigue, insomnia, anxiety, the meaning of the pain, past experiences with pain, depression, isolation, religious beliefs, and cultural expectations). *Pain tolerance* on the other hand is different for each person and varies based on many subjective factors. In reality, pain tolerance refers to the amount of pain the patient is *willing* to endure. Only the patient can relate what that tolerance level is, not the health care provider.

PHARMACOTHERAPEUTIC OPTIONS

Analgesics are usually divided into two classes on the basis of their clinical effectiveness: (1) opioid agonists and agonist-antagonist analgesics, and (2) nonopioid analgesics. Each class is distinguished by what type of pain it relieves and where in the nervous system it seems to work rather than on the potency of its analgesia. In general, opioid analgesics are used to relieve severe central pain, whereas nonopioid analgesics are given for peripheral pain. The nonopioid analgesics are discussed in Chapter 15.

Opioid Analgesics

- ❒ Codeine; (🍁) PAVERAL
- ❒ Fentanyl (FENTANYL ORALET, SUBLIMAZE, DURAGESIC)
- ❒ Hydrocodone (DUOCET, HYCODAN, HYDROGESIC, VICODIN, LORTAB ASA); (🍁) ROBIDONE, LORTAB
- ❒ Hydromorphone (DILAUDID, DILAUDID-HP)
- ❒ Levorphanol (LEVO-DROMORAN, LEVORPHAN)
- ❒ Meperidine (DEMEROL, PITHIDINE)
- ❒ Methadone (DOLOPHINE, METHADOSE)
- ❒ Morphine sulfate (DURAMORPH, MS, MSIR, MSO_4, MS CONTIN, ROXANOL); (🍁) STATEX, EPIMORPH, MORPHINE HP, MORPHITEC, M.S.S.
- ❒ Oxycodone (OXICODONE, PERCOCET, TYLOX, PERCODAN, others); (🍁) SUPEUDOL, OXYCOCET, ENDOCET, ENDODAN, OXYCODAN
- ❒ Oxymorphone (NUMORPHAN)
- ❒ Propoxyphene (DARVON, DARVOCET, WYGESIC, DARVON COMPOUND-65); (🍁) NOVO-PROPOXYN, 642, DARVON-N WITH ASA, DARVON-N COMPOUND, 692, others

Indications

The primary use of opioid analgesics is to prevent or relieve moderate to severe acute or chronic pain of various etiologies. They are the mainstay of treatment for pain caused by traumatic injuries, burns, biliary or renal colic, cancer-related pain, and pain related to postoperative states. Other uses for opioids include the treatment of acute pulmonary edema, as an obstetric analgesic during labor and delivery, and for invasive diagnostic procedures. Morphine acts as a reducer of preload in patients with myocardial infarction. A handful of the opioids (e.g., alfentanil, fentanyl, and sufentanil) are most often used as adjuncts to general anesthesia and are discussed in more depth in Chapter 16.

Most opioids are Schedule II drugs (see Chapter 1) under federal law. The pharmacologic action of opioid analgesics is similar to those of their parent compound—morphine. Morphine is the prototype by which all other opioids are measured, although they all share certain desirable and undesirable characteristics.

Pharmacodynamics

Opioids are ordinarily classified as full agonists, partial agonists, or combination agonists-antagonists. Full agonists (i.e., agonist I drugs) produce a maximal response within the cells to which they bind. Partial agonists (i.e., agonist II drugs) bind to a lesser degree, producing a reduced response. A combination agonist-antagonist activates one type of opioid receptors while simultaneously blocking another type.

All opioids, whether they are naturally occurring (e.g., morphine) or synthetic (e.g., meperidine), interact with mu (μ), kappa (K), or delta (Δ) receptors to create a variety of effects. However, only a proportion of opioid receptors are actually involved in promoting analgesia (Table 14–1). A fourth opioid receptor, or sigma (σ), has been identified, but a variety of other nonopioid drugs also appear to act at this site. Thus, it is doubtful whether this receptor is a true opioid receptor.

Although research has been successful in identifying the structure, locations, and drug specificity of opioid receptors, binding mechanisms are not yet well defined. Presumably, opioids modify the permeability and conduction of ions such as calcium and potassium, which, in turn, results in hyperpolarization of nociceptors and depression of the nervous system. Blocking calcium channels inhibits release of glutamate and substance P from primary afferent nerve terminals. The end results affect adrenergic, serotonergic, dopaminergic, and cholinergic neurotransmitter systems. In general, adrenergic drugs (e.g., amphetamine and dopamine) tend to reduce pain, whereas cholinergic and serotonergic drugs tend to cause exacerbation of pain.

Activation of opioid receptors inhibits adenyl cyclase activity. The inhibition leads to a reduction in intracellular cyclic adenosine monophosphate (cAMP). The fall in neuronal cAMP is believed to be the means by which the analgesic effect of opioids occurs.

Adverse Effects and Contraindications

The adverse effects of opioids are all direct consequences of receptor activation. The effects are largely due to the preponderance of opioid receptors in the medulla and peripheral nervous system. The incidence and severity of adverse effects increase as dosage increases.

TABLE 14–1 OPIOID RECEPTORS AND EFFECTS

Receptor	Clinical Effects	Opioid/Endogenous Peptide
Mu (μ)	Euphoria Physical dependence Respiratory depression Supraspinal analgesia	Morphine Meperidine Methadone Codeine Fentanyl Levorphanol Buprenorphine Naloxone (antagonist)
Kappa (K)	Miosis Sedation Spinal analgesia Respiratory depression	Morphine Pentazocine Naloxone (antagonist)
Delta (Δ)	Dysphoria Hallucinations Respiratory stimulation Vasomotor stimulation	Enkephalins Endorphins
Sigma (σ)	Dysphoria Hallucinations Respiratory stimulation Vasomotor stimulation	Pentazocine

Central Nervous System Effects

Opioids cross the blood-brain barrier to alter pain perception; hence, the CNS effects that are seen with opioid use. Adverse CNS effects vary from drowsiness to sleep to unconsciousness, and decreased mental and physical activity. In addition, headache, dizziness, confusion, dysphoria, unusual dreams, hallucinations, and delirium can result. Opioids also interfere with the ability to use accurate judgment, to operate machinery, and to drive.

Respiratory Effects

Medullary depression is characterized by respiratory depression. The depression ranges from slow, shallow respirations to respiratory arrest. The medullary response to carbon dioxide is reduced. Respiratory depression is noted roughly 7 minutes after intravenous (IV) administration, 30 minutes after intramuscular (IM) injection, and 90 minutes after a subcutaneous (SC) injection. Depressant effects can last from 4 to 5 hours. Respiratory depression is the most common cause of death from opioids, although there really is no upper limit on drug dosage (ceiling effects).

Death occurring secondary to opioid overdose is usually the result of respiratory depression and most often occurs in patients who have not received opioids in the past. For overdose to occur, doses well above the therapeutic level would have to be given. Accumulated doses, especially in patients with liver or renal failure and in the older adult, can cause overdose. It should be noted that equianalgesic doses of opioids produce sedative and respiratory depression effects comparable to that of morphine.

Opioid agonist-antagonists (see discussion later) cause respiratory depression to a lesser degree than do opioids. Most newer opioid analgesics were designed to be as effective as morphine but less sedating, and produce less depression and dependence. However, this effort has been less than successful.

In contrast to the multisystem adverse effects seen with opioids, they do have a clinical useful adverse effect. They exhibit antitussive activity. The antitussive activity of opioids is discussed in Chapter 48.

Cardiovascular Effects

In a supine patient, therapeutic doses of morphine or the synthetic opioids have very little effect on blood pressure and cardiac rate or rhythm. However, some patients experience orthostatic hypotension when moving from a supine position to a head-up or standing position. This hypotension is due to a direct dilating action on peripheral blood vessels caused by the opioids, which reduces the capacity of the cardiovascular system to respond to gravitational changes. Therefore, opioids are used with caution in patients who are volume depleted because the hypotensive effects are more pronounced. Increasing blood volume decreases the orthostatic changes.

Gastrointestinal Effects

A common adverse effect of opioids is constipation. Constipation is caused by diminished peristaltic contractions in the small and large intestine and delay in passage of gastric contents through the duodenum. There is also decreased lower gastrointestinal smooth muscle tone and glandular secretion and increased water reabsorption from the intestines. Tolerance does not develop to constipation as it does to the other adverse effects of opioids.

Second, biliary colic may occur as smooth muscle contraction increases the pressure within the biliary ductal system (although it happens less frequently with meperidine than with morphine). Opioids stimulate the chemoreceptor trigger zone in the medulla, especially in low doses, to produce nausea and vomiting in susceptible individuals.

Genitourinary Effects

Ureteral spasm, spasm of urinary sphincters, urinary retention or hesitancy oliguria, antidiuretic effects, and a reduced libido have been noted with opioid use. Urinary retention is especially problematic in patients with prostatic hypertrophy. Opioids also tend to prolong labor and produce respiratory depression in the neonate.

Other Effects

Severe hypersensitivity reactions to opioids are rare but, when present, usually appear as urticaria or a skin rash. Some patients experience itching or wheal formation at the site of injection, but this effect is usually a local, histamine-mediated response. Anaphylaxis is rare.

All opioids except meperidine cause pupillary constriction. Some patients may experience blurred vision, dry eyes, and lens opacities. Opioids also stimulate the release of antidiuretic hormone, prolactin, and human growth hormone.

Patients who receive a therapeutic dose of morphine several times a day develop some degree of physical dependency in approximately 2 weeks, with the dosage necessary for dependency exceeding 60 mg of morphine or its equivalent per day in some patients. Physical dependency is defined as an involuntary altered physiologic state produced by repeated administration of a drug. Continued administration of the drug is required to prevent withdrawal (abstinence) syndrome. Withdrawal symptoms include a characteristic mix of CNS and autonomic nervous system responses such as tactile hallucinations, irritability, sleeplessness, restlessness, yawning, tremor, joint and muscle pains. Anorexia, nausea, vomiting, diarrhea, dehydration, abdominal cramps, ketosis, weight loss, distorted vision, and photophobia also plague the individual. Peak severity of withdrawal symptoms occurs 36 to 72 hours after the last dose of opioid, with symptoms gradually waning over 2 to 5 weeks. Withdrawal lasting months has also been documented. Withdrawal is usually not life-threatening in an otherwise healthy individual.

Tolerance to opioids develops quickly depending on the dose, dosage frequency, and frequency of use. Tolerance is characterized by a shorter duration of pain relief, a decrease in peak analgesic effect, and an increase in the amount of opioid needed to relieve the pain. Doses that are 10 to 20 times the initial dose have been tolerated by some individuals. As a result, larger and larger doses of the drug are needed to achieve the same clinical effect. This leads to increased severity and incidence of adverse effects. When the drug is stopped, symptoms of withdrawal appear. Physical dependence, tolerance, and addiction were discussed in Chapter 10.

Contraindications

Opioids are contraindicated or must be used very cautiously in people with chronic lung disease, respiratory depression, and liver or kidney disease, and in persons with a previous hypersensitivity reaction. They should also be used with caution in patients with head injuries, increased intracranial pressure, adrenal insufficiency, Addison's disease, alcoholism, undiagnosed abdominal pain, urethral stricture, and prostatic hypertrophy. Because of the potential for neonatal respiratory depression opioids are used with caution during labor and delivery.

Pharmacokinetics

Opioids are variably absorbed from mucosal surfaces of the nose and gastrointestinal tract as well as from IM and SC injection sites. Rectal absorption can be erratic. Opioids are distributed to a variety of tissues, such as the lungs, liver, kidneys, and spleen. Skeletal muscle and fatty tissues act as storage sites, although opioid concentration in brain tissue is less that of other areas. Slow penetration of the opioid to brain sites and an effective first-pass effect influences the onset, peak, and duration of drug action.

The onset of analgesia is rapid by most routes (Table 14–2). Highly lipid-soluble drugs generally have a more rapid onset of action. The duration of action varies with the route of administration, dosage, and patient characteristics. Most opioids have a duration of action of 4 to 6 hours. The percentage of protein binding varies from 33 percent for morphine to 90 percent for methadone. Opioids are converted to metabolites to be excreted in the urine. The half-life of each of the opioids is variable.

Drug-Drug Interactions

Opioids interact with other CNS depressants such as alcohol, anesthetics, barbiturates, and sedative-hypnotics to enhance CNS depression (Table 14–3). Severe constipation and urinary retention may result with the concurrent use of tricyclic antidepressants, phenothiazines, and anticholinergic drugs. The paralyzing effects of neuromuscular blockers are enhanced in the presence of opioids. Smoking and nicotine use decrease the analgesic effect of opioids. Concurrent use of diuretics can result in additive orthostatic hypotension. Cimetadine inhibits the biotransformation of the opioids, leading to increased respiratory and CNS depression.

Dosage Regimen

Opioids are administered by mouth, IM, SC, or IV (Table 14–4). They may also be given as suppositories, by the epidural route, directly into the spinal cord (intrathecally), and transdermally. Transdermal drug delivery systems avoid the problem of fluctuating drug levels that have been associated with intermittent dosing. For example, a fentanyl transdermal patch delivers 25 to 100 mcg of fentanyl per hour for a period of 72 hours. The patient's 24-hour requirement of currently used opioid must be calculated before calculating the dosage of transdermal fentanyl.

Equianalgesia

The relative potency of analgesics is the dosage ratio of two analgesics that produce the same effect. Estimates of the relative potency afford a basis for determining the dose to be used when changing from one analgesic to another or from one administration route to another. Table 14–5 lists the equianalgesic doses of selected opioids compared with the prototype morphine. Note, for example, that 30 mg of morphine given orally is equivalent in analgesia to 300 mg of meperidine given by the same route. Also note that 10 mg of IM morphine is comparable in effect to 30 mg of morphine taken by mouth or 100 mg of meperidine given IM. Because not every patient responds the same to a given dose of opioid, the dosage and dosage frequency may need to be adjusted to gain optimum pain relief.

The duration of action for analgesics is based on the dose that produces a peak effect equivalent to that of morphine. In addition, opioids vary in the extent to which they are bioavailable. Differences in bioavailability account for the variety of oral doses identified in Table 14–5. Older drugs have a reduced bioavailability compared with newer drugs. Therefore, the dosages of newer drugs tend to be lower than those of older drugs. Further, oral equianalgesic doses are based on a single dose of the drug. Dosing requirements generally decrease once the patient has received a loading dose of the drug. However, the adverse effects of opioids tend to limit the dose that can be given and analgesic effects that can be obtained.

Opioid formulations specifically for children are generally not available. The risk of dosage errors greatly increases when a child's dose is calculated from adult dosages. Although rectal suppositories may be helpful when oral or parenteral routes are not feasible, there are disadvantages with this method. The practice of cutting adult suppositories in half or otherwise altering the formulation leads to unknown and inaccurate dosages.

Laboratory Considerations

Elevated biliary tract pressure associated with opioid use may cause increases in plasma amylase and lipase. Accurate determination of these levels may be unreliable for 24 hours in the presence of opioids.

Opioid Agonists-Antagonists

- ❐ Butorphanol (STADOL, STADOL NS)
- ❐ Buprenorphine (BUPRENEX)
- ❐ Dezocine (DALGAN)
- ❐ Nalbuphine (NUBAIN)
- ❐ Pentazocine (TALWIN, TALWIN NX)

Indications

Opioid agonists-antagonists are used for moderate to severe pain. Butorphanol, buprenorphine, and nalbuphine can be used for patients who have a true hypersensitivity to meperidine or who are intolerant to morphine. Butorphanol, nalbuphine, and pentazocine have been used for analgesia during labor, as sedation before surgery, and as a supplement in balanced anesthesia.

Pharmacodynamics

Combination agonist-antagonists activate one type of opioid receptor while simultaneously blocking another type (Fig. 14–2). However, they produce fewer adverse

TABLE 14–2 PHARMACOKINETICS OF SELECTED OPIOIDS, AGONIST-ANTAGONISTS, AND ANTAGONISTS

Drug	Route	Onset	Peak	Duration	PB(%)	$t_{1/2}$
Opioids						
Codeine	po	30–45 min	60–120 min	4 hr	50	2.5–4 hr
	IM, SC	10–30 min	30–60 min			
Fentanyl	TD	Slow	12–24 hr	24–48 hr*	79–87	13–22 hr
Hydrocodone	po	10–30 min	30–60 min	4–6 hr	UA	3.8 hr
Hydromorphone	po	30 min	90–120 min	4 hr	UA	2–4 hr
	IM	15 min	30–60 min	4–5 hr		
	IV	10–15 min	15–30 min	2–3 hr		
	SC	15 min	30–90 min	4 hr		
Levorphanol	po	10–60 min	90–120 min	4–5 hr	<50	12–16 hr
	IM	UA	60 min			
	IV	Immed	<20 min			
	SC	UA	60–90 min			
Meperidine	po	15 min	60–90 min	2–4 hr	60–80	3–8 hr
	IM	10–15 min	30–50 min			
	IV	1 min	5–7 min			
	SC	10–15 min	30–50 min			
Methadone	po	30–60 min	90–120 min	4–6 hr	90	4–6 hr
	IM	10–20 min	60–120 min	4–5 hr		
	IV	Immed	15–30 min	3–4 hr		22–48 hr†
Morphine	po	10–30 min	60–120 min	4–5 hr	33	2–3 hr
	IM	10–30 min	30–60 min			
	IV	5–10 min	20 min			
	SC	10–30 min	50–90 min			
	EP	15–60 min	—	24 hr	—	
Oxycodone	po	10–15 min	60–90 min	3–4 hr	<50	2–3 hr
Oxymorphone	IM	10–15 min	30–90 min	3–6 hr	33	2–3 hr
	IV	5–10 min	15–30 min	3–4 hr		
	SC	10–20 min	UA	3–6 hr		
Propoxyphene	po	15–60 min	120 min	4–6 hr	50	6–12 hr
Opioid Agonist-Antagonists						
Butorphanol	IM	10 min	30–60 min	3–4 hr	96	2.5–4 hr
	IV	Immed	30 min			
Buprenorphine	IM	15 min	60 min	6 hr‡	96	4–5 hr
	IV	Immed	<60 min	6 hr		
Dezocine	IM	30 min	90 min	2–4 hr	UA	1.2–7.4 hr
	IV	15 min	10 min			
Nalbuphine	IM	<15 min	60 min	3–6 hr	<30	5 hr
	IV	2–3 min	30 min	3–4 hr		
	SC	<15 min	UA	3–6 hr		
Pentazocine	po	15–30 min	60–90 min	3 hr	60	2–3 hr
	IM	15–20 min	30–60 min	2–3 hr		
	IV	2–3 min	15–30 min			
	SC	15–20 min	30–60 min			
Opioid Antagonists						
Naloxone	IM	2–5 min	UK	45 min	50	60–100 min
	IV	1–2 min		Varies§		
	SC	2–5 min				
Naltrexone	po	5–60 min	UK	Varies‖	UA	4–13 hr¶

*Duration of action of fentanyl patch after the patch is removed

†Duration of action and half-life of methadone's active metabolites with repeated dosing. May be even longer in elderly patients and patients with renal dysfunction. Extended half-life is not related to analgesic effects.

‡Respiratory depressant effects of buprenorphine occurs 1–3 hr after IM injection.

§Duration of action of naloxone varies with dose administered and route of administration.

‖Duration of action of naltrexone is dose dependent. Twenty-five milligrams can block effects of IV heroin for up to 24 hours, whereas a 100- to 150-mg dose can last 48 to 72 hours, respectively.

¶The half-life of naltrexone metabolites.

TD, Transdermal; PB, protein binding; $t_{1/2}$, elimination half-life; UK, unknown; UA, unavailable; EP, epidural; SUP, suppository.

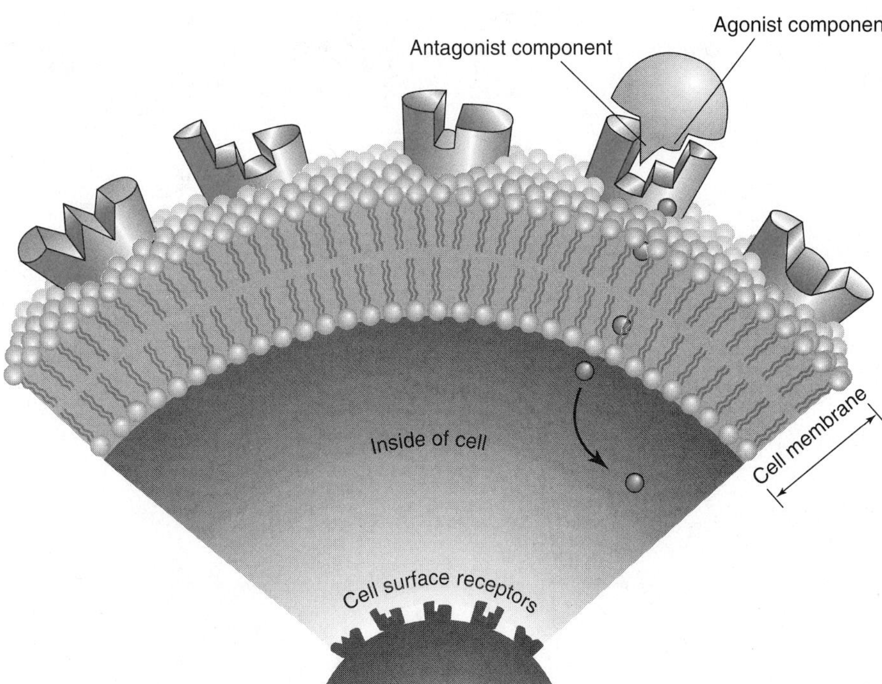

Figure 14–2 Agonist-antagonist drug receptor interactions. Combination agonist-antagonists activate one type of opioid receptor while simultaneously blocking another type. These drugs alter the perception of and response to painful stimuli while producing generalized central nervous system depression.

TABLE 14–3 DRUG-DRUG INTERACTIONS OF SELECTED OPIOIDS, AGONIST-ANTAGONISTS, AND ANTAGONISTS

Drug	Interactive Drugs	Interaction
Opioids		
Opioids	Alcohol Anesthetics Antianxiety agents Antihistamines Antipsychotic agents Barbiturates Sedative-hypnotics	Enhanced CNS depression, respiratory depression, and hypotension
	Tricyclic antidepressants Phenothiazines Anticholinergics	Severe constipation and urinary retention
	Cimetidine	May inhibit opioid biotransformation, leading to increased respiratory and CNS depression
	Diuretics	Orthostatic hypotension
	Monoamine oxidase inhibitors	CNS excitation, severe hypotension or hypertension
	Phenorphine Pentazocine	May precipitate opioid withdrawal in dependent patients
	Skeletal muscle relaxants	Enhances neuromuscular blocking action of interactive drug
	Nicotine	Decreases analgesic effect
Meperidine	Monoamine oxidase inhibitors	Additive CNS depression with hypotension and respiratory depression, or CNS stimulation with hyperexcitability and seizures
Methadone	Hydantoins	Induces biotransformation of methadone
Propoxyphene	Carbamazepine	Decreased biotransformation and increased serum concentrations of interactive drug
	Naltrexone	Withdrawal symptoms
Opioid Agonist-Antagonists		
Buprenorphine Butorphanol	Monoamine oxidase inhibitors	Increased CNS and respiratory depression, hypotension
Dezocine Nalbuphine Pentazocine	Alcohol Antihistamines Antidepressants Sedative-hypnotics	Additive CNS depression
	Opioids	Decreased effectiveness of interactive drug
Opioid Antagonists		
Naloxone Naltrexone	Opioids	Withdrawal symptoms

TABLE 14–4 DOSAGE REGIMEN FOR SELECTED OPIOIDS, AGONIST-ANTAGONISTS, AND ANTAGONISTS

Drug	Use(s)	Dosage	Implications
Opioids			
Codeine	Mild to moderate pain	*Adult:* 15–60 mg po q3–6 hr *or* 15–60 mg po IM, IV, SC q4–6 hr *Child age 6–12 yr:* 0.5 mg/kg (15 mg/m^2) po, IM, IV, SC q4–6 hr	When combined with nonopioid analgesics (aspirin, acetaminophen): #2 = 15 mg codeine, #3 = 30 mg codeine, and #4 = 60 mg codeine.
Transdermal fentanyl	Chronic pain	*Adult:* 25 mcg/hr after assessment of 24-hr opioid requirement	Transdermal fentanyl is not recommended for control of postoperative, mild, or intermittent pain. Additional short-acting opioids should be available for breakthrough pain until conversion from other opioids is successful
Hydrocodone	Moderate to severe pain	*Adult:* 5–10 mg po q4–6 hr *Child:* 0.2 mg/kg po q3–4 hr	Available in combination with acetaminophen or aspirin. May be administered with food or milk to minimize GI irritation
Hydromorphone	Moderate to severe pain	*Adult:* 2 mg po q3–6 hr. May be increased to 4 mg po q4–6 hr *or* 1–2 mg IM, SC q3–6 hr. May be increased to 3–4 mg. q4–6 hr *or* 0.5–1 mg IV q3hr *or* 0.2–30 mg/hr continuous infusion (unlabeled)	An initial bolus of two times the hourly rate in milligrams may be given, with subsequent breakthrough boluses of 50–100% of the hourly rate in milligrams.
Levorphanol	Moderate to severe pain	*Adults over 50 kg.:* 4 mg po q6–8 hr *or* 2 mg SC, IV q6–8 hr *or* 1–2 mg SC 90 minutes before surgical procedure *Adults and child under 50 kg.:* 0.04 mg/kg po q6–8 hr *or* 0.2 mg/kg SC, IV q6–8 hr	Unlabeled for use in children. Use with extreme caution in patients receiving MAO inhibitors
Meperidine	Moderate to severe pain, obstetric analgesia, preoperative sedation, adjunct to anesthesia	*Adult:* 50–150 mg po, IM, SC q3–4 hr or 15–35 mg/hr IV infusion *Child:* 1–1.8 mg/kg po, IM, SC q3–4 hr. Not to exceed 100 mg/dose	Do not confuse with morphine or hydromorphone—fatalities have occurred. May be administered with food or milk to minimize GI irritation. Local irritation is possible with repeated SC administration. Oral dose is 50% less effective as parenteral formulation
Methadone	Severe pain; suppression of opioid withdrawal symptoms	*Adults over 50 kg.:* 20 mg po q6–8 hr as analgesic *or* 15–40 mg po QD for opioid detoxification *or* 10 mg IM, SC q6–8 hr as analgesic *or* 15–40 mg. IM, SC QD for opioid detoxification *Adults and child weighing less than 50 kg:* 0.2 mg/kg po q6–8 hr *or* 0.1 mg/kg IM, SC q6–8 hr	May be administered with food or milk to minimize GI irritation. Diskettes (dispersible tablets) are to be dissolved and used for detoxification and maintenance treatment only
Morphine	Moderate to severe pain, pulmonary edema, myocardial infarction	*Adults over 50 kg:* 30 mg po, PR q3–4 hr, PRN or equivalent dose q8–12 hr as controlled-release formulation once 24-hr opioid requirement is determined *or* 10 mg IM, IV, SC q3–4 hr *or* 0.8–10 mg/hr preceded by bolus of 15 mg for continuous infusion *Adults and child weighing less than 50 kg:* 0.3 mg/kg po, PR q3–4 hr *or* 0.1 mg/kg IM, IV, SC q3–4 hr *or* 0.025–2.6 mg/kg/hr continuous infusion (unlabeled)	Larger doses may be required for chronic therapy. IV infusion rates vary greatly; up to 440 milligrams per hour have been used

effects than true opioids and have little antitussive action. These drugs alter the perception of and response to painful stimuli while producing generalized CNS depression. They have partial antagonist properties that can result in opioid withdrawal symptoms in physically dependent patients. Pentazocine tablets contain 0.5 mg of naloxone (see the discussion of naloxone that follows), which has no pharmacologic activity when taken by mouth. If the product is abused by injection, naloxone antagonizes pentazocine.

TABLE 14–4 DOSAGE REGIMEN FOR SELECTED OPIOIDS, AGONIST-ANTAGONISTS, AND ANTAGONISTS *Continued*

Drug	Use(s)	Dosage	Implications
Opioids—cont'd			
Oxycodone	Moderate to severe pain	*Adult:* 5–10 mg po q3–4 hr PRN. Controlled-release tablets q12hr *or* 10–40 mg PR q3–4 hr *Child weighing less than 50 kg.:* 0.2 mg/kg po q3–4 hr	May be administered with food or milk to minimize GI irritation. Controlled-release tablets should be taken whole, not crushed, broken, or chewed. Advise patients that empty matrix tablets may appear in the stool with controlled release formulation
Oxymorphone	Moderate to severe pain	*Adult:* 1–1.5 mg IM, SC q3–6 hr PRN *or* 0.5 mg IV q3–6 hr PRN *or* 5 mg PR q4–6 hr PRN	Suppositories should be stored in the refrigerator
Propoxyphene	Mild to moderate pain	*Adult:* 65 mg hydrochloride po q4hr *or* 100 mg napsylate q4hr PRN. Not to exceed 390 mg/day as hydrochloride or 600 mg/day as napsylate	Doses may be administered with food or milk to minimize GI irritation
Opioid Agonist-Antagonists			
Butorphanol	Moderate to severe pain, analgesia during labor, preoperative sedation, adjunct to anesthesia	*Adult:* 2 mg IM q3–4 hr PRN (range 1–4 mg) *or* 1 mg q3–4 hr IV PRN (range 0.5–2 mg) *or* 1 mg IM, IV q4–6hr for geriatric patients *or* 1 mg (1 spray intranasally in 1 nostril) q3–4hr May repeat dose in 60–90 minutes.	Instruct patient on proper use of nasal spray. Use with extreme caution in patients taking MAO inhibitors
Buprenorphine	Moderate to severe pain	*Adult:* 0.3 mg q4–6hr PRN. May repeat initial dose after 30 minutes up to 0.3 mg q4hr *or* 0.6 mg q6hr	0.6-mg doses should be given only IM in deep, well-developed muscle
Dezocine	Short-term management of moderate to severe pain	*Adult:* 10 mg IM q3–6hr PRN (range 5–20 mg) *or* 5 mg initially every 2–4hr (range 2.5–10 mg) PRN. Dosage not to exceed 120 mg/day	Coadministration with nonopioid analgesic may have additive effects and permit lower doses. Administer deep IM into well developed muscle. Avoid SC administration
Nalbuphine	Moderate to severe pain, obstetric analgesia, preoperative sedative, adjunct to anesthesia	*Adult:* 10 mg IM, SC, IV q3–4hr. Single dose not to exceed 20 mg. Total daily dose not to exceed 160 mg *or* 0.3–3 mg/kg over 10–15 min as adjunct to anesthesia	Coadministration with nonopioid analgesic may have additive effects and permit lower doses. Administer deep IM into well developed muscle.
Pentazocine	Severe pain, obstetric analgesia, preoperative sedative, adjunct to anesthesia	*Adult:* 50–100 mg po q3–4hr. Not to exceed 600 mg/day *or* 30 mg SC, IM, IV q3–4 hr as needed. Not to exceed 30 mg/dose IV or 60 mg/dose IM, SC. Not to exceed 360 mg/day SC, IM, IV	Patients requiring doses that exceed 100 mg should be switched to an opioid agonist. Patients taking concurrent MAO inhibitors should have the dosage of pentazocine reduced by 25–50% to minimize unpredictable adverse reactions. Pentazocine is not recommended for prolonged use or as first-line therapy for acute pain
Opioid Antagonists			
Naloxone	Opioid-induced CNS depression; management of refractory circulatory shock (unlabeled)	*Adult:* 0.4 mg IV, IM, SC. May be repeated every 2–3 minutes. Some patients may require up to 2 mg *Child:* 10 mcg/kg IV, IM, SC. May be repeated every 2–3 minutes. May be increased to 100 mcg (0.1 mg/kg)	IV route is preferred. May also be given by IV infusion at rate adjusted to patient response
Naltrexone	Management of opioid or alcohol dependence	*Adult:* Initial dose 25 mg po. May repeat 25-mg dose if no response. Maintenance: 50 mg po QD *or* 50 mg on weekdays and 100 mg on weekends *or* 100 mg q48hr *or* 150 mg q72hr *or* 100 mg on Monday and Wednesday and 150 mg on Friday	Patients must be opioid free for 7–10 days before starting naltrexone. Analyze urine for opioids and follow with naloxone challenge before administration of naltrexone. Assess patient for suicidal tendencies

GI, gastrointestinal; IM, intramuscular; IV, intravenous; MAO, monoamine oxidase; SC, subcutaneous.

Adverse Effects and Contraindications

Adverse effects of opioid agonist-antagonists are less common than reactions to true opioids. These drugs can precipitate withdrawal symptoms in patients who are physically dependent on a pure opioid. Common adverse effects include nausea, vomiting, light-headedness, sedation, and euphoria. Visual hallucinations, disorientation, dysphoria, and confusion can also occur. As with true opioids, respirations may be depressed with initial doses but do not worsen with increase in dosage. Insomnia and disturbed dreams can

TABLE 14–5 EQUIANALGESIA—DOSING DATA FOR OPIOID ANALGESICS

Drug	Approximate Equianalgesic Oral Dose	Approximate Equianalgesic Parenteral Dose
Opioid Agonist		
Morphine[2]	30 mg q3–4hr (around-the-clock dosing) 60 mg q3–4hr (single dose or intermittent dosing)	10 mg q3–4hr
Codeine[3]	130 mg q3–4hr	75 mg q3–4hr
Hydromorphone[2] (DILAUDID)	7.5 mg q3–4hr	1.5 mg q3–4hr
Hydrocodone (in LORCET, LORTAB, VICODIN, others)	30 mg q3–4hr	Not available
Levorphanol (LEVO-DROMORAN)	4 mg q6–8hr	2 mg q6–8hr
Meperidine (DEMEROL)	300 mg q3–4hr	100 mg q3hr
Methadone (DOLOPHINE, others)	20 mg q6–8hr	10 mg q6–8hr
Oxycodone (ROXICODONE, also in PERCOCET, PERCODAN, TYLOX, others)	30 mg q3–4hr	Not available
Oxymorphone[2] (NUMORPHAN)	Not available	1 mg q3–4hr
Opioid Agonist-Antagonist and Partial Agonist		
Buprenorphine (BUPRENEX)	Not available	0.3–0.4 mg q6–8hr
Butorphanol (STADOL)	Not available	2 mg q3–4hr
Nalbuphine (NUBAIN)	Not available	10 mg q3–4hr
Pentazocine (TALWIN, others)	150 mg q3–4hr	60 mg q3–4hr

Note: Published tables vary in the suggested doses that are equianalgesic to morphine. Clinical response is the criterion that must be applied for each patient; titration to clinical response is necessary. Because there is not complete cross tolerance among these drugs, it is usually necessary to use a lower than equianalgesic dose when changing drugs and to retitrate to response.

Caution: Recommended doses do not apply to patients with renal or hepatic insufficiency or other conditions affecting drug biotransformation and kinetics.

[1]Caution: Doses listed for patients with body weight less than 50 kg cannot be used as initial starting doses in babies less than 6 months of age. Consult the *Clinical Practice Guideline for Acute Pain Management: Operative or Medical Procedures and Trauma* section on management of pain in neonates for recommendations.

develop, especially with nalbuphine and pentazocine. Anticholinergic effects (e.g., dry mouth, blurred vision, constipation, and urinary retention) are common. Hypertension is especially problematic with nalbuphine. Hypersensitivity reactions to opioid agonist-antagonists is possible.

Parenteral use of pentazocine may lead to severe, potentially fatal reactions, including pulmonary emboli, vascular occlusion, ulceration, and abscess. Withdrawal symptoms in opioid-dependent patients can develop.

Pharmacokinetics

Absorption of opioid agonist-antagonists readily occurs with parenteral formulations. The drugs are distributed to most body tissues, including the placenta and breast milk. Some variation exists in the onset, peak, and duration of action of parenterally administered agents (see Table 14–2). With orally administered pentazocine, onset occurs 15 to 30 minutes, peaking in less than 1 to 1 ½ hours. It has a duration of action of 2 to 3 hours, with 60 percent of the drug bound to plasma proteins. Other agonists-antagonists vary in protein binding from less than 30 percent for nalbuphine to 96 percent for butorphanol and buprenorphine. Opioid agonists-antagonists are biotransformed in the liver and excreted in the urine. More than 10 percent of a butorphanol dose and a small amount of dezocine and pentazocine are eliminated via the gatrointestinal tract. The plasma half-life of these drugs varies from 2 to 13 hours.

Drug-Drug Interactions

Additive CNS depression may result when opioid agonists-antagonists are taken concurrently with other CNS depressants (see Table 14–3). Decreased effectiveness of a true opioid drug may occur in the presence of an opioid agonist-antagonist. Monoamine oxidase inhibitors used concurrently with opioid agonists-antagonists can result in unpredictable reactions including, but not limited to, increased CNS and respiratory depression and hypotension. Antihypertensive drugs and other drugs that lower blood pressure can exacerbate opioid-induced orthostatic hypotension.

Dosage Regimen

The dosage of opioid agonists-antagonists varies with the specific use and the route of administration (see Table 14–4). Patients receiving more than 100 mg of pentazocine should be switched to a true opioid. The initial dose of opioid agonists-antagonists may need to be reduced to 25 percent of the usual dose in the presence of monoamine oxidase inhibitors.

Laboratory Considerations

Agonist-antagonists can cause elevated serum amylase and lipase levels. Accurate determination of these levels may be unreliable for 24 hours in the presence of opioids.

Critical Thinking Process

Assessment

History of Present Illness

Patient self-report is the single most reliable indicator as to the existence and intensity of pain and any related psychological distress. As a rule, *pain is whatever the patient says*

Recommended Starting Dose (Adults More Than 50 kg Body Weight)		Recommended Starting Dose (Children and Adults Less Than 50 kg Body Weight)[1]	
Oral	Parenteral	Oral	Parenteral
30 mg q3–4hr	10 mg q3–4hr	0.3 mg/kg q3–4hr	0.1 mg/kg q3–4hr
60 mg q3–4hr	60 mg q2hr (intramuscular/subcutaneous)	1 mg/kg q3–4hr[4]	Not recommended
6 mg q3–4hr	1.5 mg q3–4hr	0.06 mg/kg q3–4hr	0.015 mg/kg q3–4hr
10 mg q3–4hr	Not available	0.2 mg/kg q3–4hr[4]	Not available
4 mg q6–8hr	2 mg q6–8hr	0.04 mg/kg q6–8hr	0.02 mg/kg q6–8hr
Not recommended	100 mg q3hr	Not recommended	0.75 mg/kg q2–3hr
20 mg q6–8hr	10 mg q6–8hr	0.2 mg/kg q6–8hr	0.1 mg/kg q6–8hr
10 mg q3–4hr	Not available	0.2 mg/kg q3–4hr[4]	Not available
Not available	1 mg q3–4hr	Not recommended	Not recommended
Not available	0.4 mg q6–8hr	Not available	0.004 mg/kg q6–8hr
Not available	2 mg q3–4hr	Not available	Not available
Not available	10 mg q3–4hr	Not available	0.1 mg/kg q3–4hr
50 mg q4–6hr	Not recommended	Not recommended	Not available

[2]For morphine, hydromorphone, and oxymorphone, rectal administration is an alternate route for patients unable to take oral medications, but equianalgesic doses may differ from oral and parenteral doses because of pharmacokinetic differences.

[3]Caution: Codeine doses above 65 mg often are not appropriate due to diminishing incremental analgesia with increasing doses but continually increasing constipation and other side effects.

[4]Caution: Doses of aspirin and acetaminophen in combination opioid/NSAID preparations must also be adjusted to the patient's body weight.

From the U.S. Department of Health and Human Services. (1992). *Clinical practice guidelines. Acute pain management: Operative or medical procedures and trauma* (AHCPR 92-0032). Rockville, MD: Author.

it is, existing whenever he or she says it does. Because pain is a subjective phenomenon that varies in intensity and severity, it is important that the location of the pain, onset, pattern (e.g., intermittent, continuous, or cyclical), intensity, character (e.g., sharp, dull, boring, aching, burning, or viselike), duration, and frequency of the pain be elicited. Determine how the pain affects activities of daily living. Elicit factors that precipitate, aggravate, and alleviate the patient's pain. Ask if the pain extends from where it started to other areas. Elicit information about what measures the patient has used to relieve the pain and their effectiveness.

Multiple pain complaints are common in patients with advanced disease and need to be prioritized and classified. It is imperative to clarify the patient's level of anxiety or depression and to obtain a history of previous psychiatric illness to define his or her psychological risk. Because each patient has his or her own understanding of the meaning of pain, it is useful to have the patient elaborate on this meaning. Does he or she think it represents recurrent tumor, as in the case of a patient with cancer? Is the patient convinced that it is simply arthritis? The more serious the nature of the pain diagnosis, the more likely its meaning may produce psychological distress.

Past Health History

Determine whether or not the patient has a past history or a family history of acute or chronic pain. Information on how the patient has handled previous painful events may provide insight into whether the patient is reluctant or afraid to take an opioid. Information about previously used methods of pain management that the patient has found either helpful or unhelpful should be elicited.

Physical Exam Findings

The interpretation of pain based on a patient's behavior is cumbersome because the amount of pain and responses to pain differ from person to person. Objective findings related to pain can be divided into three categories: sympathetic responses, parasympathetic responses, and behavioral responses. Although these responses are not diagnostic in and of themselves, they help provide clues to the cause of the pain. Sympathetic responses are associated with minimal to moderate pain intensity and include tachycardia, increased blood pressure and respirations, skeletal muscle tension, dilated pupils, and diaphoresis.

Parasympathetic responses are associated with intense, severe pain, or with deep pain. Objective manifestations include pallor, decreased blood pressure and heart rate, nausea and vomiting, weakness, prostration, and loss of consciousness.

Objective behavioral responses to pain include a guarded, rigid position. The patient's facial expression is drawn. The patient may cry, appear frightened, and appear restless. Moaning, sighing, grimacing, clenching of the jaws or fist, and withdrawal from others may be noted.

Diagnostic Testing

Patients usually voice an opinion about their pain level because objective measurement of pain is difficult. Although there are many pain assessment tools, three common self-report instruments are useful for adults and many children. Numeric rating scales, visual analog scales, and adjective rating scales can be used to assess pain intensity and affective distress (Fig. 14–3). These tools are easy to use and provide the patient and health care provider a way to quantify

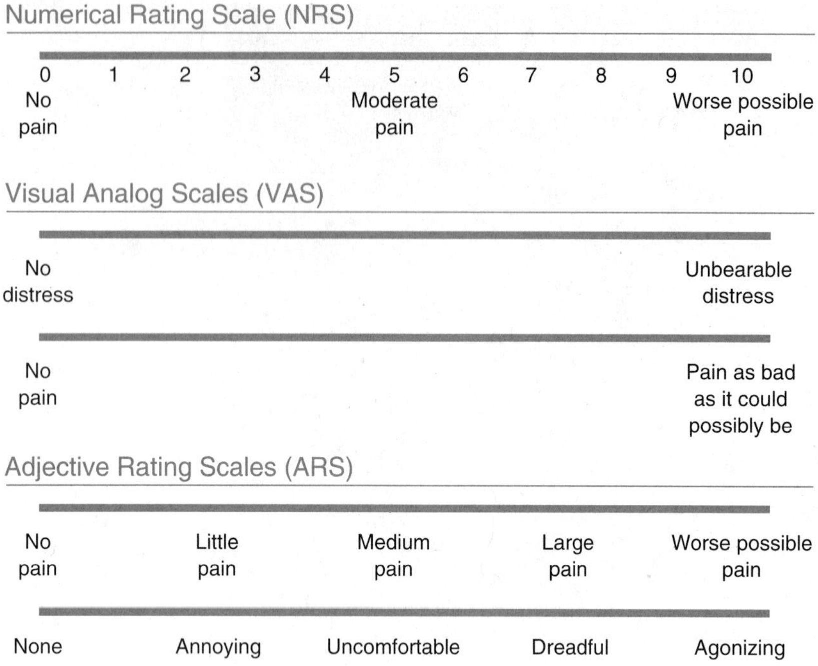

Numerical Rating Scale (NRS)

0 1 2 3 4 5 6 7 8 9 10

No pain | Moderate pain | Worse possible pain

Visual Analog Scales (VAS)

No distress | Unbearable distress

No pain | Pain as bad as it could possibly be

Adjective Rating Scales (ARS)

No pain | Little pain | Medium pain | Large pain | Worse possible pain

None | Annoying | Uncomfortable | Dreadful | Agonizing

Figure 14–3 Examples of pain assessment instruments. Numerical rating scales (NRS), visual analog scales (VAS), and adjective rating scales (ARS) can be used to assess pain intensity and affective distress. The tools quantify the pain. Visually impaired or confused patients may have difficulty using the scales.

the pain. These tools are considered valid and reliable for pain assessment as long as the end points and adjective descriptors are carefully identified. However, visually impaired or confused patients may have difficulty using the scales.

Developmental Considerations

Perinatal The gate-control theory has two important implications for childbirth. First, pain can be controlled by tactile stimulation, and second, that pain can be modified by activities that affect the CNS such as the use of back rubs, effleurage, suggestion, distraction, and physical conditioning.

Pain during the first stage of labor is, for the most part, related to dilation of the cervix. During the second stage of labor, pain is related to distention of the vagina and perineum, and pressure on adjacent structures. Uterine contractions and cervical dilatation as the placenta is expelled produce pain during the third stage of labor. The absence of crying or moaning during labor does not necessarily mean the woman is not in pain. On the other hand, crying or moaning does not necessarily mean that pain relief is desired.

Pediatric In general, pain assessment in children younger than 5 years of age is difficult to assess. Level of language development and comprehension; the confounding variables of anxiety, fear, or loneliness; the lack of a good understanding of pain phenomena; and the relative lack of valid and reliable pain assessment instruments contribute to the difficulty. Infants may cry and display muscular rigidity and thrashing behaviors. Preschoolers can be aggressive or verbally complain of discomfort. School-age children express pain verbally or behaviorally, often by displaying regression behaviors. Adolescents are often reluctant to admit that they are uncomfortable or need help.

Pain experiences of children are also influenced when the child observes the expression of pain in another child or their parent. Such observation can result in anxiety and negative social modeling that leads children to act much like the person in pain. In contrast, if the child views another child or adult coping well with the painful situation, pain expression and acting out behaviors can be reduced.

Geriatric Population studies have suggested that painful experiences occur two times more often in persons older than 60 years of age compared with younger individuals. Among institutionalized older adults, the prevalence may well be over 70 percent. Indeed, more than 80 percent of older adults suffer various forms of arthritis and most will have acute pain at some time during the course of their disease.

Pain assessment presents unique problems for older adults. Physiologic as well as psychological and cultural changes associated with aging cause pain to be perceived differently in this population. Institutionalized older adults are often stoic about pain. In addition, older adult patients often have altered presentations of common illnesses such as so-called silent myocardial infarctions and painless intra-abdominal emergencies.

The widespread belief that aging increases pain thresholds is a myth. Cognitive impairment, delirium (common among acutely ill frail older adults), and dementia represent serious barriers to pain assessment. Whether behavioral observations (agitation, restlessness, groaning) are sensitive and specific for pain assessment among the demented older adults remains uncertain. Also, visual, hearing, and motor impairments may impede the use of assessment instruments. Preliminary reports suggest that older adult patients with moderate to severe cognitive impairment are reliably able to report acute pain when it occurs or with prompting. Pain recall and integration of the pain experience over time may be less reliable, however.

Older adults, especially the frail and old-old (i.e., those older than 75), are at particular risk for both too much and too little pain management, although age-related responses are variable. Older adult patients experience a higher peak and longer duration of drug action than their younger coun-

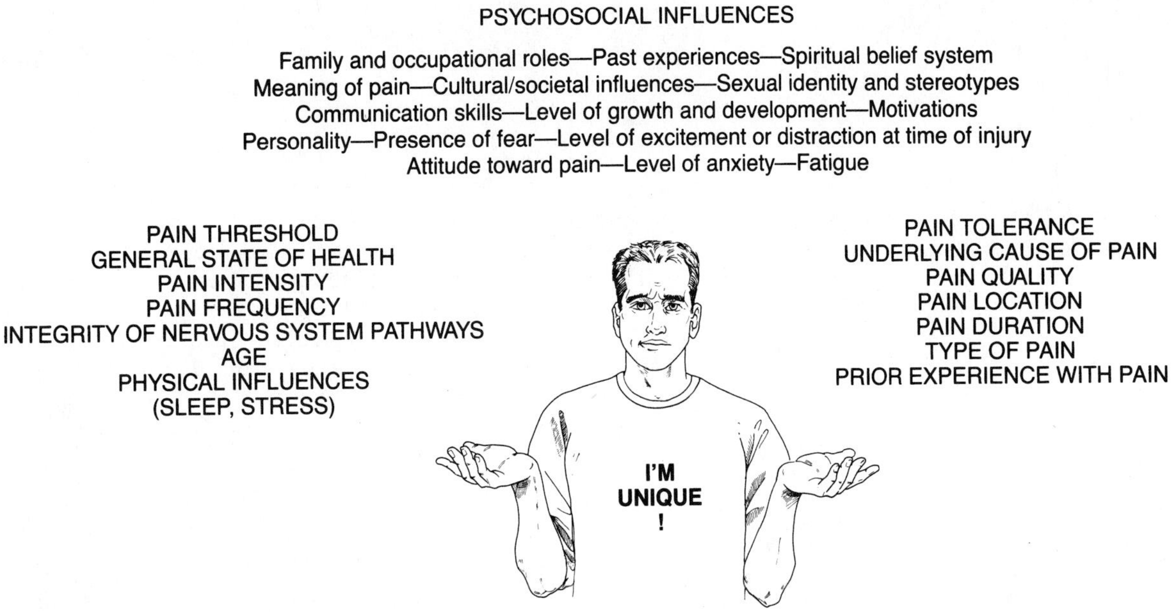

PSYCHOSOCIAL INFLUENCES

Family and occupational roles—Past experiences—Spiritual belief system
Meaning of pain—Cultural/societal influences—Sexual identity and stereotypes
Communication skills—Level of growth and development—Motivations
Personality—Presence of fear—Level of excitement or distraction at time of injury
Attitude toward pain—Level of anxiety—Fatigue

PAIN THRESHOLD
GENERAL STATE OF HEALTH
PAIN INTENSITY
PAIN FREQUENCY
INTEGRITY OF NERVOUS SYSTEM PATHWAYS
AGE
PHYSICAL INFLUENCES
(SLEEP, STRESS)

I'M
UNIQUE
!

PAIN TOLERANCE
UNDERLYING CAUSE OF PAIN
PAIN QUALITY
PAIN LOCATION
PAIN DURATION
TYPE OF PAIN
PRIOR EXPERIENCE WITH PAIN

Figure 14–4 Factors influencing responses to pain. (From Black, J.M., and Matassarin-Jacobs, E. [1997]. *Medical-surgical nursing: Clinical management for continuity of care* [5th ed., p. 363]. Philadelphia: W.B. Saunders. Used with permission.)

terparts. Age-related changes in drug distribution and elimination make the older adult more sensitive to sedation and respiratory distress.

Psychosocial Considerations

According to gate-control theory, emotional and psychological components of pain are intertwined with perceptual and reflex components. More important is the meaning of the pain. Pain perception and reactions are based heavily on expectations and learned responses. Some of these responses are culturally derived. Psychosocial factors influencing pain perception include anxiety, feelings of powerlessness, and ineffective coping mechanisms (Fig. 14–4). In addition to personality and other factors that cannot be changed (e.g., age and gender), variables that influence pain experiences include insomnia, fatigue, fear, anger, sadness, depression, mental isolation, introversion, and past experiences with pain. Factors that tend to increase pain thresholds include relief of symptoms, sleep, rest, empathy, diversion, elevation of mood, analgesics, antianxiety drugs, and antidepressants.

A particularly important factor influencing severe, chronic pain is its significance to the patient as an actual or potential loss, with associated losses of personal control and autonomy. Patients may deny severe pain for a variety of reasons, including fear of inadequate pain control or a perception that stoicism is expected or rewarded (see the Case Study—Postoperative Analgesia).

Analysis and Management

Treatment Objectives

Pain is one of the most distinctive of patient problems, one of the most troublesome to assess, and one of the most relentless to treat. This is because the total pain experience involves both the patient's perception of pain and its interpretation. However, the primary principle that applies to prevention and alleviation of pain is to remove the cause. Preventing anxiety, fear, and learned responses that augment pain and pain-related behaviors are also principles of pain management. Application of these principles in the primary treatment of pain management is directed at eliminating the pain as much and as quickly as possible using the least toxic, most effective drug, and one with the least amount of sedation. Never assume that pain is feigned by the patient.

Treatment Options

Once the underlying cause of pain has been identified and interventions do not or cannot alleviate the discomfort, pain management should begin promptly and aggressively. If the underlying cause cannot be identified, therapy should still be started but with an awareness of the patient's symptoms so as not to mask a diagnosis (e.g., abdominal pain associated with perforation of a gastric ulcer).

Pain management strategies are many and varied (Fig. 14–5). Cognitive-behavioral strategies include relaxation, distraction, imagery, and biofeedback. Physical agents such as massage or the application of heat and cold or transcutaneous electrical nerve stimulation are also effective for some patients. These strategies can be used alone or in alliance with systemic analgesics and other adjunctive drug measures.

Drug Variables

Management of mild to moderate pain should begin with nonsteroidal anti-inflammatory drugs (NSAIDs) unless otherwise contraindicated (see Chapter 15). NSAIDs decrease levels of inflammatory mediators that are generated at the site of injury. Although NSAIDs may be insufficient to control pain when used alone, they have profound dose-sparing effects and can be functional in reducing adverse effects of opioids. Furthermore, concurrent use of NSAIDs and opioids often provides more effective analgesia than either drug class used alone. Although it is plausible that NSAIDs also

Case Study Postoperative Analgesia

Patient History

History of Present Illness	AB is a 24-year-old female who was admitted to the surgical unit via the operating room and the postanesthesia care unit. She was in a motor vehicle accident and was sent to surgery from the ER for splenectomy and internal fixation of a compound fracture of the left leg. It is now 12 hours later, and AB is reporting that she is thirsty and feeling weak and "out of it" but states that her left side and leg hurt "somethin' awful." She has had three doses of 75 mg of meperidine IM since surgery, the last dose 3 hours ago, but without much relief. She refuses to cough or deep breathe, and is lying very still and rigid. She is becoming more irritable and communicates in yes or no answers only. She occasionally answers questions inappropriately. She also refuses to use the overhead trapeze due to pain from her incision and does not move unless someone turns her.
Past Health History	AB's records indicate she has a history of IV opioid drug abuse (crack) and hepatitis B since age 19 but has been drug free for the last 3 months. She has been in and out of drug abuse treatment programs since age 21. She admits to smoking 1 to 1½ packs of cigarettes a day for the past 8 years.
Physical Exam Findings	Temp 99.6°F, BP 140/92, pulse 128, respirations 28 and shallow. Urinary output over 50 mL/hr. Skin cool and clammy. Breath sounds clear to auscultation bilaterally. Abdominal and leg dressings are dry and intact.
Diagnostic Testing	CBC with differential and electrolytes WNL. Wound cultures negative. Pain assessment using numeric scale (1–10) indicates pain level of 9. AB reports her pain has been at this level since she came out of surgery.
Developmental Considerations	AB admits her sense of responsibility appropriate for this age has been lacking. She has been unable to maintain impulse control and has lacked the ability to implement realistic goals, to develop a career and has been unable to enter into mature, intimate relationships. Since she has been in a substance abuse program, she has been working on these age-appropriate behaviors.
Psychosocial Considerations	AB is reluctant to ask for pain medication, afraid that she will once again become "addicted" and that the nurses will think "bad" of her for asking. She admits to searching for the "meaning of life."
Economic Factors	AB recently returned to work after leaving a drug treatment program. She is not eligible for health insurance through her employer for another 3 months. A social worker has been contacted to explore financial alternatives with AB. It is anticipated that AB will be off work for approximately 3–4 months during rehabilitation.

Variables Influencing Decision

Treatment Objectives	• Prevention and alleviation of pain • Minimize anxiety, fear, and learned responses that may augment pain and pain-related behaviors

Drug Variables	*Drug Summary*	*Patient Variables*
Indications	Opioid analgesics are indicated for moderate to severe pain associated with trauma and postoperative states. Most any of the parenteral opioids would be acceptable for postoperative pain management. Drug selection, dose, route, and treatment regimen should be based on actual as well as anticipated pain. *Morphine* is the drug of choice for most patients. *Methadone* is a possibility for patients with a history of opioid abuse but offers no clinical advantages over morphine in pain management. Continued use of *meperidine* is also a possibility.	AB is recovering from splenectomy and internal fixation of compound fracture of her leg. She is afraid of once again becoming addicted to opioids but is reluctant to request pain medication.
Pharmacodynamics	Activation of mu opioid receptors inhibits adenyl cyclase activity leading to a reduction in intracellular cAMP. The fall in neuronal cAMP is believed to account entirely for the analgesic effect of the opioids.	There are no patient considerations that are directly related to pharmacodynamics, except that AB may have developed a tolerance to opioids owing to her history of opioid abuse. This may become a decision point.

Drug Variables	Drug Summary	Patient Variables
Adverse Effects/ Contraindications	Opioids depress CNS with the potential for respiratory depression. Appropriate dosing of opioid will minimize adverse effects and provide pain relief so patient can be more compliant with turning, coughing, and deep breathing. Methadone's most common adverse effect is sedation and confusion. The accumulation of the meperidine metabolite (normeperidine) causes effects that range from disphoria to irritable mood. These are decision points.	AB's respiratory rate is increased but shallow due to postoperative pain. Occasional inappropriate answers to questions may be due to hypoxia or drug metabolites. Appropriate pain management will provide adequate ventilation and foster mobility, and reduce likelihood of respiratory complications. This is a decision point.
Pharmacokinetics	The first-pass effect reduces the effectiveness of orally administered morphine. Morphine has high lipid solubility and, therefore, a more rapid onset of action. Meperidine metabolite is a CNS irritant that may account in part for AB's irritability.	AB's history of hepatitis may alter the first-pass effect of orally administered opioids. This will become a decision point.
Dosage Regimen	PRN dosing is possible but less effective in pain management than continuous administration that provides a more consistent serum drug level.	The ability of AB to control administration of pain medication promotes her sense of control and postoperative pain management.
Lab Considerations	AB has a history of hepatitis, which may cause increased biliary pressure and subsequent inaccurate readings for plasma lipase and amylase levels.	There are no direct patient considerations regarding laboratory testing at this time.
Cost Index*	Morphine sulfate Methadone Meperidine	Social Services department is working with patient on financial options. This is not a decision point at this time.

Summary of Decision Points

- AB is afraid of once again becoming addicted to opioids but is reluctant to request pain medication.
- AB's history of drug abuse should not deter use of pain management strategies for postoperative pain relief.
- AB's history of hepatitis may alter first-pass effect of orally administered opioids.
- PCA with morphine provides more constant and uniform analgesia, avoids first-pass effects in the liver, provides patient with a sense of control over her pain, reduces likelihood of overdose and respiratory depression, and may reduce CNS irritability secondary to meperidine metabolite.
- Appropriate pain management will foster adequate ventilation and foster mobility reducing likelihood of respiratory complications related to opioids.
- Adjunctive methods of pain management are also appropriate and can supplement opioid analgesia.

DRUGS TO BE USED

- Morphine sulfate per PCA 1 mg/hr with a lock out time of 6 minutes. Initial dose to be preceded by a bolus of 15 mg. Dosage to be titrated based on patient response. Duration of treatment approximately 72 hours then AB may be switched to a combination of NSAID and opioid oral preparation
- Adjunctive pain management strategies are to be used in conjunction with PCA

* Cost index: 1 = $ <30/mo
2 = $ 30–40/mo
3 = $ 40–50/mo
4 = $ 50–60/mo
5 = $ >60/mo

* AWP of 30 milliliters of 1 mg/mL morphine sulfate with glucose is approximately $20.

* AWP of 100-unit dose tablets of 10 mg methadone is approximately $35.

*AWP of 30 milliliters of 50 mg/mL meperidine is approximately $19.

cAMP, Cyclic adenosine monophosphate; PCA, patient-controlled analgesia; WNL, Within Normal Limits.

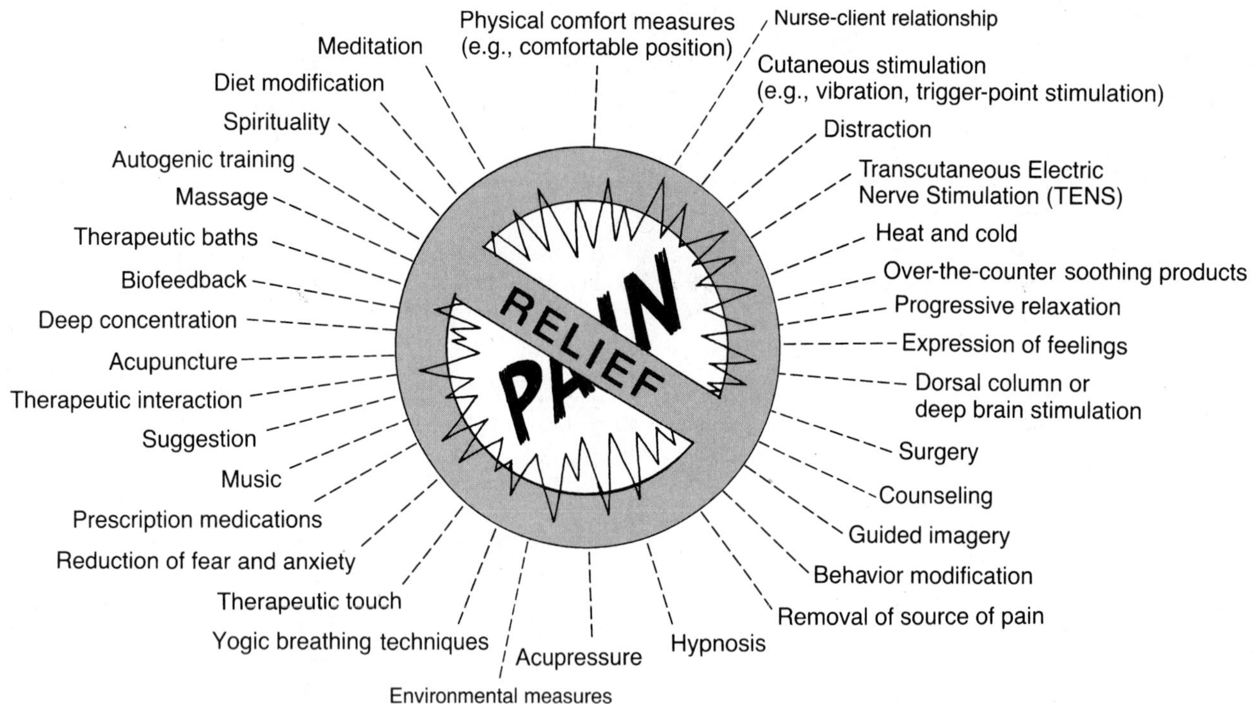

Figure 14–5 Pain management strategies. (From Black, J.M., and Matassarin-Jacobs, E. [1997]. *Medical-surgical nursing: Clinical management for continuity of care* (5th ed., p. 368]. Philadelphia: W.B. Saunders. Used with permission.)

act within the CNS in contrast to the opioids, they do not cause sedation or respiratory depression, nor do they interfere with bowel or bladder function.

Moderate to severe pain should be managed initially with an opioid. The requisites for rational opioid therapy includes several components. Knowledge of drug indications for acute and chronic pain, mechanism of action, the relationships between drug action and potentially serious adverse effects, the variability among patients with regard to pharmacokinetics, and the variability between patient and disease condition as it relates to the magnitude of effects are just a few. Drug selection, dose, route, and treatment regimen should be based also on anticipated pain. That is, drug therapy should correspond with the overall pain syndrome. Using the placebo-effect potentially present in all patients and reducing sensory input that aggravates pain provide the most effective and complete pain relief. Agonist-antagonists are not recommended for prolonged use or as first-line therapy for acute or cancer pain.

The health care provider can also take advantage of other drugs that may help reduce pain. For example, these include locally acting drugs such as capsaicin and adjunctive agents such as adrenergic agonists (e.g., clonidine), tricyclic antidepressants and selective serotonin reuptake inhibitors, carbamazepine, phenytoin, and hydroxyzine.

When opioids are used to relieve acute, severe pain associated with renal or biliary colic an antispasmodic drug (e.g., atropine) may be needed as well (see Chapter 13). Atropine, an anticholinergic drug, does not possess strong antispasmodic properties of its own. However, atropine apparently reduces the spasm-producing effects of opioid analgesics.

Morphine is the standard for opioid therapy. If it cannot be used because of hypersensitivity or an unusual reaction, another opioid such as hydromorphone can usually be substituted. There are no clinically apparent differences between hydromorphone and other opioids. Hydromorphone has an advantage over morphine in that it can be administered in smaller volumes of fluid because of its higher potency.

Meperidine should be reserved for brief treatment in patients who have demonstrated hypersensitivity or intolerance to morphine. The metabolite of meperidine is normeperidine, a cerebral irritant. Accumulation of normeperidine causes adverse effects ranging from dysphoria and irritable mood to seizures, even in young, otherwise healthy individuals.

Methadone may be an alternative to morphine for the patient with chronic pain if he or she is unable to tolerate morphine. It should be used only in patients who are allergic to all other opioids because it offers no clinical advantages over morphine for pain relief.

A fentanyl transdermal patch may be as effective as sustained-release morphine, but the dosage is more difficult to titrate. It has the advantage of a 72-hour dosing frequency but should be used only after the patient has been stabilized on a regularly dosed opioid. Fentanyl is seldom used for postoperative pain via IM or IV routes because of its short duration of action. It is, however, the drug of choice for epidural administration because it has a faster onset of action. Because of fentanyl's lipid solubility, it is easier to titrate than epidural morphine. Epidural fentanyl produces less respiratory depression, nausea and vomiting, and itching than does epidural morphine. Because of its longer duration of action, epidural morphine produces a greater incidence of late respiratory depression. Further, monitoring for up to 24 hours is necessary for patients who have received epidural morphine. This is in contrast to epidural fentanyl, in which monitoring is necessary for only about 4 hours.

Controversy

Administering Opioids to Chemically Dependent Patients

JONATHAN J. WOLFE

The World Health Organization (WHO) made pain management a priority among its programs for the 1990s. WHO studies make it clear that the needs of patients for diagnosis and treatment far exceed health care resources, particularly in the developing nations. This is particularly so for serious diseases such as cancer. However, WHO suggests that treatment of pain is a reasonable goal and one that can be achieved using inexpensive oral agents if opioid drugs form the mainstay.

In the United States, people affected by terminal diseases associated with unhealthy life-styles comprise a particularly hard-to-treat subgroup. Many patients suffering the severe deep abdominal pain associated with terminal autoimmune deficiency syndrome require pain relief that can be achieved only with opioids. However, these patients often have a long-standing history of substance abuse that includes intravenous injection of heroin and other opium derivatives.

Contemporary scholarship strongly suggests that patients in pain have almost no risk for developing opioid dependence. Such patients may paradoxically exhibit pseudoaddiction if health care providers use subtherapeutic doses of opioids. The central question revolves around the relative risk and benefit of using strong opioids (e.g., morphine, hydromorphone, and methadone) in people who have a history of drug dependence. Indeed, a patient who is actively dependent on drugs may have such severe pain that it is only relieved by opioid drugs.

The challenge facing the health care team is to decide whether an opioid constitutes effective therapy for a particular client. If it does, a plan must be devised to provide the patient with the opioid on a regular basis while minimizing the likelihood that dependence will re-emerge.

Critical Thinking Discussion

- Does the patient with a history of substance abuse have the same right to opioid therapy as the patient who has never become dependent?
- Does the patient with a history of substance abuse pose any special risk for renewed dependence during opioid therapy?
- Does the patient with a history of substance abuse pose any special risk to members of the health care team?
- What is the role of pain in preventing substance abuse?

It appears that butorphanol, buprenorphine, and nalbuphine cause less severe respiratory depression than morphine because they are partial agonists. However, if morphine (as with any other opioid) is properly titrated, there is little (if any) clinical difference between these drugs in regard to respiratory depression. Buprenorphine has a slightly longer duration of action than does morphine but is more expensive. These opioid agonist-antagonists originally appeared to have less abuse potential than true opioid agonists. However, butorphanol and pentazocine reportedly have contributed to dependence.

Determining the best route of opioid administration may be difficult. The administration route of choice for opioids is oral. The oral route is as effective as parenteral routes when the drug is used in appropriate doses. The oral route should be used if the patient tolerates oral intake. Oral formulations are also convenient and inexpensive. They are the mainstay of therapy for pain management in the ambulatory patient.

The parenteral route of choice for opioids is IV. It is suitable for titrated bolus or continuous administration, including use with patient-controlled analgesia (PCA). The disadvantage to an IV route is that it requires continual monitoring and there is a significant risk of respiratory depression with inappropriate dosing. PCA provides steady levels of analgesia and is popular with patients and nursing staff alike. It does require special infusion pumps and staff education to be effective.

IM injections have been the standard parenteral administration route in the past, but absorption is unreliable and the injections are painful. This route is generally avoided as much as possible. When a low-volume continuous infusion is needed and IV access is difficult or impossible, the SC route is preferable to IM. However, as with IM injections, SC injections are painful and absorption erratic. The SC route should be avoided when long-term repetitive dosing is needed.

Epidural and intrathecal administration routes are suitable in some circumstances and provide good analgesia. With these routes, there is a significant risk of respiratory depression. The respiratory depression is sometimes delayed in onset and requires careful monitoring, the use of infusion pumps, and a specially educated staff.

The time course to pain relief depends on the drug dose, blood level achieved, pain severity, and the patient's threshold for pain. Caution is warranted when selecting opioid dosages to be certain that excessive depression of the CNS and respiratory gas exchange is avoided.

Patient Variables

Placebos have little place in modern pain management as the sole treatment modality, albeit pain relief from placebos can frequently be equivalent to that produced by high doses of morphine. It should be noted that there is always a placebo effect for essentially all drugs, and that illness and illness behaviors provide some degree of secondary gain. A positive response to a placebo permits no diagnostic conclusion about the patient's pain. A response to placebo cannot be taken to mean that the patient is faking, that the patient's pain is not real, or that the patient is imagining some illness or symptom. Last, in most cases, patients usually tell the truth.

Relative potency estimates can be used to select the appropriate starting dose, to change the route of administration, or to change from one opioid to another. Equianalgesic doses and recommended starting doses for opioids are listed in Table 14–5. Opioid analgesia should be provided around-the-clock (ATC) or by continuous infusion rather than on an as-needed basis. It has been well established that a pro re nata (PRN) regimen is not effective for pain management and should be avoided. Further, a PRN order is not recommended because it requires the patient to communicate the presence of pain and the need for the drug. In addition, a PRN schedule promotes delays in drug administration and subsequent periods of inadequate pain relief. The best strategy that helps prevent progression of chronic pain syndrome is the appropriate and adequate treatment of acute pain.

Postoperative pain should be treated empirically because it, too, serves no useful purpose. The goal is to relieve pain without excessive sedation. Patients are better able to turn, cough, and deep breathe and implement other activities that promote recovery when they are comfortable. Postoperative pain management leads to earlier ambulation with decreased risk of deep vein thrombosis and pulmonary embolism.

Opioids should be used cautiously in patients with severe burns. A common cause of respiratory arrest in burned patients is excessive analgesia. Generally, agitation in a burned patient is interpreted as hypoxia, hypovolemia, or pain unless proved otherwise. When opioid analgesics are necessary, small IV doses should be given. Drugs given by other routes are absorbed erratically in the presence of shock and hypovolemia.

When opioids are needed for cancer pain, the primary consideration is patient comfort, not preventing drug dependency. Effective management requires that pain be relieved and prevented from recurring. With disease progression and the development of drug tolerance, larger doses and increased dosing frequency may be necessary.

Opioids are effective for the management of acute pain in most older adults. Cheyne-Stokes respirations are not unusual in the older adult during sleep. This respiratory pattern need not prompt discontinuance of an opioid unless it is associated with unacceptable levels of arterial oxygen desaturation (less than 85 percent).

Severe pain leads to intense emotional distress, and, therefore, drug therapy of the associated anxiety is frequently considered helpful (see Chapter 17). Benzodiazepines are often used for this purpose. Diazepam and lorazepam are usually the drugs of choice, providing effective antianxiety coverage over a long period. Coupled with mild amnestic effects, concurrent administration of a benzodiazepine may be beneficial in some patients. In other patients, particularly the older adult, benzodiazepines can cause distress and confusion. Special caution is in order when opioids are used with other CNS depressants or in patients who have emphysema, bronchial asthma, or any other limitations of respiratory gas exchange.

Nausea and vomiting can occur because of the action of opioids on brainstem centers. Changing the type of opioid used may stop the adverse effect, or the addition of an antiemetic drug may help. It is important to note, however, that nausea and vomiting decrease with use of analgesia. No patient should be denied pain relief because of this effect. Instead, they should simply receive treatment for the nausea and vomiting until it subsides.

Intervention

Administration

Patient-Controlled Analgesia Peaks and valleys in pain relief can be avoided by giving the drug in an ATC fashion. PCA permits intermittent self-administration of opioids. This management technique is useful for pain associated with surgery, sickle cell crises, and cancer, as well as for postoperative patient use. PCA operates under two modes: demand dosing with a fixed dose taken intermittently, or constant-rate infusion plus demand dosing.

The use of PCA begins with setting pump parameters. A loading dose is determined, along with the background infusion rate, dose to be administered per demand, the lockout interval (i.e., the minimum time between demand doses), and the maximum total dosage to be received over a specified time interval (e.g., a demand dose of 1 mg of morphine with a lockout time of 5 to 10 minutes). PCA provides constant and uniform analgesia by avoiding the potentially wide variations in serum drug levels associated with infrequent IM administration. In addition, PCA provides patients with a sense of control and, more often than not, results in less drug use than conventional IM administration. The potential addictive aspects of opioid infusions are negligible.

For the patient using PCA with morphine, 1 mg per bolus with a lockout time of 6 minutes is recommended. Some health care providers believe that 1 to 2 mg/hour permits a postoperative patient to sleep through the night. However, using a bolus with a baseline infusion may increase the amount of opioid used and adverse effects without improving pain relief. The patient should be reassessed every 1 to 2 hours, and if the pain is not well managed, the bolus dose should be increased by 25 to 50 percent. If pain relief from the bolus is adequate but the duration of pain relief is too short, the lockout time should be decreased.

For the patient using PCA with meperidine, a starting dose of 10 mg per bolus with a lockout time of 6 minutes is recommended. However, using a bolus along with a baseline infusion increases the risk of seizures. As with morphine via PCA, the patient receiving meperidine should be reassessed every 1 to 2 hours and the dosage adjusted 25 to 50 percent if pain is uncontrolled. Again, if pain relief from the bolus is adequate but duration of pain relief is too short, the lockout time should be reduced.

Rescue doses of opioids should be available for the patient with breakthrough pain or for children with poorly controlled pain who are receiving IV infusions. PCA should be considered for developmentally normal children 7 years of age and older. Request drug orders that permit the patient, child, or parent to refuse or omit the drug if they are asleep or not in pain. However, keep in mind that a steady-state drug level is necessary for a drug to be continuously effective. Interruption of an ATC schedule may cause resurgence of pain as blood levels of the drug decline.

To switch a patient to morphine from another orally administered opioid, the average daily requirement for the previous opioid should be determined and the 24-hour morphine equivalent identified. The daily morphine dosage is then divided by six, and the drug is administered every 4 hours. If the previous opioid dose was ineffective, the total daily dose of morphine can be increased by 25 to 50 percent. When titrating opioid doses, increases of 25 to 50 percent should be administered until there is either a 50-percent reduction in the patient's pain rating or the patient reports satisfactory pain relief.

Blood pressure, pulse, and respiratory rate should be assessed before and periodically during administration of an opioid. If the respiratory rate falls below 10 breaths per minute, the patients level of sedation should be assessed. Physical stimulation may be sufficient to prevent significant hypoventilation. The opioid dosage may need to be decreased by 25 to 50 percent if excessive sedation and hypoventilation develops. Initial drowsiness diminishes with continued use.

Treatment of Opioid Overdose

❒ Naloxone (NARCAN)

Naloxone is the opioid antagonist of choice when an antidote is required to reverse opioid-induced respiratory depression or coma. As a true opioid antagonist, naloxone is used to reverse CNS depression and respiratory depression due to suspected opioid overdose. It has also been used in the management of refractory circulatory shock, although it has not been approved by the Food and Drug Administration for such use.

Naloxone competitively blocks the effects of opioids including CNS and respiratory depression without producing agonist effects itself. Naloxone appears to have the highest affinity for mu (μ) receptors. As a true antagonist, naloxone has an affinity for opioid receptors but does not cause stimulation. Instead, they attach to the receptors preventing opioids, endorphins, and enkephalins from producing effects. It competitively displaces opioid already present and blocks further binding. The adverse effects of naloxone include nausea, vomiting, and occasionally, elevated blood pressure and tachycardia.

Naloxone is rapidly deactivated after oral administration owing to a significant first-pass effect in the liver. It is readily absorbed from IM and IV injection sites. Naloxone has an immediate onset of action, but the duration of action depends on the dose and route of administration. The plasma half-life of naloxone is 60 to 90 minutes with excretion via the kidneys.

True antagonists produce no significant drug-drug interactions. An opioid-dependent patient almost always experiences withdrawal symptoms if naloxone is given mixed with agonists-antagonists. The exception to this rule is nalbuphine. It can be administered before, together with, or just after administration of an opioid agonist without itself being antagonized.

When used in the treatment of overdose, a 0.4-mg ampule of naloxone is diluted in 10 ml of 0.9 percent sodium chloride. One-half milliliter (0.02 mg) of naloxone is administered by direct IV push, IM, or SC routes every 2 to 3 minutes. For patients with an overdose due to propoxyphene products, more than 0.4 mg may be used. For children and patients who weigh less than 40 kg, 0.1 mg of naloxone is diluted in 10 ml of 0.9-percent sodium chloride for a concentration of 10 mcg/mL. A dose of 0.5 mcg/kg is administered every 2 to 3 minutes.

Naloxone can also be given by continuous infusion with 2 mg of drug diluted in 500 mL, a concentration of four mcg/mL. Supplemental doses of IM or SC naloxone may be given to provide longer lasting effects. If no response occurs, the dosage may be increased to 100 mcg/kg. The dose should be titrated to avoid withdrawal, seizures, and severe pain. Patients who have been receiving opioids for longer than 1 week are remarkably sensitive to the effects of naloxone; hence, the drug should be diluted and carefully administered.

For opioid-dependent patients, withdrawal symptoms associated with naloxone develop within a few minutes to 2 hours. The severity of symptoms depends on the opioid involved, the dose of naloxone, and the degree of physical dependence. Lack of significant response suggests that symptoms may be due to a disease process or to other nonopioid CNS depressant not affected by naloxone.

❒ Naltrexone

Naltrexone, another opioid antagonist, is approved only for patients who are dependent on opioids. Unlabeled uses for naltrexone include the management of eating disorders and treatment of postconcussion syndrome. Naltrexone produces withdrawal symptoms but prevents the euphoria associated with opioid use. It does not, however, reduce the craving for the drug. Thus, treatment is less successful overall to manage opioid dependence than methadone therapy. Methadone eliminates craving for opioids while blocking euphoric effects. Naltrexone competitively inhibits the effects of opioids by binding at the opioid receptor sites.

Naltrexone is a pure antagonist with no agonist action, although it has numerous adverse effects. The major adverse effect is its ability to precipitate withdrawal symptoms. Edema, hypertension, palpitations, phlebitis, and shortness of breath have been noted. Anxiety, depression, disorientation, dizziness, headache, and nervousness illustrate the CNS adverse effects. Gastrointestinal effects such as anorexia, nausea, vomiting, diarrhea or constipation, and thirst are possible. There may be changes in libido, delayed ejaculation, and urinary frequency. Because of these numerous adverse effects naltrexone is used less often than naloxone.

Naltrexone can cause other effects, too, including dose-dependent hepatocellular damage. Thus, it should be used with caution in patients with acute hepatitis or liver failure. It is contraindicated in patients in acute opioid withdrawal and should be used with caution in patients younger than 18 years of age, and in pregnant or nursing women.

Absorption of naltrexone is rapid when taken by mouth, but like naloxone, it undergoes significant first-pass effects. About 5 percent of the drug actually reaches systemic circulation. Onset of naltrexone drug action occurs 20 to 30 minutes after administration with peak concentrations for both naltrexone and its metabolite (6-beta-naltrexol) reached in 1 hour. Its duration of action is dose dependent. In general, a 5-mg dose of naltrexone blocks the effects of 25 mg of IV opioid (e.g., heroin) for up to 24 hours. A 100- to 150-mg dose produces antagonistic effects for 48 to 72 hours. Elimination half-life of the parent drug is about 4 hours, and the elimination half-life of the metabolite is approximately 13 hours. Excretion is via the kidneys. A small portion of naltrexone is eliminated in the stool.

Candidates for therapy must be detoxified before using naltrexone. The usual adult dose of naltrexone is 25 mg orally, with an additional 25 mg given 1 hour later if no signs of drug withdrawal are present. Fifty to one hundred and fifty milligrams per day can be given per day depending on patient need.

Education

Patients should be taught to take their opioid as directed. Although this principle applies to all drugs, it is particularly important with analgesics because of potentially serious adverse effects and because analgesics may mask or enable the patient to tolerate pain for which medical attention would otherwise be required. Patients should be advised not to take any leftover medication for other disorders and not to let anyone else take their prescription.

Patients should be taught to avoid concurrent use of alcohol or other CNS depressants without first checking with the health care provider. It is suggested that patients not keep their analgesics at the bedside to prevent inadvertent overdose. They should be told not to smoke when taking an opioid because smoking when they are less alert is unsafe and it also reduces the effectiveness of opioids.

Many patients report an allergy to codeine because of a history of nausea. Instruct the patient to take the opioid analgesic with small amounts of food to reduce the potential for nausea. All patients should be advised to change positions slowly to minimize the potential for orthostatic hypotension, particularly if they are also taking antihypertensive drugs or diuretics. Hospitalized patients should be taught the reasons for raising the side rails on the bed after they have received an opioid. Side rails promote safety by serving as a reminder to stay in bed or to call for assistance.

Constipation can be prevented or at least minimized by consuming high-fiber foods, such as whole grain cereals, fruits, and vegetables; drinking 2 to 3 quarts of fluids daily, and remaining as active as possible. A bowel program should be instituted for patients receiving an opioid for longer than 24 hours. Assess bowel sounds on a regular basis. A stool softener such as ducosate sodium may be taken daily. Bulk-forming drugs such as psyllium hydrophilic muciloid (see Chapter 43) are effective for most patients, as long as adequate hydration is maintained. It is better to prevent constipation than to begin treatment after it develops.

Patients who are provided with instruction related to physiologic coping (instruction on turning, coughing, deep breathing, and ambulation) during the preoperative period reported less pain, used fewer analgesics, and had shorter lengths of stay than patients who did not receive instruction. Patients provided with procedural and sensory information as well as instructions related to physiologic coping also tended to use fewer analgesics.

Evaluation

Evaluation of the therapeutic effectiveness of opioids depends in part on the reason for use. Patients may provide a verbal statement of pain relief, demonstrate decreased behavioral manifestations of pain or discomfort, and demonstrate increased participation in the usual activities of daily living. There may be a decrease in blood pressure and pulse rate, slower and deeper respirations. The frequency of pain evaluation should be based on the knowledge of how quickly the drug works.

Psychological effects of unmanaged or undermanaged pain include fear, helplessness, anxiety, anger, and frustration. Physiologic effects include decreased thoracic movement; the normal sigh (yawn) is abolished; and there is increased splinting, reduced lung compliance, reduced lung volumes, and reduced lung capacities that may lead to atelectasis. There is often decreased mobility and an increased risk of thromboembolism. Untreated or undermanaged pain exaggerates the catecholamine response and is manifested as increased systemic vascular resistance, increased myocardial oxygen demand, and the potential for arrhythmias and hypertension. It also delays return of bowel and gastric functioning.

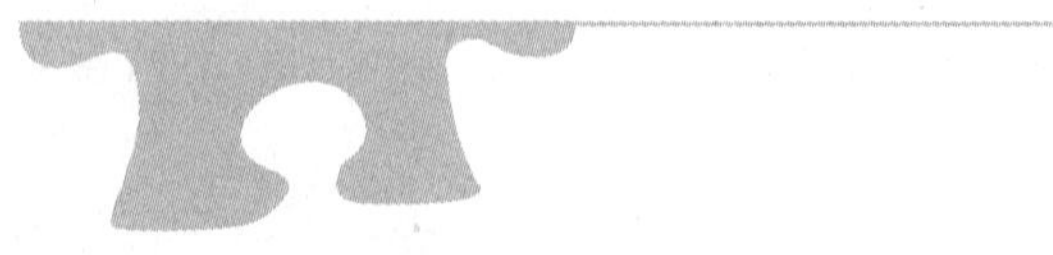

SUMMARY

- Pain is one of the most distinctive of patient problems, one of the most troublesome to assess, and one of the most relentless to treat.
- Pain is whatever the patient says it is, existing whenever he or she says it does.
- The prevalence of pain is two times greater in persons over the age of 60 compared with younger individuals. Among institutionalized older adults, the prevalence may well be over 70 percent.
- Pain perception is activated by pain-specific receptors (nociceptors) in peripheral tissues.
- Acute pain is short term, generally lasting only for the duration of tissue damage. Chronic pain is pain that lasts longer than 6 months.
- Somatic pain originates in cutaneous tissues and is well defined, localized, and of low to moderate intensity.
- Deep pain originates in bone, nerves, muscles, blood vessels, and other supporting tissues of the abdominal or thoracic regions, producing a dull, aching sensation that is hard to localize.
- Visceral pain arises from body organs. Because there are few nociceptors in body organs, pain sensations are diffuse and poorly localized.
- Neuropathic pain is related to injury or damage to nerve fibers in the periphery or damage to the CNS.
- Psychological effects of pain include fear, helplessness, anxiety, anger, and frustration.
- Physiologic effects of pain include decreased thoracic movement; the normal sigh (yawn) is abolished; and there is increased splinting, reduced lung compliance, lung volumes, and capacities that may lead to atelectasis.
- The primary treatment objective in pain management is to eliminate the pain as much and as quickly as possible using the least toxic, most effective drug, and one with the least amount of sedation.
- Effective pain management also results in earlier mobilization, shortened hospital stay, reduced cost, and improved quality of life.
- Pain management strategies and options include cognitive-behavioral strategies and physical agents.
- Management of mild to moderate pain should begin with nonsteroidal anti-inflammatory drugs (NSAIDs) unless otherwise contraindicated.
- Moderate to severe pain should be managed initially with an opioid.
- Other drugs that may help reduce pain are capsaicin, caffeine, amphetamines, adrenergic agonists, tricyclic antidepressants, carbamazepine, phenytoin, and hydroxyzine.
- Peaks and valleys in pain relief can be avoided by giving the drug on an ATC basis.
- For the patient switching to morphine from another opioid, the average daily requirement for the previous opioid should be determined and the 24-hour morphine equivalent identified before changing the drug.
- Blood pressure, pulse, and respiratory rate should be assessed before and periodically during administration of an opioid, opioid antagonist, or opioid agonist-antagonist.
- Naloxone is the antagonist of choice if an antidote is required to reverse opioid-induced respiratory depression or coma.
- Patients should be taught to take their opioid as directed because of potentially serious adverse effects and because analgesics may mask or enable the patient to tolerate pain for which medical attention is required.
- Patients should be taught to avoid alcohol and other CNS depressant drugs without first checking with the health care provider.
- Hospitalized patients should be taught the reasons for raising the side rails on the bed, to call for assistance when ambulating,

and to change positions slowly to minimize the potential for orthostatic hypotension.

- Pain relief may be assessed through verbal statements of pain relief, decreased behavioral manifestations of pain or discomfort, and increased participation in the usual activities of daily living.

BIBLIOGRAPHY

Acute Pain Management Guideline Panel. (1992). *Acute pain management: Operative or medical procedures and trauma.* AHCPR Publications No. 92-0032. Rockville, MD: Agency for Health Care Policy and Research, Public Health Service, U.S. Department of Health and Human Services.

Acute Pain Management Guideline Panel. (1992). *Acute pain management in Adults: Operative procedures. Quick reference guide for clinicians.* AHCPR Publications No. 92-0019. Rockville, MD: Agency for Health Care Policy and Research, Public Health Service, U.S. Department of Health and Human Services.

Acute Pain Management Guideline Panel. (1992). *Pain control after surgery: A patient's guide.* AHCPR Publications No. 92-0021. Rockville, MD: Agency for Health Care Policy and Research, Public Health Service, U.S. Department of Health and Human Services.

Acute Pain Management Guideline Panel. (1992). *Acute pain management in infants, children, and adolescents: Operative and medical procedures. Quick reference guide for clinicians.* AHCPR Publication No. 92-0020. Rockville, MD: Agency for Health Care Policy and Research, Public Health Service, U.S. Department of Health and Human Services.

American Pain Society. (1992). *Principles of analgesic use in the treatment of acute and cancer pain* (3rd ed.). Skokie, IL: Author.

American Pain Society. (1990). Recommendations of the American Pain Society on the principles of analgesic use in the treatment of acute and chronic cancer pain. *Clinical Pharmacology,* 9, 601–611.

American Society of Post Anesthesia Nurses. (1992). *Standards of nursing practice.* Richmond, VA: The Society.

Bonica, J. (Ed.) (1990). *The management of pain* (Vols. 1 and 2, 2nd ed.). Philadelphia: Lea & Febiger.

Bonica, J. (1980). *Pain.* New York: Raven Press.

Carr, E. (1990). Postoperative pain: Patients' expectations. *Journal of Advanced Nursing,* 15, 89–100.

Edgar, I., and Smith-Hanrahan, C. (1992). Nonpharmacological pain management. In J. Watt-Watson and M. Donovan (Eds.), *Pain management: Nursing perspective.* St. Louis: C.V. Mosby.

Gaston-Johansson, F., Albert, M., Fagan, E., et al. (1990). Similarities in pain descriptions of four different ethnic-culture groups. *Journal of Pain and Symptom Management,* 5(2), 94–100.

Gilman, A., Rall, T., Nies, A., et al. (Eds.). (1990). *Goodman and Gilman's The pharmacologic basis of therapeutics* (8th ed.) New York: Pergamon Press.

International Association for the Study of Pain. (1986). Pain terms: A current list with definitions and notes on usage. *Pain,* 3, S216–221.

Katz, J., and Melzack, R. (1990). Pain "memories" in phantom limbs: Review and clinical observations. *Pain,* 43, 319–336.

Management of Cancer Pain Guideline Panel. (1994). Management of cancer pain: Clinical practice guideline. AHCPR Publications No. 94-0592. Rockville, MD: Agency for Health Care Policy and Research, Public Health Service, U.S. Department of Health and Human Services.

McCaffery, M. (1994). Ensuring pain relief. *Nursing,* 24(9), 81–82.

McCaffery, M. (1994). How to use the new AHCPR cancer pain guidelines. *American Journal of Nursing,* 94(7), 42–47.

McCaffery, M., and Ferrell, B. (1994). Nurses' assessment of pain intensity and choice of analgesic dose. *Contemporary Nurse,* 3(2), 68–74.

McCaffery, M., and Ferrell, B. (1991). Patient age: Does it affect your pain-control decisions? *Nursing,* 21(9), 44–48.

McCarty, D., and Koopman, W. (Ed.). (1993). *Arthritis and allied conditions.* Philadelphia: Lea & Febiger.

McCormack, J., Brown, G., Levine, M., et al. (Eds.). (1996). *Drug therapy: Decision making guide.* Philadelphia: W.B. Saunders Company.

McGuire, L. (1995). Controlling phantom limb pain. *Nursing,* 25(2), 6.

McGuire, L. (1992). Comprehensive and multidimensional assessment and measurement of pain. *Journal of Pain and Symptom Management,* 7(5), 312–319.

Meinhart, N., and McCaffery, M. (1983). *Pain: A nursing approach to assessment and analysis.* Norwalk, CT: Appleton-Century-Crofts.

Melzak, R. (1987). The short form McGill pain questionnaire. *Pain,* 30, 191–197.

Melzak, R., and Wall, P. (1983). *The challenge of pain.* New York: Basic Books.

Melzak, R., and Wall, P. (1992). *The puzzle of pain.* New York: Basic Books.

Melzak, R., and Wall, P. (1965). Pain mechanisms: A new theory. *Science,* 150, 971–979.

Nash, R., Edwards, H., and Nebauer, M. (1993). Effect of attitudes, subjective norms and perceived control on nurses' intention to assess patients' pain. *Journal of Advanced Nursing,* 18(6), 941–947.

Olinski, N. (1994). Commentary on *Caveat emptor:* A critical analysis of the costs of drugs used in pain management. *AACN Nursing Scan in Critical Care,* 4(2), 24.

Pasero, C. (1994). Help for chronic pain sufferers. *American Journal of Nursing,* 94(10), 22–24.

Patterson, J. (1994). The nurse's role in pain management. *Today's OR Nurse,* 16(6), 57–58.

Payne, R. (1992). Transdermal fentanyl: Suggested recommendations for clinical use. *Journal of Pain and Symptom Management,* 7, 540–544.

Pleuvry, B., and Lauretti, G. (1996). Biochemical aspects of chronic pain and its relationship to treatment. *Pharmacologic Therapeutics,* 71, 313–324.

Reidenberg, M., and Portenoy, R. (1994). The need for an open mind about the treatment of chronic malignant pain. *Clinical Pharmacology & Therapy,* 55, 367–369.

Reilly, R. (1994). 12 steps to managing chronic pain: Chronic Pain Anonymous. *Patient Care,* 28(12), 117–121.

Schumacher, H. (Ed.). (1993). *Primer on the rheumatic diseases* (10th ed.). Atlanta: Arthritis Foundation.

Sullivan, L. (1994). Factors influencing pain management: A nursing perspective. *Journal of Post Anesthesia Nursing,* 9(2), 83–90.

Wall, P., and Melzack, R. (Eds.). (1989). *Textbook of pain* (2nd ed.). New York: Churchill Livingstone.

World Health Organization. (1990). *Cancer pain relief.* Geneva: Author.

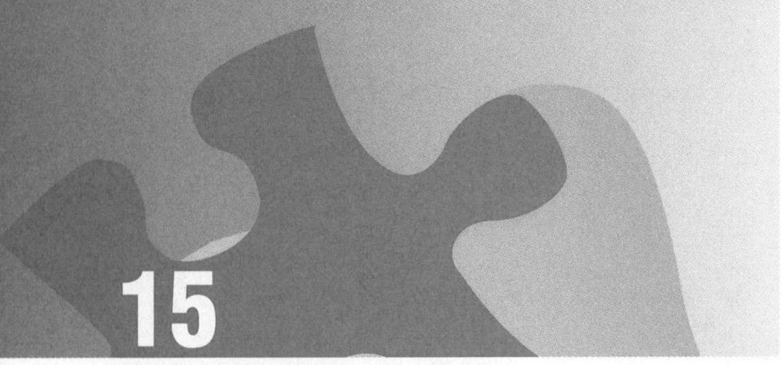

Nonsteroidal Anti-Inflammatory, Disease-Modifying Antirheumatic, and Related Drugs

Inflammation, pain, and fever are common manifestations of many conditions. Nonopioid analgesic, antipyretic, anti-inflammatory and related drugs relieve inflammation, pain, and fever. The two most important drug classes are the nonsteroidal anti-inflammatory drugs (NSAIDs), the prototype of which is aspirin; and the adrenal glucocorticosteroid hormones, the prototype of which is hydrocortisone (i.e., cortisol). Although not an anti-inflammatory drug by makeup, acetaminophen is included in this chapter because of its extensive use as an analgesic and antipyretic. Other groups of drugs discussed in this chapter are used for the prevention and treatment of gout. The drugs discussed in this chapter relieve symptoms and contribute to a patient's comfort and quality of life; they do not cure the underlying disorder producing the symptoms. To understand the actions of these drugs, an understanding of inflammation, pain, and fever is needed.

PATHOGENESIS OF INFLAMMATION

Inflammation and infection often co-exist. As a result, the two terms are often confused. Under normal circumstances, infection is always accompanied by inflammation. However, not all inflammation involves an infectious organism. Inflammation is not a pathophysiologic mechanism. However, whenever cells or body tissues are injured or killed, there is a striking, but nonspecific, response by adjacent tissues. The body uses inflammation to limit the extent and severity of injury. The inflammatory process promotes removal of dead cells, microorganisms, debris, and exudate. The response can be triggered by chemicals, heat, trauma, immune complexes, microorganisms, foreign bodies, surgery, and ionizing radiation.

Types of Inflammation

There are two broad categories of inflammation: simple acute inflammation and chronic inflammation. The *simple acute* type results in the typical signs of inflammation: pain, redness, warmth, and swelling. It is an immediate response to stressors. This type of inflammation usually resolves entirely in 8 to 10 days if no complications interfere with healing. Simple acute inflammation sometimes develops into the chronic form. *Chronic inflammation* involves the same signs as acute simple inflammation, but they are relentless and damaging, lasting weeks, months, or years.

Acute Inflammation

Chemical Response

The inflammatory response is similar regardless of cause (Fig. 15–1). Events in the process include chemical responses, vascular responses, and cellular responses. Chemical mediators are released by activated granulocytes, lymphocytes, and macrophages. The chemicals include histamine, prostaglandins (PGs), leukotrienes (LTs), cytokines, oxygen radicals, and enzymes. Histamine is the first chemical released in an inflammatory response. Histamine is widely distributed throughout the body. It is released in large amounts from mast cells and basophils during degranulation. Histamine's actions are mediated by histamine-1 (H_1) receptors. Histamine release produces venous vasodilation. If the area of vasodilation is near the body surface, there is a reddened appearance to the skin. As proteins leak through capillary walls into interstitial tissues, colloidal osmotic pressure rises and edema results. The chemicals released and the pressure of the fluid and cellular exudate on nerve endings contribute to pain. Histamine release also causes increased mucus production and bronchial constriction.

PGs contribute to vasodilation and increased vascular permeability. It is thought that PGs are responsible for the pain associated with inflammation. PGs are a group of phospholipid compounds, metabolites of arachidonic acid (Fig. 15–2). The long-chain hydroxy fatty acids stimulate a number of activities within the body (e.g., uterine and other smooth muscle contraction, lowering of blood pressure, regulation of gastric acid secretion and body temperature, platelet aggregation, and control of inflammation and vascular permeability). The PG formed depends on the specific tissue environment.

PGs arise from the cyclooxygenase (COX) metabolic pathway. There are nine types of PGs designated by the letters A to I. The degree of saturation of the side chain of each is designated by the subscript 1, 2, or 3. PgE_2, PgF_2, PgI_2 and thromboxane A_2 (TXA_2) are transiently present at the site of injury, but are nonetheless extraordinarily potent. In general, PgEs contribute to vasodilation, pain, and edema. PGs produce more erythema than histamine, and evidence suggests that PgE_2 sensitizes pain receptors to bradykinin. Aspirin and other NSAIDs block the synthesis of PGs, thereby inhibiting inflammation. The functions of other arachidonic acid metabolites are listed in Table 15–1.

Like PGs, LTs (slow-reacting substances of anaphylaxis) are mediators synthesized by mast cells. LTs are generated along the lipoxygenase pathway. This pathway generates LTA_4, LTB_4, LTC_4, LTD_4, and LTE_4. These LTs are acidic, sulfur-containing lipids that produce effects much like those of histamine, primarily smooth muscle contraction, increased vascular permeability, and neutrophil and eosinophil chemotaxis. LTB_4 is a potent chemotactic agent that causes aggregation of granulocytes. They also alter pul-

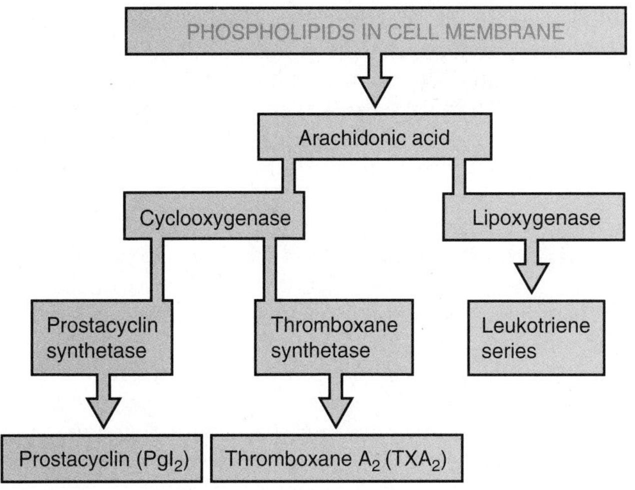

Figure 15–1 Sequence of events found with simple acute inflammation.

monary physiology. LTs are thought to be important in the later stages of the inflammatory response because they produce slower and more prolonged responses than do histamines.

Enzymes, oxidizing agents, and other metabolites from the arachidonic pathway attack lipoproteins, causing cell destruction and digestion. Neutrophils and macrophages specialize in degradation of collagen and intercellular matrix. Peptide bonds in the matrix are broken down by the enzymes collagenase, elastase, proteinase, and gelatinase.

Oxygen radicals are the most destructive of all cell enzymes or toxins. Oxidizing radicals include hydroxyl ions (OH^-), superoxide (O_2^-), and hydrogen peroxide (H_2O_2). They are formed as the result of an enzyme system present on neutrophil plasma membranes. With these oxidizing agents, neutrophils are capable of synthesizing and attacking microorganisms and increasing vascular permeability.

Vascular Response

Capillary vasoconstriction lasts from 2 seconds to 5 or 10 minutes in acute simple inflammation. The vasoconstriction produces tissue hypoxia and acidosis. The amount of vasoconstriction depends on the extent of vascular injury. Fol-

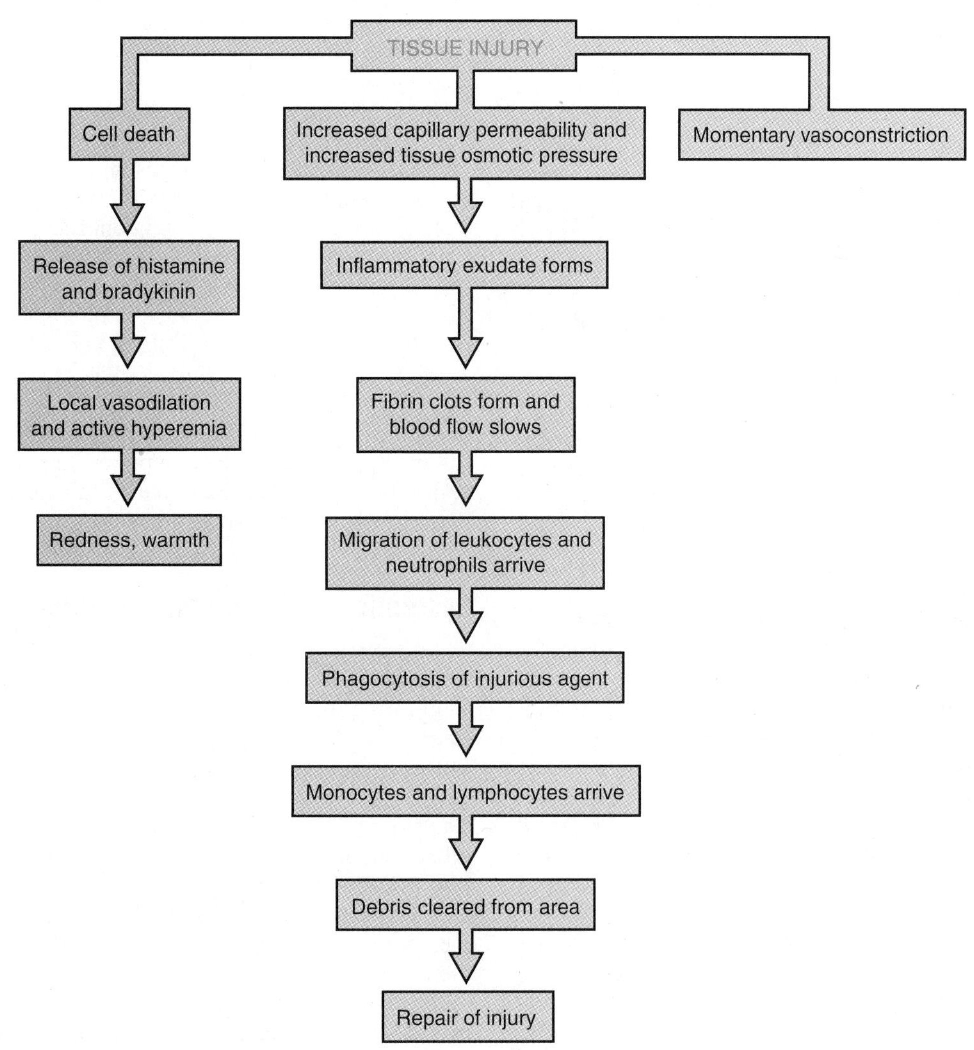

Figure 15–2 Simplified representation of the sequence of events in the synthesis of prostaglandins and leukotrienes from arachidonic acid.

TABLE 15–1 FUNCTIONS OF ARACHIDONIC ACID BYPRODUCTS

Byproduct	Functions and Effects
PgD_2	Bronchoconstriction
PgE_1, PgE_2	Hyperalgesia (along with bradykinin and histamine) Increases permeability of vasculature (along with bradykinin and histamine) Vasodilation Increases activity of gastrointestinal smooth muscle
PgI_2	Vasodilation Bronchodilation Inhibits platelet aggregation
PgD_2	Platelet aggregation and brain function
$PgF_{2\alpha}$	Increases uterine contraction Bronchoconstriction
TXA_2	Platelet aggregation Vasoconstriction Bronchodilation
LTB_4	Chemotaxis
LTC_4, LTD_4, LTE_4*	Bronchoconstriction Vasodilation

*LTC_4, LTD_4, LTE_4 make up the slow reacting substances of anaphylaxis.

lowing vasoconstriction there is a period of arteriolar vasodilation. The increased blood volume raises hydrostatic pressure within vessels. Increased pressure causes fluid to move into surrounding tissues contributing to edema.

Platelets move to the site of injury adhering to exposed vascular collagen. The intrinsic clotting cascade is stimulated, and a fibrin meshwork forms. The platelets release a number of growth factors and the fibrin clot forms within several minutes. At the same time, the remaining blood becomes thick and circulation slows.

At the same time, venous capillaries become more permeable allowing more fluid to leak into surrounding tissues. Fibrin is deposited in lymphatic channels, causing blockage of the system. The lymphatic blockage localizes the area of inflammation from the surrounding tissues and delays the spread of toxins.

Cellular Response

Neutrophils migrate through vascular endothelium (i.e., margination) into tissues by a process called *chemotaxis.* Neutrophils are lured to the area by bacterial toxins, degenerative products of inflammation, the C_{5a} complement fragment, and other substances. Neutrophils begin phagocytosis by producing collagenase which breaks down dead tissue. At the same time, they liberate endogenous pyrogens (fever-causing substances) that travel to the temperature-regulating center in the hypothalamus. Fever results, vessels dilate, more blood reaches the periphery, the patient sweats, and body temperature is returned to a normal range.

However, during febrile states, biochemical messengers are released from macrophages in the hypothalamus and the thermostatic mechanism is adjusted to a higher set point. The messengers are both endogenous and exogenous. The major endogenous pyrogen is interleukin-1 (IL-1). There are 14 known interleukins. IL-1 is a cytokine released by almost all nucleated cells. It activates growth and function of neutrophils, lymphocytes, and macrophages, and promotes the release of additional mediators that influence immune response. IL-6 and tumor necrosis factor (TNF) are also endogenous pyrogens. IL-6 is produced by many cell types including phagocytes. It mediates the acute phase response, enhances B-cell production and differentiation to antibodies, and stimulates megakaryocyte production. TNFs are released primarily by macrophages and T cells to help regulate immune response. TNF's actions are almost identical to those of IL-1. TNF and IL-1 are involved in fever production and other systemic effects of inflammation.

Known exogenous pyrogens include microorganisms and their endotoxins, certain drugs (e.g., bleomycin and colchicine), and a few steroids. Bacterial endotoxins cause release of PGs and endogenous pyrogens from neutrophils. Other arachidonic acid metabolites may also be involved in the production of fever. The reason aspirin does not reduce body temperature in patients without a fever is because no pyrogen is present to stimulate PG synthesis.

Chronic Inflammation

Chronic inflammation is self-perpetuating. It may persist for weeks, months, or even years, developing as a result of a recurrent or progressive acute inflammatory process. It may evolve also because of a low-grade smoldering response that fails to evoke an acute response.

Little is known about the mediators of chronic inflammation. However, macrophage dominance and the appearance of fibroblasts and lymphocytes signal the beginning of a chronic cellular response. Macrophages are necessary for wound healing because of their phagocytosis and débridement functions. The macrophages produce a variety of chemical mediators. Proteases help remove foreign protein from the site of injury. Tissue thromboplastin from the macrophages facilitate hemostasis and stimulate fibroblast activity necessary for healing. Because chronic inflammation involves proliferation of fibroblasts, the risk of scarring and deformity is greater than with acute inflammation. In some instances, granulation tissue replaces the normal supporting connective tissue elements or the functional parenchymal tissue of the involved structure.

Systemic Manifestations of Inflammation

Systemic signs and symptoms of inflammation vary depending on the cause and extent of tissue damage. Localized symptoms (redness, warmth, swelling, pain, and in some cases, loss of function) occur with both acute and chronic inflammation. Depending on the severity of tissue injury and the patient's vulnerability, localized inflammation can lead to systemic involvement. Fever is omnipresent in severe inflammation. Other systemic manifestations of inflammation include headache, loss of appetite, lethargy or malaise, and weakness. Leukocytosis and increased erythrocyte sedimentation rates (ESRs) also occur with systemic involvement.

Pain is a sensation of discomfort, hurt, or distress that may occur as the result of acute or chronic inflammation. It has been defined by Sternbach (1968) as a personal, private sensation of hurt. McCaffery (1979) defines pain as "whatever the experiencing person says it is and exists whenever he or she says it does". The International Association on Pain (1979) refers to pain as an unpleasant sensory and emotional experience associated with actual or potential tissue damage. Pain can be mild, moderate, or severe, acute or chronic, superficial, visceral or neuropathic in origin. (See also Chapter 14 for the original discussion of pain.)

PHARMACOTHERAPEUTIC OPTIONS

Anti-inflammatory drugs are the most widely prescribed and over-the-counter (OTC) drugs used today. Thus, it is important to understand clearly their indications for use, drug action, adverse effects, drug-drug interactions, and care implications. Serious and, at times, fatal consequences have occurred as a result of failure to recognize drug actions. This statement notwithstanding, anti-inflammatory drug use is based more on tradition and empirical results than a clear understanding of drug action.

Anti-inflammatory drugs are organized as either steroidal or nonsteroidal agents. Steroidal anti-inflammatory drugs are discussed in Chapter 52. There are two groups of NSAIDs: PG synthetase inhibitors (PSIs), and non-PG synthetase inhibitors (Non-PSIs). PSIs include salicylates, propionic acid derivatives, acetic acid derivatives, and a single phenylacetic acid drug. Non-PSIs drug groups include enolic acids and anthranilic acids.

By custom, the term NSAID refers to newer specific PSIs, exclusive of aspirin. However, using the term actually results in confusion because aspirin, the oldest NSAID, is in fact a PSI. Furthermore, many anti-inflammatory drugs are NSAIDs but are not PSIs (Table 15–2). Disease-modifying antirheumatic drugs (DMARDs) discussed in this chapter include hydroxychloroquine, methotrexate, sulfasalazine, and gold compounds. Other DMARDs include the immunosuppressant drug azathioprine, the chelating drug D-penicillamine, and the cytotoxic drug cyclophosphamide (see Chapter 30).

Nonsteroidal Anti-inflammatory Drugs

Indications

Aspirin is the prototype salicylate. There are many systemic and local uses for salicylates. Salicylates are used as analgesics in the management of headache, myalgias, osteoarthritis, ankylosing spondylitis, bursitis, tendinitis, and dysmenorrhea. Salicylates are regarded as the standard by which other drugs are compared for the treatment of rheumatoid arthritis. Because of suppression of platelet aggregation, they are also used in the management of rheumatic fever, transient ischemic attacks, coronary artery disease, and deep vein thrombosis.

The nonspecific anti-inflammatory effect of salicylates is invaluable in reducing cardiac workload for patients with severe carditis and heart failure. Aspirin has been shown to reduce the incidence of myocardial infarction in men or death in patients with unstable angina. Experience has shown that 325 mg of aspirin every other day significantly reduces the risk of fatal or nonfatal myocardial infarction, compared with an equal number of subjects receiving a placebo.

TABLE 15–2 NONSTEROIDAL ANTI-INFLAMMATORY DRUG CLASSES

Drug Class	Drug Examples
Prostaglandin Synthetase Inhibitors	
Salicylates	Aspirin (acetylsalicylic acid; ASPERGUM, ASA, BAYER ASPIRIN, ECOTRIN, EMPIRIN, others); (✱) APO-ASA, ARTHRISIN, ASTRIN, HEADSTART, RIPHEN, others
	Choline-magnesium salicylates (TRICOSAL, TRILISATE)
	Choline salicylate (ARTHROPAN)
	Diflunisal (DOLOBID)
	Magnesium salicylate (DOAN'S PILLS, MAGAN, MOBIDIN); (✱) BACK-ESE
	Salsalate DILSALCID, MONO-GESIC, SALICYLIC ACID, others)
	Sodium salicylate URACEL; (✱)
Propionic acid derivatives	Fenoprofen (NALFON)
	Flurbiprofen (ANSAID, OCUFEN)
	Ibuprofen (ADVIL, MOTRIN, EXCEDRIN IB, MIDOL IB, others); (✱) ACTIPROFEN, APO-IBUPROFEN, NOVO-PROFEN
	Ketoprofen (ACTRON, ORUDIS, ORUVAIL); (✱) ORUDIS-E, ORUDIS KT
	Naproxen (EC-NAPROSYN, NAPROSYN, ALEVE, ANAPROX, APO-NAPRO-NA; (✱) APO-NAPROXEN, NAPROSYN-E, APO-NAPRO-NA, SYNFLEX,
	Oxaprozin (DAYPRO)
Acetic acid derivatives	Etodolac (LODINE)
	Indomethacin (INDOCIN); (✱) APO-INDOMETHACIN, INDOCID, NU-INDO
	Ketorolac (TORADOL)
	Nabumetone (RELAFEN)
	Sulindac (CLINORIL); (✱) APO-SULIN, NOVO-SUNDAC
	Tolmetin (TOLECTIN); (✱) NOVO-TOLMETIN
Phenylacetic acid	Diclofenac (BOLTAREN, CATAFLAM)
Non-prostaglandin Synthetase Inhibitors	
Enolic acids	Piroxicam (FELDENE, NU-PIROX); (✱) APO-PIROXICAM, NOVO-PIROCAM
	Phenylbutazone
Anthranilic acids	Meclofenamate (MECLOFEN)
	Mefenamic acid (PONSTEL)

Myocardial ischemia due to cocaine can be treated with aspirin to decrease thrombus formation. Additional uses for aspirin and other PSIs include closure of a patent ductus arteriosus in the newborn and to treat Bartter's syndrome, a renal disorder affecting children.

Salicylates are used topically as keratolytic agents (skin-eroding product) and as counterirritants. The keratolytic effect is useful in treating warts, corns, fungal infections, and certain types of eczematous dermatitis. Methyl salicylate (oil of wintergreen) is used as a counterirritant in the treatment of inflamed muscles caused by physical exercise or viral infections. When they are placed on the skin, these drugs obscure the pain and discomfort by causing a feeling of warmth or slight burning. However, methyl salicylate is a common pediatric poison and its use is discouraged.

Salicylates are used as an antipyretic in patients for whom fever in itself may be detrimental. They are also used for patients who will be made more comfortable when a fever is lowered. The course of the patient's illness, however, can be clouded by relief of symptoms and fever reduction.

The principal indications for other NSAIDs are mild to moderate pain associated with rheumatoid arthritis and other disorders characterized by an inflammatory process. They are also used as adjuncts in the management of metastatic cancer pain, injuries (e.g., fractures), surgical procedures and some types of headaches. NSAIDs such as indomethacin, either alone or in combination with beta adrenergics, have been used to treat premature labor.

Pharmacodynamics

Salicylates and other NSAIDs are all analgesic, antipyretic, and anti-inflammatory in character. NSAIDs inhibit the synthesis and release of PGs. Salicylates irreversibly inhibit COX, the precursor to the synthesis of PG and related metabolites of arachidonic acid. When PG synthesis is blocked, the release of inflammatory mediators is inhibited. Other salicylates, such as salsalate, reversibly inhibit COX. Salicylates and salicylate-like drugs work to reduce fever by increasing heat loss through vasodilation of peripheral blood vessels, not by reducing heat production.

The mechanism and extent of antiplatelet effects differ between aspirin and the other NSAIDs. Acetylation is the introduction of one or more acetyl groups into an organic compound. When aspirin is absorbed, the acetyl portion of the compound dissociates, binding irreversibly to platelet COX. The binding prevents the synthesis of thromboxane A_2 and thus platelet aggregation is inhibited. A single dose of aspirin (325 mg or less) acetylates circulating platelets within a few minutes, but the effects are irreversible. The antiplatelet effects last for the life span of the platelet, which is about 7 to 10 days. Nonacetylated salicylates cause little or no suppression of platelet aggregation, although they are similar to aspirin (an acetylated salicylate) in most other respects. Nonacetylated salicylates bind reversibly with platelet COX, so antiplatelet effects exist only while the drug is present in the blood. For this reason, NSAIDs are not used specifically for antiplatelet activity. Chapter 36 discusses antiplatelet drugs.

Adverse Effects and Contraindications

The most common adverse effect of salicylates is gastrointestinal (GI) distress. Sometimes nausea and vomiting occur as a result of stimulation of the chemoreceptor trigger zone in the medulla. GI bleeding and subsequent iron-deficiency anemia can occur because the anti-PG effects of salicylates damage gastric mucosa. Daily use of 4 to 5 g of aspirin can cause a blood loss of 3 to 8 mL/day compared with 0.6-mL/day loss in nonaspirin users. Aspirin use is also associated with increased risk of peptic ulcer disease, although the magnitude of the problem is debatable. Data suggest that nonacetylated salicylates (e.g., diflunisal and salsalate) are associated with fewer ulcerations.

Aspirin and other salicylates do not produce sedation, physical dependence, or tolerance like opioids. However, at high doses, they stimulate the respiratory center in the medulla, increasing the rate and depth of respirations. Hyperventilation leads to respiratory alkalosis, with toxic doses directly depressing the respiratory center to cause metabolic acidosis.

Salicylates also affect uric acid elimination. Salicylate doses of 1 to 2 g/day decrease urate elimination and raise serum urate levels (*hyperuricemia*). Midrange doses of 2 to 3 g/day usually do not alter urate elimination. Doses exceeding 5 g/day actually lower plasma urate levels, thus improving gout. However, such large doses generally are not tolerated. This bimodal effect on elimination is related to the balance of reabsorption and secretion of uric acid at any given time.

Aspirin hypersensitivity or aspirin intolerance occurs in a small number of patients. Hypersensitivity is not an immune response, nor is it dose related. It may be due to blockade of the COX pathway and activation of the lipoxygenase pathway. The result is an accumulation of LTs (specifically, LTC_4, LTD_4, and LTE_4). The highest incidence of hypersensitivity is seen in middle-aged patients who have a history of asthma or nasal polyps. Symptoms of hypersensitivity include rhinitis with profuse watery secretions, bronchial constriction, hypotension, vasomotor collapse, and coma.

Large doses of aspirin (1000 to 1500 mg/day) can cause auditory and visual disturbances. These sensory responses are often accompanied by fever, changes in blood pH, and sometimes, coma. Tinnitus is an early sign of salicylate toxicity.

Contraindications to the clinical use of salicylates include peptic ulcer disease, GI or other bleeding disorders, hyperuricemia, hypersensitivity, or impaired renal function. Patients with the triad of asthma, aspirin-induced allergy, and nasal polyps are at increased risk for hypersensitivity reactions. Salicylates should also be avoided in patients who have an allergy to tartrazine (a food additive, Food and Drug Administration [FDA] yellow dye #5), and in patients with a vitamin K deficiency because of their antiplatelet effects. Large doses of salicylates should be avoided in patients with carditis. Salicylates should not be used in persons under the age of 21 years owing to the potential for *Reye's syndrome.*

Reye's syndrome, although rare, is a serious childhood illness that carries a mortality rate of 20 to 30 percent. Epidemiologic data suggest a relationship between children's viral illnesses, such as influenza or chicken pox, and the use of salicylates. Reye's syndrome is characterized pathologically by cerebral edema and fatty changes in the liver. The syndrome manifests clinically as encephalopathy and coma. Rapid progression through coma stages and high peak ammonia concentrations are associated with a more serious prognosis. Cerebral edema with increased intracranial pressure represents the most immediate threat to life.

Limit aspirin use for fever in patients with high cell turnover (i.e., cancer patients) because of the potential for uric acid build-up. Aspirin may also reduce the function of white blood cells because of its cellular inhibitory effects.

The adverse effects of NSAIDs are similar to those of salicylates and include gastric ulceration and blood loss. The inhibitory effects (i.e., vasodilation and cytoprotection) of PgE_2 and PgI_2 are lost in the presence of NSAIDs. Blood loss secondary to NSAID use may be less prevalent than with salicylates. However, like the salicylates, NSAIDs inhibit platelet aggregation and accelerate bleeding time as a result of TXA_2 inhibition. Other adverse effects include dizziness, headache, and water and sodium retention. Finally, much like the salicylates, the NSAIDs cause auditory and visual disturbances accompanied by fever and changes in blood pH. Coma occasionally occurs.

NSAID use places a fetus at risk for oligohydramnios, a deficiency of amniotic fluid. The deficiency is secondary to a decrease in fetal urine elimination. There is also a theoretic risk of premature closure of the ductus arteriosus in utero. Thus, NSAIDs are generally contraindicated during pregnancy and also during lactation.

Pharmacokinetics

NSAIDs are rapidly absorbed from the stomach and small intestine after oral administration. The principal site of absorption is the small intestine. The absorption rate is determined by many factors, including the disintegration and dissolution rates of tablets, the gastric pH, and the gastric emptying time. When aspirin is given as a rectal suppository, it is absorbed slowly and blood levels are lower than with orally administered formulations. NSAIDs are well distributed to body tissues, placental membranes, and most transcellular fluids through pH-dependent passive processes. NSAIDs are highly bound to plasma proteins, with salicylates more highly bound at low doses than at high doses. High doses of salicylates are 25 to 60 percent protein bound. Significant drug levels are found in the plasma in less than 30 minutes, with peak levels reached 2 to 4 hours after a single dose (Table 15–3). The duration of drug action ranges from 3 to 48 hours.

Biotransformation of NSAIDs occurs in the liver and many other tissues. The drug is rapidly cleared in the urine as free drug and other metabolites. Although it is variable, the elimination of free drug in the urine depends on both the dose and urinary pH. More than 30 percent of a salicylate is eliminated unchanged in an alkaline urine, whereas the amount eliminated can be as low as 2 percent in acidic urine. A small portion of some NSAIDs is eliminated via the feces.

The plasma half-life of aspirin is approximately 15 minutes. For other salicylates, the plasma half-life is 2 to 3 hours for low doses and 12 hours for large doses. The half-life of high anti-inflammatory dosages of salicylates or when there is an overdose can be as long as 15 to 30 hours.

Drug-Drug Interactions

NSAIDs interact with many other drugs (Table 15–4). NSAIDs prolong bleeding time and potentiate the effects of anticoagulants, thrombolytic drugs, plicamycin, some cephalosporins, and valproic acid. The hemorrhagic effects of salicylates are accentuated because of their platelet-inhibiting properties and by displacement of the anticoagulant warfarin from plasma proteins. Chronic use of NSAIDs with aspirin may result in increased GI distress and decreased effectiveness. The combination of alcohol and aspirin in patients on anticoagulant therapy can be lethal. NSAIDs decrease the responsiveness to diuretics and antihypertensive drugs. Chronic use of acetaminophen with NSAIDs increases the risk of adverse renal reactions. The effects of uricosuric drugs can be blocked in the presence of aspirin. Aspirin competes with the organic renal transport system to increase penicillin G concentration.

Dosage Regimen

As with all other drugs, NSAID dosages vary considerably depending on the age of the patient, the route of administration, and the condition being treated. Adult and pediatric dosages are identified in Table 15–5. Dosage regimens for severe and chronic inflammatory disorders such as rheumatic fever and rheumatoid arthritis are significantly greater than those needed for analgesia or fever reduction. Treatment regimens are also more rigorous and prolonged.

Laboratory Considerations

Salicylates may cause an elevated alanine aminotransferase (ALT; serum glutamic-pyruvic transaminase [SGPT]) aspartate aminotransferase (AST; serum glutamic-oxaloacetic transaminase [SGOT]), and alkaline phosphatase levels, especially when plasma salicylate concentrations exceed 25 mg/100 mL. Levels often return to normal despite continued drug use or dosage reduction. If severe abnormalities persist or active liver disease develops, salicylate use should be discontinued and the drug used with caution in the future. Hepatic function should be monitored before and periodically during long-term therapy. Hepatotoxicity is more likely to occur in patients with rheumatic fever, systemic lupus erythematosus (SLE), juvenile arthritis, or pre-existing hepatic disease.

Serum salicylate levels should be monitored periodically in patients with prolonged high-dose therapy. Salicylates prolong bleeding time and in large doses can prolong prothrombin times. The patient's hematocrit should be monitored periodically to assess for GI blood loss when the patient is receiving chronic salicylate therapy.

In addition, salicylates can cause false-negative urine glucose test results using enzymatic glucose testing methods (i.e., Clinistix and Tes-Tape), and false-positive urine glucose test results using the copper sulfate method (i.e., Clinitest). However, they have no effects on testing modes that are used for blood glucose monitoring. They also alter the results of serum uric acid, urine vanillylmandelic acid, protirelin-induced thyroid-stimulating hormone, urine hydroxyindoleacetic acid determinations and radionuclide thyroid imaging. Salicylates can cause reduced serum potassium and cholesterol values.

Serum potassium levels, ALT (SGPT), AST (SGOT), and alkaline phosphatase may be increased with other NSAIDs. Like salicylates, other NSAIDs can cause prolonged bleeding times that persist for some time following discontinuation of therapy. The patient's hematocrit should be periodically monitored to assess for GI blood loss.

TABLE 15–3 PHARMACOKINETICS OF SELECTED NONSTEROIDAL ANTI-INFLAMMATORY DRUGS

Drug	Route	Analgesic Action			Antirheumatic Action		PB (%)	$t_{1/2}$
		ONSET	PEAK	DURATION	ONSET	PEAK		
Salicylates								
Acetylsalicylic acid	po	15–30 min	1–3 hr	3–6 hr	—	—	90–91;	2–3 hr; 15–30 hr*
Choline magnesium salicylates	po	5–30 min	1–3 hr	3–6 hr			25–60*	2–3 hr; 15–30 hr*
Choline salicylate	po	5–30 min	1–3 hr	3–6 hr				2–3 hr; 15–30 hr*
Diflunisal	po	1 hr	2–3 hr	8–12 hr				8–12 hr
Magnesium salicylate	po	5–30 min	1–3 hr	3–6 hr				2–3 hr; 15–30 hr*
Salsalate	po	5–30 min	1–3 hr	3–6 hr				2–3 hr; 15–30 hr*
Sodium salicylate	po	5–30 min	1–3 hr	3–6 hr				2–3 hr; 15–30 hr*
Propionic Acid Derivatives								
Fenoprofen	po	30 min	1–2 hr	4–6 hr	2 days	2–3 weeks	99	2–3 hr
Flurbiprofen	po	60 min	1.5 hr	4–6 hr	—	—	> 90	5.7 hr
Ibuprofen	po	30–60 min; 7 days[†]	1–2 hr	4–6 hr	< 7 days	1–2 weeks	90–99	1.8–2.5 hr
Ketoprofen	po	30 min	0.5–2 hr	4–8 hr	—	—	99	2–4 hr
Naproxen	po	1–2 hr	2–4 hr	7–12 hr	< 14 days	2–4 weeks	99	10–20 hr
Oxaprozin	po	60 min	3–6 hr	24–48 hr	< 7 days	—	> 99	26–92 hr
Acetic Acid Derivatives								
Etodolac	po	30 min	1–2 hr	4–8 hr	—	—	99	6–8 hr
Indomethacin	po	0.5–2 hr	1–2 hr	4–6 hr	< 7 days	1–2 weeks	99	4.5 hr
Ketorolac	po	Varies	30–60 min	4–6 hr	—	—	99	2.4–8.6 hr
	IM	5–10 min	30–90 min	4–8 hr			99	5–6 hr
Nabumetone	po	1–2 hr	5 hr	24–48 hr	—	—	99	24 hr
Sulindac	po	60 min	2–4 hr	7–16 hr	< 7 days	2–3 weeks	93–98	7–8 hr; 16 hr[‡]
Tolmetin	po	Rapid	0.5–1 hr	6–8 hr	< 7 days	1–2 weeks	99	1–1.5 hr
Enolic Acids								
Piroxicam	po	15–30 min	3–5 hr; 7–12 days§	24–48 hr	7–12 days	2–3 weeks	99	30–80 hr
Phenylbutazone	po	30–60 min	2.5 hr	3–5 days	—	—	98	77–85 hr
Fenamic Acids								
Meclofenamate	po	days	2–3 weeks	days	Few days	2–3 weeks	> 99	40 min–2 hr
Mefenamic acid	po	Varies	2–4 hr	6 hr	—	—	90	2–4 hr
Phenylacetic Acid Derivatives								
Diclofenac sodium	po	60 min	2–3 hr	4–6 hr	—	—	99	1.2–1.8 hr
Others								
Acetaminophen	po	30–60 min	1–2 hr	3–4 hr	NA	NA	25¶	1.5–4 hr
	po-ER	UK	UK	Up to 8 hr				
	SUP	30–60 min	1–3 hr	3–4 hr				
Capsaicin	Top	Varies	1–2 wks	2–4 wks	NA	NA	UK	UK

* Protein binding and the half-life of low-dose and high-dose salicylates, respectively.
† The onset time of ibuprofen's analgesic and anti-inflammatory effects, respectively.
‡ Half-life of sulindac metabolites.
§ Peak blood levels and days to therapeutic effects respectively for piroxicam.
¶ Protein binding of acetaminophen is low at therapeutic dosages; 20 to 50 percent at toxic levels.
PB Protein binding; $t_{1/2}$ elimination half-life; po-ER orally administered using extended release formulation; SUP suppository; Top topical formulation; UA unavailable; UK unknown.

Other Analgesics

- ❒ Acetaminophen (DATRIL, TEMPRA, TYLENOL); (✤) APO-ACETAMINOPHEN, TEMPRO, TYLENOL
- ❒ Capsaicin (ZOSTRIX); (✤) ZOSTRIX

ACETAMINOPHEN

Acetaminophen is an analgesic and antipyretic with no anti-inflammatory properties. Its advantage in the management of discomfort and fever is that it produces minimal GI irritation and it has no effect on bleeding times, uric acid levels or respirations. Acetaminophen is a paraminophenol, although the mechanism of action is unknown. However, like the salicylates and the other NSAIDs, it is thought to act by inhibiting central and peripheral PG synthesis. Because of its weak anti-inflammatory actions, acetaminophen is not useful for treating arthritis or rheumatic fever.

Adverse drug effects are few; however, those that do exist are significant. Acute hepatic necrosis occurs with dosages of 10 to 15 g. Dosages over 25 g are usually fatal. With therapeutic dosages, 90 to 100 percent of the drug may be recovered in the urine within the first 24 hours after hepatic conjugation with glucuronic acid (about 60 percent), sulfuric acid (about 35 percent), or cysteine (about 3 percent). Small

TABLE 15–4 DRUG-DRUG INTERACTIONS OF SELECTED NONSTEROIDAL ANTI-INFLAMMATORY DRUGS

Drug	Interactive Drugs	Interaction
Nonsteroidal Anti-inflammatory Drugs		
Salicylates in general	Alcohol	Increases ulcerogenic effects of salicylates
	Anticoagulants	Increased risk of bleeding
	Corticosteroids	Decreased plasma salicylate levels Increased ulcerogenic effects
	Methotrexate	Increased effects and toxicity of methotrexate, leading to pancytopenia
	Probenecid Sulfinpyrazone	Aspirin decreases the uricosuric effects of interacting drugs
	Mannitol Citrates Sodium bicarbonate Antacids	Increased excretion of salicylates
	Penicillin-G	Increases serum concentration of interactive drug
	Sulfonylureas	Enhanced hypoglycemic effects of interacting drug
	Zidovudine	Metabolism of interactive drug inhibited
	Vancomycin Aminoglycosides Cisplatin Furosemide Bumetanide Ethacrynic acid	Increased risk for ototoxicity when given with salicylates
	Spironolactone	Decreased effectiveness of interactive drug
	Acetazolamide	May cause acetazolamide intoxication
NSAIDs in general	Cefamandole Cefotetan Maxolactam Plicamycin	May induce hypoprothrombinemia or inhibit platelet aggregation
	Acetaminophen	Increases risk of renal toxicity
	ACE inhibitors	Reduced antihypertensive effects
	Cimetidine	Increases serum concentrations of NSAID
	Gold products	Increased risk of adverse renal effects
	Hydantoins Sulfonylureas Nifedipine Verapamil	Displaces interactive drug leading to increased incidence of adverse effects
	Antihypertensives Bumetanide Furosemide	Decreased effects of interactive drug
	Oral anticoagulants Thrombolytics Glucocorticosteroids Alcohol Dextran Penicillin antibiotics Sulfinpyrazone Valproic acid	Increased risk of GI ulceration, bleeding
	Oral hypoglycemics Insulins	Increased risk of hypoglycemic effects of interactive drug
	Lithium	Increased lithium concentrations
	Beta blockers	Synthesis of renal prostaglandins inhibited leading to hypertension
	Methotrexate	Decreases tubular secretion of interactive drug leading to toxicity
	Zidovudine	Inhibits biotransformation of interactive drug leading to toxicity
Sulindac	Oral anticoagulants	Increased hypoprothrombinemic activity increases the potential for bleeding
Indomethacin	Non-amphetamine Anorexigenic drugs	May cause hypertension
Ketorolac	Salicylates	Increased plasma concentrations of interactive drug
Others		
Acetaminophen	Alcohol Hepatotoxic substances	Additive effects with increased risk of toxicity to acetaminophen
	Oral anticoagulants	Increased risk of hypoprothrombinemia and bleeding
	Barbiturates Carbamazepine Hydantoins Rifampin Sulfinpyrazone	Increased risk of hepatotoxicity and decreased therapeutic effects of interactive drug
	Aspirin	Increased risk of adverse renal effects
	Diflunisal	Increases acetaminophen levels and increases the risk of hepatotoxicity with chronic concurrent use
Capsaicin	ACE inhibitors	Increased incidence of cough from interactive drug

ACE, Angiotensin–converting enzyme; NSAID, nonsteroidal anti-inflammatory drug.

TABLE 15-5 DOSAGE REGIMEN FOR SELECTED NONSTEROIDAL ANTI-INFLAMMATORY DRUGS

Drug	Use(s)	Dosage	Implications
Prostaglandin Synthetase Inhibitors			
Salicylates			
Aspirin	Fever, pain, headache, dysmenorrhea	*Adults:* 325–975 mg po q3–4 hr PRN	Not recommended for children owing to risk of Reye's syndrome
	Rheumatic fever	*Adults:* 3.6–7.8 g po daily in three to four divided doses *Child:* 80–100 mg/kg/day po divided doses. Not to exceed 130 mg/kg/day	Take with food
	Rheumatoid arthritis	*Adult:* 3.6–5.4 g po daily in divided doses	Take with food
	Transient ischemic attacks	*Adult:* 1–1.3 g po daily in two to four divided doses	Doses may be as low as 325 mg/day in patients who are intolerant of higher doses
	Prophylaxis recurrent MI	*Adult:* 300–325 mg po daily as single dose	Doses as low as 80 mg per day may be effective
Choline-magnesium trisalicylate	Fever, rheumatoid conditions	*Adult:* 2–3 g po daily in two to three divided doses *or* 1500 mg po BID *Child over 37 kg:* 2.2 g of salicylate per day in two divided doses *Child under 37 kg:* 50 mg of salicylate per day in two divided doses	Each 500 mg tablet or 5 mL of liquid contain same amount of salicylate as 650 mg of aspirin. Tablet strength expressed in mg of salicylate: 500-mg tablet = 650 mg aspirin; 750-mg tablet = 975 mg aspirin; 1000-mg tablet = 1.3 g of aspirin
Choline salicylate	Fever, rheumatoid arthritis	*Adult:* 435–669 mg po q3hr *or* 425–870 mg po q4hr *or* 870–1305 mg q6hr PRN. As anti-inflammatory: 4.8–7.2 g po daily in divided doses	Each teaspoon contains 870 mg choline salicylate and 650 mg aspirin. 435 mg of choline salicylate is equivalent to 325 mg of aspirin
Diflunisal	Mild to moderate pain, osteoarthritis	*Adult:* 500–1000 mg. po initially followed by 250–500 mg po q8–12hr	Not indicated for fever. Takes up to 2 weeks for therapeutic effects to be reached
Magnesium salicylate	Rheumatic conditions, mild to moderate pain, fever	*Adult:* 325–1.3 g po daily in three to four divided doses	Therapeutic response in arthritis may take up to 2 weeks
Salsalate	Rheumatic conditions	*Adult:* 1500 mg po BID or 750 mg po QID. Not to exceed 4 g/day	
Sodium salicylate	Mild to moderate pain; rheumatic conditions	*Adult:* 325–650 mg po q4hr PRN. As anti-inflammatory: 3.6–5.4 g/day in divided doses *Child:* 1.5 g/m^2/day po in 4–6 divided doses. As anti-inflammatory: 80–100 mg/kg/day po in four to six divided doses	
Propionic Acid Derivatives			
Fenoprofen	Rheumatic conditions	*Adult:* 300–600 mg po three to four times daily. Not to exceed 3.2 g/day	Patients with asthma, aspirin-induced allergy and nasal polyps are at increased risk of hypersensitivity reactions
	Dysmenorrhea, mild to moderate pain	*Adult:* 200 mg po q4–6 hr	
Flurbiprofen	Rheumatic conditions	*Adult:* 200–300 mg po QD in two to four divided doses. Not to exceed 300 mg/day or 100 mg/dose	Patients with asthma, aspirin-induced allergy and nasal polyps are at increased risk of hypersensitivity reactions
	Dysmenorrhea, mild to moderate pain (unlabeled)	*Adult:* 50 mg po q4–6 hr PRN	
Ibuprofen	Rheumatic conditions	*Adult:* 300–800 mg po TID–QID. Not to exceed 3600 mg/day *Child 6 mo-12 y:* 20–40 mg/kg/day po in divided doses. Not to exceed 50 mg/kg/day	Administration in higher doses not recommended. For rapid initial effect, administer 30 minutes before or 2 hours after meals. Prophylaxis for dysmenorrhea has not shown to be effective
	Fever, mild to moderate pain, dysmenorrhea	*Adult:* 200–400 mg po q4–6hr PRN as soon as pain starts. Not to exceed 1200 mg/day *Child:* 5 mg/kg po for temp < 102.5°F or 10 mg/kg for higher temperatures. Not to exceed 40 mg/kg/day. May be repeated q4–6hr	
Ketoprofen	Rheumatic conditions	*Adult:* 150–300 mg po QD in three to four divided doses or 200 mg once daily as extended release formulation	Co-administration with opioid may produce additive analgesia thus permitting lower opioid doses
	Dysmenorrhea, mild to moderate pain	*Adult:* 25–50 mg po q6–8hr	
Naproxen	Rheumatic conditions, ankylosing spondylitis	*Adult:* 250–500 mg po BID to maximum of 1.5 g/day *or* 375–500 mg delayed-release formulation po QD *or* 275–550 mg BID to 1.65 g/day *Child:* 10 mg/kg/day po as suspension in two divided doses	Not to be confused with naproxen sodium. Caution patient to wear sunscreen and protective clothing to prevent photosensitivity reactions

TABLE 15–5 DOSAGE REGIMEN FOR SELECTED NONSTEROIDAL ANTI-INFLAMMATORY DRUGS *Continued*

Drug	Use(s)	Dosage	Implications
Propionic Acid Derivatives Continued			
Naproxen	Bursitis, tendinitis, dysmenorrhea, mild to moderate pain	*Adult:* 500 mg po initially then 250 mg po q6–8 hr PRN	
	Gout	*Adult:* 750 mg initially then 250 mg po q8hr	
Acetic Acid Derivatives			
Etodolac	Osteoarthritis	*Adult:* 400 mg po two to three times daily *or* 300 mg po three to four times daily initially then adjusted according to patient response. Range: 400–1200 mg/day	For rapid effect, administer 30 minutes before or 2 hr after meals. May be administered with food, milk, or antacids containing aluminum or magnesium to decrease GI irritation Food slows but does not reduce the extent of absorption
	Mild to moderate pain	*Adult:* 400 mg po initially then 200–400 mg po q6–8 hr. Not to exceed 1200 mg/day in patients over 60 kg or 20 mg/kg in patients < 60 Kg	
Indomethacin	Rheumatic conditions, bursitis, tendinitis, ankylosing spondylitis	*Adult:* 25–50 mg po BID-QID or 75 mg of extended-release capsule QD-BID. Not to exceed 200 mg or 150 mg of SR/day. Single bedtime dose of 100 mg may be used *Child:* 1.5–2.5 mg/kg/day po, PR in three to four divided doses. Not to exceed 4 mg/kg/day or 150–200 mg/day	Take with food. Has multiple drug-drug interactions thus use with caution and in patients with history of peptic ulcer disease
	Acute gouty arthritis	*Adult:* 100 mg initially then 50 mg po TID for relief of pain then decrease further	
Ketorolac	Short-term pain management	*Adult < 65 yr:* 20 mg po initially followed by 10 mg q4–6 hr PRN. Not to exceed 40 mg/day *or* 60 mg IM single dose *or* 30 mg q6hr *or* 30 mg IV single dose *or* 30 mg IV q6hr. Not to exceed 120 mg/day *Adults > 65 yr < 50 kg or with renal failure:* 10 mg po q4–6hr PRN. Not to exceed 40 mg/day *or* 30 mg IM single dose *or* 15 mg IM q 6hr *or* 15 mg IV single dose *or* 15 mg IV q6hr. Not to exceed 60 mg/day	Ketorolac therapy should always be given initially IM or IV. Oral therapy should be used as a continuation of parenteral therapy. Duration of ketorolac by all routes should not exceed 5 days
Nabumetone	Rheumatic conditions	*Adult:* 1000 mg po QD as a single dose or divided dose BID. May be increased up to 2000 mg/day	Use lowest effective dose during chronic therapy
Sulindac	Rheumatic conditions, acute gouty arthritis, bursitis	*Adult:* 150–200 mg po BID. Not to exceed 400 mg/day	Take with food, milk, or antacids. Food slows but does not reduce extent of absorption. Tablets may be crushed and mixed with food or fluids
Tolmetin	Rheumatic conditions	*Adult:* 400 mg po TID initially, followed by maintenance dose of 600–1800 mg/day in three to four divided doses. Not to exceed 2000 mg/day *Child > 2 yr:* 20 mg/kg initially followed by maintenance doses of 15–30 mg/kg/day in three to four divided doses. Not to exceed 30 mg/day	
Phenylacetic Acid Derivative			
Diclofenac	Ankylosing spondylitis	*Adult:* (Sodium formulation) 100–125 mg po QD in 25-mg doses QID and HS	Patients with asthma, aspirin-induced allergy, and nasal polyps are at increased risk of hypersensitivity reactions. Take with food, milk, or antacids. May take first 1–2 doses on empty stomach for more rapid onset. Administer as soon as possible after onset of menses. Prophylaxis for dysmenorrhea has not been shown effective
	Osteoarthritis	*Adult:* (Sodium or potassium formulation) 50 mg po BID-TID *or* 75 mg po BID of sodium formulation	
	Rheumatoid arthritis	*Adult:* (Sodium or potassium formulation) 50 mg po TID-QID *or* 75 mg BID sodium formulation	
	Dysmenorrhea, analgesia	*Adult:* 150 mg po TID, initial dose may be 100 mg. Not to exceed 200 mg po during first 24 hr or 150 mg/day on subsequent days	
Nonprostaglandin Derivatives			
Enolic Acid Derivatives			
Piroxicam	Rheumatic conditions	*Adult:* 10–20 mg/day as single dose or two divided doses	Begin with 10 mg/day initially for older adults
	Dysmenorrhea (unlabeled use)	*Adult:* 40 mg po initially then 20 mg/day	

Table continued on following page

TABLE 15–5 DOSAGE REGIMEN FOR SELECTED NONSTEROIDAL ANTI-INFLAMMATORY DRUGS *Continued*

Drug	Use(s)	Dosage	Implications
Anthranilic Acid Derivatives			
Meclofenamate	Rheumatoid conditions Mild to moderate pain Dysmenorrhea, excessive menstrual blood loss	*Adult:* 200–400 mg po QD in three to four divided doses *Adults:* 50–100 mg po q4–6 hr *Adults:* 100 mg po TID for up to 6 days	Caution patient to wear sunscreen and protective clothing to prevent photosensitivity reactions. Patients with asthma, aspirin-induced allergy and nasal polyps are at increased risk of hypersensitivity reactions.
Mefenamic acid	Moderate pain	*Adult:* 500 mg. po initially followed by 250 mg po q6hr PRN. Not to exceed 1 week of therapy.	Arrange for periodic ophthalmologic examination during long-term therapy
Others			
Acetaminophen	Fever, headache, myalgia, neuralgia, mild to moderate pain	*Adult:* 325–1000 mg po 4–6 hr PRN *or* 1300 mg q8hr as extended release tablets. Not to exceed 4g/day or 2.6 g/day po for chronic use *or* 325–650 mg PR q4hr PRN. Not to exceed 6 suppositories/24 hr *Child age 11–12 yr:* 480 mg po, PR q4–6 hr PRN *Child age 9–11 yr:* 400 mg po, PR q4–6 hr PRN *Child age 6–9 yr:* 320 mg po, PR q4–6 hr PRN *Child age 4–6 yr:* 240 mg po, q4–6 hr PRN *Child age 2–4 yr:* 160 mg po, PR q4–6 hr PRN *Child age 1–2 yr:* 120 mg po, PR q4–6 hr PRN *Child age 4–12 mo:* 80 mg po q4–6 hr PRN *Child age < 3 mo:* 40 mg po q4–6 hr PRN	Consult health care provider if fever lasts longer than 3 days or if over 103°F (39.5°C). Take with food or on an empty stomach. Caution patient to avoid alcohol if taking more than an occasional 1–2 doses. Avoid taking concurrently with salicylates or other NSAIDs for more than a few days. Incidence of hepatotoxicity increases with as little as 4 g/day in the presence of ethanol and/or fasting. Acute hepatic necrosis occurs with doses of 10–15 g. Doses over 25 g are usually fatal.
Capsaicin	Peripheral neuropathy	*Adult:* Apply to affected areas 3–4 times daily	Avoid getting drug in eyes or on broken or irritated skin surfaces.

GI, Gastrointestinal; MI, myocardial infarction; NSAID, nonsteroidal anti-inflammatory drug.

amounts of hydroxylated and deacetylated metabolites have also been detected. Children have less capacity for glucuronidation of the drug than do adults. A small fraction of acetaminophen is acted on by the cytochrome P_{450} enzyme system to form a highly reactive intermediate metabolite (*N*-acetyl-benzoquinoneimine). This metabolite normally reacts with sulfhydryl groups in glutathione. However, after large doses of acetaminophen, the metabolite is formed in amounts adequate to deplete hepatic glutathione. Under these circumstances, reaction with sulfhydryl groups in hepatic proteins is increased and hepatic necrosis results.

The risk of hepatotoxicity increases with as little as 4 g/day in the presence of ethanol or fasting, or both. Ethanol induces hepatic mixed function oxidase metabolism, shifting the reaction toward the more toxic metabolite. Fasting moves biotransformation of acetaminophen from one set of metabolic pathways to others by reducing the required precursor molecules. Cautious use of acetaminophen is warranted in patients with severe hepatic disease, renal disease, chronic alcohol abuse, and malnutrition. Its use is contraindicated in patients with hypersensitivity. Products containing alcohol, aspartame, saccharin, sugar, or tartrazine (FDC yellow dye #5) should be avoided in patients who have hypersensitivity or intolerance to these compounds.

Renal tubular necrosis (analgesic nephropathy) was the basis for removing the other paraminophenol, phenacetin, from the market. Because acetaminophen is a related drug, the lifetime risk of nephropathy increases with the intake of 1000 tablets, although the incidence of renal tubular necrosis is lower with aspirin.

Acetaminophen is well absorbed when taken by mouth, with peak blood levels reached in 30 to 60 minutes (see Table 15–3). Distribution is to all body tissues, with 20 to 50 percent of the drug protein bound. The manner in which acetaminophen is biotransformed depends on the dosage. At low dosages, most of the drug is biotransformed into inactive compounds. A small fraction is converted to a toxic metabolite that can harm the liver. Fortunately, the toxic metabolite usually undergoes rapid conversion to a nontoxic form. When an overdose of acetaminophen is ingested, a large quantity of the toxic metabolite is produced. The capacity of the liver to detoxify the metabolite is exceeded, and hepatic injury results.

The drug-drug interactions with acetaminophen are many (see Table 15–4). Chronic concurrent acetaminophen use with NSAIDs increases the risk of renal injury. Diflunisol increases acetaminophen blood levels and increases the risk of hepatotoxicity with chronic concurrent use. High-dose, chronic use of acetaminophen (over 2 g/day) increases the risk of bleeding in the presence of warfarin. Hepatotoxicity may be additive in the presence of other hepatotoxic drugs, including alcohol.

Acetaminophen is available as chewable tablets, granules, extended-release tablets, solutions, liquids, elixirs, and suppositories. The dosage varies from formulation to formulation. The oral adult dosage for fever, headache, myalgia, neuralgia, and mild to moderate pain is 325 to 1000 mg every 4 to 6 hours, or 1300 mg every 8 hours if an extended-release formulation is used (see Table 15–5).

Pediatric dosages vary depending on the age of the child and the formulation used, but they range from less than 40 mg every 4 to 6 hours for a child younger than three months of age to 480 mg for a child 11 to 12 years of age. Caution is warranted when using TYLENOL INFANT'S DROPS because it is a concentrated solution. Be sure to read labels closely to minimize the risk of overdose.

Acetaminophen interferes with Chemstrip G, Dextrostix, and Visidex II home blood glucose monitoring systems. The effects vary with the specific testing methods. Falsely decreased values may be noted when measured with glucose oxidase/peroxidase methods but probably not with the hexokinase/glucose-6-phosphate dehydrogenase method. Acetaminophen may cause falsely increased values with certain measurement instruments. Increased serum bilirubin, lactic dehydrogenase (LDH), liver function tests, and prothrombin time may indicate hepatotoxicity.

CAPSAICIN

Capsaicin is a newer topical analgesic used for the temporary management of pain due to rheumatoid arthritis and osteoarthritis. It has also been shown effective for pain associated with neuralgias (e.g., shingles or diabetic neuropathy). Postmastectomy pain and reflex sympathetic dystrophy syndrome has also responded to application of capsaicin, although it is not FDA approved for these uses. Capsaicin is thought to act by depleting or preventing the reaccumulation of substance P, which is responsible for transmitting pain impulses from peripheral sites to the central nervous system (CNS).

Capsaicin's adverse effects are few but include cough and transient burning at the site of administration. Hypersensitivity to capsaicin, hot peppers, or components used in preparation contraindicate its use. It should not be used near the eyes or on broken skin. Safe use during pregnancy, lactation, or in children has not been established.

The onset of drug action occurs in approximately 1 to 2 weeks, with peak effects noted in 2 to 4 weeks (see Table 15–3). For patients with head and neck neuralgias, it may take up to 6 weeks for peak effects to be reached. The duration of action of capsaicin is unknown, as is the biotransformation, elimination route, and half-life.

A thin film of capsaicin is applied to affected areas three to four times daily (see Table 15–5). Gloves should be worn during application, or hands should be washed immediately after application. If capsaicin is used on the hands for arthritis, the hands should not be washed for at least 30 minutes following application. Pain relief lasts only as long as capsaicin is used regularly. The patient should be advised that any burning usually disappears after the first few days of use but can continue for 2 to 4 weeks or longer. Patients should also be advised that burning is increased by heat, sweating, bathing in warm water, humidity, and clothing. Decreasing the number of daily applications will not lessen the amount of burning but may reduce the degree of pain relief obtained and may prolong the period of burning.

The patient with herpes zoster should be advised not to apply capsaicin cream until the lesions have completely healed. Patients should also be advised to discontinue use of capsaicin and to notify the health care provider if pain persists longer than 1 month, worsens, or if signs of infection are present.

Disease-Modifying Antirheumatic Drugs

GOLD SALTS

- ❒ Auranofin (RIDAURA)
- ❒ Aurothioglucose (SOLGANAL)
- ❒ Gold sodium thiomalate (aurothiomalate)

Indications

Gold salts are used in the management of progressive rheumatoid arthritis that is unresponsive to traditional therapies. Gold salts can relieve pain and stiffness, and for some patients, may arrest the progression of joint degeneration. These drugs do not reverse damage that has already occurred. Symptomatic improvement is seen in 60 to 70 percent of patients. About 15 percent have a remission. Auranofin has been used also as an alternative or adjunct to corticosteroids in treating pemphigus, SLE, and for patients with psoriatic arthritis who do not tolerate or respond to NSAIDs. However, it has not been FDA approved for use in these conditions. Aurothioglucose is most effective early in the course of rheumatoid arthritis in both adults and children.

Pharmacodynamics

The exact mechanism by which gold reduces symptoms and induces remission of arthritis has not been determined. It is thought that gold salts are taken up by macrophages, followed by inhibition of phagocytosis and activity of lysosomal enzymes. They decrease concentrations of rheumatoid factor and immunoglobulins, although the mechanisms are not clearly known.

Adverse Effects and Contraindications

Gold salts have a number of toxicities that limit their use. Fifteen to twenty percent of patients must discontinue treatment because of adverse effects. The most common adverse effects of gold salts are a metallic taste, stomatitis, and diarrhea accompanied by abdominal pain and cramping. Oral gold formulations cause less mucocutaneous and renal toxicity than intramuscular (IM) formulations. Some patients develop a rash, dermatitis, or dizziness. Although thrombocytopenia is a possible adverse effect, aplastic anemia and agranulocytosis are more important concerns. Interstitial pneumonitis, fibrosis, and acute tubular necrosis have been noted in patients receiving aurothioglucose. Renal toxicity, manifested as proteinuria, occurs frequently.

Toxicity and overdose become evident as a rapid decrease in hemoglobin, a white blood cell count below 4000/mm^3, eosinophil count above 5 percent, granulocyte count less than 1500/mm^3, or a platelet count under 100,000 to 150,000/mm^3. Albuminuria, hematuria, rash, dermatitis, pruritus, skin eruptions, stomatitis, persistent diarrhea, jaundice, or petechiae may also indicate toxicity.

Gold salts are contraindicated in patients with hypersensitivity to gold, in patients with severe hepatic or renal dysfunction, or in patients who have a history of heavy metal intoxication. Cautious use of gold salts is warranted in patients with a history of colitis, exfoliative dermatitis, uncontrolled diabetes mellitus, tuberculosis, congestive heart failure, SLE, and recent radiation therapy. Gold salts should not be used in debilitated patients or in women who are pregnant or lactating.

Pharmacokinetics

Orally administered auranofin is 20 to 25 percent absorbed from the GI tract (Table 15–6). Aurothioglucose and gold sodium thiomalate are rapidly absorbed following IM injection. The onset of anti-inflammatory drug action takes from 6 to 8 weeks for IM formulations to 3 to 6 months for orally administered drugs. Gold salts are widely distributed, concentrating in arthritic joints more than in uninvolved joints. They are also distributed in breast milk.

Sixty to ninety percent of gold salts are eliminated by the kidneys for up to 15 months. Up to 40 percent is eliminated in the feces. The half-life of gold salts in the blood is 3 to 26 days; however, in tissues, the half-life ranges from 40 to 128 days.

Drug-Drug Interactions

Additive bone marrow toxicity may occur when gold salts are used in conjunction with other myelosuppressive drugs such as antineoplastics. Combined use of gold salts with radiation therapy can also contribute to myelosuppression (Table 15–7).

Dosage Regimen

Gold salts are available for oral and IM use. Auranofin can be administered daily as 6 mg in one or two divided doses (Table 15–8). A total of 9 mg daily in three divided doses can be used if there is no response after 6 months of therapy at the lower dosage. The dosage should not exceed 9 mg daily. Therapy should be discontinued if the patient does not respond satisfactorily. Auranofin contains 29 percent gold.

Aurothioglucose is administered as weekly IM injections. Injections are painful, with postinjection pain common. Ten milligrams are given the first week, with the dosage increased to 25 mg the second and third week of therapy. Fifty milligrams are given the fourth and subsequent weeks. The dosage may continue at the 50-mg level every 3 to 4 weeks, as long as the patient improves without toxicity. In the absence of toxicity, monthly maintenance injections can be continued indefinitely. Tolerance to gold decreases with age. Aurothioglucose contains 50 percent gold.

Gold sodium thiomalate is also administered IM at weekly intervals at a dose similar to that of aurothioglucose. For patients with a history of mild reaction, treatment may be started at 5 mg and gradually titrated upward by 5 to 10 mg weekly or monthly until the 25- to 50-mg dosage is reached. Treatment may also continue indefinitely with this drug as long as the patient tolerates it. This drug is 50 percent gold.

Laboratory Considerations

Frequent laboratory testing and patient monitoring is required to monitor for gold toxicity. Hematologic status and liver and kidney function should be monitored before and periodically throughout therapy with gold salts. A urinalysis for protein should be obtained before each injection. Because these drugs may cause thrombocytopenia, leukopenia, and anemia, complete blood count (CBC) and platelet values should be monitored every 2 to 4 weeks. Gold salts can also cause elevated liver enzymes.

Other Disease-Modifying Antirheumatic Drugs

- ❐ Azathioprine (IMURAN); (🍁) IMURAN
- ❐ Cyclophosphamide (CYTOXAN, NEOSAR); (🍁) CYTOXAN, PROCYTOX
- ❐ Hydroxychloroquine (PLAQUENIL); (🍁) PLAQUENIL

TABLE 15–6 PHARMACOKINETICS OF SELECTED DISEASE-MODIFYING ANTIRHEUMATIC DRUGS

Drug	Route	Onset	Peak	Duration	PB (%)	$t_{1/2}$
Gold Products						
Auranofin	po	3–6 mo*	8–16 wks*	6 mo	60	26 days; 40–128 days†
Aurothioglucose	IM	6–8 wks*	1–2 mo	6 mo	85–95	3–26 days; 40–128 days†
Gold sodium thiomalate	IM	6–8 wks*	1–2 mo	6 mo	85–95	14–10 hrs; 168 hr‡
Others						
Azathioprine	po	6–8 wks	12 wks	UK	UA	3 hr
Cyclophosphamide	po	7 days	7–15 days	21 days	Low§	4–6.5 hr
Hydroxychloroquine	po	Rapid	1–2 hr	Days-wks	45	72–120 hr
Methotrexate	po, IM	4–7 days	7–14 days	21 days	50	2–4 hr
Penicillamine	po	1–3 mo	UK	1–3 mo	UA	60 min
Sulfasalazine	po	Varies	1.5–6 hr ‖	UA	UA	8.4–10.4 hr

* Peak blood levels and anti-inflammatory effects of gold products.
† Half-life of gold compound in the blood and tissues, respectively.
‡ Half-life of a single dose of gold sodium thiomalate; 14–40 hours by the third dose and up to 168 hours after the 11th dose.
§ Protein binding of cyclophosphamide is very low; however, protein binding of its active metabolites is over 60 percent.
‖ Peak effects of enteric coated sulfasalazine occur in three to 12 hours.
PB, Protein binding; $t_{1/2}$, elimination half-life; UK, unknown; UA, unavailable.

TABLE 15–7 DRUG-DRUG INTERACTIONS OF SELECTED DISEASE-MODIFYING ANTIRHEUMATIC DRUGS

Gold Compounds		
Gold compounds	Antineoplastics Radiation therapy	Additive myelosuppressive effects
Others		
Azathioprine	Antineoplastics Cyclosporine Myelosuppressive drugs	Additive myelosuppression
	Allopurinol	Inhibits the release of azathioprine increasing toxicity
	Live virus vaccines	Decreased antibody response and increased risk of toxicity
Cyclophosphamide	Rifampin Phenobarbital	Increased toxicity of cyclophosphamide
	Cocaine	Prolonged effects of interactive drug
	Allopurinol	Exaggerated bone marrow suppression
	Succinylcholine	Prolonged neuromuscular blockade
	Cytarabine Daunorubicin Doxorubicin	Cardiotoxicity may be additive
	Warfarin	Potentiates effect of interactive drug
	Live virus vaccines	Decreased antibody response and increased risk of toxicity
Hydroxychloroquine	Penicillamine	Increased risk of hematologic toxicity
	Digoxin	Increased risk of digoxin toxicity
	Urinary acidifiers	Increased renal excretion of hydroxychloroquine
Methotrexate	High dose salicylates NSAIDs Oral hypoglycemics Phenytoin Tetracyclines Probenecid Chloramphenicol	Increased risk of methotrexate toxicity
	Hepatotoxic drugs	Increased risk of hepatotoxicity
	Nephrotoxic drugs	Increased risk of nephrotoxicity
	Live virus vaccines	Decreased antibody response to interactive drug
	Asparaginase	Decreased effects of methotrexate
Penicillamine	Antineoplastics Immunosuppressive drugs Gold compounds	Increased risk of adverse hematologic effects
	Iron supplements	Concurrent administration decreases absorption of penicillamine
	Digoxin	May decrease serum levels of interactive drug
Sulfasalazine	Salicylates	Decreased effectiveness of sulfasalazine
	Glyburide Tolbutamide Warfarin	Increased effectiveness of interacting drug
	Acetaminophen	Increased risk of hepatotoxicity
	Beta blockers Cardiac glycosides	Reduced serum concentrations of interactive drug
	Cyclosporine	Additive nephrotoxicity and reduced plasma concentrations of interactive drug

- ❐ Methotrexate (FOLEX, MEXATE, RHEUMATREX); (🍁) METHOTREXATE
- ❐ Penicillamine (CUPRIMINE, DEPEN); (🍁) CUPRIMINE, DEPEN
- ❐ Sulfasalazine (AZULFIDINE); (🍁) PMS SULFASALAZINE, SALAZOPYRIN, SAS-500

AZATHIOPRINE

Azathioprine is a cytotoxic immunosuppressive drug that is used in the treatment of severe, active, erosive rheumatoid arthritis that is unresponsive to more conventional therapy. The antiarrhythmic effects of azathioprine are equivalent to those of gold salts and penicillamine (see later). Azathioprine antagonizes purine metabolism with subsequent inhibition of DNA and RNA synthesis. The benefits are the result of suppression of cell-mediated immunity and altered antibody formation. In addition to its use in arthritis, azathioprine is used to prevent organ rejection in patients receiving kidney transplants.

The most common adverse effects are fever, chills, anorexia, nausea, vomiting, and hepatotoxicity. Leukopenia, anemia, pancytopenia, and thrombocytopenia has also been noted. Serum sickness can be life-threatening. Azathioprine is teratogenic and should not be used during pregnancy. The drug may pose a small risk of malignancy.

Azathioprine is readily absorbed following oral administration. The onset of its anti-inflammatory effects occurs within 6 to 8 weeks, with peak action noted in 12 weeks. The duration of anti-inflammatory action is unknown. Azathioprine is biotransformed to mercaptopurine, which is metabolized further.

Drug-drug interactions include an additive myelosuppression with antineoplastics, cyclosporin, and myelosuppressants. Allopurinol inhibits the biotransformation of aza-

TABLE 15–8 DOSAGE REGIMEN OF SELECTED DISEASE-MODIFYING ANTIRHEUMATIC DRUGS

Gold Compounds			
Auranofin	Progressive rheumatoid arthritis resistant to conventional therapy	*Adult:* 6 mg/day po in one to two divided doses. May increase to 9 mg/day in three divided doses if no improvement occurs after 6 months	Take with meals.
Aurothioglucose		*Adult:* 10 mg IM first week, then 25 mg IM 2nd and 3rd week, then 25–50 mg/week until improvement or toxicity occurs. (Up to 1 g total.) Maintenance dose is 25–50 mg. q2 weeks for up to 20 weeks, then q3–4 weeks *Child age 6–12 yr:* 2.5 mg first week, then 6.25 mg. 2nd and 3rd week, then 12.5 mg weekly until a total of 200–250 mg has been given. Maintenance dose is 6.25–12.5 mg q3–4 weeks	Change needles after withdrawal of drug into syringe. Patient to remain recumbent for 15 minutes after injection. Closely monitor for nitritoid or allergic reaction. Injections may be followed by joint pain for 1–2 days. Never administer IV
Gold sodium thiomalate		*Adult:* 10 mg IM initially, then 25 mg IM 1 week later, followed by 25–50 mg IM weekly until improvement or toxicity occurs. Up to 1 g total, then 25–50 mg IM q2weeks for up to 20 weeks, then q3–4 weeks *Child:* 10 mg IM initially followed 1 week later by 1 mg/kg. q2weeks for up to 20 weeks, then q3–4 weeks	If patient has history of previous mild reaction: reinstitute with initial dose of 5 mg, increasing by 5–10 mg weekly or monthly until a dose of 25–50 mg is reached
Others			
Azathioprine	Severe, erosive rheumatoid arthritis unresponsive to conventional therapy	*Adult:* 1 mg/kg/day po for 6–8 weeks. Increase dose by 0.5 mg./kg. q4wk until desired response is reached or 2.5 mg/kg/day. Decrease dose by 0.5 mg./kg. q4–8 weeks to a minimum effective dose	May be administered with or after meals or in divided dose to minimize nausea
Cyclophosphamide	Severe, erosive rheumatoid arthritis unresponsive to conventional therapy	*Adult:* 1–5 mg/kg/day po, although many treatment regimens are used	Clarify dose to ensure cumulative dosage is not confused with daily dose. Errors may be fatal
Hydroxychloroquine	Severe rheumatoid arthritis and systemic lupus erythematosus	*Adult:* 400–600 mg po QD initially, then maintenance dose of 200–400 mg/day *Child:* 3–5 mg/kg/day. Not to exceed 7 mg/kg/day or 400 mg	May require up to 6 months for full benefit. Administer with food or meals
Methotrexate	Rheumatoid arthritis resistant to conventional therapy	*Adults:* Therapy is preceded by a 5–10 mg test dose. Therapy started at 7.5 mg. po weekly (2.5 mg. po q12hr for 3 doses.) Not to exceed 20 mg./week	Dosage should be decreased once desired response is obtained. Monitor liver function tests
Penicillamine	Rheumatoid arthritis resistant to conventional therapy	*Adult:* 125–250 mg/day po as single dose. May be slowly increased up to 1–1.5g/day	Monitor 24-hr urinary protein levels every 1–2 weeks in patients with moderate proteinuria. Monitor liver function tests every 6 mo during first 18 mo of therapy
Sulfasalazine	Management of rheumatoid arthritis (unlabeled use)	*Adult:* Initial: 3–4 g po daily in divided doses. Maintenance: 500 mg po QID. Dosage intervals should not exceed 8 hours	Monitor periodically for hepatitis and bone marrow suppression

thioprine, thus increasing the risk of toxicity. The dosage of azathioprine should be reduced by 25 to 33 percent with concurrent use of allopurinol. Like other DMARDs, azathioprine decreases the antibody response to live virus vaccines and increases the risk of adverse effects.

The initial dose of azathioprine for the treatment of arthritis is 1 mg/kg/day for 6 to 8 weeks. The dose may be increased by 0.5 mg/kg every 4 weeks until the desired response is elicited or 2.5 mg/kg/day is reached. The dose should then be decreased by 0.5 mg/kg every 4 to 8 weeks to the minimum effective dose.

Azathioprine decreases serum and urine uric acid, and plasma albumin levels. Renal, hepatic, and hematologic functions should be monitored before and throughout the course of therapy. Monitoring should occur weekly during the first month, bimonthly for the next 2 to 3 months, and monthly thereafter. The health care provider should be notified if the leukocyte count is less than 3000 mm^3 or the platelet count is less than 100,000 mm^3. A reduction in dosage or a temporary interruption in therapy may be warranted. Decreased hemoglobin levels may indicate bone marrow suppression. Although hepatotoxicity is rare when azathioprine is used to treat arthritis, it is indicated by increased alkaline phosphatase, bilirubin, AST (SGOT), ALT (SGPT), and amylase concentrations. Elevated liver function test values are reversible on discontinuation of azathioprine.

CYCLOPHOSPHAMIDE

Cyclophosphamide is an alkylating antineoplastic drug and a derivative of nitrogen mustard. It has been used investigationally to treat rheumatoid arthritis by interfering with DNA replication and RNA transcription. Protein synthesis is ultimately disrupted. Cyclophosphamide also has immunosuppressant action in smaller doses.

The most common adverse effects include alopecia, anorexia, nausea, vomiting, and hematuria. Thrombocytopenia is also common. Leukopenia, pulmonary fibrosis, and myocardial fibrosis are life-threatening. Adverse effects are frequent with cyclophosphamide and include hemorrhagic cystitis with the potential for bladder carcinoma, immunosuppression leading to increased risk of infection (particularly herpes zoster), suppression of gonadal function in both women and men, and long-term effects of immunosuppression with an increased incidence of lymphoma and other hematologic malignancies. Because of these adverse effects, cyclophosphamide is reserved for patients with life-threatening complications of arthritis.

The inactive drug is well absorbed from the GI tract and is converted to active metabolites by the liver. It is widely distributed. There is limited penetration of the blood-brain barrier, but the drug crosses the placental membranes and enters breast milk. Thirty percent of the drug is eliminated unchanged in the urine. There are many drug-drug interactions with cyclophosphamide. Table 15–7 identifies the interactions.

The dosage of cyclophosphamide when used for rheumatoid arthritis is 50 to 100 mg/day or 1 to 5 mg/kg/day. This drug is discussed further in Chapter 30.

Cyclophosphamide may produce false-positive results in Papanicolaou (PAP) smears and suppresses positive reactions to skin tests for *Candida,* mumps, tuberculin testing (purified protein derivative), and *Trichophyton.* CBC, differential, and platelet counts should be done before and periodically during therapy. The nadir of leukopenia occurs in 7 to 12 days, with recovery occurring in 7 to 21 days. Nadir is the time point at which the white blood cell count or platelet count is at its lowest. Leukocyte values should be maintained at 2500 to 4000 mm^3. Cyclophosphamide may also cause thrombocytopenia, with the nadir occurring in 10 to 15 days. It rarely causes anemia. Blood urea nitrogen (BUN), creatinine, and uric acid levels should also be monitored before and throughout the course of therapy to detect nephrotoxicity. Liver function tests should be monitored for evidence of hepatotoxicity and urinalysis for evidence of hematuria or inappropriate secretion of antidiuretic hormone (which is evidenced by changes in specific gravity).

HYDROXYCHLOROQUINE

Hydroxychloroquine is classified as an antiarthritic and antimalarial drug. Traditionally, the drug was reserved for patients who were unresponsive to NSAIDs. Today the drug is prescribed earlier in the management of severe rheumatoid arthritis and SLE. It is used also for the suppression and prophylaxis of malaria (see also Chapter 27 for additional information on antimalarial drugs.)

The precise anti-inflammatory mechanism of action of hydroxychloroquine is unknown. Suppression of antigens causing hypersensitivity reactions and symptoms is thought to be the underlying mechanism.

There are many adverse effects of hydroxychloroquine, but the most common include nausea, vomiting, diarrhea, corneal changes, pruritus, and bleaching of the hair. The most serious adverse effects are retinal damage, agranulocytosis, and aplastic anemia. The retinal damage may be irreversible and can produce blindness. Visual loss is directly related to drug dosage. Because retinal damage is progressive and may continue even in the absence of continued drug use, therapy should be discontinued at the first sign of retinal changes. Fatalities have occurred with the ingestion of even three or four tablets of hydroxychloroquine, so the drug should be kept out of children's reach.

Hydroxychloroquine is well absorbed following oral administration and is widely distributed in body tissues. Like the gold salts, hydroxychloroquine has a delayed onset of action. It is 45 percent bound to plasma proteins and has a half-life of 72 to 120 hours (see Table 15–6). Full therapeutic effects take 3 to 6 months to develop. Partial biotransformation takes place in the liver, with a portion of the drug eliminated unchanged in the urine. There is some indication that the drug enters breast milk.

There is increased risk of hepatotoxicity when hydroxychloroquine is administered concurrently with other hepatotoxic drugs (see Table 15–7). It may increase the risk of hematologic toxicity when concurrently taken with penicillamine. When used concurrently with drugs having dermatologic toxicity, the patient's risk of dermatitis increases. Serum digoxin levels may be increased, and urinary acidifiers may increase the renal elimination of hydroxychloroquine.

The dosage of hydroxychloroquine is expressed in milligrams of hydroxychloroquine sulfate. Two hundred milligrams approximate 155 mg of hydroxychloroquine base. The initial dose is 200 mg twice daily (see Table 15–8). Maintenance dosages range from 200 to 400 mg/day. The daily dosage should not exceed 6.4 mg/kg of body weight.

METHOTREXATE

Methotrexate, a cytotoxic immunosuppressant drug, can relieve symptoms of severe arthritis. In some cases, prolonged remission may be induced. Other uses for methotrexate are discussed in Chapter 30. Methotrexate is a folic acid antagonist. The result is inhibition of DNA synthesis and cell reproduction.

Common adverse effects of methotrexate include stomatitis, anorexia, nausea, vomiting, and hepatotoxicity. Anemia, leukopenia, thrombocytopenia, and neuropathy are also fairly common occurrences. Pulmonary fibrosis is life-threatening.

Methotrexate should be used with caution in patients with creatinine clearance rates of less than 60 mL/minute and those who are of child-bearing age. Cautious use is also warranted in patients with active infections and decreased bone marrow reserve, in older adults, and in patients with chronic debilitating illnesses.

Small doses of methotrexate are absorbed from the GI tract. Larger doses are incompletely absorbed. It is actively transported across cell membranes to be widely distributed.

The drug crosses the placenta and enters breast milk in low concentrations. Methotrexate is eliminated mostly unchanged by the kidneys.

Many drug-drug interactions are associated with methotrexate. Drugs that increase the toxicity of methotrexate are identified in Table 15–7. Additive toxicity can occur with concurrent use of other hepatotoxic and nephrotoxic drugs. Methotrexate decreases antibody response to live virus vaccines and increases the risk of adverse effects.

Methotrexate therapy is preceded by a 5- to 10-mg test dose. Methotrexate may be administered once weekly, beginning with a 5-mg dose. The dosage is gradually increased to a maximum of 15 to 20 mg (see Table 15–8).

Methotrexate may cause elevated serum uric acid concentrations. CBC and differential values should be obtained before and frequently throughout therapy. The nadir of leukopenia and thrombocytopenia occurs in 7 to 14 days. Leukocyte and thrombocyte counts usually recover 7 days after the nadirs. Renal and hepatic function should be monitored before and throughout therapy.

PENICILLAMINE

Penicillamine is an analog of the amino acid cysteine and is a chelator of heavy metals. It is used in the management of progressive rheumatoid arthritis that is unresponsive to conventional therapy. It is also used for prophylaxis and treatment of copper deposition in Wilson's disease and in the management of recurrent cystine calculi. Penicillamine has also been used as an adjunct in the treatment of heavy metal poisoning, although it has not been FDA approved for such use.

The antirheumatic effect of penicillamine is related to multiple mechanisms. It reduces immunoglobulin synthesis by monocytes and lymphocytes, inhibits polymorphonuclear leukocytes and T-cell function, and possibly protects tissues from oxygen radical damage.

The most common adverse effects of penicillamine include anorexia, oral ulcerations, epigastric pain, nausea, vomiting, diarrhea, and altered taste perception. Bone marrow depression, proteinuria, and a generalized pruritus have also been noted. Polymyositis and a myasthenic syndrome are life-threatening adverse effects.

Penicillamine is well absorbed following oral administration, although its oral bioavailability is decreased in the presence of food, antacids, and iron supplements. The onset of antirheumatic effects occurs 1 to 3 months after administration, with a duration of action of 1 to 3 months (see Table 15–6).

Drug-drug interactions are relatively few but potentially serious (see Table 15–7). When it is used with antineoplastic or immunosuppressive drugs, penicillamine increases the risk of adverse hematologic effects. Iron supplements decrease drug absorption and serum digoxin levels. Daily requirements for pyridoxine (vitamin B_6) may be increased.

Penicillamine dosages range from 125 to 250 mg as a single daily dose (see Table 15–8). The dose is slowly increased as needed to 1 to 1 1/2 g/day. No pediatric dosage has been identified.

CBC with differential, platelet counts, and urinalysis (especially for protein and cells) should be performed at least every 2 weeks during the first 6 months of therapy and monthly thereafter, and after an increase in dose. Twenty-four–hour urinary protein levels should be monitored every 1 to 2 weeks in patients with moderate proteinuria. Liver function tests should be performed every 6 months during the first 18 months of therapy.

SULFASALAZINE

Sulfasalazine has been used for years to treat inflammatory bowel disease. It is now also being used to treat rheumatoid arthritis, although it is not FDA approved for such use. Sulfasalazine blocks PG synthesis, producing anti-inflammatory effects as well as antibacterial effects.

Frequent adverse effects of sulfasalazine include anorexia, nausea, vomiting, headache, and oligospermia. Occasionally, hypersensitivity reactions, rash, urticaria, pruritus, fever, and anemia have occurred. Tinnitus, hypoglycemia, diuresis, goiter production, and photosensitivity reactions are rare. Life-threatening adverse effects can include Stevens-Johnson syndrome, hematologic toxicities, hepatotoxicity, and nephrotoxicity, although they rarely occur. Sulfasalazine should be used with caution in patients with renal failure and in patients who are pregnant or lactating. It is specifically contraindicated for patients with allergies to sulfinpyrazone, phenylbutazone, or other pyrazoles; peptic ulcer disease and symptoms of other GI inflammation; and blood dyscrasias.

Sulfasalazine interferes with a variety of cellular and mediator aspects of inflammation. The drug is split by colonic bacteria into its two component parts—sulfapyridine and 5-aminosalicylic acid. 5-Aminosalicylic acid is poorly absorbed, whereas sulfapyridine (the active component) is biotransformed in the liver by acetylation. The time of drug onset varies, with peak drug action noted in 1½ to 6 hours. Its half-life ranges from 8 hours to more than 10 hours. Fifteen percent of sulfasalazine is eliminated unchanged in the urine and the remainder as metabolites.

Drug-drug interactions include decreased effectiveness with salicylates. There may be increased drug effects noted with antidiabetic drugs (i.e., tolbutamide and glyburide) and warfarin. There is an increased risk of hepatotoxicity with acetaminophen.

The initial dosage of sulfasalazine when used for arthritis is 500 mg/day. The dosage can be increased gradually to a maximum of 2 g/day in divided doses. The drug should be administered around the clock. Dosages of more than 4 g/day increase the risk of toxicity.

Periodic monitoring of liver function and hematologic activity is necessary with sulfasalazine therapy. Urinary glucose tests using the Benedict method may be falsely elevated.

Critical Thinking Process

Assessment

History of Present Illness

The course of most disorders that require nonopioid, antipyretic, anti-inflammatory drugs are variable. Thus, a detailed description of presenting symptoms must be elicited. Determine the location, severity, and length of time the disorder has been present and what the patient has done to treat the problem. Because the inflammatory response produces pain, evaluate the patient's pain level and tolerance. Ask the patient to describe tolerable pain and what he or she desires for relief. Be sure to inquire about prescription drugs and OTC preparations used. Determine whether or not the patient has been using alternative or complementary pain relief strategies. Ask whether symptoms the patient is experiencing have been accompanied by a fever. In many cases, the patient will note that he or she has had chills even though a temperature reading was never taken. For the patient with complaints of dysmenorrhea, elicit the timing of the discomfort and what the patient has tried for relief.

Assess the activity level of the patient with rheumatoid disorders and identify which activities are most impaired by the problem. Ask also what assistance has been needed with activities of daily living. The patient should understand that fatigue or malaise is not a sign of laziness but a symptom of an underlying problem.

Past Health History

Determine whether or not the patient has a history of renal, hepatic, peptic ulcer disease, or bleeding disorders. Inquire about past drug use including prescription and OTC drugs, alcohol, and street drugs. Do not forget to ask specifically about the use of OTC analgesic, antipyretic, or anti-inflammatory drugs and herbal remedies. If the patient has previously taken an NSAID, determine his or her reaction to the drug. Did the patient obtain therapeutic effects or experience undesirable adverse effects? Ask specifically about response to aspirin because a person who is allergic to aspirin is at risk for developing cross-allergenicity to the other NSAIDs.

Physical Exam Findings

Observe for overt signs of inflammation such as redness, warmth, and edema. Note objective findings associated with pain, including changes in heart rate, blood pressure, and respirations. Vasoconstriction, pallor, sweating, restlessness, and withdrawal are also possible.

Inspect all joints and body surfaces for redness, warmth, and edema even if the patient's complaint is isolated to a single joint. There may be other sources of the inflammation. Carefully examine the joints for crepitation, deformity, subluxation, and contraction. Note muscle atrophy or decreased subcutaneous tissue. Check vital signs, paying particular attention to temperature. Patients with a fever often present with hot, dry skin and a flushed face.

Diagnostic Testing

A patient with pain or fever related to inflammation may have an elevated white blood cell count. Because objective measurement of pain and inflammation is not usually possible, patients usually express an opinion about the level of discomfort. Determine the patient's pain level using a measurement scale like those previously discussed in Chapter 14.

Developmental Considerations

Perinatal If the patient is of child-bearing age, determine whether she is pregnant or nursing before using an NSAID. DMARDs and some NSAIDs are teratogenic, and still others have not been studied during pregnancy. It is clear that any drug or chemical administered to the mother is capable of crossing placental membranes to some extent to reach the fetus. Of great concern is whether the rate and extent of drug transfer are sufficient to result in significant concentrations in the fetus. The notion that the placenta is a barrier must be discarded.

Drug use in a pregnant woman presents unique problems for the health care provider. Not only must maternal pharmacologic mechanisms be taken into account but the fetus must always be kept in mind as a potential recipient of the drug (see Chapter 6). The FDA classification system for risk factors associated with systemic drug use in pregnancy should be consulted when assessing potential use of an NSAID. The upswing in breastfeeding and markedly increased parental concerns about health needs of the fetus have contributed to increased questioning of health care providers about the safety and potential toxicity of drugs. It has also increased interest in drug and chemicals that are eliminated in breast milk.

Pediatric In general, assessing the discomfort in children younger than age 5 years is difficult because of the varying levels of language development and comprehension. However, it is not impossible. Confounding variables to assessment include anxiety, fear, or loneliness; the lack of a good understanding of pain phenomena; and the relative lack of valid and reliable assessment techniques. Infants may cry and display muscular rigidity and thrashing behaviors. Toddlers and preschoolers may be aggressive or complain verbally of discomfort. School-age children express discomfort verbally or behaviorally, often with regression to behaviors used at younger ages. Adolescents are often reluctant to admit they are uncomfortable or need help.

Geriatric Many older adults are prone to GI bleeding and ulceration, renal damage, decreased hepatic function, and CNS changes. These persons also easily develop sodium and fluid retention, which exacerbates other medical problems such as congestive heart failure. Because the older adult commonly has reduced serum protein levels, drugs that are normally highly protein bound circulate freely and can produce toxicity. Older adults often do not complain of pain, and experience a higher peak and a longer duration of drug action than their younger counterparts. Assessment tools used with older adults need to be in large print. Keep in mind the patient's educational level.

Psychosocial Considerations

A psychological assessment is important because acute or chronic inflammation, pain, and fever can cause great anxiety in both the patient and the family. Determine the meaning of symptoms to the patient. Some perceptions and reactions are heavily based on expectations and learned responses; therefore, ask about actual or potential losses the patient may be experiencing.

There is a connection between nutritional status and rheumatoid conditions; hence, dietary assessment is equally important. Ask specifically about intake of milk, cheese, and yogurt because these foods have been known to reduce joint stiffness, pain, and swelling in some patients. Foods that contain eicosopentanoic acid, a fatty acid found in fish (e.g., salmon, mackerel, tuna, rainbow trout, and sardines), may also alleviate symptoms. Ask also about cereal grains (i.e.,

Case Study Rheumatoid Arthritis

Patient History

History of Present Illness

MJ is a 73-year-old female who comes today with complaints of right hip pain. She is accompanied by her daughter, who said MJ was unable to get out of bed this morning because of the pain in her hip. MJ reports she has been getting along fine by balancing rest and exercise, and by using indomethacin several times a day for inflammation and pain. Her daughter believes that the arthritis has progressed to the point where her current medication regimen is no longer effective. Patient and daughter now requesting additional assistance in managing disease.

Past Health History

MJ has an 11-year history of rheumatoid arthritis. Her daughter indicates that the arthritis started in her left hand and gradually affected both hands, feet, and knees. She had her left knee replaced at age 60 and her right knee replaced at 65. MJ has had several regimens of physical therapy since she was originally diagnosed. She has used salicylates and other NSAIDs in the past with varying degrees of success. Indicates she is very careful to take her medicine with food or milk. MJ denies drug or food allergies, history of renal, hepatic, or GI bleeding.

Physical Exam

Range of motion is restricted in MJ's wrist, elbows, ankles, and knees. There is lateral deviation of metacarpal joints bilaterally. Generalized discomfort to right hip on palpation. Passive and active ROM limited. Crepitation noted on movement of right hip. Temperature 98^{4}°F, pulse 80 bpm.

Diagnostic Testing

Radiograph of right hip reveals arthritic changes. CBC, UA, renal function, and liver function tests within normal limits. ESR is elevated, RF positive. ANA positive.

Developmental Considerations

When MJ's husband died last year she moved to a group home. She interacts with older adults in the home and needs assistance eating because of arthritic deformities in her hands. This dependency causes a great deal of distress to MJ. She wants to remain as independent as possible in spite of her need for assistance eating.

Psychosocial Considerations

MJ and her husband lived in a mobile home; he cared for her until his death. MJ has two married daughters who have families of their own. They visit her at the home and help with her care, when possible.

Economic Factors

MJ has a limited income and would prefer to "spend my money on good food rather than on expensive medicine for my joints." She has Medicare coverage for hospitalization only lacking coverage for office visits and pharmacy needs. Her family is unable to assist her with health care costs.

Variables Influencing Decision

Treatment Objectives

- Reduce pain and inflammation while maintaining existing joint function
- Preserve quality of life and ability to carry out activities of daily living

Drug Variables	*Drug Summary*	*Patient Variables*
Indications	Ibuprofen, sulindac, oxaprozin, methotrexate, sulfinpyrazone, auranofin, gold sodium thiomalate are all indicated for rheumatoid arthritis.	MJ is 73, with a negative history of GI, renal or hepatic disease. Her condition now warrants stepwise progression of drug therapy. Patient and daughter also requesting additional assistance in managing disease.
Pharmacodynamics	NSAIDs suppress the inflammatory response as well as relieving pain. DMARDs are disease modifying, with drug action different for each agent. Rheumatoid arthritis is an inflammatory condition that should be helped by drugs in either of these drug groups. Neither group will change the underlying disease process.	MJ's disorder is characterized by inflammatory changes of joints.

Adverse Effects/ Contraindications	The most common adverse effects of NSAIDs and DMARDs are GI distress and renal and hepatic dysfunction. Bleeding times can be altered by certain drugs. Regular monitoring of laboratory parameters and patient response will help minimize adverse effects.	MJ has had little if any problems from current treatment regimen. She has no known contraindications to use of any of the NSAIDs or DMARDs. Normal changes of aging may influence drug response and increase the risk of adverse effects.
Pharmacokinetics	The onset of drug action from NSAIDs is relatively short. The onset of drug action from DMARDs may take 4 days up to 6–8 weeks. Methotrexate has shortest onset time and peak.	There are no pharmacokinetic variables other than MJ's age-related changes that will impact the decision for which drug to use.
Dosage Regimen	Dosing frequency varies from 4 times daily to once weekly depending on agent chosen.	MJ desires the simplest, least expensive drug regimen possible.
Lab Considerations	All antirheumatic drug therapies require monitoring of urinalysis, CBC, liver and renal function on a regular basis.	MJ's visiting nurse can come to the home for blood draws. This should not be a determining factor.
Cost Index*	• Ibuprofen 1 • Sulindac 1 • Sulfinpyrazone 3 • Auranofin 3 • Oxaprozin 5 • Methotrexate 5 • Gold sodium thiomalate 5	Ibuprofen may be the least expensive drug but the frequency of administration makes it less desirable. Once-a-week dosing with methotrexate or gold sodium thiomalate may be less expensive in the long run. This will be a decision point.

Summary of Decision Points

- MJ's condition warrants stepwise progression in drug therapy.
- MJ has no known contraindications to use of any of the NSAIDs or DMARDs. Normal changes of aging may, however, influence drug response and increase the risk of toxicity.
- Methotrexate has the shortest onset time and peak drug action.
- Ibuprofen may be the least expensive drug but the frequency of administration makes it less desirable. Weekly dosing with methotrexate may be less expensive in the long run.

DRUG(S) TO BE USED

- Start methotrexate therapy preceded by a 5 to 10-mg test dose. Methotrexate 2.5 mg po q12 hr for 3 doses, then 7.5 mg. weekly.
- Stop indomethacin. Start ibuprofen 600-mg tab i po QID until desired response from methotrexate is achieved.

*Cost Index: 1 = $ < 30/mo.
2 = $ 30–40/mo.
3 = $ 40–50/mo.
4 = $ 50–60/mo.
5 = $ > 60/mo.

AWP of 100, 600-mg tablets of ibuprofen is approximately $5.
AWP of 100, 150-mg tablets of sulindac is approximately $26.
AWP of 100, 200-mg tablets of sulfinpyrazone is approximately $30.
AWP of 60, 3-mg tablets of auranofin is approximately $66.
AWP of 100, 600-mg tablets of oxaprozin is approximately $122.
AWP of 100, 2.5-mg tablets of methotrexate is approximately $300.
AWP of 10 mL 50 mg/mL injectable is approximately $102.
ANA, antinuclear antibody; DMARD, disease-modifying antirheumatic drug; ESR, erythrocyte sedimentation rate; GI, gastrointestinal; NSAIDs, nonsteroidal anti-inflammatory drugs; RF, rheumatoid factor; ROM, range of motion.

wheat, oat, rye), shrimp and intake of foods containing sodium nitrate (a food preservative). These foods can trigger joint problems in some patients (see Case Study—Rheumatoid Arthritis).

Analysis and Management

Treatment Objectives

The overall treatment objectives for patients receiving nonopioid analgesics, antipyretic, anti-inflammatory drugs depend on the reason for their use. Treatment objectives for patients with disorders characterized by inflammation and pain include reducing pain and inflammation while preserving joint function, preserving the quality of life, and the patient's ability to carry out activities of daily living. The treatment objective for fever is to return body temperature to a normal range and increase the patient's comfort. Treatment objectives for the patient who has recalcitrant rheumatic disease is to relieve discomfort, slow degeneration of tissues, and maintain the quality of life as much as possible.

Treatment Options

As discussed in Chapter 14, basic interventions of care for a patient with inflammatory and inflammation-related disorders include conservative, nondrug measures such as alleviating anxiety, combating anticipatory fears related to pain, and providing physical and emotional care (e.g., meditation, relaxation, guided imagery, rhythmic breathing, and biofeedback). Balancing rest and exercise regimens, physical therapy, and appropriate use of complementary, alternative therapies (e.g., acupressure, acupuncture, hypnosis) is included in the plan of care.

Drug Variables

Nonsteroidal Anti-Inflammatory Drugs Management of mild to moderate inflammation and pain should begin with an NSAID, unless otherwise contraindicated. There are no predictive measures for deciding to which NSAID a patient will respond. All NSAIDs reduce inflammation, pain, and edema and improve movement when used in sufficient dosages.

Ibuprofen may be used for some patients when inflammation is thought to play a role in the disorder. It causes less GI irritation than does non–enteric-coated aspirin but is more expensive. However, it causes more GI distress than acetaminophen. Naproxen can also be used for its anti-inflammatory effect, and it has a convenient once or twice daily dosing schedule. However, naproxen is 20 times more potent than aspirin, whereas ibuprofen, fenoprofen and aspirin are roughly equipotent in this action. Indomethacin has a high incidence of adverse effects and drug-drug interactions, and therefore, therapy should not begin with this drug. Further, pain management should not be started with piroxicam because its long half-life does not allow the flexibility of rapid dosing. Piroxicam should be used only for maintenance therapy.

Seventy to eighty percent of patients with chronic rheumatic disorders follow a cyclic course of remissions and exacerbations. About 10 percent of patients have one to two acute exacerbations, then achieve a long-lasting remission for several years. Another 3 to 10 percent of patients have progressive inflammatory, painful disorders with no remission. These people generally respond poorly to treatment. During remission, the lowest effective dosage of an NSAID should be used to maintain control. Thus, it is important to know the onset time of anti-inflammatory drug action.

The onset of drug action occurs in about 7 days for ibuprofen, tolmetin, diclofenac, and ketoprofen, and in 14 days for sulindac, flurbiprofen, naproxen, and piroxicam. The dosage should be increased if initial drug dosages are not effective at the end of this period. If maximum dosages are also not effective in a similar time period, a different NSAID should be prescribed.

When changing drug therapies, there is little evidence that choosing a drug from another NSAID class significantly benefits the patient. It is sufficient to merely switch to another drug with a shorter half-life. The decision about which drug to use is based on potential toxicities, concomitant disease, and cost.

Further, there is no clear evidence that NSAIDs vary in their ability to cause GI distress, nephrotoxicity, and hepatotoxicity. Trends suggest that the least GI toxic NSAIDs are usually enteric-coated aspirin, ibuprofen, and salsalate (Table 15–9). The most GI toxic agents are indomethacin, tolmetin, ketoprofen, and meclofenamate.

All NSAIDs have the potential to produce nephropathy. Sulindac, piroxicam, and nabumetone generally produce the least toxic effects on the kidneys, although drug-induced nephrotic syndrome has been reported with indomethacin, ibuprofen, naproxen, fenoprofen, sulindac, and tolmetin. Fenoprofen has been implicated in 71 percent of the cases of nephrotic syndrome. Sustained-release NSAIDs appear to be as effective as regular release forms but long-term study is needed before definitive declarations can be made about efficacy and toxicity.

NSAIDs relieve symptoms rather quickly but do not retard the progression of disease. NSAIDs are generally safer than DMARDs and corticosteroids and require less vigorous monitoring. DMARDs have a delayed onset of action (typically 3 to 5 months) and, hence, are also known as slow-acting antirheumatic drugs. DMARDs may retard the progression of arthritis but are more toxic NSAIDs and require more vigorous monitoring. Corticosteroids rapidly relieve symptoms but do not retard the progression of rheumatoid arthritis. Because of the toxicity, corticosteroids are usually reserved for short-term therapy. Figure 15–3 illustrates the stepwise progression of drug selection for the patient with rheumatic disorders. As noted, NSAIDs are the initial drugs of choice. Aspirin or another salicylate are often chosen first because of their reduced cost. If the adverse effects of salicylates are intolerable, one of the newer, nonsalicylate NSAIDs may be chosen. If rheumatic symptoms cannot be controlled with an NSAID, a DMARD is warranted. Unfortunately, the DMARDs are more toxic than NSAIDs and take several months to produce effects. Because therapeutic effects are delayed, therapy with an NSAID should be continued until the DMARD has produced an adequate response. Rheumatologists have conflicting viewpoints about whether gold salts, hydroxychloroquine, methotrexate, or sulfasalazine is most effective. Azathioprine, penicillamine, and cyclophosphamide should be used only when first line DMARDs have been ineffective.

Concurrent use of opioids and NSAIDs often provide more effective analgesia than either drug class alone. Even

TABLE 15–9 RELATIVE POTENTIAL FOR NSAID-INDUCED TOXICITIES

NSAID	GI Distress	Nephrotoxicity	Hepatotoxicity
Choline salicylate	+		
Diclofenac	++	++	
Diflunisal	+++		
Enteric-coated aspirin	+		
Etodolac	+*		
Fenoprofen	++	+++	
Flurbiprofen	+++	++	
Ibuprofen	++	++	+
Indomethacin	+++	++	
Ketoprofen	+++		
Ketorolac	*		
Magnesium salicylate	+		
Meclofenamate	++		
Mefenamic acid		++	
Nabumetone	+	+	
Naproxen	++	++	+
Oxaprozin	*		
Piroxicam	+++	+	+
Salsalate	+		
Sodium salicylate	+		
Sulfasalazine	++	0	++
Sulindac	+++	+	
Tolmetin	++	+	+

+++, Considered to be the most toxic, often requires withdrawal of the drug; ++, frequent incidence of GI adverse effects, may need to add cytoprotective agent to treatment regimen; +, considered to be the least toxic, mild, usually no change in drug therapy is required; 0, no toxicity documented; GI, gastrointestinal; NSAID, nonsteroidal anti-inflammatory drug.

*Risk of GI distress to etodolac, ketorolac, and oxaprozin is not fully established.

Note: No information available for areas without designation.

when they are inadequate alone to manage pain, NSAIDs have pivotal opioid dose-sparing effects and can be used to reduce the adverse effects associated with opioids. However, NSAID dosages should be titrated to maximum and taken on a regular schedule before changing a patient from NSAIDs to opioids. If regularly scheduled NSAIDs are not effective, a combination of an NSAID with an opioid (e.g., aspirin with oxycodone) may be effective. Although it is likely that NSAIDs also act within the CNS in contrast to opioids, they do not cause sedation or respiratory depression, nor do they interfere with bowel or bladder function.

If noninflammatory mechanisms (e.g., headache or muscle aches) are thought to be causing mild pain symptoms, acetaminophen is effective, inexpensive, and produces little, if any, GI toxicity. The lifetime risk for neuropathy secondary to acetaminophen increases when 5000 tablets of acetaminophen have been taken.

Disease-Modifying Antirheumatic Drugs If DMARDs are to be used at an early stage in disease, it is important that their potential adverse effects are recognized. Treatment should be chosen to provide maximum benefit to the patient without harm. In using DMARDs and cytotoxic therapies, it

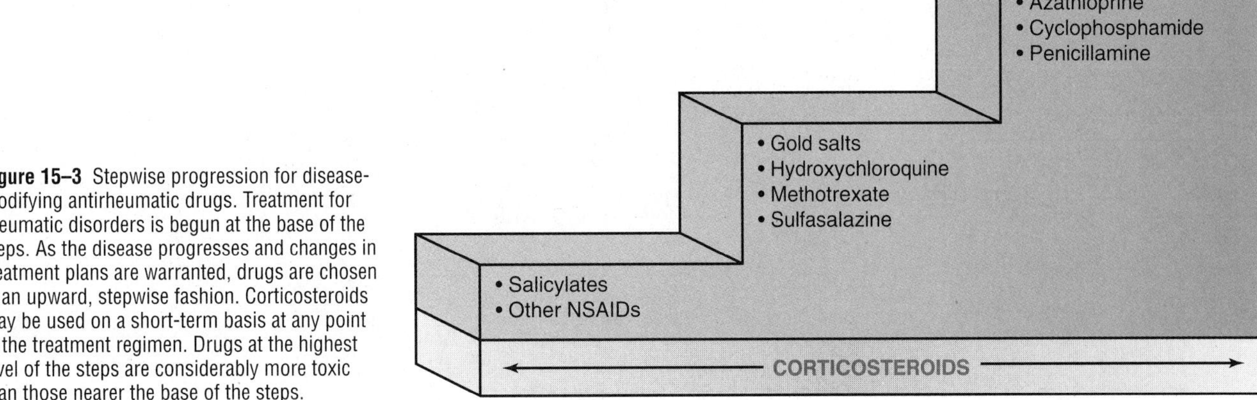

Figure 15–3 Stepwise progression for disease-modifying antirheumatic drugs. Treatment for rheumatic disorders is begun at the base of the steps. As the disease progresses and changes in treatment plans are warranted, drugs are chosen in an upward, stepwise fashion. Corticosteroids may be used on a short-term basis at any point in the treatment regimen. Drugs at the highest level of the steps are considerably more toxic than those nearer the base of the steps.

is important to try to answer three questions: (1) What drugs are available? (2) Is there a rationale for choosing one drug over another? (3) How do we tell whether the drug is working or producing adverse effects?

Methotrexate is the fastest acting of the DMARDs. Therapeutic effects can be seen as early as 3 to 6 weeks. Many rheumatologists consider methotrexate the first-line drug among the DMARDs. However, experience with methotrexate remains relatively limited, and long-term risk of toxicity is not yet clear. Table 15–10 provides an overview of relative GI, renal, and hepatic toxicity for DMARDs.

Patients with rheumatoid arthritis often remain on methotrexate for a longer period of time than with other DMARDs. Liver biopsy has been recommended in the past to monitor the presence and extent of hepatotoxicity. However, the question of when or if to biopsy the liver of patients on long-term methotrexate remains controversial. The decision to biopsy should be made on an individual basis and determined by previous hepatic disease, length of time on and dose of methotrexate, and other risk factors. Many health care providers recommend a liver biopsy after a cumulative methotrexate dose of 1.5 to 2 g or every 2 to 3 years.

Therapeutic effects of gold salts take 4 to 6 months to be noticed. Until a response to the gold salts has occurred, concurrent treatment with NSAIDs is warranted. If remission is less than complete once gold salts have reached maximum dosages, continued use of NSAIDs will be needed. Injectable gold salts are of similar efficacy to other DMARDs, including penicillamine, sulfasalazine, azathioprine, and methotrexate. Few patients remain on gold therapy for more than 5 years because of lack of or loss of efficacy and adverse effects. Because patients receiving IM gold therapy require repeated injections over a prolonged period, oral formulations are more convenient and less toxic than IM gold salts. Unfortunately, however, the oral formulation is also less effective. Many rheumatologists believe that once any toxicity has occurred, further use of gold salts should be avoided. The chances of severe toxicity can be minimized by starting therapy at low doses. If protein is found on urinalysis, gold therapy should be discontinued immediately. If the adverse effects are relatively mild, therapy can be resumed 2 to 3 weeks after symptoms have abated. Gold salts may be acceptable options for patients who are compliant with the need for regular office visits and laboratory work.

Penicillamine is about as effective as parenteral gold salts or azathioprine in the management of arthritis. There is conflicting data as to whether penicillamine prevents joint erosion in rheumatoid arthritis. More than 25 percent of patients taking penicillamine will have to discontinue the drug because of adverse effects within the first 12 months of therapy.

Sulfasalazine may be an initial choice more often in patients with reactive arthritis. Sulfasalazine would seem to have similar efficacy to gold and penicillamine, although comparative trials have not been sufficient to demonstrate differences. It is thought to retard progression of joint deterioration and may be superior to hydroxychloroquine in this regard. It may have comparable efficacy to parenteral gold salts but with less toxicity. GI adverse effects can be minimized by using enteric-coated formulations and by dividing the daily dosage. Some health care providers have noted that sulfasalazine was as effective as IM gold salts and caused less toxicity. Approximately 50 percent of patients on sulfasalazine develop adverse effects, and in the majority of cases, these occur within the first 4 months of therapy.

Patient Variables

For reasons not understood, patients often respond better to one NSAID than another. Further, some patients tolerate one NSAID better than another. Thus, to optimize therapy, treatment trials with more than one NSAID may be necessary. Because aspirin is such a familiar drug, many patients are suspicious of its efficacy. Consequently, if compliance is to be achieved, an attempt must be made to persuade patients that aspirin is in fact an effective drug. In some cases, using a prescription formulation may convince the patient that aspirin is indeed a genuine, effective drug.

There is an epidemiologic relationship between aspirin use in children and adolescents and *Reye's syndrome.* Although it is a rare but fatal disorder, Reye's syndrome is often the sequela of varicella and other viral infections. The mortality rate is between 20 to 30 percent. Reye's syndrome is characterized by encephalopathy, hepatic damage, and other serious problems. Salicylates may precipitate or accentuate this disorder but there is no equivocal proof at this time that aspirin use is a major causative factor. Nevertheless, children

TABLE 15–10 RELATIVE POTENTIAL FOR DMARD-INDUCED TOXICITIES

DMARD	GI Distress	Nephrotoxicity	Hepatotoxicity
Auranofin	+++	+	+
Aurothioglucose	+	++	+
Azathioprine	++	0	++
Cyclophosphamide	++	0	0
Gold sodium thiomalate	+	++	+
Hydroxychloroquine	++	0	0
Methotrexate	+++	0	++
Penicillamine	++	++	+
Sulfasalazine	++	0	++

+++, Considered to be the most toxic, often requires withdrawal of the drug; +, considered to be the least toxic, usually no change in drug therapy required; 0, no toxicity documented, DMARD, disease-modifying antirheumatic drug.

and adolescents who have influenza or chicken pox should abstain from the use of salicylates. Acetaminophen can be used for fever reduction and minor pain relief. It is the drug of choice for the child with febrile illness and older adults with impaired renal function (see Controversy—Salicylates and Reye's Syndrome).

Patients who are sensitive to aspirin should avoid taking NSAIDs. Acetaminophen, along with DMARDs, can be used to relieve pain for patients with rheumatic disorders. Naproxen, ibuprofen, tolmetin, and piroxicam are less likely to produce elevated liver enzymes in patients with alcohol abuse and pre-existing liver disease. The effects of fluid accumulation and edema caused by NSAID use should be considered in patients with diseases such as congestive heart failure and hypertension.

Aspirin should be used cautiously in patients taking anticoagulants because both drugs compete for plasma protein binding. Cautious use is also warranted in patients with severe hepatic damage, hyperprothrombinemia, vitamin K deficiency, and hemophilia.

Indomethacin and ibuprofen should be used cautiously in patients with cirrhosis or ascites and in patients with significantly altered hemodynamic status. These patients can experience as much as a 50-percent decrease in creatinine clearance rates when these drugs are used.

Several NSAIDs relieve pain after relatively minor surgical procedures such as dental extractions and episiotomies. Cautious use, however, is warranted because of an increased risk of bleeding. The drugs should not be given if the patient has other risk factors for bleeding. Ketorolac is the only parenteral NSAID available for postoperative patients who need to be alert, who are at risk for respiratory depression from opioids, or who are unable to tolerate opioids. In some patients, ketorolac can also be used in conjunction with opioids to decrease the amount of opioid required.

Some patients are at higher risk for adverse effects and mortality from NSAID use. These patients include older adults, those with debilitating disease, those with a history of GI ulcerations or intolerance to enteric coated aspirin, and those who abuse alcohol or use tobacco. High-dose NSAID use also contributes to a higher risk. Table 15–11 provides an overview of drugs that may be recommended for various conditions, disorders, diseases, and co-morbid states.

Evidence suggests that H_1 antagonists (e.g., cimetidine, ranitidine, and famotidine), antacids, and sucralfate do not prevent NSAID-induced ulcers (see Chapter 42). Misoprostol, a PgE_1 analog, acts on PgE_2 receptors to increase mucus formation and decrease gastric acid secretion. As a cytoprotective agent, misoprostol is helpful in reducing GI irritation from NSAIDs but it is expensive, and there is no firm evidence that it prevents ulcer complications and death. Because misoprostol stimulates uterine contractions, the drug is absolutely contraindicated in pregnancy.

Controversy

Salicylates and Reye's Syndrome: When to Use Aspirin?

JONATHAN J. WOLFE

Reye's syndrome is a grave disease that involves malignant elevation of intracranial pressure. If it is left untreated, the syndrome leads directly to irreversible brain damage or even death. Most troubling to the health care provider is the reality that Reye's syndrome is frequently an iatrogenic disease. Use of salicylates, particularly aspirin, in febrile children has been causally linked to the onset of Reye's syndrome. It is for this reason that baby aspirin has been banned from use in the United States.

The interventions required to manage Reye's syndrome are expensive. Patients are admitted to the intensive care unit to allow vigilant observance of vital signs. They may require risky invasive procedures in order to survive including induction of coma with barbiturates and the placement of an intracranial pressure monitoring device.

Clearly, prevention is the best solution for aspirin-induced Reye's syndrome. The axiom for treatment of flulike symptoms (aches, low-grade fever, headache) in children is now acetaminophen. Acetaminophen is cheap, universally available, and conveniently formulated in many strengths and dosage forms. It is difficult to imagine a reason to use any other antipyretic or analgesic in this susceptible patient population.

Critical Thinking Discussion

- At what age does a patient no longer display a significant risk for developing Reye's syndrome if treated with aspirin?
- Is it possible to draw a definite line using calendar age between various minor patients (e.g., infant, child, adolescent)? Is such an arbitrary classification possible for any drug?
- What about the time and effort that is expended in assigning blame when Reye's syndrome manifests itself in a patient?
- What is the ethical responsibility of a health care provider who has inadvertently administered aspirin to a febrile 10-year-old who subsequently presents with what appears to be Reye's syndrome?
- What safeguards ought to be in place within a health care system to prevent the use of hazardous therapies of any kind in vulnerable patient populations?
- What needs do you identify in a parent who has unknowingly administered aspirin to a child who is subsequently admitted to the intensive care unit for management of Reye's syndrome?

Intervention

Administration

NSAIDs should be administered 1 hour before or 2 hours after meals when a rapid initial effect is desired. To reduce the risk of esophageal irritation caused by NSAIDs lodging against the lining of the esophagus, a full glass of fluid or other food should be taken. Even though food delays drug absorption and decreases peak plasma levels of some of the drugs, it is probably safer to take them with food. The patient should be advised to remain upright for 15 to 30 minutes after taking the drug.

Pain relief provided by NSAIDs is subject to a ceiling effect. In other words, higher than recommended dosages may not necessarily provide additional therapeutic benefit in the treatment of pain unrelated to inflammation. Thus, the patient who omits a scheduled dose should not double the next dose but should resume the usual dosing schedule. Once pain is controlled, the average daily dosage should be decreased by 25 percent every 1 to 2 weeks until the minimum effective dose is reached. Once-daily or even as-needed dosing may be all that is required.

TABLE 15–11 INDICATIONS FOR NSAIDS IN CONDITIONS/DISORDERS/DISEASE AND CO-MORBID STATES

Conditions/ Disorders/ Disease and Co-morbid States	ACETAMINOPHEN*	ASPIRIN	DIFLUNISAL	SALSALATE	FENOPROFEN	FLURBIPROFEN	IBUPROFEN	INDOMETHACIN	KETOPROFEN	NAPROXEN	OXAPROZIN	ETODOLAC	KETOROLAC	NABUMETONE	SULINDAC	TOLMETIN	MECLOFENAMATE	MEFENAMIC ACID	DICLOFENAC	PIROXICAM
Acute gout						X		√		√		X			X					X
Acute painful shoulder						X		√				X							X	
Alcohol abuse										√										
Ankylosing spondylitis						X		√		√		X							√	
Anticoagulation therapy																√			√	
Antihypertensive therapy		√													√					
Aspirin allergy, polyps, asthma	√			√																
Aspirin, patient intolerance						√														
Bursitis, tendinitis						X		√		√		X			√					
Closure persistent ductus arteriosus								X†												
Cluster headache								X												
Compliance										√										
Congestive heart failure															√					√
Diuretic use by patient															√					√
Fever	√	√		√		X	√			X		√	√							
Gout								√												
Juvenile rheumatoid arthritis					X		X		X	√									X	
Lithium use		√													√					
Menorrhagia																	X			
Migraine																				
Abortive						X				X							X	X		
Menstrual					X				X	X							X	X		
Prophylactic					X			X	X	X										
Mild to moderate pain	√	√	√	√	√	√	√		√			√	√				√	√‡	X	
Older adult in general															√					
Osteoarthritis					√	√	√	√	√	√	√	√		√			√		√	√
Polyhydramnios								X												
Premenstrual syndrome										X								X		
Primary dysmenorrhea						X	√	X	√	√								√		X
Resistant acne vulgaris						X§														
Rheumatoid arthritis		√	√	√	√	√	√	√	√	√	√	X	√	√	√	√	√		√	√
Smoker						√														
Sunburn					X	X	X	X‖	X	X							X	X	X	

√ = FDA-labeled uses
X = Non–FDA-labeled uses
*Although acetaminophen is not considered an NSAID, it is included here because of its use as an analgesic and antipyretic.
†Intravenous indomethacin is FDA approved for this indication.
‡Mefenamic acid may be used to treat mild to moderate pain if used for less than one week.
§Ibuprofen may be used along with tetracycline for the treatment of persistent acne vulgaris.
‖Topical indomethacin may be used to prevent as well as treat sunburn.

TABLE 15–12 EXAMPLES OF OTC AND PRESCRIPTION PREPARATIONS CONTAINING SALICYLATES AND SALICYLATE-LIKE COMPOUNDS*

Examples of OTC Preparations Containing Salicylates	
Alka-Seltzer Effervescent Tablet	Buffets II Tablets
Alka-Seltzer Plus Cold Medicine	Buf-Tabs
Anacin and Anacin Maximum Strength Tablets	Carma Arthritis Strength Tablets
Arthralgen Tablets	Cope Tablets
Arthritis Pain Formula	Doan's Pills
Arthritis Strength Bufferin Tablets	Ecotrin Tablets
Arthropan Liquid	Emagrin Tablets
A.S.A. Enseals	Empirin Tablets
Ascriptin Tablets	Excedrin Tablets and Caplets
Ascriptin A/D Tablets	Maximum Bayer Aspirin
Ascriptin Extra-Strength Tablets	Mobigesic Tablets
Aspergum	Momentum Tablets
Bayer Aspirin Tablets	Pepto-Bismol Tablets and Liquid
Bayer Children's Aspirin Tablets	St. Joseph Aspirin for Adults
Bayer Children's Cold Tablets	St. Joseph Cold Tablets for Children
Bayer Timed Release 8-Hour Caplets	Stanback Powder
BC Tablet and Powder	Trigesic
Bufferin Arthritis Strength Tablets	Vanquish Caplets
Examples of Prescription Preparations Containing Salicylates	
Ascriptin with Codeine Tablets	Lanorinal Tablets
Axotal Tablets	Magan Tablets
Buff-A Comp Tablets and Capsules	Magsal Tablets
Buff-A Comp No. 3 Tablets (with codeine)	Mobidin Tablets
Darvon Compound Pulvules	Norgesic and Norgesic Forte Tablets
Darvon Compound-65 Pulvules	Percodan and Percodan-Demi Tablets
Disalcid Capsules	Robaxisal Tablets
Easprin	Soma Compound
Empirin with Codeine Tablets	Synalgos-DC Capsules
Equagesic Tablet	Talwin Compound Tablets
Fiorinal Tablets	Trilisate Tablets and Liquid
Fiorinal with Codeine	

*Not a complete listing. Other products may also contain aspirin, salicylates, and salicylamides. Occasionally, products are reformulated to add or remove salicylates.

Salicylate Toxicity Plasma salicylate levels should be measured periodically when large doses of salicylates are given for anti-inflammatory effects. Chronic administration of large doses saturates a major metabolic pathway, thereby slowing drug elimination, prolonging serum half-life, and causing drug accumulation. Drug accumulation can also occur with intentional overdose. A number of OTC and prescription preparations contain aspirin that can be easy sources of salicylate in overdose (Table 15–12). The health care provider should be aware of symptoms and signs and treatment of salicylism.

Acetaminophen Toxicity Liver damage related to acetaminophen overdose can be minimized by administering acetylcysteine. Although most effective when given shortly after acetaminophen ingestion, acetylcysteine can still provide significant protection when administered up to 24 hours after the poisoning has occurred. The health care provider should be aware of the signs and symptoms and treatment of acetaminophen toxicity.

Education

In order to fully participate in treatment, the patient must know the nature and time course of expected beneficial drug effects. With this information, the patient can help evaluate the success or failure of the treatment. Although nonopioid analgesic, antipyretic effects may become evident in a short time, in some cases, weeks or months may be required before beneficial anti-inflammatory effects are known. As previously discussed in Chapter 14, teaching nondrug measures for pain relief enhance the chance of success with drug therapy.

Just as patients must know when and how to take their drug, they must also know when to stop. Patients should be told to discontinue use of an NSAID when symptoms subside. However, in some patients, life-long treatment may be required, and still other patients may need to return for further evaluation. Patients who self-manage their NSAID or DMARD therapy should be advised as to the importance of periodic determinations of white blood cells, hemoglobin, and hematocrit levels.

Patients should be taught to notify their health care provider when they are taking OTC aspirin, ibuprofen, or other NSAIDs on a regular basis. Improvement in inflammatory disorders such as arthritis may take weeks. Patients should be advised that if one drug is ineffective, another may work because people vary in their response to drugs.

Patients on chronic aspirin therapy should be advised to terminate use 1 week before elective surgery. Because nabumetone and piroxicam have long half-lives, they should be discontinued approximately 1 week preoperatively. Most

SALICYLISM

Salicylism is a well-described syndrome that results from aspirin (or other salicylate) overdose. The overdosage required for a fatality to occur is extremely variable and depends on patient size, rate of absorption, and so forth. Mild salicylate toxicity is usually due to drug accumulation following chronic administration of 150 to 250 mg/kg body weight. Severe to lethal toxicity is found with doses exceeding 250 mg/kg. Methyl salicylate is particularly toxic in low doses, with fatalities reported following ingestion of even a single teaspoon (approximately 5 g). Toxicity is classified as mild, moderate, or severe based on plasma salicylate levels.

- *Mild toxicity:* plasma salicylate levels of 40 to 70 mg/dL.
- *Moderate toxicity:* plasma salicylate levels of 70 to 150 mg/dL.
- *Severe to lethal toxicity:* plasma salicylate levels above 150 mg/dL.

Early symptoms of salicylism include tinnitus, headache, nausea and vomiting, dizziness, and dimness of vision. The tinnitus is secondary to vasoconstriction of auditory microvasculature or to increased pressure within the labyrinth and effects on cochlear hair cells. High-frequency hearing loss is correlated with salicylate concentration but is reversible by discontinuing the drug.

Hyperventilation, an early sign of salicylate overdose, is almost always present. It is attributable to direct CNS-stimulating effects on respiratory centers and from the CO_2 that is generated by uncoupling of oxidative phosphorylation. The result is an initial respiratory alkalosis compensated in about 3 days by enhanced renal elimination of sodium and potassium bicarbonate. Compensated respiratory alkalosis in combination with the aforementioned symptoms is the usual presentation of salicylism in adults. Without intervention, respiratory alkalosis will be followed by metabolic acidosis as the patient's respiratory efforts weaken and CO_2 builds up.

Salicylism in children presents a more serious picture. Profound CNS effects occur including respiratory depression, marked hyperthermia, vomiting, diarrhea, and diaphoresis. The combined signs and symptoms produce a mixed acid-base imbalance, and respiratory and metabolic acidosis, ultimately leading to seizures, coma, and death.

The initial treatment of salicylism is directed toward reducing salicylate levels by reducing absorption and promoting elimination. Gastric lavage and activated charcoal (see Chapter 8) are often used. Hypovolemia, dehydration, and acid-base and electrolyte imbalances are corrected with IV fluids. Additional interventions may include hemodialysis, peritoneal dialysis, or exchange transfusions.

ACETAMINOPHEN TOXICITY

Acetaminophen overdose is the most common form of poisoning in children. Toxic doses in children are 150 mg/kg or greater. Toxicity from therapeutic use is rare but may occur with ingestion of approximately 150 mg/kg/day, or about double the recommended maximum therapeutic dose (90 mg/kg/day) for several days. Acetaminophen toxicity is defined as a plasma concentration of 200 mcg/mL.

Clinical manifestations of acetaminophen toxicity occur in four stages:

- *2 to 4 hours after ingestion:* nausea, vomiting, sweating, pallor
- *24 to 36 hours after ingestion:* symptoms lesson, patient's condition improves but level of toxic metabolite continues to rise
- *Days 2 to 7 after ingestion:* hepatic damage as evidenced by right upper quadrant pain, jaundice, confusion, stupor, laboratory abnormalities (increased AST [SGOT], ALT [SGPT], LDH, increased protime, hypoglycemia). Hepatic damage may be permanent.
- *After 7 days:* Patients who do not die during the stage of hepatic involvement gradually recover.

Liver damage related to acetaminophen overdose can be minimized by the timely administration of acetylcysteine (MUCOMYST). Acetylcysteine is a sulfhydryl compound that scavenges free radicals. The toxic metabolite of acetaminophen is thus inactivated. The drug is most effective when it is administered as soon as possible after the overdose. If acetylcysteine is administered 15 to 24 hours after ingestion, the incidence of severe liver damage increases to about 85 percent. Thus, the time between ingestion and treatment is critical.

First, the stomach should be emptied of its contents by inducing emesis or lavage. Acetylcysteine is available in 10- and 20-percent solutions that should be diluted to a final concentration of 1:3 for patients weighing up to 20 kg or with enough diluent to make a 5-percent solution for patients weighing more than 20 kg. It can be mixed with juice, cola, or water to increase the palatability. The initial loading dose is 140 mg/kg, followed by 70 mg/kg every 4 hours for up to 17 doses. Therapy can be discontinued when acetaminophen blood levels indicate a low risk of hepatotoxicity. Acetylcysteine has an extremely unpleasant odor, which may itself induce vomiting. If vomiting interferes with oral administration, the drug can be given through a nasogastric or orogastric tube.

other NSAIDs can be stopped 24 to 48 hours ahead of surgery.

A woman who is pregnant or who intends to become pregnant while using an NSAID or DMARD should be instructed to consult with her health care provider. These drugs may interfere with maternal and infant blood clotting and prolong the duration of pregnancy and parturition, or they may have teratogenic effects. If the mother intends to breastfeed, she should also consult with her health care provider because many of these drugs are detected in breast milk and are cleared slowly from the body of an infant.

The patient with co-morbid disorders (e.g., gastritis, ulcers, bleeding disorders, diabetes, or gout) or who is on anticoagulant therapy should discuss with the health care provider the addition of NSAIDs to the treatment regimen. Teach that acetaminophen is an effective aspirin substitute for pain or fever but not for inflammation or to prevent heart attack or stroke. Advise the patient with hypertension not to use effervescent aspirin products because of their high sodium content.

Because fever is one way the body fights infection, drug therapy may not be needed unless the fever is high or is accompanied by other uncomfortable signs and symptoms. Further, pain is not usually associated with the common cold, so analgesic-antipyretic drugs are used only for their fever-relieving characteristics. If acetaminophen use is required for more than 2 to 3 days, the health care provider should be contacted for further evaluation of the fever.

The patient should be taught to store NSAIDs and DMARDs in a closed child-proof container and keep it out of the reach of children. Additionally, it is wise to never call aspirin or other drugs "candy" because aspirin is a common cause of drug overdose in children. Further, advise the patient to discard salicylate tablets with a vinegar-like odor, a sign of salicylate deterioration.

Patients should be advised to avoid alcohol intake while they are taking NSAIDs. Alcohol intake produces synergistic effects with NSAIDs, thus increasing the risk of GI distress and bleeding. Some patients experience drowsiness and dizziness while taking NSAIDs. They should be cautioned about performing tasks that require alertness. Further, aspirin should not be taken concurrently with vitamin C products (e.g., orange juice) because it may contribute to increased gastric acidity.

Encourage the patient to report hearing changes because bilateral hearing loss of 30 to 40 decibels can occur with prolonged use of a salicylate. Reassure the patient that hearing usually returns to normal within 2 weeks after treatment is stopped.

Patients who are hypersensitive to salicylates should be advised to avoid salicylates and the other NSAIDs. Advise the patient with nasal polyps to avoid using acetylated salicylates for self-treatment of minor aches and pains because these drugs may induce an acute asthma attack. Nonacetylated salicylates may be used cautiously.

Patients should also be advised that aspirin is contained in many OTC products. In addition, there are many OTC products that contain acetaminophen, most with 500 mg of drug per tablet or capsule. Patients should be taught to read labels carefully to avoid duplicate sources of aspirin or acetaminophen and potential overdose. Overuse and overdose can be life-threatening. Patients should also be warned to avoid OTC products containing ibuprofen when they are also taking a prescription NSAID. Acetaminophen may be taken if needed for fever or pain.

Evaluation

Treatment effectiveness can be evaluated through patient reports of increased comfort and range of motion, increased mobility, and ability to perform the activities of daily living. Redness, warmth, edema, and pain are reduced or absent. If the drug is being administered for its antipyretic effects, the patient's temperature will be within the normal range. The patient is not expected to experience untoward effects of therapy. Because the health care provider has information about which activities were most impaired by the problem, this information can also be used as an indicator of improvement.

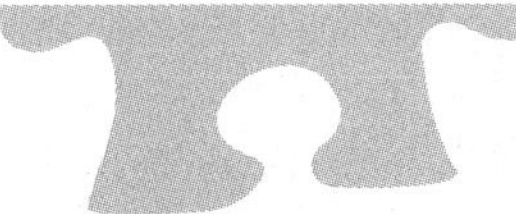

GOUT

Epidemiology and Etiology

Gout or gouty arthritis is a systemic disorder in which urate crystals deposit in joints and other body tissues. Inflammation results. Primary gout is inherited as an X-linked trait, meaning that males are affected via female carriers. About 25 percent of affected patients have a family history of gout. Eighty-five to ninety percent of patients with gout are middle aged and older men, and postmenopausal women. The peak onset of gout is between the ages of 30 and 40.

Secondary gout is caused by another disease or condition that produces elevated serum uric acid levels. It affects people of all ages. Renal insufficiency, certain antineoplastic drugs, and diuretics reduce elimination of uric acid, whereas multiple myeloma and some other cancers cause an increase in uric acid production. The end result is an imbalance between production and elimination rates.

Pathophysiology

There are four stages of primary gout: an asymptomatic hyperuricemia, acute gout, intercritical gout, and chronic gout. In *asymptomatic hyperuricemia,* there are no obvious signs and symptoms, thus the patient is usually unaware of the elevated serum uric acid levels.

Acute gout occurs as a result of an inflammatory reaction to deposits of sodium urate crystals (the end product of purine metabolism) in the synovium and other body tissues. There is a local infiltration of tissues by granulocytes, which phagocytize urate crystals. Lactate production is high in synovial tissues and in leukocytes associated with inflammation. The lactate production favors a local decrease in pH that fosters further deposition of urate crystals. Although PGs may be implicated in the pain and inflammation of gout and gouty arthritis, there is no evidence that they contribute to its pathogenesis.

With an acute attack the patient experiences excruciating pain and inflammation in one or more small joints, usually the metatarsophalangeal joint of the great toe. Seventy-five percent of all patients with gout have inflammation of the great toe joint as an initial manifestation.

Intercritical gout is a phase that can take months or years to develop. The patient is once again asymptomatic and no joint abnormalities are found on examination.

Chronic gout appears after repeated bouts of acute gout. Deposits of urate crystals develop within major organ systems, particularly the kidneys, and under the skin. Tophi, the chalky deposits of urate, typically form around the joints in cartilage, bone, bursae, subcutaneous tissues, and in the external ear (particularly the pinna). Kidney stones of urate crystals are more common in chronic gout than renal insufficiency.

PHARMACOTHERAPEUTIC OPTIONS

Antigout Drugs

- ❒ Allopurinol (LOPURIN, ZYLOPRIM)
- ❒ Colchicine (COLSALID); (🍁) NOVO-COLCHICINE

Indications

Allopurinol is effective for the treatment of both primary hyperuricemia and that which is secondary to hematologic disorders or antineoplastic therapy. It is generally used in severe chronic forms of gout characterized by one or more of the following: hyperuricemia not readily controlled by uricosuric drugs, tophaceous deposits, gouty nephropathy, renal urate stones, and impaired renal function.

Colchicine is a unique anti-inflammatory drug in that it is largely effective only against gouty arthritis. It provides dramatic relief of acute gout and is effective for prophylaxis, especially when there is frequent recurrence of attacks. Prophylaxis is indicated on initiation of long-term use of allopurinol or uricosuric drugs because acute attacks often increase in frequency during the early months of therapy.

Colchicine is also of benefit for the patient with primary biliary cirrhosis although the underlying disease may not be altered. It has also been employed to treat a variety of skin disorders including psoriasis and Behçet's syndrome (a multisystem illness characterized by lesions of the oral mucosa, genitalia, eyes, and skin). It has been approved as an orphan drug to arrest the progressive neurologic disability caused by multiple sclerosis.

Pharmacodynamics

An *antigout* drug acts to reduce the inflammatory process or to prevent the synthesis of uric acid. Allopurinol inhibits the terminal stages of uric acid synthesis. Both allopurinol and its primary metabolite alloxanthine are inhibitors of xanthine oxidase. Inhibition of this enzyme accounts for the major drug effects of allopurinol, a reduction of urates.

In contrast to allopurinol, colchicine is a particularly effective antigout drug, probably because of its effect on the mobility of granulocytes. It binds to microtubular proteins to interfere with function of the mitotic spindles and inhibits the migration of granulocytes to the inflamed area. The inhibition reduces the release of lactic acid and proinflammatory enzymes during phagocytosis. In other words, it breaks the cycle leading to inflammation. Colchicine also inhibits the release of histamine from mast cells and the secretion of insulin from beta cells of the pancreas.

Adverse Effects and Contraindications

Allopurinol's most common adverse effect is hypersensitivity. The reaction can occur even after months or years of drug use. The reaction is characterized predominantly by pruritus or an erythematous or maculopapular eruption. Occasionally, the lesions are exfoliative, urticarial, or purpuric. Fever, malaise, and muscle aches are also present. Transient leukopenia or leukocytosis and eosinophilia are rare reactions but may require stopping the drug. Other undesirable adverse effects include headache, drowsiness, nausea and vomiting, vertigo, diarrhea, and GI upset but usually do not require stopping treatment. Allopurinol is contraindicated in patients who have had serious adverse reactions, nursing mothers, and children except those who have a malignancy or certain inborn errors of purine metabolism.

Colchicine's most common adverse effect reflects drug action on rapidly proliferating epithelial cells of the GI tract, especially in the jejunum. Nausea, vomiting, diarrhea, and abdominal pain are the most common and the earliest signs of colchicine overdose. There is a latent period of several hours or more between the drug administration and the onset of symptoms. This interval is not altered by dose or route of administration. For this reason and because of individual variation, adverse effects may be unavoidable during the initial course of therapy. However, the patient remains relatively consistent in his or her response to the drug, and therefore, toxicity can be minimized or avoided during subsequent courses of therapy. The GI adverse effects may be almost completely avoided if colchicine is given IV.

Colchicine also produces a temporary leukopenia that is soon replaced by leukocytosis. Long-term administration of colchicine entails some risk of agranulocytosis, aplastic anemia, myopathy, and alopecia. Azoospermia has also been noted. It is contraindicated in patients who have severe GI disorders or creatinine clearance rates of less than 10 mL/minute. It should be used with caution in older adults and in patients who have creatinine clearance rates of 10 to 50 mL/minute. Safe use during pregnancy and lactation and in children has not been established.

Pharmacokinetics

Antigout drugs have paradoxical effects on uric acid levels. Depending on the dosage, they may either decrease or increase the elimination of uric acid. Decreased elimination usually occurs at low dosages while increased elimination is observed at higher dosages.

Allopurinol is rapidly absorbed following oral administration. Peak plasma concentrations are reached in 30 to 60 minutes (Table 15–13). It is rapidly cleared from plasma,

TABLE 15–13 PHARMACOKINETICS OF GOUT DRUGS

Drug	Route	Onset	Peak	Duration	PB (%)	$t_{1/2}$
Antigout Drugs						
Allopurinol	po	30–60 min; 24–48 hr*	1.5–4.5 hr; 1–3 wks†	18–30 hr; 1–2 wks‡	UA	1–2 hr; 18–30 hr§
Colchicine	po	20 min	0.5–2 hr	9 days	UA	20 min; 60 hr ‖
Uricosuric Drugs						
Probenecid	po	30 min	2–4 hr	5–8 hr	75	4–9 hr
Sulfinpyrazone	po	30 min	1–2 hr	4–6 hr	98–99	2.2–3 hr

* Onset times of allopurinol in the blood and therapeutic onset, respectively.
† Peak blood levels and therapeutic effects of allopurinol.
‡ Allopurinol's duration of action with effects lasting 1–2 weeks.
§ Allopurinol's half-life and half-life of metabolites, respectively.
‖ Half-life of colchicine in plasma and in white blood cells, respectively.
UA Unavailable

with approximately 20 percent of the drug eliminated in the feces in 48 to 72 hours. The half-life of allopurinol is 2 to 3 hours and is primarily converted to alloxanthine. The plasma half-life of alloxanthine is 18 to 30 hours in patients with normal renal function. Neither allopurinol or its metabolite plasma concentrations correlate well with therapeutic or toxic effects.

Colchicine is absorbed from the GI tract and then undergoes enterohepatic recirculation when more absorption may occur. It is distributed to white blood cells, where it concentrates. When it is given by mouth, the onset of colchicine occurs in 12 hours, with peak effects noted in 24 to 72 hours. Its duration of action is unknown. The plasma half-life is about 20 minutes, but the half-life in white blood cells is 60 hours. It is 30 to 50 percent protein bound. Biotransformation of colchicine takes place in the liver with elimination in the feces. Small amounts of colchicine are eliminated in the urine.

Drug-Drug Interactions

Allopurinol interferes with hepatic inactivation of other drugs including oral anticoagulants (Table 15–14). It is thought that there is an increased incidence of skin rash with concurrent administration of ampicillin. Hypersensitivity reactions have been reported in patients with compromised renal function who receive allopurinol and thiazide diuretics. Concurrent use of allopurinol and theophylline preparations leads to an increased concentration of theophylline's active metabolites. In contrast, colchicine has few drug-drug interactions. It may cause a reversible malabsorption of vitamin B_{12}.

Dosage Regimen

The initial dose of 100 mg of allopurinol is increased by 100-mg increments at weekly intervals to a maximum of 800 mg/day (Table 15–15). The usual maintenance dose for adults is 200 to 300 mg daily for those with mild gout and 400 to 600 mg for patients with moderately severe tophaceous gout. Doses exceeding 300 mg should be given in divided doses. Slow titration is recommended to prevent or minimize the risk of mobilization gout and to avoid sudden elimination of large amounts of uric acid through the kidney.

The prophylactic dose of colchicine depends on the frequency and severity of attacks. As little as 0.5 mg two to four times per week may be sufficient for some patients, whereas other patients may require as much as 1.8 mg/day. Colchicine should be given 3 days before and 3 days after surgery in patients with gout. This approach greatly reduces the very high incidence of acute attacks precipitated by operative procedures. For the treatment of acute attacks, a dose of 0.5 to 1.2 mg is given initially, followed by 0.5 to 0.6 mg every 1 to 2 hours or 1 to 1.2 mg every 2 hours until the patient experiences relief, has GI symptoms, or a total cumulative dose of 6 mg has been given. Colchicine may be used intermittently with 3 days between courses to decrease the risk of toxicity.

Laboratory Considerations

Serum uric acid levels usually begin to decrease 2 to 3 days after initiation of allopurinol therapy. Blood glucose levels should be monitored in patients receiving antidiabetic drugs because it may cause hypoglycemia. Hematologic, renal, and liver function testing should be performed before and periodically throughout therapy, especially during the first few months. Allopurinol may cause elevations in alkaline phosphatase, bilirubin AST (SGOT), and ALT (SGPT) levels. A decreased CBC and platelet level may suggest bone marrow depression. Elevated BUN, creatinine, and creatinine clearance levels may indicate nephrotoxicity. These values are usually reversed with discontinuation of therapy. Colchicine may interfere with the results of urinary 17-hydroxycorticosteroid concentrations.

Uricosuric Drugs

- ❐ Probenecid (BENEMID, PROBALAN)
- ❐ Sulfinpyrazone (ANTURANE); (🍁) ANTURAN, APO-SULFINPYRAZONE, NOVO-PYRAZONE

Indications

The use of probenecid and sulfinpyrazone for the mobilization of uric acid in chronic gout is well established. Probenecid was developed in response to a specific need. When penicillin was first developed, it was in short supply and the rapid renal elimination of the antibiotic thus had a practical significance. Researchers subsequently found an organic acid that would depress the tubular secretion of penicillin. The oral administration of probenecid in conjunction with penicillin-G results in higher, more prolonged serum concentration of the antibiotic than when penicillin is given alone. The increase in plasma is at least twofold and sometimes much greater.

TABLE 15–14 DRUG-DRUG INTERACTIONS OF GOUT DRUGS

Drugs	Interactive Drugs	Interaction
Antigout Drugs		
Allopurinol	Theophylline	Increased concentrations of interactive drug's metabolites
	Thiazide diuretics	Hypersensitivity reactions in patients with compromised renal function
	Oral anticoagulants	Increased effects of interactive drug
Colchicine	Vitamin B_{12}	May cause reversible malabsorption of interactive drug
Uricosuric Drugs		
Probenecid	Sulfonamides	Increases concentration of interactive drug in serum
Sulfinpyrazone	Probenecid	Additive effects to that of interacting drug
	Salicylates	Antagonizes effects of interactive drug
	Oral hypoglycemics	Inhibits metabolism of interacting drug

TABLE 15–15 DOSAGE REGIMEN OF GOUT DRUGS

Drug	Uses	Dosage	Implications
Antigout Drugs			
Allopurinol	Prophylaxis gouty arthritis	*Adult:* 100 mg po QD. Increase at weekly intervals based on serum uric acid level. Not to exceed 800 mg/day. Doses over 300 mg/day should be given in divided doses. Maintenance: 100–200 mg po BID-TID. Doses of less than 300 mg can be given as single daily dose	Take with milk or meals. Alkaline diet may be ordered. Large doses of alcohol decrease drug effectiveness
Colchicine	Acute gouty arthritis	*Adult:* 0.5–1.2 mg po, then 0.5–0.6 mg q1–2 hr *or* 1–1.2 mg q 2hr until relief, GI adverse effects, or a total cumulative dose of 6 mg is achieved. Prophylaxis: 0.5–0.6 mg po QD. May be used up to three times daily or as little as 1–4 times weekly. *or* 2 mg IV initially, then 0.5 mg q6hr *or* 1 mg q6hr until relief *or* cumulative dose of 4 mg has been given. Other regimens may use lower doses. Prophylaxis: 0.5–1 mg IV QD-BID	If surgery is planned, give three times daily 3 days before the procedure and 3 days after the procedure
Uricosuric Drugs			
Probenecid	Prevention of recurrences of gouty arthritis	*Adult:* 250 mg po BID × 1 week. Increase to 500 mg BID then may increase by 500 mg/day every 4 weeks. Not to exceed 3 g/day. *Child age 2–14 yr:* 25 mg/kg (700 mg/m^2) initially, then 10 mg/kg (300 mg/m^2) QID	Should not be used to treat gouty arthritis but rather for prevention. In acute attack, continue at full dose along with colchicine or NSAID. Give with food or milk
Sulfinpyrazone	Chronic gout	*Adult:* 100–200 mg po BID. May be increased to 800 mg/day	Regulate dose by monitoring serum uric acid levels

GI, Gastrointestinal.

Pharmacodynamics

In contrast to antigout drugs, *uricosuric* drugs increase the rate of uric acid secretion, thus reducing concentrations in the plasma. Probenecid and sulfinpyrazone inhibit the renal tubular reabsorption of urate, increasing the urinary elimination of uric acid, decreasing serum uric acid levels, retarding urate deposition, and promoting resorption of urate deposits. Additionally, probenecid inhibits the renal tubular reabsorption of most penicillins and cephalosporins. Sulfinpyrazone inhibits PG synthesis, which prevents platelet aggregation, but it lacks analgesic and anti-inflammatory activity.

Adverse Effects and Contraindications

Probenecid is well tolerated by most patients. Some degree of GI irritation is noted by about 2 percent of patients. The incidence of hypersensitivity, usually consisting of mild skin rashes, is between 2 and 4 percent. Serious hypersensitivity reactions are rare. Nephrotic syndrome has been reported as a toxic reaction. A large overdose results in CNS stimulation, seizures, and death from respiratory failure.

GI irritation occurs in about 10 to 15 percent of patients receiving sulfinpyrazone. Hypersensitivity reactions do occur, usually consisting of a rash with fever, but they occur less frequently than with probenecid. Depression of hematopoiesis has been demonstrated. Sulfinpyrazone is contraindicated in patients with allergies to phenylbutazone or other pyrazoles and in patients who have blood dyscrasias or a history of peptic ulcer disease. It should be used with caution in patients with renal failure or in those who are pregnant or lactating.

Pharmacokinetics

Probenecid is a highly soluble benzoic acid derivative that is completely absorbed after oral administration. Peak concentrations are reached in 2 to 4 hours. The plasma half-life is dose dependent and varies from less than 5 hours to more than 8 hours over the therapeutic range. Eighty-five to ninety-five percent of the drug is bound to plasma albumin. Biotransformation takes place in the liver, with less than 10 percent of the drug eliminated unchanged in the urine. The half-life of probenecid is 4 to 17 hours.

Like probenecid, sulfinpyrazone is well absorbed following oral administration. It is highly bound to plasma albumin (98 to 99 percent) and tends to displace other drugs that have a high affinity for the same binding sites. The half-life of the IV formulation is about 4 hours. After oral administration, its uricosuric effect may persist for as long as 10 hours. Approximately 50 percent of an oral dose appears in the urine within 24 hours 90 percent unchanged.

Drug-Drug Interactions

Probenecid increases the concentration of sulfonamide in the blood to some degree. The uricosuric action of sulfinpyrazone is additive to that of probenecid but is mutually antagonistic to that of salicylates.

Dosage Regimen

The dosage of probenecid depends on the objectives of therapy. In the treatment of chronic gout 250 mg are given twice daily for one week, following which 500 mg are given twice daily.

Sulfinpyrazone is given as 200 to 400 mg in two divided doses. The dose can be gradually increased to a maintenance dose of 400 mg/day over a period of one week, if needed. The dose is regulated by monitoring serum uric acid levels.

Laboratory Considerations

Probenecid may cause false-positive results in copper sulfate urine glucose tests (Clinitest). Glucose oxidase methods (Keto-Diastix, Tes-Tape) should be used to monitor urine glucose. CBC, serum uric acid levels, and renal function should be monitored before and routinely throughout long-term therapy. There are no significant laboratory considerations for sulfinpyrazone.

Critical Thinking Process

Assessment

The patient with gout most often complains of pain in the first metatarsophalangeal joint of the big toe. The affected joints are usually red, swollen, and exquisitely tender. Ask questions about the onset of symptoms, level of discomfort, frequency of attacks, attempts at self-treatment, and the extent to which symptoms interfere with the activities of daily living. Elicit information about concurrent drug use of thiazide diuretics and salicylates because these drugs reduce the elimination of uric acid. Diabetes mellitus and alcohol abuse also reduce uric acid secretion. Ask about the patient's fluid intake, particularly of alcohol (e.g., beer, ale, wine) and if there has been a recent, sudden loss of weight. A sudden weight loss may precipitate an acute attack of gout due to the destruction of cells.

The patient should be queried about a past history of renal disease, particularly renal calculi. Renal calculi composed of uric acid represent 5 to 10 percent of renal stones. Calcium stones are also more common in people with gout. The risk of urolithiasis is much greater in patients with a history of asymptomatic hyperuricemia or gout. Ask about treatment of previous gout episodes. Were tophi present at that time? Where were the tophi located? On the helix of the ear, extensor surfaces of forearms, or Achilles tendons? What drugs were used and how effective were they in relieving symptoms?

Serum uric acid levels or a 24-hour measurement of urine for uric acid helps determine the severity of hyperuricemia. The 24-hour measurement helps determine if the patient produces excess uric acid or if inadequate amounts of uric acid are being secreted.

Analysis and Management

Treatment Objectives

Treatment objectives in the management of gout are to decrease pain and inflammation associated with acute attacks and to prevent recurrent attacks. For control of hyperuricemia, the goal is to reduce plasma uric acid concentrations to below 6 mg/dL, although drug therapy is usually not started during an acute attack.

Treatment Options

Drug Variables

Acute Gout Several therapeutic strategies have been used to counter acute gout attacks, although drug therapy is the primary treatment modality. Colchicine or corticosteroids are effective for the symptomatic treatment. The initial drug of choice, however, is the NSAID indomethacin, an acetic acid derivative. Indomethacin is usually better tolerated than colchicine. Patients benefit more from indomethacin than from colchicine, including those for whom therapy was delayed several days after the onset of an acute attack. This is true even though colchicine has been the initial drug of choice in the past. Other NSAIDs have also been used (e.g., ibuprofen, naproxen, ketorolac) with apparently similar efficacy, but experience is much less extensive to date. The other NSAIDs can be used if the patient cannot tolerate indomethacin.

A full dosage of indomethacin (50 mg three times daily) should be used until a significant response occurs, usually in 2 to 3 days. The dosage can then be reduced to 25 mg three times daily with therapy continued for an additional 7 to 10 days until the attack has fully resolved. If there has been no response after 24 hours of treatment, an alternative drug should be tried.

Corticosteroids (i.e., prednisone) are used when indomethacin or other NSAIDs are not effective or when the patient is intolerant. They are the initial drug of choice in patients with a hypersensitivity to aspirin or for the patient with renal failure because these patients are at risk for NSAID-induced nephrotoxicity. Prednisone is given in full dosage (for 3 to 4 days) and then tapered by 5 mg/day over the next week. Intra-articular injections of corticosteroids should be considered if only the knee or ankle joint are affected.

Colchicine should be used for patients who have a history of heart failure, active peptic ulcer disease, or severe hypertension because these patients should not take a corticosteroid or NSAID. Less than 5 percent of patients fail to obtain relief with colchicine when it is given within the first few hours of an attack. Pain, swelling, and redness usually abate within 12 hours and are completely gone in 48 to 72 hours. The disadvantage to colchicine is its high incidence (80 to 100 percent) of diarrhea. If colchicine is used, it should be given one day only and then started again on day 7 if prophylactic therapy is required. This is because colchicine is eliminated slowly, its toxicity is dose related, and it has a long duration of action.

Chronic Gout The drugs used for chronic gout are different from those used for acute gout. Allopurinol represents a rational approach to therapy for chronic gout because overproduction of uric acid is a contributing factor in most patients and is characteristic of most types of secondary hyperuricemia. Probenecid and sulfinpyrazone cause uric acid to be eliminated at a rate exceeding that of formation in about two-thirds of patients. Plasma uric acid levels are thus lowered. Although IV administration of these drugs can cause a fivefold to sevenfold increase in the renal clearance of urate, continuous oral administration to patients with tophaceous gout approximately doubles the daily elimination of urates. In such patients, continuous administration prevents formation of new tophi and gradually causes reduction and even disappearance of old tophi.

Indeed, acute attacks may increase in frequency or severity during early months of therapy when urate is being mobilized from affected joints. Therefore, therapy with uricosuric drugs should not be initiated during an acute attack but may be continued if already started.

Patient Variables

It is well known that alcohol intake and starvation diets contribute to gout attacks. Because the pKa of uric acid is 5.6 and the solubility of the nonionized form is very low, maintaining the output of a large volume of alkaline urine minimizes its intrarenal deposition. This precaution is essential during the early weeks of treatment, when uric acid elimination is large, especially in patients with a history of renal disease associated with urate stones or gravel.

In patients who do not respond to uricosuric drugs because of impaired renal function, allopurinol is especially helpful. For patients with gouty nephropathy, allopurinol offers additional advantage over uricosuric drugs in that their daily elimination of uric acid is reduced rather than increased. Neither the antigout drugs nor allopurinol alters the course of the disease or supplants the use of colchicine and NSAIDs in its management.

Interventions

Administration

Antigout and uricosuric drugs should be administered after meals to minimize GI irritation. If nausea and vomiting occur, monitor intake and output and contact the health care provider. In treatment of chronic gout, the uricosuric drugs are given continually in the lowest dose that maintains satisfactory plasma uric acid concentrations.

Education

Whether or not dietary restriction of purines should be recommended is controversial. Some health care providers advocate a strict low-purine diet, whereas others believe that limiting protein foods is sufficient. Still others do not believe that dietary restrictions affect treatment outcomes. However, if purine restriction is recommended, instruct the patient to avoid the following foods: organ meats, roe, sardines, scallops, anchovies, broth and consommé, and mincemeat (see Appendix C).

Increasing fluid intake is one of the best measures to prevent urate stone formation. It also helps dilute the urine and prevent formation of sediment. Instruct patients taking uricosuric drugs to maintain oral intake sufficient to ensure a daily urinary output of at least 2 L. This may require 3000 mL of fluid intake per day. Instruct patients to limit their intake of alcohol.

Uric acid is less likely to form stones in an alkaline urine. Thus, the patient should be advised to increase his or her intake of alkaline ash foods such as citrus juices and fresh fruits (except cranberries, plums and prunes), milk, buttermilk, cream, almonds, chestnuts, and coconuts, and all vegetables (except lentils and corn). Further, for this reason, sodium bicarbonate, potassium citrate, or other alkalinizing drugs may be prescribed concurrently with probenecid (see Chapter 61).

The patient should be advised to avoid all forms of aspirin and diuretics because these drugs may precipitate a gout attack. Patients should be taught that excessive physical or emotional stress can also exacerbate the disease. Stress management techniques can be emphasized.

Evaluation

Treatment effectiveness can be demonstrated by a decrease in the pain and swelling of affected joints, a decrease in serum uric acid levels, resolution of tophi, and a subsequent decrease in the frequency of attacks. Several months of continuous therapy may be required before maximum benefits are apparent.

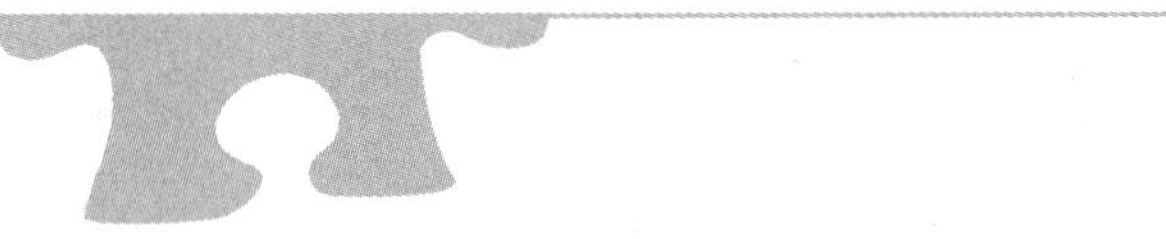

SUMMARY

- Inflammation is a nonspecific response occurring with tissue injury. Chemical mediators cause vasodilation, increased capillary permeability, chemotaxis of white blood cells, and fever.
- NSAIDs are used primarily to reduce body temperature, decrease inflammation and secondarily to relieve pain.
- Treatment options for the short-term management of fever, mild to moderate pain, and inflammatory disorders in adults include salicylates and other NSAIDs.
- Salicylates and NSAIDs are not used in children and adolescents who have viral infections or chicken pox owing to the risk of Reye's syndrome.
- Gold salts and other DMARDs are used in progressive rheumatoid disorders that are unresponsive to conventional therapies.
- NSAIDs and DMARDs are contraindicated or should be used with caution in patients with hypersensitivity, a history of peptic ulcer disease, liver disease, or renal insufficiency.
- Acetaminophen should be avoided or used with caution in patients with hepatic disease.
- Most NSAIDs, DMARDs, and antigout drugs should be taken with food or milk to minimize GI distress.
- Eighty-five to ninety percent of the patients with gout are middle-aged and older men, and postmenopausal women. The peak onset of gout is between the ages of 30 and 40 years.
- Acute gout occurs as a result of an inflammatory reaction to deposits of sodium urate crystals, the end product of purine metabolism, in the synovium and other body tissues.
- With an acute attack of gout, the patient has excruciating pain and inflammation in one or more small joints, most commonly the metatarsophalangeal joint of the great toe.
- Chronic gout appears after repeated bouts of acute gout with deposits of urate crystals developing within major organ systems and under the skin.
- The treatment goal for patients with gout include decreasing the pain and inflammation, and preventing recurrent attacks.

- Treatment options for gout include antigout drugs such as allopurinol and colchicine, uricosuric drugs such as probenecid and sulfinpyrazone, and the NSAID indomethacin.
- Increasing fluid intake is one of the best measures to prevent urate stone formation for patients with gout. Further, uric acid is less likely to form stones in an alkaline urine.
- Treatment effectiveness can be demonstrated by a decrease in the pain and swelling of affected joints, a decrease in serum uric acid levels, resolution of tophi, and a subsequent decrease in the frequency of attacks.

BIBLIOGRAPHY

Abramowicz, M. (1993). Drugs for pain. *Medical Letter on Drugs and Therapeutics,* 35(887), 1–6.

Agency for Health Care Policy and Research. (1992). *Clinical practice guidelines. Acute Pain management: Operative or medical procedures and trauma.* Washington, DC: U.S. Department of Health and Human Services, Public Health Service. Pub. No. ACHPR 92–0032.

Agency for Health Care Policy and Research. (1992). *Quick reference guide for clinicians. Acute pain management in infants, children, and adolescents: Operative and medical procedures.* Washington, DC: U.S. Department of Health and Human Services, Public Health Service. Pub. No. ACHPR 92–0020.

Alspach, G. (1994). Pain management: Dispelling some myths. *Critical Care Nurse,* 10, 13–15.

American Pain Society. (1992). *Principles of analgesic use in the treatment of acute pain and chronic cancer pain* (3rd ed.). Skokie, IL: Author.

Boyce, E. (1992). Pharmacology of antiarthritic drugs. *Clinics in Podiatric Medicine and Surgery,* 9, 327–348.

Briggs, G., Freeman, R., and Yaffe, S. (1990). *Drugs in pregnancy and lactation: A reference guide to fetal and neonatal risk.* Philadelphia: Williams & Wilkins.

Creasy, R., and Resnik, R. (1994). *Maternal-fetal medicine: Principles and practice* (3rd ed.). Philadelphia: W.B. Saunders.

Cross, S. (1994). Pathophysiology of pain. *Mayo Clinic Proceedings,* 69, 375–383.

Edgar, I., and Smith-Hanrahan, C. (1992). Nonpharmacological pain management. In J. Watt-Watson and M. Donovan (Eds.), *Pain management: Nursing perspective.* St. Louis: C.V. Mosby

Fries, J., Williams, C., and Bloch, D. (1991). The relative toxicity of nonsteroidal antiinflammatory drugs. *Arthritis and Rheumatism,* 34(11), 1353–1360.

Garcia Rodrigues, L. (1994). Risk of upper gastrointestinal bleeding and perforation associated with individual nonsteroidal antiinflammatory drugs. *Lancet,* 343, 769–772.

Gaston-Johansson, F., Albert, M., Fagan, E., et al. (1990). Similarities in pain descriptions of four different ethnic-culture groups. *Journal of Pain and Symptom Management,* 5(2), 94–100.

Gilman, A., Rall, T., Nies, A., et al. (Eds.). (1990). *Goodman and Gilman's the pharmacologic basis of therapeutics* (8th ed.). New York: Pergamon Press.

Griffin, M., Piper, J., Daugherty, J., et al. (1991). Nonsteroidal antiinflammatory drug use and increased risk for peptic ulcer disease in elderly persons. *Annals of Internal Medicine,* 11(4), 257–263.

International Association of Pain, Subcommittee on Taxonomy. (1979). Pain terms: A list with definitions and notes on usage. *Pain,* 6, 249.

Katz, J., and Melzack, R. (1990). Pain "memories" in phantom limbs: Review and clinical observations. *Pain,* 43, 319–336.

Levy, M., Spino, M., and Read, S. (1991). Colchicine: A state of the art review. *Pharmacotherapy,* 11, 196–211.

Marzinski, L. (1991). The tragedy of dementia: Clinically assessing pain in the confused, nonverbal elderly. *Journal of Obstetrics and Gynecologic Nursing,* 17(6), 25–28.

McCaffery, M. (1979). *Nursing management of the patient with pain* (2nd ed.). Philadelphia: J.B. Lippincott.

McCaffery, M., and Beebe, A. (1989). *Pain: Clinical practice manual for nursing practice.* St. Louis: C. V. Mosby.

McCarty, D., and Koopman, W. (Eds.). (1993). *Arthritis and allied conditions.* Philadelphia: Lea & Febiger.

McCormack, J., Brown, G., Levine, M., et al. (Eds.). (1996). *Drug therapy: Decision making guide.* Philadelphia: W.B. Saunders Company.

McMahon, J. (1992). Gold therapy for rheumatoid arthritis. *Annals of Internal Medicine,* 117, 169–170.

Meinhart, N., and McCaffery, M. (1983). *Pain: A nursing approach to assessment and analysis.* Norwalk, CT: Appleton-Century-Crofts.

Melzak, R., and Wall. P. (1965). Pain mechanisms: A new theory. *Science,* 150, 971–979.

Payne, R. (1992). Transdermal fentanyl: Suggested recommendations for clinical use. *Journal of Pain and Symptom Management,* 7, 540–544.

Perneger, T., Whelton, P., and Klag, M. (1994). Risk of kidney failure associated with use of acetaminophen, aspirin, and nonsteroidal antiinflammatory drugs. *New England Journal of Medicine,* 331(25), 1675–1679.

Pleuvry, B., and Lauretti, G. (1996). Biochemical aspects of chronic pain and its relationship to treatment. *Pharmacologic Therapeutics,* 71, 313–324.

Reardon, E., and Clough, J. (1992). Drug therapy in the rheumatic diseases. *Comprehensive Therapy,* 18(11), 22–25.

Recommendations of the American Pain Society on the Principles of Analgesic Use in the Treatment of Acute and Chronic Cancer Pain. (1990). *Clinical Pharmacology,* 9, 601–611.

Reidenberg, M., and Portenoy, R. (1994). The need for an open mind about the treatment of chronic malignant pain. *Clinical Pharmacology & Therapy,* 55, 367–369.

Schumacher, H. (Ed.). (1993). *Primer on the rheumatic diseases* (10th ed.). Atlanta: Arthritis Foundation.

Spilman, P., and Whelton, A. (1992). Nonsteroidal antiinflammatory drugs: Effects on kidney function and implications for nursing care. *American Nephrology Nurses' Association Journal,* 19(1), 19–26.

Sternbach, R. (1968). *Pain: A psychophysiological analysis.* New York: Academic Press.

Wall, P., and Melzack, R. (Eds.). (1989). *Textbook of pain* (2nd ed.). New York: Churchill Livingstone.

Wilcox, C., Shalek, K., and Cotsonis, G. (1994). Striking prevalence of over-the-counter nonsteroidal antiinflammatory drug use in patients with upper gastrointestinal bleeding. *Archives in Internal Medicine,* 154, 42–46.

Young, L., and Koda-Kimble, M. (1995). *Applied Therapeutics: The clinical use of drugs.* Vancouver, WA: Applied Therapeutics, Inc.

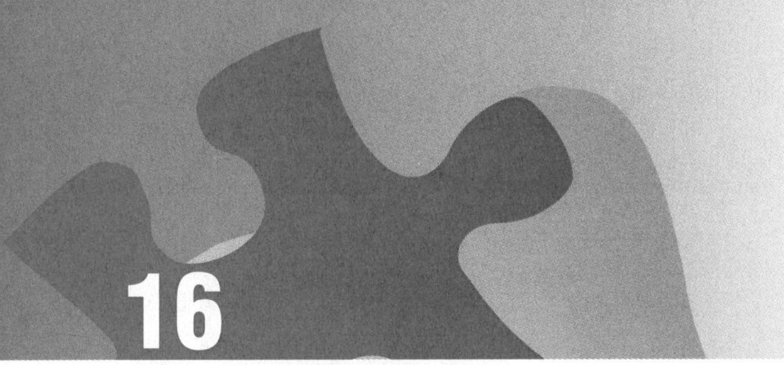

16 Anesthetic Drugs

Although not widely publicized, Dr. Crawford W. Long, a physician in rural Georgia, was the first practitioner to use inhaled vapor ether as an anesthetic in 1842. Four years later, William Morton, a Boston dentist, demonstrated the use of ether to relieve pain during surgical procedures. An eminent surgeon attending the demonstration remarked that he had "seen something today that would go around the world." Ether quickly was established as a desirable and legitimate technique during obstetric and surgical procedures across the United States and Great Britain. Thus, the American discovery of anesthesia led to a highly refined and complex process that is used to protect patients from pain.

Pharmacologic drugs used for anesthesia more closely approach the ideal—safe drugs that are easily adjusted to produce an adequate unconscious state and muscle relaxation. The patient's response to these drugs can be better monitored by sophisticated equipment. This chapter introduces the concept of the anesthetic state; includes a discussion of the stages of anesthesia, pharmacodynamics, and pharmacokinetics; and defines the types of drugs used to produce anesthesia.

The administration of anesthesia by nurses has been a recognized function of nursing for over 100 years. Nurse anesthetists were the first group of nurses to specialize beyond general duty nursing, and anesthesia care of the patient intraoperatively follows a process similar to that of other areas of nursing encompassing the duty to assess, plan, implement, and evaluate. These steps are incorporated into the Practice Standards of the American Association of Nurse Anesthetists and the International Federation of Nurse Anesthetists. These standards, which are approved by both a national and an international body, describe the foundation and expectations of nurse anesthetists worldwide.

CONCEPTS AND PRINCIPLES OF GENERAL ANESTHESIA

The term anesthesia is derived from the Greek word *anaisthesia* (*an,* without; *aisthesis,* feeling) and denotes a loss of sensation with or without loss of consciousness. It produces muscle relaxation, blocks transmission of nerve impulses, and suppresses reflexes. Although anesthetics may be used postoperatively for relief of pain, anesthesia is rarely administered as a diagnostic or therapeutic regimen. It is not used to cure but rather facilitates cure, just as nursing and dietetics facilitate cure. In the United States, anesthesia is administered by certified registered nurse anesthetists, anesthesiologists, or anesthesia assistants. Nurse anesthesia practice is considered the oldest specialty in nursing.

Classifications of Anesthesia

There are two major classifications of anesthesia: general and regional. General anesthesia blocks pain stimuli at the cerebral cortex. General anesthesia produces widespread effects by causing a drug-induced depression of the central nervous system (CNS). This physiologically altered state classically results in four states: hypnosis (unconsciousness), analgesia (insensibility to pain), amnesia (loss of memory), and muscle relaxation (relaxation or paralysis of skeletal muscle). General anesthetics are administered intravenously (IV), by inhalation, or by rectum.

Regional anesthesia, also known as local anesthesia, produces a loss of painful sensation in only one region of the body by blocking painful stimuli at their origin, along the afferent neurons, or along the spinal cord. Local anesthetics that block nerve transmission at its origin produce analgesia over specific tissue areas (e.g., topicals, or local infiltration). Drugs that block nerve transmission along afferent neurons produce analgesia over a specific area of the body (e.g., nerve blocks). Anesthetic drugs that block nerve transmission along the spinal cord produce analgesia over a specific region of the body (e.g., epidural, spinal). Local anesthetics do not result in loss of consciousness. Regional anesthetics are discussed later.

Types of General Anesthesia

Intravenous Anesthesia

Intravenous anesthesia as we know it today had its beginnings in 1934, when thiopental sodium was introduced. For many years, pentothal remained a popular choice for induction of anesthesia; however, today other drugs are also used. The patient experiences an extremely rapid induction, with unconsciousness occurring about 30 seconds after the initial IV administration. IV anesthesia is most commonly used as an induction agent before inhalation drugs are used. These drugs are potent enough, however, to be used alone for minor procedures such as dental extractions or pelvic exams. Intravenous drugs used for induction or maintenance of anesthesia are identified in Table 16–1, along with their advantages and disadvantages.

Inhalation Anesthesia

Inhalation anesthesia is a mixture of volatile liquids or gas and oxygen. These drugs exist as liquids that evaporate at room temperature. The amount of liquid evaporated is controlled by a device called a vaporizer. The amount of vapor the patient receives determines the depth of anesthesia and analgesia. When inhalation drugs are administered by mask, the gases flow into the mask through a finely calibrated vaporizer. When an endotracheal tube is used, the gases flow directly into the patient's tracheobronchial tree.

At least 19 inhaled anesthetics have been developed since the introduction of nitrous oxide (N_2O) in the mid-1800s. Figure 16–1 illustrates the historic development of inhaled anesthetics. Of those listed, only nitrous oxide, halothane,

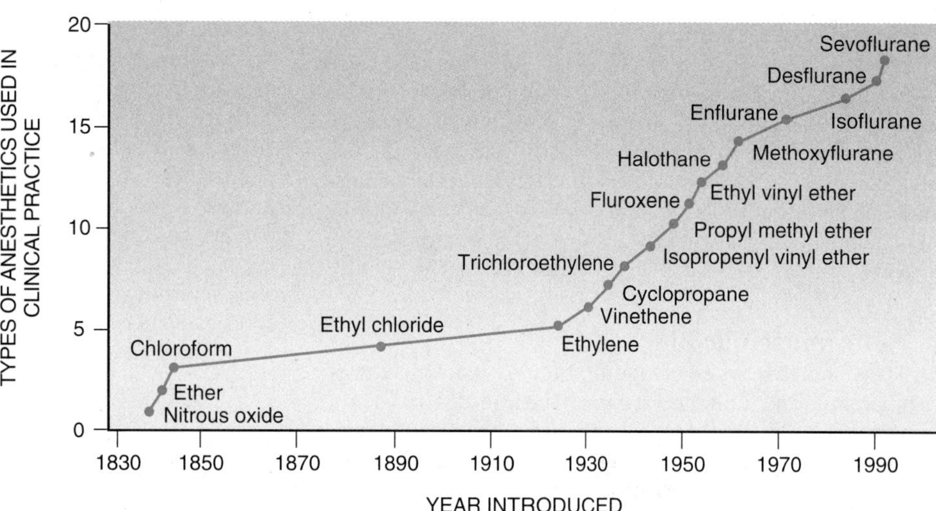

Figure 16–1 The history of inhalation anesthetics is charted through the developmental progression of inhalation anesthetics used in clinical practice since the introduction of nitrous oxide (N_2O) in the mid-1800s. (Data from Rosenburg, H., Guest, D., and Etsten, B. E. [1974]. Forane—experience with the newest inhalation agents. *Anesthesiology Review,* 1[11], 18; Eger, E. I. [1993]. *Desflurane (Suprane): A compendium and reference.* Rutherford, NJ: Healthpress Publishing Group; Stoelting, R. K., and Miller, R. D. [1994]. *Basics of anesthesia* [3rd ed.]. New York: Churchill Livingstone; Abbott Pharmaceuticals. [1995]. *History of inhalation therapy.* Chicago: Author.)

methoxyflurane, enflurane, isoflurane, desflurane, and sevoflurane are now available. Methoxyflurane is rarely used today. All of the inhaled anesthetics introduced after 1950 (except ethyl vinyl ether) have contained fluorine. Fluorination improves the solubility of volatile anesthetics. Desflurane and sevoflurane, the newest drugs to be introduced into practice, are halogenated solely with fluorine. This fluorination causes the solubility of these drugs to approach that of nitrous oxide and results in a rapid induction and smooth emergence from anesthesia.

These drugs have undergone tremendous improvement since their original introduction to clinical practice as investigators searched for an ideal anesthetic. Properties of the ideal anesthetic are as follows:

- Pleasant odor that is nonirritating to the airway
- Effective when used with high concentrations of oxygen
- Low solubility in the blood
- No organ toxicity
- Minimal cardiovascular and respiratory adverse effects
- Easily reversible cardiovascular effects without stimulant activity
- Vapor pressure and boiling point that enable the drug to be delivered using standard vaporization techniques

TABLE 16–1 INTRAVENOUS AGENTS USED FOR INDUCTION OR MAINTENANCE OF ANESTHESIA

Agents	Advantages	Disadvantages
Thiopental sodium (PENTOTHAL)	Rapid induction Cerebral vasoconstrictor	Decreased blood pressure, increased heart rate Venodilation Laryngeal reflexes not depressed Contraindicated with porphyria Hypotension with hypovolemia Vasospasm with intra-arterial injection; tissue necrosis with subcutaneous administration No skeletal muscle relaxation Shivering Anaphylaxis Laryngospasm; bronchospasm
Methohexital (BREVITAL)	Most rapid induction	Involuntary muscle movement Seizures
Etomidate (AMIDATE)	Minimal changes in blood pressure, heart rate Respiratory stability No histamine release No emergency reaction	Myoclonic movement Pain with injection Transient adrenocortical depression
Ketamine (KETALAR)	Profound analgesia Bronchodilator Hemodynamic support	Increased skeletal muscle tone Increased blood pressure and heart rate Increased cerebral blood flow and metabolic oxygen requirements Increased intracranial pressure Increased salivary gland secretion Emergency reaction; delirium, hallucinations
Propofol (DIPRIVAN)	Hypnosis Rapid induction Clear-headed, rapid recovery Less nausea, vomiting	Hypotension, tachycardia, or bradycardia Clonic myoclonic movement on emergence Pain on injection Sexual illusions

Adapted from Zaglaniczny, K., and Maree, S. (1995). Anesthesia and perioperative nursing care. In R. A. Roth (Ed.), *Perioperative nursing core curriculum* (pp. 232–233). Philadelphia: W. B. Saunders. Used with permission.

Rectal Anesthesia

Although this route for anesthesia is rarely used today, it is useful in children or when facial trauma or surgery makes it difficult to maintain an airway. Intravenous or liquid inhalation agents are instilled in the rectum via a rectal tube. Methohexital sodium is absorbed through the rectal mucosa and delivered to the CNS via the circulatory system. Because rectal anesthesia is used only during stage I anesthesia, it must be supplemented with other types of drugs.

Neuromuscular Blockade

There are two types of neuromuscular blocking drugs: depolarizing and nondepolarizing. These drugs block the transmission of nerve impulses to muscle fibers. The physiology of neuromuscular transmission is discussed in Chapter 12, but in essence, they produce temporary paralysis of voluntary muscles, including muscles that control respirations. Neuromuscular blockers are given IV to facilitate intubation, relax muscles in the surgical field, ease laryngospasms, and relax muscles for controlled mechanical ventilation. The more common neuromuscular blockers are succinylcholine, a depolarizing drug, and tubocurarine, pancuronium, vecuronium, atracurium, rocuronium, mivacurium, and cisatracurium, which are nondepolarizing drugs.

Stages of General Anesthesia

There are four stages of general anesthesia. The stages were formally described in 1920 based on observations of a patient who was receiving diethyl ether. Although not apparent with all anesthetics, all of the stages can be seen if the drug is given slowly enough. Stage I anesthesia (i.e., induction) produces a depression of the cortical areas of the brain and is characterized by loss of response to verbal commands and a loss of consciousness. The patient may be drowsy or dizzy, or may experience auditory or visual hallucinations.

Stage II anesthesia is referred to as the stage of excitement. It begins with loss of consciousness and extends through the loss of eyelid reflexes. There is a transient increase in autonomic nervous system activity with hyperreflexia, random motor activity, and irregular respirations. An exaggerated orotracheal reflex is also noted. The patient may appear to struggle at this stage.

Stage III is considered the stage of surgical anesthesia. Surgery is usually begun at this stage. It is a profound depth of anesthesia in which neurologic depression is sufficient to provide a motionless patient. Respirations are shallow but regular, and there is no blink or gag reflex. Surgical stimuli fail to produce reflex motor withdrawal and generate less intense cardiovascular, respiratory, and neuroendocrine responses. When surgery is completed and anesthesia is withdrawn, the patient moves backward through each of these three stages.

Stage IV anesthesia is characterized by an even deeper and more profound depth of anesthesia, characterized by apnea and cardiovascular collapse. These signs reflect overdose and the toxic effects of high concentrations of potent inhalation drugs and respiratory paralysis.

It is common today for a patient to receive *balanced anesthesia* (neuroleptic anesthesia). Balanced anesthesia uses several different classes of drugs from different pharmacologic classes to produce the anesthetized state. It is typically achieved through the use of an inhalation drug, oxygen, opioid, and a neuromuscular blocker (Table 16–2). Global anesthetics produce generalized depression of the CNS, whereas site-specific agents act through specific sites in the CNS or peripheral nervous systems. This approach builds on the best pharmacologic characteristics of each drug, reduces dosage requirements, minimizes adverse effects, and enhances patient safety.

Pharmacodynamics

Inhaled anesthetics produce a dose-dependent CNS depression caused by inhibition of synaptic transmission, with effects noted in the CNS, cardiovascular, respiratory, renal, hepatic, and gastrointestinal systems and the uterus. There is a dose-dependent reduction in cerebral metabolism and a dose-dependent increase in cerebral blood flow. The degree of cerebral vasodilation varies with the specific drug, but the effects occur within minutes of administration. Intracranial pressure may also be increased. If necessary, an induced

TABLE 16–2 COMPONENTS OF ANESTHESIA

	Hypnosis	Analgesia	Amnesia	Relaxation
Global Drugs				
Volatile agents	+++	+/−	+	+
Propofol	+++	0	+	+/−
Thiopental	+++	−	+	0
Nitrous oxide	+	+	+	0
Site-Specific Drugs				
Opioids	+/−	+++	0	−
Midazolam	+	0	+++	0
Muscle relaxants	0	0	0	+++

+++, primary effect; +, weaker effect; +/−, doubtful effect; 0, no effect; −, antagonist effect.

Adapted from Zaglaniczny, K, and Maree, S. (1995). Anesthesia and perioperative nursing care. In R. A. Roth (Ed.), *Perioperative nursing core curriculum* (p. 230). Philadelphia: W. B. Saunders. Used with permission.

state of hypocapnia can be used to reduce further increases in cerebral blood flow and intracranial pressure.

Inhaled anesthetics sensitize the heart to the dysrhythmic actions of catecholamines, increasing the risk of ventricular ectopy, tachycardia, or ventricular fibrillation. Halothane is more sensitizing than isoflurane, which, in turn, is more sensitizing than enflurane.

All inhaled anesthetics produce an effective bronchodilation in unconscious patients. In conscious patients, only halothane and sevoflurane are not irritating to the airways. The bronchodilation facilitates ventilation in patients with bronchospastic diseases, including asthma. Further, because the drugs cause the laryngeal and pharyngeal reflexes to be obtunded, intubation is facilitated. However, the patient is at increased risk for aspiration and aspiration pneumonitis if gastric contents are present.

Inhaled anesthetics decrease renal blood flow and the glomerular filtration rate. This effect can be offset by adequate prehydration. There is also a dose-dependent reduction in hepatic blood flow. The greatest effect is noted with halothane.

The smooth muscle of the gastrointestinal tract is relaxed in the presence of inhaled anesthetics. The drugs decrease gastric, jejunal, and colonic motility. There is also a dose-dependent relaxation of uterine smooth muscle, which can result in uterine bleeding following delivery.

The combined use of inhalation anesthetics, opioids, benzodiazepines, anticholinergics, and muscle relaxants mask many of the signs of anesthetic depth. Although it is possible to monitor exhaled concentrations and thus site concentrations of inhalation drugs through mass spectrometry, it is not possible to routinely monitor plasma concentrations of IV agents. Although they are not absolute, anesthetic depth is often monitored by the body's responses to noxious stimuli.

Sensory input obtained through the CNS can originate from somatic or visceral tissues. The patient must be conscious to perceive pain. Low concentrations of inhaled or IV anesthetics can eliminate recall or awareness of pain but still allow movement. The concentration of anesthetic required to eliminate somatic motor responses is higher than that needed to induce unconsciousness and eliminate perception of pain. The respiratory motor response to noxious stimuli can involve an increase in tidal volume and respiratory rate.

Although many advances have been made in the administration of anesthesia, the measurement of anesthetic depth is not precise. Depth of anesthesia is often measured by somatomotor reflexes or a change in those parameters controlled by the autonomic nervous system. When the somatomotor reflex is assessed, the patient moves away from the site of stimulation. Autonomic changes may include changes in cardiovascular or respiratory parameters. More elaborate but complex assessment attempts to estimate the neuroendocrine response to pain can be made by analyzing plasma catecholamine concentrations or monitoring cerebral cortical electrical responses by electroencephalograph or specialized evoked potentials. Esophageal motility has also been used to assess the adequacy of anesthetic depth. An exciting new development in measurement of anesthetic depth is a cerebral function monitor or bispectral index. Four electrodes are placed on the head, and ranges are reported on a digital readout. Bispectral index range guidelines appear in Table 16–3.

Adverse Effects and Contraindications

Of the complications associated with anesthesia, aspiration, pulmonary dysfunction, and malignant hyperthermia (MH) are among the most serious (see Perioperative Complications Associated with Anesthesia). Inhalation of acid fluid in patients with depressed airway reflexes may result in *aspiration pneumonitis* or airway obstruction. The effects range from undetectable changes in respiratory status to sudden death, depending on the amount aspirated and its acidity. The reported incidence of aspiration pneumonitis is about 1.4 to 6 per 10,000 patients, although 40 to 80 percent of patients scheduled for elective surgery may be at risk based on gastric pH and volume. Patients with gastroesophageal reflux disease (GERD) are at a greater risk, as are obese patients; patients with diabetes, peptic ulcer disease, stress or pain, or trauma; patients who have been premedicated with an opioid; ambulatory surgery patients; older adults; children; and pregnant women. The risk is also higher than average for patients with emergency esophageal, upper abdominal, and emergency laparoscopic surgery. The effects tend to be more severe if the pH of gastric contents is less than 2.5 and the volume is greater than 0.4 mL/kg of body weight.

The clinical signs of aspiration include tachypnea, wheezing, bronchospasm, tachycardia, hypotension, hypoxia, and pulmonary edema. The chest x-ray study may show lobar consolidation, but an immediate change may not be noted. Arterial blood sampling generally reveals a low PaO_2.

Treatment of aspiration pneumonitis involves correction of arterial hypoxemia with supplemental oxygen. Tracheal intubation and positive-pressure ventilation with end-expiratory pressure may be required if hypoxemia persists despite supplemental oxygen. Bronchoscopy may be required to remove the foreign material, and bronchodilators may be required for poor pulmonary compliance. Treatment with steroids remains controversial, and antibiotics are recommended only if sputum cultures indicate development of a bacterial infection.

Postoperative *pulmonary dysfunction* may be due to hypoventilation. Residual effects of anesthetics in the absence

PERIOPERATIVE COMPLICATIONS ASSOCIATED WITH ANESTHESIA

Malignant hyperthermia
Aspiration
Pulmonary dysfunction
Cardiovascular complications
Nausea and vomiting
Nerve damage
Hyperthermia
Dental damage
Corneal abrasion
Hoarseness

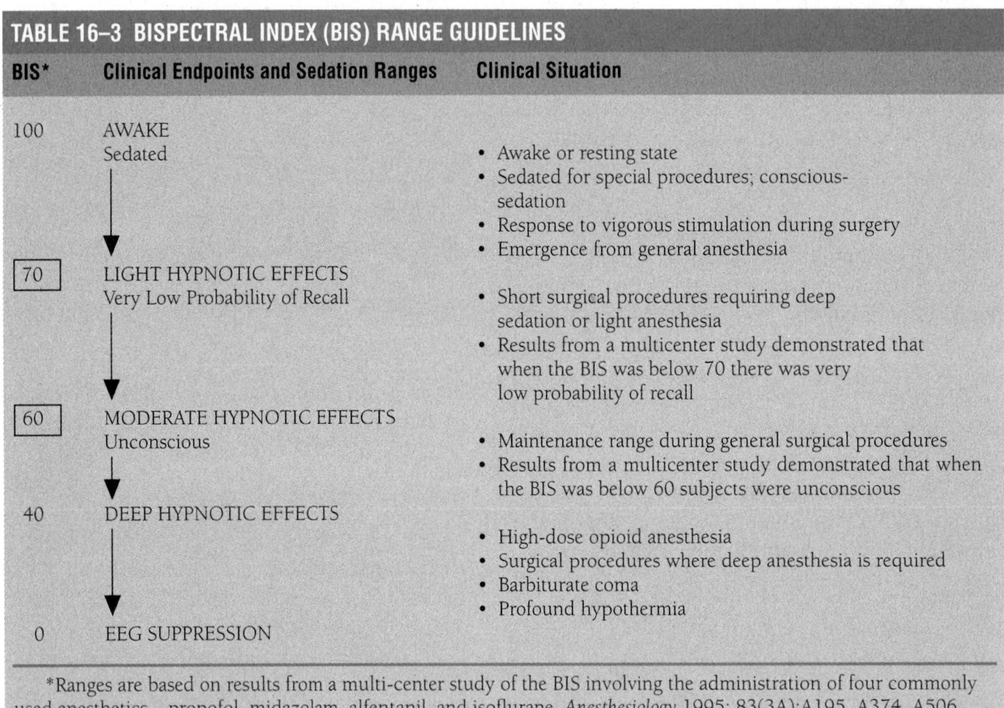

TABLE 16–3 BISPECTRAL INDEX (BIS) RANGE GUIDELINES

BIS*	Clinical Endpoints and Sedation Ranges	Clinical Situation
100	AWAKE Sedated	• Awake or resting state • Sedated for special procedures; conscious-sedation • Response to vigorous stimulation during surgery • Emergence from general anesthesia
70	LIGHT HYPNOTIC EFFECTS Very Low Probability of Recall	• Short surgical procedures requiring deep sedation or light anesthesia • Results from a multicenter study demonstrated that when the BIS was below 70 there was very low probability of recall
60	MODERATE HYPNOTIC EFFECTS Unconscious	• Maintenance range during general surgical procedures • Results from a multicenter study demonstrated that when the BIS was below 60 subjects were unconscious
40	DEEP HYPNOTIC EFFECTS	• High-dose opioid anesthesia • Surgical procedures where deep anesthesia is required • Barbiturate coma • Profound hypothermia
0	EEG SUPPRESSION	

*Ranges are based on results from a multi-center study of the BIS involving the administration of four commonly used anesthetics—propofol, midazolam, alfentanil, and isoflurane. *Anesthesiology* 1995; 83(3A):A195, A374, A506.

Note: Anesthesia is composed of many components. The BIS reflects the level of consciousness. To assess responsiveness, the degree of surgical stimulation and level of analgesia must be taken into consideration. BIS values and ranges assume that the EEG is free of artifacts that can affect its performance, i.e., EKG and EMG artifacts

Adapted from Aspect Medical Systems, Inc., (1996). *BIS range guidelines* (Appendix I) (p. 9). Natick, MA: Author. Used with permission.

of respiratory stimulation and poor patient positioning may lead to inadequate ventilatory drive. Residual neuromuscular blockade may also be responsible. Supplemental oxygen, reversal of drug effects or intubation, and positive pressure ventilation may be required.

MH is a life-threatening disorder of skeletal muscle that is believed to be due to decreased calcium reuptake by the sarcoplasmic reticulum with increased resting intracellular calcium levels. It usually occurs within 30 minutes after induction of anesthesia. Although the classic case of MH most often occurs in the operating room, it can also occur within a few hours in the postanesthesia care unit.

The early symptoms of MH are characterized by unexplained increases in expired carbon dioxide concentration, hypoxemia, acidosis, tachypnea, cyanosis, hyperkalemia, unstable blood pressure, and myoglobinuria. Tachycardia is one of the first signs of MH. Muscle rigidity is usually seen first in the masseter muscles of the jaw and may occur in the chest or extremities. Elevation in body temperature is usually a late sign and results from a hypermetabolic state of the skeletal muscle. Body temperature elevation results in an oxygen consumption of two to three times normal. If MH is not treated, the temperature may rise 1°C every 5 minutes. Temperatures of 109 to 111°F (42.8 to 44°C) have been reported. The patient develops a rosy, flushed appearance owing to the increased metabolism, which produces body heat. This heat causes vasodilation, and the skin may become mottled or cyanotic. There can be premature ventricular contractions or ventricular tachycardia on an electrocardiogram.

MH is an autosomal dominant hereditary trait, which very often is initiated by a pharmacologic trigger, most often succinylcholine. The incidence of MH is estimated to be 1 in every 15,000 pediatric surgical cases and 1 in every 50,000 adult surgical cases. Approximately 50 percent of children of MH-susceptible parents are potentially at risk. It is more frequent in male patients and in patients with muscular abnormalities such as ptosis, strabismus, and kyphoscoliosis. At one time, the mortality rate was 70 percent but this has now decreased to 10 percent with early recognition and treatment with a drug called dantrolene (DANTRIUM). Dantrolene is discussed further in Chapter 21.

Management of MH includes immediate discontinuation of all inhalation drugs and changing of the anesthesia circuit, administration of dantrolene sodium, cooling measures (surface, nasogastric, wound, rectal), hyperventilation with 100% oxygen, and correction of acid-base imbalances (e.g., sodium bicarbonate). Treatment of ventricular arrhythmias and maintenance of urinary output is undertaken, and arterial blood gases, electrolytes, and coagulation status are monitored. The patient should be observed for disseminated intravascular coagulopathy and monitored in the intensive care unit for 24 hours after such an event.

Patients known to be susceptible to MH should receive dantrolene 2.5 mg/kg IV 15 to 30 minutes before induction of anesthesia. This drug inhibits the release of calcium from the sarcoplasmic reticulum and prevents, attenuates, or reverses the metabolic and biochemical changes associated with MH crisis. A vapor-free anesthesia machine and full monitoring, including temperature and capnography, should be used. Nontriggering anesthetics (i.e., volatile anesthetics, succinylcholine) should be given. Safe drugs to be used include nitrous oxide, barbiturates, opioids, benzodiazepines, amide and ester local anesthetics, and nondepolarizing muscle relaxants.

Pharmacokinetics of Inhalation Anesthetics

The term pharmacokinetics refers to the rate of change in anesthetic concentration within the body and its component organs, tissues, and fluids, as well as its absorption, distribution, biotransformation, and elimination within the biologic system. The effectiveness of an anesthetic depends on the concentration at the effect site. The effect site concentration or therapeutic window for IV anesthesia is determined by the plasma concentration and the biotransformation of the drug. In contrast, an inhaled anesthetic moves from a vaporizer outside of the body to within the body as a result of partial pressure differences between compartments. In the gas phase, which exists between the vaporizer and the alveoli, the anesthetic concentrations and partial pressure are equal. However, once the anesthetic enters the circulation, brain, and other tissues, concentration and partial pressure are a function of solubility.

Unopposed ventilation produces a very rapid change in alveolar concentration of an inhaled anesthetic. This effect, however, is opposed by absorption or uptake of the anesthetic. The alveolar concentration that is obtained with a given anesthetic is the result of a balance between the delivery of anesthetic by ventilation and the removal of anesthetic by absorption.

Uptake is the product of three factors: solubility, cardiac output, and the alveolar-to-venous anesthetic partial pressure difference. Solubility is defined by the blood-gas partition coefficient. The coefficient represents the capacity of the blood to hold anesthetic and determines the amount of anesthetic taken up by the blood. If cardiac output is large, uptake will be larger. Alveolar-to-venous anesthetic partial pressure difference is the driving pressure that pushes anesthetic from the alveoli into the blood. If the gradient is large, absorption will be large.

The arterial-to-venous partial pressure difference is a function of tissue absorption. Uptake of the anesthetic by tissues is determined by the same three factors that determine absorption from the lungs: solubility, cardiac output, and the alveolar-to-venous anesthetic partial pressure difference. Body tissues are divided into four groups: highly perfused (liver, brain, kidney, heart, endocrine glands), moderately perfused (muscle, skin), mildly perfused (fat and bone marrow), and poorly perfused (tendons, ligaments, bone). Absorption of an anesthetic is fastest in the highly perfused, vessel-rich group of tissues and slowest in the mildly and poorly perfused groups of tissues.

The anesthetic effects of inhalation anesthetics is achieved by inhalation of the drug, uptake by the blood, and delivery to target tissue sites within the nervous system. Although these drugs are usually added after an IV induction with a barbiturate (e.g., pentathol), some patients are anesthetized by inhalation of the vapor. Anesthetic requirements (i.e., percent concentration) for inhalation drugs are judged in terms of the *minimum alveolar concentration* (MAC). MAC is defined as the concentration of an anesthetic vapor (at 1 atmosphere) that prevents skeletal muscle movement in 50 percent of patients given a painful stimulus (e.g., surgical skin incision).

The determination of MAC is made only after the drug has evenly distributed itself throughout the body. Although MAC can serve as a guide for the required concentration, it is influenced by many physiologic and pharmacologic factors. The addition of nitrous oxide to inhaled drugs lowers the MAC, as does the addition of other CNS depressants. Table 16–4 lists other factors that alter the MAC.

In addition to MAC, there are two other related terms that are important to understand. MAC-BAR represents the "minimum alveolar concentration" necessary to "block the adrenergic response" to skin incision. It can be expressed as either MAC-BAR_{50} or MAC-BAR_{95}. MAC-BAR values exceed the requirements for ablation of skeletal muscle movement with surgical stimulation. Blocking the adrenergic response requires a greater depth of anesthesia than preventing movement. The advantages and disadvantages of today's drugs are summarized in Table 16–5.

Drug-Drug Interactions

There are many drug-drug interactions with inhaled anesthetics (Table 16–6). Drugs that potentiate the effects of inhaled anesthetics and thus decrease the amount of anesthetic drug required include alcohol (in acute alcohol intoxication), ketamine, nitrous oxide, and tetrahydrocannabinol (marijuana). Aminophylline sensitizes the myocardium to

TABLE 16–4 FACTORS AFFECTING MINIMUM ALVEOLAR CONCENTRATION (MAC)

Reduced MAC	Increased MAC	No Effect
Increase in age	Hyperthermia	Duration of anesthesia
Hypoxemia	Hyperthyroidism	Gender
Hypotension	Ethanol (chronic)	Hypocapnia
Pregnancy	Monoamine oxidase inhibitors	Hypercapnia
Other CNS depressants		Hypertension
Hypothermia		
Acidosis		
Ethanol (acute)		

TABLE 16–5 INHALATION ANESTHETICS

Agent	Major Advantages	Adverse Effects, Disadvantages
Nitrous oxide (N_2O)	Amnesia, analgesia rapid onset	Low potency, diffusion hypoxia, expansion in closed gas spaces; postoperative nausea and vomiting
Halothane (FLUOTHANE)	Decreased $CMRO_2$; good induction agent for children; bronchodilator; uterine relaxant	Increased CBF, decreased blood pressure, heart rate, arrhythmias; respiratory depression, apnea; nausea, vomiting, ileus; hepatic dysfunction; trigger for malignant hyperthermia
Enflurane (ETHRANE)	Decreased $CMRO_2$; bronchodilator; less myocardial sensitization to catecholamines; no coronary steal; uterine relaxant	Increased CBF; seizure activity on EEG; hypotension, arrhythmias; respiratory depression, apnea, nausea, vomiting; occasional renal dysfunction; trigger for malignant hyperthermia
Isoflurane (FORANE)	Decreased $CMRO_2$; uterine relaxation; no organ toxicity; less myocardial sensitization to catecholamines	Trigger for malignant hyperthermia; coronary steal, hypotension, tachycardia; apnea or respiratory depression; nausea, vomiting, ileus
Desflurane (SUPRANE)	Decreased $CMRO_2$; uterine relaxation; rapid induction and emergence; no organ toxicity	Increased CBF; coughing; excitation during inhalation induction; trigger for malignant hyperthermia; hypertension, arrhythmias; respiratory depression, apnea; nausea, vomiting, ileus
Sevoflurane (ULTANE)	Decreased $CMRO_2$; rapid induction and emergencies, can be used for inhalational induction; minimal respiratory irritation	Not stable in soda lime, metabolized; trigger for malignant hyperthermia; increased CBF

$CMRO_2$, cerebral metabolic oxygen consumption rate; CBF, cerebral blood flow.
Adapted from Zaglaniczny, K., and Maree, S. (1995). Anesthesia and perioperative nursing care. In R. A. Roth (Ed.), *Perioperative nursing core curriculum* (p. 231). Philadelphia: W. B. Saunders. Used with permission.

ventricular arrhythmias when it is used in conjunction with an inhaled anesthetic. Opioids (e.g., morphine, fentanyl, sufentanil) raise the level of hypercapnia required to stimulate ventilation and sedative-hypnotics (e.g., benzodiazepines, barbiturates, phenothiazines) may depress the maximal ventilatory response to hypercapnia. Hypercapnia is the build-up of carbon dioxide in the blood.

Drugs that antagonize the effects of inhaled anesthetics and thus increase the amount of anesthetic required include the amphetamines, cocaine, chronic alcohol intoxi-

TABLE 16–6 DRUG-DRUG INTERACTIONS OF SELECTED ANESTHETICS

Drug	Interactive Drug	Interaction
Inhalation Anesthetics		
Inhalation anesthetics	Alcohol Ketamine Nitrous oxide Tetrahydrocannabinol	Potentiate the effects of inhalation anesthetics
	Aminophylline	Sensitizes the myocardium to ventricular arrhythmias
	Fentanyl Morphine Sufentanil	Raises the level of hypercapnia required to stimulate ventilation
	Barbiturates Benzodiazepines Phenothiazines	Depresses ventilatory responses to hypercapnia
	Alcohol Amphetamines Cocaine Naloxone Tetrahydrocannabinol	Antagonize the effects of inhalation anesthetics
Intravenous Anesthetics		
Midazolam Propofol	Alcohol Antihistamines Antihypertensives Nitrates Sedative-hypnotics	Additive CNS depression and increased risk of hypotension
Midazolam	Calcium channel blockers Erythromycin Ketoconazole Itraconazole	Increased midazolam levels, increased sedation, respiratory depression

CNS, Central nervous system.

cation, naloxone, and chronic tetrahydrocannabinol intoxication.

PHARMACOTHERAPEUTIC OPTIONS

Barbiturates

- ❒ Thiopental sodium (PENTOTHAL)
- ❒ Methohexital sodium (BREVITAL)

THIOPENTAL SODIUM

Thiopental sodium is an ultra short-acting thiobarbiturate that depresses the CNS and induces hypnosis and anesthesia but not analgesia. Pentothal is used for induction of general anesthesia and supplementation of regional anesthesia, as an anticonvulsant, and as a drug for reduction of elevated intracranial pressure.

The drug produces some anterograde amnesia, and airway reflexes are heightened. Pentothal is associated with respiratory depression and hemodynamic effects that include a decrease in systemic vascular resistance, arterial pressure, cardiac output, and coronary perfusion pressure. Marked hypotension can occur in a hypovolemic patient. Although histamine release is rare, anaphylaxis with cardiovascular collapse has been reported. Pentothal is contraindicated in patients with porphyria (a genetic disorder characterized by disturbance in porphyrin metabolism with resultant gastrointestinal, neurologic, and psychological symptoms).

The onset of drug action following an induction dose is 10 to 15 seconds, with a duration of action of 5 to 15 minutes. Recovery from a small dose is rapid, but high lipid solubility and slow elimination result in cumulative drug effects after repeated bolus injection or infusion.

METHOHEXITAL SODIUM

Methohexital sodium is a methylated oxybarbiturate that produces a rapid ultra short-acting anesthesia. Methohexital does not produce analgesia and has no muscle relaxant properties. This barbiturate depresses the sensory cortex, decreases motor activity, alters cerebellar function, and produces dose-dependent drowsiness, sedation, and hypnosis. These effects are thought to be mediated by enhancement of a major inhibitory transmitter in the CNS, which is gamma-aminobutyric acid. Methohexital is associated with a more rapid return to consciousness, making it especially useful in outpatient anesthesia.

Methohexital may produce excitement in older adults and children, and in other patients in the presence of pain. Induction may be associated with involuntary skeletal muscle movement and respiratory depression. Premedication with opioids reduces the incidence of excitatory phenomena. Cardiovascular effects are secondary to decreased myocardial contractility and peripheral vasodilation. Adverse reactions are rare but may include laryngospasm, bronchospasm, emergence delirium, nausea, emesis, hiccups, skeletal muscle hyperactivity, and shivering. Extravascular injection causes tissue necrosis, and intra-arterial injection may result in gangrene. Arterial injection can be managed with an arterial injection of 10 mL of 1-percent procaine, 40 to 80 mg of papaverine, or local infiltration of phentolamine (2.5 to 5 mg in 10 mL) to produce vasodilation. Methohexital is contraindicated in patients with porphyria and must be used with caution in patients with status asthmaticus.

Nonbarbiturates

- ❒ Etomidate (AMIDATE)
- ❒ Ketamine (KETALAR)
- ❒ Propofol (DIPRIVAN)

ETOMIDATE

Etomidate is a carboxylated imidazole compound that is water soluble at an acidic pH but lipid soluble at physiologic pH. Depression of the CNS is thought to be due to action at the gamma-aminobutyric acid receptor. Etomidate lowers cerebral metabolism, cerebral blood flow, and intracranial pressure. Cerebral perfusion pressure is well maintained because this drug has minimal effect on systemic blood pressure. It does not produce analgesia or trigger MH and is generally not associated with histamine release, so allergic reactions are rare. Therapeutic doses have minimal effect on myocardial contractility, cardiac output, and peripheral circulation.

Myoclonic movement occurs in about one third of patients during induction and is due to disinhibition of subcortical suppression of extrapyramidal activity. This drug should be used with caution in patients with epilepsy. Myoclonus may be reduced by premedication with a benzodiazepine or opioid. Although intraocular pressure is reduced, eye movements may be problematic for surgical procedures on the eye.

Etomidate inhibits the enzymes 17α-hydroxylase and 11β-hydroxylase. These enzymes are important in the synthesis of cortisol and aldosterone. Adrenocortical suppression may occur after a single induction dose, and it lasts for 4 to 8 hours.

Propylene glycol is a preservative of etomidate. Intravenous injection is associated with pain on injection and, on occasion, thrombophlebitis. Pain is more likely if the drug is injected into small veins.

KETAMINE

Ketamine is a phencyclidine derivative that produces rapid-acting dissociative anesthesia owing to a functional and electrophysiologic dissociation between the thalamoneocortical and limbic systems of the CNS. Analgesic effects of ketamine may be due to its effect at central and spinal opiate receptors. The unique clinical anesthetic state of catalepsy is observed with this drug. The eyes remain open with a slow nystagmic gaze, whereas corneal and light reflexes remain intact. Vocalization may occur. Varying degrees of hypertonus and occasional purposeful movements unrelated to painful stimuli are noted in the presence of adequate surgical anesthesia. Adequacy of anesthesia is based on noting the presence or absence of purposeful responses to noxious stimuli.

Ketamine generally preserves airway patency and respiratory function. Laryngeal reflexes are normal or slightly enhanced. It is a mild respiratory depressant. Salivary and tracheobronchial secretions are increased and a prophylactic antisialagogue (a drug that inhibits the flow of saliva) is required. It causes bronchodilation and has been used in the treatment and emergency intubation of pediatric patients with status asthmaticus.

A major feature that distinguishes ketamine from other IV anesthetics is stimulation of the cardiovascular system. Although it may produce myocardial depression, central sympathetic stimulation, neuronal release of catecholamines, and inhibition of neuronal uptake of catecholamines usually overrides the direct myocardial depressant effects of the drug. Hemodynamic effects include increases in systemic and pulmonary artery pressure, heart rate, and cardiac output. This advantage makes ketamine a very good choice in patients with hemodynamic compromise due to hypovolemia or cardiac tamponade. Critically ill patients with catecholamine depletion may respond to ketamine with unexpected reductions in blood pressure and cardiac output. Ketamine does not release histamine.

Postanesthetic emergence reactions have been reported with the use of ketamine. These psychic sensations have been characterized by alterations in mood and body image, dissociative or extracorporeal experiences, floating sensations, vivid dreams or illusions, or delirium. Although these sensations generally occur immediately upon awakening, flashbacks have been reported several weeks later. Ketamine is usually a poor choice for patients with a history of psychiatric illness.

The incidence of psychic disturbances with ketamine ranges from 5 to 30 percent. Factors associated with a higher incidence of reactions include age, sex, and current personality disorders. Females have a higher incidence of psychic disturbances than males, and 24 to 34 percent of reactions occur in patients over 16 years of age. There is a decreased incidence of emergence reactions when ketamine is used in conjunction with sedative-hypnotics or when it is used with benzodiazepines.

Although it is rarely used today, ketamine can be used as a premedication, for sedation or analgesia, or induction and maintenance of anesthesia. It should be used with caution in patients with severe hypertension, ischemic heart disease, aneurysms, or in patients with intracranial hypertension. It should also be used cautiously in chronic alcoholics or in acutely intoxicated patients.

PROPOFOL

Propofol is an IV induction and maintenance drug introduced into clinical practice in the United States in 1989. It exists as oil at room temperature and has a white, milky appearance. Because it has no antimicrobial properties, guidelines for handling must include strict aseptic technique, single-patient use, and use of the drug within 6 hours of opening the vial for surgical patients. Anaphylaxis has been occasionally associated with use of this drug.

Propofol produces rapid induction of anesthesia with minimal excitatory effects. It is rapidly cleared from the body. Compared with thiopental, recovery is more rapid and there is less nausea and vomiting during recovery. It reduces nausea and vomiting in high-risk patients and has been effective as a long-term infusion for refractory postoperative nausea. It is believed the drug may have direct antiemetic effects. Subhypnotic doses of propofol may be used in the postanesthesia care unit to treat postoperative nausea and vomiting, particularly if it is not of vagal origin.

Induction doses of propofol may lead to apnea and hypotension secondary to slight myocardial depression and a decrease in systemic vascular resistance. There is minimal change in heart rate. Venodilation also contributes to the 15- to 30-percent decrease in blood pressure that is occasionally observed. Hypotension is especially likely in older adults, hypovolemic, or high-risk patients who have received other CNS depressants.

Propofol injection may be associated with pain, particularly if the drug is injected into small veins. This discomfort can be minimized or eliminated by injecting the drug into a large vein or by mixing lidocaine with the induction dose of propofol. Lidocaine can also be injected before propofol. Cooling propofol to 4° C into the IV cannula immediately before administering appears as effective as 10 mg of lidocaine to 19 mL of propofol in reducing pain associated with injection.

There have been rare reports of seizures and *opisthotonos* (a form of spasm in which the head and heels are bent backward and the body bowed forward) associated with the use of propofol. These effects occur most often during emergence or in the postoperative period. Propofol-induced dyskinesias in Parkinson's disease has also been reported. Possible association between propofol and the development of postoperative pancreatitis has been reported. Sexual illusions and disinhibition are observed during propofol sedation. To avoid complications of misconduct, it is advisable to have a third party in the room at all times when this drug or any drug with central effects is given.

Since its introduction in 1989, propofol has been approved for use in monitored anesthesia care, neuroanesthesia, cardiac and pediatric anesthesia, and for sedation in the intensive care unit. Rapid onset and a rapid, clear-headed emergence make the drug very attractive today. Although a reduced incidence of postoperative nausea and vomiting is attractive, there is inconsistency regarding propofol's role in perioperative emesis (see Controversy—Appropriateness of Increased Utilization of Propofol in Anesthesia).

Opioid Agonists

- ❒ Fentanyl (SUBLIMAZE)
- ❒ Alfentanil (ALFENTA)
- ❒ Sufentanil (SUFENTA)
- ❒ Remifentanil (ULTIVA)

Opioid is a term used to describe all drugs, both synthetic and natural, that bind to opioid receptors. Synthetic opioids have almost completely replaced the use of naturally occurring narcotics in the operating room today.

Opioid receptors are classified as mu_1, mu_2, delta, kappa, and sigma. Drug interaction at mu_1 receptors provides analgesia, whereas mu_2 receptor interaction is associated with adverse effects including respiratory depression, decreased heart rate, physical dependence, and euphoria. Delta Receptor stimulation is associated with modulation of mu receptor activity. Kappa receptor stimulation leads to analgesia, sedation, respiratory depression, and miosis. Dysphoria, hypertonia, tachycardia, and tachypnea are effects of sigma recep-

Controversy

Appropriateness of Increased Utilization of Propofol in Anesthesia
JONATHAN J. WOLFE

Propofol, a newer and novel anesthetic, offers apparent advantages over other IV drugs for the induction and maintenance of anesthesia. These advantages generally include a smoother and more predictable onset of anesthesia as well as rapid recovery from anesthesia. The drug also appears to produce less incidence of perioperative nausea and vomiting. Propofol appears highly desirable from many points of view. The patient requiring surgery stands to receive superior anesthesia with less stressful induction, maintenance, and emergence. Surgery and anesthesia teams can anticipate less likelihood of patient hazard, a situation likely to promote both confidence and performance. If drug response were the only issue, propofol might quickly replace IV barbiturates and volatile anesthetics.

However, propofol carries a far higher price tag than traditional anesthetic agents. Most rapid-acting barbiturates and inhalation agents are procurable at reduced prices, simply because several generic forms of them are readily available on the market. Propofol is a patented product with a single manufacturer. Therefore, it is likely to retain a high purchase price for years to come. A surgical department may face little difficulty deciding to adopt propofol for high-risk cases, such as cardiac surgery, in which a reduction in adverse effects is desirable regardless of price. However, the decision to make the new drug broadly available may result in far greater problems.

Critical Thinking Discussion

- Does a hospital have an obligation to provide the advantages of propofol anesthesia to all patients, based on the right each person has to equal protection from adverse effects during treatment?
- Would an outpatient surgery center be justified in adopting propofol as its usual and customary agent for induction and maintenance of anesthesia, and charging higher prices to its patients and their insurance carriers, if its fewer adverse effects permitted better facility utilization, and hence higher net profits for the surgery center?
- After you have discussed an anesthesia plan using thiopental sodium for induction, a competent and well-informed patient refuses to sign the consent forms. This person instead demands that the plan be changed to propofol induction, which the patient considers to be so far superior that thiopental is not an option. The case is elective and of low risk. Your department's procedures clearly indicate that as a cost-containment matter, propofol is not to be used. How will you respond to this patient?

tor stimulation. Common opioid agonists, antagonists, and agonist-antagonists are listed in Table 16–7. Opioids are discussed in depth in Chapter 14.

FENTANYL

Fentanyl is a potent opioid agonist with an analgesic potency 75 to 125 times that of morphine. Fentanyl may be used for induction, analgesia, or as a drug to supplement other drugs. It may be added to spinal or epidural blocks and may be used postoperatively in patient-controlled analgesia. It is more lipid soluble with a rapid onset (30 seconds) and short duration of action (30 to 60 minutes). Cardiovascular stability is generally maintained, but in high doses, such as those formerly used in cardiac surgery, fentanyl can cause bradycardia and chest wall rigidity. Respiratory depression is dose dependent, potentiated by other CNS depressants, and may last longer than analgesia.

ALFENTANIL

Alfentanil is a potent opioid analgesic with a rapid onset (1 to 1½ minutes) and short duration of action (10 to 15 minutes). Small doses are used for analgesia, whereas large doses may be used for induction and maintenance of anesthesia. Alfentanil produces a deep level of analgesia and attenuates the hemodynamic response to surgical stress. Like most opioids, it reduces sympathetic tone and may produce bradycardia because of stimulation of the vagal nucleus in the medulla. This is especially true when used in combination with nonvagolytic neuromuscular blockers or if an anticholinergic has not been given. Induction doses produce respiratory depression and reduce blood pressure secondary to peripheral vasodilation. Hypotension and bradycardia are seen more often with alfentanil than with either fentanyl or sufentanil. Extreme bradycardia may be treated with atropine. Repeated doses or continuous infusions do not result in a significant cumulation. Alfentanil does not produce clinically significant changes in cerebral blood flow, cerebral metabolic rate, or intracranial pressure.

SUFENTANIL

Sufentanil is an analog of fentanyl with 5 to 7 times the analgesic potency. Cardiovascular effects are similar to those of fentanyl. Like other opioids, sufentanil may produce a dose-dependent bradycardia, which is sufficient to decrease cardiac output. Respiratory depression is due to a decrease in response of the respiratory centers in the brainstem to carbon dioxide. Skeletal muscle rigidity sufficient to interfere with ventilation may occur at higher doses. Sufentanil has no clinically significant effects on cerebral blood flow or intracranial pressure, but it does cause a decrease in the cerebral metabolic requirements for oxygen.

REMIFENTANIL

Remifentanil is a new synthetic opioid that is uniquely different from previous drugs. It is a pure agonist at mu receptors with little binding to other receptors. Because this is similar to other common synthetic opioids, pharmacologic effects such as analgesia, sedation, ventilatory depression, muscle rigidity, nausea, itching, and hemodynamic instability are easily predicted.

Remifentanil's unique characteristic is its biotransformation. Remifentanil is an ester and therefore is biotransformed by both plasma and tissue esterases. It has an onset of pharmacologic activity of approximately 1 minute, which is similar to the onset of alfentanil. Termination of opioid effect, however, is extremely rapid, making this the first truly titratable opioid.

As previously discussed, the terminal elimination half-life has been used in the past to describe offset of drug action. Terminal elimination half-life defines the time necessary to eliminate 50 percent of the drug from the body following its rapid IV injection. The terminal elimination half-life of synthetic opioids most often used in anesthesia is fentanyl, 219

TABLE 16–7 OPIOID AGONISTS, AGONIST-ANTAGONISTS, AND ANTAGONISTS

Drug	Indication	Adverse Effects
Opioid Agonists		
Fentanyl	Anesthesia Analgesia	Nausea, vomiting Delayed gastric emptying Biliary tract spasm Muscle rigidity Neonatal respiratory depression
Alfentanil	Analgesia Anesthesia	Bradycardia, hypotension Nausea, vomiting Biliary tract spasm Delayed gastric emptying
Sufentanil	Analgesia Anesthesia	Hypotension Nausea, vomiting Delayed gastric emptying Muscle rigidity
Remifentanil	Analgesia Anesthesia	Rigidity Lack of postoperative analgesia Quick awakening if infusion accidentally stopped
Agonist-Antagonists		
Butorphanol	Analgesia	Hypertension, hypotension Hallucinations Nausea, vomiting Withdrawal in opioid-dependent patient
Nalbuphine	Analgesia Anesthesia	Hypertension, hypotension, tachycardia, or bradycardia Dyspepsia Urinary urgency Pruritus Bronchospasm Withdrawal in opioid-dependent patient
Antagonists		
Naloxone	Reversal of narcotic	Tachycardia, hypertension, depression, hypotension, arrhythmia Pulmonary edema Reversal of analgesia Seizures Nausea, vomiting Sweating
Nalmefene	Reversal of narcotic	Tachycardia, hypertension, hypotension, vasodilation Reversal of analgesia Pulmonary edema Somnolence, depression, agitation, nervousness, tremor, confusion, withdrawal syndrome, myoclonus, dizziness

Adapted from Zaglaniczny, K., and Maree, S. (1995). Anesthesia and perioperative nursing care. In R. A. Roth (Ed.), *Perioperative nursing core curriculum* (p. 237). Philadelphia: W. B. Saunders. Used with permission.

minutes; sufentanil, 164 minutes; alfentanil, 90 to 111 minutes; and remifentanil, 3 to 10 minutes. Terminal elimination half-life does not always adequately predict the pharmacodynamic effects of opioids and the term context-sensitive half-time is now used to more clearly define offset of pharmacologic activity. Context-sensitive half-time is the time required for a 50-percent decrease in blood or effect site concentration after termination of an infusion rate. The context-sensitive half-times for remifentanil and alfentanil after a 3-hour infusion are approximately 3 and 47 minutes, respectively, and these times closely approximate the pharmacodynamic offset of drug effects. Even with prolonged infusions, the context-sensitive half-time of remifentanil remains constant, whereas the context-sensitive half-times for other opioids increase with duration of the infusion because of accumulation. Even when the infusion range is varied over an 80-fold range, patients awaken and can be extubated in a few minutes.

Esterase biotransformation is a well-preserved metabolic system with little variation between individuals. The circulating esterases responsible for remifentanil metabolism are distinct from those enzymes that metabolize succinylcholine or acetylcholine. The short duration of remifentanil is preserved in patients with a deficiency of pseudocholinesterase activity or in patients taking medications that inhibit plasma pseudocholinesterase (e.g., echothiophate). The pharmacokinetics of remifentanil in patients with impaired hepatic or renal function appears to be unchanged.

Remifentanil's effects on cerebral blood flow and cerebral metabolic rate for oxygen are similar to those of alfentanil. If given in equivalent doses to other opioids, hemodynamic responses are similar to the other opioids. A higher incidence of hypotension (16 percent versus 5 percent) suggests that higher doses can be given with confidence in rapid elimination. Maximum cardiovascular depression is seen after the first dose of remifentanil. The maximal cardiovascular depression can be mostly prevented by premedication with glycopyrrolate. Although remifentanil produces respiratory depression in a dose-dependent fashion, lack of accumulation and esterase biotransformation eliminates this concern 10 to 15 minutes after discontinuation of an infusion. Remifentanil does not release histamine. Although the use of this drug is associated with nausea and vomiting, the incidence is no higher than what is seen with alfentanil. The incidence of muscle rigidity, which is also comparable to what is noted with alfentanil, may be prevented by slow infusion or slow injection of bolus doses over 60 to 90 seconds.

The unique characteristics of remifentanil make it extremely useful for induction and maintenance of general anesthesia, monitored anesthesia care, and postoperative analgesia. Although remifentanil is not considered suitable as a sole drug for induction of anesthesia, it is well tolerated in combination with nitrous oxide, thiopental, or propofol. When administered with or after hypnotic drugs such as propofol, muscle rigidity is markedly reduced and the dose of the hypnotic is also reduced. When it is used for anesthetic maintenance, rapid onset and offset of drug effect results in rapid titration to meet the clinical requirements of the patient.

The use of remifentanil as part of monitored anesthesia care effectively provides patient comfort and analgesia during placement of local or regional anesthetic blocks. It can be rapidly titrated to provide patient comfort without sedation, and careful titration is associated with an adequate respiratory rate. It is associated with hemodynamic stability and is well tolerated.

Emergence from remifentanil-based anesthesia is swift and predictable. The quick offset of action, which is otherwise desirable, may result in inadequate postoperative analgesia. A transition must be made from remifentanil to some other longer acting analgesic for surgeries that result in significant pain. In select patients who have been maintained intraoperatively with infusions of this opioid, the infusion of remifentanil can be continued into the immediate postoperative setting. The use of this drug postoperatively should be under the direct supervision of an anesthesia provider.

Potentially useful implications of remifentanil's unique pharmacologic profile include cases in which profound analgesia is needed for a few minutes. It also allows the anesthesia provider to administer high-dose opioids with little risk of respiratory depression in the postoperative period. The relationship between remifentanil infusion rate and concentration is consistent with and independent of the disease state and renal or hepatic dysfunction. Disadvantages associated with the use of this drug include the necessity for administration by infusion techniques and lack of prolonged opioid effects, which may be desirable during painful procedures.

Opioid Agonist-Antagonists and Antagonists

- ❐ Butorphanol (STADOL, STADOL NS)
- ❐ Nalbuphine (NUBAIN)
- ❐ Nalmefene (REVEX)
- ❐ Naloxone (NARCAN)

Opioid agonist-antagonists bind to mu receptors, where they produce limited or no response. They do, however, provide partial agonist action at delta and kappa opioid receptors. Antagonist properties attenuate the efficacy of opioid agonists administered while the agonist-antagonist is present. Advantages of these drugs are their ability to produce analgesia with limited respiratory depression. They are sometimes used in the post-anesthesia care unit to reverse respiratory depression of narcotics without eliminating analgesia.

BUTORPHANOL

Butorphanol is a synthetic opioid agonist-antagonist with an analgesic potency 3.5 to 7 times that of morphine or 30 to 40 times that of meperidine. It has a ceiling effect for respiratory depression and analgesia at high doses or greater than 30 to 67 mcg/kg. The analgesia provided is not adequate for the performance of surgery. Its use is associated with a dose-dependent increase in sedation secondary to vascular uptake and activation of kappa receptors in the CNS. Analgesic doses increase blood pressure, pulmonary artery pressure, and cardiac output.

NALBUPHINE

Nalbuphine is also classified as an opioid agonist-antagonist. It is equal in analgesic potency to morphine and one-fourth as potent as nalorphine as an antagonist. NUBAIN is effective in reversing the ventilatory depression of opioids such as fentanyl while maintaining reasonable analgesia. Cardiovascular stability is good.

Minor changes in the structure of an opioid agonist can convert the drug into a receptor antagonist. By competitive inhibition at mu, delta, and kappa receptors, nalbuphine prevents or reverses the effects of opioids and reverses respiratory depression, sedation, and hypotension. Reversal of narcotic depression is achieved by IV or intramuscular (IM) doses. The duration of action of nalbuphine is less than that of most opioid agonists, allowing the return of respiratory depression in some patients who have received longer acting narcotics.

Adverse effects associated with the use of nalbuphine may include nausea, vomiting, hypertension, tachycardia, anxiety, hyperpnea, and discomfort. These effects may be the result of patients who have become physically dependent on opioids after receiving large doses for several hours. Pulmonary edema has been reported in patients with a history of cardiovascular disease and in healthy young adults. It was first believed that this complication was due to the administration of large doses or as much as 400 mcg. The etiology is thought to be inhibition of endogenous pain suppression pathways and unopposed nonadrenergic transmission from medullary centers that produce neurogenic pulmonary edema. The drug should be administered slowly at the lowest possible dose.

NALMEFENE

Nalmefene is a new opioid antagonist. Like naloxone, it prevents or reverses opioid effects including respiratory depression, sedation, hypotension, and analgesia. It has an elimination half-life of 10 hours compared with naloxone's 1 hour. The duration of action is approximately 8 hours when it is administered in usual doses. Clinical effects and adverse effects of nalmefene are similar to those of naloxone. Acute pulmonary edema in a young male has been reported after IV administration of the drug.

NALOXONE

Naloxone and nalmefene competitively block the effects of opioids, including CNS and respiratory depression, without producing agonist effects. They are pure antagonists with no agonist properties of their own and minimal toxicity. They are used most often to reverse the signs of opioid excess. They have a rapid onset when given IV, subcutaneously, or IM. These drugs are discussed as the antagonists to opioids in Chapter 14.

Inhalation Drugs

- Nitrous oxide
- Halothane (FLUOTHANE)
- Enflurane (ETHRANE)
- Isoflurane (FORANE)
- Desflurane (SUPRANE)
- Sevoflurane (ULTANE)

NITROUS OXIDE

Nitrous oxide is the first of the gaseous inhalational anesthetics, having been used for more than 100 years. It is still one of the most commonly used anesthetics, but now its major use is as a supplement to other inhalational or IV anesthetics. It has a very low tissue solubility, which results in rapid elimination and awakening. In addition, administration of high concentrations of a rapidly absorbed first gas will facilitate the rate of rise of alveolar concentration of a second gas. This phenomenon is called the second gas effect.

If nitrous oxide is suddenly discontinued and the patient is allowed to breathe room air, movement of large volumes of nitrous oxide from the blood to the alveoli may result in hypoxemia, which is referred to as diffusional anoxia. This transient hypoxemia can be avoided by the administration of supplemental oxygen during the first few minutes after nitrous oxide has been discontinued.

Unlike most inhaled anesthetics, nitrous oxide has a minimal effect on ventilation and does not increase $PaCO_2$. It does reduce the ventilatory drive to hypoxia, but depression of ventilation occurs only at concentrations higher than 50 percent. This is due to a direct depressant effect on the medulla and peripheral effects on intercostal muscle function. It decreases functional residual capacity and relaxes bronchial smooth muscle tone. It does not inhibit hypoxic pulmonary vasoconstriction, but it may produce increases in pulmonary vascular resistance that are exaggerated in patients with pulmonary hypertension.

Alone in a 40-percent concentration, nitrous oxide directly depresses the myocardium. When it is given to patients with heart disease, particularly in combination with opioids, it will cause hypotension and a decrease in cardiac output. Compared with other inhaled anesthetics, nitrous oxide is a sympathomimetic and has mild cardiac depressant effects. Atlhough the patient's heart rate is not usually changed, systemic vascular resistance and arterial blood pressure increase. Nitrous oxide attenuates the baroreceptor response to hypotension and hypovolemia, which is tachycardia and increased peripheral resistance.

Cerebral vasodilation produced by nitrous oxide causes an increase in cerebral blood flow and blood volume. Elevation of intracranial pressure may accompany the increase in blood volume. Hyperventilation of the lungs to a $PaCO_2$ below 30 mmHg opposes the increase in intracranial pressure. Nitrous oxide decreases cerebral metabolic rate, and increased concentrations decrease electroencephalograph wave frequency and increase voltage. This drug alters somatosensory-evoked potentials.

Because nitrous oxide is 30 times more soluble in blood than nitrogen, it exchanges with nitrogen that may be found in gas-containing areas in the body. The gas-containing area will expand as much as possible and may intensify effects of pneumothorax, bowel distention, or air embolus. Some practitioners believe that the properties of nitrous oxide increase the chance of postoperative nausea and vomiting but others disagree.

Nitrous oxide inhibits the actions of methionine synthetase, which is involved in vitamin B_{12} metabolism. Although this process may lead to bone marrow dysfunction, this is not a problem with short-term exposure. Concerns do surround individuals who are chronically exposed to nitrous oxide, however. A neuropathy that resembles vitamin B_{12} deficiency has been reported in dentists who are chronically exposed to nitrous oxide.

HALOTHANE

Halothane was introduced into clinical practice in 1956. It was the first of the halogenated liquid compounds, which form the base of all modern inhaled anesthetics. Advantages over other drugs used in 1956 included rapid induction and emergence, and lack of flammability. It is potent, however, and leads quickly to dose-dependent circulatory depression.

Alveolar hypoventilation and arterial hypercapnia occur in a dose-dependent manner when halothane is inhaled. Depression of ventilation reflects a direct depressant effect on the medulla and, possibly, peripheral effects on intercostal muscle function. Although there may be an initial increase in respiratory rate, it is insufficient to offset the decrease in tidal volume.

Other respiratory effects produced by halothane include relaxation of bronchial smooth muscle. It has no effect on pulmonary vascular resistance but may inhibit the hypoxic pulmonary vasoconstrictor response at higher concentrations.

The most prominent circulatory effect of halothane is dose-dependent arterial hypotension. The decrease in blood pressure is the result of a decrease in cardiac output. Halothane has a minor effect on systemic vascular resistance, so vasodilation is less important than cardiac output in the decline in blood pressure.

Halothane's negative inotropic effect appears to be related to alterations in intracellular calcium. Decreased influx through calcium channels, increased binding by plasma membranes, and decreased uptake by the sarcoplasmic reticulum all play a role.

Halothane decreases heart rate and may slow cardiac conduction through the atrioventricular node and His-Purkinje system. Junctional rhythms leading to reductions in blood pressure may occur. It sensitizes the myocardium to the action of epinephrine and norepinephrine, and the combination may result in serious arrhythmias. No more than 100 mcg in 10 minutes or 300 mcg/hour of epinephrine should be given to adults receiving halothane. Children tolerate higher doses of epinephrine. It does not lead to coronary vasodilation and coronary steal syndrome.

Cerebral vasodilation and increased cerebral blood flow occur with halothane. The cerebral vasculature remains responsive to carbon dioxide, and cerebral vasodilation can be prevented by hyperventilation. Halothane causes a decrease in cerebral metabolism and causes slowing and increased amplitude on the electroencephalogram.

Halothane does not depress skeletal muscle, but it does potentiate the action of nondepolarizing muscle relaxants. Uterine smooth muscle relaxation occurs in clinical doses. Although uterine smooth muscle relaxation may lead to hemorrhage following delivery, relaxation is beneficial when version (i.e., turning of the fetus) is required during delivery.

A major concern with the use of halothane involves its biotransformation. Although the major route for elimination of halothane is the lungs, approximately 20 percent is biotransformed by the cytochrome P_{450} system in the liver. The biotransformation of halothane results in the release of bromide, chloride, and trifluoroacetic acid. In some cases, hepatic dysfunction occurs.

Although the incidence of hepatic necrosis following halothane use is rare, it has occurred. The mortality rate can reach 50 percent in severe cases. The response is more likely to occur after repeated exposures and is more common in the obese patient or after a hypotensive episode. The etiology remains controversial but may involve an immune response in the face of hepatic hypoperfusion and hypoxia.

ENFLURANE

Enflurane is a halogenated hydrocarbon that is approximately one-half as potent as halothane. Like halothane, enflurane is associated with dose-dependent respiratory depression and hypercapnia. Ventilatory drive is blunted, and the response to both oxygen and carbon dioxide is impaired more than with halothane.

Moderate levels of enflurane result in a progressive decrease in blood pressure that is similar to what is seen with halothane. Profound hypotension occurs at deep anesthetic levels. The decrease in blood pressure is due to the effects on the heart and peripheral circulation. Hypotension is the result then of a decreased cardiac output and decreased systemic vascular resistance.

Cerebral blood flow is increased and cerebral vascular resistance is decreased by enflurane anesthesia. Like other volatile drugs, it causes dose-dependent decreases in cerebral metabolism and cerebral metabolic oxygen consumption.

Tonic-clonic muscle activity associated with electroencephalographic evidence of seizure activity may occur with deep levels of anesthesia in the hyperventilated and hypocapnic patient. Enflurane does not increase the incidence or severity of seizures when it is administered to epileptic patients.

Enflurane is biotransformed less than halothane. Approximately 3 percent is biotransformed by the hepatic cytochrome P_{450} enzyme system, releasing fluoride and difluoromethoxy-difluoroacetic acid. Nephrotoxicity caused by fluoride is generally not a concern under usual clinical circumstances. Some practitioners avoid this drug in patients with renal dysfunction.

ISOFLURANE

Isoflurane is an isomer of enflurane, but it undergoes minimal biotransformation and is not associated with organ toxicity. Like other volatile drugs, isoflurane impairs ventilatory drive and leads to hypercapnia. The ventilatory response to both hypoxia and hypercapnia is depressed. Like most inhalation drugs, this drug inhibits bronchoconstriction and causes bronchodilation.

Progressive dose-dependent hypotension accompanies isoflurane anesthesia but cardiac output is maintained. A decrease in systemic vascular resistance is responsible for the hypotension that may occur with the use of this drug. Tachycardia frequently occurs and is more common in young patients. Coronary arteries dilate, leading to coronary steal syndrome in approximately 25 percent of patients with coronary artery disease. Overall, it appears that isoflurane is as safe as other drugs in patients with ischemic heart disease as long as tachycardia and diastolic hypotension are avoided.

Cerebral blood flow increases secondary to cerebral dilation when isoflurane is used. Although it may cause an increase in intracranial pressure, this effect is reduced with hypocapnia. Some studies suggest some protection from ischemia or hypoxemia with isoflurane, and this has led to the popularity of use in neurosurgical procedures.

The extent of biotransformation of isoflurane is 0.2 percent, which is 1/100 that of halothane and 1/10 that of enflurane. Metabolites are insufficient to cause significant cell injury or toxicity.

DESFLURANE

Desflurane is a newer halogenated hydrocarbon with a low blood gas solubility, and thus, rapid induction and emergence from anesthesia. Because the drug boils at room temperature, special vaporizers are needed to administer the drug. The pungency of this drug increases airway irritation during inhalation induction.

Respiratory effects of desflurane are similar to that seen with isoflurane. Likewise, circulatory effects more closely follow what is seen with isoflurane, but cardiac output may be better maintained. Cerebrovascular effects are much like those observed with isoflurane also.

Biotransformation of desflurane is 0.02 percent and organ toxicity should not be associated with the use of this drug. Many perioperative events may result in hepatic dysfunction, but toxic damage associated with desflurane is extremely rare.

SEVOFLURANE

Sevoflurane is the newest inhalation drug approved for clinical use. Like desflurane, it has a low solubility in blood and tissues, and this property results in a rapid induction and emergence from anesthesia. Rapid recovery permits earlier patient assessment. It may also help hospitals reduce costs by shortening the stay in the postanesthesia care unit. Unlike desflurane, it has a pleasant, nonpungent odor and low respiratory irritability. This makes it an ideal choice for mask inductions in both children and adults. Although it leads to dose-dependent respiratory depression, overall it has the lowest frequency of respiratory changes compared with halothane, isoflurane, enflurane, and desflurane.

The cardiovascular effects of sevoflurane or decreased systemic vascular resistance and arterial blood pressure are similar to what is seen with isoflurane. It is not associated with increases in heart rate at doses up to 1.5 MAC, and coronary steal has not been reported. In pediatric cases, its use is associated with better hemodynamic stability than halothane. There are fewer ventricular arrhythmias and a lower incidence of bradycardia.

Approximately 5 percent of absorbed sevoflurane is biotransformed by cytochrome P_{450} 2E1 to hexafluoroisopropanol (HFIP) with release of inorganic fluoride and carbon dioxide. Although the potential for hepatotoxicity is of concern, it appears that sevoflurane is less capable of initiating a hepatotoxic response than halothane. This is because overall biotransformation is less, and reductive metabolism does not exist. Additionally, the organic metabolite of sevoflurane (HFIP) appears to be less reactive than trifluoroacetic acid, a metabolite of halothane. Postoperative liver function tests following sevoflurane are comparable to other volatile drugs and propofol. Sevoflurane does not exacerbate pre-existing hepatic dysfunction.

Methoxyflurane, an agent used several decades ago, was associated with elevations in serum fluoride concentrations and high-output renal failure in some patients. Because the biotransformation of sevoflurane also leads to increases in plasma fluoride, concern has been expressed about the potential for renal toxicity following procedures. Renal exposure is much less with sevoflurane, however.

Serum inorganic fluoride concentrations after exposure to sevoflurane peak within 2 hours of the end of anesthesia compared with 1 to 3 days for methoxyflurane. Levels return to baseline within 48 hours in most patients, compared with 7 days with methoxyflurane. The lack of nephrotoxicity associated with the use of sevoflurane despite levels above 50 micromols/L in 10 percent of surgical patients is possibly related to lower overall biotransformation, smaller amounts of defluorination in the kidney than methoxyflurane, and shorter periods of time the kidney is exposed to elevated plasma inorganic fluoride concentrations. Pediatric patients have approximately half the maximum concentrations of inorganic fluoride observed in adults, and the fluoride concentrations tend to return to baseline more rapidly than in adult patients.

CONCEPTS AND PRINCIPLES OF REGIONAL ANESTHESIA

Types of Regional Anesthesia

Regional anesthetics block nerve transmission at its origin, thus producing analgesia over specific tissue areas (e.g., topicals or local infiltration). Drugs that block nerve transmission along afferent neurons produce analgesia over a specific area of the body (e.g., nerve block). Anesthetic drugs that block nerve transmission along the spinal cord produce analgesia over a specific region of the body (e.g., epidural, spinal). Local anesthetics do not result in loss of consciousness. Intravenous regional anesthesia, acupuncture, hypnosis, and cryotherapy are also discussed later.

Topical Anesthesia

Topical anesthetics are applied directly to the area to be desensitized. Often, the anesthetic is available in the form of an ointment, gel, cream, powder, or solution. This form of regional anesthesia is often used for respiratory intubation or for diagnostic procedures, such as bronchoscopy, laryngoscopy, or cystoscopy. It can also be used before a rectal exam when painful hemorrhoids are present.

The drug commonly used to desensitize the eye and mucous membranes of the nose, mouth, and urethra is a 5 percent solution of cocaine. Other drugs commonly used for topical anesthesia include lidocaine and tetracaine. The onset of drug action occurs in about 2 to 8 minutes, with a duration of action of 30 to 45 minutes with lidocaine and cocaine. The duration of action of tetracaine is 30 to 60 minutes.

Local Infiltration

Local infiltration anesthesia is effected by injecting the drug into the intracutaneous and subcutaneous tissues surrounding an incision, wound, or lesion. Lidocaine is commonly used during the suturing of superficial lacerations. The drug blocks only peripheral nerve stimulation at its origin. However, caution must be used to avoid infiltrating the drug into a vein. Once a local anesthetic becomes systemic, the risk of cardiovascular collapse or seizures increases.

Field Block

A field block is evoked when a series of injections are made around the operative field, forming a barrier between the incision and the nervous system. By injecting the drug around a specific nerve or group of nerves, the entire sensory nervous system of a localized area is anesthetized. This is in contrast to infiltration anesthesia, in which only the area of the incision is injected. This type of anesthesia is used for thoracic procedures, herniorrhaphy, dental procedures, and plastic surgery. Care must be taken to avoid inadvertent IV administration.

Peripheral Nerve Block

A wide variety of peripheral nerves can be effectively blocked by injecting local anesthetic around them to provide adequate surgical anesthesia. Peripheral nerve blocks desensitize individual nerves or nerve plexuses rather than all the local nerves. The nerves most commonly blocked are those of the brachial plexus and the intercostal, sciatic, and femoral nerves. A digital nerve block anesthetizes the finger, a brachial plexus block anesthetizes the entire upper arm, and an intercostal nerve block anesthetizes the chest or abdominal wall. Onset and duration of the block are related to the drug used, its concentration and volume, and the presence of epinephrine. The drugs commonly used in peripheral nerve blocks include lidocaine, bupivacaine, and chloroprocaine. The addition of epinephrine to the anesthetic agent is not recommended for digital blocks (fingers, toes, ears, nose, penis) owing to the risk of peripheral ischemia. Complications of peripheral nerve blocks are usually caused by an inadvertent intravascular injection or an

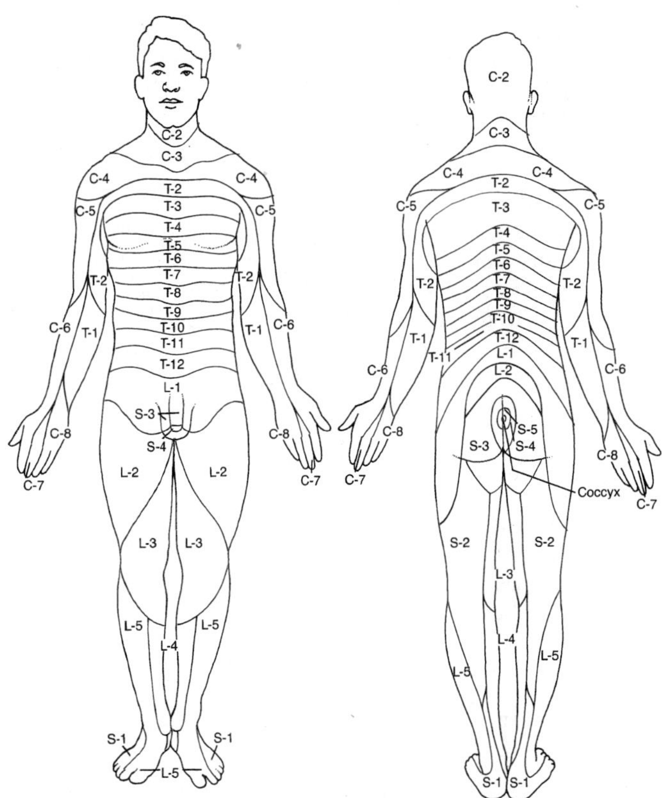

Figure 16–2 The areas of skin supplied with afferent nerve fibers by a single posterior spinal root are known as dermatomes. (From Ignatavicius, D. D., Workman, M. L., and Mishler, M. A. [1995]. *Medical-surgical nursing: A nursing process approach* [2nd ed., p. 1087]. Philadelphia: W. B. Saunders. Used with permission.)

overdose of the local anesthetic. Nerve damage from the trauma produced by the needle or compression from the volume of local anesthetic is rare.

Spinal Anesthesia

Spinal anesthesia is one of the older and most valuable of the techniques of regional anesthesia. It is the most efficient of blocks, in that a small quantity of local anesthetic injected into the spinal subarachnoid space will cause a widespread blockade of spinal nerves. It can be used for almost any kind of procedure performed below the level of the diaphragm (e.g., herniorrhaphy, appendectomy, hysterectomy).

A spinal needle is usually inserted in the L2–L3, L3–L4, or L4–L5 interspace. Autonomic nerves are the first to be affected by spinal anesthesia and the last to recover. Autonomic blockade blocks nerve fibers in the following sequence: touch, pain, motor, pressure, and proprioceptive fibers. The patient experiences a loss of sensation and paralysis of first the toes, then the feet and legs, and finally the abdomen. Recovery is in the reverse order. Spinal nerves supply specific dermatomes in the body (Fig. 16–2). Different levels of block are required for different operations: upper abdomen (T5–T6), lower abdomen (T8–T9), kidneys (T8), bladder (T10), lower limbs (T12), and perineal region (S1). Sympathetic fibers are blocked by lower drug concentrations, and, depending on the drug, may be anesthetized 2 to 6 segments higher than sensory fibers. Similarly, the level of sensory anesthesia may be 2 dermatomes higher than that of motor blockade, which requires the highest concentration of anesthetic.

Spinal anesthesia offers many advantages. First, it is relatively safe while providing excellent muscle relaxation. It does not cloud the patient's consciousness or alertness and can be used with patients who have recently eaten. This factor is advantageous because the patient will be awake to maintain the airway if vomiting occurs. However, spinal anesthesia can evoke several physiologic responses that result in complications if it is not properly managed, although systemic toxicity is never a problem. A rapid decline in blood pressure may occur after the local anesthetic is injected. This response is caused by vasodilation as the sympathetic nerves that control vasomotor tone are blocked. Peripheral pooling of blood causes reduced venous return to the heart and a decrease in cardiac output. This problem can usually be avoided by infusing a balanced salt solution immediately before the block and placing the patient in a 5-degree head-down position to improve venous return to the heart.

An inadvertently high spinal may cause paralysis of the respiratory muscles. This event necessitates immediate intubation and mechanical ventilation. Care must also be taken when positioning the patient intraoperatively to avoid neurologic damage, burns, or other trauma. Damage may occur because pain and sensory input to a portion of the patient's body are blocked.

One of the most frequent postoperative complaints following spinal anesthesia is a so-called spinal headache. The incidence is greatest in persons younger than 40 years of age. The headache is thought to be related to leakage of cerebrospinal fluid through the hole in the dura and typically occurs when the patient assumes an upright position. Various treatment modalities have been used in an attempt to relieve the headache, although this occipital headache usually resolves over 1 to 3 days. Treatment modalities for a postdural puncture headache include bedrest for 24 to 48 hours, vigorous hydration, abdominal binders, epidural infusion of saline, and an injection of 5 to 20 mL of autologous blood into the epidural space at the puncture site (known as a blood patch).

Epidural Anesthesia

The epidural space lies within the spinal canal and outside the spinal dura mater. Local anesthetic injected into the epidural space spreads both up and down the spinal canal, blocking spinal nerves as they run from the spinal cord to their respective intervertebral foramina. All modalities of nerve function—motor, sensory, and autonomic—are affected by an epidural block. Much like in spinal anesthesia, spinal nerves supply specific dermatomes in the body and different levels of blockade are required for different surgical procedures when using epidural anesthesia.

Epidural blockade is segmental, that is, it has an inferior as well as a superior limit of action. Epidural blockade begins quickest and is most intense at the level of the injection, and it diminishes as it moves inferiorly and superiorly. This means that needle and catheter insertion ideally should be as close to the dermatomal level of the surgical procedure as possible. With epidural anesthesia, the concentration of the anesthetic dictates the intensity of the blockade. Surgical epidural anesthesia usually requires intense blockade. The most commonly used agents are lidocaine (with or without epinephrine), bupivacaine, and chloroprocaine.

Compared with spinal anesthesia, epidural anesthesia requires a larger dose of local anesthetic, a larger needle for insertion, and a more subtle technique for entry into the appropriate space. The flexibility of the epidural route provides advantages for a variety of surgical procedures. There is a decreased incidence of headache, and the segmental block can be focused on the area of the surgery. There is a gradual onset of drug action with less hemodynamic changes than those seen with a spinal. Furthermore, compared with inhalation anesthesia, the autonomic response is decreased.

The disadvantages of epidural anesthesia are that it cannot be used in patients with coagulopathy, sepsis, spinal anomalies, elevated intracranial pressure, patients who are hemodynamically unstable, and in patients with advanced respiratory disease. High blocks can weaken the cough reflex. Inadvertent puncture of the dura with a large (17- to 18-gauge) epidural needle can cause a postdural puncture headache. This headache is significant in about 50 percent of patients and can be incapacitating. Treatment is the same as that used for spinal headaches.

If the anesthetic is unintentionally inserted into the subarachnoid space and the large volume of local anesthetic that is typically used for epidural anesthesia is injected as a bolus, it causes "total spinal" anesthesia. The drug moves to the brain, resulting in rapid hypotension caused by vasodilation, profound bradycardia as the vagus nerves to the heart are blocked, and a totally paralyzed and anesthetized, but awake, patient. Management includes intubation and mechanical ventilation, support of blood pressure and the cardiovascular system, and amnestic drugs until the blockade has resolved.

Epidural anesthesia can also be inadvertently injected into an epidural vein and can occur with the initial injection or any subsequent dose. Bupivacaine can cause cardiac arrest and cardiovascular collapse. Toxicity from other agents can cause sudden and profound hypotension, seizures, and tachycardia if the solution contains epinephrine. The seizures ordinarily dissipate rapidly as the anesthetic is redistributed throughout the body. A vasopressor can be used to restore blood pressure, and the patient may be paralyzed, intubated, and ventilated until the toxic effects have worn off.

Intravenous Regional Anesthesia

Intravenous regional anesthesia (i.e., Bier's block) is a simple and effective method of producing anesthesia of the limbs, both upper and lower. It is based on the notion that if the circulation to a limb is occluded and the injection of local anesthetic is made into a vein distal to that occlusion, the drug will reach the capillaries by retrograde flow and enter the extravascular space. Here it comes in contact with nerve endings and paralysis of the limb below the tourniquet is achieved for the duration of the circulatory occlusion. An inflatable tourniquet is applied around the extremity. The limb is exsanguinated of venous blood, and the cuff is inflated above systolic pressure. The local anesthetic is injected into an indwelling needle. At present, lidocaine without additives is the only local agent approved for IV regional anesthesia.

The two primary complications of IV regional anesthesia are toxicity due to accidental deflation of the cuff and tourniquet pain. Once the cuff is pressurized, a sudden deflation below arterial pressure can cause toxicity because the drug is being infused into the systemic circulation and plasma levels of the drug rise quickly. A nonelastic bandage should be wrapped around the cuff once it has been inflated to avoid accidental slippage.

Tourniquet pain may occur 20 minutes or so after the tourniquet has been inflated. If a second cuff is placed distal to the original one, the tissues beneath it will be anesthetized. The second cuff may then be inflated painlessly. Once the second cuff has been secured and inflated, the first one may be deflated. Some agencies use specially designed double cuffs.

Acupuncture

Acupuncture is the use of thin needles inserted into points on the meridians to stimulate the body's *chi*, or vital energy. This therapy is used to treat disharmony in the body, which leads to disease. Acupuncture has been used to produce regional anesthesia. Acupuncturists have identified approximately 1000 acupuncture points in the body. The mechanism of action of acupuncture to act as an anesthetic suggests that the needles stimulate the release of endorphins, or natural painkillers, in the body. The acupuncture needles are inserted along meridians, lines that connect anatomic sites on the body. Acupuncture is discussed in more depth in Chapter 60.

Hypnosis

When used as an anesthetic, hypnosis alleviates pain through relaxation, suggestion, and intense concentration on a particular object or sound to the exclusion of all other distractions. The mechanism of how hypnosis relieves pain remains unknown. One widely accepted theory is that the person's ego—that is, the part of the mind that consciously restrains instincts—is temporarily weakened under hypnosis at the person's own wish. How deeply one responds depends on many psychological and physiologic variables. However, it has been used successfully in childbirth, to set certain fractures, and with certain dental procedures. Not all patients are susceptible to hypnotic suggestion.

Cryotherapy

Cryotherapy, the use of cold to induce anesthesia, produces a very low surface temperature and thus reduces pain at the surgical site. Liquid nitrous oxide (−89.5°C), carbon dioxide (−78.5°C), and liquid nitrogen (−195.6°C), or ethyl chloride may be used. Although there are many acceptable alternatives to cryotherapy, this technique can be used in extreme life-threatening conditions and when the patient cannot tolerate a conventional form of anesthesia.

Pharmacodynamics

Regional anesthetics cause a reversible block to the conduction of impulses along nerve fibers. A propagated nerve impulse involves a wave of depolarization, followed by repolarization, passing along the nerve fiber. In the resting mode, nerve fibers are polarized, with higher concentrations of sodium ions outside than inside the cell and the reverse for potassium ions. Depolarization is caused by a flow of sodium ions through sodium channels in the nerve membrane, from the outside to the inside of nerve fibers. Repolarization involves the flow, in the reverse direction, of potassium ions. The resultant slight imbalance of ions (too much sodium inside and too much potassium outside) is corrected after repolarization by the sodium-potassium pump, which pumps sodium outside again.

The electrical spike caused by depolarization triggers the adjacent membrane, such that the sodium channels in that section of the fiber open in their turn, allowing the inward flow of sodium ions and depolarization. Thus, each depolarization and repolarization cycle that occurs triggers a similar process in adjacent membranes, and this chain of events passes along the nerve from one end to the other. In the presence of an anesthetic drug, the threshold potential is not reached, the nerve impulse or action potential is not reached, and the nerve impulse or action potential is not propagated. Conduction block in peripheral nerves progresses in the following order: peripheral vasodilation, skin temperature elevation, loss of pain and temperature sensation, loss of proprioception, loss of touch and pressure sensation, and motor paralysis.

Desensitization occurs in rank order of nerve fiber sensitivity to blockade. Nerve fibers are classified according to their function (i.e., motor, touch, pressure, proprioception, pain). Table 16–8 provides a brief overview of the types of nerve fibers and their function. B fibers, myelinated preganglionic autonomic nerves, are more sensitive to regional anesthetics than C fibers, lightly myelinated postganglionic autonomic nerves, and A delta fibers, myelinated somatic nerves. Similarly, the thinnest, least myelinated nerves are blocked first (C < B < A delta). Both A delta and C fibers are blocked by the same tissue concentrations of the drug.

Adverse Effects and Contraindications

The principal adverse effects of local anesthetics are allergic reactions and systemic toxicity. Although allergic reactions are rare, they may be life-threatening. Aminoesters are more allergenic than aminoamides because of the metabolite para-aminobenzoic acid. Local reactions may include erythema, urticaria, edema, and dermatitis. Systemic reactions include generalized erythema, urticaria, edema, bronchoconstriction, hypotension, and cardiovascular collapse. Treatment is symptomatic and supportive. Cutaneous reactions may respond to diphenhydramine, and more severe reactions may respond to epinephrine and systemic glucocorticoids such as methylprednisolone. Bronchoconstriction is treated with epinephrine, and hypotension is managed with fluids and vasopressors such as phenylephrine or inotropic drugs like dopamine.

The systemic toxicity of local anesthetics is due to an excess plasma concentration of the drug. Determinants of local anesthetic blood levels include the total dose of drug, vascularity at the injection site, addition of vasoconstrictors to the solution, local tissue binding, and tissue perfusion. Systemic absorption is greatest following intercostal nerve block, intermediate for epidural block, and least for brachial plexus block. The addition of epinephrine reduces systemic absorption by one third. The most common mechanism for excessive plasma concentration of local anesthetic is accidental intravascular injection.

Systemic toxicity of local anesthetics involves the CNS and the cardiovascular system. CNS manifestations of toxicity include numbness of tongue, lightheadedness, visual disturbances, muscular twitching, seizures, and coma. CNS toxicity is increased by hypercapnia and is decreased by barbiturates, benzodiazepines, and inhaled anesthetics. Cardiovascular toxicity can produce decreased myocardial contractility, vasodilation, and dysrhythmias. Cardiovascular toxicity is increased by acidosis, hypoxia, pregnancy, and hyperkalemia.

TABLE 16–8 CLASSIFICATION OF NERVE FIBERS

Fiber Type	Direction	Function of Fiber
A_{α}	Efferent to skeletal muscle	Motor neurons
A_{β}	Afferent from skin	Touch, pressure, and proprioception
A_{τ}	Efferent to muscle spindles	Motor neurons
B	Efferent to vascular smooth muscle	Preganglionic sympathetic neurons
C	Afferent from skin	Pain and temperature neurons
	Efferent to vascular smooth muscle	Postganglionic sympathetic neurons

A small test dose of the local anesthetic with 15 mcg of epinephrine may be given in an attempt to detect intravascular injection. A 20-percent increase in heart rate following the test dose suggests intravascular injection. Severe systemic toxicity is treated with oxygen and fluids. Seizures are controlled with diazepam, thiopental, or succinylcholine. Cardiovascular instability may be managed with antiarrhythmics, inotropes, or vasodilators.

Pharmacokinetics

Local anesthetics are divided into two classes: aminoesters and aminoamides. Examples of aminoesters are 2-chloroprocaine, procaine, and tetracaine. They are cleared from the plasma by plasma and liver cholinesterase. Aminoamides include lidocaine, prilocaine, mepivacaine, bupivacaine, ropivacaine, and etidocaine. Aminoamides are cleared by hepatic biotransformation.

As illustrated in Table 16–9, local anesthesia is classified according to its site of placement. The amount of local anesthetic that reaches a nerve depends on the proximity of the injection to the nerve. The rapidity and extent of diffusion depends on the concentration of local anesthetic injected and its lipid solubility. Systemic absorption influences the amount of local anesthetic remaining at the injection site and the duration of anesthesia. The addition of epinephrine to the local anesthetic mixture slows systemic absorption of the drug, prolongs the anesthetic effect, increases the intensity of blockade, and reduces surgical bleeding.

Drug-Drug Interactions

Because of their localized use, drug-drug interactions are rare with regional anesthetics. Drug-drug interactions, however, may occur if the drug is inadvertently given IV.

PHARMACOTHERAPEUTIC OPTIONS

Aminoesters

- Chloroprocaine (NESACAINE)
- Procaine (NOVOCAIN, others)
- Tetracaine (PONTOCAINE)
- Cocaine (many)

CHLOROPROCAINE

Chloroprocaine is a short-acting local anesthetic. Epinephrine prolongs the duration of action by reducing the rate of absorption and plasma concentration. Toxic blood concentrations produce decreased myocardial contractility and peripheral vasodilation, leading to hypotension and decreased cardiac output. It is ineffective for topical anesthesia

TABLE 16–9 LOCAL ANESTHETICS

Drug	Concentration (%)	Usual Onset	Usual Duration (h)	Maximum Single Dose (mg)
Procaine	0.5–1	Fast	0.5–1.0	1000
Chloroprocaine	0.5–1	Fast	0.5–1.0	1000
Lidocaine	0.5–1	Fast	1–2	500
Mepivacaine	0.5–1	Fast	.5–3	500
Bupivacaine	0.25–0.5	Slow	4–12	200
Peripheral Nerve Block				
Chloroprocaine	2–3	Fast	.5–1	1000+epi
Procaine	1–2	Slow	.5–1	1000
Lidocaine	1–2	Fast	1–3	500+epi
Prilocaine	1.5–2	Fast	1.5–3	600
Mepivacaine	1–2	Fast	2–3	500+epi
Bupivacaine	0.25–0.5	Slow	4–12	200+epi
Etidocaine	0.5–1.0	Fast	3–12	300+epi
IV Regional Anesthesia				
Lidocaine	0.25–0.5			500
Spinal Anesthesia				
Procaine	10	Moderate	0.5–1.0	200
Tetracaine	0.5	Fast	2–4	20
Lidocaine	5	Fast	0.5–1.5	100
Bupivacaine	0.5–0.75	Fast	2–4	20
Epidural Anesthesia				
Chloroprocaine	2–3	Fast	0.5–1	1000+epi
Lidocaine	1–2	Fast	1–2	500+epi
Prilocaine	1–3	Fast	1–2.5	600
Mepivacaine	1–2	Fast	1.0–2.5	500+epi
Bupivacaine	0.25–0.75	Moderate	2–4	200+epi
Etidocaine	1–1.5	Fast	2–4	300+epi

epi, epinephrine.

Adapted from Zaglaniczny, K., Maree, S. (1995). Anesthesia and perioperative nursing care. In R. A. Roth (Ed.), *Perioperative nursing core curriculum* (p. 242). Philadelphia: W. B. Saunders. Used with permission.

and is not recommended for IV regional anesthesia because of its high incidence of thrombophlebitis. Epidural chloroprocaine may decrease the duration of analgesia of epidural narcotics, possibly because of a specific antagonism of mu receptor–mediated analgesia. Occasional cases of severe back pain have occurred after epidural anesthesia with chloroprocaine. Contributing factors include the use of disodium edetate (EDTA), a preservative, in the formulation of chloroprocaine; large volumes or greater than 20 mL; and low pH of the commercial solution. Persistent neurologic damage or prolonged sensory or motor deficits have been reported after accidental spinal anesthesia with large doses of sodium bisulfite or methyl paraben–containing solutions. It should not be used for spinal anesthesia. Back spasms have been reported following the epidural use of chloroprocaine formulated with disodium edetate.

PROCAINE

Procaine has a rapid onset of action and short duration that depends on the anesthetic technique, type of block, concentration, and individual patient. Vasoconstrictor drugs may be added to the procaine solution to delay systemic absorption and prolong duration of action. Procaine is only weakly toxic because of rapid plasma hydrolysis. It is, however, hydrolyzed to p-amino-benzoic acid, which is responsible for the allergic reactions associated with its use in some patients.

TETRACAINE

Tetracaine is a potent, long-acting local anesthetic that is primarily used for spinal anesthetics. Its longer duration of action compared with that of the other ester anesthetics is due to a much slower rate of hydrolysis by plasma cholinesterase. High plasma levels may produce seizures and cardiovascular collapse because of decreased peripheral vascular resistance and myocardial depression.

COCAINE

Cocaine is a long-acting local anesthetic of the aminoester class. The drug is commonly used to densensitize the eye and mucous membranes of the nose, mouth, and urethra. Cocaine is a CNS stimulant, particularly of the cerebral cortex, because of the accumulating synaptic norepinephrine. Cocaine is known to inhibit the reuptake of norepinephrine at adrenergic synapses, which may account for some of its central and peripheral effects. In the CNS it potentiates neurotransmission of norepinephrine, dopamine, or serotonin. The reabsorption of the neurotransmitters is blocked, leaving circuits open that would otherwise close. Cocaine is discussed as a drug of abuse in Chapter 10. However, it does have limited medical uses.

Aminoamides

- ❒ Lidocaine (XYLOCAINE)
- ❒ Prilocaine (CITANEST)
- ❒ Mepivacaine (CARBOCAINE, POLOCAINE)
- ❒ Bupivacaine (MARCAINE, SENSORCAINE)
- ❒ Etidocaine (DURANEST)
- ❒ Ropivacaine (NAROPIN)

LIDOCAINE

Lidocaine was the first drug of the aminoamide type of local drug to be introduced. This drug remains the most versatile and most frequently used local because of its potency, rapid onset, moderate duration, and topical anesthetic activity. Lidocaine remains the only approved drug in the United States for IV regional anesthesia. It may also be used topically, for peripheral nerve block, and spinal or epidural anesthesia.

PRILOCAINE

Prilocaine is a local anesthetic equipotent to lidocaine, but it has a longer duration. It is less toxic and undergoes rapid hepatic metabolism to orthotolidine, which oxidizes hemoglobin to methemoglobin. When the dose of prilocaine exceeds 600 mg, there may be sufficient methemoglobin to cause the patient to appear cyanotic, and oxygen-carrying capacity is reduced. The unique ability of prilocaine to cause dose-related methemoglobinemia limits its usefulness. It is also useful for infiltration, peripheral nerve blockade, and epidural anesthesia.

MEPIVACAINE

Mepivacaine is similar to lidocaine in potency and speed of onset, but it has a slightly longer duration of action and lacks vasodilator activity. High plasma levels, such as what might occur in paracervical blocks, produce uterine vasoconstriction and a decrease in uterine blood flow. Additionally, the metabolism of mepivacaine is prolonged in the fetus and newborn, and the drug is generally not used in obstetric anesthesia. It is used for infiltration, peripheral nerve blocks, and epidural anesthesia. It is especially useful for brachial plexus blocks when large volumes of drug are given.

BUPIVACAINE

Bupivacaine is a long-acting local anesthetic that is capable of producing profound blockade with separation of sensory anesthesia and motor blockade. Although bupivacaine is useful for infiltration, peripheral nerve blocks, and spinal anesthesia, its major advantage appears to involve epidural analgesia for labor. Compared with other amides, intravascular injection of bupivacaine is associated with a greater degree of cardiotoxicity. This is due to slower recovery from bupivacaine-induced cardiac sodium channel blockade and greater depression of myocardial contractility and cardiac conduction.

ETIDOCAINE

Etidocaine is a long-acting local anesthetic with a rapid onset and profound sensory and motor blockade. It has been used for infiltration, peripheral nerve block, and epidural anesthesia. Doses high enough to achieve sensory anesthesia produce profound motor blockade. This property limits its use in obstetrics and for postoperative pain relief.

ROPIVACAINE

Ropivacaine possesses an onset of action similar to that of bupivacaine. Potency and duration of sensory blockade appear similar for both drugs, but ropivacaine is less potent and short acting on motor fibers. Ropivacaine appears less cardiotoxic than bupivacaine.

Critical Thinking Process

Assessment

Many variables influence the patient's physiologic and psychological response to surgery. These variables include the patient's physical and mental state, the extent of disease and co-morbid disorders, magnitude of the specific procedure, and preoperative psychological and physiologic preparations. When these variables are considered collectively, they reveal the degree of surgical risk. Fears that the patient may express concerning anesthesia should be addressed. Therefore, nursing assessment includes all of these variables.

A preoperative assessment begins with the patient's general state of health, and allergies should be elicited. Information about current drug use is important because some drugs may cause complications. For example, antibiotics, which combine with some muscle relaxants, increase the risk of postoperative respiratory depression. Antianxiety drugs lower blood pressure and increase the risk of shock. They also potentiate the effects of opioids and barbiturates. Thiazide diuretics contribute to potassium depletion. Chronic corticosteroid use impairs adrenal cortex function and thus impairs physiologic response to stress of anesthesia and surgery. Antidepressants such as monoamine oxidase inhibitors can cause hypertensive crisis when combined with anesthetics. Antiparkinson drugs can cause hypotension or hypertension when combined with anesthetics. The use of illicit drugs and alcohol abuse increase the patient's tolerance to opioids.

Specific information about co-morbid conditions, past surgical and anesthetic history, and particularly information about family history of MH should be elicited. Patient statements regarding a history of asthma and previous anesthesia problems in themselves or in family members are of special interest to the health care and anesthesia provider. In some cases, a menstrual and obstetric history should be included with the general review of systems. Question the patient carefully about smoking habits and alcohol use. Serious neurologic conditions, such as uncontrolled epilepsy or severe Parkinson's disease, increase surgical risk.

Safely preparing patients for anesthesia has traditionally included fasting for at least 6 hours preoperatively; thus, information regarding the patient's last food and fluid intake should be noted. This information is needed in order to anticipate the risk of aspiration of gastric contents during surgery and subsequent aspiration pneumonitis.

The physical exam should include height and weight, auscultation of the heart and breath sounds, blood pressure, peripheral pulses, and evaluation of venous access sites. Also included is an assessment for neurologic dysfunction, movement limitations, or abnormalities of dentition, temporomandibular joint, airway, and neck.

Laboratory tests are ordered based on the findings of the history and physical exam, and the proposed surgical procedure. Although less laboratory testing is performed today than in the past, the tests that are performed are for specific indications. For example, a prothrombin time and partial thromboplastin time are often performed to check the patient's coagulation status. A chest x-ray study is usually ordered for diagnostic purposes on some patients, such as those with cardiac disorders. Baseline blood gases and pulmonary function studies may be obtained to evaluate pulmonary function in a patient with known respiratory disease. Urinalysis and renal function tests help determine the ability of the kidneys to eliminate urea, protein wastes, and drugs. Thyroid studies are performed to evaluate the presence of hyperthyroidism or hypothyroidism. Hyperthyroidism can lead to thyroid crisis with hypertension, tachycardia, and hyperthermia, and therefore, the condition should be treated medically preoperatively. Similarly, hypothyroidism increases the risk of hypotension and cardiac arrest during anesthesia.

Analysis and Management

Treatment Objectives

The objectives for anesthetic therapy center around relief of anxiety, sedation, amnesia, analgesia, little or no emesis, aspiration prophylaxis, reduction of oral secretions, facilitation of induction, and reduction of anesthesia requirements. When using anesthesia in pregnant women, the objective is to provide maternal anesthesia without stimulating uterine activity or precipitating preterm labor. The choice of anesthesia should be made with the consideration of maintaining uteroplacental perfusion and preventing preterm labor.

Treatment Options

The decision as to which type of anesthetic to use is made largely by the anesthesia provider in consultation with the patient and the surgeon. The anesthetics to be used are determined with consideration of the following variables:

- Age of the patient, level of anxiety, and general physical condition
- Drug allergies and the presence of co-morbid disease
- Physical status (see American Society of Anesthesiologists (ASA) Classification of Physical Status)
- Patient preference (e.g., spinal versus general anesthesia)
- Patient history of previous adverse responses to anesthesia
- Magnitude of specific surgical procedure and its duration
- Technical intricacies of the procedure
- Outpatient or inpatient status

AMERICAN SOCIETY OF ANESTHESIOLOGISTS (ASA) CLASSIFICATION OF PHYSICAL STATUS

P-1: A normal, healthy patient
P-2: A patient has mild systemic disease
P-3: A patient has severe systemic disease
P-4: A patient has severe disease that is a constant threat to life
P-5: A moribund patient not expected to survive without the operation
P-6: A declared brain-dead patient whose organs are being removed for donor purposes

From the American Society of Anesthesiologists (ASA). (1997). *Manual for anesthesia department organization and management* (p. 150). Chicago: Author. Used with permission.

Drug Variables

Choices involved in the decision as to which anesthetic to use center around drugs used for induction and maintenance of anesthesia. Most adults prefer an IV induction, whereas children may elect to be anesthetized by inhalation. The choice of individual induction drugs is often made according to patient stability and preference of the anesthesia provider. For example, ketamine or etomidate may be better tolerated than thiopental or propofol in a hypovolemic trauma patient. In contrast, ketamine would not be a choice in a stable patient with coronary artery disease because of its tendency to cause tachycardia. Tachycardia in these patients increases myocardial oxygen demand and decreases myocardial oxygen supply. These changes lead to myocardial ischemia.

The decision as to which anesthesia to use for maintenance is usually based on the route of administration. Inhalation drugs can be administered as the sole drug with 100 percent oxygen. The newer drugs are associated with rapid induction and emergence with minimal risk of organ toxicity. Intravenous drugs can also have a rapid onset and short duration, and they can be used intraoperatively and postoperatively. Newer IV drugs have minimal cardiovascular effects, have no hepatic or renal toxicity, have less potential for MH, and are compatible with epinephrine. Further, IV drugs are not associated with pollution of the operating room by anesthetic gases.

Regional anesthetic techniques include spinal or subarachnoid blocks, epidural anesthetics, or caudal, brachial plexus, or interscalene blocks. Intravenous regional anesthesia is also commonly employed. These techniques are often used for procedures on the extremities or procedures below the umbilicus. Absolute contraindications to the use of spinal or epidural anesthesia include patient refusal, infection at the puncture site, uncorrected hypovolemia, and coagulation or anatomic abnormalities. Relative contraindications to the use of spinal or epidural anesthesia include bacteremia, pre-existing neurologic conditions, and patients receiving minidose anticoagulation therapy. Contraindications to peripheral nerve blocks include patient refusal or objection to being awake, local infection at block site, coagulopathy, and pre-existing peripheral vascular disease.

The relative safety of regional versus general anesthesia has been debated and remains a matter of controversy. Epidural anesthesia and analgesia appear to play a positive role in decreasing cardiovascular and pulmonary morbidity and the stress response. The incidence of thromboembolus is reduced, and there may be a reduction in blood loss as well with some regional techniques.

With the increased focus of national attention on health care and health care costs, anesthesia providers are becoming more conscious of their choice of anesthetic techniques and drugs. Compared with general anesthesia, regional or local anesthesia generally results in significant savings in hospital costs. This is in part due to shorter hospital stays and reduced need for intensive care. Significant savings can also be achieved in the selection of anesthetic drugs. Although newer induction drugs such as propofol are more expensive, they can actually reduce overall hospital costs when they are used in appropriate cases and when hospitals change protocols to allow earlier discharge. Low-flow techniques can reduce the cost of inhalation drugs 50 to 75 percent. Future decisions regarding the choice of drug must be directed to cost-versus-benefit concerns as well as the pharmacokinetics of the drug.

Patient Variables

The physical changes of pregnancy have an impact on the choice of anesthesia techniques and drugs to be used. In general, less anesthesia is required during a gravid state because of physiologic, anatomic, and hormonal changes associated with pregnancy. There is a more rapid loss of consciousness and protective airway reflexes at lower inspired concentration of IV and inhalation anesthetics. The nasal and respiratory tract mucosa becomes edematous and hyperemic during pregnancy, thus making intubation difficult. Furthermore, the pressure of the fetus on the stomach increases the risk of regurgitation and aspiration pneumonitis, thus patients should be premedicated with sodium bicitrate and a histamine$_2$ antagonist to decrease gastric acidity.

Mild increases in uterine tone have been noted postpartum but these do not appear to be clinically relevant. Halogenated gases decrease uterine resting tone, uterine muscle tension, and spontaneous uterine activity. Deep anesthesia can lead to significant decreases in maternal cardiac output and blood pressure, leading to decreased uterine blood flow. Endogenous catecholamine release from inadequate general anesthesia or airway manipulation can also decrease uterine blood flow. Uterine blood flow is also reduced in the presence of ultra short-acting barbiturate induction agents. Neonatal depression can result from placental transmission of IV depressant drugs or inhalation agents.

Halothane was commonly used in pediatric patients because it could be given by mask, was well tolerated, was less pungent than some of the other drugs, and produced less airway limitation and laryngospasm. Sevoflurane for induction by mask has largely replaced halothane in the United States. Ketamine can be used and is particularly helpful in developmentally disabled children. Regional anesthesia is sometimes used as an adjunct to general anesthesia to provide for pain management during the postoperative period.

When intubation is used for infants, bradycardia results rather than the tachycardia that is commonly found in adults. Therefore, short procedures may be carried out using a mask rather than intubating the child. The bradycardic response is the response of a mature parasympathetic nervous system but immature sympathetic innervation. Atropine is commonly used preoperatively in children to manage the bradycardia.

General anesthesia permits smooth induction and rapid recovery in the older adult. Inhalation requirements are lower because the MAC value decreases by 4 percent per year after age 40. However, drug biotransformation and clearance are delayed, requiring lower doses of barbiturates, benzodiazepines, and opioids. Moreover, the older adult is at risk of hypothermia due to the decreased proportion of body fat. It may be difficult to ventilate an edentulous patient, and arthritis may restrict the cervicospinal region and inhibit intubation. There are minimal physiologic alterations with the use of regional anesthesia in the older adult. Regional anesthesia permits rapid recovery and postoperative analgesia. It also reduces the risk of cardiovascular complications and postoperative confusion. The effects of spinal anesthesia are prolonged in the older adult, and hypotension may be pronounced. In contrast, epidural anesthesia has less impact on blood pressure and cardiovascular status. Musculoskeletal changes associated with aging may make administration of spinal anesthesia or epidural anesthesia difficult.

Intervention

Administration

Before induction of general anesthesia, the patient is generally asked to breathe 100 percent oxygen for 5 minutes or asked to take several deep breaths with oxygen. Induction may be accomplished by the IV, IM, rectal, or respiratory routes. The most commonly used induction drugs are ultra short-acting barbiturates or sedative-hypnotics such as propofol. Other IV induction drugs used in certain circumstances include ketamine, etomidate, or benzodiazepines. Inhalation inductions are popular in pediatric patients. Opioids or lidocaine may be used as adjuvants to induction drugs. Such drugs attenuate reflexes following airway stimulation and make it possible to induce consciousness with lower doses of IV hypnotic drugs.

The typical adult induction involves ventilation by mask after the patient becomes unconscious. Mask anesthesia is useful for relatively short, uncomplicated peripheral procedures, but endotracheal anesthesia is indicated when surgery involves a major body cavity; when there is risk of aspiration, a need for intraoperative or postoperative mechanical ventilation, or a need for awkward positioning; and surgery on the head and neck. Depolarizing or nondepolarizing muscle relaxants are used to establish appropriate conditions for intubation. Anesthesia is then maintained with inhalational or IV anesthetics.

If a difficult intubation is anticipated, histamine$_2$ antagonists and possibly IV metoclopramide should be started 30 minutes before induction to decrease gastric activity and volume. Nonparticulate antacids such as sodium bicitrate may be used 30 minutes before induction. Administration of atropine or glycopyrrolate decreases secretions resulting from airway stimulation. Patients with a potential for airway difficulties may be managed with a so-called rapid-sequence awake oral or blind nasal or fiberoptic laryngoscopy. Such patients include the obese or those at risk for pulmonary aspiration.

In a rapid-sequence induction, the patient is preoxygenated and then induced with a sleep dose of thiopental, ketamine, or other appropriate drug. Cricoid pressure is applied as the patient loses consciousness, and paralysis is provided by succinylcholine immediately afterward. There is no attempt to ventilate the patient at any time by mask unless intubation is impossible. In that case, cricoid pressure is maintained during mask ventilation.

If uncertainty exists about the ability to ventilate or intubate the patient after induction of general anesthesia, an awake intubation may be performed. Mild IV sedation or local anesthesia is provided by superior laryngeal nerve block, transtracheal injection, or oral spray. Laryngoscopy is performed after coating the blade with viscous lidocaine. Blind nasal intubation is useful in patients with *trismus* (motor disturbance of trigeminal nerve with difficulty in opening the mouth) or other circumstances that preclude direct laryngoscopy. Endotracheal intubation can be facilitated with the use of a fiberoptic laryngoscope or bronchoscope.

Inhalation induction by mask is the method of choice for most pediatric patients, except when rapid-sequence induction is required. Rectal methohexital can be used for children 8 months to 5 years.

In general, extubation is safest when patients are spontaneously ventilating and are able to respond to verbal commands. Sustained head lift and strong hand grip are simple ways to assess recovery from neuromuscular blockade. In some circumstances, extubation should be delayed until the patient is fully awake and stable. These cases include tracheal or maxillofacial surgery, difficulty with mask ventilation, or intubation on full stomach. Extubation may be performed under deep anesthesia to avoid coughing and straining in some cases. This technique is helpful following middle ear surgery, open eye procedures, herniorrhaphy, or transurethral resection of the prostate.

Education

The patient scheduled for any procedure that requires anesthesia must give informed consent before the procedure can be performed. The patient or legal guardian must be informed about potential risks, complications, and anesthesia alternatives. Patients should be advised in general about the anesthesia technique to be used. The expected outcome and the likelihood that the chosen anesthetic will be effective should also be addressed.

The procedure for obtaining signed consent varies from state to state and according to the policy of the health care agency. Emancipated minors (children who are younger than 18 but because of marriage or other circumstances are independent of the family) may give consent. Children under the legal age (18 in most states) who are not emancipated must have consent from their parents or legal guardian. In some cases, a court order may be needed to permit the use of anesthesia and surgery to take place.

Reassure patients receiving general anesthesia that their vital physiologic functions will be continually monitored until the effects of the drugs have dissipated. They will be kept warm and have their blood pressure, heart rate, oxygenation status, and comfort level monitored. Advise patients who are receiving regional anesthesia that the sensation and movement in the area will return once the effects of the drug have worn off.

Evaluation

The effectiveness of anesthesia includes use of appropriate techniques and anesthetic levels for the procedure and rapid emergence free of complications. The effectiveness of anesthesia in the pregnant woman can be demonstrated by the ability to carry out maternal anesthesia without stimulating uterine activity or precipitating preterm labor, and uteroplacental perfusion was maintained and preterm labor was prevented.

SUMMARY

- General anesthesia produces widespread depressive effects of the CNS. This physiologically altered state classically results in hypnosis, analgesia, amnesia, and muscle relaxation.

- General anesthetics are administered IV, by inhalation, or by rectum.
- IV anesthetics are used for rapid induction, with unconsciousness occurring about 30 seconds after the initial IV administration. Intravenous anesthesia is most commonly used as an induction agent before inhalation drugs are used.
- Regional anesthesia, also known as local anesthesia, produces a loss of painful sensation in only one region of the body by blocking painful stimuli at their origin, along the afferent neurons, or along the spinal cord.
- Inhalation anesthesia produces a dose-dependent CNS depression with effects noted in the CNS, cardiovascular, respiratory, renal, hepatic, and gastrointestinal systems and the uterus.
- The four stages of general anesthesia are induction, excitement, surgical anesthesia, and anesthetic overdose. In stage IV anesthesia, vital functions are profoundly depressed, resulting in respiratory and circulatory failure.
- The most serious complications of general anesthesia are aspiration pneumonitis, pulmonary dysfunction, and MH.
- There are many drug-drug interactions with inhaled anesthetics. Drugs that potentiate the effects of inhaled anesthetics require decreased amounts of the anesthetic drug. There are also drugs that antagonize the effects of inhaled anesthetics and thus increase the amount of anesthetic required.
- Drugs used for general anesthesia include barbiturates, nonbarbiturates, opioid agonists, opioid agonist-antagonists, antagonists, and liquid and gaseous inhalation agents.
- Regional anesthesia can include any of the following: topical anesthesia, local infiltration, field block, peripheral nerve block, spinal or epidural anesthesia, IV regional anesthesia, acupuncture, hypnosis, and cryotherapy.
- Local anesthetics that are aminoesters include chloroprocaine, procaine, tetracaine, and cocaine. Aminoamides include mepivacaine, bupivacaine, etidocaine, and ropivacaine.
- The decision as to which type of anesthetic to use is made largely by the anesthesia provider in consultation with the patient and the surgeon. The anesthetics to be used are determined with consideration of a number of patient and drug variables.
- Treatment objectives for anesthetic therapy include relief of anxiety, sedation, amnesia, analgesia, little or no emesis, aspiration prophylaxis, reduction of oral secretions, facilitation of induction, and reduction of anesthesia requirements. When using anesthesia in the pregnant women, the objective is to provide maternal anesthesia without stimulating uterine activity or precipitating preterm labor.
- Choices involved in the decision to use general anesthesia center around drugs for induction and maintenance of anesthesia.
- Compared with general anesthesia, regional or local anesthesia generally results in significant savings in hospital costs.
- Anesthesia effectiveness includes use of appropriate techniques and anesthetic levels for the procedure and rapid emergence free of complications.

BIBLIOGRAPHY

Aker, J., and Rupp, R. (1994). Standards of care in anesthesia practice. In S. Foster and L. Jardon (Eds.), *Professional aspects of nurse anesthesia practice* (pp. 89–112). Philadelphia: F.A. Davis.

American Society of Anesthesiologists. (1992). *Relative value guide: Physical status classification.* Chicago: Author.

Atanassoff, P. (1996). Effects of regional anesthesia on perioperative outcome. *Journal of Clinical Anesthesiology,* 8(6), 446–455.

Becker, K., and Carrithers, J. (1994). Practical methods of cost containment in anesthesia and surgery. *Journal of Clinical Anesthesiology,* 6(5), 388–399.

Borgeat, A., Wilder-Smith, O., and Suter, P. (1994). The nonhypnotic therapeutic applications of propofol. *Anesthesiology,* 80, 642–656.

Borgeat, A., Wilder-Smith, O., Saiah, M., et al. (1992). Subhypnotic doses of propofol possess direct antiemetic properties. *Anesthesia and Analgesia,* 74, 539–541.

Bürkle, H., Dunbar, S., Aken, H., et al. (1996). Remifentanil: A novel, short-acting, m-opioid. *Anesthesia and Analgesia,* 83, 646–651.

Butterworth, J., Strichartz, G. (1990). Molecular mechanisms of local anesthetics: A review. *Anesthesiology,* 72:722–734.

Cameron, E., Johnston, G., Crofts, S., et al. (1992). The minimum effective dose of lidocaine to prevent injection pain due to propofol in children. *Anesthesiology,* 47, 604–606.

Chick, M. (1997). Opioid agonists and antagonists. In J. J. Nagelhout and K. L. Zaglaniczny (Eds.), *Nurse Anesthesia* (pp. 441–452). Philadelphia: W. B. Saunders.

Cotter, S., Petros, A., Dore, C., et al. (1991). Low flow anesthesia. Practice, cost implications and acceptability. *Anaesthesia,* 46, 1009–1012.

Davis, L., Britten, J., and Morgan, J. (1997). Cholinesterase: Its significance in anaesthesia practice. *Anaesthesia,* 52, 244–260.

Dershwitz, M., Randel, G., Rosow, C., et al. (1995). Initial clinical experience with remifentanil, a new opioid metabolized by esterases. *Anesthesia and Analgesia,* 81, 619–623.

Egan, T., Lemmens, H., Fiset, P., et al. (1993). The pharmacokinetics of the new short-acting opioid remifentanil (G187084B) in healthy adult male volunteers. *Anesthesiology,* 48, 405–408.

Glass, P., Jhaveri, R., and Smith, L. (1994). Comparison of potency and duration of action of nalmefene and naloxone. *Anesthesia and Analgesia,* 78, 536–541.

Goodrich, P. (1991). Naloxone hydrochloride: A review. *Journal of the American Academy of Nurse Anesthetists,* 58, 14–16.

Hartung, J. (1996). Twenty-four of twenty-seven studies show a greater incidence of emesis associated with nitrous oxide than with alternative anesthetics. *Anesthesia and Analgesia,* 83, 114–116.

Henderson, C., and Reynolds, J. (1997). Acute pulmonary edema in a young male after intravenous nalmefene. *Anesthesia and Analgesia,* 84, 218–219.

Hogue, C., Bowdle, A., O'Leary, C., et al. (1996). A multicenter evaluation of total intravenous anesthesia with remifentanil and propofol for elective inpatient surgery. *Anesthesia and Analgesia,* 83, 279–285.

Hughes, M., Glass, P., and Jacobs, J. (1992). Context-sensitive half-time in multicompartment pharmacokinetic models for intravenous anesthetic drugs. *Anesthesiology,* 76, 334–341.

Hughes, N., and Lyons, J. (1995). Prolonged myoclonus and meningism following propofol. *Canadian Journal of Anaesthesia,* 42, 744–746.

Jensen, N., Fiddler, D., and Striepe, V. (1995). Anesthetic considerations in porphyrias. *Anesthesia and Analgesia,* 80, 591–599.

Kapila, A., Glass, P., Jacobs, J., et al. (1995). Measured context-sensitive half-times of remifentanil and alfentanil. *Anesthesiology,* 83, 968–975.

Kennedy, S., and Longnecker, D. (1996). History and principles of anesthesiology. In J. G. Hardman, E. Limbird, P. B. Molinoff, et al. (Eds.). *Goodman and Gilman's the pharmacological basis of therapeutics* (9th ed., (pp. 295–306). New York: McGraw-Hill.

Kent, S., Bacon, D., and Harrison, P. (1992). Sexual illusions and propofol sedation. *Anesthesiology,* 77, 1037–1038.

Krauss, J., Akeyson, E., Giam, P., et al. (1996). Propofol-induced dyskinesias in Parkinson's disease. *Anesthesia and Analgesia,* 83, 420–422.

Leisure, G., O'Flaherty, J., Green, L., et al. (1996). Propofol and postoperative pancreatitis. *Anesthesiology,* 84, 224–227.

Litwack, K. (1995). *Core curriculum for post anesthesia nursing practice* (3rd ed.). Philadelphia: W.B. Saunders.

Liu, S., Carpenter, R., and Neal, N. (1995). Epidural anesthesia and analgesia. *Anesthesiology,* 82, 1474–1506.

Martin, J., Plevak, D., Flannery, K., et al. (1995). Hepatotoxicity after desflurane anesthesia. *Anesthesiology,* 83, 1125–1129.

Martin, T., Nicolson, S., and Burgas, M. (1993). Propofol anesthesia reduces emesis and airway obstruction in pediatric outpatients. *Anesthesia and Analgesia,* 76, 144–148.

Michelsen, L., and Hug, C. (1996). The pharmacokinetics of remifentanil. *Journal of Clinical Anesthesia,* 8, 679–682.

Munday, I., Ward, P., Sorooshian, S., et al. (1995). Interaction between remifentanil and isoflurane in spontaneously breathing patients during ambulatory surgery. *Anesthesiology,* 83, A23.

Ouellette, S., and Ouellette, R. (1995). Regional anesthesia: Is it safer. *CRNA: The Clinical Forum for Nurse Anesthetists,* 6, 70–78.

Ouellette, S. (1996). Clinical aspects of CRNA practice: General anesthesia. *Nursing Clinics of North America,* 31, 623–641.

Phippen, M., and Wells, M. (1994). *Perioperative nursing practice.* Philadelphia: W.B. Saunders.

Schulman, S., Rockett, C., Canada, A., et al. (1995). Long-term propofol infusion for refractory postoperative nausea: A case report with quantitative propofol analysis. *Anesthesia and Analgesia,* 80, 636–637.

Scuderi, P., D'Angelo, R., Harris, L., et al. (1997). Small-dose propofol by continuous infusion does not prevent postoperative vomiting in females undergoing outpatient laparoscopy. *Anesthesia and Analgesia,* 84, 71–75.

Smith, I., White, P., Nathanson, M., et al. (1994). Propofol: An update on its clinical uses. *Anesthesiology,* 81, 1005–1043.

Sosia, M., Braverman, B., and Villaflor, E. (1995). Propofol but not thiopental supports the growth of *Candida albicans. Anesthesia and Analgesia,* 81, 132–134.

Splinter, W., Roberts, D., Rhine, E., et al. (1995). Nitrous oxide does not increase vomiting in children after myringotomy. *Canadian Journal of Anaesthesia,* 42, 274–276.

Sutherland, M., and Burt, P. (1994). Propofol and seizures. *Anaesthesia Intensive Care,* 22, 733–737.

Tanelian, D., Losek, P., Mody, I., et al. (1993). The role of the $GABA_A$ receptor/chloride channel complex in anesthesia. *Anesthesiology,* 78, 757–776.

Vandermeulen, E., Aken, V., and Vermylen, J. (1994). Anticoagulants and spinal-epidural anesthesia. *Anesthesia and Analgesia,* 79, 1165–1177.

Weir, P., Munro, H., and Reynolds, P. (1993). Propofol infusion and the incidence of emesis in pediatric outpatient strabismus surgery. *Anesthesia and Analgesia,* 76, 760–764.

Wicks, T. (1995). Ropivacaine: An introduction to a new local anesthetic. *CRNA: The Clinical Forum for Nurse Anesthetists,* 6, 129–134.

Zaglaniczny, K., and Maree, S. (1995). Anesthesia and perioperative nursing care. In R. A. Roth (Ed.), *Perioperative nursing core curriculum.* (pp 211–251). Philadelphia: W.B. Saunders.

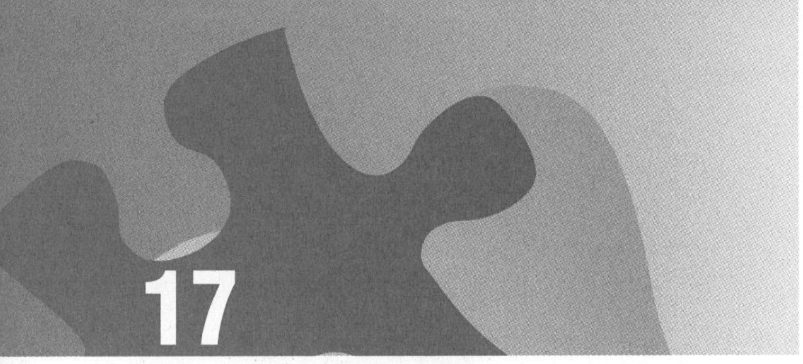

Antianxiety and Sedative-Hypnotic Drugs

The universal human emotion called *anxiety* is experienced along a spectrum of intensity. At one end of the spectrum is mild apprehension, which produces increased awareness and anticipation, such as a runner might experience before a race. At the other extreme, however, anxiety blocks awareness of surroundings, clouds judgment, and can lead to panic with complete disintegration of coping abilities. Anxiety can arise from many sources. It can be a normal reaction to stress, the adverse effects of drugs or disease processes, or a distinct psychological condition.

Sleep is defined as a period of rest in which physiologic activities and consciousness are diminished and voluntary physical activity is absent. Emotionalism and anxiety are common enemies of sleep and the most common cause of impaired sleep patterns.

Anxiety and impaired sleep patterns are common complaints, and the drugs used for treatment are widely prescribed. The distinction between antianxiety (i.e., anxiolytic, minor tranquilizer), sedative, and hypnotic effects is most often a matter of dosage. Some drugs relieve anxiety in low doses and induce sleep at higher doses. Therefore, a single drug can be considered an anxiolytic at one extreme and a hypnotic at the other.

ANXIETY

Epidemiology and Etiology

Anxiety has no gender, social, or economic boundaries. Antianxiety drugs are one of the most prescribed agents in the world today. Eleven percent of the United States population have used an antianxiety drug in the past year. Manifestations of anxiety can cause further anxiety, impair sleep, and greatly alter the patient's ability to carry out normal activities of daily living. Because anxiety is a normal part of life, health care providers must be particularly aware of the patient's ability to handle the normal stress of life.

Pathogenesis

Anxiety is an unwanted disruptive emotion. It can be discussed in three main contexts: certain drugs or disease processes, faulty neuroregulatory chemicals in the brain, or as a distinct psychiatric disease without the overlay of drugs or medical pathologies. Common anxiety-producing drugs include theophylline, corticosteroids, pseudoephedrine, epinephrine, anticholinergics, and caffeine. Additionally, illicit drugs are implicated in the pathogenesis of anxiety. These include cocaine, amphetamines, and certain hallucinogens. Various diseases and metabolic dysfunctions also produce anxiety states (see Selected Diseases, Conditions, or Drugs that Can Lead to Anxiety).

Neuroregulation of Anxiety

Neuroregulator deficiencies, receptor site antagonism, and neurotransmitter faults can all result in anxiety. Because neuroregulators cannot be studied directly, their effects must be inferred. The regulation of emotions and anxiety in the brain is extremely complex, and our understanding of their formation and inhibitions is ongoing. At present, research is focusing on the role neuroregulators play in the overall development of emotions.

Three primary structures thought to play interactive roles in the generation of emotions are the reticular activating system, the limbic system, and the hypothalamus (Fig. 17–1). The *reticular activating system* is a network of neurons that extends from the spinal cord through the medulla oblongata and pons to the thalamus and hypothalamus. It receives impulses from ascending sensory pathways, evaluates the significance of the impulses, and decides which impulses to transmit to the cerebral cortex. It excites or inhibits motor nerves controlling both reflex and voluntary movement. Stimulation of these neurons produces wakefulness and mental alertness, whereas depression causes sedation and loss of consciousness.

There are receptors in these areas and other regions of the central nervous system (CNS) that are believed to constrain anxiety. The inhibitory neuroregulator gamma-aminobutyric acid (GABA) has been studied in relation to its anxiety-inhibiting properties. It is believed that benzodiazepine receptors located in the brain play a role to inhibit anxiety and moderate sleep. Benzodiazepine-1 (BZ_1) receptors are thought to be involved with sleep mechanisms. Benzodiazepine-2 (BZ_2) receptors are associated with cognitive, memory, and sensory functions.

The limbic system of the brain involves the thalamus, hypothalamus, basal ganglia, and other structures. The function of the limbic system is to regulate emotions, such as pleasure, fear, anger, and sadness. It also regulates behaviors such as aggression, laughing, and crying. Physiologic changes in blood pressure, heart rate, respiration, and hormone secretion occur in association with emotions and behaviors.

The hypothalamus has extensive neuronal connections with higher and lower levels of the CNS and the pituitary gland. It continually collects information about the internal environment of the body, helping to maintain homeostasis by making physiologic adjustments in cardiovascular and gastrointestinal systems, levels of fluid and electrolytes, endocrine functions, and other body systems.

Psychopathology of Anxiety

The psychopathology of anxiety has been studied for years, and several theories have been proposed. The theories generally fall into three primary areas: interpersonal, behavioral, and family relationships. The interpersonal theory

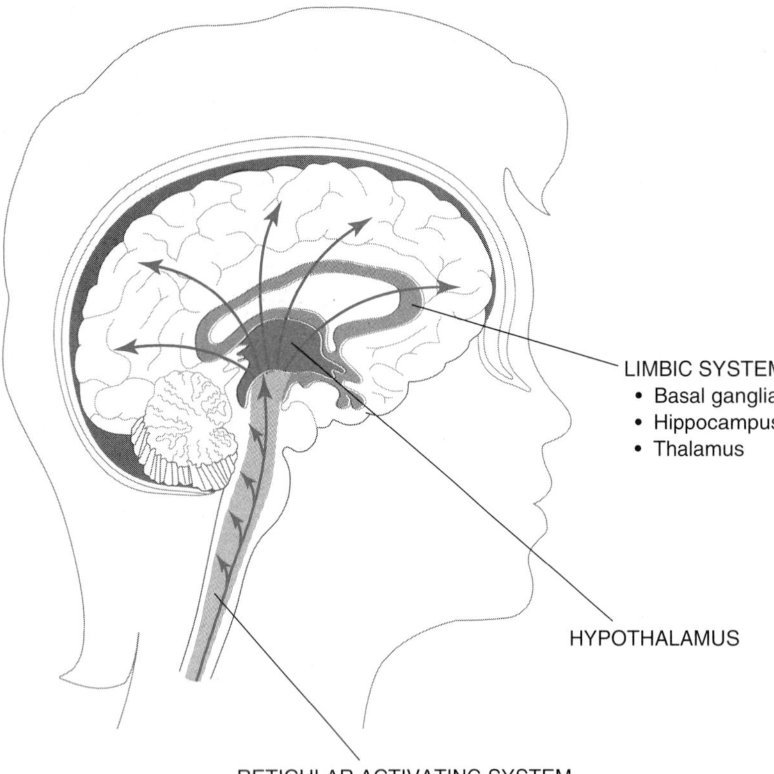

Figure 17–1 Three primary structures thought to play interactive roles in the generation of emotions are the reticular activating system (RAS), the limbic system, and the hypothalamus.

holds that fear of disapproval is the origin of anxiety. Disapproval is rooted in the fear an infant perceives as he differentiates himself from his mother. A further cause of anxiety in the interpersonal view is that negative perceptions of ability are caused by low self-esteem learned in childhood.

The behavioral theory postulates that anxiety is learned in early life when an individual is exposed to an intensely fearful situation. In some people, the experience leads to equally intense fear in similar situations. That fear, in turn, can be generalized to any fear-provoking stimulus. The person eventually experiences anxiety when he or she simply thinks about a fearful episode.

Finally, there is clear evidence that anxiety has a familial tendency. Children whose parents react with high levels of anxiety to most situations are likely to learn a similar pattern of behavior. A child learns early that any stressful situation can lead to fear and panic. This fact is important when one is working with children, older adults, or others who may have their feelings filtered or interpreted by members of their family.

SELECTED DISEASES, CONDITIONS, OR DRUGS THAT CAN LEAD TO ANXIETY

Diseases or Conditions	*Drugs*
Angina	Amphetamines
Arrhythmias	Anticholinergics
Asthma	Caffeine
Chronic airway limitation	Cocaine
Chronic pain	Corticosteroids
Congestive heart failure	Ephedrine
Fatigue	Epinephrine
Myocardial infarction	Hallucinogens
Hyperthyroidism	Levodopa
Hypoglycemia	Pseudoephedrine
Hyponatremia	Theophylline
Migraine headaches	Thyroid hormones
Mitral valve prolapse	
Seizure disorders	

Categories of Anxiety

Because anxiety is a complex emotion experienced in many ways because it has many origins, it must be properly diagnosed and categorized. The best management plans result when the health care provider has a complete understanding of the patient's diagnosis. The fourth edition of the *Diagnostic and Statistical Manual of Mental Disorders* (DSM-IV) differentiates types of anxiety. In the structure of the DSM-IV, anxiety is viewed in one of four ways: as the primary problem, as the result of a situation, as resistance to thoughts, or as the reliving of a traumatic event. Table 17–1 provides a brief overview of the key elements of various anxiety disorders. Proper diagnosis of the patient with an anxiety disorder allows the health care provider to initiate a therapeutic plan with the proper goals.

IMPAIRED SLEEP

Epidemiology and Etiology

Alterations in the sleep-wake cycle are many, varying across age groups and environmental situations. It is estimated that there are over 100 million people in the United States who have some form of sleep disorder. Sleep problems appear in-

TABLE 17–1 SELECTED ANXIETY DISORDERS

Anxiety Disorder	Key Elements
Panic disorder (with or without agoraphobia)	Attacks lead to changes in normal behaviors Feelings of smothering or doom Multiple episodes per week Not associated with a specific stimulus Palpitations, nausea, or shortness of breath Recurrent panic attacks occur without warning
Agoraphobia (without panic disorder)	Has never experienced a panic attack Fear of not being able to escape if attack occurs Intense fear of having a panic attack in public Unwillingness to leave home based on these fears
Social phobia	Examples: public speaking or using public toilets Immediate anxiety when confronted with stimulus Persistent fear of public scrutiny Realizes that the fear may be unreasonable
Specific phobia	Examples: insects, flying, tight spaces, seeing blood Immediate anxiety if stimulus is present May avoid situations if stimulus is present or anticipated Persistent fear of a discrete stimulus
Obsessive-compulsive disorder	Compulsions: intentional, repetitive actions that block or blunt the anxiety of obsessive thoughts Compulsive acts are disruptive, time consuming, and usually unwanted Obsessions: intrusive, involuntary thoughts involving violence that cause anxiety Resisting a compulsion may lead to further anxiety
Post-traumatic stress disorder (PTSD)	Ability to function normally is greatly impaired Intense anxiety surrounding recollection of event Often related to death of others or imminent death to self Person has had an experience outside range of normal human experience Recollections of event are intrusive and unwanted Sleep disturbances related to nightmares Thoughts or situations related to the event are vigorously avoided
Generalized anxiety disorder	Excessive anxiety surrounding two or more life circumstances (e.g., personal safety, finances) Duration of 6 months or longer May be associated with increased motor tension, hypervigilance, sleep disturbances, or increased autonomic activity
Anxiety (not otherwise specified)	Anxiety present but does not fit into specific category

Data from the American Psychiatric Association. (1995). *Diagnostic and statistical manual of mental disorders: DSM-IV.* Washington, D.C.: Author.

variant across countries and cultures as well. Almost one-third of the population have problems sleeping in any given year. Sleep-wake cycle disruptions are defined as patterns that occur outside the normal range for the age group or that are in conflict with environmental and sociocultural situations.

The term *impaired sleep* is nonspecific. It is used when referring to a patient who has an alteration in sleep patterns and daytime functioning. It is a more inclusive term than the concept of sleep disorders. Patients with impaired sleep exhibit a variety of alterations in the sleep-wake cycle. Impaired sleep requires a longer period to get to sleep, reduced total sleep time, reduced sleep efficiency (time asleep versus time spent trying to sleep), and increased time spent awake and in light sleep. Changes in daytime functioning and an altered sense of well-being are important components of impaired sleep.

Insomnia is a familiar disorder consisting of an inability to fall asleep easily or to remain asleep. Insomnia is reported by 40 to 50 percent of people at any given time. Among those seeking treatment, the female-to-male ratio is 2:1, and there appears to be a preponderance of cases in lower socioeconomic groups. Of the reported cases,

- 30 to 35 percent are due to psychiatric illness
- 15 to 20 percent are psychophysiologic in nature
- 10 to 15 percent are due to alcohol or drug use
- 10 to 15 percent are due to periodic limb movement disorder
- 5 to 10 percent are due to sleep apnea
- 5 to 10 percent are due to medical illness.

The incidence of impaired sleep among hospitalized patients is reported to be from 27 to 76.5 percent. Impaired sleep may be secondary to situational and environmental stressors, associated with the illness itself, or related to preexisting health problems. In many cases, the disorder decreases sleep, and in turn, the decreased sleep worsens the disorder.

There are a variety of intrinsic and extrinsic impaired sleep patterns. Intrinsic sleep disorders include insomnia, narcolepsy, sleep apnea syndrome, obstructive sleep apnea, central sleep apnea syndrome, periodic limb movement disorder, and restless legs syndrome. Extrinsic sleep disorders include arousal disorders, sleep-wake transition disorders, and other parasomnias. Additionally, sleep disorders may be secondary to medical and psychiatric disorders, including head injuries, imbalances in neurotransmitters (e.g., Parkinson's disease, depression), hormonal imbalances, respiratory and cardiovascular disorders, and gastrointestinal disorders.

Iatrogenic sleep disorders are caused by sleep deprivation, a state in which overall sensory input is decreased, or by sensory overload, or both. With sensory deprivation, there is an overall reduction in stimuli. Patients respond by becoming more sensitive to the stimuli present around them. In contrast, sensory overload is defined as a state in which the degree and nature of sensory input exceed the patient's level of tolerance. Regardless of the cause, the patient is left distressed and in a state of hyperarousal with impaired cognition and problem-solving abilities.

Pathogenesis

Components of Normal Sleep

There are two primary sleep stages that occur in a cyclical fashion: rapid eye movement (REM) sleep and non–rapid eye movement sleep (NREM) (Fig. 17–2). Sleep begins with a period of NREM sleep characterized by the sleeping posture, closed eyes, and constricted pupils. A degree of tonus remains in some muscle groups. The NREM period is followed by alternating periods of REM sleep each lasting 80 to 120 minutes each. The slower NREM sleep stages predominate during the first part of the night. REM sleep periods dominate the later hours. REM sleep accounts for about 30 percent of sleep. It should not be confused with light sleep because it generally takes a more powerful stimulus to arouse a person from REM sleep than from NREM sleep.

The Need for Sleep

Although there is an abundance of information available about the sleep cycle, the precise physiologic benefits of sleep have not been established. It is thought that sleep restores energy to the brain and the CNS, renewing balance and sensitivities among the various parts of the CNS. Sleep also influences the autonomic nervous system whereby sympathetic activity decreases and parasympathetic activity occasionally increases. Arterial blood pressure, pulse, and respirations decrease, and superficial blood vessels dilate. Oxygen consumption and the production of carbon dioxide are reduced, and metabolic rates decline. Skeletal muscles relax. Urinary outflow decreases, but gastrointestinal tract activity may increase.

Impaired sleep can result in many problems, ranging from an occasional "bad day" to complete disruption of family, work and social activities. Sleep disorders may be short term, lasting a few days, or may result in total incapacitation. Initially, daytime functioning becomes slightly impaired. However, if the sleep disorder continues, there is a progression from slight cognitive and behavioral disruptions to profound sleepiness or alertness, severe memory difficulties, and alterations in autonomic and other organ system functioning.

Many physiologic and psychological changes occur as a result of sleep deprivation. Energy mobilization decreases as

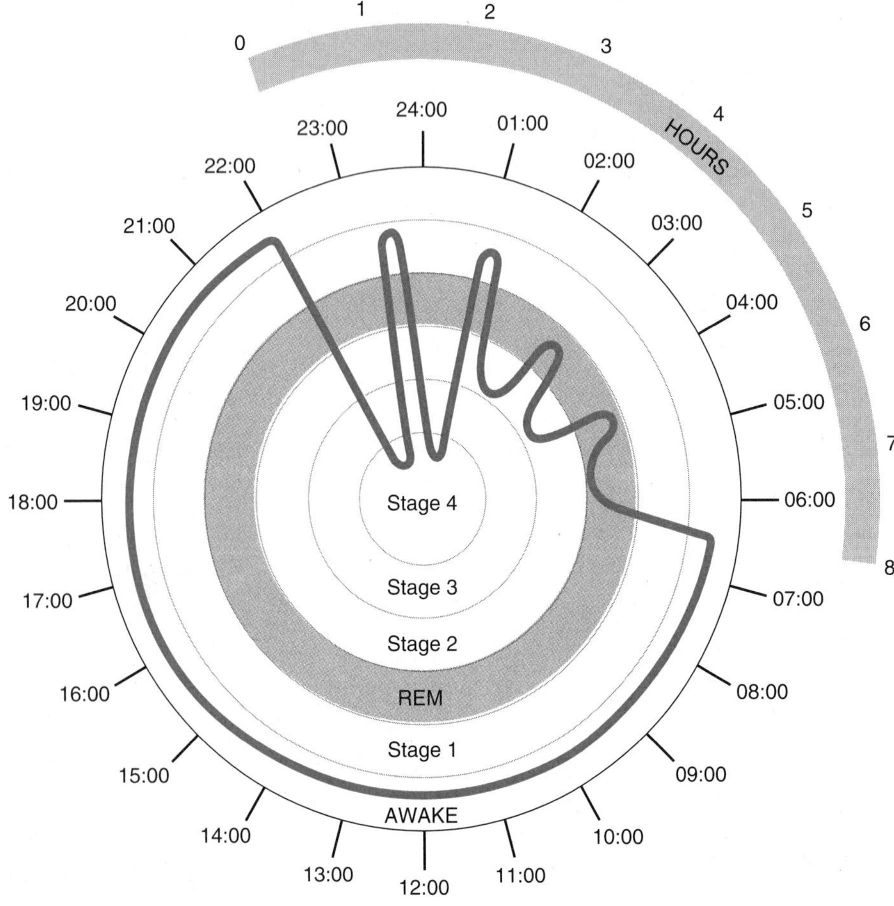

Figure 17–2 Components of normal sleep. Sleep begins with a period of NREM sleep, characterized by the sleeping posture, closed eyes, and myotic pupils. A degree of tonus remains in some muscle groups. This period is followed by alternating periods of REM and NREM sleep, each lasting 80 to 120 minutes. The slower NREM sleep stages predominate during the first part of the night, whereas REM sleep periods dominate in the later hours.

adenosine triphosphate levels in the body decrease. The stress hormones from the adrenal cortex increase in the blood and contribute to the possibility of hallucinations. Reflexes slow, and muscle coordination decreases. Equilibrium and muscle strength may be lost, with nystagmus and ptosis appearing. Respiratory efforts may diminish and arrhythmias appear. Sleep deprivation is associated with bizarre behavior and temporary neuroses or psychoses. Mental agility decreases, memory fails, attention span is limited, and sense of reality is distorted.

Although the body attempts to establish a normal equilibrium between REM and NREM sleep periods, deep sleep takes priority over dreaming sleep when there has been prolonged sleep deprivation. Deep sleep needs are met first, after which dreaming needs will be met. The outcomes of sleep deprivation can be relieved by 12 to 14 hours of sleep characterized by increased REM sleep periods. Ten days of such sleep is usually required to counteract four to five days of sleep deprivation.

PHARMACOTHERAPEUTIC OPTIONS

Benzodiazepines

SHORT-ACTING TO INTERMEDIATE-ACTING BENZODIAZEPINES

- ❒ Alprazolam (Xanax); (🍁) Apo-Alpraz, Novo-Alprazol, Nu-Alpraz
- ❒ Clonazepam (Klonopin); (🍁) Rivotril
- ❒ Lorazepam (Ativan); (🍁) Apo-Lorazepam, Novo-Lorazem
- ❒ Midazolam (Versed)
- ❒ Oxazepam (Serax); (🍁) Apo-Oxazepam, Novoxapam, Oxpam, Zapex
- ❒ Temazepam (Restoril)
- ❒ Triazolam (Halcion); (🍁) Apo-Triazo, Feb-Triazolam, Novo-Triolam, Nu-Triazo
- ❒ Zolpidem (Ambien)

LONG-ACTING BENZODIAZEPINES

- ❒ Chlordiazepoxide (Librium, Libritabs, Mitran, Reposans-10); (🍁) Apo-Chlordiazepoxide, Solium
- ❒ Clorazepate (Tranxene, Clorazetabs, Clorazecaps); (🍁) Apo-Clorazepate, GenXene, Novo-Clopate
- ❒ Diazepam (Valium, Zetran); (🍁) Po-Diazepam, Diazemuls, Vivol
- ❒ Estazolam (ProSom)
- ❒ Flurazepam (Dalmane); (🍁) Apo-Flurazepam, Novo-Flupam, Somnol
- ❒ Halazepam (Paxipam)
- ❒ Prazepam (Centrax)
- ❒ Quazepam (Doral)

Indications

Benzodiazepines are among the most widely prescribed drugs in the United States. Chlordiazepoxide and diazepam are considered the prototypes for this class. Table 17–2 provides a listing of Food and Drug Administration (FDA)–approved uses of benzodiazepines. The most frequently prescribed drugs in this class are lorazepam and alprazolam. Although zolpidem is chemically unrelated to the benzodi-

TABLE 17–2 FOOD AND DRUG ADMINISTRATION–APPROVED USES OF ANTIANXIETY AND SEDATIVE-HYPNOTIC DRUGS

Drugs	Anxiety	Insomnia	Alcohol Withdrawal	Epilepsy	Muscle Spasm	Preop Med	Anesthesia Adjunct	Panic Disorder
Benzodiazepines								
Alprazolam		X						X
Clonazepam				X				X
Clorazepate	X	X	X	X				
Chlordiazepoxide	X	X	X			X		
Diazepam	X	X	X	X	X	X		X
Estazolam		X						
Flurazepam		X						
Halazepam	X							
Lorazepam	X	X	X	X		X		X
Oxazepam	X	X	X					
Prazepam		X						
Quazepam		X						
Temazepam		X						
Triazolam		X						
Nonbenzodiazepines								
Buspirone	X							
Meprobamate	X				X			
Zolpidem		X						
Barbiturates								
Amobarbital	X					X		
Aprobarbital	X	X						
Butabarbital	X	X						
Mephobarbital	X			X				
Pentobarbital		X				X		
Phenobarbital		X		X		X		
Secobarbital		X		X		X		

azepines, it is included here because it binds to benzodiazepine receptors in the brain. Benzodiazepines are not to be used to manage the stress of everyday life.

Pharmacodynamics

Benzodiazepines act primarily at subcortical levels in the brain. Benzodiazepines assist in GABA binding at receptor sites in the brain and spinal cord to increase the effects of GABA on chloride flux (Fig. 17–3). The result is hyperpolarization of cell membranes. The result is muscle relaxation (spinal cord), antianxiety and emotional effects (limbic-cortex area), ataxia (cerebellum), and anticonvulsant activity (brain stem).

Although zolpidem is structurally unrelated to the benzodiazepines, it binds to the GABA receptor-chloride channel complex. Thus, it shares some of the properties of the benzodiazepines. Zolpidem can reduce sleep latency and awakenings, and it can prolong the duration of sleep. It does not significantly reduce the time spent in REM sleep and causes little or no rebound insomnia when treatment is discontinued. In contrast to the other benzodiazepines, zolpidem lacks antianxiety, muscle relaxant, and anticonvulsant activities.

Adverse Effects and Contraindications

To one degree or another, benzodiazepines rely on CNS depression to relieve symptoms of anxiety. For this reason, the major adverse effect of benzodiazepines is excessive sedation. Excessive sedation leads to dizziness, lethargy, ataxia, and respiratory depression. These problems are most evident in the early stages of treatment but symptoms usually subside with time. If troublesome adverse effects persist, the dosage should be adjusted accordingly.

The potential for respiratory depression caused by benzodiazepines can lead to problems in the presence of pulmonary disease, sleep apnea, or chronic airway limitation. Fatal overdosage is rare with oral benzodiazepines unless they are taken with alcohol or other CNS depressants.

There is a potential for serious behavioral disturbances in patients who use benzodiazepines. The disturbances include confusion, paradoxical agitation or excitability, amnesia, hallucinations, and vivid dreams or nightmares. In patients with pre-existing depression, benzodiazepine use may worsen the depression and foster suicidal ideation.

Idiosyncratic reactions to benzodiazepines have been reported. There are known individual cases of blood dyscrasias, rashes, and phlebitis. Patient complaints of unexplained bleeding, myalgia, calf pain, or dermatitis should be carefully evaluated.

Benzodiazepines are contraindicated in hypersensitive patients or in patients with an allergy to specific ingredients. During pregnancy, benzodiazepines must be used with extreme caution. All benzodiazepines are in either category C or D of the FDA pregnancy risks. These drugs should be used in pregnant women only when the benefits greatly outweigh risks. Infants of women who have taken benzodiazepines during pregnancy may display poor sucking, lethargy, or withdrawal symptoms at birth. Nursing mothers should also avoid using benzodiazepines because most have an active metabolite that crosses into breast milk.

Pharmacokinetics

When taken by mouth, benzodiazepines are well absorbed, with variable plasma concentrations achieved. Usually, the more rapidly absorbed the benzodiazepine, the more prompt and intense the onset of action (Table 17–3). The onset of short-acting to intermediate-acting benzodiazepines ranges from 15 to 90 minutes, with peak times reached in 1 to 2 hours. The duration of action for this group of benzodiazepines ranges from 6 to 48 hours.

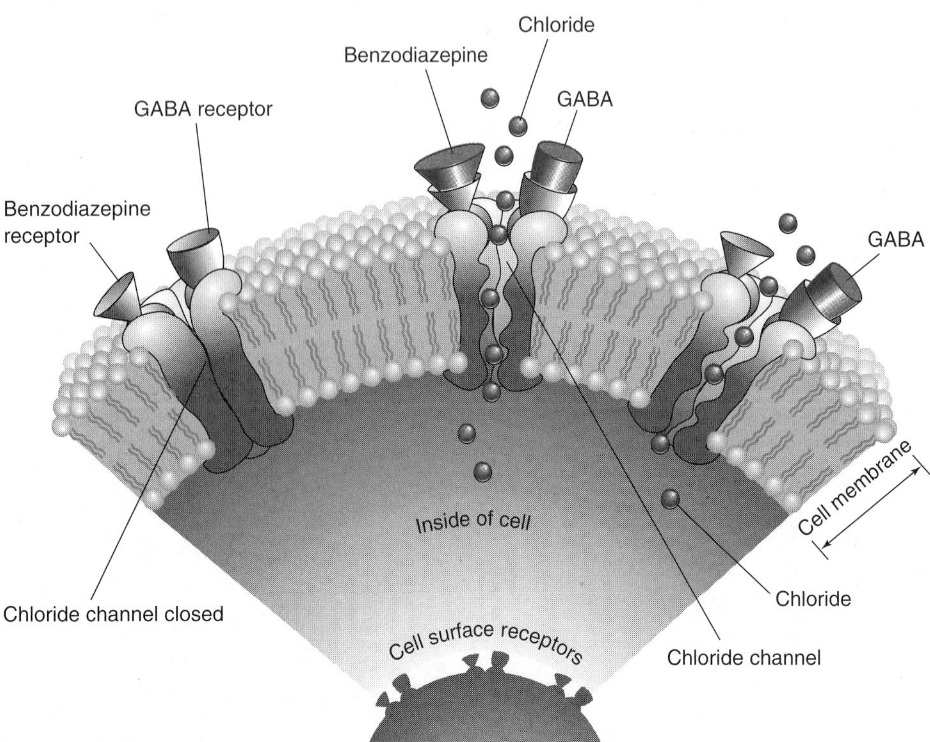

Figure 17–3 Schematic model of the GABA receptor–chloride channel complex for benzodiazepine action. The model illustrates cellular binding sites for benzodiazepines. The chloride channel complex spans the neuronal cell membrane. The channel exists in an open or closed configuration. Equilibrium between open and closed states of the chloride channel is altered by the presence of GABA. The channel is opened by GABA. The inward flow of chloride ions hyperpolarizes neurons, reducing their ability to fire. Thus, GABA is an inhibitory neurotransmitter. Binding of a benzodiazepine to the complex prolongs the time the channel remains open. GABA has no effect on channel opening in the absence of GABA.

TABLE 17–3 PHARMACOKINETICS OF SELECTED ANTIANXIETY AND SEDATIVE-HYPNOTIC DRUGS

Drug	Route	Onset	Peak	Duration	PB (%)	$t_{1/2}$*	BioA (%)
Short-Acting to Intermediate-Acting Benzodiazepines							
Alprazolam	po	15–60 min	1–2 hr	12–15 hr	71–100	12–15 hr	80
Clonazepam	po	20–60 min	1–2 hr	6–12 hr	85	18–50 hr	UA
Lorazepam	po	15–45 min	2 hr	6–8 hr	85	10–16 hr	90
	IM	15–30 min	60–90 min	>48 hr			
	IV	5–15 min	UK	>48 hr			100
Midazolam	IM	15 min	30–60 min	2–6 hr	97	1–2 hr	UA
	IV	1.5–5 min	Rapid	2–6 hr			100
Oxazepam	po	45–90 min	3 hr	6–12 hr	97	10–25 hr	92
Temazepam	po	30 min	2–3 hr†	UK	97	10–20 hr	80
Triazolam	po	15–30 min	3 days‡	UK	91	1.6–5.4 hr	44
Long-Acting Benzodiazepines							
Chlordiazepoxide	po	1–2 hr	0.5–4 hr	To 24 hr	95	5–30 hr	UA
	IM	15–30 min	1–2 hr	UK			UA
	IV	1–5 min	UK	0.25–1 hr			100
Clorazepate	po	30–60 min	1–2 hr	To 24 hr	High	48 hr	UA
Diazepam	po	15–45 min	0.5–2 hr	Variable	98	20–80 hr	85–100
	IM	15–45 min	0.5–2 hr				
	IV	1–3 min	15–30 min				
Estazolam	po	15–30 min	2 hr	6–8 hr	UA	10–24 hr	UA
Flurazepam	po	15–45 min	0.5–1 hr	7–8 hr§	97	2.3 hr†	UA
Halazepam	po	2–3 hr	1–3 hr	48 hr	97	14–34 hr	UA
Prazepam	po	UK	Days-weeks	Days	UA	5–15 hr	UA
Quazepam	po	30 min	2 hr	8 hr	95	39 hr	UA
Buspirone	po	7–10 days	40–90 min/ 7–10 days‖	UK	95	2–4 hrs	90
Chloral hydrate	po	30 min	1 hr	4–8 hr	35–41¶	8–10 hr	UA
	SUP	30–60 min	UK				
Meprobamate	po	<1 hr	1–3 hr	6–12 hr	UA	6–16 hr	UA
Paraldehyde	po	10–15 min	30–60 min	8–12 hr	UA	3.4–9.8 hr	UA
Zolpidem	po	1.5 hr	2 hrs	UK	UA	2–3 hr	UA
Short-Acting Barbiturates							
Pentobarbital	po	10–15 min	3–4 hr	3–4 hr	**	15–48 hr††	
Secobarbital	po					15–40 hr	
Intermediate-Acting Barbiturates							
Amobarbital	po	45–60 min	6–8 hr	3–4 hr		8–42 hr	
Aprobarbital	po					14–34 hr	
Butabarbital	po					34–42 hr	
Long-Acting Barbiturates							
Mephobarbital	po	>60 min	10–12 hr	10–12 hr		11–67 hr	
Phenobarbital	po					80–120 hr	

*Half-life of active metabolites: *Flurazepam:* Half-life of active metabolite may be 30 to 100 hours for desalkylflurazepam, and for the metabolite *N*-1-hydroxyethylflurazepam, it is 2 to 4 hours. *Quazepam:* Half-life of metabolites is increased in the elderly—half-life for 2-oxoquazepam is 39 hours and for *N*-desalkylflurazepam is 70 to 75 hours. *Prazepam:* Half-life of active metabolite desmethyldiazepam with multidosing is 30 to 100 hours; for oxazepam, it is 5 to 15 hours.

†Effectiveness of temazepam may be demonstrated for up to 35 days with daily administration.

‡Triazolam's maximum hypnotic response. Has a reported range of effectiveness of 1 to 42 days.

§Flurazepam reportedly effective for up to 28 days.

‖Peak serum levels of buspirone may be reached 40 to 90 minutes after oral dosing; however, it may take 7 to 10 days for relief of anxiety to be noted.

¶Half-life of the metabolite of chloral hydrate.

**Barbiturate binding to plasma proteins is a function of lipid solubility.

††Mean half-life of the short-acting, intermediate-acting, and long-acting barbiturates is dependent on the dose.

BioA, Bioavailability; PB, protein binding; SUP, suppository formulation; UA, unavailable; UK, unknown.

The more lipid-soluble benzodiazepines (e.g., diazepam) are widely distributed in the body and brain and are highly protein bound. With multiple doses, the drugs accumulate in body fluids and tissues. Saturation of storage sites permits greater serum concentrations and a longer duration of action. The accumulation in storage sites also accounts for the prolonged action of benzodiazepines after they have been discontinued.

Chlordiazepoxide, clorazepate, diazepam, flurazepam, halazepam, prazepam, and quazepam are transformed by the liver to active metabolites that may have clinical effects beyond their stated duration. Conversely, alprazolam, lorazepam, oxazepam, temazepam, triazolam, and zolpidem are transformed into weak or inactive metabolites and therefore are less likely to accumulate. Elimination of benzodiazepine and benzodiazepine-like drugs vary somewhat but essentially are eliminated via the kidneys.

Drug-Drug Interactions

Because benzodiazepines act primarily in the CNS, other CNS-active drugs either potentiate or are potentiated by these drugs (Table 17–4). Owing to plasma protein binding, other drugs interfere with the biotransformation of benzodiazepines, thereby prolonging their action. Because a primary adverse effect of benzodiazepines is sedation, concurrent use of drugs that interfere with consciousness or mental alertness (i.e., alcohol, opioids, barbiturates, psychoactive drugs) should be discouraged.

Cimetidine (but not ranitidine) reduces the plasma clearance of benzodiazepines, which, in turn, leads to increased plasma concentrations of some drugs. Cigarettes, or any nicotine use, can decrease the effectiveness of benzodiazepines.

Dosage Regimens

Dosages should initially be as low as possible and increased only after effectiveness has been evaluated. Most benzodiazepines are given orally in divided daily doses or at bedtime (Table 17–5). Additionally, intramuscular or intravenous forms of benzodiazepines are available for severe anxiety episodes, preoperative apprehension, and control of acute seizure activity.

Laboratory Considerations

Periodic blood counts and liver function testing should be performed for patients on long-term benzodiazepine therapy. There is a risk of developing jaundice and neutropenia. In the presence of chlordiazepoxide, bilirubin, AST (SGOT), ALT (SGPT), and 17-ketosteroid levels are increased. Radioactive iodine uptake is decreased. False-positive results have been noted with the Gravindex pregnancy test.

Barbiturates

SHORT-ACTING DRUGS

❒ Pentobarbital (NEMBUTAL); (✱) NOVO-PENTOBARB
❒ Secobarbital (SECONAL); (✱) NOVO-SECOBARB

INTERMEDIATE-ACTING DRUGS

❒ Amobarbital (AMYTAL); (✱) NOVAMOBARB
❒ Aprobarbital (ALURATE)
❒ Butabarbital (BUTISOL, SARISOL NO. 2)

LONG-ACTING DRUGS

❒ Mephobarbital (MEBARAL)
❒ Phenobarbital (BARBITA, LUMINAL, SOLFOTON)

Indications

The barbiturates were at one time the most commonly prescribed group of sedative-hypnotics. With few exceptions, they have been replaced by benzodiazepines. Phenobarbital is considered the prototype drug of this class. The barbiturates are commonly used as adjuncts to anesthesia and for treatment of seizure disorders; several are indicated for the treatment of insomnia. Barbiturates are only indicated for short-term use because they tend to lose their effectiveness in 14 days or less. Furthermore, barbiturates are not analgesics and should not be used to produce restful sleep when insomnia is caused by pain. However, when a barbiturate is taken concurrently with an analgesic, the sedative action is enhanced and favorably alters the patient's emotional response to the pain.

Pharmacodynamics

Barbiturates increase GABA binding to receptor sites, and in high concentrations, they may directly depress calcium-dependent action potentials and increase chloride flux without GABA (Fig. 17–4). Therefore, barbiturates result in nonselective, broader effects than those obtainable with the benzodiazepines because they also depress excitatory transmitters and nonsynaptic membranes.

The ascending reticular activating system receives stimuli from all parts of the body, relaying impulses to the cortex. Thus, wakefulness and alertness are promoted. Barbiturates cause a depression of the reticular activating system, thereby decreasing cortical stimuli. Wakefulness and alertness are accordingly decreased.

However, because barbiturates mimic GABA directly, there is no ceiling effect to the degree of CNS depression they produce. Hence, in contrast to the benzodiazepines, these drugs readily cause death when taken in excessive amounts. As dosages increase, the patient's level of consciousness progresses from sedation to sleep to general anesthesia.

At hypnotic doses, barbiturates produce modest reductions in blood pressure and heart rate. Toxic doses produce profound hypotension and shock. The reactions are the result of direct depressant effects on the myocardium and vascular smooth muscle.

Adverse Effects and Contraindications

The more frequent adverse effects of barbiturates include a hangover, ataxia, and drowsiness. Nausea, vomiting, insomnia, constipation, restlessness, headache, and fainting have also occurred. Night terrors have been reported in some patients. Patients may experience confusion, disorientation, and mental depression. Paradoxical reactions are more often seen in older adults or debilitated patients; however, patients of any age may be affected.

The more serious adverse effects of barbiturates include hypersensitivity reactions (i.e., skin rash, exfoliative dermatitis, urticaria), sore throat, fever, edema, serum sickness, apnea, bronchospasms, and Stevens-Johnson syndrome. Stevens-Johnson syndrome is an occasionally fatal inflammatory disease of children and young adults. It is characterized by fever, bullae of the skin, and ulcers of the mucous membranes of the oral cavity, nose, eyes, and genitalia.

Acute toxic effects include bradycardia, confusion, apnea, laryngospasm, ataxia, extreme weakness, and visual disturbances. Long-term barbiturate use may result in osteomalacia and rickets.

As a general rule, tolerance to one general CNS depressant bestows tolerance to all other general CNS depressants. Hence, there is cross-tolerance among barbiturates, alcohol, benzodiazepines, general anesthetics, and a number of other drugs. Tolerance to barbiturates and the other general CNS depressants does not produce significant cross-tolerance with opioids.

TABLE 17–4 DRUG-DRUG INTERACTIONS OF SELECTED ANTIANXIETY AND SEDATIVE-HYPNOTIC DRUGS

Drug	Interactive Drugs	Interaction
Benzodiazepines		
Benzodiazepines	Cimetidine Digoxin Erythromycin Fluoxetine Isoniazid Ketoconazole Metoprolol Oral contraceptives Propranolol Propoxyphene Valproic acid Zidovudine	Increases plasma half-life of benzodiazepine, particularly of alprazolam; increases risk of digoxin toxicity
	Phenytoin	May increase concentration of interactive drug
	Levodopa	Decreased plasma concentration of interactive drug; decreases effectiveness of oxazepam
	Barbiturates Rifampin Theophylline Tobacco	Increases biotransformation of benzodiazepines, decreasing their effectiveness
	Alcohol Anesthetics Antihistamines Opioids Phenothiazines Tricyclic antidepressants	Additive CNS depression
Lorazepam	Probenecid	Decreased biotransformation of lorazepam; thereby action may be increased
Nonbenzodiazepines		
Buspirone	Cimetidine MAO inhibitors	Increases buspirone effect; potential for toxicity
Chloral hydrate Meprobamate Zolpidem	Alcohol Antihistamines CNS depressants Opioids Other sedative-hypnotics	Additive CNS depression
Barbiturates		
Barbiturates	Alcohol Antihistamines Opioids Sedative-hypnotics	Additive CNS depression
	Chloramphenicol Cyclosporine Dacarbazine Glucocorticosteroids Oral contraceptives Tricyclic antidepressants Quinidine Warfarin	Induce hepatic enzyme system to increase biotransformation of interactive drugs
	Acetaminophen	May increase risk of hepatotoxicity to interactive drug
	Divalproex MAO inhibitors Valproic acid	May decrease biotransformation of phenobarbital, increasing sedation
	Cyclophosphamide	Increases risk of hematologic toxicity

CNS, Central nervous system; MAO, monoamine oxidase.

TABLE 17–5 DOSAGE REGIMENS FOR SELECTED ANTIANXIETY AND SEDATIVE-HYPNOTIC DRUGS

Drugs	Uses	Dosage	Implications
Short- to Intermediate-Acting Benzodiazepines			
Alprazolam	Anxiety disorders, panic attacks, adjunct in treatment of depression	*Adult:* 0.25–0.5 mg po TID Increase up to 3–4 mg po QD Maximum: 4 mg	Not for use under 18 yr of age. Begin with 0.25 mg BID–TID for elderly or debilitated patients.
Clonazepam	Prophylaxis of seizures Sedation, uncontrolled leg movements during sleep (unlabeled uses)	*Adult:* 0.25 mg BID. May increase by 0.5–1 mg every 3rd day, Maintenance: Not to exceed 20 mg *Child younger than 10 years of age or less than 30 kg:* Initial daily dose 0.01–0.03 mg/kg/day BID–TID, not to exceed 0.05 mg/kg/day Increase by no more than 0.25–0.5 mg every 3rd day until therapeutic blood levels are reached not to exceed 0.2 mg/kg/day	Therapeutic serum concentrations are 20–80 mcg/ml. Missed doses should be taken within 1 hr or omitted. Do not double dose. Abrupt withdrawal can cause tremors, nausea, vomiting, abdominal and muscle cramps, and status epilepticus
Lorazepam	Anxiety, insomnia, preoperative sedation, prechemotherapy antiemetic in children	*Adult:* Anxiety: 1–2 mg po BID–TID up to 10 mg daily Insomnia: 2–4 mg po HS; 1–2 mg po HS for elderly, increase PRN	Prolonged high-dose therapy may lead to psychological or physical dependence
Oxazepam	Anxiety, insomnia, alcohol withdrawal	*Adult:* 10–15 mg po TID–QID. Insomnia: 15–30 mg po HS	Drug should be tapered at the completion of therapy. Sudden cessation may lead to withdrawal
Temazepam	Short-term management of insomnia	*Adult:* 15 mg. po HS up to 30 mg	Dosage should be reduced in debilitated and older adult patients
Triazolam	Short-term management of insomnia	*Initial:* 0.25 mg po HS up to 0.5 mg	
Long-Acting Benzodiazepines			
Chlordiazepoxide	Anxiety, alcohol withdrawal	*Adult:* Anxiety: 5–25 mg po TID–QID Withdrawal: 50–100 mg po, IM, or IV repeated until agitation is controlled, up to 400 mg/day *Child older than 6 yr of age:* 5 mg po BID–QID, up to 10 mg BID–TID	Metabolites active for up to 100 hrs
Clorazepate	Anxiety, alcohol withdrawal	*Adult:* Anxiety: 15–60 mg po QD in divided doses. Withdrawal: 30 mg po BID–QID, then 15 mg po BID–QID, on first day, then gradually tapered off Maximum: 90 mg/day	May be given as a single dose of 11.25–22.5 mg at bedtime for anxiety. For elderly or debilitated patients, give 7.5–15 mg QD
Diazepam	Anxiety, alcohol withdrawal	*Adult:* Anxiety: 2–10 mg po BID–QID *or* 15–30 mg po (SR) QD *or* 2–10 mg IM/IV q3–4 hr PRN. Withdrawal: 10 mg po TID–QID first 24 hr, then decrease to 5 mg po TID–QID *Child older than 6 yr of age:* 0.1–0.8 mg/kg/day po divided every 6–8 hrs	Metabolite active for up to 200 hours. Monitor closely for excess sedation. Extremely cautious use in children.
Estazolam	Short-term management of insomnia	*Adult:* 1 mg po HS. Range: 0.5–2 mg	Assess sleep patterns before and periodically throughout therapy.
Flurazepam	Insomnia	*Adult:* 15–30 mg po HS	Dosage should be reduced in the elderly or debilitated patient.
Halazepam	Adjunct in management of anxiety	*Adult:* 20–40 mg po TID–QID	Metabolite active for up to 100 hr. Elderly: use 1/2 dose initially. Not for use in persons younger than 18 yr old.
Prazepam	Adjunct in management of anxiety	*Adult:* 10 mg po TID *or* as single HS dose of 20–40 mg Range: 20–60 mg daily	Dosage should be reduced in the elderly or debilitated patient
Quazepam	Insomnia	*Adult:* Initial dose 15 mg po HS, then titrate downward	

TABLE 17–5 DOSAGE REGIMENS FOR SELECTED ANTIANXIETY AND SEDATIVE-HYPNOTIC DRUGS *Continued*

Drugs	Uses	Dosage	Implications
Nonbenzodiazepines			
Buspirone	Anxiety	*Adult:* 10–15 mg po BID–TID Increase by 5 mg q 2–3 days Maximum: Not to exceed 60 mg daily. Usual dose 20–30 mg QD	May take up to 2 weeks for onset of action. Monitor patients closely during initial phase
Chloral hydrate	Short-term sedative-hypnotic	*Adult:* Anxiety/sedation: 250 mg po TID; 325 mg rectally TID Hypnotic: 500–1000 mg po/rectally HS *Child:* Anxiety/sedation: 8.3 mg/kg po/rectally. Up to 500 mg TID Hypnotic: 50 mg/kg po/rectally HS, up to 1 g	If suppository is too soft for insertion, chill in refrigerator for 30 minutes or run under cold water before removing foil wrapper
Meprobamate	Anxiety	*Adult:* 1200–1600 mg po QD in 2–3 divided doses *or* 800–1600 mg in two divided doses as sustained-release capsules; not to exceed 2400 mg QD *Child ages 6–12 yr:* 25 mg/kg/day in 2–3 divided doses	Use smallest effective dose. May induce psychologic or physical dependence
Zolpidem	Short-term management of insomnia	*Adult:* 10 mg po HS	Elderly or debilitated patients or patients with hepatic impairment should be started on 5 mg
Barbiturates			
Amobarbital	Preoperative sedation; situations in which sedation is required; hypnosis	*Adult:* Sedative: 30–50 mg. IV BID–TID. Hypnosis: 65–200 mg *Child older than 6 yr:* Sedation: 3–5 mg/kg IV depending on response. Hypnosis: 2–3 mg/kg/dose IM *Child younger than age 6 yr:* 3–5 mg/kg IV. Hypnosis: 2–3 mg/kg IM	Monitor respiratory status in patients receiving drug IV. Do not administer subcutaneously. Give deep IM into gluteal muscle to minimize tissue irritation. IV rate not to exceed 50 mg/minute. Titrate slowly.
Aprobarbital	Short-term sedation and sleep induction	*Adult:* Sedation: 40 mg po TID Hypnosis: 40–160 mg po at HS	Po formulations not to be taken longer than 2 weeks. Do not increase dose. Avoid other CNS depressants. Taper dosage gradually to minimize risk of seizures. Supervise ambulation and transfer of patients after administration.
Butabarbital	Short-term sedation and sleep induction	*Adult:* Sedation: 15–30 mg po TID–QID Hypnosis: 50–100 mg po at HS *Child:* Sedation: 7.5–30 mg po depending on age, weight, and sedation desired Hypnosis: based on age and weight	
Mephobarbital	Anxiety, tension, apprehension	*Adult:* Sedation: 32–100 mg po TID–QID Optimum dose: 50 mg po TID–QID *Child:* Sedation: 16–32 mg po TID–QID	
Pentobarbital	Short-term hypnosis	*Adult:* Sedation: 20 mg po TID–QID Hypnosis: 100 mg po *or* 150–200 mg IM *or* 100 mg IV to total of 500 mg *Child:* Sedative: 2–6 mg/kg/day po/IM *or* 50 mg IV *or* 2 mg/kg TID rectally	
Phenobarbital	Preoperative sedation	*Adult:* Sedation: 30–120 mg/day po/IM/IV BID–TID. Hypnosis: 100–320 mg po/IM/IV at HS *Child:* Sedative: 2 mg/kg po TID	
Secobarbital	Short-term hypnosis; preoperative sedation	*Adult:* Hypnosis: 100–200 mg IM *or* 50–250 mg IV Sedation: 1.1–2.2 mg/kg IM 10–15 minutes preoperatively *Child:* Sedation: 4–5 mg/kg IM 10–15 minutes preoperatively	

Pharmacokinetics

Barbiturates are readily absorbed via oral, rectal, and parenteral routes. The soluble sodium salts are absorbed faster than the free acids. Ultra-short-acting barbiturates are used as IV anesthetics (see Chapter 16). Sodium pentothal is an ultra-short-acting drug that acts within a few seconds to produce a state of anesthesia. The onset of short-acting drugs occurs in a relatively short period of time (10 to 15 minutes), and they reach their peak in 3 to 4 hours. Intermediate-acting drugs have an onset time of 45 to 60 minutes, reaching their peak action in 6 to 8 hours. Long-acting barbiturates require more than 60 minutes for onset and reach their peak over 10 to 12 hours (see Table 17–3).

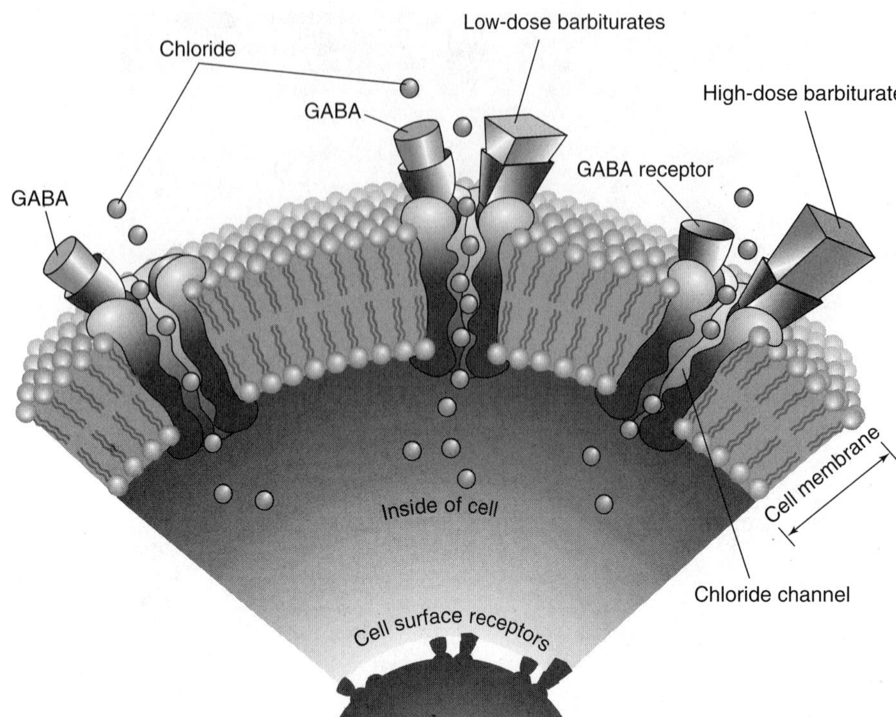

Figure 17–4 Schematic model of the GABA receptor–chloride channel complex for barbiturate action. The model illustrates cellular binding sites for barbiturates. The chloride channel complex spans the neuronal cell membrane, which exists in an open or closed configuration. Equilibrium between open and closed states of the chloride channel is altered by the presence of GABA. The channel is opened by GABA. The inward flow of chloride ions hyperpolarizes neurons and reduces their ability to fire. When barbiturates bind to the complex, the chloride channel remains open. GABA has no effect on channel opening in the absence of GABA.

The duration of action is related to the lipid solubility of the barbiturate. Drugs with the greatest lipid solubility have the longest duration of action. Conversely, those with the lowest lipid solubility have the shortest duration of action. The slower a barbiturate is altered or eliminated, the more prolonged is its action. Elimination is slow, and as administration continues, cumulative effects result.

Barbiturates also stimulate the synthesis of hepatic microsomal enzymes. As a result, barbiturates hasten their own biotransformation as well as that of many other drugs. They stimulate biotransformation by promoting the synthesis of porphyrin, a nitrogen-containing organic compound that occurs in protoplasm. Porphyrin is then converted to heme, which, in turn, is converted to cytochrome P_{450}, a key component of the microsomal enzyme system.

Drug-Drug Interactions

Increased CNS depressant effects may occur with alcohol, monoamine oxidase inhibitors, sedatives, and opioids. Oral anticoagulants, corticosteroids, griseofulvin, quinidine, oral contraceptives, and theophylline may show a decreased effect when used with barbiturates (see Table 17–4).

Dosage Regimen

The dosage of barbiturates is drug specific (see Table 17–5). They may be administered orally, IV, IM, and by rectal suppository. Oral administration is warranted for daytime sedation and to treat insomnia. Dosages should be reduced in older adults and debilitated patient.

Nonbenzodiazepine Drugs

- ❒ Buspirone (BUSPAR)
- ❒ Chloral hydrate (AQUACHLORAL); (🍁) NOVO-CHLORHYDRATE, PMS-CHLORATE HYDRATE
- ❒ Ethchlorvynol (PLACIDYL)
- ❒ Glutethimide (DORIDEN)
- ❒ Diphenhydramine (BENADRYL)
- ❒ Doxylamine (UNISOM)
- ❒ Melatonin
- ❒ Meprobamate (EQUANIL, MEPROSPAN, MILTOWN, TRANCOT); (🍁) APO-MEPROBAMATE
- ❒ Paraldehyde (PARAL)

Buspirone is the first of a new class of antianxiety drugs called axapirones. Its only indication is for the short-term management of generalized anxiety disorder. It is as effective as any other benzodiazepine for this purpose. In addition, it may be helpful for anxious patients with chronic airway limitation disorders or sleep apnea, because no respiratory depression occurs with this drug. In fact, some patients may experience an increase in their resting respiratory rate. Buspirone does not have the associated adverse effects of sedation, drowsiness, or motor retardation.

Buspirone does not act at GABA receptor sites, nor does it potentiate benzodiazepine receptor binding. It is thought to selectively antagonize 5-hydroxytryptamine (serotonin) receptors in the CNS. It does not have significant peripheral effects or anticonvulsant activity.

When a patient begins taking buspirone, it is important to note that anxiolytic effects evolve over a period of 1 to 3 weeks. Patients may mistakenly believe that the drug is ineffective because they may not feel sedated or calmed initially. This factor should be discussed with all patients before beginning buspirone therapy. It may be helpful to have the patient on a short course of a benzodiazepine concurrently until the buspirone takes effect. The benzodiazepine can be tapered and discontinued. The effectiveness of buspirone can be assessed. As long as the health care provider and patient are aware of its relatively slow onset, buspirone can be used successfully for many anxiety disorders.

Adverse effects of buspirone consist of occasional dizziness, drowsiness, and nausea. It has a low potential for abuse and does not cause withdrawal effects when abruptly discontinued. Safe use in pregnancy and use in children younger than 18 years of age has not been established.

Buspirone is well absorbed from the gastrointestinal tract, and its absorption is enhanced in the presence of food. Peak plasma levels are reached approximately 40 to 90 minutes after oral doses. It is biotransformed in the liver and eliminated in the urine. There is 95 percent plasma protein binding and, as such, may interfere with other highly protein-bound drugs (e.g., cimetidine).

Buspirone has very few interactions with other drugs. However, unlike the benzodiazepines, buspirone interacts with haloperidol and monoamine oxidase inhibitors to increase the blood pressure. It has practically no additive sedation when used with other CNS-active drugs.

The usual daily dose of buspirone is 5 mg three times daily. The recommended starting dose is 5 mg with an increase of 5-mg increments every 2 to 3 days as needed until clinical effects are achieved. The maximum recommended daily dose should not exceed 60 mg. Smaller doses are warranted in older adults and patients with renal or hepatic impairment.

Chloral hydrate is one of the oldest hypnotics and is well tolerated by most older adults. Chloral hydrate is used as a short-term sedative and hypnotic. It is also approved for preoperative use as an adjunct to anesthesia preoperatively. Much like other antianxiety and sedative-hypnotic drugs, chloral hydrate has generalized CNS depressant activity.

The most common adverse effects of chloral hydrate are excessive sedation, nausea, vomiting, diarrhea, and flatulence. It should be given with food or in capsule form because of its unpleasant taste. The development of tolerance is possible as well as physical and psychological dependency. A hangover, disorientation, headache, irritability, dizziness, and incoordination are possible.

Chloral hydrate is rapidly absorbed when taken orally, with an onset time of approximately 30 minutes. The drug is converted to an active metabolite (trichlorethanol) in the liver, with the half-life of the metabolite of 8 to 10 hours. The metabolite exerts the pharmacologic effects. There are a number of drug-drug interactions with concurrent use of chloral hydrate.

As with all other drugs, the dosage of chloral hydrate depends on the diagnosis, the age of the patient, the route of administration, and the goal of therapy. It is available as capsules and suppositories in a variety of dosages.

Ethchlorvynol and glutethimide are nonbarbiturate CNS depressants that have been used in the past as hypnotics. These drugs cause both physical and psychological dependence, and have been associated with overdose and suicide attempts. Thus, their use as sedative-hypnotics is not recommended.

Diphenhydramine and doxylamine are antihistamines approved by the FDA for sale as sleep aids without a prescription. The mild nighttime sedation that is experienced with diphenhydramine has proved to be most effective with a variety of sleep deprivation disorders. However, these drugs can cause daytime sedation, impaired performance, and troublesome anticholinergic effects such as dry mouth. Overdosage with antihistamines can cause delirium, psychosis, and urinary retention, especially in older adults. Diphenhydramine is discussed further in Chapter 46.

Melatonin has not been FDA approved for treatment of insomnia and jet lag. However, it is widely available in health food stores and is being used in self-treatment of insomnia, jet lag, and a wide variety of disorders. In some patients, melatonin has been shown to decrease both the severity and duration of jet lag symptoms. It has been recommended that the drug be taken once daily beginning 3 days before the flight and continuing for 3 days after arrival at the destination.

Melatonin has also been used for its hypnotic effects. When taken 2 hours before bedtime, melatonin was noted to decrease the time needed to fall asleep by an average of 14 minutes. It was also noted to decrease the time awake after onset of sleep by 24 minutes and to improve sleep efficiency (total time asleep as a percentage of time in bed) from 75 to 83 percent. It does not appear to increase total sleep time. Furthermore, the purity of the products sold in health food stores and the adverse effects of taking melatonin are unknown.

According to product labels, melatonin is made from bovine pineal glands, but it can also be synthesized in the laboratory. Melatonin is normally synthesized in the pineal gland from tryptophan. In healthy individuals, endogenous melatonin levels are highest during the normal hours of sleep. Levels increase rapidly in the evening, peaking after midnight, and decline toward morning. Older adults, who often suffer from insomnia, have lower serum concentrations of melatonin. People who are blind often have irregular sleep cycles and may have free-running (not 24-hour) rhythms of melatonin production.

Meprobamate, a propanediol compound, has been used for relief of anxiety and muscle tension. However, because of the likelihood it will produce tolerance, physical dependency, severe withdrawal reactions, and life-threatening toxicity, it has fallen from favor. It is used much less frequently than benzodiazepines or buspirone. Meprobamate acts in the CNS by blocking neuron impulses between the cerebral cortex and the thalamus. Its primary actions are global CNS sedation and skeletal muscle relaxation. It is not recommended for use in patients with a previous history of dependency, or for patients who are abusing alcohol or other sedative drugs.

The most common adverse effects of meprobamate are drowsiness and ataxia. Blurred vision, hypotension, anorexia, nausea, vomiting, and diarrhea have been noted. Meprobamate should be used with caution in patients with hepatic dysfunction or severe renal impairment and in patients who may be suicidal or who have been addicted to drugs in the past. Dosage reduction is recommended for older adults. It is contraindicated in patients with hypersensitivity, in comatose patients or those with pre-existing CNS depression, and in patients with uncontrolled severe pain. Safe use in pregnancy and in children has not been established.

Meprobamate is well absorbed following oral administration and is widely distributed. Onset of drug effects occurs in less than 1 hour, with peak sedation noted in 1 to 3 hours. Its duration of action is 6 to 12 hours. The onset and peak action profile of the sustained-release formulation is unknown. Meprobamate is biotransformed in the liver.

Meprobamate has significant interactions with most CNS-active drugs. Patients should be cautioned against using alcohol, sedatives-hypnotics, or other CNS-active drugs while taking meprobamate because their effect or the effect of meprobamate may be intensified.

Initial doses of meprobamate should be as low as possible and increased only after clinical effects are measured. Usual starting doses are from 400 to 800 mg twice a day, with an upper limit of 2.4 g/day. Frail elderly or debilitated patients should begin at lowered doses, and doses should be increased more slowly if needed. Therapeutic plasma levels are between 6 and 12 mcg/mL, with toxic levels being over 60 mcg/mL. Meprobamate must be tapered carefully because abrupt discontinuation can precipitate potentially dangerous withdrawal reactions. Overdose is marked by severe hypotension, coma, and potential respiratory collapse. Care consists of hemodynamic support and possible mechanical ventilation in severe cases.

Paraldehyde is a nonbenzodiazepine, nonbarbiturate drug used in some patients for alcohol withdrawal syndrome. Paraldehyde produces a nonspecific, reversible CNS depression. It is unique in that it is not dependent on kidney function for elimination. Thus, it is appropriate for the patient with impaired renal function.

The most common adverse effects include irritation of mucous membranes, gastrointestinal upset, and a strong, unpleasant breath odor for up to 24 hours after administration. Metabolic acidosis (particularly with high dosages) is possible. With prolonged use, an addiction resembling alcoholism is noted. Withdrawal symptoms are characterized by delirium tremens and hallucinations.

The onset of orally administered paraldehyde occurs in 10 to 15 minutes, with peak activity noted in 30 to 60 minutes. The duration of action varies from 8 to 12 hours. Rectally administered paraldehyde has a slow onset, with peak activity reached in 2½ hours. The duration of action is that of an orally administered dose. It is biotransformed in the liver and has a half-life of 3.4 to 9.8 hours. Paraldehyde is excreted via the bile and lungs.

All doses of paraldehyde are expressed in volume (e.g., 1 g/mL of solution). It is given in 4 to 8 mL of drug in milk or iced fruit drink to mask the taste and odor. For hypnosis, the usual dosage range is 10 to 30 mL. For sedation, 5 to 10 ml of drug is used. Delirium tremens is treated with 10 to 35 mL.

A rectal formulation of paraldehyde is available. The drug is dissolved in oil as a retention enema. Ten to 20 mL of the drug is mixed with one to two parts of olive oil or isotonic sodium chloride. Ten to 30 mL of the 1-g/ml solution is diluted as described earlier. For sedation, 5 to 10 mL of the 1-g/mL solution is used.

Pediatric dosages are based on milliliters per square meter of body surface. For hypnosis, the usual dosage is 0.3 ml/kg, or 12 ml/m^2, either orally or by rectum. For sedation, the pediatric dosage is 0.15 mg/kg, or 6 ml/m^2. The sedating dose can be given by mouth, rectally, or IM.

The drug should be used with glass implements (e.g., syringes, medicine cups) because it interacts with plastic surfaces such as syringes, glasses, and spoons. Any unused paraldehyde should be discarded. It decomposes to acetaldehyde if it is exposed to light and air.

Critical Thinking Process

Assessment

History of Present Illness

How a person with an anxiety or impaired sleep pattern presents to the health care system is important. The assessment of a patient who presents voluntarily and complains of an inability to sleep or to cope with life is very different from that of a patient on a locked psychiatric unit showing signs of panic. Much can be learned by careful observation of the patient and the symptoms. Table 17–6 reviews the levels of anxiety and their associated characteristics.

Because high anxiety levels or panic states are associated with feelings of intense fear and doom, providing a safe environment with decreased stimuli is an essential step in the assessment process. The health care provider may find it helpful to group symptoms into one of four categories: physiological, behavioral, cognitive, or affective. For example, the patient could be restless or pacing, feeling jittery, sweating, or unable to concentrate. These are all symptoms that provide early clues to the severity of the disorder and guide the diagnosis and treatment plans.

Explore stressors that may have resulted in the anxiety or impaired sleep pattern. Additionally, the patient's previous coping strategies and their effectiveness, as well as the total effect that anxiety or impaired sleep is having on a patient's life, should be addressed. When appropriate, significant others should be included in the assessment process.

An assessment of the patient's usual sleep habits and quality of sleep should be included as part of the initial assessment. Notation should be made as to the usual hour of sleep and rising times, as well as bedtime rituals or preferences that enhance sleep quality. For example, patients with chronic airway limitation or hiatal hernias may be accustomed to sleeping with several pillows or with the head of the bed elevated. If sleep quality is found to be poor, assessment should be continued and more thorough questioning conducted regarding usual bedtime activities. Information

TABLE 17–6 LEVELS OF ANXIETY

Level of Anxiety	Characteristics of Level of Anxiety
Mild anxiety	Appears calm Perceptual field broadens; perceptual abilities intensified Learning and critical thinking abilities enhanced Able to connect feelings, thoughts, and actions Focuses on present problems; cause-and-effect relationships identified
Moderate anxiety	Appears tense and restless Perceptual field narrows; perceptual abilities restricted to immediate situation Able to attend to stimuli if they are pointed out Alertness reaches its highest, most efficient level Uses ego defense mechanisms
Severe anxiety	Appears tense with increased respirations, blood pressure, and pulse Perceptual field significantly reduced Learning and critical thinking abilities reduced Unable to connect feelings, thoughts, and actions Able to focus on small aspect of problem of environment Behaviors directed at immediate relief of anxiety
Panic level	Demonstrates symptoms of helplessness, hopelessness, rage Behaviors directed at gaining or maintaining control Perceptual field distorted; details scattered, spinning Physiologic response includes hypertension and hyperventilation is possible Learning and critical thinking abilities nonexistent

about how long it takes to get to sleep, the number and perceived cause of wakenings, the regularity and consistency of sleep patterns, and the frequency and duration of naps should be elicited. Information about alcohol or caffeine intake, use of sleeping pills, or other drugs should be noted. In some cases, the patient's bed partner may report snoring, apparent pauses in breathing (apnea), and kicking movements.

Past Health History

A health history is by far the most important tool in any assessment of the patient with anxiety or sleep cycle disorders. First, it is important to ask about medical conditions. Chronic pulmonary disease, cardiac disorders, hyperthyroidism, and hypoglycemia tend to produce a relatively high level of anxiety.

The health care provider should elicit information about the drugs the patient is taking at present, both prescribed and those sold over the counter. Obtaining information about these substances is important because abrupt withdrawal itself can precipitate anxiety, particularly if the patient is physiologically dependent on the drug.

An accurate health history is more complete if the family and significant others are involved. However, inclusion of the family may, at times, be contraindicated because anxiety levels can be elevated by overly concerned family members. In cases of anxiety in children or older adults, it may be more important to involve the family because these patients are sometimes less willing or able to reflect on their circumstances. In all instances, the exam must always revolve around helping the patient feel secure in his or her environment.

Physical Exam Findings

Anxiety and impaired sleep are frequently associated with medical problems. A thorough physical exam should be made with an eye toward the discovery of underlying causes of the anxiety. The presence and severity of somatic symptoms can give the health care provider important information regarding the anxiety level of the patient. Attention should be paid to the patient's pulse rate, blood pressure, and respiratory rate. The health care provider should also observe for diaphoresis, restlessness, or trembling because these manifestations are often hallmarks of anxiety. In addition, assess for visible signs of fatigue and lack of sleep, such as reddened eyes, lack of coordination, drowsiness, and irritability.

It is beneficial to explore with the patient which symptoms are most distressing. The health care provider will be able to monitor the effectiveness of antianxiety or hypnotic therapy more accurately by referring to these baseline physical exam findings.

Diagnostic Testing

Baseline laboratory values are obtained to alert the health care provider to electrolyte imbalances suggesting underlying diseases that may lead to anxiety or impaired sleep. If endocrine abnormalities are suspected, a thyroid screen or a glucose tolerance test is indicated. A toxicology screen is called for if drug ingestion or withdrawal from drugs is suspected. There are also a number of anxiety assessment tools that can be used to assess the extent of the anxiety.

The primary diagnostic test for sleep disorders is polysomnography. Patients may be referred to a sleep center for an overnight recording of electroencephalogram, electrooculogram, and submental electromyogram using surface electrodes. Depending on the cause of the sleep disorder, a variety of other studies may be performed.

Developmental Considerations

Perinatal Pregnancy brings enormous changes to a woman's body. She must deal with alterations in body image, hormone fluctuations, the role change of becoming a mother, and normal worries about the health of her child. The chance for anxiety as a normal response or as a pathologic adjustment is apparent. The health care provider's response to the pregnant patient should be tempered with fetal safety foremost. The first trimester has the greatest risk of fetal damage from drugs. Unless benefits greatly outweigh risks, it is best to avoid antianxiety drugs during this time. Additionally, drugs used during the third trimester or during breastfeeding can lead to withdrawal symptoms in neonates, floppy baby syndrome, or poor sucking response. Nondrug therapies should be considered first.

If antianxiety drugs are used before delivery, the neonate will need to be thoroughly assessed for possible withdrawal symptoms or other potential adverse effects such as retardation or physical anomalies.

Pediatric Developmental stereotypes often lead to underestimating the prevalence of anxiety disorders in children and adolescents. In fact, anxiety disorders are more prevalent than attention deficit disorders in this age group. Children can have so-called adult anxiety disorders as well as disorders particular to children such as separation anxiety, overanxious behavior, and stranger anxiety. Children rarely have a pure anxiety disorder but instead display multiple symptoms, making diagnosis more challenging. The likelihood of substance abuse or sexual abuse should be explored. A full psychiatric review of the family is important because children with overanxious parents often learn similar behaviors. Drug therapy can decrease most symptoms but does nothing to solve the underlying cause of anxiety. Further, children are more susceptible to withdrawal problems owing to the drug's faster clearance rate in this group.

Geriatric The adjustments needed to deal with the multiple losses of independence, health, and family, which are so often encountered in the geriatric population, are conducive to anxiety. Many emotional dilemmas of the older adult can mimic or have an overlay of anxiety. Dysfunctional grieving, Alzheimer's disease, and confusion can all bear a striking resemblance to anxiety. The geriatric patient can present with somatic or behavioral symptoms similar to those noted in a younger patient but may use withdrawal more frequently as a coping mechanism. A careful geropsychiatric evaluation will help define actual pathology and allow a definitive diagnosis of anxiety to be made.

Psychosocial Considerations

Because anxiety is a normal human response, a basic task is determining whether a patient is suffering from an abnormal anxiety response or reacting to the normal stress of life. The patient can help by identifying how severely his or her life-style is affected by the anxiety level. Some areas to pursue include recent work history, family disruptions, sleeping habits, and overall satisfaction with life. The pa-

Case Study Panic Disorder

Patient History

History of Present Illness	RD is a 45-year-old white male presenting to the primary clinic with a complaint of not being able to concentrate or sleep at night. Additionally, he says that he feels that he is suffocating or blacking out. He relates that these episodes have been ongoing for at least 5 years but that their frequency and intensity have increased. Occasionally, he is unwilling to leave his home for fear that something terrible will happen.
Past Health History	RD reports overall good health with no cardiovascular or pulmonary problems. He has smoked 1 ppd for 20 years. He has been abstinent from alcohol for the past 4 months, with heavy use in the past. RD uses marijuana about twice a week but reports using no other illicit drugs. While in the Navy, RD injured his left knee and has had several arthroscopic procedures.
Physical Exam Findings	VS: pulse 90, blood pressure 146/85, respirations 22, and temperature 37° C. Lungs were clear to auscultation. He was well groomed and articulate but rarely made eye contact with the interviewer. He positioned himself so that the door to the exam room was in his sight at all times.
Diagnostic Testing	An EKG showed no cardiac abnormalities. Blood glucose was 98 mg/dL. Thyroid levels were within normal limits.
Developmental Considerations	RD is worried about his ability to compete in the real estate market with his difficulty concentrating.
Psychosocial Considerations	RD has been married for 10 years and works as a real estate agent. He reports recent sales have been slow. His childhood was described as normal, without episodes of abuse or neglect. His parents divorced when he was 10 years old, and he remembers this as a "very sad time." RD was in the Navy for 6 years and reports no episodes of imminent death or extreme danger. In the past, RD has sought therapy but reports that it was of little value, "All they did was give me drugs that put me to sleep."
Economic Factors	RD's knee injury is considered service connected, and he is therefore eligible for treatment at a local Veterans Hospital.

Variables Influencing Decision

Treatment Objective	• Minimize frequency and intensity of panic attacks to allow RD to assume his normal daily regimen with minimal sedation.

Drug Variable	*Drug Summary*	*Patient Variable*
Indications	Benzodiazepines are most commonly used for anxiety. Alprazolam is specifically approved by Food and Drug Administration for panic attacks. This will not be a decision point.	RD diagnosed with panic attacks.
Pharmacodynamics	Alprazolam and diazepam act by causing CNS depression.	Patient has expressed a desire to not feel excessively sedated. He believes that mental alertness is vital to his job. This will become a decision point.
Adverse Effects/ Contraindications	Both alprazolam and diazepam produce additive sedation in the presence of alcohol or other CNS depressants	RD has history of alcohol and marijuana use. This will become a decision point.

Case Study Panic Disorder—cont'd

Drug Variable	*Drug Summary*	*Patient Variable*
Pharmacokinetics	Both alprazolam and diazepam are similarly absorbed. Alprazolam is quicker because it does not need to be converted to an active metabolite. This will become a decision point. Alprazolam has a quick onset with a relatively short half-life that leads to less sedation. Diazepam is also quick acting but has an active metabolite that can lead to excess sedation	RD desires a quick onset when a panic attack or precipitating event is anticipated. This will become a decision point.
Dosage Regimen	The use of antianxiety drugs for more than 4 months has not proved to be effective. The problems encountered with addiction increase with prolonged use.	RD will keep in close contact with the clinic during his therapy.
Lab Considerations	With proper monitoring of behavioral changes, serum levels are rarely needed.	RD will monitor anxiety episodes, and how he responds to them as the drug dosage is changed.
Cost Index*	Alprazolam: 2 Diazepam: 1	RD is eligible for care through a local veterans' hospital so direct expense to the patient cost is not a decision point at this time.

Summary of Decision Points

- Quick onset is desired for panic attacks. Alprazolam does not need to be converted to an active metabolite before acting.
- RD desires minimal sedation and is motivated to get therapy for his anxiety disorder.
- RD has a history of alcohol and marijuana use.

DRUG TO BE USED

- Alprazolam will be started at 0.5 mg po TID
- RD will be scheduled for weekly clinic visits initially to assess the effectiveness of alprazolam
- Dosages will be titrated to effect

*Cost Index:
1 = < $30/mo
2 = $30-40/mo
3 = $40–50/mo
4 = $50–60/mo
5 = > $60/mo

AWP of 30, 0.5-mg tablets of alprazolam is approximately $19
AWP of 30, 5-mg tablets of diazepam is approximately $3

tient's perception of life-style disruption or disruptions can help guide treatment. In cases in which anxiety symptoms are severe enough to significantly alter normal daily functioning, thought should be given to pharmacologic treatment if other therapies are ineffective. Patients with phobias or post-traumatic stress disorder may have episodic interruptions in their lives. Patients with agoraphobia or generalized anxiety disorder may report severely disrupted lives and minimal functioning. How patients view their current and past interactions with the health care system is important in understanding the level of trust they will need. This is crucial information because the basis of all therapeutic relationships is trust (see the Case Study—Panic Disorder).

Analysis and Management

Treatment Objectives

Treatment objectives for the patient with anxiety disorders include a decrease in or resolution of symptoms that significantly interfere with the patient's ability to perform life's tasks. Helping the patient develop effective coping skills to deal with some aspects of the anxiety and to prevent secondary disorders such as depression or substance abuse is also an important objective. Finally, treatment objectives include preventing relapse or recurrence of the anxiety. Situation anxiety should have been previously differentiated from generalized anxiety disorders.

Treatment objectives for the patient with impaired sleep are directed at promoting sleep in the short term (i.e., 1 to 4 days). Thus, daytime disruptions such as fatigue, impaired work performance, and transient mood disturbances may be lessened. Sleep can also be promoted for up to 3 weeks while a patient is learning alternative, behavioral techniques (e.g., eliminating daytime napping, instituting relaxation exercises) to promote sleep. Drug therapy for patients with long-term sleep impairment is directed at promoting sleep as a temporary measure when there is demonstrable daytime impairment from the impaired sleep patterns.

Treatment Options

There are no specific guidelines as to when to initiate drug therapy for anxiety or impaired sleep. Treatment is usually considered when nondrug treatment modalities have been unsuccessful, if the patient is suicidal, or if symptoms of anxiety are severe, persistent, and recurrent enough to disrupt the patient's daily life. Greater response rates occur with combined behavioral and drug therapy.

Antianxiety and sedative-hypnotic drugs should not be used in place of analgesics for the patient in pain. Pain alters the patient's response to hypnotic drugs, causing an increased incidence of disorientation and paradoxical excitement. Analgesics are discussed in Chapters 14 and 15.

Controversy

Appropriate Use of Antianxiety Drugs

JONATHAN J. WOLFE

Antianxiety drugs are among the most commonly prescribed medications in the United States. They have progressed from the earliest drugs such as meprobamate (which is still popular with some health care providers and patients) to agents with far greater clinical finesse. Discovery of the benzodiazepines produced new possibilities in treating personality disorders. The progression to shorter acting drugs with enhanced potency (e.g., alprazolam) has opened pathways to more appropriate dosing regimens for special populations, particularly older adults.

However, each class of drug comes with a definable set of adverse effects. In some cases, improved pharmacokinetic profiles (e.g., shorter half-life) allow use of benzodiazepines in patients who could not tolerate previous drugs. In many cases, vigorous marketing ploys promote wider use of drugs, simply because earlier safety concerns have been met by triumphs of drug discovery.

There is a tendency in some health care settings to overuse antianxiety drugs, although it may be done with the best intentions. In every case, the autonomy and dignity of the patient require that we ask whether tranquilizers are the proper therapy.

Critical Thinking Discussion

- What concerns would you have if a 63-year-old woman who is the principal caregiver for her 82-year-old mother asked about getting a prescription for some diazepam (Valium)? The daughter states, "Mother is just driving me around the bend talking all the time about things that happened 60 years ago!"
- What role would a benzodiazepine properly play in long-term treatment of an elderly man with a 50-year history of alcohol abuse?
- At what point in the treatment of a sleep disturbance would an antianxiety drug play a proper role?
- Depression and anxiety are often unappreciated facets of the existential suffering of dying patients. What benefit might a patient in hospice care, whose physical pain is well controlled with other therapies, derive from judicious use of an antianxiety agent?

Drug Variables

There is no one best benzodiazepine or barbiturate. The ideal drug would have a rapid onset, relieve specific symptoms with minimal daytime sedation, be quickly eliminated, and have minimal withdrawal effects when discontinued. Knowledge of these factors is helpful in determining the best drug to use.

Drug selection, dose, and length of treatment should be individualized. All drugs have benefits and risks associated with onset, duration, and adverse effects. The nature and severity of symptoms experienced by the patient will guide the health care provider in the selection of the most appropriate drug.

Benzodiazepines have been considered first-line drugs for treatment *of* anxiety disorders for over 30 years. The popularity of benzodiazepines is the result of a combination of pharmacologic actions and their safety profile. Patients with anxiety may benefit from use of a benzodiazepine with a long duration of action (e.g., diazepam), but these drugs cause daytime sedation and motor impairment. Drugs with an intermediate duration of action (e.g., lorazepam or oxazepam) are preferred because rebound and hangover effects may be avoided. They also allow for easier dose titration by both the patient and the health care provider.

Evidence suggests that there is marked improvement in about 35 percent, moderate improvement with residual symptoms in about 40 percent, and no improvement in about 25 percent of the patients in whom benzodiazepines are used. However, the drugs are intended for episodic, short-term, adjunctive therapy to relieve specific symptoms. Their use on a long-term basis can lead to significant withdrawal problems (even at therapeutic doses) when they are discontinued. Clinical experience has shown that concurrent psychotherapy may reduce the time needed for drug therapy, and improved response rates may occur with combined behavioral and drug therapy.

Buspirone may be considered first-line therapy if the patient is newly diagnosed, when chronic anxiety is present with symptoms of general anxiety disorder, and there is an absence of acute precipitants. It appears to dampen anxiety rather than extinguish it. Buspirone may be an appropriate choice if sedation or psychomotor or cognitive impairment would be dangerous. Buspirone may also be appropriate for patients with a history of substance abuse, personality disorders, and obsessive-compulsive disorders.

The disadvantage of buspirone is that therapeutic effects are delayed for up to 4 weeks. Benzodiazepines, on the other hand, produce effects almost immediately. Clinical experience suggests that patients who have previously responded to benzodiazepines may not respond as well to buspirone. Patients report less dramatic effects on somatic symptoms with buspirone than the effects seen with benzodiazepines.

Patients exhibiting signs of panic disorder or high levels of anxiety will benefit from a drug with a quick onset. It is after symptoms begin to subside that nondrug interventions such as behavioral or cognitive therapy can begin. Often these patients are started on a higher dose, with the dosage being decreased as anxiolytic effects become evident. Alprazolam, chlordiazepoxide, and diazepam have shown efficacy in these instances. Alprazolam is the only benzodiazepine that is specifically approved for panic disorders. It has a relatively rapid onset and very weak metabolites, and is well tolerated in terms of sedation. Its shorter half-life may be preferred in certain cases in which the build-up of a drug could be a problem. With proper dosing and close monitoring, adverse effects are relatively predictable and controlled with dosage adjustments. When alprazolam is discontinued, it is rapidly cleared from the system. Abruptly stopping alprazolam results in rebound CNS excitation, including seizures. If cost is a major issue, high-dose diazepam or lorazepam can be used in place of alprazolam for panic disorders. Diazepam and chlordiazepoxide are similarly rapid in their onset but have active metabolites that can cause increased sedation if they accumulate. Most adverse effects appear early in therapy and decrease after a patient has adjusted to the drug.

All benzodiazepines have sedative characteristics and can be used as hypnotics as well as antianxiety drugs. They differ, however, in their pharmacokinetics, profile of adverse effects, and capacity to cause rebound insomnia. Benzodiazepines with a short duration of action (e.g., triazolam) can cause daytime anxiety and rebound insomnia. *Anterograde amnesia,* an inability to remember events that occur for a period after drug administration, appears to occur with triazolam more often than with other benzodiazepines.

Rebound insomnia is most apparent when high-potency, short-acting benzodiazepines are abruptly stopped. Longer acting benzodiazepines or zolpidem is less likely to cause rebound effects. Alprazolam is a short-acting to intermediate-acting drug, but it is not recommended for use as a hypnotic because it can be especially difficult to discontinue.

Lorazepam, oxazepam, and temazepam are equally effective in the treatment of transient situational and short-term insomnia, although there are few data on the use of lorazepam and oxazepam as hypnotics. As with other high-potency, short-acting benzodiazepines, lorazepam is associated with worse rebound effects than the less potent, longer-acting drugs. This factor may not be relevant if the drugs are used for just a few nights. Triazolam is useful for the short-term management of stress-related insomnia, when it is important to avoid daytime sleepiness. At doses of 0.25 mg or less, there is likely to be no difference between this drug and other benzodiazepines.

Unlike benzodiazepines, which tend to suppress sleep stages III and IV (deep sleep) and REM sleep, zolpidem has little effect on the relative amount of sleep in each stage. Zolpidem appears to be more efficacious as a hypnotic, with little development of tolerance, compared with benzodiazepines. Further, zolpidem's effects are not augmented by small amounts of alcohol. A hangover effect, dizziness, and a drugged feeling have been reported with zolpidem, although in doses of 5 to 20 mg, the drug did not impair memory or other mental functions the day after use. The disadvantage of zolpidem is that it is more expensive than the benzodiazepines. Short-term use of zolpidpem is not associated with significant tolerance or physical dependence, and withdrawal symptoms are minimal or absent. Thus, the abuse potential is relatively low. The safety of zolpidem in overdosage is not as clear as that of oral benzodiazepines, but no fatalities have been reported with this drug alone.

Although they have been used for years for insomnia, barbiturates are generally contraindicated in the management of insomnia. Safety factors such as tolerance, lethality in overdosage, risk of abuse, and drug-drug interactions preclude their use in most situations.

Patient Variables

Vital to successful antianxiety therapy is understanding the insight a patient has into his or her anxiety. Patients with anxiety levels bordering on panic can be expected to have minimal perception of the reasons for their distress. Lower anxiety levels can translate into heightened awareness of their condition on the part of patients. Dosages of antianxiety drugs can be proportionately adjusted to modulate higher or lower anxiety levels.

A chronic, fluctuating clinical course of anxiety raises difficult concerns regarding long-term drug management. There have been several studies describing general anxiety disorder as a chronic illness. Yet, few long-term efficacy studies have been conducted, and the efficacy of drug therapy after 6 months is unknown. The lowest effective dosage should be employed for the shortest period of time, with periodic attempts at discontinuation.

Initially, patients may be reluctant to start an antianxiety medicine. They may fear feeling sedated or worry about becoming dependent. With prolonged benzodiazepine therapy, tolerance occurs to the sedating effects but not to the anxiolytic effects. Initial and maintenance doses of benzodiazepines must be individualized. The severity of symptoms, age and health of the patient, and the anticipated length of therapy must all be taken into account before starting therapy.

Drowsiness associated with the start of antianxiety therapy often prevents patients from driving or operating machinery. These are legitimate concerns that should be addressed by the health care provider before therapy. The health care provider can then reassure the patient that adverse effects are dose related and will subside as the optimal dose is achieved. To minimize problems of withdrawal, the drug should be tapered at the end of therapy. Once therapy has begun and anxiety is reduced, most patients are compliant with doses, schedules, and limitations.

In the acute care environment, dosages and the effects produced by antianxiety drugs can be followed more closely. Initial doses can be increased quickly if the patient is in a closely monitored setting. Conversely, a patient at home or in the ambulatory care setting should have the dosage increased more slowly. Additionally, these patients require frequent follow-up visits to assess accurately how well the prescribed antianxiety drug is working.

Patients at risk for delayed drug biotransformation or elimination should be started on low dosages initially. Particular attention should be paid to persons with renal disease or hepatic impairment because active metabolites are more likely to accumulate.

Decisions to use antianxiety or sedative-hypnotic drugs in an older adult must be made only after careful evaluation of significant factors. First, diseases or drug-induced confusion must be ruled out. Second, short-acting drugs with short half-lives should be used to help prevent accumulation. The patient must be carefully monitored for signs of confusion, sedation, or ataxia during the early phase of therapy. Doses should be as low as possible initially, and increases should be made slowly. Older adults are at risk for injury because they often react more strongly to the sedative effects of antianxiety drugs. Thus, they are are at greater risk for falls and subsequent hip fractures. Careful attention to elimination pathways helps in selecting drugs that are safe for older adults or for those with hepatic or renal impairment.

The use of benzodiazepines in children is controversial at best. Most authorities agree that drug therapy should not be a first-line treatment for anxiety or sleep disorders. Behavioral, cognitive, or family therapies or psychotherapy should be initiated first. Some drugs are contraindicated in children under specific ages and require cautious use in all instances.

Intervention

Administration

Any critical decisions or judgments that are required of the patient should be made before sedative-hypnotic drugs are administered. The validity of legal documents will be in question if they are signed while the patient is under the influence of any CNS depressant drug.

Patients may take a benzodiazepine with food if gastric upset occurs when the drug is taken on an empty stomach. Sustained-release formulations should be administered intact, without crushing or chewing. If a dose is missed, it should not be doubled at the next administration time. Instead, that dose should be skipped unless its omission is realized within an hour of its usual time.

IM formulations should be avoided because they are highly alkaline and irritating to the tissues. Absorption is also erratic by this route. IV formulations should be administered slowly because apnea, hypotension, bradycardia, and cardiac arrest have been reported with rapid administration. Arteriospasm, with resultant gangrene, results from accidental intra-arterial administration. The patient who has received an IV dose of benzodiazepine should be observed closely for at least 3 hours, preferably on bedrest.

When using barbiturates, the dosage should not be increased and the drug should not be discontinued without first consulting with the health care provider. Some cases of chronic overdose arise because the patient receives prescriptions from more than one health care provider, each of whom is unaware of the others' prescription. Further, suicide is always a potential with psychoactive drugs. Usually, suicide attempts with benzodiazepines alone are rarely fatal if the victim is discovered early and supportive intervention is started promptly. Mechanical ventilation is rarely needed.

Barbiturates are highly alkaline and can cause pain and necrosis when injected IM. For this reason, IM routes are generally avoided. IV administration is reserved for general anesthesia (see Chapter 16) and emergency treatment of seizures.

Overdosage Flumazenil (ROMAZICON) is effective in reversing the effects of benzodiazepines. It is a benzodiazepine derivative that acts as a competitive antagonist at the GABA-benzodiazepine receptor. Flumazenil does not antagonize other drugs that are active at GABA sites, such as alcohol, barbiturates, opioids, or general anesthetics.

The most common adverse effects include dizziness, nausea, and vomiting. Agitation, emotional lability, headache, fatigue, confusion, somnolence, and sleep disorders have occurred. Other adverse effects include abnormal blurred vision and altered hearing. Arrhythmias, chest pain, and hypertension have also been noted. Seizures are the most life-threatening adverse effect. Flumazenil is contraindicated in patients with hypersensitivity to flumazenil or benzodiazepines, in patients receiving benzodiazepines for life-threatening medical conditions, and in patients with serious cyclic antidepressant overdosage. The use of flumazenil in patients with a long history of benzodiazepine use is also contraindicated.

Cautious use is warranted in patients with a mixed CNS-depressant overdose because the effects of the other drugs may emerge when the benzodiazepine effect is removed. Patients with a history of seizures are more likely to experience seizures when they undergo benzodiazepine withdrawal. Flumazenil may increase intracranial pressure and risk of seizures in patients with head injury. Safe use during pregnancy and lactation has not been established.

Flumazenil is 100 percent bioavailable, with drug action beginning 1 to 2 minutes after IV administration. Peak serum levels are reached in 6 to 10 minutes. The duration of action depends on the dose or concentration of benzodiazepine and the dose of the flumazenil. Flumazenil is 50 percent protein bound, but this value is decreased in patients with significant liver disease. Its half-life is 41 to 79 minutes. Elimination occurs primarily via the liver.

There are no significant drug-drug interactions with flumazenil. Administration of food during a flumazenil infusion increases drug clearance and may decrease the effect of flumazenil.

For suspected benzodiazepine overdose in adults, 0.2 mg of flumazenil is given IV over 30 seconds. If no response is noted, 0.5 mg is given over 30 seconds until a total of 3 mg is administered. For overdose in children, the package insert should be consulted. If the sedation reverses and the patient is more alert, he or she should be observed for a sufficient period of time to guard against the possibility of re-sedation. Re-sedation may occur as a result of incomplete gastric emptying of previously administered benzodiazepines. Care must be taken any time a competitive antagonist is used because its half-life and effectiveness may be shorter than those of the drug being reversed.

If a patient is physiologically dependent on benzodiazepines, reversal may precipitate an acute withdrawal reaction including seizures. In these patients, the benefits of flumazenil use must be carefully weighed against the potential risks.

Education

Successful antianxiety and sedative-hypnotic therapy depends on a close alliance between patient and health care provider. Patients must be taught that antianxiety and sedative-hypnotic drugs are useful for short-term tension relief and to promote sleep. They are not a solution to stress. Drug therapy is most effective as an adjunct, combined with other intervention modalities.

The patient should be instructed not to increase the dosage nor to abruptly stop a benzodiazepine. When tapering begins, most drugs can be safely decreased by 10 percent per day. The patient will need to be monitored for the early onset of withdrawal symptoms. If withdrawal symptoms appear, or anxiety increases the tapering should be halted until the patient stabilizes. The patient should be advised that activities requiring mental alertness (e.g., driving or using power tools) should be avoided in the early stages of therapy. The patient should be instructed to avoid alcohol, sleep-inducing over-the-counter drugs, and other CNS depressants while taking antianxiety or sedative-hypnotic drugs. Dangerous combinations of drugs are more likely to be identified if the patient purchases all drugs from the same pharmacy. Most pharmacists maintain drug profiles on their clients, monitoring records for inappropriate or potentially dangerous drug interactions.

Patients for whom sedative-hypnotics are prescribed should be cautioned about the risks inherent in their use. They should be told not to increase their dosage, nor to abruptly stop the drug without first contacting the health care provider. Additionally, supplies of the drug should be kept in a place other than the bedside table. The place chosen should be far enough away from the bedroom so that the patient is fully alert before repeating a dose. Patients who take sedative-hypnotics can develop amnesia about their use. It is thought that many cases of drug overdose arise from repeated doses taken by the patient during waking periods. In some cases, it may be necessary to place the drug supply under the supervision of a second person.

Withdrawal effects of antianxiety and sedative-hypnotic drugs are usually minimized when patients are informed about what to expect when these drugs are stopped. Of significance is that patients who have been included in the decision-making process concerning the end of drug therapy have a lower incidence of problems.

Because antianxiety and sedative-hypnotic drugs are used for adjunctive therapy, it is important that patients stay in close contact with their health care provider. Dosages and administration times may need to be adjusted in the early stages of treatment. Also, patients should be advised to inform their health care provider of any increase in sedation, lethargy, or difficulty staying awake after initial therapy has been established. In many cases, education in sleep hygiene (e.g., reducing caffeine intake, changing sleep habits, or pain relief) might be more appropriate than a sedative-hypnotic drug. Early morning wakening is one of the biologic features of depression; thus, an antidepressant may be appropriate (see Chapter 18).

Evaluation

Evaluating the efficacy of antianxiety and sedative-hypnotic drugs can be problematic because the essential characteristics of anxiety and insomnia cannot be adequately reproduced. Cognition, communication, and social relationships are difficult to assess objectively. However, clinical improvement should be evaluated and patients should report a decrease of physical symptoms. They will note better concentration and less tendency toward distraction. The sense of dread and negative anticipation is lessened, and they can begin to gain an insight into the reasons they are anxious. Furthermore, there should be no symptoms of dependency.

When impaired sleep has been the problem, the patient should report a decrease in symptoms of impaired sleep. Daytime disruptions such as fatigue, impaired work performance, and transient mood disturbances may be lessened. The patient should report that he or she is learning alternative behavioral techniques (e.g., eliminating daytime napping or practicing relaxation exercises) to promote sleep.

SUMMARY

- Anxiety and impaired sleep patterns have no social, economic, racial, or gender boundaries. Up to 11 percent of Americans suffer from some form of identifiable anxiety, and one third of the population have impaired sleep during any given year.
- Anxiety is a normal part of life, but it contributes to impaired sleep patterns. Antianxiety drugs are not intended to relieve everyday stresses or the occasional case of impaired sleep patterns.
- Anxiety can arise from three distinct sources: a response to a medical condition, faulty neuroregulation in the brain, and an identifiable psychiatric condition.
- Before initiating antianxiety therapy, the health care provider should rule out a medical condition or use of an anxiety-producing drug by the patient.
- Assessment of the level of anxiety a patient is experiencing is vital in allowing the care provider to intervene at the appropriate level.
- Use of the DSM-IV categories can assist the health care provider in identifying a patient's anxiety disorder, thus allowing greater specificity of treatment.
- Antianxiety drugs are intended to reduce the intrusive, unwanted effects of anxiety. When symptoms are modified, a patient can gain insight into the cause of the anxiety.
- First-line drugs used to treat anxiety and impaired sleep patterns are benzodiazepines. All of them have different half-lives, onset of action, and elimination pathways. Nonbenzodiazepine and nonbarbiturate drugs are also used to treat anxiety and impaired sleep pattern disorders.
- Barbiturates have fallen from favor as first-line drugs in the management of impaired sleep patterns.
- All dosages of antianxiety and hypnotic drugs need to be closely monitored during the early part of therapy. Changes are often necessary as effects are observed.
- Whenever an antianxiety or sedative-hypnotic drug is started, the next step is to plan a tapering program.
- Successful initial therapy is evidenced by a decrease in the physical manifestations of anxiety or impaired sleep patterns as noted by the health care provider and the patient.
- Patients will be able to maintain their activities of daily living as well as gain insight into the source of their anxiety and impaired sleep patterns.

BIBLIOGRAPHY

Abramowicz, M. (Ed.) (1992). Flumazenil. *Medical Letter,* 34(874), 66.

American Psychiatric Association. (1995). *Diagnostic and statistical manual of mental disorders: DSM-IV* (4th ed.). Washington, D.C.: Author.

Ashton, H. (1994). Guidelines for the rational use of benzodiazepines. *Drugs,* 48(1), 25–40.

Badger, J. (1994). Calming the anxious patient. *American Journal of Nursing,* 94(5), 46–50.

Blair, D., and Ramones, V. (1994). Psychopharmacologic treatment of anxiety. *Journal of Psychosocial Nursing and Mental Health Services,* 32(7), 49–53.

Burgess, A. (1990). *Psychiatric nursing in the community and the hospital* (5th ed.) Norwalk, CT: Appleton and Lange.

Carter, G., and Holloway, R. (1994). Treating anxiety: A collaborative approach. *Patient Care,* 28(18), 36–38, 42, 44.

Cooper, J. (1993). The use of anxiolytics and hypnotic drugs. *Nursing Homes,* 42(6), 37–39.

Coplan, J., and Tiffon, L. (1993). Therapeutic strategies for the patient with treatment-resistant anxiety. *Journal of Clinical Psychiatry,* 54(5, Suppl.), 69–74.

Derogatis, L., and Wise, T. (1989). *Anxiety and depressive disorders in the medical patient.* Washington, D.C.: American Psychiatric Press.

Dubovsky, S. (1993). Approaches to developing new anxiolytics and antidepressants. *Journal of Clinical Psychiatry,* 54(5, Suppl.), 75–82.

Farrington, E. (1993). Pediatric drug information: Flumazenil (Mazicon). *Pediatric Nursing,* 19(2), 163.

Glitz, D. (1991). 5-HT 1A partial agonists: What is their future? *Drugs,* 41, 11–18.

Glod, C. (1991). Psychopharmacology and clinical practice. *Nursing Clinics of North America,* 26(2), 375–99.

Glod, C. (1992). Xanax: Pros and cons. *Journal of Psychosocial Nursing and Mental Health Services,* 1992(6), 36–7.

Gomez, G., and Gomez, E. (1994). The use of psychotropic drugs to treat anxiety in the elderly. *Journal of Psychosocial Nursing and Mental Health Services,* 32(12), 30–34.

Hale, M. (1991). Use of antidepressants and anxiolytics in patients with heart disease. *Physician Assistant,* 15(4), 43–50.

Hauri, P., and Exther, M. (1990). Insomnia. *Mayo Clinic Proceedings,* 65, 869–882.

Hawley, C., and Tattersall, M. (1994). Comparison of long term benzodiazepine users in three settings. *British Journal of Psychiatry,* 165(6), 792–6.

Huckabee, M., and Driscoll, C. (1990). Anxiety in health and illness. *Physician Assistant,* 14(1), 19–20, 25–27, 30–32.

Kennedy, G., and Lowinger, R. (1993). Psychogeriatric emergencies. *Clinical Geriatric Medicine,* 9(3), 641–653.

Koda-Kimble, M., and Young, L. (1995). *Applied therapeutics* (5th ed.). Vancouver: Applied Therapeutics, Inc.

Markovitz, P. (1993). Treatment of anxiety in the elderly. *Journal of Clinical Psychiatry,* 54(5, Suppl.), 64–68.

News Capsules. (1993). P & T update: New approvals and dosage forms. *Hospital Formulary,* 28(3), 207.

Olin, B. (1995). *Facts and comparisons.* Philadelphia: J.B. Lippincott.

Popper, C. (1993). Psychopharmacology of anxiety disorders in children and adolescents. *Journal of Clinical Psychiatry,* 54(5, Suppl.), 52–62.

Rickels, K. (1993). Antidepressants for the treatment of generalized anxiety disorder. *Archives of General Psychiatry,* 50, 884–95.

Salzman, C. (1993). Benzodiazepine treatment of panic and agoraphobic symptoms: Use, dependence, toxicity, abuse. *Journal of Psychiatric Residency,* 27(Suppl 1), 97–110.

Sheikh, J. (1992). Anxiety disorders and their treatment. *Clinical Geriatric Medicine,* 8(2), 411–426.

Sherman, D. (1991). Evaluation and treatment of sleep disorders. *Contemporary Long-Term Care,* 14(12), 70.

Silcox, M. (1992). Flumazenil useful in reversing effects of benzodiazepines. *Journal of Emergency Nursing,* 18(4), 301.

Stoudemire, M., and Moran, M. (1993). Psychopharmacologic treatment of anxiety in the medically ill patient: Special considerations. *Journal of Clinical Psychiatry,* 54(5, Suppl.), 27–33.

Stuart, G., and Sundeen, J. (1990). *Principles and practice of psychiatric nursing* (4th ed.). St. Louis: Mosby.

Sussman, N. (1993). How to manage anxious patients who are depressed. *Journal of Clinical Psychiatry,* 54(5, Suppl.), 8–16.

Sussman, N. (1993). Treating anxiety while minimizing abuse and dependence. *Journal of Clinical Psychiatry,* 54(5, Suppl.), 44–51.

United States Pharmacopeial Convention. (1995). *Drug information for the health care professional* (15th ed.). Rockville, MD: Author.

Wise, M., and Rieck, S. (1993). Diagnostic considerations and treatment approaches to underlying anxiety in the medically ill. *Journal of Clinical Psychiatry,* 54(5, Suppl.), 22–26.

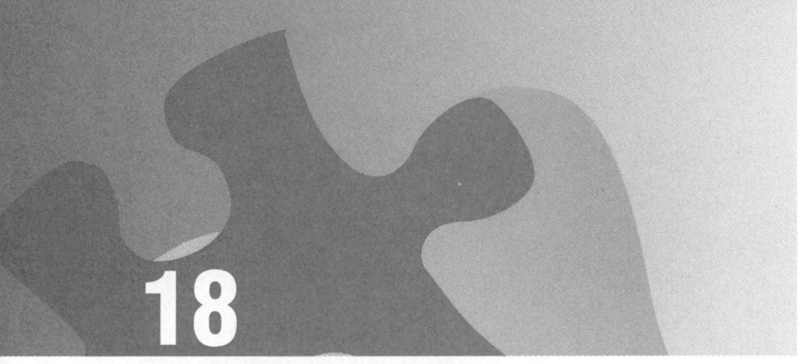

18

Antidepressant and Antimania Drugs

Mood disorders are under-recognized and undertreated severe public health and psychiatric problems. Mood disorders are so prevalent in fact that nearly 15 percent of the population of the United States will have a serious mood episode sometime during their lifetime. Depression is at least five times more common than bipolar disorder (manic-depression). Women are twice as likely as men to suffer from major depression. Mood disorders tend to be chronic in many individuals, requiring prolonged, and in some cases, life-long treatment with drugs. The social stigma surrounding mood disorders is substantial and often prevents the optimal use of current knowledge and treatments. The cost of the illness in pain, suffering, disability, and death is high.

DEPRESSION

Epidemiology and Etiology

Depression is defined as an affective disorder characterized by disturbances in emotional, cognitive, behavioral, and somatic regulation. Major depressive disorder (depression) is characterized by one or more episodes of mild, moderate, or severe clinical depression without episodes of mania or hypomania of at least 2 weeks' duration. As a primary mood disorder, depression includes both unipolar (depressive) and bipolar (manic-depressive) conditions. With *unipolar* depression, people of routinely normal moods suffer recurrent episodes of depression. With *bipolar* depression, the episodes of depression alternate with periods of mania.

At any point, 15 million Americans suffer from major depression. The prevalence of major depressive disorder in the Western industrialized nations is 2.3 to 3.2 percent for men and 4.5 to 9.3 percent for women. The lifetime risk for a major depressive disorder is 7 to 12 percent for men and 20 to 25 percent for women. The lifetime psychiatric co-morbidity rate for major depressive disorder can be as high as 43 percent. That is, up to 43 percent of patients with major depressive disorders have histories of one or more nonmood psychiatric disorders. The prevalence rates of depression based on notations in patient records by primary care providers vary from 1.5 to 4.5 percent.

Patients with major depressive disorder have substantial amounts of physical and psychological disability, as well as occupational difficulties, including loss of work time. Patients also have more physical illnesses than do other patients seen in primary care settings, and their use of health care resources is greater compared with that of other patients. Major depression is associated with an increased mortality rate, which is generally secondary to suicide and accidents. A large proportion of those who commit suicide (70 percent) have visited their primary care provider with mood or somatic complaints within the month or 6 weeks before their suicide. The mortality rate associated with depression is estimated to be 30,000 to 35,000 suicides per year. Of patients with untreated recurrent major depression, 15 percent die of suicide.

Risk Factors

Risk factors for major depressive disorder include a number of things. It is twice as likely to occur in women, with a peak onset between the ages of 20 to 40 years. It tends to run in families. If there is a family history of major depression, a person has a one and one-half to three times greater risk of having this disorder than does the general population. There is a greater incidence among separated and divorced persons. The cause and effect are unknown, but it is thought that the depression leads to separation and divorce. Depression is also more likely to be reported in unmarried men than in married men. Again, the cause is unknown; however, it is theorized that men who are depressed are less able to fulfill the role of suitor. It is more likely to be reported in married women than in unmarried women. Perhaps women with chronic low self-esteem settle for abusive and dysfunctional mates.

There is also an increased risk in women during the last trimester of pregnancy, the first 3 months after childbirth, and during the onset of menopause. All three findings suggest that fluctuations in sex hormones are important triggers for the expression of the illness. The presence of co-morbid disorders such as diabetes; pituitary, adrenal or thyroid disorders; occult malignant diseases; and neurologic, autoimmune, and nutritional deficiencies contributes to the incidence. Antihypertensive therapies are noted to increase the risk of depression. This is particularly so if the patient is treated with drugs that antagonize central biogenic amine mechanisms (i.e., norepinephrine, serotonin, and dopamine). The risk of depression also increases if the patient has had prior suicide attempts, is currently engaged in drug or alcohol abuse, or if there have been multiple stressful life events occurring within a short period of time.

Types of Depression

The *Diagnostic and Statistical Manual of Mental Disorders IV* (DSM-IV) describes several types of depression. Major depression is a single episode or recurrent incidence of mood disorder. *Primary dysthymia* (formerly called endogenous depression) has no identifiable cause. *Secondary dysthymia* (formerly called exogenous or reactive depression) may be precipitated by a number of factors such as environmental stress, adverse life events, drugs, or concurrent disease states. Regardless of the type of depression, they all share common symptoms of varying degrees and durations (see Common Symptoms of Depression).

Depression also can be categorized as an adjustment disorder with depressed mood, substance-related mood disor-

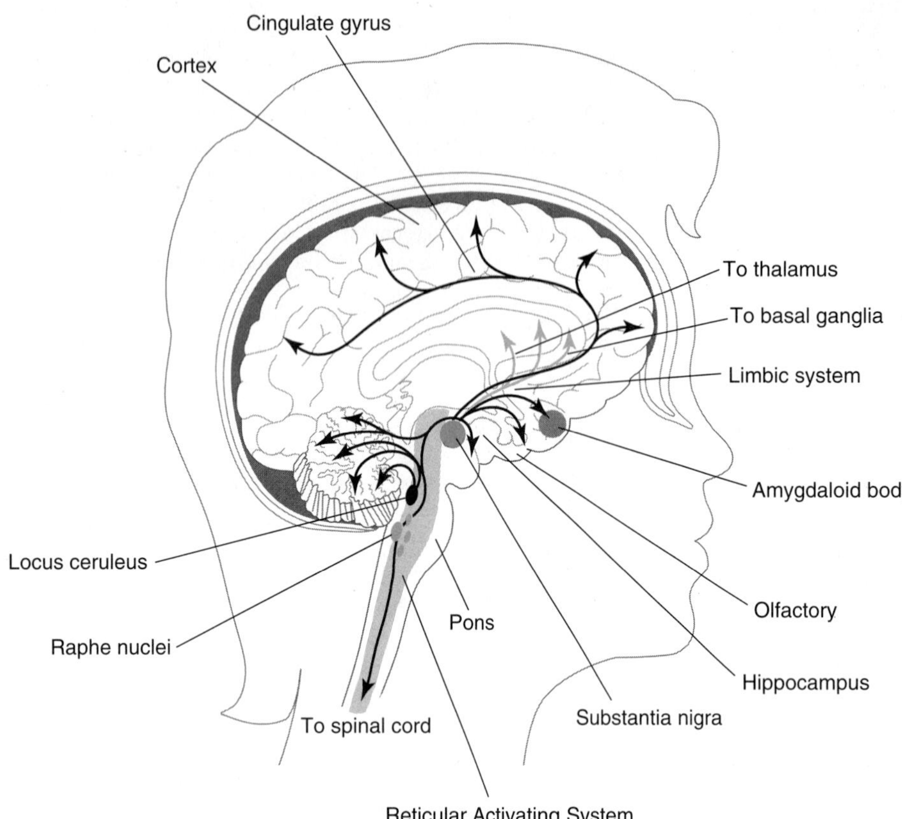

Figure 18–1 Three neurotransmitter pathways have been mapped in the brain—norepinephrine, serotonin, and dopamine. Most norepinephrine containing neurons are located in the locus ceruleus in the pons and midbrain. Serotonin is found in the nuclei of the raphe. Norepinephrine and serotonin pathways are illustrated by the black arrows. Dopamine pathways are found in the substantia nigra region and follow the blue arrows.

COMMON SYMPTOMS OF DEPRESSION

- Depressed, sad, irritable, or empty mood
- Diminished interest or pleasure in usual activities (*anhedonia*), appearance, work, or sexual activities
- Significant weight gain, or loss when not dieting, or a decrease or increase in appetite
- Sleep disorders (insomnia or hypersomnia)
- Psychomotor agitation or retardation
- Fatigue or loss of energy
- Feelings of worthlessness, or excessive or inappropriate guilt
- Diminished ability to think or concentrate, or indecisiveness
- Recurrent thoughts of death, suicidal ideation, or suicide attempt

der, dementia with depressed mood, depressive disorder due to a general medical condition, and depressive disorder not otherwise specified. This last category might include depression associated with premenstrual syndrome or any other disorder that does not meet the full criteria for the previously mentioned depression.

Pathophysiology

Mood disorders such as depression are thought to arise as a result of changes in the levels of the neurotransmitters serotonin and norepinephrine, and to a lesser extent, dopamine. Serotonergic neurons originating in the median raphe and terminating in the cortex and limbic system appear to be most involved in the regulation of mental and emotional states (Fig. 18–1). At least 14 subtypes of serotonin receptors are known to exist. Serotonin influences functions such as anxiety, sexual behavior, appetite, aggression, pain, obsessions, emesis, learning, aversion, psychosis, vasoconstriction, migraine, sleep, suicidal ideation, and circadian rhythms.

Although it is not clearly understood, the pathophysiology of depression may be viewed from five different perspectives. The *psychodynamic perspective* states that the depression involves difficulties with the formation and maintenance of self-esteem. The *cognitive perspective* views depression as the consequence rather than the origin of negative or distorted thinking. The *genetic theory* suggests there is a dominant gene with incomplete penetrance (a hereditary condition in persons who have the dominant or double recessive gene). The *neuroendocrine perspective* states that there is a link between neurotransmitter release and neurohormone activity involving hypothalamic functioning. The last perspective suggests that altered neurotransmitter metabolism is an important biochemical component of depression.

Although each type of depression varies, it generally responds to treatment with antidepressant drugs. Other organic causes are ruled out or treated before a diagnosis of depression is made.

PHARMACOTHERAPEUTIC OPTIONS

Drugs used for the treatment of depression have been available for approximately 50 years. They are derived from several chemical groups. First-generation antidepressants include tricyclic antidepressants (TCAs) and monoamine oxidase inhibitors (MAOIs). Second-generation antidepressants include selective serotonin reuptake inhibitors (SSRIs) and several miscellaneous drugs. The newer drugs, although they are chemically different from TCAs, are similar in their pharmacologic actions and antidepressant effectiveness.

Barring contraindications to drug therapy, antidepressant drugs are the first line of treatment for major depressive disorders when

- Depression is moderate to severe
- Psychotic, melancholic, or atypical features are present
- Psychotherapy by a trained, competent, psychotherapist is not available
- Maintenance treatment is planned and the patient has shown a positive prior response to treatment

Tricyclic Antidepressants

- ❒ Amitriptyline (ELAVIL, ENDEP); (✱) LEVATE, MERAVIL, NOVO-TRIPTYN
- ❒ Clomipramine (ANAFRANIL)
- ❒ Desipramine (NORPRAMIN, PERTOFRANE)
- ❒ Doxepin (ADAPIN, SINEQUAN); (✱) NOVO-DOXEPIN, TRIADAPIN
- ❒ Imipramine (TOFRANIL, TIPRAMINE, JANIMINE); (✱) APO-IMIPRAMINE, IMPRIL, NOVO-PRAMINE
- ❒ Nortriptyline (AVENTYL, PAMELOR)
- ❒ Protriptyline (VIVACTIL); (✱) TRIPTIL
- ❒ Trimipramine (SURMONTIL)

Indications

TCAs are still used as first-line drugs in the treatment of major depression. They elevate mood, increase activity and alertness, decrease morbid preoccupation, improve appetite, and normalize sleep patterns. TCAs have also been used for the treatment of chronic pain syndromes (amitriptyline, doxepin, imipramine, nortriptyline), neuropathy, migraine headache, attention deficit disorder, enuresis (imipramine), and panic disorders (doxepin). TCAs eliminate panic attacks in about 75 percent of patients. Anticipatory anxiety and phobic avoidance behaviors are not affected.

Pharmacodynamics

Antidepressant drugs appear to work by blocking presynaptic serotonin and norepinephrine reuptake (Fig. 18–2). Thus, there is an increased amount of these neurotransmitters in the synapse, prolonging and intensifying their effects. Such action is consistent with the monoamine hypothesis of depression, which asserts that depression stems from a deficiency in monoamine-mediated neurotransmission. If this is true, drugs capable of increasing the effects of monoamines would reduce symptoms of depression. The relative ability of the individual TCAs to block reuptake of serotonin and norepinephrine are summarized in Table 18–1.

It should be noted that blockade of reuptake by itself cannot fully explain the therapeutic effectiveness of the TCAs. This statement is based on the observation that clinical responses (antidepressant) and the biochemical effects (blockade) do not occur in the same time frame. In other words, the drugs block transmitter uptake within a few hours of administration, whereas relief of depression may take several weeks to develop. Therefore, it appears that an intermediary response must be occurring between the onset of the blockade and the onset of therapeutic response. What composes this intermediate response is not clear.

Adverse Effects and Contraindications

The adverse effects commonly experienced with TCAs are many and varied. However, they typically fall into several categories. Orthostatic hypotension is the most serious of the common adverse effects. It is due in part to blockade of $alpha_1$-adrenergic receptors on blood vessels. Anticholinergic adverse effects are often the most disturbing. By blocking cholinergic receptors, an array of anticholinergic effects are possible. These include blurred vision, worsening of narrow angle glaucoma, photophobia, dry mouth, constipation, urinary retention, sinus tachycardia, and mental clouding.

Cardiovascular effects of TCAs are rare in the absence of overdosage or pre-existing cardiac impairment. These drugs affect the heart by decreasing vagal influence secondary to the muscarinic blockade and by acting directly on the bundle of His to slow conduction. Both mechanisms increase the risk of arrhythmias (premature atrial and ventricular contractions, electrocardiographic ST segment depression, flattened or inverted T-waves, and the prolonged QRS segment). Congestive heart failure can be worsened.

Drowsiness, muscle tremors or twitches, paresthesias, fatigue, weakness, and seizures may occur with overdose or in patients with known seizure disorders. In addition, hallucinations, delusions, and activation of schizophrenic or manic states make up the possible neurologic adverse effects.

Adverse gastrointestinal (GI) effects include nausea, vomiting, and heartburn, as well as weight loss and gain. TCAs can also cause sexual dysfunction, which is manifested as decreased libido, reduced arousal, and impaired orgasm.

Pharmacokinetics

The majority of antidepressants are well absorbed when administered by mouth, and onset varies from 1 to 2 hours to 3 weeks (Table 18–2). All TCAs are widely distributed with effective relief of depression achieved within 2 to 6 weeks, in most cases. They are over 90-percent protein bound, with half-lives ranging from 8 to more than 67 hours. Most of the drugs are extensively biotransformed in the liver with enterohepatic recirculation and secreted into gastric juices. Some of the drugs are biotransformed to active metabolites. TCAs probably cross the placenta and enter breast milk.

Drug-Drug Interactions

Many drug-drug interactions occur with TCAs (Table 18–3). The drug groups that commonly interact with TCAs include MAOIs, direct-acting and indirect-acting sympathomimetic drugs, and central nervous system (CNS) depressants.

Dosage Regimen

The dosage regimen for TCAs is individualized (Table 18–4). The dosages of most drugs are reduced for pediatric, adolescent, and geriatric patients.

Laboratory Considerations

Amitriptyline causes an increase in aspartate transaminase (AST [SGOT]), alanine transaminase (ALT [SGPT]),

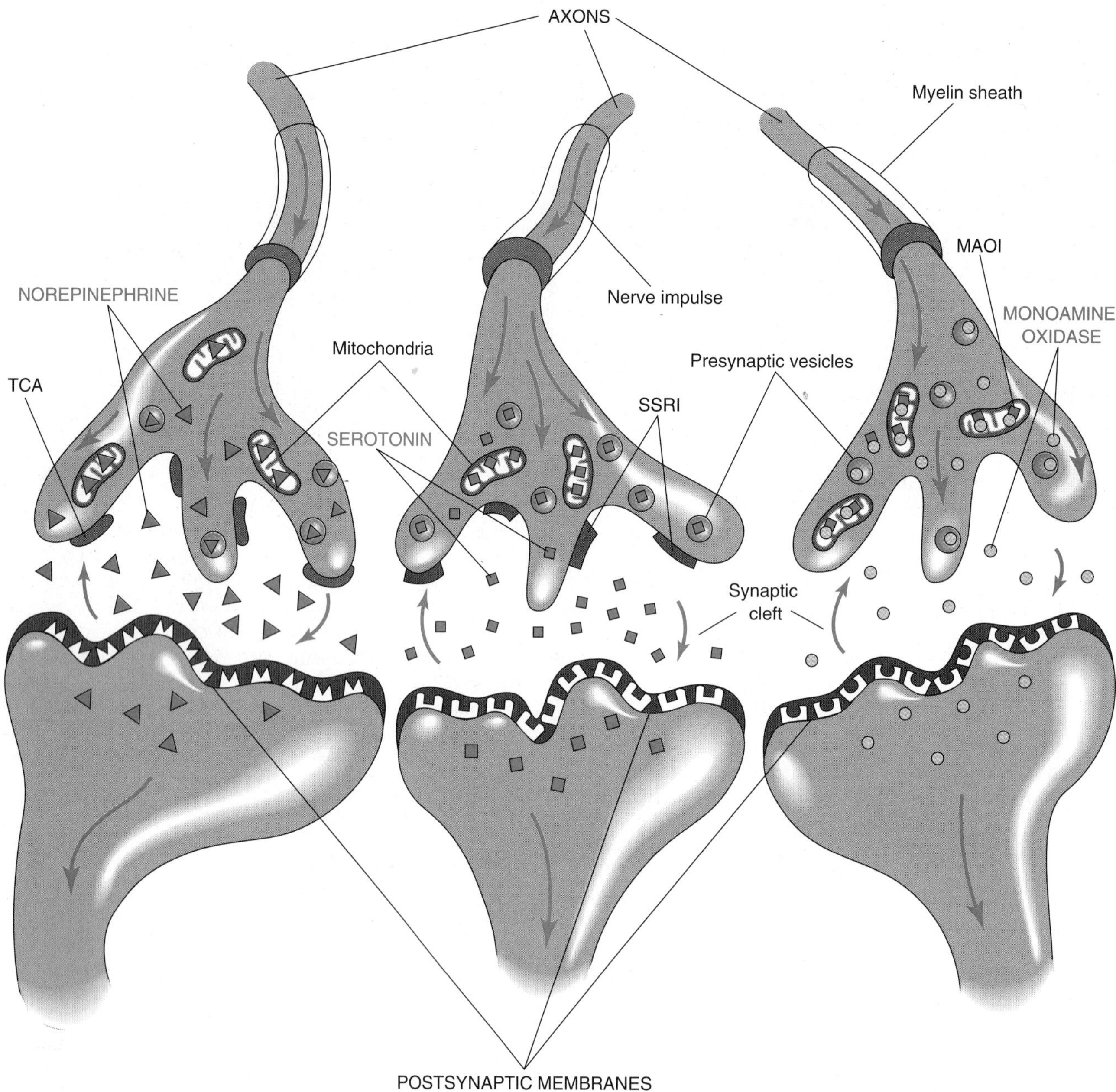

Figure 18–2 Pharmacodynamics of antidepressant drugs. Normally, norepinephrine, serotonin, and monoamine oxidase (MAO) are released from storage sites within the adrenergic nerve by the arrival of a nerve impulse. Norepinephrine is metabolized within the nerve by MAO or by catechol-O-methyltransferase (COMT) in the synapse. Most norepinephrine (NE) is taken back into the nerve and stored. Tricyclic antidepressants (TCAs) block the reuptake of norepinephrine in the synapse. Selective serotonin reuptake inhibitors (SSRIs) inhibit the reuptake of serotonin and minor amounts of norepinephrine from the synapse. Monoamine oxidase inhibitors (MAOIs) preferentially block the reuptake of monoamine oxidase, NE, and serotonin at the mitochondria level rather than in the synapse.

and serum alkaline phosphatase concentrations. Doxepin can cause elevated serum sodium levels. Imipramine and nortriptyline cause alterations in blood glucose levels.

Selective Serotonin Reuptake Inhibitors

❒ Fluoxetine (PROZAC)
❒ Fluvoxamine (LUVOX)
❒ Paroxetine (PAXIL)
❒ Sertraline (ZOLOFT)
❒ Trazodone (DESYREL)

Indications

TCAs were the mainstay of antidepressant therapy until the introduction of the SSRIs. Fluoxetine was the first SSRI released for use in the United States. It has been used by over 21 million patients world wide and is effective in treating large numbers of depressed patients. Fluoxetine is also approved for the treatment of obsessive-compulsive disorder and eating disorders. Fluvoxamine is used widely in other countries but, to date, has only received approval from the Food and Drug Administration (FDA) for the treatment of obsessive-compulsive disorder.

TABLE 18–1 NEUROTRANSMITTER REUPTAKE BLOCKADE POTENCY AND COMMON ADVERSE EFFECT PROFILES OF SELECTED ANTIDEPRESSANTS

Drug/Class	Serotonin	Norepinephrine	Anticholinergic	Sedation
Tricyclic Antidepressants				
Amitriptyline	+2	+3	+3	+3
Desipramine	0	+5	+1	+1
Doxepin	+3	+2	+3	+4
Imipramine	+3	+2	+4	+3
Nortriptyline	+2	+3	+3	+2
Protriptyline	+2	+3	+3	+1
Trimipramine	+3	+2	+4	+4
Tetracyclic Antidepressant				
Maprotiline	0	+5	+2	+4
Selected Serotonin Reuptake Inhibitors				
Fluoxetine	+4	0	0	*
Sertraline	+4	0	0	*
Trazodone	+2	0	0	+3
Monoamine Oxidase Inhibitors				
Phenelzine	†	†	0	+1
Tranylcypromine	†	†	0	+1
Miscellaneous Antidepressants				
Amoxapine	+1	+4	+2	+2
Bupropion	‡	‡	+2	*
Maprotiline	+1	+3	+3	+3

Key: + 5 strongest response, 0 none.

*Fluoxetine, sertraline, and bupropion produce moderate stimulation, not sedation.

†MAOIs do not block the uptake of transmitter. Instead they increase the intraneuronal stores at norepinephrine, serotonin, and dopamine.

‡Bupropion primarily inhibits reuptake of dopamine rather than norepinephrine or serotonin.

Paroxetine and sertraline have received approval for use in obsessive-compulsive disorder and panic attacks. SSRIs are also utilized in the treatment of anorexia nervosa, bulimia, obesity, chronic pain, fibromyalgia, migraine, attention defecit disorder, aggression, and impulsivity.

Paroxetine is the newest SSRI. Paroxetine is equally as effective as fluoxetine or sertraline and has similar adverse effects, but in some patients, it may cause a sense of calm or drowsiness.

Pharmacodynamics

SSRIs are chemically unrelated to any other class of antidepressants. The SSRIs are potent blockers of serotonin reuptake, with weak affinity for norepinephrine or dopamine blockade. They have limited affinity for alpha$_1$, alpha$_2$, beta-adrenergic, gamma-aminobutyric acid (GABA), histamine, and cholinergic receptors.

Adverse Effects and Contraindications

Although SSRIs represent a significant improvement over TCAs, they are not without adverse effects. SSRIs tend to produce excitation rather than sedation. Only about 20 percent of patients experience sedation. These effects have been referred to as "energizing adverse effects." The adverse effects of SSRIs are similar to those of other drugs in their class, although there is reduced risk of orthostatic hypotension, tachycardia, heart block, blurred vision, or dry mouth. Nausea, insomnia, sexual dysfunction (anorgasmia), ejaculatory disturbances, decreased libido, and lack of sensitivity have been noted. Priapism has been associated with the use of trazodone and can result in permanent impotence. Most adverse effects tend to be mild and well tolerated, and in some cases quickly disappear after 1 to 2 weeks of treatment.

SSRIs are contraindicated in hypersensitivity and should not be used by patients with narrow-angle glaucoma, immediately after a myocardial infarction. Caution should be used in prescribing SSRIs during pregnancy or lactation, and these drugs should be closely managed by an obstetric specialist. They should be used cautiously in older patients and those with pre-existing cardiovascular disease.

Pharmacokinetics

SSRIs are well absorbed when taken by mouth. Like the TCAs, their onset, peak, and duration of action range from 1 to 4 weeks and may require up to 12 weeks for complete effectiveness (see Table 18–2). The SSRIs are distributed throughout the body and across placental membranes. They have been found in breast milk. Most SSRIs are highly protein bound with half-lives that vary from 5 to 72 hours. The half-lives of SSRIs are prolonged in patients with hepatic impairment because they inhibit the biochemical activity of the hepatic enzymes of the cytochrome P_{450} system. The majority of these drugs are eliminated through the urine.

Drug-Drug Interactions

All SSRIs are absolutely contraindicated for concomitant use with MAOIs. The combination of SSRI and MAOI may

TABLE 18–2 PHARMACOKINETICS OF SELECTED ANTIDEPRESSANT AND MOOD STABILIZING DRUGS

	Route	Onset	Peak	Duration	PB%	$t_{1/2}$	BioA%
Tricyclic Antidepressants							
Amitriptyline	po	2–3 wk	2–6 wk	18–24 hr	>90	10–50 hr	UA
	IM	2–3 wk	2–6 wk	Days to weeks	>90	10–50 hr	UA
Clomipramine	po	2–6 wk	2 hr	12-24 hr	96	21 hr	UA
Desipramine	po	2–6 wk	4–6 hr	24 hr	>90	UA	UA
Doxepin	po	2–3 wk	6 wks	18–24 hr	>90	8–24 hr	UA
Imipramine	po	1–2 hr	2–6 wk	Weeks	>90	8–16 hr	86
	IM	1–2hr	2–6 wk	Weeks	>90	8–16 hr	UA
Nortriptyline	po	2–3 wks	6 wks	18–24 hr	>90	18–28 hr	UA
Protriptyline	po	2–6 wk	24–30 hr	12–24 hr	>90	>67 hr	UA
Trimipramine	po	2–6 wk	2 hr	8–16 hr	>90	UA	UA
Tetracyclic Antidepressant							
Maprotiline	po	2–6 wk	8–24 hr	18–24 hr	88	>51 hr	UA
Mirtazapine	po	2–6 wk	1.5 hr	12–24 hr	85	20-40 hr	50
Selective Serotonin Reuptake Inhibitors							
Fluoxetine	po	1–4 wks	6–8 hr	24-48 wk	95	1–3 days; 5–7 days*	>90
Fluvoxamine	po	2–3 wks	Dose Dependent	12-24 hr	>90	13.6–15.6 hr	UA
Paroxetine	po	1–4 wks	3-7 hr	24 hr	90	21 hr	>90
Sertraline	po	1–8 wks	6-8 hr	24 hr	98	26 hr	>90
Trazodone	po	1–2 wks	0.5–2 hr	8 hr	90	5–9 hr	UA
Monoamine Oxidase Inhibitors							
Phenelzine	po	1–4 wk	2–6 wk	2 weeks	UA	24-48	UA
Tranylcypromine	po	Days	2–3 wk	3–5 days	UA	UK	UA
Miscellaneous Antidepressants							
Amoxapine	po	1-6 wk	2–4 hr	16–24 hr	90	8 hr	UA
Bupropion	po	To 4 wk	2 hr	6-12 hr	80	14	UA
Maprotiline	po	3–7 days	1–3 wk	UK	88	51 hr	UA
Nefazodone	po	2-6 wk	48 hr	12-24 hr	99	2-4	20
Venlafaxine	po	4 days-6 wk	2-4 hr	6-8 hr	27	5 hr, 11 hr	>90
Mood Stabilizers							
Carbamazepine	po	1–2 wk	1.5 hr; 4–5 hr; 12 hr	8–12 hr	76; 57†	8–29 hr	UA
Lithium	po	1–2 wk	0.5 hr; 1–3 hr; 3–4 hr‡	6–12 hr	0	20–27 hr	UA
Valproic acid	po	4 days-2 wk	1–4 hr	8–12 hr	90–95	6-16 hr	UA

*Half life of fluoxetine is 1–3 days with the half-life of the metabolite norfluoxetine 5 to 7 days.
†Protein binding of carbamazepine in adults and children, respectively.
‡Time to peak effects of lithium tablets/capsules, syrup, and extended-release forms, respectively.
BioA, Bioavailability; PB, protein binding; $t_{1/2}$, serum half-life; UA, unavailable; UK, unknown.

result in a severe serotonergic syndrome, which is characterized by autonomic instability, rigidity, hyperpyrexia, widely fluctuating vital signs, stuporous rigidity, and possibly death (see Table 18–3). Concomitant use of paroxetine and fluoxetine with antihistamines (e.g., astemizole and terfenadine) is contraindicated. This combination can precipitate serious cardiac irregularities.

Dosage Regimen

Dosage regimens for the treatment of depression vary from drug to drug (see Table 18–4). As with the dosage regimens of TCAs, the health care provider should use the appropriate resources and references when prescribing antidepressants. Close attention should be paid to cardiovascular, hepatic, and renal status, particularly in the young and the elderly. Paroxetine and fluoxetine should be used in lower doses with patients with renal impairment, because increased concentrations may occur.

Laboratory Considerations

Proteinuria and a mild increase in AST (SGOT) may occur during sensitivity reactions to fluoxetine. It may cause hypoglycemia and hyponatremia in some patients. The complete blood count (CBC) and differential should be monitored periodically before and throughout the course of therapy, with attention to leukopenia, anemia, thrombocytopenia, or increased bleeding times.

The CBC and renal and hepatic function should be assessed before and periodically during therapy with trazodone. A slight, clinically insignificant decrease in leukocyte and neutrophil counts may occur.

TABLE 18–3 DRUG-DRUG INTERACTIONS OF SELECTED ANTIDEPRESSANT AND MOOD-STABILIZING DRUGS

Drug	Interactive Drugs	Interaction
Tricyclic Antidepressants		
Tricyclic antidepressants	Alcohol Antihistamines Barbiturates Opioids	Additive CNS depression
	MAO inhibitors	Severe hypertension or hypotension, hyperpyretic states, seizures
	Anesthetics	Tachyarrhythmias
	Anticoagulants	Increased effects of interactive drug
	Anticonvulsants	Increased seizure risk
	Aminopyrine Antipsychotics Aspirin Cimetidine Disulfiram Methylphenidate Oral contraceptives Phenothiazines Phenylbutazone Phenytoin SSRIs Steroids Thyroid drugs	Increased effects of TCA
Monoamine Oxidase Inhibitors		
Phenelzine	Amphetamines	Increased effects of MAOI
Tranylcypromine	Antihypertensive drugs Asthma drugs Cocaine Cough and cold drugs Ephedrine Methylphenidate Phenylpropanolamine Phenylephrine Tricyclic antidepressants SSRIs Sympathomimetic drugs Trazodone	Hypertensive crisis
	Meperidine	Hyperpyrexia
	Anticonvulsants	Increased CNS depression
	Insulin Sulfonylureas	Increased effect of interactive drugs
Miscellaneous Antidepressants		
Amoxapine	Clonidine MAO inhibitors	Hyperpyrexia, hypertension, seizures, death
	Antihypertensives	Decreases effects of interactive drug
	Alcohol Antihistamines Opioid analgesics Sedative-hypnotics	Additive CNS depression
	Adrenergic drugs Anticholinergic drugs	Additive effects of interactive drugs
	Cimetidine Fluoxetine Phenothiazines Oral contraceptives	Increased levels of interactive drugs
	Disulfiram	Transient delirium
Bupropion	Levodopa MAO inhibitors	Increased risk of adverse reactions of interactive drug
	Alcohol Antidepressants Benzodiazepines Phenothiazines	Increased risk of seizures with cessation of drug use.
Maprotiline	MAO inhibitors	May cause hyperpyrexia, seizures, hypertension, death
	Antihypertensives	May prevent antihypertensive effects
	Alcohol Antihistamines Clonidine Opioids Sedative-hypnotics	Additive CNS depression

Table continued on following page

TABLE 18–3 DRUG-DRUG INTERACTIONS OF SELECTED ANTIDEPRESSANT AND MOOD-STABILIZING DRUGS *Continued*		
Drug	**Interactive Drugs**	**Interaction**
Miscellaneous Antidepressants—cont'd		
Maprotiline—cont'd	Phenothiazines	Increased risk of seizures
	Adrenergics	Additive adrenergic effects, increased risk of adverse cardiovascular reactions
	Decongestants	
	Vasoconstrictors	
	Anticholinergics	Additive anticholinergic effects
	Antihistamines	
	Atropine	
	Disopyramide	
	Haloperidol	
	Phenothiazines	
	Quinidine	
	Cimetidine	Increased levels of maprotiline
	Fluoxetine	
	Oral contraceptives	
Nefazodone	Astemizole	Increased risk of toxic effects of interactive drug
Venlafaxine	Cimetidine	
	MAO inhibitors	
	Terfenadine	
	General anesthetics	Increased risk of CNS depression
Selective Serotonin Reuptake Inhibitors		
Mood Stabilizers		
Carbamazepine	Diltiazem	Increases levels of interactive drugs
	Erythromycin	
	Propoxyphene	
	Verapamil	
	MAO inhibitors	Hyperpyrexia, hypertension, seizures, death if interactive drug taken within 2 weeks
	Anticoagulants	Decreased effects of interactive drug
	Anticonvulsants	
	Barbiturates	
	Benzodiazepines	
	Doxycycline	
	Felbamate	
	Glucocorticoids	
	Oral contraceptives	
	Phenytoin	
	Quinidine	
	Acetaminophen	Increased risk of hepatotoxicity
	Dextropropoxyphene	
	Isoniazid	
	Cimetidine	Increases blood levels of carbamazepine
	Diltiazem	
	Verapamil	
Lithium	Neuromuscular blockers	Prolongs action of interactive drug
	Amphetamines	Increases risk of neurotoxicity
	Calcium channel blockers	
	Carbamazepine	
	Haloperidol	
	Molindone	
	ACE inhibitors	Increases risk of lithium toxicity
	Amiloride	
	Chlorpromazine	
	Diuretics	
	Fluoxetine	
	Methyldopa	
	NSAIDs	
	Probenecid	
	Aminophylline	Decreases effects of lithium
	Caffeine	
	Digoxin	
	Phenothiazines	
	Sodium bicarbonate	
	Sodium chloride	
	Theophyllin	
	Urea	
	Chlorpromazine	Decreased effects of interactive drug.
	Antithyroid drugs	Hypothyroid effects may be additive
	Potassium iodide	

TABLE 18–3 DRUG-DRUG INTERACTIONS OF SELECTED ANTIDEPRESSANT AND MOOD-STABILIZING DRUGS *Continued*

Drug	Interactive Drugs	Interaction
Selective Serotonin Reuptake Mood Stabilizers—cont'd		
Valproic acid	Carbamazepine	Decreases level of valproic acid
	Aspirin NSAIDs Cefamandole Cefoperazone Cefotetan Heparin Thrombolytic drugs Warfarin	Increased risk of bleeding
	Barbiturates Primidone	Decreases metabolism of interactive drug
	Alcohol Antihistamines Antidepressants Opioid analgesics MAO inhibitors Sedative/hypnotics	Additive CNS depression
	Phenytoin	Increases or decreases effects of interactive drug
	Chlorpromazine Felbamate	Increases valproic acid levels

ACE, angiotensin-converting enzyme; CNS, Central nervous system; MAO, monoamine oxidase; NSAIDs, nonsteroidal anti-inflammatory drugs; SSRIs, selective serotonin reuptake inhibitors; TCA, tricyclic antidepressant.

Monoamine Oxidase Inhibitors

- ❒ Phenelzine (NARDIL)
- ❒ Tranylcypromine (PARNATE)

MAOIs were synthesized in the early 1950s as a by-product of research into newer, more effective antituberculosis drugs. It was soon found that iproniazid had mood-elevating effects in tuberculosis patients. The patients became energized, hyperactive, and in some cases, frankly manic. As investigators assessed patient responses they concluded that iproniazid was capable of inhibiting the enzyme monoamine oxidase (MAO). Thus, MAOIs had an important impact on the development of modern biologic psychiatry.

Indications

Only two MAOIs are approved for use in the United States—phenelzine and tranylcypromine. These drugs are considered second-line or third-line antidepressants for most patients. Because their use can be hazardous, they are reserved for patients who have not responded to TCAs, SSRIs, newer drugs, or electroconvulsive therapy (ECT). However, for patients with atypical depression, MAOIs may be the drugs of first choice.

MAOIs have also been used with some success in the treatment of panic disorder, bulimia, obsessive-compulsive disorders, and agoraphobia.

Pharmacodynamics

MAO inhibitors exert their effects primarily on organ systems influenced by sympathomimetic amines and serotonin. By inhibiting intraneuronal MAO, the amount of norepinephrine and serotonin available is increased (see Fig. 18–2). The increased transmission that results in supranormal quantities is thought to be key to relief of depression. Eighty-five percent of MAO must be degradated to produce an antidepressant effect.

Phenelzine produces irreversible inhibition of intraneuronal MAO. Recovery of irreversible inhibition is a slow process requiring synthesis of new enzyme. Hence, the effects of irreversible inhibitors persist for about 2 weeks after the drug is withdrawn. In contrast, tranylcypromine produces reversible inhibition. Recovery from reversible inhibition is more rapid, occurring in 3 to 5 days. These drugs inhibit not only MAO but other enzymes as well, and they interfere with the hepatic biotransformation of many drugs.

Adverse Effects and Contraindications

The most common adverse effect associated with MAOI therapy is actually orthostatic hypotension. Restlessness, insomnia, anorexia, constipation, nausea, vomiting, dry mouth, urinary retention, impotence, drowsiness, headache, rash, dizziness, and weakness have also been noted. Other adverse effects include increased perspiration, urinary frequency, weight gain, flushing, increased appetite, numbness, paresthesias, tremor, myoclonic jerks, hyperreflexia, and muscle spasm.

Adverse effects of MAOIs are dose dependent for the most part; however, they cause severe hypertension when taken with foods containing large amounts of tyramine. Following ingestion of tyramine, there is a rapid displacement and release of norepinephrine from noradrenergic neurons, resulting in severe hypertension. The hypertensive crisis is the most serious and potentially fatal adverse effect associated with MAOI therapy. Severe headache, nausea, vomiting, sweating, neck stiffness and soreness, and mydriasis also occur. Intracranial hemorrhage can also result, which may lead to death. Tranylcypromine may produce greater CNS stimulation than phenel ine, perhaps because of its close structural similarity to amphetamine.

TABLE 18–4 DOSAGE REGIMEN FOR SELECTED ANTIDEPRESSANT AND MOOD STABILIZING DRUGS

Drug	Uses(s)	Dosage	Implications
Tricyclic Antidepressants			
Amitriptyline	Depression Chronic pain	*Adults:* 30–100 mg po QD as single HS dosage or in divided doses. Increase gradually to 150–300 mg. po QD *or* 20–30 mg IM QID. *Child 6–12 years:* 1–5 mg/kg po QD in two divided doses *Adolescents:* 10 mg po TID and 20 mg po at HS. Increase slowly to 100 mg po QD as single HS dose *Geriatric:* 25 mg po at HS. Increase up to 10 mg po TID and 20 mg HS. Daily dose not to exceed 100 mg	Dosage increases should be made at HS because of sedation. Titration may take weeks to months. IM route for short-term use only
Clomipramine		*Adults:* 25 mg po TID. Increase as tolerated to 100 mg during the first 2 weeks. Maximum: 250 mg po QD. Maintenance: Titrate to lowest effective dose (Unlabeled) *Child over ten:* 25 mg po initially. Gradually increase as tolerated during first 2 weeks. Increase dose after first 2 weeks as tolerated to maximum of 3 mg/kg or 100 mg, whichever is smaller. Maintenance: Titrate to lowest effective dose	Once maximum dose is reached, give at HS to minimize sedation. Effectiveness after 10 weeks has not been documented
Desipramine	Depression Cocaine withdrawal Eating disorders	*Adults:* 100–200 mg po QD as single dose or divided doses Gradually increase to maximum of 300 mg QD. Maintenance: At reduced dosage for at least 2 months after satisfactory response achieved *Child age 6–12 yr:* 1–5 mg/kg/day in divided doses *Geriatric:* 25–100 mg po QD initially. Not to exceed 150 mg. QD	Not recommended for children younger than age 12 years
Doxepin	Depression Chronic pain	*Adults:* 25–150 mg po QD as single HS dose or two to three divided doses. Gradually increase up to 300 mg po QD	Single dose should not exceed 150 mg
Imipramine	Depression Enuresis	*Depression Adults and Children:* 25–50 mg po TID–QID *or* 100 mg IM QD in divided doses. Not to exceed 300 mg/day *Child ages 6–12 years:* 10–30 mg po QD in two divided doses *Adolescents:* 25–50 mg po in divided doses. Not to exceed 100 mg QD *Geriatric:* 25 mg po HS initially. Up to 100 mg QD in divided doses *Enuresis:* 25 mg po QD 1 hour before bedtime. Increase by 25 mg at weekly intervals PRN to 50 mg in children younger than 12 years. In children older than age 12, increase at weekly intervals PRN to 75 mg	Total daily dose may be given at HS
Nortriptyline	Depression Chronic pain	*Adults:* 25 mg po TID-QID. Increase to 150 mg po QD *Adolescent or Geriatric:* 30–50 mg po as single daily dose or divided doses	Not recommended in children under age 18 years
Protriptyline	Depression Obstructive sleep apnea	*Adults:* 15–40 mg po QD-QID. Increase to 60 mg po QD if required. Maximum: 60 mg QD. *Adolescents or Geriatrics:* 5 mg po TID. Increase gradually if necessary	Make increases in dosage with the morning dose. Not recommended for pediatric patients. Monitor cardiovascular system closely if dosage exceeds 20 mg QD
Trimipramine	Depression associated with sleep disorders, peptic ulcer disease, dermatologic disorders	*Adults:* 75–100 mg po QD in divided doses. Increase to 150–200 mg as required. Maintenance: 50–150 mg po QD as single HS dose *Adolescent:* 50 mg po QD. Gradually increase up to 100 mg po QD *Geriatric:* 50 mg po with gradual increases up to 100 mg po QD	After satisfactory response, reduce dosage to lowest effective dose. Continue for 3 months to lessen possibility of relapse
Tetracyclic Antidepressant			
Maprotiline	Depression Bipolar disorder	*Adults:* 25 to 75 mg po QD in outpatients; 100–150 mg po QD in hospitalized patients. Increase by 25 mg increments to 150–225 mg po QD for outpatients; by 25 mg increments to 300 mg po QD for inpatients. Maintenance: reduce dosage to lowest effective level, usually 75–150 mg po QD *Geriatric over age 60:* 50–75 mg po QD for maintenance	Not recommended in children younger than age 18 years
Selective Serotonin Reuptake Inhibitors			
Fluoxetine	Depression Obesity Obsessive-compulsive disorder	*Adult:* 20 mg po QD. Increase after 2–4 weeks to maximum 20–80 mg. Administer doses over 20 mg/day on BID schedule	Safety and efficacy not established in children. Lower doses in geriatric and for renal impaired

TABLE 18–4 DOSAGE REGIMEN FOR SELECTED ANTIDEPRESSANT AND MOOD STABILIZING DRUGS *Continued*

Drug	Uses(s)	Dosage	Implications
Selective Serotonin Reuptake Inhibitors—cont'd			
Fluvoxamine	Obsessive-compulsive disorder	*Adult:* 50 mg po at HS. Increase by 50 mg increments at 4–7 day intervals. Usual range 100–300 mg po QD	Safety and efficacy not established in children
Paroxetine	Depression Obsessive-compulsive disorder Panic Disorder	*Adult:* 20 mg po QD. Increase in 2–4 weeks to maximum 20–50 mg QD	Should not be used within 14 days before or after MAOI therapy.
Sertraline	Depression Obsessive-compulsive disorder Panic Disorder	*Adults:* 50 mg po QD single dose in AM or PM. Increase at weekly intervals up to 200 mg po QD depending on response.	Should not be used within 14 days before or after MAOI therapy.
Trazodone	Depression Chronic pain Insomnia	*Adult:* 150 mg po QD in three divided doses. Increase by 50 mg po QD q3–4 days until desired response. Not to exceed 400 mg in outpatients or 600 mg in hospitalized patients. *Child 6–18 years:* 1.5–2 mg/kg/day in divided doses. Increase q3–4 days, up to 6 mg/kg/day *Geriatric:* 75 mg. po QD in divided doses initially. May be increased every 3–4 days	A larger dose may be given at bedtime to decrease daytime drowsiness and dizziness
Miscellaneous Antidepressants			
Amoxapine	Depression	*Adults:* 100–150 mg po QD in divided doses. Increase to 200–300 mg QD by end of first week. Not to exceed 300 mg daily in outpatients and 600 mg daily in divided doses in hospitalized patients. *Geriatric:* 25 mg po BID-TID. Increase to 50 mg po BID-TID. Maximum: 300 mg QD	No single dose should exceed 300 mg Once optimal dose is achieved, may give as single bedtime dose
Bupropion	Depression	*Adults:* 100 mg po BID. Increase after 3 days to 100 mg TID, after 4 weeks of treatment increase to 450 mg po in divided doses. No single dose should exceed 150 mg	Wait 6 hr between doses at 300 mg/day, or at least 4 hr between doses at 450 mg/day
Nefazodone	Depression	*Adults:* 100 mg po BID. Increase weekly up to 600 mg/day in 2 divided doses. *Elderly:* 50 mg po BID. Increase weekly as patient needs dictate	Concurrent use with terfenadine or astemizole may result in fatal adverse cardiovascular reactions. Concurrent use with MAO inhibitors should be avoided
Venlafaxine	Depression	*Adults:* 75 mg po in two to three divided doses. Increase slowly up to 225 mg/day until desired effect is achieved	Safety and efficacy not established in children or geriatric patients
Monoamine Oxidase Inhibitors			
Phenelzine	Neurotic or atypical depression Panic attacks	*Adults:* 15 mg po TID. Increase to 60-90 mg/day in divided doses, then reduce to smallest effective dose. *Geriatric:* 15 mg po QD with slow dose titration *Panic Attacks:* 15 mg po QD, increase over 2 weeks to 15 mg TID-QID.	Patient should be cautioned verbally and in writing to avoid foods containing tyramine (See Appendix C)
Tranylcypromine	Neurotic or atypical depression	*Adults:* Initial: 30 mg po QD in two divided doses. Increase after 2 weeks by 10 mg/day at 1–3 week intervals up to 60 mg/day *Geriatric:* Initial: 2.5–5 mg/ day. Increase every 3–4 days up to 45 mg/day *Panic Attacks:* 10 mg po QD initially. Increase over 2 weeks to 20–30 mg day	
Mood Stabilizing Drugs			
Carbamazepine	Bipolar disorder	*Adults:* Initial: 10–20 mg/kg/day. Usually started at 200 mg po BID-TID. Increase at 4- to 5-day intervals. Maintenance: Maximum dose: 800–1200 mg po QD	Not FDA approved for bipolar disorders
Lithium	Bipolar disorder	*Adults:* Initial: 300–600 mg po TID and increase at 5- to 7-day intervals to 900–1200 mg po BID. Maintenance: 300 mg TID-QID *or* 600 mg BID. Maximum dose not to exceed 2400 mg QD *Child:* 15–20 mg (0.4–0.5 mEq/kg/day in two to three divided doses)	300 mg lithium carbonate contains 8–12 mEq lithium Dosage listed is for tablets or capsules. The dosage for sustained-release formulations is different
Valproic acid Divalproex	Bipolar disorders Acute mania	*Adults and Elderly:* 750 mg/day in divided doses. Maximum: 60 mg/kg/day	Give in two divided doses once daily dosage exceeds 150 mg

FDA, Food and Drug Administration; MAOI, monoamine oxidase inhibitor.

Pharmacokinetics

Onset of therapeutic action produced by the MAOIs ranges from 1 to 4 weeks. Peak and duration of action are variable.

Drug-Drug Interactions

A number of drugs must be avoided while a person is receiving MAOI therapy. Most drug-drug interactions occur with indirect-acting sympathomimetic drugs (e.g., cough and cold drugs, asthma drugs, phenylpropanolamine, phenylephrine, ephedrine, and amphetamine). The interactions are secondary to inhibition of hepatic MAO (see Table 18–3). Meperidine can cause hyperpyrexia. Thus, if an analgesic is needed, a drug other than meperidine should be chosen. The use of antihypertensive drugs with MAOIs may cause excessive lowering of blood pressure. When MAOIs are taken in combination with TCAs or sympathomimetic drugs, they can produce hypertensive episodes or crises.

Drug-Food Interactions

There are a number of foods that should be avoided while the patient is receiving MAOI therapy. These are foods and beverages that contain tyramine. Foods containing high levels of tyramine that should be avoided include all aged cheeses, fermented beverages (particularly vermouth and chianti wines), pickled and smoked meats, (sausages, pepperoni, salami, bologna, liver, Spam, canned ham), soy sauce, tap beer, and broad bean pods. Any fermented meat, fish or protein food product or extracts, yeast extracts (marmite, brewer's yeast tablets), and sauerkraut should also be avoided (see Appendix C).

Dosage Regimen

The initial oral adult dosage of phenelzine is 15 mg three times daily daily (see Table 18–4). The dosage should be titrated to at least 60 mg/day as rapidly as tolerated to maximize inhibition of MAO. Total daily doses of up to 90 mg may be required. The oral dosage of tranylcypromine should be titrated to the individual's needs and tolerance but generally consists of 30 mg taken in two divided doses.

Laboratory Considerations

Serum glucose levels may be decreased in the presence of MAOIs.

Miscellaneous Antidepressants

- ❒ Amoxapine (ASENDIN)
- ❒ Bupropion (WELLBUTRIN)
- ❒ Maprotiline (LUDIOMIL)
- ❒ Mirtazapine (REMERON)
- ❒ Nefazodone (SERZONE)
- ❒ Venlafaxine (EFFEXOR)

AMOXAPINE

Amoxapine is used in the treatment of depression accompanied by anxiety. It acts by potentiating the effects of serotonin and norepinephrine in the CNS, but it has significant anticholinergic properties.

The most common adverse effects of amoxapine include drowsiness, lethargy, sedation, fatigue, hypotension, and anticholinergic effects such as dry mouth, dry eyes, blurred vision, and constipation. The most serious reaction is a remote possibility of neuroleptic malignant syndrome because amoxapine is structurally similar to some antipsychotic drugs. Extrapyramidal symptoms and tardive dyskinesia have occurred in 1 percent of patients receiving amoxapine.

Amoxapine rapidly absorbed after oral administration with peak plasma concentrations reached in 90 minutes. It is widely distributed throughout body tissues and is detected in breast milk. The plasma half-life of amoxapine is approximately 8 hours. Biotransformation takes place in the liver to two metabolites, both of which are pharmacologically active. The half-life is 30 hours. Elimination is through the urine.

BUPROPION

Like amoxapine, bupropion is used in the treatment of depression, often in conjunction with psychotherapy. The mechanism of action is unknown, but it is thought to be a weak blocker of norepinephrine, serotonin, and dopamine. It is not known to inhibit MAO. It is structurally distinct from all other antidepressants, belonging to the aminoketone class and is unrelated to tricyclic, tetracyclic, SSRIs, MAOIs, or other known antidepressants. Bupropion lacks the polycyclic rings of most other antidepressants. The chemical structure resembles that of diethylpropion, which is a sympathomimetic anorectic drug with stimulating properties.

Common adverse effects of bupropion include, agitation, anxiety, restlessness, insomnia, and weight loss. It has a significant incidence of seizures, approximately four times that of any other antidepressant. It is specifically of concern in patients with a history of seizures, head injury, anorexia, or bulimia (i.e., electrolyte imbalance) and those who are taking other drugs that may lower the seizure threshold.

Bupropion is rapidly absorbed with peak plasma concentrations occurring within 2 hours. Bupropion is widely distributed throughout the body and is 80 percent protein bound. Bupropion has two active metabolites, each with longer elimination half-lives than the parent compound. Bupropion is metabolized in the liver with elimination in the feces following a biphasic decline. The average half-life in the second phase is approximately 14 hours.

The initial adult dose of bupropion is 100 mg twice daily (morning and evening). After 3 days, the dose may be increased to 100 mg three times daily. After the fourth week of therapy, the dose may be increased to a maximum daily dosage of 450 mg taken in divided doses. No single dose should exceed 150 mg. At least 6 hours should elapse between doses at the 300-mg/day level or at least 4 hours between doses at the 450-mg/day level. Equally spaced time increments throughout the day reduce the risk of seizures. The recommended dose for the sustained release formulation is 150 mg daily for 3 days, then 150 mg twice daily thereafter.

MAPROTILINE

Maprotiline is a tetracyclic antidepressant with chemical properties similar to TCAs. It blocks only the reuptake of norepinephrine at the synapse, not serotonin. It retains some anticholinergic properties.

Although maprotiline shares the same adverse effect profile as that of TCAs, there may be a higher incidence of seizures, even in patients with no known seizure disorder. Seizures are most likely to occur when recommended doses are exceeded. Concurrent administration of other drugs known to lower the seizure threshold are to be avoided. There are a multitude of drug-drug interactions.

Maprotiline is slowly absorbed from the GI tract with peak plasma concentrations reached 8 to 24 hours after administration. Steady state is achieved in 7 days. It is metabolized in the liver to desmethylmaprotiline, which is an active compound. The plasma elimination half-life is 51 hours. One-third is eliminated in the feces and two-thirds in the urine.

The initial adult dose of maprotiline is 25 to 75 mg/day in divided doses. After the second week of therapy, the dose may be increased in 25-mg increments to be taken at bedtime. Titration should be slow, and the highest recommended dose in outpatients is 150 mg. Ocasionally, doses up to 250 mg may be required for severely depressed inpatients. Some patients may require up to 225 mg/day. The total daily dose may be given as a single dose at bedtime once the maintenance dose has been determined.

MIRTAZAPINE

Mirtazapine (Remeron) is the newest antidepressant available. It has a tetracyclic molecular structure and is chemically unrelated to SSRIs, TCAs, and MAOIs. Although its exact mechanism of action is unknown, it is thought to enhance central noradrenergic and serotonergic activity, and acts as an antagonist at presynaptic $alpha_2$ adrenergic inhibitory autoreceptors. It also blocks 5-HT2 and 5-HT3 receptors, and thus is not associated with the nausea, sexual dysfunction, nervousness, diarrhea, or insomnia that is relatively common with the use of SSRIs.

Its adverse effect profile includes weight gain and sedation, both of which are related to its affinity for histamine (H2) receptors. It is also a moderate peripheral $alpha_1$ adrenergic antagonist, which is associated with orthostatic hypotension.

Mirtazapine is rapidly absorbed following oral administration and has a half-life of 20 to 40 hours. Peak plasma concentrations are reached 2 hours after an oral dose. It has a bioavailability of 50 percent and is elimmated predominantly in the urine (75 percent) and feces (15 percent).

Women demonstrate a significantly longer half-life than men (37 hours versus 26 hours) and steady state plasma levels are reached in 5 days.

Clearance is reduced by 30 percent in patients with hepatic impairment and by 30 to 50 percent in those with moderate to severe renal impairment. Clearance in elderly men is 40 percent lower, whereas in elderly women, it is only reduced by 10 percent.

NEFAZODONE

Nefazodone is most helpful in the treatment of depression characterized by prominent anxiety and sleep disturbances. It is potent, blocking postsynaptic serotonin receptors while simultaneously inhibiting presynaptic serotonin and norepinephrine reuptake. It also antagonizes $alpha_1$ receptors.

Common adverse effects of nefazodone include headache, nervousness, insomnia, drowsiness, anxiety, tremor, dizziness and lightheadedness. GI effects may include anorexia, altered taste, nausea, vomiting, dry mouth, dyspepsia, and constipation. Postural hypotension is also possible. Sweating, rash, and pruritus have also been noted.

Nefazodone is rapidly and completely absorbed after oral administration, but it has a bioavailability of approximately 20 percent. Peak plasma concentrations occur in 1 hour. Nefazodone is subject to an extensive first-pass effect. The half-life is dose dependent, increasing from 1 hour at 50 mg to 2.4 hours at 300 mg. After multiple doses of 200 to 300 mg, the elimination half-life is increased to 3 to 4 hours. Nefazodone is extensively protein bound at 99 percent. Concurrent administration of another drug that is highly protein bound may cause increased free concentrations of the other drug or of nefazodone, possibly resulting in adverse events.

The initial adult dose of nefazodone is 100 mg twice daily. The dose may be increased weekly up to 600 mg/day in two divided doses. For older adults, the initial dose is reduced to 50 mg twice daily, but it may be increased weekly as patient needs dictate.

Smaller doses, slower titration, or daily late day dosing may be used to help patients through an initial period of sedation. Initial sedation sometimes limits nefazodone's usefulness and tolerability.

VENLAFAXINE

Venlafaxine is a drug in the newer category of serotonin-norepinephrine reuptake inhibitors. It is a phenylamine compound that is structurally unrelated to other antidepressants. It strongly inhibits the reuptake of both serotonin and norepinephrine but has no significant effect on cholinergic, histaminergic, or adrenergic receptors. It is a weak inhibitor of dopamine reuptake.

Venlafaxine has an adverse effect profile that includes nausea (especially in high or rapidly increased dosages), somnolence, nervousness, constipation, abnormal ejaculation or orgasm, dizziness, sweating, and fatigue. Venlafaxine is also associated with sustained blood pressure increases of 1 to 7 mmHg in some patients. This dose-related adverse effect occurs in approximately 13 percent of patients taking more than 300 mg/day. Only 3 percent of patients experience an increase in blood pressure at a dosage of less than 100 mg. Venlafaxine is not contraindicated in hypertensive individuals if they are well controlled on antihypertensive drugs. Venlafaxine is contraindicated in patients taking MAOIs.

Venlafaxine is well absorbed following oral administration, but undergoing extensive first-pass metabolism. Fifty-six percent of the parent compound is converted to its active metabolite O-desmethylvenlafaxine (ODV). The primary route of elimination is via the kidneys. The half-life of venlafaxine is 5 hours and that of ODV is 11 hours. Venlafaxine and ODV have low levels of protein binding, in the range of 27 percent and 30 percent, respectively. This is in contrast to the SSRIs, which are highly protein bound at 94 to 99 percent. Steady state may be reached within 24 hours.

The dosage of venlafaxine should be reduced by 25 percent in patients with renal impairment and by 50 percent in dialysis patients. A 50-percent reduction is recommended in patients with liver impairment. An extended-release preparation of venlafaxine is available, and dosing is now available on a twice-daily schedule, or in some cases, a daily schedule. A daily dose of 37.5 mg to 75 mg is usually effective for outpatients.

Critical Thinking Process

Assessment

History of Present Illness

Patients frequently complain of sad mood, feelings of emptiness or anxiety, irritability, and feeling as though they are in a black hole or bottomless pit. They often report *anhedonia* (loss of interest and pleasure in usual activities), decreased or increased appetite and weight, sleep difficulties, especially difficulty falling asleep, frequent awakening, early morning awakening with inability to return to sleep, or conversely, with excessive sleep. They may describe social isolation, demonstrate paucity of speech, and often answer questions with the phrase "I don't know." They may be fatigued, or agitated. Thoughts are slowed, vague, ruminative, and center around depressive content. An inability to focus, concentrate, or make decisions may be present. Patients may acknowledge feeling hopeless, helpless, worthless, or be excessively or even delusionally guilty. A lack of goal orientation or future orientation may be present. The patient may abuse drugs or alcohol. Social isolation is common, especially in patients with *hyperacusis* (exaggerated sensitivity and adversity to noise, voices, lights, stimulation, smells, and touch). Because of the high incidence of suicide associated with depressive disorders, the patient should be questioned directly about suicidal thoughts and impulses and his or her personal history of suicide attempts.

Patients may also present in crisis following a suicide attempt with weapons, drugs, or alcohol. Some have attempted to jump to their deaths, to hang or to maim or kill themselves in any variety of other ways. Ironically, one of the most lethal means of suicide is with overdose of TCAs. Because of their narrow therapeutic index.

Past Health History

Depression often co-exists with other medical illnesses, such as cancer, irritable bowel syndrome, endocrine disorders (e.g., diabetes or hypothyroidism), nutritional deficiencies, CNS disease (e.g., epilepsy, multiple sclerosis, stroke, Parkinson's disease, Alzheimer's disease), chronic pain, chronic infections, and connective tissue disorders (e.g., rheumatoid arthritis, fibromyalgia, polymyalgia rheumatica). Further, psychiatric disorders are closely associated with the presence of arthritis, heart disease, neurologic disorders, and chronic lung disease.

Depression can present as a single episode or, more often, tends to recur in vulnerable individuals. Therefore, it is important to determine if the patient has a history of depression. A personal or family history of depression, bipolar disorder, substance abuse, violence, panic, attention deficit disorder, obsessive-compulsive disorder, anorexia or bulimia, anxiety, or suicide attempts are all potentially important factors to note.

Physical Exam Findings

In most cases of depression, there are few exact physical exam findings. Weight gain or loss may be noted, but otherwise indications of depression are at the emotional and psychosocial levels (see the box entitled Common Symptoms of Depression).

Diagnostic Testing

Diagnosis of depression is made on the basis of DSM-IV criteria, after other treatable causes of depressive-like illness are ruled out. Testing used to rule out other diseases include CBC, liver, thyroid, and renal function testing, urinalysis, electrolytes, and vitamin B_{12} and folate levels. Serologic tests for infectious disease as well as an electocardiogram may be performed if the patient history warrants.

Various screening tools and depression scales are available to assist in making a diagnosis of depression. Among those most commonly used by psychologists are the Beck Depression Inventory and the Hamilton Depression Scale. The Zung Depression Scale is a simple screening instrument that can be used in any outpatient office by any screener.

Developmental Considerations

Perinatal Adjustment reaction with depressed mood is known as postpartum, maternal, or so-called baby blues. It occurs in at least 50 percent of all women. It is a common, short-lived, early-onset disorder depicted by mild depression, anxiety, crying episodes, headache, fatigue, and irritability. It is more severe with first births and seems related to the rapid alterations of estrogen, progesterone, and prolactin levels after birth. Women with histories of mood disorders are especially vulnerable during the postpartum period.

Pediatric Traditionally, depression was thought to occur only after the age of 15; however, in recent years, health care providers are recognizing the existence of depression in younger children. Girls are more likely to suffer from depression than boys, and it is more prevalent in adolescents than in children. Estimates of its prevalence vary considerably because of the diverse diagnostic criteria used, and the differences in presentation between children and adults.

Risk factors for depression can be genetic, environmental, and psychosocial. If one parent has a depressive disorder, the risk of depression for the offspring is 27 to 29 percent. If both parents are affected, the risk increases to 74 to 76 percent.

Psychosocial factors play a part in putting children at risk for depression. Early trauma, self-blame, rigid family dynamics, disturbance in mother-child relationships, or an unresolved loss have been reported to be precursors to depression. Other contributing factors may include loss of self-esteem, learning disabilities, chronic illness, or physical deformity.

Clinical manifestations of depression vary across the lifespan, but in essence, they are developmentally specific. During infancy, the manifestations are noted as biologic and deprivation syndromes. During early childhood (3 to 4 years of age), abnormal motor activity is most notable, with more observable episodes of sadness during the ages of 5 to 8 years. The child is not reflective in character. During late childhood (9 to 12 years of age) low self-esteem and disappointment with self are characteristic. Adolescence heralds much the same signs and symptoms as those of an adult but may also manifest as anorexia nervosa, somatization disorders, and looking at options as an inflexible all-or-none manner. It should be kept in mind that children and adolescents are also vulnerable to suicide attempts.

Case Study Major Depression

Patient History

History of Present Illness	MG is a 42-year-old white female with complaints of sad mood, intermittent crying, hypersomnia, and lack of appetite. She has decreased energy, focus, and concentration. She notes feelings of hopelessness and helplessness, anhedonia, and vague suicidal ideation. These patterns have persisted for 8 weeks.
Past Health History	MG has a history of mild depression, no drug or alcohol abuse. She is a nonsmoker. There is a family history of depression, Alzheimer's disease, and alcoholism. She has a history of head injury 4 years ago secondary to a fall but takes no medications.
Physical Exam Findings	Unremarkable. VSS.
Diagnostic Testing	MG meets DSM-IV criteria for major depression.
Developmental Considerations	MG is a healthy middle-aged woman. She is in a supportive, consistent relationship with a husband of 17 years.
Psychosocial Considerations	MG is gainfully employed in a responsible, executive position. Her degree of compliance is judged to be adequate, although she leads a very busy life, has a hectic schedule, and frequently travels on business.
Economic Factors	MG has health insurance that covers prescriptions.

Variables Influencing Decision

Treatment Objectives	• Relieve major depression. • Re-establish sleeping, eating, and normal ADL patterns.

Drug Variables	*Drug Summary*	*Patient Variables*
Indications	Antidepressants are used in the treatment of major depression.	This is a decision point because MG has been diagnosed with a major depression (unipolar without psychotic features).
Pharmacodynamics	All drugs are effective in treatment of major depression with similar efficacy.	All antidepressants have roughly equal response rates. This will not be a decision point.
Adverse Effects/ Contraindications	TCAs: Lethal in suicide attempt. Cardiotoxic potential, sedation. SSRIs: Nausea, dizziness, sexual adverse effects MAOIs: Lethal in overdose, severe dietary restrictions. If not observed, can lead to hypertensive crisis, CVA, possible death. Bupropion: Increased incidence of seizures, contraindicated with head injury, bulimia. Venlafaxine: Nausea, BP elevation	This will be a decision point due to broad variation in adverse effects. Bupropion contraindicated due to MG's history of head injury. TCAs potentially fatal in overdose, and MG does have suicidal ideation. MAOIs not practical owing to problematic adverse effects and considerable dietary restrictions, which may be difficult or impossible to follow owing to MG's business travel and hectic life.

Case Study continued on following page

Drug Variables	Drug Summary	Patient Variables
Pharmacokinetics	Drugs all have different pharmacokinetics, half-lives. Venlafaxine may have a more rapid onset of action, but requires BID-TID dosing and titration. Fluoxetine has a very long half-life and may be administered every other day, or if doses are omitted, antidepressant effect is usually not lost	All drugs have different pharmacokinetics. Half-life is important for MG because of her business travel and hectic schedule, which may lead to missed doses, at least occasionally. Fluoxetine represents a substantial advantage. MG has no serious health problems and takes no other drugs. This is a decision point.
Dosage Regimen	Antidepressant therapy is generally long term, especially when there is a history of recurrent depression or family history. All drugs would have to be continued at least 6 months following resolution of this depression	MG is autonomous and long-term compliance is not expected to be an issue since finances or motivation are not problems. This is not expected to be a decision point.
Lab Considerations	Newer drugs do not require the close monitoring as older agents. Some TCAs, especially nortriptyline, require close monitoring.	Lack of frequent laboratory monitoring would enhance compliance and safety owing to irregular schedule and travel. This will be a decision point.
Cost Index*	Fluoxetine: 3 Venlafaxine: 5 Bupropion: 4 Nefazodone: 4	MG has health insurance that covers medications with a small co-payment. This will not be a decision point.

Summary of Decision Points

- The relative lack of adverse effects of SSRIs, venlafaxine, and nefazodone compared with TCAs and MAOIs weighs heavily in their favor.
- Lack of lethality in overdose is an important advantage for newer drugs, especially in light of MG's vague suicidal ideations.
- MG's business travel, hectic life-style, and irregular schedule make a drug with a long half-life a potential benefit. These factors also bode poorly for compliance with multiple doses per day, or for observing dietary restrictions imposed with MAOIs.
- Lack of required laboratory testing with SSRIs, bupropion, venlafaxine, and nefazodone is advantageous.
- MG's history of head injury makes bupropion a relative contraindication.
- MG does have access to insurance coverage.
- MG's depression does not have psychotic features or an associated mania.

DRUGS TO BE USED

- Fluoxetine 20 mg po daily for at least 6 months following full remission of depressive symptoms.

*Cost Index:	
1	$ <30/mo
2	$ 30–40/mo
3	$ 40–50/mo
4	$ 50–60/mo
5	$ >60/mo

AWP of 90, 20-mg capsules of fluoxetine is approximately $200
AWP of 100, 25-mg tablets of venlafaxine is approximately $90
AWP of 100, 75-mg tablets of bupropion is approximately $58
AWP of 60, 100-mg tablets of nefazodone is approximately $52

ADL, Activities of daily living;
BP, blood pressure;
CVA, cerebrovascular accident;
MAOI, monoamine oxidase inhibitor;
SSRI, selective serotonin reuptake inhibitor;
TCA, tricyclic antidepressant.

Geriatric Depression is common but treatable in the elderly. Older adults who are depressed are more likely to present with somatic complaints rather than reports of depressed mood. The suicide rate increases with age and is highest among older white men. Twenty-three percent of all suicides involve older adults. Drug misuse, either in the form of overdosages or omission of dosages, may be a suicidal gesture. Self-starvation is another sign and can occur even in an institutional setting if staff members are not attentive to monitoring intake and nutritional status.

Depression in the older adult may actually be difficult to differentiate from delirium or especially dementia. Older adults with medical and neurologic illnesses, bereavement, history of depression, alcohol use, and polypharmacy are vulnerable to depressive disorders. Depression is common (25-percent incidence) in nursing home populations.

Psychosocial

Depression is still an extremely stigmatized medical disorder. There are widespread misconceptions about the cause, treatment, existence, and degree of suffering and impairment caused by depression. Depression may be erroneously regarded as merely feeling blue or a character weakness, or something the patient can recover from quickly. For this reason, many individuals are reluctant to take drugs or fear discussing the illness with their families, friends, or employers.

Patients also fear becoming dependent to antidepressants and misunderstand the need for daily dosing. Often they do not accept the idea that they have to depend on a drug, especially on a long-term basis, to help them manage something they feel they should be naturally and inherently able to manage. Some patients refer to antidepressants as "happy pills," suspecting that they will induce euphoria, which they do not. (See the Case Study—Major Depression.)

Analysis and Management

Treatment Objectives

The objectives of acute treatment for patients with depression include reduction and ultimate removal of the signs and symptoms of the depressive disorder, and to restore occupational and psychosocial functioning to that of the asymptomatic state. Objectives for the patient with chronic depression include reducing the likelihood of relapse or recurrence. To accomplish these objectives, rapid stabilization of mood, establishment of euthymia (normal mood), establishment of normal sleep and eating patterns; prevention of suicide or self-injurious behaviors; education concerning the course of depression, its biologic basis, and potential for recurrence; and drug management must also be addressed. This is necessary for both the patient and any significant others.

Treatment Options

TCAs, SSRIs, and the newer miscellaneous antidepressant drugs are all equally effective in the treatment of depression and related disorders. The newer antidepressant drugs, developed over the past decade, were planned, rational, pharmacologic undertakings. The newer drugs are designed to maximize efficiency, exercise greater selectivity in terms of the neurotransmitters affected, and eliminate the dangerous and annoying adverse effects of the earlier classes of drugs (e.g., MAOIs). The newer drugs represent a substantial improvement in safety, tolerability, and compliance potential, but they are not dramatically more effective than the TCAs or MAOIs in relieving depression.

Caution must be exercised in changing between classes of drugs, especially when MAOIs are being started or discontinued. Half-lives of other drugs and the biological changes that occur in response to MAOIs, and the continuing potential for severe drug-drug interactions, even once a drug is discontinued, are major considerations. This is particularly true with drugs having long half-lives (e.g., fluoxetine in succession with MAOIs or TCAs).

Drug Variables

There are a number of drug-related variables to be considered when choosing an antidepressant. The considerations certainly include the specific type of depression, short-term and long-term adverse effects, and the concomitant use of other nonpsychiatric drugs.

There is little basis for choosing one TCA over another, but some patients may respond better or tolerate one drug over another. Initial selection of a specific TCA is based on the patient's previous response and susceptibility to adverse effects. For example, if a patient (or close family member) responded well to a specific drug in the past, that drug should be used for recurring episodes of depression. The drug response of family members is significant because there is a distinct genetic component to depression and drug response. Imipramine and amitriptyline are the most commonly used TCAs. If therapeutic effects do not occur within about 6 weeks, the TCA should be discontinued or changed.

The SSRIs have overtaken the TCAs as drugs of first choice, however. They are considered safe, effective, have a wide therapeutic index, are not fatal in overdose, and generally produce fewer and milder adverse effects than the TCAs. The majority offer a convenient once-daily dosing schedule. Fluoxetine may even be administered every other day or three times per week due to its extremely long half-life. The biggest drawback is the potential to dampen sexual desire or response. This potential can often be ameliorated by administering cyproheptadine, yohimbine, buspirone, bupropion, or planning brief drug holidays.

Bupropion is also an effective antidepressant, but it has potentially serious adverse effects. This is especially so with larger than recommended dosages.

Because of its short half-life, venlafaxine must be dosed two to three times daily. Although this schedule creates some inconvenience and a potential issue of noncompliance, it also has some advantages. These advantages include rapid attainment of steady state and quick withdrawal from the drug should intolerable adverse effects develop. Conversely, the short half-life of venlafaxine may cause some lack of antidepressant action if one or more doses are inadvertently omitted. Patients may initially resist taking a drug two to three times daily, but if their response is dramatic and beneficial, the resistance is generally overcome.

The newer extended release formulations of both venlafaxine and bupropion make dosing much more convenient (daily or twice daily) and minimize the risks and adverse effects of these very effective drugs.

There are many disadvantages to using MAOIs. Their problematic adverse effect profile, narrow therapeutic index, considerable and cumbersome dietary restrictions, potential for hypertensive crisis, stroke, death, and drug-drug interactions significantly limit their outpatient use. It should clearly be reserved as a last choice for seriously refractory patients who are highly motivated and capable of full cooperation. These drugs should be used by a skilled health care provider who is intimately familiar with their management.

The cost of the newer drugs is similar, and surprisingly, some of the older TCAs are more expensive than newer drugs. Cost also varies substantially from pharmacy to pharmacy. The bioequivalence among generic formulations should be considered when one selects an antidepressant.

Patient Variables

The antidepressant selected should be based on patient variables: personal and family history of response to particular antidepressants, safety issues, potential for adverse effects, drug-drug interactions, the patient's ability to comply with dosing frequency requirements, any financial considerations, potential for suicide, and concomitant drug use, including those taken for nonpsychiatric problems, as well as over-the-counter (OTC) drugs (see the Controversy box—PROZAC: A Drug for all Occasions?).

Most newer drugs can be safely used with most patients. Dosage adjustments and titration steps may have to be adjusted downward for the very young, older adults, and those with hepatic or renal illness. Concomitant drug use and medical conditions should be thoroughly assessed before any antidepressant is chosen and appropriate adjustments made in the management plan.

The patient's ability to cooperate with a particular dosing schedule should be considered, because the dosing requirements of the newer drugs are variable. The patient's ability to access drugs should also be assessed. Insurance and financial resources need not be the ultimate limiting factor. Further, lack of financial resources does not necessarily mean that a less desirable or more problematic drug should be used. Health care providers, however, need to be very active partners and advocates for patients to help them obtain the drug. Drug manufacturers take seriously their responsibility to enhance access to their drugs. Local pharmaceutical company representatives are excellent resources for samples, information, patient educational materials, and research studies. They support both patients and health care providers. At least two companies (Eli Lilly and Pfizer) also have computerized patient participation programs to provide patients with information and ongoing support, as well as feedback for the health care provider.

The benefits of treating depression in elderly patients outweigh the risks of not treating or undertreating the problem. Complications of not treating depression in the elderly include chronic depression, cognitive impairment, poor resolution of medical illnesses, poor compliance with medical treatment, social dysfunction, risk of premature death from cardiac illness or cancer, and suicide.

Interventions

Administration

Therapy with antidepressants requires a certain amount of planning and preparation to enhance daily administration. Because some antidepressants may be taken up to four times daily, the patient must plan for drug administration while at work, school, away from the home, or on vacation. The patient needs to take the drug as prescribed and not on an as-needed basis. The drug should not be discontinued once the mood has improved, because doing so may cause relapse. In many cases, once an effective dose has been established, the entire daily dose can be taken at bedtime. The antidepressant may be taken with food without interfering with absorption to any great extent. Antidepressants are taken long term and, in some cases, such as patients with recurring depression, on a life-long basis.

Missed doses of drugs with short half-lives may cause some loss of antidepressant effect or some flulike withdrawal

---

Controversy

PROZAC: A Drug for All Occasions?
JONATHAN J. WOLFE

Fluoxetine (PROZAC) has aroused controversy since its debut in the United States. Some health care providers consider it a callously overprescribed drug and patients receiving it as victims of reckless prescribing. Others have ascribed impropriety to patients for demanding the drug from physicians. Bizarre behavior exhibited by some patients taking fluoxetine led to charges that the drug was inherently hazardous and played no proper role in disease management. But fluoxetine has proved to be an effective antidepressant, causing fewer adverse effects than previous generations of drugs.

Now fluoxetine is being linked to another aspect of contemporary culture—the role of prescription drugs for the treatment of obesity. Concern with physical appearance threatens to make the definition of obesity revolve around individual preference. Many patients seem to assume the central role in defining their need for drugs to control weight gain.

The withdrawal of fenfluramine and dexfenfluramine (each a component of Phen-Fen regimens for appetite suppression) from the American market occurred as a result of evidence suggesting severe cardiovascular adverse effects. Despite widespread reluctance among licensing boards to approve general use of phentermine with these drugs, remarkably large numbers of patients had accepted the treatment. The withdrawal seemed to generate a crisis and patients along with some health care providers avidly sought a replacement. Phen-Pro (phentermine and PROZAC) has been suggested as an alternative. It is instructive to note that Eli Lilly & Company, developer and marketer of PROZAC, firmly resists any promotion of its drug for use in treating obesity. Indeed, the anorexiant use of all these drug entities represents off-label use, the application of a drug to conditions that have not been clinically tested. No prudent pharmaceutical company would allow such promotion.

Critical Thinking Discussion

- What health hazards of obesity are sufficient to justify to your conscience the risk involved in prescription drug use for appetite suppression?
- What concerns do you believe underlie a patient's request for potent prescription drugs in treating obesity?
- What support can you render to the concerned patient whose Phen-Fen therapy has been suddenly cut off by removal of one drug from the market?
- Under what circumstances would you participate in patient treatment for obesity involving the use of fluoxetine?
- Would your willingness to take part in obesity treatment with fluoxetine vary with the age of your patient?

symptoms. However, patients may be directed to omit weekend doses of SSRIs with short half-lives in anticipation of sexual activity. This may actually allow for greater sexual sensation and function without significant loss of antidepressant effect and perhaps encourage the patient's compliance with ongoing administration.

Blood pressure should be carefully monitored during initiation of drug therapy with MAOIs to evaluate orthostatic hypotension or a pressor response. MAOIs should be discontinued immediately if a hypertensive crisis occurs and the patient treated with an alpha-adrenergic blocking drug, such as intravenous phentolamine. This approach will lower blood pressure and resolve the intense headache. Fever may be treated with external cooling.

Education

The importance of compliance with the treatment regimen should be reinforced, especially when drug therapy is first started because a lag time of 2 to 12 weeks may pass before the patient feels substantial benefit. Patients should also be warned at the start of therapy that it is common to have to titrate, augment, or change drugs if sufficient response is not obtained or if adverse effects limit the use of a specific drug.

Patients should be advised to avoid alcohol and other CNS depressants. Patients receiving MAOIs should also avoid OTC drugs and foods or beverages containing tyramine during therapy and for at least 2 weeks after therapy has been discontinued. Foods containing high levels of tyramine include all aged cheeses, fermented beverages (particularly vermouth and chianti wines), pickled and smoked meats (sausages, pepperoni, salami, bologna, liver, Spam, canned ham), soy sauce, tap beer, and broad bean pods. Any fermented meat, fish or protein food product or extracts, yeast extracts (marmite, brewer's yeast tablets), and sauerkraut should be avoided (see Appendix C). Patients should be warned verbally and in writing that if any signs or symptoms of hypertensive crisis occur, to proceed immediately to an emergency care center. Warning signs include intense, pounding headache; sweating; flushing; rapid heartbeat; dizziness; faintness; chest pain; and neck stiffness.

The patient should be informed that drowsiness or dizziness may occur secondary to antidepressants. Caution the patient to avoid driving or operating machinery or other activities that require alertness until response to the drug is known. Patients should also be informed about the possibility of hypotension (dizziness, lightheadedness) and be advised to sit or lie down if they occur.

A Medic-alert bracelet or necklace should be worn at all times by the patient taking MAOIs. Hostesses and restaurants should be informed of dietary restrictions. Inform the patient to notify the surgeon or dentist of the drug regimen before treatment or surgery. MAOI therapy is usually withdrawn for at least 2 weeks before the use of anesthetics.

Advise the patient that dry mouth, urinary retention, or constipation may occur with antidepressants. The health care provider should be notified if these adverse effects occur. Frequent mouth rinses, good oral hygiene, and sugarless candy or gum may diminish the dry mouth. An increase in fluid intake, fiber, and exercise may prevent constipation.

Treatment of depression with drugs alone is not optimal therapy. Emotional support and traditional psychotherapy can complement and reinforce responses to antidepressants. Thus, patients should be provided with resources and information necessary to pursue additional therapy.

Evaluation

Indications that pharmacotherapeutic interventions are successful include resolution of depression and restoration of euthymia (without invoking mania), resolution of a psychotic process if those symptoms were initially present (coadministration of an antipsychotic drug is generally required), and a therapeutic, nonproblematic physiologic response to the drug. If adverse effects develop, they are tolerable, not life threatening, and do not jeopardize compliance. Sleep, eating, and activity patterns return to normal. Suicidality resolves. The patient and family express knowledge and some degree of acceptance of depression, and they demonstrate an awareness of the nature, course, and treatment of depression.

Additionally, the patient has a means of accessing ongoing care and drug therapy and actually does access it. The patient is aware of psychosocial supports and rights as a disabled person under the Americans with Disabilities Act. Further, the patient expresses a desire to stop concomitant use of alcohol and street drugs.

BIPOLAR DISORDER

Epidemiology and Etiology

Bipolar disorder (previously known as manic-depressive disorder) is a mood disorder characterized by expansive emotional states, flight of ideas, hyperactivity, destructive behaviors, and psychotic processes. It consists of periods of depression, alternating with mania, usually separated by periods of near-normal euthymic functioning. Bipolar disorder affects at least three million people in the United States. It disrupts relationships, careers, families, contributing to billions of dollars in direct and indirect costs, and a number of deaths by suicide or recklessness.

Pathophysiology

Mania is thought to be caused by dysregulation of some of the same neurotransmitters that cause depression (i.e., serotonin, norepinephrine, dopamine, and perhaps an excitatory neurotransmitter, glutamate.) In theory, if a relative lack of neurotransmitters contributes to depression, then a relative excess may contribute to what appears to be an opposite mood state of mania.

Forms of Bipolar Disorder

Hypomania

Hypomania is an expansive, energized portion of the mood cycle, characterized by disturbances in speech, cognition, judgment, self-concept, and behavior. Hypomania is a mood state that must last at least 4 days. Accompanying this mood are other disturbances, such as inflated self-esteem, flight of ideas, distractibility, increased involvement in goal-directed activity, or psychomotor agitation. Another symptom of hypomania is excessive involvement in pleasurable activities that have a high potential for painful consequences. Hypomania may progress in some individuals to full mania, which is characterized by a more amplified and sustained version of hypomania, as well as delusions or hallucinations.

Mania

A full *manic* mood state lasts at least a week and is accompanied by the other characteristics that were noted previously. The disturbance is severe enough to cause significant impairment in social or occupational functioning. In some cases, hospitalization is required. The mood is often euphoric, and at least initially, it has an infectious quality. It is characterized by unceasing, indiscriminate enthusiasm and may be intrusive. The mood, however, may be consistently irritable or labile, alternating between euphoria and irritability.

It is common for an individual in a manic state to give advice to anyone encountered, write letters, or communicate with government officials or company presidents, offering direction. Manics may believe that they have a special relationship with famous people or religious figures, including God. Manic individuals may dress in loud clothing or wear excessive makeup, jewelry, or extreme hairstyles. There is almost invariably a decreased need for sleep, and the person may not sleep at all for days at a time. Manic speech is typically loud, pressured, tangential, nonstop, rapid, and difficult to interrupt. Irritable manics are critical and cutting. Manic individuals complain of racing thoughts that cannot be stopped or slowed down. While acutely manic, they frequently engage in reckless and dangerous activities; excessive, inappropriate, or unprotected sex; poor business investments and decisions; and buying sprees, and they may exercise poor judgment in other areas of life. These activities are all pursued despite the painful consequences the acts may cause. The patient's appetite is usually decreased, or at least the person is unable to devote any time to eating. Many thousands of calories may be expended while the patient is engaged in frantic activity, and it is common for him or her to lose weight during a manic episode. The person also does not recognize illness and resists treatment, often adamantly. Hallucinations or delusions must be present, and are the defining characteristics that delineate hypomania from full mania.

Mixed Mania

Mixed mania is characterized by a concurrent blend of mania and depression. It is estimated that approximately 40 percent of all patients with mania present with a mixture of depressed mood and hyperactivity. They report feeling dysphoric, depressed, and unhappy yet exhibit the characteristic energy associated with mania. This state is often complicated by concomitant substance abuse. It is very common to find bipolar patients (as well as psychiatric patients with any other type of mood or thought disorder) attempting to self-medicate with drugs and alcohol. Alcohol, heroin, benzodiazepines, marijuana, and sedative-hypnotics impart a sense of calmness to manic patients. Cocaine and amphetamines may be used by depressed patients to feel more energized or euthymic.

Bipolar patients may cycle only a few times within a lifetime, or they may cycle once or twice a year. Patients with rapid cycling bipolar disorder may have four or more distinct, complete cycles within a year. Some patients with ultrarapid cycling describe almost constant, quick up and down cycling.

PHARMACOTHERAPEUTIC OPTIONS

Mood-Stabilizing Drugs

- ❒ Carbamazepine (TEGRETOL, EPITOL); (✱) APO-CARBAMAZEPINE, MAZEPINE, NOVO-CARBAMAZ
- ❒ Lithium (DURALITH, ESKALITH, LITHANE, LITHONATE, LITHOTABS); (✱) CARBOLITH, LITHIZINE
- ❒ Valproic acid (DEPAKENE, DEPAKOTE)

Indications

The first-line drug used for symptomatic control of bipolar disorders is lithium. Its beneficial effects were first noted in 1949. However, because of concerns about toxicity, it was not approved for use in the United States until 1970. At present, carbamazepine and valproic acid are used for patients who fail to respond to lithium or who cannot tolerate lithium's adverse effects. These mood stabilizing drugs (i.e., carbamazepine, valproate) are most often used for the treatment of rapid-cycling bipolar disorder.

Carbamazepine is an effective treatment for acute mania and bipolar prophylaxis. During acute mania, it is ordinarily used in conjunction with an antipsychotic (see Chapter 19). When it is given to patients who have failed lithium therapy, the success rate is about 60 percent. Carbamazepine structurally resembles imipramine and other TCAs. It was first used during the 1960s for the treatment of trigeminal neuralgia and various convulsive disorders, including temporal lobe epilepsy. In the late 1960s, a series of worldwide investigations found that carbamazepine exerts potent antimanic effects. At present, it is not FDA approved for the treatment of mania but is commonly used both alone and in combination with other drugs.

Valproic acid was also originally used as an anticonvulsant drug, and in 1995, it was approved by the FDA for the treatment of mania. It has been widely used to treat seizures of various types. In 1966, the mood-stabilizing effects of valproic acid were first described. As scrutiny of the compound moved through early studies, it became clear that valproic acid consistently demonstrated some additional degree of efficacy in comparison with other drugs and improved the baseline symptoms of mania.

Pharmacodynamics

The exact mechanism of action of mood-stabilizing drugs is unknown. It is thought that carbamazepine and valproic acid may work by reducing the amount of neurotransmitters at the synapse or by increasing the levels of GABA, an inhibitory neurotransmitter. Lithium may impart some antidepressant effect by enhancement of beta receptor activity. Its antimanic properties may be related to its ability to dampen the brain's response to glutamate.

Carbamazepine has antimanic, anticholinergic, antidepressant, and sedative properties, and it is structurally related to the TCAs. Although its mechanism of antimanic action is unknown, early research focused on its ability to inhibit kindling. *Kindling* represents a process in which increasing behavioral and convulsive responses occur in response to repetition of the same stimulus, repeated over time. Some type of antikindling mechanism may be integral to its therapeutic and prophylactic effects in mania.

Adverse Effects and Contraindications

Lithium has a narrow therapeutic index and potentially lethal toxicity. The adverse effects of lithium can be categorized as those that occur at therapeutic levels and those that are most likely to occur at toxic levels. Several responses occur early in treatment at levels that are within the therapeutic range (i.e., below 1.5 mEq/L) and then usually resolve. These responses may include GI effects (e.g., anorexia, nausea, bloating, and diarrhea) and transient headache, fatigue, confusion, memory impairment, and muscle weakness in 30 percent of patients. Thirty to fifty percent of patients experience thirst and polyuria early in treatment. In 50 to 70 percent of cases, the thirst and polyuria continue with chronic lithium use.

Drug-induced fine hand tremors that interfere with writing and other motor skills may be noted. The tremors are worsened by stress, fatigue, and certain drugs such as caffeine, antidepressants, or antipsychotics. They can be reduced with the concurrent use of propranolol, a beta-blocking drug, and by dose reduction, use of divided doses, or the use of sustained-release formulations.

Although it is usually a benign state, hypothyroidism is sometimes associated with a lithium-induced goiter. Synthetic thyroid hormone is often required to restore a euthyroid state. Renal toxicity has been associated with degenerative changes in the kidney and most often is a problem in the aging individual.

Mild benign leukocytosis (10,000 to 18,000/mm^3) and dermatologic reactions such as psoriasis, acne, folliculitis, and alopecia have been noted with lithium use. These problems usually respond to a dose reduction or discontinuation. Lithium is a teratogen, and its use is discouraged during the first trimester of pregnancy. Cardiovascular abnormalities, including Ebstein's anomaly, are known to occur in the fetus.

The most serious adverse effect of lithium is intoxication (i.e., serum levels exceeding 1.5 mEq/L). The risk of intoxication is related to the magnitude and duration of exposure and individual susceptibility. Severe toxicity is associated with myoclonic jerks, seizures, impaired consciousness, coma, and ultimately, death. Renal failure and nephrogenic diabetes insipidus are common consequences of toxicity. Although toxicity usually resolves without complications once dosages are lowered or stopped, some patients die and others develop persistent neurologic disability. The most common cause of lithium accumulation in compliant patients is sodium depletion and dehydration, which reduces the volume of distribution of lithium and increases lithium levels.

Serum lithium levels of 1.5 to 2.5 mEq/L represent moderate intoxication, levels of 2.5 to 3.5 mEq/L represent severe intoxication, and levels in excess of 3.5 mEq/L are usually fatal. Even when lithium is immediately discontinued, a week or more of vigorous hydration may be required to cause levels to drop substantially.

The adverse effects of carbamazepine primarily include drowsiness and ataxia. Other adverse effects include blurred vision, blood pressure alterations, urinary hesitancy and retention, rashes, urticaria, and photosensitivity. The most severe effects include congestive heart failure, pneumonitis, hepatitis, aplastic anemia, agranulocytosis, and thrombocytopenia. Leukopenia, leukocytosis, and eosinophilia may be noted. Carbamazepine and valproic acid are also known teratogens and should be avoided during pregnancy, especially during the first trimester.

Valproic acid has been associated with indigestion, nausea, and vomiting most commonly. Hepatotoxicity is the most serious adverse effect. Other adverse effects include drowsiness, sedation, headache, dizziness, ataxia, and confusion. Anorexia, increased appetite, diarrhea, and constipation have been noted in some patients. Prolonged bleeding times, leukopenia, and thrombocytopenia can occur.

Pharmacokinetics

Lithium is rapidly and completely absorbed within the GI tract in one to two hours. It is widely distributed to many tissues and body fluids, crossing placental membranes and entering breast milk in low concentrations. It is excreted unchanged by the kidneys, and has a half-life of 20 to 27 hours (see Table 18–2).

The absorption of carbamazepine is slow, but it is almost completely absorbed from the GI tract. Peak concentration when using the oral suspension is attained in 1 1/2 hours, and with tablets, in 4 to 5 hours. It is moderately protein bound at 55 to 60 percent in children and 75 percent in adults. It is biotransformed in the liver and may induce its own metabolism as well as that of many other drugs. With repeated dosing, the half-life is 8 to 29 hours, with an average of 12 to 17 hours. Elimination is 72 percent renal and 28 percent fecal.

Valproic acid is rapidly and well absorbed from the GI tract. The divalproex sodium formulation is enteric coated, so absorption is delayed by 1 to 4 hours. Food may significantly slow the rate but not the extent of absorption. It is rapidly distributed to plasma and extracellular fluids, crossing the blood-brain barrier, placental membranes, and breast milk. Peak serum concentrations are reached 1 to 4 hours after administration of the capsule or syrup. Delayed-release capsules reach peak serum concentrations in 3 to 4 hours. Valproic acid is highly protein bound at 90 to 95 percent at serum concentrations of 50 mcg/mL. With serum concentrations of 50 to 100 mcg/mL the percentage of protein binding is 80 to 85 percent. Further, the free-fraction becomes larger, increasing the concentration gradient to the brain. It is primarily biotransformed in the liver, with minimal amounts excreted unchanged in the urine.

Drug-Drug Interactions

Of the top 200 drugs prescribed in the United States in 1994, at least 25 percent interact with lithium, 42 percent interact with carbamazepine, and 5 percent interact with valproic acid (see Table 18–3). Lithium is neither protein bound nor biotransformed by the liver. It is filtered, reabsorbed, and excreted by the kidneys. For this reason, it is the most common cause of drug-drug interactions with other drugs affecting the rate of renal clearance of lithium. Thiazide and loop diuretics, potassium-sparing diuretics, amiloride, and nonsteroidal anti-inflammatory drugs (except aspirin) create a definite reduction in renal elimination of lithium. An especially problematic combination may be lithium, carbamazepine, and diuretics because these drugs may dramatically alter normal renal function and fluid and electrolyte balance.

Dosage Regimens

For acutely manic patients, lithium therapy is started at 300 to 600 mg three times daily (see Table 18–4). The dose is adjusted at intervals of 5 to 7 days, as needed and tolerated. Maintenance doses of 300 mg three to four times daily, or 600 mg twice daily are generally adequate. The maximum daily dose should not exceed 2400 mg. Elderly or debilitated patients should be started at 300 mg daily. The regimen should be slowly increased as required and tolerated.

Carbamazepine is usually started at 200 mg two to three times per day and is increased every 4 to 5 days or until adverse effects prohibit further increases, a clinical response occurs, or desired blood levels are reached. Total daily dosage range is typically 800 to 1200 mg. The oral suspension may produce higher peak serum concentrations and should be initiated at smaller, more frequent dosages spread out over the day.

The dosage of valproic acid is 250 mg two to three times per day or 500 mg twice a day, with doses increased over two to three days to achieve the desired effect and blood levels, or until side effects prohibit further increases. For most patients, the total daily dosage ranges from 1000 to 2500 mg/day.

Laboratory Considerations

Carbamazepine may cause elevated AST (SGOT), ALT (SGPT), serum bilirubin, blood urea nitrogen, serum protein, and urine glucose levels. Thyroid function tests and serum calcium concentrations may be decreased. Further, carbamazepine may cause false-negative pregnancy test results with methods that identify the presence of human chorionic gonadotropin.

Dose-related elevations in lactate dehydrogenase and aminotransferase may occur with valproic acid. It may also interfere with the accuracy of thyroid function tests, and produce false-positive results in urine ketone tests. Occasionally, liver function tests, including serum bilirubin, may show increases.

Critical Thinking Process

Assessment

History of Present Illness

Patients with hypomania present in an energized, expansive state with elated or irritable mood, mood lability, euphoria, or dysphoria. Patients with full mania share these characteristics but display them in an even more pronounced fashion. Cognition is notable for flight of ideas, grandiosity, paranoia, and in full mania, hallucinations, delusions, and ideas of reference. Speech is rapid, circumstantial, pressured, and voluminous. Behaviorally, the patient reports a decreased need for sleep, insomnia, appetite changes, psychomotor agitation and hyperactivity, and decreased inhibitions. Intrusiveness, distractibility, hypersexuality, poor judgment, overconfidence, hyper-religiosity, demanding and critical attitude, lack of self-restraint, manipulation, and possibly, physical assault or self-injurious behaviors may also be reported.

Past Health History

The patient's past health history may be notable for episodes or mania, depression, or both. Mania may first emerge in childhood or adolescence but more commonly appears in early adulthood. It may also emerge in later life, but this is rare. The patient may also note other problems along the illness continuum, such as affective disorder–hyperactivity disorder, panic attacks, eating disorders, anxiety, and obsessive-compulsive disorder. There may also be a family history of these disorders, especially bipolar disorder. There may be a personal or family history of drug and alcohol abuse or dependence, or unrestrained sexual behaviors.

Physical Exam Findings

There are few definitive physical exam findings associated with bipolar disorders. However, a patient in the manic phase may have an elevated pulse rate and blood pressure.

Diagnostic Testing

There are no reliable laboratory tests that confirm the presence of bipolar disorder, but rather it is diagnosed by ruling out other organic causes and then by meeting DSM IV diagnostic criteria. Psychologists may administer psychometric testing to substantiate or rule out a diagnosis of bipolar disorder.

Developmental Considerations

Perinatal A decision to use mood-stabilizing drugs during pregnancy must be weighed against the risk of untreated bipolar disorder and the efficiency and teratogenic risk of the proposed drug. If therapy is continued during pregnancy, it should be carefully monitored, as physiologic and pathologic complications of pregnancy (e.g., increased glomerular filtration rate, sodium retention, edema, hypertension) can alter blood concentrations in the newborn. ECT may be a safer strategy for controlling mania in a pregnant woman. Pharmacotherapy may be resumed after delivery to reduce risk of relapse.

Pediatric The occurrence of true mánia in children is somewhat unusual, or it may be difficult to differentiate from attention deficit hyeractivity disorder, depression, oppositional defiant disorder, or other problems that are more common in children. Careful evaluation should be undertaken by qualified child experts in assessing psychiatric, psychological, medical, and neurologic bases for behavior resembling bipolar disorder.

Geriatric Older adults are at risk for mood disorders much like other population groups. The misuse, however, of psychoactive drugs may obscure an undiagnosed medical etiology, increase the risk of falls and hypotensive reactions, or allow use of drugs as a quick solution when environmental or interpersonal interventions would be far more appropriate. Because of these concerns, a set of federal guidelines have been constructed for the rational use of psychoactive

Case Study Rapid-Cycle Bipolar Disorder

Patient History

History of Present Illness	SN is a 26-year-old female with complaints of frequent, rapid mood fluctuations for the past several years. She reports at least four complete mood cycles per year. When depressed, she has feelings of irritable mood, crying, hopelessness, helplessness, insomnia, decreased appetite, and weight loss. She loses interest in usually pleasurable activities and is unable to care for her 2-year-old son. She has made a suicide attempt by ingestion of large amounts of alcohol, benzodiazepine tranquilizers, and aspirin. When her mood is elevated, she feels alternatively euphoric and irritable; may not sleep for several days at a time; has engaged in reckless activities; and exercises poor judgment in relationships, sexual encounters, and care of her child. She tends to wear excessive makeup and jewelry when manic, and spends large amounts of money and charges her credit cards beyond their limit.
Past Health History	SN past health history is unremarkable. She smokes 1 pack per day of cigarettes and drinks alcohol primarily when manic but occasionally while depressed. She has one child by vaginal delivery. She has no known allergies and no renal, hepatic, or coagulation problems. She is taking oral contraceptives.
Physical Exam Findings	VSS. Underweight woman with no physical stigmata. Otherwise the exam was unremarkable.
Diagnostic Testing	SN meets DSM-IV criteria for rapid-cycle bipolar disorder.
Developmental Considerations	Although she is a single parent, SN expresses interest in having another child before age 30.
Psychosocial Considerations	SN lives on emergency assistance from the state because she has been unable to maintain employment owing to her mood lability, poor judgment, and need to care for her child. She has a 10th grade education. Her potential for compliance is judged to be fair to good. She reports that she is highly motivated to control her mood cycling so she can be a better parent, complete her education, and start a career.
Economic Factors	SN has access to medication through her emergency assistance entitlement program.

Variables Influencing Decision

Treatment Objectives

- Correct the neurotransmitter imbalance contributing to depression
- Return the patient to optimal level of functioning.

Drug Variables	*Drug Summary*	*Patient Variables*
Indications	Lithium, carbamazepine, and valproic acid are effective in various forms of bipolar disorder. Divalproex is most effective for rapid-cycling disorders.	SN has at least four full mood cycles per year, which constitutes rapid bipolar cycling. This is a decision point.
Pharmacodynamics	All three drugs are essentially similar in terms of pharmacodynamics.	This will not be a decision point. There are no patient variables at this time that influence the decision.
Adverse Effects/ Contraindications	Lithium: Polyuria, polydipsia, GI upset, narrow therapeutic index, potential for toxicity Carbamazepine: Narrow therapeutic index, nausea, anorexia, blood dyscrasias.	This is a decision point owing to SN's impulsiveness, poor judgment, and past suicide attempt. Carbamazepine may cause anorexia, and SN is already thin and has an appetite disturbance.

Case Study continued on following page

Case Study Rapid-Cycle Bipolar Disorder—cont'd

Drug Variables	Drug Summary	Patient Variables
Adverse Effects/ Contraindications —cont'd	Valproic acid: Wide therapeutic index, potential for neurotoxicity or hepatic problems, nausea, or tremor	
Pharmacokinetics	Divalproex has the most rapid onset of action compared with lithium or carbamazepine. This will become a decision point.	SN has no variables that influence pharmacokinetics at this time.
Dosage Regimen	Treatment of bipolar disorder essentially lifelong, subject to continued cycles and relapse, even with ongoing drug regimen.	All drugs will require long-term use. This is not a decision point.
Lab Considerations	Lithium: Drug levels must be monitored frequently as are renal, LFTs, thyroid studies, and electrolytes. Carbamazepine: Levels must be monitored frequently, along with LFTs and CBC. Divalproex: Levels must be monitored periodically. LFTs and CBC should be assessed at baseline and periodically.	All drug regimens require lab monitoring. Valproate monitoring is less frequent and extensive, and is not considered a major decision point. However, because of SN's rapid cycling, she may not always comply with the need for monitoring. This will become a decision point.
Cost Index*	Generic lithium: 1 Brand name lithium: 1 Generic carbamazepine: 1 Brand name carbamazepine: 2–3 Generic divalproex: 1 Brand name divalproex: 2–3	SN's drugs are available via her emergency entitlement program. At present, this is not a decision point. However, cost may become an issue in the future, once she completes her education and enters the work force. If she does not have pharmacy coverage, affordability of drugs may become an issue.

Summary of Decision Points

- Divalproex is recognized as the most effective drug for the treatment of rapid cycling bipolar disorder.
- Impulsivity, poor judgment, past history of suicide attempt may indicate that a drug with a wide therapeutic index is safer.
- SN's insurance will cover the cost of her drug regimen. Although the drug is more expensive than others, it will also likely be more effective, potentially less lethal, and minimize other costs such as need for hospitalization or chronic dependence on public assistance programs.

DRUGS TO BE USED

- Divalproex 750 mg po QD in divided doses. Titrate rapidly to desired clinical effect or trough plasma levels of 50–125 mcg/ml. Maximum dose: 60 mg/kg/day
- If depression becomes an issue, patient will be reassessed to determine appropriate therapy.

*Cost Index:	
1	$ <30/mo.
2	$ 30–40/mo.
3	$ 40–50/mo.
4	$ 50–60/mo.
5	$ >60/mo.

AWP of 100, 250 mg enteric coated tablets of divalproex is approximately $65
AWP of 100, 250 mg capsules of divalproex is approximately $16
GI, Gastrointestinal; LFT, liver function tests.

drugs in nursing homes. Further, the physical changes of aging in older adults must be noted because elimination of these drugs is primarily through the kidneys.

Psychosocial Considerations

Patients with bipolar disorder are often oblivious to their mood cycling, although those around them are acutely aware of the situation. Manic patients are frank about missing their highs, and this factor contributes to their discontinuation of drug therapy. Therefore, they may actively resist treatment and may be particularly reluctant to have the euphoric, energized periods of mania controlled.

Bipolar patients may also be actively self-medicating their painful mood states with alcohol, street drugs, or prescription drugs such as benzodiazepines, opioids, and sedative-hypnotics. The patient and health care provider may be unaware of the underlying disorder until after the other substances are removed.

Because bipolar disorder is a life-long, unremitting, chronic medical and psychiatric disease, characterized by multiple relapses, it is common for patients to become reluctant to comply with complex or demanding drug regimens. Treatment regimens may be complicated further by annoying or dangerous adverse effects, and the need for frequent laboratory monitoring.

It may be particularly difficult for bipolar patients who lack family, social support, easily accessible community caregivers, structured housing or day programs, or financial resources to consistently comply with therapeutic regimens. Drug, dietary, or sleep hygiene practices that assist with management of the disorder and its treatment protocols are warranted.

Many bipolar patients respond very favorably to treatment and continue to live extremely productive lives. They may be very successful in their careers and personal lives, particularly if their energy and creativity can be constructively harnessed. (See Case Study—Rapid-Cycle Bipolar Disorder.)

Analysis and Management

Treatment Objectives

Treatment objectives for the patient with bipolar disorder are to correct the neurotransmitter imbalance through the appropriate use of drugs and to return the patient to an optimal level of functioning. The resolution of mood disorders is not conceptualized in terms of a cure but rather in terms of treatment, management, and prevention of relapse. Thus, rapid stabilization of mood, re-establishment of normalized sleep patterns, prevention of self-injurious acts, and long-term stabilization are necessary. Untreated or inadequately treated bipolar disorder tends to become more serious over time and more difficult to arrest.

Legislative guidelines on the use of psychoactive drugs were developed in 1987. The guidelines require that the following use of psychoactive drugs be justified in the patient's records (see Legislative Guidelines on Psychoactive Drug Usage).

Treatment Options

Drug Variables

Mania is often difficult to manage and stabilize. In acute mania, there is typically a lag time of 5 days to 3 weeks before first-line drugs effectively correct the problem. Antipsychotic drugs (see Chapter 19) are routinely used during acute mania to treat psychotic processes that may be present, as well as to provide a margin of calmness and safety for patients who are clearly out of control.

Antipsychotics are not ordinarily used as the primary therapy, but rather as an adjunct that may be tapered and eliminated as mania subsides, and primary drugs become effective. There is some evidence that newer antipsychotic drugs such as clozapine, olanzepine, and risperidone have mood-stabilizing properties as well as antipsychotic properties. Because long-term use of antipsychotic drugs carries a risk of tardive dyskinesia, antipsychotic drugs should be used only when they are absolutely necessary and in the lowest effective doses.

Anxiolytic drugs (see Chapter 17), such as the benzodiazepines, may be effective adjuncts in the management of acute mania. They offer the advantage of a more rapid antimanic response by restoring normal sleep patterns, imparting a calming effect, and eliminating or minimizing exposure to antipsychotic drugs. The benzodiazepines are helpful in controlling agitation, hyperactivity, anxiety, and sleeplessness that is associated with mania.

ECT is sometimes employed in the treatment of both depression and mania. Although the mechanism of action is unknown, it may be related to its ability to normalize neurotransmitter production, raise the seizure threshold, or decrease amygdaloid kindling. ECT is a realistic alternative for those who are unresponsive or unable to tolerate first-line drugs or who need rapid remission of acute mania owing to suicidal ideation or who are pregnant. Normal mood can then be supported by drug therapy, if indicated.

Antidepressant drugs may precipitate manic states in vulnerable individuals. Therefore, whenever possible, bipolar

LEGISLATIVE GUIDELINES ON PSYCHOACTIVE DRUG USAGE (OBRA 1987)

The following use of psychoactive drugs must be justified:

- Continuous use of hypnotic drugs for more than 30 days
- Use of two or more hypnotic drugs at the same time
- Hypnotic or anxiolytic drugs administered in excess of listed maximum doses
- Use of neuroleptic drugs in dementia unless the condition is associated with psychotic or agitated features that are subjectively disturbing to the patient or lead to agitated or dangerous behavior that interferes with patient safety or care
- Use of antipsychotics purely to control anxiety, wandering, restlessness, or insomnia
- Use of antipsychotics for less than 3 days unless to control acute episodes of agitation
- Use of two or more antipsychotic drugs at the same time
- Use of anticholinergic therapy with antipsychotic drugs in the absence of extrapyramidal symptoms
- Neuroleptic drugs administered in excess of listed maximum dosages

In addition, federal guidelines require periodic monitoring for tardive dyskinesia (using the Abnormal Involuntary Movement Scale [AIMS] assessment tool) in recognition of the older adult's vulnerability to this disorder when taking antipsychotic drugs. Patients must be provided with drug holidays, gradual dose reductions, and behavioral management in an effort to discontinue the drugs.

patients should be managed with mood stabilizer drugs alone, unless there is a clear need for the addition of antidepressants to the regimen.

The decision to use a mood-stabilizing drug should be based, at least in part, on the particular variety of mania present. Lithium is the drug of choice for euphoric, classic, milder forms of mania, but it is less likely to be effective for patients with dysphoric mania, psychotic mania, rapid-cycling bipolar disorder, co-morbid drug and alcohol abuse, or with patients who have had three or more episodes of mania. Lithium may also require up to 3 to 4 weeks to exert its full antimanic effect.

Carbamazepine may be considered an alternative drug, although it is not FDA approved for mania. Carbamazepine has a narrow therapeutic index, interacts with 47 percent of the 200 most commonly prescribed drugs, and has many potential adverse effects. However, it is efficacious in controlling mania either alone or in conjunction with other mood stabilizers.

Valproic acid (i.e., divalproex) is likely to be more effective in rapid-cycling or ultrarapid-cycling mania (up to 20 percent of bipolar disorders), mixed states (up to 40 percent of episodes), mania in the older adult, secondary mania (due to a nonpsychiatric medical condition), or episodes associated with alcohol or substance abuse and personality disorders. Mood-stabilizing drugs need to be continued indefinitely, because bipolar disorder is a recurrent disorder.

Patient Variables

A careful analysis of the patient's medical health, as well as concomitant drug use, should be undertaken before initiating a trial of any mood-stabilizing drug. The decision to use a particular drug for a particular patient is, of course, based on accurate diagnosis.

Lithium, carbamazepine, and valproic acid have been used in children, but extensive studies of the relationship of age, effects, adverse effects, and long-term effects have not been conducted. Lithium may decrease bone formation and density in children by altering parathyroid hormone concentrations. Lithium is also deposited in bone, replacing calcium, an effect that is more pronounced in immature bones.

Valproic acid places children at increased risk for serious or fatal hepatotoxicity. However, patients younger than 2 years of age are at greatest risk. The risk of hepatotoxicity increases with advancing age, with the concurrent use of anticonvulsants, and in patients with complex medical problems. Carbamazepine is likely to induce behavioral changes in children.

Lamotrigine also carries the risk of Stevens-Johnson syndrome. Children may be more at risk than adults for the potentially life-threatening rash.

Older adults usually require lower lithium dosage, lower serum concentrations, and more frequent monitoring than do younger patients. Renal clearance and rate may be decreased, as may the volume of drug distribution due to the normal changes of aging. Lithium may be more toxic to the CNS in the aging population, even when serum lithium levels are within the therapeutic range. There is also a propensity to develop lithium-induced goiter and clinical hypothyroidism. Polyuria and polydipsia may be more pronounced in the older adult.

Carbamazepine may promote confusion or agitation in the older adult. It may also cause atrioventricular heart block, syndrome of inappropriate antidiuretic hormone, and bradycardia. For younger patients and older adults, valproic acid is the safest, most effective drug for most types of mania.

For older adults on valproic acid, therapy should be started with lower daily doses and maintained at lower serum concentrations that are still within the therapeutic range. Older adults tend to have increased free drug concentrations, lowered clearance, and a reduced capacity to biotransform drugs.

When mood-stabilizing drugs are used in combination, CNS toxicity and adverse effects such as ataxia, clouded sensorium, and sedation may occur. These adverse effects may occur even when all drugs are within therapeutic range. This is true for patients of all ages, but particularly in older adults or those on complicated drug regimens.

Intervention

Administration

The use of mood-stabilizing drugs requires careful planning, administration, and monitoring. Most often, these drugs are administered two to three times daily, which requires planning to take doses while at work, school, away from home, or on vacation.

Before initiating therapy with mood-stabilizing drugs, baseline renal and thyroid function, white blood cell count (WBC) with differential, serum electrolytes, and glucose levels should be obtained. It is important to establish that a woman is not pregnant. If there is any possibility of pregnancy, a human chorionic gonadotropin pregnancy test should be completed. In addition, liver function tests, bilirubin, urinalysis, and blood urea nitrogen should be routinely performed for patients taking carbamazepine and valproic acid.

Mood-stabilizing drugs should be taken with food to minimize gastric upset. Enteric-coated or sustained-release formulations should be taken whole. They should not be broken or chewed because this practice can cause throat irritation and alter drug absorption. Liquid formulations should be shaken well before pouring, and a calibrated measuring device should be used to ensure accurate dosage. Valproic acid should not be taken with milk to prevent premature dissolution.

Therapeutic drug levels should be monitored closely throughout therapy. Lithium levels should be monitored once or twice weekly during the acute manic phase until serum concentrations have stabilized and the patient's condition has improved. Desirable lithium levels generally fall in the range of 1.0 to 1.5 mEq/L for the management of acute mania, and 0.5 to 1.0 mEq/L for maintenance regimens. Serum drug levels are measured approximately 10 to 12 hours after the previous dose. Levels of 1.5 to 2.5 mEq/L are thought to represent moderate lithium intoxication, whereas levels of 2.5 to 3.5 mEq/L indicate severe intoxication. Levels above 3.5 mEq/L are usually fatal. Lithium drug concentrations in children, adolescents, the elderly, those with chronic illnesses, and especially any renal involvement should be maintained at lower levels. Lithium levels should be repeated every 2 to 3 months during long-term therapy and more frequently in the elderly, because they are more prone to dehydration, hypothyroidism, and CNS toxicity.

Treatment of lithium toxicity is directed toward preventing further absorption and enhancing elimination of the drug from the body. Gastric lavage is warranted in acute overdose. Mild intoxication can be treated with hydration to increase urine output. Severe intoxication should be treated with hemodialysis, especially if renal function is impaired.

Most patients tolerate divalproex sodium better than valproic acid. To change a patient from valproic acid to divalproex, initiate divalproex therapy at the same total daily dose and dosing schedule as valproic acid. Once the patient is stabilized, an administration schedule of two to three times daily may be attempted.

Therapeutic levels of valproic acid range between 50 to 125 mcg/mL. However, a good correlation between daily dose, serum level, and therapeutic effects has not been established. Treatment of valproic acid overdose is supportive and is aimed at facilitating elimination by ensuring adequate urinary output. Gastric lavage is usually of little use due to rapid drug absorption.

Education

The patient and family require education concerning the course of the illness, its symptoms, and its management. One of the points that should be reinforced is the importance of compliance with the drug regimen. Patients should be aware, however, that even with complete compliance, they may be subject to periods of relapse. Sleep hygiene, regular daily routine, cognitive-behavioral therapy, group therapy, and family support are all factors that optimize functioning. Patients should be warned to report promptly any deterioration of sleep pattern because often it is the first warning sign of an impending episode of hypomania or mania. Patients may choose, for example, to avail themselves of information from drug manufacturers, advocacy groups, and the Alliance for the Mentally Ill, and to participate in employee assistance programs. Families also require information and support because the disorder impacts the entire family system, roles, relationships, responsibilities, finances, and parenting. Assisting the patient to understand that the illness does need to be an important focus, but not the only focus of life, and resuming as normal, productive and stable a life as possible is vital.

Patients need education concerning the drug regimen, adverse effects, and situations that require contacting the health care provider, or discontinuing the drug. Information concerning drug-drug interactions, especially drugs that may be given by non-psychiatric health care providers, and any OTC drug should be included. In the case of lithium, information concerning potential toxicity and fluid and electrolyte balance is important. The necessity of maintaining adequate hydration and salt in the diet, especially during periods of illness, fever, vomiting, diarrhea, or profuse sweating, should be included. Fluids should be increased during periods of hot weather to avoid dehydration.

Evaluation

Indications that pharmacotherapeutic interventions and any other measures employed have been effective include the resolution of mania or hypomania, the establishment of euthymia (normal mood), the resolution of psychotic or dysphoric symptoms (if they were present), and a therapeutic, nonproblematic physiologic response to the drug. If adverse effects develop, they are tolerable, non–life-threatening, noncompromising, and do not compel the patient to discontinue the drug.

The patient and family express knowledge and some degree of acceptance of the disorder and demonstrate an awareness of the nature, course, and treatment of the illness. Evidence should also include documentation that the patient actually has a means of accessing prescribed drugs and ongoing care and actually accesses it. Abbott Laboratories has a sample program and indigent patient program available for those who are uninsured or who cannot afford DEPAKOTE. Solvay Pharmaceuticals has a program available to supply patients with LITHOBID. The patient is aware of psychosocial supports and rights as a disabled person under the Americans with Disabilities Act. When applicable, the patient expresses a desire to stop or actually stops the use of alcohol or street drugs. The patient actually stops the use of alcohol or street drugs, or sincerely endeavors to stop.

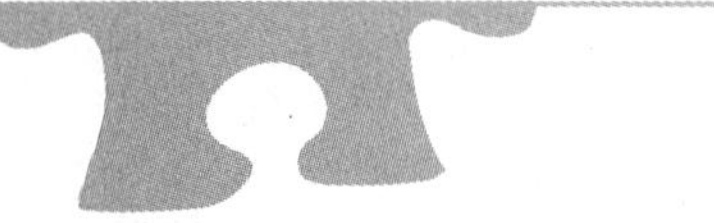

SUMMARY

- Fifteen million Americans suffer from depression, with a lifetime risk of 2.3 to 3.2 percent for men and 4.5 to 9.3 percent for women.
- Risk factors for depression include young adult (20 to 40 years of age), a positive family history, separation or divorce, chronic low self-esteem, experience with abusive relationships, third trimester of pregnancy, first 3 months after birth, and onset of menopause.
- Depression arises as a result of changes in the neurotransmitters serotonin, norepinephrine, and to a lesser extent, dopamine.
- The diagnosis of depression is made using the criteria extracted from the *Diagnostic and Statistical Manual of Mental Disorders IV.*
- Treatment objectives for acute depression include a reduction in and removal of signs of depressive disorder, and to restore occupational and psychosocial functioning.
- Objectives for chronic depression include reducing the likelihood of relapse or recurrence.
- TCAs, tetracyclic antidepressants, SSRIs, MAOIs, and a variety of miscellaneous antidepressants are useful in treating depression.
- Drug variables to consider include the specific type of depression, short-term and long-term adverse effects, and the concomitant use of other nonpsychiatric drugs.
- Patient variables include consideration of compliance and noncompliance, financial resources, age, and state of renal and hepatic functioning.
- In many cases, the entire daily dose may be taken at bedtime once the patient is stabilized on the drug. Drug holidays may be warranted or appropriate for some drugs.
- Patients should be advised that a period of 2 to 12 weeks may pass before they notice substantial benefit from drug treatment.
- Patients using MAOIs should be advised to avoid OTC drugs and foods or beverages containing tyramine to minimize the risk of hypertensive crisis.

- Effectiveness of therapy can be demonstrated by the resolution of depression and restoration of euthymia without evoking mania.
- Bipolar disorder affects at least three million people in the United States.
- Mania is thought to be caused by a relative excess of the same neurotransmitters that cause depression (i.e., serotonin, norepinephrine, and dopamine).
- Bipolar disorders include three forms: hypomania, full mania, and mixed mania.
- Diagnosis of bipolar disorder is based on criteria extracted from the *Diagnostic and Statistical Manual of Mental Disorders IV.*
- Patients present with a cycle of energized, expansive mood states, and lability alternating with depression.
- Mania may first appear in childhood or adolescence and emerge in early adulthood. A family history of bipolar disorder is common.
- Treatment objectives include correcting the neurotransmitter imbalance and returning the patient to an optimal level of functioning.
- Mood-stabilizing drugs used in the treatment of bipolar disorders include carbamazepine, lithium, and valproic acid.
- Mood-stabilizing drugs are administered two to three times daily, thus requiring planning to take doses while at work, school, away from home, or on vacation.
- The patient and serum drug levels should be closely monitored for evidence of toxicity.
- Patients should be taught that treatment is life-long in most cases and informed of the drug regimen, adverse effects, situations that require contact with the health care provider, and any OTC drugs that should be avoided.
- Effectiveness of therapy can be evaluated as the resolution of mania or hypomania, establishment of euthymia, and resolution of dysphoric symptoms.

BIBLIOGRAPHY

American Psychiatric Association. (1994). *Diagnostic and statistical manual of mental disorders* (4th ed.). Washington, D.C.: American Psychiatric Association.

Ascher, J. (1995). Bupropion: A review of its mechanism of action. *Journal of Clinical Psychiatry,* 56(9), 395–399.

Ayd, F. (1995). Nefazodone: The latest FDA approved antidepressant. *Internal Drug Therapy Newsletter,* 30(4), 17–20.

Balon, R. (1995). The effects of antidepressants on human sexuality: Diagnosis and management. *Primary Psychiatry,* 2(8), 46–51.

Bates, E., Florit, G. (1994). Interactions: Top 200 Drugs/CBZ, Lith, DVA/VPA. *Top 200 Drugs for 1994.* Gainesville, FL: Tacactiale Neuroscience Program.

Bowden, C. (1995). Predictors of response to divalproex and lithium. *Journal of Clinical Psychiatry,* 56(3), 25–30.

Bowden, C., and McElvoy, S. (1995). History of valproate for treatment of bipolar disorder. *Journal of Clinical Psychiatry,* 56(3), 3–5.

Brady, K. (1995). Valproate in the treatment of acute bipolar affective episodes complicated by substance abuse: A pilot study. *Journal of Clinical Psychiatry,* 56(3), 118–121.

Brown, D., (1995). Major depression in a community sample of African Americans. *American Journal of Psychiatry,* 152(3), 373–378.

Calabrese, J., and Woyshville, M. (1995). A medication algorithm for treatment of bipolar rapid cycling? *Journal of Clinical Psychiatry,* 56(3), 11–18.

Cardenale, V. (Ed.) (1998). *Drug topics redbook.* Montvale, NJ: Medical Economics.

Clark, D. (1995). Costs of antidepressant medicine. *Journal of Clinical Psychiatry,* 56(9), 432.

Demopulos, C., and Sachs, G. (1995). Rapid cycling: Clinical concepts. *American Society of Clinical Psychopharmacology,* 6(3), 1–3,5.

Depression Guideline Panel. (April, 1993). *Depression in primary care: Volume 1. Detection and diagnosis. Clinical practice guideline, number 5.* Rockville, MD: U.S. Department of Health and Human Services, Public Health Service, Agency for Health Care Policy and Research. AHCPR Publication No. 93-0550.

DeVane, C., and Sallee, F. (1996). Selective serotonin reuptake inhibitors in child and adolescent psychopharmacology: A review of published experience. *Journal of Clinical Psychiatry,* 57(2), 55–66.

DeVane, C. (1994). Pharmacokinetics of the newer antidepressants: Clinical relevance. *American Journal of Medicine,* 97 (Suppl 6A).

Doralswamy, P. (1995). Case studies in practical psychopharmacology. *Primary Psychiatry,* 2(8), 16–18.

Dubovsky, S., and Thomas, M. (1995). Serotonergic mechanisms and current and future psychiatric practice. *Journal of Clinical Psychiatry,* 56(Suppl 2), 38–48.

Ereshefsky, L., Overman, G., and Karp, J. (1995). Current psychotropic dosing and monitoring guidelines. *Primary Psychiatry,* (May), 42–53.

Evans, D., Byerly, M., and Greer, R. (1995). Secondary mania: Diagnosis and treatment. *Journal of Clinical Psychiatry,* 56(3), 31–37.

Fawcett, J. (1995). Compliance: Definitions and key issues. *Journal of Clinical Psychiatry,* 56(Suppl 1), 4–8.

Feiger, A. (1996). Nefazodone versus sertraline in outpatients with major depression: Focus on efficacy, tolerability, and effects on sexual function and satisfaction. *Journal of Clinical Psychiatry,* 57(Suppl), 1–10.

Feighner, J. (1994). The role of venlafaxine in rational antidepressant therapy. *Journal of Clinical Psychiatry,* 55(9, Suppl), 62–68.

Fink, M. (1995). ECT in mania: A rediscovered use. *Psychiatric Times,* 12(6), 16.

Fisher, S., Kent, T., and Bryant, S. (1995). Postmarketing surveillance by patient self-monitoring: Preliminary data for sertraline versus fluoxetine. *Journal of Clinical Psychiatry,* 56(7), 288–296.

Gelenberg, A., and Jefferson, J. (1995). Lithium tremor. *Journal of Clinical Psychiatry,* 56(7), 283–282.

Goldberg, J., Harrow, M., and Grossman, L. (1995). Course and outcome in bipolar affective disorder: A longitudinal follow-up study. *American Journal of Psychiatry,* 152(3), 379–384.

Gottschalk, A., Bauer, M., Whybro, P. (1995). Evidence of chaotic mood variations in bipolar disorder. *Archives of General Psychiatry,* 52(11), 947–959.

Gregor, K. (1994). Selective serotonin reuptake inhibitor dose titration in a naturalistic setting. *Clinical Therapeutics,* 16(2), 306–315.

Grengo, C., Kunik, M., Molinari, V., et al. (1996). The use and tolerability of fluoxetine in geropsychiatric patients. *Journal of Clinical Psychiatry,* 57(1), 12–16.

Guze, B., Richeimer, S., and Szuba, M. (1995). *The psychiatric drug handbook.* St. Louis: Mosby–Year Book.

Hirschfeld, R. (1994). Practice guidelines for the treatment of patients with bipolar disorder. *American Journal of Psychiatry,* 151(12, Suppl), 1–36.

Intercom. (1995). The experts converse: Special considerations in switching antidepressants. *Journal of Clinical Psychiatry,* 56(10) (Suppl), 1–12.

Janikack, P., Davis, J., and Preskorn, S. (1995). Update: Advances in the pharmacotherapy of depressive disorders. *Supplement to the Principles and Practices of Psychopharmacotherapy,* 1(2).

Janikack, P., Davis, J., Preskorn, S., and Ayd, F. (1995). Update: Advances in the pharmacotherapy of bipolar disorder. *Supplement to Principles and Practices of Psychopharmacotherapy,* 1(3).

Jefferson, J., and Greist, J. (1994). Lithium in psychiatry: A review. *CNS Drugs,* 1(6), 449–464.

Jefferson, J. (1995). Lithium: The present and future. *Journal of Clinical Psychiatry,* 56(1), 41–48.

Leonard, B., and Touffson, G. (1994). Focus on SSRIs: Broadening the spectrum of clinical use. *Journal of Clinical Psychiatry,* 55(10), 459–466.

McElroy, S., Keck, P., and Freidman, L. (1995). Minimizing and managing antidepressant side effects. *Journal of Clinical Psychiatry,* 56(Suppl 2), 49–55.

Montano, C. (1994). Recognition and treatment of depression in a primary care setting. *Journal of Clinical Psychiatry,* 55 (Suppl 12), 18–34.

Montgomery, S. (1994). Selective serotonin reuptake inhibitors: Meta-analysis of discontinuation rates. *International Clinical Psychopharmacology,* 9, 47–532.

Montgomery, S. (1995). Rapid onset of venlafaxine. *International Clinical Psychopharmacology,* 10(Suppl 2), 21–27.

Nemeroff, C., Devane, C., and Pollack, B. (1996). Newer antidepressants and the cytochrome P_{450} system. *American Journal of Psychiatry,* 153(3), 311–320.

Nemeroff, C. (1993). Paroxetine: An overview of the efficacy and safety of a new selective serotonin reuptake inhibitor in the treatment of depression. *Journal of American Psychiatry,* 12(6, Suppl 2), 10–17.

Neylan, T. (1995). Treatment of sleep disturbances in depressed patients. *Journal of Clinical Psychiatry,* 56(Suppl 2), 56–61.

Pray, D. (1995). Special problems in the treatment of depression. *Advances in Psychiatric Medicine* (Supplement in *Psychiatric Times*), 1–4.

Preskorn, S. (1995). Advances in antidepressant pharmacotherapy. *Psychiatric Times,* 12(6), 39–42.

Serzone (nefazodone). (June 1995). Princeton, NJ: Bristol-Myers Squibb Company.

Reynolds, C. (1994). Treatment of depression in late life. *American Journal of Medicine,* 97(6A), 39–46.

Sclar, D. (1995). Antidepressant pharmacotherapy: Economic evaluation of fluoxetine, paroxetine, and sertraline in a health maintenance organization. *Journal of International Medical Research,* 23, 395–412.

Simon, A., Ormel, J., VonKorff, M., et al. (1995). Health care costs associated with depressive and anxiety disorders in primary care. *American Journal of Psychiatry,* 152(3), 352–356.

Solomon, D., Keitner, G. (1995). Course of illness and maintenance treatments for patients with bipolar disorder. *Journal of Clinical Psychiatry,* 56(1), 5–13.

Swann, A. (1995). Mixed or dysphoric manic states: Psychopathology and treatment. *Journal of Clinical Psychiatry,* 56(3), 6–10.

Tignol, J. (1993). A double-blind randomized fluoxetine-controlled multi-center study of paroxetine in the treatment of depression. *Journal of Clinical Psychopharmacology,* 13(16, Suppl 2), 18–22.

Tollefson, G., Holman, S. (1993). Analysis of the Hamilton Depression Rating Scale Factors from a double-blind, placebo-controlled trial of fluoxetine in geriatric major depression. *International Clinical Psychopharmacology,* 8, 253–259.

United States Pharmacopeial Corporation. (1995). *Drug information for the health care professional, USPDI* (5th ed, Vol. 1). Rockville, MD: Author.

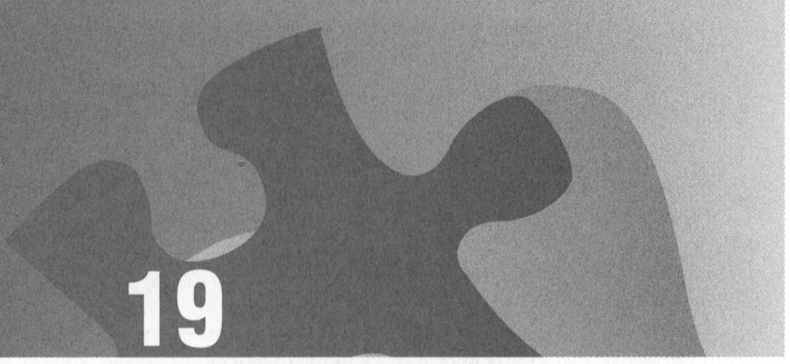

19 Antipsychotic Drugs

Interactions between the neurobiologic and endocrine systems strongly influence human functioning and behavior. Psychosis develops when these connections become dysregulated. The word *psychosis* invokes images of bizarre behaviors, loss of control, and disconnection from reality. Although such psychotic behavior is associated primarily with schizophrenia, it may also be noted with other physical and psychiatric disorders.

Throughout much of the 20th century, there was little success in the treatment of these disorders. However, in the 1950s, an accidental discovery of the antipsychotic properties of the antihypertensive drug chlorpromazine changed the course of treatment and the entire field of psychiatry. Since then, newer drugs have proved even more useful in the management of psychosis, and research is ongoing. Over the past decade, new evidence has demonstrated that individuals with primary psychotic disorders have neuroanatomy and physiology that is indeed different and out of balance.

Antipsychotic drugs assist in managing symptoms of psychosis including thought disorders, hallucinations, bizarre behaviors, agitation, and hyperactivity. The drugs do not cure psychotic disorders but do ease many of the most distressing symptoms. Although the evolution of new antipsychotic drugs has lagged considerably behind that of antianxiety drugs (see Chapter 17) and antidepressants (see Chapter 18), some promising drugs have appeared in the market place in recent years. Antipsychotic drugs are used to manage a variety of disorders including schizophrenia, schizoaffective, and schizophreniform disorders; delusional disorders; acute mania; depressive psychosis; and substance-induced psychosis. The primary use of antipsychotic drugs remains in the management of schizophrenia.

SCHIZOPHRENIA

Epidemiology and Etiology

The term *schizophrenia* is used to describe a group of psychotic disorders. The disorders are characterized by gross distortions of reality; disorganization; fragmented perception, thought and emotion; and withdrawal from social interactions. Diagnosis of schizophrenia is made based on characteristic symptoms, one or more areas of social or occupational dysfunction, and the duration of the symptoms (see DSM-IV Criteria for Schizophrenia and Related Disorders).

Schizophrenia is a chronic mental illness that is prevalent in 1 percent of the population. The onset most often occurs in young adulthood, with no differentiation by gender. Males tend to be diagnosed between the ages of 15 and 24, whereas females are often diagnosed between the ages of 24 and 34. There is no association between socioeconomic status or ethnicity. However, the disorder is so pervasive that the individual often cannot continue as a productive member of society, leading to a tendency to drift downward in socioeconomic status.

The exact etiology of schizophrenia is unknown. Alterations in dopamine transmission as well as anatomic brain differences such as enlarged ventricles are known. There appears to be a genetic link with a high concordance rate among blood relatives. Past hypotheses about poor mothering have generally been discarded as newer etiologic models that focus on biochemistry have been proposed.

Pathophysiology

The psychosis pathway reflects dysfunction of limbic system structures (i.e., hippocampus, anterior cingulate, and amygdala) in which the neurotransmitter dopamine is found (see Fig. 17–1). It has been hypothesized that excess dopamine in the brain causes psychotic symptoms. The limbic area may be hyperresponsive. It has also been hypothesized that in an effort to modulate the overactivity, the frontal areas of the brain become hyporesponsive to dopamine. The end result is major dysregulation and deficits in information processing.

Schizophrenia influences perception, thought content, thought process, affect, and day-to-day functioning. The behavioral manifestations can be grouped as positive, negative, and cognitive symptoms (see Symptoms of Schizophrenia). *Positive symptoms* are those behaviors existing in addition to or outside of the range of usual human responses (e.g., hallucinations and delusions). *Negative symptoms* are behaviors that are lessened or diminished and that are not typical of a healthy individual (e.g., flat affect, poverty of speech, attention impairment). The distinction between positive and negative symptoms is important because different psychotropic drugs tend to affect each group of symptoms differently. The cognitive symptoms, which may also be listed among the positive and negative symptoms, seem to be the least responsive to drug therapy. Examples of cognitive disturbances include looseness of association, tangentiality, circular thought process, and *neologisms* (words that have a meaning known only to the patient).

The person suffering from schizophrenia also demonstrates psychomotor and affective disturbances. Affective disturbances associated with schizophrenia include an overall reduction in emotional responsiveness, flat affect, *anhedonia* (loss of interest in normally pleasurable activities), abnormal emotions, and inappropriate responses. Psychomotor disturbances may include impulsivity, overexcitement, aggression, automatic obedience, *echopraxia* (stereotyped imitation of the movements of another person), stupor, or catalepsy.

Psychotropic drug therapy is used to manage many of these symptoms. However, it should be noted that the adverse effects of these drugs can mimic the psychosis itself.

DSM-IV CRITERIA FOR SCHIZOPHRENIA AND RELATED PSYCHOTIC DISORDERS

1. A continuous disturbance lasting at least 6 months
2. Two or more of the following symptoms lasting for a significant portion of the last month:
   - Delusions
   - Hallucinations
   - Disorganized speech
   - Grossly disorganized or catatonic behavior
   - Negative symptoms
3. One or more areas of social or occupational dysfunction
   - Work
   - Interpersonal relationships
   - Self-care

Data from American Psychiatric Association. (1994). *Diagnostic and statistical manual of mental disorders* (4th ed.) Washington DC: Author.

PHARMACOTHERAPEUTIC OPTIONS

Several different terms have been used to categorize antipsychotic drugs. The traditional antipsychotic drugs had strong neuroleptic properties and were often referred to as classic antipsychotic drugs or neuroleptics. With the advent of newer drugs that did not have the same effects and that influenced different neurochemical pathways, the terms novel or atypical antipsychotics were used. However, as ever newer drugs were developed and as the mechanisms of action of antipsychotics are further delineated, the more accepted terminology is now first-generation antipsychotics and second-generation antipsychotics.

SYMPTOMS OF SCHIZOPHRENIA

Positive Symptoms
Agitation, combativeness
Delusions, hallucinations, feelings of unreality
Hyperactivity
Insomnia
Negativism
Neologisms, racing thoughts
Paranoia, sensitivity to environmental stimuli
Rage
Terror

Negative Symptoms
Amotivation, anhedonia
Blunted affect, apathy
Disheveled appearance, poor hygiene
Emotional withdrawal
Lack of spontaneity
Poor rapport

Cognitive Symptoms
Attention deficits, memory deficits
Concrete thinking
Inability to concentrate
Inability to change cognitive set
Lack of judgment, insight
Information processing deficits
Slowed thought processing
Word salad

First-Generation Antipsychotic Drugs

- ❒ Acetophenazine (TINDAL)
- ❒ Chlorpromazine (THORAZINE, ORMAZINE); (🍁) LARGACTIL
- ❒ Chlorprothixene
- ❒ Fluphenazine (PROLIXIN); (🍁) MODECATE, MODITEN
- ❒ Haloperidol (HALDOL); (🍁) APO-HALOPERIDOL, NOVO-PERODOL, PERIDOL
- ❒ Loxapine (LOXITANE); (🍁) LOXAPAC
- ❒ Mesoridazine (SERENTIL)
- ❒ Molindone (MOBAN)
- ❒ Thioridazine (MELLARIL); (🍁) APO-THIORIDAZINE
- ❒ Trifluoperazine (STELAZINE); (🍁) APO-TRIFLUOPERAZINE
- ❒ Triflupromazine (VESPRIN)

First-generation antipsychotic drugs are classified according to potency and chemical structure and are roughly equivalent with respect to their effect on symptoms. Phenothiazines are divided into three subgroups: the aliphatic, piperidine, and piperazine types. Other antipsychotic drugs include the thioxanthenes, butyrophenone, dihydroindolone, and dibenzoxazepine. Regardless of this distinction, the drugs are similar in many ways and thus are discussed in this chapter as a whole.

Indications

Schizophrenia is the most common indication for these drugs, suppressing the symptoms associated with acute psychosis. They are also useful in the treatment of other disorders in which episodes such as schizoaffective disorder, severe mania or the acute manic phase of bipolar disorder, drug-induced psychosis, delusional disorders, Tourette's syndrome, and Huntington's chorea occur. In addition, some antipsychotic drugs possess antiemetic effects and may be used to treat severe nausea.

Pharmacodynamics

First-generation antipsychotic drugs are thought to block dopamine-2 (D_2) receptors in the postsynaptic areas. Positive symptoms of schizophrenia are affected by blocking D_2 receptors in the mesolimbic area of the brain. Blocking D_2 receptors in the chemoreceptor trigger zone (CTZ) of the medulla and the peripheral blockade of vagal influences in the gastrointestinal (GI) tract produce antiemetic effects. Blocking D_2 receptors in the nigrostriatal pathways, however, creates extrapyramidal adverse effects.

Other neurotransmitter systems are also affected by these drugs and cause many other adverse effects. Anticholinergic effects are caused by partial blockade of acetylcholine. Orthostatic hypotension results from antagonism of the alpha-adrenergic system. Alpha blockade produces sedation and raises the pain threshold. Drowsiness and weight gain result from the partial antagonism of histamine.

Adverse Effects and Contraindications

First-generation antipsychotic drugs produce a wide variety of undesired, adverse responses that affect multiple body systems (see Adverse Drug Effects of Phenothiazines). The adverse effects are drug specific but include neurologic re-

ADVERSE DRUG EFFECTS OF PHENOTHIAZINES

Neurologic
Sedation
Early-onset extrapyramidal symptoms (acute dystonia, akathisia, and parkinsonism)
Late-onset extrapyramidal symptoms (tardive dyskinesia)
Seizure disorders

Muscular
Neuroleptic malignant syndrome

Anticholinergic
Dry mouth, throat, eyes
Blurred vision
Constipation
Urinary hesitancy/retention
Temperature dysregulation

Cardiovascular
Orthostatic hypotension
ECG changes

Sexual Dysfunction
Erectile difficulty, impotence
Prolonged erection
Delayed ejaculation
Reduced libido
Changes in quality of orgasm
Anorgasmia

Allergic
Maculopapular rash
Erythema multiforme
Urticaria (generalized or localized)

Dermatologic
Photosensitivity
Pigmentary skin changes

Neuroendocrine
Amenorrhea
Galactorrhea
Gynecomastia

Hematologic
Transient leukocytosis
Transient eosinophilia
Agranulocytosis

Urinary
Incontinence
Enuresis

sponses such as sedation, extrapyramidal reactions, acute dystonia, akathisia, parkinsonism, tardive dyskinesia, seizures, and neuroleptic malignant syndrome (including diaphoresis, muscular rigidity, and hyperpyrexia). Anticholinergic effects such as dry mouth and eyes, hypotension, and changes in electrocardiogram (ECG) tracings, sexual dysfunction, allergic responses, dermatologic effects, neuroendocrine effects, hematologic effects, and urinary effects also occur.

Sedation is an adverse effect of all antipsychotics, but the degree of sedation is related to the specific drug, dose, and individual patient. Sedation usually occurs with initial administration of the drug and is experienced for the first few days of therapy. After several weeks of treatment, the patient develops a tolerance to the sedative effects.

Extrapyramidal symptoms are among the most uncomfortable adverse effects. These neuromuscular movement disorders are divided into early-onset and late-onset types. The early-onset symptoms include acute *dystonia* (impairment of muscular tonus), *parkinsonism,* and *akathisia* (motor restlessness with a feeling of muscular quivering, an urge to move about constantly, and an inability to sit still). The primary late symptom is *tardive dyskinesia* (impairment of voluntary movement). Extrapyramidal symptoms wax and wane over time and disappear during sleep. They can be aggravated by emotional stress.

Acute dystonia develops within the first days of drug treatment, with 90 percent of the cases developing by the fourth day of treatment. The involuntary tonic contractions of skeletal muscles are manifested in severe spasms of the tongue, face, neck, or back. *Oculogyric crisis* (movement of the eyeball about the anteroposterior axis) and *opisthotonos* (a form of spasm in which the head and heels are bent backward and the body bowed forward), carpopedal spasms, and dorsiflexion of the toes may also occur as part of the disorder. Dystonia can occur at any age, but it is more common in patients younger than 35 years of age. Men younger than 50 years of age are twice as likely to experience the disorder than women.

Dystonia may be seen in some patients after a short course of phenothiazines used to treat nausea and vomiting. This population of patients is often neglected with respect to dystonia, and they do not anticipate this reaction. Dystonia is a very frightening experience, with the patient presenting to the acute care setting for emergent treatment.

Parkinsonism is usually dose related. It is characterized by bradykinesia, a masklike facies, drooling, tremor, cogwheel rigidity, and a shuffling gait (Fig. 19–1). These symptoms, virtually the same as those seen with idiopathic Parkinson's disease, occur within the first month of antipsychotic therapy.

Akathisia is best described as the patient's subjective experience of restlessness. Akathisia generally occurs within the first 2 weeks of treatment. It occurs equally across ages and is seen twice as often in women.

Tardive dyskinesia usually appears more than a year after treatment. It shows itself as involuntary oral-buccal movements of the mouth, lips, and tongue, and may be accompanied by *choreiform* (rapid, involuntary) limb movements. Lip smacking, cheek puffing, and lateral jaw movements are the most commonly described triad of symptoms. Health care providers who work with patients who are taking antipsychotic drugs use a grading system for determining the severity of tardive dyskinesia. The grading system evaluates movement and posture, and is used to monitor for complications that may interrupt a patient's therapy.

Tardive dyskinesia occurs in 10 percent of patients over age 40 and in approximately 80 percent of older adults. It is seven times more common among males than females. The exact mechanism for the disorder is unknown, and at present, there is no specific treatment, other than stopping the drug. Interestingly, the symptoms may become more severe for several weeks after the drug is withdrawn. The flare up is then followed by a slow, gradual improvement over many months or years.

Anticholinergic effects, including peripheral and central nervous system (CNS) symptoms, occur secondary to

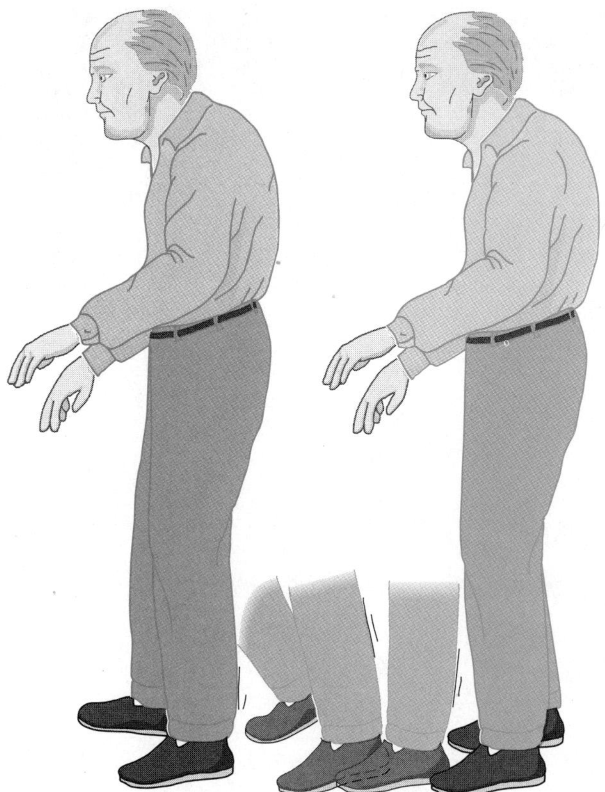

Figure 19–1 Parkinsonism is characterized by bradykinesia, a masklike facies, tremor, cogwheel rigidity, and a shuffling gait. (From Black, J.M., and Matassarin-Jacobs E. [1997]. *Medical-surgical nursing: Clinical management for the continuity of care* [5th ed., p. 879]. Philadelphia: W.B. Saunders. Used with permission.)

cholinergic blockade. The symptoms include dry mouth and eyes, blurred vision (due to ciliary muscle paresis), constipation, urinary hesitancy and retention (related to increased sphincter tone, which, in turn, requires more fluid to initiate the detrusor contraction), and disrupted thermoregulation. Urinary retention can lead to incontinence and enuresis.

There are two primary cardiovascular adverse effects. Orthostatic hypotension is related to alpha-adrenergic receptor blockade, which inhibits reflex vasoconstriction. The inhibition, in turn, causes peripheral pooling of venous blood. Orthostatic hypotension is common during the first hours or days of treatment. ECG changes include flat T waves and an increased QR interval.

Patients taking antipsychotic drugs experience a reduction in seizure threshold. This is especially true with low-potency antipsychotics and is particularly problematic in patients with a pre-existing seizure disorder, abnormal electroencephalogram (EEG), or other CNS pathology. Patients often develop tolerance to this adverse effect. In some cases, lowering the dose of antipsychotic drug or increasing the dose of the anticonvulsant drug may be necessary.

Sexual dysfunctions include disturbances in ejaculation (delayed or blocked), prolonged erection, impotence, decreased libido, and changes in the quality of orgasm or the ability to experience orgasm. The exact mechanism for these effects is unknown. The adverse effects on sexual dysfunction are possibly related to endocrine influences, the calcium channel blocking effects of the drugs, or alpha-adrenergic effects.

Allergic responses have been reported and include a maculopapular rash of face, neck, upper chest, and extremities; erythema multiforme; and localized or generalized urticaria. Five to ten percent of patients on phenothiazine therapy develop the maculopapular rash. Dermatologic adverse responses of photosensitivity or pigmentary skin changes are rare.

The neuroendocrine adverse effects associated with first-generation antipsychotic drugs include amenorrhea, galactorrhea, and gynecomastia (rare). These effects are related to increased prolactin levels, which, in turn, are secondary to dopamine blockade.

Adverse hematologic effects include transient leukocytosis and eosinophilia. These specific transient changes are of little clinical consequence. However, agranulocytosis, although especially rare with first-generation antipsychotics, requires changing the chemical class of antipsychotic used.

Given the adverse effects of phenothiazines, they are contraindicated in patients who have severe CNS depression, coma, subcortical brain damage, and seizure disorders, and in patients taking anticonvulsants. In addition, these drugs should not be used to treat persons with hepatic, renal, or cardiovascular disorders. With this in mind, the antipsychotic drugs are generally contraindicated in older adults and debilitated patients. These drugs are not recommended for children younger than 12 years of age owing to their sensitivity to extrapyramidal and neuromuscular adverse effects.

Although antipsychotics are not thought to possess abuse potential, abrupt discontinuation can cause withdrawal symptoms. Within a few days of terminating the drug, symptoms such as headache, nausea and vomiting, excessive salivation, diarrhea, and insomnia may develop. Therefore, tapering of the drug is advised.

Pharmacokinetics

Phenothiazine drugs are well absorbed when they are taken orally and parenterally. They are lipid soluble and lipophilic, readily entering the CNS and most other body tissues. In addition, many of the antipsychotic drugs are highly bound to plasma proteins. The liver is the site of drug biotransformation, with metabolites eliminated via the kidneys. Each first-generation antipsychotic drug has specific pharmacokinetic properties (Table 19–1). Peak plasma levels of the first-generation drugs are reached in 2 to 4 hours for oral administration, although they can range up to 7 days. The half-life of these drugs ranges from 1½ hours to as much as 9½ days.

Drug-Drug Interactions

Most other psychotropic drugs and drugs that affect the CNS influence the effectiveness of first-generation antipsychotics and the incidence of adverse drug responses (Table 19–2). For example, alcohol, anesthetics, antianxiety drugs, barbiturates, CNS depressants, opioids, and sedative-hypnotics potentiate the CNS depressant effects of antipsychotics, leading to lethargy, stupor, respiratory suppression, and death. Concurrent use of barbiturates may also increase muscle tremors and hypotension. Antacids, activated char-

TABLE 19–1 PHARMACOKINETICS OF SELECTED ANTIPSYCHOTIC DRUGS

Drugs	Route	Onset	Peak	Duration	PB (%)	$t_{1/2}$	Potency Ratio*
Low-Potency Antipsychotics							
Chlorpromazine	po	30–60 min	2–4 hr	4–6 hr;10–12 hr†	>90	3–40 hr	1:1
	IM	UK	2–3 hr	4–18 hr	>90		
Mesoridazine	po	UK	4–7 days‡	UK	>90	UK	UA
Thioridazine	po	Varies	2–4 hr	8–12 hr	UA	10–30 hr	1:1
Intermediate-Potency Antipsychotics							
Acetophenazine	po	2–3 hr	2–4 hr	36–48 hr	UA	10–20 hr§	UA
Loxapine	po	30 min	1.5–3 hr	12 hr	UA	3–4 hr	1:10
	IM						
Molindone	po	Varies	30–90 min	24–36 hr	UA	1.5–6 hr	1:10
Perphenazine	po	Varies	UK	UA	UA	3–5 hr	1:10
Triflupromazine	po	2 hr	2–6 hr	8–12 hr	UA	15–30 hr	
	IM	10–15 min	15–20 min	4–6 hr	UA	3–40 hr	
High-Potency Antipsychotics							
Fluphenazine HCL	po	60 min	3–5 hr	6–8 hr	>90	4.7–15.3 hr	1:50
Fluphenazine decanoate	IM	24–72 hr	24 hr	1–3 wks		6.8–9.6 days	1:50
Fluphenazine enanthate	IM	24–72 hr	48 hr	>4 wks		3.5 days	1:50
Haloperidol HCL	po	2 hr	2–6 hr	8–12 hr	92	21–24 hr	1:50
	IM	20–30 min	30–45 min	4–8 hr‖			
Haloperidol decanoate	IM	3–9 days	UK	1 month			
Thiothixene	po	Slow	1–3 hr	12 hr	UA	3–4 hr	1:25
Trifluoperazine	po	UK	2–4 hr	12–24 hr	>90	3–40 hr	1:20
Second-Generation Antipsychotics							
Clozapine	po	UK	1–6 hr¶	4–12 hr	95	9–17 hr	UA
Olanzapine	po	UA	4–5 hr			20–27 hr	UA
Risperidone	po	UK	2 hr	UK	UA	3–24 hr**	UA
Sertindole	po	UA	UA	UA	UA	UA	UA

*Potency ratio compared with 100 mg of chlorpromazine
†Chlorpromazine's duration of action for oral and extended-release formulations, respectively.
‡Steady state of mesoridazine with chronic dosing. Full therapeutic effects may take 6 weeks to 6 months to become evident.
§Hepatic half-life of acetophenazine.
‖Haloperidol's antipsychotic effects may persist for several days.
¶Peak antipsychotic effects of clozapine is several weeks.
**Half-life of risperidone for patient who is an extensive metabolizer is 3 hours, 21 hours for the metabolite 9-hydroxyrisperidone. The half-life of risperidone is 20 hours and 30 hours for 9-hydroxyrisperidone for patients who are slow metabolizers (approximately 6 to 8 percent of the white population)
PB, Protein binding; $t_{1/2}$, serum half-life; UA, unavailable; UK, unknown.

coal, and aluminum salts decrease GI absorption of the drugs, thus decreasing antipsychotic drug effectiveness. Anticholinergics decrease the antipsychotic effect and add to the anticholinergic adverse effects (e.g., blurred vision, constipation, dry mouth, and urinary retention). Tricyclic antidepressants add to the anticholinergic effects. Polymyxin B, an antimicrobial drug, has an additive effect on respiratory depression, and quinidine has an additive cardiac depressant effect.

Drugs that interfere with the absorption, biotransformation, distribution, or elimination of phenothiazines should be avoided when possible. In addition, any drugs that potentiate therapeutic effects predispose the patient to drug toxicity.

Dosage Regimen

The dosage regimen for phenothiazines varies with the individual drug. Many of the drugs can be given on a daily basis once the patient's condition is stable, thus enhancing the potential for patient compliance (Table 19–3).

Laboratory Considerations

Before initiation of antipsychotic therapy, a baseline ECG is indicated, especially for patients older than 40 years of age. Serial cardiac monitoring is warranted in patients with cardiac disease. Baseline liver function tests should be performed to provide for comparison over time. However, transitory elevations in liver enzymes may occur after initiation of drug therapy. Older adult patients, those with co-morbid conditions, or patients on multidrug therapies have increased potential for hepatotoxicity and should be carefully monitored.

A baseline complete blood count (CBC) is useful in evaluating possible transient hematologic responses to drug therapy and in monitoring the development of agranulocytosis. Any clinical signs or symptoms of an infection during the first 3 months of treatment should make the health care provider suspicious of agranulocytosis, a potentially fatal disorder.

Second-Generation Antipsychotic Drugs

- ❒ Clozapine (CLOZARIL)
- ❒ Olanzapine (ZYPREXA)
- ❒ Risperidone (RISPERDAL)
- ❒ Sertindole

TABLE 19–2 DRUG-DRUG INTERACTIONS OF SELECTED ANTIPSYCHOTIC DRUGS

Drug	Interactive Drugs	Interaction
First-Generation Antipsychotics		
Chlorpromazine	Antihypertensives	Additive hypotension
Fluphenazine	Nitrates	
Mesoridazine	Alcohol	Additive CNS depression
Thioridazine	Antidepressants	
Acetophenazine	Antihistamines	
Haloperidol	MAO inhibitors	
	Opioids	
	Sedative-hypnotics	
	General anesthetics	
	Phenobarbitol	May decrease effectiveness of chlorpromazine
	Lithium	May produce acute encephalopathy, increased excretion of lithium, and decreased absorption of chlorpromazine
	Antacids	May decrease absorption of chlorpromazine
	Absorbent antidiarrheals	
	Antithyroid drugs	Increased risk of agranulocytosis
	Bromocriptine	May decrease antiparkinson activity
	Levodopa	
	Epinephrine	Decreased vasopressor response to interactive drug
	Norepinephrine	
	Guanethidine	Decrease antihypertensive effects
	Beta blockers	May produce increased response to chlorpromazine
	Antihistamines	Increased risk of anticholinergic effects
	Tricyclic antidepressants	
	Quinidine	
	Disopyramide	
Acetophenazine	Phenytoin	Increased neurotoxicity of interactive drug
	Bacitracin	Decreased neuromuscular blockade
	Capreomycin	
	Colistimethate	
	Polymixin B	
	Metrizamide	Increased potential for seizures
Molindone	Phenytoin	Decreased absorption of interactive drug
	Tetracycline	
Perphenazine	Alcohol	Additive CNS depression
Trifluoperazine	Phenothiazines	
	Metrizamide	Increased potential for seizures
	Barbiturates	Increased risk of neuromuscular excitation and hypotension
	Antihypertensives	Decreased effect of interactive drug
Second-Generation Antipsychotics		
Clozapine	Cimetidine	Increased therapeutic and toxic effects of clozapine
	Phenytoin	Decreased therapeutic effects of clozapine
	Mephenytoin	
	Ethotoin	
Risperidone	Levodopa	Decreased antiparkinson effects of interactive drug
	Carbamazepine	Increased biotransformation of risperidone
	Clozapine	Increased effectiveness of risperidone
	Alcohol	Additive CNS depression
	Antihistamines	
	Sedative-hypnotics	
	Opiods	

CNS, Central nervous system; MAO, monoamine oxidase.

Indications

These newer, atypical, second-generation antipsychotic drugs were approved for use in the United States during the 1990s. These phenothiazines are also indicated in the treatment of schizophrenia and other psychotic disorders. They have been used as adjuncts in the management of mania and borderline personality disorder. However, they are not the first drug of choice in treatment for any of these disorders. Clozapine use is limited to patients who are nonresponsive to management with first-generation agents.

Pharmacodynamics

Second-generation antipsychotic drugs appear to have different receptor interactions than do their predecessors. Clozapine selectively acts at dopamine sites in the cortical and limbic regions of the brain, with much less effect in the

TABLE 19–3 DOSAGE REGIMEN FOR SELECTED ANTIPSYCHOTIC DRUGS

Drugs	Use(s)	Dosage	Implications
Low-Potency Antipsychotics			
Chlorpromazine	Acute and chronic psychoses particularly when accompanied by increased psychomotor activity	*Adults:* Initial: 100 mg po *or* 0.25 mg IM every 30–60 minutes until control is achieved (usually 2–3 doses) or patient does not tolerate drug. Maintenance: 300–400 mg/day as single daily dose *or* 100 mg TID Maximum: 2000 mg daily for severe psychosis *Child over 6 mo:* 0.55 mg/kg po q4–6 hr *or* 0.55 mg/kg IM q6–8 hr PRN. Not to exceed 40 mg/day ages 6 mo–5 yr, or 75 mg/day ages 5–12 yr	Administer deep IM; do not give subcutaneously. Keep patient recumbent for at least 30 minutes after IM administration to minimize hypotensive effects. Administer oral doses with full glass of water to minimize GI irritation. May color urine pink or reddish brown
Mesoridazine	Schizophrenia, behavioral problems in mental deficiency and chronic brain syndrome	*Adults:* Initial: 25–50 mg po BID–TID *or* 25 mg IM. May repeat in 30–60 minutes if necessary. Maintenance: 75–400 mg/day po *or* 25–400 mg/day IM	Do not change dosage in chronic therapy more often than weekly. Avoid prolonged exposure to sun. May color urine pink or reddish brown
Thioridazine	Acute and chronic psychoses	*Adults:* Initial: 50–150 mg po BID. Maintenance: 300–400 mg po daily as single dose. Maximum: 800 mg po daily	There is a risk of pigmentary retinopathy with doses exceeding 800 mg/day
Intermediate-Potency Antipsychotics			
Acetophenazine	Acute and chronic psychoses	*Adults:* Initial: 20 mg po TID. Maintenance: 40–80 mg po per day. Hospitalized patients: 80–120 mg po in divided doses	Doses as high as 400–600 mg/day have been used. Use lower doses and increase dose more gradually in geriatric patients
Loxapine	Psychoses, management of depression and anxiety associated with depression (unlabeled use)	*Adults:* Initial: 10–25 mg po BID *or* 12.5–50 mg IM q4–6 hr as needed and tolerated. Increase dosage after 2 weeks until appropriate response occurs. Maintenance: 100 mg. po daily in 2 divided doses. Maximum: 150 mg. daily *Adolescents:* Initial dose 10 mg BID. Maximum: 100 mg QD	Severely ill patients may require up to 50 mg/day initially, then maintenance doses up to 250 mg/day
Molindone	Acute and chronic psychoses	*Adults:* Initial: 50–75 mg/day po. Increase to 225 mg/day in three to four divided doses. Maintenance: 5–15 mg po TID–QID. Moderate symptoms: 10–25 mg po TID–QID. Severe symptoms: 225 mg/day	Use lower doses and increase dosage more gradually for geriatric patients. Pink or reddish brown urine is common, as well as yellowing of the skin and eyes
Perphenazine	Psychoses	*Adults:* Initial: 2–16 mg po BID–QID. Not to exceed 64 mg/day *or* 5–10 mg. IM. May repeat q6hr. Not to exceed 15–30 mg/day IM *Child over 12 yr:* 8 mg/day in divided doses	Keep patient recumbent for at least 30 minutes following IM administration to minimize hypotensive effects
Triflupromazine	Psychoses	*Adults:* Initial: 10–50 mg po *or* 60 mg IM BID–TID. Not to exceed 150 mg/day *Child older than 2 yr:* 0.5–2 mg/kg/day in three divided doses. May increase to 10 mg if needed. IM dose 0.2–0.25 mg/kg to a maximum of 10 mg/day	Give IM injection into large muscle mass Infrequently used
High-Potency Antipsychotics			
Fluphenazine	Acute and chronic psychoses	*Adults:* Enanthate formulation: Initial: 0.5–10 mg po *or* 2.5–5 mg IM every 30–60 minutes until control is achieved (usually 2–3 doses) or patient does not tolerate drug. Maintenance: 15 mg po daily as single dose. Maximum: 60 mg po daily. Decanoate formulation: 12.5-25 mg IM/SC q 1-3 wks	IM doses can be increased up to 100 mg; however, experience is limited with doses greater than 75 mg/2 weeks
Haloperidol	Psychoses Tourette's syndrome Hyperactivity	*Adults:* Initial: 5–10 mg po *or* 2.5–5 mg IM every 30-60 minutes until control achieved (usually 2–3 doses) or patient does not tolerate drug. Maintenance: 15 mg po as single dose *or* 0.5–5 mg po BID–TID. Maximum: 100 mg po daily *or* 2-5 mg IM q 1–8 hr not to exceed 100 mg/day *Child:* 0.05–0.15 mg/kg/day po	Consider switching to different antipsychotic drug or concurrent use of benzodiazepine once initial 20 mg dose has been reached. IM maintenance doses can be increased up to 500 mg. Experience is limited with doses greater than 300 mg/month

TABLE 19–3 DOSAGE REGIMEN FOR SELECTED ANTIPSYCHOTIC DRUGS *Continued*

Drugs	Use(s)	Dosage	Implications
Thiothixene	Psychoses	*Adults:* Initial: 10–15 mg po or 4–10 mg IM every 30–60 minutes until control is achieved (usually 2–3 doses) or patient does not tolerate drug. Generally 2–5 mg TID. Maintenance: 30 mg po daily in single dose. Maximum: 60 mg/day	Avoid prolonged exposure to sun. May color urine pink or reddish brown Discontinue drug if creatinine and BUN become abnormal or if WBC count is depressed
Trifluoperazine	Psychoses	*Adults:* Initial: 2–5 mg po BID *or* 1–2 mg IM q4–6 hr. Maintenance 15–20 mg/day po. More than 6 mg/day IM is rarely needed	Avoid prolonged exposure to sun. May color urine pink or reddish brown. Discontinue drug if creatinine and BUN become abnormal or if WBC count is depressed
Second-Generation Antipsychotics			
Clozapine	Unresponsive schizophrenia	*Adults:* Initially 12.5–25 mg. po QD–BID. Increase by 25–50 mg/day over a period of 2 weeks to a target dose of 300–450 mg/day. May increase by up to 100 mg/day once or twice weekly. Not to exceed 900 mg/day	Institute seizure precautions because drug lowers seizure threshold. Transient fevers may occur during first 3 weeks of therapy. Monitor WBC weekly during therapy and 4 weeks after stopping the drug
Olanzapine	Psychoses	*Adults:* Initial: 5–10 mg po daily. Increase to 10 mg daily within several days, adjusting by 5 mg/day thereafter at weekly intervals. Maximum: 20 mg./day	Avoid prolonged exposure to sun. Extremes in temperature should be avoided since this drug impairs body temperature regulation. Monitor patient for neuroleptic malignant syndrome
Risperidone	Psychoses	*Adults:* 1 mg po BID. Increase by 3rd day to 3 mg BID. Further increments of 1 mg BID may be made at weekly intervals. Maintenance: 4–6 mg/day. Maximum: 16 mg/day	
Sertindole	Psychoses	*Adults:* Initial: 4 mg po daily. Increase by 4 mg every 2–3 days to target dose of 20 mg/day. Maximum: 24 mg/day	

nigrostriatal region. It seems to have less affinity for D_1, D_2, and D_3 receptors, binding more with D_4 receptors. Clozapine influences serotonin-2 (S_2) receptors, as well as blocking the reuptake of norepinephrine.

Olanzapine is like clozapine in its selective effect on dopamine receptors in the mesencephalon area. It has a high affinity for serotonin receptors and D_4 receptors, as well as binding to D_1, muscarinic, alpha$_1$, and histamine-1 (H_1) receptors.

Risperidone resembles high-potency first-generation antipsychotics. It is an antagonist to S_2 and D_2 receptors as well as alpha$_1$, alpha$_2$, and H_1 receptors.

Sertindole has a preference for the limbic rather than nigrostriatal D_2 receptors. It also has a high affinity for alpha$_1$ and serotonin receptors.

Adverse Effects and Contraindications

The adverse effects of second-generation antipsychotics fall into many of the same categories as the first-generation drugs but with some distinct differences. The distinctions are in relation to the pharmacokinetic and pharmacodynamic properties of each drug. These drugs do cause sedation, and some have some extrapyramidal system or anticholinergic adverse effects, or both. Other adverse effects include agitation, headache, insomnia, nausea, rhinitis, salivation, and weight gain. Yet the relative incidence of adverse effects are different than those of first-generation agents (Table 19–4). This is one reason that new generation drugs are being used more frequently. However, because they are new, long-term effects have not been established.

Pharmacokinetics

All second-generation antipsychotic drugs are well absorbed when they are taken by mouth. They are biotransformed in the liver. Clozapine is rapidly absorbed with peak plasma concentrations seen in 6 hours (see Table 19–1). The peak plasma time for olanzapine is about 5 hours. Risperidone is rapidly absorbed, reaching its peak plasma levels within 2 hours.

Drug-Drug Interactions

Drug-drug interactions of second-generation antipsychotics are similar in many ways to first-generation drugs in that there is additive CNS depression with the concurrent use of alcohol, antihistamines, opioids, and sedative-hypnotics. Anticonvulsants and antiparkinson drugs are most affected by interaction with second-generation antipsychotic drugs (see Table 19–2).

Dosage Regimen

The recommended initial dose of clozapine is 25 mg once to twice daily for at least 3 to 6 months (see Table 19–3). The oral daily maintenance dosage range is 300 to 450 mg/day. The dosage is increased by up to 100 mg/day once or twice daily but should not exceed 900 mg/day.

The initial oral dose of olanzapine is 5 to 10 mg/day. The target dose is 10 mg administered once a day. The maximum dose should not exceed 20 mg/day.

The initial dosage range for risperidone is 0.5–1 mg/day. By day 3 of therapy, the dose is increased to 3 mg

TABLE 19–4 RELATIVE INCIDENCE OF ADVERSE EFFECTS WITH ANTIPSYCHOTIC DRUGS

Drug	Sedation	Extrapyramidal Effects*	Anticholinergic Effects	Cardiovascular Effects
Low-Potency Antipsychotics				
Chlorpromazine	+++	+	++	+++
Mesoridazine	+++	+	++	++
Thioridazine	+++	+	+++	+++
Intermediate-Potency Antipsychotics				
Acetophenazine	++	++	+	+
Loxapine	++	+++	++	++
Molindone	++	++	++	+
Perphenazine	+	+++	+	+
Triflupromazine	+++	++	++	+++
High-Potency Antipsychotics				
Fluphenazine	+	+++	+	+
Haloperidol	+	+++	+	+
Thiothixene	+	+++	+	+
Trifluoperazine	+	+++	+	+
Second-Generation Antipsychotics				
Clozapine	+++	0	0	0
Olanzapine	+++	+	+++	0
Risperidone	++	++	+	1/2+
Sertindole	0	+++	0	+

*Early extrapyramidal symptoms include acute dystonia, parkinsonism, and akathisia.

0, Essentially free of identified adverse effect; 1/2+, least incidence of adverse effects; +, lowest incidence of adverse effects; ++, medium to moderate incidence of adverse effects; +++, Highest incidence of adverse effects.

twice daily for at least 4 weeks. The maximum dosage is 16 mg/day.

No specific dosage range has been set for sertindole at this time. However, the suggested oral dosage range is from 4 to 24 mg/day. Dosing recommendations are to initiate treatment at 4 mg/day, with an increase of 4 mg every 2 to 3 days up to a target dose of 20 mg/day. Some patients may require up to 24 mg/day.

Laboratory Considerations

In addition to the baseline laboratory studies performed for the first-generation antipsychotics, patients receiving clozapine must have weekly blood monitoring. The baseline white blood cell (WBC) count for the patient on clozapine must be 3500/mm^3 or greater for therapy to continue. A differential count is warranted if the granulocyte count is greater than 1500/mm^3. If the WBC falls below 2000/mm^3 or the granulocyte count is less than 1500/mm^3, clozapine must be discontinued and the patient hospitalized in isolation for observation. Hematologist, internist, and infectious disease consultations are warranted.

Critical Thinking Process

Assessment

History of Present Illness

Initial assessment of baseline functioning and mental status are imperative to manage psychosis with antipsychotic drugs. It is necessary to obtain a thorough history of the patient before antipsychotic drugs are administered. This is especially important because drug therapy is aimed at treating symptoms and behaviors. What specific behaviors are noted? When did the psychotic behaviors begin? Was there an identifiable precipitating situation, event, or element linked to the onset of behaviors? Have the symptoms ever occurred before? If so, what was the treatment? Family members and others may need to be interviewed if patient interaction fails to provide the necessary information.

Past Health History

Identification of past health history, problems, and treatments is useful in understanding the individual nature of the patient. Additional information is gathered about family history and whether other family members have demonstrated similar behaviors or were diagnosed with a psychotic disorder. It is important to determine whether or not the patient has been on psychoactive drugs in the past. Information about the drug, dose, route, responses, and, if applicable, reason for stopping therapy is gathered. An in-depth assessment of all drugs that the patient is taking is necessary.

Physical Exam Findings

Although it may be difficult to perform a full physical exam on a psychotic individual, it is vital to establish baseline parameters. The baseline information is used to monitor progression of the disorder as well as responsiveness to the antipsychotic drug, or potential adverse effects. Keep in mind that many of the adverse effects noted while the patient is on antipsychotic drug therapy have physical manifestations. In addition, because virtually all of the antipsychotic drugs rely on the liver for biotransformation, identification of potential pre-existing hepatic disorders is needed. A neurologic exam should be performed also.

Diagnostic Testing

Although no specific diagnostic tests are required before starting antipsychotic therapy, it is prudent to gather information about liver, heart, and neurologic functioning whenever possible. CBC, liver function tests, and ECG results should be recorded. These baseline values can be used as a measuring stick to monitor patient responses to drug therapy as well as averting severe adverse responses. No specific ongoing monitoring of blood levels of first-generation antipsychotic drugs is mandated at this time. Ongoing monitoring of blood levels is mandatory if the patient is receiving clozapine because of the potential for agranulocytosis.

Developmental Considerations

Perinatal Pregnancy is a time of psychological adjustment and concern. It is a time in a woman's life that has its own distinctive developmental tasks. Family dynamics, social support, cultural influences, and whether or not the pregnancy was planned distinctly influence the mother's as well as the family's adjustment to pregnancy.

Determine whether or not the woman has a previous history of psychosis that may be now complicated by the pregnancy. During the first trimester, the woman normally feels some ambivalence about the pregnancy, even if it was planned. Discuss these feelings with the woman because she may feel the need to hide the negative feelings, thinking they are abnormal. The ambivalence usually ends by the beginning of the second trimester. Treatment of psychosis during pregnancy is complicated because many of the antipsychotic drugs are pregnancy category C drugs.

Pediatric The term childhood schizophrenia is no longer used when discussing mental disorders of childhood. Children adapting to life experiences exhibit symptoms that in an adult would be characteristic of mental illness. Psychotic behaviors generally appear after 5 years of age. Psychotic behavior in an adolescent may be obvious from childhood, or it can be triggered by a developmental crisis. Some health care providers believe that an individual must at least reach the developmental stage of adolescence before the diagnosis of schizophrenia can be made. The disease process during adolescence is noted by a gradual disintegration in several areas of mental functioning. The youth's lack of integration of thought processes is manifested most often by disturbed behavior, emotions, and speech patterns.

An adolescent is not a miniature adult, but a developing person within a family system. The individual's needs are not those of an adult, but those of an individual in an emotional and often confusing world. Thus, collect information from the parents and adolescent about the history and progress of the illness. Observations of parent-adolescent interactions and the effectiveness of those interactions with the environment are documented. Additionally, the extent to which an adolescent can distinguish self from the environment and whether there is evidence of self-mutilation or aggressive behaviors can help determine whether or not the child can distinguish between reality and fantasy. The adolescent may be unaware of anything but a growing sense of unhappiness. To an adolescent, asking for help is developmentally inconsistent with the internal drive for mastery and control. Until recently, seeking professional help also carried social stigma. Because adolescents are particularly prone to emotional disturbances, the health care provider needs to incorporate assessment of mental health as part of the database.

Geriatric An older adult's sense of self and security is threatened when it becomes necessary to adapt to various personal changes. Changes in physical status, loss of significant other, hospitalization, or movement to a long-term care facility have a profound effect on the older adult's sense of independence. Uncharacteristic behaviors may emerge, or existing personality traits may be exaggerated when a person is confined to acute-care settings, or when he or she is in a crisis state or receiving treatment and drugs. An accurate assessment of the older adult should include recent changes or new stressors, a drug history, and the use of stimulants such as caffeine, nicotine, or over-the-counter (OTC) drugs, including cold preparations.

Psychosocial Considerations

Adverse effects of many of the antipsychotic drugs may initially interfere with patient functioning. Support and education assist in the day-to-day management of the psychotic patient. Factors relating to family and social support systems are important variables in this area.

Analysis and Management

Treatment Objectives

The primary treatment objective for schizophrenia and psychotic disorders is to diminish psychotic behaviors, thus preventing harm to the patient or others, improving thought disorders, reducing the duration of inpatient hospitalization, and preventing or decreasing the severity of future exacerbations. Accomplishing these objectives permits the patient to participate more fully in psychotherapy. However, in so doing, the safety and functioning of the patient are key foci. Reduction of psychotic symptoms also facilitate the patient attaining a higher level of functioning.

Treatment Options

Antipsychotic drugs are the primary treatment modality for patients with psychosis. Whether the patient is hospitalized, is in a community-based outpatient program, or residing at home, little improvement can be made without the drugs. Maintenance drug therapy has proved valuable in preventing psychotic relapse or recurrence and rehospitalization. The relapse rate after 1 to 2 years of maintenance therapy is 16 to 30 percent compared with patients who are not receiving pharmacotherapy. Electroconvulsive therapy may also be used to control psychotic behaviors in some patients.

Drug Variables

The indications for first-generation and second-generation antipsychotic drugs are the same. The choice of drugs depends on the tolerance of the patient. Overall, the greatest distinctions between antipsychotic drugs are in their adverse effect profiles. High-potency drugs require smaller dosages to produce an effect, cause less sedation and orthostatic hypotension, and produce fewer anticholinergic effects. However, they tend to have a higher incidence of early extrapyramidal symptoms. When adverse effects become too disturbing to the patient, drug therapy is often stopped. Thus, selection of an antipsychotic drug is based on the patient's and family members' previous therapeutic response to a specific drug, differences in adverse effects, and cost. Despite the wide variety of available antipsychotic drugs, there are no convincing data that one antipsychotic drug is necessarily more effective than another.

The therapeutic dose of a drug should be maintained for at least 4 to 6 weeks at standard dosage, and the patient's response should be evaluated before use of a different drug is considered. Because first-generation antipsychotics tend to have a slow onset of action, the direct correlation between dose and therapeutic effectiveness is difficult to judge. If improvement is observed at 4 weeks, therapy is continued for an additional 2 weeks and the patient re-evaluated. The duration of therapy depends on the patient's specific diagnosis. However, in schizophrenia, maintenance therapy is usually needed to maintain patient functioning.

Patients who respond to treatment should be permitted a gradual reduction in dosage to allow for a drug holiday and to determine the need for ongoing therapy. In addition, to better manage symptoms and adverse effects, it is common to administer antipsychotic drugs as a single daily dose, which is generally given at bedtime. The drug can also be given in a split-dose regimen, with one-third of the total daily dose taken in the morning and two-thirds at bedtime.

Clozapine has been effective for patients with treatment-resistance schizophrenia and for those with negative symptomatology. The recommendation is that the patient undergo trials with at least two antipsychotic drugs to demonstrate refractoriness before considering clozapine therapy. Clozapine assists in the resolution of both positive and negative symptoms in 30 to 40 percent of treatment-resistant patients with schizophrenia. Reports also indicate reduced hospitalizations, fewer rehospitalizations, and an increased ability for patients to maintain employment. Although drug costs are high, the savings in hospitalization and minimal extrapyramidal symptoms are factors worth considering.

Clozapine produces some sedation and muscle relaxation but few extrapyramidal symptoms. However, owing to its potential life-threatening effects, patients receiving clozapine must be registered with the manufacturer and weekly blood counts monitored closely. Clozapine is not known to cause tardive dyskinesia and may, in high doses, attenuate it. Further, a 1- to 2-percent incidence of fatal agranulocytosis has been reported. The incidence may be considerably higher in Eastern European and Jewish populations. For this reason, risperidone might be considered before clozapine in patients with treatment-resistant schizophrenia.

Patient Variables

Patients with schizophrenia should receive drug therapy unless there are compelling contraindications, such as a clearly established history of lack of response or severe adverse reactions. Age and gender influence the patient's responses to antipsychotic drugs. Young men tend to be particularly susceptible to extrapyramidal or dystonic reactions. Therefore, it is best to avoid the high-potency drugs (e.g., haloperidol) in these patients. Older patients tend to have a greater number of chronic health conditions influencing their responses. Haloperidol may be chosen for older adults and for patients with cardiovascular or seizure disorders. Haloperidol is a high-potency antipsychotic with low anticholinergic effects. It produces less sedation and orthostatic hypotension than does loxapine or thiothixene. It does, however, produce a higher incidence of acute extrapyramidal or dystonic reactions. In addition, some adverse effects occur more frequently in women, whereas others occur more frequently in men. The adverse effect profile depends on the actual drug and the person's response. Fluphenazine is similar to haloperidol, and if it is found to be less expensive, fluphenazine may be chosen over haloperidol for older adults and for those with comorbid cardiovascular or seizure disorders. In most cases, use of antipsychotic drugs for children younger than 12 years of age is not recommended in most cases.

In some cases, the concurrent use of a benzodiazepine (e.g., lorazepam; see Chapter 17) and an antipsychotic drug can be effective. For example, lorazepam permits control of agitation and decreases the need for initial high doses of antipsychotics, which, in turn, decreases the likelihood of adverse effects. Further, lorazepam can be administered parenterally, which may be helpful for patients who are unwilling to take oral formulations. Other drugs that may be used for adjunctive therapy include carbamazepine, lithium, and valproic acid.

For the otherwise healthy young patient with psychosis, loxapine may be useful. Loxapine is a medium-potency antipsychotic drug that produces less sedation, has moderate anticholinergic activity, and less orthostatic hypotension than does chlorpromazine or thioridazine. It also has a lower incidence of acute extrapyramidal or dystonic reactions than higher potency drugs such as haloperidol and fluphenazine.

If sedation of the patient with psychosis is desired, chlorpromazine may be chosen. It is a low potency drug but one with high anticholinergic activity. It produces sedation and orthostatic hypotension more than the medium-potency or high-potency drugs. However, it has a low incidence of acute extrapyramidal or dystonic reactions. Thioridazine can also be used, although there is no parenteral drug form of this agent available.

No evidence suggests that higher doses of antipsychotic drugs are likely to improve psychosis more quickly. Further, higher doses increase the risk of adverse effects and should be avoided. Several days to weeks should elapse when determining patient response before the dosage is increased. In controlled, nonagitated patients, low dosages are initially used and the dosage increased every 2 weeks to minimize adverse effects and to increase the patient's acceptance of pharmacotherapy. Once the patient is tolerant of the adverse effects, a full dosage of the drug can be given at bedtime (except for loxapine). Often the patient is provided with an order for an as-needed (PRN) benzodiazepine during the initial titration of the antipsychotic drug to a maintenance dosage. If frequent doses of the PRN benzodiazepine or antipsychotic drug are needed, maintenance doses of the antipsychotic drug may need to be increased more often than every 2 weeks. Benzodiazepines are not used for long-term maintenance, and their use should be tapered within the first few weeks as the patient becomes less agitated. Tapering of therapy can usually be started after the first week of therapy.

Long-acting parenteral antipsychotic drugs are recommended for patients who are unable to manage daily dosage regimens and for the patient on maintenance therapy who is likely to be noncompliant. Depot formulations such as haloperidol decanoate or fluphenazine decanoate can be used. A calculated nonloading maintenance dose of the decanoate form may also be administered during tapering-off periods. For example, a patient has been receiving a 30-mg/day oral dose of fluphenazine. A parenteral dose 10 to 15 times that which would be calculated for a monthly dose (i.e., 300 mg/month) is administered biweekly (150 mg every 2 weeks). The previous oral dose is reduced over a period of 4 months, pending the development of adverse effects. If adverse effects develop, the reduction of the oral dose is accelerated.

Another protocol for initiating a depot regimen has been used with haloperidol decanoate. Once the patient has been stabilized on the oral form, a parenteral loading dose equal to 20 times the oral dose is administered during the month. The initial maximum dose is seldom above 100 mg, with the remaining amounts administered in the next weeks. Oral haloperidol is discontinued when the full loading dose has been reached. The maintenance dose (50 percent of the loading dose) is achieved by tapering the loading dose by 25 percent each month for 2 months. Thus, if the patient had been receiving 10 mg/day orally, a loading dose of at least 200 mg IM would be indicated, administered as 100 mg for the first dose and 100 mg 7 days later. With the administration of the second 100-mg dose, oral haloperidol would be discontinued. Oral therapy should replace parenteral therapy when the patient is able and willing to comply with a therapeutic regimen.

Intervention

Administration

Two oral dosing strategies are used for maintenance treatment: intermittent targeted treatment and continuous minimal dosing. The goal of the *intermittent targeted* strategy is to reduce total drug exposure, administering the drug only when there are active symptoms. The goal of *continuous minimal dosing* is the avoidance of relapse by providing a continuous coverage at a much lower dosage than during the acute episodes. Dose reduction may be considered once the patient has been stabilized for a 3- to 6-month period.

Typically, antipsychotic drugs are first given orally for at least 1 to 2 weeks before the patient is switched to a depot formulation. The depot form is administered, and the oral dosage tapered. At this time, no specific guidelines for tapering the oral dose have been developed. Tapering is handled on an individual basis, remaining cognizant that the steady state of the parenteral formulations is not achieved for several weeks.

The first oral dose of an antipsychotic should be given 12 to 24 hours after administration of the last parenteral dose. An intramuscular (IM) injection is the preferred route (for the most rapid effect) when prompt control of an acutely agitated patient is desired. The injection should be given in a large muscle mass. The patient should be kept recumbent for at least 30 minutes after administration to minimize the drug's hypotensive effects. If the patient refuses the injection, a liquid formulation may be used. Liquid formulations provide a more rapid response than do tablet forms. Oral formulations are to be taken with food, milk, or a full glass of water to minimize gastric irritation. Most concentrates can be diluted in 120 mL of water or fruit juice just before administration. Avoid getting the solution on the hands because it can cause contact dermatitis.

Education

The patient and support individuals who assist the patient (e.g., family or assisted living supervisor) must be taught about the psychotic disorder, its possible etiologies, the associated behaviors, and the importance of drug therapy in managing symptoms. Because some symptoms subside before others, it is helpful to educate the patient and his or her support system about which behaviors are likely to change first and how long after initiation of treatment the change will take place.

The information about possible adverse effects is necessary so that the patient does not become anxious when the responses develop. Teach the patient that many of the effects will subside in a few weeks. Also, it is imperative to instruct the patient and the support person about early and late onset adverse effects and how they might be managed. Often, there is a misunderstanding about the need to vary the dosage in a specifically supervised manner. Patients worry that varying the dosage may exacerbate symptoms. Ongoing reinforcement is especially important given the cognitive effects of schizophrenia and other psychoses. Advise the patient taking chlorpromazine, mesoridazine, thiothixene, or trifluoperazine that it may color the urine pink or reddish brown. Yellowing of the skin and eyes is common with molindone. Patients taking trifluoperazine should also be cautioned to avoid prolonged exposure to the sun to minimize photosensitivity reactions.

Institute seizure precautions for the patient on clozapine because the drug lowers the seizure threshold. Patients should be instructed about how to care for the transient fevers that may occur during the first 3 weeks of therapy. Patients should be advised to avoid extremes in temperature because olanzapine, risperidone, and sertindole impair body temperature regulation.

The adverse effects might also be managed by the concurrent administration of another drug. For example, benztropine (COGENTIN) may be administered to diminish the anticholinergic effects of haloperidol. The patient should be taught that chewing sugarless gum may assist in relieving the dry mouth associated with the drug. Frequent rinsing with cool water can refresh a dry mouth. If the patient experiences hypotensive effects, education about changing positions and rising slowly from lying or seated positions is needed.

Drug-specific instructions about withdrawal responses should be given to the patient. Patients should be cautioned not to take OTC drugs that contain interactive ingredients (e.g., antacids and drugs containing alcohol).

The patient should be advised to carry a medical alert identification that contains information about the antipsychotic management regimen. He or she should be instructed to inform all health care providers (e.g., nurses, physicians, practitioners, dentists, physical therapists) of their regimen. In so doing, monitoring for therapeutic effects and adverse drug effects and interactions can occur.

Evaluation

The effectiveness of antipsychotic therapy can be demonstrated by a decrease in the severity of psychosis and diminished symptoms. A decrease in agitation should be noted within hours of initiating therapy, and significant improvement should be seen within 24 to 48 hours. Sleep disturbances should improve within days, hallucinations within weeks, and thought disorders within 1 to 2 months. Negative symptoms such as anhedonia and restricted or blunted affect take weeks to months to improve. In some cases, negative symptoms may not improve at all. Some patients require 8 to 12 weeks of therapy at typical doses before a full response is noted. The biggest mistake health care providers make is to change drug therapy too quickly. The antipsychotic drug that provides therapeutic results with minimal adverse effects is the most effective management option. If a positive response is seen and yet intolerable adverse effects develop, the dosage can be lowered. If dosage reduction is ineffective, the drug can be stopped and the patient switched to an alternative agent. Monotherapy is recommended. There is no therapeutic advantage in combining different classes of drugs.

Patients should be monitored weekly for signs of decompensation. There is a 50-percent relapse rate at 6 months. One year after therapy is discontinued, the relapse rate is approximately 70 percent. If therapy is continued, only 40 percent of patients relapse. As a rule, after the first episode of decompensation, the patient should be treated continuously for 1 year. After a second episode, he or she should be treated continuously for at least 3 years. With a third episode of decompensation, consider treating the patient for at least 5 years before attempting a drug holiday. However, the risk of developing tardive dyskinesia increases with the length of therapy and the patient's age.

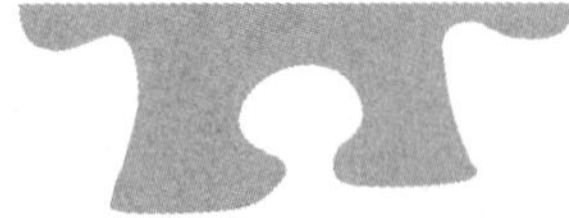

SUMMARY

- Schizophrenia is a group of psychotic disorders characterized by gross distortions of reality, disorganization, fragmented perception, thought and emotion, and withdrawal from social interactions.
- The exact etiology of schizophrenia is unknown but is thought to be related to biologic alterations in dopamine transmission and anatomic differences in the brain.
- Antipsychotic drugs assist in managing symptoms of psychosis, including thought disorders, hallucinations, bizarre behaviors and agitation, and hyperactivity.
- First-generation antipsychotic drugs block dopamine receptors in postsynaptic nerve tissues, and in the CTZ of the medulla.
- Second-generation drugs act at dopamine sites at the cortical and limbic regions of the brain with less effect in the nigrostriatal region.
- Common adverse effects of first-generation and second-generation drugs include sedation, extrapyramidal reactions (e.g., dystonia, parkinsonism, akathisia, and tardive dyskinesia), seizures, and neuroleptic malignant syndrome (e.g., diaphoresis, muscular rigidity, and hyperpyrexia).
- Orthostatic hypotension is common with the IM formulations of antipsychotic drugs.
- There are many drug-drug interactions with antipsychotic drugs, including interactions with anticholinergics, antidepressants, beta blockers, bromocriptine, catecholamines, and antiparkinson drugs.
- Assessment of the patient includes eliciting information about past medical problems and the use of psychotropic drugs by the patient and his or her family members.
- Baseline physical exam and laboratory testing should be performed before and during therapy to monitor therapeutic and adverse effects.
- The primary treatment objectives for the patient with schizophrenia are to diminish psychotic behaviors, thus preventing harm to the patient or others, improving thought disorders, reducing duration of inpatient hospitalization, and preventing or decreasing future exacerbations.
- Maintenance drug therapy is valuable in preventing psychotic relapse, recurrence, and rehospitalization.
- Therapeutic dosages should be maintained for at least 4 to 6 weeks, and the patient's response should be evaluated before use of a different drug is considered.
- Dosage is individualized based on patient response and tolerance to adverse effects because no evidence suggests that higher doses of antipsychotic drugs are likely to improve psychosis more quickly. High doses of antipsychotics increase the risk of adverse effects and should be avoided.
- Intermittent targeted treatment reduces total drug exposure by administering the drug only when there are active symptoms. Continuous minimal dosing avoids relapse by providing continuous coverage at a much lower dosage than during acute episodes.
- Patient teaching includes drug actions, interactions, anticipated therapeutic effects, adverse effects, and administration regimen.
- The effectiveness of antipsychotic therapy is demonstrated by a decrease in the severity of psychosis and diminished symptoms.

BIBLIOGRAPHY

Abramowicz, M. (Ed.). (1997). *Drugs of choice from the medical letter.* New Rochelle, NY: The Medical Letter, Inc.

Abramowicz, M. (Ed.). (1997). Drugs for psychiatric disorders. *The Medical Letter on Drugs and Therapeutics,* 39(998), 38–40.

Abramowicz, M. (Ed.). (1997). Olanzapine for schizophrenia. *The Medical Letter on Drugs and Therapeutics,* 38(992), 5–6.

American Psychiatric Association. (1994). *Diagnostic and statistical manual of mental disorders* (4th ed.). Washington, DC: Author.

Brier, A. (1995). Serotonin, schizophrenia and antipsychotic drug action. *Schizophrenia Research,* 14, 187–202.

Byerly, M., and DeVane, C. (1996). Pharmacokinetics of clozapine and risperidone: A review of recent literature. *Journal of Clinical Psychopharmacology,* 16, 177–187.

Chengappa, K., Baker, R., Schooler, N., et al. (1995). Clozapine-associated agranulocytosis: Treatment with G-CSF. *Psychopharmacology Bulletin,* 31, 556.

Cooper, J., Bloom, F., and Roth, R. (1996). *The biochemical basis of neuropharmacology.* (7th ed.). New York: Oxford University Press.

Hongifeld, G. (1996). The clozapine national registry system: Forty years of risk management. *Journal of Clinical Psychiatry,* 14, 29–32.

Johnson, D. (1990). Pharmacological treatment of patients with schizophrenia. *Drugs,* 39(4), 481–488.

Kane, J., and McGlasham, T. (1995). Treatment of schizophrenia. *Lancet,* 346, 820–825.

Kane, J. (1990). Psychopharmacologic treatment issues. *Psychiatry and Medicine,* 8(1), 111–124.

Keltner, N., and Folks, D. (1997). *Psychotropic drugs* (2nd ed.). St. Louis: Mosby–Year Book, Inc.

Liberman, J., Koreen, A., Chakos, M., et al. (1996). Factors influencing treatment response and outcome of first episode schizophrenia: Implications for understanding the pathophysiology of schizophrenia. *Journal of Clinical Psychiatry,* 57(suppl 9), 5–9.

Marder, S. (1996). Clinical experiences with risperidone. *Journal of Clinical Psychiatry,* 57(Suppl 9), 57–61.

Perry, P., Alexander, B., and Liskow, B. (1997). *Psychotropic drug handbook* (7th ed.). Washington, DC: American Psychiatric Press.

Schatzberg, A., and Nemeroff, C. (Eds.). (1995). *The American psychiatric press textbook of psychopharmacology.* Washington, DC: American Psychiatric Press.

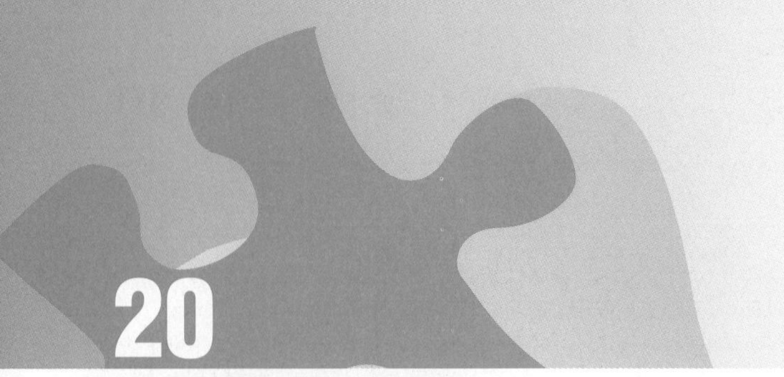

20 Central Nervous System Stimulants

Many drugs stimulate the central nervous system (CNS), but only a few are used therapeutically and their indications are limited. Three disorders are treated with CNS stimulants: narcolepsy, attention deficit—hyperactivity disorder (ADHD; formerly referred to as attention deficit disorder and hyperkinetic syndrome), and exogenous obesity. However, stimulants have a long history of use and abuse for nonmedical purposes. Coffee, tea, chocolate, cola drinks, cocaine, yerba mate, betel, mescaline, and peyote are among the CNS stimulants used in various cultures. Continuous use and abuse of CNS stimulants can result in the development of drug tolerance, drug dependence, and drug abuse.

CNS stimulants are classified according to their major effects. Psychomotor stimulants (e.g., amphetamines) primarily stimulate the cerebral cortex. Anorexiants suppress the appetite center, and analeptics (e.g., caffeine) affect centers in the medulla and brainstem.

NARCOLEPSY

Epidemiology and Etiology

Narcolepsy is a sleep disorder thought to be caused by a disturbance of the rapid eye movement (REM) sleep cycle. It occurs in 0.5 percent of adults but begins during adolescence and is more common in first-degree relatives. Although specific antigens (DR15, DQw6, and DW2) have been widely implicated, research suggests environmental factors contribute to the disorder.

Males are slightly more affected than females. Although the first episode of narcolepsy can occur at any time up to the age of 60 years, its first occurrence most frequently appears in patients in their 20s.

Pathophysiology

Symptoms of narcolepsy mimic natural experiences of the sleep-wake cycle. Falling asleep involves a shift from an alert, fully conscious responsive state to a dreamlike transition state. There is partial muscle relaxation followed by autoimagery and the complete muscle relaxation of sleep. The patient who experiences narcolepsy may have one or all of his or her natural sleep activities disturbed.

Seventy to 80 percent of patients with narcolepsy experience cataplexy. *Cataplexy* is characterized by sudden brief episodes of muscle weakness and paralysis. It is related to inhibition of the monosynaptic H-reflex and multisynaptic tendon reflexes. The neurotransmitters acetylcholine (ACh) and catecholamines help regulate REM sleep and are involved in somatic muscle tone and inhibition of deep tendon reflexes.

Sleep paralysis and hypnagogic hallucinations occur during the transition stage between wakefulness and sleep. Sleep paralysis manifests as loss of muscle tone, paralysis, and the inability to speak, although the patient is fully alert. Patients may experience paralysis at any time, but are particularly prone to attacks during emotional disturbances, such as excitement, crying, or even laughter. The patient may collapse but remain conscious, as if having a seizure, if the area of weakness is in the trunk or lower body. When only the head and neck area is involved, the patient may not show overt symptoms. The hallucinations are brief, fragmented, and dreamlike. Bizarre experiences occur while the patient is not fully awake, but not yet dreaming.

Although the preceding symptoms are the most common signs of narcolepsy, less observable symptoms are by far the most frequent. Patients may note slight buckling of the knees, but the buckling is imperceptible to an observer. The observer may notice only that the patient used a wall for support. A weakening of the jaw, similar to that accompanying the REM stage of sleep, may occur. Jaw weakness affects speech or causes wide masticatory movements or brief stutter. Patients also may complain of clumsiness, especially when they are startled or laughing. During the episodic attacks, an observer may notice the patient performing mindless and simple repetitive tasks.

Some clinicians also recognize a lesser known form of narcolepsy. Patients experiencing this form have disturbed nocturnal sleep. Although they are able to fall asleep without difficulty, they awaken after 2½ to 3 hours and may stay awake for an hour. The interval of sleeplessness is followed by yet another 2½ to 3 hours of sleep. Interestingly, treating this nighttime sleep problem has no effect on daytime somnolence.

ATTENTION DEFICIT—HYPERACTIVITY DISORDER

ADHD is one of several problems that include attention deficit disorder without hyperactivity, minimal brain dysfunction, and hyperkinesis. Diagnosis depends on patient symptoms. This section discusses ADHD because it is representative of all the others.

Epidemiology and Etiology

ADHD is found in children and is characterized by inattention, distractibility, impulsivity, and hyperactivity. The onset of symptoms occurs between the ages of 3 and 7 years. Boys are affected more often than girls by a 10:1 ratio. Symptoms must be present for 6 months before a diagnosis can be made. ADHD accounts for more referrals to child mental health services in the United States than any other singular disorder. Because other disorders (especially anxiety and depression) may cause similar symptoms, a diagnosis of ADHD must be made with care.

Although ADHD was initially conceived as a disorder of childhood, there is a growing number of adults with the disorder. Controversy continues as to whether the adult manifesting ADHD behavior is simply immature, or an individual of "bad character." Researchers who recognize adult ADHD are unsure whether the newly diagnosed adults were actually undiagnosed as children, or if there is an adult onset variety of ADHD.

Theories about the etiology of ADHD include a genetic relationship, trauma or infection in utero, nutritional deficits or allergies, an imbalance in dopamine or norepinephrine, a mutant thyroid receptor, or abnormal metabolism of the frontal lobe of the brain. A single cause of the disorder has yet to be identified.

Genetic factors are a prime suspect. First-degree relatives have a four times greater rate of ADHD compared to control subjects. Some theories propose that patients who develop ADHD have had a perinatal brain insult as a result of trauma or intrauterine infection. Head trauma, meningitis, and encephalitis are additional suspected causes.

Nutritional deficits and food allergies, particularly to certain food additives such as dyes or preservatives, have shown promise as possible causes of ADHD. Refined sugar or vitamin deficiencies also have been suggested as possible causes.

Alterations in norepinephrine and in the turnover of dopamine may be equally responsible for ADHD. What is not certain is why dopamine levels are lower in patients with ADHD than in other patients. Perhaps there is a deficiency in production, supply, or transmission of norepinephrine and dopamine. Dopamine agonists have been effective in relieving the symptoms of ADHD. This observation suggests that the patient finds relief when dopamine levels are restored. The increased firing rate of tissues in the fourth ventricle (locus ceruleus) causes increased levels of norepinephrine that in turn are available for use at the synapse.

Another theory suggests that a genetically mutant thyroid receptor might be at fault. Although some patients have improved with thyroid replacement therapy, researchers are still not able to locate the mutant thyroid receptors in a significant number of patients.

Abnormal metabolism of the frontal lobe of the brain could be a factor in the etiology of ADHD. Some children with ADHD manifest hypoperfusion of the frontal cortex, and some adults with ADHD have shown atrophy in the same area. Parents of children with ADHD, who were themselves diagnosed with ADHD, showed deficient use of glucose in the frontal cortex and some other areas.

ADHD is exacerbated by stress. Children with ADHD have lives fraught with stress. Their inattentive, impulsive behavior results in difficulties with peers and teachers. Frustrated parents often find their children difficult or impossible to deal with. Negative retorts produce low self-esteem and greater stress, which in turn propagates a worsening of symptoms.

Pathophysiology

The frontal lobe of the brain is involved in activities that include receiving, processing, storing, and retrieving information. The reticular activating system (RAS) is the "alarm clock" responsible for arousing cortical areas of the brain to receive information from sensory cortex. The connections between these structures and emotion, cognition, and behavior are not completely understood. It is known that the frontal lobe, through its communications with other areas of the brain (e.g., limbic system) initiates, sustains, inhibits, and shifts attention to organize, plan, and accomplish goals. Frontal lobe disorders are associated with disturbances in the areas of production, attention, cognition, and impulse control.

EXOGENOUS OBESITY

Epidemiology and Etiology

Obesity occurs in 35 percent of American women and 31 percent of American men. It has been defined as a body mass index (BMI) of 27 or above. The BMI is the ratio of the weight in kilograms to the height in square meters. The normal range for both men and women is a BMI between 20 and 25. An individual is considered overweight with a BMI of 25 to 30, and obese with a BMI over 30. The desirable percentage of fat to body weight in men is 9 to 18 percent of total body weight, and the ideal for women is between 18 and 28 percent.

Overweight and obesity are refractory problems in the United States. Before the industrial revolution in the United States, obesity was rare. At one time obesity was a sign of prosperity; wealthier individuals could afford excesses. In more recent times, however, obesity has been recognized as a health hazard and is especially prevalent among the poor and lower economic classes. The prevalence of obesity is 6 to 12 times more frequent in women of lower socioeconomic status than in women of the upper social classes. Black women are much more likely to be obese than white women, and 12 percent of young children are obese. Perhaps there is an over-reliance on junk foods and failure to consume natural, healthier foods. Also, it is easier and initially cheaper to prepare the tastier high fat foods, or to buy from fast food restaurants, rather than prepare healthier meals.

The shift during the 20th century from diets in which the majority of calories come from carbohydrates, to diets in which the majority of calories come from fat is a major cause of obesity. Another contributing factor is the substitution of machinery for muscle. We have progressed from a "wood-chopping" society to a society in which our most strenuous exercise may be the use of an index finger to change television channels or trigger the mouse on our computers. Evidence also points to a genetic component in the tendency toward obesity. Energy expenditure and fat distribution appear to be particularly influenced by heredity. Individuals with a family history of obesity may be viewed as having a vulnerability to obesity, with the environment playing a protective or permissive role in its ultimate development.

Pathophysiology

Obesity is either exogenous or endogenous. Exogenous obesity is defined as an imbalance between caloric intake and caloric needs. Endogenous obesity is secondary to another physical problem such as diabetes or an endocrine disorder. The underlying problem in endogenous obesity must be treated before the problem of obesity can be resolved.

Studies suggest that the resting metabolic rate of people who become obese may be slower from the beginning. Other studies suggest that children who are obese have an increased number of fat cells *(hyperplasia)*, not just larger fat cells *(hypertrophy)*. Thus, adults who were obese as children have up to three times as many fat cells as those who were of normal weight as children, which may make it easier for children to develop obesity as adults. Individuals who become obese later in life do not have an increased number of fat cells, but only much larger ones.

Whereas the accumulation of fat is around the waist in men, it tends to be in the lower body area in women. Although the exact mechanism of this phenomenon is unknown, obesity is associated with several different problems including hypertension, hyperlipidemia, carbohydrate intolerance, cardiac problems, back problems, and strokes.

PHARMACOTHERAPEUTIC OPTIONS

Psychomotor Stimulants

- ❒ Amphetamine sulfate
- ❒ Dextroamphetamine sulfate (DEXEDRINE)
- ❒ Methamphetamine (DESOXYN)
- ❒ Methylphenidate (RITALIN)
- ❒ Pemoline (CYLERT)

Indications

Psychomotor stimulants such as amphetamines promote arousal and alleviate symptoms of narcolepsy. They are particularly helpful in the management of moderate to severe ADHD. In addition to managing behavior, stimulants are thought to increase cognition, especially math and reading skills. There is also evidence that these drugs enhance memory. However, the use of psychomotor stimulants to combat fatigue and delay sleep, such as with long-distance drivers, students, and athletes, is not warranted.

Pharmacodynamics

Amphetamines have powerful CNS stimulant activities in addition to the peripheral alpha and beta actions common with indirect-acting sympathomimetic drugs. The releasing amines form storage sites in nerve terminals. The alerting, anorectic effect and at least a portion of its locomotor-stimulating action are mediated by the release of norepinephrine. Some aspects of locomotor activity and stereotypic behaviors that are induced by amphetamines are probably related to the release of dopamine from dopaminergic nerve terminals.

Disturbances in perception and overt psychotic behavior result with high doses of amphetamines. These effects are due to the release of serotonin (5-hydroxytryptamine, 5-HT) from tryptaminergic neurons and of dopamine from the mesolimbic system.

The anorectic actions produced by amphetamines are probably centered in the lateral hypothalamic feeding center. However, tolerance to the appetite suppression effects rapidly develops.

Adverse Effects and Contraindications

Psychomotor stimulants cause CNS excitation; hence their adverse effects are numerous. Tachycardia, irritability, nocturnal sleep disturbances, tremor, restlessness, amphetamine psychosis, seizures, arrhythmias, anorexia, drug tolerance, and dependency have all been associated with stimulants. They have a high potential for abuse (Chapter 9).

Adverse gastrointestinal effects include dry mouth, metallic taste, anorexia, nausea, vomiting, diarrhea, and abdominal cramps; however, these effects are unpredictable. If enteric activity is pronounced, amphetamines may cause relaxation and delay the movement of intestinal contents. If the gut is already relaxed, the opposite effect may be seen.

Psychomotor stimulants produce cardiac stimulation. Thus, they are contraindicated in patients with cardiovascular disease (e.g., hypertension, angina, arrhythmias) or hyperthyroidism. They are also contraindicated in patients who are anxious or agitated and in patients who have asthenia, psychopathic personalities, or a history of homicidal or suicidal tendencies. Patients with glaucoma should not be given psychomotor stimulants. Amphetamines in general have teratogenic effects, and their use during pregnancy should be avoided. Uterine response varies, but usually there is an increase in uterine muscle tone.

Psychomotor stimulants are not recommended for treatment of ADHD in children under the age of 6 years, or as anorexiants in children less than 12 years old. When used, psychomotor stimulants should be dosed carefully and the child closely monitored because the effects of long-term use are unknown. Suppression of height and weight has been reported as a result of appetite suppression. Psychomotor stimulants may exacerbate symptoms in children with psychosis or Tourette's syndrome.

Psychomotor stimulants should be used cautiously in the older adult. As with most other drugs, the slowed biotransformation and elimination capabilities associated with aging increase the risk of accumulation and toxicity. Older adults are likely to experience anxiety, nervousness, insomnia, and mental confusion from excessive CNS stimulation.

Pharmacokinetics

Psychomotor stimulants are rapidly absorbed after oral administration. The onset time averages 1 to 2 hours, with a duration of 4 to 10 hours (Table 20–1). Biotransformation is by the liver. The plasma half-life varies from 7 to 34 hours depending on urinary pH. Alkaline urine (as with consumption of cranberry juice) promotes reabsorption and prolongs drug action. The more acidic the urine, the faster the rate of elimination. Amphetamines cross the placental membranes and enter breast milk.

Drug-Drug Interactions

Psychomotor stimulants change insulin requirements (Table 20–2) and should be used with caution by diabetics. Amphetamines decrease the effects of antihypertensives and should not be used in combination with monoamine oxidase (MAO) inhibitors or MAO inhibitor-like drugs.

TABLE 20–1 PHARMACOKINETICS OF SELECTED CENTRAL NERVOUS SYSTEM STIMULANTS

Drug	Route	Onset	Peak	Duration	PB (%)	t½
Psychomotor Stimulants						
Amphetamine	po	1–2 hr	UK	4–10 hr	UA	7–34 hr*
Benzphetamine	po	rapid	UA	4 hr	UA	6–12 hr
Dextroamphetamine	po	1–2 hr	2 hr	2–10 hr	UA	10 hr; 6.8†
Methylphenidate	po	rapid	1–3 hr	4–6 hr; 8 hr+	UA	1–3 hr
Methamphetamine	po	1–2 hr	4–6 hr	2–10 hr	UA	10,2 hr; 6.8‡
Pemoline	po	30–45 min§	2–4 hr	8–12 hr	50	9–14 hr‖
Anorexiants						
Diethylpropion	po	UK	UK	4 hr	UK	4-6 hr
Fenfluramine	po	1–2 hr	2–4 hr	4–6 hr	UK	11–20 hr
Maxindol	po	30–60 min	UK	8–15 hr	UK	10 hr
Phenmetrazine	po	rapid	UK	4 hr	UK	UK
Phendimetrazine	po	rapid	4–6 hr	4 hr	UK	1.9–9.8 hr
Phentermine	po	UA	UA	4 hr	UA	UA
Phenylpropanolamine	po	rapid	1–2 hr	3 hr	UA	3–4 hr
Analeptics						
Caffeine	po	15 min	15–45 min	UA	UA	3–4 hr
Doxapram	IV	20–40 sec	1–2 min	5–12 min	UA	2.4–4.1 hr

*Depends on the acidity of the urine. If pH is less than 5.6, the half-life is 7 to 8 hours. Alkalinization of the urine increases the half-life, with a range between 18.6 and 33.6 hours. Every unit increase in urinary pH increases the plasma half-life by an average of 7 hours.

†Dextroamphetamine and methamphetamine: half-life in children is 6.8 hours.

‡Methylphenidate: duration of action 8 hours with extended-release formulations.

§Pemoline: onset of effects in 2 to 3 weeks. Blood levels reached in 30 to 45 minutes.

‖Pemoline: half-life follows nonlinear kinetics in children, which increases the half-life.

PB, protein binding; UA, unavailable; UK, unknown; t½, elimination half-life.

Death may occur from hypertensive crisis or cerebral hemorrhage.

Dosage Regimen

Dosages are tailored to patient needs and symptoms (Table 20–3). Most psychomotor stimulants, anorexiants, and analeptics should be used as adjuncts to other therapies and then only briefly. Tolerance may develop with long-term use; therefore, prolonged therapy is contraindicated. Therapy should be interrupted periodically and the patient's condition evaluated to determine whether continued use of the drug is necessary.

Many of the psychomotor stimulants are available as extended release or resin complexes, so the patient need take only one dose per day. Although this regimen is convenient, these formulations should never be used in the initial or subsequent titrations of the drug. The extended-release or resin complex formulations should be used only when the titration-determined daily dose is equal to, or exceeds, the dose of the extended-release form.

Laboratory Considerations

No specific laboratory monitoring is required for patients receiving psychomotor stimulants. Serum drug levels are seldom measured. A complete blood count should be done before the start of therapy. Leukopenia and anemia have been known to occur with the use of methylphenidate. Urine catecholamines should be checked before and during methylphenidate therapy to determine increased dopamine levels.

Anorexiants

- ❒ Benzphetamine (DIDREX)
- ❒ Diethylpropion (TENUATE, TEPANIL); (🍁) NOBESINE, PROPIONT, REGIBON
- ❒ Mazindol (SANOREX, MAZANOR)
- ❒ Phendimetrazine (ADIPOST, ANOREX, BONTRIL, DYREXAN-OD, PLEGINE)
- ❒ Phenmetrazine (PRELUDIN)

Indications

All anorexiants are used in the short-term management of obesity. When prescribed, they are intended to act as adjuncts to other therapies, such as behavior modification, exercise, and calorie restrictions. Treatment with an anorexiant should not exceed 6 to 12 weeks. Tolerance to the anorectic effect usually occurs within that time. Fenfluramine and phentermine had shown promise in the treatment of obesity, but have been recently withdrawn from the market because of potentially severe adverse effects.

Pharmacodynamics

The anorexiants are primarily phenethylamines, similar to amphetamines. Their mechanism of action leading to appetite suppression is unknown, but they may stimulate the satiety center in the hypothalamus. It is also thought that they act in the CNS to cause release of catecholamines from nerve terminals.

TABLE 20–2 DRUG-DRUG INTERACTIONS OF SELECTED CENTRAL NERVOUS SYSTEM STIMULANTS

Drug	Interacting Drug	Interaction
Psychomotor Stimulants		
Amphetamines	Acetazolamide	Enhances the effects of amphetamines
Dextroamphetamine	Sodium bicarbonate	
Methamphetamine	Thiazide diuretics	
	MAO inhibitors	Increases pressor response to amphetamines. Death from hypertensive crisis or intracranial hemorrhage
	Furazolidone	
	Ammonium chloride	Decreases effects of amphetamine
	Ascorbic acid	
	Haloperidol	
	Phenothiazine	
	Tricyclic antidepressants	
	General anesthetics	Increases risk of arrhythmias
	Cyclopropane	
	Halothane	
	Antihypertensive drugs	Increases risk of interacting drug
	Guanethidine	
	Methyldopa	Decreased hypotensive effect of interacting drug
	Insulin	Insulin requirements change
	Urinary acidifiers	Reduced duration of action of amphetamine
	Urine alkalinizers	Increases duration of action of amphetamines
Methylphenidate	MAO inhibitors	Increases pressor effects
	Pressor drugs	
	Guanethidine	Reduces hypotensive effects
	Bretylium	
	Coumarin anticoagulants	Reduces metabolism of methylphenidate with potential for toxicity
	Phenylbutazone anticonvulsants	
	Tricyclic antidepressants	
Pemoline	Anticonvulsants	Reduces seizure threshold
Anorexiants		
Diethylpropion	Insulin	Reduced insulin requirements
	Guanethidine	Reduced hypotensive effect of interactive drug
Fenfluramine	Alcohol	Effects may be additive. May have catecholamine depleting effects
	CNS depressants	
	General anesthetics	
	Antihypertensive drugs	Changes in blood pressure may occur in either direction
	MAO inhibitors	Hypertensive crisis
	Insulin	Reduced insulin requirements
	Alcohol	Increases psychiatric symptoms of paranoia, psychosis, and depression
Maxindol	Insulin	Reduces insulin requirements
	Guanethidine	Reduces hypotensive effects of interacting drug
	Exogenous catecholamines	Pressor effects are potentiated
	Isoproterenol	
	Norepinephrine	
	MAO inhibitors	Hypertensive crisis
Phendimetrazine	Insulin	Changes insulin requirements
Phenmetrazine		
Phentermine	Guanethidine	Reduces hypotensive effect of interacting drug
Phenylpropanolamine	Guanethidine	Reduces hypotensive effect of interacting drug
	Indomethacin	Severe hypertensive episode
	MAO inhibitors	Hypertensive crisis and intracranial hemorrhage
	Furazolidone	
Analeptics		
Doxapram	MAO inhibitors	Increased pressor effects of interactive drug
	Sympathomimetics	
	Cyclopropane	Increased effects of interactive drug
	Enflurane	
	Halothane	
Caffeine	Ciprofloxacin	Increases caffeine concentrations and may enhance adverse effects
	Cimetidine	
	Oral contraceptives	
	Disulfiram	
	Enoxacin	
	Phenylpropanolamine	
	Pipemidic acid	
	Smoking	Decreased effects of caffeine
	Aspirin	Increases metabolism of interacting drugs
	Phenobarbital	

MAO, Monoamine oxidase.

TABLE 20–3 DOSAGE REGIMENS FOR SELECTED CENTRAL NERVOUS SYSTEM STIMULANTS

Drug	Use(s)	Dosage	Implications*
Psychomotor Stimulants			
Amphetamine Dextroamphetamine	Narcolepsy	*Adult:* 5–60 mg po QD in single or 2–3 divided doses. *Child age 6–12 yr:* 5 mg po QD. Increase by 5 mg weekly based on patient response. *Child over age 12 yr:* 10 mg po QD initially. Increase by 10 mg weekly based on patient response	Give initial dose on awakening. If divided doses, give at 4–6 hr intervals. Reduce dosage, if adverse effects are intolerable. Give last daily dose early enough not to interfere with night sleep
	Exogenous obesity	*Adult:* 5–30 mg po QD in divided doses *Child over 12 yr:* 5–30 mg po QD in divided doses of 5–10 mg	Prolonged therapy is contraindicated
	ADHD	*Child over 6 yr:* 5 mg po QD–BID initially. Increase by 5 mg weekly based on patient response. Maximum: 40 mg *Child age 3–5 yr:* 2.5 mg po QD initially. Increase by 2.5 mg weekly based on patient response	Initial dose should be taken on awakening. If dividing into two to three doses, separate intervals by 4 to 6 hrs
Benzphetamine	Exogenous obesity	*Adult:* 25–50 mg po QD mid-morning or mid-afternoon. Increase to maximum of 50 mg TID	Avoid late afternoon administration. Safety and efficacy have not been established for children under 12 years.
Methamphetamine	Exogenous obesity	*Adult:* 2.5–5 mg po BID–TID before meals	Adjust dose individually, smallest dose to achieve desired effect. Do not use to combat exhaustion or fatigue
	ADHD	*Child over 6 yr:* 2.5–5 mg po initially QD–BID. Increase daily dose by 5 mg weekly to desired response. Maintenance: 20–25 mg po QD	Do not use as a substitute for sleep or as anorexiant for children younger than 12 years. Interrupt therapy and re-evaluate need for drug
Methylphenidate	ADHD	*Child over age 6 yr:* 0.25 mg/kg/day. Maximum: 2 mg/kg/day. Not to exceed 60 mg daily	Individual variations in response require careful dose adjustments. If desired response has not been achieved in 1 month after appropriate dosage adjustments, discontinue drug. Patient's improved condition may remain after drug is discontinued. Discontinue when child reaches adolescence
	Narcolepsy	*Adult:* 10 mg po BID–TID before meals. Maximum: 60 mg po QD	Do not use for normal fatigue states
Pemoline	ADHD	*Child over age 6 yr:* 37.5 mg po QD as single dose. Increase daily dose by 18.75 mg weekly to desired response. Maintenance:56.75–75 mg QD Do not exceed 112.5 mg QD	Adjust dose carefully. Response is widely varied. Expect response third or fourth week of therapy. Do not use indefinitely. Discontinue when child reaches adolescence. Patient's improved behavior may continue indefinitely after drug is terminated. Safety and efficacy have not been established in children younger than 6 years of age
Anorexiants			
Diethylpropion	Exogenous obesity	*Adult:* 25 mg po TID. May give an additional 25 mg in mid-evening if necessary	Not recommended for children younger than age 12
Fenfluramine	Obesity	*Adult:* 20 mg po TID before meals. Increase at 20 mg intervals weekly to desired response. Maximum: 40 mg TID	If initial dose is not well tolerated, reduce dose to 20 mg BID and gradually titrate upward
Maxindol	Obesity	*Adult:* 1 mg po TID before meals or 2 mg QD 1 hour before lunch	Safety and efficacy have not been established for children younger than 12 years.
Phendimetrazine	Exogenous obesity	*Adult:* 35 mg po BID-TID ac Range: 17.5 mg BID to maximum dose of 70 mg TID	Response to desired effects and tolerance is varied. Adjust dose individually, smallest dose to achieve desired effect. Not for children younger than 12 years
Phenmetrazine	Obesity	*Adult:* 25 mg po BID–TID po	Prolonged therapy and use in children are contraindicated. Sustained release provides 12-hour appetite suppression
Phentermine	Obesity	*Adult:* 8 mg po TID ac *or* 15–37.5 mg as single AM dose, 14 hours before bedtime	Not for children under 12 years
Phenylpropanolamine	Obesity	*Adult:* 25 mg po TID before meals. Timed release: 75 mg po QD. Precision release: 75 mg after meals	Precision release has 16-hour duration of action. Safety and efficacy have not been established

Table continued on following page

TABLE 20–3 DOSAGE REGIMENS FOR SELECTED CENTRAL NERVOUS SYSTEM STIMULANTS *Continued*

Drug	Use(s)	Dosage	Implications*
Analeptics			
Caffeine	Aid in staying awake, adjunct to analgesics, respiratory effects of CNS depression	*Adult:* 100–200 mg po q3–4 hr PRN. Extended release formulation: 200 mg po q3–4 hr *Respiratory depression:* 500–1000 mg IM. Do not exceed 2.5 g/day. May be given IV in severe emergency situation	Safety and efficacy in children have not been established
Doxapram	Drug-induced CNS depression	*Adult:* 2 mg/kg IV repeated in 5-minute intervals. Repeat every 1–2 hours until patient awakens. Initiate infusion at 5 mg/min. Once response is seen, 1–3 mg/min is satisfactory	If no response, continue supportive measures and repeat priming dose in 1–2 hours

*Most psychomotor stimulants, analeptics, and anorexiants should be used as adjuncts to other therapies and then only briefly. Tolerance may develop with long-term use; therefore, prolonged therapy is contraindicated. Interrupt therapy and evaluate patient's condition periodically to determine whether continued use of the drug is necessary.

Adverse Effects and Contraindications

Because of CNS stimulant actions, the most frequently reported adverse effects of anorexiants include palpitations, tachycardia, restlessness, dizziness, insomnia, weakness, fatigue, and drowsiness. Less frequently reported effects include depression, confusion, allergic skin rashes, and psychosis. Arrhythmias, dyspnea, pulmonary hypertension, hypertension, malaise, euphoria, vomiting, diarrhea, rash, and menstrual irregularities are less common. Children younger than 12 years of age should not be given anorexiant drugs.

Pharmacokinetics

The stimulants are rapidly absorbed when taken orally. Peak activity is noted in 1 to 2 hours for some agents and up to 6 hours for others. The duration of action also varies from 3 to 15 hours. Table 20–1 summarizes the pharmacokinetics of selected anorexiants. Although there are wide individual variations, the metabolites are excreted in the urine within 2 hours of administration. Acidic urine increases the elimination; alkaline urine decreases the rate of elimination.

Drug-Drug Interactions

As with the amphetamines, there are many drug-drug interactions with anorexiant drugs. Table 20–2 provides an overview of selected drug interactions. Patients who have been on MAO inhibitors within the previous 14 days should not receive anorexiants. The effects of antihypertensives may be blocked by anorexiant drugs.

Dosage Regimen

Dosage recommendations are individualized and depend on the drug used (see Table 20–3). Anorexiants are for short-term use and only as an adjunct to other therapies. When tolerance develops, the drug should be discontinued. The dosage should not be increased to achieve the same therapeutic effect.

Laboratory Considerations

Because there are wide individual variations to therapeutic responses in the pharmacologic treatment of exogenous obesity, urine and serum levels of the stimulants and anorexiants are only marginally helpful. The health care provider's own observations of the patient, the patient's weight, and patient reports are the most useful in determining success. Taking vital signs is important because of the possible side effects of the drugs.

Analeptics

- ❒ Caffeine (CAFFEDRINE, NŌDŌZ, TIREND, QUICK PEP, VIVARIN)
- ❒ Doxapram (DOPRAM)

Indications

Neither caffeine nor doxapram is used in the management of narcolepsy, ADHD, or obesity. Although caffeine is not ordinarily used in the management of medical disorders, it does stimulate the cerebral cortex to increase alertness and decrease fatigue. It is used by many persons as an aid to stay awake. Caffeine has been used as an adjunct to analgesic formulations; it also may be used in conjunction with supportive measures to treat respiratory depression related to CNS depressant overdose.

Doxapram is used in some instances to stimulate respirations and to hasten arousal in patients experiencing drug-induced CNS depression or apnea. It has been used in the treatment of apnea (associated with immaturity) when methylxanthine therapy fails, although this use is unlabeled.

Pharmacodynamics

Analeptics stimulate the CNS. Caffeine increases the calcium permeability in sarcoplasmic reticulum, promotes the accumulation of cyclic adenosine monophosphate (AMP), and blocks adenosine receptors. It stimulates the CNS, cardiac activity, secretion of gastric acid, and diuresis.

Doxapram excites peripheral carotid chemoreceptors to cause an increase in tidal volume and a slight increase in respiratory rate. This stimulation also results in pressor effects.

Adverse Effects and Contraindications

CNS adverse effects of caffeine most often include insomnia, restlessness, excitement, tachycardia, and diuresis. Headaches, light-headedness, nausea, vomiting, diarrhea, and abdominal pain also have been reported. Caffeine withdrawal is manifest as anxiety, increased muscle tension, and headache.

Caffeine is generally contraindicated in patients with a history of depression, duodenal ulcers, and diabetes mellitus, as well as in lactating women. Doxapram is contraindicated in the presence of epilepsy, head injury, cerebrovascular accident, severe hypertension, flail chest, pneumothorax, acute asthma, and pulmonary fibrosis. It is to be used cautiously during pregnancy and lactation.

Adverse effects of doxapram most often include increased reflexes and increased blood pressure. Laryngospasm, bronchospasm, and seizures have been reported and can be life-threatening. Other less common effects include headache, dizziness, disorientation, hyperactivity, diaphoresis, and flushing. Nausea, vomiting, and diarrhea can be troublesome.

Pharmacokinetics

Caffeine's effects begin within 15 minutes of oral administration and peak in 15 to 45 minutes. The duration of action is 3 to 4 hours. Caffeine is biotransformed in the liver and excreted in the urine. It crosses the placental membranes and passes into breast milk.

Because doxapram is given intravenously (IV), the time to onset is 20 to 40 seconds, with peak effects noted in 1 to 2 minutes. Its duration of action is 5 to 12 minutes. It is biotransformed in the liver and excreted in the urine. The half-life of doxapram is approximately 2 to 4 hours.

Drug-Drug Interactions

There are increased CNS effects of caffeine when it is taken with cimetidine, oral contraceptives, disulfiram, ciprofloxacin, enoxacin, and phenylpropanolamine. The effects of caffeine are diminished if it is taken while the patient is smoking.

Doxapram produces increased effects when it is given to patients who have also received halothane, cyclopropane, or enflurane anesthetics. Treatment with doxapram should be delayed at least 10 minutes after the anesthetic has been discontinued. There are increased pressor effects if doxapram is given with MAO inhibitors or sympathomimetics.

Drug-Food Interactions

Caffeine has been shown to decrease the absorption of iron if the iron is taken with, or 1 hour after, coffee or tea. There are no known drug-food interactions with doxapram.

Dosage Regimen

The usual adult dosage of caffeine is 100 to 200 mg orally every 3 to 4 hours as needed. When using a time-released formulation, 200 mg every 3 to 4 hours is recommended. If caffeine is used to counteract respiratory depression, 500 to 1000 mg of caffeine and sodium benzoate intramuscular (IM) is used. It may be given IV in a severe emergency situation, but the dosage should not exceed 2.5 g/day.

As the dosage of caffeine approaches 250 mg or more (e.g., two to three cups of coffee), the chance of potentiating CNS activity increases. Appendix D provides a listing of the amount of caffeine contained in various beverages and foods.

Doxapram is given IV for the management of drug-induced CNS depression. A priming dose of 2 mg/kg is given and the dose repeated in 5 minutes, if necessary. The dosage may be repeated every 1 to 2 hours until the patient awakens or if relapse occurs. It also may be given by intermittent IV infusion as 250 mg in 250 mL of dextrose or saline at a rate of 1 to 3 mg/minute.

Laboratory Considerations

Caffeine when used for its pharmacologic effects may cause false elevations of serum urate and urine vanillamandylic acid. A false diagnosis of pheochromocytoma or neuroblastoma may result. There are no known laboratory test interferences with doxapram.

Critical Thinking Process

Assessment

History of Present Illness

Narcolepsy is identified primarily by its symptoms. The symptoms include excessive daytime somnolence, cataplexy, sleep paralysis, and hypnagogic hallucinations (vivid auditory or visual dreams occurring at the onset of sleep). Daytime sleep attacks can be as brief as 30 seconds, or the episodes can last as long as a half hour. Daytime sleepiness can be subtle. Some patients report having difficulty focusing or note inattention while driving. Daytime sleepiness is accompanied by impaired performance and disturbances in nighttime sleeping. Although patients with narcolepsy sleep excessively, narcolepsy should not be confused with a similar sleep disorder called idiopathic hypersomnolence syndrome. A sleep diary is often helpful in establishing a pattern of signs and symptoms.

When obtaining the history of present illness for a patient with ADHD, the chief complaints usually arise from parents and teachers. They usually report the child is inattentive, easily distracted, impulsive, hyperactive, and disruptive in the classroom or with other children. In some cases, the adult will report a change in behavior with the intake of certain foods.

Patients who are obese often present with complaints of decreased exercise tolerance. They may complain of signs and symptoms attributable to many medical conditions that accompany obesity such as hypertension, diabetes, and degenerative joint disease. Hypothyroidism is common, although it is rarely the sole cause of obesity. The normal-weight or mildly obese young woman who requests a weight-loss diet or drugs should be asked about bingeing and purging behaviors. The request is the most common presentation of bulimia nervosa.

Past Health History

A history of periodic amnesia or accidents may be the presenting symptoms because of the patient's "sleep attacks" and cataplexy. A history of psychiatric disorders and medical diseases should be elicited.

Parents of a child with ADHD may report that the child has difficulty interacting with peers and teachers. Only

Case Study Attention Deficit-Hyperactivity Disorder

Patient History

History of Present Illness	TC is a 10-year-old boy with difficulty concentrating, short attention span, irritability, hyperactivity, inability to follow parent and teacher directives, distractibility, poor social skills, poor academic performance, and low frustration tolerance. His parents say that he "was born antsy" and seems to be driven by a motor that he can't turn off. His sixth grade teacher recommended TC have an evaluation by a professional health care provider for the possibility of ADHD.
Past Health History	TC has no known allergies. He had the usual childhood illnesses, but no major health problems. TC has a history of risky behaviors that have resulted in injuries. At age 5, TC climbed a 30-ft tree in the yard and had to be rescued by the local fire fighters. At 7, he dislocated his shoulder when he fell from the same tree. Last year, TC had stitches after he injured himself while chasing the family cat into the street. His symptoms have worsened over the last 3 years.
Physical Exam Findings	TC is within the low average height and weight category for his age, sex, and developmental level. The results of his physical exam were within normal limits. Weight: 75 pounds. Height: 4′6″.
Diagnostic Testing	Diagnosis of ADHD was confirmed by history and observation. TC performed several psychological tests sensitive for the ability to focus attention and to perform motor tasks, although these tests were not necessary to confirm the diagnosis of ADHD. TC's symptoms and history ruled out other possibilities to explain his symptoms, such as thyroid problems, toxins, other CNS disturbances, or metabolic problems.
Developmental Considerations	Stimulants can either suppress or stimulate growth hormones in young children. TC's social skills with peers have been adversely affected by his lack of self-control. Despite TC's poor academic performance, TC's teachers agree with his parents that TC is a bright child.
Psychosocial Considerations	TC has poor peer relations. His inability to control behavior makes him unpredictable and often the brunt of teasing by other children. As a result, TC has learned to amuse himself and to find playmates in the family's pets. TC is an only child. TC's parents have tried to compensate for his lack of friends, but when TC hangs around his parents he is quickly labeled as a "loser" by other children. Philosophically, TC's parents are not strong supporters of drug therapy for children. They waited to bring TC to treatment after exhausting many other treatment avenues to help TC.
Economic Factors	TC's parents are tenured faculty at the local university. The family has both the means and desire to provide the care they think is needed for TC.

Variables Influencing Decision

Treatment Objectives	• Control impulsive behavior, increase ability to attend and focus, improve academic and social skills.

Drug Variables	*Drug Summary*	*Patient Variables*
Indications	Both methylphenidate and dextroamphetamines are especially effective for ADHD in children.	Symptoms of TC's ADHD have not subsided with other interventions. Poor academic and social skills decrease self-esteem and undermine self-confidence. Pharmacotherapy may make it possible for TC to work more effectively. This will be a decision point.

Drug Variables	*Drug Summary*	*Patient Variables*
Pharmacodynamics	Methylphenidate: blocks the re-uptake of dopamine into dopaminergic neurons to decrease motor activity and increase attention span Dextroamphetamine: increases the release of catecholamines (NEPI) from nerve terminals, blocks reuptake of dopamine and NEPI following release into synapse	If TC does not improve with one psychomotor stimulant, another can be tried. Choose the drug that gives TC the maximum response for the minimum dose.
Adverse Effects/ Contraindications	Methylphenidate: cardiovascular, CNS, ophthalmic, GI, psychiatric, dermatologic reactions, suppression of normal weight and height gain in children with prolonged administration. Dextroamphetamine: same reactions as above with the addition of endocrine imbalances and amphetamine "zombie-like" look.	If TC has adverse reactions, another can be tried. Stimulants work in slightly different ways, and one may work better than another.
Pharmacokinetics	Pharmacokinetic parameters are similar for methylphenidate and dextroamphetamine, so this will not be a decision point.	It may take a few weeks before changes are noted in behavior even though onset times are relatively rapid.
Dosage Regimen	Each drug will need to be titrated to reach individual response with minimal or no side effects.	TC's response will be monitored by parents and teachers and the dosage titrated accordingly. Short-term use preferred by parents.
Lab Considerations	Review periodic CBCs (with differential) and platelet counts to monitor anemia and leukopenia. Check urine catecholamines before and during methylphenidate therapy to determine increases in dopamine levels.	May need to titrate higher if TC shows minimum change clinically and dopamine and norepinephrine levels are still too low. Discontinue drug if signs of hematologic adverse effects to methylphenidate. This may become a decision point.
Cost Index*	Methylphenidate: 1 Dextroamphetamine: 1	TC's parents do not believe that cost differences among the drug categories are a factor for them. Cost will not be a decision point.

Summary of Decision Points

- Nonpharmacologic therapies alone have not worked for TC.
- TC's cognition and behavior, including reports from parents and teachers, need to be continuously monitored to determine optimum response level with minimum adverse effects.
- Change medications if TC is not responding properly to the first.
- Use drug holidays to determine whether the medication can be discontinued.

DRUGS TO BE USED

- Methylphenidate 5 mg po BID—to be titrated to a maximum of 60 mg daily for up to 1 month.
- If no change in 30 days, discontinue drug and consider the use of another stimulant such as dextroamphetamine.

*Cost Index:
1 = $<30/month
2 = $30–40/month
3 = $40–50/month
4 = $50–60/month
5 = $>60/month

AWP of 100, 5 mg tablets of dextroamphetamine is approximately $20.
AWP of 100, 5 mg tablets of methylphenidate is approximately $24.

about 5 percent of children with ADHD have an associated diagnosable neurologic disorder.

The obese patient will often report a history of multiple and varied attempts at dieting. In many patients, a report of overeating in response to stress, depression, or boredom may be elicited. Approximately 30 percent of patients seeking treatment suffer from binge eating disorder. These patients tend to have more difficulty losing weight and maintaining their weight loss. They are also more likely to have a history of depression or other psychiatric disturbance. Early learning patterns and familial interactions around food and eating that perpetuate obesity also may be reported.

Physical Exam Findings

Objective data related to narcolepsy may reflect visible signs of fatigue and lack of sleep, such as induration of the eyes, lack of coordination, drowsiness, and irritability. The frequency of cataplexy experiences and their duration should be noted.

The child with ADHD may display nonlocalized, "soft" neurologic signs, motor perceptual dysfunction (e.g., poor hand-eye coordination), and electroencephalographic abnormalities. "Spot" signs are subtle. The child may have difficulty distinguishing between the left and right hands, or may have trouble standing on one foot without falling. The child is often described as "clumsy" by the parents.

Obese patients will weigh more than normal in relation to their height and body build. The patient's height and weight are measured and compared with a standardized measure for BMI. This method is inexpensive and accurate. The major disadvantage is that the percentage of body fat is not measured (e.g., the muscular athlete might appear to be obese by this method) and distribution of body fat is not obtained.

Diagnostic Testing

Several different tests can be used to diagnose and manage narcolepsy, among them the Stanford Sleepiness Scale. Other tests include the electronic pupillogram, which measures pupil diameter; the Multiple Sleep Latency Test (MSLT); and the nocturnal polysomnogram. The purpose of the polysomnogram is to find the underlying cause of the sleepiness, especially if it is disease-related. The MSLT measures the severity of the problem. Twenty-four to 36-hour sleep studies have been useful in measuring the sleep-wake cycle. The abrupt transition into REM sleep is a necessary criterion for a diagnosis of narcolepsy.

There are no definitive tests to identify or manage ADHD. The child is primarily assessed and monitored based on clinical signs and symptoms.

Few tests are routinely indicated for the obese patient. Because of the concomitant increases in the rates of non-insulin-dependent diabetes, hypercholesterolemia, and hypertriglyceridemia in the obese, however, it is prudent to obtain blood glucose levels and a fasting lipid panel.

Developmental Considerations

Narcolepsy, ADHD, and obesity frequently begin in early adult life. The impact of the disorders on the patient's interpersonal relationships can be devastating whether they occur in the perinatal, pediatric, or geriatric populations. Changes in self-image and self-esteem may be present and can be identified with sensitive questioning.

Early identification of ADHD in affected children is important, as the characteristics of the disorder significantly interfere with the normal course of emotional and psychological development. In an attempt to cope with attention deficit, many of these children develop maladaptive behavior patterns that are a deterrent to psychosocial adjustment. Their behavior evokes negative responses from others, and repeated exposure to negative feedback adversely affects the child's self-concept, especially in boys. About half the children with ADHD also have learning disorders. Most of these children have average or above-average intelligence and are often very creative.

Birth weight offers no clue to detection and prediction of childhood obesity. However, there is a high correlation in childhood adiposity with both parental adiposity and children's daytime activity levels.

Psychosocial Considerations

The psychosocial implications of narcolepsy are far reaching. The patient's daytime somnolence and ability to fall asleep or to display excessive weakness at unexpected times can lead to personal safety issues and interference with relationships with others. In some cases, the patient with narcolepsy has been detained by law enforcement officers who thought initially the individual was under the influence of illicit drugs or alcohol. The psychosocial implications of ADHD are also far reaching. It disturbs family dynamics and can contribute to disruption in social relationships.

Obesity is often a symptom in passive-dependent, compliant individuals who are readily controlled by guilt and shame. These individuals are easily influenced by outside forces that they consider more powerful than themselves (see Case Study—Attention Deficit–Hyperactivity Disorder).

Analysis and Management

Treatment Objectives

The major treatment objective for the patient with narcolepsy is to combat somnolence and aid in restoring normal function. For ADHD, treatment objectives are directed toward correction of cognitive and behavioral problems. However, pharmacotherapy by itself does not correct ADHD; it only makes the patient more receptive to treatment.

Pharmacotherapy for overweight or obese individuals becomes reasonable only for those who weigh 40 percent or more above the desired body weight. The goal is to reduce and stabilize the patient's weight at a more desirable level. The desirable level may not necessarily be within normal limits, but reduced sufficiently to lower the risk of major health problems. For patients who are less than 40 percent overweight, self-help and behavioral programs are preferable to pharmacotherapy.

The use of prescription-only appetite suppressants has been shown to significantly increase weight loss relative to placebo. However, the differences are usually modest, averaging ¼ to ½ pounds per week, with a total weight loss of 5 percent. The long-term safety of appetite suppressants has not been demonstrated, and patients tend to regain their weight when the drugs are discontinued. These drugs also may interfere with the effectiveness of behavioral interventions.

Treatment Options

Drug Variables

Clinical experience has shown that nonresponse to one psychomotor stimulant does not necessarily mean that another will not be effective. Because these drugs work through slightly different mechanisms and at different sites, one drug may provide improved efficacy over another. However, it is important not to use psychomotor stimulants for a long time, because they are intended to be an adjunct to other therapies, not a substitute for them.

Catecholamines may be involved in the control of ADHD at the level of the cerebral cortex. They increase the attention span and goal-oriented behaviors while decreasing impulsiveness, distractibility, hyperactivity, and restlessness. Overall, behavior becomes more tolerable to parents and teachers. The calming effect of amphetamines in children is not understood, however, and the long-term efficacy of both drugs is limited.

Methylphenidate, although a psychomotor stimulant, is structurally distinct from the amphetamines, but its pharmacologic effects and abuse potential are similar. Consequently, methylphenidate can be considered an amphetamine in all but name and structure.

Patient Variables

Some patients with narcolepsy respond well to nonpharmacologic therapies if their symptoms are not too severe. Others require therapy to remain alert throughout the day. Although the psychomotor stimulants are effective for many patients, they are not effective for all.

The decision to start and continue drug treatment for ADHD is difficult. Not all children who exhibit signs of ADHD should be treated with psychomotor stimulants. The decision for drug therapy depends in part on societal expectations and demands. The motivation of parents and teachers in seeking treatment for the child with ADHD should be evaluated carefully before beginning drug therapy. Because drug therapy is intended as an adjunct to other modalities, an evaluation of the interest and ability to comply with therapy should be determined; however, drug therapy is not indicated if symptoms are mild (see Controversy—Are CNS Stimulants the Answer?).

The health care provider has many options in the management of ADHD because the choice of a drug for a particular child is pragmatic. The drug of choice is the one best expected to target the symptoms. Whatever the drug chosen, the dosage should be titrated for 1 month and the results evaluated. If the first drug is not effective, a second may be tried. It is not unusual to try three different types of stimulants before finding one that is effective. When pharmacotherapy is used, drug holidays should be initiated periodically to assess the need for continuing the drug. In no case should treatment continue for more than one school year without interruption.

For patients in need of weight loss, motivation should be evaluated carefully before starting therapy. The unmotivated or ambivalent patient is unlikely to adhere to even the most excellent and well-thought out program. The psychological effects of yet another failure probably outweigh the benefits of any short-term weight loss that may be obtained. A patient with a history of drug abuse may not be a candidate for psychomotor stimulants.

Amphetamines and anorexiants have been used widely in the treatment of obesity; however, the wisdom of this strategy is at best questionable. (Some states prohibit the use of amphetamines for weight reduction.) Weight loss secondary to amphetamine use is due almost entirely to reduced food intake and only in small measure to increased energy expenditure. Amphetamines should not be provided when overeating is the result of psychological factors, because they are ineffective under these circumstances. Further, continuous weight reduction is not usually observed in obese individuals without dietary restrictions.

When health care providers consider pharmacotherapy in the treatment of obesity, it is usually after they have tried other therapies first, and when the patient is at least 40 percent overweight. Amphetamines are usually the first choice as an adjunct to other therapies in the treatment of obesity; however, they have a multitude of adverse effects and a great risk for dependence, abuse, and tolerance. Anorexiants are amphetamine-like agents. Drugs for obesity should be used short term and only as an adjunct to other therapies intended to increase exercise while decreasing caloric intake.

Controversy

Are CNS Stimulants the Answer?

JONATHAN J. WOLFE

The use of central nervous system stimulants to help control attention deficit hyperactivity disorder (ADHD) and other behavior problems has become popular in recent years. The supporters of this practice say that these drugs are a relatively inexpensive and effective way to solve undesirable behavior problems. Supporters also say that science has provided us with a tool that is reasonably safe to use.

The drugs do correct many problems quickly and avoid the cost of long-term therapy. In addition, the child gets the immediate benefit of improved social relationships, academic achievement, and behavior control, all of which increase a sense of self-esteem.

Opponents of this practice say that the science of neurophysiology and neurochemistry, although progressive, has a long way to go. Opponents believe that the use of psychoactive drugs, especially with young children, gambles that there will be no long-term adverse effects. Stimulant therapy is relatively new, and the drugs have not been used long enough to determine if there will be long-term consequences. Although it may not be as cost-effective in the short term to correct environmental circumstances that contribute to behavior problems, the long-term benefits may be much greater.

Critical Thinking Questions

- What is the economic cost to society of treating or not treating ADHD?
- Who should determine whether a child has ADHD? The parents, health care provider, social worker, school system, psychologists?
- How should the child who is receiving a CNS stimulant be monitored? How long should therapy last? Are there other management modalities that would be equally as effective?

Intervention

Administration

Blood pressure, pulse, and respirations are ordinarily monitored before administering a psychomotor stimulant, anorexiant, or analeptic drug, and periodically during therapy.

Psychomotor stimulants are usually taken on an empty stomach. Mazindol, however, may be taken with meals to reduce gastric irritation. The last dose of an amphetamine or anorexiant is usually given several hours (e.g., 6 hours) before bedtime to avoid insomnia. Additionally, the intake of large amounts of caffeine should be avoided. The dry mouth associated with psychomotor stimulants can be minimized by rinsing frequently with water or chewing sugarless gum or candy.

Anorexiants quickly become ineffective as tolerance develops. When tolerance occurs, the drug should be discontinued. Doses should not be increased to suppress appetite once tolerance has been achieved.

Treatment should be interrupted periodically to evaluate the need for continued therapy and to minimize the potential for drug tolerance. For example, a 6-week course of therapy might be followed by a 3-week discontinuation.

Education

Patients taking a psychomotor stimulant, anorexiant, or analeptic require thorough patient teaching about their disorder, the purpose and expected outcomes of drug therapy, adverse effects, and the importance of follow-up. The patient should be instructed not to increase the dosage of the prescribed drug or abruptly stop therapy without consulting the health care provider. Abrupt cessation of high doses may cause extreme fatigue and mental depression.

The patient should be informed that these drugs may impair judgment. Caution should be exercised when driving or operating machinery, and the use of alcohol should be avoided.

The patient with narcolepsy should be instructed to document the frequency and character of attacks. They may be able to counteract the effects of daytime sleepiness using a number of adjuncts or substitutes for pharmacotherapy. The strategies may include frequent short walks or other forms of exercise, avoiding large meals, caffeinated beverages, eating lunch before important meetings, and taking short naps throughout the day.

Parents should periodically monitor the child's height and inform the health care provider if growth inhibition occurs. They also should inform the health care provider of any adverse effects such as tachycardia, loss of appetite, abdominal pain, or weight loss.

Many commercial programs and support groups are available to the overweight or obese patient. In addition, the patient should be encouraged to follow through with behavior modification therapies and exercise regimens.

Evaluation

Treatment success for the patient with narcolepsy is measured by the patient's ability to stay alert and functional throughout the day. Some patients with severe narcolepsy may not overcome fatigue and sleepiness even with stimulants. In this case, success can be measured by improvement in functioning.

ADHD treatment success is determined by the child's marked improvement in behavior and cognition and in the child's ability to focus and attend. It is estimated that drug-related improvements occur in 60 to 90 percent of children. Teacher ratings of the child have noted improvement in behavior and attention span of children who are on drug therapy. These children performed better on visual-motor tasks. Although ADHD children became quieter with an increase in dosage, their academic performance declined. Thus, the child should be monitored closely so that the smallest effective dosage can be used.

Effectiveness of anorexiant therapy can be demonstrated by a decrease in appetite and subsequent decrease in weight.

SUMMARY

- Narcolepsy is a sleep disorder thought to be a disturbance of the REM sleep cycle.
- Males are more often affected than females and can occur anytime up to the age of 60 years.
- Attention deficit–hyperactivity disorder (ADHD) is one of several attention deficit problems including attention deficit disorder (without hyperactivity), minimal brain dysfunction, and hyperkinesis.
- ADHD is found in children, especially boys, and is characterized by inattention, distractibility, impulsivity, and hyperactivity. Onset of symptoms occurs between ages 3 to 7 years, with boys affected more than girls by a 10:1 ratio.
- Exogenous obesity refers to an imbalance between caloric intake and caloric needs. Endogenous obesity is secondary to another physical problem such as diabetes or an endocrine problem.
- Studies suggest that the resting metabolic rate of people who become obese may be slower from childhood. Other studies suggest that children who are obese have more fat cells, not just larger fat cells.
- Patient assessment should elicit any history of cardiovascular disease, hyperthyroidism or hypothyroidism, depression, or psychiatric illness.
- The motivation of the patient who is a candidate for psychomotor stimulant therapy and the ability of the patient to follow through with the plan of care should be determined.
- The major treatment objective for the patient with narcolepsy is to combat somnolence and aid in the restoration of normal functioning.
- The treatment objective for ADHD is to make the patient more available for treatment and to aid in the correction of the cognitive and behavioral problems.
- The goal of treatment in the overweight or obese patient is to reduce and stabilize the patient's weight at a more desirable level. The desirable level may not necessarily be within normal limits, but reduced sufficiently to lower the risk of major health problems.
- Psychomotor stimulants can be used in the management of narcolepsy, ADHD, and obesity.

- First-line drugs for patients with narcolepsy and ADHD include amphetamines and methylphenidate. These drugs increase the availability of dopamine and norepinephrine in the brain.
- All anorexiants are used as adjuncts to other therapies, such as behavior modification, exercise, and calorie restrictions, in the short-term treatment of obesity.
- Patients who take psychomotor stimulants require thorough patient teaching about their disease, drug therapy, adverse effects, and the importance of follow-up.
- The patient should be instructed not to increase the dosage of the prescribed drug, or abruptly stop therapy without consulting the health care provider.
- Treatment success for the patient with narcolepsy is measured by the patient's ability to stay alert and functional throughout the day.
- ADHD treatment success is determined by the child's marked improvement in behavior and cognition and in the ability to focus and attend.
- Effectiveness of anorexiant therapy can be demonstrated by a decrease in appetite and subsequent decrease in weight.

BIBLIOGRAPHY

American Hospital Formulary Service. (1995). *Drug information.* Bethesda, MD: American Society of Health-System Pharmacists.

Arnold, L., and Jensen, P. (1995). Attention-deficit disorders. In H. Kaplan and B. Sadock (Eds.), *Comprehensive textbook of psychiatry* (Vol. 2) (6th ed.). Baltimore: Williams & Wilkins.

American Psychiatric Association. (1994). *Diagnostic and statistical manual of mental disorders: DSM-IV* (4th ed.). Washington, D.C.: Author.

Olin, B. (1996). *Drug facts and comparisons.* St. Louis: Facts and Comparisons.

Koda-Kimble, M., and Young, L. (Eds.). (1992). *Applied therapeutics: the clinical use of drugs* (5th ed.). Vancouver: Applied Therapeutics, Inc.

Guilleminault, C. (1994). Narcolepsy syndrome. In M. Kryger, T. Roth, and W. Dement (Eds.), *Principles and practice of sleep* (2nd ed.). Philadelphia: W. B. Saunders Company.

Johnson, R., and Griffin, J. (1993). *Current therapy in neurologic disease* (4th ed.). St. Louis: Mosby.

Kryger, M., Roth, T., and Dement, W. (1994). *Principles and practice of sleep* (2nd ed.). Philadelphia: W. B. Saunders Company.

Nadeau, K. (Ed.). (1995). *A comprehensive guide to attention deficit disorder in adults.* New York: Brunner/Mazel Publishers.

United States Pharmacopeial Convention. (1994). USP DI: Drug information for the health professional (14th ed.). Rockville, MD: Author.

Wilens, T., Biederman, J., Spencer, T., et al. (1995). Pharmacotherapy of adult attention deficit/hyperactivity disorder: A review. *Journal of Clinical Psychopharmacology,* 13, 270–279.

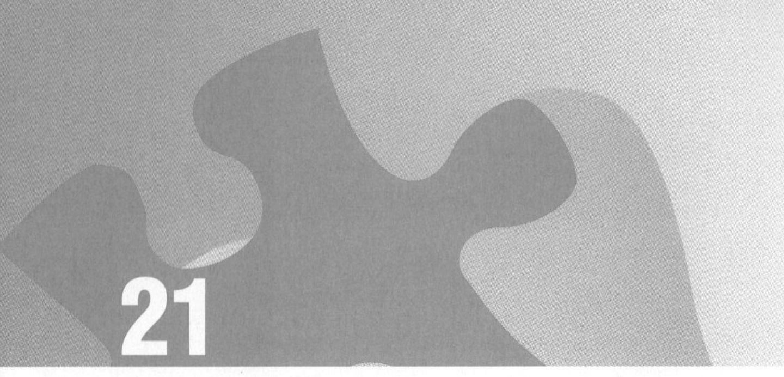

21 Skeletal Muscle Relaxants

The neuromuscular system is controlled by a complex inter-relationship between the central nervous system (CNS) and the skeletal muscles. Many disorders of the neuromuscular system result in muscle tone imbalances. Although the exact mechanisms of neuromuscular disorders are not understood, physical and drug therapy provide clues to the pathways and medical management.

Deep tendon reflexes (DTRs) are used to assess the integrity of the neuromuscular system. These muscle contractions or jerks are elicited by a quick tap with a reflex hammer to the muscle's tendon insertion. The strength of the reaction, calibrated from 0 to +4, gives the health care provider a wealth of information. A normal reaction (+2) demonstrates that neuromuscular synapses are operative and muscle fibers can contract. It also indicates that the spinal cord, dorsal root ganglion, and extrapyramidal and pyramidal systems are functional. Abnormal reactions indicate neuromuscular disorders.

SPASM VERSUS SPASTICITY

Epidemiology and Etiology

Spasms are sudden, violent, painful, involuntary contractions of a muscle or group of muscles. Most muscle spasms are related to local injury of muscles, joints, tendons, or ligaments. Specific trauma-related causes of spasms include whiplash injuries, cervical root syndrome, herniated discs, and lower back syndrome (Table 21–1). In addition, bursitis, myositis, neuritis, dislocations and fractures, muscle strains from excessive stretching or overuse, and sprains from joints with stretched or torn ligaments can also result in spasms. Although hypocalcemia or epileptic myoclonic seizure activity also produces spasms, the discussion in this chapter is limited to spasm resulting from musculoskeletal injury.

In contrast to spasm, *spasticity* involves resistance to stretching by a muscle because of abnormally increased tension. The increased muscle tone or contractions cause stiff, awkward movements. Spasticity is considered permanent and, without intervention of physical and drug therapy, frequently progresses to disabling contractures. Disorders of the CNS such as closed head injuries, cerebral palsy, multiple sclerosis, and cerebrovascular accident (stroke) are common causes of spasticity. Two-thirds of patients with multiple sclerosis have moderate to severe spasticity. Patients with spinal cord trauma, spinal tumors, poliomyelitis, hemiplegia, paraplegia, quadriplegia, and tetanus also may experience spasticity.

Pathophysiology

A delicate balance between musculoskeletal movement and body posture allows the execution of fine and gross motor skills. The physical hierarchy controlling this balance includes the motor cortex and upper motor neurons (UMNs), extrapyramidal and pyramidal systems, basal ganglia, cerebellum, descending brainstem circuitry, spinal cord, and lower motor neurons (LMNs) (Fig. 21–1). Feedback from the muscle fibers, muscle and tendon joint afferents, and thalamus helps to complete the information loop.

Motor neuron units are directly responsible for motor function and consist of one LMN unit and a cluster of muscle fibers that may include as many as 2000 muscle cells. Approximately 600,000 LMN units supply the mechanism for all skeletal muscle movement. LMN units are found in the ventral horns of gray matter of the brainstem and spinal cord. Their axons innervate the skeletal muscles of the neck, back, abdomen, and extremities. If an action potential is generated in the LMN, then, by way of the neuromuscular junction, all of the muscle cells in the motor unit fire simultaneously. Generally, fine motor skills of the hand, face, and eye are associated with small muscles and small motor neuron units, whereas gross motor skills are linked to larger muscle groups.

The stretch reflex maintains muscle tone (Fig. 21–2). Muscle tone is described as *hypotonic* (less than normal), *flaccid* (absent), or *hypertonic* (excessive, rigid, spastic, tetany). Assessment of DTRs helps determine the degree of muscle tone present.

The LMNs link spinal cord reflexes to muscles. When an LMN axon or cell body is damaged, a pattern of hyperexcitability develops that produces multiple contractions. These muscle spasms can be mild or severe, acute or chronic. Muscle spasms may also be *clonic,* characterized by alternate contraction and relaxation, or *tonic,* sustained contractions of striated muscle. Depending on their location, spasms can be aggravated by movement, sneezing, coughing, or straining. Muscle atrophy may develop as a result of long-term LMN lesions.

UMNs associated with the cerebral cortex and ventral horn of the spinal cord control the LMNs. Patterns of movement organized in the frontal cortex of the brain are carried out by the motor cortex. The basal ganglia and cerebellum provide ongoing support functions that contribute to the gracefulness and the temporal smoothness of movement (see Fig. 21–1). If the UMN system is severely injured, skilled movement is lost, but the extrapyramidal system can elicit crude movement.

Spasticity results from damage to UMNs at any of the CNS centers that control muscle tone and coordinate complex movement. Current theories postulate that spasticity may develop as the result of changes in the excitability of spinal neurons, a hypersensitivity of neuronal receptors, or the formation of new synapses. The last mechanism may account for the extended time it takes for spasticity to develop in patients with UMN lesions.

Spasticity is a velocity-dependent increase in the passive stretch resistance of a muscle or muscle group. *Clonus,* flexor spasms, mass reflexes, and a positive Babinski's sign

TABLE 21–1 COMPARISON OF SPASM AND SPASTICITY

	Spasm	Spasticity
Definition	Sudden, violent, painful, involuntary contractions of a muscle or group of muscles	Increased muscle tone or muscle contractions that cause stiff, awkward movement
Mediator	Lower motor neurons (LMNs)	Upper motor neurons (UMNs)
Etiology	Cervical root syndrome Bursitis, overuse syndromes Dislocation, fracture Epilepsy Herniated disc Hypocalcemia Myositis, neuritis Sprains, strains Whiplash injuries	Cerebrovascular accident Closed head injury Hemiplegia, paraplegia, quadriplegia Multiple sclerosis Poliomyelitis Spinal cord trauma or tumor Tetanus

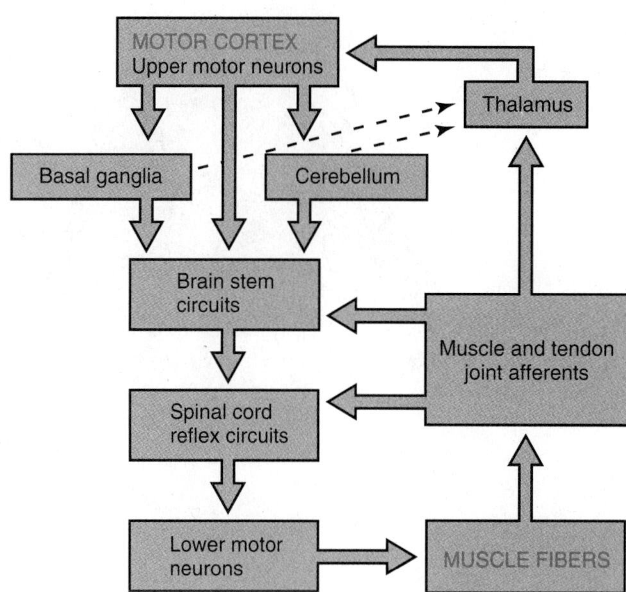

Figure 21–1 Algorithm of neural pathways controlling motor function. The hierarchy of neuromuscular control is quite complex. It begins in the motor cortex and works through motor neurons and the spinal cord to direct muscles and receive feedback information. Damage or injury to lower motor neurons (LMNs) results in the development of hyperexcitability or spasms. Damage or injury to upper motor neurons (UMNs) causes a spastic paralysis and hyperreflexia because the spinal reflex remains intact below the level of the lesion. (Adapted from Porth, C. M. [1994]. *Pathophysiology: Concepts of altered health states* [4th ed., p. 1029]. Philadelphia: J. B. Lippincott. Used with permission.)

are identifiable signs of spasticity. *Hypertonus* results from either an increase in excitatory influences or decrease in inhibitory influences. As a result, the stretch reflex is augmented and muscle fibers may lengthen in an exaggerated way (see Fig. 21–2).

Spasticity does not develop immediately after neural injury has occurred. Therefore, severity may vary throughout the progression of the disorder. A gradual increase in muscle tone triggers increases in resistance until tone is suddenly reduced resulting in a very painful *clasp-knife* phenomenon. Urinary tract infections, decubitus ulcers, and other painful stimuli can exacerbate spasticity.

Two types of spasticity have been identified. *Spinal spasticity* is characterized by a discernible loss of inhibitory influences. Hyperactive DTRs, clonus, primitive withdrawal reflexes, and a flexed posture are present. In contrast, *cerebral spasticity* produces hypoactive DTRs and increased muscle tone. Ordinarily, there are no primitive withdrawal reflexes or flexed postures with cerebral spasticity. *Dystonia* or disordered muscle tone also may be present in individuals with cerebral spasticity.

PHARMACOTHERAPEUTIC OPTIONS

Centrally Acting Drugs

- Baclofen (LIORESAL); (🍁) ALPHA-BACLOFEN
- Carisoprodol (SOMA, RELA)
- Chlorphenesin (MAOLATE)
- Chlorzoxazone (PARAFLEX, PARAFON FORTE DSC)
- Cyclobenzaprine (FLEXERIL)
- Metaxalone (SKELAXIN)
- Methocarbamol (ROBAXIN, MARBAXIN)
- Orphenadrine (NORFLEX, BANFLEX)
- Tizanidine (ZANAFLEX)

Peripherally Acting Drugs

- Dantrolene (DANTRIUM)
- Quinine (QUINAMM, QUIPHILE)

Indications

Centrally Acting Drugs

There are a variety of skeletal muscle relaxants; almost all are centrally active drugs. Skeletal muscle relaxants relieve symptoms only. Patients with pain related to flexor spasms benefit the most. As a rule of thumb, drugs used to treat acute spasm do not relieve spasticity and vice versa. Centrally acting skeletal muscle relaxants are used primarily for muscle spasms that do not promptly respond to other forms of therapy. They do not completely stop spasms, but they reduce their severity. Depolarizing and nondepolarizing skeletal muscle relaxants were discussed in Chapter 12 and are used as adjuncts to anesthesia.

Baclofen has several uses. It is used in the management of detrusor sphincter incoordination associated with spinal cord disease. When administered by an intrathecal route, it is beneficial in reducing the severe spasticity of multiple sclerosis and the spasticity of childhood cerebral palsy. Intrathecal administration produces less sedation than high doses of orally administered baclofen. Baclofen also has been used in the management of trigeminal neuralgia (tic douloureux), although this use has not been approved by the Food and Drug Administration (FDA).

Cyclobenzaprine is also used with some effectiveness in the management of fibrositis syndrome, although it is not FDA approved for such use. Orphenadrine citrate has been used in the management of quinine-resistant leg cramps (see Controversy entitled Intrathecal Baclofen in Cerebral Palsy).

Tizanidine, although it is a centrally acting drug, is indicated for spasticity.

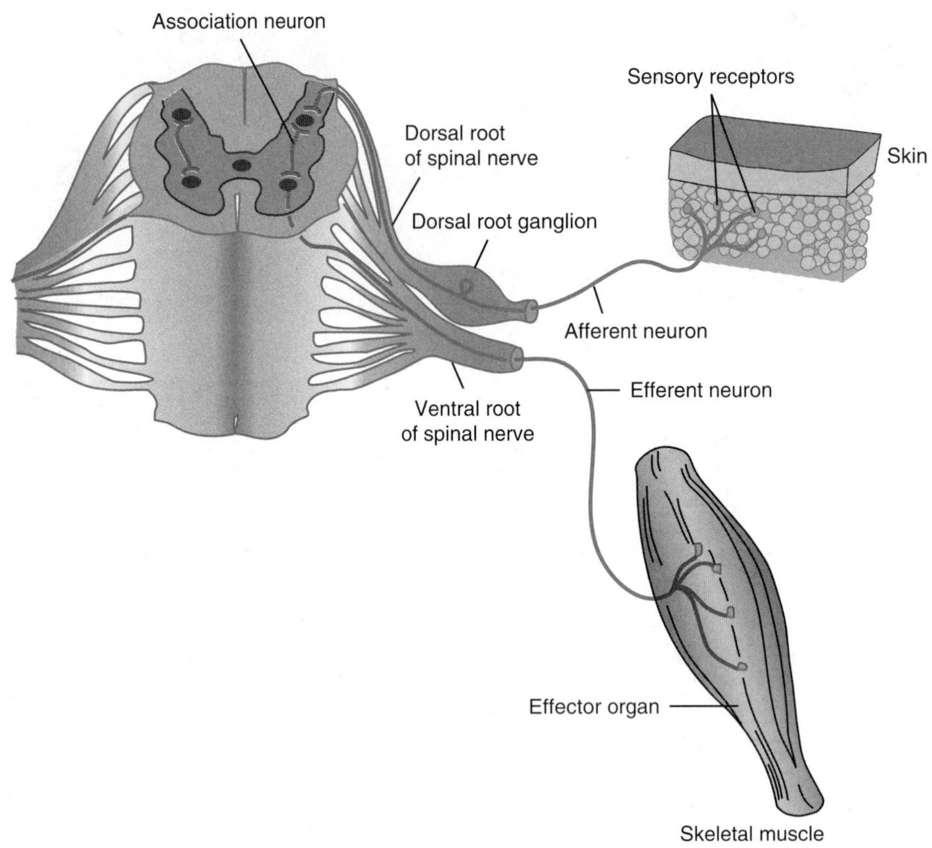

Figure 21–2 Reflex arc. The stretch reflex maintains muscle tone. When communication between sensory receptors and muscles is broken, a pattern of hyperexcitability develops that produces multiple contractions or spasms. (From Black, J. M., and Matassarin-Jacobs, E. [1997]. *Medical-surgical nursing: Clinical management for continuity of care* [5th ed., p. 701]. Philadelphia: W. B. Saunders. Used with permission.)

Peripherally Acting Drugs

Dantrolene exerts its effects directly on the peripheral skeletal muscle, hence the term peripherally acting. There are only two peripherally acting (direct-acting) skeletal muscle relaxants, dantrolene and quinine. Dantrolene is used for the symptomatic relief of spasticity caused by UMN disorders. It is also used in the preoperative and intraoperative management of malignant hyperthermia and for patients with spasticity caused by spinal cord and cerebral disease.

Quinine has been used for the relief of nocturnal leg cramps although it has generally been replaced by more effective, less toxic drugs. It has also been used alone, with pyrimethamine and sulfonamides (or with an oral tetracycline) for the treatment of chloroquine-resistant falciparum malaria (Chapter 27).

Pharmacodynamics

The exact mechanism of action for skeletal muscle relaxants is unknown. Drug action is thought to result from CNS depression of the brainstem, thalamus, basal ganglia, and spinal cord. Skeletal muscle relaxants also may block nerve impulses that cause increased muscle tone and contraction. It is unclear whether pain relief is secondary to use of skeletal muscle relaxants or occurs as a result of the sedative effects, muscular relaxation, or placebo effects.

Centrally Acting Drugs

Baclofen was developed as an oral analog of the inhibitory transmitter gamma-aminobutyric acid (GABA). Although the underlying mechanisms are not well understood, observations of CNS neurons suggest that baclofen acts as an inhibitory neurotransmitter at the spinal level. It also reduces pain in patients with spasticity by inhibiting the release of substance P in the spinal cord.

The mechanism of action of carisoprodol is also not well understood. Considered an interneuronal blocking drug, carisoprodol is chemically related to meprobamate, an antianxiety drug. Carisoprodol depresses excitatory and inhibitory neuron activity affecting muscle stretch reflexes. There are no known peripheral or autonomic effects.

In contrast, cyclobenzaprine is structurally and pharmacologically related to tricyclic antidepressants (see Chapter 18); however, its antidepressant effects are thought to be minimal. Cyclobenzaprine acts at the level of the brainstem rather than the spinal cord to reduce muscle tone and hyperactivity. Loss of muscle function does not occur.

Tizanidine reduces spasticity by increasing presynaptic inhibition of motor neurons.

Peripherally Acting Drugs

Dantrolene is unique in that it reduces muscle contractility (by 75 to 80 percent) by inhibiting calcium release from the sarcoplasmic reticulum. The blockage of calcium release is not complete, and contraction is never completely abolished. The effects are more noticeable in fast-contracting muscle fibers and depend on the frequency of nerve stimulation. Single-twitch contractions are more affected than tetanic contractions. Dantrolene does not possess GABA-

Controversy

Intrathecal Baclofen in Cerebral Palsy
JONATHAN J. WOLFE

Cerebral palsy presents vexing challenges to the patient, family, and health care provider. One of its cruelest manifestations is painful spasticity. The pain related to this element of the disease easily qualifies as malignant, for it causes intense and long-term suffering while serving no useful physiologic purpose. The patient and all concerned already know that the disease is serious with poor prognosis.

Early attempts to use baclofen, marketed as baclofen tablets, met with indifferent success. Concern about drug effects properly limited daily doses and approved durations of therapy. Even patients who were aided by baclofen therapy frequently could not sustain therapeutic levels because of the adverse effects at high dosages. Difficulties in swallowing large numbers of tablets were remedied only imperfectly by preparation of extemporaneous oral liquid formulations.

Because baclofen is a centrally acting skeletal muscle relaxant, investigation of direct injection into the intrathecal space offered a reasonable focus for research. Results in a significant number of patients have indicated that baclofen administered via this route is of genuine value. A parenteral formulation without preservatives for intrathecal injection came to market as an orphan drug under federal Food and Drug Administration (FDA) guidelines.

Therapy with intrathecal baclofen requires a trial of the drug by bolus injection. Continuous treatment requires surgical placement of a programmable infusion pump, which is refilled at intervals thereafter. Treatment exposes the patient to all the hazards of lumbar puncture, intrathecal catheter placement, and use of an implanted pump. Treatment is also quite expensive.

Critical Thinking Questions

- Do you feel that a patient with spasticity of cerebral palsy must "fail" on oral baclofen therapy before consideration of intrathecal therapy?
- What education is appropriate for a minor child and her family members to ensure proper informed consent to intrathecal baclofen therapy?
- What education is appropriate for an autonomous adult patient to ensure proper informed consent to intrathecal baclofen therapy?
- What, if any, problems do you perceive from the fact that the company sponsoring baclofen as an intrathecal injection is also a leading manufacturer and marketer of implanted programmable infusion pumps?
- What reservations would you have in evaluating continuing education materials about intrathecal baclofen therapy that were provided by the corporate sponsor of the drug? Would FDA requirements for such materials answer your reservations?

like actions. Dantrolene reduces both monosynaptic- and polysynaptic-induced muscle contractions.

Quinine, a naturally occurring substance from the bark of the cinchona tree, resembles salicylates in analgesic properties. It exerts curare-like skeletal muscle relaxation.

Adverse Effects and Contraindications

The use of centrally acting and peripherally acting skeletal muscle relaxants is almost always associated with some degree of sedation, drowsiness, light-headedness, ataxia, and dizziness. Caution should be used when the patient has preexisting co-morbid conditions that produce weakness, ataxia, or light-headedness. Other adverse effects and contraindications are drug-specific.

Headaches, sleepiness, and visual disturbances are common. Nausea, vomiting, constipation, and diarrhea have been associated with carisoprodol, chlorzoxazone, cyclobenzaprine, methocarbamol, and orphenadrine. Cyclobenzaprine has significant anticholinergic activity (e.g., dry mouth, urinary retention, blurred vision) and produces alterations in the sense of taste. Increased excitability, nervousness, and irritability have been associated with carisoprodol, chlorzoxazone, metoxalone, and orphenadrine. Chlorzoxazone is associated with severe hepatotoxicity.

Carisoprodol should not be used for patients with a history of porphyria. Porphyria is an autosomal dominant trait. Porphyrin is any of a group of nitrogen-containing organic compounds that occurs in the protoplasm and forms the basis of respiratory pigments. It increases the synthesis of porphyrin, thereby exacerbating symptoms.

Tizanidine can produce hypotension, sedation, hallucinations, somnolence, asthenia, dizziness, and dry mouth. With long-term use, bradycardia and prolonged QT intervals may occur.

Baclofen is relatively well tolerated; however, its more common adverse effects include transient drowsiness, vertigo, confusion, sleepiness, increased weakness, and nausea. Less common effects include headache, fatigue, nasal congestion, abdominal pain, anorexia, diarrhea or constipation, dysuria, urgency, urinary incontinence, and sexual dysfunction in males. Ataxia, insomnia, slurred speech, muscle stiffness, increased excitability, ankle edema, hypotension, tachycardia, and weight gain are also possible adverse effects.

Severe adverse effects of baclofen rarely occur, but include syncope, chest pain, dark urine, auditory and visual hallucinations, and tinnitus. Neuropsychiatric signs and symptoms (e.g., euphoria, depression, accommodation disorders, paresthesias) are also rare but may be difficult to discern from those of the underlying disease. An overdose of baclofen appears as visual disturbances (blurred vision, diplopia), vomiting, seizures, respiratory difficulties, and severe muscle weakness. There are no absolute contraindications to baclofen therapy other than hypersensitivity.

Dantrolene and quinine may cause dizziness, headache, confusion, euphoria, tachycardia, blurred vision, nausea, vomiting, diarrhea, pruritus, and urticaria. In addition, dantrolene may cause muscle weakness and fatigue, speech disturbances, nervousness, depression, insomnia, seizures, erratic blood pressure readings, photophobia, urinary frequency or retention, nocturnal diuresis, and erectile dysfunction. Prolonged use of dantrolene at high doses can cause hepatitis, hepatomegaly, and hepatic necrosis.

The most serious adverse effect of dantrolene is an idiosyncratic or hypersensitivity-mediated injury to the liver. When injury does occur, it ordinarily appears 3 to 12 months after the start of therapy. It is seen most often in women with multiple sclerosis. The prevalence seems high because multiple sclerosis occurs more often in women.

Quinine can cause ototoxicity, tinnitus, anxiety, acute asthmatic episodes, fever, angina, and rash. Leukopenia, thrombocytopenia, agranulocytosis, hemolytic anemia, and hypoprothrombinemia are of major concern. Toxic levels are reflected as hypotension, hypothermia, seizures, cardiovascular collapse, coma, and death.

Pharmacokinetics

The pharmacokinetics of selected skeletal muscle relaxants are identified in Table 21–2. Most drugs are readily absorbed from the gastrointestinal (GI) tract following oral administration. The bioavailability of individual drugs is not available. Baclofen and metaxalone are 30 percent protein bound, and cyclobenzaprine is 93 percent protein bound.

The time of onset for most skeletal muscle relaxants varies from 30 to 60 minutes. The onset of baclofen is long, ranging from hours to weeks. Peak times range from 1 to 4 hours. Although therapeutic serum levels are not routinely measured for patients on skeletal muscle relaxants, the level of baclofen ranges from 80 to 400 mcg/mL. The duration of action ranges from 3 to 4 hours for chlorzoxazone to 12 to 24 hours for cyclobenzaprine.

Most skeletal muscle relaxants are biotransformed in the liver and eliminated via the kidneys. Their half-lives vary a great deal from 1 hour for chlorzoxazone to 14 hours for orphenadrine. Cyclobenzaprine and methocarbamol are eliminated in the urine and feces.

In contrast to baclofen and other centrally active drugs, the absorption of dantrolene from the GI tract is slow and incomplete. Nonetheless, absorption is thought to be sufficient to provide dose-related plasma concentrations. It takes approximately 1 hour to raise blood levels, but therapeutic effects can take 1 to 2 weeks to be achieved. Peak action is reached in 5 hours, with a duration of 6 to 12 hours. Dantrolene is highly protein bound with a 100 mg dose and has a mean half-life of 6 to 9 hours.

Serum concentrations of dantrolene and its metabolites are not significantly different after a 400 mg dose than concentrations obtained after a single oral dose of 100 mg. This finding does not appear to be related to enzyme induction, but rather to capacity-limited absorption or protein binding. Dantrolene is almost entirely biotransformed by the liver, with its metabolites eliminated in the urine. The therapeutic range for dantrolene is 300 to 1100 mcg/mL for 100 mg doses.

The onset of quinine action varies when taken by mouth. Peak action is reached in 1 to 3 hours, with a duration of action of 6 to 8 hours. The bioavailability of quinine is unknown, but it is 70 to 90 percent protein bound, with a half-life of 4 to 21 hours in the healthy or convalescing patient. Serum drug concentrations vary.

Drug-Drug Interactions

Alcohol is the most commonly used drug that interacts with skeletal muscle relaxants (Table 21–3). Other interacting drugs include CNS depressants (e.g., opioids), monoamine oxidase inhibitors, antihistamines, anticonvulsants, cimetidine, levodopa, barbiturates, phenothiazines, and propoxyphene, tricyclic antidepressants, and contraceptives.

Concurrent use of dantrolene in women older than 35 years of age who are receiving estrogen replacement therapy increases the potential for hepatotoxicity. Verapamil and other calcium-channel blockers increase the risk of ventricular fibrillation and cardiovascular collapse when administered in conjunction with intravenous (IV) dantrolene.

Quinine increases digoxin levels, antagonizes the cardiac effects of cholinergic drugs, and adds to the vagolytic effects of anticholinergics. The metabolism of quinine is increased in the presence of anticonvulsants, barbiturates, and rifampin. Renal elimination of quinine is decreased by carbonic anhydrase inhibitors, sodium bicarbonate, and chronic antacid use. Warfarin may increase the hypoprothrombinemic effects.

Dosage Regimens

Determination of the optimal dosage for skeletal muscle relaxants requires careful titration. Almost all skeletal muscle relaxants can be administered orally, and some by intramuscular (IM) or IV routes (Table 21–4).

Laboratory Considerations

Serum drug levels for skeletal muscle relaxants are not ordinarily required; however, they may be desirable if the drugs are used on a long-term basis. In general, skeletal muscle relaxants produce mild elevations in aspartate aminotransferase (serum glutamic-oxaloacetic transami-

TABLE 21–2 PHARMACOKINETICS OF SELECTED SKELETAL MUSCLE RELAXANTS

Drug	Route	Onset	Peak	Duration	PB (%)	$t_{1/2}$	BioA (%)
Centrally Acting Drugs							
Baclofen	po	Hours to weeks	2–3 hr	8 hr	30	2.5–4 hr	UA
Carisoprodol	po	30 min	4 hr*	4–6 hr	UA	8 hr	UA
Chlorphenesin	po	UA	1–3 hr	UA	UA	2.5–5 hr	UA
Chlorzoxazone	po	60 min	1–2 hr	3–4 hr	UA	1–2 hr	UA
Cyclobenzaprine	po	60 min	3–8 hr	12–24 hr	93	12–24 hr	UA
Metaxalone	po	60 min	2 hr†	4–6 hr	30	2–3 hr	UA
Methocarbamol	po	30 min	2 hr	3–6 hr	UA	1–2 hr	UA
Orphenadrine	po	60 min	3 hr‡	8 hr	UA	14 hr	UA
Tizanidine	po	30 min	1–2 hr	3–6 hr	30	2.5 hr	40
Peripherally Acting Drugs							
Dantrolene	po	1 hr§	5 hr	6–12 hr	>90	6–9 hr	70
Quinine	po	Varies	1–3 hr	6–8 hr	70–90	4–21 hr	UA

*Peak drug activity for 350 mg dose of carisoprodol.
†Peak drug activity for 800 mg of metaxalone.
‡Peak drug activity for 50 mg of orphenadrine.
§Time for dantrolene to reach blood levels; therapeutic effect may take 1 to 2 weeks.
PB, protein binding; $t_{1/2}$, serum half-life; UA, unavailable; $t_{1/2}$, elimination half-life; BioA, bioavailability.

TABLE 21–3 DRUG-DRUG INTERACTIONS OF SELECTED SKELETAL MUSCLE RELAXANTS

Drug	Interactive Drug	Interaction
Centrally Acting Drugs		
Baclofen	Alcohol Antihistamines CNS depressants MAO inhibitors	Increases CNS depression; increases risk of hepatotoxicity with combination of chlorzoxazone and alcohol
Carisoprodol Chlorzoxazone Chlorphenesin Cyclobenzaprine Methocarbamol	Alcohol CNS depressants	
Chlorphenesin	Tricyclic antidepressants	Increases CNS depression; increases risk of hepatotoxicity with combination of chlorzoxazone and alcohol
Cyclobenzaprine	Phenothiazines	Potentiates anticholinergic effects
	MAO inhibitors	May precipitate hypertensive crisis
Orphenadrine	Propoxyphene	Increases confusion, anxiety, tremors
Tizanidine	Alcohol	Additive CNS depression
	Contraceptives Tylenol	Decreases clearance of tizanidine
	Antihypertensives	Additive hypotension
	Tricyclic antidepressants MAO inhibitors	Fever, convulsions
Peripherally Acting Drugs		
Dantrolene	Alcohol CNS depressants	Increases CNS depression
	Estrogens	Increases risk of hepatotoxicity
	Calcium-channel blockers	Increases risk of ventricular fibrillation
Quinine	Digoxin	Increases digoxin levels
	Anticholinergic drugs	Increases vagolytic effects
	Cholinergic drugs	Antagonizes cardiac effects
	Anticonvulsants Barbiturates Rifampin	Increases metabolism of quinine, thus decreasing efficacy
	Carbonic anhydrase inhibitors Chronic antacid use Sodium bicarbonate	Decreases renal elimination quinine, thus increasing toxicity
	Neuromuscular blockers	Increases effectiveness of neuromuscular blockers
	Warfarin	Increases hypoprothrombinemic effects

CNS, central nervous system; MAO, monoamine oxidase.

nase), alkaline phosphatase, and blood glucose levels. Methocarbamol can cause false increases in urinary 5-hydroxyindoleacetic acid (using nitrosonphthol reagent) and vanillymandelic acid (VMA) (Gitlow method) levels. Liver function tests and creatinine levels should be monitored for the patient taking dantrolene, quinine, and tizanidine quinine on a regular basis. A complete blood count should also be done for the patient taking quinine to monitor the hematologic impact of therapy.

Critical Thinking Process

Assessment

History of Present Illness

When obtaining the history of present illness, it is important to elicit information about the cause of the spasm or spastic state. Questions that may be asked include the following: Is the injury or illness related to employment or to leisure-time activities? When did the symptoms occur in relation to activities? What activities or situations aggravate or alleviate the discomfort? What has been used for self-treatment and how effective was the treatment?

Pain is the prominent symptom of muscle spasm and is usually aggravated by movement. Therefore, assessment should include the subjective descriptions of the discom-fort or pain. The location of the spasm or spasticity should be identified as precisely as possible, as well as the inten-sity, duration, and any precipitating factors. The potential for secondary gain related to spasms also should be considered.

With spasticity, the patient should be assessed for pain and impaired functional abilities (e.g., eating, dressing, bathing). Determine whether the spasticity interferes with joint and muscle mobility, as well as the ability for self-care. Factors contributing to the development of spasticity also should be elicited.

TABLE 21–4 DOSAGE REGIMEN FOR SELECTED SKELETAL MUSCLE RELAXANTS

Drug	Indication(s)	Dosage Regimen	Implications
Centrally Acting Drugs			
Baclofen	UMN disorders (multiple sclerosis, cerebral palsy, spinal cord insults, CVA)	*Adult:* 5 mg po BID–TID initially. Increase by 5 mg/dose every 3–7 days until desired response is achieved. Maintenance: Usually does not exceed 80 mg/day	If benefits are not evident after a reasonable trial period, gradually withdraw the drug. The dosage for children has not been determined. Dosage reduction may be needed in the elderly or in those with renal impairment
Carisoprodol	Relief of muscle spasm caused by inflammation and trauma.	*Adult:* 350 mg po TID–QID	Take the last dose at bedtime. Not recommended for children younger than 12 years, geriatric patients, or those with hepatic or renal impairment
Chlorphenesin	Relief of muscle spasm caused by inflammation and trauma	*Adult:* 800 mg po TID until desired effect obtained. Maintenance: Reduce dosage to 400 mg QID po or less as required	Safety for use longer than 8 weeks not established. Not recommended for children younger than 12 years, geriatric patients, or those with hepatic impairment
Chlorzoxazone	Relief of muscle spasm caused by inflammation and trauma	*Adult:* 250–500 mg po TID–QID. Increase to 750 mg po TID–QID. Reduce dosage if improvement occurs	Safe use in children has not been established. Not effective for spasticity of dyskinetic disorders
Cyclobenzaprine	Relief of muscle spasm caused by inflammation and trauma	*Adult:* 10 mg po TID. Range 20–40 mg in divided doses. Maintenance: Not to exceed 60 mg/day	Do not use longer than 2–3 weeks. Safe use in children under the age of 15 has not been established. Not effective for spasticity associated with cerebral palsy or cerebral cord disease.
Metaxalone	Relief of muscle spasm caused by inflammation and trauma	*Adult:* 800 mg po TID–QID	Safe use in children has not been established
Methocarbamol	Relief of muscle spasm caused by inflammation and trauma	*Adult:* 1.5 g po QID (up to 8 g/day) × 2–3 days Maintenance: 750 mg po q4h *or* 1 g QID, *or* 1.5 g TID	
	Adjunct for tetanus	*Adult:* 1–2 g IV. An additional dose may be given IV. Total initial dose 3 g. Dosage may be repeated q6h as necessary up to 24 g/day in divided doses. *Child:* 15 mg/kg IV q6h	IV route may be used until nasogastric tube is inserted, then change to oral formulation
Orphenadrine	Relief of muscle spasm caused by inflammation and trauma	*Adult:* 100 mg po BID *or* 60 mg IM/IV q12h	Safe use in children has not been established
Tizanidine	Relief of spasticity	*Adult:* 4 mg po q6–8 hr. Single dose not to exceed 8 mg. Increase slowly by 2–4 mg to optimal response. Not to exceed 36 mg daily	Safe use in children has not been established. Not recommended in pregnancy. Use low dose in older adults
Peripherally Acting Drugs			
Dantrolene	UMN disorders (multiple sclerosis, cerebral palsy, spinal cord insults, CVA)	*Adult:* 25 mg po QD. Increase by 25 mg BID–QID; then by increments of 25 mg BID–QID if necessary. Maintenance: Not to exceed 400 mg/day *Child:* 0.5 mg/kg BID. Increase by 0.5 mg/kg up to 3 mg/kg BID–QID. Maintenance: Not to exceed 100 mg QID	Maintain each dosage level for 4–7 days to evaluate response before increasing. Discontinue drug after 45 days if benefits not evident
	Prevention of malignant hyperthermia	*Adult & Child:* 4–8 mg/kg/day po in 3–4 divided doses 1–2 days preop. Last dose approximately 3–4 hr before scheduled surgery.	Adjust dosage to recommended range to prevent drowsiness and excessive GI irritation
	Malignant hyperthermic crisis	*Adult & Child:* 1 mg/kg IV. May repeat dosage up to cumulative dose of 10 mg/kg, followed by 4–8 mg/kg/day po in 4 divided doses for 1–3 days to prevent recurrence.	Dosage is for adults and children
Quinine	Nocturnal leg cramps	*Adult:* 260–300 mg po at HS	May be taken after evening meal and at bedtime

CVA, cerebral vascular accident; UMN, upper motor neuron; GI, gastrointestinal.

Past Health History

The past health history is helpful in determining the progress of the disease or condition and in helping to develop treatment objectives. The past health history should include a thorough history of GI disorders (e.g., peptic ulcer disease), neuromuscular, musculoskeletal, and renal disorders, and a drug history. Of significance is the patient's report of symptoms that may have been noticed several years earlier, but because they disappeared medical attention was not sought. When possible, the month and year when the patient first noticed the symptoms should be noted.

Physical Exam Findings

The clinical presentation of spasm and spasticity depends on the location of the injury in the neuromuscular system. For this reason, the physical exam should include an assessment of DTRs, Babinski, muscle strength, range of motion of joints, gait, balance, coordination, and dexterity. Muscle size, tone, symmetry, and the presence of tremor, spasms, or spasticity is noted. In patients with spasms, muscle firmness and tenderness may be noted over the affected area and are accompanied by limited movement and guarding. DTRs may be hyperactive. Adduction contractions can cause difficulties with personal hygiene, particularly of the perineal and axillary regions.

Assessment of other body systems should include neurologic symptoms such as weakness, skin color and temperature, the presence of edema, erythema, ecchymosis, or crepitus. The effect of the spasm or spasticity on urinary and bowel function also should be determined.

Diagnostic Testing

There are no definitive testing methods for spasms. An electromyogram is helpful to confirm nerve damage associated with spasticity. Magnetic resonance imaging is useful in detecting abnormalities of the spine or lesions in the gray or white matter of the brain. Radiography assists in determining the presence of fractures, dislocations, bony spurs, soft tissue swelling, and the presence of foreign objects that may be causing the spasm.

Developmental Considerations

Perinatal Skeletal muscle relaxants should not be used during pregnancy unless the anticipated benefits outweigh the risks. Most skeletal muscle relaxants cross placental membranes. Less is known about the presence of skeletal muscle relaxants in breast milk. It has been demonstrated that carisoprodol crosses into breast milk.

Pediatric Skeletal muscle relaxants are not usually needed in children, with the exception of spinal cord injuries or cerebral palsy. Most drugs are not recommended for children under age 5 years, and others are not recommended until age 12 years. When skeletal muscle relaxants are required, the dosage should be calculated on a milligram/kilogram basis.

Geriatric Spasms and spasticity are not uncommon in older adults. All skeletal muscle relaxants have adverse effects that alter the functional abilities of an older adult. Caution is warranted if dizziness or weakness is exacerbated, to prevent falls or injuries.

Psychosocial Considerations

The psychological response to spasms or spasticity is determined by the cause of the disorder, severity of symptoms, and the impact of those symptoms on life-style. Chronic or recurrent spasm and spasticity cause the patient to fear incapacitation if the symptoms cannot be managed effectively.

Considerations should be given to the potential for secondary gain associated with the patient's illness or condition. The illness or condition affects and is affected by the patient's emotional response. Emotional distress associated with spasm and spasticity can manifest as sleep disturbances, restlessness, irritability, decreased appetite, and loss of interest in daily activities. The perceived vulnerability and associated powerlessness complicate the plan of care for some patients. The sense of powerlessness stems from real and perceived losses. Losses may include employment and financial security, role status, physical or social independence, and control of home environment (see Case Study—Multiple Sclerosis and Case Study—Low Back Syndrome with Spasm).

Analysis and Management

Treatment Objectives

The decision to treat spasms and spasticity is based on the cause and issues of pain and mobility. Skeletal muscle relaxants are used to minimize or stop unwanted spasm and spasticity, with the ultimate goal of establishing normal muscle tone and function. Additionally, effective treatment regimens improve activity tolerance, range of motion, strength, and mobility.

The potential impact of spasticity on the patient's physical condition, functional status, and adaptation to disability is significant. Perceived susceptibility to disease and its seriousness influences the plan of care. Many of the skeletal muscle relaxants have unpleasant or undesirable adverse effects; therefore, the likelihood of compliance is a concern.

Treatment Options

Most spasms are self-limiting, responding rapidly to rest and physical measures. Physical measures include rest, application of cold or warm compresses, whirlpool baths, and physical therapy. Drug therapy for spasms usually involves two groups of drugs, skeletal muscle relaxants and nonsteroidal anti-inflammatory drugs (Chapter 15).

No completely satisfactory form of therapy is available to alleviate spasticity. The cornerstone of any treatment is the management of the underlying disease and physiotherapy. Measures that can be used include physical therapy for stretching, strengthening, range-of-motion exercises, assistive-adaptive devices, and hydrotherapy.

Drug Variables

Characteristics of the ideal skeletal muscle relaxant include an agent that possesses a high degree of efficacy (for specific spasm patterns), minimal adverse effects, and no clinically significant drug interactions. The drug should be formulated in oral as well as IV dosage forms, with the oral dose exhibiting a minimal first pass effect. A reasonable half-life that promotes infrequent dosing and a positive correlation between drug effectiveness and plasma concentrations are ideal. Few drugs, however, meet all of these characteristics. Because no studies indicate that any one skeletal muscle relaxant has superiority over another, drug selection is largely based on the preference of the health care provider and the patient's response.

The ability of skeletal muscle relaxants to relieve discomfort appears equal to that of salicylates and other nonsteroidal anti-inflammatory drugs. No one skeletal muscle relaxant is any more effective than any other for acute disorders. Available data, however, are more likely to support the use of cyclobenzaprine or carisoprodol.

For acute muscle spasm and pain, a drug that can be given parenterally is usually the drug of choice. Parenteral drugs are preferred for patients with orthopedic etiologies because they have greater sedative and pain-relieving characteristics. Cy-

Text continued on page 398

Case Study Multiple Sclerosis

Patient History

History of Present Illness	DL is a 40-year-old woman with a 10-year history of multiple sclerosis. Now has complaints of reduced strength and mobility, increased cutaneous, flexor and extensor spasms, and pain that started 1 month ago. Spasms disturb her sleep. States is unable to carry out routine activities of daily living and daily range of motion exercises as before. Used a cane until recently, now must use a walker. Denies recent illness, infection, unusual stress, or trauma.
Past Health History	DL has been taking alternate-day low dose prednisone for past year with general improvement in symptoms. She was actively employed until the recent change in health status. She usually follows prescribed exercise regimen and by record is a motivated patient. DL is post-menopausal; takes estrogen/progesterone daily. There are no known food or drug allergies.
Physical Exam Findings	*Height:* 5′4″. *Weight:* 125 lbs. *VS:* BP 122/72, apical pulse 72 and regular, respirations 20, temperature 98.6° F. Extensor and flexor spasms and clonus are observed. Deep tendon reflexes are exaggerated. DL has an unsteady gait and borderline muscle strength.
Diagnostic Testing	CBC, electrolytes, BUN, creatinine are WNL. CSF reflects slightly elevated WBCs, cell, and protein counts. EMG reflects slow-wave activity compared to exam 2 years ago. Repeat CT scan shows increased density in the white matter with MS plaques.
Developmental Considerations	Single, lives alone. Works as secretary-receptionist. Is age-appropriate for chronologic and developmental stage.
Psychosocial Considerations	DL copes well with disease overall. Family and employer emotionally supportive. She most fears incapacitation and has a sense of powerlessness from real and perceived losses. She has changed jobs several times in past 3 years due to MS and now perceives her financial, physical, and social independence as threatened. Interested in the theater and arts; attending shows on a regular basis with theater group.
Economic Factors	Health insurance through HMO but without pharmacy coverage. Is worried that if she changes jobs again she will lose her coverage.

Variables Influencing Decision

Treatment Objectives	• Minimize severity of spasticity • Improve activity tolerance, ROM, strength, and mobility

Drug Variables	*Drug Summary*	*Patient Variables*
Indications	UMN lesions. *Baclofen* useful with flexor and extensor spasms and spasticity of spinal origin. Preferred in patients with borderline strength. *Dantrolene* relieves spasticity also. Major utility is in nonmobile patients.	This becomes a decision point because DL diagnosed with spinal lesions of MS. Has flexor and extensor spasms and borderline strength.
Pharmacodynamics	CNS depression. Blockage of nerve impulses that cause increased muscle tone and contraction. Baclofen produces no direct relaxation in peripheral muscle strength.	This is not a decision point because all agents have similar pharmacodynamics.

Drug Variables	*Drug Summary*	*Patient Variables*
Adverse Effects/ Contraindications	Baclofen produces annoying muscle weakness, alterations in gait. Dantrolene produces weaknesses that handicap the patient more than it helps relieve spasticity. Concurrent use of estrogen increases risk of hepatotoxicity. Neither drug should be used in patients for whom spasticity is used to maintain posture and balance. Both drugs produce sedation, drowsiness, light-headedness, ataxia, dizziness.	This may be a decision point because of the potential adverse effects of baclofen and dantrolene. DL is already experiencing muscle involvement and gait disturbance. Spasticity is not used to maintain posture and balance in DL.
Pharmacokinetics	Almost all agents have similar pharmacokinetic parameters.	DL's hepatic and renal functions are intact. Because almost all agents have similar pharmacokinetics, this will not be a decision point.
Dosage Regimen	Per manufacturer's recommendations and careful titration. Oral formulations available for both baclofen and dantrolene.	DL has history of compliance with treatment regimens. Dosage regimen will not be a decision point for DL.
Lab Considerations	Skeletal muscle relaxants produce mild elevations in AST (SGOT), and alkaline phosphatase, and blood glucose levels.	DL has no history of liver disorders or diabetes. This will not be a major decision point at this time.
Cost Index*	Baclofen: 1 Dantrolene: 5	DL has health insurance through an HMO but without pharmacy coverage. This will become a decision point.

Summary of Decision Points

- Baclofen produces no direct relaxation in peripheral muscle strength and is preferred in patients with borderline strength and spasticity of spinal origin.
- DL already experiencing borderline strength and gait disturbances.
- DL is over 35 and takes estrogen, increasing her risk of hepatotoxicity if dantrolene is used.
- DL has health insurance through HMO but no pharmacy coverage.
- Employment and financial security in potential jeopardy due to physical condition.
- Baclofen the least expensive of the possible agents.

DRUGS TO BE USED

- Baclofen 5 mg po BID-TID initially. Increase by 5 mg/dose every 3–7 days until desired response achieved. Maintenance dose usually does not exceed 80 mg/day.

*Cost Index:
1 = $<30/month
2 = $30–40/month
3 = $40–50/month
4 = $50–60/month
5 = $>60/month

AWP of 100, 10 mg tablets of baclofen is approximately $14.
AWP of 100, 25 mg capsules of dantrolene is approximately $71.

Case Study Low Back Syndrome with Spasm

Patient History

History of Present Illness	SK is a 37-year-old man with complaints of low back pain described as "knifelike burning." Radiates from lumbar region to right mid-buttock and hip. Unable to sit or stand comfortably. "Any movement hurts." Was helping to unpack and transfer oversize library books to high shelf when pain occurred.
Past Health History	DJ denies history of neuromuscular, musculoskeletal, renal, or peptic ulcer disease. Has a history of acute intermittent porphyria. Has not gained or lost weight in past year. Routine exercise regimen limited to walking to and from his car and the library. Denies taking any other medications or consuming alcohol.
Physical Exam Findings	*Height:* 5′9″. *Weight:* 255 lbs. *VS:* 132/88, apical pulse 120, respirations 24, temperature 98.6° F. DJ is pacing in exam room, holding right lower back and hip. Muscle firmness and tenderness noted from L_4-S_3 on palpation and tautness of sacrospinalis and gluteal muscles. Straight leg raises aggravate the low back pain. Severe discomfort when toe walking. Unable to twist or bend at the waist without obvious discomfort. Muscle tone increased on affected side. Abdomen soft, flat, nontender. No CVA tenderness.
Diagnostic Testing	KUB, flat plate films of lower back, CT scan, and MRI are all WNL. CBC, electrolytes, BUN, creatinine, urinalysis WNL.
Developmental Considerations	Accomplishing age-appropriate developmental tasks.
Psychosocial Considerations	SK is single. Has degree in library science. Works at university library. In spare time watches videos and "veges out." Describes his life-style as that of a "couch-potato."
Economic Factors	Carries health insurance through the university policy that also includes a pharmacy plan. Workers' compensation coverage available through employer.

Variables Influencing Decision

Treatment Objectives	• Establish normal muscle tone and function. • Improve functional state and minimize discomfort.

Drug Variables	*Drug Summary*	*Patient Variables*
Indications	LMN disorders related to injury or inflammation. Skeletal muscle relaxants are used for muscle spasms that do not respond to other conservative therapies. Cyclobenzaprine less likely than carisoprodol to produce alterations in muscle function. This becomes a decision point.	SK diagnosed with low back pain with spasm secondary to lifting and turning movements. Has followed through with conservative treatment without relief. This will be a decision point.
Pharmacodynamics	All centrally active drugs act as interneuronal blockers that depress polysynaptic reflexes. There are no known peripheral or autonomic effects. Carisoprodol is chemically related to meprobamate, an antianxiety drug. Cyclobenzaprine is chemically related to tricyclic antidepressants.	Because all agents have similar pharmacodynamics, this will not become a major decision point.

Drug Variables	*Drug Summary*	*Patient Variables*
Adverse Effects/ Contraindications	All centrally active drugs can cause headaches, sleepiness, visual disturbances, sedation, drowsiness, light-headedness, ataxia. Cyclobenzaprine may cause nausea, vomiting, diarrhea or constipation, significant anticholinergic activity. Carisoprodol can cause nausea, vomiting, diarrhea or constipation, increased excitability. Cyclobenzaprine is contraindicated in patients with history of porphyria. This will become a decision point.	This is a decision point, as SK has history of intermittent porphyria.
Pharmacokinetics	All centrally active drugs have similar pharmacokinetics except for cyclobenzaprine, which has a 12–24 hour duration. All are biotransformed in liver, excreted in urine.	This is not a decision point because SK has no known liver or renal dysfunction that would cause concern.
Dosage Regimen	Per manufacturer's recommendations. Maximal treatment time 2–3 weeks.	Per patient records, SK has been compliant with previous therapies. This will not become a decision point regardless of choice of drug.
Lab Considerations	Serum drug levels not ordinarily required. No specific laboratory tests needed before or during short-term therapy.	This is not a decision point, as there are no definitive lab tests to monitor therapy.
Cost Index*	Cyclobenzaprine: 1 Carisoprodol: 1	Cost not a major decision point, although the higher the charges to insurance companies, the higher the insurance cost. SK has a co-pay pharmacy plan.

Summary of Decision Points

- SK diagnosed with low back pain with spasm secondary to lifting and turning movements.
- SK has followed through with conservative treatment without relief.
- SK has history of intermittent porphyria. Carisoprodol contraindicated with history of porphyria.

DRUGS TO BE USED

- Cyclobenzaprine 10 mg TID with food or milk for 2 weeks. Dosage not to exceed 60 mg/day.
- Supplemental ibuprofen to reduce inflammation.

*Cost Index:
1 = $<30/month
2 = $30–40/month
3 = $40–50/month
4 = $50–60/month
5 = $>60/month

AWP of 100, 10 mg tablets of cyclobenzaprine is approximately $21.
AWP of 100, 350 mg tablets of carisoprodol is approximately $8.

clobenzaprine is less likely to produce alterations in muscle function than carisoprodol, although it does have anticholinergic properties that may be bothersome.

In many cases, spasms are self-limiting and can be nicely managed with rest, physical therapy, and/or assistive devices. Most centrally acting skeletal muscle relaxants produce sedative effects and mild pain relief by reducing muscle tone and the discomfort of the spasm. If there has been tissue damage and edema, nonsteroidal anti-inflammatory drugs also may be prescribed.

Spasticity caused by spinal lesions is much more responsive to oral baclofen than spasticity caused by cerebral lesions. Baclofen is particularly useful in reducing the frequency and severity of flexor and extensor spasms, and in reducing flexor tone. Although the responses are clinically relevant, results may be limited. Benefits to the use of baclofen include less disruption of sleep, improved comfort, maintenance of an independent state of self-care, and an ability to participate in a rehabilitation program.

The most effective drug for the control of spasticity associated with multiple sclerosis is baclofen. Dantrolene and diazepam are possible alternatives. The choice of drug depends on the condition being treated, its initial or presenting status, associated illness, the drug's pharmacologic actions, and the preference of the patient and health care provider.

Dantrolene is useful because it decreases adductor muscle tone in patients with limited function. It must be used cautiously in ambulatory patients, for relief of spasticity may be associated with weakness. In turn, a patient's overall functional capacity may worsen.

The benefit of reducing spasticity versus the disadvantage of reducing muscle strength must be weighed individually. Although drugs such as baclofen and dantrolene provide variable relief of spasticity, annoying muscle weakness, alterations in gait, and a variety of other adverse effects minimize their overall usefulness. Baclofen seems to be most effective for spasticity of spinal origin. It produces no direct relaxation on peripheral muscles, and hence does not decrease muscle strength. Baclofen is preferred over dantrolene in patients with borderline strength.

Dantrolene can relieve spasticity, but the weakness it produces often handicaps the patient more than the spasticity it relieves. In view of the pharmacodynamics of dantrolene, the cause of the spasticity makes little difference. Its major utility is for nonambulatory patients whose care is made difficult by muscle contraction, and for whom relief of spasticity warrants the risk of hepatotoxicity.

Diazepam, a benzodiazepine sometimes used for its skeletal muscle relaxant properties, was discussed in depth in Chapter 17. Although diazepam may modulate spasticity, effective doses often cause intolerable drowsiness.

Patient Variables

The management of spasticity includes careful consideration of the advantages and disadvantages of spastic muscle groups and the potential consequences of treatment. For example, baclofen and dantrolene should not be used in patients for whom spasticity is used to maintain posture and balance.

The patient's subjective statements and physical exam findings are most useful in determining the management of spasm and spasticity. Special caution is needed for patients with hepatic or renal dysfunction, glaucoma, benign prostatic hypertrophy, psychiatric illness, cardiovascular disease, and emphysema, or in patients prone to drug abuse/misuse.

Hepatotoxicity is most likely to occur in people over 35 who have taken baclofen for 60 days or longer. Women over 35 who are also taking estrogen are at the highest risk. Hepatotoxicity can be prevented or minimized by administering the lowest effective dose, monitoring liver enzymes during therapy, and discontinuing the drug if beneficial effects do not occur within 45 days.

Despite their different chemical structures, all skeletal muscle relaxants are sedating and are abused primarily for this effect. At high doses, they have been described as producing a buzz (baclofen), euphoria (carisoprodol), and mood enhancement and pleasant disperceptions (orphenadrine). Carisoprodol has been abused more often than other drugs in this class, presumably because of its close similarity to meprobamate. Abusers of either of these drugs demonstrate signs of tolerance and also experience withdrawal symptoms.

The extent to which these drugs are abused is unclear, as they are often used in conjunction with other CNS depressants (e.g., alcohol, benzodiazepines, opioids). When abused, the skeletal muscle relaxants are used to prolong the effects of alcohol or an opioid, to increase the effect of the primary drug of abuse, or to achieve the same effect with a smaller dosage of alcohol or opioid. In addition, prescriptions for skeletal muscle relaxants are often easier to obtain and are less costly. Substance abusers occasionally substitute a skeletal muscle relaxant when an opioid is not available.

Health care providers today are conscious of patient's requests for opioids or benzodiazepines and are rightly concerned about the dependency potential of these drugs. However, few of the health care providers are aware of the addictive potential these drugs hold. Because skeletal muscle relaxants are not controlled, health care providers may become complacent about their use. Some of the drugs, such as carisoprodol, can even be ordered by mail through veterinary supply houses. Health care providers should be concerned about requests for frequent refills or requests for refills before the expected completion of a prescription.

Intervention

Administration

In general, the dosage of skeletal muscle relaxants should be increased gradually to reduce the likelihood of adverse effects. Baclofen, chlorphenesin, chlorzoxazone, and metaxalone should be administered with food to minimize GI distress. For ease of administration, tablet formulations can be crushed and mixed with applesauce, jelly, or other food. Relief from dry mouth caused by carisoprodol can be obtained with sips of water, ice chips, or chewing gum. The use of frequent mouth rinses and sugarless hard candy may help.

When withdrawing a patient from therapy, a gradual reduction in dosage over 2 weeks is recommended. Abrupt withdrawal (from baclofen in particular) may cause hallucinations, paranoia, nightmares, confusion, and rebound spasticity.

Education

The patient should be encouraged to comply with additional therapies prescribed for muscle spasm (e.g., rest, heat/cold, physical therapy). Correct posture and lifting techniques should be taught. Stooping rather than bending to lift objects, carrying heavy objects close to the body, and not lifting excessive amounts of weight should be stressed. Regular exercise and the use of warm-up exercises minimize the potential for injury. Strenuous exercise performed infrequently is more likely to cause acute muscle spasm.

The patient and family should be educated about the drug prescribed including the name, purpose, dose, administration times and frequency, and potential adverse effects. Missed doses should be taken within 1 hour of their scheduled time. Double doses should not be taken. If the drug is to be discontinued, the patient should be instructed not to suddenly stop the drug, but to taper the dosage as instructed.

The patient should avoid activities that require mental alertness, judgment, and physical coordination, such as operating a motor vehicle, if drowsiness occurs. Alcohol and other CNS depressants increase CNS depression and place the patient at risk for injury. Further, because many patients have postural hypotension when taking these drugs, they should be instructed to change positions slowly.

The patient also should be told not to take other drugs without the health care provider's knowledge, including nonprescription drugs. The major risks occur with concurrent use of alcohol, antihistamines, sleeping aids, or other drugs that cause drowsiness.

The patient taking baclofen should be advised that maximum benefit may not be reached for 4 to 8 weeks. The sedative effects are generally transient and usually disappear with continued therapy. Baclofen has been shown to elevate blood sugars. Patients with diabetes mellitus should be instructed to monitor their blood sugar levels more frequently.

Evaluation

Criteria that may be used to evaluate the therapeutic outcome of therapy for spasms include decreased pain and tenderness, increased mobility, and the ability to participate in the activities of daily living. When a skeletal muscle relaxant is used for the spasticity of chronic neurologic disorders, therapeutic effects include increased ability to maintain posture and balance, increased ability for self-care, improvement in strength and muscle tone, improved coordination, and ease of movement. Reduction in spasticity does not necessarily correlate with overall functional improvement.

SUMMARY

- Spasms are motor disorders involving LMNs. Spasms occur as a result of injury to peripheral muscle system structures, such as muscles, joints, tendons, or ligaments. Specific causes include whiplash injuries, cervical root syndrome, herniated discs, and lower back syndrome.
- Spasticity involves UMNs. Spasticity occurs as a result of damage to UMNs of the brain and spinal cord. Specific disorders may include multiple sclerosis, cerebral palsy, stroke, and closed head injuries.
- Impulses from the injured muscle are transmitted to the spinal cord and back, causing a reflex contraction. The reflex contraction stimulates the muscle, increasing the stimulation of the spinal cord, and thus increasing the contractions.
- The core feature of a spastic state is the exaggeration of stretch reflexes, which manifests as hypertonus. It results from either an increase in excitatory influences or a decrease in inhibitory influences.
- The clinical presentation of spasm and spasticity depends on the location of the injury to the neuromuscular system. For this reason, the physical exam should include an assessment of DTRs, Babinski's sign, muscle strength, range of motion, gait, balance, coordination, and dexterity.
- The therapeutic objectives in the treatment of spasm are relief of signs and symptoms of muscle spasm. The primary objectives in the management of spasticity are to control symptoms, reduce spasticity, prevent joint and muscle contractures, and improve the quality of life.
- As a general rule, drugs that are used to treat spasticity do not relieve acute muscle spasm and vice versa.
- The cornerstone of any treatment of patients with spasticity is the management of underlying disease and physiotherapy.
- The drugs should be administered with meals or milk to prevent GI distress, particularly baclofen, chlorphenesin, chlorzoxazone, and metaxalone.
- The dosage of skeletal muscle relaxants should be decreased gradually when the patient is withdrawing from therapy to decrease the incidence of rebound spasm or spasticity.
- The patient should be encouraged to comply with additional therapies prescribed for muscle spasm (e.g., rest, heat/cold, physical therapy).
- The patient and family should be educated about the drug prescribed including the name, purpose, dose, administration times and frequency, and potential adverse effects.
- The patient should be informed to avoid activities that require mental alertness, judgment, and physical coordination, such as operating a motor vehicle if drowsy from the drug.
- Criteria used to evaluate the therapeutic outcome of therapy for spasms include decreased pain and tenderness, increased mobility, and the ability to participate in the activities of daily living.
- Therapeutic effects of treatment for spasticity are evidenced as increased ability to maintain posture and balance, increased ability for self-care, improvement in strength and muscle tone, improved coordination, and ease of movement.

BIBLIOGRAPHY

Abel, N., and Smith, R. (1994). Intrathecal baclofen for treatment of intractable spinal spasticity. *Archives of Physical Medicine and Rehabilitation,* 75, 54–58.

American Medical Association. (1996). *Drug evaluations.* Milwaukee: Author.

Brown, P. (1994). Pathophysiology of spasticity. *Journal of Neurology, Neurosurgery and Psychiatry,* 57(7), 773–776.

Elder, N. (1991). Abuse of skeletal muscle relaxants. *American Family Physician,* 44(4), 1223–1226.

Gianino, J. (1993). Intrathecal baclofen for spinal spasticity: Implications for nursing practice. *Journal of Neuroscience Nursing, 25,* 254–264.

Hauser, S., and Doolittle, T. (1992). An anti-spasticity effect of threonine in multiple sclerosis. *Archives of Neurology, 49,* 923–926.

Katzung, B. (1995). *Basic and clinical pharmacology* (6th ed.). Norwalk, CT: Appleton and Lange.

Noth, J. (1991). Trends in the pathophysiology and pharmacotherapy of spasticity. *Journal of Neurology, 238,* 131–139.

Parziale, J., Akelman, E., and Herz, D. (1993). Spasticity: Pathophysiology and management. *Orthopedics,* 16, 801–811.

Rawlins, P. (1995). Intrathecal baclofen for spasticity of cerebral palsy: Project coordination and nursing care. *Journal of Neuroscience Nursing,* 27, 157–163.

Thompson, P. (1993). Stiff muscles. *Neurology, Neurosurgery and Psychiatry,* 56(2), 121–124.

Waldman, H. (1994). Centrally acting skeletal muscle relaxants and associated drugs. *Journal of Pain and Symptom Management,* 9, 434–441.

22 Anticonvulsants

The terms *epilepsy, seizure,* and *convulsion* are often used interchangeably. *Epilepsy,* however, is a chronic condition characterized by seizure activity. A *seizure* results from excessive stimulation of neurons in the brain leading to a sudden burst of abnormal neuron activity resulting in changes in brain function. The term applies to all types of epileptic events, and no two seizures are alike. A *convulsion* refers to spasmodic, uncontrolled contractions of the involuntary muscles or abnormal motor movement. Thus, convulsions are often a part of seizures.

Approximately 0.5 to 2 percent of the population in the United States has epilepsy. It ranks second to cerebrovascular accident as a neurologic disorder. Epilepsy can be the result of trauma sustained at birth, an inherent imbalance in central nervous system (CNS) activity, metabolic derangements, or accidents and injuries. The appearance of epilepsy in late adulthood may suggest the development of a cerebral tumor or other organic brain disease.

Seventy-five percent of those affected by epilepsy remain seizure free with the consistent use of anticonvulsant drugs. Anticonvulsants have allowed people of all ages to maintain active lives without fear of recurrent seizures.

EPILEPSY

Epidemiology and Etiology

The reported occurrence of epilepsy is low because many patients are reluctant to admit to having the disease. The stigma attached to epilepsy can lead to educational, occupational, and social discrimination. Yet 120 per 100,000 individuals in the United States will seek health care each year because of newly recognized seizures. Each year, 50 of every 100,000 individuals in the United States are diagnosed with epilepsy. This represents 125,000 new cases of epilepsy per year. Thirty percent of the newly diagnosed cases were in people under the age of 18 years.

The prevalence of active epilepsy in preschool children is about 1.5 per 1000. The onset of epilepsy is most common during childhood or after age 50 years, although its occurrence is certainly not limited to these age groups. Seventy-five percent of people have their first seizure prior to the age of 20 years.

Pathophysiology

Seizures result when an electrical discharge from a *focus* (abnormally hyperexcitable neurons) spreads to other areas of the brain. The manifestations of a particular seizure depend on the location of the focus and the neuronal connections to that focus. The neuronal connections to the focus determine to which areas of the brain seizure activity can spread. If seizure activity is confined to a very limited part of the brain, a partial or local seizure will result. If the activity is more diffuse, a generalized seizure occurs.

Seizure Classifications

Epilepsy can be classified by seizure type or by cause. Seizures that do not have a known cerebral lesion are referred to as *primary epilepsy* (idiopathic). More than 50 percent of epilepsy cases are of unknown origin. However, in some forms of primary epilepsy, a genetic basis is apparent. Primary epilepsy often appears during childhood or adolescence. *Secondary epilepsy* has a distinct cause, and cerebral abnormalities are noted. Causes of secondary epilepsy include hypoxia at birth, perinatal injuries, congenital malformations, head injury, encephalitis, brain tumors, abscesses or infections, nutritional disorders (e.g., hypoglycemia, phenylketonuria, vitamin B_6 deficiency), alcohol withdrawal, metabolic derangements, circulatory disturbances, and drug interactions.

The Commission of Classification and Terminology of the International League Against Epilepsy classified epilepsy into two broad groups: partial seizures and generalized seizures (Table 22–1). *Partial seizures* are localized to one area of the brain. *Generalized seizures* involve both hemispheres of the brain. Each seizure is a single occurrence. Single-episode seizures can be caused by such events as fever, hypoglycemia, or hyponatremia and do not mean the patient has epilepsy. The seizure type is diagnostically significant because it is the key determinant of the treatment approach.

Status epilepticus occurs when a patient has seizures in rapid succession or continuous seizures lasting 30 minutes or more. There are several types of status epilepticus, including absence status epilepticus, myoclonic status epilepticus, and tonic-clonic status epilepticus. Status epilepticus has many causes, and patients who develop it may have no previous history of epilepsy. In these cases, the cause is often related to acute brain infections, craniocerebral trauma, cerebrovascular disease, and toxic or metabolic disorders.

The most severe form of status epilepticus is the tonic-clonic form. The patient experiences an unrelenting series of tonic-clonic attacks. Loss of consciousness extends throughout the entire attack.

The sudden withdrawal of a drug or noncompliance with anticonvulsant therapy can precipitate status epilepticus. Because of the sudden withdrawal of a drug, the blood level of the drug abruptly drops and the seizure activity is no longer suppressed. Status epilepticus requires immediate intervention and aggressive treatment to prevent damage to the central nervous system.

PHARMACOTHERAPEUTIC OPTIONS

Anticonvulsant (antiseizure) drugs depress abnormal neuronal discharge. The categories from which drugs are commonly chosen for therapy include the hydantoins, barbiturates, succinimides, benzodiazepines, oxazolidine-

TABLE 22–1 TYPES OF SEIZURES WITH ASSOCIATED CHARACTERISTICS AND MANIFESTATIONS

Seizure Type	Age Group	Characteristics and Manifestations
Partial Seizures (Focal, Local)		
Simple partial seizures	Most common in older children and adults	Consciousness usually not impaired Duration: 1–2 min Functional disturbance in motor, sensory, and/or autonomic nerves and regions of the brain "Jacksonian march" and sensory symptoms (i.e., odor, taste) most common Psychic symptoms (fearful feeling, sense of *déjà vu*)
Complex partial seizures	Any age	Start as simple partial seizure and progress to impairment of consciousness (i.e., amnesia, unresponsiveness) Duration: 1–2 min with confusion lasting 1–2 min after attack Characterized by automatisms (e.g., staring; chewing; lip smacking; bizarre, purposeless motor or psychic activity; mumbled speech; unintelligible sounds) Consciousness impaired at onset Motor, somatosensory, autonomic, or psychic symptoms
Partial seizures evolving to secondary generalized seizures	Any age	Duration: minutes Simple partial seizure leading to generalized seizure activity Complex partial seizure leading to generalized seizure activity Simple partial seizure evolving to complex partial seizure and ultimately generalized seizure activity
Generalized Seizures (Convulsive or Nonconvulsive)—All Are Associated With Loss of Consciousness		
Absence seizures (petit mal)	Onset usually at 4–8 years of age; rare before age 3 or after age 15	Brief loss of consciousness, amnesia, or unawareness Duration: 10–30 sec Characterized by mild clonic movements (e.g., eye blinking, jerking movement), automatisms, changes in postural tone No postictal state after seizure Onset in childhood with approximately 40% ending in adolescence 50% supplanted by tonic-clonic seizures May occur 50–100 times per day in some people
Myoclonic seizures	Late childhood, adolescence	Characterized by single or multiple, short, abrupt muscular contractions of arms, legs, and/or torso and brief loss of consciousness Duration: 1–5 sec May be confined to face and trunk or to one or more extremities May not be classified as a seizure in some cases
Clonic seizures	Early childhood	Rare Repetitive clonic jerks that lack tonic component. Duration: seconds Movements may be symmetric or asymmetric, synchronous or asynchronous, rhythmic or dysrhythmic
Tonic seizures	Any age	Altered consciousness, tonic contraction of muscle groups with no progression to clonic movement Duration: 30 seconds to several minutes Ocular phenomena common (e.g., fixed gaze, eyelid retraction, superior ocular deviation, nystagmus, mydriasis) Autonomia (e.g., tachycardia, hypertension, respiratory distress, capillary restriction with cyanosis) Usually activated by sleep
Tonic-clonic seizures	Any age	Vague aura, loss of consciousness, sudden tonic contraction with stridor if respiratory muscle involved, rigidity May begin with shrill cry due to abrupt closure of epiglottis and secondary expulsion of air from the lungs Duration: 10–30 sec after falling to ground Tonic phase gives way to clonic phase, which lasts 30–50 sec Muscle relaxation interrupts tonic contraction with tone returning as rhythmic flexor spasms that become less frequent as seizure subsides Urinary and fecal incontinence may occur during clonic phase Amnesia after seizure
Atonic seizures	Infants and children	Characterized by abrupt, selective loss of muscle tone or of all muscle tone Duration: 10–30 sec Referred to as drop attacks if attacks are brief and patient slumps to ground; injury possible May be followed by postictal confusion
Unclassified epileptic seizures	Neonate	Seizures cannot be classified because of inadequate or incomplete data Duration: 10–30 sec "Neonatal seizures" (e.g., rhythmic eye movements, chewing or swimming movements)

Data from Santilli, N. (1996). *Managing seizure disorders: A handbook for health care professionals.* Philadelphia: Lippincott-Raven.

diones, and a variety of miscellaneous agents. Barbiturates and benzodiazepines are discussed in Chapter 17 in relation to their uses as antianxiety or sedative-hypnotic drugs. They are discussed here in relation to epilepsy. Magnesium sulfate, used to prevent or control pre-eclamptic seizures and eclamptic seizures, is discussed in Chapter 55.

Hydantoins

- ❒ Ethotoin (PEGANONE)
- ❒ Fosphenytoin (CEREBYX)
- ❒ Mephenytoin (MESANTOIN)
- ❒ Phenytoin (diphenylhydantoin, DILANTIN, DIPHENYLAN)

Indications

The hydantoins are used in generalized tonic-clonic seizures, status epilepticus, and refractory simple and complex partial seizures. Phenytoin is the most commonly used drug in this group. Ethotoin and mephenytoin are also available but are used less often. The newest drug is fosphenytoin. Fosphenytoin is used for the acute treatment of generalized convulsive status epilepticus and for the treatment of seizures occurring during neurosurgery. It is a short-term parenteral substitute for oral phenytoin. Phenytoin is a second-line drug in treating status epilepticus (see Controversy—Medication Errors from Confusing Orders and New Products).

Pharmacodynamics

The mechanisms of action of anticonvulsant drugs are not clearly understood. It is thought that anticonvulsants limit seizure propagation by altering ion (sodium, potassium, calcium) transport and by stabilizing cell membranes. Thus, they may raise the motor cortex's seizure threshold, stop or limit the seizure discharge, or reduce the spread of excitation from the seizure focus.

Hydantoins specifically modify calcium and sodium transport. They do not alter potassium transport across cell membranes. The site of action of the hydantoins, particularly phenytoin, is the motor cortex and the brainstem, where the tonic phase of tonic-clonic seizures originates. These drugs also reduce post-tetanic potentiation of synaptic transmission. This may limit detonation of cortical areas adjacent to the seizure foci and reduce sustained, high-frequency discharges.

Adverse Effects and Contraindications

The common adverse effects of ethotoin include dizziness, ataxia, sensory neuropathies, nausea, vomiting, diarrhea, nystagmus, and diplopia. The most serious adverse effects include agranulocytosis, thrombocytopenia, leukopenia, aplastic anemia, and megaloblastic anemia. It should be used with caution in patients with diabetes and in patients who slowly biotransform hydantoins. It is contraindicated in patients who are hypersensitive to hydantoins or who have blood dyscrasias, hematologic disease, or hepatic disorders or porphyria. It is a pregnancy Category C drug.

A high fosphenytoin blood level may produce ataxia, nystagmus, double vision, lethargy, slurred speech, nausea, vomiting, and hypotension. As the level increases, extreme lethargy to comatose states develop. Cautious use of fosphenytoin is warranted in patients with hypotension, porphyria, severe myocardial insufficiency, renal or hepatic disease, and hypoalbuminemia. Fosphenytoin use during pregnancy may increase the frequency of seizures. There is an increased risk of congenital malformations. It is a pregnancy Category D drug.

Mephenytoin has many of the same adverse effects as ethotoin, but in addition patients may note lethargy, exfoliative dermatitis, palpitations, tachycardia, and hypertension. Pulmonary fibrosis may develop. Mephytoin should be used with caution in patients with cardiac disorders, hyperthyroidism, diabetes, or prostatic hypertrophy. It is contraindicated in patients with hypersensitivity to sympathomimetics. It should be used with caution in patients with alcoholism, hepatic or renal disease, blood dyscrasias, congestive heart failure, respiratory depression, or diabetes. Mephenytoin is a pregnancy Category C drug. Mephenytoin is contraindicated in patients with hypersensitivity to hydantoins and in persons with sinus bradycardia and heart block.

The most common adverse effects of phenytoin are much like those of the other hydantoins. Patients under age 23 years and those taking phenytoin doses that exceed 500 mg/day are at increased risk for gingival hyperplasia. Hypertrichosis and exfoliative dermatitis, coarsened facial features, impaired cognition, dyskinesias, urinary incontinence, and thyroid disorders occur in some patients. The most serious adverse effects include agranulocytosis, encephalopathy, and coma. Phenytoin should be used with caution in patients with severe liver or cardiorespiratory disease or who are

Controversy

Medication Errors from Confusing Orders and New Products

JONATHAN J. WOLFE

Medication errors have emerged as a serious public health concern. Health care professionals have become acutely aware of the real harm and monetary cost associated with such errors. Increasingly, health care providers involved in errors find themselves subject to professional censure and discipline.

Patients as well as insurance companies are also interested in reducing drug errors. One manifestation of their participation has been the creation of the National Coordinating Council for Medication Error Reporting and Prevention (NCCMERP). This group includes founding members as diverse as the American Association of Retired Persons (AARP), American Medical Association (AMA), United States Pharmacopeia (USP), and Joint Commission on Accreditation of Healthcare Organizations (JCAHO). The Council uses a method that emphasizes finding problems in the medication handling system rather than assigning blame to individuals.

One illustration involves the introduction of fosphenytoin, a parenteral antiseizure agent. Numerous errors in practice have occurred because of confusion about dosage for this new product. First, phenytoin, a long-established generic product, remains widely available and is in many situations entirely adequate for patient needs. Second, fosphenytoin is dosed in terms of mg-PE. This means that rather than writing a prescription for a milligram dose of fosphenytoin, the prescriber is to order fosphenytoin dosed as equivalent to a milligram dose of phenytoin. The system has proved difficult to adopt smoothly in practice. Error reports have appeared from health care providers intending one dose but inadvertently ordering another. Additionally, pharmacists and nurses have prepared and administered incorrect doses when orders or prescriptions were not understood accurately.

Critical Thinking Questions

- What person in the health care system has the most immediate interest in accurate dose preparation and administration?
- What is your first concern when confronted with the possibility that an error has occurred?
- What sort of system can you imagine for classifying errors by severity or harm?
- What duty do you have to report errors or elements of your drug handling system that make errors more likely?
- What steps should drug marketers take when introducing drugs whose names or doses may be confused with similar products long established in practice?

obese. Safe use during pregnancy has not been established. It is a pregnancy Category D drug.

Fetal hydantoin syndrome can occur with the use of hydantoins, producing a wide variety of teratogenic effects. The teratogenic effects include numerous craniofacial abnormalities (e.g., cleft lip, cleft palate), hypoplasia of the digits, dislocated hips, congenital heart defects, microcephaly, and prenatal growth deficiencies.

Phenytoin hypersensitivity (fever, skin rash, lymphadenopathy) usually occurs within the first 3 to 8 weeks of therapy but may occur up to 12 weeks later. It can lead to renal failure, rhabdomyolysis, or hepatic necrosis. Phenytoin hypersensitivity can be fatal.

Pharmacokinetics

While ethotoin and mephenytoin are fairly rapidly absorbed from the gastrointestinal (GI) tract, phenytoin, depending on the formulation, is slow, variable, and often incomplete in its absorption (Table 22–2). Absorption after intramuscular administration is erratic. Hydantoins are stored in body tissues and may take up to 5 days to be re-

TABLE 22–2 PHARMACOKINETICS OF SELECTED ANTICONVULSANT DRUGS

Agent	Route	Onset	Peak	Duration	PB (%)	$t_{1/2}$	BioA (%)
Barbiturates							
Mephobarbital	po	20–60 min	6–12 hr	10–16 hr	40–60	34–52 hr	UA
Metharbital	po	20–60 min	6–8 hr	6–12 hr	40–60	48–52 hr	UA
Phenobarbital	po	20–60 min	6–12 hr	6–12 hr	40–60	37–140 hr	UA
	IM	10–30 min	UK	4–6 hr	40–60	Varies	UA
	SC						
	IV	5 min	15–30 min	4–10 hr	40–60	11–67 hr	100
Primidone	po	UA	3–4 hr	8–12 hr	19–25	5–15 hr; 10–18 hr*	60–80
Benzodiazepines							
Clonazepam	po	20–60 min	1–4 hr	6–12 hr	50–85	18–50 hr	80–98
Clorazepate	po	15 min–2 hr	1–2 hr	4–6 hr	85–98	30–100 hr	UA
Diazepam	po	30–60 min	0.5–2 hr	2–3 hr	96–99	20–100 min	UA
	IV	Immed.	15–30 min	20–60 min	85–99	20–100 hr	100
Lorazepam	IV	1–5 min	1–6 hr	6–8 hr	85	14–16 hr	83–100
Hydantoins							
Ethotoin	po	UA	UA	UA	UA	3–9 hr	UA
Fosphenytoin	IM/IV	Rapid	15–40 min	UA	High	8–15 min	100
Mephenytoin	po	30 min	UK	24–48 hr	60–68	95–144 hr	UA
Phenytoin	po	2–24 hr	1.5–3 hr; 4–12 hr†	6–12 hr; 12–36 hr†	87–95	6–42 hr†	10–90
	IV	1–2 hr	Rapid	UA	90	24–30 hr	20–90
Oxazolidinediones							
Trimethadione	po	UA	0.5–2 hr	UA	0	12–24 hr; 6–13 days‡	UA
Paramethadione	po	15–30 min	1–2 hr	4–6 hr	UA	1–3 hr; 24 hr‡	UA
Succinimides							
Ethosuximide	po	Hours	1–4 hr; 3–7 hr§	>24 hr	0–10	40–60 hr; 30 hr§	UA
Methsuximide	po	15–30 min	1–3 hr	4–6 hr	50	2–4 hr; 40–80 hr‖	UA
Phensuximide	po	Slow	1–4 hr	UA	UA	4–12 hr	UA
Miscellaneous Anticonvulsants							
Carbamazepine	po	2–4 days	2–4 hr	UK	75–90	25–29 hr	85
Phenacemide	po	UA	UA	5 hr	>95	UA	UA
Acetazolamide	po/ER	1–2 hr	3–6 hr	4–5 hr	90–95	2.4–5.8 hr	UA
	IV	2 min	15 min	4–5 hr	90–95	2.4–5.8 hr	100
Gabapentin	po	Rapid	2–4 hr	8 hr	0–3	5–7 hr	50–60
Lamotrigine	po	UK	1–4.8 hr	UK	55	24–30 hr	98–100

*Half-life of primidone and phenylethylmalonamide, respectively.

†The peak and duration of phenytoin are based on tablet and extended release formulations, respectively. The half-life averages 22 hours but is dose dependent. Its half-life is shorter in children.

‡Half-life of oxazolinidiones for parent drug and metabolite, respectively. Serum drug levels of trimethadione vary for the parent drug and metabolite.

§Peak effects and elimination half-life of ethosuximide for adults and children, respectively.

‖Elimination half-life and serum drug levels of methsuximide's parent drug and metabolite, respectively.

ER, Extended-release formulation; PB, protein binding; UK, unknown; UA, unavailable; $t_{1/2}$ elimination half-life; BioA, bioavailability

leased. Hydantoins, particularly phenytoin, are rapidly distributed to all tissues, with the highest concentrations occurring in the brain, liver, and salivary glands. The hydantoins cross the placenta and enter breast milk.

Biotransformation of hydantoins occurs in the liver. Mephenytoin is eliminated in the urine. Ethotoin is eliminated in the urine and feces and in small amounts in the saliva. Phenytoin is primarily eliminated in the bile, then reabsorbed from the GI tract, and eliminated in the urine. Approximately 5 percent of phenytoin is eliminated unchanged.

Drug-Drug Interactions

Hydantoins interact with a variety of drugs including rifampin, beta blockers, calcium channel blockers, tricyclic antidepressants, estrogens, antidiabetic drugs, and a host of other drugs. Table 22–3 provides an overview of the interactions.

Dosage Regimen

The dosage for hydantoins is dependent on the patient's age and size and on the purpose for use. Most of the drugs are initially dosed at one-fourth to one-half the total maintenance dosage (Table 22–4). Upward titration is done slowly based on therapeutic serum levels. An adult dosage of ethotoin less than 2 g/day is usually ineffective. Dilantin suspension must be well shaken. If this is not done, a subtherapeutic dose will be obtained from the top of the bottle and a supertherapeutic dose from the bottom of the bottle.

Fosphenytoin is a water-soluble prodrug of phenytoin (150 mg yields 100 mg of phenytoin). Dose, solution, concentration, and infusion rate are expressed in terms of phenytoin equivalents. Lower, less frequent dosing may be required in the older adult.

Laboratory Considerations

Serum hydantoin levels should be measured routinely throughout therapy. Therapeutic blood level values are derived from patients who have normal serum albumin levels and renal function. Patients with reduced serum albumin levels or renal disease are at risk for development of hydantoin toxicity.

Fosphenytoin and phenytoin may increase alkaline phosphatase, gamma-glutamyltransferase, and glucose levels. Ethotoin can increase serum glucose, urine glucose, bromosulfophthalein, and alkaline phosphatase levels. It will decrease the levels of urinary steroids, protein-bound iodine, dexamethasone/metyrapone tests, Schilling test, and thyroid function tests. Serum folate level, complete blood count, platelet count, serum calcium level, albumin level, serum creatinine level, urinalysis, and hepatic and thyroid function tests should be done periodically throughout the course of hydantoin therapy.

Succinimides

- ❐ Ethosuximide (ZARONTIN)
- ❐ Methsuximide (CELONTIN)
- ❐ Phensuximide (MILONTIN)

Indications

All succinimides are used to manage absence symptoms. Ethosuximide is the drug of choice for these seizures and for absence seizures that occur during pregnancy. Methsuximide is indicated for refractory absence seizures. Succinimides have been used for myoclonic and complex partial seizures, although less commonly.

Pharmacodynamics

The exact mechanism of action of succinimides is unknown. However, it is thought that they increase the seizure threshold and suppress paroxysmal spike-wave patterns in absence seizures. They depress nerve transmission in the motor cortex.

Adverse Effects and Contraindications

The adverse effects of succinimides are many but in general affect the CNS, GI tract, skin, and hematologic systems. Drowsiness, ataxia, and dizziness are common CNS adverse effects. GI adverse effects include tongue swelling, nausea, vomiting, diarrhea, gingivitis, and vague gastric upset. Eosinophilia, thrombocytopenia, aplastic anemia, bone marrow depression, leukopenia, agranulocytosis, monocytosis, and pancytopenia can be life-threatening. Stevens-Johnson syndrome, systemic lupus erythematosus, and renal damage are also possible.

Peripheral neuropathies are associated with phensuximide. Ethosuximide may cause vaginal bleeding. Nephropathies have occurred with the succinimides, and phensuximide causes the urine to be discolored.

Pharmacokinetics

The succinimides are readily and rapidly absorbed from the GI tract. They are distributed to the tissues and body water and cross placental membranes. Ethosuximide is excreted into breast milk. The steady state is reached in about 4 to 6 days in children and over a longer period in adults. Biotransformation occurs in the liver. Ethosuximide is eliminated slowly in the urine with 25 to 50 percent as unchanged drug. Small amounts are eliminated via the bile and feces. Methsuximide is eliminated in the urine with less than 1 percent as unchanged drug. Phensuximide is mainly eliminated in the urine as the parent compound and hydroxylated metabolites. Some of the drug is excreted in the bile.

Drug-Drug Interactions

As with all other drug groups, there are drug-drug interactions to be considered. Succinimides interact with hydantoins to increase serum hydantoin concentrations. Reduced primidone and phenobarbital levels have been noted with concurrent use of succinimides (see Table 22–3).

Dosage Regimen

The dosage regimen for succinimides is based on patient needs. Dosages are titrated upward at weekly intervals based on the patient's serum drug levels. Succinimides should be taken at regularly spaced intervals.

Laboratory Considerations

There are few drug-laboratory test interactions. Ethosuximide and methsuximide increase the results of Coombs'

Text continued on page 411

TABLE 22–3 DRUG-DRUG INTERACTIONS OF SELECTED ANTICONVULSANT DRUGS

Drug	Interactive Drugs		Interaction
Barbiturates			
Mephobarbital	Alcohol	MAO inhibitors	Increased CNS depression
Phenobarbital	CNS depressants		
Primidone	Posterior pituitary hormones		Cardiac arrhythmias
	MAO inhibitors		Prolonged effects of barbiturate
	Acetaminophen	Cyclosporine	Decreased effects of interactive drug
	Caffeine	Oral contraceptives	
	Theophylline	Phenothiazines	
	Oral anticoagulants	Levothyroxine	
	Chloramphenicol	Quinidine	
	Doxycycline	Tricyclic antidepressants	
	Griseofulvin		
	Furosemide		Additive orthostatic hypotension
Phenobarbital	Meperidine	Sedatives	Increased CNS depression
	Sedative-hypnotics		
	Calcium channel blockers		Reduced blood pressure
	Carbonic anhydrase inhibitors		Osteopenia
	Beta blockers	Corticosteroids	Decreased effects of interactive drug
	Digitoxin		
	Prednisone		Exacerbation of symptoms in asthmatics
Primidone	Methylphenidate	Nicotinamide	Increased serum levels of primidone
	Isoniazid		
	Sedative-hypnotics		Increased CNS depression
	Antihistamines		
	Adrenocorticotropic hormone		Decreased effects of interactive drug
	Neuroleptics		
Benzodiazepines			
Clonazepam	CNS depressants	Antihistamines	Increased CNS depression
Clorazepate	Alcohol		
Diazepam	Cimetidine		Increased effects of benzodiazepines
	Levodopa		Decreased effects of levodopa
	Rifampin		Reduced effects of benzodiazepines
	Isoniazid	Propranolol	Increased effects of benzodiazepines
	Ketoconazole	Disulfiram	
	Oral contraceptives	Fluoxetine	
	Metoprolol	Propoxyphene	
Clonazepam	Valproic acid		Absence status epilepticus
	Other anticonvulsants		Sedation
	Clozapine		Increased CNS depression
			Respiratory depression
Clorazepate	Antidepressants		Increased CNS depression
Diazepam	Valproic acid		Increased sedation
	Opioids		Increased sedation
			Respiratory depression
	Antidepressants		Increased CNS depression
	Clozapine		Respiratory depression
	Cisapride	Paroxetine	Increased serum levels of diazepam
	Erythromycin	Sertraline	
	Antacids		Delayed absorption of diazepam
Lorazepam	Loxapine		Increased risk of toxicity
	MAO inhibitors		
	Tricyclic antidepressants		
	Scopolamine		Increased sedation
			Irrational behavior
Hydantoins			
Ethotoin	Rifampin		Reduced effects of hydantoins; reduced effects of interactive drugs
Fosphenytoin	Theophylline		
Mephenytoin	Lidocaine		Additive cardiac depression with IV phenytoin, decreased concentration of IV lidocaine
Phenytoin	Propranolol		Additive cardiac depression with IV phenytoin
	Influenza virus vaccine		Increased, decreased, or no change in serum levels of phenytoin
	Estrogens		Increased effects of hydantoins, decreased effects of interactive drugs
	Tricyclic antidepressants		
	Oral anticoagulants		Greater anticoagulant effects initially, then reduced with chronic use
	Antidiabetic agents		Increased serum glucose concentrations
	Nifedipine	Verapamil	Changes in serum concentrations of both interactive drug and hydantoins
	Chlorpheniramine	Phenothiazines	Increased effects of hydantoins
	Acute ethanol ingestion	Ranitidine	
	Ibuprofen	Sulfonamides	
	Isoniazid	Salicylates	

TABLE 22–3 DRUG-DRUG INTERACTIONS OF SELECTED ANTICONVULSANT DRUGS *Continued*

Drug	Interactive Drugs		Interaction
Hydantoins *continued*			
	Metronidazole	Trazodone	
	Propoxyphene	Trimethoprim	
	Antacids	Calcium gluconate	Decreased effects of hydantoins
	Antineoplastics	Chronic ethanol use	
	Continuous-use enteral feeding solutions		
	Acetaminophen	Haloperidol	Decreased effects of interacting drug
	Cardiac glycosides	Nondepolarizing muscle relaxants	
	Dopamine	Methadone	
Oxazolidinediones			
Trimethadione	CNS depressants	Alcohol	Increased CNS depression
Paramethadione	Haloperidol	Phenothiazines	Decreased effects of oxazolidinedione and increased CNS depression
	Loxapine	Thioxanthines	
	MAO inhibitors	Tricyclic antidepressants	
Succinimides			
Ethosuximide	Isoniazid		Increased serum levels of succinimides
Methsuximide	Alcohol	Phenothiazines	Increased CNS depression; reduced effects of succinimides
Phensuximide	CNS depressants	Tricyclic antidepressants	
	MAO inhibitors		
	Haloperidol		Change in seizure pattern
			Reduced serum level of haloperidol
Miscellaneous Anticonvulsants			
Carbamazepine	Cimetidine	Verapamil	Increased serum levels of carbamazepine
	Influenza virus vaccine	Erythromycin	
	Nicotinamide	Fluoxetine	
	Propoxyphene	Isoniazid	
	Diltiazem		
	Antipsychotics		Decreased serum levels of carbamazepine
	Corticosteroids	Oral contraceptives	Reduced serum level of carbamazepine; decreased effectiveness of interacting drug
	Oral anticoagulants	Theophylline	Decreased level/effectiveness of interacting drug
	Acetaminophen	Quinidine	Decreased level/effectiveness of interacting drug
	Doxycycline	Thyroid hormones	
	Haloperidol		
	Lithium		Increased neurotoxicity
	MAO inhibitors		Hypertensive and hyperpyretic crisis
			Severe seizures
			Death
	Phenothiazines		Increased CNS depression; reduced anticonvulsant effects of carbamazepine
	Tricyclic antidepressants		
	Posterior pituitary hormones		Increased antidiuretic effects
	Vasopressin		
Valproic acid	Clonazepam		Development of absence status epilepticus
	CNS depressants	Alcohol	Increased CNS depression
	Chlorpromazine	Ranitidine	Increased half-life of valproic acid
	Cimetidine		
	Salicylates		Increased half-life and serum levels of valproate
			Increased anticoagulation effects
	Oral anticoagulants	Thrombolytic drugs	Increased risk of bleeding/hemorrhage
	Heparin	Platelet aggregation inhibitors	
	Haloperidol	Phenothiazines	Increased CNS depression
	MAO inhibitors	Tricyclic antidepressants	Lowers seizure threshold
Magnesium sulfate	Digitalis		Cardiac conduction defects leading to heart block
	Aminoglycosides		
	Nifedipine		Reduced blood pressure
	CNS depressants	Opioids	Increased CNS depression
	Neuromuscular antagonists		Increased neuromuscular blockade
Paraldehyde	CNS depressants	Alcohol	Increased CNS depression
	Disulfiram		Increased serum paraldehyde and acetaldehyde levels
Lamotrigine	Acetaminophen		Reduced half-life of lamotrigine
Gabapentin	Antacids		Reduced bioavailability of gabapentin
	Cimetidine		Reduced elimination of gabapentin leading to increased risk of toxicity of gabapentin
	Oral contraceptives		Increased norethindrone levels
Acetazolamide	Lithium		Reduced effect of lithium
	Cyclosporine		Nephrotoxicity/neurotoxicity
	Digitalis		Digitalis toxicity in presence of hypokalemia

CNS, Central nervous system; MAO, monoamine oxidase.

TABLE 22–4 DOSAGE REGIMEN FOR SELECTED ANTICONVULSANT DRUGS

Drug	Use(s)	Dosage	Implications
Barbiturates			
Phenobarbital	Tonic-clonic, partial and febrile seizures, status epilepticus	*Adult:* 60–250 mg po a single dose or two to three divided doses *or* 100–320 mg IV as needed initially to a total of 600 mg/day. For status epilepticus: 10–20 mg/kg IV *Child:* 1–6 mg/kg/day po as single dose or divided doses *or* 10–20 mg/kg IV initially followed by 1–6 mg/kg/day. Status epilepticus: 15–20 mg/kg	Note: Must be administered under direct medical supervision in a setting where supportive and resuscitative treatment can begin immediately. Therapeutic values: 10–40 mcg/mL. Time to steady state: 14–21 days. IV doses require 15–30 minutes to reach peak concentrations in the brain. Administer minimal dose and evaluate effectiveness before giving second dose to prevent barbiturate-induced CNS depression
Metharbital	Tonic-clonic, absence, and myoclonic seizures	*Adult:* 100 mg po TID. Maintenance: 600-800 mg po daily. Not to exceed 800 mg/day. *Child:* 5–15 mg/kg/day po.	Titrate until seizures are under control
Mephobarbital	Partial and generalized tonic-clonic and cortical focal seizures	*Adult:* 400–600 mg po BID-QID. *Child under age 5 yr:* 16–32 mg 3–4 times daily *Child over age 5 yr:* 32–64 mg 3–4 times daily	Timing of administration dependent on when patient's seizures usually occur
Primidone	Generalized tonic-clonic, complex partial seizures	*Adult and Child older than age 8 yr:* Titrate slowly to fixed schedule from 100 mg at bedtime to usual maintenance 125–250 mg 3–4 times daily. Not to exceed 2 g/day *Child younger than age 8 yr:* Titrate slowly by fixed schedule from 50 mg at bedtime to usual maintenance 125–250 mg 3 times daily *or* 10–25 mg/kg/day in divided doses. Not to exceed 1 g/day in divided doses	Time to steady state: 1–7 days. Therapeutic values: 5–12 mcg/mL. To switch from alternative anticonvulsant to primidone or when adding primidone to another regimen, increase the primidone dose gradually while decreasing or continuing other drug dosages to maintain seizure control. The switch to primidone should take at least 2 weeks
Benzodiazepines			
Diazepam	Termination of status epilepticus	*Adults:* 5–10 mg IV. May repeat dose q10–15 minutes for a total of 30 mg. May repeat regimen again in 2–4 hr. *Child over age 5 yr:* 1 mg q2–5 min IV for total of 10 mg. May repeat dose q2–4 hr. *Child under age 5 yr:* 0.2–0.5 mg/kg IV q2–5 min to maximum of 5 mg. May repeat q2–4 hr	Note: Must be administered under direct medical supervision is a setting where supportive and resuscitative treatment can begin immediately. IM route may be used if IV route unavailable. Maximum rate of administration is 5 mg/minute. Therapeutic level: 0.1–1.5 mcg/mL
Clonazepam	Absence seizures, myoclonic seizures	*Adult:* Initially daily dose not to exceed 0.5 mg po TID. May increase by 0.5–1 mg q3rd day. Maintenance: Not to exceed 20 mg daily *Child to age 10 yrs or 30 kg:* Initial daily dose 0.01–0.03 mg/kg/daily po. Not to exceed 0.05 mg/kg/day in 2–3 divided doses. Increase by no more than 0.25–0.5 mg po q3rd day until therapeutic blood levels are reached. Not to exceed 0.2 mg/kg/day	Time to steady state: 3–7 days. Do not abruptly stop drug. Therapeutic level: 20–80 mcg/mL
Clorazepate	Adjunctive treatment for simple partial seizures	*Adult:* 7.5 mg po TID. May increase by no more than 7.5 mg/day at weekly intervals. Not to exceed 90 mg daily *Child age 9–12 yr:* 3.75–7.5 mg twice daily initially. May increase by 7.5 mg/week. Not to exceed 60 mg/day	Time to steady state: 5 days to 2 weeks. Therapeutic values: 0.5–1.9 mcg/mL. Not recommended for child under 9 years old
Lorazepam	Status epilepticus	*Adults:* 4 mg IV. May repeat in 10–15 minutes	Give slowly—not to exceed 2 mg/minute. Therapeutic values: 50–240 ng/mL
Hydantoins			
Ethotoin	Tonic-clonic or complex partial seizures	*Adult:* 250 mg po QID initially. May increase over several days to 3 g/day in divided doses. Maintenance: 2–3 g/daily *Child:* 250 mg po BID. May increase to 250 mg po QID over several days. Maintenance: 500–1000 mg po daily. Maximum: 3 g/day (rare)	Adult doses less than 2 grs/day are usually ineffective. Doses should be spaced evenly and taken after eating. Therapeutic values: 15–50 mcg/mL

TABLE 22–4 DOSAGE REGIMEN FOR SELECTED ANTICONVULSANT DRUGS *Continued*

Drug	Use(s)	Dosage	Implications
Hydantoins *Continued*			
Fosphenytoin	Generalized seizures, status epilepticus; prevention/ treatment of seizures occurring during neurosurgery	*Adult:* Status epilepticus: 15–20 mg PE/kg IV loading dose infused at rate of 100–150 mg PE/minute. Nonemergent seizures: 10–20 mg PE/kg as one time loading dose IM or at less than 150 mg PE/minute. Maintenance: 4–6 mg PE/kg/day at less than 150 mg PE/minute.	Dose, concentration solution, infusion rate expressed in terms of phenytoin equivalents (PE). Therapeutic value: 10–20 mcg/mL. Not approved for children
Mephenytoin	Tonic-clonic, simple and complex partial seizures	*Adult:* 50–100 mg po daily initially. Increase by 50–100 mg at weekly intervals. Maintenance: 200–600 mg po daily in 3 divided doses. Maximum: 800 mg daily *Child:* Titrate slowly from 50–100 mg daily to 3–15 mg/kg/day po in 3 divided doses. Maintenance: 100–400 mg daily	For patients refractory to less toxic anticonvulsants. Therapeutic values: 25–40 mcg/mL parent drug plus metabolite
Phenytoin	Tonic-clonic, simple and complex partial seizures	*Adult:* 1 g or 20 mg/kg loading dose as extended release capsules in 3–4 divided doses at 2 hour intervals or as 400 mg, then 300 mg q2hr for two doses. Maintenance: 300–400 mg daily *Older adult:* 3 mg/kg/day po in divided doses *Child:* 5 mg/kg/day po in two to three divided doses. Maintenance: 4–8 mg/kg/day in two to three divided doses. Maximum: 300 mg/day	Note: Loading dose must be administered in a setting where serum phenytoin levels can be rapidly monitored. Loading doses should be avoided in patients with hepatic or renal disease. Maintenance doses are usually started 24 hours later. Limit IM injections to one/week. Therapeutic values: 10–20 mcg/mL. Maintenance doses for patients unable to use oral route may be utilized for up to one week. Adjust dosage upward for IM then decrease when returning to oral route
	Termination of status epilepticus	*Adult:* 15–20 mg/kg IV. Rate not to exceed 25–50 mg/minute followed by 100 mg q6–8 hr. *Child:* 15–20 mg/kg at 1–3 mg/kg/minute	Note: Must be administered under direct medical supervision in a setting where supportive and resuscitative treatment can begin immediately. Administer by slow IV push using undiluted solution or dilute 50 mg/ml in 50–100 mL normal saline. Should not be infused in any glucose-containing solutions. IM route not recommended due to crystallization at injection site causing delayed and erratic absorption
Succinimides			
Ethosuximide	Absence seizures; myoclonic and complex partial seizures (rare)	*Adult and Child older than age 6 yr:* 250 mg po BID. Increase by 250 mg as needed every 4–7 days up to 1.5 g/day in two divided doses *Child age 3–6 years:* Titrate up from 250 mg daily in two divided doses to effect (up to 20 mg/kg/day in divided doses). Do not exceed 1 g/day	Administer with food to decrease GI effects. Time to steady state: 4–10 days. Therapeutic levels: 40–100 mcg/mL. Do not abruptly discontinue
Methsuximide	Absence seizures	*Adult:* 50–100 mg po daily initially. Increase by 50–100 mg at weekly intervals. Maintenance: 200–600 mg/day in divided doses. Maximum: 800 mg/day *Child:* 3–15 mg/kg/day po in three divided doses. Maintenance: 100–400 mg/day in three divided doses	Therapeutic levels: 0.04–0.08 mcg/mL for parent drug and 10–40 mcg/mL for the metabolite. Take with food. Do not abruptly discontinue
Phensuximide	Absence seizures	*Adult and Child:* 500 mg po two to three times daily. Increase dosage by weekly intervals as necessary. Maintenance: 1.5 g/day po in divided doses. Maximum: 3 g/day	Take with food. Do not discontinue abruptly. Therapeutic values: 10–20 mcg/mL
Oxazolidinediones			
Paramethadione	Absence seizures	*Adults:* Titrate from 300 mg po TID. Increase by 300 mg daily at weekly intervals. Not to exceed 600 mg po four times daily *Child over age 6 yr:* 300–900 mg/day in divided doses three to four times daily	Give with milk or juice to cover taste/ smell and to decrease GI symptoms. Wear dark glasses if photosensitivity occurs. Avoid driving and other activities that require alertness until effects of drug are known. Therapeutic values of trimethadione: 12 mcg/mL/l mg/kg of daily dose
Trimethadione	Absence seizures	*Adults:* 300 mg po TID. May increase by 300 mg/day at weekly intervals. Not to exceed 600 mg po QID	

Table continued on following page

TABLE 22–4 DOSAGE REGIMEN FOR SELECTED ANTICONVULSANT DRUGS *Continued*

Drug	Use(s)	Dosage	Implications
Trimethadione *(continued)*		*Child:* 20–50 mg/kg/day in divided doses every 6–8 hr. May increase by 150–300 mg/daily at weekly intervals	
Miscellaneous Anticonvulsants			
Valproic acid	Tonic-clonic, myoclonic, absence, and complex partial seizures	*Adult and Child:* Multidrug therapy: 15 mg/kg/day po. Monotherapy: 5–15 mg/kg/day po. Increase by 5–10 mg/kg/day po at weekly intervals. Maintenance: 30–60 mg/kg/day po in two to three divided doses *Child over 20 kg:* Dose must be individualized	Time to steady state: 2–7 days. Therapeutic value: 50–100 mcg/mL. Divide doses if daily dose is greater than 250 mg
Acetazolamide	Tonic-clonic and refractory absence seizures	*Adult:* Multidrug therapy: 250 mg/day po. Monotherapy: 4–30 mg/kg/day po in 1–4 divided doses or 250–500 mg IM/IV. May repeat in 2–4 hr. (Range: 375–1000 mg/day po) Maximum: 1 g/day *Child:* 4–30 mg/kg/day in one to four divided doses. Not to exceed 1 g/day	The sustained release preparation is not appropriate for use as an anticonvulsant. If parenteral route needed, administer only by direct IV
Carbamazepine	Tonic-clonic, complex partial, and mixed seizures	*Adult:* 200 mg po BID (tablets) *or* 100 mg po QID (suspension) initially. Increase by 200 mg/day q7days until therapeutic levels are reached. Not to exceed 1.2 g/day *Child age 6–12 yr:* 100 mg po (tablets BID *or* 50 mg po QID (suspension). Increase dose by 100 mg/day at weekly intervals until therapeutic levels reached. Not to exceed 1 g/day *Child under age 6:* Not established. Must be individualized	Therapeutic values: 4–12 mcg/mL. Extended-release formulations given once to twice daily. Also available as tablets, chewable tablets, suspension. Dosage not to exceed 1 g/day in 12–15 year olds
Gabapentin	Adjunct therapy for partial seizures in adults with or without secondary generalized seizure activity	*Adult and Child over 12 yr:* 300 mg po at bedtime on first day, 300 mg po BID on second day, 300 mg po TID on third day. Maintenance: 900–1800 mg/day in three divided doses	Rapid titration may be continued until desired effects are obtained. Doses should not be more than 12 hours apart. Therapeutic values: 2–3 mcg/mL
Lamotrigine	Adjunct therapy for partial, tonic-clonic, and absence seizures in adults; Lennox-Gastaut syndrome	*Adult and Child over age 16 yrs on multidrug therapy with carbamazepine, phenobarbital, phenytoin, or primidone:* 50 mg/day as a single dose for first 2 weeks, then 50 mg twice daily for next 2 weeks, then increase by 100 mg/day on a weekly basis to maintenance dose of 300–500 mg/day in two divided doses. *Child 2–16 years:* 2 mg/kg/day BID for 2 weeks, then 5 mg/kg/day po BID for 2 weeks, then 10 mg/kg/day po BID for 2 weeks *Adult and Child over age 16 years on multidrug therapy with carbamazepine, phenobarbital, phenytoin, or primidone and valproic acid:* 25 mg every other day for first 2 weeks, then 25 mg/day for next 2 weeks, then increase by 25–50 mg/day every 1–2 weeks to maintenance of 100–150 mg/day in two divided doses	Do not double doses. Do not abruptly discontinue. Discontinue gradually over a period of 2 weeks unless safety concerns require a more rapid withdrawal. Caution patient to wear sunscreen to prevent photosensitivity reactions. Concurrent use with valproic acid results in a twofold increase in lamotrigine levels and a decrease in valproic acid levels. Therapeutic levels: 1–4 mcg/mL

CNS, central nervous system; GI, gastrointestinal; IM, intramuscular.

test. All patients taking succinimides should have a complete blood count with differential and liver enzyme testing on a regular basis throughout therapy.

Barbiturates

❒ Mephobarbital (MEBARAL)
❒ Metharbital (GEMONIL)
❒ Phenobarbital (LUMINAL, SOLFOTON)

Indications

While barbiturates all possess anticonvulsant effects, the long-acting barbiturates (phenobarbital, mephobarbital, and metharbital) are the only ones used to provide oral anticonvulsant action in subhypnotic doses. They were discussed in relation to their sedative-hypnotic effects in Chapter 17. Mephobarbital is used for partial and generalized tonic-clonic seizures. It is often used as a replacement drug for phenobarbital when there is paradoxical excitement in children or ongoing sedation or behavior changes in adults. It can be used as a monotherapeutic drug or with other anticonvulsant drugs.

Metharbital is used in the management of tonic-clonic, absence, and myoclonic seizures. It is usually used as a replacement drug for phenobarbital in patients with tonic-clonic seizures.

Phenobarbital is used in the prevention and treatment of tonic-clonic, simple, and complex partial seizures. It is also used for fever-induced seizures and status epilepticus. Its long-term use for febrile seizures is controversial, and it is ineffective for absence seizures.

Pharmacodynamics

Barbiturates are thought to potentiate the inhibitory action of gamma-aminobutyric acid. By depressing impulse transmission from the thalamus to the cortex, barbiturates reduce the excitability of neurons and raise the seizure threshold.

Adverse Effects and Contraindications

The barbiturates produce CNS depression. The most common adverse effects include drowsiness, dizziness, lethargy, and behavioral changes. GI adverse effects include constipation. Rashes and urticaria have been noted. Angioedema and serum sickness are the most life-threatening adverse effects. Adverse effects of mephobarbital include all of those just mentioned plus agranulocytosis, thrombocytopenia, and megaloblastic anemia (with long-term therapy). Respiratory depression, apnea, laryngospasm, and bronchospasm have been noted with mephobarbital use. Erythema multiforme and coma may occur with phenobarbital use. (Coma may be an intentionally induced effect in treating status epilepticus.)

Phenobarbital is contraindicated in patients with porphyria or hypersensitivity to this drug or to primidone. Phenobarbital and primidone must be used with caution in patients with nephritis or pulmonary insufficiency. Patients with respiratory depression or obstruction, asthma, congestive heart failure, severe anemia, hepatic dysfunction, hypoadrenalism, hypothyroidism, or depression or those experiencing acute or chronic pain must use phenobarbital with caution. Impaired memory occurs in some children taking phenobarbital.

A hydantoin-like syndrome has occurred when phenobarbital is administered during pregnancy. The newborn may present with withdrawal symptoms as well.

Pharmacokinetics

Barbiturates are absorbed from the GI tract in varying degrees (approximately 50 percent for mephobarbital to 90 percent for phenobarbital) in 20 to 60 minutes (see Table 22–2). Distribution of barbiturates occurs throughout all tissues and fluids, particularly the brain, cerebrospinal fluid, liver, and kidneys. The barbiturates all readily cross the placenta and can be found in breast milk. Biotransformation occurs slowly, chiefly in the liver, with elimination occurring predominantly in the urine. Mephobarbital and metharbital are eliminated almost entirely as metabolites. Phenobarbital is eliminated 25 to 50 percent unchanged in the urine.

Drug-Drug Interactions

Drug-drug interactions with barbiturates are many. Table 22–3 provides an overview of the interactions. Barbiturates interact with other CNS depressant drugs to increase the CNS depression. The effects of certain drugs, such as acetaminophen, oral anticoagulants, some antibiotics, tricyclic antidepressants, oral contraceptives, and xanthines, are reduced. Orthostatic hypotension can occur with concurrent use of furosemide.

Dosage Regimen

The dosage regimen for barbiturates is individualized (see Table 22–4). IV doses of phenobarbital require 15 to 30 minutes to reach peak concentrations in the brain. Administer a minimal dose and evaluate effectiveness before giving a second dose to prevent barbiturate-induced CNS depression. The timing of mephobarbital administration is dependent on when the patient's seizures usually occur.

Laboratory Considerations

Patients on prolonged phenobarbital therapy should have hepatic and renal function and complete blood count periodically monitored. Serum folate concentrations should be monitored periodically during therapy because these drugs increase folate requirements. Phenobarbital may cause decreased serum bilirubin concentrations in neonates, in patients with congenital nonhemolytic unconjugated hyperbilirubinemia, and in patients with epilepsy. Serum phenobarbital levels should be monitored. Therapeutic levels of phenobarbital range from 10 to 40 mcg/ml.

Benzodiazepines

- ❒ Clonazepam (KLONOPIN); (🍁) PMS-CLONAZEPAM, RIVOTRIL
- ❒ Clorazepate (GEN-XENE, TRANXENE); (🍁) APO-CLORAZEPATE, NOVO-CLOPATE
- ❒ Diazepam (VALIUM)
- ❒ Lorazepam (ATIVAN)

Benzodiazepines are discussed in Chapter 17 for their use as antianxiety sedative-hypnotic drugs. They are also used in the management of epilepsy. Clonazepam and clorazepate have been approved for the treatment of absence and myoclonic seizures. Clorazepate is used concurrently with other anticonvulsant drugs for the treatment of partial simple seizures. Diazepam and lorazepam are currently used for the treatment of status epilepticus.

Benzodiazepines act at many levels to depress the CNS. Their effects are most likely related to potentiation of gamma-aminobutyric acid activity. They have anticonvulsant properties owing to enhanced presynaptic inhibition. Receptor sites include the spinal cord, hypothalamus, hippocampus, substantia nigra, cerebellar cortex, and cerebral cortex.

Sedation, restlessness, aggression, irritability, hallucinations, and agitation may occur with clonazepam and diazepam. Dysuria may also be noted. Extrapyramidal effects and dystonias have been noted. Impaired memory may be seen with oral benzodiazepines.

Benzodiazepines should be used cautiously in patients with chronic respiratory conditions and in children, older adults, and those patients who are in a debilitated state. They should also be used with caution in anyone who has a tendency toward physical or psychological dependency. Clonazepam and clorazepate must be used with care in patients who have acute angle-closure glaucoma. Benzodiazepines are contraindicated in patients with hypersensitivity to clonazepam and other benzodiazepines and in patients with severe liver disease, or with optic nerve or retinal disease.

The benzodiazepines are rapidly and well absorbed from the GI tract. Little is known about the distribution of oral benzodiazepines. They are thought to cross the blood-brain barrier, and they are known to cross the placenta. Benzodiazepines are eliminated extensively into breast milk. Biotransformation occurs in the liver and elimination via the kidneys, with less than 1 percent eliminated as unchanged drug.

Diazepam is slowly and erratically absorbed when administered intramuscularly. IV effects of diazepam are very rapid. Because distribution to the brain occurs seconds after IV injection, immediate anticonvulsant effects are obtained. Redistribution to tissues occurs fairly rapidly, causing the central effects of IV benzodiazepines to quickly diminish. The dosages for these drugs are listed in Table 22–4.

Valproates

- ❐ Divalproex sodium (DEPAKENE, DEPAKOTE)
- ❐ Valproic acid

Valproates are used in the treatment of complex partial and absence seizures. Although not approved by the Food and Drug Administration for such use, divalproex and valproic acid have been used in the treatment of partial seizures with complex symptomatology, myoclonic seizures, and tonic-clonic seizures. Valproates are discussed in Chapter 18 for their use as mood-stabilizing drugs. Valproates increase the level of gamma-aminobutyric acid, an inhibitory neurotransmitter in the CNS.

Valproic acid has been most commonly associated with indigestion, nausea, and vomiting. Hepatotoxicity and pancreatitis are the most serious adverse effects. Other adverse effects include anxiety, irritability, and confusion. Anorexia, increased appetite, diarrhea, and constipation have been noted in some patients. Prolonged bleeding times, anemia, and thrombocytopenia can occur. Valproates should be used with caution in patients with bleeding disorders, hypoalbuminemia or a history of liver or renal disease, and organic brain disease. Safe use during pregnancy and lactation has not been established. They are contraindicated in patients with hypersensitivity and hepatic impairment. Some formulations of valproates contain tartrazine and should be avoided in patients with known hypersensitivity.

Valproic acid is rapidly and well absorbed from the GI tract. The divalproex sodium formulation is enteric coated so absorption is delayed by 1 to 4 hours (see Table 22–2). Food may significantly slow the rate but not the extent of absorption. It is rapidly distributed to plasma and extracellular fluids, crossing the blood-brain barrier, placental membranes, and breast milk. Peak serum concentrations are reached 1 to 4 hours after using the capsule and syrup. Delayed-release capsules reach peak serum concentrations in 3 to 4 hours. Valproic acid is highly protein bound at 90 to 95 percent at serum concentrations of 50 mcg/ml. With serum concentrations of 50 to 100 mcg/ml, the percentage of protein binding is 80 to 85 percent. Furthermore, the free fraction becomes larger, increasing the concentration gradient to the brain. It is primarily biotransformed in the liver, with minimal amounts eliminated unchanged in the urine. Therapeutic valproate values are 50 to 100 mcg/ml. Table 22–4 identifies drug dosages for patients using the drug for seizure activity.

Dose-related elevations in lactate dehydrogenase and aminotransferase may occur with valproic acid. It may also interfere with the accuracy of thyroid function tests and produce false-positive results in urine ketone tests. Occasionally, liver function tests, including serum bilirubin, may show increases. Serum calcium levels may be decreased. Complete blood count, platelet count, and bleeding time should be monitored prior to and throughout therapy. These drugs may cause leukopenia and thrombocytopenia. Liver function tests and serum ammonia concentrations should also be monitored for evidence of hepatotoxicity.

Miscellaneous Anticonvulsants

- ❐ Acetazolamide (DIAMOX); (🍁) CETAZOLAM, APO-ACETAZOLAMIDE, NOVO-ZOLAMIDE
- ❐ Carbamazepine (EPITOL, TEGRETOL); (🍁) APO-CARBAMAZEPINE, MAZEPINE, NOVO-CARBAMAZ, PMS-CARBAMAZEPINE
- ❐ Gabapentin (NEURONTIN)
- ❐ Lamotrigine (LAMICTAL)
- ❐ Trimethadione (TRIDIONE)
- ❐ Paraldehyde
- ❐ Primidone (MYSOLINE); (🍁) APO-PRIMIDONE, MYSOLINE, SERTAN
- ❐ Paramethadione

ACETAZOLAMIDE

Acetazolamide, a carbonic anhydrase inhibitor (Chapter 39), is used as an adjunct in managing tonic-clonic and refractory absence seizures. Its usefulness is limited, however, owing to the rapid development of tolerance to its action. It is thought that by inhibiting carbonic anhydrase, thus lowering the serum pH, excessive neuronal discharge and seizure activity are reduced.

Only a few adverse effects have been associated with carbonic anhydrase inhibitors. The most notable is the loss of potassium leading to hypokalemia. In large doses, acetazolamide produces weakness, paresthesias, and metabolic acidosis. Hypersensitivity reactions are rare. When they do occur they manifest as fever, rash, bone marrow suppression, or sulfonamide-like renal lesions. Some patients experience dysuria and GI symptoms such as nausea, vomiting, anorexia, and constipation. In the glaucoma patient, as intraocular pressure is reduced, transient myopia may be noticed.

Patients with pre-existing fluid and electrolyte imbalances such as hyponatremia, hyperkalemia, and hyperchloremic acidosis should not receive carbonic anhydrase inhibitors because they worsen these conditions. Furthermore, carbonic anhydrase inhibitors are contraindicated in patients with severe pulmonary obstruction. A recurrence of calculi may occur in patients with a history of calcium-containing renal stones. Calculus formation is due to decreases in urinary citrate. In addition, teratogenic changes have been demonstrated in animals; therefore, these drugs should not be used during pregnancy. They are Food and Drug Administration pregnancy Category C.

Acetazolamide is well absorbed orally and with IV administration. It is distributed to body tissues, crosses the blood-brain barrier, and is found in the kidneys and erythrocytes. The onset time of acetazolamide is 1 to 2 hours with the tablet and extended-release formulations, respectively (see Table 22–2). IV onset is within 2 minutes. Acetazolamide crosses the placenta and is eliminated into breast milk. From 70 to 100 percent of the unchanged drug is eliminated within 24 hours by the kidneys.

Acetazolamide interacts with lithium to decrease lithium effects. Concurrent use with digitalis may cause a toxicity to the cardiac glycoside. Nephrotoxicity and neurotoxicity have been noted in the presence of cyclosporine.

The dosage of acetazolamide varies depending on whether it is being used as monotherapy or as an adjunct with other anticonvulsants. In general, the sustained-release formulation is not appropriate for use as an anticonvulsant.

Serum electrolytes, complete blood count, and platelet counts should be monitored periodically throughout therapy. Acetazolamide may decrease potassium, bicarbonate, and white and red blood cell counts. It may cause increased serum chloride levels. False-positive results for urine protein and 17-hydroxycorticosteroid values have been noted. Blood ammonia, bilirubin, uric acid, urobilinogen, and calcium levels can be increased.

CARBAMAZEPINE

Carbamazepine is one of the drugs of choice in the management of tonic-clonic seizures. It is also used to manage complex partial and mixed seizures. It is ineffective for absence and myoclonic seizures in adults. Carbamazepine decreases synaptic transmission in the CNS by affecting sodium and calcium channels in neurons.

Restlessness, aggression, irritability, and agitation may occur with carbamazepine. When children take carbamazepine they may demonstrate an inability to attend to tasks. Carbamazepine causes many renal effects, including renal failure, glycosuria, and urinary frequency and water retention (due to stimulation of antidiuretic hormone). Depression may occur in patients on carbamazepine. Mood disturbances can be seen in children on carbamazepine. Dystonias may be seen with carbamazepine, particularly when it is combined with phenytoin. The CNS adverse effects include syncope, dizziness, confusion, ataxia, and, most serious, encephalopathy. Additional visual effects include photosensitivity, nystagmus, and visual changes.

Serious conditions associated with carbamazepine include aplastic anemia, agranulocytosis, systemic lupus erythematosus, thrombophlebitis, arrhythmias, cardiac conduction disturbances, and heart failure. Carbamazepine is contraindicated in patients with hypersensitivity, bone marrow depression, blood dyscrasias, and atrioventricular heart block. It can be used cautiously with patients who are recovering alcoholics and in those with behavioral problems, cardiac disease, metabolic disorders, renal and hepatic impairments, diabetes, or increased intraocular pressure.

Carbamazepine is slowly and erratically absorbed after oral administration. Absorption is rapid on a full stomach. Distribution to tissues is wide and very quickly found in the brain, cerebrospinal fluid, bile, and saliva. Carbamazepine crosses placental membranes and can be found in the fetus, with accumulations in the liver and kidneys. The drug can be found in breast milk. Biotransformation occurs in the liver, and elimination occurs with approximately 72 percent in the urine and 28 percent in the feces (see Table 22–2).

Carbamazepine interacts with numerous drugs that will increase the serum levels of carbamazepine. In the presence of a significant number of drugs, the serum levels of carbamazepine will be reduced.

GABAPENTIN

Gabapentin is used as an adjunct therapy for adults with partial seizures, with or without generalization. It is ineffective for absence seizures. Its mechanism of action is unknown. It appears to affect the transport of amino acids across neuronal membranes.

The most common adverse effects are somnolence and ataxia, although weakness, malaise, vertigo, depression, and anxiety have occurred. Nystagmus, abnormal vision, hypertension or hypotension, dyskinesias, respiratory symptoms, hematuria, urinary frequency, pruritus, angioedema, eczema, anorexia, flatulence, gingivitis, and muscle pain are possible. Gabapentin is to be used with caution in patients with renal insufficiency and in the elderly, in whom sedation is a concern. Safe use during pregnancy (Category C) and lactation has not been established. The drug is contraindicated with hypersensitivity.

Approximately 50 to 60 percent of gabapentin is absorbed after oral administration. The drug crosses the blood-brain barrier and is readily distributed into the cerebrospinal fluid. The drug is not appreciably biotransformed and is eliminated almost entirely unchanged via the kidneys (76 to 81 percent) with the remainder in the feces.

Drug-drug interactions with gabapentin are few. Antacids may decrease the absorption of gabapentin.

The dosage of gabapentin is titrated over 3 days from 300 mg once daily to 300 mg three times daily. Rapid titration may be continued until the desired effects are obtained. Doses should not be more than 12 hours apart.

Gabapentin therapy may cause anemia, thrombocytopenia, leukopenia, and an increase in bleeding time. Thus, laboratory monitoring of the complete blood count, differential, and platelets is warranted prior to and throughout therapy. Gabapentin may cause a false-positive reading when the Ames N-Multistix SG dipstick test for urinary protein is used. The sulfosalicylic acid precipitation procedure should be used instead.

LAMOTRIGINE

Lamotrigine is used as adjunct treatment of partial, tonic-clonic, and absence seizures in adults. Although not yet approved by the Food and Drug Administration for use in patients under 16 years of age, it has been cited as useful in Lennox-Gastaut syndrome. Lennox-Gastaut syndrome is a complex form of epilepsy marked by early childhood onset, poorly controlled multiple seizure types, slow-spike electroencephalographic (EEG) waves, and a high incidence of mental retardation. Lamotrigine appears to act by stabilizing neuronal membranes via inhibition of sodium channels.

The most common adverse effects of lamotrigine include ataxia, dizziness, headache, somnolence, nausea, vomiting, rash, arthralgias, and photosensitivity. Lamotrigine has also elicited allergic reactions, infections, hematuria, and complaints of dyspnea, pharyngitis, cough, and rhinitis. Anxiety and depression may occur in those taking lamotrigine. Lamotrigine should be used with caution in patients with renal impairment or cardiac disease.

Lamotrigine is rapidly and completely absorbed after oral administration and distributed to the tissues and saliva. Its time to onset and duration of action are unknown. Biotransformation occurs in the liver and kidneys. The majority is eliminated in the urine with a small amount in the feces.

Lamotrigine, when used concurrently with carbamazepine, may result in decreased levels of lamotrigine and increased levels of an active metabolite of carbamazepine. Lamotrigine levels are decreased in the presence of phenobarbital, phenytoin, or primidone. Concurrent use with valproic acid raises lamotrigine levels and decreases valproic acid levels.

The dosage of lamotrigine is based on its polypharmaceutical relationship with other anticonvulsants. The dosage is different when the drug is taken concurrently with carbamazepine, phenobarbital, phenytoin, or primidone from when it is taken with the same drugs *and* valproic acid (see Table 22–4).

Oxazolidinediones

- ❒ Paramethadione
- ❒ Trimethadione (TRIDIONE)

OXAZOLIDINEDIONES

The oxazolidinediones, trimethadione and paramethadione, are used today only for absence seizures refractory to succinimides. The mechanisms of action of oxazolidinediones are not well understood. The seizure threshold in the basal ganglia and the cortex is raised with a reduction in the synaptic response to repetitive low-frequency stimulation.

The adverse effects of trimethadione include drowsiness, nausea, and vomiting, although other CNS and GI effects have been noted. The most severe CNS effects include encephalopathy and coma. Exfoliative dermatitis, thrombocytopenia, leukopenia, neutropenia, aplastic anemia, bone marrow depression, and systemic lupus erythematosus have been noted. Oxazolidinediones have caused nephrosis and proteinuria. Hiccups have been observed. Hepatic dysfunction and dyskinesia have been observed with paramethadione.

Oxazolidinediones are contraindicated in patients with hypersensitivity, hematologic disturbances, and hepatic or renal disease. They should be used with caution in patients with optic nerve or retinal disease, intermittent porphyria, and myasthenia gravis. Trimethadione (Pregnancy Category D) is thought by many to be the riskiest for the fetus of all anticonvulsants.

Paramethadione and trimethadione are rapidly absorbed from the GI tract. They are freely and uniformly distributed throughout the tissues and body water. They cross the placental barrier, but it is unknown whether they are excreted into breast milk. Biotransformation by demethylation occurs in the liver, with slow elimination by the kidneys, almost entirely as the metabolite, dimethadione.

PARALDEHYDE

Paraldehyde is used rarely in the treatment of status epilepticus and seizures occurring with tetanus or alcohol withdrawal refractory to other anticonvulsants. Paraldehyde's mechanism of action is unknown; however, it is likely related to its CNS depressant effects. Paraldehyde was discussed in Chapter 17 for its antianxiety effects.

PRIMIDONE

Primidone is a prophylactic drug used for partial seizures. It is a management drug for tonic-clonic and simple partial seizures and is believed by many to be the drug of choice for complex partial seizures. Primidone is used as monotherapy or as polytherapy (usually with phenytoin or carbamazepine). It decreases neuronal excitability and increases the seizure threshold in the motor cortex.

The most common adverse effects of primidone are drowsiness, ataxia, vertigo, lethargy, and anorexia. Systemic lupus erythematosus, blood dyscrasias, megaloblastic anemia, and hypersensitivity reactions are possible. Phenobarbital toxicity may increase when it is used with primidone, causing additive sedation. Primidone must be used with caution in patients with renal impairments, hepatic dysfunction and pulmonary insufficiency. It is contraindicated in patients with porphyria.

The bioavailability of primidone is 60 to 80 percent when absorbed from the GI tract. It is widely distributed, crossing placental membranes and entering breast milk. Primidone's time to onset is 4 to 7 days, with peak activity noted in 7 to 10 days. Its duration of action is 8 to 12 hours. It is converted to phenobarbital and another active metabolite (phenylethylmalonamide) by the liver. Fifteen to forty percent of primidone is eliminated unchanged in the urine. The half-life is 3 to 24 hours.

Newer Anticonvulsant Drugs

Other anticonvulsant drugs now in different stages of clinical trials are eterobarb, a long-acting barbiturate; topiramate; stiripentol; tiagabine (for treating simple and complex partial and tonic-clonic seizures); and vigabatrin, an alternative treatment for partial seizures.

Critical Thinking Process

Assessment

History of Present Illness

Because alterations in consciousness often accompany seizures, information about patient activities before, during, and after the seizure may be obtained from family or friends. If the patient remembers the events before, during, or after a seizure, obtain the data from the patient. Establish a trend in the patient's behavior before the seizure as well as during and after. Ask about the course and duration of the seizure activity. Where in the body did the seizures begin? Do the seizures travel through the body? Does the muscle tone seem tense or limp? Were color changes noted in the face or lips, or was there a loss of consciousness? Did the patient experience an aura before the seizure? Were there precipitating events? After the seizure, does the patient sleep or have any confusion, weakness, headache, or muscle ache? How have the seizures affected the patient's life?

Past Health History

The patient's past health history provides information about allergies, injuries, previous illnesses, and hospitalizations. Knowledge of prenatal, birth, and developmental history, family history, and history of previous trauma is necessary. Conditions to be noted include syncope, either cardiac, vasovagal, or reflex in adults; vertigo and periodic syndromes in children (including childhood migraine headaches), hyperventilation or breath-holding, staring spells, and daydreaming; and narcolepsy or sleep apnea and pseudo-seizures. A drug history is important to obtain because there are many drugs that interact with anticonvulsants.

Physical Exam

Seizures are classified by clinical symptoms and electrophysiologic data. The clinical symptoms observed during the seizure and those functional deficits found upon physical exam such as weakness, sensory and thought process disturbances, and reflex alteration are essential to the classification of seizures.

The physical exam is important in determining neurologic deficits that may contribute to seizure activity. Signs of localized brain abnormality may be detected and may include weakness, sensory disturbance, and reflex alteration, as well as altered thought processes or memory. A thorough neurologic exam is necessary to help distinguish between types of seizures. The exam should include evaluation of cranial nerves, muscle strength, cerebellar function, sensory system, deep tendon reflexes, and level of consciousness.

Diagnostic Testing

The diagnosis of a seizure disorder is based on data collected from careful patient observation, comprehensive health history, and clinical exam. Other diagnostic tests that may reveal neurologic abnormalities and structural lesions include EEG, routine skull radiographs, magnetic resonance imaging, and computed tomography scans. The EEG, computed tomography, and magnetic resonance imaging are of value in localizing the pathologic processes associated with epilepsy. In some forms of epilepsy, there are EEG patterns during and between seizure attacks.

Developmental Considerations

Perinatal There are many factors that must be considered in the treatment of epilepsy in women. This is particularly true for women of childbearing age, when epilepsy may be influenced by hormones, contraception, fertility, pregnancy, and sexuality. Hormones can affect the seizure threshold and seizure by altering the excitability of the neurons. Fertility may be adversely affected, as well as the effectiveness of oral contraceptives.

Although most women receiving anticonvulsants deliver normal children, approximately two to three times the number of birth defects occur in pregnancies during which the mother (and sometimes the father) takes anticonvulsant drugs. The risk to women, particularly in pregnancy, requires careful planning, monitoring, and special interventions to safeguard both the mother and infant.

Pediatric Epilepsy in infancy, childhood, and adolescence is complex to diagnose and treat because of the cause, ages, and need for family involvement. The majority of children with epilepsy can lead normal, active lives. However, for some, their seizure disorder can be disabling and can lead to social, emotional, and academic problems. When this occurs, children need additional resources from family, school, and community.

Seizures in newborns do not conform to the international classification of epileptic seizures. Seizures in newborns are caused by identifiable metabolic or infectious conditions. They may also be associated with perinatal complications such as electrolyte disorders, cerebral infarction, meningitis, septicemia, brain malfunctions, or hypoxic-ischemic disease.

The epilepsies in infancy range from benign to severe, with those beginning during the first year of life having the poorest prognosis. Infants may also have seizures due to transient causes, have normal clinical and EEG findings, and do not develop epilepsy.

The outcome of neonatal seizures is dependent on the cause. Generalized seizures are more common than partial seizures in young children. However, children over 10 years of age who develop epilepsy usually have partial seizures.

The most common epileptic syndromes in infants and young children are febrile seizures and encephalopathic epilepsy. There is some controversy about categorizing febrile seizures as a form of epilepsy. Febrile convulsions occur in 3 to 4 percent of all children and are usually benign. The convulsions occur between the ages of 6 months and 6 years in children whose temperature is elevated from any cause other than a CNS insult. Brain damage is almost never a consequence, but can occur when febrile convulsions are prolonged. Febrile seizures do not cause epilepsy, but are recognized as a common antecedent.

Encephalopathic epilepsies in infants and young children are associated with a cerebral disorder and mental retardation. They are referred to as West's syndrome (infantile spasms) and Lennox-Gastaut syndrome (myoclonic-astatic epilepsy of early childhood). The most common epilepsies affecting older children and adolescents are partial seizures. However, they may experience generalized epilepsies with absence seizures. Benign partial epilepsies account for more than one-third of all cases of epilepsy that begin in childhood.

Geriatric The treatment of seizure disorders in older adults is very complex. They may have diseases and conditions that increase their vulnerability to seizures. They are susceptible to organ failure, metabolic disturbance, infection, CNS lesions, falls, trauma, alcohol withdrawal, and the adverse effects of polypharmacy. Epilepsy in the older adult is sometimes complicated by other problems related to aging. Management with anticonvulsant drugs takes special assessment, intervention, and evaluation skills, as well as an understanding of the health needs of the older adult.

Psychosocial Considerations

There are numerous psychosocial considerations related to epilepsy. Of major concern are the negative attitudes and stigma associated with the disorder. The fear of having a seizure affects patients' life-styles and may affect social, academic, and/or vocational career. For parents, family, or friends, seeing their loved one have a seizure is a frightening experience. Feelings of guilt, anger, isolation, and frustration are not uncommon. Of greatest consequence is the sense of loss and grief associated with the vulnerability of having a potentially life-long disability. Epilepsy can influence a patient's self-esteem and self-confidence, and as a result, decisions regarding education, driving a car, participating in sports, and childrearing may be affected. Most states require that the patient be seizure free in order to obtain a driver's license (see Case Study—Epilepsy).

TABLE 22–5 TREATMENT OPTIONS FOR SEIZURES

Type of Seizure	First-Line Drugs	Alternative Drugs
Partial Seizures (Focal Seizures)		
Simple partial seizures	Carbamazepine	Gabapentin (adjunct)
Complex partial seizures	Phenytoin	Lamotrigine (adjunct)
	Valproic acid	Phenobarbital
		Primidone
		Valproic acid
Generalized Seizures (Convulsive and Nonconvulsive Types)		
Absence seizures	Ethosuximide	Clonazepam
	Valproic acid	Lamotrigine
Atonic seizures	Valproic acid	Clonazepam
Myoclonic seizures		Felbamate (adjunct)
Status epilepticus	Diazepam	Lorazepam
	Phenytoin	Lidocaine
	Phenobarbital	
Tonic-clonic seizures	Carbamazepine	Phenobarbital
	Phenytoin	Primidone
	Valproic acid	

Analysis and Management

Treatment Objectives

The treatment objectives for epilepsy are to prevent, or at least reduce to the greatest extent possible, the number and/or severity of seizures, while assisting the individual to maintain the highest level of independent functioning achievable.

Although anticonvulsant drugs may control seizures, they do not cure the underlying disorder. In cases where epilepsy is found not to be the cause of seizures, the condition that lowers the seizure threshold and/or precipitates a seizure (e.g., hypoglycemia, electrolyte imbalances, fever, exposure to toxins, and drug overdoses or withdrawal) must be controlled in addition to treating the seizures themselves. It is important to diagnose the etiology of seizures as early as possible because this may influence the choice of drug and duration of therapy.

Treatment Options

The treatment choice of anticonvulsant drug(s) is dependent on a variety of factors:

- Type or pattern of seizures
- Age of the patient
- Family history
- Response to any previously used anticonvulsant drug and any untoward or adverse effects of the drug
- Accurate diagnosis of seizure type—partial, generalized, or unclassified epileptic seizures

Pharmacologic options include a selection of drugs from the classification of anticonvulsant drugs: barbiturates, benzodiazepines, hydantoins, succinimides, and other miscellaneous anticonvulsants. Treatment options for the main types of seizures are summarized in Table 22–5. The treatment option chosen should be based on the importance of controlling the seizures using the fewest number of anticonvulsant drugs possible, with minimal adverse effects. Drug therapy for epilepsy reduces the risk of trauma arising from seizures (e.g., headbanging, falling, and prolonged periods of anoxia with status epilepticus and/or aspiration and its complications). Surgical intervention is an increasingly available option for those who have seizures that are not effectively managed with drugs.

It is usually not necessary to begin therapy for the first seizure unless computed tomography or magnetic resonance imaging scan detects a lesion or an epileptic focus is seen on the EEG. Therapy should be started when there is a history of recurrent seizures (more than one) that cannot be explained by drug or alcohol use, cardiac arrhythmias, metabolic disorders, or other cause.

For approximately 5 percent of people with epilepsy, surgery may be an approach to control the disease. Criteria for surgical intervention include failure of previous medical approaches with anticonvulsants and localization of the focus of abnormal discharge being surgically accessible. Surgery is most beneficial for people whose seizures originate from clearly delineated, unilateral, anterior temporal lobe foci.

Drug Variables

Approximately 80 percent of all patients with epilepsy experience control of their disease or show a significant reduction in the severity of the seizures with appropriate anticonvulsant therapy. The efficacies of the various drugs vary according to the age at onset, type, and severity of the disease and the serum anticonvulsant level.

Unfortunately, all anticonvulsant drugs may cause a variety of toxic effects. Because of this, seizures are ideally controlled with the use of a single drug. Only when a monotherapeutic regimen fails is polytherapy attempted. This often occurs when a patient simultaneously experiences two or more types of seizures.

Generalized Seizures Valproic acid is effective and better tolerated than phenytoin or carbamazepine for the treatment of generalized seizures. Phenytoin and carbamazepine have been associated with a greater incidence of CNS adverse effects than the valproates. Valproic acid is also useful if the patient has a generalized tonic-clonic and absence seizures because valproic acid works on both types of seizures.

Case Study Epilepsy

Patient History

History of Present Illness	PS is a 29-year-old woman who underwent emergency surgery, during which she showed marked and sudden changes in neurologic functioning and experienced seizures. She was found to have a basal ganglion hematoma with infarct.
Past Health History	PS has no significant health history and no past history of seizures. She has a 2-month-old infant. Her pregnancy and delivery were uncomplicated. PS found the past 2 months physically and emotionally stressful.
Physical Exam Findings	PS experienced generalized seizures of the tonic-clonic type. Through the physical exam, signs of localized brain abnormalities can be detected. A comprehensive neurologic examination was conducted.
Diagnostic Testing	EEG: altered electrophysiologic activity of the brain and abnormal waveforms
Developmental Considerations	PS has special concerns that are associated with childbearing and childrearing.
Psychosocial Considerations	The fear of seizures may affect PS's confidence and self-image. This could raise questions about intimacy, sexual activity, and parenting. A plan for child care may necessitate additional support and safety measures. Breastfeeding is not appropriate with anticonvulsant drugs because the drugs enter breast milk.
Economic Factors	The cost of anticonvulsant medication, additional support for child care, and physical therapy will be necessary.

Variables Influencing Decision

Treatment Objective	• Provide maximum control of seizures with minimal adverse effects.

Drug Variables	*Drug Summary*	*Patient Variables*
Indications	Prevention of seizures typically associated with epilepsy	PS has experienced seizures resulting from a basal ganglion hematoma with infarct.
Pharmacodynamics	Phenobarbital potentiates inhibitory action of gamma-aminobutyric acid, depressing impulse transmission from the thalamus to the cortex, reducing excitability of neurons and raising the seizure threshold. Phenytoin acts on the motor cortex, limiting detonation of the cortical areas adjacent to the seizure foci. The drug modifies sodium and calcium transportation.	The two agents, one a barbiturate and the other a hydantoin, have different pharmacodynamics but are used in tonic-clonic seizure types. This may influence the selection of anticonvulsant for PS.
Adverse Effects/ Contraindications	Phenobarbital: drowsiness, dizziness, lethargy, nausea, vomiting, rash, and behavioral changes, such as excitability and irritability. Phenytoin: nystagmus, blurred or double vision, gingival hyperplasia, ataxia, skin rash, folate deficiency. Considered the least-sedating anticonvulsant.	PS must be advised on both the adverse effects and the achievement of activities of daily living, including child care. Both drugs are classified as pregnancy Category D agents. Genetic counseling and neurologic consultation may be considered.

Case Study continued on following page

Drug Variables	*Drug Summary*	*Patient Variables*
Pharmacokinetics	Phenobarbital provides oral anticonvulsant action in subhypnotic doses. Up to 90% of the drug is absorbed from the GI tract in 20–60 min. Peak: 6–12 hr. Duration: 6–12 hr. Steady-state blood level: 14–21 days. Phenytoin: absorbed slowly and often incompletely from the stomach and small intestine. Highest concentrations are found in the brain, liver, and salivary glands. Peak: 1.5–3 hr (prompt release), 4–12 hr (extended release). Duration: 6–12 hr (prompt release); 12–36 hr (extended release). Steady-state blood level: 7–21 days.	The onset, peak, and duration of each anticonvulsant's action vary from one drug to another and from one patient to another. The peak action of phenytoin is less than that of phenobarbital; the duration is approximately the same, while the steady-state blood level can be achieved earlier with phenytoin.
Dosage Regimen	Initial dosages for both medications are similar. Phenytoin can be given in a loading dose, and the time to steady state is approximately half that for phenobarbital. Phenobarbital has the longest half-life of all the standard anticonvulsant drugs.	PS desires a simple dosing regimen to enhance her compliance.
Lab Considerations	Blood studies should include complete blood count, liver function tests, renal function tests, serum total cholesterol, high-density lipoprotein cholesterol, triglycerides, and calcium and folate levels. Urinalysis should be obtained. Ongoing serum drug level monitoring is essential.	Monitoring of PS's lab tests is essential to carefully screen for signs and symptoms related to serious blood dyscrasias, hepatoxicity, or renal damage.
Cost Index*	Phenobarbital: 1 Phenytoin: 1	Treatment may be extensive, so cost may be a factor in the selection of the drug of choice.

Summary of Decision Points

- Type of seizure and treatment of generalized seizures; tonic-clonic type differs from others.
- Concerns associated with childbearing and childrearing years.
- Potential adverse effects associated with the treatment of epilepsy.
- Half-life influences compliance and tolerance of adverse effects.

DRUG TO BE USED

- Phenytoin 20 mg/kg loading dose to be followed by 300 mg daily. Titration based on response.

*Cost Index:

1 = $<30/mo.
2 = $30–40/mo.
3 = $40–50/mo.
4 = $50–60/mo.
5 = $>60/mo.

AWP of 100, 100-mg tablets of phenobarbital is approximately $7.
AWP of 100, 100-mg capsules of phenytoin is approximately $7.

Many health care providers prefer carbamazepine over phenytoin as initial therapy. Fewer adverse effects, easier dose titration, and fewer cosmetic adverse effects have been documented with carbamazepine over phenytoin. On the other hand, carbamazepine is more expensive than phenytoin and must be dosed twice daily compared with once-daily dosing for phenytoin.

Phenytoin is the drug of choice if an IV route is required. Phenytoin causes more cosmetic effects than carbamazepine (e.g., hirsutism, coarsening of facial features, and gingival hypertrophy). Phenytoin may also cause a greater incidence of cognitive effects than carbamazepine. Ethotoin is not as effective as, but is less toxic than, phenytoin.

Phenobarbital should be used only if valproic acid, phenytoin, and carbamazepine have been ineffective. Maximum drug effects may not be seen for up to 30 minutes after administration. The drug should be given time to work before a second dose is administered to avoid overdose. Although an efficacious agent, phenobarbital has a greater potential for causing sedation and behavioral disturbances than other agents.

Absence Seizures Ethosuximide is as effective as valproic acid in the management of absence seizures. It is preferred because of the risk of serious hepatotoxicity and pancreatitis with valproic acid, although the risk of hepatotoxicity with valproic acid is much lower for adults than for children. Valproic acid can be used if there is a contraindication to the use of ethosuximide or if the drug is ineffective. Many patients can be successfully managed with ethosuximide, although GI distress appears to be dose related and most patients better tolerate a twice daily regimen.

Methsuximide is as effective as ethosuximide but slightly more toxic; thus, it is used to treat absence seizures refractory to other anticonvulsants. Because it is not as likely to exacerbate tonic-clonic seizures, it is the best succinimide to give concurrently with other anticonvulsant drugs used for mixed seizures. Phensuximide is the least toxic of the succinimides but slightly less effective in its treatment of absence seizures.

Clonazepam is an effective alternative for absence seizures in patients who do not tolerate or respond to first-line drugs. Clonazepam is a second-line drug because of its CNS and behavioral adverse effects.

Myoclonic Seizures Valproic acid is the drug of choice for myoclonic seizures. It is also the most effective agent for juvenile myoclonic epilepsy. Patients with juvenile myoclonic epilepsy generally require lower doses than adults. Clonazepam has also been used for myoclonic seizures with success.

Partial Seizures Carbamazepine and phenytoin are equally efficacious, and the decision to choose one of these drugs is similar to that in generalized seizures. Carbamazepine has fewer adverse effects and an easier dosing regimen. Valproic acid is not as effective as carbamazepine and phenytoin, although it is an alternative for patients who do not respond to or cannot tolerate these two drugs. Phenobarbital should also be used if the other drugs are ineffective.

Status Epilepticus Lorazepam, a benzodiazepine, is the first drug of choice of many health care providers, although diazepam is as effective and less expensive. Lorazepam distributes out of the CNS slowly and has a longer duration of action than diazepam (even with its shorter half-life). When given IV, diazepam causes more irritation than does lorazepam, and it is absorbed erratically when administered as an intramuscular injection. Diazepam continues to be effective for 1 to 2 days after stopping drug therapy owing to its long duration of action.

Fosphenytoin or phenytoin should be started as soon as possible after the initial dose of a benzodiazepine. Once the patient's history is determined, phenytoin may not be needed. However, it is best to give the patient phenytoin initially and then decide in 12 to 24 hours whether the patient requires maintenance therapy with this drug. Phenobarbital can be used if the patient is still seizing 1 hour after the loading dose of phenytoin.

Patient Variables

No drug used to prevent or treat seizure disorders is without adverse effects. For this reason, there is a high rate of noncompliance with anticonvulsant drugs. Toxic effects of the anticonvulsant drugs appear to be influenced by many factors, including dosage and duration of therapy, age of the patient, concurrent use of other anticonvulsant drugs, and other diseases.

Caution must be taken to ensure drug compliance, monitoring of blood levels necessary to ensure a steady level of drug in the blood stream, and prevention of complications such as status epilepticus. Special consideration is necessary in the treatment of children and the older adult. When drug therapy is used during pregnancy, the mother and the fetus must be monitored very closely.

When anticonvulsants must be used during pregnancy, monotherapy is preferable. Monitoring of blood levels with as-needed dosage adjustments and stabilization is mandatory. For absence seizures, ethosuximide is the drug of choice. Carbamazepine, although linked with some malformations (such as spina bifida, retarded growth, and congenital heart defects) and thought by some not to be recommended for use in pregnancy, is considered one of the safest drugs for seizures during pregnancy.

All patients with the potential for alcohol withdrawal syndrome should receive prophylactic anticonvulsant therapy to reduce the signs and symptoms of withdrawal and to prevent further withdrawal seizures. All alcohol withdrawal seizures should be treated because they can become life-threatening events.

If seizures are frequent enough, the frequency of seizures should be used as a guide to determine when to increase the dosage or change drug therapy. If seizures are infrequent, therapy is usually continued until steady-state drug levels within the therapeutic range are achieved.

Intervention

Administration

Drug treatment typically begins with one anticonvulsant drug, with the dosage increased gradually until seizures are controlled, clinical manifestations of toxicity are experienced, or serum drug levels reach the high end of the therapeutic range without controlling the seizures. In most cases, seizures can be controlled by a single drug. In cases where this is not true, other anticonvulsant drugs should be tried—each alone—before polytherapy. Combining drugs does not appear to be as effective as monotherapy, because drug-drug interaction decreases effectiveness.

Arriving at an appropriate dosage of the anticonvulsant drugs will involve trial and error, because drug absorption and elimination vary widely from one patient to another. In determining what dosage is appropriate, therapy is started at low levels (often one-fourth to one-third of the recommended therapeutic dosage) of a single drug and slowly increased or decreased to achieve the desired effect. Optimally, a balance between the best seizure control and the least toxic/adverse effects is the objective of anticonvulsant therapy. Most minor adverse effects diminish after a few weeks; however, if CNS depression or other intolerable toxic effects persist, doses will need to be reduced or another drug substituted.

Anticonvulsant drugs should be taken regularly as prescribed, at the same time of the day, and with meals to decrease the risk of GI upset. Oral suspensions and extended-release drugs are available. Anticonvulsant drugs administered parenterally should be given with caution. In some cases, cardiac monitoring is required for patients receiving IV anticonvulsant drugs.

For patients on enteral feedings, 2 hours should elapse between the feeding and phenytoin administration. If the drug is given via a nasogastric tube, the tube should be flushed with 2 to 4 ounces of water before and after administration. The chewable phenytoin tablets and phenytoin sodium capsules are not bioequivalent. They should not be used interchangeably. Furthermore, capsules labeled "extended" may be used for once-daily dosing. Those labeled "prompt" may result in toxic serum concentrations if they are used for once-daily dosing. However, abrupt discontinuation of hydantoins after long-term use may precipitate seizure activity.

Education

Development of a drug plan that either prevents or arrests the seizures usually requires weeks of drug trial, error, and adjustment. During this time the patient must be compliant. Observation of the effects of the drug and documentation of any seizure activity are essential. Anticonvulsant drugs require time to take effect and to attain an acceptable level in the blood. Once the seizure disorder is controlled with anticonvulsant drugs, major risk factors are noncompliance, lack of medical supervision, and discontinuation of the drug. These actions can increase the incidence of status epilepticus.

No drug used to treat epilepsy is without adverse effects, and a high rate of noncompliance associated with anticonvulsant drugs can occur. Patients taking anticonvulsant drugs over an extended period of time need to know the adverse effects of the drug, including neurologic symptoms, gastrointestinal disturbances, visual disturbances, blood dyscrasias, and hepatic and renal impairment. Reinforcement of the risk/benefit ratio is essential to ensure that the patient understands and accepts the importance of compliance with the treatment plan.

Patients also need to be aware of how epilepsy can impact their daily lives and to take several precautionary steps when on drug therapy. These steps include knowledge of:

- Epilepsy and how it affects their lives and the lives of family members and friends
- Care required during a seizure and keeping a journal of all seizure activity
- Adequate diet, fluid intake, sleep, and moderate recreation and exercise
- Contraindication of alcoholic beverages and other substances
- Wearing a Medic-Alert bracelet and identification with pertinent information
- Legal protection under the law regarding employment
- The availability of resources such as the Epilepsy Foundation of America

The duration of treatment with anticonvulsants is influenced by several considerations, including the probability of the patient's remaining seizure free without drugs, the adverse consequences of recurrent seizures, and the adverse effects of long-term anticonvulsant drug therapy. In some cases the patient with epilepsy can have therapy discontinued. There are a number of factors to consider in this regard. It is recommended that the patient be seizure free for at least 4 years. The decision to discontinue drug therapy should be made with careful consideration of the patient's desire and motivation, along with the likelihood of success and the risks associated with the recurrence of a seizure (including also the possible loss of driver's license). Patients should be advised not to drive during the withdrawal period and for 3 to 4 months thereafter. This restriction makes it difficult for some patients to try withdrawal.

Before withdrawal from therapy, patients should be taught that about 33 percent (a low risk) will experience relapse. If a seizure occurs, the patient and health care provider will know that the drug is still necessary. Recurrence of seizures usually occurs within the first 6 months. Patients at low risk for recurrence include those with primary epilepsy, seizure onset between the ages of 2 and 35 years, and a normal EEG. The longer the patient remains seizure free, the less likely seizures are to recur.

Patients at high risk can have a 50 percent chance of recurrence. High-risk patients include those who have partial complex seizures and seizures with an identifiable lesion. Patients with a history of frequent seizures or status epilepticus, multiple seizure types, persistently abnormal EEG, and the development of altered cognition are poor candidates for drug withdrawal.

The patient should be taught that drugs will be withdrawn one at a time, withdrawing the least effective or most toxic agent first. The dosage should be decreased slowly over 3 to 6 months until the drug is completely withdrawn. Allow time for a new steady state to be reached before continuing with dosage reductions. If the patient remains seizure free for 1 month, the second drug can be discontinued in the same manner, and so on. If seizures recur, therapy will be restarted using the last drug that was withdrawn.

Evaluation

The goal of successful treatment with anticonvulsant drugs is to prevent or at least reduce to the greatest extent possible the number and/or severity of seizures. Accurate diagnosis of the seizure type, drug administration and compliance, and helping the patient deal with any adverse side effects of the drug are essential to achieving this goal. The influence of epilepsy on the patient's life-style and well-being is an important component in the care and support of the patient and his or her family and is essential for treatment success.

SUMMARY

- Epilepsy is a recurrent, paroxysmal neurologic disorder characterized by seizures that occur when the brain is subjected to abnormal, excessive discharges by localized and/or generalized neurons.
- More than 2 million people in the United States are currently affected by epilepsy. Seventy-five percent of people have their first seizure before the age of 20 years.
- Seizures classified as primary are of unknown origin. Seizures classified as secondary have a diagnosed cause.
- The pathogenesis of seizures varies greatly across the life cycle.
- Status epilepticus is a medical emergency that occurs when a patient has seizures in rapid succession or continuous seizures lasting at least 30 minutes.
- The diagnosis of epilepsy is made on the basis of clinical data, historical information, and observation.
- Complete physical exam including a detailed neurologic exam and skull radiography is essential.
- EEG, computed tomography, and magnetic resonance imaging provide important information regarding the electrophysiologic activity of the brain.
- The treatment objective is to prevent or at least reduce to the greatest extent possible the number and/or severity of seizures, while assisting the patient in maintaining the highest level of individual functioning achievable.
- An effort to eliminate factor(s) that may cause or precipitate seizures should be made.
- Effectiveness of therapy can be demonstrated by absence of seizures and improved quality of life.

BIBLIOGRAPHY

Abramowicz, M. (1994). Gabapentin: A new anticonvulsant. *Medical Letter on Drugs and Therapeutics,* 36(921), 39–40.

Abramowicz, M. (1995). Drugs for epilepsy. *Medical Letter on Drugs and Therapeutics,* 37(947), 37–40.

Aldredge, B., Knutsen, A., and Ferriero, D. (1994). Antiepileptic drug hypersensitivity syndrome: In vitro and clinical observations. *Pediatric Neurology,* 10, 169–171.

Anderson, G., and Ritland, S. (1995). Life threatening intoxication with sodium valproate. *Clinical Toxicology,* 33, 279–284.

Barratt, E. S. (1993). The use of anticonvulsants in aggression and violence. *Psychopharmacology Bulletin,* 29(1), 75–81.

Bourgeois, B. F. D. (1995). Antiepileptic drugs in pediatric practice. *Epilepsia,* 36(Suppl. 2), S34–S45.

Brodie, M. (1990). Established anticonvulsants and treatment of refractory epilepsy. *Lancet,* 336, 350–354.

Committee on Drugs. (1994). The transfer of drugs and other chemicals into human milk. *Pediatrics,* 93(1), 137–150.

Dilorioc, H. (1995). Self-management in persons with epilepsy. *Journal of Neuroscience Nursing,* 27(6), 338–343.

Donaldson, J. (1990). The pregnant epileptic fetal risks from anticonvulsant therapy. *Journal of the American Medical Association,* 264, 1044.

Dupuis, R., and Massari, J. (1991). Anticonvulsants: Pharmacotherapeutic issues in the critically ill patient. *AACN Clinical Issues,* 2(4), 641–656.

Ellenhorn, M., Schonwald, S., Ordog, G., et al. (1997). *Ellenhorn's medical toxicology: Diagnosis and treatment of human poisoning* (2nd ed.). Baltimore: Williams & Wilkins.

French, J. (1994). The long-term therapeutic management of epilepsy. *Annals of Internal Medicine,* 120, 411–422.

Gilman, A., Rall, T., Nies, A., et al. (1990). *Goodman and Gilman's the pharmacological basis of therapeutics* (8th ed.). New York: Pergamon Press, Inc.

Goa, K., Ross, S., and Chrisp, P. (1993). Lamotrigine: A review of its pharmacological properties and clinical efficacy in epilepsy. *Drugs,* 46, 152–176.

Goldfrank, L., Flomenbaum, N., and Lewen, N. (1994). *Goldfrank's toxicologic emergencies* (5th ed.). Norwalk, CT: Appleton and Lange.

Haddad, L., Shannon, M., and Winchester, J. (1998). *Clinical management of poisoning and drug overdose* (3rd ed.). Philadelphia: W.B. Saunders.s

Keltner, N., and Folks, D. (1993). *Psychotropic drugs.* St. Louis: Mosby–Year Book.

Lacy, C., Armstrong, L., Ingrim, N., et al. (1996). *Drug information handbook: 1996–1997* (4th ed.). Cleveland: Lexi-Comp, Inc.

Laxer, K. (1994). Treating epilepsy. *Western Journal of Medicine,* 161, 309–319.

Long, J., and Rybacki, J. (1995). *The essential guide to prescription drugs.* New York: Harper Perennial.

Margolis, S. (ed.). (1993). *The Johns Hopkins handbook of drugs.* New York: Rebus.

McEvoy, G. (ed.) (1994). *AHFS drug information 94.* Bethesda: American Society of Hospital Pharmacists.

Meadow, R. (1991). Anticonvulsants in pregnancy. *Archives of Disease in Childhood,* 66:62–65.

Olin, B. (ed.). (1996). *Drug facts and comparisons* (5th ed.). St. Louis: A. Wolters Kluwer Co.

Polaski, A., and Tatro, S. (1996). *Luckmann's core principles and practice of medical-surgical nursing.* Philadelphia: W. B. Saunders Co.

Recommendations of the Epilepsy Foundation of America's Working Group on Status Epilepticus. (1993). Treatment of convulsive status epilepticus. *Journal of the American Medical Association,* 270:854–859.

Santilli, N. (1996). *Managing seizure disorders: A handbook for health care professionals.* Philadelphia: Lippincott-Raven Publishers.

Takemoto, C., Hodding, J., and Kraus, D. (1996). *Pediatric dosage handbook 1996–1997* (3rd ed.). Cleveland: Lexi-Comp, Inc.

Vestermark, V., and Vestermark, S. (1991). Teratogenic effect of carbamazepine. *Archives of Disease in Childhood,* 66(5), 641.

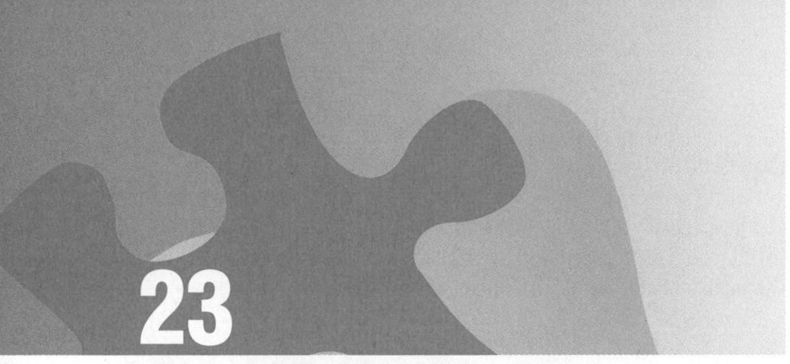

23

Antiparkinsonian and Myasthenia Gravis Drugs

Neurons are the basic structural and functional units of the nervous system. They respond to physical and chemical stimuli, conduct impulses, and release specific chemical regulators called neurotransmitters. All neurons use neurotransmitters to contact other cells and neurons. Neurons are classified according to structure or function. Motor impulses originate in the central nervous system (CNS) and are conducted via motor, or efferent, neurons to a muscle or gland. Sensory impulses originate in sensory receptors and are conducted by sensory, or afferent, neurons to the CNS. When a nerve is stimulated, neurotransmitters are released at the axon. The release of acetylcholine (ACh) at the neuromuscular junction causes muscle cell contraction. The neurotransmitters move into the synapse, where some are decomposed by cholinesterase. Neurotransmitters cross the synapse to occupy specific receptors on the next neuron or cell.

Parkinson's disease is characterized by extensive deterioration of neurons within the basal ganglia of the brain. These neurons are normally needed to synthesize the neurotransmitter dopamine. Myasthenia gravis, a degenerative neuromuscular disorder, involves a defect in ACh-generated transmission of impulses from nerve to muscle cells at the neuromuscular junction.

PARKINSON'S DISEASE

Epidemiology and Etiology

Parkinson's disease, also known as paralysis agitans, is a clinical syndrome characterized by tremor, weakness of resting muscles, bradykinesia (slowness of movement), and postural disorders. Parkinson's disease plagues people of all races and occurs throughout the world. In the United States, the prevalence ranges from 100 to 150 cases per 100,000 individuals. The annual incidence is 20 per 100,000 but increases with age. The onset of this degenerative neurologic disease generally occurs between the ages of 50 and 70 years. An onset prior to 40 years is very uncommon. The lifetime risk of developing Parkinson's disease is estimated to be 1 to 2 percent. The rate of progression is variable.

Parkinson's disease may be classified as primary or secondary. Primary Parkinson's disease results from deterioration of neurons in the basal ganglia of the substantia nigra, but its etiology is unknown. It does not show a familial pattern. Epidemiologic data suggest vascular, viral, and metabolic factors as possible causes. Much research has also been directed at the possibility of environmental toxins.

Secondary parkinsonism is caused by disorders such as infection, tumor, trauma, and drug intoxication. Drug-induced Parkinson's disease is the most common secondary type and is often reversible. Table 23–1 provides an overview of drugs associated with secondary parkinsonism. Acute parkinsonism has developed in a few drug abusers exposed to the synthetic narcotic "designer drug" *N*-methyl-4-phenyl-1,2,3,6-tetrahydropyridine (MPTP). Poisoning with manganese, carbon monoxide, mercury, methanol, or cyanide produces clinical abnormalities similar to those of Parkinson's disease. Parkinson symptoms have been seen in patients recovering from attempted suicide by drug overdose, during which there is a presumed hypoxic/ischemic injury from respiratory depression and hypotension. In addition, repeated head trauma may result in Parkinson symptoms. Some boxers have developed pugilistic Parkinson's disease.

Pathophysiology

Symptoms of Parkinson's disease result from widespread destruction of that portion of the substantia nigra that sends dopamine-secreting nerve fibers to the caudate nucleus and putamen (Fig. 23–1). Dopamine normally inhibits the excitatory signals produced by ACh. Depletion of dopamine, and thus an excess of cholinergic activity, in the basal ganglia is associated with tremor, rigidity, and akinesia. Symptoms appear when dopaminergic activity is reduced to 20 percent of normal. Studies of the effects of MPTP suggest that the enzyme monoamine oxidase B (MAOB) and free radicals in the form of superoxide or peroxide may be involved in the pathogenesis of neuronal destruction and dopamine depletion. MAOB, found in the brain, regulates the concentration of dopamine by causing the breakdown of dopamine. Monoamine oxidase A (MAOA), found in the gut, regulates the entry into the body of the naturally occurring precursors of dopamine and norepinephrine that are present in the diet.

Tremor is usually the first symptom to appear. It is an asymmetric, regular, rhythmic tremor. The *resting tremor* of eight to ten cycles per second disappears with voluntary movement and reappears when the limb is at rest. The tremor produces a pronation-supination motion of the forearm. With voluntary movement, the tremor is temporarily blocked, because other motor control signals arriving in the thalamus override the abnormal signals from the basal ganglia. A parkinsonian tremor is quite different from the tremor seen with cerebellar disease, for the former occurs during all waking hours. Although it is most prominent in the hands, the tremor may also involve the tongue, jaw, eyelids, and feet.

A movement of the thumb against the fingers is also seen. This *pill-rolling tremor* occurs at four to six cycles per second and may begin asymmetrically in an upper extremity. It becomes bilateral as the disease progresses.

Rigidity, a state of involuntary contraction of all skeletal muscles, seems to take over as the disease worsens, impeding active and passive movement. It is present during the entire arc of movement of a joint. *Cogwheel rigidity* is a jerky, ratcheting movement demonstrated on passive motion, usually at the wrist or elbow.

TABLE 23–1 DRUGS KNOWN TO CAUSE SECONDARY PARKINSONISM

Antiemetics	Metoclopramide (REGLAN) Procloperazine (COMPAZINE) Trimethobenzamide (TIGAN)
Antihypertensives	Methyldopa (ALDOMET) Diazoxide (HYPERSTAT) Reserpine (RESERPINE)
Antipsychotics	Droperidol (INAPSINE) Fluphenazine (PROLIXIN, PERMITIL) Haloperidol (HALDOL) Lithium (ESKALITH, LITHANE); (🍁) DURALITH, LITHIZINE Perphenazine (TRILAFON) Trifluoperazine (STELAZINE) Thiothixine (NAVANE)

Bradykinesia, one of the cardinal symptoms of Parkinson's disease, is probably the most crippling of all symptoms. It is a general slowness characterized by difficulty initiating movement and an inability to perform rapid repetitive movements. The severity of bradykinesia may fluctuate markedly throughout the day.

Hypokinesia is an abnormally diminished motor response to a stimulus. It is seen in patients with Parkinson's disease when they sit or lie down for long periods without an accompanying shift in weight. There is a decreased tendency to cross the legs when sitting, to gesture with the hands when talking, or to swing the arms when walking.

The combination of rigidity and bradykinesia results in a number of characteristic signs. *Masked facies* (loss of facial expression), decreased frequency of blinking, fixed flexion of the trunk, neck, and extremities, a slow and hesitant gait, and postural instability are seen. *Micrographia* (handwriting that gets progressively smaller), dysarthria, dysphagia, and general poverty of movement also are noted. Other common clinical features of the disease are constipation, depression, intellectual impairment, orthostatic hypotension, bladder instability, eczema, and peripheral neuropathy.

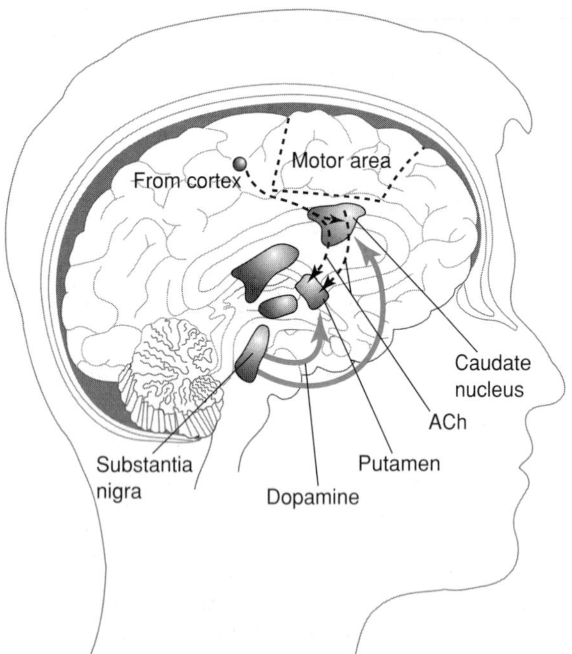

Figure 23–1 Neural pathways secrete dopamine and acetylcholine (ACh) in the basal ganglia, which constitute the motor axis of the central nervous system.

PHARMACOTHERAPEUTIC OPTIONS

Because there is no universal antiparkinsonian drug, no single drug will alleviate all symptoms and disabilities of Parkinson's disease. Most drugs either enhance dopaminergic transmission or impede cholinergic transmission. Unfortunately, precise delivery of the right dose and drug to counteract the disease is not always possible. Often, drugs are given by trial and error until the drug that is most effective with the fewest adverse effects is found.

Dopaminergic Drugs

- ❐ Carbidopa/levodopa (SINEMET)
- ❐ Levodopa (L-dopa) (DOPAR, LARODOPA)

Indications

Dopaminergic drugs are the mainstay of drug treatment for Parkinson's disease and are more effective than other drugs currently available. Levodopa and carbidopa/levodopa combination drugs are the treatment of choice for moderate and severe cases of Parkinson's disease.

The therapeutic effect of the levodopa drugs is the relief of tremor and rigidity. These agents are also recommended for the management of idiopathic, postencephalitic, and symptomatic parkinsonism associated with cerebral arteriosclerosis.

Pharmacodynamics

Levodopa is a precursor of dopamine. Dopamine in itself is unable to cross the blood-brain barrier. Levodopa, however, crosses the blood-brain barrier and is converted to dopamine. It is believed that dopamine restores the normal balance between inhibition and excitation in the caudate nucleus and putamen. Carbidopa is a decarboxylase inhibitor that allows a greater concentration of levodopa to reach the brain and decreases its peripheral adverse effects.

Adverse Effects and Contraindications

The most common adverse effects of dopaminergic drugs are involuntary movements such as *dystonia* and nausea and vomiting, with or without abdominal pain. The majority of patients on long-term therapy develop abnormal involuntary movements. A dry mouth, dysphagia, ataxia, increased hand tremors, numbness, weakness, and faintness have been noted. Agitation and anxiety have occurred in some individuals. Cardiac arrhythmias can develop in patients who have pre-existing rhythm disturbances. The adverse effects of dopaminergic drugs are reversible and can generally be controlled by a reduction in dosage.

When carbidopa is combined with levodopa, adverse effects occur more rapidly than when levodopa is used alone. Dyskinesias may require dosage reduction.

Patient taking levodopa often exhibit the *"on-off" phenomenon.* Patient response suddenly wanes after an improvement in clinical status, and the loss of therapeutic effect manifests as an abrupt onset of akinesia. The phenomenon is most often associated with long-term treatment. It usually occurs after 2 to 3 years of treatment and increases in frequency after 5 years. The phenomenon affects 90 percent of patients treated for 10 or more years with dopaminergics.

Contraindications to the use of the dopaminergic drugs include hypersensitivity, narrow-angle glaucoma, blood dyscrasias, hypertension, coronary sclerosis, and concurrent use of monoamine oxidase (MAO) inhibitors. Levodopa should be avoided in patients with malignant melanoma, because the drug may activate this form of skin cancer. Cautious use is warranted in patients with a history of cardiac disease (e.g., myocardial infarctions, arrhythmias), of psychiatric disorders (e.g., psychosis, neurosis, convulsions), or of ulcer disease, in patients with renal, hepatic, or endocrine diseases, and in patients with bronchial asthma or emphysema who are taking sympathomimetic drugs.

Safe use of dopaminergics during pregnancy and lactation and in children less than 12 years of age has not been established. Dopaminergics may be used during pregnancy only if the benefits outweigh the risks. Geriatric patients have a reduced tolerance to the drug and may require a lower dose.

Pharmacokinetics

Levodopa is well absorbed when taken orally, achieving peak serum levels within 30 to 120 minutes (Table 23–2). Absorption occurs in the duodenum and the proximal area of the small bowel. Peak plasma levels are reached in 30 minutes to 2 hours but may be delayed in the presence of food. The rate of absorption depends on the rate of gastric emptying, gastric pH, and the length of time the drug is exposed to degradative enzymes. Bioavailability is reduced by 20 to 30 percent with the controlled-release form of levodopa; thus, more drug must be given to produce a satisfactory clinical response. Levodopa does enter breast milk.

The liver and the periphery biotransform approximately 95 percent of levodopa. The plasma half-life ranges from 1 to 4 hours. The short half-life requires the patient to take multiple daily doses of levodopa to maintain even intermittently effective plasma levels. The drug is eliminated primarily in the urine.

Use of the combination carbidopa/levodopa reduces the amount of levodopa required by approximately 70 percent. The combination of drugs increases plasma levels and the plasma half-life of levodopa.

Drug-Drug Interactions

Table 23–3 illustrates the drug-drug interactions of the dopaminergic drugs. Levodopa interacts with several other drugs. When antacids and metoclopramide are given concurrently with levodopa, bioavailability is increased. Phenytoin and methionine both reduce the effectiveness of levodopa, whereas pyridoxine reverses the effect of levodopa. Hypertension is seen when MAO inhibitors or tricyclic antidepressants are taken concurrently with levodopa.

Dosage Regimen

Individual needs and responses to therapy vary widely. The optimal daily dosage of levodopa is determined by careful titration. Initially, levodopa is administered at 500 to 1000 mg daily, divided into two or more doses (Table 23–4). The dose is gradually increased as tolerated every 3 to 7 days in increments not to exceed 750 mg/day. The dosage should not exceed 8 g/day except in unusual circumstances. Therapeutic response may not be noted for 6 months.

The combination carbidopa/levodopa drugs are used quite frequently. SINEMET-10/100 has a 1:10 ratio of carbidopa to levodopa. About 75 mg of carbidopa is needed to achieve full peripheral decarboxylation, and thus concentrate the levodopa in the brain.

The usual oral dose of carbidopa/levodopa is 10 mg carbidopa and 100 mg levodopa three to four times daily, or 25

TABLE 23–2 PHARMACOKINETICS OF SELECTED ANTIPARKINSONIAN DRUGS

Drug	Route	Onset	Peak	Duration	PB (%)	$t_{1/2}$	BioA (%)
Dopaminergics							
Levodopa	po	2–3 wk	0.5–2 hr	5–24 hr	30	1–3 hr	UK
Carbidopa/levodopa	po	UK	UK	5–24 hr	36	1–4 hr	UK
Anticholinergics							
Biperidin	po	15–30 min	1–1.5 hr	UK	UK	18–24 hr	29
Benztropine	po	1–2 hr	Days	24 hr	UK	UK	UK
Ethopropazine	po	30 min	UK	4 hr	UK	UK	UK
Procyclidine	po	30–45 min	1–2 hr	4–6 hr	UK	11–12 hr	52–97
Trihexyphenidyl	po	60 min	2–3 hr	6–12 hr	UK	5–10 hr	100
Dopamine Agonists							
Amantadine	po	48 hr	2 wks	12–24 hr	67	9–37 hr	50–90
Bromocriptine	po	30–90 min	1–3 hr	6–24 hr	90	3–7 hr*	UK
Pergolide	po	UK	1–2 hr	5–9 hr	90	24–72 hr	UK
MAOB Inhibitor							
Selegiline	po	2–3 d	UK	Weeks	UK	Varies†	45

*Initial phase $t_{1/2}$ of bromocriptine is 3–7 hours, with a terminal phase of 50 hours.
†Half-lives of each of the three metabolites of selegiline range from 2 to 20.5 hours.
UK, Unknown; PB, protein binding; $t_{1/2}$ elimination half-life; BioA, bioavailability.

TABLE 23–3 DRUG-DRUG INTERACTIONS WITH SELECTED ANTIPARKINSONIAN DRUGS

Drug	Interactive Drugs	Interaction(s)
Dopaminergics		
Levodopa	Antacids Metoclopramide	Increased effectiveness of levodopa due to increased bioavailability
Carbidopa/levodopa	Anticholinergics	Postural hypotension
	Antihypertensives Benzodiazepines Haloperidol Metoclopramide Papaverine Phenothiazines Reserpine	Decreased effectiveness of interactive drugs
	MAO inhibitors Tricyclic antidepressants	Hypertensive reactions
	Pyridoxine (large doses) Phenytoin Methionine	Decreased effects of carbidopa/levodopa
	Sympathomimetics	Increased risk of arrhythmias
Anticholinergics		
Trihexyphenidyl and centrally acting antimuscarinic drugs	Antacids Antidiarrheals	Decreased absorption of anticholinergic drug
	Antimuscarinic drugs	Increased risk, severity of CNS, peripheral atropine–like effects; possible muscarinic poisoning syndrome
	Antipsychotic drugs	Increased antimuscarinic effects Decreased effectiveness of interacting drug Worsening of psychoses
	General CNS depressants	Increased CNS depression
Dopamine Agonists		
Amantadine	Benztropine Levodopa Orphenadrine Trihexyphenidyl	Increased effectiveness of interactive agent
	Amphetamine and amphetamine-like drugs	Increased effectiveness of amantadine
	Hydrochlorothiazide/triamterene	Increased blood level of amantadine
Bromocriptine	Antihypertensive drugs	Increased drop in blood pressure
	Phenothiazines	Decreased effects of bromocriptine
	Antihistamines Haloperidol Methyldopa Reserpine Tricyclic antidepressants	Decreased effectiveness of bromocriptine
	Antihistamines Alcohol Narcotics Sedative-hypnotics	Increased CNS depression
	Levodopa	Increased neurologic deficits
Pergolide	Haloperidol Metoclopramide Phenothiazines	Decreased effects of interactive drugs
MAOB Inhibitor		
Selegiline	Fluoxetine Meperidine Opioids	Adverse effects such as excitation, sweating, rigidity, hypertension, or hypotension; fatalities are also possible
	Carbidopa/levodopa	Initial increase in effectiveness of interacting drug
	Alcohol	Increased hypotension and sedative effects of selegiline
	Chloroprothixene Haloperidol Metoclopramide Phenothiazines Reserpine (large doses) Thiothexene	Decreased effects of selegiline
	Antihypertensive drugs	Increased risk of hypotension

CNS, Central nervous system. MAO, monoamine oxidase.

TABLE 23–4 DOSAGE REGIMENS FOR SELECTED ANTIPARKINSONIAN DRUGS			
Drug	**Use(s)**	**Dosage**	**Implications**
Dopaminergics			
Levodopa	Idiopathic Parkinson's disease Postencephalitic parkinsonism Symptomatic parkinsonism related to CNS injury by carbon monoxide and manganese intoxication	*Initial:* 0.5–1 g po QD in 2 or more divided doses. May increase by 0.75 g po QD every 3–7 days. Not to exceed 8 g po q 24 hr.	Safety in pregnancy and children younger than 18 years has not been established
Carbidopa/levodopa	Idiopathic Parkinson's disease Postencephalitic parkinsonism Symptomatic parkinsonism related to CNS injury by carbon monoxide and manganese intoxication	*Initial:* 25 mg carbidopa/100 mg levodopa po TID *or* 10 mg carbidopa/100 mg levodopa po TID–QID. May increase by 1 tab per day or every other day as necessary until dosage of 8 tablets is reached *Controlled-release form:* 1 tablet po BID at intervals of not less than 6 hr. Usual dose: 2–8 tabs po q4–8h while awake	Safety in pregnancy and children younger than 18 years not established Doses and dosing intervals may be altered on basis of response
Anticholinergics			
Trihexyphenidyl	All forms of parkinsonism Adjunct to levodopa Drug-induced extrapyramidal disorders	*Initial:* 1–2 mg first day. May increase by 2 mg q3–5D. *Maintenance:* 5–15 mg po QD in divided doses. Extended-release form may be given q12–24h.	For tolerance over long-term therapy, dose may be increased or changed When being discontinued, dose should be tapered over 1 week
Biperiden	Adjunct for all forms of parkinsonism, drug-induced extrapyramidal effects, and acute dystonic reactions	*Initial:* 2 mg po TID–QID *or* 2 mg IM/IV. May repeat q30 min. Not to exceed 8 mg/24 hr *Maintenance:* Not to exceed 16 mg/day	For tolerance over long-term therapy, dose may be increased or changed When being discontinued, dose should be tapered over 1 week
Benztropine	Adjunct for all forms of parkinsonism Control of extrapyramidal disorders (except tardive dyskinesia) due to neuroleptic drugs	*Initial:* 1–2 mg po QD. Range: 0.5–6 mg QD. Give 1–2 mg IM/IV in emergency situations	Oral route preferred. Has cumulative action Contraindicated in children younger than 3 years
Ethopropazine	Adjunct for all forms of parkinsonism Control of extrapyramidal disorders due to CNS drugs such as reserpine and phenothiazines Drug of choice for major tremors	*Initial:* 50 mg po QD–BID. May increase by 10 mg per dose q2–3 days until optimal effect reached. *Maintenance:* 100–600 mg po QD.	Has high incidence of adverse effects
Procyclidine	Relief of rigidity related to parkinsonism (rather than tremor)	*Initial:* 2.5 mg po TID after meals. May increase if tolerated to 5 mg TID and HS.	Contraindicated in pediatric patients When drug is being dicontinued, dose should be tapered over 1 week
Dopamine Agonists			
Amantadine	All forms of parkinsonism	*Initial:* 100 mg po QD–BID. *Maintenance:* Total dose should not exceed 400 mg	Reported to increase susceptibility to German measles When drug is being discontinued, dose should be tapered over 1 week
Bromocriptine	Idiopathic or postencephalitic Parkinson's disease Adjunct to levodopa	*Initial:* 1.25–2.5 mg po QD. May increase by 2.5–5 mg on alternate days *Maintenance:* 2.5–100 mg po QD in divided doses. Usual dosage range: 10–40 mg QD. Not to exceed 300 mg QD.	Safety during pregnancy and in children younger than 15 years not established
Pergolide	Solely as adjunct to dopaminergic agents in treatment of Parkinson's disease, in those with dyskinesia and increasing "on-off" episodes	*Initial:* 0.05 mg po QD. May increase by 0.1–0.15 mg po every 3rd day over 2 weeks. Dosage may then be increased by 0.25 mg every 3rd day until desired response is obtained. Total dose given in 3 equal doses at 6–8 hr intervals *Maintenance:* 3 mg/24 hr. Not to exceed 5 mg/24 hr	Safety during pregnancy and lactation and in children not established
MAOB Inhibitor			
Selegiline	Adjunct for carbidopa/levodopa in Parkinson's disease	*Initial:* 5 mg po QD–BID *Maintenance:* 5 mg po after breakfast and lunch	Dose of carbidopa/levodopa may be decreased after introduction of selegiline

mg carbidopa and 100 mg levodopa three times a day. The dose is gradually increased, depending on the patient's history, mental impairment, and individual response. The optimal dose is reached when the smallest dose necessary to control symptoms and decrease disability is reached. A 25 mg carbidopa/250 mg levodopa combination formulation is also available.

For patients who have difficulty with nausea and vomiting when the dose is 10 mg carbidopa and 100 mg levodopa, an additional 25 mg of carbidopa may be given with the first dose each day. Additional doses of 12.5 or 25 mg of carbidopa may be given during the day with each dose. For patients are taking 25 mg carbidopa/250 mg levodopa, 25 mg carbidopa may be given with any dose for optimum therapeutic response.

For patients who cannot tolerate multidose regimens, there is now a new sustained-release form of levodopa (SINEMET CR contains 50 mg of carbidopa and 200 mg of levodopa). More stable blood levels of carbidopa/levodopa prevent the sudden and unpredictable "on-off" phenomenon. In fact, it has been reported that some patients show more improvement while taking fewer daily doses of this formulation.

Laboratory Considerations

Patients on long-term levodopa and carbidopa/levodopa therapy require periodic monitoring, consisting of complete blood count and both hepatic and renal function studies. Blood urea nitrogen (BUN), creatinine, and uric acid levels are lower during concomitant administration of carbidopa and levodopa than with levodopa alone.

Levodopa formulations may cause an increase in serum levels of alanine transaminase (serum glutamate-pyruvate transaminase), aspartate transaminase (serum glutamic-oxaloacetic transaminase), alkaline phosphatase, lactate dehydrogenase, protein-bound iodine, and bilirubin. The Coombs' test has occasionally become positive with extended levodopa therapy. Elevations of uric acid have occurred with the calorimetric testing method but not with the uricase method.

Levodopa interferes with results of urine glucose and urine ketone testing. The Clinitest and Ketostix methods of testing urine glucose and ketones may produce false-positive results. The Tes-Tape method for urine glucose evaluation may have false-negative results in patients on levodopa therapy.

Anticholinergics

- ❒ Benztropine (COGENTIN); (♣) APO-BENZTROPINE, PMS-BENZTROPINE
- ❒ Biperiden (AKINETON)
- ❒ Ethopropazine (PARSIDOL)
- ❒ Procyclidine (KEMADRIN); (♣) PROCYCLID, PMS-PROCYCLIDINE
- ❒ Trihexyphenidyl (ARTANE); (♣) APO-TRIHEX

Indications

Anticholinergics are useful early in the course of Parkinson's disease more to control tremor by relaxing smooth muscle than for treatment of the other manifestations of the disease. They are a reasonable treatment choice in middle-aged patients who have tremor but little rigidity or bradykinesia. Anticholinergics are useful in controlling salivation and drooling but may cause a dry mouth. These drugs are also the choice agents for treating *akathisia* (extrapyramidal reactions) arising from antipsychotic drugs. Trihexyphenidyl is the only anticholinergic used as an adjunct to carbidopa/levodopa therapy. The adverse effects of anticholinergics have limited their usefulness and are particularly problematic in patients older than 70 years.

Anticholinergic drugs are also used in the management of bradyarrhythmias and of nausea and vomiting associated with motion sickness and vertigo (see Chapter 13). Selected drugs are used to decrease gastric secretory activity and to increase esophageal sphincter tone. Some anticholinergic drugs are used as ophthalmic mydriatics (see Chapter 62).

Pharmacodynamics

Anticholinergic drugs work on the theory that as Parkinson's disease progresses, dopaminergic activity decreases, cholinergic activity becomes dominant, and motor dysfunction results. Anticholinergic drugs act by competitively inhibiting the action of ACh at postsynaptic muscarinic receptors. The receptors are found in smooth muscle, cardiac muscle, and parasympathetic-innervated glands as well as in the brain. This mechanism restores the cholinergic-dopaminergic balance in the striatum.

Adverse Effects and Contraindications

Adverse CNS effects of anticholinergic drugs include headache, nervousness, disorientation, dizziness, weakness, insomnia, and fever in children. Adverse effects are more common in older adults and are generally more disabling. Cardiovascular effects include tachycardia and palpitations. Nausea, vomiting, dry mouth, constipation, heartburn, dysphagia, paralytic ileus, and urinary retention or hesitancy in men with prostatic hypertrophy and impotence have been noted. Suppression of glandular secretions including lactation, decreased perspiration, heat prostration, and flushed skin can be troublesome in some patients. Dilated pupils, blurred vision, photophobia, and exacerbation of acute angle-closure-glaucoma has also been documented with anticholinergic drugs.

The adverse effects of anticholinergic drugs are most often seen when they are taken with other CNS-active drugs, such as antipsychotics, antihistamines, and antidepressants. Anticholinergic drugs are contraindicated in patients with hypersensitivity, acute angle-closure glaucoma, acute hemorrhage, tachycardia secondary to cardiac insufficiency or thyrotoxicosis, Down's syndrome, asthma, and chronic lung disease. Anticholinergic drugs are also contraindicated in patients with bronchial asthma or emphysema who are currently taking sympathomimetic drugs.

Cautious use of anticholinergic drugs is warranted in patients with severe or chronic renal, cardiac, pulmonary, or hepatic disease. Caution should be used in prescribing such agents for infants, children, and older adults, who are at higher risk for adverse effects. Anticholinergics should also be used with caution in patients with prostatic hypertrophy and intestinal obstruction, owing to the drugs' spasmolytic action on smooth muscle. Safe use of anticholinergics during pregnancy and lactation has not been established (Pregnancy category C).

Pharmacokinetics

Few pharmacokinetic data are available for anticholinergic drugs. Table 23–2 provides an overview of known data. Anticholinergics are well absorbed when taken by mouth. The extent of distribution, biotransformation, and elimination are unknown.

Drug-Drug Interactions

Anticholinergic drugs exhibit additive or antagonistic effects with other antiparkinsonian drugs and other anticholinergics (see Table 23–3). The concurrent use of an anticholinergic and amantadine increases the incidence of the anticholinergic's adverse effects. The effects disappear when the anticholinergic dosage is reduced. Serum digoxin levels may be raised by anticholinergics when digoxin is administered as a slow-dissolution oral tablet. Concurrent use of haloperidol and an anticholinergic worsens schizophrenic symptoms and reduces serum concentrations of the haloperidol.

When anticholinergic drugs are combined with levodopa, gastric motility may decrease, increasing the deactivation of levodopa and reducing intestinal absorption. A reduction in levodopa's efficacy may thus be noted. Therapeutic effects of phenothiazines may be diminished with concurrent use of anticholinergic agents.

Additive anticholinergic effects may be noted with drugs that share anticholinergic properties, such as antihistamines, quinidine, disopyramide, and tricyclic antidepressants. Antacids and antidiarrheals decrease the absorption of anticholinergic drugs.

Dosage Regimen

The dosage regimen of anticholinergics for Parkinson's disease varies with the specific drug, the severity of symptoms, the age of the patient, whether the drug is used in conjunction with another agent, and how long the patient has been using anticholinergics. Acquired tolerance is not a problem, but progression of the disease leads to an apparent loss of efficacy in many patients. Table 23–4 provides an overview of the anticholinergic drugs and their recommended dosages.

Dopamine Agonists

- ❒ Amantadine (SYMMETREL)
- ❒ Bromocriptine (PARLODEL)
- ❒ Pergolide (PERMAX)

Indications

Bromocriptine is currently the most popular dopamine agonist drug. It is currently useful for both postencephalitic and idiopathic parkinsonism. Bromocriptine has also been used to prevent lactation following childbirth and to correct infertility and amenorrhea in women with high prolactin levels.

Pergolide is used solely as an adjunct to carbidopa/levodopa in the treatment of patients who experience intolerable dyskinesia and/or increasing "on-off" episodes when taking levodopa alone.

As natural or synthetic compounds that directly activate dopamine receptors, dopamine agonists are capable of producing an acute antiparkinsonian effect equal to that of levodopa. Dopamine agonists were developed as a result of the "on-off" phenomenon, the waning of therapeutic effects associated with long-term therapy.

Pharmacodynamics

Amantadine's mechanism of action is unknown. It appears to have both presynaptic and postsynaptic actions at the remaining dopaminergic terminals. Amantadine enhances the synthesis of dopamine in the presynaptic storage vessels and inhibits re-uptake in the synapse.

Bromocriptine and pergolide have similar actions. They serve as substitutes for dopamine by directly stimulating dopamine receptor cells in the corpus striatum. In turn, the deficiency of dopamine is offset, diminishing rigidity, tremor, and sluggish movements.

Adverse Effects and Contraindications

The adverse drug effects of dopamine agonists are similar to those of levodopa but are more prominent and occur more frequently. The effects are usually additive.

Orthostatic hypotension and gastrointestinal (GI) disturbances secondary to dopamine agonists result from peripheral and central dopaminergic effects. Central dopaminergic effects include confusion, hallucinations, and dyskinesia. They tend to worsen if the dose of the agonist or the levodopa (in the combination) is not reduced. Dyspnea may be noted with dopaminergic drugs. The cause is uncertain, although it is thought to be a combination of dopaminergic and idiosyncratic mechanisms. Cardiac arrhythmias, angina, and erythromelalgia (bilateral vasodilation, particularly of the extremities, with burning pain, increased skin temperature, and redness), all have been linked to the dopamine agonists. Hot environments may cause a lowering of blood pressure.

Amantadine's most common adverse drug reactions are dizziness, ataxia, insomnia, hypotension, and skin mottling. Amantadine is contraindicated in patients with hypersensitivity. This drug may increase the patient's susceptibility to rubella infections. Its safe use during pregnancy and lactation has not been established.

Bromocriptine's most common adverse effects are nausea, vomiting, dyspepsia, hypotension, hallucinations, psychosis, and dyskinesis. Leg cramps often occur in patients on long-term therapy. Bromocriptine should be used cautiously in patients with liver disease, owing to the drug's poor biotransformation in the liver and elimination via the biliary tract. It should also be used cautiously in patients with a history of cardiac disorders. The neurologic and psychiatric disturbances caused by bromocriptine may last 2 to 6 weeks after therapy is discontinued. Thickening of the pleura and pleural effusion have been noted in patients on long-term bromocriptine therapy.

The adverse reactions to pergolide are similar to those to bromocriptine and include nausea, hallucinations, dyskinesia, sedation, and postural hypotension. Pergolide should be used cautiously in patients with coronary artery disease, angina, heart rhythm disorders, Raynaud's syndrome, and seizure disorders. Long-term use of pergolide may produce dyskinesias. A sudden withdrawal can cause confusion, paranoid thinking, and severe hallucinations.

Safe use of dopamine agonists in children and during pregnancy has not been established. The potential benefits should be judged to outweigh the potential risks before dopamine agonists are administered to children or pregnant patients.

Pharmacokinetics

Amantadine is well absorbed from the GI tract. Its initial onset is 48 hours, and its duration of action is 12 to 24 hours (see Table 23–2). It is distributed to various body tissues and fluids, including the CNS and breast milk. Amantadine is eliminated unchanged in the urine.

Bromocriptine is poorly absorbed from the GI tract. It has an onset time of 30 to 90 minutes, peaking in 1 to 3 hours. It is 90 percent protein bound, with a duration of action of 6 to 24 hours. Bromocriptine is completely biotransformed in the liver and eliminated in the feces. Its half-life is 3 to 7 hours in the initial phase and up to 50 hours in the terminal phase.

Pergolide is well absorbed when taken by mouth, although distribution throughout the body is unknown and the onset of action questionable. This drug is 10 to 1000 times more potent than bromocriptine on a milligram-to-milligram basis in vitro. Pergolide peaks in 1 to 2 hours, with an average duration of 5 to 9 hours. It has a half-life of approximately 24 to 72 hours. Biotransformation occurs in the liver, and metabolites are eliminated primarily in the urine.

Drug-Drug Interactions

Anticholinergic effects (dry mouth, blurred vision) are increased by the concurrent use of antihistamines, phenothiazines, quinidine, and tricyclic antidepressants (see Table 23–3). Amphetamine and amphetamine-like stimulant drugs amplify the effects of amantadine by causing excess stimulation and adverse behavioral effects. The combination diuretic hydrochlorothiazide-triamterene has been noted to raise blood levels of amantadine.

Bromocriptine taken concurrently with antihypertensive drugs can cause an excessive drop in blood pressure. When bromocriptine is taken with phenothiazines, the effects of bromocriptine are reduced. Antihistamines, alcohol, opioids, and sedative-hypnotics have been known to cause additional CNS depression when taken with bromocriptine. Levodopa and bromocriptine taken together can produce additional neurologic effects in the patient with Parkinson's disease. Concurrent administration of pergolide with dopamine antagonists, such as phenothiazines, metoclopramide, and haloperidol, should be avoided.

Dosage Regimen

Amantadine is available in both capsules and syrup. The usual adult antiparkinsonian dose is 100 mg once or twice daily (see Table 23–4). The total daily dosage should not exceed 400 mg. The actual dose and administration schedule are determined with the patient's renal function in mind.

Bromocriptine is available in both capsules and tablets. Initially, 1.25 to 2.5 mg is administered once daily. The maintenance dose is 2.5 to 100 mg daily in divided doses. The dose can be increased by 2.5 to 5 mg on alternate days until the desired effect is reached. The usual dosage range, however, is 30 to 90 mg per day in three divided doses. The total daily dosage should not exceed 100 mg.

Pergolide is available in tablets only. The initial dose is 0.05 mg daily for the first 2 days. The dosage is gradually increased by 0.1 to 0.15 mg every third day over the next 2 weeks. If the optimal response is not achieved in that period, the dose is increased by 0.25 mg every third day until optimal response is observed. The usual dose is 3 mg/day in three divided doses given every 6 to 8 hours. The dosage should not exceed 5 mg/day.

Laboratory Considerations

Amantadine has a plasma drug level of 0.2 mcg/L when it is given in therapeutic doses. Serum levels of the other dopamine agonists are not known.

Amantadine increases liver enzymes and may increase BUN. Periodic evaluations of the white blood cell count, liver function, and renal function tests should be done with amantadine.

Bromocriptine can cause elevations in BUN and in serum, alanine transaminase (serum glutamate-pyruvate transaminase), aspartate transaminase (serum glutamic-oxaloacetic transaminase), creatine phosphokinase, alkaline phosphatase, and uric acid levels. However, the elevations are usually not clinically significant. Reductions in prolactin and growth hormone serum levels have been noted.

Pergolide can cause a marked reduction in blood prolactin levels. This appears to be its only effect on laboratory values.

Monoamine Oxidase B Inhibitor

❒ Selegiline (ELDEPRYL)

Indications

Selegiline is indicated as an adjunct to carbidopa/levodopa in all stages of Parkinson's disease. It is more effective when used early in the disease. This drug is useful for patients who have moderate to severe limitations and/or disabilities. Its use may help patients avoid the complications associated with long-term, high-dose levodopa therapy.

Pharmacodynamics

The mechanism of action for selegiline is not completely understood, but this drug is thought to irreversibly inhibit MAOB activity. By blocking MAOB, selegiline prevents the breakdown of dopamine, a desirable effect in patients with Parkinson's disease. There is evidence that selegiline increases dopaminergic activity by interfering with dopamine re-uptake at the synapses and by mediation through its metabolites. Enhancement of several neurotransmitters and interference with neuron uptake have been seen in two of selegiline's principal metabolites. Further, evidence strongly suggests that selegiline may prevent the formation of cytotoxic free radicals, which play a role in initiating the destruction of dopamine-producing cells in the brain. When taken with carbidopa/levodopa, selegiline may slow the loss of these important brain cells and, hence, the progression of the disease.

Adverse Effects and Contraindications

Selegiline has no life-threatening or irreversible adverse effects, although it does exert numerous, troublesome effects on every body system. Adverse CNS, cardiovascular, genitourinary, GI, musculoskeletal, endocrine, metabolic, and visual effects have been noted. Once the drug dosage is lowered or discontinued, the adverse effects cease.

Selegiline is contraindicated in patients with hypersensitivity. Concurrent opioid or meperidine therapy may result in fatal reactions. Cautious use of selegiline is warranted with doses greater than 10 mg/day because of the higher risk of hypersensitivity reactions with foods containing tyramine. Safe use of this agent during pregnancy or lactation or in children has not been established.

Pharmacokinetics

Selegiline appears to be well absorbed following oral administration, with 45 percent bioavailability. It is widely distributed. Selegiline is a long-acting drug with an onset time of 2 to 3 days. Peak and duration of action are unknown. It is rapidly metabolized into three metabolites: *N*-desmethydeprenyl, amphetamine, and methamphetamine. The half-lives of the metabolites differ, ranging from 2 to 20.5 hours (see Table 23–2). Because new MAOB enzyme synthesis must occur for a patient to regain activity, it takes several weeks for the clinical effects of selegiline to fully disappear.

Drug-Drug Interactions

Selegiline is contraindicated for use with meperidine and other opiates, as well as with fluoxetine (see Table 23–3). There have been reports of fatal interactions, including excitation, sweating, rigidity, hypertension or hypotension, and coma. Excessive drop in blood pressure has been noted when selegiline is taken with antihypertensive drugs.

Drug-Food Interactions

Hypertensive crisis occurs when doses of selegiline greater than 10 mg/day are taken concurrently with tyramine-containing foods (see Appendix C). The earliest symptom of a hypertensive crisis is a severe headache. Phentolamine, an alpha-adrenergic blocking drug, may be given to lower blood pressure during the crisis. Interestingly, MAOB isozymes lack the notable interaction that occurs with the ingestion of foods containing tyramine.

Dosage Regimen

The initial dose of selegiline is 5 mg once or twice a day (see Table 23–4). The usual maintenance dose is 10 mg/day in two divided doses that are taken after breakfast and again after lunch.

Critical Thinking Process

Assessment

History of Present Illness

Key information to be obtained for the patient with Parkinson's disease includes why the patient came to the hospital/clinic and when the symptoms started. What does the patient think caused the symptoms? Has the patient experienced these symptoms in the past? When? Complaints of interference with the activities of daily living precede the recognition of parkinsonism by months or years.

Past Health History

The past health history should elicit information about any drug, toxin, or food allergies and the reaction the patient exhibited. Past or present alcohol or drug use, current drugs taken, and any exposure to environmental toxins should be noted. Information related to history of renal, hepatic, cardiovascular, or GI disorders should also be elicited.

Physical Exam Findings

Parkinson's disease is defined solely by clinical signs and symptoms, especially physical signs. To evaluate the severity of the disease, the health care provider must perform an exam. However, the exam may not reveal a patient's ability to perform outside the office and to carry out the activities of daily living. Nonetheless, a thorough assessment is required so that proper intervention can be undertaken.

Careful questioning and visualization of the patient during the interview may reveal changes in speech and facial expression, arm swing, and gait. The exam can reveal valuable clues as to the extent of interference with activities of daily living. Assessment of the neurologic system may be the greatest diagnostic aid. Other areas of importance are the musculoskeletal system, head and neck, and skin.

The patient's mental status along with observable characteristics of Parkinson's disease provides a broad picture of the problems the patient is experiencing. Commonly, the patient with Parkinson's disease is emotionally labile, demonstrates a depressed affect, is easily upset, and shows signs of paranoia. When questioned, the patient may respond slowly owing to cognitive impairments. The same impairments may be evident as delayed reaction time in the completion of a requested task. Evidence of dementia and acute confusion are common in the older adult with this disease.

Observation of the posture and gait of the patient is helpful. Because the postural reflexes are lost, postural abnormalities may occur as early signs. The patient may experience involuntary flexion of the head and neck. When walking or standing, the patient exhibits a flexed, "stooped" posture. There is also truncal rigidity, noted when the patient attempts to change position from sitting to standing. The patient tends to move the body as a unit and may be unable to correct position when changing from one position to another or merely when rolling over. A characteristic propulsive gait is noted in patients with Parkinson's disease. The patient may be slow to initiate the walk but may spontaneously break into a run. When pushed forward or backward, the patient may actually have difficulty stopping quickly.

Typically, the arms are flexed at the elbows, with the wrists slightly dorsiflexed and the fingers adducted and flexed at the metacarpophalangeal joint. During walking, the arm swings are decreased or absent. There may be difficulties with handwriting (micrographia), using kitchen utensils, grooming, and fastening buttons. Rapid repetitive movements, such as tapping of the fingers or pronation and supination of the hand, are common.

Examination of the head and face shows the patient to have a masklike facial expression owing to limited facial

Case Study Parkinson's Disease

Patient History

History of Present Illness	DP is a 75-year-old woman with complaints of a general feeling of stiffness, mild to moderate tremors in both arms, and increasing difficulty dressing and eating. Her family noticed that her handwriting has changed and her speech is slower than normal. She does not exercise but has started to lose weight.
Past Health History	DP denies allergies to food or medications. Her last physical exam 6 years ago was unremarkable. She has mild arthritis and takes ASA for discomfort. She denies a history of hospitalizations, illnesses, smoking, or consumption of alcohol. *Current meds:* ASA gr. X PRN for shoulder and knee discomfort (requires about 4 tablets/week).
Physical Exam	*Height:* 5′1″>. *Weight:* 93 lb (5 lb below usual). *VSS:* Afebrile. Slight pill-rolling movements of the thumb against the fingers in the left hand. Mild to moderate resting tremors and rigidity noted bilaterally. Low-pitched, poorly articulated speech, lacks modulation.
Diagnostic Testing	Chest x-ray, ECG, MRI, CBC, and electrolytes within normal limits.
Developmental Considerations	Age-related physiologic changes to body systems.
Psychosocial Considerations	DP retired from working in a grocery store at the age of 55. Currently living in retirement community with husband, who is in good health. She has an attentive daughter and 2 grandchildren who live within 5 miles. They visit often. Sister out of town.
Economic Factors	DP has access to both a medical facility and a pharmacy. Husband provides transportation as needed. Through her insurance and retirement benefits, the majority of her medical bills and prescriptions are paid.

Variables Influencing Decision

Treatment Objectives

- Reduce symptoms and enhance the quality of life.
- Maintain function and independence for as long as possible.
- Provide patient with lowest possible dosage that is effective in controlling symptoms.

Drug Variables	*Drug Summary*	*Patient Variables*
Indications	Dopaminergics are indicated for patients with idiopathic PD: in patients with bradykinesia, for impairments in balance and gait, hand dexterity, and oral and written communication.	This is a decision point. DP has not been previously treated for PD. Symptoms are now starting to interfere with ADLs.
Pharmacodynamics	The four drug groups have different mechanisms of action but are directed at increasing dopamine levels in the CNS.	This will not be a decision point, because all drug groups have similar mechanisms of action.
Adverse Effects/ Contraindications	All four drug groups have a variety of troublesome as well as serious adverse effects.	This is not a decision point, because all drug classes have a broad variety of adverse effects.

Drug Variables	*Drug Summary*	*Patient Variables*
Pharmacokinetics	Vary with individual drug. Most are excreted through kidneys in the urine.	Since there are few pharmacokinetic data available on the drugs, this will not be a decision point. However, DP's impaired renal function associated with aging will have an impact on drug elimination by the kidneys that could potentially lead to toxicity.
Dosage Regimen	Follow manufacturer's recommendations based on patient response. Presence of carbidopa with levodopa allows a 60–80% reduction in the oral dose of levodopa required for therapeutic effects.	DP is able to take drugs orally. Knowledgeable and expected to be compliant with drug regimen at this time.
Laboratory Considerations	The drugs in the four groups cause alterations in CBC, liver, and renal function tests.	This may be a decision point, because accurate liver and renal function tests are necessary to monitor therapy.
Cost Index*	Benztropine: 1 Carbidopa/levodopa: 4 Amantadine: 1 Selegiline: 5	DP's insurance covers the cost of her drug regimen; therefore, this will not be a major decision point.

Summary of Decision Points

- Anticholinergic drugs (benztropine) tend to control tremor better than other manifestations of Parkinson's disease and are a reasonable treatment choice initially in middle-aged patients with little rigidity or bradykinesia.
- Dopaminergic drugs (carbidopa/levodopa) are the mainstay of drug treatment for PD and are more effective than the other drugs currently available.
- Presence of carbidopa with levodopa allows a 60–80% reduction in the oral dose of levodopa required for therapeutic effects.
- Results of studies involving the efficacy of amantadine are conflicting.
- There appears to be no difference in efficacy among benztropine, trihexyphenidyl, and pro-cyclidine.

DRUG TO BE USED

- Low-dose carbidopa/levodopa: ½ of scored 25 mg carbidopa/100 mg levodopa tablet initially. Increase dosage by ½ tablet at weekly intervals until improvement or toxicities are noted. Switch to a 10:1 formulation once total daily dose of 200 mg levodopa is reached.

*Cost Index:
1 = $ < 30/mo.
2 = $ 30–40/mo.
3 = $ 40–50/mo.
4 = $ 50–60/mo.
5 = $ > 60/mo.

AWP of 100, 0.5-mg tablets of bentropine is approximately $3.
AWP of 100, 25-mg carbidopa/100-mg levodopa tablets is approximately $45.
AWP of 60, 5-mg tablets of selegiline is approximately $130.
AWP of 100, 100-mg tablets of amantadine is approximately $10.

muscle movements. A blank expression, decreased blinking, and characteristic stare are all common. Unfortunately, these effects are associated with other head and neck symptoms, such as difficulties in swallowing and chewing. Drooling may be noted as the disease progresses. In addition, the patient's speech may become softer and less distinct.

Other "red flags" in the physical exam center on hypothalamic function, including both autonomic and neuroendocrine systems. Autonomic symptoms include diaphoresis, orthostatic hypotension, and constipation. Neuroendocrine dysfunction accounts for the excessively oily skin, especially on the face.

Severity Scales Many scales have been developed to rate the severity of Parkinson's disease. These weighted numerical scales are based on an evaluation of the signs and symptoms. Each of the scales differs in which symptoms are evaluated and the value assigned to each. A relatively common scale developed by Hoehn and Yahr divides the disease into five stages, as follows:

Stage 0—No visible disease.
Stage I—Disease involves only one side of the body.
Stage II—Disease involves both sides of the body but does not impair balance.
Stage III—Disease impairs balance or walking.
Stage IV—Disease markedly impairs balance or walking.
Stage V—Disease results in complete immobility.

Stages 0 through II constitute mild disease. Stage III is moderate disease, and stages IV and V constitute marked or advanced disease. There are gray areas between the successive stages.

Diagnostic Testing

There are no laboratory tests to confirm or refute the clinical diagnosis of Parkinson's disease. Chemistry tests are most commonly used to seek treatable causes of dementia with parkinsonism, especially hypothyroidism. Imaging or laboratory techniques are useful to rule out other disorders.

Although unreliable in diagnosing idiopathic parkinsonism, magnetic resonance imaging has proven to be the single most useful means of looking for other etiologies. Computed tomography is also useful. If a computed tomography scan shows calcification of the basal ganglia, the possibilities of hyperparathyroidism and hypoparathyroidism should be investigated through measurements of blood calcium, phosphorus, and parathormone levels.

Developmental Considerations

Perinatal Antiparkinsonian drugs should not be used during pregnancy unless the anticipated benefits outweigh the risks arising from failure to treat Parkinson's disease. It is not known whether antiparkinsonian drugs cause fetal harm or affect reproductive capacity. Rodent studies have shown that antiparkinsonian drugs produced alterations in fetal and postnatal growth and viability.

Pediatric Antiparkinsonian drugs are usually not needed in children. Further, the safety and efficacy of antiparkinsonian drugs have not been established for this age group. Juvenile parkinsonism may occur but is usually associated with Wilson's disease, progressive lenticular degeneration, or Huntington's chorea.

Geriatric If frail older adults are receiving multiple drugs for non-neurologic purposes, such drugs influence response to antiparkinsonian therapy. Existing dementia should be noted as well as occasional confusion before the start of any drug therapy. Normal changes of aging alter the biotransformation and elimination of antiparkinsonian drugs, increasing the risk of adverse effects.

Psychosocial Considerations

Coping strategies of the patient and family are important to note. The patient may have periods of irritability, depression, or anger; mood swings; or periods of feeling useless. Additional feelings of inadequacy and frustration result. Reassurance and encouragement are very much needed from those around the patient (see Case Study—Parkinson's Disease).

Analysis and Management

Treatment Objectives

Management of the patient with Parkinson's disease is aimed at maintaining function and independence and reducing the symptoms and disabilities caused by the disease as much as and for as long as possible. This may be accomplished by maintaining a balance between dopaminergic and cholinergic activity in the basal ganglia. In general, 85 percent of patients with early, mild Parkinson's disease can achieve at least 50 percent improvement in level of function with appropriate drug therapy.

Treatment Options

Numerous strategies can be chosen for the management of Parkinson's disease according to the etiology. Table 23–5 provides an overview of possibilities. Currently, no available drugs have been proved to modify the disease process or to affect its natural progression. Most drugs either lessen or reverse the symptoms by replacing the chemicals needed for neural transmission and movement. Treatment should be individualized.

Drug Variables

Dopaminergics The combination of carbidopa with levodopa is now the most effective preparation available for treatment of Parkinson's disease. The combination of carbidopa (the dopa-decarboxylase inhibitor component) with levodopa concentrates levodopa in the brain and minimizes the adverse effects of dopamine. The addition of carbidopa allows a 60 to 80 percent reduction in the therapeutic oral dose of levodopa. The combination reduces nausea and other peripheral adverse effects. It also is available in more useful dosages and formulations.

The benefits of using a dopaminergic begin to decrease, and adverse drug reactions become more severe, the longer the patient is taking the drug. Loss of control of a previously levodopa-responsive symptom should not be interpreted as loss of levodopa effect or evidence of disease progression. Recurrence of symptoms previously under control should trigger a search for other treatable etiologies, such as drug interactions, difficulties with drug absorption, and other illnesses associated with Parkinson's disease (e.g., dehydration). Pyridoxine (vitamin B_6) rapidly reverses the therapeutic effects of levodopa, and its use should be limited. It is

TABLE 23–5 DRUG THERAPY INDICATIONS FOR TYPES OF PARKINSON'S DISEASE AND PARKINSONISM

Drug	Idiopathic Disease	Drug-Induced Extrapyramidal Symptoms	Chemical/Drug-Induced Disease	Arteriosclerotic Disease	Postencephalitic Disease
Dopaminergics					
Carbidopa/levodopa	X		X		X
Levodopa	X		X	X	X
Anticholinergics					
Biperiden	X	X	X	X	X
Benztropine	X	X	X	X	X
Ethopropazine	X	X	X	X	X
Procyclidine	X	X	X	X	X
Trihexyphenidyl	X	X	X	X	X
Dopamine Agonists					
Amantadine		X	X		
Bromocriptine	X				X
Pergolide				Adjunctive use only	
MAOB Inhibitor					
Selegiline				Adjunctive use only	

also necessary to limit the intake of pyrimidine from all sources for any patient taking levodopa.

Anticholinergics Anticholinergics have historically been used as first-line treatment for mild Parkinson's disease in which tremor was the predominant symptom and the patient had good cognitive functioning. Today, with the introduction of levodopa and decarboxylase inhibitors, the anticholinergics have been moved to second-line drugs. They are used as adjuncts when tremors remain a problem. Trihexyphenidyl is the only anticholinergic used as an adjunct to carbidopa/levodopa therapy.

There appears to be no difference among benztropine, trihexyphenidyl, and procyclidine with respect to efficacy. However, benztropine may have greater sedative effects than other anticholinergics. Trihexyphenidyl is more stimulating than the other drugs.

Dopamine Agonists Dopamine agonists produce acute antiparkinsonian effects equal to those of levodopa. However, studies of the efficacy of amantadine have conflicting results. Some health care providers note an initial decline in benefits followed by stabilization, whereas others report vast initial improvement. Except in a few patients, the effect of amantadine is minimal and wears off quickly.

Nevertheless, amantadine is rated as superior to anticholinergic drugs but inferior to levodopa in patient response. When levodopa is added to an amantadine regimen, there is a lower incidence of long-term adverse effects than with anticholinergic drugs. Improvements are noted for the first few months, but the patient returns to a baseline response in a short time.

Bromocriptine does not produce early, serious fluctuations or the "on-off" phenomenon as long as patients have not previously received levodopa. Dyskinesia is seen much less commonly and is less severe in patients taking bromocriptine alone. Bromocriptine may be added to a treatment regimen for a patient with unstable, fluctuating response patterns. It can also be used when additional intervention (e.g., alterations in dosage intervals or dosage reduction, use of sustained-release levodopa formulations) is ineffective in minimizing the fluctuations.

Pergolide is the newest dopamine agonist that in combination with carbidopa/levodopa may benefit patients with advanced Parkinson's disease. However, its adverse effects limit its use, so it should be used only by health care providers with extensive experience in the management of Parkinson's disease. When a patient is taking both levodopa and pergolide, the daily dosage of levodopa should be reduced and the additional relief of parkinsonian symptoms noted. A significant reduction in the long-term adverse effects of levodopa has also been observed with concurrent therapy.

Monoamine Oxidase B Inhibitor Selegiline can be added to levodopa therapy as an adjunct to antiparkinsonian therapy when the patient's condition deteriorates. Dosages of levodopa (with carbidopa) greater than 700 mg by mouth daily may be used. At doses higher than 20 to 25 mg, selegiline begins to lose its MAOB selectivity. Like the nonselective MAO inhibitors, selegiline can produce a potentially fatal hypertensive crisis. Reduction in levodopa dosage is usually not practical unless selegiline is added late in therapy.

Patient Variables

Parkinson's disease progresses from minimal dysfunction to severe disability in 3 to 10 years if left untreated. Treatment generally retards but will not completely halt progression of the disease. It may, however, prolong independent functioning and longevity by 5 to 15 years. Treatment is not warranted for patients with early, mild symptoms that produce no disability. Drug therapy is started when disability interferes with the patient's social, emotional, or work life.

Therapy for Parkinson's disease is life long. Persons with pre-existing cardiac or psychiatric illness are especially susceptible to the adverse effects of antiparkinsonian drugs. For some patients, the risks of adverse effects may outweigh the benefits of therapy. Patients are treated with each drug (increasing the dosages weekly) until either the desired effects are achieved or the adverse effects become intolerable. If a partial response is seen with the initial drug, the drug should be continued and additional drugs in the sequence added as needed.

Intervention

Administration

Blood pressure and pulse should be taken throughout the treatment regimen. This intervention is necessary because some of the antiparkinsonian drugs have a tendency to cause orthostatic hypotension and/or hypertension.

Dopaminergic Drugs Excessive gastric acidity can cause erratic gastric emptying and decrease the absorption of levodopa. Gastric emptying, and consequently the absorption of levodopa, can be accelerated by taking the drug with antacids or warm liquids and by chewing the tablets before swallowing. Food has less effect on the absorption of the controlled-release preparations than on that of the regular levodopa formulations, a benefit to patients with erratic absorption.

When carbidopa/levodopa capsules are opened or tablets crushed, the drug should be used immediately because levodopa oxidizes in the presence of moisture. Carbidopa/levodopa should be taken with food to minimize GI irritation.

It is thought that protein-restricted diets minimize the fluctuations (decreased response to levodopa at the end of each day or at various times of the day) that occur in some patients. Total dietary protein should be lowered from the average daily intake of 1.6 g/kg to the recommended daily allowance of 0.8 g/kg. Dietary protein may be divided into portions eaten throughout the day or may be consumed in the evening meal.

To alleviate the "on-off" phenomenon, the dose should be kept low or saved entirely for severe cases. The notion of "starting low and going slow" definitely applies to antiparkinsonian drugs. The use of "drug holidays" from levodopa may be dangerous and is generally not recommended. Abrupt cessation of levodopa therapy may precipitate a serious hyperpyretic state similar to neuroleptic malignant syndrome.

Overdose with levodopa is possible. The symptoms include muscle twitching, facial grimacing, eye twitching, exaggerated protrusion of the tongue, behavioral changes, and blepharospasm. Overdose of the levodopa drugs should be treated immediately with gastric lavage. The airway should be maintained and IV fluids given carefully.

Anticholinergic Drugs Anticholinergic drugs are taken by mouth with food or meals to minimize gastric irritation. The tablets may be crushed and administered with food if the patient has difficulty swallowing. The sustained-release capsules should not be broken, crushed, or chewed.

Excessive dosage of anticholinergics may cause dry mouth, burning sensation of the mouth, difficulty in swallowing, restlessness, tachycardia, increased respiration, muscle incoordination, dilated pupils, paralysis, tremors, seizures, hallucinations, and death. If overdosage is suspected, gastric lavage or induction of emesis followed by activated charcoal is the treatment of choice. Anticholinergic effects can be reversed by administering one of the anticholinesterase drugs physostigmine or neostigmine methylsulfate. Artificial respiration should be instituted for paralysis of respiratory muscles.

Dopamine Agonists Amantadine produces insomnia in some patients so it is best not administered near bedtime. Divided doses of this drug will help reduce the number of CNS adverse effects. Amantadine, bromocriptine, and pergolide may be taken with or following meals. Capsules may be opened for administration, if necessary.

A small initial dose of pergolide is used for patients older than 60 years. Close observation is needed because of such patients' greater susceptibility to adverse effects, including confusion, agitation, hallucinations, and postural hypotension.

Overdosage with dopamine agonists manifests as increased severity of adverse effects. The serum blood levels should be checked and the drug withheld or the dose lowered to maintain optimal effects. Acute overdosage is treated by induction of emesis or gastric lavage followed by activated charcoal.

Monoamine Oxidase B Inhibitor Selegiline is given as an adjunctive treatment with carbidopa/levodopa. The usual dose of 5 mg should be taken with breakfast and lunch. An attempt to reduce the dose of carbidopa/levodopa by 10 to 30 percent may be made after 2 to 3 days of selegiline therapy.

Education

Antiparkinsonian drugs should be taken as prescribed to achieve maximum therapeutic effects while minimizing adverse effects. The patient and family should be taught what the drug is, why it is being taken, the correct dosage, and the warning signs of adverse effects. The patient should be told not to abruptly discontinue the drug. A sudden withdrawal of the drug could cause a drastic increase in parkinsonian symptoms and deterioration of control. The patient should also be taught that if a dose is missed, a double dose should never be taken. It is better to wait 2 to 4 hours (depending on the drug) before taking the second dose.

The patient and the family should be taught that antiparkinsonian drugs may cause drowsiness or dizziness. The patient should avoid driving or other activities that require alertness until the response to the drug is known. The patient should be cautioned to make position changes slowly to minimize orthostatic hypotension. Also, the patient should be warned that perspiration may decrease, so that overheating could occur during hot weather. Patients should remain indoors in an air-conditioned environment during hot weather.

The patient should be advised to increase activity, bulk, and fluid in the diet as much as possible to minimize the constipating effects of the drugs. Further, the importance of maintaining a low-protein diet when taking carbidopa/levodopa should be taught. The daily protein intake can be divided among all meals, with the majority consumed in the evening. Most antiparkinsonian drugs are recommended to be taken with or shortly after food or milk to lessen GI irritation.

Instruct the patient that frequent rinsing of mouth, good oral hygiene, and use of sugarless gum or candy may decrease the dry mouth associated with antiparkinsonian drugs. The patient should notify the health care provider if dryness persists. Saliva substitutes may be required. A dentist should be notified if mouth dryness interferes with denture use. Also, the patient should apprise the dentist of the drug regimen before undergoing oral surgery or dental work. Giving a dose of meperidine for pain or sedation to a patient who is taking selegiline could be disastrous because the mechanism of action of selegiline is not clear.

Alcohol should be avoided by a patient taking antiparkinsonian drugs. The combined effects of the drug and alcohol may exaggerate the blood-pressure–lowering and sedative effects of the drug. Patients taking levodopa should avoid multivitamins, because vitamin B_6 (pyridoxine) interferes with the action of levodopa.

Patients should be informed that harmless darkening of urine and sweat may occur with some antiparkinsonian drugs. They should also be taught to monitor themselves for skin lesions that might be new or changed, which could indicate malignant melanoma.

Patients with diabetes who are taking carbidopa/levodopa should be taught to perform fingerstick glucose monitoring rather than testing of urine, because false results are possible with Clinitest and Ketostix.

Support groups and psychotherapy for patients with Parkinson's disease and their families have proved very beneficial. Patients should be encouraged to pursue as many of their pre-disease activities as possible.

Evaluation

The management of Parkinson's disease is guided by the impact of the patient's symptoms on activities of daily living. The patient should be seen at regular intervals, every 2 to 6 months, to monitor response to therapy and assess for adverse effects. Therapeutic effectiveness of antiparkinsonian therapy is noted as a decrease in symptoms. Therapeutic effects usually become evident after 2 to 3 weeks of therapy but may require up to 6 months in some patients.

Patients whose disease has not responded to 300 mg of levodopa (with carbidopa) taken four times daily are not likely to respond to higher dosages. If the patient reaches a daily dosage of 1200 mg of levodopa (with at least 75 mg of carbidopa) with no response, the diagnosis of Parkinson's disease should be revisited.

MYASTHENIA GRAVIS

Epidemiology and Etiology

Myasthenia gravis is a degenerative neurologic disease characterized, as its name implies, by "grave muscle weakness" (without atrophy). It presents as muscular weakness and fatigue that worsens with exercise and improves with rest. Although the weakness and easily fatigued extremities were identified in the 1600s, drug therapies were not discovered until the 1930s. The cause of myasthenia gravis is unknown, but 80 percent of people with the generalized form have elevated acetylcholine (ACh) antibody titers.

Myasthenia gravis may appear at any age, with two peaks of onset. Between the ages of 20 and 30 years, women are most often affected; after the age of 50 years, men are more often affected. Myasthenia gravis associated with a tumor of the thymus gland has a tendency to appear at a later age and is rare in patients younger than 30. The overall incidence of myasthenia gravis is 0.4 per 100,000. The prevalence is 0.5 to 5.0 per 100,000.

Pathophysiology

The functional physiologic defect of myasthenia gravis appears to be a lack of ACh or an excess of cholinesterase at the neuromuscular junction. Thus, nerve impulses fail to produce normal muscle contraction. Normal neuromuscular transmission is mediated by ACh stored within nerve terminals. In the presence of a nerve impulse, a large amount of ACh is released, resulting in depolarization and production of an action potential. The action potential travels along the muscle to cause contraction. In myasthenia gravis, the same amount of ACh is released, but receptor sites are blocked, either directly or indirectly, by immunoglobulin G antibodies (Fig. 23–2). The antibodies fix to receptor sites, blocking the binding of ACh. The electrical impulse to the muscle is diminished, thus causing a weak contraction.

The life of the ACh receptor is also diminished in myasthenia gravis, from a normal of 7 days to an average life span of 1 day. The body attempts to compensate by increasing the number of ACh receptors.

Types of Myasthenia Gravis

Five distinct types of myasthenia gravis have been identified: neonatal, congenital, juvenile, adult, and drug-induced.

The *neonatal* form appears in approximately 15 percent of children born to women with myasthenia gravis. It is secondary to passive transfer of myasthenia gravis–specific immunoglobulin G from the mother and is usually transient. Newborn infants have carried myasthenic symptoms for 7 to 14 days after birth. However, once antibodies in the blood are gone, symptoms also disappear. Interestingly, it is thought that these patients develop antibodies to their own ACh-activated ion channels, supporting the notion that myasthenia gravis is an autoimmune disorder. Myasthenia gravis can be life-threatening during the first 2 weeks after birth. It is characterized by generalized weakness with poor muscle tone, sucking ability, and cry. Respiratory depression and arrest may occur.

Congenital myasthenia gravis may be evident at birth as dysphagia, respiratory distress, and generalized muscle weakness. More commonly, the disease manifests during the first 2 years of life and is characterized by ptosis or ophthalmoplegia.

Juvenile myasthenia gravis is rare but closely resembles adult and drug-induced myasthenia gravis. *Drug-induced* myasthenia gravis can be caused by a number of different drugs (Table 23–6). The drugs trigger antibody production to ACh receptors in patients treated for rheumatic disorders. In approximately 70 percent of the patients who develop myasthenia gravis while taking the disease-modifying antirheumatic drug penicillamine, remission occurs within a year of stopping the drug.

Stages of Myasthenia Gravis

Stage 1 myasthenia gravis occurs the first 5 to 7 years of the disease. Symptoms involve extraocular muscles of the eye. *Ptosis* (drooping eyelids), blurred vision, and/or *diplopia* (double vision) are characteristic. Visual symptoms are found in approximately 50 percent of persons affected with myasthenia gravis. Ptosis is caused by paresis of the levator palpebrae superioris muscle. It can affect only one eyelid, with the disease limited to this muscle group. Bright sunlight can precipitate ptosis and blurred vision. The symptoms may subside for months or years, with relapses following remissions.

Stage 2 myasthenia gravis is divided into two substages, A and B, but is characterized by ocular manifestations. It

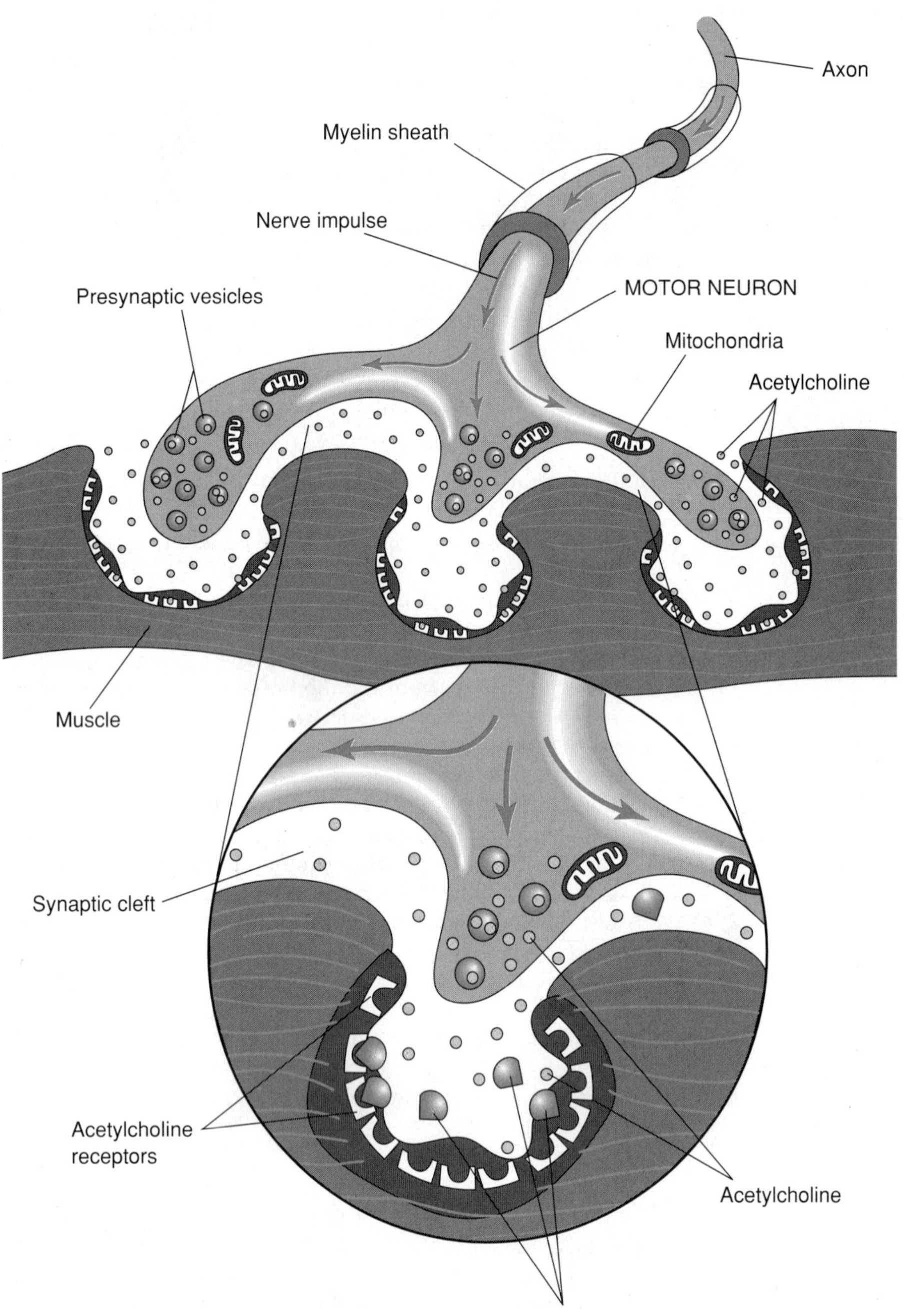

Figure 23–2 Myasthenia gravis. Synaptic vesicles normally contain large amounts of acetylcholine (ACh). ACh is released, accumulates within the synaptic cleft, and stimulates postsynaptic neurons. The result is a large depolarization and the production of an action potential. In myasthenia gravis, the same amount of ACh is present but it is not available to the membrane receiving the impulse. IgG antibodies fix to receptor sites in postsynaptic membranes and block the binding of acetylcholine. More ACh is exposed to acetylcholinesterase breakdown. The electrical impulse from the nerve to the muscle is diminished, and the muscle contraction is weak.

lasts about 15 years or to a point in the disease at which respiratory reserve diminishes. Temporary improvement may be achieved with immunosuppressive drugs. Stage 2 is more prevalent among males and responds best to corticosteroid drugs.

Stage 2A is mild and generalized, with slow progression. It is responsive to drug therapy. Muscle involvement in stage 2A comprises weakness of the facial and levator palpebrae muscles, giving the patient a masklike, expressionless appearance. The patient has droopy eyes and full lips with the underlip slightly everted. When the patient attempts to smile, a snarl appears instead. The jaw sags when muscles of mastication are involved. Further, the patient may hold a hand under the chin to support the head if flexor muscles of the neck are involved. Laryngeal muscle involvement results in a nasal sound to the voice or difficulty in articulation. Aphonia, an inability to produce vocal sounds, may develop with severe involvement.

Weakness of arm, hand, and leg muscles is seen in about 20 percent of newly diagnosed patients. The upper extremities are usually affected before the lower, and the proximal muscles before the distal. When muscles of respiration are affected, the patient has an impaired ability to cough and swallow, predisposing to aspiration and pneumonia.

Stage 2B is seen most often in the juvenile patient and is moderately generalized, with severe skeletal and bulbar involvement. Its response to drug therapy is less satisfactory.

Stage 3 of myasthenia gravis is termed the "burnout" stage. It is ordinarily reached 14 to 20 years after the onset of the disease. A stage 3 designation applies to patients who

TABLE 23–6 DRUGS KNOWN TO EXACERBATE MYASTHENIA GRAVIS

Antibiotics	Clindamycin Colistin Gentamicin Kanamycin Lincomycin Neomycin Oxytetracycline Polymyxin B Streptomycin Tetracyclines Tobramycin Trimethoprim-sulfamethoxazole
Disease-modifying antirheumatic drugs	Chloroquine D-Penicillamine
Anticonvulsants	Magnesium sulfate Phenytoin Trimethadione
Cardiovascular drugs	Beta blockers Calcium channel blockers Disopyramide Lidocaine Oxyprenolol Procainamide Quinine Quinidine
Hormonal drugs	ACTH Corticosteroids Oral contraceptives Thyroid hormones
Psychoactive drugs	Lithium Phenothiazides Chlorpromazine
Anesthetics	Chloroform Chlorprocaine Curare Ether Fluothane Halothane Tetracaine Trichloroethylene Tubocurarine
Sedatives	Antihistamines Barbiturates Opioids

have presented with the ocular symptoms but who rapidly progressed to severe disability and respiratory problems. There is a high incidence of muscular atrophy and reduced response to cholinesterase inhibitor drugs in this stage.

The clinical symptoms vary from patient to patient. The onset of symptoms in myasthenia gravis is usually insidious but may be sudden in some cases. Emotional upset, febrile illness, or even extreme physical exertion may precipitate onset of symptoms. Pregnancy and postpartum states are typical times when a woman may first experience symptoms. Another time might be when there is an abnormal response to a muscle relaxant used during general anesthesia.

Variability in the strength of voluntary muscles throughout the day is characteristic of myasthenia gravis. It may be worse in the morning or evening, with symptoms fluctuating in severity from day to day. Symptoms can be exacerbated by heat, stress, or repetitive tasks and may worsen during periods of menstruation, pregnancy, and infection. Simple tasks such as brushing the teeth or combing the hair may trigger muscle weakness, requiring the patient to stop and rest. Recovery after rest is often incomplete. Once the muscles are involved, the patient cannot perform sustained or repeated muscle contractions such as walking or keeping the eyelids open.

PHARMACOTHERAPEUTIC OPTIONS

Cholinesterase Inhibitors

- ❒ Ambenonium chloride (MYTELASE)
- ❒ Edrophonium chloride (ENLON, REVERSOL, TENSILON)
- ❒ Neostigmine (PROSTIGMIN)
- ❒ Pyridostigmine (MESTINON, REGONOL)
- ❒ Tacrine hydrochloride (COGNEX)

Indications

Cholinesterase inhibitors (i.e., anticholinesterase drugs) are used in the diagnosis and treatment of myasthenia gravis. They effectively and rapidly restore muscle strength in the majority of patients. Because the drugs do not increase the production of ACh, they are effective only as long as the transmitter is released at motor nerve endings and ACh receptors are intact. In stage 3 myasthenia gravis, this may not be so.

Edrophonium is useful primarily as a diagnostic aid in myasthenia gravis. A test dose is given and muscle strength assessed. If there is no improvement, a second dose is given. Improvement in muscle strength suggests the diagnosis of myasthenia gravis. Further, edrophonium and neostigmine are useful in determining whether a patient with confirmed myasthenia gravis is in cholinergic or myasthenic crisis. After a dose of the drug is given, the patient in cholinergic crisis becomes temporarily worse (a negative test), whereas the patient in myasthenic crisis has a temporary improvement in muscle strength (a positive test). Edrophonium has also been used in the treatment of supraventricular tachyarrhythmias. Tacrine hydrochloride is also used in the treatment of mild to moderate dementia of the Alzheimer's type.

Ambenonium has the potential for serious adverse effects; therefore, it is useful when the patient cannot tolerate pyridostigmine or neostigmine. Ambenonium is not a bromide salt, making it a better choice than either neostigmine or pyridostigmine for patients allergic to bromide.

Topical application of cholinesterase inhibitors is useful in improving the function of extraocular muscles and eyelids. The reversibly acting drugs may be alternated with mydriatics to break adhesions between the lens and the iris.

Cholinesterase inhibitors are also used to reverse the effects of nondepolarizing neuromuscular blocking drugs used in surgery. Neostigmine is used to reverse the effects of tubocurarine (see Chapter 16). Physostigmine is used to antagonize the toxic CNS effects of antimuscarinic drugs, tricyclic antidepressants, antihistamines, and benzodiazepines, and also to reduce the respiratory depressant, but not the analgesic, effects of opiates.

Pharmacodynamics

Cholinesterase inhibitors act by decreasing the amount of acetylcholinesterase, thereby stopping the destruction of available ACh. More ACh is available to the neuron for a longer time. The longer exposure time allows for increased interactions between ACh and the receptor sites that are not blocked.

Adverse Effects and Contraindications

Gastrointestinal and respiratory adverse effects are most common with cholinesterase inhibitors. Nausea, vomiting, abdominal cramps, diarrhea, excess salivation, dysphagia, and flatulence have been documented. Respiratory adverse effects may be potentially serious and include excessive oral, pharyngeal, and bronchial secretions. Bronchospasm, laryngospasm, dyspnea, and respiratory depression are most serious. Cardiovascular adverse effects are bradycardia, tachycardia, hypotension, electrocardiographic changes, atrioventricular block, nodal rhythms, and cardiac arrest in susceptible patients. The musculoskeletal, CNS, genitourinary, and dermatologic systems are also affected by cholinesterase inhibitors in a variety of ways. Miosis, lacrimation, hyperemia of conjunctiva, double vision, and visual changes have also been noted.

The cholinesterase inhibitors are contraindicated in the patient with mechanical obstruction of the GI or genitourinary tract, peritonitis, history of bromide sensitivity, urinary bladder outlet obstruction, or hypersensitivity. They should be used cautiously in patients with a history of ulcer disease, bronchial asthma, Parkinson's disease, epilepsy, cardiac disease, hypotension, bradycardia, and hyperthyroidism, and during lactation. When administered intravenously, these drugs may cause uterine irritability during the third trimester of pregnancy.

Pharmacokinetics

The clinical pharmacokinetics of cholinesterase inhibitors vary from drug to drug (Table 23–7). The drugs are lipid soluble and do not enter the CNS to affect central cholinergic function.

Ambenonium given by mouth has an onset of 20 to 30 minutes, with a duration of action of 3 to 8 hours. The bioavailability, peak action, and half-life are unknown.

The onset of action and duration of orally administered neostigmine is 2 to 4 hours. However, it is poorly absorbed from the GI tract, with a bioavailability of only 1 to 2 percent. When given IV, neostigmine is 100 percent bioavailable. The onset time is 10 to 30 minutes, with a duration of 2 to 4 hours. Neostigmine has a half-life of 0.4 to 1.2 hours. It is biotransformed in the liver and eliminated in the urine.

Pyridostigmine has an oral bioavailability of 10 to 20 percent, higher than that of neostigmine. Peak plasma levels of pyridostigmine occur 1 to 2 hours after oral administration, with a duration of action of 3 to 6 hours.

Edrophonium is short acting. Given intramuscularly (IM), it has an onset time of 2 to 10 minutes and a duration of 5 to 30 minutes. When this drug is given IV, the onset is very rapid—within 30 to 60 seconds—but the duration is only 5 to 10 minutes. Edrophonium is biotransformed in the liver, with a half-life of 5 to 10 minutes. The route of elimination is unknown.

Drug-Drug Interactions

Table 23–8 summarizes the drug-drug interactions of cholinesterase inhibitors. The drugs with the greatest interactions are atropine, guanethidine, procainamide, quinidine, and quinine. These drugs, when used concurrently, decrease the effect of the cholinesterase inhibitors. The actions of neostigmine may be antagonized by any drug that has anticholinergic properties (e.g., antihistamines, antidepressants). With concomitant alcohol use, weakness and unsteadiness are exacerbated.

Dosage Regimen

Dosage regimens for the cholinesterase inhibitors vary with the drug used (Table 23–9). Ambenonium is formulated as caplets. It is administered to adults at 5 mg three to four times daily. The dosage is increased every 1 to 2 days according to patient response. Children are given 0.3 mg/kg daily in divided doses, increasing to a maximum daily dose of 1.5 mg/kg.

TABLE 23–7 PHARMACOKINETICS OF SELECTED MYASTHENIA GRAVIS DRUGS

Agent	Route	Onset	Peak	Duration	PB (%)	t½	BioA (%)
Anticholinesterase Drugs							
Ambenonium	po	20–30 min	UK	3–8 hr	30	UK	UK
Edrophonium	IM	2–10 min	UK	5–30 min	UK	UK	UK
	IV	30–60 sec	UK	5–10 min	UK	UK	100
Neostigmine	po	45–75 min	UK	2–4 hr	15–25	40–60 min	1–2
	IM	10–30 min	20–30 min	2–4 hr	UK	50–90 min	UK
	IV	10–30 min	20–30 min	2–4 hr	UK	40–60 min	100
Pyridostigmine	po	30–45 min	UK	3–6 hr	UK	3–7 hr	11–17
	ER	30–60 min	UK	6–12 hr	UK	3–7 hr	UK
	IM	15 min	UK	2–4 hr	UK	3–7 hr	UK
	IV	2–5 min	UK	2–3 hr	UK	1–9 hr	100
Corticosteroid							
Prednisone	po	60 min	1–2 hr	1–2 days	70–75	3–4 hr	80–90
Immunosuppressants							
Azathioprine	po	Days–weeks	UK	Days–weeks	30	3–5 hr	30–90
Cyclosporine	po	UK	3.5 hr	UK	90	19–27 hr	10–60

UK, Unknown; ER, extended-release; BioA, bioavailability; PB, protein binding; t½, elimination half-life.

TABLE 23–8 DRUG-DRUG INTERACTIONS WITH SELECTED MYASTHENIA GRAVIS DRUGS

Drug	Interactive Drugs	Interaction(s)
Anticholinesterase Agents		
Neostigmine	Antihistamines	Action of neostigmine may be antagonized
Pyridostigmine	Antidepressants	
	Atropine	
	Haloperidol	
	Phenothiazines	
	Antiarrhythmic drugs	Neostigmine prolongs action
	Succinylcholine	
	Decamethonium	
Pyridostigmine	Demecarium	Additive toxicity
	Echothiophate	
	Isoflurophate	
	Quanadrel	Decreased antimyasthenic effects
	Guanethidine	
	Trimethophan	
Ambenonium	Aminoglycosides	Decreased action of ambenonium
	Anesthetics	
	Antiarrhythmics	
	Corticosteroids	
	Magnesium	
	Mecamylamine	
	Polymyxin B	
	Succinylcholine	
	Succinylcholine	Increased action of succinylcholine
Corticosteroid		
Prednisone	Barbiturates	Decreased action of prednisone
	Colestipol	
	Ephedrine	
	Phenytoin	
	Rifampin	
	Theophylline	
	Anticoagulants	Decreased effects of interacting drug
	Anticonvulsants	
	Antidiabetic agents	
	Cholinesterase inhibitors	
	Salicylates	
	Somatrem	
	Alcohol	Increased adverse effects of prednisone
	Amphotericin B	
	Cyclosporine	
	Digitalis	
	Diuretics	
	Indomethacin	
	Salicylates	
	Estrogens	Increased action of prednisone
	Ketoconazole	
	Indomethacin	
	Macrolide antibiotics	
	Oral contraceptives	
	Salicylates	
Immunosuppressive Drugs		
Azathioprine	Allopurinol	Inhibited metabolism of azathioprine
	Antineoplastics	Additive myelosuppression
	Myelosuppressive drugs	
Cyclosporine	Amphotericin B	Increased risk of nephrotoxicity
	Aminoglycosides	
	Erythromycin	
	Fluoroquinolones	
	Ketoconazole	
	NSAIDs	
	Melphalan	
	Sulfonamides	
	Anabolic steroids	Blood levels and risk of toxicity of cyclosporine are increased
	Calcium channel blockers	
	Cimetidine	
	Danazol	
	Erythromycin	
	Fluconazole	
	Ketoconazole	

Table continued on following page

TABLE 23–8 DRUG-DRUG INTERACTIONS WITH SELECTED MYASTHENIA GRAVIS DRUGS *Continued*

Drug	Interactive Drugs	Interaction(s)
Immunosuppressive Drugs *Continued*		
Cyclosporine	Miconazole	
Continued	Azathioprine	Additive immunosuppression
	Cyclophosphamide	
	Glucocorticoids	
	Verapamil	
	Barbiturates	May decrease the effect of cyclosporine
	Carbamazepine	
	Phenytoin	
	Rifampin	
	Sulfonamides	
	ACE inhibitors	Increased risk of hyperkalemia
	Potassium-sparing diuretics	
	Potassium supplements	
	Digoxin	Increased risk of digoxin toxicity
	Neuromuscular blocking drugs	Prolonged action of interactive drugs
	Imipenem/cilastatin	Increased risk of seizures
	Live virus vaccines	Decreased antibody response to interactive drug
	Lovastatin	Increased risk of rhabdomyolysis

ACE, Angiotension-converting enzyme; NSAIDs, nonsteroidal anti-inflammatory drugs.

Neostigmine is available in both tablet and injection. Because of its low bioavailability, 1 mg of neostigmine given parenterally is equivalent to 15 mg given orally. The usual initial dose for adults is 15 to 30 mg per day taken every 3 to 4 hours. Maintenance doses can be as high as 375 mg/day, if needed. Most patients with myasthenia gravis are maintained on 75 to 150 mg/day. The child's dose is half that for the adult.

Pyridostigmine is available as a syrup and as tablets and prolonged-action tablets. Adults initially receive 60 to 120 mg six to eight times daily, with a maintenance dose of up to 1500 mg/24 hours. The average daily dose is 600 mg/day. Prolonged-action tablets contain 180 mg of pyridostigmine, and the patient takes 540 mg once or twice a day. Children are given either the syrup or the tablets at a dose of 7 mg/kg/day given five to six times throughout the day.

Edrophonium is used for diagnostic purposes only. It is given IM or IV. The dosage used varies from 1 to 2 mg and may be repeated in 30 minutes if there is no response to the first dose. The dosage in children and infants varies according to the patient's weight.

Corticosteroids

Indications

Corticosteroids are useful in the patient with myasthenia gravis who is older than 50 years and cannot be managed with cholinesterase inhibitors, whose thymus gland has been removed, or who has pure ocular myasthenia gravis. These agents also benefit the patient with severe generalized myasthenia gravis. In many cases, the disease goes into remission and the possibility of relapse is minimized in response to corticosteroids.

The usual course of treatment extends over 2 years. Corticosteroids are customarily given in high doses initially, and then, when improvement is seen, the regimen is changed to alternate-day therapy. The dosage is gradually reduced to the smallest effective maintenance level in order to have fewest possible adverse effects. Corticosteroids are intended for short-term use, and it has been suggested that they are more beneficial in adolescents and young females.

Pharmacodynamics

Corticosteroids are thought to somehow protect ACh receptor sites from immunologic attack by immunoglobulin G, thus increasing the amount of ACh available at the site. Another hypothesis is that the drugs reduce the total number of circulating antibodies and the degradation of the receptor sites, thereby increasing the effectiveness of ACh. Overall, the corticosteroid drugs suppress the patient's immune response.

Adverse Effects and Contraindications

The adverse effects of adrenal corticosteroids are many and varied, and some may be life threatening. Chapter 52 contains a thorough discussion of the corticosteroids.

Corticosteroids are contraindicated in active, untreated infections, because these drugs mask infection. They are also contraindicated in patients who are lactating or who have psychoses, Cushing's syndrome, active tuberculosis, congestive heart failure, varicella, or peptic ulcer disease. These drugs should be used cautiously during pregnancy and in children, because their safety has not been established. Corticosteroids should also be used cautiously in patients with diabetes, hypertension, chronic nephritis, seizure disorders, hepatic or renal disorders, and thrombophlebitis.

Pharmacokinetics

Corticosteroids are well absorbed when taken orally. The onset of action for oral prednisone is approximately 1 hour,

TABLE 23–9 DOSAGE REGIMENS FOR SELECTED MYASTHENIA GRAVIS DRUGS			
Drug	**Use(s)**	**Dosage**	**Implications**
Cholinesterase Inhibitors			
Ambenonium	Improvement of muscle strength in myasthenia gravis	*Initial:* 5 mg po TID–QID. Increase dose every 1–2 days as needed.	Drug of choice for patients allergic to bromide
Edrophonium	Diagnosis of myasthenia gravis Differentiation of myasthenic from cholinergic crisis	*Adult:*2 mg IV initially. If no response, give 8 mg more. May repeat in 30 minutes. *Child 34 kg:* 1 mg IV. If no response, give 1 mg q30–45 min to a total of 10 mg *Child > 34 kg:* 2 mg IV. If no response, give 1 mg q30–45 min to a total of 10 mg	Patient may feel flushed, dizzy, hypotensive immediately after injection If cholinergic response occurs, give atropine
Neostigmine	Improvement of muscle strength in myasthenia gravis Reversal of neuromuscular nondepolarizing neuromuscular blockers	*Adult:* 15–30 mg po initially in divided doses *or* 0.5–2 mg q1–3 hr IM/IV Maintentance: 75–150 mg/day. May go as high as 375 g/day *Child:* 2 mg/kg/day in divided doses	Dose may be increased daily until desired response achieved
Pyridostigmine	Improvement of muscle strength in myasthenia gravis Reversal of nondepolarizing neuromuscular blockers	*Adult:* 60–120 mg po initially 6–8 times/day *or* 2 mg IM/IV. May repeat q2 hr. Average dose: 600 mg/day. Maintenance doses up to 1500 mg daily *Child:* 7 mg/kg/day in 5–6 divided doses	Dose may be increased daily until desired response achieved
Corticosteroid			
Prednisone	Adjunct in treatment of myasthenia gravis	*Adult:* 20–25 mg po daily	Alternative-day therapy or a single daily dose may be used for maintenance Dosage should be tapered when being discontinued
Immunosuppressive Drugs			
Azathioprine	Myasthenia gravis	*Adult:* 1 mg/kg/day. Maximum dose of 2.5 mg/kg/day	Contraceptive use is recommended for up to 12 weeks after therapy is discontinued
Cyclosporine		*Adult:* 14–18 mg/kg/day po *or* 5–6 mg/kg/day IV. Maintenance dose is 5–10 mg/kg/day	Microemulsion products (NEORAL) and other formulations of cyclosporine (SANDIMMUNE) are not interchangeable

peak drug levels being reached within 1 to 2 hours. The duration of the drug's action may be as long as 1 to 2 days. Prednisone is biotransformed in the liver to prednisolone and has a half-life of more than 200 minutes.

In contrast, when prednisone is given IM, it is absorbed very slowly from the injection site and produces a duration of action of up to 4 weeks. Prednisone is about three to five times more potent than cortisone or hydrocortisone.

Drug-Drug Interactions

Table 23–8 lists the drug-drug interactions of the corticosteroid drugs. These drugs may have additive or antagonistic effects when combined with many other drugs. A patient with diabetes who is taking a corticosteroid may develop hyperglycemia and may need to adjust antidiabetic drug dosage. The dose of prednisone may have to be increased for a patient who is also taking an antacid, a barbiturate, phenytoin, or rifampin.

Prednisone taken concurrently with an oral anticoagulant increases the effect of the anticoagulant. Hypoprothrombinemia results. This combination also increases the risk of hemorrhage owing to the vascular effects of the corticosteroids.

Women using oral contraceptives should be warned that corticosteroids can cause a loss of contraceptive action. In addition, estrogen increases the anti-inflammatory effect of corticosteroids by reducing its breakdown in the liver.

Dosage Regimen

The dosage of corticosteroids is highly individualized and based on patient response. A patient may respond better to one type of corticosteroid than to another. Treatment should always start with the minimum effective dose for the shortest time. Long-term use of corticosteroids has the potential for serious adverse effects.

The oral dosage of prednisone is 2.5 to 15 mg two to four times daily (see Table 23–9). The maintenance dose may be given as a single daily dose or every other day. The dose is gradually decreased by 5 to 10 mg every 4 to 5 days to establish a maintenance dose. Children are given 0.1 to 0.15 mg/kg daily. Dosage should be gradually tapered when the drug is being discontinued. Corticosteroids should never be abruptly withdrawn.

Laboratory Considerations

The corticosteroid drugs play havoc with laboratory test results. The corticosteroids decrease the white blood cell count, as well as serum potassium, calcium, uric acid, protein-bound iodine, and thyroxine concentrations. On the other hand, they may increase serum glucose (especially in patients with diabetes), amylase, sodium, cholesterol, and lipid values. Males may have a decrease in sperm production and count when taking corticosteroids.

Immunosuppressants

❒ Azathioprine (IMURAN)
❒ Cyclosporine (SANDIMMUNE)

Indications

Although approved by the Federal Drug Administration for use in myasthenia gravis, immunosuppressive therapy with azathioprine is directed toward reducing antireceptor antibody production. Azathioprine is also useful for myasthenia gravis that is not responsive to corticosteroids. Cyclosporine is useful in patients with myasthenia gravis in whom corticosteroid drug therapy and azathioprine treatment are limited by the adverse effects and/or the lack of improvement.

Pharmacodynamics

Azathioprine is an analog of the antineoplastic drug mercaptopurine. In myasthenia gravis, it appears to affect T-cell proliferation and the synthesis of antibodies.

Cyclosporine is a fungal peptide with potent immunosuppressive activity. It inhibits normal immune responses by inhibiting interleukin-2, a factor necessary for initiation of cytotoxic T-cell activity. It inhibits both T helper cell and T suppressor cell activity.

Adverse Effects and Contraindications

Azathioprine therapy is limited by its adverse effects, the most serious and limiting of which is bone marrow suppression. Symptoms common to bone marrow suppression include macrocytic anemia, thrombocytopenia, pancytopenia, and leukocytopenia. Bruising and bleeding may also occur as a result. Allergic reactions to azathioprine include rashes and serum sickness. Azathioprine can cause mild taste alterations when given IV.

Cyclosporine's most common adverse effects are tremor, gingival hyperplasia, diarrhea, hypertension, renal dysfunction, hirsutism, and acne. Hepatotoxicity can be life threatening. This drug is contraindicated in patients who have a hypersensitivity to cyclosporine and polyoxyethylated castor oil, are lactating, or are using potassium-sparing diuretics. Caution should be used in administering cyclosporine to patients with hepatic and renal problems, untreated infections, and malabsorption disorders as well as during pregnancy. The agent's safety and efficacy in children have not been established.

Immunosuppressant drugs are contraindicated in pregnancy unless the potential benefits outweigh the risks. Long-term use of immunosuppressants in children decreases growth and development. Further, the drugs mask signs of infection (fever, inflammation). With long-term use of such drugs, the patient's adrenal function can become suppressed, leading to hypotension, weight loss, weakness, nausea and vomiting, anorexia, lethargy, confusion, and restlessness.

Pharmacokinetics

Azathioprine is readily absorbed from the GI tract, with a bioavailability of 80 to 90 percent. Thirty percent of the drug is bound to plasma proteins. The onset of action of oral azathioprine is at 6 to 8 weeks, with a peak of 12 weeks (see Table 23–9). It is biotransformed to mercaptopurine and metabolites. Azathioprine is eliminated through the kidneys, with minimal elimination of unchanged drug.

Cyclosporine is erratically absorbed after oral administration but is widely distributed to extracellular fluid and blood cells. The plasma peak level is reached 3½ hours after administration, although absorption may be delayed or impaired by food. This drug crosses the placenta and enters breast milk. Cyclosporine is biotransformed by the liver, and the inactive metabolites are eliminated mainly through the bile. The half-life is approximately 19 hours in adults and 7 hours in children.

Drug-Drug Interactions

Azathioprine is partially metabolized by xanthine oxidase. Allopurinol, an inhibitor of this enzyme, increases the potential for toxicity by decreasing the biotransformation of azathioprine in the liver. The dosage of azathioprine should be reduced by 75 percent when allopurinol is taken concurrently. The effects of tubocurarine are decreased. After prolonged therapy with corticosteroids, muscle wasting may occur. Myelosuppression increases in a patient taking both azathioprine and other antineoplastic or myelosuppressive drugs. Captopril, when given concurrently with azathioprine, worsens the patient's leukopenia. Erythromycin increases the absorption of azathioprine.

Cyclosporine interacts with many drugs. Nephrotoxicity may occur when this drug is given concurrently with any nephrotoxic drugs such as amphotericin B or any of the nonsteroidal anti-inflammatory drugs (NSAIDs). Drugs that reduce biotransformation of cyclosporine (e.g., diltiazem, verapamil) increase the concentration of cyclosporine. The risk of lymphoma and immunosuppression rises when cyclosporine is taken with other immunosuppressants. Corticosteroids increase immunosuppression through the suppression of lymphocytes. Infection and malignancy may also occur with the concurrent use of the corticosteroids.

Dosage Regimen

The recommended maintenance dose of azathioprine in an adult or child is 1 mg/kg/day, with a maximum dose of 2.5 mg/kg/day (see Table 23–9). Actual dosage is based on patient response. Intermittent parenteral azathioprine is infused at 20 mg/mL over 20 to 60 minutes.

Adults and children should initially take 14–18 mg/Kg/day of cyclosporine orally, or 5–6 mg/kg/day IV. A change to an oral formulation as soon as possible is recommended. The maintenance dosage is 5–10 mg/kg/day. Children may require larger or more frequent dosing because of faster clearance.

Laboratory Considerations

Azathioprine specifically affects renal, hepatic, and hematologic functions. Serum and urine uric acid and plasma albumin all may fall. Increases in serum alkaline phosphatase, bilirubin, aspartate aminotransferase (serum glutamic-oxaloacetic transaminase), alanine aminotransferase (serum glutamate-pyruvate transaminase), and amylase all signal hepatotoxicity. Bone marrow depression may be suspected when there is a decrease in hemoglobin. A leukocyte count less than 3000/mm^3 or a platelet count less than 100,000/mm^3 may indicate the need to decrease dosage.

Serum drug levels should be evaluated frequently when a patient is taking cyclosporine. Keeping serum trough levels between 250 and 800 mcg/mL or plasma levels between 50 and 300 mcg/mL per 24 hours after a dose is given has been shown to lessen adverse effects.

Laboratory studies that may be affected when the patient is taking cyclosporine are BUN, total bilirubin, serum creatinine, uric acid, alkaline phosphatase, serum potassium, cholesterol, low-density lipoprotein, and apolipoprotein B. Laboratory values for all these tests will be increased.

Critical Thinking Process

Assessment

History of Present Illness

The medical history is important for the patient in whom myasthenia gravis is suspected. Often, the exacerbations are precipitated by factors such as stress, infection, menstruation, and pregnancy. The patient's and family's description of symptoms is important, along with the duration of the symptoms. There may be some deviations from normal voice, eye, and facial function.

The patient may complain of symptoms that interfere with day-to-day activities and of the need for frequent rest periods. The examiner should ask the patient to identify the specific areas or body parts that are weak. When the weakness started (slowly or suddenly), its progress, whether it affects one or both sides of the body, and whether it interferes with activities such as combing hair, eating, swallowing, or walking should also be investigated.

Past Health History

The past health history is important in identifying factors that have contributed to the current state of the patient's health. The health care provider should elicit information regarding past operations, anesthetics received, allergies, history of exposure to toxins or food, and the reaction noted. Past drug and alcohol use, history of rheumatoid arthritis, and any vision changes within the past few years are important to note.

Physical Exam Findings

Patients with myasthenia gravis present with a characteristic picture. The health care provider should note the presence of a nasal voice or aphonia, changes in facial expressions, ptosis, or a snarl instead of a smile. A sagging jaw and an inability to hold up the head suggest the presence of neck muscle involvement.

The temperature, pulse, respiration, and blood pressure should be checked. A patient's inability to hold the thermometer in the mouth without help is relevant. The ability to chew and swallow should be evaluated. An important clue to dietary problems may be any weight loss experienced over the past few months. An eye exam contributes valuable information as to whether the patient has ocular palsy.

Any muscle weakness during the physical exam should be noted. The health care provider should distinguish between proximal and distal weakness. Does the patient tire easily after performing a simple act such as combing hair? If leg muscles are involved, the health care provider should evaluate the risk of falls by noting the gait.

It is important to note any weakness of cough, attacks of dyspnea following exertion, difficulty clearing the respiratory tract, and skin color changes. In severe disease, respiratory muscle weakness may lead to ventilatory failure.

Diagnostic Testing

Pulmonary function tests, nerve conduction tests, and nerve stimulation tests are helpful in determining the baseline status. Laboratory testing should include a lupus screen (to rule out lupus erythematosus); tests for antinuclear antibodies, rheumatoid factor, and antithyroglobulin antibodies; a tuberculin test; and a fasting blood sugar measurement. Approximately 5 percent of patients with myasthenia gravis have thyrotoxicosis. Serum anti–ACh receptor antibody titers may be elevated.

In most cases, the diagnosis of myasthenia gravis is obvious from the history and physical exam findings. However, edrophonium testing can confirm the diagnosis of myasthenia gravis and help monitor for worsening of symptoms. The procedure for edrophonium testing is as follows:

- A 2-mg dose of edrophonium is given IV.
- The patient is observed for an increase in muscle strength within 1 to 3 minutes.
- If no response occurs, another 8 to 10 mg of edrophonium is given over the next 2 minutes.
- Muscle strength is again assessed. If an increase in the muscle strength occurs within 10 to 30 seconds, myasthenia gravis is diagnosed.

Immediately following the edrophonium dose, the patient may complain of feeling dizzy, flushed, or faint and may experience a drop in blood pressure. However, because the drug action is short-lived, these effects rarely last longer than 5 minutes.

Electromyography is helpful in demonstrating the fatigability of affected muscles. A 10 percent or more decrease in amplitude during progressive stimulation generally indicates defective neuromuscular transmission.

Approximately 10 to 15 percent of persons with myasthenia gravis have a tumor of the thymus gland. Routine anteroposterior and lateral chest x-ray studies, chest computed tomography, and, possibly, magnetic resonance imaging have been useful in identifying a thymoma.

Developmental Considerations

Perinatal The pregnant patient with myasthenia gravis should be in the care of a neurologist who specializes in neuromuscular disease. No specific effects of pregnancy on myasthenia gravis have been documented; however, either significant improvement in symptoms or drastic worsening may occur. Labor proceeds as in the nonmyasthenic patient. Sedatives and opioid analgesics should be used sparingly and with careful measurement of vital capacities. The obstetrician should have injectable cholinesterase inhibitors avail-

Case Study Myasthenia Gravis

Patient History

History of Present Illness	DD is a 56-year-old white man in moderate distress with complaints of blurred vision and an inability to open his left eye. It was first noticed when he returned home from sailing 2 days ago. Reports bright sunlight worsens the "droopy eyelid." He has noticed more fatigue recently than in the past. He states, "I'm just getting older." He jogs 2 miles/day, down from 5 miles/day 3 months ago. He follows a low-cholesterol diet.
Past Health History	DD is allergic to aspirin and penicillin. He has no food allergies. His last physical exam was 1 year ago. He denies hospitalizations but has been told he has borderline high cholesterol. He denies history of alcohol, smoking, or drugs. He is currently taking no routine medications.
Physical Exam	*Height:* 5′11″. *Weight:* 165 lb (no recent weight loss or gain). VSS. *Lg. Snellen:* 20/200 corrected OU; ptosis of left eye noted. *Neuromuscular:* Weakness noted in lifting and movement of the left shoulder only. Remainder of exam unremarkable.
Diagnostic Testing	Edrophonium test positive—shoulder felt much better with improved strength and less ptosis, diplopia. CT of chest and chest x-ray negative for thymoma. EKG: sinus bradycardia at a rate of 56 bpm. Anti–ACh receptor antibody titer elevated.
Developmental Considerations	DD is 56 years old with age-related physiologic changes to body systems. He has had no disabilities until recently.
Psychosocial Considerations	DD is currently working as the manager of a local discount store. He is married, and his wife is in excellent health. He is very health conscious and visits his physician semiannually for a complete physical.
Economic Factors	DD has access to both the medical facility and the pharmacy. He is able to drive without difficulty and has a late model automobile. He has excellent health insurance through his employer. His prescriptions require a $10 co-pay.

Variables Influencing Decision

Treatment Objectives	• Alleviate current ocular problems and muscular weakness and worsening fatigue. • Achieve maximal benefit (muscle strength and endurance) with least adverse effects.

Drug Variables	*Drug Summary*	*Patient Variables*
Indications	Myasthenia gravis	DD diagnosed with stage 1 myasthenia gravis. This will become a decision point.
Pharmacodynamics	Cholinesterase inhibitors stop destruction of available ACh. Corticosteroids protect receptors from destruction by immunoglobulin G. Immunosuppressants depress immune response.	This may be a decision point owing to the early stage of the disease.
Adverse Effects/ Contraindications	All three drug groups have a variety of troublesome as well as serious adverse effects.	This is not a decision point, because all drug classes have a broad variety of adverse effects.

Case Study Myasthenia Gravis—cont'd

Drug Variables	Drug Summary	Patient Variables
Pharmacokinetics	Vary with the individual drug. Most are eliminated through the urine.	This may be a decision point because of the variety of onset times. Biotransformation and excretion variables are not a decision point.
Dosage Regimen	Follow manufacturer's recommendations and patient response.	DD is able to take drugs orally at this time. Knowledgeable and expected to be compliant with drug regimen at this time. This is not a decision point at this time.
Laboratory Considerations	All three drug groups are biotransformed in the liver and excreted through the urine. Liver and renal function testing would be appropriate.	This will not be a decision point because DD is an otherwise healthy male and sees the health care provider on a routine basis.
Cost Index*	Pyridostigmine: 2 Prednisone: 1 Azathioprine: 5 Cyclosporine: 5	Because DD's drugs are available for a $10 copay, this will not be a decision point.

Summary of Decision Points

- Pyridostigmine is the initial drug of choice for nonprogressive eye muscle weakness and mild limb muscle weakness.
- Pyridostigmine, coupled with prednisone, increases the possibility of remission.

DRUGS TO BE USED

- Pyridostigmine 600 mg po in divided dosages spaced to provide maximum relief. Optimal control may require supplementation with the more rapidly acting syrup.
- Low-dose prednisone based on patient response to pyridostigmine.

*Cost Index:

1 = $<30/mo.
2 = $ 30–40/mo.
3 = $ 40–50/mo.
4 = $ 50–60/mo.
5 = $ >60/mo.

AWP of 100, 60-mg tablets of pyridostigmine is approximately $39.
AWP of 100, 5-mg tablets of prednisone is approximately $3.
AWP of 100, 50-mg tablets of azathioprine is approximately $120.
AWP of 30, 50-mg tablets of cyclosporine is approximately $81.

able in case of myasthenic crisis and for use during labor, when nausea may preclude oral administration.

The second stage of labor is associated with muscle fatigue and increased risk of myasthenic crisis. The vaginal route is the preferred method of delivery. Cesarean section is thought to be too stressful, with the potential to precipitate myasthenic crisis. An epidural anesthetic is best to decrease fatigue and provide adequate anesthesia.

Pediatric It is very rare for a myasthenic mother to have more than one child affected with the disease. Neonatal myasthenia gravis develops in approximately 10 to 12 percent of babies born of myasthenic mothers. No prenatal prognostic factors or test has yet identified babies at risk for this problem. The pediatrician should be equipped with full resuscitation equipment at birth, and the child should be closely monitored for 12 to 72 hours. The infant may have poor muscle tone and a weak cry and may be unable to take a bottle because of a decrease in muscle tone. Breastfeeding, however, is not advised, because the antibodies of myasthenia gravis cross into the breast milk. Breastfeeding prolongs the myasthenic state for the neonate.

Geriatric The older adult is not immune to myasthenia gravis, although the disease is more likely to have been diagnosed earlier in life. However, older adults are more prone to complications and more frequent crisis situations than younger populations. Stress factors tending to precipitate crisis in the older adult include complications of immobility, fractures secondary to falls, sepsis, pneumonia, and a generalized poor state of health.

The natural decline of kidney function in the aging adult warrants the administration of smaller drug dosages to prevent drug accumulation. Further, some patients may not have the mental capacity and/or proper vision to take the drug as scheduled and in the proper dosage.

Psychosocial Considerations

A patient's adjustment to myasthenia gravis depends on the extent of loss of independence, the resultant body changes, and the mere nature of the disease. Factors such as age, gender, available support systems, and occupation all play important roles in the patient's ability to cope with the disease. Social adjustment may change dramatically over the course of the disease from minimal to overall maximal adjustment.

The generalized weakness and fatigue associated with myasthenia gravis contribute to social isolation and changes in body image. Neck and shoulder muscle weakness and loss of fine motor control add to the problem. The patient may become frustrated with the changes. Rest is critical after periods of activity (see Case Study—Myasthenia Gravis).

Analysis and Management

Treatment Objectives

The primary treatment objective does not include a cure for myasthenia gravis. Rather, the objective is to achieve the maximum muscle strength and endurance possible with the fewest adverse effects (excessive salivation, sweating, nausea, diarrhea, abdominal cramps, or tachycardia).

Treatment Options

Drug Variables

Because cholinesterase inhibitors provide only transient, symptomatic relief of myasthenia gravis, they are of limited use in most cases of moderate to severe disease. Pyridostigmine is the initial drug of choice for nonprogressive eye muscle weakness and mild limb muscle weakness. Use of pyridostigmine in conjunction with prednisone increases the possibility of remission and is probably the best treatment regimen.

Corticosteroid drugs (usually prednisone) are widely used in the management of myasthenia gravis. These agents reduce the levels of serum ACh receptor antibodies. However, clinical improvement can occur even when there is no significant decrease in antibody levels. Corticosteroids can temporarily worsen symptoms; however, such a response is followed by gradual improvement in muscle strength. Once peak improvement is reached and maintained for several weeks, the dosage of both prednisone and cholinesterase inhibitor may be gradually decreased to the smallest effective maintenance level. A low-maintenance dose of alternate-day prednisone may be effective for many months or years.

Immunosuppressant drugs are useful in reducing corticosteroid requirements and can produce improvement or remission when used alone. Immunosuppressives are believed to be slightly less toxic overall than long-term corticosteroid therapy. Use of immunosuppressives prevents prolonged use of cholinesterase inhibitors, promotes remission, and minimizes the possibility of relapse. When azathioprine is used in combination with corticosteroids, a lower corticosteroid dose may be given, reducing the adverse effects of corticosteroids.

Remission can occur in 30 to 50 percent of patients treated with azathioprine, although the benefits may take 3 months to appear and a year to maximize. It is common to administer this drug to a patient with advanced myasthenia gravis for 12 to 36 months to prevent a relapse of symptoms.

Cyclosporine is used for patients in whom the corticosteroids and immunosuppressive therapy are limited by adverse effects and/or lack of optimal response. Its benefit is similar to that of azathioprine, but cyclosporine acts more promptly, usually within 1 to 3 months.

Patient Variables

The myasthenic stage and the extent of disability determine the therapeutic regimen. The drug regimen for each patient is individualized and is developed on a trial-and-error basis for the most part. The optimal dose and administration schedule will fluctuate during periods of stress.

Like therapy for Parkinson's disease, therapy for myasthenia gravis is life long. A treatment regimen for myasthenia gravis should be planned around the patient's life-style and disability. Persons with pre-existing neuromuscular disorders are especially susceptible to the adverse effects of drugs used for myasthenia gravis. Even the most perfect drug regimen is ineffective if the patient is unable or unwilling to comply with the therapy because of its impact on life-style.

The postpartum period may be associated with exacerbations of myasthenia gravis. Drug dosages need to be adjusted as the mother returns to her pre-pregnant state. Breastfeeding is not advised for patients with a myasthenic exacerbation, for those receiving high doses of cholinesterase inhibitors, and for those with high circulating antibody titers.

Children with seizure disorders, bronchial asthma, urinary tract infections, or severely impaired kidney function should use myasthenia gravis drugs with caution. The dosage and administration schedule must be modified for such patients.

Blood pressure and vital signs should be checked for all myasthenia gravis patients before beginning any drug therapy and periodically thereafter. The presence of either hypotension or hypertension helps determine whether one drug is better than another. Elevation in temperature may indicate an infection, thus contraindicating the use of an immunosuppressant drug at that time.

Intervention

Administration

The importance of taking an antimyasthenic drug as prescribed cannot be overstated. The risk of a myasthenic crisis or cholinergic crisis increases with improper dosing or with improper administration. All drugs used in the management of myasthenia gravis should be taken with food or milk. Doses should be evenly spaced to minimize gastric distress and adverse effects. In older adults, it is often helpful to have a family member oversee the treatment regimen.

Myasthenic crisis is the sudden onset of muscular weakness. It can be caused by a late dose or inadequate dosing with an cholinesterase-inhibiting drug. Symptoms are noted

TABLE 23–10 COMPARISON OF CHOLINERGIC AND MYASTHENIC CRISES

	Cholinergic Crisis	Myasthenic Crisis
Cause	Excessive cholinesterase inhibitor drug	Insufficient cholinesterase inhibitor drug
Signs and symptoms	Nausea, vomiting, diarrhea, abdominal cramps, blurred vision, pallor, facial muscle twitching, pupillary miosis, hypotension	Tachycardia, tachypnea, elevated blood pressure, anoxia, cyanosis, bladder and bowel incontinence, decreased urinary output, absence of cough or swallow reflexes

approximately 3 hours after the dose was due (Table 23–10). Myasthenic crisis manifests as an inability to swallow or speak; weakness of respiratory, laryngeal, pharyn-geal and bulbar muscles; and sudden respiratory distress. The patient in myasthenic crisis is in danger of respiratory arrest. Extreme quadriparesis or quadriplegia may also be noted.

Symptoms of *cholinergic crisis* arise within 1 hour of an excessive dose of a cholinesterase inhibitor. The clinical picture is much like that of myasthenic crisis but includes other symptoms. Intestinal motility increases, with episodes of diarrhea and complaints of cramping. Fasciculations, bradycardia, pupillary constriction, increased salivation, and increased sweating are noted. As in myasthenic crisis, the patient is at risk for respiratory arrest. Testing with edrophonium may determine whether the patient is in myasthenic or cholinergic crisis.

Antimyasthenic drugs given IV are fast acting and peak very quickly compared with those given by mouth. Before drug administration, it is important that the patency of the IV line be double checked. The concentration of the solution, administration time, possible drug-drug interactions, and the desired patient response are also important.

Education

Patients with myasthenia gravis and their families should be taught strategies that facilitate chewing and swallowing and thus help prevent weight loss and aspiration. Remaining upright while eating, using thick liquids, and eating a soft diet all reduce the risk of aspiration. Small, frequent meals with high-calorie snacks may help minimize weight loss. Patients should be encouraged to take small bites and eat slowly. As the disease worsens, patients may require tube feedings.

Impaired verbal communication is often an area of frustration. It may be necessary to identify effective communication strategies before impairment becomes severe. The patient may be taught to lip read or to use sign language or an erasable board.

Visual difficulties compound the other problems. Ptosis and ocular palsy lead to the patient's inability to close the eyes, increasing the risk of corneal abrasions. If necessary, the patient should be taught to use a patch and shield to protect the eyes. The eyes also have a tendency for excessive dryness. Artificial tears can be used to keep the eyes moist. Alternating eye patches may help to relieve diplopia.

The patient and family should be taught to identify measures that will help prevent or modify fatigue and to incorporate those measures into daily activities. The patient should be assisted in planning to alternate activities with periods of rest. Activities that can be completed in short periods of time or divided into several segments are desirable; for example, read one chapter of a book at a time, or avoid scheduling two energy-draining activities for the same day. Conserving energy through rest, planning, and priority setting helps prevent or alleviate fatigue.

The patient and family should be informed of the names of the drugs prescribed along with the dose, the benefits, and the possible adverse effects. Proper administration technique for the dosage form should be stressed to both patient and family. They should also be taught to recognize symptoms of cholinergic and myasthenia gravis crises. The importance of taking drugs on time—not too late or too early—and how to intervene in a crisis situation should also be explained.

Both patients and families should be aware that it may take weeks or months before the full benefits of a particular drug are seen. Patients should be advised to avoid immunizations while taking immunosuppressants, which decrease the effectiveness of any therapy that enhances immunity.

Women of childbearing age and their partners should be instructed that immunosuppressant drugs may interfere with the effectiveness of contraceptives. Safe use of immunosuppressant drugs during pregnancy has not been established. Further, women should be advised to avoid conception for at least 4 months after drug therapy with immunosuppressants.

If extended-release formulations are prescribed, the patient should be instructed not to crush the tablets or to take them less often than every 6 hours. The patient should also be advised not to take other drugs without first contacting the health care provider, in order to avoid or minimize potential drug interactions.

Further, the patient should be advised to wear a form of "medical alert" identification and to carry written information regarding their prescribed drugs and dosages. It is also important for the patient to carry a list of drugs contraindicated for persons with myasthenia gravis (see Table 23–6). Patients and families can be referred to local, state, and/or national myasthenia gravis support groups for additional information.

Evaluation

Drug therapy for myasthenia gravis is considered successful if the patient experiences improved muscle strength and endurance with few troublesome adverse effects. The highest possible level of functioning should be achieved. The patient and family should be able to identify community resources that will help them maintain an effective level of functioning. The patient should also be able to identify measures that will help prevent or modify fatigue.

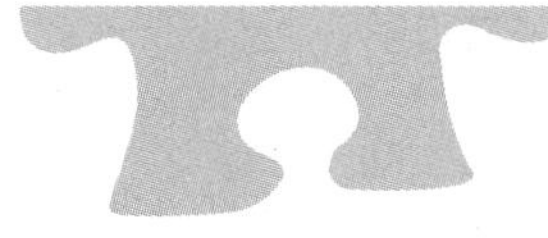

SUMMARY

- Epidemiologic data suggest vascular, viral, and metabolic factors as possible causes of Parkinson's disease. The possibility of an environmental contributor, such as toxins found in the workplace or used in industry, is also being explored.
- Parkinson's disease is characterized by a large deterioration of neurons within the basal ganglia. These neurons are normally needed to synthesize the neurotransmitter dopamine.
- Diagnosis of Parkinson's disease is based on the history and physical exam. There are no laboratory tests to confirm or refute the clinical diagnosis.
- Treatment is aimed at abolishing, as far as possible, the symptoms and disabilities caused by the disease.
- There is no universal antiparkinsonian drug; therefore, there is no single drug to alleviate all symptoms and disabilities.
- Drugs are given by trial and error until the most effective drug that exhibits the fewest adverse effects is found.
- Dopaminergic drugs such as levodopa and combination carbidopa/levodopa are generally the drugs of choice for initial therapy.
- Anticholinergic drugs are useful for patients with minimal symptoms. Dopamine agonists and MAOB inhibitors are more useful in the treatment of moderate to severe disease.
- Therapeutic effectiveness of antiparkinsonian drug therapy is noted as a decrease in signs and symptoms, and the effects usually become evident after 2 to 3 weeks of therapy. In some patients, drug effects may take up to 6 months to be noticed.
- Myasthenia gravis is a disorder of voluntary muscles characterized by muscle weakness and fatigability.
- Onset of myasthenia gravis occurs between 20 and 30 years of age in women and after 50 years of age in men.
- Myasthenia gravis is an autoimmune disease resulting from a defect in nerve impulse transmission at the neuromuscular junction. Immunoglobulin G antibody is secreted against ACh receptors, blocking the binding of the neurotransmitter.
- Clinical manifestations include weakness of the muscles of the face and throat but may involve muscles of the diaphragm and chest wall.
- The diagnosis of myasthenia gravis is based on a history of illness, symptoms, diagnostic tests, and physical exam results. The onset of clinical symptoms is usually insidious, varying from patient to patient.
- The diagnosis of myasthenia gravis is confirmed using the cholinesterase inhibitor edrophonium. Improved muscle strength indicates a positive test and the diagnosis of myasthenia gravis.
- Treatment options for myasthenia gravis include cholinesterase inhibitors, corticosteroid drugs, and immunosuppressants.
- Cholinesterase inhibitors decrease the breakdown of ACh. They provide transient symptomatic relief and are most useful for nonprogressive eye muscle weakness and mild limb muscle weakness.
- Corticosteroids protect ACh receptor sites and are given early in large doses until improvement is seen.
- Immunosuppressants reduce corticosteroid requirements and produce improvement and remission when used alone.
- Cyclosporine is used for patients in whom use of corticosteroids and immunosuppressants is limited by adverse effects and/or lack of optimal response.
- Vital signs, neuromuscular status, ptosis, diplopia, chewing difficulties, dysphagia, gait, muscle strength of arms and legs, and respiratory status should be assessed before and throughout the course of treatment.
- The patient in either myasthenic or cholinergic crisis is in danger of respiratory arrest.
- The patient and family should be taught strategies that will facilitate chewing and swallowing and thus help prevent weight loss and aspiration.
- Drug therapy is considered successful if the patient experiences improved muscle strength and endurance with few troublesome adverse effects.

BIBLIOGRAPHY

Ahlskog, J. (1992). Parkinson's disease: Update on pharmacologic options to slow progression and treat symptoms. *Hospital Formulary,* 27, 146–161.

American Parkinson Disease Association. (1991). *Parkinson's disease handbook: A guide for patients and their families.* New York: Author.

Aminoff, M. (Ed.). (1995). *Neurology and general medicine.* New York: Churchill Livingstone.

Burke, M. (1993). Neuromuscular complications. *Journal of Perinatal Nursing,* 7(1), 11–21.

Chipps, E., Clanin, N., and Campbell, V. (1992). *Mosby's clinical nursing series: Neurologic disorders.* St. Louis: Mosby–Year Book.

Eadie, M. (1992). *Drug therapy in neurology.* Edinburgh: Churchill Livingstone.

Fowler, S., and Bergen, M. (1993). Continuous duodenal infusions of levodopa. *The Journal of Neuroscience Nursing,* 23(5), 317–320.

Guyton, A. (1991). *Textbook of medical physiology* (8th ed.). Philadelphia: W. B. Saunders.

Huber, S., and Cummings, J. (1992). *Parkinson's disease: Neurobehavioral aspects.* Oxford: Oxford University Press.

Kastrup, E. (Ed.). (1996). *Drug facts and comparisons.* St. Louis: Facts and Comparisons, Inc.

Koller, W., and Paulson, G. (Eds.). (1995). *Therapy of Parkinson's disease* (2nd ed.). New York: Marcel Dekker, Inc.

Koller, W., and Hubble, J. (1990). Levodopa therapy in Parkinson's disease. *Neurology,* 40 (Suppl. 3), 40–47.

Langtry, H., and Clissold, S. (1990). Pergolide: A review of its pharmacological properties and therapeutic potential in Parkinson's disease. *Drugs,* 39, 491–506.

Lavin, M., and Rifkin, A. (1991). Prophylactic antiparkinson drug use. I. Initial prophylaxis and prevention of extrapyromidal side effects. *Journal of Clinical Pharmacology,* 31(8), 763–768.

Long, J. (1992). *The essential guide to prescription drugs.* Harper Perennial: Harper Collins.

McCance, K., and Huether, S. (1998). *Pathophysiology: The biologic basis for disease in adults and children* (3rd ed.). St. Louis: C.V. Mosby.

Nutt, J., Hammerstad, J., and Gancher, S. (1992). *Parkinson's disease: 100 maxims in neurology* (Vol. 2). St. Louis: Mosby–Year Book.

Paulson, G. (1993). Management of the patient with newly-diagnosed Parkinson's disease. *Geriatrics,* 48(2), 30–40.

Pearce, J. (1992). *Parkinson's disease and its management.* Oxford: Oxford University Press.

Schneider, J., and Gupta, M. (1993). *Current concepts in Parkinson's disease research.* Seattle: Hogrefe and Huber.

Wright, R. (1992). Myasthenia. In Klawans, H., Goetz, C., and Tanner, C. (Eds.). *Textbook of clinical neuropharmacology and therapeutics* (2nd ed.). New York: Raven Press.

Unit IV

Drugs Influencing the Immune System

THE IMMUNE SYSTEM

The human immune system is a highly complex network of cells and molecules that interact to protect our bodies from foreign agents. Amazingly, this defense system is capable of recognizing and remembering harmful exogenous molecules, and differentiating them from normal cells and necessary proteins. As cell research continues to evolve, laboratory scientists and health care providers work to understand disease and the body's response.

The arrival of antimicrobial, immunotherapeutic, and antineoplastic therapy has been the most dramatic advance in health care during this century. Antimicrobial drugs interfere with metabolism, resulting in inhibition of growth or death of the organism. Immunotherapeutic drugs, such as vaccines and sera, offer a deliberate attempt to protect humans against disease by stimulating active or passive immunity. Antineoplastic therapy is used in the management of cancer to interfere with the growth, reproduction, or metabolism of neoplastic processes. Increasing knowledge of immune function is making it possible to develop drugs and treatments that offer greater accuracy and increased confidence for improved patient outcomes.

FUNCTIONAL ORGANIZATION OF THE IMMUNE SYSTEM

The vast majority of organisms that commonly reside in or on the body do so without causing disease, and many are actually beneficial. Such organisms normally compete with and prevent infection by pathogenic organisms. Unfortunately, in many cases, the organisms function as parasites, living at the expense of their human host. *Subclinical infections* cause no apparent response in the host and, thus, are accompanied by no objective manifestations. On the other hand, *clinical infections* cause overt injury and are marked by a variety of symptoms that range from mild to fatal.

Infectious states account for approximately 20 percent of all acute and chronic diseases seen in ambulatory care settings, with as many as 70 percent of these being acute respiratory tract illnesses. Of all the diseases affecting humans, the vast majority of infections are preventable and curable. The specific diseases that grasp the attention of health care providers, and occasionally the public, shift from time to time, but the challenges of dealing with infectious processes endure.

One requirement for the development of any infection is that the pathogen adhere to, colonize, or invade the host and proliferate. It is not surprising then that human beings have evolved an elaborate set of defense mechanisms. Strong intact host defenses prevent microbial invaders from entering the body or destroy pathogenic organisms that gain entry. Conversely, impaired host defenses may be unable to guard against pathogen invasion.

The bone marrow produces stem cells from which the active cells of the immune system, that is the *leukocytes* or white blood cells, evolve. There are two stem cell lines: (1) the myeloid stem cells that produce granulocytes and monocytes and (2) the lymphoid stem cells that produce T lymphocytes (T cells) and B lymphocytes (B cells) (see Figure 29–3).

There are three different types of *granulocytes:* neutrophils, eosinophils, and basophils. The *neutrophils,* also referred to as polymorphonuclear leukocytes, make up 60 percent of the circulating leukocytes. They are responsible for phagocytosis and chemotaxis, and are essential for the nonspecific immune response. *Eosinophils* make up 1 to 4 percent of the white blood cells and are responsible for allergic reactions and the destruction of parasitic organisms. *Basophils* make up 1 percent of the total leukocyte count and are thought to bring anticoagulant substances to inflamed tissues. Increased numbers of basophils are found during the healing phase of inflammation.

Agranulocytes are made up of lymphocytes and monocytes. Monocyte and macrophage receptors are nonspecific for antigens. They recognize all foreign antigens and can quickly respond. Macrophages are monocytes that leave the circulation to reside in the tissues. They aid white blood cells in phagocytosis and chemotaxis, and also process and present antigens, which, in turn, activate the T and B cells. The lymph nodes, alveoli, spleen, tonsils, and liver accumulate significant quantities of agranulocytes.

Host defense mechanisms are classified as nonspecific or specific. *Nonspecific mechanisms* most often represent the body's first encounter with an invading organism. The nonspecific mechanisms include physical barriers, chemical barriers, phagocytosis, and the inflammatory process. *Specific mechanisms* of immune defense include the body's ability to produce humoral and cell-mediated antibodies.

Nonspecific Defenses

The first line of nonspecific defenses includes physical barriers, chemical defenses, and the body's normal flora. Physical barriers begin with intact skin and mucous membranes, skin oil, cilia of the respiratory tract, cough and gag reflexes, gastrointestinal and genitourinary tract peristalsis, and the mechanical flushing action of tears, mucus, and saliva. Chemical defenses are found in the secretions within tears, saliva, digestive juices, perspiration, urine, vaginal secretions, and the enzymes that are a part of all body functions.

The second line of defense is the body's inflammatory response, which neutralizes and destroys many pathogens. This protective process involves vascular, chemical, and cellular physiologic responses. The vascular response is evoked after pathogens gain entrance into the body and cause cell injury (see Chapter 15). The vascular response lasts up to 10 minutes, producing hypoxia and acidosis of the tissues. Momentary vasoconstriction is immediately followed by a chemically induced (e.g., histamine, kinin, plasmin, serotonin, prostaglandin) vasodilation. The vasodilation increases the volume of blood to the affected area, causing redness and heat. The increased blood volume and greater hydrostatic pressure enhance capillary permeability, which facilitates fluid entry to the cell and locally dilutes toxins and organisms. Fluid exudate, consisting primarily of serous fluid, moves from the capillaries to the interstitial spaces, and lost protein further contributes to the resulting edema.

Another step in the inflammatory response is cellular exudation, in which the white blood cells migrate through capillary walls into injured tissue. Neutrophils ingest bacteria and dead tissue cells, and die. Proteolytic enzymes are released to liquefy dead cells (e.g., neutrophils, bacteria). Phagocytosis continues to digest and remove bacteria and damaged tissue.

The inflammatory response generates four cardinal symptoms of inflammation: redness and warmth from the hyperemia, edema caused by fluid exudate, pain from fluid exudate pressure and chemical irritation of nerve endings by bradykinin and prostaglandin, and loss of function from swelling and pain. An acute inflammatory response is usually short lived, lasting less than 2 weeks.

Specific Defenses

Third-line defenses include specific humoral or cell-mediated immune responses that are triggered by exposure to an antigen. The immune system recognizes the foreign invaders—bacteria, virus, fungi, protozoa, parasite, or protein—and rapidly synthesizes and delivers immune products to the infection site, differentiates and directs specific action against the invaders, and deactivates the involved body mechanism. Lymphocytes recognize and react to the antigens and expand in numbers to attack more efficiently. However, it may take up to 7 days to generate an adequate response. Subsequent exposure results in faster and more comprehensive lymphocyte response.

The humoral immune system produces antibodies directed against certain organisms. These antibodies serve to inactivate or eradicate the invading organism as well as to protect against future infection by that organism. Resistance to other organisms is mediated by the action of specifically sensitized T cells. The various components of the immune system work both independently and together to protect against infection.

The homeostatic mechanisms of immunity are basic to human survival in a world swarming with potentially harmful organisms. The immune system is sometimes compared with a double-edged sword. On one hand, humans are dependent on the immune system for survival, and on the other, they are vulnerable to conditions arising from states of immunodeficiency or hypersensitivity disorders.

Active and Passive Immunity

Immunity in human beings may be attained in two ways—actively or passively. *Active immunity* is generated by the body's own immune system as a result of active exposure to infection or by vaccination. Antibodies are produced that correspond to the specific antigen, protecting the body against future exposure to the same antigen. *Passive immunity* involves the transfer of plasma containing preformed antibodies from an immunized individual to a nonimmunized individual. Passive transfer occurs across placental membranes or in the shift of breast milk from mother to fetus. Other methods of transfer include direct injection of antibodies such as human or animal immune globulin (see Chapter 28).

The functioning of the immune system is greatly influenced by age. The immune response has not yet developed in newborns and very young children. The aging process alters the immune system of the older adult by decreasing the ability to respond to antigenic stimulation. The thymus gland decreases in size, weight, and function in older adults, thereby causing a decrease in the antibody titer, production of thymosis hormone, T cells, cell-mediated immunity, response to bacterial antigens, and promptness in the repair of damaged tissue. Additionally, the aging process leads to a decreased B-cell response and a change in cellular composition of the spleen and lymph nodes that also contributes to a decline in immunity.

DETERMINANTS OF INFECTION

The transport of pathogens to the body is an essential characteristic of infection. However, the mere presence of a pathogen does not mean that an infection will necessarily occur. Development of an infection requires the cyclic interaction of six elements—a susceptible host, a pathogen, a reservoir or a source for pathogen growth, a portal of exit from the reservoir, a mode of transmission, and a portal of entry to the host.

Pathogenic Organisms

Bacteria

Several factors determine the pathogenicity of bacteria. The presence of flagella, commonly found on gram-negative rods, promotes motility. Fimbriae, also common in gram-negative rods, appear to aid in bacterial adherence to host tissues. Some bacteria produce a capsule that enables the cell to escape phagocytosis. Still others possess the ability to form spores in situations of inadequate nutritional supply. The spores are resistant to destruction by temperature or chemicals and, therefore, allow the bacterial cells to survive until conditions become more favorable.

Bacteria may cause disease in virtually every organ system, and infections range from the simple invasion of intact skin to localized visceral infection involving the lungs, kidneys, spleen, or heart. Widespread invasion of the blood stream may occur via the lymphatic channels if local phagocytic mechanisms are overwhelmed. Bacterial seeding may lead to endotoxemia, septicemia, and even death given the right circumstances. Antibacterial drugs are discussed in Chapter 24.

Viruses

Viral diseases are the most common of human infections. Once thought to be confined to the childhood years, viral infections have increasingly been recognized in adults as a cause of morbidity and death. They include infectious diseases such as hepatitis, autoimmune deficiency syndrome, and other sexually transmitted diseases. Viruses also are considered possible etiologic agents in cancer, affecting immunosuppressed patients and the older adult.

Until recently, viruses were thought to be the simplest pathogens producing infection in humans. They are divided into two groups according to the type of nucleic acid they contain: ribonucleic acid (RNA) or deoxyribonucleic acid (DNA). They are submicroscopic, filterable organisms that are entirely dependent on host cells for protein synthesis and replication. They are, therefore, obligate intracellular parasites. Once it is within the cells, the virus sheds its coat, allowing its nucleic acid to use cellular machinery of the host to reproduce or to integrate into the host cell.

Viruses have developed several mechanisms for evading host defenses. By multiplying within host cells, viruses can avoid cytotoxic antibodies and other extracellular host defenses. Viral infections historically have been considered almost entirely community acquired. It has become apparent that certain viral pathogens are associated with nosocomial transmission. Antiviral drugs are discussed in Chapter 25.

Chlamydiae

Chlamydiae fall between viruses and bacteria in complexity but are also obligate intracellular parasites. Unlike viruses, these organisms contain both DNA and RNA, have a cell wall, and contain ribosomes. Chlamydiae organisms are unable to synthesize compounds such as adenosine triphosphate and thus depend on energy from the host cell to survive. These organisms are easily engulfed by phagocytes; however, they possess an unusual ability to proliferate within the phagosome. Chlamydial antigens prevent phagosome-lysosome fusion, and the organism is thus protected from normal host defenses. Through a long developmental cycle, the chlamydiae develop inclusion bodies, which nearly fill entire host cells. Reproduction occurs in the inclusion bodies, with the new organisms continually infecting susceptible host cells.

Fungi

Of the more than 50,000 species of fungi, approximately 50 are generally recognized as being pathogenic in humans. Fungi are organisms that live in soil enriched by decaying nitrogenous matter. They are capable of maintaining a separate existence by a parasitic cycle in humans or animals. Humans become accidental hosts through the inhalation of spores or by introduction into the tissues through trauma.

Most fungi exist in a yeast form, round to ovoid cells that may reproduce by budding, or a mold form, a complex of tubular structures that grow by branching or extension. The cell walls of fungi are primarily composed of polysaccharide, which permits cell synthesis even in the presence of antimicrobial drugs. Antifungal drugs are discussed in Chapter 25.

Mycobacterium

Mycobacterium diseases such as tuberculosis and leprosy can manifest as local lesions or disseminate to other parts of the body. Exposure to *Mycobacterium tuberculosis* or *Mycobacterium leprae* bacilli occurs primarily through airborne droplets. Both tuberculosis and leprosy are communicable diseases. The degree of communicability depends on the number and virulence of discharged bacilli, adequacy of ventilation, exposure of the bacilli to the sun or ultraviolet light, and opportunities for aerosolization. Antimycobacterial drugs are discussed in Chapter 26.

Mycoplasmas

Mycoplasmas are the smallest, least complex free-living organisms. In contrast to viruses and chlamydiae, Mycoplasmas can grow on cell-free media and produce disease without intracellular penetration. Like other bacteria, these organisms have a cell membrane but no cell walls. Thus, antimicrobial drugs that act on cell walls have no effect on Mycoplasmas. This group of three major species includes pathogens that produce pharyngitis, pneumonia, nongonococcal urethritis, pyelonephritis, and pelvic inflammatory disease.

Rickettsiae

Rickettsiae are small, gram-negative coccobacilli organisms that structurally resemble bacteria, but on the average, are only one-tenth to one-half as large. They are obligate intracellular pathogens that produce disease in humans through the bite of an insect vector such as a tick, flea, or mite. Culture of these organisms is virtually impossible except in reference laboratories. Rickettsiae produce a group of illnesses characterized by fever, headache, and rash. Because most of these illnesses are transmitted by an insect vector, they are frequently limited by climate and to a lesser extent by geographic location.

Protozoa

More than 65,000 species of protozoa have been identified, although only a few are human pathogens. Protozoal organisms can cause localized gastrointestinal illness such as amebiasis and giardiasis, genitourinary tract infection such as trichomoniasis, or widespread infection of the blood stream and hematopoietic system. *Pneumocystis carinii* pneumonia is thought to be caused by a protozoa.

Helminths

Diseases due to *helminths* (worms) are among the most prevalent in developing nations, but are less common causes of illness in the United States. The largest and most complex of human pathogens, the helminths are visible to the eye and can be divided into three categories: flukes (trematodes), tapeworms (cestodes), and roundworms (nematodes). Helminths infect humans via ingestion, penetration of the skin, or injection by an insect vector. Manifestations of helminth infection vary widely, from the local pruritus of enterobiasis (pinworm infestation), to diarrhea associated with trichinosis, to life-threatening bladder, intestinal, or liver disease that may be associated with schistosomiasis, a parasitic disease caused by infestation with blood flukes. Antiprotozoal and anthelmintic drugs are discussed in Chapter 27.

PHARMACOLOGIC IMPLICATIONS

Treatment of infectious disease depends on the taxonomy to which the organism belongs, because different classifications of antimicrobial agents are used for treating different organisms. Antimicrobial drugs help cure or alleviate most infections; however, antimicrobials alone do not necessarily rid the body of the organisms. Drugs are viewed as adjuncts to other nonpharmaceutical treatments such as handwashing, wound débridement, or pulmonary hygiene.

When antimicrobial therapy is contemplated, a number of factors should be taken into consideration: the infecting organism, either suspected or confirmed; the sensitivity of the particular organism to antimicrobial agents; the site of the infection and the status of the individual's host defenses;

the pharmacokinetics of the particular antimicrobial under consideration; and the status of the individual's renal and hepatic functioning. Also, the clinical evaluation of antimicrobial effectiveness is an important consideration.

In addition, antiviral and antifungal agents, immunotherapeutic therapy, and antineoplastic drugs continue to become effective tools for pharmacologic intervention.

Identification of the Infecting Organism

Most of the available antimicrobial drugs have a specific effect on a limited range of organisms. The drug to be used for a given infectious process is best chosen after the infecting organism has been identified. It is desirable to have culture and sensitivity (susceptibility) reports before initiating antimicrobial therapy. However, it is impractical in some circumstances to wait for these reports. In acute, life-threatening situations, therapy must be initiated without delay. In these situations, the antimicrobial drug chosen for initial therapy is based on tentative identification of the organism. When positive identification of the offending organism is difficult, *broad-spectrum* antimicrobial drugs, or several different drugs, can be prescribed for concurrent administration. Widespread use of broad-spectrum antimicrobials, however, almost invariably leads to emergence of resistant strains of the organism. On the other hand, the sicker the individual, and the less certainty there is regarding the responsible pathogen, the more important initial empiric broad-spectrum coverage becomes.

Sensitivity and Resistance

Sensitivity testing determines the ability of a particular antimicrobial drug to limit growth or kill the organism. The term intermediate or *partially resistant,* or *moderately susceptible,* means that the strain tested is not completely inhibited by therapeutic concentrations of a specific drug. Many health care providers rely more on published reports of the drug's effectiveness against the isolated organism than on the sensitivity report because sensitivity is an *in vitro* test (in glass) and the antimicrobial agent will be working *in vivo* (in the body).

Antimicrobial drugs exert their bactericidal or bacteriostatic effects in one of four major ways. Unlike host cells, bacteria are not isotonic with body fluids. Their contents are under high osmotic pressure and their viability depends on the integrity of the cell walls. Furthermore, a drug that inhibits any step in the synthesis of the cell wall causes it to weaken and the cell to lyse. Antimicrobial drugs having this action are *bactericidal.* Disruption or alteration of membrane permeability results in leakage of essential bacterial metabolic components. These drugs may be either bactericidal or *bacteriostatic.* Last, antimicrobial drugs act by inhibiting the synthesis of essential metabolites. Drugs that work in this manner structurally resemble physiologic compounds and act as competitive inhibitors in a metabolic pathway. As a general rule, these drugs are considered bacteriostatic.

Resistance refers to the ability of a particular organism to resist the effects of a specific antimicrobial drug. There are several mechanisms by which drug resistance develops. The resistance mechanisms include (1) the development of altered receptors or enzymes that interact with the drug, (2) a decrease in the drug concentration reaching receptors, (3) inactivation or enhanced destruction of the drug, (4) synthesis of resistant biotransformation pathways, and (5) failure of biotransformation. Organisms may develop one or all of these mechanisms simultaneously. As a general rule, organisms resistant to a certain drug tend to be resistant to other chemically and structurally related antimicrobial drugs in the same class, a phenomenon known as *cross-resistance.*

Site and Host Defenses

Although an organism may have been identified, it is also important to consider the location of the infection when determining selection and dosage of an antimicrobial drug. Deep-seated and bacteremic infections generally require higher doses of antimicrobials than superficial infections of the skin. A particular antimicrobial drug may not reach the necessary body compartment in sufficient concentrations to be effective. Thus, it is important to select an antimicrobial drug that can penetrate the appropriate tissues in concentrations sufficient to inhibit or destroy the pathogens.

No antimicrobial drug will cure an infectious process if host defense mechanisms are inadequate. Such drugs act only on the causative organisms and have no effect on the defense mechanisms of the body. Many infections do not require drug treatment and are adequately combated by individual defense mechanisms, including antibody production, phagocytosis, interferon production, fibrosis, or gastrointestinal rejection. Host defense mechanisms, however, may be diminished, requiring supportive therapy of various types to ensure adequate oxygenation, fluid and electrolyte balance, and optimal nutrition for antimicrobial therapy to be effective. In some circumstances, appropriate surgical intervention may be required in addition to an antimicrobial drug.

Pharmacokinetics

Knowing the factors that influence absorption, distribution, biotransformation, elimination, toxic effects, and spectrum of antimicrobial activity is vital to successful therapy. Drug concentration at the site of infection must be sufficient to inhibit or kill the pathogen. Understanding that lipid-soluble drugs penetrate most membranes more readily than more ionized compounds is also important. Additionally, using drugs that are eliminated unchanged in the urine may be particularly effective in the presence of renal insufficiency.

Renal and Hepatic Function

The primary organs of elimination for most antimicrobial drugs are the kidneys and the liver. In patients with impaired renal or hepatic function, the dose of most antimicrobial agents must be reduced or the dosage interval increased. Antimicrobial drugs for which no dosage reduction is required in renal insufficiency are select penicillins, cephalosporins, and antifungal drugs.

Antimicrobial Therapy

Clinical evaluation of potential toxicities associated with antimicrobial therapy is important. For some antimicrobial drugs, the ratio of effective to toxic concentrations is narrow (i.e., narrow therapeutic index). Thus, serum levels of the drug must be monitored to ensure appropriate dosing. Although the technique of monitoring antimicrobial serum activity shortly after (peak) and just before (valley or trough) antimicrobial drug administration is not well standardized, the dosage is often adjusted to maintain serum bactericidal titers of at least 1:8 in treating certain types of infection.

Antiviral and Antifungal Drugs

Antiviral drugs must be designed to target specifically one of the steps in the molecular mechanism between host cell reception and reproduction of the virus. In the absence of natural or stimulated immunity, an antiviral drug may block protein reception at the cell wall, interfere with DNA or RNA replication, or destroy enzymes necessary to viral metabolism. Often, these drugs must be prescribed for ongoing regimens because they do not eradicate the virus, but rather only control the disease process. The recent ability to describe the molecular anatomy of viruses is helping researchers produce more effective chemotherapeutic agents.

Most fungus infections are superficial skin diseases and can be easily treated because the antifungal drugs may destroy the fungal cell wall. Systemic infections, however, prove more difficult because the level of drug needed to reach the site of infection is often toxic. Longer regimens of carefully monitored drug levels are often necessary.

Immunologic Protection

The body's ability to establish immunologic resistance to pathogenic organisms and foreign substances is a vital part of homeostasis and is critical to the ability to stay healthy. The susceptibility of humans to infection by microorganisms reflects both innate and acquired characteristics.

Natural immunity is a nonspecific response to foreign invaders, regardless of the composition of the invader. Natural mechanisms, such as physical and chemical barriers, and biologic response modifiers are the basis for natural immunity. The inflammatory response is a major component of the natural immune system that is elicited in response to tissue injury or invading organisms. When natural immunity is inadequate to provide protection, artificial immunity may be gained by either providing the antibodies or stimulating antibody production (see Chapters 28 and 29).

Tumor immunology is a science that examines the immune system's recognition of and response to cancer cells. The underlying assumption is that cancer cells are formed continuously throughout the lifetime. Immune surveillance works to destroy cancer cells before they can grow into clinically detectable masses. Cell cycle kinetics provide a basis for understanding antineoplastic therapy (see Chapter 30).

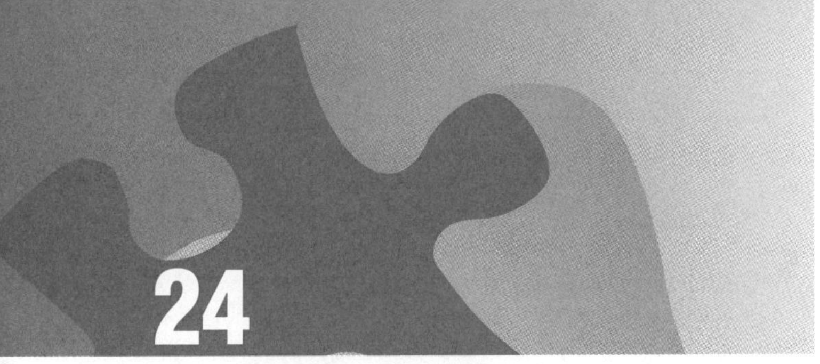

24 Antibiotic Drugs

An *antibiotic* is a chemical substance produced by a microorganism that has the ability, in dilute solutions, to kill or inhibit the growth of microorganisms. Antibiotics that are sufficiently nontoxic to the host are used as chemotherapeutic agents in the treatment of infectious disease caused by bacterial pathogens including prokaryotes, spirochetes, and mycoplasms. Antibiotics are the indicated drug therapy in infectious conditions to inhibit the growth or destroy one or more causative pathogens. Generally, one antibiotic is sufficient. However, in some instances multidrug antibiotic therapy is needed to eradicate the infectious process. For example, the United States Centers for Disease Control and Prevention and many health care providers recommend the combination of an aminoglycoside (e.g., gentamicin) with clindamycin, a miscellaneous antibiotic, as a regimen for the treatment of acute pelvic inflammatory disease.

Infections have been a great concern throughout world history. During the first half of this century, infections were among the most common causes of death. The discovery and application of sulfonamides and penicillins offered the first real pharmaceutical armamentarium against infectious disease, specifically bacterial infections. In the 1980s, new bacterial infections such as Legionella emerged, and during the 1990s, there has been a worldwide resurgence of preventable bacterial diseases.

Many factors have contributed to the global resurgence of infectious disease. Among them are the development of strains of bacteria resistant to antibiotics, larger populations of immunocompromised individuals, increases in the number and complexity of invasive medical procedures, and the prolonged survival of patients with chronic debilitating diseases. Indeed, the issue of drug resistance has provoked an ongoing re-examination of the use of antibiotics and antibacterial therapies. Drug resistance has developed in part because of a lack of knowledge regarding treatment regimens appropriate for specific infections, how organisms mutate, and the existence of other pathogenic organisms. As microbiochemistry continues to evolve, health care providers can access information providing them with a clearer understanding of the complex interactions of microorganisms as well as new drugs designed to target specific diseases.

BACTERIAL INFECTION

Epidemiology and Etiology

Infection is responsible for the mortality of many individuals. People at the extremes of age, the very young or very old, and the critically or chronically ill are particularly susceptible to infections. Additional factors that influence exposure and resistance to infection include the patient's general health, nutritional status, hormonal balance, co-morbid conditions, living environment, drug use, hygiene, and sexual practices. Immunocompromised patients are another group with increased susceptibility to infection and infectious diseases.

During the past decade, gram-positive bacteria have gradually emerged as the most frequent causes of *nosocomial* infections, those acquired during hospitalization. Nosocomial infections caused by staphylococcal isolates are significant agents of infection in large teaching hospitals, smaller community hospitals, and extended care facilities. *Staphylococcus aureus* is the most common cause of skin and wound infection and bacteremia as well as the second most frequent cause of lower respiratory infection in nosocomial disease. Each year in the United States, approximately 2 million patients of the 40 million hospitalized will acquire a nosocomial infection. Patients in some intensive care units have a 25 to 70 percent chance of such infection, most often caused by drug resistant organisms. Nosocomial infections extend a hospital stay by an average of 7 days, raising associated hospital costs approximately $6000. Furthermore, the number of deaths related to nosocomial infections is estimated at 60,000 to 70,000 per year.

In the United States, enterococci have become the third most common organism causing nosocomial infections (after *S. aureus* and *Escherichia coli*). These organisms are associated with wound infections, infections of the urinary tract, septicemia, and endocarditis.

Community-acquired infections that are resistant to multiple antibiotics have also become prevalent. The incidence of salmonella, shigella, *Mycobacterium tuberculosis,* and *Streptococcus pneumonia* has increased. *S. pneumonia* causes several potentially life-threatening infections. Each year in the United States, there are over 6,000 cases of pneumococcal meningitis, 500,000 cases of pneumonia, 55,000 cases of bacteremia, and 6 million cases of inner ear infection. In addition to young children and older adults, patients with splenic dysfunction or those who have human immunodeficiency virus (HIV) infection are at high risk for these infections.

Pathophysiology

Bacteria are known as *prokaryotes.* Prokaryotes are single-celled organisms that differ from all other organisms *(eukaryotes)* in that they lack a true nucleus and organelles (i.e., mitochondria, chloroplasts, lysosomes). Prokaryotes are approximately the size of the eukaryotic mitochondria, about 1 nanometer in diameter. There is some evidence that they may be the evolutionary ancestors of mitochondria. Their genetic material consists of a single loop of double stranded DNA, whereas the genetic material in eukaryotes consists of multiple chromosomes. Most bacteria have a rigid cell wall outside of a cytoplasmic cell membrane. The cell wall is primarily composed of a dense layer of peptidoglycan, a network of polysaccharide chains with polypeptide cross-links.

The structure and synthesis of the cell wall determine the shape of the organism. A spherical bacterium is called a *coccus*. When the cocci divide into chains, they are referred to as *streptococci*. Some species do not always completely separate when the cells divide and characteristically occur in pairs known as *diplococci*. When they appear in clusters, they are known as *staphylococci*. A rod-shaped organism is called a *bacillus*. *Fusiform bacilli* have tapered ends, whereas *filamentous bacilli* are shaped like long threads or spirals *(spirochetes)*.

The external structures of bacteria consist of flagella (whiplike organelles), pili (minute filamentous appendages), and a capsule (a layer of gelatinous material around the cell). The capsule protects the organism from phagocytosis. Various types of pili are involved in conjugation and the adherence of bacteria to mucosal surfaces. The rotary action of flagella permit the organism to travel through a liquid environment like a propeller.

Bacteria are classified as *gram positive* or *gram negative* based on their reaction to Gram's stain. Gram-positive bacteria stain purple when flushed with a primary basic dye (e.g., crystal violet). Bacteria that do not take the purple stain are counter stained with safranin O, a red dye. The shape of the organism and its staining characteristics are used in combination to describe the bacteria.

Each bacterium has a well-defined set of criteria needed for growth, including light, humidity, temperature, and atmosphere. Bacteria can be divided into obligate *aerobes,* those that require oxygen, or obligate *anaerobes,* which grow only in the absence of oxygen. *Facultative* anaerobes can adapt to either environment.

However, bacteria are highly adaptable, with cell division taking place every 20 minutes. Because of this frequency of cell division, bacteria have a very high rate of population growth and evolution. Genetic material can be transferred between bacteria by three processes—transformation (absorption of naked DNA), transduction (transfer by a virus), and conjugation (transfer by independently replicating DNA molecules called plasmids that are inserted into the bacterial DNA).

The different bacteria affect various organs and systems of the body. Staphylococci are generally found on the skin. When the skin surface is breached, staphylococci usually produce a local infection with inflammation and pus formation. Disseminated infection from staphylococci is rare. Streptococci infections, however, are often serious and tend to resist localization, spreading through the circulation. Infections caused by streptococci include sore throat, rheumatic fever, and scarlet fever.

Bacteria can cause disease by producing toxins, causing inflammation, or provoking a hypersensitivity reaction. *Exotoxins* are exceedingly powerful poisons produced by some gram-positive bacteria; *endotoxins* are components of the outer membrane of gram-negative cell walls and are released by cell lysis.

Bacteria can be transmitted directly or indirectly. *Direct transmission* involves contact between two people (e.g., touching, kissing, sneezing, sexual contact). *Indirect transmission* of infection involves vectors (e.g., air, water, milk, food, soil). Inanimate objects such as needles, eating utensils, and urinary catheters may serve as vectors. Although organisms are prevalent throughout the environment, some are also resident in the human body. Normal flora inhabit the skin, mucous membranes of the respiratory and gastrointestinal (GI) tracts, and the vagina.

Ordinarily, endogenous microflora do not cause disease. The human body serves as a host to some parasitic flora, and the organisms live together in a symbiotic relationship. Normal flora, however, can be pathogenic under conditions such as immunosuppression. Infection may ensue when such flora are displaced from usual habitats and transferred to another site. For example, *E. coli* commonly inhabits the GI tract but may cause infection when it colonizes in the urinary tract.

PHARMACOTHERAPEUTIC OPTIONS

The primary management of infection is pharmacotherapy. Several classifications of antibiotics have been developed over the past 25 years. Current classifications of antibiotics include the sulfonamides, penicillins, cephalosporins, tetracyclines, aminoglycosides, macrolides, and several other miscellaneous pharmacotherapeutic drugs. The antibiotic selected for treatment of an infection should be the most effective in eradicating the causative organisms and yet create the least harmful adverse effects.

Sulfonamide Drugs

- ❒ Sulfacytine (RENOQUID)
- ❒ Sulfadiazine (MICROSULFON)
- ❒ Sulfamethizole (THIOSULFIL FORTE)
- ❒ Sulfamethoxazole (GANTANOL, UROBAK); (🍁) APO-SULFAMETHOXAZOLE
- ❒ Sulfasalazine (AZULFIDINE); (🍁) PMS SULFASALAZINE EC, SALZOPYRIN, S.A.S. ENEMA, S.A.S. ENTERIC-500, S.A.S.500
- ❒ Sulfisoxazole
- ❒ Trimethoprim-sulfamethoxazole (TMP-SMZ; BACTRIM, co-trimoxazole, SEPTRA)

Indications

Sulfonamides were once a major treatment modality for infection and originally were active against a wide range of gram-positive and gram-negative bacteria. However, at present, their usefulness is limited due to the development of resistant strains of many bacteria. Sulfonamides are indicated for the treatment of urinary tract infections, otitis media, and bronchitis. Furthermore, sulfonamides are used in the treatment of malaria, ulcerative colitis, dermatitis herpetiformis, chlamydia, nocardiosis, gonorrhea, and protozoal infections (e.g., toxoplasmosis, *Pneumocystis carinii* pneumonia). Sulfonamides are also used prophylactically in patients with a history of rheumatic fever, in penicillin-allergic patients, children infected with human immunodeficiency virus, granulocytopenic patients, and in patients with traveler's diarrhea.

Pharmacodynamics

Sulfonamides are *bacteriostatic* against a wide range of bacteria, including pneumococci, *E. coli, Streptococcus pyogenes, Streptococcus pneumoniae, Haemophilus influenzae, Ducreyi, Nocardia, Actinomyces, Calymmatobacterium granulomatis,* and

Chlamydia trachomatis. Protozoa susceptible to sulfonamides include *Plasmodium falciparum* and *Toxoplasma gondii.*

Sulfonamides inhibit bacterial growth by acting as antimetabolites of para-aminobenzoic acid (PABA), which organisms require to produce folic acid. Folic acid, in turn, is required for the production of bacterial intracellular proteins. The sulfonamides enter the reaction instead of PABA, competing for the enzyme involved and causing the formation of nonfunctional derivatives of folic acid. Thus, sulfonamides stop growth, development, and multiplication of new bacteria but do not kill mature, fully formed bacteria.

Some bacteria are able to alter their metabolic pathways to use precursors or other forms of folic acid, thereby developing resistance to the antibacterial action of sulfonamides. Once resistance to one sulfonamide develops, cross-resistance to others is common.

Adverse Effects and Contraindications

The most common adverse effects of sulfonamides include headache, anorexia, nausea, vomiting, diarrhea, and rash. Other adverse effects include urticaria, weakness, flushing, vertigo, stomatitis, glossitis, abdominal pain, photosensitivity, peripheral neuritis, oliguria, anuria, crystalluria, uric acid kidney stones, and exacerbations of gout.

The more serious adverse effects of sulfonamides involve hemolytic anemia, thrombocytopenia, convulsions, hepatic necrosis, and renal failure. *Stevens-Johnson syndrome* is the most serious form of cutaneous sensitivity and has been noted with all sulfonamides. It manifests as erythema and ulceration of mucous membranes (eyes, mouth, urethra). Serum sickness and drug fever are also noted. Patients with acquired immunodeficiency syndrome are more likely to develop rashes secondary to sulfonamide therapy than patients without acquired immunodeficiency syndrome.

Acute hemolytic anemia results from increased destruction of red blood cells. The anemia is most likely to occur in patients taking a sulfonamide whose red blood cells have been sensitized because of a glucose-6-phosphate dehydrogenase deficiency. When red blood cells are challenged by one of several sulfonamides, glutathione is depleted, Heinz bodies form, and glucose use is inhibited.

Agranulocytosis or aplastic anemia can occur in patients taking a sulfonamide because of the direct toxic effects of the drug on the bone marrow. Also rare but serious is focal or diffuse necrosis of the liver secondary to direct toxicity or hypersensitivity. These reactions are rare; however, should they develop, prompt discontinuation of the offending drug is essential.

Sulfonamides are contraindicated in patients who have blood dyscrasias, porphyria, uric acid kidney stones, during or within 2 or 3 weeks of an acute gout attack, excessive elimination of uric acid (over 1000 mg/day), or in patients who have a creatinine clearance less than 50 mg/minute. Cautious use of sulfonamides is suggested for patients with a history of peptic ulcer disease because these drugs tend to irritate the gastric mucosa.

Sulfonamides are also contraindicated during pregnancy and lactation, and in infants younger than 2 months of age (unless the infant is being treated for congenital toxoplasmosis). The primary danger of using sulfonamides during pregnancy occurs when these drugs are given close to delivery. The sulfonamides compete with bilirubin for binding to plasma albumin. In utero, the fetus clears free bilirubin through the placental circulation. However, after birth, this mechanism is no longer available and unbound bilirubin is free to cross the blood-brain barrier. Kernicterus may result.

Pharmacokinetics

The pharmacokinetics of sulfonamides are identified in Table 24–1. Most sulfonamides are well absorbed following oral administration and are distributed throughout all body tissues with good penetration of pleural, peritoneal, synovial, and ocular fluids. They cross placental membranes and the blood-brain barrier, diffusing into cerebrospinal fluid (CSF). The largest percentage of sulfonamides are eliminated by the kidneys; therefore, dosage adjustments are necessary in patients with renal insufficiency.

Drug-Drug Interactions

Table 24–2 lists drug-drug interactions of selected sulfonamide drugs. The most common drug-drug interactions involve anticoagulants, oral hypoglycemic drugs, and phenytoin.

TABLE 24–1 PHARMACOKINETICS OF SELECTED SULFONAMIDE ANTIBIOTICS

Drug	Route	Onset	Peak	Duration	PB (%)	$t_{1/2}$	BioA (%)
Sulfacytine	po	UA	UA	UA	UA	UA	UA
Sulfadiazine	po	Varies	3–6 hr	UA	32–56	13 hr	70–100
Sulfamethizole	po	Varies	3–6 hr	UA	UA	UK	UA
Sulfamethoxazole	po	1 hr	3–4 hr	UA	65	7–12 hr	70–100
Sulfasalazine	po	1 hr	1.5–6 hr	UK	UA	5–10 hr	10–15
Sulfamethoxazole/ trimethoprim	po	Rapid	1–4 hr	UK	65; 50*	10–13 hr 8–10 hr†	UA
Sulfisoxazole	po	UK	2–4 hr	UK	90	5–8 hr	70–100
	IV	Immed	End of inf				100
	IV	Rapid	End of inf	UA	< 10	2–3 hr	100

*Protein binding of sulfamethoxazole/trimethoprim, respectively.

†Half-life of trimethoprim and sulfamethoxazole, respectively.

PB, Protein binding; $t_{1/2}$, elimination half-life; NA, not applicable; UA, unavailable; UK, unknown; BioA, bioavailability.

TABLE 24–2 DRUG-DRUG INTERACTIONS OF SELECTED ANTIBIOTICS

Drug	Interactive Drugs		Interaction
Sulfonamides			
Sulfonamides	Oral anticoagulants		Increases risk of hypoprothrombinemia
	Acetohexamide	Glyburide	Increased risk of hypoglycemia
	Chlorpropamide	Tolbutamide	
	Glipizide	Tolazamide	
	Phenytoin		Increased risk of toxicity to interactive drug
	Cephalosporins	Penicillin G	Prolongs antibiotic blood levels
	Salicylates		Decreases uricosuric activity
	Methotrexate	Sulfonylureas	Increased action of interactive drug
	Nitrofurantoin		Decreased efficacy and increased risk of toxicity of interactive drug
	Alcohol		Increased blood urate levels
Penicillins			
Penicillins	Aminoglycosides	Warfarin	Increased bactericidal effects of interactive drug
	Clavulanate		
	Probenecid	Sulfinpyrazone	Delays renal elimination of penicillin, thus increasing blood levels
	Oral contraceptives	Rifampin	Decreased activity of interactive drug
	NSAIDs		Increased penicillin action and half-life
	Potassium-sparing diuretics		Increased risk of hyperkalemia
	Colestipol		Decreased blood levels of penicillin
Cephalosporins			
Cephalosporins	Alcohol		Disulfiram-like reaction
	Probenecid		Increased cephalosporin concentration
	Nephrotoxic drugs		Increased nephrotoxicity
Tetracyclines			
Tetracyclines	Antacids	Iron preparations	Decreased antibacterial action of tetracycline
	Antidiarrheal drugs	Cimetidine	
	Aminoglycosides	Penicillins	
	Barbiturates	Phenytoin	Decreased half-life of doxycycline
	Carbamazepine		
	Oral anticoagulants	Methoxyflurane	Decreased activity of interactive drug
Aminoglycosides			
Aminoglycosides	Furosemide	Ethacrynic acid	Increased nephrotoxicity and ototoxicity of aminoglycoside
	Penicillins		Inactivation of aminoglycoside
	Neuromuscular blockers	General anesthetics	Increased neuromuscular blockade
	Oral anticoagulants	Nephrotoxic drugs	Increased activity of interactive drug
	Ototoxic drugs		
	Neurotoxic drugs		
Fluoroquinolones			
Fluoroquinolones	Theophylline		Increased serum levels of interactive drug and risk of toxicity
	Antacids	Sucralfate	Decreased absorption of fluoroquinolone
	Bismuth subsalicylate	Zinc salts	
	Iron salts		
	Warfarin		Increased effects of interactive drug
	Antineoplastic drugs		Decreased serum levels of fluoroquinolone
	Cimetidine		Interactive drug interferes with elimination of fluoroquinoline
	Glucocorticoids		Concurrent use may increase the risk of tendon rupture
	Nitrofurantoin	Probenecid	Interactive drug antagonizes ciprofloxacin
Ciprofloxacin	Foscarnet		Concurrent use may increase risk of seizures
Sparfloxacin	Amiodarone	Disopyramide	Increased risk of serious adverse cardiovascular effects
	Astemizole	Quinidine	
	Bepridil	Sotalol	
	Aluminum	Magnesium	Absorption of fluoroquinolone is decreased with concurrent use
	Antacids	Multivitamins with zinc	
	Iron	Sucralfate	
Enoxacin	Digoxin		Increased serum levels of interactive drug
Macrolides			
Macrolides	Carbamazepine	Triazolam	Increased risk of toxicity of interactive drug
	Cyclosporine	Warfarin	
	Theophylline	Digoxin	
	Midazolam		
	Ergotamine		Increased ischemia, dysesthesia, peripheral vasospasm

TABLE 24–2 DRUG-DRUG INTERACTIONS OF SELECTED ANTIBIOTICS *Continued*

Drug	Interactive Drugs		Interaction
Macrolides *continued*			
Imipenem/cilastatin	Penicillins	Cephalosporins	Antagonizes the action of interactive drug
	Aminoglycosides		Inactivation of interactive drug
	Probenecid		Increased blood levels of imipenem/cilastatin
	Ganciclovir		Increased risk of seizures
Clindamycin	Chloramphenicol	Erythromycin	Decreased action of interactive drug
Chloramphenicol	Oral hypoglycemics	Phenytoin	Increased effects of interactive drug
	Oral anticoagulants		
	Phenobarbital	Rifampin	Decreased chloramphenicol levels
	Folic acid	Vitamin B_{12}	Delayed response to interactive drug
	Antineoplastics		Additive bone marrow depression
	Acetaminophen		Increased risk of toxicity
Miscellaneous Antibiotics			
Vancomycin	Aspirin	Cisplatin	Additive ototoxicity and nephrotoxicity
	Aminoglycosides	Loop diuretics	
	Cyclosporine		
	Nondepolarizing neuromuscular blockers		Enhances neuromuscular blockade
	Anesthetics		Increased risk of histamine flush in children

NSAIDs, Nonsteroidal anti-inflammatory drugs.

Dosage Regimen

The sulfonamides fall into two major categories: systemic sulfonamides and sulfonamides used for local effects (e.g., burns). The systemic sulfonamides are more widely used and are identified in Table 24–3. Topical sulfonamides are discussed in Chapter 64.

Laboratory Considerations

Serum levels of alkaline phosphatase, transaminase, creatinine, and bilirubin may be elevated when taking sulfonamides. A false-positive urinary glucose test result is possible when using Benedict's method for testing.

Penicillins

PENICILLINASE-SENSITIVE PENICILLINS

❒ Penicillin G sodium
❒ Penicillin G benzathine (BICILLIN)
❒ Penicillin G potassium (PFIZERPEN, others)
❒ Penicillin G procaine (WYCILLIN, others)
❒ Penicillin V (V-CILLIN, PEN-VEE K, VEETIDS, others)

PENICILLINASE-RESISTANT PENICILLINS

❒ Cloxacillin (CLOXAPEN, TEGOPEN); (🍁) APO-CLOXI, NOVO-CLOXIN, CLOXILEAN, ORBENIN
❒ Dicloxacillin (DYCILL, DYNAPEN, PATHOCIL)
❒ Methicillin (STAPHCILLIN)
❒ Nafcillin (NAFCIL, NALLPEN, UNIPEN)
❒ Oxacillin (BACTOCILL, PROSTAPHLIN)

AMINOPENICILLINS

❒ Amoxicillin (AMOXIL, many others)
❒ Ampicillin (OMNIPEN, FOTACILLIN, many others)
❒ Bacampicillin (SPECTROBID)

ANTIPSEUDOMONALS

❒ Carbenicillin (GEOPEN, GEOCILLIN)
❒ Mezlocillin (MEZLIN)
❒ Piperacillin (PIPRACIL)
❒ Ticarcillin (TICAR)

PENICILLIN AND BETA-LACTAMASE INHIBITOR COMBINATIONS

❒ Amoxicillin/clavulanate (AUGMENTIN)
❒ Ampicillin/sulbactam (UNASYN)
❒ Piperacillin/tazobactam (ZOSYN)
❒ Ticarcillin/clavulanate (TIMENTIN)

Indications

Infectious conditions in which penicillins are used include respiratory and GU tract infections, skin, soft tissue, bone, joints, and intra-abdominal infections. More specific conditions in which penicillins are considered the drug of choice include tetanus, meningitis, pneumonia, Lyme disease, anthrax, botulism, gas gangrene, gonorrhea, syphilis, and bacterial septicemia.

Penicillins are used prophylactically for patients with bacterial endocarditis who are undergoing dental procedures or minor upper respiratory tract surgery. Penicillins are generally administered 30 to 60 minutes before the procedure and again 6 hours later. Penicillin is also used prophylactically for pneumococcal infections and long-term, continuous prophylaxis of recurrent rheumatic fever. Rheumatic fever prophylaxis drug therapy is usually initiated as soon as a diagnosis of active rheumatic fever or rheumatic heart disease is formulated.

Pharmacodynamics

Penicillins are classified according to their spectrum of activity. The classifications include natural penicillins, which are penicillinase sensitive; narrow-spectrum penicillins, which are penicillinase resistant; aminopenicillins (broad-spectrum penicillins); and antipseudomonal penicillins (extended-spectrum penicillins).

Penicillin-sensitive penicillins are active against aerobic, gram-positive organisms, including various species of

TABLE 24-3 DOSAGE REGIMEN FOR SELECTED SULFONAMIDES

Drug	Dosage	Implications
Sulfonamides		
Sulfacytine	*Adult:* 500 mg po initially then 250 mg QID	Short-acting. Rapidly absorbed and eliminated
Sulfadiazine	*Adult:* 2–4 g po initially then 2–4 g daily in 4–6 divided doses. *Child over 2 mo:* 75 mg/kg po initially then 150 mg/kg/day in 4–6 divided doses. Maximal dose 6g/day. Rheumatic fever prophylaxis in child under 30 kg: 500 mg po QD. Rheumatic fever prophylaxis in child over 30 kg: 1 g po QD	Therapeutic blood levels are 10–15 mg/100 mL. Low solubility, short acting, rapidly eliminated
Sulfamethizole	*Adult:* 500 mg–1 g po TID–QID *Child over 2 mo:* 30–45 mg/kg/day in 4 divided doses	Highly soluble, rapidly absorbed, rapidly eliminated
Sulfamethoxazole	*Adult:* 2 g po initially then 1–2 g BID–TID *Child over 2 mo:* 50–60 mg/kg po initially then 25–30 mg/kg q12hr. Maximum: 75 mg/kg	Absorbed and eliminated more slowly than sulfisoxazole. More likely to cause high blood levels and crystalluria than sulfisoxazole
Sulfasalazine	*Adult:* 3–4 g po in 3–4 divided doses. Maximum: 8 g/day. *Child over 2 yr:* 40–50 mg/kg in 4 divided doses followed by 30 mg/kg/day in 4 divided doses. Not to exceed 2 g/day	May permanently stain contact lenses yellow. Poorly absorbed. Does not alter GI normal flora
Sulfisoxazole	*Adult:* 2–4 g po/IV/SC in divided doses q4–6 hr then 4–8 g/day po in 4–6 divided doses. Vaginitis: 2.5–5 g of 10% vaginal cream BID *Child over 2 mo:* 75 mg/kg then 150 mg/kg/day in 4–6 divided doses. Not to exceed 6 g/day	Fluid intake should be at least 1200–1500 mL/day if drug taken orally to minimize crystalluria
Trimethoprim (TMP)/ sulfamethoxazole (SMZ)	*Adult:* 160 mg TMP/800 mg SMZ po q12hr *or* 8–10 mg/kg TMP/50 mg/kg SMZ IV q6–12 hr in divided doses *Child over 2 mo:* 4–6 mg/kg TMP/20–30 mg/kg SMZ po q12 hr *or* 8–10 mg/kg TMP/50 mg/kg SMZ IV q6–12 hr in divided doses *Adult and child over 2 mo:* PCP: 3.75–5 mg/kg TMP/18.75–25 mg/kg SMZ po q6hr	Fluid intake should be at least 1200–1500 mL/day to minimize crystalluria Phlebitis possible with IV route

GI, Gastrointestinal.

streptococci, enterococci, and nonpenicillinase-producing staphylococci. They are also active against certain gram-negative organisms such as nonpenicillinase-producing strains of *Neisseria gonorrhoea* and *Neisseria meningitides,* and certain anaerobic oral flora. Furthermore, penicillin-sensitive penicillins are highly effective against *Actinomyces israelii, Pasteurella multocida, Listeria monocytogenes,* and *Treponema pallidum.*

Penicillinase-resistant penicillins are narrow spectrum antibiotics that are effective against staphylococcal infections including *Staphylococcus aureus* and *Staphylococcus epidermidis.* Numerous gram-positive and gram-negative bacteria produce beta-lactamase enzymes (penicillinase, cephalosporinase) that open the beta-lactam ring and inactivate antibiotics. An intact beta-lactam ring is essential for antibacterial activity. Penicillinase-resistant drugs preserve the beta-lactam ring by attaching a protective chain around it, preventing the penicillinase from destroying or inactivating the antibiotic. However, certain bacteria such as *S. aureus* and *S. epidermidis* are becoming increasingly resistant and are able to survive the activity of penicillinase-resistant peniclins (and cephalosporins) and a few other drugs that are known as beta-lactam antibiotics. The resistant microorganisms are referred to as methicillin-resistant *S. aureus* (MRSA) or methicillin-resistant *S. epidermidis* (MRSE). However, both organisms are becoming increasingly resistant to this class of penicillins.

Aminopenicillins are broad-spectrum antibiotics that are effective against many of the same organisms as penicillin G but are also active against certain gram-negative bacilli. This group of antibiotics has enhanced activity with gram-negative urinary tract pathogens (see Chapter 40) and *Enterococcus faecalis.* Nonpenicillinase-producing strains of *H. influenzae* type B are also sensitive to aminopenicillins.

Antipseudomonal, extended-spectrum penicillins have enhanced effectiveness against gram-negative bacilli, especially *Pseudomonas aeruginosa,* while retaining activity similar to that of the aminopenicillin antibiotics. Mezlocillin and piperacillin are effective against *P. aeruginosa* and other enteric gram-negative rods. Mezlocillin also is effective against the *Klebsiella* species. The antipseudomonal penicillins are often used as monotherapy or in combination with an aminoglycoside (discussion follows) to treat nosocomial gram-negative infections.

The addition of beta-lactamase inhibitors such as clavulanate, sulbactam, and tazobactam to certain aminopenicillins and certain antipseudomonal penicillins has broadened the spectrum of penicillins. These extended-spectrum penicillins are bactericidal against gram-positive and gram-negative aerobes, anaerobes, and enterococci that may be resistant to other antibiotics.

An organism's cell wall is normally stiff, penetrable, and meshlike, lying outside the cytoplasmic membrane. The osmotic pressure within the organism's cytoplasmic membrane is very high, creating a strong gradient that takes up water and swells. If it were not for the stiff cell wall, water would be absorbed to such a degree that the organism would burst. Penicillins act by weakening the organism's cell wall, causing excessive amounts of water to be taken up and rupturing the cell wall (Fig. 24–1). The organism's cell wall is weakened through two mechanisms: autolysis and inhibition of transpeptidases. Autolysis is carried out by bacterial enzymes that cleave the strong bond that forms the cell wall so as to permit growth and division. Furthermore, by simultaneously inhibiting transpeptidases, the penicillins disrupt cell wall synthesis and promote its active destruction.

Thus, penicillin antibiotics are typically *bactericidal* only to organisms that are actively growing and dividing. Because human cells lack a cell wall, the penicillins have virtually no direct effect on host cells.

Adverse Effects and Contraindications

Penicillins are the most common cause of drug allergy, although penicillin G is the least toxic of all. Less than 10 percent of patients receiving penicillins experience allergic responses. Allergic reactions vary from minor rashes to life-threatening anaphylaxis. The severe reactions are most likely to occur with parenteral use.

Immediate penicillin reactions occur 2 to 30 minutes after drug administration. Hypersensitivity is generally manifested by nausea, vomiting, pruritus, tachycardia, severe dyspnea, diaphoresis, stridor, vertigo, loss of consciousness, and peripheral circulatory failure. Because of cross-sensitivity,

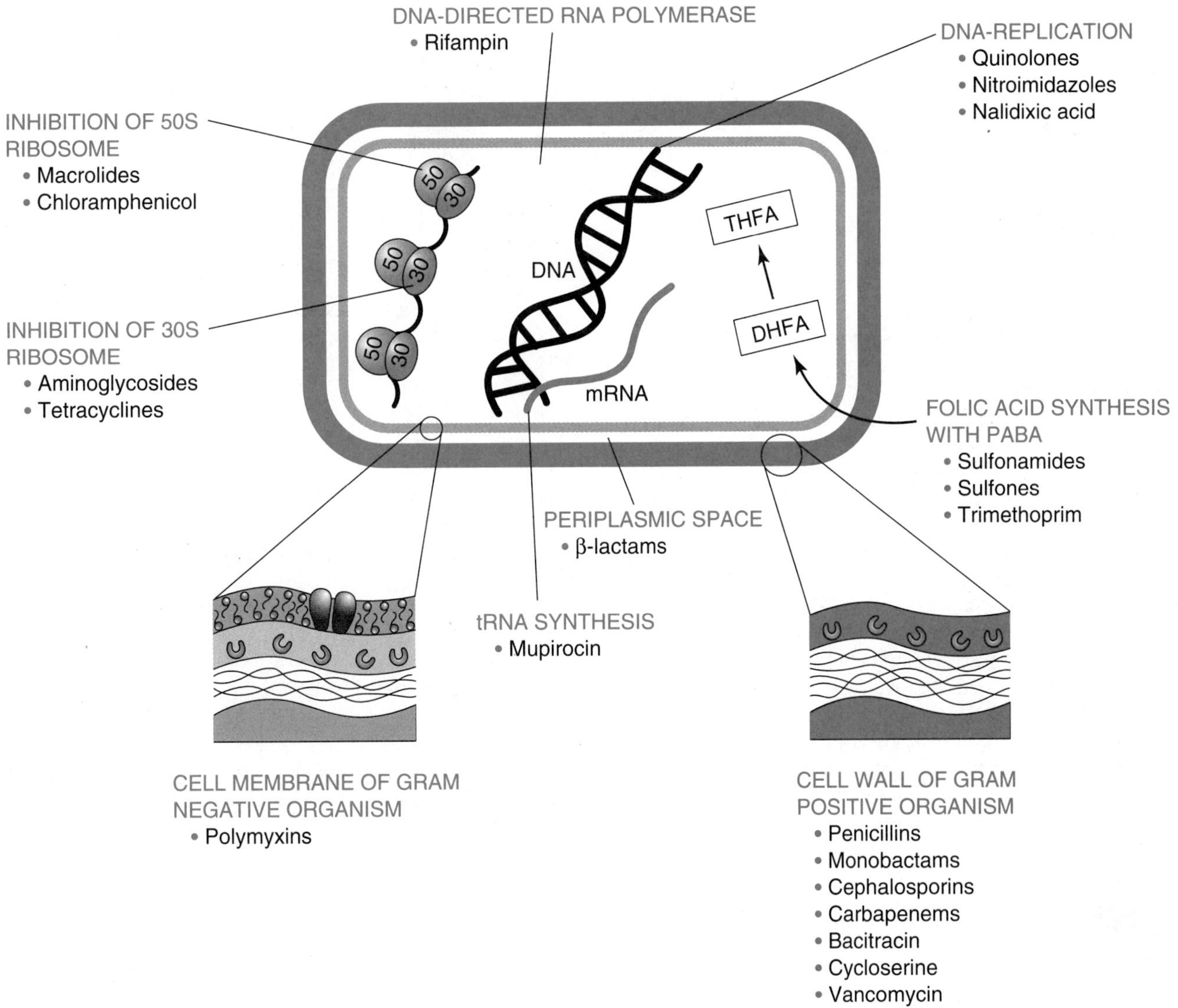

Figure 24–1 Site and mechanism of action of antibiotics. Gram-negative bacteria have a cell membrane; gram-positive bacteria have a cell wall. Drugs interfering with the production of bacterial cell walls are toxic to bacteria but harmless to the host. Further, the bacterial ribosome is sufficiently different from human ribosomes, making bacterial ribosomes good targets for antibacterial drug action.

patients allergic to one penicillin are generally considered allergic to all penicillins. Additionally, 5 to 10 percent of penicillin-sensitive patients display a cross-sensitivity to cephalosporins because of the close structural similarity between the two types of drugs. Accelerated reactions occur 1 to 72 hours after administration. Late reactions may take days or even weeks to develop.

Other adverse effects noted from penicillins include heartburn, anorexia, abdominal pain, and mild-to-severe diarrhea. Taste alterations, sore mouth, and discolored or sore tongue (black, furry tongue) have also been noted.

Penicillins may cause neurologic, nephrologic, or hematologic toxicities. Neurotoxic reactions are manifested as lethargy, twitching, confusion, dysphasia, hyperreflexia, agitation, depression, hallucinations, convulsions, and coma. Signs of nephropathy include fever, macular rash, eosinophilia, proteinuria, hematuria, leukocyturia, and eosinophiluria, which can progress to renal failure. Hematologic toxicity is reflected in altered hematologic findings such as neutropenia, thrombocytopenia, and prolonged bleeding time.

Penicillins are contraindicated in patients with a history of allergic reaction to any penicillin. In addition, cautious use is indicated in patients with an allergy to cephalosporins, during pregnancy, and in patients with anemia, thrombocytopenia, granulocytopenia, or bone marrow depression.

Pharmacokinetics

Penicillins are well absorbed following oral administration; however, penicillin G is unstable in acid, and the majority of an oral dose is destroyed in the stomach. Food slows gastric emptying, thus prolonging exposure of the penicillin to gastric acid. Accordingly, in order to produce blood levels comparable to those of parenteral formulations, the oral dose must be four to five times greater and the drug taken on an empty stomach.

All forms of penicillin may be given intramuscularly (IM). However, the various penicillin salts (sodium, potassium, procaine, benzathine) are absorbed at different rates. For example, the absorption of sodium and potassium formulations of penicillin G is rapid, with peak blood levels reached 15 minutes after injection (Table 24–4). In contrast, procaine and benzathine formulations are slowly absorbed. The procaine and benzathine formulations are preferred as depot agents.

Penicillins are distributed well to most tissues and body fluids. In the absence of inflammation, penetration of meninges, joints, and eye fluids is poor. Conversely, in the presence of inflammation, the absorption of penicillins into CSF, joints, and the eyes is enhanced.

Penicillins are slightly biotransformed in the liver and eliminated primarily unchanged in the urine. Ninety percent of renal elimination is through active tubular secretion, with the remainder from glomerular filtration. As with many other drugs, renal insufficiency prolongs the half-life and increases the risk of penicillin toxicity. Renal elimination can be prolonged with the use of another drug that competes with penicillin for active tubular transport (i.e., probenecid). Probenecid was used to prolong the effects of penicillin during the time when penicillin was both scarce and expensive. Concurrent use is rare because penicillins are now readily available and inexpensive.

Drug-Drug Interactions

Table 24–2 lists drug-drug interactions of selected penicillin drugs. The majority of drug-drug interactions are with antigout drugs (probenecid, sulfinpyrazone), potassium-sparing diuretics, aminoglycosides, anticoagulants, rifampin, and colestipol.

Dosage Regimen

Dosage regimens of penicillins vary based on the type and severity of infection and the desired route of administration. Penicillin salts (sodium, potassium, procaine, and benzathine) differ with regard to routes of administration. Penicillin G sodium is administered IM or intravenously (IV), the potassium formulation is given by mouth, benzathine is given orally or IM, and procaine formulations are only administered IM (Table 24–5). It should be noted that dosages of penicillin G formulations are prescribed in units (1 unit = 0.6 mcg). Other penicillin formulations are prescribed in milligrams or grams.

Laboratory Considerations

Penicillins may cause false laboratory results for some diagnostic tests. For example, penicillins cause false-positive urinary glucose test results when the copper sulfate method (Clinitest) is used. Penicillins also cause elevated serum uric acid concentrations and an elevated value for urine specific gravity.

Cephalosporins

FIRST-GENERATION CEPHALOSPORINS

- ❒ Cefadroxil (DURICEF)
- ❒ Cefazolin sodium (ANCEF, KEFZOL, ZOLICEF)
- ❒ Cephalexin (KEFLEX, KEFTAB); (🍁) NOVO-LEXIN
- ❒ Cephalothin sodium (KEFLIN); (🍁) CEPORACIN
- ❒ Cephapirin sodium
- ❒ Cephradine (VELOSEF)

SECOND-GENERATION CEPHALOSPORINS

- ❒ Cefpodoxime (VANTIN)
- ❒ Cefaclor (CECLOR)
- ❒ Cefamandole (MANDOL)
- ❒ Cefmetazole (ZEFAZONE)
- ❒ Cefonicid sodium (MONOCID)
- ❒ Ceforanide
- ❒ Cefotetan (CEFOTAN)
- ❒ Cefoxitin sodium (MEFOXIN)
- ❒ Cefprozil (CEFZIL)
- ❒ Cefuroxime axetil (CEFTIN)
- ❒ Cefuroxime sodium (KEFUROX, ZINACEF)
- ❒ Loracarbef (LORABID)

THIRD-GENERATION CEPHALOSPORINS

- ❒ Cefdinir (OMNICEF)
- ❒ Ceftibuten (CEDAX)
- ❒ Cefixime (SUPRAX)
- ❒ Cefoperazone (CEFOBID)
- ❒ Cefotaxime (CLAFORAN)
- ❒ Ceftazidime (FORTAZ, TAZICEF, TAZIDIME)
- ❒ Ceftizoxime (CEFIZOX)

TABLE 24–4 PHARMACOKINETICS OF SELECTED PENICILLINS

Drug	Route	Onset	Peak	Duration	PB (%)	$t_{1/2}$	BioA (%)
Penicillinase-Sensitive Penicillins							
Penicillin G sodium	IM	Rapid	1–3 hr	UA	60	0.7 hr	0
	IV	Immed	Rapid	UA	60	0.7 hr	100
Penicillin G benzathine	IM	Delayed	12–24 hr	1–4 wks	UA	30–60 min	0
Penicillin G procaine	IM	Delayed	1–4 hr	1.5 hr	UA	30–60 min	0
Penicillin G potassium	po	1 hr	1 hr	UA	UA	30–60 min	UA
	IM	Rapid	15–30 min	UA	UA	30–60 min	0
	IV	Immed	End of inf	UA	UA	30–60 min	100
Penicillin V	po	Rapid	0.5–1 hr	UA	80	0.5 hr	60
Penicillinase-Resistant Penicillins							
Cloxacillin	po	30 min	30 min–2 hr	UA	93	0.5 hr	49
Dicloxacillin	po	30 min	1–2 hr	UA	96	0.8 hr	UA
Methicillin	IM	Rapid	0.5–1 hr	6 hr	40	0.4 hr	Min
	IV	Immed	0.5–1 hr	6 hr	40	0.4 hr	100
Nafcillin	po	Rapid	0.5–1 hr	UA	80	0.5–1.5 hr	Low
	IM	Rapid	0.5–1 hr	UA	80	0.5–1.5 hr	0
	IV	Immed	End of inf	UA	80	0.5–1.5 hr	100
Oxacillin	po	Rapid	30–60 min	UA	90	20–50 min	33
	IM	Rapid	30 min	UA	90	20–50 min	0
	IV	Immed	End of inf	UA	90	20–50 min	100
Aminopenicillins							
Amoxicillin	po	30 min	1–2 hr	UA	20	1–1.3 hr	80
Ampicillin	po	Rapid	1.5–2 hr	UA	20	1–1.3 hr	50
	IM	Rapid	1 hr	UA	20	1–1.3 hr	0
	IV	Immed	End of inf	UA	20	1–1.3 hr	100
Bacampicillin	po	Rapid	1.5–2 hr	UA	20	1–1.3 hr	50
Antipseudomonal Penicillins							
Carbenicillin	po	30 min	30 min–2 hr	UA	UA	0.8–1 hr	UA
	IV	Immed	30 min–2 hr	UA	UA	0.8–1 hr	100
Mezlocillin	IM	Rapid	5 min	Variable	30	0.7–1.3 hr	0
	IV	Immed	End of inf	Variable	30	0.7–1.3 hr	100
Piperacillin	IM	Rapid	0.5–1 hr	UA	19	0.5–1.2 hr	0
	IV	Immed	End of inf	UA	19	0.5–1.2 hr	100
Penicillin/Beta-Lactamase Inhibitor Combinations							
Ampicillin/sulbactam	IM	Rapid	1–2 hr	UA	20	1–1.3 hr	50
	IV	Immed	End of inf	UA	20	1–1.3 hr	100
Amoxicillin/clavulanate	po	30 min	1–2 hr	UA	20	1–1.3 hr	80
Piperacillin/tazobactam	IM	Rapid	30–50 min	4–6 hr	16; 30	0.7–1.2 hr	80
	IV	Rapid	End of inf	4–6 hr	16; 30	0.7–1.2 hr	100
Ticarcillin/clavulanate	IV	UK	30–45 min	4 hr	50	1–1.3 hr	100

PB, Protein binding; $t_{1/2}$, elimination half-life; UA, unavailable; UK, unknown; BioA, bioavailability.

❒ Ceftriaxone (ROCEPHIN)
❒ Moxalactam (MOXAM)

FOURTH-GENERATION CEPHALOSPORIN
❒ Cefepime (MAXIPIME)

Indications

Cephalosporins are indicated for infections caused by susceptible organisms that have invaded the respiratory, urinary, and biliary tracts; skin; soft tissue; and bone. Cephalosporins are also used in serious conditions such as septicemia, meningitis, endocarditis, peritonitis, acute pelvic inflammatory disease, and gonorrhea.

Prophylactic use of cephalosporins is indicated in perioperative patients who are undergoing surgical procedures associated with a high risk of infection. Examples of such procedures include biliary, cardiovascular, obstetric, gynecologic, orthopedic, or potentially contaminated surgery.

Pharmacodynamics

Cephalosporins are categorized into four generations based on their order of development. Each generation differs significantly with respect to its spectra. In general, there is increasing activity against gram-negative organisms and anaerobes with each generation, increasing destruction of beta-lactamase, and increasing ability of the drug to enter CSF. Cefoxitin and cefotetan are technically cephamycins derived from a different fungus; they are included here because of their similarities to the group.

First-generation cephalosporins are active against gram-positive cocci including *S. aureus* (except MRSA), *S. epidermidis, S. pyogenes, S. agalactiae,* and *S. pneumoniae.* First-generation cephalosporins have limited action against gram-negative bacteria and do not reach effective concentrations in CSF.

Second-generation cephalosporins are active against organisms that are susceptible to the first-generation cephalosporins and gram-negative organisms, including most strains of *H. influenzae, Enterobacter, Klebsiella, E. coli,*

TABLE 24–5 DOSAGE REGIMEN FOR SELECTED PENICILLINS

Drug	Dosage	Implications
Penicillinase-Sensitive Penicillins		
Penicillin G sodium	*Adult:* 600,000–3 million units/day po *Child:* 25,000–90,000 units/kg/day in divided doses q6–8 hr	Note that penicillin dosages are identified in units rather than mg or g
Penicillin G potassium	*Adult:* 300,000–8 million units IM daily *or*-6–20 million units IV daily by continuous or intermittent infusion q2–4 hr *Child:* 50,000–250,000 units/kg/day IM/IV in divided doses q4hr	Up to 60 million units/day has been given in certain serious infections
Penicillin G benzathine	***Infection:*** *Adult:* 1.2–2.4 million units IM as a single dose *or* 400,000–600,000 units q4–6 hr *Child:* 25,000–90,000 units/kg/day po in 3–6 divided doses *or* 50,000 units/kg IM as a single dose ***Syphilis:*** *Adult:* 2.4 million units IM in each buttock as a single dose *Child:* 50,000 units/kg IM as a single dose ***Prophylaxis rheumatic fever:*** *Adult and Child:* 1.2 million units IM q4wk *or* 600,000 units every 2 wk	1 mg = 1600 units. Never give suspension IV. May cause embolism or toxic reactions
Penicillin G procaine	***Infection:*** *Adult:* 600,000–1.2 million units/day IM as single dose or 2 divided doses ***Gonorrhea:*** *Adult:* 4.8 million units at 2 different sites	1 g probenecid po precedes penicillin in the treatment of gonorrhea. 1 mg = 1600 units
Penicillin V	*Adult:* 125–500 mg po 4–6 times daily *Child:* 15–50 mg/kg/day po in three to six divided doses	
Penicillinase-Resistant Penicillins		
Cloxacillin	*Adult & Child over 20 kg:* 250–500 mg po q6hr *Child over 1 mo and under 20 kg:* 12.5–25 mg/kg/day in divided doses q6hr Maximum: 4 g/day	Acidic juices decrease absorption
Dicloxacillin	*Adult and Child over 40 kg:* 125–500 mg po q6hr. Up to 6 g/day *Child under 40 kg:* 12.5–25 mg/kg/day in divided doses q6hr Maximum: 4 g/day	Acidic juices decrease absorption.
Methicillin	*Adult:* 1 g IM q4–6 hr *or* 1–2 g in 50 mL sodium chloride infused over 5–10 min q4hr *Child:* 100–300 mg/kg/day IM in four divided doses q6hr	
Nafcillin	*Adult:* 500 mg–2 g IM q4–6 hr. Maximum dose for serious infections: 12 g *Child:* 50–100 mg/kg/day po in four divided doses 100–300 mg/kg/day IM/IV in divided doses q4–6 hr	
Oxacillin	*Adult and Child over 40 kg:* 500 mg–2 g po/IM/IV q4–6 hr Maximum: 12 g/day *Child under 40 kg:* 50–100 mg/kg/day po/IM/IV in four divided doses q6hr	
Aminopenicillins		
Amoxicillin	*Adult and child over 20 kg:* 250–500 mg po q8hr *Child under 20 kg:* 20–40 mg/kg/day in divided doses q8hr	1 g probenecid accompanies single dose amoxicillin
Ampicillin	*Adult and child over 20 kg:* 250–500 mg po/IM/IV q6hr. Doses up to 2 g/4 hr may be given IV for severe infections *Child under 20 kg:* 25–100 mg/kg/day in divided doses q6hr	
Bacampicillin	*Adult and child over 25 kg:* 400–800 mg po q12hr *Child under 20 kg:* 12.5–25 mg/kg q12hr	

and some strains of *Proteus.* Each of the drugs has a somewhat different antimicrobial spectrum; therefore, susceptibility tests must be performed for each drug rather than for the entire group. None of the second-generation drugs is active against *P. aeruginosa,* and they do not reach effective concentrations in CSF.

Third-generation cephalosporins are active against organisms susceptible to the first- and second-generation

TABLE 24-5 DOSAGE REGIMEN FOR SELECTED PENICILLINS *Continued*

Drug	Dosage	Implications
Antipseudomonal Penicillins		
Carbenicillin	*Adult:* 382–764 mg po q6hr	Administer on empty stomach
Mezlocillin	*Adult:* 150–200 mg/kg/day IM/IV in 4–6 divided doses. Usual adult dose 3 g q4hr *or* 4 g q6hr *Child age 1 mo–12 yr:* 50–75 mg/kg IM/IV in 6 divided doses q4hr	
Piperacillin	*Adult:* 150–200 mg/kg/day IM/IV in divided doses q4–6hr. Usual adult dose 3–4 g q4–6 hr. Maximum daily dose 24 g *Child:* Safe use in children under 12 not established	1 g probenecid po precedes piperacillin for treatment of uncomplicated gonococcal infections
Ticarcillin	*Adult:* 1–2 g IM/IV q6hr. *Child under 40 kg:* 50–200 mg/kg/day IM/IV q6–8 hr	Injections should not exceed 2 g
Penicillin/Beta-Lactamase Inhibitor Combinations		
Ampicillin/sulbactam	*Adult and child over 12 yr:* 250 mg–2 g IM/IV q6hr or 250–500 mg po q6hr *Child under 12 yr:* 25–50 mg/kg/day po *or* 25–100 mg/kg/day IM/IV	
Amoxicillin/clavulanate	*Adult:* 250–500 mg amoxicillin/125 mg clavulanic acid po q8hr *Child under 40 kg:* 20–40 mg/kg/day amoxicillin equivalent po q8hr	
Piperacillin/tazobactam	*Adult:* 3.375 g IV q6hr *Child:* Safe dosage not established	
Ticarcillin/clavulanate	*Adults:* 3.1 g IV q4–6 hr *Child under 60 kg:* 200–300 mg/kg/day IV in divided doses q4–6 hr	

cephalosporins and further extend the spectrum of activity against gram-negative organisms. Third-generation cephalosporins are also active against unusual strains of enteric organisms such as *Citrobacter, Enterobacter, Morganella, Providencia,* and *Serratia.* Some third-generation cephalosporins are effective against *P. aeruginosa,* although drug-resistant strains emerge when a cephalosporin is used alone for treatment of a pseudomonal infection. The third-generation drugs reach clinically effective concentrations in the CSF. The newest third-generation cephalosporin cefdinir has antimicrobial activity similar to cefpodoxime.

Fourth-generation cephalosporins have a greater spectrum of antibiotic activity and greater stability against beta-lactamase enzymes compared with third-generation drugs. They are active against both gram-positive and gram-negative organisms. In addition, the only fourth-generation available at this time retains activity against strains of *Enterobacteriaceae* and *P. aeruginosa* that have developed resistance to third-generation drugs.

Cephalosporins are bactericidal. Although the exact mechanisms of action have not been fully explained, cephalosporins are thought to inhibit mucopeptide synthesis. This interference results in the formation of defective cell walls and bacterial cell death.

Adverse Effects and Contraindications

Cephalosporins are usually tolerated well and are one of the safest groups of antimicrobial drugs. The most common systemic adverse effects involve hypersensitivity reactions with rash, pruritus, fever, chills, urticaria, joint pain or inflammation, edema, erythema, and eosinophilia. Immediate hypersensitivity reactions with bronchospasm and anaphylaxis are uncommon. Because of the structural similarity of cephalosporins to penicillins, penicillin-sensitive patients may experience cross-allergenicity. For patients with mild penicillin allergy, cephalosporins can be used with minimal concern. In practice, the incidence of cross-allergenicity is only 5 to 10 percent. However, because of the potential for anaphylaxis, patients with a history of severe allergy to penicillins should not be given cephalosporins.

Cefamandole, cefoperazone, cefotetan and moxalactam cause bleeding tendencies. They cause a reduction in prothrombin levels by interfering with the metabolism of vitamin K. In addition, moxalactam impairs platelet aggregation. Because moxalactam alters bleeding through two mechanisms, bleeding can be considerably more severe than with the other three drugs. The hematologic reactions are particularly dangerous in older adults, in debilitated and malnourished patients, and in those with severe renal insufficiency.

Common GI adverse effects of cephalosporins include anorexia, nausea, vomiting, and diarrhea. Additional GI adverse effects consist of decreased salivation, taste alteration, dyspepsia, glossitis, flatulence, and abdominal pain. Other adverse effects that have been noted include vertigo, hallucinations, malaise, fatigue, nightmares, headache, hepatic dysfunction, menstrual irregularities, vaginitis, genital pruritus, and vaginal moniliasis. Nephrotoxicity is associated with cephalothin.

Cephalosporins can cause an overgrowth of nonsusceptible organisms, resulting in a *superinfection.* Clinically significant superinfections due to *Pseudomonas, Candida,* and *Enterococci* are more often associated with third-generation drugs. In rare situations, cephalosporins have caused drug-induced pseudomembranous colitis due to overgrowth with

Clostridium difficile. The cephalosporin drug should be stopped and the patient treated, if necessary, with oral vancomycin or metronidazole.

Pharmacokinetics

Ten cephalosporins can be administered by mouth. However, many of the cephalosporins (e.g., cefamandole, cefazolin, cefonicid, cefoperazone, ceftriaxone) are not readily absorbed from the GI tract and must be administered parenterally. Cephalosporins are variously bound to plasma proteins, with half-lives ranging from less than one hour to over 10 hours (Table 24–6).

Only third-generation cephalosporins are distributed to the CSF in sufficient quantities to produce bactericidal effects. For example, ceftriaxone passes easily through the blood-brain barrier and can be used to treat meningitis. Notably, only one third-generation cephalosporin, cefoperazone, is unable to produce therapeutic concentrations in the CSF.

TABLE 24–6 PHARMACOKINETICS OF SELECTED CEPHALOSPORINS

Drug	Route	Onset	Peak	Duration	PB (%)	$t_{1/2}$	BioA (%)
First-Generation Cephalosporins							
Cephalexin	po	15–30 min	1 hr	6–12 hr	6–15	0.5–1.2 hr	UA
Cephalothin	IM	Rapid	30 min	UA	65–79	0.5–1 hr	0
	IV	Immed	End of inf	UA	65–79	0.5–1 hr	100
Cephapirin	IM	Rapid	30 min	UA	44–50	0.6 hr	0
	IV	Immed	End of inf	UA	44–50	0.6 hr	100
Cefazolin	IM	Rapid	1–2 hr	Variable	74–86	1.5–2.5 hr	0
	IV	10 min	End of inf	Variable	74–86	1.5–2.5 hr	100
Cefadroxil	po	Rapid	1.5–2 hr	UA	15–20	1.5–2 hr	90
Cephradine	po	Rapid	1 hr	UA	6–20	0.7–2 hr	> 90
	IM	Rapid	1 hr	UA	6–20	0.7–2 hr	> 90
	IV	Immed	End of inf	UA	6–20	0.7–2 hr	100
Second-Generation Cephalosporins							
Cefaclor	po	15 min	30–60 min	UA	25	0.6–0.9 hr	High
Cefamandole	IM	Rapid	30–120 min	UA	65–75	0.5–2.1 hr	0
	IV	Immed	End of inf	UA	65–75	0.5–2.1 hr	100
Cefmetazole	IV	Rapid	End of inf	UA	80	0.8–1.8 hr	100
Cefonicid	IM	Rapid	60 min	UA	98	4.5 hr	0
	IV	Immed	End of inf	UA	98	4.5 hr	100
Ceforanide	IM	Rapid	1 hr	UA	80	2.9 hr	0
	IV	Immed	2 hr	UA	80	2.9 hr	100
Cefotetan	IM	Rapid	1–3 hr	UA	88	3–5 hr	0
	IV	Immed	End of inf	UA	88	3–5 hr	100
Cefoxitin	IM	Rapid	20–30 min	Variable	73	0.7–1.1 hr	0
	IV	Immed	End of inf	Variable	73	0.7–1.1 hr	100
Cefuroxime	po	Rapid	2 hr	UA	UA	1.3 hr	UA
	IM	Rapid	15–60 min	UA	UA	1.3 hr	0
	IV	Immed	End of inf	UA	UA	1.3 hr	100
Cefprozil	po	UK	1.5 hr	UA	36	1.3 hr	95
Cefpodoxime	po	UK	2–3 hr	12 hr	21–29	2–3 hr	UA
Loracarbef	po	Rapid	1 hr	8–12 hr	25	0.8–1.1 hr	79
Third-Generation Cephalosporins							
Cefdinir	po	Slow	2–4 hr	UA	UA	1.7 hr	20–25
Ceftibuten	po	Rapid	2–3 hr	24 hr	65	2–2.4 hr	UA
Cefixime	po	15–30 min	1 hr	12 hr	65–70	3–4 hr	30–50
Cefoperazone	IM	Rapid	1–2 hr	UA	82–93	1.6–2.6 hr	0
	IV	5 min	End of inf	UA	82–93	1.6–2.6 hr	100
Cefotaxime	IM	Rapid	0.5 hr	UA	13–38	0.9–1.7 hr	0
	IV	Rapid	End of inf	UA	13–38	0.9–1.7 hr	100
Ceftazidime	IM	Rapid	1 hr	UA	5–24	30–60 min	0
	IV	Immed	End of inf	UA	5–24	30–60 min	100
Ceftizoxime	IM	Rapid	0.5–1.5 hr	UA	30	1.5–2 hr	0
	IV	Immed	End of inf	UA	30	1.5–2 hr	100
Ceftriaxone	IM	Rapid	1–2 hr	6–8 hr	58–95	5.4–10.9 hr	0
	IV	Immed	End of inf	6–8 hr	58–95	5.4–10.9 hr	100
Moxalactam	IM	Rapid	30 min–2 hr	6–8 hr	25	1.5–2.5 hr	UA
	IV	Immed	5 min	6–8 hr	25	1.5–2.5 hr	100
Fourth-Generation Cephalosporins							
Cefepime	IM	30 min	1.5–2 hr	10–12 hr		102–138 min	
	IV	Immed	5 min	10–12 hr		102–138 min	100

PB, Protein binding; $t_{1/2}$, elimination half-life; UA, unavailable; UK, unknown; BioA, bioavailability.

Most of the cephalosporins are eliminated through the kidneys. Only two drugs, cefoperazone and ceftriaxone, are eliminated by nonrenal routes, and therefore, they can be used with relative safety in patients with significant renal impairment.

Drug-Drug Interactions

Table 24–2 lists drug-drug interactions of selected cephalosporin drugs. As with penicillins, probenecid delays the renal excretion of some cephalosporins and therefore prolongs their effects. Cefamandole, cefoperazone, and cefotetan will induce a disulfiram-like reaction when taken with alcohol. As previously discussed, the disulfiram effect is brought about by accumulation of acetaldehyde and can be dangerous. Furthermore, drugs that promote bleeding (i.e., anticoagulants, nonsteroidal anti-inflammatory drugs, thrombolytics) may place the patient at risk if they are used concurrently with cephalosporins.

Dosage Regimen

The dosage regimens for selected cephalosporins are noted in Table 24–7. With the exception of cefoperazone and ceftriaxone, the dosages of most cephalosporins should be reduced in patients with significant renal impairment. Generally, cephalosporin drug treatment is continued for a minimum of 48 to 72 hours after the patient achieves an asymptomatic state. Perioperative prophylaxis is usually discontinued within 24 to 48 hours after surgery.

Laboratory Considerations

Prothrombin times should be monitored for appropriate dosage adjustment when oral anticoagulants are administered in conjunction with cephalosporins. Peak and trough laboratory values should be drawn periodically throughout therapy.

Cephalosporins have been noted to cause transient increases in blood urea nitrogen (BUN), alanine aminotransferase (ALT; serum glutamic-pyruvic transaminase [SGPT]), aspartate aminotransferase (AST; serum glutamic-oxaloacetic transaminase [SGOT]), alkaline phosphatase, LDH, and bilirubin levels. They may cause false-positive results for Coombs' test and urine glucose when tested with the copper sulfate method (Clinitest). Thus, urine glucose testing should be performed using glucose enzymatic tests (i.e., Clinistix or Tes-Tape). Cefotetan can cause falsely elevated serum and urine creatinine concentrations. Serum samples should not be drawn within 2 hours of drug administration.

Tetracyclines

- ❐ Doxycycline (DORYX, DOXY, MONODOX, VIBRAMYCIN, VIBRA-TABS); (🍁) APO-DOXY, DOXYCIN, NOVO-DOXYLIN
- ❐ Minocycline (MINOCIN)
- ❐ Oxytetracycline (TERRAMYCIN)
- ❐ Tetracycline (ACHROMYCIN V, PANMYCIN, SUMYCIN, TETRACYN); (🍁) NOVO-TETRA

Indications

Tetracyclines are broad-spectrum antibiotics that are valuable for treating several uncommon infections. The extensive use of tetracyclines in the past resulted in increased bacterial resistance. As a result, they are now rarely the drug of first choice for common bacterial infections. Disorders for which tetracyclines are considered first-line drugs include Rocky Mountain spotted fever, typhus fever, Q fever (rickettsial infections), trachoma, lymphogranuloma venereum, urethritis, cervicitis *(C. trachomatis)*, pneumonia *(Mycoplasma pneumoniae)*, peptic ulcer disease *(Helicobacter pylori)*, brucellosis *(Brucella)*, and cholera *(Vibrio cholera)*. Tetracycline has also been used to treat Lyme disease *(Borrelia burgdorferi)*, but it is not approved by the Food and Drug Administration for such use. Other diseases in which tetracyclines render effective treatment include sinusitis, tularemia, anthrax, yaws, plague, tetanus, rat-bite fever, tropical sprue, and cystitis. Tetracycline is also effective for acne. Doxycycline appears to be effective prophylaxis in individuals traveling to most countries where malaria is prevalent.

Pharmacodynamics

Tetracyclines are bacteriostatic, entering microbial cells by passive diffusion and an active transport system. They obstruct the synthesis of protein by competing for the binding of the 30S subunit site of the RNA ribosome to diminish the essential functions of growth and repair. Tetracyclines may be bactericidal in high concentrations or against highly susceptible organisms.

The exact action of tetracycline on acne has not been fully clarified. Tetracyclines seem to inhibit the growth of *Propionibacterium acnes* on the skin surface and reduce the concentration of free fatty acids in sebum. Sebum is believed to cause the inflammatory acne lesions (e.g., papules, pustules, nodules, and cysts).

Adverse Effects and Contraindications

GI effects appear more often after oral administration of tetracyclines but may also appear after IM and IV administration. The most common adverse effects of tetracyclines are primarily nausea, vomiting, diarrhea, and photosensitivity. Lightheadedness, dizziness, vertigo, and vestibular reactions are common with minocycline.

Tetracyclines bind to calcium in bones and teeth, resulting in yellow or brown discoloration. The intensity of tooth discoloration is related to the total cumulative dose. The staining is darker with prolonged and repeated treatment. The risk of discoloration is less with doxycycline and oxytetracycline than with other tetracyclines. Hypoplasia of tooth enamel may also occur.

Tetracyclines taken after the fourth month of pregnancy can cause staining of deciduous teeth in offspring. Discoloration of permanent teeth occurs when tetracyclines are taken by patients 4 months to 8 years of age. The drugs should be avoided if at all possible by children younger than 8 years of age. In premature infants, tetracyclines also suppress long-bone growth. Bone growth can be depressed up to 40 percent after prolonged exposure to tetracyclines. The effects are reversible on discontinuation of treatment.

All tetracyclines have the potential to cause fatty infiltration of the liver. It appears that dosages over 2 g/day, tetracyclines given by IV infusion, and use during pregnancy have been associated with the likelihood of developing a toxic hepatic reaction.

TABLE 24–7 DOSAGE REGIMEN FOR SELECTED CEPHALOSPORINS

Drug	Dosage	Implications
First-Generation Cephalosporins		
Cephalexin	*Adult:* 250–500 mg po q6hr. Increase to 4 g q6hr if necessary for severe infections *Child:* 25–50 mg/kg/day po in two divided doses q12hr	Somewhat less active against penicillinase-producing staphylococci than cephalothin
Cephalothin	*Adults:* 250 mg–2 g IM/IV q4–6 hr depending on severity of infection *Child:* 80–160 mg/kg/day IM/IV q4 hr	The first cephalosporin. May cause superinfection
Cephapirin	*Adult:* 500 mg-1g IM/IV q4–6hr *Child:* 40–80 mg/kg/day IM/IV in 3–4 divided doses	More active against *Escherichia coli* and *Klebsiella* than cephalothin
Cefazolin	*Adult:* 0.25–2 g IM/IV q6–8 hr. Up to 12 g/day *Child over 1 mo:* 25–50 mg/kg/day in divided doses q6–8 hr. Up to 100 mg/kg/day	Do not use if solution is cloudy or contains precipitate
Cefadroxil	*Adult:* 1–2 g po BID *Child:* 30 mg/kg/day po in two divided doses q12 hr	A derivative of cephalexin but with longer half-life and reduced dosing frequency
Cephradine	*Adult:* 250–500 mg po q6hr *or* 500–1000 mg q12 hr *or* 2–4 g/day IM/IV in four divided doses *Child over 9 mo:* 25–50 mg/kg/day po in divided doses q6–12 hr *or* 50–100 mg/kg/day IM/IV in divided doses q6hr	Reconstituted parenteral doses may vary in color from light straw to yellow. Color changes do not alter potency
Second-Generation Cephalosporins		
Cefaclor	*Adult:* 250–500 mg po q8hr *Child over 1 mo:* 20–40 mg/kg/day po in divided doses q8–12 hr	Suspension is stable for 14 days if refrigerated
Cefamandole	*Adult:* 0.5–2 g IM/IV q4–6 hr. Up to 12 g/day for life-threatening infections *Child:* 50–150 mg/kg/day in 4–6 divided doses q4–6 hr	Major clinical use for treatment of gram-negative infections caused by organisms resistant to other cephalosporins
Cefmetazole	*Adult:* 2 g IV q6–12 hr × 5–14 days. Surgical prophylaxis: 1–2 g IV 30–90 min before surgery. May repeat 8 and 16 hr later for total of 3 doses	Similar to cefoxitin in antibacterial spectrum
Cefonicid	*Adult:* 1 g IM/IV q24hr. Surgical prophylaxis: 1 g IM/IV 1 hr before surgery	Spectrum similar to other second-generation cephalosporins. Not approved for use in children
Ceforanide	*Adult:* 0.5–1 g IM/IV q12hr. Surgical prophylaxis: 0.5–1 g IM/IV 1 hr before surgery *Child:* 20–40 mg/kg/day in divided doses q12hr	Has long half-life and can be given twice daily
Cefotetan	*Adult:* 1–2 g IM/IV q12 hr × 5–10 days. Maximum: 3 g q12hr in life-threatening infections Prophylaxis: 1–2 g IV 30–60 min before surgery	Highly resistant to beta-lactamase enzymes. Effective against most organisms except *Pseudomonas*
Cefoxitin	*Adult:* 1–2 g IM/IV q 6–8 hr *Child:* 80–160 mg/kg/day IM/IV in divided doses q4–6hr. Maximum: 12 g/day	The first cephamycin. More active against gram-negative organisms and less active against gram-positive organisms
Cefuroxime	*Adult:* 250–500 mg po q12 hr *or* 750 mg–1.5 g IM/IV q8hr. Surgical prophylaxis: 1.5 g IV 30–60 min before skin incision and then 750 mg IM/IV q8hr if procedure is prolonged *Child over 3 mo:* 50–100 mg/kg/day IM/IV in divided doses q6–8 hr. Bacterial meningitis: 200–240 mg/kg/day IV in divided doses q6–8hr. Reduce to 100 mg/kg/day with clinical improvement	
Cefprozil	*Adult:* 250–500 mg po q12–24 hr *Child:* 15 mg/kg po q12hr	Similar to cefaclor and cefuroxime
Cefpodoxime	*Adult:* 200 mg po q12hr *Child:* 10 mg/kg po q12hr.	Some activity against staphylococci (except MRSA) Similar to cefixime
Loracarbef	*Adult and child over 13 yr:* 200–400 mg po q12hr. *Child 6 mo to 12 yr:* 15–30 mg/kg/day po in divided doses q12 hr *Uncomplicated cystitis:* *Adult:* 200 mg po q24hr	No significant drug-drug interactions
Third-Generation Cephalosporins		
Ceftibuten	*Adult and child over 40 kg:* 400 mg po QD × 10 days. CrCl 30–49 mL/min: 200 mg po q24hr. CrCl 5–29 mL/min: 100 mg po q24hr *Child 10 kg:* 5 mL po daily *Child 20 kg:* 10 mL po daily *Child 40 kg:* 20 mL po daily	Use oral suspension for children 90 mg/mL
Cefdinir	*Adult:* 300 mg po q12 hr *or* 600 mg po q24hr *Child:* 7 mg/kg po q12hr *or* 14mg/kg po q24hr	Some health care providers are concerned about once daily use of a drug with such a short half-life. Older, better established drugs are preferred

TABLE 24–7 DOSAGE REGIMEN FOR SELECTED CEPHALOSPORINS *Continued*

Drug	Dosage	Implications
Third-Generation Cephalosporins *Continued*		
Cefixime	*Adult and child over 12 yr or over 50 kg:* 400 mg po as single dose *or* 200 mg po q12 hr *Child:* 8 mg/kg/day as single dose or in two divided doses q12hr	Use suspension only when treating otitis media
Cefoperazone	*Adult:* 1–2 g/day IM/IV in divided doses q12 hr	Safe use in children has not been established. Active against gram-negative organisms resistant to previous cephalosporins
Cefotaxime	*Adult:* 1–2 g IM/IV q6–12 hr. Up to 2 g q4hr *Child over 1 mo:* 50–180 mg/kg/day IM/IV in divided doses q4–6 hr *Infant 1–4 weeks:* 50 mg/kg IV q8hr *Infant 0–1 wk:* 50 mg/kg IV q12 hr	Administer over 30 minutes. Change IV sites q48–72 hr to prevent phlebitis
Ceftazidime	*Adult and Child over 50 g:* 1–2 g IM/IV q8–12hr. Maximum: 8 g/24 hr *Child over 1 mo:* 30–50 mg/kg/day IM/IV in divided doses q8hr *Neonates 1–4 wk:* 30 mg/kg IV q12hr.	Active against most gram-negative and gram-positive bacteria. Some activity against *Pseudomonas* resistant to second-generation cephalosporins
Ceftizoxime	*Adult:* 1–2 g IM/IV q8–12hr. Uncomplicated gonorrhea: 1 g IM as a single dose *Child over 6 mo:* 50 mg/kg IM/IV q6–8 hr. If necessary, increase to total daily dose of 200 mg/kg	Dosage must be reduced with even mild renal insufficiency (CrCl < 80 mL/min). Broader gram-negative and anaerobic activity. Active against *Bacteroides fragilis*
Ceftriaxone	*Adult:* 1–2 g/day IM/IV. Surgical prophylaxis: 1 g IV/IM 30 min–2 hr before surgery *Child:* 50–75 mg/kg/day IM/IV. Maximum: 2 g daily in divided doses q12hr. Meningitis: 100 mg/kg/day IM/IV. Maximum: 4 g daily in divided doses q12 hr	Reconstituted parenteral doses may vary in color from light straw to yellow. Color changes do not alter potency
Moxalactam	*Adult:* 2–4 g IM/IV q12hr *Child 1 mo–12 yr:* 50 mg/kg IV q6–8 hr *Neonate to 1 wk:* 50 mg/kg IV q12hr *Neonate 1–4 wk:* 50 mg/kg IV q8hr	Spectrum similar to that of cefotaxime but better activity against anaerobic bacteria. Penetrates CSF
Fourth-Generation Cephalosporin		
Cefepime	*Adult:* 0.5–1 g IM/IV q12hr × 7–10 days. Renal impairment: CrCl 30–60 mL/min: 1 g q24hr. CrCl 11–29mL/min: 0.5 g q24hr. CrCl < 10 mL/min: 250–500 mg q24 hr.	Safe dosage in children has not been established

CrCl, Creatinine clearance; CSF, cerebrospinal fluid; MRSA, methicillin-resistant *Staphylococcus* aureus.

Photosensitivity reactions occur most often with doxycycline. The onset of photosensitivity occurs within a few minutes to several hours after sun exposure and may last 1 or 2 days after tetracycline has been discontinued. Additional photosensitivity effects include an exaggerated sunburn and paresthesia (e.g., tingling and burning of the nose, hands, and feet). Minocycline appears to be the least likely to cause the sunburn reaction, although a blue-gray or muddy brown pigmentation, accentuated in sun-exposed areas of the skin, has been noted.

Tetracyclines can lead to superinfection because of alterations in the normal flora of the respiratory tract, GI tract, and vagina. *Candida* superinfections are more likely to occur with prolonged therapy and in debilitated patients.

Pharmacokinetics

The absorption of orally administered tetracyclines is incomplete but can be enhanced by taking the drugs on an empty stomach. Food appears to interfere less with the absorption of doxycycline and minocycline. Alterations in gastric pH (e.g., after antacid administration) may also decrease the absorption of tetracyclines.

Doxycycline and minocycline are the most lipid soluble forms and, thus, are distributed to various tissues, crossing the blood-brain barrier and placental membranes. Fetal plasma concentrations reach 60 percent of the level in the maternal circulation. The drugs are also found in breast milk. Tetracyclines as a class undergo enterohepatic recirculation and are eliminated in the urine and feces (Table 24–8).

Drug-Drug Interactions

The primary drug-drug interactions associated with tetracyclines include antacids, dairy products and iron, and oral contraceptives (see Table 24–2). The absorption of tetracycline is decreased when taken concurrently with compounds containing magnesium, calcium, aluminum, or iron. The net effect is a decrease in the antibacterial efficacy of tetracycline. Tetracyclines have also been reported to decrease the efficacy of oral contraceptives because they undergo the same enterohepatic recirculation as tetracyclines. There appears to be interference with the hydrolytic process, thus reducing or abolishing the reabsorption of the oral contraceptive drug. The risk of pregnancy can be significant.

TABLE 24–8 PHARMACOKINETICS OF SELECTED TETRACYCLINES

Drug	Route	Onset	Peak	Duration	PB (%)	$t_{1/2}$	BioA (%)
Tetracycline	po	1–2 hr	2–4 hr	UA	20–67	6–12 hr	60–80
Doxycycline	po	1–4 hr	1.5–4 hr	To 12 hr	25–93	14–24 hr	93
	IV	Immed	End of inf	To 12 hr	25–93	14–24 hr	100
Minocycline	po	Rapid	2–3 hr	UA	55–88	15–20 hr	90
	IV	Immed	End of inf	UA	55–80	15–20 hr	100

PB, Protein binding; $t_{1/2}$, elimination half-life; UA, unavailable; BioA, bioavailability.

Dosage Regimen

The dosage regimen of tetracyclines varies based on the reason for their use (Table 24–9). Tetracyclines may be administered by mouth or parenterally. The IV route should be employed only when oral therapy cannot be tolerated or has proved inadequate. IM injections are painful, and the route is rarely used.

Laboratory Considerations

Tetracyclines may cause a false-positive result in urine glucose measurement using the copper sulfate method (Benedict's reagent, Clinitest) and a false-negative result in urine glucose measurement using glucose oxidase reagent (e.g., Clinistix, Tes-Tape). A false elevation is also noted in fluorometric determinations of urine catecholamines. Tetracyclines can cause BUN levels to be elevated, depending on the dose.

Aminoglycoside Drugs

- ❒ Amikacin sulfate (AMIKIN)
- ❒ Gentamicin sulfate (GARAMYCIN, GENTAMICIN); (✱) ALCOMICIN; CIDOMYCIN
- ❒ Kanamycin sulfate (KANTREX)
- ❒ Neomycin sulfate (MYCIFRADIN, MYCIGUENT)
- ❒ Netilmicin (NETROMYCIN)
- ❒ Paromomycin (HUMATIN)
- ❒ Streptomycin sulfate
- ❒ Tobramycin sulfate (NEBCIN, TOBREX)

Indications

Aminoglycosides are narrow-spectrum antibiotics. They are indicated for serious, systemic infections of the blood stream, respiratory tract, bones and joints, skin and soft tissue, and intra-abdominal area caused by susceptible aerobic, gram-negative organisms. In the United States, eight aminoglycosides are approved by the Food and Drug Administration for clinical use.

Gentamicin, tobramycin, and amikacin are the most common. Paromomycin is used only for its local effects within the intestine to treat intestinal amebiasis and tapeworm infestations. Neomycin is the most toxic aminoglycoside. It can cause severe damage to the kidneys and inner ear. Because of its toxicity, neomycin is not used parenterally but is used for topical treatment of eye, ear, and skin infections. Oral neomycin is used to suppress the normal flora of the bowel in preparation for intestinal surgery. A few aminoglycosides are administered topically to the eye or to the skin. These are discussed in Chapters 62 and 64, respectively.

Aminoglycosides are inactive against fungi, viruses, and most anaerobic infections. Because they are very potent antibiotics, aminoglycosides cause harsh adverse effects. They are reserved for situations in which less toxic drugs have

TABLE 24–9 DOSAGE REGIMEN FOR SELECTED TETRACYCLINES

Drug	Dosage	Implications
Doxycycline	*Adult:* 100–200 mg/day po/IV QD or in divided doses q12hr *Child over 8 yr:* 2.2–4.4 mg/kg/day po/IV QD or in divided doses q12hr	Avoid use of dairy products, antacids, sodium bicarbonate, iron supplements, calcium supplements, antidiarrheal drugs within 1–3 hours of oral tetracyclines. Avoid extravasation if drug is given IV
Minocycline	*Adult:* 100–200 mg po initially then 100 mg q12hr *or* 50 mg q6hr *or* 200 mg IV initially then 100 mg IV q12hr up to 400 mg/day *Child over 8 yr:* 4 mg/kg po initially then 2 mg/kg q12hr *or* 4 mg/kg IV initially then 2 mg/kg q12hr	
Tetracycline	*Adult:* 1–2 g/day in divided doses q6–12 hr Chronic acne treatment: 500 mg–1 g/day for 3 wk, then decreased to 125 mg–1g/day. *Child over 8 yr:* 25–50 mg/kg/day in divided doses q6–12 hr.	

proved ineffective and for very serious, life-threatening infections.

Pharmacodynamics

Aminoglycosides are bactericidal, primarily targeting *P. aeruginosa, E. coli, Klebsiella, Serratia,* and *Proteus mirabilis.* Although the exact mechanism of action has not been fully determined, aminoglycosides seem to penetrate susceptible bacterial cell walls, binding to the 30S ribosome. As a result, the synthesis of proteins necessary for bacterial function and replication is inhibited. All aminoglycosides carry multiple positive charges. As a result, these drugs are not absorbed from the GI tract and, therefore, must be administered parenterally.

Adverse Effects and Contraindications

Adverse effects most commonly associated with aminoglycosides include nausea, vomiting, and diarrhea. Other undesirable adverse effects consist of syncope, vertigo, skin rash, fever, headache, neuromuscular blockade, paresthesia, and superinfection. Hypersensitivity symptoms manifest as a rash, urticaria, stomatitis, pruritus, generalized burning, fever, and eosinophilia.

The most serious adverse effects associated with aminoglycosides are neurotoxicity, nephrotoxicity, and ototoxicity. Neurotoxicity manifests as neuromuscular blockade, respiratory depression, and paralysis. Most episodes of neuromuscular blockade occur following intrapleural or intraperitoneal instillation of aminoglycosides. The risk of paralysis is more likely to occur with concurrent use of neuromuscular blocking drugs, aminoglycosides, and general anesthetics. Nephrotoxicity usually manifests as acute tubular necrosis with proteinuria, oliguria, WBCs or casts in urine, hematuria, elevated BUN, and serum creatinine.

Ototoxicity is caused by damage to the eighth cranial nerve and is manifested by vestibular symptoms (e.g., vertigo, ataxia, nystagmus) and auditory symptoms (e.g., tinnitus and varying degrees of hearing impairment). Factors that increase the risk of ototoxicity include renal dysfunction, concurrent use of a drug that has ototoxic properties of its own, and the use of excessive doses of aminoglycosides for longer than 10 days.

Owing to their potential nephrotoxic effects, aminoglycosides are contraindicated in patients with known renal impairment. Aminoglycosides present an increased risk of nephrotoxicity in infants. Aminoglycosides are also contraindicated in patients with allergy to bisulfites because most of the parenteral formulations contain this allergen. Products containing benzyl alcohol should be avoided in neonates. Cross-sensitivity among aminoglycosides may occur. These drugs should be administered cautiously to patients with myasthenia gravis and other neuromuscular disorders because muscle weakness may be escalated.

Pharmacokinetics

The pharmacokinetics of aminoglycosides are identified in Table 24–10. They are poorly absorbed when taken by mouth; thus, most aminoglycosides are given parenterally. Aminoglycosides are largely distributed in extracellular fluids. Sufficient concentrations occur in peritoneal fluids, making them useful for treating peritonitis. Similarly, periocular injections may be indicated for serious eye infections. The low CSF concentrations following parenteral administration require direct injection of these antibiotics into the CSF. Distribution to amniotic fluid and fetal plasma occurs; thus, aminoglycosides should be used only if their potential benefit outweighs the risk. They are eliminated from the body via glomerular filtration. There is little tubular secretion and no hepatic biotransformation.

Drug-Drug Interactions

Table 24–2 lists drug-drug interactions of selected aminoglycoside drugs. Aminoglycosides are inactivated when they are given concurrently with penicillins. There is increased nephrotoxicity and ototoxicity when aminoglycosides are given with ethacrynic acid or furosemide. The activity of oral anticoagulants is increased.

Dosage Regimen

Aminoglycosides may be given by several different routes. Owing to poor GI absorption, aminoglycosides are generally given IM or IV (Table 24–11). Furthermore, because of the multiple toxicities associated with aminoglycosides, dosages are cal-

TABLE 24–10 PHARMACOKINETICS OF SELECTED AMINOGLYCOSIDES

Drug	Route	Onset	Peak	Duration	PB (%)	$t_{1/2}$	BioA (%)
Amikacin	IM	Rapid	0.75–1.5 hr	8–12 hr	4	2–3 hr	0
	IV	Immed	End of inf	8–12 hr	4	2–3 hr	100
Gentamicin	IM	Rapid	0.5–2 hr	8–12 hr	< 10	2–3 hr	0
	IV	Immed	End of inf	8–12 hr	< 10	2–3 hr	100
Kanamycin	IM	Rapid	1–2 hr	UA	< 10	2–3 hr	0
	IV	Rapid	End of inf	UA	< 10	2–3 hr	100
Neomycin	po	Varies	1–4 hr	6–8 hr	UA	2–3 hr	UA
	IM	Rapid	1–2 hr	6–8 hr	UA	2–3 hr	0
Netilmicin	IM	Rapid	1–2 hr	UA	10	2–3 hr	0
	IV	Immed	1–2 hr	UA	10	2–3 hr	100
Streptomycin	IM	Rapid	1–2 hr	UA	30	2–3 hr	0
Tobramycin	IM	Rapid	1 hr	UA	< 10	2–3 hr	0
	IV	Immed	End of inf	UA	< 10	2–3 hr	100

PB, Protein binding; $t_{1/2}$, elimination half-life; UA, unavailable; BioA, bioavailability.

TABLE 24–11 DOSAGE REGIMEN FOR SELECTED AMINOGLYCOSIDES

Drug	Dosage	Implications
Amikacin	*Adult and older child:* Initial loading dose: 5–7.5 mg/kg then 7.5 mg IM/IV q12hr *Neonate:* 10 mg/kg IV initially then 7.5 mg/kg IV q12hr	Peak and trough levels checked with third dose. Peak: 20–30 mcg/mL. Trough: < 10 mcg/mL. Used primarily for infections resistant to other aminoglycosides. Has broader spectrum than other aminoglycosides
Gentamicin	*Adult:* Initial loading dose: 1.5–2 mg/kg then 3–5 mg/kg/day IM–IV in divided doses q8hr *Child:* 6–7.5 mg/kg/day IM–IV in divided doses q8hr *Infant and neonate:* 2.5 mg/kg/day IM–IV q8–16 hr *Premature infant and neonate < 1 wk:* 2.5 mg/kg IM–IV q12–24 hr	Peak and trough levels checked with third dose. Peak: 5–8 mcg/mL. Trough: < 2 mcg/mL. Combined with ticarcillin, it inhibits emergence of resistant bacteria that may occur when either drug is used alone
Kanamycin	*Adult and child:* Serious infection: 15 mg/kg/day IM/IV in 2–3 divideddoses. Suppression of GI bacteria: 1 g po q1hr × 4 doses then 1 g po q6hr × 36–72 hr	Peak and trough levels checked with third dose. Occasionally used to decrease GI flora before surgery
Neomycin	*Adult:* Suppression of GI bacteria: 1 g po q1hr × 4 doses then 1 g q4hr × 5 doses	Poorly absorbed from GI tract. Toxic levels may accumulate in presence of renal failure
Netilmicin	*Adult:* Initial loading dose: 1.5–2 mg/kg then 2–3.3 mg/kg/day IM/IV in 2–3 divided doses q12 hr *Child 6 wk to 12 yr:* 1.8–2 mg/kg/day in 2–3 divided doses, q8–12 hr	Peak and trough levels checked with third dose Peak: 4–12 mcg/mL. Trough: < 4 mcg/mL. Similar in spectrum to gentamicin. Less active against *Pseudomonas.*
Paromomycin	*Adult:* 25–35 mg/kg/day po in 3 divided doses × 5–10 days. Repeat in 2 weeks if necessary	Not absorbed from GI tract and unlikely to cause ototoxicity and nephrotoxicity. Systemic absorption may occur in presence of inflammation of GI tract
Streptomycin	*Adult:* 15 mg/kg/day IM to maximum of 1 g *or* 25–30 mg/kg 2–3 times weekly. Maximum: 1.5 g/dose *Child:* 20–40 mg/kg/day IM in two divided doses q12 hr to maximum of 1 g/day	The first aminoglycoside. Less favored today because of CN VIII nerve damage and emergence of resistant organisms
Tobramycin	*Adult and child:* Initial loading dose: 1.5–2 mg/kg then 3–5 mg/kg/day IM/IV q24 hr *or* 1.5–2.5 mg/kg IM/IV q12 hr *or* 1–1.7 mg/kg IM/IV q8hr *Neonates 1 wk or less:* Up to 4 mg/kg/day IM/IV in 2 divided doses q12 hr	Peak and trough levels checked with third dose. Peak: 5–8 mcg/mL. Trough: < 2 mcg/mL. Similar in spectrum to gentamicin. Used when penicillins or less toxic drugs are contraindicated

CN, Cranial nerve; GI, gastrointestinal.

culated based on milligrams per kilograms of body weight rather than using a fixed dosage. Two major dosing schedules are used—one involving multiple daily doses and one involving a single daily dose. The multiple dose regimen has been used for many years and the guidelines are well established.

An initial loading dose is given to achieve therapeutic serum levels rapidly. The dosage is based on body weight (milligrams per kilogram) and the desired peak serum drug level. If the patient is obese, lean or ideal body weight should be used because aminoglycosides are not significantly distributed to body fat. Serum drug levels are vital to maintenance dosage calculation and adjustment, especially in patients with compromised renal function. For gentamicin and tobramycin, peak levels above 10 to 12 mcg/mL and trough levels above 2 mcg/mL for prolonged periods have been associated with nephrotoxicity. For accuracy, peak and trough levels must be drawn at the correct times. Serum drug levels can be used to adjust dosages in patients with impaired renal failure, or the time interval between doses can be adjusted based on creatinine clearance levels.

Greater interest has been shown in once-daily or extended- interval aminoglycoside dosing. Once-daily dosing has evolved as information about therapy with aminoglycosides has increased. Two factors have contributed to the interest in once-daily dosing: concentration-dependent bactericidal effects and postantibiotic effects. The concentration-dependent effects mean that the drugs are most effective in killing organisms with a large dose and high peak serum concentrations. The postantibiotic effects mean that aminoglycosides continue killing organisms even with low serum concentrations. These two factors permit dosage regimens high enough to achieve high peak serum levels and optimal killing of organisms. The 24-hour period between doses permits the patient to eliminate the drug to very low serum levels for about 6 hours. During this low serum drug level period, the postantibiotic effect is active and there is minimal drug accumulation in the body. There are several reported advantages to this regimen. Antibacterial effects are enhanced, there is less nephrotoxicity, reduced need for peak and trough drug levels, and reduced health care provider time for administration.

Laboratory Considerations

Aminoglycosides may cause increased BUN, AST (SGOT), ALT (SGPT), serum alkaline phosphatase, bilirubin, creatinine, and LDH concentrations. They may cause decreased serum calcium, magnesium, potassium, and sodium concentrations.

Fluoroquinolones

- ❒ Ciprofloxacin (CIPRO); (🍁) DALACIN
- ❒ Enoxacin (PENETREX)
- ❒ Levofloxacin (LEVAQUIN)

TABLE 24–12 PHARMACOKINETICS OF SELECTED FLUOROQUINOLONES

Drug	Route	Onset	Peak	Duration	PB (%)	$t_{1/2}$	BioA (%)
Ciprofloxacin	IV	Rapid	End of inf	12 hr	UA	3–4.8 hr	100
	po	1 hr	1–2.3 hr	12 hr	UA	3–4.8 hr	UA
Enoxacin	po	Rapid	1–3 hr	UK	40	3–6 hr	90
Lomefloxacin	po	Rapid	UK	UK	10	8 hr	95–98
Norfloxacin	po	Rapid	2–3 hr	12 hr	10–15	6.5 hr	30–40
Ofloxacin	po	Rapid	1–2 hr	12 hr	20–25	5–7 hr	89
	IV	Rapid	End of inf	12 hr	20–25	5–7 hr	100
Sparfloxacin	po	Rapid	3–6 hr	24 hr	45	20 hr	92

PB, Protein binding; $t_{1/2}$, elimination half-life; UA, unavailable; UK, unknown; BioA bioavailability.

❒ Lomefloxacin (MAXAQUIN)
❒ Norfloxacin (CHIBROXIN, NOROXIN)
❒ Ofloxacin (FLOXIN)
❒ Sparfloxacin (ZAGAM)

Indications

Fluoroquinolones are the newest classification of broad-spectrum antibiotics. They are chemically related to nalidixic acid, a narrow-spectrum antibiotic used only for urinary tract infections. Fluoroquinolones used for urinary tract infections are discussed in Chapter 40.

Fluoroquinolones are indicated for a variety of infections caused by gram-negative and other organisms. They can be used to treat infections of the respiratory tract, GU and GI tracts, as well as infections of bones and joints, and skin and soft tissues. They are also being used to treat multidrug-resistant tuberculosis (see Chapter 26), infections caused by atypical mycobacteria (e.g., *Mycobacterium avium*) in patients with acquired immunodeficiency syndrome, and fever in neutropenic patients with cancer.

Pharmacodynamics

In contrast to nalidixic acid, fluoroquinolones are active against aerobic gram-negative (*Enterobacteriaceae, P. aeruginosa*) and some gram-positive bacteria (e.g., *S. aureus, S. epidermidis, E. faecalis*). The drugs are not useful against infections caused by anaerobes and have poor activity against *S. pneumoniae*.

Fluoroquinolones act by interfering with deoxyribonucleic acid (DNA) gyrase. DNA gyrase is the enzyme responsible for the stranding of bacterial DNA synthesis, as well as bacterial growth and replication.

Adverse Effects and Contraindications

Common adverse effects of fluoroquinolones include nausea, vomiting, diarrhea, abdominal pain, and restlessness. An unpleasant taste in the mouth, decreased appetite, dry mouth, and photophobia have been reported. The most serious adverse effects include seizures. Bone and cartilage toxicities (e.g., tendon rupture) are rarely noted. However, until further studies are conducted, it seems prudent to avoid this drug in pediatric patients whose skeletal growth is incomplete. Hypersensitivity is uncommon, but anaphylaxis has occurred. Superinfections such as vaginitis have developed due to *Candida* overgrowth. Crystalluria has been reported with large doses.

Fluoroquinolones are contraindicated in patients with hypersensitivity. Cross-allergenicity among fluoroquinolone agents may occur. These drugs should not be used during pregnancy or lactation, or in persons under the age of 18. Fluoroquinolones should be used with caution in patients with underlying CNS pathology and renal impairment. Older adults and dialysis patients are at greater risk for tendon rupture.

Pharmacokinetics

Fluoroquinolones are well absorbed when taken orally and are widely distributed throughout body tissues and fluids such as saliva, nasal and bronchial secretions, sputum, bile, lymph, and peritoneal fluid. (Table 24–12). The bioavailability of fluoroquinolones varies from 70 percent for ciprofloxacin to 98 percent for lomefloxacin. Protein binding varies from 20 to 40 percent for ciprofloxacin to 10 to 15 percent for norfloxacin. The onset of drug action is rapid, but the duration of drug action is unknown. The majority of fluoroquinolones are biotransformed in the liver and eliminated unchanged through the urine. A small percentage of lomefloxacin is eliminated unchanged in the feces.

Drug-Drug Interactions

There are many drug-drug interactions with fluoroquinolones. Fluoroquinolones interfere with the biotransformation of caffeine, warfarin, and theophylline because of effects on hepatic cytochrome P_{450} enzymes. The serum concentration of these drugs is thus increased, resulting in possible toxicity (see Table 24–2).

Dosage Regimens

Dosages should be adjusted in patients with creatinine clearance values of less than 30 mL/minute. Dosage recommendations are identified in Table 24–13.

Laboratory Considerations

Fluoroquinolone use leads to infrequent laboratory abnormalities. Eosinophilia, leukopenia, and elevated ALT (SGPT), AST (SGOT), BUN, and serum creatinine may occur after use but are all reversible with discontinuation of the drug.

Macrolide Drugs

❒ Azithromycin (ZITHROMAX)
❒ Clarithromycin (BIAXIN FILMTABS)
❒ Dirithromycin (DYNABEC)
❒ Erythromycin base (E-BASE, E-MYCIN, ERYC, ERY-TAB, PCE); (🍁) APO-ERYTHRO-E-C, ERYBID, ERYTHROMID, ILOTYCIN GLUCEPTATE, NOVO-RYTHRO

TABLE 24–13 DOSAGE REGIMEN FOR SELECTED FLUOROQUINOLONES

Drug	Dosage	Implications
Ciprofloxacin	*Adult:* 250–750 mg po q12hr *or* 200–400 mg IV q12hr over 60 minutes	Fluid intake should be at least 2000–3000 mL/day to minimize crystalluria
Enoxacin	*Adult:* 200–400 mg po q12hr × 7–14 days. Gonorrhea: 400 mg po as a single dose	Used only for UTI and uncomplicated gonorrhea
Levofloxacin	*Adult:* 250–500 mg po/IV once daily	Infuse IV dose slowly over 60 minutes. Broad spectrum
Lomefloxacin	*Adult:* 400 mg po once daily. Surgical prophylaxis: 400 mg po as single dose 2–6 hr before surgery	Much like ciprofloxacin. Useful as prophylaxis before transurethral surgical procedures
Norfloxacin	*Adult:* 400 mg po BID	Used only for UTI and uncomplicated gonorrhea
Ofloxacin	*Adult:* 200–400 mg po/IV q12 hr × 7–10 days. Gonorrhea: 400 mg po as a single dose	Much like ciprofloxacin
Sparfloxacin	*Adult:* 400 mg po initially then 200 mg po q24 hr × 10 days	May be administered without regard to food. Encourage patient to maintain fluid intake of at least 1500–2000 mL/day to prevent crystalluria.

- ❒ Erythromycin estolate (ILOSONE); (🍁) NOVO-RYTHRO
- ❒ Erythromycin ethylsuccinate (E.E.S., ERY-PED); (🍁) APO-ERYTHRO-ES
- ❒ Erythromycin lactobionate (ERYTHROCIN)
- ❒ Erythromycin stearate (ERYTHROCIN STEARATE); (🍁) APO-ERYTHRO-S, NOVO-RYTHRO

Indications

Macrolides are indicated for susceptible infections located in the upper and lower respiratory tract, skin, and soft tissue; pertussis; diphtheria; intestinal amebiasis; pelvic inflammatory disease; nongonococcal urethritis; syphilis; legionnaires' disease; and rheumatic fever. They have variable activity against anaerobic gram-negative organisms. Macrolides are not considered suitable for prophylaxis use. Erythromycin formulations are used less often today because of microbial resistance and the development of newer macrolides. Ophthalmic and topical formulations are discussed in Chapters 62 and 64, respectively.

Pharmacodynamics

Macrolides are effective against *Mycoplasma pneumoniae, Legionella pneumophila, Treponema pallidum* (syphilis), *Campylobacter jejuni,* and *C. trachomatis* (Chlamydia). They control the development or reproduction of bacteria; hence, they are considered bacteriostatic. However, macrolides may be bactericidal in high concentrations or against highly susceptible organisms. Macrolides are thought to inhibit protein synthesis by penetrating the wall of sensitive bacteria. They reversibly bind to the 50S ribosomal subunit to inhibit polypeptide chain formation. The ribosomal binding fails to occur in resistant bacteria.

Azithromycin and clarithromycin are also active against the atypical mycobacteria that cause *Mycobacterium avium* complex disease. This disease is an opportunistic infection that occurs primarily in people with HIV infection.

Adverse Effects and Contraindications

The most common adverse effects of macrolides include dose-related abdominal pain and cramping, nausea, vomiting, diarrhea, stomatitis, flatulence, anorexia, heartburn, and pruritus ani. A reversible mild acute pancreatitis has been noted. Adverse effects not related to dose include hypersensitivity reactions (e.g., skin rash, drug fever, eosinophilia) and hepatotoxicity (e.g., cholestatic jaundice). Hepatotoxicity occurs with the estolate and ethylsuccinate forms of erythromycin.

Other adverse effects of erythromycin involve palpitations, chest pain, headache, vertigo, somnolence, tinnitus, and bilateral hearing loss. Hearing loss occurs 36 hours to 1 week following IV administration, but it is reversible 24 hours to 2 weeks after the drug is discontinued. Recovery time is not dose related. Concomitant use of other ototoxic drugs increases the potential for ototoxicity.

Pharmacokinetics

Erythromycin base and stearate formulations are susceptible to inactivation by gastric acid. For this reason, enteric coating and alterations to the chemical structure of the estolate and ethylsuccinate formulations were made to decrease acid inactivation. Macrolides are widely distributed to most body tissues and fluids, except the brain and CSF. Penetration into the prostate gland is approximately 40 percent of the simultaneous serum concentration. Bronchial secretions, middle ear, and sinus fluids reach drug levels that are in excess of the inhibitory concentrations of several pathogens causing community-acquired pneumonias, otitis media, or acute sinusitis. They cross the placental membranes, attaining fetal plasma concentrations 20 percent that of maternal circulation. Erythromycin concentrates in the liver and is eliminated mainly via the bile. Some of the drug is also eliminated in urine.

Clarithromycin and azithromycin are well absorbed from the GI tract and are not inactivated by gastric acids. Food may decrease the absorption of azithromycin by 50 percent; therefore, the drug is usually administered at least 1 hour before or 2 hours after a meal. Clarithromycin is widely distributed, with high concentrations being deposited in the nasal mucosa, tonsils, and lungs. Serum concentrations are relatively low for azithromycin, but both drugs penetrate polymorphonuclear leukocytes and macrophages. Tissue concentrations last for days. The half-life of azithromycin is

TABLE 24–14 PHARMACOKINETICS OF SELECTED MACROLIDES

Drug	Route	Onset	Peak	Duration	PB (%)	$t_{1/2}$	BioA (%)
Azithromycin	po	UK	2.5 hr	24 hr	7–50	25–68 hr	37
Clarithromycin	po	UK	2–4 hr	6–8 hr	42–72	4.3 hr	55
Dirithromycin	po	UK	2–4 hr	6–8 hr	15–30	2–36 hr; 16–65 hr*	10
Erythromycin formulations	po	1 hr	1–4 hr	UA	70–90	1.4–2 hr	60
Imipenem/ cilastatin	IM IV	UK Rapid	UK 30–60 min	UA	20	1–1.3 hr	0 100

*Half-life and terminal half-life of dirithromycin, respectively.
PB, Protein binding; $t_{1/2}$, elimination half-life; UA, unavailable; UK, unknown; BioA, bioavailability.

much longer than that of erythromycin or clarithromycin. About 20 percent of clarithromycin is eliminated unchanged in the urine. Azithromycin is hepatically biotransformed, with only 6 percent of the dose recovered unchanged in the urine (Table 24–14). Dirithromycin is eliminated primarily in bile.

Drug-Drug Interactions

Table 24–2 lists drug-drug interactions of selected macrolide drugs. Macrolides may inhibit the metabolism of other drugs metabolized by the liver. Relatively few studies that examine other macrolide-drug interactions are available.

Dosage Regimen

The dosage regimen for macrolides depends on the type of infection (Table 24–15). Erythromycin is available in oral and parenteral formulations. Oral erythromycins and azithromycin should be administered on an empty stomach. Parenteral formulations of erythromycin are reserved for se-

TABLE 24–15 DOSAGE REGIMEN FOR SELECTED MACROLIDES

Drug	Dosage	Implications
Azithromycin	*Adult:* Respiratory and skin infections: 500 mg po on first day then 250 mg po QD × 4 more days (total dose of 1.5 g). Nongonococcal urethritis or cervicitis: 1 g po single dose *Child over 6 mo:* Acute otitis media: 10 mg/kg po as single dose on first day then 5 mg/kg po once daily × 4 days *Child over 2 yr:* Pharyngitis/tonsillitis: 12 mg/kg po once daily × 5 days *or* 7.5 mg/kg q12 hr. Not to exceed 500 mg po q12 hr	Food decreases absorption by 43%
Clarithromycin	*Adult:* 250–500 mg po q12 hr × 7–14 days *Child:* 7.5 mg/kg q12 hr. Not to exceed 500 mg q12hr	May take without regard to meals
Dirithromycin	*Adult:* 500 mg po daily × 7, 10, or 14 days based on purpose for its use	Safe dosage in children has not been established
Erythromycin base	*Adult:* 250–500 mg po q6–12hr. For severe infections dosage may increase to 4 g daily in divided doses *Child:* 30–50 mg/kg/day in divided doses q6–12hr. For severe infections may increase to 100 mg/kg/day in divided doses	
Erythromycin estolate	*Adult and child over 25 kg:* 250 mg po q6hr. Maximum: 4 g/day *Child 10–25 kg:* 30–50 mg/kg/day po in divided doses *Child under 10 kg:* 10 mg/kg/day po in divided doses q6–12 hr	
Erythromycin ethylsuccinate	*Adult:* 400 mg po QID. For severe infections, up to 4 g or more daily in divided doses *Child:* 30–50 mg/kg/day po in four divided doses q6hr. For severe infections, 60–100 mg/kg/day po in divided doses	
Erythromycin lactobionate	*Adult and child:* 15–20 mg/kg/day IV in divided doses. For severe infections, up to 4 g po daily.	
Erythromycin stearate	*Adult:* 250 mg po q6hr *or* 500 mg po q12hr. For severe infections, up to 4 g po daily	

vere infections and are rarely used. (Two hundred fifty milligrams of base, estolate, or stearate equals 400 mg of erythromycin ethylsuccinate.) Clarithromycin may be taken without regard to meals. Dirithromycin should be taken within 1 hour of meals to enhance absorption.

Laboratory Considerations

Macrolides may cause several altered test results. Elevations may be noted in AST (SGOT), ALT (SGPT), and alkaline phosphatase concentrations. Catecholamines, 17-hydroxycorticosteroids, and 17 ketosteroids may be falsely elevated. Clarithromycin also alters liver function tests and rarely causes elevated prothrombin time, BUN, and serum creatinine levels. It may occasionally cause a decrease in the number of WBCs. In addition, azithromycin may cause a decreased platelet count. Serum albumin, chloride, hematocrit, hemoglobin, neutrophils, platelet counts, and total protein levels may be decreased in the presence of dirithromycin. Dirithromycin can cause elevation of alkaline phosphatase, ALT (SGPT), AST (SGOT), bands, basophils, total bilirubin, creatinine, leukocytes, monocytes, and uric acid levels.

Miscellaneous Antibiotics

- ❒ Aztreonam (AZACTAM)
- ❒ Clindamycin (CLEOCIN)
- ❒ Chloramphenicol (CHLOROMYCETIN)
- ❒ Imipenem/cilastatin (PRIMAXIN)
- ❒ Meropenem (MERREM)
- ❒ Vancomycin (VANCOCIN, VANCOLED)
- ❒ Teicoplanin (TARGOCID)
- ❒ Quinupristin-dalfoprostin (SYNERCID)

AZTREONAM

Aztreonam is a monobactam, the only drug in its class, with activity against aerobic gram-negative rods (e.g., *E. coli, K. pneumoniae, Proteus* species, *Enterobacter* species, and *P. aeruginosa*). It is effective against *N. gonorrhoeae* and *H. influenzae* but has no activity against anaerobic or gram-positive organisms. Aztreonam is used to eliminate urinary tract infections, lower respiratory tract infections, septicemia, and abdominal and gynecologic infections caused by susceptible organisms. Its ability to preserve normal gram-positive and anaerobic flora may be an advantage over most other antibiotic drugs.

Aztreonam has the same adverse effect profile as that of penicillins and cephalosporins. Cross-allergenicity with other beta-lactam drugs is minimal to nonexistent. Seizures are the most serious adverse effect.

Aztreonam is readily and almost completely absorbed following oral administration. Distribution is rapid following administration, with penetration to CSF in patients with meningitis. Small amounts of the drug are biotransformed in the liver, with 70 to 80 percent of the drug eliminated unchanged in the urine. Pharmacokinetics, drug-drug interactions, and dosage regimens are noted in Tables 24–2, 24–16, and 24–17.

CLINDAMYCIN

The indications for clindamycin are limited due to its potential to cause severe antibiotic-associated colitis. It is indicated only for gram-negative and gram-positive anaerobic infections located outside the CNS. Clindamycin is indicated for the treatment of serious respiratory infections (e.g., empyema, pneumonia, and lung abscess), serious skin and soft tissue infection, septicemia, intra-abdominal infections, and infections of the female pelvis and genital tract (e.g., endometritis, pelvic cellulitis, nongonococcal tubo-ovarian abscess, pelvic inflammatory disease, bacterial vaginosis, bacterial endocarditis, toxoplasmosis, and acne). Susceptible organisms include *B. fragilis, Fusobacterium, Clostridium perfringens,* and anaerobic streptococci. Its actions are usually bacteriostatic, but it may produce bactericidal effects if the target organism is particularly sensitive. Drug resistance can be significant with *B. fragilis.* Clindamycin is also used prophylactically against bacterial endocarditis if the patient is allergic to penicillin or does not tolerate erythromycin. Clindamycin is also used in patients who are having dental procedures or minor respiratory tract surgery.

The most notable adverse effect of clindamycin is the antibiotic-associated diarrhea and pseudomembranous colitis. These adverse effects are not unique to clindamycin and are noted with other broad-spectrum antibiotics (e.g., ampicillin, cephalosporins). It alters the normal colonic flora to

TABLE 24–16 PHARMACOKINETICS OF SELECTED MISCELLANEOUS ANTIBIOTICS

Drug	Route	Onset	Peak	Duration	PB (%)	$t_{1/2}$	BioA (%)
Aztreonam	IM	Rapid	60 min	6–12 hr	56–60	1.5–2.2 hr	UA
	IV	Rapid	End of inf	6–12 hr	56–60	1.5–2.2 hr	100
Clindamycin	po	Rapid	1.5–2 hr	UA	93	2–3 hr	>90
	IM	Rapid	90 min	UA	93	2–3 hr	0
	IV	Rapid	End of inf	UA	93	2–3 hr	100
Chloramphenicol	po	15 min	1–3 hr	UA	60	1.5–3.5 hr	UA
	IV	Rapid	End of inf	UA	60	1.5–3.5 hr	100
Imipenem/	IM	UK	UK	UA	20	1–1.3 hr	UA
cilastatin	IV	Rapid	30–60 min	UA	20	1–1.3 hr	100
Meropenem	IV	Rapid	End of inf	8 hr	2	1 hr	100
Vancomycin	po	UA	1 hr	To 12 hr	52–56	4–6 hr	<1
	IV	Immed	End of inf	To 12 hr	52–56	4–6 hr	100
Teicoplanin	IV	Immed	End of inf	To 12 hr	52–56	>100 hr	100

PB, Protein binding; $t_{1/2}$, elimination half-life; UA, unavailable; UK, unknown; BioA, bioavailability.

TABLE 24–17 DOSAGE REGIMEN FOR SELECTED MISCELLANEOUS ANTIBIOTICS

Drug	Dosage	Implications
Aztreonam	*Adults:* 0.5–2.0 g IM/IV q6–12 hr. For serious infections: 2 g IM/IV q6–8 hr	Administer IM injections into large, well-developed muscle. Intermittent infusions should be given over 20–60 minutes. Warn patient drug may cause taste alteration or superinfections
Clindamycin	*Adults:* 150–450 mg po q6hr *or* 300–900 mg/day IM-IV in two to four divided doses. Up to 4.8 g/day IV *Child:* 8–25 mg/kg/day po in divided doses q6–8 hr Children <10 kg should receive at least 37.5 mg po q8hr *Child over 1 mo:* 20–40 mg/kg/day IM-IV in three to four divided doses (350–450 mg/m^2/day) *Neonates to 1 mo:* 15–20 mg/kg/day IM-IV in divided doses q6–8 hr *Neonates under 1 mo:* 15–20 mg/kg/day IM-IV in three to four divided doses	Single IM doses over 600 mg are not recommended
Chloramphenicol	*Adult:* 50–100 mg/kg po/IV in four divided doses q6hr *Child and full-term infants over 2 wks:* 50 mg/kg/day po in three to four divided doses q6–8 hr	Monitor serum levels weekly, especially in low-birth-weight infants, patients with impaired metabolic function, and patients receiving other drugs biotransformed by the liver. Therapeutic level: 10–25 mcg/mL. Concentrations over 25 mcg/mL increase risk of reversible bone marrow depression and gray baby syndrome
Imipenem/cilastatin	*Adults:* 250 mg–1 g IV q6hr *or* 500 mg–1 g q8hr *or* 500–750 mg IM q12 hr	Administer over 20–60 minutes
Meropenem	*Adult:* 1 g IV q8hr as bolus injection over 3–5 minutes or infusion over 15–30 minutes. *Child over 3 mo:* 20–40 mg/kg IV q8hr. Maximum 2 g q8hr	Reduce dosage in patients with CrCl rate less than 50 mL/min. Do not admix with other antibiotics
Vancomycin	*Serious systemic infections:* *Adults:* 500 mg/kg IV q12 hr over 60–90 minutes *Child:* 40 mg/kg/day in divided doses q6–12 hr. *Neonates under 1 mo:* 15 mg/kg IV initially then 10 mg/kg IV q8hr *Neonates younger than 1 wk:* 15mg/kg IV initially then 10 mg/kg q12hr *Endocarditis Prophylaxis in Penicillin-Allergic Patients* *Adults:* 1 g IV single dose 1 hour before procedure *Child:* 20 mg/kg IV as single dose 1 hour before procedure *Pseudomembranous Colitis:* *Adults:* 0.5–2.0 g/day po in divided doses q6–8 hr *Child:* 40 mg/kg/day po in divided doses q6–8 hr. Not to exceed 2 g/day *Neonates:* 10 mg/kg/day po in divided doses	Do not administer rapidly or as a bolus to minimize risk of thrombophlebitis, hypotension, and *redneck syndrome.* Oral formulation stable for 14 days if refrigerated
Teicoplanin	*Adult:* 6 mg/kg/day IM/IV up to 30 mg/kg for serious staphylococcal infections	Dosage should be reduced in patients with renal impairment

CrCl, Creatinine clearance.

allow overgrowth of *C. difficile,* producing a powerful toxin that results in the diarrhea. If a patient on clindamycin develops persistent diarrhea, the drug should be stopped or may be continued only with frequent observation of the patient. A metallic taste may develop from high IV doses of clindamycin. Clindamycin may lead to sensitivity reactions of skin rash, urticaria, pruritus, fever, hypotension, and contact dermatitis. A few anaphylactoid reactions have been reported. Superinfection (e.g., *Candida*) is common with clindamycin. Additionally, caution should be used in patients with a history of colitis, renal, or hepatic impairment.

Much like erythromycin, clindamycin inhibits bacterial protein synthesis by binding to the 50S ribosomal subunit. Oral administration results in complete absorption, with significant concentrations of the drug found in bile, pleural, and peritoneal fluids. However, in the absence of inflammation, penetration of the CSF is poor, and in the presence of common bile duct obstruction, no drug is detected. It readily crosses placental membranes. Both the parent drug and its metabolites are eliminated in the bile and urine. Pharmacokinetics, drug-drug interactions, and dosage regimens are noted in Tables 24–2, 24–16, and 24–17, respectively.

Clindamycin may lead to the following alterations in laboratory results: increased bilirubin, alkaline phosphatase, AST (SGOT), transient leukopenia, neutropenia, eosinophilia, thrombocytopenia, and agranulocytosis. Therefore, liver, renal, and blood cell counts should be performed periodically.

CHLORAMPHENICOL

Chloramphenicol use is limited to the treatment of skin, intra-abdominal, CNS, meningitis, bacteremia, and soft tissue infections when less toxic drugs cannot be used. It is a broad-spectrum drug with activity against meningococcal, pneumococcal, and *H. meningitis* in penicillin-allergic patients, anaerobic brain abscess, *Bacteroides fragilis* infections, rickettsial infections, and brucellosis when tetracyclines are contraindicated, and *Klebsiella* and *Haemophilus* infections that are resistant to other drugs. It is the drug of choice only in typhoid fever. *Pseudomonas* is resistant to this drug. Chloramphenicol is rarely used in infections caused by gram-positive organs because of the effectiveness and low toxicity of penicillins, cephalosporins, and macrolides. Chloramphenicol acts by interfering with microbial protein synthesis.

Chloramphenicol produces two major adverse effects. There is an idiosyncratic hypersensitivity reaction that is irreversible and a fatal aplastic anemia that is reported to occur in one out of 40,000 courses of therapy. These effects are unpredictable, independent of serum drug levels, unrelated to dosage, and may occur more often during prolonged therapy or in patients with previous chloramphenicol exposure.

Anemia also occurs even with a normal-appearing bone marrow. The anemia is predictable, reversible, correlates with serum drug concentrations, and is a dose-related effect. It can be minimized by maintaining serum drug levels below 25 mcg/mL. Patients with anemia, leukopenia, or thrombocytopenia during therapy should be suspected of having a drug-related toxicity, and a dosage reduction should be considered.

Chloramphenicol is well absorbed when taken by mouth, with peak serum concentrations similar to those found after IV administration. It is well distributed to most body tissues and fluids, penetrating ocular fluid and CSF (over 50 percent), even in the presence of inflammation. Chloramphenicol crosses placental membranes and enters breast milk. Repeated administration of high doses of chloramphenicol to neonates leads to accumulation of large amounts of drug and interference with tissue respiration. This effect is known as *gray baby syndrome* and is characterized by abdominal distention, cyanosis, and circulatory collapse. Pharmacokinetics, drug-drug interactions, and dosage regimens are noted in Tables 24–2, 24–16, and 24–17, respectively.

IMIPENEM/CILASTATIN

There are two carbapenems on the market: imipenem/cilastatin and meropenem. Imipenem/cilastatin has the broadest antibacterial action of any beta-lactam antibiotic and is extremely potent against staphylococci and streptococci, with variable activity against *Enterococci, Proteus, Enterobacter-Klebsiella-Serratia,* and *Pseudomonas.* In addition, it maintains activity against *H. influenzae, N. meningitides, N. gonorrhoea, B. fragilis, Peptostreptococcus,* and *Fusobacterium.* It is not effective for MRSA. The primary use of imipenem/cilastatin is treatment of infections caused by organisms that are resistant to other drugs.

Adverse effects of imipenem/cilastatin are the same as those occurring with other beta-lactam antibiotics. Patients allergic to penicillins should be considered to be allergic to imipenem/cilastatin. Infrequent reactions have included drug fever, urticaria, pruritus, and other rashes. Seizures have been noted in 1.5 percent of patients and appear to be more common in older adults with renal insufficiency and in patients with head injury, intracranial neoplasm, or a history of seizures or alcohol abuse. The most common adverse effects include nausea, vomiting, and diarrhea. Hypotension may or may not occur. It is unpredictable and may occur inconsistently in the same patient. Slowing the infusion may be the only intervention necessary.

A unique feature of imipenem is that it is inactivated in the kidney by an enzyme found in the proximal tubular cells. The postexcretory biotransformation can be prevented by co-administering the enzyme inhibitor cilastatin. Cilastatin has virtually no antibacterial activity of its own, but by inhibiting the enzyme activity, the amount of bacterially active imipenem eliminated in the urine is markedly increased, enabling imipenem's use in urinary tract infections.

Imipenem/cilastatin is not absorbed by mouth and, thus, is only available for IV or IM use. The drug is well distributed to most tissues and body fluids, and penetrates inflamed meninges. Approximately 50 percent of the dose is eliminated by the kidneys via glomerular filtration, 25 percent by tubular secretion, and approximately 25 percent by nonrenal routes. Pharmacokinetics, drug-drug interactions, and dosage regimens are noted in Tables 24–2, 24–16, and 24–17, respectively.

MEROPENEM

Meropenem is the newest carbapenem. It has a broad spectrum of activity and may be used as empirical monotherapy before culture results are available. It is used most often in the treatment of intra-abdominal infections and bacterial meningitis in pediatric patients older than 3 years of age. It has been used for hospital-acquired pneumonia and febrile neutropenia, although the drug is not approved by the Food and Drug Administration for these uses.

Meropenem is reported to be effective against penicillin-susceptible staphylococci and *S. pneumoniae,* most gram-negative aerobes *(E. coli, H. influenzae, Klebsiella pneumoniae, Pseudomonas),* and some anaerobes including *B. fragilis.* Compared with imipenem/cilastatin, meropenem offers no additional clinical advantages and is more expensive.

The most common adverse effects of meropenem have not yet been identified, although there is evidence that the drug may cause nausea, constipation, diarrhea, glossitis (children only), rash, pruritus, dizziness, and headache. Pseudomembranous colitis, apnea, and seizures are the most serious adverse effects to be identified to date.

Meropenem is completely bioavailable following IV administration. The drug is widely distributed to body tissues and fluids, entering the CSF in bactericidal levels when the meninges are inflamed. Three-fourths of the drug is eliminated unchanged through the kidneys, with the remaining drug eliminated as an inactive metabolite.

Probenecid is the only identified drug-drug interaction at this time. It decreases the renal elimination of meropenem and increases serum drug levels. BUN, AST (SGOT), ALT (SGPT), LDH, serum alkaline phosphatase, bilirubin, and creatinine may be transiently elevated. Hemoglobin, hematocrit, and WBC concentration may be decreased. Meropenem may cause a positive direct or indirect Coombs' test. Pharmacokinetics, drug-drug interactions, and dosage regimens are noted in Tables 24–2, 24–16, and 24–17, respectively.

VANCOMYCIN

Use of vancomycin, a narrow-spectrum bactericidal drug, has increased because of the development of MRSA and MRSE, and endocarditis caused by *S. viridans* (in patients allergic to or with infections resistant to penicillins or cephalosporins), or *Enterococcus faecalis* (with an aminoglycoside). Vancomycin is indicated in the treatment of rickettsial, chlamydial, mycoplasmal, gonorrheal, and spirochetal infections. It is also active against gram-positive bacteria such as streptococci, staphylococci, pneumococci, enterococci, and *Clostridia*.

Because of vancomycin's widespread use, vancomycin-resistant enterococci are being encountered more often, particularly in critical care units. Treatment options for infections caused by these organisms are very limited. To reduce the spread of vancomycin-resistant enterococci, the Centers for Disease Control and Prevention recommend limiting the use of vancomycin. Their specific recommendations are as follows:

- Avoid or minimize use in the empiric treatment of febrile patients with neutropenia (unless the prevalence of MRSA or MRSE is high)
- Metronidazole is the preferred initial treatment for *Clostridium difficile* colitis
- Avoid or minimize use of vancomycin as surgical prophylaxis, for low-birthweight infants, intravascular catheter colonization or infection, and peritoneal dialysis

Vancomycin therapy can lead to serious adverse effects such as ototoxicity, nephrotoxicity, and anaphylaxis. Vancomycin may also lead to hypersensitivity and superinfections. This potent drug is contraindicated in children younger than 8 years old and in women who are pregnant or lactating. Vancomycin binds with calcium in the body, preventing normal bone growth. In a small child or fetus, vancomycin causes hypoplasia of the teeth enamel.

Red-neck or red-man syndrome is unique to vancomycin and is related to rapid infusion of large doses. It is characterized by fever, chills, paresthesias, and erythema at the base of the neck and upper back. It may be followed by hypotension. It usually begins 10 minutes after the start of the infusion, resolving 15 to 20 minutes after the infusion is stopped. Patients on IV vancomycin may also note thrombophlebitis, neutropenia, and thrombocytopenia.

Vancomycin acts in both a bactericidal and bacteriostatic manner. It is distributed throughout various body fluids and interferes with cell membrane synthesis. It enters the CSF only in the presence of inflammation. Approximately 90 percent of an IV dose is eliminated by the kidneys. Eosinophilia and leukopenia are transient with vancomycin. Pharmacokinetics, drug-drug interactions, and dosage regimens are noted in Tables 24–2, 24–16, and 24–17.

TEICOPLANIN

Teicoplanin is a newer drug similar to vancomycin, and like vancomycin, it is active only against gram-positive organisms. It is reported to be as effective as vancomycin in the treatment of infections caused by streptococci and staphylococci, and it may be useful in some enterococcal infections that are resistant to vancomycin. It has potential use for patients with MRSA, MRSE, and enterococcal infections. Concurrent use of teicoplanin with the aminoglycoside gentamicin can increase its bactericidal action.

Teicoplanin disrupts cell wall synthesis to cause cell lysis and death. Like vancomycin, and unlike cephalosporins, aztreonam, imipenem/cilastatin, meropenem, and vancomycin, it does not have a beta-lactam ring.

Teicoplanin is essentially devoid of adverse effects. It does not cause the histamine release (flushing, tachycardia, hypotension, erythematous rash of the face, neck, chest, and extremities) that vancomycin does, and it can be given once daily for most infections. Interestingly, patients allergic to beta-lactam antibiotics do not have a cross-allergenicity to teicoplanin.

Teicoplanin is not absorbed from the GI tract; thus, oral administration is reserved for intestinal infections. Following IV administration, teicoplanin is well distributed to body tissues and body fluids with the exception of the CSF. Teicoplanin is eliminated almost entirely through the kidneys.

QUINUPRISTIN/DALFOPROSTIN

Quinupristin/dalfoprostin is the first of a new class of antibiotics, called *streptogramins,* to be introduced in 20 years. The first streptogramin, called pristinamycin, was isolated from an Argentine soil sample. It was difficult to manufacture and for years was outranked by vancomycin. The two molecules act synergistically to prevent bacteria from multiplying, and together they are bactericidal.

Critical Thinking Process

Assessment

History of Present Illness

The patient who is admitted to an emergency room with an infection typically presents with the five cardinal signs and symptoms of infection. The cardinal signs and symptoms of infection include swelling, redness, pain, heat, and loss of function. Many times the cardinal signs and symptoms are ignored by the patient. If there is a wound, local signs and symptoms may reveal purulent drainage and a foul odor. Although systemic signs and symptoms such as fever and malaise may occur, medical attention is generally sought because the pain has become unbearable or the loss of function has seriously affected the patient's activities of daily living.

Past Health History

A thorough health history may reveal previous hypersensitivity reactions to a particular antibiotic. The patient should be questioned for clues regarding general health, nutritional status, hormonal balance, co-morbid disease, living conditions, drug use, hygiene, sexual practices, and environmental exposure to microorganisms (potential pathogens). It is important to document the patient's previous encounters with infectious conditions such as hypersensitivity reactions.

Physical Exam Findings

The physical exam of a patient with an infection usually reveals the cardinal signs and symptoms of infection. A thorough exam of body surfaces is necessary for the possible detection of infection traveling indirectly from a distant body site (e.g., a total joint replacement of the hip may fail as a result of a cut finger that became infected).

A surgical incision or traumatic wound may exhibit the redness and heat from the vascular response and the excessive blood volume in the affected area. Swelling, due to enhanced capillary permeability from increased hydrostatic pressure and fluid exudation, is usually seen in an infected area. Although serous fluid is lost initially, protein is lost later, leading to further edema. As the fluid exudate causes pressure, pain is felt from ischemia or from chemical irritation of nerve endings by bradykinins and prostaglandins. The physical exam may reveal a loss of function of the involved body part, which can result from swelling and pain.

Diagnostic Testing

Vital signs may reveal systemic signs and symptoms of infection (e.g., fever and tachycardia). Traditionally, culture and sensitivity tests are performed to determine the causative organism. Sensitivity testing determines whether the organisms are strain resistant.

The monitoring of many toxicities is very important. Many antibiotics have harsh adverse effects such as nephrotoxicity and ototoxicity. Therefore, once drug therapy is started, close monitoring is necessary to prevent a toxicity from reaching the irreversible stage. Monitoring for nephrotoxicity includes the following: BUN, serum creatinine, proteinuria, azotemia, and intake and output measurement. Ototoxicity is monitored with audiometric tests.

Developmental Considerations

Perinatal The physiologic changes that occur during pregnancy alter the pharmacokinetics of drugs in general. Dosages of appropriate antibiotics may need to be altered due to the increase in overall body fluids, and changes in drug absorption and renal function. When assessing pregnant women, attention should be given to length of gestation because many drugs can be safely given only during a specific period.

Pediatric The immaturity of body systems of the fetus, neonate, and child should be considered when assessing the pediatric patient who requires antibiotic therapy. Because most drugs are biotransformed in the liver and eliminated through the kidneys, there is the potential for accumulation and toxicity.

Geriatric Much like the immature systems found in pediatric patients, the aging process affects the hepatic and renal system of older adults by decreasing function. The potential for hepatotoxicity and renal toxicity increases as function decreases.

Psychosocial Considerations

In most cases, infections are short-term, subacute conditions that are easily treated on an outpatient basis. However, in some cases, hospitalization is required for serious, potentially life-threatening infections. The impact of psychosocial variables should be noted when planning patient drug regimens.

Overall, the psychosocial considerations associated with antibiotics are minimal. Teenagers and some adults who have severe, unrelenting acne may be treated with antibiotics. Effective treatment with tetracycline improves self-image and self-esteem. However, it should be noted that although tetracyclines are beneficial drugs, they may also lead to undesirable adverse effects such as tooth discoloration, skin discoloration, and an exaggerated sunburn. These adverse effects may affect psychosocial relationships because people, in general, are sensitive regarding their appearance.

The cost of antibiotics has risen sharply and presents a hardship to many individuals, especially older adults and those who are disadvantaged. Additionally, many antibiotics require expensive laboratory follow-up testing. Peak and trough testing may be necessary for the assurance of achieving an adequate dosage for therapeutic effectiveness and avoidance of drug toxicity. Laboratory testing is also needed to provide early detection of pertinent adverse effects (e.g., blood dyscrasias, nephrotoxicity). Because health care insurance systems are in flux and many payment systems are inadequate, the high cost of antibiotics is of major economic concern (see Case Study—Soft Tissue Infection).

Analysis and Management

Treatment Objectives

The objectives of antibiotic therapy are to ameliorate the signs and symptoms of infection, prevent sepsis and death, and prevent complications associated with therapy. Achievement of the treatment objectives is promoted by accurate diagnosis, accurate administration of pharmacologic therapy, and close monitoring for toxicities.

Treatment Options

Before antibiotic therapy is begun, the target area of infection should be cultured to identify the specific pathogen. The causative pathogen is then tested for antibiotic sensitivity. *Sensitivity* testing indicates which antibiotic is most likely to kill the specific causative pathogen effectively. Because it requires 48 to 72 hours to obtain results from culture and sensitivity testing, additional factors, including a drug's ability to penetrate infected tissue, toxicity, and cost, are needed to guide antibiotic selection.

Because certain pathogens are known to be associated with a specific site of infection, therapy often can be directed against these organisms. Although a number of antibiotics can be considered, clinical efficacy, adverse effect profile, pharmacokinetic disposition, and cost considerations ultimately guide the choice of therapy. Once a drug has been selected, the dosage must be based on patient size, site of infection, route of elimination, and other factors such as the likelihood of drug resistance (see Controversy—Antibiotics and Drug Resistance).

Drug Resistance

During the last few years in the United States, antibiotic-resistant strains of *S. pneumoniae* and *Mycobacterium tuberculosis,* and vancomycin-resistant enterococci infections have

Case Study Soft Tissue Infection

Patient History

History of Present Illness	LM is an 82-year-old white male with complaints of a puncture wound on the bottom of his right foot. He reports that it is red, swollen, warm, and painful. He stepped on a nail outside of his barn 5 days ago. He also complains of fever and malaise. He is accompanied by a daughter-in-law.
Past Health History	LM has an allergy to penicillin and cephalosporins (anaphylaxis). Does not remember when he had his last tetanus shot. He has had diabetes mellitus for 25 years and takes Humulin NPH insulin 25 units BID. LM also had a recent myocardial infarction and is on warfarin therapy. LM has been unable to ambulate for 2 days due to the pain in his foot. Daughter-in-law reports that LM has consumed large quantities of water his whole life, which makes it difficult to monitor for polydipsia.
Physical Exam	LM has noticeable edema on the bottom of his right foot with redness. The area is warm to touch. LM's vital signs are stable except for tachycardia and a fever of 100.2°F.
Diagnostic Testing	WBC: 14,000. Wound culture, foot: polymicrobic. BUN: 20 mg/dL. Creatinine: 1.3 mg/dL. Creatinine clearance: >50 mL/min. HbA_{1c}: 12%. FBS: 326 mg/dL.
Developmental Considerations	LM may have impaired renal function due to aging process.
Psychosocial Considerations	LM lives alone on his small farm with occasional assistance from two sons. His degree of compliance is unknown. One son wants LM to move into his home until his foot heals.
Economic Factors	LM has limited income, surviving on Social Security. LM is unable to drive and needs assistance to the medical clinic for follow-up visits.

Variables Influencing Decision

Treatment Objectives

- Ameliorate signs and symptoms of infection.
- Prevent sepsis and death.
- Prevent complications such as tissue necrosis, local extension of infection, bone destruction, loss of limb, thrombophlebitis.

Drug Variables	*Drug Summary*	*Patient Variables*
Indications	Confirmed soft tissue wound infection with polymicrobic organisms requires antimicrobial therapy.	LM has post-traumatic, polymicrobic wound infection of right foot. Febrile with sepsis. History of type 1 diabetes.
Pharmacodynamics	Traumatic polymicrobic wound infections are sensitive to ampicillin/sulbactam, or ticarcillin/clavulanate, or piperacillin/tazobactam, or imipenem/cilastatin, or meropenem as first-line drugs. Organisms also sensitive to ciprofloxacin and clindamycin but these are second-line drugs. These will become decision points.	LM does not remember his last tetanus shot. LM has anaphylaxis allergy to penicillins and cephalosporins. These will become decision points.
Adverse Effects/ Contraindications	Imipenem/cilastatin: nausea, vomiting, diarrhea are most common. Phlebitis at IV site. Anaphylaxis and seizures possible. Cross-sensitivity to penicillins and cephalosporins. Ciprofloxacin: restlessness, nausea, vomiting, diarrhea, abdominal pain are most common.	This is decision point because of LM's previous allergy to penicillin and cephalosporins. Imipenem/cilastatin or ciprofloxacin may be drugs of choice.

Case Study continued on following page

Drug Variables	*Drug Summary*	*Patient Variables*
Pharmacokinetics	Imipenem/cilastatin: completely bioavailable when given IV with a rapid onset of action. IM injections well absorbed. No drug-drug interactions with current meds. Ciprofloxacin: completely bioavailable when given IV with a rapid onset of action. May need to decrease warfarin dose in presence of this drug.	LM's febrile status with evidence of sepsis and history of type 1 diabetes indicates need for hospitalization and IV antibiotic. Recent MI necessitates continuation of warfarin therapy. These will become decision points.
Dosage Regimen	Minimum treatment duration for antibiotic therapy should be 10 days or 3 days past return to afebrile status for patients who are immunocompromised.	LM's diabetes compromises his immune status. This will become a decision point.
Lab Considerations	Both imipenem/cilastatin and ciprofloxacin may cause increased AST (SGOT), ALT (SGPT), LDH, bilirubin, alkaline phosphatase, BUN, and creatinine levels. Ciprofloxacin may cause crystalluria.	Periodic PT times are needed because of LM's anticoagulant therapy. LM's BUN and creatinine on high end of normal range. This will become a decision point.
Cost Index*	Imipenem/cilastatin: 5 Ciprofloxacin: 5	LM has Medicare Parts A and B. His drugs as well as hospitalization would be funded. Although both ciprofloxacin and imipenem/cilastatin are expensive, there are few choices for LM; therefore, cost is not a major decision point.

Summary of Decision Points

- Traumatic polymicrobic wound infection is sensitive to imipenem/cilastatin. LM has allergies to penicillins and cephalosporins. Organisms also sensitive to ciprofloxacin and clindamycin but these are second-line drugs.
- Patient's diabetes requires additional consideration because of nephropathy and neuropathy.
- LM's febrile status with evidence of sepsis and history of type 1 diabetes indicates need for hospitalization and IV antibiotic. Recent MI necessitates warfarin therapy.
- Possible cross-allergenicity to imipenem/cilastatin essentially contraindicates use of this drug.
- LM's diabetes compromises his immune status thus influencing the duration of therapy.
- LM's BUN and creatinine on high end of normal range.
- Pharmacokinetics is considered in regard to the patient's age with associated renal impairment.

DRUGS TO BE USED

- Ciprofloxacin 400 mg IV q12 hr
- Tetanus immune globulin (TIG)
- Tetanus and diphtheria (Td) toxoid

*Cost Index:
1 = $ <30/mo.
2 = $ 30–40/mo.
3 = $ 40–50/mo.
4 = $ 50–60/mo.
5 = $ >60/mo.

AWP of 24 doses of 400 mg/200 mL premixed IV ciprofloxacin is approximately $750.
AWP of 25 doses of 500 mg imipenem/cilastatin powder for IV use is approximately $700.
AWP of single, 1 mL, IM dose of tetanus immune globulin is approximately $62.
AWP of single, 0.5 mL, IM dose of tetanus and diphtheria toxoids (Td) is approximately $2.

Controversy

Antibiotics and Drug Resistance
JONATHAN J. WOLFE

The availability of antibiotics probably enhanced the reputation of traditional medicine among patients as much as any advance since anesthesia. Health care providers who had previously been powerless in the face of infectious disease found a new power. No longer limited to comforting the patient and offering supportive care, they were able to apply remedies that through understandable scientific processes struck at the root cause of illness. The lay public proved quick to applaud the accomplishments of antibiotic therapy.

Decades have passed since sulfanilamide, penicillin, and other classic antibiotics appeared. Patients and health care providers alike have come to accept antibiotics as commonplace. One result has been unthinking and even irrational use of this class of drugs. Patients frequently demand an antibiotic prescription, even if the underlying cause of discomfort and fever is a viral disease. Health care providers frequently choose to cover the possibility of a bacterial infection by ordering broad-spectrum antibiotics. This may reduce opportunistic infections and return clinic visits.

The hazard is that inappropriate use of antibiotics promotes drug resistance. Bacteria exhibit resistance in several ways. The classic scenario is that susceptible organisms die out, beneficial commensal organisms also die out, and resistant organisms overgrow in the absence of these two classes of bacteria. More threatening is that organisms may, through plasmid transfer, share the genetic basis for drug resistance. When this occurs, bacteria exhibit drug resistance even before exposure to a particular antibiotic. When such strains become established in a health care facility, they exacerbate all the hazards of nosocomial infections.

Critical Thinking Discussion

- What is the most common setting in which your patients receive prescriptions for antibiotics?
- When antibiotics are prescribed prophylactically (a reasonable practice), what steps are important to ensure that appropriate drug therapy has been used?
- What is the chief outcome appropriate to the use of an antibiotic?
- Failure of patients to complete courses of antibiotic therapy may lead to drug resistance. What counseling and follow-up are appropriate to ensure that patients use antibiotics as directed?

emerged. The resistance of these strains to antibiotics is similar to the MRSA and MRSE, which appeared within 2 years after the semisynthetic penicillin was developed in the 1960s. MRSA is resistant to methicillin, nafcillin, oxacillin, and cephalosporins. In the 1980s, ciprofloxacin was useful in the treatment of serious MRSA infections, but resistance developed within 1 year. The current antibiotic of choice for MRSA infections is vancomycin.

When a strain of bacteria is exposed for the first time to an antibiotic, the effect produced is what is anticipated: retardation of bacterial growth. However, as drug therapy continues, bacterial growth resumes and the organisms now present are unaffected by the same concentration of drug that was originally inhibitory or lethal. The organisms accomplish the resistance by undergoing spontaneous mutation. In the presence of the antibiotic, the mutants that are insensitive to the drug survive and multiply, giving rise eventually to an entirely new drug-resistance population. Thus, the drug permits survival of the least susceptible organisms. For example, in the United States in 1940 and 1941, over 70 percent of patients with gonorrhea were rapidly cured with the use of various sulfonamide drugs. Four years later, the same drugs failed in 70 percent of patients. Fortunately, penicillin became available and proved to be successful in treating this drug-resistance problem. As a general rule, organisms resistant to a drug in a particular class tend to be equally insensitive to chemically related drugs (i.e., those drugs in the same class). However, they remain sensitive to chemically dissimilar drugs.

There are three primary mechanisms that account for drug resistance. The most common include elaboration of specific inactivating enzymes. For example, there are two primary factors contributing to bacterial resistance to penicillin—the inability of the penicillin to reach the penicillin-binding proteins and inactivation by bacterial enzymes. The inability to reach protein-binding proteins is related to the envelope that surrounds gram-positive and gram-negative bacteria. Inactivation of penicillin is caused by beta-lactamase, enzymes that cleave the beta-lactam ring of penicillin.

The primary mechanism of resistance to cephalosporins is the production of beta-lactamase, enzymes that render these drugs inactive. In some cases, bacterial resistance results from production of altered protein-binding proteins that have a low affinity for cephalosporins. MRSA produce the unusual proteins and are resistant to cephalosporins as a result.

Bacterial resistance may also occur when a drug that acts intracellularly significantly reduces its rate of entry to the cell, rendering the cell resistant to drug action. Changes in the permeability of the cell membrane decrease the rate of passive diffusion, whereas changes in a carrier system may diminish the rate of facilitated diffusion or active transport. In either case, the result is a lowered concentration of drug within the microbial cell. Malarial parasites have become resistant to antimalarial drugs through this mechanism just as some organisms have become resistant to tetracyclines (see Chapter 26).

The third primary mechanism by which organisms develop resistance is related to genetic modifications of specific proteins responsible for idiosyncratic drug responses. Genetic modification may be responsible for drug resistance when an alteration occurs in a protein that is the specific target for a drug causing growth inhibition or cell growth. If the drug cannot interact with the altered protein, organisms containing the genetic modification will survive at the expense of the others. For example, sulfonamide drugs inhibit the growth of sensitive bacteria by competing with PABA for binding sites on the enzyme, catalyzing the first step in the synthesis of folic acid. In resistant bacteria, the sulfonamide drugs can no longer interact effectively with the enzyme and consequently do not inhibit the incorporation of PABA into folic acid, an essential vitamin.

The more antibiotics are used, the faster drug-resistance organisms emerge. Furthermore, not only do antibiotics promote emergence of drug-resistant organisms but they also promote overgrowth of normal flora. Because drug use increases the resistance of normal flora, and because the organisms can transfer resistance to other organisms, every effort should be made to avoid the use of antibiotics in patients who do not actually need them.

Superinfection is defined as a new infection that appears during the course of treatment for a primary infection. It can develop because antibiotics eliminate the inhibitory influence of normal flora. Broad-spectrum antibiotics are more likely than narrow-spectrum antibiotics to cause superinfection. Superinfections can be difficult to treat because they are, by definition, caused by organisms that are drug-resistant.

Strategies to Reduce Resistance Several strategies help delay drug resistance. Most importantly, antibiotics should be used only when they are truly indicated. It is estimated that 95 percent of antibiotic use is unnecessary and inappropriate. Secondly, narrow-spectrum drugs should be used whenever possible. Conventional use of broad-spectrum drugs is discouraged. In addition, newer antibiotics should be retained for situations in which older drugs are too dangerous or ineffective. Extensive use of the newer antibiotics will only expedite their obsolescence.

The appropriate duration of use also reduces drug resistance. The duration of use may vary from a single dose to weeks, months, or even years in some cases. For most acute infections, the average duration of treatment is 7 to 10 days or until the patient has been afebrile and symptomatic for 48 to 72 hours.

Drug Variables

Because there are many classifications of antibiotics, the selection process revolves around several variables. For any given infection, however, there is usually one drug that is superior to the alternatives (Table 24–18). The specific drug may be superior for several reasons, such as because it has greater efficacy, lower toxicity, or narrower spectrum. Factors that may rule out a first-line drug include patient allergy, inability of the drug to reach the site of infection, and atypical susceptibility of the patient to the toxicity of the first-line drug.

Appropriate considerations include the location of the infection and the offending organism, the spectrum of activity against the organisms, potential drug resistance, potential for hypersensitivity and harm to the patient due to age or physical state (e.g., health, pregnancy, lactation), and the speed with which the drug's action is needed.

Antibiotics may be selected based on the area of absorption. Aminoglycosides, macrolides, and penicillins seem to be active against respiratory tract, bone, joint, skin, and soft tissue infections specifically. Sulfonamides seem to be active against otitis media, bronchitis, gout, arthritis, ulcerative colitis, urinary tract infections, and malaria. Tetracyclines can be used effectively for pertussis, meningitis, gas gangrene, tetanus, and acne. Sexually transmitted diseases may be treated with macrolides, penicillins, sulfonamides, and tetracyclines. In addition, cephalosporins are frequently given for prophylaxis of infection in perioperative patients, and penicillins are considered common prophylaxis for patients with bacterial endocarditis having dental procedures or minor surgery.

Several antibiotic classifications cause hepatotoxicity or nephrotoxicity. Therefore, knowledge about the metabolism and elimination is very important. Also, drug half-life is an important factor. When a drug has a high percentage of protein binding, which is influenced by the serum albumin level, it is in the body for an extended time period. Conversely, a low percentage of protein binding would lead to a faster elimination.

Prophylaxis When they are used prophylactically for surgery, antibiotics should be given before the scheduled operation. Appropriate timing of administration provides for effective tissue concentrations during the procedure should contamination occur. The choice of the drug depends on the organisms most likely to enter the operative site. A first-generation cephalosporin (e.g., cefazolin) is commonly used, most often as a single preoperative dose. Postoperative antibiotics are warranted with dirty, traumatic wounds or ruptured viscera.

Patients with a history of congenital or valvular heart disease and those with prosthetic valves are especially susceptible to bacterial endocarditis. Bacterial endocarditis can develop following surgery, dental procedures, or other work that may cause bacteria to enter the blood stream. Hence, these patients should receive prophylactic antibiotic treatment before undergoing such procedures.

There is some evidence that antibiotic prophylaxis reduces the risk of infection in patients with severe neutropenia. However, antibiotic therapy also escalates the risk of infection caused by fungi. By killing off normal flora, whose presence restrains fungal growth, antibiotics encourage fungal invasion.

Multidrug Therapy Multidrug antibiotic therapy is indicated when the infection is known or thought to be caused by multiple organisms. A second indication is a serious infection in which a combination of drugs would be synergistic. The likely emergence of drug-resistant organisms may also warrant combination therapy. A fourth indication is fever or other evidence that the patient is immunosuppressed. There are, however, disadvantages to multidrug therapy. There is an increased risk of allergic and toxic reactions, as well as possible antagonism of antibiotic effects. There is also an increased risk of superinfection and the increased cost. For these reasons, multidrug therapy should be employed only when clearly warranted.

Patient Variables

The patient's past health history may provide insight to the appropriate selection of antibiotic therapy. Location of the infection in the body is important because some antibiotic classifications are effective on specific body tissue or fluid. Pertinent variables that have an impact on treatment options include age, adverse effects, accessibility for close monitoring, and physical state.

Therefore, many antibiotics are contraindicated in older adults, or at least they should be administered with caution. Older adults also have diminished renal as well as hepatic function that may limit the use of a specific drug or classification of drugs.

Adverse effects such as hypersensitivity to prior administration of a specific antibiotic should be foremost in the consideration of available treatment options. Some antibiotics may be administered with more ease if the patient is in the hospital setting because the patient is accessible for close laboratory monitoring.

Antibiotic use in patients with renal insufficiency or failure must be undertaken with caution. Dosage reduction may be necessary for some drugs. Dosage calculations are usually based on creatinine clearance rates. The formula for

TABLE 24–18 SELECTED EXAMPLES OF FIRST-LINE ANTIMICROBIAL DRUGS FOR INFECTIONS

	Organism	First-Line Drugs	Second-Line Drugs
Gram-Positive Cocci			
Staphylococcus	*aureus,* (nonpenicillinase producing)	Penicillin G Penicillin V	Cefazolin, vancomycin imipenem/cilastatin
	aureus, (penicillinase producing)	Nafcillin	Cefazolin, vancomycin, amoxicillin/clavulanic acid
	MRSA	Vancomycin, with/without rifampin and/or gentamicin	Trimethoprim/sulfamethoxazole, minocycline
Streptococcus	*pyogenes* group A, C, and G	Penicillin G Penicillin V	Cefazolin, vancomycin, erythromycin
	group B	Penicillin G Ampicillin	
	viridans group	Penicillin G with/without gentamicin	Cefazolin, vancomycin
	bovis	Penicillin G	Cefazolin, vancomycin
	faecalis (endocarditis and other severe infections)	Penicillin G Ampicillin with gentamicin	Vancomycin with gentamicin
	faecalis (uncomplicated UTI)	Ampicillin Amoxicillin	Nitrofurantoin, fluoroquinolones
	anaerobius	Penicillin G	Clindamycin, cefazolin, vancomycin
	pneumoniae	Penicillin G Penicillin V	Erythromycin, cefazolin, vancomycin, chloramphenicol
Gram-Negative Cocci			
Neisseria	*gonorrhoeae*	Ceftriaxone	Penicillin G, amoxicillin, spectinomycin, cefoxitin, trimethoprim/sulfamethoxazole, chloramphenicol, a fluoroquinolone
	meningitidis	Penicillin G	Cefuroxime, chloramphenicol
Enteric Gram-Negative Bacilli			
Bacteroides	Oropharyngeal strains	Penicillin G	Metronidazole, clindamycin, cefoxitin
	GI strains	Metronidazole	Clindamycin, imipenem, ticarcillin/clavulanic acid
Campylobacter	*jejuni*	Fluoroquinolones Ciprofloxacin	Tetracycline, gentamicin
Escherichia coli		First-generation cephalosporin	Ampicillin with or without gentamicin, ticarcillin/clavulanic acid, trimethoprim/sulfamethoxazole
Enterobacter species		Imipenem/cilastatin	Ciprofloxacin, trimethoprim/sulfamethoxazole, a third-generation cephalosporin
Helicobacter	*pylori*	Tetracycline + metronidazole + bismuth subsalicylate	—
Klebsiella	*pneumoniae*	Cefotaxime	Gentamicin, tobramycin, amikacin
Proteus, indole positive	Indole positive, *Providencia rettgeri, Morganella morganii*	Cefotaxime, ceftizoxime, ceftriaxone	Gentamicin, fluoroquinolones, trimethoprim/sulfamethoxazole
	mirabilis	Ampicillin	First-generation cephalosporin, trimethoprim/sulfamethoxazole
Salmonella	*typhi*	Ceftriaxone	Trimethoprim/sulfamethoxazole, ampicillin, amoxicillin, chloramphenicol
	other strains	Ceftriaxone, cefotaxime	Trimethoprim/sulfamethoxazole, ciprofloxacin, chloramphenicol, ampicillin
Serratia		Cefotaxime, ceftizoxime, ceftriaxone	Gentamicin, amikacin, imipenem
Shigella		Fluoroquinolones	Trimethoprim/sulfamethoxazole, ciprofloxacin, ampicillin, ceftriaxone
Yersinia	*enterocolitica*	Trimethoprim/sulfamethoxazole	Fluoroquinolones, gentamicin, tobramycin
Gram-Positive Bacilli			
Clostridium	*difficile*	Vancomycin, metronidazole	Bacitracin
	perfringens	Penicillin G	Metronidazole, chloramphenicol
	tetani	Penicillin G	Tetracyclines
Corynebacterium	*diphtheriae*	Erythromycin	Penicillin G
Listeria	*monocytogenes*	Ampicillin with or without gentamicin	Trimethoprim/sulfamethoxazole

Table continued on following page

TABLE 24–18 SELECTED EXAMPLES OF FIRST-LINE ANTIMICROBIAL DRUGS FOR INFECTIONS *Continued*

	Organism	First-Line Drugs	Second-Line Drugs
Other Gram-Negative Bacilli			
Acinetobacter		Imipenem	Trimethoprim/sulfamethoxazole, tobramycin, gentamicin
Bordatella	*pertussis*	Erythromycin	Trimethoprim/sulfamethoxazole, ampicillin
Gardnerella	*vaginalis*	Metronidazole	Ampicillin
Haemophilus	*ducreyi*	Ceftriaxone, erythromycin	Trimethoprim/sulfamethoxazole
	influenzae (meningitis, epiglottitis, arthritis, other serious infections)	Cefotaxime, ceftriaxone	Cefuroxime, chloramphenicol
	upper respiratory infections, bronchitis	Trimethoprim/ sulfamethoxazole	Ampicillin, amoxicillin
Legionella	*pneumophila*	Erythromycin with rifampin	Trimethoprim/sulfamethoxazole
Pseudomonas	*aeruginosa* (UTI)	Ciprofloxacin	Piperacillin, ceftazidime, imipenem/ cilastatin, carbenicillin, ticarcillin
	aeruginosa (other infections)	Ticarcillin, mezlocillin, piperacillin with tobramycin, gentamicin or amikacin	Tobramycin, gentamicin or amikacin plus ceftazidime, imipenem or aztreonam
Chlamydiae			
Chlamydia	*trachoma*	Tetracycline (oral plus topical)	Sulfonamides (oral plus topical)
	(urethritis, cervicitis)	Erythromycin, doxycycline	Azithromycin, ofloxacin, sulfisoxazole
	lymphogranuloma venereum	Doxycycline	Erythromycin
Mycoplasma			
Mycoplasma	*pneumoniae*	Erythromycin, tetracycline	Clarithromycin
	Ureaplasma Urealyticum	Erythromycin	Tetracycline, clarithromycin
Rickettsiae			
Rocky Mountain spotted fever		Tetracycline	Chloramphenicol, fluoroquinolones
Spirochetes			
Treponema	*pallidum*	Penicillin G	Tetracycline

GI, Gastrointestinal; MRSA, methicillin-resistant *Staphylococcus aureus*; UTI, urinary tract infection.

calculating creatinine clearance is found in Appendix D. In general, antibiotic use in patients with renal dysfunction falls into one of the following categories:

- Antibiotics that should not be given unless the infecting organism is sensitive only to a particular drug (e.g., tetracyclines except doxycycline)
- Antibiotics that are not used unless the infection is caused by organisms resistant to safer drugs (e.g., aminoglycosides, carbenicillin, cephalexin)
- Antibiotics requiring dosage reduction (e.g., penicillin G, ampicillin, methicillin, oxacillin, most cephalosporins, and trimethoprim-sulfamethoxazole)
- Antibiotics that require little or no dosage adjustment (e.g., cloxacillin, dicloxacillin, nafcillin, erythromycin, doxycycline, clindamycin, and chloramphenicol)

Antibiotics that are biotransformed by the liver must be reduced in dosage for patients with severe liver disease. Drugs specifically affected include erythromycin, clindamycin, and chloramphenicol.

Perinatal Antibiotic therapy in perinatal patients should be undertaken carefully owing to the potential for teratogenicity. The general principles of perinatal antibiotic therapy are as follows. Sulfonamides are contraindicated during the last 3 months of pregnancy due to the danger of kernicterus to the neonate. If premature delivery is expected, these drugs should not be administered at any time during the third trimester. Sulfonamides may be administered earlier in pregnancy to treat urinary tract infections.

Penicillins, first-generation and second-generation cephalosporins, and erythromycins are safe to use during pregnancy in patients who are not allergic. However, there is a paucity of clinical experience with the newer drugs and these drugs should be considered only when another, better-studied antibiotic cannot be used. Preparations of the erythromycin estolate ester should be avoided altogether.

Tetracyclines are contraindicated during pregnancy. They cross placental membranes and are deposited in fetal teeth and bones. It has also been noted that there is an increased incidence of toxicity from tetracycline during pregnancy that is characterized by hepatic necrosis, pancreatitis, renal damage, and in extreme cases, death.

The aminoglycosides are given during pregnancy only when serious gram-negative infections are present. Gentamicin is preferable to tobramycin, amikacin, or netilmicin because it has been more extensively studied.

Antibiotics enter breast milk and may affect the nursing infant. For example, sulfonamides reach levels in breast milk that are sufficient to cause kernicterus. As a general guideline, antibiotics and all other drugs should be avoided in women who are breastfeeding.

Pediatric General principles of pediatric antibiotic therapy include the following. Penicillins, cephalosporins, and erythromycins are generally considered safe for most age groups but should be used cautiously in neonates due to immature renal function. The safety of some drugs (e.g., imipenem/cilastatin, aztreonam, clarithromycin, azithromycin, ciprofloxacin) has not been established in children younger than 12 years of age.

Aminoglycosides may cause nephrotoxicity and ototoxicity in any patient population. Neonates are at higher risk due to immature renal function. Tetracyclines are contraindicated in children younger than 8 years of age because of the adverse effects on bones and teeth.

Geriatric General principles of geriatric antibiotic therapy include the following. Penicillins, cephalosporins, and erythromycins are generally considered safe. However, hyperkalemia may occur with large IV doses of penicillin and is more likely to occur in patients with impaired renal function. Cephalosporins may aggravate existing renal dysfunction, especially when they are given with other nephrotoxic drugs. Clarithromycin and azithromycin have not been used extensively in older adults but appear to be relatively safe. The dosage of cephalosporins, clarithromycin, and azithromycin may need to be reduced.

Aminoglycosides and tetracyclines are contraindicated in the presence of renal dysfunction if less toxic drugs are available. Older adults are at high risk of nephrotoxicity and ototoxicity from these drugs.

Intervention

Administration

Before the first dose of an antibiotic, a culture and a sensitivity test is usually performed. A culture reveals the causative pathogen, and sensitivity testing provides information about the appropriate antibiotics to use. If a drug is administered before the culture and sensitivity tests are performed, the results may be skewed.

Antibiotic therapy is often begun with a loading dose. A loading dose is used to begin the bacteriostatic or bactericidal action against the pathogens. After the loading dose, the patient requires a maintenance dose to continue the offensive action for the purpose of eradicating the pathogens.

Many antibiotics can be administered by a combination of routes (oral, IM, IV). Before administration, the health care provider should check thoroughly that the route ordered is correct for the individual drug. Several antibiotics that are taken by mouth (e.g., cephalosporins, sulfonamides) commonly cause GI distress. To decrease the uncomfortable GI distress, many oral antibiotics may be taken at mealtimes with food, despite the absorption delay. However, tetracyclines should not be taken with dairy products, antacids, sodium bicarbonate, iron, or antidiarrheal drugs due to the binding effect, which results in reduced antibiotic action. Tetracycline administration needs to be spaced 2 to 3 hours apart from the intake of food or drugs.

Many IM antibiotics result in irritation of localized tissue. To reduce potential tissue irritation, the IM drug needs to be properly diluted according to the manufacturer's recommendations. Other measures that can be used to reduce local tissue irritation from an IM injection include the selection of a large muscle site (e.g., dorsal gluteal), rotation of injection sites, and use of the Z-track technique.

Antibiotics frequently cause vein irritation when they are administered by the IV route. To reduce IV site irritation, the drug needs to be diluted and administered in the time frame recommended by the manufacturer. The IV insertion site should be assessed frequently for signs and symptoms of inflammation (e.g., redness, tenderness) so that the site can be changed as needed.

Because hypersensitivity is common with the administration of many different antibiotics (e.g., penicillin), the health care provider should be prepared for an anaphylactic reaction. Especially when administering penicillins, the patient should be observed closely for at least 30 minutes for detection of a possible allergic reaction. When anaphylaxis occurs, basic management includes IV administration of epinephrine and maintenance of an airway. Further emergency measures may require the use of oxygen, steroids, vasopressors, or cardiopulmonary resuscitation.

While a patient is on antibiotic therapy, laboratory testing of peaks and troughs can be performed to determine drug effectiveness and to monitor for toxicity. The trough is measured before drug administration to determine blood level of the antibiotic. Thirty to sixty minutes after drug administration, the peak serum drug level is measured to monitor therapeutic and toxic levels.

To avoid a high risk for nephrotoxicity that results from antibiotics, patients should be kept well hydrated, the concurrent use of diuretics should be avoided, and the administration of antibiotics should be limited to 10 days or less. Signs and symptoms of nephrotoxicity need to be detected early, and the dosage must be decreased or discontinued in older adults.

Education

Patients should be taught about their drugs. Knowledge is helpful in improving the patient's compliance with the dosage regimen. It is important that patients understand that antibiotics are to be taken precisely as prescribed in dosage, frequency, and for the specified time (usually 10 days) even though symptoms may abate before the full course of therapy is completed. For example, if the antibiotic is prescribed every 12 hours, it should be taken as much as possible every 12 hours or the antibiotic blood level will not be maintained adequately to fight the pathogens. If the antibiotic blood level drops because of a late dose or discontinuing the drug too soon, the pathogens have an opportunity to increase in virulence or become resistant to the drug.

If a dose is missed, it should be taken as soon as remembered unless it is almost time for the next dose. The health care provider should be contacted before other drugs are used to avoid drug-drug interactions. Advise the patient that sharing the antibiotic with friends or family members can be dangerous.

Patients should be instructed to report any signs or symptoms of allergic response. Some antibiotics may initially cause dizziness; thus, caution is warranted when driving or operating machinery until the patient's response to the drug is known. Patients with antibiotic allergies should be advised to wear some form of identification (e.g., Medic Alert) to inform health care personnel of the allergy. Carrying the identification in a wallet or purse is usually not helpful if emergency care is needed.

In addition, patients should be taught what signs and symptoms to report to the health care provider. Patients should watch for signs and symptoms of serious adverse effects and toxicities such as blood dyscrasias (e.g., bruising, bleeding), nephrotoxicity (e.g., oliguria), and ototoxicity (e.g., tinnitus, dizziness). Advise the patient to notify the health care provider if GI reactions are severe or persistent. Evidence of superinfection (e.g., diarrhea, vaginal or anal itching, black furry appearance of the tongue) should be reported. Superinfection by *Candida* can usually be managed by discontinuing the antibiotics or by administering an antifungal drug.

Because the effects of contraceptives are reduced when taking many of the antibiotics, patients should be advised to use a second form of birth control during treatment and for up to 2 weeks after completing the drug regimen.

Sulfonamides Patients taking sulfonamides should be instructed to take them on an empty stomach with a full glass of water. Erythromycin estolate, ethylsuccinate, and enteric-coated formulations may be taken without regard to meals. A minimum of 8 to 10 glasses of water should be consumed daily to minimize the crystallization of sulfonamides. Alkalinization of the urine (e.g., with sodium bicarbonate tablets) can also be beneficial. Advise the patient to avoid prolonged exposure to sunlight, to wear protective clothing, and to apply a sunscreen to exposed skin.

Penicillins Patients should be instructed to take oral penicillins with a full glass of water 1 hour before or 2 hours after meals. Penicillin V, amoxicillin, amoxicillin/clavulanate, and bacampicillin can be taken with meals. They should also be informed to report any signs of allergic response (e.g., skin rash, itching, hives). They should be told that, as a rule, a history of penicillin allergy contraindicates further use of penicillins.

Cephalosporins Patients should be advised to take oral cephalosporins with food if gastric upset occurs. Oral suspensions should be refrigerated. Advise the patient that IM injections are frequently painful. Alcohol or alcohol-containing products (cough or cold medications) should be avoided because of the disulfiram-type reactions that may develop.

Tetracyclines Patients should be instructed about the interference of certain foods and drugs with tetracyclines. Tetracyclines should be taken on an empty stomach and with a full glass of water. GI upset may be minimized by taking the drug with food, although absorption will be delayed. Doxycycline and minocycline may be taken with food. The absorption of tetracyclines, however, is reduced by milk products, calcium and iron supplements, magnesium-containing laxatives, and most antacids. Instruct the patient to separate the ingestion of the antibiotic and these products by at least 2 hours. The patient should be told to avoid prolonged exposure to sunlight, to wear protective clothing, and to use sunscreen on exposed skin.

Aminoglycosides Patients receiving aminoglycosides should be informed of the symptoms of ototoxicity (e.g., hearing loss, tinnitus, nausea, unsteadiness, dizziness, vertigo). Instruct them to notify the health care provider should they occur.

Macrolides Patients taking erythromycin should be instructed to take oral formulations on an empty stomach with a full glass of water. If GI upset occurs, however, the drug may be taken with food. Patients taking the estolate, ethylsuccinate, and enteric-coated formulations can do so without regard to meals. The health care provider should be notified if GI reactions are severe or persistent. The patient should also be instructed about the early signs of blood dyscrasias (e.g., sore throat, fever, pallor) or liver injury (e.g., abdominal pain, jaundice, darkened urine, pale stools) and to notify the health care provider should they occur. The patient should discontinue the drug immediately at the first sign of hypersensitivity (e.g., rash).

Evaluation

Antibiotic effectiveness is assessed by monitoring clinical responses and laboratory results. The frequency of monitoring is proportional to the severity of the infection. Important clinical indicators of effective treatment include a reduction in fever and resolution of the signs and symptoms of infection, vital signs return to normal for the patient, the WBCs return to normal limits, and a culture and sensitivity test is negative for the offending organism. Further proof may include an increase in appetite, energy level, and general sense of well-being.

SUMMARY

- Patients particularly susceptible to infection and infectious diseases include the extremes of age, either the very young or the very old, as well as the immunocompromised individual.
- Factors contributing to susceptibility include an individual's general health, nutritional status, hormonal balance, concurrent diseases, living conditions, drug use, hygiene, and sexual practices.
- Infection begins when a pathogenic organism is transmitted to a susceptible host and is allowed to flourish.
- Nonpathogenic normal flora can cause an infection under certain conditions such as immunosuppression and displacement.
- First-line defenses against infection include physical barriers, chemical defenses, and normal flora. The second-line defense is the body's inflammatory response. The third-line defense is the immune response involving antigen-antibody action.
- Patients with infections may present with signs and symptoms of localized swelling, redness, pain, heat, loss of function, and foul odor or purulent drainage in the case of a wound.
- Systemic signs and symptoms of infection include fever, tachycardia, and malaise.
- Patients should be questioned thoroughly regarding past health history, past hypersensitivity reactions, general health status, nutritional state, hormonal balance, co-morbid disease, living conditions, drug use, hygiene, sexual practices, and environmental exposure to potential pathogens.
- A culture and sensitivity test determines the specific causative microorganism and drug sensitivities.
- The objectives of antibiotic therapy include amelioration of signs and symptoms of infection, prevention of sepsis, and prevention of complications.
- Treatment options involve several classifications: sulfonamides, penicillins, cephalosporins, tetracyclines, aminoglycosides, macrolides, and several miscellaneous drugs.

- Antibiotic selection may also depend on patient variables such as age, potential adverse effects, and physical state (pregnancy or lactation).
- Drug resistance develops when bacterial growth resumes and is unaffected by the same concentration of a drug that was originally inhibitory or lethal.
- Prophylaxis is appropriate for patients with a history of congenital or valvular heart disease and those with prosthetic valves or artificial joints.
- Multidrug therapy is indicated when the infection is known or thought to be caused by multiple organisms, when the combination would be synergistic, if there is an expected emergence of drug-resistant organisms, and if there is fever or other evidence the patient is immunosuppressed.
- Patient variables related to the decision for a particular antibiotic include hypersensitivity, renal insufficiency, hepatic disease, and perinatal, pediatric, and geriatric considerations.
- Antibiotics causing GI distress should be given with food except for tetracyclines, which should not be given with chelating substances.
- To prevent IM antibiotics from irritating tissue, proper dilution, use of a large muscle, and rotation of sites are helpful.
- Because antibiotics given IV frequently cause vein irritation, the IV drug needs to be diluted and given over the proper time frame. The insertion site needs to be assessed frequently and to be changed as needed.
- The health care provider should observe the patient closely, especially during the first 30 minutes, for hypersensitivity and anaphylaxis.
- Patients should be taught about their antibiotic regimen to improve compliance and minimize interference with certain foods or alcohol. They also need to be advised about the need to have adequate hydration, avoidance of sun when taking tetracyclines and sulfonamides, the necessity of an additional form of birth control, and signs and symptoms to report.
- Therapeutic and toxic antibiotic blood levels are monitored by peak and trough testing.
- Evidence of successful antibiotic therapy includes the elimination of signs and symptoms of infection, vital signs that are within normal limits, WBCs within normal limits, and a negative culture and sensitivity.
- Further proof of a noninfectious state includes an increase in appetite, energy level, and an improved general sense of well-being.

BIBLIOGRAPHY

American Medical Association. (1996). *Drug evaluations annual.* Chicago: Author.

Beam, T. Jr., (1994). Anti-infective drugs in the prevention and treatment of sepsis syndrome. *Critical Care Nursing Clinics of North America,* 6(2), 275–293.

Black, J., and Matassarin-Jacobs, E. (1997). *Luckmann and Sorensen's medical-surgical nursing: A psychophysiologic approach* (5th ed.). Philadelphia: W.B. Saunders.

Bullock, B. (1996). *Pathophysiology: Adaptations and alterations in function* (4th ed.). Philadelphia: J.B. Lippincott.

Continuing Education Forum. (1995). Rational antibiotic selection. *Journal of the American Academy of Nurse Practitioners,* 7(11), 557–569.

Corwin, E. (1996). *Handbook of pathophysiology.* Philadelphia: J.B. Lippincott.

Copstead, L. (1995). *Perspectives on pathophysiology.* Philadelphia: W.B. Saunders.

Cunha, B. (1994). Intensive care, not intensive antibiotics. *Heart & Lung,* 23(5), 361–362.

Gants, N., Daye, D., and Weart, W. (1995). Antibiotics '95: Back to basics. *Patient Care,* 29 (1), 68–82.

Gaynes, R. (1995). Antibiotic resistance in ICUs: A multifaceted problem requiring a multifaceted solution. *Infection Control and Hospital Epidemiology,* 16(6), 328–330.

Grinbaum, R., de Mendonca, J., and Cardo, D. (1995). An outbreak of handscrubbing-related surgical site infections in vascular surgical procedures. *Infection Control and Hospital Epidemiology,* 16(4), 198–202.

Gullo, S. (1993). Implanted ports: Technologic advances and nursing care issues. *Nursing Clinics of North America,* 28(4), 859–871.

Hardman, J., Limbird, L., Molinoff, P., et al. (1996). *Goodman and Gilman's the pharmacological basis of therapeutics* (9th ed.). New York: McGraw-Hill.

Hassay, K. (1995). Effective management of urinary discomfort. *Nurse Practitioner,* 20(2), 36–44.

Hecht, A., Siple, J., Deitz, S., et al. (1995). Diagnosis and treatment of pneumonia in the nursing home. *Nurse Practitioner,* 20(5), 24–39.

Hofland, S., and Mort, J. (1994). Infections in long-term care facilities: Issues for practice. *Geriatric Nursing,* 15(5), 260–264.

Hoppe, B. (1995). Central venous catheter–related infections: Pathogenesis, predictors, and prevention. *Heart & Lung,* 24(4), 333–337.

Ignatavicius, D., Workman, M., and Mishler, M. (1995). *Medical-surgical nursing: A nursing process approach* (2nd ed.). Philadelphia: W.B. Saunders.

Israel, D., and Polk, R. (1992). Focus on clarithromycin and azithromycin: Two new macrolide antibiotics. *Hospital Formulary,* 27, 115–134.

Johannsen, J. (1994). Chronic obstructive pulmonary disease: Current comprehensive care for emphysema and bronchitis. *Nurse Practitioner,* 19(1), 59–67.

Kollef, M. (1994). Antibiotic use and antibiotic resistance in the intensive care unit: Are we curing or creating disease? *Heart & Lung,* 23(5), 363–366.

Lam, S., Singer, C., Tucci, V., et al. (1995). The challenge of vancomycin-resistant enterococci: A clinical and epidemiologic study. *American Journal of Infection Control,* 23(3), 170–180.

Lilley, L., Aucker, L., (1998). *Pharmacology and the nursing process.* St. Louis: Mosby.

Lortholary, O., Tod, M., Cohen, Y., et al. (1995). Aminoglycosides. *Medical Clinics of North America,* 79(4), 761–787.

McCraney, S., Rapp, R. (1993). Antibiotic agents in critical care. *Critical Care Nursing Clinics of North America,* 5(2):313–323.

McGowan, J. (1995). Antibiotic-resistant bacteria and healthcare systems: Four steps for effective response. *Infection Control and Hospital Epidemiology,* 16(2), 67–70.

Osterholm, M., MacDonald, K. (1995). Antibiotic-resistant bugs: When, where, and why? *Infection Control and Hospital Epidemiology,* 16(7), 382–384.

Phipps, W., Cassmeyer, V., Sands, J., and Lehman, M. (1995). *Medical-surgical nursing: Concepts and clinical practice* (5th ed.). St. Louis: Mosby.

Polaski, A., and Tatro, S. (1996). *Luckmann's core principles and practice of medical-surgical nursing.* Philadelphia: W.B. Saunders.

Preston, S., and Briceland, L. (1995). Single daily dosing of aminoglycosides. *Pharmacotherapy,* 15(3), 297–316.

Ronk, L. (1995). Surgical patients with multiantibiotic-resistant bacteria. *AORN Journal,* 61(6), 1023–1027.

Rush, K., Haller, L. (1995). Patient factors and central line infection. *Clinical Nursing Research,* 4(4), 397–410.

Shannon, M., Wilson, B., and Stang, C. (1995). *Drugs and nursing implications* (8th ed.). Norwalk, CT: Appleton & Lange.

Shea, K., and Cunha, B. (1995). *Escherichia coli* sternal osteomyelitis after open heart surgery. *Heart & Lung,* 24(2), 177–178.

The Hospital Infection Control Practices Advisory Committee, Hospital Infections Program, National Center for Infectious Diseases, U.S. Department of Health and Human Services, Public Health Service, Centers for Disease Control and Prevention. (1995). Recommendations for preventing the spread of vancomycin resistance: Recommendations of the hospital infection control practices advisory committee. *American Journal of Infection Control,* 239(2), 87–92.

Wade, W., McCall, C., and Tyson, D. (1994). Aminoglycoside dosing in the critical care patient: A case report of tertiary level pharmaceutical care. *Heart & Lung,* 23(3), 259–262.

Wiessner, W., Casey, L., and Zbilut, J. (1995). Treatment of sepsis and septic shock: A review. *Heart & Lung,* 24(5), 380–389.

Young, L., and Koda-Kimble, M. (1995). *Applied therapeutics: The clinical use of drugs* (6th ed.). Vancouver, WA: Applied Therapeutics.

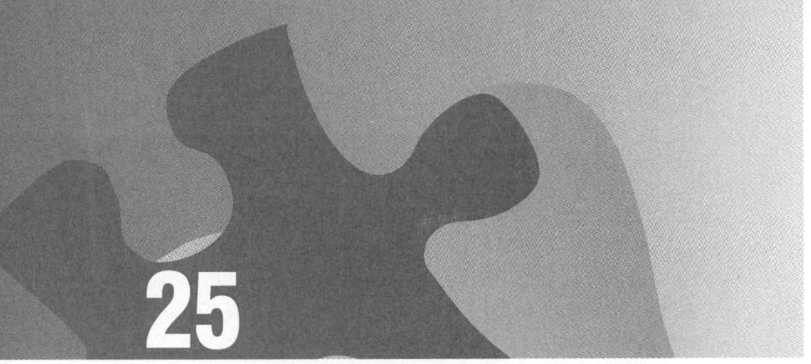

25 Antiviral and Antifungal Drugs

Infectious diseases caused by viruses range in severity from upper respiratory ailments produced by relatively benign adenoviruses to the progressive acquired immunodeficiency syndrome (AIDS) associated with retroviruses. While viral agents differ greatly in size and shape, infectious outcomes, and specific mechanisms of action, they all rely on susceptible host cells to accomplish metabolism and replication. Therefore, the formulation of antiviral drugs has proved more complex than the development of antibiotics and antifungals, both of which work by disrupting the pathogen's cell membrane, nuclear division, or nuclear acid synthesis. Instead, antivirals must target one of the steps in the molecular mechanism between host cell reception and virion reproduction.

Indeed, a virus may attack and damage cells, and as a consequence their host tissues, in a variety of ways. In the absence of natural or acquired immunity (see Chapter 28), a virus binds to specific proteins on the host cell wall surface. Such receptors are not present on all cell surfaces, which presents another natural line of defense against the viral invader. Viruses are categorized as either DNA or RNA depending on their method of replication once inside the host cell. The host cell's ability to reproduce may be altered or lost; protein synthesis may be disrupted; lysosomal enzymes may destroy the cell; associated cells may be changed or damaged by the viral infections. In the case of human immunodeficiency virus (HIV), the retrovirus uses a reverse transcriptase enzyme to help insinuate its viral DNA into the host cell's chromosomes, thus allowing replication of HIV in the host cell's progeny.

Antiviral drugs are used to treat a wide range of viral infections, including cytomegalovirus (CMV) infections, genital herpes infection, herpes zoster (shingles), varicella zoster, and respiratory syncytial virus (RSV) infections. However, viral infections are difficult to cure because antiviral agents do not effectively destroy their target, and most (though not all) viral diseases are self-limiting and of short duration. Many viruses depend on enzymes to reproduce and can quickly mutate in the presence of drug therapy.

In 1981, United States public health officials published a report of a new unknown infectious disease. The initial cases were thought to represent a geographically localized epidemic; however, a global pandemic soon became apparent. Acquired immunodeficiency syndrome is now rapidly becoming the largest lethal epidemic in history. This HIV infection is a serious, debilitating, and eventually fatal disease. Patients develop any number of opportunistic infections as the immune system becomes progressively compromised.

Several recent developments provide reasons for optimism. The virus's molecular anatomy can now be described, new classifications of antiviral drugs have emerged, and patients with AIDS are living longer. The hope continues that HIV infection may soon be treated like other chronic diseases with attendant gains in quality of life and survival.

Fungal infections are common in immunocompromised individuals (e.g., HIV-infected patients). These infections are often associated with severe illness; however, fungal infections contracted as a result of inhalation of airborne spores, oral ingestion, or implantation under the skin may range in intensity from mild, superficial lesions to life-threatening systemic disease. Systemic fungal infections, such as coccidioidomycosis, crytococcosis, aspergillis, and histoplasmosis, are especially difficult to treat. Balance must be maintained between the high dosage of systemic antifungal drugs required to reach the site of infection and their toxicity. Dermatophytoses (e.g., tinea pedis, tinea capitus) and candidiasis are common, and although they are possible in HIV patients, these conditions also develop in individuals with other immunocompromised disorders such as diabetes. Fungal infections of the skin also occur in otherwise healthy individuals and are treated with topical antifungal drugs (see Chapter 64).

HIV INFECTION

Epidemiology and Etiology

Globally through 1996 an estimated 29.4 million people worldwide have been infected with the HIV virus. Approximately 8.4 million have gone on to develop AIDS. Adults living with HIV/AIDS are estimated at 21.8 million worldwide. Forty-two percent of this group are women, and the proportion of women is growing globally. There are over 830,000 children living with HIV/AIDS.

Worldwide, heterosexual intercourse is responsible for 75 percent of all adult HIV infections. Vertical transmission from mother to child accounts for more than 90 percent of all HIV infections worldwide in infants and children. By the year 2000 an estimated 40 million people worldwide will be infected with HIV, and 90 percent of these will appear in developing countries.

The HIV was isolated and identified as the etiological agent of AIDS in 1983. An international committee on the taxonomy of viruses recommends the term *HIV* be used because of confusion that has been caused by different names for the same virus. For example, HIV-1 is the predominant cause of HIV infection in the United States, whereas, HIV-2 is the predominant cause of HIV infection in West Africa.

Pathophysiology

HIV infection is caused by a retrovirus, a group of RNA viruses that are so called because they carry the enzyme reverse transcriptase. The HIV retrovirus selectively destroys the cluster designation 4 (CD4) antigen that is found on T helper cells. The cluster designation refers to a number of

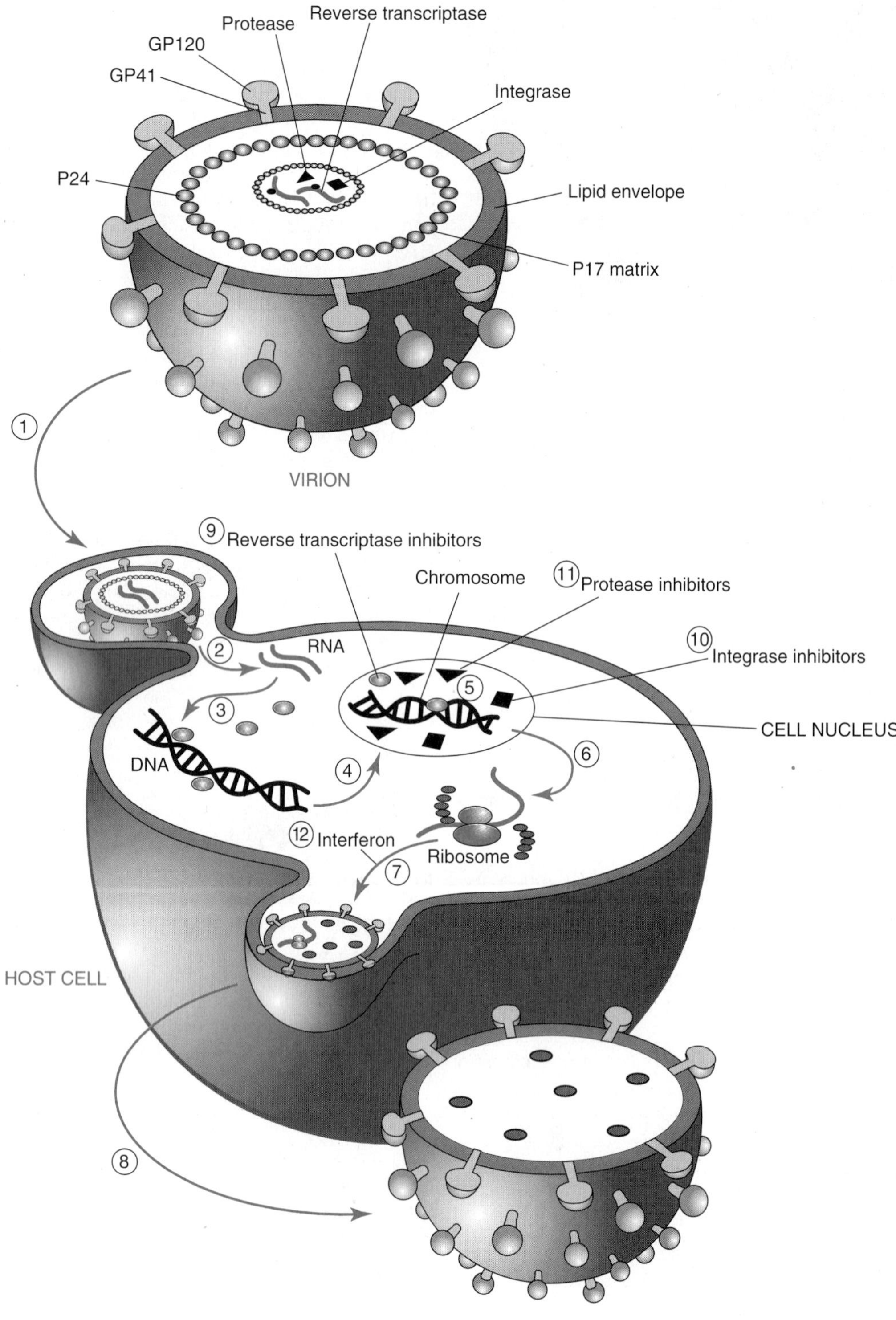

Figure 25–1 Life cycle of the complete infectious viral particle or virion with sites of drug action identified.

1. Attachment and injection of virion into the core of susceptible host cell.
2. Uncoating of viral RNA
3. Reverse transcriptase converts single-stranded viral RNA to double-stranded DNA
4. Entrance of DNA into host cell's nucleus
5. Viral DNA integrated as provirus into host's own DNA. Integrase enzyme splices DNA into the host cell's chromosomes
6. New viral RNA is translated into viral protein precursors at ribosomes
7. Newly made proteins fold together to form new virion
8. Budding and release of new virion
9. Nucleoside reverse transcriptase inhibitors prevent transcription of viral RNA to DNA. Non-nucleoside reverse transcriptase inhibitors bind directly to HIV viral reverse transcriptase to disrupt the active center of the enzyme
10. Integrase inhibitors
11. Protease inhibitors inhibit viral protease and prevent processing of PR 160, the precursor to all structural proteins and viral enzymes
12. Interferon keeps virus from reassembling itself and budding out of the cell

cell surface markers expressed by leukocytes and used to distinguish cell lineages, developmental stages, and functional subsets of antigens.

A surface protein in the viral envelope of HIV, GP120, binds to CD4 receptor sites on the surface of the lymphocyte (Fig. 25–1). Once attached to the CD4 receptor, the virus sheds its protein coat and gains entry into the cytoplasm of the cell. Macrophage and microglial cells have CD4 surface receptor sites that provide targets for the HIV as well. Macrophages are more resistant to cytopathic consequences of HIV infection than CD4. It is thought that macrophages play critical roles in the persistence of an HIV infection by providing reservoirs of chronically infected cells. Once inside the cell, reverse transcriptase enables the virus to reproduce its genetic material within a human cell.

Retroviruses use only RNA as their genetic material within the cell. The reverse transcriptase enzymes force the human DNA to produce viral RNA. If the infected host cell reproduces, the HIV DNA will be duplicated and passed on to the two daughter cells. The host cell now has a new set of genetic instructions, enzymes, and structural proteins. Viral enzymes promote the movement of viral particles out to the periphery of the cell and emerge from the host cell to infect other cells.

HIV invasion activates both cellular and humoral immune responses. Humoral immunity produces antibodies with B lymphocytes. Cellular immunity activates a subset of T cells called cytotoxic or killer T cells. T-helper cells, which are now capable of HIV replication, modulate both cellular and humoral immunity.

Both humoral and cellular immune responses are initiated simultaneously. Cellular immune mechanisms involve the activation of killer T cells, which can be specifically directed by helper T cells to bind other cells and destroy them. Killer T cells bind to infected T helper cells and either directly or indirectly cause their own destruction.

After initial infection the level of T helper cells drops and then is maintained at a steady state. The initial immune response is followed by a continuous state of viral replication, and destruction and replacement of T helper cells. Ongoing HIV replication with an incompletely effective host antiviral immune response is responsible for the secondary manifestations of the disease (i.e., wasting, dementia).

In the latter stages of the HIV growth cycle, two key viral gene products, the gag gene and the gag-pol gene, are translated as polyproteins and form an immature viral bud. These precursor polyproteins are cleaved by a viral pol-encoded aspartic proteinase to yield the final structural proteins of the mature virion core. The polyproteins also activate reverse transcriptase necessary for the next round of infection. Functional proteinase is essential for release of infectious virus.

High levels of HIV replication have been demonstrated during all stages of HIV infection. The lymph nodes serve as a major reservoir for the virus. The network of dendritic cells with lymphoid tissue acts as a filter, trapping free virus and infected CD4 cells. This reservoir of free virus infects large numbers of previously uninfected CD4 lymphocytes as they flow through the lymph nodes. The architecture of the lymph nodes and entrapment of HIV virus breaks down. This releases more free virus in the blood. The thymus is also an early target of HIV infection and damage. The thymus limits effective T-cell production in younger patients.

Mathematical modeling has demonstrated that the population of HIV *virions,* the complete viral particles that infect other living cells, is cleared over two days. New virions and CD4 cells turn over at a rate of about 10 percent per day. Thus, early treatment may be beneficial.

HIV is also capable of infecting monocytes by attaching to CD4 receptors. Infected monocytes move into body tissues, where they differentiate into macrophages. HIV is able to replicate in infected macrophages without budding. This allows the cell to remain intact while becoming an HIV factory. Localized inflammatory responses cause the macrophage to rupture, allowing HIV virions to move out into the surrounding tissues. Skin, lungs, bone marrow, and central nervous system (CNS) tissues are directly infected.

With an HIV infection a point is reached at which the body's steady state can no longer be maintained. Too many CD4 cells are destroyed to continue to regulate immune response. The stage is set for the development of life-threatening opportunistic infections. The average length of time from initial HIV infection to the development of opportunistic infections is about 10 years.

Transmission

Sexual contact with an infected partner is the most common mode of HIV transmission. Sexual activity provides an opportunity for contact through blood, semen, vaginal, and cervical secretions since these secretions contain sufficient concentrations of HIV to transmit infection. The most risky form of intercourse is unprotected anal intercourse. The risk of infection is greater for the receptive partner due to prolonged contact with semen.

HIV infection by exposure to blood through sharing of contaminated needles is the next most common mechanism of transmission. Any used parenteral equipment is potentially contaminated with HIV.

Routine screening of blood donors was implemented in 1985 along with testing for the presence of HIV antibodies. Transfusion recipients account for a small portion of newly reported cases of AIDS. HIV infection is now unlikely but still possible. Clotting factors derived from pooled plasma prior to 1985 have also been implicated in the transmission of HIV.

HIV has been transmitted to health care workers after exposure to HIV-infected body fluids. The average risk of occupational HIV infection from all types of percutaneous exposures to HIV infected blood is 0.3 percent, or one in three hundred. The risk is higher if the exposure is caused by a blood-filled, large-bore needle with blood from a person whose HIV status is unknown. Injuries from instruments previously used in an infected patient's vein or artery pose increased risk. Infected or source patients near death with AIDS or patients with symptoms of acute HIV infection usually have higher amounts of HIV in their blood and may represent increased risk. Studies suggest that percutaneous exposures involving larger blood volumes and high HIV blood titers may increase the risk of percutaneous exposures above 0.3 percent.

The risk of occupational HIV exposure after mucous membrane eye, nose, or mouth and skin exposures to HIV-infected blood is 0.1 percent or one in a thousand. Risk from these exposures may be increased depending on the volume of blood present, integrity of mucous membranes and skin, and HIV titers in the blood.

The risk after exposure of the skin to HIV-infected blood is estimated at less than 0.1 percent or one in a thousand. A small amount of blood on intact skin probably poses no risk at all. There have been no cases to date of HIV transmission due to an exposure involving a small amount of blood on intact skin. The risk may be higher if the skin is damaged by a recent cut or if the contact involves a large area of skin or is prolonged.

Perinatal transmission from an HIV-infected mother to an infant can occur during pregnancy, at the time of delivery, or after birth through breastfeeding. The most common route for vertical transmission is in utero through maternal-placental circulation. Inoculation of the infant may occur during labor or the birth process. Infants at risk include the first-born twin, premature infants, and infants with neonatal bacterial infections.

Mothers at highest risk to transmit HIV to infants include those with advanced HIV disease, lower antibody titer to GP120, prolonged complicated labor, and continued illicit drug use.

Clinical Course of HIV Infection

Primary HIV infection may occur within two to six weeks of initial exposure and seroconversion. This acute viral syndrome is characterized by flulike symptoms that last 1 to 4 weeks (average 2 weeks). Complete clinical recovery with reduced plasma levels of HIV RNA plasma viremia follows.

The symptoms of primary HIV infection that are most common include fever; adenopathy; pharyngitis; maculopapular erythematous rash, which may involve the palms and soles of the feet; mucocutaneous ulcerations involving the mouth, esophagus, or genitals; myalgia; diarrhea; headache; and nausea and vomiting.

The high level of viremia during the acute illness is associated with dissemination of the virus to the CNS and lymphatic tissue. Lymph nodes, spleen, tonsils, and adenoids serve as the major reservoir of HIV burden and predication. Nonlymphoid organ infection with high levels of HIV occurs in late-stage disease.

The presence of symptomatic virus with asymptomatic seroconversion and illness greater than 2 weeks correlates with more rapid progression to AIDS. The level of plasma viremia during the acute HIV syndrome does not predict outcome. Qualitative immune response does.

Seroconversion with positive HIV serology takes place at 6 to 12 weeks following needle stick injuries. More than 95 percent of patients seroconvert within 6 months.

Early HIV disease represents the period from seroconversion to 6 months following HIV transmission. Clinical studies show a considerable variation in CD4 cell count and viral burden. At 6 months the viral burden establishes a set point, which shows minimal variation when followed over a period of years in the absence of antiviral therapy. This set point strongly correlates with prognosis.

During the period of *asymptomatic infection,* the patient has no clinical findings on physical exam except for persistent generalized lymphadenopathy. Persistent generalized lymphadenopathy is defined as enlarged lymph nodes involving at least two noncontiguous sites other than inguinal nodes. The patient remains generally healthy. Vague symptoms include fatigue, headaches, low-grade fevers, and night sweats. Demyelinating peripheral neuropathies resembling Guillain-Barré may occur. The follicular dendritic cells filter and trap free virus and infected CD4 cells. The viral burden in peripheral blood is low. As the disease progresses, the lymph node architecture is disrupted and more HIV is released. The rate of CD4 decline correlates with viral burden. The patient may be unaware of the infection during this asymptomatic phase, creating a tremendous public health problem.

Toward the end of the asymptomatic phase and before a diagnosis of AIDS, the CD4 lymphocyte drops below 500 to 600 cells/mL and *early symptomatic disease* develops. This phase was initially called AIDS-related complex (ARC).

Early symptoms include persistent fevers, recurrent night sweats, chronic diarrhea, headaches, and fatigue. Other conditions include idiopathic thrombocytopenia purpura, listeriosis, cervical dysplasia, and oral hairy leukoplakia.

The most common early infection associated with HIV is oral candidiasis. This fungal infection rarely causes problems in the healthy adult. Vaginal candidiasis that is persistent, frequent, and difficult to manage may occur as well. These oral lesions may provide the earliest indications of HIV.

Neurologic manifestations can occur at any time during the course of HIV infection. Many HIV-infected patients develop neurologic symptoms at this point. Headaches, aseptic meningitis, cranial nerve palsies, myopathies, painful peripheral neuropathies, opportunistic infections, or adverse effects of medications develop.

A diagnosis of AIDS cannot be made until the HIV-infected patient meets case definition criteria established by Centers for Disease Control. At least one condition indicative of severe immunosuppression, especially of defective cell-mediated immunity, should be observed. A CD4 lymphocyte cell count of less than $200/mm^3$ is included in the criteria. The median CD4 count at the time of an AIDS-defining complication is $67\ mm^3$.

Advanced HIV infection is defined as a CD4 cell count of less than $50\ mm^3$. These patients have a medium survival time of 12 to 18 months. All patients who die of HIV-related complications are in this CD4 cell count stratum. The survival after an AIDS-defining complication is 1 year.

Long-term survivors are people who have lived eight or more years after a diagnosis of an AIDS-defining disease. Long-term survivors have all the clinical manifestations of HIV infection and require antiviral treatment as well as prophylaxis and treatment of opportunistic infections. Improved survival is attributed to the introduction in the late 1980s of antiretroviral drugs. Prophylactic drug therapy to prevent opportunistic infections, many of which are fungal in origin, has also improved survival.

Dramatic advances continue to evolve in clinical research and treatment of HIV. The availability of more numerous and potent drugs to inhibit HIV replication has led to therapeutic approaches involving combinations of antiretroviral drugs that provide nearly complete suppression of detectable HIV replication in many HIV-infected persons.

PHARMACOTHERAPEUTIC OPTIONS

Protease Inhibitors

- ❒ Indinavir (CRIXIVAN)
- ❒ Nelfinavir (VIRACEPT)
- ❒ Ritonavir (NORVIR)
- ❒ Saquinovir (INVIRASE)

Indications

Protease inhibitors are indicated in the treatment of HIV infection as part of combination therapy and appear to be the most effective antiretroviral drugs currently available. When used in combination, viral loads can be reduced to an undetectable level.

Pharmacodynamics

Protease inhibitors are by design selective, competitive inhibitors of HIV protease. Protease inhibitors are structural analogs of the HIV protease cleavage site; function of the enzyme is inhibited. By interfering with the formation of essential proteins and the enzyme's reverse transcriptase, integrase, and protease, the maturation of HIV virus is blocked. The result is formation of nonfunctional, immature, noninfectious virions.

Protease inhibitors are active in both acutely and chronically infected cells. Protease inhibitors are also active with chronically infected monocytes and macrophages that are not affected by reverse transcriptase inhibitors. Early stages of the HIV replication cycle are not affected.

Adverse Effects and Contraindications

The most common adverse effects of indinavir include headache, nausea, and abdominal pain. Nephrolithiasis, including flank pain with or without hematuria, was observed in 40 percent of patients receiving indinavir. Nephrolithiasis appears to be dose related, occurring more frequently in patients receiving greater than 2.4 g daily.

Neutropenia occurred in less than 2 percent of patients receiving indinavir alone or in combination. Anemia and thrombocytopenia have also been reported. Lymphadenopathy and splenic disorders occur in less than 2 percent of patients. Spontaneous bleeding episodes have also been reported in patients with hemophilia who were receiving a protease inhibitor. Patients presented with hematomas and hemarthroses, although a causal relationship has not been established.

The most common adverse effect with nelfinavir is diarrhea. Anorexia, dyspepsia, epigastric pain, gastrointestinal (GI) bleeding, hepatitis, pancreatitis, and ulcerations of the mouth have been noted. Dyspnea, pharyngitis, sinusitis, renal calculus, and sexual dysfunction have also been reported.

Studies of patients who received saquinavir alone or as combination therapy reported few adverse reactions. Headache reported as mild was the most common, along with nausea, diarrhea, and abdominal pain. Mental confusion, acute myeloblastic leukemia, hemolytic anemia, and Stevens-Johnson syndrome have been reported, although they are rare.

The most common adverse effects associated with ritonavir include asthenia, anorexia, nausea, vomiting, diarrhea, and abdominal pain. Taste perversion and circumoral and peripheral paresthesia have also been noted with ritonavir.

Gout, avitaminosis, dehydration, glycosuria, and hypercholesterolemia have been noted in less than 2 percent of patients taking ritonavir. Anemia, ecchymosis, leukopenia, lymphadenopathy, lymphocytosis, and thrombocytopenia have been reported. Cardiovascular adverse effects were noted in less than 2 percent of patients but include syncope, postural hypotension, tachycardia, and palpitations. CNS adverse effects that have been reported in a small percentage of patients taking ritonavir include abnormal dreams, agitation, aphasia, ataxia, convulsions, diplopia, emotional lability, and paralysis.

Protease inhibitors may also contribute to increases in blood sugar in HIV patients. Patients who have reported the development of diabetes while on protease inhibitors have been able to control blood sugars with oral drugs or insulin.

Resistance is a problem with protease inhibitors and is the major obstacle to the long-term efficacy of antiretroviral therapy. Two types of resistance occur, genotypic and phenotypic. In genotype resistance the viral genetic material mutates. In phenotype resistance the virus becomes less sensitive to the drug. Cross resistance with protease inhibitors is also possible when viral strains resistant to one protease inhibitor may also be resistant to others as well. Nelfinavir has less of a problem with cross resistance than other protease inhibitors. Cross resistance between ritonavir and zalcitabine or nonnucleoside reverse transcriptase inhibitors is highly unlikely because the drugs have different target enzymes.

Pharmacokinetics

Indinavir is rapidly absorbed in a fasting state following oral administration, with 60 percent of the drug bound to plasma proteins. It is biotransformed in the liver, with less than 20 percent eliminated unchanged in the urine. Indinavir has a rapid onset of action, with peak blood levels reached in 0.8 hours (Table 25–1). The duration of action is 8 hours. Therapeutic levels of indinavir are 0.05 mcg to 10 mcg/mL.

Nelfinavir is also well absorbed following oral administration but has a higher protein binding (98 percent) that indinavir. Peak plasma concentrations averaged 3 to 4 mg/mL. Trough concentrations drawn 11 hours after the previous evening dose were 1 to 3 mcg/mL. Nelfinavir is extensively biotransformed by the liver, with the metabolites eliminated in the urine (75 percent) and the feces (15 percent).

Ritonavir appears to be well absorbed following oral administration with a plasma protein binding of 98 to 99 percent. Food promotes the absorption of ritonavir. It is unknown if ritonavir crosses the placenta or is distributed into human milk. Peak plasma concentrations average 11.2 mcg/mL and trough concentrations average 3 to 3.7 mcg/mL, although the relationship between plasma ritonavir concentrations and therapeutic effects of the drug has not been determined. Like nelfinavir, ritonavir is extensively biotransformed by the liver, with one metabolite maintaining antiviral activity. A small percentage (3.5 percent) is eliminated in the urine.

TABLE 25–1 PHARMACOKINETICS OF SELECTED ANTIVIRAL DRUGS

Drug	Route	Onset	Peak	Duration	PB (%)	$t_{1/2}$	BioA (%)
Protease Inhibitors							
Indinavir	po	Rapid	0.8 hr	8 hr	60	1.5–2 hr	30
Nelfinavir	po	Rapid	2–4 hr	8 hr	98	3.5–5 hr	20–80
Ritonavir	po	Rapid	4 hr	12 hr	98–99	3–5 hr	60–70
Saquinavir	po	UK	2 hr	7 hr	90	1–2 hr	4
Nucleoside Reverse Transcriptase Inhibitors							
Didanosine	po	Rapid	0.5–1.0 hr	UA	<5	1.6 hr; 0.8 hr*	20–25
Lamivudine	po	Rapid	0.9 hr	12 hr	<36	3–6 hr; 2 hr†	86; 66†
Stavudine	po	Rapid	0.5–1.0 hr	3–5 hr	<5	3.0 hr	82; 78‡
Zalcitabine	po	Rapid	1–2 hr	8 hr; 3 hr§	<4	2.6–10 hr	85
Zidovudine	po	Rapid	0.5–1.5 hr	8 hr; 3 hr	34–38	0.8–1.2 hr; 1–1.8 hr	52–75
Non-Nucleoside Reverse Transcriptase Inhibitors							
Delavirdine	po	Rapid	1 hr	UA	98	5.8 hr	85
Nevirapine	po	Rapid	4 hr	UA	60	24–45 hr	93
Nucleoside Analogs							
Acyclovir	po	UK	1.5–2.5 hr	UA	9–33	2.5–3.3 hr	15–20
	IV	Immediate	End of inf	UA	9–33	2.5–3.3 hr	100
Famciclovir	po	Rapid	1 hr	8–12 hr	20	2.1–3 hr	77
Ganciclovir	po	UA	UA	UA	1–2	2.5–3.6 hr	3–9
	IV	Immediate	1 hr	UA	1–2	3–7.3 hr	100
Ribavirin	INH	Rapid	60–90 min	UK	IS	24 hr; 9.5 hr; 40 days‖	NA
Valacyclovir	po	UK	1.5–2.5 hr	8 hr	13.5–17.9¶	2.5–3.3 hr; 14 hr¶	54
Miscellaneous Antiviral Drugs							
Amantadine	po	48 hr	1–4 hr	UK	67	9–37 hr	67
Cidofovir	IV	Immediate	End of inf	UK	6	17–65 hr	100
Foscarnet	IV	Immediate	End of inf	NA	14–17	3 hr; 90 hr**	100
Rimantadine	po	Rapid	6–7 hr	NA	40	20–65 hr	UA

*Half-life of the active metabolites of didanosine for adult and child, respectively.
†Half-life and bioavailability of lamivudine for adult and child, respectively.
‡Half-life and bioavailability of stavudine for adult and child, respectively.
§Duration of action and half-life of zalcitabine for adult and child, respectively.
‖Elimination half-life of ribavirin and RBC, respectively.
¶Elimination half-life of valacyclovir is 2.5 to 3.3 hours. The half-life may extend (as acyclovir) to as much as 14 hours in patients with renal impairment.
**The long elimination half-life of foscarnet may reflect release of the drug from bone.
BioA, bioavailability; IS, insignificant; NA, not applicable; PB, protein binding; $t_{1/2}$, elimination half-life; UA, unavailable; UK, unknown.

Saquinavir is incompletely absorbed following oral administration. It undergoes a significant first-pass effect, leaving 4 percent of the drug bioavailable for distribution to tissues. Peak plasma concentrations average 90.4 ng/mL in healthy individuals and 253.3 ng/mL in HIV-infected patients; however, the relationship between saquinavir concentrations and therapeutic effects has not been determined. Saquinavir is mostly biotransformed in the liver, with small amounts eliminated unchanged in the urine.

Central nervous system penetration for all of the protease inhibitors is low. This fact provides justification for the use of CNS-penetrating nucleoside antiviral drugs with protease inhibitors.

Drug-Drug Interactions

Clinically important drug interactions may occur when protease inhibitors are administered concomitantly with some other drugs (Table 25–2). Biotransformation of protease inhibitors is mediated by the P_{450} isoenzyme CYP3A4. Drugs that induce this isoenzyme reduce plasma concentrations of the drug. Conversely, concomitant administration of drugs that inhibit the P_{450} isoenzyme CYP3A4 isoenzyme result in decreased biotransformation, causing their levels to rise. Dosage adjustments and close monitoring of patients is thus required.

Indinavir should not be taken concurrently with astemizole, cisapride, ergot alkaloids, hismanal midazolam, or triazolam due to the possibility of cardiac arrhythmias or prolonged sedation.

Rifampin is a potent inducer of isoenzyme CYP3A4, causing marked reduction in plasma concentrations of indinavir. The manufacturer of indinavir recommends that rifampin and indinavir not be administered concomitantly. Concomitant administration of indinavir and isoniazid increased plasma levels of isoniazid by 13 percent but does not affect indinavir levels.

Concomitant administration of indinavir and clarithromycin results in a 29-percent increase in plasma levels of indinavir and a 53-percent increase in plasma levels of clarithromycin. Dose adjustments are probably not necessary.

Indinavir concomitantly administered with quinidine sulfate increases indinavir plasma levels by 10 percent. There is some evidence that coadministration of indinavir enhances the CD4 cell response to interleukin 2.

Anticonvulsants such as phenytoin may decrease nelfinavir plasma concentrations. Coadministration of rifabutin

TABLE 25–2 DRUG-DRUG INTERACTIONS OF SELECTED ANTIVIRAL DRUGS		
Drug	**Interactive Drug**	**Interaction**
Protease Inhibitors		
Indinavir	Astemizole Cisapride Hismanal Midazolam Triazolam	May cause cardiac arrhythmias and excessive sedation
	Didanosine	Reduces absorption of indinavir
	Fluconazole Rifampin	Reduces serum levels of indinavir
	Ketoconazole Isoniazid Oral contraceptives Rifabutin Saquinavir	Increase plasma levels of interactive drug
Nelfinavir	Rifabutin	Decreases metabolism and may increase effects of interactive drug
	Carbamazepine Oral contraceptives Phenobarbital Phenytoin Theophylline Zidovudine	Reduce plasma concentration and effectiveness of interactive drug
	Cisapride Erythromycin Midazolam Indinavir Ritonavir Saquinavir Triazolam Warfarin	Increase plasma concentration and effectiveness of interactive drug
	Ketoconazole	Increases plasma concentration of nelfinavir
Ritonavir	Amiodarone Astemizole Bepridil Bupropion Cisapride Clozapine Encainide Flecainide Meperidine Piroxicam Propafenone Propoxyphene Quinidine Rifabutin	Produce large increases in serum levels and effects of interactive drug
	Disulfiram	May cause disulfiram-like reaction if used concurrently
	Alprazolam Clorazepate Diazepam Estazolam Flurazepam Midazolam Triazolam Zolpidim	Increase serum levels and risk of excessive sedation and respiratory depression
	Selected opioids Selected NSAIDs Selected antiarrhythmics Selected antimicrobials Many antidepressants Selected antiemetics Selected beta blockers Many calcium channel blockers Selected antineoplastic drugs Selected glucocorticoids Selected antilipemic drugs Selected immunosuppressants Selected antipsychotic drugs Methamphetamine Saquinavir Warfarin	May increase blood levels and effects of interactive drugs. (Check individual drugs to be used concurrently prior to administration.)
	Protease inhibitors	Synergistic effects if used concurrently
	Oral contraceptives Zidovudine Sulfamethoxazole Theophylline	May decrease blood levels of interactive drugs

Table continued on following page

TABLE 25–2 DRUG-DRUG INTERACTIONS OF SELECTED ANTIVIRAL DRUGS *Continued*

Drug	Interactive Drug	Interaction
Protease Inhibitors *Continued*		
	Ergotamine	Ergot toxicity
	Dihydroergotamine	
Saquinavir	Astemizole	Increase plasma concentration of saquinavir
	Calcium channel blockers	
	Clindamycin	
	Dapsone	
	Quinidine	
	Triazolam	
	Ketoconazole	
	Ritonavir	
	Carbamazepine	Decrease plasma concentration of saquinavir
	Dexamethasone	
	Phenobarbital	
	Phenytoin	
	Rifampin	
Nucleoside Reverse Transcriptase Inhibitors		
Didanosine	Dapsone	Decrease gastric absorption of interactive drug
	Fluoroquinolones	
	Itraconazole	
	Ketoconazole	
	Tetracycline	
	Antacids	Increases bioavailability of didanosine
	Zalcitabine	Reoccurrence or exacerbation of neuropathy
	Alcohol	May increase risk of pancreatic toxicity
	Clotrimazole	
	Diuretics	
	Pentamidine	
Lamivudine	Trimethoprim/Sulfamethoxazole	Increases serum levels of lamivudine
	Zidovudine	Increases serum levels of zidovudine
Stavudine	Chloramphenicol	Increases risk of peripheral neuropathy
Zalcitabine	Cisplatin	
	Dapsone	
	Didanosine	
	Disulfiram	
	Ethionamide	
	Ethambutol	
	Glutethimide	
	Gold	
	Hydralazine	
	Isoniazid	
	Lithium	
	Metronidazole	
	Nitrofurantoin	
	Phenytoin	
	Vincristine	
	Zalcitabine	
	Zidovudine	Possible viral antagonism
Zalcitabine	Antacids	Decrease bioavailability of zalcitabine
	Alcohol	Increase risk of pancreatitis
	Asparaginase	
	Azathioprine	
	Estrogens	
	Furosemide	
	Methyldopa	
	Nitrofurantoin	
	Pentamidine	
	Sulfonamides	
	Tetracyclines	
	Thiazide diuretics	
	Valproic acid	
	Pentamidine	May increase risk of pancreatic toxicity
	Aminoglycosides	Decrease renal clearance of zalcitabine and increase risk of peripheral neuropathy
	Amphotericin B	
	Foscarnet	
	Ribavirin	May antagonize antiviral activity of zalcitabine
	Zidovudine	Synergistic antiviral activity
	Probenecid	Increases blood levels of zalcitabine
Zidovudine	Acyclovir	Synergistic antiviral activity
	Didanosine	

TABLE 25–2 DRUG-DRUG INTERACTIONS OF SELECTED ANTIVIRAL DRUGS *Continued*

Drug	Interactive Drug	Interaction
Nucleoside Reverse Transcriptase Inhibitors *Continued*		
	Foscarnet	
	Ganciclovir	
	GM-CSFs	
	Interferon alfa	
	Zalcitabine	
	Zidovudine	
	Ganciclovir	Antagonize antiviral activity. Increase risk of hematologic toxicity
	Ribavirin	
	Acyclovir	Additive neurotoxicity
	Fluconazole	Increase risk of zidovudine toxicity
	Phenytoin	
	Probenecid	
	Trimethoprim	
	Acetaminophen	Decrease levels of zidovudine
	Clarithromycin	
	Phenytoin	Increase levels of zidovudine
	Trimethoprim	
Non-Nucleoside Reverse Transcriptase Inhibitors		
Nevirapine	Rifampin	Decrease bioavailability of nevirapine
	Rifabutin	
	Protease inhibitors	Reduce plasma levels of interactive drug
	Oral contraceptives	
Delavirdine	Alprazolam	Increase plasma levels of interactive drug
	Antiarrhythmics	
	Astemizole	
	Dihydropyridine CCBs	
	Clarithromycin	
	Cisapride	
	Dapsone	
	Ergot alkaloids	
	Midazolam	
	Quinidine	
	Warfarin	
	Antacids	Decreased absorption of delaviradine
	Didanosine	
Nucleoside Analogs		
Acyclovir	Amphotericin B	Synergistic effects
	Probenecid	Increases serum levels of acyclovir
	Nephrotoxic drugs	May increase risk of nephrotoxicity
	Methotrexate (intrathecal)	May increase risk of CNS adverse effects
	Zidovudine	
Famciclovir	Cimetidine	Increase serum levels of famciclovir
	Probenecid	
	Digoxin	Increase plasma levels of digoxin and risk of toxicity
	Theophylline	Decreases renal clearance of famciclovir
Ganciclovir	Amphotericin B	Increase risk of bone marrow depression
	Antineoplastic drugs	
	Dapsone	
	Flutocytosine	
	Immunosuppressive drugs	
	Other nucleoside analogs	
	Pentamidine	
	Pyrimethamine	
	Radiation therapy	
	Didanosine	Antagonize antiretroviral activity of interactive drug
	Zidovudine	
	Foscarnet	Additive or synergistic activity
	Probenecid	Increases risk of toxicity to ganciclovir
	Imipenem/cilastatin	Increases risk of seizures
	Amphotericin B	Increase risk of nephrotoxicity
	Cyclosporine	
	Nephrotoxic drugs	
Ribavirin	Zalcitabine	Antagonize antiviral activity of ribavirin and potentiate hematologic toxicity
	Zidovudine	
	Didanosine	Potentiates action of interactive drug
Valacyclovir	Cimetidine	Increase levels of acyclovir component of valacyclovir
	Probenecid	
	Zidovudine	Increases drowsiness and lethargy

Table continued on following page

TABLE 25–2 DRUG-DRUG INTERACTIONS OF SELECTED ANTIVIRAL DRUGS *Continued*

Drug	Interactive Drug	Interaction
Miscellaneous Antiviral Drugs		
Amantadine	Antihistamines Disopyramide Phenothiazines Quinidine Tricyclic antidepressants	Increase anticholinergic effects of amantadine
	Hydrochlorothiazide/triamterene	Decreases urinary elimination of amantadine and increases plasma concentrations
	Antihistamines Phenothiazines Tricyclic antidepressants	Increase anticholinergic effects
	Alcohol	Increases risk of CNS depression
	CNS stimulants	Increase risk of CNS stimulation
Cidofovir	Aminoglycosides Amphotericin B Foscarnet Pentamidine	Increase risk of nephrotoxicity with concurrent use
	Acetaminophen Acyclovir ACE inhibitors Barbiturates Benzodiazepines Bumetanide Methotrexate Famotidine Furosemide NSAIDs Theophylline Zidovudine	May interact with probenecid that is required for concurrent use
Foscarnet	Parenteral pentamidine	May cause severe life-threatening hypocalcemia
	Imipenem	Increases risk of seizures
	Didanosine	Decreases elimination of foscarnet
	Amphotericin B Aminoglycosides	Increase risk of nephrotoxicity
Rimantadine	Acetaminophen Aspirin Cimetidine	Slightly decrease plasma levels of rimantadine

ACE, angiotensin converting enzyme;
CCBs, calcium channel blockers;
CNS, central nervous system;
GM-CSFs, granulocyte-macrophage colony stimulating factors;
NSAIDs, nonsteroidal anti-inflammatory drugs.

with nelfinavir resulted in a 32-percent decrease in nelfinavir plasma levels and a 20-percent increase in rifabutin levels. It is recommended that the dose of rifabutin be reduced to one half the usual dose when administered with nelfinavir. Coadministration of rifampin and nelfinavir is contraindicated. Rifampin increases nelfinavir plasma levels by 80 percent.

Coadministration of ritonavir with nelfinavir resulted in a 152-percent increase in nelfinavir plasma levels and a 392 percent increase in saquinavir. Nelfinavir coadministered with oral contraceptives resulted in a 47-percent decrease in ethinyl estradiol and an 18 percent decrease in norethindrone plasma concentrations. Nelfinavir coadministered with zidovudine and lamivudine resulted in a 35-percent decrease in zidovudine.

Ritonavir exhibits a high affinity for several isoforms of the cytochrome P_{450} enzyme system, including CP3A, CYP2D6, CYP2C9, CYP2C19, CYP2A6, CYP1A2, and CYP2EI. Concomitant use of some drugs is contraindicated with ritonavir because of potentially serious or life-threatening adverse effects, including arrhythmogenic, hematologic, neurologic, or other toxicities that could occur as a result of increased plasma concentrations of the drug. Other drugs may be used concomitantly with ritonavir as long as dosage adjustments of either drug is made. A drug handbook should be consulted regarding the numerous drug-drug interactions with ritonavir.

Tobacco use in patients receiving ritonavir may decrease ritonavir plasma levels. Ritonavir capsules and oral solution contain alcohol. Concomitant administration with disulfiram may produce reactions. Absorption of ritonavir from capsules was higher when given with meals.

Patients receiving saquinavir should not receive astemizole or cisapride. Concomitant use may precipitate prolonged QT intervals, ventricular tachycardia, torsades de points, and death. Patients receiving saquinavir with calcium channel blockers, clindamycin, dapsone, quinidine, and triazolam should be monitored for toxicity because of the increased plasma levels of these drugs.

The antiviral effects of saquinavir and dideoxynucleoside antiviral drugs such as didanosine, lamivudine, stavudine, zalcitabine, and zidovudine are synergetic against HIV. The combination of saquinavir and zidovudine may be active against some strains of zidovudine-resistant HIV. Concomitant administration of ritonavir and saquinavir results in substantially increased saquinavir levels.

Drug-Food Interactions

Administration of indinavir with grapefruit juice results in a decrease in indinavir plasma levels. In contrast, the bioavailability of saquinavir is increased when it is administered with grapefruit juice.

Dosage Regimen

The dosage of protease inhibitor drugs varies with the specific agent (Table 25–3). Indinavir should be taken 1 hour before or after a low-fat meal. In contrast, saquinavir should be taken within 2 hours of a high-fat meal.

Laboratory Considerations

Patients receiving indinavir may experience asymptomatic hyperbilirubinemia. This is reflected by elevations in alanine aminotransferase (ALT; serum glutamic-pyruvic transaminase [SGPT]) and aspartate aminotransferase (AST; serum glutamic-oxaloacetic transaminase [SGOT]).

Nelfinavir has been associated with increases in alkaline phosphatase, amylase, creatine phosphokinase, lactic dehydrogenase, AST (SGOT), ALT (SGPT), hyperlipidemia, hyperuricemia, hypoglycemia, and abnormal liver function tests.

Ritonavir has been associated with alterations in triglyceride levels, AST (SGOT), ALT (SGPT), oral glucose tolerance tests, creatine phosphokinase (CPK), and uric acid levels. Lab testing should be done prior to initiating ritonavir therapy to establish baseline readings. The patient should be monitored for clinical signs and symptoms of hepatic dysfunction during therapy.

Saquinavir may cause anemia, thrombocytopenia, and elevated liver enzymes. The patient should be monitored for hematologic and hepatic function prior to and during therapy. Therapeutic levels of drugs administered should be monitored concurrently.

Nucleoside Reverse Transcriptase Inhibitors

- ❒ Didanosine (VIDEX, dideoxyinosine [DDI])
- ❒ Lamivudine (EPIVIR, [3TC])
- ❒ Stavudine (ZERIT, [D4T])
- ❒ Zalcitabine (HIVID, dideoxycytidine [DDC])
- ❒ Zidovudine (RETROVIR, azidothymidine [ZVD]); (🍁) APO-ZIDOVUDINE, NOVO-AZT

Indications

Nucleoside reverse transcriptase inhibitors were the first drugs used against HIV infection and remain the mainstays of treatment. They are indicated for the management of HIV infection as a component of combination antiretroviral therapy. Didanosine is approved only for HIV infection. Because monotherapy with any retroviral drug can rapidly lead to resistance, didanosine should always be used in combination with at least one other antiretroviral drug. For example, didanosine may be combined with zidovudine or stavudine and a protease inhibitor.

To date the only drug shown to reduce the risk of perinatal HIV transmission is zidovudine. Zidovudine is also indicated for the management of HIV-related thrombocytopenia but is not FDA approved for this use at this time. In addition, zidovudine is the only drug with established merit in reducing HIV transmission from needle stick injuries.

Pharmacodynamics

As the name implies, nucleoside reverse transcriptase inhibitors are chemical relatives of naturally occurring nucleosides. Antiretroviral activity is the result of suppressing synthesis of viral DNA by reverse transcriptase. Reverse transcriptase is an essential enzyme that the HIV needs to transform its RNA genetic material into DNA. These drugs prevent the spread of HIV to new cells but do not interfere with viral replication in cells that are already infected.

Didanosine inhibits viral replication by incorporation of its active metabolites into the viral DNA.

Lamivudine is converted to its active form after uptake by the cells. It then suppresses HIV replication by causing premature termination of the growing DNA strand. The active metabolite of lamivudine also inhibits the RNA- and DNA-dependent polymerase activities of reverse transcriptase.

Combination therapy of lamivudine and zidovudine results in a significant decrease in viral load and in some cases an increase in CD4 counts. The combination of drugs produces synergistic retroviral activity and delays the emergence of viral mutations that confer resistance to zidovudine.

Stavudine is a synthetic pyrimidine nucleoside analog. It inhibits HIV reverse transcriptase by competing with the natural substrate deoxythymidine triphosphate. Further, stavudine inhibits synthesis of viral DNA by causing DNA chain termination. This occurs because stavudine lacks the three hydroxyl groups necessary for DNA longation. Stavudine also inhibits cellular DNA polymerase beta and gamma and markedly reduces mitochondrial DNA synthesis.

Zalcitabine inhibits the replication of the HIV retrovirus by interfering with the viral RNA-directed DNA polymerase. It is an analog of cytidine, a naturally occurring nucleoside. It is active in vitro against HIV and hepatitis B but inactive against herpes simplex 1 and herpes simplex 2 viruses.

Zidovudine interferes with the HIV virus–dependent DNA polymerase reverse transcriptase, thus exerting a virustatic effect. Following incorporation of zidovudine into the viral DNA chain, DNA synthesis is terminated. Zidovudine has bactericidal effects against some gram-negative bacteria, particularly *Enterobacteriaceae.* At concentrations exceeding 1.9 mcg/mL, zidovudine reportedly inhibits *Giardia lamblia.*

Strains of HIV have emerged that may be resistant to zidovudine. Resistance appears to be a function of both the duration of therapy and the severity of the HIV infection. Resistance is more likely to develop in patients with advanced disease. Zidovudine-resistant HIV variants have been shown to persist in infected persons and to replicate well enough to be transmitted from one person to another. Zidovudine acts synergistically with a number of other anti-HIV agents, including didanosine, zalcitabine, and interferon alpha, thus inhibiting HIV replication.

TABLE 25–3 DOSAGE REGIMENS OF SELECTED ANTIVIRAL DRUGS

Drug	Uses	Dosage	Implications
Protease Inhibitors			
Indinavir	HIV	*Adult:* 800 mg po q8hr	Take one hour before or after low-fat meals
Nelfinavir	HIV	*Adult:* 750 mg po q8hr *Child:* 20–30 mg/kg/dose	Take with food
Ritonavir	HIV	*Adult:* 600 mg po q12hr	Start with 300 mg po BID and gradually increase dose if patient complains of nausea
Saquinavir	HIV	*Adult:* 600 mg po q8hr. Combination therapy: 400–600 mg q8hr	Take within 2 hours of high-fat meal
Nucleoside Reverse Transcriptase Inhibitors			
Didanosine	HIV	*Adult weighing more than 60 kg:* 200 mg po BID *Child BSA 1.1–1.4 m^2:* 100 mg po q12hr *Child BSA 0.8–1 m^2:* 75 mg po q12hr *Child BSA 0.5–0.7 m^2:* 50 mg po q12hr *Child BSA less than 0.4 m^2:* 25 mg po q12hr	Monitor patient for restless leg syndrome. Take on empty stomach. Monitor intake and output. Dosage modification required if CrCl less than 60 mL/min
Lamivudine	HIV	*Adult:* 150 mg po BID *Child:* 4 mg/kg po BID. Maximum: 150 mg po BID	Used in combination therapy. Dosage is reduced in patients with CrCl rates less than 50 mL/min
Stavudine	HIV	*Adult weighing more than 60 kg:* 20–40 mg po BID *Adult 40–60 kg:* 15–30 mg po BID *Adult weighing less than 40 kg:* 10–20 mg po BID *Child:* 1 mg/kg po q12hr. Not to exceed 40 mg po q12hr	May be taken with or without food. Take a missed dose as soon as possible. Do not double doses. Avoid concurrent use of OTC drugs. Dosage modification required in patients with renal failure
Zalcitabine	HIV	*Adult:* 0.75 mg po q8hr. *CrCl 20–50 mL/min:* 0.75 mg po BID. *CrCl less than 10 mL/min:* 0.75 mg po QD	
Zidovudine	HIV	*Symptomatic adult and child older than 13 yr:* Monotherapy: 100 mg po q4hr (600 mg/day) *or* 1–2 mg/kg IV q4hr Combination therapy: 200 mg zidovudine with zalcitabine 0.75 mg po q8hr *Asymptomatic adult:* 100 mg po q4hr while awake (500 mg/day) *Symptomatic child 3 mo–12 yr:* 180 mg/m^2 po q6hr (120 mg/m^2 po q6hr if granulocytopenic). Not to exceed 200 mg po q6hr *or* 120 mg/m^2 IV q6hr. IV dose not to exceed 160 mg *Pregnant adult over 14 wks:* Prevention of HIV maternal/fetal transmission: 100 mg po 5 times daily until onset of labor *Pregnant adult during labor and delivery:* 2 mg/kg IV over 1 hr, then continuous infusion of 1 mg/kg/hr until umbilical cord is clamped *Infants:* 1.5 mg/kg IV q6hr until able to take po, then 2 mg/kg po q6hr started within 12 hr of birth and continued for 6 weeks	Change from IV to oral therapy as soon as possible. IV infusion should be administered at a constant rate over 1 hour. Avoid rapid infusion or bolus injection. Monitor CBC every 2–4 weeks during initial therapy. Anemia may appear 2–4 weeks after initialization of therapy. Granulocytopenia usually occurs after 6–8 weeks of therapy
Non-Nucleoside Reverse Transcriptase Inhibitors			
Delavirdine	HIV	*Adult:* 400 mg po TID	Used in combination therapy. Disperse tablets in 3 ounces of water and stir
Nevirapine	HIV	*Adult:* 200 mg po QD for 14 days, then 200 mg po BID	Lead-in therapy helps reduce incidence of rash. If therapy is interrupted for longer than 7 days, restart at 200 mg po daily
Nucleoside Analogs			
Acyclovir	Initial outbreak of genital herpes	*Adult:* 200 mg po q4hr while awake	Acyclovir treatment should be started as soon as possible after symptoms appear and within 24 hours of herpes zoster outbreak
	Prophylaxis genital herpes	*Adult:* 400 mg po BID × 12 months	
	Chickenpox	*Adult and child age 2–12 yr:* 20 mg/kg po Maximum: 800 mg QID × 5 days.	
	Mucosal/cutaneous herpes, severe genital herpes	*Adult:* 5 mg/kg/IV q8hr *Child younger than 12 yr:* 250 mg/m^2 IV q8hr × 7 days	Do not administer IM, SC, or rapid IV. Administer via infusion pump over at least 1 hr to minimize renal tubular damage. Maintain adequate hydration and urine output. Space doses evenly around the clock. Dosage is reduced in patients with renal impairment
	Herpes simplex encephalitis	*Adult:* 10 mg/kg IV q8hr × 10 days *Child 6 mo–12 yr:* 500 mg/m^2 IV q8hr × 10 days	
	Varicella zoster	*Adult:* 10 mg/kg IV q8hr × 7 days *Child:* 500 mg/m^2 IV q8hr × 7 days	
Famciclovir	Herpes zoster	*Adult:* 500 mg po q8hr × 7 days	Reduce dosage if renal impairment
	Herpes genitalis	*Adult:* 125 mg po BID × 5 days	

TABLE 25–3 DOSAGE REGIMENS OF SELECTED ANTIVIRAL DRUGS *Continued*

Drug	Uses	Dosage	Implications
Nucleoside Analogs *Continued*			
Ganciclovir	Treatment of CMV	*Adult:* 5 mg/kg IV q12 hr × 14–21 days	Do not give if neutrophil count is less than 500/mm³ or platelet count less than 25,000/mm³
	CMV disease prevention	*Adult:* 5 mg/kg IV q12hr × 7–14 days	Check IV site q15 min. Monitor blood pressure BID
	Maintenance CMV infection	*Adult:* 5 mg/kg IV × 7 days, then 1 g po TID *or* 500 mg po 6 times daily given q3hr	Visual exam recommended periodically. Take with food
Ribavirin	CMV infection	*Infant and child:* 300 mL of 20 mg solution delivered via inhalation mist 12–18 hr/day × 3–7 days	Administer using infant aerosol generator. Monitor gas exchange and ventilation. Assess breath sounds frequently
Valacyclovir	Herpes zoster in immunocompetent patients	*Adult:* 1 g po TID × 7 days	Treatment should be started as soon as possible after onset of signs and symptoms of disease. Most effective if started within 48 hours of onset of rash. Efficacy if started after 72 hours unknown
Miscellaneous Antiviral Drugs			
Amantadine	Influenza A infection	*Adult and child older than 12 yr:* 200 mg po QD as a single dose *or* 100 mg po BID *Child 9–12 yr:* 100 mg po q12hr *Child 1–9 yr:* 1.5–3 mg/kg po q8hr *or* 2.2–4.4 mg/kg q12hr. Not to exceed 150 mg/day	Dose reductions necessary in patients with renal impairment. If dose is missed, do not take within 4 hours of the next dose. Assess patient for mental status changes. Advise caution operating machinery until drug effects are known. Abrupt withdrawal can result in neurolept malignant syndrome
Cidofovir	CMV retinitis	*Adult:* 5 mg/kg IV. Probenecid must be administered po with each cidofovir dose. Two grams must be administered 3 hr prior to cidofovir dose and 1 g administered at 2 and 8 hr after the completion of the 1-hr cidofovir infusion for a total of 4 grams	IV infusion administered once weekly for 2 consecutive weeks. Maintenance given as IV infusion once every 2 weeks. To minimize potential nephrotoxicity, probenecid and IV saline rehydration must be administered along with cidofovir infusion. Check serum creatinine and urine protein levels prior to administration
Foscarnet	HIV retinitis	*Adult:* 90 mg/kg IV q12hr *or* 60 mg/kg IV q8hr. Maintenance: 90–120 mg/kg/day IV	A pump must be used to control infusion rate. Adequate hydration prior to and during therapy must be established to minimize renal toxicity. No other drug may be given through the same IV line. Check serum calcium level and electrolytes if patient complains of perioral tingling, numbness, and paresthesia. Advise patient drug is not a cure for CMV retinitis. Advise patient to get regular ophthalmologic exams
	Herpes simplex infection in patient with AIDS	*Adult:* 40–60 mg/kg IV q8hr × 2–3 wks May be followed by 50 mg/kg/day for 5–7 days/wk up to 15 weeks	Must be diluted to 12 mg/mL if administered via peripheral line. May be given via central line in standard 24 mg/mL solution undiluted
	Acyclovir-resistant herpes simplex infection in immunocompromised patients	*Adult:* 40 mg/kg IV q8–12hr for up to 3 wks	
Rimantadine	Influenza A prophylaxis	*Adult and child older than 10 yr:* 100 mg po BID *Geriatric:* 100 mg po daily *Child:* 5 mg/kg/day po as a single dose. Not to exceed 150 mg/day	Do not drive or perform tasks that require alert response if dizziness or decreased concentration occurs

CMV, cytomegalovirus; HIV, human immunodeficiency virus; OTC, over the counter.

Adverse Effects and Contraindications

The most common adverse effects of didanosine are headache, rhinitis, cough, anorexia, nausea, vomiting, abdominal pain, chills, fever, liver function abnormalities, and peripheral neuropathy. Transient morbilliform rash and mild erythematous macular eruptions have been reported. Less than 15 percent of patients have experienced loss of taste, stomatitis, CNS depression, alopecia, facial edema, bronchitis, cerebrovascular disorders, and vision and hearing problems.

The major adverse effects associated with didanosine are peripheral neuropathy and potentially fatal pancreatitis. The incidence is 3 to 17 percent. Didanosine does not appear to be associated with substantial myelosuppression. Although it is rare and a causal relationship has not been established, hepatic failure of unknown etiology has occurred in patients receiving didanosine.

Retinal depigmentation has been reported in a few children receiving didanosine in doses greater than 300 mg/m^2 daily. Patients with renal impairment or hepatic impairment may be at increased risk of adverse effects because of decreased clearance of didanosine. Didanosine is contraindicated in patients with hypersensitivity, in lactating females, and in patients with phenylketonuria since the tablets contain phenylalanine. It should be used with caution in patients with a history of gout, in patients on sodium-restricted diets (tablets contain 264.5 mg of sodium), and in patients with a history of seizures or renal impairment.

The most common adverse effects of lamivudine used in combination with zidovudine include fatigue, headache, photophobia, insomnia, malaise, cough, anorexia, nausea, vomiting, diarrhea, musculoskeletal pain, neuropathy, and paresthesia.

The major adverse effects noted with lamivudine include vasculitis and neutropenia. Long-term effects of lamivudine are unknown. Lamivudine is contraindicated in patients with hypersensitivity or who are lactating. It should be used with caution in older adults and patients with impaired renal function. Pancreatitis has been noted in both adults and children receiving lamivudine. The drug should be used in children only if there is no other alternative. Safe use during pregnancy has not been established.

The most common adverse effect of stavudine is peripheral neuropathy. Stavudine-related neuropathy may resolve if the drug is withdrawn promptly. Symptoms may worsen temporarily following therapy discontinuation. Stavudine therapy may be reconsidered at a lower dose if symptoms completely resolve.

Other adverse effects include weakness, headache, insomnia, anorexia, diarrhea, arthralgia, myalgia, and anemia. Pancreatitis is possible although rare. Safe use during pregnancy and lactation has not been established. Stavudine is contraindicated in patients with hypersensitivity. It should be used cautiously in patients with a history of alcohol abuse, liver disease or hepatic failure, and peripheral neuropathy. Safe use during pregnancy and lactation and in children has not been established. Breastfeeding should be avoided by HIV-infected mothers due to transmission of the virus in breast milk.

The most common dose-limiting adverse effects of zalcitabine include ulcerations of mucous membranes and peripheral neuropathy. Patients with any sign of peripheral neuropathy should discontinue zalcitabine, and if improvement occurs the drug may be restarted at 50 percent of the previous dose. Headache and fatigue are the most common CNS adverse effects of zalcitabine. Confusion, tremors, amnesia, somnolence, hypertonia, and tremor occur in less than 1 percent of patients. Deafness, ototoxicity, and tinnitus also occurred in fewer than 1 percent of patients. Pharyngitis has been reported in 5 percent of patients receiving zalcitabine, and coughing, dyspnea, cyanosis, fever, and flulike symptoms in 1 percent of patients. Stomatitis and aphthous esophageal ulcers may occur and require interruption of treatment with zalcitabine.

Asymptomatic maculopapular eruptions and erythematous macules accompanied by fever, malaise, and pruritus have been reported in a large percentage of patients receiving zalcitabine. The rash was dose related and involved the trunk and extremities. The fever, malaise, and pruritus resolved in many patients with continued zalcitabine therapy. Occasionally, the rash was severe enough to discontinue zalcitabine therapy. Leukopenia, neutropenia, thrombocytopenia, and anemia occur in 5 percent of patients on zalcitabine.

Zalcitabine is contraindicated in patients with hypersensitivity. It should be used with caution in patients with a history of pancreatitis or any risk factor for pancreatitis. Zalcitabine should be discontinued immediately if nausea, vomiting, or abdominal pain suggestive of pancreatitis occur. Zalcitabine may exacerbate pre-existing hepatic dysfunction. Zalcitabine should be used with caution in patients with impaired hepatic function, pre-existing liver disease, increased liver enzyme concentrations, hepatitis, or a history of alcohol use. It should also be used with caution in patients with baseline cardiomyopathy or history of heart failure. Safe use of zalcitabine in pregnancy, lactation, or children has not been established.

The most common adverse effects noted with zidovudine are headache, weakness, nausea, diarrhea, and abdominal pain. Esophageal ulceration, local in origin, has been reported in patients who swallowed their nightly doses of zidovudine while in a recumbent position. The frequency and severity of adverse effects associated with the use of zidovudine are greater in patients with more advanced disease at the time of initiation of therapy. Zidovudine may cause fingernail discoloration. A dark, bluish discoloration at the base of the nail may be noted 2 to 6 weeks after therapy.

The major adverse effect of zidovudine is bone marrow toxicity, resulting in severe anemia and granulocytopenia. Forty percent of patients required blood transfusions or drug modification. Patients with low serum folate or B_{12} levels are at greater risk for bone marrow toxicity. Myopathy is an infrequent complication of advanced disease with zidovudine treatment that exceeds more than 1 year.

Rare occurrences of lactic acidosis in the absence of hypoxemia and severe hepatomegaly with steatosis have been reported with the use of nucleoside reverse transcriptase inhibitors. Consider lactic acidosis whenever a patient receiving zidovudine develops unexplained tachypnea or dyspnea or there is a fall in serum bicarbonate level. Zidovudine therapy should be suspended under these circumstances. Exercise caution in administering zidovudine to any patient with hepatomegaly, hepatitis, or other known risk factor for liver disease.

Pharmacokinetics

The absorption of oral didanosine is variable and depends on dose, gastric PH, and the presence of food in the GI tract. Didanosine is rapidly degraded at an acidic pH. Buffered preparations facilitate absorption. The presence of food in the GI tract decreases the rate and extent of absorption of didanosine. Peak plasma concentrations of didanosine are dose dependent (see Table 25–1). Didanosine is distributed to cerebral spinal fluid, with levels 21 percent of the plasma levels in adults. It crosses the placenta and is distributed to cord blood and amniotic fluid. Didanosine is eliminated in the urine through glomerular filtration and active tubular secretion.

Lamivudine is rapidly absorbed following oral administration. The drug's bioavailability in adults is 86 percent and in children 66 percent. The mechanism for diminished bioavailability in infants and children is unknown. Lamivudine is distributed to extravascular spaces with some penetration of CSF. There is minimal biotransformation of lamivudine (less than 5 percent). The drug is mostly eliminated unchanged in the urine.

Stavudine is well absorbed following oral administration. Stavudine distributes into extravascular spaces, crossing the blood-brain barrier and entering red blood cells and plasma equally. Plasma protein binding is negligible. Stavudine is biotransformed in the liver, with about 40 percent eliminated unchanged in the urine. The remainder is eliminated through nonrenal means, perhaps through degradation and salvage by other pyrimidine pathways.

Zalcitabine is well absorbed (80 percent) following oral administration. The presence of food in the GI tract may decrease the rate and absorption of oral zalcitabine. The drug is distributed into intracellular fluids, crossing the blood-brain barrier. The remainder of distribution is unknown. Time to peak concentration is 1 to 2 hours. Peak plasma concentrations increase linearly with dose. Zalcitabine is stable in plasma and resistant to first-pass effects by the liver. Seventy percent of zalcitabine is eliminated by the kidneys.

Zidovudine is well absorbed following oral administration with wide distribution. It crosses the blood-brain barrier, entering the CNS. Zidovudine is rapidly biotransformed by the liver. As a result of first-pass effects, the average bioavailability ranges from 52 to 75 percent. Zidovudine is cleared by the kidneys, indicating glomerular filtration and active tubular secretion. CSF levels are 60 percent of serum levels.

Zidovudine crosses the human placenta and is distributed into cord blood, amniotic fluid, as well as fetal liver, muscle, and CNS tissue.

Drug-Drug Interactions

Concomitant administration of an oral antacid increases the oral bioavailability of didanosine (see Table 25–2). Buffers present in the didanosine preparation may decrease the gastric absorption of dapsone, ketoconazale, quinoline, itraconazale, and tetracycline. Each didanosine tablet contains 15.7 mEq of magnesium hydroxide, which may impose an excessive magnesium load on patients with renal impairment.

Individuals who must restrict their intake of phenylalanine should be informed that didanosine tablets contain aspartame, which is metabolized in the GI tract as a phenylalanine.

Patients with a history of peripheral neuropathy during didanosine or zalcitabine therapy may be at increased risk of exacerbation or recurrence of neuropathy. Didanosine should be used cautiously in patients receiving other drugs associated with pancreatic toxicity, such as pentamidine and clotrimazole.

Coadministration of lamivudine and zidovudine results in an increase of 39 percent of zidovudine. The coadministration of lamivudine with trimethoprim/sulfamethoxazole results in an increase of 44 percent lamivudine, a decrease of 29 percent in oral clearance, and a decrease of 30 percent in renal clearance.

Stavudine should be used with caution with other drugs that cause peripheral neuropathy, such as cisplatin, disulfiram, ethionamide, ethambutol, isoniazid, phenytoin, vincristine, glutethimide, gold, hydralazine, and long-term use of metronidazole. Dapsone, lithium, chloramphenicol, and didanosine may also cause peripheral neuropathy. Concurrent use of stavudine with zidovudine is not recommended due to possible viral antagonism.

The concomitant use of zalcitabine and other drugs associated with pancreatic toxicity could increase the risk of pancreatitis. If parenteral pentamidine is used to treat *Pneumocystis carinii* pneumonia, zalcitabine therapy should be discontinued. Zalcitabine should not be reinitiated until 1 to 2 weeks after parenteral pentamidine therapy has been completed.

Drugs with nephrotoxic potential, such as aminoglycosides, amphotericin B, and foscarnet, may decrease renal clearance of zalcitabine. The drug may also increase the risk of peripheral neuropathy and other zalcitabine toxicities. Ribavirin may antagonize the antiretroviral activity of zalcitabine. Zidovidine and zalcitabine are synergetic against HIV virus. Concomitant use of probenecid decreases the elimination of zalcitabine by inhibiting renal tubular secretion of zalcitabine.

Acyclovir, didanosine, foscarnet, interferon alpha, ganciclovir, and zalcitabine potentiate the antiviral effect of zidovudine. Concomitant use of zalcitabine does not appear to increase the hematologic toxicity of zidovudine. Combined use of ganciclovir and zidovudine increases the risk of hematologic toxicity. Ganciclovir may antagonize the antiviral activity of zidovudine. Ribavirin and ganciclovir antagonize the antiviral activity of zidovudine.

Fluconazole appears to interfere with the biotransformation and clearance of zidovudine. Biosynthetic granulocyte-macrophage colony-stimulating factors (GM-CSFs) may potentiate the antiretroviral activity of zidovudine.

Dosage Regimen

The dosage regimen for nucleoside reverse transcriptase inhibitors is identified in Table 25–3. These drugs must also be used in combination to reduce drug resistance.

Laboratory Considerations

Didanosine may increase alkaline phosphatase, AST (SGOT), ALT (SGPT), bilirubin, amylase, lipase, triglycerides, and uric acid levels. Diarrhea from the buffer contained in didanosine may decrease serum potassium levels.

Patients receiving didanosine therapy should have complete blood counts (CBCs), uric acid, and hepatic function monitored throughout therapy. Serum potassium levels should also be monitored periodically and throughout treatment.

Lamivudine may cause neutropenia, thrombocytopenia, and anemia in susceptible patients. It may cause elevated AST (SGOT), ALT (SGPT), hemoglobin, and bilirubin levels.

Mild to moderate increases in AST (SGOT) and ALT (SGPT) occur with stavudine. These parameters return to normal following interruption of therapy. Stavudine may also cause increases in amylase and lipase levels. CBCs with differential, prothrombin time, and CD4 counts and hepatic and renal function tests should be done prior to and throughout therapy.

Patients receiving zalcitabine drug therapy should have CBC and liver function studies done prior to and periodically during therapy. Zalcitabine may cause leukopenia and anemia and increase AST (SGOT), ALT (SGPT), and alkaline phosphatase levels. Serum amylase, lipase, triglyceride, and calcium levels should be monitored throughout zalcitabine therapy. Rising serum amylase, lipase, and triglyceride and decreasing calcium levels may indicate pancreatitis. Baseline assessment measurements should be made in patients with a prior history of pancreatitis, increased amylase levels, and alcohol abuse and in those patients receiving total parenteral nutrition. Zalcitabine should be discontinued if serum amylase is elevated by 1.5 to 2 times the normal limits.

Zidovudine may increase the mean corpuscular volume (MCV). Patients receiving zidovudine therapy should have CBC monitoring every 2 weeks during the first 8 weeks of therapy. If zidovudine is well tolerated, a CBC may be performed monthly and then every 3 months in patients who are asymptomatic.

Non-Nucleoside Reverse Transcriptase Inhibitors

❐ Delavirdine (RESCRIPTOR)
❐ Nevirapine (VIRAMUNE)

Indications

Delavirdine is indicated for the treatment of HIV infection as combination therapy. Nevirapine is indicated in combination with nucleoside reverse transcriptase inhibitors for the treatment of HIV infection. It is approved only for treating infection caused by HIV-1. The drug is not active against HIV-2. Nevirapine is recommended as an alternative to the preferred grouping.

Pharmacodynamics

Non-nucleoside reverse transcriptase inhibitors differ from nucleoside inhibitors in structure and mechanism of action. They are not structurally related to the naturally occurring nucleosides.

Delavirdine binds directly to reverse transcriptase to block RNA-dependent and DNA-dependent DNA polymerase activities. Delavirdine does not compete with the template primer or deoxynucleoside triphosphates.

Delavirdine may confer cross resistance to other non-nucleoside reverse transcriptase inhibitors when they are used alone or in combination. The potential for cross resistance between delavirdine and protease inhibitors is low because of the different enzyme targets involved. The potential for cross resistance between these drugs and nucleoside reverse transcriptase inhibitors is also low because of the different binding sites on the viral reverse transcriptase and their distinct mechanisms of action.

Nevirapine binds directly to reverse transcriptase and blocks the RNA-dependent and DNA-dependent DNA polymerase activities by causing a disruption of the enzyme's catalytic site. The activity of nevirapine does not complete with template or nucleoside triphosphates. Rapid emergence of HIV strains that are cross resistant to these drugs has been observed. Monotherapy with nevirapine is associated with a rapid and high-level resistance with reverse transcriptase mutations. Nevirapine must be used in combination with two nucleoside reverse transcriptase inhibitors or protease inhibitors. Data on cross resistance between non-nucleoside and nucleoside reverse transcriptase inhibitors is limited.

Adverse Effects and Contraindications

The most frequent adverse events related to non-nucleoside reverse transcriptase inhibitors are rash, fever, nausea, headache, and abnormal liver function tests. The skin involvement is ordinarily benign, with maculopapular and erythematous rash with or without pruritus. It is located on the face, trunk, and extremities. The drug should be discontinued if the rash is severe or is accompanied by fever, blisters, mucous membrane involvement, conjunctivitis, edema, arthralgias, or malaise. These symptoms may indicate that the patient is developing Stevens-Johnson syndrome (erythema multiforme). Hospitalization may be required for these patients. The likelihood of a rash can be minimized by using a low dosage initially and then increasing the dose if no rash occurs. Other adverse effects include drug-induced hepatitis. If liver function tests are moderately or severely impaired, the drug should be discontinued. Safe use of non-nucleoside reverse transcriptase inhibitors has not been established in pregnant women, lactation, or children.

Headache, fatigue, nausea, vomiting, and diarrhea may be seen in 2 percent of patients taking delavirdine. Cardiovascular adverse effects are rare but include syncope, bradycardia, tachycardia, and vasodilation. Anemia, bruising, neutropenia, and prolonged partial thromboplastin time may be seen. Safe use during pregnancy and lactation and in children younger than 16 has not been established.

Pharmacokinetics

Delavirdine is rapidly absorbed following oral administration, with peak plasma concentrations reached in 1 hour (see Table 25–1). Absorption is increased 20 percent when delavirdine is administered as a slurry prepared by allowing the drug to disintegrate in water. Food reduces absorption by 20 percent. Patients with achlorhydria should take delavirdine with acidic beverages. Delavirdine does not cross the blood-brain barrier and is extensively (98 percent) bound to plasma proteins, primarily albumin. Delavirdine is biotransformed by the hepatic CYP3A cytochrome enzyme, indicating that it inhibits its own biotransformation as well as that of indinavir, nelfinavir, and saquinavir.

More than 90 percent of nevirapine is absorbed after oral administration both in the presence and absence of food. Peak plasma concentrations are attained within 4 hours. Nevirapine is widely distributed, readily crossing placenta membranes and entering breast milk. Cerebrospinal fluid levels are 45 percent of plasma levels. Nevirapine is biotransformed by cytochromes of the CYP3A family to hydroxylated metabolites that are eliminated in the urine. Nevirapine autoinduces hepatic cytochrome P_{450} enzymes, reducing its own plasma half-life to 2 to 4 weeks from 45 hours to 25 hours. Patients with hepatic or renal disease may have altered pharmacokinetics.

Drug-Drug Interactions

Delavirdine induces the cytochrome P_{450} enzyme system and thereby increases serum levels of other drugs, including indinavir, saquinavir, clarithromycin, dapsone, ergot alkaloids, dihydropyridine calcium channel blockers, quinidine, and warfarin. Because of this inhibition, astemizole, alprazolam, midazolam, triazolam, and cisapride are contraindicated. Antacids and didanosine decrease the absorption of delavirdine.

Nevirapine also induces the cytochrome P_{450} enzyme system and thereby decreases blood levels of other drugs (see Table 25–2). Because of this, the effects of nevirapine used with protease inhibitors or oral contraceptives are of special concern. Rifampin and rifabutin decrease nevirapine levels by inducing the cytochrome P_{450} enzyme system.

Dosage Regimen

The dosage regimen for non-nucleoside reverse transcriptase inhibitors is identified in Table 25–3. Delavirdine also must be used in combination therapy.

Laboratory Considerations

Laboratory abnormalities noted with delavirdine therapy include neutropenia, anemia, thrombocytopenia, increased ALT (SGPT), AST (SGPT), amylase, and bilirubin. Hyperkalemia, hypocalcemia, hyponatremia, and hypophosphatemia may also occur. Patient evaluation prior to initiation of therapy should include CBC, prothrombin time, partial thromboplastin time, electrolytes, and renal and liver function studies.

Laboratory abnormalities noted after nevirapine administration include decreased neutrophils, decreased platelets, increased ALT (SGPT), AST (SGOT), glutamyltransferase (GGT), and total bilirubin levels. Baseline laboratory data should be obtained before drug therapy and periodically throughout therapy.

Nucleoside Analogs

- ❒ Acyclovir (ZOVIRAX); (🍁) AVIRAX
- ❒ Famciclovir (FAMVIR)
- ❒ Ganciclovir (CYTOVENE)
- ❒ Ribavirin (VIRAZOLE)
- ❒ Valacyclovir (VALTREX)

Indications

Nucleoside analogs are indicated for a number of viral infections that are non-HIV in origin. Acyclovir is the drug of choice for infections caused by herpes simplex viruses and the herpes zoster virus. Of these, the herpes viruses are most sensitive, followed in turn by varicella zoster. Most strains of cytomegalovirus (CMV) are resistant to acyclovir.

Acyclovir is used parenterally and ophthalmically as the drug of choice for treatment of recurrent herpes simplex 1 and 2 infections in immunocompromised adults and children. Acyclovir is also used parenterally for herpes-zoster infections, for herpes simplex encephalitis in patients older than 6 months of age, and in patients with an initial, severe outbreak of genital herpes. Oral acyclovir is indicated for genital herpes, herpes zoster, CMV pneumonia, and retinitis. Topical formulations may also be used to treat genital herpes and nonthreatening herpes simplex infections.

Famciclovir is indicated for the treatment of localized herpes zoster. Famciclovir may prevent the appearance of new herpes zoster lesions, decrease viral shedding, reduce pain, and promote healing. Famciclovir may also be used in the treatment of genital herpes infection.

Ganciclovir has two approved indications: the treatment of CMV retinitis in immunocompromised patients (including those with AIDS), and the prevention of CMV infection in transplant patients considered at risk for viral infection. Ganciclovir has also been used for the treatment of other CMV infections of the GI tract or for the treatment of CMV pneumonitis, hepatitis, and viremia.

Ribavirin is used via nasal and oral inhalation for the treatment of severe lower respiratory tract infections caused by respiratory syncytial virus (RSV) in hospitalized infants and children. Unfortunately, the benefits of treatment are most often minimal and the cost is high (over $1400/day). Ribavirin is also used for the treatment of infections caused by various strains of influenza A and B virus. Ribavirin is effective orally and parenterally for the treatment of Lassa fever virus infection. It has also been used, albeit in a limited number of patients, for the treatment of Korean hemorrhagic fever with renal syndrome caused by the Hanta virus. Ribavirin is inactive against the Ebola and Marburg viruses.

Valacyclovir is a prodrug form of acyclovir. It is indicated for the oral treatment of herpes zoster and recurrent genital herpes in immunocompetent adults.

Pharmacodynamics

Acyclovir is a synthetic purine nucleoside analog with inhibitory activity against herpes virus, although the inhibitory action is highly selective. The enzyme thymidine kinase of normal uninfected cells does not effectively use acyclovir as a substrate. However, thymidine kinase encoded by herpes simplex virus or varicella zoster on the Epstein-Barr virus converts acyclovir into acyclovir monophosphate, a nucleotide analog. The monophosphate is further converted into diphosphate and triphosphate by cellular enzymes. Acyclovir triphosphate interferes with herpes simplex virus DNA polymerase to inhibit DNA replication. Acyclovir triphosphate can be incorporated into growing chains of DNA by viral DNA polymerase. When incorporation occurs the DNA chain is terminated.

Famciclovir is a synthetic, acyclic purine nucleoside analog derived from guanine. Famciclovir is a prodrug of penciclovir triphosphate, a compound that inhibits viral DNA polymerase. Replication of viral DNA is thus inhibited. It exhibits no antiviral activity until hydrolyzed to penciclovir and its active metabolites.

Ganciclovir interferes with DNA synthesis for incorporation into viral DNA and viral DNA chains. The active form of ganciclovir, ganciclovir triphosphate, inhibits viral DNA polymerase. Ganciclovir is incorporated into growing DNA chains as a false nucleotide, resulting in formation of a mutant DNA chain and thus inhibiting viral replication.

Ribavirin appears to exert antiviral activity by interfering with DNA and RNA synthesis and viral replication. The antiviral activity of the drug results principally in an intracellular virustatic effect.

Valacyclovir is a prodrug of acyclovir. Valacyclovir is the hydrochloride salt of L-valyl ester of the antiviral drug. Valacyclovir is rapidly converted to acyclovir, which has inhibitory action against herpes 1 and herpes 2 viruses. The inhibitory activity is highly selective due to the affinity for the enzyme thymidine kinase. The viral enzyme converts acyclovir into acyclovir monophosphate, a nucleotide analog. The monophosphate is further converted to diphosphate by cellular guanylate kinase and into triphosphate by cellular enzymes. Triphosphate stops the replication of herpes viral DNA by competitive inhibition of viral DNA polymerase, incorporation and termination of the growing viral DNA chain, and inactivation of the viral DNA polymerase.

Adverse Effects and Contraindications

Adverse reactions to acyclovir are generally minimal following parenteral and oral administration. The most frequent adverse effects of parenteral acyclovir are local reactions at the injection site following inadvertent extravasation of acyclovir IV solutions. Headache, dizziness, diarrhea, nausea, and vomiting are also frequently reported.

Impaired renal function may occur with rapid IV injection and renal failure with oral administration. Pre-existing renal disease or concurrent rise of other nephrotoxic drugs increases the risk of acyclovir-induced renal impairment. It is important to maintain hydration of patients receiving acyclovir. Precipitation of acyclovir crystals in the renal tubules can cause decreased creatinine clearance and increased BUN and serum creatinine concentrations. Renal tubular damage may cause renal failure.

Thrombocytosis, thrombocytopenia, transient leukopenia and lymphopenia, and bone marrow hypoplasia are rare in patients receiving IV acyclovir. Leukopenia has also been reported with oral administration. Parenteral acyclovir therapy can cause signs and symptoms of encephalopathy.

Acyclovir is contraindicated in patients with hypersensitivity to the drug. It should be used with caution in patients who have underlying neurologic abnormalities and in patients with serious renal, hepatic, or electrolyte abnormalities or substantial hypoxia. Acyclovir is not teratogenic, but the potential exists for chromosomal damage at high doses. The CDCP recommends the use of acyclovir during pregnancy only for life-threatening disease.

The most frequent adverse reactions associated with famciclovir are headache and nausea. Dizziness, insomnia, somnolence, and paresthesia may be seen occasionally. Diarrhea, abdominal pain, dyspepsia, flatulence, constipation, and vomiting have been reported. Fatigue, pain, fever, rigors, pharyngitis, and sinusitis have been noted in a small number of patients. Confusion, delirium, disorientation, and confusional states have been reported in older adults but are rare.

Famciclovir is contraindicated in patients with hypersensitivity to the drug. It should be used with caution in patients with impaired renal function (creatinine clearance less than 60 mL/min) who have herpes zoster or less than 40 mL/min in patients who have herpes genitalis. Safe use during pregnancy and lactation and in children under the age of 18 has not been established.

Anorexia, nausea, vomiting, diarrhea, GI bleeding, and abnormal liver function tests have been reported with ganciclovir therapy. Impaired renal function is frequent in patients receiving ganciclovir for prevention of CMV infection following transplantation.

Neutropenia with an absolute neutrophil count less than 1000/mm^3, which is potentially fatal, is the most common dose-limiting adverse effect of ganciclovir. Neutropenia occurs in 25 to 50 percent of patients. Neutropenia usually occurs within the first 2 weeks of treatment but may occur at any time. Patients with HIV are at greater risk for neutropenia than healthy individuals. Thrombocytopenia occurs frequently in patients receiving ganciclovir.

Retinal detachment can develop as a consequence of ganciclovir-induced resolution of retinitis and has been reported in 30 percent of patients. The detachment is thought to result from the hastening of the involutional stage of the disease, in which the retina thins as necrotic tissue is mobilized and edema resorbs. These changes predispose the retina to tears and detachment.

Adverse CNS effects of ganciclovir range in severity from headache to coma. The most common adverse effect, confusion, occurs in 1 to 3 percent of patients. Localized inflammation, phlebitis, and pain at the site of IV infusion may occur and are related to the high pH of the infusion solution. Fever, rash, malaise, cardiac arrhythmias, decreased blood glucose, dyspnea, alopecia, hyponatremia, and inappropriate secretion of antidiuretic hormone (SIADH) are rare.

Ganciclovir may adversely affect spermatogenesis and fertility. Barrier contraceptive methods should be employed for at least 90 days after therapy has been discontinued. Safe use during pregnancy and lactation and in children has not been established. Ganciclovir is teratogenic.

Ribavirin inhalation therapy in patients who require assisted respiration may result in mechanical problems caused by precipitation of the drug in respiratory apparatus, including endotracheal tubes and other tubing. The precipitation may result in inadequate assisted respiration and altered gas exchange. Deaths have been reported in mechanically ventilated children receiving ribavirin. Excessively high pulmonary pressures and diminished oxygenation appeared to be responsible for the death. Prolonged courses of inhalation therapy with ribavirin could potentially affect respiratory tract physiology due to biochemical changes.

Serious adverse effects noted with ribavirin therapy include cardiac arrest, hypotension, bradycardia, and cardiac glycoside intoxication. Reversible anemia, reticulocytoses, and hemolytic anemia have been reported. Ribavirin-induced anemia seems to result from hemolysis of erythrocytes and inhibition of the late stages of erythrocyte maturation in bone marrow. The stem cells do not appear to be affected.

Rash and erythema of the eyelids and conjunctivitis may occur with ribavirin inhalation therapy. The most frequent adverse effects noted to date in health care personnel exposed to aerosolized ribavirin include eye irritation and headache. Nasal irritation, pharyngitis, lacrimation, nausea, dizziness, fatigue, rash, bronchospasm, and nasal congestion have been reported. Because of the uncertainties about potential risk, procedures to minimize environmental exposure to aerosolized ribavirin should be developed. Ribavirin may cause fetal toxicity when administered to pregnant women and has been shown toxic during lactation.

The most common adverse effects of valacyclovir include headache and nausea. Weakness, abdominal pain, anorexia, constipation, and diarrhea have also been reported.

Valacyclovir is contraindicated in patients with known hypersensitivity or intolerance to valacyclovir or acyclovir and in patients who are immunocompromised. Death has resulted from valacyclovir therapy in patients with HIV infection and in bone and renal transplant patients. The cause of death was thrombocytopenic purpura/hemolytic uremic syndrome. This syndrome has not been seen in immunocompetent patients receiving valacyclovir. Further, valacyclovir should be used with caution in patients with acute renal failure (creatinine clearance less than 50 mL/min) and in patients who have glomerulonephritis. Renal tubular damage may be seen. Safe use of valacyclovir during pregnancy and lactation and in children has not been established.

Pharmacokinetics

Acyclovir is poorly absorbed from the GI tract. It is estimated that only 15 to 30 percent of orally administered acyclovir is absorbed (see Table 25–1). Peak plasma concentrations are usually reached within 1.5 to 2.5 hours. Steady-state peak and trough concentrations are not proportional over the oral dosing range. Peak and trough plasma concentrations averaged 1.44 mcg/mL and 0.55 mcg/mL in immunocompromised patients.

Acyclovir is widely distributed in body tissues and fluids, including the brain, kidneys, saliva, uterus and vaginal mucosa, cerebrospinal fluid, and herpetic vesicular fluid. Acyclovir is also distributed in semen. Acyclovir is able to cross the placenta and is distributed in breast milk. Acyclovir is partially biotransformed by cellular enzymes and eliminated in the urine.

The bioavailability of famciclovir is 77 percent. Delayed absorption is noted with food in the gastrointestinal tract. Famciclovir is rapidly converted in the intestinal wall and liver to penciclovir, the active compound. The distribution sites of famciclovir are unknown. Penciclovir is eliminated in the urine.

Ganciclovir is poorly absorbed (5 to 9 percent) from the GI tract. Plasma ganciclovir concentrations required for therapeutic antiviral activity are unknown. Ganciclovir is widely distributed in tissues, crossing the blood-brain barrier and demonstrating good ocular distribution following IV administration. Ganciclovir may be distributed in human milk and crosses the placenta. Ganciclovir is eliminated unchanged in the urine.

Ribavirin is absorbed systemically from the respiratory tract following nasal and oral inhalation. Peak plasma concentrations occur at the end of the inhalation period. The highest ribavirin concentrations are found in the respiratory tract and red blood cells. Ribavirin is slowly distributed into CSF. Ribavirin is biotransformed in the liver and eliminated in the urine.

Valacyclovir is rapidly absorbed from the gastrointestinal tract. Fifty-four percent of valacyclovir reaches systemic circulation as acyclovir. The drug is rapidly and completely converted to acyclovir and L-valine by first-pass effect and hepatic biotransformation. Peak plasma valacyclovir concentrations are generally less than 0.5 mcg/mL at all doses within 1.5 hours. The plasma half-life ranges from 2.5 to 3.3 hours but can extend to as much as 14 hours in patients with renal impairment. Valacyclovir is widely distributed to body tissues, including CSF, saliva, and major body organs. Valacyclovir crosses the placenta and is excreted in breast milk.

Drug-Drug Interactions

Acyclovir has an increased half-life when probenecid is administered 1 hour before acyclovir (see Table 25–2). Amphotericin B has been shown to potentiate the action of acyclovir. Nephrotoxic drugs may increase renal toxicity. Zidovudine and intrathecal methotrexate may increase the risk of central nervous system side effects.

Concurrent use of famciclovir with probenecid or other drugs that are eliminated by active tubular secretion may result in increased plasma concentrations of the active metabolite penciclovir. Famciclovir plasma levels are also increased in the presence of cimetidine. Renal clearance of penciclovir is decreased by 12 percent with coadministration with theophylline. The plasma levels of digoxin are increased by 19 percent when administered with famciclovir.

Ganciclovir antagonizes the antiretroviral activity of zidovudine and didanosine against HIV. Concomitant use of zidovudine with ganciclovir can increase the risk of bone marrow depression. Foscarnet has exhibited additive or synergistic activity with ganciclovir. Drugs that inhibit renal tubular secretion may interfere with renal clearance of ganciclovir. Patients receiving immunosuppressive drugs may require decreased doses or temporary withdrawal during ganciclovir therapy to prevent excessive bone marrow suppression. Concomitant use of ganciclovir and other potentially nephrotoxic drugs in transplant recipients has been associated with renal impairment. Generalized seizures have occurred in patients during combined therapy with imipenem/cilastatin.

Ribavirin may potentiate the action of didanosine against HIV. Ribavirin antagonizes the antiviral activity of zidovudine and zalcitabine against HIV.

Probenecid and cimetidine increase blood levels of acyclovir during valacyclovir therapy. Zidovudine may cause increased drowsiness and lethargy when concomitantly used with valacyclovir.

Dosage Regimen

Table 25–3 identifies the various uses and dosages for nucleoside analog drugs. Dosage reduction is required in patients with renal insufficiency.

Laboratory Considerations

Acyclovir may increase blood urea nitrogen (BUN) and serum creatinine levels. Decreased creatinine clearance may indicate renal failure. Monitor BUN and creatinine levels prior to and throughout therapy.

Prior to initiation of therapy with ganciclovir the CBC, electrolytes, and hepatic and renal function of the patient should be evaluated. Patients receiving ganciclovir should have neutrophil and platelet counts performed at least every other day during twice weekly therapy and weekly thereafter. Do not administer ganciclovir if the neutrophil count is less than 500/mm^3 or if platelet count is less than 25,000/mm^3. Recovery begins 3 to 7 days after discontinuation of therapy. Granulocytopenia usually occurs within the first 2 weeks of therapy but may occur at any time. Renal function should be monitored frequently, with serum creatinine or creatinine clearance checked every 2 weeks throughout therapy. Older adults should have renal function closely monitored. Ganciclovir may cause abnormal liver function studies. Periodic monitoring of AST (SGOT), ALT (SGPT), and serum bilirubin is indicated. The drug may also cause a decrease in blood glucose levels.

Miscellaneous Antiviral Drugs

❒ Amantadine (SYMADINE, SYMMETREL)
❒ Cidofovir (VISTIDE)
❒ Foscarnet (FOSCAVIR)
❒ Rimantadine (FLUMADINE)

Indications

Amantadine is used in the prevention and treatment of respiratory tract infections due to influenza A virus, although chemoprophylaxis with amantadine is not a substitute for vaccination. Antiviral prophylaxis may be considered for high-risk patients when influenza virus vaccine is contraindicated. Chemoprophylaxis and treatment of respiratory tract illness caused by influenza A virus is indicated for high-risk patients who have underlying co-morbid conditions such as cardiovascular, pulmonary, metabolic, neuromuscular, or immunodeficiency disease and for health care providers. Amantadine is also used as initial therapy or as adjunct therapy with anticholinergic drugs in the treatment of all forms of Parkinsonism (see Chapter 23).

Cidofovir is indicated for the treatment of CMV retinitis in patients with HIV infection. The safety and efficacy of cidofovir have not been established for treatment of other CMV infections, such as pneumonitis, gastroenteritis, or CMV infections in non-HIV infected patients. Foscarnet is indicated for the treatment of CMV retinitis in patients with HIV. It is also used in the management of acyclovir-resistant mucocutaneous herpes simplex viral infections. Foscarnet has also been used in a limited number of patients with AIDS for the management of acyclovir-resistant varicella zoster infections. Foscarnet may decrease the duration of viral shedding and time required for crusting and healing of lesions, and the duration of positive cultures in AIDS patients with herpes simplex infections that did not respond to oral or parenteral acyclovir therapy. Other antiviral drugs used for ophthalmic conditions are discussed in Chapter 62.

Rimantadine is indicated for the treatment of influenza A infection in adults. Rimantadine is also used for the prophylaxis of influenza A virus infection in adults and children and as an adjunct to influenza vaccine for high-risk individuals. Chemoprophylaxis with rimantadine is not a substitute for vaccination. Prophylaxis with rimantadine may be indicated

- In unvaccinated children and adults at high risk because of co-morbid cardiovascular, pulmonary, metabolic, or neuromuscular diseases
- In unvaccinated older adults or hospitalized patients following a demonstrated outbreak of influenza A
- When there is an extensive outbreak of influenza A in a community
- When antigens contained in the current vaccine do not closely match the viral strain
- When a poor antibody response to the vaccine is expected in HIV patients with advanced disease

Pharmacodynamics

The exact mechanism of action of the antiviral activity of amantadine is not fully understood. Amantadine produces a virustatic effect early in the viral replication cycle, possibly by inhibiting the uncoating of the virus particle. Absorption of the virus to and penetration into cells does not appear to be affected by amantadine. RNA-dependent polymerase activity is not inhibited. To prevent infection, amantadine must be present in the tissues before exposure to the virus. It appears that the amino acid sequence in the transmembrane portion of the M_2 protein of the virus is susceptible to amantadine.

Cidofovir suppresses CMV replication by selective inhibition of viral DNA synthesis. There is selective inhibition of CMV DNA polymerase by cidofovir diphosphate, the active intracellular metabolite of cidofovir. Incorporation of cidofovir into the growing viral DNA chains results in reductions in the rate of viral DNA synthesis. CMV variants with reduced susceptibility to cidofovir have been identified.

Foscarnet is an organic analog of inorganic pyrophosphate that inhibits replication of all known herpes viruses in vitro, including CMV. Foscarnet exerts its antiviral activity through a selective inhibition at pyrophosphate binding sites on virus-specific DNA polymerases at concentrations that do not affect cellular DNA polymerases. It also prevents viral replication by inhibiting reverse transcriptase.

Rimantadine has a virustatic effect early in the viral replication cycle, possibly inhibiting the uncoating of the virus particle. Absorption and penetration of the virus into cells does not appear to be affected by the drug, and RNA-dependent RNA polymerase activity is not inhibited. The inhibitory effect of rimantadine depends on the concentration of both the drug and the virus. There is evidence that the amino acid sequence in the transmembrane portion of the M_2 protein of the virus is susceptible to rimantadine. This protein is incorporated into the plasma membranes of influenza A but not B.

Adverse Effects and Contraindications

The most common adverse effects of amantadine include dizziness, ataxia, insomnia, and livedo reticularis. Livedo reticularis is a semipermanent bluish mottling of the skin of the legs and hands and may result from abnormal capillary permeability associated with vasoconstriction. It is accompanied by lowered skin temperature, decreased peripheral blood flow, and a depletion of catecholamines in peripheral nerve endings. The edema is not associated with an increase of total body water. Occasionally orthostatic hypotension, peripheral edema, and leukopenia have been reported with the use of amantadine. Congestive heart failure, hypertension, urinary retention, decreased libido, dyspnea, rash, and visual disturbances are rare.

Many of the adverse effects of amantadine are manifested as CNS or psychic disturbances, which are usually dose related and reversible. Symptoms usually appear within a few hours to days after initiation of amantadine therapy or after an increase in dose. Dizziness, insomnia, nervousness, anxiety, and impaired concentration are among the most frequent CNS adverse effects. The older adult is more affected than younger patients. Less than 5 percent of patients report psychosis, abnormal thinking, amnesia, hyperkinesia, weakness, and slurred speech. Forgetfulness, a sense of drunkenness or detachment, drowsiness, tremor, mood changes, and lingual facial dyskinesia or seizures have been reported although they are rare. Patients with a history of mental or behavioral disorders may be at greatest risk of adverse CNS effects from amantadine therapy.

In addition and although rare, suicide attempts have been reported in patients receiving amantadine. Suicide ideation or attempts have been reported in both patients with or without a prior history of psychiatric disorders. Amantadine can exacerbate psychiatric disorders or substance abuse in susceptible individuals. Patients with suicidal tendencies may exhibit abnormal mental states, including disorientation, confusion, depression, personality changes, agitation, aggressive behavior, hallucinations, paranoia, or other psychotic reactions.

Amantadine is contraindicated in patients with hypersensitivity. It should be administered with caution in patients with liver disease or a history of recurrent eczema, uncontrolled psychosis or severe psychoneurosis, epilepsy, or seizures and in patients receiving drugs with CNS activity. Amantadine should be used with caution in patients with renal impairment, congestive heart failure, peripheral edema, or orthostatic hypotension. The safety and efficacy of amantadine during pregnancy and lactation and in children younger than 1 year has not been established.

The most common adverse effects of cidofovir include headache, weakness, dyspnea, anorexia, nausea, vomiting, diarrhea, abdominal pain, fever, chills, alopecia, rash, infection, and proteinuria. Anemia and thrombocytopenia may occur with cidofovir administration. Asthma, bronchitis, coughing and dyspnea, amblyopia, conjunctivitis, and ocular hypotony have also been noted with cidofovir therapy. Neutropenia and granulocytopenia have been observed.

The major toxicity of cidofovir is renal impairment. Dose-dependent nephrotoxicity is the major dose-limiting toxicity related to cidofovir. Proteinuria may be an early indicator of cidofovir-related nephrotoxicity. Continued administration of cidofovir leads to additional proximal tubular cell injury that may result in glycosuria; decreases in serum phosphate, uric acid, and bicarbonate levels; and elevations in serum creatinine. Patients with these adverse effects occurring concurrently and meeting a criteria of Fanconi's syndrome have been reported. Renal function may not return to baseline after discontinuation of cidofovir.

Cidofovir is contraindicated in patients with hypersensitivity to cidofovir, probenecid, or sulfonamides. It is also contraindicated in patients with serum clearance rates greater than 1.5 mg/dL, creatinine clearance rates of less than 55 mL/min, or urine proteins exceeding 100 mg/dL (over 2+ proteinuria). Concurrent use of foscarnet, amphotericin B, aminoglycoside antibiotics, nonsteroidal anti-inflammatory drugs, or IV pentamidine is also contraindicated. Cidofovir should be used with caution during pregnancy and in children. Use during breastfeeding is not recommended in HIV-infected women. Any condition that increases the risk of dehydration warrants extreme caution in the use of cidofovir.

Adverse effects to foscarnet occur frequently and can be serious. Patients receiving foscarnet usually have serious comorbid disease and are frequently being treated with other drugs concurrently. The most common adverse effect of foscarnet is renal impairment. Renal impairment occurs in most patients and may require dose adjustments or discontinuance of the drug. Patients vary in their sensitivity to foscarnet-induced nephrotoxicity. Initial renal function may not be predictive of the potential for drug-induced renal impairment. Renal impairment is most likely to become clinically evident during the second week of induction therapy but may occur at any time. Elevations in serum creatinine are usually reversible following discontinuation or dose adjustments of foscarnet.

Foscarnet has the propensity to chelate divalent metal ions and alter serum concentrations of calcium and magnesium, potassium, or phosphate, which may contribute to the risk of cardiac disturbances and seizures. The drug has thus been associated with the development of hypocalcemia, hypophosphatemia, hyperphosphatemia, hypomagnesemia, and hypokalemia. There appears to be a dose-related decrease in ionized serum calcium, which may not be reflected in total serum calcium. Seizures are usually related to renal failure and hypocalcemia.

Headache, seizures, fatigue, malaise, paresthesia, dizziness, confusion, and anxiety have been reported with foscarnet. Anemia has been noted in 33 percent of patients. The anemia is manageable with transfusions. Leukopenia and thrombocytopenia are seen less frequently. GI adverse effects include nausea, vomiting, diarrhea, and esophageal ulceration, although ulceration is rare. Visual abnormalities have been reported in patients with cytomegalovirus retinitis receiving foscarnet. Ocular pain, conjunctivitis, diplopia, retinal detachment, and visual field defects may occur and may represent progression of the retinitis.

Foscarnet is contraindicated in patients with hypersensitivity to the drug. It should be used with caution in patients with renal impairment and in patients with a history of seizures. Safe use during pregnancy and lactation and in children under the age of 18 years has not been established.

The most common adverse effects of rimantadine involve the GI tract and nervous systems. The signs and symptoms that have been reported included anorexia, nausea, vomiting, dry mouth, insomnia, dizziness, headache, nervousness, and fatigue.

Rimantadine is contraindicated in patients with hypersensitivity to rimantadine or amantadine. It should be used cautiously in patients with a history of seizures and in older adults or patients with severe hepatic or renal disease. Safe use during pregnancy has not been established.

Pharmacokinetics

Amantadine is rapidly and completely absorbed from the GI tract. Mean peak serum concentrations of 0.3 mcg/mL are noted 1 to 4 hours after an oral dose. Steady-state blood concentrations of 0.68 to 1.01 mcg/mL are reached after 4 to 5 days of therapy. Amantadine is distributed into saliva, nasal secretions, and breast milk and crosses placental membranes. CSF concentrations of amantadine are one half the blood concentration. It appears that amantadine concentration in lung tissues is higher than that in the blood.

Intravenous administration of cidofovir results in 100-percent bioavailability (see Table 25–1). The drug is less than 6 percent bound to plasma or serum proteins over the cidofovir concentration range of 0.25 to 25 mcg/mL. CSF concentrations were undetectable 15 minutes after the end of a 1-hour infusion. Renal tubular secretion contributes to the elimination of cidofovir.

Foscarnet absorption is essentially complete with IV administration with variable penetration (15 to 70 percent) into CSF. There is evidence that it may concentrate in and be slowly released from bone. Foscarnet is 14 to 17 percent bound to plasma proteins. Eighty to ninety percent of foscarnet is eliminated unchanged in the urine. Urinary elimination occurs by tubular secretion and glomerular filtration.

Rimantadine is readily absorbed from the GI tract following oral administration. Food does not appear to affect absorption. The time to peak serum concentration is approximately 6 hours. Rimantadine is extensively biotransformed in the liver, with less than 25 percent of the dose eliminated unchanged in the urine. The half-life of rimantadine ranges from 13 to 65 hours depending on hepatic and renal status.

Drug-Drug Interactions

Administration of amantadine in patients receiving drugs with anticholinergic activity may result in increased adverse anticholinergic effects (tricyclic antidepressants, antihistamines, phenothiazines). Amantadine should be administered with caution to patients receiving other CNS stimulant drugs. Hydrochlorothiazide plus triamterene may decrease urinary excretion of amantadine with increased plasma concentrations of amantadine. Alcohol may enhance the CNS effects of amantadine (see Table 25–2).

Concurrent use of cidofovir with aminoglycosides, amphotericin B, foscarnet, or pentamidine increases the risk of nephrotoxicity. Acetaminophen, acyclovir, angiotensin converting enzyme (ACE) inhibitors, barbiturates, benzodiazepines, bumetanide, methotrexate, famotidine, furosemide, nonsteroidal anti-inflammatory drugs (NSAIDs), theophylline, and zidovudine increase the risk of drug-drug interaction with probenecid. Probenecid is required to be used concurrently with cidofovir to reduce the risk of nephrotoxicity.

Concurrent administration of foscarnet with pentamidine may cause severe hypocalcemia. Amphotericin B, didanosine, aminoglycosides, and pentamidine may increase the risk of nephrotoxicity. A possibility of seizure may occur with imipenem. Zidovudine may increase the risk of anemia. Concurrent use of didanosine decreases the elimination of foscarnet.

Administration of cimetidine, aspirin, and acetaminophen may slightly decrease the plasma levels of rimantadine.

Dosage Regimen

Symptoms of influenza may be less severe and disappear more rapidly if amantadine is given within 24 to 48 hours after the onset of symptoms (see Table 25–3). To minimize the emergence of resistant strains of virus to amantadine, antiviral treatment should be discontinued after 3 to 5 days or 24 to 48 hours after the disappearance of signs and symptoms. Abrupt withdrawal after long-term use can result in neurolept malignant syndrome.

Cidofovir is administered IV once weekly for 2 weeks and then every 2 weeks. It must be administered with probenecid to reduce the risk of nephrotoxicity. Two grams of probenecid is given orally 3 hours before IV administration of cidofovir and then 1 g is given 2 hours and 8 hours following completion of the infusion. Saline prehydration is mandatory with cidofovir. Zidovudine therapy should be temporarily discontinued or decreased by 50 percent on the days of cidofovir therapy due to the effects of probenecid on zidovudine.

It is recommended that 75 to 100 mL of normal saline with 5 percent dextrose and water be given before the first infusion of foscarnet to establish diuresis. After the first dose of foscarnet, the hydration fluid may be given concurrently with each infusion of foscarnet. The rate of infusion of foscarnet may cause a transient decrease in ionized serum calcium concentrations. Slowing the rate of infusion may decrease or prevent symptoms.

Laboratory Considerations

There are no significant altered lab values noted with amantadine or rimantadine therapy. However, before the initiation of therapy and before each treatment with cidofovir, renal function should be monitored, including serum creatinine, urine protein, and white blood cell counts. In patients with proteinuria, administer IV hydration and repeat the test. Monitor serum phosphate, uric acid and bicarbonate, and creatinine. CBC and neutrophil counts should be done before and during therapy with cidofovir. Periodically monitor the patient's intraocular pressure, visual acuity, and ocular symptoms.

Foscarnet may alter electrolytes, particularly serum calcium and phosphate concentrations. Foscarnet may decrease magnesium and potassium levels. Increases may be seen in AST (SGOT), ALT (SGPT), alkaline phosphatase, bilirubin, and creatinine. Before initiation of foscarnet therapy, patients should have renal function studies and a CBC with differential performed. Monitor serum creatinine before and two to three times weekly during induction therapy and at least weekly during maintenance therapy. Twenty-four-hour urine collection for creatinine clearance should be done before and periodically throughout therapy. If the creatinine clearance value drops below 0.4 mL/min/kg, foscarnet may need to be discontinued.

Critical Thinking Process

Assessment

History of Present Illness

Demographic data to be collected includes date, patient's name, age, gender, race or ethnic origin, birthplace, marital status, and occupation. This data may elicit information relevant to identified risk factors correlated with HIV infection. This information assists in the diagnosis and individualization of a treatment plan specific to meet the patient's needs.

A chronologic record of the reason why the patient is seeking care should be obtained. Many patients with acute retroviral syndrome after initial infection may be asymptomatic, but a significant majority develop an abrupt onset febrile illness that resembles acute mononucleosis or influenza. Early HIV infection and acute retroviral syndrome presents with a wide range of clinical features unique to each individual patient. The patient remains generally healthy, but the most common complaints are fatigue, myalgia or arthralgia, pharyngitis, sore mouth, nausea, vomiting, diarrhea, headache, and weight loss. Complaints of night sweats and low-grade fevers are not uncommon. For many patients these symptoms of early HIV infection go undetected.

Early symptomatic HIV infection may present some years later. The median time between HIV infection and early symptomatic infection is 10 years or more. The patient with early symptomatic infection may complain of oral candidiasis or thrush. As the disease progresses to AIDS, opportunistic diseases occur. Numerous infections and a variety of malignancies, wasting, and dementia occur. All too often the first indication of HIV infection for some patients is the onset of opportunistic infections such as *Pneumocystis carinii* pneumonia, oral candidiasis, or vaginal fungal infections.

Past Health History

The past health history provides information about childhood illnesses, accidents, injuries, hospitalizations, operations, obstetric history, immunizations, allergies, current medications, and foreign travel. It is important to note any operative procedures that may have included the administration of blood between 1977 and 1985. The presence of hemophilia or other blood diseases is significant.

The drug history should include information about prescribed drugs, over-the-counter (OTC) drugs, and herbal remedies. Information related to alcohol use and illicit drug use is critically important. Compatibility, synergy, and adverse effects of drugs in current use are important. The use of any immunosuppressant drugs is critically important to note.

Substance abuse and the incidence of HIV infection is high among people who use IV drugs and their sexual partners. A detailed drug history should contain all of the information necessary to assess past risk of HIV exposure. Information about the drugs used, pattern of drug use, shared needle use, or participation in drug treatment programs should be elicited.

Obtaining a complete and accurate sexual health history is critically important. Information needs to be gathered to determine past risk as well as future risk for infection with HIV, and education needs of the patient. Questions that relate to current sexual partner, past sexual partners, numbers of sexual relationships, kinds of sexual activity, history of sexually transmitted disease, homosexual or bisexual activity, and sexual relationships with persons who used IV drugs are necessary.

The immunization history should include a review of immunizations for hepatitis B, influenza, and the basic childhood series or diphtheria-tetanus-pertussis (DTP), measles-mumps-rubella (MMR), and polio. History of infectious diseases should include chickenpox, shingles, tuberculosis, mononucleosis, Epstein-Barr virus, dermatitis, and any parasitic infections.

Physical Exam Findings

The physical exam begins with the patient's general overall appearance. Note the patient's height and weight. Specific signs to look for include recent weight loss, fever, chills, and night sweats. Look for specific signs that may indicate any underlying conditions. The baseline physical exam should cover each of the systems most likely to be affected by HIV infection or the opportunistic infections associated with HIV. These systems include neuropsychiatric, neurologic, musculoskeletal, cardiorespiratory, GI, genitourinary tract, dermatologic, and head, eyes, ears, nose, and throat (HEENT). Many patients who complain of no symptoms at baseline will have some abnormalities noted on physical examination or laboratory evaluation.

Diagnostic Testing

The laboratory testing used in the diagnosis of HIV includes enzyme-linked immunosorbent assay (ELISA), Western blot, immunofluorescence assay, and polymerase chain reaction (PCR). ELISA detects antibodies to HIV but does not detect HIV directly. ELISA results are reported as positive, negative, or indeterminate. If the ELISA is positive or indeterminate, a repeat test is done. If the specimen is repeatedly ELISA positive, a more specific confirming test such as the Western blot or indirect immunofluorescence assay is done. Blood that is reactive in all three steps is reported as HIV positive.

The Western blot is able to detect HIV antibodies and identifies the individual viral components to which antibodies are reactive. If the ELISA is either positive or indeterminate but the Western blot is negative, the ELISA is considered falsely positive and the patient is not infected with HIV. The indirect immunofluorescence assay may be used as a substitute for a Western blot and may be able to clarify the results of indeterminate Western blot findings but requires significant time, expense, and expertise to perform.

PCR is a technique for HIV detection that identifies the presence of HIV genetic material. PCR detects the presence of proviral DNA using genetic probes specific for the nucleotide sequences of HIV proviral DNA. Proviral DNA copies are generated from viral RNA through an enzyme-mediated process. The copies are found in the cytoplasm of the cell or as part of the host cell genome.

The laboratory testing used to monitor HIV infection and guide management decisions includes viral loads (plasma HIV RNA assays) and CD4 counts. Viral loads reflect the magnitude of HIV replication and predict the rate of CD4 cell destruction.

CD4 counts indicate the extent of HIV-induced immune damage the patient has sustained. CD4 counts are necessary to determine the risk of disease progression and when to initiate or modify antiretroviral treatment regimens. The CD4 count is calculated based on the percentage of CD4 cells in the total lymphocyte count. The normal CD4 count is approximately 800 to 1100 cells/mm^3 with a range of approximately 500 to 1400 cells/mm^3, approximately 40 percent of the total number of lymphocytes. A CD4 count of less than 500/mm^3 is considered abnormally low. A count below 200/mm^3 is a criterion for diagnosing AIDS in HIV-infected patients. CD4 cell counts less than 22 cells/mm^3 or less than 14 percent place the patient at risk for developing an opportunistic infection. Patients with full-blown AIDS may have a CD4 count as low as 5 to 10 cells/mm^3 and a percentage of 1 to 2 percent of all lymphocytes. Both CD4 counts and percentages reflect immune status, not HIV activity.

Viral load testing measures the amount of HIV RNA or genetic material in plasma. Viral load determinations are an important prognostic marker of disease progression and when used appropriately provide a valuable tool in the management of individual patients. Three tests are currently used to measure viral load: reverse transcriptase polymerase chain reaction (RT-PCR), branched-chain DNA (bDNA), and nucleic acid sequence-based amplification (NASBA).

RT-PCR is a modification of DNA PCR. This technique measures the quantity of HIV RNA genetic material in plasma. Sensitivity for detecting viral RNA in plasma is close to 100 percent, and reliability makes the technique excellent for quantification of viral burden over time.

Branched DNA is a sensitive, reproducible, rapid, quantitative means of measuring HIV RNA levels in plasma. This assay rapidly detects changes in virus levels and permits health care providers to respond with changes in therapy.

In each of the three viral load tests, results are reported in copies/mL. Fewer than 10,000 copies/mL indicates a low risk for clinical progression, 10,000 to 100,000 indicates a moderate risk, and more than 100,000 copies indicates a high risk. It is important to note that the values obtained using the RT-PCR may be as much as two times higher than those obtained using the bDNA. Thus, to interpret the results accurately, the health care provider must know which test was employed.

Developmental Considerations

Perinatal Various processes are involved in the perinatal transmission of HIV infection to newborns. Virus transmission has been documented in utero by direct transplacental hematogenous spread in utero, by ascending infection of amniotic fluid, iatrogenically by direct invasive methods used for diagnosis (such as scalp monitoring), and through breastfeeding.

Maternal characteristics that may increase risk factors related to transmission include increased maternal viremia, declining maternal health due to advanced disease, and immunosuppression. Asymptomatic women transmit HIV at a much lower rate than women with AIDS. Prolonged complicated labor and clinical chorioamnionitis and continued illicit drug use also increase the risk of perinatal HIV transmission.

Intrauterine transmission is believed to be responsible for a significant amount of transmission. The rate of infection may be as high as 50 to 70 percent. Placental factors include cell susceptibility to virus infection, developmental stage of the placenta, and integrity of the placenta. Maternal viral virulence, virus phenotype, and genotype are being studied as well.

Intrapartum factors resulting in HIV infections include extended time from rupture of membranes, invasive fetal monitoring, the route of delivery, first-born twin, and gestational age at delivery. It is theorized that direct exposure to virus in blood or secretions during labor and delivery results in higher risk of infection. Many infants swallow secretions in the birth process. There are reports of twins in whom the first twin through the birth canal was infected and the second was not. Cesarean section is associated with a slightly lower infection rate. This finding supports the concept that cleansing of the birth canal and immediate washing of the infant could interrupt virus transmission.

Fetal factors that affect susceptibility to infection include gestational age at birth, the development of the immune system of the fetus, and breastfeeding. Infants born before 34 weeks' gestation have an increased risk of infection. HIV has been found in the cellular and cell-free faction of breast milk, although there has been no correlation to date between maternal disease and HIV in breast milk.

Pediatric Most new pediatric infection is acquired perinatally. Identification of HIV-infected infants soon after delivery or during the first few weeks following their birth provides opportunities for the treatment of primary HIV infection.

Initial testing is recommended within the first 48 hours of life because nearly 40 percent of infected infants can be identified at this time. Interpretation of CD4 counts among children must consider age as an important variable. CD4 and percentage values in healthy infants who are not infected with HIV are considerably higher than those observed in uninfected adults and slowly decline to adult values over the first 6 years of life. While the CD4 count changes with age, the CD4 percent that defines each immunologic category does not. For this reason a change in CD4 percentage, not the number, may be a better marker to identify disease progression in children. Adult guidelines for antiretroviral therapy are appropriate for older children and adolescents.

Children are dependant on caregivers for the administration of drug therapy. The environment as well as the willingness of the caregiver to adhere to a complex multidrug regimen should be evaluated. Absorption of some antiretroviral drugs is affected by food. It can be difficult to juggle drug administration times around infant feedings. The adolescent has developmental issues that are unique as well. Concrete thought processes make it difficult to adhere to a drug treatment regimen when the adolescent generally feels well. Adolescents also do not want to be different from their peers.

Geriatric HIV infection is often overlooked in older adults because health care providers often do not consider this population to be at risk. Risk factors most often associated with HIV transmission in the older adult include sexual contact, blood transfusions prior to 1985, and illicit drug use.

Many factors relate to the increased risk of the older adult becoming infected through sexual activity. Older adults often do not use condoms. Pregnancy is no longer an issue, and older adults do not view themselves at risk for sexually transmitted diseases. Changes occur in the vagina (e.g., reduced lubrication, friable tissues) and immune response that make older women more susceptible to transmission of disease. Older men who have been with prostitutes are at risk for transmission of disease. Elderly gay men may be at increased risk after the death of a long-term mate or a change to a younger partner.

HIV infection in the older adult has been called the great imitator because it can present as dementia that is mistaken for Alzheimer's disease or other chronic illness. Subtle differences between Alzheimer's disease and related dementias and HIV dementia also make patient assessment difficult. In addition, other symptoms, such as fatigue, weakness, anorexia, and weight loss, occur in many comorbid conditions, other than HIV infection, that the patient may have.

Currently the only way to slow down the progression of HIV infection is with antiretroviral drug therapy. Older adults are generally more prone to adverse effects from drugs than younger patients. Older patients are also more prone to adverse effects of drugs secondary to polypharmacy. Renal insufficiency may make older patients less tolerant of drugs. Nephron mass and renal blood flow decrease with age, which may affect the dosing of drugs eliminated by the kidneys. Lean muscle mass decreases, while the proportion of body fat increases. This may lengthen the effects of fat-soluble medications. It is important to note if older adults' cognitive status, hearing, and visual acuity will enable them to hear, understand, read, and follow directions with regard to drug therapy.

Psychosocial Considerations

Current social history and prejudices constitute a large portion of what preoccupies HIV-infected people. Health care providers should focus vital information on issues that relate to housing, family and community support, family dynamics, employment, and health insurance. It may be necessary to remove system barriers to treatment in order to stabilize patients' lives prior to the initiation of drug therapy.

Economic realities provide a blunt boundary line for this disease. Many people at high risk for HIV infection belong to lower socioeconomic groups. Often these patients do not have health insurance or access to health care.

The current demographic, social, and economic realities make HIV care challenging and sometimes exasperating. Noncompliance seems to be a major impediment to maximal benefit from medical intervention. There are large numbers of patients who are lost to follow-up, with as many reasons for those losses as there are patients. Patients often lack transportation or have no stable address or phone, suffer from psychiatric illness, use illicit drugs, or may be incarcerated. Some are embarrassed because they are unable to pay bills and purchase the required drugs. Many patients need constant social service interventions to ensure continuity of care. A psychosocial history will uncover problems with coping and stress management. Additionally, the health care provider should determine if the patient has a history of depression, suicidal tendencies, isolation, insomnia, or any other emotional problems. The kind of social supports the patient has in place will either facilitate or hinder treatment.

The complexity of HIV disease is related to its chronic nature. The problems associated with HIV infection are exacerbated by trauma related to the physical deterioration and social attitudes surrounding HIV infection. HIV causes increasing physical disability. Often the patient experiences cyclical problems that compound one another. The health care system is often difficult to navigate, and all of this taxes the patient's ability to cope (see Case Study—HIV Infection).

Analysis and Management

New information on HIV pathogenesis, viral load monitoring, and the impact of potent antiretroviral drug regimens is emerging at a rapid pace. Recommendations for treatment should be continuously reevaluated in order to synthesize the latest developments in basic science, drug development, and clinical investigation. Recent evidence suggests that early treatment of HIV infection slows disease progression and, according to some mathematical models, may eradicate HIV. Early diagnosis of acute primary HIV infection is important for explaining a patient's often undiagnosed acute illness. Early diagnosis is also important in counseling, preventing further transmission, elucidating the natural history of HIV infection, and starting early treatment with drug therapy. Diagnosis of HIV infection is often missed at the initial clinical encounter with the health care provider. Although most patients seek medical attention during their acute illness, only 25 percent are diagnosed at that time. Health care providers must consider the possibility of HIV infection in all patients who have symptoms consistent with acute retroviral syndrome.

Treatment Objectives

The goal of early therapy is to maximally suppress viral loads to undetectable levels, suppress viral replication, preserve immune function, prolong health and life, and decrease the risk of drug resistance due to early suppression of viral replication. Any patient with less than 500 CD4 cells/mm^3 or greater than 10,000 (bDNA) or 20,000 (RT-PCR) copies of HIV RNA/mL of plasma should be offered therapy.

Treatment Options

Drug Variables

HIV treatment and care requires a close alliance between patient and health care provider. Patients should be included in a process of shared decision making prior to the initiation of drug therapy. The goal of this process is to analyze the risks and benefits of different treatment options together. Both patient and health care provider need to take the time to explore how available drug therapies fit into a person's home life, work life, and perception of self. It is important for the health care provider to look into all of the patient's circumstances so that the patient is given every opportunity for success in combination therapy.

The current state of knowledge indicates that combination therapy of two or more drugs rather than monotherapy should be used to fight the rapid replication of HIV virus. The best opportunity to accomplish maximal suppression of virus replication, minimize the risk of drug-resistant HIV variants, and maximize immune system protection is to use combinations of effective antiviral drugs in patients with no prior history of anti-HIV therapy.

Multidrug therapy exerts constant maximal suppression of HIV replication and is the best approach to minimize the risk of drug-resistant variants. Multidrug therapy should be initiated with all drugs started simultaneously. Antiretroviral therapies should not be added sequentially. Sequential introduction of antiretroviral drugs increases the likelihood of incomplete suppression of HIV replication and increases the chance of viral mutations.

Preferred initial drug therapy would include one highly active protease inhibitor and two nucleoside reverse transcriptase inhibitors. The combination of drugs produces a

Case Study HIV Infection

Patient History

History of Present Illness	JDS is a 43-year-old man with a recent history of newly diagnosed HIV infection. He presents with fatigue, night sweats, dyspnea, and dry cough.
Past Health History	JDS has no known allergies. He has never been treated with antiretroviral therapy. Vegetarian diet. Nonsmoker, nondrinker.
Physical Exam	BP 124/82, heart rate 128, respiratory rate 32, O_2 Sat room air: 90%. Temp 103.2°F. Weight loss 40 lb over last 3 months. No skin lesions, no masses, decreased breath sounds, clear, dry cough. Neurologic exam negative. Cranial nerves intact.
Diagnostic Testing	CXR: diffuse infiltrates. Bronchial washings pending, PPD negative, CD4 count 128, WBC: 5.8, RBC: 3.35, Hgb: 10.6, Hct: 30, Lymph 15, Viral load pending, K 3.9, BUN 10, Cr .7
Developmental Considerations	Early diagnosis of HIV undetected. HIV a disease of young people. Renal function adequate.
Psychosocial Considerations	JDS is married and divorced and now lives alone. He suspects his HIV infection may have been heterosexual transmission. Currently on leave from job. Support system includes sister.
Economic Factors	Health plan will cover prescriptions presently. Co-payment plans of $5.00 per prescription.

Variables Influencing Decision

Treatment Objectives	• Maintain immune function as near normal state as possible. • Prevent disease progression and prolong survival. • Preserve quality of life by effectively suppressing HIV replication.

Drug Variables	*Drug Summary*	*Patient Variables*
Indications	The combination of zidovudine, lamivudine, and ritonavir during early-stage disease produces significant and sustained reduction of viral load as well as an increase in CD4 count. The same combination in late-state disease with CD4 cell counts of less than 50 cells/mm^3 usually lowered mortality rates. Triple therapy demonstrates a benefit over double nucleoside therapy in both viral load and clinical benefit.	Chest x-ray consistent with PCP. JDS's CD4 count below 200/mm^3. Dry cough, dyspnea.
Pharmacodynamics	Bactrim is bacteriostatic. Zidovudine and lamivudine are virustatic by interfering with HIV virus–dependent polymerase reverse transcriptase. Ritonavir interferes with the formation of essential proteins and reverse transcriptase thus blocking maturation of the HIV virus.	There are no specific patient variables that influence clinical decision-making.
Adverse Effects/ Contraindications	Bactrim: Rash, GI upset, *C. difficile* diarrhea, leukopenia, neutropenia, anemia, ataxia, hyperkalemia. Zidovudine: Bone marrow suppression, anemia, GI upset. Lamivudine: Minimal toxicity. Headache, nausea, and anemia, neutropenia may be noted. Ritonavir: Nausea and vomiting.	JDS is newly diagnosed with HIV. He has not had an antiviral drug at this point that would have caused adverse effects. There are no known patient variables to the use of these drugs.

Drug Variables	*Drug Summary*	*Patient Variables*
Pharmacokinetics	Zidovudine: half-life 3 hours, CNS levels 60% serum levels, renal excretion, hepatic biotransformation. Lamivudine: half-life 12 hours, 10% CNS penetration, renal excretion. Ritonavir: half-life 3–5 hours, potent inhibitor of cytochrome P_{450} enzyme can produce large increases of drugs that are metabolized by that pathway.	JDS has normal BUN, Cr level. Has never been treated with antiretrovirals before.
Dosage Regimen	Zidovudine: 300 mg every 12 hours. Lamivudine: 150 mg every 12 hours. Ritonavir: 600 mg every 12 hours with food.	Compliance with therapy would be enhanced if a twice-daily drug could be used rather than one requiring administration every 4 hours. This will become a decision point.
Lab Considerations	CBC, LFTs, BUN, creatinine, electrolytes. Prior to initiation of treatment. CD4 count, plasma load baseline testing one month apart before treatment is initiated and then every 3–4 months.	JDS's sister will transport him to the clinic for laboratory work. This will not be a decision point.
Cost Index*	Zidovudine: 5 Lamivudine: 5 Ritonavir: 5	JDS's health plan will help to cover cost of pharmacotherapy.

Summary of Decision Points

- The variety of adverse effects associated with multidrug therapy requires close monitoring.
- The best time to initiate therapy is during the acute stage of the infection.
- Therapy should be initiated in any patient who is symptomatic or when CD4 count is less than 500 cells/mm^3 or viral load is greater than 5000 copies/mL.
- When changing drug therapy, never change a single drug but at least two at a time.
- Do not use didanosine with zalcitabine because of overlapping side effects.
- Never use zalcitabine as monotherapy. It is most effective when used with zidovudine in antiretroviral naive patients.
- Switching to stavudine after greater than 6 months of zidovudine therapy increases CD4 count and slows clinical progression.
- Therapy should be changed when toxicity or intolerance occurs or there is evidence of drug failure. Choose drugs that have not been taken before.

DRUGS TO BE USED

- Bactrim 5 mg/kg IV for 21 days
- Zidovudine 100 mg po q4hr around the clock
- Ritonavir 600 mg po BID with food
- Lamivudine 150 mg po BID

*Cost Index:

1 $<30/mo.
2 $30–40/mo.
3 $40–50/mo.
4 $50–60/mo.
5 $>60/mo.

AWP of 1, 150-mg tablet of lamivudine is $4 or $240 monthly.
AWP of 1, 100-mg tablet of zidovudine is $2 per tablet or $360 monthly.
AWP of 1, 100-mg capsule of ritonavir is $2 per capsule or $720 monthly.

sustained reduction of viral load in the majority of patients who comply with the regimen. Saquinavir is not recommended here because of poor bioavailability due to hard gel capsules.

Protease Inhibitor	Nucleoside Reverse Transcriptase Inhibitors
• Indinavir	-plus - Zidovudine -and- Didanosine
• Nelfinavir	-plus - Stavudine -and- Zalcitabine
• Retonavir	-plus - Zidovudine -and- Lamivudine
• Saquinavir	-plus - Stavudine -and- Lamivudine
• Saquinavir	-plus - Stavudine -and- Didanosine

The hard-gelatin capsule formulation of saquinavir moves this drug to a second-line agent. Further, high-level viral resistance to lamivudine develops within 2 to 4 weeks if partially suppressive treatment regimens are used. Optimal use of lamivudine is in drug combinations that reduce viral load to less than 500 copies/mL. Additionally, of the two non-nucleoside reverse transcriptase inhibitors available, only nevirapine has been shown effective in combination with nucleoside reverse transcriptase inhibitors.

Alternative multidrug combinations may include nevirapine plus two nucleoside reverse transcriptase inhibitors. The combination of nelfinavir plus zidovudine and didanosine has shown dramatic improvements in overall health and well-being and sharp reductions in viral load. These alternative groupings do not achieve the goal of suppressing viremia to below detectable levels as consistently as multidrug therapy using two nucleoside reverse transcriptase inhibitors and a protease inhibitor.

Monotherapy with any of the available antiretroviral drugs is not recommended for initiation of treatment of HIV disease. Viral resistance usually emerges within weeks to months with monotherapy. Monotherapy causes a transient decrease in plasma viral load but compromises future effective therapies by selecting for viral mutants that are resistant to one or more antiretroviral drugs. One exception to the use of monotherapy is the use of zidovudine specifically for the purpose of reducing the risk of perinatal HIV transmission in pregnant women who have high CD4 counts and low viral loads and who have decided not to initiate antiretroviral therapy. This time-limited use of zidovudine has important benefits to infants and is not likely to compromise the mother's ability to benefit from combination antiretroviral therapy in the future.

Advanced-stage HIV patients being maintained on an antiretroviral regimen should not have therapy discontinued during an acute opportunistic infection or malignancy unless there are concerns about drug toxicity, intolerance, or drug interactions.

Changing Drug Regimens Decisions to alter therapy are based on individual responses to drug therapy. It is important not to abandon a specific therapeutic regimen too soon. Each decision to alter therapy may limit future alternative options. Because there are only nine antiretroviral drugs presently available, options for changing therapeutic regimens are clearly limited.

There are four primary reasons for changing therapeutic regimens: treatment failure, drug toxicity, patient noncompliance, and use of a suboptimal drug regimen. However, before the decision is made to change antiretroviral therapy based on viral loads, the test should be repeated using the same type of test. Treatment failure is identified when (1) viral loads fail to drop by 10-fold (1 log) within the first 4 weeks of treatment, (2) the viral load fails to drop to undetectable levels within the first 4 to 6 months of therapy, (3) the viral load rebounds after falling to an undetectable level, (4) CD4 counts continue to drop despite antiretroviral therapy, and (5) clinical symptoms continue to progress in the presence of antiretroviral therapy.

Increasing viral loads in a person receiving antiretroviral therapy may be due to a number of factors. Increased levels of HIV replication may indicate the emergence of HIV drug-resistant variant, incomplete adherence to antiretroviral therapy, decreased absorption of antiretroviral drugs, altered drug biotransformation, drug-drug interactions, or intercurrent infection.

The degree of plasma HIV increase should be considered before changing therapy. Any patient with any reproducible significant increase (defined as threefold or greater from the nadir of viral load not attributable to intercurrent infection, vaccination, or test methodology) should be considered for changing therapy. Persistent, declining CD4 counts measured on two separate occasions and clinical deterioration are additional reasons to consider changing therapy.

Changes in drug regimen should include complete replacement of the regimen with different drugs that the patient has not taken before. Ideally, if the patient has been taking a protease inhibitor and two nucleoside reverse transcriptase inhibitors, the replacement regimen would consist of a new protease inhibitor and two new nucleoside reverse transcriptase inhibitors. Avoid changing from one protease inhibitor to another protease inhibitor. Also avoid changing from one non-nucleoside reverse transcriptase inhibitor (e.g., nevirapine) to another non-nucleoside reverse transcriptase inhibitor (e.g., delavirdine). Cross resistance is possible. Although clinical benefit has been demonstrated using two nucleoside reverse transcriptase inhibitors, initial virus suppression is not sustained in most patients. Consultation with an HIV expert is strongly recommended when changing therapeutic drug regimens. To date there is limited experience with multidrug therapy made up of two protease inhibitors or a protease inhibitor and a non-nucleoside reverse transcriptase inhibitor. Because the protease inhibitors indinavir and ritonavir have shown cross resistance, these drugs should not be substituted for each other. Similarly, the non-nucleoside reverse transcriptase inhibitors nevirapine and delavirdine should not be substituted for each other because of cross resistance.

Suboptimal therapy is defined as a failure to suppress viral loads to an undetectable level. Additionally, suboptimal treatment also occurs when treatment is undertaken using single or dual nucleoside reverse transcriptase inhibitors. The new drugs are intended to replace the old drugs. They are not taken in addition to the old drugs.

Patients who become toxic to a specific drug in the treatment regimen should have that drug discontinued. The toxic drug should be replaced with one of equal efficacy that is from the same class. For example, if a patient were to become toxic to zidovudine, that drug should be discontinued and replaced with another nucleoside reverse transcriptase inhibitor such as lamivudine. Changing one drug is considered correct procedure when toxicity is the reason for altering the treatment regimen. When resistance or suboptimal treatment is the reason, all drugs should be changed.

Long, slow recovery of the immune system with continued viral shutdown is being reported with the use of highly active antiretroviral regimens (HAART). It does appear that slow recovery of the immune function is possible as long as the virus is kept in check.

Patient Variables

Therapy should be considered for all patients with HIV infection and detectable plasma HIV RNA who request it and are committed to lifelong adherence to necessary treatment. Therapy is also recommended for patients who are symptomatic with HIV disease or who have CD4 counts below 500/mm^3 and particularly for patients below 350/mm^3. The potential toxicities of therapy, quality of life, and ability to adhere to a complex antiretroviral drug regimen need to be balanced with the anticipated clinical benefit of maximal suppression of HIV replication.

People with HIV infection must be considered at risk for progressive disease. The potential benefit of treatment of patients with viral loads persistently below detection is not known. High levels of CD4 counts in the absence of therapy are at low risk for disease progression in the near future.

Patients with late-stage disease have been shown to benefit from appropriate antiretroviral therapy with decreased risk of further disease and death. Antiretroviral therapy can benefit patients even when CD4 increase is not seen. Discontinuation of antiretroviral therapy may be considered if drug therapies do not suppress HIV replication or if drug toxicities outweigh the anticipated clinical benefit.

Women should receive optimal antiretroviral therapy regardless of pregnancy status, according to the most recent guidelines from the Department of Health and Human Services. Treatment decisions are based on the future health of the mother as well as the prevention of perinatal transmission to the fetus and ensuring the health of the fetus and neonate. To date the only drug that has demonstrated the ability to reduce the risk of perinatal HIV transmission is zidovudine. Zidovudine is administered orally at 14 weeks gestation and continued throughout pregnancy. Zidovudine is then administered IV during the intrapartum period and to the newborn for the first 6 weeks of life. If combination antiretroviral therapy is administered to pregnant women, zidovudine should be included as a component of therapy in the intrapartum period and zidovudine should be administered to the neonate. Zidovudine therapy has been shown to be effective in reducing perinatal HIV transmission regardless of maternal viral load.

Women receiving antiretroviral therapy at the time pregnancy is diagnosed should continue their therapy. If antiretroviral therapy is discontinued during the first trimester of pregnancy for any reason, all drugs should be discontinued simultaneously. Once the antiviral regimen is reinstituted, all drugs should be started simultaneously.

The choice of which antiretroviral drug to administer to pregnant women requires consideration of pharmacokinetics and safety of antiretroviral drugs in pregnancy. It is important to note the potential effects of drugs on the fetus and newborn. Placental passage of the drug and preclinical data indicate potential teratogenicity, mutagenicity, or carcinogenicity. Some drugs have positive findings on one or more of these tests; however, data collection in the Pregnancy Registry has shown no evidence to this point of increased risks of birth defects in infants.

The pharmacokinetics of only zidovudine and lamivudine have been evaluated in infected women. Both are well tolerated at the usual adult doses and cross the placenta, achieving concentrations in cord blood similar to that observed in maternal blood at delivery. All the nucleoside reverse transcriptase inhibitors except didanosine have been classified as FDA pregnancy category C. Didanosine has been classified as category B. Of the non-nucleoside reverse transcriptase inhibitors, only nevirapine has been evaluated in pregnant women. Nevirapine is well tolerated after a single dose given to pregnant infected women in labor. It crossed the placenta, reaching neonatal blood concentrations equivalent to that in the mother. Data on multiple dosing during pregnancy is not available. Studies on the use of other non-nucleoside reverse transcriptase inhibitors in pregnancy have not been conducted.

Studies of combination therapy with protease inhibitors in pregnant infected women are in progress. There is currently no data available regarding safety and tolerance in pregnancy. Indinavir and ritonavir both have significant placental passage. Indinavir is associated with adverse effects of hyperbilirubinemia and renal stones that theoretically could be problematic for the neonate if indinavir is administered shortly before delivery. This risk is due to the immaturity of the metabolic enzyme system of the neonatal liver. A prolonged half-life leading to extended drug exposure in the newborn may lead to potential exacerbation of physiologic neonatal hyperbilirubinemia. Immature renal function and the inability of the neonate to ensure adequate hydration voluntarily may lead to high drug concentrations or delayed elimination and higher concentrations. However, these concerns are at present theoretical.

Antiviral therapy is recommended for HIV-infected children with clinical symptoms of HIV infection or evidence of immune suppression regardless of age or viral load. The majority of children with HIV infection will have clinical symptoms early in life. Many health care providers will initiate therapy in all HIV-infected infants under 12 months of age as soon as a confirmed diagnosis is established, regardless of clinical status, immunologic status, or viral load. A growing number of adolescents are long-term survivors of perinatal or blood product HIV infection as children and have a unique clinical course.

Other clinicians would defer the initiation of therapy and carefully monitor the clinical, immunologic, and virologic status of the patient. The viral load indicative of increased risk for disease progression is not well defined in children. Any child with a viral load greater than 100,000 copies/mL would be at high risk and should be started on antiretroviral therapy. Any child with viral loads that demonstrate a significant increase of more than 0.5 to 0.7 log 10 on repeat testing should be offered antiretroviral therapy.

Combination therapy is recommended for all infants, children, and adolescents who are treated with antiretroviral drugs. Zidovudine may be appropriate in infants of indeterminate HIV status during the first 6 weeks of life to prevent perinatal transmission. Infants who are identified as HIV infected while receiving zidovudine chemoprophylaxis should be changed to a combination antiretroviral drug regimen.

Occupational Exposure The current recommendations for chemoprophylaxis after occupational exposure to HIV are determined by type of exposure and source material. Provisional postexposure chemoprophylaxis recommendations have been developed as guidelines to manage known occupational exposures to HIV. Most occupational exposures do not result in infection transmission, and the potential toxicity of antiretroviral drugs must be carefully considered when prescribing postexposure prophylaxis (PEP). Patients with occupational exposures to source patients with unknown HIV status should be considered for the initiation of PEP on a case-by-case basis.

PEP should be recommended for health care workers who experience exposure to individuals with a high risk for HIV transmission. For exposures with a lower but non-negligible risk, PEP should be offered, balancing the lower risk against the use of drugs having uncertain efficacy and toxicity. For exposures with negligible risk PEP is not justified. Table 25–4 identifies the chemoprophylaxis recommendations for persons with occupational HIV exposure.

Chemoprophylaxis should consist of zidovudine therapy in all cases of postexposure chemoprophylaxis. Lamivudine is added for additional antiretroviral activity or for the presence of HIV zidovudine (ZVD)-resistant strains. Protease inhibitors are added to the chemoprophylaxis regimen for highest-risk occupational exposures. Chemoprophylaxis should be initiated immediately after the exposure, preferably within 1 to 2 hours of the exposure. For high-risk occupational exposures, initiation of therapy after longer intervals may be considered. The optimal duration for chemoprophylaxis regimen is unknown but should probably be prescribed for 4 weeks based on tolerance.

Health care workers considering postexposure chemoprophylaxis should have baseline testing done before the initiation of therapy. Baseline testing should include a chemistry panel to include creatinine, CBC with differential, liver enzymes, and pregnancy testing. Baseline tests such as HIV antibody test and hepatitis B and C should also be performed. HIV antibody testing should be performed periodically for at least 6 months postexposure. If postexposure prophylaxis is used, drug toxicity monitoring should be performed.

Intervention

Administration

Before initiating antiretroviral therapy, a detailed discussion between the patient and his or her primary caretaker is necessary to assess the patient's ability and willingness to commit to a complex, costly, and potentially toxic drug regimen. This is very important in asymptomatic patients at an early stage of illness in whom the ability to maintain a long-term adherence to the regimen is a major challenge.

Pharmacologic treatment is life-long with multiple classifications of drugs. Schedules that require fewer daily doses make life easier for patients. Multidrug therapy should be maintained at recommended doses. Underdosing should be avoided. Antiretroviral drug resistance is less likely to occur if all antiretroviral therapy is temporarily stopped than if it the dosage is reduced or if one component is withheld.

Education

Psychologists believe that the biggest predictor of compliance with prescribed drug protocols is the amount of chaos in someone's life. There is a need to approach HIV patients holistically. For many, the circumstances are such that the patient has neither the capacity nor the will to be compliant with drug therapy. Patients do not persist in treatment for varying reasons. It is difficult for some patients to adhere to drug treatment when they are symptom free, especially if the drugs have adverse effects that interfere with activities of daily living. The cost of drugs for many patients is significant.

Adequate information enables patients to make informed choices about life-style issues they may be faced with (see

TABLE 25–4 RECOMMENDATIONS FOR OCCUPATIONAL HIV EXPOSURE CHEMOPROPHYLAXIS

Type of Exposure	Source	Prophylaxis	Therapy
Percutaneous (highest risk)	Blood	Recommend	Zidovudine + lamivudine + indinavir
Percutaneous (increased risk)	Blood	Recommend	Zidovudine + lamivudine +/− indinavir
Percutaneous (no increased risk)	Blood	Offer	Zidovudine + lamivudine
Percutaneous	Fluid containing visible blood, or other potentially infectious fluid or tissue	Offer	Zidovudine + lamivudine
Mucous membrane	Blood	Offer	Zidovudine + lamivudine +/− indinavir
Mucous membrane	Fluid containing visible blood, or other potentially infectious fluid or tissue	Offer	Zidovudine +/− lamivudine
Mucous membrane	Other body fluid such as urine	Not offer	—
Skin (increased risk, high HIV titer, prolonged contact, extensive area, area without skin integrity)	Blood	Offer	Zidovudine + lamivudine +/− indinavir

Data from the United States Public Health Service, 1996.

HIV INFORMATION RESOURCES

- HIV Telephone Consultation Service, 1-800-933-3413
- AIDS Clinical Trials Information Service (ACTIS), 1-800-TRIALS-A (874-2572) (English and Spanish)
- The American Foundation for AIDS Research, 1-800-39AMFAR (392-6327)
- AIDS Treatment Data Network, 1-212-268-4196
- AIDS Treatment News, 1-800-TREAT 1-2 (893-2812)
- National AIDS Hotline, 1-800-342-AIDS (342-2437) (English), 1-800-344-SIDA (344-7432) (Spanish), 1-800-AIDS-TTY (243-7889) (hearing impaired)
- National Association of People with AIDS, 1-202-898-0414
- Hemophilia and AIDS/HIV Network for Dissemination of Information (HANDI), 1-800-42-HANDI (424-2634)
- National Pediatric HIV Resource Center, 1-800-362-0071
- Antiretroviral Pregnancy Registry, Post Office Box 13398, Research Triangle Park, NC 27709-3398, 1-919-483-9437, 1-800-722-9292 x 39437, FAX 1-929-315-8981
- HIV Post Exposure Prophylaxis (PEP) Registry, 1-888-737-4448

HIV Information Resources). Information helps patients adhere to a treatment program. In the absence of a vaccination, education and behavioral change are the only effective tools for prevention of HIV infection. Educational messages should be specific to the patient's needs, culturally sensitive, and age specific.

Once the decision has been made to begin therapy, specific information concerning drug administration, expected outcomes, and adverse effects needs to be discussed with the patient and his or her family. The patient should be informed that antiretroviral drug therapy is not a cure for HIV infection, nor does therapy reduce the risk of transmission of HIV to others through sexual contact, blood contamination, or contact with body fluids. Indeed, multidrug therapy, at this time, is lifelong.

The patient should be instructed to take the drugs exactly as prescribed. In some cases (e.g., zidovudine), therapy is required around the clock, even if sleep is interrupted. The importance of compliance with therapy, not taking more than the prescribed amount, and not discontinuing a drug without first consulting with the health care provider must be strongly emphasized. In most cases, missed doses should be taken as soon as the patient remembers, unless it is almost time for the next dose. But doses should not be doubled. The patient should be cautioned not to share the drugs with others. OTC drugs should be avoided without first contacting the health care provider.

The impact of drug therapy on the overall monthly cost of HIV care is significant, adding significantly to the cost of illness. The patient should be informed that there are compassionate-use drug programs that have been put in place to offer assistance with the economic realities of care (Table 25–5).

The health care provider must be clear when teaching patients about their drug regimen. Some drugs must be taken on an empty stomach, others must be taken with water, while some drugs are to be mixed with juice, milk, or formulas (e.g., Ensure, Advera). For example, patients with achlorhydria require an acidic beverage when taking their drug delavirdine for maximum benefit. In contrast, patients using the powdered formulation of didanosine should be advised to mix the powder with water (not fruit juice or acid-containing beverages). Some drugs, such as retonavir, may be mixed with chocolate milk, Ensure, or Advera to improve the taste. The patient should be instructed on the proper storage of the drugs. Some drugs (e.g., indinavir) are sensitive to moisture; others need to be stored in the refrigerator; while some may be kept at room temperature.

The health care provider should instruct the patient to call promptly if evidence of adverse effects appear. Some of the drugs may cause drowsiness and blurred vision (e.g., didanosine); thus the patient should be cautioned to avoid driving or other activities that require alertness until the response to the drugs is known. Frequent oral rinses, sugarless gum or candy, and good oral hygiene may help relieve the dry mouth associated with some of the drugs. If dry mouth persists longer than 2 weeks, advise the patient to contact the health care provider or dentist regarding use of saliva substitutes. Adequate fluid intake, at least 1 to 2 L of water, should be taken to reduce the risk of adverse effects (e.g., kidney stones with lamivudine). Similarly, the health care provider should be sure the patient understands which drugs should be taken with meals and which should be taken on an empty stomach. It is often necessary to use a drug box that will conveniently organize the days or weeks

TABLE 25–5 EXAMPLES OF COST FOR MULTIDRUG THERAPY

Drug	Dosage	Monthly Cost	Compassionate Assistance
Protease Inhibitors			
Indinavir	Two, 400-mg capsules q8hr	$2/capsule × 6 capsules/day = $360/mo	Merck and Company, Inc. 800-850-3430
Nelfinavir	Three, 250-mg tablets q8hr	$2/tablet × 9 tablets/day = $540/mo	Agouran Pharmaceuticals 619-622-3000
Retonavir	Six, 100-mg capsules q12hr	$2/capsule × 12 capsules/day = $720/mo	Abbott Pharmaceuticals 800-659-9050
Saquinavir	Three, 200-mg capsules q8hr	$2/capsule × 9 capsules/day = $540/mo	Roche Laboratories 800-282-7780
Nucleoside Reverse Transcriptase Inhibitors			
Didanosine	One, 150-mg tablet q12hr 1, One, 100-mg tablet q12hr	$3/150 mg capsule × 2 capsules/day = $180 $2/100 mg capsule × 2 capsules/day = $120 → $300/mo	Bristol Myers 800-272-4878
Lamivudine	One, 150-mg tablet q12hr	$4/tablet × 2 tablets/day = $240/mo	Glaxo-Wellcome 800-722-9294
Stavudine	One, 20-mg tablet q12hr	$4/tablet × 2 tablets/day = $240/mo	Bristol Myers 800-272-4878
Zalcitabine	One, 750-mg tablet q12hr	$2/tablet × 2 tablets/day = $120/mo	Roche Labs 800-282-7780
Zidovudine	One, 100-mg tablet q4hr	$2/tablet × 6 tablets/day = $360/mo	Glaxo-Wellcome 800-722-9294

Controversy

Ethical Challenges in HIV Treatment of the Homeless
MAUREEN MCDONALD

The standard of care for HIV-infected patients has become combination antiretroviral therapy using a protease inhibitor. The cost of these drugs often approaches $12,000 to $15,000 per year. New therapeutic advances raise many ethical challenges, including questions related to equal access to medical care, limits of patient autonomy, medical paternalism, and threats to public health caused by poor drug compliance.

Controversy exists over whether the new drugs should be made available to homeless patients, who make up a substantial subset of the urban poor. There are reasons for caution in prescribing protease inhibitors for the homeless. These drugs require specific regimens for storage and administration. Combination therapy with protease inhibitors must be timed around meals. Some drugs are taken with meals and others on an empty stomach. Ritonavir needs to be refrigerated. And patients must continually be monitored for adverse effects as well as undergo frequent blood testing. Adherence to treatment is thought to be poor enough in this patient group to disrupt the effectiveness of therapy. Noncompliance is known to lead to the development of drug resistance in viruses. Additionally, the cost of protease inhibitors may well be spent in other interventions that have the potential for greater success.

The homeless population has an HIV infection rate of 8 to 20 percent. The prevalence of mental illness, alcoholism, and drug abuse also is high in this group of patients. Prior to the initiation of combination drug therapy for HIV infection, patients should be stabilized with respect to housing, contact with the health care system, chemical dependency, and mental illness. Patients can then be informed of the risks and benefits of treatments. Physicians, nurses, social workers, dietitians, and others involved as caregivers for these patients should work as a team to facilitate holistic treatment.

Access to therapy should never be based on broad social characteristics such as mental illness, homelessness, or drug use. However, these conditions should trigger a careful, individualized assessment of the ability of individual patients to comply with treatment regimens. Remediation of social conditions that undermine a patient's capacity for compliance should be the initial step in treatment. Provision of housing may do more to increase life expectancy than initiation of drug therapy.

Critical Thinking Discussion

- What issues of social justice exist concerning the availability of combination antiretroviral drug therapy?
- Should requirements for supervised administration of HIV treatment regimens exist for populations of patients that may be noncompliant?
- Can our society choose to restrict successful therapies to select groups of patients? On an economic basis? On a public health basis?

medications as to administration time. Also inform the patient to contact the health care provider if they are taking oral contraceptives. An alternative, nonhormonal method of birth control may be required.

Avoidance of temperature extremes may also be necessary when taking some drugs. The patient should be advised to change position slowly to minimize orthostatic hypotension that is associated with some antiretroviral drugs. Additionally, if diarrhea occurs secondary to drug therapy, it can usually be controlled with OTC drugs (e.g., loperamide), but the patient should first contact the health care provider before instituting antidiarrheal therapy.

Patients should be cautioned to avoid crowds and people with known infections. They should use a soft toothbrush, exercise caution when using toothpicks or dental floss, and have dental work performed before therapy, when possible. The importance of regular follow-up examinations and laboratory testing to determine progress and to monitor for adverse effects should be emphasized (see Controversy—Ethical Challenges in HIV Treatment of the Homeless).

Evaluation

The goal of therapy in treating HIV infection is to control viral replication. This preserves the immunocompetence of the patient and prevents the emergence of viral resistance. It also sustains the effectiveness of the combination regimen. The effectiveness of drug therapy can be demonstrated by decreasing viral load values, increasing CD4 counts, and general improvement of health status. Benefits of therapy for specific populations of patients and in various settings can be measured by population-based morbidity and mortality data. AIDS research is a dynamic field, and information about care and treatment advances may be obtained from a variety of resources.

FUNGAL INFECTIONS

Epidemiology and Etiology

Few fungi are capable of causing disease in humans but, when present, can range from mild, superficial infections to life-threatening systemic infections. Systemic fungal infections occur much less frequently than superficial infections but are significantly more dangerous. Systemic, opportunistic mycoses have become more common, largely because of AIDS, the use of immunosuppressant drugs to treat cancer patients and organ transplant recipients, the use of indwelling IV catheters for prolonged IV therapy or parenteral nutrition, more frequent implantation of prosthetic devices, burns, and wide spread use of broad-spectrum antibiotics.

Immunocompromised patients such as newborns and those with malignancies, leukemia, or an HIV infection are at most risk for fungal infections. Further, conditions such as pregnancy, diabetes mellitus, and the use of oral contraceptives increase the glycogen content of vaginal secretions, predisposing the patient to a fungal infection.

Pathophysiology

Fungi are free-living, highly organized cells containing a nucleus bounded by a nuclear membrane. Fungi have a rigid cell wall and contain a spore stage somewhere in their life cycle. They occur naturally in soil, water, air, and on plants. Fungi can be separated into two groups, yeasts and molds. Dimorphic fungi are capable of growing as yeasts at one temperature and as molds at another temperature.

As dimorphic organisms, fungi exhibit two different growth phases, forming typical mycelial colonies on laboratory culture media but forming small, yeastlike structures in the tissues. The oval-shaped, single-celled yeast organism reproduces by *budding*. The buds separate from the parent cell and mature into identical daughter cells. Mold reproduction, on the other hand, involves a three-step process. In the first stage, a spore produces branches called *hyphae*. As the hyphae grow and mass together, they are called *mycelium*. Mycelia break away from the parent structure to become a free-standing mold. The spore form most readily spreads infection and is commonly identified with asymptomatic colonization of the tissues. The mycelium form seems to be associated with symptomatic infections.

Similar to the bacterial pathogens of humans, fungi can produce disease only if they can grow at the temperature of the infected body site. For example, a number of fungal pathogens called *dermatophytes* are incapable of growing at core body temperature. The infection is limited to the cooler cutaneous surfaces. Diseases caused by dermatophytes are referred to as *superficial mycoses*. Superficial mycoses include *tinea pedis* (a chronic, superficial fungal infection of the skin of the foot), *tinea corporis* (ringworm, skin areas excluding scalp, face, hands, groin, and feet), *tinea cruris* (groin, commonly known as jock itch), *tinea manus* (hand), *tinea capitis* (a fungal infection of the scalp), and *tinea unguium* (or onychomycosis, nails).

Dimorphic organisms include a number of human pathogens, such as the agents of aspergillosis, cryptococcosis, histoplasmosis, and coccidioidomycosis (i.e., San Joaquin fever, desert fever, desert rheumatism). Patients with HIV are at high risk for these infections. Aspergillosis is characterized by inflammatory, granulomatous lesions in the skin, ear, orbit, nasal sinuses, and sometimes the bones and meninges. A tumor-like granulomatous mass may form in the bronchus or pulmonary cavity. The organism may also disseminate to the brain, heart, and kidneys.

Cryptococcosis most often causes a respiratory infection that resembles pneumonia or tuberculosis. Other organs may be involved, however, including the bones, liver, spleen, kidneys, and especially subcutaneous tissues. Cutaneous cryptococcosis is characterized by pustules, ulcerations, and abscesses. The organism can be isolated from old pigeon nests and pigeon droppings.

Histoplasmosis is endemic in many parts of the world. Most infections are asymptomatic or produce minimal symptoms, and thus treatment is not sought. Clinically evident symptoms include those of an acute, influenza-like respiratory infection. The disease occasionally occurs as a rapidly fatal infection involving the liver, spleen, and other organs. Healed lung lesions may calcify and be confused with the lesions of tuberculosis. The fungus causing histoplasmosis is found in the soil and organic debris, especially around chicken houses, bird roosts, and caves inhabited by bats.

Coccidioidomycosis usually occurs as an acute, self-limiting respiratory infection but may occur as a chronic, diffusion disease involving almost any body part. The fungus causing this infection grows in hot, dry areas, especially in the southwestern United States, Mexico, and in parts of Central and South America. The disease occurs in a primary and a secondary form. The primary form is due to inhalation of windborne spores. It varies in severity from that of the common cold to symptoms resembling influenza. The secondary form is virulent and severe. It is a progressive, granulomatous disease that results in involvement of cutaneous and subcutaneous tissues, viscera, CNS, and lungs.

Systemic fungal infections, by definition, are caused by organisms capable of growth at core body temperature that lead to serious infections of deep tissues. Two factors normally keep fungi from colonizing in deep tissues: an intact immune system and competition for nutrients provided by normal bacterial flora. However, alterations in either of these components by disease states or antibiotic therapy can upset the balance, permitting fungal overgrowth and setting the stage for opportunistic infections.

PHARMACOTHERAPEUTIC OPTIONS

There are four main classes of antifungal drugs: the polyene macrolides, the antifungal azoles, the allylamines, and a nuclear acid synthesis inhibitor. In addition, there are two other miscellaneous drugs, griseofulvin and amolorfine (see General Classifications of Antifungal Drugs). These drugs can be applied in systemic or topical regimens, as indicated by the level of infection.

Systemic Antifungal Drugs

❒ Amphotericin B (FUNGIZONE, ABELCET)
❒ Ketoconazole (NIZORAL)
❒ Itraconazole (SPORANOX)
❒ Fluconazole (DIFLUCAN)
❒ Miconazole (MONISTAT IV)
❒ 5-Flucytosine (ANCOBON, 5-FC)

GENERAL CLASSIFICATIONS OF ANTIFUNGAL DRUGS

Polyene Macrolides
- Amphotericin B
- Nystatin
- Natamycin

Azoles
Imidazoles
- Butaconazole
- Clotrimazole
- Econazole
- Ketoconazole
- Terconazole
- Tioconazole

Triazoles
- Fluconazole
- Itraconazole

Allylamines
- Naftifine
- Terbinafine

Nuclear Acid Synthesis Inhibitor
- Flucytosine

Miscellaneous Antifungal Drugs
- Amorolfine
- Griseofulvin

Indications

Amphotericin B is a broad-spectrum antifungal drug available for systemic and topical use. Amphotericin B is the drug of choice for most systemic mycoses. Before the availability of this drug, systemic fungal infections were usually fatal.

Amphotericin B can used topically in the treatment of cutaneous or mucocutaneous infections caused by *C. albicans*, such as perleche, intertriginous candidiasis, diaper rash, and paronychia. In patients with coexisting intestinal candidiasis, nystatin may be administered orally in conjunction with topical amphotericin B, to prevent the recurrence of candidial infection of the skin and mucous membranes. Amphotericin B has also been used in the treatment of oral candidiasis (thrush). Amphotericin B has also been used as a local irrigant for the treatment of candidial cystitis and vaginitis. In addition, it has been used intrapleurally for the treatment of histoplasmal pleural effusions, and intrabronchially for the treatment of pulmonary aspergillosis. Amphotericin B has been given by nebulization to patients with pulmonary coccidioidomycosis.

Ketoconazole is an oral alternative to amphotericin B for the treatment of disseminated and mucocutaneous candidiasis, chromomycosis (a chronic fungal infection of the skin, producing wartlike nodules or papillomas that may ulcerate), coccidioidomycosis, and histoplasmosis.

Itraconazole is used in the treatment of aspergillosis and also for pulmonary and extrapulmonary blastomycosis, histoplasmosis, and topically for onychomycosis. Because of its broad antifungal spectrum, it has also been used for other systemic fungal infections, including coccidioidomycosis, cryptococcosis (the most common fungus infection of the CNS), and sporotrichosis, and for superficial fungal infections.

Fluconazole is used primarily to treat oropharyngeal and esophageal candidiasis and meningitis caused by *Cryptococcus neoformans* and *Coccidioides immitis*. It is also approved as oral therapy for vaginal candidiasis.

Miconazole is used primarily for the topical treatment of superficial mycoses. In some cases it is also used for the treatment of severe, disseminated pulmonary infections.

5-Flucytosine is used to treat serious infections caused by the *Candida* species and *Cryptococcus neoformans*. However, because resistance is common, 5-flucytosine is almost always used in combination with amphotericin B.

Pharmacodynamics

Systemic antifungal drugs are usually fungistatic in action but in high concentrations may be fungicidal. They exert antifungal activity by binding to ergosterol in the fungal cell membranes (Fig. 25–2). As a result of this binding, the cell membrane is no longer able to function as a selective barrier, and permeability to potassium and other cellular constituents is increased. For a cell to be susceptible to the drug, its cytoplasmic membranes must contain sterols. Since bacterial membranes do not contain sterols, they are not affected.

Amphotericin B, a polyene macrolide, is active against a broad spectrum of fungi as well as some protozoa. Emergence of resistant strains of fungi is rare, although it has been noted with long-term therapy. In all cases of drug resistance, the fungal membranes were lacking ergosterol. Like amphotericin B, ketoconazole is effective for most systemic mycoses. In addition, it is active against the fungi that cause superficial infections (e.g., dermatophytes, *Candida* species). Drug resistance is rare.

Azole antifungal drugs (i.e., imidazoles and triazoles) inhibit fungal ergosterol synthesis in cell membranes. They also interfere with fungal oxidative enzymes (predominately the 14α-demethylase microsomal P_{450} enzyme), resulting in accumulation of 14α-methyl sterols. This interference disrupts the packing of acyl chains of phospholipids, inhibiting fungal growth and interfering with membrane-bound enzyme systems. Triazoles have greater selectivity against fungi than imidazoles. Resistance to azole drugs is rare, but resistant strains of *Candida* have been recovered from AIDS patients who have chronic mucocutaneous candidiasis.

Allylamines (i.e., terbinafine, naftifine) interfere with ergosterol synthesis by inhibiting enzyme systems. Naftifine inhibits the enzyme squalene epoxidase. Terbinafine prevents ergosterol synthesis by inhibiting squalene epoxidase, resulting in accumulation, disruption of the fungal cell membrane, and cell death.

Flucytosine interferes with nucleic acid synthesis by inhibiting the enzyme thymidylate synthesis. It is active in cells that can transport it into the fungal cell via cytosine permease, where it is converted to 5-fluorouracil, an antimetabolite. 5-Fluorouracil then is biotransformed and incorporated into RNA or biotransformed further to a potent thymidylate synthetase inhibitor. As a result, DNA synthesis within the fungal cell is disrupted.

Griseofulvin is thought to interfere with microtubule function or nucleic acid synthesis and polymerization. It inhibits dermatophyte growth but has no effect on the fungi that produce deep mycoses or *Candida*.

Adverse Effects and Contraindications

The most common adverse effects of amphotericin B include headache, nausea, vomiting, diarrhea, fever, and chills. Hypotension, hypokalemia, and nephrotoxicity have also been reported. Nephrotoxicity occurs because amphotericin B is directly cytotoxic to kidney cells. Renal impairment occurs in almost all patients receiving amphotericin B. The extent of kidney damage is related to the total dose administered during the course of therapy. In most cases, renal function returns to within normal limits following discontinuation of the drug. Residual renal impairment is likely with doses that exceed 4 g. Hypokalemia may occur as a result of kidney damage.

Other adverse effects associated with amphotericin B include delirium, hypotension or hypertension, wheezing, and hypoxia. IV infusion of amphotericin B is associated with a high incidence of phlebitis. Bone marrow depression has occurred that resulted in normocytic, normochromic anemia. Although rare, amphotericin B has caused rash, seizures, arrhythmias, acute liver failure, and nephrogenic diabetes insipidus. Hypersensitivity reactions to amphotericin B are the most life-threatening; hence the need for a test dose before administration.

Amphotericin B is contraindicated in patients with hypersensitivity. It should be used with caution in patients with electrolyte abnormalities. Safe use during pregnancy and lactation has not been established.

The most common adverse effects of ketoconazole are nausea and vomiting. Other adverse effects are relatively

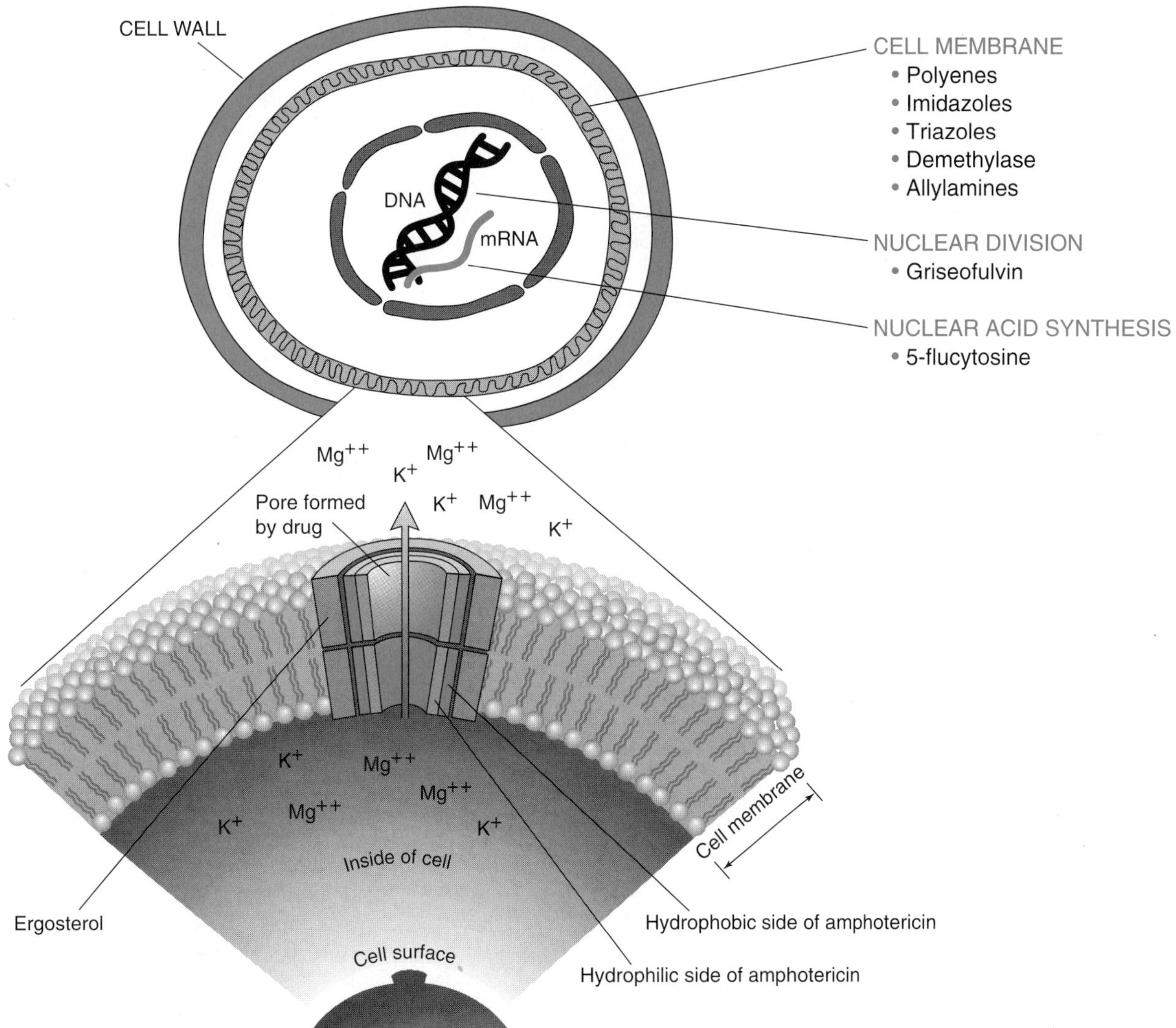

Figure 25–2 Sites and mechanism of antifungal drug action. Polyene macrolides (e.g., amphotericin) bind to membrane ergosterol, imidazoles (e.g., ketoconazole) and triazoles (e.g., fluconazole) inhibit the cytochrome P_{450} enzyme system, and allylamines (e.g., naftifine, terbinafine) prevent ergosterol synthesis. Demethylase blocks the synthesis of ergosterol. Ergosterol binding damages the fungal cell membrane, with subsequent leakage of ions.

mild and include headache, rash, itching, dizziness, fever, chills, constipation, diarrhea, and photophobia. Gynecomastia has been reported. Hepatotoxicity is rare but potentially serious. Fatal hepatic necrosis has occurred.

Ketoconazole is contraindicated in patients with hypersensitivity. It should be used with caution in patients with a history of liver disease, achlorhydria, or hypochlorhydria or in patients who abuse alcohol.

The most common adverse effect of itraconazole is nausea, although many other adverse effects have been reported. Other adverse effects include fatigue, malaise, headache, somnolence, dizziness, tinnitus, and fever. Hypertension, edema, anorexia, flatulence, diarrhea, abdominal pain, a decreased libido, and impotence have been noted. Rhabdomyolysis, hypokalemia, adrenal insufficiency, toxic epidermal necrolysis, and albuminuria are reported.

Itraconazole is contraindicated in patients with hypersensitivity or who are lactating. Cross sensitivity with other azole antifungals (i.e., miconazole, ketoconazole) may occur. It should be used with caution in patients with hepatic impairment and in patients with achlorhydria or hypochlorhydria. Safe use during pregnancy and lactation has not been established.

The most common adverse effects of IV miconazole are phlebitis and pruritus. Other adverse effects include drowsiness, dizziness, anxiety, headache, blurred vision, dry eyes, nausea, vomiting, diarrhea, a bitter taste in the mouth, anemia, and hyponatremia. The drug is contraindicated in patients with hypersensitivity to the drug or hypersensitivity to castor oil or parabens.

The most common adverse effects of 5-flucytosine include nausea, vomiting, diarrhea, leukopenia, and pancytopenia. Other adverse effects of 5-flucytosine that have been reported include dizziness, drowsiness, confusion, photosensitivity, anemia, and thrombocytopenia.

Pharmacokinetics

The absorption of amphotericin B from the GI tract is poor, but the drug is 100 percent bioavailable following IV administration (Table 25–6). It is distributed to sterol-containing membranes of various body tissues but has poor penetration into CSF. Levels about half those noted in plasma are achieved in aqueous humor and in peritoneal, pleural, and joint fluids. Elimination of the drug is very prolonged, being detectable in the urine up to 7 weeks after the drug is discontinued.

The absorption of ketoconazole from the GI tract is pH dependent. Increasing the pH of the stomach decreases absorption. It is widely distributed, although penetration of the CNS is unpredictable and minimal. The drug crosses placental membranes and is found in breast milk. Ketoconazole is partially biotransformed by the liver and eliminated in the feces.

Absorption of itraconazole is enhanced in the presence of food. Tissue concentrations are higher than plasma concentrations. The drug does not enter CSF but has been noted in breast milk. Itraconazole is biotransformed by the liver and eliminated in the feces. Hydroxyitraconazole, the major metabolite, has antifungal activity.

Miconazole is poorly absorbed following oral administration. It is widely distributed following IV administration, although penetration of CSF is poor. Intrathecal administration would be needed in the treatment of meningitis. Miconazole is mostly biotransformed by the liver.

5-Flucytosine is well absorbed from the GI tract following oral administration. It is widely distributed, crossing the blood-brain barrier and the placental membranes. The majority of the drug (80 to 90 percent) is eliminated unchanged in the urine.

Drug-Drug Interactions

Drug-drug interactions with amphotericin B include those that increase the risk of nephrotoxicity (Table 25–7). Drugs likely to increase the risk of nephrotoxicity include aminoglycosides and cyclosporine. Diuretics, glucocorticoids, mezlocillin, piperacillin, and ticarcillin may potentiate hypokalemia.

There are many drug-drug interactions with ketoconazole. Drugs that increase gastric pH may decrease the absorption of ketoconazole. Additive hepatotoxicity is possible with other hepatotoxic drugs, including alcohol. Serious arrhythmias have occurred with the concurrent use of astemizole or cisapride.

Like other systemic antifungal drugs, itraconazole has many drug-drug interactions. Used concurrently with astemizole or cisapride, there is an increased risk of ventricular arrhythmias and torsades de pointes.

Drug-drug interactions with IV miconazole include enhanced anticoagulant activity in the presence of warfarin. Concurrent use of rifampin or isoniazid decreases blood levels and effectiveness of miconazole.

Drug-drug interactions with 5-flucytosine include antineoplastic drugs, radiation therapy, amphotericin B, and cytarabine. Additive bone marrow depression occurs with other bone marrow depressant drugs, such as antineoplastics, amphotericin B, cytarabine, and radiation therapy. Amphotericin B may increase toxicity to 5-flucytosine but may also increase its antifungal activity. Cytarabine may decrease antifungal activity.

Dosage Regimen

Table 25–8 contains dosage regimens for selected antifungal drugs. The dosage of systemic amphotericin B is individualized based on the severity of the patient's infection. An optimal dosage has not been established. A test dose of 1 mg is given IV followed by an initial dose of 0.25 mg/kg. The dosage is increased daily to 0.5 mg/kg. In some cases, 1 mg/kg/day is given or 1.5 mg/kg every other day. Systemic treatment is prolonged; 6 to 8 weeks is common. In some cases treatment may last for 3 or 4 months. Kidney damage

TABLE 25–6 PHARMACOKINETICS OF SELECTED ANTIFUNGAL DRUGS

Drug	Route	Onset	Peak	Duration	PB (%)	$t_{1/2}$	BioA (%)
Selected Systemic Antifungal Drugs							
Amphotericin B	IV	Rapid	End of inf	20–24 hr	90–95	24–48 hr; 15 days*	100
Fluconazole	po	Slow	1–2 hr	2–4 days	11–12	20–50 hr	90
	IV	Immediate	1 hr	2–4 days	11–12	20–50 hr	100
Flucytosine	po	Rapid	2 hr	UK	2–4	2.5–6 hr	80
Griseofulvin	po	4 hr	4–8 hr	2 days	UA	9–24 hr	UA
Itraconazole	po	Rapid	1.5–5 hr	12–24 hr	99	21–64 hr	55
Ketoconazole	po	Rapid	1–4 hr	24 hr	99	8 hr	75
Miconazole	IV	Rapid	End of inf	8 hr	90	0.4, 2.1, 24 hr†	50
Selected Topical Antifungal Drugs							
Butoconazole	Vaginal cream	Rapid	UK	24 hr	NA	21–24 hr	NA
Ciclopirox	Topical	1 wk	UK	12 hr	NA	1.7 hr	NA
Clotrimazole	Vaginal cream/tablets	Rapid	UK	24 hr	NA	NA	NA
Miconazole	Vaginal cream/suppositories	Slow	6 days	8 hr	NA	21–24 hr	NA
Naftifine	Topical	7 days	UA	UA	UA	2–3 days	NA
Nystatin	Vaginal tablets	Rapid	UK	6–12 hr	NA	NA	NA
Terconazole	Vaginal cream	3 days	6.6 hr	24 hr	NA	4–11 hr	NA
Tioconazole	Vaginal ointment	Rapid	UK	24 hr	NA	20–25 hr	NA
Triacetin	Topical	1 wk	UK	8–12 hr	NA	NA	NA

*The half-life of amphotericin B is biphasic, with the initial phase lasting 24 to 48 hours and the terminal phase 15 days.
†Plasma concentrations of miconazole decline triphasically with sequential biologic half-lives.
BioA, bioavailability; PB, protein binding; $t_{1/2}$, elimination half-life; NA, not applicable; UA, unavailable; UK, unknown.

TABLE 25–7 DRUG-DRUG INTERACTIONS OF SELECTED ANTIFUNGAL DRUGS

Drug	Interactive Drug	Interaction
Amphotericin B	Aminoglycosides	Increase risk of renal toxicity
	Capreomycin	
	Colistin	
	Cisplatin	
	Cyclosporine	
	Furosemide	
	Methoxyflurane	
	Pentamidine	
	Polymyxin B	
	Vancomycin	
	Corticosteroids	Sodium retention, potassium depletion
	Tubocurarine	Enhances effects of muscle relaxants
	Digitalis	Increases risk of digitalis toxicity with hypokalemia
	Flucytosine	Synergistic effect with greater toxicity of flucytosine
	Antineoplastic agents	Increase renal toxicity, bronchospasm, hypotension
	Diuretics	May potentiate hypokalemia
	Corticosteroids	
	Mezlocillin	
	Piperacillin	
	Ticarcillin	
	Norfloxacin	Possible enhancement of antifungal activity
Fluconazole	Coumarin	Increases prothrombin times
	Cyclosporine	Increases cyclosporine concentrations in renal transplant recipients
	Astemizole	Cardiac arrhythmias
	Phenytoin	Increases phenytoin levels
	Rifampin	Decreases plasma levels of fluconazole
	Tolbutamide	Hypoglycemia. Increase plasma concentrations of antidiabetic agents
	Glyburide	
	Glipizide	
	Thiazide diuretics	Increase fluconazole plasma concentrations
Flucytosine	Amphotericin B	Synergistic effect. Increases toxicity of flucytosine
	Norfloxacin	Enhances antifungal activity of antifungal agents
	Cytarabine	Antagonizes antifungal activity of flucytosine
Griseofulvin	Alcohol	May cause flushing and tachycardia
	Barbiturates	May decrease activity of griseofulvin
	Oral anticoagulants	May decrease hypoprothrombinemic effects of oral anticoagulants
	Oral contraceptives	May decrease efficacy of oral contraceptives
Ketoconazole	Alcohol	Sunburnlike reaction may occur. Increased risk for hepatotoxicity
	Astemizole	Increase risk of serious arrhythmias due to increased plasma concentrations of interactive drug
	Cisapride	
	Triazolam	Increases peak and prolonged half-life of triazolam
	Sulfonylureas	Severe hypoglycemia
	Antacids	Increase gastric pH and decrease absorption of ketoconazole
	Antimuscarinics	
	Didanosine	
	Histamine-2 antagonists	
	Lansoprazole	
	Omeprazole	
	Alcohol	Concurrent administration may cause severe liver disease
	Hepatotoxic drugs	
	Isoniazid	May decrease serum levels of ketoconazole
	Rifampin	
	Warfarin	Enhances activity of interactive drug
	Cyclosporin	May increase blood levels and toxicity of interactive drug
	Glucocorticoids	
	Phenytoin	Alters the biotransformation of interactive drug
	Theophylline	May decrease serum levels and effectiveness of interactive drug
Itraconazole	Midazolam	Prolonged sedation may occur
	Triazolam	
	Antacids	Absorption may be decreased
	Histamine-2 antagonists	
	Drugs that increase gastric pH	
	Cardiac glycosides	Increases risk of glycoside toxicity in presence of hypokalemia

Table continued on following page

TABLE 25–7 DRUG-DRUG INTERACTIONS OF SELECTED ANTIFUNGAL DRUGS *Continued*

Drug	Interactive Drug	Interaction
	Astemizole Cisapride	May increase risk of serious arrhythmias
	Carbamazepine Isoniazid Phenytoin Phenobarbital Rifampin	Increase biotransformation of itraconazole
	Cyclosporine Phenytoin Tacrolimus Oral hypoglycemic drugs Warfarin	Decrease biotransformation of and increase effects of interactive drug
Miconazole	Warfarin	Enhances anticoagulation effects
	Isoniazid Rifampin	Decrease blood levels and effectiveness of miconazole
Flucytosine	Antineoplastic drugs Radiation therapy	Additive bone marrow depression
	Amphotericin B	May increase toxicity but also increase antifungal activity of flucytosine
	Cytarabine	Decreases antifungal activity
Griseofulvin	Alcohol	CNS depression, tachycardia, flushing
	Oral contraceptives Phenobarbital Warfarin	Decrease blood levels of oral contraceptives
Clioquinol	Antimalarials Iodides	May produce cross sensitivity to other hydroxyquinoline and quinoline derivatives

can be minimized by infusing 1 L of normal saline on the day of amphotericin B administration.

IV infusion of amphotericin B frequently produces headache, fever, chills, rigors, and nausea. Mild reactions can be minimized by pretreating the patient with diphenhydramine and aspirin or acetaminophen. Meperidine can be given if rigors occur. Hydrocortisone can be used to decrease fever and chills if other measures fail.

Ketoconazole should be administered with meals or snacks to minimize nausea and vomiting. It should not be administered within 2 hours of taking an OTC drug, histamine-2 antagonist, or antacid.

Miconazole is administered IV as well as by bladder instillation. A continuous bladder irrigation for mycoses can be used concurrently with IV administration.

5-Flucytosine is administered by mouth in both adults and children. To reduce the likelihood of nausea and vomiting, administer capsules a few at a time over a 15-minute period.

Laboratory Considerations

CBC, platelets, BUN, and creatinine should be measured every other day while increasing dose, and then twice weekly. Biweekly potassium and magnesium levels should be done. If the BUN exceeds 40 mg/mL or the serum creatinine exceeds 3 mg/100 mL, the dosage of amphotericin B should be decreased or discontinued until renal function improves. Amphotericin B may cause decreased hemoglobin, hematocrit, and magnesium levels.

Liver function tests should be monitored in the patient taking ketoconazole or itraconazole prior to and monthly for 3 to 4 months, and then periodically throughout therapy. Ketoconazole may increase the AST (SGOT), ALT (SGPT), alkaline phosphatase, and bilirubin concentrations. The drug should be discontinued if even minor abnormalities occur.

Hematocrit, hemoglobin, and serum electrolytes should be monitored periodically throughout IV therapy. IV miconazole may cause abnormalities in tests of serum lipid concentrations.

Adverse effects of 5-flucytosine are more common with serum levels that exceed 100 mcg/mL. Thus, serum levels should be monitored throughout therapy. Hematologic function should also be regularly measured. Because 5-flucytosine is administered concurrently with amphotericin B in many cases, it is important to monitor renal function.

Topical Antifungal Drugs

❒ Amphotericin B (FUNGIZONE)
❒ Amorolfine
❒ Butoconazole (FEMSTAT)
❒ Clotrimazole (GYNE-LOTRIMIN, FEM CARE, FEMIZOLE-7, MYCELEX G, MYCELEX-7, MYCELEX TWIN PAK); (🍁) CANESTEN, CLOTRIMADERM
❒ Carbol-fuchsin (CASTELLANI'S PAINT)
❒ Ciclopirox (LOPROX)
❒ Clioquinol (VIOFORM)
❒ Clotrimazole (LOTRIMIN, LOTRIMIN AF, MYCELEX, MYCELEX OTC); (🍁) CANESTEN, CLOTRIMADERM, MYCLO, NEO-ZOL
❒ Econazole (SPECTAZOLE)
❒ Haloprogin (HALOTEX)
❒ Ketoconazole (NIZORAL)
❒ Miconazole (MICATIN, MONISTAT-DERM, PRESCRIPTION STRENGTH DESENEX, ZEASORB-AF, MICONAZOLE-7, MONISTAT-3, MONISTAT-7)
❒ Naftifine (NAFTIN)
❒ Nystatin (MYCOSTATIN, NILSTAT, NYSTEX); Nadostine, Nyaderm
❒ Oxiconazole (OXISTAT)

TABLE 25–8 DOSAGE REGIMEN FOR SELECTED ANTIFUNGAL DRUGS

Drug	Use(s)	Dosage	Implications
Selected Systemic Antifungal Drugs			
Amphotericin B	Systemic mycoses	*Adult:* 0.25 mg/kg IV. Increase daily doses slowly to 0.5 mg/kg. Can give up to 1 mg/kg/day *or* 1.5 mg/kg/every other day *Child:* 0.25 mg/kg. Increase by 0.25 mg/kg every other day to maximum of 1 mg/kg/day	Fungicidal. Give a test dose before giving drug. Monitor patient closely after test dose and during first 1–2 hours of each infusion. Monitor BP and pulse q15 min. Adequate hydration may minimize nephrotoxicity
	Cutaneous and mucocutaneous candidial infections	*Topical:* Apply 3% lotion, cream, or ointment to affected areas 2–4 times/day. Duration of therapy may be 1–3 weeks	Avoid use of occlusive dressings and ointment formulations. Nail infections may require several months of therapy or longer
	Candidial cystitis	Continuous bladder irrigation of 50 μg/mL *or* 5–50 mg in 1000 mL NS	Some health care providers may use concentrations of 5–10 μg/mL
	Histoplasmal pulmonary effusions	*Adult:* 15–20 mg with 25 mg of hydrocortisone sodium succinate given intrapleural	Addition of steroid reduces inflammation
	Ophthalmic candidial infections	*Adult:* One drop to affected eye q30 min	If no improvement within 24–48 hours, repeat injection will not be beneficial
Flucytosine	Mycoses caused by *Candida* species and *Cryptococcus neoformans*	*Adult:* 12.5–37.5 mg/kg po q6hr *Child:* 12.5–37.5 mg/kg po q6hr *or* 375–562.5 mg/m^2 q6hr	This dosage may require 10 or more capsules/dose. Nausea and vomiting can be reduced by taking drug over 15-minute period
Ketoconazole	Mucocutaneous and disseminated candidiasis, coccidioidomycosis, histoplasmosis	*Adult:* 200–400 mg po as single daily dose *Child older than 2 yr:* 3.3–6.6 mg/kg/day as single dose	Administer with meals or snacks to minimize nausea and vomiting. Do not administer histamine-2 antagonists within 2 hr of ketoconazole
Itraconazole	Blastomyces, histoplasmosis	*Adult:* 200 mg po QD. May be increased by 100 mg/day up to 200 mg po BID	Administer with meal or snack to minimize nausea and vomiting and to increase absorption. Do not give with antacids or other drugs that increase gastric pH
	Aspergillosis	*Adult:* 200 mg po QD-BID for a minimum of 3 months	
	Onychomycosis	*Adult:* 200 mg/day for 3–6 mo	
Fluconazole	Oropharyngeal candidiasis	*Adult:* 200 mg po initially, then 100 mg daily for at least 2 weeks	Because bioavailability of oral and IV formulations is similar, doses are equal. Infuse IV at maximum rate of 200 mg/hr
	Esophageal candidiasis	*Adult:* 200 mg po/IV initially then 100 mg QD for at least 3 wks *or* 2 wks following improvement in symptoms	
	Other candidiasis	*Adult:* 50–400 mg/day IV	
	Vaginal candidiasis	*Adult:* 150 mg po as single dose	
Griseofulvin	Tinea pedis, onychomycosis	*Adult:* 500 mg microsize tabs po q12hr *or* 250–375 mg ultramicrosize tabs po q12hr *Child weighing more than 23 kg:* 125–250 mg microsize tabs po q12hr *or* 250–500 mg microsize tabs po QD *or* 62.5–165 mg ultramicrosize tabs po q12hr or 125–330 mg ultramicrosize tabs po QD *Child weighing more than 14–23 kg:* 62.5–125 mg microsize tabs po q12hr *or* 250 mg microsize tabs po QD *or* 31.25–82.5 mg ultramicrosize tabs po q12 hr *or* 62.5–165 mg ultramicrosize tabs po QD	Concurrent use of topical drug is usually required. Ultramicrosize 250–330 mg formulation provides serum concentration equal to that of microsize 500 mg formulation of griseofulvin. Administer with or after high-fat meals to minimize GI irritation and increase absorption. Advise females to use supplemental form of birth control while using this drug and until next menstrual period. Notify health care provider if pregnancy is suspected. Advise patient to avoid alcohol

Table continued on following page

TABLE 25–8 DOSAGE REGIMEN FOR SELECTED ANTIFUNGAL DRUGS *Continued*

Drug	Use(s)	Dosage	Implications
Selected Systemic Antifungal Drugs *Continued*			
Miconazole	Disseminated pulmonary fungal infections	*Adult:* 200–3600 mg/day IV in divided doses q8hr *Child age 1–12 yr:* 20–40 mg/kg/day in divided doses q8hr. Not to exceed 15 mg/kg/dose	Monitor IV site closely for phlebitis. Administer over 30–60 minutes at rate of 100 mg/hr. Nausea and vomiting may be reduced by slowing the rate, avoiding administration at meal time, or administering antiemetic or antihistamine prior to infusion
	Bladder mycoses	*Adult:* 200 mg q6–12hr by continuous bladder irrigation	Bladder irrigation may be used concurrently with IV administration for bladder mycoses
Selected Topical Antifungal Drugs			
5% Amorolfine nail lacquer	Onychomycosis	*Adult:* Apply to affected fingernails or toenails once *or* twice weekly	Nails should be cleaned and filed down before application. Allow lacquer to dry for 3 minutes
0.25% Amorolfine	Tinea pedis	*Adult:* Apply to affected skin area once daily in evening for 2–3 weeks	Feet should be clean and dry before application
Butoconazole	Vulvovaginal candidiasis	*Nonpregnant adult:* One applicator intravaginally qHS × 3 days *Pregnant patients:* One applicator intravaginally qHS × 6 days	Therapy with butoconazole should be continued during menstruation. Pregnant women should insert the vaginal applicator gently. If there is resistance the woman should contact her physician
1% Ciclopirox	Tinea pedis, tinea cruris, tinea corporis, tinea versicolor, cutaneous candidiasis	*Adult and child:* Rub sufficient amount of topical cream *or* lotion to affected area of skin twice daily in the morning and evening for two to four weeks	Occlusive dressings should not be used. Adult incontinent diapers are an occlusive dressing and should not be used with therapy. Advise patient that shoes and socks should be changed at least once daily
3% Clioquinol	Tinea pedis, tinea cruris	*Adult and child:* Apply to affected area 2–4 times daily for 4 weeks	Cleanse affected area with soap and water before applying drug. Change shoes and socks daily
Clotrimazole	Superficial mycoses	*Adult:* Apply to affected areas (1%) twice daily	Occlusive dressings should not be applied
	Vulvovaginal infections	*Adult:* One applicator intravaginally qHS × 7–14 days or 2 vaginal tablets nightly for 3 nights *or* 1,500-mg vaginal tablet as a single bedtime dose	Advise patient that sexual partner may experience burning and irritation of penis or urethritis. Advise partner to use condoms
	Oropharyngeal candidiasis	*Adult:* One lozenge (10 mg) 5 times daily *or* every 3 hours for 14 days	Patient's physical and mental condition must enable him or her to dissolve lozenge in the mouth
1% Econazole	Tinea cruris, tinea corporis, tinea pedis, tinea versicolor	*Adult and child:* Apply sufficient cream to cover the affected area once daily	Use for the full prescribed time
	Cutaneous candidiasis	*Adult and child:* Apply to affected area twice daily	If no improvement is noted after recommended treatment, notify primary care provider
Ketoconazole	Tinea corporis, tinea cruris, tinea versicolor, tinea pedis, cutaneous candidiasis	*Adult and child:* Apply to affected areas and surrounding skin once *or* twice daily for two weeks	A treatment of 4–8 weeks is necessary if the cream is used for the treatment of tinea pedis
Miconazole	Tinea pedis, tinea cruris tinea corporis	*Adult and child:* Apply to affected area twice daily	Tinea pedis should be treated for one month to prevent reoccurrence

TABLE 25–8 DOSAGE REGIMEN FOR SELECTED ANTIFUNGAL DRUGS *Continued*

Drug	Use(s)	Dosage	Implications
Selected Topical Antifungal Drugs *Continued*			
Miconazole *(continued)*	Vulvovaginal candidiasis	*Adult:* One 200-mg suppository intravaginally qHS × 3 days *or* 100-mg suppository intravaginally qHS × 7 days	Consult with primary health care provider if condition persists for longer than 7 days
Naftifine	Tinea pedis, tinea cruris, tinea corporis	*Adult and child:* Apply cream to affected area once daily *or* the gel twice daily. May use up to 4 weeks	Warn patient to avoid contact with eyes or mucous membranes
Nystatin	Oropharyngeal candidiasis	*Adult and child:* 1–2 pastilles (200,000–400,000 units) dissolved in mouth 4–5 times daily. Maximum: 14 days. *or* 4–6 mL (100,000 units/mL) QID as swish and swallow *Child:* 2 mL (100,000 units/mL) po QID (1 mL on each side of mouth)	The suspension should be retained in the mouth for as long as possible before swallowing. Patient must allow lozenges to dissolve in their mouth
	Intestinal candidiasis	*Adult:* 1–2 tablets (500,000 units/tab) po TID	Not for systemic mycoses. Continue treatment for at least 48 hours after clinical cure
	Superficial candidial infections	*Adult and child:* Apply to affected area several times daily	Occlusive dressings should be avoided
	Vulvovaginal candidiasis	*Adult:* 1–2 tablets inserted high into vagina once *or* twice daily	Therapy should be continued during menstruation
Oxiconazole	Tinea pedis, tinea cruris, tinea corporis	*Adults:* Apply to affected area once daily in the evening × 2 weeks	Tinea pedis should be treated for 1 month to reduce the possibility of recurrence
Terbinafine	Tinea pedis	*Adult:* Apply to affected area BID × 2 weeks	Improvement may continue for 2–6 weeks after completion of therapy. Not recommended for children
	Tinea cruris, tinea corporis	*Adult:* Apply 1–2 times daily × 1–4 weeks	
Terconazole	Vulvovaginal candidiasis	*Adults:* One applicator (0.8%) cream intravaginally qHS × 3 days *or* 1 suppository (80 mg) intravaginally qHS × 3 days *or* 1 applicator (0.4%) cream intravaginally qHS × 7 days	Inform patient that terconazole may interact with diaphragms and latex condoms. Advise patient to wear cotton underwear. Not recommended for children
1% Tolnaftate	Tinea pedis, tinea corporis, tinea cruris	*Adults:* Apply cream sparingly to affected area and massage in BID × 4 wks. Apply powder in shoes and socks if feet are infected. Maintenance and prophylaxis: Apply powder once daily	Treatment should be continued for 2–3 weeks after symptoms have subsided to prevent reoccurrence
1% Oxiconazole	Tinea pedis, tinea cruris, tinea corporis	*Adult:* Apply to affected area QD *or* BID	Use for 2 weeks for cruris and corporis, 4 weeks for pedis. Reevaluate if no improvement

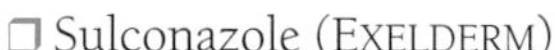

- ❐ Sulconazole (EXELDERM)
- ❐ Terbinafine (LAMISIL)
- ❐ Terconazole (TERAZOL-3, TERAZOL-7)
- ❐ Tioconazole (VAGISTAT); (✽) GYNE-TROSYD
- ❐ Tolnaftate (ABSORBINE ANTIFUNGAL, ABSORBINE JR ANTIFUNGAL, AFTATE, BREEZE MIST AEROSOL, DESENEX SPRAY, GENASPOR, NP 27, QUINSANA PLUS, TINACTIN, TING)
- ❐ Triacetin (FUNGOID, ONY-CLEAR NAIL)
- ❐ Undecylenic acid compound (CALDESENE, CRUEX, DECYLENES, DESENEX CREAM, DESENEX FOAM, DESENEX POWDER, others)

Indications

Topical antifungal drugs are used for a variety of cutaneous fungal infections, including cutaneous candidiasis, tinea pedis, and tinea corporis. Undecylenic acid is used only for tinea infections. Amphotericin B is used only for candidial infections, although newer agents may be more effective. Antifungal drugs used for ophthalmic conditions are discussed in Chapter 62.

Pharmacodynamics

Topical antifungal drugs act in a fashion much like that of systemic antifungal drugs. Clotrimazole, econazole, miconazole, nystatin, and oxiconazole affect the synthesis of ergosterol, an essential component of the fungal cytoplasmic membrane. Leakage of cellular contents results. Undecylenic acid also contains zinc undecylenate, which acts as an astringent. Some drugs, such as triacetin, have antibacterial characteristics.

Adverse Effects and Contraindications

The most common adverse effects of topically administered antifungal drugs include burning, itching, stinging, redness, and local hypersensitivity reactions. Some agents may stain hair, skin, and fabric. Carbol-fuchsin topical solution should not be applied to eroded skin or over extensive areas because contact sensitivity may occur.

Clotrimazole vaginal tablets have produced mild burning occasionally. Rarely reported adverse effects with clotrimazole vaginal tablets include skin rash, vulval irritation, lower abdominal cramps, bloating, slight cramping, dyspareunia, and slight urinary frequency.

Topical gentian violet is usually well tolerated but may cause irritation or sensitivity reactions and ulceration of mucous membranes. Esophagitis, laryngitis, or tracheitis may result from swallowing a solution of gentian violet, and laryngeal obstruction has been reported following frequent and prolonged use of gentian violet in the treatment of oral candidiasis. Tattooing of the skin may occur where gentian violet is applied to granulation tissue. Gentian violet should not be used on ulcerative lesions of the face.

Adverse effects reported in patients receiving topical ketoconazole as a shampoo include increased hair loss, skin irritation, abnormal hair texture, scalp pustules, dry skin, pruritus, and oiliness or dryness of hair and scalp. In some patients with permed hair, loss of curl occurred. Headache, fever, and a flulike syndrome with fever, chills, headache, and hypotension have occurred in patients taking terconazole.

Patients using terconazole for vulvovaginal candidiasis may complain of headache and body pain. Other vaginal adverse effects include irritation, sensitization, and vulvovaginal burning. Vaginal antifungal drugs are contraindicated in persons with hypersensitivity to active ingredients, additives, preservatives, or other components of the formulations. Butoconazole is specifically contraindicated in the first trimester of pregnancy. Safe use of terconazole during lactation has not been established.

Sodium sulfite is contained in some topical preparations (e.g., ketoconazole) and may cause allergic-type reactions, including anaphylaxis and life-threatening or less severe asthmatic episodes in certain susceptible individuals. Sulfite sensitivity tends to occur more frequently in asthmatic individuals. The preservatives ethylenediamine, parabens, and thimerosal that are contained in nystatin have been associated with a high incidence of contact dermatitis.

Topical antifungal drugs are contraindicated in patients who are hypersensitive to the ingredients, additives, preservatives, or bases. Clioquinol contains iodine and should not be used in patients with iodine sensitivity. Topical drugs should be used with caution during pregnancy and lactation and in children. Safe use of ciclopirox, haloprogin, naftifine, terbinafine, and undecylenic acid has not been established in these populations.

Pharmacokinetics

Most topical antifungal drugs are minimally absorbed through the skin or mucous membranes (see Table 25–6). Clioquinol is rapidly and extensively absorbed and may affect thyroid function. The distribution of topical drugs is unknown since the action is primarily localized. Biotransformation of the drugs is not known. Biotransformation and elimination routes are not known.

Antifungal drugs used for vulvovaginal candidiasis, such as nystatin, miconazole, and tioconazole, are minimally absorbed. Five percent of butoconazole is absorbed, 3 to 10 percent of clotrimazole, and 5 to 15 percent of terconazole is absorbed following intravaginal administration. Distribution sites are unknown because drug action is primarily localized to the vaginal tract and perineal areas. The onset of drug action is rapid, with the duration of drug action 24 hours.

Drug-Drug Interactions

There are few drug-drug interactions with topical antifungal drugs. However, if sufficient ketoconazole is absorbed through the skin, it may increase the risk of ventricular arrhythmias when used with astemizole (see Table 25–7). Concurrent cyclosporine use with topical antifungal drugs may contribute to nephrotoxicity. Topical administration of clioquinol may produce cross sensitivity to other hydroxyquinoline and quinoline derivatives, such as certain antimalarials, and occasionally to iodides. There are no known drug-drug interactions with vaginal antifungal drugs.

Dosage Regimen

Dosage regimens of topical antifungal drugs are identified in Table 25–8. Application frequency ranges from once daily to four times daily. Duration of therapy can vary from 1 week to as much as 4 weeks or more.

The dosage regimen for vaginal antifungal drugs varies somewhat with the formulation. In most cases, one applicator of the vaginal creams, tablets, or suppository is used at bedtime for a period of 3 to 7 days. Clotrimazole may also be dosed as two vaginal tablets nightly for three nights, or one 500-mg vaginal tablet as a single bedtime dose. The cream formulation of clotrimazole must be used for 7 to 14 days. Applicators are supplied for vaginal administration. Tioconazole vaginal ointment is administered as a single bedtime dose. Nystatin therapy should be continued for 2 weeks.

Laboratory Considerations

Laboratory confirmation of onychomycosis by microscopy, culture, and histological evaluation of nail clippings and subungual debris is necessary before initiating therapy. Elevated AST (SGOT) concentrations have been reported in patients receiving clotrimazole lozenges. Thus, liver function tests should be conducted periodically during oral therapy, particularly in patients with pre-existing hepatic impairment.

Percutaneously absorbed clioquinol contains iodine, which may interfere with certain thyroid functions tests, such as protein-bound iodine. The manufacturer recommends that at least one month elapse between discontinuance of topical clioquinol therapy and performance of thyroid function tests. Clioquinol may produce false positive results in the ferric chloride test for phenylketonuria when clioquinol is present in urine or on the diaper.

Controversy

Using Topical Antifungal and Antiviral Drugs

JONATHAN J. WOLFE

A central problem to the use of both antifungal and antiviral drugs relates to the nature of infections caused by the pathogens. In both cases, patients may be slow to commence therapy, and then prove reluctant to treat the infections for as long as needed. This problem is particularly true when topical preparations of such drugs are needed.

Fungi are notoriously slow growing. They therefore usually prove difficult to kill, since the most susceptible microorganism is typically one in the process of cell division. This means that the patient must treat fungi for weeks or even months in order to eradicate the problem. Many fungi represent cosmetic defects in the eye of the sufferer. The patient may easily become discouraged and stop treatment in the face of continued disfigurement. It is difficult to promote best drug therapy under such circumstances.

Various topical antifungals have been available for years. Some, such as gentian violet and silver nitrate, are of ancient origin. Topical drugs to treat viral infections, however, are of more recent origin. Canker sores of the nose, lip, and buccal mucosa are both disfiguring and painful. Patients may try inappropriate treatment, like products containing camphor, for a time but usually request more effective drugs to deal with viral infections. It is difficult to refuse such requests. It also proves difficult to prevent patients from sharing topical antivirals with friends who exhibit similar lesions.

Critical Thinking Discussion

- Is drug resistance a serious matter when considering the use of topical antifungal drugs? Justify your answer, based on the history of fungi to exhibit drug resistance.
- One feature of viruses is their incredible variance from one year to the next. Based on the frequent changes encountered in viruses, do they appear to offer a greater or lesser hazard for developing resistance if frequently treated with antiviral drugs?
- What supportive instruction can you offer to the patient discouraged by the persistence of a prominent cold sore on the upper lip?
- One problem with systemic antifungal drugs is liver toxicity. What methods would you employ to encourage a patient suffering from alcoholism who has become discouraged over a persistent and unsightly fungal infection of her toenails?

Critical Thinking Process

Assessment

History of Present Illness

Initial questions to be elicited from a patient with a dermatologic complaint should include when and where the disorder began (see Controversy—Using Topical Antifungal and Antiviral Drugs). Establishing the time of onset helps determine if the problem is acute or chronic or if relapse has occurred. Knowledge about the site of the initial lesion and if there is pruritus may also be helpful. The distribution and development of individual lesions are often characteristic; therefore, information regarding any changes in the lesions should be elicited. Determining if the patient has had any other symptoms helps distinguish systemic from localized problems. Information about what has been done to treat the disorder should be noted because many types of lesions are altered by therapies, some for the better, some for the worse.

The patient should also be asked about the effect of sunlight on the disorder because several disorders may result from photosensitivity. Questions about possible exposure to others with a similar skin condition helps elicit information about contagious illness. Asking patients what they think may be causing the problem may provide some insight into the cause. Often, however, the patient guesses incorrectly.

Other factors to be considered are the patient's profession and home and workplace environments. It is important to understand what the patient comes in contact with and to what extent. For example, does the patient work around chemicals? What is the home environment like? Are there pets, plants, or flowers in the home or workplace? Patient-determined or health care provider-prescribed factors that may have alleviated the condition and the patient's psychologic response to the problem should also be noted.

Ask also about the patient's self-care habits. Determine the frequency with which soaps, lotions, abrasives, and cosmetics are used. Elicit information about drugs that are in current use. HIV-infected patients may have a long list of such drugs.

Past Health History

Patients should be asked if they have had a similar problem in the past. This question may help reveal a recurrent condition. They should also be asked about the presence of other types of skin lesions or rashes and other illnesses they now have or had in the past. The background check helps the health care provider find clues that contribute to the antifungal condition and the patient's response to treatment.

Physical Exam Findings

A differential diagnosis of a superficial fungal disorder is based on one feature—the appearance of the skin lesion. Therefore, inspection and palpation are essential when evaluating skin lesions. Examination should be accomplished by comparing the left side of the body to the right using a good light source.

Lesions should be inspected for the following variables: color, size, shape, margin characteristics, location and distribution (localized or generalized), texture, temperature, and odor. The arrangement (clustered, linear, annular, or dermatomal), whether the lesions are primary or secondary (see also Chapter 64), and if there is evidence of healing should also be noted. Descriptions of the lesions need to be specific, using the metric system for measurement.

Some superficial lesions are moist while others are dry and scaling. They also may appear inflamed or discolored. Skin lesions are likely to be observed in the perineal and intertriginous areas. They are usually moist, inflamed, pruritic areas with vesicles and pustules. Oral lesions appear as white patches that adhere to the buccal mucosa. Vaginal infection causes a cheesy vaginal discharge, burning, and itching. Intestinal infection appears as diarrhea.

Primary lesions develop without any preceding skin changes. In many cases primary lesions are not seen; thus, the health care provider must depend on the patient to describe how the lesion looked when it first appeared. Primary lesions include macules, papules, patches, plaques, nodules, wheals, vesicles, bullae, and pustules. Dermatologic diagnoses rely heavily on these primary lesions.

Secondary lesions result from changes in primary lesions and are influenced by scratching or infection. These changes may be brought about by the patient or the patient's environment and often occur in the epidermal layer of skin. Secondary lesions include scales, crusts, lichenification, keloids, scars, excoriations, atrophy, ulcers, and fissures.

The patient with cryptococcosis, coccidioidomycosis, and histoplasmosis often complains of a cough, fever, malaise, and other pulmonary manifestations.

Diagnostic Testing

Fungal cultures are done to identify the specific type of fungus. Superficial infections can be diagnosed by microscopy and culture of skin scrapings, plucked (not cut) hairs, or nail clippings. Systemic infections are diagnosed by microscopy and culture of blood, spinal fluid, sputum, urine, feces, exudate, pus, and tissue biopsy. Gram's stain or potassium hydroxide (KOH) testing determines the presence of mycelial fragments, arthrospores, and budding yeast cells. The use of a Wood lamp helps determine the presence of a fungus. When used in a darkened room, infected hair will fluoresce a bright yellow-green. Serologic tests are mainly available only in speciality laboratories but help establish the diagnosis of many mycoses.

Skin testing is of limited significance in histoplasmosis and coccidioidomycosis. Positive tests have no diagnostic value in ringworm and *Candida* infections. Skin testing is useful only if a patient has recently visited an endemic area for the first time but may be of value for *Aspergillus* hypersensitivity.

Developmental Considerations

Perinatal Except for vaginal infections secondary to *Candida,* mycotic infections in healthy pregnant women are uncommon. Disseminated candidiasis, cryptococcosis, aspergillosis, and histoplasmosis occur as opportunistic infections in immunocompromised patients. Pregnancy predisposes the women to dissemination of an otherwise acute, self-limited respiratory infection. Vulvovaginal candidiasis is common during pregnancy, as evidenced by the characteristic curdy, white, itchy discharge.

Neither the incidence nor the severity of cryptococcal or histoplasmal infections is known to be affected by pregnancy. In contrast, coccidioidomycosis can be very severe in pregnancy, and disseminated infections usually are fatal if left untreated. Oral candidiasis is common in infants who pass through a birth canal affected with *Candida.* Fetal loss may be as high as 50 percent in instances where the fungus invades the placenta. Infants born to mothers with cryptococcosis are without illness, indicating the absence of placental transfer of the fungus. Data on the effects, if any, of maternal histoplasmosis on the fetus are scarce.

Pediatric Children have an increased risk of systemic toxicity from topically applied drugs for two reasons. First, because of their greater surface area to weight ratio, a given amount of applied drug represents a greater dose (in mg/kg) compared with adults. Second, at least in preterm neonates, the permeability of the skin is increased (see Chapter 7).

Geriatric Physiologic changes of aging affect the skin. Progressive impairment of the peripheral vascular circulation alters the cutaneous response to physical trauma, cold, or infection. In contrast to pediatric patients, the skin of older adults is less permeable to drugs, perhaps because of the altered lipid content and loss of subcutaneous tissue (see Chapter 8). Changes in the CNS modify the perception of itching and pain, and atrophy of the reticuloendothelial system may impair the immune response. Also, emotional factors are certainly important and may prolong or exacerbate a skin disorder.

Psychosocial Considerations

Skin diseases are visible and, therefore, have a profound psychological effect. Visually or physically disabling chronic skin disorders have been associated with chronic unemployment, poor mental health, and even suicide. Further, there are a variety of cultural attitudes toward illness. In light of this, it is best not to assume, based on someone's ethnicity, that a certain idea or belief is held about their illness. Stereotyping inhibits an effective patient-health care provider relationship. It is better to ask patients how they feel about the condition and to individualize care.

Socioeconomic considerations cannot be ignored. Compliance with a treatment plan and return for follow-up care are influenced by social expectations or financial ability to pay for desired drugs and treatments. Further, many topical therapies are expensive and cost is a factor that influences patient compliance with the treatment plan.

At every pharmacy, the cost to the patient is calculated using a specific formula. Usually, a pharmacy charge is added to the result. One large prescription is usually less costly (although not necessarily inexpensive) than the same amount of drug given using refills, since the pharmacy charge is added to each refill. This may be particularly true with inexpensive drugs where the pharmacy charge may be most of the patient cost.

Analysis and Management

Treatment Objectives

Treatment objectives for the patient with a fungal infection include controlling symptoms (e.g., local pain, altered taste, dysphagia, itching, visual lesions), avoiding preventable adverse effects secondary to the use of systemic drugs, and preventing reinfection.

Treatment Options

There are many antifungal drugs and formulations that can be used to manage many skin problems. The decision as to which agents to use includes whether the lesion is dry or moist, pruritic, or inflammatory; whether there is an infectious agent; and the location and spread of the lesion. In general, it is better for the health care provider to be thoroughly familiar with a few dermatologic drugs and treatment methods than to attempt to use a great many. Naturally, the course of some endogenous skin diseases cannot be altered. However, steps can be taken to prevent their occurrence and to minimize their effects.

Drug Variables

Treatment of fungal infections is related to the type and location of fungi and includes both topical and systemic antifungal drugs. The major drugs used for systemic therapy are certain azoles (i.e., ketoconazole, itraconazole, fluconazole) and amphotericin B, 5-flucytosine, and griseofulvin. Topical antifungal drugs most often used include clotrimazole, miconazole, nystatin, and amphotericin B. Each antifungal drug has a distinct spectrum of antifungal activity and specific therapeutic uses. Because of the vast number of drugs available, it would be impossible to discuss them all. Further, not all generic topical drugs are equivalent to their brand name counterparts, either in potency or in the presence of ingredients that may cause further irritation or allergy.

Topical drugs should be used initially for oropharyngeal candidiasis because they are associated with less toxicity and less potential for drug interactions. Clotrimazole is the preferred initial treatment of oropharyngeal candidiasis. It may be better tolerated than nystatin; however, clotrimazole is more expensive than nystatin. Nystatin is equally as effective as clotrimazole but may be less well tolerated. Unfortunately, compliance with either nystatin or clotrimazole may be poor, and this may mandate a change to systemic antifungal therapy such as ketoconazole, fluconazole, or itraconazole.

Public Health Service guidelines currently do not recommend routine primary prophylaxis against mucocutaneous candidiasis in HIV-infected patients. Poor evidence exists to support a recommendation for or against prophylaxis, and there are currently no clinical trials to support or refute this recommendation. However, primary prophylaxis against mucocutaneous candidiasis may be considered in HIV-infected infants and children with severe immunosuppression. Severe immunosuppression is defined by age-adjusted criteria such as a CD4 percentage less than 15 percent and a CD4 count less than 750/mm^3 in children younger than 1 year of age, less than 500/mm^3 in children 1 to 5 years of age, and 200/mm^3 in children 6 years of age or older. If primary prophylaxis is used with these children, oral clotrimazole is preferred, with oral ketoconazole or fluconazole considered as alternatives.

The Centers for Disease Control and Prevention recommend that vulvovaginal candidiasis be treated intravaginally with an imidazole derivative antifungal drug such as clotrimazole. Single-dose regimes may be used for uncomplicated mild or moderate vulvovaginal candidiasis. Severe or complicated vulvovaginal candidiasis require 3- to 7-day regimens. Longer regimens are recommended in pregnant women.

Ketoconazole is the preferred drug for the initial treatment of esophageal candidiasis because it is less expensive than fluconazole. However, it is not as well tolerated and is somewhat less effective than fluconazole. Itraconazole and ketoconazole both given as oral therapy result in similar response rates for both esophageal and oropharyngeal candidiasis. Fluconazole can be used if there is failure to achieve symptomatic improvement after 5 to 7 days of therapy using ketoconazole. It may also be used initially if a drug interaction may be more likely to result in failed therapy with ketoconazole or itraconazole (e.g., rifampin, histamine-2 antagonists, and omeprazole).

The response rate to topical therapy usually decreases with repeated episodes, as evidenced by an increased amount of time needed to achieve symptomatic relief with each new episode as well as a shortening of the symptom-free interval between episodes. In this case, it is useful to change to systemic antifungal therapy. Systemic therapy may be warranted if persistent symptoms are severe enough to warrant the increased expense and potential adverse effects or drug interactions of the systemic drugs. A combination of topical and systemic therapy is not recommended, as it usually does not increase efficacy. There is information to suggest that itraconazole oral solution may be effective in fluconazole-resistant oropharyngeal candidiasis. Patients who do not respond to itraconazole solution should be considered for therapy using amphotericin B.

Management of the patient with a fungal disorder may require monitoring of systemic parameters as well as monitoring of skin lesions. Because the primary effect of most antifungal drugs is to prevent colonization of new organisms, any drug should be used for a minimum of 4 weeks to eradicate the infection. Many fungal infections of the nails begin in the matrix, and cure thus consists of eradication of the organism from that protected site. Treatment can take 6 to 12 months for fingernails and 12 to 24 months for toenails. The success rate, however, is probably less than 60 percent.

Patient Variables

United States Public Health Service states that intermittent or long-term prophylaxis may be considered for patients who have frequent or severe recurrences of candidial infections. Several factors should be considered when initiating therapy, such as the impact of recurrences on the patient's well-being and quality of life, the need for prophylaxis against other fungal infections, the cost of prophylaxis, drug toxicities, and drug interactions. Oral fluconazole is the drug of choice for prophylaxis. Alternative drugs include oral ketoconazole, oral itraconazole, or topical therapy with oral nystatin or oral clotrimazole.

Only nystatin vaginal tablets are recommended for vulvovaginal candidiasis during the first trimester of pregnancy. Amphotericin B is the drug of choice for most systemic fungal infections. Data concerning the use of amphotericin B during the first trimester of pregnancy are scarce. Women with coccidioidomycosis and cryptococcosis have been successfully treated during the second and third trimesters without harm to the fetus. Although the teratogenicity of 5-flucytosine is unknown, the drug has been used in the treatment of disseminated candidiasis and cryptococcosis. Ketoconazole has been useful in the treatment of coccidioidomycosis, candidiasis, and histoplasmosis. However, because the drug is given for extended periods of one or more years, it should not be used in pregnancy without first obtaining appropriate consultation.

The Centers for Disease Control and Prevention (CDCP) states that treating the partner of a woman with vulvovaginal candidiasis is not necessary unless candidial balanitis is present or chronicity is a problem.

Intervention

Administration

Small amounts of the drug should be applied to the affected area. Avoid the use of occlusive dressings unless directed by the health care provider since the dressings increase the absorption of the drug.

Education

The patient and family should be informed that systemic fungal infections are not contagious; however, superficial fungal infections are highly contagious. A likely source of infection can be given if the species of fungus is known. For example, treatment of pets or use of prophylactic antifungal dusting powder after swimming may be helpful to prevent reinfection.

The risk of cryptococcosis can be reduced by wearing masks when working in and around old pigeon nests and droppings. Rodent burrows are the reservoir for coccidioidomycosis. The fungus can be transmitted to humans, cattle, cats, dogs, horses, burros, sheep, swine, coyotes, chinchillas, llamas, and other animal species given the appropriate temperature, moisture, and soil requirements. The patient can be told to avoid dusty occupations, such as road building. The risk of histoplasmosis can be reduced by teaching the patient to avoid old chicken houses, caves harboring bats, and starling and blackbird roosts.

Tinea infections can be prevented by educating the patient, especially parents, about the danger of acquiring the infection from infected children as well as from dogs, cats, and other animals. The fungus is transmitted by direct skin-to-skin contact or indirect contact, especially from the backs of theater seats, barber clippers, toilet articles such as combs and hairbrushes, or clothing and hats contaminated with hair from infected persons or animals.

Tinea cruris and tinea corporis infections can be prevented with thorough laundering of towels and clothing with hot water and fungicidal agents. Tinea cruris occurs most often in males, who need to be reminded that the fungus can be transmitted by direct or indirect contact with the skin lesions of infected persons or inanimate objects. General cleanliness in showers and dressing rooms of gymnasiums and frequent hosing and rapid draining of shower rooms may help.

Onychomycosis is transmitted presumably by direct contact with skin or nail lesions of infected persons and possibly from contaminated floors and shower stalls. Even so, patients need to be advised that there is a low rate of transmission, even to close family associates. The patient and family members should be advised that cleanliness and the use of a fungicidal agent for disinfecting floors in common use and frequent hosing and rapid draining of shower rooms reduce organism growth.

Fungal infection can be spread by sharing towels and hairbrushes. Careful attention to drying and ventilation of intertriginous areas can help prevent candidiasis. The importance of handwashing also should be emphasized repeatedly. Parents of children with a fungal infection should be taught how to care for the child. In some cases, the child may need to stay home from school until the treatment regimen is established and the child is responding. Systemic infections are not contagious.

Pregnant women should be advised that therapy is required if they develop vulvovaginal candidiasis during their third trimester of pregnancy. Treatment helps to prevent neonatal candidiasis. *Candida* is often a part of normal human flora. Patients who are immunocompromised should be advised to contact their health care provider as soon as possible for early detection and treatment of oral, esophageal, or urinary candidiasis to prevent systemic spread. In addition, patients who are neutropenic or otherwise immunocompromised should be advised to decrease their exposure to environmental fungi. For example, soil-containing plants should be disposed of or removed from the patient's immediate environment. Regular inspection of air conditioning systems should also be performed.

Evaluation

Treatment effectiveness can be demonstrated by a decrease in skin irritation and resolution of infection. Early relief of symptoms may be seen in 2 or 3 days. However, for *Candida*, tinea cruris, and tinea corporis, 2 weeks of therapy are needed. For tinea pedis, therapeutic response may take as much as 3 to 4 weeks. Treatment effectiveness for vulvovaginal candidiasis can be evaluated by a decrease in skin irritation and vaginal discomfort. Therapeutic response is usually observed after 1 week. Recurrent fungal infections may be a sign of systemic illness.

SUMMARY

- The mechanism of action for viral infections allows either DNA or RNA viruses to take over a susceptible host cell and use it for metabolic functions and to replicate new virions, which then systemically spread the disease.
- The success of antiviral agents depends on the integrity of the patient's immune system.
- HIV infection presents clinically in stages: primary infection or HIV seropositive but asymptomatic, those who are HIV seropositive and symptomatic, and patients whose disease has progressed to AIDS.
- The pathogenicity of HIV appears to be a function of the destruction and disruption of CD4 cells, which are central to the maintenance of immunocompetency.
- Non–AIDS-defining opportunistic infections begin to appear as the CD4 count drops below 500/mm^3. AIDS-defining opportunistic infections develop as the CD4 count falls below 300/mm^3.
- The primary objectives of therapy are to decrease symptoms, slow the progression of the disease, and improve and prolong the quality of life.
- All patients with acute primary HIV disease or advanced, symptomatic HIV disease should receive multidrug therapy. Multidrug therapy with a protease inhibitor and two nucleoside reverse transcriptase inhibitors is recommended. Monotherapy is contraindicated because of the high risk of resistance.

- Categories of drugs that are used in the treatment of HIV infection include protease inhibitors, nucleoside reverse transcriptase inhibitors, and non-nucleoside reverse transcriptase inhibitors.
- Protease inhibitors are the most effective antiretroviral drugs available. They act by binding HIV protease and thereby preventing the enzyme from cleaving HIV polyproteins. The enzymes and structural proteins of HIV remain nonfunctional, and therefore the virus remains immature and noninfectious.
- All protease inhibitors inhibit cytochrome P_{450} and, therefore, can suppress biotransformation of other drugs, causing their serum levels to rise.
- Nucleoside reverse transcriptase inhibitors suppress HIV replication by incorporating into the growing strand of viral DNA by reverse transcriptase to prevent strand growth and by competing with natural nucleoside triphosphates for binding to reverse transcriptase and thereby competitively inhibiting the enzyme.
- Non-nucleoside reverse transcriptase inhibitors act by causing direct noncompetitive inhibition of reverse transcriptase by binding to its active center.
- Zidovudine is the only drug approved to reduce the risk of perinatal HIV transmission. Thus, zidovudine should be one of the agents used in multidrug therapy regimens.
- In most cases, the principles that guide antiretroviral therapy in adults also apply to children and adolescents.
- The primary laboratory tests employed to monitor HIV infection and to guide therapy are viral loads (plasma HIV RNA) and CD4 counts. Viral load counts indicate the magnitude of HIV infection and predict the rate of CD4 destruction. CD4 counts indicate how much damage the immune system has already suffered.
- Viral loads are the best measurement for predicting clinical outcomes. If the viral load is high, the prognosis if poor. If the viral load is low, the risk of disease progression is significantly reduced. Therefore, the goal of antiretroviral therapy is to decrease the viral load to levels that are undetectable.
- Changing antiretroviral drug regimens is necessary when there is (1) failure of the viral load to drop to an undetectable level, (2) a rebound in viral load after falling to an undetectable level, (3) continued decline of CD4 counts, and (4) continued progression of clinical disease.
- If treatment failure is caused by drug resistance, the preferred response is to change all drugs in the regimen. The drugs used should be ones the patient has not previously taken or that have a cross resistance.
- Patients should remain under close clinical supervision by a care provider experienced in the treatment of HIV-associated diseases.
- Information regarding HIV/AIDS information resources, clinical trials, and treatment regimens should be available to the health care provider and patient, as appropriate.
- Infections caused by fungi are called mycotic infections or mycoses. They can be either superficial or systemic.
- Candidiasis, a common mycosis, is defined as an infection of the skin or mucous membrane with any species of *Candida,* but chiefly *Candida albicans.*
- Candidiasis infection often presents clinically as oral candidiasis, intertrigo, vulvovaginitis, paronychia, or onychomycosis.
- Broad-spectrum antibiotics such as the penicillins, tetracyclines, and cephalosporins eliminate the normal protective vaginal flora, thereby permitting an overgrowth of *Candida.*
- Immunosuppressed states (as in newborns, malignancies, leukemia, and HIV infection), pregnancy, and diabetes mellitus may also predispose the patient to a candidial infection.
- Microscopic demonstration of hyphae and/or yeast cells in infected tissue or body fluids is the single most important diagnostic test for candidiasis.
- Management objectives for the patient with fungal infections include controlling symptoms, avoiding preventable adverse effects secondary to the use of systemic drugs, and preventing reinfection.
- Ketoconazole, itraconazole, fluconazole, amphotericin B, 5-flucytosine, and griseofulvin are used to treat systemic fungal infections. Because these drugs have the potential for toxicity, hospitalization of the patient is required for treatment.
- Clotrimazole, miconazole, nystatin, and amphotericin B are used as topical treatment for superficial fungal infections.
- The duration of therapy depends on the formulation and dosage employed, dosage schedule, severity of the infection, and degree of patient compliance.
- The CDCP states that treatment of the partner is not necessary unless candidial balanitis is present or chronicity is a problem.
- The higher hormone levels found in pregnancy result in a higher glycogen content in the vagina and increase the incidence of vulvovaginal candidiasis.
- Only nystatin is recommended for vulvovaginal candidiasis during the first trimester of pregnancy. Miconazole and clotrimazole are relatively safe for use only during the second and third trimesters of pregnancy.
- Factors that influence the absorption of topical dermatologic drugs include the degree of skin hydration and humidity, occlusion, drug concentration, and the site of administration.
- All symptomatic pregnant patients should be treated aggressively to avoid neonatal candidiasis (thrush).
- Measures that help prevent reinfection should be taught.

BIBLIOGRAPHY

Alrabiah, F., and Sacks, S. (1996). New antiherpes virus agents. *Drugs,* 52 (1), 17–36.

Bangsberg, D., Tulsky, J. P., Hecht, F. M., et al. (1997). Protease inhibitors in the homeless. *The Journal of the American Medical Association,* 278 (1), 63–65.

Batt, M. (1994). Update of mycobacterial issues for the acquired immune deficiency syndrome era. *Journal of Intravenous Nursing,* 17 (45), 217–219.

Barrick, B., and Vogel, S. (1996). Application of laboratory diagnostics in HIV nursing. *Nursing Clinics of North America,* 31 (1), 41–55.

Bartlett, J. (1997). Recommendations for antiretroviral therapy: A comparison of IAS-USA and Department of Health and Human Services Guidelines. *The Hopkins HIV Report,* September.

Bartlett, J. (1997) *Medical management of HIV* (2nd ed.). Baltimore: John Hopkins University Press.

Bechtel-Boenning, C. (1996). State of the art antiviral treatment of HIV infection. *Nursing Clinics of North America,* 31 (1), 1–13.

Bennett, J. (1996). Antifungal agents. In J. Hardman, L. Limbird, P. Molinoff, et al. (Eds.), *Goodman and Gilman's the pharmacologic basis of therapeutics* (9th ed.). New York: McGraw-Hill.

Boland, M. (1996). Overview of perinatally transmitted HIV infection. *Nursing Clinics of North America,* 31 (1), 155–165.

Carpenter, C. C., Fischl, M. A., Hammer, S. M., et al. (1997). Antiretroviral therapy for HIV infection in 1997. Updated recommendations of the International AIDS Society—USA panel. *The Journal of the American Medical Association,* 277 (24), 1962–1969.

Case Definitions for Infectious Conditions Under Public Health Surveillance (1997). *Morbidity and Mortality Weekly Report,* 46, RR10.

Cavert, W. (1997). Assessing effects of potent combination therapy on tissue viral load. *The AIDS Reader,* 7 (4), 123–125.

Chaisson, R. (1997). 1997 Revisions to Guidelines for Prevention of Opportunistic Infections. Baltimore: *The John Hopkins University HIV Report,* 9 (3).

Cotton, D. (1996). To treat or not to treat: Approaches to antiretroviral therapy. *AIDS Clinical Care,* 8 (1).

Cotton, D. (1996). Optimism rises on combination therapy and protease inhibitor data. *AIDS Clinical Care,* 8 (3).

Cotton, D. (1996). The use of protease inhibitors. *AIDS Clinical Care,* 8 (5).

Cotton, D. (1996). New antiretroviral therapy guidelines. *AIDS Clinical Care,* 8 (10).

Cotton, D. (1997). Nonnucleoside reverse transcriptase inhibitors. *AIDS Clinical Care,* 9 (10).

De Santis, M., Noria, G., Caruso, A., et al. (1995). Guidelines for the use of zidovudine in pregnant women with HIV infection. *Drugs,* 50 (1), 43–47.

Dudley, M., Graham, K., Kaul, S. (1992). Pharmacokinetics of stavudine in patients with AIDS or AIDS-related complex. *Journal of Infectious Diseases,* 166 (3), 480–485.

El-Sadr, W., Oleske, J., Agins, B., et al. (1994). *Evaluation and Management of Early HIV Infection.* Clinical Practice Guideline No. 7. AHCPR Publication No. 94-0572. Rockville, MD: Agency for Health Care Policy and Research, Public Health Service, U.S. Department of Health and Human Services.

El-Sadr, W., Oleske, J., Agins, B., et al. (1994). *Managing Early HIV Infection: Quick Reference Guide for Clinicians.* AHCPR Publication No. 94-0573. Rockville, MD: Agency for Health Care Policy and Research, Public Health Service, U.S. Department of Health and Human Services.

Filler, S., and Edwards, S. (1995). When and how to treat serious candidal infections: Concepts and controversies. *Current Clinical Topics in Infectious Disease,* 15, 1–8.

Goa, K., and Barradell, L. (1995). Fluconazole: An update of its pharmacodynamic and pharmacokinetic properties and therapeutic use in major superficial and systemic mycosis in immunocompromised patients. *Drugs,* 50 (4), 658–690.

Gray, M. (1996). Antiviral medications. *Orthopaedic Nursing,* 15 (6), 82–91.

Gulick, R. M., Mellors, J. W., Havlir, D., et al. (1997). Treatment with indinavir, zidovudine, and lamivudine in adults with human immunodeficiency virus infection and prior antiretroviral therapy. *The New England Journal of Medicine,* 337 (11), 734–739.

Jones, R., and Gelone, S. (1997). Antiretroviral drugs to fight AIDS. *Hospital Medicine,* 33 (8), 31–33, 37–38, 40–42, 45.

Lea, A., and Faulds, D. (1996). Ritonavir. *Drugs,* 52 (4), 541–545.

Moyle, G. (1996). Use of viral resistance patterns to antiretroviral drugs in optimizing selection of drug combinations and sequences. *Drugs,* 52 (2), 169–175.

Olin, B. (ed.) (1997). *Drug facts and comparisons.* St. Louis: Facts and Comparisons.

Perry, C., and Faulds, D. (1996). Valacyclovir. *Drugs,* 52 (5), 754–772.

Porche, D. (1997). Postexposure prophylaxis after an occupational exposure to HIV. *Journal of the Association of Nurses in AIDS Care,* 8 (1), 83–87.

Provisional Public Health Service Recommendations for Chemoprophylaxis after Occupational Exposure to HIV. (1996). *Morbidity and Mortality Weekly Report,* 45 (22), 468–479.

Quinn, T. (1997). Acute primary HIV infection. *Journal of the American Medical Association,* 278, 58–63.

Richman, D. (1996). New Strategies to Combat HIV Drug Resistance. *Hospital Practice,* 31 (8), 47–58.

Senak, M. (1997). Predicting antiviral compliance: Physicians responsibilities vs patients rights. *Journal of the International Association of Physicians in AIDS Care,* June, 6 (6), 45–48.

Ungvarski, P. (1997). Update on HIV Infection. *American Journal of Nursing,* 97 (1), 44–62.

Wortley, P. (1997). AIDS in women in the United States. *Journal of the American Medical Association,* 278 (11), 911–916.

Yarchoan, R., Mitsuya, H., and Broder, S. (1992). The immunology of HIV infection: Implications for therapy. *Aids Research and Human Retroviruses,* 8 (6), 1023–1031.

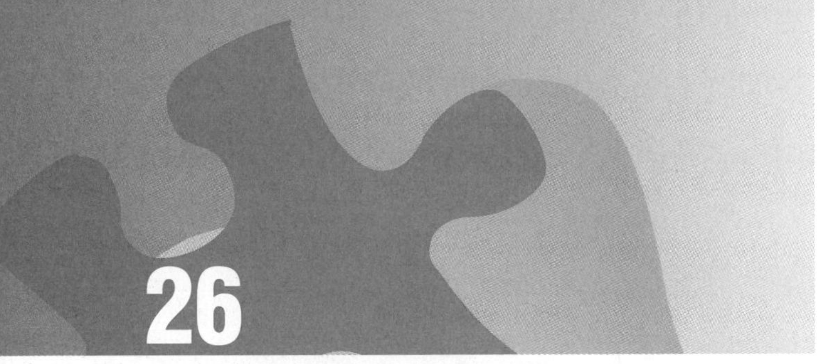

26

Antitubercular and Antileprotic Drugs

Tuberculosis (TB) and leprosy (Hansen's disease) remain a major concern to public health officials throughout the world. The mycobacterial organisms that cause tuberculosis, *Mycobacterium tuberculosis,* and leprosy, *Mycobacterium leprae,* are slow-growing microbes. The infections they cause require multiple-drug regimens and prolonged therapy.

Few primary care providers are called upon to treat TB and leprosy. The development of effective treatment regimens, however, has permitted most patients to be managed within the community rather than in acute care settings.

TUBERCULOSIS

Epidemiology and Etiology

In the 1900s, tuberculosis was the leading cause of death in the United States and Europe. From 1953, when statistics on TB were first reported, until 1985, there was a decline in the number of cases reported in the United States. However, since 1986, the prevalence of TB has increased nearly 16 percent. Today, approximately 8 million people worldwide are affected with TB.

Approximately 66 percent of the cases of TB in the United States today occur among ethnic minorities. The largest increase has occurred in males 25 to 44 years old and, to a lesser extent, children younger than 15 years. The Hispanic, black, and Asian populations are most often affected.

Two primary factors are associated with the rise in TB. The most important is the epidemic of human immunodeficiency virus (HIV) infection and acquired immune deficiency syndrome (AIDS). Persons with AIDS are highly susceptible to opportunistic respiratory infections, including TB. Tuberculosis is ordinarily diagnosed before or at the same time as the AIDS. Because of the overlap of risk groups, the index of suspicion for TB should be high in HIV-infected persons. Similarly, the index of suspicion for HIV infection should be high in persons diagnosed with TB.

Tuberculosis is also on the rise because of greater numbers of drug-resistant strains of the tubercular bacillus. Drug therapy that is too short contributes to the development of resistant strains. The Centers for Disease Control and Prevention recognizes the following groups as having a higher incidence of TB:

- Patients with medical factors that increase their risk of developing active disease (e.g., persons with HIV)
- Racial or ethnic populations (e.g., Native Americans, Alaskan Natives, Hispanics, blacks, Asians, and Pacific Islanders)
- Intravenous drug users and those who abuse alcohol
- Emigrants to the U.S. who were born in countries where TB is endemic
- Members of low-income populations who do not receive routine medical evaluations
- People living in close environments with persons suspected or known to have TB
- Residents of nursing homes, correctional facilities, mental institutions, and other long-term care facilities
- The homeless population

Persons commonly infected with tuberculosis have prolonged, close exposure to an infected person who is not yet diagnosed. Expiratory efforts, such as coughing, sneezing, laughing, talking, and singing, provide exposure to the bacilli through aerosolization (i.e., an airborne route). Bacilli contained in droplets are very small (1 to 5 mm) and are carried by air currents over large areas and for long periods. Once bacilli are inhaled and deposited in alveoli, infection develops and spreads to other organs and tissues. Certain areas of the body favor multiplication of the bacillus, including the upper lobes of the lungs, bones, kidneys, and brain.

The incubation period from infection to demonstrable primary lesions or profound tuberculin reaction is 4 to 12 weeks. The subsequent risk of progressive pulmonary or extrapulmonary TB is greatest the first year or two after infection, but may persist for a lifetime as a latent infection. In theory, as long as viable bacilli are present in sputum, the disease remains communicable. Communicability depends on the number and virulence of the bacilli, adequacy of ventilation, exposure of the bacilli to the sun or ultraviolet light, and opportunities for aerosolization.

Forms

Tuberculosis occurs in three forms: primary, reactivation, and miliary. The appearance of a lung infection with no known prior exposure to the organism is referred to as *primary* TB. Activation of cell-mediated immunity leads to resolution of primary infections in most persons, but they remain at risk for reactivation for life. Children with primary TB are generally not infectious.

Reactivation or secondary TB results when dormant bacilli become endogenously active or the person is again exposed to TB. Reactivation TB occurs anytime, even years after the primary event, at sites seeded with bacilli at the time of primary infection. Seeded areas are most commonly found in the upper lobes of the lungs, perhaps because of the relatively high oxygen tension.

Miliary TB (disseminated disease), more common in older adults, occurs when bacilli are dispersed throughout other organs and tissues of the body. The bacilli produce lesions resembling tiny seeds.

Pathophysiology

Progression of TB occurs in two stages. The first is a primary infection, or active disease. The patient has a positive TB skin test, a normal chest x-ray study, and sputum cultures negative for acid-fast bacilli. Ninety percent of those infected with TB never develop active disease, because they have an intact immune system. The American Thoracic Society has graded TB to aid in evaluation and determination of appropriate pharmacotherapy; the grading system is summarized in Table 26–1.

Primary Infection

Once bacilli are inhaled and multiply, they cause nonspecific, exudative pneumonitis and necrosis. The inflammatory response brings neutrophils and alveolar macrophages to the area. Bacilli are taken up and killed by the neutrophils and macrophages. However, in certain situations, the bacilli multiply within the phagocytes, because they are resistant to the cell's destructive action. Monocytes from the blood are attracted to the infected area but are unable to kill the bacilli. The multiplying bacilli disperse from the original pulmonary site with extensive hilar lymph node involvement. In addition, the spillover from lymphatic vessels to the blood stream causes infection in lung apices and in other organs and tissues. The process ordinarily resolves within a few weeks as a result of cell-mediated immunity. Coincidental to the resolution, a marked increase in the ability of macrophages to inhibit multiplication of the bacilli develops.

Reactivation

Endogenous reactivation of dormant bacilli may occur. It is often related to poor nutritional status, type I diabetes mellitus, long-term steroid therapy, and other debilitating diseases. *Necrosis,* a conspicuous feature of reactivation, is due to tissue destruction following the inflammatory reaction. The resultant granulomatous area is surrounded by collagen, fibroblasts, and lymphocytes, thus sealing off colonies of bacilli. The lesion, referred to as *Ghon's tubercle,* prevents the spread of organisms. The necrotic areas calcify, and the organism remains dormant for life. If, however, the disease progresses, *caseation necrosis* (liquefaction) may occur. Caseation occurs as infected tissues within the tubercle die, forming a cheese-like material. The liquid material empties into a bronchus, whereby the evacuated area becomes a cavity *(cavitation)* (Fig. 26–1). The cheese-like material spreads the bacilli to new areas of the lung.

Miliary Tuberculosis

If the immune system is compromised, or if there is an erosion of Ghon's tubercles, bronchogenic spread may occur. When a blood vessel is affected, the bacilli spread hematogenously. These changes are referred to as *miliary* tuberculosis. Active disease develops because macrophages and lymphocytes do not function or survive in necrotic areas, and therefore, the value of cell-mediated immunity is lost. The patient may be acutely ill, with fever, dyspnea, and cyanosis, or chronically ill, with systemic manifestations such as weight loss, fever, and gastrointestinal (GI) disturbances. In addition, generalized lymphadenopathy, hepatomegaly, and splenomegaly may be present.

Pleural effusions form with the release of caseous material into the pleural cavity. Pleuritis develops from a superficial lesion that involves the pleura. Acute pneumonia can also be found when large numbers of bacilli are discharged from a liquefied lesion into the lung or lymph node. The meninges, bones and joint tissues, kidneys, and genital tracts may also be involved.

In cavities, oxygen tension is fairly high, the medium is neutral or slightly alkaline, and multiplication of bacilli is active. In closed caseous lesions, the oxygen tension is low and the medium neutral, so bacillus replication is slow and intermittent. The intracellular environment of macrophages is acidic, so multiplication of bacilli is relatively slow.

TABLE 26–1 GRADING OF TUBERCULOSIS

Grade	Classification	Associated Findings
0	No tuberculosis, no exposure, no infection	Negative tuberculin test
1	Exposure to tuberculosis, no infection	History of exposure Negative tuberculin test
2	Tuberculosis infection, no active disease	Significant reaction to tuberculin skin test Negative bacteriologic studies No x-ray findings compatible with TB No clinical evidence of TB
3	Tuberculosis, active disease	Positive bacteriologic studies *or* a significant reaction to tuberculin skin test and clinical or x-ray evidence of active disease
4	Tuberculosis, no active disease	History of previous episode of TB *or* abnormal, stable x-ray findings in a person with a significant reaction to tuberculin skin test Negative bacteriologic studies (if done) No clinical or x-ray evidence of active disease
5	Tuberculosis suspected	Diagnosis pending

Data from the American Thoracic Society. (1990). Diagnostic standards and classification of tuberculosis. *American Review of Respiratory Diseases,* 142(3), 725–735.

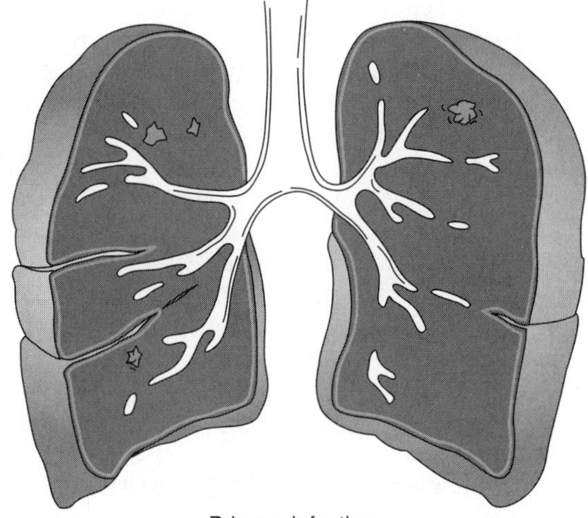

Primary infection

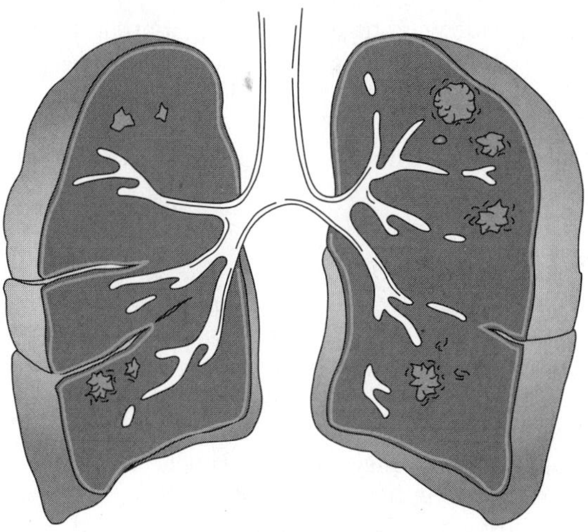

Cavitation of a caseous tubercle

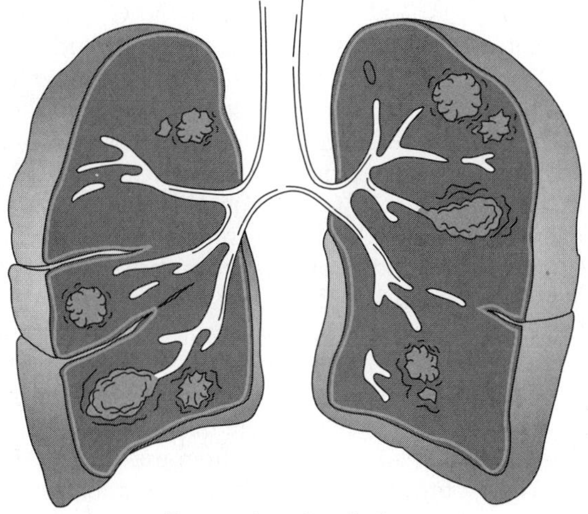

Progression of cavitations

Figure 26–1 Tubercular lesions may occur in any lobe of the lung. Lesions in various stages of development and resolution are noted: primary infection, cavitation of a caseous tubercle, and progression of the cavitations with erosion into bronchi. Cavitations are illustrated as empty areas.

PHARMACOTHERAPEUTIC OPTIONS

Primary treatment for TB is pharmacotherapy and consists of first-line and/or second-line antitubercular drugs. First-line drugs include isoniazid, rifampin, ethambutol, and pyrazinamide. These drugs provide the most effective antitubercular activity with an acceptable degree of toxicity. Second-line drugs, such as cycloserine, capreomycin, ethionamide, and kanamycin, provide acceptable antimicrobial activity but with excessive toxicity. With the re-emergence of multidrug-resistant strains of *M. tuberculosis,* the use of second-line drugs has gained even greater importance. Newer drugs are currently in clinical trials.

First-Line Drugs

- ❒ Ethambutol (EMB), (MYAMBUTOL); MYAMBUTOL, ETIBI (🍁)
- ❒ Isoniazid (INH) (LANIAZID); Isotamine, (🍁) PMS-ISONIZAID
- ❒ Pyrazinamide (PZA); (🍁) PMS-PYRAZINAMIDE, TEBRAZID
- ❒ Rifampin (RIF), (RIFADIN, RIMACTANE); (🍁) RIFADIN, RIMACTANE, ROFACT
- ❒ Streptomycin

Indications

Persons who have been exposed to TB (close contacts, HIV-infected persons with significant reactions to a TB test, and newly infected persons) but who have not developed active disease are candidates for prophylaxis with isoniazid (see Recommendations for Isoniazid Prophylaxis). The benefits of prophylaxis are prevention of active disease and minimization of the spread of infection.

Pharmacodynamics

Isoniazid is a potent bactericidal drug. The precise mechanism of action is unknown, although several hypotheses have been proposed. The hypotheses include effects of the organism on lipids, nucleic acid biosynthesis, and glycolysis. It is also believed that isoniazid as well as ethambutol inhibit synthesis of mycolic acids, important constituents of the mycobacterial cell wall. Because mycolic acids are unique to mycobacteria, this action explains the high selectivity of isoniazid. Bacterial resistance develops when ethambutol is given as monotherapy.

Rifampin inhibits DNA-dependent RNA polymerase, leading to suppression of RNA synthesis. Bactericidal action results in destruction of both multiplying and inactive bacilli.

Ethambutol inhibits the synthesis of metabolites in growing mycobacterial cells, thereby impairing cell metabolism. It arrests cell multiplication, causing cell death.

Pyrazinamide, a synthetic pyrazine analog of nicotinamide, has bacteriostatic and bactericidal effects. This drug requires an acidic environment to be effective.

Streptomycin is essentially bactericidal in the extracellular, alkaline environment. The longer therapy is continued, the higher the incidence of bacterial resistance. Approximately 80 percent of patients treated with streptomycin alone harbor insensitive bacilli after 4 months of treatment.

RECOMMENDATIONS FOR ISONIAZID PROPHYLAXIS

1. HIV-infected persons with significant reactions to a TB test.
2. Household members and other close contacts of patients with active pulmonary TB.
3. Newly infected persons (i.e., those with a TB skin test conversion during the previous 2 years).
4. People with a history of TB and inadequate chemotherapy.
5. People with a TB skin test and an abnormal chest x-ray consistent with previous (nonprogressive) disease.
6. People who demonstrate significant reactions to a TB test and who are at special risk of developing active disease because of factors such as:
   - Silicosis
   - Diabetes mellitus
   - Certain hematologic and reticuloendothelial diseases (leukemia, Hodgkin's disease)
   - End-stage renal disease
   - Conditions associated with substantial weight loss or chronic undernutrition, including postgastrectomy states, intestinal bypass surgery, chronic peptic ulcer disease, chronic malabsorption syndromes, and carcinomas of the oropharynx and upper GI tract that inhibit adequate nutritional intake
   - Long-term therapy with adrenal corticosteroids or immunosuppressive therapy
   - Age less than 35 years

Adverse Effects and Contraindications

Generally, first-line antitubercular drugs are less toxic than second-line drugs. Reactions to first-line drugs may be related to patient age, dose, or the length of therapy.

Isoniazid is associated with two major adverse effects: peripheral neuritis and hepatitis. Peripheral neuritis occurs in about 2 percent of patients receiving 5 mg/kg/day who are not concurrently taking pyridoxine (vitamin B_6). Pyridoxine prevents the development of peripheral neuritis, especially in patients with diabetes mellitus, alcoholism, and malnutrition, even if therapy lasts as long as 2 years.

Severe hepatic injury leading to death may occur in some patients taking isoniazid. The risk of hepatitis is greater in patients who are older than 35 years and/or consume alcohol on a daily basis. Prodromal symptoms of hepatitis are anorexia, nausea and vomiting, malaise, fatigue, and weakness. When isoniazid and rifampin are given concurrently, the incidence of hepatotoxicity is fourfold that seen with isoniazid therapy alone. Isoniazid is contraindicated in the presence of allergy, liver disorders, and pregnancy (Category C). Its cautious use is warranted in the presence of renal dysfunction and during lactation.

The most common adverse effects associated with rifampin are nausea, vomiting, diarrhea, flatulence, and abdominal pain. A red-orange discoloration of the urine, feces, saliva, sputum, sweat, and tears also occurs. Other less common reactions include a flu-like syndrome, hypersensitivity with pruritus and rash, and thrombocytopenia. Rifampin is contraindicated in the presence of allergy to any rifamycin, acute hepatic disease, and during lactation. Cautious use is warranted during pregnancy (Category C) because teratogenic effects have been reported in preclinical studies.

The most significant adverse effect associated with ethambutol is optic neuritis. The presence of optic neuritis appears to be dose related, with signs and symptoms such as decreased visual acuity, loss of red-green color detection, diminished visual fields, or loss of vision. Other adverse reactions are acute gout episodes, peripheral neuritis, and skin rash. Contraindications to the use of ethambutol include allergy, optic neuritis, and pregnancy (Category B). Ethambutol should be used cautiously in the presence of impaired renal function and in children.

A dose-related hepatotoxicity is the most serious adverse effect associated with pyrazinamide. Arthralgia is another common reaction, occurring in about 40 percent of patients receiving pyrazinamide. Contraindications to the use of pyrazinamide are acute hepatic disease, pregnancy (Category C), and lactation. Cautious use of this drug is warranted in the presence of gout, diabetes mellitus, or acute intermittent porphyria.

The most significant adverse effect associated with streptomycin is ototoxicity. Damage to the eighth cranial nerve (CN VIII) results in vertigo, loss of hearing, nausea, and vomiting. High dosage and a lengthy treatment regimen raise the risk for ototoxicity. The risk of nephrotoxicity increases in patients with renal failure. Contraindications to streptomycin include allergy to aminoglycosides; herpes, vaccinia, varicella, and fungal infections; and pregnancy (Category C) or lactation. Cautious use is warranted in older adults or patients with diminished hearing, decreased renal function, dehydration, or neuromuscular disorders.

Pharmacokinetics

Isoniazid is rapidly absorbed after oral administration. It is readily distributed into all body tissues and fluids, including cerebrospinal fluid and breast milk, reaching peak effects in 1 to 2 hours (Table 26–2). It penetrates well into caseous material. Drug concentration is initially higher in plasma and muscle than in infected tissue. However, muscle retains the drug for a long time in quantities above those required for bacteriostasis. Biotransformation of isoniazid occurs in the liver. The half-life is 1 to 4 hours; approximately 75 to 95 percent of isoniazid is eliminated in the urine within 24 hours, mostly as metabolites.

Rifampin is rapidly absorbed from the GI tract on an empty stomach. Bioavailability is between 90 and 95 percent. Rifampin is distributed to most body tissues and fluids, including breast milk and cerebrospinal fluid. It peaks in 2 to 4 hours, with a duration of action of 24 hours. Up to 60 percent of the drug is eliminated in the feces, with 30 percent in the urine. The half-life is approximately 3 hours.

Pyrazinamide and ethambutol are rapidly absorbed from the GI tract. Distribution of pyrazinamide occurs throughout most body tissues and fluids, including cerebrospinal fluid, lungs, and liver. Seventy percent of pyrazinamide is excreted in the urine. Approximately 65 percent of ethambutol is eliminated via the urine, and another 20 percent via the feces. Streptomycin is rapidly absorbed after intramuscular injection but is not absorbed from the GI tract. It diffuses into most organs, with higher concentrations found in tuberculous cavities. Streptomycin is eliminated almost entirely by the kidneys.

Drug-Drug Interactions

Table 26–3 lists drug-drug interactions of selected antitubercular drugs. A large number of other drugs can interact with antitubercular drugs.

TABLE 26–2 PHARMACOKINETICS OF SELECTED ANTITUBERCULAR AND ANTILEPROTIC DRUGS

Drug	Route	Onset	Peak (hr)	Duration	PB (%)	$t_{1/2}$	BioA (%)	Serum Levels (mcg/mL)
First-Line Antitubercular Drugs								
Isoniazid	po	rapid	1–2	UK	0	1–4 hr	UK	3–7
Rifampin	po	rapid	2–4	24 hr	88–90	1.5–5 hr	90–95	6–10
Pyrazinamide	po	rapid	2	UK	UK	9–10 hr	UK	20–50
Ethambutol	po	rapid	2–4	24 hr	UK	3–4 hr	69–85	1–5
Streptomycin	IM	rapid	1–2	UK	34–62	2–3 hr	UK	5–25
Second-Line Antitubercular Drugs								
Ethionamide	po	rapid	3	UK	10	2–3 hr	100	1–5
Cycloserine	po	rapid	3–4	12 hr	0	10 hr	70–90	10–30
Kanamycin	IM	rapid	1–2	UK	UK	2.5 hr	UK	22
Capreomycin	IM	rapid	1–2	UK	UK	4–6 hr	UK	20–45
Antileprotic Drugs								
Dapsone	po	slow	2–8	8–12 days	70–90	22–30 hr	70–80	0.1–0.7
Clofazimine	po	varies	1–6	5 days	UK	10 days	42–62	0.7–1

UK, Unknown; PB, protein binding; $t_{1/2}$, elimination half-life; BioA, bioavailability.

TABLE 26–3 DRUG-DRUG INTERACTIONS OF SELECTED ANTITUBERCULAR AND ANTILEPROTIC DRUGS

Drug	Interactive Drug(s)	Interaction
Antitubercular Drugs		
Isoniazid	Alcohol	Increased hepatotoxicity
	Alfentanil	Prolonged duration of alfentanil
	Carbamazepine	Increased serum level and toxicity of carbamazepine Increased isoniazid hepatotoxicity
	Disulfiram	Increased central nervous system effects
	Rifampin	Increased risk of hepatotoxicity
	Phenytoin	Increased phenytoin serum levels
	Cycloserine	Increased central nervous system effects
	Aluminum antacids	Decreased isoniazid absorption
	Corticosteroids	Decreased isoniazid effectiveness
Rifampin	Oral anticoagulants	Decreased effectiveness of anticoagulants
	Cardiac glycosides	Decreased serum levels of digoxin and digitoxin
	Quinidine	Decreased serum levels of quinidine
	Verapamil	Decreased serum level of verapamil—reversal of verapamil's cardiac effects
	Oral contraceptives	Decreased effectiveness of oral contraceptives with estrogen
	Cyclosporine	Increased metabolism of cyclosporine
	Phenytoin	Increased elimination of phenytoin—reduction of its effect
Pyrazinamide	Antigout agents	Increased serum levels of ethambutol and uric acid
	Neurotoxic agents	Increased risk of optic neuritis
	Streptomycin	
	Other ototoxic agents	Increased risk of ototoxicity
	Other nephrotoxic agents	Increased risk of nephrotoxicity
	Neuromuscular blockers	Increased neuromuscular blocking effect
Capreomycin	Other ototoxic and nephrotoxic agents	Additive effects of ototoxicity and nephrotoxicity
	Cycloserine	
	Isoniazid	Additive adverse central nervous system effects
	Ethionamide	
	Phenytoin	Inhibition of phenytoin biotransformation
	Ethionamide	Increased risk of neurotoxicity
	Other neurotoxic agents	
Kanamycin	Penicillins	When used concomitantly, drugs are inactivated, especially in patients with altered renal function
	Cephalosporins	
	Neuromuscular blockers	Increased risk of respiratory paralysis
Antileprotic Drugs		
Dapsone	Rifampin	Decreases blood levels of dapsone
	Clofazimine	Transient increase in urinary elimination of dapsone
	Hemolytics	Increased risk of agranulocytosis, aplastic anemia, and blood dyscrasias
	Dideoxyinosine	Decreased absorption of dapsone
	Trimethoprim	Increased serum levels of dapsone
Clofazimine	Rifampin	Decreased rate of rifampin absorption and delayed time to reach peak serum concentrations of rifampin
	Isoniazid	Increased serum and urinary concentrations of clofazimine

Drug-Food Interactions

Patients on isoniazid therapy should avoid consuming Swiss or cheshire cheese, fish (tuna, skipjack), and, possibly, tyramine-containing foods (see Appendix C). When such foods are taken concurrently with isoniazid, redness or itching of the skin, warmth, palpitations, diaphoresis, chills, cold clammy sensations, headache, or lightheadedness may result. There are no known drug-food interactions with rifampin, pyrazinamide, or streptomycin.

Dosage Regimen

The American Thoracic Society and Centers for Disease Control and Prevention recommend that initial treatment for tuberculosis be given as a 6-month regimen (short course). The daily use of antitubercular drugs for a period of 6 months helps eliminate actively multiplying extracellular bacilli, rendering the sputum noninfectious.

Treatment during the second phase is designed to eliminate intracellular bacilli. The regimen involves daily or twice-weekly therapy with isoniazid and rifampin. If isoniazid resistance is suspected, ethambutol should be substituted in the regimen. Rifampin is also recommended for isoniazid resistance, along with ethambutol, given for at least 12 months. Pyrazinamide may also be used on a short-term basis (Table 26–4).

An alternative short course (9 months) uses isoniazid and rifampin alone. The two drugs are taken daily for 1 month, and then either daily or biweekly for 8 months more.

Laboratory Considerations

Desired therapeutic serum drug levels for first-line antitubercular drugs are found in Table 26–2. Isoniazid, rifampin, pyrazinamide, and streptomycin cause elevations of liver enzymes—alanine transaminase (serum glutamic pyruvate transaminase), aspartate transaminase (serum glutamic-oxaloacetic transaminase), and bilirubin—in approximately 10 to 20 percent of patients. Therefore, liver enzymes should be closely monitored.

Treatment with rifampin also requires monitoring of complete blood count before and during therapy. Rifampin

TABLE 26–4 DOSAGE REGIMENS FOR ANTITUBERCULAR DRUGS

Drug	Use*	Dosage	Implications
ATS and CDCP Guidelines for 6-Month Regimen*			
Isoniazid	Active disease	*Adult:* 5 mg/kg po or IM daily *Child:* 10–20 mg/kg po or IM daily Maximum dose 300 mg daily	Initial treatment of tuberculosis except in drug resistance or toxicity
Rifampin	Active disease	*Adult:* 10 mg/kg po daily *Child:* 10–20 mg/kg daily Maximum dose 600 mg daily	May cause orange discoloration of urine, feces, sputum, sweat, tears
Pyrazinamide	Active disease	*Adult and child:* 15–30 mg/kg po daily for 2 mo Maximum dose 2 g daily	Maintain high fluid intake
Streptomycin	Active disease	*Adult:* 15 mg/kg IM daily *Child:* 20–40 mg/kg IM daily for 2 mo Maximum dose 1 g daily	Used initially when isoniazid resistance occurs in patients over age 60 Limit dose to 10 mg/kg, with maximum 750 mg daily
Ethambutol	Active disease	*Adult and child:* 15–25 mg/kg po daily for 2 mo Maximum dose 2.5 g daily	Either ethambutol or streptomycin initially used when isoniazid resistance occurs; not recommended for very young children
Second-Line Antitubercular Drugs			
Cycloserine	Failure of first-line drugs	*Adult and child:* 15–20 mg/kg po daily or 500 mg po BID	Give equal doses twice a day
Capreomycin	MDR-TB	*Adult and child:* 15–30 mg/kg IM daily or up to 1 g for 60–120 days	Should not be used together with streptomycin or kanamycin
Ethionamide	Failure of first-line drugs	*Adult and child:* 15–20 mg/kg po daily	Concomitant use of pyridoxine is recommended
Kanamycin	Failure of first-line drugs	*Adult and child:* 15–30 mg/kg IM daily	Dose reduction necessary in patients with impaired renal function

*Joint statement by American Thoracic Society (ATS) and Centers for Disease Control and Prevention (CDCP). These drugs are used in combination with other antitubercular agents. Maximum daily dose for second-line antitubercular drugs is 1 for adults and children.

MDR-TB, multidrug-resistant tuberculosis.

and isoniazid interfere with the determination of vitamin B_{12} and folate levels. Further, prothrombin time should be monitored more frequently in patients receiving rifampin. Patients who are taking concurrently phenytoin and rifampin should have careful monitoring of phenytoin levels.

Serum uric acid levels may be increased in the presence of pyrazinamide and ethambutol. Measurements of blood urea nitrogen, creatinine, and urine specific gravity as well as urinalysis should be monitored routinely, especially for patients with impaired renal function.

Second-Line Drugs

- ❒ Cycloserine (SEROMYCIN)
- ❒ Capreomycin (CAPASTAT)
- ❒ Ethionamide (TRECATOR-SC)
- ❒ Kanamycin (KANTREX)
- ❒ Amikacin (AMIKIN)

Indications

Second-line drugs are used only for treatment of drug-resistant organisms. Each second-line drug has advantages and disadvantages. First, the second-line drugs are especially useful in the treatment of multidrug-resistant TB. However, they are less effective than first-line drugs, and they have greater toxicity. Amikacin is extremely active against several mycobacterial species and may become an important drug for treatment of disease caused by nontuberculous mycobacteria.

Pharmacodynamics

Cycloserine, as an analog of D-alanine (a nonessential amino acid occurring in proteins and found at high levels in plasma), inhibits mycobacterial cell wall synthesis. There is no cross resistance between cycloserine and other antitubercular drugs.

Capreomycin is an antimycobacterial cyclic peptide simplified from *Streptomyces capreolus.* It inhibits RNA synthesis, thereby decreasing the replication of tubercle bacilli. Bacterial resistance to capreomycin develops when it is given alone, and the resistant organisms show cross resistance to kanamycin.

Ethionamide provides a bacteriostatic action against the tubercle bacilli. A congener of thioisonicotinamide, ethionamide is considered more effective than the parent compound. As with capreomycin, resistance can develop.

Kanamycin and amikacin, both aminoglycoside drugs, were previously discussed in Chapter 22. These two drugs interfere with protein synthesis in the bacillus's cell. They bind to a ribosomal subunit, causing inaccurate sequences to form in the protein chain. The outcome is death of the bacillus. Aminoglycosides are most often a pregnancy category D drug.

Another drug has been used in the past in the treatment of TB but has lost favor among care providers in recent years. Para-aminosalicylic acid (PAS), an analog of para-aminobenzoic acid (PABA), is bacteriostatic with action similar to that of sulfonamide antibiotics. It is likely that the enzymes responsible for the biosynthesis of folate are quite exacting in their capacity to distinguish various analogs from the true metabolite.

Adverse Effects and Contraindications

The most common adverse effects of cycloserine involve the central nervous system. Seizures have been known to occur when cycloserine is used concomitantly with isoniazid or ethionamide. Ingestion of alcohol further increases the likelihood of seizures. Some neurologic effects may be prevented by using pyridoxine (vitamin B_6) with cycloserine. Because limited information is available to date on the use of cycloserine during pregnancy (Category C), a specific indication is necessary for it to be considered.

Capreomycin's most common adverse effects are ototoxicity and nephrotoxicity, although hepatic dysfunction has also been evident in some patients. Leukocytosis, leukopenia, eosinophilia, and hypokalemia have also been demonstrated in patients taking capreomycin.

The concomitant use of capreomycin with other ototoxic and nephrotoxic drugs, including streptomycin and kanamycin, should be avoided. The risk-benefit ratio for capreomycin use during pregnancy (Category C) should be based on available data. Its safe use in the pediatric population has not been established.

The most common adverse effects of ethionamide are GI disturbances, including anorexia, nausea, and vomiting. Some patients develop a metallic taste in the mouth. Less common effects are hepatitis and optic and peripheral neuritis. Ethionamide may increase the risk for neurotoxicity when used with other neurotoxic drugs.

Pharmacokinetics

Cycloserine and ethionamide are rapidly absorbed from the GI tract following oral administration. Both are distributed throughout most body tissues and fluids. There is no appreciable blood-brain barrier to the drugs, and cerebrospinal fluid concentrations in all patients are approximately the same as plasma concentrations. Peak serum levels of ethionamide are present in 3 hours, with nearly 100 percent bioavailability (see Table 26–2). Approximately 35 percent of the antibiotic is biotransformed. The majority of ethionamide is eliminated in the urine as inactive metabolites. Sixty to 70 percent of cycloserine is eliminated unchanged in the urine over a period of 72 hours.

Capreomycin is poorly absorbed from the GI tract and must be given by intramuscular injection. Peak serum levels are reached in 1 to 2 hours. Elimination of capreomycin occurs primarily through the urine.

Kanamycin is rapidly absorbed following intramuscular injection, with peak levels found in about 1 hour. Elimination is through urine and feces. Nephrotoxicity and ototoxicity occur with prolonged use and high dosages. Peak serum levels are about 22 mcg/mL. Use of kanamycin with neuromuscular blocking drugs results in a greater risk for respiratory paralysis.

Dosage Regimen

Because second-line antitubercular drugs are potentially ototoxic and nephrotoxic, no two drugs from this group should be given concurrently. Further, these drugs should not be used in combination with streptomycin.

Cycloserine is given orally to adults at 15 to 20 mg/kg daily or up to 500 mg twice daily (see Table 26–4). Optimum therapy can be obtained with serum drug level measurements of 25 to 30 mcg/mL. Higher serum drug levels are found in patients with renal impairment. Increased aspartate transaminase (serum glutamic-oxaloacetic transaminase) levels have been reported in patients with liver disease. Dosage adjustments may be required on the basis of renal function tests and serum drug levels.

Capreomycin dosage ranges from 15 to 30 mg/kg intramuscularly daily to a maximum dose of 1 g. In patients with normal renal function, peak serum capreomycin levels range from 20 to 45 mcg/mL. Renal impairment associated with capreomycin use results in increased blood urea nitrogen and decreased creatinine clearance as well as electrolyte disturbances. Eosinophilia occurs often during therapy with capreomycin but usually subsides when the dose is reduced.

Ethionamide's daily oral dosage range is 15 to 20 mg/kg. Peak serum levels range from 1 to 5 mcg/mL. Serum levels should be monitored, especially in patients with hepatic dysfunction.

The antitubercular dose of kanamycin is 15 to 30 mg/kg intramuscularly daily. Patient monitoring should include renal function tests, auditory exams, and vestibular function tests.

Laboratory Considerations

Increased aspartate transaminase (serum glutamic-oxaloacetic transaminase) levels have been reported in patients with liver disease who are taking cycloserine. Dosage adjustments may be required on the basis of renal function tests and serum drug levels.

Renal impairment associated with capreomycin use results in increased blood urea nitrogen and decreased creatinine clearance levels as well as electrolyte disturbances. Eosinophilia occurs often during therapy with capreomycin but usually subsides when the dosage in reduced.

Ethionamide therapy results in increased alanine transaminase (serum glutamate pyruvate transaminase) and aspartate transaminase (serum glutamic-oxaloacetic transaminase) levels. These levels should be measured before and during therapy.

Newer Antitubercular Drugs

Ofloxacin (FLOXIN) and ciprofloxacin (CIPRO, CILOXAN) are fluoroquinolones (see also Chapter 24) useful in the treatment of tuberculosis when other drugs have failed. The new macrolide antimicrobial drugs, clarithromycin (BIAXIN) and azithromycin (ZITHROMAX), are being studied for use against TB.

Rifabutin (MYCOBUTIN) is a newly approved first-line drug used to prevent disseminated *Mycobacterium avium* complex (MAC) disease in patients with advanced HIV infection. It is a combination of isoniazid and rifampin. Much like rifampin, rifabutin appears to inhibit DNA-dependent RNA polymerase in susceptible organisms. It is active against most strains of *M. tuberculosis*.

Rifabutin is well absorbed following oral administration, but absorption is decreased in about 20 percent of HIV-positive patients. It is widely distributed to body tissues and fluids, with a half-life of 45 hours. Its onset is rapid, with peak serum levels reached in 2 to 4 hours. The drug is metabolized by the liver, with less than 5 percent eliminated unchanged in the urine.

Although adverse effects are uncommon with ribafutin it can cause pressure in the chest. The drug also produces a brown-orange discoloration of body fluids. There is an increased risk for hepatitis. Its drug-drug interactions are similar to those of rifampin but also include greater biotransformation and reduced effectiveness of opioid analgesics, oral hypoglycemic drugs, oral anticoagulants, estrogens, and oral contraceptive drugs. Patients should be counseled to use an alternative, nonhormonal form of contraception throughout any antitubercular therapy.

Rifabutin is available as a single capsule, thereby enhancing compliance. It may be administered without regard to meals, although high-fat meals reduce the rate but not the extent of absorption. Once-daily dosing with 300 mg has been recommended. If GI distress develops, twice-daily dosing with 150 mg may be suggested.

Critical Thinking Process

Assessment

History of Present Illness

The patient's chief complaint and description of symptoms are important to document. Characteristically, patients with TB present with progressive symptoms of fatigue, lethargy, nausea, anorexia, weight loss, irregular menses, low-grade fevers, and night sweats. A cough accompanied by the production of mucoid, mucopurulent, and/or bloody sputum may also be noticed. Tight, dull, aching chest pain may accompany the cough. The chest pain may also be pleuritic, occurring as a result of inflammation to the parietal pleura. The signs and symptoms have often been attributed to the "flu" and ignored by the patient. The patient may seek medical attention only after chest pain or hemoptysis appears.

Past Health History

The patient and family's past health history provides valuable information that helps in selecting appropriate treatment of the TB. Tuberculosis has an insidious onset; therefore, early detection depends on subjective findings rather than presentation of symptoms. The health care provider should inquire about the patient's country of origin and any travel to foreign countries in which TB is endemic. It is also important to note previous testing for TB and the results of that testing.

The patient's drug history is vital, and accurate information must be obtained, preferably through medical records. It should be determined whether the patient has received the bacille Calmette-Guérin (BCG) vaccine. This vaccine contains attenuated bacilli and is routinely given in foreign countries to increase resistance to TB. BCG vaccination of uninfected persons is thought to induce sensitivity in more than 90 percent of those vaccinated. Recipients of the BCG vaccine have a positive skin test and should be evaluated for TB through use of a chest x-ray. Protection given by the BCG may persist for as long as 20 years.

Diagnostic Testing

In most instances, three sputum samples are obtained for acid-fast smear. A positive sputum culture confirms the diagnosis of TB. Once pharmacotherapy is started, sputum samples are again obtained to monitor the effectiveness of therapy.

A TB skin test (Mantoux's test) is useful for screening groups at high risk for developing TB. A small amount (0.1 mL) of intermediate-strength purified protein derivative (PPD) containing 5 tuberculin units is administered intradermally in the forearm, and the site is evaluated 48 to 72 hours after injection. An area of induration measuring 10 mm or more in diameter is considered a positive reaction. A positive reaction does not suggest active disease, but rather indicates exposure to the bacilli or dormant disease and the development of antibodies. Interpretation of TB skin test results is as follows. A 15-mm or larger area of induration is considered positive in all persons. A 10-mm or larger area of induration is considered positive in persons who:

- Were born in high-prevalence areas in countries in Asia, Africa, Latin America, and Oceania
- Are intravenous drug abusers
- Belong to any of the medically underserved, low-income populations, including high-risk racial or ethnic minorities (blacks, Hispanic Americans, Native Americans, Eskimo Americans) and the homeless
- Reside in long-term care facilities (e.g., prisons, mental institutions) or congregate living settings
- Have medical conditions reported to increase the risk of TB—silicosis, gastrectomy, jejunoileal bypass, 10 percent or greater loss of body weight, chronic renal failure, diabetes, high-dose corticosteroid use, immunosuppressive therapies, hematologic disorders (e.g., leukemia, lymphoma), and other malignancies
- Work in health care.

A 5-mm or greater area of induration is considered positive in patients who:

- Are known to be HIV positive or with unknown HIV status and high-risk factors for infection
- Have or have had close or recent contact with patients who have confirmed active TB
- Have chest x-rays consistent with old, healed TB.

Once a skin test is positive, chest x-ray is essential to rule out clinically active TB or to detect old, healed lesions. Nodules, calcifications, cavities, and hilar enlargement (enlarged mediastinal lymph nodes) may be seen in the upper lobes. Routine skin tests and chest x-rays are no longer recommended in these patients. They should be advised to seek medical attention if they develop symptoms suggestive of TB.

In adults older than 50 years, a two-step testing procedure is recommended. The patient is retested in 1 to 2 weeks if the first test was negative. A positive second test indicates that the patient was previously infected.

Mycobacterium avium is the organism responsible for the disease in patients with HIV. It is difficult to identify TB in HIV-positive patients, in whom the skin test may be negative. The negative finding is due to a weak immune response. In addition, sputum cultures may remain negative for acid-fast bacilli.

In the United States, it is mandatory for health care providers to report newly diagnosed cases of TB to state public health officials as well as patients who discontinue treatment prematurely. Detailed records of therapy must be kept, including changes in the drug regimen, all bacteriologic reports, and the results of sensitivity testing.

Developmental Considerations

Perinatal Active disease during pregnancy has been associated with an increase in hypertensive disorders of pregnancy. Higher rates of spontaneous abortion are seen in pregnant patients who have active TB.

Although it is possible for the disease to be transmitted via the placenta to cause fetal/neonatal infection, congenital tuberculosis is rare. When it does occur, however, pneumonia and death can result.

Pediatric The incidence of TB has risen significantly in children, with a 36.1 percent increase in children up to 4 years old. A 34.1 percent rise has been noted in children ages 5 to 14 years. The increases have been attributed in part to the many tuberculosis-positive persons emigrating to the United States.

Children are susceptible to both types of TB, *M. tuberculosis,* and *Mycobacterium bovis.* The bovine type is a common source of infection in children in parts of the world where TB in cattle is not controlled or pasteurization of milk is not practiced. The morbidity and mortality of TB are higher in girls than in boys, particularly in later childhood and adolescence.

Geriatric The incidence of TB is higher among the older adult population (65 years of age and older) than in any other group, except for persons in developing countries who have HIV. In the older adult population, some persons were infected many years before antitubercular drugs were available. These persons may have been hosts to the dormant bacilli for any years. Tuberculosis among older adults is reactivated by several factors, including diabetes mellitus, poor nutrition, long-term corticosteroid therapy, smoking, alcohol, and immunosuppression. Older adult residents of long-term care facilities are at greater risk than older adults in the general population. Careful screening for TB is required in all long-term care facilities.

Psychosocial Considerations

As recently as the 1960s, patients with TB were often confined for months or years in sanatoriums for treatment. Today, TB is still viewed as "shameful" by many in the general population. The patient with suspected TB may be aware of a nonspecific anxiety or nervousness associated with the altered state of health. The health care provider should take this factor into consideration when interacting with the patient. Each aspect of the treatment regimen should be explained to the patient. Most treatment failures occur because patients neglect to take their medication, discontinue it prematurely, or take it irregularly. (See Case Study—Active Tuberculosis.)

Analysis and Management

Treatment Objectives

Treatment objectives for the patient with TB are to eliminate the infectious state as quickly as possible and to maintain consistently negative sputum cultures thereafter. Preventing drug-resistant strains of TB from forming and

Case Study Active Tuberculosis

Patient History

History of Present Illness	LR is a 70-year-old black female with intermittent, dull chest pain for 2 months. Other symptoms are fatigue, night sweats, and bloody sputum.
Past Health History	LR has no known allergies. She has been on a 6-month regimen of methotrexate for seropositive rheumatoid arthritis. She admits to a daily consumption of 16 oz of alcohol and has a 25 ppy smoking history. LR's diet is deficient in vitamins C and E.
Physical Exam	LR has experienced an unintended 10-lb weight loss in the last 3 months. VSS: Febrile. Respirations are labored with productive cough, hemoptysis.
Diagnostic Testing	*Chest x-ray:* interstitial infiltrates, hilar enlargement, and cavitation in left upper lobe. *Sputum culture* × *3:* positive for acid-fast bacilli. *Mantoux (PPD):* positive with 12 cm of induration. *Liver function tests:* within normal limits.
Developmental Considerations	LR may have less effective hepatic and renal function associated with aging.
Psychosocial Considerations	LR lives on social security disability income in a group home. Her level of compliance is unknown. The care provider within the home monitors drug compliance as needed for residents.
Economic Factors	LR has access to any required drug therapy through a state funding program. Also, LR's health care transportation is provided.

Variables Influencing Decision

Treatment Objectives	• Render patient noninfectious • Prevent bacilli replication and resistance • Reduce organism count

Drug Variables	*Drug Summary*	*Patient Variables*
Indications	Prophylaxis (as indicated) and active disease	LR has active tuberculosis. Will be a decision point.
Pharmacodynamics	All four agents are bactericidal to active and dormant bacilli. Multidrug therapy reduces probability of organism resistance.	Because all four agents have similar pharmacodynamics, this will not be a decision point.
Adverse Effects/ Contraindications	Isoniazid: Hepatotoxicity; peripheral neuritis, secondary to pyridoxine deficiency. Rifampin: Nausea, vomiting, diarrhea, red-orange color to body fluids. Ethambutol: Dose-dependent optic neuritis. Pyrazinamide: Hepatotoxicity, arthralgia.	Will be a decision point owing to broad variation in adverse effects. LR's alcohol intake may be a contraindication to isoniazid and pyrazinamide.
Pharmacokinetics	All four agents have similar onset and peak. Duration of action varies from 6 to 24 hours.	Since all four agents in general have similar pharmacokinetics, this will not be a decision point. However, LR's impaired renal function associated with aging may have an impact on the elimination of the drugs by the kidneys that could potentially lead to toxicity.

Drug Variables	*Drug Summary*	*Patient Variables*
Dosage Regimen	Per American Thoracic Society, Centers for Disease Control and Prevention, and manufacturer's recommendations, mimimum duration of therapy is 6 months, most often 6–9 months.	Because LR will have someone to monitor her dosage regimen and compliance, this will not be a major decision factor.
Laboratory Considerations	Complete blood count, liver function tests, blood urea nitrogen, creatinine, uric acid, and urinalysis prior to initiating drug therapy and every 1–2 months thereafter. Serum drug levels every 1–2 months.	This may be a decision point owing to impaired renal function associated with aging.
Cost Index*	Isoniazid: 1 Rifampin: 5 Ethambutol: 4 Pyrazinamide: 2	As LR's drugs are available through state funding, cost is not a major decision point.

Summary of Decision Points

- The variety of adverse effects associated with multiple-drug therapy requires close monitoring.
- Pharmacokinetics in general is not a major consideration; however, LR's alcohol intake and changes in renal function due to aging increase the potential for hepatotoxicity and nephrotoxicity.
- Laboratory testing of liver and renal function is an important component owing to potential for hepatotoxicity and nephrotoxicity.

DRUGS TO BE USED

- Isoniazid, rifampin, ethambutol, and pyrazinamide × 2 months, then isoniazid and rifampin × 4 months; to be continued 3–6 months after sputum cultures are negative.
- Supplemental pyridoxine (as appropriate) to minimize potential for peripheral neuritis.

*Cost Index:
1 = <$30/mo.
2 = $30–40/mo.
3 = $40–50/mo.
4 = $50–60/mo.
5 = >$60/mo.

AWP of 100, 100-mg tablets of isoniazid is approximately $4.
AWP of 100, 300-mg capsules of rifampin is approximately $165.
AWP of 100, 400-mg tablets of ethambutol is approximately $162.
AWP of 100, 500-mg tablets of pyrazinamide is approximately $97.

avoiding a reactivation of the TB are equally important. To accomplish these objectives, treatment is designed to eradicate three replicating populations of bacilli: those in cavitary lesions, those in closed caseous lesions, and those existing within macrophages.

Treatment Options

Drug Variables

There are two main principles of antitubercular therapy. First, the therapy must consist of two or more drugs to which the bacilli are sensitive. Second, treatment must continue for at least 3 to 6 months after the sputum becomes negative. This practice sterilizes the lesions and prevents relapse. Because there are three different populations of bacilli, antitubercular drugs differ in their bacteriostatic/bactericidal activity. Further, because *M. tuberculosis* is slow growing and the disease is often chronic, patient compliance, drug toxicity, and the development of bacterial resistance present special therapeutic problems.

Active Disease In the United States, initial intensive therapy is accomplished using a combination of isoniazid, rifampin, pyrazinamide, and ethambutol. Streptomycin is added to the regimen if resistance is suspected. A large proportion of organisms from Latin American, African, and Asian immigrants have been found resistant to isoniazid. Two or more drugs are used to treat active disease, because the combination provides additive antitubercular activity, and because one drug minimizes or delays the development of resistance to the other.

The choice of drugs used depends on the organism load and the susceptibility of the mycobacterial strain. Short-term therapy covers 6 to 9 months, whereas conventional therapy typically lasts 18 to 24 months. The most common regimen recommended by the American Thoracic Society and the Centers for Disease Control and Prevention consists of four-drug combination therapy. Therapy is initiated over a 2-month period using isoniazid, rifampin, ethambutol, and pyrazinamide. It is then followed by two-drug therapy using isoniazid and rifampin for 4 months longer. However, alternative time-variable treatment regimens demonstrate efficacy equal to that of short-term therapy. An equally efficacious treatment option is to use combination therapy twice to three times a week, rather than daily.

Another alternative course of treatment consists of isoniazid and rifampin taken daily for 1 month. The second phase of therapy consists of a daily or biweekly dose of isoniazid and rifampin for 8 months. Therapy is continued for a period of 3 to 6 months after sputum cultures are negative.

In patients with HIV infection, a four-drug treatment regimen is recommended. Ethambutol is preferred over pyrazinamide. The length of treatment is individualized according to the patient's response to therapy.

Treatment for multidrug-resistant TB should be given on an individual basis after a thorough review of the patient's previous therapy and current sensitivity testing has been done. Treatment for multidrug-resistant TB often involves the use of four to seven antitubercular drugs. Bacteria resistant to first-line and second-line drugs are used for 24 months or longer, until sputum cultures are negative.

Second-line drugs are similar in several respects. They are all used only for treatment of disease caused by resistant organisms or by nontuberculous mycobacteria. They all must be given parenterally and have similar pharmacokinetics and toxicities. Because second-line drugs are potentially ototoxic and nephrotoxic, no two drugs from this group should be used together, nor should any of these drugs be used in combination with streptomycin.

Prophylaxis Generally, the benefits of prophylaxis outweigh the risks of hepatotoxicity, the primary toxicity of isoniazid. However, prophylaxis is contraindicated in persons who have liver disease or have had serious adverse reactions to isoniazid in the past. Persons older than 35 years should not be routinely treated, because the risk of isoniazid-induced liver damage increases significantly with age. Prophylaxis should be reserved for TB-positive persons who have other factors placing them at increased risk (e.g., diabetes, leukemia, drug-induced immunosuppression). Prophylaxis for a pregnant woman should be postponed until after delivery.

Patient Variables

Patient as well as drug variables identified during assessment should be taken into account in the planning of treatment objectives. Not all data obtained from the history, physical exam, and laboratory tests are relevant to a drug regimen. However, relevant data do include information that affects compliance, pharmacokinetic parameters, and the evaluation of treatment effectiveness and adverse effects. Compliance with the treatment regimen and the patient's response are both influenced by the physiologic as well as the developmental and psychosocial aspects of the disease.

Developmental changes associated with the perinatal, pediatric, and geriatric patient are vital to effective drug therapy. All pregnant women with active TB should receive antitubercular therapy, but it may be prudent to postpone prophylaxis until after delivery. The risks and benefits of antitubercular therapy should be discussed with the pregnant patient. She should understand that problems associated with not treating the TB far outweigh the possible risks to her and her unborn child. Isoniazid, rifampin, and ethambutol have not been shown to have teratogenic effects. Streptomycin, capreomycin, and kanamycin should not be used during pregnancy because of documented fetal ototoxicity. The safe use of pyrazinamide and cycloserine during pregnancy has not been established. Pregnant women receiving antitubercular therapy should not be discouraged from breastfeeding. Toxicity among breastfed infants is rare.

Drugs may accumulate in a child's system as a result of immature hepatic and renal functioning. Pediatric patients generally have a higher percentage of body water, thereby influencing dosage amount and frequency and, thus, the potential for ineffective drug levels and/or toxicity. Nonetheless, they should be treated with the appropriate regimen at dosages calculated for their size.

At the opposite end of the spectrum is the older adult. The physical changes of aging affect biotransformation and elimination of drugs by the kidneys that can lead to toxicity. Further, distribution of drugs that are highly protein bound is influenced by the level of albumin in the serum. Rifampin, for example, is 88 to 90 percent protein bound, so its time in the body is extended. On the other hand, isoniazid has little to no protein binding, so more free drug is available to act on the mycobacterium.

Intervention

Administration

Therapy using antitubercular drugs requires special considerations. For example, when isoniazid is prescribed without supplemental pyridoxine (vitamin B_6), the patient should be monitored early for vitamin B_6 deficiency. The signs and symptoms of deficiency are irritability, seborrhea-like skin lesions, weakness, hypochromic microcytic anemias, impaired immune responses, and seizures (in infants). If isoniazid is taken with food or antacids, absorption may be decreased. All four drugs should be taken at the same time each day, and a high fluid intake maintained.

Rifampin, ethambutol, and pyrazinamide should be administered 1 to 2 hours after meals for best absorption and to reduce GI irritation. If the patient has difficulty swallowing the rifampin capsules, they may be opened and the drug mixed with applesauce or jelly before administration.

Directly observed therapy is recommended by the Advisory Council for the Elimination of Tuberculosis in areas where patients do not complete at least 90 percent of the recommended therapy. Directly observed therapy requires that another person actually watch the patient as the prescribed drugs are taken. This approach is feasible for patients taking their drugs on daily, twice-weekly, or thrice-weekly regimens. It improves compliance in both rural and urban settings and is cost effective even though it requires additional resources. (See Controversy—Directly Observed Therapy.)

Controversy

Directly Observed Therapy for Tuberculosis
SANDRA FRANKLIN

The incidence of tuberculosis (TB) declined for 30 years after the introduction of antitubercular drugs. Unfortunately, tuberculosis re-emerged as a serious threat to public health in the mid-1980s. The significant rise in tuberculosis can be attributed in part to the increased prevalence of human immunodeficiency virus (HIV) infections, but resurgence of TB has been documented in a variety of health care settings.

Standard treatment regimens for tuberculosis involve self-administration of specific drugs for a period of several months. However, approximately one-third of patients with active disease do not follow the prescribed treatment regimen. Their disease then relapses.

Current protocols promote directly observed therapy (DOT) as an effective alternative to the standard self-administration strategy. DOT requires that patients receive and swallow their drugs under supervision. Implementation of DOT has demonstrated a significant decrease in the frequency of primary drug resistance, as well as reductions in rates of acquired drug resistance and relapse.

Management costs for DOT and standard antitubercular therapy are comparable. The costs for one patient who fails standard treatment regimens and develops multidrug-resistant tuberculosis far outweigh the cost of implementing DOT for several hundred patients.

Critical Thinking Discussion

- What factors make self-administration of drug difficult for patient?
- What is primary drug resistance? What is acquired drug resistance?
- What constitutes a relapse of tuberculosis? Why is this a public health menace as well as a problem for the patient?

Education

Patients should be taught to cover the mouth and nose when coughing or sneezing. Persons in close contact with those who cannot or will not cover their mouths or who are coughing should wear masks. Patients who have primary TB or whose sputum is bacteriologically negative, but who do not cough and are known to be receiving adequate pharmacotherapy, need not be isolated. Hospitalization is necessary only for patients with severe illness and for whom medical or psychosocial circumstances make treatment at home difficult or impossible.

Most patients need careful instruction in order to manage their drug regimens properly. Compliance is a key factor in the success of drug treatment for TB, especially among specific high-risk populations. Patients should be questioned on a regular basis about adherence to drug regimens.

Spot urine and serum drug level testing and diligent record keeping should be done to validate compliance. Patients should be advised to keep clinic appointments for drug dispensing, laboratory testing, and follow-up physical exams. Public health officials should be notified if appointments are not kept. It may be beneficial to offer incentives for improved compliance, such as taxi fare to and from the clinic, food vouchers, or free day care.

Preventive treatment may be indicated for close contacts of patients with TB. BCG vaccination of tuberculin-negative household contacts, especially infants and children, may be warranted under special circumstances. Continuing exposure to untreated or ineffectively treated persons with sputum-positive TB may require additional intervention strategies.

Patients should be taught to recognize the signs and symptoms of hepatitis and optic neuritis. Signs and symptoms of hepatitis (yellow eyes and skin, nausea and vomiting, anorexia, fatigue or weakness, or dark urine) and of optic neuritis (eye pain, blurred vision, and/or loss of vision), and hearing disturbances and/or dizziness, tinnitus, or vertigo should be readily reported to the health care provider. Regular ophthalmologic examinations aid in the detection and follow-up of optic neuritis. Patients receiving rifampin should be warned that the drug may turn body fluids and urine a red-orange and should be reassured that it is harmless. Patients should wear glasses instead of contact lenses to prevent discoloration of lenses while taking rifampin.

Evaluation

Indications that the infection is under control should be monitored. Diminished cough and sputum production, decreased fever and night sweats, amelioration of anorexia with a concomitant weight gain, and fewer bacilli in sputum specimens are all evidence of improvement. Successful therapy is further noted as an absence of observable bacilli in the sputum and in sputum cultures. Once sputum cultures are negative, usually in 3 to 6 months, therapy should continue for 3 to 6 months longer. The patient's liver function parameters and electrolyte values should remain within normal limits. Optic neuritis is closely followed through ophthalmologic examinations. Serum uric acid levels should remain within normal limits, and patient records should indicate that the patient is keeping follow-up appointments.

LEPROSY

Epidemiology and Etiology

Leprosy (Hansen's disease) is a chronic bacterial infection occurring in approximately 12 million people worldwide. However, 95 percent of the population have a natural immunity to leprosy. In the 5 percent susceptible to infection, leprosy occurs as a result of altered cell-mediated immunity. The areas of the world where leprosy is endemic are South and Southeast Asia including the Philippines, Indonesia, some Pacific islands, India, Bangladesh, Myanmar (Burma), Indonesia, and tropical Africa. The disease also occurs in the colder climates of Tibet, Nepal, Korea, and Siberia. Small numbers (300 to 500 per year) of cases currently occur in the United States. Cases have been reported in California, Hawaii, Texas, Florida, Louisiana, New York City, and Puerto Rico. The rise in leprosy in the United States has been attributed to immigration from endemic areas.

THE SPECTRUM OF LEPROSY—RIDLEY-JOPLIN CLASSIFICATION

Paucibacillary Forms

Patients with the most intact immune response who are able to self-heal or to localize the disease. Patients with a BI (bacterial index; see below) of 0 on skin scrapings at all sites at the time of diagnosis and only rare bacilli on biopsy specimens (World Health Organization) are classified as having paucibacillary leprosy, which has three forms:

- Indeterminate
- Tuberculoid
- Borderline tuberculoid

Multibacillary Forms

Patients with the least intact immune response whose disease becomes generalized; patients with the following bacterial index (BI; see below) at the times of diagnosis are classified as having the following forms of multibacillary leprosy:

- BI 2–3+: Mid-borderline
- BI 3–5+: Borderline lepromatous
- BI 6+: Lepromatous (LL)

Bacterial Index (BI)

A semilogarithmic scale ranging from 0 (indicating no bacilli in 100 oil immersion fields) to 6+ (indicating more than 1000 organisms per oil immersion field); specimens are obtained from biopsy sections and skin scrapings.

Pathophysiology

Mycobacterium leprae (M. leprae), is a slow-growing bacillus. Humans are the only proven reservoir of significance, and although the exact mode of transmission is not clearly understood, household or prolonged close contact appear to be important. The bacillus grows best in cooler parts of the body. The areas affected typically are the skin, peripheral nerves, nasal mucosa, upper airway, and the eyes. It is widely believed that disease transmission occurs when bacilli are spread from the respiratory tract of infected persons to the respiratory tract of susceptible persons. Millions of bacilli are liberated daily in the nasal secretions of untreated lepromatous patients. Bacilli remain viable for at least 7 days in dried nasal secretions. Cutaneous ulcerations may also shed large numbers of bacilli. In children younger than 1 year, transmission is presumed to have been transplacental.

Forms

The three forms of paucibacillary leprosy are indeterminate, tuberculoid, and borderline tuberculoid (see The Spectrum of Leprosy). At one end of the spectrum is *indeterminate* leprosy, occurring very early in the course of the infection. Macular skin lesions reflect limited cellular response on biopsy and thus do not reveal the specific type of leprosy. Of the population with indeterminate leprosy, 75 percent heal spontaneously; the remainder progress to other forms of leprosy.

Tuberculoid leprosy is characterized by one or a few macular skin lesions. The lesions are usually hypopigmented on dark-skinned persons and erythematous on light-skinned persons. There are losses of hair and of sensation at skin lesions. Sensory changes include alterations in the perception of light touch, pain, and temperature. The incubation period for tuberculoid leprosy ranges from 9 months to 20 years, with an average of 4 years.

The lesions of *borderline tuberculoid* leprosy appear in greater numbers. These lesions are more symmetric and are associated with a loss of sensation and hair.

The three forms of multibacillary leprosy are mid-borderline, borderline lepromatous, and lepromatous. The lesions of *mid-borderline* leprosy are numerous and have a raised plaque appearance with punched-out areas. Loss of sensation is variable in these lesions. With *borderline lepromatous* leprosy, the skin lesions occur in greater numbers and are similar to the mid-borderline form. However, the macular, papular, or nodular lesions tend to have a shiny appearance and are bilaterally symmetric.

Patients with the *lepromatous* form of leprosy have markedly impaired cell-mediated immunity. This form is characterized by diffuse or ill-defined localized infiltration of the skin, which becomes thickened, glossy, and corrugated (Fig. 26–2). Skin lesions are too numerous to count, with smooth, shiny erythematous areas. Sensory loss occurs late with lepromatous leprosy. The incubation period of lepromatous leprosy ranges from 18 months to 40 years. As the

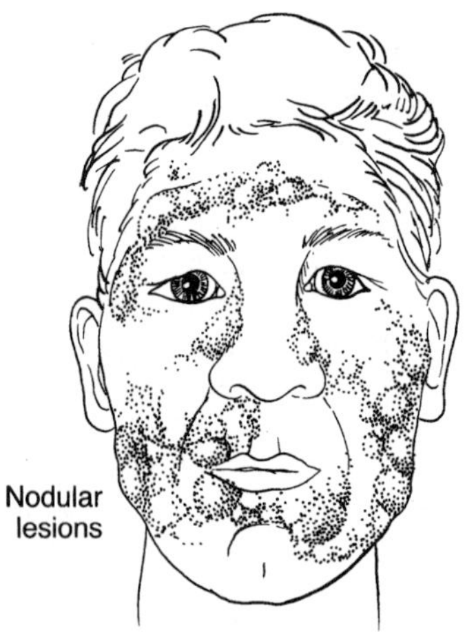

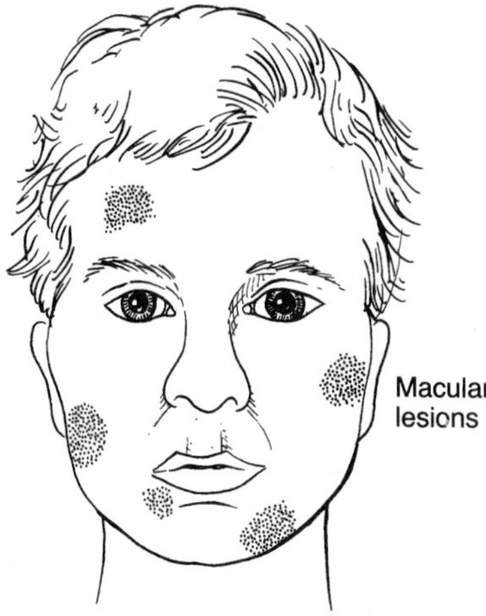

Figure 26–2 Comparison of lepromatous and tuberculoid forms of leprosy. Lepromatous leprosy (LL) is characterized by diffuse or ill-defined localized infiltration of the skin. The lesions become thickened, glossy, and corrugated. Skin lesions are too numerous to count, with smooth, shiny erythematous areas. Tuberculoid (TT) leprosy is characterized by one or a few macular skin lesions produced by a granulomatous reaction. The lesions are usually hypopigmented on dark-skinned persons, and erythematous on light-skinned persons. There is hair loss and a loss of sensation at skin lesions produced by a granulomatous reaction. (From Cotran, R., Kumar, V., and Robbins, S. [1994]. *Pathologic basis of disease* [5th ed.] Philadelphia: W.B. Saunders. Used with permission.)

lepromatous form progresses, large nerve trunks are involved, and anesthesia, atrophy of the skin and muscle, absorption of small bones, ulceration, and spontaneous amputations may occur. Earlobes may enlarge, and the face develops deep lines characteristic of *leonine facies*. Eyebrows and eyelashes disappear. Nasal stuffiness and epistaxis, along with a saddle-nose deformity, may occur as a result of damage to the nasal mucosa and cartilage.

Differences in cell-mediated immunity may account for the various forms of leprosy. Host resistance to *M. leprae* is more prominent in the indeterminate and tuberculoid forms, but much less prominent in the lepromatous form.

Leprotic reactions—manifestations of delayed hypersensitivity to the *M. leprae* organism—occur in approximately 50 percent of patients during therapy. Type 1, or "reversal," reactions are seen in the tuberculoid and mid-borderline forms of leprosy. Type 2 reactions, seen in borderline lepromatous and lepromatous forms, are characterized by the appearance of raised, tender, intracutaneous nodules, severe constitutional symptoms, and high fever. A type 2 reaction may be triggered by several conditions but is most often associated with therapy. It is thought to be an Arthus-type reaction related to the release of microbial antigens in patients harboring large numbers of bacilli.

PHARMACOTHERAPEUTIC OPTIONS

First-Line Drugs

❒ Clofazimine (LAMPRENE)
❒ Dapsone (DDS); (✤) AVLOSULFON
❒ Rifampin (RIF) (RIFADIN, RIMACTANE); (✤) RIFADIN, RIMACTANE, ROFACT

Indications

Dapsone is among the oldest and most widely used antileprotic drugs, remaining the drug of choice for all sulfone-sensitive strains of leprosy. According to World Health Organization guidelines, clofazimine is used in conjunction with dapsone and rifampin for the treatment of multibacillary leprosy. In National Hansen's Disease Center regimens, dapsone is used in conjunction with rifampin for the treatment of paucibacillary and multibacillary forms of leprosy due to sulfone-resistant strains. The anti-inflammatory effects of clofazimine are useful for the treatment of leprotic reactions associated with multibacillary forms of leprosy.

Rifampin and ethionamide were discussed previously in this chapter as antitubercular drugs. Rifampin is also useful in the treatment of all forms of leprosy.

Ethionamide has been found useful in the treatment of multibacillary leprosy. However, it is weakly bactericidal to the *M. leprae* organism.

Pharmacodynamics

Dapsone is a synthetic sulfone with bacteriostatic properties. A sulfone is a compound containing two hydrocarbon radicals attached to the $—SO_2—$ group. The mechanism of action of the sulfones is similar to that of the sulfonamide antibiotics. They interfere with the bacterial synthesis of folic acid. Dapsone and sulfonamide antibiotics possess approximately the same ranges of antibacterial activity, and both are agonized by para-aminobenzoic acid (PABA).

The exact mechanism of action of clofazimine is unclear. The drug binds with mycobacterial DNA to inhibit the multiplication and growth of the *M. leprae* organism. Cross resistance to dapsone or rifampin has not been demonstrated.

Adverse Effects and Contraindications

The overall incidence of adverse reactions to dapsone and rifampin treatment regimens is approximately 0.4 percent. The most common adverse effect of dapsone is a dose-dependent hemolytic anemia. The anemia occurs in patients who receive a daily dose of 200 mg or more. The hematologic effects are most severe with patients who have a glucose-6-phosphate dehydrogenase deficiency. A syndrome similar to mononucleosis has occasionally occurred. Signs and symptoms of the syndrome are skin rashes, fever, jaundice, hepatitis, methemoglobinemia, and anemia.

Hypersensitivity reactions to dapsone are manifested by a variety of skin rashes. If the reaction is severe, it may be necessary to discontinue the drug. GI and central nervous system adverse effects have also occurred. Hepatic adverse effects include jaundice and hepatitis. Blurred vision, tinnitus, and fever also may occur.

The most serious adverse effects of clofazimine are dose-related GI problems. At doses of 100 mg or less, nausea, vomiting, or diarrhea may be present. More serious effects occur with higher doses of several months' duration. The more serious adverse effects include abdominal pain, perhaps related to the accumulation of the drug in the small intestine. On rare occasions, bowel obstruction, GI bleeding, and splenic infarction have been reported.

Clofazimine contains a red-hued dye that leads to discoloration of the skin and conjunctiva in 75 to 100 percent of patients. The skin changes from red to a brown-black discoloration, with the skin lesions also affected. The skin discoloration is reversible, but it may take several months or years to disappear completely. Many patients find the skin discoloration unacceptable. Tears (38 to 57 percent), sweat, sputum, urine, and feces are also discolored. In addition to discoloration, 8 to 38 percent of patients experience itching and dry skin.

Pharmacokinetics

Dapsone is slowly absorbed from the GI tract following oral administration, with a 93 to 100 percent bioavailability. Absorption occurs best in an acid environment. It is well distributed throughout the body, including the skin, kidneys, liver, and muscle. Dapsone's onset of action occurs in 8 hours, and its duration of action is 3 weeks (see Table 26–2). Fifteen percent of dapsone is eliminated through the kidneys, with a urinary pH of 6 to 7. Seventy-three to 74 percent of dapsone is bound to plasma proteins. The half-life ranges from 15 to 28 hours.

Clofazimine is absorbed in the body at variable rates. The rate of absorption depends on several factors, including the site of administration, the dose, and whether food is present in the GI tract. The bioavailability ranges from 42 to 62 percent. The drug's onset of action varies a great deal from patient to patient, but its duration of action is measured in months, because it tends to accumulate in fatty tissues, the cells of the reticuloendothelial system, and the small intestine. Clofazimine is eliminated very slowly from the body, primarily through the feces. The drug has a half-life of nearly 70 days.

Drug-Drug Interactions

Table 26–3 lists drug-drug interactions of antileprotic drugs. Although the drug-drug interactions are fewer than those found with antitubercular drugs, it is important that the interactions be noted before these agents are used.

Dosage Regimen

Both the National Hansen's Disease Center and the World Health Organization recommend dapsone for use in the treatment of sulfone-sensitive paucibacillary leprosy. A daily oral dose of 100 mg for 6 months is recommended for the indeterminate and tuberculoid types (Table 26–5). Therapy must be continued for 3 years after negative skin tests are documented. For the borderline tuberculoid type of leprosy, the drug is continued at the same dose for 5 years after negative skin tests.

Dapsone therapy for multibacillary forms is a daily oral dose of 100 mg for approximately 2 years, until skin tests are negative. For sulfone-sensitive, mid-borderline type, a daily oral dose of 100 mg for 3 years is indicated. The drug is continued for 10 years after negative skin tests. For the borderline lepromatous and lepromatous types, the drug is continued indefinitely.

For the treatment of multibacillary forms of leprosy, the World Health Organization recommends a daily oral dose of clofazimine 50 mg self-administered, and 300 mg given once a month, supervised. Doses in excess of 300 mg should not be given. Clofazimine should be taken with food or milk to maximize absorption.

For patients with pary forms of leprosy, the oral dose of rifampin is 600 mg, once a month for 6 months. For patients with multibacillary forms of leprosy, the oral dose is 600 mg once a month, for a minimum of 2 years or until skin tests are negative. Monthly administration is preferred because there are no significant toxic effects and the monetary expense to the patient is greatly reduced. Directly

TABLE 26–5 DOSAGE REGIMENS FOR ANTILEPROTIC DRUGS

Drug	Use	Dosage	Implications
Dapsone	*WHO Recommendation*		
	Paucibacillary form	*Adult:* 100 mg po QD for 6 mo *Child:* 1–2 mg/kg po QD for 6 mo	Self-administered in adults, in combination with rifampin
	Multibacillary form	*Adult:* 100 mg po QD for a minimum of 2 yr *Child:* 1–2 mg/kg po daily for a minimum of 2 yr	Or given until skin tests are negative Self-administered in adults, combined with rifampin
	*NHDC Recommendation**		
	Paucibacillary form due to sulfone-sensitive strains	*Adult:* 100 mg po QD 6 mo, given with rifampin	For indeterminate and tuberculoid forms, drug is continued for 3 yr after negative skin tests For borderline tuberculoid form, drug is continued for 5 yr after negative skin test
	Multibacillary form due to sulfone-sensitive strains	*Adult:* 100 mg po QD for 3 yr, given with rifampin	For mid-borderline form, drug is continued for 10 yr after negative skin test For borderline and lepromatous forms, drug is continued indefinitely
Rifampin	*WHO Recommendaiton*		
	Paucibacillary form	*Adult:* 600 mg po monthly for 6 mo	Supervised, in combination with dapsone
	Multibacillary form	*Adult:* 600 mg po monthly for patients > 35 kg; 450 mg for patients < 35 kg *Child:* 10 mg/kg po monthly	Supervised, in combination with dapsone and clofazimine Drug is given for 2 yr
	*NHDC Recommendation**		
	Paucibacillary form due to sulfone-sensitive strains	*Adult:* 600 mg po monthly for 6 mo	In combination with dapsone
	Multibacillary form due to sulfone-sensitive strains	*Adult:* 600 mg po monthly for 3 yr	In combination with dapsone
	For sulfone-resistant strains	*Adult:* 600 mg po monthly for 3 yr	In combination with clofazimine
Clofazimine†	*WHO Recommendaiton*		
	Multibacillary forms	*Adult:* 50 mg po QD and 300 mg monthly *Child:* 50 mg po given on alternate days, supplemented by 200 mg monthly	Self-administered. Supervised, given for 2 yr or until skin tests are negative Supervised, given for 2 yr
	NHDC Recommendation		
	Paucibacillary due to sulfone-resistant strains	*Adult:* 50–100 mg po QD	In place of dapsone, given in the same regimen
	Multibacillary forms due to sulfone-resistant strains	*Adult:* 50–100 mg po QD indefinitely	In combination with rifampin

*The NHDC (National Hansen's Disease Center) regimens have no recommendations for pediatric dosages.

†For WHO (World Health Organization) regimens, when clofazimine is unacceptable to patients, ethionamide 250–375 mg po daily may be given to adults for self-administration. For NHDC regimens, when clofazimine is unacceptable to patients, ethionamide 250 mg po daily along with rifampin 600 mg po daily may be given to adults.

observed therapy is recommended to ensure patient compliance.

The World Health Organization and the National Hansen's Disease Center both recommend ethionamide for patients with multibacillary forms of leprosy who refuse to take clofazimine. The World Health Organization recommends a daily oral dose of 250 to 375 mg, self-administered, for a minimum of 2 years or until skin tests are negative. The National Hansen's Disease Center recommended dose of ethionamide is 250 mg by mouth daily, taken indefinitely.

Laboratory Considerations

Desired therapeutic serum levels of dapsone are 0.1 to 7 mcg/mL. As a result of its long half-life, dapsone may be present in the body up to 3 weeks after it is discontinued.

Dapsone has been shown to decrease the platelet count and hemoglobin levels by 1 to 2 g/dL, and to increase the reticulocyte count by 2 to 12 percent. As a result, complete blood counts are recommended at regular intervals during the first few weeks of therapy and then every 3 to 6 months.

Dapsone has also been associated with increased serum levels of alkaline phosphatase, aspartate transaminase (serum glutamic-oxaloacetic transaminase), alanine transaminase (serum glutamate pyruvate transaminase), lactate dehydrogenase, and bilirubin. These values should be monitored before and during therapy. Methemoglobinemia may be present, so hemoglobin levels should be monitored if patients develop cyanosis, headache, fatigue, and/or shortness of breath.

Therapeutic serum levels of clofazimine average 0.7 mcg/mL for patients receiving 100 mg daily, and 1 mcg/mL for patients receiving 300 mg daily. To date, there is no correlation between serum concentrations and therapeutic effects of the drug.

The erythrocyte sedimentation rate may be raised in the presence of clofazimine. The serum albumin, aspartate transaminase (serum glutamic-oxaloacetic transaminase), bilirubin, and blood glucose levels may also be increased. The serum potassium level is reduced.

Newer Antileprotic Drugs

Fluoroquinolones have shown new promise in the treatment of leprosy. As mentioned in the discussion of tuberculosis, floxacin and ciprofloxacin are thought to be bactericidal. Single-dose and multiple-dose regimens are being utilized in clinical trials.

Critical Thinking Process

Assessment

History of Present Illness

The patient's history provides pertinent information about the course of the disease. The health care provider should elicit specific information about signs and symptoms related to skin lesions, contact with individuals known to have the disease, contact with armadillos (a naturally acquired leprosy has been found in armadillos), and immigration from or living for extended periods in endemic areas. Specific information to be obtained about the skin lesions includes time since the appearance of the lesions, their location, characteristics, and quantity, and any associated manifestations. The health care provider should ask specifically about loss of sensation, the patient's reaction to skin lesions, and any use of home remedies.

Past Health History

The past health history provides information about allergies and injuries, hospitalizations not already described, and drug history. Patients with leprosy may have a history of sensorimotor dysfunction leading to deformities that predispose to accidents or injuries. A detailed family history may identify the source of the infection. A thorough drug history including allergies is necessary to determine the appropriate drugs to treat the infection.

Physical Exam Findings

Clinical diagnosis of leprosy is based on complete examination of the skin. During the physical exam, the patient's need for privacy should be respected. All skin areas need to be examined, especially those where skin lesions commonly occur (i.e., face, ears, and extremities). The skin lesions are characteristically nonpruritic, and are hypopigmented in dark-skinned persons and erythematous in light-skinned persons. The number, type, location, and characteristics of any lesions must be documented. Any sensorimotor dysfunction, such as loss of sensation, muscular weakness, or deformity, is important to note. The patient should be examined for edema, particularly of the face, hands, and feet. Peripheral nerve trunks (ulnar nerve at the elbow, peroneal nerve at the head of the fibula, and the great auricular nerve) should be examined bilaterally to compare size, extent of softness, hardness, or firmness, and tenderness.

The patient should also be examined for signs of leprosy reactions. In type 1 reactions, signs of neuritis should be sought. With type 2 reactions, the examiner should watch for signs of painful skin lesions, fever, inflammation of the eyes, arthritis, lymphadenopathy, and glomerulonephritis.

Diagnostic Testing

Mycobacterium leprae is rarely found in smears made from quiescent lesions but may appear during activity. *M. leprae* is demonstrable in the lepromatous form of the disorder when Virchow's cells are present.

The lepromin skin test helps identify the form of leprosy a patient has and the prognosis for that patient. Lepromin (a preparation of killed *M. leprae*) is injected intradermally, and the reaction is evaluated 4 weeks later. The presence of a nodule and a 3-mm or larger area of induration denotes a positive response in the tuberculoid and borderline tuberculoid forms of leprosy. In contrast, the lepromatous and borderline lepromatous forms demonstrate a negative response to the lepromin test. With mid-borderline and indeterminate forms, the results are variable; the response demonstrates the patient's tendency toward either the tuberculoid or the lepromatous end of the immunologic spectrum and is of prognostic value.

Developmental Considerations

Perinatal Transmission of the disease from an untreated, infected mother to an infant is not uncommon. Pregnancy

Case Study Leprosy

Patient History

History of Present Illness	MF is a 30-year-old white female with symmetric "red spots that don't itch or hurt" on arms and face near the eyes, and in nares. States they first appeared 6 weeks ago.
Past Health History	Denies allergies to food or drugs. Only hospitalization was at age 16 for appendectomy.
Physical Exam	Macular, erythematous lesions on forearms and left forehead near eyes. Lesions within nares apparent. Loss of hair and sensation in and around all affected areas.
Diagnostic Testing	Skin smears confirm *M. leprae*. Lepromin skin test positive. Sulfone sensitivity testing confirms sensitivity to dapsone.
Developmental Considerations	Worried about changes in self-image caused by presence of lesions.
Psychosocial Considerations	Currently active-duty military who just returned from a remote 4-year assignment in Southeast Asia. Single and lives on base in the barracks. Drinks 1–2 beers/week but denies other drug use.
Economic Factors	Military health care system provides pharmacy services to patient without cost while on active duty.

Variables Influencing Decision

Treatment Objectives
- Render patient noninfectious
- Prevent spread of infection

Drug Variables	*Drug Summary*	*Patient Variables*
Indications	Dapsone, rifampin, and clofazimine combinations for paucibacillary and multibacillary forms. With no documented dapsone resistance, dapsone should be used with rifampin to prevent *M. leprae* from multiplying.	Patient diagnosed with borderline lepromatous (BL), one of the multibacillary forms of leprosy. Dapsone in combination with rifampin appropriate for multibacillary, sulfone-sensitive strain of *M. leprae*.
Pharmacodynamics	Dapsone and clofazimine are bacteriostatic. Rifampin is bactericidal. Combinations of dapsone and rifampin are effective and avoid development of mycobacterial resistance.	Since a combination of bactericidal and bacteriostatic drugs will be used, this will not become a decision point.
Adverse Effects/ Contraindications	Dapsone: Dose-dependent hemolytic anemia, jaundice, hepatitis. Rifampin: Nausea, vomiting, diarrhea, red-orange color to body fluids. Clofazimine: Dose-dependent nausea, vomiting, diarrhea, abdominal pain, brown-black discoloration to skin lesions and body fluids.	Will be a decision point owing to broad variation in adverse effects, although overall side effects at 0.4%. Since drugs produce color changes to body fluids, MF's self-image may be affected.
Pharmacokinetics	Pharmacokinetic parameters are all different for each of the three drugs.	Because all three drugs have different pharmacokinetics, this may be a decision point. The long serum half-life of dapsone (30 hr) creates a wide therapeutic margin.

Case Study Leprosy—cont'd

Drug Variables	Drug Summary	Patient Variables
Dosage Regimen	Per National Hansen's Disease Center, the World Health Organization, and manufacturer's recommendation, minimum duration of rifampin therapy is 3 years after skin tests are negative for BL form of leprosy, but therapy with dapsone may continue indefinitely.	Compliance with long-term therapy may be of concern. While on active duty, MF will have oversight by care provider, so this is not a decision point. May become an issue if MF leaves military service.
Laboratory Considerations	Complete blood count and liver-function studies should be done before therapy is initiated and periodically during treatment. Periodic skin smears and lepromin skin testing should also be done.	Military health care system will perform skin smears, lepromin testing, complete blood count, and liver function testing while patient on active duty in military.
Cost Index*	Dapsone: 1 Rifampin: 1 Clofazimine: 1	Military health care system will provide drug therapy without cost to patient while she is on active duty. Concern would be that if patient is discharged, rifampin is relatively expensive even if taken monthly.

Summary of Decision Points

- Because of the emergence of dapsone-resistant strains of *M. leprae,* combination therapy is recommended.
- Dapsone remains drug of choice for all sulfone-sensitive strains of leprosy.
- Emotional support of patient vital, because these drugs produce color changes of body fluids and patient already has body image concerns.
- Lab monitoring vital, because dapsone is associated with an increase in liver function parameters and decreases in reticulocyte, hemoglobin, and platelet values.

DRUGS TO BE USED

- Dapsone, 100 mg daily unsupervised with rifampin 600 mg once/month supervised; dapsone is continued indefinitely, rifampin for 3 years.

*Cost Index:
1 = < $ 30/mo.
2 = $ 30–40/mo.
3 = $ 40–50/mo.
4 = $ 50–60/mo.
5 = > $ 60/mo.

AWP of 30, 100-mg tablets of dapsone is approximately $11.
AWP of 2, 300-mg capsules of rifampin is approximately $4.
AWP of 30, 50-mg capsules of clofazimine is approximately $5.

and the subsequent 6 months of lactation are said to result in an exacerbation in about one-third of patients with leprosy. The fetal effects are said to include low birth weight, small placenta, and a high incidence of infant mortality.

Pediatric Leprosy can manifest at any age, but it is seldom seen in children younger than 3 years. The age-specific incidence peaks during childhood in most developing countries. Up to 20 percent of cases appear in children younger than 10 years. Because leprosy is most prevalent in poorer socioeconomic groups, this figure may simply reflect the age distribution of the high-risk population. The gender ratio of leprosy manifesting during childhood is 1:1, although males predominate by a 2:1 ratio in adulthood manifestation. The physiologic immunodeficiency of the newborn may lead to an early colonization with the bacillus.

Geriatric The immunosuppression found in the older adult causes infections to be a significant risk factor for this age group. Thymic mass is steadily lost, so that serum activity of thymic hormones is almost undetectable. With the decline in T-cell activity and the presence of higher numbers of immature T cells in the thymus, a significant decline in cell-mediated immunity occurs. Thus, T lymphocytes are less able to proliferate in response to *M. leprae*.

Psychosocial Considerations

The social stigma associated with leprosy has been noted throughout history. The Hebrew word "leper" (from Greek translations) meant someone who was an outcast from society. Dating back to biblical times, the castigation of persons with leprosy is gradually being replaced with the attitude that leprosy is a disease, not a social stigma. Even today, though, the word leprosy has negative connotations. A person with leprosy has been characterized as one who is "a morally or spiritually harmful influence."

Leprosy has been identified as a disease affecting the body of the patient and the mind of the public. The attitudes of health care providers toward patients with leprosy can influence public opinion.

Analysis and Management

Treatment Objectives

The objective of treatment is to render the patient noninfectious, thereby preventing the spread of the disease. To achieve this objective, the patient should be given the correct dose and combination of drugs for an appropriate duration and, if necessary, should be supervised to ensure compliance.

Treatment Options

Drug Variables

The principal treatment for leprosy is pharmacotherapy. Treatment recommendations for leprosy, according to the World Health Organization and the National Hansen's Disease Center, consist of dapsone, rifampin, and clofazimine. Clinical evidence suggests that in most instances, infectiousness is lost within 3 months of continuous and regular treatment with antileprotic drugs, or within 3 days of treatment with rifampin.

Because of the emergence of dapsone-resistant strains of *M. leprae,* combination drug therapy is recommended. The use of combination drug therapy rapidly decreases a patient's infectious state and reduces the likelihood that resistant strains will develop. With a long half-life (30 hours), the serum concentration of dapsone remains high for days, thus creating a wide therapeutic margin. As a result, *M. leprae* bacilli are prevented from multiplying, even when there is moderate resistance to the drug.

Rifampin, in combination with other antileprotic drugs, is recommended for all forms of leprosy. It has a rapid effect, and a single dose of 600 mg has been found to kill 99 percent of the bacilli, thus rendering the patient noninfectious. The bactericidal effect of ethionamide appears sooner than that of dapsone but later than that of rifampin.

The appearance of bactericidal effects of clofazimine is between those of dapsone and rifampin. However, it takes approximately 50 days for clofazimine's bactericidal activity to occur. Concurrent use of clofazimine with rifampin may decrease the rate of absorption of rifampin. This factor becomes an important consideration if the response to leprosy treatment is poor.

In 1982, the World Health Organization recommended a shortened drug regimen for leprosy. A short-term regimen is more feasible than long-term therapy (possible life-long) in most developing countries. In the United States, the National Hansen's Disease Center recommends a longer regimen of drug therapy than that suggested by the World Health Organization.

Patient Variables

Infectious patients need not be hospitalized, provided that (1) there is compliance with the treatment plan and adequate supervision, (2) the home environment meets specific conditions, and (3) the local health officer concurs in the disposition of the case. Patient as well as drug variables identified during assessment should be taken into account in the planning of the treatment regimen. Not all data obtained from the history, physical exam, and laboratory findings are relevant to a drug regimen. However, relevant data include information that affects treatment objectives, compliance, pharmacokinetic parameters, evaluation of treatment effectiveness, and adverse effects. Compliance with the treatment regimen and the patient's response are both influenced by the physiologic as well as the developmental and psychosocial aspects of the disease.

Developmental changes seen in the perinatal, pediatric, and geriatric patient are vital to effective drug therapy. Pharmacotherapy for leprosy should be undertaken with caution during pregnancy. Studies have demonstrated no adverse effects on the fetus from dapsone. However, because of the risk for tumor development in animal studies, dapsone is not recommended for nursing mothers. The patient should make an informed decision regarding whether to discontinue nursing the infant or taking the drug. The risk-benefit ratio of the use of rifampin should be thoroughly explained. Rifampin is secreted in breast milk and has tumorigenic effects similar to those of dapsone.

Clofazimine is not recommended during the first trimester of pregnancy or for use in nursing mothers. Infants born to mothers taking this drug have darkened skin tones that gradually fade within the first year.

Ethionamide is not recommended in pregnant or lactating women with leprosy. It crosses the placenta to cause developmental abnormalities.

Studies in the pediatric population are limited at present. The available data suggest no specific problems with dapsone or rifampin. Clofazimine has been used with a limited number of children, although no pediatric dose has been established. Ethionamide may be used if other antileprotic drugs are unavailable. Children receiving antileprotic drugs should be followed closely and observed for adverse effects, including hepatic impairment.

Intervention

Administration

Dapsone should be taken with food if GI upset occurs. The prescription instructions should be followed carefully. Efficacy depends on prolonged use. Dapsone should not be used if the patient is allergic to sulfonamide preparations.

To maximize absorption, clofazimine should be taken with food or milk. Like dapsone, clofazimine is needed for a prolonged period. The drug should be protected from moisture and heat. In patients who experience abdominal pain, diarrhea, or colic, the dosage may need to be reduced. If reactional leprosy episodes occur (worsening of leprosy activity related to therapy), the use of other antileprotic drugs, analgesics, corticosteroids, or surgery may be necessary.

The absorption of rifampin is reduced when the drug is taken with food. It should be taken either 1 hour before or 2 hours after a meal, followed by a full glass (240 mL) of water. If GI irritation becomes a problem, rifampin can be administered with food. Capsules may be opened and their contents mixed with applesauce or jelly for patients with difficulty swallowing. A pharmacist can compound a syrup for patients unable to swallow the solid formulation.

As previously stated, infectious patients need not be hospitalized, provided that (1) there is compliance with the treatment plan and adequate supervision, (2) the home environment meets specific conditions, and (3) the local health officer concurs in the disposition of the case.

Education

The patient and family should be given written instructions about all drugs, including the name, the prescribed dose, the reason for taking the drug, its adverse effects, and when to call the health care provider. The patient should be reminded about the importance of completing the entire drug regimen, which may take years. If the patient misses a dose of antileprotic drugs, the patient should take that dose as soon as possible but should not take a double dose. The adverse effects of the drugs, particularly skin discoloration and serious GI problems, should be discussed with the patient.

Support and encouragement are warranted to help the patient deal with the changes in skin pigmentation. The health care provider should reassure the patient that skin color changes are usually reversible but may take several months to years to disappear. There have been reports of suicides by patients due to severe depression about the pigmentation effects. The patient should be informed of the support groups available to help with this issue.

Patients taking clofazimine who experience dry, itchy skin may find relief by using an oil or an emollient with urea. Patients should be informed of all adverse effects related to clofazimine, including skin color changes and changes in the color of body fluids, to ensure compliance with the drug regimen.

Evaluation

Symptoms that indicate resolution of the infection should be monitored. Improvement of skin lesions and an improvement in cell-mediated immunity status should be noted. Resolution of skin lesions may take 8 to 12 weeks, depending on the severity of the disease.

Determined by the type of leprosy, some treatment regimens may last as long as 10 years, and others for life.

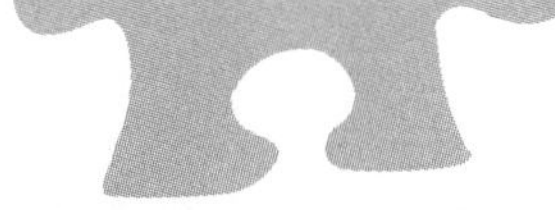

SUMMARY

- The highest incidences of TB are in males 25 to 44 years and in children younger than 15 years, as well as in the Native American, Hispanic, black, Asian, and Oceania populations.
- Noncompliance, crowded institutional settings, increasing numbers of homeless persons, substance abuse, the emigration of infected persons, and lack of access to health care have contributed to the rising incidence of TB.
- Two primary factors have been associated with the rise in TB: the epidemic of human immunodeficiency virus infection (HIV) and acquired immune deficiency syndrome (AIDS), and the development of growing numbers of drug-resistant strains of the tubercular bacillus.
- The extent of communicability of TB depends on the number and virulence of discharged bacilli, adequacy of ventilation, exposure of the bacilli to the sun or ultraviolet light, and opportunities for aerosolization.
- The appearance of a lung infection with no known prior exposure to the organism is referred to as *primary TB*. *Reactivation TB* applies when dormant bacilli become endogenously reactive or the individual has a repeated exposure to the TB.
- In *miliary TB* (disseminated disease), more common in older adult patients, bacilli are dispersed throughout body organs and tissues.
- The objectives of treatment are eliminating the patient's infectious state and preventing the development of drug-resistant strains of TB.
- First-line antitubercular drugs are isoniazid, rifampin, ethambutol, and pyrazinamide. Streptomycin may be an option in some cases.
- Second-line antitubercular drugs are cycloserine, capreomycin, kanamycin, and ethionamide.
- Short-term therapy takes place over 6 to 9 months, whereas conventional therapy typically lasts 18 to 24 months.
- Patients with TB may present with progressive symptoms of fatigue, lethargy, nausea, anorexia, weight loss, irregular menses, night sweats, and low-grade fevers.
- A positive sputum culture for acid-fast bacilli confirms the diagnosis of TB.
- An area of induration measuring 10 mm or more in diameter on the Mantoux test indicates exposure to TB and the production of antibodies against the bacillus.
- Nursing care of patients receiving antitubercular drugs includes educating the individual and/or family about the importance of adhering to the prescribed medication regimen.
- Because therapy for tuberculosis is complex and lengthy, drug toxicity, poor patient compliance, and the development of microbial resistance present significant problems.
- To achieve treatment objectives, the patient should be given the correct dose and combination of drugs for an appropriate period of time, and, if necessary, should be supervised to ensure compliance.
- Successful antitubercular therapy is noted as an absence of observable mycobacteria in the sputum and as the failure of sputum cultures to yield colonies of bacilli.
- An estimated 12 million patients worldwide have leprosy.
- The diagnosis of leprosy is based on the presence of skin lesions with a loss of sensation, enlarged peripheral nerves, and acid-fast bacilli in skin smears.
- *Mycobacterium leprae (M. leprae),* a slow-growing bacillus, causes leprosy.
- Humans are the only reservoir of proven significance, and although the exact mode of transmission is not clearly known, household and prolonged close contacts appear to be important.

- The incubation period for leprosy ranges from 9 months to 20 years, with an average of approximately 4 years for the tuberculoid form, and twice that for lepromatous leprosy.
- Paucibacillary leprosy comprises indeterminate, tuberculoid, and borderline tuberculoid forms. Multibacillary leprosy comprises mid-borderline, borderline lepromatous, and lepromatous forms.
- Differences in cell-mediated immunity may account for the various forms of leprosy.
- The objectives of treatment are to render patients noninfectious and to prevent spread of disease.
- Treatment options for leprosy primarily are dapsone, rifampin, and clofazimine.
- Dapsone is considered the drug of choice for all forms of leprosy caused by sulfone-sensitive strains. Clofazimine is especially potent against sulfone-resistant strains of *M. leprae.* Ethionamide may be used as a substitute for clofazimine in the treatment of multibacillary forms of leprosy.
- Specific information to elicit about skin lesions includes the length of time since the onset of lesions, as well as their location, characteristics, and quantity, associated loss of sensation, the patient's response to the skin lesions, and the use of home remedies.
- Patients with leprosy may have a history of sensorimotor dysfunction that leads to deformities and predisposes the patient to accidents or injuries.
- The skin lesions are characteristically nonpruritic, being hypopigmented in dark-skinned persons and erythematous in light-skinned persons.
- Patients should understand that the key to controlling leprosy is to prevent the spread of the disease. This may require a life-long commitment by the patient to comply with therapy.
- To achieve treatment objectives, the patient should be given the correct dose and combination of drugs for an appropriate period of time and, if necessary, should be supervised to ensure compliance.
- Symptoms that indicate resolution of the infection should be monitored.

BIBLIOGRAPHY

American Thoracic Society. (1994). Treatment of tuberculosis and tuberculosis infection in adults and children. *American Journal of Respiratory and Critical Care Medicine,* 149, 1359–1374.

American Thoracic Society. (1990). Diagnostic standards and classification of tuberculosis. *American Review of Respiratory Diseases,* 142(3), 725–735.

Antimycobacterial agents. (1994). In *Drug evaluations.* Chicago: American Medical Association.

Bayer, R., and Wilkinson, D. (1995). Directly observed therapy for tuberculosis: History of an idea. *Lancet,* 345(4), 1545–1548.

Benenson, A. (Ed.) (1990). *Control of communicable diseases in man.* (15th ed.). Washington, DC: American Public Health Association.

Bloom, B., and Murray, C. (1992). Tuberculosis: Commentary on a recurrent killer. *Science,* 257, 1055–1078.

Boutotte, J. (1993). TB: The second time around. *Nursing '93,* 22(5),42–49.

Brausch, L., and Bass, J. (1993). The treatment of tuberculosis. *Medical Clinics of North America,* 77(6), 1277–1286.

Drugs for tuberculosis. (1995). *The Medical Letter on Drugs and Therapeutics,* 37(954), 67–70.

Dutt, A., and Stead, W. (1993). Tuberculosis in the elderly. In Mahler, D. (Ed.). *Pulmonary disease in the elderly.* New York: Marcel Dekker.

Ellard, G. (1991). The chemotherapy of leprosy. Part 2. *International Journal of Leprosy,* 59(1), 82–90.

Goodless, D., and Johnson, A. (1990). Hansen's disease update. *Journal of Florida Medical Association,* 77(5), 520–525.

Gray, M. (1993). Medications for a growing concern: Tuberculosis. *Orthopaedic Nursing,* 12(2), 75–79.

Iseman, M. (1993). Directly observed treatment of tuberculosis: We can't afford not to try it. *New England Journal of Medicine,* 328(8), 576–578.

Iseman, M. (1993). Treatment of multidrug-resistant tuberculosis. *The New England Journal of Medicine,* 329(11), 784–791.

Jereb, J., Kelly, G., Dooley, S., et al. (1991). Tuberculosis morbidity in the United States: Final data, 1990. In CDC Surveillance Summaries. *Morbidity and Mortality Weekly Report,* 40(No.SS-3), 23–27.

Lancaster, E. (1993). Tuberculosis comeback: Impact on long-term care facilities. *Journal of Gerontological Nursing,* 19(7), 16–21.

Lordi, G., and Reichman, L. (1993). Drug resistance to tuberculosis: The new face of an old enemy. *Drug Therapy,* 23(3), 17.

Lordi, G., and Reichman, L. (1991). Treatment of tuberculosis. *American Family Physician,* 44(1), 219–224.

McMahon-Casey, K. (1993). Fighting MDR-TB. *RN,* 56(9), 26–31.

McEvoy, G. (Ed.) (1994). Drug information. American Hospital Formulary Service. Bethesda, MD: American Society of Hospital Pharmacists.

O'Brien, L., and Bartlett, K. (1992). TB plus HIV spells trouble. *American Journal of Nursing,* 92(5), 28–34.

Peloquin, C. (1993). Pharmacology of the antimycobacterial drugs. *Medical Clinics of North America,* 77(6), 1253–1262.

Peloquin, C. (1992). Therapeutic drug monitoring: Principles and applications in mycobacterial infections. *Drug Therapy,* 22(7), 31.

Starke, J. (1992). Current chemotherapy for tuberculosis in children. *Infectious Disease Clinics of North America,* 6(1), 215–238.

Srinivasan, H. (1993). *Prevention of disabilities in patients with leprosy: A practical guide.* Geneva: World Health Organization.

Takayama, K., Schnoes, H., Armstrong, E., et al. (1975). Site of inhibitory action of isoniazid in the synthesis of mycolic acids in *Mycobacterium tuberculosis. Journal of Lipid Research,* 16, 308–317.

Thangaraj, R., and Yamalkar, S. (1987). *Leprosy for medical practitioners and paramedical workers.* (2nd ed.). Basel: Ciba-Geigy Limited.

U.S. Centers for Disease Control. (1990). Screening for tuberculosis and tuberculosis infection in high-risk populations, and the use of preventative therapy for tuberculosis infection in the United States. *Morbidity and Mortality Weekly Report,* 39(RR-18), 1–12.

U.S. Congress, Office of Technology Assessment. (1993). *The continuing challenge of tuberculosis.* Washington, DC: U.S. Government Printing Office.

Weis, S., Slocum, P., Blais, F., et al. (1994). The effect of directly observed therapy on the rate of drug resistance and relapse in tuberculosis. *New England Journal of Medicine,* 330, 1179–1184.

World Health Organization. (1988). *A guide to leprosy control.* (2nd ed.) Singapore: Macmillan.

World Health Organization. (1991). *WHO model prescribing information—drugs used in mycobacterial diseases.* Geneva: World Health Organization.

Yoshikawa, T. (1992). Infectious diseases. *Clinics in Geriatric Medicine,* 8(4),761–773.

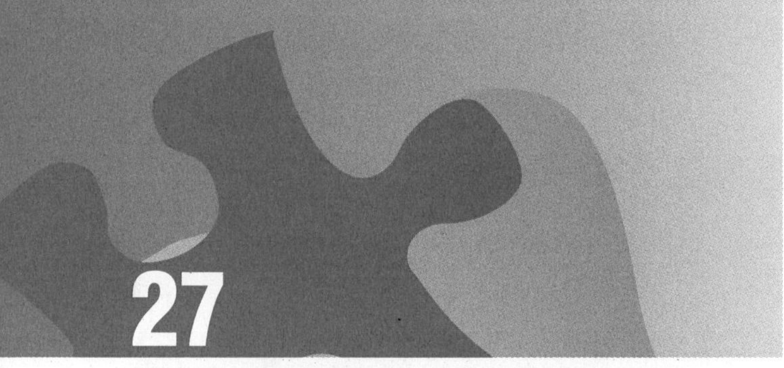

27 Anthelmintic, Antimalarial, and Antiparasitic Drugs

Helminthic, parasitic, and malarial diseases account for major health problems throughout the world, particularly in developing countries. Health care providers have become more familiar with the diseases as a group because of increased travel and immigration from endemic regions. Although major infestations are more commonly associated with tropical climates, outbreaks are becoming universal in distribution.

HELMINTHIASIS

Epidemiology and Etiology

Helminthiasis, an infestation of parasitic worms, is a major health problem in many parts of the world, affecting more than 2 billion people. In the United States, more than 60 million people are estimated to harbor a helminthic parasite.

Parasitic worms can be divided into three groups: nematodes (roundworms), cestodes (flatworms and tapeworms), and trematodes (flukes) (Table 27–1). Relatively unchanged from the beginnings of organic life forms, these creatures live dependently by sharing the body juices of plants, animals, and humans. The presence of worms, most often in the gastrointestinal (GI) tract, bladder, lungs, and liver of a human, is called an "infestation" rather than an "infection."

Roundworm Infestation

Roundworm (nematode) infestations are the most common helminthic disease in the world. They occur most often in tropical regions, where the prevalence often exceeds 50 percent. The prevalence and intensity of infestations are usually highest in children between the ages of 3 and 8 years. Distribution in the United States is limited to the Southeastern states.

Trichinosis (infection with *Trichinella spiralis*), also an intestinal roundworm infestation, occurs worldwide but with variable incidence. It is most often associated with inadequately cooked meat, especially pork. Necropsy results obtained in the mid-20th century revealed a prevalence of 16.7 percent in the United States. The age-adjusted rate is now 2 percent or less. Cases are usually sporadic, and outbreaks localized.

Roundworm infestations, particularly trichinosis, produce variable clinical disorders, from an occult infestation to a fulminating, fatal disease, depending on the number of larvae ingested. The infestations are transmitted through ingestion of contaminated food and water. Live worms, passed in feces and occasionally from the mouth or nose, are often the first-recognized sign of infestation. Some patients have pulmonary manifestations (i.e., sneezing, coughing, fever, eosinophilia, pulmonary infiltration). Serious bowel obstructions, particularly in children, or obstruction by one or more adult worms of the bile duct, pancreatic duct, and appendix may occur. In time, the larvae wall off in the tissues, remaining in the body for 10 years or longer.

Hookworm Infestations

Hookworm infestations are widely endemic in tropical and subtropical countries (e.g., Far East, Southeast Asia, South Pacific, Africa) where sanitary disposal of human feces is not practiced and the soil, moisture, and temperature conditions favor larvae development. They may also occur in temperate climates under the same conditions. The specific agent varies with geographic locale.

Hookworm is spread by ova-containing feces from infected people. Ova develop into larvae after deposition on the soil. Upon contact (usually through the foot), larvae burrow through the skin to cause a characteristic dermatitis. They pass through lymphatics and blood stream to the lungs, enter the alveoli, and migrate to the trachea and pharynx. They are then swallowed, reaching the small intestine, where they attach to the mucosa. Adult hookworms typically produce eggs in 6 to 7 weeks.

Tapeworm Infestations

Six varieties of tapeworms infest humans. *Diphyllobothrium latum* (fish tapeworm) is the largest, growing up to 10 meters in length. The fish tapeworm is a segmented flatworm. The head has hooks or suckers that attach to tissues and a number of segments (proglottids) that in some cases may extend 20 to 30 feet in the bowel. This worm has no digestive tract, so it depends on nutrients that are intended for the host. Upon ingestion, the larvae mature to adulthood in the intestine and travel to extraintestinal sites such as liver, muscle, and eye tissues.

Diphyllobothrium latum tapeworms are prevalent in the waters of northern Michigan and Minnesota as well as Canada, and are found in raw gefilte fish. Contamination of bodies of fresh water by raw sewage increases the risk for infestation. Infestation is acquired by exposure to parasitic cysts contained in smoked or uncooked fresh-water fish (e.g., sushi, sashimi, or ceviche). The worms reach maturity in 3 to 6 weeks and survive for up to 20 years.

The beef tapeworm *(Taenia saginata)* and pork tapeworm *(Taenia solium)* are found in contaminated, raw, or improperly cooked beef and pork, respectively. The pork tapeworm is commonly found in Central and South America, India, and Mexico. Although rare in the United States, an infestation of the pork tapeworm is more serious, because it produces larvae that enter the circulation and migrate to other body tissues (i.e., muscles, liver, lungs, brain). The beef tapeworm is found more often in the Middle East, Kenya, Ethiopia, South America, Mexico, and Russia.

TABLE 27–1 SELECTED HELMINTHS

Infestation or Condition	Helminths	Geographic Distribution	Source or Route of Transmission
Roundworms (Nematodes)			
Ascariasis	*Ascaris lumbricoides*	Warm, moist climates	Eggs, vegtables, soil, feces
Pinworms	*Enterobius vermicularis*	Common in children in U.S.	Feces or soil to food, hand to mouth
Uncinariasis	*Ancylostoma duodenale* *Necator americanus* (Hookworm)	Europe, Italy, Asia, North Africa, Middle and Far East, South America	Feces to soil to skin
Strongyloidiasis	*Strongyloides stercoralis* (Threadworm)	Most tropics, southern U.S.	
Trichuriasis	*Trichuris trichiura* (Whipworm)	Rare in U.S.	Feces to soil to food
Trichinosis	*Trichinella spiralis* (Pork roundworm)	Northern hemisphere	Meat, usually pork
Intestinal Tapeworms (Cestodes)			
Diphyllobothriasis	*Diphyllobothrium latum* (Fish tapeworm)	Northern Michigan, Canada	Fresh-water fish
Taeniasis	*Taenia saginata* (Beef tapeworm)	Middle East, Kenya, Ethiopia, South America, Mexico, Russia	Raw beef
	Taenia solium (Pork tapeworm)	Central and South America, India, Mexico	Raw pork
Hymenolepiasis	*Hymenolepis nana* (Dwarf tapeworm)	Southern U.S.	Eggs
Tissue Tapeworms			
Cystic hydatid disease	*Echinococcus granulosus*	Sheep pastures, Alaska, Utah, Arizona, Nevada	Dog feces
Alveolar hydatid disease	*Echinococcus multilocularis*	Primarily northern hemisphere	Dog feces
Cysticercosis	*Cysticercus cellulosae*	Mexico, Central and South America, India, China	*T. solium* eggs in feces-contaminated food and soil
Flukes (Trematodes)			
Intestinal	*Fasciolopsis buski* *Heterophyes* *Metagonimus*	Rare in U.S.	Water, plants, fresh-water fish
Hepatic	*Fasciola hepatica* *Clonorchis sinensis*	Common in sheep pastures	Water, plants, fresh-water fish
Pulmonary	*Paragonimus westermani* Other *Paragonimus* species	Africa, Orient, South America, Near East, rare in U.S.	Contaminated crabs, crayfish
Blood	*Schistosoma japonicum*	Orient, Africa, South America, Near East	Water contaminated with forked-tail larvae from snails
	Schistosoma mansoni	Africa, West India, South America, Middle East	
	Schistosoma mekongi	Japan, China, Philippines	

Threadworm Infestation

As with other helminthiases, infestations of threadworms (*Strongyloides stercoralis* or other *Strongyloides* spp.) are found throughout tropical and temperate climates. Their prevalence is not accurately known, although the incidence is greater in institutions where personal hygiene is poor. *S. fulleborni* has been reported only in Africa and Papua New Guinea.

Threadworms enter the body and are carried to the lungs. They penetrate capillary walls, enter alveoli, and ascend from the trachea to the epiglottis. They then descend into the digestive tract and burrow into the mucosa of the duodenum and upper jejunum. The female lays eggs, but the male is eliminated in the feces. The eggs hatch into larvae that can penetrate all body tissues. The period from penetration of the skin to evidence of larvae in the feces is about 2 weeks. The time until symptoms appear is indefinite and variable.

Pinworm Infestation

Pinworm *(Enterobius vermicularis)* infestation is the most common parasitic worm infestation in the United States. The highest prevalence is in school-age children, followed by preschoolers. The incidence is lowest in adults, except for mothers of infected children. Infection often occurs in more than one family member. In some groups, it reaches nearly 50 percent prevalence. Figures are higher in domiciliary institutions.

Pinworm infestation is caused by direct transfer of infective eggs by hand from the anus to the mouth of the same or another person. They may also be transmitted indirectly through clothing, bedding, food, or other contaminated articles.

Pinworm eggs become infective within a few hours after being deposited at the anus by migrating gravid females. Larvae from ingested eggs hatch in the small intestine (Fig. 27–1). Young worms mature in the cecum and upper portions of the

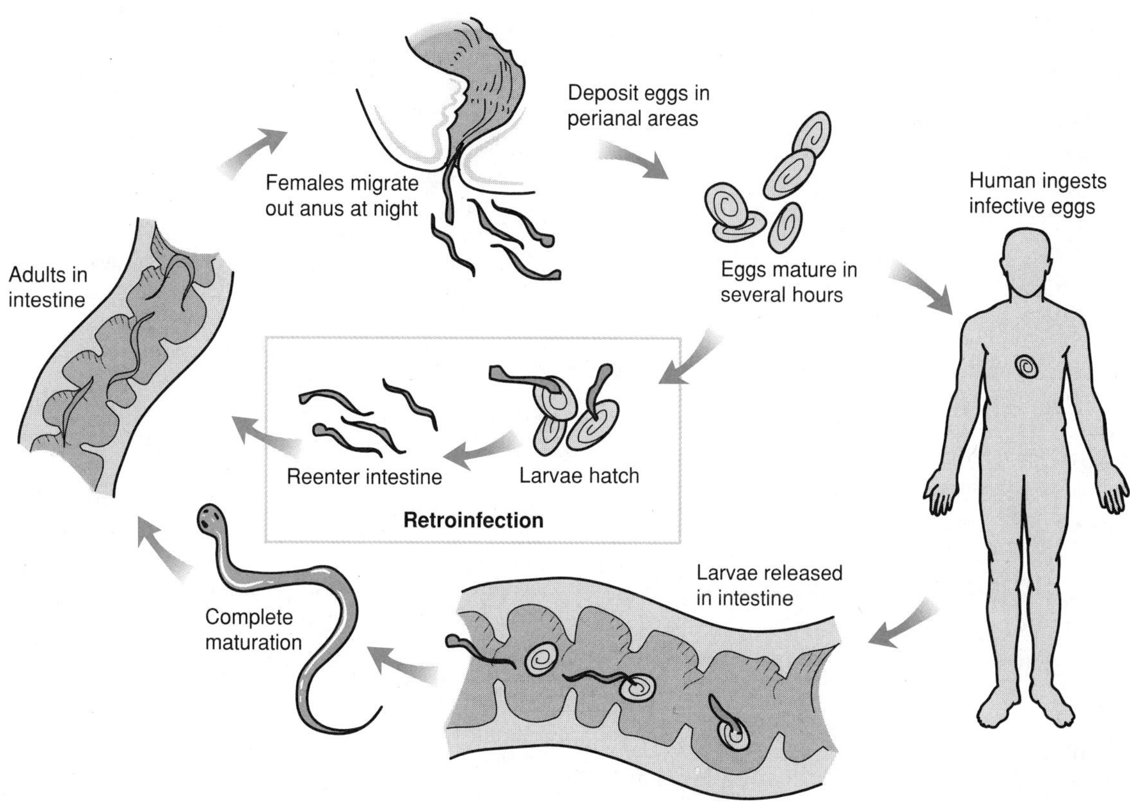

Figure 27–1 Life cycle of *Enterobius vermicularis.* Pinworm infestation is caused by direct transfer of infective eggs by hand from the anus to the mouth of the same or another person. Larvae from ingested eggs hatch in the small intestine. Young worms mature in the cecum and upper portions of the colon. (From Mahon, C. R., and Manuselis, G., Jr. [1995]. *Textbook of diagnostic microbiology* [p. 781]. Philadelphia: W. B. Saunders. Used with permission.)

colon. Gravid worms may actively migrate from the rectum to enter adjacent orifices. Their life cycle takes 2 to 6 weeks to complete. The eggs survive less than 2 weeks outside the body. Symptomatic disease with high worm loads results from successive reinfections within months of the initial exposure.

Trematodes

Trematodes are the "flukes" of the worm world. They utilize snail hosts as intermediaries but are also found as cercariae (the free-swimming larval stage in the development of a fluke). These worms develop within sporocysts that parasitize snails or bivalve mollusks. They emerge from the mollusk either to enter their final host directly or to encyst in an intermediate host that is eaten by the final host. For example, the cercariae of the species *Clonorchis sinensis* are eaten by fish, which in turn are eaten by humans. The cercariae invade the intestinal tract. They can live in the human liver for 20 to 50 years, continually passing eggs into the feces. These organisms even live through the pickling process used to preserve many varieties of fish.

Trematodes are cosmopolitan and common in many watery areas of the world, such as Asia, Japan, central and south China, Thailand, Africa, South America, and the West Indies. They are relatively rare in the United States.

Their pattern of infestation consists of penetration of the skin followed by migration to the hepatic portal circulation or into the duodenum. From these locations, they migrate to the bladder or intestines or to the bile ducts or pancreas, respectively.

Symptoms of trematode infestation are diverse, ranging from asymptomatic with findings only at autopsy to swimmer's itch, a benign form of schistosomiasis. The penetrating cercariae cause fever, urticaria, eosinophilia, hepatosplenomegaly, and lymphadenopathy. When the adults reach their appointed location, symptoms such as cystitis and chronic diarrhea arise. It is not uncommon to diagnose ascites of unknown etiology in a patient in whom an infestation has been overlooked.

Pathophysiology

Helminthic infestations usually do not cause clinical manifestations, although they may be detrimental for a number of reasons. Heavy infestations produce nutritional deficits, particularly in children. Host tissues can be traumatized, thus predisposing the patient to bacterial infection. Toxic substances produced by the helminth may be absorbed by the host. In large numbers, helminths cause obstruction of lymphatic channels and massive edema. Intestinal obstruction and blood loss may also occur.

PHARMACOTHERAPEUTIC OPTIONS

Anthelmintics

❒ Diethylcarbamazine citrate (HETRAZAN)
❒ Mebendazole (VERMOX); (🍁) NEMASOLE

- ❐ Niclosamide (NICLOCIDE); (✽) YOMESAN
- ❐ Oxamniquine (VANSIL)
- ❐ Piperazine citrate (ANTEPAR, VERMIZINE)
- ❐ Praziquantel (BILTRICIDE)
- ❐ Pyrantel pamoate (ANTIMINTH, PIN-X, REESE'S PINWORM); (✽) COMBANTRIN, HELMEX
- ❐ Thiabendazole (MINTEZOL); (✽) MINTEZOL

Indications

The anthelmintic of choice is based on the specific infestation. Diethylcarbamazine is used to treat tropical pulmonary eosinophilia caused by filariasis, infestation by a long nematode that lives in lymphatic vessels and organs, circulatory system, connective tissues, and serous cavities. Mebendazole and pyrantel pamoate are considered broad spectrum and are effective in the treatment of roundworms, hookworms, and pinworms. They are less effective for tapeworm infestations. An analog of pyrantel is effective against whipworm.

Niclosamide is indicated for the treatment of intestinal tapeworm infestations but is ineffective against the cysticercosis of *Diphyllobothrium latum* or *Echinococcus granulosus*. Surgical incisions must be used to remove the cysts from tissues. Oxamniquine is used in the treatment of *Schistosoma mansoni* infestations. Piperazine is effective against roundworm and pinworm infestations. Thiabendazole is used most often against threadworms and pinworms. Praziquantel is recommended for schistosomiasis.

Pharmacodynamics

Some anthelmintics act directly or indirectly in the host to affect the parasite. Some work to "starve the worm to death" or to paralyze it through destruction of its central nervous system. Others interfere with production of adenosine triphosphate in the helminth or act on specific enzymes in the worm itself, not touching the host's structures.

Other substrates affected by anthelmintic drugs are glycogen, glucose, and phosphorylase phosphatase. In the choice of drug to use, the substrate component should be taken into consideration. For example, pyrantel pamoate is a neuromuscular blocking drug that releases acetylcholine. Inhibiting cholinesterase produces seizures in the helminth.

Niclosamide inhibits the oxidative phosphorylation of the worm, killing the scolex (head) and proximal segments on contact. The host's normal digestive system destroys the residue, so the scolex may not be found on exam of the feces.

The actions of praziquantel, piperazine, and oxamniquine are unclear. These agents seem to kill the helminth by causing a hyperpolarization of its muscles. The worms are then dislodged and expelled in the feces. The mechanism of action against *Enterobius* is not understood.

Thiabendazole suppresses production of eggs or larvae and their subsequent development. It does so by inhibiting a helminth-specific enzyme.

Adverse Effects and Contraindications

The adverse effects associated with anthelmintic drugs vary with the specific agent. Those effects occurring most often are diarrhea, vomiting, nausea, transient abdominal pain, fever, pruritus, and skin rash.

Reversible neutropenia may occur with mebendazole, especially when larger than usual doses are given to treat echinococcosis or trichinosis. Systemic adverse effects are rare. Niclosamide and praziquantel can cause hypersensitivity reactions.

Niclosamide has been associated with abdominal cramps, loss of appetite, diarrhea, constipation, and a bad taste in the mouth. Oral mucus membrane irritation occurs at all dosage levels. Drowsiness, headache, and weakness have also been recorded, as well as fever, sweating, palpitations, edema of the extremities, irritability, and backache. These effects are transitory and do not require discontinuation of the drug.

Oxamniquine may cause transient pulmonary infiltration, liver function test abnormalities, eosinophilia, hallucinations, and seizures in some patients. It should not be given to patients with epilepsy, decompensated heart failure, or renal disease. Although there is no evidence that oxamniquine is teratogenic or carcinogenic, compounds related to it are.

Piperazine can cause muscular incoordination or weakness, vertigo, dysphasia, confusion, and myoclonic contractions. These effects usually disappear when the drug is discontinued. It may also induce or exacerbate epileptic seizures in susceptible patients. For these reasons, piperazine is contraindicated in patients with renal or hepatic insufficiency and with epilepsy.

Large doses of praziquantel are associated with headache and malaise. Because the drug is chemically related to sedative and antianxiety drugs, drowsiness is relatively common. A syndrome consisting of headache, hyperthermia, seizures, intracranial hypertension, and/or arachnoiditis develops in many patients given praziquantel for neurocysticercosis, especially in patients with multiple brain cysts. This syndrome is presumed to be the result of an inflammatory process from dead or dying organisms. The symptoms may be prevented by prior and/or concurrent corticosteroid therapy. Because destruction of parasites within the eye causes irreparable lesions, praziquantel is contraindicated in the treatment of ocular cysticercosis.

Adverse effects noted with thiabendazole include tinnitus, conjunctival injection, blurred vision, hypotension, syncope, anaphylaxis, numbness, seizures, and transient leukopenia. A few cases of erythema multiforme and Stevens-Johnson syndrome have been reported.

Pharmacokinetics

The pharmacokinetics of many of the anthelmintic drugs are unknown. The pharmacokinetics of the remainder vary from drug to drug (Table 27–2). The absorption of mebendazole is minimal (2 to 10 percent), owing to its low aqueous solubility. Oral bioavailability is also low because of a significant first pass effect. Distribution sites are unknown, although biotransformation takes place in the liver. More than 95 percent is eliminated in the stool, and small amounts in urine.

The onset of action of oxamniquine is rapid, with peak serum concentrations reached in 3 hours. The presence of food in the GI tract retards absorption and reduces plasma concentrations. The elimination half-life is 1 to 2½ hours, and 70 percent of a dose is eliminated in the urine.

The pharmacokinetics of piperazine are limited, although the drug is rapidly absorbed from the small intestine. A sub-

TABLE 27–2 PHARMACOKINETICS OF SELECTED ANTHELMINTIC, ANTIMALARIAL, AND ANTIPARASITIC DRUGS

Drug	Route	Onset	Peak	Duration	PB (%)	$t_{1/2}$	BioA (%)
Anthelmintics							
Mebendazole	po	UK	1.5–7.5 hr	UK	95	2.5–5.5 hr†	2–3
Oxamniquine	po	Rapid	3 hr	UK	UK	1–2.5 hr	UK
Piperazine	po	UK	UK	UK	UK	UK	UK
Praziquantel	po	Varies	1–2 hr	UK	UK	0.8–1.5 hr; 4–5 hr*	< 80
Pyrantel pamoate	po	UK	1–3 hr	UK	UK	2.5–9 hr	2–10
Thiabendazole	po	Rapid	1–2 hr	UK	UK	UK	UK
Antimalarials							
Chloroquine	po	3–3.5 hr	UK	UK	50–60	Dose specific; 30–60 days	UA
Mefloquine	po	1–2 hr	1–2 hr	UK	85	2–3 wk	UK
Quinine	po	1–3 hr	1–3 hr	UK	80	11 hr	UK
Primaquine	po	Rapid	3 hr	UK	100	6 hr	UK
Sulfadoxine-pyrimethamine	po	Rapid	2.5–6 hr; 1.5–8 hr	UK	UK	100–230 hr; 50–150 hr	UK
Antiparasitic							
Sodium stibogluconate	IM IV	Rapid	UK	UK	UK	2 hr; 33–76 hr†	100

*Half-life is 4–5 hours for the praziquantel metabolites.
†Two-phase elimination half-life of sodium stibogluconate. Terminal phase reflects conversion of pentavalent to trivalent form and accounts for accumulation and slow release of the drug during multiple dosing.
NA, Not applicable; UA, unavailable; UK, unknown; PB, protein binding; BioA, bioavailability.

stantial amount is eliminated unchanged in the urine within 24 hours.

Praziquantel varies in its onset of action but peaks 1 to 3 hours after administration. The anthelmintic activity of metabolites is less than that of the parent drug. Serum half-life is 0.8 to 1.5 hours for the unchanged drug, and 4 to 5 hours for its metabolites. High plasma concentrations are associated with a higher incidence of adverse effects in patients with hepatic disease.

Pyrantel pamoate is slowly and poorly absorbed when taken by mouth. Its peak serum concentration time is 1 to 3 hours. Most of an oral dose is eliminated unchanged in the feces, with a small percentage eliminated through the urine.

Thiabendazole is rapidly absorbed after oral administration, with peak serum levels occurring in 1 to 2 hours. The drug is almost completely biotransformed in the liver. More than 90 percent of the conjugates (sulfate and glucuronide) are recovered from urine in 24 hours.

Drug-Drug Interactions

There are few drug-drug interactions with the anthelmintics. The interactions most commonly noted are identified in Table 27–3.

Dosage Regimens

Because of the relative specificity of some anthelmintic drugs, accurate diagnosis is necessary for optimal therapy. However, this may be less essential with broader-spectrum drugs such as mebendazole, pyrantel pamoate, and praziquantel. Dosage regimens are given in Table 27–4.

The patient taking niclosamide should have a saline purge such as magnesium sulfate 1 to 2 hours after drug administration, to prevent the development of cysticercosis in the intestinal tract. Moreover, the purge provides a good possibility of expulsion of an intact scolex.

Laboratory Considerations

Depending on the specific infestation, the stool should be recultured in 1 week to 3 to 6 months to determine whether the infestation has cleared. Stool specimens for intestinal, liver, and blood flukes are collected at 1 week, and 1, 6, and 12 months following treatment. A stool specimen is collected 1 month following treatment for lung flukes, and 1 and 3 months following treatment for tapeworms.

Stool specimens should not be contaminated with water, urine, or chemicals, which might destroy the parasite. Cure is not accomplished unless the stool is negative for eggs and worms after 3 months. Blood and tissue samples are also obtained periodically to monitor patient progress.

Critical Thinking Process

Assessment

History of Present Illness

The history of the present illness is important to assessing any complaints that may suggest infestation. The patient may report abdominal cramps, diarrhea (true diarrhea is liquid stool with a frequency exceeding five times in 5 hours), malaise, coughs, itching, rash, blood in stool, or seeing the proglottids or scolex of an adult worm. Contact with family or friends who have recently been treated for infestation should also be noted.

Past Health History

The examiner should elicit information about travel to, or residence in, endemic areas. In addition, information about the patient's food habits helps pinpoint the source of infestation. Eating raw or exotic meats (e.g., walrus, seal, moose)

TABLE 27-3 DRUG-DRUG INTERACTIONS OF SELECTED ANTHELMINTIC, ANTIMALARIAL, AND ANTIPARASITIC DRUGS

Drug	Interactive Drugs	Interaction
Anthelmintics		
Mebendazole	Insulin Oral hypoglycemics	Increased secretion of insulin, potential for hypoglycemia increases
	Carbamazepine Phenytoin	Decreased plasma concentration of mebendazole when latter is used in large doses
	Cimetidine	Increased serum concentration of mebendazole
Pyrantel pamoate	Piperazine citrate	Antagonistic to each other
Antimalarials		
Chloroquine	Highly protein-bound drugs	Decreased effects of other highly protein-bound drugs
	Cimetidine	Increased effects of chloroquine
	Magnesium trisilicate	Decreased absorption of both drugs
Mefloquine	Chloroquine	Higher risk of seizures
	Quinine Quinidine	Higher risk of cardiac toxicity and seizures
Quinine	Mefloquine	Increased incidence of seizures and electrocardiogram abnormalities
	Digoxin Digitoxin Amiodarone Verapamil	Increased serum levels of interacting drug
	Neuromuscular blockers Succinylcholine	Respiratory difficulties if taken concurrently
	Oral anticoagulants	Increased anticoagulant effects
	Antacids Sodium bicarbonate	Increased cardiac depressant effects
	Phenobarbital Hydantoins Rifampin	Decreased quinine levels
Primaquine	Hemolytic drugs Immunosuppressants	Increased risk of bone marrow depression
Antiparasitic		
Malathion	Aminoglycosides Cholinesterase inhibitors Endrophonium Succinylcholine	Increased cholinesterase inhibition

and fishing or swimming in snail-infested locations, such as swamps or undrained ponds, should alert the health care provider to the potential for infestation.

Physical Exam Findings

In addition to a routine physical, the exam must include observation of skin as well as anal folds.

Diagnostic Testing

Laboratory identification of helminths can be made through examination of freshly passed stool, taken in early mornings on 3 to 5 consecutive days. The frequency of stool collection is guided by expectations of worm load. Light infestations may not demonstrate eggs or larvae in some stool samples. Heavy infestations may demonstrate adult worms in the first stool sample. In roundworm infestations, adult worms are vomited or coughed up. Muscle biopsy can be taken after the fourth week if there is diffuse myositis from inoculation with *Trichinella* species.

Blood, tissue fluid, or skin snips are better scanned when they are fresh. Immunologic techniques for identification include the complement fixation test, the immunofluorescent antibody test, and the enzyme-linked immunosorbent assay.

Requests for laboratory testing must include information about the suspicion of helminths to be sure a correct diagnosis is made. The immunofluorescent antibody test and the enzyme-linked immunosorbent assay are not routinely available except in special parasitology laboratories.

Laboratory requests for examination of fresh stool specimens for ova and parasites must have clear directions as to the type of parasite expected. It is not unusual to confuse hookworm larvae with *Strongyloides* larvae if the specimen is not examined within one-half hour after being taken.

Developmental Considerations

Helminthic infestations occur in any age group. Pinworm infestations are more common in the preschool or school-age child.

Psychosocial Considerations

The primary psychosocial implication of an infestation is embarrassment if the condition becomes public knowledge. Use of public facilities to toilet, bathe, or wash clothes may be limited or nonexistent for homeless, indigent, or mentally troubled wanderers who present with symptoms. Investigations of the patient's home, family members, and living conditions, such as laundry, cleanliness, personal habits, food preparation, and elimination facilities, must be conducted with decorum and consideration. Use of public health departments and other public resources can be invaluable for support and education of an individual with an infestation.

TABLE 27–4 DOSAGE REGIMEN FOR SELECTED ANTHELMINTIC, ANTIMALARIAL, AND ANTIPARASITIC DRUGS

Drug	Use(s)	Dosage	Implications
Anthelmintics			
Mebendazole	Whipworm, hookworm, Roundworm	*Adult or child:* 100 mg po BID × 3 days	Regimen may be repeated in 2 weeks if treatment unsuccessful Safe use in children younger than 2 years has not been established
	Pinworm	*Adult or child:* 100 mg po × 1 dose	
Niclosamide	Beef tapeworm, fish tapeworm	*Adult:* 2 g po × 1 dose *Child: 11–34 kg:* 1 g po on the first day, then 1 tablet po for the next 6 days *Child: > 34 kg:* 1.5 g po on day 1, then 1 g for next 6 days	Repeat dose if stool culture is positive 7 days after therapy Reculture 4 days after treatment and periodically for 3 months Safety in children younger than 2 years has not been established
	Dwarf tapeworm	*Adult:* 2 g po QD × 7 days *Child: 11–34 kg:* 1 g po on the first day, then 0.5 g po for the next 6 days *Child: > 34 kg:* 1.5 g po on day 1, then 1 g for next 6 days	Not systemically absorbed Safety in children younger than 2 years has not been established
Oxamniquine	Threadworm	*Adult:* 12–15 mg/kg po × 1 dose *Child: < 30 kg:* 20 mg/kg po in 2 divided doses with 2–8 hr between doses	A reddish-orange discoloration of the urine may occur
Piperazine citrate	Roundworm	*Adult:* 3.5 g po QD × 2 days *Child:* 75 mg/kg po QD × 2 days Maximum daily dose 3.5 g	May repeat after 1 week interval for severe infestations
	Pinworm	*Adult or child:* 65 mg/kg po QD × 7 days Maximum daily dose 2.5 g	
Pyrantel pamoate	Roundworm, pinworm	*Adult or child:* 11 mg/kg po one time only Maximum dose 1 g	May be mixed with juice or milk
Praziquantel	Schistosomiasis, hermaphroditic infections	*Adult:* 40–75 mg/kg TID × 1 day *Child:* 40–60 mg/kg TID × 1 day	Although approved by Food and Drug Administration, drug is considered experimental for these purposes
	Fish tapeworm, beef tapeworm, pork tapeworm	*Adult or child:* 5–10 mg/kg × 1 dose	
	Dwarf tapeworm	*Adult:* 5–10 mg/kg × 1 dose *Child:* 25 mg/kg × 1 dose	
	Cysticercus cellulosae	*Adult or child:* 50 mg/kg/day in 3 doses × 15 days	
Thiabendazole	Pinworms	*Adult or child <150 lb:* 10 mg/kg BID × 1 day; Repeat in 7 days to reduce risk of re-infection (or 2 doses/day for 2 successive days)	Urine may have unusual odor
Antimalarial			
Chloroquine HCl	*P. vivax, P. ovale, P. malariae,* Chloroquine-susceptible *P. falciparum*	*Adult:* 160–200 mg chloroquine base IM q6hr if necessary. Not to exceed 800 mg chloroquine base. Treatment by mouth should be started as soon as practicable and continued until a course of approximately 1.5 grams of base in 3 days is completed *Child:* 5 mg chloroquine base/kg. May repeat q6hr, however total dose should not exceed 10 mg base/kg	Treatment regimen must be precisely followed. Infants and children are extremely susceptible to overdosage of this drug. Severe deaths and reactions have occurred
Chloroquine phosphate	*P. vivax, P. ovale, P. malariae,* Chloroquine-susceptible *P. falciparum*	*Adult:* Prophylaxis: 500 mg (300 mg base) po on exactly the same day each week and then continued for up to 8 weeks after leaving the endemic area. Treatment: 1 g (600 mg base) followed by additional 500 mg (300 mg base) after 6-8 hours and a single dose of 500 mg (300 mg base) on each of 2 consecutive days *Child:* 5 mg base/kg. Dosage should not exceed adult dose regardless of weight	The dosage of chloroquine phosphate is often expressed or calculated as the base. Each 500 mg tablet is equivalent to 300 mg base. The treatment dosage represents a total dose of 2.5 g of chloroquine phosphate or 1.5 g base in 3 days
Mefloquine	Multidrug-resistant *P. falciparum*	*Adult:* Prophylaxis: 250 mg po once weekly. Treatment: 1250 mg po as a single dose. *Child:* 25 mg/kg base po × 1 dose	Centers for Disease Control and Prevention should be contacted for current prophylaxis regimen. Prophylaxis should begin 1 week before departure to endemic area, should always be taken on the same day each week, and therapy continued for an additional 4 weeks after leaving endemic area. Tablets should not be taken on an empty stomach

Table continued on following page

TABLE 27–4 DOSAGE REGIMEN FOR SELECTED ANTHELMINTIC, AND ANTIPARASITIC DRUGS *Continued*

Drug	Use(s)	Dosage	Implications
Antimalarial *Continued*			
Primaquine	*P. vivax*, *P. ovale*, *P. malariae*, *P. falciparum*	*Adult:* 26.3 mg (15 mg base) po QD × 14 days *Child:* 0.5 mg/kg/day po (0.3 mg/kg base) po QD × 14 days. Maximum dose: 15 mg/kg base/dose	Begin treatment during the last 2 weeks of, or following a course of suppression with, chloroquine or a comparable drug. Combination therapy with chloroquine phosphate to eliminate erythrocytic forms of the parasite
Quinine sulfate	*P. vivax*, *P. ovale*, *P. malariae*, Chloroquine-resistant *P. falciparum*	*Adult:* Chloroquine-resistant malaria: 650 mg po q8hr × 5–7 days. Chloroquine sensitive malaria: 600 mg po q8hr × 5–7 days *Child:* Chloroquine-resistant malaria: 25 mg/kg po q8hr × 5–7 days. Chloroquine sensitive malaria: 10 mg/kg po q8hr × 5–7 days	Duration of therapy may be shortened if drug is taken concurrently with other antimalarial drugs.
Sulfadoxine-pyrimethamine	Chloroquine-resistant *P. falciparum*	*Adult:* 3 tablets po as single dose (500 mg sulfadoxine, 25 mg pyrimethamine)	Presumptive treatment of travelers in remote areas who suspect infestation or infection but do not have ready access to medical attention
Antiparasitic			
Stibogluconate sodium	Cutaneous leishmaniasis	*Adult:* 20 mg/kg IV/IM QD × 20 days	Cure rates are high if treatment recommendations are followed
	Systemic or mucocutaneous leishmaniasis	*Adult:* 20 mg/kg IV/IM QD × 30 days	

Analysis and Management

Treatment Objectives

The primary treatment objective for helminthic infestations is to kill or destroy the adult worm, thus reducing the worm load. Because most anthelmintics are highly effective against specific parasites, the organism must be accurately identified before treatment is started.

The life cycles of many helminths are complex, offering a formidable challenge to disease eradication and even to drug treatment. Consultation with a pharmacist, public health department, and/or the Centers for Disease Control and Prevention (CDC) will be helpful. Light infestations—those that require stool concentrations to find the eggs or worms—do not usually require treatment.

Treatment Options

Drug Variables

A key to eradication of infestation is to use anthelmintic drugs that interfere with the life cycle of adult parasites. Antibiotics are not appropriate for the treatment of infestations. Because helminths feed on the substrates of the nutrition process in the body, the drug chosen must be effective in blocking parasitic dependence.

Choice of treatments for cestode infestations is between two drugs, niclosamide and praziquantel. If no hypersensitivity has occurred with praziquantel, and the patient history is negative for previous infestation, this agent may be a better choice. There are relatively fewer adverse reactions with praziquantel than with niclosamide.

Treatment options for intestinal nematode infestations are mebendazole, thiabendazole, and diethylcarbamazine. (The recommendation to use diethylcarbamazine is based on limited clinical trials.) Albendazole, a benzimidazole derivative similar to mebendazole, is a broad-spectrum drug with activity against intestinal nematodes. It has shown activity against *Ascaris lumbricoides, Necator americanus, Ancylostoma duodenale,* and *Enterobius vermicularis.* In contrast to mebendazole, however, it also has some activity against *Strongyloides* and *Trichinella.* Unfortunately, albendazole is not yet approved for use in the United States. It is available in France and the United Kingdom.

Treatment for trichinosis is complicated by the fact that the disease often goes unnoticed until the helminth has invaded muscle. During the enteral phase, the adult worms are highly susceptible to thiabendazole, the drug of choice.

For the treatment of all infections caused by *Schistosoma* species, praziquantel is the drug of choice. As a broad-spectrum agent, it is efficacious against a variety of both trematodes and cestodes. It is usually effective in a single oral dose and has limited adverse effects, making it attractive as an anthelmintic.

In some cases, the initial regimen using the drug of choice does not effect a cure, and alternative treatment options are hazardous. Retreatment with the first drug should be undertaken before another anthelmintic drug is prescribed.

Many of the anthelmintic drugs are not routinely available in the United States. In some cases, the drugs may be available only through the Parasitic Disease Drug Service at the CDC in Atlanta, Georgia.

Patient Variables

Patients who have infestations are often reluctant to discuss the problem. They may have used home remedies for a long time before seeking professional help, and they are often socially unacceptable in behavior and attitude. They may not divulge personal information that would assist in their treatment and in the prevention of additional infestations.

Neonates are not to be treated for infestations. If neonatal infestation is identified, a neonatologist or pediatrician should be consulted. The neonate's systems are still developing, and competition for nutritional substrates by the worm can cause severe complications. In such a circumstance, the family must be considered the source of infestation, their living conditions scrutinized, and large-scale treatment considered. Most anthelmintic drugs are contraindicated for children less than 30 lbs or younger than 3 years.

Intervention

Administration

The drug regimen for specific infestations must be followed closely in order for treatment to be successful. The half-life of some drugs is enhanced when they are taken with fatty foods. Further, gastric irritation can be mini-mized if the drugs are taken with food. If necessary, tablets may be crushed and mixed with applesauce or other food for administration. The chewable tablets of niclosamide should be followed with a small amount of water. Chewing praziquantel tablets can cause gagging and vomiting because of their bitter taste. Oral suspensions of thiabendazole should be shaken well and the calibrated measuring device used to ensure accurate dosage. In most cases, no dietary restrictions, laxatives, or post-treatment enemas are necessary.

Education

The compliance and dependability of the person being treated are crucial factors for successful elimination of the parasites. Careful instructions must be given for time of return visits, for submission of specimens, and for taking of medications.

The importance of meticulous hygiene, that is, washing hands before eating and after toileting, and keeping hands or objects away from the mouth, should be emphasized. Toilet facilities should be disinfected daily. The patient should be instructed to take frequent showers rather than baths, and to change clothing, bed linens, and towels daily to prevent re-infection. The importance of follow up with the health care provider cannot be stressed enough.

Because niclosamide, praziquantel, pyrantel pamoate, and thiabendazole may cause drowsiness and dizziness, the patient should be advised about driving a motor vehicle or operating machinery. The patient should also be warned that oxamniquine causes a harmless reddish-orange discoloration of the urine.

Travelers must be cautioned regarding the reservoir for helminths when they are visiting other countries. This is particularly important if their travel takes them to underdeveloped areas with primitive facilities for elimination, eating, or drinking.

Evaluation

For most patients with helminthic infestation, three stool samples examined after the completion of therapy should be negative. After roundworm infestation, the patient's stool samples should be free of ova, larvae, or worms 2 to 3 weeks after completion of therapy. Specimens from a patient with flukes should be negative for several months before the patient is considered cured. For pinworm infestation, perianal swabs should be negative for 7 days.

MALARIAL PARASITES

Epidemiology and Etiology

Malaria remains the world's most devastating human infection, affecting more than 200 million people and causing more than 2 million deaths annually. The disease is caused by exposure to *Plasmodium falciparum, Plasmodium vivax, Plasmodium ovale,* and/or *Plasmodium malariae.* The causative organisms have different biologic patterns, and all affect humans. The species with the highest morbidity and mortality in humans is *P. falciparum,* posing the greatest risk to immunocompromised persons and children younger than 5 years.

Although the *Anopheles* mosquito–borne infection has been virtually eradicated in the United States, emigration from and travel to endemic regions constitutes a continuing health concern. In the 1950s, attempts to eradicate the infectious organism failed, primarily because of the development of resistance to insecticides and antimalarial drugs. Since 1960, transmission of malaria has risen and the degree of resistance to drugs has increased.

Pathophysiology

Malarial parasites were named *Plasmodium* because of their affinity for erythrocytes (red blood cells; RBCs) in the plasma. The life cycle of the malarial infection must be appreciated in order to understand the actions and uses of antimalarial drugs (Fig. 27–2).

The parasite (sporozoite) invades an RBC traveling to the liver, where it resides and multiplies asexually. This stage of development is known as the exoerythrocytic stage and is largely asymptomatic. The parasite (now known as a merozoite) invades the RBCs. It multiplies to such an extent in each blood cell that the RBC cannot contain it; the cell then bursts, and the merozoites are freed. Two to 4 weeks after exposure, the symptoms of malaria are evident. The patient's fever cycles correspond with the bursting of erythrocytes.

The *P. vivax, P. ovale,* and *P. malariae* organisms are exoerythrocytic, persisting in the liver (as hypnozoites) for years and periodically seeding the body system. It is unusual for more than 1 percent of the RBCs to become infested except in *P. falciparum* infection, in which more than 50 percent of the RBCs can show the parasite.

Symptoms of the infestation appear after an incubation period of 10 to 35 days, often with a break period of flulike symptoms. *P. vivax* and *P. ovale* cause less severe but abrupt attacks, consisting of shaking chills, fever, and sweats, as well as irregular, intermittent fevers. Headache may precede the first chill. Rigors occur at 48-hour intervals and last 1 to 8 hours with no symptoms in between.

P. falciparum infection begins with a chilly sensation rather than a shaking chill, and the temperature rises and falls with lysis. The episodes may last 20 to 36 hours, with prominent headache and increasing prostration. In a patient with fever of 104°F or higher, and a severe headache with drowsiness, delirium, or confusion, cerebral malaria should be suspected.

Infection with *P. malariae* begins with a severe paroxysm that recurs in 72 hours.

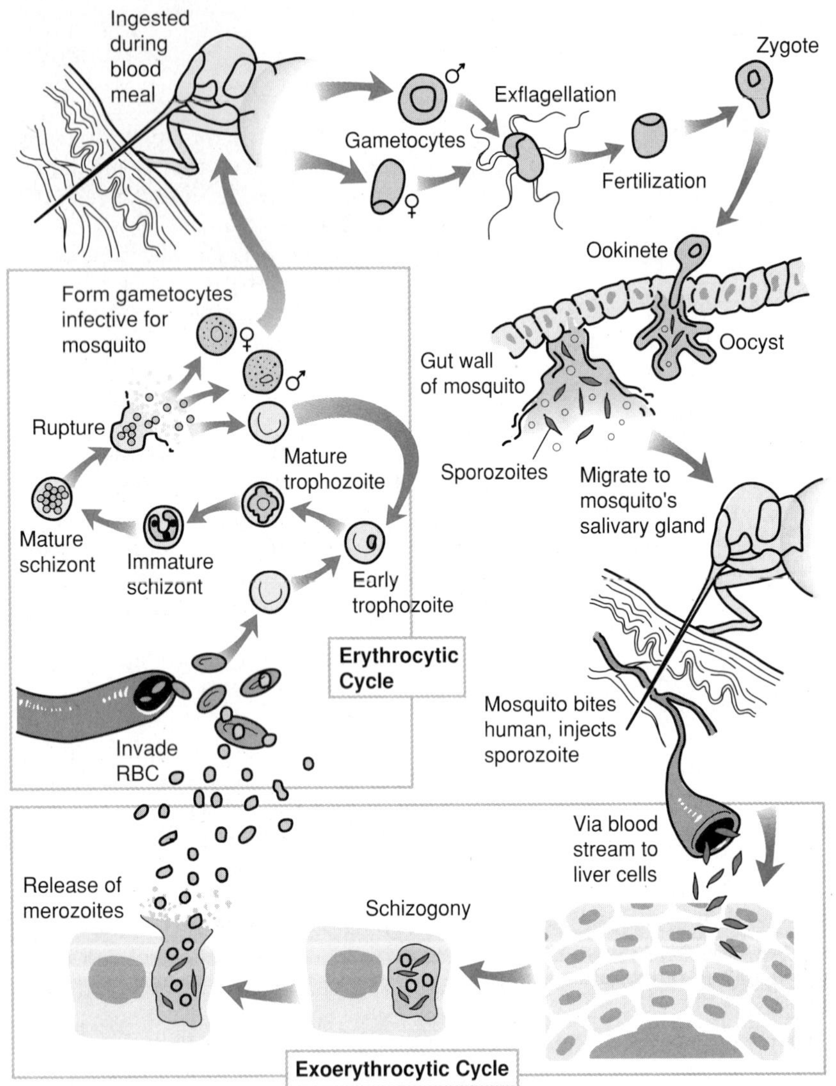

Figure 27–2 Life cycle of *Plasmodium.* The organism is transmitted to the bloodstream of humans by the bite of anopheline mosquitoes. The sporozoites migrate to the liver, where they develop and multiply and ultimately invade red blood cells. (From Mahon, C. R., and Manuselis, G., Jr. [1995]. *Textbook of Diagnostic Microbiology* [p. 754]. Philadelphia: W. B. Saunders. Used with permission.)

The severity of rigors in malaria is related to the number of species present, differences in the strains, and the immunity of the subject. Chronic malaria exists in residents of hyperendemic areas of the world. The paroxysms of chronic malaria are shorter and lighter than those seen with an acute attack.

PHARMACOTHERAPEUTIC OPTIONS

Antiparasitics

- ❒ Chloroquine (ARALEN)
- ❒ Mefloquine (LARIAM, MEPHAQUIN)
- ❒ Primaquine phosphate
- ❒ Quinine sulfate (QUINAMM); (🍁) NOVO-QUININE
- ❒ Sulfadoxine-pyrimethamine (FANSIDAR)

Indications

Antimalarial drugs can be categorized according to the stage of the parasite they affect and the particular malarial strain involved. Drugs acting primarily on plasmodia in the liver include pyrimethamine and primaquine. Pyrimethamine is used extensively in combination with sulfadoxine because of the synergistic effects it produces. Uses of the combination drug sulfadoxine-pyrimethamine include prophylaxis (even in pregnant women) against the *P. falciparum* species. In combination with quinine, it has been used in the treatment of acute malarial attacks resulting from chloroquine-resistant strains. It has also been used for prophylaxis against *P. ovale* and *P. vivax*.

Primaquine also has prophylactic activity, but it is seldom used for this purpose because of its toxicity. Primaquine is the only antimalarial drug clinically employed to eradicate tissue forms of plasmodia that cause relapse.

Chloroquine, quinine, and related derivatives, such as mefloquine, have been used for clinical or suppressive cure of malaria and to destroy sexual erythrocytic forms of plasmodia.

Chloroquine has been the mainstay of prophylaxis against malarial infection. It is given, before exposure, to people living in or traveling to an endemic area. Chloroquine is not so much a prophylactic drug as a suppressant of clinical symptoms once the person has been exposed to the parasite. This agent is not effective against the tissue forms of malaria, so it will not cure infections caused by *P. ovale* or

P. vivax. It is the drug of choice for all chloroquine-sensitive strains of malaria. The *P. falciparum* species has shown resistance to the drug. Chloroquine is safe for use during pregnancy. Use of mefloquine in infants or in women of childbearing age is not recommended.

Quinine is the oldest antimalarial drug. It has been used to treat malarial fevers since 1633. Mefloquine hydrochloride is a structural derivative of quinine. One of the newer antimalarial drugs, it is used only for the treatment of chloroquine-resistant *P. falciparum*. Because resistance to this drug is already occurring, limitations on its use are prudent.

Pharmacodynamics

The mechanism of action of chloroquine is unclear, but there are two possibilities. It is known that chloroquine (1) binds to a product of heme breakdown that is highly lytic to RBCs and (2) accumulates into the acidic lysosome compartments of the parasite. As a weak base, chloroquine neutralizes these compartments. The parasite thus cannot utilize protein substances involved in heme breakdown, an operation essential for its survival. The action of quinine is thought to be similar to that of chloroquine.

Mefloquine's action is also unknown, although, like chloroquine and quinine, it concentrates in the lysosome compartments of the parasite.

Little is known about the mechanism of action of primaquine, especially why it is more active against tissue forms and gametes than against asexual forms of plasmodia. There is some evidence that the drug itself accounts for the antimalarial activity.

Pyrimethamine-sulfadoxine is a folic acid antagonist acting selectively to inhibit plasmodial dihydrofolate reductase. This enzyme is important to the cellular biosynthesis of proteins. The *Plasmodium* enzyme is much more sensitive to this drug than its mammalian counterparts.

Adverse Effects and Contraindications

Chloroquine is associated with relatively mild adverse effects, including headache, nausea, and visual disturbances (blurring, diplopia). Prolonged treatment may cause a lichenoid skin eruption, toxic myopathy, cardiomyopathy, and peripheral neuropathy in a few patients. The conditions subside promptly when the drug is discontinued. When chloroquine has been used for treatment of diseases other than malaria, prolonged high doses have resulted in irreversible retinopathy. Doses larger than 5 g are usually fatal. Chloroquine is contraindicated in patients with psoriasis or porphyria, which may be exacerbated by the drug.

Mefloquine produces a dose-related nausea, vomiting, abdominal pain, and dizziness. Rare manifestations of central nervous system toxicity, such as disorientation, hallucinations, seizures, and depression, are seen.

Primaquine is fairly innocuous when given in therapeutic doses to white patients. Mild to moderate cramping and occasional epigastric distress occur in some people given larger doses. Mild anemia, methemoglobinemia, and leukocytosis have been observed.

Quinine, when given in full therapeutic dosages, produces a typical dose-related cluster of symptoms termed *cinchonism*. In mild form, cinchonism consists of tinnitus, headache, nausea, and disturbed vision. When the drug is continued or after large single doses, GI, cardiovascular, and dermal manifestations may appear. Hearing and vision are particularly affected. This drug is contraindicated in patients with a history of glucose-6-phosphate dehydrogenase deficiency.

The visual manifestations of cinchonism are blurred vision, altered color perception, photophobia, diplopia, night blindness, constricted visual fields, scotomata, and mydriasis. Functional impairment of the eighth cranial nerve results in tinnitus, decreased auditory acuity, and vertigo.

Gastrointestinal symptoms result from the local irritant effect of quinine, but nausea and emesis also have a central origin. Vomiting, abdominal pain, and diarrhea result from the irritation.

The cardiovascular adverse effects of quinine are qualitatively related to those of its isomer, quinidine. Therapeutic doses of quinine have little, if any, effect on the normal heart or blood pressure. When given as an intravenous bolus, quinine sometimes causes alarming and even fatal hypotension.

When taken at a dosage of 25 mg once weekly, pyrimethamine alone causes no significant adverse effects, except occasional skin rashes and depression of hematopoiesis. Excessive doses produce a megaloblastic anemia that resembles folic acid deficiency. The anemia readily reverses upon discontinuation of the drug or administration of leucovorin (folinic acid). In rare cases, Stevens-Johnson syndrome, toxic epidermal necrosis, serum sickness–type reactions, urticaria, exfoliative dermatitis, and hepatitis have been associated with sulfadoxine-pyrimethamine. The combination drug is teratogenic in laboratory studies.

Adverse effects of atovaquone are most commonly headache, insomnia, weakness, nausea, vomiting, and diarrhea. Fever and rash have also been noted. Use of the drug is contraindicated in hypersensitivity. Its safe use during pregnancy and lactation has not been established.

Pharmacokinetics

Chloroquine is absorbed in the GI tract, with peak plasma levels reached in 1 to 2 hours (see Table 27–2). The drug is well distributed to all body tissues, with concentration in the RBCs. It is eliminated in the urine as a metabolite (diethylchloroquine) and has a half-life of 3.1 hours with a 250-mg dose, of 42.9 hours with a 500-mg dose, and of 312 hours with a 1-g dose. Any unabsorbed drug is eliminated in the feces, although it can remain in urine for years after the drug is stopped.

Mefloquine is rapidly absorbed when taken by mouth, with a bioavailability exceeding 85 percent. It is extensively bound (98 percent) to plasma proteins. Tissue concentrations are relatively high for extended periods. Peak plasma concentrations are attained in a few hours and then slowly decline, with an elimination half-life of 2 to 3 weeks. Several metabolites are formed with biotransformation. Elimination is primarily through the feces.

Quinine is readily absorbed (80 percent bioavailability) when taken orally, even in patients with diarrhea. Peak plasma concentrations occur 1 to 3 hours after a single oral dose. With termination of therapy, plasma concentrations fall, with a half-life of about 11 hours. Plasma concentrations of 8 to 15 mg/L are clinically effective and are generally nontoxic. About 90 percent of the drug is bound to plasma proteins. Quinine is extensively biotransformed in the liver, only about 10 percent of the dose being eliminated unchanged in the urine. There is no accumulation of the drug with continued administration. Renal elimination is twice as rapid when the urine is acidic as when it is alkaline.

Primaquine absorption reaches almost 100 percent after oral administration. The plasma concentration after a single dose reaches a maximum in 3 hours and then falls, with an elimination half-life of 6 hours. The drug is rapidly biotransformed, with only a small fraction eliminated as the parent drug. Its three metabolites have considerably less antimalarial activity but greater hemolytic activity than the parent compound.

Sulfadoxine-pyrimethamine is well absorbed in the GI tract following oral administration. Peak serum concentrations are reached in 2 to 6 hours with a 500-mg dose. Distribution is throughout the kidney, lungs, liver, and spleen. Elimination half-life averages 111 hours.

Drug-Drug Interactions

Drug-drug interactions are relatively few with anthelmintic drugs. Table 27–3 provides a brief overview.

Dosage Regimen

The dosage regimen for each of the antimalarial drugs varies a great deal. Table 27–4 lists selected dosage regimens.

Critical Thinking Process

Assessment

History of Present Illness

The patient with malaria usually presents with a history of fever and chills at 48-hour intervals with *P. vivax* and *P. ovale,* and at 72-hour intervals with *P. malariae.* By contrast, patients with *P. falciparum* infection typically have irregular fever and chills and rarely present with a regular cycle of symptoms. Diarrhea is a common complaint among children with *P. falciparum* infection.

Past Health History

The health care provider should elicit information about travel to or residence in endemic areas. Information regarding exposure to mosquitos, the use of mosquito netting when sleeping and the application of mosquito repellents should be noted.

It is also important to note any pre-existing conditions or drugs taken by the patient that would influence the choice of drug treatment—specifically, a history of myasthenia gravis, thrombocytopenic purpura, or cardiac arrhythmias, glucose-6-phosphate dehydrogenase deficiency, psoriasis or porphyria, convulsive disorders, and blood dyscrasias. In a patient with any of these disorders, specific antimalarial drugs may be contraindicated or at least should be used with caution. A thorough drug history should be obtained to minimize the potential for drug-drug interactions.

Physical Exam Findings

In addition to a general physical exam, ophthalmic and neurologic exams should be done. The findings will be used, in part, as a baseline for drug monitoring. Attention should be given to signs and symptoms of dehydration and electrolyte imbalance.

Diagnostic Testing

Identification of plasmodia in serial blood smears is definitive for malaria. If the health care provider suspects a drug-resistant strain of *P. falciparum,* the laboratory order forms should be marked accordingly. A commercial kit is available for the diagnosis of *P. falciparum* infection. The identification of the type of plasmodium is important for therapy. In some cases, the patient is infected with more than one strain of plasmodia. Baseline laboratory tests, including complete blood count, platelet count, electrolyte and glucose-6-phosphate dehydrogenase measurements, and renal and liver function tests should be done before initiation of drug therapy.

Developmental Considerations

Malaria in the perinatal and pediatric populations requires special considerations. Many of the antimalarial drugs are contraindicated in children who are younger than 3 years or weigh less than 30 lbs.

Psychosocial Considerations

About 10 percent of blacks, 5 to 10 percent of Sephardic Jews, Greeks, Iranians, Chinese, Filipinos, and Indonesians have G6PD deficiency. There is evidence that G6PD is essential for metabolism in the plasmodia, so persons with this genetic deficiency are believed to have some natural immunity to malaria.

Malaria tends to be a chronic disease. Treatment may be long term or recurrent. Because antimalarial drugs cause discomfort and are somewhat hazardous, patients may have difficulty complying with their drug regimen. (See Case Study—Malaria.)

Analysis and Management

Treatment Objectives

Treatment objectives for malaria are to reduce or eliminate signs and symptoms of malaria and to decrease patient discomfort. Prevention of drug-related complications is also important.

Treatment Options

Drug Variables

During the past decade, the malaria parasite has become resistant to antimalarial drugs that have been used for its prevention and cure. Even chloroquine, once the drug of choice, may not be reliable in some cases.

Antibiotics are not usually effective against the malarial parasites; however, sulfonamides, tetracyclines, and chloramphenicol have been shown to be active against malaria. They are most useful when administered in combination with either quinine or pyrimethamine to treat drug-resistant strains of parasites. Doxycycline is used as an alternative when mefloquine cannot be tolerated or is contraindicated. Antibiotics are discussed in more detail in Chapter 24.

A malaria vaccine is not available, although it is hoped that this goal will ultimately be achieved. Because the three

Case Study Malaria

Patient History

History of Present Illness	JD is a 26-year-old female missionary trainee, recently (1 week) returned from 3-month stay with the Klong tribes of Thailand. Has faithfully taken prophylaxis for malaria, and will complete 5 more weeks of therapy. Complains of general malaise, fevers ranging from subnormal to 38 °C, headaches, intermittent cold sensations, and myalgia. Thinks she may have the flu, because her companions have also been ill.
Past Health History	Health good, passed full physical prior to the church appointment 9 months ago. Denies history of diabetes, hypertension, cancer. Family health history benign. Mother and father alive and well, as are two siblings.
Physical Exam Findings	WNL (within normal limits) except for temp. elevation of 37.8 °C. Pulse and respirations WNL. Skin intact, pink, clear. Nail beds clear, no clubbing. Deep tendon reflexes WNL. Abdomen benign, bowel sounds present. Lungs clear to auscultation.
Diagnostic Testing	Suspect malarial parasite from travel history. Blood tests to determine presence of *Plasmodium*. Will obtain 3 samples and ask for identification of parasite, if found. Ask for sensitivity of parasite to chloroquine.
Developmental Considerations	Determine whether patient is pregnant or expecting to become so in very near future.
Psychosocial Considerations	JD voices concerns about the type of illness and chronicity, the need for continual drug therapy, and obligations to church program in Thailand.
Economic Factors	Therapy and laboratory fees will probably be paid by church insurance. Infestation may be considered a job-related illness with long-term implications

Variables Influencing Decision

Treatment Objectives

- Cure infestation if this is acute attack.
- Prevent chronic state if this is *P. viva* or *P. ovale*.

Drug Variables	*Drug Summary*	*Patient Variables*
Indications	Malaria caused by *P. vivax* or *P. ovale*. Drug-resistant malaria.	JD diagnosed with *P. ovale* malaria. Reports she faithfully followed prophylaxis regimen.
Pharmacodynamics	Chloroquine stays in system for months to years. Pyrimethamine is cleared in less than 24 hours and is a folic acid inhibitor. Sulfadoxine stays in system for at least a week, acts in synergy with pyrimethamine. Primaquine interferes with DNA production, leaves system in less than 24 hours.	There are no patient variables applicable to pharmacodynamics.
Adverse Effects/ Contraindications	Mild, reversible. Prolonged treatment with chloroquine can cause blurred vision and retinopathy, which are mild, reversible. Prolonged treatment with pyrimethamine can cause folic acid deficiency. Sulfadoxine causes all the severe reactions seen with the sulfonamides.	JD's history negative for other health problems, and she denies history of sensitivity to sulfa. This will become a decision point.

Case Study continues on following page

Drug Variables	Drug Summary	Patient Variables
Pharmacokinetics	Chloroquine stays in system for months to years. Pyrimethamine is cleared in less than 24 hours. Sulfadoxine stays in system for at least 1 week.	JD has intact, functional hepatic and renal functions. This will not become a decision point.
Dosage Regimen	Specific to drug chosen.	This will not be a decision point, because JD's compliance has been good.
Laboratory Considerations	Monitoring of drug therapy requires 3 blood samples.	JD has agreed to go to the lab daily for 3 days. This will become a decision point.
Cost Index*	Chloroquine: 1 Sulfadoxine-primethamine: 1	Drug cost to be covered by JD's worker's compensation insurance.
Summary of Decision Points	• Suspect drug-resistant strain of malaria, since species is endemic in Thailand. • JD faithfully followed prophylaxis while in Thailand. • JD denies sensitivity to sulfonamides.	
DRUG TO BE USED	• Chloroquine 600 mg base po followed by 300 mg po 6 hours later and again on days 2 and 3. • Sulfadoxine-pyrimethamine tabs 3 as single dose (500 mg sulfadoxine, 25 mg pyrimethamine).	

*Cost Index
1 = $>30/mo.
2 = $30–40/mo.
3 = $40–50/mo.
4 = $50–60/mo.
5 = $>60/mo.

AWP of 6 tablets of chloroquine is approximately $23.
AWP of 3 tablets of sulfadoxine-pyrimethamine is approximately $11.

major parasitic stages in humans are antigenically distinct, a successful vaccine will likely need to contain at least three parasite antigens (sporozoite, merozoite, and gametocyte). A vaccine that limited the magnitude of the parasitemia could have a marked effect on survival, even if it had no effect on the incidence of infection, because severe morbidity and mortality are associated with high parasitemias.

Patient Variables

Alternative drugs, although available for the treatment of malaria, are not fully effective, require difficult dosage schedules, cause serious adverse effects, or are too expensive. For example, the average wholesale price of mefloquine is more than $6.00 per tablet.

Intervention

Administration

Regardless of the drug chosen for treatment, compliance with the regimen is important. Patients should be instructed to take the drug exactly as prescribed. Sustained-release drug forms should not be crushed or chewed. Most antimalarial drugs should be taken with food to minimize GI upset.

A calendar can be prepared for the patient taking the antimalarial drugs for prophylaxis, with the dosage days marked. Mefloquine, for example, should be taken the same day each week, beginning 1 week before exposure and continuing for 4 weeks after the traveler has returned to a malaria-free area.

Education

Because of growing drug resistance, greater emphasis is placed on reducing exposure to the anopheline mosquito, especially in hyperendemic areas such as Africa. Strategies that are successful and should be considered include the application of insect repellents that contain DEET (diethyltoluamide) and the use of netting impregnated with pyrethrin (insecticide) over the bed for protection during sleep. DDT (dichlorodiphenyltrichloroethane) is no longer effective in most regions of the world because of widespread resistance. Exposed nonimmune persons should be advised to consider malaria prophylaxis, to use insect repellents, and otherwise to reduce their exposure to the anopheline mosquito.

Prophylaxis for malaria can begin 1 week before travel and continue daily for 4 weeks after the patient leaves the area. Updated recommendations on malaria prophylaxis may be obtained 24 hours a day, 7 days a week through the CDC.

Persons who harbor the sexual forms of plasmodia are called *carriers*. It is from the carriers that mosquitos receive the forms of the parasite that perpetuate the disease. Carriers should be advised to avoid giving blood, because it is possible that the recipient of their blood will contract malaria or become a carrier. A growing number of malaria cases have been associated with transfusion of infected blood. Any person who has had malaria or has been exposed to the disease by visiting a region where it is prevalent must be disqualified as a blood donor.

Evaluation

Treatment effectiveness for the patient with malaria is evidenced by the absence of clinical signs and symptoms, by negative cultures, and by lack of adverse drug effects. If fever persists after adequate antimalarial therapy, the diagnosis must be re-evaluated.

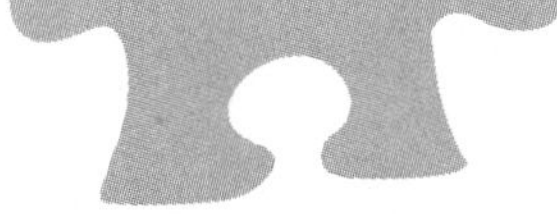

ECTOPARASITES

Ectoparasites are insects that live on the outer surface of the body. Strictly speaking, the term encompasses fungal infections of the skin as well as infestations by mites and lice. In practice, it refers only to mites and lice. Treatment of ectoparasitic infestations includes the use of scabicides and pediculicides, as listed below:

- ❒ Crotamiton (EURAX)
- ❒ Lindane (SCABENE)
- ❒ Malathion (OVIDE)
- ❒ Permethrin (NIX, ELIMITE)

Scabies

Scabies is a highly communicable disease caused by the itch mite, *Sarcoptes scabiei*. It is transmitted from one person to another by close contact. Transmission between bed partners is common and does not require body contact. Infestation occurs most often in the sides of the fingers, interdigital webs, flexor surfaces of wrists, elbows, skin around the nipples, and penis. Other lesions, including erythematous papules, lichenified patches, and pustules, can occur on the abdomen, thighs, and buttocks. In infants and young children, the mites burrow in the palms and soles, and papular lesions may be seen on the scalp, face, and neck. (See Case Study—Scabies.)

Intense pruritus begins 2 to 6 weeks after the first exposure. Definitive diagnosis is often difficult because of excoriations. Itching occurs almost exclusively at night, when the pests move around. Nits (eggs) and egg cases may be seen with the naked eye. The head and neck are usually exempt from infestation. Diagnosis depends on observing the mite in skin scrapings, by gently raising the top of the burrow with a sterile needle and looking with a magnifier. In most cases, 10 to 15 mites are present.

The drug of choice for treatment is the scabicide crotamiton. It is massaged into the skin from the chin down, with attention to body creases and folds. It is reapplied in 24 and 48 hours and then washed from the body surface (crotamiton requires two applications for one treatment). Two applications usually eradicate most infestations. In resistant cases, it may be applied again 1 week later. Permethrin (5 percent in dermal cream) in a single-dose regimen of 8 to 14 hours has been used with success. One percent lindane cream or lotion is often used in an 8- to 12-hour treatment for adults, followed by thorough washing. The patient should be advised that the pruritus and dermatitis may persist for days after adequate treatment. Lindane is contraindicated for infants and pregnant women. Chrysanthemum sensitivity must be assessed if permethrin is prescribed.

All the patient's household and intimate contacts should be treated to prevent recurrence or continued transmission. Clothing, especially undergarments, bedding, and towels should be laundered in hot water. As with other parasitic diseases, the patient should be advised regarding strategies to minimize exposure.

Lice

Pediculosis is an infestation of the body with lice. The incidence of infestation has been increasing in North America and western Europe. It was once thought that overcrowding, poor hygiene, lack of laundry and bathing facilities, and general uncleanliness promoted the infestation. This assumption, however, has proved to be untrue. The infestation is transmitted from one person to another by close contact or through sharing of combs, clothing, or towels.

There are three varieties of infestation. Observation of nits or lice in the hair and scalp confirms the diagnosis of head lice *(pediculosis capitis)*. They are found most often over the postauricular and occipital regions of the head. Nits attached to the seams of clothing, often in undergarments, indicate the presence of body lice *(pediculosis corporis)*. Body lice are usually not found directly on the body. Nits or lice attached to pubic hairs indicate pubic (crab) lice *(pediculosis pubis)*. Pubic infestations are found only in postpubertal individuals. Less commonly, lice are found on axillary hair, beards, mustache, eyebrows, and eyelashes. Common signs and symptoms are pruritus and, occasionally, sky-blue macules on the inner thighs or lower abdomen.

The drug of choice is the pediculicide lindane, although malathion and permethrin are being used more commonly because of their ovicidal effect. An organophosphate pediculicide, malathion has been shown to destroy lindane-resistant lice by inhibiting cholinesterase. Permethrin has a high cure rate (up to 90 percent) in treating head lice, after only a single application. It acts on the louse's nerve cell membranes to disrupt the sodium channel, thereby delaying

Case Study Scabies

Patient History

History of Present Illness	GB is a 76-year-old immunocompromised male, debilitated, dehydrated resident of a nursing home specifically for retarded persons and mentally ill. Has been bound in a private room. Admitted to acute care psych unit with reports of a fine rash on all body. Rash first noted 3 weeks after admission to medical floor for physical assessment and hydration with IV fluids. All information obtained from patient's chart. Patient is uncommunicative and incontinent of stool; has sheath catheter in place for urine drainage. There is no family in this area. No treatment for rash recorded. Rash area with crusting.
Past Health History	Diagnosis of severe schizophrenia with aphasia. Documented war trauma on old chart. Has been a long-time resident of nursing home.
Physical Exam Findings	Chest wheezes, crackles, severe dehydration with cachexia, poor muscle tone, and turgor. Stage II decubiti on left ischial crest and sacrum. Fresh dressings in place. Soft fleece pads on elbows, heels. Patient lying on sheepskin. Oral cavity dry and sticky. Perineal area clean, urine scant and dark. Heavy scalp involvement with nits/eggs.
Diagnostic Findings	Skin/hair scraping to view with magnification. Lab request for identification of mites/eggs/cases.
Developmental Considerations	None specific, although GB has physiologic changes of aging.
Psychosocial Considerations	Recommend social worker and dietician confer with nurses and physician for correlation of all treatments and diet supplements, frequency, supply, and administration. May need agency aides for one/one care. Will investigate source of possible lice infestation in nursing home, personnel, and acute care personnel.
Economic Factors	Patient is military veteran receiving a Veterans' Administration pension. This resource will be used.

Variables Influencing Decision

Treatment Objective	• Clear infestation of pediculus capitis.

Drug Variables	*Drug Summary*	*Patient Variables*
Indications	Active infestation of scabies	GB is severely debilitated and has scabies infestation of scalp.
Pharmacodynamics	Available drugs are scabicidal	There are no patient-related variables for pharmacodynamics.
Adverse Effects/ Contraindications	Least toxic drug may be malathion for this patient. Lindane is known to be absorbed via the skin with CNS toxicity; it is contraindicated in patients with allergy to chrysanthemums. Pyrethrin may be a problem in shampoo, as it could get into the eyes, mouth, and nose, with resultant CNS involvement.	GB is elderly, has thin skin, and is immunocompromised. Nursing personnel who care for patient must also be monitored for their compliance with drug therapy and their risk of infestation. GB also has an allergy to chrysanthemums.
Pharmacokinetics	Potential for greater transdermal absorption due to age.	Age-related changes in subcutaneous tissues may increase potential for toxicity. This will be a decision point.

Case Study Scabies—cont'd

Drug Variables	*Drug Summary*	*Patient Variables*
Dosage Regimen	Three applications of crotamiton lotion. Permethrin cream is a single-dose regimen. Lindane cream or lotion is also a single dose regimen.	Agency staff to administer. There is no compliance issue with GB. This will not be a decision point.
Laboratory Considerations	There are no specific laboratory considerations with the use of the available drugs for limited usage.	There are no specific patient considerations with the use of available drug for limited usage.
Cost Index*	Crotamiton lotion: 5 Permethrin cream: 1 Lindane lotion: 1	Permethrin and lindane in VA formulary. Crotamiton not available through VA pharmacy service. VA health care system will provide drug. This is a decision point.

Summary of Decision Points

- GB has a heavy infestation of pediculosis capitis.
- Scabies should be suspected in immunocompromised patient.
- GB is allergic to chrysanthemums; thus, lindane lotion is contraindicated.
- Cost of crotamiton high and drug not in VA formulary.

DRUG TO BE USED

- Permethrin 5% cream as single-dose regimen of 8–14 hours.

*Cost Index
1 = $<30/mo.
2 = $30–40/mo.
3 = $40–50/mo.
4 = $50–60/mo.
5 = $>60/mo.

AWP of 480 mL of 10% crotamiton lotiion is approximately $70.
AWP of 60 G of 5% permethrin cream is approximately $18.
AWP of 480 mL of 1% lindane lotion is approximately $13.

repolarization and paralyzing the parasite. Lindane is a chlorinated hydrocarbon.

One effective treatment regimen for head lice is a shampoo with permethrin (1 percent) cream rinse. A 5-minute, 1 percent lindane shampoo of the pubic area can be used for pubic infestations. After treatment, lice and nits can be removed using a metal comb with teeth 0.1 mm apart. Moisture or oil rinses may make this easier. Wet hair should not be exposed to open flame or to hair dryers on high setting. Mechanical removal is recommended for facial and pubic louse infestations. Lindane should be used with caution in infants, children, and pregnant women.

Preventing recurrence of lice involves treatment of human contacts and materials. Pillow cases, hats, scarves, and other items should be washed or cleaned. Infested combs and brushes should be cleaned and boiled or soaked for 1 hour in 1 percent lindane or 2 percent Lysol. Away from the body, head and body lice survive only about 3 days, 10 days maximum.

Sexual partners of persons with pubic lice should be treated and bedding, towels, and clothing washed or dry cleaned. Pubic lice do not survive longer than 24 hours away from the body. Transmission via toilet seats is unlikely. Fumigation is generally unnecessary, although vacuuming is helpful to remove stray lice and shed hairs with affixed nits. As with other parasitic diseases, the patient should be advised about strategies to minimize exposure.

PROTOZOAL DISORDER

Leishmaniasis

❒ Stibogluconate sodium (PENTOSTAM)
❒ Meglumine antimoniate (GLUCANTIME)

Leishmaniasis is a name given to a spectrum of diseases caused by a variety of protozoal species. The infection occurs on all continents except Australia and probably affects at least 100 million people. Uncommon in the United States, the parasite is common in India, the Middle East, and Central and South America. The annual incidence is estimated at more than 12 million cases. Military veterans of Desert Storm, the Sudan campaigns, African assignments, or Central American service must be suspect if symptoms dictate.

The disorder is transmitted to humans most often by the bites of infected female phlebotomine sandflies. The flagellated extracellular organisms live in the GI tract and saliva of the insect vector, which passes infection on to humans during a blood meal. Once in the host, the organisms multiply in macrophages and in cells of the reticuloendothelial system. The three species cause distinct disease and differ in their geographic distribution and species of vector. *Leishmania donovani* causes visceral leishmaniasis (kala-azar); *Leishmania tropica* causes cutaneous leishmaniasis (oriental sore); and *Leishmania braziliensis* causes mucocutaneous leishmaniasis.

Leishmania donovani is responsible for the most significant clinical disease. All internal organs may be affected, but the liver, spleen, and bone marrow are most involved. Active disease manifests as fever, pronounced splenomegaly, emaciation, and pancytopenia. The fever may be intermittent and irregular. Lymph nodes may be enlarged. If left untreated, this form of leishmaniasis is always fatal. In contrast, *L. tropica* and L. braziliensis are usually self-limiting, but facial and head lesions can be disfiguring. Recovery from leishmaniasis due to *L. donovani* or *L. tropica* provides a lasting immunity.

Treatment of leishmaniasis is difficult, because the available drugs are quite toxic and not very effective. Treatment has most often relied on antimonial compounds (heavy metals) such as sodium stibogluconate sodium and meglumine antimoniate. Stibogluconate sodium is available in the United States through the CDC and is also used in Europe, Africa, and India. It appears to act by inhibiting parasitic enzyme systems and is given only intravenously or intramuscularly. Meglumine antimoniate is available in Latin America, France, and Francophonic countries in Africa.

To treat cutaneous leishmaniasis, a 20 mg/kg daily dose of stibogluconate sodium should be given for 20 days. If a cure rate of 95 percent or higher is reached, the dosage may be decreased or a shorter time period tried. For mucocutaneous and systemic leishmaniasis, the World Health Organization recommends 20 mg/kg for 30 days. Children's dosages are the same as adults'. About 80 percent of the drug is eliminated via the kidneys after intravenous injection within 6 hours. The pharmacokinetic behavior is the same whether the drug is given intravenously or intramuscularly.

Because stibogluconate sodium is a heavy metal, it is considered a fairly toxic drug. Its main adverse effects are pain at the injection site, joint pain, and GI upset. In some cases, hepatic failure and renal failure have occurred. This agent's principal disadvantages, however, are related to the long courses of treatment, the necessity for parenteral administration, and its relatively high cost.

Pentamidine is recommended for the 15 percent of cases of East African (Sudan) kala-azar that are unresponsive to stibogluconate sodium. Pentamidine produces hypotension by an unknown mechanism. Patients with cardiac disorders should be closely observed while under treatment. Pentamidine can also have hypoglycemic and diabetic effects. Other effects of pentamidine are inhibition of platelet aggregation and inhibition of cholinesterase in laboratory analysis.

Amphotericin B, although an antifungal drug, is another excellent but toxic alternative for the treatment of mucosal leishmaniasis (see Chapter 25).

SUMMARY

- Helminthiasis, an infestation of parasitic worms, is a major health problem in many parts of the world.
- The presence of worms is called an "infestation" rather than an "infection."
- Roundworms, hookworms, tapeworms, threadworms, and pinworms make up the bulk of the causative agents. Trematodes are the "flukes" of the worm world.
- A variety of drugs are used in the treatment of infestation and act directly or indirectly to interfere with the life cycle of the adult parasite.
- Assessment of the patient includes gathering information related to travel to or residence in endemic areas as well as eating habits.
- The primary treatment objective is to kill or destroy the adult worm, thus reducing the worm load.
- Compliance and dependability of the patient being treated are crucial factors for successful elimination of the parasites.
- Although the *Anopheles* mosquito has been virtually eradicated in the United states, malaria remains the world's most devastating human infection.
- Malarial parasites are of four types and are called *Plasmodium* because of their affinity for erythrocytes.
- Antimalarial drugs are categorized according to the stage of the parasite they affect and the particular malarial strain involved.
- The pharmacodynamics of antimalarial drugs are unclear, but they appear to bind to a product of heme breakdown that is highly lytic to RBCs and to accumulate in the acidic lysosome compartments of the parasite.
- As with infestations, the patient history should elicit travel to or residence in endemic areas.
- Treatment objectives for malaria include a reduction in or elimination of signs and symptoms, and decreasing patient discomfort.
- Few drugs are available for the treatment of malaria, and what is available is in danger of becoming ineffective in treatment.
- Prophylaxis and treatment regimens should be followed closely to prevent adverse drug effects as well as to promote efficacy.
- Ectoparasites live on the outer surfaces of the body as infestations by mites and lice. The two most common infestations are scabies and pediculosis.
- Scabies and pediculosis are highly communicable and are caused by the itch mite and lice, respectively.
- The drug of choice for the treatment of scabies is crotamiton, but permethrin and lindane are also effective.
- For pediculosis, the drug of choice is lindane, although malathion and permethrin are also useful.
- Leishmaniasis is a spectrum of diseases caused by a variety of protozoal species. The disease is transmitted to humans by the bites of infected female sandflies.
- The three principal *Leishmania* species cause distinct diseases and differ in geographic distribution and species of vector.
- Treatment for leishmaniasis relies most often on antimonial compounds (heavy metals).

BIBLIOGRAPHY

Beadles, D., McElroy, P., Oster, C., et al. (1995). Impact of transmission intensity and age on *Plasmodium falciparum* density and associated fever: Implications for malarial vaccine trial design. *Journal of Infectious Disease,* 172, 1047–1054.

Berg, R. (Ed.) (1993). *APIC curriculum for infection control practice.* Dubuque, Iowa: Kendall Hunt Publishing Co.

Braude, A., Davis, C., and Fierer, M. (Eds.). (1986). *Infectious diseases and medical microbiology.* (2nd ed.). Philadelphia: W.B. Saunders.

Clark, J., Friesen, D., and Williams, W. (1992). Management of an outbreak of Norwegian scabies. *American Journal of Infection Control,* 20(4), 217–220.

McCarthy, J., Guinea, A., Weil, G., et al. (1995). Clearance of circulating filarial antigen as a measure of the microfilaricidal activity of diethylcarbamazine in *Wuchereria bancrofti* infection. *Journal of Infectious Disease,* 172, 521–526.

Sanford, J., Gilbert, D., Gerberding, J. et al. (Eds.). (1994). *Guide to antimicrobial therapy.* Dallas: Roche Laboratories.

Schulman, M., Doherty, P., Zinc, D., et al. (1994). Microbial conversion of invermectin by *Saccharopolyspora erythraea:* Hydroxylation at C-27. *Journal of Antibiotics,* 47(3), 372–375.

Tellier, R., and Keystone, J. (1992). Prevention of traveler's diarrhea. *Infectious Disease Clinics of North America,* 6(2), 333–354.

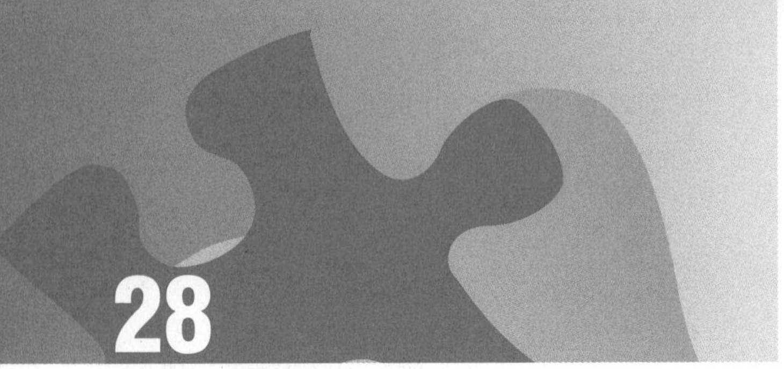

28

Sera, Vaccines, and Immunizing Drugs

Vaccines are one of the most effective disease prevention tools available in the world. Widespread immunization of children in the United States has led to more than 90 percent reduction in all childhood diseases. The effectiveness of immunization campaigns has been demonstrated through a measurable reduction in the *incidence* of vaccine-preventable infectious disease in this country.

Prevalence rates of vaccine-preventable diseases are one of the traditional measures of the quality and effectiveness of a nation's overall health care delivery system. Immunizations are considered the most basic of all preventive health care strategies.

The long-term goal of immunization programs is eradication of disease. The immediate goal is prevention of disease in individuals and groups. In order to achieve these goals, participation in immunization programs must be a high priority for people of all ages—children, adolescents, and adults. Factors interfering with these goals must be addressed. Cultural barriers, adverse effects, and contraindications must be considered in the design of an effective immunization campaign.

Health care providers are able to play an active role in immunization programs when they understand immunity and the types of drugs used as well as the indications and current recommendations for vaccines. Knowledge of administration and vaccine reactions is also required. Additionally, they should be familiar with the legislative and societal concerns associated with this important component of health promotion and disease prevention (see Terminology Associated with Immunization).

Recommendations for vaccinating infants, children, and adults are based on characteristics of immunobiologics, scientific knowledge about the principles of active and passive immunity, and the epidemiology of diseases. In the United States, these recommendations are developed by the Advisory Committee for Immunization Practices (ACIP) of the Food and Drug Administration, with input from the Centers for Disease Control and Prevention and the American Academy of Pediatrics. In Canada, The *Canadian Immunization Guide* from the National Advisory Council on Immunization is used to determine immunization schedules.

IMMUNITY

Immunity is a state in which the host is resistant to a specific disease. Immunity may be natural, as when the host lives in an environment filled with organisms without becoming ill. *Active immunity* is the production of antibody or other immune responses through the administration of a vaccine or toxoid. It prepares the individual for future challenges. *Acquired immunity* develops after the host has contracted the illness, or when the host is injected with a vaccine or a toxoid.

The terms vaccination and immunization are often used interchangeably to refer to active immunization, although they are technically not synonymous. The administration of an immunobiologic (vaccination) cannot be equated with the development of immunity.

Passive immunity provides temporary immunity through the administration of preformed antibodies. It provides protection for those hosts already, or about to be, exposed. Passive immunity is achieved by introducing antibodies produced by someone other than the host (e.g., breastfeeding). Three types of immunobiologics are utilized to provide passive immunity: human immune globulin (IG), specific immune globulin preparations, and antitoxins.

Antigen and Antibody Response

Active immunity is the basis for development of most immunizations and vaccines. With the injection of an antigen, the immune system of the patient responds by producing antibodies. It is often assumed that active immunization provides life-long protection, but in reality, it does not. Periodic boosters are needed with many vaccinations to further stimulate antibody production to maintain active, acquired immunity.

The success of most vaccines in establishing an antigen-antibody response depends on the humoral response of the immune system. The introduction of an antigen stimulates a response independent of T lymphocytes (T cells) that can occur only through B-lymphocyte (B-cell) mediation. The B-cell response is very poor or completely absent in children younger than 1 year. Consequently, for an immune response to occur in this age group, a T cell–dependent antibody response must be initiated. In this process, T cells stimulate the development of antibodies. T cell–dependent antigens can be converted from T cell–independent antigens through chemical linkage of the antigen to a carrier protein. Polysaccharide antigens, which are connected to a carrier protein, are considerably less immunogenic in younger children than protein antigens. Connecting a polysaccharide antigen with a protein antigen (e.g., diphtheria, tetanus) significantly increases the immunity in this age group. *Haemophilus influenzae,* meningococcal, and pneumococcal vaccines are in this group of antigens. Repeated immunizations offer assurance of a uniform population response to the antigen.

The antigens used in a vaccine depend on the disease for which they are providing protection. Many immunizations contain live virus, which after inoculation stimulates an active infection in the host without the adverse effects. Live viruses tend to be more effective in providing immunity. Inactivated preparations, those containing killed viruses, do not replicate in the host and therefore must contain sufficient amounts of antigen to stimulate the desired response. Maintenance of long-term immunity with these immunizations usually requires boosters at regular intervals.

TERMINOLOGY ASSOCIATED WITH IMMUNIZATION

Active immunity—The production of antibody or other immune responses through the administration of a vaccine or toxoid.
Acquired immunity—Develops after a host has contracted an illness, or when injected with a vaccine or a toxoid.
Antisera—A serum containing antibodies. Usually obtained from an animal that received the antigen, either by injection into the tissues or blood or by infection.
Antitoxins—A specific antibody manufactured in the body in response to the presence of a toxin.
Attenuated vaccine—The change in virulence of an organism induced by passage through another host species, decreasing its virulence for the native host and increasing it for the new host. The basis for the development of live vaccines.
Incidence—The number of new cases of a specific disease occurring during a certain period.
Immunity—A state in which the host is resistant to a specific disease.
Live virus—Stimulates an active infection in the host without producing the adverse effects.
Immunization—Used when referring to active immunization.
Passive immunity—Achieved by introducing antibodies produced by someone other than the host.
Prevalence—The total number of cases of a specific disease in existence in a given population at a given time.
Sera—The blood serum from persons or animals whose bodies have built antibodies, called antisera or immune serum. Used when person has already been exposed or contracted the disease. Pleural for serum.
Seroconversion—The change of a serologic test from negative to positive, indicating the development of antibodies in response to immunization or infection.
Trivalent—The number of antigen binding sites possessed by an antibody molecule.
Toxoid—A toxin treated by heat or chemical agent to destroy its deleterious properties. The toxin's pathogenic quality is destroyed but its antigenic properties remain.
Vaccine—A suspension of live or attenuated organisms administered for the purpose of establishing active immunity to an infectious disease.
Vaccination—Used when referring to active immunization.

IMMUNIZING PRODUCTS

Vaccines

A *vaccine* is a suspension of live or *attenuated* microorganisms administered for the purpose of establishing active immunity to an infectious disease. There are two general classes of vaccines, viral and bacterial. Viral vaccines include

- Live, attenuated viruses (e.g., measles, mumps, rubella, oral poliovirus vaccines)
- Inactivated nonliving whole virus (e.g., influenza, rabies, inactivated poliomyelitis vaccines)
- Antigenic components of the virus particle (e.g., influenza "split-virus" vaccine, hepatitis B vaccine)

Vaccines containing live, attenuated viruses produce a mild or subclinical infection that results in long-term active immunity. For example, two doses of live oral poliovirus vaccine (OPV) and two doses of measles-mumps-rubella (MMR) vaccine are currently recommended to ensure *seroconversion*. Replication of the virus in the recipient is necessary to the induction of immunity.

Inactivated viral vaccines must contain a sufficient amount of antigen to induce the desired immune response, because the organisms in these preparations cannot replicate in the host. Repeated dosing is usually necessary to provoke long-term immunity. The immunization schedule for inactivated vaccines usually consists of two to three doses, with booster doses used to maintain the immunity.

In contrast to viral vaccines, bacterial vaccines are prepared from any of the following sources:

- Whole bacteria (e.g., pertussis vaccine)
- Purified products of whole-cell vaccine (e.g., acellular pertussis vaccine)
- Purified capsular polysaccharides of certain bacteria (e.g., pneumococcal and meningococcal vaccines)
- Purified polysaccharides conjugated to protein carriers to improve immunogenicity (e.g., *H. influenzae* type B [Hib] vaccine)

Live, attenuated bacterial vaccines act much like live virus vaccines. They stimulate the production of various antibodies. Those that play a protective role are directed against antigens on the surface of the bacterial cell or its exotoxin. Coating bacterial surface antigens with antibodies either renders the organisms susceptible to phagocytosis, lysis, and aggregation or interferes with the function of critical bacterial surface structures. Inactivated bacterial vaccines are usually given in two to four doses. Polysaccharide vaccines provide long-term protection, usually after a single dose (except in children younger than 2 years).

Live attenuated viral vaccines should not be given to patients with acquired immune deficiency syndrome, other immune diseases, or impairment of immune systems due to leukemia, lymphoma, corticosteroid or antineoplastic drugs, or radiation therapy. The virus may replicate and cause infection in these individuals.

Certain vaccines (i.e., diphtheria-tetanus-pertussis [DTP], MMR, poliovirus, hepatitis B, Hib) are routinely used for pediatric immunization, whereas others (e.g., rabies, influenza, meningococcal, pneumococcal, bacille Calmette-Guérin [BCG], plague, typhoid, cholera, yellow fever) are used primarily for patients at high risk. Most vaccines are intended for use in healthy individuals, although some may be safe and effective in persons with underlying diseases or conditions.

All vaccines contain similar major constituents. Each has an active component specific for a disease or an ill-defined constituent. The active component is contained in a suspension, usually normal saline or water. Trace amounts of chemicals serve as preservatives, stabilizers, and antimicrobial agents. Adjuvants (e.g., aluminum compounds) are used to increase the antigenicity of the vaccine and to prolong its stimulatory effects. Identification of these components is necessary so that potential hypersensitivity can be identified before immunization.

Toxoids

Toxoids, like vaccines, stimulate active immunity without causing disease. During the preparation of toxoids, the toxin's pathogenic quality is destroyed but its antigenic properties remain. Some toxoids are precipitated or absorbed with chemicals that cause them to remain in the tissues longer. The absorbed formulation increases the production of antibodies, making the response long-lasting. Nevertheless, toxoids can produce painful, localized reactions. The adverse effects, which are more pronounced in adults and older children, may necessitate the use of smaller initial doses.

Antitoxins

Antitoxins are used when a person has been exposed to an organism that secretes toxins. Antitoxins are obtained through the injection of an animal such as a horse with a purified toxin. After antibodies have had time to develop, blood is withdrawn from the animal and prepared for clinical use. Antitoxins provide passive immunity. Examples of antitoxins are those for tetanus, botulism, diphtheria, gas-gangrene, and rabies. Antitoxins are used for prophylaxis as well as therapeutic purposes. The disadvantage of antitoxins is related to the hypersensitivity that many people have to horse serum.

Sera

Sera are used to prevent infectious disease or to relieve symptoms of the disease after suspected or actual exposure. They provide passive immunity. Human serum immune globulin is used to reduce the severity of disease or to prevent certain diseases after exposure. It is a sterile, concentrated protein solution (15 to 18 percent) composed primarily of the immunoglobulin (Ig) fraction with trace amounts of IgA or IgM. It contains specific antibodies in proportion to the infection and immunization experience of the population from which it is derived. Peak serum levels of antibodies are achieved 48 to 72 hours after inoculation. The dosage of immune globulin is based on body weight. Immune globulin is indicated as replacement therapy for antibody deficiency disorders, hepatitis A, and measles prophylaxis. Adverse effects include discomfort and pain at the site of administration.

Antisera

Animal antisera (antibodies of animal origin) are derived from the sera of horses. They are used in those illnesses for which specific immune globulins of human origin are unavailable (i.e., diphtheria and botulism). Each patient receiving animal serum is tested for sensitivity by means of a scratch or intradermal test before administration of the serum. If sensitivity is evident, desensitization should be undertaken because anaphylaxis is probable. Other reactions that may occur as a result are acute febrile reactions, serum sickness including fever, urticaria, maculopapular rash, arthritis, or arthralgia, and lymphadenopathy (1 to 3 weeks after administration), and anaphylaxis.

DISEASES AND DRUGS

Diphtheria, Tetanus, and Pertussis

Diphtheria

Diphtheria is an acute bacterial infection of the tonsils, pharynx, larynx, nose, and, occasionally, other mucus membranes. The skin and sometimes the conjunctivae or genitalia are affected. Diphtheria results from infection by *Corynebacterium diphtheriae,* which produces a potent endotoxin. The characteristic diphtheria lesion is marked by a patch or patches of an adherent grayish membrane with surrounding inflammation. Late effects, which appear 2 to 6 weeks after absorption of the toxin, include cranial and peripheral motor and sensory nerve palsies and myocarditis. The mortality rates (5 to 10 percent) for noncutaneous diphtheria have changed little in 50 years.

Diphtheria occurs in colder months in temperate zones. It affects primarily nonimmunized children younger than 15 years but may also be found in adults whose immunization was neglected. Formerly a prevalent disease, diphtheria has largely disappeared in areas with effective immunization programs.

Extensive study of the disease led to the use of an antitoxin in the late 1800s and a toxin-antitoxin mixture by the 1920s. In developed countries, the incidence of diphtheria has declined markedly since 1920, when the first vaccine became available.

Recovery from a clinical attack of diphtheria is not always followed by lasting immunity. Immunity is often acquired through inapparent infection. Prolonged active immunity can be induced by toxoid. Diphtheria vaccine provides active immunity and is most often administered in combination with tetanus, or with tetanus and pertussis.

Tetanus

Tetanus is a bacterial infection whose symptoms result from the action of the *Clostridium tetani* exotoxin, *tetanospasmin.* The exotoxin invades devitalized tissue. The disease is characterized by painful muscular contractions, primarily of the masseter and neck muscles. Trunk muscles may be involved secondarily. The organism is rarely recovered from the site of infection, and typically, there is no detectable antibody response. Fifty to 90 cases of tetanus and 20 to 30 deaths are reported annually in the United States. About 60 percent of the cases occur in persons older than 60 years. Tetanus is more common in areas where contact with animal feces is likely and immunization inadequate.

The bacilli *C. tetani* are large, gram-positive, nonencapsulated rods with terminal spores. They require strict anaerobic conditions for growth and toxin elaboration. The spores are very resistant to destruction, living in the soil. Although recognized as a disease around 4 BC, it was not until the late 1800s that the organism was isolated and a toxoid developed.

Childhood immunizations with DTP, adult immunization with Td, and careful wound management have reduced the incidence of tetanus. Susceptibility to the disease is directly related to immunization status. The primary immunization series is given in infancy, and booster doses are needed every 10 years (Table 28–1).

Pertussis

Pertussis (commonly known as whooping cough) is an acute bacterial infection that involves the respiratory tract. It is caused by the gram-negative bacillus *Bordetella pertussis.* The initial catarrhal stage (inflammation of mucus membranes with free discharge) has an insidious onset with an irritating cough that gradually becomes paroxysmal. The stage

TABLE 28–1 DOSAGE REGIMEN FOR SELECTED SERA, VACCINES, AND OTHER IMMUNIZING DRUGS

Drug	FRM*	IMM	P/Tr	Dosage	Implications
Vaccines					
Diphtheria-tetanus-pertussis vaccine (DTP)	T	A	P	*Child younger than 7 yr:* #1 0.5 mL IM at age 2 mo. #2 0.5 mL IM at age 4 mo. #3 0.5 mL IM at age 6 mo. #4 0.5 mL IM 6–12 mo later Booster: 0.5 mL IM at age 4–6 yr (entry to school)	Efficacy: High Duration: 10 yr
Diphtheria-tetanus–whole cell pertussis vaccine (DTwP, TRI-IMMUNOL)	T	A	P	*Child younger than 7 yr:* #1 0.5 mL IM at age 2 mo. #2 0.5 mL IM at age 4 mo. #3 0.5 mL IM at age 6 mo. #4 0.5 mL IM at age 4–6 yr (entry to school)	DTP and DTaP are used until age 7. After age 7, Td is used. A booster of Td is required every 10 yr. Efficacy: High Duration: 10 yr.
Diphtheria-tetanus–acellular pertussis vaccine (DTaP, ACEL-IMMUNE, TRIPEDIA)	T	A	P	*Child younger than 7 yr:* #1 0.5 mL IM at age 2 mo. #2 0.5 mL IM at age 4 mo. #3 0.5 mL IM at age 6 mo. #4 0.5 mL IM at age 4–6 yr (entry to school)	Decreases serious adverse effects associated with the whole-cell vaccine. Efficacy: High Duration: 10 yr
Diphtheria-tetanus–whole cell pertussis with *Haemophilus influenzae* type B conjugate vaccine (DTwP-HIBTITER, TETRAMUNE)	T/IBV	A	P	*Child 2 mo to 5 yr:* #1 0.5 mL .initially #2 0.5 mL 2 mo later. #3 0.5 mL 4 mo after first dose. #4 0.5 mL 9–12 mo later	Not recommended for children who experienced active *Haemophilus influenzae* type B infection within the last 24 months. Contraindicated in children over age 7
Haemophilus influenzae type B polysaccharide vaccine (HIBTITER, PEDVAXHIB, PROHIBIT)	IBV	A	P	*Child to 6 yr:* #1 0.5 mL IM at age 2 mo. #2 0.5 mL IM at age 4 mo. #3 0.5 mL IM at age 6 mo. #4 0.5 mL IM at age 12–15 mo	If initial dose given after age 18 mo, only one dose (PROHIBIT) needed. HIBTITER not for this use. A minimum of 1 mo. between immunizations is required regardless of age. Contraindicated in febrile illness or active infection
Hepatitis A vaccine (HAVRIX)	IVV	A	P	*Adult:* #1 1 mL IM. #2 1 mL IM 6–12 mo later. *Child:* #1 0.5 mL IM age 2–18 yr. #2 0.5 mL IM 1 mo later. #3 0.5 mL IM 6–12 mo after first dose	Can be given concurrently with other other travel vaccines without interfering with immune responses. Contraindicated in patients with bleeding disorders or febrile illness Efficacy: 80–98% Duration: 10 yr 1 mL = 1440 ELISA units
Hepatitis B vaccine (ENERGIX B)	IVV	A	P	*Neonates to 10 yr whose mothers are HBsAg negative:* #1 0.5 mL IM at birth #2 0.5 mL IM at age 1–2 mo. #3 0.5 mL IM 4 mo after second dose Booster: 0.5 mL IM × 1 dose *Child older than 10 yr and Adults:* #1 1 mL initially. #2 1 mL 1 mo later. #3 1 mL 5 mo after second dose. Booster: 1 mL × 1 dose *Dialysis patients:* 2 mL initially, and at 1, 2, and 6 mo after first dose.	Dialysis patients should receive special formulation of 40 mcg. surface antigen/mL Efficacy: 96% children 88% adults Duration: Unknown 20 mcg = 1 mL
Hepatitis B vaccine (RECOMBIVAX HB)	IVV	A	P	*Neonates to 10 yr whose mothers are HBsAg negative:* #1 0.25 mL IM at birth. #2 0.25 mL IM at 1–2 mo. #3 0.25 mL IM 4 mo after second dose. *Child age 11–19 yrs:* #1 0.5 mL initially. #2 0.5 mL 1 mo later #3 0.5 mL 5 mo after second dose. *Dialysis patients:*1 mL IM × 3 doses initially and at 1 mo and 6 mo after first dose	Booster: one dose of 1 mL if antibody level less than 10 million units/mL 1–2 months after the third dose of schedule. Dialysis patients should receive special formulation of 40 mcg. surface antigen/mL Efficacy: 96% children 88% adults Duration: Unknown 10 mcg = 1 mL

Table continued on following page

TABLE 28–1 DOSAGE REGIMEN FOR SELECTED SERA, VACCINES, AND OTHER IMMUNIZING DRUGS *Continued*

Drug	FRM*	IMM	P/Tr	Dosage	Implications
Vaccines *Continued*					
Energix B		A		*Child 0 to 19 years:* #1 0.5 mL initially #2 0.5 mL 1 mo later #3 0.5 mL 4 mo after second dose *Adults over 19 years:* #1 1 mL initially #2 1 mL 1 mo later #3 1 mL 4 mo after second dose	
Influenza vaccine (FLUOGEN, FLU-ZONE, FLUSHIELD, FLUVIRIN, FLU-IMMUNE, INFLUENZA VIRUS, VACCINE)	IVV	A	P	*Child to 3 yr:* 0.25 mL IM × 1 dose *Adult and child older than 3 yr:* 0.5 mL IM × 1 dose	Maximum antibody protection occurs in 2 wk. Children younger than 9 yr not previously immunized need two doses at least 1 month apart. Nasal spray under development Contraindicated in patients with allergy to eggs and those with a history of Guillain-Barré syndrome. Efficacy: 60–75% Duration: 1 mo
Measles, mumps, rubella vaccine (M-M-R II)	LAVV	A	P	*Child to age 12 yr:* Total volume of reconstituted vial given SC at: #1 age 12–15 mo #2 age 4–6 yr (entry to school) or age 11–12 yrs	Combination agent preferred over single agents. Contraindicated in persons with allergies to eggs or neomycin Efficacy: 95% Duration: Years to life
Measles vaccine (rubeola, ATTENUVAX)	LAVV	A	P	*Adult and child:* 0.5 mL SC × 1 dose.	Usually given with mumps and rubella vaccines. May invalidate TB test if given within 6 weeks of immunization Efficacy: 95% Duration: Years to life 0.5 mL = 1000 $TCID_{50}$
Measles-rubella vaccine (M-R-VAX II)	LAVV	A	P	*Child:* Total volume of reconstituted vial SC	A mixture of live attenuated rubeola virus and rubella virus
Meningococcal vaccine (MENOMUNE-A/C/Y/W-135)	IBV	A	P	*Adult and child:* 0.5 mL SC × 1 dose.	Not for routine immunization Efficacy: 90%; variable in young children. Effectiveness drops to 67% after 3 years. Duration: 3 yr
Mumps vaccine (MUMPSVAX)	LAVV	A	P	*Adult and child older than 12 mo:* 0.5 mL SC × 1 dose	Efficacy: High Duration: 10 yr 0.5 mL = 20,000 $TCID_{50}$
Mumps-rubella vaccine (BIAVAX II)	LVV	A	P	*Child older than 12 mo:* Total volume of reconstituted vial SC	A mixture of mumps and rubella virus strains. Used less often than MMR
Rubella vaccine (MERUVAX II)	LAVV	A	P	*Adult:* 0.5 mL SC × 1 dose	Efficacy: 95% Duration: 6–15 yr 0.5 mL = 1000 $TCID_{50}$
Pneumococcal vaccine (PNEUMOVAX 23, PNU-IMUNE 23)	IBV	A	P	*Adult and child older than 2 yr:* 0.5 mL SC/IM × 1 dose	Not recommended for children younger than 2 yr because they may be unable to produce adequate antibody levels
Polio oral trivalent vaccine [Sabin] (OPV, ORIMUNE)	LAVV	A	P	*Adult and child:* #1 0.5 mL PO at 2 mo #2 0.5 mL PO at 4 mo #3 0.5 mL PO at 6–18 mo Booster: 0.5 mL PO at age 4–6 yr (entry to school)	Duration: Years to life
Poliomyelitis vaccine [Salk] (IPV)	KVV	A	P	*Adult:* #1 0.5 mL SC initially. #2 0.5 mL SC 1–2 mo later. #3 0.5 mL SC 6–12 mo after second dose. *Child:* #1 0.5 mL SC at 2 mo #2 0.5 mL SC at 4 mo #3 0.5 mL SC 6–12 mo after second dose. Booster: 0.5 mL × 1 dose at age 4–6 yr (entry to school)	IPV now recommended for first two doses followed by OPV. OPV can still be given as noted in table. IPV can be given instead of OPV as noted in table IPV booster for those who have not received OPV every 5 yr Efficacy: 90%
Rabies human diploid cell vaccine (HDCV, IMOVAX)	KVV	A	P	*Pre-exposure prophylaxis in adult:* #1 1.0 mL IM initially. #2 1.0 mL IM 1 wk later. #3 1.0 mL IM 4 wk after first dose. Booster: 1.0 mL every 2 yr.	Boosters recommended every 2 yr for people identified as high risk. Rabies immunoglobulin (RIG) is administered at the same time as the initial dose of HDCV vaccine

TABLE 28–1 DOSAGE REGIMEN FOR SELECTED SERA, VACCINES, AND OTHER IMMUNIZING DRUGS *Continued*

Drug	FRM*	IMM	P/Tr	Dosage	Implications
Vaccines ***Continued***					
Rabies vaccine (absorbed, RVA)				*Post-exposure prophylaxis in adult:* #1 1.0 mL IM initially. #2 1.0 mL IM on day 3 after injury. #3 1.0 mL IM on day 7. #4 1.0 mL IM on day 14. #5 1.0 mL IM on day 28.	Duration: 1 yr
Tetanus-diptheria vaccine (Adult type, Td)	T	A	P	*Adult and child:* First visit: 0.5 mL IM 4 wk later: 0.5 mL IM 6–12 mo later: 0.5 mL IM Booster: 0.5 mL IM	Reactions are usually mild. Td booster recommended every 6–10 yr
Tetanus-diptheria vaccine (Pediatric type, DT)	T	A	P	*Adult and child to 7 yr:* #1 0.5 mL IM initially #2 0.5 mL IM 4 wk later #3 0.5 mL IM 1 yr later Booster: 0.5 mL IM at age 4–6 yr (entry to school)	Routine administration for children up to 6 yr in whom pertussis vaccine is contraindicated
Varicella vaccine (VARIVAX)	LAVV	A	P	*Healthy adult and child with no history of disease:* 2 doses 4–8 wk apart for persons past their 13th birthday 1 dose for those under 13 yrs	Can be given along with MMR, using separate syringes and injection sites Efficacy: 95–97% 1–12 yr 79% 13–17 yr
Toxoids					
Tetanus toxoid	T	P	P	*Adult and child, fluid formulation:* #1,2,3 0.5 mL IM/SC at 4–8 wk intervals #4 0.5 mL 6–12 mo later. Booster: 0.5 mL every 10 yr *Adult and child, absorbed formulation:* #1,2,3 0.5 mL IM/SC at 4–8 wk intervals. Booster: 0.5 mL every 10 yr	Fluid formulation: 0.5 mL. = 4–5 Lf of toxoid. Absorbed formulation: 0.5 mL. = 5–10 Lf of toxoid Duration: 10 yr
Antitoxins					
Botulism antitoxin	KAT	P	Tr	*Adult and child:* Consult package insert for instructions regarding route of administration and dose	Provides passive immunity. Test for hypersensitivity to horse serum preceding administration of antitoxin. Available from the CDCP
Diptheria antitoxin	KAT	P	P/Tr	*Adult and child:* Prophylaxis: 10,000 units IM Treatment: 20,000–120,000 units IM	Used in conjunction with antibiotics to eliminate bacterial but do not eliminate bacterial toxins
Tetanus antitoxin	AT	P	P	*Adult and child:* 3000–5000 units IM/SC	
Sera					
Cytomegalovirus human immune globulin (CMV-IGIV, CYTOGAM)	S	P	T	*Adult and child:* 150 mg/kg IV infusion within 72 hr of transplant. 100 mg/kg 2–8 wk after transplant. 50 mg/kg 12–16 wk after transplant	Provides passive immunity against CMV
Hepatitis B immune globulin (human, H-BIG, HYPER-HEP, HEP-B-GAMMAGEE)	S	P	P	*Newborns:* 0.5 mL IM within 24 hr after birth. Repeat at 3 and 6 mo *Adult and child:* 0.06 mL/kg as soon as possible after exposure. Repeat dose in 1 mo	Not for treatment of fulminant acute or chronic active hepatitis B Effective: 70–80% after second dose 94–98% after third dose
Immune serum globulin (gamma globulin, ISG, GAMMAR, GAMASTAN)	S	P	P/Tr	*Adult and child with hepatitis exposure:* 0.02–0.04 mL/kg IM × 1 dose *Adult and child with measles exposure:* 0.25 mL/kg IM given within 6 days of exposure × 1 dose *Adult and child with varicella exposure:* 0.6–1.2 mL/kg IM × 1 dose *Pregnant women with rubella exposure:* 0.55 mL/kg × 1 dose *Bacterial infections:* 0.5–3.5 mL/kg IM.	Routine use in early pregnancy is not recommended. Produces adequate serum levels of IgG in 2–5 days
Immune serum globulin (IGIV, GAMIMUNE, SANDOGLOBULIN)	S	P	Tr	*GAMIMUNE:* 100–200 mg/kg IV q mo *SANDOGLOBULIN:* 200 mg/kg IV q mo *ITP:* 400 mg/kg IM daily × 5 days	If clinical response or serum level of IgG is insufficient, GAMIMUNE may be given more often or dosage increased to 400 mg/kg or SANDOGLOBULIN dose may be increased to 300 mg/kg

Table continued on following page

TABLE 28–1 DOSAGE REGIMEN FOR SELECTED SERA, VACCINES, AND OTHER IMMUNIZING DRUGS *Continued*

Drug	FRM*	IMM	P/Tr	Dosage	Implications
Sera *Continued*					
Rabies immune serum globulin (RIG, HYPERAB, IMOGAM)	S	P	P	*Adult and child:* 20 units/kg IM as soon as possible after exposure	One-half of dose may be infiltrated around the wound Duration: 21 days
Antirabies equine serum	KAT	P	P	*Adult and child:* 55 units/kg IM as soon as possible after exposure	Used only if human rabies immuneglobulin not available. Half of dose may be infiltrated around the wound
Rh_0 human immune globulin (GAMULIN RH, HYPRHO-D, RHOGAM)	S	P	P	*Obstetric use:* 1 vial IM for every 15 mL fetal packed RBC volume within 72 hr after delivery, miscarriage, or abortion *Transfusion mishap:* 1 vial IM for every 15 mL of Rh-positive packed RBC volume	Consult package insert for blood typing and drug administration procedures 1 vial = 300 mcg
Tetanus immune globulin (human, TIG, HYPER-TET)	S	P	P	*Prophylaxis adult and child:* 250 units IM× 1 dose *Clinical disease in adults and children:* 3000–6000 units IM × 1 dose	Tetanus toxoid should be given at the same time to initiate active immune response. Preferred to tetanus antitoxin, because does not cause allergic reaction and has longer duration of action
Varicella-zoster immune globulin (human, VZIG)	S	P	P	*Adult and child:* 125 units/kg IM up to a maximum of 625 units as soon as possible after exposure. Minimal dose: 125 units	May be used in other children younger than 15 yr and adults on an individual basis. Not for immunocompromised individuals. Only for individuals with significant risk factors Duration: More than 1 mo

A, Active; AT, antitoxin; CDCP, Centers for Disease Control and Prevention; FRM, formulation; IMM, immunity; IBV, inactivated bacterial vaccine; IVV, inactivated viral vaccine; KAT, killed antitoxin; KBV, killed bacterial vaccine; KW, killed viral vaccine; LAVV, live attenuated viral vaccine; LA/L, live attenuated/live; Pa, passive; RBC, red blood cell; S, sera; T, toxoid; $TCID_{50}$, tissue culture infectious dose; Tr, treatment; V, vaccine

*Formulation; sera, vaccine, toxoid, antitoxin, vaccine.

usually develops within 1 to 2 weeks and lasts 1 to 2 months or longer. Paroxysmal coughing episodes commonly end with the expulsion of clear, tenacious mucus, followed by vomiting. Adults and infants less than 6 months of age often do not have the typical "whoop."

Complications of the disease include pneumonia, seizures, and encephalitis. Approximately 90 percent of deaths are among children younger than 1 year, with 75 percent in those younger than 6 months. Morbidity and mortality are higher in females. In nonimmunized populations, especially patients with underlying malnutrition and multiple enteric and respiratory infections, pertussis is the most lethal disease of infants and young children. Pneumonia is the most common cause of death.

Susceptibility to the disease increases in adolescence and adulthood as immunity wanes. Adults who contract the disease do not suffer the severe complications of childhood illness and provide a reservoir by which the disease can be transmitted to susceptible children. Because pertussis in adults commonly goes undiagnosed and because subclinical cases can occur, adults can be a common source of infection.

Standard pertussis vaccines were introduced in the 1950s, resulting in a marked decline in the incidence of pertussis. The disease is on the rise again, however, largely owing to lack of immunization. Significant adverse reactions to this vaccine have been reported and have stimulated efforts to provide a less allergenic vaccine. An *acellular vaccine* is currently being used. DTaP (acellular pertussis vaccine) is administered on the same schedule as whole cell pertussis.

Simultaneous vaccination against diphtheria, tetanus, and pertussis (DTP) during infancy and childhood has been a routine practice in the United States since the late 1940s. Vaccination provides protection against diphtheria and tetanus for approximately 10 years. Protection for pertussis lasts somewhat less than that but is of less concern, because the severity of pertussis disease decreases with age. DTP or DTaP is administered in infancy at 2 months, 4 months, and 6 months of age with a booster at least 6 months after the initial series. A booster at age 4 to 6 years, before the child enters school, is recommended.

After age 7, pertussis is no longer advised. Tetanus-diphtheria (Td) boosters are recommended every 10 years throughout life. For children younger than 7 years with a contraindication to pertussis, diphtheria-tetanus vaccine (DT) is administered instead of DTP on the same schedule. DT has the same concentration of diphtheria toxoid as DTP and DTaP.

Td is routinely administered to adults to provide immunity against both tetanus and diphtheria. Antibody levels wane 10 years after administration. The Td vaccine is formulated with a lower "adult" dose of diphtheria toxoid, because adverse reactions to that component increase with age. Td has 2 units of diphtheria per dose, in contrast to pediatric formulations that contain 6.7 to 12.5 units per dose.

Human tetanus immune globulin is used to prevent tetanus in patients with wounds possibly contaminated with *C. tetani.* It is also recommended for patients whose immunization history is uncertain or includes fewer than two immunizing doses of tetanus toxoid. It is used also in the treatment of tetanus. Human tetanus IG is a solution of globulins from the plasma of people hyperimmunized with tetanus toxoid. Tetanus toxoid should be given at the same time as the IG formulation to initiate active immunization.

Adverse Effects and Contraindications

Both local and systemic affects can occur with administration of DTP vaccine. Most reactions occur within 48 hours of vaccine administration. Local effects include redness, swelling, and pain at the site of injection. A nodule may be palpable at the injection site. Sterile abscesses rarely occur. Local reactions occur most commonly, with mild systemic reactions less common, and neurologic reactions least common. Systemic effects include fever, drowsiness, persistent and inconsolable crying in infants, anorexia, vomiting, collapse, and seizures.

Rare but serious acute neurologic illness (e.g., encephalopathy, status epilepticus) have been anecdotally reported following the administration of diphtheria-tetanus–whole-cell pertussis vaccines. Whether this is a cause or coincidentally related is difficult to determine conclusively. Serious acute neurologic illnesses may occur during the first year of life. It is difficult to determine before vaccination if infants are neurologically normal. This fact makes it difficult to assess with certainty whether the recipient was neurologically impaired before receiving the vaccine. There does not appear to be a causal relationship between DTP vaccination and serious acute neurologic illness or permanent neurologic injury.

The ACIP further states that DTP vaccination is contraindicated in patients who have had an immediate anaphylactic reaction, encephalopathy occurring within 7 days after vaccination that is not related to another cause, and any acute, severe, central nervous system disorder occurring within 7 days following vaccination. Contraindications also include major alterations in consciousness, unresponsiveness, and generalized or focal seizures persisting longer than a few hours with failure to recover within 24 hours.

Haemophilus Influenzae Type B

Before the introduction of a vaccine, *Haemophilus influenzae* type B was the leading cause of bacterial infection in preschool children, with an estimated 12,000 cases of meningitis occurring annually. As many as 6 percent of meningitis patients died, and up to 30 percent of survivors suffered permanent damage, which ranged from mild hearing loss to profound mental retardation. *H. influenzae* infection is seen most often in children between the ages of 3 months and 3 years.

H. influenzae are gram-negative organisms consisting of both encapsulated and nonencapsulated strains. The virulence of the bacterium is attributed to its outer capsule, which triggers an unusual immune response that is difficult for infants to handle. Nonencapsulated strains are common constituents of upper respiratory flora and can cause otitis media, sinusitis, and bronchitis.

The major component of *H. influenzae* B (Hib) vaccine is a capsular polysaccharide. The polysaccharide is T cell independent, because it does not stimulate a T-cell memory response. It is attached to a protein to enhance its immunogenicity in infants, who have more immature immune systems. Infants younger than 7 months require multiple doses of Hib conjugate to reach protective levels of anticapsular antibody. Hib vaccine is administered simultaneously with DTP at 2, 4, and 6 months of age, with a booster given at age 15 to 18 months.

The first Hib vaccines licensed for use in the United States contained polyribosyl ribitol phosphate (PRP) and were effective against type B strains in children at 18 months of age. Because most Hib invasive disease occurs in infants and children younger than 18 months, a vaccine using the PRP polysaccharide attached to protein carriers was developed and licensed for use in infants. Four conjugate vaccines are now available for use in infants. All have similar efficacy. The carrier proteins used in three of these are derived from the toxoids used in DTP vaccine.

In 1993, a vaccine was developed that combined diphtheria-tetanus–whole cell pertussis and Hib vaccines. It appears to provide similar protection against diphtheria, pertussis, tetanus, and *H. influenzae* disease as well as the individual vaccines.

Hib vaccine is given at 2-month intervals beginning at 2 months of age. A booster is recommended at 12 to 15 months of age. The vaccination series should be completed using the same Hib conjugate vaccine. If different vaccines are administered, a total of three Hib conjugate vaccine injections is adequate. A single dose of any one of the conjugate vaccines may be administered in nonvaccinated children aged 15 to 59 months. Hib conjugate vaccines may be administered simultaneously with DTP, oral polio vaccine, measles-mumps-rubella, influenza, and hepatitis B vaccines. The diphtheria-tetanus–whole-cell pertussis/Hib conjugate vaccine may be administered along with OPV, inactivated poliomyelitis vaccine (IPV), MMR, influenza, and hepatitis B vaccines.

Adverse Effects and Contraindications

Adverse reactions to polysaccharide conjugate vaccines are rare. These vaccines are considered the safest of all vaccine products. Swelling, redness, and pain at the injection site have been reported but usually resolve in 12 to 24 hours. Systemic reactions such as fever and irritability are uncommon.

Vaccination with Hib conjugate vaccine is contraindicated in persons known to have had anaphylaxis following a prior dose of the vaccine. Contraindications and precautions for diphtheria-tetanus–whole-cell pertussis/Hib type B conjugate vaccine are the same as those for DTP. Allergy to thimerosal contraindicates the use of Hib vaccine.

Hepatitis A

Hepatitis A (HAV) occurs worldwide and is spread by the fecal oral route. It is caused by an RNA virus, a member of the picornavirus group (a positive-strand RNA virus). HAV is an acute febrile illness characterized by fever, malaise, anorexia, nausea, and abdominal discomfort. Jaundice follows these symptoms within a few days. The disease varies in severity from a mild illness lasting 1 to 2 weeks to a severe disabling disease lasting several months. The mortality rate is low (0.6 percent). When death occurs, it is usually in an older patient with fulminant disease. In infants and preschool children, most infections either are asymptomatic or cause mild nonspecific symptoms without jaundice.

Hepatitis A vaccine is prepared in human cell culture, purified, and inactivated. It is licensed for use in persons 2 years of age and older, for travelers going to endemic areas, and other high-risk groups. Many adults in the United States are naturally immune to hepatitis A. Testing for antibodies is less expensive than two doses of the vaccine.

The usual adult dosage of hepatitis A vaccine is 1 mL (1440 EL.U./mL) given intramuscularly, followed by a booster 6 to 12 months later. The pediatric formulation contains 720 EL.U./mL. Recommendations for administration to children age 2 to 18 years comprise two 0.5-mL intramuscular doses given 1 month apart, followed by a booster 6 to 12 months later. The vaccine is given by intramuscular injection into the deltoid muscle and can be administered simultaneously with other vaccines and toxoids.

Adverse Effects and Contraindications

Mild injection site soreness occurs in about 50 percent of adults and 15 percent of children. Transient headache, fatigue, fever, malaise, anorexia, and nausea have been reported but are uncommon. Safe use of the HAV vaccine in pregnancy has not been established.

The administration of immune globulin (IG) (commonly called gamma globulin) is recommended for those who are exposed and have close household contact with a patient who has hepatitis A, measles, or varicella. IG provides immediate antibodies to the recipient. When there is an outbreak of hepatitis A in child care facilities, administration of IG is recommended for employees in contact with the child and for children in the same room as the index case. In child care facilities where children are not yet toilet trained, all employees and children enrolled in the facility should receive IG. Household contacts of persons with hepatitis A should also receive IG. IG prophylaxis is also recommended for all susceptible travelers to developing countries.

Hepatitis B

Hepatitis B virus (HBV) is a double-stranded DNA virus that causes a wide spectrum of infections, ranging from asymptomatic seroconversion to clinical hepatitis with jaundice, arthralgias, arthritis, or macular rashes. Complications of hepatitis B infection include fulminant hepatitis, cirrhosis, and hepatocellular carcinoma. Transmission occurs by exposure to blood and body fluids and through sexual contact. Chronic HBV infection, which is seen in the carrier state, occurs in as many as 90 percent of infants who become infected through perinatal transmission, and in 6 to 10 percent of others who acquire HBV infection. Chronic carriers are at increased risk for liver disease or primary hepatocellular carcinoma in later life.

Pre-exposure immunization of susceptible persons is the most effective means of preventing HBV transmission. HBV vaccination is recommended for all infants as part of the routine childhood immunization schedule. For persons not immunized in infancy, immunization before adolescence is recommended. Groups at risk for the development of HBV infection include

- Users of intravenous drugs
- Heterosexual people with multiple partners
- Homosexual men
- People with occupational exposure to blood and blood products
- Staff of institutions and residential child care programs for the developmentally disabled
- Patients receiving hemodialysis
- Sexual or household contacts of persons with acute or chronic infections
- International travelers who plan to spend more than 6 months in areas with high rates of HBV infection.

Because the first HBV vaccine was derived from the plasma of homosexual men, many potential recipients refused immunization. The original vaccine is no longer produced. Two types of hepatitis vaccine are currently licensed for use in the United States. They were created using recombinant DNA technologies and were licensed by the Food and Drug Administration in 1989. They are considered safe and highly effective.

The American Academy of Pediatrics recommends that all infants and adolescents be vaccinated against hepatitis B. All recipients receive an initial dose followed by a second dose in 1 to 2 months, and a third dose 4 to 6 months after the first.

Hepatitis B immune globulin (HBIG) is a solution of immunoglobulins that contains antibodies to hepatitis B surface antigen (HBsAg). It is used in specific situations in which nonimmunized patients have been exposed to HBV. HBIG is used in the prevention of perinatal HBV infection in infants born to HBsAg-positive mothers, and is given concurrently with HBV vaccination within 12 hours of birth. Other candidates for HBIG are susceptible sexual partners of persons with acute HBV infection, household contacts having identifiable blood exposure to persons with acute HBV infection, susceptible infants (younger than 12 months) who were exposed to a caregiver with acute HBV infection, and an individual exposed through percutaneous or permucosal contact. All of these individuals should receive HBV vaccination series.

Adverse Effects and Contraindications

Pain at the injection site and a temperature higher than 37.7 °C are the most commonly reported adverse effects. Allergic reactions after hepatitis B vaccination have been reported but are rare. Pregnancy is not a contraindication for immunization against hepatitis B, but the vaccine is contraindicated in patients hypersensitive to thimerosal.

Influenza

Influenza is an acute viral disease of the respiratory tract that manifests as acute onset of fever, cough, headache, myalgia, sore throat, coryza, and prostration. It is spread by way of airborne droplets and direct contact. The common cold, croup, viral pneumonia, and undifferentiated acute respiratory disease may be caused by the influenza virus.

Influenza derives its significance from the speed with which epidemics evolve, the widespread morbidity, and the seriousness of complications. Viral and bacterial pneumonias are most notable. During major epidemics, severe disease and deaths occur predominantly among older adults and persons debilitated by chronic disease (e.g., cardiac, pulmonary, renal, or metabolic), anemia, or immunosuppression.

Three types of influenza virus are identified, A, B, and C. Type A virus has been associated with widespread epidemics and pandemics. Type B is associated with regional or widespread epidemics, and Type C has been associated with sporadic cases and minor localized outbreaks. Type A virus causes most annual epidemics, whereas epidemics caused by Type B appear every 2 to 3 years. Mixed A and B epidemics also occur. Clinical attack rates during epidemics range from 10 to 30 percent of the general population, to more than 50 percent in closed populations (e.g., nursing homes, boarding schools).

Influenza vaccine helps prevent disease caused by influenza virus types A and B. Influenza is caused by a changeable virus, and the vaccine-induced immunity wanes within a few months. Annual vaccination is required. New vaccine is produced each year containing the inactivated particles of the viral strains expected to cause disease that year. Each year's vaccine is trivalent, containing two strains of Type A and one strain of Type B. Whole virus, subvirion, and purified-surface-antigen preparations are available. Any of these may be used for adults, but only the subvirion or purified-surface-antigen preparations should be used for children.

Influenza vaccine is recommended for any person at least 6 months of age who is considered at high risk for complications of influenza. Children less than 9 years of age who have never before received influenza vaccine should receive two doses at least 4 weeks apart to ensure adequate immune response.

Persons who are susceptible to influenza-related complications include

- People 65 years of age or older
- Residents of nursing homes and other institutional facilities
- Adults and children with chronic disorders of the pulmonary or cardiovascular system
- Adults and children who required regular medical follow-up or hospitalization during the preceding year because of chronic metabolic diseases, renal dysfunction, hemoglobinopathies, or immunosuppression
- Children and teenagers who are receiving long-term aspirin therapy and may be at risk for developing Reye's syndrome
- People in contact with high-risk groups, such as health care providers, employees of nursing homes and chronic care facilities, providers of home care, and household members of persons in high-risk groups.

The optimal time for vaccination is mid-October to mid-November. The incidence of influenza ordinarily peaks between late December and early March.

Adverse Effects and Contraindications

The most common adverse effects of influenza immunization are localized reactions at the injection site lasting up to 2 days. Fever, malaise, myalgia, and other symptoms occur uncommonly starting 6 to 12 hours after vaccination. Anaphylaxis may occur in persons with hypersensitivity to some vaccine component.

The use of influenza vaccine is contraindicated in persons known to have a hypersensitivity to eggs, because the vaccine is grown in chick embryos. Adults with acute febrile illnesses should not be vaccinated until symptoms have disappeared. Minor acute illnesses in children do not contraindicate use of the influenza vaccine.

Measles, Mumps, and Rubella

Measles

Measles (rubeola, "hard measles," "14-day measles") is an acute, highly communicable viral disease. It is characterized by a prodromal fever, cough, coryza, conjunctivitis, and pathognomonic enanthem (Koplik's spots) on the buccal mucosa. An erythematous maculopapular rash appears in 3 to 7 days; it begins on the face, becomes generalized, and lasts 4 to 7 days. The disease is more severe in infants and adults than in children. Complications of the disease may result from viral replication or bacterial superinfection and include otitis, bronchopneumonia, encephalitis, diarrhea, and subacute sclerosing panencephalitis.

In persons in the United States who received inactivated measles vaccine before 1968, viral infection may cause severe atypical manifestations, including pneumonitis, pleural effusion, and peripheral edema. There is a predilection for an atypical rash on extremities that resembles the rash of Rocky Mountain spotted fever.

Measles is transmitted through direct contact and by airborne particles. It was extremely contagious before widespread immunization program for preschool and young school-age children appeared. Since 1963, when measles vaccine was licensed, the incidence has decreased dramatically in all age groups. In the late 1980s, the incidence of measles began to increase, especially in preschool children. Outbreaks also occur in vaccinated adolescents in junior and senior high schools and on college campuses.

Mumps

Mumps is also an acute viral disease characterized by fever and swelling and tenderness of one or more salivary glands. It usually affects the parotid and sometimes the sublingual or submaxillary glands. In addition to swelling of the salivary glands, encephalitis, and orchitis after puberty (20 to 30 percent) can occur with this disease. Oophoritis occurs in about 5 percent of females affected after puberty. Sterility is extremely rare. Central nervous system involvement is common; it can occur early or late in the disease and usually results in an aseptic meningitis, almost always without sequelae. The mortality rate of mumps averages 1.4 percent. Mumps infection during the first trimester of pregnancy may cause spontaneous abortion, but there is no firm evidence that mumps during pregnancy causes congenital malformations.

Mumps most often occurs during the winter and spring seasons. Infection is spread by droplet. Nevertheless, the incidence of mumps has declined with the introduction of the mumps vaccine in 1967. The decline has occurred in all age groups, but with effective pediatric and preschool immunization programs, the greatest risk of infection has shifted toward older children, adolescents, and young adults.

Rubella

Rubella (German measles, "3-day measles") is a mild febrile viral disease caused by an RNA virus. It is characterized by a diffuse, punctate, and maculopapular rash, generalized lymphadenopathy, and a slight fever. The rash sometimes resembles that of measles or scarlet fever, although up to 50 percent of infections occur without evident rash. Children usually present with few or no constitutional symptoms. Adults may have a prodromal period of low-grade fever, headache, malaise, mild coryza, and conjunctivitis before rubella develops 1 to 5 days later. Postauricular, occipital, and posterior cervical adenopathy usually precedes the rash by 5 to 10 days.

Rubella is a significant disease because of its ability to produce anomalies in the developing fetus. Congenital rubella syndrome occurs in more than 25 percent of infants born to women who acquired rubella during the first trimester of pregnancy. The risk of a single congenital defect falls to 10 to 20 percent by the 16th week. Defects are rare when maternal infection develops after the 20th week of gestation.

Measles-mumps-rubella vaccine (MMR) is a trivalent live virus vaccine that was first licensed in 1968. It produces serum antibody levels in approximately 95 percent of patients. The incidence of the three diseases declined dramatically until 1986, when the incidence of measles and mumps began to rise. Through the remainder of the 1980s and into the early 1990s, the incidence of measles remained high. More than half of the cases occurred in individuals older than 5 years, many of whom had already been immunized. Before this time, it was recommended that children receive one dose of MMR administered at 15 months of age. Following the outbreaks in the late 1980s, immunization recommendations were changed to include a second dose of MMR, either when the child starts school (ages 4 to 6 years) or before entry into the seventh grade. This schedule reduced the outbreaks of measles.

Children whose mothers received MMR vaccination as children were found to have a lower level of passive antibodies to measles, which waned by the time the child was 1 year of age. As a result, the recommended age for the initial MMR immunization has been changed from 15 months to 12 to 15 months, with a second immunization given between 4 and 6 years.

MMR is given as two 0.5-mL subcutaneous vaccinations. The first dose is given between the age of 12 and 15 months. In high risk areas, the recommendation is to administer the vaccine at 12 months of age. In some cases, the first dose may be given as early as 6 months of age. The second dose is administered either upon the child's entry into school (4 to 6 years) or at 11 to 12 years. The risk of contracting measles increases substantially after entry into middle school.

Susceptible persons exposed to measles should be vaccinated within 72 hours. Measles immunoglobulin is an alternative for patients considered too young to receive the vaccine or when the period since exposure exceeds 72 hours.

Measles vaccine is a sterile preparation of live, attenuated rubeola virus. It is usually given as a combination product containing mumps and rubella vaccines. It should not be given for 3 months after administration of immune serum globulin, plasma, or whole blood.

Measles and rubella vaccines are mixtures of live attenuated rubeola virus and rubella virus. They are recommended for use in young, nonimmunized women and health care providers.

Adverse Effects and Contraindications

Five to 15 percent of recipients develop a fever 7 to 12 days after vaccination. The fever lasts 1 to 2 days. Five percent of recipients report a transient rash. Less common adverse effects are encephalitis and transient thrombocytopenia.

MMR vaccine is contraindicated in patients with a previous anaphylactic reaction to rubeola vaccine or eggs, and in patients with altered immune status (not including human immunodeficiency virus infection). MMR also contains trace elements of neomycin, so it should not be given to patients allergic to neomycin. It should be used with caution in patients who have received immune globulin within the previous 3 months.

Pneumococcal Infection

Pneumococcal pneumonia is an acute bacterial infection characterized by a sudden onset of shaking chills, fever, pleural pain, dyspnea, a productive cough with "rusty" sputum, and leukocytosis. The onset is less precipitous in the older adult, and a chest x-ray provides the first evidence of the infection. In infants, vomiting and seizures may be the initial manifestations of pneumococcal pneumonia.

The mortality rate, formerly 20 to 40 percent among hospitalized patients, has declined to 5 to 10 percent with antimicrobial therapy. The mortality rate remains 20 to 40 percent among patients with substantial underlying co-morbid diseases.

The current pneumococcal vaccine formulation is composed of purified, capsular polysaccharide antigens of 23 pneumococcal serotypes. The 23 strains of pneumococci cause approximately 85 to 90 percent of the serious pneumococcal infections in the United States. Like other polysaccharide antigens, some pneumococcal serotypes have limited immunogenicity in children younger than 2 years. Prophylactic administration of pneumococcal vaccines has been proven effective in older children and adults.

Pneumococcal vaccine is specifically recommended for two groups of patients: (1) children older than 2 year who have sickle cell disease, functional or anatomic asplenia, nephrotic syndrome or chronic renal failure, immunosuppression, human immunodeficiency virus infection, or cerebral spinal fluid leaks and (2) persons older than 65 years, especially those who are immunocompromised or who have chronic illnesses.

The current 23-valent vaccine can be administered to patients who previously received the 14-valent preparation 6 or more years ago. It should be administered only one time, except in persons with certain medical problems. Protection begins about the third week after vaccination and lasts many years.

Adverse Effects and Contraindications

Injection site tenderness occurs with the administration of pneumococcal vaccine. Fever, myalgia, and severe local reactions are very uncommon. Anaphylaxis is rare. As with many other vaccines, hypersensitivity to thimerosal or phenol contraindicates the use of pneumococcal vaccine.

Poliomyelitis

Poliomyelitis is an acute viral infection with a severity ranging from asymptomatic infection through nonspecific febrile illness, aseptic meningitis, and paralytic disease to death. It is related to an enterovirus and is caused by poliovirus types 1, 2, and 3. It is transmitted by the fecal-oral route where sanitation is poor and during epidemics. It is less commonly transmitted by the respiratory route. The virus is detectable more easily and for longer periods in feces than in pharyngeal secretions. The ingested virus multiplies first in the gastrointestinal tract, with viremia following. Invasion of the central nervous system and selective involvement of motor neurons results in flaccid paralysis, most commonly of the lower extremities.

Highly contagious, poliomyelitis is more common in infants and young children but causes paralysis more often in older individuals. Poliomyelitis is rare in the United States at this time. Of the cases that do exist, most have been associated with the administration of the oral vaccine. Polio is still prevalent in developing countries and is a potential threat to travelers in those regions. The mortality rate for paralytic cases varies from 2 to 10 percent in different epidemics. The mortality rate increases markedly with age. The incidence of asymptomatic infections and minor illness usually exceeds 100 times that of paralytic cases, especially when infection occurs in early life.

Before 1955, more than 20,000 cases of paralytic poliomyelitis occurred every year, leaving half its victims with neurologic complications. Paralytic polio was virtually wiped out in the United States with the introduction of the Salk vaccine. The Sabin vaccine, a superior strain of live virus, was available for use in 1960.

National immunization policy calls for the use of the oral polio vaccine (Sabin) for the general public. Oral polio vaccine (OPV), a live attenuated trivalent vaccine, may be used for primary immunization of children. It induces mucosal immunity by colonizing the gastrointestinal tract with the polio virus. OPV is easy to administer, is well accepted by patients, results in herd immunity, and has eliminated disease in the United States. The growth and excretion of attenuated vaccine virus via the gastrointestinal tract results in spread of the vaccine to nonvaccinated contacts, thereby immunizing them as well and increasing the level of shared immunity.

OPV may be administered as a series to infants at 2, 4, and 6 months of age. Two doses produce an antibody response in more than 90 percent of recipients. The third dose can be administered any time between ages 6 and 18 months. A fourth booster is administered upon the patient's entry into school. OPV can be administered simultaneously with other vaccines. ACIP also recommends two doses of IPV at 2 months and 4 months, followed by two doses of OPV at 12 to 18 months of age and at 4 to 6 years of age.

Routine primary immunization of previously nonvaccinated or partially vaccinated adults is not recommended. The exception is in an outbreak of a wild-type virus, or exposure to OPV from household contacts. Routine primary immunizations should be considered for the following individuals:

- Travelers to areas where poliomyelitis is epidemic or endemic
- Members of communities experiencing disease caused by wild poliovirus
- Laboratory workers who handle specimens containing poliovirus
- Health care workers in close contact with patients who have poliovirus.

Because the risk of contracting polio is slim with the killed virus (IPV), some public health experts propose returning to the Salk vaccine for routine administration. Herd immunity for a given population requires that 80 percent of the community be effectively immunized. However, outbreaks have occurred in countries where the Salk vaccine is the only formulation used. Poliomyelitis continues to be a problem in other parts of the world, and because of increased mobility of people, "imported poliomyelitis" still poses a significant threat.

IPV induces seroconversion rates equal to those of OPV after only three doses. Persons in whom OPV is contraindicated are candidates for IPV. Candidates for IPV are patients who have immunodeficiency disorders (including human immunodeficiency virus infection), are household contacts of persons with immunodeficiency disease, have altered immune states, are immunosuppressed because of therapy, or are parents of immunodeficient children.

The use of IPV in the primary immunization of children is recommended by ACIP. Either of two schedules is recommended for use in infants/children:

- Two doses of IPV @ 2 months and 4 months followed by 2 doses of OPV at 12 to 18 months and 4 to 6 years of age.
- Four doses of IPV at 2 months, 4 months, 12 to 18 months, and 4 to 6 years of age.

Primary immunization with IPV is recommended and preferred in nonimmunized adults, because the risk of vaccine-associated paralysis after OPV is slightly higher in adults. Two doses of IPV should be given 1 to 2 months apart and a third dose given 6 to 12 months later. Partially immunized adults at risk for exposure may receive either IPV or OPV.

Adverse Effects and Contraindications

OPV has been associated with paralysis in recipients and their contacts. The greatest risk of paralysis occurs with the first dose of vaccine. The risk of paralysis is extremely small—1 in 700,000 with the first dose, and 1 in 6.9 million with subsequent doses. The risk is slightly higher in previously nonvaccinated adults than in children.

OPV is contraindicated in patients with immunodeficiency disorders and in household contacts of persons who are immunosuppressed, because of the theoretical risk of paralytic disease. Pregnancy is not an absolute contraindication to administration of OPV, although IPV is preferred if immunization is needed during pregnancy.

No serious adverse effects of the currently available IPV have been documented. Trace amounts of streptomycin and neomycin are found in IPV, so its use in patients with sensitivity to those antibiotics is contraindicated.

Rabies

Rabies is an almost invariably fatal acute viral encephalomyelitis. Its onset is often heralded by a sense of apprehension, headache, fever, and malaise. Indefinite sensory changes are often referred to the site of the animal bite wound. The RNA virus is found in the saliva of animals such as skunks, bats, and raccoons. These rodents in turn may infect domestic animals (dogs most often in the United States), from which infections in most humans occur. There are an estimated 30,000 deaths worldwide annually, almost all in developing countries. Rabies is uncommon in developed countries. At present, the only locales free of rabies are Australia, New Zealand, New Guinea, Japan, Hawaii, Taiwan and the Pacific Islands, the United Kingdom, Ireland, mainland Norway, Sweden, Portugal, and some of the West Indies and Atlantic islands.

Immunization involves the use of human diploid cell vaccine, an inactivated virus. Rabies vaccine, adsorbed, is a newer inactivated virus vaccine. Either vaccine can be given as a pre-exposure control measure or as postexposure treatment.

Pre-exposure immunization is recommended for persons in high-risk groups, such as veterinarians, animal handlers, and people living in endemic areas. The schedule is the same for each of the preparations, three injections given on the day of injury (day 1), day 7, and day 28. Immunity develops 7 to 10 days after immunization and lasts 1 year or longer.

Post-exposure immunization is used prophylactically for people who have been bitten by potentially rabid animals or who have scratches or abrasions exposed to animal saliva (e.g., animal licking a wound), urine, or blood. Prompt treatment prevents the rabies virus from entering the neural tissue. Rabies immune globulin and either human diploid cell vaccine or rabies vaccine, adsorbed, should be given concurrently to bridge the time between onset of treatment and active antibody production of the vaccine. Rabies IG is obtained from the plasma of people hyperimmunized with rabies vaccine. It is not useful in the treatment of clinical rabies.

Serum antibody titers decline 2 years after the primary series. Booster vaccinations of either vaccine produce an effective response but are associated with significant allergic reactions in about 6 percent of recipients. Boosters are not routinely recommended except for persons whose risk of exposure is likely to be continuous or frequent. In such individuals, rabies antibody titers should be obtained at 6-month intervals and boosters used to maintain antibody concentrations.

Adverse Effects and Contraindications

Systemic reactions such as headache, nausea, abdominal pain, muscle aches, and dizziness have been reported with rabies vaccinations. Rare neurologic illness resembling Guillain-Barré syndrome that resolves without sequelae has been noted. Immune complex–like reactions have been noted in persons receiving booster doses of human diploid cell vaccine. These manifest as generalized urticaria, arthralgia, arthritis, angioedema, nausea, vomiting, fever, and malaise. Pregnancy is not a contraindication to the use of post-exposure vaccine.

Varicella

Varicella (chickenpox) is an acute, generalized viral illness characterized by a sudden onset of slight fever, mild constitutional symptoms, and skin eruptions. The maculopapular rash lasts a few hours then changes to vesicles for 3 to 4 days, leaving a granular scab over the lesions. The lesions occur in crops, with several stages of maturity present at the same time. Lesions tend to be more abundant on skin surfaces that are covered with clothing than on exposed body parts. Mild, atypical, and asymptomatic infections occur. Varicella in children is a self-limiting, contagious disease spread by direct contact, droplet nuclei, and aerosols from vesicles or respiratory tract secretions. In adults, the fever and constitutional symptoms may be severe.

Varicella develops primarily in children younger than 8 years. By age 12, only 10 percent of children are still at risk for this disease. The number of adults contracting varicella appears to be increasing in the United States as a result of immigration from tropical countries. Although adults account for only 2 percent of varicella cases, they carry a 50 percent mortality rate, with 25 percent of deaths occurring in immunocompromised patients.

Herpes zoster (shingles) is caused by the reactivation of a latent varicella-zoster virus. About 15 percent of people who have had varicella develop zoster. The incidence of zoster in immunocompromised patients and older adults is related to a decline in cellular immunity. The vesicles of zoster have an erythematous base and are restricted to skin areas supplied by the sensory nerves of a single or associated group of dorsal root ganglia. Lesions appear in an irregular fashion along nerve pathways, are usually unilateral, and are deeper seated and more closely aggregated than those of chickenpox. Histologically, the two disorders are identical. Severe pain and paresthesias are common with zoster. Zoster occurs primarily in adults, although there is evidence to suggest that almost 10 percent of children being treated for a malignant process are prone to develop zoster. Persons who have human immunodeficiency virus or are immunosuppressed are also at increased risk.

Varicella vaccine, the newest on the market, is a live attenuated vaccine. It is 95 percent effective in preventing chickenpox, but not as protective as live virus vaccines (e.g., measles vaccine). The risk of zoster is considerably reduced in patients receiving the vaccine. Seroconversion occurs in 97 percent of susceptible children aged 1 to 12 years, but in only 79 percent of recipients aged 13 to 17 years.

A single dose of varicella vaccine is recommended for healthy children between the ages of 1 and 12 years. Two doses of varicella vaccine are given 4 to 8 weeks apart for children 13 years and older. Vaccination is recommended for healthy adults and adolescents with no history of the disease. Varicella vaccine can be given simultaneously with MMR at separate injection sites. Data are not yet available on simultaneous administration of the new vaccine with other childhood vaccinations.

Varicella-zoster human immune globulin is used to prevent or decrease the severity of varicella infections in children younger than 15 years who are immunosuppressed because of illness (e.g., lymphoma, leukemia) or drug therapy (e.g., antineoplastic or corticosteroid drugs), and who have had significant exposure to varicella or herpes zoster. The antibodies it provides last about 1 month or longer.

Adverse Affects and Contraindications

Pain and erythema at the site of injection are the main adverse effects of the vaccination. A generalized varicella-like rash may occur. The virus can be transmitted from immunized individuals to others, but it does not become more virulent. Varicella pneumonia is the most common serious complication in adults.

Varicella vaccine is contraindicated in patients who are immunodeficient or are receiving high dose steroids. Pregnancy is a contraindication to administration of varicella vaccine. The use of salicylates for 6 weeks after immunization is not recommended because of the association among varicella, salicylates, and Reye's syndrome.

TRAVEL-RELATED IMMUNIZATIONS

The increased risk of contracting infectious diseases during international travel results from two primary factors: the close proximity of individuals in transportation, and exposure to exotic infectious agents through contact with foreign populations and natural environments. The number and kind of immunizations needed are determined by the patient's itinerary. The health care provider must consider the geographic location, style of accommodation, and planned activities when determining which immunizations are needed. The patient's age, prior immunization history, allergies, and general health must also be taken into account. The efficacy and adverse effects of vaccines are important considerations.

National vaccine recommendations are formulated by the ACIP. The Centers for Disease Control and Prevention provides recommendations and position statements on administration of vaccines for travel. The World Health Organization regulates vaccine requirements for entry into member countries. Currently, yellow fever vaccine is the only required immunization for international travelers. The International Certificates of Vaccination, a document in booklet form, validates the immunization status of international travelers (Table 28–2).

Cholera

Cholera is an acute bacterial disease caused by *Vibrio cholerae*. It is characterized by sudden onset, profuse painless watery stools, occasional vomiting, rapid dehydration, acidosis, and circulatory collapse. Cholera is transmitted by the fecal-oral route in environments where hygienic preparation of food and sanitary disposal of human wastes are lacking. Asymptomatic infection is much more common than clinical illness. In severe untreated cases, death can occur within a few hours. The mortality rate can exceed 50 percent, but with proper treatment, the rate falls below 1 percent. Cholera presents a continuing health risk in Asia, Africa, and Latin America.

Cholera immunization (an inactivated whole-cell bacterial vaccine) is not highly efficacious. It provides only about 50 percent protective immunity when the series of two doses are received. Booster doses are required at 6-month intervals in cases of continued exposure. Cholera vaccine is no longer required by the World Health Organization for entry into any country, but some individual countries still require a validated cholera vaccination for admission.

Japanese Encephalitis

Japanese encephalitis is a mosquito-transmitted, acute inflammatory viral disease of short duration that involves the brain, spinal cord, and meninges. It is prevalent in many areas of subcontinental India and Asia, occurring from June to September in temperate zones and throughout the year in tropical zones of the Far East. The disease occurs primarily in young children and adults older than 65 years. Japanese encephalitis carries a high mortality and morbidity rate, and therefore, vaccination is considered for travelers. The risk when traveling to urban areas and staying for a brief period is low. Detailed information on vaccine recommendations is available from the Centers for Disease Control and Prevention.

The Japanese encephalitis vaccine is an inactivated vaccine derived from the brain of an infected mouse. The recommended immunization series consists of three doses of 1 mL each administered subcutaneously on day 0, day 7, and day 30. The schedule is the same for children, but the dose is 0.5 mL. Vaccination is about 78 percent effective after the second dose, and 99 percent effective after the third dose. Onset of drug action is after the second dose.

Meningococcus

Meningococcal meningitis is an acute bacterial disease characterized by sudden onset of fever, intense headache, nausea and vomiting (often), stiff neck, and, commonly, a petechial rash. The infection may be asymptomatic, may be restricted to the nasopharynx, or may cause upper airway symptoms. It can cause meningococcal pneumonia, can be invasive with acutely ill septicemic patients, or can be meningeal. The mortality rate exceeds 50 percent, but with early diagnosis, modern therapy, and supportive measures, the rate drops below 10 percent.

Meningococcal vaccine has been given to military recruits in the United States since 1971. It is recommended for travelers going to areas with recognized epidemic disease, such as Nepal, the New Delhi region of India, Kenya, Tanzania, Saudi Arabia, and sub-Saharan Africa. Routine immunization for civilians is not recommended.

The meningococcal vaccine currently available is a quadrivalent polysaccharide that induces immunity against serogroups A, C, Y, and W-135. A single dose provides protection for 3 years. Vaccine efficacy is variable in young chil-

TABLE 28–2 TRAVEL IMMUNIZATIONS

Drug	FRM*	IMM	P/Tr	Dosage	Implications
Cholera	IBV	A	P	*Child 6 mo to 4 yr:* 0.2 mL SC/IM × 1 dose *Child 5–10 yr:* 0.3 mL SC/IM × 1 dose. *Adult and child older than 10 yr:* 0.5 mL × 2 doses 1 wk to 1 mo apart. Booster in 6 mo depending on exposure	Repeat dose every 6 mo as long as risk is present. Administer yellow fever vaccine at least 3 wk apart from cholera, since may decrease antibody formation Efficacy: 50% Duration: 3–6 mo
Japanese encephalitis vaccine (JE-VAX)	IVV	A	P	*Child younger than 3 yr:* 0.5 mL SC on days 1, 7, and 30. *Adult and child older than 3 yr:* 1 mL SC on days 1, 7, and 30. Booster in 1–3 yr, depending on exposure	Do not travel within 10 days of vaccination. Effectiveness: 78% after second dose, 99% after third dose
Plague vaccine	IBV	A	P	*Adult and child:* #1 1 mL IM initially. #2 0.2 mL IM 4 wk later. #3 0.2 mL IM in 3–6 mo. Booster: Every 6 mo × 5 doses, then every 12–24 mo	Contraindicated in patients with sensitivity to beef, protein, soy, casein, Use of vaccine Increases chances of recovery in epidemic situations. Continue drug regimen as long as danger of exposure exists Duration: Several months
Bacille Calmette-Guérin (TICE BCG)	LA/L	A	P	*Adult and child:* 0.2–0.3 mL topically followed by multiple puncture gun/disc	Do not administer SC/ID, or IV. Conduct post-vaccination TB test in 2–3 mo. Repeat dose in 2–3 mo if still TB negative. Patient should avoid persons with active TB for 6–12 wk after immunization
Typhoid vaccine	IBV	A	P	*Adult and child older than 10 yr:* #1 0.5 mL SC or 0.1 mL ID initially. #2 0.5 mL SC or 0.1 mL ID 4 wk later. Booster: 3 yr later *Oral formulation (Ty21a):* 1 capsule every other day × 4 capsules Booster: 5 yr later. *Child to 10 yr:* #1 0.25 mL SC or 0.1 mL ID initially #2 0.25 mL SC or 0.1 mL ID 4 wk later	Concurrent use with antibiotics or within 7 days of antibiotic use should be avoided Efficacy: 70–90% Duration: 3 yr
Yellow-fever (YF-VAX)	LAVV	A	P	*Adult and child older than 6 mo:* 0.5 mL SC × 1 dose. Booster: Every 10 yr	Caution with allergy to chicken or egg products. Contraindicated in patients who are immunosuppressed, in children younger than 6 mo, and during pregnancy Effectiveness: 100% after 7–10 days

A, Active; AT, antitoxin; CDCP, Centers for Disease Control and Prevention; FRM, formulation; IMM, immunity; IBV, inactivated bacterial vaccine; IVV, inactivated viral vaccine; LAVV, live attenuated viral vaccine; LA/L, live attenuated/live.

*Formulation; sera, vaccine, toxoid, antitoxin, vaccine.

(Data from the Advisory Committee on Immunization Practices, the Centers for Disease Control and Prevention, the American Academy of pediatrics, and the American Academy of Family Practice. (1998). Recommended Childhood Immunization Schedule—United States, January–December 1998 (RE9807). *Pediatrics,* 101(1), 134–135.)

dren, so a second dose administered 2 to 3 years after the first is recommended. The vaccine's effectiveness drops to about 67 percent after 3 years.

Plague

Plague (bubonic plague), a bacterial disease caused by *Yersinia pestis,* a gram-negative bacillus, is transmitted from rodents and their fleas to animals and people. It is characterized by lymphadenitis in nodes receiving drainage from the site of the flea bite. Plague occurs more often in lymph nodes in the inguinal area and less commonly in axillary and cervical nodes. The nodes become edematous, inflamed, tender, and suppurative. Fever is ordinarily present. Secondary pulmonary involvement results in pneumonia, mediastinitis, or pleural effusion.

Plague occurs most commonly in parts of the western United States, part of South America, Africa, and Asia. Those at risk for exposure include field biologists and people who reside or work in rural mountainous areas.

An inactivated whole-cell bacterial vaccine is available for persons who are at high risk for contracting the disease. Primary immunization consists of three doses of vaccine; the second and third doses are given 1 and 4 months after the first and are followed by a booster given 3 to 6 months after the third dose. Boosters are indicated every 6 months until a total of five doses are given, then every 12 to 24 months as long as danger of exposure exists. Adverse effects include pain, redness, and induration at the site of injection. Systemic symptoms, including fever, headache, and malaise, may occur after repeated doses.

Tick-Borne Encephalitis

Tick-borne encephalitis is a viral disease spread by ticks in central and eastern Europe during the months of April to

September. Human infection results from the bite of an infected *Ixodes persulcatus* tick, which is found in forested areas of endemic regions.

Vaccination against tick-borne encephalitis is not available in the United States. A vaccine manufactured in Austria is available in Europe. The immunization schedule consists of three doses given subcutaneously on day 0, day 30, and day 180. Boosters are given at 3- and 5-year intervals for continuing risk of exposure.

Tuberculosis

Tuberculosis is caused by *Mycobacterium tuberculosis,* an acid-fast bacillus (see Chapter 26). Exposure in developing countries usually occurs as a result of prolonged contact with respiratory droplets from infected persons. For travelers, the best approach to tuberculosis prevention is pretravel and post-travel tuberculin testing rather than immunization.

Bacillus Calmette-Guérin (BCG) vaccine is widely used outside North America for immunization against tuberculosis. The World Health Organization recommends a single dose at birth, and most of the world's children receive BCG vaccine according to varying schedules. The BCG vaccine is approved by the American Academy of Pediatrics for children who will be living in areas where tuberculosis is prevalent. The United States has not endorsed the use of BCG vaccine for prevention of tuberculosis.

BCG vaccine may be considered for uninfected children who are at unavoidable risk of exposure and for whom other methods of prevention and control are not feasible. BCG can be given to infants from birth to 2 months of age without tuberculin testing. Thereafter, BCG is given only to children who have a negative Mantoux test. The vaccine is contraindicated in people with immunosuppression. Pregnancy is considered a relative contraindication.

Typhoid

Typhoid is a systemic bacterial disease caused by *Salmonella typhi.* It is characterized by an insidious onset of sustained fever, headache, malaise, anorexia, bradycardia, splenomegaly, rose spots on the trunk, nonproductive cough, constipation (more often than diarrhea), and lymphadenopathy. Although this disease rarely occurs in the United States, the typhoid that does occur is contracted through international travel. The risk of transmission is particularly high in Mexico, Peru, India, Chile, and Pakistan. Typhoid vaccine is recommended for persons who expect to consume food and water at nontourist facilities in endemic areas. It is not routinely recommended in the United States or for foreign travel.

Two injectable typhoid vaccines are available in the United States, a parenteral heat-phenol-inactivated vaccine (typhoid vaccine) and a newer capsular polysaccharide vaccine. Typhoid vaccine can be administered to children as young as 6 months. The primary series requires two doses given 4 weeks apart and followed by a booster every 3 years.

The capsular polysaccharide vaccine can be given to children 2 years or older who require one dose (25 mcg or 0.5 mL) for primary immunization, followed by a booster every 2 years. The injectable, inactivated vaccine has more troublesome adverse effects than the ViCPS: injection site soreness, headache, low-grade fever, and general malaise for 1 to 2 days following immunization.

The oral typhoid formulation contains a live, attenuated strain of *S. typhi*. Its efficacy is comparable to that of the injectable vaccine. The primary series consists of four capsules taken every other day over the course of a week. A booster is required after 5 years. Oral typhoid vaccine cannot be taken with antibiotics or within 7 days after concluding an antibiotic course. It is not recommended for children younger than 6 years, immunocompromised individuals, or pregnant women. Adverse effects of this oral vaccine are fewer than from the injectable vaccine.

Yellow Fever

Yellow fever is a serious and potentially fatal viral infection of short duration and varying severity. It is characterized by a sudden onset of fever, chills, headache, backache, generalized muscle pain, prostration, nausea, and vomiting. It is transmitted by the *Aedes aegypti* mosquito in tropical and subtropical regions of the world. The mortality rate among indigenous populations of endemic regions is less than 5 percent. The mortality rate can exceed 50 percent among nonindigenous groups and during epidemics. Although the disease is now rare, many countries have retained an entrance requirement for yellow fever immunization despite years of having had no reported cases.

Yellow fever vaccine is a live attenuated viral vaccine prepared from vaccine virus strain 17D. A single dose of vaccine is given subcutaneously for primary immunization. The onset of immunity is 10 days. Boosters are required at 10-year intervals. Contraindications to the vaccine are allergy to eggs and immunosuppression due to underlying disease. It is not recommended for use in children younger than 6 months because of a higher incidence of adverse effects. It is also contraindicated in pregnancy, except when travel to a highly endemic area cannot be avoided.

Critical Thinking Process

Assessment

History of Present Illness

For persons who present for routine immunizations, a history of present illness is irrelevant. In most cases, these are considered well-person visits. Nonetheless, for certain immunizations, information about allergies to egg protein, sulfites, thimerosal, neomycin, or other components of the immunizing agent are elicited.

For patients exposed to infectious disease, the health care provider should determine the extent of exposure and when it occurred, as well as whether it was related to household contacts or to a brief, casual contact. For patients with wounds, the health care provider should determine how and when the wound was sustained and what was done for treatment.

Past Health History

The patient should be asked to bring the immunization record to the appointment. The health care provider should determine whether the patient has had previous immunizations and has had any allergic reaction. Because some immunizations may not be given in close proximity to others, attention should be paid to the dates of previous immunizations. For example, immune globulin should not be given 3 months before or 2 weeks after a live viral vaccine. IG does not, however, appear to interfere with the immune response to oral polio vaccine or to yellow fever vaccine.

Further, many vaccines are not administered to a patient with an acute infection or to anyone who is immunosuppressed. In addition, patients who may be at risk for disease exposure should be identified. The risk groups include persons traveling to foreign countries, health care workers, immigrants to this country, older adults, and the chronically ill. For international travelers, information about the geographic itinerary, month, and duration of travel in each country is elicited. The location of the travel (i.e., urban or rural) should also be noted.

Physical Exam Findings

The patient's temperature should be taken before administration of an immunizing agent. The presence of a fever may preclude vaccination; however, a minor, afebrile illness does not contraindicate an immunization.

Diagnostic Testing

No true laboratory tests are require before immunization. However, the antigens contained in vaccines and antisera may cause hypersensitivity reactions. Certain constituents of vaccines (e.g., egg protein, neomycin) may cause allergic reactions, and individuals known to have severe allergies should not receive vaccines containing them.

An intracutaneous skin test preceded by a conjunctival test must be performed before injection of any animal serum, regardless of whether the patient has previously received the serum species. A negative conjunctival or skin test, however, does not guarantee that hypersensitivity is absent. It only suggests that sensitivity is probably lacking. Test results can be false in the presence of antihistamines.

In the patient for whom pregnancy status is questionable, a pregnancy test should be done before immunizations are given. For pregnant women not known to be immunized against rubella, serum antibody titers should be measured to determine resistance or susceptibility to the disease.

Developmental Considerations

The risk of not receiving childhood immunizations is offset by the benefit they provide. Immunizations for children and older adults with chronic illnesses should be used with an awareness of potential adverse effects.

Psychosocial Considerations

The health care provider should suspect that a child may not have been properly immunized if one or both parents have less than a high-school education or if there are three or more siblings. Member of families that are economically disadvantaged or who seek health care at public clinics also may not have full immunization.

Analysis and Management

Treatment Objectives

National Health Objectives for the Year 2000 include achieving a 90 percent primary immunization rate for children younger than 2 years and an increase to at least 80 percent for U.S. children (age 2 to 12 years) who have received all of their screening and immunization services. Similarly, at least an 80 percent immunization rate is sought for babies younger than 18 months.

Treatment Options

Recommendations for infant, child, and adult immunizations are influenced by the age-specific risks for disease and for complications, the ability of persons of a given age to respond to the vaccine, and potential interference with the immune response by passively transferred maternal antibodies. Benefits and risks associated with the use of all immunobiologics should also be considered, because no vaccine is completely safe or completely effective.

The benefits of immunization range from partial to complete protection against the consequences of the infection. The risks vary from common, minor, and inconvenient effects to rare, severe, and life-threatening conditions. Benefits, costs, and risks must be considered in achieving optimal protection against infectious diseases. Recommendations attempt to minimize the risk by providing specific advice on dose, route, and timing of vaccines, and by delineating circumstances that warrant precaution in, or abstention from, administration of a particular vaccine.

In the United States, the Committee on Infectious Diseases appointed by the American Academy of Pediatrics and the Public Health Service's ACIP, in collaboration with the Centers for Disease Control and Prevention, review immunization data, provide recommendations, and publish updated information. The American Academy of Pediatrics and its publications address pediatric and general practice in conjunction with public health. Thus, there may be some differences between its recommendations and those of the ACIP in its journal, *Morbidity and Mortality Weekly Report* (MMWR). Table 28–3 provides an overview of the currently recommended immunization schedules.

Drug and Patient Variables

For routine immunizations, combined antigenic preparations are preferred (e.g., DTP, MMR). Single antigenic formulations are recommended when other components in the formulation are contraindicated. Immunization for adults should be individualized, with age, physical health, and possible allergic reactions taken into account. For example, pertussis immunization may be inappropriate because the risk of reactions to the vaccine outweighs the protection it provides, particularly in older adults. Live attenuated viral vaccines (e.g., MMR, oral polio) should not be given to people who are immunocompromised (e.g., human immunodeficiency virus, leukemia, lymphoma) or who are taking corticosteroid or antineoplastic drugs, and in whom the viruses can reproduce and cause infection. If such a patient is exposed to varicella, immune globulin or varicella-zoster immune globulin may be given for passive immunization.

To offset the reluctance of adults to be immunized against hepatitis B, the ACIP has recommended that children receive the hepatitis B vaccine at 2, 4, 6, and 15 months of age. This regimen is suggested even though persons affected by this disease are usually adolescents or adults. Hepatitis immunization programs are the first to prevent illness (and possibly death) in adults by directing the immunization toward children. The effectiveness of the program will not be

TABLE 28–3 IMMUNIZATION SCHEDULES

Age or Time	HBV	DTap or DTP	OPV or IPV	Hib	MMR	Td	PPD
Recommended Immunization Schedule for Healthy Infants and Children							
Birth–12 hr	√						
1–2 mo	√						
2 mo		√	√	√			
4 mo		√	√	√			
6 mo		√		√			
6–18 mo	√		√				
12–15 mo				√*	√		√
15–18 mo		√					
4–6 yr		√	√		√†		
11–12 yr					√		
14–16 yr						√	
Recommended Immunization Schedules for Infants and Children Not Immunized as Above							
First visit	√	√	√				√
1 mo later	√				√‡		
2 mo after first visit		√	√	√			
4 mo after first visit	√	√	√				
10–16 mo after last dose		√	√	√			
4–6 yr		√	√				
14–16 yr		√					√

*Hib #3 may be needed at 12–15 months if not received at age 6 months.
†MMR #2 given at age 11–12 years if not given at age 4–6 years (entry to school).
‡MMR not given before age 15 months. Hib used for children between the ages of 18–60 months.
Data from the Advisory Committee on Immunization Practices, the Centers for Disease Control and Prevention, the American Academy of Pediatrics and the American Academy of Family Practice. (1998). Recommended Childhood Immunization Schedule–United States, January–December 1998 (RE9807). *Pediatrics,* 101(1), 134–135.

apparent until the vaccinated children reach adolescence or adulthood.

Intervention

Storage

Immunizing drugs are stored according to manufacturer's directions to maintain efficacy of vaccines and other biologic preparations. Most are stored in the refrigerator (not on the door) at temperatures ranging from 35.6 to 46.4 °F (2 to 8 °C). Some vaccines (e.g., MMR) require protection from light. If immunizing agents are to be transported, ice packs and polystyrene foam containers should be used. Polio vaccines should be transported with dry ice only. Most immunizing agents are mixed just before use.

Administration

The health care provider should read the package insert before administering any immunization. The vaccine and diluent should be inspected for particulate matter or discoloration. The solution should be discarded if precipitate or discoloration is present.

Persons administering vaccines should take basic precautions to minimize the risk of spreading disease. In general, patients are instructed to wait 30 minutes after the vaccination so they may be observed for allergic reactions.

When multiple vaccines are administered simultaneously, each drug should be given at a different site, using separate needles and syringes. The only exception to this is PRP-T, or Hib conjugate vaccine, which can be mixed with DTP vaccine. If two injections are administered in the same limb, the injection sites are separated by 1 to 2 inches so that local reactions do not overlap.

Timing of Administration Some vaccines require more than one dose for development of an adequate antibody response. Others require periodic reinforcement (booster doses) to maintain protection. The ACIP recommends the interval between administration of doses and vaccines. Longer than recommended dosage intervals do not reduce antibody concentrations. Administering doses of a vaccine or toxoid at less than the recommended minimum intervals may decrease the antibody response and should be avoided. When administered too frequently, some vaccines reduce the rates of local or systemic reactions in some recipients.

Many commonly used vaccines and immunizations can be administered safely and effectively when given simultaneously. Others can be administered on the same day but not at the same anatomic site. Killed vaccines can be administered simultaneously at separate sites. Local or systemic reactions can be accentuated when killed vaccines are administered simultaneously. Live and inactivated vaccines may be administered simultaneously (Table 28–4). Simultaneous administration of routine vaccinations does not interfere with the immune response to these vaccines.

Inactivated vaccines generally do not interfere with the immune response to other inactivated vaccines or to live vaccines. Yellow fever and cholera vaccines are an exception to this rule. Immune response to one live virus vaccine might be impaired if it is administered within 30 days of another live virus vaccine. Whenever possible, live virus vaccines should be administered at least 30 days apart.

Administration of immune globulin can inhibit the immune response to live vaccines for 3 months or more.

TABLE 28–4 USE OF LIVE AND KILLED VACCINES

Antigen	Example of Antigen	Recommended Interval Between Doses
2 or more killed antigens	Measles, mumps, rubella, polio	None May be administered together or at any interval
Killed and live antigens	—	None May be administered together or at any interval
2 or more live antigens	Influenza, pertussis	Minimum of 4-wk interval if agents not administered simultaneously

Therefore, MMR and its individual components should be administered 3 months after administration of immune globulin. Immune globulin formulations interact less with inactivated vaccines and toxoids than with live vaccines. Therefore, they can be administered simultaneously or at any interval between. They should be administered at different sites and using the standard recommended dose of corresponding vaccine.

Education

Many people think that certain diseases have been eradicated and are no longer a threat, so it is not unusual for patients or parents to resist recommendations to have immunizations. Others fear serious adverse effects, are deterred by the cost of the vaccine, or say they do not have the time for successive vaccinations or boosters. Public education is vital so that people understand the need for prevention and the reasons for seeking health care in the event of injury, animal bite, or exposure to various contagious diseases.

The vaccine recipient should be advised that adverse reactions have been reported for all vaccines. The reactions are usually local and transient, but they can be systemic, and either immediate or delayed. Local inflammatory reactions at the injection site are the most common. Fever, rash, and hypersensitivity occur uncommonly. Most reactions resolve within 48 hours and can usually be effectively managed with symptomatic treatment. This information is transmitted through informed consent statements and patient education materials. Signature sheets for informed consent are also available.

Seeking information about travel immunizations is an important part of travel preparation. Individuals traveling to high-risk areas should be instructed to contact their health care provider, health department, and/or travel clinic for guidance regarding any required immunizations. Information about vaccinations is also available from the Centers for Disease Control and Prevention via the Internet. In addition, patients traveling in areas where there is serious endemic disease (e.g., cholera) should be cautioned to not drink untreated water or to eat raw fish or uncooked or unpeeled fruits and vegetables.

Evaluation

Evaluation of the benefits of immunization is difficult to ascertain directly. However, if universal immunization of infants is successful, there will be a dramatic decline in the transmission of infectious diseases. Greater attention to the vaccination of high-risk individuals would accelerate the decline. Compliance with recommended immunization regi-

Controversy

Immunization Policy Issues

JONATHAN J. WOLFE

Immunization is possibly the best response to communicable disease, because it is proactive. Successful immunization prevents disease and all its sequelae. Immunization, however, is not a perfectly benign process. Although patients rarely suffer harm from vaccines, adverse reactions include anaphylaxis. Occasionally, a patient may unaccountably contract the disease that the vaccine seeks to prevent. Also, people with incompetent immune systems are at some risk if immunized with live attenuated virus preparations. The benefits to health, however, clearly outweigh the risks.

People's acceptance of an immunization program is important, too. Sometimes, religious convictions stand in the way of receiving vaccines. At other times, fear of even the slightest risk of harm prevents participation. Many people refuse to submit their minor children to the risks associated with immunization. Indeed, the press may exacerbate the problem by reporting rare adverse events without adequately presenting the countervailing benefit. Stories about people harmed by vaccines make gripping headlines and television sound bites. The long-term benefits of disease-free health are less obvious to readers and listeners.

Health care reform, with its suggestions of rationing care, adds urgency to the discussion of immunization. Public and private payers alike want to know where the right of individuals to refuse immunization infringes on the right of the majority to lower health care costs resulting from responsible preventive care. All children and adults may one day be required to participate in immunization programs before they are allowed to use public buildings, schools, and transportation.

Critical Thinking Discussion

- The discovery and preparation of vaccines was watched and welcomed as a sign of progress in the late 19th century and on through the advent of the Salk poliomyelitis vaccines in the 1950s. Why has the public perceptions of vaccines changed?
- To what extent do you think concerns about legal liability for the harmful effects of vaccines inhibit wider immunization?
- What particular issues of individual autonomy must be respected in any debate about immunization?
- Physicians are no longer the sole source for vaccination. What do you consider to be the proper role for nurses in vaccination? For advanced practice nurses? For pharmacists?
- What harm can you foresee to our society if immunization coverage were to fall to low levels?
- What geographic areas of the United States are at greatest risk from low levels of immunization?
- What one vaccine is most important to discover and make available in the next 10 years?

VAERS

VACCINE ADVERSE EVENT REPORTING SYSTEM
24 Hour Toll-free information line 1-800-822-7967
P.O. Box 1100, Rockville, MD 20849-1100
PATIENT IDENTITY KEPT CONFIDENTIAL

For CDC/FDA Use Only
VAERS Number ________
Date Received ________

Patient Name: ________
Last First M.I.
Address ________
City State Zip
Telephone no. (____)________

Vaccine administered by (Name): ________
Responsible Physician ________
Facility Name/Address ________
City State Zip
Telephone no. (____)________

Form completed by (Name): ________
Relation to Patient ☐ Vaccine Provider ☐ Patient/Parent ☐ Manufacturer ☐ Other
Address *(if different from patient or provider)* ________
City State Zip
Telephone no. (____)________

1. State
2. County where administered
3. Date of birth __/__/__ mm dd yy
4. Patient age
5. Sex ☐ M ☐ F
6. Date form completed __/__/__ mm dd yy

7. Describe adverse event(s) (symptoms, signs, time course) and treatment, if any

8. Check all appropriate:
☐ Patient died (date __/__/__) mm dd yy
☐ Life threatening illness
☐ Required emergency room/doctor visit
☐ Required hospitalization (______days)
☐ Resulted in prolongation of hospitalization
☐ Resulted in permanent disability
☐ None of the above

9. Patient recovered ☐ YES ☐ NO ☐ UNKNOWN

10. Date of vaccination __/__/__ mm dd yy Time ______ AM PM
11. Adverse event onset __/__/__ mm dd yy Time ______ AM PM

12. Relevant diagnostic tests/laboratory data

13. Enter all vaccines given on date listed in no. 10

	Vaccine (type)	Manufacturer	Lot number	Route/Site	No. Previous doses
a.					
b.					
c.					
d.					

14. Any other vaccinations within 4 weeks prior to the date listed in no. 10

	Vaccine (type)	Manufacturer	Lot number	Route/Site	No. Previous doses	Date given
a.						
b.						

15. Vaccinated at:
☐ Private doctor's office/hospital ☐ Military clinic/hospital
☐ Public health clinic/hospital ☐ Other/unknown

16. Vaccine purchased with:
☐ Private funds ☐ Military funds
☐ Public funds ☐ Other /unknown

17. Other medications

18. Illness at time of vaccination (specify)

19. Pre-existing physician-diagnosed allergies, birth defects, medical conditions (specify)

20. Have you reported this adverse event previously? ☐ No ☐ To health department ☐ To doctor ☐ To manufacturer

Only for children 5 and under
22. Birth weight ____ lb. ____ oz.
23. No. of brothers and sisters

21. Adverse event following prior vaccination (check all applicable, specify)

	Adverse Event	Onset Age	Type Vaccine	Dose no. in series
☐ In patient				
☐ In brother or sister				

Only for reports submitted by manufacturer/immunization project
24. Mfr. / imm. proj. report no.
25. Date received by mfr. / imm. proj.
26. 15 day report? ☐ Yes ☐ No
27. Report type ☐ Initial ☐ Follow-Up

Health care providers and manufacturers are required by law (42 USC 300aa-25) to report reactions to vaccines listed in the Table of Reportable Events Following Immunization. Reports for reactions to other vaccines are voluntary except when required as a condition of immunization grant awards.

Form VAERS -1

Figure 28–1 Vaccine Adverse Event Report Food and Drug Administration (Law 42 USC 300aa-25) requires that a report be filed whenever a recipient of an immunization experiences an adverse reaction to vaccines listed in Table 28–5. (From Vaccine Adverse Event Reporting System. (1997). *The reportable events table.* Rockville, MD: Author.)

TABLE 28–5 REPORTABLE EVENTS

Event	Interval*
DTP, Pertussis, Combined DTP/polio	
Anaphylaxis or anaphylactic shock	24 hr
Encephalopathy or encephalitis	7 days
Shock-collapse, or hypotonic-hyporesponsive collapse	7 days
Residual seizure disorder	No limit
Acute complications or sequelae of above events (including death)	No limit
Events described in manufacturer's package insert as contraindications to additional doses of vaccine	See package insert
MMR, DT, Td, Tetanus Toxoid	
Anaphylaxis or anaphylactic shock	24 hr
Encephalopathy or encephalitis	15 days
Residual seizure disorder	15 days
Acute complications or sequelae of above events (including death)	No limit
Events described in manufacturer's package insert as contraindications to additional doses of vaccine	See package insert
Oral Polio Vaccine	
Paralytic poliomyelitis in a nonimmunodeficient recipient	30 days
In an immunocompromised recipient	6 months
In a vaccine-associated community case	No limit
Any acute complication or sequelae of above events (including death)	No limit
Events described in manufacturer's package insert as contraindications to additional doses of vaccine	See package insert
Inactivated Polio Vaccine	
Anaphylaxis or anaphylactic shock	24 hours
Acute complication or sequelae of above events (including death)	No limit
Events described in manufacturer's package insert as contraindications to additional doses of vaccine	See package insert

*Interval between immunization and event.

Data from Vaccine Adverse Event Reporting System. (1997). The Reportable Events Table. Rockville, MD: Author.

mens is an important variable in determining the patient's understanding of immunizations.

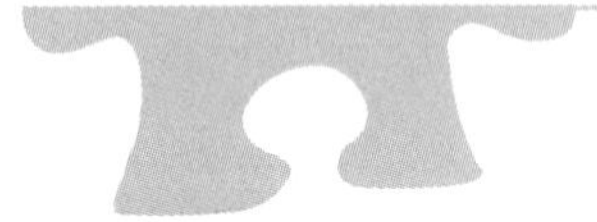

LEGAL IMPLICATIONS OF IMMUNIZATIONS

Customary medical practice in most states includes providing information to parents and patients about the benefits and risks of preventive procedures such as immunizations. Benefits and risks of vaccines should be explained before the administration of the vaccines. Disclosure of information through the use of prepared informed consent statements have been developed for most vaccines and include space for a signature. Patient understanding of the major benefits and rare adverse effects of immunizations is crucial to the success of immunization programs. (See Controversy—Immunization Policy Issues.)

On the other hand, there has been a shortage of MMR and Hib vaccines because drug manufacturers are fearful of product liability suits. The federal government has intervened and now accepts responsibility under the National Childhood Vaccine Injury Act of 1986. Under this legislation, provisions are made for one time payment to families of children who have had significant adverse reactions following the administration of vaccines as an alternative to civil litigation under the traditional tort system. A report of the adverse reaction must be submitted and an agreement not to pursue litigation is made before payment.

The Food and Drug Administration requires that a Vaccine Adverse Event Report (Fig. 28–1) be filed whenever an immunization recipient experiences an adverse reaction to any vaccine (Table 28–5) (Law: 42 USC 300aa-25). Low-grade allergic responses occur when a vaccine is made from killed bacteria grown in artificial media. Viruses grown in living animal tissues cause a higher rate of allergic reactions.

Immunization Records

Health care providers who administer one or more of the vaccines covered by the National Childhood Vaccine Injury Act of 1986 must ensure that the recipient's permanent medical records include the date the vaccine was administered, the vaccine manufacturer, the vaccine lot number, and the name, address, and title of the person administering the vaccine. The ACIP recommends that this information be kept for all vaccinations. In addition, it is recommended that parents establish a permanent immunization record for each newborn child and that it be continuously updated.

It is not unusual for a health care provider to encounter people without adequate documentation of immunizations.

Immunizations should not be postponed for lack of records. Such persons should be considered susceptible, and an appropriate immunization schedule initiated.

SUMMARY

- Sera, vaccines, and other immunizing agents are capable of producing active and passive immunity.
- Active acquired immunity develops when antibodies are formed by the host after exposure to modified pathogens or toxins.
- Passive immunity develops when the host is given antibodies from another individual or animal.
- Success of most vaccines in establishing antigen-antibody response depends on the humoral response of the immune system.
- Vaccines are a suspension of live or attenuated microorganisms administered for the purpose of establishing active immunity to an infectious disease.
- There are two general classes of vaccines, bacterial and viral vaccines.
- The bacterial toxins pathogenic quality is destroyed but its antigenic properties remain. Like vaccines, they stimulate active immunity without causing disease.
- Antitoxins are used when a person has been exposed to an organism that secretes toxins. Antitoxins provide passive immunity.
- Sera provides passive immunity. Examples are human serum immune globulin and hepatitis immune globulin.
- Antisera are antibodies of animal origin and are used when immune globulins of human origin are unavailable for a specific illness.
- Diseases for which vaccinations may be recommended for travel include cholera, Japanese encephalitis, meningococcus, plague, tuberculosis, typhoid, and yellow fever.
- The specific drug to be used for active immunity depends on disease endemicity, degree of exposure, season, and length of time exposed.
- The patient history should include a thorough immunization history and physical exam, including body temperature.
- Treatment objectives follow the National Health Objectives for the Year 2000 as outlined by the U.S. Preventive Services Task Force.
- The Centers for Disease Control and Prevention has a recommended immunization schedule developed under the guidance of the Advisory Committee for Immunization Practices.
- Interventions associated with immunizing drugs include attention to storage, administration methods, and timing.
- Nursing care of the patient comprises education about the recommended immunization schedule, administering the prescribed agent, and monitoring for allergic responses.
- Universal immunization of infants and other at risk individuals will produce a dramatic decline in the transmission of infectious diseases.
- The federal government accepts responsibility for adverse reactions under the National Childhood Vaccine Injury Act of 1986.
- The Food and Drug Administration requires that a Vaccine Adverse Event Report system form be completed whenever an immunization recipient experiences an adverse reaction to specific vaccines.
- Health care providers must ensure that the recipient's permanent medical records indicate the date each vaccine was administered, the vaccine manufacturer, the vaccine lot number, and the name, address, and title of the person administering the vaccine. The ACIP recommends that this information be kept for all vaccinations.
- It is not unusual for a health care provider to encounter persons without adequate documentation of immunizations. Immunizations should not be postponed for lack of records.

BIBLIOGRAPHY

Abramowicz, M. (ed.) (1995). Varicella vaccine. *The Medical Letter,* 37(951), 55–57.

Abramowicz, M. (ed.) (1995). Hepatitis A vaccine. *The Medical Letter,* 37(950), 51–52.

Ad Hoc Working Group for the Development of Standards for Pediatric Immunization Practices. (1993). Standards for pediatric immunization practices. *Journal of the American Medical Association,* 269, 1817–1822.

Arnold, P., and Schlenker, T. (1992). The impact of health care financing on childhood immunization practices. *American Journal of Diseases in Children,* 146(6), 728–732.

Atkinson, W., Watson, J., Hadler, S. (1994). Acceptability of immunizations given in other countries. *The Pediatric Infectious Disease Journal,* 13(11), 1026–1027.

Ball, T. (1995). Immunizations: Toddler documentation gap. *Clinical Pediatrics,* 34(1), 54–56.

Centers for Disease Control and Prevention. (1997). Recommended childhood immunization schedule in the United States, 1997. *Journal of the American Medical Association,* 277(5), 371–372.

Centers for Disease Control. (1991). Diphtheria, tetanus, and pertussis: Recommendations for vaccine use and other preventive measures. *Morbidity and Mortality Weekly Report,* 40(RR-10), 1–23.

Centers for Disease Control. (1994). General recommendations on immunization. *Morbidity and Mortality Weekly Report,* 43(RR-1), 8–31.

Centers for Disease Control. (1991). Haemophilus b conjugate vaccines for prevention of *Haemophilus influenzae* type B disease among infants and children two months of age and older: Recommendations of the immunization practices advisory committee (ACIP). *Morbidity and Mortality Weekly Review,* 40(RR-1), 1–8.

Centers for Disease Control. (1995). Licensure of inactivated hepatitis A vaccine and recommendations for use among international travelers. *Morbidity and Mortality Weekly Report,* 44(29), 559–561.

Centers for Disease Control. (1994). Prevention and control of influenza part I: Vaccines. Recommendations of the Advisory Committee on Immunization Practices. *Morbidity and Mortality Weekly Report,* 43(RR-9), 1–5.

Centers for Disease Control. (1995). Progress toward elimination of *Haemophilus influenzae* type B disease among infants and children. *Morbidity and Mortality Weekly Report,* 44(29), 545–549.

Centers for Disease Control. (1995). Recommended childhood immunization schedule: United States, 1995. *Morbidity and Mortality Weekly Report,* 44(RR-5), 1–8.

Centers for Disease Control. (1993). Recommendations for use of Haemophilus B conjugate vaccines and a combined diphtheria, tetanus, pertussis, and Haemophilus B vaccine: Recommendation of the Advisory Committee on Immunization Practices (ACIP). *Morbidity and Mortality Weekly Report,* 42(RR-13), 1–15.

Centers for Disease Control. (1990). Rubella prevention: Recommendations of the Immunization Practices Advisory Committee (ACIP). *Morbidity and Mortality Weekly Report,* 39(RR-15), 1–17.

Centers for Disease Control. (1993). Tuberculosis control laws: United States, 1993. *Morbidity and Mortality Weekly Report,* 42(RR-15), 1–13.

Centers for Disease Control. (1994). Typhoid immunization. *Morbidity and Mortality Weekly Report,* 43(RR-14), 1–7.

Centers for Disease Control. (1993). Use of vaccines and immune globulins for persons with altered immunocompetence: Recommendations of the Advisory Committee on Immunization Practices (ACIP). *Morbidity and Mortality Weekly Review,* 42(RR-4), 1–12.

Committee on Infectious Diseases. (1994). *1994 redbook: Report of the committee on infectious diseases.* (23rd ed.). Elk Grove Village, IL.: American Academy of Pediatrics.

D'Angio, C. Maniscalco, W., and Pichichero, M. (1995). Immunologic response of extremely premature infants to tetanus, *Haemophilus influenzae,* and polio immunizations. *Pediatrics,* 96(1), 18–22.

Daly, J., Johnston, W., and Chung, Y. (1992). Injection sites utilized for DPT immunizations. *Journal of Community Health Nursing,* 9(2), 87–94.

Edwards, K. (1993). Pediatric immunizations. *Current Problems in Pediatrics,* 23(5), 186–205.

Freed, G., Bordley, C., and Defriese, G. (1993). Childhood immunization programs: An analysis of policy issues. *The Milbank Quarterly,* 71(1), 65–96.

Fulginiti, V. (1992). How safe are pertussis and rubella vaccines? A commentary on the Institute of Medicine report. *Pediatrics,* 89(2), 153–157.

Ganiats, T., Bowersox, M., and Ralph, L. (1993). Universal neonatal hepatitis B immunization: Are we jumping on the band wagon too early? *Journal of Family Practice,* 36(2), 147–149.

General Recommendations on Immunization: Recommendations of the Advisory Committee on Immunization Practices (ACIP). (1994). *Morbidity and Mortality Weekly Report,* 43(RR-1), 1–38.

Hinman, A. (1993). What will it take to fully protect all American children with vaccines? An update. *American Journal of Diseases of Children,* 147(5), 536–537.

Hinman, A., Orenstein, W., and Mortimer, E. (1992). When, where, and how do immunizations fail? *American Family Physician,* 2(6), 805–811.

Holt, D. (1992). Recommendations, usage, and efficacy of immunizations for the elderly. *Nurse Practitioner,* 17(3), 51–59.

Howson, C., and Finebirg, H. (1992). The ricochet of magic bullets: Summary of the Institute of Medicine report, adverse effects of pertussis and rubella vaccines. *Pediatrics,* 89(2), 318–323.

Huston, R. (1993). Problems with vaccination coverage in the United States. *Clinical Pediatrics,* 32(3), 163–166.

Hymel, T., Sherman, J., Pope, S., and Kelleher, K. (1993). Inadequate immunizations: Identification using clinic charts. *Clinical Pediatrics,* 32(3), 156–160.

Kefalas, M. (1993). American children and immunizations: Part I, how bad is it? *Journal of Pediatric Nursing,* 8(6), 345–347.

Kefalas, M. (1993). American children and immunizations: Part II, how bad is it? *Journal of Pediatric Nursing,* 8(6), 403–405.

Kum-Nji, P., James, D., and Herrod, H. (1995). Immunization status of hospitalized preschool children: Risk factors associated with inadequate immunization. *Pediatrics,* 96(3), 434–438.

Landwirth, J. (1990). Medical-legal aspects of immunization. *Pediatric Clinics of North America,* 37(3), 771–783.

Lannon, C., Brack, V., Stuart, J., et al. (1995). What mothers say about why poor children fall behind on immunizations. *Archives of Pediatric and Adolescent Medicine,* 149(10), 1070–1075.

Lyznicki, J., and Rinaldi, R. (1994). Childhood immunizations and the vaccines for children program. *Archives of Family Medicine,* 3(8), 728–730.

Mulligan, M., and Stiehm, R. (1994). Neonatal hepatitis B infection: Clinical and immunologic considerations. *Journal of Perinatology,* XIV(1), 2–9.

National Vaccine Advisory Committee. (1991). The measles epidemic: The problems, barriers, and recommendations. Journal of the American Medical Association, 266(11), 1547–1552.

Petry, J. (1993). Immunization controversies. *Journal of Family Practice,* 36(2), 141–143.

Salsberry, P., Nickel, J., and Mitch, R. (1993). Why aren't preschoolers immunized? A comparison of parents' and providers' perceptions of the barriers to immunizations. *Journal of Community Health Nursing,* 10(4), 213–224.

Spaulding, S., and Kugler, J. (1991). Influenza immunization: The impact of notifying patients of high risk status. *The Journal of Family Practice,* 33(5), 495–498.

Task Force on Adult Immunization. (1994). Adult immunization 1994. *Annals of Internal Medicine,* 121(7), 540–541.

United States Department of Health and Human Services. (1991). *Healthy people 2000: National health promotion and disease prevention objectives.* Washington, DC: U.S. Government Printing Office.

Williams, I., Milton, J., Farrell, J., et al. (1995). Interaction of socioeconomic status and provider practices as predictors of immunization coverage in Virginia children. *Pediatrics,* 96(3), 439–445.

Zell, E., Dietz, V., Stevenson, J., et al. (1994). Low vaccination levels of US preschool and school-age children. *Journal of the American Medical Center,* 271(11), 833–839.

Zimmerman, R., and Burns, I. (1994). Childhood immunization guidelines: Current and future. *Primary Care,* 21(4), 693–715.

Zimmerman, R., and Clover, R. (1995). Adult immunizations: A practical approach for clinicians: Part I. *American Family Physician,* 51(4), 859–863.

Zimmerman, R., and Clover, R. (1995). Adult immunizations—a practical approach for clinicians: Part II. *American Family Physician,* 51(4), 1139–1148.

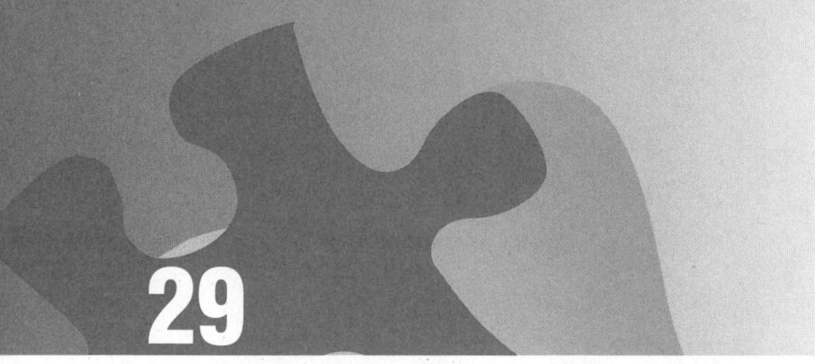

29 Biologic Response Modifiers

The relationship between the immune system and cancer has been explored for more than a century. William Coley, a surgeon who practiced in New York in the late 1800s, is credited with the first use of specific drugs that modified the immune system. In the late 1960s, the concept of *immunotherapy,* stimulating the body's immune system to fight disease, emerged. Many clinical trials using bacterial extracts such as bacillus Calmette-Guérin (BCG) and *Cornybacterium parvum* were conducted. However, the results of the trials were inconsistent, and disappointed researchers turned their attention elsewhere.

Biologic response modifiers (BRMs) are produced through biotechnology. These drugs are designed to elicit a response that uses the patient's own biologic mechanisms to fight disease. Two developments in the mid- to late-1970s fostered the development of BRMs: hybridoma and recombinant DNA technology. Hybridoma technology allows the production of monoclonal antibodies by using the antigen-antibody reaction to advantage (Fig. 29–1). A monoclonal antibody is produced by hybridizing B cells from the spleens of mice that have been injected with a specific antigen with immortal plasma cells (B cells) from a plasma cell tumor. The result is a hybridoma, a B cell clone that is both antigen-specific and capable of indefinite proliferation. Hybridoma tumors are kept alive in the mouse while the desired clones are cultured and frozen. The monoclonal antibodies are purified and readied for use. Today's generation of monoclonal antibodies has created new therapeutic and diagnostic possibilities, particularly in the treatment of cancer and early detection of viral infections.

The fundamental components of recombinant DNA technology are the bacterial plasmids, small, circular sections of self-replicating DNA. Plasmids can be removed from or inserted into bacteria without severely disrupting bacterial growth or reproduction.

DNA technology withdraws a plasmid from the bacterial host and exposes it to restrictive enzymes. The enzymes cut the plasmid's DNA at a precise site in the nucleotide sequence (Fig. 29–2). For example, the common enzyme *EcoRI* (named for the bacteria that produce it, *Escherichia coli*) cuts a strand of the plasmid's DNA where the nucleotide sequence G-A-A-T-T-C is found. Human DNA also can be exposed to *EcoRI* and cut at the same site. The pieces of human DNA and bacterial DNA can then be recombined. The plasmid, which now contains human genes in addition to its own, is then reintroduced into the bacterium where it divides and replicates, copying itself and the recombinant DNA. Through cell division, millions of bacterial clones are formed, all containing the same human gene. The human gene directs protein synthesis in the bacteria, resulting in production of human proteins by the bacteria. Because protein enzymes are responsible for most chemical reactions within cells, the ability to replicate specific proteins becomes extremely important to the understanding and manipulation of cell activity and the most basic elements of body function.

BRMs can be organized into two categories: immunostimulants and immunosuppressants. Immunostimulants augment the immune response by stimulating cells of the reticuloendothelial system (e.g., monocytes, macrophages) to initiate action against foreign invaders. Interferons (IFN), BCG, and methanol-extracted residue of BCG are examples of immunoaugmenting drugs. Other immunostimulants enhance or inhibit T lymphocyte (T cell) and B cell production and stimulate secretion of a variety of cytokines. Examples of some of these drugs include interleukins (ILs), colony-stimulating factors (CSFs), epoetin alfa (EPO), and tumor necrosis factors (TNFs). Restorative drugs such as levamisole and thymosin stimulate or restore depressed antigenic responses and cellular immune function.

The influence exerted by immunostimulants varies with the type of immunity modulated and the therapeutic results that are expected. Patients receiving immunostimulants artificially acquire either active or passive immunity to specific foreign proteins or antigens. Chapter 28 discusses the immunostimulating effects of vaccinations.

The major immunosuppressant drug groups include cytotoxins, T-helper cell suppressors, lymphocyte antibodies, and corticosteroids. These drugs inhibit or suppress immune response. Examples of cytotoxins include TNFs and lymphotoxins. Corticosteroids are discussed in Chapter 52.

PATHOGENESIS

BRMs act along with the immune system to destroy tumor cells. When the immune system is functioning normally, foreign invaders are recognized and destroyed. However, the immune response requires the interaction of many different cells with differing actions. Each cell within the immune system begins life in the bone marrow as a pluripotent stem cell. The maturation of each cell is depicted in the hematopoietic cascade (Fig. 29–3).

The primary cell of the immune response is the lymphocyte. Lymphocytes originate in the liver and spleen of the fetus and the bone marrow of the child or adult as lymphocyte precursors or stem cells. To become immunocompetent, they must migrate through the lymphatics and blood vessels and then through lymphoid tissues in various parts of the body. While passing through these tissues, they mature and undergo changes that commit them to one of two cellular lines. The lymphocytes that migrate through one set of lymphoid tissues are referred to as B cells. When B cells encounter antigens, they are stimulated to mature into plasma cells that produce antibodies (i.e., IgG, IgM, IgA, IgE). B cells are responsible for humoral immunity.

Lymphocytes migrating through the thymus gland become T cells. T cells become sensitized to and recognize specific antigens, which they then directly attack. Cytotoxic T cells attack antigens directly and destroy cells bearing for-

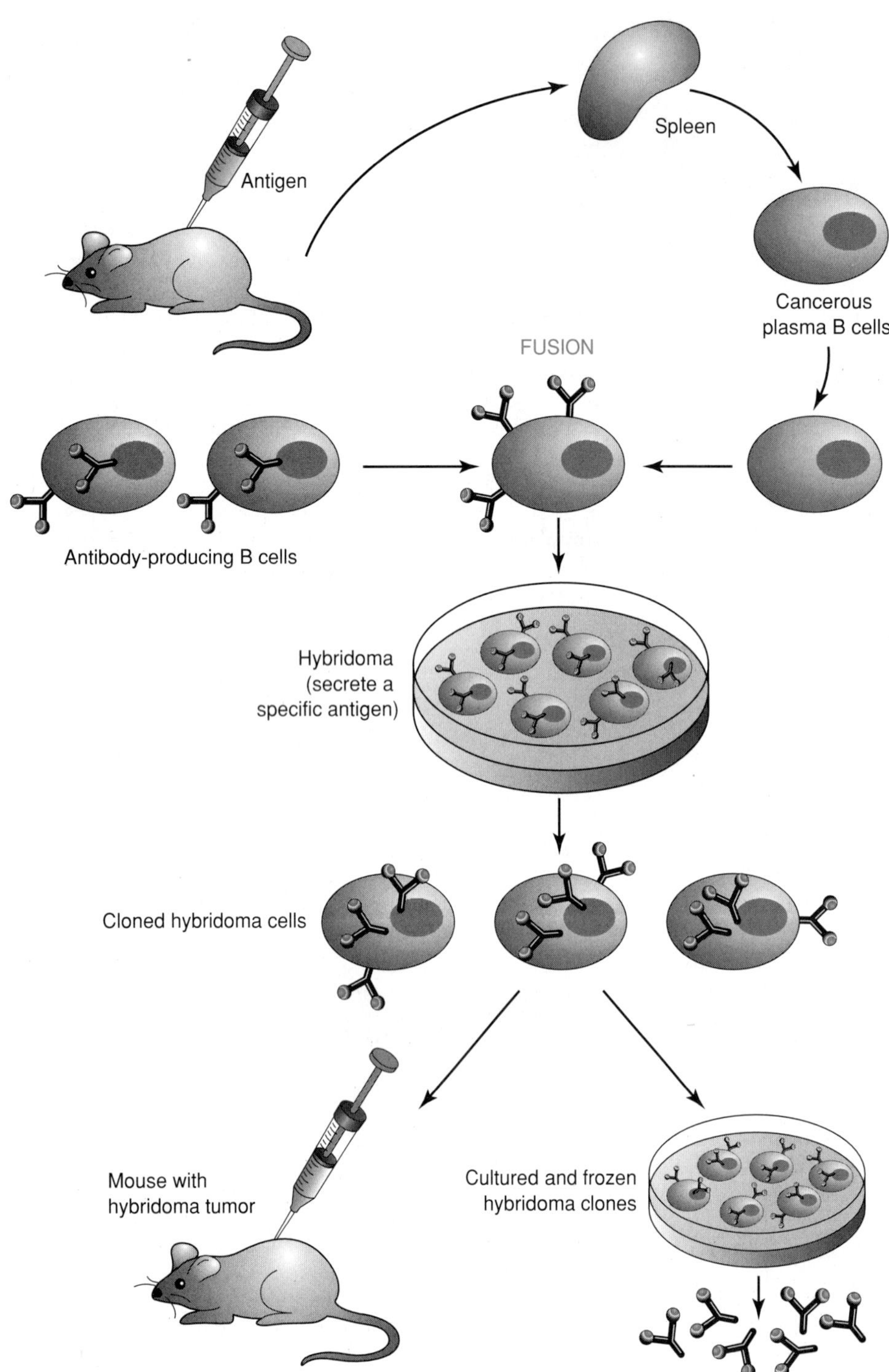

Figure 29–1 Hybridoma technology. Monoclonal antibodies are produced by hybridizing B cells from the spleens of mice that have been injected with a specific antigen and B cells from a plasma cell tumor. The result is hybridoma that is both antigen specific and capable of indefinite proliferation.

eign antigens such as virally infected cells, tumors, or foreign grafts. Cytotoxic T cells secrete *cytokines*, chemical messengers with many different actions. Cytokine is a general term for cell-derived factors that mediate interactions between cells. Those produced by lymphocytes are referred to as *lymphokines* and those produced by the monocyte-macrophage cells are called *monokines*. Some of these factors are called *interleukins,* indicating service as regulatory signals between various leukocytes. Table 29–1 provides an overview of specific cytokines, the cell source, and main function.

Helper T cells and suppressor T cells control both humoral and cell-mediated immune processes. Memory cells induce the secondary immune response. Lymphokine-producing cells transfer delayed hypersensitivity (Td) and secrete lymphokines that activate other cells such as macrophages. The Td cell phenotype is most likely a subset of T-helper cells. T-helper cells produce lymphokines that trigger macrophage activity, but do not appear to mediate any other function.

Another specialized lymphocyte, the natural killer (NK) cell appears to have undergone only partial commitment to the T-cell lineage. NK cells do not bind to antigens and do

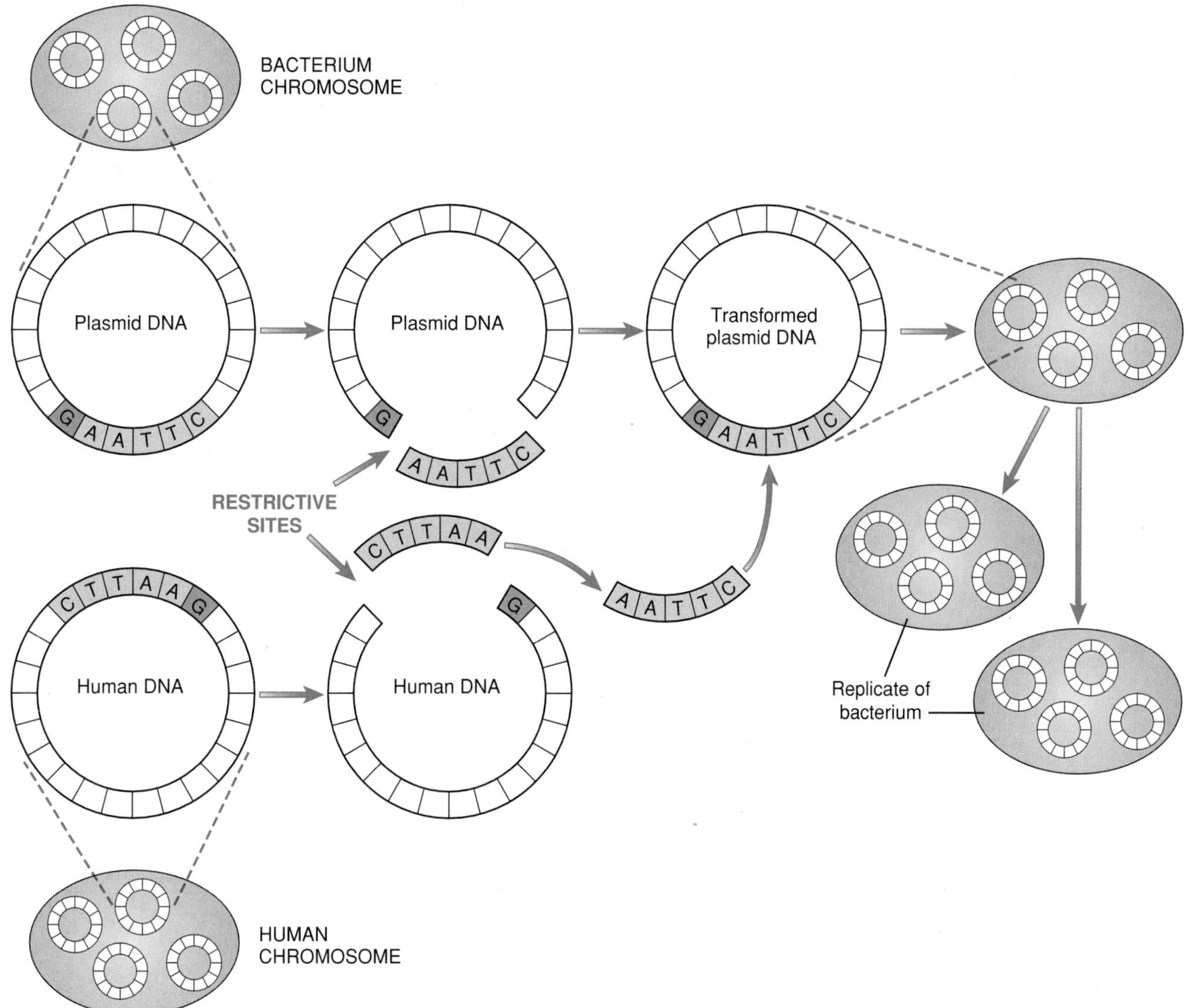

Figure 29–2 Recombinant DNA technology. Human DNA and plasmid DNA from a bacterium (e.g., *Escherichia coli*) are cleaved by a restrictive enzyme. The enzymes cut both DNA fragments at a precise site in the nucleotide sequence, for example, where the nucleotide sequence G-A-A-T-T-C is found. The human DNA is then recombined with bacterial DNA. The plasmids, which now also contain human genes, are introduced back into the bacterium where it divides and replicates, copying itself and the recombinant DNA. (G, Guanine; A, adenine; T, thymine; C, cytosine.)

not proliferate by immunization with antigen. The NK cell recognizes yet undefined chemical changes on the surface of virally infected cells or malignant cells, binding and killing the target cell by mechanisms similar to those of the cytotoxic T cell. The success of the overall immune response depends on the interaction between humoral and cell-mediated responses.

The myeloid stem cell also produces erythrocytes, granulocytes (a type of white blood cell), macrophages, and megakaryocytes (platelets). Each lineage produces a mature functioning cell following the same maturation process.

PHARMACOTHERAPEUTIC OPTIONS

Interferons

- ❒ Interferon alfa-2a (ROFERON-A); (🍁) ROFERON-A
- ❒ Interferon alfa-2b (INTRON A); (🍁) INTRON A
- ❒ Interferon alfa-n3 (ALFERON N)
- ❒ Interferon beta-1a (AVONEX)
- ❒ Interferon beta-1b (BETASERON)
- ❒ Interferon gamma-1b (ACTIMMUNE)

IFN was the first BRM to be discovered and studied. The development of all other biotherapy agents is based on this prototype. The first IFN was discovered in the 1940s. A protein substance isolated in 1957 appeared to inhibit viral activity in cells exposed to a virus. The protein was named interferon. Since IFN was first discovered, three different types of IFNs have been identified. Alpha-IFN (leukocyte, type I) is produced normally by leukocytes, beta-IFN (fibroblast, type I) by fibroblasts, and gamma-IFN (macrophage-activating factor) by lymphocytes. Within the alpha-IFN class there are 14 different subclasses. The nucleotide sequence of each of the subclasses is slightly different.

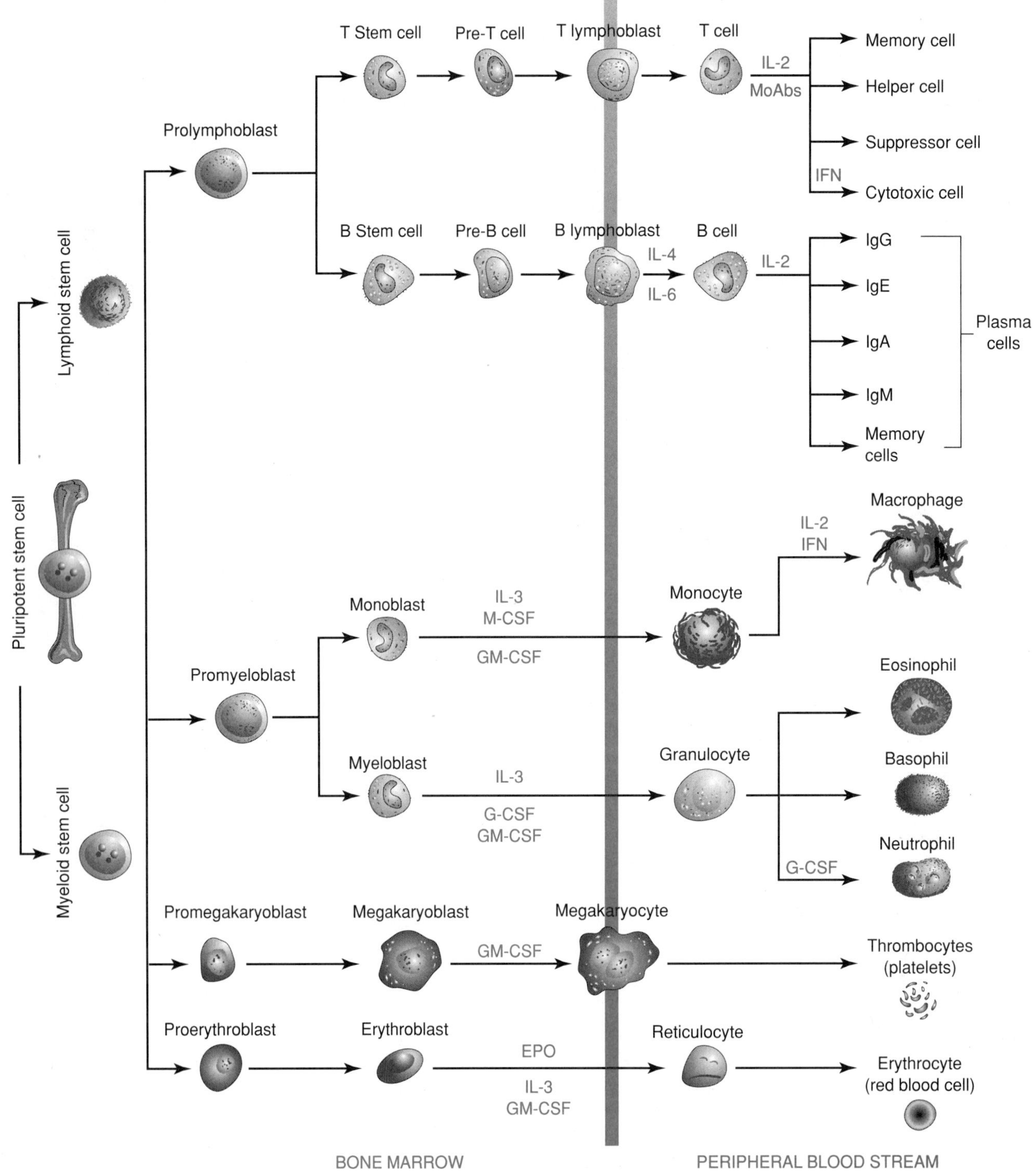

Figure 29–3 Hematopoietic cascade. Blood cell production occurs in the liver and spleen of the fetus; however, it occurs in the bone marrow in an adult. The process involves proliferation and differentiation. Each type of cell is derived from a stem cell undergoing mitosis in response to specific biochemical signals. The pathway by which natural killer (NK) cells develop is unknown. Biologic response modifiers work at various stages of the hematopoietic cascade. (GM-CSF, Granulocyte-macrophage colony–stimulating factor; G-CSF, granulocyte colony–stimulating factor; M-CSF, macrophage colony–stimulating factor; IFN, interferon; IL, interleukin.)

Indications

Alpha-IFNs are indicated for the treatment of both malignant and nonmalignant diseases including hairy cell leukemia, Kaposi's sarcoma, renal cell carcinoma, malignant melanoma, hepatitis C, and chronic hepatitis B. It is also used for selected cases of condylomata acuminata involving external surfaces of the genital and perianal areas, chronic myelogenous leukemia, non-Hodgkin's lymphoma, and cutaneous T-cell lymphomas. Juvenile laryngeal papilloma or papillomatosis also has been treated with alpha-IFN. The response to IFN treatment with each of these diseases is evaluated differently.

TABLE 29–1 IMMUNOSTIMULANTS

Cytokine	Cell Source	Main Functions
Interleukins		
IL-1 (alpha and beta)	Macrophages	T-cell and B-cell activation
IL-2 (T-cell growth factor)	T-helper cells, NK cells	T-cell and NK cell activation and proliferation
IL-3 (multiple colony-stimulating factor)	T cells, mast cells, NK cells	Stem cell proliferation and differentiation, increased NK cells
IL-4 (B-cell growth factor)	T cells, mast cells	B-cell differentiation and increased IgE reactions; T-helper$_2$ cell differentiation
IL-5	T cells, macrophages	T-cell, B-cell, and eosinophil differentiation and activation
IL-6	T cells, B cells, monocytes, fibroblasts, endothelial cells	B-cell differentiation; increased hematopoiesis, increased inflammatory response
IL-7	Stromal cells, bone marrow, thymus	B-cell proliferation and differentiation
IL-8 (monocyte-derived neutrophil chemotactic factor)	Macrophages, monocytes, endothelial cells	Triggers neutrophil and lymphocyte chemotaxis
IL-9	T-helper cells	T-cell and mast cell growth factor, maturation of erythroid progenitors
IL-10	T-helper cells	Inhibition of T-helper$_1$ cells; increased cytotoxic T-cell differentiation, induces MHC antigen expression, decreased cytokines
IL-11	Fibroblasts	Increased B-cell and monocyte function; decreases some inflammatory cytokines
IL-12	Macrophages	T-helper$_1$ cell production and differentiation
IL-13	Activated T cells	Increased expression of genes in nerve and intestinal cells; increased osteoclasts; increased progenitor cells in bone marrow
IL-14	T cells	B-cell growth factor
IL-15	Macrophages	T-cell and NK cell activation and proliferation
IL-16	CD_8 cells, T cells	Chemotaxic factor and growth factor for CD_4 T cells; eosinophil chemotaxis
IL-17	T-helper cells	Increases IL-6 and IL-8
Colony-Stimulating Factors		
G-CSF	Monocytes, fibroblasts	Myeloid growth factor
GM-CSF	T cells	Eosinophil activation
M-CSF	Monocytes, lymphocytes, fibroblasts, endothelial cells, epithelial cells	Myelocytic growth factor
Interferons		
Gamma-IFN	T cells, NK cells	Inhibition of T-helper$_2$ cells, macrophage activation; MHC class I and II induction
Beta-IFN	Fibroblasts, macrophages, epithelial cells	Antiviral protection; increases IL-6 and IL-8
Alpha-IFN	Macrophages	NK cell activation; MHC class I induction; decreased B-cell proliferation, IL-8, tumor growth
Tumor Necrosis Factors		
TNF-alpha	Macrophages, lymphocytes, fibroblasts, endothelial cells	Activation of macrophages, granulocytes, and cytotoxic T cells
TNF-beta	T cells	Tumor cell cytotoxicity; increased macrophages, phagocytosis, B-cell proliferation

IL, Interleukins; G-CSF, granulocyte colony-stimulating factor; GM-CSF, granulocyte-macrophage colony-stimulating factor; M-CSF, macrophage colony-stimulating factor; IFN, interferon; TNF, tumor necrosis factor; MHC, major histocompatibility complex; NK, natural killer.

Alfa-2a IFN also has been used as an orphan drug in the treatment of chronic myelogenous leukemia, advanced colorectal cancer, esophageal carcinoma, metastatic malignant melanoma, and renal cell carcinoma. Its unlabeled uses include the treatment of malignant and viral conditions, as well as asymptomatic human immunodeficiency viral infection and symptomatic human immunodeficiency virus (HIV) infection.

Alfa-2b IFN also has been used in the management of similar disorders. In addition, it is classified as an orphan drug in the treatment of ovarian and invasive cervical cancer, laryngeal papillomatosis, and carcinoma in situ of the urinary bladder. Alfa-2b IFN also is used as maintenance therapy for patients with multiple myeloma.

Alfa-n3 IFN is used in the refractory treatment of condylomata acuminata. Its other uses are much like that of the other alpha IFNs.

Beta-1a and beta-1b IFNs are used to reduce the frequency of clinical exacerbations of relapsing, remitting multiple sclerosis, acquired immune deficiency syndrome (AIDS), Kaposi's sarcoma, renal cell carcinoma, malignant melanoma, and acute hepatitis C. In addition, beta-1a IFN has been used as an unlabeled use in the treatment of cutaneous T-cell lymphoma.

Gamma-IFN, the newest agent, is used for chronic granulomatous disease. It is functionally related to the other IFNs but has different immunomodulatory effects.

Pharmacodynamics

Alpha-IFN and beta-IFN are antiviral agents that enhance NK-cell activity. They activate cytotoxic T-cell activity and phagocytic activity of macrophages and NK cells (see Fig. 29–3). Alpha-IFN is produced by a number of different cells (e.g., B cells, T cells, NK cells, null cells, and macrophages). Their target cells are the same.

Alpha- and beta-IFNs also have antiproliferative and antitumor effects. Although the exact mechanism remains unclear, the antiproliferative effects of IFNs include inhibition of DNA and protein synthesis in tumor cells, as well as stimulation of human lymphocyte antigen (HLA) and tumor-associated antigen expression on tumor cell surfaces.

After cancer cells have been exposed to IFN, observable changes occur in the appearance and behavior of malignant cells. They look and behave more like normal cells. IFN is also thought to have an inhibiting effect on cell growth by prolonging the phases of the cell cycle (see Chapter 30). The immunomodulating effects are produced by direct interaction of IFNs with T cells, which, in turn, stimulates the cell-mediated immune response.

Gamma-IFN generates toxic oxygen metabolites within phagocytes for enhanced killing of microorganisms such as *Staphylococcus aureus* or *Mycobacterium avium*. This IFN also has other biologic activities such as enhanced activity of macrophages, enhanced antibody-dependent cytotoxicity, and increased activity of NK cells. Gamma-IFN also induces the production of T-suppressor cell factor. There is increasing evidence that gamma-IFN can be characterized as IL-like in activity and interactions.

Adverse Effects and Contraindications

A variety of well-defined adverse effects are associated with IFNs, all of which are dose dependent. The most common is a flulike syndrome with fever, chills, malaise, headache, mild anorexia, myalgias, arthralgias, xerostomia, taste alterations, weight loss, and pervasive fatigue. Neurologic alterations may occur over time, including slowed thinking, poor concentration, and decreased short-term memory and attention span. Myelosuppression, neutropenia, mild anemia, paranoia, and psychoses are also possible.

With high dose IFN, the patient may experience hypotension, tachycardia, somnolence, confusion, and peripheral neuropathies. Rare acute hypersensitivity reactions have been reported with urticaria, angioedema, bronchoconstriction, and anaphylaxis.

Pharmacokinetics

The serum concentration of subcutaneous (SC) and intramuscular (IM) IFNs is generally comparable with a serum half-life of 2 to 8.5 hours and biotransformation 16 hours after injection. When administered intravenously (IV) the concentration peaks at 30 minutes, with a half-life of 2 hours. Undetectable levels of IFN occur 4 hours after administration (Table 29–2).

Drug-Drug Interactions

The interaction of IFNs with other drugs is not fully understood. Caution should be used when IFNs are administered with other myelosuppressive drugs (Table 29–3). The combination may result in profound neutropenia and increased risk of infection. IFN used in combination with theophylline drugs results in reduced drug biotransformation.

Dosage Regimen

Because IFN is a protein, it would be destroyed by digestive enzymes if taken by mouth; therefore, it must be administered either IM or SC (Table 29–4). Each US Food and Drug Administration (FDA) approved IFN has a different dosage regimen. Alfa-2a IFN and alfa-2b IFN are not interchangeable drugs. Alfa-2a IFN is packaged with a diluent that contains sodium chloride, albumin, and phenol. Alfa-2b IFN is diluted with sterile or bacteriostatic water for injection.

Laboratory Considerations

IFNs may increase aspartate aminotransferase (AST [SGPT]), alanine aminotransferase (ALT [SGOT]), alkaline phosphatase, and lactate dehydrogenase (LDH) values. Hemoglobin, hematocrit, white blood cell count, and platelet counts may decrease in the presence of IFNs. Prothrombin times may be falsely elevated in patients taking alfa-3n IFN. Blood urea nitrogen (BUN), creatinine, calcium, and glucose values may be falsely increased in patients taking beta-1a and beta-1b IFNs. No significant alterations are seen as a result of gamma-IFN.

Interleukins

❒ Aldesleukin (Interleukin-2, IL-2, PROLEUKIN)

Interleukins (ILs) are a group of chemical messengers produced in the body. One of the best known is IL-1. It was originally described in the early 1960s. The action of each IL is unique, but many have actions shared by other ILs as well. The production of one IL often produces a cascade of other ILs and cytokines. Fourteen ILs are currently identified. Each is assigned a number according to the order of discovery. The only FDA approved agent is interleukin-2 (IL-2). Other interleukins (e.g., IL-3, IL-4, IL-5, IL-6, IL-8, IL-10, IL-12) are also in clinical trials and may be ready for use in the near future.

Indications

IL-2 is indicated for patients with metastatic renal cell carcinoma. IL-2 also has been used in the treatment of Kaposi's sarcoma along with zidovudine, treatment of metastatic melanoma along with cyclophosphamide, treatment of non-Hodgkin's lymphoma along with lymphokine-activated killer (LAK) cells, and in the treatment of HIV infection. IL-2 is not FDA approved for these uses, however. Aldesleukin has recently been used in the management of multiple sclerosis.

Pharmacodynamics

IL-2 has multiple immunoregulatory functions. It acts as a growth and differentiation factor for cytotoxic T cells, T-helper cells, T-suppressor cells, and NK cells (Fig. 29–3). It induces lymphokine production by T cells and monocytes. There is enhancement of NK cell activity. IL-2 also induces

TABLE 29–2 PHARMACOKINETICS OF SELECTED BIOLOGIC RESPONSE MODIFIERS

Agent	Route	Onset	Peak	Duration	PB (%)	$t_{1/2}$	BioA (%)
Interferons							
Interferon alpha-2a	IM	Rapid	3–4 hr*	Weeks	UA	3.7–8.5 hr	UA
	SQ	Slow	7.3 hr	UA			UA
	IV	Immed	30 min	Minutes		2 hr	100
Interferon alpha-2b	IM/SQ	Varies†	6–8 hr; 3–5 days to 4–8 wk‡	UK	UA	2–7 hr	UA
Interferon alpha-n3	Intralesion	Varies	UA	UA	UA	6–8 hr	UA
Interferon beta-1a	IM	Varies	3–15 hr	4 days	UA	10 hr	UA
Interferon beta-1b	SQ	Rapid	1–8 hr	UK	UK	8 min–4.3 hr	50
Interferon gamma-1b	SQ	Slow	4–7 hr	UK	UK	2.9–5.9 hr	89
Interleukins							
Interleukin-2	IV	5 min	13 min	3–4 hr	UA	30–120 min	100
Colony- and Cell-Stimulating Factors							
Epoetin alfa (EPO)	IV/SQ	7–14 days	5–24 hr§	24 hr	UA	4–13 hr‖	100
Filgrastim (G-CSF)	IV/SQ	UK	2–8 hr	4 days¶	UA	3.5 hr	100
Sargramostim (GM-CSF)	IV	UK	2 hr	6 hr	UA	12–17 min; then 2 hr	100
Monoclonal Antibodies							
Muromonab-CD3	IV	UK	3 days	3–14 days	UA	18 hr	100
Satumoab pendetide	IV	UK	48–96 hr	UK	UK	UK	100
Miscellaneous Biologic Response Modifiers							
Levamisole	po	UK	1.5–2 hr	UK	UA	3–4 hr	UA
Lymphocyte immune globulin	IV	Rapid	UA	UA	UA	3–9 days	100
Mycophenolate	po	Rapid	0.8–1.3 hr	NA	UA	17.9 hr**	UA
Rh_o(D) immune globulin	IM	Rapid	5–10 days	UK	UA	30 days	UA
	IV	††1–2 days	5–7 days	30 days	UA	24 days	100
Cyclosporine	po	UK	3–4 hr	UK	90	19–27 hr	20–50
	IV		End of infusion				100
Tacrolimus	IV	Rapid	UA	UA	UA	10–11 hr	Varies

*Alpha-2a interferon's effects on blood counts. Clinical response may take 1 to 3 months to onset.
†Alpha-2b interferon's onset of clinical response is 1 to 3 months; onset of effects on platelet counts unknown; onset of changes in liver function tests seen in approximately 2 weeks.
‡Alpha-2b interferon's peak effects on platelet counts seen in 3 to 5 days, 4 to 8 weeks for intralesional route.
§Therapeutic serum levels of epoetin alfa are not routinely measured.
‖Epoetin alfa: Clinically significant increases in the reticulocyte count occur in 7 to 10 days, with a rise in hematocrit and hemoglobin usually occurring in 2 to 6 weeks. Peak effects, which is the targeted hematocrit level, may be achieved in 8 weeks with adequate dosing.
¶Filgrastim (G-CSF) return of neutrophil count to baseline.
**The half-life of mycophenolate's metabolite, mycophenolic acid (MPA).
††When Rh_o(D) immune globulin is used for idiopathic thrombocytopenic purpura, platelet counts start to rise in 1 to 2 days, peak after 5 to 7 days, and last for 30 days.
G-CSF, Granulocyte colony-stimulating factor; GM-CSF, granulocyte-macrophage colony-stimulating factor; PB, protein binding; $t_{1/2}$, serum half-life; NA, not applicable; UK, unknown; UA, unavailable; IM, intramuscular; SQ, subcutaneous; IV, intravenous.

LAK cells and induces gamma IFN. IL-2 supports the growth of macrophages, as well as B and T cells. The exact antitumor effects of IL-2 are unknown.

IL-2 is also well known from its first identification as a T-cell growth factor. The growth-enhancing function was crucial in the original studies of some of the retroviruses. Chapter 25 discusses antiretroviral drugs.

Adverse Effects and Contraindications

The adverse effects associated with IL-2 are dose dependent, self-limiting, and usually reversible within 2 to 3 days after therapy is stopped. The adverse effects, however, are quite significant. The most frequent adverse effects include mental status changes, fever, chills, nausea, vomiting, diarrhea, gastrointestinal (GI) bleeding, oliguria and anuria, sinus tachycardia, respiratory failure, ventricular arrhythmias, and myocardial ischemia or infarction.

Occasional adverse effects include headache, dizziness, weight gain, urinary tract infection, and infection at injection sites or at catheter tips. Dry skin, sensory disorders, dermatitis, arthralgia, myalgia, weight loss, conjunctivitis, hematuria, and proteinuria are possible but rare.

Capillary leak syndrome is a common and serious complication of IL-2 administration. Plasma proteins and fluid leak into extravascular spaces resulting in a loss of vascular tone. The loss of vascular tone leads to hypotension and decreased organ perfusion 2 to 12 hours after the start of the IL-2 infusion. Clinical evaluation should eliminate patients with significant cardiac, pulmonary, renal, hepatic, or central nervous system (CNS) impairment. Because IL-2 can in-

TABLE 29–3 DRUG-DRUG INTERACTIONS OF SELECTED BIOLOGIC RESPONSE MODIFIERS

Drug	Interactive Drugs	Interaction
Interferons		
Interferon alfa-2a Interferon alfa-2b Interferon alfa-n3 Interferon gamma-1b	Myelosuppressive drugs Radiation therapy	Profound neutropenia Increased risk of infection
Interferon alfa-2a	Aminophylline	Decreases metabolism and increases blood levels of interactive drug; toxicity
Interferon alfa 2b	Zidovudine	Increased risk of neutropenia
Interferon alfa-n3	Alcohol CNS depressants	Enhanced CNS depressant effects of either drug
Interleukin (IL)		
Interleukin-2	Antianxiety drugs Antiemetics Opioids Sedatives	Additive CNS effects
	Aminoglycosides Antineoplastic drugs Indomethacin	Potential for organ toxicity is increased
	Corticosteroids NSAIDs	Reduces antitumor effectiveness of IL-2
	Antihypertensives Beta blockers	Increased potential for hypotension
Colony-Stimulating Factors		
Epoetin alfa	Anticoagulants	May increase need for anticoagulation during dialysis
Filgrastim	Antineoplastic drugs	Increased risk of neutropenia
Sargramostim	Lithium Corticosteroids	May potentiate myeloproliferative effects of sargramostim
Monoclonal Antibodies		
Muromonab-CD3 Satumoab pendetide	Immunosuppressant drugs	Increased risk of infection, lymphoproliferative disorders
	Live virus vaccines	Increased adverse effects of interactive drug, decreased antibody response
Miscellaneous Biologic Response Modifiers		
Cyclosporine	Amphotericin B Aminoglycosides Erythromycin Fluoroquinolones Ketoconazole NSAIDs Melphalan Sulfonamides	Increased risk of nephrotoxicity
	Anabolic steroids Calcium-channel blockers Cimetidine Danazol Erythromycin	Blood levels and risk of cyclosporine toxicity increase

crease symptoms of CNS disease, the patient must be neurologically stable before the start of therapy.

Continued treatment with IL-2 is contraindicated if the patient experienced serious adverse effects during a prior course of therapy. Effects that contraindicate continued therapy include sustained ventricular tachycardia, uncontrolled cardiac arrhythmias, recurrent angina, intubation exceeding 72 hours, pericardial tamponade, renal dysfunction requiring dialysis longer than 72 hours, coma or psychoses exceeding 48 hours, uncontrolled seizures, bowel ischemia or perforation, and GI bleeding requiring surgery.

Pharmacokinetics

High plasma concentrations of IL-2 are reached after IV infusion with rapid distribution to extravascular and extracellular spaces. IL-2 is quickly biotransformed to amino acids in the cells lining the proximal convoluted tubules. Its metabolites are eliminated in the urine.

Drug-Drug Interactions

IL-2 affects CNS functioning. Therefore, interactions can occur with concomitant use of IL-2 with opioids, antiemet-

TABLE 29–3 DRUG-DRUG INTERACTIONS OF SELECTED BIOLOGIC RESPONSE MODIFIERS *Continued*

Drug	Interactive Drugs	Interaction
Miscellaneous Biologic Response Modifiers *Continued*		
	Fluconazole Ketoconazole Miconazole Oral contraceptives	
	Azathioprine Corticosteroids Cyclophosphamide Verapamil	Additive immunosuppression
	Barbiturates Carbamazepine Phenytoin Rifampin Sulfonamides	Decreased effects of cyclosporine
	ACE inhibitors Potassium-sparing diuretics Potassium supplements	Additive hyperkalemia
	Digoxin	Increased risk of toxicity to interactive drug
	Neuromuscular blockers	Prolonged action of interactive drug
	Imipenen/cilastin	Increased risk of seizures
	Live virus vaccines	Decreased antibody response and increased risk of adverse reactions
	Lovastatin	Increased risk of rhabdomyolysis
Levamisole	Antineoplastic drugs Radiation therapy	Increased bone marrow suppression
	Alcohol	Dilsulfiram-like reaction
	Phenytoin	May increase blood levels and risk of toxicity to interacting drug
	Warfarin	May increase effects of interactive drug
Mycophenolate	Acyclovir Ganciclovir	Compete with metabolite for renal excretion; increased risk of toxicity to mycophenolate
	Aluminum antacids Cholestyramine Colestipol Magnesium antacids	Decrease the absorption of mycophenolic acid (MPA)
Tacrolimus	Aminoglycosides Cisplatin Cyclosporine	Increased risk of toxicity
	Antifungal drugs Calcium-channel blockers Cimetidine Danazol Erythromycin	Increased blood levels of tacrolimus
	Carbamazepine Phenobarbital Phenytoin Rifampin	Decreased blood levels of tacrolimus

CNS, central nervous system; NSAIDs, nonsteroidal anti-inflammatory drugs; ACE, angiotensin-converting enzyme.

ics, sedatives, or antianxiety drugs. Beta blockers and other antihypertensive drugs may cause additive hypotension. Organ toxicity may be enhanced with the use of nephrotoxic drugs such as aminoglycosides or indomethacin, or antineoplastic drugs that are myelotoxic, cardiotoxic, or hepatotoxic. The use of corticosteroids is contraindicated because they can reduce the antitumor effectiveness of IL-2.

Dosage Regimen

The optimum dosage for IL-2 is still under investigation. A course of IL-2 therapy consists of two, 5-day treatment

TABLE 29–4 DOSAGE REGIMEN FOR SELECTED BIOLOGIC RESPONSE MODIFIERS			
Drug	**Use(s)**	**Dosage**	**Implications**
Interferons (IFN)			
Interferon alfa-2a	Hairy cell leukemia	*Adults:* 3 MIU SC/IM QD × 16–24 wk. Maintenance: 3 MIU 3 × weekly. Do not use 36 million unit vial.	Alpha 2a-IFN is not interchangeable with alpha-2b IFN. The diluents are different. Give antipyretic and antihistamine PRN for fever and flulike symptoms. Have patient avoid sources of infection. Adjust dose or hold as ordered for dose-limiting adverse effects. Have patient pace activities in presence of fatigue. Monitor patients with history of cardiopulmonary disease for adverse effects. Assess for and have patient report signs of fluid overload.
	Chronic myelogenous leukemia	*Adults:* 9 MIU SC/IM daily	
	Kaposi's sarcoma	*Adults:* 36 MIU SC/IM 3 times weekly × 10–12 wk. May give 3 MIU on day 1; 9 MIU on day 2; 18 MIU on day 3; then begin 36 MIU/day for remainder of 10–12 wk. Maintenance: 36 MIU/day 3 × weekly.	
Interferon alfa-2b	Hairy cell leukemia	*Adults:* 2 MIU/m^2 SC/IM 3 × weekly	
	Condyloma acuminata	*Adults:* 10 MIU/1 mL per wart 3 times weekly for 3 wk	
	Chronic hepatitis B	*Adults:* 30–35 MIU/wk (5 MIU/day SC/IM -OR-10 MIU 3 times weekly) for 16 weeks	
	Hepatitis C	*Adults:* 3 MIU SC/IM 3 times weekly for up to 6 months (at least 1 year for chronic disease)	
Interferon alfa-n3	Condyloma acuminata	*Adults:* 250,000 IU (0.05 mL) into wart twice weekly for up to 8 weeks. Maximum: 2.5 MIU (0.5 mL) per session	Do not repeat for 3 months after initial 8 weeks of treatment unless warts enlarge or new warts appear
Interferon beta-1a	Relapsing-remitting multiple sclerosis	*Adult:* 30 mcg IM once weekly	
Interferon beta-1b	Relapsing-remitting multiple sclerosis	*Adult:* 8 MIU (0.25 mg) SC every other day	
Interferon gamma-1b	Chronic granulomatous disease	*Adults and Child with BSA over 0.5 m^2:* 50 mcg/m^2 (1.5 MIU/m^2) SC three times weekly *Adults and Child with BSA under 0.5 m^2:* 1.5 mcg/kg/dose SC three times weekly	Do not shake vial before administration
Colony-Stimulating Factors			
Epoetin alfa	Anemia in dialysis-dependent ESRD	*Adults:* 50–100 units/kg SC/IV three times weekly.	Adjust dose by 25 units/kg/dose to maintain hematocrit at desired level.
	Antineoplastic-induced anemia	*Adults:* 150 units/kg SC 3 times weekly. May increase after 2 months up to 300 units/kg three times weekly.	
	Anemia in ZVD-treated patients with HIV	*Adults:* 100 units/kg SC/IV three times weekly for 2 months. May increase by 50–100 units/kg q1–2mo up to 300 units/kg three times weekly.	Therapeutic response in reticulocyte count should appear in 1–2 weeks.
Filgrastim	Antineoplastic-associated neutropenia in patients with nonmyeloid malignancy. Prolonged myelosuppression after bone marrow transplantation	*Adults:* 5 mcg/kg/day SC in a single dose. May increase by 5 mcg/kg in each treatment cycle. Give daily for up to 2 weeks until the absolute neutrophil count (ANC) is 10,000/m^3.	Response to G-CSF is much greater with SC than IV therapy

TABLE 29–4 DOSAGE REGIMEN FOR SELECTED BIOLOGIC RESPONSE MODIFIERS *Continued*

Drug	Use(s)	Dosage	Implications
Sargramostim	Autologous bone marrow transplant; acceleration of myeloid recovery in patients with non-Hodgkin's lymphoma, acute lymphoblastic leukemia, bone marrow transplantation failure or engraftment delay	*Adult:* 250 mcg/m²/day IV over 2 hours. When used for myeloid recovery purposes, may be repeated in 7 days with dosage increased to 500 mcg/m²/day × 14 days. Length of treatment may vary depending on specific diagnosis and patient response.	Start infusion 2–4 hours after autologous bone marrow infusion, not less than 24 hours after last dose of antineoplastics and 12 hours after last dose of radiotherapy, bone marow transplant failure, or engraftment delay.
Interleukin			
Aldesleukin	Metastatic renal cell cancer	*Adults:* 600,000 IU/kg IV q8h × 14 doses. Therapy consists of two 5-day treatment cycles for a total of 28 doses.	A 9-day rest period should separate treatment cycles. Bring to room temperature before administration.
Monoclonal Antibodies			
Muromonab-CD3	Acute allograft rejection in renal, cardiac/hepatic transplantations	*Adults:* 5 mg/day IV over 1 minute or less for 10–14 days *Child under 12 yr:* 0.1 mg/kg/day rapid IV push for 10–14 days	Has no advantage over other antirejection drugs for prevention of rejection.
Satumoab pendetide	Detection of extrahepatic lesions; staging of ovarian and colorectal cancer	*Adult:* 1 mg IV over 5 minutes	Optimal time for imaging is 48–96 hr after administration.
Miscellaneous Biologic Response Modifiers			
Levamisole	Adjunct for colorectal cancer; advanced malignant melanoma (unlabeled use)	*Adults:* 50 mg po q8h for 3 days every 2 weeks with fluorouracil 450 mg/m²/day for 5 days initially, then followed 28 days later by fluorouracil 450 mg/m² once weekly. Repeat course of therapy every 14 days for 1 year.	Initiate therapy no earlier than 7 days and no later than 30 days after surgery. Fluorouracil therapy should be started no earlier than 21 days and no later than 35 days after surgery. Check monographs for specific information regarding regimen.
Lymphocyte immune globulin	Acute graft rejection; aplastic anemia	*Adults:* 10–30 mg/kg/day IV	Drug mixed with saline and infused through a central line over a period of 4 hours or more
Mycophenolate	Allogenic renal transplantation	*Adult:* 1g po BID	Therapy to be started within 72 hours of transplantation
Rh_o(D) immune globulin	Prevent isoimmunization in Rh negative women exposed to Rh positive blood in the process of labor and delivery, abortions, miscarriages, or amniocentesis	*Adults following delivery:* 300 mcg IM within 72 hr of delivery. *Adult before delivery:* 300 mcg IM at 28th week gestation *Termination of pregnancy (less than 13 weeks gestation):* 50 mcg IM within 72 hr *Termination of pregnancy (over 13 weeks gestation):* 300 mcg IM within 72 hr	Check formulation carefully. Rh_o(D) immune globulin is for IM use only. Rh_o(D) immune globulin IV is for IM *or* IV use.
	Management of idiopathic thrombocytopenic purpura (ITP)	*ITP:* 50 mcg/kg IV initially. If hemoglobin less than 10 g/dL reduce dose to 25–40 mcg/kg	Further dosing and frequency determined by clinical response. Each dose may be given as a single dose or in two divided doses on separate days.
Cyclosporine	Prevent rejection of solid organ transplantations	*Adult and Child:* 12–15 mg/kg/day po for 1–2 weeks. Taper dose by 5% weekly to maintenance dose of 5–10 mg/kg/day. -OR- 2–6 mg/kg/day (1/3 the oral dose) IV initially.	First dose should be given before the transplantation. Change from IV to po formulation as soon as possible. Children may require larger or more frequent dosing because of faster rate of clearance.
Tacrolimus	Prevent rejection of organ transplantations	*Adult and Child:* 0.15 mg/kg/day IV × 3 days then 0.15 mg/kg BID	Give with food to reduce GI upset.

MIU, Million International Units; BSA, body surface area; ESRD, end-stage renal disease; ZVD, zidovudine SC, subcutaneous; IV, intravenous; G-CSF, granulocyte colony-stimulating factor; GI, gastrointestinal.

cycles separated by a 9-day rest period. IL-2 is administered over 15 minutes as an IV infusion. The recommended dose is 600,000 IU/kg every 8 hours for 14 doses. There is a minimum rest period between courses of 7 weeks from hospital discharge. If there is a response, the patient continues with the next course. Evaluation for response is determined 4 weeks after treatment, and then immediately before the next course. The short half-life of IL-2 (30 to 120 minutes) necessitates frequent, short-dosing schedules.

Laboratory Considerations

IL-2 may increase bilirubin, BUN, serum creatinine, transaminase, and alkaline phosphatase results. Laboratory values of magnesium, calcium, phosphorus, potassium, and sodium may decrease.

Colony-Stimulating Factors

- ❐ Epoetin alfa (EPO, EPOGEN)
- ❐ Filgrastim (G-CSF, NEUPOGEN)
- ❐ Sargramostim (GM-CSF, colony-stimulating factor alpha), pluripoietin, LEUKINE, PROKINE)

Colony-stimulating factors (CSFs) are hormone-like proteins that stimulate the growth of hematopoietic cells. They are a group of polypeptide hormones produced in the body that direct cells to proliferate and differentiate in the bone marrow. A steady supply of cells for the peripheral blood circulation is thus maintained.

CSFs exert their effects on cells of the hematopoietic cascade, and each is named for the mature cell produced. Some CSFs have multilineage effects; that is, they are influenced by several cell lines. Others are lineage restricted, stimulating cell division and maturation in only one cell line.

Four of the CSFs that are active on myeloid cells have been cloned and the recombinant product introduced into pharmacotherapy. The recombinant products include granulocyte colony-stimulating factor (G-CSF), granulocyte-macrophage colony-stimulating factor (GM-CSF), macrophage colony-stimulating factor (M-CSF), and interleukin-3 (IL-3). The largest clinical experience has been with G-CSF and GM-CSF. Epoetin alpha was the first CSF to be developed.

Indications

To date, CSFs have been used for iatrogenically induced bone marrow dysfunction, antiviral therapy for AIDS, myelosuppression related to antineoplastic therapy, and bone marrow transplantation. They also have been used in the management of intrinsic bone marrow dysfunction states such as myelodysplasia, congenital cyclic neutropenia, aplastic anemia, and other states of bone marrow infiltration such as hairy cell leukemia.

G-CSF is indicated for patients undergoing myelosuppressive antineoplastic therapy including those with delayed engraftment of the marrow cells after bone marrow transplantation. GM-CSF is indicated for specific patients undergoing autologous bone marrow transplantation, that is, patients with non-Hodgkin's lymphoma, Hodgkin's disease, and acute lymphocytic leukemia.

Epoetin alfa, the first CSF approved by the FDA, was first approved for patients with end-stage renal disease who are on dialysis (see Chapter 41) and are transfusion dependent, and for patients with HIV infection who are receiving myelosuppressive therapy. It was later used for patients with chronic anemia resulting from cancer or cancer therapy. Epoetin alfa decreases the need for transfusion support.

Pharmacodynamics

CSFs increase the production of granulocytes and monocytes by stimulating stem and precursor cell replication and maturation. The precise location where the drugs exert their action is unclear.

G-CSF is lineage specific, responsible for the proliferation, maturation, and differentiation of the neutrophil; but it is also known to have effects on early stem cells (Fig. 29–3). In contrast, GM-CSF has broader activity because of its multilineage effects. It stimulates monocytes, eosinophils, neutrophils, and megakaryocyte growth in vitro. IL-3 appears to act earlier than GM-CSF in stem cell development. It stimulates platelet and basophil production in vivo. M-CSF affects only mononuclear phagocyte development activity by interacting with specific cell surface receptors.

Endogenous epoetin alfa is secreted by the kidney in response to decreased circulation or anemia. Epoetin carries the message to the bone marrow to produce more red blood cells (RBCs). It has the same biologic effects as the endogenous form. It stimulates the division and maturation of committed progenitors (immature erythroid cells) in the bone marrow to produce a greater number and faster maturation of RBCs.

Adverse Effects and Contraindications

G-CSF is generally well tolerated, with bone pain being the most common adverse effect. The bone pain appears to be related to extensive bone marrow regeneration but is transient, usually of short duration, and is easily managed with acetaminophen. Bone pain occurs most often in patients receiving high doses via IV routes. It is seen less frequently with low dose, subcutaneous routes. Alopecia, nausea, vomiting, diarrhea, fever, and fatigue are also common. An exacerbation of pre-existing inflammatory conditions and possibly an increase in spleen size has been noted. Occasionally, anorexia, dyspnea, headache, cough, and skin rash have occurred.

The development of psoriasis, hematuria/proteinuria, thrombocytopenia, arrhythmias, myocardial infarction, and osteoporosis is rare with G-CSF but is possible. Chronic administration of G-CSF occasionally produces chronic neutropenia and splenomegaly. Adult respiratory distress syndrome can occur in septic patients.

GM-CSF may cause a few more adverse effects than G-CSF, including bone pain, rash, pruritus, myalgia, fatigue, anorexia, diarrhea, malaise, phlebitis, and thrombosis. Peripheral edema, weight gain, shortness of breath, fever, and leukocytosis occasionally occur. At doses higher than 16 mcg/kg/day, capillary leak syndrome with pericardial and pleural effusions and edema have been seen. Eosinophilia has developed and may represent a toxicity; therefore, laboratory monitoring should include baseline, then twice weekly complete blood count (CBC), platelets, differential, and reticulocyte count.

Adverse effects of epoetin alfa include hypertension, headache, tachycardia, nausea, vomiting, edema, diarrhea, shortness of breath, hyperkalemia, skin reaction at the injection site, and clotted IV access devices. Rare adverse effects are seizures, cerebrovascular accident, transient ischemic attacks, and myocardial infarction.

Hypertension must be controlled before epoetin alfa therapy, because blood pressure can increase early in treatment from the increasing hematocrit. If a rapid response occurs, such as an increase of four percentage points in the hematocrit in 2 weeks, the dose is reduced to prevent hypertension. Known hypersensitivity to albumin or mammalian cell-derived products is a contraindication to epoetin alfa therapy.

Pharmacokinetics

Knowledge of the pharmacokinetics of CSFs is limited. G-CSF is well absorbed after SC administration. Its distribution, biotransformation, and elimination are unknown. GM-CSF peaks in 2 hours when given IV with a duration of action of 6 hours. Its biotransformation site is unknown.

In patients with chronic renal failure, IV administration of epoetin alfa has a half-life of 4 to 13 hours. Detectable levels remain for 24 hours if therapeutic dosages are given. The drug peaks 5 to 24 hours after SC administration. In healthy individuals, plasma epoetin alfa levels are 0.01 to 0.13 U/mL, with a 100- to 1000-fold increase during periods of hypoxia or anemia.

Drug-Drug Interactions

Simultaneous use of G-CSF with antineoplastic drugs may produce adverse effects on rapidly proliferating neutrophils. Use should be avoided 24 hours before and 24 hours after antineoplastic therapy. There is known drug-drug interaction of epoetin alfa with any other drug. Lithium and corticosteroids may increase the effects of GM-CSF.

Dosage Regimen

The treatment regimen for G-CSF is started at least 24 hours after the last dose of antineoplastic therapy and discontinued at least 24 hours before the next scheduled dose of antineoplastic drug. When used for myelosuppression, the initial dose is 5 mcg/kg/day. The dosage may be increased by 5 mcg/kg for each antineoplastic treatment cycle until the absolute neutrophil count exceeds 10,000 cells/mm^3.

When G-CSF is used for bone marrow transplantation, 10 mcg/kg/day is used. The dose is adjusted daily during the period of neutrophil recovery and is regulated based on neutrophil response.

GM-CSF is given for 21 days, or until the bone marrow has recovered. Recovery is defined as an absolute neutrophil count over 20,000 cells/mm^3 or a platelet count that exceeds 500,000 cell/mm^3. The usual adult dose is 250 mcg/m^2/day as a 2-hour infusion. It should be started 2 to 4 hours after autologous bone marrow infusion and not less than 24 hours after the last dose of antineoplastic therapy, or not less than 12 hours after the last radiation therapy treatment. GM-CSF therapy should be discontinued if blast cells appear or the underlying disease progresses.

Epoetin alfa can be administered IV or SC three times a week. The dosage varies with the indication. Laboratory values are assessed twice a week until stable. When the hematocrit reaches 30 to 33 percent, the dose is decreased by 25 percent to avoid exceeding the target level of 36 percent. If the hematocrit rises too quickly, the dose is held until the hematocrit begins to decrease. The epoetin alfa is then restarted with a 25 percent reduction in dosage. Laboratory values are assessed twice a week for another 4 to 6 weeks after changes in dosage.

If a five to six point increase in hematocrit is not achieved after 8 weeks of epoetin alfa therapy, the dose is increased by 25 U/kg three times a week, every 4 to 6 weeks until a response is seen. A delayed or inadequate response may be due to iron deficiency, underlying processes (e.g., infection, inflammation, malignancy), occult blood loss, underlying hematologic disease, hemolysis, or vitamin deficiency (e.g., folic acid or vitamin B_{12}).

Laboratory Considerations

Laboratory values for alkaline phosphatase, LDH, uric acid, and leukocytes may be elevated in the presence of G-CSF. Albumin levels may decrease in the presence of GM-CSF, with elevations noted in bilirubin, creatinine, and liver enzymes. Epoetin alfa may cause a decrease in bleeding time, iron concentration, and serum ferritin values. It may increase BUN, creatinine, phosphorus, potassium, sodium, and uric acid values.

Monoclonal Antibodies

- ❐ Muromonab-CD3 (ORTHOCLONE OKT3)
- ❐ Satumomab pendetide (CYT-103, ONCOSCINT)

The basis for cancer therapy using an antigen-antibody response is the knowledge that all cells, including tumor cells, have antigens unique to that cell. This uniqueness is referred to as *specificity.* Antibody therapy utilizes this characteristic to target certain cells for destruction. The "bullets" are monoclonal antibodies (MoAbs) programmed to destroy the target cells.

There are two classifications of MoAbs: unconjugated and conjugated. Unconjugated MoAbs are used alone, whereas conjugated MoAbs are combined with another drug such as antineoplastics, toxins, or radioisotopes. The immunoconjugates use the MoAb bullet to deliver the toxic drug directly to the tumor cell.

Unconjugated MoAbs are usually formed from mouse (i.e., murine) antibodies and have been used investigationally to directly treat certain cancers. The results have been inconsistent for a variety of reasons, and there are significant adverse effects (most notably anaphylaxis). Further, antibodies develop quickly to the MoAbs. Thus, results with MoAbs have been somewhat disappointing and remain investigational.

Indications

MoAbs are high-molecular-weight proteins produced by a clone of cells and are meant to attack one specific antigen. They are used in diagnosing or screening cancers, monitoring disease progression, and as therapeutic agents in the management of cancer.

Satumomab pendetide is useful for detection of extrahepatic tumor lesions and staging of patients with known colorectal and ovarian carcinoma. This drug combines a murine MoAb with the radioisotope indium (^{111}In).

There are specific indications for use of this drug in patients with colorectal carcinoma. In conjunction with other tests, radioisotope imaging permits complete staging of the cancer before surgery. There is an ability to evaluate the extent of extrahepatic disease in patients being considered for curative resection of primary, recurrent, and metastatic disease, and to identify patients who may not be surgical candidates. Imaging using ^{111}In also may be useful in following patients at risk for recurrent disease. The applications in ovarian cancer are similar. Muromonab-CD3 is indicated for acute allograft rejection in patients undergoing renal and cardiac/hepatic transplantation.

Pharmacodynamics

There is evidence that MoAbs may interfere with cellular proliferation by one or two mechanisms. MoAbs may block graft rejection by binding to CD3 receptors on mature circulating T cells and medullary thymocytes (see Fig. 29–3). This action blocks the ability of cells to recognize foreign antigens, thereby inhibiting the generation and function of cytotoxic T cells responsible for graft rejection. Further, they may incite an inflammatory response through recognition of a specific portion of antibody.

Adverse Effects and Contraindications

Multiple possible adverse effects are associated with MoAbs, although most occur in less than 1 percent of patients. Flulike symptoms are common and include fever, chills, headache, nausea, vomiting, diarrhea, and general malaise. The adverse effects often decrease with subsequent injections. Less frequent adverse effects include reversible thrombocytopenia, marked hypotension, chest pain, pulmonary edema in fluid-overloaded patients, aseptic meningitis, and an acute decline in the glomerular filtration rate.

Patients can develop human antimurine antibody (HAMA) after injection with any murine MoAb. If repeated injection with the MoAb is necessary, the HAMA can result in allergic or anaphylactic reactions. Because satumomab pendetide is administered one time only, the implications of HAMA use are unclear. There are no data regarding the repeated use of this drug.

Satumomab pendetide should not be used in patients with previous hypersensitivity to the radioisotope or other products of murine origin. Appropriate shielding of the radioactive solution is necessary to minimize exposure by personnel. The use of this MoAb to evaluate patients with suspected ovarian or colon cancer is not recommended, nor is it intended to be a screening test.

There are no data regarding administration of ^{111}In during pregnancy. In general, it is recommended that radioisotope exams be administered to women of child-bearing age during the first few days post menses. There are no data regarding use of ^{111}In in children.

Pharmacokinetics

MoAbs are well absorbed after IV administration. The distribution of muromonab-CD3 is approximately with distribution similar to that of albumin. Trough levels of muromonab-CD3 after 5 mg/day rise over the first 3 days and then average 900 mcg/mL on days 3 to 14. Therapeutic levels exceeding 800 mcg/mL block the function of cytotoxic T cells.

The optimal time for satumoab pendetide disease-staging imaging is 48 to 96 hours, although adequate images can be obtained as early as 24 hours and late as 96 hours after administration. Elimination of the MoAb is through the kidneys and is relatively slow at 5 mL/hour. However, there is minimal radioactivity detected in the urine 72 hours after injection. The minimal level suggests significant detachment of the isotope from the MoAb before elimination.

There is minimal reactivity of the MoAb portion of satumoab pendetide in normal adult tissue. ^{111}In localizes to malignant colorectal and ovarian tissues, with 97 percent reactivity to common epithelial ovarian tumors and 83 percent reactivity with colorectal adenocarcinomas.

Drug-Drug Interactions

Drug-drug interactions with MoAbs include increased risks of infection and lymphoproliferative disorders in the presence of immunosuppressant drugs. Vaccines formulated with live virus may increase the adverse effects and produce decreased antibody response to the vaccine.

Dosage Regimen

Muromoab-CD3 is administered as an IV bolus in a dose of 5 mg/day for 10 to 14 days. The patient should be weighed before administration to be sure the weight is within 3 percent of baseline to avoid fluid overload and pulmonary edema.

Satumoab pendetide is available as an already "linked" preparation. It also can be prepared at the time of administration by adding ^{111}In chloride. The recommended dosage is 1 mg administered IV over 5 minutes. The injection is followed by appropriate imaging techniques.

Laboratory Considerations

The administration of ^{111}In may interfere with other murine antibody-based immunoassays. For example, the assays for carcinoembryonic antigen (CEA) or CA-125, which are used to identify the presence of colon and ovarian carcinomas, respectively, may be elevated.

Miscellaneous Biologic Response Modifiers

- ❒ Tumor necrosis factor
- ❒ Levamisole (ERGAMISOLE)
- ❒ Lymphocyte immune globulin (ATGAM)
- ❒ Mycophenolate (CELL CEPT)
- ❒ Rh_o (D) Immune Globulin (RHIG, RHOGAM, GAMULIN RH, HYPRHO-D, WENRHO SD, RHECONATE)
- ❒ Cyclosporine A (cyclosporine, cyclosporine A, SANDIMMUNE, NEORAL)
- ❒ FK 506
- ❒ Cyclophosphamide (CYTOXAN, NEOSAR)
- ❒ Azathioprine (IMURAN)
- ❒ Tacrolimus (PROGRAF)

TUMOR NECROSIS FACTOR

TNF is an investigational drug being studied for the management of metastatic adenocarcinoma of the colon and rectum, liver, and urinary bladder. It is also being used experimentally for non–small cell lung cancer, renal cell cancer and malignant melanoma. Clinical trials are still underway to determine tumor response, extent of immunomodulation, therapeutic dosage, route of administration, and expected adverse effects of TNF. Studies continue as to the effectiveness of TNF in regional therapy such as isolated limb perfusion for melanoma and IV administration for a variety of tumors. In combination with antineoplastic drugs, the TNF is believed to produce the highest possible cell kill of malignant cells.

TNF is a naturally occurring tumoricidal protein produced by monocytes. It is thought to exert a direct effect on tumor cells by binding with receptors on the cell surface. Although the exact mechanism is unclear, it is thought that TNF may cause capillary endothelial damage supplying the tumor and cause hemorrhage. Drug action occurs at the G_2 phase of the cell cycle (see Chapter 30), producing immediate cell death and cytostasis (arrest of growth). Some tumor cells are resistant to the effects of TNF.

Another possible mechanism is that the TNF may augment and increase NK cell cytolytic activity, and increase the number of B cells and polymorphonucleocytes. Perhaps TNF incites an inflammatory response by stimulating macrophage cytotoxicity or by inducing the release of IL-1 by monocytes.

The toxicities of TNF are similar to those of IFN. An acute flulike syndrome is most common. Hypotension is possible. Chronic effects include fatigue and malaise. The adverse effects are dose dependent and resolve quickly after discontinuation of the TNF. There may be local skin reactions if the TNF is administered IM or SC. Further, TNF enhances coagulation and depressed anticoagulation.

The serum half-life of IV TNF is approximately 7 hours. The half-life is affected by the route of administration and dosage. TNF can be administered IV, IM, or SC.

Different routes of administration are being studied, including intraperitoneal and arterial. No specific dosage has been identified at this time. TNF causes an elevation in liver function tests and a transient increase in blood counts. Coagulation studies may be elevated.

LEVAMISOLE

Levamisole is an antineoplastic, immunomodulating drug. It is used as adjunct therapy after surgery for colorectal cancer (along with fluorouracil). It has been used for advanced malignant melanoma, although it is not FDA approved for this use. Levamisole returns leukocyte function to normal levels after antineoplastic therapy or surgery, including the formation of antibodies, T-cell response, phagocytosis, and chemotaxis.

The most common adverse effects of levamisole include fatigue, stomatitis, nausea, vomiting, diarrhea, dermatitis and alopecia, anemia, leukopenia, and thrombocytopenia. CNS impairment is rare but includes ataxia, blurred vision, confusion, mental status changes, paresthesias, seizures, tardive dyskinesia, and tremors. Agranulocytosis is the most life-threatening adverse effect. Levamisole should be used with caution in patients with bone marrow depression, other chronic debilitating diseases, and in patients of childbearing age. Safe use during lactation and in children has not been established.

Levamisole is rapidly absorbed after oral administration, although its distribution is unknown. It is extensively biotransformed in the liver and has a half-life of 3 to 4 hours.

LYMPHOCYTE IMMUNE GLOBULIN

Lymphocyte immune globulin is a lymphocyte-selective, polyclonal antibody, immunosuppressive drug. It is utilized primarily to treat allograft rejection related to renal transplantation, but also for the management of aplastic anemia.

Polyclonal antibodies are formulated using human lymphocyte suspensions to immunize animals. The formulation is referred to as antithymocyte serum (ATS) when derived from the thymus gland. Antilymphocyte serum (ALS) or antilymphocyte globulin (ALG) is derived from thoracic duct lymphocytes, splenic cells, or peripheral blood lymphocytes. Lymphocyte immune globulin is formulated by immunizing horses with human T cells. By modifying T-cell activity, the cell-mediated immune response is impaired.

Lymphocyte immune globulin's adverse effects include fever, chills, itching, erythema, and hemolysis in about 5 percent of patients. Anaphylaxis is possible. Because patients who receive this drug are also being treated with other immunosuppressive agents, allergic reactions to the equine protein are not as frequent or as severe as would otherwise be expected. To minimize the risk of anaphylaxis, the patient is skin-tested before the first dose. Intradermal skin testing is done using 0.1 mL of a 1:1000 dilution in normal saline, and the patient is monitored for 30 minutes to 1 hour. A positive skin test is distinguished by the presence of erythema or an area of induration that exceeds 10 mm in diameter at the site of administration.

The usual adult dose when used for transplantation rejection is 10 to 15 mg/kg/day for up to 14 days after transplantation. If used in the management of aplastic anemia, the drug is administered at a dose of 10 to 20 mg/kg/day for 8 to 14 days. The drug should be kept at room temperature before administration and infused through a central line, vascular shunt, or arterial venous fistula, using an in-line filter. Drug-induced phlebitis can occur if the drug is infused through peripheral veins. Lymphocyte immune globulin should be given over 4 to 12 hours, with the patient continually monitored for adverse effects.

MYCOPHENOLATE

Mycophenolate is an immunosuppressant used in the prevention of rejection in patients who have undergone allogenic renal transplantation. It is used in conjunction with cyclosporine and glucocorticoids. Mycophenolate inhibits inosine monophosphate dehydrogenase, an enzyme required for synthesis of guanine nucleotides, which are necessary for DNA synthesis. This results in suppression of both T- and B-cell proliferation and impairment of immune responses that may promote rejection of transplanted organs.

The most common adverse effects include diarrhea, vomiting, leukopenia, and sepsis. GI bleeding is the most life-threatening adverse effect. There is an increased risk of malignancy. Mycophenolate should be used with caution in patients with active serious pathology of the GI tract, severe chronic renal impairment, delayed graft function following transplantation, and in patients of child-bearing age. Safe use in children has not been established.

Mycophenolate is rapidly hydrolyzed to mycophenolic acid (MPA), its active metabolite, after oral administration. Its distribution is unknown. The time of onset is rapid, with peak blood levels of the metabolite reached in 0.8 to 1.3 hours. Its duration of action is unknown. MPA is extensively biotransformed, with less than 1 percent eliminated unchanged in the urine. Some enterohepatic recirculation of MPA occurs. When mycophenolate is administered with food, peak blood levels of MPA are significantly decreased.

The usual adult dose of mycophenolate is 1 g taken two times a day. Therapy should be started within 72 hours after transplantation.

Mycophenolate may cause increased serum alkaline phosphatase and other liver function tests. It also may cause hypercalcemia or hypocalcemia, hyperuricemia, hyperlipidemia, hypoglycemia, and hypoproteinemia. The patient's hepatic, hematopoietic, and renal status should be monitored periodically during therapy. Neutropenia occurs most frequently 31 to 180 days after transplantation. If the actual neutrophil count is less than 1000/mm^3, the dosage should be reduced or the drug discontinued.

RH$_O$(D) IMMUNE GLOBULIN

Rh$_o$(D) immune globulin is a human antibody directed at the D antigen of the Rh system. It is used to prevent isoimmunization (sensitization) in Rh-negative women who are exposed to Rh-positive blood in the process of labor and delivery, abortion, ectopic pregnancy, version, trauma, fetomaternal hemorrhage, chorionic villi sampling, or amniocentesis. It should be noted, however, that many other blood antigens trigger the development of antibodies. For example, idiopathic thrombocytopenic purpura (ITP) is a disorder that results in a reduced number of platelets. The cause is unknown. RhIG has been used for the management of this disorder because it helps to increase platelet counts and decrease the episodes of bleeding.

When the mother is Rh-negative with an Rh-positive fetus, the mother's immune system responds by producing anti-Rh$_o$(D) antibodies. During subsequent pregnancies these antibodies cross placental membranes to enter fetal circulation. The anti-Rh$_o$(D) antibodies attack the RBCs of the Rh-positive fetus to cause hemolysis. RhIG grants passive immunity by coating fetal Rh-positive cells as they enter maternal circulation. The coating prevents the maternal immune system from identifying the cells as foreign, thereby preventing antibody formation. Administration of RhIG has decreased the incidence of hemolytic disease of the newborn (i.e., erythroblastosis fetalis) by 70 percent.

The most common adverse effects of RhIG are irritation at the injection site, fever, lethargy, and myalgia. Anemia is possible when the drug is used in the management of ITP. The drug is contraindicated in patients with previous immunization with this drug and in Rh$_o$(O)-positive/D^u-positive patients. It should be used with caution in patients with previous hypersensitivity reactions to immune globulins or thimerosal and in patients with ITP who have a pre-existing anemia.

Little is understood about the pharmacokinetics of RhIG. The drug is well absorbed from IM administration sites, but its distribution, biotransformation, and elimination are unknown. The half-life of RhIG is approximately 30 days when given IM and 24 days when given IV.

RhIG is available in an IM and an IM/IV formulation. The dosage is different for the two formulations; labels should be checked carefully. Table 29–4 provides information about the recommended dosages. Keep in mind that the drug is given to the mother and not the infant. The drug is administered IM into the deltoid muscle within 72 hours of delivery. When the IV formulation is used, the administration rate is 3 to 5 minutes.

The blood type of the mother and newborn should be determined to identify the need for the drug. The mother must be Rh$_o$(D) negative and D^u negative. The infant must be Rh$_o$(D) positive. If there is any doubt regarding the infant's blood type or if the father is Rh$_o$(D)-positive, the drug should be administered. An infant born to a woman previously treated with RhIG during the antepartum period may have a weakly positive direct Coombs' test on cord or infant blood.

The Kleihauer-Betke test, which quantifies the amount of fetal blood entering maternal circulation, is used as the basis for RhIG dosage. One unit of RhIG (i.e., 300 mcg) neutralizes 30 mL of fetal whole blood or 15 mL of fetal RBCs. For most vaginal deliveries, this is more than enough RhIG. However, if the quantity of fetal blood entering maternal circulation exceeds this amount, a larger dose of RhIG may be necessary to prevent an antibody response. Situations that may require a larger dose include cesarean birth, manual removal of the placenta, breech birth, stillbirth, placenta previa, or abruptio placenta.

The patient receiving RhIG for ITP should have platelet counts, RBC counts, hemoglobin levels, and reticulocyte levels monitored to determine the effectiveness of therapy.

CYCLOSPORINE

Cyclosporine is a fungus-derived peptide. It is used most often to prevent the rejection of solid organ transplantations. It is a potent immunosuppressor of T-helper cells and acts by blocking the synthesis and secretion of IL-2 (IL-2 is required for the proliferation and growth of antigen-stimulated cells). It impairs cell-mediated responses without destroying the effector lymphocyte. It has minimal to no effect on T-suppressor cells, B cells, granulocytes, or macrophages. Further, it does not prevent immune cells already present and activated by an antigen from maturing and differentiating. Therefore, the drug is of little use in the management of chronic transplantation rejection.

The most common adverse effects of cyclosporine include oral candidiasis, hyperplasia of the gums, headache, hirsutism, tremors, and headache. Hirsutism and gingival hyperplasia are seen in 10 to 30 percent of patients who receive cyclosporine, but these reactions rarely affect therapy. Life-threatening adverse effects include hepatotoxicity, albuminuria, hematuria, proteinuria, and renal failure. Treatment with cyclosporine is associated with an increased incidence of infections, but this problem is generally less prominent than with other immunosuppressive drugs. There is a relatively low incidence of malignancies in patients treated with cyclosporine alone. However, when cyclosporine is used in combination with other agents, the drug causes malignant lymphomas with an unusually high incidence of brain metastases.

The use of cyclosporine is contraindicated in hypersensitivity and in patients on disulfiram therapy or who have a known alcohol intolerance (IV and oral liquid dosage formulations contain alcohol). Cautious use is warranted in patients with severe liver or kidney disease, active infection, and in children.

Cyclosporine is erratically absorbed after oral administration, with a significant first pass effect by the liver. The oral bioavailability of cyclosporine varies from 20 to 50 percent. The microemulsion products (NEORAL) have greater bioavailability. Cyclosporine is widely distributed, primarily into extracellular fluid and blood cells. It crosses placental membranes and enters breast milk. It reaches peak concentrations in plasma within 3 to 4 hours. About 60 to 70 percent of the drug in whole blood is contained in RBCs. Despite their small contribution to blood volume, leukocytes contain 10 to 20 percent of circulating cyclosporine. It is extensively biotransformed in the liver and eliminated in the bile. Small amounts are eliminated unchanged in the urine. The half-life of cyclosporine is 19 to 27 hours. There are many drug-drug interactions of cyclosporine (see Table 29–3).

Many cyclosporine regimens are used. The microemulsion formulation (NEORAL) and other formulations (SANDIMMUNE) are not interchangeable. Table 29–4 identifies the most common dosages.

About 50 percent of patients taking cyclosporine will have elevated hepatic transaminase activities or concentrations of bilirubin in the plasma. These abnormalities generally disappear if dosage is reduced or the drug is discontinued. Cyclosporine may cause increased serum potassium, uric acid, and serum lipid levels. Serum cyclosporine levels should be monitored periodically during therapy and the dosage adjusted daily. The guidelines for desired serum levels vary among institutions.

FK-506

FK-506 is a newly described macrolide antibiotic whose functions are similar to cyclosporine; however, it is 50 to 100 times more potent than cyclosporine. It has been used as a primary immunosuppressant after liver transplantation. It also has been used to suppress T-cell activity after kidney, heart, heart-lung, pancreas, lung, small intestine, and islet-cell transplantations. FK-506 inhibits cell-mediated immune response by blocking the production of IL-2 and other lymphokines. It has a powerful hepatotrophic effect; that is, it fosters regeneration and repair of the liver. It is more potent than cyclosporine, and its adverse effects appear to be fewer than those of cyclosporine. FK-506 has caused serious vasculitis and renal damage in some animal species.

CYCLOPHOSPHAMIDE

Cyclophosphamide is an alkylating drug with extremely potent humoral immunosuppressive properties. It is used to treat a variety of disorders including Hodgkin's disease, malignant melanoma, leukemia, mycosis fungoides, neuroblastoma, ovarian and breast cancers, glomerulonephritis, autoimmune blood dyscrasias, and systemic lupus erythematosus. Additional information about cyclophosphamide can be found in Chapters 15 and 30, where its use as a disease-modifying antirheumatic drug and antineoplastic, respectively, is discussed.

AZATHIOPRINE

Azathioprine (combined with prednisone) has been the mainstay of attempts to suppress rejection of transplanted organs for the last 20 years. It has made renal transplantation possible. Azathioprine is a prodrug that is cleaved to mercaptopurine. This purine analog is subsequently converted to mercaptopurine-containing nucleotides that exert action on the synthesis and utilization of RNA and DNA precursors.

Hematologic toxicity appears as thrombocytopenia and leukopenia. Nausea and vomiting are common but ordinarily do not restrict therapy. Although hepatic toxicity is rare, a severe hepatic veno-occlusive disease has been seen in some patients with transplants.

Prophylactic antirejection therapy using azathioprine is usually initiated 1 to 2 days before transplantation. The total daily dosage is 3 to 10 mg/kg, with a maintenance dose of 1 to 3 mg/kg. Azathioprine is discussed in Chapter 15.

TACROLIMUS

Tacrolimus is a macrolide immunosuppressant used in organ transplantation to prevent rejection. Much like cyclosporine and FK-506, it acts by inhibiting T-cell activity.

The most common adverse effects of tacrolimus include headache and tremors. Nausea, vomiting, diarrhea, constipation, hypertension, insomnia, paresthesia, fever and chills, a rash, and flushing also may be noted. The metabolic adverse effects include hirsutism, hyperglycemia, hyperkalemia, hyperuricemia, hypokalemia, and hypomagnesemia. The life-threatening adverse effects of tacrolimus include anemia, leukocytosis, thrombocytopenia, albuminuria, hematuria, proteinuria, and renal failure. Pleural effusion and atelectasis also have been noted. Tacrolimus is contraindicated in hypersensitivity to this drug or to some kinds of castor oil. It should be used with caution in patients with renal disease, diabetes, hyperkalemia, and in patients with hyperuricemia or gout, lymphomas, pregnancy, or lactation. Safe use in children under 12 years of age has not been established.

Tacrolimus is administered IV and is extensively biotransformed. It is 75 percent protein bound and has a half-life of 10 to 11 hours. It is eliminated in the urine.

Known drug-drug interactions of tacrolimus include the risk of increased toxicity with concurrent use of aminoglycosides, cisplatin, or cyclosporine. There may be increased blood levels of antifungal drugs, calcium-channel blockers, cimetidine, danazol, and erythromycin. Carbamazepine, phenobarbital, phenytoin, and rifampin blood levels may be decreased in the presence of tacrolimus. The effect of live virus vaccines is diminished.

The usual dose of tacrolimus for adults and children is 0.15 mg/kg/day IV for 3 days. The patient should then be switched to an oral formulation at 0.15 mg/kg given twice a day.

Investigational Biologic Response Modifiers

Other biologic response modifiers include desoxyspergualin, a guanidine derivative with immunosuppressive properties. Its clinical use is limited to the management of organ transplantation rejection. RS61443 is a purine antagonist. It has been compared to azathioprine in efficacy; however, bone marrow suppression is not as profound.

Examples of other drugs currently under investigation include T10B9, 1A-3A, 33B.1, and OKT4A. The extensive use and success of the monoclonal antibody muromonab-CD3 have ignited greater interest in the development of new monoclonal antibodies that have fewer adverse effects.

Critical Thinking Process

Assessment

History of Present Illness

The history of the patient's present illness is obtained with attention to the integrity of the patient's immune system. Particularly note any treatment with antineoplastic drugs, other immunosuppressant or immunostimulant drugs, or radiation therapy. An affirmative response may suggest prior organ injury or circumstances that contribute to chronic fatigue or nutrition problems.

Past Health History

Past history includes other medical conditions for which the patient has received treatment and concurrent conditions that may make the patient more susceptible to side effects. A history of cardiac disease, GI disorders, renal disease, alcohol abuse, liver disease, or mood swings and depression indicates a higher risk for severe side effects of BRMs. Ask about allergies, including food, drugs, insect, or pollen sensitivities. Determine how the allergies affect the patient and what measures are ordinarily used to diminish the allergic response. Ask specifically about sneezing, sniffling, rhinitis, nasal stuffiness, itching of the throat, wheezing, and frequent cough.

Physical Exam Findings

BRMs can affect every organ system in the body. Adverse effects can be acute (anaphylaxis) or chronic (fatigue), constitutional (fever, chills), or system specific (hypotension). Therefore, a complete physical exam is required before beginning BRM therapy. Include in the exam an emphasis on those systems expected to benefit from BRM therapy. Inspect all lymph node regions. Look for visible nodal enlargement or color abnormalities. Palpate superficial lymph nodes of the head and neck, axilla, and inguinal and popliteal regions. Blood pressure should be assessed in both lying and standing positions to rule out hydration problems that may be magnified by the effects of certain BRMs. Intake and output measurements provide insight into the possibility of fluid deficit or excess.

Diagnostic Testing

Common laboratory testing includes a CBC, RBC indices, white blood cell count with differential, platelet count, activated partial thromboplastin time, and immunoelectrophoresis. In some cases, a bone marrow aspiration may be done. A chest radiograph and electrocardiogram help establish a baseline of pulmonary and cardiac function (see box entitled Recommended Baseline Testing for Patients Receiving BRMs).

RECOMMENDED BASELINE LABORATORY TESTING FOR PATIENTS RECEIVING BRMS

- Complete blood count, differential, platelets
- Prothrombin time, partial prothrombin time
- Blood urea nitrogen, creatinine
- Sodium, potassium, chloride, carbon dioxide
- Serum albumin
- Alkaline phosphatase, lactate dehydrogenase (LDH), serum glutamic-oxaloacetic transaminase (AST, [SGOT]), serum glutamic-pyruvic transaminase (ALT, [SGPT]), and bilirubin
- Urinalysis

Developmental Considerations

Perinatal The use and effects of BRMs during pregnancy are unclear. They are generally not recommended for use during pregnancy or lactation. To prevent undesirable complications to the fetus or newborn child, determine whether the patient is pregnant or nursing before administering BRMs.

Pediatric BRMs are ordinarily not used in persons under the age of 18. However, if the patient is an infant, ask if the child is breastfed or bottle-fed. Breastfeeding introduces antibodies to the infant's GI tract, conferring some immunity. For all children, determine which immunizations they have received (e.g., measles, mumps, pertussis).

Geriatric Increasing age is identified as a risk factor for the constitutional, cardiovascular, and neurologic side effects of BRMs. Headache, fever, chills, fatigue, malaise, and weakness are more pronounced in older patients. Older patients are more likely to have pre-existing cardiovascular dysfunction as well.

Psychosocial Considerations

Determine potential sources of infections in the home. Ascertain the age of all household members. Does anyone in the home have a chronic, low-grade infection (e.g., bronchitis)? Is the home generally free of major allergens? Ask about the patient's workplace environment. Is the patient exposed to substances that affect the immune system?

Lifelong compliance by the patient is necessary with most immunosuppressant treatment regimens. Unfortunately, these drugs often cause undesirable clinical responses that contribute to the patient discontinuing drug use or to reducing the dosage. Early detection of noncompliance may allow alterations in the type or amount of drug prescribed and contribute to improved compliance.

Determine the patient's social network and support system. Quality of life is a great issue with BRM administration that cannot be ignored. There is a significant incidence of adverse effects because BRM therapy often continues for months to years, and fatigue is a significant adverse effect of many BRMs. Fatigue diminishes the patient's ability to work and participate in activities of daily living, even though the person is still able to perform self-care. Increased tumor response and survival do not directly correlate with enhanced quality of life.

BRM drugs are expensive. Prices are established to offset the high cost of years of research and development. The technology used to produce the products (hybridoma and recombinant DNA) is expensive as well. For example, one hospitalization for 14 doses of IL-2 therapy can easily exceed $30,000.00; one course of an antineoplastic drug with the additional support of a TNF can increase the cost of treatment by $2500.00. The cost of sargramostim to the pharmacist is more than $4000.00.

Analysis and Management

Treatment Objectives

Treatment objectives for the patient receiving BRMs depend somewhat on the reason for use of the drug. In general, the major objective is to decrease the risk of organ toxicities and constitutional adverse effects of the BRMs. For example, for patients receiving G-CSFs, the objective is to abate the risk of infection by accelerating the recovery of neutrophils after high-dose antineoplastic therapy. For patients taking GM-CSFs, the therapeutic objective is to hasten myeloid recovery in patients who have received an autologous bone marrow transplantation subsequent to high-dose antineoplastic therapy. The treatment objective for the patient receiving ILs may be to reduce the size of the tumor. The objective for patients receiving epoetin alfa is the restoration and maintenance of erythrocyte counts. For all patients receiving BRMs, early detection and treatment of infection (should it occur) are paramount.

Treatment Options

Drug Variables

Antineoplastic drugs are generally administered to treat patients with cancer. However, because of the unique nature of BRMs, concurrent biotherapy is being used more often and for a wider range of disorders. BRMs may provide immunomodulatory, direct antitumor, and other biologic effects (Fig. 29–4). The purpose of clinical studies is to establish the maximum tolerated dose, determine a dose-response relationship, and identify the dose-toxicity relationship.

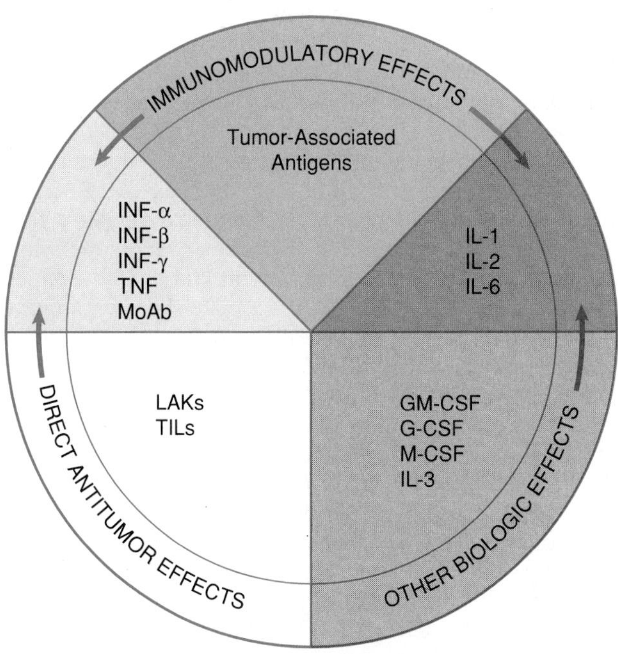

Figure 29–4 Action of biologic response–modifying drugs. Biologic response modifiers have more than one drug action, including immunomodulatory, direct antitumor, and other biologic effects. (GM-CSF, Granulocyte-macrophage colony stimulating factor; G-CSF, granulocyte colony-stimulating factor; M-CSF, macrophage colony-stimulating factor; TNF, tumor necrosis factor; MoAb, monoclonal antibody; LAKs, lymphocyte activated killer cells; IL, interleukin.)

BRMs have made it possible to successfully control rejection of transplanted tissue without compromising all immune functions in the host. The branch of the immune system that must be controlled is cell-mediated immunity. Certain drugs, such as IFN or IL-2, are used as conventional treatment for cancer with the expected response of tumor shrinkage.

The advantages of using monoclonal antibodies over conventional antisera (antibody-containing sera) are that a single antibody of known antigenic specificity is generated rather than a mixture of different antibodies and that monoclonal antibodies have a single, constant binding affinity. Further, the monoclonal antibody can be diluted to a uniform titer because the actual concentration of antibody is known. The monoclonal antibody can also be refined easily to homogeneity. They can be chosen for a specific antigenic determinant of a virus and manufactured in large amounts. As a result of hybridoma technology, the health care provider can order tests for viral antigens that are specific and diagnostic and detect disease early in its course. Currently, satumoab pendetide is the only MoAb approved for diagnostic purposes.

CSFs reduce inpatient hospital stays, antibiotic use, febrile days, and transfusion requirements. These benefits are reflected in reduction in the cost of treatment and improvement in the quality of life.

The use of BRMs has raised many economic issues because characteristics of this classification of drugs go beyond current applications for reimbursement. The first economic consideration in the use of BRMs is the investigational status of most of the drugs. Approximately 14 BRMs are FDA approved, but many more are used in clinical trials. FDA indications are usually narrow, whereas clinical applications are quite broad. Reimbursement is frequently refused when use is outside approved FDA indications (see Controversy—Biologic Response Modifiers: New and Overused).

Patient Variables

Many of the BRMs are administered as self-injections. This method is generally not covered by insurance, as it assumes the patient can be taught to give the drug. However, all patients are not able and willing to administer the drug to themselves or do not have another person who can assist. In addition, many patients are too ill to reliably take the drug but not sick enough to be hospitalized.

There have been few studies on pregnant women receiving BRMs. Adverse effects have been documented in animal studies, and certain BRMs may be secreted in breast milk. It is recommended that BRMs be used in pregnant or lactating women only if the benefits clearly outweigh the risks. Menses have resumed in some patients treated with epoetin alfa. The possibility of pregnancy should be discussed with the patient. Many of these drugs have not been studied in persons less than 18 years old; therefore, use of BRMs is not recommended in this population.

There is an increased risk of adverse effects in older adults. With increasing age, the patient may experience alterations in hepatic and renal function, decreasing cardiovascular function, altered neurosensory function, and decreased integrity of tissue, skin, and mucous membranes. All

Controversy

Biologic Response Modifiers: New and Overused?

JONATHAN J. WOLFE

Biologic response modifiers represent the closest approach in pharmacology to finding the Holy Grail. These agents, which include the interferons, are as nearly ideal for their purpose as any product so far discovered. The interferons are naturally produced within the healthy body in response to the presence of foreign substances. This is true of the alpha, beta, and gamma interferons. Their discovery was remarkable enough in itself, but their synthesis for medical use adds to their attraction. The commercially available interferon products result from recombinant DNA technology in which genes specific for their synthesis are spliced into the genetic material of microorganisms. The resulting product is remarkably free of extraneous substances that can produce side effects. Any adverse effects from the biologic response modifiers are likely to be specific to the active drug itself.

Biologic response modifiers, like other recent drug discoveries, have come at high cost for research and production. They have also been eagerly anticipated before their appearance on the market. A variety of forces propelled their rapid and broad adoption in patient care. On the one hand, practitioners have avidly applied them because they offered the chance for improved outcomes with lower risk. Patients and their families have demanded their use as the best chance to overcome serious illness. Finally, drug companies have widely promoted their use, both to recover costs of discovery and to reap the profits that sustain their large-scale enterprises. Inevitably, promotion has also sought to broaden the market share for each company's product as a means to competitive advantage.

Earlier products used to modify biologic responses remain in common use. These include the corticosteroids, which the new products have in some areas eclipsed. They also include older products such as anti-inflammatory and antiemetic drugs. The challenge is to use the established drug where appropriate, while adopting the new drugs for the uses where improved outcomes justify the greater cost.

Critical Thinking Discussion

- Once a drug is approved by the Food and Drug Administration for marketing in the United States, it may be prescribed legally by any physician for any use the prescriber judges to be appropriate. What reservation (if any) would you have about administering a regimen of alpha interferon to a patient with a tumor refractory to other chemotherapy, if the drug were approved for use in leukemias?
- What concern would you have about the use of a new and expensive biologic response modifier in an otherwise healthy patient whose acute nausea and vomiting could reasonably be managed with traditional antiemetics?
- What issues related to social justice can you identify that would operate if the next generation of biologic response modifiers were formulated from the DNA of a single patient and matched only that one person? Such a DNA-customized drug might cost $50,000 for a single dose.

of these changes place the older person at more risk for the adverse effects of BRM therapy. Every patient must be assessed individually for the appropriateness of BRM therapy.

Intervention

Administration

Administration of BRMs includes all the usual factors: knowledge of the route, correct dosage, drug formulation, storage, and transport. The unique characteristics of biologic drugs are considered as well. The dosages of BRMs vary according to the disease being treated and the expected therapeutic effects. Because dosage units are not necessarily standardized, different formulations are not interchangeable unless approved by the health care provider and pharmacist.

BRM therapy ordinarily involves the use of many other drugs to reduce or minimize the adverse effects of the biologic drug. Strategies that may be recommended to minimize or prevent the flulike symptoms include the use of acetaminophen or indomethacin to reduce fever. Meperidine may be used to reduce the shaking chills (rigors). Histamine antagonists (e.g., ranitidine, cimetidine) may be used for prophylaxis of GI irritation and bleeding. Antiemetics and antidiarrheal drugs also may be useful. Patients with indwelling catheters should receive prophylactic antibiotic therapy for *S. aureus*. The patient taking MoAbs may require premedication with an antihistamine, acetaminophen, and glucocorticoids to alleviate undesirable clinical responses.

Most BRMs require refrigeration and tolerate room temperatures only for short periods after reconstitution. This has implications for home administration, as improper storage could mean administration of inactive drug. In turn, there may be no evidence of tumor response, biologic activity, or expected adverse effects.

In general, BRMs are less stable than chemical drugs. They are more difficult to reconstitute and may need to be administered more quickly after reconstitution. The drugs should not be shaken during preparation so as to preserve their biologic activity. Be aware of which BRMs require skin testing before administration.

The route of drug administration can be oral, IV, IM, or SC. The most appropriate route of administration and the setting (e.g., hospital, outpatient clinic, home) where the BRM is given are determined by the treatment schedule and patient condition. Some BRMs can be taken with food, but others cannot. Thus, it is important to check the package insert for information. Drugs that are to be given on an empty stomach should be taken 1 hour before or 2 hours after a meal. Further, some oral formulations (e.g., cyclosporine) must be measured with a dropper and then diluted in a glass container. It is important to use proper technique when preparing the drug for administration and to know which drug formulations can be crushed, can be chewed, can have the capsule opened, or must be taken whole.

Drugs given IV should be infused through a large vessel and the site closely monitored for extravasation of the drug. Drug monographs should be checked for proper administration times and requirements for an in-line filter. A drug given IM should be administered in a large muscle. Site rotation techniques used with insulin or heparin administration are recommended when BRMs are given by IM or SC routes.

Be sure to check the results of laboratory testing before administering a BRM. Assess patients who are at high risk for organ or drug toxicities.

Education

Patients receiving BRMs have the same educational needs with regard to their drug therapy as do other patients. Information and the ability to participate in self-care activities increase self-esteem and enhance coping ability. The basic function of the immune system, the mechanism of action of the specific drug taken, and the desired therapeutic results should be addressed. The expected adverse effects, both of the specific BRM and the adverse effects of combination therapy (BRM plus antineoplastic drug, or more than one BRM), and administration techniques also should be covered. The importance of laboratory testing and follow-up with the health care provider cannot be overemphasized. Be sure the patient and family know when to contact the health care provider. Patients also should be advised to avoid driving or operating hazardous machinery if blurry vision or drowsiness occurs. The female patient should be taught to use contraceptive measures during BRM treatment and for 12 weeks after ending therapy.

The family must be considered a resource for the patient. The patient often needs a partner and coach to tolerate the physical and emotional strain of BRM therapy. In addition, it is important to teach the family to identify and report adverse effects that the patient may be unable to recognize (e.g., neurologic changes).

Because the patient is at risk for infection while taking immunosuppressing BRMs, teach the patient and family to monitor specifically for signs and symptoms of infection. Patients should be taught how to take their temperature. They also should be advised to avoid persons who have just received immunizations that contain live vaccine. Advise patients to wear a mask that covers the mouth and nose if they anticipate exposure to someone who has recently received oral polio vaccine. Some patients may need to avoid exposure to house plants and animals. In some cases, the immunocompromised patient may need to be isolated to reduce the risk of contracting an infection. Conscientious handwashing is required of all who come in contact with the patient.

Patient and family knowledge about what constitutes adequate nutrition is vital. Encourage the patient to consume high-quality dietary nutrients and to avoid as much as possible "empty" calories. Use of supplemental vitamins and minerals may need to be considered for some patients. Protein supplements also may be warranted.

Evaluation

The effectiveness of BRM therapy is specific to the disorder under treatment. For example, therapeutic effectiveness may be demonstrated by immunosuppression of an autoimmune disorder or the absence of graft rejection for patients who have undergone transplantation. Tumor regression and decreased spread of a malignancy can be noted as early as 4 weeks after completion of the first course of IL therapy and may continue for up to 12 months after the start of therapy. The patient taking ILs for relapsing-remitting multiple sclerosis may see a decrease in the frequency of relapse, further providing evidence of drug effectiveness. Normalized blood parameters may provide evidence of therapeutic response. The time to hematopoietic response is due to the interval required for the maturation of immature cells to become fully mature and to be released into the peripheral circulation. The rate and extent of a hematopoietic response are influenced by available iron stores, baseline hematocrit, and presence of concurrent medical problems.

SUMMARY

- Biologic response modifiers (BRMs) are produced through hybridoma and recombinant gene technologies.
- BRMs act in conjunction with the immune system to destroy tumor cells, influence chronic granulomatous disease and multiple sclerosis, and in the treatment of the hematologic adverse effects of autologous bone marrow transplantation.
- BRMs have more than one of the following actions: cytotoxicity, immunomodulation, or other biologic effects.
- There may be one or more pharmacotherapeutic objectives for the use of BRMs, depending on the disease or condition for which it is used.
- The development of all biotherapy agents is based on the prototype drug interferon. Colony-stimulating factors (CSFs) (e.g., epoetin alfa), interleukins (e.g., aldesleukin), monoclonal antibodies (satumoab pendetide), and tumor necrosis factor (TNF) were developed later.
- Other FDA approved CSFs include granulocyte colony-stimulating factor (G-CSF), and granulocyte-macrophage colony-stimulating factor (GM-CSF).
- Monoclonal antibodies are highly specific to lymphocyte membrane antigens. Polyclonal antibodies impair cell-mediated immune responses, specifically T-cell activity.
- BRMs tend to be more effective when the disease entity or tumor mass is quantitatively small. For this reason, they are used in combination with other drugs or treatment modalities.
- Because BRMs can affect every body system, a full physical and psychosocial assessment is required before treatment.
- Administration and patient education must be tailored for the individual BRM being administered.
- Quality of life is a great issue with the use of BRMs. There is a significant incidence of adverse effects because BRM therapy often continues for months to years.
- Increased tumor response and survival do not directly correlate with enhanced quality of life.

BIBLIOGRAPHY

American College of Obstetricians and Gynecologists (ACOG). (1990). *Prevention of D isoimmunization.* Technical Bulletin 147. Washington, DC: Author.

Amgen, Inc. (1990). *Colony stimulating factors: A review.* Thousand Oaks, CA: Author.

Bender, C. (1994). Cognitive dysfunction associated with biological response modifier therapy. *Oncology Nursing Forum, 21,* 515–523.

Brophy, L., and Sharp, E. (1991). Physical symptoms of combination biotherapy: A quality of life issue. *Oncology Nursing Forum,* 18, 25–30.

Doweiko, J., and Goldberg, M. (1991). Erythropoietin therapy in cancer patients. *Oncology,* 5, 31–37.

Hanson, L., Hermanson, J., Lee, J., et al. (1990). Helpful hints in caring for patients receiving biotherapy. Rigors associated with outpatient tumor necrosis factor. *Administration Oncology Nursing Forum,* 17(6), 963.

Hogan, C. (1991). Coping with biotherapy: Physiological and psychosocial concerns. *Oncology Nursing Forum,* 18, 19–23.

Hynes, M., Bournes, L., Brish, A., et al. (1990). Managing side effects associated with IL-2 therapy. *Oncology Nursing Forum,* 17, 963–964.

Jassak, P. Biotherapy. (1993). In S. Groenwald, M. Frogge, M. Goodman, et al. (Eds.), *Cancer nursing: Principles and practice* (3rd ed.). Boston: Jones and Bartlett.

Jusko, W., Kung, L., and Schmelter, R. (1992). Immunopharmacokinetics of In-111 CYT-103 in ovarian cancer patients. In R. Maguire, and D. Van Nostrand (Eds.), *Diagnosis of colorectal and ovarian carcinoma: Application of immunoscintigraphic technology.* New York: Marcel Dekker, Inc.

Nabi H., and Doerr, R. (1992). Radiolabeled monoclonal antibody imaging (immunoscintigraphy) of colorectal cancer: Current status and future perspectives. *American Journal of Surgery,* 163, 448–456.

Piascik, M. (1991). Research and development of drugs and biologic entities. *American Journal of Hospital Pharmacies, 48,* S413.

Reiger, P. (Ed.). (1994). *Biotherapy: A comprehensive overview.* Boston: Jones & Bartlett.

Robinson, K., and Posner, J. (1992). Patterns of self-care needs and interventions related to biologic response modifier therapy: Fatigue as a model. *Seminars in Oncology Nursing,* 8, 17–22.

Rumsey, K., and Rieger, P. (Eds.). (1992). *Biological response modifiers: A self-instruction manual for health professionals.* Chicago: Precept Press, Inc.

Rust, D., Bell, D., Colao, D., et al. (1990). Symptom management for patients receiving biotherapy. *Oncology Nursing Forum,* 17(6), 964.

Shelton, B., and Sargent, C. (1990). Neurologic toxicity management with BRMs. *Oncology Nursing Forum,* 17(6), 964–965.

Straw L., and Conrad, K. (1994). Patient education resources related to biotherapy and the immune system. *Oncology Nursing Forum,* 21, 1223–1228.

Tenenbaum, L. (1994). *Cancer chemotherapy and biotherapy* (2nd ed.). Philadelphia: W.B. Saunders Company.

Wolf, B. (1996). Overview of therapeutic drug monitoring and biotechnologic drugs. *Therapeutic Drug Monitoring,* 18, 402–404.

Wordell, C. (1991). Biotechnology update. *Hospital Pharmacy,* 26, 897–900.

Wujcik, D. (1991). Overview of colony-stimulating factors: Focus on the neutrophil. A case management approach to patients receiving G-CSF. In R. Johnson (Ed.), *A Case Management Approach to Patients Receiving G-CSF.* Pittsburgh: Oncology Nursing Press.

Wujcik, D. (1993). An odyssey into biologic therapy. *Oncology Nursing Forum,* 20, 879–897.

Xistris, D. (1992). Reimbursement of biotherapy: Present status, future directions: Perspectives of the office-based oncology nurse. *Seminars in Oncology Nursing,* 8, 8–12.

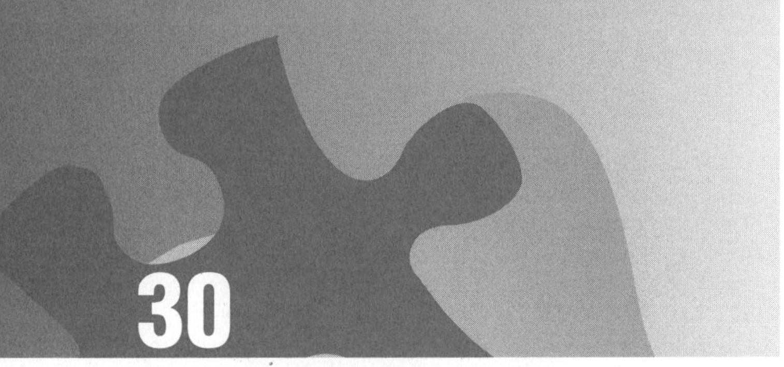

30 Antineoplastic Drugs

Cancer is no longer considered an immediate death sentence because of modern treatment options. Today, malignant diseases that were previously considered incurable can be cured. According to the National Cancer Institute's Surveillance, Epidemiology, and End Results (NCI-SEER) program, a significant improvement can be seen in 5-year survival trends, ranging from 39 percent in the 1960s to more than 50 percent in the 1990s. However, cancer remains the second leading cause of death in the United States, preceded only by cardiovascular disease. The rate of occurrence for certain types of neoplastic disease, including breast, lung, and skin cancer, continues to increase. Antineoplastic therapy is the treatment of choice for hematolymphatic malignancies and solid tumors that have undergone regional or distant metastasis. The ultimate goal of antineoplastic therapy is to provide cure, control, or palliation of disease.

CANCER

Epidemiology and Etiology

The occurrence, distribution, and outcomes of malignant diseases reflect varying patterns, depending upon gender, age, geographic location, and socioeconomic status. Cancers of the lung are equally likely to occur in men and women and account for the highest rates of mortality in both genders. In women, the leading sites of fatal cancers are the lung, breast, colon, and rectum, while the lung, prostate, colon, and rectum are the leading sites in men. Age-adjusted death rates over the last few decades show a steady increase in cancer death rates for both genders, which may be due, at least in part, to improved detection and diagnosis of the disease.

The exact cause of cancer remains unknown. There is evidence to suggest that cellular genes, normally responsible for cellular metabolism, division, and growth, convert to malignant *oncogenes* (gene found in chromosomes of tumor cells) that cause uncontrolled cell growth and replication. Various substances have been identified as *carcinogenic* (cancer causing) or able to promote the development of cancer.

Tobacco remains the most important known carcinogen in the United States. Approximately 30 percent of all cancer deaths could be avoided with the elimination of tobacco. Diets high in animal fat tend to be associated with an increased incidence of colorectal, prostate, endometrial, and breast cancer. A correlation appears to exist between excessive alcohol intake and the development of cancers of the oropharynx, esophagus, and liver.

For certain types of tumors, cancer may have an infectious component. Primary hepatocellular carcinoma has been linked with hepatitis B viral infections. The Epstein-Barr virus has been associated with Burkitt's lymphoma, which is a form of undifferentiated malignant lymphoma.

In addition to the Epstein-Barr virus (EBV), a member of the Herpes group associated with nasopharyngeal cancer, herpes simplex II virus and human papilloma virus have both been linked to cancer of the cervix. Human T-cell leukemia-lymphoma virus is associated with leukemias and lymphomas.

Exposure to environmental, chemical, and industrial agents has also been shown to increase the risk of cancer. Uranium, nickel, and beryllium are carcinogenic in animals and are probable causative agents in the development of lung cancer in miners. Radiation exposure is capable of inducing cancers of the breast, thyroid gland, and bone marrow. Asbestos exposure has been directly correlated in exposed individuals to the development of mesothelioma, a malignant tumor composed of cells that line the pleura, pericardium, and peritoneum.

Physical carcinogens can produce altered DNA structure and create chromosomal alterations and translocations. Ultraviolet rays of the sun can cause skin cancer. Ionizing radiation (x-ray therapy, radon gas, nuclear power) is associated with cancers of the lung, bone, liver, thyroid, thymus, and breast. Leukemia has been reported following exposure to radioactive gas as the result of atomic bomb blasts in Nagasaki and Hiroshima during World War II and, more recently, near the site of nuclear reactors at Three Mile Island and in Chernobyl, Russia. A smaller number of leukemias and some solid tumors have been attributed to high-dose radiation therapy. If a radiation-induced solid tumor develops, it is usually located in the anatomic region to which radiation therapy was delivered.

The earliest chemical carcinogens to be identified were tobacco snuff (1759) and soot (1775). Today, it is well known that tars and other carcinogens are emitted by a cigarette, and cigarette smokers can be at a tenfold increased risk for cancer over nonsmokers. The risk increases with the number of cigarettes and length of time smoked. Secondhand smoke, or passive smoking, has been implicated as a cause of lung cancer in those indirectly exposed to tobacco smoke, including children, spouses, and fellow workers. To date, smoking is known to be a causative factor of cancer of the lung, larynx, oral cavity, bladder, kidney, colon, and cervix and has been implicated in some leukemias. Other chemical carcinogens include crude petroleum, coal tar, and polycyclic aromatic hydrocarbons, which are formed by cooking noncarcinogenic hydrocarbons in food and oil to high temperatures. Heavy consumption of alcohol is related to cancers of the oral cavity, esophagus, and liver and may be synergistic or additive to the effects of tobacco use.

Some drugs, including antineoplastics, have been associated with increased risk for some cancers. Alkylating agents interact with DNA directly or indirectly. Unopposed estrogen therapy or oral contraceptives containing only estrogen do not cause cancer, but may allow potentially neoplastic changes to take place, increasing the risk for endometrial cancer.

High dietary fat intake has been associated with increased incidence of many solid tumors. Cancers of the breast, prostate, colon, and rectum are more common in the Western world and higher economic groups, where dietary fat intake is higher. Studies have shown a rise in cancer incidence in females from oriental countries after migration to the United States and increases in dietary fat intake. The role of fat in colon cancer is supported by both the increased incidence with dietary change and the potential relationship of fat consumption to bile acids, which are known to be mutagenic. Cancer of the ovaries, endometrium, prostate, and pancreas is also related to high fat intake, but the evidence is not conclusive.

Neoplasia have been attributed to abnormalities in one or more genes regulating growth and differentiation. Women with a family history of breast cancer are at higher risk for breast cancer. Chromosomal disorders often precede some neoplasms. Retinoblastoma may be inherited as an autosomal dominant trait. People with xeroderma pigmentosum, an autosomal recessive disease of the skin, have a higher incidence of skin cancers than the general population.

Pathophysiology

Cancer is characterized by both uncontrolled cell proliferation and impaired differentiation. Tumors are neoplastic or new growths of cells. Benign tumors do not *metastasize* or spread from their original location. Malignant tumors spread by direct extension into surrounding tissues, via the lymphatic system, and hematogenously via blood circulation.

Cancer cells proliferate only when the normal capacity to identify and repair mutations in the genome is lost. A *genome* is a complete set of hereditary factors contained in the haploid set (one-half) of chromosomes. Except for the germ cells of the gonads, each body cell is programmed for a limited number of cell divisions. The program involves telomeres that are located at the ends of the chromosome and produced and maintained by telomerase, an enzyme in both germ and embryonic cells. Telomeres pair and align at mitosis. They normally lose function during development since a portion of the telomere is lost with each cell division. Telomeric loss serves as a cellular clock. In contrast, cancer cells re-express telomerase, which allows continued proliferation. Loss of normal cell cycle controls causes ongoing expression of the enzyme. As many as 95 percent of cancer cells express the telomerase enzyme, making it a potential target for drug intervention.

Physical characteristics of tumor cells are described in terms of cell cycle time, doubling time, and growth fraction. The cell cycle involves a series of events during which both neoplastic and normal cells grow and reproduce. Rapidly growing cancers are more susceptible to antineoplastic drugs than slower-growing cancers. The term *growth fraction* refers to the percentage of cells that are actively proceeding through the cell cycle (dividing) at any given time. During the early stages of tumor expansion, the growth fraction is high, and the tumor doubling time is rapid.

Tumor growth is best described by gompertzian kinetics (Table 30–1) rather than logarithmic growth. The log kill hypothesis assumes that drugs kill a constant fraction of tumor cells, related to the log number of cells, and not a constant number of cells. Log kill varies with cell growth rate; thus, there is a gradual decrease in log kill in the late stages of tumor growth when cells stop cycling. Early return of slow-growing tumors occurs because the log kill is small. Late return of rapid-growing tumors may occur despite effective treatment if too few courses of treatment are given.

Doubling time is the period required for a tumor mass to increase twofold. When tumor volume is low and the cells are rapidly dividing, a relatively high proportion of cells undergo division. As a result, tumor cells that are rapidly dividing are more sensitive to antineoplastic drugs (e.g., antimetabolites). Similarly, a tumor with a relatively vigorous doubling time (e.g., testicular cancer [21 days], Ewing's sarcoma [22 days]) is more sensitive to antineoplastic therapy than tumors with a slow doubling time (e.g., colon cancer [96 days], breast cancer [129 days], adenocarcinoma of the lung [134 days]).

The larger the tumor cell population, the longer the tumor doubling time. Larger tumors have a less efficient blood supply than smaller tumors, divide more slowly, and may respond more favorably to drugs that are effective in any phase of the cell cycle (e.g., alkylating drugs). For this reason, cell cycle nonspecific drugs are likely to be more effective against slow-growing cancers. In contrast, drugs that are cell cycle specific tend to be effective against rapid-growing cancers. Unfortunately, as the tumor burden increases, the patient becomes more and more debilitated and less able to withstand antineoplastic therapy. The patient's ability to withstand therapy is related to the fact that normal cells also have a high growth fraction. This is why the gastrointestinal (GI) tract, hair follicles, and the bone marrow experience the most toxicity when exposed to antineoplastic drugs.

TABLE 30–1. GOMPERTZIAN GROWTH KINETICS

Cell Burden	Number of Cells Present	Clinical Response
10^0	1	Clinical disease undetectable by physical exam
10^5	100,000	
10^9	1,000,000,000	Clinical symptoms begin to appear*
10^{10}	10,000,000,000	Regional spread of cancer cells
10^{11}	100,000,000,000	Metastasis of cancer cells
10^{13}	10,000,000,000,000	Cancerous process likely to be lethal

*A cell burden of 10^9 is typically the smallest tumor physically detectable. The patient has approximately one billion cancer cells at this point, equivalent to a tumor the size of a small grape and weighing 1 g. Clinical symptoms usually begin to appear.

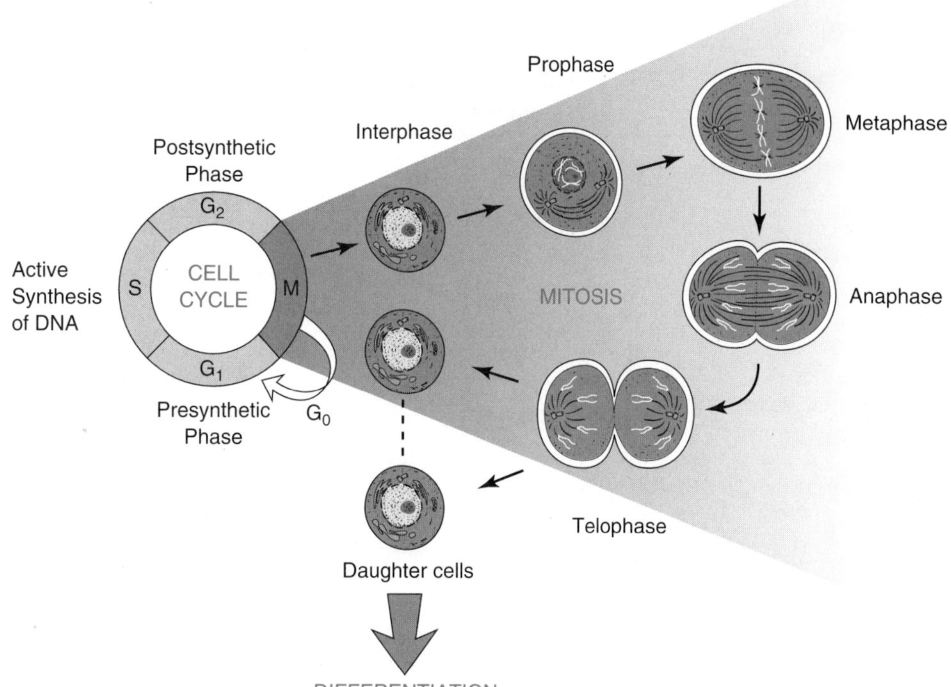

Figure 30–1. The cell cycle represents the interval from the midpoint of mitosis to the ensuing end point of mitosis, where a daughter cell is produced. The phases include synthesis (S), in which DNA is synthesized in the cell's nucleus; gap-2 (G_2), in which RNA and protein synthesis occurs (construction of mitotic apparatus); mitosis (M), where both nuclear and cytoplasmic division take place; and gap-1 (G_1), the postmitotic period between the M phase and the start of DNA synthesis, when RNA and protein synthesis is increased and cell growth occurs.

Cell Cycle Concepts

Understanding the basic processes of cellular proliferation is essential to an understanding of the mechanisms of action of antineoplastic drugs. At any given time, tissue cells are either actively dividing, differentiating, or dormant. The term *cell cycle* describes the series of events during which both neoplastic and normal cells grow and reproduce. *Cell cycle time* is defined as the period required for the cell to complete one complete cycle, from mitosis to mitosis. Cell cycles vary depending on the type of tissue which accounts for differences in response by specific cell types to antineoplastic drugs.

Cell Cycle Phases

Four distinct phases of the cell cycle are recognized. During the first phase of the cell cycle, gap 1 (G_1), proteins, RNA, and enzymes required for synthesis of DNA are formed (Figure 30–1). The G_1 phase may be virtually absent, as in embryonic cells, or so prolonged that is produces dormancy (G_0).

In the synthesis (S) phase, DNA is formed and chromosomes double within the cell as a preliminary step to mitosis. The activity of replicative enzymes such as thymidine kinase, DNA polymerase, dihydrofolate reductase, ribonucleotide reductase, RNA polymerase II, and topoisomerases I and II is increased during the S phase. The synthesis phase may last 10 to 20 hours depending on the cell type. Many antineoplastic drugs cause direct damage to the DNA code during this phase, thereby decreasing the cell's ability to replicate.

In the gap 2 (G_2) phase, the second period of RNA and protein synthesis, the mitotic spindle forms. This phase lasts 1 to 8 hours, and the DNA complement is twice the normal number of chromosomes.

During mitosis (M), the parent cell divides into two new daughter cells. Each daughter cell contains the same number and kind of chromosomes as the parent cell. This phase may last only 30 to 60 minutes. After mitosis, cells will either return to the G_1 phase or go into the resting stage (G_0).

Antineoplastic drugs that target the cell cycle are classified according to their mechanism of action and how they act within a specific phase of the cell cycle. Drugs that are characterized as *cell cycle specific* (CCS) act on cells that are undergoing specific phases in cell production (see Summary of Cell Cycle Activity for Selected Antineoplastic Drugs). These drugs include most subcategories of antimetabolites that act specifically in the S phase of the cell cycle, and mitotic inhibitors, specific to late G_2 and M phases. For example, the antimetabolite agent methotrexate is most effective in the S phase of the cell cycle. It binds with folic acid reductase, thus inhibiting synthesis of DNA and RNA. *Cell cycle nonspecific* (CCNS) drugs act on the cell, whether it is dividing or in a resting state. CCNS drugs include alkylating drugs (e.g., cyclophosphamide, chlorambucil) and antitumor antibiotics (e.g., mitomycin, doxorubicin, daunorubicin) as well as the other drugs. These drugs are active regardless of the specific phase of the cell cycle.

Combination drug regimens, which act in different phases of the cell cycle, have been shown to yield an improved tumor cell kill when compared to single drug regimens. In addition, multidrug treatment regimens have been shown to decrease the risk of developing a drug-resistant tumor cell line.

Concept of Cell Kill

The effects of antineoplastic drugs on cancer cells follow the concept of first-order kinetics. This concept refers to the destruction of a constant percentage of cancer cells, not a

SUMMARY OF CELL CYCLE ACTIVITY FOR SELECTIVE ANTINEOPLASTIC DRUGS

Cell Cycle Specific Drugs	*Cell Cycle Nonspecific Drugs*
Phase S	Alkylating Drugs
Antimetabolites	• Busulfan
• Cytarabine	• Carboplatin
• Fluorouracil	• Carmustine
• Hydroxyurea	• Chlorambucil
• Methotrexate	• Cisplatin
• Thioguanine	• Cyclophosphamide
Phase G_2	• Ifosfamide
Antitumor Antibiotic	• Lomustine
• Bleomycin	• Mechlorethamine
Mitotic Inhibitors	• Melphalan
• Etoposide	• Streptozocin
• Teniposide	
Phase M	Antitumor Antibiotics
Vinca Alkaloids	• Dactinomycin
• Vinblastine	• Daunorubicin
• Vincristine	• Doxorubicin
• Vindesine	• Idarubicin
Taxanes	• Mitomycin
• Paclitaxel	• Mitoxantrone
Phase G_1	• Plicamycin
• L-Asparaginase	
Adrenocorticosteroids	
• Prednisone	

constant number, regardless of the number of cells present. To eradicate all viable cancer cells, the antineoplastic agent or drug combination must be administered at repeated intervals over time until the drug, along with the patient's immune system, destroys all cancer cells. According to the *cell kill hypothesis,* if the cancer contains one million cells and the treatment regimen has a 90 percent kill rate, the first course of therapy would theoretically destroy 90 percent of tumor cells, leaving 10 percent unaffected. The second dose would kill 90 percent of the remaining cells, leaving 10 percent, and so on until one cell remains. The body's immune response would then destroy the final remaining cell. This hypothesis explains why most antineoplastic treatment regimens consist of multidrug therapy administered at regular intervals over a period of months or years.

The degree of cell kill is directly proportional to the dose administered. Ideally, with each additional course of therapy, the dose remains the same, even though the cancer may be getting progressively smaller. The patient must be able to tolerate the same level of drug toxicity if therapy is to continue. This theory provides useful insight into applications and antineoplastic treatment strategies but fails to account for variations in the tumor's responsiveness to treatment.

Tumor Cell Resistance

Tumor cell heterogeneity is important because it can be linked to the emergence of antineoplastic-resistant tumor cells. The origin of these heterogeneous subsets is thought to be predictable and due to random mutational events. A tumor mass contains subsets of cells whose characteristics vary greatly, including their responsiveness to antineoplastic therapy.

Tumor cell resistance may be temporary or permanent. Factors related to *temporary resistance* include alterations in the bioavailability, biotransformation, or elimination of the drug; the presence of tumor in sanctuary sites; limited drug diffusion; alteration in cell kinetics; host toxicity; and the blood supply of the tumor. A *sanctuary site* is defined as an area in the body that is not readily perfused by antineoplastic drugs.

Permanent resistance is genetically based. There may be changes in the tumor cell itself, such as a genetic mutation. The probability of having at least one drug-resistant cell is the yield of the mutation rate and the size of the tumor. Thus, the likelihood of cure in a patient having a large tumor is diminished. At least one resistant mutation may have occurred. The mechanisms associated with permanent drug resistance include defective drug transport or biotransformation, transformed nucleotide pools, increased drug activation, altered repair of DNA, gene amplification, altered target proteins, and multidrug resistance. In some cases, cancer cells can repair DNA damage caused by the antineoplastic drug or decrease permeability to prevent drug activation. Tumor cell resistance can also occur because of the inability of a tumor to convert a drug to its active form or its ability to inactive a drug. The larger the tumor mass (i.e., the greater the heterogenicity), the greater the likelihood of the existence of drug-resistant clones and multi-drug-resistant clones. Fortunately, tumor cell mutation resulting in resistance to one drug does not usually result in resistance to other drugs of different classes. This provides rationale for combination drug therapy.

Tumor cell resistance can be intrinsic or acquired. *Intrinsic resistance* is resistance to a specific drug without any prior exposure to that drug. *Acquired resistance* develops after the start of therapy and represents a change in the tumor cells themselves.

PHARMACOTHERAPEUTIC OPTIONS

Research is ongoing regarding the therapeutic uses of antineoplastic drugs. Although comparatively few drugs have been discovered within the last decade, new combinations of drugs and higher dosages have yielded promising results in the outcome of cancer treatment. The categories of drugs that may be used in the treatment of cancer include alkylating drugs, which interact directly with DNA, and those that interfere with the synthesis of DNA precursors, such as antimetabolites, antitumor antibiotics, mitotic inhibitors, a variety of miscellaneous drugs, and hormones and hormone antagonists.

Alkylating Drugs

ALKYL SULFONATES

❒ Busulfan (MIELUCIN, MYLERAN, SULFABUTIN); (🍁) MYLERAN

ETHYLENIMINES

❒ Triethylenethiophosphoramide/thiotepa (thiotepa, THIOPLEX, TESPA)

NITROGEN MUSTARDS

❒ Altretamine (Hexamethylmelamine, HEXALEN, NEXISTAT, HMM); (🍁) HEXALEN

❒ Cyclophosphamide (CYTOXAN, NEOSAR); (✽) CYTOXAN, PROCYTOX
❒ Chlorambucil (LEUKERAN); (✽) LEUKERAN
❒ Ifosfamide (IFEX); (✽) IFEX
❒ Mechlorethamine (MUSTARGEN); (✽) MUSTARGEN
❒ Melphalan (ALKERAN); (✽) ALKERAN

METAL SALTS
❒ Carboplatin (PARAPLATIN); (✽) PARAPLATIN-AQ
❒ Cisplatin (PLATINOL, PLATINOL AQ, CIS, DDP); (✽) PLATINOL-AQ

NITROSOUREAS
❒ Carmustine (BCNU, BICNU, GLIADEL); (✽) BICNU
❒ Lomustine (CEENU, GLIADEL); (✽) CEENU
❒ Streptozocin (ZANOSAR); (✽) ZANOSAR

TRIAZENES
❒ Dacarbazine (DTIC-DOME); (✽) DTIC

Indications

Alkylating drugs include an alkyl sulfonate, an ethylenimine, nitrogen mustards, metal salts, nitrosureas, and a triazine. The wide variety of applications for alkylating drugs will be discussed under Dosage Regimen.

Pharmacodynamics

Alkylating drugs are CCNS agents. Nevertheless, some alkylating drugs seem more cytocidal to cells in particular phases of the cell cycle (e.g., nitrosoureas in G_1 or G_2, and mechlorethamine, which is most active in phase M and G_1). As a group, alkylating drugs produce intermediates that readily form covalent bonds with negatively charged cellular substances. One of the reactions is alkylation of the 7-nitrogen of guanine in DNA, which can lead to miscoding and cross-linking between two DNA strands. For example, the alkyl sulfonate drug busulfan substitutes an alkyl group for a hydrogen ion in tumor cells, resulting in alkylation of DNA. Alkylation of DNA results in a monofunctional or bifunctional reaction. Monofunctional alkylating reactions occur when the alkyl has only one reaction site and can only bind with the DNA in one place. Monofunctional reactions result in miscoding of DNA. However, alkylating drugs may attack DNA in double-stranded form, forming cross-links or chemical bonds between the strands. Normally, strands of DNA must unwind and separate during replication, but cross-linking prevents this and blocks DNA replication. Cross-linking of DNA produces the most injurious effects; therefore, bifunctional reactions are more likely to result in cell death.

Tumor resistance to alkylating drugs is often multifactorial. Resistance may be the result of decreased membrane transport (e.g., for melphalan and cisplatin) or it may be bound by glutathione in the cytoplasm and inactivated. The alkylating drug can also be biotransformed to an inactive agent (e.g., by enzymes such as aldehyde dehydrogenase I).

Adverse Effects and Contraindications

Alkylating drugs are toxic to tissues that have a high growth fraction. Thus, the hematopoietic system is very susceptible to the effects of these drugs. Lymphocytes are more sensitive to the destructive action of the nitrogen mustards and relatively resistant to the effects of busulfan, an action that is considered responsible for the immunosuppressive effects observed with cyclophosphamide. Busulfan is more toxic to granulocytes and in combination with chlorambucil closely simulates the hematologic effects of whole-body radiation.

Nausea and vomiting occur with all alkylating drugs but can be especially severe with cisplatin and mechlorethamine and are presumably the result of central nervous system (CNS) stimulation. Seizures, progressive muscular paralysis, and various cholinomimetic effects have been observed. Teratogenesis and gonadal atrophy are common but variable according to the specific drug, its administration schedule, and route of administration. In women, amenorrhea of several months duration sometimes follows a course of therapy with alkylating drugs. Impairment of spermatogenesis may be noted in men. Damage to hair follicles is much more pronounced with cyclophosphamide than with other nitrogen mustards, frequently resulting in alopecia. This effect is usually reversible, even with continued therapy.

Therapy with alkylating drugs also carries a major risk of leukemogenesis (induction or development of leukemia) and carcinogenesis. Other adverse effects include destruction of the beta cells of the pancreas with streptozocin, causing diabetes mellitus. Alopecia develops with cyclophosphamide and interstitial pneumonitis with busulfan and the nitrosoureas. Cyclophosphamide and ifosfamide cause renal and bladder toxicities.

Cyclophosphamide should be used with caution in patients who have undergone radiation therapy or other antineoplastic therapy and in patients with leukopenia, thrombocytopenia, or hepatic or liver disease. It should also be used with caution in patients with malignant infiltration of the bone marrow. Giving the drug at bedtime increases the risk of cystitis.

Aluminum can react with cisplatin and carboplatin, resulting in precipitation and decreased drug potency. Thus, needles and IV equipment containing aluminum should be avoided. Carboplatin carries a greater risk of neurotoxicity in patients older than 65 years of age and thus should be used with caution.

Pharmacokinetics

Alkylating drugs are prodrugs whose cellular uptake is by active transport into cells via physiologic transporters (for nitrogen mustards) or passively (for nitrosoureas). For example, mechlorethamine uses the choline transporter, melphalan the L-glutamine transporter, and cisplatin the methionine transporter.

Alkylation sites are widespread and include enzymes, cell membranes, and nucleotides, accounting for the adverse as well as therapeutic effects. Except for cyclophosphamide, the alkylating drugs have very short half-lives in plasma (Table 30–2). Alkylating agents are generally biotransformed in the liver and eliminated by the kidneys.

A unique feature of nitrosoureas is their high lipid solubility. The high lipid solubility allows them to enter the brain and cerebrospinal fluid more effectively than most other antineoplastic drugs.

Drug-Drug Interactions

Drug-drug interactions with alkylating drugs are many (Table 30–3). All of the alkylating drugs interact with other

TABLE 30–2. PHARMACOKINETICS OF SELECTED ANTINEOPLASTIC DRUGS

Drug	Route	Onset	Peak	Duration	PB (%)	$t_{1/2}$	BioA (%)
Alkylating Drugs							
Altretamine	po	UK	3–4 wks	6 wks	6; 25; 50*	4.7–10.2 h	UA
Busulfan	po	10–15 days	Weeks	1 mo†	UA	2.5 h	UA
Carboplatin	IV	UK	21 days	28 days	High	2.6–5.9 h	100
Carmustine	IV	Days	4–5 wks	6 weeks	High	15–30%	100
Chlorambucil	po	7–14 days	7–14 days	14–28 days	99	1.5 h	UA
Cisplatin	IV	UK	18–23 days	39 days	90	30–100 h	100
Cyclophosphamide	po	7 days	7–15 days	21 days	>60	4–6.5 h	UA
Dacarbazine‡	IV	16–20 days	16 days	3–5 days	Low	5 h	100
Ifosfamide	IV	UK	7–14 days	21 days	UA	15 h	100
Lomustine	po	UK	4–7 wks	1–2 wks	50	1–2 days	UA
Mechlorethamine	IV	Immediate	UK	UK	UK	UK	100
Melphalan	po	5 days	2–3 wks	5–6 wks	<30	1.5 h	UA
Streptozocin	IV	UK; 17 days§	1–2 wks; 35 days§	UK	UA	35–40 min	100
Thiotepa	IV	10–30 days	14 days	21 days	UA	UK	100
Antimetabolites							
Cladribine	IV	UK	UK	5 wks‖	UA	5.4 h	100
Cytarabine	IV	24 h; 15–24 h¶	24 days	12 days; 25–34 days	15	1–3 h	100
Fludarabine	IV	UK	13–16 days	UK	UA	10 h	100
Fluorouracil	IV	1–9 days	9–21 days	30 days	UA	20 h	100
Gemcitabine	IV	Immediate	30 min	UA	UA	42–70 min	100
Mercaptopurine	po	7–10 days	14 days	21 days	20	45 min; 2.5 h; 10 h**	10–15
Methotrexate	po/IV	4–7 days	7–14 days	21 days	35	8 h	100
Pentostatin	IV	4–7 mo	UK	7.7–35.1 mo††	4	6 h	100
Thioguanine	po	7–10 days	14 days	21 days	UA	11 h	30
Antitumor Antibiotics							
Bleomycin	IV	Immediate	10–20 min	UA	UA	2 h	100
Dactinomycin	IV	7 days	14 days	21–28 days	UA	36 h	100
Daunorubicin	IV	7–10 days	10–14 days	21 days	UA	18.5 h; 26.7 h‡‡	100
Doxorubicin	IV	10 days	14 days	21–24 days	UA	16.7 h	100
Idarubicin	IV	UK	10–14 days	21 days	97; 94§§	4–46 h	100
Mitomycin	IV	3–8 wks	4–8 wks	3 months	UA	50 min	100
Mitoxantrone	IV	10 days	10 days	21 days	78	5.8 days	100
Plicamycin	IV	UK	7–10 days	3–4 wks	UA	UK	100
Mitotic Inhibitors							
Docetaxel	IV	Immediate	8 days	7 days	94–97	11.1 h	100
Etoposide	po/IV	7–14 days	9–16 days	20 days	97	3–12 h	100¶¶
Irinotecan	IV	UK	UK	UK	30–68	6 h	100
Paclitaxel	IV	UK	11 days	3 wks	89–98	5.3–17.4 h	100
Teniposide	IV	UK	16–18 days	15 days	99	5 h	100
Topotecan	IV	Days	11 days	7 days	35	2–3 hr	100
Vinblastine	IV	5–7 days	10 days	7–14 days	75	24 h	100
Vincristine	IV	UK	4 days	7 days	75	10.5–155 h	100
Vinorelbine	IV	UK	7–10 days	7–14 days	UA	28–44 h	100
Miscellaneous							
Hydroxyurea	po	7 days	10 days	21 days	UA	3–4 h	UA
L-asparaginase	IV	Immediate	UK	23–33 days	UA	8–30 h	100
Mitotane	po	2–4 wks	6 wks	UK	UA	18–159 h	30–40
Pegaspargase	IV	Immediate	UK	14 days	UA	5.7 days	100
Procarbazine	po	14 days	2–8 wks	28–42 days	UA	10 min	100

*Protein binding of altretamine, pentamethylmelamine, and tetramethylmelamine metabolites, respectively.
†Recovery from busulfan may take up to 20 months.
‡Onset, peak, and duration of dacarbazine effects on white blood cells and platelets, respectively.
§Onset of and peak effects on blood counts and tumor response for streptozocin, respectively.
‖Cladribine time to normalization of blood counts.
¶Onset and duration of cytarabine's phase 1 and 2 effects on white blood cell count.
**Mercaptopurine has a triphasic half-life.
††The duration of inhibition of adenine diaminase lasts over 1 week following administration of pentostatin.
‡‡Half-life of daunorubicin and its metabolite, respectively.
§§Protein binding of idarubacin and its metabolite, respectively.
¶¶Bioavailable of oral and IV etoposide, respectively.
PB, Protein binding; $t_{1/2}$, elimination half-life; NA, not applicable; UA, unavailable; UK, unknown; BioA, bioavailability.

TABLE 30–3. DRUG-DRUG INTERACTIONS OF SELECTED ANTINEOPLASTIC DRUGS

Drug	Interactive Drug	Interaction
Alkylating Drugs		
Alkylating drugs in general	Antineoplastic drugs Radiation therapy	Additive bone marrow suppression
	Live virus vaccines	May decrease the antibody response to and risk of adverse effects of interactive drug
Carboplatin, cisplatin	Aminoglycosides Amphotericin B Vancomycin	Increased risk of nephrotoxicity of cisplatin and carboplatin
	Aminoglycosides Furosemide	Increased risk of ototoxicity
Carmustine	Smoking	Increased risk of pulmonary toxicity
Cyclophosphamide	Phenobarbital Rifampin	May increase the toxicity of cyclophosphamide
	Allopurinol	May exaggerate bone marrow depression
	Succinylcholine	Prolonged neuromuscular blockade
	Diuretics	Increased risk of leukopenia
	Insulin	Increased risk of hypoglycemia
	Cytarabine Daunorubicin Doxorubicin	Additive cardiotoxicity
	Warfarin	May potentiate effects of interactive drug
	Adrenocorticosteroids Azathioprine Chlorambucil Cyclosporine Mercaptopurine	Increased risk of infection and further development of neoplasms
	Probenecid Sulfinpyrazone	Hyperuricemia and gout may develop
	Cocaine	Prolongs the effects of cocaine
Dacarbazine	Phenobarbital Phenytoin	May increase biotransformation of dacarbazine and decrease effectiveness
Melphalan	Carmustine	Increased risk of pulmonary toxicity
	Cyclosporin	Increased risk of renal failure
	Nalidixic acid	Increased risk of enterocolitis
Streptozocin	Aminoglycosides	Increased risk of nephrotoxicity
	Phenytoin	Increased risk of toxicity to streptozocin
	Doxorubicin	Increased risk of toxicity to doxorubicin
Thiotepa	Succinylcholine	Prolonged neuromuscular blockade
Antimetabolites		
Methotrexate	Aspirin NSAIDs	Decreased renal elimination of methotrexate and increased risk of toxicity
	Leucovorin	Decreased methotrexate cytotoxicity
	Probenecid	Increased methotrexate protein displacement and increased toxicity
	Sulfonamides	Additive enzyme inhibition and increased toxicity
Floxuridine	Dexamethasone	Decreased floxuridine hepatotoxicity
Fluorouracil	Allopurinol	Decreased fluorouracil toxicity
	Cimetidine	Increased serum concentration of fluorouracil
	α-Interferon Leucovorin Methotrexate	Increased toxicity to fluorouracil
Cytarabine	Digoxin	Decreased serum levels of interactive drug
Mercaptopurine	Allopurinol	Biotransformation of mercaptopurine inhibited with increased risk of toxicity
	Non-depolarizing muscle relaxants	Decreased neuromuscular blockade
	Warfarin	Potentiates or antagonizes activity
Thioguanine	Myelosuppressants	Increased risk of toxicity, bleeding, hepatotoxicity
Antitumor Antibiotics		
Antitumor antibiotics in general	Antineoplastic drugs Radiation	Increased risk of pulmonary and hematologic toxicity
	Live virus vaccines	May decrease antibody response and increase risk of adverse effects
Bleomycin	Cisplatin	Decreased elimination of bleomycin and increased risk of toxicity
Dactinomycin	Doxorubicin	May increase the risk of cardiotoxicity
Daunorubicin	Cyclophosphamide	Increased risk of cardiotoxicity
Doxorubicin	Cyclophosphamide	May increase risk of hemorrhagic cystitis from cyclophosphamide
	Mercaptopurine	May increase risk of hepatitis from mercaptopurine
	Cyclophosphamide Radiation	May increase risk of cardiotoxicity
Mitomycin	Vinblastine Vincristine	Increased risk of respiratory toxicity

Table continued on following page

TABLE 30–3. DRUG-DRUG INTERACTIONS OF SELECTED ANTINEOPLASTIC DRUGS *Continued*

Drug	Interactive Drug	Interaction
Antitumor Antibiotics *Continued*		
	Vindesine	
	Vinorelbine	
Plicamycin	Aspirin	Increased risk of bleeding
	Cephalosporins (some)	
	Dextran	
	Heparin	
	NSAIDs	
	Sulfinpyrazone	
	Thrombolytic drugs	
	Valproic acid	
	Warfarin	
	Aminoglycosides	Increased risk of hepatotoxicity
	Amphotericin B	
	Vancomycin	
	Nephrotoxic drugs	Increased risk of nephrotoxicity
Mitotic Inhibitors		
Mitotic inhibitors in general	Antineoplastic drugs	Additive bone marrow depression
	Radiation therapy	
	Live virus vaccines	May decrease antibody response and increase risk of adverse effects
Docetaxel	Cyclosporine	May significantly alter the effects of docetaxel
	Ketoconazole	
	Erythromycin	
	Troleandomycin	
Irinotecan	Laxatives	May exacerbate diarrhea
	Diuretics	May increase the risk of dehydration if diarrhea occurs
	Dexamethasone	May increase the risk of hyperglycemia and lymphocytopenia if interactive drug is used as antiemetic
	Prochlorperazine	May increase the risk of akathisia if given the same day
Mitoxantrone	Dactinomycin	Increased risk of cardiomyopathy with previous use of interactive drugs
	Doxorubicin	
	Idarubicin	
Paclitaxel	Ketoconazole	May inhibit biotransformation of paclitaxel and increase the risk of serious toxicity
Teniposide	Antineoplastic drugs	Increased myelosuppression
	Radiation	
	Sodium salicylate	
	Sulfamethizole	
	Tolbutamide	
Topotecan	G-CSF	Prolonged neutropenia
Vinblastine	Mitomycin	Bronchospasm may occur in patients previously treated with interactive drug
Vincristine	L-Asparaginase	May decrease hepatic biotransformation of vincristine
Vinorelbine	Cisplatin	Increased risk and severity of myelosuppression
	Mitomycin	Increased risk of acute pulmonary reactions
	Radiation to chest	
Miscellaneous		
Hydroxyurea	Antineoplastic drugs	Additive bone marrow suppression
	Radiation	
	Live virus vaccines	May decrease antibody response and increase risk of adverse effects
L-Asparaginase	Vincristine	Decreases hepatic clearance of vincristine
	Methotrexate	Effects of methotrexate are diminished
	Prednisone	Increased toxicity to L-asparaginase
Mitotane	Phenytoin	Hepatic cytochrome enzyme stimulated with decreased effectiveness of interactive drugs
	Warfarin	
	Alcohol	Additive CNS depression
	Antihistamines	
	Antidepressants	
	Opioids	
	Sedative-hypnotics	
	Spironolactone	May block the effects of mitotane in Cushing's disease
Pegaspargase	Anticoagulants	May alter response to interactive drug
	Antiplatelet drugs	
Procarbazine	Alcohol	Additive CNS depression
	Antidepressants	
	Antihistamines	
	Opioids	
	Sedative-hypnotics	
	Alcohol	Disulfiram-like reaction

TABLE 30–3. DRUG-DRUG INTERACTIONS OF SELECTED ANTINEOPLASTIC DRUGS *Continued*

Drug	Interactive Drug	Interaction
Miscellaneous *Continued*		
	Antidepressants Levodopa Local anesthetics Guanethidine Guanadrel Reserpine Sympathomimetic amines Vasoconstrictors	Increased risk of severe hypertensive episodes since procarbazine contains some monoamine oxidase inhibitory properties
	Meperidine Opioid analgesics	Severe paradoxical reactions
	Carbamazepine Fluoxetine MAO inhibitors Tricyclic antidepressants	Increased risk of seizure and hyperpyrexia
	Antineoplastic drugs Radiation	Additive bone marrow suppression
	Insulin Oral hypoglycemic drugs	May potentiate hypoglycemia

CNS, Central nervous system; G-CSF, granulocyte colony stimulating factor; NSAIDs, nonsteroidal anti-inflammatory drugs; MAO, Monoamine oxidase.

antineoplastic drugs and radiation therapy to increase the risk of bone marrow suppression. The antibody response to live virus vaccines is decreased and the risk of adverse effects to the alkylating drug increases. Cyclophosphamide carries the largest number of drug-drug interactions.

Dosage Regimen

Alkylating drug dosages are usually based on the patient's body weight (mg/kg) or surface area (mg/m^2). The usual doses listed for individual drugs apply only if monotherapy is used (Table 30–4). With multidrug therapy, the dosage of each drug is individualized based on patient needs. The dosage is reduced in the presence of bone marrow suppression (as evidenced by leukopenia or thrombocytopenia) and in the presence of liver or kidney impairment.

Laboratory Considerations

Alkylating drugs cause bone marrow suppression; therefore, careful attention must be paid to monitoring blood cell counts. White blood cell counts less than 500/mm^3, platelet counts less than 50,000/mm^3, and hematocrit values less than 28 mg/dL must be reported to the health care provider. Additionally, liver function tests, BUN, and creatinine must be carefully monitored because these drugs are biotransformed in the liver and eliminated by the liver and kidneys. Any alteration in the functioning of these organs could alter the action and toxicity of the alkylating drug.

Serum alanine aminotransferase (ALT; serum glutamic-pyruvic transaminase [SGPT]), aspartate aminotransferase (AST; serum glutamic-oxaloacetic transaminase [SGOT]), bilirubin, alkaline phosphatase, lactate dehydrogenase (LDH), uric acid levels, BUN, creatinine, and electrolyte values should be monitored prior to and periodically throughout alkylating drug therapy. Busulfan may cause elevated uric acid levels and produce false-positive cytology results of breast, bladder, cervix, and lung tissues. Carboplatin may cause decreased serum sodium, potassium, calcium, and magnesium concentrations. Cisplatin may cause positive Coomb's test. Cyclophosphamide may suppress positive reactions to skin tests for *Candida,* mumps, *Trichophyton,* and tuberculin purified protein derivative (PPD) tests. It may also produce false-positive results in PAP smears. Melphalan may cause elevated 5-hydroxyindoleacetic acid (5-HIAA) concentrations as a result of tumor breakdown. Serum glucose levels should be monitored prior to and after the initial dose of streptozocin due to the risk of hypoglycemia and then periodically throughout therapy.

Antimetabolites

FOLIC ACID ANALOGS

- ❒ Methotrexate (FOLEX, MEXATE, MEXATE AQ, MTX, RHEUMATREX); (❋) FOLEX, MEXATE

PURINE ANALOGS

- ❒ Cladribine (LEUSTATIN)
- ❒ Fludarabine (FLUDARA); (❋) FLUDARA
- ❒ Mercaptopurine (PURINETHOL); (❋) PURINETHOL
- ❒ Pentostatin (NIPENT)
- ❒ Thioguanine (LANVIS); (❋) LANVIS

PYRIMIDINE ANALOGS

- ❒ Cytarabine (ARA-C, CYTOSAR-U, TARABINE); (❋) CYTOSAR
- ❒ Fluorouracil (ADRUCIL, EFUDEX); (❋) ADRUCIL, EFUDEX, FLUOROPLEX
- ❒ Gemcitabine (GEMZAR); (❋) GEMZAR

Indications

Antimetabolites structurally resemble naturally occurring metabolites within a cell. The antimetabolite drugs are divided into three categories: folic acid analogs, purine analogs, and pyrimidine analogs. The names of these subclasses are derived from the metabolite affected by the antimetabolite agent.

TABLE 30–4. DOSAGE REGIMEN OF SELECTED ANTINEOPLASTIC DRUGS*

Drug	Use(s)	Dosage	Implications
Alkylating Drugs			
Busulfan	CML, ANLL	4–8 mg/day po for several weeks	Administer either 1 hour before or 2 hours after meals
Carboplatin	Ovarian, head and neck, testicular, and lung cancers	360 mg/m^2 IV on day 1 of therapy	Do not confuse with cisplatin. Do not use aluminum needles or equipment during preparation or administration, because the aluminum reacts with the drug
Carmustine	Brain tumors, multiple myeloma, Hodgkin's disease, non-Hodgkin's lymphoma, melanoma, colorectal, stomach, liver cancers	150–200 mg/m^2 IV q6wks as a single dose or divided daily injections (75–100 mg/m^2 on 2 successive days)	Withhold dose and notify health care provider if platelet count is less than 100,000/mm^3 or leukocyte count is below 4000/mm^3. Anemia is usually mild
Chlorambucil	CLL, malignant lymphomas, breast cancer, hair cell leukemia, multiple myeloma, ovarian, testicular, trophoblastic neoplasms	4–8 mg/m^2/day po × 3–6 weeks	Neutrophil count may decrease for 10 days after the last dose. Administer either 1 hour before or 2 hours after meals
Cisplatin	Testicular, ovarian cancer, transitional cell bladder cancer, cancers of the brain, adrenal cortex, breast, endometrium, cervical, and uterine cancer, trophoblastic neoplasms, head and neck, esophagus, lung, melanoma, non-Hodgkin's lymphoma, osteosarcoma, prostate, stomach	Dosages vary depending on condition Testicular cancer: 20 mg/m^2/day IV × 5 days q3 weeks for 3 courses	Used concurrently with other drugs for testicular cancer. Withhold drug if WBC is less than 4000/mm^3 or platelet count is less than 100,000/mm^3
Cyclophosphamide	Non-Hodgkin's lymphoma, Hodgkin's disease, myeloma, cutaneous T-cell lymphoma, neuroblastoma, adenocarcinoma of ovary and breast, ALL, ANLL, bladder, cervical, endometrium, CML, Ewing's sarcoma, head and neck, lung, osteosarcoma, testicular, Wilm's tumor, sarcomas, prostate, rhabdomyosarcoma, retinoblastoma, trophoblastic neoplasms	1–5 mg/kg/day po *or* 60–120 mg/m^2 *or* 40–50 mg/kg IV in divided doses over 2–5 days up to 100 mg/kg initially, then 10–15 mg/kg IV q7–10 days *or* 3–5 mg twice weekly High-dose bone marrow transplant: 1.8–7 g/m^2	Administer oral drug on empty stomach. Adjust dose with renal function
Dacarbazine	Malignant melanoma, Hodgkin's disease, islet cell carcinoma, neuroblastoma, soft tissue sarcoma	Malignant melanoma: 2–4.5 mg/kg/day IV × 10 days. Repeat at 4-week intervals Hodgkin's disease: 150 mg/m^2/day IV × 5 days. Repeat every 4 weeks. Used concurrently with other drugs	Platelet counts should be monitored throughout therapy. Solution is colorless or clear yellow. Do not use solution that has turned pink
Altretamine	Persistent or recurrent ovarian cancer	240–320 mg/m^2/day po	Single-agent use for this disorder
Ifosfamide	Germ cell testicular cancer	1.2 g/m^2/day IV × 5 days. Coadminister with mesna. May repeat cycle q3 weeks	Used in combination with other agents. Mesna helps to prevent drug-induced hemorrhagic cystitis
Lomustine	Brain tumors, Hodgkin's disease, breast, lung, colorectal, kidney, melanoma, myeloma, non-Hodgkin's lymphoma	100–130 mg/m^2 po q6–8 weeks	Considered secondary therapy and used in combination with other antineoplastic drugs for Hodgkin's disease. Myelosuppression is cumulative
Mechlorethamine	Hodgkin's disease, lymphosarcoma, CML, CLL, polycythemia vera, mycosis fungoides, bronchogenic cancer, palliative treatment of metastatic cancer resulting in effusion, brain tumors	Hodgkin's disease: 6 mg/m^2 IV on day 1 and 8 of a 28-day cycle Other neoplasms: 0.4 mg/kg given as single dose *or* in divided doses of 0.1–0.2 mg/kg/day. May repeat course in 3–6 weeks	Nausea and vomiting may occur 1–3 hours after therapy. Vomiting may persist for 8 hours. Nausea may persist for 24 hours. Parenteral antiemetic drugs should be given 30–45 minutes before therapy
Melphalan	Multiple myeloma, nonresectable epithelial ovarian cancer, breast, testes, thyroid	0.1–0.15 mg/kg/day po × 2–3 weeks. May be taken in divided doses or as a single daily dose	Reduce dose with hepatic or renal impairment
Steptozocin	Metastatic islet cell cancer, carcinoid tumors, Hodgkin's disease, pancreatic carcinoma	500 mg/m^2 IV × 5 consecutive days every 6 weeks until maximum benefit reached *or* 1000 mg/m^2 IV weekly for 2 weeks, then dosage adjusted depending on patient response	Solution is pale gold. Do not use if dark brown. IV dextrose should be readily available as hypoglycemia may occur in response to initial dose

TABLE 30–4. DOSAGE REGIMEN OF SELECTED ANTINEOPLASTIC DRUGS* *Continued*

Drug	Use(s)	Dosage	Implications
Alkylating Drugs *Continued*			
Thiotepa	Adenocarcinoma of breast or ovary, intracavitary effusions, superficial papillary bladder cancer, lymphoma, Hodgkin's disease, lung cancer	0.3–0.4 mg/kg IV rapid infusion at intervals of 1–4 weeks	May also be administered by intracavitary or intravesicular routes. Discontinue or reduce dose at first sign of sudden large decrease in leukocyte or platelet count
Antimetabolites			
Cladribine	Hairy cell leukemia, advanced cutaneous T-cell lymphoma, CLL, non-Hodgkin's lymphoma, AML, mycosis fungoides or Sezary syndrome, autoimmune hemolytic anemia	0.09–0.1 mg/kg/day IV × 7 days	Monitor platelet count throughout therapy. Avoid administering IM injections and taking rectal temperatures. Anemia may occur. Transfusions of platelets and RBCs may be necessary
Cytarabine	ANLL, ALL, CML, meningeal leukemia, Hodgkin's and non-Hodgkin's lymphoma	200 mg/m^2 IV over 24 hours *or* 100 mg/m^2 daily by continuous infusion × 5–10 days	May also be administered subcutaneously and by intrathecal route
Fludarabine	B-cell CLL that is unresponsive to standard therapy, non-Hodgkin's lymphoma	25 mg/m^2 daily × 5 days. Repeat course every 28 days	Assess for mental status changes throughout therapy and up to 60 days following therapy. Therapy may be discontinued if neurotoxicity occurs
Fluorouracil	Carcinoma of stomach, colon, rectum, breast, pancreas, bladder, cervix, endometrium, esophagus, head and neck, islet cell, liver, lung, ovary, prostate	12 mg/kg/day IV × 4 consecutive days up to 800 mg or until toxicity develops or 12 days of therapy has been reached. May repeat at 1-month intervals	If toxicity develops, 15 mg/kg once per week can be given until toxicity subsides
	Premalignant actinic keratoses and superficial skin cancers	Apply topical cream to affected area BID × 3–6 weeks	Inspect involved skin before and throughout the course of therapy
Floxuridine	GI adenocarcinoma metastatic to liver, ANLL, ALL, bladder, brain, breast, cervix, gall bladder, head and neck, kidney, ovary, prostate	0.1–0.6 mg/kg/day by intra-arterial route	Close attention to intra-arterial IV site is vital
Gemcitabine	Locally advanced metastatic cancer of pancreas in patients who have previously received fluorouracil	1000 mg/m^2 IV over 30 minutes once weekly for up to 7 weeks or until bone marrow suppression requires withholding treatment. Subsequent cycles of once weekly × 3 consecutive weeks out of 4 can be given after 1 week of rest from treatment	Patients who require further therapy and have not experienced severe toxicity may be given 25% larger dose with careful monitoring
Mercaptopurine	Remission induction and maintenance therapy for ALL, ANLL, CML, non-Hodgkin's lymphoma	80–100 mg/m^2/day po × 5 days	Reduce dose in presence of hepatic or renal dysfunction
Methotrexate	Choriocarcinoma, hydatidiform mole prophylaxis and treatment of meningeal lymphocytic leukemia, breast cancer, epidermoid cancers of head and neck, lung cancer, non-Hodgkin's lymphoma, osteosarcoma, psoriasis (severe, recalcitrant, disabling), rheumatoid arthritis (second- or third-line treatment), ANLL, bladder, brain, cervix, cutaneous T-cell lymphoma, esophagus, kidney, myeloma, ovary, prostate, rhabdomyosarcoma, stomach, testes	Trophoblastic neoplasms: 15–30 mg/day po/IM/IV × 5 days. Repeat q12 weeks for 3–5 courses Leukemia induction: 3.3 mg/m^2/day IM/IV Leukemia maintenance: 20–30 mg/m^2 twice weekly Rheumatoid arthritis: 2.5–5 mg po q12 hr × 3 doses each week or 7.5 mg po once weekly	May also be given by intrathecal route
Pentostatin	Hairy cell leukemia	4 mg/m^2 IV every other week	May be administered undiluted. Monitor for anaphylaxis
Thioguanine	ALL, CML, remission induction, consolidation, and maintenance therapy for ANLL	80–100 mg/m^2 po QD at HS	May also be divided into two doses and given 12 hours apart
Antitumor Antibiotics			
Bleomycin	Disseminated nonseminomatous testicular cancer, disseminated seminomatous testicular cancer, Hodgkin's disease, squamous cell head and neck cancers, skin, penis, cervix, vulva	10–20 units/m^2 IM/IV/SC once or twice weekly for a total dose of 300–400 units *or* 15 units/m^2/day IV over 24 hours × 4–5 days Intra-arterial infusion for squamous cell cancer of head and neck: 30–60 units/day IV over 1–24 hours	Used in combination with vinblastine and cisplatin (VBP) for testicular cancers. Also used in combination with doxorubicin, vinblastine, and dacarbazine (ABVD) as alternatives to mechlorethamine, vincristine, procarbazine, and prednisone (MOPP) for Hodgkin's disease

Table continued on following page

TABLE 30–4. DOSAGE REGIMEN OF SELECTED ANTINEOPLASTIC DRUGS* ***Continued***

Drug	Use(s)	Dosage	Implications
Antitumor Antibiotics ***Continued***			
Bleomycin *Continued*		Intrapleural infusion for malignant pleural effusion: instill 15–120 units in 100 mL of 0.9% sodium chloride and allow to dwell × 24 hours	
Dactinomycin	Wilms' tumor, rhabdomyosarcoma, Ewing's sarcoma, osteosarcoma, Kaposi sarcoma, choriocarcinoma, testicular carcinoma	0.01–0.015 mg/kg/day IV × 5 days every 4–6 weeks *or* 0.5 mg/m^2 IV once a week × 3 weeks *Children:* 0.01–0.015 mg/kg/day IV × 5 days *or* a total dose of 2.5 mg/m^2 IV in divided doses over 7 days. May repeat every 4–6 weeks	Used in combination with surgery, radiation, and combinations with vincristine for Wilm's tumor Is also used in combination with chlorambucil and methotrexate in metastatic testicular cancer, although it is not as satisfactory as the VBP combination
Daunorubicin	ALL, AML	30–60 mg/m^2/day IV × 3 days. Repeat at 3–6 week intervals	Do not confuse with doxorubicin. Administer over at least 2–3 minutes. Rapid administration may cause facial flushing or erythema along the vein
Doxorubicin	Hodgkin's disease, non-Hodgkin's lymphoma, ALL, AML, osteogenic sarcoma, Ewing's sarcoma, rhabdomyosarcoma, metastatic thyroid cancer, endometrium, ovary, testes, prostate, stomach, lung, pancreas, bladder, neuroblastomas, Wilm's tumor	20 mg/m^2/week IV	May also be given by intra-arterial and intraperitoneal routes
Idarubicin	Induction therapy in adults with AML	12 mg/m^2 IV daily × 3 days	Given by slow IV injection in combination with cytarabine
Mitomycin	Disseminated adenocarcinoma of stomach or pancreas	10–20 mg/m^2 IV q6–8 weeks	Ensure patency of IV. Extravasation may cause severe tissue necrosis
Plicamycin	Hypercalcemia, hypercalciuria	0.015–0.025 mg/kg/day IV × 3–4 days. May repeat at 1-week intervals	Ensure patency of IV. Extravasation may cause irritation and cellulitis. Apply ice to site to prevent pain and swelling
Mitotic Inhibitors			
Amsacrine	AML	—	Severe toxicity limits use
Docetaxel	Advanced breast cancer	60–100 mg/m^2 IV over 1 hour every 3 weeks	An analog of paclitaxel
Etoposide	Refractory testicular tumors, small cell lung cancer, Kaposi's sarcoma	50–100 mg/m^2/day IV × 5 days	Used in combination with cyclophosphamide for small cell lung cancer
Irinotecan	Colon and breast cancer, small cell lung cancer, leukemia	125 mg/m^2 IV weekly × 4	Monitor closely for early and late onset diarrhea. Avoid extravasation
Mitoxantrone	ANLL induction	12 mg/m^2/day on days 1, 2, and 3 with cytarabine given over 24 hours on days 1–7	Cytarabine is given as continuous infusion
Paclitaxel	Advanced ovarian cancer, breast cancer, advanced non-small-cell cancer, squamous cell carcinoma of the head and neck	135 mg/m^2 IV over 24 hours every 3 weeks *or* 175 mg/m^2 IV over 3 hours every 3 weeks	Monitor vital signs frequently, especially during first hour of 24 hours of infusion. Monitor cardiovascular status
Teniposide	Refractory ALL in children	165 mg/m^2 IV in combination with 300 mg/m^2 cytarabine twice weekly × 8–9 doses	Avoid contact with skin. Use Luer-Lok tubing to prevent accidental leakage Do not use polyvinyl chloride IV bags
Topotecan	Refractory colorectal cancer, head and neck cancers, malignant glioma	1.5 mg/m^2 IV × 5 days every 21 days	Monitor platelet count. Anemia commonly occurs. Assess IV site for extravasation
Vinblastine	Testicular cancer (VBP), Hodgkin's disease (ABVD as alternative to MOPP), breast cancer, neuroblastomas, histiocytosis X, Kaposi sarcoma, lymphomas refractory to alkylating drugs and choriocarcinomas refractory to methotrexate	2 mg/m^2/day IV × 5 days *or* as part of VBP regimen, 4–8 mg/m^2 days 1 and 2. Repeat cycle q21–28 days	Administer over 15 to 30 minutes. Administering over a longer period or with more diluent may increase irritation of the vein
Vincristine	ALL, Hodgkin's disease, Burkitt's lymphoma, rhabdomyosarcoma, lung, breast, cervical carcinoma, neuroblastoma, Wilm's tumor	*Adults:* 0.4–1.4 mg/m^2 IV q7 days as a single dose *Child weighing more than 10 kg:* 1.5–2 mg/m^2 IV q7 days as a single dose	Do not administer SC, IM, or IT. Intrathecal administration is fatal. Overwrap of solution should remain in place until immediately before administration

TABLE 30–4. DOSAGE REGIMEN OF SELECTED ANTINEOPLASTIC DRUGS* *Continued*

Drug	Use(s)	Dosage	Implications
Mitotic Inhibitors ***Continued***			
Vinorelbine	Unresectable advanced non-small-cell lung cancer	30 mg/m^2 IV as a single dose, given once weekly or with cisplatin 120 mg/m^2 on days 1 and 29 and then every 6 weeks	Used in combination with cisplatin. Reduce dose with hepatic impairment
Miscellaneous			
Hydroxyurea	CML, malignant melanoma, metastatic or inoperable ovarian cancer, head and neck cancer	Intermittent therapy: 80 mg/kg po as single dose q3 days Continuous therapy: 20–30 mg/kg/day po as a single dose Concomitant therapy with radiation: 80 mg/kg po as single dose q3 days	Used in combination with radiation therapy for head and neck cancers
L-Asparaginase	Remission induction in pediatric ALL	Example of regimen: L-asparaginase 1000 IU/kg/day IV × 10 days starting day 22	Used in combination with vincristine 2 mg/m^2 IV once weekly on days 1, 8, and 15 and prednisone 40 mg/m^2/day in 3 divided doses × 15 days, then 20 mg/m^2 × 2 days, 10 mg/m^2 × 2 days, 5 mg/m^2 × 2 days, then 2.5 mg/m^2 × 2 days
Mitotane	Palliation of inoperable cancer of adrenal cortex	2–6 g/day po in divided doses TID or QID	Premedication with an antiemetic drug may be required
Pegaspargase	ALL patients who are sensitive to asparaginase	2500 IU/m^2 IM (preferred route) *or* IV q14 days	Assess patient for previous hypersensitivity to L-asparaginase
Procarbazine	Advanced Hodgkin's disease (MOPP), primary and metastatic brain tumors, small-cell lung cancer	2–4 mg/kg/day po × 7 days. Maintain dose at 4–6 mg/kg/day until WBC count falls below 4000 mm^3 or platelets drop below 100,000 mm^3; then stop drug	May resume treatment once hematologic recovery has occurred

*Health care providers are advised to consult definitive sources of information for uses and appropriate dosages of antineoplastic drugs. Some drugs are not yet FDA approved for the identified uses.

Abbreviations: ABVD, Doxorubicin, bleomycin, vinblastine, dacarbazine; ALL, acute lymphocytic leukemia; AML, acute myelocytic leukemia; ANLL, acute nonlymphocytic leukemia; CML, chronic myelocytic leukemia; GI, gastrointestinal; MOPP, mechlorethamine, vincristine (ONCOVIN), procarbazine, prednisone; VBP, vinblastine, bleomycin, cisplatin; WBC, white blood cell.

The antimetabolites have been used to treat the entire spectrum of cancers. The effectiveness of the individual drugs varies with the different kinds of cancer.

Pharmacodynamics

Antimetabolites are CCS within the S phase. To be effective, the drugs that are S-phase specific must be present for an extended period. The antimetabolites are structural analogs (i.e., folic acid, pyrimidine, purines) of important, naturally occurring metabolites within a cell. The cell incorporates the folic acid, pyrimidine (e.g., cytosine, thymine, uracil), or purine (e.g., adenine, guanine, hypoxanthine) analog into itself during cellular metabolism, disrupting critical metabolic processes. Thus, the neoplastic cell is unable to continue dividing, resulting in cell death. For example, methotrexate competitively inhibits dihydrofolate reductase, the enzyme that reduces dihydrofolic acid to tetrahydrofolic acid. Tetrahydrofolic acid is then transformed to a variety of coenzymes that are required for one-carbon transfer reactions. The reaction most sensitive to lack of a coenzyme is the conversion of deoxyuridylate to thymidylate, an essential component of DNA. By inhibiting dihydrofolate reductase, methotrexate causes an intracellular accumulation of inactive oxidized folates, leading to inhibition of protein synthesis, thymidylate, DNA, and RNA.

Various therapeutic strategies have been recommended to avoid selection of resistant cells and heighten the effects of methotrexate. A technique known as LEUCOVORIN RESCUE (Jaffee regimen) is commonly used. Some neoplastic cells are resistant to methotrexate because they lack the transport mechanism required for active uptake of the drug. By giving mammoth doses, the drug is forced into the cells via passive diffusion. However, since this strategy also subjects normal cells to extremely high levels of methotrexate, these cells are also affected by the drug. In order to save the normal cells, leucovorin is given. Leucovorin bypasses the metabolic impedance caused by methotrexate, thus permitting normal cells to synthesize thymidylate and other compounds. Cancer cells are not affected because leucovorin uptake requires the same transport system as methotrexate, a transport system that these cells lack.

Tumor resistance to methotrexate occurs as a result of decreased uptake of methotrexate or an increased synthesis of dihydrofolate reductase. Resistance may also occur as a result of the synthesis of a modified form of dihydrofolate reductase that has a reduced affinity for the drug.

Pyrimidine analogs, because of their structural similarity to naturally occurring pyrimidines (i.e., cytosine, thymine, uracil), act in several ways. They can inhibit the biosynthesis of pyrimidines, inhibit the biosynthesis of DNA and RNA, and undergo incorporation into DNA and RNA. All of the pyrimidine analogs are prodrugs that must be converted to active metabolites for drug action to take place. Cytarabine is a nucleoside analog of cytosine. It is a prodrug that requires phosphorylation to produce the active monophosphate product and subsequently a triphosphate. Gemcitabine is a cytidine analog, similar to cytarabine in that it is a prodrug, is deaminated, and is activated by cytidine deoxyribose kinase. It too inhibits DNA synthesis. The triphosphate form of gemcitabine is retained intracellularly much longer than cytarabine. Gemcitabine is active throughout the cell cycle.

Purine analogs (i.e., adenine, guanine, hypoxanthine), like the pyrimidines, are bases used in the biosynthesis of nucleic acids. The purine analogs act to reduce purine levels in tumor cells. This reduction is achieved in a number of ways. The ribonucleotide 6-mercaptopurine inhibits de novo purine biosynthesis, thus inhibiting the first step in purine synthesis. It does this by mimicking the purine nucleoside, glutamine 5-phosphoribosylpyrophosphate aminotransferase. Azathioprine, a widely used immunosuppressant, is a prodrug of mercaptopurine (see also Chapter 15).

Adverse Effects and Contraindications

The toxic effects of antimetabolites primarily involve the bone marrow, epithelial lining of the GI tract, and hair follicles. Nausea, vomiting, and stomatitis occur with many of the antimetabolite drugs. Death can result from intestinal perforation and hemorrhagic enteritis, particularly with methotrexate. High doses can cause direct injury to the kidneys. Neurologic symptoms, including ataxia, confusion, and coma, may occur. Patients taking fludarabine, methotrexate, or pentostatin are at risk for pulmonary hypersensitivity and pulmonary fibrosis. Pentostatin has also been linked with anaphylaxis and myocardial infarction. It causes a dose-related profound immunosuppression due to T-cell cytolysis, somnolence, and coma. Approximately 30 to 40 percent of patients have decreased renal function after receiving pentostatin. Hepatotoxicity is possible with mercaptopurine.

Methotrexate should be used with caution in patients with peptic ulcer disease, ulcerative colitis, impaired renal or hepatic function, aplasia, leukopenia, thrombocytopenia, bone marrow suppression, or anemia. Fluorouracil should be used with caution in patients who have undergone high-dose pelvic radiation or therapy with alkylating drugs. The administration of live virus vaccines during treatment with fluorouracil should be avoided since it suppresses normal defense mechanisms and may increase replication of the virus, causing adverse effects.

Pharmacokinetics

Intravenous administration of antimetabolite drugs results in complete bioavailability. Orally administered drugs are variably absorbed following administration (see Table 30–2). The drugs are widely distributed, with some of the drugs minimally crossing the blood-brain barrier. Antimetabolites are generally biotransformed in the liver and excreted in the kidneys.

Drug-Drug Interactions

Drug-drug interactions with antimetabolite drugs are identified in Table 30–3. In many cases, antimetabolite drugs increase the risks of myelosuppression when they are used with other antineoplastic drugs.

Dosage Regimen

Although there is no exact way to determine precisely when a drug is likely to be most effective (i.e., kill the largest number of cancer cells), information has been obtained empirically. Thus, dosage recommendations and schedules should be followed as closely as possible for maximal effectiveness. Like with the alkylating drugs, antimetabolite drug dosages are usually based on the patient's body weight (mg/kg) or surface area (mg/m^2) (see Table 30–4). The usual doses listed for individual drugs apply only if monotherapy is used. With multidrug therapy, the dosage of each drug is individualized based on patient needs. The dosage is reduced in the presence of bone marrow suppression (as evidenced by leukopenia or thrombocytopenia) and in the presence of liver or kidney impairment.

Laboratory Considerations

Antimetabolites produce myelosuppression; thus routine monitoring of complete blood count (CBC), white blood cell (WBC), and platelet counts is important prior to and periodically throughout therapy. Serum ALT (SGPT), AST (SGOT), bilirubin, alkaline phosphatase, LDH, uric acid levels, BUN, creatinine, and electrolyte values should be monitored prior to and periodically throughout antimetabolite drug therapy. Urinary pH should be monitored for patients taking high-dose methotrexate therapy and every 6 hours during leucovorin rescue. Urine pH should be kept above 7.0 to prevent renal damage. Bone marrow aspiration and biopsy may be required every 2 to 3 months for patients receiving pentostatin to assess response to therapy. Fluorouracil may cause an increase in urinary excretion of 5-HIAA. Cytarabine may cause increased uric acid concentrations. Patients with high tumor burdens who are undergoing antineoplastic therapy may also have elevated uric acid levels.

Antitumor Antibiotics

ANTHRACYCLINES
- ❒ Daunorubicin (CERUBIDINE)
- ❒ Doxorubicin (ADRIAMYCIN PFS, ADRIAMYCIN RDF, RUBEX, ADR)
- ❒ Idarubicin (IDAMYCIN)

ANTHRACENEDIONES
- ❒ Mitoxantrone

CHROMOMYCINS
- ❒ Dactinomycin (COSMEGEN)

MISCELLANEOUS ANTITUMOR ANTIBIOTICS
- ❒ Bleomycin (BLENOXANE)
- ❒ Mitomycin (MUTAMYCIN)
- ❒ Plicamycin (MITHRACIN)

Indications

Antitumor antibiotics are derivatives of soil fungus and have some anti-infective activity; however, they are too toxic for this use. The three categories of antitumor antibiotics include the anthracyclines, chromomycins, and miscellaneous drugs.

Pharmacodynamics

The anthracyclines and chromomycins are CCNS drugs. The antitumor antibiotics produce their effects by forming complexes with DNA, thereby inhibiting DNA activity through the process of intercalation. Bleomycin is phase specific to the G_2 and S phases. All active bleomycin compounds bind reduced iron (Fe^{2+}) so their molecular action is not directed at tissues. It acts by producing breaks in single- and double-stranded DNA. These breaks are reflected as DNA chromosomal gaps, deletions, and fragments. These result from a secondary action in which free radical formation from Fe^{2+}-bleomycin-oxygen forms an intercalated complex between DNA strands. The complex catalyzes the reduction of molecular oxygen to superoxide or hydroxyl radicals. This reduction causes breaks in the DNA strands and inhibition of DNA synthesis. There appears to be inhibition of RNA and protein synthesis as well.

Although dactinomycin is a CCNS drug, its activity seems to be greatest in phase G_1 of the cell cycle. It intercalates between adjacent base pairs in DNA and becomes bound to DNA. The intercalation process distorts DNA structure, which in turn prohibits RNA polymerase from using DNA as a template. The result is inhibition of RNA synthesis.

Daunorubicin and doxorubicin are produced by the fungus *Streptomyces peucetius*. The two drugs differ only slightly in chemical structure. These compounds intercalate with DNA, affecting DNA and RNA synthesis. Single- and double-strand breaks occur, as does sister chromatid exchange. Scission of DNA is thought to be mediated either by action of topoisomerase II or by the generation of free radicals. As would be expected of drugs that inhibit DNA function, maximal toxicity occurs during the S phase of the cell cycle. At low concentrations of drug, tumor cells will proceed through the S phase and die in phase G_2.

Free radical formation via electron reduction is a second cytotoxic mechanism. All anthracyclines are quinones capable of producing free radicals, which damage membranes, proteins, and lipids. Glutathione and catalase detoxify the free radical quinones, and the lack of catalase in cardiac tissue is the basis for anthracycline cardiotoxicity. Enzymatic defenses (e.g., superoxide dismutase, catalase) are believed to play an important role in protecting cells against the toxicity of daunorubicin and doxorubicin. Further, it appears that enzymatic defenses can be enhanced with the exogenous intake of antioxidants (e.g., alpha tocopherol).

Mitomycin activity is dependent on bioreductive alkylation under anaerobic, reducing conditions. It needs to be reduced at quinone sites to form unstable intermediates that react monofunctionally at a position on guanine. It is therefore a prodrug. Free radical formation under aerobic conditions may lead to single-strand breaks in DNA, or these may result from unsuccessful alkylation repair.

Mitoxantrone acts by interacting with topoisomerase II and DNA, resulting in breaks in DNA strands. It does not produce free radicals like some other agents.

Adverse Effects and Contraindications

The anthracyclines can cause pulmonary and cardiac toxicities, which are major dose-limiting factors. Anaphylaxis can occur with any of the antitumor antibiotics, particularly if the drug is a derivative of a naturally occurring substance. Alopecia, stomatitis, nausea, and vomiting are also common adverse effects. Most of the antitumor antibiotics are also vesicants. Vesicants are drugs with the potential to cause severe tissue damage when they leak (extravasate) from the vein.

The adverse effects of dactinomycin include nausea, vomiting, stomatitis, dose-limiting myelosuppression, and dermatologic manifestations. As a radiation sensitizer, dactinomycin can produce a severe radiation recall injury.

The adverse effects of daunorubicin and doxorubicin include myelosuppression, mucositis, and stomatitis. Stomatitis is especially likely with doxorubicin and with a continuous infusion rather than with bolus dosing. Cardiotoxicity often leads to irreversible heart failure. Patients with comorbid heart disease, hypertension, and cardiac radiation therapy are at high risk. Cardiotoxicity is a function of peak dose levels.

The adverse effects of bleomycin are confined to the lungs and skin. Pulmonary toxicity is the major problem and is manifested as subacute or chronic interstitial pneumonitis and later pulmonary fibrosis.

Mitoxantrone is an anthracenedione that is less cardiotoxic than anthracyclines. Other adverse effects include extravasation injuries, alopecia, nausea, and a dose-limiting myelosuppression. Overall, the adverse effect profile is much more favorable than that for anthracyclines, especially as it relates to cardiotoxicity. Cardiotoxicity is just as severe as that seen with anthracyclines, but occurs less often.

Pharmacokinetics

The pharmacokinetics of the antitumor antibiotics vary greatly depending on the individual drug. Bleomycin is not absorbed from the GI tract; thus it is given most often IV. It is widely distributed, with concentrations in the skin, lung, peritoneum, kidneys, and lymphatics. Sixty to seventy percent of the drug is eliminated via the kidneys.

IV administration of any antitumor antibiotic results in complete bioavailability. The times of drug onset vary from approximately 1 week to as much as 8 weeks. Peak drug activity is reached in approximately 10 to 14 days. The duration of drug action averages 21 days, although the half-lives of these drugs vary greatly (see Table 30–2).

Drug-Drug Interactions

As with the other antineoplastic drugs, interactions with antitumor antibiotics can be significant if the drugs are used concurrently with other antineoplastic drugs or in patients who are receiving radiation therapy (see Table 30–3). Receipt of live virus vaccines may increase the risk of adverse effects due to inadequate antibody response. The risk of cardiotoxicity increases in patients taking dactinomycin with doxorubicin, daunorubicin with cyclophosphamide, and doxorubicin with cyclophosphamide or radiation. Plicamycin used concurrently in patients with drugs that interfere with platelet function or clotting factors increases the risk of bleeding.

Dosage Regimen

Like alkylating drugs and antimetabolites, the dosages of antitumor antibiotics are calculated based on body weight or body surface area. Table 30–4 provides a selected listing of the antitumor antibiotics along with their uses.

Laboratory Considerations

Antitumor antibiotics produce dose-limiting myelosuppression; thus, routine monitoring of CBC, WBC, and platelet counts is important prior to and periodically throughout therapy. Serum ALT (SGPT), AST (SGOT), bilirubin, alkaline phosphatase, LDH, uric acid levels, BUN, creatinine, and electrolyte values should be monitored prior to and periodically throughout antineoplastic drug therapy.

Mitotic Inhibitors

VINCA ALKALOIDS

- ❒ Vinblastine (VELBAN, VELSAR)
- ❒ Vincristine (ONCOVIN, VINCASAR PFS, VCR)
- ❒ Vindesin (ELDISINE)
- ❒ Vinorelbine (NAVELBINE)

TAXANES

- ❒ Paclitaxel (TAXOL)
- ❒ Docetaxel (TAXOTERE); (🍁) TAXOTERE

TOPOISOMERASE I INHIBITORS

- ❒ Irinotecan (CAMPTOSAR)
- ❒ Topotecan (HYCAMTIN)

TOPOISOMERASE II DERIVATIVES

- ❒ Etoposide (VP-16, VEPESID)
- ❒ Teniposide (VM-26, VUMON)

Indications

Mitotic inhibitors are derivatives of plant extracts and may be grouped into three classes: vinca or plant alkaloids, taxanes, and podophyllotoxins. Vincristine, vinblastine, and vindesin are derived from the periwinkle plant, *Vinca rosea,* and are widely used today. Etoposide and teniposide are semisynthetic compounds derived from podophyllotoxin, a derivative of the mandrake plant. Paclitaxel and docetaxel are derivatives obtained from the bark and needles of yew trees.

Pharmacodynamics

Vinca alkaloids enter cells by nonsaturable energy-dependent membrane transport. They bind to tubulin, inhibiting the formation and assembly of the microtubular components of the mitotic spindle. The inhibition leads to arrest of mitosis in the metaphase portion of the cell cycle. The microtubules are the filaments that move chromosomes during cell division. In the absence of the microtubules, the distribution of chromosomes to daughter cells becomes random, leading to cell death. Although the vinca alkaloids act throughout the cell cycle, they are particularly effective in the last phase or G_2/M phase of the cell cycle. Tumor resistance to vinca alkaloids involves mutations in tubulin-binding sites.

Taxanes, such as paclitaxel and docetaxel, promote the assembly of microtubules but inhibit the disassembly of these structures by stabilizing the tubulin polymers. By inhibiting disassembly of the microtubules, the division in the tumor cells in the M and G_2 phases of the cell cycle is effectively stopped.

Topoisomerase I and II are nuclear enzymes that cleave one (topoisomerase I) or two (topoisomerase II) strands of DNA to allow the DNA to unwind and separate the intertwined segments of DNA. Topoisomerase enzymes are necessary for the completion of mitosis.

Irinotecan and topotecan are topoisomerase I inhibitors that act by creating reversible single-strand breaks in DNA. The drugs bind to the DNA-topoisomerase I complex, thereby preventing repair of strand breaks caused by topoisomerase. Cytotoxicity is believed to result from impaired DNA replication. Thus, the drug effects are manifest during the S phase of the cell cycle.

Structurally, etoposide and teniposide are semisynthetic epipodophyllotoxins. They act by inhibiting topoisomerase II, a DNA enzyme that is responsible for initiating the separation of daughter DNA strands before mitosis. This activity results in permanent cross-linking of DNA strands and eventual cell death. Topoisomerase II plays a key role in the tertiary structure of chromatin. The predominant isoform is tightly cell cycle regulated (i.e., increased in the S phase and increased even further in the M phase). This enzyme can be elevated in neoplastic cells independently of increased proliferation.

Adverse Effects and Contraindications

In terms of adverse effects, vinblastine and vinorelbine are more likely to cause bone marrow suppression and vincristine is more likely to cause peripheral neuropathy. Neutropenia develops in about half of patients treated with vinca alkaloids. Other adverse effects of vinca alkaloids include alopecia, constipation, nausea, and vomiting. Like vinblastine and vincristine, vinorelbine can cause local tissue necrosis if extravasation occurs.

The common adverse effects of topoisomerase I inhibitors include nausea, vomiting, and peripheral neuropathy. Early symptoms of peripheral neuropathy include numbness and paresthesia in the fingers and toes. Higher doses may result in paresthesias, muscle cramps, loss of deep tendon reflexes, and gait disturbances. Failure to reduce the dosage or discontinue the drug may result in permanent neurological damage. Autonomic neuropathy may be manifested as severe constipation, urinary retention or incontinence, and cranial nerve damage, which will eventually resolve after the drug is discontinued. Neurologic damage may also be seen with vinblastine but occurs only with high dosages. Peripheral neuropathy may be more problematic if these drugs are administered in combination with other neurotoxic agents, such as cisplatin.

In addition, topotecan can cause alopecia, nausea, vomiting, diarrhea, stomatitis, abdominal pain, and headache. Two types of diarrhea can occur with irinotecan, early and late. Early diarrhea occurs in half of the patients treated with topotecan, manifesting within 24 hours of the onset of the infusion. Late diarrhea occurs in about 88 percent of the patients, developing 24 hours or more after the infusion. Late diarrhea can be prolonged, causing severe dehydration and electrolyte imbalance.

Serious thrombocytopenia is uncommon in patients treated with irinotecan, although neutropenia occurs 54 percent of the time and anemia 61 percent of the time. Sepsis secondary to neutropenia has resulted in death. Irinotecan can also cause nausea, vomiting, asthenia, alopecia, abdominal discomfort, anorexia, fever, and weight loss. Less common adverse effects include stomatitis, dyspepsia, headache, cough, rhinitis, insomnia, and rash.

The adverse effects of topoisomerase II inhibitors include myelosuppression, especially a dose-limiting neutropenia, but also oral mucositis. Toxicity depends a great deal upon the regimen used. Myelosuppression and toxicity are not cumulative. Other adverse effects of etoposide include alopecia and peripheral neuropathy. Early adverse effects include nausea, vomiting, diarrhea, and fever. Hypotension can occur with rapid IV administration.

Severe hypersensitivity reactions (urticaria, angioedema, bronchospasm, hypotension) have occurred in patients receiving teniposide. Secondary leukemias have developed within 8 years of initial drug exposure. Other adverse effects include nausea, vomiting, diarrhea, and alopecia.

Myelosuppression is the major dose-limiting toxicity for the taxanes. Allergic reactions may occur with any naturally derived substance but are most frequently seen with paclitaxel and docetaxel.

Pharmacokinetics

Vinca alkaloids are poorly absorbed when given by mouth, so they are only given IV (see Table 30–2). They are extensively bound to plasma proteins or tissues but either do not penetrate the blood-brain barrier or do so poorly. Plasma clearance is multiphasic. The vinca alkaloids are primarily biotransformed in the liver and eliminated in the feces, with a small amount eliminated in the urine.

Etoposide and teniposide are well absorbed following IV administration. The drugs are rapidly distributed but do not appear to enter the CSF to a significant degree. Some biotransformation of etoposide takes place in the liver, with the drug eliminated unchanged in the kidneys. About half of teniposide is eliminated via the kidneys, with 10 percent or less eliminated in the stool.

Paclitaxel and docetaxel are completely bioavailable when given IV. The distribution of both drugs is unknown. Both drugs are highly protein bound, with peak drug action noted in 8 to 11 days. The duration of the drugs' effects on blood cell counts ranges from 1 to 3 weeks. Paclitaxel and docetaxel are extensively biotransformed in the liver, with elimination in the stool.

Drug-Drug Interactions

Drugs that interact with the mitotic inhibitors are identified in Table 30–3. Mitotic inhibitors interact with other antineoplastic drugs or radiation therapy to increase myelosuppression. Live virus vaccines given to patients taking a mitotic inhibitor may not produce the desired response, and the risk of adverse effects of the vaccine is increased.

Dosage Regimen

Dosage regimens of antineoplastic drugs are prescribed according to body weight or body surface area. Dosage regimens will also vary according to the age and performance status of the client, as well as diagnosis and treatment protocol. Currently accepted uses and standard dosages are provided in Table 30–4.

Laboratory Considerations

Mitotic inhibitors produce dose-limiting myelosuppression; thus routine monitoring of CBC, WBC, and platelet counts is important prior to and periodically throughout therapy. Serum ALT (SGPT), AST (SGOT), bilirubin, alkaline phosphatase, LDH, uric acid levels, BUN, creatinine, and electrolyte values should be monitored prior to and periodically throughout antineoplastic drug therapy.

Miscellaneous Antineoplastic Drugs

- ❒ Hydroxyurea (HYDREA)
- ❒ L-Asparaginase (ELSPAR)
- ❒ Mitotane (LYSODREN)
- ❒ Pegaspargase (ONCASPAR, PEG-L-ASPARAGINASE)
- ❒ Procarbazine (MATULANE); (🍁) NATULAN

Not all antineoplastic drugs can be neatly categorized into a major classification group, either because the exact mechanism of action is unknown or the chemical structure poorly understood.

HYDROXYUREA

Hydroxyurea is used in the treatment of myeloproliferative disorders, primarily chronic myelocytic leukemia. Hydroxyurea is ordinarily used in combination with radiation therapy in cancers of the head and neck. In some patients hydroxyurea has produced temporary remission of malignant melanoma and metastatic or inoperable ovarian cancer. The drug is CCS for the S phase of the cell cycle and acts by inhibiting the enzyme ribonucleoside diphosphate reductase. This enzyme normally catalyzes the conversion of RNA to DNA. In the absence of the nucleotides, DNA cannot be made.

Myelosuppression is the major adverse effect, although bone marrow recovery occurs quickly after therapy is discontinued. Adverse effects and toxicities of hydroxyurea also include neutropenia, anorexia, nausea and vomiting, alterations in liver function, hyperpigmentation of the skin, and radiation recall reactions.

Hydroxyurea produces additive bone marrow suppression when used with other agents that suppress bone marrow function. It may also decrease the antibody response to and increase the risk of adverse reactions to live virus vaccines.

L-ASPARAGINASE

L-Asparaginase is ordinarily used along with vincristine and prednisone to induce remission of acute lymphocytic leukemia. It is an enzyme derived from culture of either *Escherichia coli* or *Erwinia carotovora* (a plant parasite). L-Asparaginase acts by depriving susceptible cells of asparagine, an essential nutrient. L-Asparaginase catalyzes the hydrolysis of the amino acid asparagine to aspartic acid and ammonia. Thus, the amount of asparagine available to tumor cells is reduced. Most normal tissues synthesize what asparagine they need. The lymphoblast in patients with acute lymphocytic leukemia appears to lack the enzyme asparagine synthetase and cannot convert aspartic acid to asparagine (but it does require asparagine for growth). The asparagine-depleting action interferes with the synthesis of tumor proteins, DNA, and RNA. The drug is probably CCS for the G_1 phase of the cell cycle, but its usefulness is limited by acute hypersensitivity reactions, which are more likely to occur with repeated treatments.

Because normal tissues as well as leukemic cells are sensitive to L-asparaginase, a variety of adverse effects may occur.

L-Asparaginase does not cause alopecia or stomatitis and is rarely associated with bone marrow suppression. However, about 40 percent of patients experience hypersensitivity reactions that range from urticaria to anaphylactic shock. Emergency life support equipment should be readily available before this drug is administered. The incidence of anaphylaxis is greater with IV administration than with IM routes. Neurotoxic reactions are caused by inhibition of protein synthesis in the brain. Reverse encephalopathy, with manifestations ranging from confusion to coma, occurs in about 25 percent of patients.

Thrombosis and hemorrhage have been reported with L-asparaginase because of the drug's effects on clotting factors. Pancreatitis may progress to severe, even fatal, hemorrhagic pancreatitis. Liver function tests are elevated but return to normal when the drug is discontinued. Acute renal insufficiency can be fatal.

L-Asparaginase may negate the antineoplastic activity of methotrexate and enhance the hepatotoxicity of other hepatotoxic drugs. Additive hypoglycemia has been reported when L-asparaginase is used with glucocorticoids. The concurrent IV use of L-asparaginase with or immediately preceding vincristine may result in increased neurotoxicity and hyperglycemia. As with other antineoplastic drugs, L-asparaginase may alter the patient's response to live vaccines by decreasing antibody response and increasing the risk of adverse reactions.

MITOTANE

Mitotane is a structural analog of two insecticides, dichlorodiphenyldichlorothane (DDD) and dichlorodiphenyltrichloroethane (DDT). It is used in the palliation of inoperative carcinoma of the adrenal cortex. The drug is selectively toxic to tumor cells, but normal cells are also damaged. This isomer of the pesticide DDT acts to inhibit corticosteroid biosynthesis. The drug is indicated for the treatment of inoperable adrenal cortical cancer. Adverse reactions and toxicities of this drug include anorexia, nausea, vomiting, diarrhea, skin rash, and gynecomastia in males. Patients receiving this drug should be well hydrated to prevent nephrotoxicity, and periodic monitoring of renal function and CBCs should be done.

The primary adverse effects of mitotane include depression, sedation, lethargy, vertigo, and dizziness. Anorexia, nausea, vomiting, diarrhea, and rash also occur. Adrenal insufficiency develops because of the action of mitotane on the adrenal cortex. Corticosteroid replacement therapy may be necessary. Mitotane does not cause inflammation of the GI tract or bone marrow depression.

Mitotane stimulates hepatic cytochrome enzymes, which may decrease the effectiveness of phenytoin and warfarin. Additive CNS depression is likely if mitotane is used with other CNS depressants, such as alcohol, antihistamines, antidepressants, opioids, or sedative-hypnotics. Spironolactone may block the effects of mitotane in Cushing's syndrome.

PEGASPARGASE

Pegaspargase is used with other drugs in the treatment of acute lymphoblastic leukemia in patients who have had a previous hypersensitivity reaction to L-asparaginase. Pegaspargase consists of L-asparaginase bound to polyethylene glycol (PEG). The two drugs are essentially very similar. They have the same mechanism of drug action and produce the same spectrum of adverse effects, including liver and kidney dysfunction, pancreatitis, coagulopathy, and hypersensitivity reactions.

The polyethylene glycol-pegaspargase depletes asparagine, which leukemic cells cannot synthesize. Normal cells are able to produce their own asparagine and thus are less likely to be affected by asparaginase. Binding to polyethylene glycol renders asparaginase less antigenic, and therefore the drug is less likely to induce hypersensitivity reactions.

As with other antineoplastic drugs, hematologic adverse effects are possible, including leukopenia, pancytopenia, thrombocytopenia, decreased fibrinogen levels, and increased thromboplastin levels. Paresthesia, myalgia, arthralgia, and extremity pain are also common. Seizures and pancreatitis are the most life-threatening adverse effects. Pegaspargase used in conjunction with anticoagulants or antiplatelet drugs increases the risk of bleeding and the response to other drugs that are biotransformed by the liver may be altered.

Pegaspargase may alter the response to anticoagulants or antiplatelet drugs. It may also alter the response to other drugs that are biotransformed by the liver.

PROCARBAZINE

Like dacarbazine, procarbazine is a nonclassical alkylating drug. In and of itself, procarbazine is not cytotoxic or mutagenic. However, it is activated in the liver to an azo intermediate, which is then converted to alkylating azoxy compounds. The molecular mechanism of action is DNA alkylation. Procarbazine is thought to disrupt chromatin arrangement and interfere with mitosis. This drug is used as adjunct therapy and for palliation of Hodgkin's disease and inoperable carcinoma of the adrenal cortex.

The adverse effects of procarbazine include bone marrow suppression, nausea, vomiting, dermatitis, and neuropathies. Mylosuppression occurs following oral, but not parenteral, administration of the drug. Nausea and vomiting are significant. Hypertensive crisis is possible in the presence of tyramine-containing foods (e.g., cheese, red wine) because procarbazine inactivates the enzyme monoamine oxidase. Neurotoxicity is worse when the drug is given IV because of higher peak levels. Neurotoxicity is manifest as somnolence, confusion, mood changes, and paresthesias. Hypersensitivity responses have also been reported.

Phenytoin and phenobarbital increase both the clearance and antitumor effects of procarbazine by accelerating production of its cytotoxic metabolites. It is a monoamine oxidase inhibitor, and patients receiving this therapy should be cautioned to avoid foods high in tyramine.

Hormones and Hormone Antagonists

Hormones used in antineoplastic therapy include androgens, antiandrogens, estrogens, antiestrogens, adrencocorticosteroids, adrenocorticosteroid inhibitors, gonadotropin-releasing hormone analogs, and progestins (see Hormones and Hormone Antagonists). Hormones and hormone antagonists exert beneficial effects by altering the hormonal envi-

HORMONES AND HORMONE ANTAGONISTS

Androgens
- Fluoxymesterone (HALOTESTIN)
- Testolactone (TESLAC)

Antiandrogens
- Bicalutamide (CASODEX)
- Flutamide (EULEXIN)
- Nilutamide (NILANDRON)

Estrogens
- Diethylstilbestrol (DES) (STILBESTROL)
- Ethinyl estradiol (ESTINYL, others)

Antiestrogens
- Anastrazole (ARIMIDEX)
- Tamoxifen (NOLVADEX)

Adrenocorticosteroids
- Prednisone (METICORTEN, others)

Adrenocorticosteroid inhibitors
- Aminoglutethimide (CYTADREN)

Gonadotropin-releasing hormone analogs
- Leuprolide (LUPRON)
- Goserelin acetate (ZOLADEX)

Progestins
- Medroxyprogesterone (PROVERA, DEPO-PROVERA)
- Megestrol acetate (MEGACE)

ronment that promotes cancer growth. The primary indications for these drugs are cancers of the breast, endometrium, and prostate. In addition, the adrencocorticosteroids are used against lymphomas and certain leukemias.

The sex hormones such as estrogens (e.g., diethylstilbestrol, ethinyl estradiol), progestins (e.g., medroxyprogesterone, megestrol), and androgens (e.g., fluoxymesterone, testolactone, estramustine) are useful in cancers of the breast and prostate gland. Estrogens change the hormonal environment of the tumor. *Estrogens,* such as diethylstilbestrol and other estrogens, are second-line drugs for treating prostate cancer. Benefits stem from suppressing androgen production, which prostate cells need to survive. Estrogens suppress androgen production, acting in the pituitary to suppress the release of interstitial cell-stimulating hormone. In the absence of this hormone, production of androgens by the testes declines.

Progestins, such as medroxyprogesterone, are used in the treatment of metastatic endometrial carcinoma. They promote palliation and tumor regression. The exact mechanism by which progestins suppress tumor growth is unknown. The basic pharmacology of estrogens and progestins is discussed in Chapter 54.

Androgens are used for the palliative management of estrogen-receptive metastatic breast cancer in postmenopausal women. It should be noted, however, that tamoxifen is the preferred drug for this indication. The basic pharmacology of androgens is discussed in Chapter 53.

Antiestrogenic drugs (e.g., tamoxifen, anastrazole) compete with estrogen for binding sites in breast tissues. Tamoxifen is a nonsteroidal antiestrogen drug that competes with estradiol for binding to estrogen receptors on the cancer cell membrane. The binding interferes with the cell's use of estrogen needed for tumor growth. It appears that estrogen receptor-positive tumors treated with tamoxifen are arrested in the G_0 and G_1 phase of the cell cycle, immediately after mitosis.

Tamoxifen is also thought to inhibit the production of several growth factors that stimulate tumor cell growth, including growth factor A, epidermal growth factor, and insulin-like growth factor. It also enhances the production of transforming growth factor B, an inhibitor of breast tumor cell growth. Tamoxifen may also act as a pure antiestrogen or as an estrogen depending on the target organ and other factors. The estrogen agonist effect is thought to offer some protection against osteoporosis and cardiovascular disease in postmenopausal women.

Anastrazole is the newest antiestrogenic drug. It is used in the treatment of advanced breast cancer in postmenopausal women whose disease has progressed despite tamoxifen therapy. It acts by inhibiting the enzyme aromatase, which is partially responsible for conversion of precursors to estrogen. By lowering levels of circulating estrogen, the progression of estrogen-sensitive breast cancer may be halted.

Antiandrogenic drugs such as flutamide act either to inhibit the uptake of androgen or to inhibit the nuclear binding of androgen in target tissues. Bicalutamide competitively inhibits the action of androgens by binding to androgen receptors in target tissue. Accordingly, the effects of androgen on androgen-sensitive tissues are reduced.

Gonadotropin-releasing hormone analogs such as goserelin and leuprolide are alternative therapies (e.g., orchiectomy, estrogen) for men with advanced prostate cancer. They are synthetic analogs of luteinizing hormone releasing hormone. They increase the production of luteinizing hormone and follicle-stimulating hormone in the pituitary gland, resulting in transient increases in testosterone and dihydrotestosterone in males. With prolonged administration, luteinizing hormone and follicle-stimulating hormone receptors are downregulated in the pituitary gland. Eventually gonadotropin secretion is reduced, ultimately decreasing testosterone to castration levels. The drug effects persist for up to 3 years. The drugs are as effective as an orchiectomy (surgical removal of the testicles) in lowering testosterone levels.

Adrenocorticosteroids interfere with the mitosis of lymphocytes and lymphoid proliferation, resulting in cell death. This may result in glucose deprivation. Adrenocorticosteroids are CCS active in phase G_1 of the cell cycle. They are used to induce remission in children with acute lymphocytic leukemia, to relieve the complications of cancer and cancer treatment, such as nausea, vomiting, hypercalcemia, hemorrhagic thrombocytopenia, and intracranial metastasis, and are components of various antineoplastic regimens. They are used for palliation and symptom relief because they reduce pain and fever and increase appetite, strength, and sense of well-being. They are used at times in radiation therapy to reduce edema in the mediastinum, brain, and spinal cord.

The *adrencocorticosteroid-inhibitor* drug, aminoglutethimide, is useful in patients with advanced prostatic cancer and produces a state that mimics an adrenalectomy.

Antineoplastic Drugs on the Horizon

Angiogenesis inhibitors (e.g., angiostatin, endostatin) are the newest class of antineoplastic drugs on the horizon. It is presently known that when cancer cells are still very small (1 to 2 mm diameter) they do not need blood vessels to survive. However, in order to grow to any size at all, they need a sufficient blood supply that will provide the needed nutrients. To do so, tumor cells convince nearby capillaries to extend outward, thus carrying the required nutrients to the tumor cells. Angiogenesis inhibitors are thought to block the construction of the new capillaries, thereby preventing the tumor cells from receiving nutrients. As a result, the tumor may stop growing, shrink, or in some cases regress to a microscopic dormant lesion (see Figure 30–2).

Angiostatin, a potent naturally occurring inhibitor of angiogenesis and growth of tumor metastasis, is generated by proteolysis of plasminogen. To date, it is known that in a defined cell-free system, plasminogen activators (e.g., tissue plasminogen activator [tPA], streptokinase) in combination with *N*-acetyl-L-cysteine, D-penicillamine, captopril, L-cysteine, or reduced glutathione, generate angiostatin from plasminogen. It is also known that human prostate carcinoma cells possess enzymes that convert plasminogen to angiostatin. Endostatin is produced by hemangioendothelioma. It specifically inhibits endothelial proliferation and potently inhibits angiogenesis and tumor growth. Using a sustained release method, *Escherichia coli*–derived endostatin appears to cause primary tumors to regress.

In addition to angiostatin and endostatin, a number of other drugs are being investigated for their effects on blood vessels. Marimastat, synthesized in the laboratory, appears to block the activity of enzymes that are needed to build tumor blood vessels. Neovastat, derived from the cartilage of spinydogfish sharks, appears to inhibit the activity of enzymes involved in the growth of tumor blood vessels cells. SU-5416 seems to prevent a blood vessel growth factor in the tumor cells from binding to its receptor site. Combretastatin, originally derived from the African bush willow, is thought to destroy the tumor's cells in the blood vessel.

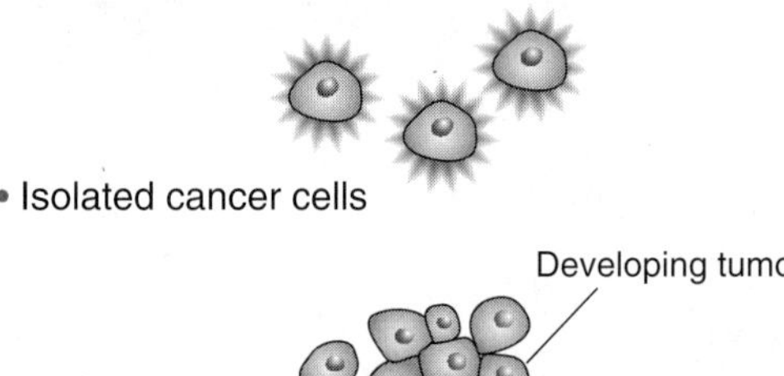

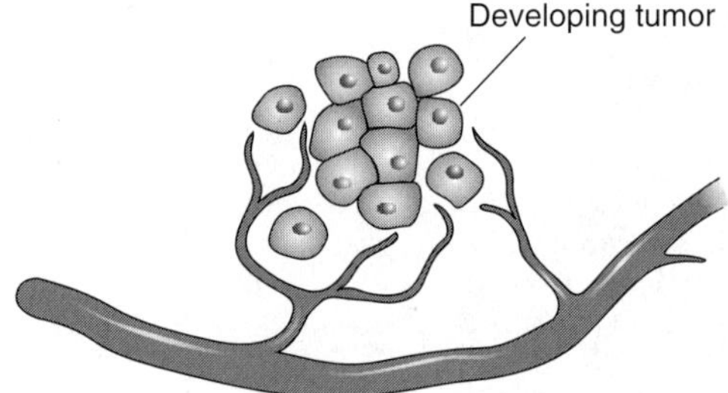

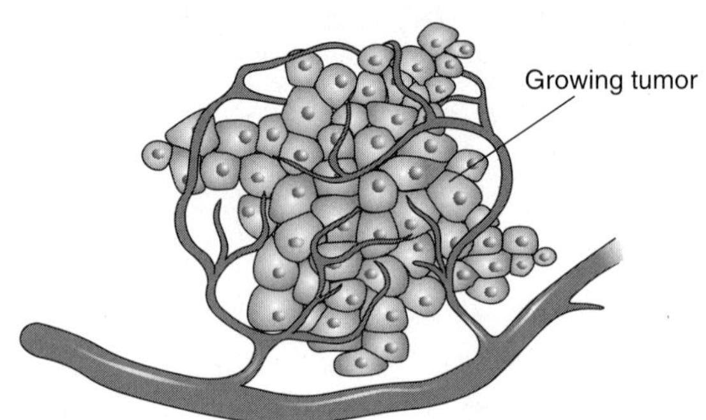

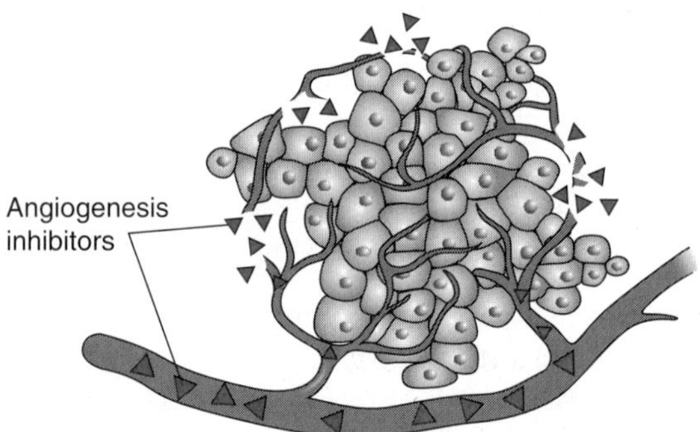

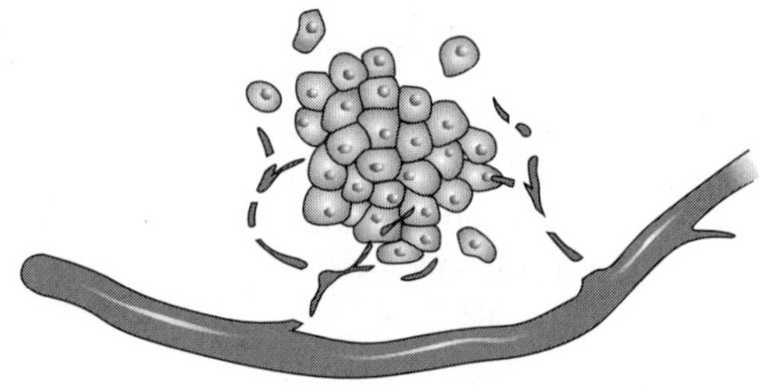

Figure 30–2. Angiogenesis-inhibiting drugs currently under investigation such as angiostatin and endostatin act by preventing the formation of the capillary network that nourishes the malignant tumor and provides access to the circulatory system.

Critical Thinking Process

Assessment

Prior to initiating antineoplastic treatment, it is important that a comprehensive history be obtained, which provides information about the patient's physical, psychological, and emotional status. Antineoplastic therapy is a rigorous treatment that may cause many toxic and adverse reactions. In order to provide safe and effective therapy, patients must be screened for any preexisting organ disease, physical, or psychosocial concerns that would impact their ability to tolerate therapy.

History of Present Illness

Assessment data should include when the present illness occurred, as well as any presenting symptoms that led to the diagnosis. Any surgeries, diagnostic studies, or previous treatment for the illness should also be recorded in detail. If possible, obtain the patient's consent to request records from other institutions where treatment was provided.

Past Health History

Detailed information regarding past health history must be obtained. Surgeries, infectious diseases, and chronic illnesses and medical conditions must be listed in detail in the patient's records. Chronic illnesses that may lead to or cause impaired organ function may require changes in dosages or treatment protocols. Information regarding all drugs used on a routine basis should also be listed because of the potential for adverse drug interactions. Instances of anaphylactic reactions have been reported; thus it is important to ask about prior sensitivity. Further, information about previous drugs used or drug therapies received is important because second malignancies have developed in some patients treated with antineoplastic drugs, especially alkylating agents. Additionally, the patient's past history may hold clues to the present illness, as many cancers are found more frequently following some nonmalignant disorders.

Physical Exam Findings

The person with cancer may appear to be in perfect health, with only mild signs and symptoms, or may be diagnosed in a later stage of the disease, with local and systemic alterations. A comprehensive baseline physical exam is important when evaluating the patient who will be receiving antineoplastic therapy. This data must be recorded in the patient's permanent record, where it can then serve as a basis for comparison and further evaluation after the patient begins a treatment regimen.

Diagnostic Testing

Diagnostic testing is initially directed toward obtaining a diagnosis and determining the extent and spread of the patient's cancer. During the initial evaluation period, the patient may require biopsies, surgery, radionucleotide scans, and radiologic studies. After the diagnosis is obtained, further diagnostic testing will be directed toward assessing the patient's ability to tolerate drug therapy without suffering lethal consequences.

Depending upon the nature of the drug or drugs and anticipated toxicities, a CBC and serum chemistry panel is obtained as a part of the screening process. Evaluation of cardiopulmonary, hepatic, and renal status is also done.

Developmental Considerations

Perinatal Malignant diseases that occur in pregnancy, in order of decreasing frequency, include breast cancer, hematopoietic malignancy, melanoma, gynecologic cancer, and bone tumors. The glandular hyperplasia of the breast that accompanies pregnancy makes recognition of suspicious breast masses difficult. However, when matched for age and stage of cancer, survival rates of breast cancer found during pregnancy are no different from the nonpregnant state. Survival is generally not improved by terminating the pregnancy. However, it may be appropriate to avoid the risk of fetal exposure to either antineoplastic drugs or radiation therapy. Treatment recommendations for pregnant women will vary but depend on the location of the cancer, stage of the disease, gestational age of the pregnancy, and maternal health in general.

Pediatric A comprehensive baseline assessment is particularly important for the pediatric patient. A child diagnosed with cancer may be an extraordinary stressor for the family unit, and the health care provider must be prepared to give the extra time needed to provide patient and family teaching and emotional support. The parents and child must be given detailed information on the implications of the diagnosis, adverse effects and toxicities associated with antineoplastic therapy, and desired therapeutic effects. It is particularly important that the parents understand the potential for late effects of antineoplastic drugs, including sterility, hypogonadism, growth retardation, and cognitive impairment.

Geriatric Older adults may suffer from impaired communication ability, sensory deficits, and decreased cognitive function. There is an increased incidence of organ damage due to changes associated with age and chronic disease. Obtaining a comprehensive health history may be difficult, particularly if the patient is a poor historian. In this instance, a comprehensive physical exam and evaluation are imperative in order to avoid an excessively toxic therapeutic regimen.

Psychosocial Considerations

Patients who are faced with a potentially fatal illness exhibit a wide array of coping behaviors. It is the responsibility of the health care provider to determine which patients exhibit ineffective or harmful coping mechanisms that require psychological intervention and counseling and to determine the social support available to the patient. Social support as well as coping skills have been well documented as important factors in the successful completion of treatment regimens.

A diagnosis of cancer may have devastating economic effects on the patient and family members. Inability to work may lead to loss of insurance coverage, which then jeopardizes the patient's access to life-saving medical care. Basic insurance coverage may be insufficient to cover the cost of cancer therapy, placing the patient's home, savings, and financial earnings at risk. Most patients with a diagnosis of cancer can benefit from a referral to social services for assistance with their financial affairs.

Analysis and Management

Treatment Objectives

Choices of antineoplastic therapies must be guided by the most realistic and achievable treatment objectives. The three major goals of antineoplastic therapy are cure, control, and palliation. An increasing number of cancers are curable, particularly if they are identified and treated before metastasis has occurred.

Cure is defined as eradication of all clinically detectable cancer, giving the patient treated the same life expectancy as an individual who does not have cancer. Highly proliferative tumors (e.g., pediatric acute lymphocytic leukemia, Hodgkin's disease, neuroblastoma, testicular carcinoma, choriocarcinoma) are often curable. Cure must not be achieved, however, at the cost of a poor quality of life or disabling treatment-related symptoms.

The common reference points used to predict the likelihood of cure and to judge the results of therapy are 5- and 10-year survival rates without evidence of disease. Advanced solid tumors are not generally curable using antineoplastic therapies.

Control of the disease is the next objective. When the disease is found to be incurable, prolongation of life is the next objective. Given the variety of drugs and treatment options available, it is often possible to control metastatic disease for many months or years while providing an optimal quality of life for the patient.

Palliation is the third and final objective. Palliation is defined as providing relief of distressing symptoms (e.g., pain, hypercalcemia) and maintaining function as near normal as possible when it is no longer possible to achieve a remission. When cure or control are no longer possible, relief of symptoms may still be achieved by antineoplastic therapy, particularly if doses are adjusted to minimize toxicities.

Treatment Options

When planning an antineoplastic treatment regimen, variables to be considered include the size and stage of the tumor, growth rate, and heterogeneity of the tumor. *Neoadjuvant therapy* (primary antineoplastic therapy, induction therapy) is used prior to other therapies (e.g., surgery, radiation therapy) in an attempt to decrease tumor size and bulk and increase surgical resectability of the tumor. Many solid tumors have micrometastatic disease and are considered systemic diseases incurable by surgery alone. This fact justifies the use of antineoplastic therapy in combination with surgery or radiation therapy. Administration of adjuvant antineoplastic therapy is therefore based on the biologic behavior of certain cancers that metastasize early in the course of the disease. The goal of *adjuvant therapy* is to eradicate possible micrometastatic deposits when they are most susceptible.

Drug Variables

Selection of the appropriate antineoplastic treatment regimen involves a complex series of decisions that must consider the type of tumor, the cell types involved, and the degree of cellular differentiation. Tumors that microscopically display the least number of normal cellular characteristics tend to grow more rapidly, spread more readily, and impose more lethal consequences on the host. Because of their cellular characteristics, poorly differentiated tumors tend to be more responsive to drug therapy in the short term than slow-growing, well-differentiated cancers. The growth fraction of the tumor, or number of cells that are cycling at any given time, will also affect how the tumor responds to therapy.

The stage of the tumor must also be considered when evaluating treatment options. Patients with extensive metastatic disease may not be candidates for antineoplastic therapy, because dosages required to eradicate the disease may cause lethal toxicities.

Antineoplastic therapy damages cancer cells and healthy cells. The ultimate goal of antineoplastic therapy is to limit damage to healthy cells while yielding a 100 percent kill rate to cancer cells. An intermittent schedule of drug therapy allows normal cells to repair and grow between doses of chemotherapy. During the break from therapy, however, the cancer cells also have time to repair damage produced by the antineoplastic drug. For intermittent therapy to be successful, healthy cells must be able to repair damage and repopulate faster than the cancer cells. If the cancer cells repopulate faster than normal cells, intermittent therapy will fail.

A treatment regimen that uses multiple drugs is generally more successful than regimens that employ a single agent. Antineoplastic drugs chosen for combination regimens should be individually effective against the targeted neoplasm and minimize toxicity to normal cells, produce minimally overlapping toxicities, and possess different mechanisms of actions.

Administering multiple drugs that have different mechanisms of action and different toxicities produces greater cell kill than monotherapy. The dose of an individual drug is limited by the toxicity the patient can tolerate. Choosing drugs with minimal or no overlapping toxicities allows the maximum tolerated dose of each drug to be administered. Increased cell kill is additionally produced because the combination of drugs assaults the cancer cells by a variety of mechanisms rather than one action produced by a single drug.

Experience demonstrates that cancer cells are capable of developing temporary and permanent drug resistance. The degree and type of drug resistance will depend upon the blood supply and nutrients available to the tumor, the bioavailability of the drug, and the presence of tumor in sanctuary sites. Permanent drug resistance is genetically based and is the result of random cell mutations. The greater the mutation rate, the less likely it is that cure or control of the disease will occur. Tumor cells may possess innate resistance to a specific drug without having previous exposure to the agent. Tumor cells may also acquire drug resistance after exposure to the drug and may develop cross resistance to other antineoplastic agents.

Toxicities associated with antineoplastic therapy may adversely impact almost any body organ, but in general are a reflection of damage to rapidly dividing cells. Normal tissue with a high growth fraction, such as the GI mucosa, bone marrow, hair follicles, and reproductive system, is most likely to be damaged. The damage varies in severity depending upon the drugs administered, drug dosages, treatment protocol, and the patient's health status prior to the start of treatment.

Myelosuppression Myelosuppression is a general term used to describe the suppressive effects of cytotoxic agents on the bone marrow. As a consequence of disease or therapy, patients may experience neutropenia, thrombocytopenia, and anemia to varying degrees. Since the life span of the leukocyte is very brief (12 hours), leukopenia occurs frequently. The time after antineoplastic drug administration when the white blood cell or platelet count is at the lowest point is referred to as the *nadir*. For most myelosuppressive drugs, the nadir occurs within 7 to 14 days after drug administration (Table 30–5). Knowledge of the blood count nadirs helps the health care provider predict when the patient is at greatest risk for infection and bleeding.

An absolute neutrophil count (ANC) is calculated by multiplying the WBC by the percentage of neutrophils in the differential (ANC = WBC × % neutrophils). For example, if the WBC is 1200 cells/mm^3 and the neutrophil count is 34 percent, the ANC is 408 cells/mm^3. A patient is considered neutropenic if his or her absolute neutrophil count is 1000 cells/mm^3 or less. The frequency of infection increases as the ANC falls below 500 cells/mm^3 and the longer the patient remains neutropenic. A normal leukocyte count is 4000 to 10,000 cells/mm^3.

Thrombocytopenia increases the patient's risk of bleeding if the platelet count falls below 20,000 cells/mm^3. Fatal CNS hemorrhage or massive GI bleeding can occur when the platelet count falls below 10,000 cells/mm^3. Some controversy exists as to whether patients should receive prophylactic transfusions when their platelet count falls below a certain level or when the patient is actively bleeding. Most health care providers will transfuse the patient in order to keep the platelet count above 20,000 cells/mm^3. A normal platelet count is 140,000 to 440,000 cells/mm^3.

TABLE 30–5. EFFECTS OF SELECTED ANTINEOPLASTIC DRUGS ON NADIR AND RECOVERY

Antineoplastic Drug	WBC Nadir (Days)	WBC Recovery (Days)	Platelet Nadir (Days)	Comments
Alkylating Drugs				
Busulfan	7–10	24–54	10–30	—
Carmustine	35–42	42–56	28–35	Myelosuppressive effects are cumulative, delayed, and prolonged
Chlorambucil	7–14	28–42	7–14	—
Cisplatin	18–23	29	14	—
Cyclophosphamide	8–14	18–25	10–25	Somewhat platelet sparing
Dacarbazine	10–14	24	14–28	—
Ifosfamide	10–15	18	Platelet sparing	—
Lomustine	42	60	28	Myelosuppressive effects are cumulative, delayed, and prolonged; thrombocytopenia is more common than leukopenia
Mechlorethamine	6–8	14–28	10–14	—
Melphalan	10–12	28–42	7–14	Thrombocytopenia secondary to melphalan is more common than leukopenia
Streptozocin	14	21	14	Myelosuppression secondary to streptozocin is not usually dose limiting
Thiotepa	10–14	28	14–28	—
Antimetabolites				
Cytarabine	12–14	22–24	12–15	Somewhat platelet sparing
Fludarabine	3–25	UA	2–32	—
Fluorouracil	9–14	20–30	7–17	—
Mercaptopurine	7–14	14–21	10–14	—
Methotrexate	7–14	14–21	5–12	—
Thioguanine	14–28	28–35	14	—
Antitumor Antibiotics				
Dactinomycin	14–21	21–25	10–14	—
Daunorubicin	8–10	21	10–14	Myelosuppression is profound and dose limiting
Doxorubicin	10–14	22	14	—
Idarubicin	10–15	21	10–14	—
Mitomycin	21–28	28–42	30	Effects are cumulative and prolonged
Mitoxantrone	10–14	21	8–16	Myelosuppression is profound and dose limiting
Mitotic Inhibitors				
Docetaxel	8	7	UA	—
Etoposide	7–14	21	9–16	—
Paclitaxel	11	15–21	Platelet sparing	—
Teniposide	16–18	15	16–18	—
Topotecan	11	18	15	—
Vinblastine	5–9	14–21	4–10	—
Vincristine	4–10	7–14	Platelet sparing	—
Vindesine	7	14	7	—
Vinorelbine	7–10	7–14	Platelet sparing	—
Miscellaneous Antineoplastic Drugs				
Hydroxyurea	7	14–21	Somewhat platelet sparing	—
L-Asparaginase	4–7	10–14	5–10	Somewhat platelet sparing; myelosuppression is seldom a problem
Procarbazine	25–36	35–50	21	Myelosuppression is prolonged and delayed

UA, Unavailable.

Data from Goodman, M. (1992). *Cancer: Chemotherapy and care*. Princeton, NJ: Bristol-Myers Squibb Co.; and Hodgson, B., and Kizior, R. (1998). *Saunders nursing drug handbook 1999*. Philadelphia: W.B. Saunders.

Anemia is a reduction in the concentration of hemoglobin and circulating red blood cell (RBC) mass. Anemia leads to tissue hypoxia due to impaired oxygen-carrying capacity. Anemia is manifested as a drop in hemoglobin, hematocrit, or RBC count. Dehydration may raise the hematocrit, thus masking an anemia. A normal hemoglobin is 13 to 16 g/dL in males and 12 to 15 g/dL in females. The patient is anemic if the values fall below 13 or 12 g/dL, respectively. Severe anemia can result in hypotension and myocardial infarction. One unit of blood will usually raise the hemoglobin 1 g/dL.

Patients are able to tolerate varying degrees of anemia or may be reluctant to accept transfusions. However, packed RBCs may be required to relieve anemia that is producing symptoms. Erythropoietin may be ordered to elevate or maintain the RBC level and decrease the need for transfusions (see Chapter 41).

Gastrointestinal Effects Antineoplastic therapy can cause nausea, vomiting, diarrhea, stomatitis, oral mucositis, aversion to food, changes in taste and smell, diarrhea, and constipation. The emetic potential of a particular antineoplastic drug regimen depends on the drugs given, the dose and route of administration, and the patient's susceptibility to emesis (see Antineoplastic Drugs Commonly Associated with Nausea and Vomiting). Uncontrolled nausea and vomiting can result in anorexia, malnutrition, dehydration, metabolic imbalances, psychological depression, and reduced immunity.

ANTINEOPLASTIC DRUGS COMMONLY ASSOCIATED WITH NAUSEA AND VOMITING

Drugs with an almost certain (90%) risk of nausea and vomiting

Alkylating Drugs
- Cisplatin
- Cyclophosphamide
- Dacarbazine
- Mechlorethamine

Antimetabolites
- Cytarabine

Drugs with a high (60–90%) risk of nausea and vomiting

Alkylating Drugs
- Carboplatin
- Carmustine
- Lomustine
- Streptozocin

Antitumor Antibiotics
- Dactinomycin
- Daunorubicin
- Doxorubicin

Drugs with a moderate (30–60%) risk of nausea and vomiting

Alkylating Drugs
- Altretamine
- Ifosfamide

Antimetabolites
- Pentostatin

Antitumor Antibiotics
- Idarubicin
- Mitomycin
- Plicamycin

Mitotic Inhibitors
- Etoposide
- Mitoxantrone
- Topotecan

Miscellaneous Antineoplastics
- L-Asparaginase
- Procarbazine

Drugs with a low (0–30%) risk of nausea and vomiting

Alkylating Drugs
- Busulfan
- Chlorambucil
- Melphalan
- Thiotepa

Antimetabolites
- Cytarabine
- Fludarabine
- Fluorouracil
- Floxuridine
- Methotrexate
- Mercaptopurine
- Thioguanine

Antitumor Antibiotics
- Bleomycin

Mitotic Inhibitors
- Paclitaxel
- Vinblastine
- Vincristine
- Vindesine
- Vinorelbine

Miscellaneous Antineoplastics
- Hydroxyurea

Three patterns of nausea and vomiting are associated with antineoplastic therapy. Once the patient has experienced nausea and vomiting, anticipatory nausea and vomiting may occur before the administration of the next treatment regimen. Acute posttherapy nausea and vomiting occur within the first 24 hours after drug administration. Delayed nausea and vomiting persists or develops 24 hours after drug administration. The health care provider responsible for drug administration must be thoroughly familiar with antiemetic agents and adjunct measures that can be used to control nausea and vomiting.

Stomatitis or oral mucositis is a consequence of delayed cell renewal caused by antineoplastic drugs. What is seen in the mouth is present throughout the GI tract. The drugs most commonly associated with stomatitis are the antimetabolites, the antitumor antibiotics, and the mitotic inhibitors (i.e., vinca alkaloids). Oral lesions associated with antineoplastic therapy may be so severe that patients are unable to eat, drink, speak, or swallow their own oral secretions. Severe stomatitis may be a dose-limiting toxicity for the patient.

Diarrhea is most often associated with antimetabolite drugs. Constipation is frequently the effect of vinca alkaloids on peristalsis. Other causes of constipation include opioid use, immobility, decreased fluid and fiber intake, tumor invasion of the GI tract, and depression.

Dermatologic Effects Dermatologic toxicities of antineoplastic drugs include alopecia, skin and nail hyperpigmentation, and onycholysis of the nails. Toxicities and adverse effects gradually resolve with cessation of treatment. The extent of hair loss depends on the specific drug, dosage, and mode of administration. Alopecia is temporary. Hair regrowth often occurs before antineoplastic therapy ends, although the hair color and texture may change. Scalp hypothermia decreases blood flow to the hair follicles, thereby reducing contact between the drug and epithelial cells. It is rarely used today owing to the risk of creating a sanctuary site for metastatic disease. Scalp hypothermia is contraindicated in patients with brain tumors or metastatic disease to this area.

Hyperpigmentation of the nail bed, mouth, gums or teeth, and along veins used for IV therapy is not uncommon. The hyperpigmentation usually occurs 2 to 3 weeks after therapy and continues for 10 to 12 weeks following discontinuance. Photosensitivity may result in acute sunburn after just a short exposure to the sun. Radiation recall may occur in patients who received radiation therapy weeks or months prior to the administration of antineoplastic drugs. Skin effects occur in the area previously radiated and range from redness, shedding, or peeling to blisters and oozing. Once the skin heals, it is permanently darkened.

Reproductive Effects The effects of antineoplastic therapy on gonadal function and reproduction capacity can be temporary or permanent. The effects on gonadal function vary with respect to the patient's age at the time of therapy, the drugs administered, and total dosage. Azoospermia, oligospermia, and sterility have been documented in males. Amenorrhea, manifestations of menopause, and sterility have been noted in females.

Patient Variables

Host factors that may influence treatment outcome include immune function, nutritional status, psychologic status, availability of supportive care, and social support. Patients who are relatively asymptomatic and able to carry out normal activities of daily living are more likely to have positive outcomes from therapy compared to the patient who is bedridden, cachectic, and dependent on others for care.

Administration of antineoplastic drugs during the first trimester of pregnancy increases the risk of spontaneous abortion and fetal malformations. Second- and third-trimester exposure to antineoplastic drugs may result in low birth weight or prematurity. Contraceptives should be used for birth control during therapy and for up to 2 years following completion of therapy.

Intervention

Administration

For the most part, all antineoplastic drugs are carcinogenic, teratogenic, and mutagenic. The primary exposure routes are absorption through the skin, inhalation, and ingestion through contaminated food and surfaces. Preparation and administration of antineoplastic drugs should be performed only by specially trained health care providers. Personnel should be familiar with the Occupational Safety and Health Administration (OSHA) guidelines, Oncology Nursing Society (ONS) guidelines, and individual agency policies.

Preparation of antineoplastic drugs should occur in a low traffic area away from patients. Work surfaces should be covered with plastic-backed, absorbent pads. Nonabsorbent gowns, with long sleeves, elastic cuffs, and back closures, and powder-free latex gloves should be worn during preparation of antineoplastic drugs. They should be prepared under a Class II, biologic safety cabinet with a vertical laminar air flow system. If a biologic safety cabinet is not available, a respirator with a high-efficiency filter should be worn during preparation. No eating, drinking, or application of make-up should be allowed in this area. Drugs should be prepared and stored following the manufacturer's guidelines regarding solution compatibility, sensitivities, and stability.

Selection of the administration site is an important consideration when using antineoplastic drugs. Large veins in the forearm are the preferred sites. If a drug does extravasate in this area, there is maximum soft tissue coverage to prevent functional impairment. Vesicants and irritants should not be administered through veins in the hands, in the antecubital fossa, or over bony prominences (see Antineoplastic Vesicant and Irritant Drugs). Extravasation in these areas can lead to destruction of nerves and tendons, resulting in loss of function. Veins that are damaged or sclerosed and sites that have been damaged by burns, grafts, surgery, amputation, and mastectomy should be avoided. An extravasation kit, containing agency-approved antidotes, should be kept at the patient's side whenever a vesicant is being administered. Blood return and infusion site should be monitored before, during, and after drug administration.

Central venous access devices (e.g., Hickman or Groshong single-lumen catheters, Port-A-Cath Dual-Lumen Venous Access System, OmegaPort, Infusaid Microport) are recommended for continuous infusion of vesicants. Because the termination site is in a large central vein, hyperosmolar solutions can be safely administered, and rapid dilution and dispersion of irritating drugs will occur.

Regional administration of antineoplastic drugs includes topical, intrathecal, intracavitary, and intra-arterial routes. Although intra-arterial routes pose some risk, major organs or tumor sites receive maximal exposure with limited serum drug levels. As a result, systemic adverse effects are minimal.

Almost all antineoplastic drugs are given in relatively high doses, on an intermittent or cyclic schedule. This appears to be more efficacious than low doses given continuously or massive doses given only once. It also causes less immunosuppression and provides for drug holidays, during which normal tissues can repair themselves from antineoplastic drug-induced damage. Fortunately, normal cells are repaired quicker than neoplastic cells. Subsequent doses are usually administered as soon as tissue repair becomes evident, usually while leukocyte and platelet counts return to acceptable levels.

Multidrug therapies should follow the recommended schedule precisely since safety and efficacy may be schedule dependent (Table 30–6). When antineoplastic therapy is used as an adjuvant to surgery, it is started as soon as possible and given in maximal doses (as tolerated), just as if advanced disease were present. Therapy is continued for several months to a year.

In general, most nausea and vomiting can be successfully controlled with careful administration of antiemetic therapy in conjunction with the drug treatments. Antiemetics are ordinarily administered 6 to 12 hours before therapy and are continued every 4 to 6 hours for at least 12 to 24 hours, or for as long as manifestations persist.

Education

Patients should be given a complete explanation of their treatment regimen, including adverse effects, before informed consent is obtained for antineoplastic drug administration. Care should be taken to mention not only the life-threatening and pathology-producing adverse effects, but also the adverse effects that produce discomfort and embarrassment. In the past, oncology patients could rely on health care professionals to monitor their health status. Drug administration, however, is quickly becoming the domain of outpatient and home settings, and it is imperative that patients know how to monitor their own health status.

Antineoplastic drug regimens typically induce periods of low white blood cell and platelet counts. Patients should become familiar with normal cell counts and learn to monitor their own cell counts. The risk of infection can be reduced by teaching patients to avoid potential sources. These sources include individuals with a cold or flu and live plants

ANTINEOPLASTIC VESICANT AND IRRITANT DRUGS

Vesicants
- Dacarbazine
- Dactinomycin
- Daunorubicin
- Doxorubicin
- Idarubicin
- Mechlorethamine
- Mitomycin
- Paclitaxel
- Platinol
- Vinblastine
- Vincristine
- Vinorelbine

Irritants
- Carmustine
- Plicamycin
- Streptozocin

TABLE 30–6. EXAMPLES OF COMBINATION ANTINEOPLASTIC DRUG REGIMENS

Regimen	Disorder	Drug*	Route	Schedule
ABVD	Hodgkin's disease	Doxorubicin (**A**DRIAMYCIN)	IV	Days 1 and 15
		Bleomycin	po	Days 1 and 15
		Vinblastine	IV	Days 1 and 15
		Dacarbazine	IV	Days 1 and 15
		Drug-free period		Days 16 through 27
				Repeat cycle every 28 days
MOPP	Hodgkin's disease	**M**echlorethamine	IV	Days 1 and 8
		Vincristine (**O**NCOVIN)	IV	Days 1 and 8
		Procarbazine	po	Days 1 through 14
		Prednisone	po	Days 1 through 14
		Drug-free period		Days 15 through 28
				Repeat cycle every 28 days
BACOP	Non-Hodgkin's lymphoma	**B**leomycin	IV	Days 15 and 22
		Doxorubicin (**A**DRIAMYCIN)	IV	Days 1 and 8
		Cyclophosphamide	IV	Days 1 and 8
		Vincristine (**O**NCOVIN)	IV	Days 1 and 8
		Prednisone	po	Days 15 through 28
CAF	Breast cancer	**C**yclophosphamide	po	Days 1 through 14
		Doxorubicin (**A**DRIAMYCIN)	IV	Days 1 and 8
		Fluorouracil	IV	Days 1 and 8
				Repeat every 28 days
CMF(P)	Breast cancer	**C**yclophosphamide	po	Days 1 through 14 or
			IV	Day 1 only
		Methotrexate	IV	Days 1 and 8
		Fluorouracil	IV	Days 1 and 8
		Prednisone	po	Days 1 through 14
		Drug-free period		Days 15 through 28
				Repeat cycle every 28 days for 10 cycles
FAM-BCNU	Gastric adenocarcinoma	**F**luorouracil	IV	Days 1, 8, 29, and 36
		Doxorubicin (**A**DRIAMYCIN)	IV	Days 1 and 29
		Mitomycin	IV	Days 30 through 56
		Carmustine (**BCNU**)	IV	2 days every 6 weeks
				Repeat cycle every 8 weeks

*The drug regimen abbreviations seen in the leftmost column are derived from the first letter (printed in bold) of each drug used in that specific combination treatment. These are six examples of the numerous drug combinations used to treat neoplastic disorders.

and flowers (sources of microscopic fungus, bacteria, and insects). Patients receiving antineoplastic therapy should be advised against receiving live virus vaccines until months after antineoplastic therapy has been discontinued. In addition, persons in close contact with the patient should not receive oral polio vaccine, because the live virus is excreted by the person receiving it, and it can then be transmitted to the patient. Additionally, patients need to understand the importance of reporting the early signs and symptoms of infection (low-grade temps, sore throat, cough). The single most important practice that can be undertaken to prevent infection, however, is for all health care workers, patients, families and friends to practice strict hand washing.

Low platelet counts are an additional risk factor for patients receiving antineoplastic drugs. The potential for hemorrhage can be minimized by teaching patients to avoid aspirin and other over-the-counter (OTC) drugs that prolong clotting times, to substitute electric shavers for razors (decreases the risk of nicks and cuts), refrain from using suppositories (may cause tears to rectal tissue), hold pressure over cuts and venipuncture sites for 5 to 10 minutes, and avoid intramuscular injections as much as possible. Most importantly, patients need to understand the signs and symptoms of internal bleeding and report these symptoms immediately.

Patients who are thrombocytopenic should avoid any aspirin-containing products or drugs that inhibit platelet activity, and may require activity restrictions or bedrest in order to decrease the risk of injury. Blood counts must be scrutinized closely before a patient undergoes surgery or any invasive procedure.

The patient with stomatitis will require education regarding the prevention of infection, frequent gentle mouth care, and measures to relieve pain, maintain comfort, and promote hygiene.

Patient education is essential when administering antineoplastic therapy. With proper education, many patients in the home are able to self-administer the drugs and adjunctive regimens (e.g., antiemetics, antidiarrheals) and properly identify significant adverse effects. Instruction sheets for most chemotherapy drugs are available in English or Spanish from the National Cancer Institute.

Evaluation

The success of antineoplastic therapy is evaluated based on the patient's response to treatment. Relatively standardized criteria have been developed to evaluate the efficacy of antineoplastic therapy. The criteria include survival rates, degree of response or remission, duration of response, and degree of toxicity. *Complete response* generally refers to the complete disappearance of all evidence of disease for 1 month or longer following completion of therapy. *Partial response* is usually defined as a reduction in measurable tumor mass of 50 percent or more of its original size for 1 month or more. Moreover, there is no evidence of new disease, and the patient subjectively improved. *Improvement* refers to a reduction in measurable tumor mass by 25 to 50 percent of its original size with subjective improvement in patient status. *Stable disease* is tumor regression of 25 percent or less with or without subjective patient improvement. *Disease progression* refers to clinical evidence of advancing disease during antineoplastic therapy. Assuming that an adequate trial of antineoplastic therapy has been conducted, disease progression indicates a treatment failure.

These anticipated outcomes vary significantly depending upon the patient's physical status, specific diagnosis, and extent of disease. The ultimate goal of antineoplastic therapy is to achieve a cure, without unreasonable toxicities and adverse reactions. When cure is impossible, antineoplastic drugs are a valuable tool in prolonging life and minimizing the suffering associated with a diagnosis of cancer. The health care provider must be knowledgeable about the antineoplastic drugs and their toxicities in order to ensure the patient's safety, minimize adverse effects, and assist the patient to cope with a life-threatening illness.

SUMMARY

- Cell cycle specific drugs are effective only during a specific phase of the cell cycle (i.e., S, G_2, M, G_1).
- Cell cycle nonspecific drugs are effective throughout the cell cycle, including G_0.
- Alkylating drugs include an alkyl sulfonate, ethylenimines, nitrogen mustards, nitrosoureas, metal salts, and a triazine.
- Alkylating drugs act by causing interstrand and intrastrand cross-linkages in DNA, thus blocking replication. They are CCNS drugs, although in some cases cells appear to be more sensitive in one phase than another.
- Bifunctional alkylating drugs form cross-links in DNA and thus prevent DNA replication.
- Antimetabolite drugs are important natural metabolites and include folic acid analogs, pyrimidine analogs, and purine analogs.
- Antimetabolite act in phase S of the cell cycle to interfere with DNA synthesis.
- The antitumor antibiotics produce their effects by forming complexes with DNA, thereby inhibiting DNA activity through the process of intercalation.
- Mitotic inhibitors act by interfering with assembly of the microtubular components of the mitotic spindle.
- Hormones used in antineoplastic therapy include androgens, antiandrogens, estrogens, antiestrogens, adrencocorticosteroids, adrenocorticosteroid inhibitors, gonadotropin-releasing hormone analogs, and progestins.
- Hydroxyurea is CCS for the S phase of the cell cycle. It acts by inhibiting the enzyme that normally catalyzes the conversion of RNA to DNA. In the absence of the nucleotides, DNA cannot be made.
- L-Asparaginase catalyzes the hydrolysis of the amino acid asparagine to aspartic acid and ammonia. Thus, the amount of asparagine available to tumor cells is reduced. The asparagine-depleting action interferes with the synthesis of tumor proteins, DNA, and RNA.
- Mitotane is selectively toxic to tumor cells. This isomer of the pesticide DDT acts to inhibit corticosteroid biosynthesis.
- Pegaspargase consists of L-asparaginase bound to polyethylene glycol. The polyethylene glycol-pegaspargase depletes asparagine, which leukemic cells cannot synthesize.
- Procarbazine is thought to disrupt chromatin arrangement and interfere with mitosis.
- Angiogenesis inhibitors are thought to block the construction of the new capillaries, thereby preventing the tumor cells from receiving nutrients.
- The three major goals of antineoplastic therapy are cure, control, and palliation. Cure is defined as eradication of all cancer, giving the patient treated the same life expectancy as an individual who does not have cancer.
- Controlling the disease and prolonging life are necessary when cancer is found to be incurable.
- Palliation provides relief of symptoms and maintenance of function as near normal as possible when it is no longer possible to achieve a remission.
- Neoadjuvant therapy (primary antineoplastic therapy, induction therapy) is used prior to other therapies in an attempt to decrease tumor size and bulk and increase surgical resectability of the tumor.
- The goal of adjuvant therapy is to eradicate possible micrometastatic deposits when they are most susceptible.
- Selection of the appropriate antineoplastic treatment regimen involves a complex series of decisions that must consider the type of tumor, the cell types involved, and the degree of cellular differentiation.
- Toxicities associated with antineoplastic therapy are a reflection of damage to rapidly dividing cells. Normal tissue with a high growth fraction, such as the GI mucosa, bone marrow, hair follicles, and reproductive system, are most likely to be damaged.
- Host factors that may influence treatment outcome include immune function, nutritional status, psychologic status, availability of supportive care, and social support.
- The time after antineoplastic drug administration when the WBC or platelet count is at the lowest point is referred to as the nadir. For most myelosuppressive drugs, the nadir occurs within 7 to 14 days after drug administration.
- Complete response generally refers to the complete disappearance of all evidence of disease for 1 month or longer following completion of therapy.
- Partial response is usually defined as a reduction in measurable tumor mass of 50 percent or more of its original size for 1 month or more.
- Improvement refers to a reduction in measurable tumor mass by 25 to 50 percent of its original size with subjective improvement in patient status.
- Stable disease is tumor regression of 25 percent or less with or without subjective patient improvement.
- Disease progression refers to clinical evidence of advancing disease during antineoplastic therapy.

BIBLIOGRAPHY

Berman, A., Chisholm, L., deCarvalho, M., et al. (1993). Programmed instruction: Cancer chemotherapy; Intravenous administration. *Cancer Nursing*, 16(2), 145–160.

Bickell, R., and Harris, A. (1996). Mechanisms and therapeutic implications of angiogenesis. *Current Opinions in Oncology*, 8(1), 60–65.

Bonadonna, G., Valagussa, PL., Moliterni, A. (1995). Adjuvant cyclophosphamide, methotrexate, and fluorouracil in node-positive breast cancer. *New England Journal of Medicine,* 332(14), 901–906.

Busollini, F., Montovani, A., Persico, G. (1997). Molecular mechanism of blood vessel formation. *Trends in Biochemical Sciences,* 22(7), 251–256.

Chabner, B., and Longo, D. (1996). *Cancer chemotherapy and biotherapy* (2nd ed.). Philadelphia: Lippincott-Raven.

Charette, J. (1995). Contemporary approaches of chemotherapy. *Critical Care Nursing Clinics of North America,* 7(1), 135–142.

Darnell, J., Lodish, H., Baltimore, D. (1995). *Molecular cell biology* (3rd ed.). New York: W. H. Freeman and Company.

Devita, V., Hellman, S., Rosenberg, S. (1993). *Cancer: Principles and practice of oncology* (4th ed.). Philadelphia: J. B. Lippincott.

Fisher, D., Knobf, M., Durivage, H. (1993). *The cancer chemotherapy handbook* (4th ed.). St. Louis: Mosby Yearbook, Inc.

Fuerst, M. (1996). Multidrug resistance. *Cope,* 12(2), 34–35.

Gately, S., Twordowski, P., Stack, M., et al. (1997). Mechanism of cancer-mediated conversion of plasminogen to the angiogenesis inhibitor angiostatin. *Proceedings of the National Academy of Sciences,* 94(20), 10868–10872.

Hardman, J., Limbird, L., Molinoff, P., et al. (1996). *Goodman and Gilman's the pharmacological basis of therapeutics* (9th ed). New York: McGraw-Hill.

Lake, T., and Jenkins, J. (1993). Programmed instruction: Cancer chemotherapy; clinical trials. *Cancer Nursing,* 16(6), 486–497.

Levy, W., Meadows, B., Quint-Kasner, S., et al. (1993). Programmed instruction: Cancer chemotherapy; chemotherapy agents: Part I. *Cancer Nursing,* 16(4), 321–336.

Madeya, M. (1996). Oral complications from cancer therapy: Parts 1 and 2. *Oncology Nursing Forum,* 23(5), 801–821.

O'Reilly, M., Boehm, T., Shing, Y., et al. (1997). Endostatin: An endogenous inhibitor of angiogenesis tumor growth. *Cell,* 88(2), 277–285.

O'Reilly, M. (1997). Angiostatin: An endogenous inhibitor of angiogenesis and of tumor growth. *EXS (Supplement to Experientia),* 79, 273–294.

Quint-Kasner, S., Chisholm, L., deCarvalho, M., et al. (1993). Programmed instruction: Cancer chemotherapy: Basic principles. *Cancer Nursing,* 16(1), 63–78.

Quint-Kasner, S., Levy, W., Meadows, B., et al. (1993). Programmed instruction: Cancer chemotherapy: Chemotherapy agents: Part II. *Cancer Nursing,* 16(5), 398–418.

Rhodes, V., Johnson, M., McDanial, R. (1995). Nausea, vomiting, and retching: The management of symptoms experience. *Seminars in Oncology Nursing,* 11(4), 256–265.

Tenenbaum, L. (ed.) (1994). *Cancer chemotherapy and biotherapy: A reference guide.* (2nd ed.). Philadelphia: W. B. Saunders.

Zetter, B. (1998). Angiogenesis and tumor metastasis. *Annual Review in Medicine,* 49, 407–424.

Unit V

Drugs Influencing the Cardiovascular System

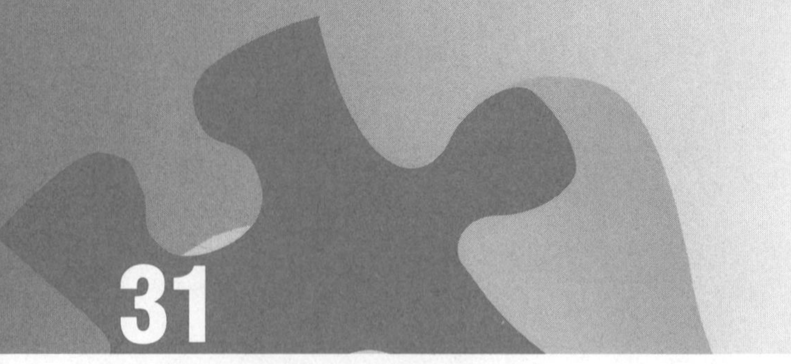

31 Inotropic Drugs

Disorders of the cardiovascular system are many and varied. In addition, the terminology associated with cardiovascular drugs can be confusing. A clear understanding of this terminology is necessary to appreciate the action and effects of cardiovascular drugs.

Cardiovascular drugs can have inotropic, chronotropic, or dromotropic actions. Drugs with *positive inotropic* effects increase the contractile forces of the heart, causing the ventricles to empty more completely, thus improving cardiac output. Positive inotropic drugs include digoxin, a cardiac glycoside, and adrenergic drugs such as dobutamine, dopamine, epinephrine, and isoproterenol (see Chapters 11 and 34). Drugs with *negative inotropic* effects weaken or decrease the force of myocardial contraction. Negative inotropic drugs include lidocaine, quinidine, and propranolol (see Chapter 33).

Drugs with chronotropic action affect the heart rate. Drugs with *positive chronotropic* effects, such as norepinephrine, accelerate the heart rate by increasing the rate of impulse formation at the sinoatrial (SA) node. Drugs with *negative chronotropic* effects (e.g., propranolol) slow the heart rate by decreasing the rate of impulse formation.

Drugs with dromotropic action affect conduction velocity, the speed with which impulses from the SA node pass through conduction pathways. Phenytoin, which has a *positive dromotropic* effect, increases conduction velocity. Drugs with *negative dromotropic* effects, such as the calcium channel–blocking drug verapamil, decrease conduction velocity.

HEART FAILURE

Heart failure is defined as a state in which the heart is unable to pump enough blood to meet the metabolic needs of the body at rest or during exercise. Impairment of cardiac function is responsible for failure of the heart to pump blood at a volume commensurate with venous return—hence, the term *failure*. The term *congestive heart failure* refers to the circulatory overload secondary to heart failure. Pump failure results in hypoperfused tissues followed by pulmonary and vascular congestion. In addition, fluid overload secondary to activation of the body's compensatory mechanisms compounds the difficulty. As cardiac performance deteriorates, blood backs up behind the failing ventricles, causing venous distention and edema—hence, the descriptive term *congestive*. Other terms used to denote heart failure include *cardiac decompensation, cardiac insufficiency,* and *ventricular failure.*

Heart failure can be related to a variety of causes and a spectrum of clinical manifestations. Normally, the pumping action of the left and right sides of the heart complement each other, producing a continuous blood flow. However, as a result of pathologic conditions, one side may fail while the other side continues to function normally for a period of time. With prolonged strain, the functional side of the heart also eventually fails, resulting in biventricular failure (low output failure). Biventricular failure may be unresponsive to treatment because myocardial disease renders the myocardium unable to contract more forcefully no matter what the stimulus.

Epidemiology and Etiology

Cardiovascular disorders are a leading cause of morbidity and mortality in all industrialized nations. According to the American Heart Association, approximately 4.7 million Americans have heart failure, and there are about 400,000 new cases diagnosed each year. The incidence of heart failure after the age of 65 approaches 10:1000 people. Heart failure is the most common cause of in-hospital mortality in patients with cardiovascular disease. It is responsible for one-third of all deaths in patients who have had a myocardial infarction (MI). The etiologies of heart failure can be divided into three groups: abnormal loading, abnormal muscle function, and conditions that precipitate or exacerbate heart failure. When the heart is overloaded with blood, there is excessive stretch of myocardial muscle fibers *(preload).* The increased preload lessens the force and efficiency of ventricular contraction. Conditions that contribute to increased preload include valvular regurgitation, hypervolemia, congenital defects (i.e., septal defects), patent ductus arteriosus, and heart failure.

Afterload is the systemic pressure that opposes left ventricular ejection, that is, the tension the heart must overcome for sufficient ventricular emptying to occur—how hard the heart must pump to force blood into the circulation. Afterload is determined by the vascular tone of the arterioles, the elasticity of the aorta and large arteries, the thickness and size of the ventricle, the presence of aortic stenosis, and the viscosity of the blood. Elevated peripheral vascular resistance and high blood pressure require the ventricles to work harder. With prolonged high pressure, the ventricles eventually fail. Conditions that contribute to increased afterload include aortic and mitral valve stenoses, pulmonary valve stenosis, pulmonary hypertension, high peripheral vascular resistance, and systemic hypertension. In 75 percent of the cases, hypertension preceded the heart failure.

Intrinsic conditions that contribute to abnormal muscle function include MI, myocarditis, cardiomyopathy, and ventricular aneurysm. These disorders impair function of myocardial muscle fibers and reduce ventricular emptying and stroke volume. Extrinsic conditions can also cause abnormal function of the heart muscle. Constrictive pericarditis (an inflammatory, fibrotic process of the pericardial sac) and cardiac tamponade (accumulation of fluid or blood in the pericardial sac) hamper ventricular filling and contractility. Because the pericardium encompasses the entire heart, compression decreases ventricular relaxation, thereby increasing diastolic pressure and hampering forward blood flow through the heart.

Emotional or physical stress increases the workload of the heart by increasing sympathetic nervous system activity. Fever and infection increase the oxygen demands of body tissues. Thyrotoxicosis increases the body's metabolic rate, thus accelerating heart rate and myocardial workload. Anemia reduces the oxygen-carrying capacity of the blood, necessitating increased cardiac output to meet the body's needs for oxygen. Pregnancy, like thyrotoxicosis and anemia, increases the metabolic needs of the body and increases the workload. Thiamine (vitamin B_1) deficiency, often associated with excessive use of alcohol, interferes with cardiac function by decreasing contractility, increasing the heart rate, and causing ventricular dilation. Pulmonary diseases such as chronic airway limitation (previously known as chronic obstructive pulmonary disease), severe pulmonary embolism, and primary pulmonary hypertension produce sizeable resistance to right ventricular emptying. The resistance can lead to right ventricular hypertrophy and heart failure.

Heart failure can also be precipitated or exacerbated by hypervolemia. Expanded circulatory volume increases venous return to the heart and in turn increases preload. Possible causes of hypervolemia include poor renal function, underlying cardiac disease, corticosteroid therapy, and excessive intake of sodium.

Physiology and Pathophysiology

To understand the relationship of preload and afterload to heart failure and how inotropic drugs influence body systems, a review of anatomy and physiology is necessary. The cardiovascular system functions simply to deliver oxygen, nutrients, and other substances to body cells and assist in removing the waste products of cellular metabolism. Any disease, condition, or drug that influences these basic functions affects overall cardiovascular function. The kidneys, often viewed as merely organs of elimination, are essential to the cardiovascular system in that they regulate blood volume, composition, and pressure.

Cardiac Function

The heart is viewed as two pumps functioning synchronously to serve the pulmonary and peripheral circulations. The right side of the heart pumps blood through the lungs. The left side of the heart pumps blood through the peripheral circulation. The heart's position within the chest cavity changes with each respiration, moving vertically during inspiration as the diaphragm descends and horizontally as the diaphragm ascends during expiration.

Each of the pulsatile two-chamber structures is made up of an atrium and a ventricle. Conceptually, the atria are primer pumps that increase the effectiveness of ventricular output by as much as 25 percent. The heart can continue to operate, however, even without the additional 25 percent. This is because the heart normally has the ability to pump 300 to 400 percent more blood than is required by the resting body. When the atria fail, the difference may go unnoticed unless the person exercises; then shortness of breath and other acute signs of heart failure may appear.

The ventricles, on the other hand, supply the main force that propels blood through the pulmonic valve into pulmonary circulation and through the aortic valve into peripheral circulation. The two pump systems are serially connected; thus the output of the right ventricle becomes the input for the left ventricle.

For the two pumps to be effective they must operate in tandem with each other. The atria contract while the ventricles are relaxed, allowing blood to flow freely and rapidly from the atria to the ventricles. Driven by the left ventricle, pressures are greatest in the peripheral circulation. This explains why the muscle of the left ventricle is several times thicker than that of the right ventricle, which sends blood only through the low-pressure pulmonary circulation. When the ventricles contract, the atria are relaxed and filling with blood.

During systole the ventricles contract, and blood is ejected. The mitral and tricuspid valves close (S_1 heart sound), preventing the backflow of blood into the atria. The aortic and pulmonic valves open, permitting forward flow of blood into the pulmonic and systemic circulations. During diastole the ventricles relax, and atria contract. This allows the ventricles to fill. The aortic and pulmonic valves close (S_2 heart sound), and the mitral and tricuspid valves open.

The volume of blood that is ejected from the left ventricle into the aorta (in 1 minute) is referred to as *cardiac output*. Because the blood transports oxygen and other substances to all body tissues, cardiac output is probably the most important circulatory measurement.

Cardiac output is determined by the stroke volume and the heart rate (beats per minute [bpm]). In a resting adult, the *stroke volume,* the amount of blood ejected during each ventricular contraction, averages 70 to 75 mL of blood. The average heart rate is 75 bpm. The average cardiac output, then, in a resting adult may be calculated as follows:

$$\text{Cardiac output} = \text{stroke volume} \times \text{heart rate (bpm)}$$

$$\text{CO} = 70\ \text{mL} \times 75\ \text{bpm} = 5250\ \text{mL/min or } 5.25\ \text{L/min}$$

Any factor that increases the stroke volume or heart rate increases cardiac output. Stroke volume is increased by circulating catecholamines, certain drugs, and sympathetic nervous system stimulation. For example, during mild exercise stroke volume may be increased to 100 mL/contraction and the heart rate 100 bpm due to sympathetic stimulation. The cardiac output then is 10 L/min. During more vigorous exercise the stroke volume may be 112 mL/contraction with the heart rate at 120 bpm. Cardiac output then would be 13.44 L/min. Factors that decrease the stroke volume or heart rate, such as hypoxemia and acidosis, tend also to decrease cardiac output.

Stroke volume is dependent on three factors: preload, the intrinsic contractility of the myocardium, and the afterload. Preload is measured by the degree of stretch of ventricular muscle fibers at the onset of contraction. The larger the preload, the greater the stroke volume, until a point is reached when the muscle is so stretched that it can no longer contract.

According to Starling's law, the force of the contraction is determined primarily by the length of muscle fibers and is proportional to the amount of blood remaining in the ventricle at the end of diastole. The situation is somewhat like stretching a rubber band; the more it is stretched, the harder it contracts. To monitor preload, the index of left ventricular end diastolic pressure is used. Knowledge of pressure changes is important because excessive left ventricular filling pressures cause blood to back up into pulmonary circulation where it forces plasma out through vessel walls. That fluid accumulation in lung tissues is *pulmonary edema.*

End diastolic volume refers to the volume of blood left in the ventricle following contraction and is determined by two additional factors: the quantity of venous blood returning to the heart and the strength of the atrial contraction pumping blood into the ventricles. When the preload decreases, the amount of blood in the ventricles at the end of diastole decreases, and therefore stroke volume is decreased. When other factors are held constant (heart rate, contractility, and afterload), the force of muscle contraction is directly proportional to the preload.

End systolic volume is determined principally by arterial pressure and the force of ventricular contraction. Arterial pressure in the aorta and pulmonary trunk just prior to ventricular systole is the pressure that must be overcome for the pulmonic and aortic valves to open. If arterial pressure is significantly elevated, the resistance prevents the ventricles from pumping as much as they should, and stroke volume decreases.

Compensatory Mechanisms

Heart failure can have an abrupt onset, or it can be the result of a slow, insidious, progressive disease process. In an attempt to maintain adequate cardiac output the body triggers three primary compensatory mechanisms: sympathetic nervous system stimulation, ventricular dilation, and ventricular hypertrophy. Because of an inadequate stroke volume and cardiac output, the baroreceptor reflexes stimulate the sympathetic nervous system to release epinephrine and norepinephrine. The increased sympathetic nervous system activity increases the heart rate and contractility to raise cardiac output. Arteriolar constriction increases blood pressure and decreases blood flow to the periphery and increases blood flow to vital organs. Venous constriction improves venous return to the heart and increases preload. Venous vasoconstriction occurs in an attempt to increase venous blood flow to the heart. The arteriolar vasoconstriction, however, has a downside in that it increases the afterload and increases myocardial oxygen requirements.

In addition to sympathetic stimulation of the heart rate and stroke volume, the failing heart attempts to compensate via Starling's law either by ventricular dilation or by hypertrophy to increase cardiac output. Ventricular dilation and increased contractility create greater wall tension, but also increase myocardial oxygen consumption. Similarly, hypertrophy of the heart muscle increases the amount of working muscle mass and their contractile powers. There are tradeoffs, however. Eventually, ventricular hypertrophy becomes inadequate as the elastic elements of muscle fibers are strained. The overstretched muscle fibers create increased contractile forces. The dilation and hypertrophy result in a decrease in coronary blood flow. Hypertrophied ventricles become stiff, requiring greater left end diastolic pressures to achieve adequate filling.

The mechanism of fluid retention and subsequent elevation of left end diastolic pressure in patients with heart failure is multifactorial. As cardiac output falls, blood flow to the kidneys also falls. The juxtaglomerular apparatus in the kidneys interprets this as a decreased volume. The kidneys release renin, which interacts with angiotensinogen to form angiotensin, a potent vasoconstrictor. The angiotensin causes the adrenal cortex to release aldosterone, which in turn causes sodium retention that increases blood volume and further increases arterial pressure. The posterior pituitary senses the increased osmotic pressure (due to sodium and water retention) and subsequently secretes antidiuretic hormone. Antidiuretic hormone increases water reabsorption in the distal convoluted tubules and collecting ducts of the nephron. The process is cyclical, creating a downward spiral of the patient's condition.

When the compensatory mechanisms function properly to provide adequate cardiac output, the patient has compensated heart failure. When the compensatory mechanisms can no longer assist in maintaining cardiac output, and therefore adequate tissue perfusion, the patient has decompensated heart failure. Even with treatment, the prognosis for decompensated heart failure is poor and may even be fatal.

Classification of Heart Failure

There are several different classifications of heart failure. This discussion is limited to the three that apply to chronic heart failure: left ventricular failure versus right ventricular failure, forward failure versus backward failure, and acute versus chronic failure.

Left Ventricular Failure Versus Right Ventricular Failure

The basis of left ventricular failure versus right ventricular failure is the fact that blood accumulates behind the chamber that first fails. Because contractility is altered, there is an accumulation of blood in the left ventricle, left atrium, and pulmonary circulation—hence, left ventricular heart failure. However, because the cardiovascular structures make up a closed system, failure of one ventricle frequently progresses to failure of the other. Although it is common for right-sided heart failure to follow left-sided failure, the reverse is rare (Fig. 31–1). Right ventricular heart failure is most often caused by pulmonary vasoconstriction due to hypoxia from chronic airway limitation (e.g., chronic bronchitis or emphysema). Right-sided failure due to pulmonary disease is referred to as *cor pulmonale.*

Forward Versus Backward Failure

Forward heart failure is characterized by inadequate cardiac output in a forward direction (i.e., toward systemic circulation). It leads to a decrease in the perfusion of vital organs. Backward failure is usually caused by some mechanical cardiac obstruction, such as valvular stenosis. Damming of blood behind the failing chamber causes increased pressure upstream from one or both ventricles.

Acute Versus Chronic Failure

Acute versus chronic failure is also sometimes referred to as *high-output versus low-output* heart failure, respectively.

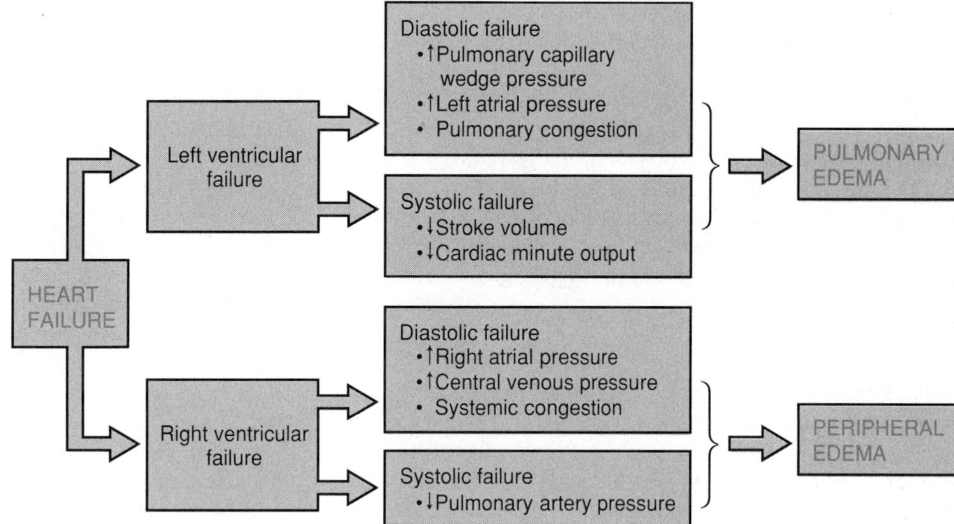

Figure 31–1 Compensatory mechanisms associated with right and left ventricular failure.

Acute failure occurs when the heart is unable to meet the accelerated needs of the body. Causes of acute failure include sepsis, Paget's disease, anemia, thyrotoxicosis, arteriovenous (AV) fistula, pregnancy, and acute MI. The underlying symptoms of chronic heart failure develop slowly because the various compensatory mechanisms are in operation. Chronic failure occurs in most forms of heart disease. The underlying problem is related to ineffective ventricular pumping and low cardiac output related to the increased metabolic needs of body tissues. Patients may have a superimposed acute heart failure caused by an aggravating factor such as uncontrolled atrial fibrillation.

PHARMACOTHERAPEUTIC OPTIONS

In 1785, William Withering published his famous book, *An Account of the Foxglove and Some of Its Medical Uses: With Practical Remarks on Dropsy and Other Diseases.* Heart failure was referred to as *dropsy* at the time because of the edema. Digitalis, the prototype drug, is derived from the dried leaf of the purple or white foxglove and has been used therapeutically for many years. The term *digitalis* is sometimes used to designate the entire class of digitalis glycosides. Natural sources include the flowers of the lily of the valley and the Christmas rose, the bulb of a marine plant known as *squill,* and the venom of certain toads. The expense of purifying the latter substances prevents their direct clinical use. At this time, there are no synthetic sources of the cardiac glycosides. Indeed, the most current drugs used in the treatment of heart failure do include the cardiac glycosides but also phosphodiesterase inhibitors, angiotensin-converting enzyme (ACE) inhibitors, diuretics, and vasodilators. This chapter focuses exclusively on the cardiac glycosides and phosphodiesterase inhibitors. Chapter 33 discusses vasodilators in depth, Chapter 34 discusses ACE inhibitors, and Chapter 39 discusses the diuretics.

Cardiac Glycosides

❒ Digoxin (LANOXIN, LANOXICAPS); (🍁) NOVO-DIGOXIN
❒ Digitoxin (CRYSTODIGIN); (🍁) DIGITALINE

Indications

Cardiac glycosides, alone or in combination with diuretics and vasodilators, have conventionally been used in the management of heart failure. In addition, cardiac glycosides are used to control the ventricular rate of patients with atrial fibrillation, atrial flutter, and paroxysmal atrial tachycardia. The drugs in a sense are palliative in that they improve cardiac functioning without treating the underlying cause.

Pharmacodynamics

Each of the cardiac glycoside preparations has an aglycone (the noncarbohydrate group of a glycoside molecule) that is conjugated with one to four different sugar molecules. The sugar molecules act to modify the water and lipid solubility, potency, and pharmacokinetic properties of the resulting glycoside. All of the glycosides are potent in very small doses, and their therapeutic effects on the heart are qualitatively similar.

The exact mechanism of cardiac glycoside activity is unknown. However, it is thought that positive inotropic effects are produced by inhibiting the Na^+-K^+-ATPase enzyme. This enzyme normally hydrolyzes adenosine triphosphate (ATP) to provide the energy needed for the Na^+-K^+ pump to release sodium and transport potassium into the cardiac cell during repolarization. By binding specifically to the Na^+-K^+-ATPase complex, glycosides inhibit the active transport of sodium and potassium. With the complex inhibited, more calcium is allowed to enter the cell, rendering it more irritable, with a more forceful contraction. The increased inotropic action thus increases cardiac output, which reduces preload and, secondarily, the left ventricular end diastolic pressure. At the same time, there is no overall increase in oxygen consumption. ATPase is further inhibited when serum potassium or serum magnesium levels are low, possibly leading to arrhythmias.

In addition, the glycosides produce negative chronotropic and dromotropic effects by influencing three electrophysical properties of cardiac muscle tissue: automaticity, conduction velocity, and the refractory period. Low to moderate doses of cardiac glycoside slow the heart rate because the SA node depolarizes less often. Conduction through the

AV node and the bundle of His is depressed due to an increase in the refractory period of the AV node and increased vagal tone.

By increasing the stroke volume and improving ventricular emptying, the glycosides act indirectly to decrease heart size. On the other hand, toxic levels of a glycoside preparation directly increase automaticity, increasing the rate of action potential formation and spontaneous depolarization. This is one of the mechanisms responsible for glycoside-induced ectopic pacemakers. Antiarrhythmic drugs are discussed in Chapter 33.

Adverse Effects and Contraindications

Most adverse effects associated with cardiac glycosides are symptoms of toxicity. There are two primary causes of cardiac glycoside toxicity: improper dosing and the concurrent administration of diuretics. Some diuretics promote potassium loss. However, potassium loss can have a number of other causes. These include vomiting or diarrhea, steroid or laxative use, concurrent use of certain extended-spectrum penicillins (e.g., carbenicillin, ticarcillin, piperacillin, mezlocillin), and amphotericin B, an antifungal drug. Poor dietary intake of potassium, the continuous use of potassium-free intravenous (IV) solutions, and dialysis may also contribute to low serum potassium levels.

Various other factors predispose the patient to toxicity. The most obvious cause of toxicity is the administration of too large a dose of glycoside. The overdosage, however, may result from a health care provider's decision, the patient independently increasing the dosage, or increased absorption of the drug. For example, increased absorption may occur as the result of changes from one formulation to one with greater bioavailability. Rapid IV administration can also produce toxicity. A decreased renal elimination rate can increase serum concentrations of the drug to a toxic level. Hypothyroidism increases the likelihood of glycoside toxicity because elimination of the glycoside is depressed and because the heart is more sensitive to glycosides.

Serum concentrations of digitalis that are associated with toxicity typically cause rhythm disturbances. The therapeutic effect of slowing conduction through the AV node, although beneficial and desirable in most cases of heart failure, can produce varying degrees of arrhythmias and heart block. Premature ventricular contractions are among the most common glycoside-induced arrhythmias and are usually described by the patient as "skipped beats." Premature ventricular contractions can be caused by one of several causes, however, and are not specific for glycoside toxicity. Bradycardia, a slowing of the pulse rate to 60 bpm or less, is an extension of the drug's therapeutic action of slowing AV nodal conduction and of SA nodal suppression.

Additionally, abnormally large concentrations of serum calcium may also contribute to toxicity. A hypercalcemic state can result from sustained bedrest, multiple myeloma, parathyroid disease, or iatrogenic calcium supplements. A low serum magnesium level, commonly found in persons who abuse alcohol, produces effects similar to those of hypercalcemia.

The earliest sign of chronic toxicity is anorexia, but this is often overlooked. Diarrhea may also be noted and, in rare cases, is the only gastrointestinal manifestation of toxicity. Abdominal discomfort often accompanies the other symptoms. Because adverse effects are caused, at least in part, by stimulation of the chemoreceptor trigger zone in the medulla, nausea occurs with parenteral as well as oral forms of the drug. The presence of these symptoms raises a suspicion of glycoside toxicity. The gastrointestinal effects are usually self-limiting and disappear with continued therapy.

Toxic symptoms may also appear in other body symptoms. Headache, drowsiness, fatigue, and confusion are common adverse effects that may occur early in treatment. Generalized muscle weakness and fatigue may be particularly prominent. The central nervous system adverse effects are most common in older adults.

Visual disturbances appear as blurred vision or double vision. White borders or halos may appear on dark objects (hence the term *white vision*), and the objects may appear frosted. Color vision may be disturbed, with the colors green and yellow most commonly affected (chromatopsia). In some cases red, brown, and blue colors are also affected.

Gynecomastia, although rare, can be seen in both genders. It is related to the steroid component of the glycoside and is more common with digoxin. Other less common adverse effects include pruritus, mental depression, and respiratory depression.

Contraindications to cardiac glycosides include hypersensitivity, uncontrolled ventricular arrhythmias, AV block, idiopathic hypertrophic subaortic stenosis, constrictive pericarditis, and known alcohol intolerance. These drugs should be used with caution in patients with electrolyte abnormalities who have had a recent MI and in older adults because of a particular sensitivity to toxic effects.

Pharmacokinetics

The majority of cardiac glycosides are completely absorbed from the gastrointestinal tract, primarily the jejunum. The extent of the absorption varies with the specific drug formulation. Digoxin tablets are 60 to 85 percent absorbed, whereas liquid-filled capsules are 90 to 100 percent absorbed and elixirs approximately 75 to 80 percent absorbed. Digoxin administered by intramuscular (IM) injection is approximately 80 percent absorbed; however, the IM route is not recommended due to pain and irritation.

Peak plasma levels are reached in an otherwise healthy person in 6 to 8 hours when the drug is administered orally (Table 31–1). If a loading dose is not given, it can take up to a full week before steady-state plasma concentrations are achieved.

Absorption of digitoxin is over 90 percent because it is more lipid soluble than digoxin. Because of its long half-life (5 to 7 days), steady-state concentrations are attained more slowly than with digoxin and recovery from a toxic state may be extended.

Cardiac glycosides are slowly, but widely, distributed throughout the body. The highest concentrations are found in the heart, kidneys, liver, intestine, stomach, and skeletal muscle. Serum levels are not significantly altered by body fat concentration. However, heart failure itself may slow the rate at which steady-state distribution is attained. Differences in tissue protein binding between digoxin and digitoxin account for, in part, the differences in therapeutic levels. At equilibrium, serum concentrations in cardiac tissues

TABLE 31–1 PHARMACOKINETICS OF SELECTED INOTROPIC DRUGS

Drug	Route	Onset	Peak	Duration	PB (%)	t½	BioA (%)	Serum Level
Cardiac Glycosides								
Digoxin	po	0.5–2 hr	6–8 hr	2–4 days	20–30	26–52 hr	57–83	0.5–2 mcg/mL
	IV	5–30 min	1–5 hr			32–48 hr	100	
Digitoxin	po	0.5–2 hr	4–12 hr	2–3 weeks	97	5–7 days	>90	14–26 mcg/mL
Phosphodiesterase Inhibitors								
Amrinone	IV	2–5 min	10 min	30 min to 2 hr	10–49	3.6–5.8 hr	80–100	3.7 mcg/mL
Milrinone	IV	Immediately	5–15 min	8 hr	UA	2.3 hr	100	UA

UA, unavailable; PB, protein binding; BioA, bioavailability, t½, elimination half-life.

are 15 to 30 times those of plasma. Cardiac glycosides cross the blood-brain barrier and placental membranes and are found in breast milk. Biotransformation of cardiac glycosides takes place in the liver, with 14 percent of the administered dose transformed by hepatic enzymes. Digoxin is eliminated almost entirely unchanged by the kidneys. Digitoxin on the other hand is primarily biotransformed by the liver. Some of the metabolites retain cardiac activity.

The half-life of orally administered digoxin (26 to 52 hours) is dependent on adequate renal function and the oral formulation used. At any given maintenance dose, there is a close correlation between creatinine clearance and the concentration of digoxin in the plasma. Digoxin is excreted almost totally unchanged by the kidneys.

Drug-Drug Interactions

Drug-drug interactions with glycosides are many (Table 31–2). Additive, synergistic, and even antagonistic effects may occur. Biotransformation of cardiac glycosides can be

TABLE 31–2 DRUG-DRUG INTERACTIONS OF SELECTED INOTROPIC DRUGS

Drug	Interactive Drug	Interaction
Digoxin Digitoxin	Adrenocorticosteroids Amphotericin-B Loop and thiazide diuretics Mezlocillin Piperacillin Ticarcillin	Increased risk of hypokalemia that can lead to digoxin toxicity
	Amiodarone Anticholinergics Cyclosporine Diflunisal Diltiazem Hydroxychloroquine Propafenone Quinidine Spironolactone Verapamil	Increased serum levels leading to increased risk of toxicity
	Beta blockers Diltiazem Disopyramide Quinidine Verapamil	Additive bradycardia
	Antacids Antidiarrheals Cathartics Cholestyramine Colestipol Oral aminoglycosides	Decreased absorption and effectiveness of cardiac glycoside
	Magnesium sulfate Succinylcholine Thyroid preparations	Increased risk of arrhythmias and cardiac toxicity
	Phenobarbital Phenylbutazone Phenytoin Rifampin Thyroid preparations	Decreased effectiveness of digitoxin
	Indomethacin	Decreased excretion of glycoside
Amrinone	Cardiac glycosides	Additive inotropic effects
	Disopyramide	Exaggerated hypotension

enhanced with the concurrent administration of hepatic enzyme-inducing drugs such as phenobarbital, rifampin, and phenytoin.

Drug-Food Interactions

The concurrent ingestion of a high fiber meal may decrease the absorption of the cardiac glycoside. Milk, cheeses, yogurt, and ice cream should be avoided for at least 2 hours before and after taking digoxin because these foods reduce its absorption.

Dosage Regimens

Digitalizing Doses

For rapid effects, a larger initial loading dose *(digitalizing dose)* is administered several times (e.g., every 4 to 8 hours IV or every 6 hours orally) over 12 to 24 hours. Digitalization allows saturation of plasma proteins and other body tissues before therapeutic serum concentrations are achieved. Nomograms and formula calculations are available to estimate digoxin dosage. However, most calculations are based on the patient's body weight (Table 31–3). In a given situation, load-

TABLE 31–3 DOSAGE REGIMENS OF SELECTED INOTROPICS

Drug	Age	Dosage	Implications
Cardiac Glycosides			
IV digoxin	Neonate	*Loading dose:* 20–30 mcg/kg in divided doses Q6–8 hr. *Maintenance dose:* 20–30% of initial dose in 2 divided doses/day	Monitor apical pulse for 1 full minute prior to administering a cardiac glycoside. Withhold dose and notify health care provider if pulse rate is below 60 bpm or over 110 bpm in an adult or less than 90 bpm in an infant. Before administering an initial loading dose determine if the patient has taken any digitalis preparations in the previous 2–3 weeks. For rapid digitalization, the initial dose is higher than the maintenance dose; ¼ to ½ of the total digitalizing dose is given initially. The remainder of the dose to be administered in the increments at 4–8 hr intervals. Use caution whenchanging formulations. They are not equivalent
	1–24 mo	*Loading dose:* 30–50 mcg/kg in divided doses Q6–8 hr. *Maintenance dose:* 25–35% of initial dose given in 2–3 divided doses/day	
	2–5 years	*Loading dose:* 25–35 mcg/kg in divided doses Q6–8 hr. *Maintenance dose:* 25–35% of initial dose given in 2–3 divided doses/day	
	5–10 years	*Loading dose:* 15–30 mcg/kg in divided doses Q6–8 hr. *Maintenance dose:* 25–35% of initial dose given in 2–3 divided doses/day	
	Adults and children over 10	*Loading dose:* 8–12 mcg/kg in divided doses Q4–8 hr (Q6–8 hr in children). *Maintenance dose:* 25–35% of initial dose given in 2–3 divided doses/day	
Digoxin tablets/elixir	Neonates	*Loading dose:* 25–35 mcg/kg in divided doses Q6–8 hr. *Maintenance dose:* 25–35% of initial dose as a single daily dose	
	1–24 mo	*Loading dose:* 35–60 mcg/kg in divided doses Q6–8 hr. *Maintenance dose:* 25–35% of initial dose as a single daily dose	
	2–10 years	*Loading dose:* 30–40 mcg/kg in divided doses Q6–8 hr. *Maintenance dose:* 20–30% of initial dose as a single daily dose	
	Adults	*Loading dose:* 8–12 mcg/kg. Give ½ dose initially, the remainder Q4–8 hr. *Maintenance dose:* 15–25% of initial dose as a single daily dose	
Oral digitoxin	Adults	*Loading dose:* 1.2–1.6 mg/kg in divided doses/day. *Maintenance dose:* 50–300 mcg daily	
Phosphodiesterase Inhibitors			
IV amrinone	Neonate	*Loading dose:* 3–4.5 mg/kg in divided doses followed by infusion at 3–5 mcg/kg/min	Protect drug from light and avoid mixing with glucose-containing solutions. Blood pressure, pulse, electrocardiogram, respiratory rate, cardiac index, pulmonary wedge pressure, and central venous pressure should be monitored frequently during therapy. Hypokalemia should be corrected before administration. Change position slowly to minimize drug-induced hypotension
	Infants	*Loading dose:* 3–4.5 mg/kg in divided doses followed by infusion at 10 mcg/kg/min	
	Adults	*Loading dose:* 0.75 mg/kg over 2–3 min. Start infusion of 5–10 mcg/kg/min. May give another bolus 30 min after start of therapy. Not to exceed 10 mg/kg total daily dose	
IV milrinone	Adults	*Loading dose:* 50 mcg/kg over 10 minutes followed by infusion at 0.5 mcg/kg/min. Range: 0.375–0.75 mcg/kg/min	Monitor the electrocardiogram, blood pressure, respirations, and heart rate continually during therapy. The risk of ventricular arrhythmias is increased in patients with a history of arrhythmias, electrolyte disturbances, and abnormal digoxin levels or who have vascular catheters inserted

ing doses are somewhat relative depending on age, body size, medical condition of the patient, the particular glycoside, and the route of administration.

Maintenance Doses

Maintenance doses are based on the patient's renal function and individual response and on the proportion of daily losses. In general, however, doses required for atrial arrhythmias are higher than those for inotropic effects. In patients taking digoxin who have normal renal function, this is approximately 35 percent of the total body store. For those on digitoxin, it is approximately 10 percent. Whether the desired effect has been obtained can be evaluated through careful and frequent observation of the patient. Electrocardiograms and plasma drug levels are helpful in adjusting the dose. Evaluation of therapeutic response includes noting changes in the signs and symptoms of failure, such as weight loss, reduced venous pressure, and improved exercise tolerance.

Laboratory Considerations

Serum electrolytes and hepatic functions should be evaluated periodically throughout glycoside therapy. Hypokalemia, hypomagnesemia, and hypercalcemia make the patient more susceptible to toxicity. There are no known drug-laboratory test alterations with glycosides.

Phosphodiesterase Inhibitors

- ❐ Amrinone (INOCOR)
- ❐ Milrinone (PRIMACOR)

AMRINONE

Presently, amrinone lactate is the only phosphodiesterase inhibitor approved for use in the United States for the short-term management (2 to 3 days) of heart failure in patients who have not responded to diuretics, digoxin, or vasodilators. The drug was discovered in a search for positive inotropic drugs that had a better therapeutic/toxic ratio than digoxin. When given to digitalized patients, amrinone increases stroke volume and cardiac output, decreases left ventricular end diastolic pressure and pulmonary artery wedge pressure, promotes vasodilation, and increases exercise tolerance.

Amrinone does not inhibit Na^+-K^+-ATPase. Instead, the effects result from intracellular accumulation of cyclic adenosine monophosphate secondary to inhibition of phosphodiesterase III, the enzyme that normally degrades cyclic adenosine monophosphate. In so doing, it reduces preload and afterload through a direct effect on vascular smooth muscle. The phosphodiesterase inhibitors do not stimulate alpha or beta receptors or provoke the release of histamine or prostaglandins. They are considered nonglycoside, noncatecholamine drugs that relax vascular tone, thus decreasing peripheral and pulmonary vascular resistance and dilating coronary vessels. They also have been evaluated as substitutes for cardiac glycosides in the treatment of heart failure that is unresponsive to glycosides, diuretics, or vasodilators.

The most common adverse effects of amrinone are arrhythmias, thrombocytopenia, and tachyphylaxis. Dyspnea, nausea, vomiting, diarrhea, hepatotoxicity, hypokalemia, fever, and hypersensitivity reactions are also possible adverse effects. The drug is contraindicated in patients with hypersensitivity to amrinone or bisulfates and in patients with idiopathic hypertrophic subaortic stenosis. It should be used with caution in patients with atrial fibrillation or flutter because it can increase ventricular response. In this case, pretreatment with a cardiac glycoside may be necessary. Amrinone should also be used with caution in patients who have had recent aggressive diuretic therapy and in pregnancy and lactation. Safe use in children under age 18 years has not been established.

Amrinone is available only as an IV injection. Amrinone is 100 percent bioavailable when given IV. The distribution sites of amrinone are unknown, although it is 10 to 49 percent bound to plasma proteins. Onset of amrinone's inotropic effects is 2 to 5 minutes, with peak effects noted in approximately 10 minutes. The effects of amrinone can last up to 2 hours after the infusion is discontinued. Its half-life is approximately 3.6 hours, but this value may be increased to approximately 5.8 hours in patients with heart failure. One-half of a dose of amrinone is biotransformed in the liver. Sixty-three percent of the drug is eliminated in the urine as both parent compound and metabolites. Approximately 18 percent is eliminated in the stool.

Drug-drug interactions with amrinone are few but can be significant. There may be additive inotropic effects when amrinone is used concurrently with cardiac glycosides. Hypotension may be exaggerated in the presence of disopyramide.

Amrinone therapy is initiated with a dosage of 0.75 mg/kg over 2 to 3 minutes, followed by a maintenance infusion of 5 to 10 mcg/kg/min. The recommended maximal daily dose should not exceed 10 mg/kg. The dosage is adjusted according to patient response. Tachyphylaxis (rapid development of tolerance) develops within the first 72 hours.

Platelet counts, serum electrolytes, liver enzymes, and hepatic and renal function should be evaluated periodically throughout therapy. If the platelet count drops below $150{,}000/mm^3$ the health care provider should be promptly notified. Increased liver enzymes may indicate hepatotoxicity. Amrinone may also cause decreased serum potassium levels.

MILRINONE

Milrinone is also used for the short-term management of heart failure unresponsive to conventional therapy with cardiac glycosides, diuretics, and vasodilators. It has been shown to increase myocardial contractility and to decrease preload and afterload through a direct dilating effect on vascular smooth muscle. Its actions overall are similar to those of amrinone. In recent studies of patients with moderately severe heart failure, the combination of milrinone and digoxin was no more effective than digoxin alone.

Adverse effects of milrinone include headache, tremor, hypotension, hypokalemia, thrombocytopenia, angina pectoris, and chest pain. Its life-threatening effects include supraventricular arrhythmias and ventricular arrhythmias. Recent evidence suggests that there may be an increased mortality rate associated with milrinone therapy.

Milrinone is contraindicated in patients with hypersensitivity, severe aortic or pulmonary valvular heart disease, and hypertrophic subaortic stenosis. It should be used cautiously in patients with a history of arrhythmias, electrolyte imbalances, and abnormal digoxin levels. Insertion of vascular catheters causes increased risk of ventricular arrhythmias. Safety during pregnancy and lactation or in children has not been established.

Milrinone is 100 percent bioavailable, although its distribution is unknown. From 80 to 90 percent of milrinone is eliminated unchanged in the urine, with a half-life of 2.3 hours. The half-life is increased in patients with renal impairment.

A loading dose of milrinone 50 mcg/kg is followed by an infusion of 0.5 mcg/kg/min. The dosage range is from 0.375 to 0.75 mcg/kg/min. Overdose manifests as hypotension. When this occurs, the dosage should be decreased or the drug discontinued.

Laboratory testing of electrolytes and renal function is required frequently during milrinone therapy. Hypokalemia should be corrected prior to administration to reduce the risk of arrhythmias. As with amrinone, platelet counts should also be monitored throughout therapy.

Critical Thinking Process

Assessment

History of Present Illness

The most common symptoms of heart failure are shortness of breath, often exertional at first and progressing to orthopnea, paroxysmal nocturnal dyspnea, and resting dyspnea. A more subtle and often overlooked symptom is a chronic nonproductive cough. Patients may also complain of fatigue, weakness, memory loss and confusion, palpitations, anorexia, and insomnia. With right-sided failure, the patient may complain of weight gain, peripheral edema, abdominal distention, gastric distress, anorexia, or nausea (Table 31–4).

Past Health History

The past health history helps reveal the life-long health record of the patient. The patient should be asked about childhood and infectious diseases, major illnesses, and hospitalizations. A drug history should be done with attention to the use of antihypertensives, diuretics, vasodilators (antianginal drugs), cardiac glycosides, anticoagulants, bronchodilators, contraceptives, and steroids. Corticosteroids cause hypertension and increase fluid retention. Contraceptives increase the risk of thrombophlebitis. Noncardiac drugs can also have profound effects on cardiovascular performance. For example, tricyclic antidepressants and other psychoactive drugs can potentiate arrhythmias. Cocaine increases the heart rate, contractility, blood glucose levels, and peripheral vasoconstriction. It also potentiates the effects of circulating catecholamines.

Several other factors can predispose the patient to heart failure or may worsen its state. Elicit information from the patient regarding past history of anemia, thyrotoxicosis, pulmonary disease, excessive sodium intake, and corticosteroid administration. Anemia requires increased cardiac output to meet the body's need for oxygen. Thyrotoxicosis increases the metabolic needs of the body, accelerating the heart rate and the workload of the heart. Pulmonary disease (e.g., chronic airway limitation, pulmonary emboli, primary pulmonary artery hypertension) increases pressure in the pulmonary system, producing sizeable resistance to the emptying of the right ventricle. An excess in circulating blood volume can result from poor renal function, cardiac disease, drugs (e.g., corticosteroids), or excessive intake of sodium. Overadministration of parenteral fluids may aggravate preexisting heart failure. Infections and fever increase the oxygen demands of body tissues, and strenuous physical and emotional stress increase sympathetic nervous system tone and release of catecholamine. Stress increases heart rate, myocardial contractility, and blood pressure. Additionally, past MI, arrhythmias, and rheumatic carditis also increase the workload of the heart.

Physical Exam

The patient with acute onset heart failure appears acutely ill, but is usually well nourished. In severe failure, peripheral pulses may be weak and thready, and the extremities are cool. Patients may exhibit air hunger when lying flat. The

TABLE 31–4 SUMMARY OF CLINICAL MANIFESTATIONS OF HEART FAILURE

	Signs	Symptoms
Decreased cardiac output	Decreased blood pressure, pulse pressure Pulsus alternans Tachycardia Supraventricular rhythms S_3 and S_4 present	Anxiety and fear Dizziness Syncope Decreased exercise tolerance, fatigue Chest pain
Pulmonary congestion (left ventricular failure)	Dyspnea Orthopnea Paroxysmal nocturnal dyspnea Nocturia	Cough with frothy sputum Tachypnea Bibasilar crackles Increased PADP, PAWP
Systemic congestion (right ventricular failure)	Nausea Indigestion Weakness	Vomiting Jugular vein distention Peripheral and sacral edema Hepatosplenomegaly, ascites Abdominal distention Increased RAP

RAP, right arterial pressure; PADP, pulmonary artery diastolic pressure; PAWP, pulmonary artery wedge pressure.

patient with chronic heart failure often appears malnourished and sometimes even cachectic.

Physical exam findings of patients with heart failure include decreased blood pressure and pulse pressure, pulsus alternans, tachycardia, and supraventricular electrocardiographic rhythms. The classic physical exam findings of left-sided heart failure are crackles, an S_3 gallop, tachypnea, bibasilar crackles, and an increase in pulmonary arterial diastolic and wedge pressures.

Crackles are absent in right-sided failure. Characteristic findings of patients with right-sided heart failure include vomiting, jugular vein distention, peripheral and sacral edema, hepatosplenomegaly, ascites and abdominal distension, and an increased right atrial pressure.

Diagnostic Testing

Several diagnostic tests are useful in evaluating the patient with heart failure. Electrocardiography, exercise electrocardiography (stress testing), echocardiography, chest x-ray, ventriculography (multigated blood pool imaging [MUGA scan]), and cardiac catheterization are sometimes useful. Echocardiography provides information about chamber size and functional ability. A chest x-ray may reveal prominent pulmonary vasculature, evidence suggestive of interstitial edema (Kerley B lines), pleural fluid in fissures, and evidence of pleural effusion.

Developmental Considerations

Perinatal The incidence of heart disease in pregnant women ranges from 0.5 to 2 percent; however, heart failure still ranks high among the causes of death during pregnancy. Rheumatic fever, once responsible for 88 percent of cardiac disease during pregnancy, is now on the decline, responsible for only about 50 percent of cardiac disease cases in pregnancy. Congenital disease now plays a more prominent role. However, because of increases in total body water and changes in cardiovascular, renal, and hormonal function, the woman with a pre-existing disorder can develop heart failure. In addition, a pregnancy with pre-existing cardiac disease increases the woman's risk for thromboembolism, palpitations, and fluid retention. Drug therapy will depend on the specific cardiac abnormality. Although digoxin crosses placental membranes, it does not affect fetal cardiac function. However, this passage into fetal circulation can decrease maternal concentrations and require dosage adjustment. It should also be kept in mind that, just as myocardial contractility is increased, uterine contractility can be affected, leading to preterm labor. Thus, the benefit of inotropic drugs should be balanced with the potential for harm to the mother and the fetus.

Pediatric Heart failure in the pediatric population is most often the result of a surgically correctable structural abnormality. For example, septal defects can cause large left-to-right shunts, resulting in a volume load on the right ventricle. Obstruction to flow from the left ventricle, such as coarctation of the aorta (narrowing), can cause increased pressure inside the ventricle. Heart failure can also be caused by arrhythmias, anemia, myocardial disease (e.g., myocarditis), sepsis, or hypertension. In addition to the usual symptoms of heart failure, the child may experience failure to thrive and feeding difficulties.

Geriatric Heart failure in the older adult is a fairly common occurrence that increases with age. The physical changes of aging and co-morbid diseases such as hypertension, coronary artery disease, bronchitis, and pneumonia influence the incidence of heart failure with advanced age. Associated edema, shortness of breath, and orthopnea reduce activity tolerance. The problem is common in older adults because of age-related changes. The age-related changes, such as reduced elasticity and lumen size of vessels and an increase in blood pressure interfering with the blood supply to the heart muscle makes the heart work harder. The decreased cardiac reserves of the older adult limit the heart's ability to withstand effects of disease or injury. Symptoms of heart failure in older patients include confusion, insomnia, wandering during the night, agitation, depression, anorexia, nausea, weakness, dyspnea, orthopnea, weight gain, and bilateral ankle edema. The management of heart failure in the older adult is basically the same as in middle-aged adults.

Psychosocial Considerations

The psychosocial impact of heart failure on the patient should be assessed. If the patient smokes, inquire about the duration of the smoking habit and the number of cigarettes smoked daily. Cigarette smoking increases the risk of coronary artery disease, worsens hypertension, and contributes to heart failure.

There is no conclusive evidence that caffeine or alcohol intake increases the risk of heart disease. Nevertheless, caffeine increases the heart rate and blood pressure, both of which raise the myocardial workload and can precipitate heart failure. As heart failure worsens, patients may find that their activities of daily living and social activities are restricted due to dyspnea, chest pain, or peripheral edema. Furthermore, the social isolation that results may significantly affect the patient's ability to cope with his or her disease (see Case Study—Chronic Heart Failure with Digoxin Toxicity).

Analysis and Management

Treatment Objectives

The overall management objectives for heart failure include improving hemodynamics, identifying and correcting precipitating factors, relieving symptoms, and improving exercise tolerance and the patient's quality of life. Symptom relief, improved exercise tolerance, and improved quality of life can be enhanced with the use of digoxin, ACE inhibitors, and diuretics. Prolonged survival has been demonstrated with ACE inhibitors. Hemodynamics can be improved with drugs that reduce preload, including cardiac glycosides, ACE inhibitors, diuretics, and nitrates (see Chapter 32).

Drug therapy should be considered in all patients after symptomatic heart failure is documented and acute reversible precipitating factors are removed. Symptoms that warrant drug therapy include decreased exercise tolerance, orthopnea, shortness of breath, and nocturnal polyuria. Drug therapy should be started immediately for patients in acute failure.

The underlying cause of heart failure should be treated. If arrhythmias precipitated the failure, the arrhythmias should be treated accordingly. When the underlying cause is hypertension, antihypertensive drugs are helpful. Surgery may be required if valvular or septal defects are the contributing factors to heart failure.

Case Study Chronic Heart Failure With Digoxin Toxicity

Patient History

History of Present Illness	MB is a 70-year-old black male admitted for evaluation of increasing fatigue and ankle edema. Until recently he was able to remain active. During the past month, the persistent dyspnea confined him to his home. He reports that the dyspnea awakens him at night, and he sits by an open window to "catch his breath." He reports he has "lost my good appetite." He feels the medicines he started 6 weeks ago are not working. Records indicate previous nondrug therapies have failed.
Past Health Illness	MB had an acute MI 5 years ago with subsequent development of chronic heart failure. Since then he has had occasional premature ventricular contractions. Current medicine: benazepril 20 mg po BID, furosemide 20 mg po QD. Although he has a history of CAD, he attributes an otherwise healthy state to the fact that he never drank or smoked and he always eats nutritious meals, including salads. "They are easy to fix and easy for my wife and I to eat. They are also cheaper than some other things."
Physical Exam	Height: 5′8″. Weight: 135 lb. (Up 9 lb from usual weight.) Blood pressure 130/70, respirations 28, temperature 98.6°F. Bibasilar breath sounds within normal limits on auscultation. 1+ pitting edema of ankles, liver enlargement. Pale, but no evidence of cyanosis. Presence of S_3 gallop.
Diagnostic Testing	Chest x-ray: left ventricular enlargement with congestion of pulmonary vasculature, fluid level more prominent right side than left. Electrocardiogram reflects atrial fibrillation with apical rate of 124 bpm. Eight premature ventricular contractions per minute were noted. Sodium 131 mEq/L, potassium 3.8 mEq/L, chlorine 91 mEq/L, blood urea nitrogen 35 mg%, creatinine 1.6 mg%. Thyroid-stimulating hormone within normal limits.
Developmental Considerations	Age-related changes in cardiovascular, gastrointestinal, and renal function. MB reports he is "simply waiting for his turn to meet God."
Psychosocial Considerations	MB retired 3 years ago after 40 years as a railroad mechanic. On several occasions he has expressed concern that he will become a burden to his wife, who is 74 years old and physically unable to assume the responsibility for his care. He feels that if he needs changes in his medicine that he wants to go to once-daily dosing so he will remember to take it. MB has one son and daughter who live nearby. They visit their parents regularly and help with transportation to grocery store, medical appointments, and so forth.
Economic Considerations	MB is covered by Medicare and a railroad supplemental insurance policy that includes pharmacy coverage. He and his wife live on his railroad retirement income.

Variables Influencing Decision

Treatment Objective

- Enhance cardiac performance.
- Identify and correct precipitating factors
- Relieve symptoms of CHF

Drug Variables	*Drug Summary*	*Patient Variables*
Indications	Digoxin: Most effective with dilated heart, low ejection fraction, S_3 gallop, and history of CAD. Benazepril: Reduces mortality and improves functional status with all stages of CHF. Furosemide: Effective for moderate to severe CHF.	MB has dilated heart, low ejection fraction, an S_3 gallop, and history of CAD. He remains symptomatic in spite of ACE inhibitors and diuretic. These become decision points.

Drug Variables	*Drug Summary*	*Patient Variables*
Pharmacodynamics	Digoxin: Slows ventricular rate through AV node. Benazepril: Causes mixed preload and afterload reduction. Furosemide: Decreases plasma volume and increases elimination of sodium and water. Decreases preload. Adding digoxin may help to relieve symptoms through different mechanisms.	MB remains symptomatic in spite of ACE inhibitors and diuretic. This becomes a decision point.
Adverse Effects/ Contraindications	Digoxin and furosemide: Electrolyte abnormalities, increased risk of toxicity related to hypokalemia. Benazepril: Benign cough most common.	MB's serum potassium level is low at this time. Must replace potassium if choose to continue furosemide and add digoxin. This becomes a decision point.
Pharmacokinetics	Pharmacokinetics of benazepril, furosemide, and digoxin vary; however, digoxin has narrow therapeutic index that may contribute to digoxin toxicity if not closely monitored.	Potential for digoxin toxicity due to age-related changes in renal function and concurrent use of furosemide. This may become a decision point.
Dosage Regimen	Use drug options when possible that require once-daily dosing only to foster compliance.	MB has been compliant with drug therapy to date but requests once-daily dosing if possible. This becomes a decision point.
Lab Considerations	Electrolytes and serum drug levels will need to be checked on regular basis for therapeutic effects and to monitor for digoxin toxicity.	MB's son will transport him for required lab monitoring. This will not become a decision point.
Cost Index*	Digoxin: 1 Benazepril: 1 Furosemide: 1	Cost somewhat of a concern but uses AARP pharmacy services for routine drugs to keep cost of out-of-pocket expenses down.

Summary of Decision Points

- Patients who demonstrate the best response to cardiac glycosides are those who have a dilated heart, a low ejection fraction, and an S_3 gallop on auscultation. MB has all three findings.
- Glycosides are most appropriate for low-output ventricular failure caused by CAD. MB has documented history of CAD and MI.
- MB's serum potassium level is low at this time. Must replace potassium if choose to continue furosemide and add digoxin.
- Continued use of ACE inhibitor reduces risk of mortality and improves functional status in patients with all stages of CHF.
- MB requests once-daily dosing if possible so he will remember to take his medicine.

DRUGS TO BE USED

- Change benazepril to 40 mg po QD and furosemide to 20 mg po QD.
- Add digoxin 0.125 mg po QD—titrate based on patient response.

*Cost Index:
1 = $<30/mo.
2 = $30–40/mo.
3 = $40–50/mo.
4 = $50–60/mo.
5 = $>60/mo.

AWP of 30, 0.125-mg tablets of digoxin is approximately $5.
AWP of 30, 40-mg, tablets of benazepril is approximately $20.
AWP of 30, 20-mg, tablets of furosemide is approximately $1.
AARP = American Association of Retired Persons
CAD = Coronary artery disease
CHF = Chronic heart failure

Treatment Options

Drug Variables

Heart failure is a clinical syndrome that results in symptomatic deterioration, functional impairment, and shortened life-span. The syndrome is complicated in that both peripheral and cardiac effects contribute to the progression of heart failure. In the periphery, elevations in sympathetic nervous system activity and the renin-angiotensin system increase afterload, further contributing to salt and water retention. The cardiac abnormalities include remodeling of the heart and down-regulation of beta receptors. Health care providers must be aware of this duality when considering the potential benefits of therapeutic advances and current treatment recommendations. Figure 31–2 provides an algorithm outlining currently recommended drug management strategies (see Controversy—Inotropics: Expectations and Limits).

Cardiac Glycosides The drugs used in the management of heart failure have undergone significant changes in recent years. The use of cardiac glycosides is no longer considered obligatory, and it has become clear that not everyone with heart failure should receive a glycoside. Patients with mild to moderate heart failure may respond sufficiently to nondrug measures, such as sodium restriction and rest. If nondrug measures are ineffective, drug therapy is warranted. If intensive therapy is required, a combination of cardiac glycosides, diuretics, and ACE inhibitors may be warranted.

The effectiveness of cardiac glycosides in treating heart failure depends in part on the cause of the failure and the severity of cardiac damage. The best response to cardiac glycosides is seen in patients who have a dilated heart, a low ejection fraction, and an S_3 gallop on auscultation. Cardiac glycosides are most appropriate for low-output ventricular failure caused by coronary artery disease, hypertension, and cardiac myopathies. They are less effective in high-output failure caused by thiamine deficiency, thyrotoxicosis, and anemia and in mechanical disturbances such as rheumatic heart disease and other valvular disorders. Cardiac glycosides are also less effective in the treatment of right-sided failure.

Because cardiac glycosides act by improving contractility, they are useful only in patients with decreased systolic left ventricular function and heart failure. Many patients with heart failure have normal systemic left ventricular function but diastolic dysfunction because of a thickened left ventricle. This is the case in patients with hypertensive cardiomyopathy.

Digoxin is ideal for slowing the ventricular rate in patients with atrial fibrillation because it increases the refractory period of the AV junction and consequently slows conduction at this site. It blocks atrial impulses from reaching the ventricle. However, cardiac glycosides will not convert fibrillating atria into normally contracting ones. Synchronized cardioversion is the intervention of choice for converting atrial fibrillation to normal sinus rhythm.

ACE Inhibitors Improved survival with ACE inhibitor therapy (e.g., captopril, enalapril, lisinopril, benazepril) (see Chapter 32) has been demonstrated in patients with mild to severe heart failure. Captopril is not ordinarily used for patients with acute heart failure. It is started after diuresis has been initiated with a loop diuretic. Captopril is preferred in

---

Controversy

Inotropics: Expectations and Limits

JONATHAN J. WOLFE

Cardiotonic glycosides derived from the plant genus *Digitalis* have established the classic definition of inotropic agents. Their therapeutic use was established by William Withering in the eighteenth century. These drugs slow the pulse rate and simultaneously strengthen the force of cardiac contraction, thus providing a significant advantage in therapy that continues to have value today. As with most drugs, even these classic inotropic agents present a mixed effect. The challenge now is to use them rationally in an era that offers the health care provider a broad choice of agents, some of which are clearly superior for a given patient.

The advent of intravenous agents has allowed rescue of patients once beyond the reach of treatment. While amrinone represents an almost pure inotropic agent among injectable drugs, dopamine and dobutamine are often considered as inotropes because of their predominant effect. The ability to resuscitate patients or help high-risk patients make a smooth transition through surgery and recovery with the aid of these drugs means that many more patients survive to require chronic therapy.

What drugs ought to be used for the long haul? The issue of choice is clouded by cost. Digoxin is an inexpensive, elegant, and universally available product. However, it is not proper to try every patient who requires inotropic therapy on cardiotonic glycosides. The precision of diagnosis possible with present-day technology allows clear sorting of patients into categories whose best treatment is discoverable. The standard of practice has carried us far beyond the day of the stethoscope and monitoring of edema in the extremities. The same parallel exists in drug choice.

Certain patients must avoid inotropics in favor of other drugs. The calcium channel–blocking agents and the ACE inhibitors have established themselves for monotherapy, as well as for multiple-drug therapy. The addition of new drugs allows increased sophistication in treatment, but obliges vigilance in balancing the elements of a particular drug regimen.

Critical Thinking Discussion

- Your patient has been stable on digoxin for 11 years. Her dosage has required little adjustment, except to decrease the dose around her eightieth birthday. Her general health is good, with only age-related decrease in renal function. A new calcium channel–blocking agent has come to market that may benefit her. What concerns do you have in regard to cost, compliance, and outcome for this patient?
- The 18-month-old boy about to be discharged from your post-surgery care unit has done well since closure of his ventricular septal defect. He was smoothly digitalized after surgery and now receives oral liquid digoxin every 12 hours. What three points are most important for you to make in teaching his parents about giving this drug?
- A 64-year-old man who has been your patient presents to the clinic complaining of nausea, dizziness, and visual disturbance. He has been taking digoxin 250 mcg orally once daily without incident for the past 10 months. The only remarkable element of his history today is that he has decided to use vitamin and mineral supplements in order to bolster his health, as advised by a new book he has bought at the Herbal Boutique at the nearby mall. What mineral would you be most concerned to find he is taking in megadose quantities?

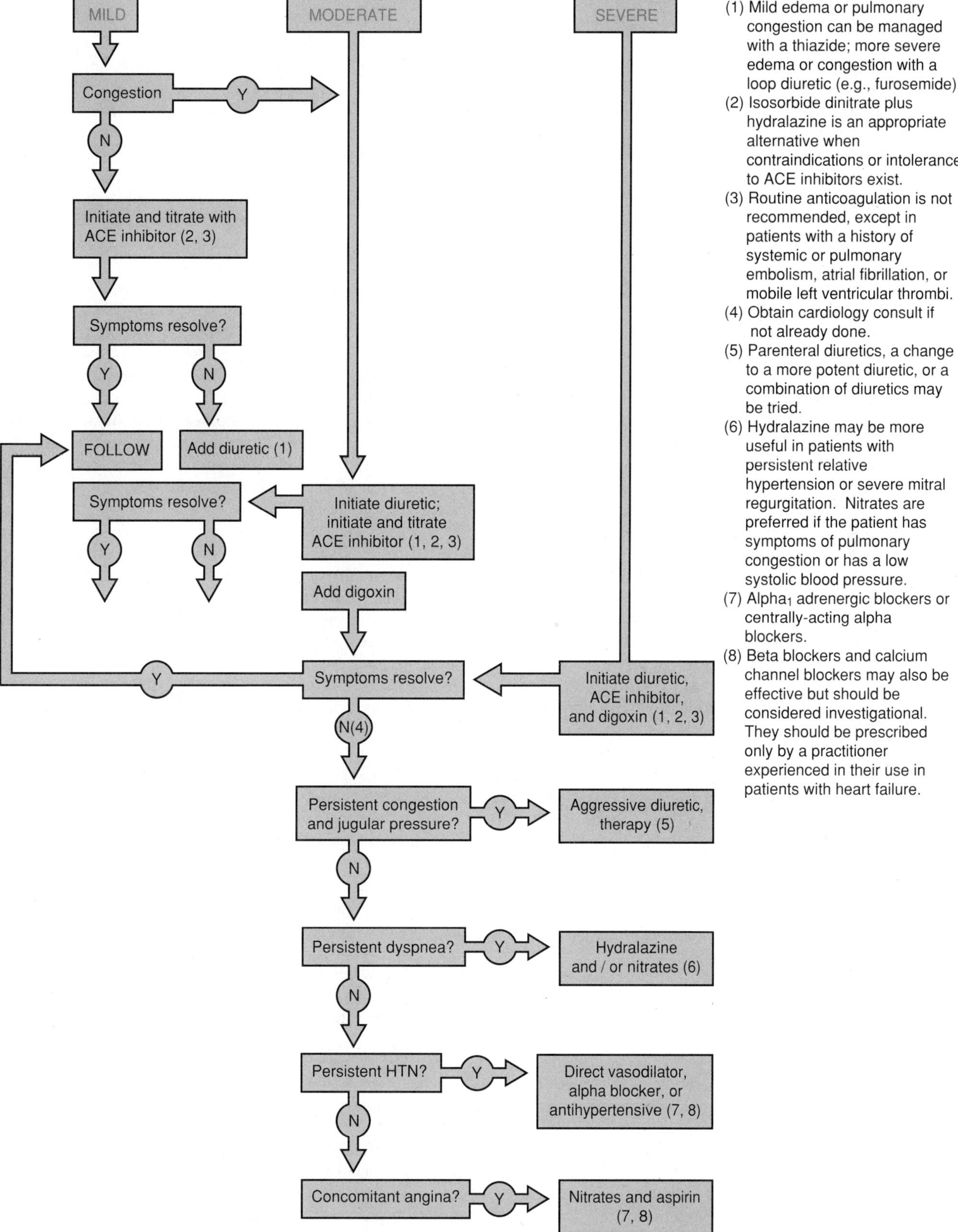

(1) Mild edema or pulmonary congestion can be managed with a thiazide; more severe edema or congestion with a loop diuretic (e.g., furosemide).
(2) Isosorbide dinitrate plus hydralazine is an appropriate alternative when contraindications or intolerance to ACE inhibitors exist.
(3) Routine anticoagulation is not recommended, except in patients with a history of systemic or pulmonary embolism, atrial fibrillation, or mobile left ventricular thrombi.
(4) Obtain cardiology consult if not already done.
(5) Parenteral diuretics, a change to a more potent diuretic, or a combination of diuretics may be tried.
(6) Hydralazine may be more useful in patients with persistent relative hypertension or severe mitral regurgitation. Nitrates are preferred if the patient has symptoms of pulmonary congestion or has a low systolic blood pressure.
(7) $Alpha_1$ adrenergic blockers or centrally-acting alpha blockers.
(8) Beta blockers and calcium channel blockers may also be effective but should be considered investigational. They should be prescribed only by a practitioner experienced in their use in patients with heart failure.

Figure 31–2 Suggested drug management of heart failure. These guidelines are for patients with symptomatic left ventricular dysfunction. Asymptomatic patients with left ventricular dysfunction (ejection fraction less than 40 percent) should be treated with an ACE inhibitor. Drug treatment should follow initial evaluation, and if symptoms persist, adherence should be assessed and the treatment reevaluated. (Adapted from Clinical Practice Guidelines #11. U.S. Department of Health and Human Services, Public Health Services. Agency for Health Care Policy and Research AHCPR, Publication #94-0612, June, 1994.)

the acute care setting because it has a faster onset than other ACE inhibitors. The more rapid onset of captopril permits easier titration, and, if adverse effects occur, they are less prolonged. Concern does exist, however, with the use of ACE inhibitors in the context of diuresis because they can cause a clinically important drop in blood pressure and an increase in serum creatinine levels. The systolic blood pressure should not be allowed to fall below 90 mmHg.

The concurrent use of ACE inhibitors with a cardiac glycoside appears to provide greater benefits than either drug alone, at least for acute heart failure. Although the mechanisms of action of ACE inhibitors and cardiac glycosides differ, the overall effect is that of vasodilation, thus decreasing both preload and afterload. ACE inhibitors have now become the standard of therapy for heart failure regardless of severity.

No evidence exists to support the use of ACE inhibitors alone in the management of acute or chronic heart failure. These drugs are best used concomitantly with loop diuretics. Because ACE inhibitors reduce aldosterone secretion, they are helpful in maintaining a normal serum potassium level in patients who are receiving diuretics.

Once the patient is stable, an ACE inhibitor should be chosen for long-term therapy based on dosing frequency and cost. All ACE inhibitors are thought to be equally efficacious. However, captopril and enalapril have been shown to provide greater survival benefits than the other agents. In addition, all ACE inhibitors except captopril can be given once daily and can be used for patients with both heart failure and hypertension because they treat both disorders and prolong survival.

Diuretics Management of heart failure has included treatment of fluid retention with diuretics (Chapter 39), although their effect on mortality has not been addressed. Diuretics are often used alone in patients with acute failure (i.e., pulmonary edema) to mobilize interstitial lung fluid and to promote a rapid diuresis. Preload is thus decreased. Loop diuretics (e.g., furosemide) also have vasodilatory effects that reduce afterload in acute left-sided failure. Intravenous loop diuretics are used when a rapid diuretic response is needed.

Loop diuretics should be chosen over thiazide diuretics because they have a faster onset, are more effective, provide greater diuresis, and leave fewer metabolic changes when used in equivalent natriuretic doses. Although thiazide diuretics are less expensive than loop diuretics, they can be a problem for patients with diabetes because they tend to increase blood glucose levels. Thiazide diuretics may be helpful when mild heart failure co-exists with hypertension. The diuretic effect versus the antihypertensive effect of thiazides is not always maintained for extended periods. Furthermore, ACE inhibitors, in the absence of loop diuretics, may be ineffective.

Potassium-sparing diuretics (e.g., spironolactone) should be used only in addition to other diuretics. They are useful in some cases for patients who experience persistent hypokalemia despite the use of ACE inhibitors. Spironolactone is preferred because it is more potent than other potassium-sparing agents. When spironolactone is used in combination with an ACE inhibitor, the patient should be monitored for hyperkalemia.

Vasodilators Although vasodilator drugs have long been used for other purposes, their use in heart failure is relatively recent. Venous dilator drugs such as nitroglycerine (Chapter 32) and other nitrates act to decrease preload. Arterial vasodilators such as hydralazine decrease afterload, and prazosin dilates both arteries and veins to decrease preload and afterload. The combined use of vasodilators and diuretics, however, without a cardiac glycoside may not be effective because of the development of tolerance to vasodilators and the progression of the underlying disease. At the same time, if diuretics and vasodilators result in satisfactory clinical response, long-term treatment without a cardiac glycoside is reasonable. The combination of nitrate with hydralazine reduces heart size, improves exercise tolerance, and reduces mortality.

Short-acting nitrates (e.g., sublingual nitroglycerine) may be useful in reducing preload in patients with acute failure but who are slow to respond to diuretics. Nitroglycerine should be used if the loop diuretic does not reduce symptoms within 30 minutes of the first IV dose. Nitroglycerine should be used with caution, however, because there is a danger of decreasing preload, which leads to decreased cardiac output. Nitroprusside, another nitrate, is useful in patients who have acute failure and severe hypertension because it balances arterial and venous effects. Nitrates may prolong survival but should only be used in patients who are intolerant to ACE inhibitors.

Newer direct-acting vasodilators (e.g., glosequinan, epoprostenol) have demonstrated improved exercise tolerance but have an adverse effect on mortality. Although novel drugs such as xamoterol, pimobendan, and vesnarinone have produced improved hemodynamics and improved symptoms in some cases, they are not advisable at present due to increased mortality related to treatment or a high incidence of adverse effects. Beta blockers, used judiciously, may improve functional capacity as well as mortality and may be an important supplement to current conventional treatment. The new generation of beta blockers (see Chapters 11, 33, and 34) with vasodilating properties, such as carvedilol and bucindolol, appear promising in the treatment of heart failure.

Beta Blockers and Calcium Channel Blockers Beta blockers, particularly the new drugs carvedilol and bucindolol, and calcium channel blockers may also be effective in the management of heart failure. Their use should be considered investigational, however. They may be a useful adjunct in patients who have heart failure due to underlying hypertensive heart disease. Patients with diastolic dysfunction may respond to these drugs because they relax the heart during diastole. In contrast, patients with systolic dysfunction may experience a worsening of the heart failure.

Patient Variables

The drugs chosen for the treatment of pediatric heart failure are based on the child's symptomatology and the severity of the heart failure. Infants require higher dosages of digoxin than adults because of increased renal clearance. The dosage regimen must be individualized according to the degree of maturity of the infant. Because the dose of digoxin is determined in part by the child's weight, an increase in dosage will usually be necessary following a weight gain.

Although there is considerable controversy about how much cardiac glycoside crosses placental membranes, no evidence currently exists that there are harmful fetal effects. It should be kept in mind that, because of the expansion of maternal blood volume and the increased glomerular filtration rate during pregnancy, a larger dosage of cardiac glycoside may be necessary to maintain therapeutic serum levels as the pregnancy progresses. This can be achieved by adjusting the dosage. Desirable maternal serum levels of digoxin fall between 1 and 2 mcg, though daily doses of 0.5 to 1 mg are not uncommon.

In general, the older adult has reduced renal function, thereby necessitating a reduction in the dosage of digoxin. Blood levels of cardiac glycoside and metabolites after a single dose have been reported to be two times higher in the older adult than in younger patients, primarily because of decreased renal clearance. Correspondingly, the half-life of digoxin can be 50 percent greater in the older adult than in his or her younger counterpart. Patients taking a cardiac glycoside who enter a nursing home may also receive a diuretic or a potassium supplement, or both. Thus, the older adult must be closely followed to ensure maintenance of therapeutic drug levels and to avoid unrecognized hypokalemia and cardiac glycoside toxicity.

Chronic digoxin use is of no clinical value in many patients. Thus, recognizing patients with chronic heart failure in whom the cardiac glycoside may be safely discontinued is an important issue. Cautious, step by step withdrawal of the cardiac glycoside should be considered if

- The drug was originally prescribed to treat heart failure related to MI, pneumonia, or surgery-induced failure and clinical signs of failure have not reappeared
- Heart failure was essentially due to diastolic dysfunction; a cardiac glycoside is not likely to produce improvement in the presence of a normal left ventricular ejection fraction
- Heart failure is not present, and there is a vague history of prior symptoms

Intervention

Treatment of acute heart failure begins with positioning of the patient. A high Fowler's position with the legs maintained in a dependent position as much as possible reduces pulmonary venous congestion and relieves dyspnea. Note that, although the legs may be edematous, elevation increases venous return to the heart, thus adding to its workload.

Oxygen administration by mask or cannula (in high concentrations) relieves hypoxia and dyspnea and improves oxygen–carbon dioxide exchange. Physical and emotional rest allows the patient to conserve energy and decreases the need for additional oxygen. The amount of rest is dependent on the severity of the heart failure. A patient with severe heart disease is most often on bedrest with limited activity. A patient with mild heart failure may be ambulatory with restrictions placed on strenuous activities. For both mild and severe failure, rest periods should be planned between activities.

Administration

Drug labels should be read carefully when preparing a dose of any cardiac glycoside. Owing to name similarity, especially between digoxin and digitoxin, care must be taken to avoid giving one drug for another. Dosage and potencies differ.

The patient's apical and radial pulse should be taken for 1 full minute before administering each dose. Bradycardia is an adverse effect and an indication of toxicity. The drug should be omitted and the health care provider notified if the pulse, taken before a scheduled dose, is less than 60 bpm, over 110 bpm, unusually irregular, or under 90 bpm in children.

Oral cardiac glycoside formulations can be administered without regard to meals. However, if gastrointestinal irritation occurs, they can be taken with food or milk. Tablets can be crushed and administered with food or fluids if the patient has difficulty swallowing. A calibrating measuring device should be used for liquid formulations. Do not alternate between dosage forms. The bioavailability of capsules is not equal to tablets or elixir.

Intramuscular administration of a cardiac glycoside is not recommended; however, when necessary, one should be given into the gluteal muscle and the area massaged well to reduce painful local reaction. No more than 2 mL of digoxin should be administered at any one IM site. IV formulations can be given by direct IV or each milliliter may be diluted in sterile water, saline, or lactated Ringer's solution for injection. IV formulations should be administered immediately after mixing. It should be given over at least 5 minutes with the patient on a cardiac monitor. The excipient (i.e., propylene glycol) used in its diluent has a toxic effect on cardiac conduction if given too rapidly. Be sure to check package inserts for dilution information.

Rapid digitalization is reserved for the patient in acute distress. It is best accomplished in controlled environments equipped for continuous assessment of cardiac function and prompt treatment of serious arrhythmias. With rapid digitalization, drug toxicities become quickly evident. Intravenous administration may be particularly hazardous. Before administering the initial loading dose, determine if the patient has taken any cardiac glycoside preparation in the preceding 2 to 3 weeks.

Slow digitalization may be accomplished on an outpatient basis with therapeutic levels gradually established over a period of 1 to 2 weeks. This period equates somewhat to the fifth half-life of the drug. For example, digoxin has a half-life of 26 to 52 hours. It would thus take approximately 7 days for digitalization to occur with digoxin. Digitoxin, on the other hand, whose half-life is 5 to 7 days, would require about 1 month to reach therapeutic levels.

Cardiac Glycoside Toxicity

Toxicity can be life threatening and is relatively common, occurring in 10 to 20 percent of patients receiving cardiac glycoside preparations. The overall incidence of toxicity is uncertain, but it has been estimated that approximately 25 percent of hospitalized patients taking a cardiac glycoside show some signs and symptoms. The only difference between the few cardiac glycosides is the duration of action. For example, digoxin is rapidly eliminated, and thus the duration of toxicity is comparatively shorter than that of digitoxin. It is important, therefore, to understand the signs and symptoms that point to toxicity.

Heart rates below 60 bpm in adults and below 90 bpm in children are considered undesirable and generally contraindicate further drug administration until the patient's heart rate improves. Likewise, an excessive prolongation of the P-R interval (indicating depressed AV conduction rate), a shortened Q-T interval, and an altered P wave also require evaluation before giving another dose.

It is important to note that not all rhythm disturbances are associated with high serum or tissue concentrations of cardiac glycosides and are not necessarily manifestations of toxicity. Low plasma concentrations of a cardiac glycoside, though, do not preclude the possibility of drug-induced arrhythmias. Serum concentrations provide a crude, although useful, guide to the likelihood of efficacy and toxicity. A good rule of thumb when evaluating a new rhythm disturbance in a patient receiving a cardiac glycoside is to assume it is drug-induced until proven otherwise.

When toxicity is diagnosed, the drug is discontinued. If the toxicity is severe, the timely administration of antigen-binding fragments of digoxin-specific antibody (DIGIBIND) may be appropriate (Table 31–5). The antibody, produced in sheep, acts antigenically to unbind the cardiac glycoside, decreasing the concentration of free drug available to interact with myocardial membranes. Total plasma concentration of the cardiac glycoside rises markedly because of binding to the antibody, but the fraction of free drug in the plasma is reduced to extremely low levels. DIGIBIND is readily eliminated in the urine.

Education

Patients should be taught the name of the drug, the dosage, and the reason for its use. Encourage patients to carry the information in written form. They should be taught how to take a radial pulse and to do so at least once daily. They should be advised to take the drug at the same time each day to maintain more consistent blood levels and to assist in remembering to take the drug. If a dose is missed, it should be taken as soon as remembered; the dosage should not, however, be doubled. The health care provider should be contacted if doses for 2 or more days are missed. Also advise the patient to avoid concurrent use of other drugs without first checking with the health care provider and to avoid taking antacids or antidiarrheal drugs within 2 hours of the glycoside. The patient should be instructed to keep digoxin tablets in their original container and not to mix them in pill containers with other medications.

Treatment of heart failure with cardiac glycosides and diuretics often requires concurrent use of potassium supplements. The patient should be advised as to which foods are good sources of potassium (see Appendix C).

One of the most common causes for exacerbation of heart failure is noncompliance with a low sodium diet, but control of excessive salt and water retention can be achieved through salt restriction. Sodium in the average American diet usually far exceeds the recommended daily allowance of intake. Approximately 4 g of sodium is contained in the av-

TABLE 31–5 DIGIBIND (Digoxin immune antibody–binding fragment)

Indications	Management of serious life-threatening overdose of digoxin or digitoxin
Pharmacodynamics	Binds to unbound digoxin and digitoxin in serum
Adverse effects/contraindications	Hypokalemia, reemergence of atrial fibrillation, congestive heart failure
Pharmacokinetics	Absorption: 100% Distribution: Widely distributed Onset: Variable, 30 minutes Biotransformation: Liver Duration of action: 2–6 hours Elimination: Kidneys
Dosage	When digoxin or digitoxin dosage is unknown: 800 mg (20 vials) When dosage of digoxin or digitoxin is known (tablets, oral solution, IM formulations): DIGIBIND dose (mg) = ingested glycoside dose (mg) × 0.8 × 40 When dosage is known for digitoxin tablets, digoxin capsules, or IV digoxin: DIGIBIND dose (mg) = ingested glycoside dose (mg) × 40

Single ingestion of digoxin overdose in adults and children:

Quantity Ingested*	DIGIBIND (mg)	No. DIGIBIND
25	340	8.5
50	680	17
75	1000	25
100	1360	34
150	2000	50
200	2680	67

When adult serum digoxin concentration and weight in kg is known:

Wt (kg)	Serum digoxin concentration (ng/mL)						
	1	2	4	8	12	16	20
40	0.5	1	2	3	5	6	8
60	0.5	1	2	5	7	9	11
70	1	2	3	5	8	11	13
80	1	2	3	6	9	12	15
100	1	2	4	8	11	15	18

Implications	• Serum levels prior to administration of DIGIBIND • Continuously monitor ECG and VS prior to treatment • Patients with atrial fibrillation may develop a rapid ventricular response as a result of elevated digoxin or digitoxin levels • Monitor serum potassium levels since they may drop rapidly, especially during the first few hours of administration • Treat hypokalemia promptly • Skin test patients if there is a history of allergy to DIGIBIND or sheep proteins

*Number of 0.25-mg digoxin tablets or 0.2-mg capsules ingested.

erage 10 g of table salt consumed daily. A 4-g salt diet can be obtained by avoiding salty foods and not adding salt at the table. For people with more severe disease, a 2-g sodium diet may be prescribed that requires food be prepared without salt. It is unusual to restrict fluid intake except when severe heart failure with dilutional hyponatremia results. Patients should also be advised to check with their care provider before using salt substitutes.

Occasionally, parents may experience difficulty complying with prescribed drug administration times for their children. The problem is more likely to occur in a very busy household with several children or when the infant or child is receiving several drugs. An exploration of the parents' understanding of drug therapy and of their support systems may help to identify any knowledge deficits.

Evaluation

Once diet and drug therapy are initiated, there should be improvement in clinical symptoms such as dyspnea, orthopnea, and fatigue. The evaluation of cardiac glycoside therapy should be based on the information obtained from the patient database. Generally the evaluation criteria include sufficient knowledge of the disease process and treatment regimen to actively participate in the plan of care; maintenance of a therapeutic blood level; reduction in symptoms; compliance with dietary modifications; and an understanding of, and compliance with, an exercise regimen.

The effectiveness of drug and nondrug therapies can be demonstrated by an increase in cardiac output. Therefore, a decrease in the severity of the heart failure with fewer signs and symptoms of pulmonary congestion (dyspnea, orthopnea, cyanosis, cough, hemoptysis, crackles, anxiety, and restlessness) results. The pulmonary symptoms that developed with the heart failure were the result of events initiated by insufficient cardiac output. The improved strength of myocardial contraction reverses the potentially fatal chain of events.

Fewer signs and symptoms of peripheral congestion (absence of pitting edema, decreased abdominal girth, and weight loss) are indicators of more effective right heart function. An increased activity tolerance indicates a more adequate blood supply to tissues. Diuresis and decreasing edema result from the improved circulation and renal blood flow.

A reduction in heart rate toward more normal levels in patients with heart failure is an expected and desirable response to cardiac glycosides, but an excessive decrease in heart rate is possible. Therapeutic levels of glycosides also alter certain aspects of the electrocardiogram. They cause a narrowing of the QRS complex, depress or invert the T waves, and slow the heart rate.

SUMMARY

- Approximately 4.7 million Americans have heart failure, with more than 400,000 new cases diagnosed yearly.
- Heart failure arises when the pumping action of the heart is impaired and cardiac output falls below venous return.
- With left-sided failure, there is an accumulation of blood in the left ventricle, atrium, and pulmonary circulation. With right-sided failure, blood backs up in systemic circulation.
- Common signs and symptoms of left-sided failure include shortness of breath, orthopnea, paroxysmal nocturnal dyspnea, chronic nonproductive cough, fatigue, weakness, memory loss, confusion, diaphoresis, palpitations, anorexia, and insomnia.
- Right-sided failure is characterized by complaints of weight gain, peripheral edema, abdominal distention, gastric distress, anorexia, and nausea.
- In many cases the patient with heart failure has a history of anemia, thyrotoxicosis, pulmonary embolism, respiratory infection, excessive sodium intake, corticosteroid administration, MI, and rheumatic carditis.
- Treatment objectives are to enhance cardiac performance, identify and correct precipitating factors, and relieve symptoms.
- Drug management of heart failure includes use of ACE inhibitors, diuretics, vasodilators, and cardiac glycosides.
- ACE inhibitors are shown to reduce mortality rates and improve the quality of life.
- Diuretics, used alone or in combination with other drugs, decrease plasma volume and preload.
- Venous and arterial vasodilators have recently been used to treat chronic heart failure. They act to decrease preload, afterload, or a combination of preload and afterload.
- Glycosides decrease the workload of the heart, improve cardiac contractility, and increase renal blood flow and are most effective for patients with a dilated heart, a low ejection fraction, and an S_3 gallop.
- Glycosides produce positive inotropic effects and negative dromotropic and chronotropic effects.
- An initial loading or digitalizing dose is used if a rapid response is desired.
- If the pulse rate is below 60 bpm or over 110 bpm, the health care provider should be notified and the drug withheld.
- The potential for digoxin toxicity increases in the presence of diuretics. The patient should be closely monitored for hypokalemia and signs and symptoms of toxicity.
- DIGIBIND may be used to manage severe digoxin toxicity.
- The intensity of care varies with the patient's baseline status, type of drug used, route of administration, and concomitant use of other drugs.
- Patients should be advised to continue nondrug therapies (e.g., low sodium diet, rest) while receiving drug therapies for heart failure.
- The effectiveness of drug therapy can be demonstrated by an increase in cardiac output and therefore a decrease in the severity of the heart failure with fewer signs and symptoms of pulmonary congestion.
- Therapeutic levels of glycosides produce a narrowing of the QRS complex, depress or invert the T waves, and slow the heart rate.

BIBLIOGRAPHY

Abramowicz, M. (Ed.) (1993). Drugs for chronic heart failure. *Medical Letter,* 35, 40–42.

Baker, D., Koustam, M., Bottorff, M., et al. (1994). Management of heart failure: Pharmacologic treatment. *Journal of the American Medical Association,* 272, 1361–1366.

Bonarjee, V., and Dickstein, K. (1996). Novel drugs and current therapeutic approaches in the treatment of heart failure. *Drugs,* 51(3), 347–358.

Brown, K. (1993). Boosting the failing heart with inotropic drugs. *Nursing,* 23(4), 34–43.

Carson, P. (1996). Pharmacologic treatment of congestive heart failure. *Clinical Cardiology,* 19(4), 271–277.

Cohn, J. (1992). The prevention of heart failure: a new agenda. *New England Journal of Medicine,* 327, 725–727.

Dracup, K. (1996). Heart failure secondary to left ventricular systolic dysfunction: Therapeutic advances and treatment recommendations. *Nurse Practitioner,* 21(9), 61, 65–68.

Gilbert, E., and Harmon, J. (1993). *Manual of high risk pregnancy and delivery.* St. Louis: C. V. Mosby.

McGhie, A., and Golstein, R. (1992). Pathogenesis and management of acute heart failure and cardiogenic shock: Role of inotropic therapy. *Chest,* 102(suppl. 2), 626S–632S.

Meissner, J., and Gever, L. (1993). Reducing the risks of digitalis toxicity. *Nursing,* 23(7), 46–51.

Miller, M. (1994). Current trends in the primary care management of chronic congestive heart failure. *American Journal of Primary Health Care,* 19(5), 64–70.

Pfeffer, M. (1992). Effect of captopril on mortality and morbidity in patients with left ventricular dysfunction after myocardial infarction: results of the survival and ventricular enlargement trial. *New England Journal of Medicine,* 327, 669–677.

Reddy, S., Benatar, D., and Gheorghiade, M. (1997). Update on digoxin and other oral positive inotropic agents for chronic heart failure. *Current Opinions in Cardiology,* 12(3), 233–241.

Sarter, B., and Marchlinski, F. (1992). Redefining the role of digoxin in the treatment of atrial fibrillation. *American Journal of Cardiology,* 69, 71G–81G.

Sasayama, S. (1997). Inotropic agents in the treatment of heart failure: despair or hope? *Cardiovascular Drug Therapy,* 10(6), 703–709.

Stanley, R. (1990). Drug therapy for heart failure. *Journal of Cardiovascular Nursing,* 4, 17–34.

Swedburg, K., et al. (1992). Effects of the early administration of enalapril on mortality in patients with acute myocardial infarction: results of the Cooperative New Scandinavian Enalapril Survival Study II (CONSENSUS II). *New England Journal of Medicine,* 327, 678–684.

Withering, W. (1977). An account of the foxglove and some of its medical uses: with practical remarks on dropsy and other diseases. (Reprint of 1785 edition.) Wakefield, NH: Longwood Publishing Group.

Yontz, L. (1994). Congestive heart failure: early recognition of congestive heart failure in the primary care setting. *Journal of the American Academy of Nurse Practitioners,* 6(6), 273–278.

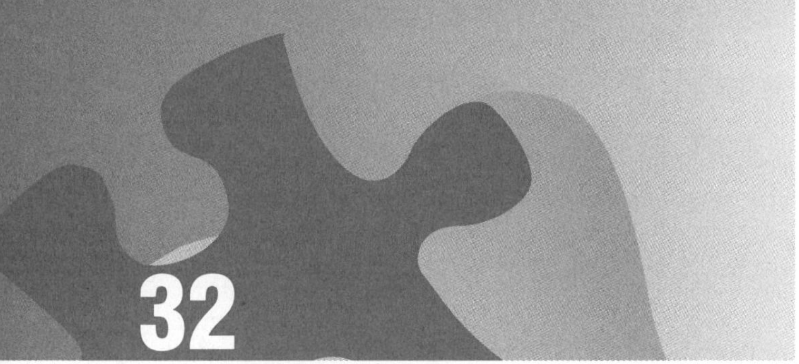

32 Antianginal Drugs

Coronary arteries supply blood flow to the heart muscle that adequately meets tissue demands in healthy people. If sufficient oxygen extraction does not take place, coronary arteries dilate to increase the flow of oxygenated blood to the myocardium. However, a variety of pathologic mechanisms can interfere with the ability of the coronary arteries to dilate, thereby contributing to myocardial ischemia and anginal pain.

Anginal pain is dramatic in onset, usually intensifying during exercise and dissipating with rest. This chapter discusses antianginal drugs, those agents used in the management of *angina pectoris,* chest pain caused by transient myocardial ischemia. The drugs used in the management of angina are separated into three categories: organic nitrates, beta blockers, and calcium channel blockers. The purpose for using these groups of drugs for relief of anginal pain is to improve the balance between myocardial oxygen supply and demand.

PATHOPHYSIOLOGY OF ANGINA PECTORIS

Epidemiology and Etiology

The term angina pectoris is derived from the Latin words *angere,* meaning "to choke," and *pectoralis,* referring to the chest or breast. The angina sensation was first described in 1772 by Dr. William Heberden and is still accurate today. Although angina has many characteristics, the term is used to describe a sensation of choking or strangling in the chest area accompanied by anxiety or fear of death. The chest pain of angina is a sensory response to a transient lack of oxygen.

Angina pectoris is common, although its incidence is not documented. Angina pectoris is not a disease in and of itself, but in most cases a symptom of coronary artery disease (CAD) (Fig. 32–1). Angina can also occur in patients with normal coronary arteries but is less common. Any condition that increases myocardial contractility or heart rate (e.g., exercise, stress, anemia, polycythemia, hyperthyroidism) raises the risk of an anginal episode. Left ventricular hypertrophy, caused by disorders that increase systemic vascular resistance (e.g., aortic stenosis, heart failure, high systolic blood pressure) can also contribute to an anginal episode. Hypercholesterolemia, defined as excess cholesterol in the blood, and smoking are also known risk factors for the development of angina, hypertension, acute myocardial infarction (MI), and sudden coronary death.

Physiology and Pathophysiology

Oxygen Supply Versus Demand

Coronary arteries ordinarily supply the myocardium with blood during diastole, thus meeting its metabolic needs. When oxygen demand increases, the vessels dilate to supply the heart muscle with more blood. The hemodynamic mechanisms responsible for alterations in total and regional coronary blood flow are not clearly understood; however, it is known that relaxation of vascular smooth muscle reduces cardiac workload. Notwithstanding, as the vessels become narrowed by atherosclerotic plaques, the vessels cannot dilate. As the vessels become more occluded, the growing mass of plaque accumulates platelets, fibrin, and cellular debris. Platelet aggregates release prostaglandins (thromboxane A_2) capable of causing vessel spasm. Thromboxane A_2 is a vasoconstrictor capable of causing spasm of coronary arteries. Ironically, thromboxane A_2 also promotes platelet aggregation, resulting in a vicious circle of vasoconstriction and platelet build-up in vessel walls.

Smoking has been traced to the development of atherosclerosis, although the mechanism by which it increases plaque build-up is uncertain. Nicotine may enhance platelet adhesiveness, thereby raising the risk of clot formation within the arteries and contributing to an ischemic episode. Further, the carbon monoxide in smoke reduces the oxygen content of arterial blood. Also, nicotine stimulates the release of epinephrine and norepinephrine. These catecholamines in turn raise heart rate and peripheral vascular resistance. As a result, blood pressure, cardiac workload, and oxygen demand increase.

Disorders of coronary blood vessels, the circulation, or the blood may lead to deficits in the balance of oxygen supply and demand. Disorders of coronary vessels, in addition to atherosclerosis, include arterial spasm and coronary arteritis. Atherosclerosis and arterial spasm increase resistance to blood flow. Coronary arteritis is an inflammation of the coronary arteries due to an infection or autoimmune disorder.

Disorders of the circulation include hypotension and aortic stenosis or insufficiency. Hypotension can be caused by potent antihypertensive drugs, blood loss, spinal anesthesia, or other factors that lessen venous return to the heart. Aortic stenosis or insufficiency lowers the filling pressure of the coronary arteries.

Conditions that increase oxygen demands on the heart include exercise, cold, emotion, digestion of a large meal, anemia, hypoxemia, polycythemia, and hyperthyroidism. Exercise, cold, and emotion increase catecholamine release and thus the heart rate. Digestion of a large meal shunts blood toward the gastrointestinal tract and away from other structures. Anemia and hypoxemia cause a reduction in perfusion of the myocardium. Polycythemia increases the viscosity of the blood, which slows blood flow through coronary arteries. Hyperthyroidism stimulates activity of the thyroid gland, which in turn increases the production of thyroid hormones. Excess thyroid hormones raise blood pressure, myocardial contractility, heart rate, and cardiac output. In addition, rhythm disturbances such as premature ventricular contractions, atrial fibrillation, and paroxysmal atrial tachycardia associated with hyperthyroidism are possible contributors to anginal pain.

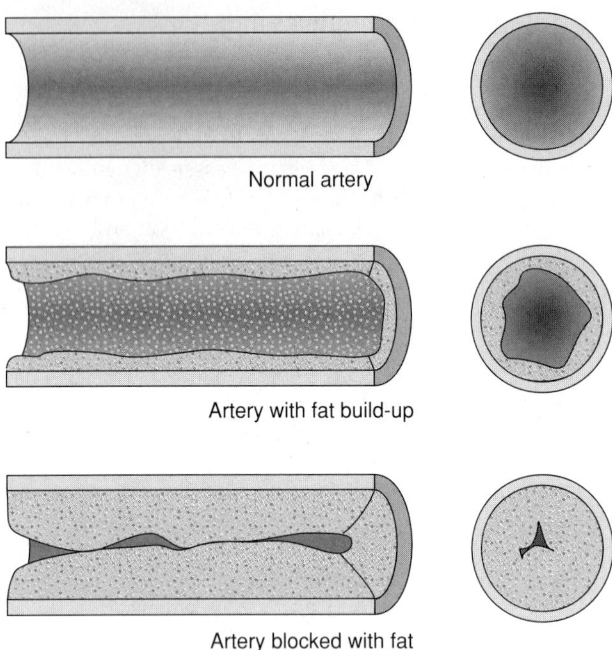

Figure 32–1 Schematic drawing of the stages of atherosclerotic plaque formation. Cross section of a normal artery and an artery altered by disease. The affected artery is obstructed by a mass of platelets, red blood cells, and cholesterol bodies and is indicative of coronary heart disease. With progressive disease the artery becomes almost completely obstructed.

Myocardial Ischemia

Myocardial ischemia, then, occurs when either oxygen demand or oxygen supply is altered. In some patients, the coronary arteries are able to supply adequate blood when the patient is at rest. However, when the person exercises or is otherwise taxed in some fashion, angina develops. Myocardial cells become ischemic within 10 seconds of a coronary artery occlusion. Within several minutes, the heart loses its ability to contract, thus impairing pump function and depriving the myocardium of the glucose necessary for aerobic metabolism. Anaerobic metabolism takes over, with an accumulation of lactic acid. As lactic acid accumulates, anginal pain develops. The pain may also be related to an abnormal stretching of ischemic tissues. The abnormal stretching irritates nerve endings. Afferent sympathetic fibers, entering the spinal cord from levels C3–T4, account for the variety of locations and for the radiation pattern of anginal pain (Fig. 32–2).

Myocardial cells remain viable for approximately 20 minutes under ischemic conditions. If blood flow is restored, aerobic metabolism resumes, contractility is restored, and cellular repair begins. Myocardial infarction occurs if coronary arteries are unable to compensate for the lack of oxygen.

Forms of Angina

Angina pectoris typically takes one of three forms: stable angina (classic, stable exertional, or predictable angina), unstable angina (acute coronary insufficiency, intermittent coronary syndrome, crescendo, or preinfarction angina), or variant angina (Prinzmetal's or vasospastic angina).

The chest pain of *stable angina* is paroxysmal and tends to build gradually, usually in response to a predictable level of emotional stress or exertion. The pain reaches maximum intensity before dissipating. It is brought on by known stimuli and causes characteristic sensations with each episode. Some patients with stable angina have episodes of discomfort in the morning. Figure 32–3 shows that in some patients with chronic stable angina, both silent and symptomatic episodes of angina clearly had a peak incidence in the morning and early afternoon hours. The frequency gradually declined beginning in the late afternoon and was lowest in the early morning. Angiographic studies have suggested that coronary arterial lumens are smaller in the morning than at other times of the day. An electrocardiogram completed in these early morning hours may show a depression of the ST segment. Correction of the precipitating event, rest, and/or the administration of nitrates usually terminates the anginal pain.

Unstable angina is defined as a change in the stability of a previously established pattern of pain or a new onset of severe angina. In some cases, the attack may waken the patient at night. Unstable angina is seldom predictable. The onset and course of pain differ with each attack, increasing in both frequency and duration (up to 30 minutes). Symptoms of unstable angina may be only partially relieved by rest or vasodilating drugs.

Variant angina is chest pain due to vasospasm of coronary vessels. This type of angina is not necessarily associated with atherosclerosis. The chest pain is similar to that of stable angina but lasts longer and may occur at rest. Attacks may be cyclical, occurring at the same time of the night, and often during the rapid eye movement phase of sleep (nocturnal angina). Smoking, alcohol, or cocaine use may precipitate spasm.

Three other terms are often used to refer to angina. *Angina decubitus* is paroxysmal chest pain that occurs when the patient reclines and lessens when the patient sits or stands. *Intractable angina* refers to chronic, incapacitating chest pain; this type of angina is often unresponsive to intervention. *Postinfarction angina* occurs after an MI, when residual ischemia may cause anginal episodes.

PHARMACOTHERAPEUTIC OPTIONS

The major drug categories used in the management of angina pectoris are opioids, nitrates, beta blockers, calcium channel blockers, and antiplatelet drugs. Opioids were discussed in Chapter 14. Antiplatelet drugs are discussed in Chapter 36. The nitrates, beta blockers, and calcium channel blockers are discussed here as they relate to the management of angina pectoris.

Nitrates

- ❒ Amyl nitrite (ASPIROL, VAPOROLE)
- ❒ Erythrityl tetranitrate
- ❒ Isosorbide dinitrate (ISORDIL, SORBITRATE, DILATRATE-SR, ISDN, ISO-BID, ISORDIL, SORBITRATE SA); (✤) APO-ISDN, CEDOCARD-SR, CORONES
- ❒ Isosorbide mononitrate (IMDUR, ISMO, MONOKET)
- ❒ Nitroglycerin (NITROSTAT, NITROBID IV, NITROSTAT IV, NITROLINGUAL, NITROGLYN, NITROBID, NITROSPAN, NITROL, NITRONG, NITRODISC, TRANSDERM-NITRO, NITROGARD)
- ❒ Pentaerythritol tetranitrate

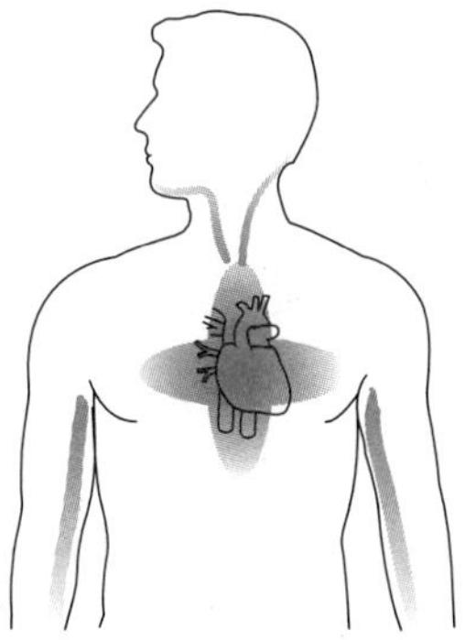

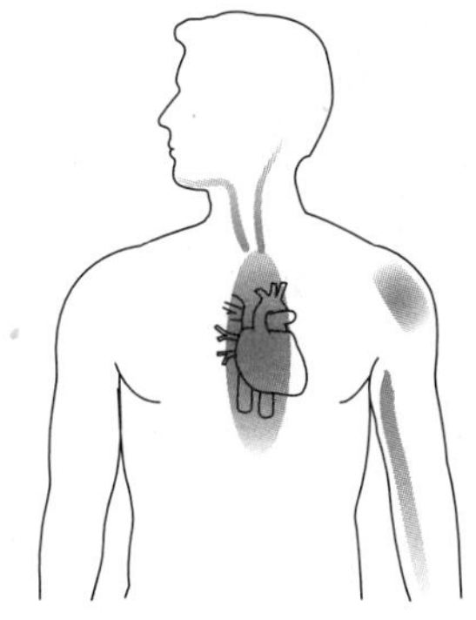

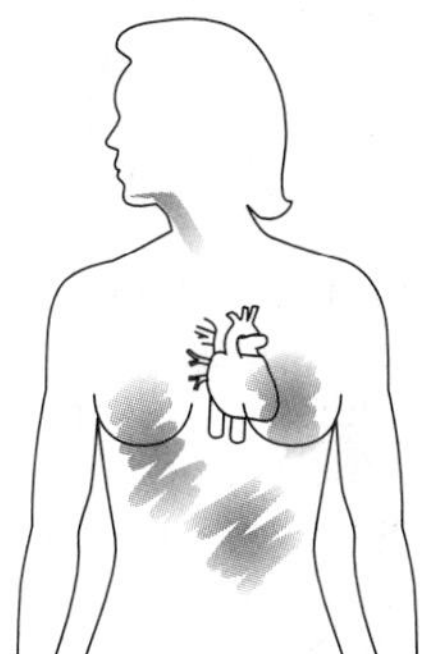

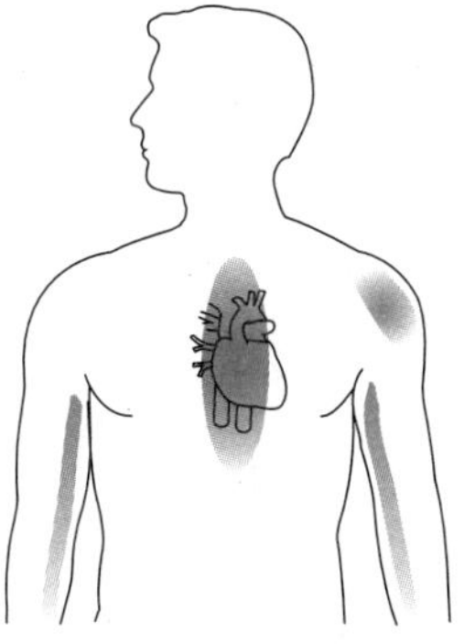

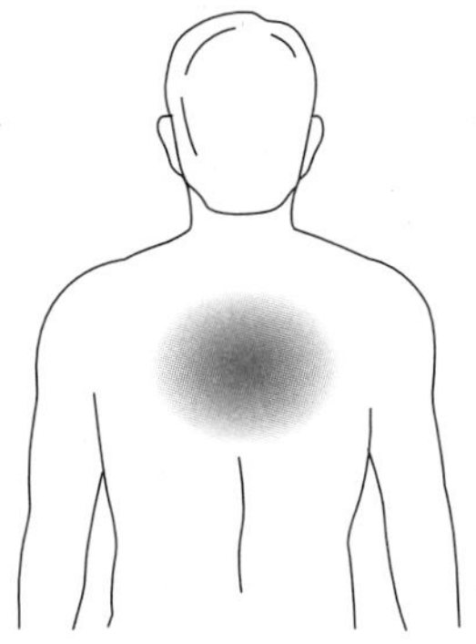

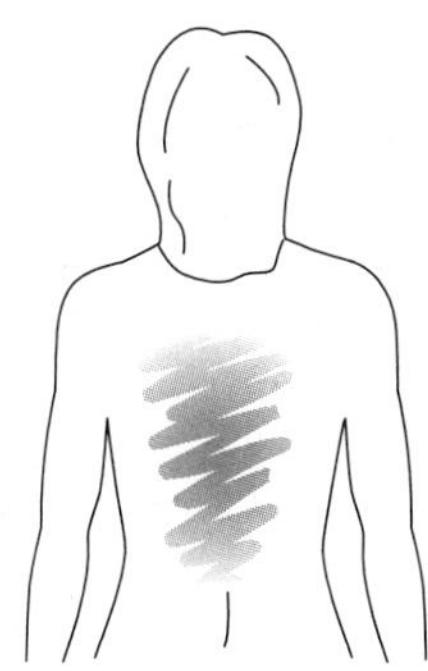

Figure 32–2 Common sites of anginal pain *(shaded areas)*. The locations of the pain are similar in males and females.

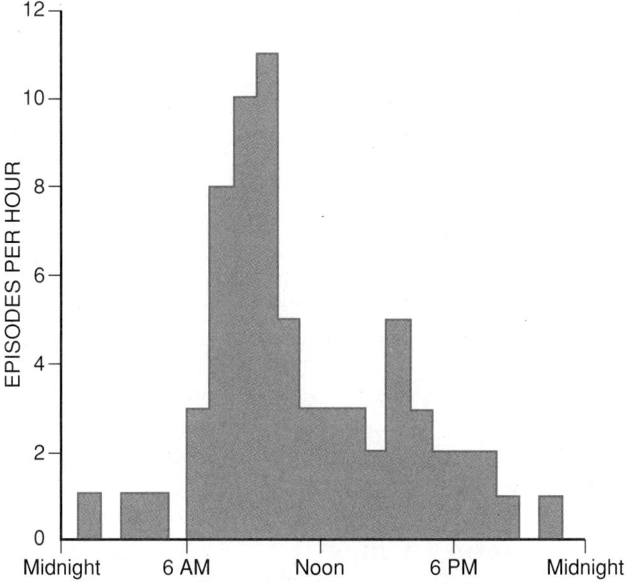

Figure 32–3 Distribution of ischemic episodes. Some patients with chronic stable angina, both silent and symptomatic episodes of angina, clearly have a peak incidence in the morning and early afternoon hours. The frequency gradually declines in the late afternoon and is lowest in the early morning. (Adapted from Nademanee, K., Intarachot, V., Josephson, M., et al. [1987]. Circadian variations in occurrence of transient overt and silent myocardial ischemia in chronic stable angina and comparison with Prinzmetal's angina in men. *American Journal of Cardiology,* 60, 498. Used with permission.)

Indications

Nitroglycerin, the short-acting ester of nitric acid, has been the drug of choice against anginal attacks since 1867. Today, nitrates remain the major weapon for immediate relief of acute angina, for prevention of angina when an attack is anticipated, and for long-term prevention of chronic anginal attacks. The nitrates can be used alone or with beta blockers and calcium channel blockers. Nitrate products may also be used to increase the exercise capacity of patients with coronary artery disease.

Pharmacodynamics

Of the general mechanisms by which nitrates reduce myocardial ischemia, their ability to reduce the oxygen demand appears to be the most important. Low-dose nitrates preferentially cause dilation of veins over arterioles, resulting in a pooling of blood in the periphery. In turn, there are decreases in venous return to the heart and filling of the left ventricle (preload). Decreasing venous return to the heart in turn reduces left end-diastolic pressure and volume, and oxygen consumption. In addition, a reduction in preload generates a higher pressure gradient across the ventricular wall. The higher pressure gradient favors subendocardial perfusion. With the reduced filling of the left ventricle, the workload of the heart is also reduced. The heart therefore requires less oxygen, and angina is relieved. Nitrates do not directly change the inotropic (e.g., force) or chronotropic (i.e., rate) state of the heart.

Independent of autonomic nervous system activity, nitrates also dilate arteries through direct action on arterial smooth muscle. Most resistance to the ejection of blood from the left ventricle occurs in the arterioles. The greater the arteriolar constriction, the more resistance to ejection from the left ventricle. Nitrates decrease the afterload by dilating arterioles. Thus, the energy required for the heart to pump blood is reduced. Systemic vascular resistance is usually unaffected, the heart rate is unchanged or slightly increased, and pulmonary vascular resistance and cardiac output are reduced. The apparent selectivity of some nitrates for different vascular beds may relate to differences in bioavailability and cellular biotransformation of the drugs.

Adverse Effects and Contraindications

In general, the adverse effects of nitrates are almost all secondary to their action on the cardiovascular system. The decreased afterload produced by arteriolar dilation causes hypotension. The reduced preload and cardiac output result in worsened hypotension, which is most noticeable when the patient assumes an upright position. Transient episodes of dizziness, weakness, and other symptoms of postural hypotension may develop, particularly when the patient stands immobile. Hypotension occasionally progresses to a loss of consciousness, especially when accompanied by alcohol ingestion. Even with the most severe syncopal episode, positioning and other strategies that facilitate venous return to the heart are the only therapeutic measures needed.

Approximately 50 percent of patients receiving nitrates for acute angina attacks experience flushing and a pounding headache after administration. The headache is probably caused by dilation of meningeal blood vessels. Such headaches usually disappear after several days of continued treatment and often can be effectively controlled through reduction of the nitrate dose. They occur less commonly with long-term, prophylaxis therapy.

Other adverse effects are blurred vision, dry mouth, and increased peripheral edema. Methemoglobinemia (a condition in which more than 1 percent of hemoglobin in the blood has been oxidized to the ferric form) occurs with large, continuous doses of nitrates. The principal sign of methemoglobinemia is cyanosis, which occurs because the oxidized hemoglobin is unable to transport oxygen.

Organic nitrates occasionally produce a rash. A rash is seen most often with pentaerythritol tetranitrate. The drug rash caused by isosorbide mononitrate is reported less often than with isosorbide dinitrate. There is also less flushing and halitosis with the mononitrate formulation of isosorbide.

Pharmacokinetics

Nitrates are well absorbed following oral, buccal, sublingual, or topical administration. The onset, peak, and duration of action vary with the route of administration. Table 32–1 summarizes the pharmacokinetics of nitrates. Orally administered nitrates are rapidly biotransformed in the liver, leading to decreased bioavailability. An extensive first pass effect limits the usefulness of oral therapy in most cases. As a consequence of reduction hydrolysis, nitrates are transformed from lipid-soluble organic esters to more water-soluble dinitrated metabolites and inorganic nitrites. Elimination is through the kidneys.

Drug-Drug Interactions

The drug-drug interactions associated with nitrates usually result in additive hypotension. When nitrates are used concurrently with drugs that have anticholinergic properties (antihistamines, antidepressants, and phenothiazines), the absorption of sublingual and buccal nitroglycerin formulations is reduced (see Table 32–2).

Dosage Regimen

The drug regimen required for angina is determined by the frequency and intensity of anginal episodes as well as by the patient's response to therapy. Nitrates are available in a variety of multiple formulations.

Immediate Therapy

Sublingual or buccal forms of nitroglycerin usually relieve acute anginal pain in approximately 3 to 5 minutes. The usual dose of sublingual nitroglycerin is 0.15 to 0.3 mg (gr 1/200 to gr 1/150), although the tablets contain as much as 0.6 mg of nitroglycerin. The generally accepted dose is 1 tablet every 5 to 10 minutes to a maximum of 3 tablets. Failure of the third dose to relieve pain should be considered an indication of possible MI, and medical assistance should immediately be sought.

A newer, and allegedly more convenient, dosage form is a lingual spray. It delivers nitroglycerin from a pressurized container, releasing a metered dose of 0.4 mg with each activation. As with the sublingual tablets, no more than 3 metered doses are recommended within 15 minutes. If chest pain persists and does not change, the patient should seek immediate medical attention.

Sublingual tablets and lingual sprays may also be used prophylactically. The patient is instructed to use 1 nitroglycerin tablet or metered spray before engaging in an activity known to cause anginal pain (i.e., mild to moderate exercise, sexual activity). This strategy often prevents angina by producing adequate vasodilation and decreasing myocardial oxygen demand.

Intravenous nitroglycerin has an immediate onset and can be titrated to prevent, treat, and stop acute anginal attacks. Titration is carefully performed according to the patient's tolerance and therapeutic response. With low-dose therapy, titration by up to 10 to 20 mcg/minute may be done. In high-dose therapy, titration dosages may be as high as 20 to 50 mcg/minute. Titration is continued until the desired fall in systolic blood pressure and/or until relief of chest pain is accomplished. Because of its rapid degradation, nitroglycerin can be titrated quickly and safely. Continuous monitoring of hemodynamic parameters—arterial pressure, pulmonary artery pressures, and pulmonary capillary wedge pressures—is extremely important and should be done throughout drug administration.

Long-Term Therapy

Long-acting nitrates act too slowly to be useful for acute anginal attacks. They are most often used for prophylaxis. Nitroglycerin ointment is a 2 percent topical preparation in a lanolin base. Its doses are measured by the inch, with 1 inch of ointment containing 15 mg of nitroglycerin. The dosage is titrated according to the patient's response and blood pressure. The dosage is more likely to be consistent if

TABLE 32–1 PHARMACOKINETICS OF SELECTED ANTIANGINAL DRUGS

Drug	Route	Onset	Peak	Duration	PB (%)	$t_{1/2}$	BioA (%)
Nitrates*							
Nitroglycerin	SL	1–3 min	3–5 min	30–60 min	60	1–4 min	12–64
	IV	1–2 min	UK	3–5 min			100
	Buccal	2–4 min	UK	3–5 hr			UA
	Ointment	30–60 min	UK	2–12 hr			52–92
	TD	30–60 min	UK	18–24 hr			52–92
	po/SR	40–60 min	3–4 hr	4–8 hr			<1
	TL	2 min	UK	30–60 min			UA
Isosorbide dinitrate,	SL or chewable	2–5 min	30–60 min	1–2 hr		50 min, 5 hr†	22–38‡
isosorbide mononitrate	po	15–40 min	UK	4–6 hr		UA	8–36‡
	SR	Slow	3–4 hr	8–12 hr		UA	UA
Erythrityl tetranitrate	SL	5 min	15 min	2–4 hr		UA	UA
	po	15–30 min	1 hr	6 hr		UA	UA
Pentaerythritol	po	20–60 min	3–4 hr	4–5 hr		UA	UA
tetranitrate	SR	30–60 min	UK	8–12 hr		UA	UA
Amyl nitrite	Inh	30 sec	UK	3–5 min		UA	UA
Nonselective Beta Blockers§							
Propranolol	po	30 min	60–90 min	6–12 hr	90	3.4–6 hr	16–36
	po/ER	UK	6 hr	24 hr	90	3.4–6 hr	UA
	IV	2 min	1 min‖	4–6 hr	90	3–6 hr	100
Nadolol	po	>5 days	2–4 hr	24 hr	30	16–18 hr	29–39
Selective Beta Blockers§							
Atenolol	po	60 min	2–4 hr	24 hr	<5	6–9 hr	26–86
Metoprolol	po	30–60 min	90 min	24 hr	12	3–7 hr	24–52
	IV	Immediate	20 min	5–8 hr	12	3–4 hr	100
Calcium Channel Blockers							
Amlodipine	po	UK	UK	24 hr	UA	30–50 hr	64–90
Bepridil	po	8 days††	UK	24 hr	UA	42 hr‡‡	UA
Isradipine	po	<2 hr	2–3 hr	12 hr	95	8 hr	64–90
Felodipine	po	60 min	2–4 hr	Up to 24 hr	99	11–16 hr	UA
Verapamil	po	30 min	1–2 hr	4–8 hr	83–92	3–7 hr	UA
	SR	UK	5–7 hr	24 hr	83–92	4–12 hr	UA
Nifedipine	po	20 min	30 min	2.5–3 hr	92–98	2–5 hr	UA
Diltiazem	po	30 min	2–3 hr	4–8 hr	70–85	3–5 hr	UA
Nicardipine	po	20 min	0.5–2 hr	8 hr	>95	2–4 hr	UA

*Cardiovascular effects of nitrates.
†Half-life values for isosorbide dinitrate and isosorbide mononitrate, respectively.
‡Bioavailability calculations from single doses, because systemic clearance may be reduced with long-term use of isosorbide formulations.
§Because beta blockers are not used for relief of acute anginal pain, their onset of action is difficult to measure.
‖Antianginal effects of propranolol are manifest at 15–90 mcg/mL to achieve a 50% decrease in exercise-induced cardioacceleration.
¶To achieve a 30% reduction in exercise-induced cardioacceleration.
**To achieve a 10% decrease in resting heart rate.
††Onset of steady-state antianginal effects with long-term dosing of bepridil.
‡‡Half-life of bepridil following cessation of multiple dosing.
ER, extended release; Inh, Inhaled; IV, Intravenous; NA, Not applicable; po, by mouth; SL, Sublingual; SR, sustained release; TD, Transdermal patch; TL, Translingual spray; UA, Unavailable; UK, Unknown; PB, protein binding; t½, elimination half-life; BioA, bioavailability.

the patient actually measures the drug onto the specially marked paper that comes with the nitroglycerin. The paper, not the hand, is used to spread the ointment on the skin surface, where it is slowly absorbed, producing anginal prophylaxis for approximately 3 to 6 hours. Topical formulations can be applied anywhere on the body surface, but the skin should be clean, dry, and free of hair.

Transdermal, controlled-release nitrates currently are compounded in one of two ways, as a matrix or as a reservoir (Fig. 32–4). TRANSDERM-NITRO is a reservoir formulation. The drug migrates to the absorption site through a rate-controlled permeable membrane. NITRO-DUR and NITRODISC are matrix formulations; the nitrate is slowly dispersed through the polymer matrix to the absorption site.

Several manufacturers market transdermal patches. Each product is available in doses ranging from 20 to 187.5 mg, with a release rate of 2.5 to 15 mg/24 hours. Table 32–3 provides the recommended dosages for the various forms of nitrates.

Laboratory Considerations

All nitrates cause falsely elevated serum cholesterol levels. Nitrates also increase urine concentrations of catecholamines and vanillylmandelic acid. Excessive doses may raise methemoglobin values.

Beta Blockers

NONSELECTIVE

- ❒ Labetalol (NORMODYNE, TRANDATE)
- ❒ Nadolol (CORGARD); (🍁) SYN-NADOLOL

TABLE 32–2 DRUG-DRUG INTERACTIONS OF SELECTED ANTIANGINAL DRUGS

Drug	Interactive Drugs	Interaction
Nitrates		
Nitrates	Antihypertensives	Additive hypotension
Nitroglycerin	Alcohol	
	Beta blockers	
	Calcium channel blockers	
	Diuretics	
	Haloperidol	
	Phenothiazines	
	Antihistamines	Decreased absorption of sublingual and buccal nitroglycerin
	Tricyclic antidepressants	
Beta Blockers		
Atenolol	Antacids	Decreased aborption from GI tract
Metoprolol	Nonsteroidal anti-inflammatory drugs (salicylates, indomethacin)	Decreased hypotensive effects
Nadolol		
Propranolol	Barbiturates	Increased biotransformation of beta blocker
	Calcium channel blockers	Increased drug and toxic effects of both drugs
	Cardiac glycosides	Increased bradycardia and atrioventricular nodal depression
	Cimetidine	Decreased biotransformation of beta blocker.
		Increased ability of beta blocker to reduce pulse rate
	Clonidine	Increased antihypertensive and bradycardia effects
	Insulin	Hypoglycemia, hyperglycemia
	Oral hypoglycemics	May mask tachycardia as a sign of hypoglycemia (other symptoms still present)
	Lidocaine	Increased plasma levels of lidocaine
		May potentiate toxicity and produce additive cardiac depression
	Rifampin	Inhibits response to propranolol and metoprolol
	Albuterol	Hypertension and reflex bradycardia from unopposed alpha effects and increased vagal tone
	Dobutamine	
	Dopamine	
	Epinephrine	
	Isoproterenol	
	Metaproterenol	
	Terbutaline	
	Ritodrine	
Calcium Channel Blockers		
Amlodipine	Cimetidine	Decreased hepatic clearance of calcium channel blocker
Bepridil		
Diltiazem	Calcium salts, vitamin D	Decreased response to calcium channel blocker
Felodipine		
Isradipine	Digoxin	Increased serum digoxin level
Nicardipine	Disopyramide phosphate	Causes myocardial depression
Nifedipine	Other beta blockers	
Verapamil	Carbamazepine	Enhances action of interacting drug
	Cyclosporine	
	Nondepolarizing blockers	

❒ Pindolol (VISKEN); (✱) NOVO-PINDOL, SYN-PINDOLOL

❒ Propranolol (INDERAL, INDERAL LA); (✱) APO-PROPRANOLOL

SELECTIVE

❒ Acebutolol (SECTRAL); (✱) MONITAN

❒ Atenolol (TENORMIN); (✱) APO-ATENOLOL, NOVO-ATENOL

❒ Metoprolol (LOPRESSOR, TOPROL XL); (✱) BETALOC, BETALOC DURULES, LOPRESOR, LOPRESOR SR, NOVO-METOPROL

Indications

Beta blockers constitute a major treatment modality for angina, second only to nitrates. The drugs currently approved by the U.S. Food And Drug Administration for use as antianginal drugs are the nonselective beta blockers propranolol and nadolol, and the cardioselective drugs atenolol

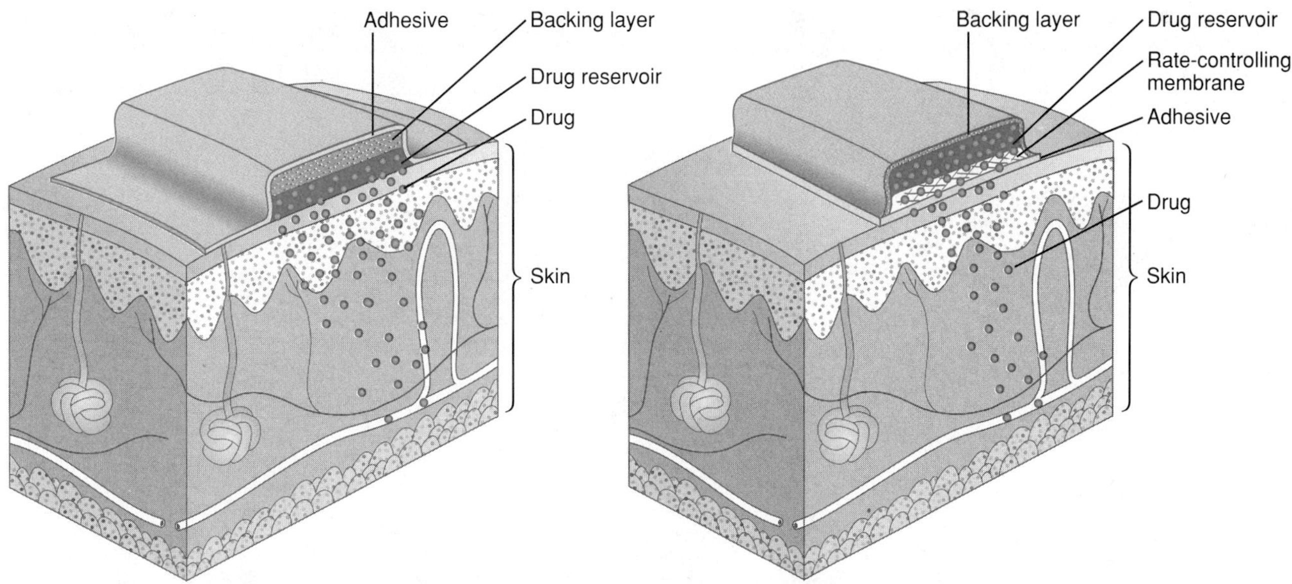

Figure 32–4 Schematic drawing of transdermal drug delivery systems. *Left,* In matrix formulations, the drug is slowly dispersed through the polymer matrix to the absorption site. *Right,* In reservoir delivery systems, the drug migrates to the absorption site through a rate-controlling permeable membrane.

and metoprolol. Beta blockers are effective in reducing the severity and frequency of exertional angina attacks. Acebutolol, labetalol, and pindolol have not been approved by the U.S. Food And Drug Administration for angina, but they are occasionally prescribed.

Patients taking a beta blocker for angina usually note improved exercise tolerance and report a decrease in the number and severity of attacks. The beta blockers are also used for the treatment of hypertension, migraine headaches, anxiety, pheochromocytoma, arrhythmias, and open-angle glaucoma associated with hyperthyroidism. The uses of beta blockers as antiarrhythmics and antiglaucoma drugs are discussed in Chapters 11, 33, and 62.

Pharmacodynamics

Beta blockers, the most widely used adrenergic antagonists, reduce the oxygen requirements of the myocardium by preventing stimulation of sympathetic nervous system receptors, inhibiting catecholamine action at these sites, and reducing contractility, sinus node rate, and atrioventricular conduction velocity (negative dromotropic action). These actions, in turn, raise the exercise tolerance of patients with reduced coronary blood flow. The competitive blocking action occurs not only at adrenergic nerve receptors but also in the adrenal medulla. Drug action at these two sites accounts for the widespread effects of beta blockers. Certain beta blockers (e.g., propranolol, metoprolol) can also produce central nervous system activity, with effects exerted at the vasomotor center of the brain stem.

Selective beta blockers preferentially act on $beta_1$-adrenergic receptor sites. The principal effects are slowing of the heart rate (negative chronotropic effect), reduction in the force of the contraction (negative inotropic effect), and suppression of impulse conduction through the atrioventricular node. Because of the blockade, these agents decrease the workload of the heart and, thereby, oxygen demand. Oxygen demand is brought into balance with oxygen supply, and anginal pain is prevented. In contrast, nonselective beta blockers act on both $beta_1$- and $beta_2$-adrenergic receptors, preventing not only cardiac excitement but also bronchiolar dilation.

Adverse Effects and Contraindications

The most common adverse reactions to beta blockers occur when the drug is started. Hypotension, bradycardia, and bronchospasm are potentially harmful. Because of the negative inotropic effect and greater preload produced by beta blockers, heart failure may be precipitated or exacerbated. The rapid discontinuance of a beta blocker may precipitate an anginal attack, hypertension, arrhythmias (especially atrioventricular block), or an acute MI.

Although occurring most often with propranolol, adverse central nervous system effects of the beta blockers include dizziness, fatigue, lethargy, confusion or depression, and decreased libido. The gastrointestinal reactions—nausea, vomiting, and diarrhea—are usually transient.

Significant bronchoconstriction may result from blockade of beta-adrenergic receptors. Although this reaction is more likely to occur with the nonselective drugs (i.e., nadolol, propranolol), it can also occur with high doses of the selective drugs atenolol and metoprolol. Beta blockers are contraindicated in variant angina. The deleterious effect of beta blockers on variant angina is probably due to an increase in coronary resistance caused by the unopposed effects of catecholamines on alpha-adrenergic receptors. Nonselective beta blockers are also contraindicated in patients with heart failure, acute bronchospasm, some forms of valvular heart disease, bradyarrhythmias, and heart block. In low dosages, metoprolol and atenolol can induce full cardiac beta blockade without causing wheezing in patients who have pulmonary disease. At larger doses, selective beta blockers may become nonselective and may block both cardiac and bronchial beta-adrenergic receptors. They should be used cautiously in pregnant and lactating fe-

TABLE 32–3 DOSAGE AND ADMINISTRATION OF SELECTED ANTIANGINAL DRUGS

Drug	Use(s)	Dosage	Implications
Nitrates			
Nitroglycerin	Acute unstable angina, acute myocardial infarction, angina prophylaxis, adjunct in congestive heart failure	*Adult:* 0.15–0.6 mg (gr. 1/100 –gr. 1/400) sublingual formulation. May repeat q5min for 15 minutes for acute attack	
		Adult: 5 mcg/min by IV drip. Increase by 5 mcg/min q3–5 min to 20 mcg/min, then increase by 10–20 mcg q3–5min (25–500 mcg/mL). Titrate based on blood pressure and pulse measurement	Low-dose therapy—titrate up by 10–20 mcg High-dose therapy—titrate up by 20–50 mcg Continue to titrate until desired fall in systolic BP and/or chest pain relief occurs
		Adult: 1–2 (0.4 mg) lingual sprays. May repeat q5min for 15 minutes for acute attack	Highly flammable. Spray onto oral mucosa. Do not inhale or swallow spray
		Adult: 2.5–6.5 mg extended-release capsules po q8–12 hr *or* 1.3–6.5 mg extended-release tablets q8–12 hr	Take on empty stomach. Do not chew. Monitor BP carefully
		Adult: 1/2-inch to 5-inch ribbon (7.5–75 mg) of topical ointment q3–4 hr	Rotate sites. Do not touch ointment with hands. Cover with plastic wrap for better absorption
		Adult: 1 transdermal patch q24 hr	Release rate 2.5–15 mg/24 hr. Rotate sites. Remove patch before defibrillation to avoid arcing. Wash site when patch is removed
		Adult: 1–3 mg extended-release buccal tablets q3–5hr while awake	Take tablet after meals. Talking and tongue movement may dislodge tablet. Hot liquids may increase dissolution
Isosorbide dinitrate: (ISORDIL, ISO-BID)		*Adult:* 2.5–10 mg po PRN. Initial dose not to exceed 5 mg. May repeat q5–10 min × 3 doses	Do not crush or chew tablets
ISORDIL, TEMBIDS		*Adult:* 40 mg po q6–12 hr	Do not chew
Pentaerythritol tetranitrate PERITRATE		*Adult:* 10–20 mg po QID. Titrate up to 40 mg QID	Take on empty stomach.
		Adult: 30–80 mg po (SR) q12 hr	Do not crush or chew tablet
Amyl nitrite		*Adult:* 0.18–0.3 mL (2–5 mg)	Crush between fingers
Erythrityl tetranitrate		*Adult:* 5–30 mg po or buccal TID. Titrate as needed	Chewable tablet. Take on empty stomach
Nonselective Beta Blockers			
Propranolol	Chronic exertional angina	*Adult:* 10–20 mg po TID–QID. Increase q3–7days till desired effect achieved. Maintenance: 160 mg/day in divided doses	Contraindicated in patients with respiratory disorders. Abrupt withdrawal may result in life-threatening arrhythmias
	Myocardial infarction	*Adult:* 180–240 mg po QD in 3–4 divided doses.	
Nadolol	Chronic exertional angina	*Adult:* 40 mg po QD. Increase q3–7days till desired effect achieved. Maintenance: 80–240 mg po QD	

males, because they may cause fetal bradycardia and hypoglycemia.

Pharmacokinetics

Only oral beta blockers are used to treat angina. These drugs have varying pharmacokinetic properties, which are listed in Table 32–1.

Drug-Drug Interactions

Drug-drug interactions with beta blockers are numerous and are summarized in Table 32–2. Cimetidine increases the beta blocking effects of propranolol by slowing its hepatic clearance and elimination. Adrenergic agonists, which stimulate beta receptors, can reverse the bradycardia induced by beta blockers.

Dosage Regimen

Table 32–3 identifies the dosage regimens for beta blockers used in the management of angina pectoris. As with most drugs, the dosage for the individual formulations varies. For the initial treatment of chronic exertional angina, 40 mg of nadolol is given. It may be increased by 40 mg daily every 3 to 7 days until symptoms are controlled or a daily maximum of 240 mg is reached. Nadolol dosage can also be titrated until exercise-induced heart rate is decreased by 15 percent.

The dosage of propranolol is 10 to 20 mg three to four times daily. The dosage may be increased every 3 to 7 days until the desired effects are achieved. Maintenance dosage should not exceed 160 mg/day in divided doses.

Atenolol is given at 50 mg daily. Increases of 50 mg can be made until symptoms are controlled or a maximum daily

TABLE 32–3 DOSAGE AND ADMINISTRATION OF SELECTED ANTIANGINAL DRUGS *Continued*

Drug	Use(s)	Dosage	Implications
Selective Beta Blockers			
Atenolol	Angina hypertension	*Adult:* 50 mg po QD. Increase by 50 mg/day q3days until desired effect is achieved	Can also be titrated until exercise-induced heart rate is decreased by 15%. Reduce dosage to 50 mg QOD in renal failure
	Myocardial infarction	*Adult:* 5 mg IV q2min × 3 doses; then 5 mg po q6hr × 48 hr; then 100 mg q12hr	Withhold if apical pulse rate before administration is less then 50 beats per min
Metoprolol	Exertional angina, hypertension	*Adult:* 100–450 mg po single dose or BID. Increase q7days as needed up to 450 mg/day. Extended-release form is given once daily	When used for angina, the total daily dosage should be administered in divided doses. Hypotensive effects may persist for up to 4 wk after discontinuation
Calcium Channel Blockers			
Amlodipine	Prinzmetal's angina	*Adult:* 5–10 mg po QD Maintenance: 2.5–10 mg po QD	May take without regard to meals
Verapamil	Angina	*Adult:* 80–120 mg po TID *or* 120–240 mg QD of sustained-release formulation. Increase in daily or weekly intervals as needed Maintenance: 240–480 mg po QD *or* 5–10 mg IV. May repeat with 10 mg after 30 minutes	Initial dose lower in patients with hepatic impairment or poor left ventricular function, or in the elderly
Bepridil	Exercise-induced angina	*Adult:* 200 mg po QD. Increase after 10 days to 300 mg QD. Maintenance dose not to exceed 400 mg/day	May be administered with meals if gastrointestinal distress is a problem
Diltiazem	Prinzmetal's angina; exercise-induced angina	*Adult:* 30–120 mg po TID–QID *or* 60–120 mg BID as sustained-release capsules *or* 180–240 mg daily as CD or XR capsules. Maintenance: Not to exceed 360 mg daily	Useful addition if beta blocker and nitrates are not effective. Usually the best-tolerated calcium channel blocker
Isradipine	Angina, essential hypertension	*Adult:* 2.5 mg po BID. Increase at 3–4-wk intervals up to 10 mg BID	Limit consumption of caffeine
Felodipine	Angina, hypertension	*Adult:* 5 mg/day po. May increase every 2 weeks. Usual daily dose 5–10 mg. Not to exceed 20 mg daily	Start older adults at 2.5 mg/day
Nicardipine	Stable angina, hypertension	*Adult:* 20 mg po TID. Increase after 3 days to maximum dose of 30 mg TID if needed. Maintenance: 20–40 mg po TID *or* 60 mg (SR) BID	Absorption may be increased by concurrent administration of a high-fat meal
Nifedipine	Prinzmetal's angina	*Adult:* 10–30 mg po TID *or* 30–90 mg QD of extended-release formulation *or* 10 mg SL Maintenance: Not to exceed 180 mg of oral agent of 120 mg of sustained-release formulation	Sublingual formulation may be repeated in 15 minutes if necessary, although this route has not been approved by U.S. Food and Drug Administration

dose of 200 mg is reached. If the intravenous (IV) formulation of atenolol is required, 5 mg of the drug is administered IV every 2 minutes for three doses. The drug is then administered as 5 mg orally every 6 hours for 48 hours, and lastly as 100 mg every 12 hours. The drug should be withheld if the apical pulse rate before administration is less than 50 beats per minute.

Metoprolol may be administered as a single oral dose of 100 to 450 mg. It can also be administered twice daily. The dosage can be increased every 7 days as needed up to 450 mg/day. Extended-release forms are administered once daily.

Laboratory Considerations

Selective and nonselective beta blockers may increase blood urea nitrogen, serum lipoprotein, and potassium, triglyceride, and uric acid levels. Antinuclear antibody titers and blood glucose levels may also be raised. Metoprolol may cause elevations in serum alkaline phosphatase, lactate dehydrogenase, alanine transaminase (serum glutamate pyruvate transaminase), and aspartate transaminase (serum glutamic-oxaloacetic transaminase) levels.

Calcium Channel Blockers

- ❒ Amlodipine (NORVASC)
- ❒ Bepridil (VASCOR)
- ❒ Diltiazem (CARDIZEM, CARDIZEM SR, CARDIZEM CD, DILACOR XR)
- ❒ Felodipine (PLENDIL)
- ❒ Isradipine (DYNACIRC)
- ❒ Nicardipine (CARDENE, CARDENE SR)
- ❒ Nifedipine (ADALAT, ADALAT CC, PROCARDIA, PROCARDIA XL)
- ❒ Verapamil (CALAN, CALAN SR, ISOPTIN, ISOPTIN SR, VERELAN)

Indications

Verapamil is considered the prototype drug and was the first calcium channel blocker approved for use in the United States. Calcium channel blockers are used alone or with other agents in the management of angina and hypertension, as well as of arrhythmias (see Chapter 34). Although the following uses are not approved by the U.S. Food and Drug Administration, some calcium channel blockers have been used for the prevention of migraine headaches, to treat arrhythmias and heart failure, and in the management of cardiomyopathy. Bepridil, the newest calcium channel blocking drug, is used only for the management of angina. The clinical use of these drugs varies with the manner in which each affects the heart.

Pharmacodynamics

Calcium channel blockers produce antianginal effects by mechanisms different from those of nitrates or beta blockers. Nifedipine and amlodipine have the greatest peripheral arterial vasodilating effect, verapamil has a moderate effect, and diltiazem has the least effect on peripheral vasculature. Nifedipine appears to complement the antianginal action of nitrates and beta blockers.

Physiologically, cardiac tissue is rapidly depolarized by the rapid influx of sodium ions. The depolarization is quickly followed by a slow inward current of calcium. The calcium channel blockers, by inhibiting calcium entry into cardiac and smooth muscle cells, dilate peripheral arteries and arterioles. The pacer cells of the sinoatrial and atrioventricular nodes are depolarized primarily by calcium. Myocardial contractility is decreased, as are atrioventricular nodal conduction and heart rate.

Adverse Effects and Contraindications

Because calcium channel blockers decrease afterload and the force of ventricular contraction, they sometimes predictably cause hypotension. Arrhythmias (e.g., bradycardia, tachycardia) and chest pain can occur as the result of inhibition of sinoatrial and atrioventricular nodes, particularly with verapamil and diltiazem. The depressant action on myocardial contractility can contribute to the onset or worsening of heart failure. Peripheral edema is possible and is more likely to occur with amlodipine and nifedipine. Peripheral edema is less likely to occur with bepridil and verapamil.

The predictable vasodilating effect of calcium channel blockers can result in dizziness, headache, flushing, and weakness, especially with nicardipine and nifedipine. Other possible adverse effects of calcium channel blockers are dry mouth, anorexia, dyspepsia, nausea (bepridil), vomiting, constipation, diarrhea, and abnormal liver function values. Some patients complain of weight gain, muscle cramps, and joint stiffness.

A rash or dermatitis, pruritus, and urticaria have been reported with calcium channel blockers, particularly nifedipine, but are less likely to occur with verapamil. Stevens-Johnson syndrome, another adverse effect, can be life threatening. Sexual dysfunction, urinary frequency, polyuria, dysuria, and nocturia are possible. Shortness of breath, dyspnea, congestion, cough, and epistaxis have occurred in susceptible patients.

There are a number of contraindications to the use of calcium channel blockers. Hypersensitivity, sick sinus syndrome, and second- or third-degree heart block (unless a pacemaker is in place) contraindicate use of these drugs. Patients with blood pressure less than 90 mm Hg should avoid bepridil, diltiazem, and verapamil. A recent MI or the presence of pulmonary congestion contraindicates diltiazem. Verapamil is contraindicated in patients with heart failure, severe ventricular dysfunction, cardiogenic shock, severe bradycardia, or hypotension.

Calcium channel blockers should be used with caution in patients with severe hepatic or renal dysfunction, patients with a history of serious ventricular arrhythmias or heart failure, and older adults. The safe use of these agents during pregnancy and lactation has not been established.

Pharmacokinetics

Although each of the calcium channel blockers has different chemical structures, they produce similar effects. The absorption of calcium channel blockers varies considerably, from 64 to 90 percent. Isradipine, felodipine, and nifedipine are well absorbed following oral administration, but they are extensively biotransformed, decreasing their bioavailability. The calcium channel blockers are significantly bound to plasma proteins. All of the drugs have a relatively rapid onset of action, reaching peak serum levels in 1 to 2 hours. Specific information on pharmacokinetics can be found in Table 32–1.

Drug-Drug Interactions

Like many other drugs, calcium channel blockers interact with a variety of other agents (see Table 32–2). For example, cimetidine decreases the hepatic clearance of calcium channel blockers. Disopyramide and beta blockers can produce additive myocardial depression when given along with calcium channel blockers.

Dosage Regimen

The dosages of other calcium channel blockers are given in Table 32–3. Caution should be used in administering oral versus sustained-release formulations of the same drug, because the dosages are different. None of the drug dosages are interchangeable.

Laboratory Considerations

Total serum calcium levels are not affected by calcium channel blockers. Hypokalemia increases the risk of arrhythmias, and thus, potassium levels should be corrected before these agents are used, especially in patients to be given bepridil. Calcium channel blockers such as nifedipine may increase creatine kinase, lactate dehydrogenase, aspartate transaminase (serum glutamic-oxaloacetic transaminase), and alanine transaminase (serum glutamate pyruvate transaminase) levels, and may produce a positive Coombs' test. Liver function values generally return to normal on discontinuation of therapy. Although the aspartate transaminase level is always increased in acute myocardial infarction, the alanine transaminase level does not necessarily rise proportionately. Nifedipine can cause positive antinuclear antibody and direct Coombs' test results. Nimodipine may occasionally decrease platelet counts.

Critical Thinking Process

Assessment

History of Present Illness

The patient with angina may present with pain anywhere in the chest, neck, arms, or back. The most common location is the retrosternal region. The pain, lasting 3 to 5 minutes, commonly radiates to the left arm but may also radiate bilaterally, to the mandible, and/or to the neck (see Fig. 32–2). Patients often demonstrate Levine's sign— a clenched fist placed over the sternum—to explain the location of their discomfort. The patient should be asked to rate the chest discomfort on a scale of 1 to 10. In many cases, the discomfort is commonly mistaken for indigestion.

The patient's perception of the pain is elicited, including the sensation, location, radiation, and duration. For example, does the chest pain occur with exertion or rest? What makes the discomfort better, and what makes it worse? Does the patient take nitroglycerin or other drugs for relief?

Past Health History

If the chest pain is present at the time of the interview, further history-taking activities are delayed until pain relief is initiated. When the patient is more comfortable, information regarding possible stress-related symptoms, such as chest pain, rapid pulse, palpitations, hyperventilation, diarrhea, constipation, anorexia, and diaphoresis, is obtained. Information about drug history, family history, and modifiable risk factors for CAD is also obtained. Eating habits, life-style, and physical activity levels should also be documented.

The health care provider should determine pre-existing conditions that may require cautious use of a nitrate, beta blocker, or calcium channel blocker. Such pre-existing conditions are asthma, heart block, depleted intravascular fluid volume, low systolic blood pressure, pregnancy, and lactation.

Physical Exam Findings

Diaphoresis, dyspnea, vomiting, dizziness, weakness, palpitations, and pallor may accompany anginal pain. However, the presence of these manifestations without chest pain is significant. Chest pain may be mild or even absent in 15 to 25 percent of patients with an MI.

High-priority assessments for the patient with suspected angina or MI are blood pressure and apical pulse measurements. Skin color, temperature, and turgor, jugular vein distention, heart rate and rhythm, heart sounds, and peripheral pulses should also be noted, and a respiratory assessment performed. If angina or an uncomplicated MI is occurring, the skin will be warm, with peripheral pulses palpable. In patients with complicated angina or MI, cardiac output may be reduced, manifesting as cool, diaphoretic skin.

An S_3 gallop may be present, often indicating heart failure, a serious and common complication of MI. The presence of an S_4 heart sound is a common finding in patients who have had a previous MI or hypertension. Respiratory rate and rhythm should be noted. Auscultation of breath sounds may reflect crackles or rhonchi, and wheezes in the presence of congestive heart failure.

Diagnostic Testing

No laboratory tests can confirm a diagnosis of angina. Serum enzyme determinations are not helpful in assessing angina, although an absence of serum enzymes indicates that the patient has not had an MI. If possible, an electrocardiogram should be done to assess for arrhythmias.

An MI can be confirmed by the presence of abnormally high levels of cardiac enzymes and isoenzymes. Enzymes that assist in the diagnosis and monitoring of cardiac status are lactate dehydrogenase and creatine kinase. Creatine kinase is the most sensitive and reliable indicator of MI. An elevated white cell count appears on the second day after an MI.

Other diagnostic testing applicable for the patient with angina includes thallium scans that use radioisotope imaging to assess for ischemia. Exercise tolerance testing (stress testing) to assess for electrocardiographic changes consistent with angina may also be done.

Developmental Considerations

Pregnancy is normally accompanied by significant physiologic changes in the maternal cardiovascular system—blood volume, cardiac output, pulse, blood pressure, and peripheral vascular resistance (see Chapter 6). In the majority of patients, these changes present no significant risk to maternal or fetal well-being. However, certain patients experience a sudden decompensation of heart function during pregnancy.

Both the myocardium and the myometrium of the uterus possess alpha-adrenergic and beta-adrenergic receptors. The smooth muscle of the uterus contracts in response to alpha-adrenergic stimulation and relaxes with beta-adrenergic stimulation. Secondary uterine effects should be considered in patients treated with cardiac drugs that cause either type of stimulation. Further, there is controversy regarding the safety of beta blockers in pregnancy. There is some evidence that propranolol may lower umbilical blood flow. Report of an increased incidence of growth retardation, delayed neonatal respirations, bradycardia, hypoglycemia, and blunting of accelerations of intrapartum fetal heart rate have been described with beta blockers. Whether these phenomena are dose related or are caused by the underlying cardiac disease is unclear. No clear evidence exists to suggest that beta blockers are teratogenic.

Pediatric An estimated 400,000 babies are born with congenital heart disease in the United States each year. Of these, about one-third become critically ill during their first year of life, one-third develop problems later in childhood or as young adults, and one-third never experience serious handicaps. Management of heart disease in children is primarily surgical.

Geriatric Physiologic changes in the cardiovascular system manifest a variety of ways in the older adult. The efficiency and contractile strength of the myocardium declines, resulting in a 1 percent per year reduction in cardiac output. Stroke volume is thought to decrease by 0.7 percent yearly. The systolic and diastolic phases of the myocardial cycle are prolonged. Ordinarily, older adults adjust to these changes without much difficulty. However, when unusual demands are placed on the heart (e.g., shoveling snow, running to catch a bus), the changes become more evident. Pulse rates

Case Study Angina Pectoris

Patient History

History of Present Illness	JS, a 49-year-old male, presents to the clinic accompanied by his wife. He complained of chest pain after shoveling snow this morning but is in no acute distress at this time. He reports that the pain radiated to his jaw and left arm. It was relieved with rest and two nitroglycerin tablets. During the attack, he complained of being dizzy, anxious. His wife noticed he was breathing rapidly and that he looked pale.
Past Health History	JS first experienced nonradiating chest pain 3 years ago. A stress test showed ischemic ST and T wave changes with exercise. He was diagnosed with exercise-induced angina and prescribed nitroglycerin tablets, 0.3 mg. SL PRN chest pain. He reports taking the nitroglycerin 2 or 3 times during the past year. He has been on a low-cholesterol diet and taking clofibrate 500 mg po TID. Uses albuterol inhaler PRN for the reactive airway disease he has had since childhood. JS smokes cigarettes, ½ pack per day. He has a strong family history for coronary artery disease and hypercholesterolemia.
Physical Exam	VS: BP 168/90, apical pulse 94 and irregular, respirations 26, temp 37°C. Dyspnea noted. Breath sounds clear bilaterally. PMI palpable at 5th ICS, MCL. $S_1 > S_2$ at the apex. No murmur or S_3 or S_4 heart sounds noted on auscultation. Peripheral pulses strong bilaterally. No carotid, aortic, renal artery, or femoral artery bruits noted.
Diagnostic Testing	CBC: Within normal limits. Cardiac enzymes/isoenzymes: Unremarkable. Cholesterol: 240 mg/dL; HDL: 35 mg/dL; triglycerides: 180 mg/dL. ECG: Slight ST segment elevation.
Developmental Considerations	JS has 3 children under the age of 10. The 7-year-old boy is developmentally disabled and has been having behavioral difficulties at school recently. JS's wife does not work outside the home.
Psychosocial Considerations	JS is a self-employed accountant who has been spending long periods at the office owing to tax season. He remains an active coach for the local basketball team.
Economic Factors	JS considers he has an upper-middle-class family with no unusual financial stressors. The family has health insurance through a local PPO but no pharmacy coverage.

Variables Influencing Decision

Treatment Objectives

- Enhance cardiac performance.
- Decrease the duration and intensity of anginal attacks.
- Improve work capacity.

Drug Variables	*Drug Summary*	*Patient Variables*
Indications	Nitrates, beta blockers, and calcium channel blockers all useful to treat angina. Combination of nitrates and beta blockers is effective for exercise-induced angina.	JS has diagnosis of exercise-induced angina and reactive airway disease.
Pharmacodynamics	Nitrates, beta blockers, and calcium channel blockers reduce oxygen consumption through different means. Concurrent use recommended.	JS has exercise-induced angina.
Adverse Effects/ Contraindications	Hypotension most commonly associated wtih antianginal drugs. Nonselective beta blockers are contraindicated in patients with respiratory disorders.	Cautious use of beta blockers is needed due to JS's history of reactive airway disease. This is a decision point.

Case Study Angina Pectoris—cont'd

Drug Variables	*Drug Summary*	*Patient Variables*
Pharmacokinetics	The pharmacokinetics for antianginal drugs vary with the specific agent and formulation. Nadolol may negate the effects of beta-adrenergic bronchodilators. No identified problem with metoprolol.	Long-acting and short-acting agents most appropriate for JS. JS uses beta-adrenergic bronchodilator PRN. This is a decision point.
Dosage Regimen	Per manufacturer's recommendations. Once-daily dosing would promote compliance.	JS would prefer drug with once/day dosing because of his busy schedule. This will be a decision point.
Laboratory Considerations	No specific lab tests used to monitor drug effectiveness.	No specific variable here, so there is no decision point.
Cost Index*	Nitroglycerin SL tablets: 1 Metoprolol: 1 Atenolol: 1	Atenolol is cheaper overall as initial drug of choice compared with metoprolol. JS has no pharmacy coverage. This will be a decision point.
Summary of Decision Points	• Nonselective beta blockers contraindicated in patients with history of reactive airway disease. Will need to use cardioselective agent. • JS uses a beta-adrenergic bronchodilator PRN. Nadolol will negate the effects of bronchodilator. No identifiable problem with metoprolol. • Long-acting and short-acting agents most appropriate for JS. • JS has no pharmacy coverage. Atenolol cheaper overall, based on dosage regimen, than metoprolol.	
DRUGS TO USED	• Nitroglycerin 0.3 mg SL tablets PRN chest pain × 3 tablets. If no relief, health care provider will be contacted • Atenolol 50 mg po QD. Will titrate dose according to patient response in 3–7 days.	

*Cost Index	
1	$<30/mo.
2	$ 30–40/mo.
3	$ 40–50/mo.
4	$ 50–60/mo.
5	$>60/mo.

AWP of 100, 0.3-mg sublingual tablets of nitroglycerin is approximately $7.
AWP of 100, 50-mg tablets of metoprolol is approximately $21.
AWP of 100, 50-mg tablets of atenolol is approximately $9.

may not reach the levels of younger persons, and tachycardia lasts longer. There is some disagreement among health care providers as to when the normal elevation becomes hypertension. In some older adults, the blood pressure may remain stable while tachycardia progresses to anginal episodes and heart failure.

Resistance to peripheral blood flow increases by 1 percent each year. Decreased elasticity of the arteries is responsible for vascular changes to the heart. Because of the rigidity of vessel walls and narrowing of lumens, more force is required to move blood through the vessels, increasing the risk of angina. These changes also lead to a higher diastolic blood pressure. Further, there is a decrease in the ability of the aorta to distend, in turn raising systolic pressure. Vagal tone increases, and the heart becomes more sensitive to carotid sinus stimulation. Reduced sensitivity of the baroreceptors potentiates orthostatic hypotension.

Psychosocial Considerations

Denial is a common early reaction to the chest discomfort associated with angina or MI. On the average, the patient with an acute MI waits more than 2 hours before seeking care. Thus, the patient's perceived susceptibility to anginal pain, and perhaps to myocardial infarction and its subsequent limitations, influences the overall plan of care. Further, the likelihood of compliance with a plan of care is also determined by the ratio of perceived benefits of compliance versus risks of nonaction.

Fear, anxiety, and anger are common reactions of patients and family members to this situation. The health care provider must assess behavioral patterns that stem from these reactions. For example, a patient may not report recurrent chest pain because of fear (see Case Study—Angina Pectoris).

Analysis and Management

Treatment Objectives

The primary treatment objective in the management of angina is to enhance cardiac performance, thereby restoring the balance between myocardial oxygen supply and demand. This objective may be accomplished by reducing the duration and intensity of symptoms, preventing attacks, and improving work capacity (even though angina may occur). The ultimate outcome is to prevent or delay the onset of MI. Diseases or conditions that predispose an individual to angina should be treated as part of a comprehensive therapeutic program.

Treatment Options

Drug Variables

The choice of antianginal drugs and route of administration is made with consideration of the desired onset of therapeutic effects, the suitability of various routes of administration for the particular patient, the need for stable drug concentration, co-morbid conditions, and the likelihood of tolerance or toxicity. The ideal antianginal drug establishes a balance between coronary blood flow and the metabolic demands of the heart. It would produce local effects by acting directly on coronary vessels rather than on other organ systems, and would promote oxygen extraction by the heart from arterial circulation. The drug would be effective taken orally and would have sustained action. The ideal drug would also have an absence of tolerance. No drug currently meets the ideal. Table 32–4 provides a summary of the systemic effects of nitrates, beta blockers, and calcium channel blockers.

When relief of acute anginal pain is the desired goal, a rapid onset of drug action is necessary, and the duration of action is less important. In comparison, for angina prophylaxis, the duration of action and the predictability of effect are the key issues. The rapidity of onset and the duration of action of any nitrate are directly related to the route of administration.

All patients with suspected or proven angina should receive drug therapy in an attempt to reduce the severity and frequency of anginal symptoms and thereby enhance the quality of life and minimize the risk of MI. Because nitrates, beta blockers, and calcium channel blockers are useful in the treatment of angina, and each reduces oxygen consumption through different means, concurrent therapy may be advised in some patients.

Nitrates Nitrates reduce the rise in left ventricular end-diastolic pressure associated with beta blockade by increasing venous capacitance. They are effective and inexpensive drugs of first choice for patients who have heart failure or impaired left ventricular function (i.e., ejection fraction less than 40 percent). They can be used in such patients even when mitral regurgitation is present. Nitrates are also used as first-line drugs for patients with chronic airway limitation, diabetes, and intermittent claudication (Table 32–5). They are second-line drugs for patients with hypertension and Raynaud's phenomenon. Nitrates are not ordinarily recommended for patients who have angina and concomitant migraine headaches. Sublingual nitroglycerin should be available to any patient with suspected anginal symptoms. It is useful as prophylaxis before planned exercise that may bring on symptoms.

The sublingual and buccal formulations can be used for all patients with chronic stable angina. Nitroglycerin tablets and sprays are equally effective. They have a similar onset time, but the effects of the buccal form last only as long as the tablet remains intact (approximately 5 hours). The onset and duration of action of the lingual spray are comparable to those of sublingual nitroglycerin tablets. Nitrate tablets, such as isosorbide dinitrate, are longer acting than sublingual forms of nitroglycerin and, when used in adequate doses, are effective in reducing the incidence of anginal attacks.

The nitrate drug of choice for long-term treatment depends on the presence or absence of other co-morbid disease, adverse effects, and cost. Nitroglycerin spray is more expensive per dose than the tablets. However, if nitroglycerin is used infrequently, the spray may be more cost effective, because nitroglycerin tablets are outdated in 6 months but the lingual spray is good for approximately 3 years.

Oral nitrates have a long history of safety and effectiveness as well as low cost. Because the oral nitrates lack serious adverse effects, they should be used in patients in whom

TABLE 32–4 COMPARISON OF EFFECTS OF NITRATES, BETA BLOCKERS, AND CALCIUM CHANNEL BLOCKERS ON CARDIAC FUNCTION

Response	Nitrates	Beta Blockers	Calcium Channel Blockers
Coronary blood flow	↑	↑ or NC	↑
Coronary vessel resistance	↓	↑ or NC	↓
Coronary spasms	↓	↑ or NC	↓
Collateral blood flow	↑	NC	↓
Heart rate	↓	↓	↑, ↓, NC
Myocardial contractility	NC	↓	↓
Systolic blood pressure	↓	↓	↓
Ventricular volume	↓	↑	↓ or NC

↑, Increased; ↓, Decreased; NC, No change.

TABLE 32–5 INITIAL TREATMENT OF ANGINA BASED ON CO-MORBID CONDITION

Co-Morbid Condition	Nitrate	Beta Blocker	Calcium Channel Blocker
Chronic airway limitation	1st	NR	2nd
Diabetes mellitus	1st	NR	2nd
Heart failure	1st	NR	NR
Hypertension	2nd	1st	3rd
Hyperthyroidism	NA	1st	NA
Intermittent claudication	1st	1st	1st
Migraine	NR	1st	2nd
Raynaud's phenomenon	2nd	NR	1st

NR, Not recommended.

1st, First choice drug; 2nd, alternative drug; 3rd, possible alternative drug if patient is unable to tolerate the alternative drug; NA, not applicable.

Note: Where no drug of choice is identified, there may be no specific recommendation.

beta blockers are ineffective or are not tolerated. The advantages of isosorbide mononitrate over the dinitrate formulation are that it does not require conversion in the body from dinitrate to mononitrate form and that it has proven efficacy in dosages that tend to circumvent tolerance. There is little evidence to suggest that isosorbide dinitrate tolerance is circumvented after the second and third doses. Further, drug rash, flushing, and halitosis have not been reported with isosorbide mononitrate as they have with isosorbide dinitrate.

The greatest benefit of an IV nitrate is generated when it is administered within 4 hours of the onset of symptoms. However, it also offers benefits when given as along as 8 hours following onset of symptoms. Its effects include decreases in anginal episodes, ventricular ectopic beats, and left ventricular failure.

Topical nitrates may be useful for the patient with nocturnal and unstable angina, because they have a longer duration of action than sublingual and lingual formulations. The disadvantage, however, is that topical formulations are often messy and have a relative short duration of action, necessitating repeated application.

Topical formulations are available as pastes and patches. Paste formulations come in a tube, much like toothpaste, with a specially designed paper applicator. The drug is measured (by the inch) onto the paper applicator and then applied to the skin surface. The only advantage of a topical formulation over oral nitrates is that the effects can be stopped relatively quickly by simply wiping the drug off the skin.

Both the reservoir and matrix patch systems offer steady-state plasma levels within the therapeutic range over 24 hours, thus making only one application per day necessary. The disadvantage of the reservoir system is "dose dumping" if the seal is punctured or broken. Dose dumping does not occur with the matrix system. Both systems achieve plasma steady-state levels in approximately 2 hours. However, transdermal formulations must be removed for 10 to 12 hours each day to avoid development of tolerance.

NITRATE TOLERANCE Tolerance to nitrates develops with sustained, long-term use. Patients appear to develop tolerance not just to specific nitrates but to the entire classification of drugs. Nitroglycerin patches become ineffective when they are left in place and reapplied on a daily basis, and they will remain ineffective even if the dosage is progressively increased. Patches that deliver 10 mg or more of nitroglycerin remain effective if they are removed for a period of 10 to 12 hours each day. Intermittent treatment results in reproducible cardiovascular effects, whereas long-term, repeated exposure to high-dose nitrates leads to a decrease in the magnitude of most of the pharmacologic effects. The therapeutic implications of this phenomenon are likely to proliferate as higher dosages of oral and transdermal formulations become more prevalent. The extent of the tolerance to the drug is related to the amount and frequency.

To minimize tolerance, nitrate therapy should be individualized, using the lowest effective dose and an intermittent dosing schedule. Drug holidays—brief periods of no therapy—may be sufficient to avoid the development of tolerance. Although such actions may minimize tolerance, there is a disadvantage to nitrate-free periods. The shortest drug-free period that enables maintenance of nitrate effectiveness is unknown. Thus, in some patients, symptoms may worsen toward the end of the drug-free interval. Tolerance has not been reported with buccal forms of nitroglycerin, possibly because of the drug-free interval at night.

Beta Blockers Beta blockers should be first-line therapy, in conjunction with sublingual nitroglycerin, for patients with angina who have no co-morbid conditions. Beta blockers can be used as first-line agents in patients who have hypertension, hyperthyroidism, intermittent claudication, or migraine headaches. Beta blockers may be chosen over nitrates to treat both angina and hypertension using a single drug. Their use is generally contraindicated in patients with chronic airflow limitation, diabetes mellitus, heart failure, or Raynaud's phenomenon. However, when introduced slowly, beta blockers can improve, not worsen, heart failure.

Concurrent use of beta blockers and nitrates reduces coronary vascular resistance associated with beta blockade. Beta blockers (e.g., atenolol, nadolol) are effective and inexpensive, can be given once daily, and lower the likelihood of arrhythmia, reinfarction, and even sudden cardiac death after MI. Beta blockers can be used for patients in whom coronary vasospasm plays a role in the development of anginal pain during exercise and at rest. The additive benefit is primarily a result of one drug's blocking the adverse effects of the other on myocardial oxygen consumption. Beta blockers inhibit the reflex tachycardia and higher contractile force that are sometimes associated with nitrates.

Nadolol, a nonselective beta blocker with low lipid solubility, may be used initially, because it has proven effectiveness and several advantages over propranolol. The absorption of nadolol is consistent, and it can be given once daily. Nadolol also offers distinct advantages in that it blocks catecholamine-induced ($beta_2$) arrhythmias and hypokalemia. Acebutolol, another selective beta blocker, and atenolol can be used instead of nadolol if they are found to be less expensive, or if the patient has a problem with cold extremities. Cold extremities can be worsened by antagonizing $beta_2$-adrenergic receptors.

Calcium Channel Blockers Calcium channel blockers are useful additions to antianginal therapy if nitrates and beta blockers are ineffective. All calcium channel blockers are equally effective as antianginal agents. Diltiazem is usually the best tolerated, however, and should be chosen over other agents unless there are significant price differences. Calcium channel blockers are expensive and usually must be taken more than once a day. Sustained-release formulations are recommended, because they are more convenient than, and usually not much different in price from, the regular-release products.

In patients with stable angina that is inadequately controlled with nitrates and beta blockers, the use of a calcium channel blocker with a beta blocker may provide some improvement, specifically the dihydropyridines nifedipine and nicardipine. Only the dihydropyridines should be used in conjunction with a beta blocker. The beta blocker lessens the reflex tachycardia caused by the nifedipine. During exercise, the combined use of nifedipine and propranolol achieves lower heart rate and blood pressure than are observed when either drug is taken alone. Nifedipine may be useful if the reduction in afterload exceeds the negative inotropic effect.

Calcium channel blockers are more effective than beta blockers in the patient with Prinzmetal's angina, although they are more expensive. Calcium channel blockers may be considered first-line drugs in the patient with intermittent claudication or Raynaud's phenomenon. They are often second-line drugs for the patient with chronic airway limitation, diabetes, or migraines. Calcium channel blockers can be used for patients with angina and hypertension who are unable to take beta blockers. Because they depress left ventricular function, calcium channel blockers should not be used in patients with heart failure, particularly those with left ejection fractions less than 30 percent.

Variant angina, however, is best treated with nitrates and calcium channel blockers so as to reduce the vasospasm of the coronary arteries. The combination of a nitrate and a calcium channel blocker may provide greater relief of severe stable or variant angina than can be obtained with either drug alone. Calcium channel blockers are as effective as nitrates and may even be preferred to beta blockers in the therapeutic management of variant or unstable angina. Nitrates reduce preload, whereas calcium channel blockers reduce afterload. The net effect on reduction of oxygen demand is additive. It should be noted, however, that excessive vasodilation may occur. The steps by which the antianginal therapeutic regimen progresses are summarized in Figure 32–5.

Cardiac glycosides (e.g., digoxin) may be indicated if the patient with angina has pre-existing heart failure that is contributing to difficulties in oxygen supply, demand, and extraction. The opioid morphine offers analgesia and lowers myocardial oxygen demand by reducing preload. Peak respiratory depression occurs 10 minutes after the dose, but if

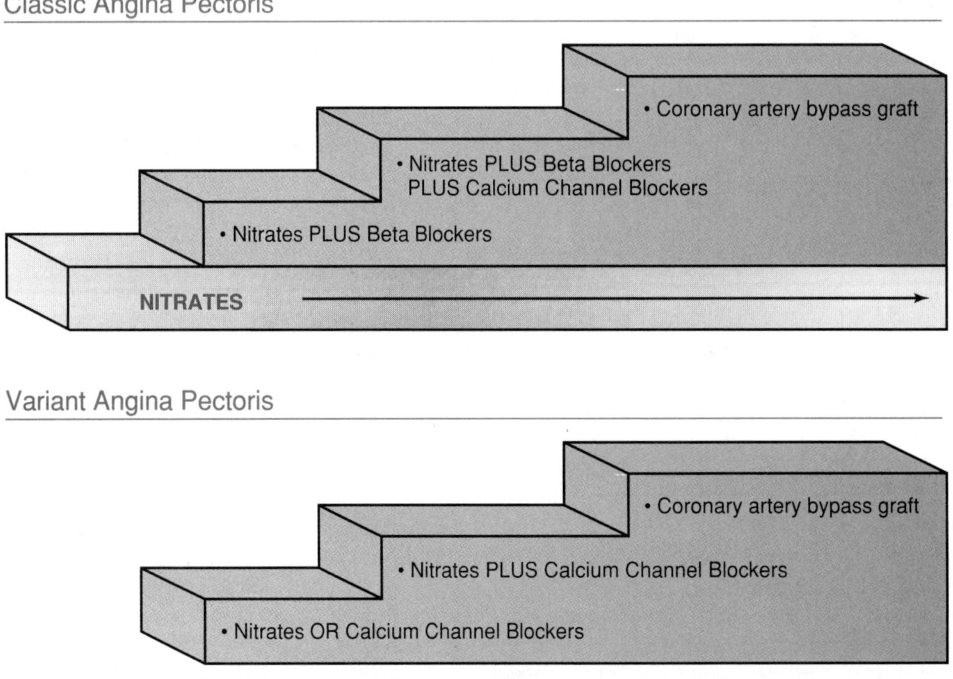

Figure 32–5 Recommended progression of antianginal therapeutic regimens, for both classic and variant angina pectoris.

the patient is still in pain 5 minutes after the initial dose, it is highly unlikely that respiratory depression will occur at 10 minutes. The patient should be given morphine (2 mg) every 5 minutes until the pain is relieved. The disadvantage of morphine, though, is that it blocks the perception of pain, an important indicator of the severity of ischemia.

The anticoagulant heparin (see Chapter 36) should be available for all patients with acute anginal pain at rest (symptomatic proven unstable angina) to prevent thrombus formation. Antiplatelet drugs, fibrinolytics (see Chapter 37), antihypertensives (see Chapter 34), and cholesterol-lowering drugs (see Chapter 35) may also be useful in the management of angina. Antiplatelet drugs (e.g., aspirin) interfere with platelet aggregation by inhibiting the formation of thromboxane A_2. When used to treat patients with unstable angina, aspirin lowers the risk of developing an acute MI and reduces mortality by 50 percent. Aspirin currently is the only antiplatelet drug recommended for the prevention of acute MI in patients with unstable angina, because no other antiplatelet drug has been found to be as effective. In the management of unstable angina, aspirin should be used only in addition to nondrug interventions. Antiplatelet drugs are discussed further in Chapter 36.

A 10 percent reduction in cholesterol reduces the risk of CAD by 20 percent. A 6 mmHg reduction in diastolic blood pressure lowers the risk of CAD by 10 percent. Further, there is a 50 percent reduction in the progression of unstable angina to MI with the daily use of aspirin. All men and women with angina should take aspirin daily.

Patient Variables

The management strategies chosen should take into consideration the psychosocial, cultural, economic, and religious background of the patient. Compliance may be improved by using drugs that simplify the regimen, such as those requiring once-daily dosing, that come in a lingual spray, or that require little psychomotor skill for application. For example, the use of transdermal nitroglycerin may be less bothersome, and therefore the patient more compliant, than the use of a nitroglycerin paste. In assessment of the overall benefit of therapeutic intervention, improvement in life-style should be judged not only from the ability of the patient to sustain normal activities without symptoms but also on the basis of the inconvenience caused by treatment.

The patient's clinical response to therapy should be considered when any drug is prescribed. Drug response may vary greatly, because no two people have identical physiologic or psychologic compositions. Maintenance drug therapy should be considered for patients who are psychologically distressed by recurrent anginal episodes or who have symptoms more than two or three times a week.

Intervention

Administration

Before administration of an antianginal drug, the patient's blood pressure and pulse should be taken. They should be taken again at the onset of drug action. For an acute anginal episode, the first nitrate dose is administered with the patient sitting or lying down. The patient is instructed to place the sublingual drug form under the tongue until the tablet dissolves. Up to three sublingual tablets or three lingual sprays can be used within 15 minutes, if necessary. If chest pain is not relieved with rest and the nitroglycerin, an MI should be assumed to be occurring until proven otherwise. The patient should be kept quiet and the emergency medical system contacted.

For hospitalized patients, sublingual nitroglycerin should be left at the bedside. Sublingual tablets and lingual sprays should be within reach so they can be used immediately, if necessary. An adequate supply should be available and a record kept of when and how much the drug is used.

Long-acting antianginal drugs should be administered at regularly spaced intervals to maximize their effectiveness in preventing angina attacks. When oral nitrates and topical preparations are used concurrently, the patient is encouraged to stagger administration times, in order to minimize the possibility of additive hypotension and headache.

Nitroglycerin paste is applied with the special paper applicator. The patient should avoid applying the drug to hairy or irritated skin surfaces. Transdermal nitroglycerin should be applied at the same time each day, and the paste or patch removed at same time each night, as directed. This routine promotes drug effectiveness and consistent drug absorption, and minimizes tachyphylaxis.

Patients should be carefully assessed when alternating manufacturer products or when changing dosage forms. For example, if a patient is changing from nitroglycerin ointment (containing 12.5 to 15 mg per inch) to a transdermal form, the smallest dose size of the transdermal patch should be used, and the dosage appropriately titrated.

Intravenous nitroglycerin should be diluted according to manufacturer's instructions, and should be titrated as needed. Blood pressure and pulse should be checked every 5 to 15 minutes during dose titration and every hour thereafter. The flow rate should be adjusted according to patient response—a drop in systolic blood pressure of 20 mmHg or relief of pain. It should be noted, however, that intravenous nitroglycerin binds to the polyvinyl chloride plastic that is used in most intravenous solution bags and infusion sets. So much drug can bind to the plastic that very little reaches the patient's circulation. Anticipate the need for dosage increases if polyvinyl chloride infusion sets are used. The tubing that comes with intravenous nitroglycerin from the manufacturer is made of special plastic with which the drug does not bind and should be used when possible. Nitroglycerin solutions should be stored in a glass bottle and used within 24 hours.

Nitrate Toxicity Nitrate overdose causes dose-dependent hypotension and reflex tachycardia. A simultaneous increase in oxygen demand and a decrease in oxygen supply contribute to myocardial ischemia and possible MI. Severe hypotension may also cause cerebral ischemia and stroke. Proper management includes temporarily stopping the nitrate, because the drug's short duration of action usually allows blood pressure to rise in a relatively short period. If an intentional overdose was taken orally, induced emesis and other measures to decrease drug absorption may be indicated. Vasopressors may be indicated to correct excessive hypotension. However, they should be used with caution to avoid coronary artery vasoconstriction that can further aggravate angina. Epinephrine should not be used, as it may lower myocardial blood flow and oxygen supply by reducing diastolic pressure and almost always increases oxygen demands by causing tachycardia. Oxygen therapy is indicated to help overcome inadequate tissue oxygenation. Oxygen improves saturation and assists in meeting tissue oxygenation needs. It helps also to relieve the dyspnea associated with ischemic episodes.

Education

The patient should be instructed as to the need for smoking cessation, dietary management of hypercholesterolemia, stress reduction, and regular exercise.

The patient should be advised to stop smoking at once. Stopping smoking lowers the risk of CAD by 37 percent. Smoking raises carboxyhemoglobin levels in the blood, reducing the amount of oxygen available to the myocardium and possibly precipitating an anginal episode. Patients who are exposed for 2 hours to smoke not only suffer elevations in carboxyhemoglobin concentrations but also experience shortened exercise time and increased heart rate and blood pressure. Second-hand smoke ("passive smoking") should also be avoided.

Patients with angina should lose excess weight. They should be encouraged to eat small meals, avoid high-calorie and high-cholesterol foods, abstain from gas-forming foods, and rest for short periods after eating. In addition, a high-fiber diet is recommended. It not only prevents constipation and other gastrointestinal ailments but also decreases the number and severity of anginal episodes. Diets high in fiber also lower serum cholesterol and triglyceride levels. CAD is less common in patients with a high intake of dietary fiber than in those with a low intake. High-fiber diets can also decrease hypertension.

Strenuous exercise is known to precipitate an anginal attack but may be effectively managed with appropriate exercise limitations and patient education. Exercise does enlarge heart volume and mass, increase capillary vascularity, and decrease heart rate—all of which may protect the myocardium from the effects of ischemic damage. However, the patient with documented evidence of ischemic heart disease should be cautioned against engaging in strenuous exercise, because it raises myocardial oxygen demand.

Patients who lead active, hectic lives should be advised to adjust activities to below the level that precipitates anginal episodes. They should try for brief rest periods throughout the work day, an early bedtime, and longer or more frequent vacations. The health care provider should help patients who are anxious and nervous to understand the importance of counseling. Relaxation exercises and other stress reduction techniques may be used to reduce the incidence of angina.

In spite of compliance with nondrug therapies, some patients continue to experience angina and require frequent monitoring. Antianginal drugs are most often taken on an outpatient basis, so the patient should be instructed to recorded the number and severity of anginal episodes, along with the effectiveness and total number of nitroglycerin tablets taken daily. Information from the patient is important to monitoring therapeutic and adverse effects of drug therapy.

The patient should also be instructed as to proper storage of antianginal preparations. Sublingual formulations are effective for a period of 5 to 6 months when stored in a dark, cool location. Lingual sprays are viable for up to 3 years. Tablets are inactivated by light, heat, air, and moisture; they should be stored at room temperature in an amber glass container with a tight-fitting lid. Patients should be advised not to transfer the drug to other containers and to discard unused nitroglycerin tablets 6 months after opening the container.

The patient and family should be reminded that antianginal drugs should be taken only as prescribed. Family members should be kept informed about the location and proper use of the drugs in case the patient needs help taking them. Dosage of these drugs is individualized to maximize therapeutic effects and minimize adverse reactions. Abrupt discontinuance of antianginal drugs has been associated with increases in anginal episodes and possible MI.

Sublingual tablets are dissolved slowly under the tongue. The patient is advised not to eat, drink, or smoke while an undissolved tablet remains in the mouth. Some nitroglycerin tablets cause a tingling or slight burning sensation when placed under the tongue. For many years, the tingling/burning sensation was used as an indicator of the drug's "freshness." This sign cannot be regarded as an indicator that the drug will be effective. Older patients may not experience the tingling, even with new nitroglycerin tablets. Patients who doubt the potency of their drug should have their prescription refilled and then should discard the old drug.

Patients should be taught to seek medical attention immediately if acute chest pain is not relieved with rest and sublingual nitroglycerin. In addition, the patient or family members should be taught how to recognize and report signs and symptoms of hypotension and to minimize the effects of orthostatic hypotension.

Patients must swallow sustained-release formulations. Tablets should not be chewed or taken sublingually, and capsules should not be opened. Patients using long-acting antianginal drugs should have a sublingual dosage form on hand at all times.

Transdermal ointment should be carefully measured, preferably using the special paper applicators. A disposable applicator stick, rubber gloves, or both can be used to spread the drug evenly over 2 to 3 square inches of skin area. The application site is covered with plastic wrap, if instructed. Application sites should be rotated. Most patients are instructed to remove transdermal patches at bedtime, to wipe off any remaining drug, and to reapply a fresh patch upon awakening. All transdermal patches can be worn during bathing, showering, and swimming.

The patient should avoid concurrent use of other drugs without checking with the health care provider. Over-the-counter decongestants, cold remedies, and diet pills stimulate the heart, constrict blood vessels, and may contribute to anginal episodes.

The patient should be instructed not to abruptly discontinue an antianginal drug. These agents should be discontinued slowly over several days to prevent rebound angina, hypertension, arrhythmias, and acute MI.

Evaluation

The patient with angina will report a decrease in the frequency and severity of anginal attacks along with improved activity tolerance. If the nitrates were administered for heart failure, the patient demonstrates a clearing of peripheral edema and lung fields, and improvements in urinary output and blood pressure. Pulmonary artery and pulmonary capillary wedge pressures are within normal limits.

The patient using beta blockers and calcium channel blocking drugs as antianginal treatment have a decrease in the frequency and severity of anginal attacks. Beta blockers have been shown to prevent myocardial reinfarction. Calcium channel blockers are thought to reduce the need for nitrate therapy.

The patient should be able to correctly identify his or her drug, proper administration technique, and dose. Signs and symptoms of hypotension, ways to minimize orthostatic changes, and the importance of keeping follow-up appointments should be identified.

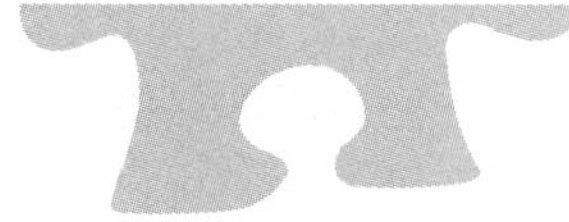

SUMMARY

- Coronary artery disease secondary to atherosclerosis is the most common cause of angina pectoris.
- Risk factors for the development of angina are coronary artery disease, hypertension, hypercholesterolemia, smoking, and lack of regular exercise.
- Atherosclerotic plaque may narrow the lumen, decreasing elasticity and impairing dilation of coronary arteries, and resulting in impaired blood flow to the myocardium, especially when exercise or other factors increase cardiac workload and the demand for oxygen.
- Angina pectoris arises when there is an imbalance between the supply of and demand for oxygen.
- Angina typically takes one of three forms: stable angina (classic, stable exertional, predictable), unstable angina (acute coronary insufficiency, crescendo, preinfarction), and variant angina (Prinzmetal's, vasospastic).
- Classic angina pain is located in the retrosternal region, but the pain may occur anywhere in the chest, neck, arms, or back. It commonly radiates to the left arm, mandible, or neck.
- Levine's sign is often displayed when patients explain the location of their discomfort.
- Associated signs and symptoms are diaphoresis, dizziness, dyspnea, vomiting, weakness, palpitations, and pallor. In some patients with a myocardial infarction, chest pain is minimal or absent.
- The goals of therapy with antianginal drugs are to decrease the duration and intensity of pain during an attack, reduce the frequency of attacks, and improve work capacity.
- Nondrug measures used for prevention and treatment of angina include stress management, smoking cessation, adequate and timely rest periods, and avoidance of circumstances known to precipitate an attack.
- Drug measures used in the treatment of angina pectoris include single as well as combination therapy with nitrates, beta blockers, and/or calcium channel blockers.
- Choice of antianginal drug and route of administration are made with consideration of the onset of effects, suitability of the route for that patient, need for stable drug concentrations, and likelihood of tolerance or toxicity.
- Combination therapy has been advocated, because selected drugs in each of the drug categories are useful in treating of angina and reducing oxygen consumption.
- The patient's blood pressure and pulse should be measured before administration of an antianginal drug and again at the onset of drug action. The first dose of nitrate should be administered with the patient sitting or lying down.
- Sublingual tablets should be allowed to dissolve slowly under the tongue. The patient should be advised not to eat, drink, or smoke while an undissolved tablet remains in the mouth.
- Patients taking long-acting nitrates must have a supply of a short-acting nitrate on hand in case of angina attack requiring more nitrate.
- Intermittent treatment using transdermal patches minimizes the potential for tolerance to nitrates.
- The patient should be monitored for toxicities associated with nitrates, beta blockers, and calcium channel blockers.
- Patients should know the name of their antianginal drug, its correct use and adverse effects, and when to seek medical attention if chest pain is unrelieved.
- Therapeutic effects of antianginal therapy are demonstrated by patient reports of a decrease in the frequency and severity of anginal attacks along with improved activity tolerance.

BIBLIOGRAPHY

Brouwer, J., Viersma, J., van Veldhuisen, D., et al. (1995). Usefulness of heart rate variability in predicting efficacy (metoprolol vs. diltiazem) in patients with stable angina pectoris. *American Journal of Cardiology,* 76(11), 759–763.

Diodati, J., Theroux, P., Latour, J., et al. (1990). Effects of nitroglycerine at therapeutic doses on platelet aggregation in unstable angina pectoris and acute myocardial infarction. *American Journal of Cardiology,* 66(7), 683–688.

Cairns, J. (1995). Medical management of unstable angina. *Lancet,* 346(8991/8992), 1644.

Freedman, S. (1994). Stable angina: Diagnosis and management. *Modern Medicine: Journal of Clinical Medicine,* 37(10), 30–34.

Gollub, S. (1993). Combination medical therapy in treatment of angina pectoris. *Hospital Formulary,* 28(1), 34.

Lewis, J. (1983). Protective effects of aspirin against acute myocardial infarction and death in men with unstable angina: Results of a Veterans Administration Cooperative Study. *New England Journal of Medicine,* 309(7), 396–403.

Lung-Johansen, P. (1992). Hemodynamic effects of adrenergic blocking agents. *Cleveland Clinic Journal of Medicine,* 59(2), 193.

Marshall, J. (1992). Chest pain in patients with normal coronary arteries: A new look at potential causes. *Postgraduate Medicine,* 91(6), 213–216.

Temkin, L. (1989). High dose monotherapy and combination therapy with calcium channel blockers for angina: A comprehensive review of literature. *American Journal of Medicine,* 86(1A), 23–27.

US Department of Health and Human Services, Public Health Service, Agency for Health Care Policy and Research. (1994). *Clinical practice guideline: Diagnosing and managing unstable angina.* Rockville, MD: Author.

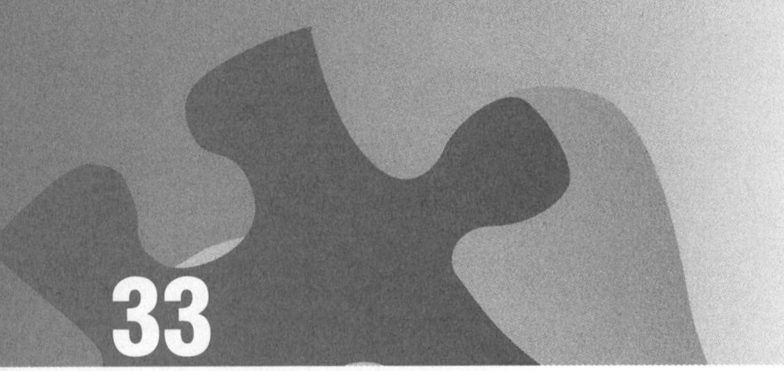

33 Antiarrhythmic Drugs

Antiarrhythmic drugs are used for the prevention and treatment of cardiac arrhythmias. An *arrhythmia,* also known as a *dysrhythmia,* is defined as an abnormal, disordered, or disturbed rhythm—any deviation from normal sinus rhythm (NSR). An abnormality may involve alterations in the heart rate or rhythm or both. There are two basic rhythm disturbances: *tachyarrhythmias,* seen as irregularities of heartbeat combined with a rapid rate, and *bradyarrhythmias,* which are rhythm irregularities that decrease heart rate. This chapter primarily discusses tachyarrhythmias. To aid in understanding arrhythmias and antiarrhythmic drugs, a review of the physiology of cardiac conduction and contractility is necessary.

ARRHYTHMIAS

Epidemiology and Etiology

Arrhythmias are common in patients with cardiac disorders, but also occur in people with normal hearts. Abnormalities of cardiac rhythm and conduction can cause sudden cardiac death or can present as symptomatic (with syncope, dizziness, or palpitations) or asymptomatic. The irregularities may be mild or severe, acute or chronic, episodic or relatively continuous.

Although a variety of diseases and disorders can cause arrhythmias, the most common cause is myocardial infarction (MI) secondary to coronary artery disease (CAD). The incidence of MI in patients with CAD is approximately 90 percent. Rhythm disturbances occur in approximately 90 to 95 percent of all individuals experiencing an MI. Other causes of arrhythmias include electrolyte imbalance, hypoxia, and drug toxicity. Multiple predisposing factors account for arrhythmias. These factors include sympathetic nervous system (SNS) stimulation, metabolic disturbances (e.g., lactic acidosis caused by compromised tissue perfusion or hyperthyroidism), and hemodynamic abnormalities (e.g., a reduction in coronary perfusion associated with hypertension). Rhythm disturbances are dangerous to the extent that they reduce cardiac output so that perfusion of the brain or myocardium is impaired, or they tend to deteriorate into more serious arrhythmias with the same consequences.

Physiology and Pathophysiology

Cardiac Electrophysiology

The electrophysiologic characteristics of cardiac muscle include excitability, automaticity, conductivity, and refractoriness. Normally, these characteristics result in effective myocardial contraction and distribution of blood throughout the body. Each cardiac cycle consists of four events: stimulation from an electrical impulse, transmission of the impulse to conductive or contractile tissue, contraction of atria and ventricles, and relaxation of atria and ventricles. During relaxation, the atria and ventricles refill with blood in preparation for the next cycle.

Excitability is the ability of cardiac muscle cells to respond to an electrical stimulus. Differences in intracellular and extracellular ion concentrations create electrical and concentration gradients for ionic movement across myocardial membranes. At rest, the inside of the myocardial cell is more negative than the outside. This *resting membrane potential* results from differences in sodium and potassium concentrations on either side of cell membranes. Potassium is primarily concentrated in the intracellular space, whereas sodium is more concentrated in the extracellular space.

Automaticity is the ability of the heart to generate an electrical impulse. The ability of the heart to generate an impulse depends on the movement of sodium and calcium ions into the myocardial cell and the movement of potassium ions out of the cell. When the myocardial cell is stimulated to a certain threshold, the membrane potential changes. The movement of ions changes the membrane potential from a state of electrical neutrality to an energized state. This change in the membrane potential is known as an *action potential.* The action potential is made up of two phases, the depolarization and repolarization phases. Depolarization, the discharge of the electrical energy, results in myocardial muscle contraction.

Some of the cells in the conduction system of the heart depolarize in response to the entry of calcium ions rather than the entry of sodium ions. These calcium-responsive cells are found primarily in the sinoatrial (SA) and atrioventricular (AV) nodes. The conduction of an electrical impulse generated by calcium is slower than that produced by a change in sodium. In general, activation of the SA and AV nodes depends on a slow depolarizing current through calcium channels. Activation of the atria and ventricles depends on a rapid depolarizing current through sodium channels. These two types of conduction tissues are often called *slow* and *fast* channels, respectively.

Following myocardial muscle contraction there is a period of decreased excitability during which the cell cannot respond to a new stimulus. During this refractory period sodium and calcium ions return to the extracellular space, and potassium ions return to the intracellular space. Muscle relaxation occurs, and the cell prepares for the next cycle of electrical activity and contraction.

Conductivity is the ability of the heart to convey electrical impulses along and across cell membranes. The systematic, rhythmic transmission of impulses results in effective myocardial muscle contraction. Normally, electrical impulses originate in the SA node. The impulses are transmitted to the atria where they cause atrial contraction. Impulses continue through conduction pathways to the AV node, the bundle of His, bundle branches, and Purkinje fibers, resulting in ventricular contraction.

Refractoriness is the inability of the heart to respond to new stimuli while it is still in a state of contraction from a previous stimulus. Refractoriness develops as a result of inactivation of sodium channels during depolarization. Thus, the heart does not respond to restimulation during the action potential, reducing the likelihood of tetanic contractions. Refractoriness normally prevents uncontrolled rapid myocardial contractions, helping to preserve heart rhythm.

Origin of Disturbances

Arrhythmias emanate from disruptions in electrophysiology, including the spontaneous initiation of an impulse (automaticity), the conduction of the impulse (conductivity), or both. Arrhythmias can originate in any part of the conduction system: the SA node, atria, AV node, bundle of His, bundle branches, Purkinje fibers, or ventricles. Table 33–1 provides examples of arrhythmias according to their site of origin and mechanism. Electrophysiologic alterations are represented by changes in the configuration of the electrocardiogram (ECG).

Automaticity Disturbances

A disturbance in the spontaneous initiation of an electrical impulse increases or decreases heart rate and rhythm. The SA node is the pacemaker of the heart because it holds the highest level of automaticity. It normally produces a rhythm of 60 to 100 beats/min (bpm). A decrease in the automaticity of the SA node produces sinus bradycardia (heart rate below 60 bpm). Sinus bradycardia frequently occurs in young adults and well trained athletes and is common at night. An increase in automaticity produces sinus tachycardia (heart rate above 100 bpm).

On the other hand, an arrhythmia can be the result of an ectopic focus. An *ectopic focus* is a shift in the site of impulse formation from the SA node to another site within the myocardium. For example, if the SA node fails to fire, other sites in the atria can fire. If the atria do not initiate a beat, it can begin in the AV node, and if the AV node does not initiate a beat, one can start in the ventricles. If the ectopic focus depolarizes at a rate faster than the SA node, the ectopic focus becomes the dominant pacemaker. Ectopic foci indicate myocardial irritability and potentially serious impairment of cardiac function. Ectopic foci can be activated by hypoxia, ischemia, hyperkalemia, hypocalcemia, increased catecholamine activity, digitalis toxicity, and administration of atropine.

Conduction Disturbances

Altered conduction probably accounts for more arrhythmias than changes in automaticity. Conduction can be too rapid or too slow. Conduction disturbances result from a delay or block of impulse formation or from what is referred to as the *re-entry phenomenon* (Fig. 33–1). Under normal circumstances, an electrical impulse moves down the conduction pathway until it reaches recently excited tissue that is refractory to stimulation. This causes the impulse to be extinguished. Re-entry is a phenomenon whereby an impulse continues to re-enter an area of the heart rather than becoming extinguished. For a re-entry phenomenon to occur an obstacle must be present within the normal conduction pathway. The obstacle permits electrical conduction in one direction only, thus causing a circuitous movement of the impulse. The obstacle is ordinarily an area of damage. The damage can be caused by electrolyte imbalance, impaired cellular metabolism, cardiac glycoside toxicity, ischemia, beta-blocking drugs, increased atrial preload, scarring of conduction pathways, compression of the AV node by scar tissue, AV nodal inflammation, excessive vagal stimulation of the heart, MI (particularly an inferior location), and valvular surgery.

Combined Disturbance

Combined automaticity and conduction disorders are observed when several arrhythmias are noted at a given time. For example, a combined disorder may be premature atrial contractions (PACs), a disturbance in automaticity, and first-degree AV block, a conduction disturbance.

TABLE 33–1 EXAMPLES OF ARRHYTHMIAS ACCORDING TO SITE OF ORIGIN AND MECHANISM

Automaticity Disturbances	Conduction Disturbances
Atrial Arrhythmias	
Sinus tachycardia	Premature atrial contraction
	Paroxysmal atrial tachycardia
	Atrial flutter
	Atrial fibrillation
AV Node Arrhythmias	
Premature junctional contractions	First-degree atrioventricular heart block
Junctional escape rhythm	Second-degree atrioventricular heart block
Premature junctional tachycardias	Mobitz Type I block (Wenckebach phenomenon)
	Mobitz Type II block
	Third-degree atrioventricular heart block
Ventricular Arrhythmias	
Premature ventricular contraction	Right bundle branch block
Ventricular tachycardia	Left bundle branch block
Ventricular fibrillation	Ventricular asystole
Torsades de pointes	

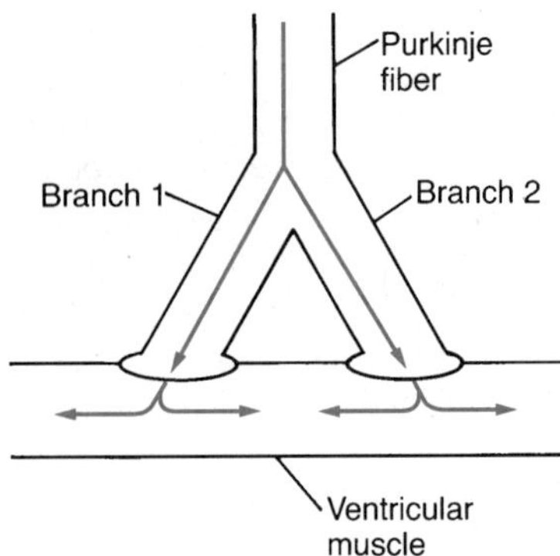

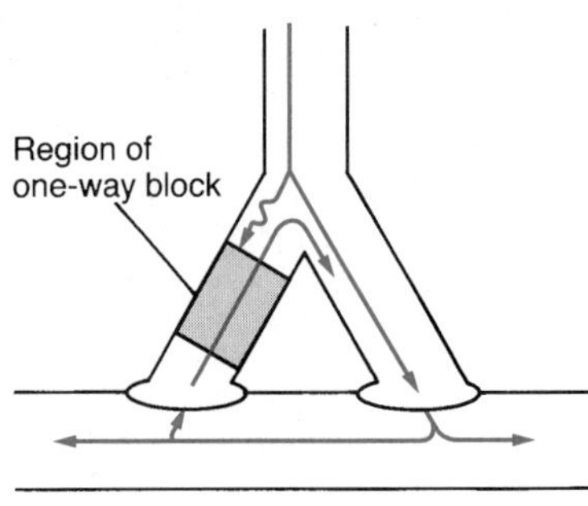

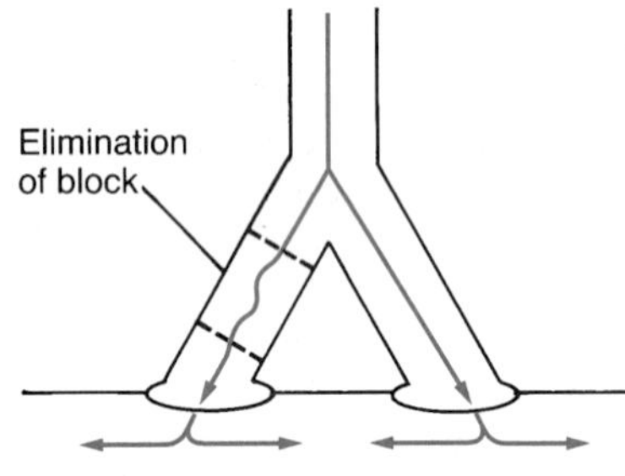

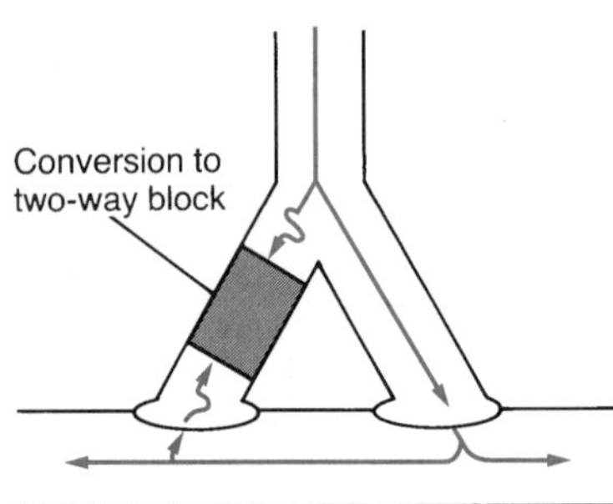

Figure 33–1 Re-entry phenomenon is the result of a barricade (e.g., myocardial muscle damage) located in the normal conduction pathway. The electrical impulse continues to re-enter an area of the heart rather than becoming extinguished. The damaged area permits conduction in only one direction, causing a circular movement of the impulse. (From Lehne, R. A. [1998]. *Pharmacology for nursing care* [3nd ed., p. 500]. Philadelphia: W. B. Saunders. Used with permission.)

Types of Arrhythmias

Most arrhythmias are classified according to site and mechanism (see Classifying an Arrhythmia). For example, sinus tachycardia is a common arrhythmia. The term *sinus* refers to the site, and *tachycardia* refers to the mechanism of the arrhythmia.

Atrial Arrhythmias

Atrial arrhythmias are viewed along a continuum of rate acceleration and a progressive reduction in atrial function: PAC, atrial tachycardia (a rate of approximately 150 bpm), atrial flutter (a rate of about 300 bpm), and atrial fibrillation (quivering, uncoordinated activity). To protect the ventricles from responding to extreme rates, the AV node does not conduct atrial impulses at rates exceeding 180 bpm.

PACs are recognized by the presence of premature P waves that differ in appearance, size, or shape. Atrial tachycardia is characterized by P waves that become lost in the preceding T wave. The PR and QRS intervals may be normal. Atrial flutter is identified by inverted or bidirectional P waves that produce a saw-tooth pattern. Only every second or third impulse is conducted in atrial flutter. Atrial fibrillation is characterized by erratic or no P waves, an irregular RR interval, and a baseline that appears to be irregular and undulating (Fig. 33–2). The hemodynamic response to atrial arrhythmias depends on ventricular rate and myocardial contractility.

Atrial arrhythmias are usually significant only in the presence of underlying heart disease. In CAD, atrial tachycardia increases myocardial oxygen consumption and shortens diastole. As a result, anginal pain may occur. With aortic valvular disease or hypertrophic myopathies, atrial flutter or atrial fibrillation decreases ventricular filling by as much as 30 percent; thus cardiac output is severely impaired. Atrial fibrillation and flutter may also lead to the formation of thrombi in the atria.

CLASSIFYING AN ARRHYTHMIA

- What is the site and the type (mechanism) of the arrhythmia?
- Is it atrial (supraventricular) or ventricular?
- Is it passive (due to escape) or active (due to enhanced automaticity)?
- Is impaired conduction the problem?

Nodal Arrhythmias

Nodal arrhythmias consist of tachycardia, with increased workload for the heart, or bradycardia from heart block. Heart block involves impaired conduction of the electrical impulse through the AV node. With first-degree heart block, conduction is impaired, but not significantly. The ECG reveals a regular P wave followed by a QRS complex. The PR interval is prolonged beyond normal. With second-degree heart block, every second, third, or fourth impulse is blocked and does not reach the ventricles (a 2:1, 3:1, or 4:1

block). Atrial and ventricular rates thus differ. Second-degree heart block may interfere with cardiac output or progress to third-degree block. Third-degree block is the most serious because no atrial impulses can pass the AV node to reach the ventricles. As a result, the ventricles beat independently of the atria at a rate of 30 to 40 bpm. The slow ventricular rate severely reduces cardiac output.

Ventricular Arrhythmias

Occasional premature ventricular contractions (PVCs) occur in everyone and are rarely significant. However, PVCs occurring after an acute MI, those that occur more than five times per minute, and those that are coupled, grouped, or multifocal or that occur during the resting phase of the cardiac cycle are considered life threatening. These arrhythmias may lead to ventricular tachycardia, ventricular flutter, or ventricular fibrillation. Ventricular tachycardia increases myocardial oxygen consumption and shortens diastole. Ventricular flutter or fibrillation results in ineffective myocardial contraction. As a result, there is little to no cardiac output. Death results unless effective cardiopulmonary resuscitation or defibrillation is instituted.

PHARMACOTHERAPEUTIC OPTIONS

There is no universal antiarrhythmic drug that is effective for all arrhythmias. In recent years, an increasing number of antiarrhythmic drugs have been classified based on their fundamental mechanism of action. Antiarrhythmic drugs discussed in this chapter include

- Class I drugs that block sodium channels
- Class II drugs that block beta-adrenergic receptors
- Class III drugs that usually block potassium channels
- Class IV drugs that block calcium channels

Table 33–2 provides a summary of antiarrhythmic drug classifications, their mechanisms of action, indications, and expected therapeutic ECG changes. Each group has a different mechanism of action that suppresses arrhythmias. The majority of antiarrhythmic drugs are used to treat tachyarrhythmias and as such are myocardial depressants.

The ideal antiarrhythmic drug would have five distinct characteristics: (1) the drug would have a high degree of efficacy for a well-defined group of arrhythmias; (2) cardiac and extracardiac adverse effects would be minimal, with no clinically significant drug interactions; (3) oral dosage forms would exhibit minimal first-pass effects and would be available as an IV formulation; (4) the drug would have a reasonable half-life, thereby permitting infrequent dosing and promoting patient compliance; and (5) the drug would have a positive correlation between efficacy and plasma concentration. To date, not one antiarrhythmic drug meets all of these criteria. These characteristics, however, can be used when surveying the advantages and disadvantages of the various drugs.

TABLE 33 2–SUMMARY OF ANTIARRHYTHMIC DRUG CLASSIFICATIONS*

Drug	Indications
Class I: Drugs with local anesthetic effects and membrane stabilizing properties. Tend to suppress automaticity by lowering the action potential needed to trigger spontaneous depolarization. Prolong effective refractory periods so that premature stimulation is less likely to occur	
Class I_A	Atrial flutter, atrial fibrillation (conversion or prophylaxis), premature atrial contractions, premature ventricular contractions, ventricular tachycardia
Disopyramide	
Procainamide	
Quinidine	
Class I_B	Ventricular arrhythmias only, including premature ventricular contractions, ventricular tachycardia, ventricular fibrillation
Lidocaine	
Mexiletine	
Phenytoin	
Tocainide	
Class I_C	Severe ventricular arrhythmias only
Flecainide	
Propafenone	
Other Class I	Life-threatening ventricular arrhythmias, including sustained ventricular tachycardia. (Shares properties of I_A, I_B, and I_C drugs)
Moricizine	
Class II: Antagonize catecholamine-induced electrophysiologic effects. Suppress automaticity and the rate of impulse conduction	
Acebutolol	Premature ventricular contractions
Esmolol	Atrial fibrillation, atrial flutter, sinus tachycardia
Propranolol	Sinus tachycardia, paroxysmal supraventricular tachycardia, atrial flutter, atrial fibrillation
Class III: Selectively prolong the action potential duration. Have little or no effect on spontaneous depolarization. No membrane stabilizing effects	
Amiodarone	Life-threatening ventricular tachycardia or ventricular fibrillation resistant to other drugs, supraventricular tachycardia
Sotalol	Ventricular tachycardia, ventricular fibrillation
Bretylium	
Class IV: Block the slow inward movement of calcium to slow impulse conduction; prolong refractory period, particularly of the AV node	
Diltiazem	Paroxysmal supraventricular tachycardia; atrial fibrillation or flutter
Verapamil	Paroxysmal supraventricular tachycardia

*Antiarrhythmic drugs are placed in classifications based on major electrophysiologic effects on the heart. Drugs in the same class or subclass share common effects, but otherwise are so different that a prototype cannot be identified.

Normal Sinus Rhythm

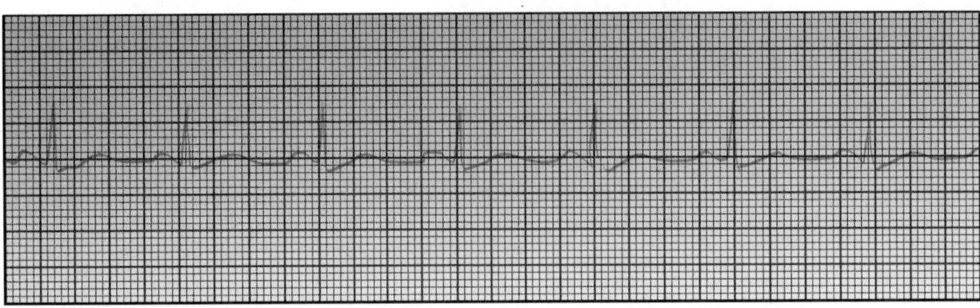

Atrial Flutter

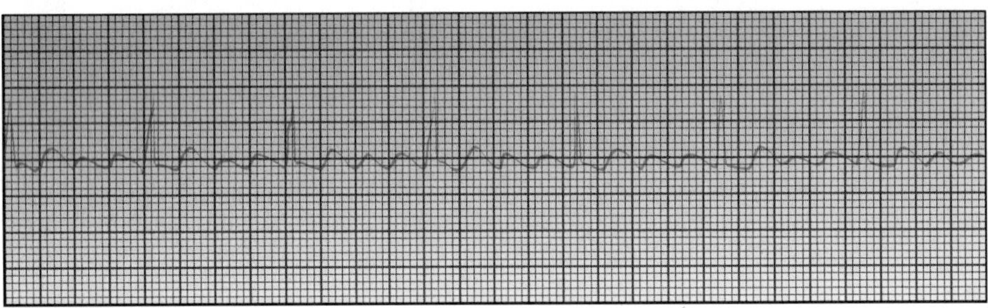

Ventricular Tachycardia

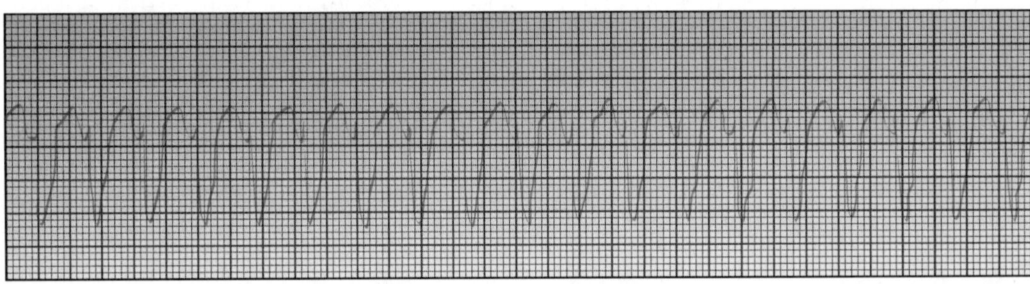

Torsades de Pointes

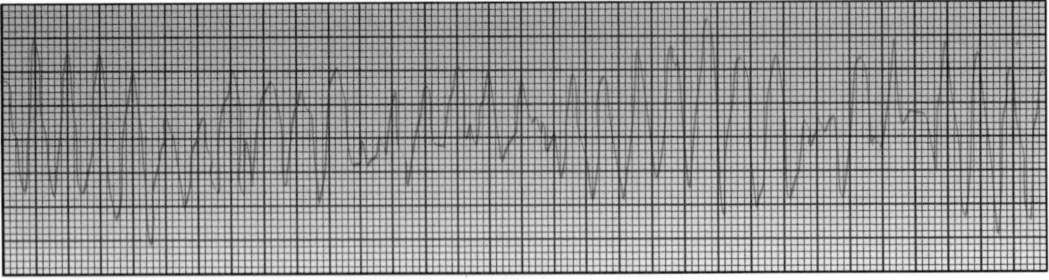

Figure 33–2 See legend on oppoite page

Class I Antiarrhythmics

Class I antiarrhythmics are similar in structure and action to local anesthetics. They are divided into subclasses based on the type of sodium channel blockade they produce. Three subclasses are further defined by the effects of the drugs on the Purkinje fiber action potential. Class I_A drugs slow the rate of rise of the action potential and prolong its duration, thus slowing conduction and increasing refractoriness. Class I_B drugs shorten the duration of the action potential. They do not affect conduction or refractoriness. Class I_C drugs prolong the rise of the action potential and slow repolarization, thus slowing conduction and prolonging refractoriness, but more so than Class I_A drugs.

Class I_A Antiarrhythmics

- ❒ Disopyramide (NORPACE, NORPACE CR); (♣) RHYTHMODAN, RHYTHMODAN LA
- ❒ Procainamide (PROCAN SR, PROMINE, PRONESTYL, PRONESTYL-SR)
- ❒ Quinidine gluconate (QUINAGLUTE, QUINALAN)
- ❒ Quinidine sulfate (QUINIDEX EXTENTABS, QUINORA); (♣) APO-QUINIDINE, NOVO-QUINIDIN

Indications

Class I_A antiarrhythmics have powerful direct effects on most types of myocardial cells. Although there is no one overall prototypical antiarrhythmic, quinidine is considered a prototype of sorts for Class I_A drugs. It is the most widely used Class I_A antiarrhythmic, and it is effective in the management of a wide variety of atrial and ventricular arrhythmias, including premature atrial contractions, premature ventricular contractions, ventricular tachycardia, and paroxysmal atrial tachycardia. Quinidine is also used as prophylaxis against atrial flutter and fibrillation.

With the advent of cardioversion, quinidine and procainamide are now used as prophylaxis in the management of atrial flutter and fibrillation. Of the patients scheduled for cardioversion who are medicated 1 to 2 days before the procedure, approximately one-third with atrial fibrillation and a similar number who have atrial flutter will convert to NSR before cardioversion. However, the majority of patients still require cardioversion. Maintenance therapy with quinidine or procainamide helps to prevent recurrence of the arrhythmia.

Disopyramide is also used for the suppression and prevention of unifocal and multifocal PVCs and ventricular tachycardia. It has also been used for the prevention and treatment of supraventricular tachyarrhythmias, although it has not been approved by the Food and Drug Administration for such use.

Pharmacodynamics

Class I_A drugs produce local anesthetic effects by virtue of their ability to block neuronal sodium channels. These drugs slow the rate of rise of the action potential in phase 0 depolarization and slow conduction velocity in Purkinje fibers. Class I_A drugs tend to suppress automaticity by lowering the pacemaker potential needed to provoke spontaneous depolarization. Refractory periods are prolonged, and premature electrical stimulation is less likely to occur. The shift in the threshold is due to blocking of fast sodium channels and slowing of the reactivation rate. Indirectly, quinidine also possesses strong anticholinergic properties. There is little effect on the heart rate, but the drugs exert a direct negative inotropic effect.

Responses to Class I_A antiarrhythmic drugs can include an increased pulse rate, a widening of the QRS complex, and prolongation of the PR and QT intervals. Effects on the QRS complex and the QT interval are caused by slowing conduction through the bundle of His, Purkinje fibers, and ventricular fibers. Prolongation of the PR interval is caused by slowing the conduction through the AV node.

Figure 33–2 Electrocardiographic (ECG) pattern. A normal ECG pattern of the sinus rhythm is recognized by impulse waves arbitrarily designated by the letters P, Q, R, S, and T. The P wave represents depolarization of atria, and is present and upright. P waves are all shaped alike. The PR interval is the time it takes for the impulse to spread from atria to ventricles—a duration greater than three but less than five small squares. The time interval is the same for all beats. The QRS complex reflects ventricular depolarization. All of the QRS complexes are shaped alike, with a duration of not more than 2½ small squares. Ventricular repolarization is represented by the T wave. The ST segment represents completion of ventricular depolarization. Electrical systole is represented by the QT interval. Note the regularly spaced R-R interval. The time and voltage lines found on ECG paper are explained as follows:

Horizontal Axis	Vertical Axis
One small box equals 0.04 second	One millimeter equals 0.1 mV.
Five small boxes equal 0.2 second	Five millimeters equal 0.5 mV.
Twenty-five small boxes equal 1 second	Ten millimeters equal 1 mV.
Each large block equals 0.2 second	

Rhythm is the distance between QRS complexes and should not vary by more than three small squares. The rate averages three to five large squares between QRS complexes or 60 to 100 bpm.

Atrial fibrillation can be recognized by an erratic or no P wave, an irregular R-R interval, and a baseline that appears to be irregular and undulating. Because of atrial disorganization, there is no atrial kick.

Ventricular tachycardia is recognized by a rapidly occurring series of premature ventricular contractions (three or more), with no normal beats in between. The P wave and PR interval are absent and QRS complex widened. Ventricular tachycardia can progress to fibrillation at any time.

Torsades de pointes is recognized by prolonged QT intervals and broad flat T waves in the preceding sinus rhythm; the QRS complex is wide and bizarre. This pattern may precede ventricular fibrillation and sudden death. (From Black, J. M., and Matassarin-Jacobs, E. [1997]. *Medical-surgical nursing: Clinical management for the continuity of care* [5th ed., pp. 1296, 1300, 1306, 1309]. Philadelphia: W. B. Saunders; and Phillips, R.E., and Feeney, M.K. [1990]. *The cardiac rhythms: A systematic approach to interpretation* [3rd ed., p. 393]. Philadelphia: W. B. Saunders. Used with permission.)

Adverse Effects and Contraindications

The most common adverse effects associated with quinidine include nausea, vomiting, diarrhea, and abdominal pain. Disopyramide predisposes the individual to constipation. Disopyramide and procainamide exert anticholinergic effects that cause dry mouth and eyes, blurred vision, and urinary hesitancy. Furthermore, procainamide is likely to cause urinary retention because of its potent antimuscarinic effects. Both quinidine and disopyramide are hepatotoxic.

Life-threatening adverse effects of quinidine include widened QRS complex, heart block, ventricular flutter, ventricular fibrillation, acute hemolytic anemia, agranulocytosis, respiratory depression, vascular collapse, and torsades de pointes (see Fig. 33–2). Torsades de pointes is an atypical rapid ventricular tachycardia with periodic waxing and waning of amplitude of the QRS complexes on the ECG. It is either self-limiting or progresses to ventricular fibrillation. Hyperkalemia enhances the effects of quinidine, whereas hypokalemia reduces the drug's effectiveness.

Cinchonism is a constellation of adverse effects characterized by tinnitus, hearing loss, headache, vertigo, dizziness, lightheadedness, disturbed vision, nausea, and vomiting. These adverse effects can occur after a single dose of quinidine. If the adverse effects are severe, diplopia, photophobia, and altered color perception may occur.

Quinidine is generally contraindicated in patients with hypersensitivity, conduction defects, and cardiac glycoside toxicity. It should be used cautiously in patients with heart failure or severe liver disease. Safe use in pregnancy or lactation or in children has not been established. The extended release formulations, in particular, should not be used in children.

The most common adverse effect of procainamide is a lupus-like syndrome. The syndrome is characterized by arthralgia, myalgia, skin rash, and the development of antinuclear antibodies (ANAs). It affects about 50 percent of patients receiving high dose therapy for a year or longer. Treatment is usually discontinued because of the possibility of pleural effusion and potentially lethal pericardial tamponade. In some cases, a corticosteroid drug is added to the treatment regimen to permit continued use of procainamide. Patients who are rapid acetylators are less likely to develop the syndrome. Procainamide can also cause myelosuppression and agranulocytosis.

Life-threatening adverse effects of procainamide include ventricular fibrillation, torsades de pointes, and agranulocytosis (with repeated use). Evidence of bone marrow dysfunction usually occurs during the first 3 months of therapy. Some health care providers consider the extended release formulation of procainamide to be particularly responsible for these problems.

Procainamide is contraindicated in patients with hypersensitivity, AV block, or myasthenia gravis and in patients who are sensitive to tartrazine (FDC yellow dye No. 5), which is present in some oral formulations. It should be used with caution in patients with MI or cardiac glycoside toxicity, heart failure, or renal or hepatic insufficiency. Cautious use is also warranted in older adults. Safe use during pregnancy or lactation or in children has not been established.

The most common adverse effects of disopyramide include anticholinergic effects such as dry mouth, blurred vision, constipation, and urinary hesitancy and retention. Life-threatening adverse effects include hypotension, heart block, torsades de pointes, cardiogenic shock, and respiratory distress (e.g., laryngospasm).

Disopyramide is contraindicated in patients with hypersensitivity, cardiogenic shock, second- and third-degree heart block, or sick sinus syndrome who do not have a pacemaker. It should be used with caution in patients with left ventricular dysfunction, decompensated heart failure, and hepatic or renal insufficiency. Cautious use is also warranted in older men with prostatic enlargement and in patients with glaucoma or myasthenia gravis. Safe use during pregnancy or lactation has not been established.

Pharmacokinetics

Table 33–3 provides an overview of the pharmacokinetics of antiarrhythmic drugs. There are three quinidine salts: quinidine sulfate, quinidine gluconate, and quinidine polygalacturonate. The active drug content is different for each formulation, as are the absorption and time to peak plasma levels.

Quinidine is rapidly absorbed when taken by mouth. Peak responses to quinidine sulfate occur in 1 to 3 hours. Peak antiarrhythmic effects of quinidine gluconate occur 3 to 4 hours after oral administration. Quinidine polygalacturonate peaks in 6 hours. Approximately 70 to 95 percent of the drug is bound to albumin, other plasma proteins, and hemoglobin. Quinidine is extensively biotransformed in the liver to several metabolites. Whether the metabolites possess antiarrhythmic activity remains controversial. In patients with hepatic insufficiency, the unbound fraction may be significantly increased. In patients with cirrhosis, the elimination half-life may be prolonged. The effect of renal dysfunction on disposition of quinidine also remains controversial. An alkaline urine retards drug elimination, whereas urinary acidification facilitates elimination of quinidine.

Seventy-five to 90 percent of procainamide is absorbed from the gastrointestinal (GI) tract. Plasma levels reach about 50 percent of peak in 30 minutes, 90 percent of peak antiarrhythmic effect in 60 minutes, and peak effects at 90 to 120 minutes. Food and extremes in gastric pH hasten or delay drug absorption. Procainamide is well distributed through all body tissues, with a plasma protein binding of 15 percent. Procainamide is extensively biotransformed in the liver by the enzyme *N*-acetyltransferase to *N*-acetylprocainamide (NAPA). Acetylation of procainamide occurs primarily as a first-pass effect after oral administration. The rate of biotransformation varies widely and is under genetic control. Patients who are rapid acetylators have higher plasma concentrations of the metabolite NAPA and eliminate greater quantities of NAPA in the urine than patients who are slow acetylators. Both procainamide and NAPA are eliminated via active tubular secretion as well as by glomerular filtration.

Disopyramide is also well absorbed from the GI tract with 90 percent bioavailability. Peak plasma concentrations are reached within about 2 hours of an oral dose. Sustained release formulations peak in about 4.9 hours. Disopyramide is bound to plasma proteins, but binding ranges from 35 to 90 percent, depending on plasma concentration. The hepatic biotransformation of disopyramide is not clear. About 50 percent is eliminated in the urine as unchanged drug and 30 percent as metabolites. The plasma half-life ranges from 4 to

TABLE 33-3 PHARMACOKINETICS OF SELECTED ANTIARRHYTHMIC DRUGS

Drug	Route	Onset	Peak	Duration	PB (%)	$t_{1/2}$	BioA (%)	Plasma Level
Class I_A Antiarrhythmics								
Quinidine sulfate	po	30 min	1–3 hr	6–8 hr	70–95	6–8 hr	70–73	2–7 mcg/mL.
Quinidine gluconate	po	UK	3–5 hr	6–8 hr	75–95	6–8 hr	70–73	Toxicity: 5–8 mcg/mL
Quinidine polygalacturonate	po	UK	6 hr	8–12 hr	65–95	6–8 hr	70–73	
Procainamide	po	30 min	30–120 min	3–4 hr	15–20	2.5–4.7 hr*	75–90	3–10 mcg/mL
Disopyramide	po/SR	0.5–3.5 hr	2.5–4.9 hr	1.5–12 hr	35–95	4–10 hr	90	2–4 mcg/mL
Class I_B Antiarrhythmics								
Lidocaine	IV	Immed	Immed	10–20 min	60–80†	7–30 min; 90–120 min‡	100	2–5 mcg/mL
	IM		15 min	90 min			35	
Mexiletine	po	30–120 min	2–3 hr	8–12 hr	50–70	10–12 hr	90	1–2 mcg/mL
Phenytoin	po	Slow	1.5–12 hr	UK	90	Dose dependent	90–93	10–20 mcg/mL
	IV	Immed	Immed			Dose dependent	90–93	10–20 mcg/mL
Tocainide	po	30–60 min	1–2 hr	8–12 hr	10	11–23 hr	100	3–10 mcg/mL
Class I_C Antiarrhythmics								
Flecainide	po	UK	2–3 hr	12 hr	32–47	11–14 hr	95	0.2–1 mcg/mL. Toxicity: >1.0 mcg/mL
Propafenone	po	Hours	4–5 days§	Hours	97	2–17 hr§	3–11	NA
Other Class I Antiarrhythmics								
Moricizine	po	UK	30–120 min	8–12 hr	95	1.5–3.5 hr	35	NA
Class II Antiarrhythmics								
Acebutolol	po	60 min	4–6 hr	10 hr	26	3–4 hr; 8–13 hr‖	<50	UK
Esmolol	IV	5 min	10–30 min	20–30 min	55	5–23 min	UK	NA
Propranolol	po	30 min	60–90 min	6–12 hr	93	3–5 hr	25	50–100 mcg/mL
Class III Antiarrhythmics								
Amiodarone	po	1–3 weeks	UK	Weeks to months	96	13–107 days¶	35–65	1–2.5 mcg/mL
	IV	2 hr	UK	UK			100	
Bretylium	IV (VF)	Minutes	End of infusion	6–24 hr	Neg	5–10 hr	100	0.5–1.5 mcg/mL
	IV (VT, PVCs)	20 min to 6 hr	6–9 hr					
Sotalol	po	UK	2–3 hr	UK	50	10–15 hr	100	UK
Class IV Antiarrhythmics								
Diltiazem	po/SR	30 min	2–3 hr	6–8 hr; 12 hr**	70–80	3.5–9 hr	UK	0.025–1 mcg/mL
	IV	2–5 min	UK	UK			100	
Verapamil	IV	1–5 min††	3–5 min	2 hr	90	4.5–12 hr	100	80–300 mcg/mL
	po/SR	1–2 hr	30–90 min‡‡	3–7 hr			UK	
Unclassified Antiarrhythmics								
Adenosine	IV	Immed	UK	1–2 min	UA	<10 sec	100	NA
Ibutilide	IV	Immed	UA	UA	UA	2–12 hr	100	NA

*Over 90% of patients taking procainamide are considered extensive metabolizers so half-life is 2–10 hr. In slow metabolizers the half-life is 10–32 hr.
†Protein binding of lidocaine depends on blood levels.
‡The half-life of lidocaine is biphasic, with the initial phase lasting 7–30 min and the terminal phase 90–120 min.
§Peak drug action with chronic dosing of propafenone. Plasma concentrations have limited usefulness because of variability between rapid (2–10 hr) and slow (10–32 hr) metabolizers.
‖Half-life of acebutolol and the metabolite, respectively.
¶The half-life of amiodarone is biphasic.
**Duration of drug action for rapid release and sustained release formulations of diltiazem.
††Onset of antiarrhythmic effects and hemodynamic effects of verapamil is 3–5 min following injection and persist for up to 20 min.
‡‡Peak concentration of a single dose of verapamil. Effects of multiple doses may not be evident for 24–48 hr.
BioA, Bioavailability; Neg., negligible; Immed., immediately; UA, unavailable; UK, unknown; VF, ventricular fibrillation; VT, ventricular tachycardia; PVCs, premature ventricular contractions; SR, sustained release formulation; PB, protein binding; $t_{1/2}$, elimination half-life.

10 hours, with a mean of 6.7 hours. A small percentage of the drug is eliminated in the feces.

Drug-Drug Interactions

Class I_A antiarrhythmic drugs exhibit additive or antagonistic effects with other antiarrhythmics as well as with anticholinergic drugs. When quinidine is used concurrently with digoxin, mechanisms occur by which serum digoxin concentration nearly doubles. Quinidine biotransformation is inhibited in the presence of cimetidine and induced by phenytoin, phenobarbital, and rifampin (Table 33–4).

Procainamide interacts with cimetidine and ranitidine to block its tubular secretion and increase the bioavailability. Procainamide also interacts with other antiarrhythmics, antihypertensives, nitrates, neuromuscular blockers, anticholinesterase, and anticholinergic drugs.

Disopyramide also has numerous drug-drug interactions. Phenytoin, rifampin, and phenobarbital induce biotransformation of disopyramide, thereby increasing its elimination and perhaps lowering its therapeutic effects. Procainamide and lidocaine used concurrently cause a widening of the QRS complex or QT prolongation. Concurrent use of procainamide and the antibiotic erythromycin can increase the risk of arrhythmias.

Drug-Food Interactions

Foods that alkalinize the urine may increase serum quinidine levels and increase the risk of toxicity. These foods include cheeses, fish, meats, poultry, cranberries, breads and cereals, plums, prunes, and eggs (see Appendix C).

Dosage Regimen

Quinidine formulations have different concentrations of active drug. For this reason they are not interchangeable without appropriate dosage adjustment. The sulfate salt contains 83 percent quinidine base. Quinidine gluconate and quinidine polygalacturonate contain 62 and 60 percent active drug, respectively.

Laboratory Considerations

Because of the narrow therapeutic index and toxicity potential of Class I_A antiarrhythmic drugs, serum blood levels should be closely monitored. Therapeutic serum levels of these drugs are identified in Table 33–3. Quinidine increases creatine kinase values. Serum potassium levels should be monitored, particularly if the patient has received a cardiac glycoside in conjunction with quinidine treatment.

Disopyramide can cause increased values in aspartate aminotransferase (AST; serum glutamic-oxaloacetic transaminase [SGOT]), alanine aminotransferase (ALT; serum glutamic-pyruvic transaminase [SGPT]), bilirubin, lipids, blood urea nitrogen (BUN), and creatinine. Blood glucose values may be decreased in the presence of disopyramide.

Procainamide causes increased liver function tests and alkaline phosphatase values and a positive Coombs' test. A complete blood count (CBC) should be monitored every 2 weeks during the first 3 months of therapy. Neutropenia, leukopenia, and thrombocytopenia rarely occur; however, therapy should be discontinued if leukopenia occurs. ANAs should be periodically monitored during prolonged therapy or if symptoms of lupus-like reactions occur. Procainamide therapy is discontinued if a steady increase in ANA titers occurs.

Class I_B Antiarrhythmics

- ❒ Lidocaine (ANESTACON, BAYLOCAINE, LIDOPEN, XYLOCAINE); (✱) ZYLOGARD
- ❒ Mexiletine (MEXITIL)
- ❒ Phenytoin (diphenylhydantoin, DPH, DILANTIN, DIPHENYLAN)
- ❒ Tocainide (TONOCARD)

Indications

Although there are fewer indications for Class I_B drugs, they are more effective in treating acute ventricular arrhythmias and cause fewer adverse reactions. Class I_B drugs are most effective when used in the treatment or palliation of both acute and chronic arrhythmias, including PVCs and ventricular tachycardia. They are generally ineffective in treatment of atrial arrhythmias.

Lidocaine is the drug of choice for treating serious ventricular arrhythmias associated with acute MI, cardiac surgery, cardiac catheterization, cardioversion, and cardiac glycoside toxicity. There is no evidence of a teratogenic potential with lidocaine, so it can be safely administered in pregnancy as the drug of choice for acute ventricular tachycardias.

Mexiletine and tocainide are oral analogs of lidocaine. They are used to suppress ventricular arrhythmias, including frequent PVCs and ventricular tachycardia. Phenytoin is commonly used for arrhythmias associated with cardiac glycoside toxicity, although it has not been approved by the Food and Drug Administration for this use.

Pharmacodynamics

Lidocaine decreases depolarization, automaticity, and excitability of the ventricles during diastole. It has little effect on atrial tissues and therefore is of little use for atrial arrhythmias.

Mexiletine and tocainide shorten the duration of action potential and decrease the effective refractory period (ERP) in the bundle of His and Purkinje fibers. These effects are mediated by blocking sodium transport across myocardial cell membranes.

Phenytoin decreases abnormal ventricular automaticity to shorten the refractory period, QT interval, and duration of action potential. Automaticity is decreased, and conduction through the AV node is improved. With the exception of phenytoin, class I_B drugs exert no significant action on the autonomic nervous system. Most of the effects of phenytoin arise from actions within the central nervous system (CNS). Vagal nerve activity is tempered, and the outgoing traffic from the myocardium is reduced.

Adverse Effects and Contraindications

Class I_B antiarrhythmics have fewer adverse cardiac effects than do those in Class I_A. The most common adverse effects of lidocaine include drowsiness, confusion, and stinging at the administration site. Although serious adverse

Text continued on page 706

TABLE 33–4 DRUG-DRUG INTERACTIONS OF SELECTED ANTIARRHYTHMIC DRUGS

Drug	Interactive Drug	Interaction
Class I_A Antiarrhythmics		
Quinidine	Amiodarone	Increased blood levels of quinidine and risk of toxicity
	Alcohol	Additive hypotension
	Antihypertensives	
	Nitrates	
	Digoxin	Increased blood levels of interactive drug and risk of toxicity
	Procainamide	
	Propafenone	
	Tricyclic antidepressants	
	Cimetidine	Increased risk of quinidine intoxication
	High dose antacids	
	Potassium-wasting diuretics	
	Reserpine	
	Sodium bicarbonate	
	Verapamil	
	Phenobarbital	Quinidine biotransformation enhanced leading to subtherapeutic levels
	Phenytoin	
	Rifampin	
	Verapamil	Significant hypotension in patients with obstructive cardiomyopathy
	Neuromuscular blockers	Increased risk of thrombocytopenia, bleeding
	Warfarin	
	Lidocaine	Possible increased CNS stimulation
Disopyramide	Anticholinergics	Increased intensity of atropine-like side effects
	Antiarrhythmics	Additive cardiac toxicity effects
	Verapamil	
	Erythromycin	Increased disopyramide levels and risk of arrhythmias
	Phenytoin	Decreased blood levels of disopyramide
	Phenobarbital	
	Rifampin	
	Quinidine	Increased risk of disopyramide toxicity when high doses of disopyramide are used
	Warfarin	Increased anticoagulant effect of warfarin
	Cimetidine	Increased blood levels of disopyramide
Procainamide	Antiarrhythmics	Additive or antagonistic effects
	Lidocaine	Additive neurologic toxicity
	Antihypertensives	Additive hypotensive effects
	Nitrates	
	Neuromuscular blockers	Potentiated effects of interactive drug
	Anticholinesterase drugs	Antagonized effects of interactive drug
	Antihistamines	Additive anticholinergic effects
	Antidepressants	
	Atropine	
	Haloperidol	
	Phenothiazines	
	Cimetidine	Increased effects of procainamide
	Quinidine	
	Ranitidine	
	Trimethoprim	
Flecainide Procainamide	Alcohol	Increased or decreased response to antiarrhythmic agents depends on whether alcohol consumption is acute or long-standing
	Amiodarone	Increased blood levels of amiodarone
	Cimetidine	Cimetidine increases blood level and half-life of procainamide due to decreased metabolism of antiarrhythmic
Class I_B Antiarrhythmics		
Lidocaine	Beta blockers	May decrease biotransformation of lidocaine and increase risk of toxicity
	Cimetidine	
	Phenobarbital	
	Phenytoin	Additive cardiac depression and toxicity
	Procainamide	
	Propranolol	
	Quinidine	
Mexiletine	Antacids	May slow absorption of mexiletine
	Atropine	
	Opioids	
	Metoclopramide	May speed absorption of mexiletine
	Phenytoin	May increase biotransformation and decrease effectiveness of mexiletine
	Phenobarbital	
	Rifampin	
	Smoking	
	Cimetidine	May slow biotransformation and increase risk of toxicity
	Antiarrhythmics	Additive cardiac effects

Table continued on following page

TABLE 33–4 DRUG-DRUG INTERACTIONS OF SELECTED ANTIARRHYTHMIC DRUGS *Continued*

Drug	Interactive Drug	Interaction
Class I_B Antiarrhythmics *Continued*		
	Alkalinizing drugs	Increased reabsorption and blood levels
	Acidifying drugs	Increased excretion and decreased blood levels
Tocainide	Antiarrhythmics	Additive cardiac effects
	Beta blockers	May precipitate heart failure
	Cimetidine	May decrease blood levels of tocainide
	Rifampin	
Phenytoin	Barbiturates	May stimulate biotransformation and decrease effectiveness of interactive drugs
	Chronic alcohol abuse	
	Warfarin	
	Cyclosporin	May stimulate phenytoin biotransformation and decrease blood levels
	Digitoxin	
	Methadone	
	Oral contraceptives	
	Streptozocin	
	Theophylline	
	Benzodiazepines	May decrease phenytoin biotransformation and increase blood levels
	Chloramphenicol	
	Cimetidine	
	Disulfiram	
	Felbamate	
	Fluconazole	
	Influenza vaccine	
	Isoniazid	
	Ketoconazole	
	Metronidazole	
	Miconazole	
	Omeprazole	
	Succinamides	
	Sulfonamides	
	Alcohol	Additive CNS depression
	Antihistamines	
	Opioids	
	Sedative-hypnotics	
	Warfarin	May alter the effectiveness of interactive drug
	Antacids	May decrease absorption of orally administered phenytoin
	Carbamazepine	May increase or decrease phenytoin plasma levels
	Valproic acid	
	Felbamate	Decreased blood level of interactive drug
Class I_C Antiarrhythmics		
Flecainide	Antiarrhythmics	Increased risk of arrhythmias
	Calcium channel blockers	
	Beta blockers	Additive myocardial depressant effects
	Disopyramide	
	Verapamil	
	Amiodarone	Doubled serum flecainide levels
	Digoxin	Increased serum digoxin levels by 15–25%
	Beta blockers	Increased levels of both flecainide and beta blocker
	Acidifying drugs	Increased renal elimination and decreased effectiveness of flecainide
	Alkalinizing drugs	Promote reabsorption and increase risk of toxicity
Propafenone	Digoxin	Increased serum digoxin levels by 35–85%
	Metoprolol	Increased blood levels of interactive drugs
	Propranolol	
	Quinidine	Inhibits biotransformation of propafenone
	Local anesthetics	May increase risk of CNS adverse effects
	Warfarin	May increase risk of bleeding
	Cyclosporin	May increase blood levels and risk of nephrotoxicity
	Rifampin	May decrease serum drug levels and effectiveness of propafenone
Other Class I Antiarrhythmics		
Moricizine	Theophylline	Decreased concentrations of interactive drug
	Cimetidine	Decreased clearance and increased blood levels of moricizine
	Digoxin	
	Propranolol	
Class II Antiarrhythmics		
Acebutolol	Antihypertensives	Increased hypotension
Esmolol	Diuretics	
	Phenothiazines	
	Sympathomimetics	Inhibit effects of acebutolol

TABLE 33–4 DRUG-DRUG INTERACTIONS OF SELECTED ANTIARRHYTHMIC DRUGS *Continued*

Drug	Interactive Drug	Interaction
Class II Antiarrhythmics *Continued*		
	Xanthines	
	Insulin	Prolonged effects of interactive drug
	Neuromuscular blockers	
	Oral hypoglycemics	
	NSAIDs	Decreased antihypertensive effect of acebutolol
	Cimetidine	May increase plasma concentration of acebutolol
Esmolol	MAO inhibitors	May cause significant hypertension
	Digoxin	Increased serum digoxin levels
	Morphine	Increased serum level of esmolol
Propranolol	General anesthesia	May cause additive myocardial depression
	IV phenytoin	
	Verapamil	
	Cardiac glycosides	Additive bradycardia
	Alcohol	Additive hypotension
	Antihypertensives	
	Nitrates	
	Amphetamines	May result in unopposed alpha-adrenergic stimulation leading to excessive hypertension and bradycardia
	Cocaine	
	Ephedrine	
	Epinephrine	
	Norepinephrine	
	Phenylephrine	
	Pseudoephedrine	
	Thyroid hormones	Decreased effectiveness of propranolol
	Beta-adrenergic bronchodilators	Altered effectiveness of interactive drugs
	Insulin	
	Oral hypoglycemics	
	Theophylline	
	Dopamine	Decreased beneficial $beta_1$ cardiovascular effects of interactive drugs
	Dobutamine	
	Anticholinergics	May increase risk of hypertension
	MAO inhibitors	
	Cimetidine	Increased risk of toxicity to propranolol
	Anticholinergics	
	NSAIDs	May decrease antihypertensive action
Class III Antiarrhythmics		
Amiodarone	Cyclosporine	Increased blood levels of interactive drug and risk of toxicity
	Digoxin	
	Flecainide	
	Lidocaine	
	Mexiletine	
	Phenytoin	
	Procainamide	
	Quinidine	
	Warfarin	
	Cimetidine	Increased amiodarone levels
	Cholestyramine	Decreased amiodarone blood levels
	Phenytoin	
	Beta blockers	Increased risk of bradyarrhythmias, sinus, arrest, or AV block
	Calcium channel blockers	
Bretylium	Antidepressants	Initial cardiac stimulation; pressor response is reduced
	Dopamine	Enhanced action of interactive drugs
	Norepinephrine	
	Antiarrhythmics	Additive or antagonistic effects to bretylium
	Antihypertensives	Increased risk of hypotension
	Cardiac glycosides	Possible increased severity of glycoside-induced arrhythmias
Sotalol	Antiarrhythmics	May increase prolonged QT interval
	Astemizole	
	Phenothiazines	
	Tricyclic antidepressants	
	Terfenadine	
	Digoxin	May increase proarrhythmic effects
	Calcium channel blockers	May increase effect on AV conduction and blood pressure
	Insulin	May mask signs and symptoms of hypoglycemia, prolong effects of interactive drugs
	Oral hypoglycemics	
	Sympathomimetics	May inhibit effects of interactive drug
	Clonidine	May potentiate rebound hypertension after discontinuance of clonidine

Table continued on following page

TABLE 33–4 DRUG-DRUG INTERACTIONS OF SELECTED ANTIARRHYTHMIC DRUGS *Continued*

Drug	Interactive Drug	Interaction
Class IV Antiarrhythmics		
Diltiazem	Alcohol	Additive hypotension when used concurrently
	Antihypertensives	
	Fentanyl	
	Nitrates	
	Quinidine	
	NSAIDs	Decreased antihypertensive effects
	Digoxin	Increased serum levels of interactive drug
	Beta blockers	May result in bradycardia, conduction defects, or heart failure
	Digoxin	
	Disopyramide	
	Phenytoin	
	Phenobarbital	May increase biotransformation and decrease effectiveness of diltiazem
	Phenytoin	
	Cimetidine	May decrease biotransformation and increase risk of toxicity to diltiazem
	Propranolol	
	Carbamazepine	May decrease the biotransformation of and increase the risk of toxicity to interactive drug
	Cyclosporin	
	Prazosin	
	Quinidine	
Verapamil	Rifampin	May decrease effectiveness of interactive drug
	Nondepolarizing neuromuscular blockers	Increased muscle-paralyzing effects of interactive drug
	Calcium	Decreased effectiveness of verapamil with concurrent use
	Vitamin D	
	Lithium	Altered serum levels of interactive drug
Unclassified Antiarrhythmics		
Adenosine	Methylxanthines	May decrease effect of adenosine
	Dipyridamole	May increase effect of adenosine
	Carbamazepine	May increase degree of heart block caused by adenosine
Ibutilide	Amiodarone	Additive antiarrhythmic action
	Bretylium	
	Disopyramide	
	Moricizine	
	Procainamide	
	Quinidine	
	Sotalol	
	Histamine-1 receptor antagonists	May prolong QT interval
	Phenothiazines	
	Tetracyclic antidepressants	
	Tricyclic antidepressants	

MAO, Monoamine oxidase; NSAIDs, nonsteroidal anti-inflammatory drugs.

effects of lidocaine are uncommon, high dosages can produce cardiovascular depression (i.e., bradycardia, somnolence, hypotension, arrhythmias, heart block, cardiovascular collapse, cardiac arrest).

Lidocaine is contraindicated in patients with hypersensitivity or advanced AV block. It should be used cautiously in patients with liver disease or heart failure, those weighing less than 50 kg, and those who are older adults. Respiratory depression, shock, and heart block also require cautious use. Safe use during pregnancy and lactation has not been established.

The most common adverse effects of mexiletine include dizziness, nervousness, tremor, heartburn, nausea, and vomiting. Arrhythmias, palpitations, chest pain, blood dyscrasias, headache, changes in sleep habits, fatigue, confusion, and edema have been noted. The most serious adverse effect is hepatic necrosis.

Mexiletine is contraindicated in patients with hypersensitivity, cardiogenic shock, or second- or third-degree heart block (if a pacemaker has not been inserted) and during lactation. It should be used with caution in patients with sinus node or intraventricular conduction abnormalities, hypotension, heart failure, or severe hepatic involvement. Safe use during pregnancy and in children has not been established.

There are numerous common adverse effects of tocainide, including lightheadedness, vertigo tremor, headache, hallucinations, mood changes, restlessness, sedation, and blurred vision. Hypotension, tachycardia or bradycardia, palpitations, heart failure, arrhythmias, anorexia, nausea, vomiting, and diarrhea are also noted. The most serious adverse effects of tocainide include seizures, pulmonary fibrosis, and agranulocytosis.

Tocainide is contraindicated in patients with hypersensitivity or advanced heart block. It should be used with caution in patients with heart failure and hepatic or renal impairment. As with the other drugs in this class, cautious use is warranted in patients with heart disease and hepatic or renal dysfunction. Safe use during pregnancy or lactation and in children has not been established.

The most common adverse effects of phenytoin include nystagmus, ataxia, diplopia, gingival hyperplasia, nausea, hypotension, hypertrichosis, and skin rashes. Life-threatening adverse effects include aplastic anemia, agranulocytosis, and Stevens-Johnson syndrome.

Phenytoin is contraindicated in patients with hypersensitivity to the drug or to propylene glycol (injection only), alcohol intolerance (injection and liquid only), sinus bradycardia, and heart block. There are a number of patients in whom phenytoin should be used with caution, including those with severe liver, severe cardiac, or respiratory disease, older adults, obese patients, and pregnant patients. Fetal hydantoin syndrome may result if used chronically, and hemorrhage in the newborn may occur if the drug is used at term. Safe use during lactation has not been established.

Pharmacokinetics

Lidocaine is well absorbed from the GI tract; however, it is subject to extensive first-pass effect. Only about one-third of the drug reaches the general circulation. Systemically, it is widely distributed throughout the body to concentrate in adipose tissue. It crosses the blood-brain barrier and placental membranes. Lidocaine is variably bound to plasma proteins depending on blood level of the drug. Lidocaine biotransformation takes place in the liver. The clearance of lidocaine approximates the rate of hepatic blood flow and is thus sensitive to changes in blood flow. It is important to note that lidocaine has a pronounced redistribution phase as well as a metabolic phase. This is why the effects of a bolus dose of lidocaine are short lived. Prolonged infusions of lidocaine reduce drug clearance.

Mexiletine is readily absorbed after oral administration and is approximately 90 percent bioavailable. Peak blood levels are reached in 2 to 3 hours. Mexiletine is 50 to 70 percent protein bound with a relatively low first-pass effect. Urinary acidification accelerates elimination, whereas alkalinization retards elimination of the drug.

Tocainide is completely absorbed after oral administration, with peak plasma concentrations occurring within 1 to 2 hours. It is 50 percent bound to plasma proteins with a duration of action of 8 to 12 hours. The half-life of tocainide in plasma is 11 to 23 hours, but this value may be increased twofold in patients with renal or hepatic disease. Tocainide undergoes little first-pass effect, with oxidative deamination converting tocainide to inactive metabolites. Severe liver disease or reduced hepatic perfusion decreases the rate of biotransformation. About 40 percent of tocainide is excreted unchanged in the urine.

Phenytoin is slowly absorbed from the GI tract and erratically and unreliably absorbed when given IM. The bioavailability differs among the formulations. About 90 percent is bound to plasma proteins, with less binding found in patients with uremia. Distribution takes place quickly, with biotransformation taking place through hepatic hydroxylation. The enzyme system responsible for phenytoin biotransformation becomes saturated at therapeutic concentrations of the drug; hence, the half-life of phenytoin is dose dependent. Unexpected toxicity may occur in some patients.

Drug-Drug Interactions

Class I_B drugs can exhibit additive or antagonistic effects when administered with other antiarrhythmic drugs. Few drug interactions have been reported with lidocaine. Basic drugs displace lidocaine from its binding sites. Plasma concentrations are higher in patients who are concurrently receiving cimetidine or propranolol (see Table 33–3).

Biotransformation of mexiletine can be increased with concurrent administration of phenytoin or rifampin. Drugs that drastically alter urinary pH may affect blood levels of mexiletine. Alkalinization increases the reabsorption and blood levels of mexiletine. Acidification increases drug elimination and decreases effectiveness.

Additive cardiac effects occur with concurrent use of tocainide and other antiarrhythmics. Concurrent use of beta blockers may precipitate heart failure in susceptible patients. Cimetidine and rifampin may decrease blood levels of tocainide. Numerous drug-drug interactions occur with phenytoin and are too numerous to discuss here.

Drug-Food Interactions

Phenytoin decreases the absorption of folic acid. Foods that alter urinary pH may affect the serum levels of mexiletine. Concurrent administration of enteral tube feedings may decrease the absorption of phenytoin.

Dosage Regimen

Information on dosage and administration of Class I_B antiarrhythmic drugs is found in Table 33–5. Lidocaine is available in concentrations ranging from 20 to 200 mg/mL. A single IV dose of lidocaine can terminate ventricular arrhythmias. The usual adult dose is 50 to 100 mg (approximately 1 mg/kg), injected at a rate of 25 to 50 mg/min. This dose produces effective antiarrhythmic blood levels of about 2 to 5 mcg/mL. If necessary, the dose can be repeated in 3 to 5 minutes. Once sinus rhythm has stabilized, an IV infusion of 1 to 4 mg/min is started. Higher doses or faster administration can cause excessive myocardial depression and CNS stimulation. If IV administration of lidocaine is impossible, IM injections can be used, but it may take about 15 minutes to reach effective blood levels. The IM dosage can be repeated at 60- to 90-minute intervals, if necessary.

An oral loading dose of 400 mg of mexiletine is usually given initially, followed by 200 mg 8 hours later, then 200 to 400 mg every 8 hours. If the patient's arrhythmia is controlled on less than 300 mg every 8 hours, the same daily dose can be administered at 12-hour intervals. Some patients may require dosing every 6 hours. Reduced dosage may be required for individuals with hepatic impairment.

Because it has chemical and therapeutically similar effects, tocainide has often been referred to as an oral lidocaine. For the treatment of life-threatening ventricular tachycardia and PVCs, an initial oral loading dose of 400 mg is recommended, followed by 400 mg every 8 hours. Maintenance therapy ranges from 1200 to 1800 mg daily in divided doses. The daily maintenance dosage should be reduced to less than 1200 mg in individuals with renal or hepatic impairment. A dosage protocol for children has not been established.

The usual dose of phenytoin for adult patients with arrhythmia is 50 to 100 mg IV every 10 to 15 minutes until the arrhythmia is abolished or 15 mg/kg has been given. Administration of an IV bolus of phenytoin should not exceed 50 mg/min. The administration rate may be as low as 5 to 10 mg/min in patients who develop hypotension, are on sympathomimetic drugs, have cardiovascular disease, or are older adults. The IV formulation of phenytoin has a pH of approximately 12 and can cause severe phlebitis. Life-threatening arrhythmias should not be treated with IM phenytoin because absorption is too sporadic.

Laboratory Considerations

In view of the potential for toxicity, serum blood levels of antiarrhythmic drugs should be closely monitored. Therapeutic serum lidocaine levels range from 2 to 5 mcg/mL. Drug levels should be monitored periodically throughout prolonged or high dose therapy. Lidocaine has been shown to increase creatine phosphokinase values.

Serum mexiletine concentrations should be monitored during dosage adjustment. The incidence of adverse effects is greater with concentrations of mexiletine above 2 mcg/mL. Mexiletine may occasionally cause positive ANA test results as well as a transient increase in AST (SGOT) concentrations. A thrombocytopenia may occur a few days after initiation of therapy. Blood counts return to normal about 1 month after discontinuation of therapy.

CBC, white blood cell count with differential, and platelet counts should be monitored weekly during the first 3 months of tocainide therapy. Blood counts should be performed promptly if the patient develops signs of infection (i.e., fever, chills, sore throat, stomatitis), bleeding, or bruising. Leukopenia, agranulocytosis, and thrombocytopenia usually occur after 2 to 12 weeks. These values usually return to normal about 1 month after therapy is discontinued.

Phenytoin may cause increased serum alkaline phosphatase and glucose levels. CBC and platelets, serum calcium, urinalysis, and hepatic and thyroid testing should be done prior to therapy. Serum folate levels should be monitored. Glucose, alkaline phosphatase, and bromosulfophthalein laboratory values are elevated with phenytoin, with decreased values for the dexamethasone suppression test, metyrapone (cortisol), protein-bound iodine, and urinary steroids. Serum phenytoin levels should be routinely monitored. Therapeutic blood levels are 10 to 20 mcg/mL.

Class I_C Antiarrhythmics

❒ Flecainide (TAMBOCOR)
❒ Propafenone (RHYTHMIN)

Indications

Class I_C drugs are used in managing severe refractory ventricular arrhythmias, including ventricular tachycardia, paroxysmal supraventricular tachycardia, paroxysmal atrial flutter, and paroxysmal atrial fibrillation. Class I_C drugs should be reserved for hospitalized patients with malignant ventricular arrhythmias, symptomatic heart failure, sinus node dysfunction, or heart block.

Pharmacodynamics

Class I_C drugs primarily block the inward movement of sodium through the fast sodium channel of the myocardial membrane. Spontaneous depolarization is thus decreased. Unlike Class I_A drugs, Class I_C drugs do not produce a significant change in the ERP or in the action potential duration.

Flecainide produces a dose-related decrease in intracardiac conduction and has minor effects on the ERP, repolarization, or action potential duration. Its effect on intra-atrial and AV conduction is less pronounced than its effect on intraventricular conduction. Although flecainide has little effect on normal SA or AV nodes or atrial cells, it depresses conduction and function of dysfunctional cells. Flecainide also increases the endocardial pacing threshold and exerts negative inotropic effects. It does not interfere with autonomic nervous system control of the heart. Flecainide is similar to procainamide except that it lacks the lupus-like syndrome seen frequently with procainamide.

Propafenone has weak beta-blocking actions. Like flecainide, propafenone prolongs intracardiac conduction, produces minor effects on the ability of the heart to be restimulated, and has little effect on normal SA node function. It may, however, overpower SA node function in patients with a diseased node. It also lengthens AV nodal functioning and the ERP. Furthermore, propafenone modifies pacing and sensing thresholds of artificial pacemakers.

Adverse Effects and Contraindications

Class I_C drugs produce similar adverse cardiac effects. Proarrhythmic effects occur in about 8 to 15 percent of patients with malignant ventricular arrhythmias. The most common adverse effects of flecainide include dizziness, nervousness, headache, fatigue, tremor, blurred vision, and nausea. Flecainide increases the pacing threshold so that pacemaker-dependent patients may need their pacemakers reprogrammed. New or worsening heart failure occurs in a small but significant percentage of patients receiving flecainide. Thrombocytopenia and exfoliative dermatitis can occur. The life-threatening adverse effects of flecainide include arrhythmias, heart failure, palpitations, chest pain, edema, and ECG changes. SA node dysfunction and second- or third-degree AV heart block can occur. Unlike class I_A drugs, flecainide less commonly causes GI or urinary tract distress.

Flecainide is contraindicated in patients with hypersensitivity or cardiogenic shock. It should be used with caution in patients with heart failure, pre-existing sinus node dysfunction, second- or third-degree heart block (without a pacemaker), and renal impairment. Safe use during pregnancy and lactation or in children has not been established.

The most common adverse effects of propafenone include a metallic taste in the mouth, GI distress (i.e., constipation, nausea, vomiting), dizziness, fatigue, and conduction abnormalities. Exacerbation of heart failure and proarrhythmic effects (e.g., supraventricular arrhythmias) is possible. Agranulocytosis is rare but has occurred.

Pharmacokinetics

Flecainide is almost completely absorbed after oral administration. Peak plasma concentrations occur in about 3 hours. Absorption is prolonged in the presence of food but its bioavailability is not altered. Flecainide is moderately bound to plasma proteins. It is biotransformed in the liver with the metabolites exerting little or no antiarrhythmic activity. The half-life ranges from 12 to 30 hours. Flecainide is eliminated unchanged by the kidneys; however, the drug can accumulate in patients with renal failure.

Although propafenone is almost completely absorbed from the GI tract, the bioavailability is reduced because of an extensive first-pass effect. Peak concentrations in plasma occur in about 4 to 5 days with chronic dosing. Propafenone undergoes extensive oxidative biotransformation with 11 metabolites produced. Two of the 11 metabolites have known antiarrhythmic properties. Because of the variability between rapid metabolizers (2 to 10 hours) and slow metabolizers (10 to 32 hours), plasma concentration measurements have limited usefulness in adjusting dosage. Overall, the pharmacokinetic properties of propafenone are dose dependent. For example, an increase in dosage from 300 to 900 mg/day may result in as much as a 10-fold increase in plasma concentrations.

Drug-Drug Interactions

Evidence suggests that cimetidine, digoxin, and propranolol all have the potential to cause clinically important drug interactions with flecainide and propafenone. Cimetidine increases blood levels due to the decreased biotransformation of flecainide. Propafenone modestly increases serum digoxin levels. It should be used cautiously with propranolol, metoprolol, and warfarin because the levels of these drugs may rise. Propafenone may have additive beta-blocking effects, so it is contraindicated for individuals with bronchospastic disorders. Quinidine can inhibit the biotransformation of propafenone.

Drug-Food Interactions

Patients on a strict vegetarian diet consume foods that increase the urinary pH to over 7. The rise in pH causes increased flecainide blood levels. Conversely, foods or beverages that decrease the urinary pH to less than 5 increase renal elimination of flecainide and may decrease its effectiveness. Foods altering urinary pH are identified in Appendix C.

Dosage Regimen

The dosages of Class I_C drugs vary. To reduce the incidence of adverse effects, initial dosing with flecainide should be low, for example, 100 mg orally twice daily for 4 days. The dosage may then be increased every 4 days in increments of 100 mg/day up to a maximum of 400 to 600 mg in divided doses. Previous antiarrhythmic therapy (except lidocaine) should be withdrawn two to four half-lives before starting flecainide.

The usual oral adult dose of propafenone is 150 mg every 8 hours. The dosage may be gradually increased at 3- to 4-day intervals as required up to 300 mg every 8 to 12 hours. Pre-existing hypokalemia or hyperkalemia should be corrected before instituting propafenone therapy. Table 33–5 provides a summary of dosages for Class I antiarrhythmic drugs.

Laboratory Considerations

The therapeutic serum level for flecainide is 0.2 to 1.0 mcg/mL. The probability of toxicity exists with serum levels exceeding 1.0 mcg/mL. Creatine phosphate levels are elevated in the presence of flecainide or propafenone. Renal, pulmonary, and hepatic functions and CBC should be evaluated periodically for patients on long-term therapy. It should be noted also that flecainide may cause elevations in serum alkaline phosphatase during prolonged therapy. Propafenone may cause elevated ANA titers that are usually asymptomatic and reversible.

Other Class I Antiarrhythmics

Moricizine (ETHMOZINE) is a Class I antiarrhythmic that shares many of the properties of other Class I drugs, but it does not cleanly fit into the existing subclasses. It is used in the management of life-threatening ventricular arrhythmias such as sustained ventricular tachycardia that has not responded to other drugs. Its antiarrhythmic effects are similar to those of Class I_A drugs, but its uses and adverse effects are more similar to those of Class I_C drugs. Moricizine suppresses abnormal automaticity and prolongs the PR and QRS intervals and AV nodal, bundle of His, and Purkinje fiber conduction times by blocking sodium channels in myocardial tissues. The drug has minimal effects on the amplitude of the action potential and on normal automaticity.

The most common adverse effects of moricizine include anxiety, dizziness, euphoria, headache, perioral numbness, fatigue, and nausea. Arrhythmias are the most life-threatening adverse effects. Moricizine is contraindicated in patients with hypersensitivity, cardiogenic shock, second- or third-degree heart block, or bundle branch block (unless a pacemaker is present). It should be used with caution in patients with electrolyte disturbances, heart failure, and se-vere renal or hepatic dysfunction. Extreme caution should be used in patients with sick sinus syndrome. Safe use during pregnancy or lactation or in children has not been established.

Moricizine is well absorbed but rapidly biotransformed following oral administration. Peak plasma concentrations are usually reached in 30 minutes to 2 hours. Administration after a meal delays the rate of absorption but not the extent of absorption. Moricizine is 95 percent bound to plasma proteins. Less than 1 percent of the unchanged drug is eliminated in the urine. The metabolites may have antiarrhythmic action.

Class II Antiarrhythmics

- ❒ Acebutolol (SECTRAL); (🍁) MONITAN, SECTRAL
- ❒ Esmolol (BREVIBLOC)
- ❒ Propranolol (INDERAL, INDERAL LA); (🍁) APO-PROPRANOLOL, DETENSOL, NOVO-PRANOL, PMS-PROPRANOLOL

Indications

Beta-blocking drugs make up Class II antiarrhythmics and include acebutolol, esmolol, and propranolol. Acebutolol is used primarily in the management of PVCs. Esmolol is an ultra short-acting drug used for the rapid, short-term control of ventricular rate in patients with supraventricular arrhythmias and sinus tachycardia. Propranolol is used in the management of paroxysmal supraventricular tachycardia, atrial fibrillation, atrial flutter, and sinus tachycardia associated with excessive catecholamine release.

TABLE 33–5 DOSAGE REGIMEN OF SELECTED ANTIARRHYTHMIC DRUGS

Drug	Use(s)	Dosage	Implications
Class I_A Antiarrhythmics			
Quinidine sulfate	Broad spectrum: suppression of chronic supraventricular and ventricular arrhythmias	*Adult:* PACs or PVCs: 200–300 mg po Q6–8hr *or* 300–600 mg of extended release formulation Q8–12hr. Maintenance not to exceed 3–4 g/day. *PSVT:* 400–600 mg po Q2–3hr until arrhythmia terminated. *Fibrillation:* 200 mg po Q2–3hr × 5–8 doses, then increase at daily intervals if necessary. *Child:* 6 mg/kg or 180 mg/m^2 5 times daily	Patient is usually digitalized before starting therapy. A test dose of a single 200-mg quinidine sulfate tablet may be administered before therapy to check for intolerance. Give drug on empty stomach. Do not allow extended release formulations to be opened, crushed, broken, or chewed. Sulfate formulation is 83% quinidine. Gluconate formulation is 62% quinidine. Polygalacturonate formulation is 60% quinidine
Quinidine gluconate		*Adult:* 324–660 mg po Q6–12hr as extended release formulation *or* 325–650 mg po Q6hr if not extended release	
Quinidine polygalacturonate		*Adult:* 275–825 mg po Q3–4hr × 3–4 doses that may be increased by 137.5–275 mg every 3rd or 4th dose until arrhythmia controlled. Maintenance: 275 mg po Q8–12hr. *Child:* 8.25 mg/kg or 247.5 mg/m^2 5 times daily	
Procainamide	Broad spectrum: suppression of chronic supraventricular and ventricular arrhythmias	*Adult: Atrial arrhythmias:* 1.25 g po loading dose, then 750 mg 2 hr later, then 0.5–1 g Q2–3hr. Maintenance: 0.5–1 g po Q4–6hr or 1 g Q6hr as extended release formulation. *Ventricular arrhythmias:* 50 mg/kg/day in divided doses Q3hr or Q6hr for extended release formulation. *Child:* 12.5 mg/kg (375 mg/m^2) 4 times daily	Not interchangeable with quinidine. Produces lupus-like syndrome. Use lower doses or longer dosing intervals for older adults and patients with renal, hepatic, or cardiac insufficiency
Disopyramide	Broad spectrum: used for ventricular arrhythmias	*Adults >50 kg:* 300 mg po loading dose followed by 150 mg Q6hr as extended release formulation *or* 300 mg po Q12hr as extended release formulation. Maintenance: Not to exceed 800 mg po QD in divided doses. *Adults <50 kg:* 200 po Q6hr or 200 mg po Q12hr as extended release formulation. *Child age 12–18 years:* 6–15 mg/kg/day in divided doses Q6hr. *Child age 4–12 years:* 10–15 mg/kg/day in divided doses Q6hr. *Child age 1–4 years:* 10–20 mg/kg/day in divided doses Q6hr. *Child <1 year:* 10–30 mg/kg/day in divided doses	Loading dose should be eliminated in patients with cardiomyopathy or decompensated heart failure. Dosage must be reduced in renal insufficiency. Give drug on empty stomach. Do not allow extended release formulations to be opened, crushed, broken, or chewed. If necessary drug may be mg po loading dose followed by 100 mg prepared as a suspension using 100-mg capsules and cherry syrup
Class I_B Antiarrhythmics			
Lidocaine	Narrow spectrum: ventricular arrhythmias associated with acute MI, cardiac surgery, cardiac catheterization, cardioversion, cardiac glycoside toxicity	*Adult:* 1–2 mg/kg IV. Not to exceed 50–100 mg as single bolus over 2 min. Continuous drip: 1–4 mg/min. Maximum: 300 mg/hr. *Child:* 1 mg/kg followed by IV drip of 20–50 mcg/kg/min	Preferred drug for digitalis-induced ventricular arrhythmias. Lidocaine formulations that also contain catecholamines must never be given IV
Mexiletine	Narrow spectrum: ventricular arrhythmias including ventricular tachycardia and PVCs	*Adult:* Initial: 400 mg po loading dose, then 200 mg 8 hr later, then 200–400 mg Q8hr. If controlled on less than 300 mg Q8hr, can give same daily dose at 12-hr intervals. Not to exceed 1200 mg/day	Continuous ECG monitoring required to determine increased PR or QRS intervals. Give with food or milk. Reduced dosage is necessary for patients with hepatic disease
Tocainide	Narrow spectrum: multifocal and unifocal PVCs, ventricular tachycardia	*Adult:* 400 mg po loading dose. Maintenance: 1200–1800 g/day in divided doses Q8hr. Twice daily dosing may be used in some patients	Give with food or milk. Administer dopamine if circulatory depression occurs, diazepam or thiopental for seizures. Safe use in children has not been established

TABLE 33–5 DOSAGE REGIMEN OF SELECTED ANTIARRHYTHMIC DRUGS *Continued*

Drug	Use(s)	Dosage	Implications
Class I_B Antiarrhythmics *Continued*			
Phenytoin	Narrow spectrum: digitalis-induced ventricular arrhythmias	*Adult:* 50–100 mg IV Q10–15min until arrhythmia has been abolished or 15 mg/kg has been given. Administer at a rate not to exceed 50 mg over 1 min. Administration rate may be as low as 5–10 mg/min in some patients who develop hypotension, are on sympathomimetic drugs, have cardiovascular disease, or are older adults	Not a first-line agent. Lidocaine preferred. Rapid administration may result in severe hypotension, cardiovascular collapse, or CNS depression
Class I_C Antiarrhythmics			
Flecainide	Supraventricular and ventricular arrhythmias only	*Adult: Ventricular tachycardia:* 100 mg po Q12hr initially. Increase by 50 mg BID until response is obtained or maximum total daily dose of 400 mg is reached. *PSVT/PAF:* 50 mg po Q12hr initially. Increase by 50 mg BID until response obtained or maximum total daily dose of 300 mg is reached	Some patients may require Q8hr dosing. Administer with meals if GI distress occurs. Previous antiarrhythmic therapy (except lidocaine) should be withdrawn 2–4 half-lives before starting flecainide. Administer dopamine for circulatory depression if necessary, diazepam or thiopental for seizures
Propafenone	Ventricular arrhythmias	*Adult:* 150 mg po Q8hr. Increase as required up to 300 mg Q8–12 hr. Allow 3–4 days before increasing interval	Pre-existing hypokalemia or hyperkalemia should be corrected prior to instituting therapy
Other Class I Antiarrhythmics			
Moricizine	Life-threatening ventricular arrhythmias refractory to other drugs	*Adult:* 600–900 mg/day given Q8hr. Within this range the dosage may be adjusted by 150 mg/day every 3 days as required and tolerated. Some patients may tolerate Q12hr dosing, not to exceed 900 mg/day	Therapy should be initiated in a hospital with facilities for cardiac monitoring. Previous antiarrhythmic therapy should be withdrawn 1–2 half-lives before starting moricizine. Dosage adjustments should be 3 days apart due to the long half-life of moricizine
Class II Antiarrhythmics			
Acebutolol	Premature ventricular contractions	*Adult:* 200 mg po Q12hr initially. Increase gradually to a maximum daily dose of 600–1200 mg BID	Always check apical pulse before administering. If less than 60 bpm, hold drug. May be given without regard to meals
Esmolol	Atrial fibrillation, atrial flutter, sinus tachycardia	*Adult:* Loading dose of 500 mcg/kg over 1 min, followed by a 4-min maintenance infusion of 50 mcg/kg/min. May repeat loading dose if necessary. Maintenance: 100 mcg/kg/min over 4 min	Not to be used longer than 48 hr. Continuously monitor ECG. Titration of drug is complex. Check manufacturer's instructions before drug administration
Propranolol	PSVT, atrial fibrillation, atrial flutter, sinus tachycardia associated with excessive catecholamine release	*Adult:* 1–3 mg slow IV push not to exceed 1 mg/min. May be repeated after 2 min if necessary and again in 4 hr if needed **OR** 10–30 mg po TID-QID. Do not administer more frequently than Q4hr. Maintenance: 10–80 mg po TID-QID. *Child:* 10–100 mcg/kg up to 1 mg/dose. May be repeated Q6–8hr if needed	Double check dosage and route before administration. IV doses are much smaller than po doses. Patients receiving IV propranolol must have continuous ECG monitoring and may have PCWP or CVP monitoring during and for several hours after administration
Class III Antiarrhythmics			
Amiodarone	Life-threatening, recurrent ventricular arrhythmias, supraventricular tachycardia, ventricular fibrillation resistant to other drugs	*Adult:* Loading dose 800–1600 mg/day for 1–3 weeks, then 600–800 mg/day in 1–2 doses for 1 mo, then 400 mg/day maintenance dose **OR** 150 mg IV over 10 min (150 mg/min), followed by 360 mgover next 6 hr (1 mg/min), 540 mg then over the next 18 hr (0.5 mg/min). *Child:* 10 mg/kg/day (800 mg/1.72 m^2/day) × 10 days or until response or adverse effects occur, then 5 mg/kg/day (400 mg/1.72 m^2/day) for several weeks, then decreased to 2.5 mg/kg/day (200 mg/1.72 m^2/day) or lowest effective dose	Therapeutic effects delayed 5–30 days unless loading doses are given. Effects persist for several weeks after drug is discontinued. Continue IV infusion at 0.5 mg/min until oral therapy is initiated. Conversion to initial oral therapy: if duration of infusion was less than 1 week, oral dose should be 800–1000 mg/day; if duration of infusion was 1–3 weeks, oral dose should be 600–800 mg/day; if IV infusion extended past 3 weeks, oral dose should be 400 mg/day

Table continued on following page

TABLE 33–5 DOSAGE REGIMEN OF SELECTED ANTIARRHYTHMIC DRUGS *Continued*

Drug	Use(s)	Dosage	Implications
Class III Antiarrhythmics *Continued*			
Bretylium	Ventricular tachycardia, drug-resistant ventricular fibrillation	*Adult: Ventricular fibrillation:* 5 mg/kg IV push over 1 min. If necessary, increase to 10 mg/kg and repeat every 15–30 min until 30 mg/kg has been given if required. *Other ventricular arrhythmias:* Dilute and infuse 5–10 mg/kg IV Q6–8hr. May also be given as continuous infusion at 1–2 mg/min. *Child: Ventricular fibrillation:* 5 mg/kg followed by 10 mg/kg Q15–30 min to a total of 30 mg/kg. *Other ventricular arrhythmias:* 5–10 mg/kg Q6hr (unlabeled uses)	Arrhythmias usually resolve in minutes. Infuse in diluted solution. Contraindicated in patients with digitalis-induced arrhythmias. When discontinuing therapy, the dosage should be gradually reduced over 3–5 days with close ECG monitoring. Notify health care provider if systolic blood pressure less than 75 mmHg or patient symptomatic. Dopamine, dobutamine, or norepinephrine and volume replacement may be necessary. Safety and efficacy in children have not been established
Sotalol	Life-threatening ventricular arrhythmias, sustained supraventricular tachycardia	*Adult:* 80 mg po BID. May increase gradually at 2–3 day intervals to a range of 240–320 mg/day. Not to exceed 480–640 mg/day	Increase dosage interval if CrCl is less than 60 ml/min. Dosing more than BID usually not necessary due to long half-life. Patients who develop anaphylaxis may be more resistant to epinephrine. Safety and efficacy in children have not been established
Class IV Antiarrhythmics			
Diltiazem	Paroxysmal supraventricular tachycardia, atrial flutter, atrial fibrillation	*Adult:* 30–120 mg po TID-QID **OR** 60–120 mg BID if sustained release formulation used. Maximum: 360 mg/day **OR** 0.25 mg/kg IV. May repeat in 15 min with a dose of 0.35 mg/kg. May follow with continuous infusion at 10 mg/hr (range 5–15 mg/hr) for up to 24 hr	Most often used for prophylaxis. Do not allow sustained release formulation to be opened, crushed, broken, or chewed. Empty tablets that appear in the stool are not significant
Verapamil		*Adult:* 80–120 mg po Q6–8hr. Dose may be increased as needed **OR** 120–240 mg/day of extended release formulation. May be increased as needed to 480 mg/day **OR** 5–10 mg (75–150 mcg/kg). May repeat with 10 mg after 30 min. *Child over 16 years:* 4–8 mg/kg/day po in divided doses. *Child age 1–16 years:* 100–300 mcg/kg. May repeat after 30 min. Initial dose not to exceed 5 mg. Repeat dose not to exceed 10 mg. *Child under 1 year:* 100–200 mcg/kg IV. May repeat after 30 min	Contraindicated in digitalis toxicity because it worsens heart block. Do not use IV form with IV propranolol because of potential for fatal bradycardia and hypotension. The patient should remain recumbent for at least 1 hr following IV administration to minimize hypotensive effects. Contact health care provider if pulse rate less than 50 bpm
Unclassified Antiarrhythmics			
Adenosine	Paroxysmal supraventricular tachycardia, Wolff-Parkinson-White syndrome	*Adult:* 6 mg IV over 1–2 sec. If first dose does not convert arrhythmia within 1–2 min, give 12 mg. May repeat 12 mg dose in 1–2 min if no response has occurred	Administer directly into vein or in proximal IV line. Follow by rapid saline flush. Assess cardiac performance via continuous ECG monitoring
Ibutilide	Rapid conversion atrial fibrillation, atrial flutter of recent onset	*Adults over 60 kg:* 1 mg IV over 10 min. If arrhythmia still present 10 min after initial infusion, a second 1-mg infusion may be given 10 min after completion of first infusion. *Adults under 60 kg:* 0.1 mg/kg given over 10 min. If arrhythmia still present 10 min after initial infusion, a second dose may be given 10 min after completion of first infusion	Continuously monitor ECG for at least 4 hr following infusion or until QT interval has returned to baseline. Patients with atrial fibrillation that lasts more than 2–3 days duration may be treated with anticoagulants for at least 2 weeks before ibutilide therapy

CrCl, creatinine clearance; PCWP, pulmonary capillary wedge pressure; CVP, central venous pressure; PSVT/PAF, paroxysmal supraventricular tachycardia/paroxysmal atrial fibrillation

Class II antiarrhythmic drugs are not considered initial drugs of choice to treat arrhythmias. This is in part because of their multiple effects and because of possible breakthrough ectopy. The use of these drugs with other antiarrhythmics remains to be evaluated.

Pharmacodynamics

Class II antiarrhythmic drugs exert antiarrhythmic effects by antagonizing SNS stimulation of beta receptors in the heart. Blockade of beta receptors in the SA node and ectopic pacemakers decreases automaticity. All beta blockers cause a substantial increase in the ERP of the AV node. This action is the basis for the use of these drugs as antiarrhythmic drugs.

Acebutolol predominantly blocks $beta_1$ receptors to slow sinus heart rate and decrease cardiac output and blood pressure. In large doses it may block $beta_2$ receptors, thus increasing airway resistance. It slows AV conduction and reduces the rate of spontaneous firing of the SA node.

Esmolol also selectively blocks $beta_1$ receptors to slow the heart rate, decrease cardiac output, and lower blood pressure. The exact mechanism for reducing blood pressure is unknown but esmolol may block peripheral adrenergic receptors, thus decreasing sympathetic output from the CNS or by decreasing renin release from the kidney. Its antiarrhythmic effect is due to blocking stimulation of cardiac pacemaker potentials.

Propranolol is a nonselective beta blocker with effects on both $beta_1$ and $beta_2$ receptors. It also has substantial local anesthetic (membrane stabilizing) actions. It has no intrinsic sympathomimetic activity. Like acebutolol and esmolol, propranolol blocks $beta_1$ receptors, thus slowing the heart rate, decreasing cardiac output, and reducing the blood pressure. However, by blocking $beta_2$ receptors located in the respiratory tract, airway resistance is increased.

Class II antiarrhythmic drugs also exert a significant negative inotropic effect. By decreasing myocardial oxygen demand, myocardial ischemia is decreased. As ischemia abates, myocardial cells lose their automaticity and suppress atrial and ventricular ectopy.

Adverse Effects and Contraindications

The most common adverse reactions to Class II antiarrhythmics usually occur with initial use of the drugs. Because they inhibit SA node stimulation, Class II drugs may produce bradycardia.

The most common adverse effects include mild, transient hypotension, dizziness, nausea, diaphoresis, headache, cold extremities, fatigue, constipation, and diarrhea. Insomnia, flatulence, urinary frequency, and impotence or decreased libido occasionally occur. A rash, arthralgia, myalgia, confusion (especially in the older adult), and a change in taste can occur but are rare. An overdose can produce profound bradycardia and hypotension. Acebutolol may precipitate heart failure or MI in patients with cardiac disease, thyroid storm in patients with thyrotoxicosis, and peripheral ischemia in patients with peripheral vascular disease. Hypoglycemia may occur in patients with previously controlled diabetes. Thrombocytopenia is possible but rare.

Esmolol is generally well tolerated. The most common adverse effects are transient and mild, including hypotension, dizziness, nausea, diaphoresis, headache, cold extremities, and fatigue. IV infusions of esmolol cause inflammation and induration at the injection site in about 80 percent of individuals. Somnolence and confusion occasionally occur. Bronchospasm, bradycardia, and peripheral ischemia are rare.

The adverse effects of IV propranolol are more common and more severe than with oral dosage forms, especially in the elderly and azotemic patients. Bradycardia is frequent. A Raynaud-type peripheral vascular insufficiency, dizziness, and fatigue occur occasionally. Although rare, sedation, behavioral change, hypotension, GI upset, peripheral skin necrosis, rash, and rhythm and/or conduction disturbances have occurred.

Beta blockers are contraindicated in patients with hypersensitivity, sinus bradycardia, second- or third-degree heart block, cardiogenic shock, heart failure, asthma, and chronic airway limitation and during lactation. These drugs should be used with caution in patients with diabetes, thyrotoxicosis, and hepatic or renal impairment.

There is controversy regarding the safety of beta blockers in pregnancy. Reports of an increased incidence of growth retardation, delayed neonatal respirations, bradycardia, hypoglycemia, and blunting of accelerations of the intrapartum fetal heart rate have all been described. Whether this phenomenon is dose related or caused by the underlying disease for which the therapy is indicated is unclear. No evidence exists to suggest that beta blockers are teratogenic.

Pharmacokinetics

Acebutolol has an onset time of 90 minutes, with peak concentrations reached in 3 to 8 hours. The bioavailability of acebutolol is less than 50 percent, with a half-life of 3 to 4 hours. Its duration of action ranges from 24 to 30 hours. Elimination is through the kidneys and feces.

Esmolol has an onset time of 5 minutes and is quickly and widely distributed, with peak concentrations reached in 10 to 30 minutes. It is about 55 percent bound to plasma proteins, with a duration of action of 20 to 30 minutes. Esmolol has a half-life of 5 to 23 minutes. Most of the esmolol dose is biotransformed to an inactive metabolite that is eliminated in the urine.

Propranolol is almost completely absorbed from the GI tract after oral administration, but an extensive first-pass effect reduces bioavailability to about 25 percent. Peak plasma concentrations are seen 60 to 90 minutes after administration. As with lidocaine, the hepatic extraction of propranolol is high and elimination is significantly reduced when hepatic blood flow decreases. Propranolol may decrease its own rate of elimination by decreasing cardiac output and hepatic blood flow, particularly in individuals with left ventricular dysfunction. Ninety-three percent of the drug is bound to plasma proteins. Hepatic disease decreases the plasma protein bound fraction of propranolol and increases the amount of free drug in the circulation. Hyperthyroidism increases the clearance of propranolol by the liver. The half-life of propranolol is 3 to 5 hours. Propranolol is eliminated through the urine and feces.

Drug-Drug Interaction

Class II antiarrhythmic drugs interact with a number of other drugs, sometimes increasing and at others decreasing the drug effects. For example, phenothiazines, antihypertensive drugs, and diuretics may potentiate hypotension. Cimetidine decreases propranolol biotransformation, thus increasing plasma concentrations. Concurrent use of verapamil, a Class IV drug, with beta blockers creates additive myocardial depression. Anticholinergics potentiate the pressor effects of beta blockers, causing hypertension and reducing the efficacy of the beta blockers. Esmolol interacts with digoxin to increase serum digoxin concentration and with morphine to increase the blood level of esmolol.

Dosage Regimen

Acebutolol is given orally with an initial dose of 200 mg twice daily. The dosage is gradually increased to a maximum daily dosage of 600 to 1200 mg administered in divided doses. The apical pulse should be checked prior to administering acebutolol and the drug held if the pulse is less than 60 bpm. The drug may be given without regard to meals.

Esmolol is only administered IV with a loading dose of 500 mcg/kg over 1 minute. This dose may be followed by a 4-minute maintenance infusion of 50 mcg/kg/min. The maintenance infusion may be titrated up to 300 mcg/kg/min in 50-mcg/kg increments every 5 to 10 minutes until the desired response occurs. After control of the ventricular rate is achieved, long-term oral therapy is started with an appropriate drug. As with other IV administered antiarrhythmic drugs, the blood pressure and ECG should be continuously monitored.

The initial dose of propranolol for acute arrhythmias is 1 to 3 mg given by slow IV push. The dose may be repeated if necessary after 2 minutes and again in 4 hours. When possible, the patient is started on oral propranolol therapy with doses ranging from 10 to 30 mg three to four times daily. Note that IV doses are much smaller than po doses, so be sure to check the package label carefully. Patients receiving IV propranolol must have continuous ECG monitoring and may have pulmonary capillary wedge pressure or central venous pressure monitoring during and for several hours after administration. The duration of action of propranolol can be extended by the administration of large doses because beta-blocking drugs have a greater margin of safety than do most antiarrhythmic drugs.

Laboratory Considerations

Laboratory values that may be altered in the presence of acebutolol are numerous. Acebutolol may increase ANA titers, AST (SGOT), ALT (SGPT), bilirubin, alkaline phosphatase, lactate dehydrogenase, BUN, creatinine, potassium, uric acid, lipoproteins, and triglycerides. There are no significant laboratory values altered with esmolol. Propranolol may cause increased ANA, glucose, BUN, potassium, serum lipoproteins, triglycerides, and uric acid levels. Beta-blocking drugs in general may mask the signs and symptoms of hypoglycemia and potential insulin-induced hypoglycemia in some patients.

Class III Antiarrhythmics

- ❒ Amiodarone (CORDARONE); (✱) CORDARONE
- ❒ Bretylium (BRETYLOL); (✱) BRETYLATE
- ❒ Sotalol (BETAPACE); (✱) SOTACOR

Indications

Amiodarone, bretylium, and sotalol are used to treat ventricular arrhythmias. Because of its long half-life and life-threatening adverse effects, amiodarone is indicated only for recurrent ventricular fibrillation and recurrent, hemodynamically unstable sustained ventricular tachycardia. Treatment should always be started in the hospital with efficacy and response assessed.

Bretylium is currently recommended only for the treatment of life-threatening ventricular arrhythmias that fail to respond to adequate doses of a first-line antiarrhythmic drug (e.g., lidocaine, procainamide). Use of bretylium should be limited to critical care units. It should not be used in circulatory shock. The associated release of catecholamines could increase myocardial oxygen consumption in an individual with ischemic heart disease.

Sotalol is apparently safer than amiodarone and may be a good first-line drug in the treatment of malignant ventricular arrhythmias. Sotalol appears to be effective in the treatment of sustained supraventricular tachycardia and atrial fibrillation and in some patients with Wolff-Parkinson-White syndrome. Sotalol can reduce cardiac function in patients dependent on SNS activity to maintain a normal cardiac output.

Because of their adverse effects, class III drugs are considered to be second- or third-line drugs. These drugs may convert unidirectional block to bidirectional block, but they have little or no effect on depolarization.

Pharmacodynamics

While all of the drugs in this class possess diverse pharmacologic properties, they all share the common property of prolonging the action potential duration and refractoriness in Purkinje fibers and ventricular muscle, thus decreasing the automaticity rate of ventricular ectopic foci. The exact mechanism of action of Class III antiarrhythmics that is most responsible for the antiarrhythmic effects remains uncertain.

Amiodarone, a benzofuron derivative (much of the drug is iodine), also causes potent sodium and calcium channel blockade. It prolongs repolarization, reduces the automaticity of the SA node, increases conduction time and refractoriness of the AV node, and reduces conduction velocity in the myocardium and Purkinje fibers. Amiodarone may decrease intracardiac conduction, as shown by increased PR and QT intervals. The QRS complex may be unchanged or increased. Amiodarone also decreases myocardial oxygen demand and enhances cardiac performance because it relaxes vascular smooth muscle and decreases systemic and coronary vascular resistance. It is also a weak, noncompetitive, alpha- and beta-blocking drug.

Bretylium does not prolong the PR and QT intervals. Although bretylium can transiently increase myocardial contractility by releasing norepinephrine, it can also cause orthostatic hypotension through blockade of sympathetic cardiovascular reflexes. Both amiodarone and bretylium produce some degree of peripheral and coronary vasodilation.

Sotalol prolongs the action potential, ERP, and QT interval. It decreases automaticity presumably by blocking $beta_1$- and $beta_2$-adrenergic receptors. It lengthens the action potential duration in myocardial fibers without producing significant effects on membrane responsiveness or conduction through Purkinje fibers. Conduction through the AV node is significantly reduced. Sotalol is also thought to terminate reentry arrhythmias by markedly prolonging refractoriness without affecting the propagation of the electrical impulse. At therapeutic drug levels, sotalol decreases heart rate.

Adverse Effects and Contraindications

The adverse effects of Class III antiarrhythmics vary widely and commonly lead to discontinuance of the drug. More than 75 percent of individuals treated with amiodarone for 1 to 2 years experience adverse effects, and 25 to 33 percent of this number discontinue treatment. Hypotension, nausea, and anorexia are not uncommon. In 20 to 40 percent of individuals amiodarone also causes CNS reactions, including malaise, fatigue, tremor, involuntary movements, ataxia, abnormal gait, lack of coordination, dizziness, and paresthesia. Corneal microdeposits occur in almost all patients receiving the drug; however, only about 10 percent experience vision disturbances. The deposits will disappear with the reduction in dosage or drug discontinuance. Peripheral neuropathy and proximal myopathy may occur.

The adverse effects of amiodarone of greatest concern, however, are exacerbations of arrhythmias, worsening of heart failure, pulmonary fibrosis, and pneumonitis. Symptomatic pulmonary toxicity occurs in 10 to 15 percent of patients treated for 1 to 3 years. Death results in about 10 percent of patients with pulmonary involvement. Pulmonary toxicity is characterized by cough and progressive dyspnea. The disorder is thought to result from indirect toxicity (i.e., hypersensitivity pneumonitis) or direct toxicity (i.e., interstitial alveolar pneumonitis). Pre-existing pulmonary disease does not seem to increase the risk of pulmonary toxicity. However, patients with pulmonary disease have a poor prognosis if pulmonary toxicity does develop. Substantial increases in low-density lipoprotein concentrations are frequently observed.

Because amiodarone contains iodine, which is ultimately released into systemic circulation, it inhibits the conversion of thyroxine to triiodothyronine (T_3). It can cause hypothyroidism or hyperthyroidism, with the latter a greater threat to cardiovascular status.

Hypotension is the principal adverse effect of bretylium. The hypotension occurs as the result of peripheral vasodilation caused by adrenergic blockade. The hypotension is most often postural; however, marked supine hypotension can occur. It can also precipitate a torsades de pointes episode. Rapid IV administration can cause nausea and vomiting. In addition, bradycardia, diarrhea, swelling, tenderness of the parotid gland (especially at mealtime), and vertigo have all been reported.

The most common adverse effects of sotalol include bradycardia and palpitations. Anxiety, nervousness, nausea, vomiting, diarrhea, constipation, nightmares, transient hypotension, heart failure, bronchospasm, peripheral ischemia (i.e., cold hands, feet), and unusual tiredness or weakness have also been noted. Although rare, skin rashes, chest pain, and depression may occur. The most severe adverse effects include hypoglycemia, prolonged QT interval, torsades de pointes, ventricular tachycardia, and premature ventricular complexes.

Pharmacokinetics

Absorption of orally administered amiodarone is slow and variable, with 35 to 65 percent of the drug bioavailable. The time to peak plasma concentrations after an oral or IV dose is unknown. Amiodarone is distributed to and accumulates slowly in body tissues. High drug levels are reached in body fat, muscle, liver, lungs, and spleen. During long-term treatment with amiodarone, the active metabolite accumulates in the plasma, and its concentration may exceed that of the parent compound. Amiodarone is biotransformed in the liver. One metabolite, *N*-desethylamiodarone, has antiarrhythmic activity. Amiodarone is eliminated from the body via the bile. The half-life is biphasic, with a mean of 53 days. It can be detected in plasma for up to 9 months after administration.

Bretylium's erratic GI absorption mandates that it be administered IV or IM. The drug accumulates in sympathetic ganglia and postadrenergic neurons with negligible protein binding. It has an immediate onset with IV administration, with peak concentrations reached at the end of the infusion. The average duration of action is 6 to 24 hours, with a half-life of 5 to 10 hours. More than 90 percent is eliminated through the kidneys as unchanged drug.

Sotalol is rapidly absorbed after oral administration, with a bioavailability of nearly 100 percent. Maximum plasma concentrations are reached 2 to 3 hours after administration, with approximately 50 percent of the drug bound to plasma proteins. The half-life is 12 hours. Sotalol is almost entirely eliminated in the urine as unchanged drug.

Drug-Drug Interactions

Amiodarone increases the plasma concentrations and effects of cyclosporine digoxin, flecainide, lidocaine, mexiletine, phenytoin, procainamide, quinidine, and warfarin. Amiodarone also increases the likelihood of bradycardia, sinus arrest, and AV block when beta blockers or calcium channel blockers are concurrently administered. Because of slow elimination rates, the potential for interactions and other adverse effects persists for many weeks after amiodarone is discontinued.

There is a possibility of increasing the severity of drug-induced arrhythmias when bretylium is used in the presence of cardiac glycosides. Additive or antagonistic effects of bretylium can be noted when other antiarrhythmic drugs are present. Dopamine and norepinephrine drug actions are enhanced. There is an increased risk of hypotension when bretylium is used concurrently with antihypertensive drugs.

Antiarrhythmics, astemizole, phenothiazines, and tricyclic antidepressants are likely to cause an increased prolonged QT interval when sotalol is also used. Digoxin may cause increased risk of proarrhythmic effects. Calcium channel blockers increase AV nodal conduction and blood pressure in the presence of sotalol. The signs and symptoms of hypoglycemia may be masked and the effects of insulin prolonged. Sotalol may potentiate rebound hypertension if the patient has been on clonidine, even after clonidine has been discontinued.

Dosage Regimen

Because it takes amiodarone several months to reach full effect, loading doses of 800 to 1600 mg/day are administered for 1 to 3 weeks in the hospital, with continuous ECG monitoring. A gradual decrease in dosage to 600 to 800 mg/day for 1 month is recommended, with an oral maintenance dose of 400 mg/day. Treatment effectiveness is evaluated after 2 to 8 weeks. Long-term effective treatment has been associated with plasma concentrations of 1.0 to 2.5 mcg/mL.

Bretylium is diluted to a concentration of 10 mg/mL or less and a 5-mg/kg bolus given over 60 seconds initially. The arrhythmia should resolve in minutes. If necessary, a second loading dose of 10 mg/kg may be given up to three times. Present indications limit the use of bretylium to a 5-day period.

The usual oral dosage of sotalol is 80 mg twice daily. The dose may be gradually increased at 2- to 3-day intervals but should not exceed 480 to 640 mg/day. Dosing more than twice daily is usually not necessary because of the long half-life of sotalol.

Laboratory Considerations

Amiodarone may cause elevated ALT (SGPT), AST (SGOT), and alkaline phosphatase concentrations. Liver, lung, thyroid, and neurologic functions should be monitored before and periodically throughout therapy. ANA titer concentrations may be elevated, but the patient is not usually symptomatic. The long elimination half-life of amiodarone causes persistent drug effects long after dosage adjustment or the drug is discontinued.

Bretylium produces decreased laboratory values of urinary epinephrine, norepinephrine, and vanillylmandelic acid. Sotalol may cause elevations in serum potassium, uric acid, lactate dehydrogenase, glucose, lipoproteins, triglyceride levels, and BUN. Hepatic and renal function and CBC should be routinely monitored in patients receiving prolonged sotalol therapy. Correct hypokalemia and hypomagnesemia prior to initiating therapy with sotalol.

Class IV Antiarrhythmics

- ❒ Diltiazem (CARDIZEM, CARDIZEM SR, CARDIZEM CD, DILACOR XR); (🍁) APO-DILTIAZ, NOVO-DILTAZEM, SYN-DILTIAZEM
- ❒ Verapamil (CALAN, CALAN SR, ISOPTIN, ISOPTIN SR, VERELAN); (🍁) NOVO-VERAMIL, NU-VERAP

Indications

Although there are other calcium channel blockers, verapamil and diltiazem are the only drugs in this class approved by the Food and Drug Administration for the treatment of arrhythmias. Diltiazem and verapamil are approved for the temporary management of rapid ventricular rate in atrial fibrillation and atrial flutter and paroxysmal supraventricular tachycardia. Verapamil has been used successfully in the transplacental cardioversion of fetal paroxysmal atrial tachycardia.

Pharmacodynamics

Class IV drugs are calcium channel blockers in that they inhibit calcium movement across cell membranes of cardiac and vascular smooth muscle. The inhibition of calcium movement slows the conduction rate between the atria and ventricles and greatly increases the ERP of the AV node. Diltiazem and verapamil slow the spontaneous firing of pacemaker cells in the SA node. However, heart rate slows minimally because this direct effect is balanced by increased reflex sympathetic activity resulting from arterial vasodilation. Depression of the AV node is responsible for slowing the ventricular response to atrial flutter or fibrillation and termination of paroxysmal supraventricular tachycardia. Neither verapamil nor diltiazem has cholinergic or beta-blocking properties. Verapamil does, however, have appreciable alpha-adrenergic blocking activity.

Adverse Effects and Contraindications

The most common adverse effects of diltiazem therapy are peripheral edema, facial flushing, dizziness, headache, asthenia (i.e., weakness, loss of strength), and bradycardia. Diarrhea, constipation, and a rash are possible although rare. Occasionally, patients may note hypotension, pruritus, burning at an IV injection site, vasodilation, atrial flutter, bradycardia, and diaphoresis. The most severe adverse effects include second- and third-degree AV heart block, increased frequency and duration of anginal pain, and heart failure.

Diltiazem is contraindicated in patients with sick sinus syndrome, second- or third-degree AV block (except in the presence of a pacemaker), severe hypotension (systolic blood pressure less than 90 mmHg), acute MI, and pulmonary congestion. Cautious use is warranted in patients with renal or hepatic disorders.

The most common adverse effect of verapamil is constipation. Dizziness, hypotension, peripheral edema, bradycardia, headache, and fatigue are frequent occurrences. Hypotension, bradycardia, dizziness, and headache are occasionally noted when verapamil is given IV. Severe tachycardia is rare, although verapamil can increase ventricular rate because of reflex increases in SNS activity.

Verapamil is contraindicated in patients with sick sinus syndrome, second- or third-degree AV block (except in the presence of a pacemaker), severe hypotension (systolic blood pressure less than 90 mmHg), acute MI, and pulmonary congestion. In addition, verapamil is contraindicated in patients with cardiogenic shock and severe heart failure (unless secondary to supraventricular tachycardia). Cautious use is warranted in patients with renal or hepatic disorders.

IV use of calcium channel blockers is contraindicated in patients who have hypotension, severe heart failure, sick sinus syndrome, AV block, atrial fibrillation, Wolff-Parkinson-White syndrome, or ventricular tachycardia.

Pharmacokinetics

The onset of diltiazem's oral and sustained release formulations is 30 minutes after administration. Drug effects peak in 2 to 3 hours, with a 6- to 8-hour duration. The sustained release formulation has a 12-hour duration of action. It has a half-life of 3.5 to 9 hours.

The antiarrhythmic effects of IV verapamil begin in 1 to 5 minutes, with peak action occurring in 3 to 5 minutes. Hemodynamic effects begin 3 to 5 minutes following injection and persist for up to 20 minutes. Verapamil has a 2-hour duration of antiarrhythmic action. When taken by mouth, verapamil onset is in 1 to 2 hours, with peak antiarrhythmic effects occurring in 30 to 90 minutes. The onset of the sustained release formulation is unknown, but the drug peaks in 5 to 7 hours with a 24-hour duration of action.

Drug-Drug Interactions

The major interaction with Class IV antiarrhythmics is with digoxin, with the clearance of digoxin being reduced. The negative inotropic effect of verapamil could negate some of the advantages from the positive inotropic action of digoxin, thereby requiring a dosage adjustment. The main reason for this is the additive effect of these drugs on the SA or AV node. Additionally, verapamil interacts with digoxin in a manner not unlike the quinidine-digoxin reaction in which digoxin serum levels are increased. Concurrent use of verapamil or diltiazem with antihypertensive drugs that depress the SA node can intensify sinus bradycardia. Highly protein bound drugs could displace or be displaced by calcium channel blockers.

Dosage Regimen

Oral doses of diltiazem are 30 to 120 mg 3 to 4 times daily or 60 to 120 mg twice daily as sustained release capsules. Maximum dosage of oral diltiazem is 360 mg/day.

To convert a paroxysmal supraventricular tachycardia to normal sinus rhythm, an IV dose of 5 to 10 mg of verapamil is given over 10 to 15 minutes. A second dose may be given if necessary 30 minutes later. Verapamil can be administered as a continuous infusion at the rate of 0.1 mg/min. To prevent the recurrence of paroxysmal supraventricular tachycardia or to control the ventricular response to atrial fibrillation, oral doses of 240 to 480 mg/day are given in divided doses.

Laboratory Considerations

Total serum calcium levels are not affected by calcium channel blockers. Serum potassium levels should be monitored periodically throughout therapy because hypokalemia increases the risk of arrhythmias. Renal and hepatic functions should be monitored during long-term therapy. Hepatic enzyme levels may increase after several days of therapy but return to normal on discontinuation of the drug.

Unclassified Antiarrhythmics

- ❒ Adenosine (ADENOCARD, ADENOSCAN)
- ❒ Ibutilide (CORVERT)

ADENOSINE

Adenosine is an unclassified antiarrhythmic drug used in the management of paroxysmal supraventricular tachycardia, including arrhythmias associated with Wolff-Parkinson-White syndrome. It is ineffective for other arrhythmias. Do not confuse adenosine (ADENOCARD) with *adenosine phosphate.*

Adenosine is a naturally occurring component of all body cells that is an important physiologic mediator in different organ systems. It is produced in myocardial cells by dephosphorylation of adenosine monophosphate and by degradation of *S*-adenosylhomocysteine. Adenosine acts to slow calcium movement into cells by decreasing impulse formation in the SA node, conduction through the AV node, and to depress left ventricular function.

The frequent adverse effects of adenosine include facial flushing, headache, new arrhythmias (e.g., PVCs, sinus bradycardia), pain in the chest/arm/jaw/throat, and shortness of breath. Cough, dizziness, nausea, and numbness/tingling in the arms are occasionally noted. Adenosine is contraindicated in patients with second- or third-degree heart block or sick sinus syndrome (except with functioning pacemaker), atrial flutter or fibrillation, and ventricular tachycardia. It should be used with caution in patients with heart block, arrhythmias at the time of conversion, asthma, and hepatic or renal failure. Safe use during pregnancy and lactation and in children is unclear.

Absorption of adenosine is essentially complete after IV administration. It is taken up by erythrocytes and vascular endothelium and rapidly converted to inosine and adenosine monophosphate. Adenosine has a short duration of action. Its serum half-life is less than 10 seconds; thus it must be given as a rapid bolus injection, preferably through a central venous IV line. If given slowly, it is eliminated before it can reach cardiac tissues and exert cardiac action. The dosing regimen of adenosine is identified in Table 33–5. Doses greater than 12 mg decrease blood pressure by decreasing peripheral vascular resistance.

IBUTILIDE

Ibutilide is a newer antiarrhythmic drug used for the recent onset of atrial fibrillation or atrial flutter. Arrhythmias of longer duration are less likely to respond to therapy. Ibutilide prolongs both atrial and ventricular action potential durations and increases both atrial and ventricular refractory periods. Ibutilide activates the slow, inward movement of sodium, producing mild slowing of sinus rate and AV conduction. There is a dose-related prolongation of the QT interval.

Ibutilide is generally well tolerated. The most common adverse effect is an occasional episode of ventricular extrasystole, ventricular tachycardia, headache, hypotension, and postural hypotension. Overdosage results in CNS toxicity and may exaggerate expected prolongation of repolarization. It may worsen existing arrhythmias or produce new arrhythmias. Bundle branch block, AV block, bradycardia, and hypertension are rare. Ibutilide is contraindicated in patients with hypersensitivity. Cautious use is warranted in patients with abnormal liver function or heart block.

Ibutilide is widely distributed following IV administration. Most of a dose is biotransformed, with the metabolites eliminated in the urine and feces. The half-life is 2 to 12 hours, with a mean of 6 hours. Patients with atrial fibrillation of over 2 to 3 days duration must be treated with anticoagulants for at least 2 weeks prior to ibutilide therapy. The patient should be observed with continuous ECG monitoring for at least 4 hours following the infusion or until the QT interval has returned to baseline. If any arrhythmic activity is noted, ECG monitoring should be continued.

Critical Thinking Process

Assessment

History of Present Illness

The reason for the hospitalization or clinic visit should be determined. The patient's perception of the problem, its onset, recent stressors, life changes, or other precipitants should be elicited. When obtaining a history from a patient with suspected or confirmed arrhythmias, the health care provider obtains information related to heart failure, CAD, rheumatic fever, congenital defects, history of cardiac arrest, and use of cardiac drugs, diuretics, or potassium supplements. Identify conditions or risk factors that may precipitate arrhythmias, including hypoxia, electrolyte imbalances, acid-base imbalance, ischemic heart disease, valvular heart disease, respiratory disorders, excessive ingestion of caffeine-containing beverages, smoking, emotional upset, and febrile illness.

Subjective information that should be elicited includes chest pain, palpitations, shortness of breath, dizziness, syncopal episodes, confusion, and diaphoresis. If the symptoms were experienced previously, the patient should be queried as to the length, frequency, and tolerance of each episode. Mild arrhythmias may be perceived by the individual as palpitations or skipped beats. More severe manifestations may reflect decreased cardiac output and other hemodynamic changes.

Past Health History

The patient's past health history includes allergies and the physiologic response to the allergy, concomitant disease or illnesses, and drug history. Information about hypomagnesemia (often related to excessive alcohol intake), hypoxia related to an underlying respiratory disorder, hypertension, thyrotoxicosis, obesity, and diabetes mellitus is also elicited.

Physical Exam Findings

The physical exam should include an assessment of vital signs. Severe arrhythmias may produce manifestations that reflect decreased cardiac output and other hemodynamic changes. The manifestations can include hypotension, bradycardia, tachycardia, and irregular pulse (e.g., pulsus alternans, bigeminal pulse, pulse deficit). Shortness of breath, dyspnea, and cough from impaired respiration should be noted. Syncope or mental confusion from reduced cerebral blood flow may be noted. Urinary output should be assessed because oliguria from decreased renal blood flow is possible.

Physical assessment findings may also reveal a heart rate below 50 or above 140 bpm, an extremely irregular heart rate, a first heart sound that varies in intensity, the sudden appearance of heart failure, shock and angina pectoris, and a slow regular heart rate that does not change with activity or drug therapy. Arrhythmias that compromise cardiac output are reflected in part as a change in the characteristics of peripheral pulses.

Diagnostic Testing

Electrolyte levels, acid-base balance, serum drug levels, and ECG changes should be evaluated. The key to arrhythmia interpretation is the analysis of the form and relationships of the P wave, the PR interval, and the QRS complex. The ECG should be analyzed with regard to its rate and rhythm, the site of the dominant pacemaker, and the configuration of the P and QRS waves. ECG findings should be correlated with clinical observations of the patient. ECG changes reflective of severely compromised cardiac output should be reported immediately before presenting signs and symptoms cause further deterioration of the patient's condition.

Blood drawn for routine serum drug levels is done approximately 30 minutes to 1 hour after an antiarrhythmic drug has been administered for a peak level and immediately before the next dose for a trough level. Any abnormalities should be corrected because most antiarrhythmic drugs are less effective in the presence of acid-base imbalance or electrolyte disturbances, particularly those related to potassium.

Developmental Considerations

Perinatal Pregnancy is normally accompanied by significant physiologic changes in the maternal cardiovascular system. Pregnancy-related changes in blood volume, cardiac output, pulse, blood pressure, and peripheral vascular resistance are discussed in Chapter 6. In the majority of individuals, these changes pose no significant threat to maternal or fetal well being and are well tolerated. Even in women with pre-existing rheumatic heart disease and with most forms of congenital heart disease, the physiologic changes of pregnancy do not result in a significant threat. However, sudden cardiac decompensation may occur in certain individuals during pregnancy. Included in this group are individuals with previously diagnosed cardiac dysfunction as well as those who demonstrate decompensation for the first time during pregnancy. It is important to have a clear understanding of the normal changes of pregnancy so that normal complaints can be well managed. Symptoms that suggest significant underlying cardiac dysfunction can then be recognized as early as possible.

Pediatric Antiarrhythmic drugs are needed less often in children than in adults. Supraventricular tachycardias are the most common arrhythmias in children. The onset of supraventricular tachycardia is often sudden, and the duration is variable. Infants and young children with this arrhythmia may be unable to communicate the rapid heart rate, and the clinical course can progress to heart failure. Important signs of arrhythmia in the infant and young child include poor feeding, extreme irritability, and pallor.

Geriatric During the third and fourth decades of life, pacemaker cells decrease in number as myocardial fat, collagen, and elastin fibers increase. This change affects the SA node, which shows evidence of acceleration through the sixth decade. The number of SA cells at age 75 is 10 percent of what existed at age 20 years. Similarly, the AV node and the bundle of His lose a number of conductive cells into the fourth decade and the left bundle between the fifth and seventh decades. Alteration in the excitation and contraction mechanisms is an adaptive rather than a degenerative change because they maintain contractile function of the aged heart. The majority of rate irregularities in the older adult are attributed to myocardial damage.

Psychosocial Considerations

A patient's psychological response to an arrhythmia is determined by the severity of symptoms and the impact of the arrhythmia on life-style. Chronic or recurrent arrhythmias often cause the patient to fear incapacitation or even death if the arrhythmia recurs or cannot be effectively managed. For this reason, the patient's compliance with the plan of care is often enhanced.

There is evidence that significant short- and long-term emotional distress occurs in patients with ventricular fibrillation and subsequent cardiac resuscitation. The distress manifests as sleep disturbances, restlessness, irritability, and a strong identification with having been dead. Other evidence suggests that long-term emotional disturbances are rare. The perceived vulnerability and powerlessness complicate the plan of care. For some patients, the sense of vulnerability is alleviated by surgery (e.g., coronary artery bypass graft) because it is perceived as curative or by their ability to attribute the arrhythmia to a specific correctable cause (i.e., potassium imbalance). The sense of powerlessness stems from real and perceived losses. The losses may include, for example, a loss of employment and financial security, role status, physical or social independence, and short-term memory and a lack of control over their illness (see Case Study—Atrial Fibrillations).

Analysis and Management

As with the patient who takes cardiac glycosides or antianginal drugs, the perceived susceptibility to disease and its seriousness influences the plan of care. Because many of the antiarrhythmic drugs have unpleasant or undesirable adverse effects, the likelihood of compliance is also an important consideration. It is necessary to work with the patient and family members, when appropriate, to ensure their cooperation. Once the importance of continued medical treatment and follow up is understood, the majority of patients are usually compliant. The fact that the patient is often recovering from a life-threatening event, such as an MI, also motivates compliance.

Treatment Objectives

There are three general objectives for the management of arrhythmias. These include abolishing the abnormal rhythm, restoring normal sinus rhythm, and preventing a recurrence of the arrhythmia. Overall desired outcomes of antiarrhythmic therapy include maintained cardiac output, increased activity tolerance, and reduced fear and anxiety.

Treatment Options

There is a general consensus among health care providers that appropriate treatment for arrhythmias includes also treating the underlying disease processes contributing to the arrhythmia. These disease processes include cardiovascular (i.e., MI) and noncardiovascular (i.e., chronic pulmonary disease) disorders. Other conditions that predispose the patient to arrhythmias (i.e., hypoxia, electrolyte imbalance) should be prevented or treated. Help the patient to stop smoking and to avoid overeating, excessive coffee intake, and other habits that may cause or aggravate arrhythmias.

Intervention using an antiarrhythmic drug is appropriate when the patient has an acute arrhythmia that is producing life-threatening rhythm disturbances. The patient is hospitalized in a coronary care unit and placed on telemetry. After the acute phase has resolved, the need for antiarrhythmic therapy may end. In spite of this, there is some disagreement about the appropriateness of long-term antiarrhythmic therapy for patients with recurrent symptomatic episodes. Rational antiarrhythmic therapy requires that the health care provider possess the knowledge, skill, and ability to

- Accurately identify the arrhythmia
- Understand the mechanisms causing the arrhythmia
- Interpret the ECG and hemodynamic effects of an arrhythmia
- Understand antiarrhythmic drug actions, including the desired onset of drug action, the suitability of the various routes of administration, the need for a stable serum concentration, the likelihood of tolerance or toxicity
- Expect that the drug's therapeutic effects outweigh the potential adverse effects

The therapeutic/toxic ratio of most antiarrhythmics is relatively narrow; therefore, knowledge of pharmacokinetics is important to avoid toxic peak and subtherapeutic trough concentrations. It should be remembered, however, that therapeutic response to one drug in a particular class does not guarantee a therapeutic response to another drug of the same class.

Drug Variables

The general trends and recommendations for the management of arrhythmias are identified in Table 33–6. Note that the premature atrial contractions are usually not treated with antiarrhythmic drugs. Quinidine has long been used to prevent the recurrence of atrial fibrillation. However, some health care providers are questioning this approach because up to 50 percent of patients have recurrences of the arrhythmia within 1 year. There is also some evidence that the mortality rate may be increased with the use of quinidine. A cardiac glycoside may be the first-line drug for the management of both acute and chronic atrial flutter and fibrillation. Quinidine has been used in some patients with chronic PACs. Although the actions of quinidine and procainamide are similar, quinidine is generally preferred for long-term therapy because of the drug-induced lupus syndrome that can develop with procainamide. To prevent a drug-induced increase in ventricular rate, patients with atrial arrhythmias are often pretreated with a cardiac glycoside prior to receiving quinidine.

Not infrequently, propranolol and digoxin may successfully control the ventricular rate in patients with atrial flutter or fibrillation when maximal doses of digoxin alone do not. This additive effect may result because digoxin increases vagal tone, while propranolol blocks beta-adrenergic influences on the AV node. Verapamil or diltiazem may be preferred for slowing the ventricular rate in atrial flutter or fibrillation, although digoxin has long been used for this purpose. These drugs can also be used to treat paroxysmal supraventricular tachycardia. Although approved by the Food and Drug Administration only for the treatment of refractory arrhythmias, amiodarone and sotalol are being used more often for prophylaxis of atrial fibrillation.

Lidocaine is a first-line drug in the management of cardiac glycoside-induced arrhythmias. Phenytoin is a second-line drug for this purpose. Lidocaine is also the drug of choice for management of PVCs and ventricular tachycardia. Mexiletine and tocainide may be useful because they can be given by mouth.

Propranolol, acebutolol, and esmolol are not drugs of first choice for the initial treatment of most arrhythmias. However, they may be useful in combination with other antiarrhythmics in treating a variety of arrhythmias. Refractory life-threatening ventricular arrhythmias (e.g., ventricular tachycardia) may be managed with amiodarone, bretylium, flecainide, propafenone, and sotalol.

The proarrhythmic effects of some antiarrhythmic drugs are of special concern in patients with compromised left

Case Study Atrial Fibrillation

Patient History

History of Present Illness	BG is an 82-year-old white male in moderate distress with complaints of increasing dyspnea and fatigue. The dyspnea has progressively worsened over the past month, and he is now confined to home. He walks 1 mile per day. He sleeps with two pillows but awakens at night with complaints of dyspnea, sitting by the open window "to catch my breath." He follows a 1500-mg sodium diet.
Past Health History	BG denies allergies to food or medications. He had a mitral valve replacement at age 64 and a myocardial infarction at age 75 without sequelae. His last ECG was 2 weeks ago. He denies history of other hospitalizations, illness, consumption of alcohol, or smoking. Current medications: digoxin 0.125 mg po QD; furosemide 20 mg QD; K-lor, 15 mEq po QD.
Physical Exam Findings	Height: 5′8″. Weight: 155 lbs (9 lbs above usual). Vital signs: Blood pressure 160/70, respirations 28, increasing to 32 with minimal exertion; apical pulse 120 bpm resting and 130 to 140 bpm with exertion; radial pulse 104 bpm. Bibasilar fine crackles on auscultation. Diaphragmatic excursion 4 cm. Gallop rhythm on auscultation of the heart with variation in intensity of S_1. Liver 5 cm below costal margin. Skin pale without cyanosis.
Diagnostic Testing	Chest x-ray: Left ventricular enlargement and fluid at both bases and congestion of the pulmonary vasculature. ECG: Atrial fibrillation with rate of 124 bpm and occasional PVCs. Lytes: Na^+ 130 mEq/L; K^+ 3.6 mEq/L; Cl^- 92 mEq/L; BUN 34 mg/100 mL; creatinine 1.3 mg/100 mL.
Psychosocial Considerations	BG retired at age 75. He visits his health care provider only when necessary and takes little preventative care. He believes in natural foods and always eats nutritious meals. He has expressed on several occasions concern that he will become a burden to his 74-year-old wife, who is physically unable to assume responsibility for his care. They have an adult son and daughter who live six blocks away.
Developmental Factors	BG is likely to have age-related physiologic changes to body systems such as cardiac, renal, GI.
Economic Factors	Lives on social security and retirement benefits. Has Medicare parts A and B. Uses AARP pharmacy mail services for routine drugs. Will need to obtain new drug from local pharmacy until response to therapy is determined; therefore cost is greater than what he pays through AARP.

Variables Influencing Decision

Treatment Objectives

- Restore normal sinus rhythm.
- Prevent development of other arrhythmias.
- Prevent or reduce frequency of recurrent episodes of atrial fibrillation.
- Maintain adequate tissue perfusion and cardiac output.

Drug Variables	*Drug Summary*	*Patient Variables*
Indications	Quinidine: Preferred for long-term therapy but has tendency to cause cinchonism and questionable increase in mortality. Propranolol: Combined with digoxin effectively blocks catecholamine influences on AV node. Useful if rate not controlled with digoxin and/or is excessively rapid during exercise. Proven long-term effects on postinfarction mortality. Verapamil: Minimally slows heart rate because the slowing of SA firing is offset by increased reflex sympathetic activity, resulting in arterial vasodilation. Used in patients who do not respond to digoxin and beta blockers.	BG diagnosed with atrial fibrillation but has existing mild chronic heart failure also. Need to treat to reduce potential for decompensation. Increased risk of systemic emboli. History of previous MI and mitral valve replacement.
Pharmacodynamics	Classes produce effects through a variety of drug-specific actions. Mechanism not a specific decision point.	Antiarrhythmic actions will restore normal sinus rhythm and reduce blood pressure and pulse. This is not a specific decision point.

Drug Variables	Drug Summary	Patient Variables
Adverse Effects/ Contraindications	Quinidine: Tendency for cinchonism. Questionable increase in mortality. Increases potential for digoxin toxicity. Propranolol: Contraindicated in presence of respiratory disorders. Depression and bradycardia common. Verapamil: Bradycardia, hypotension, edema most common. Potential for sinus arrest.	BG has no history of respiratory disorders.
Pharmacokinetics	Vary with specific drug. Desire relatively rapid onset of action. Most antiarrhythmics can be administered at intervals equal to the elimination half-life of the drug after an initial loading dose.	BG is stable at this time. Physical changes of aging may contribute to this as a decision point because dosing based in part on elimination half-life. Oral formulation acceptable. BG is on digoxin but takes drug 1 hour before meals.
Dosage Regimen	Quinidine: Requires multiple dosing throughout day. Propranolol: Less expensive than verapamil and can be used once daily. Sustained release formulation available so once-daily dosing possible. Verapamil: Requires multiple dosing throughout day.	Able to take drugs by mouth but BG is more likely to be compliant with therapy with once-a-day dosing if available. May need to decrease dosage of digoxin due to potential for additive bradycardia with concurrent use of propranolol. These will become decision points.
Lab Considerations	Serum drug levels are of secondary importance if the response to the chosen drug is appropriate and adverse effects are absent. CBC, lytes, and liver and renal function tests should be monitored while taking antiarrhythmics.	BG visits health care provider only as needed. Monitoring therapeutic and adverse responses may become difficult. This becomes a decision point.
Cost Index*	Quinidine: Tablets: 1 Propranolol: Tablets: 1 Verapamil: Tablets: 1	Patient states he is not sure if he can afford "any more medicine" on his present income. Family unable to assist.

Summary of Decision Points

- Propranolol and digoxin combination effectively controls ventricular rate by blocking beta-adrenergic influences on AV node. Also helps minimize chance of sudden death related to previous MI.
- Therapeutic and toxicity responses monitored by patient rather than serum drug levels.
- Pharmacokinetics similar overall so no major influence on decision.
- May need to decrease dosage of digoxin due to potential for additive bradycardia with concurrent use of propranolol.
- Quinidine and verapamil increase potential for digoxin toxicity, especially in presence of furosemide.

DRUGS TO BE USED

- Continue digoxin but decrease dosage to 0.125 mg po QOD
- Continue furosemide at present dosage level.
- Add propranolol 20-mg tablets po TID. Titrate based on patient response but monitor patient closely because both propranolol and digoxin suppress AV conduction.

*Cost Index:
1 = $<30/mo.
2 = $30–40/mo.
3 = $40–50/mo.
4 = $50–60/mo.
5 = $>60/mo.

AWP of 100, 200-mg tablets of quinidine is approximately $12
AWP of 100, 20-mg tablets of propranolol is approximately $2.
AWP of 100, 40-mg tablets of verapamil is approximately $29.
AWP of 100, 0.125-mg tablets of digoxin is approximately $10.
AWP of 100, 20-mg tablets of furosemide is approximately $3.

TABLE 33–6 RECOMMENDATIONS FOR THE MANAGEMENT OF ARRHYTHMIAS

	Acute Antiarrhythmic Therapy		Chronic Antiarrhythmic Therapy	
Diagnosed Arrhythmia	FIRST-LINE DRUGS	ALTERNATIVE DRUGS	FIRST-LINE DRUGS	ALTERNATIVE DRUGS
Premature atrial contractions	Usually not treated		Quinidine	Disopyramide Procainamide
Atrial flutter, fibrillation	(Cardioversion) Digoxin	Verapamil Propranolol Class I_A drug	Diltiazem Verapamil	Amiodarone Digoxin with or without quinidine Verapamil
Paroxysmal atrial tachycardia	Verapamil	Digoxin Propranolol	Digoxin Verapamil	Amiodarone Quinidine
Atrioventricular nodal tachycardias	Verapamil	Diltiazem Adenosine	Digoxin or propranolol or esmolol	Class I_A, I_C, II Verapamil
Premature ventricular contractions	Beta blocker	Disopyramide Procainamide Quinidine	Disopyramide Procainamide Quinidine	Procainamide Disopyramide Amiodarone
Ventricular tachycardia	(Cardioversion) Lidocaine	Bretylium Disopyramide Procainamide Quinidine	Sotalol Disopyramide or procainamide or quinidine	Amiodarone Flecainide Mexiletine Propranolol

From Smith, C., and Reynard, A. (1995). *Essentials of Pharmacology.* Philadelphia: W. B. Saunders Company. Used with permission.

ventricular function or who have sustained ventricular arrhythmias. Although they are effective drugs and are usually well tolerated, in some cases the arrhythmia is worsened. Although all antiarrhythmic drugs may cause arrhythmias, flecainide has been shown to increase the incidence of sudden death and total mortality. Class I_C drugs may also aggravate heart failure.

Patient Variables

Identifying the circumstances in which the arrhythmia occurs helps determine if acute or chronic, long-term therapy is required. For example, the appearance of ventricular fibrillation in a patient with an acute MI may not require long-term therapy to alleviate the arrhythmia because the chance of recurrence is negligible. However, patients who have disabling symptoms such as dizziness, orthostatic hypotension, or palpitations may benefit from long-term therapy. Note that rhythm disturbances that are well tolerated in persons with structurally normal hearts may not be tolerated in those with heart disease.

Antiarrhythmic drugs should not be used during pregnancy unless the anticipated benefits outweigh the risks arising from failure to treat the arrhythmia or the possible risks to the fetus. Arrhythmias otherwise treated with quinidine or procainamide should also be treated during pregnancy without fear of adverse reaction to the fetus or newborn. Fetal hydantoin syndrome occurs in approximately 10 percent of fetuses chronically exposed to phenytoin. Lidocaine has been reported to increase uterine tone and to decrease uterine blood flow when used as an anesthetic drug in a paracervical block. Fetal bradycardia, either secondary to direct myocardial suppression or secondary to changes in uterine perfusion and tone, has also been reported. There is no evidence of a teratogenic potential with lidocaine, and it may be safely administered in pregnancy as the drug of choice for certain acute ventricular tachyarrhythmias.

As with adults, the drugs chosen for the pediatric patient should be used only when clearly indicated. Supraventricular tachycardias (often occurring with anxiety, fever, or hypovolemia) are the most common arrhythmias in children. Propranolol, quinidine, or verapamil may be used as prophylaxis or treatment. Lidocaine may be used to treat ventricular arrhythmias precipitated by cardiac surgery or cardiac glycoside toxicity. The child should be closely monitored because all of the antiarrhythmic drugs can cause adverse effects, including hypotension and the development of new arrhythmias.

Cardiac arrhythmias are not uncommon in older adults but, in general, only arrhythmias causing symptoms of circulatory impairment should be treated. Hypotension and heart failure may occur from the myocardial depressant effects of antiarrhythmic drugs. Cautious use is required, and dosage generally needs to be reduced to compensate for heart disease or impaired drug elimination processes (see controversy Antiarrhythmics: Good Versus Harm).

Intervention

Administration

The health care provider should check the blood pressure and apical pulse before each dose of antiarrhythmic drug. Withhold the dose and report to the health care provider if marked changes are noted in the rate, rhythm, or quality of pulses. Hypotension and bradycardia related to antiarrhythmic therapy are most likely to occur when drug therapy is being initiated or altered. These signs are more likely to occur with IV drug formulations than with oral dosage forms and may indicate the need for dosage adjustment. Continuous cardiac monitoring should be maintained during IV administration of antiarrhythmic drugs.

IV formulations are administered via a free-flowing peripheral vein with attention to concentration, administration

Controversy

Antiarrhythmics: Good Versus Harm

JONATHAN J. WOLFE

On the surface, the concept of adding an antiarrhythmic drug to therapy in the patient with a history of MI appears reasonable and natural. This is so because we recognize that the post-MI patient is most vulnerable to development of dysrhythmias. These irregularities of heart function constitute a leading cause of mortality in the recovery phase after surviving an MI.

Reality has proven that antiarrhythmics are problematic in actual practice. Part of the difficulty arises from their nature. Local anesthetic agents represent the most potent antiarrhythmics, but they are best administered parenterally. This is not practical for long-term treatment, and indeed use of lidocaine infusions is best ended as soon as possible. None of these drugs is free of hazard.

The search for an ideal orally administered antiarrhythmic has produced several classes of such agents. The best-studied and still first-line drug is quinidine. The advent of sustained release dosage forms has simplified compliance once an effective dose is established. The patient who cannot tolerate quinidine may be tried on procainamide and other drugs. Meta-analysis does not yet permit certainty about the relative value of drugs in Classes I, I_A, and III. In each case the practitioner must also consider the interactions of these drugs with other agents the patient likely will use.

The antiarrhythmics remind us powerfully that there are no pure drugs. In every case significant side effects accompany even the most valuable product. The patient with pre-existing cardiac disease and the patient who has survived an MI must be monitored closely in assessing the risk and benefit of add-on drug therapy.

Critical Thinking Discussion

- Your patient has survived an MI, extensive cardiopulmonary resuscitation, and a stay in the intensive care unit. In addition to being depressed, this 64-year-old-man is extremely apprehensive and fearful of dying. He has searched the Internet for information about cardiac arrhythmias. Now he returns to the clinic demanding a prescription for flecainide. What is your first response? Do you feel that it is proper for patients to request particular treatments?
- An 80-year-old woman in your cardiac care unit has just been cardioverted for the fourth time in 2 days. She has significant co-morbid conditions (diabetes mellitus, chronic renal failure, and hypertension). Her orders include prophylactic IV boluses of lidocaine 50 mg for treatment of PVCs or other arrhythmias. Is she at significant risk for this complication? Is a continuous infusion of lidocaine appropriate for her?
- A 72-old-man cared for in your clinic has been taking amiodarone for 2 weeks. His history includes two previous MIs. His wife calls, reporting that she found him dead in the back yard. She had not seen him for an hour. The emergency medical team was unable to resuscitate him from the unwitnessed arrest. His wife asks if the new drug caused him to die. What is your response?

time, drug-drug interactions, and patient response. The majority of IV antiarrhythmics should be infused via an infusion pump. Be sure to read package labeling carefully. Use only solutions labeled "for cardiac arrhythmias," and do not use solutions that also contain epinephrine. Lidocaine solutions containing epinephrine are used for local anesthesia only. They should *never* be given IV in the management of arrhythmias because the epinephrine can aggravate or cause new arrhythmias. Furthermore, rapid injection (less than 30 seconds) produces transient blood levels several times higher than therapeutic range limits. Therefore, there is greater risk of toxicity without a concomitant increase in therapeutic effectiveness.

With the exception of adenosine, IV antiarrhythmics should be administered in a peripheral vein to allow mixing with blood. Injection into systemic circulation is hazardous because a high drug concentration develops locally within the heart.

When changing from another antiarrhythmic therapy to mexiletine, give the first dose 6 to 12 hours after the last dose of quinidine, 3 to 6 hours after the last dose of procainamide, or 8 to 12 hours after the last dose of tocainide. When changing from parenteral lidocaine, decrease the lidocaine dose or discontinue the lidocaine 1 to 2 hours after administration of mexiletine or administer lower doses of mexiletine.

It is recommended that oral antiarrhythmic drug formulations be administered with food to decrease GI irritation. In addition, the drugs should be given at evenly spaced time intervals to maintain adequate blood levels.

Knowledge as to when peak plasma levels are reached for the various antiarrhythmic drugs may be helpful in determining when therapeutic effects are most likely to appear. However, there are many other factors that influence therapeutic effects, including the dose, frequency of administration, presence of conditions that alter drug biotransformation, arterial blood gases, serum electrolyte levels, and myocardial status. Serum drug levels are identified in Table 33–3, but they must be interpreted in light of the patient's clinical response to therapy. Antiarrhythmic drugs can accumulate in patients with renal or hepatic dysfunction, so patients should be carefully monitored for signs and symptoms of increasing impairment. Drug dosages may need to be adjusted based on these data.

Because some antiarrhythmics have proarrhythmic effects, the health care provider should be alert to the development of new arrhythmias. For example, a torsades de pointes arrhythmia may develop in patients receiving quinidine, procainamide, disopyramide, amiodarone, or sotalol. Women are more at risk for torsades de pointes than men, especially during administration of cardiovascular drugs that prolong depolarization. Liquid protein diets and electrolyte disturbances (e.g., hypokalemia, hypomagnesemia) may also precipitate development of this arrhythmia. By prolonging the QT interval, certain noncardiac drugs such as some antihypertensives, antibiotics, diuretics, antihistamines, tricyclic antidepressants, and phenothiazines may also set the stage for torsades de pointes. This arrhythmia may manifest as unexplained syncope. This arrhythmia and other proarrhythmic events often occur within a few days of initiating antiarrhythmic therapy, but they may also develop unexpectedly later in the course of long-term treatment.

Education

As with all drugs, antiarrhythmics should be taken as prescribed, with the dosage regimen individualized to maximize therapeutic effects and minimize adverse reactions. The patient and/or the family should be taught the name of the drug, the dose, and the reason it is needed. Patients should also be taught a proper administration technique for the dosage form they are receiving. Abrupt discontinuance of antiarrhythmic drugs has been associated with reappearance of arrhythmia. Encourage the patient not to miss a dose and to carry information regarding the prescribed drugs in written form. For patients on several drugs, the health care provider should stress the risks of multidrug therapy, such as the potential for drug-drug interactions, altered drug responses, and increased risk of adverse effects. The patient should also wear a form of Medic-alert identification.

Teach the patient and family members to recognize and report signs and symptoms of bradycardia, hypotension, arrhythmia, heart failure, pulmonary and peripheral embolism, and cardiac arrest. Teach the patient to avoid sudden changes in position to reduce the severity of postural hypotension. Blood pressure should be monitored frequently, particularly in patients with known ventricular dysfunction or hypertrophy. The antiarrhythmic drug may need to be discontinued if severe hypotension occurs. The patient's intake and output and weight should be monitored for indications of heart failure (i.e., shortness of breath, edema, weight gain, intake greater than urinary output, fatigue).

Advise patients to notify their health care provider or dentist of their drug regimen prior to dental treatment or surgery. Advise patients to avoid concurrent use of other medications without first checking with their health care provider to minimize potential drug-drug interactions. In addition, advise patients to avoid alcohol, smoking, excess sodium intake, caffeine, and sunlight (for those on amiodarone). They should be cautioned to avoid hazardous activities until the effects of the antiarrhythmic drug are known. Encourage patients to keep follow-up appointments with their health care provider.

Evaluation

Criteria that may be used to evaluate the therapeutic outcome of antiarrhythmic therapy include the following: (1) the impulse is generated at the SA node; (2) conduction occurs within a uniform, normal time period; (3) contraction takes place at regular, equally spaced intervals at a rate of 60 to 100 bpm in an adult and 130 to 160 bpm in a newborn; and (4) AV and intraventricular conduction take place via the appropriate conduction tissues. The data required for evaluating the therapeutic effectiveness relate to cardiac output, activity tolerance, fear and anxiety, tissue perfusion status, compliance or lack of compliance with the treatment regimen, and incidence of absence of complications resulting from antiarrhythmic therapy.

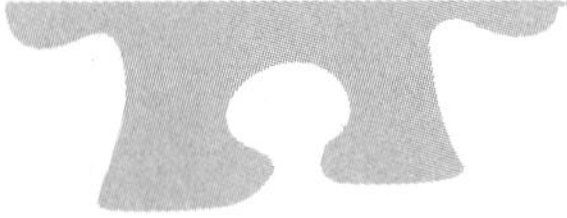

SUMMARY

- Cardiac arrhythmias, the most common complication of MI, arise from disruptions in the spontaneous initiation of an impulse (automaticity), the conduction of the impulse (conductivity), or both.
- Arrhythmias may originate in any part of the conduction system: SA node, atria, AV node, bundle of His, Purkinje fibers, bundle branches, or ventricular tissues.
- Atrial arrhythmias are viewed along a continuum of rate acceleration and a progressive reduction in atrial function: premature atrial contractions, atrial tachycardia (a rate of approximately 150 bpm), atrial flutter (a rate of about 300 bpm), and atrial fibrillation (quivering, uncoordinated activity).
- Nodal arrhythmias involve tachycardia with increased workload for the heart or bradycardia from heart block. Heart block involves impaired conduction of the electrical impulse through the AV node.
- Ventricular arrhythmias may progress to ventricular tachycardia, ventricular flutter, ventricular fibrillation, or asystole.
- Subjective information that should be elicited includes chest pain, palpitations, shortness of breath, dizziness, syncopal episodes, confusion, or diaphoresis. If the symptoms were experienced previously, the patient should be queried as to the length, frequency, and tolerance of each episode.
- A determination of cardiac rhythm and regularity and the presence of extra beats or skipped beats should be noted as well as the rate, rhythm, amplitude, and symmetry of peripheral pulses.
- Management of the patient with an arrhythmia is focused on relieving the acute episode of cardiac irregularity, establishing normal sinus rhythm, and prevention of further attacks.
- A determination should be made as to whether the arrhythmia should be treated before antiarrhythmic therapy is instituted. (Any arrhythmia that may cause symptomatic hypotension or sudden death should be treated.)
- Certain antiarrhythmic drugs are known to be more effective for one type of arrhythmia than another. Much of antiarrhythmic drug therapy remains a trial-and-error proposition.
- Even drugs within the same classification may vary in their electrophysiologic effects, and, when one drug is unsuccessful in a particular individual, another drug from the same class may be effective.
- It is important to remember that the potential adverse effect of any antiarrhythmic drug is an exacerbation of the arrhythmia or the development of new rhythm disturbances.
- Class I antiarrhythmic drugs (quinidine, procainamide, disopyramide) depress cardiac action by blocking the sodium channel in the myocardial membranes. They exert negative inotropic, chronotropic, and dromotropic effects. Class I drugs are used to treat or prevent the recurrence of tachyarrhythmias but themselves can cause arrhythmias and decreased output.
- Class II antiarrhythmic drugs (propranolol, esmolol, acebutolol) are beta-blocking drugs. Class II drugs are used for certain arrhythmias, hypertension, and a variety of other disorders.
- Class III antiarrhythmic drugs (amiodarone, bretylium, sotalol) are used in the treatment of life-threatening ventricular arrhythmias that are resistant to other drugs. Class III drugs alter the cardiac arrhythmia by slowing heart action, prolonging the duration of the action potential, or prolonging myocardial repolarization.
- Class IV antiarrhythmic drugs (verapamil, diltiazem) are calcium channel blockers.
- Although maintenance therapy to prevent the recurrence of arrhythmias is prescribed for nonhospitalized individuals, therapy is usually initiated within an acute care facility in which cardiovascular functioning can be closely monitored.

BIBLIOGRAPHY

Abernathy, D., and Andrawis, N. (1993). Critical drug interactions: A guide to important examples. *Drug Therapy,* 10, 15.

DiMarco, J. (1994). Adenosine. *Cardiology Review,* 2(1), 33–41.

Dubin, D. (1970). *Rapid interpretation of EKG's: A programmed course* (4th ed.). Tampa: Cover Publishing Company.

Fette, C., and Enger, E. (1996). Using amiodarone to tame cardiac arrhythmias. *Nursing,* 26(3), 32y–32BB.

Fleischer, D., Sheth, N., and Kou, J. (1990). Phenytoin interaction with enteral feedings administered through nasogastric tubes. *Journal of Parenteral Enteral Nutrition,* 14, 513–516.

Grant, A., and Wendt, D. (1992). Block and modulation of cardiac Na^+ channels by antiarrhythmic drugs, neurotransmitters and hormones. *Trends in Pharmacological Sciences,* 13(9), 352–358.

Green, H. (1992). Clinical significance and management of arrhythmias in the heart failure patient. *Clinical Cardiology,* 15(9 suppl), 1–13.

Griffith, M., Linker, N. Garrah, C., et al. (1990). Relative efficacy and safety of intravenous drugs for termination of sustained ventricular tachycardia. *Lancet,* 336(8716), 670–673.

Hampton, J. (1994). Choosing the right beta blocker. *Drugs,* 48(4), 549–568.

Hine, L., Laird, N., Hewitt, P. et al. (1989). Meta-analysis of empirical long term antiarrhythmic therapy after myocardial infarction. *Journal of the American Medical Association,* 262(21), 3037–3040.

Hohnloser, S., and Woosley, R. (1994). Sotalol. *New England Journal of Medicine,* 331(1), 31–38.

Morton, P. (1994). Update on new antiarrhythmic drugs. *Critical Care Nursing Clinics of North America,* 6(1), 69–74.

Nattel, S. (1993). Comparative mechanisms of action of antiarrhythmic drugs. *American Journal of Cardiology,* 72(11), 13F–17F.

Olin, B. (ed.) (1996). *Drug facts and comparisons* (51st ed.). St. Louis: Facts and Comparisons.

Pharand, C., and Chow, M. (1992). Sotalol: a class II antiarrhythmic agent with beta blocking activity. *Hospital Formulary,* 27(11), 1093.

Pritchett, E., Wilkinson, W., Clair, W., et al. (1993). Comparison of mortality in patients treated with propafenone to those treated with a variety of antiarrhythmic drugs for supraventricular arrhythmias. *American Journal of Cardiology,* 72(1), 108–110.

Schoenbaum, M. (1995). Recognizing torsades de pointes. *American Journal of Nursing,* 95(2), 54.

Shenasa, M., Borggrefe, M., Haverkamp, W., et al (1993). Ventricular tachycardia. *Lancet,* 341(8859), 1512–1519.

Stahl, L. (1995). How to manage common arrhythmias in medical patients. *American Journal of Nursing,* 95(3), 36–41.

Steinbeck, G., Andreson, D., Bach, P., et al (1992). A comparison of electrophysiologically guided antiarrhythmic drug therapy with beta blocker therapy in patients with symptomatic, sustained ventricular tachyarrhythmia. *New England Journal of Medicine,* 327(14), 987–992.

Yacone-Morton, L. (1995). Antiarrhythmics. *RN,* 58(4), 26–35.

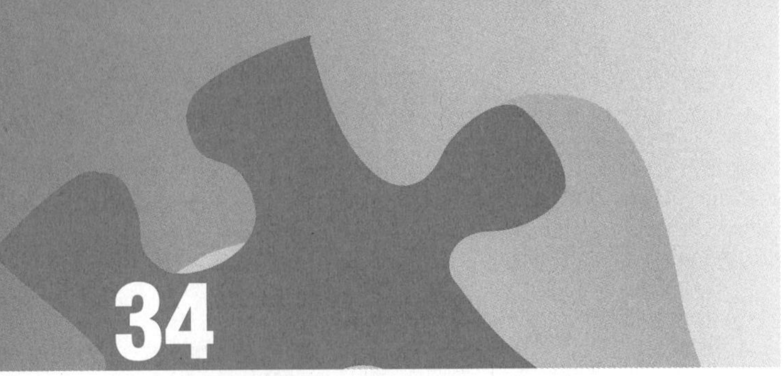

34 Antihypertensive Drugs

Hypertension is generally defined in an adult as a resting systolic blood pressure over 140 mmHg or a diastolic pressure over 90 mmHg, or both. If the condition is left untreated, hypertension leads to deadly complications such as heart and renal disease, blindness, and stroke. The condition is often referred to as the silent killer. The prevention, detection, evaluation, and management of hypertension are major public health challenges. Public education programs and the development of successful drug therapies have reduced the mortality rate of hypertension in the last several decades.

DETERMINANTS OF BLOOD PRESSURE

The principal determinants of blood pressure include cardiac output and peripheral vascular resistance. Cardiac output is equal to *stroke volume,* which is the quantity of blood in milliliters ejected with each heartbeat, multiplied by the heart rate. Normal cardiac output is about 5.5 L/min. An increase in cardiac output or peripheral vascular resistance increases the mean arterial blood pressure.

Cardiac Output

Cardiac output is influenced by the heart rate, the force of myocardial contraction, blood volume, and venous return to the heart. An increase in any of these factors increases cardiac output and, therefore, blood pressure. In contrast, when these factors are reduced, the blood pressure falls. Drugs that alter these factors include diuretics, beta blockers, and peripheral vasodilators. Diuretics decrease blood volume. Beta blockers decrease the heart rate and force of myocardial contraction. Vasodilators reduce venous return.

Peripheral Vascular Resistance

Peripheral vascular resistance is regulated by autonomic reflexes involving baroreceptors located in the carotid sinuses, the aortic arch, and in the wall of thoracic and neck vessels. Normally, the arterial system is compliant and dilates as arterial pressure and blood flow increase. As blood pressure rises, the baroreceptors send impulses to the vasomotor center in the brain. The baroreceptors respond to cause vasodilation and lowering of blood pressure. Afferent impulses from baroreceptors stimulate parasympathetic activity, leading to a reduction in heart rate and contractility.

The vasomotor center, a cluster of neurons in the medulla, maintains control of blood pressure by altering cardiac output and blood vessel diameter. Impulses are transmitted along sympathetic vasomotor fibers to arteriolar smooth muscle, and vascular tone is maintained. Increases in sympathetic activity cause vasoconstriction and the blood pressure increases. Decreases in sympathetic activity cause vasodilation and lower blood pressure.

Hormones

Hormones influence blood pressure by acting directly on the vasomotor center or on vascular smooth muscle. For example, epinephrine and norepinephrine are released by the adrenal medullae in response to low mean arterial pressure. The effects of these hormones are the same as direct sympathetic nervous system stimulation: vasoconstriction, increased heart rate, and increased myocardial contractility. These mechanisms work to raise blood pressure.

The kidneys release renin when blood pressure falls and renal perfusion is reduced. Renin acts on the enzyme *angiotensinogen* to produce *angiotensin I,* an inactive substance. *Angiotensin-converting enzyme* (ACE), found primarily in the vasculature of the lungs, converts angiotensin I to *angiotensin II,* a potent vasoconstrictor. Angiotensin II, in turn, promotes renal retention of sodium and water by stimulating the release of aldosterone from the adrenal medullae.

Antidiuretic hormone, produced in the hypothalamus and released by the posterior pituitary gland, also stimulates the kidneys to conserve water. Antidiuretic hormone released in large amounts causes vasoconstriction. In addition, the kidneys work to maintain blood pressure through regulation of fluid volume. Increases in fluid volume that result in higher pressures cause the kidneys to filter more fluid. When fluid volume decreases the kidneys conserve fluid.

Atrial natriuretic peptide hormone is released from myocytes in the atria in response to stimulation of stretch receptors by excess blood volume. Release of atrial natriuretic peptide acts as an aldosterone-antagonist to increase the glomerular filtration rate and the elimination of sodium and water, and to cause vasodilation. In addition, atrial natriuretic peptide inhibits the secretion of renin, aldosterone, and vasopressin.

Other substances such as endothelium-derived factors, histamines, kinins, prostacyclin, and various metabolites have the ability to produce local vasoconstriction. At this time, the exact mechanism of action and the clinical significance of these agents is not clear. Endothelin, a peptide, is released in response to low blood flow. It enhances calcium entry into vascular smooth muscle, causing an increase in blood pressure. Nitric oxide is a short-acting vasoactive substance secreted by endothelial cells. Nitric oxide is released in response to high blood flow rate and secretion of acetylcholine. Nitric oxide acts through the cyclic guanosine monophosphate (cGMP) second messenger system to cause systemic and local vasodilation.

HYPERTENSION

Epidemiology and Etiology

Fifty to sixty million adults in the United States have hypertension. This figure represents 25 percent of the adult population. Further, 31 percent of the population do not know they have hypertension and only 55 percent of persons with a diagnosis of hypertension take antihypertensive drugs. Approximately 21 percent of patients with hypertension have blood pressure that is not under control (i.e., less than 140/90 mmHg). Additionally, 11 months after antihypertensive therapy is started, half of the patients stop taking their drugs. Hypertension is responsible for over 30,000 deaths annually. However, there is evidence that the morbidity and mortality associated with hypertension decreases when the disorder is effectively managed.

Classifications of Hypertension

A classification scheme for blood pressure has been developed by the Sixth Joint National Committee on Detection, Evaluation, and Treatment of High Blood Pressure (JNC VI) and has redefined the disorder for persons older than 18 years of age. The scheme is based on the understanding that as both systolic and diastolic blood pressure increase, so does the risk of cardiovascular complications. Optimal blood pressure readings with respect to cardiovascular risk are less than 130 mmHg systolic and less than 85 mmHg diastolic. A diagnosis of hypertension is assigned when the patient's blood pressure exceeds 140/90 mmHg on two or more visits following an initial screening (Table 34–1). Unusually low readings should be evaluated for their clinical significance.

Risk Factors

Several variables are associated with hypertension. Nonmodifiable factors contributing to the risk for hypertension include age, gender, family history, and ethnicity. First-degree relatives (i.e., parents, sibling) of patients with hypertension have a three times greater risk of developing the disorder.

The onset of hypertension ordinarily occurs between the ages of 25 and 55 years. A diagnosis of hypertension is uncommon before the age of 20. However, compared with normotensive children, children younger than 16 years of age with blood pressure readings in the 90th percentile have three times the relative risk of developing hypertension as an adult (Table 34–2). Further, the younger the patient when hypertension is detected the greater the reduction in life expectancy.

Hypertension has been reported to be two to three times more common in women who are taking oral contraceptives, particularly in women who are also smokers. Men are affected more often by hypertension than women until women reach menopause. After menopause, women are affected more often than men.

An increase in blood pressure with increased age is primarily attributable to arteriosclerosis. The rise in systolic blood pressure accounts for the isolated systolic hypertension often seen in the older adult.

Modifiable factors associated with the development of hypertension include stress, socioeconomic and nutritional status, obesity, smoking, alcohol use, and physical inactivity. A high salt intake, decreased calcium intake, large family size, and crowding are also associated risk factors.

The incidence of hypertension in Native Americans is the same or higher than the general population. Among Hispanics, blood pressure is generally the same as or lower than that of whites, despite a high incidence of obesity and type 2 diabetes. The incidence of hypertension among Hispanics is thought to be high, but no confirmation data are available for this group. Hypertension is rare in non-Western societies. The prevalence of hypertension among blacks is among the highest in the world. Compared with whites, hypertension develops earlier in life, and blood pressure elevation is much higher in blacks. Blacks have a higher incidence of stage 3 hypertension than whites, causing a greater burden of hypertension complications. The earlier onset, higher prevalence, and increased rate of stage 3 hypertension is accompanied by an 80-percent higher mortality rate from stroke, a 50-percent higher rate of heart disease, and a 320-percent incidence of hypertension-related end-stage renal disease than that of the general population.

TABLE 34–1 CLASSIFICATION OF BLOOD PRESSURE STAGES*

Stage	Systolic (mmHg)		Diastolic (mmHg)
Optimal†	Less than 120		Less than 80
Normal	Less than 130		Less than 85
High Normal	130–139	or	85–89
Hypertension†			
Stage 1	140–159	or	90–99
Stage 2	160–179	or	100–109
Stage 3	Over 180	or	Over 110

*Based on an average of two or more readings taken at each of two or more visits following an initial screening in adults over age 18. The patient is not taking antihypertensive drugs and is not acutely ill.

†Optimal blood pressure with respect to cardiovascular risk is less than 120/80 mmHg. However, unusually low values should be evaluated for clinical significance. When systolic and diastolic pressures fall into different categories, the higher category should be used to classify the patient's blood pressure status. For example, 182/102 would be classified as stage 3 hypertension.

From Joint National Committee on Detection, Evaluation, and Treatment of High Blood Pressure. (1997). The sixth Report of the Joint National Committee on the Prevention, Detection, Evaluation, and Treatment of High Blood Pressure (JNC VI). *Archives of Internal Medicine*, 157(21), 2417.

Types of Hypertension

A number of different terms are used in an attempt to describe the various types of hypertension (see Terms Associated with Hypertension). These terms include primary hypertension, secondary hypertension, isolated systolic hypertension, pre-eclampsia, and malignant hypertension.

Primary Hypertension

Primary hypertension (idiopathic hypertension, essential hypertension) is the most common form, affecting 90 to 95 percent of patients. The cause is unknown, although a variety of physiologic mechanisms are under investigation for their role in high blood pressure. The renin-angiotensin-aldosterone system and mechanisms controlling sodium elimination are of particular interest. This system is usually activated in response to low renal perfusion. There is a renal retention of sodium and water, which increases vascular volume, renal perfusion, and blood pressure. Additionally, 15 percent of patients with hypertension have high levels of renin activity. With situations of hypovolemia and sodium deficiency, renin activity is stimulated, thus causing sodium and water retention and vasoconstriction.

In contrast, 30 percent of patients with hypertension, including blacks, have low renin levels. The low renin level is linked to sodium excess, which reduces renin activity. However, the effect is the same as in patients with high renin activity. There is increased vascular volume and elevated blood pressure.

Aldosterone is released when the renin-angiotensin-aldosterone system is stimulated. In response to aldosterone, the kidneys retain sodium ions and excrete potassium ions. The possibility of reducing blood pressure by increasing potassium intake rather than restricting sodium is being evaluated.

Vascular endothelium is now thought to be a hormone-producing endocrine gland in its own right. Endothelial cells produce a variety of vasoactive substances. There may be an excess of vasoactive substances that produce vasoconstriction. A deficit of these substances may result in high blood pressure.

The role of vasopressin in the development of primary hypertension has also been explored. A heightened sensitivity in blacks to vasopressin has been identified. This knowledge may help, in part, to explain some of the ethnic variability in blood pressure.

Type 2 diabetes mellitus (non–insulin-dependent diabetes mellitus) has been recognized as a risk factor for primary hypertension. The prevalence of hypertension in these patients is as high as 50 percent. Obesity in patients with type 2 diabetes explains part of the increased risk of hypertension. Type 2 diabetes, obesity, and hypertension may be accompanied by insulin resistance and hyperinsulinemia. Hypotheses being explored for the hypertensive mechanisms of insulin resistance include increased release of norepinephrine, sodium retention, and increased vascular tone. The increased vascular tone may be related to sodium transport mechanisms in the blood vessels. Blood pressure declines in black patients who have diabetes as the blood sugar levels are reduced (independent of a change in antihypertensive drugs).

Secondary Hypertension

Secondary hypertension affects less than 5 to 10 percent of persons with the disease. Secondary hypertension is related to an identifiable cause (see Common Causes of Secondary Hypertension) and usually develops before age 35 years or after age 55 years. Renal, adrenal, vascular, and neurologic disorders, pheochromocytoma, and exogenous compounds (e.g., certain drugs) are primarily responsible for secondary hypertension.

Isolated Systolic Hypertension

Isolated systolic hypertension is defined as systolic blood pressure greater than or equal to 140 mmHg, with diastolic blood pressure less than 90 mmHg. It occurs in approximately 10 percent of persons aged 65 to 74 years and in 24 percent of patients older than 80 years of age. Decreased distensibility of the aorta and large arteries occurs as arteriosclerosis progresses with age. The reduced distensibility of arteries causes an elevated systolic blood pressure without an increase in diastolic blood pressure.

Pre-eclampsia

Pre-eclampsia is characterized by elevated blood pressure, proteinuria, and edema. Several theories have been proposed for its cause. An increased sensitivity to angiotensin II, hormonal changes that increase vasoconstriction, and a tendency toward reduced calcium intake during pregnancy may combine to cause a hypertensive state. Generalized vasospasm, perhaps due to an imbalance in the production of thromboxane A_2 (a vasoconstrictor) and prostacyclin (a vasodilator), may contribute to high blood pressure.

Pre-eclampsia most often develops after the 20th week of gestation in susceptible women, although it can occur earlier in the pregnancy. An onset of pre-eclampsia during the second trimester is associated with increased risk of maternal and fetal harm. The disorder occurs during first and subsequent pregnancies, with blood pressure returning to normal between pregnancies.

TERMS ASSOCIATED WITH HYPERTENSION

Term	Definition
Primary hypertension	Hypertension characterized by a slow, progressive elevation in blood pressure over several years. Etiology is unknown
Secondary hypertension	Hypertension related to underlying renal or endocrine cause. Known etiology
Resistant hypertension	Diastolic blood pressure readings that are consistently above 90 mmHg while under treatment with antihypertensive drugs
Malignant hypertension	Severely elevated diastolic blood pressure over 140 mmHg associated with papilledema. A medical emergency
Isolated systolic hypertension	Systolic blood above 160 mmHg in patients over the age of 60
Complicated hypertension	Arterial hypertension of any cause in which there is evidence of cardiovascular damage related to BP elevation
White-coat hypertension	Elevated blood pressure when taken by health care provider but which is normal when measured outside of the health care environment
Refractory hypertension	Hypertension that fails to respond to therapy
Pre-eclampsia	Blood pressure elevation 15 mmHg above normal pressure during pregnancy and characterized by increased blood pressure, albuminuria, and edema.

Malignant Hypertension

Malignant hypertension is a rapidly progressing, potentially fatal form of hypertension. In this form of hypertension, the diastolic pressure exceeds 120 mmHg. Approximately 1 percent of all patients with hypertension develop this form. If the condition is left untreated, the 1-year mortality rate for malignant hypertension is almost 90 percent. Males, middle-age adults, and blacks are most likely to develop this form of hypertension. The most common mechanism of the disorder is bilateral renal artery stenosis. Severe emotional stress, excessive salt intake, or abrupt discontinuance of antihypertensive drug therapy may trigger a hypertensive crisis. Further, any disease or condition that produces high blood pressure can result in this accelerated form of high blood pressure.

End-organ damage is associated with all forms of hypertension. Any organ can be damaged, but the kidneys are affected most often (see End-Organ Pathology with Hypertension). Damage to afferent arterioles produces thick, stiffened arterioles that are less responsive to changes in perfusion. Renal failure may result. Other end-organ damage that results from arterial destruction includes severe retinopathy, encephalopathy, heart failure, and dissecting aortic aneurysm.

PHARMACOTHERAPEUTIC OPTIONS

Drugs from a number of different classifications are used in the management of chronic hypertension. The drug groups include ACE inhibitors, angiotensin II inhibitors, diuretics, alpha blockers, beta blockers, combined alpha and beta blockers, calcium channel blockers, and direct-acting peripheral vasodilators.

Angiotensin-Converting Enzyme Inhibitors

❒ Benazepril (LOTENSIN)
❒ Captopril (CAPOTEN)
❒ Enalapril (VASOTEC)
❒ Fosinopril (MONOPRIL)
❒ Lisinopril (PRINIVIL, ZESTRIL)
❒ Moexipril (UNIVASC)
❒ Quinapril (ACCUPRIL)
❒ Ramipril (ALTACE)
❒ Trandolapril (MAVIK)

Indications

ACE inhibitors are effective as monotherapy for patients with all types and degrees of hypertension and cardiac failure. ACE inhibitors are effective in patients with normal and low plasma renin activity and in patients with renin-dependent forms of hypertension. They are among the first-line drugs in the treatment of hypertension because of their efficacy and tolerability.

ACE inhibitors are recommended when the use of diuretics and beta blockers are contraindicated. There is compelling evidence to indicate that ACE inhibitors reduce proteinuria associated with diabetic nephropathy and help slow the progression of neuropathy. Early administration of ACE inhibitors may decrease the incidence, duration, and inducibility of ventricular arrhythmias during the course of ischemic myocardial injury. ACE inhibitors salvage ischemic myocardium, improve left ventricular function, reduce neurohumoral activity, and lessen the likelihood of electrolyte abnormalities.

COMMON CAUSES OF SECONDARY HYPERTENSION

Systolic and Diastolic Hypertension
- Coarctation of the aorta
- Cushing's syndrome
- Diabetes mellitus
- Pheochromocytoma
- Chemicals and drugs—Antidepressants, appetite suppressants, cyclosporin, erythropoietin, glucocorticoids, monoamine oxidase inhibitors, mineralocorticoids, nasal decongestants, nonsteroidal anti-inflammatory drugs, oral contraceptives, phenothiazines, sympathomimetics, tyramine

Isolated Systolic Hypertension
- Aging, with associated aortic rigidity
- Decreased peripheral vascular resistance
- Anemia
- Aortic valvular insufficiency
- Thyrotoxicosis

END-ORGAN PATHOLOGY IN HYPERTENSION

Kidneys
- Accelerated atherosclerosis, decreased renal perfusion
- Increased renin aldosterone, increased blood pressure
- Edema
- Decreased cellular oxygenation with resultant damage to renal parenchyma and renal filtration
- Renal insufficiency, prerenal azotemia
- Nephrosclerosis, renal failure

Eyes
- Retinal vascular sclerosis
- Exudates
- Blurring of vision, spots before eyes
- Blindness
- Hemorrhage

Brain
- Accelerated atherosclerosis, decreased cerebral perfusion
- Cerebral ischemia, transient ischemic attacks, stroke
- Weakened blood vessels, aneurysms
- Hemorrhage

Cardiovascular
- Coronary artery disease
- Increased myocardial workload
- Left ventricular hypertrophy, heart failure
- Decreased myocardial perfusion and ischemia, angina, myocardial infarction
- Sudden death

Peripheral
- Increased atherosclerosis

Vessel
- Weakened arterial walls, aneurysms
- Intermittent claudication, peripheral vascular disease
- Gangrene

Pharmacodynamics

ACE inhibitors reduce arterial pressure by preventing the generation of hemodynamically active angiotensin II from its inactive angiotensin I (Fig. 34–1). Angiotensin II is one of the most potent vasoactive substances known. It directly affects smooth muscle and stimulates the synthesis and secretion of aldosterone.

Hemodynamically ACE inhibitors reduce blood pressure as a result of arteriolar dilation and reduced total peripheral resistance. Heart rate and cardiac output do not increase in response, but renal blood flow improves. Glomerular filtration rates remain stable, suggesting that reduced glomerular hydrostatic pressure results from efferent glomerular arteriolar dilation.

Studies indicate that the entire renin-angiotensin system exists in vascular walls and in cardiac myocytes. This fact may explain the effectiveness of ACE inhibitors in patients with normal and low plasma renin activity and in patients who have had a removal of the kidney.

Beneficial effects of ACE inhibitors include improved responsiveness to insulin and no elevation in lipid levels. They significantly reduce left ventricular hypertrophy in patients with hypertension. The renal protection offered by ACE inhibitors has been demonstrated in patients with scleroderma crisis and diabetic nephropathy.

ACE inhibitors, however, have a paradoxical effect on renal function. On one hand, they cause renal vasodilation, preventing the slow deterioration of glomerular filtration; reduce proteinuria; and improve morbidity and mortality in diabetic nephropathy. On the other hand, in states of low renal artery stenosis, severe heart failure, and severe sodium and volume depletion, they can worsen renal function and even precipitate acute renal failure. The usual interpretation is that in severe heart failure, renal artery stenosis, and sodium and volume depletion, renal function is angiotensin dependent.

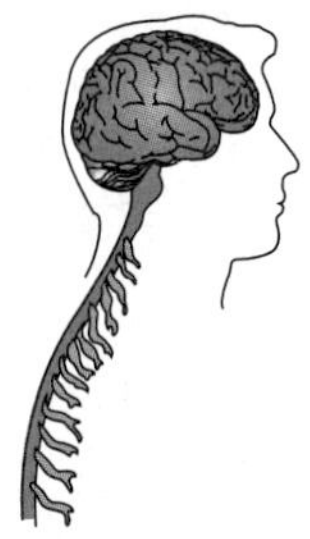

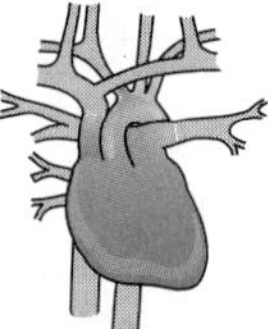

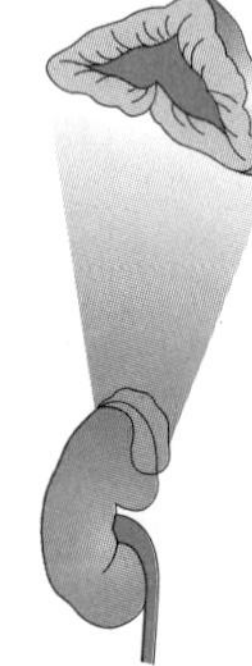

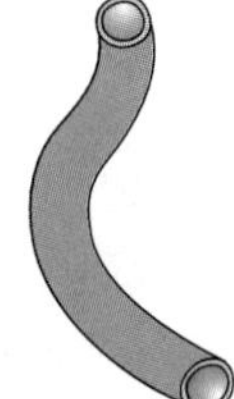

Figure 34–1 Sites of action of antihypertensive drugs. Note that some antihypertensive drugs act at more than one site. For example, beta blockers act on the heart as well as on the kidneys. Angiotensin II inhibitors act on the adrenal medullae and the vasculature.

Adverse Effects and Contraindications

ACE inhibitors are usually well tolerated and have a low incidence of adverse effects. A nonproductive cough occurs in 10 percent of patients, but it usually subsides several days after the drug is discontinued. Under normal circumstances, ACE is responsible for the breakdown of kinins. ACE inhibitors interfere with the breakdown of kinin, causing an inflammatory response in respiratory tissues and the subsequent cough. However, the cough can be confused with an exacerbation of chronic airway limitation. The incidence of coughing is higher in women than in men. Angioedema of the face, extremities, lips, tongue, glottis, and larynx has been reported in patients on ACE inhibitors.

ACE inhibitors can cause hypotension in patients who have been volume depleted or salt depleted as a result of prolonged diuretic therapy, dietary salt restrictions, dialysis, diarrhea, or vomiting. Although such circumstances are rare, ACE inhibitors have been associated with a cholestatic jaundice syndrome that progresses to fulminant hepatic necrosis and death. The mechanism of this syndrome is not understood.

In patients with severe heart failure whose renal function depends on activity of the renin-angiotensin aldosterone system, treatment with an ACE inhibitor has been associated with oliguria and progressive azotemia. On rare occasions, renal failure and death have occurred.

ACE inhibitor use during the second and third trimesters of pregnancy can cause injury and death to a developing fetus. ACE inhibitors are pregnancy category D drugs whose use should be discontinued as soon as possible once pregnancy is detected.

Sudden and potentially life-threatening anaphylactoid reactions have been reported in some hemodialysis patients on ACE inhibitors who use high-flux membranes.

ACE inhibitors should not be used in conjunction with supplemental potassium therapy or with potassium-retaining drugs because severe hyperkalemia may result as a consequence of reduced aldosterone levels.

Pharmacokinetics

The onset time following oral administration of an ACE inhibitor is less than 60 minutes except for ramipril, which has an onset time of 1 to 2 hours (Table 34–2). The bioavailability of the various drugs ranges from 13 percent for moexipril to 100 percent for intravenous (IV) enalapril. ACE inhibitors and their metabolites are well distributed, entering breast milk in small amounts. Ramipril does not appear to enter breast milk. Enalapril and its metabolite cross the blood-brain barrier in small amounts.

The majority of ACE inhibitors are biotransformed in the liver to active metabolites. Benazepril is converted to the active metabolite benazeprilat. Fifty percent of captopril is biotransformed by the liver to inactive compounds, with the remainder eliminated unchanged through the kidneys. Fosinopril is converted to the active metabolite fosinoprilat, with 50 percent eliminated through the kidneys and 50 percent through the stool. One hundred percent of lisinopril is eliminated by the kidneys. A small amount of moexipril is eliminated in the urine. The majority of moexipril is eliminated through the feces. Quinapril is biotransformed in the liver, gastrointestinal (GI) mucosa, and tissues to quinaprilat, the active metabolite. A large amount of the drug is eliminated through the urine, with the remainder eliminated in the stool. Ramipril is biotransformed to ramiprilat, the active metabolite, with 60 percent eliminated by the kidneys and 40 percent through the stool.

The half-life of ACE inhibitors varies from less than 3 hours to as much as 24 hours for the newest drug trandolapril. The half-life of all ACE inhibitors is increased in the presence of renal impairment.

Drug-Drug Interactions

The drug-drug interactions of ACE inhibitors are many (Table 34–3). The antihypertensive effects of ACE inhibitors may be decreased if they are taken with nonsteroidal anti-inflammatory drugs. Antacids decrease absorption of captopril and most other ACE inhibitors. Other antihypertensives and diuretics increase the risk of hypotension. Concurrent use of potassium supplements, potassium-sparing diuretics, and cyclosporine increases the risk of hyperkalemia. Increased serum lithium levels and symptoms of lithium toxicity have been reported in patients receiving concomitant ACE inhibitors. Simultaneous administration of tetracycline with quinapril reduces the absorption of tetracycline by approximately 37 percent because of the high magnesium content of quinapril.

Dosage Regimen

As with all other drugs, the dosage regimen for ACE inhibitors is drug specific and patient specific (Table 34–4). Most dosages range from 1 to 2 mg/day for trandolapril to 25 mg/day for captopril. The dosage for an individual drug is reduced for the patient also taking a diuretic. A precipitous drop in blood pressure during the first 1 to 3 hours following the first dose of an ACE inhibitor may require volume expansion with normal saline but is seldom an indication for stopping therapy.

Laboratory Considerations

ACE inhibitors may cause increased potassium levels and transiently elevated blood urea nitrogen (BUN) and creatinine levels, whereas sodium levels may be decreased. They can cause elevated aspartate aminotransferase (AST; serum glutamic-oxaloacetic transaminase [SGOT], alanine aminotransferase (ALT; serum glutamic-pyruvic transaminase [SGPT), alkaline phosphatase, serum bilirubin, uric acid,

TABLE 34–2 PHARMACOKINETICS OF SELECTED ACE INHIBITORS AND ANGIOTENSIN II INHIBITORS

Drug	Route	Onset	Peak	Duration	PB (%)	$t_{1/2}$	BioA (%)
ACE Inhibitors							
Benazepril	po	30 min	2–4 hr	24 hr	97; 95†	10–11 hr*	37
Captopril	po	15–60 min	60–90 min	6–12 hr	25–30	<3 hr	75
Enalapril	po	60 min	4–6 hr	24 hr	50–60†	11 hr*	60
	IV	15 min	1–4 hr	6 hr		11 hr*	100
Fosinopril	po	<60 min	2–6 hr	24 hr	95†	11.5 hr*	36
Lisinopril	po	60 min	6 hr	24 hr	0	12 hr	25
Moexipril	po	<60 min	3–6 hr	To 24 hr	50†	12 hr*	13+
Perindopril	po	UK	UK	UK	UK	UK	UK
Quinapril	po	<60 min	2–4 hr	To 24 hr	97†	1–2 hr	60
Ramipril	po	1–2 hr	4–6.5 hr	24 hr	73; 56†	13–17 hr*	50–60
Trandolapril	po	UA	60 min	UA	UA	16–24 hr	UA
Angiotensin II Inhibitors							
Irbesartan	po	UA	UA	UA	UA	UA	UA
Losartan	po	Varies	1–3 hr	UA	UA	2h; 6–9 hr‡	UA
Valsartan	po	Varies	1–3 hr	UA	UA	2h; 6hr‡	UA

*The half-life of metabolites.
†Protein binding of ACE inhibitor's active metabolite.
‡Half life of losartan and valsartan is biphasic.
ACE, Angiotensin-converting enzyme; BioA, bioavailability; PB, protein binding; $t_{1/2}$, elimiination half-life; UA, unavailable; UK, unknown.

TABLE 34–3 DRUG-DRUG INTERACTIONS OF SELECTED ACE INHIBITORS AND ANGIOTENSIN II INHIBITORS

Drug	Interactive Drugs	Interaction
ACE Inhibitors		
ACE Inhibitors	Alcohol Antihypertensives Diuretics Nitrates Phenothiazines	Excessive or additive hypotension
	Cyclosporin Potasium-sparing diuretics Potassium supplements	Hyperkalemia possible with concurrent use
	Indomethacin NSAIDs	Response to ACE inhibitor may be blunted
	Antacids	Absorption of ACE inhibitor may be decreased
	Digoxin Lithium	Increased risk of toxicity of interactive drug
	Allopurinol	Increased risk of hypersensitivity reactions
	Capsaicin	Increased incidence of cough
Captopril	Probenecid	Decreases elimination and increases level of captopril
Enalapril	Rifampin	Decreased effectiveness of enalapril
Quinapril	Tetracycline	Decreased absorption of interactive drug
Angiotensin II Inhibitors		
Irbesartan Losartan Valsartan	Phenobarbital	Decreased serum levels and effectiveness of interactive drug
	Cimetidine	Increases losartan levels and drug effectiveness
	Potassium supplements Potassium-sparing diuretics	Increases the risk of hyperkalemia

ACE, Angiotensin-converting enzyme; NSAIDs, nonsteroidal anti-inflammatory agents.

and glucose levels. Antinuclear antibody testing may be positive. Captopril may cause false-positive test results for urine acetone.

Renal function tests should be done before treatment with captopril. In patients with prior renal disease or patients receiving dosages higher than 150 mg/day of captopril, urine should be checked for protein. A complete blood count (CBC) and differential should be performed before starting therapy, then every 2 weeks for 3 months, and periodically thereafter. Therapy should be discontinued if the neutrophil count is less than $1000/mm^3$. Although such cases are rare, ACE inhibitors can produce a slight decrease in hemoglobin and hematocrit.

Fosinopril may cause a false low serum digoxin level when the Digi-lab RIA kit is used. Other testing kits should be used to monitor digoxin levels.

Angiotensin II Inhibitors

❒ Irbesartan (AVAPRO)
❒ Losartan (COZAAR)
❒ Valsartan (DIOVAN)

Indications

The outstanding success of the ACE inhibitors in the treatment of hypertension and cardiovascular diseases has led to interest in alternative ways to block the renin-angiotensin system. The development of specific, selective, angiotensin II receptor antagonists has been an important advance. Losartan is the prototype of this new type of cardiovascular drug. Thus far, losartan has been approved for use only in essential hypertension. Other potential uses include diabetic nephropathy and other forms of glomerulonephropathy, restenosis after coronary angioplasty, and atherosclerosis. Further, clinical studies have demonstrated that losartan is successful in lowering blood pressure in patients with renal insufficiency without worsening creatinine clearance. Valsartan and irbesartan are FDA approved for use only in hypertension at this time.

Pharmacodynamics

The ACE inhibitors block the conversion of angiotensin I to angiotensin II; however, angiotensin II is also formed by other enzymes that are not blocked by ACE inhibitors. In contrast, angiotensin II inhibitors block the binding of angiotensin II to specific tissue receptors found in vascular smooth muscle and the adrenal glands. This action blocks the vasoconstrictive effect of the renin-angiotensin system and the release of aldosterone, leading to a decline in blood pressure. Like the ACE inhibitors, angiotensin II inhibitors improve insulin sensitivity and reduce plasma levels of catecholamines.

Adverse Effects and Contraindications

The most frequently reported adverse effects of losartan are fatigue, headache, dizziness, insomnia, nasal congestion, sinus disorders, and cough. However, the frequency of cough with losartan is significantly lower than that seen with ACE inhibitors. Valsartan rarely, if ever, causes a cough. Losartan also appears to produce less angioedema than is associated with the ACE inhibitors. Diarrhea, dyspepsia, and elevated liver enzymes and renal function tests have been noted. Muscle cramps, myalgia, and back and leg pain have been documented.

TABLE 34–4 DOSAGE REGIMEN FOR SELECTED ACE INHIBITORS AND ANGIOTENSIN II INHIBITORS

Drug	Dosage	Implications*
ACE Inhibitors		
Benazepril	*Adults:* Initial: 5–10 mg po daily. Increase gradually to maintenance dose of 20–40 mg/day as single dose or two divided doses	Initiate therapy at 5 mg/day if patient also on diuretics
Captopril	*Adults:* Initial: 12.5–25 mg po BID–TID. May be increased at 1–2 week intervals up to 150 mg TID. Usual dose: 50 mg po TID. Maximum: 450 mg/day	Administer on empty stomach. Tablets may have a sulfurous odor. Initiate therapy at 6.25–12.5 mg BID–TID daily for patients taking diuretics
	Child: Initial: 0.3 mg/kg TID. May be increased by 0.3 mg/kg q8–24 hr	Initiate therapy at 0.15 mg/kg in children who are receiving diuretics or who have renal impairment
Enalapril	*Adults:* Initial: 5 mg po QD *or* 0.625–1.25 mg IV q6hr. Increase dose based on patient response. Usual oral dosage range 10–40 mg/day in one to two divided doses	Initiate therapy at 2.5 mg po/day *or* 0.625 mg IV for patients taking diuretics. May administer IV undiluted over 5 minutes or as slow intermittent infusion
Fosinopril	*Adults:* Initial: 10 mg po QD. Increase based on patient response. Dosage range 20–40 mg daily. Maximum: 80 mg/day	Monitor for neutropenia and agranulocytosis
Lisinopril	*Adults:* 10 mg po QD. May increase to 20–40 mg/day.	Initiate therapy at 5 mg/day in patients receiving diuretics.
Moexipril	*Adults:* Initial: 7.5 mg po QD. May be increased as needed. Usual dose: 7.5–30 mg/day in one to two divided doses	Take on empty stomach. Initiate therapy at 3.75 mg in patients receiving diuretics
Quinapril	*Adults:* Initial: 5–10 mg/day. May be increased at 2-week intervals. Dosage range: 20–80 mg/day in one to two divided doses	Initiate therapy at 5 mg/day in patients receiving diuretics
Ramipril	*Adults:* Initial: 2.5 mg po QD. Increase slowly to 20 mg/day in one to two divided doses	Capsules may be opened and added to apple sauce, apple juice, or 4 ounces of water to administer. Initiate therapy at 1.25 mg/day in patients receiving diuretics
Trandolapril	*Adults:* Initial: 1–2 mg po QD. Usual dosage: 2–4 mg/day.	Initiate therapy at 0.5 mg/day in patients receiving diuretics
Angiotensin II Inhibitors		
Irbesartan	*Adults:* Initial: 150 mg po QD	Volume-depleted patients should be stabilized before administration of irbesartan
Losartan	*Adults:* 50 mg po QD alone *or* 25 mg QD when used in combination with other antihypertensives. Range: 25–100 mg po QD–BID	May take without regard to meals
Valsartan	*Adults:* 80 mg po QD. Gradually increase to 320 mg daily	No adjustment is recommended for concurrent use of a diuretic, old age, or mild-to-moderate liver disease or renal insufficiency

*A precipitous drop in blood pressure one to three hours following the first dose of ACE inhibitor may require volume expansion with normal saline but is not normally an indication for stopping therapy. Discontinuing diuretic therapy or increasing salt intake 1 week before initiation of therapy decreases the risk of hypotension. Monitor the patient closely for at least 1 hour after blood pressure has stabilized. Resume diuretics if blood pressure is not controlled.

Clinical experience thus far indicates no clinically significant age, gender, or ethnicity-related differences in the overall safety profile of angiotensin II inhibitors. There is no evidence of rebound hypertension if the drug is withdrawn suddenly. Losartan does not alter lipids, glucose, or other metabolic parameters.

Pharmacokinetics

Pharmacokinetic parameters are best understood for losartan at this time. The pharmacokinetic parameters of irbesartan and valsartan are still being evaluated. Angiotensin II inhibitors are well absorbed from the GI tract, independent of food intake, reaching peak plasma concentrations in 3 to 6 weeks. Blood pressure reduction with losartan is biphasic and occurs several hours after the peak plasma concentration of the parent drug is reached. Losartan has a significant first-pass effect in the liver, with a resulting bioavailability of 33 percent. The active metabolite of losartan has a terminal half-life of 6 hours. Losartan and its metabolite actively engage angiotensin II receptors before undergoing oxidation and conversion to glucuronic acid conjugates in the liver. Because of the long half-life of the metabolite, losartan is effective for 24 hours with a once-daily dosing regimen. Overall elimination of the compound and the metabolite is one third renal and two thirds biliary.

Drug-Drug Interactions

To date, no clinically significant drug-drug interactions have been noted with losartan, although concurrent use of cimetidine increases losartan levels. Phenobarbital used with losartan produces decreased levels of losartan. Evidence suggests that concurrent use of angiotensin II antagonists with potassium supplements or potassium-sparing diuretics should be avoided to minimize the risk of hyperkalemia. Whether nonsteroidal anti-inflammatory agents interact with angiotensin II antagonists as they do with ACE inhibitors is not yet known.

Dosage Regimen

As with most other antihypertensive drugs, angiotensin II inhibitors are given on a once-daily dosage schedule. Volume depletion should be corrected before patients receive irbesartan. A lower dose of losartan should be used when this drug is given concurrently with another antihypertensive. The dosage of angiotensin II inhibitors should be adjusted slowly according to patient response.

Laboratory Considerations

Laboratory considerations for angiotensin II antagonists are similar to those of ACE inhibitors. Although such cases are rare, losartan can cause elevations in BUN and creatinine. Minimal decreases in hemoglobin and hematocrit are usually insignificant. Angiotensin II inhibitors occasionally cause elevated liver enzymes and serum bilirubin levels.

Diuretics

Diuretics are the mainstay for patients with hypertension. They reduce blood pressure when they are used alone or in combination with other antihypertensive drugs. Classifications of diuretics used in the management of hypertension include thiazides and thiazide-like drugs, loop diuretics, and potassium-sparing drugs (aldosterone antagonists). The basic pharmacology of diuretics is discussed in Chapter 39.

Thiazide and Thiazide-Like Diuretics

Thiazides (e.g., hydrochlorothiazide and chlorothiazide) are the most commonly used class of drugs. They are most effective against hypertension in patients with normal renal function. They decrease blood pressure by reducing blood volume and arterial resistance. The initial antihypertensive effects are the result of reduced blood volume. The long-term effects of these drugs are the result of changes in sodium balance and decreased sensitivity of the vessels to norepinephrine because of the sodium change.

Loop Diuretics

Loop diuretics (e.g., furosemide and bumetanide) are approximately 10 times as potent as thiazides, producing much greater diuresis. Like thiazides, loop diuretics reduce blood pressure by reducing blood volume. They have no effect on vasculature. Loop diuretics, however, are not routinely used in the management of hypertension because the amount of fluid lost is greater than is needed or desired. However, loop diuretics are used for patients who need greater diuresis than thiazides can provide (e.g., patients with heart failure).

Potassium-Sparing Diuretics

Potassium-sparing diuretics (e.g., spironolactone) are also used in the management of hypertension, although they are not as effective as other antihypertensive drugs. The diuresis produced by these drugs is relatively small. These drugs can, however, play an important role in balancing potassium loss caused by thiazides or loop diuretics. Because of a significant risk of hyperkalemia, concurrent use of potassium-sparing diuretics with ACE inhibitors or potassium supplements should be avoided. Many potassium-sparing diuretics have been combined with thiazides (e.g., spironolactone and hydrochlorothiazide).

Alpha-Adrenergic Blockers

- ❐ Doxazosin (CARDURA)
- ❐ Phenoxybenzamine (DIBENZYLINE)
- ❐ Phentolamine (REGITINE); (🍁) ROGITINE
- ❐ Prazosin (MINIPRESS)
- ❐ Terazosin (HYTRIN)

Alpha blockers are discussed in Chapter 11. The primary indication for this group of drugs is mild to moderate hypertension. First-generation alpha blockers (i.e., phenoxybenzamine and phentolamine) have limited usefulness for the treatment of most ambulatory patients with hypertension. However, they may be administered by continuous IV infusion in patients with pheochromocytoma crises or in patients with pressor crises related to clonidine withdrawal.

Alpha blockers selectively block postsynaptic stimulation of $alpha_1$ receptors, resulting in dilation of both arterioles and veins. Peripheral vascular resistance is decreased, thus reducing blood pressure.

The most significant adverse effect of alpha blockers is orthostatic hypotension. It can be particularly severe with the initial dose of the drug. Significant hypotension continues with subsequent dosing although it is less profound.

Beta-Adrenergic Blockers

SELECTIVE BETA BLOCKERS

- ❐ Acebutolol (SECTRAL); (🍁) MONITAN
- ❐ Atenolol (TENORMIN); (🍁) APO-ATENOLOL, NOVO-ATENOL
- ❐ Betaxolol (KERLONE)
- ❐ Bisoprolol (ZEBETA)
- ❐ Metoprolol (LOPRESSOR, TOPROL-XL); (🍁) BETALOC, LOPRESSOR, NOVO-METOPROL

NONSELECTIVE BETA BLOCKERS

- ❐ Carteolol (CARTROL)
- ❐ Nadolol (CORGARD); (🍁) SYN-NADOLOL
- ❐ Penbutolol (LEVATOL)
- ❐ Pindolol (VISKEN); (🍁) NOVO-PINDOL, SYN-PINDOLOL
- ❐ Propranolol (INDERAL); (🍁) APO-PROPRANOLOL, DETENSOL, NOVO-PRANOL, PMS-PROPRANOLOL
- ❐ Timolol (BLOCADREN); (🍁) APO-TIMOL, NOVO-TIMOL

COMBINED $ALPHA_1$/BETA BLOCKER

- ❐ Carvedilol (COREG)
- ❐ Labetolol (NORMODYNE, TRANDATE)

Indications

Selective, nonselective, and combined alpha and beta blockers are among the most widely used antihypertensive drugs, second only to diuretics. They are also used in the management of angina pectoris, tachyarrhythmias, myocardial infarction, and glaucoma. Beta blockers are discussed in Chapter 11. They are discussed here in relation to hypertension therapy only. Chapter 62 discusses the use of beta blockers for the treatment of glaucoma.

Propranolol, a nonselective agent, is the oldest beta-blocking drug and is considered the prototype of this class. In addition to its use in hypertension, angina pectoris, tachyarrhythmias, and myocardial infarction, it is used in the management of hypertrophic obstructive cardiomyopathies, pheochromocytoma, and hyperthyroidism and in the prevention of migraine headaches.

Pharmacodynamics

The exact mechanism by which beta blockers reduce blood pressure is not clear. Nonselective beta blockers (e.g., propranolol) block both $beta_1$ (cardiac) and $beta_2$ (smooth muscle of the bronchi and blood vessels). Beta-selective drugs (e.g., atenolol, metoprolol) have more effect on $beta_1$ receptors than on $beta_2$ receptors.

Beta blockers in general appear to impede the action of catecholamines at adrenergic receptors. $Beta_1$ blockade reduces the heart rate (negative chronotropic effect), the force of myocardial contraction (negative inotropic effect), and the velocity of impulse conduction through the AV node (negative dromotropic effect). The automaticity of ectopic pacemakers is also decreased as well as the blood pressure in supine and standing positions. They also provide blockade of $beta_1$ receptors on the juxtaglomerular apparatus of the kidneys to reduce the release of renin. Thus, angiotensin II–mediated vasoconstriction and aldosterone-mediated volume expansion are reduced and blood pressure is reduced.

In addition to the above-mentioned actions, some of the nonselective drugs improve exercise tolerance in patients with hypertrophic obstructive cardiomyopathy and decrease tachycardia and arrhythmias in patients with pheochromocytoma. They also act to reduce heart rate, cardiac output, and tremor in patients with hyperthyroidism. The drug action of propranolol in treating migraine headaches is unknown.

Labetolol is a combination $alpha_1$ and beta blocker. It promotes arteriolar and venous dilation through $alpha_1$ blockade. Heart rate and myocardial contractility are reduced by blocking $beta_1$ receptors in the heart. Labetolol also suppresses the release of renin by blocking $beta_1$ receptors in the juxtaglomerular apparatus of the kidneys.

Carvedilol competitively blocks $alpha_1$, $beta_1$, and $beta_2$ receptors. It also has some *intrinsic sympathomimetic activity* (ISA) at $beta_2$ receptors. Drugs with intrinsic sympathomimetic activity have a chemical structure similar to catecholamines. As a result, they can block some beta receptors and stimulate others. Both the alpha- and beta-blocking actions contribute to the blood pressure–lowering effects of the drug. Beta blockade prevents the reflex tachycardia seen with most alpha-blocking drugs and significantly decreases plasma renin activity.

Adverse Effects and Contraindications

Blockade of $beta_1$ receptors is associated with adverse effects such as bronchoconstriction, peripheral vasoconstriction, and interference with glycogenolysis. Compared with the nonselective beta blockers, selective beta blockers cause less bronchospasm, less peripheral vascular insufficiency, and less impairment of glucose metabolism.

TABLE 34-5 PHARMACOKINETICS OF SELECTED BETA BLOCKERS

Drug	Rte	Onset	Peak	Duration	PB (%)	$t_{1/2}$	BioA (%)
Selective Beta Blockers							
Acebutolol	po	60 min	4-6 hr	10 hr	26	3-4 hr; 8–13 hr*	<50
Atenolol	po	60 min	2-4 hr	24 hr	6-16	6-9 hr	50–60
Betaxolol	po	3–4 hr	7–14 days†	24 hr	50–55	15–20 hr	UA
Bisoprolol	po	UK	1–4 hr	24 hr	24 hr	26–33	80
Metoprolol	po/ER	15 min; UK	UK; 6–12 hr‡	UK; 6–12 hr	12	3–7 hr	UK
	IV	Immed	20 min	5–8 hr	12	3–7 hr	100
Nonselective Beta Blockers							
Carteolol	po	UK	1–3 hr	>24 hr	23–30	6–8 hr; 8–12 hr§	85
Nadolol	po	To 5 days	6–9 days	24 hr	4–30	10–24 hr	30
Penbutolol	po	60 min	1.5–3 hr‖	24 hr	80–98	5 hr	UA
Pindolol	po	7 days	2 wks	8–24 hr	40	3–4 hr	UA
Propranolol	po	30 min	60–90 min	6–12 hr	93	3–5 hr	25
Timolol	po	UK	1–2 hr‖	12–24 hr	<10	3–4 hr	UA
Combined Alpha and Beta Blockers							
Carvedilol	po	60 min	3–4 hr	8–10 hr	98	5–9 hr	UA
Labetolol	po	20–120 min	1–4 hr	8–12 hr	50	3–8 hr	25
	IV	2–5 min	5–15 min	2–24 hr	50	3–8 hr	100

*Acebutolol's half-life is biphasic.
†Betaxolol's peak cardiovascular effects with multiple dosing.
‡Metoprolol's maximal cardiovascular effects on blood pressure with chronic therapy may not occur for 1 week. Hypotensive effects may persist for up to 4 weeks after the drug is discontinued.
§Carteolol's half-life of parent drug and metabolite respectively.
‖Penbutolol and timolol's peak cardiovascular effects following a single dose. Full effects not seen until after several weeks of therapy.
BioA, Bioavailability; PB, protein binding; UA, unavailable; UK, unknown.

As useful as beta blockers are overall, they should not be used in patients with a history of sick sinus syndrome, heart failure, or second- or third-degree heart block. This is because blockade of $beta_1$ receptors in the heart reduces myocardial contractility and AV conduction, and produces bradycardia. Blockade of $alpha_1$ receptors produces postural hypotension.

Beta blockers should also be avoided in patients with asthma or chronic airway limitation. They are potentially hazardous to the patient because they block $beta_2$ receptors in the lungs, which causes constriction of the bronchioles. Beta blockers must be used with caution in diabetics receiving hypoglycemic treatment because they inhibit the usual sympathetic responses to hypoglycemia. Furthermore, beta blockers should not be used in patients with a history of depression because their drug actions can have an adverse effect on the central nervous system. They also can cause bizzare dreams, insomnia, depression, and sexual dysfunction. Beta blockers can precipitate labor in eclamptic states.

Pharmacokinetics

The pharmacokinetics of beta blockers are identified in Table 34–5. Most of the drugs taken by mouth have varying bioavailabilities ranging from 25 percent to as much as 100 percent for metoprolol and labetolol given IV. The high protein binding of some drugs and a long duration of action increase the likelihood of once-daily dosing for some patients. Most beta blockers are biotransformed by the liver. The remainder are eliminated via the kidneys.

Drug-Drug Interactions

The drug-drug interactions of beta blockers are identified in Table 34–6. All beta blockers, both selective and nonselective drugs, interact with a wide variety of drugs. The unopposed alpha-adrenergic stimulation caused by concurrent use of amphetamines, cocaine, ephedrine, epinephrine, norepinephrine, phenylephrine, and pseudoephedrine can lead to excessive hypertension and bradycardia. Most nonsteroidal anti-inflammatory drugs cause decreased antihypertensive action of beta blockers.

Dosage Regimen

Once-daily dosing with antihypertensive drugs is common. There are selected drugs that must be given on a twice-daily basis. Dosages should be increased slowly at no less than weekly intervals. Some drugs (e.g., pindolol) may be titrated upward every 2 to 3 weeks as needed.

Laboratory Considerations

Nonselective beta blockers may cause increased BUN, serum lipoproteins, potassium, triglyceride, uric acid levels, ANA, and blood glucose levels. Acebutolol, metoprolol, and labetolol specifically may cause increased serum alkaline phosphatase, LDH, AST (SGOT), and ALT (SGPT) levels.

Centrally Acting Alpha Agonists

- ❒ Clonidine (CATAPRES); (🍁) DIXARIT
- ❒ Guanabenz (WYTENSIN)
- ❒ Guanfacine (TENEX)
- ❒ Methyldopa and methyldopate (ALDOMET); (🍁) APO-METHYLDOPA, DOPAMET, NOVO-MEDOPA

Centrally acting alpha agonists are discussed in Chapter 11. Guanabenz and guanfacine are used in the treatment of

TABLE 34-6 DRUG-DRUG INTERACTIONS OF SELECTED BETA BLOCKERS

Drug	Interactive Drugs	Interaction
Selective Beta Blockers		
Beta blockers in general	General anesthesia Phenytoin (IV) Verapamil	May cause additive myocardial depression
	Cardiac glycosides	Additive bradycardia
	Alcohol Antihypertensives Nitrates	May cause additive hypotension
	Amphetamines Cocaine Ephedrine Epinephrine Norepinephrine Phenylephrine Pseudoephedrine	May result in unopposed alpha-adrenergic stimulation, leading to excessive hypertension, bradycardia
	Thyroid preparations	May decrease effectiveness of beta blocker
	NSAIDs	Concurrent use may decrease antihypertensive action of beta blockers
	Insulin Oral hypoglycemics	May alter effectiveness of interactive drug
	Dopamine Dobutamine Theophylline	May decrease the effectiveness of interactive drug
	MAO inhibitors	Concurrent use may result in hypertension
Labetolol Propranolol Timolol	Cimetidine	May increase toxicity from beta blocker

NSAIDs, Nonsteroidal anti-inflammatory drugs; IV, intravenous; MAO, monoamine oxidase.

TABLE 34-7 DOSAGE REGIMEN OF SELECTED BETA BLOCKERS

Agent	Dosage	Implications
Nonselective Beta Blockers		
Acebutolol	*Adult:* 400 mg po QD as a single dose or in two divided doses. May be increased as needed. Range: 400–800 mg/day	Monitor blood pressure and pulse frequently during dosage adjustment period and periodically throughout therapy. Apical pulse should be taken before administering selective beta blockers. Drug should be withheld and the health care provider notified if the pulse rate is less than 50 bpm. Metoprolol should be taken with meals. Instruct patient to take drug at the same time each day (daily dosing usually taken at bedtime) even if the patient is feeling well. Do not skip or double up on missed doses. Diabetics should closely monitor blood glucose levels. Reinforce need for weight loss, sodium reduction, regular exercise, limited alcohol intake, and smoking cessation. Extended-release products should be given once daily.
Atenolol	*Adult:* 25–50 mg po QD initially. May be increased after 2 weeks to 50–100 mg QD	
Betaxolol	*Adult:* 10 mg po QD initially. May be increased to 10 mg after 1–2 weeks. Maximum: 20 mg/day.	
Bisoprolol	*Adult:* 5 mg po QD initially. May be increased to 10 mg QD. Range 2.5–20 mg/day.	
Metoprolol	*Adult:* 100 mg po QD as a single dose or in two divided doses. May be increased q7days as needed, up to 450 mg/day.	
Selective Beta Blockers		
Carteolol	*Adult:* 2.5 mg po QD initially. May be increased as needed up to 10 mg/day.	
Nadolol	*Adult:* 40 mg po QD initially. May increase by 40–80 mg/day q7days as needed, up to 320 mg/day.	
Penbutolol	*Adult:* 20 mg po QD	
Pindolol	*Adult:* 5 mg po BID initially. May be increased by 10 mg/day q2–3 weeks as needed up to 45–60 mg/day.	
Propranolol	*Adult:* 40 mg po BID initially. May be increased as needed. Range 120–240 mg/day *or* 80 mg extended release capsules QD. Increase as needed *Child:* 0.5–1 mg/kg/day in two to four divided doses. May be increased as needed. Maintenance: 2–4 mg/kg/day in two divided doses	
Timolol	*Adult:* 10 mg po BID initially. May be increased q7days as needed. Maintenance: 10–20 mg BID up to 60 mg/day.	
Combined $Alpha_1$ and Beta Blockers		
Carvedilol	*Adult:* 6.25 mg po BID initially. May be increased q7–14 days up to 25 mg BID.	
Labetolol	*Adult:* 100 mg po BID initially. May be increased by 100 mg BID q2–3 days as needed. Range: 400–800 mg/day in two to three divided doses.	

mild to moderate hypertension. Methyldopa is not generally considered a first-line drug for the management of hypertension, although it is widely used, particularly for hypertension that develops during pregnancy.

Centrally acting alpha agonists operate within the brainstem to subdue sympathetic outflow to the heart, kidneys, and peripheral vasculature. The result is a decrease in systolic and diastolic blood pressure and a reduction in systemic vascular resistance. They also slow the pulse rate slightly. The alpha agonists also work to increase the negative feedback at the synaptic junction, resulting in decreased release of norepinephrine at this point.

The adverse effects of centrally acting alpha agonists include drowsiness, sedation, dizziness, weakness, sluggishness, dyspnea, and restlessness. Nervousness, hallucinations, and depression may also occur. Adverse effects associated with the GI tract include dry mouth, constipation, abdominal pain, and pseudo-obstruction of the large bowel. Hepatitis, hyperbilirubinemia, and sodium retention with weight gain has been noted. Impotence and loss of libido are not uncommon.

Adrenergic Neuronal Blockers

- ❒ Guanadrel (HYLOREL)
- ❒ Guanethidine (ISMELIN)
- ❒ Reserpine (SERPASIL); (🍁) NOVO-RESERPINE

Adrenergic neuronal blockers are not first-line drugs for hypertension. When they are used, they are administered concurrently with other drugs (e.g., diuretics) to increase their effectiveness and to prevent the development of resistance.

Guanethidine has limited use in hypertension because of the profound orthostatic hypotension that results. It can be used either alone or in conjunction with a thiazide diuretic or hydralazine in the treatment of moderate to severe hypertension. Guanadrel was introduced in recent years for use in patients with less severe hypertension. Reserpine has been used in combination with other antihypertensives (e.g., thiazides) in the management of mild to moderate hypertension. It us used less commonly today owing to its potentially severe adverse effects.

Adrenergic neuronal blockers act by depleting catecholamine stores and 5-hydroxytryptamine in many organs. Depression of sympathetic function results in decreased heart rate and lowering of arterial blood pressure. Guanethidine inhibits the release of epinephrine, whereas reserpine causes depletion of norepinephrine. Guanadrel acts by slowly displacing norepinephrine from its storage sites in nerve endings. Thus, the release of norepinephrine normally produced by nerve stimulation is blocked, leading to reduced arteriolar vasoconstriction. In addition, reserpine interferes with the binding of serotonin at receptor sites.

The adverse effects of adrenergic neuronal blockers vary with the specific drug used, although most cause nasal stuffiness is a result of vascular congestion. Depression to the point of suicide is a major concern and thus limits the use of this group of drugs. The major adverse effects of guanadrel are bronchospasm and heart failure. Fatigue, headache, peripheral edema, GI upset and urinary symptoms have been reported.

Orthostatic hypotension is the major adverse effect of guanethidine. It results from decreased sympathetic tone to veins.

Reserpine can also cause a Parkinson-like syndrome. Respiratory depression, seizures, and hypothermia are also possible.

Adrenergic neuronal blockers are contraindicated in patients with a history of depression, pheochromocytoma, and heart failure. They should be used with caution in patients with diabetes mellitus, impaired renal or hepatic function, recent myocardial infarction (MI), peripheral vascular disease, asthma, and patients taking monoamine oxidase inhibitors.

Calcium Channel Blockers

DIHYDROPYRIDINES

- ❐ Amlodipine (NORVASC)
- ❐ Felodipine (PLENDIL); (🍁) RENEDIL
- ❐ Isradipine (DYNACIRC, DYNACIRC CR)
- ❐ Nicardipine (CARDENE, CARDENE SR)
- ❐ Nifedipine (ADALAT CC, PROCARDIA XL)
- ❐ Nisoldipine (SULAR)

BENZOTHIAZEPINE

- ❐ Diltiazem (CARDIZEM, CARDIZEM SR, CARDIZEM CD, DILACOR, TIAZAC)

DIPHENYLALKYLAMINE

- ❐ Verapamil (CALAN, CALAN, SR, COVERA HS, ISOPTIN SR, VERELAN); (🍁) APO-NIFED, NOVO-NIFEDIN, NU-NIFED

The basic pharmacology of calcium channel blockers is discussed in Chapter 32. Although there are several other calcium channel blockers, those listed earlier are used predominantly in the management of hypertension. The drugs used most often include verapamil, diltiazem, and nifedipine. The newest agents are mibefradil and nisoldipine. Sublingual nifedipine has been used in emergent situations to reduce the blood pressure; however, the FDA has not approved this administration route. Further, the short-acting calcium channel blockers are not approved for the management of hypertension owing to the risk of MI.

All calcium channel blockers available in the United States block calcium influx in vascular smooth muscle, along the myocardial conduction system, and in the myocardium. Arteriolar vasodilation results. Mibefradil, the newest calcium channel blocker, produces coronary and peripheral vasodilation without decreasing myocardial contractility or causing reflex tachycardia. Although the newest antihypertensive drug on the market, early reports suggest that mibefradil may be associated with a dose-related decrease in heart rate. The bradycardia seems to occur whether mibefradil is used as monotherapy or in combination with beta blockers. In susceptible patients, the decrease in sinus node activity may result in severe sinus bradycardia or sinus arrest.

With the exception of mibefradil, calcium channel blockers cause vasodilation. The vasodilation is most profound with nifedipine. The incidence of reflex tachycardia is minimal with diltiazem and verapamil. However, because of their ability to compromise cardiac performance, diltiazem and verapamil must be used with caution in hypertensive patients who have a history of bradycardia, heart failure or AV block.

Direct-Acting Peripheral Vasodilators

- ❐ Diazoxide (HYPERSTAT, PROGLYCEM)
- ❐ Hydralazine (APRESOLINE)
- ❐ Minoxidil (LONITEN, ROGAINE)
- ❐ Nitroprusside

Indications

Direct-acting peripheral vasodilators are also used in the management of hypertension. Diazoxide is administered IV for rapid reduction of blood pressure in hospitalized patients with hypertensive crisis. Diazoxide is commonly used with a diuretic such as furosemide to counteract diazoxide-induced sodium and water retention. Diazoxide is also used orally to elevate blood glucose in hypoglycemic patients with hyperinsulinism caused by pancreatic islet cell adenoma or carcinoma, extra pancreatic malignancy, and other conditions.

Hydralazine is indicated for use in essential hypertension. Hydralazine can be used in early malignant hypertension that persists after sympathectomy.

Minoxidil is used in the management of severe symptomatic hypertension. It can be used for hypertension associated with end-organ damage that is refractory to other drug therapy. Use of minoxidil in mild cases of hypertension is not recommended.

Nitroprusside is used for rapid reduction of blood pressure in a hypertensive crisis and is consistently effective even in refractory hypertension. Nitroprusside is used to produce controlled hypotension during surgery to reduce blood loss.

Pharmacodynamics

Direct-acting peripheral vasodilators produce prompt reduction of blood pressure by relaxing smooth muscle of the arterioles. Cardiac output increases as blood pressure is reduced. Coronary blood flow and cerebral blood flow are maintained, while renal blood flow is increased. Diastolic pressure is affected more with hydralazine than systolic pressure. Postural hypotension is minimized through preferential dilation of arterioles over other vasculature.

Hydralazine increases renin activity in plasma. Increased renin activity leads to the production of angiotensin II. The result is stimulation of aldosterone and consequent sodium reabsorption. Hydralazine maintains or increases renal and cerebral blood flow.

Nitroprusside is potent and rapid acting, with effects similar to those of nitrates. The mechanism of action involves interference with the influx and intracellular activation of calcium. It relaxes vascular smooth muscle, promoting vasodilation. Thus, both arterial and venous blood pressure are lowered, reducing preload and afterload.

Adverse Effects and Contraindications

Adverse effects of centrally acting peripheral vasodilators vary with the specific drug. The adverse effects of diazoxide include sodium and water retention, which can lead to heart failure. Shock levels of hypotension, angina, myocardial ischemia, and infarction can occur. Atrial and ventricular arrhythmias and electrocardiographic changes have been noted. Transient cerebral ischemia may occur, and occasionally, cerebral infarction has been noted. Neurologic findings include throbbing headaches, dizziness, lightheadedness, lethargy, euphoria, momentary hearing loss, and weakness. Hyperglycemia may occur in diabetic patients and transient hyperglycemia in nondiabetic patients. Renal adverse effects include decreased urinary output, nephrotic syndrome, hematuria, increased nocturia, proteinuria, and azotemia.

Intravenous diazoxide is contraindicated in patients with coarctation of the aorta and arteriovenous shunt, and in patients known to be hypersensitive to diazoxide, thiazide diuretics, or sulfonamide-derived drugs. Diazoxide should be used cautiously in patients with diabetes mellitus, impaired cerebral or cardiac circulation, impaired renal function, and uremia. Caution should be used in patients taking corticosteroids or estrogen-progestin combinations. Safe use of diazoxide during pregnancy has not been established. Intravenous use during labor can cause cessation of uterine contractions.

Adverse effects of hydralazine include headache, tremors, dizziness, anxiety, palpitations, reflex tachycardia, angina, shock, and rebound hypertension. Adverse effects associated with the GI tract include anorexia, nausea, vomiting, and diarrhea. Sodium and water retention, urinary retention, and impotence have been noted. Blood dyscrasias including a reduction in hemoglobin and red cell counts, leukopenia, and agranulocytosis may also occur with hydralazine. Therapy should be discontinued if blood dyscrasias develop.

Common adverse effects of minoxidil include drowsiness, dizziness, and sedation. Potentially life-threatening effects include severe rebound hypertension, heart failure, pulmonary edema, pericardial effusion, pericarditis, thrombocytopenia, and leukopenia. The possibility of minoxidil-associated cardiac damage cannot be excluded, with changes in the direction and magnitude of T waves noted on the electrocardiogram. An initial decrease in hematocrit, hemoglobin, and red blood cell count can occur. Respiratory adverse effects include bronchitis and upper respiratory infection. Fluid volume expansion with sodium and water retention is common with minoxidil.

Dermatologic adverse effects of minoxidil include temporary edema and hypertrichosis. Elongation, thickening, and enhanced pigmentation of body hair can be seen 3 to 6 weeks after initiation of therapy. The changes are first noticed on the temples and between the eyebrows, extending to other parts of the face, scalp, back, arms, and legs. Other adverse effects include Stevens-Johnson syndrome, rash, and bullous skin eruptions

Hydralazine and minoxidil should be avoided in hypertensive patients with a history of MI, angina pectoris, cardiac failure, dissecting aortic aneurysm, or renal disease. Hydralazine is also contraindicated in patients with coronary artery disease, rheumatic heart disease, and tachycardia. The myocardial stimulation produced by hydralazine can cause myocardial ischemia and anginal attacks. In doses greater than 300 mg/day, hydralazine produces a clinical picture resembling that of systemic lupus erythematosus.

Adverse effects of nitroprusside include profound hypotension, nausea, retching, abdominal pain, nasal stuffiness, and diaphoresis. Restlessness, headache, dizziness, and muscle twitching occur. Retrosternal discomfort, palpitations, an increase or transient lowering of pulse rate, electrocardiogram changes, decreased platelet aggregation, and methemoglobinemia have been noted. Further, nitroprusside use has occasionally resulted in accumulation of lethal amounts of cyanide. Cyanide toxicity is most likely to occur in patients with liver disease who have low levels of thiosulfate, a co-factor needed for cyanide detoxification. The risk of cyanide poisoning can be minimized by avoiding prolonged use of nitroprusside.

Nitroprusside is contraindicated in persons with known hypersensitivity or compensatory hypertension related to an arteriovenous shunt or coarctation of the aorta. Nitroprusside should be avoided in patients with increased intracranial pressure. Cautious use is warranted in patients with hepatic insufficiency, hypothyroidism, severe renal impairment, hyponatremia, and in older adults with low vitamin B_{12} plasma levels or Leber's optic atrophy.

Pharmacokinetics

Oral formulations of direct-acting peripheral vasodilators are well absorbed from the GI tract. The onset of action ranges from immediate for nitroprusside given IV to 60 minutes for diazoxide (Table 34–8). Peak action is reached in 15 to 30 minutes for IV hydralazine and 8 to 12 hours for diazoxide.

Diazoxide and hydralazine are highly bound to plasma proteins. Minoxidil does not bind to plasma proteins. The known metabolites of minoxidil exert much less pharmacologic effect than minoxidil itself. Fifty percent of diazoxide is biotransformed in the liver, with 50 percent eliminated unchanged in the urine. Hydralazine is mostly biotransformed by the GI mucosa and liver. Biotransformation of nitroprusside occurs rapidly in the liver and tissues to cyanide and subsequently by the liver to thiocyanate. It has a half-life of 2 minutes.

Drug-Drug Interactions

There are several drug-drug interactions with direct-acting peripheral vasodilators (Table 34–9). Because diazoxide is highly bound to serum proteins, it can be expected to displace other substances that are also protein bound.

The effects of hydralazine are enhanced in the presence of alcohol, other antihypertensives, monoamine oxidase in-

TABLE 34–8 PHARMACOKINETICS OF SELECTED DIRECT-ACTING PERIPHERAL VASODILATORS

Drug	Route	Onset	Peak	Duration	PB (%)	$t_{1/2}$	BioA (%)
Diazoxide	IV	Immed	5 min	3–12 hr	>90	21–45 hr	100
Hydralazine	po	45 min	2 hr	3–8 hr	87	2–8 hr	UA
	IM	10–30 min	1 hr				UA
	IV	10–20 min	15–30 min				100
Minoxidil	po	30 min	2–3 hr	2–5 days	0	4.2 hr	UA
Nitroprusside	IV	Immed	Rapid	1–10 min	UA	2 min	100

BioA, Bioavailability; PB, protein binding; UA, Unavailable; $t_{1/2}$, elimination half-life.

hibitors, and nitrates. Nonsteroidal anti-inflammatory drugs reduce the antihypertensive response of hydralazine. Beta blockers can decrease the tachycardia caused by hydralazine. Metoprolol and propranolol, in particular, can cause an increase in the blood levels of hydralazine and vice versa. The pressor response of epinephrine is reduced in the presence of hydralazine.

Dosage Regimen

The dosage regimen for direct-acting vasodilators is individualized based on patient response. Table 34–10 provides an overview of the dosage regimens.

Laboratory Considerations

Diazoxide may cause increased serum glucose, BUN, alkaline phosphatase, AST (SGOT), sodium, and uric acid levels. It may cause decreased creatinine clearance, hematocrit, and hemoglobin values.

Hydralazine may cause a positive direct Coombs' test. CBCs, electrolytes, and antinuclear antibodies (ANA) titer determinations are indicated before and periodically throughout prolonged therapy.

Minoxidil elevates BUN, serum creatinine, alkaline phosphatase, plasma renin activity, and sodium levels. Decreased red cell, hemoglobin, and hematocrit counts may also occur. Hematologic and renal values usually return to pretreatment levels with continued therapy. Renal and hepatic function, CBC, and electrolytes should be monitored before and periodically throughout therapy.

Nitroprusside may cause a decrease in bicarbonate concentrations, $PaCO_2$, and pH and an increase in lactate concentrations. Monitoring blood thiocyanate levels is recommended in patients receiving prolonged nitroprusside therapy or in patients with severe renal dysfunction. Thiocyanate levels should not exceed 1 mmol/L. Plasma cyanogen levels should be determined after 1 to 2 days of therapy in patients with impaired hepatic function. Serum

TABLE 34–9 DRUG-DRUG INTERACTIONS OF DIRECT-ACTING PERIPHERAL VASODILATORS

Drug	Interactive Drugs	Interaction
Diazoxide	Diuretics	Concurrent use potentiates hyperglycemia, hyperuricemia, and hypotensive effects
	Phenytoin	Increases biotransformation of interactive drug
	Corticosteroids	May increase hyperglycemia
	Estrogen/progesterone	
	Phenytoin	
	Warfarin	Increases effects of interactive drug
	Insulin	May alter effects of interactive drug
	Oral hypoglycemics	
Hydralazine	Alcohol	Produces additive or exaggerated hypotension
	Antihypertensives	
	MAO inhibitors	
	Nitrates	
	Epinephrine	Pressor response of interactive drug is reduced
	NSAIDs	Decreases antihypertensive response
	Beta blockers	Decreases tachycardia caused by hydralazine
	Metoprolol	Increases blood levels of hydralazine; hydralazine increases blood levels of interactive drugs
	Propranolol	
Minoxidil	Guanethidine	Severe hypotension
	NSAIDs	Decreases antihypertensive effects of minoxidil
	Alcohol	Additive hypotension
	Antihypertensives	
	Nitrates	
Nitroprusside	Antihypertensives	Increased hypotensive effects
	Ganglionic blockers	
	General anesthetics	

MAO, Monoamine oxidase; NSAIDs, nonsteroidal anti-inflammatory agents.

TABLE 34–10 DOSAGE REGIMEN FOR SELECTED DIRECT-ACTING PERIPHERAL VASODILATORS

Drug	Use(s)	Dosage	Implications
Diazoxide	Hypertensive crisis	*Adults and Child:* 1–3 mg/kg (not to exceed 150 mg/dose) IV every 5–15 min until blood pressure is lowered to desired level. May be repeated q4–24 hr	Administer undiluted over 30 seconds or less only into a peripheral vein to prevent arrhythmias
Hydralazine	Moderate to severe hypertension	*Adults:* Initial: 10 mg po QID *or* 20–40 mg IM/IV repeated as needed. May increase after 2–4 days to 25 mg po QID for remainder of first week. May increase to 50 mg po QID up to 300 mg/day *Child:* 0.75 mg/kg/day po in 4 divided doses *or* 0.1–0.2 mg/kg/day IM/IV q 4–6 hr, as needed. May gradually increase to 7.5 mg/kg/day QID	Twice-daily dosing may be used once maintenance dose is established. Administer with meals to enhance absorption. Inject IV formulation through Y-tubing or 3-way stopcock
Minoxidil	Severe symptomatic hypertension/ refractory hypertension	*Adults:* Initial: 5 mg po QD. Increase at 3-day intervals to 10 mg/day then 20 mg/day, then 40 mg/day in two divided doses. Usual dose: 10–40 mg/day. *Child under 12 yr.:* Initial: 0.2 mg/kg/day. May increase gradually at 3 day intervals until desired response reached. Usual dose: 0.25–1 mg/kg/day in one to two divided doses	Doses of 100 mg/day have been used in adults. For rapid blood pressure control in children doses may be adjusted every 6 hr. Daily dose not to exceed 50 mg. May be administered without regard to meals or food. Discontinue drug gradually to prevent rebound hypertension
Nitroprusside	Hypertensive crisis	*Adults and Child:* Initial dose started as 0.25–0.3 mcg/kg/min. May increase as needed up to 10 mcg/kg/min. Usual dose 3 mcg/kg/min. Not to exceed 10 min of therapy at 10 mcg/kg/min	Drug effects are quickly reversed within 1–10 min by decreasing infusion rate or temporarily discontinuing the infusion. Monitor plasma thiocyanate levels and ECG in patients on prolonged infusions

ECG, Electrocardiogram.

methemoglobin concentrations should be monitored in patients receiving over 10 mg/kg of nitroprusside or patients who exhibit signs of impaired oxygen delivery despite adequate cardiac output and arterial $PaCO_2$.

Critical Thinking Process

Assessment

History of Present Illness

Evaluation of patients with hypertension is directed at uncovering correctable secondary causes of hypertension and establishing a pretreatment baseline in patients who have no end-organ damage. When symptoms do bring patients to seek health care, they often relate to the elevated pressure itself, vascular disease, or the underlying disease process of secondary hypertension.

Hypertension usually remains asymptomatic until the patient experiences severe blood pressure elevations (e.g., 220/110 mmHg). Complaints often associated with hypertension include fatigue, an early morning occipital and pulsating headache that goes away as the day progresses, lightheadedness, flushing, epistaxis, chest pains, visual and speech disturbances, and dyspnea. Complaints of impotence have also been noted.

Specific symptoms of secondary causes of hypertension can often aid in the diagnosis. For example, intermittent claudication from lower extremity ischemia may be related to coarctation of the aorta. Other symptoms of secondary hypertension include hirsutism and easy bruising (Cushing's syndrome), excessive diaphoresis, sustained or intermittent hypertension, paroxysmal headaches, palpitations, anxiety attacks, nausea and vomiting (pheochromocytoma), hypokalemia, muscle weakness, cramps, polyuria, paralysis, nocturia (primary hyperaldosteronism), and flank pain (renal or renovascular disease).

Life-style factors that may contribute to hypertension should be identified. Diet, physical activity, family status, stress level, work, and educational level should be included in the database. Factors that may impact treatment should also be noted. In men, a sexual history documents pretreatment level of sexual functioning.

Past Health History

The past health history provides information about childhood illnesses, accidents, injuries, hospitalizations, operations, obstetric history, immunizations, allergies, and all prescription and nonprescription drugs taken. Information related to alcohol use and illicit drug use is obtained. A drug history is obtained to determine allergies.

When asked, patients with essential hypertension may report a strong family history for hypertension, along with instances of intermittent elevations of blood pressure noted in previous blood pressure readings. Smoking, diabetes mellitus, lipid disorders, and a strong family history of early deaths due to cardiovascular disease should be noted in the health history. This information is used in part to determine the patient's risk factors for hypertension or the risk of end-organ damage, or both.

Physical Exam

Blood pressure reading should be verified at two subsequent office visits before the confirmation of a diagnosis of hypertension. Blood pressure and pulse should be measured in both arms with the patient supine, seated, and standing.

Postural changes can occur with pheochromocytoma, with diabetic autonomic neuropathy, in hypertensive patients using tricyclic antidepressants, and in older adults. A rise in diastolic pressure when the patient goes from supine to standing position is consistent with essential hypertension. A fall of blood pressure in the absence of antihypertensive drugs suggests secondary forms of hypertension. Verification of elevated blood pressure values should be made in different settings also (e.g., clinic or workplace).

The initial physical exam of the patient with hypertension should include an assessment of end-organ damage and identification of signs suggesting a specific secondary cause. Signs of end-organ damage include arteriolar narrowing, arteriovenous compression, hemorrhages, exudates, or papilledema on funduscopic exam. Carotid bruits and distended jugular veins in the neck, a loud aortic second sound, precordial heave, arrhythmia, or early systolic click on cardiac exam may suggest cardiovascular end-organ damage. Diminished or absent peripheral arterial pulses, peripheral edema, abdominal aortic aneurysm, and an abnormal neurologic assessment may also be noted with end-organ damage.

Signs suggestive of secondary hypertension include abdominal or flank masses (polycystic kidneys), absence of femoral pulses (coarctation of aorta), tachycardia, diaphoresis, orthostatic hypotension (pheochromocytoma), abdominal bruits (renovascular disease), truncal obesity, ecchymoses, pigmented striae (Cushing's syndrome), and enlarged or nodular thyroid gland (hyperthyroidism).

Diagnostic Testing

Diagnostic testing is important to assess for end-organ damage, to identify patients at high risk for developing cardiovascular complications, to determine if other cardiovascular complications exist, and to screen for possible secondary causes of hypertension. Routine tests for all newly diagnosed hypertensive patients include hemoglobin and hematocrit, chemistry panel (i.e., potassium, creatinine, fasting glucose, calcium, and uric acid), cholesterol, fasting lipid panels, urinalysis, and electrocardiogram. When specific secondary causes of hypertension are suspected, a chest x-ray study, dexamethasone suppression test (Cushing's syndrome), urinary metanephrine and vanillylmandelic acid levels (pheochromocytoma), intravenous pyelogram, renal scan, or angiography (renal vascular disease) and plasma renin activity levels (primary aldosteronism or renovascular disease) may be ordered. By obtaining these laboratory tests, the patient's cardiovascular risk and potential for complications associated with antihypertensive therapy can be assessed.

Developmental Considerations

Perinatal Hypertension is a serious complication of pregnancy. The risk to both mother and neonate can be reduced by appropriate assessment, therapy, and supervision. Hypertension may be an indication of underlying maternal disease aggravated by pregnancy. Hypertension may also be the first sign of pre-eclampsia.

The incidence of chronic hypertension in pregnant women ranges from 1 to 5 percent. The rates are higher in older women, obese women, and black women.

During normal pregnancy, systolic pressure changes very little. Diastolic pressure decreases by 10 mmHg in early pregnancy and rises to pre-pregnancy levels in the third trimester. The initial fall is due to general vasodilation that occurs with pregnancy. An increase in renin and aldosterone levels occurs in normal pregnancy.

Chronic hypertension during pregnancy may be mild or severe. Diagnostic criteria for hypertension in pregnancy include a rise of blood pressure of 20 to 30 mmHg from preconception values or first trimester values and an absolute level of blood pressure greater than 140/90 mmHg at any stage of pregnancy. Severe hypertension is present when blood pressure readings are greater than 170/110 mmHg.

Pregnant women with chronic hypertension are at risk for superimposed pre-eclampsia and abruptio placentae. Accelerated hypertension may result in disseminated intravascular coagulation and resultant end-organ damage to the mother. Fetal death or intrauterine growth restriction may occur as a result of uteroplacental insufficiency from hypertension. Hypertension is often associated with increased risks of fetal growth restriction and can cause both maternal and fetal problems. Control of moderate and severe hypertension results in lower rates of perinatal morbidity and mortality.

Pediatric The prevalence of hypertension in children varies from 0 to 13 percent. Frequent causes of persistent hypertension in children are renal hypertension and coarctation of the aorta. Children have a higher risk of hypertension if both parents are hypertensive. There is a striking increase in sustained new hypertension between the ages of 15 and 25 years. It is not clear if hypertensive adolescents continue to be hypertensive as adults. Premature labeling of adolescents as hypertensive may interfere with some career choices and the ability to obtain life insurance later. However, children whose blood pressure is consistently above the 95 percentile for height, weight, and age should be closely evaluated and treated.

Criteria used for categorizing hypertension in adults is not applicable to children. Blood pressure normally increases in children at a rate of 1½ mmHg systolic and 1 mmHg diastolic values per year. Blood pressure readings level off at 18 to 20 years of age (Table 34-11).

Compliance with treatment regimens can be a major problem with adolescents who are asymptomatic. They often do not want to be different from peers with diet and lifestyle.

TABLE 34–11 AVERAGE BLOOD PRESSURES BY SELECTED AGES IN GIRLS AND BOYS

	Girls		Boys	
Age/Year	50TH PERCENTILE	90TH PERCENTILE	50TH PERCENTILE	90TH PERCENTILE
1	91/54	105/67	90/56	105/69
3	91/56	106/69	92/55	107/68
6	96/57	111/70	96/57	111/70
9	100/61	115/74	101/61	115/74
12	107/66	122/78	107/64	121/77
15	111/67	126/82	114/65	129/79
18	112/66	127/80	121/70	136/84

Data from the National High Blood Pressure Education Program Working Group on Hypertension Control in Children and Adolescents, 1996. Update on the 1987 task force report on high blood pressure in children and adolescents. A working group report from the National High Blood Pressure Education Program. *Pediatrics* 98(4 Pt 1), 649–658.

Geriatric The prevalence of hypertension among older adults is extremely common. Among Americans aged 60 and older, elevated blood pressure occurs in about 60 percent of whites, 71 percent of blacks, and 61 percent of Hispanics. Especially among older adults, systolic blood pressure is a more accurate predictor of adverse events (i.e., coronary artery disease, heart failure, stroke, and end-stage renal disease) than is diastolic blood pressure. Primary hypertension is the most common form of hypertension in older adults.

Blood pressure must be measured with special care in older adults because some persons have *pseudohypertension,* a falsely high blood pressure reading, due to excessive vascular stiffness. In addition, older persons with hypertension and excessive variability in systolic blood pressure values may have white-coat hypertension. Additionally, older adults are more likely to experience orthostatic changes in blood pressure than younger patients. Thus, blood pressure readings should always be measured with the patient standing as well as in the seated or supine positions.

The older adult is at increased risk for adverse drug effects because of the physiologic changes associated with aging. These changes can affect the concentration and distribution of drugs. The effects of drugs at their sites of action may also be affected. Renal blood flow decreases with age, which affects the dosing of drugs that are eliminated by the kidneys. Lean muscle mass decreases, whereas the proportion of fat in the body increases. This factor may extend the effects of fat-soluble drugs.

Further, older adults often take multiple drugs obtained from several different physicians. Eye drops might not be mentioned when patients are asked to list drugs taken. Yet ocular drugs (e.g., beta blockers) may cause significant systemic effects.

Psychosocial Considerations

Cultural values and beliefs influence how a person defines health and health care. It is important to understand these cultural beliefs and incorporate cultural sensitivity into delivery of care.

Patients cope differently with a diagnosis of hypertension. Acceptance, denial, and retreat are some reactions. It is important to allow patients to express fears and feelings in a nonjudgmental, empathetic atmosphere. Changes in attitudes and beliefs about self, illness, treatment, and relationships with family and health care providers are important to note. Identifying present life stressors that may be affecting the patient is helpful.

Further, patients may not comply with their treatment regimen for a variety of reasons. For some patients, it is difficult to realize that treatment now, when they feel well, will prevent future complications. For others, the drugs interfere with their quality of life. The idea of life-long treatment is a difficult adaptation for some people. The cost of drugs may also be an issue for patients who have to pay for their drugs out of their pocket (see Case Study—Hypertension).

Analysis and Management

Treatment Objectives

The immediate goal of antihypertensive therapy is to reduce arterial pressure, minimize organ damage, and prolong life. The goal of prevention and management of hypertension is to reduce morbidity and mortality by the least intrusive means possible. This goal can be accomplished by achieving and maintaining the systolic pressure below 140 mmHg and diastolic pressure under 90 mmHg while controlling modifiable risk factors for cardiovascular disease. Treatment interventions to levels below 140/90 may prevent stroke, preserve renal function, and prevent or slow progression of heart failure. Drug therapy used appropriately can enhance the patient's quality of life.

Treatment Options

Hypertension is a multifactorial disease. Yet, no clinically useful indicators (e.g., age, race, renin status) are available to guide which drug will be effective for a specific patient. Individualizing therapy is essential to attain a successful outcome of antihypertensive therapies, although there is a 60 to 80 percent chance the patient will respond to a particular drug group. Life-style changes should be included in the treatment plan as early as possible.

Life-style Changes Although life-style changes are discussed in this section on treatment options, life-style changes are not an option. They are extremely important aspects of the management plan, particularly for patients with dyslipidemia or diabetes. Life-style changes have been

Case Study Hypertension

Patient History

History of Present Illness	MD is a 57-year-old white asymptomatic female who presents for a routine employment physical. She is anticipating a mid-life career change.
Past Health History	No known allergies. Nonsmoker, nondrinker. Was diagnosed with non–insulin-dependent diabetes 10 years ago. Blood sugars poorly controlled by diet. Quit smoking 7 years ago but gained 50 lbs. Stopped smoking because of an exacerbation of her asthma. Denies prevous personal or family history of cardiovascular disease and renal or hepatic disorders, although patient is a poor historian. Medical records indicate patient not always compliant with recommended treatment plans regardless of state of health. MD reports she is perimenopausal. Her last physical and eye exams were 2 years ago. Reports no regular exercise program.
Physical Exam	Height: 5'5". Weight: 182 lbs. Today's B/P 210/118 right arm sitting and 206/114 left arm sitting. Apical pulse 100 and regular. Previous three readings ranged from 152/88 to 194/96. Apical pulse 82 and regular. PMI not discernable. No lifts, heaves, thrills, or murmurs noted. Negative for extra heart sounds. No carotid bruits noted. Breath sounds clear to auscultation bilaterally. Abdomen negative for bruits or palpable masses. Pulses +2 all four extremities, no peripheral edema. Neurologic exam negative. Funduscopy unremarkable.
Diagnostic Testing	Chest x-ray studies unremarkable. Urinalysis: glycosuria, no protein. CBC: unremarkable. Hgb: 12.9, Hct: 42.0. Serum calcium 9.0 mg/dL. Chloride: 102 mmol/L. Blood sugar: 180 mg/dL. BUN: 14 mg/dL. Creatinine: 1.0 mg/dL. Uric acid: 4.8 mg/dL. ALT (SGPT): 28 U/L, AST (SGOT): 34 U/L. Total cholesterol: 228 mg/dL. HDL: 46 mg/dL. LDL: 147 mg/dL. ECG: normal sinus rhythm.
Developmental Considerations	MD lives with her husband, who is a traveling architect. Their three adult children have recently moved into an apartment of their own. Husband and wife feel "like their nest is empty."
Psychosocial Considerations	MD's preferred health care provider is naturopath. She would prefer to receive all health care from this individual, particularly because he will be able to meet all of her health care needs with naturopathy.
Economic Factors	MD is covered for prescriptions under her current health plan. Co-payments range from \$5–\$10 per drug. MD is an accountant and does not rely on her husband for income.

Variables Influencing Decision

Treatment Objectives

- Reduce arterial pressure safely and effectively
- Prevent adverse effects and maintain quality of life
- Minimize end-organ complications such as stroke, cardiovascular disease, and renal failure

Drug Variables	*Drug Summary*	*Patient Variables*
Indications	Diuretics, beta blockers, calcium channel blockers, ACE inhibitors, angiotensin II antagonists, and sympatholytic drugs are indicated in the treatment of elevated systolic and diastolic blood pressures.	This will become a decision point because MD's blood pressure has exceeded 140/90 on her last three readings. Further, lab values reflect probable atherosclerosis.
Pharmacodynamics	Each drug category has different mechanisms of action.	There are no pharmacodynamic parameters impacting MD's treatment decision at this time.

Drug Variables	*Drug Summary*	*Patient Variables*
Adverse Effects/ Contraindications	Thiazides are contraindicated in poorly controlled diabetes and severe hyperlipidemia. Beta blockers are contraindicated in diabetes and asthma and worsen elevated triglyceride levels. Calcium channel blockers can cause decrease in regional myocardial perfusion and sick sinus syndrome. Ace inhibitors can cause bronchial irritation. Angiotensin II antagonists apparently have less angioedema and respiratory adverse effects than ACE inhibitors. These will become decision points in MD's treatment.	MD has a history of diabetes and asthma. She has no history of congestive heart failure, heart block, renal or hepatic disease. MD's LDL and triglyceride levels are elevated. These will become decision points.
Pharmacokinetics	The onset of most antihypertensive drugs is within one hour with peak action reached in 2–6 hours. The duration of action is approximately 24 hours, thus permitting once-daily dosing in many cases. All drugs are biotransformed in the liver.	MD's liver function tests are within normal limits. Renal function unimpaired at this time. This is a decision point.
Dosage Regimen	Many antihypertensives can be given as a once daily dose. This will become a decision point.	Once-daily dosing desired since MD has previous history of noncompliance. This will become a decision point.
Lab Considerations	CBC, renal and hepatic function, lipids, and glucose values should be monitored prior to initiating therapy and periodically thereafter.	MD may initially comply with follow-up for laboratory testing but long-term monitoring will be difficult. This is a decision point.
Cost Index*	Nifedipine: 2 Lisinopril: 5 Losartan: 5	MD has a co-payment for pharmacy needs but otherwise should be able to afford cost of drugs and follow-up care.

Summary of Decision Points

- MD's blood pressure has exceeded 140/90 on her last three readings.
- Diuretics and beta blockers contraindicated because of MD's history of diabetes and asthma, and elevated triglyceride levels.
- MD's liver function and renal function tests are within normal limits at this time.
- Once daily dosing warranted with MD's history of noncompliance. Calcium channel blockers, ACE inhibitors, and angiotensin II antagonists can be given as once daily dose.
- MD may initially comply with follow-up for laboratory testing but long-term monitoring will be difficult.

DRUGS TO BE USED

- Losartan 50 mg po once daily at bedtime. Can be increased to 50–100 mg/day if necessary.
- Life-style modifications related to diet, exercise, stress reduction.

*Cost index

1 = $< 20/mo
2 = $ 20–30/mo
3 = $ 30–40/mo
4 = $ 40–50/mo
5 = $ 50

AWP of 100 tablets of 5 mg. lisinopril is approximately $78.
AWP of 100 tablets of 10 mg. nifedipine is approximately $13.
AWP of 100 tablets of 50 mg. losartan is approximately $66.

shown to prevent hypertension, are effective in lowering blood pressure, and can reduce cardiovascular risk factors at little cost and with minimal risk. Even if changes in life-style are not sufficient to reduce blood pressure, the changes may reduce the need for multidrug therapy.

A reduction in weight of even 10 pounds reduces blood pressure in a large proportion of overweight patients. Further, weight loss augments the blood pressure–lowering effects of antihypertensive drugs and can significantly reduce cardiovascular risk factors.

Sodium intake is linked to blood pressure elevation. Patients with hypertension or diabetes, older adults, and blacks are more sensitive to changes in sodium intake than other persons in the general population. A diet with a moderately reduced sodium intake (daily intake of no more than 2.4 g of sodium or 6 g of sodium chloride) has also been associated with reduced need for antihypertensive drugs, reduced diuretic-caused potassium loss, and possible regression of left ventricular hypertrophy.

Regular aerobic activity enhances weight loss and functional health status, reduces cardiovascular risk factors, and other causes of morbidity and mortality. Blood pressure can be reduced by 30 to 45 minutes of moderately intense exercise carried out daily.

Excessive alcohol intake causes resistance to antihypertensive drugs and is a risk factor for stroke. Patients should limit their daily intake to no more than one ounce of ethanol (i.e., 24 ounces of beer, 10 ounces of wine, or 2 ounces of 100-proof whiskey). A daily intake of ½ ounce of alcohol or less is advised for women and lighter weight persons. It should also be noted that significant hypertension can develop in patients with heavy alcohol intake who abruptly stop consumption.

There is some evidence that increased intake of potassium, calcium, and magnesium may protect against hypertension. There is also evidence that these electrolytes improve blood pressure control in patients with hypertension. An intake of approximately 90 mmol/day of potassium is thought to be adequate. Recommendations for calcium and magnesium intake have not been identified. Supplemental potassium intake may be required, particularly for patients who are receiving a potassium-losing diuretic. Potassium supplementation, however, is contraindicated in patients who are taking ACE inhibitors or angiotensin II–inhibiting drugs, or in patients with renal dysfunction.

Dyslipidemia is a significant independent risk factor for coronary artery disease. However, diets varying in total fat and the proportion of saturated to unsaturated fats have had little, if any, direct effect on blood pressure. In some patients, a large intake of omega-3 fatty acids may lower blood pressure. However, some patients experience abdominal discomfort with a large intake of these fatty acids. Further, some health care providers advise hypertensive patients to avoid caffeine intake. Although caffeine may raise blood pressure acutely, tolerance to the pressor effects of caffeine develops quickly. There has been no direct relationship found between caffeine intake and hypertension.

Tobacco use in any form should be avoided by hypertensive patients. Patients who continue to smoke while on antihypertensive therapy will not receive the full benefit of therapy. The cardiovascular benefits of discontinuing tobacco use can be seen in all age groups within a year of stopping. Smokers should be repeatedly and unambiguously advised to stop smoking. However, interventions directed at minimizing weight gain after stopping smoking are often required.

Drug Variables

Fewer than one third of hypertensive patients have their disease effectively managed. Suboptimal treatment by the health care provider is the most common cause of unresponsiveness. Other causes of unresponsiveness include drug intolerance, undiagnosed secondary causes of hypertension, and patient noncompliance.

The decision to start antihypertensive drug therapy requires careful consideration of several variables including the

- Stage and degree of blood pressure elevation
- Presence of clinical cardiovascular or other risk factors
- Presence of end-organ damage
- Safety profile of the specific drug or drugs
- Efficacy and convenience of specific drug or drugs
- Potential for drug-drug interactions
- Treatment costs, including laboratory testing and follow-up visits to health care provider.

The ideal antihypertensive drug should be effective as monotherapy, with minimal adverse effects. Once-daily dosing should provide 24-hour blood pressure control, with 50 percent of peak effects remaining at the end of the 24 hours. Long-acting drugs are preferred over short-acting agents for several reasons:

- Adherence to therapy is greater with once-daily dosing
- For some antihypertensive drugs, fewer tablets are required, thus the cost to the patient is lower
- Control of hypertension is continuous and smooth rather than intermittent
- There is a reduced risk of sudden death, heart attack, and stroke caused by abrupt increases in blood pressure after arising.

In spite of these ideal aspects, even the most ideal drug is less than 70-percent effective on a long-term basis. Yet 80 percent of compliant patients eventually achieve adequate control with the use of one or two drugs. Only a small number of patients will require multidrug therapy.

Current management approaches to hypertension, as reported in the Sixth Report of the Joint National Committee on the Prevention, Detection, Evaluation, and Treatment of High Blood Pressure (JNC VI, 1997), calls for diuretics and beta blockers as initial therapy for uncomplicated hypertension (Fig. 34–2). As shown in Table 34–12, there are some unequivocal reasons for using specific drugs in certain clinical situations. In most other situations, the choice of drug is individualized, using the drug that is most suitable to the patient's needs. Diuretics and beta blockers cause a 40-percent relative reduction in the frequency of fatal and nonfatal strokes over 5 years of treatment. Evidence also suggests that diuretics and beta blockers reduce the incidence of cardiovascular complications of hypertension (i.e., sudden death, stroke, MI, left ventricular hypertrophy, renal failure) (see Controversy—Initial Use of Diuretics and Beta Blockers).

If the initial drug of choice does not adequately control the blood pressure after reaching the full dose, two options for

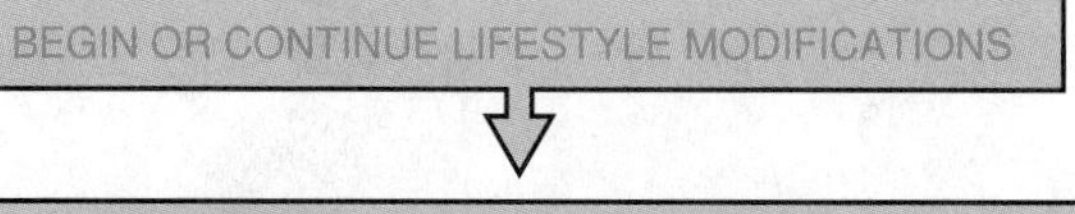

If blood pressure is not at goal (<140/90 mmHg)
Patients with diabetes or renal disease should have lower blood pressure goals

INITIAL DRUG CHOICES (Unless contraindiicated)

Uncomplicated Hypertension
(Based on randomized controlled trials)
- Diuretics
- β-Blockers

Compelling Indications
(Based on randomized controlled trials)

Diabetes Mellitus (Type I) with Proteinuria
- ACE Inhibitors

Heart Failure
- ACE Inhibitors
- Diuretics

Isolated Systolic Hypertension (Older persons)
- Diuretics preferred
- Long-acting Dihydropyridine Calcium Antagonists

Myocardial Infarction
- β-Blockers (Non-ISA)
- ACE Inhibitors (With Systolic Dysfunction)

The following drugs have additional specific indications: ACE Inhibitors, Angiotensin II Receptor Blockers, α-Blockers, α-β-Blockers, β-Blockers, Calcium Antagonists, Diuretics

Start with a low dose of a long-acting once-daily drug and titrate dose; low-dose combination may be appropriate

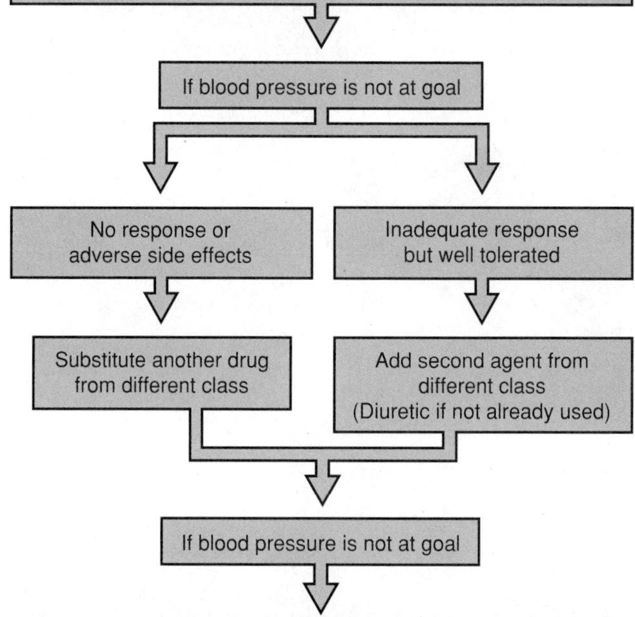

Figure 34–2 An algorithm for antihypertensive therapy replaces the stepwise approach to therapy used previously. The new algorithm includes compelling indications for use of certain drug groups for specific patients. (Adapted from the Sixth Report of the Joint National Committee on Prevention, Detection, Evaluation and Treatment of High Blood Pressure [1997]. *Archives of Internal Medicine*, 157 [21], 2430.)

subsequent therapy should be considered. If the patient is tolerating the drug of first choice, a second drug from a different class may be added. If the patient is having significant adverse effects or there is no response to the first drug, an agent from a different class can be substituted. Using two drugs from the same classification is not advised. If a diuretic was not used as a first-line agent, it should be used as the second-step drug because it enhances the effects of the first drug. The dosages of both drugs should be kept low to minimize adverse effects. If addition of the second drug controls blood pressure, an attempt to withdraw the first drug may be considered.

There is an increasing number of combination antihypertensive drugs on the market. Common drug combinations include

- Thiazide diuretic with beta blockers (e.g., chlorthalidone plus atenolol; hydrochlorothiazide plus bisoprolol; hydrochlorothiazide plus metoprolol)
- Thiazide diuretic with ACE inhibitors (e.g., hydrochlorothiazide plus benazepril; hydrochlorothiazide plus captopril)
- Thiazide diuretic with angiotensin II inhibitor (e.g., hydrochlorothiazide plus losartan)
- Thiazide diuretic with alpha blocker (e.g., polythiazide and prazosin)
- Thiazide diuretic with alpha agonist (e.g., methyldopa and hydrochlorothiazide)
- Thiazide diuretic with potassium-sparing diuretic (e.g., hydrochlorothiazide with spironolactone; hydrochlorothiazide with amiloride)
- ACE inhibitors with calcium channel blockers (e.g., benazepril and amlodipine; enalapril and diltiazem)

Although combination antihypertensive drugs are convenient, many health care providers prefer to adjust the dosage of each drug individually. When optimum maintenance doses coincide to the ratio of drugs in a fixed combination formulation, taking fewer tablets may help improve compliance with antihypertensive therapy.

Patient Variables

The JNC VI guidelines stress that drug choice should be based on what is most likely to benefit the individual patient. Factors to consider include

- Patient age and ethnicity
- Severity of disease and extent of end-organ damage
- Concurrent risk factors and co-morbid disease
- General life-style, including diet and exercise patterns
- Impact of hypertension and drug therapy on the quality of life (physical state, emotional well-being, sexual and social functioning, cognitive acuity)
- Previous responses to drug therapy, if any.

TABLE 34–12 PERCEIVED ADVANTAGES AND DISADVANTAGES OF ANTIHYPERTENSIVE DRUGS

Perceived Advantages	Perceived Disadvantages
ACE Inhibitors (Benazepril, Captopril, Enalapril, Fosinopril, Lisinopril, Quinapril, Ramipril, Trandolapril)	
Effective in older adult patients who have low cardiac output,* reduced total blood volume, high peripheral vascular resistance, low plasma renin activity, and high catecholamine activity (unequivocal indication) Slows development of nephropathy in type I diabetes (unequivocal indication) Increases survival after MI in patients who have heart failure or left ventricular dysfunction (unequivocal indication) May reduce proteinuria when used in combination with nondihydropyridine calcium channel blockers more than either drug alone Improves responsiveness to insulin and does not elevate lipid levels Well tolerated and highly effective alone or with diuretics May cause less pedal edema when used in combination with dihydropyridine calcium channel blockers than calcium channel blockers used alone Acceptable for patients with bronchospastic disease Use of generic formulations acceptable	Concurrent NSAID use blunts action of ACE inhibitor and may accelerate renal failure Less effective in blacks (although not necessarily ineffective) and in patients with low renin states May increase sodium and potassium levels, produce dry cough, angioedema, and tracheobronchial irritation Cough contributes to likelihood of noncompliance Patients with renovascular hypertension with renal perfusion that is maintained by high levels of angiotensin II and who have creatinine levels exceeding 3 mg/dL may develop acute renal failure Patients with high renin levels (i.e., volume depleted, using diuretics, renovascular disease) may experience excessive hypotension Although rare, associated with cholestatic jaundice that can progress to fulminant hepatic necrosis and death
Angiotensin II Inhibitors (Irbesartan, Losartan, Valsartan)	
Produces hemodynamic effects similar to that of ACE inhibitors while avoiding adverse effect of dry cough Useful in patients who are unable to tolerate ACE inhibitors Improves insulin sensitivity and reduces plasma levels of catecholamines Losartan does not alter lipids, glucose, or other metabolic parameters Generic formulations acceptable	May increase sodium, potassium levels, cough, angioedema, tracheobronchial irritation Decreases blood pressure if patient has low pre-existing volume, is on diuretics, has heart failure, or renal failure. Concurrent NSAID use may accelerate renal failure Usually more expensive since they are newest drugs on the market May be less effective (but not ineffective) for blacks.
Diuretics (*Thiazides:* Chlorthalidone, Chlorothiazide, Hydrochlorothiazide. *Thiazide-like:* Indapamide, Metolazone. *Loop Diuretic:* Bumetanide, Ethacrynic acid, Furosemide, Torsemide. *Potassium-sparing:* Amiloride, Spironolactone, Triamterene.)	
Effective in blacks with hypertension characterized by low cardiac output, expanded total blood volume,* and high peripheral vascular resistance Reduces mortality and morbidity associated with hypertension, MI, heart failure, renal failure (unequivocal indication) Relative reduction in frequency of fatal and nonfatal strokes (unequivocal indication) Have long, proven track record of effectiveness Effective for blacks and others with low-renin states, and older adults Enhances effects of other antihypertensive drugs without producing adverse metabolic effects Thiazides may produce positive benefits in patients with osteoporosis Loop diuretics produce greater diuresis than thiazides and do not promote vasodilation compared to thiazides Bumetanide less likely to cause hypercalcemia than other loop diuretics Indapamide produces little or no hypercholesterolemia Metolazone and indapamide may be effective in patients with impaired renal function when thiazides are not Considerably less expensive than other drugs Generic formulations acceptable	Cannot use in patients with symptomatic gout, poorly controlled diabetes, or severe hyperlipidemia May potentiate digoxin toxicity Increases risk of death if patient has baseline ECG abnormalities Cannot use potassium-sparing diuretics concurrently with ACE inhibitors or potassium supplements due to risk of hyperkalemia Amount of fluid lost with loop diuretics is greater than needed or desirable in most cases NSAIDs blunt the action of diuretics reducing effectiveness
Centrally Acting Alpha Agonists (Clonidine, Guanabenz, Guanfacine, Methyldopa)	
Decreases sympathetic nervous system outflow to reduce heart rate and peripheral vascular resistance Guanfacine produces fewer withdrawal symptoms than clonidine Methyldopa preferred for hypertension during pregnancy Generic formulations acceptable	Abrupt discontinuation causes rebound hypertension Significant sedation, dry mouth, depression Impotence possible Concurrent NSAID use may accelerate renal failure
Beta Blockers (*Beta Selective:* Acebutolol, Atenolol, Betaxolol, Bisoprolol, Metoprolol. *Beta Nonselective:* Carteolol, Nadolol, Penbutolol, Pindolol, Propranolol, Timolol. *Alpha/Beta Selective:* Carvedilol, Labetolol.)	
Effective for young patients with hypertension who have a high cardiac output, normal total blood volume. normal peripheral vascular resistance, and high plasma renin activity (unequivocal indication)	Cannot use for patients with diabetes, asthma, heart failure (except for carvedilol), peripheral vascular disease, second-degree or third-degree heart block

TABLE 34–12 PERCEIVED ADVANTAGES AND DISADVANTAGES OF ANTIHYPERTENSIVE DRUGS *Continued*

Perceived Advantages	Perceived Disadvantages
Beta Blockers (*Beta Selective:* Acebutolol, Atenolol, Betaxolol, Bisoprolol, Metoprolol. *Beta Nonselective:* Carteolol, Nadolol, Penbutolol, Pindolol, Propranolol, Timolol. *Alpha/Beta Selective:* Carvedilol, Labetolol.) *Continued*	
Decreased incidence of sudden death, stroke, MI, renal failure, and left ventricular hypertrophy associated with hypertension (unequivocal indication) Appropriate for patients with migraine headaches May have favorable effects for patients with angina, atrial tachycardia, atrial fibrillation, essential tremor, hyperthyroidism Less likely to delay recovery from hypoglycemia or cause severe hypertension when hypoglycemia leads to an increase in circulating catecholamines Labetolol decreases blood pressure more promptly than other drugs because of nonselective beta and alpha blockade Labetolol equally effective in blacks and whites, and does not elevate serum lipid levels Generic formulations acceptable	Drugs with nonintrinsic sympathomimetic action worsen GI upset and triglyceride levels. May mask signs of hypoglycemia Can cause insomnia, depression, bizarre dreams, sexual dysfunction (impotence) Concurrent NSAID use blunts effects of beta blockers Becomes less effective as dosage is increased
Calcium Channel Blockers (*Diphydropyridines:* Amlodipine, Felodipine, Isradipine, Nicardipine, Nifedipine, Nimodipine. *Benzothiazepine:* Diltiazem. *Diphenylalkylamine:* Verapamil)	
Effective in older adult patients who have low cardiac output, reduced total blood volume, high peripheral vascular resistance, low plasma renin activity, and high catecholamine activity Decreases left ventricular hypertrophy Limited to no effect on insulin sensitivity, glycemic control, lipids, potassium, and calcium levels May use in blacks, and those with chronic airflow limitation, variant angina, arrhythmias Decreased incidence of drug-induced orthostatic hypotension Effective for isolated systolic hypertension in older adults Diltiazem and verapamil modestly reduce blood pressure following non–Q wave MI and after MI with preserved left ventricular dysfunction Verapamil, diltiazem, and amlodipine cause little or no change in heart rate Generic formulations acceptable	Cautious use with concurrent beta blockers needed because they can alter AV conduction Cannot use short-acting calcium channel blockers for hypertension, in patients with heart failure, sick sinus syndrome, second or third degreee heart block Can cause reflex tachycardia and ischemic events, especially with immediate-release nifedipine, diltiazem, and verapamil May be associated with stroke, angina, vascular problems (specifically isradipine) Dihydropyridine formulations cause initial reflex tachycardia
Alpha Blockers (*Alpha selective:* Doxazosin, Phenoxybenzamine, Phentolamine, Prazosin, Terazosin, *Alpha/Beta Selective:* Carvedilol, Labetalol)	
Causes vascular dilation and reduces peripheral vascular resistance Increases peak urine flow in men with benign prostatic hypertrophy Have no effects on lipid levels Less tachycardia than with direct-acting peripheral vasodilators May increase HDL/total cholesterol ratio Improves responsiveness to insulin Provide symptomatic relief from prostatism Generic formulations acceptable	Can produce significant orthostatic hypotension, especially in elderly with first dose (first dose phenomenon) Can cause stress incontinence in women Concurrent NSAID use may accelerate renal failure
Adrenergic Neuronal Blockers (Guanethidine, Guanadrel, Reserpine)	
Reduces catecholamine release to decrease peripheral vascular resistance, cardiac output, and systolic blood pressure (more than diastolic)	Exacerbates or causes depression Increased vasodilation and orthostatic hypotension with exercise, alcohol use, hot environment Decreases libido, may cause diarrhea
Direct-Acting Vasodilators (Diazoxide, Hydralazine, Minoxidil, Nitroprusside)	
No significant venous dilation so little orthostatic hypotension Diazoxide and hydralazine are acceptable for use during pregnancy Generic formulations acceptable	Need concurrent use of beta blocker and diuretic, or centrally acting drugs to help offset adverse effects Stimulates reflex sympathetic action of cardiovascular system and fluid retention Lupus-like syndrome with hydralazine, hirsutism with minoxidil

*Most prominent diagnostic finding of this age group.

ACE, Angiotensin-converting enzyme; ECG, electrocardiogram; GI, gastrointestinal; MI, myocardial infarction; NSAID, nonsteroidal anti-inflammatory drug.

Controversy

Initial Use of Diuretics and Beta Blockers

JONATHAN J. WOLFE

The Sixth Report of the Joint National Committee on Prevention, Detection, Evaluation, and Treatment of High Blood Pressure (JNC VI) advocates choosing diuretics and beta blockers for initial treatment in patients when life-style changes are inadequate for blood pressure control. However, not all authorities agree with these recommendations. At present, diuretics and beta blockers are the only agents for which long-term data are available. The advantages over the long term cannot be compared with those of the newer drugs because of the limitations of previous studies.

Critics have questioned the scientific basis on which JNC VI selected diuretics and beta blockers as preferred agents. Studies used as a basis for these recommendations do not include high-risk populations, women, or blacks. Critics of JNC VI go on to argue that the guidelines underplay the importance of flexibility for patients with other diseases or risk factors. Flexibility in treatment regimens becomes an important issue when increasingly aggressive strategies are used by managed care programs and insurers to control what health care providers prescribe.

Direct costs are among the easiest medical costs to calculate. As insurers take steps that range from offering financial incentives to requiring prior authorization for the prescription of certain drugs, they encourage health care providers to use lower cost drugs, especially low-dose diuretics and beta blockers. JNC VI guidelines are cited as the rationale.

The second controversy that occurs is the practice of giving sublingual nifedipine for hypertensive emergencies and urgencies. The practice of puncturing a nifedipine capsule and expressing the contents under the tongue is common. However, this practice is neither safe nor effective. Nifedipine is not absorbed sublingually. Most absorption takes place in the intestinal mucosa. Serious, even fatal adverse effects have been reported when nifedipine was administered for acute treatment of severe hypertension. Uncontrolled reduction in blood pressure with sublingual nifedipine can result in coma, stroke, myocardial infarction, acute renal failure, and death. Given the seriousness of adverse effects and lack of documentation as to its benefit, the use of nifedipine capsules for hypertensive emergencies should be abandoned.

Critical Thinking Discussion

- Critique of the Sixth Report of the Joint National Committee on Prevention, Detection, Evaluation, and Treatment of High Blood Pressure (JNC VI, 1997). How will you interpret and use the results of this report?
- Is there reasonable evidence in this report to warrant discontinuing the practice of using sublingual nifedipine? Why or why not? What additional information, if any, do you need to make an informed decision about using nifedipine by the sublingual route?
- Does the report provide sufficient support for the unequivocal use of beta blockers, diuretics, and ACE inhibitors for selected groups of patients? How does the health care provider individualize therapy in light of the compelling indications for drugs in these categories?

Consider using drugs that have been proved to reduce mortality and morbidity (i.e., beta blockers, and diuretics). Remember, however, that reducing blood pressure with multidrug therapy does not necessarily equate with an equal reduction in end-organ damage.

The JNC VI continues to recommend that all patients with stage 1 and stage 2 hypertension seriously attempt to make alterations in their life-style before drug therapy is instituted. JNC VI also recommends that patients who have systolic blood pressures exceeding 160 mmHg after complying with vigorous life-style changes receive drug therapy (even when diastolic blood pressure is normal). Patients with pressures ranging from 140 to 159 mmHg may be candidates for drug therapy, particularly when there is evidence of end-organ damage. However, rigidly controlled hypertension (i.e., diastolic pressure less than 85 mmHg) may result in a fatal MI. The goal of therapy should be a systolic pressure between 140 and 155 mmHg and a diastolic pressure between 85 and 95 mmHg. Blood pressure readings within these ranges realize the greatest reduction in mortality and morbidity, and are consistent with patient safety and tolerance.

Appropriate drug therapy may be beneficial for some patients more than others. Patients with diabetes (especially those with nephropathy) or heart failure may benefit most from an ACE inhibitor. For patients with elevated lipid levels, an ACE inhibitor, alpha blocker, or calcium channel blocker may be a good choice.

In white and black patients, diuretics have proved to reduce the mortality and morbidity associated with hypertension. Thus, diuretics should be the drug of first choice in this population unless there are conditions prohibiting their use. Calcium channel blockers and alpha and beta blockers are also effective in lowering blood pressure. Monotherapy with beta blockers or ACE inhibitors is less effective, but not necessarily ineffective. The addition of diuretics markedly improves patient response in this population. Black patients often require multidrug therapy because of the higher incidence of stage 3 hypertension in this population group.

A beta blocker without intrinsic sympathomimetic activity may be indicated for hypertensive patients who also have a history of angina or migraine headaches. They have also proved effective in reducing mortality and morbidity in patients who have had an MI. ACE inhibitors are used for patients with diabetic nephropathy or left ventricular systolic dysfunction.

If they are taken before pregnancy occurs, diuretics and most other antihypertensive drugs (except ACE inhibitors and angiotensin II inhibitors—pregnancy category D agents) may be continued. Methyldopa has been most extensively evaluated and is recommended for women whose hypertension is first diagnosed during pregnancy. The use of beta blockers in early pregnancy has been associated with fetal growth retardation. However, beta blockers (e.g., atenolol and metoprolol) can be effective alternatives and are considered safe for use during the latter half of pregnancy.

Diuretics are recommended for chronic hypertension if they are prescribed before pregnancy or if the patient appears to be salt sensitive. They are not recommended for use in patients with pre-eclampsia. Hydralazine, a direct-acting vasodilator, is the parenteral drug of choice based on its long history of safety and effectiveness. The aim of antihypertensive therapy in the pregnant woman is to keep mean arterial pressure below 120 mmHg but not less than 105 mmHg. Hypotension may result in acute placental insufficiency.

Although the recommendations for choice of drugs are similar in children and adults, dosages of antihypertensives should be smaller and adjusted very carefully for children. ACE inhibitors and angiotensin II inhibitors should not be used in sexually active females or during pregnancy owing to the potential for fetal harm. Antihypertensive therapy in older adults should begin with life-style modifications. Older adults ordinarily respond to weight loss and a modest reduction in salt intake. If blood pressure values do not respond, drug therapy is warranted. The starting dose of antihypertensive drugs should be about half of that used in young patients. Thiazide diuretics or beta blockers in combination are recommended because they reduce morbidity and mortality. When compared with each other, diuretics (e.g., hydrochlorothiazide with amiloride) are superior to the beta blocker atenolol.

In older adults with isolated systolic hypertension, the drug of choice is diuretics because they significantly reduce multiple end-organ complications. The goal of treatment is the same as in young patients; a systolic value less than 140 mmHg and a diastolic value under 90. Albeit, an interim goal of systolic values less than 160 mmHg may be acceptable in patients who have marked systolic hypertension. However, any reduction in blood pressure confers benefit and the closer the blood pressure is to normal, the greater the benefit. Antihypertensive drugs that exaggerate orthostatic changes in blood pressure (i.e., high-dose diuretics, alpha blockers, peripheral vasodilators) or drugs that cause cognitive dysfunction (i.e., central sympathomimetics) should be used with caution.

Intervention

Administration

Drug treatment of primary hypertension is usually lifelong. Thus, it is important to use a flexible approach to drug therapy. Patients respond differently to individual drugs or combinations of drugs. Further, simplified drug regimens make life easier for patients and increase compliance with treatment plans. Monotherapy with once-daily or twice-daily dosing is likely to achieve adequate blood pressure control in the compliant patient. However, effective dosages of antihypertensive drugs are often lower than those recommended in most texts. For example, drug therapy in the older adult should begin at one half the normal starting dose. Titration dosages should be small and spaced at longer intervals than those used for a younger patient.

Abruptly stopping antihypertensive drugs may result in withdrawal syndrome characterized by sweating, palpitations, headache, tremulousness, and rebound hypertension. Withdrawal syndrome may precipitate CHF and MI in patients with cardiac disease, a thyroid storm in patients with thyrotoxicosis, and peripheral ischemia in patients with peripheral vascular disease. Hypoglycemia may occur in patients with previously controlled diabetes.

Education

It is important to develop and implement a teaching plan that is individualized for each patient. Teaching the patient how to monitor blood pressure at home enables the patient to become a more active participant in care, treatment goals are reinforced, and compliance is enhanced. Advise the patient to check his or her blood pressure weekly and report significant changes to the health care provider. Reinforce the notion that hypertension may not produce symptoms but is a chronic disease that requires life-long interventions. Patient beliefs about personal susceptibility to complications of hypertension, treatment effectiveness, and consequences of nontreatment should be discussed. Patients should be helped to understand that drug therapy controls, but does not cure, hypertension.

The importance of life-style modification should be stressed, including the importance of a low sodium–low fat diet, weight reduction, adequate potassium and calcium intake, limited alcohol consumption, smoking cessation, and increased physical activity. However, not all patients are motivated to make the necessary life-style changes that are required for the management of hypertension. Patients who believe that they play an active part in controlling their disease are more likely to comply with treatment. Patients are likely to comply with treatment regimens when they understand the plan, it makes sense to them, and the plan is consistent with their own beliefs. Adequate information enables the patient to make informed choices about life-style changes.

Hypertension and obesity frequently co-exist. Thus, dietary recommendations should be given to all hypertensive patients. Weight control also permits reduced dosages of antihypertensive drugs in patients receiving drug therapy. Dietary restriction of cholesterol and saturated fats is advised and helps reduce the incidence of arteriosclerotic complications. Excessive alcohol intake is related to noncompliance with the antihypertensive treatment program and should be avoided.

Sodium restriction continues to be controversial. Sodium intake greater than 70 to 100 mEq/day (2360 mg) plays a role in elevating blood pressure in some patients with essential hypertension. In other patients, sodium restriction may limit drug effectiveness. Thus, mild sodium restriction is the most practical approach. Teaching the patient to eliminate, or at least restrict, the use of frozen, canned, or processed foods can reduce sodium intake considerably. A diet with moderately high calcium intake and magnesium supplementation may be beneficial in lowering blood pressure and reducing the risk of osteoporosis. The patient should be advised to avoid caffeine and tobacco intake as well.

A long-term regular exercise program can help control abnormally elevated arterial blood pressure. Blood pressure will increase if the patient returns to a sedentary life-style after as little as 3 months of exercise. Subsequent blood pressure readings will still be lower than pre-exercise levels, however. Isotonic exercises (e.g., jogging or walking) reduce blood pressure by 30 to 50 percent. Isometric exercises (e.g., weight lifting) may raise arterial pressure. Exercise lowers blood pressure in blacks more dramatically than in whites. In older adults, low-intensity training has resulted in a 20-mmHg decrease in systolic pressure and a 12-mmHg fall in diastolic pressure. An individualized exercise plan should be reviewed with the patient, and continuing encouragement should be provided.

Patients should be taught stress management techniques because these methods have been shown to decrease catecholamine release, oxygen consumption, respiratory rate, heart rate, and acute blood pressure elevation. Use of a combination of biofeedback and stress management techniques have been shown to be better than either strategy alone.

Patient education about the treatment regimen should be written and include identification of prescribed drugs by

TABLE 34-13 RECOMMENDATIONS FOR FOLLOW-UP BASED ON INITIAL BLOOD PRESSURE MEASUREMENTS FOR ADULTS

Initial Blood Pressure Reading		Recommended Follow-up*
SYSTOLIC (mmHg)	DIASTOLIC (mmHg)	
Less than 130	Less than 85	Recheck in 2 years
130-139	85-89	Recheck in 1 year†
140-159	90-99	Confirm within 2 months‡ Advise about life-style changes
160-179	100-109	Evaluate or refer to health care provider within 1 month
Over 180	Over 110	Evaluate or refer to health care provider immediately or within 1 week based on clinical situation

*If systolic and diastolic values are different, follow recommendations for shorter follow-up period. For example, a measurement of 136/80 should be evaluated in 1 year rather than 2 years.

†Modify the follow-up schedule according to reliable information about past blood pressure measurements, other cardiovascular risk factors, or target organ disease.

‡Provide advice about life-style modifications.

From Joint National Committee on Detection, Evaluation, and Treatment of High Blood Pressure. (1997). The Sixth Report of the Joint National Committee on the Prevention, Detection, Evaluation, and Treatment of High Blood Pressure (JNC VI). *Archives of Internal Medicine*, 157 (21), 2418.

both generic and trade names, the mechanism or mechanisms of action, and adverse effects. The patient should know the dosing frequency and what to do if a dose is forgotten. He or she should be encouraged to contact the health care provider before using over-the-counter cold remedies because many of these products contain sympathomimetic ingredients. Instruct the patient to continue taking the prescribed drug, even if he or she is feeling well, because abrupt withdrawal can cause rebound hypertension. Also, advise the patient to inform other health care providers and dentists of the diagnosis of hypertension and treatment regimen before treatment or surgery.

Although education has a substantial effect on the patient's knowledge and a positive effect on compliance, the effect of knowledge tends to diminish over time. It is beneficial to reinforce education at periodic intervals. Dialogue between the health care provider and the patient tends to reinforce treatment goals and positive behaviors.

Evaluation

Evaluation of the patient with hypertension is based on whether blood pressure has been reduced and end-organ damage prevented or minimized. Patients whose diastolic blood pressures exceed 115 mmHg should be re-evaluated after 48 hours of therapy to ensure that at least a 5- to 10-mmHg drop in pressure has occurred. Patients whose pressures fall below this number may be followed up in 1 to 2 weeks. Blood pressure should be rechecked every 4 weeks, after each dosage change, or until it is controlled. Once the blood pressure is controlled, the patient is ordinarily monitored two to four times yearly. If blood pressure remains controlled and there are no co-morbid conditions, a serum creatinine, blood sugar, cholesterol values, and urinalysis should be checked a minimum of every 5 years (Table 34–13).

The patient should be reassessed if the blood pressure has not decreased after 4 to 8 weeks of therapy. The present drug should be stopped and treatment restarted with a different drug at low dosage. If the blood pressure has decreased but not to the level desired, and if the patient has no adverse drug effects, the initial drug can be continued but a second drug added at low dosage. The dosage of the second drug is titrated based on patient response. If, however, the patient's pressure has been reduced but is not to the desired level *and* they are experiencing adverse effects, *or* if they cannot tolerate the treatment regimen, the drug should be discontinued and another started. Another option for the patient who is responding to drug therapy is to decrease the dosage to a tolerable level of adverse effects. If the patient is still unable to tolerate the adverse effects, the drug should be stopped and the patient changed to another agent.

Step-down therapy should be considered for patients whose blood pressure has been well controlled during the previous few visits. Fifty percent of patients remain stable. The drug dosage for these patients can be reduced by 50 percent and the patient re-evaluated in 2 weeks. If they remain stable, the dosage may be decreased another 50 percent and again the patient evaluated in 2 weeks. If the patient is stable at this point, the drug may be discontinued and the patient again evaluated in 2 weeks. Patients who may successfully withdraw from antihypertensive therapy include patients

- Whose blood pressure has been well controlled over the last few visits with the health care provider
- With a pretreatment diastolic blood pressure less than 100 mmHg
- With no evidence of end-organ disease
- Who have been on monotherapy only
- Who have lost weight, are following a sodium restricted diet, have decreased their alcohol intake, and have increased their exercise regimen.

SUMMARY

- Twenty-five percent of the adult population have hypertension, and a significant number of people remain undiagnosed.
- The morbidity and mortality associated with hypertension decreases when hypertension is managed effectively.
- The exact etiology of essential hypertension is unknown; several theories suggest complex hormonal and neural mechanisms.
- Modifiable risk factors for hypertension include stress, socioeconomic factors, nutrition, obesity, smoking, alcohol, and

physical activity. Nonmodifiable risk factors include age, sex, family history, and ethnicity.

- The initial evaluation of the patient is directed at detection of correctable forms of secondary hypertension and determining baseline patient status.
- The majority of patients with essential hypertension have no specific symptoms. Presenting symptoms are often related to end-organ damage.
- Blood pressure and pulse should be measured in both arms with the patient supine, seated, and standing using a standardized technique.
- The goal of treatment is to reduce arterial blood pressure, minimize organ damage, and prolong life.
- Drug groups that are used to treat hypertension: ACE inhibitors, angiotensin II inhibitors, beta blockers, diuretics, calcium channel blockers, centrally acting drugs, and direct-acting vasodilators.
- It is important incorporate life-style changes, individualized drug therapy, patient education, and follow-up into the treatment plan.

BIBLIOGRAPHY

Abrams, J., Vela, B., Coultas, D., et al. (1995). Coronary risk factors and their modification: Lipids, smoking, hypertension, estrogen, and the elderly. *Current Problems in Cardiology,* 20(8), 586–600.

Abramowicz, M. (Ed.). (1995). Drugs for hypertension. *The Medical Letter on Drugs and Therapeutics,* 37(949), 45–50.

Alderman, M., Elliot, W., Oparil, S., et al. (1994). Addressing multiple risks in hypertension therapy. *Patient Care,* 15, 64–76.

Alderman, M., Grimm, R., Swales, J., et al. (1995). Treating hypertension: Which drugs first? *Patient Care,* 15, 72–99.

Amsterdam, E., Weart, C., and Weber, M. (1997). ACE inhibitors and beta blockers: Casting a wider net. *Patient Care,* 31(20), 92–123.

Barron, H., and Amidon, T. (1996). Options in antihypertensive drug therapy. *Symposium,* 100(4), 89–94.

Black, H., Dluhy, R., and Prisant, L. (1997). Getting to the source of refractory hypertension. *Patient Care,* 31(17), 14–39.

Bottorff, J., Johnson, J., Ratner, P., et al. (1996). The effects of cognitive-perceptual factors on health promotion behavior maintenance. *Nursing Research,* 45(1), 30–36.

Bravo, E. (1995). Individualizing drug therapy for the hypertensive patient. *Hospital Practice,* 15, 97–108.

Brogden, R., and Sorkin, E. (1995). Drug Evaluation. *Drugs,* 49(4), 618–649.

Devine, E., and Reifschneider, E. (1995). A meta-analysis of the effects of psychoeducational care in adults with hypertension. *Nursing Research,* 44(4), 237–243.

Eaton, L., Buck, E., and Catanzaro, J. (1996). The nurse's role in facilitating compliance in clients with hypertension. *Medsurg Nursing,* 5(5), 339–359.

Farrehi, P., Santinga, J., and Eagle, K. (1995). Syncope: Diagnosis of cardiac and noncardiac causes. *Geriatrics,* 50(1), 24–30.

Frampton, J., and Peters, D. (1995). Ramipril: An updated review of its therapeutic use in essential hypertension and heart failure. *Drug Evaluation,* 49(3), 440–466.

Freis, E., and Papademetriou, V. (1996). Current drug treatment and treatment patterns with antihypertensive drugs. *Drugs,* 52(1), 1–16.

Gallery, E. (1995). Hypertension in pregnancy. *Practical Therapeutics,* 49(4), 555–562.

Gandhi, S., and Santiesteban, H. (1996). Resistant hypertension. *Symposium,* 100(4), 97–107.

Girvin, B., and Johnston, D. (1996). The implications of noncompliance with antihypertensive medication. *Drugs,* 52(2), 1–8.

Goode, G., Miller, J., and Heagerty, A. (1995). Hyperlipidaemia, hypertension, and coronary heart disease. *Lancet,* 345 (8946), 362–364.

Gregoire, J., and Sheps, S. (1996). Hypertension in lung patients: Which drugs to choose, which to avoid? *Consultant,* 36(4), 690–693.

Gold, G., and Fishman, P. (1995). Hypertension: Special concerns in managing the older patient. *Geriatrics,* 50(11), 39–46.

Goldberg, A., Dunlay, M., and Sweet, C. (1995). Systemic hypertension: Safety of losartan potassium. *The American Journal of Cardiology,* 75, 793–795.

Grossman, E., Messeril, F., Grodzicki, T., et al. (1996). Should a moratorium be placed on sublingual nifedipine capsules given for hypertensive emergencies and pseudoemergencies? *Journal of the American Medical Association,* 276(16), 1328–1330.

Hirschl, M. (1995). Guidelines for the drug treatment of hypertensive crises. *Drugs,* 50(6), 991–1000.

Hupert, N. (1997). Syncope: A systematic search for the cause. *Patient Care,* 15, 136–152.

Irby, B., and Hallisey, R. (1996). Pharmacologic management of mild-moderate hypertension. *Drug Therapy,* VI(5), 1–3.

Johnston, C. (1995). Angiotensin receptor antagonists: Focus on losartan. *Lancet,* 346 (8987), 1407.

Joint National Committee on Detection, Evaluation, and Treatment of High Blood Pressure. (1997). The Sixth Report of the Joint National Committee on the Prevention, Detection, Evaluation, and Treatment of High Blood Pressure (JNC VI). *Archives of Internal Medicine,* 157(21), 2413 –2446.

Kaplan, N. (1995). Resistant hypertension: What to do after trying the usual. *Geriatrics,* 50(5), 24–38.

Kitamura, K., Kangawa, K., Matsuo, H., et al. (1995). Adrenomedullin: Implications for hypertension research. *Drugs,* 49(4), 485–495.

Leonetti, G., and Cuspid, C. (1995). Choosing the right ACE inhibitor. *Drugs,* 49(4), 516–535.

Liu, J., and Devereux, R. (1996). How to manage cardiovascular complications during hypertensive crisis. *The Journal of Critical Illness,* 11(9), 586–601.

Loggie, J., and Sardegna, K. (1997). Latest standards for hypertension in teens. *Patient Care,* 15, 121–135.

Marieb, E. (1995). *Human Anatomy and Physiology* (2nd ed.). Redwood City, CA: Benjamin/Cummings Publishing Co., Inc.

National High Blood Pressure Education Program Working Group on Hypertension Control in Children and Adolescents. (1996). Update on the 1987 task force report on high blood pressure in children and adolescents: A working group report from the National High Blood Pressure Education Program. *Pediatrics,* 98, 649–658.

Noble, S., and Sorkin, E. (1995). Spirapril: A preliminary review of its pharmacology and therapeutic efficacy in the treatment of hypertension. *Drugs,* 49(5), 750–766.

Pinkquish, M. (1995). Practical briefings. *Patient Care,* 15, 16–21.

Plosker, G., and Faulds, D. (1996). Nisoldipine coat-core. *Drugs,* 52(2), 159–305.

Reynolds, E., and Baron, R. (1996). Hypertension in women and the elderly. *Postgraduate Medicine,* 100(4), 58–70.

Salom, I., and Davis, K. (1995). Prescribing for older patients: How to avoid toxic drug reactions. *Geriatrics,* 50(10), 37–44.

Setaro, J., and Moser, M. (1995). Hypertension: What to include in a cost-effective office workup. *Consultant,* 35(7), 957–964.

Sibai, B. (1996). Treatment of hypertension in pregnant women. *Drug Therapy,* 335(4), 257–265.

Steigerwalt, S. (1995). Unraveling the causes of hypertension and hypokalemia. *Hospital Practice,* 30(7), 67–79.

Weir, M. (1996). Angiotensin-II receptor antagonists: A new class of antihypertensive agents. *American Family Physician,* 53(2), 589–594.

Will, P., Demko, T., George, D. (1996). Prescribing exercise for health: A simple framework for primary care. *American Family Physician,* 53(2), 579–585.

Zellner, C., and Sudhir, K. (1996). Lifestyle modifications for hypertension. *Postgraduate Medicine,* 100(4), 75–79.

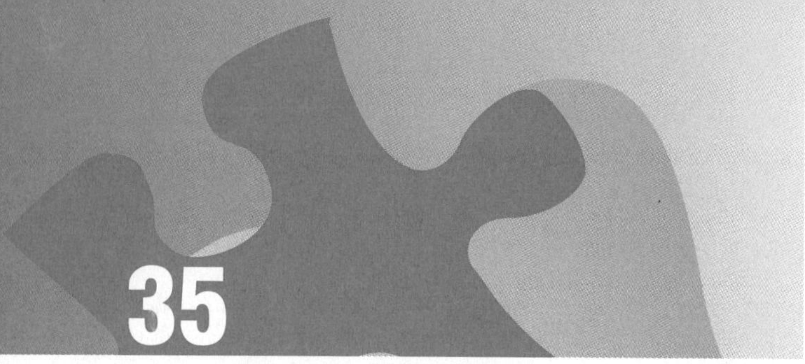

35 Antilipemic Drugs

Diseases of the heart and blood vessels are the principal cause of death in the industrialized countries of the world. In the United States, more people die from heart and blood vessel disease than any other illness, including cancer. More than three-fourths of deaths resulting from cardiovascular disease can be attributed to hyperlipoproteinemia and resultant atherosclerosis. Effective treatment for hyperlipoproteinemia must be directed at causative factors and prevention rather than reversal, because it is a slowly developing disorder. Clinical investigation has shown that vigorous drug therapy slows progression, and in some cases produces regression, of atherosclerotic lesions that lead to coronary artery disease.

HYPERLIPOPROTEINEMIA

Epidemiology and Etiology

Hyperlipidemia is a general term for elevated concentrations of any or all of the lipids contained in plasma. *Hyperlipoproteinemia* is an excess of the lipoproteins in the blood, which is due to a disorder of lipoprotein metabolism. It may be acquired or hereditary. The acquired form occurs secondary to another disorder or as a result of environmental factors (e.g., diet, smoking). The hereditary form has been classified into five phenotypes on the basis of clinical features, enzymatic abnormalities, and serum lipoprotein patterns.

Hyperlipoproteinemia has reached epidemic proportions in the United States. Twenty percent of adults older than 20 years have total serum cholesterol values exceeding 240 mg/dL, a level associated with greater risk of coronary artery disease (CAD). Risk factors associated with hyperlipoproteinemia are variables of age, gender, genetic factors, diet, exercise, weight, smoking, co-morbid diseases, and specific drugs. Table 35–1 provides an overview of CAD risk factors.

Pathophysiology

Cholesterol is a waxy, fatlike substance found in all animal fats and oils. Cholesterol can enter the body in the form of dietary fat; it is also manufactured by the liver from saturated fats. Cholesterol is an important component of cell membranes, bile acids, myelin sheath, and other body components as well as a precursor of steroid hormones and vitamin D. The liver produces about 1000 mg of cholesterol per day, enough for the body to maintain its required functions. The highest rate of cholesterol synthesis occurs between midnight and 5 AM.

The production of atherogenic lipoproteins and atheromatous plaque involves both an exogenous and an endogenous pathway (Fig. 35–1). The exogenous pathway follows absorption of dietary fat from the intestine to the tissue and back to the liver. Essentially no feedback mechanism exists within the exogenous pathway. The endogenous pathway, however, can exert feedback inhibition through receptors on cell surfaces. The endogenous pathway follows the formation of lipoproteins within the liver through metabolism in other parts of the body and return to the liver.

Fats are not water soluble. In order to facilitate transportation of lipids from the liver through the blood stream to other tissue, cholesterol and triglycerides are bound to specialized proteins called apoproteins. The resultant *lipoproteins* move through the plasma, distributing and picking up the lipid components. Lipoproteins are classified according to density, a reflection of relative protein and lipid content: chylomicrons, very-low-density lipoprotein (VLDL), intermediate-density lipoprotein, low-density lipoprotein (LDL), and high-density lipoprotein (HDL) (Fig. 35–2).

The four major classes of apoproteins are A (apos A-I, A-II, A-III, A-IV), B (apos B-48, B-100), C (apos C-I, C-II, C-III), and E (Table 35–2). *Apoproteins* are responsible for metabolic interactions and sometimes act as catalysts for enzymatic reactions (e.g., lipoprotein lipase) that allow the transfer of lipid agents to and from cells. Other apoproteins serve as cellular receptors for the metabolism of lipoproteins.

Chylomicrons

Absorbed dietary fats form *chylomicrons,* which carry large quantities of triglycerides throughout the body. Triglycerides are synthesized primarily from carbohydrates in the liver and make up 85 to 95 percent of each chylomicron. Cholesterol esters (a compound formed from an alcohol and an acid by removal of water) make up 3 to 5 percent of the chylomicron. Triglycerides are removed from the chylomicrons by the action of the enzyme lipoprotein lipase. Patients deficient in this enzyme or its co-factors (insulin and apo C-II) have very high triglyceride levels and a greater risk of pancreatitis. Chylomicrons have the lowest density of all lipoproteins; they can be found floating on a plasma specimen left in the refrigerator overnight.

Very-Low-Density Lipoproteins

Very-low-density lipoproteins contain about 75 percent triglycerides and 25 percent cholesterol. VLDLs transport triglycerides from the liver and intestines to capillary beds that service adipose and muscle cells. VLDLs also serve as acceptors of cholesterol transferred from HDL, possibly accounting for the inverse relationship between HDL cholesterol and VLDLs. When the triglycerides have been removed from the VLDLs, the remaining remnants, which now contain about 45 percent cholesterol, are the intermediate-density lipoproteins. VLDLs are not known to be atherogenic.

Intermediate-Density Lipoproteins

Intermediate-density lipoproteins are formed when VLDL loses its triglycerides. The remnant intermediate-density lipoproteins are either taken up by the liver through

TABLE 35–1 RISK FACTORS FOR CORONARY ARTERY DISEASE OTHER THAN HIGH LDL LEVELS

Variables	Comments
Positive Risk Factors	
Age >45 years for males	Men have higher total cholesterol levels than women until age 50
Age >55 years for females without estrogen replacement	Women have a higher proportion of cholesterol as HDL than men There is an increase in LDL levels with the onset of menopause
Definitive myocardial infarction or sudden death in first-degree male relative before age 55 or in female first-degree relative before age 65	Monogenic mechanisms account for a small fraction of patients with hyperlipidemia. Familial hypercholesterolemia affects 5 percent of the general population
Current cigarette smoking (especially if over 10/day)	Reduces HDL cholesterol levels
HDL<35 mg/dL	Proved to contribute to CAD
Treated or untreated systolic blood pressure >140 mmHg or diastolic blood pressure >90 mmHg	Other components all contribute to development of hypertension and thus increase the risk for CAD related to hyperlipidemia
Diet high in saturated fats	Raises total and LDL cholesterol levels
Treated or untreated diabetes mellitus	Elevates triglycerides, LDL, and total cholesterol levels
Negative Risk Factor†	
HDL level >60 mg/dL*	Proved to be protective against CAD

*Obesity is not listed as a separate risk factor, because it operates through a variety of other risk factors that are included (e.g., hypertension, hyperlipidemia, low HDL levels, diabetes). Obesity (i.e., 130 percent above ideal body weight) elevates triglyceride levels more than cholesterol levels and decreases HDL levels. Both obesity and inactivity are targets for intervention.

†Net risk status is determined by adding the number of positive risk factors and then subtracting one risk factor if HDL level exceeds 60 mg/dL. High HDL levels protect against CAD.

CAD, Coronary heart disease; HDL, high-density lipoprotein; LDL, low-density lipoprotein.

Adapted from the Summary of the Second Report of the National Cholesterol Education Program Adult Treatment Panel. (1993). *Journal of the American Medical Association,* 269 (23), 3015–3023.

apo E receptors or are converted to LDL by an intravascular process that removes much of the remaining triglycerides. Intermediate-density lipoproteins are about 70 percent cholesterol. In normally healthy individuals, intermediate-density lipoprotein is not found in significant amounts.

Low-Density Lipoproteins

Low-density lipoproteins are responsible for supplying cholesterol to the tissues and therefore carry proportionally more cholesterol than other lipoproteins. High levels of LDLs, "the bad cholesterol," have been clearly implicated in atherogenesis. The core of LDLs is composed almost entirely of cholesterol esters (50 percent), a relatively small amount of triglyceride (7 to 10 percent), and the surface coat contains only one apoprotein, B-100. Also, although most LDL receptors are found in the liver, extrahepatic tissues (e.g., endothelial cells, lymphoid cells, smooth muscle cells, adrenal glands) use the receptor-dependent pathways to obtain the cholesterol needed for the synthesis of cell membranes and hormones. The extrahepatic tissues regulate cholesterol uptake by adding or deleting LDL receptors. Serum LDL levels are increased in persons who consume large amounts of saturated fats or cholesterol, have defects in either their LDL receptors or in the structure of LDL apoprotein apo B, or have a familial form of increased LDLs. LDL can become trapped in the arterial vasculature when serum levels are extremely high. The association of serum cholesterol with CAD is predominantly a reflection of LDL levels.

Many of the mechanisms by which LDL increases the risk for atherosclerosis occur beneath the arterial wall. After traversing the tunica intima, LDL is oxidized by endothelial and smooth muscle cells. Oxidation of LDLs results in an accumulation of circulating monocytes, which take up the modified LDLs via alternative scavenger receptors. The monocytes become lipid-filled macrophages that further oxidize LDLs. Continued oxidation of LDLs appears to inhibit macrophage motility, and the first visible lesion of atherosclerosis, the fatty streak, appears. The return of LDLs from peripheral tissues to the liver involves HDLs.

TABLE 35–2 MAJOR CLASSES OF LIPOPROTEINS

Lipoprotein Class	Major Lipid	Major Apoproteins
Chylomicrons and chylomicron remnants	Dietary triglycerides	A-I, A-II, B-48, C-I, C-II, C-III, E
Very-low-density lipoproteins	Endogenous triglycerides	B-48, C-I, C-II, C-III, E
Intermediate-density lipoproteins	Cholesterol esters, triglycerides	B-100, C-III, E
Low-density lipoproteins	Cholesterol esters	B-100
High-density lipoproteins	Cholesterol esters	A-1, A-II

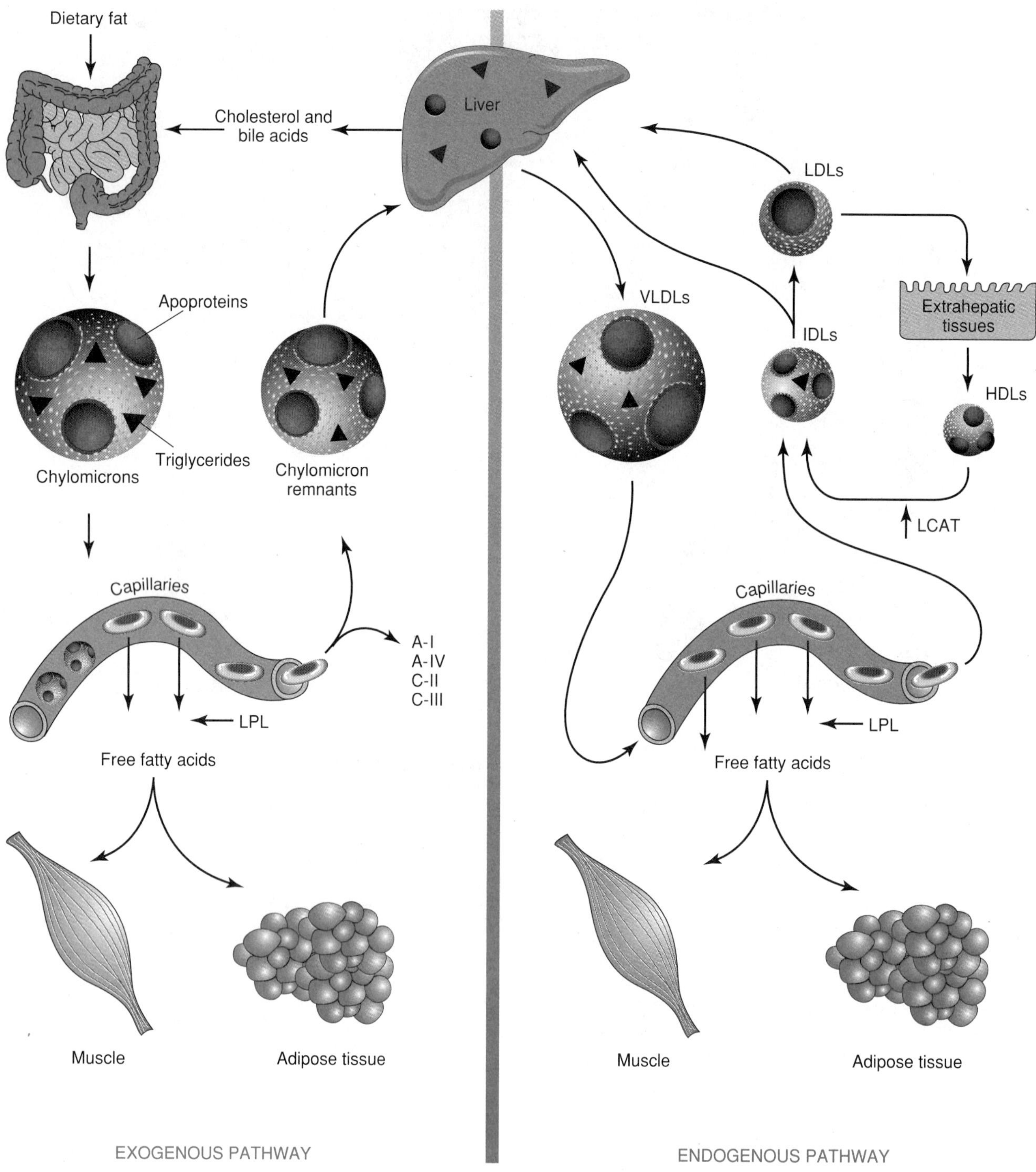

Figure 35–1 Metabolic pathways for lipoproteins. This diagram shows the exogenous and endogenous pathways that allow the transportation of lipids, in the form of plasma-soluble lipoproteins, from the intestine and liver to body tissues and back to the liver. Apoproteins, which bind with cholesterol and triglycerides to form lipoproteins, sometimes act as catalysts for enzymatic reactions. Apoproteins A-1, A-IV, C-II, and C-III activate lipolytic enzymes to remove lipids from lipoproteins; Lecithin-cholesterol acyltransferase (LCAT) converts high-density lipoprotein (HDL) to intermediate-density lipoprotein (IDL) and low-density lipoprotein (LDL) for return to the liver. LPL, Lipoprotein lipase; VLDL, Very-low density lipoprotein.

High-Density Lipoproteins

High-density lipoproteins, the good cholesterol, are synthesized in the liver. HDLs contain relatively little lipid and much protein, and thus are the smallest and most dense of the lipoproteins. There are two subfractions of HDL, HDL_2 and HDL_3. HDL_2 concentration is the single most powerful indicator of CAD risk. HDLs are thought to function in peripheral tissues as acceptors of free cholesterol. The cholesterol (17 to 20 percent) is esterified and stored in the central core of the HDL. HDLs are made up of 1 to

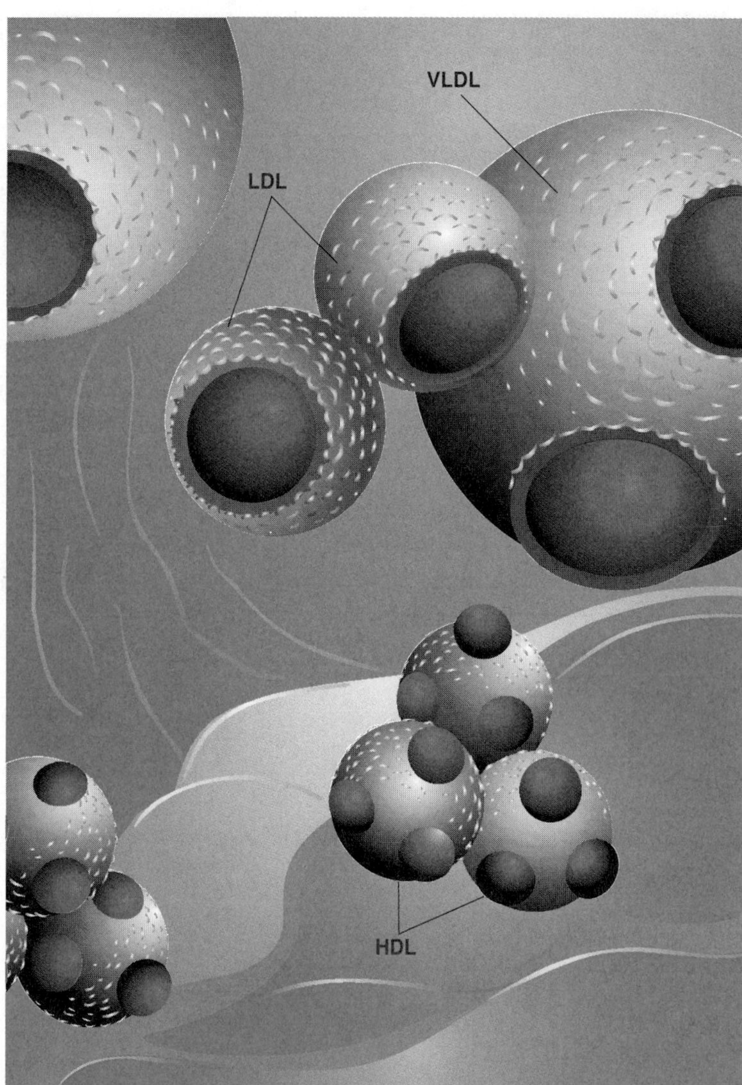

Figure 35–2 Density and function of lipoproteins. Lipoproteins—very-low density (VLDL), low-density (LDL), and high-density (HDL)—are classified according to density, which reflects protein and lipid content. Lipids are transported in plasma as components of these particles. The larger VLDL particles contain a higher percentage of lipid and are less dense, whereas the smaller HDL particles have less lipid and a higher percentage of protein, and are more dense. VLDLs and LDLs transport cholesterol and triglycerides away from the liver to organs and tissues. HDL particles move cholesterol toward the liver and away from tissues.

7 percent triglycerides. A reverse transport system from the periphery to the liver may explain why patients with very high HDL levels have a lower risk for CAD, even if LDL levels are elevated. In addition to the protective effect of reverse transport, HDLs may be beneficial because they inhibit binding of LDL to matrix proteins, oxidation of LDL, and receptor uptake of oxidized LDL. Women have higher levels of HDL than men, in part because of higher estrogen levels. Exercise increases HDLs, whereas obesity, hypertriglyceridemia, and smoking are associated with lower HDL levels.

Types of Hyperlipoproteinemia

The Frederickson-Levy classification identifies five major types of hyperlipoproteinemia (Table 35–3). They are essentially organized according to underlying cause and characteristic lipid and lipoprotein values. Type IIA, IIB, and III hyperlipoproteinemias have a positive correlation with CAD. The risk of CAD from Type IV and V hyperlipoproteinemias is unclear at this time. There is no known increase in the incidence of CAD with Type I hyperlipoproteinemia.

PHARMACOTHERAPEUTIC OPTIONS

Several different medical therapies are currently available in the United States for treatment of hyperlipidemia. They are bile acid resins, fibric acid derivatives, and HMG-CoA (3-hydroxy-3-methylglutaryl coenzyme A) reductase inhibitors. In addition, nicotinic acid, probucol, and clofibrate are available. All of these drugs can reduce LDL levels. In some patients, a combination of drugs may be required.

Bile Acid Resins

- ❐ Cholestyramine (QUESTRAN, QUESTRAN LIGHT, CHOLYBAR)
- ❐ Colestipol (COLESTID)

Indications

Bile acid resins are approved for use in the treatment of Type II hypercholesterolemia. When used in conjunction with a low cholesterol diet, they can reduce LDL levels by 15 to 20 percent. They are useful for patients who have a low risk for CAD but in whom diet therapy alone has failed to re-

TABLE 35–3 CLASSIFICATION OF HYPERLIPOPROTEINEMIAS

		Abnormality							
Type	**Common Name**	Chyl†	Chol*	VLDL‡	LDL§	HDL‖	TriG	**CAD Risk**	**Etiology**
I	Exogenous hypertriglyceridemia	↑	N	NC	↓	↓	↑↑	Not known	Dietary fat not cleared from plasma
IIA	Familial hypercholesterolemia	—	↑	NC	↑	↓	N	Yes	Autosomal dominant defect
IIB	Combined hyperlipidemia	—	↑	↑	↑	NC	↑	Yes	Autosomal dominant defect
III	Familial dysbetahyperlipoproteinemia	↑	↑	↑	↑¶	NC	↑	Yes	Autosomal recessive defect
IV	Endogenous hypertriglyceridemia	—	N or ↑	↑	NC	NC or ↓	↑	Unclear	Excessive carbohydrate intake
V	Mixed hypertriglyceridemia	↑	↑	↑	NC	NC or ↓	↑↑	Unclear	Possible metabolic defect

*Cholesterol. Most cases of elevated cholesterol values are multifactorial: genetics, nutrition, and metabolic disease.
†Chylomicrons: 85–95% triglycerides, 3–5% cholesterol esters, 1% free cholesterol, 8% phospholipids, 1% protein.
‡Very-low-density lipoproteins: 64–80% triglycerides, 7–14% cholesterol esters, 6% free cholesterol, 18% phospholipids, 7% protein.
§Low-density lipoproteins: 7–10% triglycerides, 40–50% cholesterol esters, 7% free cholesterol, 23% phospholipids, 21% protein.
‖High-density lipoproteins: 1–7% triglycerides, 17–20% cholesterol esters, 2% free cholesterol, 26% phospholipids, 46% protein.
¶Beta VLDL particles.
CAD, Coronary artery disease; N, normal; NC, no change; TriG, triglycerides.

duce LDL levels. By lowering plasma LDL levels, the bile acid resins significantly decrease morbidity and mortality from CAD.

Pharmacodynamics

Cholestyramine and colestipol are quaternary ammonium anion-exchange resins that act indirectly to reduce LDL levels by binding bile salts in exchange for chloride ions. These drugs form an insoluble complex with the bile acids in the intestine. The bile acid–drug complex prevents the reabsorption of the bile acids, thus increasing their elimination. In an attempt to compensate for the loss of bile salts, the liver raises the rate of bile acid synthesis. LDLs provide the cholesterol necessary for the synthesis of bile acids. To benefit from the presence of LDL, liver cells increase the number of LDL receptors, thereby enlarging their capacity for LDL uptake. The resultant increase in LDL uptake is the mechanism responsible for lowering LDL levels. The ability of liver cells to increase their numbers of LDL receptors is vital for the therapeutic effects of bile acid resins to be realized. Patients genetically incapable of increasing the number of LDL receptors on their liver cells are unable to benefit from bile resins.

Adverse Effects and Contraindications

Because the bile acid–binding resins are not absorbed from the gastrointestinal (GI) tract, there are no systemic adverse effects. However, bile acid resin therapy is not without problems. Resins are insoluble powders with the consistency of fine sand. They must be mixed with fluids to be ingested. They tend to cause bloating, nausea, indigestion, flatulence, and constipation. Because of the exchange of chloride ions for bile acids, greater chloride absorption can result in a hyperchloremic metabolic acidosis. Further, excess fat may appear in the stool because of the binding of bile acids by the resins and the resultant loss of their emulsifying action. Although it is possible that bile acid resin therapy may interfere with the absorption of fat-soluble vitamins (A, D, E, K), there is some disagreement as to whether vitamin supplementation is warranted.

The use of bile acid resins is contraindicated in patients with complete or partial biliary obstruction. They should be used cautiously in patients with steatorrhea or pre-existing constipation. These drugs can be used in the treatment of hypercholesterolemia in children and pregnant women, although clear-cut data as to the safety of their long-term use in children or their use during pregnancy and lactation are not available.

Pharmacokinetics

Bile acid resins are not absorbed in the GI tract. The onset of hypocholesterolemic effects occurs in 24 to 48 hours (Table 35– 4). Peak action is achieved in 1 to 3 weeks, with a duration of action for cholestyramine of 2 to 4 weeks, and for colestipol, 4 weeks. Once bound to the bile acids, the drugs are eliminated in the feces. The dose-response curves for bile acid resins are not linear, and when given in doses above the maximum recommended doses, these drugs have demonstrated little additional cholesterol-lowering effect.

Drug-Drug Interactions

Bile acid resins diminish the absorption of many orally administered drugs (Table 35–5). The resulting decrease in absorption of antibiotics, cardiac glycosides, folic acid, and warfarin reduces their effects. The effect of bile acid resins on many other drugs has not been well studied.

TABLE 35–4 PHARMACOKINETICS OF SELECTED ANTILIPEMIC DRUGS

Drug	Route	Onset	Peak	Duration	PB (%)	t½	BioA (%)
Bile Acid Resins							
Cholestyramine	po	24–48 hr	1–3 wk	2–4 wk	NA	UK	0
Colestipol	po	24–48 hr	4 wk	4 wk	NA	UK	0
Fibric Acid Derivatives							
Gemfibrozil	po	2–5 days*	4 wks*	Mo	95	1.3–1.5 hr	UA
Fenofibrate	po	Varies	3–6 hr	Wks	UA	15 h	UA
HMG-CoA Reductase Inhibitors							
Atorvastatin	po	Rapid	1–2 hr	UA	>95	20 hr	30
Cerivastatin	po	UA	1–3 hr	UA	99	2–3 hr	60
Fluvastatin	po	Slow	UA	4–6 wk	>95	UK	30
Lovastatin	po	3 days	2–4 hr; 4–6 wks†	UA	95	1–2 hr	30
Pravastatin	po	1 hr	1–1.5 hr; wks‡	48 hr	50	77 hr	34
Simvastatin	po	1 hr	1.3–2.4 hr	UA	95	UA	85
Other Antilipemic Drugs							
Nicotinic acid	po	Hours-days	1 hr; UK‖	UK	UK	1 hr	UA

*Time for gemifibrozil's onset and reduction of triglyceride–VLDL levels, respectively.
†The biphasic peaks of lovastatin and pravastatin, respectively.
‡Clinical effects of pravastatin take 4 to 6 weeks.
‖Peak drug levels of niacin are reached in one hour, however, its peak effects on lipids is unknown.
NA, Not applicable; UA, unavailable; UK, unknown.

Dosage Regimen

Cholestyramine is given as 4 g one to six times daily to a maximum dose of 24 g daily (Table 35–6). The drug should be taken before meals. Chewable bar formulations of cholestyramine contain 50 calories each; thus, calorie intake may be a problem for patients on reduction diets. Pediatric dosages are based on cholesterol levels more often than on kilograms of body weight.

Initial dosage of colestipol is 5 g once or twice daily. The dosage is gradually increased to 15 to 30 grams per day in two to four divided doses.

Laboratory Considerations

Serum cholesterol and triglyceride levels should be evaluated before initiation of therapy and periodically throughout the treatment period. Transient elevations of alkaline phosphatase, aspartate aminotransferase (AST [SGPT]), and chloride levels have been reported with bile resin drugs. Decreases in serum calcium, sodium, and potassium levels have been noted, but they are not severe enough for the drug to be discontinued. Bile acid resins can also cause prolonged prothrombin times.

Fibric Acid Derivatives

❒ Clofibrate (ATROMID-S); (✱) CLARIPEX
❒ Fenofibrate
❒ Gemfibrozil (LOPID)

Indications

Gemfibrozil is used to treat Types III, IV, and V hyperlipoproteinemia. Some health care providers believe that it is also effective for Type IIB. Clofibrate is rarely used today because of its association with unexplained high death rates and an increased incidence of cholelithiasis requiring surgery. A higher incidence of malignant liver tumors has also been reported. This first-generation fibric acid derivative has now been virtually replaced by gemfibrozil.

Gemfibrozil is currently approved by the U. S. Food and Drug Administration for treatment of patients with triglyceride concentrations exceeding 750 mg/dL. High triglyceride levels pose a risk not only for atherogenesis but more often for the development of pancreatitis. Gemfibrozil decreases serum triglyceride levels by 40 to 55 percent and VLDL levels by 40 percent, with variable reductions in total cholesterol. It increases HDL levels by 17 to 25 percent. Gemfibrozil does not reduce LDL levels.

Fenofibrate was recently approved by the U. S. Food and Drug Administration for use in patients with hypertriglyceridemia (Types IV and V). It is used as adjunctive therapy in patients who are at risk for pancreatitis and whose very high triglyceride elevations do not respond adequately to determined efforts at dietary control.

Pharmacodynamics

Gemfibrozil also causes an alteration in the rate of synthesis of specific lipoproteins (i.e., C-II, C-III) with activation of extrahepatic lipoprotein lipase. Synthesis of apoproteins (i.e., A-I, A-II) and, thus, formation of HDL particles increase. There is no explanation for how gemfibrozil raises HDL levels. However, because triglycerides make up the primary core of VLDLs, there is some speculation that the ability of gemfibrozil to reduce triglyceride production may be the mechanism by which this drug lowers LDL levels.

Fenofibrate inhibits the biosynthesis of LDL and VLDL, which are responsible for triglyceride development in the liver. It helps mobilize triglycerides from tissues and in-

TABLE 35–5 DRUG-DRUG INTERACTIONS OF SELECTED ANTILIPEMIC DRUGS

Drug	Interactive Drugs	Interaction
Bile Acid Resins		
Cholestyramine	Acetaminophen	Decreased absorption of interactive drug
Colestipol	Amiodarone	
	Antibiotics	
	Cardiac glycosides	
	Corticosteroids	
	Fat-soluble vitamins	
	Folic acid	
	Iron preparations	
	Methotrexate	
	Naproxen	
	Phenobarbital	
	Phenylbutazone	
	Piroxicam	
	Propranolol	
	Thiazide diuretics	
	Thyroxine	
	Ursodiol	
	Oral anticoagulants	
	Warfarin	
Fibric Acid Derivatives		
Gemfibrozil	Warfarin	Increased effects of interactive drug
	Lovastatin	Increased risk of myositis, myalgia
Fenofibrate	Anticoagulants	Increased effects of interactive drug
	Insulin	
	Sulfonylureas	
	Probenecid	Increased toxicity of fenofibrate
	Rifampin	Decreased effects of fenofibrate
HMG-CoA Reductase Inhibitors		
Atorvastatin	Cholestyramine	Additive cholesterol-lowering effects
Fluvastatin	Colestipol	
Lovastatin	Azole antifungals	Increased risk of myopathy, rhabdomyolysis
Pravastatin	Cyclosporin	
Simvastatin	Erythromycin	
	Gemfibrozil	
	Niacin	
	Digoxin	Increased serum drug levels of interactive drug
	Warfarin	
Fluvastatin	Cimetidine	Increased fluvastatin levels
	Omeprazole	
	Ranitidine	
Other Antilipemic Drugs		
Nicotinic acid	Lovastatin	Increased risk of myopathy, rhabdomyolysis
	Guanethidine	Additive hypotension
	Guanadrel	
	Probenecid	Large doses may decrease uricosuric effects of interactive drugs
	Sulfinpyrazone	

creases the elimination of neutral sterols. It also has antiplatelet effects.

Adverse Effects and Contraindications

Gemfibrozil is generally well tolerated. Its most common adverse effect is GI disturbance, followed by fatigue, eczema, rash, vertigo, and headache. Head, neck, or extremity pain, anemia, leukopenia, and hyperglycemia (particularly in patients receiving insulin or oral antihyperglycemic drugs) are uncommon. Cholecystitis, cholelithiasis, acute appendicitis, pancreatitis, and malignancy rarely occur.

The most common adverse effects of fenofibrate are nausea, vomiting, dyspepsia, stomatitis, gastritis, increased risk of cholelithiasis, and weight gain. Impotence, decreased libido, dysuria, proteinuria, and oliguria have been noted. Skin rashes, urticaria, pruritus, dry hair and skin, and alopecia are possible. Flulike symptoms, including myalgias and arthralgias, are also common. Hematuria, pulmonary emboli, leukopenia, and eosinophilia have been documented and are the most life-threatening adverse effects.

Contraindications to the use of fibric acid derivatives are hepatic or renal disease and primary biliary cirrhosis. The drugs should be used cautiously in patients with a history of peptic ulcer disease.

Pharmacokinetics

The onset of triglyceride-VLDL reduction from gemfibrozil takes 2 to 5 days, although the drug reaches peak

TABLE 35–6 DOSAGE REGIMEN FOR SELECTED ANTILIPEMIC DRUGS

Drug	Type(s) of Hyperlipoproteinemia	Dosage	Implications
Bile Acid Resins			
Cholestyramine	II	*Adult:* 4 g po 1–6 × daily. Maximum: Not to exceed 24 g/day. *Child:* 2 g BID intially. Increase as needed and tolerated up to 8–24 g/day in two or more divided doses. Pediatric dosage based on cholesterol level rather than body weight	Take before meals. Mix powder with 4–6 oz of water, milk, fruit juice or other noncarbonated beverage, and shake vigorously. Cholebars contain 50 calories/each, so calorie intake may be a problem for patients on reduction diet
Colestipol	II	*Adult:* 15–30 g/day in two–four divided doses. Increase to 30 g/day as single or divided doses	Take before meals. Can be mixed in a large glass with water, juice, or carbonated beverages. Powder is allowed to sit on fluid for 1–2 min to hydrate before mixing. Should be stirred slowly. Should not be taken dry
Fibric Acid Derivatives			
Gemfibrozil	III, IV, V	*Adults:* 600 mg po BID. Maximum: 1500 mg daily	Take 30 min before breakfast and dinner
Fenofibrate	IV, V	*Adult:* 100 mg po in divided doses. *Child:* Safety and efficacy in pediatric patients has not been established	Used most often for patients at risk for pancreatitis
HMG-CoA Reductase Inhibitors			
Atorvastatin	IIA, V	*Adult:* 10 mg po QD. Range: 10–80 mg/day. Maximum: 80 mg/day	Once-daily dose is taken at bedtime
Cerivastatin	IIA	*Adult:* 0.2–0.3 mg po QD	May be taken with or without food. Once-daily dose is taken at bedtime
Fluvastatin	IIA, IIB	*Adult:* Initial, 20 mg po QD; maintenance, 20–40 mg po *Child:* Safety and efficacy not established	Once-daily dose is taken at bedtime
Lovastatin	II	*Adult:* 20 mg po QD. Increase at 4-week intervals to a maximum of 80 mg/day in single or divided doses	Initial, once-daily dose is taken with the evening meal
Pravastatin	IIA, IIB	*Adult:* 10–20 mg po QD. Geriatric patients start at 10 mg po QD. Increase at weekly intervals to a maximum of 40 mg/day	Once-daily dose is taken at bedtime
Simvastatin	IIA, IIB	*Adult:* 5–10 mg po QD. Start with 10 mg/day for patients with LDL values >190 mg/dL. Increase at 4-week intervals to a maximum of 40 mg/day	Patients on concurrent cyclosporin should not receive more than 10 mg daily
Other Antilipemic Drugs			
Nicotinic acid	II, III, IV, V	*Adult:* 250–500 mg po QD. Increase at weekly intervals to 1.5–2 g/day. After 2 months, can increase to 3–4 g. Maximum: 6 g/day	Once-daily dose is taken after the evening meal

blood levels in 1 to 2 hours. It is 95 percent protein bound with a half-life of 1.5 hours (see Table 35–4). Biotransformation takes place in the liver with elimination in the urine.

Fenofibrate is well absorbed when taken by mouth, with varying times of onset. Its serum levels peak in 3 to 6 hours, and its duration of action is measured in weeks. It has a half-life of 15 hours and is eliminated in the urine.

Drug-Drug Interactions

As with other antilipemic drugs, there are drug-drug interactions for fibric acid derivatives (see Table 35–5). The action of warfarin is enhanced in the presence of gemfibrozil; thus, it is wise to monitor liver function and prothrombin times periodically when the two drugs are used concurrently. Increased bleeding tendencies have been noted if oral anticoagulants are given with fenofibrate. A dosage reduction of as much as 50 percent is often required.

Dosage Regimen

Gemfibrozil is given at 600 mg twice daily, 30 minutes before meals (see Table 35–6). The maximum dose of gemfibrozil is 1500 mg daily. Fenofibrate is prescribed as 100 mg orally daily.

Laboratory Considerations

Fibric acid derivatives increase the results of liver function, creatine phosphokinase, bromsulfophthalein (BSP), and thymol turbidity tests. In addition, gemfibrozil raises glucose levels and may cause a mild reduction in hemoglobin, hematocrit, and white blood cell measurements. Gemfibrozil may also decrease serum potassium concentration.

HMG-CoA Reductase Inhibitors

- ❒ Atorvastatin (LIPITOR)
- ❒ Cerivastatin (BAYCOL)
- ❒ Fluvastatin (LESCOL)
- ❒ Lovastatin (MEVACOR)
- ❒ Pravastatin (PRAVACHOL)
- ❒ Simvastatin (ZOCOR)

Indications

HMG-CoA reductase inhibitors are effective for most patients with hypercholesterolemia, decreasing total plasma cholesterol and LDL levels by 20 to 45 percent. There is emerging evidence of their ability to affect plaque progression, even when used alone. HDL levels increase 8 to 23 percent in response to these agents.

Pharmacodynamics

These drugs are selective inhibitors of the enzyme HMG-CoA reductase. HMG-CoA reductase is an enzyme required in the initial and rate-limiting step in cholesterol synthesis. They lower total cholesterol, LDL, and apo B lipoprotein levels by inhibiting HMG-CoA reductase and cholesterol synthesis in the liver.

The decrease in cholesterol synthesis is met by an up-regulation of cellular LDL receptors. As greater catabolism of LDL occurs, plasma concentrations of LDL fall, and less LDL is available. The reason for the greater effect of these drugs on hepatic HMG-CoA reductase is that 90 percent of the drug is extracted on the first pass through the liver.

Adverse Effects and Contraindications

Headache is the most common adverse effect noted with HMG-CoA reductase inhibitors. Additionally, up to 10 percent of patients have GI symptoms, consisting of diarrhea, constipation, dyspepsia, flatulence, abdominal pain or cramps, and nausea.

Myalgias have been reported in a small percentage of patients. Specifically, 30 percent of immunosuppressed patients who received lovastatin developed myositis within 1 year of starting the drug. If the HMG-CoA reductase inhibitor is not withdrawn, myositis can progress to rhabdomyolysis, possibly associated with acute renal failure.

Hepatotoxicity has been reported in a small percentage of patients taking HMG-CoA reductase inhibitors, although jaundice and other clinical signs were absent. Cautious use of these drugs is warranted in patients with liver disease and in those who consume alcohol to excess. Possible adverse consequences of long-term suppression of cholesterol synthesis are not known.

HMG-CoA reductase inhibitors are contraindicated in patients who are hypersensitive, because cross-sensitivity among agents may occur. They are also contraindicated in patients with active liver disease. Their cautious use is warranted in patients with a history of liver disease, alcoholism, severe acute infection, hypotension, major surgery, trauma, severe metabolic, endocrine or electrolyte disorders, uncontrolled seizure activity, visual disturbances, or myopathy. There is no compelling reason to use these drugs during pregnancy. Women of child-bearing age should be advised about the potential for fetal harm and warned against becoming pregnant while taking these drugs. HMG-CoA reductase inhibitors are also contraindicated during lactation.

Pharmacokinetics

HMG-CoA reductase inhibitors differ in their bioavailability and in the effect of food on their absorption. Food reduces the bioavailability of these drugs (except lovastatin and simvastatin) but not their efficacy. All of these drugs are subject to significant first pass effects (60%) by the liver.

Maximum plasma levels for most HMG-CoA reductase inhibitors occur in approximately 1 to 2 hours, although their cholesterol-lowering effects may take several weeks. Plasma concentrations are lower with evening than with morning drug administration; however, LDL reduction is the same regardless of the time of day the drug is taken.

Some metabolites of these drugs are also active HMG-CoA reductase inhibitors. The drugs and their metabolites are primarily eliminated in the bile following hepatic and extrahepatic biotransformation. Small amounts (less than 20 percent) of the unchanged drugs are eliminated in the urine.

Drug-Drug Interactions

Niacin, erythromycin, gemfibrozil, cyclosporin, and azole antifungal drugs interact with HMG-CoA reductase inhibitors to raise the risk of myopathy and rhabdomyolysis (see Table 35–5). Warfarin and digoxin doses may need to be adjusted owing to their increased serum drug levels. When an HMG-CoA reductase inhibitor is co-administered with an antacid, the plasma concentration of the inhibitor is reduced but not its ability to reduce LDL levels.

Dosage Regimen

The dosage for HMG-CoA reductase inhibitors varies with the specific agent, although fluvastatin, pravastatin, and simvastatin are administered once daily at bedtime (see Table 35–6). These three drugs may be administered without regard to food. Lovastatin, on the other hand, should be administered with food, because its administration on an empty stomach decreases absorption by as much as 30 percent. Initial once-daily doses are administered with the evening meal. If needed, the dosages of these drugs can be increased at 4-week intervals.

Laboratory Considerations

Pronounced and persistent increases in serum transaminase occur in a small percentage of adult patients who receive HMG-CoA reductase inhibitors for longer than 12 months. In a patient who develops muscle tenderness during therapy, creatine phosphokinase levels should be monitored. If these levels are markedly increased or myopathy occurs, therapy should be discontinued.

Liver function tests, including aspartate transaminase (serum glutamic-oxaloacetic transaminase) should be monitored before therapy starts; then every 4 to 6 weeks after the first 3 months of therapy; and then every 6 to 12 weeks for the remainder of the first year or after an increase in dosage; and then every 6 months. If aspartate transaminase (serum glutamic-oxaloacetic transaminase) levels increase to three times normal, the drug should be discontinued. HMG-CoA reductase inhibitors may also raise alkaline phosphatase and bilirubin levels.

Nicotinic Acid

❒ Niacin (Nia-Bid, Niacor, Nico-400, Nicobid, Nicolar, Nicotinex, Nicotinic acid, Slo-Niacin)

Indications

The lipid-lowering effects of nicotinic acid (niacin) were shown more than 30 years ago. Because it lowers both LDL and VLDL, nicotinic acid has been used successfully in a variety of hyperlipidemic conditions. It is the drug of choice for patients at risk for pancreatitis and for those with concurrent elevations of LDL and VLDL. Nicotinic acid reduces plasma triglyceride and total cholesterol levels by 30 to 40 percent and 15 to 20 percent, respectively. LDL levels may be reduced by 20 percent or more. A significant rise in HDL (approximately 15 percent) is also reported.

Pharmacodynamics

Nicotinic acid is a water-soluble vitamin of the B complex that is incorporated into the coenzymes niacinamide adenine dinucleotide and nicotinamide adenine dinucleotide phosphate, which are required for many oxidative-reduction reactions. Both these coenzymes act as hydrogen carriers for glycogenolysis, tissue respiration, and lipid metabolism.

The action of nicotinic acid in lowering lipid levels is independent of its vitamin activity. It also acts as a vasodilator in pharmacotherapeutic doses (more than 250 mg/day). The mechanism by which it lowers cholesterol levels and affects vasodilation is unclear at this time. However, the greater clearance of chylomicrons and VLDL from the plasma decreases LDL and an increases HDL. Central to the action of nicotinic acid is its ability to inhibit the release of free fatty acids from fatty tissue stores.

Adverse Effects and Contraindications

The adverse effects of nicotinic acid include intense flushing and pruritus of the trunk, face, and arms. The flushing is mediated by the release of prostaglandin E_1 and histamine and can be partially inhibited by the ingestion of 325 mg of aspirin 30 to 60 minutes before administration of the nicotinic acid. The flushing usually decreases with prolonged administration, but this tolerance may not occur in warm climates.

The gastrointestinal adverse effects of nicotinic acid include dyspepsia, vomiting, and diarrhea. Activation of peptic ulcer disease has been documented. The GI problems are due, at least in part, to the increases in GI motility and gastric acid secretion stimulated by the released histamine. Less common adverse effects are acanthosis nigricans, vascular-type headaches, orthostatic hypotension (especially in older adults), and reversible blurred vision resulting from macular edema. Nicotinic acid inhibits the tubular elimination of uric acid, thus predisposing the patient to hyperuricemia and gout. There also appears to be a higher incidence of cardiac arrhythmias, including but not limited to atrial fibrillation. Anaphylaxis is more likely with intravenous use of nicotinic acid.

Elevations in plasma glucose levels, attributed to the rebound in fatty acid concentrations, may occur after each dose of nicotinic acid in susceptible individuals. The larger amounts of free fatty acids may compete with the use of glucose by peripheral tissues.

Hepatotoxicity may manifest as cholestatic jaundice with marked elevations of serum transaminases. Fulminant hepatic failure has been reported when patients were changed from immediate-release formulations to sustained-release formulations.

Niacin is contraindicated in patients with known hypersensitivity, hepatic dysfunction, or active peptic ulcer disease. Some formulations may contain tartrazine (FD&C yellow dye #5) and should be avoided in patients with aspirin allergy. Nicotinic acid should be used cautiously in patients with arterial bleeding, gout, glaucoma, and diabetes mellitus.

Pharmacokinetics

Niacin is well absorbed in the intestine following oral administration. It is widely distributed following rapid conversion to niacinamide. (Niacinamide has no effect on lipid levels). When it is taken by mouth, peak drug concentrations are reached within 1 hour, but the time to peak effects on lipid levels is unknown (see Table 35–4). The half-life of niacin in plasma is approximately 1 hour. Large doses of nicotinic acid are eliminated unchanged in the urine.

Drug-Drug Interactions

Large doses of nicotinic acid may decrease the uricosuric effects of probenecid or sulfinpyrazone and produce an increase in uric acid levels (see Table 35–5). There is a higher risk of myopathy with concurrent use of lovastatin. Additive hypotension is associated with the concurrent use of adrenergic neuronal blocking drugs (guanethidine, guanadrel).

Dosage Regimen

The oral dosage regimen for nicotinic acid in the treatment of hypercholesterolemia is 250 to 500 mg daily (see Table 35–6). It may be increased to 1.5 to 2 g at weekly intervals. The patient's ability to tolerate nicotinic acid may be increased by starting therapy at low doses (e.g., 100 to 250 mg three times daily during or just after meals) and administering aspirin before the first dose of the day. After 2 months the dosage can be increased to 3 to 4 g if warranted and the patient is tolerant. The total dosage should not exceed 6 g per day. The higher doses increase both the lipid-altering effect and the incidence of adverse effects. The drug should be administered after the evening meal for best results.

Sustained-release formulations of nicotinic acid should be initiated at 1,500-mg tablet daily and the dosage gradually increased to a maximum of 6 g per day.

Laboratory Considerations

Serum cholesterol, triglycerides, serum glucose, uric acid, and liver function values should be monitored before and periodically throughout therapy, especially with prolonged high-dose therapy. The health care provider should be notified if the aspartate transaminase (serum glutamic-oxaloacetic transaminase), ALT (serum glutamate pyruvate transaminase), or LDH becomes elevated.

Nicotinic acid may increase serum prothrombin times and decrease serum albumin levels. High-dose therapy may cause falsely elevated values for catecholamine and urine glucose if they are measured using the copper sulfate method (Clinitest).

Miscellaneous Antilipemic Drugs

ESTROGENS

In postmenopausal women, estrogen replacement therapy is effective in lowering LDL levels and raising HDL levels. Thus, there is an attendant reduction in the risk of CAD. There is some suggestion that mortality from cardiovascular disease can be reduced by as much as 70 percent in users of estrogen compared with women who do not take estrogen. Nonetheless, use of unopposed estrogen significantly raises the risk of endometrial cancer. Thus, for women who have not had a hysterectomy, hormonal replacement therapy should include both an estrogen and a progestin. The addition of progestin does not appear to significantly reduce the benefits of estrogen, but this impression has not been confirmed. Chapter 54 discusses estrogens and progestins in depth.

OMEGA-3 FATTY ACIDS

The clinical utility of omega-3 fatty acids is greater in patients with elevated triglyceride levels (i.e., hyperlipoproteinemia Types IIB, III, IV, and V). Omega-3 fatty acids, contained in fish oils, produce a sustained reduction in plasma triglyceride levels by inhibiting VLDL and apo B-100 synthesis and decreasing postprandial lipemia. The effects on LDL or apo B and HDL levels are not as clear, but the effect on LDL appears to be dose dependent. Higher doses produce greater effects on lipid levels.

Omega-3 fatty acids affect many steps in atherogenesis, most notably as precursors of the prostaglandins that interfere with blood clotting. Ingestion of large quantities of omega-3 fatty acids can cause prolonged bleeding time, because they inhibit platelet activity. This inhibition has led to concern about spontaneous or excessive bleeding in some patients. A prolonged bleeding time is common to Eskimo populations, who ordinarily have high dietary intake of omega-3 fatty acids and a low incidence of CAD. Other risks associated with omega-3 fatty acids are vitamin A and vitamin D toxicity from fish oil contained in cod liver oil, and increased weight gain from the 9 calories per gram of fish oil.

Critical Thinking Process

Assessment

History of Present Illness

Most patients with lipid disorders display no overt signs and symptoms for decades. An MI or stroke is often the first sign of a lipid problem. Thus, patients should be screened for CAD risk factors at an early age, before these problems arise. Each risk factor identified is thought by some health care providers to double the risk of CAD. For example, a 45-year-old (1 risk factor) male who smokes (2) and has diabetes (3), hypertension (4), and a low HDL level (5) will have a 30-fold increase (5 risk factors; $2 \times 2 \times 2 \times 2 \times 2 = 32$) in risk for CAD compared with a female with no risk factors. Some health care providers "subtract" one risk factor in persons with an HDL level exceeding 50 mg/dL, and two risk factors for patients with an HDL level exceeding 70 mg/dL.

A diet history should be obtained from the patient, especially in regard to fat consumption. Saturated fat intake raises LDL levels more than cholesterol intake. Polyunsaturated fats lower LDL and HDL values. Monounsaturated fat lowers LDL but does not affect HDL levels.

Past Health History

The patient should be queried about a history of constipation, peptic ulcer disease, gallstones or biliary obstruction, steatorrhea, iodism, impaired renal function, and bleeding disorders. Information on previously diagnosed heart disease in the patient or a first-degree family member is also significant.

A drug history is important, owing to the possible drug-drug interactions that can occur with the use of antilipemic drugs. Particular attention should be paid to drugs that may increase lipid levels. A history of allergy to fungal by-products should be specifically noted for patients who are candidates for HMG-CoA reductase inhibitors, which are derived from fungi.

Physical Exam Findings

Most lipid disorders are detected through laboratory determinations. Although uncommonly, patients with extremely high levels of chylomicrons or triglycerides (more than 1000 mg/dL) may complain of eruptive xanthomas and xanthelasma, especially over the buttocks and Achilles and patellar tendons, and on the backs of the hands. The presence of xanthomas usually indicates genetically based hyperlipoproteinemia.

In patients with extremely high triglyceride levels (more than 2000 mg/dL), the appearance of cream-colored blood vessels in the fundus of the eye (lipemia retinalis) and retinal arteriovenous crossing changes may be seen. Arcus senilis may also be seen.

Assessment of typical changes related to decreased oxygen supply, such as pallor around the lips and nail beds, rubor of the skin, thickened or clubbed nails, dry skin, or loss of hair on the extremities, should be noted. Arterial obstruction secondary to the build-up of atheromatous plaques contributes to these signs.

Diagnostic Testing

A lipid profile should be performed for any patient who is symptomatic or asymptomatic and has risk factors for CAD. Determinations of total cholesterol, LDL, and HDL levels allow for a reasonable estimate of CAD risk. Decisions about which tests to order for a particular patient require consideration of test accuracy, cost, and availability as well as the significance and presence of other CAD risk factors. Results obtained with desktop analyzers using finger-stick blood samples are often erroneous.

Correct preparation of the patient for evaluation of lipids is important. The patient should be advised to abstain from alcohol for 48 hours before testing. A 12-hour fast before testing is required, although water may be taken. Smoking should be avoided. These preparations help to minimize transient increases in lipid levels that occur following a heavy meal or alcohol ingestion. A further precaution is that cholesterol and HDL levels are ordinarily not performed immediately after an MI.

An average of two separate cholesterol/triglyceride readings should be taken 1 to 8 hours apart. If the results differ by more than 30 mg/dL, a third reading should be taken and the average value of the three readings used. An HDL level exceeding 60 mg/dL is considered a negative risk factor.

The ratio of total cholesterol to HDL cholesterol should be calculated. A ratio lower than 4.5 is desirable. As a rule of thumb, for every 10-mg/dL rise in total cholesterol levels, there is a 10 percent increase in risk for CAD. Although not routinely measured, apo B is a major component of LDL and is a more sensitive indicator of CAD in men than standard cholesterol measures. Apo A, a major component of HDL, is a much more sensitive predictor of CAD in women.

If the patient is hypothyroid with a normal cholesterol level, the possibility of a laboratory error should be considered. Patients with hypothyroidism generally have elevated total cholesterol levels.

Developmental Considerations

Perinatal Metabolic changes associated with pregnancy elevate cholesterol, lipoproteins, and triglycerides. The cholesterol level can increase by as much as 40 to 60 percent. The higher lipid levels needed for cellular metabolism, carbohydrates, lipids, proteins, vitamins, and inorganic substances are derived from ingested foods. These substrates are used to form new cells and synthesize new substances, and are also burned as fuel for energy.

During pregnancy, the use of glucose accelerates because of rapid fetal cell and organ growth. In addition, maternal sensitivity to insulin is diminished. As a result, pregnancy is said to produce a diabetes-like state. This diabetes-like state may contribute to the upset in lipid values, at least during the pregnancy. Although pregnancy occurs most often in young, healthy individuals, the risk of lipid disorders, especially those that are genetically determined, remains.

Pediatric Childhood cholesterol levels appear to be a major population predictor for adult cholesterol levels. Current evidence indicates that a presymptomatic phase of atherosclerosis begins during childhood. Children who exhibit cholesterol levels in the upper percentiles of normal seem to have a higher risk of retaining cholesterol levels in the upper percentiles of normal into adulthood. The more seriously affected children are customarily those for whom dietary and possibly drug management is warranted. On the other hand, children whose cholesterol levels are in the lower percentiles of normal are unlikely to have elevated cholesterol values as adults.

Geriatric Cholesterol levels have been reported to gradually increase with age in both men and women. Women have high levels of HDL in all age groups. Postmenopausal women have a drop in estrogen that triggers a rise in cholesterol levels. With changes in lipid metabolism, cholesterol levels rise to a maximum at 65 years and then decrease, but never as low as that in young adults. LDL and HDL levels in combination with systolic blood pressure are significant in predicting coronary risk in the elder adults. Triglyceride values also rise with age. The increase is greater in females than males at 50 years. The triglyceride level then decreases in men and rises significantly higher with age in women.

Older adults often have diabetes, impaired liver function, or other conditions that also raise blood lipid levels. They are also likely to have cardiovascular and other disorders for which they are taking drugs. For example, diuretics such as hydrochlorothiazide and chlorthalidone may be taken for hypertension or heart failure, but they can increase cholesterol levels by 10 percent. Beta blockers, such as propranolol, and estrogens can increase triglyceride levels by 25 to 50 percent.

Psychosocial Considerations

Stress and coronary prone (type A) behaviors can markedly elevate LDL and total cholesterol values in susceptible individuals. In some cases, low self-esteem contributes to stress, the tendency toward type A personality, smoking behaviors, and obesity, all of which are risk factors for lipid disorders.

Alcohol intake is related to triglyceride elevations but has little effect on total cholesterol. There is some evidence that moderate ingestion of alcohol causes HDL levels to rise. However, research has also suggested that alcohol has little effect on the protective fraction of HDLs (see Case Study—Hyperlipoproteinemia).

Analysis and Management

Treatment Objectives

The ultimate goal for treatment of hyperlipoproteinemia is to prevent the progression of coronary atherosclerosis and reduce the risk of CAD and other vascular disorders. The immediate goal is to reduce LDL levels while keeping the management regimen affordable.

For primary prevention (in patients with no established CAD), the target LDL level is less than 160 mg/dL in patients with fewer than two CAD risk factors, and less than 130 mg/dL in patients with two or more CAD risk factors (Table 35–7). For secondary prevention (in patients with established CAD), the target LDL level is less than 100 mg/dL.

Effective reduction in CAD risk requires identifying and aggressively treating all CAD risk factors responsive to intervention, including smoking, hypertension, diabetes, and obesity. The approach to treatment is guided by an assessment of total CAD risk, not just the lipid abnormality. For a given degree of LDL elevation, the threshold for initiation of therapy decreases and the intensity of therapy increases as CAD risk rises. Dietary modification, complemented by weight reduction and exercise, is the core of lipid management, with drug therapy reserved for patients at highest risk.

Treatment Options

Life-Style Changes Dietary management for patients with hyperlipoproteinemia should precede and accompany drug therapy. It remains the cornerstone of treatment, effective for both treatment and prevention of lipid disorders. Decreases in the intake of cholesterol and saturated fat in controlled settings can reduce total cholesterol and LDL levels by up to 30 percent. The reductions average about 10 percent, however, when a similar intensive treatment regimen is prescribed for outpatient use. The argument for dietary therapy as the initial step in treatment is based on the following con-

Case Study Hyperlipoproteinemia

Patient History

History of Present Illness	MM, a 56-year-old male, presents for follow-up of hyperlipoproteinemia, type II diabetes mellitus, and hypertension. His last visit was 6 months ago, at which time dietary interventions and an exercise regimen were prescribed. He reports today feeling "a little sluggish" recently but attributes it to stress in the workplace, the need for a part-time second job, and perhaps an elevation in his blood pressure. His work requires him to travel three to four times a month, and he admits to noncompliance with the previously prescribed diet and exercise regimen. He reports smoking cigarettes 1–2 packs/day for last 30 years, and consuming 3–4 oz of alcohol daily for the past 5–6 months. He has been taking hydrochlorothiazide 50 mg po QD, and potassium chloride 20 mEq po QD, since diagnosed with hypertension 3 years ago. He takes glipizide 5 mg po QD for his diabetes.
Past Health History	MM has a positive family history for heart disease and hypertension. His father died at 53 of an MI. Mother is alive and well. Brother has diabetes mellitus and a history of alcoholism. Except for hypertension, MM has an otherwise negative past health history.
Physical Exam	BP 158/88, pulse 100, respirations 24; temp, 98.6° F. Height, 5.9″; weight, 188 lb (up 25 lb from previous visit). Remainder of exam unremarkable.
Diagnostic Testing	Complete blood count, electrolytes, blood urea nitrogen, creatinine, and thyroid function tests are within normal limits. Total cholesterol, 260 mg/dL; LDL, 159 mg/dL; HDL, 34 mg/dL; triglycerides, 559 mg/dL; FBS, 180 mg/dL; hemoglobin A_{1c}, 11.0% (poor control).
Developmental Considerations	MM is attempting to support family with two sons in their late teens and to care for his aging mother, who is trying to remain independent at home.
Psychosocial Considerations	MM admits he is a type A personality with a strong drive (i.e., need) to be the breadwinner in the family. His wife died 10 years ago in a motor vehicle accident.
Economic Factors	MM has health insurance and pharmacy coverage for his sons but does not carry his own insurance because of the expense. Is concerned about the cost of his own health care needs but feels unable to obtain personal health insurance at this time. Pays cash for visits to health care provider and hopes hospitalization will not be necessary.

Variables Influencing Decision

Treatment Objectives	• Prevent the progression of coronary atherosclerosis and reduce the risk of coronary artery disease • Reduce LDL cholesterol levels while keeping the treatment regimen affordable • Improve adherence to concurrent dietary and exercise regimen

Drug Variables	*Drug Summary*	*Patient Variables*
Indications	The following drugs are indicated in the treatment of type II hyperlipoproteinemia: bile acid resins, HMG-CoA reductase inhibitors, and nicotinic acid.	MM diagnosed with Type II hyperlipoproteinemia (combined hyperlipidemia) and has multiple risk factors for CAD. Dietary and exercise regimen has failed. On hydrochlorothiazide which increases LDL levels. This is a decision point.
Pharmacodynamics	Antilipemic drugs work to reduce serum cholesterol and LDL levels, or to increase HDL levels through various mechanisms.	No direct pharmacodynamic considerations influence the decision to use a specific antilipemic drug for MM. This will not be a decision point.

Drug Variables	*Drug Summary*	*Patient Variables*
Adverse Effects/ Contraindications	Adverse effects vary with specific drug to be chosen, but adverse effects in general include gastrointestinal distress. Most are contraindicated in patients with hepatic, renal, or biliary disease.	MM has no contraindications to therapy. Will need to monitor for adverse effects regardless of the drug used.
Pharmocokinetics	Antilipemic drugs have various onset, peak, and duration times, protein binding, and half-lives.	No direct pharmacokinetic considerations influence the decision to use a specific antilipemic drug. This will not be decision point.
Dosage Regimen	Once-daily dosing possible with all antilipemic drugs but requires long-term therapy.	MM more likely to comply with a once-daily regimen, but long-term regimen may become a problem. This will be a decision point.
Laboratory Considerations	Lipid profile necessary to monitor therapy, although can be done on an every 3–6 month basis on basis of patient status.	Cost of lab monitoring may be a decision point, since MM has no health insurance.
Cost Index*	Cholestyramine: 5 Colestipol: 5 Fluvastatin: 5 Pravastatin: 5 Lovastatin: 5 Simvastatin: 5 Nicotinic acid: 1	Need to use least expensive treatment option owing to self-pay status of patient, and easiest formulation to promote compliance. This will be a decision point.

Summary of Decision Points

- MM has multiple risk factors for hyperlipoproteinemia and CAD, and has failed to follow dietary and exercise regimen. Taking hydrochlorothiazide, which increases LDL levels.
- MM more likely to be compliant if a once-daily drug regimen is utilized.
- Need to use least expensive treatment option owing to self-pay status of patient, and easiest formulation to promote compliance.
- Dramatic difference in drug costs among bile acid resins, HMG-CoA reductase inhibitors, and niacin.
- Need to continue to encourage dietary and exercise regimen, smoking cessation, weight loss, and control of hypertension.

DRUGS TO BE USED

- Discontinue hydrochlorothiazide and potassium chloride. Start spironolactone 25 mg po QD.
- Continue glipizide 5 mg po QD for diabetes with regular monitoring of blood glucose and hemoglobin A_{1c} levels.
- Nicotinic acid 250 mg po QD after evening meal × 1 week; then 500 mg po QD × 1 week; then increase dosage at weekly intervals to 1.5 g on basis of patient response.
- Add a bile acid resin (e.g., cholestyramine) if necessary to enhance cholesterol-lowering effects.

Cost Index: 1 = $ < 30/mo.
2 = $ 30–40/mo.
3 = $ 40–50/mo.
4 = $ 50–60/mo.
5 = $ > 60/mo.

AWP of 90, 5-gram/packets of colestipol powder is approximately $107.
AWP of 90, 4-gram/packets of cholestyramine powder is approximately $121.
AWP of 100, 20-mg capsules of fluvastatin is approximately $108.
AWP of 100, 20-mg pravastatin tablets is approximately $190.
AWP of 100, 20-mg lovastatin tablets is approximately $214.
AWP of 100, 5-mg simvastatin tablets is approximately $180.
AWP of 100, 500-mg nicotinic acid tablets is approximately $4.

TABLE 35–7 GENERAL GUIDELINES FOR DRUG MANAGEMENT OF HYPERLIPOPROTEINEMIA

Regimen	History of CAD	Risk Factors Present	Present LDL Level	LDL Treatment Goal
Dietary	No	<2	>160 mg/dL	<160 mg/dL
	No	2 or more	>130 mg/dL	<130 mg/dL
	Yes	NA	>100 mg/dL	<100 mg/dL
Drug	No	<2	>190 mg/dL*	<160 mg dL
	No	2 or more	>160 mg/dL*	<130 mg/dL
	Yes	NA	>130 mg/dL*	<100 mg/dL

*LDL level despite strict adherence to prescribed dietary regimen.
CAD, Coronary artery disease; LDL, low-density lipoprotein; NA, not applicable.

siderations: (1) diet is the most physiologic approach, (2) the change in life-style should be life-long, (3) no drugs are without known or potential adverse effects, and (4) in most cases, drug therapy is expensive. (see Controversy—Diet versus Drugs in Treating Hyperlipidemia.)

It is recommended that all Americans adopt the Phase I dietary plan published by the American Heart Association (Table 35–8). This plan has the following features:

- Total fat as a percentage of total calories is reduced from an average of 40 or 45 percent to 30 percent.
- Saturated fat intake is restricted to 10 percent or less of caloric intake.
- Polyunsaturated fat is increased to 10 percent of calories.
- Dietary intake of cholesterol is reduced from 500 mg per day to no more than 300 mg per day.
- Protein intake is held constant.

Step I dietary modifications do not require a dramatic alteration in the patient's eating habits and can be readily adopted by most persons. However, Step II dietary modifications require more effort, because they go beyond eliminating obvious sources of fat and cholesterol. Step II dietary modifications are indicated for patients who are already utilizing a Step I diet at the time of diagnosis, who do not achieve adequate results with Step I dietary management, or who have established CAD. If these limitations fail to reduce lipid levels to the desired range, a Phase III dietary modification may be necessary.

Renewed emphasis on exercise and weight reduction as complements to dietary therapy are essential components of a comprehensive nondrug treatment program. They are helpful not only in correcting lipid abnormalities but also in reducing other CAD risk factors. For example, exercise raises HDL levels, lowers blood pressure, and improves the efficiency of peripheral oxygen extraction. Weight loss efforts lower fat intake, reduce the risk of diabetes, and decrease myocardial workload. Exercise performed on a regular basis reduces LDL and elevates HDL. Thus, the risk of CAD is reduced. In addition, patients should be advised to quit smoking.

Nonprescription dietary supplements are no substitute for dietary modification. Nonetheless, they are popular with patients, even though they can be expensive. There is some evidence that omega-3 fatty acids, available in fish oils, may be useful, but they are too limited to serve as the basis for dietary recommendations. Antioxidant vitamins such as vita-

Controversy

Diet Versus Drugs In Treating Hyperlipidemia

JONATHAN J. WOLFE

Health care providers universally recognize the central role of hyperlipidemia in cardiovascular disease. This set of diseases poses difficulties in treatment. On the one hand, a minority of patients have an inherited metabolic predisposition to high levels of cholesterol or triglycerides. However, dietary and life-style interventions may not suffice for persons with familial hyperlipidemia. They may meet tragically early cardiac deaths if their disorder is not diagnosed and aggressively treated.

In the United States, many people expose themselves to predictable disorders simply by rejecting a healthful diet and reasonable levels of exercise. This second group of patients would not seem to need lipid-lowering drugs. Indeed, their unhealthy life-style choices may also expose them to hepatic dysfunction related to therapy with lipid-lowering drugs. The issue becomes one of the cost and risk of using lipid-lowering drugs versus the cost and risk of cardiovascular disease. Are we, as a society, more apt to choose a drug than to alter our comfort index by adopting a low-fat diet and regular exercise plan?

In addition, nontraditional approaches to hyperlipidemia are available from a thriving dietary supplement industry. These dietary supplements exist outside U. S. Food and Drug Administration regulation; a product may be legally marketed so long as no therapeutic claims are made about it. Advice touting such dietary supplements for health promotion has proliferated in print and broadcast media, advertising, and busy retail outlets.

Critical Thinking Discussion

- Why do you think patients are quick to seek alternatives to traditional medicine in preventing cardiovascular disease related to elevated serum lipids?
- Why do you think patients so commonly prefer to take drugs rather than to alter their life-style choices regarding diet and exercise?
- What counseling would you provide to a patient who presents for a routine check-up and volunteers that she has stopped taking prescription drugs for hypercholesterolemia, but now takes an herbal tea that has the same effects and for lower cost?
- Why do patients consider herbal and other natural products to be safer than mainstream pharmaceuticals?
- What issues of social justice are involved when a patient on a fixed income says he no longer complies with drug treatment regimens because it means a choice between buying groceries for the last 10 days of the month or buying his medication?

TABLE 35–8 DIETARY GUIDELINES FOR HEALTHY AMERICANS

Dietary Component	Average Intake	Step I Diet	Step II Diet
Dietary cholesterol	500 mg	<300 mg	200–250 mg
Total fat (as % of total calories)	40–45	30% or less	30% or less
Saturated fat	17	8-10%	<7%
Monounsaturated fat	18	To 15%	To 15%
Polyunsaturated fat	7	To 10%	To 10%
Carbohydrates (as % total calories)	40–45	55% or more	55% or more
Protein (as % total calories)	15–20	Approx 15%	Approx 15%

Data from the American Heart Association: Stone, N., Nicolosi, R., Kris-Etherton, P., et al. (1996). Summary of the scientific conference on the efficacy of hypocholesterolemic dietary interventions. *Circulation,* 94, 3388–3391; and Krauss, R., Deckelbaum, R., Ernst, N., et al. (1996). Dietary guidelines for healthy American adults. *Circulation,* 94, 1795-1800.

min C, vitamin E, and beta carotene do not lower cholesterol levels. However, they may increase LDL resistance to oxidative change and thus reduce the risk of injury to vasculature. Additional study is needed, but daily doses of 400 IU of vitamin E, 0.5 to 1 g of vitamin C, and 25 mg of beta carotene appear safe and perhaps may prove beneficial. Garlic supplements (one-half to one clove/day) can produce a 5 to 10 percent reduction in serum cholesterol.

Psyllium (found in METAMUCIL and other products) has also been shown to be effective in some patients at a dose of 10 g per day. Psyllium lowers LDL and total cholesterol levels an average of 5 to 10 percent. It is a logical drug of choice to treat moderately elevated LDL levels (130 to 159 mg/dL) when HDL levels are above 45 mg/dL, especially in older adults. Psyllium promotes bowel regularity, sometimes causes flatulence, but has no serious adverse effects. Psyllium is discussed in more depth in Chapter 43.

Drug Variables

The range of available drugs is extensive, and they vary greatly in cost, effect on cholesterol fractions, efficacy, and adverse effects. No drugs currently available are effective in lowering all types of hyperlipoproteinemia, and all have adverse effects. Drug therapy is started when diet therapy and exercise for 3 to 6 months have been ineffective. Conditions known to increase serum lipid levels (i.e., diabetes, hypothyroidism, liver disease, long-term corticosteroid use) may impose the need for drug therapy. Thus, clinical decisions regarding drug therapy are based on a number of factors, as follows:

- Cholesterol and triglyceride levels
- The nature of the patient's lipoprotein abnormality
- The presence of co-morbid disease or conditions
- CAD risk factors
- Drug mechanism of action and adverse effects

The best management regimen is one that addresses and fits well into the patient's overall clinical state. A high level of individualization is necessary. The patient should always be involved in treatment decisions and should be told of the absolute benefits and risks of the various management options.

Bile Acid Resins Bile acid resins have been used as first-line therapy for hyperlipoproteinemias for many years and have an established safety record. Though not as effective as other pharmacotherapeutic interventions (e.g., HMG-CoA reductase inhibitors, nicotinic acid), they are effective for patients with a low CAD risk but in whom diet alone fails to lower LDL to desired levels. Bile acid resins are not as cost-effective as the HMG-CoA reductase inhibitors or nicotinic acid, but they are effective when used in combination to treat high-risk patients with severe hypercholesterolemia. There is some evidence that combination therapy reduces LDL levels to such an extent that there may be actual regression of atherosclerotic plaque.

Although bile acid resins primarily lower LDL levels, they also modestly increase HDL levels (Table 35–9). A variable but transient rise in triglycerides is in patients whose triglyceride levels already exceed 250 mg/dL. The rise is secondary to increases in triglyceride production and VLDL triglyceride content and size. Cholesterol levels managed with bile acid resins start to decline 48 hours after the start of therapy but may take 1 year to stabilize. Bile resin therapy is usually discontinued if the patient's clinical response remains poor after 3 months.

TABLE 35–9 LIPID-LOWERING EFFECTS OF SELECTED ANTILIPEMIC DRUGS

Drug	Total Cholesterol (%)	LDL (%)	HDL (%)	Triglycerides (%)
Bile acid resins	↓15–30	↓15–35	↑10–38	↑5–40
Fibric acid derivatives	↓2–10	↓5–18	↑17–25	↓40–50
HMG-CoA reductase inhibitors	↓20–45	↓20–45	↑8–23	↓8–25
Nicotinic acid	↓15–30	↓15–30	↑10–30	↓30–40
Probucol	↓10–20	↓10–15	↓10–15	NE

HDL, High-density lipoprotein; LDL, low-density lipoprotein; NE, no significant effect.

Bile acid resins raise triglycerides and are therefore not particularly useful in the treatment of mixed lipid disorders. They may be used, however, in combination with gemfibrozil or nicotinic acid for patients who develop myositis with a combination of gemfibrozil and lovastatin.

HMG-CoA Reductase Inhibitors Second-line drugs to date, HMG-CoA reductase inhibitors are quickly moving to first-line status by virtue of their effectiveness, patient acceptability, and increasingly favorable safety records. They are more effective than all other drugs (except nicotinic acid) in lowering total cholesterol, VLDL, LDL, and triglyceride levels. They also have proven efficacy in reducing cardiovascular mortality and morbidity. Further, they are better tolerated than bile acid resins or nicotinic acid. HMG-CoA reductase inhibitors can be chosen for patients who cannot take or tolerate nicotinic acid. The least expensive of these agents can be chosen, because they are equal in effectiveness and patient tolerance.

The major drawbacks to the use of HMG-CoA reductase inhibitors are cost and the lack of data on their long-term safety. Although these agents are expensive, the selection of a specific drug may be based on price, as already mentioned, because they all have similar efficacy. However, when cost is considered as a function of LDL-lowering capacity, only nicotinic acid is more cost effective. All of the HMG-CoA reductase inhibitors are similar in effectiveness and adverse effects, but lovastatin appears to be either as effective or more effective than other currently available drugs.

Nicotinic Acid Nicotinic acid should be considered a first-line agent for patients with hypercholesterolemia in whom cost is a limiting factor, because it is less expensive than bile acid resins and HMG-CoA reductase inhibitors. Nicotinic acid is also chosen when agents from those two drug groups are ineffective or not well tolerated. However, the effect of nicotinic acid on cholesterol lowering can be enhanced by coadministration of bile acid resins. A full dose of nicotinic acid reduces LDL concentrations by 15 to 30 percent. When nicotinic acid is taken in combination with one of the bile acid resins, however, a 60 to 70 percent reduction is often reported. The adverse effects (e.g., intense flushing, pruritus) of this drug limit its acceptance and usefulness.

Nicotinic acid is not as effective in reducing triglycerides as fibric acid derivatives. It is much less expensive, however, and should be considered if fibric acid derivatives are not effective or not tolerated.

Nicotinic acid is recommended for the treatment of combined hypercholesterolemia and hypertriglyceridemia. Assuming it is tolerated, it has proven efficacy in reducing cardiovascular disease, lowering triglycerides, raising HDL, and lowering LDL. It is also the least expensive of the drug options.

Fibric Acid Derivatives Fibric acid derivatives generally reduce LDL levels less than bile acid resins, nicotinic acid, or HMG-CoA reductase inhibitors, and in some cases may even raise the levels. Therefore, they should be considered for the treatment of hypercholesterolemia only if all other drugs have failed. Evidence suggests that gemfibrozil can actually raise LDL levels in patients with very elevated triglyceride levels, but decreases LDL levels in patients with normal or moderately elevated triglyceride levels. However, there are apparent inconsistencies in gemfibrozil's effects, which may be related to triglyceride levels.

Fibric acid derivatives are recommended in the treatment of hypertriglyceridemia because of their proven efficacy in reducing the incidence of cardiovascular disease and their main effect on triglycerides. Unless there is significant cost advantage, gemfibrozil should be used rather than fenofibrate, because there are no long-term studies evaluating fenofibrate's effect on cardiovascular morbidity and mortality.

If after 3 months of treatment with any of the antilipemic drugs, the drug is tolerated and there has been at least a 15 percent decrease in lipids but not to the desired level, the first drug can be continued and a second-line drug added. If, on the other hand, the patient is not tolerating the drug, or there is less than a 15 percent decrease in total cholesterol levels, the first drug should be stopped and a second-line drug started. In either case, the patient should be monitored as if it is the first use of the drug.

Patient Variables

Drug therapy in adult men younger than 35 years with no history of coronary or atherosclerotic disease and with fewer than two risk factors should be considered only when LDL levels exceed 220 mg/dL despite a 6-month trial of intensive dietary management and exercise. For men older than 35 years with no risk factors, drug therapy is recommended if the LDL is higher than 190 mg/dL or the total cholesterol is higher than 260 mg/dL after a 6-month trial of intensive dietary management and exercise.

Drug therapy for premenopausal and postmenopausal women should be considered only when LDL levels exceed 220 mg/dL despite a 6-month trial of intensive dietary management and exercise. Because of the low incidence of CAD in premenopausal women, drug therapy is often delayed until after menopause. The health care provider should be aware that the relationship between CAD and cholesterol levels is less consistent in women older than 65 years than in other groups.

No data support or refute drug therapy in patients older than 65 years, although moderate dietary modification and exercise should not be discouraged. Some health care providers suggest that older adults who are not of advanced physiologic or chronologic age and who do not have heart failure, dementia, or cancer should receive antilipemic therapy in a fashion similar to that of middle-aged patients. Older adults with advanced physiologic or chronologic age or with severe life-limiting illness are generally not candidates for aggressive drug or nondrug therapy.

Patients with hypertriglyceridemia or a mixed lipid disorder (hypercholesterolemia and hypertriglyceridemia) should be considered for drug therapy only if they are symptomatic with xanthomas or pancreatitis. There is no evidence yet to support the treatment or screening of patients with asymptomatic triglyceride elevations.

Patients with hypothyroidism, nephrotic syndrome, or liver disease have increased total cholesterol and LDL levels. Similarly, patients taking thiazide diuretics may have increased LDL levels. The concurrent use of beta blockers with antilipemic drugs generally reduces HDL levels and of estrogen increases HDL levels. Estrogen replacement therapy also increases triglyceride levels.

Over-the-counter drugs are often a preferred choice for antilipemic therapy for many patients, because they are inexpensive, safe, and effective. Prescription drugs, especially HMG-CoA reductase inhibitors and bile acid resins, are expensive.

The balance among potential benefits, adverse effects, cost, and compliance should be weighed carefully before prescription drugs are used. Further, patients who are homozygous for the absence of LDL receptors may not benefit from these drugs.

Intervention

Administration

The bile acid resins cholestyramine and colestipol are formulated as powders for suspension and should be mixed with any liquid or any food with a high-moisture content. Cholestyramine should be mixed with 4 to 6 oz of water, milk, fruit juice, or other noncarbonated beverage before administration. Colestipol can be mixed with water, juice, carbonated beverages, highly fluid soups, cereals, applesauce, or crushed pineapple. The powder should be allowed to sit on the fluid for 1 to 2 minutes before being mixed in. These drugs should not be taken dry. Food also helps disguise the taste and grainy texture of the drugs. Bile acid resins should not be taken concurrently with other drugs, particularly acidic drugs, because of their ability to bind with them. Other drugs should be administered 1 hour before or 4 to 6 hours after a bile acid resin.

HMG-CoA reductase inhibitors should be taken in the evening, because the highest rates of cholesterol synthesis are between midnight and 5 AM. They may be taken without regard for meals.

Fibric acid derivatives should be taken 30 minutes before meals. If GI upset occurs, gemfibrozil or fenofibrate can be taken with meals.

Timed-release tablets and capsules of nicotinic acid should be swallowed whole, without crushing, breaking, or chewing. They should be administered with meals or milk to minimize GI irritation.

Education

Patient education and discussion with family members are vital to foster an understanding of the importance of long-term commitment to therapy. Explanations of the lipid disorder, consequences, treatment regimens, and required life-style modifications are important. The patient should be advised that antilipemic drugs are used in conjunction with dietary restrictions of fat, cholesterol, calories, and alcohol. The importance of exercise, smoking cessation, weight reduction, and control of co-morbid diseases should be included in the teaching.

It is important to work with the members of the patient's household who cook and shop for groceries, so that they understand how to select and prepare "heart-healthy" meals. Eating less saturated fat and cholesterol can usually lower total cholesterol levels by 10 to 20 percent. Less pork and beef should be eaten, and more fish, chicken, turkey, and nonfat or low-fat milk. Minimal amounts of other whole-milk dairy products, such as cheese, butter, ice cream, and sour cream, are acceptable. Margarines and cooking oils that contain polyunsaturated oil products (e.g., safflower, corn, soybean) or monounsaturated oil products (e.g., olive oil) should be used. Oat bran, consumed as cereal or muffins, helps reduce total cholesterol and LDL levels an average of 5 to 10 percent.

As with all drugs, the patient should be instructed to take a prescribed antilipemic drug exactly as instructed and not to skip doses or to double up on missed doses. If a dose is missed, it should be taken as soon as remembered. The importance of regular follow-up visits and laboratory evaluations should be stressed.

Constipation is possible with bile resins and other antilipemic drugs. Thus, explaining the importance of fluids and bulk in the diet as well as exercise, stool softeners, and laxatives (if necessary) is vital. The patient should be told to contact the health care provider if constipation, nausea, flatulence, and heartburn are persistent, or if the stools become frothy and foul-smelling. The patient should also be told to report unusual bleeding or bruising, petechiae, or black, tarry stools. Treatment with vitamin K may be necessary.

Evaluation

The prognosis for patients with lipid disorders can be greatly improved by lasting life-style changes and, in many cases, long-term drug therapy. Drug therapy for hyperlipoproteinemia can continue for many years and possibly a lifetime. Thus, the health care provider should consider reducing or stopping drug therapy if the desired LDL cholesterol level is maintained for a period of 2 years, to re-establish the diagnosis, and to check the efficacy of nondrug measures. Dietary therapy should continue. Total cholesterol levels should be measured 4 to 6 weeks after drugs are stopped and again at 3 months. If the levels are again elevated, therapy should be restarted.

SUMMARY

- Hyperlipoproteinemia is an increase in the concentration of protein/lipid complexes in the blood, containing cholesterol, triglycerides, and phospholipids.
- Hyperlipoproteinemia is a problem of epidemic proportions in the United States and a major risk factor for CAD.
- Elevations in total cholesterol and LDL levels and a reduction in HDL cholesterol are strongly positive independent risk factors for the development of CAD in persons younger than 65 years.
- The lipoproteins are usually divided into five classes on the basis of their density, a reflection of relative protein and lipid content.
- The five major types of hyperlipoproteinemia are essentially organized according to their underlying cause and characteristic lipid values.
- Most patients with lipid disorders display no overt signs and symptoms for decades. An MI or stroke often is the first sign of a lipid problem.
- Patients should be screened for CAD risk factors before cardiovascular problems arise.
- The ultimate goal for treatment of hyperlipoproteinemia is a reduction in CAD risk.
- The immediate treatment goal is a reduction in LDL cholesterol levels.
- Diet, exercise, smoking cessation, and drug therapy effectively reduce total and LDL cholesterol levels and raise HDL levels.
- The patient should be advised that antilipemic drugs are used in conjunction with dietary restrictions of fat, cholesterol, calories, and alcohol.

- Treatment options for hyperlipoproteinemia include bile acid resins, HMG-CoA reductase inhibitors, fibric acid derivatives, and a small number of miscellaneous drugs. Each group carries its own advantages and disadvantages for the individual patient.
- Patient education and discussion with family members are vital to foster an understanding of the importance of a long-term commitment to therapy.
- Explanations of the disorder, consequences, treatment regimens, and the importance of life-style modifications are vital to successful management.
- Patients should be taught how and when to take their antilipemic drug, because some agents should be taken on an empty stomach and some may require the presence of food to enhance absorption.
- The prognosis for patients with lipid disorders can be greatly improved by lasting life-style changes and, in many cases, long-term drug therapy.
- The health care provider may consider reducing or stopping drug therapy if the desired LDL cholesterol level is maintained for a period of 2 years, to re-establish the diagnosis, and to check the efficacy of nondrug measures.

BIBLIOGRAPHY

Abramowicz, M (1998). Cerivastatin for hypercholesterolemia. *The Medical Letter on Drugs and Therapeutics*, 40 (1018), 13–14.

Betteridge, D., Durrington, P., Fairhurst, G., et al. (1994). Comparison of lipid lowering effects of low dose fluvastatin and conventional dose gemfibrozil in patients with primary hypercholesterolemia. *American Journal of Medicine,* 96(6), 45S-54S.

Carter, B., and Bakht, F. (1990). Therapy for hypercholesterolemia. *Primary Care,* 17(3), 479–493.

Cerrato, P. (1993). OTC interactions: Vitamins and minerals. *RN,* 56(6), 28–33.

Eaker, E., Johnson, D., Loop, F., et al. (1992). Heart disease in women: How different? *Patient Care,* 26(3), 191–204.

Expert Panel on Detection, Evaluation, and Treatment of High Blood Cholesterol in Adults. (1993). Summary of the Second Report of the National Cholesterol Education Program (NCEP). *Journal of the American Medical Association,* 269(23), 3015–3023.

Hunninghake, D., Stein, E., and Dujovne, C. (1993). The efficacy of intensive dietary therapy alone or combined with lovastatin in outpatients with hypercholesterolemia. *New England Journal of Medicine,* 328(17), 1213–1219.

Joint National Committee on Detection, Evaluation, and Treatment of High Blood Pressure. (1997). The Sixth Report of the Joint National Committee on Detection, Evaluation, and Treatment of High Blood Pressure. *Archives of Internal Medicine,* 157(21), 2413–2446.

Kafonek, S., and Kwiterovich, P. (1990). Treatment of hypercholesterolemia in the elderly. *Annals of Internal Medicine,* 112(10), 723–725.

Klag, M., Ford, D., Mead, L., et al. (1993). Serum cholesterol in young men and subsequent cardiovascular disease. *New England Journal of Medicine,* 328(5), 313–318.

Koda-Kimbell, M., and Young, L. (1995). *Applied therapy: The clinical use of drugs.* Vancouver, BC: Applied Therapeutics, Inc.

Kupecz, D. (1997). Atorvastatin: A new agent for hyperlipidemia. *Nurse Practitioner: The American Journal of Primary Health Care,* 22(11), 87–88.

McKenney, J. (1993). New guidelines for managing hypercholesterolemia: National Cholesterol Education Program. *American Pharmacy,* NS33(7), 24–32.

Milander, M., and Kuhn, M. (1992). Lipid-lowering drugs. *AACN:* Clinical Issues in Critical Care Nursing. 3(2), 494–506.

New Drugs/Drug News. (1994). New triglyceride-lowering drugs. *Pharmacy and Therapeutics,* 19(3), 218.

Santinga, J., Rosman, H., Rubenfire, M., et al. (1994). Efficacy and safety of pravastatin in the long-term treatment of elderly patients with hypercholesterolemia. *American Journal of Medicine,* 96(6), 509–515.

Schell, M. (1990). Cholesterol, lipoproteins, lipid profiles: A challenge in patient education. *Focus on Critical Care,* 17(3), 203–211.

Spreuill, B. (1991). Managing hyperlipidemia in the elderly. *Clinical Consultation,* 10(3), 1.

Summary of the Second Report of the National Cholesterol Education Program (1994). Fluvastatin for lowering cholesterol. *The Medical Letter,* 36, 45–46.

United States Pharmacopeial Convention. (1994). *USP DI: Drug information for the health care professional.* (14th ed.). Rockville, MD: Author.

Witztum, J. (1996). Drugs in the treatment of hyperlipoproteinemias. In J. Hardman, L. Limbird, and P. Malinoff, et al. (eds.). *Goodman and Gilman's The pharmacological basis of therapeutics* (9th ed.). New York: McGraw-Hill.

Wones, R. (1990). Screening, diagnosis, and treatment of hypercholesterolemia. *Primary Care,* 16(1), 479–497.

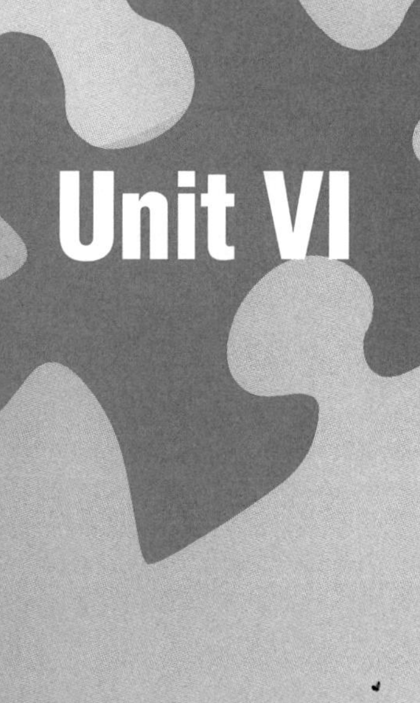

Drugs Influencing the Hematologic System

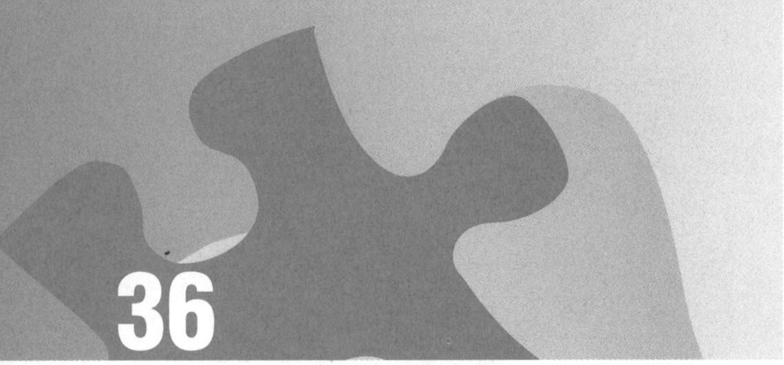

36 Anticoagulant and Antiplatelet Drugs

Blood clots are a defense mechanism that protects the body from excessive bleeding. The cascade of biochemical events that produces a stable fibrin-platelet plug or clot is the result of enzymatic triggers that respond instantly when blood vessels or tissue are compromised. However, clot formation may also occur as a result of hypercoaguability of the blood. And clots, regardless of origin, can obstruct blood flow through a vessel and increase the risk of tissue necrosis. An *embolus* or mobile mass of clotted blood that has broken off from a plug can lodge in a variety of organs, block blood flow, and even cause death. Drugs discussed in this chapter disrupt normal *hemostasis,* the arrest of bleeding or interruption of blood flow, thereby causing a significant risk of hemorrhage. Unlike thrombolytic drugs, which are used to dissolve blood clots, anticoagulant and antiplatelet drugs prevent the development or extension of clots.

THROMBOEMBOLIC DISEASE

Epidemiology and Etiology

Thromboembolic disease refers to the development of thrombophlebitis or thromboembolism. *Thrombophlebitis* is the inflammation of a vein associated with the formation of a *thrombus* (blood clot). It most often involves the greater or lesser veins of the lower extremity. Thrombus formation obstructs blood flow through both superficial and deep veins, and is usually attributed to *Virchow's triad:* venous stasis, damage to venous epithelium, and a hypercoagulable state. Two of the three factors must be present for thrombi to form.

Venous stasis is usually associated with restricted mobility or a lack of the use of calf muscles. Other conditions contributing to venous stasis include prolonged bedrest, surgery with general, spinal, or epidural anesthesia that lasts longer than 30 minutes, pregnancy, obesity, paralysis, and heart failure.

Damage to venous epithelium can be caused by intravenous (IV) injections, inattentive care of IV insertion sites, chemical injury from sclerosing drugs, x-ray studies requiring IV contrast media, certain antibiotics, thromboangiitis obliterans (Buerger's disease), fractures, and dislocations. The combination of venous stasis and a hypercoagulable state results in thrombus formation.

Hypercoagulable states often accompany neoplasms, particularly visceral and ovarian tumors. Estrogen therapy, the use of oral contraceptives, and high dosages of vitamin E increase the risk of a hypercoagulable state. Dehydration and blood dyscrasias raise platelet counts, reduce fibrinolysis, increase clotting factors or blood viscosity, and contribute to the risk of thrombus formation (see Risk Factors Associated with Thromboembolic Disease). There are a number of consequences of thromboembolic disease but the most frequent are stroke and myocardial infarction (MI).

Superficial thrombosis of upper extremities is rare. Deep vein thrombosis (DVT) of the lower extremities occurs in a significant number of hospitalized patients. DVT is more common in women (especially during pregnancy) and in older adults. It is estimated that 50,000 to 100,000 deaths occur annually from its major consequence, pulmonary embolus (PE). The mortality rate associated with untreated PE ranges from 25 to 42 percent. Survival rates are as high as 92 percent when the patient is adequately treated.

An MI is caused by a sudden blockage of one of the branches of a coronary artery. The blockage may be caused by a thrombus in the coronary artery (coronary thrombosis), sudden progression of atherosclerotic changes, or prolonged constriction of coronary arteries. The blockage can be extensive enough to cause necrosis of myocardial tissues or severe enough to interfere with cardiac function or cause immediate death.

The mortality rate associated with acute MI ranges as high as 30 to 40 percent. A substantial number of deaths take place before the patients reach the hospital. Approximately 80 percent of patients who do reach the hospital survive. Most in-hospital deaths from MIs occur during the first 3 to 4 days after the onset of the blockage. The person who has had an MI is at a high risk for recurrence.

Cerebrovascular accident (stroke) is a disturbance in cerebral circulation caused by a thrombus, embolus, or hemorrhage. Stroke is the most common disease of the nervous system in the 60- to 90-year-old age group and the third highest cause of death in the United States. Each year, 500,000 Americans experience an acute stroke. Of that number, 30 percent were preceded by transient ischemic attacks (TIAs) in the previous 3 to 5 years. Many of the patients affected have a history of hypertension or diabetes mellitus. TIAs are transient, temporary episodes of neurologic dysfunction that is manifest by contralateral weakness of the lower portion of the face, fingers, hands, arms, and legs. Transient dysphagia and some sensory impairment is also noted.

Cerebral embolism is the second most common cause of stroke. Patients who experience a stroke secondary to embolism are usually younger. Most often, the embolus originates from a thrombus in the heart. The myocardial thrombus is usually related to rheumatic heart disease with mitral stenosis and atrial fibrillation.

Pathophysiology

Thrombus development begins when red blood cells, white blood cells, platelets, and fibrin adhere to exposed collagen fibers in the affected vessel. The most common site of thrombus formation is the valve cusps of veins, where venous stasis allows blood products to accumulate. Increased

RISK FACTORS ASSOCIATED WITH THROMBOEMBOLIC DISEASE

- Abdominal and pelvic surgery, surgery on long bones
- Advanced age (particularly patients older than 40 years of age)
- Bedrest, prolonged travel without limited mobility
- Cardiovascular disease (atrial fibrillation, heart failure, MI, hypertension, stroke)
- Cigarette smoking
- Dehydration or malnutrition
- Diabetes mellitus
- Estrogen therapy or use of oral contraceptives
- Excessive intake of vitamin E
- Fractured hip
- Intravenous therapy, venous catheterization
- Joint arthroplasty
- Neoplasms, especially hepatic and pancreatic
- Obesity
- Pregnancy, particularly the postpartum period
- Previous history of thrombophlebitis, varicose veins
- Selected blood dyscrasias (polycythemia vera)
- Sepsis
- Surgery lasting more than 30 minutes with general, spinal, or epidural anesthesia
- Trauma, spinal cord injury

numbers of blood cells and fibrin collect to produce an even larger clot with a tail that eventually occludes the lumen of the vein.

Two pathways exist for blood coagulation to take place: the intrinsic pathway and the extrinsic pathway (Fig. 36–1). Certain clotting factors, or proteins, are necessary for the pathways to produce a fibrin clot (Table 36–1). The intrinsic pathway requires several minutes for fibrin to be produced. The intrinsic pathway involves the blood or damage to blood vessels. The intrinsic pathway is stimulated when factor XII comes in contact with a foreign surface. This contact begins a cascade of reactions, resulting in activation of factor X, leading to the common pathway, and to the conversion of prothrombin to thrombin and, finally, fibrinogen to a fibrin.

In contrast, the extrinsic pathway produces fibrin in seconds, much more quickly than the intrinsic pathway, by skirting the beginning stages of the cascade. The extrinsic pathway begins with tissue damage outside the vessel. Damaged tissues circulate factor III, or thromboplastin, which launches the clotting cascade to form activated factor X and the concluding pathway of clot development. In addition, a platelet plug forms when a vessel wall is injured as a result of collagen stimulation. When platelet adhesion occurs, adenosine diphosphate, thrombin, thromboxane A_2 (TXA_2), and prostaglandin H_2 are released into circulation. Platelets collect at the site of injury, forming a weak clot in an attempt to repair the injured site. The addition of fibrin results in the stable fibrin-platelet plug (Fig. 36–2).

Most thrombi have long tails that can detach and travel in the vascular system. A mobile thrombus is known as an *embolus*. The embolus circulates until it lodges at a site such as a pulmonary artery. Thus, *embolization* results in damage at a site distant from the initial thrombus. A PE results in sudden occlusion of the pulmonary artery with disruption of blood supply to the lung parenchyma. The obstruction of blood flow through the pulmonary artery leads to an increase in alveolar dead space. Vasoactive and bronchoconstrictive substances are released from the blood clot, which further intensifies the ventilation-perfusion imbalance. Left untreated, the patient experiences right ventricular heart failure with reduced cardiac output and shock due to the increased workload required of the heart.

An MI results when a coronary artery is occluded, blocking blood flow to the heart muscle. Cellular death and necrosis results when cells and tissues are deprived of oxygen and nutrients for more than 20 to 45 minutes. Hence, it is vital to prevent such an occurrence as much as possible.

A stroke is an abrupt impairment of brain function resulting from the interruption of the blood flow to an area of the brain. There are two basic types of stroke—thrombotic and hemorrhagic. Thrombotic strokes are the most common and are usually caused by arteriosclerosis and slowing of cerebral blood flow. Blood clots causing embolic strokes usually originate in the left side of the heart. In both the thrombotic and embolic strokes, the result is an obstruction in blood supply to the brain, causing a transient or permanent impairment of movement, thought, recall, speech, or sensation. The clinical symptoms depend on the vascular territory involved (e.g., carotid or vertebrobasilar artery).

TABLE 36–1 COMMON NAMES FOR COAGULATION FACTORS

Factor	Common Name
I	Fibrinogen
II	Prothrombin
III	Tissue thromboplastin
IV	Calcium
V	AC-Globulin
VII	Prothrombin conversion accelerator, stable factor
VIII	Antihemophilic factor
IX	Christmas factor, plasma thromboplastin component
X	Stuart-Prower factor
XI	Plasma thromboplastin antecedent
XII	Hageman factor
XIII	Fibrin-stabilizing factor

PHARMACOTHERAPEUTIC OPTIONS

Anticoagulants

- ❒ Ardeparin (NORMIFLO)
- ❒ Dalteparin (FRAGMIN)
- ❒ Enoxaparin (LOVENOX)
- ❒ Heparin calcium and heparin sodium (CALCIPARINE, LIQUAEMIN SODIUM,); (🍁) HEPALEAN, HEPARIN LEO
- ❒ Warfarin (COUMADIN); (🍁) WARNERIN, WARFILONE

Indications

Warfarin, a coumarin derivative, is the prototype and the oldest oral anticoagulant. It is the most frequently used oral anticoagulant employed in the long-term prevention and prophylaxis of thrombosis. It is also used in the prophylaxis and treatment of atrial fibrillation, PE, and MI. Although warfarin is not approved by the Food and Drug Admin-

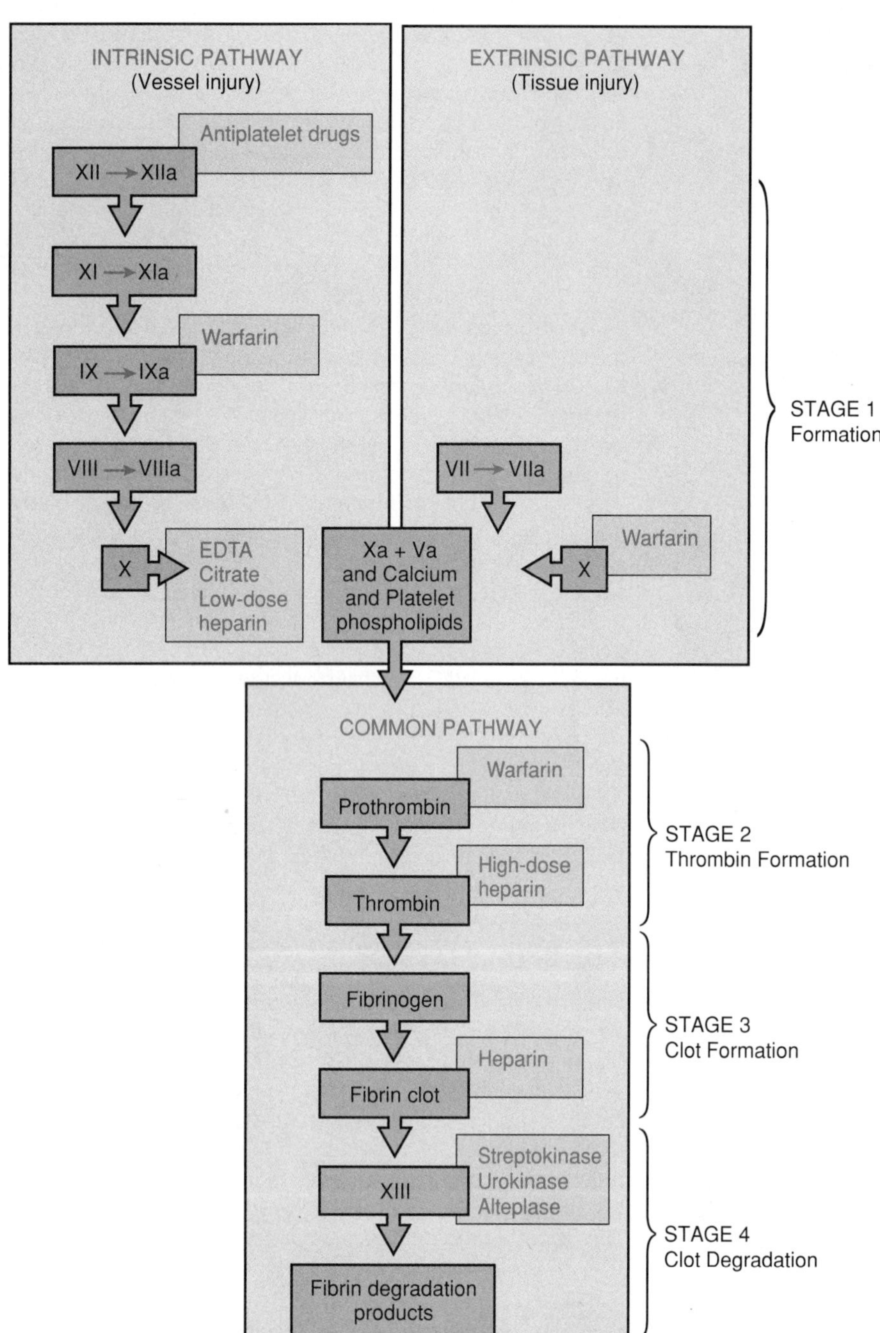

Figure 36–1 Coagulation cascade. The coagulation cascade is a series of enzymatic reactions that produces a fibrin blood clot. Damage to blood vessels or, in some cases, hypercoagulability of the blood initiates the intrinsic pathway. The extrinsic pathway is activated by tissue injury. Both sequences activate factor X, Stuart-Prower factor, leading to a common pathway and fibrin clot formation. Anticoagulant and antiplatelet drugs can act at a variety of locations during the cascade. Thrombolytic drugs act at stage 4 of the coagulation cascade and cause a breakdown of the fibrin clot into fibrin degradation products.

istration (FDA), it has also been used in the prevention of recurrent transient ischemic attacks and recurrent MI, and as an adjunct to therapy in small cell carcinoma of the lung.

Heparin, a parenteral anticoagulant, is used for the prevention and treatment of venous thrombosis, and PE, and in the treatment of atrial fibrillation with embolization. It is also used in the diagnosis and treatment of disseminated intravascular coagulation (DIC) and for prevention of clotting in blood samples and heparin locks, and during dialysis procedures. It has been used as an adjunct in the treatment of acute coronary occlusion, prevention of left ventricular thrombi and strokes after an MI, and in the prevention of cerebral thrombosis in patients with an evolving stroke.

Enoxaparin is a low-molecular-weight heparin used in the prevention of DVT following hip or knee replacement and general surgical procedures. Dalteparin is used in the prevention of DVT for at-risk patients undergoing abdominal surgery. The newest low-molecular-weight heparin is ardeparin. It is indicated for prevention of thrombosis for patients having orthopaedic surgery.

Pharmacodynamics

Anticoagulants hinder clot formation in general by inhibiting specific clotting factors. Anticoagulant drugs offer no benefit in dissolving a formed clot but are effective in preventing thrombus formation because they decrease the coagulability of blood.

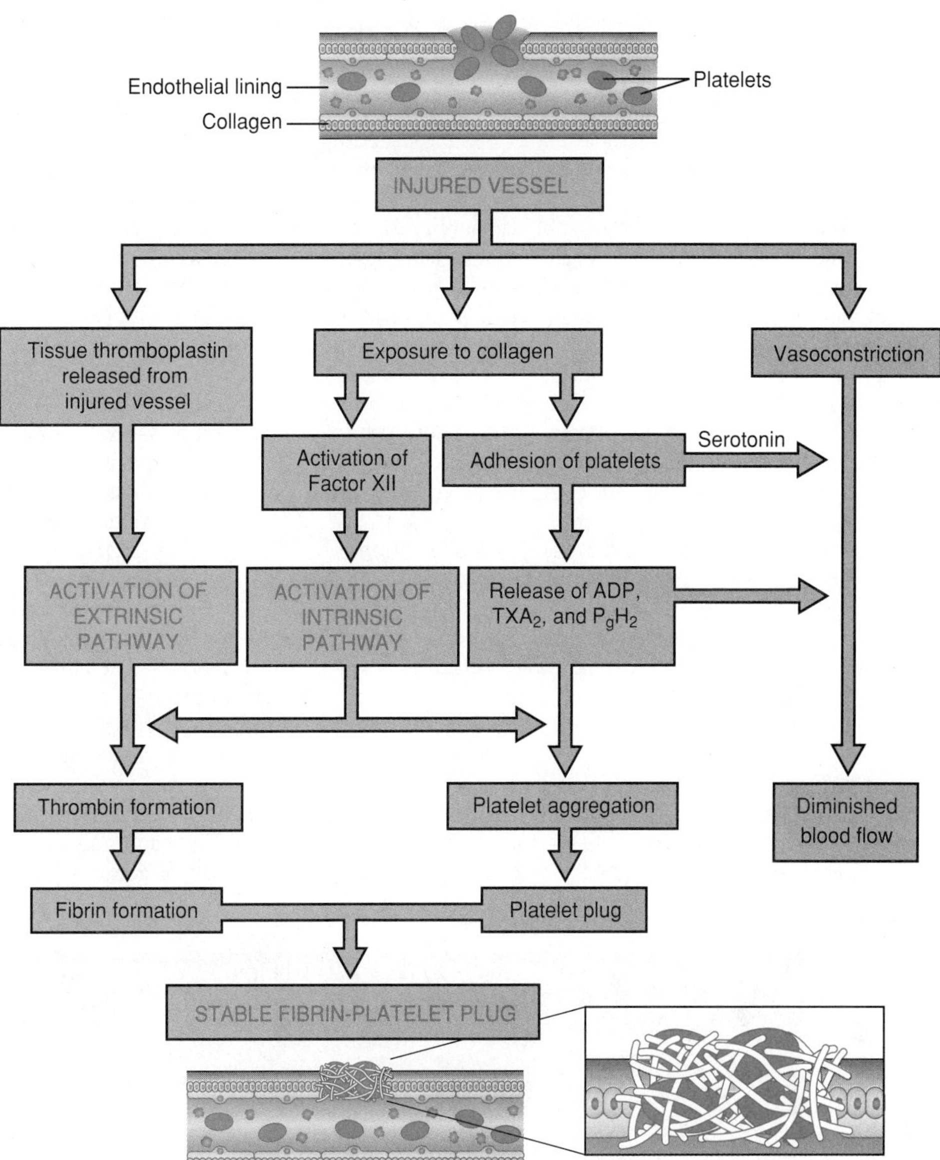

Figure 36–2 Events leading to formation of stable fibrin-platelet plug. When the endothelial lining of a blood vessel is damaged, physical and biochemical mechanisms work together to produce a stable fibrin-platelet plug and prevent blood loss. The activation of Factor XII combined with continually circulating platelets in the blood stream leads to the coagulation cascade and aggregation of a stable fibrin-platelet plug.

Warfarin suppresses coagulation activity by interfering with the production of vitamin K–dependent clotting factors in the liver. By reducing the amount of available vitamin K, clotting factors II, VII, IX, and X are reduced.

Heparin, on the other hand, acts on circulating clotting factors to inhibit thrombus formation. It potentiates the effects of antithrombin III, and in low doses, heparin prevents the conversion of prothrombin to thrombin by its effects on factor Xa. In higher doses, it neutralizes thrombin, thus preventing the conversion of fibrinogen to fibrin.

Enoxaparin and dalteparin inhibit thrombus formation by blocking factor IIA. Enoxaparin also blocks factor Xa, thus preventing clot formation.

Adverse Effects and Contraindications

Bleeding is the principal complication of anticoagulant use, occurring in approximately 10 percent of patients. The danger of bleeding increases as the dosage of the anticoagulant increases and with the addition of other platelet-altering drugs (e.g., aspirin). Other potentially unfavorable reactions to warfarin include gastrointestinal (GI) disturbances, skin necrosis, dermatitis, hair loss, urticaria, fever, and orange-red urine discoloration.

Warfarin is contraindicated for patients with vitamin K deficiency, hemorrhagic disorders, hepatic or renal disease, diabetes, subacute bacterial endocarditis, uncontrolled hypertension, visceral carcinoma, and severe thrombocytopenia. Patients requiring indwelling catheters and those undergoing lumbar puncture, regional anesthesia, and surgery of the eye, brain, or spinal cord should avoid warfarin.

Warfarin is used cautiously in patients with bleeding tendencies such as hemophilia; patients with increased capillary permeability, dissecting aneurysm, duodenal, gastric or esophageal ulcers, and severe hypertension; and in women contemplating abortion. Warfarin should also be used with caution in patients with heart failure, diarrhea, fever, thyrotoxicosis, senile psychosis, or depression. Warfarin administration during pregnancy and lactation is contraindicated. Warfarin crosses the placental barrier and can result in fetal injury, such as malformation, central nervous system defects, optic atrophy, hemorrhage, and death. Warfarin also enters breast milk and should not be used during lactation.

The adverse effects of heparin are similar but less extensive than those of warfarin. Bleeding tendencies, thrombocytopenia, hyperkalemia, and hair loss are possible. In addition, suppression of renal function occurs with high-dose, long-term therapy.

The contraindications of heparin are also similar to those of warfarin. It should be avoided in patients with severe thrombocytopenia or uncontrolled bleeding. Any patient who cannot be regularly monitored, who is in labor or in the immediate postpartum period, or who has had recent surgery or injury should also avoid heparin. It may be used as prophylaxis in low doses. Women over age 60 who are at high risk for hemorrhaging require cautious use of heparin. If an anticoagulant is needed during pregnancy, heparin may be used because it does not cross the placental membranes.

The adverse effects, contraindications, and precautions of enoxaparin, dalteparin, and ardeparin are similar to those of heparin. They are contraindicated in the presence of hypersensitivity, thrombocytopenia, and uncontrolled bleeding. In addition, these drugs are contraindicated for patients with an allergy to pork.

Pharmacokinetics

Warfarin is readily absorbed from the GI tract after oral administration. Ninety-five to ninety-seven percent of warfarin binds to serum albumin (Table 36–2). Its anticoagulant effects begin 8 to 12 hours following administration, but peak effects do not appear for 48 to 72 hours. The slow drug onset and peak effects are delayed because this oral anticoagulant has no effect on existing clotting factors in the blood. That is, until clotting factors present in the circulation at the time the drug is administered break down, the anticoagulant effect of warfarin will not be evident. It takes 6 to 60 hours for of existing clotting factors to decay, depending on which clotting factors are involved. Once the patient has stopped taking warfarin, the anticoagulant effect may remain for up to 120 hours as a result of the long half-life of warfarin (36 to 48 hours).

Heparin, on the other hand, is a protein destroyed by enzymes in the GI tract; therefore, parenteral administration is necessary. It is well absorbed following subcutaneous (SC) administration and does not cross the placenta or enter breast milk. It has a rapid onset of action when given IV. It takes 20 to 60 minutes for the drug effects to onset when it is given SC. Heparin peaks in 5 to 10 minutes when it is given IV and in 2 to 4 hours when it is given SC. It appears to be biotransformed and removed by the reticuloendothelial system (i.e., lymph nodes and spleen) with a half-life of 1 to 2 hours. The half-life lengthens with increasing dosage. The duration of action lasts from 2 to 6 hours for IV routes and 8 to 12 hours when given SC.

The pharmacokinetics of enoxaparin, dalteparin, and ardeparin are also identified in Table 36–2. They are administered SC and have onset times of 20 to 60 minutes; peak action is reached 3 to 5 hours after administration, with a duration of action of 12 hours. The low-molecular-weight

TABLE 36–2 PHARMACOKINETICS OF SELECTED ANTICOAGULANT AND ANTIPLATELET DRUGS

Drugs	Route	Onset	Peak	Duration	PB (%)	$t_{1/2}$	BioA (%)
Anticoagulants							
Ardeparin	SC	20–60 min	3–5 hr	12 hr	High	UA	92
Dalteparin	SC	20–60 min	3–5 hr	12 hr	High	UA	92
Enoxaparin	SC	20–60 min	3–5 hr	12 hr	High	4.5 hr	92
Heparin	SC	20–60 min	2–4 hr	8–12 hr	High	1–2 hr*	100
	IV	Immediate	5–10 min	2–6 hr	High	1–2 hr*	100
Warfarin	po	Slow	0.5–3 days	2–5 days	95–97%	0.5–3 days	85–99
Antiplatelet Drugs							
Aspirin	po	5–30 min	15 min –2 hr	3–6 hr	Vary	2–3 hr; 15–30 hr †	Vary
Dipyridamole	po	Varies	75 min	3–4 hr	UA	10 hr	30–60
	IV	Immediate	6.5 min	30 min	UA	10 hr	100
Pentoxifylline	po	2–4 wks	8 wks	UK	UA	25–50 min	UA
Sulfinpyrazone	po	Varies	1–2 hr	4–6 hr	98%	3 hr‡	100
Ticlodipine	po	48 hr	7 days	14 days	High	12.6; 4–5 days§	80
Anticoagulant Antagonists							
Protamine sulfate	IV	30–60 sec	UK	2 hr‖	UA	UK	100
Phytonadione	po	6–12 hr	UK	UK	UA	UA	UA
	SC/IM	1–2 hr	3–6 hr¶	12–24 hr	UA	UA	100

*Half life of heparin increases with increasing dosage.
†Half life of aspirin with low doses and large doses repectively.
‡Half life of parahydroxysulfinpyrazone 1 hour, up 10 to 13 hours for sulfide metabolite.
§Half life of ticlopidine with single dose 12.6 hr, with multiple dosing 4–5 days.
‖Duration of action of protamine sulfate depends on body temperature.
¶Peak action of phytonadione for control of hemorrhage when given SC/IM. Duration of drug action of phytonadione to achieve normal PT value.
PB, Protein binding; $t_{1/2}$, elimination half-life; N/A, not applicable; UA, unavailable; UK, unknown; BioA, bioavailability..

TABLE 36–3 DRUG-DRUG INTERACTIONS OF SELECTED ANTICOAGULANT AND ANTIPLATELET DRUGS

Drug	Interactive Drugs		Interaction
Anticoagulants			
Warfarin	Acetaminophen	Amiodarone	Increased effects of anticoagulant
	Androgens	Aspirin	
	Bumetanide	Cephalosporins	
	Chloral hydrate	Clofibrate	
	Chloramphenicol	Cimetidine	
	Co-trimoxazole	Danazol	
	Disulfiram	Erythromycin	
	Ethacrynic acid	Famotidine	
	Furosemide	Glucagon	
	Meclofenamate	Mefenamic acid	
	Metronidazole	Moxalactam	
	Nalidixic acid	Nizatidine	
	Oxyphenbutazone	Phenylbutazone	
	Quinidine	Quinine	
	Ranitidine	Salicylates	
	Sulfinpyrazone		
	Aminogluthethimide	Barbiturates	Decreased effects of anticoagulants
	Carbamazepine	Colestyramine	
	Ethchlorvynol	Glutethimide	
	Griseofulvin	Rifampin	
	Oral contraceptives	Vitamin E	
	Vitamin K		
	Phenytoin		Increased effects of interactive drug
	Methimazole		Altered effects of warfarin
	Propylthiouracil		
Heparin	Antiplatelet drugs	Cephalosporins	Increased effects of heparin
	NSAIDs	Penicillins	
	Probenecid	Salicylates	
	Oral anticoagulants		
	Nitroglycerin		Decreased effects of heparin
Ardeparin	Oral anticoagulants	Cephalosporins	Increased effects of enoxaparin
Enoxaparin	Penicillins	Salicylates	
Dalteparin			
Antiplatelet Drugs			
Aspirin	Oral anticoagulants	Heparin	Increased effect of interactive drugs
	Insulin	Methotrexate	
	Sulfonylureas	Valproic acid	
	Beta blockers	Captopril	Decreased effect of interactive drugs
	Furosemide	Probenecid	
	Spironolactone	Sulfinpyrazone	
	Alcohol	Corticosteroids	Increased risk of GI ulceration
	NSAIDs	Phenylbutazone	
	Ammonium chloride	Ascorbic acid	Increased serum salicylate levels
	Furosemide	Methionine	
	Carbonic anhydrase inhibitors		
	Acetazolamide	Antacids	Decreased serum salicylate levels
	Alkalinizers	Corticosteroids	
	Methazolamide		
Dipyridamole	Theophylline		Decreased coronary vasodilation effects
Pentoxifylline	Cimetidine		Increased effects of pentoxifylline
Sulfinpyrazone	Salicylates		Decreased effects of sulfinpyrazone
	Acetaminophen	Glyburide	Increased effects of interacting drug
	Tolbutamide	Warfarin	
Ticlopidine	Digoxin		Decreased effects of interacting drug
	Aspirin	Theophylline	Increased effects of interacting drug
	Cimetidine		Increased effects of ticlopidine
	Antacids		Decreased effects of ticlopidine

heparin drugs cross placental membranes and enter breast milk.

Drug-Drug Interactions

Numerous drug interactions can occur with warfarin and heparins. The anticoagulation effects may be either increased or decreased. Table 36–3 summarizes drug-drug interactions for anticoagulants.

Drug-Food Interactions

Alterations in vitamin K levels alter the effects of warfarin. A diet high in green leafy vegetables reduces the effectiveness of warfarin. There are no major drug-food interactions with the parenteral anticoagulants unless the foods are used in excess.

Dosage Regimens

Patient response to warfarin is unpredictable. To avoid bleeding complications, the dosage must be adjusted according to results of laboratory tests. Drug dosages are adjusted based on the International Normalized Ratio (INR) value every week for the first month and then once a month. The patient on warfarin may initially receive 10 to 15 mg daily with subsequent maintenance doses based on INR values (Table 36–4). The risk of bleeding, the main complication of anticoagulant therapy, usually is not increased when

TABLE 36–4 DOSAGE REGIMENS FOR SELECTED ANTICOAGULANT AND ANTIPLATELET DRUGS

Drug	Use(s)	Dosage	Implications
Anticoagulants			
Ardeparin	Prevention of thrombosis in knee replacement	*Adult:* 50 units/kg SC BID starting 12–24 hr after surgery	Safety and efficacy in children not established
Dalteparin	Prevention of DVT after general surgery, orthopaedic surgery, venous thromboembolism	*Adult:* 2500 units SC each day starting 1–2 hr before surgery and repeating once daily for 5–10 days postoperatively	Dosage for general surgery patients based on potential for thrombus formation. Safety and efficacy in children not established
Enoxaparin	Prevention of DVT after hip replacement, general surgery, or orthopaedic surgery	*Adult:* 30 mg SC BID as initial dose as soon as possible after surgery, not more than 24 hr. Treatment continued throughout postop period. Up to 14 days may be needed	Dosage for general surgery patients based on potential for thrombus formation
Heparin	Prevention of DVT, pulmonary embolism	*Adult: General anticoagulation:* 5000 units IV loading dose then 10,000–20,000 units SC, followed by 8000–10,000 units q8 hr or 15,000–20,000 units q12 hr *Intermittent IV:* 10,000 units IV then 5000–10,000 units q4–6 hr *Continuous IV:* 5000 units IV loading dose then 20,000–40,000 units/day *Postoperative Prophylaxis:* 5000 units SC 2 hr before surgery and q8–12 hr thereafter for 7 days or until patient ambulatory *Child:* 50 units/kg IV bolus then 100 units/kg IV q4 hr, or 20,000 units/m^2 by continuous IV infusion	Dosage determined by PTT or APTT values
Warfarin sodium	Prevention of thrombus formation	*Adult:* 10–15 mg po QD. Dosage increase based on laboratory values. Maintenance dose 2–10 mg po QD based on laboratory values	Determined by PT and INR values. Lower doses usually needed for elderly
Antiplatelet Drugs			
Aspirin	TIAs in men	*Adult:* 650 mg po BID *or* 325 mg po QID	Low doses do not significantly change laboratory values
	Myocardial infarction	*Adult:* 300–325 mg po QD	
Dipyridamole	After valvular surgery	*Adult:* 75–100 mg po QID	Used as an adjunct to warfarin therapy
Pentoxifylline	Intermittent claudication	*Adult:* 400 mg po TID	Tablets should not be crushed, broken, or chewed
Sulfinpyrazone	Decreases incidence of sudden death after MI; rheumatic mitral stenosis to decrease chance of systemic embolism	*Adult:* 100–200 mg po BID. Increase up to 800 mg po QD in two divided doses	Safety and efficacy in children not established
Ticlopidine	Reduce risk of CVA. Unlabeled uses: Intermittent claudication, chronic arterial occlusion, subarachnoid hemorrhage, AV shunts or fistulas, open heart surgery, CABG, primary glomerulonephritis, sickle cell disease	*Adult:* 250 mg po BID	Safety and efficacy in children younger than age 18 years not established
Anticoagulant Antagonists			
Protamine sulfate	Acute management heparin overdose, neutralize heparin after dialysis and other procedures	*Adult:* 1 mg/1000 units of heparin IV if given within 30 minutes of heparin dose. If past 30 minutes, give 0.5 mg/100 units of heparin	Further doses determined by PTT or APTT values
Phytonadione	Hypoprothrombinemia	*Adult:* 2.5–10 mg po/SC/IM in 12–48 hr if necessary *or* 6–8 hr after parenteral dose. Maximum dose: 25–50 mg *Child:* 5–10 mg po/SC/IM *Infants:* 1–2 mg po/SC/IM	Monitor PT before and throughout therapy

the INR is in the target range of 2 to 3. Higher INRs are associated with a greater risk of bleeding.

Heparin may be given SC, intermittent IV, or continuous IV infusion. In contrast to warfarin, heparin is dosed based on the partial thromboplastin time (PTT) or activated partial thromboplastin time (APTT). The therapeutic dosage range is usually a PTT or APTT value 1½ to 2 times the normal. For cardiac surgery patients, the ratio may range from 1½ to 2½ times the normal. If the APTT is too high the dosage is decreased. If the APTT is too low the dosage is increased.

Unlike heparin, the dosages of low-molecular-weight heparins are not monitored using the PTT and APTT values. Monitoring of PTT and APTT values are not necessary because the low doses used in the prophylaxis do not notably alter involved coagulation factors.

The recommended initial dosage of enoxaparin is 30 mg SC twice daily as soon as possible after surgery but not more than 24 hours later. Treatment is usually continued throughout the postoperative period. Up to 14 days of therapy may be needed.

Patients at low risk for thrombus formation who are having general surgery may receive 2500 units of dalteparin SC 1 to 2 hours before surgery and then once daily afterward. If they are a high-risk patient 5000 units of dalteparin SC 10 to 12 hours before surgery may be given with the frequency reduced to once daily in the postoperative period. The recommended dose of dalteparin, when used for patients undergoing orthopaedic surgery, is as 5000 units 8 to 12 hours before surgery and once daily starting 12 hours postoperatively.

Ardeparin is the newest low-molecular-weight heparin, and it is given as 50 units/kg twice daily starting 12 to 24 hours after orthopaedic surgery.

Laboratory Considerations

The red-orange discoloration of urine caused by warfarin may interfere with the results of some laboratory tests. Heparin, enoxaparin, dalteparin, and ardeparin may cause increased alanine aminotransferase (ALT; serum glutamic-pyruvic transaminase [SGPT]) and aspartate aminotransferase (AST; serum glutamic-oxaloacetic transaminase [SGOT]) levels and thyroid function test results. Heparin also causes prolonged sulfobromophthalein (BSP) levels and a false-negative ^{125}I fibrinogen uptake. Heparin alters blood gas results, specifically carbon dioxide, bicarbonate, and base excess values. Further, heparin decreases serum triglyceride and cholesterol levels and increases plasma free fatty acid concentrations.

Antiplatelet Drugs

- ❒ Aspirin (ASA, ECOTRIN, EMPIRIN, ZORPRIN); (🍁) APO-ASA, ENTROPHEN
- ❒ Dipyridamole (PERSANTINE); (🍁) APO-DIPYRIDAMOLE
- ❒ Pentoxifylline (TRENTAL)
- ❒ Sulfinpyrazone (ANTURANE)
- ❒ Ticlopidine (TICLID)

Indications

Antiplatelet drugs are used primarily in the prevention of arterial thrombus. Aspirin is the most commonly used antiplatelet drug and is used to reduce the risk of recurrent TIAs or stroke in men with a history of TIA due to fibrin platelet emboli. Aspirin has also been used to reduce the risk of death or nonfatal MI in patients with a history of infarction or unstable angina pectoris.

Dipyridamole is thought to be effective for long-term therapy of angina pectoris, although it is no longer approved by the FDA for this use. It has been used in conjunction with warfarin to prevent thromboembolism in patients with prosthetic heart valves. Although it is considered unlabeled, dipyridamole has also been used in the prevention of myocardial reinfarction, reduction of post-MI mortality, and with aspirin to prevent occlusion of coronary artery bypass grafts.

Pentoxifylline is used in the management of intermittent claudication. Its unlabeled uses include cerebrovascular insufficiency and to improve psychopathologic symptoms.

Sulfinpyrazone is not approved by the FDA as an antiplatelet drug, although it has been used to decrease the incidence of sudden death in the post-MI patient. It has also been used to decrease the frequency of systemic embolism for the patient with rheumatic mitral stenosis. It is FDA approved for the treatment of chronic and intermittent gouty arthritis (see Chapter 15).

Ticlopidine is used for the prevention of thrombotic stroke in patients who have experienced the precursors of stroke and in patients who have had a completed thrombotic stroke. Its use has been reserved for patients who are intolerant of aspirin because the adverse effects of ticlopidine may be life-threatening. Its unlabeled uses include intermittent claudication, chronic arterial occlusion, subarachnoid hemorrhage, management of arteriovenous shunts or fistulas in patients with uremia, open heart surgery, coronary artery bypass grafts, primary glomerulonephritis, and sickle cell disease.

Pharmacodynamics

Aspirin prevents thrombus formation by preventing the production of TXA_2. TXA_2 is a substance that causes blood vessel constriction and platelet aggregation.

Dipyridamole also inhibits platelet aggregation. However, how it accomplishes this task is not completely understood. It is believed that dipyridamole stimulates the release of prostacyclin and inhibits the formation of TXA_2. Dipyridamole may also prevent the release of adenosine diphosphate, further decreasing the ability of platelets to aggregate. The drug decreases coronary vascular resistance and increases coronary blood flow without increasing myocardial oxygen consumption.

Pentoxifylline inhibits red blood cell and platelet aggregation and local hyperviscosity. It also decreases fibrinogen concentration in the blood, although the precise mechanism is unknown.

Ticlopidine inhibits platelet aggregation by inhibiting fibrinogen binding and platelet-platelet interaction by modifying the function of platelet membranes. The drug's effects are irreversible for the life of the platelet.

Adverse Effects and Contraindications

The most common adverse effects of aspirin include heartburn, dyspepsia, nausea, and GI bleeding. Other possible adverse effects include an increased risk for bruising, thrombocytopenia, agranulocytosis, leukopenia, neutropenia, and hemolytic anemia. Acute salicylate overdose is possible and manifests as respiratory alkalosis, hyperpnea, tachypnea, confusion, asterixis, seizures, tetany, and metabolic acidosis. Fever, coma, cardiovascular collapse, and dose-related renal and respiratory failure are possible.

Few adverse reactions are associated with dipyridamole. Hypotension may occur. GI disturbances, flushing or pruritus of the skin, headache, and dizziness may develop but are rare. These symptoms, however, subside when the drug is discontinued. Fatal and nonfatal MIs, ventricular fibrillation, and bronchospasm have been documented.

The most common adverse effects of pentoxifylline include dizziness, headache, nervousness, dyspepsia, nausea, vomiting, and hand tremors. Thrombocytopenia and pancytopenia have also been documented.

Upper GI disturbances are common adverse effects of sulfinpyrazone. Blood dyscrasias are also possible.

The most common adverse effects of ticlopidine are nausea and diarrhea. In addition, the patient may experience rash, purpura, and pruritus.

Pharmacokinetics

Primary absorption of aspirin takes place in the small intestine. The absorption of enteric-coated aspirin formulations may be unreliable and rectal absorption is slow and variable. Distribution is rapid and wide, crossing the placenta and entering breast milk. It is extensively biotransformed by the liver. The effects of aspirin onset in 5 to 30 minutes, with peak effects reached in 15 minutes to 2 hours. The duration of action is 3 to 6 hours, with a half-life of 2 to 3 hours at low doses and 15 to 30 hours for higher doses (see Table 36–2).

Orally administered dipyridamole has a variable onset time. It is 30- to 60-percent absorbed after oral administration and is widely distributed. Peak effects are reached in 75 minutes, with a duration of action of 3 to 4 hours. The half-life of the drug is approximately 10 hours. Biotransformation takes place in the liver, with elimination in the feces.

Pentoxifylline is well absorbed following oral administration, with an improvement in blood flow noted in 2 to 4 weeks. The drug's distribution sites are unknown. Peak actions are reached in 8 weeks. It is biotransformed in the liver and by red blood cells. The half-life varies from 25 to 50 minutes.

Sulfinpyrazone is also well absorbed following oral administration, but its distribution to tissues is not known. The onset time varies, but peak effects are noted 1 to 2 hours after administration, with a duration of action of 4 to 6 hours. It is 98-percent protein bound. The half-life varies from 1 to 13 hours for its metabolites.

Over 80 percent of ticlopidine is absorbed following oral administration, although its distribution sites are unknown. Antiplatelet effects have an onset time of less than 48 hours, reaching a peak in 7 days and having a duration of action of 2 weeks. The drug is extensively biotransformed by the liver. Minimal elimination of the unchanged drug occurs by the kidneys. The half-life of a single dose of ticlopidine is approximately 12.6 hours, while the half-life with multiple dosing is 4 to 5 days. Drug effects continue for up to 14 days after the drug is discontinued.

Drug-Drug Interactions

Several serious drug interactions are possible with antiplatelet drugs (see Table 36–3). For example, when antiplatelet drugs are administered concurrently with anticoagulants, there is an increased risk for hemorrhage. In addition, when aspirin is given with steroids and nonsteroidal anti-inflammatory drugs or dipyridamole, the potential for bleeding and GI irritation is enhanced.

Drug-Food Interactions

Alcohol intake in conjunction with dipyridamole may potentiate hypotension. In addition, serum salicylate levels may be enhanced when dipyridamole is taken with foods such as cheese, cranberries, and fish, which acidify the urine. Furthermore, absorption of ticlopidine is enhanced when it is administered with food.

Dosage Regimens

The recommended dosage of aspirin for the treatment of men with a history of TIAs is 650 mg twice daily or one 325-mg tablet four times a day. When used for MI prophylaxis the dosage is commonly 300 to 325 mg/day (see Table 36–4).

The dose of dipyridamole is 75 to 100 mg four times daily. It is used most often as an adjunct to warfarin therapy.

Pentoxifylline 400 mg is administered with food three times daily. The controlled-release tablets should not be crushed, broken, or chewed.

The daily dosage of sulfinpyrazone is not identified in most drug references because it has not been approved as an antiplatelet drug. The dosage commonly used to decrease the incidence of sudden death after MI is 200 mg orally three to four times daily.

Ticlopidine is usually administered with food in dosages of 250 mg twice daily.

Laboratory Considerations

Aspirin prolongs bleeding time for 4 to 7 days and, in large doses, may cause prolonged PT, false-negative urine glucose test results using Clinistix or Tes-Tape, or a false-positive urine glucose test result with the copper sulfate method (Clinitest).

Critical Thinking Process

Assessment

History of Present Illness

The patient with a DVT usually complains of pain in the calf muscle at rest or during exercise or pain in the thigh. Patients may have a history of previous DVT or other associated risk factors. A sudden onset of chest pain, dyspnea, or rapid breathing may indicate pulmonary embolism.

Patients with a pulmonary embolism should be assessed for the recent onset of any of the following symptoms: dyspnea, substernal chest pain, hemoptysis, palpitations, pleuritic pain, and apprehension. As with DVT, risk factors should also be elicited.

Patients having an MI note chest pain as their most frequent complaint. Determine the patient's perception of the pain, its location and radiation to other sites, the quality of the pain, onset and duration, and factors that alleviate or aggravate the pain. Elicit feelings of uneasiness or impending doom; fear of death and the possibility of denial or depression; and the presence of associated symptoms such as dyspnea, nausea, dizziness, and sleep disturbances.

Subjective data to be elicited from the patient with a suspected stroke include the presence, nature, and location of a headache or sensory deficits, presence of diplopia or blurred vision, and complaints of an inability to think clearly. The patient's perception of what is happening is also important to note.

Past Health History

The past health history provides information regarding existing disorders that can predispose the patient to the development of thrombosis. In addition, the patient's family history may provide information helpful in identifying individuals who may be more likely to develop thrombosis. The patient's history should include any risk factors associated with thrombophlebitis and thromboembolism (see Risk Factors Associated with Thromboembolic Disease).

Physical Exam Findings

Clinical manifestations of thrombosis vary according to the size and location of the thrombus and the adequacy of collateral circulation. The patient with superficial thrombophlebitis may have a palpable, firm, SC cordlike vein. The area surrounding the vein may be tender to the touch, reddened, and warm. A mild systemic fever and leukocytosis may be present. Deep vein thrombophlebitis may produce no symptoms, or it may generate unilateral edema, pain, warm skin, and a fever greater than 100.4°F (38°C).

Patients are also examined for signs of predisposition to thrombus formation, such as hypertension, atrial fibrillation, heart murmurs, or infectious diseases of the heart. Extremities are examined for the presence of peripheral pulses as well as temperature, pallor, and mottling.

Pulmonary embolism may cause tachypnea and tachycardia. Chest auscultation may reveal rales, wheezes, and pleural friction rubs and increased S_2. Unilateral leg edema and pain may represent thrombophlebitis, which may be the origin of a PE.

Physical exam findings of the patient with an MI may include crackles or audible wheezes and a rapid pulse that may be barely perceptible. The blood pressure usually falls, and the patient may collapse. Heart sounds (S_1 and S_2) are often faint. An S_4 and, at times, an S_3 heart sound, which indicates left ventricular failure, can often be heard. A soft systolic murmur may be heard at the apex.

Objective data to be collected for the patient with a suspected stroke include motor strength, paresis, paralysis, any change in the level of consciousness, signs of increased intracranial pressure, and the presence or absence of aphasia. The patient's respiratory rate and depth should also be noted.

Diagnostic Testing

A complete blood cell count, platelet count, hemoglobin and hematocrit should be conducted as a baseline. A baseline PT, PTT, or APTT should also be performed. Because many of the anticoagulant and antiplatelet drugs provide an elevation in liver function tests, it is important to establish a baseline for those values also.

Diagnostic testing for the patient with a suspected MI can be divided into three categories: nonspecific indicators of tissue necrosis and inflammation, electrocardiogram, and serum enzymes. Nonspecific indicators of MI include leukocytosis and an elevated erythrocyte sedimentation rate. The electrocardiogram may indicate characteristic changes, depending on the location of the MI. It should be noted that the electrocardiogram does not always provide definitive evidence of an ischemic process. Serum enzymes such as creatine kinase, AST (SGOT), and lactic acid dehydrogenase are valuable diagnostic indicators of MI. It should be noted however, that enzyme elevations are not solely specific to myocardial damage.

A CT scan may show the occurrence of a stroke but often not until several days after the onset. A lumbar puncture may be performed and may reveal elevated spinal fluid pressure. If blood is noted in the spinal fluid, hemorrhage has occurred. CT scans may be used before a lumbar puncture if the patient is in a coma and the severity of increased intracranial pressure is unknown. After a TIA, a cerebral angiogram or digital subtraction angiogram may be obtained to discover blocked or occluded vessels.

Developmental Considerations

Perinatal The risk of thromboembolic disease in pregnancy is approximately 6 times greater than the nonpregnant state, with 3 to 12 occurrences per 1000 pregnancies. The true incidence may be significantly higher in the postpartum period. Risk factors for thromboembolic disease during pregnancy, in addition to those previously identified, include:

- Advanced maternal age (older than 40 years)
- Collagen-vascular disease
- Grand multiparity (more than four previous term pregnancies)
- Homocystinuria (predisposes to arterial and venous thrombosis)
- Nephrotic syndrome
- Cesarean section or instrumented delivery

Pregnancy-related alterations in the coagulation system may also predispose the patient to thrombus and related complications. Treatment for DVT and PE in pregnancy centers on anticoagulation. The incidence of TIA and stroke are relatively rare in pregnancy.

Pediatric The incidence of thromboembolic disease in the pediatric population is not all that uncommon. When needed, consideration should be given to the infant or child's immature body systems that are required for drug absorption, distribution, biotransformation, and elimination. The potential for drug accumulation and toxicity exists in this patient population.

Geriatric In contrast to the pediatric population, the use of anticoagulant and antiplatelet drugs in the geriatric population has its own risks. Normal changes of aging impact the use, required monitoring, and therapeutic effectiveness of the drugs.

Case Study Deep Vein Thrombosis

Patient History

History of Present Illness	GR is a 65-year-old white male who is having a left hip replacement.
Past Health History	GR has no known allergies. He has been treated for atherosclerosis and mild hypertension for the past 2 years. He also smokes 1 pack of cigarettes per day. He states that he has had pain in his left leg for the past several months that limits his mobility. Current meds: furosemide 20 mg po QD; K-Lor 20 mEq po QD.
Physical Exam	VSS. Left dorsalis pedis and posterior tibial pulses are weak. GR has poor eyesight and is unable to read small print.
Diagnostic Testing	Preoperative PT, INR, and PTT within normal limits. BUN, creatinine within normal limits.
Developmental Considerations	GR has changes of aging related to hepatic and renal function.
Psychosocial Considerations	GR lives alone and is on Social Security income. GR is unable to drive owing to his poor eyesight. He has four adult children who live in another state. Relies on friends for transportation.
Economic Factors	GR has a small retirement pension in addition to social security benefits.

Variables Influencing Decision

Treatment Objectives

- GR will not develop deep vein thrombosis while recovering from hip replacement surgery.

Drug Variables	*Drug Summary*	*Patient Variables*
Indications	Prophylaxis postoperative hip replacement. The drug of choice is parenteral agent during immediate postoperative period, followed by oral agent for several months. Enoxaparin drug of choice for hip replacement.	GR has large number of risk factors for development of DVT postoperatively. He is also visually impaired. This will become a decision point.
Pharmacodynamics	All drugs are anticoagulants that interfere with the synthesis of or act on circulating clotting factors.	Because the drugs have similar pharmacodynamics, this will not be a decision point.
Adverse Effects/ Contraindications	Warfarin: Use cautiously in patients having regional anesthesia. Heparin and enoxaparin: Use caution with known kidney and liver diseases.	Will be a decision point owing to variations in adverse effects.
Pharmacokinetics	Oral drugs have slower onset and peak. Warfarin has many drug-drug interactions that may interact with GR's other meds. This will become a decision point.	GR is taking loop diuretic. Prolonged duration of action may be decision point.
Dosage Regimen	Enoxaparin and heparin are administered parenterally. Warfarin is an oral anticoagulant.	GR lives alone and has poor eyesight that may restrict his use of parenteral drug. This is a decision point.

Drug Variables	*Drug Summary*	*Patient Variables*
Lab Considerations	Heparin requires PTT or APTT monitoring. Warfarin requires PT and INR.	GR no longer drives so may have difficulty returning for follow-up laboratory work. This may become a decision point.
Cost Index*	Warfarin: 1 Heparin: 1 Enoxaparin: 3	GR has supplemental insurance that will pay drug costs. This will still be a decision point.

Summary of Decision Points

- Drug of choice is parenteral agent during immediate postoperative period, followed by oral agent for several months.
- Warfarin has many drug-drug interactions that may interact with GR's other meds (i.e., furosemide).
- GR's poor eyesight may restrict his ability to use parenteral agent after discharge.
- GR no longer drives, so he may have difficulty returning for follow-up laboratory work.
- Supplemental insurance will help pay drug costs.

DRUGS TO BE USED

- Enoxaparin 30 mg SC BID × 14 days or until GR is discharged.
- Warfarin po QD dose titrated to PT and INR values. To continue for 3 months postoperatively.

*Cost Index:
1 = $ < 30/mo.
2 = $ 30–40/mo.
3 = $ 40–50/mo.
4 = $ 50–60/mo.
5 = $ > 60/mo.

AWP of 10, 30-mg/mL prefilled syringes of enoxaparin is approximately $158.
AWP of 10, 5000 units/mL prefilled syringes of heparin is approximately $8.
AWP of 100, 5-mg tablets of warfarin sodium is approximately $59.

Psychosocial Considerations

As with any other health problem, the availability of health care to selected populations may be limited. Further, family health beliefs and practices may restrict or reduce the use of contemporary medicine.

Anticoagulant and antiplatelet drugs themselves are relatively inexpensive with the exception of some of the low-molecular-weight heparins. The inpatient treatment that may be initially required, however, is expensive. Further, older adults are most likely to require preventive treatment for thrombus formation. If cost is a concern, the patient should be referred to social services for assistance (see Case Study—Deep Vein Thrombosis).

Analysis and Management

Treatment Objectives

Treatment objectives for the patient at risk for thrombus formation are directed toward prevention or progression of thromboembolic disease, regardless of the site or sequelae. In addition, treatment is directed at speedy resolution of pain, inflammation, patient discomfort, and reduction in morbidity and mortality.

Treatment Options

Drug Variables

Preventive intervention for thromboembolic disease is primarily pharmacotherapy. The specific drug used depends on the location of the thrombus and the administration route most likely to be tolerated by the patient. The occurrence and recurrence of thromboembolic disease can be decreased to less than 5 percent if adequate anticoagulation is maintained. Twenty-nine to forty-seven percent of patients have a recurrence of the DVT unless adequate anticoagulation is maintained after the initial treatment regimen has been completed.

In most cases, heparin is the drug of choice for acute conditions. In the case of DVT or PE, heparin is continued for a minimum of 5 days or until the patient's condition stabilizes. Owing to the shorter hospital stays of today, warfarin therapy is also initiated at the same time and the heparin continued until an INR value of 2 to 3 (a PT ratio of 1.3 to 1½ times the control value) is achieved. Warfarin therapy may be continued for 3 months with the first episode of DVT or PE, for 1 year with a second episode, or indefinitely as long as there is a continued risk of embolism.

Compared with standard heparin, low-molecular-weight heparin has more predictable anticoagulant activity, better bioavailability, and a longer half-life. Therefore, laboratory monitoring is not required. They differ in half-life and inhibition of specific factors in the coagulation cascade. Their dosages also differ, although they are generally administered in fixed doses adjusted for body weight. Further, it has been shown that patients with proximal DVTs can be effectively treated at home with low-molecular-weight heparin.

All patients with an MI receive some type of anticoagulant or antiplatelet drug to decrease the incidence of systemic thromboembolism. Drug therapy decreases further coronary artery thrombosis and extension of mural thrombosis. Heparin therapy should be instituted even in patients who do not receive thrombolytic therapy (see Chapter 37). Once the patient is taken off heparin, warfarin is continued for about 3 months and aspirin therapy continued indefinitely.

Drug therapy for cerebral thromboembolic disease should be started as soon as possible after a diagnosis of TIA is made. Anticoagulation for a patient with a progressing thrombotic stroke and progressive neurologic deficits should be used only after hemorrhage has been ruled out by CT scan. If the patient has not stabilized after 48 hours of anticoagulant therapy, drug therapy should be halted and the clinical condition reassessed.

Antiplatelet drug therapy should be considered when nondrug measures such as diet, exercise, and removal or avoidance of risk factors have been ineffective. Patients with diabetes mellitus, angina pectoris, heart failure, and hyperlipidemia should have their condition stabilized before initiation of drug therapy. In selected cases, patients with signs and symptoms extending over 12 months may have a better response to antiplatelet therapy than those with symptoms of shorter duration. Improvement should be noted in 2 to 4 weeks after treatment is started. If an improvement of at least 25 to 50 percent is not evident after 8 weeks, drug therapy should be discontinued and the patient's condition reassessed. If improvement does occur at 8 weeks, it is usually continued for approximately 6 months, followed by a 2-month drug-free period.

Patient Variables

SC heparin prophylaxis should be considered for patients who are immobilized for more than 3 days, who are obese, or who have signs of chronic venous insufficiency. In addition, conditions that alter metabolic rate (e.g., hyperthyroidism, fever) cause an increase in the effectiveness of warfarin because the patient's responsiveness to warfarin is intensified.

The ability of the patient to adhere to the prescribed treatment regimen must be taken into account. The patient must safely administer long-term anticoagulant or antiplatelet therapy at home. The patient must also understand and be able to comply with the laboratory testing required for adequate monitoring of therapeutic as well as adverse effects.

Intervention

Administration

Parenteral anticoagulant solutions should be colorless to slightly yellow. Do not use solutions that contain particulate matter. SC injections are given using a 25- to 27-gauge, ⅜- to ⅝-inch needle. The dose to be administered should be double checked with a second licensed health care provider before administration. The preferred injection site for heparin is the lower abdomen. Unlike other injections, aspiration does not precede drug administration. Aspiration or massage of the injection site may cause unnecessary bruising. Injection sites should be rotated to facilitate drug absorption. Hematoma formation is possible with IM injection and, therefore, should be avoided. When venipunctures and injections are unavoidable, pressure should be applied to the site to minimize bleeding.

When heparin is given IV, loading doses usually precede a continuous infusion. An infusion pump should be used to ensure dosage accuracy. Because there are numerous possible drug-drug interactions with heparin, the nurse should check for Y-site and additive compatibilities and incompatibilities before administration. The IV site should be checked for patency and evidence of inflammation according to hospital policy.

Inpatients on anticoagulation therapy should be readily identified through the use of appropriate signage, wrist band, or other identification technique. Outpatients who are on anticoagulant therapy should carry Medic-Alert identification at all times. The patient should also be capable of self-care to avoid injury and reduce the risk for injury.

Dosage Monitoring Because PT test results vary greatly from laboratory to laboratory, an INR is included with PT results. INR values are not dependent on the laboratory methods. The standard method of determining therapeutic PT values (PT ratios between 1½ to 2 times the control value) is converted to a value that takes into consideration the sensitivity of the reagent used as well as the instrumentation. The INR is derived by multiplying the PT ratio by a correction factor specific to the thromboplastin preparation being used in the test.

The goal of warfarin treatment is to raise the INR value to an adequate therapeutic level. An INR of 2 to 3 is sufficient for the majority of patients. However, some patients require an INR value of up to 4½ for adequate anticoagulant effects to occur. Table 36–5 provides a comparison of normal and therapeutic values of warfarin and heparin. Table 36–6 provides a brief overview of recommended ranges of PT-derived values for monitoring oral anticoagulant therapy. If the INR is too low, the warfarin dosage should be increased. During the first 2 to 3 days of therapy, it is desirable to increase the PT by only 1 to 2 seconds/day.

TABLE 35–5 COMPARISON OF COAGULATION TESTS

Drug	Test*	Normal Values	Therapeutic Value†
Warfarin	PT	10–14 seconds	15–28 seconds
Heparin	PTT	30–45 seconds	45–90 seconds
	APTT	16–25 seconds	24–50 seconds

*Normal ranges for PT vary with the type of thromboplastin used. Normal ranges for PTT and APTT vary with phospholipid used.

†Therapeutic value calculated as 1.5 to 2 times the normal value.

PT, Prothrombin time; PTT, partial thromboplastin time; APTT, activated partial thromboplastin time. APTT is a more sensitive test than PTT. APTT values over 100 seconds signify spontaneous bleeding.

TABLE 36–6 RECOMMENDED PROTHROMBIN TIME-DERIVED VALUES

Condition Under Treatment*	Observed PT Ratio†	INR‡
Acute myocardial infarction	1.3–1.5	2.0–3.0
Atrial fibrillation		
Valvular heart disease		
Tissue heart valves		
Mechanical heart valves	1.5–2.0	3.0–4.5
Venous thrombosis§	1.3–1.5	2.0–3.0
Treatment of pulmonary embolism	1.3–1.5	2.0–3.0
Prevention of systemic embolism	1.3–1.5	2.0–3.0
Recurrent systemic embolism	1.5–2.0	3.0–4.5

*For prevention of systemic embolism.

†Observed PT ratio: Ratio of patient's PT to a control PT value. In this particular case, the reagent used to determine the control PT value is one of the preparations of rabbit brain thromboplastic employed in the United States. Had a different preparation of thromboplastin been used, the observed PT ratio could be very different.

‡An international normalized ratio (INR) is calculated from the observed PT ratio. The INR is equivalent to the PT ratio that would have been obtained if the patient's PT had been compared to a PT value obtained using the International Reference Preparation, a standardized human brain thromboplastin prepared by the World Health Organization. In contrast to PT ratios, INR values are comparable from one laboratory to the next throughout the United States and the rest of the world.

§For prophylaxis DVT in high-risk surgical patients and for treatment of DVT.

INR, International Normalized Ratio; PT, prothrombin time.

Adapted from Lehne, R. A. (1998). *Pharmacology for nursing care.* (3rd ed., p. 540). Philadelphia: W. B. Saunders. Used with permission.

Changes greater than 1 to 2 seconds/day indicate that the dosage is too high and the daily warfarin dosage needs to be reduced, usually by about 50 percent (see Controversy—Anticoagulation Therapy).

Therapeutic values of heparin therapy are similar to those of warfarin. The PTT and APTT therapeutic range is usually 1½ to 2 times the normal value. Blood is drawn to establish baseline levels and then 6 hours after the start of the infusion or dosage change. If the patient's baseline is already elevated, heparin should be held until the lab values normalize. Patients on low-dose heparin therapy may not require routine laboratory monitoring. The exceptions to this are for patients who are malnourished, those who have had prior coagulation difficulties, or those who are receiving broad-spectrum antibiotics (e.g., cephalosporins).

Management of Overdose Withholding one or more doses of warfarin is usually sufficient if the patient's PT value is excessively prolonged or if minor bleeding occurs. If overdose occurs and anticoagulation needs to be reversed, the administration of phytonadione (vitamin K_1) can be used. Phytonadione is an antagonist to warfarin. It may be administered orally, SC, or IM. The dosage and route of phytonadione is dependent on the patient's situation and the severity of bleeding. Ten to twenty milligrams given orally is ordinarily used for mild bleeding. The anticoagulation actions of warfarin should normalize within 24 hours following phytonadione administration. Five to fifty milligrams of parenteral phytonadione is administered for severe bleeding.

Controversy

Anticoagulation Therapy

JONATHAN J. WOLFE

Anticoagulation is well established as valuable therapy. Ambulatory anticoagulant therapy using warfarin has demonstrated its worth in prophylaxis against cardiac disease and stroke. When it is properly monitored, this therapy is safe and effective and certainly less risky than embolization of the heart, lungs, or brain.

Monitoring anticoagulant therapy, however, presents special challenges. On one hand, it involves proper acquisition of clinical specimens through blood drawing. These samples must be correctly handled both in the clinic and laboratory. Once results are known, they are correlated with the clinical status of the patient and the desired therapeutic outcomes. For this reason, reliance on prothrombin time (PT) has been replaced by use of the International Normalized Ratio (INR). This test uses the International Sensitivity Index (ISI) as an exponent to relate a particular patient's PT (versus mean normal PT) to the sensitivity of the reagent used. It is a rugged and readily applied system that minimizes differences among laboratories and operators.

The other special challenge derives from the effect of both drugs and diet on warfarin pharmacokinetics. Drug interactions may bring the patient to disastrously low or high levels of anticoagulation, depending on the drugs involved. Seasonal variations in diet involving greatly increased or decreased intake of vegetables rich in vitamin K may similarly send INR values sharply out of control. Therefore, patients must be educated about the seriousness of possible drug and diet interactions when they are taking warfarin.

Critical Thinking Discussion

- What problems had to be overcome in order to secure acceptance of INR as the successor to decades of reliance on PT?
- What information about dietary habits should you elicit from a patient who is to be placed on anticoagulant therapy?
- What cautions should you give patients who will be taking anticoagulants about consulting other physicians or having prescriptions filled in multiple pharmacies?
- What cautions are appropriate in choosing how to respond to a reported INR that is far out of line with a patient's past history?
- What assurance would you offer a reluctant patient who has been told that warfarin is really rat poison?

The effects of phytonadione can last up to 168 hours. Therefore, if warfarin administration needs to be restarted, resistance to its anticoagulant effects will occur until the effects of the drug have subsided. If phytonadione does not control bleeding or if quicker results are needed, clotting factor levels may be increased by administering plasma or clotting factor concentrates (see Chapter 38).

The antagonist to heparin and low-molecular-weight heparins is protamine sulfate. The dosage of protamine sulfate is calculated based on the amount of heparin given and the time interval since administration, but in general, 1 mg of protamine sulfate is given for every 100 units of heparin to be neutralized. The antagonistic effects begin with the administration of the drug and last for up to 2 hours. However, because of the short half-life of heparin overdose can often be treated by withholding the drug.

The antagonist to ticlopidine, which is an antiplatelet drug, is IV methylprednisolone. Methylprednisolone is a short-acting systemic glucocorticoid (see Chapter 52). It should be available in the event excessive bleeding occurs.

Education

The patient and family should be provided with written instructions about all drugs they are receiving, including the name, prescribed dose, reasons for receiving the drug, and adverse effects. They should be advised to take the drug exactly as prescribed and at the same time each day. If a dose is missed, it should be taken as soon as remembered that day. Double doses should not be taken. The health care provider should be notified of any missed doses at the time of check-up or laboratory testing.

The patient should be instructed to notify the health care provider if signs of bleeding or bruising occur. These signs include bleeding gums, black tarry-looking stools, nosebleeds, excessively heavy menstrual flow, or hematuria. They should also be instructed to avoid alcohol and over-the-counter drugs, especially those containing aspirin, ibuprofen, or other nonsteroidal anti-inflammatory drugs without first consulting with the health care provider or pharmacist.

Caution the patient to avoid IM injections, contact sports, and other activities that may lead to injury. Instruct the patient to use a soft toothbrush, not to floss, and to shave with an electric razor during anticoagulant therapy. Also, advise the patient to notify dentists or other health care providers of the anticoagulation therapy. Emphasize the importance of frequent follow-up lab tests to monitor coagulation factors.

For patients taking aspirin for antiplatelet therapy, they should be advised that one over-the-counter aspirin preparation is generally as good as another. They need not pay a high price to get the desired effects. Most oral antiplatelet drugs as well as warfarin should be taken with food or after meals to avoid GI upset. Further, if postural hypotension occurs, as is sometimes the case with dipyridamole, the patient should be instructed to change positions slowly or to lie down for a short time after taking the drug to reduce the risk of falling. Patients should also be informed that exacerbation of gout or renal stones may occur with sulfinpyrazone. Consuming plenty of fluids (2 to 3 L/day) should minimize this problem.

Evaluation

Clinical response to parenteral anticoagulant therapy is indicated by a PTT or APTT that is 1½ to 2 times the normal, without signs of bleeding. Clinical response to oral anticoagulants can be evaluated using the desired INR range. Antiplatelet therapy is considered successful if the patient experiences no further signs and symptoms of the disorder and negative sequelae have been avoided. The prevention and control of thromboembolic disease and its associated complications is evidence of overall treatment success.

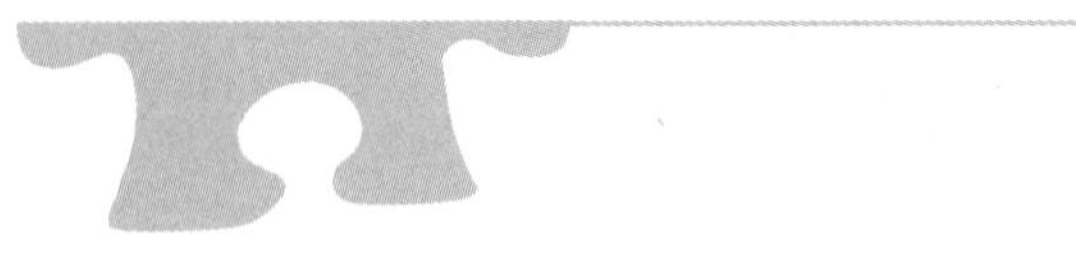

SUMMARY

- DVT develops in a significant number of hospitalized patients. It is estimated that 50,000 to 100,000 deaths occur annually from its major consequence, PE. The mortality rate associated with untreated PE ranges from 25 to 42 percent.
- An MI may be caused by formation of a thrombus in the coronary artery, sudden progression of atherosclerotic changes, or prolonged constriction of the arteries. The mortality rate associated with an acute MI ranges as high as 30 to 40 percent.
- Cellular damage from an MI occurs because the cells are deprived of oxygen and nutrients resulting from the obstructed flow of blood.
- Thrombosis is the most frequent cause of stroke. The most frequent cause of cerebral thrombosis is atherosclerosis and is seen most often in the 60- to 90-year-old age group. Many of these persons have a history of hypertension or diabetes mellitus.
- Thrombus development begins when red blood cells, white blood cells, platelets, and fibrin adhere to exposed collagen fibers in the affected vessel.
- The intrinsic pathway and extrinsic pathway require certain clotting factors to produce a fibrin clot.
- The goal of anticoagulant and antiplatelet therapy is to prevent the formation and progression of intravascular blood clots and their sequelae.
- Treatment options for thromboembolic disease include oral anticoagulants, such as warfarin, and parenteral anticoagulants, such as ardeparin, dalteparin, enoxaparin, and heparin.
- Antiplatelet drugs that may be used in the management of thromboembolic disease include aspirin, dipyridamole, pentoxifylline, sulfinpyrazone, and ticlopidine.
- Antiplatelet drugs are used primarily for prevention of arterial thrombus.
- Patient assessment includes evaluation of risk factors for thromboembolic disease and the presence of related signs and symptoms.
- PT and INR values monitor therapeutic and potentially adverse effects of oral anticoagulants. PTT or APTT values monitor heparin therapy.
- Protamine sulfate and phytonadione are the antagonists to heparin and warfarin, respectively. They are used in the event of dosage excess or if there is a need to quickly reverse the effects of the anticoagulant.
- Signs and symptoms of bleeding are monitored during administration of anticoagulants and antiplatelet drugs.
- Care of the patient receiving anticoagulant and antiplatelet drugs includes education about the drug's purpose and possible adverse effects, noting primarily the potential for bleeding.
- Successful preventive treatment of thrombus formation is noted by the absence of thrombus formation. Successful therapeutic treatment is noted by a PT, PTT, or APTT value that ranges between 1½ to 2 times the normal value. INR values range from 2.0 to 3.0.

BIBLIOGRAPHY

Butler, M. (1995). Use of anticoagulants in hospital and community. *Nursing Times*, 91(13), 36–37.

Catania, U. (1994). Monitoring Coumadin therapy. *RN*, 57(2), 29–34.

Corbett, J., and Kinney, C. (1995). Anticoagulants during pregnancy. *MCN: The American Journal of Maternal/Child Nursing*, 20(1), 56.

Drug watch: Fatal neutropenia from ticlopidine. (1995). *American Journal of Nursing*, 95(2), 55.

Farrington, E. (1994). Warfarin drug interactions. *Pediatric Nursing*, 20(1), 56.

Fowler, S. (1995). Deep vein thrombosis and pulmonary emboli in neuroscience patients. *Journal of Neuroscience Nursing*, 27(4), 224–228.

Ginsberg, J. (1996). Management of venous thromboembolism. *New England Journal of Medicine,* 335, 1816–1828.

Gupta, M. (1995). Pharmacist consult: Seven steps for administering enoxaparin. *Nursing,* 25(9), 72.

Hull, R., Raskob, G., Pineo, G., et al. (1997). Subcutaneous low-molecular-weight heparin vs warfarin for prophylaxis of deep vein thrombosis after hip or knee implantation: An economic perspective. *Archives of Internal Medicine,* 157, 298–303.

Hyers, T., Hull, R., and Weg, J. (1992). Antithrombotic therapy for venous thromboembolic disease. *Chest,* 102(4 Suppl), 408S–425S.

Inconsistencies in anticoagulant monitoring. (1994). *Emergency Medicine,* 26(2), 80.

Mallet, L. (1993). Aspirin and ticlopidine often lead forces in battle against stroke. *Provider,* 19(10), 55.

Meade, T., and Miller, G. (1995). Combined use of aspirin and warfarin in primary prevention of ischemic heart disease in men at high risk. *American Journal of Cardiology,* 75(6), 23B–25B.

Moccia, J. (1996). Pulmonary embolism: Targeting an elusive enemy. *Nursing,* 26(4), 26–32.

Raimer, F., and Thomas, M. (1995). Clot stoppers: Using anticoagulants safely and effectively. *Nursing,* 25(3), 34–45.

Sparks, K. (1996). Are you up to date on weight-based heparin dosing? *American Journal of Nursing,* 96(4), 33–36.

The Columbus Investigators. (1997). Low-molecular-weight heparin in the treatment of patients with venous thromboembolism. *New England Journal of Medicine,* 337, 657–662.

Wilson, B. (1994). Enoxaparin and a new look at clot prevention. *Medsurg Nursing,* 3(1), 66–67.

Workman, M. (1994). Anticoagulants and thrombolytics: What's the difference? *AACN Clinical Issues in Critical Care Nursing,* 5(1), 26–35.

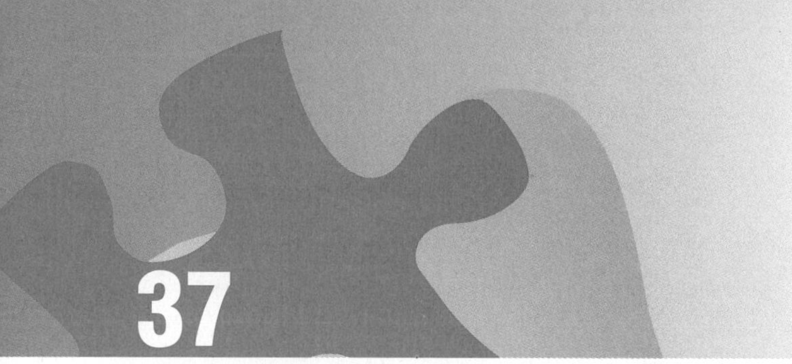

37 Thrombolytic and Sclerosing Drugs

Thrombolytic therapy was first introduced in 1958 for the treatment of myocardial infarction (MI). It met with little success. It was believed that thrombosis was a secondary problem and not a primary problem associated with MI. In the last two decades, there has been a resurgence of interest in thrombolytic therapy for use during coronary angiography. The realization that in many cases thrombosis is a primary cause of infarction has also added to the interest. Thrombolytic therapy is now the standard of care for patients with acute MI, and it is emerging as a treatment modality for other disease processes related to thrombosis (e.g., pulmonary embolus [PE], deep vein thrombosis [DVT], and peripheral arterial occlusive disease). It has also been used in the treatment of cerebral thrombosis.

Sclerosing drugs are used primarily for the treatment of bleeding esophageal varices and uncomplicated superficial varicose veins of the lower extremities.

CARDIOVASCULAR DISORDERS

Myocardial Infarction

Epidemiology and Etiology

Since 1940, MI has been the leading cause of death in the United States. Approximately 1.5 million cases occur annually in the United States as a result of MI. One-third of these patients die. MI affects the arteries that provide blood, oxygen, and nutrients to the myocardium. Death of myocardial tissue results from a sudden cessation of oxygen supply to the muscle. The cause of MI is usually related to atherosclerosis or narrowing of the coronary vessels due to a build-up of plaque. However, approximately 80 percent of MIs are the direct result of an embolus.

Pathophysiology

The heart muscle receives its nutritive and oxygen-carrying blood supply through two major vessels located on the surface of the heart, the right and left coronary arteries (Fig. 37–1). These arteries originate from the aorta and divide into smaller arterioles that penetrate the heart muscle. The left coronary artery is divided into two parts. The left anterior descending artery supplies blood to the anterior surface of the left ventricle, and the left circumflex artery supplies blood to the lateral wall of the left ventricle. The right coronary artery supplies the inferior aspect of the left ventricle and the right ventricle. The right coronary artery also supplies the posterior aspect of the right and left ventricles. However, in about 20 percent of the population, the left circumflex artery supplies blood to the posterior portion of the heart. An obstruction in any one of these vessels impedes the flow of blood carrying oxygen and nutrients to that area of the myocardium.

In patients with coronary artery disease (CAD), atherosclerotic plaque builds up slowly over time. Because plaque has a rough surface, platelets begin to adhere, fibrin is deposited, and blood cells become trapped. A clot eventually forms that occludes the vessel. In some cases, the clot can break away and travel to a smaller vessel, where it will cause an occlusion.

Immediately after an acute coronary vessel occlusion, blood flow ceases to the area beyond the occlusion. There are small amounts of collateral blood flow available from surrounding vessels. However, in areas with no oxygen available to the affected tissues, cells die.

Infarction is a dynamic process that occurs over several hours. Obvious physical changes do not begin in the heart muscle until approximately 6 hours after the infarct. The infarcted area appears blue and swollen. Approximately 48 hours later, neutrophils invade to remove necrotic cells and the area turns gray with yellow streaks. Granulation tissue forms at the edges by the eighth to tenth day after the infarct. Over the next 2 to 3 months, the necrotic area is reduced to a shrunken, thin, firm scar. The presence of scar tissue permanently changes the structure and the function of the ventricle, which, in turn, increases morbidity and mortality.

Thromboembolic Disease

Epidemiology and Etiology

PE is an obstruction of a pulmonary artery by a thrombus originating in the venous system or the right side of the heart. Any substance can cause a PE. Ordinarily it is caused by a blood clot that has broken loose from a DVT. The populations at risk for thromboembolic disease were discussed in Chapter 36. DVT and PE are responsible for more than 250,000 hospitalizations and approximately 50,000 deaths each year in the United States. The immediate cause of death in the patient who develops PE is right-sided heart failure.

Pathophysiology

Stasis of blood flow, damage to the endothelial lining of the vessel, and changes in the mechanics of coagulation are the three primary causes of DVT (Virchow's triad). Once a clot has formed in a vessel, blood flow past the clot is likely to break it loose. Free-flowing clots are called *emboli.* When the embolus is dislodged, it is transported to the right ventricle and then to the pulmonary arterial system, where it becomes lodged and obstructs circulation.

Platelets accumulate behind the embolus, triggering the release of serotonin and thromboxane A_2, which, in turn, causes vasoconstriction. Circulation decreases further. An imbalance results in areas where the lung is ventilated but not perfused. This results in hypoxemia. The larger the vessel affected, the more serious the consequences. By defini-

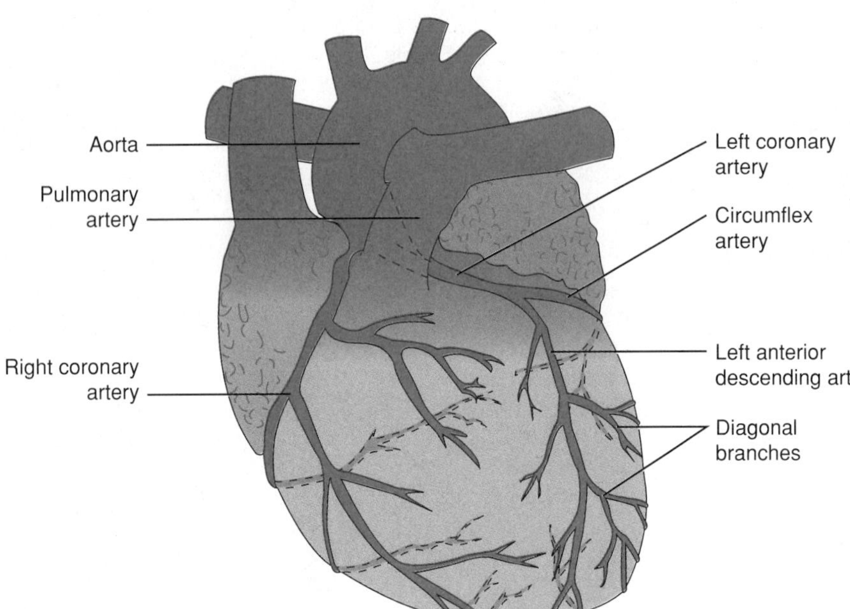

Figure 37–1 Right and left coronary arteries through which the heart muscle receives its major blood supply. (From Black, J.M., and Matassarin-Jacobs, E. [1997]. Medical-surgical nursing: Clinical management for continuity of care [5th ed., p. 1194]. Philadelphia: W. B. Saunders. Used with permission.)

tion, a massive PE obstructs more than 50 percent of blood flow to the lungs.

A hemodynamic consequence of this process is an increase in pulmonary vascular resistance. The increased resistance is due to a decrease in the size of the pulmonary vascular bed, resulting in greater pulmonary arterial pressures. In turn, an increase in the right ventricular workload is needed to maintain pulmonary blood flow. However, when myocardial work load requirements exceed capacity, right ventricular failure occurs. There is a subsequent decrease in cardiac output, and shock may occur.

Peripheral Arterial Occlusion

Epidemiology and Etiology

Arterial occlusions occur more commonly in the lower extremity than in the upper extremity; however, cerebral, mesenteric, and renal arteries can be involved. Emboli originating in the arterial system or that come from the left side of the heart are the usual causes. Predisposing factors for arterial thrombosis are the same as those for CAD. Whereas chronic peripheral vascular disease is a slow process, the onset of arterial occlusion may be sudden.

Pathophysiology

Arterial emboli most often develop in the chambers of the heart as a result of atrial fibrillation or atrial flutter. Inadequate emptying of the atrium allows blood flow to stagnate and predisposes to clotting. If clots detach, they are propelled from the heart into the arterial system and become lodged when they reach an area smaller in size than the embolus. The result is the immediate cessation of blood flow below the area of occlusion. Clots typically lodge at arterial bifurcations and in narrowed vessels. Secondary vasospasm that occurs contributes to the ischemia.

Thrombosis with emboli formation may also develop in an artery with advanced atherosclerosis because of roughening of the atheromatous plaque. A clot is formed on the wall of an artery in a mechanism similar to that of venous thrombosis formation. A part of the thrombus may break loose and travel to a vessel smaller than the size of the embolus.

A third site for formation of arterial thrombosis is an arterial aneurysm. An aneurysm, a weakness in the intima of an artery, provides for stasis of blood with eventual clotting. The force of the arterial pressure can propel the clot from the aneurysm into arterial circulation.

Cerebrovascular Accident

Epidemiology and Etiology

A cerebrovascular occlusion (stroke, cerebrovascular accident [CVA]) is a sudden loss of brain function resulting from a disruption in the blood supply to a part of the brain. It is the primary neurologic problem, not only in the United States but in the world. Although the number of stroke-related deaths has declined in the past several years, CVA remains the third leading cause of death in the United States and the number one cause of death in the world. It also leaves a large number of people disabled each year. Treatment of CVAs in the United States exceeds $15 billion per year.

There are three major causes of CVAs. Ischemic strokes are divided into those caused by a thrombus and those that are caused by emboli. Embolic CVAs are more common in patients with a history of valvular disease, prosthetic valve replacements, atrial fibrillation, ischemic heart disease, or rheumatic heart disease. A hemorrhagic CVA produces bleeding into the brain. It generally results from a ruptured saccular aneurysm, rupture of an arteriovenous malformation, or more commonly, hypertension.

Pathophysiology

Embolic CVAs are abrupt in development with steady progression of symptoms. The embolus tends to lodge in the middle cerebral artery or one of its branches. As it occludes the vessel, ischemia occurs in brain tissue supplied by the affected artery. Brain dysfunction results. Ischemia leads to hypoxia or anoxia and hypoglycemia. These processes cause death of the neurons, glia, and vasculature in the involved areas. Further, brain metabolism is disrupted in the involved area and in the opposite hemisphere.

Catheter Occlusions

Central venous access devices may, on occasion, become occluded by fibrin clots and other plasma proteins. Occlusion can be a serious potential complication of central venous access device catheters.

Clots normally form when thrombin, an enzyme made from prothrombin, converts fibrinogen to fibrin. The conversion typically occurs in response to trauma to the vascular wall. Insertion of a large catheter would cause such trauma. The body's natural response is for activated plasminogen to form plasmin, a proteolytic enzyme that dissolves the clot and keeps fibrinogen from making new fibrin. This process cannot occur within the lumen of a central venous catheter. Therefore, blood adhering to the catheter wall has a tendency to form fibrin clots.

PHARMACOTHERAPEUTIC OPTIONS

First-Generation Thrombolytics

- ❐ Streptokinase (STREPTASE, KABIKINASE)
- ❐ Urokinase (ABBOKINASE)

Second-Generation Thrombolytics

- ❐ Alteplase (recombinant tissue plasminogen activator [tPA], ACTIVASE)
- ❐ Anistreplase (anisoylated plasminogen streptokinase activator complex [APSAC], EMINASE)

Third-Generation Thrombolytics

- ❐ Reteplase recombinant (RETAVASE)

Indications

Thrombolytic therapy is indicated in the treatment of MI, PE, DVT, CVA, and arterial occlusions. Thrombolytics are also used to restore patency to occluded central venous catheters. Different drugs have been found to be more beneficial in some conditions than in others. Streptokinase, the prototype thrombolytic, was the first drug widely available for clinical use.

With prompt use of thrombolytic drugs and reperfusion following an MI, there is a reduction in the size of the infarct, improvement in left ventricular function, and reduction of mortality. A thrombolytic drug is indicated for the patient who has chest pain consistent with an MI for at least 30 minutes but not longer than 6 hours and who has at least 0.1 mV of ST-segment elevation in at least two contiguous electrocardiographic leads. Figure 37–2 shows the changes in electrocardiographic patterns associated with ischemia, injury, and infarction.

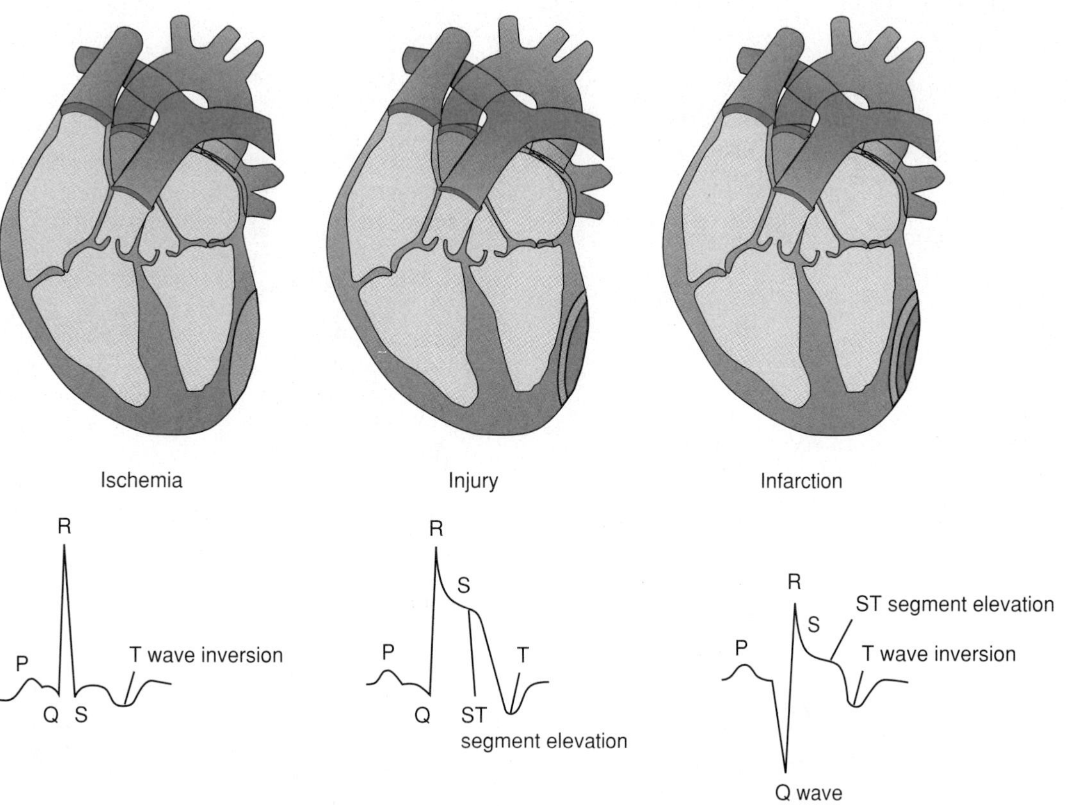

Figure 37–2 The changes in electrocardiograph patterns associated with ischemia, injury, and infarction show how ST segment elevation progresses through each stage. (From Black, J. M., and Matassarin-Jacobs, E. [1997]. *Medical-surgical nursing: Clinical management for continuity of care* [5th ed., p. 1261]. Philadelphia: W. B. Saunders. Used with permission.)

Thrombolytic therapy has been indicated in the treatment of acute massive PE. Rapid dissolution of the clot helps normalize the patient's hemodynamic status. It is also indicated in the treatment of DVT. Alteplase has been approved by the Food and Drug Administration (FDA) for use in computed tomography (CT)–confirmed ischemic CVA.

Urokinase has been used successfully to restore patency to occluded central venous catheters when the occlusion is the result of a fibrous clot. Streptokinase can be used to restore patency to occluded arteriovenous cannulae.

Restoring patency of occluded AV shunts is another possible use for thrombolytics. Urokinase has been used in a pulse spray method via a multi-sidehole catheter placed in a crisscross pattern in the graft.

Suggested possible future uses of thrombolytics include treatment of cerebral emboli with intra-arterial injection of urokinase and prevention of fibrin build-up in peritoneal dialysis catheters. The treatment of thrombosis of prosthetic valves in the left side of the heart is also being explored.

Pharmacodynamics

Unlike anticoagulants, which prevent the formation or extension of blood clots, thrombolytic drugs dissolve thrombi after formation. They convert plasminogen to plasmin which in turn degrades fibrin present in the clots. Streptokinase combines with plasminogen to form activator complexes that then convert plasminogen to plasmin.

Urokinase is a protein initially isolated from human urine. It activates plasminogen directly. Because it is not a derivative of streptococci, as is streptokinase, there is less incidence of allergic reaction with urokinase than with streptokinase.

Thrombolytics activate plasminogen directly. Fibrinogen levels are decreased for 24 to 36 hours after therapy. Direct and indirect effects of thrombolysis are prolonged because of the drug's extended presence in the circulation and because of the elevated concentrations of fibrinogen degradation products in the plasma.

Alteplase is fibrin specific. Once it is injected into the circulation, it binds to fibrin in a thrombus and converts the trapped plasminogen to plasmin. There is less effect on circulating plasminogen.

Anistreplase is an active complex of streptokinase and plasminogen. Like alteplase, anistreplase was developed initially as a clot-specific drug; however, it seems to work equally well on systemic plasminogen conversion. Anistreplase is an inactive derivative of a fibrinolytic enzyme, with the center of the activator complex temporarily blocked by an anisoyl group. In solution, the anisoyl group is removed and the enzymatically active lys-plasminogen streptokinase complex is activated.

Reteplase, the newest thrombolytic drug, is a recombinant protein derived from tissue plasminogen activator. It, too, catalyzes the conversion of plasminogen to plasmin, with the activation stimulated by the presence of fibrin. Plasmin then degrades the fibrin matrix of the thrombus. Reteplase has a lower affinity for fibrin, which may result in better clot penetration.

Adverse Effects and Contraindications

Overall, bleeding represents the most common complication of thrombolytic therapy, occurring in 8 to 16 percent of patients. Bleeding may occur in the gastrointestinal (GI) tract, genitourinary tract, and retroperitoneal, ocular, or intracranial spaces. Bleeding from puncture sites may also occur.

Bleeding is more common in women than in men. Major bleeding severe enough to require a blood transfusion occurs in 12 to 15 percent of patients. Hemorrhagic CVAs, which occur in one-half to one percent of patients, is the single most dreaded complication associated with thrombolytic therapy. The risk of intracranial hemorrhage is higher in patients receiving thrombolytics for the treatment of CVA than those receiving them for the treatment of MI. Hemorrhagic bleeding occurs most often with the accelerated alteplase protocol. Drug-induced hypotension occurs infrequently but is reported more frequently with streptokinase and anistreplase.

Other adverse effects of thrombolytic drugs include reperfusion arrhythmias, nausea and vomiting, and hypersensitivity reactions. Hypersensitivity reactions most commonly occur with streptokinase, with symptoms ranging in severity from minor breathing difficulty to bronchospasm, periorbital swelling, or angioneurotic edema. Other milder allergic effects such as urticaria, itching, flushing, nausea, headache, and musculoskeletal pain have been observed. Anaphylaxis is rare. Approximately 33 percent of patients experience an increase in temperature.

Cross sensitivity of anistreplase with streptokinase may occur. Streptokinase is a bacterial protein that can be antigenic. It can cause a hypersensitivity response in any patient who has been treated for streptococcal infection during the previous year. These patients develop streptococcal antibodies that neutralize the streptokinase, causing severe allergic reactions.

Because thrombolytic therapy carries serious risks, care must be taken to exclude patients who are at high risk for complications and those in whom the risks outweigh the benefits that they would receive (see Contraindications to Thrombolytic Therapy and Contraindications to Thrombolytic Therapy for Acute Ischemic Stroke).

Thrombolytic therapy is generally contraindicated during pregnancy. Urokinase has been classified as pregnancy category B. The remaining thrombolytics are category C drugs.

Pharmacokinetics

Information on the pharmacokinetics of thrombolytic drugs is incomplete. Streptokinase has an immediate action, with peak action reached in 30 to 60 minutes. The duration of action is 4 to 12 hours. It is cleared from the circulation by antibodies. The half-life of streptokinase is 23 minutes (Table 37–1). Streptokinase does not cross placental membranes, but the antibodies produced in response to the streptokinase do cross over to the fetus.

Urokinase has an immediate onset, peaking by the end of the infusion. Urokinase crosses the placental membranes and may pass into breast milk. It has a duration of action of up to 12 hours. It is biotransformed and eliminated primarily by the liver; however, small amounts are eliminated in the urine. The half-life of the drug is 20 minutes or less but is prolonged if there is liver impairment.

Alteplase is rapidly absorbed via IV routes with an immediate onset of action. Alteplase crosses the placental barrier and may pass into breast milk. It peaks in 5 to 10 minutes, with a duration of action of 2½ to 3 hours. Biotransformation

CONTRAINDICATIONS TO THROMBOLYTIC THERAPY

Absolute Contraindications

- Active internal bleeding
- Aneurysm
- Arteriovenous malformation
- Cerebral surgery or trauma in the previous 2 months
- History of CVA
- Intracranial neoplasm
- Known bleeding diathesis
- Severe uncontrolled hypertension
- Spinal surgery in the previous 2 months

Relative Contraindications

- Acute pericarditis
- Age greater than 75 years
- Cerebrovascular disease
- Chronic renal failure
- Diabetic hemorrhagic retinopathy
- Hemorrhagic ophthalmic conditions
- Hypertension
- Liver dysfunction
- Mitral stenosis with atrial fibrillation
- Occluded AV cannula at an infected IV site
- Patients on anticoagulants
- Pregnancy or recent delivery
- Prolonged cardiopulmonary resuscitation
- Recent GI or genitourinary bleeding
- Septic thrombophlebitis
- Subacute bacterial endocarditis
- Trauma or surgery within previous 10 days

CONTRAINDICATIONS TO THROMBOLYTIC THERAPY FOR ACUTE ISCHEMIC STROKE

Absolute Contraindications

- Evidence of intracranial hemorrhage on pretreatment evaluation
- Suspicion of subarachnoid hemorrhage
- Intracranial surgery within the previous 14 days
- Serious head trauma within previous 3 months
- CVA within previous 3 months
- History of intracranial hemorrhage
- Uncontrolled hypertension (e.g., systolic BP over 185 mmHg or diastolic over 110 mmHg)
- Blood glucose value under 50 or over 400 mg/dL
- Seizure at onset of CVA
- Active internal bleeding
- Gastrointestinal or urinary bleeding within the past 21 days
- Intracranial neoplasm, AV malformation, or aneurysm
- Known bleeding diathesis including but not limited to current use of anticoagulant with a prothrombin time exceeding 15 seconds; administration of heparin within 48 hours preceding onset of CVA; an elevated aPTT upon arrival at health care facility
- Platelet count under 100,000 mm^3
- Recent MI

Ablative Contraindications

Patients with severe neurologic deficit over 22 on National Institute of Health Scale

Patients with early infarct signs on CT scan (e.g., substantial edema, mass effect, or midline shift)

takes place in the liver, with small amounts eliminated in the urine.

The onset of anistreplase is immediate, with peak effects reached in 45 minutes. Like alteplase, anistreplase crosses the placenta and may pass into breast milk. Its duration of action is 4 to 6 hours. Biotransformation occurs in the plasma, with inactivation caused by binding to plasmin inactivators. The half-life is 70 to 120 minutes.

The half-life of reteplase is approximately 13 to 16 minutes. It is biotransformed in the liver and eliminated in the urine. It is not known whether it is excreted in human milk. The safety and efficacy of use in children has not been established.

Drug-Drug Interactions

The concurrent administration of antiplatelet drugs, anticoagulants, dipyridamole, indomethacin, and phenylbutazone increases the risk of bleeding. The use of low-dose aspirin with thrombolytics has been shown to reduce the incidence of reinfarction and CVA. The addition of aspirin seems to produce a slight increase in the incidence of minor bleeding but not in major bleeding.

Dosage Regimen

Dosage regimens for thrombolytic drugs are different for each drug depending on the patient's diagnosis (Table 37–2). Caution should be used when checking dosages because some references list dosages based on body weight in pounds rather than in kilograms per pound.

Laboratory Considerations

Before beginning thrombolytic therapy, a baseline hematocrit, platelet count, fibrinogen level, thrombin time, partial thromboplastin time (PTT) (or activated partial thrombo-

TABLE 37–1 PHARMACOKINETICS OF THROMBOLYTIC DRUGS

Drug	Route	Onset	Peak	Duration	PB (%)	$t_{1/2}$	BioA (%)
Alteplase	IV	Immediate	5–10 min	2.5–3 hr	UA	5 min	100
Anistreplase	IV	Immediate	45 min	4–6 hr*	UA	70–120 min	100
Reteplase	IV	Immediate	5–10 min	UA	UA	13–16 min	100
Streptokinase	IV	Immediate	30–60 min†	4–12 hr	UA	23 min	100
Urokinase	IV	Immediate	End of infusion	Up to 12 hr	UA	20 min	100

*Systemic hyperfibrinolytic state may persist for 48 hours with the use of anistreplase.

†Clearance and thrombolytic activity of streptokinase appears to decline with continuous infusion; BioA, bioavailability; PB, protein binding; $t_{1/2}$, elimination half-life; UA, unavailable.

TABLE 37–2 DOSAGE REGIMEN FOR THROMBOLYTIC DRUGS

Drug	Use(s)	Dosage	Implications
Alteplase	Ischemic stroke	*Adults:* 0.9 mg/kg. Maximum: 90 mg with 10% of dose given as bolus over 1 minute followed by infusion lasting 60 minutes	Must be given within 3 hours of ischemic stroke
	Acute myocardial infarction	*Standard dosage regimen:* *Adults over 65 kg:* 10 mg IV bolus over 2 minutes, followed by 50 mg over next hour, then 20 mg over next hour, and 20 mg over the third hour *Adults under 65 kg:* 0.075–0.125 mg IV bolus over first 1–2 minutes, followed by 0.25 mg/kg over the next hour, then 0.25 mg/kg over the third hour *Accelerated dosage regimen:* *Adults over 65 kg:* 100 mg administered as a 15-mg IV bolus, followed by 50 mg over next 30 minutes, then 35 mg over next 60 minutes *Adults below 65 kg:* 15-mg IV bolus, followed by 0.75 mg/kg over next 30 minutes (not to exceed 50 mg) and then 0.5 mg/kg over next 60 minutes (not to exceed 35 mg)	Doses greater than 150 mg have been associated with an increased risk of intracranial bleeding. Use infusion pump for drug administration
	Pulmonary embolism	*Adults.* 100 mg IV over 2 hours	To be followed by heparin therapy
Anistreplase	Acute myocardial infarction	*Adults:* 30 units IV over 2–5 minutes	History of strep infection may contraindicate use
Reteplase	Acute myocardial infarction	*Adults:* 10 units IV over 2 minutes followed by a second bolus after 30 minutes	
Streptokinase	Acute myocardial infarction	*Adults:* 250,000 units over 30 minutes followed by 100,000 units/hour × 24–72 hours	History of strep infection contraindicates use of streptokinase
	Deep vein thrombosis, pulmonary embolism, arterial embolism or thrombosis	*Adults:*250,000 IU. IV loading dose over 30 minutes followed by 100,000 IU/hr for 24 hours for pulmonary emboli, 72 hours for recurrent pulmonary emboli or deep vein thrombosis	
	Arteriovenous cannula occlusion	*Adults:* 100,000–250,000 IU into each occluded limb of cannula, clamp for 2 hours, then aspirate	Flush line with normal saline after aspiration
Urokinase	Pulmonary emboli, deep vein thrombosis	*Adults:* 4400 IU/kg loading dose over 10 minutes followed by 4400 IU/kg/hr for 12–24 hours	Some references list dosage based on body weight in pounds rather than kilograms. Check dosage carefully
	Arteriovenous cannula occlusion	*Adults:* 5000 IU./ml. solution injected into cathether, then aspirated. May repeat every 5 minutes for 30 minutes. Volume to be instilled is equal to or slightly less than volume of catheter	If no result, may cap and leave in catheter for 30–60 minutes, then aspirated

TABLE 37–3 LABORATORY TEST RESULTS AFTER THROMBOLYTIC THERAPY

Laboratory Test	Results
Protime	Increased
Activated partial thromboplastin time	Increased
Thrombin time	Increased
Fibrinogen level	Decreased
Plasminogen level	Decreased

plastin time, APTT), and prothrombin (PT) time should be drawn. Abnormalities in these laboratory values may prevent the patient from being considered as a candidate for thrombolytic therapy. During therapy, there will be an increase in the thrombin time, PTT, and PT, which should normalize within 12 to 24 hours. There will be a decrease in the fibrinogen and plasminogen levels (Table 37–3).

Critical Thinking Process

Assessment

History of Present Illness

Careful assessment of the patient is critical for the prompt treatment of acute MI. The symptoms of an acute MI include chest pain or pressure that usually radiates to the left arm, neck, or jaw that is unrelieved by nitroglycerin. The pain is usually accompanied by associated symptoms such as nausea, shortness of breath, diaphoresis, or a feeling of impending doom.

The patient with a PE presents with a history of chest pain and a sudden onset of shortness of breath. He or she may have a history of known DVT or risk factors associated with DVT.

Patients with a CVA have a variety of symptoms depending on the location of the cerebral infarction. The most common symptoms are changes in mental status, weakness, or partial paralysis of one side of the body and slurred speech or aphasia.

Past Health History

Past health history is crucial in the determination of proper candidates for thrombolytic therapy. It is imperative to note whether the patient has any of the relative or absolute contraindications to thrombolytic therapy (see the section on Contraindications). In addition, determine whether or not the patient has had a streptococcus infection in the past, as well as any previous administration of streptokinase or anistreplase. Identify allergies to any other medications. It is important to know whether or not the patient is also taking anticoagulants, antiplatelet drugs, or indomethacin because these drugs may cause an increased risk for bleeding if thrombolytic drugs are used concurrently.

Physical Exam Findings

Symptoms found during the physical exam are often the first indicators that a potentially lethal incident has occurred. Detections of subtle changes in the patient are the most important keys to early diagnosis and lead to rapid treatment decisions.

The patient who presents with an acute MI appears to be in obvious distress. The skin may be cool and clammy. The skin color may be pale or cyanotic. The blood pressure may be decreased, and the pulse and respiratory rate may be increased.

DVT is manifested by pain in the effected extremity. The affected extremity is usually warm to the touch and may be reddened. Homans' sign may be present, although it is absent in about 50 percent of patients. The affected extremity may be measurably larger than the unaffected one.

The patient with a PE exhibits signs and symptoms that include a sudden, marked shortness of breath, tachycardia, chest pain, and hemoptysis. A feeling of panic so intense that it may cause panic and a fear of impending death is also common.

Signs and symptoms exhibited by the patient with peripheral arterial occlusive disease are pain, pulselessness, pallor, paresthesia, and paralysis of the affected extremity. These are the classic 5 Ps of arterial obstruction.

CVA should be considered in any patient who presents with a sudden deterioration in level of consciousness or who has focal neurologic deficits. Symptoms of acute ischemic stroke and hemorrhagic stroke often overlap, so clinical presentation cannot be relied on for treatment decisions. Further diagnostic testing must be performed.

A baseline physical assessment should be conducted to monitor for treatment effectiveness as well as complications related to the thrombolytic therapy. Assessment of the patient's mental status, level of consciousness and orientation, cardiac status including heart rhythm, and respiratory status must be performed before the beginning of therapy. Physical exam findings may also help identify the patient at risk for the complications.

Diagnostic Testing

An elevated creatine kinase (CK) with a myocardial band (MB) isoenzyme greater than 10 percent of the total is diagnostic of an acute MI. However, CK isoenzymes are not available immediately and the decision to treat with thrombolytics must be made before the enzyme results return. Electrocardiographic changes along with unrelieved chest pain are used as the definitive criteria for administration of thrombolytic therapy. Criteria for therapy is an electrocardiogram that exhibits ST-segment elevation of 1-mm duration in two contiguous leads.

A newer test, thrombus precursor protein (T_PP), is able to detect the formation of a blood clot. Earlier detection permits earlier diagnosis and treatment with thrombolytics.

Patients who present with suspected PE should be diagnosed with a ventilation-perfusion lung scan to obtain a correct diagnosis. There are diagnostic tests available for DVT, but because of the classic signs and symptoms, physical exam findings are usually enough to make a diagnosis.

When a patient presents with a CVA, it is impossible to differentiate an embolic stroke from a hemorrhagic stroke without the use of a CT scan or magnetic resonance imaging. A follow up with a lumbar puncture or cerebral angiography must be performed if any doubt remains after the CT study. Very little change is seen on a CT scan in the early stages of an embolic event. If the CT shows massive edema, midline shift, or a mass this may be an indication that the time interval has been longer than first thought or that the CVA is massive. These findings would put the patient at higher risk for intracranial hemorrhage.

Developmental Considerations

Safety and efficacy of thrombolytic drugs have not been established for perinatal, lactating, or pediatric patients. Further, patients 75 years of age or older are at higher risk for bleeding due to cerebrovascular disease. The older adult population is also at a higher risk for the disease processes that are typically treated with thrombolytic therapy.

Psychosocial Considerations

MI, PE, and CVA are generally considered to be urgent to emergent conditions that may warrant treatment with thrombolytics. It is a frightening experience not only for the patient but also for the family. Emotional support is essential at these times. Because the health care system is tuned to the

Case Study Acute Myocardial Infarction

Patient History

History of Present Illness	JH is a 40-year-old obese white male who is admitted with complaints of substernal chest pain radiating to the left arm. The pain began approximately 1 hour ago. The ambulance crew has administered three nitroglycerin tablets without relief.
Past Health History	JH is a two pack/day smoker. He has a history of adult-onset diabetes mellitus and is on tolbutamide. His last cholesterol measurement was 465. He has no known allergies and has no previous hospital admissions. However, he thinks that he has had strep throat on several occasions in the past year.
Physical Exam	Skin is moist. Respirations are 28/min and slightly labored. Lungs are clear. B/P: 100/70, apical pulse 76/min and irregular. Monitor shows sinus rhythm with PVCs.
Diagnostic Testing	CK isoenzymes have been drawn. An ECG has been done and shows ST-segment elevation in leads II and III, and AVF.
Developmental Considerations	JH is a middle-aged adult completing the tasks of generativity vs. stagnation. A myocardial infarction may have an impact on his role in the family, his earning capacity, and his social relationships.
Psychosocial Considerations	JH is an accountant for a very successful firm. He usually works 50–60 hours per week.
Economic Factors	JH has insurance that will cover a large percentage of his hospitalization. He also has money available in savings to cover a short convalescence.

Variables Influencing Decision

Treatment Objectives	• To restore the patency of the occluded vessel, prevent myocardial damage, and preserve myocardial function.

Drug Variables	*Drug Summary*	*Patient Variables*
Indications	Streptokinase, urokinase, alteplase, and anistreplase are indicated for use with MI. Urokinase is more effective in the treatment of PE and in restoring patency to occluded catheters.	JH has had no previous MIs. At this point, he has viable heart muscle. It has been approximately 2 hours since the onset of symptoms. This will become a decision point.
Pharmacodynamics	All thrombolytics act to break down clots already formed.	There are no pharmacodynamics that relate directly to JH's MI.
Adverse Effects/ Contraindications	There are relative and absolute contraindications for all thrombolytics. There is an increased risk of allergic reaction with streptokinase and anistreplase in patients with streptococci exposure.	JH meets none of the criteria for contraindications; however, he has a history of strep throat. This will become a decision point.
Pharmacokinetics	The onset for all drugs is immediate; however, alteplase peaks sooner (within 5–10 minutes).	There are no pharmacokinetic considerations for JH's care.
Dosage Regimen	The accelerated protocol for alteplase has been shown to have a better patency rate than other thrombolytics.	JH has no previous history of MI. This may be a decision point.

Case Study Acute Myocardial Infarction—cont'd

Drug Variables	Drug Summary	Patient Variables
Lab Considerations	Laboratory considerations are the same for all drugs. Baseline Hct, thromboplastin time, APTT, and PT should be drawn. Lab results will be monitored until results normalize.	JH will be hospitalized during drug therapy so this will not be a decision point. He is readily accessible to laboratory personnel.
Cost Index*	Streptokinase: 5 Urokinase: 5 Anistreplase: 5 Alteplase: 5	Because JH has a history of strep throat, the streptokinase and anistreplase cannot be used. This will be a decision point.

Summary of Decision Points

- JH has had no previous damage to the myocardium. Prompt therapy with an effective agent can prevent damage and preserve myocardial function.
- JH has a history of strep throat. Because of the possibility of allergic reactions and anaphylactic shock, JH will not be a candidate for streptokinase or anistreplase.

DRUG TO BE USED

- Accelerated protocol alteplase: 100 mg administered as IV bolus, followed by 50 mg over next 30 minutes, and then 35 mg over next hour

*Cost Index:
1 = $<30/mo
2 = $30-40/mo
3 = $40-50/mo
4 = $50-60/mo
5 = $>60/mo

AWP of streptokinase is less than $300/dose.
AWP of urokinase is approximately $500/dose.
AWP of anistreplase is approximately $2500/dose.
AWP of alteplase is approximately $2500/dose.

emergence of the situation, the psychosocial aspects are often overlooked. Extra care should be taken to address these needs (see Case Study—Acute Myocardial Infarction).

Analysis and Management

Treatment Objectives

Treatment objectives for the patient receiving a thrombolytic include opening the occluded artery as soon as possible and maintaining patency after blood flow is re-established. Preventing ischemia-related arrhythmias and minimizing the loss of tissues are also treatment objectives.

Treatment Options

Drug Variables

There are advantages and disadvantages to each of the thrombolytic drugs. Patients who meet the selection criteria for the administration of thrombolytics must also be carefully screened for contraindications before the decision is made to treat the patient with a thrombolytic. There is little risk of antigen-antibody response with alteplase; however, there is an increased risk for cerebral bleeding. Reteplase is also indicated for the treatment of the patient with an acute MI. The primary advantage of reteplase is the simple method of administration, thus allowing for quicker initiation of therapy and decreased opportunity for dosage errors.

Thrombolytics have been shown to decrease the mortality rate associated with PE. They must be administered within a few hours of the onset of symptoms to produce the beneficial effect. Therefore, prompt recognition of the patient who has experienced a PE is essential. Any of the thrombolytics except anistreplase can be used. Anistreplase is FDA approved only for the treatment of acute MI.

Streptokinase and urokinase are the two drugs available to treat arterial occlusive disease. Streptokinase is the one most commonly used and is the drug recommended for thrombolytic treatment of DVT. Urokinase has been most extensively studied, and although it is used almost exclusively for restoring patency to occluded central venous lines, there are dosage recommendations for MI, DVT, and PE also.

Alteplase is the only thrombolytic drug presently recommended in the treatment of ischemic stroke. It must be administered within 3 hours of onset of symptoms and only after hemorrhagic stroke has been ruled out.

There are several variables that must be considered when making the decision to use thrombolytics in the instances when more than one may be indicated. The risks of allergic reactions, increased risk of intracerebral bleed, and the efficacy of each drug must be considered. In the studies that have been performed to determine the "best" thrombolytic, several concurrent therapies have been recommended. The administration of low-dose aspirin with concurrent use of thrombolytics has been shown to increase the efficacy of the drug in treating MI. The accelerated alteplase protocol has a higher patency rate when IV heparin is used in conjunction with the alteplase. The greatest advantage of alteplase seems to be prevention of valvular damage and consequent venous insufficiency, as well as postphlebotic syndrome.

The systemic use of thrombolytics in arterial occlusion has been disappointing because bleeding complications have outweighed the benefits. However, local intra-arterial thrombolytic therapy with urokinase has emerged as an alternative to surgery in the treatment of selected patients. It is important to remember that thrombolytics used in the treatment of DVT may break up the clot and cause emboli to be released into the circulation. To be most effective, therapy must begin within 5 days of the onset of the symptoms.

Streptokinase is probably the least expensive of the four drugs, and alteplase is the most expensive. Careful consideration must be given to the drug to be used and the comparable cost of that drug. The accelerated protocol of alteplase has shown to be more effective than streptokinase. However, there is a greater risk of cerebral bleeding with alteplase than with streptokinase.

Patient Variables

The patient must be screened carefully for contraindications to thrombolytic therapy. When a patient falls into the category of relative contraindications, the risks must be weighed carefully against the benefits before a treatment decision is made.

Although there is no age limit indicated in the contraindications, the age of the patient must be considered when deciding whether the benefits of thrombolytic therapy outweigh the risks.

The drug of choice for patients who have previously received streptokinase, who have been given anisoylated plasminogen streptokinase activator complex, or who have been treated for a streptococcal infection within the previous year is alteplase. These patients develop streptococcal antibodies that neutralize the streptokinase, causing severe allergic reactions. Careful consideration must also be given to the time that has lapsed from the onset of symptoms to the beginning of treatment, especially in the patient with an acute MI and acute ischemic CVA. Once tissue death has occurred, even though patency of the vessel is restored, there is little that can be done to improve function of the affected tissues. Therefore, the risks associated with late use of thrombolytic therapy heavily outweigh possible benefits.

Intervention

Administration

The time to treatment of acute MI is 6 hours from onset of chest pain. There is a correlation between the amount of time that elapses before therapy and the risk for cardiac rupture. Initiation of thrombolytic therapy for acute MI may begin in the emergency department or in a prehospital setting. The earlier therapy is started after onset of symptoms, the better the chance of preserving myocardial tissue.

Health care facilities that administer thrombolytics must have access to cardiac catheterization labs. Institutions that do not have catheterization labs begin treatment for patients who fit the established protocol and then transfer the patient to a facility that can provide coronary angiography and angioplasty.

Initiation of thrombolytic therapy for the treatment of acute ischemic CVA cannot begin until the possibility of a hemorrhagic CVA has been ruled out. Facilities that do not have the ability to perform CT scans must transfer the patient to a facility that does before treatment can be begun. The time to treatment for acute ischemic CVA is within 3 hours from the onset of symptoms.

Administration of thrombolytics in the treatment of PE should begin as soon as possible after the onset of symptoms. Therapy may be started up to 7 days after the thrombotic event.

Baseline vital signs should be obtained before drug administration for comparison during treatment. An increase in heart rate and a decrease in blood pressure may be an indication of bleeding. Document the patient's hematocrit and hemoglobin before administering the thrombolytic drug. Assess for abdominal and back pain, which may indicate internal bleeding. Note changes in the color of urine and stool. Assess for neurologic changes indicative of intracranial bleeding.

The possibility of bleeding exists up to 24 hours after thrombolytic therapy has been discontinued. Any unnecessary venipunctures or injections should be avoided during that time. When they are necessary, pressure should be applied manually for 10 minutes at venous sites and 30 minutes at arterial sites. Pressure dressings are then applied. Avoid venipunctures in noncompressible sites such as subclavian or internal jugular sites. Type and cross match the patient for possible blood replacement.

Observe the patient for signs and symptoms of allergic reactions (rash, dyspnea, fever, changes in facial color, swelling around the eyes, and wheezing). Allergic reactions are more common in the patient who is receiving streptokinase or anistreplase. If severe allergic manifestations occur the drug is discontinued and the patient treated with epinephrine, antihistamines, and steroids.

Careful monitoring and management of blood pressure are necessary, especially for the patient with an acute CVA. An elevated blood pressure is likely to contribute to the development of intracranial bleeding and can worsen ischemia. Frequent monitoring of the patient's neurologic status is imperative. If there is a sudden decrease in level of consciousness, cerebral hemorrhage should be suspected. If the thrombolytic drug is being used to treat a PE, the patient should be monitored for indications that the clot has been lysed. If used for the treatment of DVT, monitor closely for symptoms of PE.

Patients who receive thrombolytics for the treatment of MI are usually maintained on heparin and nitroglycerin drips following treatment. Later, the patient is started on aspirin to decrease platelet aggregation at the site.

Education

Explain thrombolytic therapy and possible complications to the patient and family before starting treatment. Instruct the patient to report any adverse effects, such as lightheadedness, dizziness, palpitations, or nausea. Explain the probability that bruising will occur as a result of the therapy, and therefore, bedrest and minimal handling of the patient are required. The patient should be instructed to notify the health care provider if pain develops or intensifies.

Community education regarding the signs and symptoms of a heart attack and stroke and the importance of the need to seek help immediately should be a high priority for health care providers. It is common for patients having an MI to put off getting help as they work through their denial of what is happening. However, the sooner they seek help, the greater benefit thrombolytic therapy will be.

Risk factors and preventive measures for MI, PE, and DVT should also be taught to the community because most of these disease processes can be prevented or decreased. Certain risk factors have been linked to the occurrence of CAD. Major risk factors include advancing age, male gender, family history of heart disease, diabetes mellitus, smoking, elevated blood pressure, elevated serum cholesterol, excess weight, excess alcohol intake, sedentary life-style, and left ventricular hypertrophy. All risk factors, with the exception of age, gender, and family history of heart disease, can be modified somewhat to reduce the risk of cardiovascular disease and decrease the associated mortality. The risk factors of CAD are the same factors that are linked with peripheral artery occlusive disease. Essentially, it is the same disease process, only in different vessels.

Evaluation

The patient receiving thrombolytic therapy should be evaluated for the effectiveness of treatment. In general, therapy is deemed effective if the patency of the vessel is restored, circulation to the area beyond the occlusion is restored, and the viability of tissues maintained. Indications of effective treatment in the patient with an acute MI include cessation of chest pain, onset of reperfusion arrhythmias, resolution of ST-segment elevation, and a peak in the creatine kinase value at 12 hours. The patient who is treated for a PE should experience resolution of the chest pain and a return of pulmonary hemodynamics to a normal range. Patients with occluded arteries or veins should note a cessation of the accompanying symptoms. The desired outcome for the patient with a CVA is that there is minimal or no disability at 3 months.

VARICOSITIES

Varicose Veins

Epidemiology and Etiology

Varicosities are most frequently found in the saphenous veins in the lower extremities. It is estimated that varicose veins affect one in five persons worldwide. They are most prevalent in women and in persons whose occupations require prolonged standing or sitting. There are two major types of varicose veins—primary and secondary. Primary varicosities are those in which the superficial veins are dilated. The valves may or may not be incompetent. The primary form tends to be familial and is probably caused by a congenital weakness of the veins. Secondary varicosities are usually the result of a previous injury such as thrombophlebitis of a deep femoral vein with subsequent valvular incompetence. Secondary varicosities may also occur in the esophagus (esophageal varices), in the anorectal area (hemorrhoids), and as abnormal arteriovenous connections.

Pathophysiology

Varicosities develop most often as a result of increased hydrostatic pressure or obstruction of venous blood flow. Continually elevated venous pressure weakens venous walls. The constant pressure also prevents the valves from closing completely. As pressure elevation continues valves are damaged and the veins become tortuous and enlarged. There is an accompanying increase in the capillary pressure, and perfusion is decreased. Painful weak muscles and edema ensue. Stasis ulcers and gangrene can develop.

Esophageal Varices

Epidemiology and Etiology

Esophageal varices are dilated tortuous veins that are usually found in the submucosa of the lower esophagus; however, they may develop more proximally or extend into the stomach. Esophageal varices are a complication of cirrhosis of the liver. They are one of the major causes of death in the patient with cirrhosis. The mortality rate resulting from an initial esophageal bleed is 45 to 50 percent.

Pathophysiology

Esophageal varices are almost always related to portal hypertension. There is a back flow of blood into esophageal vessels and an increased amount of pressure within the vessels. The vessels become tortuous, brittle, and bleed easily. Varices usually produce no symptoms until the pressure suddenly increases, and then massive hemorrhage can occur.

Factors that contribute to hemorrhage include straining, coughing, sneezing, heavy lifting, vomiting, poorly chewed foods, or irritating foods or fluids. Salicylates and any drugs that erode esophageal mucosa may increase the risk of bleeding.

PHARMACOTHERAPEUTIC OPTIONS

Sclerosing Drugs

- ❐ Ethanolamine oleate (ETHAMOLIN)
- ❐ Morrhuate sodium (SCLEROMATE)
- ❐ Sodium tetradecyl sulfate (SOTRADECOL)

Indications

Intravenous injection of sclerosing drugs is indicated in the treatment of superficial varicose veins of the lower extremities. Other possible uses for sclerosing drugs include treatment of internal hemorrhoids, closure of hernial rings, and the removal of condylomata acuminata. Sclerosing of varicose veins is an adjunct to, rather than a primary treatment for, varicosities. There have been some cases in which sclerosing drugs were used in place of surgery for varicose veins; however, the risk-to-benefit ratio must be heavily weighed.

Endoscopic sclerotherapy is indicated in both acute and chronic cases of esophageal varices. Prophylactic sclerotherapy may be performed on distended nonbleeding veins.

Morrhuate sodium and sodium tetradecyl sulfate are used in both the treatment of varicose veins and esophageal varices. Ethanolamine oleate is not recommended for the treatment of varicose veins.

Pharmacodynamics

Sclerosing drugs thrombose and obliterate distended veins. The drugs traumatize the endothelial lining, causing thrombosis and eventual sclerosing (hardening). In the treatment of varicose veins, the drug causes an inflammation of the intima of the vessel with subsequent formation of a thrombus. The clot occludes the vein and fibrous tissue develops obliterating the vein.

Adverse Effects and Contraindications

A common adverse effect of sclerosing drugs for treatment of varicose veins is burning or cramping at the injection site. Sloughing of tissue occurs if the drug is allowed to extravasate. Mild systemic responses include headache, dizziness, nausea, and vomiting. Significant adverse effects include urticaria, tissue sloughing and necrosis, and anaphylaxis. Allergic reactions may occur within a few minutes of the injection. Allergic reactions are more common when therapy is reinstituted after an interval of several weeks.

After endoscopic sclerotherapy the patient may experience chest pain for up to 72 hours. The pain is not cardiac in nature but related to the procedure. Pleural effusion or infiltrate is a complication associated with the use of sclerosing drugs. Esophageal perforation, ulceration, and strictures have also been noted. Overdosage or overtreatment of esophageal varices may result in severe necrosis of the esophagus. Local reactions include esophagitis, tearing of the esophagus, and sloughing of the mucosa.

Sclerosing drugs are contraindicated in patients with a known hypersensitivity to the drug, acute superficial thrombophlebitis, valvular or deep vein incompetency, and large superficial veins that communicate freely with deep veins. Embolism can occur as late as 4 weeks after an injection. Sclerosing drugs are also contraindicated in patients with underlying arterial disease; varicosities caused by abdominal and pelvic tumors, uncontrolled diabetes mellitus, thyrotoxicosis, tuberculosis, a neoplasm, asthma, sepsis, blood dyscrasias, or acute respiratory or skin disease; and in bedridden patients. Continued use of the drug is contraindicated when a local reaction occurs. The sclerosing drugs are classified as pregnancy category C. It is not known whether they are excreted in human breast milk.

Pharmacokinetics

Sclerosing drugs are usually cleared from the circulation within minutes via the portal vein. There seems to be a delayed response, especially with ethanolamine oleate, and complete sclerosing and obliteration of the vein may take up to 2½ months.

Drug-Drug Interactions

There are few documented drug-drug interactions with sclerosing drugs. Heparin is incompatible and therefore should not be mixed in the syringe with a sclerosing drug.

Dosage Regimen

The usual dosage of ethanolamine oleate for esophageal varices is 1.5 to 5 mL per varix, with a maximum dose of 20 mL per session. The dosage should be decreased in patients with a history of liver or heart disease. The drug may be administered at the time of the bleed and repeated at 1 week, 6 weeks, 3 months, and 6 months after the initial dose. It is indicated for the prevention of recurrent bleeding of esophageal varices. It should not be used as a prophylactic therapy.

The dosage of morrhuate sodium depends on the size of the varicosed vein. The usual dose for obliteration of small to medium-sized veins is 50 to 100 mg (1 to 2 mL) of a 5-percent solution. The dosage for larger vessels is 150 to 250 mg (3 to 5 mL). The injection may be repeated at 5- to 7-day intervals as needed.

The dosage for sodium tetradecyl sulfate also depends on the size of the varicosed vein, although the strength of the solution also varies with the size of the varicosity being treated. A 1-percent solution is used for small to medium varicosities, and a 3-percent solution is used for larger veins. The dosage is kept small, with 0.5 to 2 mL used for each injection. It is preferred that the quantity of a single dose not exceed 1 mL. The maximum dosage should not exceed 10 mL.

Laboratory Considerations

No laboratory test can be used to monitor the effectiveness or possible adverse effects of sclerosing drugs. Because there is a significant risk for DVT and PE with the administration of sclerosing drugs, the degree of valvular incompetency should be evaluated by angiography or Doppler venous examination before injection.

Critical Thinking Process

Assessment

History of Present Illness

The patient with varicose veins may present with a history of pain, muscle weakness, and edema if there has been valvular damage. Esophageal varices appear much like upper GI bleeding with abdominal pain, nausea, and vomiting. Because bleeding from esophageal varices is an emergency situation, time should not be wasted trying to differentiate between the two disorders.

Past Health History

A previous history of sclerosing drug injections, vein stripping, or phlebitis is an important assessment parameter because obliteration of too many vessels can occlude venous circulation. Other data to be noted from the past health history is that of recurrent DVT.

Factors associated with the onset of varicose veins include pregnancy, obesity, abdominal tumors, and standing for long periods. The patient should be questioned about a family history of varicose veins because there is a genetic tendency toward primary varicosities. A history of cirrhosis or known alcoholism should immediately indicate the origin of esophageal varices.

Physical Exam Findings

The patient with varicose veins has tortuous veins in the lower extremities. If there has been valvular damage, there may also be swelling and pain in the extremity. Secondary varicosities may occur in areas other than the legs.

Portal hypertension with esophageal varices may be indicated by dilated abdominal veins, ascites, and hemorrhoids. The patient will be in acute distress and shock, with acute bleeding from esophageal varices.

Diagnostic Testing

The Trendelenburg test is used to help diagnose varicose veins. The patient is placed in a supine position with the legs elevated. A tourniquet is placed above the knee after the legs have been elevated. As the patient sits up, normal veins will fill from the distal end. However, if varicosities are present, the veins fill from the proximal end. A venogram and phlebogram may be performed to assess for adequate circulation before a sclerosing procedure is done.

Diagnosis of esophageal varices is made by endoscopic examination. During an acute bleeding episode, diagnosis is usually made by history and physical exam because there is no time for an endoscopy.

Developmental Considerations

The disease processes for which sclerosing drugs are indicated are not found in children. The normal changes associated with pregnancy may predispose the woman to varicosities in the lower extremities. These varicosities usually do not require sclerotherapy. Both esophageal varices and peripheral varicosities are typically progressive states that occur when the primary problem has been present over a prolonged period of time. Hence, the older population may be at increased risk given the associated risk factors for the disorders.

Psychosocial Considerations

The psychosocial considerations related to peripheral varicosities may be significant. The disease can be exacerbated in patients whose employment requires excessive periods of standing or sitting. If the patient is unable to work because of the discomfort or because the varicosities are unsightly, feelings of powerlessness and changes in self-image may impact their state of wellness.

Esophageal varices is often a complication of cirrhosis of the liver, which, in turn, may be the result of chronic alcohol use. Often, these patients have not admitted to themselves or others just how extensive their drinking problem is until they are diagnosed with cirrhosis. The efficacy of sclerotherapy for patients with habitual alcohol use is less than would otherwise be desired. Another important psychosocial aspect to be considered is the high mortality rate associated with bleeding and the fear and anxiety experienced by these patients.

Analyses and Management

Treatment Objectives

The objective of treatment of varicose veins is directed toward improving circulation, relieving discomfort and swelling, and avoiding complications. The objective of sclerotherapy for esophageal varices is to control the bleeding and avoid hemorrhage. It does not eliminate the possibility that the varicosities will recur.

Treatment Options

Drug Variables

There seems to be less incidence of anaphylaxis with ethanolamine oleate than with the other two drugs, even though it is still a possible adverse effect. Ethanolamine oleate requires a much longer course of therapy than the other two drugs, putting the patient at risk for complications for an extended period of time. It also is rapidly diffused through the vein to produce an extravascular inflammatory response that is not present with the other two drugs. Further, ethanolamine is not recommended for the treatment of varicose veins. Sclerosing drugs control active esophageal bleeding in 70 to 80 percent of patients having one treatment and in 90 to 95 percent with an additional injection.

Patient Variables

Typically, sclerotherapy is used as an adjunct to surgery. However, patients who are at very high risk for surgery may be possible candidates for treatment solely with sclerosing drugs. Because the use of sclerosing drugs has not been studied during pregnancy, sclerotherapy should be used only when it is absolutely necessary and the benefits greatly outweigh risks.

Intervention

Administration

The sclerosing drugs used for varicose veins are administered directly into the sclerosed veins. Care must be taken to avoid extravasation because of the possibility of necrosis of the surrounding tissues. The minimal effective volume should be used at each injection site. It is recommended that a small test dose be given first and the patient observed before the full dose is administered in order to ascertain hypersensitivity before proceeding.

Sclerosing drugs are introduced via endoscopy for the treatment of bleeding esophageal varices. Before the therapy is performed, baseline vital signs and informed consent should be obtained. Vital signs are then monitored throughout the procedure. A sedative is usually administered before the procedure. The patient may be taken to the GI laboratory, or if the patient's condition is critical, the procedure can be performed at the bedside. The patient's throat is sprayed with a topical anesthetic. A dose of the sclerosing drug is injected through a flexible injector into the varicosity. The procedure usually takes about an hour. After treatment, the patient is observed for bleeding from perforation of the esophagus, aspiration pneumonia, and esophageal stricture.

Education

As with all interventions, patient education is vital to the success of the treatment. The patient should be told what to expect during the procedure and what unusual sensations or adverse effects may occur. They should also be advised of the behaviors and or activities that should be avoided after therapy and when to return for follow-up care.

Prevention is a key factor related to varicose veins. The patient who is predisposed to varicose veins should be taught to avoid occupations that require prolong periods of standing or sitting. They should also avoid wearing tight girdles or garters and not cross the legs at the knee. Any activity that increases venous stasis or increases pressure in the venous system in the lower extremities can lead to the formation of varicose veins. Patients who are obese have a higher incidence of varicose veins, so dietary teaching about weight loss may be warranted.

The patient with esophageal varices should be taught to avoid alcohol, nonsteroidal anti-inflammatory drugs, and irritating foods. These substances can irritate varices and cause bleeding. After sclerotherapy for esophageal varices, achiness and feeling of stiffness develop and may persist for 48 hours. Varices have a tendency to recur, so the need for follow-up endoscopy must be stressed. Assistance finding support groups for patients who use alcohol should be offered.

Evaluation

After treatment for varicose veins, the vein should be hard and swollen for 2 to 4 hours. After the first 24 hours, the vein should remain hard and tender to touch. The surrounding skin is be a light bronze color, which is a temporary condition. However, there may be a permanent but barely discernible discoloration that will remain along the path of the sclerosed vein.

When sclerosing drugs are administered for esophageal varices, bleeding should stop within 2 minutes after the introduction of the drug. If bleeding continues, a second injection attempt is made below the bleeding site. The health care provider should conduct a follow-up examination to determine whether or not assistance with alcohol abuse has been obtained.

SUMMARY

- Thrombolytic drugs are used in the treatment of MI, DVT, PE, peripheral arterial occlusion, CVAs, and occluded central venous catheters.
- Each thrombolytic drug acts in a different fashion to dissolve thrombi after formation.
- Assessment of the patient should include special attention to a history of streptococcal infection within the previous year.
- The patient history should include a drug history with particular attention to drug allergies and any previous thrombolytic therapy.
- Treatment objectives include opening the occluded artery as soon as possible, maintaining patency after flow is re-established, and prevention of complications related to bleeding.
- First-generation thrombolytic drugs include streptokinase and urokinase. Second-generation drugs include alteplase and anistreplase. Reteplase is the newest thrombolytic drug.
- Close attention should be paid to relative and absolute contraindications of thrombolytic drugs.
- Patient monitoring during thrombolytic therapy should include hematocrit, hemoglobin, thrombin time, partial thromboplastin time, prothrombin time values, and other laboratory testing specifically required for the disorder being treated.
- In general, therapy is deemed successful if the patency of the vessel is restored, circulation to the area beyond the occlusion is restored, and the viability of tissues is maintained.
- Sclerosing drugs are used in the management of varicose veins or esophageal varices to occlude tortuous, weakened veins.
- Sclerosing drugs act to thrombose and obliterate distended veins by traumatizing the endothelial lining of the vessels.
- Treatment objectives for varicose veins are directed toward improvement of circulation, relief of discomfort and swelling, and avoidance of complications of sclerotherapy.
- Treatment objectives for esophageal varices are to control bleeding and prevent hemorrhage.
- There is less incidence of anaphylaxis with ethanolamine oleate than with morrhuate sodium or sodium tetradecyl sulfate.
- Sclerosing drugs for varicose veins are administered directly into the affected vein. Drugs used in the treatment of esophageal varices are introduced via endoscopy.
- Patients receiving sclerotherapy for esophageal varices require close physiologic monitoring before, during, and after treatment because bleeding can occur for up to 24 hours after the treatment is completed.
- The peripheral varicosity should be hard along the path of the vein after sclerotherapy.
- Bleeding esophageal varices should resolve 2 minutes after introduction of the sclerosing drug.

BIBLIOGRAPHY

Abramowicz, M. (1996). Alteplase for thrombolysis in acute ischemic stroke. *The Medical Letter,* 38(987), 99–100.

Abramowicz, M. (1997). Reteplase (Retavase). *The Medical Letter,* 39(995), 17–18.

Adams, H., Brott, T., Furlan, A., et al. (1996). Guidelines for thrombolytic therapy for acute stroke: A supplement to the guidelines for the management of patients with acute ischemic stroke. *Stroke,* 27(9), 1711–1718.

Amato, T. (1996). Thrombolytic therapy in a 79 year old man with massive pulmonary embolism and unstable hemodynamic status. *Journal of Emergency Nursing,* 22(1), 14–17.

Apple, S. (1996). New trends in thrombolytic therapy. *RN,* 59(1), 30–34.

Cannon, C., and Goldhaber, S. (1995). The importance of rapidly treating patients with acute myocardial infarction. *Chest,* 107(3), 598–600.

Goldhaber, S., Agnelli, G., and Levine, M. (1994). Reduced dose bolus alteplase vs. conventional alteplase infusion for pulmonary embolism thrombolysis: An international multicenter randomized trial. The Bolus Alteplase Embolism Group. *Chest,* 106(3), 718–724.

Goldhaber, S. (1995). Contemporary pulmonary embolism thrombolysis. *Chest,* 107(1), 45S–51S.

Gunnar, R., Passamani, E., Bourdillon, P., et al. (1990). Guidelines for the early management of patients with acute myocardial infarction. Report of the American College of Cardiology/American Heart Association Task Force on Assessment of Diagnostic and Therapeutic Cardiovascular Procedures. *Journal of American College of Cardiology,* 2, 249–292.

Habib, G. (1995). Current status of thrombolysis in acute myocardial infarction. *Chest,* 107, 225–232.

Ignatavicius, D., Workman, M., and Mishler, M. (1995). *Medical-surgical nursing: A nursing process approach* (2nd ed.). Philadelphia: W. B. Saunders.

Kumpe, D., Cohen, M., and Durham, J. (1992) Treatment of failing and failed hemodialysis access sites: Comparison of surgical treatment with thrombolysis/angioplasty. *Seminars in Vascular Surgery,* 5(2), 118–127.

Lemmon, P., Kalman, J., and Sefcik, K. (1994). Tissue plasminogen activator: The nurse's role. *Critical Care Nurse,* 14(6), 22–31.

Lewis, S., Collier, I., and Heitkemper, M. (1996) *Medical-surgical nursing: Assessment and management of clinical problems (4th ed.)* Mosby: St. Louis.

Majoros, K., and Moccia, J. (1996). *Embolism: Targeting an elusive enemy*. *Nursing,* 26(4), 26–31.

Mounsey, J., Skinner, J., Hawkins, T., et al. (1995). Rescue thrombolysis: Alteplase as adjunct treatment after streptokinase in acute myocardial infarction. *British Heart Journal,* 74(4), 348–353.

Northsea, C. (1994). Using urokinase to restore patency to double lumen catheters. AANA *American Association of Nurse Anesthesia Journal,* 21(5), 261–264.

Prewitt, R., Shia, G., Schick, U., et al. (1995). Intravenous administration of recombinant tissue plasminogen activator. *Chest,* 107(4), 1146–1151.

Roberts, A., Valji, K., Bookstein, J., et al. (1993). Pulse spray pharmacomechanical thrombolysis for treatment of thrombosed dialysis access grafts. *The American Journal of Surgery,* 166(99), 221–226.

Rogers, S., and Sherman, D. (1993). Pathophysiology and treatment of acute ischemic stroke. *Clinical Pharmacology,* 12, 359–376.

Saul, L. (Ed.). (1991). *Activase therapy in acute myocardial infarction and acute massive pulmonary embolism: Nursing care guidelines.* New Jersey: SynerMed.

Smalling, R., Bode, C., Kalbfleisch, J., et al. (1995). More rapid, complete, and stable coronary thrombolysis with bolus administration of reteplase compared with alteplase infusion in acute myocardial infarction. *Circulation,* 91(11), 2725–2732.

The National Institute of Neurological Disorders and Stroke rt-PA Stroke Study Group (1995). Tissue plasminogen activator for acute ischemic stroke. *New England Journal of Medicine,* 333(24), 1581–1587.

Topol, E. (1993). An international randomized trial comparing four thrombolytic strategies for acute myocardial infarction. *The New England Journal of Medicine,* 329(10), 673–682.

Wagstaff, A., Gillis, J., Goa, K. (1995). Alteplase: A reappraisal of its pharmacology and therapeutic use in vascular disorders other than acute myocardial infarction. *Drugs,* 50(2), 289–316.

Wall, T., Phillips, H., III, Stack, R., et al. (1990). Results of high dose intravenous urokinase for acute myocardial infarction. *American Journal of Cardiology,* 65(3), 124–131.

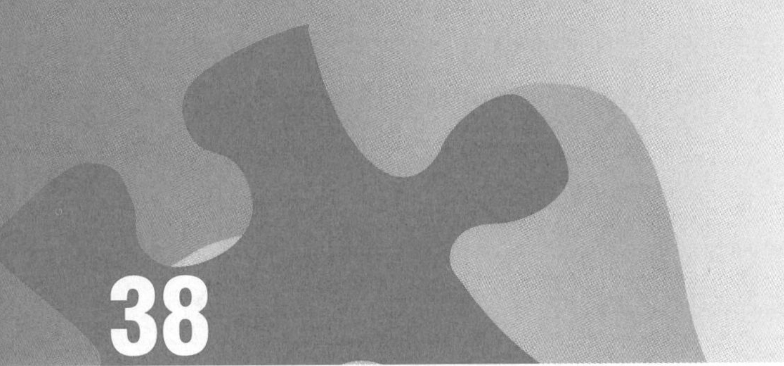

38 Blood and Blood Products

In the mid-17th century, Denis, a physician in the court of Louis XIV, performed the first blood transfusion when he successfully administered lamb's blood to a 15-year-old boy using a quill and an animal's bladder. The French physician's subsequent attempts at animal to human transfusion and the efforts of other physicians were not successful and, in fact, resulted in a number of fatalities. These failures and the demonstrated risk of mortality led the French Parliament, with the backing of the Church, to ban further animal-to-human transfusions. Knowledge associated with blood transfusions remained stagnant until 1818, when an English physician, Blundell, using human blood, successfully transfused moribund women suffering with puerperal hemorrhages.

Early in the 20th century, the individual efforts of Landsteiner, Ottenberg, and Epstein led to the development of the ABO typing and matching system for blood donors and recipients, thus decreasing the number of incompatible transfusions. In 1940, Landsteiner and Weiner pinpointed the anti-Rh antigen as the cause of hemolytic disease of the newborn due to alloimmunization during gestation. Thus, Rh factor determination joined the ABO matching system in defining donor and recipient compatibility. By the late 1940s, the medical community had discovered how to save blood for future use with the addition of sodium citrate as an anticoagulant. This discovery set the stage for the development of blood banks.

BLOOD AND BLOOD PRODUCT USE

According to the American Association of Blood Banks (AABB), about eight million volunteers donate close to 14 million units of blood, including approximately one million autologous units used for self-transfusion, each year in the United States. Unfortunately, fewer than 5 percent of healthy Americans who are eligible to donate blood do so. Blood banks separate most of these units of blood into various components. For example, each unit of whole blood may be separated into four components: red blood cells (RBCs), platelets, granulocytes, and plasma. Separating whole blood into its components allows specific problems to be treated with specific blood components.

Annually, more than 12 million units of RBCs, five million units of platelets, and two million units of plasma are administered in the United States. Health care providers in the United States transfuse more than four million patients per year. Up to 19 percent of all patients receiving antineoplastic drugs require RBC transfusions for anemia.

Blood and its components are living tissue in the form of cellular products. The administration of blood components is actually a transplant of cells from donor to recipient. Blood banks carefully screen donors and perform laboratory tests to ensure safe, compatible transfusions. Current donor screening protocols used by the American Red Cross include an extensive, confidential, and private interview with its donors. Donors may complete a confidential exclusion process indicating that the blood collected should not be used for transfusion due to reasons the donor found too sensitive to disclose during the interview portion of the screening process. In addition to testing donor blood to identify the donor's ABO group and Rh type, the AABB requires that blood banks test a sample from each donation intended for the following: allogenic (same species to same species) use for antibodies to human immunodeficiency virus (anti-HIV), hepatitis B surface antigen, antibody to hepatitis B core antigen, antibody to hepatitis C virus, and antibody to human T-cell lymphotropic virus type I. Blood banks also test donor blood for syphilis. In spite of the extensive screening process, the risk of transmitting infectious diseases and transfusion-related complications is always present. It is because of this ever-present potential for disease transmission and the limited blood supply that the American Red Cross and the AABB, in conjunction with the Food and Drug Administration, strongly recommend that blood products be used only in patient conditions that cannot be remedied with other pharmacotherapeutic methods.

COMPOSITION OF BLOOD AND BLOOD PRODUCTS

Blood is one of the three main fluids in the body. The other two are intracellular fluid (the fluid within cells) and extracellular fluid (the fluid around cells). Whole blood consists of cells and plasma. The cellular components represent about 45 percent of the total blood volume and consist of erythrocytes (RBCs), leukocytes (white blood cells [WBCs]), and platelets (Fig. 38–1). Plasma, the liquid part of blood, makes up the other 55 percent of the volume. Plasma consists of 90 percent water and 10 percent solutes. Some of the solutes present in blood plasma are true solutes or crystalloids. *Crystalloids* are solute particles less than 1 nm in diameter (e.g., ions or glucose). Other solutes in plasma are colloids. *Colloids* are particles from 1 to about 100 nm in diameter (e.g., proteins of all types). Proteins represent the largest quantity of all solutes present in plasma. Other solutes include food substances, such as glucose, amino acids, and lipids; products of biotransformation, such as urea, uric acid, creatinine, and lactic acid; respiratory gases such as oxygen and carbon dioxide; and regulatory substances, such as hormones, enzymes, and other substances.

Blood, the intravascular fluid, supplies oxygen, transports nutrients, waste, and hormonal messengers to each of the 60 billion cells in the body, as well as defends the body against foreign material. There are close to 30 trillion blood cells in an adult. Each cubic millimeter of blood contains 4.5 to 5.5 million RBCs and an average total of 7500 WBCs. Because both RBCs and WBCs are continually being destroyed,

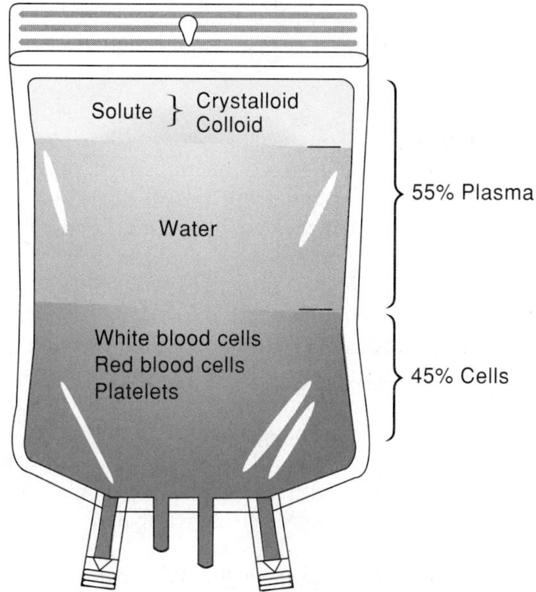

Figure 38–1 A unit of whole blood is composed of 55 percent plasma, of which 90 percent is water and 10 percent solute, and 45 percent red blood cells, white blood cells, and platelets.

the body must continue to produce new ones. About 2.5 million RBCs die every second, at the same time about 2.5 million new ones are created.

Hematopoiesis takes place primarily in the red bone marrow of axial skeletal bones and the proximal heads of the femur and humerus. Most cells mature in the bone marrow, but some mature in the thymus, spleen, lymph nodes, and tonsils. Within the red marrow are parent cells and other earliest forms of blood cells. The earliest forms of blood cells are divided into stem cells, which can mature and differentiate into all the hemopoietic cells or form new stem cells, and progenitor cells, which can become mature differentiated cells but cannot form new stem cells.

BASIC IMMUNOHEMATOLOGY PRINCIPLES

Immunohematology is the scientific discipline that deals with the body of knowledge associated with the antigens and antibodies of the blood. Because the transfusion of incompatible blood triggers life-threatening reactions in the body, it is important to understand the basics of RBC (antigen) and plasma (antibody) compatibilities.

Antigens

An *antigen* stimulates the formation of an antibody. Some antigens occur naturally in the body, whereas others are acquired. Antigens in the different blood typing systems are called *agglutinogens*. Agglutinogens are hereditary and are located on the surface of the RBC. Agglutinogens are also components of WBCs and are soluble in the plasma.

Two of the most important antigens associated with blood compatibility are found in the ABO system: antigen A and antigen B. The presence or absence of these two antigens determines an individual's blood group. People with antigen A have blood type A, and those with antigen B have blood type B. Some individuals have both antigens A and B on their red cells and consequently have blood type AB. People with neither antigen A nor B on their red cells have blood type O.

There are other groups of antigens important in the understanding of immunohematology. These are the Rhesus, or *Rh system*, antigens. The Rh system consists of almost 50 different RBC antigens. The most important of these antigens, for the purpose of this basic discussion, is D. The presence or absence of the D antigen on the RBC is one of the factors that determines if a person is Rh positive or Rh negative.

Human leukocyte antigens (HLA) are on the surface of lymphocytes and other nucleated cells. They are important to immunity and, at times, compatibility. HLA antigens determine the degree of histocompatibility between transplant recipients and donors. Because blood is a living organism, the transfusion of blood is essentially a transplant and some patients may reject their transfusions because of the presence of incompatible HLAs on the surface of white cells present in the blood product.

Exposure to HLAs through multiple or frequent transfusions may cause some patients to develop antibodies to donor platelets or RBCs, making HLA-matched donations necessary. Other indications for HLA matching include patients receiving WBC transfusions and patients with a history of refractory febrile transfusion reactions.

Antibodies

Antibodies are proteins (immunoglobulins) that float freely in the plasma. Like antigens, some antibodies occur naturally in the body. Other antibodies develop in response to stimulation by an antigen that the individual does not have. The body recognizes the antigen as foreign, and the immune system responds by producing an antibody.

Antibodies may be classified as either complete or incomplete. A complete antibody is one that agglutinates cells in a saline medium without the presence of other proteins. This process is very direct. When the reaction occurs during a transfusion, it takes place in the patient's vascular system, causing intravascular hemolysis.

There are many different antigens on an RBC, but the most clinically significant ones are those that determine blood group and type. In the ABO system, antibodies A and B are complete. The antibodies that make up the ABO antibody system in plasma are naturally occurring. Their names derive from the antigens with which they react. Anti-A and anti-B react with antigen A and antigen B, respectively. RBC antigens and their corresponding antibodies do not exist naturally in the same person. Therefore, an individual with type A blood, that is a person with antigen A on the RBC, does not normally have anti-A antibody in the plasma.

In contrast to a complete antibody, an incomplete antibody can not cause agglutination by itself, and the type of agglutination it causes is not a direct process. Incomplete antibody agglutination requires mediation or assistance of other body mechanisms. In incomplete antibody agglutination, the antibody coats the RBC. The body then recognizes the cell as defective and hides it away in either the liver or the spleen until the reticuloendothelial system destroys it.

Because this process takes place outside of the vascular system, it is known as extravascular hemolysis.

Unlike anti-A and anti-B, the anti-Rh antibody is not naturally occurring. People with Rh-positive blood do not have anti-Rh antibodies in their serum; if they did, the antibodies would destroy their RBCs. The Rh antigen is very immunogenic (i.e., capable of initiating the body's immune responses) and, therefore, is likely to stimulate antibody formation. A person with Rh-negative blood transfused with Rh positive blood will develop anti-Rh antibodies after the exposure to the Rh(D) antigen. The reaction generally does not occur on the initial exposure because the Rh antibodies develop slowly. Once sensitized, this person will probably experience a transfusion reaction and associated hemolysis of the RBCs with the next exposure.

Transfusion is not the only opportunity for Rh-negative people to be exposed to Rh-positive antigens. An Rh-negative woman who is pregnant with an Rh-positive fetus is exposed to the Rh antigen during her pregnancy. Until 30 years ago, a subsequent pregnancy with an Rh-positive fetus precipitated the development of anti-Rh antibodies that attacked the RBCs of the fetus. This phenomenon is known as hemolytic disease of the newborn. Giving human Rh_0(D) immune globulin (RhoGAM) by intramuscular injection within 72 hours of delivery, miscarriage, or abortion prevents the formation of anti-Rh antibodies and prevents the disorder. The injection reduces the formation of anti-Rh (anti-D) to 1 to 2 percent. There is evidence that the formation of anti-Rh can be decreased to 0.1 percent by administering two doses of the immune globulin, one at 28 weeks' gestation and the other 72 hours after delivery. Although this drug was developed for the treatment of hemolytic disease of the newborn, it is now also given after transfusion of an Rh-positive blood product to an Rh-negative recipient.

When blood banks determine compatibility of donor blood for transfusion, they perform an indirect Coombs' test to determine whether the patient has antibodies in the serum that may react with the red cells in the transfusion. Sometimes this test identifies weak variants (subantigens) of the Rh(D) factor. These antigens are less immunogenic than Rh(D). One of these antigens is the D^u antigen. Blood banks test donor blood for the D and the D^u antigen before determining an individual's Rh status. Individuals with the D antigen are Rh-positive donors and Rh-positive and Rh-negative recipients. Individuals with the subantigen, called D^u, are Rh-positive donors but are Rh-negative recipients.

There are other clinically significant Rh antigens, but these are less immunogenic and, therefore, are less likely to produce hemolytic reactions. These antigens are frequently important in establishing paternity.

Simply put, RBCs should not be given to recipients with matching antibodies in their plasma, and plasma should not be given to recipients with matching antigens on their RBCs.

PHARMACOTHERAPEUTIC OPTIONS

Whole Blood

Whole blood consists of RBCs; plasma, which contains plasma proteins (e.g. globulins, antibodies); stable clotting factors; and anticoagulant or preservative. Laboratory processing removes most of the platelets and WBCs. Any remaining platelets and WBCs are usually not viable after a few days.

Indications

Whole blood is used to treat acute, massive blood loss requiring the oxygen-carrying properties of RBCs along with the volume expansion provided by plasma. Patients with symptomatic anemia and hypovolemia due to large blood volume deficit, enough to be associated with shock (a loss of 25 to 30 percent of circulating blood volume or more), are candidates for transfusion with whole blood. When the patient does not exhibit signs of hypovolemia, a transfusion with RBCs only is the treatment of choice. Neonates, infants, or adults who require exchange transfusions receive whole blood that is less than 7 days old to ensure that any cellular breakdown associated with the blood unit's age will not cause potentially dangerous electrolyte imbalances in the recipient. Whole blood should not be considered a source of viable platelets, WBCs, or the labile coagulation factors V and VIII. Patients requiring these components are better managed with the actual component or derivative.

At times, units of whole blood may be modified by the blood bank. The plasma is removed, the platelets or cryoprecipitate is collected, and the plasma is returned to the unit of red cells. Whole blood modified in this manner is useful for patients who are hemorrhaging and in need of red cells, volume expansion, and oncotic proteins. It is always recommended that coagulation factors be replaced by using the appropriate components (platelets, fresh frozen plasma [FFP], or cryoprecipitate).

Pharmacodynamics

A transfusion of whole blood immediately provides the recipient with the oxygen-carrying capability of RBCs. Whole blood is also an intravascular volume expander and source of proteins with oncotic properties and some stabile coagulation factors. Whether it is modified or not, a unit of whole blood contains enough hemoglobin to raise an anemic adult's hematocrit by about 3 percentage points. Only when the donor and recipient are ABO identical should whole blood be used. ABO compatibility allows the recipient and donor profiles outlined in Table 38–1.

A traditional unit of whole blood contains approximately 500 mL (+/− 10 percent), of which 240 to 275 mL is plasma and 62 mL is anticoagulant. The hematocrit of whole

TABLE 38–1 ABO-Rh COMPATIBILITY WITH WHOLE BLOOD

	Donor Blood Type					
Recipient Blood Type	A	B	O	AB	Rh+	Rh−
A	X					
B		X				
O			X			
AB				X		
Rh+					X	X
Rh−						X

blood is about 35 to 40 percent. Anticoagulant solutions used in whole blood include Anticoagulant Heparin Solution, Anticoagulant Citrate Dextrose Solution, Anticoagulant Citrate Phosphate Dextrose Solution, Anticoagulant Citrate Phosphate Dextrose Adenine Solution, and Citrate Phosphate Double Dextrose Solution. The label of the blood unit lists the volume of the unit (+/− 10 percent) and the anticoagulant solution used.

Adverse Effects and Contraindications

Many of the adverse effects associated with the administration of whole blood such as disease transmission, hemolytic transfusion reactions, and graft-versus-host disease (GVHD) are also associated with the administration of other blood products and are addressed at the end of the discussion of each type of product. Circulatory overload and metabolic complications are primarily associated with whole blood and RBC transfusions, and are discussed in this section.

Circulatory Overload

Patients with cardiac or pulmonary compromise may experience circulatory overload manifested by heart failure. Elderly patients, those of small stature, or patients with chronic severe anemia are at particular risk when RBC mass is decreased and plasma volume is increased. Additionally, each unit of whole blood contains about 56 mEq of sodium, which may lead to pulmonary edema in patients with cardiopulmonary compromise who require rapid or multiple-unit infusions.

Metabolic Derangement

Patients requiring massive transfusions, especially those with liver disease, are at risk for citrate toxicity due to the complexing of ionized calcium by the anticoagulant in the blood unit. The citrate-induced hypocalcemia (intestinal cramping, muscle twitching, decreased urine output, possible renal failure) is a rare occurrence, unless the patient with severe liver disease receives more than 1 unit of blood every 5 minutes. The patient may note tingling of the fingertips or muscular cramping. If the condition is left untreated, the patient may experience seizures, cardiac arrhythmias, or cardiac arrest. Metabolic alkalosis may also develop as citrate is converted to pyruvate and bicarbonate.

Unless the patient is experiencing severe symptoms of hypocalcemia, treatment consists of slowing or discontinuing the transfusion. This situation will eventually correct itself without further intervention. If the patient is experiencing severe symptoms, the health care provider may order a slow infusion of calcium chloride. Careful screening and monitoring of patients at risk for hypocalcemia are the only means of prevention.

RBCs in storage break down and leak potassium into the plasma. After 3 weeks of storage, potassium levels in donor plasma may reach 18 to 30 mEq/L. This is normally not a problem for patients receiving 1 to 2 units of blood because the potassium level is ordinarily self-correcting. However, if large quantities of RBCs are given, particularly to patients with renal disease, signs and symptoms of hyperkalemia can appear. Laboratory data will show high serum potassium levels and an electrocardiogram will exhibit high, peaked T-waves and wide QRS complexes. If the condition is left untreated, the patient's cardiac status can deteriorate to bradycardia and asystole.

To decrease potassium levels, the physician may order sodium polystyrene sulfonate. Depending on the patient's condition, this cation-exchange resin may be administered orally or as a retention enema. When the patient is expected to receive large quantities of blood, requesting that the blood bank use the freshest blood available decreases the potential for hyperkalemia.

Coagulopathies

Some patients may hemorrhage as a result of platelet loss and deficiency of labile plasma coagulation factors (factors V and VIII) in stored whole blood. Factors V and VIII begin to degrade after 24 hours. These coagulopathies can usually be prevented by administering platelets and FFP or by only using fresh units (less than 24 hours old) of unaltered whole blood.

Hypothermia

Hypothermia occurs when patients receive large quantities of cold blood products or when cold blood is rapidly administered through a central intravenous line. The patient exhibits shaking chills, hypotension, and cardiac arrhythmias. If the condition is left untreated, the patient's condition may proceed to cardiac arrest. Treatment includes stopping the transfusion, warming the patient with blankets, and if tolerated, encouraging warm liquids. Monitor the patient's vital signs. An ECG will detect arrhythmias. For patients in need of massive, rapid transfusions, warming the blood to 37°C with automatic blood warmers prevents hypothermia.

Patients with anemias that are treatable with drugs such as iron, vitamin B_{12}, recombinant erythropoietin, or folic acid, and whose condition permits sufficient time for these measures to promote erythropoiesis are not candidates for blood transfusions. Whole blood is not considered first-line treatment to expand circulating volume because of the risks of complications, disease transmission, and the limited blood supply. The use of crystalline solutions such as 0.9-percent sodium chloride solution or lactated Ringer's, or colloids such as albumin or plasma protein fraction are the treatments of choice in hypovolemia. They are safer alternatives. In coagulation deficiencies, the appropriate coagulation products and derivatives are superior to whole blood.

Dosage Regimen

The number of units or volume of the transfusion depends on the patient's clinical condition. Unless the patient's condition dictates otherwise, the infusion should begin at a rate not to exceed 5 mL/minute for the first 15 minutes of the transfusion. During this initial period, the patient requires close observation because some life-threatening reactions may occur after only a small volume of incompatible blood is infused. After the first 15 minutes, the remainder of the transfusion should be infused as quickly as necessary to correct and maintain homeostasis. The pediatric infusion rate is initially 20 mL/kg, followed by the volume required for stabilization. Patients who do not tolerate a rapid administration rate should be considered candidates for treatment with RBCs rather than with whole blood.

Red Blood Cells

Blood banks prepare a unit of packed red blood cells (PRBCs) by removing the plasma from a unit of whole blood using centrifugal or gravitational separation of red cells from the plasma. These processes remove most of the platelets along with the plasma. The red cell concentrate has the same RBC mass as a unit of whole blood, but only 20 to 30 percent of the plasma and a much smaller quantity of leukocytes and platelets.

Two major types of RBC products are available: RBCs with CDPA-1 solution (anticoagulant-preservative only) that has a final hematocrit no higher than 80 percent, and RBCs with 100 mL of additive solution (AS-1, AS-3, or AS-5). The final hematocrit is usually 55 to 60 percent. The health care provider may also find a unit of PRBCs with adenine-saline added or leukocyte-poor RBCs. The label on the unit describes the exact additions, deletions, or preparation technique used.

As the name indicates, leukocyte-poor preparations are units of RBCs in which the number of WBCs has been reduced to less than 5×10^8 through centrifugation (removal of residual buffy coat), filtration (passage through a microaggregate or leukocyte depletion filter), washing, freezing, or sedimentation. At least 80 percent of the RBCs remain. Washing RBCs with saline solution removes 99 percent of the plasma, 80 to 95 percent of the WBCs, and 100 percent of the platelets from a unit.

Indications

RBCs are used to increase the oxygen-carrying capacity in anemic patients without the need for volume expansion. Symptomatic patients who have deficient oxygen-carrying capacity without hypovolemia are candidates for RBC transfusion. Patients with heart failure, older adults, debilitated patients, and those with normal or expanded plasma volumes who cannot tolerate rapid shifts of blood volume receive PRBCs. In some cases, RBCs may be used for exchange transfusions, but as with whole blood, these cells must be less than 7 days old to avoid potential electrolyte imbalances.

Leukocyte-poor RBCs are used to prevent recurrence of febrile, nonhemolytic transfusion reactions caused by donor WBC antigens reacting with recipient WBC antibodies. Leukocyte-poor RBCs is the preparation of choice for patients who require multiple transfusions and consequently may become HLA alloimmunized (e.g., patients with leukemia or aplastic anemia). Washed or frozen deglycerolized RBCs may be used to reduce the incidence of urticarial and anaphylactic reactions. Washed RBCs may be indicated for patients with paroxysmal nocturnal hemoglobinuria or other conditions that require the transfusion of RBCs with minimal amounts of plasma.

Irradiated blood products are used to prevent post-transfusion GVHD in patients receiving blood products containing viable WBCs. Irradiated blood products are indicated for Hodgkin's or non-Hodgkin's lymphoma, acute leukemia, congenital immunodeficiency syndromes, low-birthweight neonates, intrauterine transfusions, and bone marrow transplants.

Pharmacodynamics

Unlike whole blood, RBC transfusions must be ABO compatible but not ABO identical because most of the plasma, and therefore, the ABO alloantibodies have been removed. ABO compatibility allows the donor and recipient profiles outlined in Table 38–2. RBCs have a volume of about 300 mL, with a hematocrit of 65 to 80 percent.

TABLE 38–2 ABO-Rh COMPATIBILITY WITH PACKED RED BLOOD CELLS

	Donor Blood Type					
Recipient Blood Type	A	B	O	AB	Rh+	Rh−
A	X		X			
B		X	X			
O			X			
AB	X	X	X	X		
Rh+					X	X
Rh−						X

RBCs with additive solution (AS) contain red cells with 90 percent of the plasma removed and 100 mL of a special solution containing the necessary preservative to increase the shelf life (42 days) and decrease viscosity. RBCs with CPDA-1 solution have a 35-day shelf life. Because of the presence of additional preservative solution, the AS units have a higher volume and lower hematocrit than do RBCs with CPDA-1 solution.

Irradiated blood products have been exposed to a measured amount of radiation, thereby rendering the donor lymphocytes incapable of replication. Irradiated blood products are identified on the bag label. The product carries no radiation risk to the health care provider or the recipient. Products that contain no viable RBCs such as FFP and cryoprecipitate require no radiation.

Adverse Effects and Contraindications

In general, the same adverse effects associated with whole blood transfusions are found with RBCs, but there is a reduced risk of febrile nonhemolytic reactions and circulatory overload. However, as in the case of whole blood, hypovolemia without significant deficit in red cell mass is best treated with other volume expanders and not RBCs.

RBCs should not be used for volume expansion, in place of a hematinic drug, to enhance wound healing, or to improve the general well-being of the patient.

Dosage Regimen

As with whole blood, the number of units to be transfused depends on the patient's clinical condition. The rate of administration and clinical interventions are the same as for whole blood, beginning at 5 mL for the first 15 minutes and then proceeding as rapidly as the patient tolerates the infusion and as clinically indicated. One unit is usually infused over a period of 2 to 3 hours. Pediatric infusions should be started at 10 mL/kg, with the dose not to exceed more than 15 mL/kg. Pediatric infusion rates are 2 to 5 mL/kg/hour. RBC units may be aliquoted by the laboratory into several bags that contain small volumes.

Plasma

The blood product known as plasma may be plasma, liquid plasma, or FFP. Plasma and liquid plasma are the clear portions of blood that have been separated from the cells by centrifugation or sedimentation. Anticoagulants have been added. Plasma is stored frozen, whereas liquid plasma is refrigerated. Plasma and liquid plasma contain the stable coagulation factors.

FFP is separated from a fresh unit of whole blood (less than 6 hours old) and frozen. It is 91 percent water, 7 percent protein (i.e., albumin, globulins, antibodies, clotting factors), and 2 percent carbohydrate. When FFP is frozen within 6 hours of collection, it can be stored for up to one year without loss of labile (factor V, VIII) and nonlabile coagulation factors.

Indications

Plasma and liquid plasma are indicated for the treatment of stable clotting factor deficiencies for which no concentrates are available. In some cases, even when clotting factor concentrates are available, plasma is the blood product of choice. Use of plasma keeps patient exposure to multiple-donor products to a minimum. Factors V and VIII are not present in either plasma or liquid plasma, and neither blood product should be used in an attempt to replace these labile coagulation factors.

FFP is used to control bleeding in patients with a demonstrated deficiency who require labile plasma coagulation factors and blood volume expansion. It is essential in the management of idiopathic thrombocytopenic purpura (ITP).

Pharmacodynamics

Plasma and liquid plasma provide the patient with nonlabile clotting factors such as fibrinogen and factor IX. Cross matching is not required before transfusing plasma or liquid plasma, but the transfusion must be compatible with the patient's donor or recipient ABO status (Table 38–3). Rh compatibility is not an issue because blood cells are not part of the transfusion, and consequently, the Rh(D) antigen and subantigens are not present.

A cross match between donor and recipient is not required to use FFP, but the plasma must be ABO compatible with the recipient's cells. One unit of FFP contains about 250 mg of fibrinogen, although there is great variability from one donor to another. One unit of FFP raises the recipient's plasma fibrinogen level about 10 mg/dL. Therefore, FFP is not the first choice in the treatment of hypofibrinogenemia.

A unit of plasma or liquid plasma usually contains between 180 and 300 mL of anticoagulated plasma. The volume is identified on the container label. Each milliliter contains 2 to 4 mg of fibrinogen.

TABLE 38–3 ABO-Rh COMPATIBILITY OF FRESH FROZEN PLASMA

	Donor Blood Type					
Recipient Blood Type	A	B	O	AB	Rh+	Rh−
A	X		X			
B		X		X		
O	X	X	X	X		
AB				X		
Rh+					X	X
Rh−					X	X

Adverse Effects and Contraindications

Plasma and liquid plasma have the same adverse effects as those of whole blood. FFP is an isotonic volume expander, so the patient receiving more than 1 unit should be monitored closely for fluid overload. The adverse effects and hazards are similar to those associated with whole blood administration.

Plasma carries the same risk of disease transmission (except for cytomegalovirus [CMV]) as whole blood. Plasma or liquid plasma used as a volume expander is contraindicated if the volume can be safely replaced with other methods such as 0.9-percent sodium chloride, Ringer's lactate, albumin, and plasma protein fraction. FFP should not be used for volume expansion, as a nutritional supplement, prophylactically with massive blood transfusion, or prophylactically in patients following cardiopulmonary bypass.

Dosage Regimen

The individual patient's clinical situation determines the volume of the treatment. Knowlege of the patient's size and serial laboratory assays of coagulation function assists in determining the dosage.

FFP should be used within 24 hours after thawing if the therapeutic objective is to provide labile coagulation factors. The rate of administration is 200 mL/hour, or more slowly if circulatory overload is a potential problem. The infusion rate for pediatric patients who are hemorrhaging is dictated by the clinical situation. When FFP is used for pediatric clotting deficiency, the infusion rate is 1 to 2 mL/minute.

Platelets

Platelets are plasma components found in pooled or single donor units. Each bag of platelets prepared from an individual unit of whole blood contains approximately 5.5×10^{10} platelets suspended in 20 to 70 mL of plasma. Pooled platelets are obtained via *plasmapheresis* from whole blood of multiple, random donors. To approximate the number of platelets available in a unit of pooled platelets, multiply the number of platelet bags by 5.5×10^{10}. The number of bags of platelets in the pool will be indicated on the bag.

Single donor platelets are concentrates harvested from a single volunteer donor. Single donor platelets are collected using a procedure known as *hemapheresis*. Units of hemapheresed platelets usually contain at least 3×10^{11} platelets (equivalent to about 5 to 6 units of pooled random donor units) suspended in 200 to 500 mL of plasma. This product contains lymphocytes in varying numbers depending on which blood cell separator was used for the collection and whether the separation was performed after collection to remove RBCs and most lymphocytes.

In some cases, the patient may require HLA-matched platelets. Platelets for these patients are obtained by apheresis from a donor who is an HLA-match to the recipient. HLA antigens, which are located on all nucleated cells of the body and most of the circulating body cells, play a vital role in tissue transplantation.

Indications

Platelets are used to control or prevent bleeding associated with deficiencies in platelet number or function. Platelets are used prophylactically in patients who have platelet counts less than 10,000 to 20,000/μL. They are also administered if there is evidence of bleeding with platelet counts less than 50,000/μL.

Patients with thrombocytopenic bleeding or bleeding due to decreased platelet production receive platelet transfusions. Patients receiving antineoplastic therapy or who have leukemia require multiple, repeated platelet infusions. The multiple infusions place the patients at risk for alloimmunization to the donors' leukocytes and platelets. It is believed that with increased exposure to multiple donors, the recipient's risk of alloimmunization increases and the recipient can become refractory to the platelet transfusions. In these patients, the use of single donor hemapheresed platelets decreases the patient's exposure to foreign leukocyte antigens from 6 to 1.

Single donor platelets may reduce the risk of transmission-related disease and HLA-antibody formation by decreasing the number of donor exposures. Patients who are unresponsive to pooled and single donor platelets may respond to HLA-matched platelets (but only if the HLA antibodies are the primary cause of platelet destruction). However, perfectly HLA-matched platelets from unrelated donors are rare. This is a limited match in that the donor and recipient have only certain HLA antigens in common, but in many cases, using HLA-matched platelets allows the patient to receive treatment. A family member such as a sibling is the most likely suitable match for platelets but this matching should be avoided if the family member plans to donate bone marrow for use by the patient. The blood sample for HLA matching should be drawn before any immunosuppressive therapy because leukopenia can make HLA typing more difficult.

Patients with a history of febrile, nonhemolytic reactions may require leukocyte-poor platelets. Special filters are available for this purpose. Filters specifically designed for platelet administration should not be used. Removal of leukocytes reduces the risk of alloimmunization and risk of CMV transmission.

It is best to give platelets from Rh-negative donors to Rh-negative females of child-bearing age. If that is not possible, administration of RhoGAM should be considered when Rh-positive platelets must be transfused.

Pharmacodynamics

Normal hemostasis requires platelets. Platelet masses physically occlude breaks in small blood vessels like a patch. Platelets are also a source of phospholipids required for blood coagulation.

Factors V and VIII are bound to platelets and may contribute to hemostasis in patients receiving multiple transfusions, in patients with disseminated intravascular coagulopathy (DIC), or in patients who are deficient in factor V. Each unit of platelets raises the platelet count of a nonbleeding 70 kg adult by 5000 to 10,000/μL. A bag of pheresed platelets is equivalent to five to eight bags of platelets.

Adverse Effects and Contraindications

Patients who require multiple or frequent platelet infusions may become refractory to treatment. When the patient becomes refractory, platelet counts no longer respond to the infusion. Instead, previously acquired HLA antibodies destroy the infused platelets. Experience suggests that it is not the number of donor exposures but rather the number of allogenic donor leukocytes that causes HLA alloimmunization and platelet refractoriness. Other causes of platelet refractoriness include DIC, ITP, hypersplenism, fever, and sepsis.

Immunization to RBC antigens may occur due to the presence of some red cells in pheresed platelet concentrates. Platelets incompatible with recipient RBCs may cause a positive direct antiglobulin test and possible low-grade hemolysis due to isoagglutinins in the plasma.

Platelet concentrates contain few RBCs. Hence, ABO compatibility is not required. However, ABO red cell compatibility can enhance platelet recovery and survival. Rh compatibility should be considered, particularly in Rh-negative females of child-bearing age. If it is impossible to use platelets from Rh-negative donors, consideration should be given to immunization with RhoGAM in this population of recipients.

Platelets should not be transfused to patients with ITP (unless there is life-threatening bleeding), prophylactically with massive blood transfusion, or prophylactically in patients following cardiopulmonary bypass.

Dosage Regimen

The patient's clinical situation determines the number of platelet concentrate units to be administered. The usual adult dose for a bleeding patient with a platelet count below 20×10^9/L is six to eight bags. The patient may require a repeat dose in 1 to 3 days because transfused platelets have a life-span of only 3 to 4 days. Another acceptable dosage calculation is to infuse 1 unit of platelets per 10 kg of patient body weight. Platelet infusions may be administered as rapidly as tolerated but should be completed within 4 hours.

The average pediatric dose of platelet concentrates is 1 unit/7 to 10 kg of body weight. The infusion rate is determined by volume tolerance, but the total amount should be infused within 4 hours. Plasma volume may be reduced if circulatory overload is a potential problem.

Granulocytes

Granulocyte infusions are administered infrequently. This cellular product is obtained from a single donor by centrifugation hemapheresis and must be maintained at room temperature. The product generally contains other leukocytes and platelets and 20 to 50 mL of RBCs. The cells are suspended in 200 to 300 mL of anticoagulant and plasma. Granulocyte infusions contain at least 1.0×10^{10} granulocytes.

Indications

Pheresed granulocytes are indicated as supportive therapy for patients with acquired neutropenia (usually less than 0.5×10^9/L) or WBC dysfunction who are suffering from a documented gram-negative infection unresponsive to antibiotics or other treatments. These patients are very ill and may or may not have the bone marrow capacity to generate granulocytes on their own. The clinical course of those who will not recover bone marrow function is generally not altered with the use of granulocyte infusions. Only CMV-seronegative granulocytes should be given to profoundly immunosuppressed CMV-seronegative recipients (e.g., bone marrow transplant recipients). The long-term benefits of granulocyte infusions remain questionable and continue to be evaluated.

Pharmacodynamics

Granulocytes are phagocytes that migrate toward and kill bacteria. An infusion of granulocytes will not cause the patient's granulocyte count to increase. This may be due to prior immunization to leukocyte antigens and subsequent sequestration of the granulocytes by the body. It may also be due to consumption of the granulocytes as they fight the infection.

Because the granulocyte product contains a considerable number of RBCs and plasma, cross matching of donor to recipient is necessary. Pretransfusion testing for granulocyte transfusions is ordinarily the same as for RBC transfusion (Table 38–4).

Adverse Effects and Contraindications

It is not unusual for patients receiving granulocyte infusions to exhibit febrile, nonhemolytic reactions. Chills, fevers, and pulmonary insufficiency may be avoided with slow administration and pretreatment; however, patients may experience these adverse effects in spite of interventions. Pretreatment with meperidine, acetaminophen, or antihistamines may help avoid some of the adverse effects. The same types of reactions and hazards associated with the administration of whole blood may occur with granulocyte infusions.

Granulocyte infusions are contraindicated in the treatment of infections responsive to antibiotics. Only patients whose conditions have not responded to trials of broad-spectrum antibiotics are candidates for treatment with granulocytes.

The systemic antifungal drug amphotericin B should not be administered within 4 hours of granulocyte transfusion. Pulmonary insufficiency has been seen with concurrent administration of granulocytes and amphotericin B.

Dosage Regimen

Ideally, granulocytes are administered within 6 hours of harvesting but the product must be infused within 24 hours of collection. The recommended dosage is 3×10^8 cells/kg per infusion. The unit is administered over 4 hours (based on a 200-mL volume) through a standard infusion set. Depth-type microaggregate or leukocyte reduction filters remove granulocytes and are not appropriate for administering this blood product.

Other regimens are documented, and more research is necessary to determine the most efficacious therapy. When the decision is made that granulocyte infusion is appropriate, the patient should receive daily infusions of the product until the infection is cured, the patient's fever abates, or the absolute granulocyte count returns to at least 0.5×10^9/L.

Cryoprecipitate

Cryoprecipitate is a plasma component essential in the treatment of certain types of hemophilia. It is prepared by thawing FFP and recovering the precipitate. On the average, each bag of cryoprecipitated antihemolytic factor (AHF) contains 80 to 120 units of factor VIII (antihemophilic factor), 250 mg of fibrinogen, and 20 to 30 percent of the factor XIII present in the original unit.

Indications

Cryoprecipitate is used to control bleeding caused by deficiency of Factor VIII (i.e., hemophilia A), von Willebrand's factor, factor XIII, and fibrinogen. It is occasionally used to control bleeding in uremic patients.

Cryoprecipitate AHF is also indicated in the treatment of hypofibrinogenemia. This deficiency may be caused by an inherited coagulopathy or DIC. Cryoprecipitate is the only source of concentrated fibrinogen available.

Pharmacodynamics

Cryoprecipitated AHF assists in controlling bleeding in patients with coagulopathies associated with deficits of factors VIII, XIII, fibrinogen, and von Willebrand's factor (AHF-VWF) by replacing selected clotting factors.

Cryoprecipitate contains a small volume of plasma and no RBCs. Cross matching and Rh determination is preferred but not required (Table 38–5).

Adverse Effects and Contraindications

Adverse effects of cryoprecipitate are similar to those described for whole blood. Adverse effects may include allergic reactions, transmission of infectious diseases, and bacterial contamination.

TABLE 38–4 ABO-Rh COMPATIBILITY FOR GRANULOCYTE INFUSIONS

	Donor Blood Type					
Recipient Blood Type	A	B	O	AB	Rh+	Rh−
A	X		X			
B		X	X			
O			X			
AB	X	X	X	X		
Rh+					X	X
Rh−						X

TABLE 38–5 ABO-Rh COMPATIBILITY FOR CRYOPRECIPITATE

	Donor Blood Type					
Recipient Blood Type	A	B	O	AB	Rh+	Rh−
A	X			X		
B		X		X		
O	X	X	X	X		
AB				X		
Rh+					X	X
Rh−					X	X

Dosage Regimen

The dosage of cryoprecipitate is calculated on plasma volume. Eight to ten bags supply 2 g of fibrinogen (hemostatic dose). The formula for calculating the appropriate number of bags of cryoprecipitate needed is included in Appendix E.

When treating bleeding patients with hemophilia, a rapid infusion of 10 mL/min of factor VIII as a loading dose yields the desire effect; this infusion is followed by a smaller maintenance dose every 8 to 12 hours. After surgery, a regimen of therapy for 10 days or more may be necessary. Patients with circulating antibodies to factor VIII require larger doses. Managing and monitoring cryoprecipitated AHF responses in factor VIII–deficient patients require periodic plasma factor VIII:C assays. Smaller doses of cryoprecipitated AHF usually control the bleeding time of patients with von Willebrand's disease. Fibrinogen assays are necessary to monitor patients with hypofibrinogenemia.

Critical Thinking Process

Assessment

History of Present Illness

The symptoms and complaints of the patient who presents with blood loss depend on the rapidity with which the loss occurred, the volume of loss, and the ability of the patient's compensatory mechanisms to maintain homeostasis. Details such as the onset of present symptoms and any precipitating factors are important information for the health care team.

Patients with bleeding disorders may present with a history of bleeding following minor surgical procedures, dental procedures, childbirth, or other trauma. They may have a family history of bleeding. The patient may state that bleeding has occurred from multiple sites without any history of trauma. Before treating the patient with a bleeding disorder, the health care provider determines whether the bleeding disorder is due to a platelet disorder and the etiology of the disorder.

The examiner should determine whether the patient has had a recent viral or bacterial infection, particularly involving the upper respiratory tract. Autoimmune thrombocytopenic purpura, also know as ITP, frequently follows upper respiratory infections or other viral infections.

High doses of penicillin and aspirin or other nonsteroidal anti-inflammatory drugs may lead to defective platelet activation. Myeloproliferative disorders and cancer can cause thrombocytosis. In thrombocytosis, the number of platelets is adequate but they function poorly and aggregate abnormally. Cytotoxic drugs (cytosine arabinoside, daunorubicin, cyclophosphamide, busulfan, methotrexate, and 6-mercaptopurine), thiazides, and ethanol cause thrombocytopenia due to decreased platelet production. Other drugs (sulfonamides, quinidine, isoniazid, sedative-hypnotics, chlorpromazine, and digoxin) lead to thrombocytopenia by destroying platelets.

Past Health History

When caring for the patient with acute blood loss, begin by obtaining as complete a past medical history as the patient's condition will allow. A history of jaundice, blood loss, alcohol abuse, diarrhea, or chronic diseases may assist in determining the cause of the patient's symptoms. Attempt to get a thorough drug history because many drugs contribute to or exacerbate bleeding (see Drugs Contributing to Bleeding Disorders). Allergy and transfusion history, as well as any history of coagulopathies, provide the health care provider with information about the patient's potential risks for adverse effects should blood or blood product infusion be necessary. The patient presenting with acute blood loss secondary to major trauma will likely be unable to assist with a history and all initial efforts when dealing with the patient in this condition are directed at maintaining the patient's airway, breathing, and circulation.

Physical Exam Findings

Before there are discernible changes in vital signs, the patient with hypovolemia will display restlessness, thirst, and generalized anxiety such as that seen in dehydration. Urinary output is reduced. Patient's with blood loss via the gastrointestinal (GI) tract may complain of black tarry stools. Blood in the GI tract functions as an effective cathartic, and the patient may have diarrhea. The stool may first appear as black and tarry, proceed to maroon-colored loose stools, and then become liquid frank blood.

A loss of at least 10 percent of circulating volume is usually necessary before there is a decrease in systolic blood pressure. In advanced blood loss, as the patient's blood pressure and cardiac output fall, the heart rate increases as the body attempts to compensate for the fall in cardiac output. The patient may exhibit postural changes in blood pressure. Mucous membranes and the extremities will be pale and cool due to vasoconstriction as the body shunts blood away from the periphery to the vital organs. There may also be peripheral edema and systolic ejection murmurs. Vital signs reflect the patient's volume status.

DRUGS CONTRIBUTING TO BLEEDING DISORDERS

Semisynthetic penicillins
Cephalosporins
Dipyridamole
Thiazides
Alcohol
Quinidine
Chlorpromazine
Sulfonamides
Isoniazid (INH)
Rifampin (RIF)
Methyldopa
Phenytoin
Barbiturates
Warfarin
Heparin
Nonsteroidal anti-inflammatory drugs
Acetylsalicylic acid

Patients with platelet defects generally experience bleeding immediately after trauma. Bleeding may be evident on the skin in the form of petechiae (less than 3 mm) or ecchymoses (greater than 3 mm). Other common areas of bleeding in platelet disorders are the mucous membranes, nose, and GI or urinary tracts. Patients with platelet disorders may have hepatosplenomegaly due to increased platelet destruction. A rectal exam determines the presence of blood in the GI tract.

Diagnostic Testing

Laboratory studies include a complete blood count with differential, platelet count, and reticulocyte count. Additionally, prothrombin (PT), activated partial thromboplastin (APTT), and bleeding times assist in determining the etiology of the patient's symptoms. Blood for type and cross match or type and hold are drawn and sent to the laboratory to prepare for transfusion, if it becomes necessary.

Initially, the patient's hemoglobin and hematocrit may be falsely high because the compensatory vasoconstriction evoked by hypovolemia initially prevents the extravascular fluids from replacing the intravascular fluid loss. Eventually, the hemoglobin and hematocrit fall. Reticulocyte counts in acute blood loss are elevated.

Laboratory studies in patients with platelet-associated bleeding disorders include a complete blood count and platelet count. Platelet counts of less than 100,000/mm^3 are associated with mildly prolonged bleeding times. Platelet counts of less than 50,000/mm^3 result in easy bruising. Patients whose platelet counts are less than 20,000/mm^3 are at increased risk for spontaneous bleeding. PT assesses the function of the extrinsic coagulation system. APTT aids in assessing the function of the intrinsic coagulation system. The clotting cascade is discussed in Chapter 36 (see Figure 36–1).

Determination of bleeding time is used in diagnosing patients with bleeding disorders. Patients with prolonged bleeding times (over 9 minutes) in the presence of normal platelet counts have a qualitative platelet defect. In the patient with thrombocytopenia, a bone marrow biopsy is helpful in determining whether the patient has bone marrow aplasia due to malignancy or fibrosis. If the bone marrow biopsy reveals an increase in megakaryocytes, ITP is the likely diagnosis.

Developmental Considerations

Perinatal In pregnancy, fibrinogen, platelet adhesiveness, and factor VIII are increased. Antithrombin III and the activators of plasminogen are decreased. Plasminogen itself is increased. Therefore, the equilibrium of coagulation and fibrinolysis is skewed toward procoagulation.

DIC is a secondary disorder that may occur in the pregnant woman (as well as patients with surgical, infectious, hemolytic, and neoplastic disorders) as a result of an abruptio placenta, intrauterine fetal death (especially if longer than 5 weeks in duration), pre-eclampsia and eclampsia, postpartum hemorrhagic sepsis, a rapid traumatic labor and delivery, or amniotic fluid embolism. These disorders cause infusion of tissue extract from injured tissues, severe injury to endothelial cells, red cell or platelet injury, build-up of bacterial debris or endotoxins, immune reactions, and thrombocytopenia. All of these factors activate the intrinsic coagulation sequence in some way. Paradoxically, the intravascular clotting ultimately produces hemorrhage because of rapid consumption of fi-brinogen, platelets, prothrombin, and clotting factors V, VIII, and X.

The tendency toward excessive bleeding can appear suddenly and, with little warning, rapidly progress to severe or even fatal hemorrhage. Signs of DIC include continued bleeding from a venipuncture site, occult and internal bleeding, and in some cases, profuse bleeding from all orifices. Other less obvious and more easily missed signs of bleeding are generalized sweating, cold and mottled fingers and toes (due to capillary thrombi and hypoxia), and petechiae.

Pediatric The etiology of bleeding disorders in children is similar to that of an adult, although there are some disorders that are seen more often in children. For example, von Willebrand's disease is a hereditary bleeding disorder characterized by a factor VIII deficiency and low levels of factor VIII–related antigen. In addition, a functional component of the factor VIII molecule that is required for platelet adhesion to vascular subendothelium is reduced. This factor results in prolonged bleeding time because the platelets fail to adhere to the walls of ruptured vessels. von Willebrand's disease can be mild, moderate, or severe.

There is an increased tendency toward bleeding from mucous membranes. The most common symptom is frequent nosebleeds, followed by gingival bleeding, easy bruising, and menorrhagia in females. Unlike hemophilia, it affects both males and females because its inheritance is autosomal dominant.

Hemophilia is an X-linked recessive disorder and may be mild, moderate, or severe. The most common pattern of transmission is between an unaffected male and a trait-carrier female. The two most common forms of the disorder are factor VIII deficiency (hemophilia A, or classic hemophilia), and factor IX deficiency (hemophilia B, or Christmas disease). Factor VIII deficiency accounts for about 75 percent of the cases.

Bleeding in hemophilic patients is variable, depending on the level of deficiency of the clotting factor. Approximately 60 percent of children with hemophilia A or B are severely affected and may have spontaneous bleeding without any recognized trauma. Soft tissue bleeding from the neck, lower face, and tongue may cause grave consequences if it is not treated. Hematuria and GI bleeding are likely. *Hemarthrosis,* bleeding into the joints, can lead to painful stiffening and permanent disability. The leading cause of death, however, is intracranial bleeding. Hemorrhagic complications can be avoided or minimized with early and adequate factor replacement therapy.

Geriatric Patients with chronic illnesses, particularly older adults, are at increased risk for fluid volume deficit because of impaired recognition of thirst or an inability to obtain fluids, inadequate maintenance of chronic conditions (e.g. hyperglycemia), or inadequate monitoring of therapeutic regimens (e.g. diuretic-induced hypotension).

The older adult who presents with bruising requires the health care provider to differentiate between a bleeding disorder or senile purpura, the bleeding under the skin associated with increased capillary fragility due to the aging process.

Psychosocial Considerations

In addition to cultural heritage, religion plays a vital role in a patient's perception of health and illness. An integral component of culture, religious beliefs may influence a patient's explanation of the cause of illness, perception of its severity, and the choice of health care providers. In times of crisis, religion may influence the course of action believed to be appropriate.

Blood and blood products are generally acceptable to Hindus, Mennonites, Seventh-Day Adventists, Unitarians, and followers of Islam. There is no restriction to the use of blood and blood products according to the Mormon doctrine.

Catholicism, according to the Roman Rite, permits the use of blood and blood products as along as they are used for the good of the whole person. There is a prohibition in Judaism against ingesting blood (e.g. blood sausage, raw meat). However, this does not apply to receiving blood transfusions. Blood and blood products are not ordinarily used by members of the Church of Christ (Christian Scientists).

Jehovah's Witnesses must refuse blood in any form and agents in which blood is an ingredient. Blood volume expanders are acceptable if they are not derivatives of blood. Mechanical devices for circulating the blood are acceptable as long as they are not primed with blood initially. The determination of Jehovah's Witnesses to abstain from blood is based on scriptural references and precedents in the history of Christianity. Courts of justice have often upheld the principle that each person has a right to bodily integrity, yet some health care providers and hospital administrators have turned to the courts for legal authorization to force blood to be used as a medical treatment for an individual whose religious convictions prohibit the use of blood. In some cases, children have been made wards of the court so that they could receive blood when a life-threatening medical condition occurred.

Other patients may refuse blood or blood product transfusions due to their fear of contracting infectious diseases. In all cases, the health care providers explain to patients in terms that they can understand the potential outcomes related to their decisions and support these patients in their informed decisions.

Analysis and Management

Treatment Objectives

Treatment objectives for patients with fluid volume deficits are to reverse hypovolemia, restore fluid volume, and prevent ischemic complications. To accomplish these objectives, the treatment options include surgical or medical management of the patient. Both of these options may include the use of blood and or blood products, other colloids or crystalloid solutions (see also Chapter 57). The guiding principal in clinical decision-making is to use the least extreme measure to accomplish treatment objectives safely. When electing the type of infusion to use, blood and blood products are always considered an extreme measure.

Treatment Options

Homologous blood transfusion is the transfer or transplantation of living tissue from one person to another. All homologous blood products carry the risk of disease transfusion and transfusion reactions. Although the development of sensitivity screening has reduced the incidence of disease transmission, it has not eliminated transmission. Patients continue to have a high level of anxiety related to disease transmission by homologous blood.

In contrast, autologous blood is considered the safest type of blood for transfusion in most patients for a variety of reasons, including elimination of disease transmission and elimination of transfusion reactions. In addition, the quality of autologous blood is morphologically, physiologically, and biochemically superior to that of homologous blood.

Drug Variables

Patients who have experienced minor blood loss (less than 10 percent) and whose conditions are stable may receive colloids such as plasma protein fractions (PLASMANATE) and synthetic plasma expanders such as hetastarch to replace volume. If bleeding has been arrested and the patient is not exhibiting life-threatening symptoms such as shortness of breath or chest pain, replacing the oxygen-carrying capacity of RBCs over time by using erythropoietin alpha is appropriate (see Chapter 41).

Table 38–6 provides an overview of the blood components, along with their indications and implications. Treatment options for the patient with platelet disorders depend on the underlying cause of the platelet disorder. Not all platelet disorders are curable, and some may require long-term treatment. Patients with platelet disorders secondary to drugs may require dosage adjustment or a change of drugs. An evaluation of the risks and benefits associated with continued treatment with these drugs is necessary for patient well-being.

Patient Variables

Patients displaying signs and symptoms of hypovolemia require no special considerations related to age because the treatment goals for patients with these serious symptoms are not age related.

Patient signs and symptoms that warrant whole blood transfusion include blood loss with hypotension, tachycardia, shortness of breath, pallor, and low hemoglobin and hematocrit. Patients with major blood loss who are symptomatic for hypoxia and hypovolemia require immediate replenishment of volume and oxygen-carrying capacity. The health care provider may request whole blood in very severe cases of major trauma or a combination of PRBCs, plasma, platelets, and crystalloid solutions when these infusions will successfully treat the individual patient's condition.

Indications for platelet transfusion include patients who are actively bleeding with a platelet count of less than 50,000/mm^3 or a qualitative defect. Patients who require surgery and whose platelet counts are less than 50,000/mm^3 (less than 90,000/mm^3 if the surgery is on the central nervous system or the eye) receive platelets. Platelet transfusions are also appropriate for patients with chronic thrombocytopenia whose platelet counts are between 10,000 and 20,000/mm^3 owing to decreased platelet production.

Patients with disorders related to increased destruction of platelets such as ITP receive only a transitory benefit from platelet infusions because the patient's immune system destroys the transfused platelets in the same manner that it destroys the patient's platelets. Options for the patient with ITP who is bleeding or who has a platelet count of less than 20,000/mm^3 include treatment with prednisone (1 to 2

TABLE 38–6 OVERVIEW OF BLOOD COMPONENTS

Product	Indications	Implications
Whole blood	Symptomatic anemia with large volume deficit. Restores oxygen-carrying capacity of blood as well as circulatory volume	Must be ABO identical. Observe for volume overload in infants and older adults. Infuse as rapidly as tolerated
Red blood cells	Symptomatic anemia. Restores oxygen-carrying capacity of blood	Must be ABO compatible. Infuse as rapidly as tolerated but complete in 4 hours
Leukocyte-poor red blood cells	Restores oxygen-carrying capacity for patients with febrile reactions from leukocyte antibodies	Must be ABO compatible. Infuse as rapidly as tolerated but complete in 4 hours
Fresh frozen plasma	Deficit of labile and nonlabile plasma coagulation factors and ITP	Should be ABO compatible. Infuse as rapidly as tolerated but complete in 4 hours
Platelets	Bleeding from thrombocytopenia or platelet function abnormality	ABO compatibility not required although when done enhances platelet recovery and survival. Do not use microaggregate filters. Follow manufacturer instructions. Infuse in less than 4 hours
Granulocytes	Neutropenia with infection	Must be ABO compatible. Do not use depth-type microaggregate filters. Observe carefully for reactions
Cryoprecipitate	Hemophilia A, von Willebrand's disease, hypofibrinogenemia, factor XIII deficiency	ABO compatibility is preferred but not required. Frequent, repeated doses may be necessary. Infuse as rapidly as tolerated but within 4 hours

ITP, idiopathic thrombocytopenic purpura.
Adapted from Booker, M. F., and Ignatavicius, D. D. (1996). *Infusion therapy: Techniques and medications* (p. 298). Philadelphia: W.B. Saunders.

mg/kg/day) or methylprednisolone (1 g/day) for 3 days. Infusions of prednisone or methylprednisolone increase the patient's platelet count and arrest bleeding. Intravenous doses of immunoglobulin G (IgG) (1 g/kg/day) can also transiently increase the platelet count. Other nonsurgical options include low doses of antineoplastic drugs such as danazol, vincristine, vinblastine, cyclophosphamide, or azathioprine. Surgical interventions include splenectomy.

Intervention

Administration

The responsibilities when hanging blood and blood components include inspection of the product and container for defects, positive identification of the patient, and verifications of the product and its expiration date. Additionally, compatibility between the patient and the donor must be confirmed and the patient's informed consent obtained. Review the patient's chart for evidence of previous transfusion reaction and the orders for the transfusion.

The patient will require an intravenous (IV) site with a cannula large enough to accommodate the blood component to be administered. Inspect the patient's current IV for patency and intactness. Determine that the IV catheter is an 18- or 19-gauge cannula, which facilitates transfusion flow and prevent hemolysis of RBCs. Restart the IV if necessary. After obtaining the unit of product from the blood bank, the transfusion should begin within 30 minutes unless the product is held in a controlled cooling device that meets the specifications of the American Association of Blood Banks. No single unit of blood product should infuse for more than 4 hours, and platelets should be infused as rapidly as possible.

For routine administration of blood, a standard blood filter with a minimum pore size of 170 microns is recommended. If the patient requires three or more units of blood or the blood product is over 5 days old, microaggregate blood filters with pore sizes of 30 to 40 microns are effective in removing any tiny clots or debris that may have developed during storage.

Patients with a history of severe febrile transfusion reactions may benefit from leukocyte-depleting filters. If the patient requires the rapid infusion of multiple units of blood or if there is a history of cold agglutinins (antibodies that agglutinate RBCs more efficiently at temperature below 37°C), a blood warmer should be used. This device will warm the blood to 37°C and avoid making the patient hypothermic.

Under no circumstances should any drugs be mixed with the blood product. The only solution appropriate for administration with blood or blood products is 0.9-percent sodium chloride solution. Additive solution RBCs do not need to be diluted before transfusion. Units without additive solution may be viscous and require dilution with 0.9-percent sodium chloride. A 19-gauge or larger needle is used to achieve optimal flow rate. Unless the patient's condition dictates otherwise, the infusion of RBCs or whole blood begins at a rate of 5 mL/minute for the first 15 minutes of the infusion. During that time and throughout the transfusion, observe the patient very closely, monitoring vital signs and any signs of a transfusion reaction. After this initial period, the transfusion should proceed as quickly as possible.

The patient's clinical situation determines the number of platelets to be administered. The usual dose in a bleeding adult with a platelet count of less than 20,000/mm^3 is six to eight bags. The responsibility for inspection of the product container and positive identification of the unit and the patient are the same when hanging platelets as when hanging other blood products. Pretreatment with antihistamines, meperidine, or acetaminophen helps most patients avoid febrile reactions. Because platelets are fragile, handle the bag carefully and administer the infusion as rapidly as the patient tolerates. Monitor vital signs carefully. Filters must be appropriate for platelet administration. Check the package insert for information on the appropriate use of filters.

The use of leukocyte-reduction filters will decrease the patient's risk of alloimmunization to HLA. If the situation is such that the patient will likely require multiple platelet transfusions over a period of time, it is prudent to use a leukocyte-reduction filter with the patient's first platelet infusion.

Strict adherence to verification before blood or blood product administration greatly reduces the risk of infusing the wrong blood type. With another registered nurse at the bedside, verify the blood product and the patient's identity by comparing the laboratory blood record with the

- Patient's name and identification number, both verbally and against the patient's wristband
- Blood unit number on the blood bag label
- Blood group and Rh type on the blood bag label
- Type of blood component with the health care provider's order
- Expiration date noted on the blood bag label

Many blood banks have pediatric packs of blood available in 50 to 100 mL for infusing to children. Agency protocol should be followed for blood administration. If the patient is an older adult with cardiac failure, careful assessment is required in order to prevent fluid overload. PRBCs are frequently infused to limit the volume being infused.

Although such cases are rare, transfusions can result in fatal reactions. Approximately 30 people in the United States die each year as a direct result of blood product transfusion. Death is not the only adverse effect patients suffer as a direct result of transfusions. Each year, 10 to 15 percent of patients receiving transfusions experience adverse reactions, with 1 percent experiencing serious adverse effects. By law, when complications from the transfusion of blood or blood components result in death, the blood bank must notify the Food and Drug Administration by phone within 24 hours and a file a written report of the investigation of the reaction with the Food and Drug Administration within 7 days.

Transfusion Reactions Adverse effects of blood transfusions are categorized as immediate and delayed effects. *Immediate effects* may be immunologically mediated and result in intravascular or extravascular hemolysis. Other immediate adverse effects include febrile nonhemolytic reactions, transfusion-related acute lung injury, allergic reactions with or without anaphylaxis, and bacterial sepsis. *Delayed effects* may also be immunologically mediated as in GVHD or posttransfusion purpura. Infections with bacterial, protozoal, or viral agents are other potential delayed reactions. Table 38–7 provides an overview of immunologic reactions to blood transfusions.

Since 1985, all donated blood has been tested for antibodies to HIV by enzyme-linked immunosorbent assay, a procedure that has been found to be greater than 99-percent accurate in detecting potentially infectious units of blood. These efforts translate to a 1 in 400,000 chance of acquiring HIV per unit of blood product transfused in the United States. HIV transmission via transfusion remains a major problem in developing countries due to lack of donor screening.

The HIV retrovirus infects and kills CD4-positive lymphocytes (helper T cells), destroying the immune system. The resultant immunodeficiency renders the patient vulnerable to opportunistic infections. Clinical manifestations of HIV infection include weight loss, diarrhea, fever, lymphadenopathy, Kaposi's sarcoma, and opportunistic infections.

Hepatitis has been a common hazard for patients receiving transfusions for over 40 years. Before 1980, the risk for hepatitis C (NANB hepatitis) transmission among those receiving multiple transfusions was 7 to 10 percent. Although the incidence of hepatitis has dramatically decreased since the advent of specific tests for hepatitis B and hepatitis C virus and the use of alanine aminotransferase (ALT; serum glutamic-pyruvic transaminase [SGPT]), hepatitis remains the most common transfusion-related infection.

Hepatitis may be transmitted via RBCs, platelets, FFP, cryoprecipitate, Rh_0(D) immune globulin, or clotting factors. The disease is manifested by elevated liver enzymes, anorexia, fatigue, malaise, dark urine, fever, and jaundice. The disease usually runs a 4- to 6-week course.

Education

Explain the transfusion procedure to the patient. Advise the patient that vital signs will be taken before initiation of the transfusion and a consent form will need to be signed. Instruct the patient to report signs and symptoms of adverse transfusion reactions. Frequently, it is the patient who will report a problem before the health care provider is able to discern it on physical assessment. The health care provider should instruct the patient to report low back pain, fever, chills, tachycardia, tachypnea, dizziness, urticaria, itching, pain at the IV site, or nausea. Any of these signs and symptoms should alert the health care provider to potential problems with the patient's infusion.

Evaluation

Patients who have received whole blood will likely have resolution of symptoms of hypovolemic shock and anemia. If a patient is actively bleeding, the hematocrit and hemoglobin may fluctuate due to rapid fluid shifts. In a nonbleeding adult, 1 unit of whole blood should increase the hematocrit by 3 percentage points and the hemoglobin by 1 g/dL.

A transfusion of RBCs provides resolution of symptoms of anemia. As with whole blood, in a nonbleeding adult, 1 unit of RBCs or additive solution RBCs should increase the hematocrit by 3 percentage points and the hemoglobin by 1 g/dL.

Treatment effectiveness of plasma infusions is assessed by monitoring coagulation function, which is measured by the PT, international normalized ratio, APTT, or by specific factor assays.

A transfusion of platelets to a bleeding patient yields a cessation of bleeding, correction of prolonged bleeding times, and an increase in the patient's platelet count. One unit of platelets should raise the peripheral platelet count of a 70-kg adult by 5000 to 10,000/μL and an 18-kg child by 20,000/mm^3 if the underlying cause of thrombocytopenia is resolved or controlled. To assess therapeutic effects, a platelet count should be performed within 1 hour of the transfusion.

The expected outcome of granulocyte infusion is improvement in or resolution of the infection. No increase in peripheral WBC count is usually seen following granulocyte infusion in adults; however, an increase may be seen in chil-

TABLE 38–7 IMMUNOLOGIC REACTIONS TO BLOOD TRANSFUSION

Cause	Characteristic	Manifestations	Implications
Immediate Reactions			
Intravascular hemolytic reaction	Incompatibility between the recipient's plasma and the donor's RBCs	Chills, fever, low back pain, flushing, tachycardia, tachypnea, hypotension, vascular collapse, hemoglobinuria, hemoglobinemia, bleeding, acute renal failure, shock, cardiac arrest, death	Treat shock. Draw blood samples for serologic testing. Maintain BP with IV colloid solutions. Give diuretics to maintain urine flow. Measure urinary output
Extravascular hemolytic reaction	Sensitization to an incompatible antigen through a previous transfusion or pregnancy	Fever, hemoglobinuria, hyperbilirubinemia. Continued fall in hemoglobin 4 to14 days after the transfusion or continued anemia	Rarely preventable. A complete and accurate transfusion history given to the blood bank may assist in identifying patients at risk
Febrile, nonhemolytic reaction (most common)	Antigen-antibody response of HLA antigens on donor leukocytes reacting with the patient's antibodies	Sudden chills, fever (rise in temperature greater than 2°F), headache, flushing, anxiety, muscle pain	Do not restart transfusion. Give antipyretics as prescribed. Do not give aspirin to thrombocytopenic patients. Self-limiting. Leukocyte-poor products or leukocyte-depleting filters are indicated for patients with a recurrent history of febrile nonhemolytic transfusion reactions
Transfusion-related acute lung injury	Anti-HLA antibodies in the donor's plasma react with antigens on the recipient's WBCs or platelets	Fever (to 104°F), chills possible, cyanosis. Pulmonary edema in severe cases.	Symptom relief. Antipyretics. Oxygen and IV steroids if pulmonary edema present. Symptoms usually abate in 48 hours. Use leukocyte-poor products or leukocyte-depleting filters to prevent recurrence
Allergic reactions (mild to anaphylaxis	Sensitivity to donor's IgA antibody	Urticaria, itching, flushing. Chills and fever at times. Bronchospasm, dyspnea, pulmonary edema.	Antihistamines if mild. Epinephrine and corticosteroids, if severe. Donors with allergies should be eliminated from the donor pool. These patients will require frozen or washed red blood cells and IgA-deficient plasma for future transfusions
Acute nonimmunologically mediated hemolytic reactions	Administration of a hypotonic fluid with the transfusion product, bacterial infection of the patient or contamination of the donor's blood, acute hemolytic anemia from any cause, or improper handling of the blood product by the blood bank	Fever, chills, hemoglobinuria. Disseminated intravascular coagulation and renal failure in severe cases	Treat shock. Draw blood samples for serologic testing. Maintain BP with IV colloid solutions. Give diuretics to maintain urine flow. Measure urinary output
Transfusion-related bacterial sepsis	Contamination of blood or blood product with bacteria	Rigors, fever, nausea, vomiting, diarrhea, chest or back pain, hypotension, tachycardia, dyspnea, cyanosis. May progress to respiratory failure, acute respiratory distress syndrome, disseminated intravascular coagulation and death	Peripheral blood smears positive for hemolysis, a positive Gram stain of a sample from the suspected blood unit and an elevated WBC count differentiates bacterial sepsis from acute hemolytic reactions. Antibiotic therapy warranted
Delayed Reactions			
Graft-versus-host disease	Immunodeficient person receives lymphocytes and these lymphocytes begin to reject cells 4 to 30 days after transfusion	High fever, skin rash, diarrhea, possibly jaundice. Death	Symptomatic treatment and supportive care based on the body systems involved. Irradiation of RBCs or removal of all plasma from the product may prove beneficial
Delayed hemolytic reaction	Sensitization to RBC antigen, not ABO system. Anamnestic immune response occurs 7 to 14 days after transfusion	Fever, chills, back pain, jaundice, anemia, hemoglobinuria	Antipyretics. Monitor adequacy of urinary output. Do more specific type and cross match when giving blood

dren. An improvement in the patient's clinical condition due to resolution of the infection is the only measure of treatment effectiveness.

SUMMARY

- Blood administration is a transplant of living cells from donor to recipient.
- Whole blood consists of 45 percent cells (WBCs, RBCs, and platelets) and 55 percent plasma, of which 90 percent is water.
- The antigens of the ABO system, antigen A and antigen B, are hereditary and determine a persons blood type.
- The antibodies anti-A and anti-B are complete antibodies and cause intravascular hemolysis in the presence of antigen A and antigen B, respectively.
- The indication for whole blood is patients with symptomatic anemia and hypovolemia due to large volume deficit. Patients with symptomatic anemia who do not require volume replacement are candidates for RBCs.
- Patients whose conditions are treatable with diet and drugs are not candidates for blood or blood product administration.
- Plasma and liquid plasma are indicated for the treatment of stable clotting factor deficiencies for which no concentrates are available, or for volume expansion when blood volume cannot adequately and safely be replaced with 0.9-percent sodium chloride, albumin, or plasma protein fraction.
- Patients who require multiple platelet transfusions are at risk for alloimmunization to donors' leukocytes and platelets. These patients require HLA-matched platelets.
- Granulocyte infusions are indicated for supportive therapy in patients with neutropenia who are suffering from a documented gram-negative infection not responsive to antibiotic therapy.
- Patients with von Willebrand's factor deficiency require treatment with cryoprecipitated AHF because commercially prepared factor VIII does not contain sufficient amounts of VWF.
- Adverse blood transfusion reactions may be separated into immediate and delayed effects.
- Immediate effects are immunologically mediated and result in intravascular or extravascular hemolysis. Other immediate adverse effects include febrile nonhemolytic reactions, transfusion-related acute lung injury, allergic reactions, and bacterial sepsis.
- Delayed effects may be immunologically mediated as in GVHD or infections with bacterial, protozoal, or viral agents.

BIBLIOGRAPHY

Andrews, M., and Boyle, J. (1995). *Transcultural concepts in nursing care* (2nd ed.). Philadelphia: J.B. Lippincott.

Booker, M. F., and Ignatavicius, D. D. (1996). *Infusion therapy: Techniques and medications.* Philadelphia: W.B. Saunders.

Brettler, D., and Levine, P. (1994). Clinical manifestations and therapy of inherited coagulation factor deficiencies. In R. Coleman, J. Hirsh, V. Maider, et al. (Eds.), *Hemostasis and thrombosis: Basic principles and clinical practice* (3rd ed.). Philadelphia: J.B. Lippincott.

Fischer, H. E. (1993). Blood donor screening and prevention of transfusion-associated hepatitis C virus infection. *Current Issues in Transfusion Medicine.* Jan–Mar.

Gelb, A., and Leavith, A. (1997). Crossmatch compatible platelets improve corrected count increments in patients who are refractory to randomly selected platelets. *Transfusion,* 37(6), 624–630.

Greene, J. N., Sinnott, J. T., Wyckoff, J. A. et al. (1995). Bacterial infection following blood transfusion: Some bad blood bugging you? *Infections in Medicine,* 12(4), 165–170.

Hoehns, B., Skelly, K., and Graber, M. A. (1997). *University of Iowa family practice handbook.* Philadelphia: Mosby.

Hoyer, L. W. (1994). Hemophilia A. *New England Journal of Medicine,* 330(1), 38–47.

Intravenous Nurses Society. (1998). *Revised intravenous nursing standards of practice.* Belmont, MA: Author.

Lucas, K. G. (1996). Another look at granulocyte transfusion in neutropenic patients with cancer. *Infections in Medicine,* 13(2), 79–80, 82, 92, 129.

Menitove, J. E. (1997). Standards for blood banks and transfusion services (18th ed.). Arlington, VA: American Association of Blood Banks.

Myhre, B. A. (1990). The first recorded blood transfusion: 1656–1668. *Transfusion,* 30(4), 358–362.

Nishino, M, Yoskioka, A. (1997). The revised classification of von Willebrand disease including the previously masqueraded female hemophilia A (type 2N). *International Journal of Hematology,* 66(1), 21–30.

Schiffer, C. A. (1991). Prevention of alloimmunization against platelets. *Blood,* 77(1), 1–4.

Skillings, J. R., Sridhar, F. G., Wong, C. et al (1993). The frequency of red cell transfusions for anemia in patients receiving chemotherapy: A retrospective cohort study. *American Journal of Clinical Oncology,* 16(1), 22–25.

Surgenor, D. M., Wallace, E. L., Hao, S. H., et al. (1990). Collection and transfusion of blood in the United States, 1982–1988. *New England Journal of Medicine,* 322(23), 1642–1651.

U.S. Department of Health and Human Services, Public Health Service. (1993). Institute of Medicine Executive Summary: Research Report Leukemia, NIH Publication #94–329. Washington: Author.

Weir, J. A. (1995). Blood component therapy. In J. Terry, L. Baronowski, R. Lonsway, et al. (Eds.), *Intravenous therapy: Clinical principles and practice.* Philadelphia: W.B. Saunders.

Unit VII

Drugs Influencing the Renal and Urinary Systems

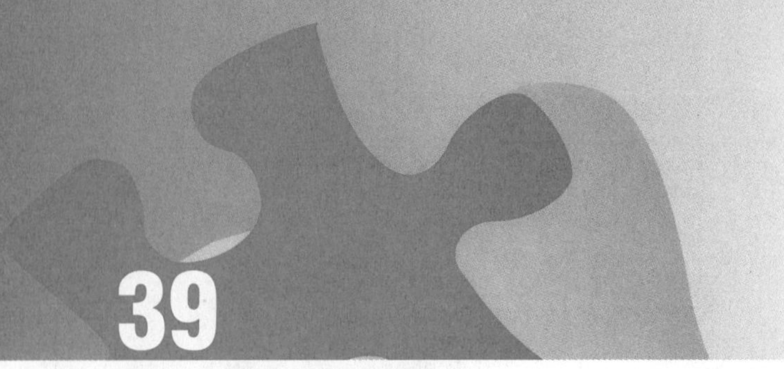

39 Diuretic Drugs

The discovery and clinical application of diuretics is one of the most significant advances in modern medicine. These drugs were among the first synthetic medications used in the clinical setting. Although there is a long history of effectively treating fluid volume excess with diuretics, many of the early drugs are no longer used. Today's drugs are safer as well as more potent and effective. In order to appreciate how diuretics work in the management of fluid volume excess, it is essential to understand how fluids function within the body and, in particular, the filtration and elimination activities of the kidney.

RENAL FUNCTION

Body fluids function in a variety of ways to promote health and wellness. They serve as media for the transport of substances to, from, and across cell membranes. They are the media with which most metabolic reactions take place. Body fluid provides lubrication for body parts and assists in heat regulation.

A chemical equilibrium must be maintained if these functions are to occur. The equilibrium is reflected in normal urine volume, composition, distribution, and pH of body fluids. Equilibrium is achieved through fluid, electrolyte, and acid-base balance. The volume and composition of body fluid is controlled by three processes: glomerular filtration, tubular reabsorption, and tubular secretion.

Urine formation begins with filtration of the plasma by the glomerulus. Renal blood flow equals about 25 percent of cardiac output, or about 1200 mL/minute (660 mL/minute plasma flow). The glomerular filtration rate (GFR) is approximately 125 mL/minute. Water and crystalloids are readily filtered, whereas blood cells and large molecules such as proteins are restrained by the filtration membrane. As fluid is forced through the glomeruli, plasma proteins (primarily albumin) remain in the circulation, maintaining *oncotic pressure* (the sum of protein osmotic pressure and osmotic pressure of obligate cations). Albumin tends to pull water into the blood vessels.

Hydrostatic pressure, the pressure a solution exerts against the wall of its container, is maintained by the contraction of the heart. Blood vessels have a greater hydrostatic pressure than that of interstitial spaces, therefore, there is a tendency for water to be forced out. At the arterial end, nutrients diffuse out of blood vessels. At the venous end, owing to oncotic pressure, water and waste products diffuse into blood vessels.

Three classes of substances are filtered at the glomerulus: electrolytes, nonelectrolytes, and water. The electrolytes that are filtered include sodium, potassium, calcium, magnesium, bicarbonate, chloride, and phosphate. The ultrafiltrate contains electrolytes and other small molecular weight solutes, including 25,200 mEq of sodium/day. Nonelectrolytes that are filtered include glucose, amino acids, and the metabolic end products of protein metabolism: urea, uric acid, and creatinine.

After passing through the glomerulus, the filtrate travels through renal tubules, where 99 percent of it is reabsorbed. The composition of the reabsorbed filtrate approximates the composition of the extracellular fluid. In the reabsorptive process, sodium passively enters the tubule cells down an electrochemical gradient. Sodium also moves against a concentration gradient into the blood by active transport using adenosine triphosphate. Adenosine triphosphate moves sodium out of the cell and potassium into it across the basilar membranes. In addition, sodium diffuses back into peritubular capillaries through pericellular pathways. The mechanisms for its reabsorption are associated with recapturing the filtrate.

Tubular secretion refers to the active and passive processes that move substances from the peritubular capillary into interstitial fluid and then into the tubular lumen. Thus, substances that are secreted are eliminated from the body.

In a healthy individual, these processes work well and equilibrium is maintained. However, alterations in the volume, composition, distribution, or pH of body fluids cause disequilibrium and, in some cases, illness. The disequilibrium can occur as a result of disorders of intake, elimination, or regulation of body fluid components, or as a part of a pathophysiologic response to other disease states. A fluid shift from the extracellular compartment to the interstitial compartment results in edema.

Fluid volume excess, also referred to as *edema,* results from a number of disease states and may be organized according to the mechanisms involved (see Common Causes of Edema with Underlying Mechanisms). Alterations in cardiac, renal, hepatic, or endocrine function are primary etiologies, although edema may be seen with other states such as the edema associated with pregnancy and premenstrual tension. Edema may also be drug induced.

FLUID VOLUME EXCESS

Epidemiology and Etiology

A number of disorders and states can result in fluid volume excess (edema). *Fluid volume excess* is defined as increased fluid retention in the intravascular and interstitial spaces. The body systems most often involved with disorders producing fluid volume excess are the heart, liver, and kidneys.

The etiology of heart failure can be divided into three groups. The first group includes conditions that result in direct damage to the heart (e.g., myocardial infarction, myocarditis, myocardial fibrosis, ventricular aneurysms). The second group includes conditions that result in ventricular overload, and the third group are conditions that lead to

COMMON CAUSES OF EDEMA WITH UNDERLYING MECHANISMS

Mechanism	*Disorders and States*
Increased capillary pressure	• Allergic responses • Cardiogenic pulmonary edema • Environmental heat stress • Heart failure • Hepatic obstruction • Increased levels of ACTH • Idiopathic edema in women • Inflammation • Pregnancy • Premenstrual sodium retention • Prolonged standing • Thrombophlebitis
Increased capillary permeability	• Immune responses • Neoplastic diseases • Noncardiogenic pulmonary edema • Tissue injury and burns
Decreased colloidal osmotic pressure	• Liver disease • Protein-losing enteropathy • Starvation
Obstruction of lymphatic flow	• Infection or disease of lymph nodes • Surgical removal of lymph nodes
Drug-induced	• NSAIDs: Ketoprofen, flurbiprofen, naproxen, phenylbutazone, tolmetin • Antihypertensives: Diltiazem, labetolol, nifedipine, pindolol • Hormones: Androgenic steroids, corticosteroids, estrogens • Others: Estramustine, etretinate, interferon alfa-2a, phenothiazines, tamoxifen

ACTH, Adrenocorticotropic hormone; NSAIDs, nonsteroidal anti-inflammatory drugs.

ventricular constriction (e.g., cardiac tamponade, constrictive cardiomyopathies, pericarditis).

Severe liver problems can result from a variety of causes such as infective organisms, neoplastic growths, toxic agents, and trauma. The pathologic states that result can be categorized as focal or diffuse.

Nephrotic syndrome (nephrosis) has been associated with allergic reactions, systemic disease, circulatory problems, and pregnancy. Glomerular disease is the most common precipitating event in adults. Fifty to seventy-five percent of adults who develop nephrosis progress to renal failure within 5 years. No specific treatment exists for nephrotic syndrome. Diuretics may be prescribed but are often ineffective.

Pathophysiology

Edema is caused by a disruption in Starling forces. Edema can be the result of an increase in capillary hydrostatic pressure, capillary permeability, or interstitial oncotic pressure, or it may be due to a decrease in plasma oncotic pressure.

Edema indicates an excess amount of sodium, which is accompanied by an obligatory water load. The sodium excess may serve as either an initiating event or as a secondary factor in the development of edema. Excess sodium levels are most often caused by increased retention or a decreased ability to eliminate the ion. The sodium and water retention is often a compensatory mechanism serving to restore and maintain circulatory volume while fluid accumulates in interstitial spaces. Retention of sodium and water is illustrated in conditions such as cardiac failure, liver disease, and nephrotic syndrome (Fig. 39–1).

Heart Failure

Heart failure begins when the heart is unable to maintain effective pumping action. Compensation for ineffective pumping is via the sympathetic nervous system. This leads to an increased heart rate, decreased cardiac contractility, and constriction of the peripheral arteries. Vasopressin, which is released through sympathetic stimulation, leads to a constriction of the arteries.

A decrease in peripheral arterial blood flow and renal blood flow results. Decreased perfusion of the kidney leads to the release of renin and the conversion of circulating angiotensin I to angiotensin II. Angiotensin II is a powerful vasoconstrictor that stimulates the adrenal gland to release aldosterone. Aldosterone, in turn, stimulates the kidney to reabsorb sodium and water. Thus, blood pressure is maintained by constricting the blood vessels and increasing intravascular volume. In the process, GFR also decreases, resulting in the retention of sodium and water.

As the process continues, a point is reached at which the compensatory mechanisms no longer work. The circulatory and respiratory systems become overloaded with increasing hydrostatic pressure, causing edema, either in the pulmonary tissues or in peripheral tissues.

As pulmonary edema develops, it inhibits oxygen and carbon dioxide exchange at the alveolar capillary membranes. There is a mild increase in respiratory rate and a decrease in both PaO_2 and $PaCO_2$. If pulmonary venous pressure continues to increase, more fluid moves into the interstitial lung spaces than the lymphatic drainage system can handle. The patient has severe tachypnea and worsening blood gases. Alveolar edema develops even further as pulmonary venous pressure increases. As the disruption at the alveolar-capillary membranes worsens, the alveoli and airways become flooded with fluid.

Clinical signs and symptoms of pulmonary edema are unmistakable. The patient is agitated, cold and clammy, and has severe dyspnea. There is orthopnea, the use of accessory muscles, and a respiratory rate greater than 30 breaths/minute. There may be wheezing and coughing with the production of frothy, blood-tinged sputum. The heart rate and blood pressure may be elevated or at shock level depending on the severity of the condition.

The process may progress to affect the right ventricle also. The hydrostatic pressure of the venous system increases, leading to peripheral edema. The edema of right-sided heart failure is seen in the lower extremities as pitting

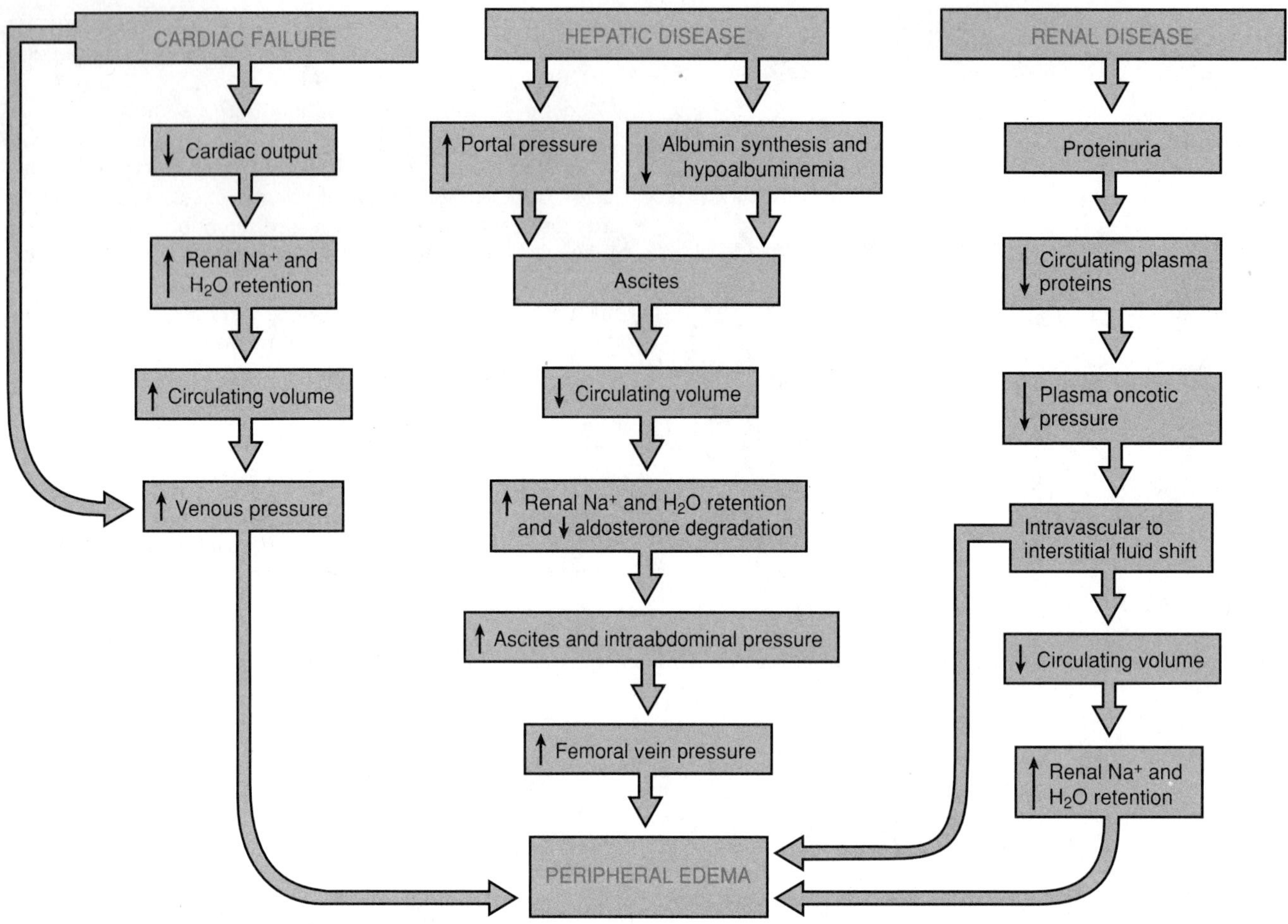

Figure 39–1 Edema is a primary manifestation of alterations in capillary hemodynamics and sodium and water balance caused by cardiac failure, hepatic disease, and renal disease. (Adapted from Groer, M. W., and Shekleton, M. E. [1989]. *Basic pathophysiology: A holistic approach* [3rd ed., p. 799]. St Louis: Mosby. Used with permission.)

edema. Right-sided heart failure can progress to hepatomegaly. Liver lobules become congested, with venous blood causing impaired liver function. Eventually, liver cells die, fibrosis occurs, and cirrhosis can develop.

Hepatic Disease

Much like heart failure, liver disease is characterized, in part, by a disruption in capillary hemodynamics. There is increased pressure within the portal vein, which, in turn, causes increased hydrostatic pressure. Additionally, albumin synthesis is decreased and hypoalbuminemia develops. The result of these changes is *ascites,* an accumulation of fluid within the peritoneal cavity. As the accumulation of fluid progresses, the patient develops hypovolemia and the kidneys are underperfused. When kidney perfusion decreases, renin and angiotensin activities are initiated and the degradation of aldosterone is decreased. The response is to retain sodium and water, further contributing to the accumulation of fluid in the abdomen and to increases in intra-abdominal pressure. The ascites and abdominal pressure increases cause increased femoral vein pressure, leading to peripheral edema.

Peripheral edema and ascites are but two of the complications of liver disease. In time, jaundice, gastrointestinal (GI) distress, skin lesions, hematologic disorders, endocrine disturbances, and peripheral neuropathies also appear.

Renal Disease

Nephrotic syndrome, also known as renal edema, is not a single disease entity but a constellation of symptoms that involve the loss of protein in the urine. Damaged glomeruli permit sodium and plasma proteins to leak into the tubules to be lost in the urine. In some cases, protein loss can exceed 3 g/day. Increased permeability of glomerular membranes is responsible for the massive loss of protein in the urine.

The loss of circulating plasma proteins reduces plasma oncotic pressure. There is a fluid shift from the extracellular compartment to interstitial spaces, thereby reducing circulating volume. The kidneys respond by increasing the retention of sodium and water. Peripheral edema results.

Hypoalbuminemia, hyperlipidemia, and hyperlipiduria are seen in patients with nephrotic syndrome. Generalized edema results from the hypoalbuminemia, and this condition, in turn, leads to hypoperfusion of the kidney. Poor perfusion of the kidney stimulates the renin-angiotensin-aldosterone response. Water and sodium are retained, and the formation of edema is continued.

PHARMACOTHERAPEUTIC OPTIONS

Diuretics are classified by their chemical structure and site of action. Classification by chemical structure is of limited value, however, in understanding pharmacodynamics. Classifying diuretics based on the major site of action is the traditional and more helpful approach. Because inhibition of sodium reabsorption in a given portion of the nephron affects electrolyte elimination, the site of action provides information as to the relative potency of the drug.

Carbonic anhydrase inhibitors (CAIs) act in the proximal tubules and loop diuretics in the thick ascending limb of the loop of Henle. The early distal tubule or the cortical portion of the diluting segment constitutes the site of action for thiazides and thiazide-like agents. The potassium-sparing diuretics act in the late distal and early collecting tubules. Two other classifications of diuretics include the osmotics and the xanthines (Fig. 39–2). Additionally, other classes of diuretics are now obsolete—the organic mercurial diuretics and the acid-forming salts.

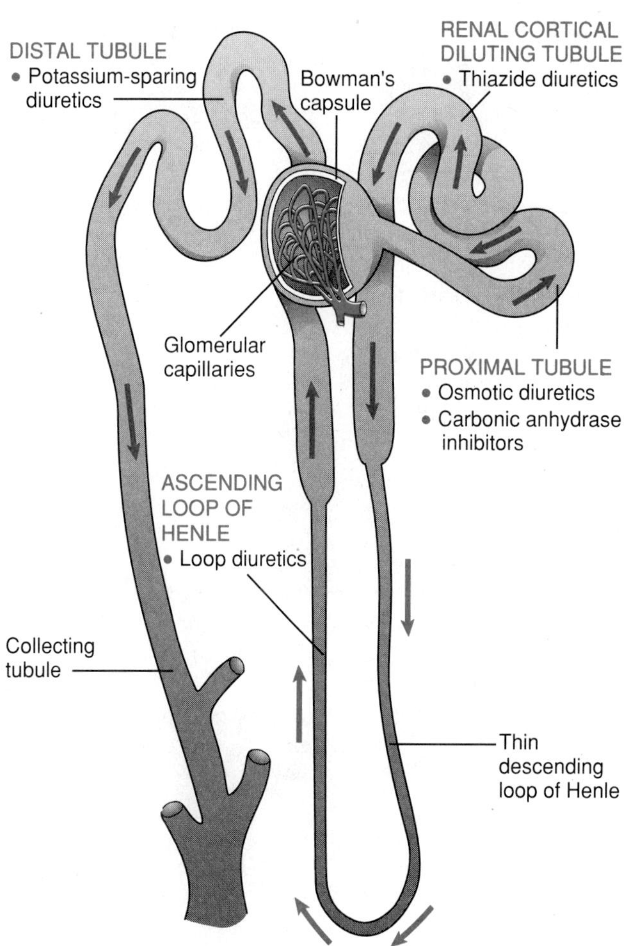

Figure 39–2 Sites of drug action. Carbonic anhydrase inhibitors act in the proximal tubules and loop diuretics in the ascending limb of the loop of Henle. The early distal tubule or the cortical portion of the diluting segment constitutes the site of action for thiazides and thiazide-like diuretics.

Carbonic Anhydrase Inhibitors

- ❒ Acetazolamide (DIAMOX); (♣) ACETAZOLAM
- ❒ Methazolamide (NEPTAZANE)
- ❒ Dichlorphenamide (DARANIDE)
- ❒ Ethoxozolamide

Indications

CAIs have been effectively used for disorders unrelated to renal function. In grand mal and petit mal epilepsy, sodium movement into cerebrospinal fluid is related to carbonic anhydrase activity of the glial and choroid plexus cells. By inhibiting enzyme activity, less sodium enters the cerebrospinal fluid and the rate of spinal fluid formation is decreased.

The most common use of CAIs is to reduce intraocular pressure in the management of glaucoma. Inhibition of carbonic anhydrase lowers the rate of aqueous humor formation by 45 to 60 percent, thus decreasing intraocular pressure. All of the CAIs have been used in the treatment of wide-angle and chronic glaucoma, and to reduce intraocular pressure after cataract surgery.

The alkaline diuresis that occurs with CAIs is beneficial in the treatment of overdose and poisoning with organic acids such as salicylates or phenobarbital. The production of alkaline urine also facilitates the elimination of uric acid and is sometimes helpful in treating hyperuricemia associated with clinical gout. Acetazolamide is also effective in ameliorating the symptoms of high-altitude pulmonary edema.

Acetazolamide is seldom a first-line diuretic. It is chosen when the addition of a proximally acting drug is warranted. It is used primarily in patients with pre-existing metabolic alkalosis, such as in patients with heart failure who have been previously treated with more distally-acting drugs. The proximal tubular action is advantageous when acetazolamide is given concurrently with a distally acting drug to produce a sequential blockade of nephron sites.

Pharmacodynamics

CAIs are derived from sulfonamide antibiotics. They bind to carbonic anhydrase, the enzyme found in the brush border of the proximal tubules' epithelial cells. They act through noncompetitive inhibition of renal carbonic anhydrase. The inhibition causes decreased production of hydrogen ions that would be exchanged for sodium. The result is elimination of sodium, potassium, chloride, and bicarbonate in the urine. Most of the sodium and chloride escaping from proximal tubules is subsequently reabsorbed in the ascending limb. However, there is an increase in the delivery of sodium bicarbonate to the distal tubule. Here, bicarbonate acts as a nonreabsorbable anion and further increases the elimination of sodium and potassium. Urine volume increases, and the normally acid urine becomes alkaline.

The diuretic effect of CAIs is limited because of the systemic hyperchloremic acidosis that occurs. In an acid environment, the effect of CAIs is decreased or absent and a refractory response develops within a few days.

Adverse Effects and Contraindications

Only a few adverse effects have been associated with CAIs. The most notable is potassium loss leading to hypokalemia. In large doses, acetazolamide produces drowsiness and paresthesias. Hypersensitivity reactions are rare. When they do occur, fever, rash, bone marrow suppression, or sulfonamide-like renal lesions are noted. Some patients experience GI upset such as anorexia, nausea, vomiting, and constipation. In the glaucoma patient, transient myopia may be noted as intraocular pressure is reduced.

Patients with pre-existing fluid and electrolyte imbalances such as hyponatremia, hyperkalemia, and hyperchloremic acidosis should not receive CAIs because they worsen these conditions. Further, CAIs are contraindicated in patients with severe pulmonary obstruction. A recurrence of calculi may occur in patients with a history of calcium-containing renal stones. Calculus formation is due to decreases in urinary citrate. In addition, teratogenic changes have been demonstrated in animals; therefore, these drugs should not be used during pregnancy (they are Category C drugs).

Pharmacokinetics

CAIs are well absorbed when they are taken orally. The onset, peak, and duration of action of CAIs are different for each drug (Table 39–1). The onset times range from 30 minutes to 4 hours, with peak ranges of 2 to 12 hours. The duration of action ranges from 6 to 24 hours. Increasing the drug dose does not increase the diuretic effect. CAIs are eliminated through the kidneys.

Drug-Drug Interactions

Alkalinization of the urine by CAIs promotes reabsorption of other drugs such as quinidine, amphetamine, ephedrine, flecainide, and pseudoephedrine (Table 39–2). Patients receiving a combination of these drugs need to be monitored for signs of toxicity.

Patients taking digoxin may develop toxicity because of a hypokalemic state. Patients on salicylates may develop severe metabolic acidosis and salicylate toxicity. Drugs that are effective in an acid urine are ineffective if used concurrently with acetazolamide.

Dosage Regimens

The dosage for CAIs depends on the specific drug and its use (Table 39–3). The oral effective dose of acetazolamide, whether it is given orally or parenterally, is 250 to 375 mg/day. Alternate-day therapy may be used in some cases. For its metabolic acidosis effects, it is administered every 8 hours. When it is used for chronic simple glaucoma, the dosage ranges between 250 to 1000 mg/day in divided doses. Because acetazolamide is an alkaline solution, it is painful if it is given intramuscularly. The intravenous (IV) route is the preferred parenteral route.

Methazolamide is usually given to adults in 25- to 100-mg doses orally two to three times per day. The dose of dichlorphenamide is 100 to 200 mg orally for the initial

TABLE 39–1 PHARMACOKINETICS OF SELECTED DIURETICS

Drug	Route	Onset	Peak	Duration	PB (%)	$t_{1/2}$	BioA (%)
Carbonic Anhydrase Inhibitors							
Acetazolamide	po	1 hr	2–4 hr	6–12 hr	Highly	13 hr	UA
	SR	2 hr	8–12 hr	18–24 hr	UA	UA	UA
Dichlorphenamide	po	1 hr	2–4 hr	6–12 hr	UA	UA	UA
Methazolamide	po	2–4 hr	6–8 hr	10–18 hr	UA	14 hr	UA
Loop Diuretics							
Bumetanide	po	30–60 min	1–2 hr	4–6 hr	95	1–1.5 hr	100
	IV	Minutes	15–30 min	0.5–1 hr	95	UA	100
Ethacrynic acid	po	30 min	2 hr	6–8 hr	95	30–70 min	UA
	IV	5 min	15–20 min	2 hr	95	UA	100
Furosemide	po	60 min	1–2 hr	6–9 hr	95	2 hr	60
	IV	5 min	30 min	2 hr	95	UA	100
Thiazides							
Bendroflumethiazide	po	1–2 hr	6–12 hr	6–12 hr	UA	3–3.9 hr	UA
Benzthiazide	po	2 hr	4–6 hr	6–12 hr	UA	UA	UA
Chlorothiazide	po	2 hr	4 hr	6–12 hr	95	1–2 hr	10
	IV	15 min	30 min	6–12 hr	UA	UA	100
Cyclothiazide	po	6 hr	7–12 hr	18–24 hr	UA	UA	UA
Hydrochlorothiazide	po	2 hr	4 hr	6–12 hr	65	1–2 hr	UA
Hydroflumethiazide	po	1–2 hr	3–4 hr	18–24 hr	UA	17 hr	UA
Methyclothiazide	po	2 hr	6 hr	24 hr	UA	UA	UA
Polythiazide	po	2 hr	6 hr	24–48 hr	UA	25 hr	UA
Trichlormethiazide	po	2 hr	6 hr	24 hr	UA	2–7 hr	UA
Thiazide-Like Diuretics							
Chlorthalidone	po	2 hr	4–6 hr	24–72 hr	UA	40 hr*	UA
Metolazone	po	1 hr	2 hr	12–24 hr	33	8 hr	UA
Quinethazone	po	2 hr	6 hr	18–24 hr	UA	UA	UA
Potassium-Sparing Drugs							
Amiloride	po	2 hr	6 hr	24 hr	40	6–9 hr	20
Spironolactone	po	8 hr	2–4 hr	48 hr	90	17–22 hr	UA
Triamterene	po	2–4 hr	2–4 hr	72 hr	60	2–4 hr	UA
Osmotic Drugs							
Mannitol	IV	30–60 min	*IOP:* 30–60 min *Diuresis:* 6–12 hr	4–8 hr	UA	15 min–1.5 hr	UA
Urea	IV	15 min	*IOP:* 1–2 hr *Diuresis* 6–12 hr	5–6 hr	UA	3–4 hr	UA

*Chlorthalidone is sequestered in red blood cells; the $t_{1/2}$ is longer if blood rather than plasma is analyzed;.

BioA, Bioavailability; IOP, intraocular pressure; PB, protein binding; SR, sustained release; UA, unavailable;.$t_{1/2}$, elimination half-life.

TABLE 39–2 DRUG-DRUG INTERACTIONS OF SELECTED DIURETICS

Drugs	Interactive Drugs	Interaction
Carbonic anhydrase inhibitors	Thyroid agents	Decreased uptake of thyroidal iodine
	Methenamine	Alkalinization of urine interferes with action of interactive agent
	Salicylates	Severe metabolic acidosis and salicylate toxicity
	Quinidine Amphetamines Ephedrine, pseudoephedrine Flecainide	Alkalinization of the urine promotes reabsorption of interactive agent
Loop diurectics	Oral hypoglycemic drugs	Increased potential for hyperglycemia
	Aminoglycoside Cisplatin	Increased potential for ototoxicity
	Lithium carbonate Salicylates	Decreased elimination of lithium and salicylates; lithium toxicity, salicylate toxicity
	Digoxin	Increased potential for digoxin toxicity related to potassium loss
	NSAIDs	Decreased antihypertensive and diuretic effect of diuretic
	Neuromuscular blocking drugs	Increased effects of neuromuscular blockade
	Phenytoin	Decreased absorption and effectiveness of furosemide
	Theophyllines	Increased diuresis from furosemide
Thiazide and thiazide-like diuretics	Antihypertensive agents	Increased action of the antihypertensive agent
	Digoxin	Increased potential for digoxin toxicity due to potassium loss
	Oral hypoglycemic drugs Insulin	May cause hyperglycemia and hyponatremia, resulting in thiazide resistance
	Corticosteroids ACTH	Increased loss of potassium
	Probenecid	Decreased uric acid elimination; may precipitate gout
	Lithium carbonate Salicylates	Decreased elimination of lithium, salicylates; lithium toxicity, salicylate toxicity
	NSAIDs	Decreased antihypertensive effect of thiazide
	Depolarizing skeletal muscle relaxants	Increased responsiveness to skeletal muscle relaxants
	Methenamine	Methenamine requires acid urine to be effective, thiazides cause alkaline urine
	Anion exchange resins	Decreased absorption of thiazides if taken concurrently
Potassium-sparing diuretics	Other potassium-sparing diuretics and potassium supplements ACE inhibitors	Increased risk of hyperkalemia
	Digoxin	Decreased elimination of digoxin; digoxin toxicity
	Salicylates	Decreased effectiveness of spironolactone
	Antihypertensives	Increased effectiveness of antihypertensive
	Norepinephrine	Decreased vascular response to norepinephrine
Osmotic diuretics	Lithium	Decreased effectiveness of lithium in presence of mannitol

ACE, Angiotensin-converting enzyme; ACTH, adrenocorticotropic hormone; NSAIDs, nonsteroidal anti-inflammatory drugs.

dose but can be repeated in 100-mg doses every 12 hours until the desired effect is achieved. A maintenance dose of 25 to 100 mg may be given once to three times per day.

Laboratory Considerations

Patients receiving concurrent glycoside cardiac therapy should have digoxin levels monitored. Because patients on CAIs are at risk for fluid and electrolyte disturbances, acid-base balance and fluid-electrolyte balance should be monitored. Acetazolamide has caused elevations in blood glucose and glycosuria in patients with a history of diabetes.

Loop Diuretics

❒ Bumetanide (BUMEX)
❒ Ethacrynic acid (EDECRIN)
❒ Furosemide (LASIX,); (🍁) APO-FUROSEMIDE, NOVO-SEMIDE, LASIX

Indications

Furosemide, the prototype loop diuretic, is one of the top 10 prescription drugs, the second most prescribed diuretic, and the most commonly used loop diuretic. Loop diuretics are often referred to as high-ceiling diuretics because they are the most potent diuretics available.

TABLE 39–3 DOSAGE REGIMENS OF SELECTED DIURETICS

Drug	Use	Dosage	Implications
Carbonic Anhydrase Inhibitors			
Acetazolamide	Pre-existing metabolic alkalosis, grand and petit mal epilepsy, acute and chronic glaucoma, decrease IOP after cataract surgery, overdose of organic acids (e.g. salicylates, phenobarbital)	*Adult: Diuresis.* 250–375 mg/day po daily or every other day. *Alkalosis:* 250–375 mg po q8hr. *Glaucoma:* 250–1000 mg po/day in divided doses	Use caution if giving other drugs whose elimination is inhibited by alkaline urine
Methazolamide	Open-angle glaucoma, preoperatively in narrow-angle glaucoma, concurrent with miotic, osmotic agents	*Adult:* 50–100 mg po BID–TID	Give in morning to avoid sleeplessness. Potassium replacement if serum potassium level less than 3.0 mEq/L
Dichlorphenamide	Open-angle glaucoma, preoperatively in narrow-angle glaucoma, concurrent with miotic, osmotic agents	*Adult:* 100–200 mg po. May repeat in 100-mg doses q12hr until desired response achieved. Maintenance: 25–100 mg po QD–TID	Cautious use in renal or hepatic disorders
Loop Diuretics			
Bumetanide	Edema, hypertension	*Adult:* 0.5–2 mg po single daily dose. May repeat q4–5 hr up to 10 mg/day. Maintenance: intermittently with 1–2 day rest periods	Not FDA approved for use in children. Use cautiously in patients with hepatic cirrhosis and ascites, and in those with depressed renal function. Supplemental potassium or use of potassium-sparing diuretics may be used to prevent hypokalemia. May be substituted for furosemide in sensitive patients
Ethacrynic acid	Acute pulmonary edema, other forms of edema	*Adult: Acute pulmonary edema:* 50–100 mg IV over several minutes *or* 50–200 mg po QD or on alternate days. *Other forms of edema:* May use up to 200 mg po BID *Child: Edema:* 25 mg po. Gradually increase by 25-mg increments until therapeutic effect achieved	Use cautiously in patients with electrolyte imbalance, azotemia, or oliguria. If these disorders develop drug may be discontinued
Furosemide	Acute pulmonary edema, other forms of edema, hypertensive crisis, acute and chronic renal failure, hypertension, hypercalcemia	*Adult: Pulmonary edema:* 40 mg IV. May repeat q2hr PRN. *Other forms of edema:* 20–80 mg po QD–BID up to 600 mg QD *or* 20–40 mg IV. May repeat q2hr until therapeutic effect is achieved *Hypertension:* 20–80 mg po QD–BID *or* 20–24 mg IV *Hypertensive crisis:* 100–200 mg over 1–2 minutes. *ARF:* 100–200 mg IV over 1–2 minutes. *CRF:* 80–120 mg po QD *Child:* 1–2 mg/kg po q6–8 hr *or* 1 mg/kg IM/IV. Increase by 1 mg/kg after 2 hours. Maximum of 6 mg/kg/day	Can cause profound water and electrolyte depletion. Use cautiously in patients with cardiogenic shock complicated by pulmonary edema. Use cautiously in patients with anuria and hepatic coma
Thiazide Diuretics			
Bendroflumethiazide	Edema of cardiac, renal or hepatic failure; hypertension	*Adult:* 5–20 mg po QD in divided doses. Maintenance: 2.5–5 mg po QD *Child:* 0.1–0.4 mg/kg QD in 1–2 doses. Maintenance:0.05–0.1 mg/kg in 1–2 doses	Use cautiously in severe renal disease or impaired hepatic function
Benzthiazide		*Adult: Edema:* 50–200 mg po QD in divided doses *Hypertension:* 50 mg po QD–BID *Child:* 1–4 mg/kg QD or in three divided doses	Use cautiously in patients with severe renal disease or impaired hepatic function
Chlorothiazide		*Adult: Edema:* 500 mg or 2 g po/IV QD in divided doses *Hypertension:* 500 mg to 1 g po/IV QD in divided doses *Child less than 6 mo:* Up to 30 mg/kg QD in divided doses *Child older than 6 mo:* 2.2 mg/kg po/IV QD in divided doses	May not be administered IM or SC. Use cautiously in patients with severe renal disease

TABLE 39–3 DOSAGE REGIMENS OF SELECTED DIURETICS *Continued*

Drug	Use	Dosage	Implications
Thiazide Diuretics *continued*			
Cyclothiazide		*Adult:* 1–2 mg po QD. Maintenance: 1 mg po QD 2–4 times/week *Child:* 0.02–0.04 mg/kg po QD. Maintenance: Reduce dosage for maintenance	Use cautiously in patients with severe renal disease or impaired hepatic function
Hydrochlorothiazide		*Adult: Edema:* 25–200 mg po QD or intermittently *Hypertension:* 25–100 mg po QD or in divided doses *Child less than 6 mo:* 3.3 mg/kg po QD in two divided doses *Child over 6 mo:* 2.2 mg/kg po QD in two divideed doses	Increase or decrease dose based on patient response. Use cautiously in patients with severe renal disease, impaired hepatic function, and progressive hepatic disease
Hydroflumethiazide		*Adult: Edema:* 25–100 mg po QD in divided doses. Maintenance: 25–200 mg po intermittently or on alternate days *Hypertension:* 50–100 mg po QD–BID. Maintenance: 25–200 mg po on alternate days. Up to maximum of 200 mg QD *Child:* 1 mg/kg po QD	Use cautiously in patients with severe renal disease, impaired hepatic function, and progressive hepatic disease
Methyclothiazide		*Adult:* 2.5–10 mg po QD	Long-acting drug. Pediatric dosage not determined
Polythiazide		*Adult: Edema:* 1–4 mg po daily. *Hypertension:* 2–4 mg po QD *Child:* 0.02–0.08 mg/kg po QD	Long-acting drug. Use cautiously in severe renal disease, impaired hepatic function, and allergies
Trichlormethiazide		*Adult: Edema:* 1–4 mg po QD in divided doses *Hypertension:* 2–4 mg po QD *Child over 6 mo:* 0.07 mg/kg po QD in two divided doses	Long-acting drug
Thiazide-Like Diuretics			
Chlorthalidone	Edema, hypertension.	*Adult: Edema:* 50–100 mg po QD *or* 100 mg on alternate days. *Hypertension:* 25–100 mg po QD *or* 100 mg 3 times/week or on alternate days. Maintenance edema/hypertension: May require up to 200 mg/day for therapeutic effect. *Child:* 2 mg/kg po three times weekly	Long-acting drug. Use cautiously in patients with severe renal disease, impaired hepatic function, and progressive hepatic disease
Metolazone	Hypertension and edema secondary to heart failure, hepatic disease, renal disease	*Adult: Edema of CHF:* 5–10 mg po QD *Renal/hepatic disease:* 5–20 mg po QD *Hypertension:* 2.5–5 mg po QD	Effective even if GFR is less than 20 mL/minute. Pediatric dosage not established. Use cautiously in patients with hyperuremia, impaired renal or hepatic function
Quinethazone	Edema	*Adult:* 50–100 mg po QD. May be increased up to 200 mg/day	Pediatric dosage not established. Use cautiously in severe renal disease, impaired hepatic function, and allergies
Potassium-Sparing Drugs			
Amiloride	Adjunct to thiazide or loop diuretics in hypertension or edema associated with heart failure. Maintenance of serum potassium levels in patients with hypokalemia	*Adult:* 5–10 mg po QD with food. Increase by up to 20 mg/day	Pediatric dosage not determined. Contraindicated in patients with elevated serum potassium levels
Spironolactone	Refractory edema, idiopathic edema, cirrhosis, nephrotic syndrome, hirsutism, primary aldosteronism	*Adult: Edema:* 25–200 mg po QD *Essential hypertension:* 50–100 mg po QD. May be given as a single dose or in two divided doses. Maintenance: dosage adjusted up to 400 mg po QD based on patient's response *Child: Edema:* 3.3 mg/kg po QD in divided doses	Use cautiously in patients with fluid and electrolye disturbances, renal insufficiency, and hepatic disease

Table continued on following page

TABLE 39–3 DOSAGE REGIMENS OF SELECTED DIURETICS *Continued*

Drug	Use	Dosage	Implications
Potassium-Sparing Drugs *continued*			
Triamterene	Adjunct to other diuretics for hypertension, edema associated with heart failure, cirrhosis, nephrotic syndrome, idiopathic edema, steroid-induced edema, and edema of hyperaldosteronism	*Adult:* 100 mg po BID up to 300 mg/day *Child:* 4 mg/kg po QD in two divided doses. Increase up to 6 mg/kg/day. Maintenance: not to exceed 30 mg/day	Use cautiously in patients with hepatic disease, diabetes mellitus, pregnancy and lactation
Osmotics			
Mannitol	Oliguria, acute renal failure, increased intraocular and intracranial pressure. To induce diuresis in treatment of drug intoxication	*Adult: Diuresis:* 50–100 g IV of a 5–25% solution over 24 hours. *Prevent ARF or oliguria:* 50–100 g of a 5–25% solution over 24 hours. *IIOP/IICP:* 1.5–2 g/kg IV of a 15–20% solution. Give 1–1.5 hours before surgery *Drug intoxication:* Up to 200 g IV of a 5–10% solution. May repeat once if response is not adequate (IV rate: 30–50 mL/hour) *Child:* Above-mentioned doses can be used in children over 12 years of age	Contraindicated in patients with severe pulmonary edema, heart failure, progressive renal disease and anuria. Solution crystallizes, especially at low temperatures. Do not use solution when crystals are present
Urea	IICP and IIOP, prevent acute renal failure from surgery or trauma	*Adult:* 1–1.5 g/kg IV in a 30% solution infused over 1.5–2 hrs. Maximum dose not to exceed 120 g/day *Child over age 2 yr:* 0.5–1.5 g/kg IV in a 30% solution infused over 1.5–2 hrs	Contraindicated in patients with severe renal and hepatic impairment, severe dehydration, and active intracranial bleeding. Use cautiously in pregnancy, lactation, in patients with cardiac disease and sickle cell disease with CNS involvement

ARF, Acute renal failure; CHF, congestive heart failure; CNS, central nervous system; FDA, Food and Drug Administration; GFR, glomerular filtration rate; IICP, increased intracranial pressure; IIOP, increased intraocular pressure; IOP, intraocular pressure.

Loop diuretics are indicated in the management of edema related to cardiac, renal, or hepatic disease. Their rapid action and effectiveness have made them the drugs of choice in the treatment of cardiogenic pulmonary edema resulting from left-sided heart failure. Because of their efficacy, they are sometimes useful in the early stages of renal failure, probably because of their ability to increase renal prostaglandin levels.

Furosemide is useful specifically in the first 24 hours of acute oliguric renal failure. Volume depletion is corrected first, and then diuresis is initiated. In some clinical settings, the patient may require low-dose dopamine, a sympathomimetic drug, and mannitol, an osmotic drug, in addition to furosemide. If a patient does not respond to the treatment, it is usually because of insufficient intravascular volume expansion and a dose of diuretic that is too high.

The ability of loop diuretics to inhibit calcium reabsorption makes them useful in hypercalcemic crises. Loop diuretics may also be used in hypertensive patients who are unresponsive to thiazides. Loop diuretics may be used in combination with potassium-sparing diuretics to prevent hypokalemia. Furosemide is used in conjunction with mannitol to treat severe cerebral edema.

Pharmacodynamics

Loop diuretics are a group of dissimilar chemical compounds that have similar mechanisms and sites of action. In order for a loop diuretic to be effective, some degree of renal function must exist. Loop diuretics are secreted by the proximal tubule and travel to the loop of Henle.

Loop diuretics have a direct action on the ascending limb of the Loop of Henle, inhibiting sodium and chloride reabsorption. A dose-dependent diuresis is produced that is characterized by increased water, sodium, potassium, chloride, calcium, and magnesium elimination. Twenty to twenty-five percent of the sodium filtered is eliminated. The increased potassium loss is primarily due to the increase in volume flow rate through distal tubules and increased delivery of sodium to the sodium-potassium exchange pumps.

Further, loop diuretics decrease left ventricular filling pressure and increase venous capacitance. Increased renal vasodilation permits an increase in the inner cortical and medullary blood flow. Increased medullary flow leads to a decrease in medullary hypertonicity and decreased water reabsorption in the collecting ducts. Evidence suggests that this is a prostaglandin-induced process. The use of loop diuretics leads to increased amounts of the vasodilator prostaglandin E_2 by inhibiting the enzyme prostaglandin dehydrogenase. Prostaglandin E_2 also acts directly on the ascending limb to inhibit chloride transport. Hence, hemodynamics seem to improve even before significant diuresis has occurred.

Adverse Effects and Contraindications

Most adverse effects and contraindications to the use of loop diuretics are related to fluid and electrolyte imbalances due to excessive diuresis. Volume contraction and loss of electrolytes leads to hypovolemia, hyponatremia, hypokalemia, hyperuricemia, and hyperglycemia. Because potassium is lost along with the water, hypokalemia frequently is a problem. If a patient is also taking digoxin, there is an additional risk for digoxin toxicity (see Chapter 29) and development of arrhythmias.

Ototoxicity may occur as a result of electrolyte alterations in the inner ear. The potential for ototoxicity is greater with ethacrynic acid and less so with furosemide. Bumetanide is the least toxic of the three drugs. The potential for toxicity is of particular concern in patients who concurrently receive other ototoxic drugs. In general, ototoxicity is a reversible effect, disappearing on withdrawal of the drug. Permanent hearing loss has been reported with ethacrynic acid.

Hyperuricemia is related, in part, to the contraction of fluid volume. However, it is also due to interference with the elimination of uric acid by the organic acid excretory transport system.

A decrease in glucose tolerance has been reported occasionally. The rationale for its development is unclear. However, it may be associated with diuretic-induced hypokalemia or insulin activity.

Occasionally, allergic reactions, photosensitivity, leukopenia, anemia, granulocytopenia, and thrombocytopenia occur. Allergic reactions manifest as skin eruptions, exfoliative dermatitis, and jaundice.

Loop diuretics must be used cautiously in pregnant women. Only when the potential benefits significantly outweigh the risks would the drug be indicated. The safe use of bumetanide in children younger than 18 years of age has not been established.

Pharmacokinetics

In general, loop diuretics maintain their efficacy in patients with impaired renal function. They are well absorbed with a steep dose-response curve, have a rapid onset of action, are widely distributed, and are over 90-percent protein bound (see Table 39–1). Peak concentrations are attained within ½ to 2 hours, with a duration of action of 30 minutes to 9 hours. Although loop diuretics are extensively bound to plasma proteins, they have a strong affinity for the organic acid excretory transporter, accounting for the relatively short half-lives. Furosemide is eliminated essentially unchanged through the kidneys. Loop diuretics cross the placental membranes and also appear in breast milk.

Bumetanide is structurally related to furosemide and is comparable in activity and maximal effects, but it is considerably more potent on a weight basis. Bumetanide is biotransformed by the liver. One-third of ethacrynic acid is eliminated in the bile and the remainder through the kidneys.

Drug-Drug Interactions

There are a number of drugs that interact with loop diuretics resulting in fluid and electrolyte imbalance, altered renal function, and enhancement of the other drugs' effects (see Table 39–2). Loop diuretics interact with oral hypoglycemic drugs to increase the potential for hyperglycemia. When they are used with aminoglycosides, cisplatin, or other drugs with ototoxicity potential, they may cause additive ototoxicity. Patients taking lithium carbonate or salicylates may experience a decrease in drug elimination, resulting in lithium or salicylate toxicity.

Loop diuretics used in conjunction with cardiac glycosides can lead to electrolyte disturbances that predispose the patient to hypokalemia-induced arrhythmias. When they are used with nonsteroidal anti-inflammatory drugs, the antihypertensive and diuretic characteristics of loop diuretics are inhibited. Furosemide interacts with neuromuscular blocking drugs to enhance neuromuscular blockade and with phenytoin to decrease the absorption and effectiveness of furosemide.

Dosage Regimens

Because of their efficacy and potency, initial doses of loop diuretics should be relatively low (see Table 39–3). Although loop diuretics are effective in renal impairment, higher than normal doses may be needed when GFRs fall as low as 2 mL/minute.

For edema or hypertension, an initial oral furosemide dose of 20 to 80 mg is given once or twice daily. When given IV, 20 to 40 mg is used. The dosage may be increased if needed by 20 to 40 mg at 2-hour intervals to a total daily dose of 600 mg. For pediatric use, the dose is 1 to 2 mg/kg of body weight, given at 6- to 8-hour intervals, or 1 mg/kg intramuscularly (IM) or IV. The maximum pediatric dose is 6 mg/kg.

In the management of pulmonary edema, furosemide is given at frequent intervals so that urine flow rates can be titrated to the desired level while avoiding excessively rapid volume depletion. An initial dose of 40 mg IV is recommended. The dose may be repeated in 2 hours if there is no response. The pediatric dose is 1 mg/kg IV. The pediatric dose may increased by 1 mg/kg after 2 hours. However, the use of IV furosemide in children may predispose the child to episodes of diarrhea. The diarrhea is secondary to the sorbitol that is present in the parenteral solution.

For most conditions, the dosage of loop diuretic is reduced as blood pressure falls. Therapy should be continued until the lowest possible dose of furosemide is reached that is compatible with maximum symptom relief.

Oral bumetanide is given in doses of 0.5 to 2.0 mg every 4 to 5 hours up to a maximum of 10 mg/24 hours. Bumetanide dosage should be checked with extreme caution since it is 40 times more potent than furosemide.

Laboratory Considerations

Loop diuretics have effects on digoxin, warfarin, and lithium that can lead to toxicity. Patients taking these drugs need to have serum digoxin, warfarin, and lithium levels monitored. With concurrent use of theophylline and furosemide, theophylline levels should be monitored.

Electrolytes, renal and hepatic functioning, and glucose and uric acid levels should be monitored before and periodically throughout the course of therapy. These patients may develop metabolic alkalosis, hypokalemia, hyponatremia, and hypochloremia because potassium, sodium, and chloride are lost. Calcium and magnesium levels may reflect hypocalcemia and hypomagnesemia. Glucose and uric acid levels may also be elevated.

Thiazide and Thiazide-Like Diuretics

- ❒ Bendroflumethiazide (NATURETIN)
- ❒ Benzthiazide (AGUATAG, AQUAPRES, EXNA, MARAZIDE, PROAQUA, URAZIDE)
- ❒ Chlorothiazide (DIURIL)
- ❒ Chlorthalidone (HYGROTON, THALITONE); (🍁) APO-CHLORTHALIDONE
- ❒ Hydrochlorothiazide (ESIDRIX, HYDRODIURIL)
- ❒ Hydroflumethiazide (DIUCARDIN, SALURON)
- ❒ Methyclothiazide (AQUATENSEN, ENDURON)
- ❒ Metolazone (ZAROXOLYN, MYKROX)
- ❒ Polythiazide (RENESE)
- ❒ Quinethazone (HYDROMOX)
- ❒ Trichlormethiazide (METAHYDRIN, NAQUA)

Indications

Thiazide and thiazide-like diuretics are sulfonamide derivatives, developed approximately 30 years ago in an attempt to find a more potent diuretic to replace CAIs. Thiazides are often the first choice in treating salt-sensitive patients, and they are frequently used to control the edema associated with pre-existing hypertension, right-sided heart failure, and chronic hepatic or renal disease. Their beneficial effects are present after the excess fluid volume has been removed. Increased sodium and water elimination is accompanied by weight loss and a slightly negative state of sodium balance. The antihypertensive effect persists even though a return in sodium balance occurs. Along with sodium restriction, thiazides are usually sufficient to control mild to moderate hypertension. They tend to potentiate antihypertensive drugs by one-third to one-half.

Fixed combinations of thiazide diuretics and antihypertensives are available, primarily for the management of hypertension. The combined agents include thiazides with angiotensin-converting enzyme (ACE) inhibitors, alpha or beta blockers, centrally acting antihypertensives, electrolytes, monoamine oxidase inhibitors, potassium-sparing diuretics, rauwolfias, vasodilators, and combinations of thiazide, rauwolfia, and a vasodilator (see Combination Diuretics).

COMBINATION DIURETICS

Thiazide or thiazide-like diuretic in combination with	
ACE inhibitors	• Captopril with hydrochlorothiazide (CAPOZIDE)
	• Enalapril maleate with hydrochlorothiazide (VASERETIC)
	• Lisinopril with hydrochlorothiazide
Alpha blocker	• Prazosin with polythiazide (MINIZIDE)
Beta blockers	• Atenolol with chlorthalidone (TENORETIC)
	• Labetalol HCL with hydrochlorothiazide (NORMOZIDE)
	• Metoprolol with hydrochlorothiazide (LOPRESSOR HCT)
	• Nadolol with bendroflumethiazide (CORZIDE)
	• Pindolol with hydrochlorothiazide
	• Propranolol with hydrochlorothiazide (INDERIDE)
	• Timolol with hydrochlorothiazide (TIMOLIDE)
Centrally acting antihypertensives	• Clonidine with chlorthalidone (COMBIPRESS)
	• Guanethidine with hydrochlorothiazide (ESIMIL)
	• Methyldopa with chlorothiazide (ALDOCLOR)
	• Methyldopa with hydrochlorothiazide (ALDORIL)
Electrolyte	• Potassium chloride with bendroflumethiazide (NATURETIN)
MAO inhibitor	• Pargyline with methyclothiazide
Potassium-sparing diuretics	• Amiloride with hydrochlorothiazide (MODURETIC)
	• Spironolactone with hydrochlorothiazide (ALDACTAZIDE, SPIRACTAZIDE)
	• Triamterene with hydrochlorothiazide (DYAZIDE, MAXZIDE)
Rauwolfias	• Deserpidine with hydrochlorothiazide
	• Deserpidine with methyclothiazide (ENDURONYL)
	• Reserpine withchlorothiazide
	• Reserpine with chlorthalidone (REGROTON, DEMI-REGROTON)
	• Reserpine with benzthiazide (EXNA-R)
	• Reserpine with hydrochlorothiazide (HYDROPRES, HYDROSINE)
	• Reserpine with hydroflumethiazide (SALAZIDE, SALUTENSIN)
	• Reserpine with trichlormethiazide (DIURESE, METATENSIN No. 2)
	• Reserpine with methyclothiazide (DIUTENSEN-R)
	• Reserpine with quinethazone (HYDROMOX)
	• Reserpine with polythiazide (RENESE)
	• Reserpine, potassium chloride, with bendroflumethiazide
	• Reserpine, potassium chloride, with flumethiazide
Vasodilator	• Hydralazine with hydrochlorothiazide (APRESAZIDE APRESOLINE-ESIDRIX, H-H)
Rauwolfia and vasodilator	• Reserpine, hydralazine HCL with hydrochlorothiazide
	• UNIPRES, (SER-AP-ES, SERPAZIDE, TRI-HYDROSERPINE, HYDROPRES)

ACE, Angiotensin-converting enzyme; MAO, monoamine oxidase.

In addition, thiazides are the only drugs available to decrease urine volume in patients with nephrogenic diabetes insipidus, in whom the drugs produce a fall in urine volume and a rise in urine osmolarity. The drug-induced contraction of fluid volume is associated with a decrease in GFR and an increase in proximal reabsorption. The reabsorption results in a decrease in the delivery of the filtrate to the distal nephron. More filtrate is reabsorbed than would have been without the thiazide. Thiazides do not cure diabetes insipidus, although improved fluid balance is achieved.

The disadvantage of thiazides include a relatively low potency and resistance to its effects in the presence of renal impairment. Furthermore, they have no therapeutic value in patients with a GFR of less than 25 to 30 mL/minute.

Pharmacodynamics

Thiazide and thiazide-like diuretics act by inhibiting the reabsorption of sodium and chloride in the early distal tubule and diluting segment of the ascending Loop of Henle, increasing the elimination of sodium and water. They have a relatively moderate potency and lead to elimination of 5 to 8 percent of the filtered load. Sodium and chloride ions pass into the collecting ducts, taking water with them. The exact mechanism that causes this process remains unclear. Potassium is also lost.

A minor degree of carbonic anhydrase inhibition is created. The elimination of bicarbonate ions is increased, along with loss of additional sodium ions. However, this action lasts for only a few days. During this time, elimination of ammonium, urates, and calcium is decreased.

Adverse Effects and Contraindications

The most common adverse effects of thiazide and thiazide-like diuretics are electrolyte imbalances. The increased quantity of sodium reaching the distal tubule site is the main reason for the potassium loss in the urine. Serum potassium levels can fall below 3.0 to 3.5 mEq/L with long-term therapy. In addition, serum sodium, chloride, and magnesium levels fall. In contrast to the loop diuretics, serum calcium levels may be elevated with thiazides due to the increased protein-bound fraction of calcium.

Like uric acid, thiazides occupy the organic acid transport system, and competition may result in hyperuricemia and gout in susceptible people. In addition, contraction of plasma volume also serves to increase uric acid reabsorption in the proximal tubule.

Although hyperlipidemia and hyperglycemia have been reported with thiazides, such increases are relatively small and their clinical significance is controversial. There may be interference with the conversion of proinsulin to insulin. Thiazides have also been reported to reduce libido and cause impotence.

Some patients experience GI upset, including nausea, vomiting, constipation, jaundice, and even pancreatitis when taking thiazides. Blood dyscrasias have also been reported that include leukopenia, thrombocytopenia, agranulocytosis, and aplastic anemia.

Mild dizziness, headache, and paresthesias have been seen. In the case of overdose, lethargy, and even coma may occur. Cardiac function and respiratory rate are not significantly depressed, although orthostatic hypotension unrelated to volume changes may be experienced.

Thiazide diuretics exhibit cross-allergenicity with sulfonamide drugs. Allergic reactions such as urticaria are usually mild, although anaphylaxis has occurred. Use of thiazide diuretics during pregnancy is not recommended because they cross the placental membranes (it is a Category B drug). Newborns may develop thrombocytopenia and bone marrow depression. The drugs also appear in breast milk.

Pharmacokinetics

Thiazides are readily, but incompletely, absorbed by the GI tract. The drugs are variably plasma protein bound, ranging from 65 percent for hydrochlorothiazide to 95 percent for chlorothiazide.

Onset of drug action, peak effects, and the duration of action vary with the various drugs (see Table 39–1). Generally, the onset of action occurs within 1 hour of oral intake. Depending on drug elimination rate, the duration of action can last from 24 to 48 hours with a few exceptions. IV chlorothiazide lasts for 2 hours, polythiazide action from 24 to 48 hours, and chlorthalidone action from 24 to 72 hours. They all differ in plasma and biologic half-life. Thiazide elimination is delayed in patients with heart failure, impaired renal function in which the GFR is less than 20 mL/minute, or in any disorder that results in reduced blood flow to the kidneys.

Much depends on the lipid solubility of thiazides and their volume of distribution. There is a flat dose-response curve, which means that the toxic and therapeutic levels never meet. As a result, the thiazide and thiazide-like diuretics have a wide margin of safety. The greater volume of distribution leads to a lower renal clearance and longer duration of action. Although chlorthalidone has a slightly longer duration of action than others, no real benefit is achieved because thiazide diuretics are all dosed once daily and are well tolerated.

The differences in thiazides appear to be proportional to plasma protein binding and the degree of reabsorption in the renal tubule. They differ also in their degree of biotransformation and elimination. For example, hydrochlorothiazide is eliminated unchanged, whereas polythiazide is extensively biotransformed.

Drug-Drug Interactions

Thiazide and thiazide-like diuretics potentiate the actions of antihypertensive drugs, especially those with actions at ganglionic or peripheral adrenergic sites (see Table 39–2). Patients on digoxin may be more susceptible to digoxin toxicity because of the potassium loss. The situation is worsened when thiazides are used concurrently with corticosteroids or adrenocorticotropic hormone. Thiazide diuretics enhance the effects of depolarizing skeletal muscle relaxants such as tubocurarine, a drug frequently used in surgery. Lithium elimination is decreased by thiazides, predisposing the patient to lithium toxicity. Because thiazide diuretics produce an alkaline urine, the effectiveness of methenamine is decreased. Anion exchange resins delay the absorption of thiazides if they are taken concurrently.

Dosage Regimens

The dosage of thiazide and thiazide-like diuretics should be individually adjusted (see Table 39–3). The drug may be administered daily as a single dose as when treating edema, or in divided doses when treating hypertension. Use of any of the thiazides warrant caution in patients who have renal or hepatic disease.

Laboratory Considerations

Laboratory considerations include monitoring serum electrolytes (especially potassium), blood glucose, blood urea nitrogen, and serum uric acid levels before and periodically throughout therapy. Some thiazide diuretics are not as effective in patients with blood urea nitrogen and creatinine levels higher than twice normal. The thiazide diuretics may cause increased serum cholesterol, low-density lipoprotein and triglyceride concentrations.

Thiazide diuretics interact with digoxin and lithium; thus, serum levels of digoxin and lithium should be monitored on a regular basis to reduce the risk of toxicity.

Calcium levels may rise due to the decrease in calcium elimination. In a few patients who have been on long-term therapy, both hypercalcemia and hypophosphatemia have occurred. The imbalance may lead to suppression of parathyroid gland activity. In these patients, calcium, phosphate, and parathyroid hormone levels may need to be monitored. For accurate results, the thiazide drug should be stopped before obtaining tests for parathyroid function.

Potassium-Sparing Diuretics

❐ Amiloride (MIDAMOR)
❐ Spironolactone (ALDACTONE)
❐ Triamterene (DYRENIUM)

Indications

Potassium-sparing drugs are weak diuretics when they are used alone. However, their ability to protect against potassium loss has made them beneficial as adjunct therapy with other, more effective drugs. They are generally used in combination with a thiazide diuretic or an antihypertensive drug. These drugs preserve both hydrogen and potassium, counteracting the metabolic alkalosis produced when sodium and potassium are eliminated with chloride.

Spironolactone and triamterene are used to treat primary aldosteronism and edema secondary to cirrhosis, nephrotic syndrome, idiopathic edema, and hirsutism. Although once widely used in the treatment of hypertension, spironolactone has lost its popularity because of its adverse effects (i.e., hyperkalemia, gynecomastia). Breast cancer and fibroadenomas have been reported in a few male patients during and after spironolactone therapy. No cause-and-effect relationship has been established, however.

These drugs are contraindicated in patients with anuria or renal impairment and severe hepatic function. They should be used with caution in patients with diabetes mellitus and in patients who are either pregnant or lactating.

Pharmacodynamics

Potassium-sparing diuretics act on the distal renal tubules to inhibit distal sodium-potassium exchange. The result is an increase in the elimination of 2 to 3 percent of filtered sodium and chloride. The small percentage eliminated is due to the modest amounts of water and solutes delivered to the area.

This class of diuretics is divided into two categories based on their effectiveness in the presence of aldosterone, because a portion of the sodium-potassium exchange in the distal tubule is aldosterone dependent and a portion is aldosterone independent. Competitive antagonism of aldosterone results in inhibition of the sodium-potassium exchange. Spironolactone is the major aldosterone antagonist. It is effective when mineralocorticoid activity is high, but it has little activity in the absence of aldosterone. Because spironolactone is a competitive inhibitor, its action is overcome by higher concentrations of aldosterone. Calcium elimination is increased through the direct effect of aldosterone on tubular transport mechanisms.

The aldosterone-independent sodium-potassium exchange is inhibited by triamterene and amiloride, drugs that directly block the uptake of sodium into the distal tubule cell. Triamterene is effective from the peritubular side. Amiloride acts at the luminal surface of the tubule cell. The voltage-dependent process results in a decrease in sodium permeability and sodium loss without potassium loss.

Adverse Effects and Contraindications

Because of the potassium-sparing characteristics, there is an increased potential for hyperkalemia with chronic use. Other general reactions include headache, dizziness, orthostatic hypotension (related to volume depletion), dry mouth, and sore throat. Megaloblastic anemia and folic acid deficiency are sometimes seen with triamterene use. In rare instances, agranulocytosis has occurred with spironolactone. Both spironolactone and amiloride may cause GI distress.

Spironolactone may also contribute to breast tenderness and menstrual abnormalities in women and gynecomastia in men. Some men who take spironolactone have reported impotence. All three agents have the potential to induce hyperchloremic acidosis.

Hypersensitivity reactions may occur in some patients who receive potassium-sparing diuretics. The reactions may include urticaria, pruritus, rash, erythematous eruptions, and photosensitivity. Anaphylaxis has been reported.

Pharmacokinetics

All potassium-sparing diuretics are given by mouth and are absorbed by the GI tract (see Table 39–1). Their onset of action is relatively rapid, and the duration of action increases with multiple doses.

The absorption of spironolactone is variable in the GI tract. The bioavailability of spironolactone is 90 percent. It is widely distributed in body fluid and tissues. The onset of drug action is 2 to 4 hours. Spironolactone is a steroid derivative that is extensively biotransformed by the liver, where it is converted to the metabolite canrenone. Both the spironolactone and metabolite are 90-percent protein bound in the plasma. The metabolites of spironolactone appear in both the urine and bile.

Absorption of triamterene is somewhat erratic, and maximum benefit may not be seen for several days after the start of therapy. About 60 percent of the drug is protein bound. Onset of action is within 2 to 4 hours. The drug is biotransformed in the liver and eliminated through the kidneys.

Only about 20 percent of amiloride is absorbed. The drug is not biotransformed but is eliminated unchanged through the kidneys. Its slow onset and long duration of action permits single dosing during the day. With the exception of patients with renal failure, the drug does not accumulate.

Drug-Drug Interactions

The potassium-sparing diuretics have few drug-drug interactions (see Table 39–2). Those that have occurred are related the use of potassium supplements. Drug-drug interactions have also been noted in patients who are receiving a second potassium-sparing diuretic or an ACE inhibitor.

Patients receiving concurrent antihypertensive drugs may require a reduction in the dose of their antihypertensive drug. Spironolactone can decrease the elimination of cardiac glycosides and contribute to digoxin toxicity. Salicylates reduce the effectiveness of spironolactone. Spironolactone reduces the vascular response to norepinephrine.

Dosage Regimens

The amiloride dose for adults is 5 to 10 mg by mouth, with dosages increased to 20 mg/day. The initial adult dose of spironolactone for hypertension is 50 to 100 mg/day by mouth and 25 to 200 mg for edema. The dose may be adjusted upward to 400 mg/day in divided doses (see Table 39–3).

The initial adult dose of triamterene is 100 mg by mouth. The dosage may be adjusted upward to a maximum of 300 mg/day as needed. The usual pediatric dose of triamterene is 4 mg/kg of body weight given in two divided doses. The dosage may be increased to 6 mg/kg/day as needed but should not exceed 30 mg/day.

Laboratory Considerations

Electrolyte and acid-base balance should be monitored. Patients taking digoxin should have digoxin levels drawn before and periodically throughout therapy to monitor for toxicity.

Osmotic Diuretics

- ❐ Mannitol (OSMITROL)
- ❐ Urea (UREAPHIL, UREVERT)

Indications

Osmotic diuretics are low-molecular-weight substances that remain in renal tubules to increase plasma osmolality, glomerular filtrate, and tubular fluid. Their primary use is in preventing acute renal failure. When the GFR falls, as with surgical procedures with large blood loss, there is more complete reabsorption of tubular fluid, which can lead to anuria. Maintenance of tubular flow also prevents the precipitation of toxins, as in drug overdose, in the kidneys. Decreased tubular flow also favors precipitation of compounds having low solubility and may cause physical damage to the nephrons. In drug overdose, increasing the urine flow rate increases drug elimination. Mannitol is the most commonly used osmotic diuretic.

Osmotic diuretics are also useful in conditions requiring dehydration of cells. For example, intraocular and intracranial pressure elevations can be alleviated by the use of mannitol. Water is drawn toward the osmotically active drug in the plasma.

Osmotic diuretics are not used in the management of heart failure because the addition of osmolar substances to the plasma may contribute to edema. Expansion of the extracellular fluid is undesirable as well as risky.

Pharmacodynamics

Osmotic diuretics are inert nonelectrolyte substances that contribute nonabsorbable osmolar particles to the tubular fluid and obligate water. They increase the osmolality of plasma. Osmotics have no specific cellular receptors. The presence of the additional solute and the resulting increase in tubular flow rate interferes with the reabsorption of filtrate and normal urinary concentration. The result is elimination of large amounts of solute and water. Although sodium and water reabsorption is inhibited in the proximal tubule, there are also major effects noted in the thick ascending limb of the loop of Henle.

Adverse Effects and Contraindications

The common adverse effects of osmotic diuretics include a transient expansion of plasma volume and an increase in extracellular osmolality. These increases can result in circulatory overload. Patient responses include tachycardia, electrolyte imbalance, volume depletion, and cellular dehydration. The degree of volume expansion is dose dependent.

Other adverse effects of osmotic diuretics include headache, nausea, and vomiting. Mannitol can produce rebound elevations of intracranial pressure 8 to 12 hours after diuresis. Chest pain, blurred vision, rhinitis, thirst, and urine retention have been reported. The osmotics cause local irritation at the IV site. If extravasation occurs, thrombophlebitis may result.

In patients with renal impairment, the osmotic diuretic may accumulate in the blood, causing dangerous shifts in salt and water balance. The use of osmotic diuretics is contraindicated in severely renal impaired patients. Urea is contraindicated in patients with liver impairment because high levels of urea place additional demands on liver function. Other contraindications to osmotic diuretics include active intracranial bleeding and marked dehydration. Safe use of the drugs during pregnancy, lactation, or in children has not been established.

Pharmacokinetics

Mannitol and urea are distributed rapidly when administered IV (see Table 39–1). They are filtered by the glomeruli and eliminated unchanged in the urine. The elimination rate is reduced in patients with renal insufficiency.

The onset of osmotic drug action occurs within 15 minutes. Diuresis occurs within 1 to 3 hours when mannitol is used and within 1 to 2 hours if urea is administered. Peak drug concentrations are reached 30 minutes to 1 hour after the administration of urea and 1 to 2 hours after mannitol is given. The duration of action ranges from 3 to 8 hours for mannitol and 3 to 10 hours for urea.

Drug-Drug Interactions

There are no significant drug interactions with the use of osmotic diuretics. Mannitol enhances the elimination of lithium, decreasing its effectiveness (see Table 39–2).

Dosage Regimens

Osmotic diuretics are given IV (see Table 39–3). The dosage of mannitol, when used for diuresis, is 50 to 100 g of a 5- to 25-percent solution administered over a 24-hour period. For the prevention of acute renal failure during surgery, or for the treatment of oliguria, the total adult dose is 50 to 100 g. In the treatment of intraocular pressure or intracranial pressure elevations, a 15- to 20-percent solution is infused over 30 to 60 minutes at 1.5 to 2 g/kg. When mannitol is used for the treatment of drug intoxication, 200 g of a 5- to 10-percent solution is administered over a 24-hour period.

The average adult dose of urea is 1 to 1.5 g/kg of a 30-percent solution given over 1.5 to 2 hours. The maximum dose should not exceed 120 g/day. The dose for children older than 2 years of age is 0.5 to 1.5 g/kg of a 30-percent solution infused over 1.5 to 2 hours. For children younger than two years of age, the dose is 0.1 to 0.5 g/kg of a 30-percent solution infused over 1.5 to 2 hours.

Laboratory Considerations

Mannitol increases the elimination of lithium; thus, patients should have lithium levels monitored. Because osmotic diuretics create the potential for fluid and electrolyte disturbances, serum electrolyte levels should be monitored before and periodically throughout therapy.

Other Diuretics

XANTHINES

Xanthines which include theophylline, theobromine, and caffeine are the most common over-the-counter diuretics. Although xanthines produce a mild diuresis compared with other diuretics, they are seldom used as diuretics. The xanthines are extensively used in the treatment of asthma, bronchitis, emphysema, and neonatal apnea. Their exact mechanism of action is unclear; however, xanthines produce cardiac stimulation and renal arteriolar vasodilation. Renal plasma flow and the GFR are increased. Xanthines also inhibit sodium and chloride reabsorption in the proximal convoluted tubule. Theophylline is more potent than either theobromine or caffeine.

Adverse reactions to xanthines are related to central nervous system stimulation and GI disturbances that lead to vomiting and dehydration. Cardiovascular toxicities manifest as palpitations, hypotension, and circulatory collapse. There are many drug-drug interactions with xanthines. Chapter 46 discusses xanthines in relation to their bronchodilator effects.

AQUARETICS

Aquaretics as a class of diuretics are rarely discussed. They are thought to be useful in diseases characterized by abnormal antidiuretic hormone levels (e.g., syndrome of inappropriate secretion of antidiuretic hormone [SIADH], cirrhosis, and psychogenic polydipsia). As antagonists to ADH receptors, aquaretics interfere with water reabsorption, causing water elimination out of proportion to solute concentrations. The tetracycline antibiotic demeclocycline is an aquaretic. Other tetracyclines have not been shown to be as effective.

Newer Diuretics

Newer loop diuretics have been introduced to the marketplace. They include piretanide, muzolimine, and xipamide. They differ from each other primarily in their pharmacokinetic characteristics. They have a longer duration of action than the loop diuretics previously mentioned. The potency of piretanide is intermediate to that of furosemide and bumetanide. Negligible amounts of muzolimine are eliminated in the urine. It has a half-life of approximately 13 hours.

Indapamide (LOZOL) is structurally similar to furosemide and bumetanide, but it is different in that it has prolonged diuretic action. It provokes sodium elimination despite renal impairment. Additionally, it has vasodilator, antihypertensive effects that are independent of any drug-induced sodium elimination. It is extensively biotransformed, with only 5 percent eliminated unchanged in the urine. It is 80-percent bound to plasma proteins and sequestered in red blood cells.

Critical Thinking Process

Assessment

History of Present Illness

The patient who reports symptoms related to fluid volume excess should be asked the following questions:

- Has there been a change in the amount, color, or odor of the urine?
- Has there been dysuria, frequency, urgency, hesitation, incontinence?
- Do you awake from sleep to void?
- Has there been unusual swelling around the eyes, or in the hands or feet?
- Has their been an unexplainable change in your weight?
- Are rings, wrist watch, or shoes too tight?
- Do you have leg swelling that increases during the day and decreases at night?
- Do your legs feel more swollen after you have been up during the day?

Further, patients with fluid volume excess often report edema, headache, anorexia, nausea, vomiting, and abdominal pain. Reports regarding changes in mental status include mood and personality changes, restlessness, confusion, and anxiety. Some patients may report shortness of breath or shallow respirations.

When evaluating symptoms, determine when they began. Does the patient consider them to be mild, moderate, or severe in nature? Is there something that aggravates or provokes the symptoms, and does the patient have methods for lessening or alleviating the symptoms?

Past Health History

The past medical history may reveal a pre-existing condition that contraindicates the use of certain diuretics or that requires special caution. A thorough history includes any known electrolyte imbalance, hypertension, cardiac disease, hepatic or renal dysfunction, diabetes, pregnancy and lactation, and allergies.

Patients with a history of diabetes, hypertension, congestive heart failure, liver disease, or renal disease likely has a history of diuretic therapy, or the patient may be taking a drug that interacts with the diuretic that may be prescribed. The past medical history also includes any major diagnostic procedures and the dates they were performed.

Physical Exam Findings

Physical assessment of the patient who requires a diuretic should include a baseline assessment of neurologic, cardiovascular, respiratory, renal, skin, and nutritional parameters. Each system is assessed to detect real and potential problems that may compromise diuretic therapy.

Assessment of the patient's neurologic status should include orientation, mental status, cranial nerve testing, deep tendon reflexes, muscle strength, and hearing. Neurologic deficits may also be attributed to other medical conditions such as uncontrolled diabetes or encephalopathy related to hepatic disease.

Assessment of the patient's cardiovascular status includes, at minimum, blood pressure (lying, sitting, and standing), heart rate and rhythm, heart sounds, and peripheral pulses. Capillary refill should be noted, as well as the skin color, temperature, and turgor. A baseline electrocardiogram may also be appropriate. Changes in cardiovascular status indicative of fluid overload would be an increased heart rate, the presence of an S_3 heart sound, blood pressure changes, jugular venous distention, and an increase in central venous pressure and pulmonary artery wedge pressure.

The respiratory assessment should include rate, depth, and pattern. The presence of adventitious breath sounds (e.g., crackles, wheezes, rales, rubs), if any, should be noted. Assessment of renal status includes fluid intake and output, and any changes in weight.

Skin assessment includes temperature, color, and turgor, as well as the presence and degree of edema. Edema is first seen in the submalleolar spaces in the ambulatory patient, and overlying the sacrum, flanks, and lateral thighs of a bedridden patient. When pressure is applied with a finger to an edematous area, the small depression that is left usually disappears within 30 seconds. The pitting edema can be quantified further by measuring the depth of the depression in millimeters. The depression of one-plus (1+) edema is approximately 2 mm in depth and is usually considered minimal edema. Two-plus (2+) edema is marked edema with a depression depth of 4 mm. Three-plus (3+) edema is 6 mm in depth and four-plus (4+) edema is massive with a depth of 8 mm. When edema is seen in all body tissues, it is called *anasarca.*

Extremity circumference should be measured bilaterally. Comparisons, made from side to side, assist in determining and documenting the extent of the edema.

Local swelling that is firm and nonpitting is the major sign of capillary edema. The swelling is due to the increased protein content of the edematous fluid. A severe form of such swelling is common in patients with lymphedema and is usually unilateral rather than bilateral.

Diagnostic Testing

Before and throughout diuretic therapy, the patient should have hemoglobin, hematocrit, electrolytes, glucose, blood urea nitrogen, creatinine, serum protein levels, uric acid, cholesterol, and triglyceride levels measured. A patient's hemoglobin and hematocrit values are decreased with fluid volume excess due to hemodilution. Potassium levels, and in some cases, sodium and chloride levels may be decreased. An elevated glucose level may be of concern in the patient with diabetes. An elevated blood urea nitrogen and creatinine suggest alterations in renal function. Elevated uric acid levels have been identified in 65 to 70 percent of patients treated with diuretics. However, clinical gout rarely occurs and then only in susceptible individuals. Cholesterol and triglyceride levels should be monitored for elevations, particularly with prolonged diuretic usage. Patient's experiencing pulmonary edema related to fluid volume excess will have alterations in arterial blood gas values, particularly pH and pCO_2.

A urinalysis is also a helpful parameter. The volume of urine should be documented, as well as urine specific gravity, urine osmolality, and electrolytes. A random sample may be obtained for a quick analysis or a 24-hour collection may be needed to determine the specific nature of a renal problem.

A chest x-ray study may help reveal pulmonary congestion. Patients with hypokalemia may have flattened T waves on electrocardiogram.

Developmental Considerations

Perinatal Diuretics are not readily used in pregnancy. Water is retained during pregnancy to increase blood volume and to aid in providing nutrients to the fetus. There are recognized physiologic benefits to the fluid (see Chapter 6). There is no evidence supporting the notion that diuretics prevent the development of hypertension in pregnancy. In general, before diuretics are used, the effects of the drug must be weighed against the potential risk to the fetus. Furthermore, many diuretics are contraindicated in lactating patients because the diuretic passes into breast milk, exposing the infant to the drug.

Pediatric In infants and children, the most common causes of heart failure are congenital heart disorders and rheumatic fever. These two conditions result in decreased renal blood flow and urinary insufficiency. Pediatric dosage considerations include the age and size of the child, with attention directed toward the reasons a diuretic is necessary. Dosage should be calculated on a milligram-per-kilogram-of-body-weight basis.

Geriatric The geriatric population requires special consideration. Owing to altered physiology and underlying diseases, older adults, are more sensitive to diuretics and tend to experience more adverse effects than younger people. The renal function of the older adult is diminished because of the normal changes of aging, and thus, he or she may be unable to handle shifts in electrolyte balance. For this reason, serum electrolyte levels (especially potassium) should be checked at least every 3 to 4 months.

Compliance with a drug regimen implies a few economic considerations. The older adult frequently has a fixed income and Medicare does not pay for drugs. Older adults are generally taking several drugs at any given time and may not be able to afford all of them. This group of patients sometimes exhibits poor nutritional status or a change in their condition because they are using their financial resources for drugs rather than for food. Furthermore, many of the lower cost food choices are high in sodium. Failure to restrict sodium intake increases the potential for fluid volume excess and electrolyte imbalance.

Psychosocial Considerations

In some instances, diuretics have been abused by those seeking quick weight loss. The abuse of diuretics has been observed in some obese individuals and in athletes who must meet a weight limit. The diuretic is used before weigh-in, and then the athlete attempts to rehydrate before the competition. The use of diuretics for weight control is not justified in the absence of edematous conditions. Some patients, however, receive diuretics from more than one health care provider or from an authorized source (see Case Study—Fluid Volume Excess).

Analysis and Management

Treatment Objectives

Diuretics bring about a negative fluid balance, mobilize excessive extracellular fluid, and reduce fluid volume excess. Treatment objectives for the patient with fluid volume excess are to improve hemodynamics, improve exercise tolerance and the quality of care, and to prolong survival.

Treatment Options

Drug Variables

The use of combination therapy rather than a single drug is based on the principle of sequential blockade of nephron sites. For example, a diuretic that works at the loop of Henle or in the early distal tubules combined with one that works at the late distal tubules reduces the loss of potassium caused by loop and thiazide diuretics. The combination diuretics are most often used for patients who develop resistance to one diuretic, or when it is desirable to nullify potassium loss by adding a drug that acts at another site (see the section on Combination Diuretics).

There are several drug groups, in addition to diuretics, that may be used in the management of fluid volume excess related to heart failure. ACE inhibitors and digoxin have been shown to provide symptom relief, improve exercise tolerance, and enhance the quality of life. ACE inhibitors, in combination with hydralazine and isosorbide, have been shown to prolong survival, although ACE inhibitors have been found to be superior to either hydralazine or isosorbide alone. Diuretics, ACE inhibitors, digoxin, and nitrates all reduce preload. ACE inhibitors with digoxin improve cardiac output; however, the use of ACE inhibitors in the absence of furosemide may be ineffective.

Furosemide, a loop diuretic, is usually preferred over thiazide diuretics because it is more effective, has a broader dose-response curve, a faster onset, provides greater diuresis, and causes less metabolic changes than do thiazides when it is given in equivalent natriuretic doses. These variables allow for greater accuracy in titrating a dose to a particular patient, and there are fewer GI adverse effects.

Hydrochlorothiazide is useful only when heart failure exists concomitantly with hypertension. The diuretic effect of hydrochlorothiazide is not always maintained for an extended period. Metolazone, on the other hand, is useful in diuretic-resistant states. Even in low doses, when metolazone is combined with furosemide, a dramatic diuresis may occur.

Potassium-sparing diuretics such as spironolactone are used only in addition to other diuretics. They are especially useful when hypokalemia persists despite the use of ACE inhibitors. Spironolactone is preferable to the other potassium-sparing diuretics because it has the most diuretic effects.

Patient Variables

Nowhere in the health care arena is the axiom "treat the underlying cause" more important than in the treatment of edematous states. General measures used to promote mobilization of edematous fluid include bedrest and moderate sodium restriction (i.e., 1 to 2 g of sodium chloride per day). The use of a diuretic is adjunctive to specific other therapies.

Some patients may be at risk for hypokalemia, an inevitable consequence of the effective action of thiazide and loop diuretics. Patients with high circulating aldosterone levels, such as those noted in primary hyperaldosteronism, are already eliminating too much potassium. Patients with heart disease who are taking digoxin may experience arrhythmias related to hypokalemia. High doses of long-acting diuretics may be a problem because the patient is already potassium depleted. Concurrent therapy with corticosteroids, carbenoxolone, or potent laxatives further contributes to potassium loss. Further, hypokalemia impairs glucose tolerance in patients with diabetes.

Drug therapy should be considered in patients with mild to moderate congestive heart failure after symptomatic heart failure is documented and acute reversible precipitating factors are ruled out. Symptoms warranting therapy include shortness of breath, decreased exercise tolerance, orthopnea, and nocturnal polyuria.

Pre-existing conditions that necessitate the cautious use of diuretics include a history of gout, renal calculi, and seizure disorders. Furthermore, the fact that most patients receive diuretics for a chronic condition provides them with extended exposure to the drugs, increasing the potential for fluid and electrolyte imbalances, and toxicity.

Intervention

Administration

Most diuretics should be taken with meals to avoid GI upset. All diuretics are best taken in the morning or early afternoon so the effects are complete before the patient's normal sleep time. Some patients may be able to take the diuretic on an alternate-day regimen or several times a week rather than on a daily basis. If the dosage regimen seems to interfere with sleep patterns or if there appears to be no improvement in the patient's condition, a review of the drug regimen may be needed.

When IV loop diuretics are used, they should be given slowly, following the manufacturer's recommendations for administration time. Large doses of furosemide are given at a rate no faster than 4 mg/minute. Slow administration rates decrease the risk of ototoxicity. Further, furosemide is light sensitive and must be stored in light-resistant containers. Discolored (yellow) injectable furosemide solutions should not be used.

Education

In treating the patient on diuretic therapy, there are a number of goals. To reach these goals effectively, patient co-

Case Study Fluid Volume Excess

Patient History

History of Present Illness	JR is a 60-year-old white male in moderate distress who reports recurring dyspnea and increased edema in his lower extremetries. The patient had noted a gradual increase in shortness of breath on exertion, orthopnea, nocturia, and peripheral edema. Patient states that he is compliant with his medication regimen but has problems staying on his sodium-restricted diet. Patient did not have complaints of chest pain or diaphoresis.
Past Health History	JR denies allergies to food or medications. He has a history of previous hospitalizations for cardiomyopathy, and congestive heart failure, the last of which was 4 weeks ago. No known history of hypertension. He has a past history of smoking but stopped 2 years ago. Patient denies alcohol use. Current medications: enalapril 5 mg po QD; digoxin 0.25 mg po QD.; furosemide 80 mg po BID. Has documented history of noncompliance with planned treatment regimens.
Physical Exam	Height: 5'11" Admission weight: 189 pounds (20 pounds up since discharged from hospital), *VS:* BP 118/82, respirations 24/min, apical heart rate 96 bpm and regular. Wet crackles at the bases of the lungs, distended jugular veins, and 4+ peripheral edema extending to the mid-thigh. S_3 heart sound present.
Diagnostic Testing	Laboratory findings unremarkable except for BUN of 52 mg/dL and plasma creatinine of 2.2 mg/dL.
Developmental Considerations	In the elderly, illnesses that appear relatively minor may precipitate decompensation that can rapidly progress to a severe state. Warning signs warrant special attention such as those patients with congestive heart failure and a history of prolonged weight gain of as little as 1 pound per week.
Psychosocial Considerations	JR retired at age 58 from the postal service secondary to health problems. Receives retirement benefits from the postal service and from retired military service. Visits his health care provider on a regular basis. Patient first began having health problems at age 52. Before this time, he rarely sought medical care. Patient is married with two children and six grandchildren. Patient receives much emotional support from his family.
Economic Factors	JR is eligible for medications through the Veterans Administration.

Variables Influencing Decision

Treatment Objectives

- Relieve symptoms of fluid volume excess
- Improve exercise tolerance and the quality of life
- Improve hemodynamics and prolong survival

Drug Variables	*Drug Summary*	*Patient Variables*
Indications	Diuretics promote the loss of sodium and water, and are indicated in patients with heart failure, renal, and hepatic disease. Furosemide causes less metabolic changes than do thiazides. Thiazides appropriate if CHF exists with hypertension.	JR diagnosed with congestive heart failure but not hypertension. This becomes a decision point.
Pharmacodynamics	Loop diuretics act rapidly in comparison to thiazide and thiazide-like diuretics. Potassium-sparing diuretics act on the distal renal tubules	JR has problems staying on a sodium-restricted diet. Loop diuretics remain effective in circumstances in which salt intake is high.

Case Study continued on following page

Case Study Fluid Volume Excess—cont'd

Drug Variables	*Drug Summary*	*Patient Variables*
Adverse Effects/ Contraindications	Most diuretics put the patient at risk for fluid and electrolyte imbalance. Imbalance increases the potential for toxic effects of other drugs.	JR needs careful monitoring of fluid and electrolyte imbalance due to history of noncompliance with planned treatment modalities.
Pharmacokinetics	Loop diuretics are well absorbed with a steep dose-response curve, have a rapid onset of action, and are widely distributed.	JR had a 20-pound weight gain and was experiencing worsening signs and symptoms of congestive heart failure. A fast-acting drug was indicated.
Dosage Regimen	Patient initially received diuretic in a single oral dose, but response was not as desired. Dose changed to IV and to BID until most of edema was resolved without adverse effects. Medication changed back to po. Patient compliant at this time with taking medication.	Patient did not respond as quickly as desired to oral medication but had a good response to IV drug. Maintenance dose of furosemide was increased.
Lab Considerations	Serum electrolytes must be followed closely and corrective measures implemented when necessary. Serum levels of drugs that interact with the specific diuretic must be followed.	Initial findings of increased BUN and creatinine were indicative of decreased renal blood flow related to congestive heart failure. Major consideration during diuresis is the loss of potassium. JR is on digoxin and would be subject to digoxin toxicity.
Cost Index*	Furosemide: 1 Enalapril: 2 Digoxin: 1	Patient does not pay for medications as he is eligible to receive medications from the VA.

Summary of Decision Points

- Loop diuretics are very efficient in manageing edema caused by congestive heart failure and remain effective in circumstances where salt intake is high.
- Thiazides have diminished efficacy in treating edema of congestive heart failure without hypertension.
- Potassium-sparing diuretics have a weak effect on sodium excretion.
- JR's edema was well controlled in the hospital setting but recurred after discharge. Increased sodium intake, increased exertion, and time spent in an upright position played a contributory role in this recurrence.

DRUGS TO BE USED

- Furosemide 80 mg po BID initially. Increase dosage every 3–4 days until desired clinical response obtained.
- Continue concurrent use of ACE inhibitor (i.e., enalapril) and cardiac glycoside (i.e., digoxin)

*Cost Index:
1 $ < 30/mo.
2 $ 30–40/mo.
3 $ 40–50/mo.
4 $ 50–60/mo.
5 $ > 60/mo.

AWP of 100, 80 mg tablets of furosemide is approximately $5.
AWP of 100, 5 mg tablets of enalapril is approximately $82.
AWP of 100, 0.25 mg tablets of digoxin is approximately $9.

operation is most important. Compliance is best encouraged by teaching the patient about the disease process and the drug used to treat the problem. Family members or significant others should be included in the teaching. Information to be included in the teaching plan include the name of the drug, the dose, why the drug is being given, and what can be expected to occur as a result of taking the drug. The patient also needs to be aware of any special precautions and adverse effects. Patients must be advised to expect an increase in urinary frequency, and in the amount of urine produced. In the hospital setting for the patient on bedrest, the bedpan or urinal needs to be readily available. For the ambulatory patient, bathroom facilities should be readily available.

The patient should be instructed to take the drug early in the day. By taking it early, the drug has dissipated before bedtime, thus avoiding interruption of sleep patterns. The patient should be advised to remain close to bathroom facilities the first few hours after taking the drug. Patients who are incontinent may require information on how to manage the problem. A patient caught in an embarrassing situation is not likely to be as compliant with drug therapy.

At times, the peak period of drug activity interferes with work or leisure plans. Patients should be helped to adjust their schedule so as not to be caught in an embarrassing situation. Statistically, diuretics are associated with urinary incontinence, particularly in older adult women.

The importance of sleep patterns are twofold. The first consideration is the timing of administration of the diuretic. Because of the increased frequency of urination, it is important for the patient to take their medication early in the day. If it is taken close to bedtime, it will cause frequent nocturia. Sleep disturbances may also occur as a result of the patient's disease process.

Patients on diuretics are at risk for electrolyte imbalance; therefore, it is important that they recognize the signs and symptoms that may occur with these disturbances. Rapid heart rate, rapid respirations, dizziness, muscle weakness, abdominal cramps, nausea, and vomiting are all symptoms that should be reported.

Postural hypotension can occur in patients taking diuretics. This problem may be related to the drug itself or to hypovolemia. It is important that the patient sit up a few minutes before standing to minimize these effects. Advise patients to protect themselves from the sun and to report any episodes of delayed sunburn or the development of a rash.

With the exception of the potassium-sparing diuretics, potassium is depleted with diuretic therapy. Therefore, dietary teaching is an important part of the patient teaching plan. A dietitian may assist with the teaching in some cases. Hypokalemia can be avoided by consuming foods high in potassium and by using potassium supplements. In patients on potassium-sparing diuretics or ACE inhibitors, these same foods need to be avoided or eaten only in moderation. Salt substitutes are high in potassium and should be avoided also. The patient should be taught to identify and avoid foods high in sodium content (see Appendix C). Fast foods, canned foods, and prepackaged foods are often high in sodium and sugar. Many of the foods that are beneficial for the patient to prepare and consume, however, require more time and effort in preparation and are more costly.

The patient should also be given guidelines to help him or her identify the response to therapy. Daily weights can be used to monitor diuretic response. The patient should be instructed to weigh on the same scale first thing in the morning, after voiding but before eating, and while wearing similar clothing. The patient should have an idea of her target weight and when to notify the health care professional if changes are noted. A weight gain of more than 2 pounds daily should be reported; in older adults, 1 pound/week may be significant. Continuous weight gain should always be evaluated.

Evaluation

Evaluation of the effectiveness of diuretic therapy is based on the treatment objectives that were determined before treatment. In most cases, the criteria include an informed patient and family who understand the disease processes and the treatment regimen; a reduction in symptoms as a result of compliance with the plan of care; dietary controls; and minimum adverse effects related to therapy. The decrease in uncomfortable symptoms such as swollen feet and legs, puffy hands, or dyspnea on exertion may be sufficient incentive to comply with the regimen.

With effective therapy, the patient's urine output increases, electrolyte balance is corrected or maintained, and edema is decreased. If these goals are not reached, realistic goals within the limits of the patients illness should be collaboratively set with the patient and the family.

The patient should be evaluated for fluid volume deficit as well as for drug resistance. In the face of a shrunken intravascular volume, the part of the tubular system not affected by the diuretic reacts by reabsorbing more sodium. For this reason, it is important to obtain answers to the following questions:

- Is the patient compliant with sodium restriction?
- Are the optimal drug and dosage being used?
- Is complete bedrest required?
- Are there any electrolyte imbalances that should be corrected?
- Is the patient's general cardiovascular status optimal?
- Are inotropic drugs being used judiciously?

Signs of fluid deficit should also be evaluated, particularly if the patient has overresponded to the diuretic therapy. Changes in blood pressure or vital signs may be the first indication that the patient is experiencing excessive diuresis. Orthostatic hypotension may be a problem, putting the patient at a greater risk of falling. Other signs and symptoms of fluid volume deficit include poor skin turgor, dry skin and mucous membranes, weight loss, tachycardia, reduced urine output, and rapid respirations.

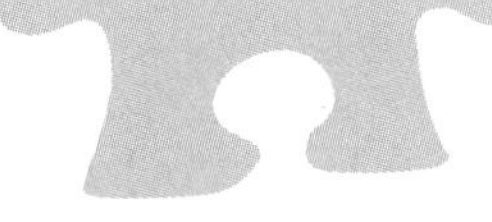

SUMMARY

- The volume and composition of body fluid is controlled by three processes: glomerular filtration, tubular reabsorption, and tubular secretion.

- Electrolytes filtered through the glomeruli include sodium, potassium, calcium, magnesium, bicarbonate, chloride, and phosphate.
- Nonelectrolytes that are filtered include glucose, amino acids, and the metabolic end products of protein metabolism: urea, uric acid, and creatinine.
- Alterations in cardiac, renal, hepatic, or endocrine function are primary etiologies of edema. Other causes include pregnancy, premenstrual tension, and drug-induced.
- Fluid volume excess results in an abnormal accumulation of fluid in tissues or cavities of the body, resulting in swelling.
- Patients with fluid volume overload exhibit signs and symptoms of fluid overload, which include peripheral and periorbital edema, a bounding pulse, pulmonary rales, and dyspnea without exertion.
- Heart failure decreases renal blood flow, which, in turn, decreases the GFR, resulting in the retention of sodium and water.
- Liver disease increases the pressure within the portal vein. Along with decreased albumin synthesis, decreased oncotic pressure results, which leads to underperfused kidneys, which, in turn, respond by retaining sodium and water.
- The damaged glomeruli of nephrotic syndrome hold back sodium and permit plasma proteins to leak into the tubules. Generalized edema results from hypoalbuminemia, and this problem, in turn, leads to hypoperfusion of the kidney.
- Physical assessment should include a baseline assessment of neurologic, cardiovascular, respiratory, renal, skin, and nutritional parameters. Each system is assessed to detect real and potential problems that may compromise diuretic therapy.
- Before and throughout diuretic therapy, hemoglobin and hematocrit, electrolytes, glucose, blood urea nitrogen, creatinine, serum protein levels, uric acid, cholesterol, and triglyceride levels should be measured.
- The renal function of older adults is diminished due to normal changes of aging, and thus, they may be unable to handle electrolyte shifts related to diuretic therapy or their underlying disease.
- Treatment goals include improved hemodynamics, improved exercise tolerance and the quality of life, and prolonged survival.
- The use of a single agent versus combination therapy is based on the principle of sequential blockade of nephron sites.
- Combination therapy is most often used for patients who develop resistance to one diuretic or when it is desirable to nullify potassium loss by adding a drug that acts at a different site.
- Dietary restriction of salt and adequate intake of potassium are essential.
- Loop diuretics are usually preferred over thiazides because they are more effective, have a broader dose-response curve, a faster onset, provide greater diuresis, and cause less metabolic changes when given in equivalent natriuretic doses.
- Hydrochlorothiazide is useful only when heart failure exists concomitantly with hypertension. The diuretic effect of hydrochlorothiazide is not always maintained for an extended period.
- Potassium-sparing diuretics such as spironolactone are used only in addition to other diuretics. They are especially useful if hypokalemia persists despite the use of ACE inhibitors.
- Patients at risk for hypokalemia include those with high circulating aldosterone levels; patients with cardiac disease who are taking digoxin or those with diabetes; or those on long-acting diuretics or who are receiving concurrent corticosteroids, carbenoxolone, or potent purgatives.
- All diuretics are best if taken in the morning or early afternoon so the effects are complete before the patient's normal sleep time.
- Information to be included in the teaching plan are the name of the drug, the dose, why the drug is being given, and what can be expected to occur as a result of taking the drug.
- Hypokalemia can be avoided by consuming foods high in potassium and the possible use of potassium supplements. In patients on potassium-sparing diuretics or ACE inhibitors, these same foods need to be avoided or eaten only in moderation. Teach the patient to identify and avoid foods high in sodium content.
- Patients on diuretics are at risk for fluid and electrolyte imbalance; therefore, it is important that they recognize the signs and symptoms of disturbances and be aware of appropriate interventions.
- Effectiveness of diuretic therapy can be evaluated by accurately monitoring physical exam parameters, blood pressure, weight, fluid and electrolyte balance, and laboratory values.

BIBLIOGRAPHY

Beare, P., and Myers, J. (1994). *Adult health nursing* (2nd ed.). St. Louis: Mosby.

Brown, S. (1991). Management of hypertension in patients with diabetes. *Physician Assistant,* 15(10), 52–60.

Bobak, I., and Jensen, M. (1991). *Essentials of maternity nursing* (3rd ed.). St. Louis: Mosby.

International Conference on Diuretics. (1993). Diuretics IV: Chemistry, pharmacology, and clinical applications. In J. Puschett and A. Greenburg (Eds.), *Proceedings of the Fourth International Conference on Diuretics.* The Netherlands: Elsevier Science Publications.

Jacob, L. (1996). Diuretic Agents. In L.S. Jacob (Ed.), *The national medical series for independent study: Pharmacology* (4th ed.). Malvern, PA: Harwal Publishing.

Jessup, M., Lakatta, E., Leier, C., et al. (1992). Managing CHF in the older patient. *Patient Care,* 26(16), 65–80.

Kollick, K. (1992). Diuretics. *AACN Clinical Issues,* 3(2), 472–482.

Lancaster, L. (1995). The pharmacologic aspects of renal failure. In *Core curriculum for nephrology nursing* (3rd. ed.). Pitman, NJ: Anthony J. Jannetti, Inc.

Mendyka, B. (1992). Fluid and electrolyte disorders caused by diuretic therapy. *AACN Clinical Issues,* 3(3), 672–680.

Pillitteri, A. (1992). *Maternal and child nursing.* Philadelphia: J.B. Lippincott.

Rose, B. (1991). Diuretics. *Kidney International,* 39, 336–352.

Suki, W., and Eknoyan, G. (1992). Physiology of diuretic action. In D. Seldin, and G. Giebisch (Eds.), *The kidney: Physiology and pathophysiology.* New York: Raven Press.

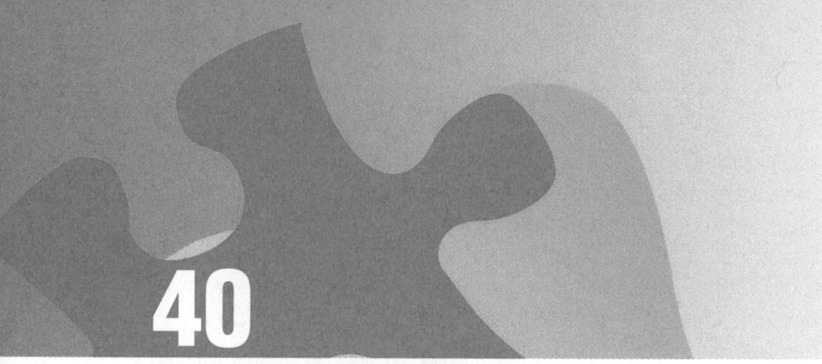

40 Urinary Antimicrobial and Related Drugs

Urinary tract infection (UTI, cystitis) is a common health problem among all age groups. It is estimated that dysuria, urgency, and frequency, characteristic of upper and lower (UTI), account for more than 6 million patient visits to health care providers annually. It is a particular scourge among women of child-bearing age. In the past, terms such as acute, chronic, and recurrent have been commonly used to describe the spectrum of UTIs. These words have been replaced by terminology considered more descriptive of the clinical presentation of a UTI (see Commonly Confused Terms). To enhance pharmacotherapeutic management, the current terminology for classifying UTIs must be understood.

A 7- to 10-day course of an appropriate urinary antimicrobial drug was once considered the standard treatment for an acute UTI. However, in recent years considerable effort has been devoted toward decreasing the emergence of resistant organisms. Attention also has been directed at simplifying management, improving cost-effectiveness, and enhancing patient compliance by investigating the efficacy of shorter dosage regimens. At present, most children and adults presenting with uncomplicated acute UTI are treated with a 3-day course of a culture-sensitive urinary antimicrobial drug. Single-dose therapy, although attractive, is generally considered less effective in fully eradicating bacteria than are 3-, 5-, or 7-day regimens.

A variety of antimicrobial drugs are available for the treatment of UTI. The focus of this chapter is the treatment of UTI with fluoroquinolones, sulfonamides, or urinary tract antiseptic drugs. These drug groups target the urinary system and have proved efficacious against the bacteria that typically cause UTIs. They are also among the most widely prescribed drugs for UTIs. Beta-lactam antibiotics, including penicillin and cephalosporin drugs, and tetracyclines are also used for treatment of UTI. Information about these drugs is found in Chapter 25. Selection of any antimicrobial drug for the treatment of UTI depends primarily on thorough analysis of urine specimen culture and sensitivity testing results.

URINARY TRACT INFECTIONS

Epidemiology and Etiology

UTIs encompass a variety of conditions including cystitis, pyelonephritis, urethritis, and catheter-related bacteriuria. The incidence of UTIs depends on the patient's age and gender. UTIs are more common in women than in men because of the relative shortness of the female urethra. By the age of 30 years, half of all women will have endured at least one UTI. Twenty to thirty percent of women experience a UTI in their lifetime, and 40 percent will have a recurrence, i.e., more than two episodes in 6 months or three episodes in 1 year. Overall, UTIs are more prevalent in females up to the age of 50.

The occurrence of UTI in nonpregnant women correlates with the commencement of sexual activity. The use of a diaphragm or spermicidal gel for birth control tends to increase susceptibility to bacteriuria. In many instances women with a symptomatic UTI often report having had intercourse 24 to 48 hours before the onset of symptoms. Other factors commonly linked to the development of UTIs, but not scientifically substantiated, include inadequate fluid intake, the use of occlusive undergarments or tight-fitting pants, frequent tub baths, the use of bubble bath or tampons, and wiping from the back to front after urination or defecation. Because users of oral contraceptives also have an increased risk of UTI, the higher prevalence rates may reflect estrogen-mediated dilation of the urethra. Another risk factor for the development of UTI is the voluntary retention of urine for an hour or longer beyond one's usual strong urge to urinate. This practice contributes to a pattern of infrequent bladder emptying, repeated bladder overdistention, and urinary stasis.

UTIs become a problem in men after the age of 50 because of prostate enlargement and urinary stasis. Although UTI is far less prevalent in men—about 25 times so—when it occurs in men, it is almost always a more serious condition than in women.

The significance of bacteriuria in elderly people is in question. The prevalence of UTI increases in older adulthood, with bacteriuria present in approximately 6 to 8 percent of women over the age of 60 and 20 percent of women over 80. There is also an increased prevalence of bacteriuria in 1 to 3 percent of men between 60 and 65 years of age. The rate of infection increases to over 10 percent for men over 80 years of age. Institutionalization dramatically increases the prevalence of bacteriuria among both genders because of functional deficits and co-existing illnesses such as cerebrovascular accident, Alzheimer's disease, and Parkinson's disease.

Fifty percent of severely impaired institutionalized elderly have bacteriuria, and the rate rises to nearly 100 percent with long-term indwelling catheterization. The presence of pyuria has been used traditionally to differentiate infection from colonization in the elderly patient, but this is not helpful, as virtually all patients who have bacteriuria also have pyuria.

Factors contributing to bacteriuria in non-institutionalized elderly women include the decreased effect of estrogen on the urinary tract mucosa, ineffective bladder emptying with increased residual urine, and the presence of cystocele, rectocele, and bladder diverticula. The primary factors contributing to bacteriuria in non-institutionalized elderly men include lower urinary tract obstructions such as urethral strictures and benign prostatic hyperplasia. These conditions result in increased residual urine and persistent bacterial prostatitis. Risk factors common to older adults of both genders include prior bladder catheterization, previous an-

COMMONLY CONFUSED TERMS

- **Acute urinary tract infection:** Symptomatic infection caused by a single pathogen. For most persons the occurrence will be their first documented urinary tract infection.
- **Unresolved bacteriuria:** The presence of bacteria in the urine after initial treatment for urinary tract infection is completed.
- **Bacterial persistence:** Recurrence of infection by the same organism several days after antimicrobial therapy has been discontinued and urine culture shows sterile urine.
- **Reinfection:** Recurrence of infection by a different pathogen after a previous infection has been eradicated. It is estimated that 80 to 95 percent of all recurrent infections are reinfections.
- **Uncomplicated urinary tract infection:** An afebrile infection, usually of the lower urinary tract, in a young, sexually active, nonpregnant, immunocompetent woman with no known structural abnormalities or urinary dysfunction.
- **Complicated urinary tract infection:** Infection occurring in patients who have structural or functional abnormalities of the urinary tract, or who have co-existing illness.

tibiotic use, alterations in cognition, and diseases that compromise the immune system such as cancer or diabetes. In fact, diabetes itself appears to predispose patients to UTI. The risk of bacteriuria in diabetic women is approximately three times that in nondiabetic women.

Finally, there are conditions that predispose persons of all ages to UTIs. Included in this category are urinary tract instrumentation (67 percent) or surgery, the presence of urinary calculi, neurogenic voiding dysfunction, pre-existing chronic renal disease, immunosuppression, and malnutrition. Because risk factors are shared by many and bacteriuria frequently resolves spontaneously as well as after therapy, the cumulative prevalence of bacteriuria is actually higher. Chronic, asymptomatic infection is a potential source of disseminated infection, such as endocarditis.

Pathophysiology

UTIs are classified as lower urinary tract infections (e.g., cystitis) and upper urinary tract infection (e.g., pyelonephritis). Cystitis is predominantly a localized infection, whereas pyelonephritis produces systemic symptoms as well as the dysuria, frequency, and urgency commonly associated with cystitis.

Cystitis

Although the lower urinary tract is constantly exposed to pathogenic bacteria, a symptomatic infection requiring treatment may not always result. Several host defense mechanisms work to protect the bladder from bacterial invasion. Regular, spontaneous voiding with complete bladder emptying promptly clears invading bacteria and is the urinary tract's principal line of defense against infection. Another important defense is the natural antibacterial properties of urine to many common urinary pathogens. Extremes in urinary pH, high urine osmolality, and concentrations of urea nitrogen and ammonium are considered intrinsic factors that inhibit bacterial growth. The presence of specific antibodies (IgA and IgG) and antibacterial enzymes (lysozyme and lactoferrin) in the urine is also thought to deter bacteria. The integrity of the mucosal lining of the bladder also acts as a defense against bacterial invasion. An intact bladder wall readily resists bacterial invasion. However, when the mucosa is altered from its normal state by situations such as infrequent voiding, repeated overdistention, obstruction, pregnancy, or ischemia, it is more susceptible to bacterial adherence and infection.

Current evidence suggests that most episodes of UTI in adult women are secondary to ascending infection (Fig. 40–1). Bacteria reach the bladder primarily by traveling upward from the urethra. Infection of the lower urinary tract in females is typically caused by bacteria that first colonize the vaginal introitus. With sexual activity, bacteria are forced through the characteristically short female urethra to reach the bladder. In males, bacteria colonize the urethra and can infect not only the bladder but also the epididymis and prostate.

Under normal circumstances, organisms do not navigate the length of the male urethra, and the organisms that do settle into the male urinary tract tend to be different from those that plague women. In men, an antibacterial substance produced by the prostate acts as a natural defense, thus prohibiting the further migration of pathogenic organisms into the bladder. Men with a history of bacterial prostatitis appear to be more susceptible to cystitis because zinc, a key component of prostatic secretions, is either present in significantly reduced amounts or absent. Symptomatic men are always assumed to have a complicated infection.

Bacteria must adhere to mucosal cells to colonize and infect the lower urinary tract. Bacterial cells typically possess long, filament-like appendages called pili or fimbriae that bind the bacteria to the mucosal cell. Bacterial adherence also requires the availability of receptors in host cells. Adherence further depends on host susceptibility, as well as the strains, numbers, and virulence of the bacteria. On occasion, the number of bacteria alone can sometimes overwhelm intrinsic defense mechanisms of the urinary tract and produce infection.

Microorganisms that commonly cause lower urinary tract infection are frequently normal inhabitants of the intestinal tract. *Escherichia coli* causes about 90 percent of acute UTIs. Other urinary tract pathogens are listed in Table 40–1.

Pathologic changes in the bladder in the early stages of an acute infection include edema, hyperemia, and neutrophil infiltrates. Eventually the surface of the bladder takes on a granular texture and the tissue becomes friable. Hemorrhagic and visible ulcerations containing exudate appear. With bacterial persistence, the submucosal layer of the bladder becomes involved, causing the bladder wall to become thick, fibrotic, and inelastic.

Pyelonephritis

Pyelonephritis usually results from bacteria ascending up the ureters to the kidneys. On rare occasions, bacteria spread to the kidney through the blood stream from a distant focus of infection such as infections of the teeth, gums, ears, or throat. More unusual, although possible, is the lymphatic spread of bacteria from the large intestines to the kidney.

Pyelonephritis is often secondary to an established infection in the bladder. The migration of bacteria to the kidney

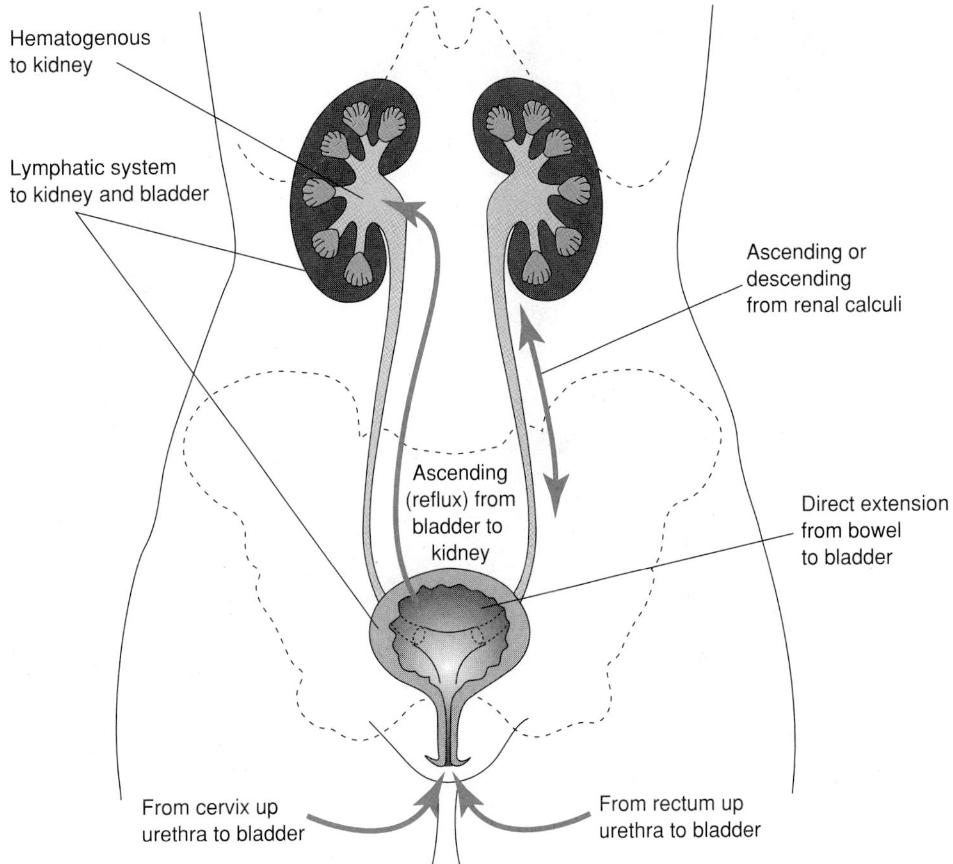

Figure 40–1 Route for bacteria entering the female urinary tract.

is facilitated by vesicoureteral reflux, ineffective ureteral peristalsis, susceptibility of the renal medulla to infection, and bacterial virulence. *E. coli, Klebsiella, Proteus, Enterobacter, Pseudomonas, Serratia,* and *Citrobacter* are pathogens commonly cultured from the urine of someone with pyelonephritis. On occasion, *Streptococcus faecalis* and *Staphylococcus aureus* are the infection-causing organisms.

Pathologic changes with acute pyelonephritis include a kidney that is grossly enlarged, with yellow-colored abscesses found throughout the renal parenchyma. Mucosal surfaces of the renal pelvis and calices are congested, thickened, and covered by exudate. With bacterial persistence, the kidney becomes scarred and pitted. Fibrosis and thinning are evident in portions of the parenchyma. In some instances, glomeruli become fibrotic and the tubules atrophied.

PHARMACOTHERAPEUTIC OPTIONS

Fluoroquinolones

- ❒ Ciprofloxacin(CIPRO); (🍁) CILOXIN
- ❒ Enoxacin (PENETREX)
- ❒ Lomefloxacin (MAXAQUIN)
- ❒ Norfloxacin (NOROXIN, CHIBROXIN)
- ❒ Ofloxacin (FLOXIN)

Indications

Fluoroquinolones are recommended for use in adults who have uncomplicated and complicated UTIs. Because of their ability to achieve high therapeutic levels in urine, fluoroquinolones are particularly effective against bacteria infecting the urinary tract. Urinary pathogens sensitive to the fluoroquinolones include Enterobacteriaceae, gram-positive organisms such as staphylococci, some enterococci, and most strains of *Pseudomonas aeruginosa.* Enoxacin and lomefloxacin are effective against similar gram-positive and gram-negative organisms. Enoxacin, however, is not effective against *Haemophilus influenzae* or *S. aureus.* Lomefloxacin is effective against methicillin-susceptible and methicillin-resistant strains of *S. aureus.*

Although fluoroquinolones offer a broad spectrum of activity and are safe and clinically effective against many community-acquired organisms, concerns have been raised about the emerging resistance of *S. aureus, P. aeruginosa,* and *Serratia marcescens* to ciprofloxacin. For this reason, the use of oral fluoroquinolones should be restricted to persons who have complicated UTIs caused by organisms resistant to other antimicrobials, persons unable to tolerate other oral agents, persons for whom parenteral drugs may be the only alternative, and persons with infections for which other oral agents have failed.

Pharmacodynamics

Fluoroquinolones are chemically related to nalidixic acid, a narrow-spectrum antibiotic used only for UTIs. They are bactericidal. Fluoroquinolones work by inhibiting DNA gyrase (an enzyme) and interfering with DNA replication, repair, and transcription. When given in high concentrations, fluoroquinolones cause a dose-dependent inhibition of RNA

TABLE 40–1 URINARY TRACT ANTIMICROBIALS AND SUSCEPTIBLE ORGANISMS

Drug Class	Susceptible Organisms
Fluoroquinolones	
Ciprofloxacin	Enterobacteriaceae
Enoxacin	Staphylococci
Lomefloxacin	Some enterococci
Norfloxacin	*Pseudomonas. aeruginosa*
Ofloxacin	
Sulfonamides	
Sulfacytine	*E. coli*
Sulfamethizole	*Klebsiella*
Sulfamethoxazole	*Enterobacter*
Sulfisoxazole	*Staphylococcus aureus*
	Proteus mirabilis
	Proteus vulgaris
	Staphylococcus saprophyticus
Urinary Tract Antiseptics	
Cinoxacin	*E. coli*
	Klebsiella
	Enterobacter
	P. mirabilis
	P. vulgaris
Methenamine	*E. coli*
	Klebsiella
	Enterobacter
	P. mirabilis
	Proteus morganii
	Serratia
	Citrobacter
Nalidixic acid	*Proteus*
	Klebsiella
	Enterobacter
Nitrofurantoin	*E. coli*
	Enterococci
	Klebsiella (select strains)
	Enterobacter
	S. aureus
Trimethoprim	*E. coli*
	P. mirabilis
	Klebsiella pneumoniae
	Enterobacter
	S. saprophyticus
Trimethoprim-sulfamethoxazole	*E. coli*
	M. morganii
	P. mirabilis
	P. vulgaris
	Klebsiella
	Enterobacter
Antibiotic	
Aztreonam	*E. coli*
	Serratia
	Klebsiella
	Enterobacter
	Shigella
	Providencia

synthesis that results in decreased bactericidal activity. These drugs also tend to exhibit distinct postantibiotic effects for gram-negative and gram-positive bacteria. This means that bacterial growth does not occur for several hours following transient exposure to the drug. This property enables fluoroquinolones to be given in the short dosage regimens now recommended for UTI.

Adverse Effects and Contraindications

Overall, fluoroquinolones are fairly well tolerated by most persons. Gastrointestinal (GI) symptoms are reported in 3 to 13 percent of patients and are the most frequently occurring adverse effects. Typical complaints include dry mouth, nausea, vomiting, dyspepsia, diarrhea, abdominal pain, and flatulence. Central nervous system (CNS) manifestations occur in 1 to 7 percent of patients and include headache, dizziness, fatigue, insomnia, agitation, restlessness, and hallucinations. Skin disorders usually present as either a rash or pruritus and occur in less than 2 percent of patients.

The effectiveness of varying doses of ciprofloxacin for the treatment of uncomplicated, acute, symptomatic UTI and the frequency of adverse effects do not change with high or low drug dosages.

Long-term use of fluoroquinolones has been associated with cartilage erosion and joint disease in juvenile animal models. Therefore, these drugs are not recommended for children or women who are pregnant (Category C) or breastfeeding.

Pharmacokinetics

Fluoroquinolones are rapidly absorbed from the GI tract but with some degree of variability (Table 40–2). Ofloxacin is highly absorbed, ciprofloxacin and enoxacin are moderately absorbed, and norfloxacin is absorbed least well. Ciprofloxacin, enoxacin, and ofloxacin are widely distributed, with high concentrations achieved in the urine and in most tissues including the kidneys and prostate. Norfloxacin does not produce high serum concentrations, but it does concentrate well in the urine and GI tract.

The time of onset of fluoroquinolones is rapid, with peak levels reached in 1 to 2 hours for most drugs. The duration of action varies a great deal, from 6 hours to more than 48 hours. Protein binding does not significantly vary and ranges from 10 to 15 percent for norfloxacin to 40 percent for ciprofloxacin and enoxacin. The half-life is similar for most fluoroquinolones, ranging from 3 to 6 hours.

Enoxacin is biotransformed to five metabolites and excreted via the kidneys. The elimination of ofloxacin is primarily via renal excretion. Ciprofloxacin is eliminated via renal, biliary, and transintestinal routes, whereas norfloxacin undergoes biotransformation in the liver followed by biliary (30 percent) and renal (40 to 50 percent) excretion.

Drug-Drug Interactions

Fluoroquinolones interact with a number of other drugs including cimetidine, digoxin, foscarnet, and anticoagulants. Toxicity to these drugs is possible because of increased serum concentrations. Table 40–3 lists drug-drug interactions for fluoroquinolones most commonly used for the treatment of UTI.

Dosage Regimen

The dosage regimen for fluoroquinolones varies with the specific drug and whether the UTI is complicated or uncomplicated, acute or persistent. The minimum effective dose of ciprofloxacin is 100 mg twice a day for 3 days (Table 40–4). This dosing schedule produces a bacterial and clinical response equivalent to a regimen of 250 mg twice a day for 3 days. When used for complicated UTIs, ciprofloxacin is taken 7 to 10 days. Enoxacin is administered for 3 to 7 days for uncomplicated UTIs. For complicated UTIs, it is used for up to 14 days. Lomefloxacin is given for daily for 10 days for

TABLE 40–2 PHARMACOKINETICS OF SELECTED URINARY ANTIMICROBIAL AND RELATED DRUGS

Drug	Route	Onset	Peak	Duration	PB (%)	$t_{1/2}$	BioA (%)	Serum Level
Fluoroquinolones								
Ciprofloxacin	po	Rapid	1–2 hr	To 24 hr	20–40	3–4 hr	70	1.2 mcg/mL*
Enoxacin	po	Rapid	1–3 hr	To 48 hr	14–40	3–6 hr	90	0.93 mcg/mL*
Lomefloxacin	po	Rapid	1–1.5 hr	8–10 hr	10	8 hr	95–98	UA
Norfloxacin	po	Rapid	1 hr	12–24 hr	10–15	3–4.5 hr	30–40	0.8 mcg/mL*
Ofloxacin	po	Rapid	1–2 hr	To 36 hr	32	4–5 hr	98	1.5 mcg/mL*
Sulfonamides								
Sulfamethizole	po	Rapid	Varies	†	90	<4 hr	UA	5–15 mg/mL
Sulfamethoxazole	po	Rapid	2 hr	To 24 hr	70	10 hr	100	38 mcg/mL*
Sulfisoxazole	po	Rapid	1–4 hr	48 hr	85	4.6–7.8 hr	82–100	127–211 mcg/mL
Urinary Antiseptics								
Cinoxacin	po	Rapid	1–2 hr	10–12 hr	60–80	1–1.5 hr	UA	15 mcg/mL
Methenamine	po	<30 min	2 hr	To 6 hr	NA	3–6 hr	UA	Negligible
Nalidixic acid	po	Rapid	1–2 hr	UK	90–93	1–2.5 hr	UA	20–50 mcg/mL
Nitrofurantoin	po	Rapid	30 min	6–12 hr	60	20–60 min	>40‡	<1 mcg/mL
Trimethoprim	po	Rapid	1–4 hr	24 hr	44	8–10 hr	100	1.0 mg/mL*
Antibiotic								
Aztreonam	IM	Rapid	60 min	6–12 hr	UA	1.5–2.2 hr	UA	UA
Urinary Analgesic								
Phenazopyridine	po	UK	5–6 hr	6–8 hr	UA	UK	UA	NA
Urinary Antispasmodics								
Flavoxate	po	Slow	UA	6 hr	UA	2–3 hr	UA	NA
Hyoscyamine	po	UA	UA	UA	UA	3.5 hr	UA	NA
Oxybutynin	po	30–60 min	3–6 hr	6–10 hr	UA	UA	UA	NA

*Peak serum level based on single minimum dosage; serum concentrations increase proportionally with higher dosages.
†Sulfamethizole's duration of action with 80 percent renal clearance in 8 hours; 98 percent in 15 to 24 hours.
‡Bioavailability of nitrofurantoin increases to 40 percent when given with food.
PB, protein binding; $t_{1/2}$, elimination half-life; NA, not applicable; UA, unavailable; UK, unknown, BioA, bioavailability.

uncomplicated infections. A 14-day regimen is recommended for complicated UTIs. Seven to 10 days of treatment with norfloxacin is required for uncomplicated UTIs and 10 to 21 days for complicated UTIs. Ofloxacin is given for 3 days for uncomplicated UTIs and 10 days for complicated UTIs.

Laboratory Considerations

Because fluoroquinolones are reported to increase the effect of anticoagulants, regular monitoring of prothrombin time is recommended. Patients taking fluoroquinolones concurrently with theophylline are at risk for developing theophylline toxicity; therefore, serum theophylline levels should be checked frequently.

Sulfonamides

- ❐ Sulfacytine (RENOQUID)
- ❐ Sulfamethizole (THIOSULFIL FORTE, UROBIOTIC-250)
- ❐ Sulfamethoxazole (GANTANOL, UROBAK)
- ❐ Sulfamethoxazole with trimethoprim (BACTRIM)
- ❐ Sulfisoxazole (GANTRISIN); (🍁) STERINE

Indications

Sulfonamides are frequently prescribed for the treatment of uncomplicated acute UTI caused by community-acquired organisms such as *E. coli, Klebsiella, Enterobacter, S. aureus, Proteus mirabilis, Proteus vulgaris,* and *Staphylococcus saprophyticus*. Sulfacytine is the newest sulfonamide used for UTIs. Sulfonamides are ineffective for treating UTIs caused by *P. aeruginosa*. For patients with a first-time UTI, sulfonamides are often the ideal drugs because of their ease of administration, low cost, safety profile, and effectiveness. Sulfonamides are discussed in Chapter 24.

Pharmacodynamics

Sulfonamides are bacteriostatic. Most gram-positive and gram-negative urinary pathogens are sensitive to the broad-spectrum activity of sulfonamides. Sulfonamides act by competitively inhibiting para-aminobenzoic acid (PABA), a necessary element in bacterial folate synthesis. By blocking the synthesis of dihydrofolic acid, a decrease in tetrahydrofolic acid results, which interferes with the synthesis of purines, thymidine, and DNA in the organism. Therefore, the bacteria most sensitive to sulfonamides are those that synthesize their own folic acid.

Sulfacytine and sulfamethizole are considered short-acting sulfonamides, whereas sulfamethoxazole and sulfisoxazole are considered intermediate-acting sulfonamides, with a greater degree of solubility in urine. Alkaline urine tends to enhance the efficacy of sulfonamides. The presence of pus, necrotic tissue, and serum interferes with the activities of the sulfonamides because PABA is present in such materials.

Adverse Effects and Contraindications

The most common adverse effect associated with sulfonamides is hypersensitivity, including complaints of generalized skin eruptions, urticaria, pruritus, photosensitivity, and periorbital edema. Other adverse effects occur infrequently

TABLE 40–3 DRUG-DRUG INTERACTIONS OF SELECTED URINARY ANTIMICROBIAL AND RELATED DRUGS

Drugs	Interactive Drugs	Interaction
Fluoroquinolones		
Ciprofloxacin Enoxacin Lomefloxacin Norfloxacin Ofloxacin	Aluminum antacids Bismuth subsalicylate Iron salts Sucralfate Zinc salts	Interferes with GI absorption of fluoroquinolones
	Anticoagulants	Increases effects of anticoagulant
	Antineoplastic agents	Decreases serum levels of fluoroquinolones
	Caffeine	Decreases clearance of ciprofloxacin Increases effects of caffeine
	Cimetidine	Interferes with elimination of fluoroquinolones
	Cyclosporine	Increases risk of neurotoxicity
	Digoxin	Increases drug levels of digoxin with enoxacin
	Foscarnet	Increases risk of seizures
	Nitrofurantoin	Antagonizes antibacterial effect of norfloxacin
	Probenecid	Decreases renal clearance of fluoroquinolone
	Theophylline	Decreases renal clearance of interacting drug
Sulfonamides		
Sulfamethizole Sulfamethoxazole Sulfisoxazole	Methotrexate Oral anticoagulants Oral hypoglycemics Phenytoin Zidovudine	Increased risk of toxicity from interactive drug
	Barbiturate anesthetics	Sufisoxazole may enhance anesthetic effect of thiopental
	Cyclosporine	Reduces immunosuppressive effects of interactive drug
	Methenamine	Increased risk of crystalluria
Urinary Tract Antiseptics		
Cinoxacin	Probenecid	Decreased elimination of cinoxacin
Methenamine hippurate Methenamine mandelate	Acetazolamide Sodium bicarbonate	Decreased effectiveness of methenamine
	Sulfonamides	Sulfonamides may precipitate with concurrent use
Nalidixic acid	Oral anticoagulants	Enhances effects of anticoagulants
Nitrofurantoin	Antacids	Decreases absorption of nitrofurantoin
	Anticholinergic drugs	Increases bioavailability of nitrofurantoin
	Probenecid	Increases serum levels of nitrofurantoin with high doses of interactive drug
Trimethoprim	Antineoplastic drugs	Increases risk of bone marrow depression
	Methotrexate	Increases risk of folate deficiency
	Phenytoin	Increases effects of interactive drug
	Rifampin	Increases elimination of interactive drug
Antibiotic		
Aztreonam	Furosemide Probenecid	Increases levels of aztreonam
	Cefoxitin Imipenem	Decreases effects of both drugs
	Aminoglycosides	Increases risk of nephrotoxicity
Urinary Tract Antispasmodics		
Hyoscyamine	Antacids Antidiarrheals	May decrease absorption of hyoscyamine
	Anticholinergics	May increase effects of hyoscyamine
	Ketoconazole	May decrease absorption of interactive drug
	Wax matrix of potassium chloride	May increase severity of GI lesions
Oxybutynin	Alcohol CNS depressants	Potentiates effects of oxybutynin

CNS, Central nervous system; GI, gastrointestinal.

but include headaches, nausea, vomiting, abdominal pain, blood dyscrasias, crystalluria, hematuria, drug fever, and chills.

Stevens-Johnson syndrome is a severe and sometimes fatal form of erythema multiforme. The syndrome represents a skin and mucous membrane reaction in which macular, bullous, papular, or vesicular lesions develop in the oral and anogenital mucosa, eyes, and viscera. The characteristic lesion is the iris, bull's eye, or target lesion. It consists of a central papule with two or more concentric rings. Constitutional symptoms such as malaise, headache, fever, arthralgia, and conjunctivitis are also seen with this syndrome. Sulfonamides should not be used in infants less than 2 months old or in women during the third trimester of pregnancy (Category C and Category D at term). However, these drugs apparently can be used safely by breastfeeding mothers because sulfonamide excretion into breast milk will not adversely affect the healthy full-term infant. They are

TABLE 40–4 DOSAGE REGIMEN FOR SELECTED URINARY ANTIMICROBIAL AND RELATED DRUGS

Drug	Use(s)	Dosage	Implications
Fluoroquinolones			
Ciprofloxacin	Uncomplicated and complicated UTI in adults	*Uncomplicated:* 100 mg po q12h × 3 days *Complicated:* 250–500 po-IV q12h × 7–10 days	Most effective for UTI caused by gram-negative bacilli resistant to other antimicrobial agents and as oral treatment for *P. aeruginosa* UTI
Enoxacin		*Uncomplicated:* 200 mg po q12h × 3–7 days *Complicated:* 400 mg po q12h up to 14 days	Same as above. No parenteral formulation available. Best reserved for oral treatment of complicated UTI
Lomefloxacin		*Uncomplicated:* 400 mg po QD × 10 days *Complicated:* 400 mg po QD × 14 days	Continue for 2 days after signs and symptoms have disappeared
Norfloxacin		*Uncomplicated:* 400 mg po q12h × 7–10 days *Complicated:* 400 mg po q12h × 10–21 days	Same as above
Ofloxacin		*Uncomplicated:* 200 mg po-IV q12h × 3 days *or* 200 mg po-IV q12h × 7 days *Complicated:* 200 mg po-IV q12h × 10 days	Three-day regimen for UTI due to *E. coli* or *K. pneumoniae;* 7-day regimen for UTI due to other organisms
Sulfonamides			
Sulfacytine	Uncomplicated acute UTI	*Adult:* 500 mg initially, then 250 mg po QID × 10 days	Not recommended for use in children under age 14 years
Sulfamethizole		*Adult:* 0.5–1.0 g. po TID-QID up to 10 days *Child over 2 mo:* 30–45 mg/kg/day po in four divided doses up to 10 days	Recommended for UTI caused by *E. coli, S. aureus, P. mirabilis, Klebsiella, Enterobacter, P. vulgaris*
Sulfamethoxazole		*Adult:* 2 g po then 1 g po BID × 3–7 days *Child over 2 mo:* 50–60 mg/kg, then 25–30 mg/kg BID × 3–7 days. Not to exceed 75 mg/kg/day	Same as above. Resistant organisms often emerge when drug is used repeatedly for persistent bacteriuria or reinfection. Combination therapy with trimethoprim decreases emergence of resistant strains
Sulfisoxazole		*Adult Initial:* 2–4 g po, then 4–8 g/day po in four to six divided doses × 3–7 days *Child over 2 mo:* 75 mg/kg po, then 25 mg po q4h *or* 37.50 mg/kg q6h	Child maintenance dose should not exceed 6 g/day
Urinary Antiseptics			
Cinoxacin	Uncomplicated acute UTI, persistent bacteriuria, and reinfection in adults; prophylactic therapy	*Acute UTI:* 1 g/day po in two to four divided doses × 7–14 days *UTI Prophylaxis:* 250 mg HS (up to 5 months)	Not active against *Pseudomonas,* enterococci, or staphylococci in UTI. Not for use in prepubertal children. Dose should be decreased for persons with impaired renal function
Methenamine hippurate	Long-term suppression or elimination of bacteriuria	*Adult and Child over 12 yr:* 1 g po BID *Child 6–12 yr:* 0.5–1.0 g po BID	Effective only in acid urine with pH range of 5–6. Patient compliance needed to maintain acid urine
Methenamine mandelate		*Adult:* 1 g po QID after meals and HS *Child 6–12 yr:* 0.5 g po QID *Child under 6 yr:* 0.25 g/14 kg po QID	
Nalidixic acid	Uncomplicated acute UTI, persistent bacteriuria, and reinfection	*Adult:* 500 mg po q8h × 3 days *or* 1 g po QID × 7–14 days. Total dose not to exceed 4 g/day *Adult Maintenance:* 2 g/day *Child 3 mo–12 yr:* 55 mg/kg/day in 4 equally divided doses × 7–14 days *Child Maintenance:* 33 mg/kg/day × 7–14 days	Underdosage during treatment for acute UTI may predispose to emergence of bacterial resistance. Ineffective against *S. saprophyticus*
Nitrofurantoin	Uncomplicated acute UTI, persistent bacteriuria, reinfection, and bacteriuria in pregnancy	*Adult:* 50–100 mg po q8h × 3 days *or* 100 mg po q12h × 7–10 days as extended-release formulation *Adult Maintenance:* 50–100 mg po HS *Child over 1 mo:* 0.75–1.75 mg/kg/day po q6h *Child Maintenance:* 1 mg/kg/day in single or two divided doses (unlabeled)	For treatment of lower UTI, use for at least 1 week, and for at least 3 days after culture confirms sterile urine. Ineffective against *Proteus* species. Ineffective for treatment of pyelonephritis and other related renal infections

Table continued on following page

TABLE 40–4 DOSAGE REGIMEN FOR SELECTED URINARY ANTIMICROBIAL AND RELATED DRUGS *Continued*

Drug	Use(s)	Dosage	Implications
Urinary Antiseptics *Continued*			
Trimethoprim	Uncomplicated acute UTI; long-term prophylactic treatment of bacteriuria	*Acute:* 300 mg po daily × 3 days *or* 100 mg po q12h × 3–7 days *or* 200 mg po q24h × 10 days *Prophylaxis:* 100 mg po qHS every other night or after intercourse (unlabeled)	Reduced dosage for patients with renal impairment. Effectiveness not established for children younger than age 12
Trimethoprim-sulfamethoxazole	Uncomplicated acute UTI, persistent bacteriuria, reinfection and long-term prophylactic treatment of bacteriuria	*Adult/Acute:* two DS tablets po single dose, *or* 1 DS tablet po q12h × 3 days *Adult/Persistent or Reinfection:* 1 DS tablet po q12h × 7 days *Adult/Prophylaxis:* 1/2 single-strength tablet qHS every other night or after intercourse *Child/Acute:* trimethoprim 6–12 mg/kg and 30–60 mg/kg sulfamethoxazole po in two divided doses q12h up to 10 days *Child/Prophylaxis:* trimethoprim 1–2 mg/kg/day and 5–10 mg/kg/day sulfamethoxazole po qHS	Single-strength tablets contain 80 mg trimethoprim and 400 mg sulfamethoxazole. Double-strength tablets contain 160 mg trimethoprim and 800 mg sulfamethoxazole. IV formulations are available
Antibiotic			
Aztreonam	Drug-resistant UTI	*Adult:* 500 mg–1 g IM q8–12 h Infuse dose over 20 minutes if given IV	May have cross-allergenicity with penicillins or cephalosporins
Urinary Analgesic			
Phenazopyridine	Symptomatic relief of UTI symptoms	*Adult:* 200 mg po TID × 2 days *Child:* 4 mg/kg TID × 2 days	Administer drug with or after meals to decrease GI irritation. Do not crush or chew tablet
Urinary Antispasmodics			
Flavoxate	Symptomatic relief of dysuria, urgency, nocturia, suprapubic pain, frequency, incontinence	*Adult and Child over age 12:* 100–200 mg po TID–QID. Reduce dose when symptoms improve	Safety and efficacy in pediatric patients have not been established
Hyoscyamine		*Adult:* 0.125–0.25 mg po TID–QID *or* extended-release formulation 0.375–0.75 mg po q12h	Instruct patient to void before administering drug to reduce risk of urinary retention
Oxybutynin		*Adult:* 5 mg po BID–TID. Not to exceed 20 mg/day *Child over 5 years:* 5 mg po BID–TID. Not to exceed 15 mg/day	Advise patient that drug decreases ability to perspire. Avoid strenuous activity in warm climate to avoid overheating. Avoid other CNS depressants

contraindicated in patients with a hypersensitivity to sulfa or other chemically related drugs.

Pharmacokinetics

Seventy to 100 percent of orally administered sulfonamide is rapidly absorbed from the GI tract to be distributed throughout all body tissues. Bioavailability ranges from 82 to 100 percent, with a half-life of less than 4 hours for sulfamethizole to 10 hours for sulfamethoxazole (see Table 40–2). Onset times are rapid, with peak blood levels reached in 1 to 4 hours. The duration of action varies depending on the drug but is generally over 24 hours. Biotransformation occurs in the liver primarily through acetylation, with elimination through the kidneys.

Most sulfonamides are reabsorbed to some extent by the kidney. Some of the sulfonamides and especially their acetyl derivatives are relatively insoluble in neutral or acid media. Thus, as the kidney concentrates urine (which becomes more acidic), there is a danger that the sulfonamide will precipitate, causing crystalluria, hematuria, renal stones, and even renal failure. Small amounts of sulfonamides are also eliminated in other bodily secretions such as stool, bile, and breast milk.

Drug-Drug Interactions

Table 40–3 lists drug-drug interactions for the sulfonamides that are most commonly used for UTIs. Sulfonamides increase the risk of toxicity from oral anticoagulants, oral hypoglycemic drugs, phenytoin, methotrexate, and zidovudine. When sulfonamides are used concurrently with methenamine, there is an increased risk of crystalluria. Concurrent use of sulfonamides with methotrexate contributes to increased bone marrow depression.

Dosage Regimen

A 3-day regimen is suggested for patients with a first-time UTI. Treatment may extend up to 7 days for patients with UTIs characterized as bacterial persistence or reinfection. An initial 2-g loading dose of sulfamethoxazole is required to quickly establish therapeutic concentration of the drug in the urine (see Table 40–4). One gram of sulfamethoxazole is then taken twice daily.

An initial loading dose of 2 to 4 g of sulfisoxazole is recommended. Maintenance doses of 750 to 1500 mg should be taken every 4 hours. The oral dose of sulfamethizole is 0.5 to 1 g. The initial dose of sulfacytine is 500 mg followed by 250 mg four times a day. The duration of treatment using sulfamethizole and sulfacytine is 10 days.

Laboratory Considerations

Sulfonamides are known to produce false-positive results when testing for urinary glucose using Benedict's solution. Sulfisoxazole, in particular, may interfere with urine dipstick test results and may produce false-positive results with sulfosalicylic acid tests for proteinuria. In addition, because sulfonamides enhance the action of warfarin, close monitoring of prothrombin times is warranted.

Urinary Tract Antiseptics

- ❒ Cinoxacin (CINOBAC)
- ❒ Methenamine (HIPREX, MANDELAMINE, MANDAMETH, URISED, UREX); (🍁) HIP-REX
- ❒ Nalidixic acid (NEGGRAM)
- ❒ Nitrofurantoin (FURADANTIN, MACROBID, MACRODANTIN); (🍁) NOVO-FURAN
- ❒ Trimethoprim (PROLOPRIM, TRIMPEX)
- ❒ Trimethoprim-sulfamethoxazole (BACTRIM, COTRIM, SEPTRA)

Indications

Urinary tract antiseptics exert antibacterial action in the urine but have little or no systemic antibacterial action. Cinoxacin is recommended for the treatment of initial uncomplicated, acute UTI, and some instances of persistent bacteriuria and reinfection. Microorganisms usually susceptible to cinoxacin include *E. coli, Klebsiella, Enterobacter, P. mirabilis,* and *P. vulgaris* (see Table 40–1).

Methenamine is used for long-term prophylaxis or as suppressive therapy for patients at risk for bacterial reinfection. This drug is not appropriate for the treatment of acute, symptomatic infection but instead should be used after the UTI has been eradicated with another culture-sensitive antimicrobial. Methenamine is effective against *E. coli, Klebsiella, Enterobacter, P. mirabilis, Proteus morganii, Serratia,* and *Citrobacter.*

Nalidixic acid may be used for primary treatment of uncomplicated, acute UTI and for prolonged treatment of persistent bacteriuria or episodes of reinfection. It is particularly effective in treating UTIs caused by gram-negative bacteria including *E. coli,* most strains of *Proteus, Klebsiella,* and *Enterobacter.*

Nitrofurantoin can be used for primary treatment of uncomplicated acute UTI and is among the few drugs considered safe for the treatment of acute UTI during pregnancy. In most patients, however, it is more effective when used for prolonged treatment for persistent bacteriuria or episodes of reinfection caused by *E. coli,* enterococci, some strains of *Klebsiella* and *Enterobacter,* and *S. aureus.* Nitrofurantoin is not recommended for the treatment of pyelonephritis or perinephric abscess and is ineffective against *Proteus.*

Trimethoprim, given alone or in combination with sulfamethoxazole, is recommended for the initial treatment of uncomplicated, acute UTI. It is also used for prolonged treatment of persistent bacteriuria or episodes of reinfection. Bacteria often susceptible to trimethoprim include *E. coli, P. mirabilis, Klebsiella pneumoniae, Enterobacter,* and *S. saprophyticus.* Bacteria susceptible to the combination drug trimethoprim-sulfamethoxazole include *E. coli, M. morganii, P. mirabilis, P. vulgaris, Klebsiella,* and *Enterobacter.*

Pharmacodynamics

The pharmacodynamics of urinary tract antiseptics vary with the individual drug. Cinoxacin is bactericidal. A quinolone-type antiseptic, cinoxacin is chemically related to nalidixic acid and acts by inhibiting DNA replication. It is active within the full range of urinary pH (4.5 to 8.0).

Nalidixic acid is also bactericidal, acting through interference with DNA and RNA synthesis in susceptible gram-negative organisms. Like cinoxacin, it is effective over the full range of urinary pH.

Methenamine exerts bactericidal effects by decomposing in the urine to produce ammonia and formaldehyde. Bacteria are sensitive to the formaldehyde when urine concentrations rise above 20 mcg/mL. For methenamine to be effective, a urinary pH of less than 5.5 must be maintained. The combination of methenamine and acid salts (hippurate and mandelate) helps maintain urinary pH in the desired range.

Unlike cinoxacin, nalidixic acid, and methenamine, nitrofurantoin is bacteriostatic in low concentrations but bactericidal in concentrations above 10 mcg/mL. It inhibits bacterial acetyl coenzyme A activity with subsequent disruption of cell wall formation.

Trimethoprim inhibits dihydrofolate reductase by blocking the production of tetrahydrofolic acid from dihydrofolic acid. Trimethoprim is effective because it binds much more strongly to bacterial dihydrofolate reductase than to human dihydrofolate reductase. Trimethoprim's interference with bacterial metabolism results in inhibition of bacterial biosynthesis of nucleic acids and proteins. When trimethoprim is combined with sulfamethoxazole, there is a two-step synergistic inhibition of bacterial biotransformation of dihydrofolic acid. The combination of trimethoprim and sulfamethoxazole is more effective in delaying the emergence of bacterial resistance than when either drug is used separately.

Adverse Effects and Contraindications

The reported incidence of adverse effects associated with cinoxacin is approximately 4 percent. GI symptoms include nausea, anorexia, vomiting, abdominal cramps/pain, diarrhea, and distorted taste. Symptoms associated with hypersensitivity include rash, urticaria, pruritus, edema, angioedema, and eosinophilia. These adverse effects are among the most common complaints. The rate of occurrence of headaches, dizziness, and other CNS symptoms is less than 1 percent. Thrombocytopenia is rare. Cinoxacin is not recommended for use during pregnancy (Category B) because of the risk of arthropathy in the developing fetus.

Nalidixic acid may result in a variety of adverse effects. Among the most common are drowsiness, weakness, headache, dizziness, vertigo, abdominal pain, nausea, vomiting, diarrhea, hypersensitivity, and photosensitivity. Visual disturbances such as sensitivity to bright lights, altered color perception, double vision, focusing difficulty, and diminished visual acuity are troubling but infrequent occurrences that can be eliminated by decreasing dosage or discontinuing the drug. Because of the risk of seizures, nalidixic acid should not be administered to persons with a convulsive disorder. This drug also should be avoided in women during the first trimester of pregnancy but may be given during the second and third trimesters. It should be discontinued at the first sign of labor to avoid high serum drug levels in the neonate after birth (Category B).

Adverse effects reported with methenamine include nausea, vomiting, cramps, and anorexia. Genitourinary symptoms such as dysuria, frequency/urgency, hematuria, and proteinuria also may be experienced. When taken in large doses, methenamine can cause crystalluria. Methenamine is contraindicated in patients with renal insufficiency, severe dehydration, or severe hepatic insufficiency. Although empirical evidence suggests that methenamine may be safely administered to women during the last trimester of pregnancy (Category C), caution should be exercised and the drug given to pregnant women only if clinically necessary.

Anorexia, nausea, and vomiting are the predominant adverse reactions associated with nitrofurantoin. Toxicity is associated with prolonged use of the drug. Rare but potentially serious adverse effects include pulmonary fibrosis, peripheral neuropathy, and acute/chronic hepatic injury. Because of the severity and irreversible nature of these conditions, patients taking nitrofurantoin should be monitored continually and carefully for early signs of adverse reaction. Nitrofurantoin is not recommended for patients with renal impairment, anemia, diabetes, electrolyte imbalance, vitamin B deficiency, or debilitating disease. Although nitrofurantoin is generally regarded as safe for use during pregnancy, it is contraindicated in pregnant women at term and during labor and delivery (Category B). Nitrofurantoin should be used with caution in patients with peripheral neuropathy because it may worsen the condition. In patients with pulmonary disease, the drug may cause a pulmonary reaction, including pneumonitis. Nalidixic acid should be used with caution in patients with a history of seizures or CNS injury.

The most frequent adverse dermatologic effects of trimethoprim include rashes, pruritus, and exfoliative dermatitis. Other potential adverse effects include epigastric distress, nausea, vomiting, and thrombocytopenia. Trimethoprim is contraindicated in patients with a hypersensitivity to the drug and in patients with folate deficiency–induced megaloblastic anemia. It is not recommended for use during pregnancy (Category C) and should be used with caution in breastfeeding mothers, as trimethoprim interferes with folic acid biotransformation.

Pharmacokinetics

Cinoxacin is rapidly absorbed after oral administration. A 30 percent decrease in peak serum concentration results when it is taken concurrently with food. Cinoxacin is excreted by the kidneys, with 97 percent of the drug present in the urine within 24 hours of ingestion (see Table 40–2).

Nalidixic acid is quickly absorbed, undergoing biotransformation in the liver to hydroxynalidixic acid before being rapidly excreted by the kidney. Approximately 4 percent of the drug is also excreted in the feces. Impaired renal function may significantly alter renal excretion of nalidixic acid. The result is an increase in serum concentration levels of the drug and a decrease in urine drug levels.

Methenamine is absorbed quickly after oral administration. It undergoes biotransformation in the liver and is excreted in the urine. The effectiveness of methenamine depends on an adequately maintained urine concentration of formaldehyde. Urinary pH is easily altered by an increase in urinary pH, an increased fluid intake and high urine output, and the length of time that urine is retained in the bladder. Peak urine concentrations of formaldehyde usually occur 2 hours after a single dose of methenamine hippurate, and 3 to 8 hours after a single dose of methenamine mandelate. Formaldehyde levels in the urine should stabilize at a constant level within 2 to 3 days after treatment is initiated.

Orally administered nitrofurantoin is fully absorbed from the GI tract. The microcrystalline form of nitrofurantoin (i.e., MACRODANTIN) dissolves slower; therefore, the rate of absorption is slower. When nitrofurantoin is taken with food, its bioavailability is enhanced and there is less GI upset. Biotransformation occurs rapidly before the drug is excreted by way of the kidneys. As much as 30 to 50 percent of the drug is excreted unchanged in the urine. An alkaline urine decreases the antimicrobial activity of nitrofurantoin.

Oral trimethoprim is rapidly absorbed, achieving higher peak urine concentration than serum levels within the first 4 hours of a single dose. Less than 20 percent of the drug undergoes biotransformation. Approximately 80 percent of trimethoprim is excreted unchanged. Excretion of trimethoprim is primarily through the urine, but about 4 percent of the drug is excreted in the feces. When trimethoprim is combined with sulfamethoxazole, there is a synergistic effect; yet pairing these two drugs does not affect the biotransformation or excretion patterns of either.

Drug-Drug Interactions

Table 40–3 lists drug-drug interactions for commonly used urinary tract antiseptics. Many of the urinary tract antiseptics interact with probenecid to decrease the elimination of the urinary tract antiseptics.

Dosage Regimen

Cinoxacin, when used for the treatment of uncomplicated, acute UTI, bacterial persistence, and episodes of reinfection, should be administered in two to four divided doses to equal a total daily dosage of 1 g (see Table 40–4). No evidence suggests that cinoxacin is effective for short-course therapy; therefore, treatment should be maintained for 7 to 14 days or until follow-up urine cultures are negative. A low daily dosage of cinoxacin also may be used for long-term prevention of bacteriuria.

Nalidixic acid should be administered to achieve a total daily dosage of 4 g. For many patients, however, this dosage level is associated with a high incidence of adverse affects. As an alternative, nalidixic acid can be administered as a 500-mg dose every 8 hours. This regimen seems to be better tolerated while maintaining the optimal bactericidal effect of the drug. After the initial treatment period, the dosage of nalidixic acid may be reduced to 2 g or less per day for prolonged or suppressive treatment.

For suppressive or preventive therapy for UTIs, a total daily adult dose of 1 g of methenamine should be administered in two divided doses. Methenamine may be administered safely to children 6 to 12 years of age, but in lesser amounts.

Nitrofurantoin may be administered as a 3-day regimen for treatment of uncomplicated, acute UTI and symptomatic bacteriuria during pregnancy. The usual dose is 50 mg every 8 hours. For instances of persistent bacteriuria or reinfection, treatment should continue for 7 to 10 days. Patients who require long-term prophylaxis may safely take a lower dose of nitrofurantoin nightly for many months. In fact, it can be used for the duration of pregnancy, if necessary.

A 3-day regimen of oral trimethoprim, either alone or in combination with sulfamethoxazole, is as effective as the 7-day regimen but with fewer adverse effects and at a much lower cost. Dosing options for the 3-day course of treatment with trimethoprim may range from 300 mg taken once a day to 100 mg taken every 12 hours. As preventive therapy, 100 mg of trimethoprim taken every night or every other night is generally effective.

For single-dose therapy with trimethoprim-sulfamethoxazole to be effective, treatment must be initiated immediately at the onset of irritative voiding symptoms. Two double-strength (DS) tablets of trimethoprim-sulfamethoxazole is the suggested single dose. One DS tablet every 12 hours is the recommended dose for 3-day therapy.

Laboratory Considerations

Cinoxacin may cause the following laboratory values to abnormally elevated: blood urea nitrogen (BUN), aspartate aminotransferase (AST; serum glutamic-oxaloacetic transaminase [SGOT]), alanine aminotransferase (ALT; serum glutamate-pyruvate transaminase [SGPT]), serum creatinine, alkaline phosphatase, hemoglobin, and hematocrit. Methenamine may cause false elevations of 17-hydroxycorticosteroids, catecholamines, and vanillylmandelic acid (VMA). A false decrease may occur in the determination of 5-hydroxyindoleacetic acid (5-HIAA).

Nalidixic acid and nitrofurantoin cause false-positive reactions for urine glucose when the test is performed using Benedict's or Fehling's solution. Nalidixic acid causes CLINITEST reagent tablets to produce a false-positive urine glucose. It also falsely elevates urinary 17-keto- and ketogenic steroids. Trimethoprim interferes with serum methotrexate assays if measurement is performed using procedures other than radioimmunoassay.

Antibiotics

The primary antimicrobial drugs used to treat UTIs include ampicillin, amoxicillin, and cephalosporins. These drugs are discussed in Chapter 24. They are used to treat UTIs sensitive to their antibacterial action such as against *E. coli*. Ampicillin causes a maculopapular rash in approximately 10 to 15 percent of patients; therefore, amoxicillin combined with potassium clavulanate (AUGMENTIN), a beta-lactamase inhibitor, reduces the incidence of rash. The presence of potassium clavulanate reduces the incidence of resistant organisms. The effectiveness of this drug is reportedly equivalent to that obtained with sulfonamides.

AZTREONAM

Aztreonam (AZACTAM) is a newer, monobactam antibiotic effective against many aerobic gram-negative bacteria such as *E. coli, Serratia, Klebsiella, Enterobacter, Shigella,* and *Providencia.* It is ineffective against *S. aureus, Enterococcus,* and *Bacteroides fragilis.* Aztreonam inhibits bacterial cell wall synthesis, resulting in lysis of bacterial cells. Because of its beta-lactamase stability, it is effective in treating infections caused by drug-resistant or virulent pathogens.

Adverse effects of aztreonam are few but include nausea, vomiting, diarrhea, and rashes. When the drug is given intravenously (IV), altered taste may occur. Phlebitis and pain at an intramuscular (IM) injection site also occur. The use of aztreonam is contraindicated in patients with hypersensitivity or who are sensitive to penicillins or cephalosporin antibiotics. It should be used with caution in patients with a creatinine clearance rate of less than 30 mL/min/1.73 m^2. Safe use during pregnancy and lactation as well as in children has not been established.

Aztreonam is well absorbed after IM and IV administration to be widely distributed. It crosses the placenta and enters breast milk in low concentrations. It is moderately bound (56 to 60 percent) to plasma proteins. Small amounts of aztreonam are biotransformed in the liver, with 65 to 75 percent of the drug excreted unchanged in the urine. The half-life of aztreonam is relatively short. Serum levels of aztreonam are increased in the presence of furosemide or probenecid. The usual adult dose of aztreonam when used for UTIs is 500 mg to 1 g given either IM or IV every 8 to 12 hours.

Urinary Tract Analgesic

PHENAZOPYRIDINE

Phenazopyridine (PYRIDIUM, AZO-STANDARD, UROGESIC, URODINE) is a nonopioid urinary tract analgesic that provides relief of UTI symptoms such as pain, itching, burning, urgency, and frequency. It is intended for short-term use only because the underlying reason for the irritation should be determined and appropriately treated. Phenazopyridine's exact mechanism of action is unknown, but it appears to produce topical analgesic and local anesthetic effects on the urinary tract mucosa. It has no antimicrobial activity.

Adverse effects of phenazopyridine are few but include headache, vertigo, nausea, abdominal pain, cramps or gas, and a rash. Its most common adverse effect is the bright reddish-orange color it produces in the urine. Phenazopyridine also causes a blue to purple skin discoloration, due to methemoglobinemia, and hemolytic jaundice. It is contraindicated in patients with glomerulonephritis, severe hepatitis, renal insufficiency, renal failure, uremia, and a glucose-6-phosphate dehydrogenase (G6-PD) deficiency. Safe use during pregnancy and lactation has not been established.

Phenazopyridine is well absorbed after oral administration; onset time to urinary analgesia is unknown. Peak effects are reached in 5 to 6 hours, with a duration of action of 6 to 8 hours. It is biotransformed in the liver and other body tissues. Almost 90 percent is excreted by the kidneys within 24 hours. No significant drug-drug interactions are noted with phenazopyridine. A total of 200 mg of phenazopyridine is administered three times a day for 2 days. The dosage for children is 4 mg/kg three times a day for 2 days. Concurrent urinary antimicrobial therapy must be continued for the full duration of therapy.

Phenazopyridine interferes with urine tests based on color reactions (glucose, ketones, bilirubin, steroids, protein). Glucose enzymatic testing methods (CLINISTIX, TES-TAPE) should be used to test urine glucose concentrations.

Urinary Tract Antispasmodics

- ❒ Flavoxate (URISPAS)
- ❒ Hyoscyamine (ANASPAZ, LEVSIN, LEVSINEX)
- ❒ Oxybutynin (DITROPAN)

FLAVOXATE

Flavoxate is a urinary tract antispasmodic agent. It is used for the symptomatic relief of dysuria, urgency, nocturia, frequency, and incontinence associated with cystitis. It also has been used in the management of prostatitis, urethritis, and urethrocystitis. It acts by relaxing the detrusor muscle and other smooth muscle by cholinergic blockade. It produces anticholinergic, local anesthetic, and analgesic effects.

Flavoxate is generally well tolerated. Common adverse effects are usually mild and transient. Drowsiness, dry mouth, and throat are common. Occasionally, constipation, difficult urination, blurred vision, dizziness, headache, photophobia, nausea, vomiting, and abdominal pain have occurred. Confusion, hypersensitivity, increased intraocular pressure, and leukopenia are rare occurrences. Flavoxate should be used cautiously in patients with glaucoma and is contraindicated in hypersensitivity, pyloric or duodenal obstruction, obstructive intestinal lesions or ileus, achalasia, GI bleeding, and obstructive uropathies of the lower urinary tract.

Flavoxate is well absorbed when taken by mouth; however, the onset of drug action is relatively slow. Duration of drug action is approximately 6 hours, with a half-life of 2 to 3 hours. Drug excretion is through the urine.

The usual oral dose for adults and children over age 12 years is 100 to 200 mg three to four times a day. The dosage should be reduced once symptoms improve. The safety and efficacy have not been established for patients under age 12 years.

HYOSCYAMINE

Hyoscyamine sulfate is an anticholinergic agent used as an aid in controlling spastic bladder. It also is used as an adjunct in the treatment of GI hypermotility, neurogenic bowel syndrome, and visceral spasm. Hyoscyamine inhibits the action of acetylcholine at postganglionic (muscarinic) receptor sites, thus reducing the motility of the urinary and GI tracts.

As discussed in Chapter 13, there are numerous contraindications and warnings with the use of anticholinergics. The most frequent adverse effects include dry mouth (sometimes severe), decreased sweating, and diaphoresis. Occasionally there may be blurred vision, bloating, urinary hesitancy, and drowsiness (with high dosage), headache, intolerance to light, loss of taste, nervousness, flushing, insomnia, impotence, and mental confusion. Toxic dosages produce adverse effects in the cardiac, respiratory, and CNS systems.

Hyoscyamine is well absorbed from the GI tract to be widely distributed. It is 50 percent protein bound. Biotransformation is primarily through the liver, with a half-life of 3 to 4 hours. Excretion is primarily in the urine.

Hyoscyamine interacts with antacids, and antidiarrheal drugs may decrease drug absorption. When anticholinergic drugs are taken concurrently with hyoscyamine, anticholinergic drug effects will be enhanced. Hyoscyamine may decrease the absorption of ketoconazole. There are no significant laboratory considerations.

The usual adult oral dose of hyoscyamine is 0.125 to 0.25 mg taken three to four times a day. If the extended-release formulation is used, the dose is 0.375 to 0.75 mg taken every 12 hours. For children, the dose is based on weight and taken every 4 hours.

OXYBUTYNIN

Oxybutynin is a urinary antispasmodic used in the treatment of urinary symptoms such as frequent urination, urgency, nocturia, and incontinence. It is often used for patients with urinary symptoms associated with neurogenic bladder. Oxybutynin is a tertiary amine that acts by inhibiting the action of acetylcholine at postganglionic receptors. It has direct spasmolytic action on smooth muscle, including smooth muscle of the genitourinary tract, without affecting vascular smooth muscle. The therapeutic effects, then, are an increased bladder capacity and a delayed desire to void.

The therapeutic effects of oral oxybutynin are associated with a high incidence (up to 80 percent) of adverse effects. The effects are typically antimuscarinic in nature (e.g., dry mouth, constipation, drowsiness, blurred vision) and are often dose-limiting. Other adverse effects of oxybutynin are numerous, affecting most body symptoms. CNS adverse effects include dizziness, insomnia, weakness, and hallucinations. Mydriasis, increased intraocular pressure, cycloplegia, and photophobia are possible. Tachycardia, palpitations, and hyperthermia can occur. Further, nausea, vomiting, and a bloated feeling also have been noted. Oxybutynin is contraindicated in patients with hypersensitivity, glaucoma, intestinal obstruction or atony, toxic megacolon, paralytic ileus, severe colitis, myasthenia gravis, acute hemorrhage with shock, and obstructive uropathy.

Oxybutynin is rapidly absorbed after oral administration but undergoes an extensive first-pass metabolism. It is 6 percent bioavailable in healthy volunteers. Drug action onset is 30 to 60 minutes, with peak action noted in 3 to 6 hours. The duration of urinary antispasmodic effects is 6 to 10 hours. An active metabolite of oxybutynin, *N*-desethyl oxybutynin, has pharmacologic properties similar to those of the parent compound but occurs in much higher concentrations. It appears, therefore, that the effect of oral oxybutynin is largely exerted by the metabolite. The presence of an active metabolite may also explain the lack of correlation between plasma oxybutynin concentrations and adverse effects. The half-life is also unknown.

There may be additive anticholinergic effects when oxybutynin is taken concurrently with other drugs having anticholinergic effects, including antidepressants, phenothiazines, disopyramide, and haloperidol. Additive CNS depression occurs when oxybutynin is taken along with other CNS depressive agents such as alcohol, antihistamines, antidepressants, opioids, and sedative hypnotics. Concurrent use with haloperidol may result in tardive dyskinesia and decreased haloperidol levels. Serum digoxin levels may be increased.

The usual oral adult dosage for oxybutynin is 5 mg two to three times a day. The dosage should not exceed 20 mg/day. Children's dosages are the same as for an adult; however, the total daily dosage should not exceed 15 mg/day.

Critical Thinking Process

Assessment

History of Present Illness

Urinary frequency, urgency, and dysuria are classic symptoms of acute cystitis. Patients with these symptoms often describe an overwhelming urge to urinate more often than every 2 or 3 hours, and sometimes as frequent as every 15 to 30 minutes. The act of voiding is typically associated with suprapubic discomfort and/or a burning sensation at the start of, during, or end of urination. The female patient may describe pain or burning along the entire length of the urethra, whereas the male patient may notice discomfort only in the distal urethra. Reports of fever, chills, a dull ache or tenderness in the flank, or hematuria may suggest an upper UTI.

Development of a UTI, especially in women, is often related to sexual intercourse within the previous 24 to 48 hours. Careful questioning of the patient may reveal that on the day intercourse occurred, a hectic or unusual schedule caused her to take in fewer fluids and void much less frequently than would be customary. The patient also may report that the act of intercourse itself was more prolonged or repetitive than usual, and that voiding after intercourse was delayed until many hours afterward.

The health care provider should elicit a sexual history specifically focusing on a new sexual partner, a partner who has a penile discharge, or recent urethritis, mucoid vaginal discharge, or a gradual onset of symptoms. A recent history of chlamydial urethritis, gonorrhea, or exposure should also be checked.

Past Health History

The health care provider should elicit information about the patient's normal voiding patterns (day and nighttime), type and amount of fluid typically consumed in a 24-hour period, and previous treatment for any urinary, gynecologic, or GI disorders. Determine also if the patient has a history of hepatic or renal impairment, because urinary tract antiseptics should be used with caution in these patients.

Determine if the patient has a history of blood dyscrasias, G6PD deficiency, or porphyria, as these disorders contraindicate the use of sulfonamides. Information about contraceptive use (specifically the diaphragm, spermicidal gel/foam, and condom), personal hygiene habits (frequency of tub baths, direction of wiping after elimination), tampon use, and information about the type of undergarments usually worn also should be elicited.

The patient presenting with a reinfection of the lower urinary tract should be questioned about length of time between this and the previous episode of acute infection and the number of infections treated within the last year. Detailed information should be obtained about previous drug therapy for UTIs including drug names, duration of treatment, and treatment efficacy. All patients should be questioned about known hypersensitivity or adverse reaction to urinary antimicrobials and related agents. A thorough drug history is also important, as many drugs cause varying degrees of urinary retention or obstructive, irritative symptoms (Fig. 40–2).

Physical Exam Findings

Acute cystitis is unique in that there are no specific physical findings to distinguish the condition. Exam of the patient should begin with a determination of body temperature followed by percussion of the costovertebral angle (CVA) for tenderness. The health care provider may evoke pain or tenderness in the suprapubic region to deep palpation or percussion; however, the absence of such a response in no way rules out the diagnosis of an acute infection.

Patients who complain of dysuria without frequency or urgency, for example, may actually have vulvovaginitis or urethritis. Thus, a pelvic exam may be warranted in patients in whom the possibility of sexually transmitted diseases exists.

Diagnostic Testing

Urinalysis is essential. A clean-catch, midstream urine specimen should be collected. Female patients may be catheterized to obtain a urine sample, but the clean voided specimen is preferred because it eliminates the risk of contaminating bladder urine with urethral bacteria. When assessing for the presence of bacteria in infants, paraplegics, and adult patients absolutely unable to produce a voided specimen, suprapubic bladder aspiration is considered a safe method for obtaining uncontaminated urine.

Nitrite testing for bacteriuria by dipstick has a sensitivity of greater than 90 percent, but the specificity is variable, ranging from 35 to 85 percent. Dipstick tests for leukocyte esterase activity as a marker for pyuria are more sensitive (72 to 97 percent) but less specific (64 to 82 percent). The finding of pyuria (greater than two to five white blood count [WBC] per high-power field on exam of spun sediment) is indicative of UTI and predictive of response to antimicrobial therapy. The absence of pyuria suggests a vaginal cause for the symptoms. A urinalysis negative for bacteria does not necessarily mean that the patient is not experiencing an acute inflammation of the bladder any more than the presence of large numbers of microscopic bacteria is always a predictor of a positive urine culture.

Pyuria and hematuria are considered reliable indicators of UTI, especially when they are correlated with complaints of frequency, urgency, and dysuria. Patients without pyuria usually do not have a UTI. If there is no pyuria, the health care provider should question the diagnosis of UTI until culture results prove otherwise. It is also important to remem-

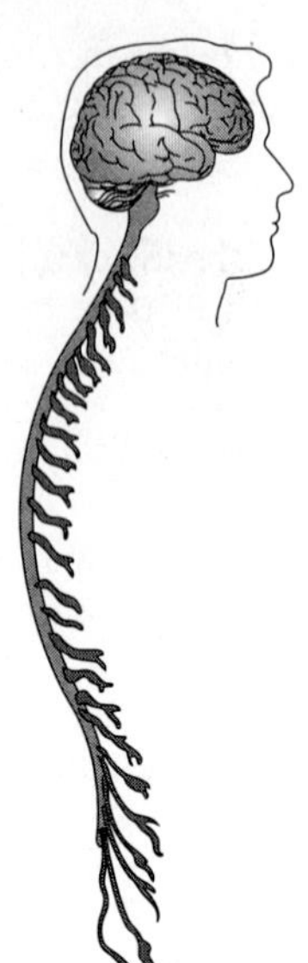

- Baclofen
- Carbamazepine
- Clonazepam
- Opioids and opioid-like drugs
- Phenytoin

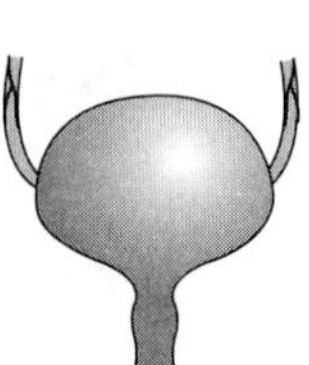

- Anticholinergics
- Antihistamines
- Antiparkinson drugs
- Beta adrenergic drugs
- Calcium channel blocking drugs
- Diuretics
- Ganglionic blocking drugs
- Muscle relaxants
- Prostaglandin inhibitors
- Phenothiazines
- Tricyclic antidepressants

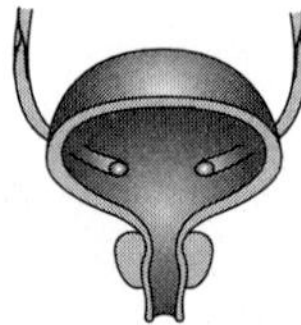

- Alpha adrenergic agonists
- Amphetamines
- Beta adrenergic blocking drugs
- Estrogen combinations
- Levodopa
- Tricyclic antidepressants

Figure 40–2 Drugs associated with varying degrees of urinary retention and obstruction.

ber that other diseases of the urinary tract can cause pyuria and hematuria without bacteriuria.

A urine culture is considered diagnostic when there are greater than 100,000 (10^5) colony-forming units (CFU) of a single pathogen per milliliter of urine. The urine culture should be considered contaminated when the growth of multiple organisms is reported. Contaminated urine usually contains fewer than 10,000 (10^4) CFU/mL. However, a count of 100 to 10,000 CFU/mL may be clinically significant, especially if a single known organism has been isolated and the patient is symptomatic, because frequent voiding slows the doubling or incubation time for bacteria in the urine. Low bacterial counts in an asymptomatic patient suggest that the urine specimen was contaminated and point to the need for retesting. Persistent pyuria with a negative culture can signal tuberculosis as a cause of UTI.

Urine collected for culture should be sent to the laboratory or refrigerated immediately. If promptly refrigerated, specimens can be cultured up to 24 hours after collection. Exposure to room temperature for longer than 1 hour after collection allows excessive multiplication of bacteria, contributing to inaccurate results.

Other diagnostic tests, imaging procedures, and cystoscopy are not indicated for patients with a first-time, uncomplicated, acute infection. However, patients with persistent bacteriuria or frequent episodes of reinfection require further assessment.

Developmental Considerations

Perinatal UTIs frequently occur in the second trimester of pregnancy and are considered a common complication. Increasing levels of progesterone and an enlarging uterus induce physiologic changes in both the upper and lower portions of the urinary tract, creating an environment favoring the development of bacteriuria. The highest prevalence of UTIs is among women of lower socioeconomic groups who have a high parity, a history of UTI, and sickle cell disease or sickle cell trait.

Asymptomatic bacteriuria, defined as repeated recovery of greater than 10^5 CFU/mL in voided urine, occurs in approximately 5 percent of pregnancies. Without prophylaxis, 25 to 40 percent of pregnant women with untreated asymptomatic bacteriuria will develop pyelonephritis. The risk of bacteriuria is greatest between the ninth and seventeenth weeks of gestation.

Untreated asymptomatic bacteriuria can result in preterm labor. Women with bacteriuria are also twice as likely to deliver a low-birth-weight infant. The relative risk of perinatal infant mortality is estimated to be 1:6. If a pregnant women develops an acute UTI, especially with high fever, amniotic fluid infection may develop and retard the growth of the placenta.

Pediatric During the first 6 months of life, all healthy girls and boys are susceptible to UTIs. This is due in part to immature immune systems and intense bacterial colonization of the periurethral area in females and the foreskin in males. Uncircumcised infants seem to have significantly more UTIs than circumcised infants. By 4 months of age, UTIs are 10 times more common in girls than in boys. Pyelonephritis is usually preceded by cystitis. The risk of developing an acute pyelonephritis before puberty is approximately 3 percent for girls and 1 to 2 percent for boys. Beyond the newborn and infant periods, the prevalence of UTI in childhood and adolescence is less than 1 percent. However, the increased incidence of UTI in girls continues throughout childhood and extends into adulthood.

Children troubled by bacterial persistence or repeated reinfection are thought to have some pathophysiologic predisposition to UTI. Additionally, congenital conditions such as vesicoureteral reflux, ureteropelvic junction obstruction, megaureter, and spina bifida contribute to the incidence of urinary infection in children. Other factors such as the use of bubble bath and constipation also have been suggested as contributing factors in the development of UTIs. Scientific evidence supporting these factors as causal is limited.

Geriatric The incidence of asymptomatic bacteriuria is increased in the elderly. Long-term use of an indwelling urinary catheter almost guarantees such a situation. Further, there is increased incidence of bacteremia and death in these patients. Atypical presentations of UTI in the elderly are common. Blunted fever response, anorexia, nausea, vomiting, and abdominal pain may be present. Confusion and changes in behavior also are common. Fever, chills, and flank pain in the elderly are considered medical emergencies because septicemia may develop.

Dosage amounts of all antimicrobial agents may need to be decreased for elderly patients in proportion to age-related changes in the glomerular filtration rate. Colonization with Enterobacteriaceae occurs postmenopausally and is believed to account for much of the increased risk of UTI seen in this age group. Estrogen-deficient tissues are more susceptible to colonization by *E. coli*.

Psychosocial Considerations

Because the onset of symptoms so closely coincides with sexual intercourse, young women with acute postcoital (honeymoon) UTIs are often embarrassed and may be reluctant to seek help. It is important that these patients understand that the development of a UTI is commonly associated with normal sexual activity and does not imply that the patient engaged in unusual or abnormal sexual acts (see Case Study—Acute Urinary Tract Infections).

Analysis and Management

Treatment Objectives

Treatment objectives for all patients with a UTI focus on the prompt eradication of symptomatic infection, identification and correction of predisposing factors, prevention of reinfection, and subsequent ascending progression of the disease to the kidneys. Antimicrobial drugs selected should have the ability to achieve higher urine than serum concentrations for a prolonged period. They should also be selected based on the susceptibility of bacterial cells to specific drugs. Other factors to be considered when assembling a therapeutic plan include the location and severity of infection, patient gender, and underlying co-morbid conditions. Finally, the antimicrobial drug chosen should thwart the development of clinically significant bacterial resistance and demonstrate a clinical response with few adverse reactions, all at a reasonable cost.

Treatment Options

Drug Variables

An important consideration in choos-ing therapy for UTIs is the ability of the drug to selectively affect bacterial cells. In vitro testing has established which organisms are most likely to be susceptible to a given drug. However, factors such as an institution's bacterial environment, the presence of a structural or functional urinary tract abnormality, and the accuracy of culture techniques and sensitivity testing create a certain degree of unpredictability.

Empirical treatment of an initial, uncomplicated, acute UTI may be best accomplished with trimethoprim-sulfamethoxazole because of this drug's proven efficacy against *E. coli* (Fig. 40–3). However, careful consideration also should be given to using a fluoroquinolone. Fluoroquinolones have shown good activity against a variety of gram-negative organisms, most importantly *P. aeruginosa*. The choice of the most appropriate antimicrobial drug should ultimately be based on urine culture and sensitivity testing results.

To successfully treat a UTI, the antimicrobial drug must achieve a higher urine than serum concentration. Antimicrobial agents used to treat UTIs often demonstrate urinary levels several hundred times greater than serum levels. Based on the single criterion of urine concentration, sulfamethizole would be an optimal treatment choice, as it achieves a mean urinary level of 700 mcg/mL, with 95 percent of the dose excreted in the urine (Table 40–5).

The ability of an antimicrobial drug to thwart the development of clinically significant bacterial resistance should be of concern. Most urinary antimicrobial drugs typically act on a single cellular target. However, little bacterial resistance to nitrofurantoin has developed in more than 30 years of use, apparently because of the ability of the drug to attack multiple sites within the bacterial cell. Experts concerned about the development of resistance recommend that fluoro-

TABLE 40–5 URINARY LEVELS OF SELECTED ANTIMICROBIAL DRUGS

Drug	Dosage	Urinary Antimicrobial Concentration (mcg/mL)	Eliminated in Urine (%)
Cinoxacin	500 mg single dose	300	97
Ciprofloxacin	500 mg single dose	160–700	40–50
Enoxacin	NA	NA	>40
Methenamine	1 g	25–85%*	90
Nalidixic acid	4 g/24 hr	75	79 (5% active)
Nitrofurantoin	50–100 mg single dose	50–250	42
Norfloxacin	400 mg single dose	>200	26–32
Ofloxacin	200 mg single dose	220	70–80
Sulfamethizole	1 g/24 hr	700	95 (85% active)
Trimethoprim	100 mg/12 hr	92	55
Trimethoprim (TMP)/ sulfamethoxazole (SMZ)	160 TMP/800 SMZ/ 12 hr	150/400	55/50 (0/37% active)

*Formaldehyde concentration in urine.
NA, data not available for enoxacin.

Case Study Acute Urinary Tract Infections

Patient History

History of Present Illness	LW is a 26-year-old African-American woman who is alarmed because her urine appears to have blood in it. She complains of burning when she urinates, suprapubic discomfort, and the need to go to the bathroom every 30 to 60 minutes. States her symptoms have intensified over the last 24 hours. She reports having had intercourse with a new partner 2 days ago.
Past Health History	The patient states she usually voids every 4 to 5 hours during the day, and rarely at night. Denies history of genitourinary or gynecologic problems, and practices good hygiene habits. Diaphragm and spermicidal gel are used for contraception. No known allergies.
Physical Exam	Temp 98.6° F. Exam unremarkable, except for some discomfort when deep palpation of suprapubic region performed. No costovertebral angle tenderness. Pelvic exam unremarkable.
Diagnostic Testing	Dipstick of urine reveals presence of nitrites and leukocytes. Microscopic examination of urinary sediment shows numerous white and red blood cells. Culture reveals *E. coli*.
Developmental Considerations	Sexually active for about 6 years.
Psychosocial Considerations	Employed as a second grade public school teacher. Single and lives alone in an apartment. Patient feels her symptoms may be related to recent sexual activity and is extremely embarrassed about needing to contact her health care provider. Admits to being relatively noncompliant with taking medicine—"it's too much trouble."
Economic Factors	Enrolled in a health care plan through her employer; all drug prescriptions require a co-payment of $10.

Variables Influencing Decision

Treatment Objectives	• Relieve symptoms of irritative voiding brought on by acute UTI.

Drug Variables	*Drug Summary*	*Patient Variables*
Indications	Ciprofloxacin, sulfisoxazole, nitrofurantoin, trimethoprim, and trimethoprim-sulfamethoxazole are all indicated for treatment of uncomplicated acute UTI.	LW has classic symptoms of uncomplicated, acute cystitis caused by *E. coli*. No known allergies. This will become a decision point.
Pharmacodynamics	Ciprofloxacin is broad-spectrum bactericidal. Sulfisoxazole and nitrofurantoin are bacteriostatic. Trimethoprim-sulfamethoxazole causes inhibition of bacterial metabolism of dihydrofolic acid. Will become a decision point because ciprofloxacin has significant post-antibiotic effect yet potent bactericidal properties causing resistant pathogens to emerge. Trimethoprim-sulfamethoxazole is more effective in delaying emergence of bacterial resistance.	There are no individual pharmacodynamic considerations for LW except that she has a history of noncompliance with drug therapies. This will become a decision point.

Drug Variables	*Drug Summary*	*Patient Variables*
Adverse Effects/ Contraindications	Ciprofloxacin: nausea, vomiting, abdominal pain, dyspepsia, diarrhea, headache Sulfisoxazole: hypersensitivity reactions common Nitrofurantoin: anorexia, nausea, and vomiting Trimethoprim: rashes, pruritus, and exfoliative dermatitis Trimethoprim-sulfamethoxazole: anorexia, nausea and vomiting, allergic skin reactions	Since LW has no known allergies, particularly to sulfa drugs, this will become a decision point.
Pharmacokinetics	All drugs are rapidly absorbed and excreted in varying amounts by the kidneys. The ability of the drug to achieve a therapeutic concentration in the urine will become a decision point.	The rapid-acting nature of the drugs and their relatively long duration of action contribute to their ability to provide LW with a short course of therapy. This will become a decision point.
Dosage Regimen	Studies show that uncomplicated acute UTI can be treated effectively with a 3-day course of an appropriate urinary antimicrobial drug. Trimethoprim-sulfamethoxazole may be used for single-dose therapy, but only if taken at first sign of infection.	Ciprofloxacin has been shown to be as effective as trimethoprim-sulfamethoxazole for treatment of uncomplicated acute UTI when administered as part of 3-day regimen. LW desires the shortest possible treatment regimen. This aspect will become a decision point.
Lab Considerations	For treatment of first-time acute UTI, urinalysis findings should be correlated with patient symptoms	Urine specimen for culture and sensitivity should be obtained for patients with persistent bacteriuria or episodes of reinfection. This is LW's first UTI of record.
Cost Index*	Ciprofloxacin: 5 Nitrofurantoin: 3 Sulfisoxazole: 2 Trimethoprim: 1 Trimethoprim/sulfamethoxazole: 3	Not a decision point because drug co-payment will be LW's only expense for pharmacologic treatment of UTI.

Summary of Decision Points

- Ciprofloxacin has significant postantibiotic effects yet potent bactericidal properties, causing resistant pathogens to emerge.
- Trimethoprim-sulfamethoxazole is more effective in delaying emergence of bacterial resistance.
- The rapid-acting nature and relatively long duration of action of these drugs contribute to their ability to provide LW with a short course of therapy.
- Uncomplicated acute UTI can be treated effectively with a 3-day course of urinary antimicrobial.
- 3-day regimen of ciprofloxacin is as effective as trimethoprim-sulfamethoxazole for treatment of uncomplicated, acute UTI.

DRUGS TO BE USED

- Trimethoprim-sulfamethoxazole DS one tablet po every 12 hours for 3 days
- Ciprofloxacin 100 mg po every 12 hours × 3 days if infection becomes recurrent

*Cost Index based on 3-day regimen:

1 = < $2
2 = $2–5
3 = $5–10
4 = $10–15
5 = >$15

AWP of ciprofloxacin is approximately $17.
AWP of sulfisoxazole is approximately $5.
AWP of nitrofurantoin is approximately $6.
AWP of trimethoprim is approximately $2.
AWP of double-strength tablets of trimethoprim-sulfamethoxazole is approximately $8.

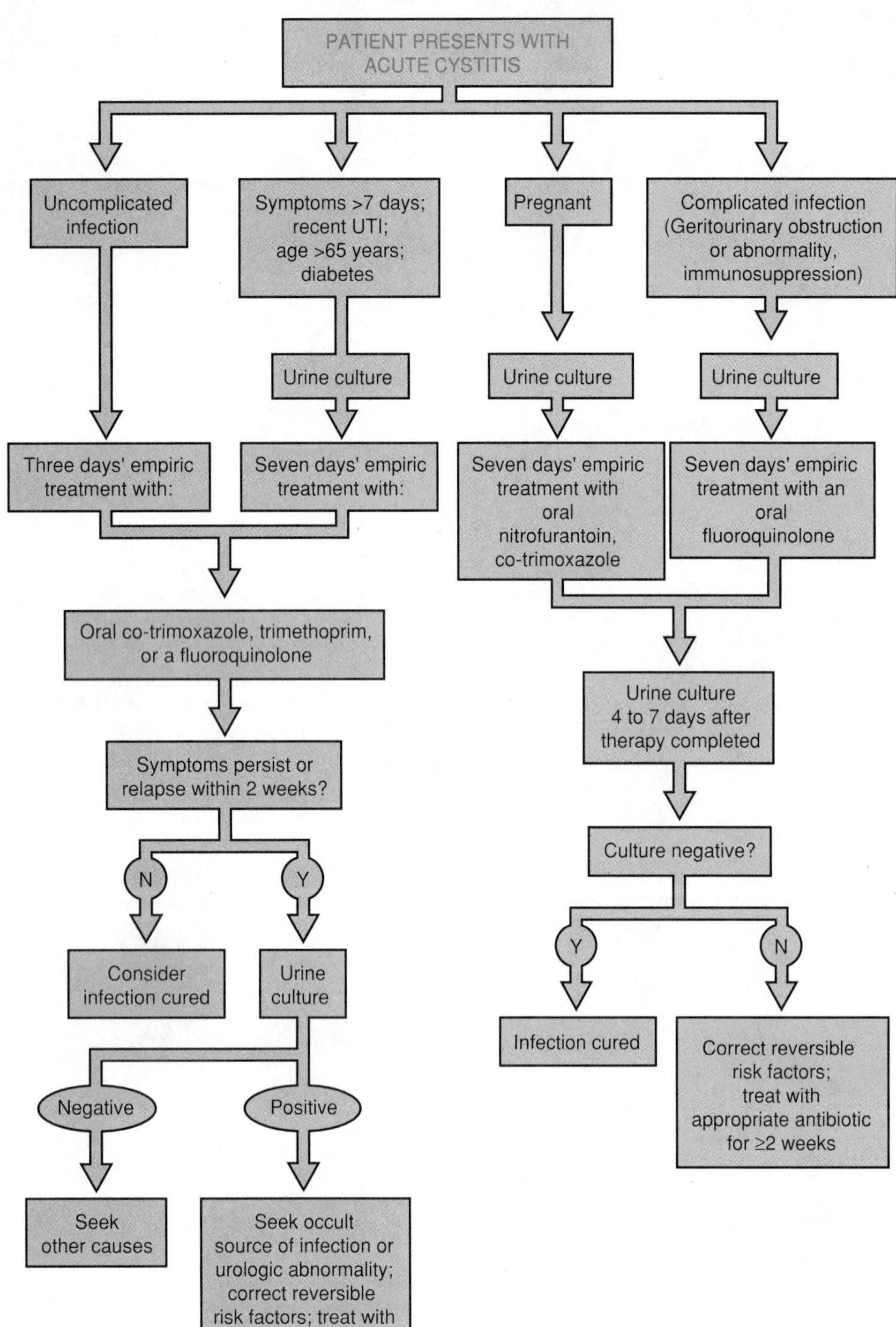

Figure 40–3 Management algorithm for acute cystitis. (Reproduced with permission. Adapted from Hooton, T. M. A simplified approach to urinary tract infection. *Hospital Practice* 1995; 30[2]:23. © 1995 The McGraw-Hill Companies, Inc.)

quinolones not be used to treat uncomplicated UTI if feasible alternatives exist. Further, it has been estimated that 15 to 20 percent of all pathogens causing uncomplicated, acute cystitis show in vitro resistance to nitrofurantoin, whereas 33 percent show resistance to sulfonamides, with 5 to 15 percent resistance to trimethoprim and trimethoprim-sulfamethoxazole. However, the combination of trimethoprim-sulfamethoxazole has synergistic effects that limit the emergence of resistant bacterial strains.

Numerous studies have evaluated the overall effectiveness and safety of various fluoroquinolone dosing regimens compared to other urinary antimicrobial drugs. Current evidence suggests that single-dose therapy of any fluoroquinolone drug is less effective (75 to 96 percent bacterial response) than 3-, 5-, and 7-day regimens of sulfonamides (92 to 100 percent bacterial response) in eradicating uncomplicated, acute UTIs. However, ciprofloxacin is as effective as trimethoprim-sulfamethoxazole and superior to nalidixic acid or trimethoprim alone, and it is better than trimethoprim-sulfamethoxazole for the treatment of complicated UTIs.

Amoxicillin and ampicillin, typically reserved for pregnant patients, have met with significant bacterial resistance in some geographic areas and have been known to alter the normal intestinal flora. Although regional and environmental factors have some bearing on the development of bacterial resistance, practice patterns also have an effect. All too often the doses of antimicrobial drugs are too high, treatment periods are too long, and the antimicrobial spectrum is too broad. This is especially true for fluoroquinolones, which have caused the emergence of bacterial resistance at a rate far greater than anticipated. For this reason, the minimum effective dosage and shortest treatment regimen of other equally effective drugs should be utilized.

The newer sulfonamides have an increased solubility, and precipitation is less of a problem compared with older agents. Sulfisoxazole is quite soluble even in acid urine. The problem of solubility, however, can be managed by using combination therapy with small doses of two or three different sulfonamides. In this way, the saturation point of each drug is not reached and each drug remains in solution.

Although sulfacytine and sulfamethizole are exclusively labeled for treatment of UTIs, they are used less often because their short duration of action necessitates increased dosing frequencies for a longer time. Of all the drugs available to treat UTI, most agree that trimethoprim-sulfamethoxazole is the best choice for single-dose therapy. The pathogens most commonly implicated in uncomplicated cystitis (primarily *E. coli* and *Klebsiella*) are ordinarily sensitive to trimethoprim-sulfamethoxazole. This drug provides a convenient twice daily dosing frequency and is less expensive than newer drugs. Ciprofloxacin can be used if the patient is allergic to trimethoprim-sulfamethoxazole. Ciprofloxacin should be used rather than norfloxacin for upper urinary tract infections (i.e., pyelonephritis) with systemic manifestations.

Some health care providers suggest that methenamine should be used only when suppressive therapy with other antimicrobial drugs has failed. Because there is little risk of toxicity with prolonged use with methenamine, treatment may continue for 6 months or longer. In women with a history of frequent episodes of urinary reinfection, cinoxacin may be used continuously for preventive therapy for up to 5 months.

The practice of treating UTIs with an appropriate antimicrobial for 3 days, or in some cases with a single dose, has dramatically decreased the cost of treating this condition. Some antimicrobial agents cost considerably more than others but may have an efficacy equal to that of less costly agents, even when treatment is limited to 3 days. In all cases, selection of an appropriate antimicrobial for treatment of UTI should be guided first by urine culture and sensitivity reports, second by the overall efficacy and risk of adverse reactions, and third by the cost-effectiveness of the treatment.

Patient Variables

Perhaps the most important patient-related variable to consider when choosing an antimicrobial is the type of infection. Patients with a first-time or an occasional, acute UTI require an antimicrobial agent that will effectively treat the infection using a single-dose or 3-day regimen. Patients with bacterial persistence or frequent episodes of reinfection may require treatment for the traditional 7 to 14 days. Patients needing suppressive or prophylactic therapy require a drug that can be administered in small dosages over an extended time.

The intensity and duration of drug therapy should correlate with the patient's clinical symptoms. The patient's age should be considered when assessing the appropriateness of specific therapies. For example, fluoroquinolones are used only in adults, trimethoprim is not recommended for use in children under age 12, and nitrofurantoin is reported to cause more serious adverse reactions in older adults. Patients who are allergic to sulfonamides are likely to respond well to nitrofurantoin, a drug that has high concentrations in the urine and low serum levels. Remember, however, that patients with G6-PD deficiency are at risk of hemolytic anemia secondary to nitrofurantoin. Trimethoprim as a single entity or a cephalosporin can be prescribed for these patients. Intravaginal use of topical estrogen helps prevent recurrent UTI in postmenopausal women.

Another patient-related variable to consider is whether the infection is classified as uncomplicated or complicated. The health care provider should expect the patient with an uncomplicated UTI to respond quickly to treatment; however, the patient with a complicated infection will require closer monitoring and prolonged treatment to ensure that bacteria are completely eradicated. Low-dose, long-term prophylaxis should be used in women who experience more than three symptomatic, recurrent infections in a year. In these cases, reinfection with the same or a different organism should be considered.

For men, a treatment course of 7 to 10 days is warranted; the longer course is also warranted if the patient has a complicated UTI, low socioeconomic class (more likely to have "silent" renal infection), urologic abnormalities, or renal disease or kidney stones.

When treating a UTI in a pregnant woman, there are two goals: prevention of renal infection in the mother and prevention of adverse effects in the fetus, including premature delivery, low birth weight, and fetal infection. The key to achieving these goals is immediate treatment of the mother. Concern for the safety of the mother and fetus and the results of urine culture and sensitivity testing should guide the drug selection. Because of its long history of safe use in pregnancy, nitrofurantoin should be used initially. Effective treatment also has been safely achieved with beta-lactam antibiotics such as penicillins and cephalosporins. Ciprofloxacin and other fluoroquinolones, although quite effective, should not be used during pregnancy.

Sulfonamides are often used but should be avoided, particularly late in the third trimester. These drugs tend to raise the level of free bilirubin in the serum, thus increasing the risk of kernicterus in the neonate. The wide use of trimethoprim-sulfamethoxazole in pregnancy is debatable, as it interferes with folic acid biotransformation. Fluoroquinolones should be avoided entirely because they can cause abnormalities in the development of cartilage in the fetus.

For asymptomatic bacteriuria in pregnant women, a 3-day treatment regimen is acceptable. A single dose of trimethoprim-sulfamethoxazole is adequate for women without urinary tract abnormalities after short-term catheterization. Catheter-related infections should be treated for 5 days. Prophylaxis for recurrent lower UTIs extends for 6 months. Treatment is then discontinued and the patient reassessed.

Children with an uncomplicated UTI seem to respond as well as adults to 3-day treatment with oral culture-sensitive antimicrobial drugs. However, if they are severely ill, with a high fever, unable to tolerate oral fluids, or infected with a highly resistant organism, treatment should first begin with the parenteral form of a broad-spectrum antimicrobial drug. Treatment should continue until the child is able to take adequate fluids and an oral agent. Once the patient can tolerate an oral formulation, therapy should continue for approximately 10 days. Because children are sometimes less tolerant of acute symptoms, systemic analgesia with acetaminophen, warm sitz baths, or warm abdominal compresses may be needed for pain relief.

Studies have demonstrated no benefit from treating asymptomatic UTI in elderly patients, except when there is a history of renal disease or urinary tract abnormalities, when the patient is to undergo an invasive genitourinary procedure, or if there is evidence of sepsis. UTI symptoms, a change in mental status, loss of appetite, increased WBC count, or fever indicates the need for a urine culture.

Elderly men and women with symptomatic UTI do not respond well to short-course therapy and should be treated for 7 to 14 days. A fluoroquinolone is usually the drug of choice. Institutionalized older adults are exposed to a wide range of organisms; therefore, a broad-spectrum antibiotic is recommended. Reduced doses are often warranted because the older adult is more vulnerable to adverse effects. Regardless of the dose prescribed, renal function needs to be monitored. Nitrofurantoin is associated with more serious adverse reactions in elderly patients and should be used with caution. It should also be used with caution in patients with peripheral neuropathy because it may worsen the condition. Finally, nitrofurantoin may cause a pulmonary reaction, including pneumonitis in patients with pre-existing pulmonary disease.

The use of fluoroquinolones to treat UTI in elderly patients has become increasingly popular, although no studies demonstrate their superiority over other oral agents for this population. Thus, fluoroquinolones should be used in the elderly only when infection is caused by an organism resistant to other oral agents. Fluoroquinolone serum levels of geriatric patients are usually 50 percent higher than those of their younger counterparts. Trimethoprim-sulfamethoxazole is an effective broad-spectrum antimicrobial agent that can be used for initial treatment and long-term prophylactic therapy of UTI in the elderly.

Indiscriminate use of broad-spectrum antimicrobial drugs to treat asymptomatic bacteriuria invites the emergence of resistant organisms, especially among institutionalized elderly patients, who tend to harbor gram-negative organisms in the oropharynx. On occasion, suppressive drugs such as methenamine or acidifying drugs such as vitamin C are used. Morbidity secondary to UTI has not been widely studied, but these infections account for only a small number of hospital admissions. It should be noted that less than 1 percent of nursing home deaths are attributed to UTIs.

Adjuvant drugs such as urinary antiseptics and antispasmodic agents can be used to treat symptoms associated with UTI. Phenazopyridine, an azo dye available over the counter or by prescription, is a topical anesthetic. Antispasmodic drugs such as hyoscyamine or oxybutynin may prove helpful for patients who, despite a few days of antimicrobial therapy, are still experiencing urgency.

Intervention

Administration

Adequate fluid intake is extremely important for the patient taking a urinary antimicrobial drug. The patient with a UTI should consume approximately 2000 mL/24 hr. A higher fluid intake compromises the efficacy of the prescribed antimicrobial by making the urine too dilute. Water is preferred over other types of beverages, and in most instances a full glass of water should be consumed with each oral dose of the drug.

Drugs that should be consumed with food include methenamine, nalidixic acid, nitrofurantoin, and sulfonamides. Fluoroquinolones should be taken at least 2 hours after meals or on an empty stomach. Cinoxacin and trimethoprim may be administered without regard for meal times.

Because most urinary antimicrobial agents are excreted by the kidneys and have higher urine than serum concentrations, attention to renal function is required. Aging patients and those with renal insufficiency require either reduced dosages and/or lengthened dosage intervals to avoid retaining the drug and developing nephrotoxicity. On the other hand, urine must be carefully monitored to ensure that the bacteria are being effectively eliminated, as the inhibitory action of the antimicrobial agent is dependent on an adequate urine level.

Education

First and foremost, patients should be taught about nonpharmacologic approaches that help keep the bladder healthy. Remind patients to drink enough fluid to keep the bladder well flushed, but not excessive amounts that will cause the drug to be diluted. Dark, concentrated urine suggests a need for better hydration. Advise the patient to void when the urge arises rather than waiting for a more convenient opportunity. Patients should wipe from front to rear after urinating or having a bowel movement. Wearing cotton underwear and avoiding prolonged periods in wet swimming suits also minimize risk of UTIs. Urinating after intercourse and rinsing well after lathering up in the shower also help reduce the risk. Advise postmenopausal women to consider estrogen replacement, as estrogen-deficient tissues are more susceptible to colonization.

Some women can correlate episodes of UTI with sexual intercourse, recent diaphragm or spermicide use, and even a recent pelvic exam. Patients who recognize any of these associations can be instructed to take a single small dose of an antibiotic—any of those mentioned are suitable—with a large glass of water after intercourse.

The risk of infection also can be reduced by using intermittent catheterization rather than an indwelling catheter, or an external drainage device, such as a condom catheter. Make sure that all patients dependent on catheters maintain an adequate fluid intake. Indwelling catheters should be changed every 4 to 6 weeks to prevent incrustations and bacterial overgrowth.

Regular and complete bladder emptying should be stressed to all patients. A regular schedule of bladder emptying will allow the urinary system to re-establish its natural defense against infection. For female patients, voiding before and soon after intercourse is important. Patients who rely on a diaphragm and spermicide for contraception should consider using other methods if they are prone to UTI. Other teaching points include the importance of regular and adequate hygiene, use of a shower instead of a tub for bathing, use of cotton rather than synthetic underwear, discontinuing the use of feminine hygiene sprays, and reconsidering the use of the diaphragm and spermicidal gel for contraceptive purposes. Patients also should be taught to be alert to the signs and symptoms of UTI and to seek treatment promptly if they occur.

A dilute urine coupled with regular bladder emptying is a preventive strategy that patients should adopt as a life-long habit. Acidification of the urine inhibits the growth of many urinary tract organisms and enhances the effects of several urinary antiseptics. Thus, patients should be encouraged to consume large amounts of fluids. Fluids that increase urine acidity, such as cranberry, blueberry, or prune juice, should be selected; 300 mL of cranberry juice decreases bacteria counts. A nondialyzable polymeric substance found in cranberries, as well as in blueberries, prevents bacteria from clinging to bladder mucosa. Vitamin C also acidifies the urine, thus enhancing anti-infective therapy. Eating more protein, plums, or prunes helps make the urine more acidic. The patient should be advised to avoid most citrus fruits and juices, milk and other dairy products, and other alkalinizing foods. Over-the-counter products such as ALKA-SELTZER and sodium bicarbonate, which alkalinize the urine, should be avoided. Other fluids to avoid that may irritate the bladder include alcohol and caffeine products. A summary of the various aspects of patient teaching is provided in Strategies for Preventing UTIs.

Middle-aged and older adults are often fearful of being diagnosed with cancer and need to be reassured that there is no relationship between the classic symptoms of acute UTI and cancer. Male patients must be helped to understand that an underlying condition, such as benign prostatic hyperplasia, may in fact be the cause for infection and that further assessment is required. Because the discomfort associated with an acute UTI resolves quickly once treatment is initiated, patients of all ages have a tendency to discontinue treatment or engage in self-determined alternative dosing and disregard information about the prevention of future infections. Thorough patient education is required.

Patients should be taught the importance of completing the entire course of treatment. Although shorter dosage regimens have significantly enhanced patient compliance, there is still a tendency to discontinue the drug once UTI symptoms have resolved. Emphasize to patients that the infection could persist and symptoms recur without strict adherence to the treatment regimen. To enhance compliance, explain to the patient and/or caregiver the premise underlying the action of all urinary antimicrobials, that is, the ability to achieve a therapeutic concentration in the urine.

Patients also should be taught about the potential adverse effects of their prescribed drugs. Signs and symptoms of a hypersensitivity reaction, particularly if a sulfonamide has been prescribed, should be provided along with suggested strategies for managing a hypersensitivity response.

Patients who require long-term suppressive or prophylactic therapy should be taught the importance of taking their medication just before going to bed. Urinary antimicrobial agents used for this purpose are more effective when they are able to reach peak urine concentration levels during the longest natural period of urinary retention (i.e., while the patient sleeps). Patients taking methenamine for suppressive therapy should be taught to monitor the pH of their urine to ensure the effectiveness of the drug. An adequate fluid intake of at least 2000 mL/24 hr should be maintained even after antimicrobial therapy has been discontinued.

Patients taking phenazopyridine should be advised that there will be a reddish orange discoloration to the urine and that it may stain clothing or bedding. A sanitary napkin can be worn to avoid clothing stains. Patients also should be advised that the drug will cause staining of soft contact lenses. Eye glasses should be worn during the period that phenazopyridine is taken.

STRATEGIES FOR PREVENTING UTI

- Make regular urination a habit (i.e., at 3- to 4-hour intervals), avoid long waits.
- Increase fluid intake, especially water, to a minimum of six to eight glasses daily.
- Avoid bladder irritants such as caffeine, alcohol, and carbonated beverages.
- Avoid prolonged bicycling, motorcycling, horseback riding, and traveling involving long periods of sitting, which can contribute to irritation of the urethral meatus.
- Practice good hygiene, including wiping from front to back after urination and bowel movements.
- Avoid bubble bath, perfumed soap, feminine hygiene sprays, or products containing hexachlorophene.
- Be aware that vigorous or frequent sexual activity may contribute to urinary tract infection.
- Urinate before and after intercourse to empty the bladder and cleanse the urethra.
- Do not ignore vaginal discharge or other signs of vaginal infection.
- Avoid wearing nylon pantyhose, tight slacks, or any clothing that traps perineal moisture and prevents evaporation.
- Complete prescribed drug regimens even though symptoms are diminished.
- Do not use drugs left over from previous infections.
- Drink cranberry, blueberry, or prune juice to acidify the urine and relieve symptoms.
- Use Credé's maneuver to facilitate bladder emptying when appropriate.
- Prevent constipation through the use of bowel management programs: diet, activity, fluids, and toileting.
- When an indwelling catheter is required, use the smallest size possible; maintain a closed sterile drainage system and unobstructed urine flow.
- Re-evaluate frequently the need for indwelling catheters and remove as soon as possible.

Evaluation

Relief of irritative voiding symptoms, the absence of urine odor, and the return of urine to its characteristic clear, light yellow color, provide strong evidence that a UTI has been effectively treated. Nonetheless, a follow-up urine culture should be performed to ensure that the urine has been rendered sterile. The ideal time to perform the "test of cure" culture is about 4 to 7 days after the completion of drug therapy.

For initial and infrequent lower UTIs, cultures are not needed as long as treatment is successful. If signs and symptoms persist after initial treatment, urine cultures should be obtained to verify sensitivity of the offending organism. Follow-up cultures are mandatory in children, pregnant patients with recurrent symptoms of upper UTIs, and patients who are at high risk for renal damage (even if they are asymptomatic) within 1 to 2 weeks of completion of treatment.

Urgency, frequency, and dysuria should disappear after 24 to 48 hours if appropriate therapy has been instituted. If a patient experiences a relapse after a 3-day or 7- to 10-day antimicrobial course, treatment should be reinstituted for 2 weeks. If the patient experiences another relapse after 2 weeks, treatment should be reinstituted for 6 weeks. If the patient experiences relapse after 6 weeks, treatment should continue for 6 months.

Women caught in a cycle of recurrent, uncomplicated infections can benefit from suppressive drug therapy, although some of the drugs discussed may not be FDA approved for prophylaxis. The goal is to prevent infection by changing the microbial balance in the vagina and rectum. Suppressive tactics should be evaluated after the first 3 to 6 months. Stop preventive therapy, obtain a urine culture, and assess the frequency of subsequent UTIs. Patients who continue to have recurrent infections should receive prophylactic therapy for an extended period; 1 to 2 years is not unusual.

Follow-up urinalysis and urine cultures are recommended for all children treated for UTI. A child requiring long-term preventive or prophylactic therapy for UTI should receive a different antimicrobial drug from that used to treat the acute infection.

SUMMARY

- Both symptomatic and asymptomatic bacteriuria is a common phenomenon with well-defined risk factors.
- The prevalence of UTI is greater in females than in males and tends to increase with age.
- Children older than 6 months of age who are troubled by persistent bacteriuria in the absence of any congenital condition may have a pathophysiologic predisposition to UTI.
- The prevalence of UTI in women of child-bearing age is primarily related to sexual activity, use of the diaphragm and/or spermicidal gel, inadequate hygiene, and poor voiding habits.
- Institutionalized elderly have a higher prevalence of UTIs than non-institutionalized elderly because of functional deficits, co-existing illnesses, and greater exposure to microorganisms.
- The primary factor contributing to bacteriuria in older females is the decreased effect of estrogen on the urinary tract mucosa. The primary factor contributing to bacteriuria in elderly men is benign prostatic hyperplasia.
- Bacteria enter the urinary system primarily by ascending from the urethra. In rare instances, the mode of entry may be by hematogenous or lymphatic spread.
- Regular, spontaneous voiding, the antibacterial properties of urine, and an intact bladder wall are the urinary tract's intrinsic defense mechanisms.
- Pyelonephritis is often secondary to an established infection in the bladder.
- Microorganisms infecting the urinary tract are frequently normal inhabitants of the intestinal tract. *E. coli* causes about 90 percent of acute UTIs.
- Urinary frequency, urgency, dysuria, and sometimes hematuria are classic signs of acute UTI. Voiding may be as frequent as every 15 to 30 minutes and associated with suprapubic discomfort or urethral burning. Flank pain also may be reported.
- The urine is often cloudy and blood-tinged with a foul odor. The presence of pyuria and hematuria is indicative of UTI.
- A urine culture is diagnostic of UTI when it has greater than 100,000 CFU/mL of a single pathogen. A culture reporting 100 to 10,000 CFU/mL may be clinically significant if a single pathogen is isolated and the patient is symptomatic.
- The objectives of treatment are the prompt eradication of symptoms of UTI and the prevention of disease progression to the kidneys.
- The choice of an appropriate antimicrobial agent for the treatment of UTI should be based on culture and sensitivity reports, overall efficacy of the drug and risk of adverse reactions, and the cost-effectiveness of treatment.
- Sulfamethizole, trimethoprim, trimethoprim-sulfamethoxazole, and nitrofurantoin are equally effective, less costly alternatives to ciprofloxacin for the treatment of acute cystitis.
- The use of oral fluoroquinolones should be reserved for the treatment of complicated UTI caused by bacteria resistant to other antimicrobial agents, or for instances when a parenteral drug is needed or other agents have failed.
- To avoid the emergence of resistant pathogens, the urinary antimicrobial drug selected should be administered at the minimum effective dosage.
- A full glass of water should be consumed with each oral dose of a urinary antimicrobial drug. Total fluid intake should approximate 2000 mL/24 hr.
- Patients should be taught to complete the entire course of treatment, the need for regular bladder emptying and adequate hygiene, and the importance of recognizing signs and symptoms of UTI.
- Evidence that the UTI has been treated effectively include the patient's verbalization of the relief of frequency, urgency, and dysuria; the absence of urine odor; and the return of urine to its clear, light-yellow color.
- "Test of cure" urine cultures should be performed 4 to 7 days after treatment is completed to ensure that urine has been rendered sterile.

BIBLIOGRAPHY

Avorn, J., Monane, M., Gurwitz, J., et al. (1994). Reduction of bacteriuria and pyuria after ingestion of cranberry juice. *Journal of the American Medical Association, 271*(10), 751–754.

Bailey, R. (1993). Management of lower urinary tract infections. *Drugs, 45*(Suppl 3), 139–144.

Bint, A., and Hill, D. (1994). Bacteriuria of pregnancy: An update on significance, diagnosis, and management. *Journal of Antimicrobial Chemotherapy, 33*(Suppl A), 93–97.

Donabedian, H., O'Donnell, E., Drill, C., et al. (1995). Prevention of subsequent urinary tract infections in women by the use of anti-adherence antimicrobial agents: A double-blind comparison of enoxacin with co-trimoxazole. *Journal of Antimicrobial Chemotherapy, 35*, 409–420.

Fillet, H., and Rowe, J. (1992). The aging kidney. In J. Brocklehurst, R. Tallis, and H. Fillet (Eds.), *Textbook of geriatric medicine and gerontology* (4th ed.). Edinburgh: Churchill Livingstone.

Fuselier, H., Hanno, P. Kupin, W., et al. (1997). Cystitis: Not always a simple problem. *Patient Care, 31,* 34–47.

Giroux, J. (1995). Urinary tract infections in adults. In K. Karlowicz (Ed.), *Urologic nursing: Principles and practice.* Philadelphia: W. B. Saunders.

Gottlieb, P. (1995). Comparison of enoxacin versus trimethoprim-sulfamethoxazole in the treatment of patients with complicated urinary tract infections. *Clinical Therapeutics, 17,* 493–502.

Hatton, J., Hughes, M., and Raymond, C. (1994). Management of bacterial urinary tract infections in adults. *Annals of Pharmacotherapy, 28,* 1264–1272.

Hellerstein, S. (1995). Urinary tract infections: Old and new concepts. *Pediatric Clinics of North America, 42,* 1433–1457.

Hendershot, E. (1995). Fluoroquinolones. *Infectious Disease Clinics of North America, 9,* 715–730.

Hodgman, D. (1994). Management of urinary tract infections in pregnancy. *Journal of Perinatal and Neonatal Nursing, 8,* 1–11.

Hooton, T., Scholes, D., Hughes, J., et al. (1996). A prospective study of risk factors for symptomatic urinary tract infection in young women. *The New England Journal of Medicine, 335*(7), 468–474.

Hooton T. (1995). A simplified approach to urinary tract infection. *Hospital Practice, 30*(2), 23–30.

Iravani, A., Tice, A., McCarty, J., et al. (1995). Short-course ciprofloxacin treatment of acute uncomplicated urinary tract infections in women. *Archives of Internal Medicine, 155,* 485–494.

Kinningham, R. (1993). Asymptomatic bacteriuria in pregnancy. *American Family Physician, 47,* 1232–1238.

Kunin, C. (1994). Chemoprophylaxis and suppressive therapy in the management of urinary tract infections. *Journal of Antimicrobial Chemotherapy, 33*(Suppl. A), 51–62.

Louie, T. (1994). Ciprofloxacin: An oral quinolone for the treatment of infections with gram-negative pathogens. *Canadian Medical Association Journal, 150,* 669–676.

MacDonald, T. (1994). The economic evaluation of antibiotic therapy: Relevance to urinary tract infection. *Journal of Antimicrobial Chemotherapy, 33*(Suppl.A), 137–145.

McOsker, C., and Fitzpatrick, P. (1994). Nitrofurantoin: Mechanism of action and implications for resistance development in common uropathogens. *Journal of Antimicrobial Chemotherapy, 33*(Suppl. A), 23–30.

Mikhail, M., and Anyaegbunam, A. (1995). Lower urinary tract dysfunction in pregnancy: A review. *Obstetrical and Gynecological Survey, 50,* 675–683.

Naber, K. (1996). Fluoroquinolones in urinary tract infections: Proper and improper use. *Drugs 52*(Suppl 2), 27–33.

Nicolle, L. (1994). Urinary tract infection. In P. O'Donnell (Ed.), *Geriatric urology.* Boston: Little, Brown.

Nicolle, L. (1994). Urinary tract infection in the elderly. *Journal of Antimicrobial Chemotherapy, 33*(Suppl. A), 99–109.

Nygaard, I., Johnson, J. (1996). Urinary tract infections in elderly women. *American Family Physician, 53,* 175–182.

Ponte, C., and Fisher, M. (1993). Use of fluoroquinolones: Practical considerations. *American Family Physician, 47*(5), 1243–1249.

Schaeffer, A. (1992). Infections of the urinary tract. In P. Walsh, A. Retik, T. Stanley, et al. (Eds.), *Campbell's urology* (5th ed.). Philadelphia: W. B. Saunders.

Shortliffe, L. (1995). The management of urinary tract infections in children without urinary tract abnormalities. *Urologic Clinics of North America, 22,* 67–73.

Swedish Urinary Tract Infection Study Group. (1995). Interpretation of the bacteriologic outcome of antibiotic treatment for uncomplicated cystitis: Impact of the definition of significant bacteriuria in a comparison of ritipenem acoxil with norfloxacin. *Clinical Infectious Disease, 20,* 507–513.

Thomson, K., Sanders, W., and Sanders C. (1994). USA resistance patterns among UTI pathogens. *Journal of Antimicrobial Chemotherapy, 33*(Suppl. A), 9–15.

Vercaigne, L., and Zhanel, G. (1994). Recommended treatment for urinary tract infection in pregnancy. *The Annals of Pharmacotherapy, 28*(2), 248–251.

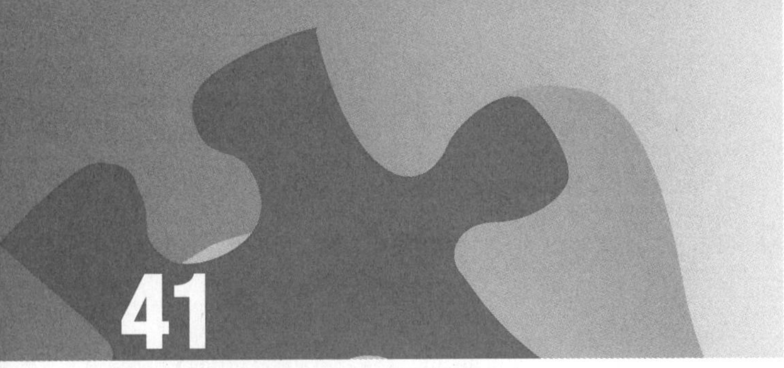

41 Drugs Used in Renal Dysfunction

The kidneys play a major role in maintaining physical well-being by eliminating metabolic waste products; regulating fluids, electrolytes, and the balance of acids and bases in the body; and secreting hormones related to their endocrine function. As a consequence, impairment of renal function is accompanied by major disturbances in biochemical and physiologic functions.

Drug therapy in patients with impaired renal function is complex. Caregivers should examine four major associated factors because treatment may include multidrug therapy. First, the deterioration of renal functioning results in major changes in the bioavailability, distribution, biotransformation, and activity of drugs. Most drugs or their metabolites are at least partially removed by the kidneys; therefore, reduced renal function influences both therapeutic and toxic responses. Second, drugs may adversely affect renal function as a result of a physiologic alteration in renal blood flow (RBF) and glomerular filtration rate (GFR), or by causing parenchymal injury. Third, there are increasing numbers of drugs being used to prevent or retard the progression or development of acute renal failure (ARF). Drug therapy has been used in an attempt to retard the progression of chronic renal failure (CRF), specifically in the treatment of diabetic nephropathy. Finally, several drugs can be used to manage the complications related to loss of renal function.

RENAL FAILURE

Epidemiology and Etiology

Acute Renal Failure

ARF is defined as a sudden, rapid, partial, or complete loss of renal function that occurs over a matter of hours or, at most, a few days. It may be *oliguric* (less than 500 mL of urine/day) or *nonoliguric* (more than 800 mL/day) and usually, but not always, is accompanied by azotemia. *Azotemia* is a build-up of nitrogenous waste in the blood. ARF was first recognized as a clinical entity during World War II and has been a persistent worldwide health problem ever since.

ARF can occur in seriously ill people of any age, gender, or community, and in any hospital unit or extended care facility. Numerous renal insults can cause ARF, but the acute syndrome, unlike the chronic condition, is usually reversible. One potentially preventable cause of hospital-acquired ARF is the inappropriate use of antibiotics. The development of hospital-acquired ARF results in extended hospital stays that are frequently in the intensive care setting. The problem adds significantly to the costs of the initial condition that required hospitalization.

The etiologies of ARF are divided into three groups based on anatomic location: prerenal, intrarenal, and postrenal (Fig. 41–1 and Table 41–1). Prerenal causes of ARF include loss of circulating volume or shifts in circulating volume, decreased cardiac output, decreased peripheral vascular resistance, and renal vascular obstruction.

Acute tubular necrosis (ATN) is the most common cause of intrarenal (parenchymal) azotemia and of ARF in general. ATN is basically ARF that is due to ischemia or toxins, or both. The volume of urinary output produced is related to the number of injured nephrons and the location of the injury (i.e., cortex versus the medulla). Approximately 50 percent of patients with ATN have oliguric renal failure, and 50 percent have nonoliguric renal failure.

Other causes of ATN include acute medullary or cortical necrosis and acute interstitial nephritis. In addition, any prerenal factor that causes renal ischemia is an etiology of intrarenal azotemia. Although prerenal ARF is the most common, intrarenal causes of ARF are the most serious, with the greatest morbidity and a mortality rate of approximately 50 percent. Approximately 10 to 20 percent of adults and 50 percent of children with intrarenal factors have pre-existing parenchymal disease. ARF may also be caused by trauma, severe muscle exertion, certain genetic conditions, infection disease, metabolic disorders, glomerulonephritis, or vascular lesions.

Postrenal factors contributing to ARF are those causing obstruction or disruption of the drainage system. Postrenal obstruction is the major cause of postrenal azotemia, accounting for 2 to 15 percent of all cases of ARF and the second most common cause of ARF in infants. Common causes of postrenal obstruction in the newborn are related to congenital anomalies (e.g., ureteropelvic stricture). In the older adult, prostatic disease is the most common cause of postrenal obstruction, and in the female, it is pelvic cancer. Traumatic and surgical injuries may also contribute to postrenal ARF.

Most patients who survive ARF experience full return of renal function. However, infection develops in 80 percent of patients and is of particular concern in patients with diabetes, trauma, and those who have had surgery. Gastrointestinal (GI) bleeding occurs in approximately 25 percent of patients with ARF. The prognosis is better for patients with nonoliguric ARF than those with the oliguric form. The use of specific diuretics may improve the prognosis by increasing urinary output, but the use of diuretics does not improve renal function.

Chronic Renal Failure

CRF can develop insidiously over many years, or it can occur as a result of ARF from which the patient fails to recover. The etiology of CRF is complex and multifaceted. More than 100 different disease processes can contribute to progressive loss of renal function. Diabetes mellitus and hypertension represent over 60 percent of the causes of end-stage renal disease (ESRD) in the United States. Further-

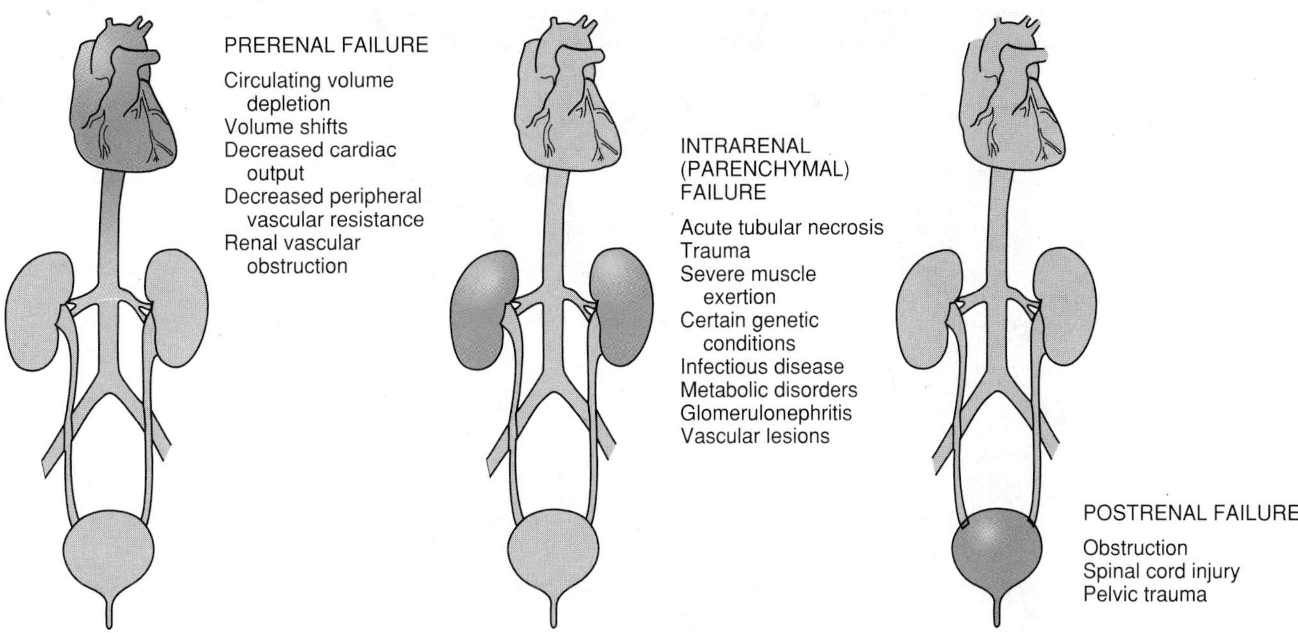

Figure 41–1 Anatomic location of prerenal, intrarenal, and postrenal failure. (From Black, J. M., and Matassarin-Jacbos, E. [1997]. *Medical-surgical nursing: Clinical management for continuity of care* [5th ed., p. 1637]. Philadelphia: W. B. Saunders. Used with permission.)

more, it is estimated that 70 to 90 percent of patients with renal failure are hypertensive, with about 30 percent requiring antihypertensive therapy. The third most common cause of CRF is glomerulonephritis, an inflammation of the glomeruli that frequently follows streptococcal infections of the upper respiratory tract. Acute glomerulonephritis can completely resolve or progress to chronic glomerulonephritis and eventual renal failure.

In patients with CRF, the kidney is unable to remove metabolic wastes and excessive water from the circulation. When renal failure progresses to ESRD, kidney impairment is permanent. The incidence of CRF is continually growing in the United States as a result of our increasing ability to prolong life using technical replacements for renal function. It is estimated that approximately 30 percent of the population undergoing hemodialysis has diabetes, and that 25 to 50 percent of patients with insulin-dependent diabetes will develop ESRD within 10 to 20 years of beginning insulin therapy. Renal disease can also develop in the non–insulin-dependent patient. The incidence of proteinuria is about 25 percent after 20 years of diabetes. Furthermore, thousands of additional people who have diabetes are in various stages of renal insufficiency.

Genetics play a major role in the development of ESRD. The incidence of renal failure in the black population is four times as great as in the white population. In addition, blacks have a 6.2 times greater chance of developing ESRD secondary to hypertension. Focal and segmental glomerulosclerosis that occurs in association with intravenous (IV) drug use and acquired immunodeficiency syndrome is the most common cause of renal failure in young black adult males. These figures represent a 10 times greater risk for developing CRF than whites. Hispanics and Native Americans are also at increased risk for renal failure secondary to type II diabetes mellitus. The exact role socioeconomic factors play in predisposing these populations to an increased risk of ESRD is unclear.

Pathophysiology

The kidneys receive 20 to 25 percent of the cardiac output every minute and are very sensitive to changes in blood supply. A number of prerenal and intrarenal events can cause a critical fall in RBF. When RBF is diminished, the nutrients and oxygen for basic renal cellular metabolism and tubular transport systems are also diminished. Further, when RBF decreases, the fundamental driving force for filtration is reduced. The decline in RBF is further reduced by release of vasoconstrictive hormones, including angiotensin, vasopressin, and catecholamines. The result is a crucial fall in RBF, and glomerular filtration can no longer be maintained. In addition, there is a resultant rise in blood urea nitrogen (BUN) and creatinine levels and a fall in urinary output. Correcting the factors that contribute to reduced RBF helps re-establish adequate circulation, thereby preventing ischemic injury.

Acute Renal Failure

ARF is characterized by an initial oliguric phase, followed in 10 to 14 days to a few weeks by a diuretic phase. Problems seen during the oliguric phase include an inability to eliminate solute loads, regulate electrolytes, and eliminate metabolic waste products. During the diuretic phase, large amounts of fluids (4 to 5 L/day) and electrolytes are lost. The recovery phase may take as long as 6 months to a year before renal function returns to a normal range.

Prerenal Factors

When ARF occurs from prerenal factors, blood flow to the kidneys is reduced. In most cases, poor systemic perfu-

TABLE 41–1 CAUSES OF RENAL FAILURE

Prerenal Factors	
Hypovolemia	Hemorrhage, burns, shock, excessive sweating, GI losses, peritonitis, nephrotic syndrome, diuretics, diabetes insipidus
Altered peripheral vascular resistance	Antihypertensive drugs, sepsis, drug overdose, anaphylaxis, neurogenic shock
Cardiac disorders	Congestive heart failure, myocardial infarction, cardiac tamponade, arrhythmias
Renal artery disorders	Emboli, thrombi, stenosis, aneurysm, occlusion, trauma
Drug-induced	ACE inhibitors, NSAIDs
Hepatorenal syndrome	
Intrarenal Factors	
Inflammatory processes	Bacterial, viral, pre-eclampsia
Immune processes	Autoimmunity, hypersensitivity, rejection
Trauma	Penetrating (e.g., knife, bullet), nonpenetrating (e.g., fall, crushing injury, motor vehicle accident, sports injury)
Obstruction	Neoplasm, stones, scar tissue
Systemic and vascular disorders	Diabetes mellitus, systemic lupus erythematosus, sickle cell disease, multiple myeloma, renal vein thrombosis
Drug-induced	Anesthetics, antimicrobials, NSAIDs, antineoplastics, contrast media
Nephrotoxins	Tumor toxins, heme pigments (e.g., hemoglobin, myoglobin), pesticides, fungicides, organic solvents, heavy metals, mushrooms, snake venom
Postrenal Factors	
Obstruction	Congenital anomalies (e.g., ureteropelvic stricture), benign prostatic hypertrophy, pelvic cancer, trauma, surgical injury

ACE, Angiotensin-converting enzyme; GI, gastrointestinal; NSAIDs, nonsteroidal anti-inflammatory drugs.

sion exists and circulating blood volume, peripheral vascular resistance, and cardiac output are diminished. The body's adaptive mechanisms shunt blood to vital organs, such as the heart and brain, and away from the musculoskeletal, splenic, and renal areas. The kidneys respond to decreased perfusion through autoregulation and the release of renin.

Dilation of afferent arterioles and vasoconstriction of efferent arterioles help maintain glomerular hydrostatic pressures. The autoregulatory mechanism, however, is restricted by the degree and the duration of renal hypoperfusion, and the functional state of the arterioles. If the arterioles are affected by a vascular disorder (e.g., diabetes mellitus or chronic hypertension), they may be unable to change tone adequately and thus autoregulation is incomplete.

The renin-angiotensin-aldosterone system is also stimulated by renal hypoperfusion. Activation of the renin-angiotensin-aldosterone system causes peripheral vasoconstriction, increased potassium elimination, and sodium reabsorption. The resulting increase in plasma osmolality stimulates hypothalamic osmoreceptors, causing the release of antidiuretic hormone (ADH). The presence of ADH, in turn, causes further vasoconstriction and water reabsorption from distal tubules. With increased sodium and water reabsorption, tubular flow rates decrease, enhancing the reabsorption of urea.

The patient's urinary output will be decreased, the urine will be concentrated and will contain little sodium. Plasma osmolality, sodium, and BUN levels are increased, and potassium levels are decreased. Plasma creatinine levels usually do not rise because creatine clearance is a function of glomerular filtration, which is maintained at this time.

Intrarenal Factors

In contrast to prerenal mechanisms, intrarenal factors result in damage to renal parenchyma. The two most common insults related to intrarenal ARF are ischemia and toxins. Although the initial affront results in injury to the glomeruli, tubules, or interstitial cells, surrounding tissues also become quickly involved. In general, the sequence of events occurring in response to renal ischemia are vasoconstriction, decreased GFR, and tubular dysfunction. Vasoconstriction is mediated by angiotensin II which causes renal vasoconstriction. The prostaglandins also act as antagonists to angiotensin II, thereby altering the degree of vasoconstriction. Renal vasoconstriction is also enhanced by the presence of ADH.

Several factors cause the decrease in GFR. Decreased RBF contributes to decreased GFR, but even if RBF is improved, the GFR remains reduced. Cell debris, sloughed microvilli, and the formation of casts cause tubular obstruction and increased hydrostatic pressure in Bowman's capsule and a decrease in GFR. Furthermore, persistent local or systemic vasoconstriction decreases the GFR.

The extent of tubular dysfunction relates to the duration of ischemia. Sixty minutes of ischemia produces prompt necrosis, but it is mostly reversible in time. Ninety to one hundred and twenty minutes of ischemia produces irreversible damage. Injury to basement membranes causes increased tubular permeability, with leakage of tubular fluid into the interstitium and capillaries. Debris clogs tubular lumens to impair the flow of tubular fluids.

The eventual outcome of vasoconstriction, decreased GFR, and tubular dysfunction is an inability of the nephron to sustain its ability to transport substances, concentrate urine, maintain acid-base balance, and eliminate waste.

Toxic ATN is different from ischemic ATN in that the initial mechanism is injury to tubule cells. The onset is more insidious because some degree of tubular damage has occurred before clinical manifestations become evident. The kidney is vulnerable to toxins for several reasons. First, the kidneys are repeatedly exposed to everything in the blood. The liver detoxifies many substances that the kidneys eliminate, but with liver disease, the kidneys become overloaded with substances that have not been detoxified. The renal cortex contains enzymes that change nontoxic substances (especially drugs) to toxic compounds, and the countercurrent mechanism concentrates toxic as well as body substances. Thus, patients at most risk for toxic ATN are those with hepatic or renal dysfunction, or both.

Postrenal Factors

Obstruction can occur within the genitourinary tract or outside the tract to compress urinary structures. The initial physiologic change is an increase in pressure within the collecting ducts to the point of obstruction. In turn, there is increased pressure within tubular lumens. The increased intratubular pressure counteracts normal glomerular filtration pressures, and glomerular filtration ceases. With chronic obstruction, the tubular capabilities of urinary concentration, solute reabsorption, and urinary acidification are decreased.

With long-term obstruction, dilatation of urinary tract structures occurs proximal to the site of obstruction. The medulla is almost completely destroyed, and the cortex thins. Subsequent destruction of renal parenchyma results in loss of renal function.

Chronic Renal Failure

CRF is characterized by histologic evidence of irreversible renal damage. Three stages characterize CRF. Initially, there is diminished renal reserve without accumulation of metabolic wastes. The unaffected kidney compensates for the decreased function of the diseased kidney. The next stages are mild (40 to 80 percent of normal function), moderate (15 to 40 percent), or severe (2 to 20 percent) renal insufficiency. In these stages, metabolic waste accumulates in the blood because the healthier kidney can no longer compensate for the loss of function of the other kidney. Ultimately, the patient enters ESRD. Excessive amounts of nitrogenous wastes accumulate in the blood, and the kidneys are unable to maintain homeostasis. Severe fluid and electrolyte imbalances occur. Unless some form of dialysis is started, ESRD is fatal. The time from onset of disease to total loss of renal function can be variable but usually represents a period of 5 to 10 years.

Multiple system dysfunction occurs as renal failure progresses, leading to anemia, uremia, disorders of calcium and phosphorus biotransformation, and acidosis. Anemia, an expected complication of advanced renal failure, primarily results from the inability of diseased kidneys to manufacture erythropoietin. However, it can be further aggravated by deficiencies of iron and certain vitamins. Although iron deficiency is not uncommon in renal failure alone, it is common in patients who are maintained on hemodialysis for long periods of time. The anemia is a consequence of continued blood sampling for diagnostic studies and losses associated with the procedure. Owing to recombinant DNA technology, the anemic state can now largely be prevented and cured with epoetin alfa.

The uremic state is associated with abnormal platelet function that manifests as prolonged bleeding times and a predisposition to bleeding. A number of abnormal mechanisms contribute to the potential for bleeding. Platelet factor III activity is decreased, there are decreased levels of thromboxane A_2, increased levels of the platelet inhibitor prostacyclin, and suboptimal activity of factor VIII (von Willebrand's factor). The defects in platelet function can be partially corrected by repeated dialysis. Cryoprecipitate has been previously used to correct abnormal bleeding times. Desmopressin acetate (DDAVP), a synthetic analog of ADH, has been used. Both cryoprecipitate and DDAVP increase von Willebrand's factor concentrations and shorten bleeding times.

Disorders of calcium and phosphorus biotransformation, including hypocalcemia, hyperphosphatemia, secondary hyperparathyroidism, bone disease, and metastatic calcification, are common findings in patients with advanced renal failure. These disturbances are largely a consequence of the kidneys' inability to eliminate phosphate, synthesize the active metabolite of vitamin D ($1,25[OH]_2D_3$), and eliminate hydrogen ions. Retention of phosphorus results in hyperphosphatemia, promoting soft tissue calcification and suppression of serum calcium levels. The hypocalcemia, in turn, causes secondary hyperparathyroidism and promotes bone disease. The hyperparathyroid state is further intensified by an inability of the diseased kidney to synthesize $1,25(OH)_2D_3$. $1,25(OH)_2D_3$ normally exerts a suppressive effect on parathyroid hormone synthesis. Therapy is directed at normalizing serum phosphorus levels and suppressing the hyperparathyroid state. This goal can be accomplished by the administration of phosphate binding drugs and calcitriol, a vitamin D supplement.

Acidosis represents a compounding factor in the genesis of bone disease. The patient with CRF has a positive hydrogen ion balance as a result of the inability to eliminate diet-derived acids adequately. The retained hydrogen ions are thought to be buffered by bone salts, resulting in the dissolution of bone crystals. Orally administered sodium bicarbonate effectively corrects chronic acidosis and thus prevents the dissolution of bone salts.

PHARMACOTHERAPEUTIC OPTIONS

The management of a patient with renal failure ordinarily includes multidrug therapy, diet therapy, and dialysis in some form. Managing drug therapy in patients with renal disease is a complex endeavor because of the numerous drugs used. As the patient's renal function deteriorates, adjustments in dosage are repeatedly required.

There are a variety of drug classes used in the management of renal failure, including angiotensin-converting enzyme (ACE) inhibitors, antianemic drugs, iron supplements, antihemorrhagic drugs, phosphate binders, vitamin D supplements, heavy metal antagonists (chelating drugs), systemic antacids, loop diuretics, vasopressors, and cation exchange resins.

Angiotensin-Converting Enzyme Inhibitors

❒ Captopril (CAPOTEN)

Indications

The major objectives in the management of patients with CRF are to slow or prevent the progression of renal failure to ESRD and to alleviate the complications and consequences of advanced renal failure. The most common ACE inhibitor approved by the Food and Drug Administration for these purposes is captopril (see also Chapter 34). Captopril is most useful in patients with type I diabetic nephropathy who have decreasing renal function, but it is also thought to exert similar beneficial effects in all types of proteinuric renal diseases.

Pharmacodynamics

Captopril alters intrarenal hemodynamics by blocking the conversion of angiotensin I to angiotensin II. By blocking angiotensin II formation, efferent arteriolar vasoconstriction is reduced, the permeability of the glomerular basement membrane is reduced, and sodium is reabsorbed from the proximal tubules. The blood pressure is normalized, and thus, the rate of functional deterioration in proteinuric renal disease is decreased.

Adverse Effects and Contraindications

Adverse effects of ACE inhibitors include skin rash, hypotension, and angioedema, which can, in turn, cause airway obstruction and cough.

A major adverse effect noted in patients with renal failure is hyperkalemia. Hyperkalemia secondary to the use of captopril results from reduced circulating aldosterone concentrations and a reduced GFR. A loss of taste perception may also occur and is usually reversible in 2 to 3 months.

Captopril is contraindicated in patients with hypersensitivity. Cross-hypersensitivity among ACE inhibitors may occur. Use during pregnancy may cause fetal malformation or death, and hypotension, oliguria, or hypokalemia may occur in the newborn. Captopril should be used cautiously in patients with renal impairment, hepatic impairment, hypovolemia, hyponatremia, aortic stenosis, and cerebrovascular or cardiac insufficiency; older adults; and patients receiving concurrent diuretic therapy. Safety during lactation and in children has not been established.

Pharmacokinetics

The pharmacokinetics of captopril are identified in Table 41–2. Seventy-five percent of captopril is absorbed following oral administration, but bioavailability is decreased in the presence of food. Twenty-five to thirty percent is bound to plasma proteins, with 50 percent biotransformed by the liver to inactive compounds. Fifty percent of the drug is eliminated unchanged by the kidneys.

Drug-Drug Interactions

There are several drug-drug interactions with captopril as well as other drugs used in the treatment of renal failure (Table 41–3). The concurrent use of nonsteroidal anti-inflammatory drugs (NSAIDs), especially indomethacin, may reduce the antihypertensive effect of captopril by inhibiting the synthesis of renal prostaglandin or causing sodium and water retention. Concurrent use of diuretics and some antihypertensive drugs produces additive hypotensive effects. Any antihypertensive drug that causes renin release or that affects sympathetic activity also has an additive effect. Dosage adjustment of antihypertensives may be required when these drugs are used concurrently with captopril or when one or the other drug is discontinued. Antacids have been reported to decrease the effect of captopril and should be administered separately.

Dosage Regimen

The oral dose of captopril used to prevent progression of renal failure is 25 mg three times daily (see Table 41–3). Safe use in pediatric patients has not been established. Furthermore, neonates are more susceptible to the hemodynamic effects of captopril and, therefore, are at risk for oliguria and neurologic abnormalities. This drug is also not recommended for use during the last two trimesters of pregnancy because ACE inhibitors have been shown to cause injury and death in the developing fetus. Older adults tend to have lower plasma renin activity that makes them less sensitive to hypotensive effects. However, this sensitivity may be offset somewhat by the decreased metabolic and elimination capacity. Captopril is removed with hemodialysis, and therefore, dosage adjustment is required for control of hypertension.

Laboratory Considerations

There is a higher incidence of life-threatening neutropenia and agranulocytosis in patients with impaired renal function. Therefore, it is recommended that white blood cell determinations (i.e., total and differential) be obtained before starting therapy and monitored periodically thereafter. ACE inhibitor therapy should be discontinued if the neutrophil count is less than $1000/mm^3$.

BUN and creatinine levels should be measured because captopril, as a consequence of reducing glomerular filtration pressure, can cause the BUN and creatinine to be transiently increased. Patients who may have elevated levels are those who are volume or sodium depleted, who have bilateral renal artery stenosis, or who had a rapid reduction in chronic or severe hypertension. The health care provider should monitor white blood cell counts (i.e., total and differential) before the initiation of therapy and periodically throughout the course of therapy.

Captopril may cause an elevation of serum potassium levels due to a drug-induced reduction of aldosterone production and the elevated potassium of ESRD. Therefore, frequent monitoring of serum potassium levels is recommended, especially when there is concurrent use of

TABLE 41–2 PHARMACOKINETICS OF SELECTED DRUGS USED TO TREAT RENAL DYSFUNCTION*

Drug	Route	Onset	Peak	Duration	PB (%)	$t_{1/2}$	BioA (%)
ACE Inhibitor							
Captopril	po	15–60 min	0.5–1.5 hrs	6–12 hrs	25–36	1.5–2 hrs	65
Antianemic							
Epoetin alfa	IV/SC	7–14 days	2–6 weeks†	2 weeks	UA	4–13 hrs	UA
Iron Supplements							
Ferrous formulations	po	4 days	7–10 days‡	2–3 months	UA	UK	UA
Iron dextran	IM	Slow	1–2 weeks	Months	UK	6 hrs	UK
Antihemorrhagic Drug							
Desmopressin acetate	IV/SC	Min	15–30 min	90–120 min	UA	75 min	100
	IN	1 hr	1–5 hrs	8–20 hrs	UA	75 min	10–20
Phosphate-Binding Drugs							
Aluminum hydroxide§	po	Hrs–days	Days–weeks	Days	UA	UK	UA
Calcium salts	po	UK	UK	UK	45	UK	UK
	IV	Immed	Immed	0.5–2 hr	45	UK	100
Vitamin Supplement							
Calcitriol	po	2–6 hrs	2–6 hrs	1–5 days	Variable	3–8 hr	UK
Heavy Metal Antagonist							
Deferoxamine	IM/IV/SC	UK	UK	UK	UA	1 hr	UK
Loop Diuretic							
Furosemide	po	30–60 min	1–2 hrs	6–8 hr	95	30–60 min	60
	IV	5 min	30 min	2 hrs	95	UA	100
Vasopressor							
Dopamine	IV	1–2 min	10 min	Dur of inf	UA	2 min	100
Systemic Antacid							
Sodium bicarbonate	po	Immed	30 min	1–3 hrs	UA	UK	UK
	IV	Immed	Rapid	UK	UA	UK	100
Cation-Exchange Resin							
Sodium polystyrene sulfonate	po	2–12 hrs	UK	6–24 hrs	UA	UK	0
	PR	2–12 hrs	UK	4–6 hr	UA	UK	0

*Therapeutic serum drug levels for these renal drugs are not routinely measured.

†Epoetin alfa: Peak effect, which is the targeted hematocrit level, may be achieved in 8 weeks with adequate dosing. Elevation in red blood cell count lasts for approximately 2 weeks following discontinuation of the drug.

‡Peak levels and the amount of iron absorbed are approximately in linear relationship to dose ingested.

§Hypophosphatemic effects of aluminum hydroxide given orally.

PB, Protein binding; $t_{1/2}$, elimination half-life; UK, unknown; UA, unavailable; IN, intranasal; BioA, bioavailability.

potassium-containing medications, potassium supplements, and salt substitutes containing potassium.

Antianemics

❒ Epoetin alfa (erythropoietin, EPO, EPOGEN, PROCRIT)

Indications

Anemia universally accompanies chronic renal disease. In fact, hematocrit values of 16 to 22 percent were common in the days before epoetin alfa was available. Epoetin alfa is now a well-accepted drug for the treatment of the anemia associated with CRF. It is used for patients who are not on dialysis, as well as for those undergoing the various dialytic therapies. Epoetin alfa is not a substitute for blood transfusions and is not intended as an emergency treatment for severe anemia or blood loss. However, it has decreased the transfusion dependency of many patients with CRF. Patients treated with this drug have an increase in hematocrit, improved energy, and less fatigue. Other favorable outcomes include improvements in cardiovascular status and cognitive function, exercise tolerance, and quality of life.

Epoetin alfa is also indicated for the management of anemia secondary to zidovudine therapy in human immunodeficiency virus–infected patients. Patients with nonmyeloid malignancies who have anemia secondary to antineoplastic therapy may also be candidates for epoetin alfa.

Pharmacodynamics

Epoetin alfa induces erythropoiesis by stimulating the division and differentiation of erythroid progenitor cells. Reticulocytes are released from the bone marrow and mature to erythrocytes. Clinically significant increases in the reticulocyte count occur in 7 to 10 days, with a rise in hemoglobin and hematocrit occurring in 2 to 6 weeks. However, the increased hemoglobin and hematocrit levels increase blood viscosity and peripheral vascular resistance. Blood pressure increases in 25 to 30 percent of patients, and thus, changes in antihypertensive therapy may be required. Furthermore, increased red blood cell (RBC) volume shortens bleeding time. Hemodialysis patients may require increased anticoagulation to prevent blood clotting in the dialyzer or vascular access device.

TABLE 41–3 DRUG-DRUG INTERACTIONS OF SELECTED DRUGS USED TO TREAT RENAL DYSFUNCTION

Drug	Interactive Drug	Interaction
ACE Inhibitor		
Captopril	Indomethacin	Decreased antihypertensive effect of captopril
	Antihypertensives Diuretics	Increased hypotensive effects
	Antacids	Decreased absorption of captopril
Antianemic		
Epoetin alfa	Heparin	May increase the requirement for heparin anticoagulation during dialysis
Iron Supplements		
Ferrous fumarate, gluconate, sulfate, iron dextran	Ciprofloxacin Enoxacin Norfloxacin Ofloxacin Penicillamine	Decreased effects of interactive drug
	Levodopa	Decreased effects
	Chloramphenicol Vitamin E	Impairs hematologic response to iron therapy
	Tetracycline	Decreased absorption of interactive drug
	Antacids	Inhibits absorption of iron by forming insoluble compounds
	Vitamin C	May slightly increase absorption of oral iron preparations
Antihemorrhagic Drugs		
Desmopressin acetate	Chlorpropamide Clofibrate Carbamazepine	May enhance the antidiuretic response to desmopressin acetate
	Demeclocycline Lithium Norepinephrine	May diminish the antidiuretic response to desmopressin acetate
Phosphate-Binding Drugs		
Calcium preparations	Ciprofloxacin Digitalis preparations Fluoroquinolone antibiotics Iron salts Phenytoin Tetracyclines	Decreased absorption of interactive drugs
	Cardiac glycosides	Hypercalcemia increases the risk of glycoside toxicity
	Antacids	Chronic use may lead to milk-alkali syndrome
	Atenolol Calcium channel blocking drugs	Excessive amounts of calcium may decrease the effects of interactive drugs
	Thiazide diuretics	Concurrent use may result in hypercalcemia
	Sodium polystyrene sulfonate	May decrease the ability of interactive drugs to decrease serum potassium levels
Aluminum hydroxide	Chlorpromazine Digitalis preparations Fluoroquinolone antibiotics Iron salts	Absorption of interactive drug may be decreased
	Calcium citrate Sodium citrate	Markedly enhanced absorption of aluminum leading to toxicity
	Amphetamine Mexiletine Quinidine	Interactive drug levels may be increased if enough aluminum hydroxide is ingested such that urinary pH is increased
	Salicylates	Interactive drug blood levels may be decreased
Vitamin Supplement		
Calcitriol	Magnesium containing antacids	Increased risk of hypermagnesemia
	Cholestyramine Mineral oil	Decreased absorption of fat-soluble vitamins
	Thiazide diuretics	Increased risk of hypercalcemia
	Barbiturates Hydantoin Primidone	Increased biotransformation of calcitriol and decreased effects
Heavy Metal Antagonist		
Deferoxamine	Ascorbic acid	May increase effectiveness of deferoxamine but also may increase cardiac iron toxicity

TABLE 41–3 DRUG-DRUG INTERACTIONS OF SELECTED DRUGS USED TO TREAT RENAL DYSFUNCTION *Continued*

Drug	Interactive Drug	Interaction
Loop Diuretic		
Furosemide	Oral hypoglycemic drugs	Increased potential for hyperglycemia
	Aminoglycoside	Increased potential for toxicity
	Cisplatin	
	Lithium carbonate	Decreased secretion of lithium, salicylate, increased risk of toxicity
	Salicylates	
	Digoxin	Increased potential for digoxin toxicity related to potassium loss
	NSAIDs	Decreased antihypertensive effect of furosemide
	Neuromuscular blocking drugs	Increased effects of neuromuscular blockade
	Phenytoin	Decreased absorption and effectiveness of furosemide
	Theophylline	Increased diuresis from furosemide
Vasopressor		
Dopamine	Beta blockers	Decreased therapeutic effects of dopamine
	General anesthetics	Increased risk of arrhythmias
	Monoamine oxidase inhibitors	Increased intensity and prolongs cardiac stimulant and vasopressor effects of dopamine
	Phenytoin	May cause sudden hypotension and bradycardia
Cation-Exchange Resin		
Sodium polystyrene sulfonate	Magnesium and calcium containing antacids and laxatives	Increased risk of metabolic alkalosis
	Cardiac glycosides	Increased risk of glycoside toxicity
Systemic Antacid		
Sodium bicarbonate	Ketoconazole	Decreased absorption of interacting agent
	Demeclocycline	Increased excretion of interacting agent
	Doxycycline	
	Lithium	
	Methacycline	
	Salicylates	
	Sulfonylureas	
	Tetracyclines	
	Flecainide	Decreased excretion of interacting agent
	Mexiletine	
	Quinidine	
	Anorexiants	Increased effects of interacting agents
	Sympathomimetics	
	Amphetamines	Increased half-lives and duration of action of interacting agent
	Ephedrine	
	Pseudoephedrine	

Adverse Effects and Contraindications

Hypertension is the most common adverse effect of epoetin alfa. Headache, transient rashes, and thrombotic events (in patients on dialysis) are also possible. Female patients may have a resumption of menses and fertility may be restored; therefore, the risk of pregnancy should be evaluated. If pregnancy is desired, there should be a thorough evaluation of currently prescribed medications that could be injurious to the fetus. Contraceptive methods should be used for women in whom pregnancy is to be avoided.

Although they are rare, seizures are the most serious adverse effect, occurring in about 1.1 percent of the patients receiving epoetin alfa. If the hematocrit increases more than four points in a 2-week period, the likelihood of a hypertensive reaction and seizures increases.

Epoetin alfa is contraindicated in patients with hypersensitivity to albumin or mammalian cell–derived products or in those with uncontrolled hypertension. It is also contraindicated in patients with erythropoietin levels exceeding 200 mU/mL. The drug should be used cautiously in patients with a history of seizures. Safe use during pregnancy, lactation, or in children has not been established.

Pharmacokinetics

Epoetin alfa is well absorbed following subcutaneous (SC) and IV administration, although its distribution, biotransformation, and elimination are unknown (see Table 41–2). An increase in reticulocyte count is observed in 7 to 14 days with peak activity noted in 2 to 6 weeks. The increase in RBC counts lasts for approximately 2 weeks following discontinuation of the drug. The half life of epoetin alfa is 4 to 13 hours.

Drug-Drug Interactions

There are few drug-drug interactions with epoetin alfa. The drug may increase the requirement for heparin anticoagulation in patients on dialysis (see Table 41–3).

Dosage Regimen

Before starting therapy, the patient's iron status should be evaluated because the efficacy of epoetin alfa is decreased when iron stores are insufficient to promote erythropoiesis. Furthermore, iron deficiency may occur with the use of epoetin alfa due to an internal shift of iron stores to RBCs during the correction of acute anemia or the external loss of RBC iron during both the acute and maintenance phases of therapy. Because iron is necessary for continued RBC production, virtually all patients receiving epoetin alfa eventually require supplemental iron. A poor initial response or loss of response may be due to other factors, such as infection, iron deficiency, or occult bleeding. Serum ferritin levels should be greater than 100 ng/mL and transferrin saturation greater than 20 percent. If iron stores fall below these levels, the patient should receive supplemental iron before starting epoetin alfa. Oral iron preparations may be adequate for peritoneal dialysis patients; however, hemodialysis patients may require parenteral iron because there is a continuous loss of blood with the hemodialysis procedure (1 mL of blood loss is equal to 1 mg of iron loss).

The usual initial dose of epoetin alfa for patients on dialysis is 50 to 100 units/kg IV three times weekly (Table 41–4). It may be given either IV or SC for patients who are not on dialysis. If the hematocrit does not rise by five or six points or the hematocrit level has not reached the target range of 30 to 35 percent after 8 weeks of therapy, the dosage is increased by 25 units/kg. In patients not on dialysis, epoetin alfa should be used only when the hematocrit falls below 30 percent. The individual response to therapy is variable, so higher doses may be needed in some patients. The maintenance dose is achieved by increasing the dose by 25 units/kg/month until the hematocrit reaches the desired level. Hemoglobin and hematocrit levels should be measured twice weekly until a maintenance dose is established. The hematocrit level declines 2 weeks after discontinuing the drug.

Lower doses of epoetin alfa are required when the SC route is used because of the longer half-life of SC administered drug. The variable absorption from SC sites makes the response less predictable. Safe use in pediatric patients has not been established.

Laboratory Considerations

Epoetin alfa has been reported to cause an increase in white blood cell and platelet counts, and it may decrease bleeding times. It has also been shown to cause elevations in BUN, creatinine, phosphorus, potassium, sodium, and uric acid. It is unclear if the elevations are the result of drug action, the efficacy of dialysis, or if the elevations are caused by noncompliance with dietary restrictions. The patient should also be monitored for an additional 2 to 6 weeks following a change in dosage or until the hematocrit has stabilized. Once it is stable, the hematocrit should be monitored at monthly intervals throughout the course of therapy.

Iron Supplements

- ❐ Ferrous fumarate (FEMIRON, FEOSTAT, FUMASORB, FUMERIN, HEMOCYTE, IRCON); (🍁) PALAFER
- ❐ Ferrous gluconate (FERGON, FERRALET, SIMRON); (🍁) APO-FERROUS GLUCONATE
- ❐ Ferrous sulfate (FEOSOL, FEROSPACE, FER-IN-SOL, FER-IRON, FERO-GRADUMET FILMTABS, FERRALYN, FERRA-TD, MOL-IRON, SLOW FE); (🍁) APO-FERROUS SULFATE, FERO-GRAD, PMS-FERROUS SULFATE
- ❐ Iron dextran (IMFERON, INFED)

Indications

Patients on dialysis are prone to iron deficiency because of repeated blood testing, surgical interventions, and blood loss during the dialysis procedure. A minority of dialysis patients will have an increase in hematocrit and symptomatic improvement with correction of iron deficiency alone. However, iron is a necessary component of erythropoiesis. Therapy with epoetin alfa will be hindered if patients do not have adequate iron stores. Iron dextran, a parenteral form, is used when iron deficiency has been documented in patients who received oral iron supplementation previously.

Pharmacodynamics

Iron is an essential mineral found in hemoglobin, myoglobin, and a number of enzymes, and it is necessary for effective erythropoiesis and for transport and utilization of oxygen. It elevates serum iron concentration and is then converted to hemoglobin or trapped in the reticuloendothelial cells for storage and eventual conversion to a usable form of iron. Parenteral iron enters the blood stream and organs of the reticuloendothelial system (i.e., liver, spleen, bone marrow), where it is separated from the dextran complex and becomes part of the body's iron stores.

Adverse Effects and Contraindications

Oral iron preparations are usually well tolerated, although nausea, epigastric pain, constipation, diarrhea, abdominal cramping, GI bleeding, and black stools may result. Contact irritation of the throat may occur with oral formulations, particularly liquids. Hypotension is the most common adverse effect of parenterally administered iron supplements. Headache, dizziness, syncope, tachycardia, urticaria, flushing, arthralgias, and phlebitis have also been reported. Seizures and anaphylaxis are the most serious adverse effects.

Iron supplements are contraindicated in patients with primary hemochromatosis, hemolytic anemias, and other anemias not associated with iron deficiency. They should be used with caution in patients with peptic ulcers, ulcerative colitis, or regional enteritis, whose conditions may be aggravated. Some products contain alcohol or tartrazine and should be avoided in patients with known intolerance or hypersensitivity. Indiscriminate use of iron supplements may lead to iron overload. Patients with autoimmune disorders and arthritis are more susceptible to allergic reactions. Extreme caution should be used when administering iron supplements to patients with severe liver impairment.

Pharmacokinetics

The pharmacokinetics of iron preparations are identified in Table 41–2. In general, only five to 10 percent of dietary iron is absorbed. In deficiency states, this may increase to 30 percent. Therapeutically administered oral iron may be 60-percent absorbed. Iron supplements are well absorbed following IM administration. Iron remains in the body for many months, crossing the placenta and entering breast milk. It is over 90-percent protein bound. Iron supplements are mostly recycled, with small daily losses occurring through desquamation, sweat, urine, and bile.

TABLE 41–4 DOSAGE REGIMEN OF SELECTED DRUGS USED TO TREAT RENAL DYSFUNCTION

Drug	Use(s)	Dosage	Implications
ACE Inhibitor			
Captopril	Slow or prevent progression of ESRD in type I diabetes, proteinuric renal disease	*Adult:* 25 mg po TID	Discontinue if neutrophil count < 1000/mm^3. Safe use in pediatric patients has not been established
Antianemic			
Epoetin alfa	Anemia related to chronic renal failure	*Adult:* 50–100 units/kg IV/SC three times weekly. Increase by 25 units/kg if Hct does not rise by 5–6 points or has not reached the target range of 30–35% after 8 weeks of therapy. Maintenance: Decrease dose by 25 units/month until desired levels are achieved	Target hematocrit range for patients on dialysis: 30–35%. If patient is not on dialysis, drug should be used only when hematocrit is less than 30%
	Anemia secondary to zidovudine therapy	*Adult:* 100 units/kg IV/SC 3 times weekly for 8 weeks. If inadequate response, may increase by 50–100 units/kg every 4–8 weeks, up to 300 units/kg three times weekly	Determine endogenous serum erythropoietin level before administration. Patients with levels exceeding 500 mU/mL may not respond to therapy. Monitor Hct weekly during dosage adjustment
	Anemia secondary to antineoplastic therapy	*Adult:* 150 units/kg SC three times weekly. May increase after 8 weeks up to 300 units/kg three times weekly	Patients with lower baseline erythropoietin levels may respond more rapidly. Not recommended if erythropoietin levels exceed 200 mU/mL
Iron Supplements			
Ferrous fumarate	Iron supplementation. Prevention and treatment of iron deficiency anemia, iron replacement for blood loss	*Adult:* Prophylaxis: 200 mg po daily. Therapeutic: 200 mg po TID–QID. Controlled release capsules may be given twice daily. *Child:* Prophylaxis: 3 mg/kg/day po. Therapeutic: 3–6 mg/kg po TID	Approximately 6–10 months may be required to raise iron stores before desired response achieved. Ferrous fumarate contains 106 mg elemental iron, gluconate 38 mg, and sulfate 96 mg. Ascorbic acid enhances absorption of iron in ratio of 200 mg ascorbic acid/30 mg iron
Ferrous gluconate		*Adult:* Prophylaxis: 325 mg po daily. Therapeutic: 325–650 mg po QID. Sustained-release capsules may be given twice daily *Child:* Prophylaxis: 8 mg/kg/day po. Therapeutic: 16 mg/kg po TID	
Ferrous sulfate		*Adult:* Prophylaxis: 300–325 mg po daily. Therapeutic: 300 mg po BID–QID. Timed release tablets may be given twice daily. *Child:* Prophylaxis: 5 mg/kg/day po. Therapeutic: 10 mg/kg po TID	
Iron dextran		*Adult and Child over 15 kg:* Total dose (mL) = 0.0476 × weight (kg) × (14.8 − hemoglobin) + 1 mL/5 kg weight up to 14 mL for iron stores. Divided and given in small daily doses IM/IV until total is reached. Not to exceed 100 mg/day. *Child:* Total dose (mL) = 0.0476 × weight (kg) × (12 − hemoglobin) + iron stores (not to exceed 25 mg/day in children under 5 kg; 50 mg/day in children under 10 kg; or 100 mg/day in others	Test doses of 0.5 mL (25 mg) should be given prior to therapy. Give only Z-track into the upper outer quadrant of the buttocks. Continuous IV infusion has been used but is not FDA approved. See Appendix E for information on dosage calculation. Total daily dose should not exceed 1.4 g in adults
Antihemorrhagic Drug			
Desmopressin acetate	Bleeding associated with uremia; prevention of post-renal biopsy bleeding	*Adult and Child over 3 mo:* 0.3 mcg/kg IV diluted in 50 mL 0.9% NaCl. Administer over 15–30 minutes. May repeat as needed *or* 1 intranasal spray (150 mcg) in each nostril in adults and children over 50 kg. In adults and children under 50 kg, use 1 intranasal spray (150 mcg) in one nostril *Child less than 10 kg:* 0.3 mcg/kg diluted in 10 mL of saline and infused over 15–30 minutes. May repeat as needed	Reduction in bleeding usually occurs within 1 hour and lasts about 4 hours. Tachyphylaxis may occur if used more frequently than every 24–48 hours

Table continued on following page

TABLE 41–4 DOSAGE REGIMEN OF SELECTED DRUGS USED TO TREAT RENAL DYSFUNCTION *Continued*

Drug	Use(s)	Dosage	Implications
Phosphate-Binding Drugs			
Calcium acetate, calcium carbonate	Reduce serum phosphorus levels in uremia; secondary hyperparathyroidism; reduce severity of bone disease in uremic patients. Prevent development of metastatic calcification	*Adult:* Amount necessary to control serum phosphate and calcium levels	Dosages adjusted to maintain serum phosphorus levels of 3.5–6 mg/dL. Separate administration of aluminum hydroxide and other oral drugs by at least 1–2 hours. Shake liquid preparations well before pouring. Tablets must be thoroughly chewed before swallowing to prevent entering small intestine in undissolved form. Follow with glass of water or juice
Aluminum hydroxide		*Adult:* 1.9–4.8 g (30–40 mL) of regular suspension *or* 15–20 mL of concentrated suspension po TID–QID. *Child:* 50–150 mg/kg/day po in 4–6 divided doses. Titrate to normal serum phosphate levels	
Vitamin D Supplement			
Calcitriol	Correction of hypocalcemia or uremia	*Adult:* Prophylaxis: 0.5–3 mcg po QD. Larger doses have been used. Hyperparathyroidism on dialysis: 2–3 mcg IV 3 ×/wk on conclusion of dialysis treatment. Chronic peritoneal dialysis: 1–3 mcg three times weekly *Child 1–5 yr:* 0.25–0.75 mcg po QD *Child over 6 yr:* 0.5–2 mcg po QD	Dosage is limited by the development of hypercalcemia. Oral formulations may be administered without regard to meals. May be mixed with juice, cereal, or food. Also observe patient closely for evidence of hypocalcemia. Monitor BUN, creatinine, alkaline phosphatase, parathyroid hormone levels, urinary calcium and creatinine ratio, 24-hour urinary calcium periodically during therapy
Heavy Metal Antagonist			
Deferoxamine	Acute iron toxicity; treatment of chronic iron overload. Unlabeled use: Management of aluminum accumulation in bone in renal failure and aluminum-induced dialysis encephalopathy	*Adult:* Acute toxicity: 15 mg/kg/hr IV up to 90 mg/kg/8 hr (not to exceed 6 g/day) *or* 90 mg/kg IM initially, then 45 mg/kg (up to 1 g/dose) q4–12 hr (not to exceed 6 g/day). Chronic overload: 0.5–1 g IM/IV/ intraperitoneal routes QID *or* 1–2 g/day SQ. Not to exceed 15 mg/kg/ day. *Adult and Child older than 3 years:* 20–40 mg/kg/day by continuous SC infusion given over 8–24 hr *Child younger than 3 years:* Acute/ chronic overload: 10 mg/kg/hr IV. Not to exceed 6 g/24 hr or 2 g/dose	An increase in plasma aluminum or iron levels 12–24 hours following deferoxamine administration reflects binding to the drug. Spacing of dose determined by severity of signs and symptoms. Signs and symptoms take 2–3 months to correct. Use of a pump is recommended for continuous IV infusion.
Loop Diuretic			
Furosemide	Acute and chronic renal failure; hypertensive crisis related to ARF	*Adult:* CRF: 80–120 mg po QD *or* 240–500 mg IV q4–6hr PRN until desired response is achieved. Hypertensive crisis related to ARF: 100–200 mg IV over 1–2 min *Child:* 2 mg/kg po as a single dose. Increase by 1–2 mg/kg q6–8 hr, then 1–2 mg/kg/day up to 5–6 mg/kg/day *or* 1 mg/kg IV. May increase by 1 mg/kg q 2hr. Not to exceed 6 mg/kg	Can cause profound water and electrolyte depletion. Use cautiously in patients with anuria and hepatic coma. Doses up to 6 g/day have been used
Vasopressor			
Dopamine	Hemodynamic imbalances associated with renal failure	*Adult:* 0.3–5 mcg/kg/min IV. Increase by 5–10 mcg/kg/min IV to a rate of 20–50 mcg/kg/min	Check urine output frequently if doses exceeding 16 mcg/kg/min are needed. Safety and efficacy in children have not been established
Cation-Exchange Resin			
Sodium polystyrene sulfonate	Treatment of hyperkalemia secondary to ARF and CRF	*Adult:* 15 g po QD–QID *or* 30–50 g as enema q6h in appropriate vehicle and retained for 30–60 min *Child:* Calculate dosage based on exchange ratio of 1 mEq potassium per gram of resin	Exchange ratio approximately 15 mEq potassium/15 mEq sodium. Patients should have one to two watery stools each day during the course of therapy

TABLE 41–4 DOSAGE REGIMEN OF SELECTED DRUGS USED TO TREAT RENAL DYSFUNCTION *Continued*

Drug	Use(s)	Dosage	Implications
Systemic Antacids			
Sodium bicarbonate	Treatment of metabolic acidosis associated with renal failure	*Adult:* 2–5 mEq/kg over 4–8 hr IV. Acidosis of CRF: 1 g TID. Maintenance 1 g TID *Child:* 0.5–1 mEq/kg	Rate and dosage determined by ABGs and estimate of base deficit.
Sodium citrate		*Adult:* 10–30 mL solution diluted in water po QID	Adjust dosage based on urine pH. Contains 1 mEq sodium and 1 mEq bicarbonate/mL of solution.

ABGs, Arterial blood gases; FDA, Food and Drug Administration; PR, per rectum.

Drug-Drug Interactions

Iron preparations may decrease the antimicrobial actions of fluoroquinolone antibiotics if they are taken concurrently (see Table 41–3). The absorption of iron is decreased when it is taken with antacids, and the effectiveness of levodopa is decreased. Serum iron levels may increase when iron preparations are taken with chloramphenicol. Because there are no physiologic means of removing toxic amounts of iron from the body, a heavy metal antagonist (e.g., deferoxamine) may be needed to chelate the iron.

Dosage Regimen

Dosage regimens of ferrous formulations are identified in Table 41–4. Ferrous fumarate formulations contain 106 mg elemental iron, ferrous gluconate formulations contain 38 mg elemental iron, and ferrous sulfate formulations contain 96 mg elemental iron. Ascorbic acid taken concurrently enhances absorption of iron in a ratio of 200 mg ascorbic acid per 30 mg iron.

When the dosage is expressed in milligrams of elemental iron, the usual adult dosage is 50 mg orally three times daily for adults. For children, 4 to 6 mg/kg/day of elemental iron is given in three divided doses daily. One to two milligrams per kilogram per day is used for infants, and 30 to 60 mg/day of elemental iron is used during pregnancy.

Because parenteral iron can cause allergic reactions, an IM or IV test dose of 25 mg (0.5 mL) of elemental iron should be given before starting therapy. If no adverse reaction occurs, the therapeutic dose can be administered.

The total dose of parenteral iron should not exceed 1.4 g in adults. Iron dextran is not usually given to infants younger than 4 months of age because sepsis has been reported following IM injection. Furthermore, it has been suggested that the repletion of iron stores may serve as a growth medium for certain microorganisms.

Laboratory Considerations

Iron levels of patients on dialysis (especially those receiving epoetin alfa) should be evaluated monthly. Total serum iron, iron-binding capacity, and ferritin levels should be monitored until the target hematocrit value is reached. Thereafter, iron studies should be performed every 2 to 3 months. An iron saturation of less than 20 percent and serum ferritin levels less than 60 mcg/mL are consistent with iron deficiency. Similarly, lack of hemoglobin and hematocrit response to epoetin alfa, and microcytic RBCs are also strongly suggestive of iron deficiency. Occult blood in stools may be obscured by the black coloration of iron in stool. Guaiac test results may occasionally be false positive.

Antihemorrhagic Drugs

❒ Desmopressin acetate (DDAVP, STIMATE)

Indications

DDAVP is effective in reversing the bleeding disorder present in uremia and is useful for the prevention of postrenal biopsy bleeding. It is also used in the management of diabetes insipidus caused by a deficiency of vasopressin and to control bleeding in certain types of hemophilia and von Willebrand's disease (factor VIII deficiency).

Pharmacodynamics

DDAVP is a synthetic polypeptide that is structurally related to the posterior pituitary hormone ADH. The mechanism for antihemorrhagic action is unclear, but it is thought to increase factor VIII activity and to produce direct effects on vessel walls. The antidiuretic effect increases the permeability of the collecting duct, thereby enhancing water reabsorption by the nephrons.

Adverse Effects and Contraindications

The major adverse effects of DDAVP are dose related. It can cause mild hypertension and excess water retention. Less bothersome adverse effects include rhinitis, headache, nausea, and abdominal or stomach cramps. Large IV doses can cause tachycardia. Water intoxication and hyponatremia are possible, along with phlebitis at the IV site.

Desmopressin is contraindicated in patients with hypersensitivity to DDAVP or hypersensitivity to chlorobutanol, and in patients with type IIB or platelet-type (pseudo) von Willebrand's disease. It should be used with caution in patients with angina pectoris or hypertension. Safe use during pregnancy and lactation has not been established.

Pharmacokinetics

Ten to twenty percent of DDAVP is absorbed from the nasal mucosa when the drug is administered intranasally, and it is 100-percent bioavailable when given IV (see Table 41–2). Distribution sites are unknown. DDAVP is biotransformed by the kidney with a half-life of 75 minutes. The onset of drug effects when DDAVP is given intranasally is 1 hour, with peak activity noted in 1 to 5 hours. The intranasal form of DDAVP has a duration of action of 8 to 20 hours. The onset of drug action occurs within minutes of IV administration. Peak effects are noted in 15 to 30 minutes, with a duration of action of 3 hours.

Drug-Drug Interactions

DDAVP used in the presence of chlorpropamide, clofibrate, or carbamazepine may elicit an enhanced diuretic response (see Table 41–3). Demeclocycline, lithium, or norepinephrine may diminish the antidiuretic response to desmopressin.

Dosage Regimen

The dosage and route of administration for DDAVP vary with the reason for use (see Table 41–4). It can be given either by intranasal or parenteral routes (IV/SQ). The parenteral route is usually recommended, although intranasal administration has also been used for antihemorrhagic action. The SC or IV dose is 0.3 mcg/kg. For IV use, the prescribed dose is diluted in 50 mL of 0.9 percent sodium chloride and infused slowly over 15 to 30 minutes. For children weighing less than 10 kg, the usual dosage is 0.3 mcg/kg diluted in 10 mL of saline and infused over 15 to 30 minutes. The dosage may be repeated as needed; however, tachyphylaxis may occur if it is used more frequently than every 24 to 48 hours. The antihemorrhagic effect of IV desmopressin occurs within minutes, peaks in 15 to 30 minutes, and lasts approximately 3 hours. Reduction in bleeding usually occurs within 1 hour and lasts for about 4 hours.

Laboratory Considerations

DDAVP may cause a concentrated urine with an increase in specific gravity and osmolality. As a result of water retention, hyponatremia and a decrease in serum osmolality may occur in patients with normal renal function. These effects are minimal in patients with chronic renal disease.

Phosphate-Binding Drugs

- ❒ Calcium acetate (PHOS-EX, PHOSLO)
- ❒ Calcium carbonate (CALTRATE, MAALOX ANTACID CAPLETS, NEPHRO-CALCI, OS-CAL, ROLAIDS, TUMS, TITRILAC, others); (🍁) APO-CAL, CALCITE, CALSAN, MYLANTA LOZENGES, NU-CAL
- ❒ Aluminum hydroxide (ALTERNA GEL, ALU-CAP, ALU-TAB, AMPHOJEL, BASALJEL, DIALUME, NEPHROX)

Indications

Phosphate-binding drugs are used in renal failure to normalize serum phosphorus levels, and decrease the severity of secondary hyperparathyroidism and the incidence and severity of bone disease. The major calcium compounds include calcium carbonate and calcium acetate. Aluminum hydroxide may be used as a phosphate binder in adults when calcium compounds are found to be ineffective. Overall, the use of aluminum hydroxide as a phosphate binder is largely discouraged.

Pharmacodynamics

Calcium salts prevent absorption of dietary phosphorus from the GI tract by combining with phosphorus to form the insoluble compound calcium phosphate. Aluminum hydroxide binds phosphate in the GI tract to lower serum phosphate levels.

Adverse Effects and Contraindications

The major adverse effects of calcium salts are mild GI complaints such as diarrhea, gas, and constipation. Hypercalcemia may also occur but is unusual if the patient takes the calcium compounds with meals and they are not receiving vitamin D supplements. Arrhythmias have been noted with excess calcium intake. The phosphate depletion that results in bone disease can be induced with excessive use of phosphate binders.

Calcium salts are contraindicated in patients with hypercalcemia, renal calculi, or ventricular fibrillation. They should be used cautiously in patients receiving cardiac glycosides, and in patients who have severe respiratory insufficiency, or renal or cardiac disease.

Aluminum is retained in uremic patients and causes severe skeletal, hematopoietic, and neurologic toxicity. Children with renal failure should not receive aluminum-containing phosphate binding compounds because of the risk of aluminum toxicity.

Aluminum hydroxide is contraindicated in patients with severe abdominal pain of unknown cause. It should be used with caution in patients with hypercalcemia or hypophosphatemia. Use during pregnancy is generally considered safe, although chronic high-dose therapy should be avoided.

Pharmacokinetics

Absorption of calcium salts from the GI tract requires the presence of vitamin D. One hundred–percent bioavailability is noted with oral administration. Calcium salts are 45-percent bound to plasma proteins and readily enter extracellular fluids. Elimination is mostly through the feces, with only 20 percent eliminated by the kidneys. The half-life of calcium salts is unknown (see Table 41–2).

With chronic use, small amounts of aluminum are absorbed systemically. When aluminum is absorbed, it is widely distributed, and with chronic use, it concentrates in the central nervous system. Aluminum is mostly eliminated in the feces.

Drug-Drug Interactions

Calcium compounds prevent the absorption of other elements (e.g., iron), antibiotics (i.e., tetracyclines, fluoroquinolone antibiotics), and digitalis preparations and should not be taken concurrently (see Table 41–3). Calcium acetate should not be given with other calcium supplements.

Aluminum hydroxide should not be taken concurrently with compounds containing citrate (i.e., sodium citrate, calcium citrate) because they markedly enhance the absorption of aluminum, leading to toxicity. Aluminum hydroxide also interacts with many other drugs.

Drug-Food Interactions

Foods such as cereals, spinach, or rhubarb may decrease the absorption of calcium salts when taken concurrently.

Dosage Regimen

Dosages of calcium salts are expressed in milligrams, grams, or milliequivalents of calcium. Administer calcium salts in the amount necessary to control serum phosphate and calcium levels. The dosage is adjusted to maintain serum phosphorus levels at 3.5 to 6 mg/dL (see Table 41–4).

Aluminum hydroxide is dosed at 1.9 to 4.8 g (30 to 40 mL of regular suspension or 15 to 20 mL of concentrated suspension) orally three to four times daily. Children's dosages are 50 to 150 mg/kg/day orally in four to six divided doses.

Laboratory Considerations

The efficacy and safety of the phosphate binders are determined by monitoring serum phosphorus and calcium levels. Serum phosphorus levels should be maintained between 3.5 and 6 mg/100 mL and serum calcium levels between 8 and 11 mg/100 mL. Plasma aluminum levels should be monitored in patients receiving aluminum-containing binders. If aluminum levels exceed 25 mcg/L, the dose should be either reduced or the drug discontinued.

Vitamin D Supplement

❐ Calcitriol (ROCALTROL)

Indications

Calcitriol, a fat-soluble vitamin and a synthetic form of vitamin D_3, is well accepted in the treatment of CRF. It replaces a hormone that can no longer be synthesized by the diseased kidney. Calcitriol is also effective, especially when given IV, in suppressing parathyroid hormone production and improving bone disease that results from secondary hyperparathyroidism. To achieve maximum suppression of parathyroid hormone levels and improve bone disease, a treatment regimen of a year or more may be needed. The desired outcome is reduced bone pain, elimination of fractures, and improvement of muscle strength.

Pharmacodynamics

Calcitriol is a synthetic steroid hormone identical to that synthesized by the renal proximal tubule cells. Calcitriol is the active form of vitamin D and binds to receptors in the small intestine to promote the production of a calcium-binding protein. The calcium-binding protein is essential for the absorption of dietary calcium and phosphorus.

Adverse Effects and Contraindications

Hypercalcemia is the primary adverse effect associated with calcitriol. However, because of the relatively short duration of action of calcitriol, any hypercalcemia associated with its administration is of brief duration and is usually associated with minimal symptoms. Manifestations of hypercalcemia include weakness, nausea, vomiting, and muscle and bone pain.

Calcitriol is contraindicated in patients with hypersensitivity, hypercalcemia, vitamin D toxicity, and during lactation (in large doses). It should be used with caution in patients with sarcoidosis and hyperparathyroidism, and in those receiving cardiac glycosides. Safe use of large doses during pregnancy has not been established.

Pharmacokinetics

Calcitriol is readily absorbed from the small intestine following oral administration. It is bound in the serum to alpha globulins. The onset of drug action occurs in 2 to 6 hours, with a duration of action of 1 to 2 days (see Table 41–2). Its plasma half-life is 3 to 8 hours, with biotransformation and degradation occurring partly in the kidney. It is eliminated primarily through biliary mechanisms.

Drug-Drug Interactions

Barbiturates, primidone, and hydantoin may reduce the effect of calcitriol by accelerating its biotransformation (see Table 41–3). Calcitriol-induced hypercalcemia potentiates the effect of cardiac glycosides, causing arrhythmias. Aluminum hydroxide precipitates bile acids in the small intestine, decreasing absorption of calcitriol and other fat-soluble vitamins. Additionally, calcitriol promotes the absorption of phosphorus from dietary sources, resulting in hyperphosphatemia.

Dosage Regimen

The usual oral dose of calcitriol for patients who are hypocalcemic during chronic dialysis is 0.5 to 3 mcg/day (see Table 41–4). Larger doses have been used. Most dialyzed patients with secondary hyperparathyroidism respond to 2 to 3 mcg/day IV three times a week, given at the end of dialysis. For treatment of secondary hyperparathyroidism in patients on chronic peritoneal dialysis, it can be administered in an oral dose of 1 to 3 mcg three times weekly. The dosage of calcitriol, however, is limited by the development of hypercalcemia.

The usual oral dose of calcitriol for children ages 1 to 5 years is 0.25 to 0.75 mcg/day. For children older than 6 years of age, the usual oral dose is 0.5 mcg/day.

Laboratory Considerations

The efficacy of calcitriol therapy can be documented by suppression of parathyroid hormone levels, normalization of serum calcium, and reduction of alkaline phosphatase levels. Histologic and radiologic evidence of improved hyperparathyroid bone disease can also be documented. Serum calcium levels should be monitored monthly because of the possibility of hypercalcemia. Overdosage is associated with a serum calcium times phosphate ($Ca \times PO_4$) level of greater than 70 and an elevated BUN, alanine aminotransferase (ALT; serum glutamic-pyruvic transaminase [SGPT]) and aspartate aminotransferase (AST; serum glutamic-oxaloacetic transaminase [SGOT]). A fall in alkaline phosphatase levels may also signal the onset of hypercalcemia. Serum phosphorus levels should also be closely monitored to prevent hyperphosphatemia and production of soft tissue calcification. Calcitriol may also cause elevated serum cholesterol levels.

Heavy Metal Antagonist

❐ Deferoxamine (DESFERAL)

Indications

Deferoxamine, a heavy metal antagonist, is effective in alleviating bone pain, muscle weakness, and the anemia that results from iron and aluminum toxicities. It is also used in the management of secondary iron overload syndrome associated with multiple transfusion therapy. Musculoskeletal symptoms and anemia are ordinarily corrected in 2 or 3 months. Aluminum neurotoxicity is more resistant to treatment, with 6 months to 1 year of continuous therapy required before improvement is noted.

Pharmacodynamics

Deferoxamine has a strong affinity for trivalent iron and aluminum, forming soluble stable complexes that are readily eliminated by the kidney or removed with dialysis. Theoretically, 100 mg of deferoxamine is capable of binding 8.5 mg of ferric iron or 17 mg of aluminum.

Adverse Effects and Contraindications

The most common adverse effects of deferoxamine are fever, tachycardia, diarrhea, and abdominal discomfort. A red coloration to the urine, anaphylactic reactions, auditory neurotoxicity, and ocular toxicity have also been reported. Hypotension, shock, skin rash, hives, itching, and wheezing can result and are often due to a too-rapid infusion of deferoxamine. Because deferoxamine is a naturally occurring iron siderophore (a macrophage containing hemosiderin), it acts as a growth factor for *Yersinia* and *Rhizopus* (mucormycosis). In susceptible individuals, deferoxamine increases the proliferation and virulence of these organisms, resulting in severe, often fatal, infection.

Pharmacokinetics

Deferoxamine is poorly absorbed by the GI system following oral administration; therefore, it must be given IM or SC. It is rapidly biotransformed by tissue and plasma enzymes, with a serum half-life of approximately 1 hour (see Table 41–2). The chelated complexes that are formed have an extended plasma half-life. Elimination is totally dependent on either renal function or removal by dialysis. Thirty-three percent of iron is removed through biliary elimination.

Drug-Drug Interactions

Ascorbic acid improves the chelation action for iron and increases the amount of iron eliminated (see Table 41–3). However, deferoxamine should be used judiciously because concurrent use enhances tissue iron toxicity, especially in the heart, causing cardiac decompensation.

Dosage Regimen

Deferoxamine can be administered either IM, IV, SC, or intraperitoneal. The usual IV dose for acute iron ingestion is 15 mg/kg/hour, up to 90 mg/kg initially, then 45 mg/kg up to a 1-g dose every 4 to 12 hours (see Table 41–4). Dosage should not exceed 6 g/day. The spacing of dosage is determined by the severity of symptoms associated with the toxicity. The recommended dose for uremic children is 15 mg/kg/hour IV, not to exceed 6 g in 24 hours or 2 g per dose. Maximum IV infusion rate is 15 mg/kg/hour. Rapid infusion may cause hypotension, erythema, urticaria, wheezing, convulsions, tachycardia, or shock.

Deferoxamine is used in conjunction with induction of emesis or gastric aspiration and lavage with sodium bicarbonate for acute iron ingestion. A trial dose should be administered 2 to 4 hours after the acute ingestion but after the GI tract has been cleansed. The urine is monitored for color change. Orange-rose–colored urine indicates significant iron ingestion.

Laboratory Considerations

Serum deferoxamine levels are not directly monitored. However, an increase in plasma aluminum or iron levels 12 to 24 hours following deferoxamine administration reflects binding to the drug. Liver function studies should be monitored to assess damage from iron poisoning.

Diuretics

❒ Furosemide (LASIX); (🍁) APO-FUROSEMIDE, FUROSIDE, LASIX SPECIAL, MYROSEMIDE, NOVO-SEMIDE
❒ Mannitol (OSMITROL)

Diuretics are mostly used in patients with established renal failure for the conversion of oliguric ATN to nonoliguric ATN. Loop diuretics (e.g., furosemide) and osmotics (e.g., mannitol) are most often used, although the efficacy of diuretics in renal failure varies. Owing to reduction in renal function, large doses are usually required. Diuretics should be administered only after vital signs are stabilized and extracellular fluid volume is optimized.

Loop diuretics are used in the early stages of renal insufficiency and in the ATN type of ARF. The nonoliguric form of ATN rarely requires dialysis and has a better prognosis than oliguric ATN. Osmotic diuretics are used for the prevention of radiocontrast media-induced ATN.

Although diuretics have some effect on RBF, possibly by increasing prostaglandin synthesis, their major therapeutic efficacy is in improving tubule flow rate. The increased flow rate is thought to wash out debris, mostly tubule cells that were sloughed off as a result of the initial injury. However, the debris can obstruct the lumen of low flow nephrons, further compromising GFR. Additionally, by decreasing tubule sodium reabsorption, loop diuretics decrease oxygen demands and biotransformation of the tubule cells. Although these drugs may not improve renal function, they can increase diuresis and facilitate patient management. As kidney function deteriorates, diuretics become increasingly nephrotoxic and are seldom used in patients with ESRD after dialysis has been initiated. Diuretics are discussed in greater detail in Chapter 39.

Cation-Exchange Resins

❒ Sodium polystyrene sulfonate (KAYEXALATE, SPS)

Sodium polystyrene sulfonate is a cation-exchange resin used in the treatment of hyperkalemic states in both ARF and CRF (see also Chapter 45). When used as an enema, the cation-exchange resin trades sodium ions for potassium in the large intestine and, to a lesser extent, other cations (e.g., calcium and magnesium), which are then eliminated in the feces. Almost 100 percent of the administered dose is eliminated. In contrast with oral administration of the resin, sodium ions are exchanged for hydrogen ions in the stomach. The hydrogen ions are subsequently exchanged for potassium cations in the large intestine, where there is a high concentration of potassium. Sodium polystyrene sulfonate is nonabsorbable and not biotransformed. The exchange efficiency is approximately 33 percent. For each gram of resin used, approximately 1 mEq of potassium is exchanged for an equal amount of sodium.

Concurrent use of antacids and laxatives that contain magnesium should be avoided due to the risk of metabolic alkalosis. However, the risk is decreased with rectal administration. Because sodium polystyrene sulfonate exchanges sodium for potassium, fluid retention may occur. Hypokalemia enhances cardiac glycoside toxicity. Sodium polystyrene sulfonate may be administered either orally or rectally.

The usual oral dose of sodium polystyrene sulfonate is 15 to 40 g, administered four times daily. Rectal administration is recommended when the patient is receiving nothing by mouth or is vomiting, or if there is an upper GI tract disorder. However, the rectal route is less effective in reducing potassium levels than the oral method of administration. Further, constipation, fecal impaction, and colonic necrosis have been reported either as the result of the omission of cleansing enemas before or after the resin enema or because of failure to give sorbitol with the oral formulation.

Serum electrolytes, including calcium and magnesium levels, should be monitored when therapy continues for more than one day. Serum potassium levels should be monitored at least daily to determine the effectiveness of therapy. Bicarbonate levels should be monitored at least weekly with chronic therapy, especially if the resin is prescribed concurrently with laxatives and antacids.

Vasopressors

❒ Dopamine (INTROPIN)

Low-dose dopamine has been used to improve RBF, GFR, and renal salt and water elimination. In hypotensive states associated with increased renal vasoconstriction, dopamine improves RBF, thereby reducing oliguria and preventing the development of ARF. Additional uses of dopamine are discussed in Chapter 11.

Dopamine has two distinct actions. It stimulates adrenergic receptors to cause vasoconstriction and acts on dopaminergic receptors to cause vasodilation. In addition, dopamine causes a decrease in sodium reabsorption and increases the rate of sodium elimination in the urine (a natriuretic effect).

Low-dose dopamine (0.5 to 2 mcg/kg/minute IV) causes renal vasodilation. In so doing, it increases RBF, GFR, and sodium elimination, with minimal effect on the vasoconstrictive adrenergic receptors. There are few adverse effects with low-dose dopamine. However, at doses of 2 to 10 mcg/kg/minute, dopaminergic and beta-adrenergic receptors are stimulated, producing cardiac stimulation and greater renal vasodilation. Hypotension and arrhythmias are potentially problematic at higher doses.

Systemic Antacids

❒ Sodium bicarbonate (CITROCARBONATE, NEUT, SODA MINT)

❒ Sodium citrate (BICITRA, ORACIT, SHOHL MODIFIED SOLUTION)

Sodium bicarbonate is a systemic alkalizing agent used for the treatment of metabolic acidosis caused by renal failure. The logic for the use of sodium bicarbonate in the treatment of ARF also applies to the treatment in CRF. By increasing plasma bicarbonate levels, excess hydrogen ions are buffered and blood pH is raised, thus reversing the clinical manifestations of acidosis. The increase in serum pH results in translocation of potassium from the extracellular pool and a corresponding acute fall of plasma potassium levels (see also Chapter 42). However, administration of sodium bicarbonate can result in modest sodium and fluid retention. The retention of sodium and fluids has the potential for aggravating a hypertensive state and edema formation.

Correction of acidosis results in improvement of GI symptoms associated with uremia. In addition, by buffering the retained dietary acids, sodium bicarbonate saves bone buffers and retards the development of renal osteodystrophy. Chronic correction of acidosis in uremia is accomplished by the oral administration of either sodium bicarbonate or sodium citrate. Both are equally effective in correction of the acidotic state. However, because of citrate's ability to enhance the absorption of some toxic elements, namely aluminum, bicarbonate is the preferred drug.

Sodium bicarbonate is always administered IV for acute acidosis. Generally, the initial dose is 2 to 5 mEq/kg administered IV over 4 to 8 hours. However, some calculation is required. Bicarbonate replacement is calculated based on the difference between actual plasma bicarbonate and the desired bicarbonate levels. With acute acidosis, the volume of distribution of bicarbonate is assumed to be 50 percent of body weight. In most cases, half of the calculated bicarbonate deficit is initially replaced. Replacement therapy is monitored by serial determinations of serum CO_2 content and arterial pH.

The acidosis of CRF is ordinarily managed with the oral administration of sodium bicarbonate. One gram of sodium bicarbonate given three times daily is adequate to control the chronic acidosis of uremia in adults. Chronic maintenance therapy for children is 0.5 to 1 mEq/kg of body weight.

Sodium citrate dosage is calculated based on urinary pH. For adults, 10 to 30 mL of solution is diluted in water and administered four times daily. In children, 5 to 15 mL of solution is diluted in water and given four times daily.

Critical Thinking Process

Assessment

History of Present Illness

The history of present illness should address each of the body systems that are commonly implicated in renal failure, including the genitourinary system; GI tract; and neurologic, cardiovascular, respiratory, and dermatologic systems. Often, symptoms associated with renal failure are mistakenly interpreted by the patient as the flu or some other infection.

The frequency of voiding, urine quantity, the appearance of the urine, and any difficulty starting or controlling urination should be described. This information helps identify the stage of renal dysfunction, determine the cause of renal damage, and monitor treatment. Patients with chronic lower urinary tract obstructive disease (e.g., prostatic disease) may relate a long history of strangury, frequency, urgency, nocturia, incontinence, hesitancy, and decreased stream size. With more advanced renal disease, the patient experiences increasing symptoms associated with the uremic state.

A change in the taste of food, nausea, and vomiting often accompany renal failure as a result of azotemia and nervous system disruptions, drug therapies, and changes in diet and fluid intake. Excessive intake of high-protein foods and sodium contributes to electrolyte imbalance and accelerates the build-up of metabolic wastes. Diarrhea and constipation are also common symptoms and the result of a build-up of metabolic and nitrogenous waste.

Neurologic complaints such as excitement and insomnia may alternate with weakness and lassitude with periods of extreme drowsiness. The patient may complain of a short attention span and peripheral neuropathies, with numb, weak extremities, particularly of the hands. Neurologic disruptions also generate complaints of headache and muscle twitching, which can progress to convulsions and coma in severe cases.

Excessive fluid intake contributes to cardiovascular overload and eventually results in peripheral edema, pulmonary edema, and heart failure. Complaints of edema, dizziness, weakness, lethargy, and abnormal bleeding may be indications of worsening renal failure. Symptoms reported by the patient may also be related to the hypertension associated with certain types of ARF and are the result, in part, of altered function of the renin-angiotensin-aldosterone system. Anemia associated with renal failure may be evidenced in complaints of weakness, pallor, lethargy, shortness of breath, and dizziness.

Past Health History

The patient may report a history of renal calculi, difficulty voiding, or acute abdominal or flank pain secondary to a distended bladder or ureteral stone. A positive history of hypertension, diabetes, systemic lupus erythematosus, cancer, tuberculosis, and many other disorders can contribute to or worsen renal function. Frequently, there is a recent history of infection; severe trauma; a complicated surgical procedure; an episode of sepsis; or the administration of nephrotoxic drugs, such as contrast media, antimicrobials, or antineoplastic drugs.

Furthermore, some over-the-counter drugs can be precipitating or aggravating factors in the development or worsening of renal failure; therefore, a thorough drug history is important. A history of analgesic abuse (most notably NSAIDs) is associated with both ARF and CRF. Occupational exposure to some trace elements such as cadmium and lead can also result in CRF. Furthermore, a history of IV drug abuse represents an additional risk factor.

Family history is also relevant in assessing the patient with renal disease. A patient with a family history of diabetic nephropathy and hypertension places the patient at additional risk for renal failure. Similarly, patients with a family history of hereditary renal disease (e.g., Alport's syndrome, polycystic kidney disease), and recessive or sex-linked diseases (e.g., Fabry's disease, tuberous sclerosis, medullary cystic disease, type I glycogen storage disease, cystinosis, oxalate nephropathy) frequently know of another family member with a similar condition.

Physical Exam Findings

The patient's height, weight, and vital signs should be noted, with attention directed toward fluid balance. A measurement of fluid intake and urinary output should be included. Any recent, unintended weight gain or edema may suggest cardiovascular overload and fluid retention. Fluid overload is supported by the presence of shortness of breath, activity intolerance, increased jugular pulsations, crackles on pulmonary auscultation, and the presence of edema. In contrast, volume depletion is seen as orthostatic changes in blood pressure and pulse, poor skin turgor, and dry mucous membranes. A pericardial friction rub may also be present.

The normal flora of the mouth is altered in uremia. The ammonia generated from the hydrolysis of urea contributes to a breath odor that smells like urine. It also causes uremic stomatitis (mouth inflammation). With advanced uremia, the patient's skin develops a sallow appearance because of the presence of urochrome pigments. Skin excoriations are the result of severe pruritus, although the cause of the pruritus is unknown. In advanced renal failure, a dusting of urea crystals (uremic frost) from evaporated perspiration is sometimes seen on the face and eyebrows. Evidence of bleeding from the nose, gums, vaginal tract, GI tract, or skin surfaces may be indicative of decreased erythrocyte production, thrombocytopenia, and a resultant defect in platelet activity.

Assessment of other body systems should include neurologic evaluation because myoclonic jerks, asterixis, and hyperreflexia may also be noted with renal disease.

Diagnostic Testing

Renal function is evaluated by measuring the GFR. Although it is an indirect measurement, creatinine clearance (CrCl) is the most commonly used clinical means of estimating GFR. It is classically measured with a blood test and a timed urine collection; however, this combination of tests may not always be possible. Alternatively, CrCl can be estimated from serum creatinine determination alone using the Crockcroft and Gault equation (see Appendix E). The normal CrCl for men is 140 ± 27 mL/minute, and for women, it is 112 ± 20 mL/minute.

Like CrCl, BUN is a measure of renal function. However, unlike creatinine, the production rate of urea varies as a result of the ingestion of dietary protein, and the catabolic status of the patient. In addition, urea clearance depends on urine flow. Thus, urea clearance fluctuates, making it a less reliable marker of GFR.

Urinalysis can be of value in establishing and monitoring the patient with parenchymal renal disease. The majority of renal diseases, whether acute or chronic, will have abnormalities consisting of increased numbers of white blood cells or red cells, casts, and proteins. Chronic renal disease causes hematuria and proteinuria, and the urine may become cloudy with heavy sediment. In ESRD, the urine becomes more dilute and clear, which reflects the diminished GFR of a diseased kidney. Serum electrolytes, bicarbonate, and hemoglobin should also be evaluated.

Patients with uremia are frequently anemic and acidotic, and have electrolyte disturbances and alterations in calcium and phosphorus balance. Therefore, a complete blood count, serum bicarbonate, electrolytes, phosphate, and calcium levels should be serially evaluated. Owing to the proteinuria accompanying some CRF states, serum albumin may be low. Urinary protein elimination should be measured and serum albumin determined. In addition, glomerular and vascular causes of ARF produce serologic abnormalities that include alterations in serum complement levels. Circulating immune complexes, antiglomerular basement membrane antibodies, and antinuclear cytotoxic antibodies may also be present.

Renal ultrasound is valuable in documenting the status of the ureters, pelvis, calyceals, and bladder. The noninvasive procedure usually takes about 30 minutes and can be used safely in patients in renal failure. No special preparation is required before or after the ultrasound other than explanation of the procedure to the patient.

Developmental Considerations

Perinatal Pregnancy is normally accompanied by physiologic changes in the systemic circulation and urinary system. The systemic circulatory and renal alterations of pregnancy were described in Chapter 6. Several changes are noted in the urinary system, including a rather marked increase in the GFR and dilatation of the collecting system. With these changes, the pregnant patient is at greater risk for renal failure.

In general, renal disease is not affected by pregnancy if it is mild and the patient is not hypertensive at time of conception. However, in the presence of renal disease and hypertension, pregnancy is often complicated with worsening hypertension or a decline in renal function, or both.

Renal disease can be caused by a urinary tract infection before or during pregnancy, can be the result of other diseases such as diabetes, or can occur during pregnancy from complications such as pre-eclampsia, HELLP (hemolysis, elevated liver enzymes, low platelets) syndrome, or abruptio placental. Treatment of sudden ARF during pregnancy resembles that of the nonpregnant population. The aim is to retard the development of uremic symptoms, restore acid-base and electrolyte balance, and volume homeostasis.

Pediatric Chronic kidney disease affects children in many of the same ways it affects adults. However, because the child's body, character, and personality are still forming, the effects on maturation are even more pronounced. Furthermore, because childhood illness often results in stunted physical, psychological, and educational development, it is generally true that the older the child is when he or she becomes ill, the better the chances are of having established a secure sense of self.

Growth failure is an important consequence of childhood renal disease. The growth rate may be somewhat improved with control of acidosis and calcitriol supplementation. Recombinant human growth hormone has been used in children with uremia and in those with transplants who experienced substantially increased growth rates. In addition, adequate peritoneal dialysis, especially continuous cycle-assisted peritoneal dialysis, is the therapy of choice for improved growth rate. However, none of the above-mentioned therapies produce catch-up growth.

The recurrent hospitalizations and lengthy treatment regimens often make the child's reintegration to school and social activities a challenge. The return to school and activities, however, helps minimize the depression, isolation, and low self-esteem associated with chronic illness. The child needs encouragement to assume as much responsibility for self-care as possible. The child's ability to cope with what may be a complex drug regimen can foster self-esteem and improve the outcomes of the treatment regimen. However, the age and maturity of the child will determine the degree to which they participate in their drug therapies.

Geriatric The effects of normal aging result in a decrease in the size and function of the kidneys, and a subsequent decrease in GFR and tubular function. Owing to the physiologic changes of aging, older adults are more susceptible to dehydration, hypotension, fever, and acute renal insufficiency. Advanced age also represents an additional risk factor for the development of ARF secondary to antimicrobial use (e.g., aminoglycosides) as well as radiocontrast drugs.

The incidence of ESRD increases dramatically with advanced age. Between the ages of 20 and 44, the incidence of ESRD is 91 per million population, compared with 680 per million population between ages of 65 and 75 years. The etiology of renal failure also changes with aging.

As a consequence of social, financial, psychological, and co-morbidity factors, older patients frequently do not cope well with chronic dialytic and drug therapies that are associated with renal failure. These factors result in chronic fatigue, depression, concerns regarding quality of life, and suicidal ideations. Over 40 percent of patients 65 years and older discontinue dialysis for the above-mentioned reasons.

Psychosocial Considerations

In assessing psychosocial factors that influence the patient and his or her family, it is important for the health care provider to inquire about their understanding of the diagnosis, implications, and treatment regimens (e.g., diet, drugs, dialysis). The coping mechanisms used by the patient and family members should also be noted because family relations, social activities, work patterns, body image, and sexual activities are altered by renal disease. Introducing a life-threatening illness such as ESRD to the already stressful demands placed on the contemporary family system taxes coping mechanisms. Role changes are common in these families such that spouses often take on the role responsibilities of the sick partner while maintaining their own role. This leads to reduced rest and leisure for the spouse and lowers physical reserve. Major changes in thinking and living must be made, and at the same time, relationships must be maintained and nurtured.

The psychosocial support required is determined by the reversibility and severity of the underlying disease or condition responsible for producing renal failure. Further, complex drug regimens and any associated medical or surgical conditions determine whether the patient and the family is compliant with the plan of care.

Other factors to be considered when assessing the patient are the health beliefs about what is considered a healthy state and personal beliefs related to religious and cultural practices. Additionally, past compliance with medical regimens and family support are important factors in the assessment and planning process.

It is essential to identify any barriers to the teaching-learning process, including the physical, psychological, and maturational readiness of the patient. The patient's educational level, reading ability, attitude toward learning, and cultural values that affect health care decisions should be noted. The existence of language barriers, the patient's degree of motivation, and his or her previous compliance with medical care are important considerations when developing the interdisciplinary teaching plan.

Compliance with drug therapy is further impacted by the expense of the required drug regimens. Patients with little or no financial resources will have difficulty obtaining their drugs and complying with the plan of care. Federal, state, and local resources may provide assistance with the cost of therapy. The End Stage Renal Disease Program, a part of Medicare, was initiated in 1972 to relieve kidney patients of the catastrophic costs of dialysis by covering 80 percent of the costs of service. It does not cover the cost of drugs.

Analysis and Management

Treatment Objectives

The primary objective in the management of renal failure is prevention. The avoidance or removal of nephrotoxic drugs, along with rapid correction of cardiovascular alterations that lead to renal ischemia, will prevent or minimize progression of the disease. Once renal failure has developed, however, treatment objectives are directed at supporting the patient and maintaining existing system functioning. Achieving and maintaining acceptable fluid and electrolyte balance, and minimizing the risk of complications from fluid and electrolyte imbalances are also relevant objectives. Maintenance of adequate nutritional status and compliance with the plan of care are also desirable outcomes.

One of the risk-reduction objectives listed in the *Healthy People 2000* document of the United States Public Health Service and the Department of Health and Human Services relates to ESRD. The objective is to reverse the increase in ESRD (requiring maintenance dialysis or transplantation) to attain an incidence of no more than 13 per 100,000 cases (Baseline: 13.9/100,000 in 1987).

Treatment Options

Drug Variables

Knowledge of the pharmacokinetics and many other factors is required for the appropriate pharmacotherapeutic management of the patient with renal failure. An estimate of the degree of renal function and the effects of renal impairment on drug elimination and half-life should be made. The effects of dialysis on drug removal and the appropriate method for altering drug doses or dosage intervals to achieve desired blood levels are also important factors to be considered.

Recent studies strongly suggest that ACE inhibitors (e.g., captopril) are highly effective in decreasing the progression of diabetic nephropathy. Because over 30 percent of the annual rate of ESRD are patients with diabetes, there is a major impact on ESRD programs. In addition, there is reasonable evidence that other types of proteinuric renal disease may also benefit from the use of ACE inhibitors. Because the average cost of treating a patient with ESRD is over $50,000 annually, preventive therapy with ACE inhibitors at the recommended dose would be less than $1500 annually. Furthermore, it has been estimated that the use of captopril with Type 1 diabetic nephropathy could reduce national health costs by over three billion dollars over the next 10 years.

In contrast, recent advances in therapies directed at improving the quality of life of patients with ESRD have done little to improve rehabilitation but have markedly increased costs. For example, epoetin alfa, an antianemic drug, has increased the annual cost of treating a patient with ESRD by $5000 to $7000. It is also estimated that the cost of recombinant human growth hormone for treatment of growth failure in children with renal disease will be even more expensive than epoetin alfa.

Patient Variables

The patient with renal failure responds to many drugs differently from the patient with healthy kidneys. Because of these variations in response, a variety of therapeutic regimens may provide the best results. The major patient variable encountered in pharmacotherapy is the degree of renal impairment. Because many drugs are eliminated through the kidneys, the potential for toxicity is increased as renal function decreases. If patients with slower than normal elimination rates (e.g., those with renal disease and older adults) are given normal doses of drugs, excessive accumulation and toxicity can occur. Toxicity is potentially preventable with proper modification of dose.

Intervention

Administration

Drug administration regimens are modified based on the degree of functional impairment by using interval extension and dose reduction strategies. Using the *interval extension method,* the time between each dose is lengthened while the dose remains the same. The interval extension method is useful for drugs with wide therapeutic ranges and long plasma half-lives. With the *dose reduction method,* the size of the individual dose is reduced but the interval between each dose remains unchanged. The dose reduction method is preferred when constant blood levels of a drug are required, and for drugs with narrow therapeutic ranges and rather short half-lives. At times, a combination of these two methods is employed to achieve maximum therapeutic benefits. Guidance regarding dosage reduction and interval modification for most drugs can be found in a number of books, including *Drug Prescribing in Renal Failure,* published by the American College of Physicians.

Measurement of peak and trough serum drug levels is useful in documenting the effectiveness of the dosing schedule. The levels are indicators of drug elimination and reflect potential drug accumulation. Peak levels are most useful when they are obtained 30 minutes to 1 hour after the third dose of the drug. Trough levels are obtained immediately before the next dose. Reliable clinical assessment of changes in the patient's condition and knowledge of drug interactions must be used to aid in the interpretation of test results. Further, several principles should be used when adjusting dosages for patients with renal failure:

- The loading dose given to a patient with renal insufficiency is usually the same as the initial dose of a drug given to a patient with normal renal function

- The maintenance dose of a drug for patients with renal insufficiency can be adjusted using the interval extension or dose reduction method
- In patients with substantial edema or ascites, the initial dose may be somewhat higher than that usually given to achieve desired blood levels

The importance of consistency in obtaining peak and trough values cannot be overstated. Regardless of the sampling procedure used, it is important that the same time interval between sampling and dose administration be used consistently when comparing results from serial samples on the same patient.

Furthermore, there are a number of considerations regarding drug administration in renal failure. Drugs that are to be taken on an empty stomach should be taken 1 hour before or 2 hours after meals to enhance absorption. Drugs should not be stopped without first checking with the health care provider. Over-the-counter drug use should be avoided, especially cough, cold, and allergy preparations that may contain ingredients that interact with the drugs used in the treatment regimens.

Iron preparations should be taken with meals if GI discomfort is severe, but milk, eggs, coffee, and tea should be avoided because they alter absorption of the iron. Liquid iron preparations should be mixed with water or juice to mask the taste and given through a straw to prevent staining of the teeth. The patient should be informed that the iron will turn the stool dark green or black. Periodic monitoring of hematocrit and hemoglobin levels should be done to monitor effectiveness and prevent possible toxicity.

Intranasal formulations of DDAVP should be administered by drawing the solution into the flexible calibrated tube that is supplied with the drug. The patient is instructed to insert one end of the tube into the nostril and to blow into the other end to deposit the solution deep into the nasal cavity. Inappropriate administration technique can lead to nasal ulcerations. The nasal solution and injectable formulations should be stored in the refrigerator.

Phosphate-binding drugs should be taken 1 to 3 hours after meals and at bedtime, or as prescribed by the health care provider. Other drugs should not be taken within 1 to 2 hours of the phosphate binder. Encourage the patient to chew the phosphate-binding (e.g., calcium carbonate) tablets thoroughly before swallowing and follow with a glass of water or milk. Patients should be reminded to avoid magnesium-containing antacid preparations due to the possibility of magnesium toxicity. Serum calcium and phosphorus levels should be measured before beginning therapy with the vitamin D supplement and calcitriol, and at least weekly during therapy to monitor for hypercalcemia.

Deferoxamine is used most often in the acute care environment. When an IV route is required, the drug should be infused slowly, preferably using an infusion pump. Pain at the injection site with SC or IM forms is common.

Furosemide should be taken with food or milk to prevent GI upset. The dosage of the diuretic may be reduced with the concurrent use of antihypertensives. It should be administered early in the day so that increased urination will not disturb sleep. IV use should be avoided if oral routes are at all possible. Oral solutions of furosemide should be refrigerated.

Extreme caution should be used in calculating and preparing dopamine for IV infusion. Small errors in dosage can cause serious adverse effects. The drug should always be diluted before use if it is not prediluted. The large veins of the antecubital fossa are preferred to veins in the hands or ankle. The initial dosage should be reduced by 1/10 in patients who have been on monoamine oxidase inhibitors. Phentolamine, an alpha-adrenergic blocking drug, should be available in case extravasation occurs. If required, infiltration with 10 to 15 mL of saline containing 5 to 10 mg of phentolamine is effective in reducing tissue damage.

Sodium polystyrene sulfonate is administered in a suspension of 3 to 4 mL of a 70-percent sorbitol syrup per gram of resin and mixed with either food or liquid to improve palatability. Liquid vehicles include warm water, 1-percent methylcellulose, or 5- to 10-percent dextrose in water, in addition to the sorbitol. The osmotic cathartic effect of sorbitol hastens the elimination of potassium and prevents constipation and, more importantly, fecal impaction.

For rectal use, 30 to 50 g of resin is mixed with 100 to 200 mL of an aqueous solution (i.e., 25-percent sorbitol, 1-percent methylcellulose, or 10-percent dextrose) and instilled at least 20 cm into the colon as a retention enema following a cleansing enema. Following instillation, the tubing is flushed with 100 to 200 mL of a non–sodium-containing solution to ensure complete instillation of the solution. The enema should be retained for at least 30 to 60 minutes and up to 4 to 10 hours, followed by a non–sodium-containing cleansing enema. The resin should not be administered as a thick paste because it is less effective in that form.

Serum potassium levels should be checked before the administration of sodium bicarbonate. The risk of metabolic acidosis is increased in states of hypokalemia, and the dosage of sodium bicarbonate may need to be reduced. Dosage should be adjusted based on arterial blood gases and patient response. Complete correction of acid-base imbalance within the first 24 hours should be avoided because of the increased risk of metabolic alkalosis. In most cases, drug interactions with sodium bicarbonate may be avoided by not administering other oral medications within 1 to 2 hours.

Education

The most important role of the health care provider for the patient and family with renal failure is patient teaching. The majority of patients receive their care on an outpatient basis. Therefore, whenever possible, the patient should be encouraged to take the major responsibility for compliance with the treatment plan. However, owing to the changes in cognitive functioning of the patient with renal failure or the level of understanding due to age limitations, it is important to involve family members in the teaching process.

The family should be involved in the plan of care from the beginning, and their goals and objectives for treatment should be taken into consideration. Not only should they be educated about the medical regimen but also the consequences if they choose not to comply with the prescribed treatment plan. Ongoing patient and family support, along with management by the health care provider, are of primary importance in assisting the patient to achieve his or her personal goals.

Both the patient and family should have a thorough understanding of the consequences of renal disease in order to adjust to the numerous limitations of renal failure. An understanding of the reasons for dietary restrictions, drug regimens, and adherence to the dialysis schedule, when applic-

TABLE 41–5 DRUG DOSING OF ANTIBIOTICS IN PATIENTS WITH RENAL DYSFUNCTION

Drug	Method of Dose Adjustment	CrCl > 50 mL/min	CrCl 10–50 mL/min	CrCl < 10 mL/min	H - P*
Aminoglycosides					
Amikacin	Dose	60–90%	30–70%	20–30%	H & P
	Interval	12 hr	12–18 hr	24 hr	
Gentamicin	Dose	60–90%	30–70%	20–30%	H & P
	Interval	8–12 hr	12 hr	24 hr	
Netilmicin	Dose	60–90%	30–70%	20–30%	H & P
	Interval	8–12 hr	12 hr	24 hr	
Tobramycin	Dose	60–90%	30–70%	20–30%	H & P
	Interval	8–12 hr	12 hr	24 hr	
Cephalosporins					
Cephalexin	Interval	6 hr	6–8 hr	6–12 hr	H
Cefadroxil	Interval	8 hr	12–24 hr	24–48 hr	H
Cephradine	Dose	—	50%	25%	H & P
Cephapirin	Interval	6 hr	6–8 hr	12 hr	H & P
Cefazolin	Interval	8 hr	12 hr	18–48 hr	H
Cefaclor	Dose	—	50%	33%	H
Cefmetazole	Interval	12 hr	24 hr	48 hr	H
Cefotetan	Interval	12 hr	24 hr	48 hr	H
Cefoperazone	Interval	—	—	—	H
Ceftriaxone	Dose	—	—	—	No
Ceftazidime	Interval	8–12 hr	8–12 hr	18–24 hr	H
Tetracyclines					
Doxycycline	Interval	12 hr	12–18 hr	18–24 hr	No
Minocycline	Dose	—	—	—	No
Fluoroquinolones					
Norfloxacin	Interval	—	24 hr	24 hr	H & P
Ciprofloxacin	Interval	—	12 hr	24 hr	H & P
Ofloxacin	Dose	—	50%	25–50%	H & P
Penicillins					
Amoxicillin	Interval	6 hr	6–12 hr	12–16 hr	H
Ampicillin	Interval	6 hr	6–12 hr	12–16 hr	H
Carbenicillin	Interval	8–12 hr	12–24 hr	24–48 hr	H & P
Cloxacillin	Dose	—	—	—	No
Dicloxacillin	Interval	—	—	—	No
Methicillin	Interval	4–6 hr	6–8 hr	8–12 hr	No
Oxacillin	Dose	—	—	—	No

able, is necessary for acceptance and compliance with the medical regimen.

All patients with decreased renal function must limit their protein consumption to some degree because the accumulation of nitrogenous waste products from protein metabolism is the primary cause of uremia. Protein is restricted based on the degree of renal insufficiency and the severity of the symptoms. The GFR, albumin, creatinine, and BUN levels are often used as a guide to safe levels of protein consumption.

Low-protein diets are usually deficient in vitamins, and water-soluble vitamins are removed from the blood during dialysis. In addition, anemia is a chronic problem owing to the limited iron content of low-protein diets and decreased erythropoietin production by the kidneys. For these reasons, all patients with renal failure are given some type of vitamin and mineral supplement. The patient should be taught to take the vitamin and mineral supplements after dialysis rather than before because they will be dialyzed out of the body if taken before and the patient would receive no benefit.

Phosphate-binding drugs, often referred to by the patient as antacids, are necessary because the metabolism of calcium and phosphorus is altered in renal failure. The patient should be taught the purpose of these drugs and to avoid preparations containing magnesium. The patient's inability to metabolize magnesium predisposes him or her to dangerous levels of magnesium toxicity. Further, the patient should be taught to monitor for signs and symptoms of hypophosphatemia, including muscle weakness, anorexia, malaise, tremors, and bone pain.

The importance of taking antihypertensive drugs (see Chapter 34) on a regularly scheduled basis should be emphasized. Uncontrolled elevations in blood pressure further compromise renal perfusion and worsen renal failure.

Diuretics are often used in the early stages of renal failure and should be taken early in the day to avoid disturbing sleep. The diuresis produced is useful in treating fluid overload in patients who still have some urinary function. Careful intake and output records should be kept because as kidney function deteriorates, these drugs become increasingly nephrotoxic. Diuretics are seldom used in patients with ESRD after dialysis has been initiated.

Because a large percentage of patients with renal failure also have diabetes, patient teaching should include the need for close monitoring of blood glucose levels. As renal disease

TABLE 41–5 DRUG DOSING OF ANTIBIOTICS IN PATIENTS WITH RENAL DYSFUNCTION *Continued*

Drug	Method of Dose Adjustment	CrCl > 50 mL/min	CrCl 10–50 mL/min	CrCl < 10 mL/min	H - P*
Penicillins *Continued*					
Penicillin G	Dose	—	75%	20–50%	H
	Interval	6–8 hr	8–12 hr	12–16 hr	—
Piperacillin	Interval	4–6 hr	6–8 hr	8 hr	H
Ticarcillin	Interval	6–8 hr	12–24 hr	12–24 hr	H & P
Miscellaneous					
Aztreonam	Dose	—	50–75%	25%	—
Chloramphenicol	Dose	—	—	—	H
Clindamycin	Dose	—	—	—	No
Erythromycin	Dose	—	—	—	No
Metronidazole	Dose	—	—	50%	H
	Interval	8 hr	—	—	—
Trimethoprim/sulfamethoxazole	Interval	12 hr	12 hr	24 hr	H
Vancomycin	Interval	24–72 hr	72–240 hr	240 hr	No
Antifungal					
Amphotericin B	Interval	24 hr	24 hr	24–36 hr	No
Flucytosine	Dose	50%	30–50%	20–30%	H & P
Fluconazole	Dose	—	50%	25%	H
Ketoconazole	Dose	—	—	—	No
Itraconazole	Dose	—	—	—	UK
Miconazole	Dose	—	—	—	No
	Interval	6 hr	12–24 hr	24–48 hr	H & P
Antituberculosis					
Ethambutol	Dose	—	50%	30–50%	H & P
	Interval	24 hr	24–36 hr	48 hr	—
Isoniazid	Dose	—	—	65–75%	H & P
Rifampin	Interval	—	—	—	No
Antivirals					
Acyclovir	Interval	8 hr	24 hr	48 hr	H
Amantadine	Interval	12–24 hr	48–72 hr	168 hr	No
Ganciclovir	Dose	50%	25%	25%	H
	Interval	24 hr	24 hr	24 hr	—

CrCl, Creatinine clearance; H, removed by hemodialysis; P, removed by peritoneal dialysis; Interval, hours between dosing; UK, unknown. Dosage is given as percentage administered to an adult with normal renal function.

progresses, the patient with diabetes requires a decrease in insulin dosage because insulin is partially biotransformed by the kidneys. Urinary glucose measurements may be inaccurate owing to the renal disease and, if possible, should not be used.

Patients with uremia are particularly sensitive to the respiratory depressant effects of opioid analgesics and should be taught to use them with caution. The effects of opioids often last much longer in patients with renal failure than in persons with healthy kidneys. Because opioids are biotransformed by the liver and not the kidneys, dosage recommendations are often the same regardless of kidney function. The patient should also be taught to avoid aspirin because it is normally eliminated by the kidneys and may rapidly build to toxic levels and prolong bleeding time.

Infection related to altered immune, nutritional, and biochemical states represents an additional cause of morbidity and mortality in patients with renal failure. Meticulous handwashing is essential, and the patient should be taught to avoid contact with people with known infections. It is important that patients understand aseptic technique and that it be used with all necessary invasive procedures. Additionally, invasive procedures by the health care provider should be avoided whenever possible, especially the use of indwelling catheters. Antibiotics (see Chapter 24) are used prophylactically before any dental procedures to prevent pericarditis, which may result if oral bacteria enter the circulation. The patient should be taught to discuss the need for antibiotics and the preferred protocol because it varies with the patient's needs and the preference of the health care provider. Drug dosing with antibiotics is based on the degree of renal dysfunction (Table 41–5).

Patients and their families should be informed of the various resources that are available. Home care nurses are often required to monitor the patient's status and evaluate maintenance of the prescribed treatment regimen. Social service personnel are usually involved because of the complex process of paying for the required care and in applying for financial aid. Physical and occupational therapists often work with patients who have renal failure, depending on their needs. The patient and family may benefit from joining support groups or obtaining other services locally. Resources such as The National Kidney Foundation and the American Kidney Fund are good initial contacts.

Evaluation

Successful achievement of treatment objectives is indicated by a number of factors. The patient is free from peripheral edema, hypertension, respiratory distress, and other signs of fluid and electrolyte imbalance. There are no signs of infection, and the patient is feeling more rested and less fatigued. Blood pressure is maintained within an acceptable range. There are no signs of bleeding; anorexia, nausea, and pruritus are controlled; and there is no muscle cramping. The patient demonstrates mental clarity and an ability to perform activities of daily living independently and safely. Any co-morbid illness, including heart failure, anemia, and dehydration, is controlled or resolved. Furthermore, the patient should be able to correctly describe the nature of his or her illness, treatment and drug regimens, and plans for follow-up care.

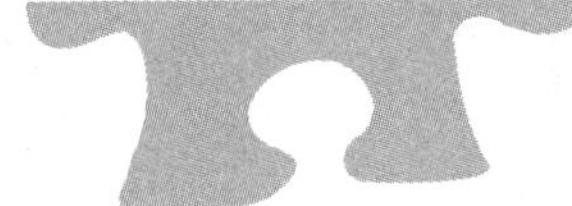

SUMMARY

- Prerenal factors associated with ARF cause hypoperfusion, intrarenal factors cause injury to renal parenchyma, and postrenal factors obstruct urine flow.
- The most common cause of ARF is renal hypoperfusion, and the second most common cause is nephrotoxins.
- Three stages characterize CRF: diminished renal reserve without accumulation of metabolic wastes; mild (40 to 80 percent of normal function), moderate (15 to 40 percent), or severe (2 to 20 percent) renal insufficiency, and finally, ESRD.
- Multiple system dysfunction occurs as renal failure progresses, leading to anemia, uremia, disorders of calcium and phosphorus biotransformation, and acidosis.
- With ARF, there is usually a recent history of infection, severe trauma, a complicated surgical procedure, an episode of sepsis, or the administration of nephrotoxic drugs, such as contrast media, antimicrobials, or antineoplastic drugs.
- Fluid overload is supported by the presence of increased jugular pulsations, crackles on pulmonary auscultation, and the presence of edema.
- CrCl, BUN, and urine analyses are useful determinants of renal functioning.
- In general, renal disease is not affected by pregnancy if it is mild and the patient is not hypertensive at time of conception.
- Chronic kidney disease affects children in many of the same ways it affects adults. However, because the child's body, character, and personality are still forming, the effects on maturation are even more pronounced.
- The normal aging process results in a decrease in the size and function of the kidneys, and a subsequent decrease in GFR and tubular function. Therefore, the elderly are more susceptible to acute renal insufficiency.
- The objectives in the management of renal failure are prevention, removal of nephrotoxic drugs, rapid correction of cardiovascular alterations leading to renal ischemia, and reduction of the severity and duration of established ARF.
- The management of a patient with renal failure includes drug therapy, diet therapy, and dialysis in some form.
- Adjust the drug dosage to correlate with the severity of the patient's renal failure by using the interval extension and dose reduction methods.
- Captopril, an ACE inhibitor, is most useful in decreasing functional deterioration in Type 1 diabetic renal disease, but it is also thought to exert similar beneficial effects in all types of proteinuric renal diseases.
- Epoetin alfa is a well-accepted drug for the treatment of the anemia associated with CRF.
- Because iron is necessary for continued RBC production, virtually all patients receiving epoetin alfa eventually require supplemental iron.
- DDAVP, an antihemorrhagic agent, is effective in reversing the bleeding disorder present in uremia and is useful for the prevention of postrenal biopsy bleeding.
- Phosphate-binding drugs (calcium carbonate) normalize serum phosphorus levels and decrease the severity of secondary hyperparathyroidism and the incidence and severity of bone disease.
- Calcitriol, a vitamin D supplement, is effective in suppressing parathyroid hormone production and improving bone disease resulting from the secondary hyperparathyroidism.
- Deferoxamine mesylate, a heavy metal antagonist, is effective in alleviating bone pain, muscle weakness, and the anemia that results from iron and aluminum toxicities.
- Furosemide, a loop diuretic, is used primarily in the ATN type of ARF to convert oliguric ATN to nonoliguric ATN and in the early stages of renal insufficiency.
- In hypotensive states associated with increased renal vasoconstriction, dopamine, a vasopressor, may improve RBF, preventing the development of ARF and reducing oliguria.
- Sodium polystyrene sulfonate, a cation-exchange resin, is used in the treatment of hyperkalemic states in both ARF and CRF.
- Sodium bicarbonate is a systemic alkalizing agent used for the treatment of metabolic acidosis caused by the impaired acid elimination in renal failure.
- Evaluation of patient outcomes includes a patient that is free of peripheral edema, hypertension, respiratory distress, or other signs of fluid and electrolyte imbalance. Also, the patient should demonstrate mental clarity and an ability to perform his or her activities independently and safely.

BIBLIOGRAPHY

Beaufils, M. (1994). Angiotensin-converting enzyme inhibition and diabetic nephropathy. *Journal of Cardiovascular Pharmacology*, 19(Suppl 6), S33.

Bennett, W., Aronoff, G., Golper, T., et al. (1991). *Drug prescribing in renal failure* (2nd ed.). Philadelphia: American College of Physicians.

Bernstein, J., and Erk, S. (1990). Choice of antibiotics, pharmacokinetics, and dose adjustments in acute and chronic renal failure. *Medical Clinics of North America*, 74(4), 1059–1077.

Black, J., and Matassarin-Jacobs, E. (1997). *Medical-surgical nursing: clinical management for continuity of care* (5th ed.). Philadelphia: W.B. Saunders Company.

Byers, J., and Goshorn, J. (1995). How to manage diuretic therapy. *American Journal of Nursing*, 95(2), 38–44.

Daugirdas, J., and Ing, T. (1994). *Handbook of dialysis*. (2nd ed.). Boston: Little, Brown and Company.

DeSoi, C., and Umans, J. (1992). Principles of drug therapy in renal failure. *Hospital Formulary*, 27(2), 164–180.

Dolleris, P. (1992). Diuretic and vasopressor usage in acute renal failure: A synopsis. *Critical Care Nursing Quarterly*, 14(4), 28–31.

Eberst, E., and Berkowitz, L. (1994). Hemostasis in renal disease: Pathophysiology and management. *American Journal of Medicine,* 96(2), 168–179.

Eschbach, J., and Adamson, J. (1993). Anemia in renal disease. *In* R. Schrier and C. Gottschalk (Eds.), *Disease of the kidney.* Boston: Little, Brown and Company.

Horl, W. (1992). Optimal route of administration of erythropoietin in chronic renal failure patients: Intravenous versus subcutaneous. *Acta Haematologia,* 87(Suppl 1), 16–19.

Lewis, E., Hunsicker, L., and Bain, R. (1993). The effect of angiotensin-converting enzyme inhibition on diabetic nephropathy. *New England Journal of Medicine,* 329(20), 1456–1462.

Loffel, L., McGill, J., and Gans, D. (1995). The beneficial effect of angiotensin-converting enzyme inhibition with captopril on diabetic nephropathy in normotensive IDDM patients with microalbuminemia. *American Journal of Medicine,* 99(5), 497–505.

Lui, S., Law, C., Ting, S., et al. (1991). Once weekly versus twice weekly subcutaneous administration of recombinant human erythropoietin in patients on continuous ambulatory peritoneal dialysis. *Clinical Nephrology,* 36, 246–251.

USPDI (1992) Drug information for the health care professional (12th ed.). Kingsport, TN: Arcata Graphics.

Vitting, K. (1994). Principles of drug therapy in the geriatric renal patient. *Geriatric Nephrology and Urology,* 4(1), 43–47.

Weisberg, L., Kurnik, P., and Kurnik, B. (1994). Risk of radiocontrast nephropathy in patients with and without diabetes mellitus. *Kidney International,* 45(1), 259–265.

Wiegman, T., Herron, K., and Chonko, A. (1994). Effect of angiotensin-converting enzyme inhibition on renal function and albuminuria in normotensive type I diabetic patients. *Diabetes,* 41(1), 62.

Zappacosta, A. (1991). Weekly subcutaneous recombinant human erythropoietin corrects anemia of progressive renal failure. *American Journal of Medicine,* 91(3), 229–232.

Unit VIII

Drugs Influencing the Gastrointestinal System

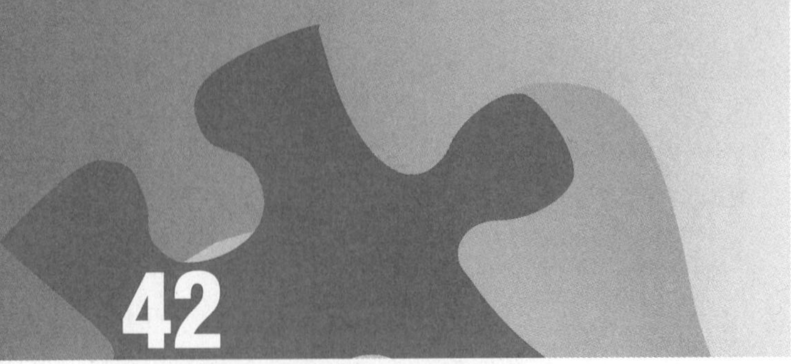

42 Peptic Ulcer and Hyperacidity Drugs

Management of hyperacidity and peptic ulcer disease often relies on four groups of drugs: antacids that neutralize gastric acids; drugs that inhibit gastric acid production, including H_2 antagonists, proton pump inhibitors, and prostaglandins; prokinetic agents that stimulate gastric motility; and cytoprotective agents. Optimum management for peptic ulcers and hyperacidity, however, requires a knowledge of basic gastrointestinal (GI) physiology and the pathophysiology of hyperacidity states.

Hyperacidity is defined as an excess of gastric secretions or the presence of gastric secretions that have a pH less than 2.0. Hyperacidity may be acute or chronic, episodic, or a relatively continuous problem, but it is not associated with erosion of the gastric mucosa. Hyperacidity is clinically significant because it predisposes the patient to gastric and intestinal irritation, the development of ulcerations, and the potential for perforation. If the etiologies of hyperacidity can be identified, appropriate interventions may be able to reduce or even eliminate the need for drug therapy.

In contrast to hyperacidity, *peptic ulcer disease* (PUD) is defined as a break in the continuity of the gastric mucosa. It may develop in any part of the GI tract that comes in contact with hydrochloric (HCL) acid and pepsin. PUD is clinically significant because of the loss of integrity of the gastric or duodenal walls, the actual or potential hemorrhage, and the impact on nutritional balance.

PEPTIC ULCER DISEASE AND HYPERACIDITY

Epidemiology and Etiology

Reliable data regarding the prevalence of hyperacidity and PUD is difficult to obtain because of the remitting and relapsing characteristic of the disorders, although they generally appear in middle to late life. Eighty percent of the cases of PUD occur in the duodenum between the ages of 45 and 54. The remainder of PUD cases occur in the stomach between the ages of 55 and 65. Both duodenal and gastric ulcers occur more often in men than in women, but the frequency varies with the patient's age. No significant ethnic variations have been identified.

No firm prevalence figures exist on the occurrence of PUD in children. Technology has revealed, however, that 1 to 2 percent of hospitalized pediatric patients have peptic ulcerations. Male children are affected more frequently than female children. PUD is more common in late school-age children and adolescents than in younger children.

The lifetime incidence for PUD is approximately 10 percent, with a cost to society that exceeds one billion dollars per year. It causes the loss of many productive hours of work and has been the subject of millions of dollars in research.

Fifty to eighty percent of the adult population worldwide who have PUD are infected with the gram-negative organism *Helicobacter pylori,* previously classified as *Campylobacter pylori*. If the condition is left untreated, it can persist for decades. However, only 10 to 20 percent of these patients go on to develop peptic ulcer disease or neoplasia, although many more have low-grade gastritis.

Risk Factors

There are several risk factors strongly associated with hyperacidity and the development of PUD, although the factors associated with acquisition of *H. pylori* remain under investigation. There appears to be a positive relationship with better economic conditions in childhood; however, it is thought that a positive relationship exists with crowded conditions and growing up in rural areas. The mode of transmission is uncertain, although contact with animals and contaminated sewage are possibilities.

Other factors less strongly associated with PUD include a strong family history of PUD in first-degree relatives. Persons with type O blood group have been shown to have a 30 percent greater risk for duodenal ulcers than those with other blood types. The capacity to secrete mucopolysaccharide blood group substances into salivary and GI secretions is an inherited trait. Twenty to forty percent of patients with duodenal ulcers have a positive family history, with a 50 percent concordance in identical (monozygotic) twins, compared with a 14 percent concordance in fraternal (dizygotic) twins. Nonsecretors of the blood group substances are 50 percent as likely to develop duodenal ulcers than secretors.

Patients with *H. pylori* infections may develop clinical disease that involves different strains and virulence of the organism. The virulent strains of *H. pylori* that cause cytotoxicity and peptic ulcers are associated with the vacA gene, but this relationship is not unequivocal. Dietary habits have not been shown to play a significant role in the development of PUD or its recurrence, although the age at which the host acquired the infection and environmental factors may contribute to its development.

A number of diseases have been associated with PUD, including Laennec's cirrhosis (alcoholic cirrhosis), chronic pancreatitis, chronic lung disease, Zollinger-Ellison syndrome, chronic renal failure, and hyperparathyroidism. The association of these diseases to PUD relates to the hypercalcemia that develops. Hypercalcemia stimulates gastrin secretion, and therefore, acid secretion.

Occasionally, PUD develops as an acute response to medical or surgical stressors. *Stress ulcerations* are frequently seen in patients who have sustained head injuries (Cushing's ulcers) or burns (Curling's ulcers); in patients who have experienced respiratory failure, major surgical procedures, or shock; and in those who are septic. In addition, PUD is more likely to appear with the long-term use of drugs that irritate gastric mucosa. Nonsteroidal anti-inflammatory drugs

(NSAIDs) increase the risk of recurrence and of GI complications two to six times, depending on the dose, half-life of the drug, dosing frequency, and duration of use. Further, the rate of ulcer recurrence and complications increases more than threefold with continued cigarette smoking.

Pathophysiology

Although defined as peptic ulcers, gastric and duodenal ulcers are distinctly different in their etiology and incidence. A gastric ulcer is a break in the gastric mucosa that extends into the muscularis mucosae. In contrast, a duodenal ulcer is a chronic break in the duodenal mucosa that extends through the muscularis mucosae. Chronic ulcers of long duration erode through the muscular wall and form fibrous tissue. The development of the ulcer may be due to an imbalance of HCL acid relative to the stomach's natural protective barriers (e.g., prostaglandins). Ulcerogenic drugs, such as aspirin and aspirin-like compounds, inhibit the synthesis of mucus and prostaglandin and cause abnormal cellular permeability. Furthermore, corticosteroids reduce the protective effects of gastric mucus and decrease the rate of mucous cell renewal. Lipid-soluble cytotoxic drugs can pass through the protective gastric barrier to destroy it.

Hyperacidity and PUD can be an acute or chronic problem. Acute ulcers are associated with superficial erosion and minimal inflammation. They are of short duration and quickly resolve when the cause is identified and removed. It may be continuously present for months or reappear intermittently throughout a person's life. Chronic ulcers are at least four times as common as acute erosions.

Gastric Ulcers

Gastric ulcers can appear in any portion of the stomach but are most often found on the lesser curvature in close proximity to the antral junction (Fig. 42–1). Gastric ulcers arise as a result of backward diffusion of acid or pyloric sphincter dysfunction. Normally, a thick, tenacious barrier of gastric mucus acts as the first line of defense against autodigestion, protecting the stomach from mechanical trauma and chemical agents. Although the exact nature is not understood, the mucosal barrier permits very little backward diffusion of hydrogen ions from the lumen to the blood. Even with the large concentration gradient that exists (gastric acid has a pH of 1 to 2, the blood, 7.45), there is little movement of acids back into the tissues. Increased backward diffusion injures the gastric epithelium.

In addition to mucosal and epithelial barriers, tissue resistance to ulceration also depends on an abundant vascular supply and continued, rapid regeneration of epithelial cells. Gastric ulcers are usually slow to heal, in part, because of poor circulation to the ulcerative site. Further, gastric epithelial cells are normally replaced every 3 days. Failure of the replacement mechanism may also play a part in the pathogenesis of PUD.

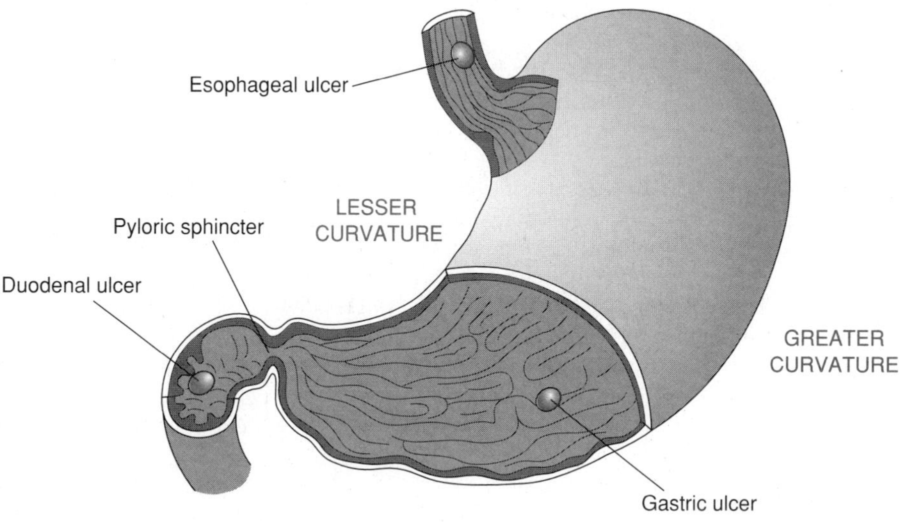

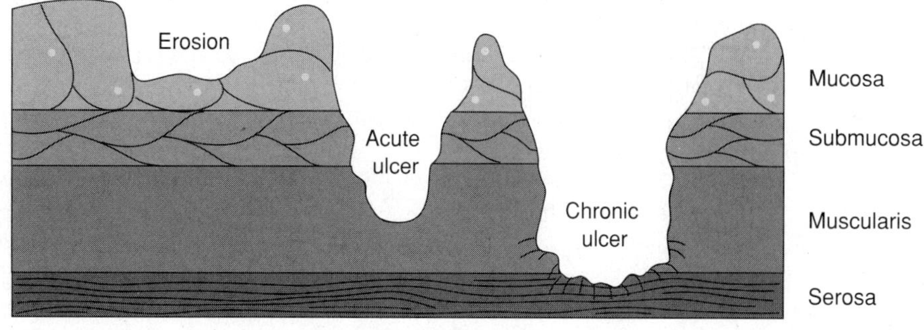

Figure 42–1 Location and depth of ulcerations. Gastric ulcerations are most often located on the lesser curvature of the stomach. Duodenal ulcers are located in the first portion of the duodenum, usually within 2 cm of the pyloric ring. Acute lesions that do not extend through the muscularis are called erosions. Chronic ulcers may erode through the mucosa, submucosa, and muscularis to the serosa.

Duodenal Ulcers

Most peptic ulcers occur downstream from the source of acid secretion. Approximately 98 percent of duodenal ulcers are located in the first portion of the duodenum within 2 centimeters of the pyloric ring. Duodenal ulcers are associated with increased numbers of parietal cells in the stomach, elevated gastrin levels, and rapid gastric emptying. The resistance of the duodenum to ulcer formation is thought to be a function of Brunner's glands (located in the intestinal wall), which produce a highly alkaline, viscid, mucoid secretion that neutralizes the acid chyme. Hypersecretion of HCL acid and pepsin appears to be the most important pathogenic factor in the development of duodenal ulcers, although an inadequate secretion of bicarbonate by the duodenal mucosa may also be related.

Other factors thought to contribute to ulcer formation include failure of the feedback mechanism, in which acid in the gastric antrum inhibits gastrin release. Thus, after eating, serum gastrin levels remain high longer than normal, stimulating acid secretion. It has been postulated that high serum gastrin levels are caused by the *H. pylori* organism. Rapid gastric emptying overcomes the buffering capacity of the bicarbonate-rich pancreatic secretions, which contribute to inflammation.

Stress Ulcerations

Stress ulcerations associated with head injury are characterized by marked hyperacidity. The ulcer results from decreased mucosal blood flow and hypersecretion of acid caused by vagal overstimulation. The shock, anoxia, and sympathetic response produced by the precipitating event decreases mucosal blood flow and contribute to ischemia. On the other hand, stress ulcers associated with shock, sepsis, burns, or drugs are not characterized by the hypersecretion of gastric acid. The mucosal lining degenerates because the metabolism of the mucosal cells declines in response to reduced arterial blood flow. Acid diffuses back into the mucosa, causing inflammation, ulceration, hemorrhage, and necrosis.

Most often, stress ulcerations become known only when they cause bleeding, the primary clinical manifestation of stress ulcers. The bleeding may be slight or, if a vessel is perforated, amount to hundreds of milliliters of blood. Stress ulcerations sometimes carry more than a 50 percent mortality rate. Because of this high rate, much attention is directed toward preventing their development in patients at high risk.

Complications

Intractability

Intractability simply means that conservative management of hyperacidity and PUD failed to control patient symptoms adequately. Intractability is the most common complication of PUD. One third of all patients with ulcers have a single episode of intractability with no recurrence. Sleep is interrupted by the pain, time is lost from work, hospitalization may be required, or patients are just unable to follow the treatment regimen. Intractability is the most common reason for recommending surgery.

Perforation

Approximately 5 percent of all ulcers perforate, accounting for about 65 percent of deaths from PUD. Perforation arises when an ulcer infiltrates serosal surfaces, spilling the gastric or duodenal contents into the peritoneal cavity. Perforations are usually found on the anterior wall of the duodenum or stomach, because this area is covered only by peritoneum. Within minutes of the perforation, a chemical peritonitis develops as a result of escaping gastric acid, pepsin, food, air, saliva, bile, pancreatic juices, and bacteria. A bacterial peritonitis then develops 6 to 12 hours after the perforation, followed by a paralytic ileus. The intensity of the peritonitis is proportional to the amount and duration of the spillage through the perforation.

Hemorrhage

Bleeding is a common complication of PUD, occurring in more than 25 percent of patients at some time during the course of the disease. The most common site of hemorrhage is the posterior wall of the duodenal bulb. The left gastric artery may be penetrated by a gastric ulcer and the superior pancreatic-duodenal artery by a duodenal ulcer.

Although approximately 75 percent of patients who have massive upper GI hemorrhage will spontaneously stop bleeding, the cause must be identified and treatment initiated immediately. In spite of advances in intensive care, intravascular monitoring, and fiberoptic endoscopy, there has been little change in the mortality rate. The mortality rate has remained approximately 10 percent for the past 40 years.

Gastric Outlet Obstruction

Obstruction of the gastric outlet is the result of inflammation and edema, pylorospasm, or scarring in about 5 percent of patients. It is most common in patients with duodenal ulcers, but occasionally occurs when a gastric ulcer is located close to the pyloric sphincter. The patient with gastric outlet obstruction generally reports a long history of ulcer pain.

PHARMACOTHERAPEUTIC OPTIONS

Nonsystemic Antacids

ALUMINUM COMPOUNDS

- ❒ Aluminum hydroxide (ALTERNAGEL, ALU-CAP, AMPHOJEL, ALU-TAB, BASALJEL, DIALUME, NEPHROX)
- ❒ Dihydroxyaluminum sodium carbonate (ROLAIDS)

MAGNESIUM COMPOUNDS

- ❒ Magaldrate (RIOPAN); (✱) IOSOPAN, RIOPAN PLUS
- ❒ Magnesium hydroxide (MILK OF MAGNESIA)
- ❒ Magnesium oxide (URO-MAG)

CALCIUM COMPOUNDS

- ❒ Calcium carbonate (TITRALAC)

COMBINATION COMPOUNDS

- ❒ Aluminum hydroxide and magnesium hydroxide (MAALOX, MYLANTA, WINGEL, GELUSIL, DI-GEL, others); (✱) DIOVOL, GELUSIL, NEUTRALCA-S
- ❒ Aluminum hydroxide and magnesium trisilicate (GAVISCON)

Indications

Nonsystemic antacids include aluminum, magnesium, and calcium compounds. The most commonly used antacids are combinations of aluminum hydroxide and magnesium hydroxide. Antacids are the initial drugs of choice for patients with nonulcer dyspepsia and gastroesophageal reflux disease (GERD). They are used on an as-needed basis for symptom relief, but only if the patient describes symptomatic relief after use.

Antacids decrease the incidence of intractable pain and worsening of ulcer symptoms. Further, recurrence is decreased when long-term maintenance therapy with antacids (and H_2 antagonists, proton pump inhibitors, and prostaglandin) is used. Although calcium compounds apparently are as effective as aluminum or magnesium compounds and have a rapid onset of action, they are rarely used in the management of PUD.

Sodium bicarbonate, a systemically absorbed antacid, is discussed in more depth in Chapter 61. It is potent, but its effects are brief, and the potential for electrolyte imbalance is greater than with nonsystemic antacids. An ideal antacid is one that decreases acidity, is effective for prolonged periods, is pleasant to take by mouth, is not constipating or cathartic in effect, and does not cause systemic effects.

Pharmacodynamics

Antacids are basic substances that neutralize the HCL acid secreted by parietal cells of the stomach, increase gastric pH, and inhibit the conversion of pepsinogen to pepsin (Fig. 42–2). The anions from the antacid combine with the acidic hydrogen cations to increase the pH of stomach contents. They do not neutralize all of the stomach acid and usually do not increase the pH above 4.0 or 5.0. By increasing the pH from 1.0 to 2.0, 90 percent of gastric acid is neutralized. By increasing the pH to 3.0, 99 percent of the gastric acid is neutralized.

A change in gastric pH also affects the activity of pepsin. Pepsin activity is greatest at a pH of 1.5 to 2.5. By increasing the pH, proteolytic activity is reduced, becoming minimal at a pH above 4.0. However, it is thought that by raising gastric pH, the potential for bacterial growth increases.

By increasing the pH and decreasing pepsin activity, symptomatic relief and healing is facilitated. Neither the amount, nor the duration of neutralization required for optimal healing is known. Most health care providers recommend that the gastric pH be maintained between 3.0 and 3.5 during the course of treatment.

Adverse Effects and Contraindications

Antacids differ in the amounts needed to raise gastric pH and in their adverse effects. Aluminum compounds in and of themselves generally have a low neutralizing capacity and a slow onset; therefore, large doses are required. Ingestion of large amounts of aluminum-based antacids over a long period of time causes hypophosphatemia and osteomalacia. The aluminum combines with phosphates in the GI tract, preventing phosphate absorption. Because they have been known to cause constipation, aluminum compounds are often found in combination with magnesium. Further, aluminum concentrates in the central nervous system (CNS) and contributes to encephalopathy, anemia, and anorexia.

Magnesium compounds have a high neutralizing capacity and a rapid onset, but may cause diarrhea and hypermagnesemia. Because magnesium is excreted by the kidneys, it is contraindicated in patient's with anuria. The use of magnesium compounds is also contraindicated in patients with hypermagnesemia, hypocalcemia, heart block, and women in active labor. They should be used cautiously in patients with renal insufficiency. Magnesium hydroxide also has the potential to cause drowsiness, hypothermia, decreased respiratory rates, bradycardia, arrhythmias, hypotension, flushing and sweating, decreased deep-tendon reflexes, and paralysis.

Antacids may cause hypersecretion of gastric acid (acid rebound) and milk-alkali syndrome (i.e., alkalosis and azote-

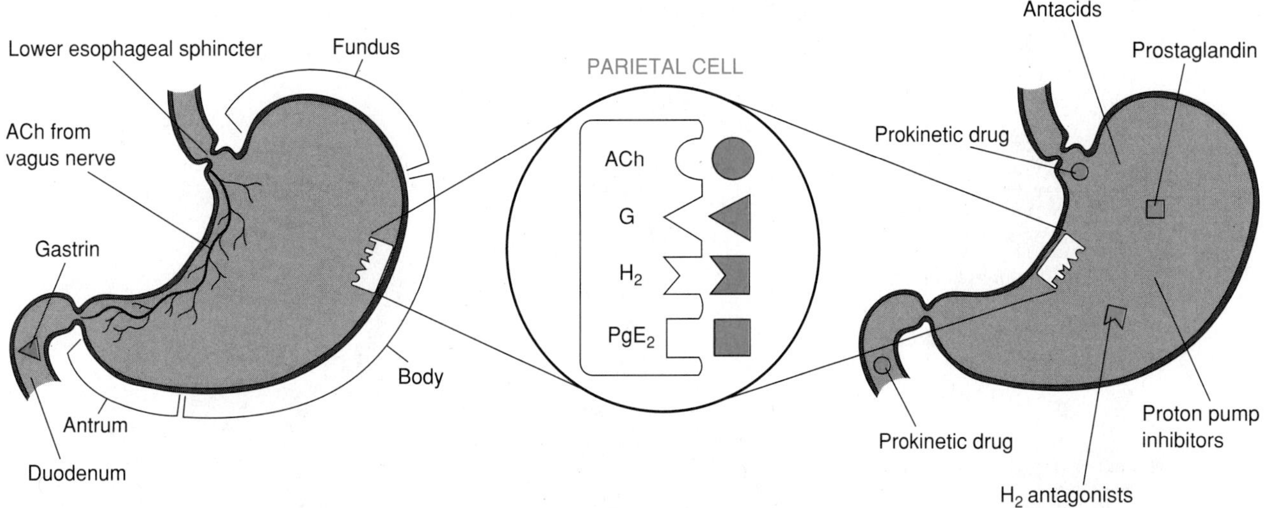

Figure 42–2 Sites of gastrointestinal drug action. Secretion of hydrochloric acid from the parietal cells of the stomach is controlled by duodenally released gastrin (G), acetylcholine (ACh) from the parasympathetic nervous system, and histamine. Gastrin and acetylcholine act through histamine to cause release of hydrochloric acid. Histamine is a powerful stimulant of gastric acid secretion.

Prokinetic agents cause ACh release and increase lower esophageal sphincter tone, gastric motility, and gastric emptying time. Antacids neutralize gastric acid and inhibit the conversion of pepsinogen to pepsin. Prostaglandins (PgE_2) inhibit the secretion of gastric acid and increase mucous and bicarbonate production. Proton pump inhibitors block the final step in the production of gastric acid. H_2 antagonists block histamine action at H_2 receptors and reduce pepsin secretion. Cytoprotective drugs provide a physical barrier to protect the mucosa from contact with hydrochloric acid, pepsin, and bile.

mia). They should be used cautiously in patients with cardiac disease, severe respiratory insufficiency, and renal disease. Furthermore, calcium formulations should not be used in patients with renal calculi, ventricular fibrillation, or hypercalcemia.

Most antacids are formulated to minimize sodium content. All antacids that contain more than 0.2 mEq of sodium per dose must be labeled with the amount.

Sodium bicarbonate, when used in excessive amounts as an antacid, can cause edema, metabolic alkalosis, hypernatremia, hypokalemia, hypocalcemia, gastric distention, flatulence, and tetany. The routine use of sodium bicarbonate for indigestion and gastric irritation should be avoided.

Pharmacokinetics

Table 42–1 provides an overview of the pharmacokinetics of selected antacids. In general, antacids are nonabsorbable. However, with chronic use, 15 to 30 percent of magnesium and smaller quantities of the aluminum are absorbed. The absorbed magnesium and aluminum are widely distributed, crossing the membranes of the placenta. They are also found in breast milk.

The onset of most of the antacids range from 3 to 30 minutes. Aluminum has a delayed onset and magnesium an immediate onset, with peak effects of both generally reached in 30 minutes. The duration of the effects of the antacid depends on whether the drug is taken on an empty stomach or with food. The acid-neutralizing effects of antacids last approximately 30 minutes to 1 hour when taken on an empty stomach, and approximately 3 hours when taken after meals. The neutralizing capacity of antacids is identified in Table 42–2. The aluminum and magnesium antacids are eliminated through the feces.

Drug-Drug Interactions

Most significant drug-drug interactions alter the effects of other drugs rather than those of the antacid (Table 42–3). For example, they may decrease the absorption of H_2 antagonists, decrease the effects of beta blockers such as atenolol, decrease absorption of metronidazole and other antibiotics, and decrease the renal excretion and increase the toxicity of quinidine. Magnesium and aluminum salts decrease the absorptive characteristics of digoxin, tetracyclines, phenothiazines, iron salts, isoniazid, fluoroquinolones, and other drugs. Salicylate levels may also be decreased in the presence of antacid-caused alkaline urine. The elimination of flecainide and amphetamines are markedly reduced, and toxicity is possible with large antacid doses and an alkaline urine. Further, antacids remove the enteric coating on drugs, thereby increasing the drug's premature release in the stomach.

Dosage Regimen

Antacid dosages, including the frequency of administration, depend primarily on the purpose for use, the buffering capacity of the antacid, and the patient's response. Generally speaking, aluminum-containing antacids are the least potent and calcium carbonate the most potent. Calcium antacids are safe only for intermittent use.

TABLE 42–1 PHARMACOKINETICS OF SELECTED PEPTIC ULCER AND HYPERACIDITY DRUGS

Drug	Route	Onset	Peak	Duration	PB (%)	$t_{1/2}$	BioA (%)
Nonsystemic Antacids							
Aluminum hydroxide	po	15–30 min	30 min	30 min–3 hr	UK	UK	UK
Magnesium hydroxide	po	Immed	30 min	60 min	UK	UK	UK
Calcium carbonate	po	3–5 min	UK	UK	UK	UK	UK
Histamine-2 Antagonists							
Cimetidine	po	Varies	1–1.5 hr*	UK	19	2–3 hr	55–68
	IV/IM	Rapid	<1.5 hr*	UK	19	2–3 hr	100
Ranitidine	po	Varies	1–3 hr	8–12 hr	15	2–3 hr	50–60
	IM	Rapid	15 min	8–12 hr	15	2–3 hr	100
	IV	Immed	5–10 min	8–12 hr	15	2–3 hr	100
Famotidine	po	Slow	1–3 hr†	6–12 hr	17	1.3–2.6 hr	45–50
	IV	<1 hr	0.5–3 hr†	8–15 hr	17	1.3–2.6 hr	100
Nizatidine	po	Varies	1–2 hr†	UA	35	1.5 hr	90
Proton Pump Inhibitors							
Lansoprazole	po	Rapid	UK	>24 hr	97.5	8–10 hr	35–40
Omeprazole	po	<60 min	<2 hr	72–96 hr	70–76	0.5–1 hr	UA
Prostaglandin							
Misoprostol	po	30 min	UK	1–2 hr	30	20–40 min	UA
	IV	1–3 min	Immed				100
	IM	10–15 min	UK				UA
Prokinetic Drugs							
Cisapride	po	30–60 min	70 min	UK	97.5	8–10 hr	35–40
Metoclopramide	po	30–60 min	UK	1–2 hr	30	2.5–5 hr	UA
	IM	10–15 min	UK				
	IV	1–3 min	Immed				100
Cytoprotective Drug							
Sucralfate	po	30 min	UK	5 hr	UA	6–20 hr	5

*Concentrations of cimetidine that inhibit gastric acid secretion by 50% and 90%, respectively.
†Concentration of famotidine or nizatidine that inhibit gastric secretion by 50%.
PB, Protein binding; $t_{1/2}$, elimination half-life; NA, not applicable; UK, unknown; UA, unavailable; BioA, bioavailability.

TABLE 42–2 NEUTRALIZING CAPACITY OF SELECTED ANTACIDS*

	Ingredient (mg/5 mL)					
Brand Name of Drug	$AL(OH)_3$ IN MG	$MG(OH)_2$ IN MG	$CaCO_3$	SIMETH	NA CONTENT	**Acid-Neutralizing Capacity (mEq/5 mL)**
ALTERNAGEL	600	0	0	—	<2.5	16
ALUDROX	307	103	0	—	2.3	12
AMPHOJEL	320	0	0	—	<2.3	10
BASALJEL	400†	†	†	—	2.9	12
DI-GEL	200	200	0	20	<5	—
GAVISCON	31.7‡	‡	‡	—	4	13
GELUSIL	200	200	0	25	0.7	12
GELUSIL-M§	300	200	0	25	1.2	15
MAALOX	225	200	0	0	1.4	13
MILK OF MAGNESIA	0	390	0	0	0.12	14
MYLANTA	200	200	0	20	0.7	13
MYLANTA II	400	400	0	40	1.1	25
WINGEL	180	160	0	0	—	10

*Many of these antacid preparations are also available in solid dosage forms (i.e., tablets). Although the composition of these forms is often similar to that of suspensions, there are variations.

†BASALJEL: $Al(OH)CO_3$ equivalent to 400 mg of $AL(OH)_3$

‡GAVISCON: $AL(OH)_3$ plus 137 $MgCO_3$ plus sodium alginate

§Therapeutic concentrate of GELUSIL; M, medium strength

Simeth, simethicone.

Commonly, 5 to 30 mL or one to two tablets (500 to 1500 mg) of aluminum hydroxide or magnesium hydroxide are taken 1 hour and 3 hours after meals and at bedtime (Table 42–4). Although this routine is effective and rational, gastric acid is only buffered intermittently rather than continuously. When it is used as an antacid, the usual dose of calcium carbonate is 0.5 to 2 g by mouth 1 hour and 3 hours after meals and at bedtime.

For a patient with a nasogastric tube in place, the antacid dosage may be titrated by aspirating stomach contents, determining the pH with Nitrazine paper, and then basing the dose on the pH. Most gastric acid is neutralized at a pH above 3.5, with most pepsin activity eliminated at a pH above 5. If the pH is less than 5, the frequency or dosage of the antacid may be increased.

To prevent stress ulcerations in seriously ill or injured patients and to treat acute GI bleeding, nearly continuous neutralization of gastric acid is desirable. The dosage and frequency of administration must be sufficient to neutralize 50 to 80 mEq of gastric acid each hour. This may be accomplished by hourly administration of an antacid or through a continuous *intragastric* drip.

Laboratory Considerations

With chronic antacid use, serum phosphate, calcium, and electrolyte levels should be monitored periodically. Hypercalcemia increases the risk of cardiac glycoside toxicity, and hypocalcemia can create tetany, cardiac arrhythmias, and other adverse effects. Serum osmolarity, acid-base balance, and renal function testing may also be warranted depending on the patient's response to therapy.

Histamine-2 Antagonists

- ❐ Cimetidine (TAGAMET); (♣) APO-CIMETIDINE, NOVO-CIMETINE, PEPTOL
- ❐ Ranitidine (ZANTAC); (♣) APO-RANITIDINE, ZANTAC-C
- ❐ Famotidine (PEPCID)
- ❐ Nizatidine (AXID)

Indications

H_2 antagonists, also referred to as H_2-blocking drugs, are used in the short-term management of active duodenal ulcers and benign gastric ulcers. In low doses, H_2 antagonists can be used for duodenal ulcer prophylaxis, and in the prevention and treatment of acute stress ulcerations, esophagitis resulting from GERD, and Zollinger-Ellison syndrome.

Cimetidine is the drug of choice for the initial treatment of stress-induced upper GI bleeding in critically ill patients because it has the fewest adverse effects. H_2 antagonists heal more than 90 percent of duodenal ulcers and more than 70 percent of gastric ulcers.

Pharmacodynamics

Histamine is found in most body tissues and is normally released in response to certain stimuli (e.g., tissue injury, allergic reactions). Once released, it produces a number of effects, including a strong stimulation of gastric acid secretion. In addition, vagal stimulation causes the release of histamine from the cells in the gastric mucosa. The histamine then acts on parietal cell receptors (H_2 receptors) to increase production of HCL acid.

These drugs inhibit the action of histamine at the H_2 receptors, inhibiting gastric acid secretion and reducing total pepsin output. The resultant decrease in acid permits healing of ulcerated areas. The drugs are highly selective and have little to no effect on H_1 or other receptors. H_1 antagonists, the typical antihistamines, are discussed in Chapter 47. H_1 antagonists prevent or reduce the effects of histamine but do nothing to block the production of gastric acid.

TABLE 42–3 DRUG-DRUG INTERACTIONS OF SELECTED PEPTIC ULCER AND HYPERACIDITY DRUGS

Drug	Interactive Drug		Interaction
Nonsystemic Antacids			
Aluminum hydroxide	Allopurinol		Decreased pharmacologic effects of interactive drug
Magnesium hydroxide	Corticosteroids	Isoniazid	
	Diflunisol	Penicillamine	
	Digoxin	Phenothiazines	
	Fluoroquinolones	Ranitidine	
	Iron	Tetracyclines	
	Amphetamines	Salicylates	Increased pharmacologic effects of interactive drugs
	Benzodiazepines		
	Amphetamines	Quinidine	Reduced elimination of interactive drug and increased risk of toxicity
	Flecainide		
	Enteric coated drugs		Premature release of interactive drug
Magnesium hydroxide	Nitrofurantoin	Penicillamine	Decreased pharmacologic effect of interactive drug
	Tetracyclines		
Calcium carbonate	Digoxin		Increased potential for glycoside toxicity
Histamine-2 Antagonists			
Cimetidine	Antimetabolites	Alkylating agents	Increased risk of decreased WBC count
	Benzodiazepines	Propranolol	Prolongs half-life of interactive drug, thereby increasing its effects
	Digitoxin	Quinidine	
	Mexiletine	Theophylline	
	Nifedipine	Tricyclic antidepressants	
	Phenobarbital	Warfarin	
	Phenytoin		
Ranitidine	Tricyclic antidepressants		Increased effects of interactive drug
	Warfarin		
	Diazepam		Decreased effects of interactive drug
	Lidocaine	Nifedipine	Decreased clearance; potential toxicity
Famotidine	Antacids	Ketoconazole	Decreased absorption of interactive agents
Nizatidine	Salicylates		Increased salicylate levels in patients taking over 3900 mg/day
	Antacids		Decreased absorption of nizatidine
Proton Pump Inhibitors			
Lansoprazole	Diazepam	Warfarin	Decreased metabolism of interactive agent
Omeprazole	Phenytoin		
	Esters of ampicillin	Iron salts	Interferes with absorption of drugs requiring acid pH
	Ketoconazole		
Lansoprazole	Sucralfate		Decreases the absorption of lansoprazole
Prostaglandin			
Misoprostol	Magnesium-containing antacids		Increases risk of diarrhea
Prokinetic Drugs			
Metoclopramide	Alcohol	Opioids	Additive CNS depression
	Antidepressants	Sedative hypnotics	
	Antihistamines		
	Insulin		May require insulin adjustment
	Orally administered drugs		May affect GI absorption of other orally administered drugs
	General anesthesia		Exaggerated hypotension
	Haloperidol	Phenothiazines	Increased risk of extrapyramidal reactions
	Anticholinergics	Opioids	May antagonist GI effects of metoclopramide
	Cyclosporine		Increased absorption and risk of toxicity from interactive drug
	MAO inhibitors		Increased risk of hypertensive episode
	Succinylcholine		Increased neuromuscular blockade
Cisapride	Anticholinergics		Decreases effects of cisapride
	Alcohol	Benzodiazepines	Accelerates the sedative effects of interactive drugs
	Anticonvulsants	Digoxin	May alter effects of drugs that have narrow therapeutic margins
	Cimetidine	Ranitidine	Increases plasma levels of cisapride
	Ketoconazole		Increases blood levels and risk of arrhythmias from cisapride
	Itraconazole		
Cytoprotective Drug			
Sucralfate	Fat soluble vitamin	Tetracycline	Decreases the absorption of interacting agent
	Phenytoin		
	Antacids		Decreases effectiveness of sucralfate
	Fluoroquinolones		Decreases absorption with concurrent use

CNS, Central nervous system; GI, gastrointestinal; MAO, monoamine oxidase; WBC, white blood cell.

TABLE 42–4 DOSAGE REGIMEN OF SELECTED PEPTIC ULCER AND HYPERACIDITY DRUGS			
Drug	**Uses**	**Dosage**	**Implications**
Nonsystemic Antacids*			
Aluminum hydroxide	Hyperacidity, GERD, PUD, gastritis, esophagitis, hiatal hernia, stress ulcerations	*Adult:* 5–30 mL *or* 2 tablets (500–1500 mg) po 1 hr and 3 hrs pc & HS *Child:* 5–15 mL po q1–2 hr	For PUD continue use 4–6 weeks after symptoms disappear
Magnesium hydroxide		*Adult:* 5–15 mL liquid *or* 650–1300 mg as tablets QID	For adults and children older than age 12 years
Calcium carbonate		*Adult:* 0.5–2 g po 1 hr and 3 hrs pc and HS	Taken hourly for first 2 weeks when used in treatment of acute PUD
Histamine-2 Antagonists†			
Cimetidine	Active PUD, Zollinger-Ellison syndrome, stress ulcerations, erosive GERD, esophagitis	*Adult:* 800 mg po QD HS *or* 300 mg po QID ac and HS *or* 400 mg po BID	Continue therapy for 4–8 weeks. Individualize dosage. Not recommended for children under 16 years
Ranitidine		*Adult:* 150 mg po BID *or* 300 mg po QD at HS *or* 50 mg IM/IV q6-8hr or by intermittent IV infusion	Continue therapy for 4–8 weeks. Dosage not to exceed 400 mg/day
Famotidine		*Adult:* 40 mg po/IV HS *or* 20 mg po/IV BID. Maintenance: 20–40 mg po HS	Full dosage therapy not to exceed 6–8 weeks. Doses up to 160 mg q6hr have been used for hypersecretory syndrome
Nizatidine		*Adult:* 300 mg po QD at HS *or* 150 mg po BID. Maintenance: 150 mg po at HS	Safety and efficacy in children not established. Reduce dosage in older adults or patients with renal impairment
Proton Pump Inhibitors			
Lansoprazole	Erosive esophagitis, active duodenal ulcers, hypersecretory states	*Adult: Erosive esophagitis:* 30 mg po before meals × 8 weeks. *Duodenal ulcers:* 15 mg before meals × 4 weeks. *Hypersecretory conditions:* 60 mg once daily. May be increased up to 90 mg BID if necessary.	Give in divided doses if dosage exceeds 120 mg/day. Advise patients to avoid alcohol, aspirin-containing products, other NSAIDs, and foods that may cause increased GI irritation
Omeprazole	Hyperacidity, PUD, GERD	*Adult: GERD:* 20–40 mg po QD × 4–8 wks. *Maintenance healing erosive gastritis* 20 mg po QD. *Hypersecretory states:* 60 mg po QD initially. May increase up to 120 mg TID.	Continue GERD therapy for 4–8 weeks. Doses over 80 mg should be given in divided doses
Prostaglandins			
Cisapride	Nocturnal symptoms associated with GERD. Gastroparesis (Unlabeled use)	*Adult:* 10–20 mg po QID 15 min ac and HS. Other regimens include 5 mg TID, 10 mg BID, or 20 mg at HS.	Advise patient to avoid alcohol or other depressants since drug may enhance sedative effects
Misoprostol	Antineoplastic drug-induced emesis, small bowel intubation, GERD, gastroparesis. Hiccoughs (Unlabeled use)	*Adult: Antineoplastic drug-induced emesis:* 1–2 mg/kg IV 30 min before therapy. Additional doses of 1–2mg/kg may be given q2hr × 2 doses, then q3hr × 3 additional doses. *Small bowel intubation:* 10 mg IV *Gastroparesis:* 10 mg po 30 min ac and HS *or* 15 mg PR 30–60 min ac and HS. *GERD:* 10–15 mg po 30 min ac and HS up to four times daily, not to exceed 0.5 mg/kg/day. A single dose of 20 mg may be used in situations likely to provide symptoms *Postoperative nausea and vomiting:* 10–20 mg IM *Hiccoughs:* 10–20 mg po QID. May be preceded by a single 10 mg IM dose	Adults who are sensitive to drug effects may respond to doses as small as 5 mg. Monitor for tardive dyskinesia, which may occur after a year or more of continued therapy. Dystonic reactions may occur within minutes of IV infusion and stop within 24 hours of drug discontinuation. Dystonia may be treated with 50 mg of diphenhydramine IM or 1 mg/kg IV 15 minutes before metoclopramide IV infusion. Extrapyramidal effects may occur at any age but are more common in children and young adults
Cytoprotective Drug			
Sucralfate	PUD, prevention of PUD secondary to NSAID use	*Adult: Ulcers:* 1 g po QID 1 hr ac and HS or 2 g BID *Ulcer prophylaxis:* 1 g BID 1 hour before meals. *GERD:* 1 g QID ac and HS (unlabeled) *Child: GERD:* 500–1g QID ac and HS (unlabeled)	Take on empty stomach. Avoid antacids within ½ hr of drug. If NG administration is required, consult pharmacist since protein-binding properties of sucralfate have resulted in formation of a bezoar when administered with enteral feedings and other drugs

*Combinations of aluminum hydroxide and magnesium hydroxide are more commonly used for antacid effects than single formulations.
†Dosage regimen of histamine-2 antagonists varies with specific use and patient response.
GERD, Gastroesophageal reflux disease; NSAIDS, nonsteroidal anti-inflammatory disease; PUD, peptic ulcer disease.

Adverse Effects and Contraindications

There are few adverse effects associated with H_2 antagonists, although dizziness, somnolence, headache, confusion, and hallucinations have been noted. Diarrhea is the most common GI adverse effect. Cimetidine in particular may act as an antiandrogen and cause reversible impotence and gynecomastia, which are disturbing to male patients.

There are no absolute contraindications to the use of H_2 antagonists except a history of allergy. However, the drugs should be used with caution in pregnant or lactating women, children, older adults, and in patients with impaired renal or hepatic function (see Controversy—Self-Medication with Histamine-2 Antagonists).

Pharmacokinetics

As a group, H_2 antagonists are rapidly and well absorbed following oral administration. Peak plasma concentrations are achieved via the oral route within 1 to 2 hours (see Table 42–1). First-pass hepatic biotransformation limits the bioavailability of cimetidine, ranitidine, and famotidine to about 50 percent, whereas the oral bioavailability of nizatidine is approximately 90 percent. The elimination half-life of cimetidine, ranitidine, and famotidine is approximately 2 to 3 hours, whereas nizatidine's half-life is 1 to 3 hours. The drugs in large part are eliminated unchanged in the urine. However, the half-life of ranitidine is significantly prolonged in patients with liver disorders.

Controversy

Self-Medication with Histamine-2 Antagonists

JONATHAN W. WOLFE

The advent of cimetidine as an intravenous medication in 1976 was universally acclaimed. Here was a drug that had no known adverse effects and could essentially rescue patients with gastric ulcerations from bleeding. Gone was the need for partial to total gastric resection, which too often led to dumping syndrome. Gone also were the desperate and often futile interventions (e.g., iced gavage with levarterenol) against uncontrollable hemorrhage. The commercial success of the drug has served as a benchmark for every product since that time.

The intervening years have brought change. The adverse effects of the original H_2 blocker have become clear. The effect of cimetidine on the cytochrome P_{450} enzyme systems in the liver embargoes its use in combination with many drugs. The recognition of cimetidine effects on mentation, particularly in older patients, limits its use. Newer, more selective H_2 antagonists have come to market (e.g., ranitidine). They offer better adverse effect profiles. And as the patents have expired for these drugs, their costs have decreased and are now comparable to that of cimetidine.

Perhaps the most stunning change has been the appearance of over-the-counter (OTC) forms of the H_2 blocking drugs. What once was a miracle infusion in the intensive care unit is now hanging on racks in service stations next to breath mints and chewing gum. Indeed these wonder medications are advertised on television as the answer to heartburn.

Critical Thinking Discussion

- When cimetidine was introduced, patients were cautioned to take it regularly rather than in response to symptoms. Why do we now have OTC products for PRN use?
- How do you respond to a patient who tells you that rather than pay for a new prescription for ranitidine 300 mg, he will just take four 75 mg OTC tablets at bedtime "when the pain is bad." Should you document this statement in the patient's medical record?
- What hazard is posed when the patient chooses to use OTC H_2 antagonists for 6 weeks before seeing a physician?
- What restrictions on the OTC sale of H_2 antagonists would you consider reasonable?

Drug-Drug Interactions

Drug-drug interactions of H_2 antagonists are many (see Table 42–3). All drugs that inhibit gastric acid secretion alter the bioavailability and absorption rate of certain drugs secondary to changes in gastric pH. Cimetidine, but not the other agents, inhibits the activity of cytochrome P_{450} enzymes, thereby slowing the biotransformation of many drugs that are substrates for hepatic mixed-function oxidases. Thus, the concurrent use of cimetidine will prolong the half-life of a host of drugs. Such interactions require either dosage reduction or interval extension strategies.

Dosage Regimen

H_2 antagonists are generally well tolerated and can be administered in doses well in excess of those needed to produce an effect. Thus, despite their short plasma half-lives, these drugs may often be taken only once or twice daily.

The oral dosage of cimetidine, when used for the treatment of active PUD, is 800 mg daily at bedtime (see Table 42–4). Alternatively, 300 mg may be taken four times a day with meals, or 400 mg twice daily. The treatment regimen usually extends over 4 to 8 weeks. A dose of 400 mg may be taken at bedtime for the prevention of recurrence of duodenal ulcers. Solutions are available for intravenous (IV) or intramuscular (IM) use.

The usual oral dose of ranitidine for the treatment of active duodenal ulcers is 150 mg twice daily, or 300 mg at bedtime. Injectable solutions are available for IV or IM use every 6 to 8 hours.

Famotidine, when used for acute duodenal ulcers, is administered orally or by IV route in 40-mg doses at bedtime, or alternatively, 20 mg twice daily. Full-dose therapy should not exceed 6 to 8 weeks. Doses of up to 160 mg every 6 hours have been used for hypersecretory syndromes. Oral suspensions are available for those who cannot manage the tablet form.

The recommended oral dose of nizatidine is 150 mg twice daily or 300 mg at bedtime. Maintenance doses are 150 mg orally at bedtime. There are no parenteral formulations of nizatidine at this time.

Laboratory Considerations

A complete blood count and differential should be monitored periodically throughout therapy. White blood cell counts should be monitored while on cimetidine, especially if other drugs known to cause neutropenia are taken. H_2 blockers may cause a transient increase in liver function tests and in serum creatinine. Serum prolactin concentrations may be increased following IV bolus cimetidine. It may also cause decreased parathyroid hormone concentrations. False-negative results of allergy tests may be noted; therefore, cimetidine should be discontinued 24 hours before testing. Further, false-negative results for urine protein has been noted with ranitidine. Nizatidine has caused false-positive results on tests for urobilinogen.

Proton Pump Inhibitors

❒ Lansoprazole (PREVACID)
❒ Omeprazole (PRILOSEC)

Indications

Current indications for omeprazole and its fluorinated counterpart lansoprazole include the short-term treatment of active PUD, erosive gastritis, GERD, and Zollinger-Ellison syndrome. Omeprazole is thought to be more effective than the H_2 antagonists in the management of duodenal ulcers but at present should be used only for patients who do not respond to H_2 antagonists. It appears that healing occurs in 88 to 100 percent of patients with duodenal ulcers after 6 weeks of treatment. However, the high cost and unknown long-term effects of omeprazole transfer it to a second-line regimen at the present time. Further, most patients respond satisfactorily to other less expensive drugs.

Pharmacodynamics

Proton pump inhibitors suppress gastric acid secretion by irreversibly binding with the hydrogen-potassium-adenosine triphosphatase enzyme (H^+-K^+-ATPase) proton pump system that controls hydrogen secretion from the parietal cell into the secretory canals. Thus, the final step in the production of gastric acid is blocked. These drugs inhibit gastric acid secretion by more than 90 percent and frequently produce achlorhydria.

Proton pump inhibitors are inactive prodrugs that are converted at acid pH in the parietal cell to sulfenamide, which combines covalently with sulfhydryl groups on the H^+-K^+-ATPase. Proton pump inhibitors are formulated as enteric-coated drugs to prevent sulfenamide formation in the stomach. Sulfenamide, unlike omeprazole, does not readily cross biologic membranes, and therefore, it accumulates in the parietal cells. Because of this and the unique nature of the pump, proton pump inhibitors have little action on ion pumps elsewhere in the body.

Adverse Effects and Contraindications

The most frequent adverse effects of omeprazole include headache, dizziness, nausea, vomiting, diarrhea, and abdominal pain. Symptoms of upper respiratory infection may also be noted. A rash, inflammation, urticaria, pruritus, alopecia, and dry skin have been demonstrated. Omeprazole should be used with caution in patients who are pregnant or lactating. Safe use in children has not been established.

Fewer adverse effects are associated with lansoprazole. Drowsiness, nausea, and abdominal pain have been reported. Lansoprazole should be used with caution in elderly patients, patients with severe hepatic impairment, and in pregnant or lactating patients. Safe use in children has not been established.

Pharmacokinetics

Lansoprazole is well absorbed (80 percent) following oral administration. Its distribution is unknown (see Table 42–1). Biotransformation to inactive metabolites is extensive in the liver. The drug is converted intracellularly to at least two other antisecretory compounds. The half-life is less than 2 hours, although it is increased in older adults and in patients with impaired liver function.

Omeprazole is well absorbed when taken by mouth, with uptake into gastric parietal cells. It is 70- to 76-percent bound to plasma proteins. The drug onsets within 1 hour of administration. Acid-inhibiting effects occur within 2 hours. The duration of action is 72 to 96 hours. Omeprazole is extensively biotransformed by the liver. The half-life of omeprazole is ½ to 1 hour longer for patients with liver disease. Seventy-five percent of the administered dose is eliminated in the urine, with about 25 percent eliminated in feces. When the drug is discontinued, the effects persist for 3 to 5 days, until the gastric parietal cells synthesize additional H^+-K^+-ATPase enzymes.

Drug-Drug Interactions

Lansoprazole interacts with sucralfate to decrease the absorption of lansoprazole. Lansoprazole may also decrease the absorption of drugs requiring acid pH including ketoconazole, ampicillin esters, iron salts, and digoxin.

Omeprazole decreases the biotransformation and increases the effects of diazepam, phenytoin, and warfarin (see Table 42–3). It interferes with the absorption of other drugs that require an acidic gastric pH to be effective. Examples of such drugs include ketoconazole, esters of ampicillin, and iron salts. Omeprazole has been safely used concurrently with antacids.

Dosage Regimen

When proton pump inhibitors are used for the short-term treatment of erosive esophagitis, the usual dose is 30 mg daily before meals. Treatment usually lasts for about 8 weeks.

When these drugs are used to treat gastric hyperacidity and GERD, a 20-mg daily dose of omeprazole used for 4 to 8 weeks is recommended (see Table 42–4). It should be taken before meals. For patients with Zollinger-Ellison syndrome, a 60-mg dose taken once daily is recommended. The dosage may be increased to 120 mg three times daily, if needed. Doses that exceed 80 mg/day should be administered as divided doses.

Laboratory Considerations

Serum levels of theophylline may be elevated in the presence of lansoprazole. Serum drug levels of omeprazole are not measured routinely.

Omeprazole has been shown to elevate serum levels of alanine aminotransferase (ALT; serum glutamic-pyruvic transaminase [SGPT]) and aspartate aminotransferase (AST; serum glutamic-oxaloacetic transaminase [SGOT]), alkaline phosphatase, and bilirubin levels. Low blood sugar levels may also be noted. This drug may also cause serum gastrin concentrations to increase during the first 1 to 2 weeks of therapy. Serum gastrin levels return to normal after discontinuation of the drug. A complete blood count and differential should be monitored periodically throughout therapy.

Lansoprazole is also known to cause increased liver function tests and gastrin levels, but it may also cause an abnormal albumin/globulin ratio, hyperlipidemia, and increased or decreased cholesterol levels.

Prostaglandins

❒ Misoprostol (CYTOTEC)

Indications

Misoprostol is a synthetic form of prostaglandin E. It is used to prevent gastric ulcerations secondary to the use of NSAIDs. There is no evidence that misoprostol prevents ulcer complications and death. Misoprostol may also be used for patients at high risk for GI bleeding, such as the elderly, debilitated patients, or patients with a history of PUD.

Pharmacodynamics

The protective ability of misoprostol is attributed to its ability to inhibit gastric acid secretion (antisecretory effect). Misoprostol also increases bicarbonate and mucus production (cytoprotective effects).

Adverse Effects and Contraindications

Misoprostol is generally well tolerated. The most common adverse effects include nausea, flatulence, diarrhea, and abdominal pain in 10 to 40 percent of patients. It is important to note that misoprostol is not recommended for use with women of child-bearing age unless consistent, effective birth control methods are used. The greatest risk of prostaglandin therapy is that of abortion, excessive bleeding, spotting, cramping, hypermenorrhea, and dysmenorrhea.

Pharmacokinetics

Misoprostol is well absorbed following oral administration and is rapidly converted to its active form. Its onset time is approximately 30 minutes, with a duration of action of 3 hours. Plasma steady state is achieved within 2 days. The half-life is 20 to 40 minutes. Misoprostol undergoes biotransformation in the liver and is eliminated by the kidneys (see Table 42–1).

Drug-Drug Interactions

No known drug interactions exist with natural or synthetic prostaglandin drugs. It should be noted, however, that an increased risk of diarrhea exists when misoprostol is taken with a magnesium-containing antacid.

Dosage Regimen

The usual adult dose of misoprostol is 200 mcg four times daily, with or after meals and at bedtime. It may also be administered twice daily in 400 mcg doses, with the last dose at bedtime. If the patient is unable to tolerate the 400 mcg dose, the dosage may be decreased to 100 mcg daily.

Prokinetic Drugs

❒ Cisapride (PROPULSID)
❒ Metoclopramide (REGLAN)

Indications

Prokinetic drugs are used in conjunction with proton pump inhibitors and H_2 antagonists in the management of GERD. Cisapride is used in the management of nocturnal heartburn associated with GERD. It has also been used to manage gastroparesis due to diabetes, pseudo-obstruction, and other causes.

Metoclopramide is used to prevent antineoplastic drug-induced emesis. Postsurgical and diabetic gastric stasis is also effectively treated with metoclopramide. These drugs also facilitate small bowel intubation in radiographic procedures and is used in the prevention and treatment of postoperative nausea and vomiting when nasogastric suctioning is undesirable. Although it is not approved by the Food and Drug Administration (FDA) for such use, metoclopramide has also been used as treatment for hiccoughs.

Pharmacodynamics

Cisapride enhances the action of acetylcholine at the myenteric plexus. It also increases the strength of esophageal peristalsis and increases the lower esophageal sphincter pressure. It is a substituted benzamide, with antagonistic actions at 5-hydroxytryptamine$_3$ receptors while stimulating 5-hydroxytryptamine$_4$ (serotonin) receptors.

Metoclopramide is a dopamine type 2 receptor antagonist and a 5-HT_4 receptor stimulant. Drug action is thought to result in the release of acetylcholine, increased gastric motility, and an increased rate of gastric emptying. These effects plus the ability to increase lower esophageal sphincter tone also helps reduce symptoms of GERD. There is little evidence to date that metoclopramide heals an eroded esophagus. Metoclopramide also has anticholinergic and CNS effects as a result of dopamine blockade.

Adverse Effects and Contraindications

The adverse effects of cisapride include headache, dizziness, fatigue, and depression. Rhinitis, pharyngitis, diarrhea, abdominal pain, dyspepsia, vomiting, flatulence, and constipation have also been noted. Dehydration, back pain, and myalgia is possible in susceptible individuals.

Pharmacokinetics

The pharmacokinetics of prokinetic drugs is identified in Table 42–1. Note that the drugs act relatively quickly to promote esophageal and gastric emptying. Cisapride is rapidly absorbed following oral administration, although its bioavailability is only 35 to 40 percent. It is extensively biotransformed (over 90 percent) in the liver, with a half-life of 8 to 10 hours.

Metoclopramide is also well absorbed from the GI tract, from rectal mucosa, and from IM administration sites. It is widely distributed to body tissues and fluids, crossing the blood-brain barrier and placental membranes. It is partially biotransformed in the liver, with 25 percent of the original drug eliminated unchanged in the urine. Metoclopramide has a relatively short half-life at 2.5 to 5 hours.

Drug-Drug Interactions

Prokinetic drugs interact with a variety of other drugs (see Table 42–3), although the interactions differ somewhat between metoclopramide and cisapride. For example, metoclopramide interacts with CNS depressants, including alcohol, antidepressants, antihistamines, opioids, and sedative-hypnotics to cause additive CNS depression. Cisapride does not interact with CNS depressants except for benzodiazepines and alcohol.

Dosage Regimen

The dosage regimens for prokinetic drugs are identified in Table 42–4. Because these drugs are used for a variety of purposes, the doses and dosages should be checked carefully before administration.

Laboratory Considerations

Metoclopramide may alter liver function test results. It may also cause increased serum prolactin and aldosterone concentrations. There are no known laboratory considerations with cisapride.

Cytoprotective Drug

❒ Sucralfate (CARAFATE)

Indications

Sucralfate, as a locally acting drug, has been used in the management of PUD and hyperacidity when patients are unable to tolerate H_2 antagonists or omeprazole. It may also be used when H_2 antagonists have been ineffective.

Sucralfate is the preferred drug for stress ulcerations. It is less expensive than parenteral H_2 antagonists, is not likely to increase the chance of nosocomial pneumonia, and does not require measurement of gastric pH on a regular basis. A 4- to 8-week treatment regimen is recommended to ensure healing.

Pharmacodynamics

Sucralfate, as the only approved drug in this group, has been shown to heal gastric and duodenal ulcerations by forming a protective barrier between the gastric acid, pepsin, and bile salts and the gastric or duodenal wall. It reacts with gastric acid to form a thick exudate at the ulcer site or sites. The barrier formed thus decreases tissue damage at the ulcer site.

Adverse Effects and Contraindications

The adverse effects of sucralfate that are most often reported include dry mouth and constipation. Nausea, indigestion, and gastric discomfort have been noted in some patients.

Pharmacokinetics

Only 5 percent of sucralfate is absorbed systemically. It is well tolerated, producing few adverse effects. The onset of drug action is within 30 minutes, with a duration of drug action lasting as long as 5 hours. The half-life of sucralfate ranges from 6 hours to as long as 20 hours.

Drug-Drug Interactions

Drug-drug interactions with sucralfate include phenytoin, fat-soluble vitamins, tetracyclines, and antacids. Antacids decrease the effectiveness of the sucralfate, whereas the absorption of phenytoin, fat-soluble vitamins, and tetracyclines is increased. The absorption of fluoroquinolones is reduced with concurrent use of sucralfate.

Dosage Regimen

One gram of sucralfate is taken four times a day on an empty stomach, 1 hour before meals, and at bedtime (see Table 42–4). The tablets should not be crushed or chewed. By taking the drug before meals, it has time to form the protective coating over the ulcer before a high level of gastric acidity is reached. It requires an acidic environment to be effective.

If a nasogastric route is required, consultation with a pharmacist is needed. Information about the amount and type of diluent needed is necessary because sucralfate is insoluble and a *bezoar* may form. If antacids are prescribed, they should not be administered within 1 hour of the sucralfate.

Laboratory Considerations

There are little or no laboratory considerations associated with sucralfate. It is a locally acting drug and therefore has little systemic effects.

Critical Thinking Process

Assessment

History of Present Illness

The reason for the hospitalization or clinic visit should be determined. The patient's perception of the problem, its onset, recent stressors, life-style changes during the previous 2 years, and any other precipitating factors should be evaluated. The health care provider should elicit information about recent fever; nausea; vomiting; burning or indigestion; tarry stools, changes in bowel patterns (constipation or diarrhea), or abdominal cramping; recent weight changes; and bleeding from other sites.

The patient should also be questioned about respiratory or cardiovascular disease, current traumas, burns, and recent intake and output values. Activities or factors that precipitate, exacerbate, or alleviate symptoms should be noted. For example, a common activity that often alleviates epigastric pain for a short time is eating.

It is common for patients with PUD to have no pain or other symptoms because gastric and duodenal mucosae do not have pain sensory fibers. The pain of gastric ulcers is located high in the epigastrium and occurs spontaneously 1 to 2 hours after meals. It is often described as a burning, gaseous pain. The pain occurs when the stomach is empty and when food has been ingested. If the ulcer has eroded through the gastric mucosa, food tends to aggravate rather than alleviate the pain. Some patients do not experience pain until a perforation or hemorrhage has occurred.

The pain of duodenal ulcers usually occurs 2 to 4 hours after meals, when the stomach is empty, and is described as burning or cramplike. The pain is located in the midepigastrium, beneath the xiphoid process. The pain is relieved by antacids and sometimes by foods that neutralize and dilute gastric acid. Some patients claim that their symptoms are worse in the spring and fall of the year, thus supporting the seasonal trend in occurrence. Ulcers located on the posterior aspect of the duodenum may manifest as back pain.

Lack of symptoms does not necessarily indicate the absence of an ulcer. Asymptomatic ulcers are common, especially in older adults and in patients who are on chronic

NSAIDs therapy. It is estimated that 30 to 50 percent of peptic ulcer complications occur in asymptomatic patients.

It is difficult to determine based on the sudden onset of symptoms whether gastric or duodenal ulcer is the cause of perforation. The clinical characteristics of perforation are the same for both types of ulcers. Perforation is characterized by a sudden and dramatic onset of severe, upper abdominal pain that quickly spreads through the abdomen. There may be shoulder pain if the spillage irritates the phrenic nerve. The abdominal muscles are rigid and boardlike, with rapid, shallow respirations. Nausea and vomiting is uncommon.

Past Health History

Information important in the assessment of a patient complaining of GI distress includes the patient's and family's past medical history, allergies, drug history, concomitant diseases or illnesses, and associated risk factors.

If the patient reports having chronic allergies, the health care provider should investigate the type of allergies, the physiologic effect on the patient, all drugs used in the treatment of allergies, and the patient's reactions to the drugs. H_2 blockers are frequently used in the management of allergies but have no effect on GI histamine receptors and the GI tract's ability to secrete gastric acid. Steroids are also used in allergy treatment and may cause GI upset.

Specific drugs may produce GI discomfort; therefore, the health history should include the patient's current and past use of medication. It should include use of over-the-counter (OTC) drugs, prescription drugs including chemotherapy and radiation, vitamin and mineral supplements, and the use of household items such as baking soda, laxatives and enemas, and items ingested based on cultural beliefs such as paint chips, specific herbs, and other items. The use of aspirin, aspirin-containing products, NSAIDs, corticosteroids, and anticoagulants place the patient at greater risk for bleeding episodes. Because many OTC drugs contain aspirin, it is not unusual for the patient to deny taking aspirin but self-medicate with products such as ALKA-SELTZER, BUFFERIN, or EXCEDRIN. Therefore, a careful history of all commonly used medications is, necessary.

Physical Exam Findings

Before the start of the physical, it is important to have the patient identify the area causing most pain and for the examiner to avoid that area until the end of the exam. It is also necessary to assess any acute or chronic signs briefly that may dictate the need for urgent interventions.

The more acute the abdominal pain, the greater the likelihood of perforation. If the pain is acute, the response needs to be immediate, without a thorough history or assessment. If the patient complains of chills or is febrile, the situation is more acute in that sepsis may be occurring. The absence of liver dullness may indicate an air viscus from perforation.

The patient's vital signs rarely provide clues to the cause of chronic abdominal pain, but close monitoring helps identify early changes in condition. Inspection of the abdomen usually does not provide significant data regarding peptic ulcer and hyperacidity. However, note whether the patient has any scars that may indicate previous abdominal surgery and whether the patient is guarding the abdomen. Alteration in bowel sounds and muscle spasms are unusual in most cases of hyperacidity and PUD. The health care provider may be able to detect air in the stomach and bowels by listening for tympanic sounds over these areas. No abdominal pain on coughing or rebound tenderness should exist unless peritoneal irritation is present.

Diagnostic Testing

Laboratory tests are normal in patients with uncomplicated PUD but are ordered to exclude ulcer complications or confounding disease states. Anemia may occur with acute blood loss from a bleeding ulcer or, less commonly, from chronic blood loss. An elevated serum amylase level in a patient with severe epigastric pain suggests ulcer penetration into the pancreas. A fasting serum gastrin level to screen for Zollinger-Ellison syndrome is obtained in some patients. H_2-antagonist therapy should be discontinued 24 hours before gastrin levels are measured.

Given the importance of *H. pylori* in the pathogenesis of PUD, testing for this organism should be performed in all patients with PUD. In patients for whom an ulcer is diagnosed by endoscopy, gastric mucosal biopsies should be obtained for both a rapid urease test and histology. The histology specimen is discarded if the urease test is positive.

A gastric analysis may also be used to determine the acidity of gastric secretions in a basal state (without stimulation) and the maximal secretory state (with stimulation of gastric secretions). Elevated levels of free hydrochloride may indicate either a duodenal or gastric ulcer or Zollinger-Ellison syndrome. It has been suggested that the reason for the low level of acid recovered by gastric analysis in patients with gastric ulcer is increased backward diffusion rather than lower production.

In patients with a history of PUD or when an ulcer is diagnosed by upper GI x-ray studies, noninvasive assessment for *H. pylori* with urease breath testing or serologic testing is usually performed. Serologic tests may be helpful in the initial diagnosis of *H. pylori* but are not reliable in documenting eradication. The FDA-approved breath test, MERETEK UBT, can be used to test for eradication but may cost about $300. To use the test, the patient drinks a liquid containing ^{13}C (which is not radioactive) and breathes into a container, which is then sent to the laboratory. In the presence of *H. pylori,* bacterial urease hydrolyzes the urea, releasing $_{13}CO_2$, which can be detected by mass spectrometer. This new test appears to be highly specific but can yield five- to 10-percent false-negative results.

Liver enzyme studies help identify liver problems, such as cirrhosis, that may complicate the treatment for PUD or hyperacidity. A serum amylase is frequently ordered if posterior penetration of the pancreas by an ulcer is suspected. Urine and stool are routinely tested for occult blood.

Any emesis from the patient should be tested for the presence of blood. The color and consistency of the emesis and obvious blood should also be noted. Vomiting may occur in response to excessive pain or may reflect intra-abdominal irritation. A coffee-ground appearance to the emesis suggests that blood has been in the stomach long enough to interact with HCL acid. On the other hand, bright red blood indicates active bleeding of the esophageal mucosal lining or cardiac portion of the stomach.

Developmental Considerations

Perinatal The perinatal patient has unique considerations. Nausea and vomiting during the first trimester is usually caused by the body's response to human chorionic gonadotrophin secreted by the implanted fetus and reactions to changes in carbohydrate metabolism (see Chapter 6). However, the perinatal patient's gastric contents become more acidic during pregnancy as a result of elevated gastrin levels produced by the placenta. During the second and third trimesters, several GI symptoms are attributable to the physical pressure from the growing uterus, as well as the smooth muscle relaxation triggered by elevated progesterone levels. Relaxation of the cardiac sphincter frequently causes heartburn as the gastric contents from the stomach move into the lower esophagus. Gastric emptying time and intestinal motility are also delayed, which lead to frequent complaints of constipation and bloating.

Pediatric In children, ulcers may occur in the stomach or duodenum and are characterized as multiple and superficial. Ulcers are frequently related to events such as trauma and burns, but they may also accompany sepsis, and respiratory, renal, or hepatic failure. Primary ulcers occur mostly in children with genetic predisposition to PUD. They are most often solitary and deep in the gastric antrum or duodenum. Stress is a major factor in the development of ulcers in children.

Considerations regarding hyperacidity and PUD in children additionally include support and reassurance of the parents. Parents are usually less concerned at the site of gastric bleeding than at esophageal bleeding, which is more red, and may not even note tarry stools that are suggestive of blood. Parents should be reassured that the situation is rarely as dramatic as it appears, and the parents' knowledge of diet, ulcers, and stress management should be assessed. Chronic abdominal pain or weight loss may be the only signs of primary PUD. The abdominal pain may be nonspecific, but epigastric pain, especially if it penetrates to the back and is relieved temporarily by eating, points to the possibility of an ulcer. The presence of anemia or occult stool blood are further indications of possible PUD.

In children, upper GI contrast studies are less effective if the children are not able to cooperate fully, and because of this, endoscopic exams of infants and children are more frequent. In most cases, the best treatment for hyperacidity and PUD in children is prevention. Children at risk should be treated prophylactically. Children with chronic ulcers should receive histamine antagonists.

Geriatric Although peptic ulcers occur most frequently at younger ages, the incidence is on the rise in older adults. Ulcer development in the older adult is an insidious process diagnosed only by upper GI x-ray studies. An older adult experiencing a major body insult, whether medical or psychological, is at risk for ulcer development, particularly if a preexisting gastritis is present. In addition to stress, diet, and genetic predisposition as causes, other factors are believed to account for the increased incidence of ulcers in the aged. Longevity, more precise diagnostic evaluation, and the fact that ulcers can be a complication of chronic airway limitation disorders also increase the incidence.

Early symptoms commonly associated with peptic ulcers may not be as evident in the older patient. Epigastric pain is not a prominent feature. More frequently, the outstanding symptoms the older adult exhibits include poorly localized pain, decreased appetite, decreased general energy level, melena, weight loss, vomiting, and anemia. Even with a perforation, symptoms may be vague. Regardless of the etiology, the consequences of GI bleeding are much more severe in the elderly.

Psychosocial Considerations

A patient's diet has a direct effect on the GI tract mucous membranes. The quality of mucosal tissue has a direct relationship to the amount of protective resistance the mucous membranes provide. Dietary choices have both a direct and indirect effect on the mucosal tissue integrity. Food choices that cause topical irritation of the membranes include alcohol and caffeine. The patient's use of salt and sugar substitutes should be noted. Fluid and fiber intake should also be noted. Anorexia and weight loss should be discussed and recorded. Poor nutrition contributes to the occurrence of peptic ulcers.

Milk and other protein foods were thought to be buffers against gastric acids; however, they also induce gastric secretions. High-calcium foods and proteins have been shown to increase gastric acid secretion more than carbohydrates and fats. Any form of fat tends to suppress gastric secretions. The sight, smell, and taste of foods triggers gastric acid production more than herbs or spices. No significant change in gastric pH occurs in the presence of herbs and spices, except with black pepper. A regular diet, with sufficient dietary fiber, has been shown to be beneficial for gastric and intestinal health.

It is also necessary to assess the patient's use of alcohol and cigarettes. Alcohol and cigarettes irritate the mucosal lining of the GI tract and may contribute to ulcer formation. It may also be helpful to assess the relationship that food and drink have to the patient. Does the patient eat alone? What percentage of income is spent on food? Is help required for meal preparation or transportation?

The stressor or stressors that exist in the patient's life and the coping mechanisms used to respond should be determined. The amount of stress necessary to affect a patient's physiology is idiosyncratic. A person's perception of the stressor and methods of handling stress are, for a large part, a product of their environment.

The effectiveness of a patient's support network may be an indicator of the level of stress a patient may be experiencing. If the patient has an effective support network and uses the network, studies have shown that the patient experiences a lower level of overall stress than a patient without a support network.

A regular employment pattern is important because it relates to the ability of the patient to meet life's needs. An individual looks to employment to satisfy any number of needs, such as the need to be productive, to provide for individual and family financial needs, to meet social needs, and more. When an imbalance exists between the patient's needs and the job's ability to meet those needs, stress results. A patient's activity level is an additional factor in the overall data. It is important to evaluate the patient's employment and activity level from the patient's perspective and the effect on the patient's state of health.

A patient's educational level has an indirect effect on the patient's health as it relates to stress and seeking medical care. If a low education level results in poverty, the consistent stress level that is present in such cases has a chronic effect on peptic ulcers and hyperacidity. Studies have shown

Case Study Peptic Ulcer Disease

Patient History

History of Present Illness	NJ, a 72-year-old female reports to the medical clinic today and reports increasing weakness, dark stools, and epigastric tenderness for past 48 hours. Has tried an occasional dose of MAALOX with relief of the epigastric pain. She presented to the dentist with an abscessed tooth 2 weeks ago. She had been taking two aspirins several times a day for the discomfort. The dentist prescribed a 14-day regimen of penicillin V to reduce the infection and propoxyphene to relieve the pain. She is finishing the last of the 14-day antibiotic regimen today. Considers self otherwise healthy.
Past Health History	Past history negative for peptic ulcer disease. She reports she does not smoke or drink alcohol, nor does she take any other drugs on a routine basis. Remainder of past medical history unremarkable.
Physical Exam	VSS. Height: 5′3″. Weight: 145 lbs. Bowel sounds present all four quadrants. No bruits noted. Epigastric area tender to light and deep palpation. No masses noted.
Diagnostic Testing	CBC and electrolytes, WNL. Stool for occult blood positive. UGI reflects small ulcer on posterior aspect of duodenal bulb. *Helicobacter pylori* organisms absent on analysis.
Developmental Considerations	NJ was worried that she would be admitted to the hospital for the abdominal pain and not be able to help her husband on the family farm.
Psychosocial Considerations	NJ is a housewife who lives on a farm with her husband of 50 years. Her husband was hospitalized 3 months ago with CHF. Although his condition improved, NJ worried about him a great deal. NJ has two grown daughters who live nearby. NJ is active in community and church affairs.
Economic Factors	NJ and her husband are self-employed with the family farm. They carry only catastrophic health insurance and have no pharmacy coverage. NJ is worried about the cost of treatment.

Variables Influencing Decision

Treatment Objectives	• Ameliorate symptoms, promote ulcer healing, prevent complications, and prevent recurrence of PUD.	
Drug Variables	***Drug Summary***	***Patient Variables***
Indications	Drug therapy with antacids or H_2 antagonist indicated for PUD. Promotes healing and decreases pain. Antibiotics appropriate to treat if have confirmation of *H. pylori* infection. Combination drug therapy does not appear to be effective in prevention of PUD recurrence. These factors will become a decision point.	NJ diagnosed with small peptic ulcer. *H. pylori* organisms are absent.
Pharmacodynamics	Antacids neutralize gastric acid. H_2 antagonist decreases acid secretion. Antibiotics manage *H. pylori* infection.	Antacids are useful if patient experiences relief with their use. This will become a decision point.
Adverse Effects/ Contraindications	Few adverse effects with PRN antacids and H_2 antagonists. Confusion most common adverse effects of cimetidine.	PRN antacid has few adverse effects for NJ. Potential for adverse effects to H_2 antagonist is small. NJ does not have a history of confusion.
Pharmacokinetics	Most H_2 antagonists and many antibiotics require dosage reduction in patients with renal impairment and the elderly. All H_2 antagonists have equivalent efficacy.	NJ has intake renal function but does have age-related changes in renal and hepatic function. This will be a decision point.

Case Study Peptic Ulcer Disease—cont'd

Drug Variables	*Drug Summary*	*Patient Variables*
Dosage Regimen	PRN antacids simple regimen to manage. H_2 antagonist BID will help to manage daytime ulcer pain. Once daytime pain is relieved, can take H_2 at HS.	NJ requests the most simple regimen possible due to responsibilities and schedule of farm activities.
Lab Considerations	Follow-up of stool for occult bloods necessary as well as CBC. Baseline renal function testing performed before starting therapy. May need repeat UGI at later date.	NJ understands importance of follow-up testing and is able to return for same. Baseline renal function tests desirable due to changes of aging.
Cost Index*	Antacid: 1 Cimetidine: 5 Omeprazole: 5	NJ understands importance of compliance but is concerned about cost of drugs. This will become a decision point.

Summary of Decision Points

- Antibiotic therapy can be delayed until after the first relapse because there is no evidence of *H. pylori* at this time.
- Combination drug therapy does not appear to be effective in preventing the recurrence of PUD.
- Cimetidine is the initial drug of choice for PUD. It has few adverse effects, can be taken once daily, and is less expensive than other H_2 antagonists.
- Antacids are useful if NJ experiences relief with their use.
- The simplest regimen will promote better long-term compliance with treatment plan.
- Cimetidine is cheaper than other H_2 antagonists, although it may be expensive on a long-term basis. Omeprazole the most expensive.

DRUGS TO BE USED

- Antacid of choice PRN.
- Cimetidine 800 mg pō BID × 6 weeks.

*Cost Index:
1 = $ < 30/mo.
2 = $ 30–40/mo.
3 = $ 40–50/mo.
4 = $ 50–60/mo.
5 = $ > 60/mo.

AWP of 353 mL of magnesium/aluminum hydroxide combination is approximately $4.
AWP of 100, 400 mg tablets of cimetidine is approximately $100.
AWP of 100, 20 mg tablets of omeprazole is approximately $350.

that patients with lower educational levels are less informed regarding the benefits of medical care, fewer are covered by health insurance, and are less likely to be compliant with follow-up care.

The patient's past experiences with the health care system should be evaluated because it affects patient care management. The point at which the patient sought medical care, the patient's level of trust in health care providers, the degree of compliance with the long-term and short-term plan of care, and the integration of life-style changes into the patient's life are all-important. Awareness of the patient's past experiences may permit a more appropriate plan of care that will provide maximum benefit for the patient (see Case Study—Peptic Ulcer Disease).

Analysis and Management

Treatment Objectives

The primary objective in the treatment of hyperacidity disorders and PUD is to ameliorate symptoms and promote healing. Complications should be prevented, and the potential for recurrence of PUD should be minimized when possible.

Treatment Options

Drug Variables

In general, duodenal ulcers are treated with night-time acid suppression, whereas gastric ulcers and GERD usually require 24-hour acid suppression. With this principle in mind, pharmacotherapeutic options available include the nonsystemic antacids, H_2 antagonists, proton pump inhibitors, prostaglandin, or a cytoprotective drug. A combination of these agents may be used in some circumstances.

To lessen the recurrence of PUD associated with *H. pylori* infection, treatment regimens must involve elimination of the organism. Recurrence of duodenal ulceration after healing can be as high as 80 percent within 1 year when elimination of *H. pylori* is not part of treatment. The recurrence rate is less than 5 percent when *H. pylori* is eradicated. If eradication of the organism is not part of the treatment, recurrence can still be reduced by maintenance doses of acid secretion inhibitors.

At the present time, there are two primary types of treatment regimens for *H. pylori*–associated PUD. Treatment may consist of antibiotics and bismuth subsalicylate or antibiotics combined with either a proton pump inhibitor or an H_2 antagonist. The drug combinations, duration of therapy, and doses are emerging questions (see Treatment Options for PUD). The effectiveness of different drug combinations in eradicating *H. pylori* depends on the antibacterial activity of the drugs and the resistance patterns of the organisms, the patient's history of exposure to antibiotics, and the patient's ability to tolerate the drug's adverse effects and to take a large number of pills. For many patients, better tolerated, shorter treatment regimens that require fewer pills per day may prove to be more effective than more complicated regimens with higher eradication rates.

The classic triple therapy includes 1 week of bismuth, metronidazole, and either tetracycline or amoxicillin. This regimen eliminates *H. pylori* in 90 percent of patients and heals the ulcers in virtually all patients. However, this regimen contributes to noncompliance because of the adverse effects of the drugs. Furthermore, there is a chance for rapid development of resistance to clarithromycin and metronidazole, and there is the undesirable disulfiram-like reaction when alcohol is taken concurrently with metronidazole. Bacterial resistance rarely occurs to tetracycline and not at all to amoxicillin. These adjunct drugs are discussed in Chapters 24 and 25. Bismuth is discussed further in Chapter 43.

Both metronidazole and tetracycline cause mild GI upset. Amoxicillin may cause diarrhea. Bismuth subsalicylate temporarily turns the tongue and stool black, and can cause tinnitus. Clarithromycin can also cause GI symptoms, although they are less frequent than those seen with metronidazole or tetracycline. Clarithromycin can cause taste disturbances that some patients find intolerable.

In contrast, dual therapy includes omeprazole given with a single antibiotic, usually either clarithromycin or amoxicillin. However, omeprazole has also been used with both antibiotics or as quadruple therapy with both antibiotics plus metronidazole. It has been suggested that omeprazole plus a single antibiotic are as effective as triple drug therapy.

Otherwise healthy patients with a classic history of uncomplicated GERD can be treated empirically, employing step 1 and 2 measures (see Stepwise Progression for Treatment of Esophageal Reflux). In many cases, these measures will suffice. If the patient fails to respond or if the reflux is complicated by dysphagia, weight loss, anemia, or if the stool tests positive for occult bleeding, then, a more comprehensive diagnostic evaluation is indicated.

The choice of antacid for uncomplicated hyperacidity problems depends on characteristics of both the patient and

TREATMENT OPTIONS FOR PEPTIC ULCER DISEASE

Active* Helicobacter pylori*–Associated Ulcer (Use one of the following four regimens)*

Omeprazole 20 mg po BID × 7 days and
metronidazole 500 mg po BID and
clarithromycin 500 mg po BID

Omeprazole 20 mg po BID × 7 days and
amoxicillin 1 g po BID and
clarithromycin 500 mg po BID

Omeprazole 20 mg po BID × 7 days and
amoxicillin 1 g po BID and
metronidazole 500 mg po BID

Omeprazole 20 mg po BID × 7 days plus
bismuth subsalicylate 2 tablets po QID plus
tetracycline 500 mg po QID plus
metronidazole 250 mg po QID

Then continue treatment for next 4 to 8 weeks with proton pump inhibitor or H_2 antagonist to promote ulcer healing†

Uncomplicated, Active, Duodenal Ulcer not Attributed to* Helicobacter pylori *infection (Use one of the following three regimens)

Omeprazole 20 mg, or lansoprazole 15 mg po once daily × 4 weeks

Cimetidine 800 mg, or ranitidine 300 mg, or nizatidine 300 mg, or famotidine 20 mg po QD at HS × 6 weeks

Sucralfate 1 g po QID

***Uncomplicated, Active, Gastric Ulcer not Attributed to* Helicobacter pylori** (Use one of the following two regimens)

Omeprazole 20 mg po BID or lansoprazole 30 mg po QD × 6 to 8 weeks

Cimetidine 400 mg, or ranitidine 150 mg, or nizatidine 150 mg, or famotidine 20 mg po BID × 8 to 12 weeks

Prevention of NSAID-Induced Ulcers (Use one of the following two regimens)‡

Misoprostol 100 to 200 mcg po QID

Proton pump inhibitor po BID (for high-risk patients intolerant of misoprostol)

Chronic Maintenance Therapy§

Cimetidine 400 to 800 mg, or ranitidine 150 to 300 mg, or nizatidine 150 to 300 mg, or famotidine 20 to 40 mg po at HS

*Give omeprazole before meals and the antibiotics and bismuth with meals. Avoid metronidazole-based treatment regimens in areas of known metronidazole resistance or in patients who have failed a course of treatment that included metronidazole. The choice among the regimens should be based on convenience, potential for toxicity, and cost.

†All H_2 antagonists have equivalent efficacy and toxicity. If the patient is taking other drugs that interact with cimetidine, ranitidine, famotidine, or nizatidine may be chosen, whichever is the least expensive. All four of these drugs are available over the counter in half the prescription dosage for the treatment of heartburn.

‡Prophylaxis for NSAID-induced ulcer is reserved for high-risk patients (i.e., prior ulcer disease or ulcer complications, use of corticosteroids or anticoagulants, patients older than age 70).

§Chronic maintenance therapy is indicated in patients with recurrent ulcers who are *H. pylori* negative or in whom attempts at elimination of the organism have failed, and in patients with a history of ulcer complications.

STEPWISE PROGRESSION FOR TREATMENT OF ESOPHAGEAL REFLUX

Step 1

- Avoid foods high in fat or carbohydrates (chocolate can be particularly problematic because it is high in both elements)
- Lose weight if obese
- Avoid large meals near bedtime or before exercise
- Elevate the head of the bed with 6-inch blocks under the bedposts (pillows are not sufficient for elevation)
- When possible, avoid drugs that decrease lower esophageal sphincter tone (e.g., theophylline, calcium channel blockers, meperidine, anticholinergics)
- When possible, avoid drugs that may injure esophageal mucosa (e.g., tetracycline, wax matrix potassium supplements, NSAIDs)
- Avoid caffeine, coffee, and cigarettes
- Administer antacids after meals and at bedtime

Step 2

- Add an oral H_2 antagonist

Step 3

- Add omeprazole but limit therapy to no more than 3 to 6 months (drug of choice for erosive esophagitis)

Step 4

- Add metoclopramide, cisapride, or bethanechol, or consider antireflux surgery (e.g., fundoplication, crural tightening) for incapacitating refractory disease

drug. The most commonly used antacids are combinations of aluminum hydroxide and magnesium hydroxide. Although the basic anions in antacids include carbonate, bicarbonate, citrate, phosphate, or trisilicate, the hydroxide formulation is most commonly used. Aluminum-based antacids are used by patients with chronic renal failure and hyperphosphatemia to decrease the absorption of phosphates contained in food products.

As a general rule, single compound antacids are preferable to combinations. However, combination antacids have several advantages over single-ingredient products. Combining an antacid with a laxative effect (e.g., magnesium hydroxide) with one having a constipating effect (e.g., aluminum hydroxide) tends to prevent or reduce the incidence of diarrhea or constipation. Furthermore, by combining rapid-acting and slow-acting formulations, antacids prolong the neutralization of gastric acid. Combinations usually also permit smaller dosages of individual ingredients, thereby preventing or reducing adverse effects.

Antacid suspensions usually act more rapidly than chewable tablets; however, suspensions have not proved to be more effective in neutralizing gastric acid. Chewable tablets may be more convenient in some circumstances but should be thoroughly chewed in order to increase the surface area of drug available to neutralize gastric acid.

Some antacids contain ingredients such as simethicone. Simethicone does not affect gastric acidity but instead is an antiflatulent. It is reported to decrease the surface tension of gas bubbles, thereby reducing GI distention and abdominal discomfort. Simethicone does not, however, prevent the formation of gas. Simethicone has an immediate onset of action with antiflatulent effects lasting up to 3 hours. There is no systemic absorption, and the drug is eliminated unchanged in feces.

Patient Variables

Prevention of PUD may be primary, secondary, or tertiary. For persons at high risk for the development of PUD, identification of contributory factors should be carried out. Once those factors have been identified, the person can take primary preventative action. Smoking, although not a primary cause of PUD or of hyperacidity, has an irritating effect on the mucosa, increases gastric motility, and delays mucosal healing. The combination of inadequate rest and smoking accelerates ulcer development.

Secondary prevention involves the detection and treatment of the disease early in its course. For example, the use of aspirin and NSAIDs should be discontinued when possible. Interventions are aimed at detecting problems early in their course so that prompt treatment can forestall the serious consequences of advanced disease. When irritating drugs must be continued, enteric-coated or highly buffered preparations are more suitable.

Tertiary prevention of PUD is time intensive. The healing and subsequent cure of PUD requires many weeks of therapy. Although the pain may be alleviated in less than a week, healing is much slower. Complete healing may take four weeks to as many as 12 weeks depending on ulcer size and treatment regimen.

Because recurrence of PUD is common, interruption or discontinuation of therapy can have detrimental results. The patient may stop the antacid when they sense the ulcers have healed, or if therapy is continued, it is done so intermittently based on reappearance of symptoms. Decisions regarding the most appropriate drug therapy should be made in light of the total patient, and in most cases, more than one approach is combined to provide the patient maximum healing capability in the shortest time period.

Intervention

Administration

It is important that PUD and hyperacidity drug therapies be administered on time, for the full duration of therapy, and that other medications be administered at other times.

When using tablet forms of antacids, a full glass of water should follow ingestion of the tablets. Furthermore, in most cases, antacids decrease the absorption of drugs taken concurrently. Therefore, it is recommended that the ingestion of other drugs be separated by at least 1 hour. To ensure healing, antacids, when used to treat PUD, should be continued for 4 to 8 weeks after all symptoms have disappeared. The healing period is variable, depending upon the depth, number, and location of ulcers. Some antacids contain large amounts of sodium and should be used cautiously in patients on sodium restriction.

The minimal acceptable pH with antacid therapy is 3.5. For patients with acute disease, the goal may be a pH of 7 (neutral). To titrate therapy adequately, gastric pH is first measured, and the results recorded. The antacid is then administered through the nasogastric tube, the tube clamped for 15 minutes, and the pH of gastric secretions retested. If the pH is below 7, a comparable amount of antacid may again be instilled, and the process repeated until a neutral pH is attained. Antacids are then administered on a regular or intermittent basis to maintain a neutral pH.

Education

The successful management of hyperacidity and PUD depends on the patient's compliance with diet, drugs, and postural measures. A thorough explanation of the mechanisms of reflux and its aggravating factors help provide a rational basis for patient action. The patient and family members, as appropriate, should be taught the name of the drug, the dose, purpose for taking the drug, benefits anticipated from therapy, and the time period over which pharmacotherapy is anticipated. The use of other potentially ulcerogenic drugs should be avoided.

Patients should be helped to realize that no single measure will alleviate the discomfort of reflux, but when all of the interventions are performed together, relief is extremely likely. Nondrug measures, such as relaxation and stress management help prevent or minimize symptoms and are often as effective as drugs when they are used concurrently. There is no practical way to avoid psychological stress because it is a part of everyday life, but it is possible to reduce the stress.

Diet therapy has little role in the prevention or treatment of hyperacidity and PUD. Although many patients consider milk an alkali, it has little effect on the pH of gastric secretions. In addition, the calcium and protein content of dairy products stimulate gastric acid secretion. A treatment regimen that includes the frequent ingestion of dairy products may actually aggravate PUD. Avoiding highly spiced foods, gas-forming foods and caffeine-containing beverages may help relieve symptoms and promote healing. Smoking should also be avoided.

For patients bothered by diarrhea or constipation as a result of antacid use, suggesting the use of a combination antacid product may help. A high-fiber diet and consuming 2000 to 3000 mL of fluid daily also help in preventing constipation.

Patients must be encouraged to comply with therapy and continue with follow-up care for at least 1 year. The patient and family should also be instructed that any change in symptoms or the appearance of blood, tarry stools, or coffee-ground emesis signals the need to contact the health care provider. It is also critical that the patient be instructed to take the drug for the full duration of therapy. Halting therapy when symptoms improve is a major cause for exacerbation of symptoms.

Evaluation

As with all patient care, perceived susceptibility to disease and its seriousness influences treatment outcomes. The need for long-term drug regimens should raise questions regarding the patient's commitment to the plan of care. It is necessary to work with the patient and family members, as appropriate, to solicit support and cooperation from all parties. A plan that is relevant to the patient increases the level of compliance.

The primary determination of pharmacotherapeutic effectiveness is in the healing of peptic ulcers and a reduction in hyperacidity. In the case of most drugs used for PUD and hyperacidity, the effectiveness is demonstrated by the relief of gastric pain and irritation and ulcer healing.

The patient and family should be able to articulate an understanding of the treatment regimen and demonstrate an acceptable degree of compliance. In evaluating the patient's response to the regimen, the health care provider would expect to find fewer complaints of abdominal pain and discomfort, and few or no complaints of adverse drug effects.

For the patient who is of child-bearing age, the patient should be knowledgeable about contraceptives and should select an appropriate form of contraception to use during misoprostol therapy.

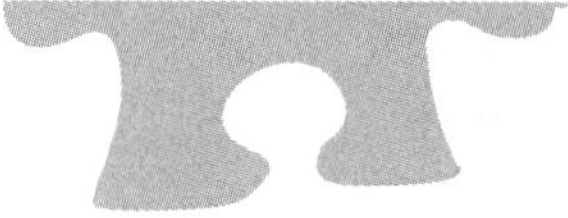

SUMMARY

- PUD is characterized by circumscribed areas of mucosal inflammation and ulceration caused by excessive secretion of gastric acid, disruption of the protective mucosal barrier, or both. *H. pylori* has been identified as an etiologic factor in PUD in both adults and children.
- Risk factors associated with PUD and hyperacidity include smoking, the use of NSAIDs, corticosteroids, and other gastric irritants.
- Duodenal ulcers are the most common and are associated with increased numbers of parietal cells (acid secreting), the presence of *H. pylori* organisms, and elevated gastrin levels.
- Gastric ulcers generally develop in the antrum of the stomach and tend to become chronic. Gastric secretions may be increased or decreased, with pain occurring after eating. *H. pylori* is usually not present.
- Stress ulcerations develop suddenly after severe illness, neural injury, or trauma and are related to overstimulation of the vagal nuclei. Ulceration follows mucosal damage related to decreased blood flow to the gastric mucosa.
- Complications associated with PUD and hyperacidity include intractability, perforation, hemorrhage, and gastric outlet obstruction.
- A history of recurrent epigastric discomfort, ½ to 1 hour after meals and early in the morning hours is typical. The discomfort is relieved with food or antacids. Nausea may also be present. A history of recurrent vomiting, hematemesis, or melena in patients with a history of recurrent epigastric discomfort suggests complications of PUD.
- Lack of symptoms does not necessarily indicate the absence of an ulcer.
- The primary objective in the treatment of hyperacidity and PUD is to ameliorate symptoms and promote healing.
- In general, duodenal ulcers are treated with night-time acid suppression, whereas gastric ulcers and GERD usually require 24-hour acid suppression.
- Pharmacotherapeutic treatment of PUD and hyperacidity include antacids, H_2 antagonists, proton pump inhibitors, prostaglandin, and a cytoprotective agent.
- Antacids raise the pH of gastric secretions to a level less acidic or neutral. They do not coat the stomach lining.
- H_2 antagonists inhibit the action of histamine at the H_2 receptors, thus decreasing gastric acid secretion and reducing total pepsin output.

- Proton pump inhibitors bind with the H^+-K^+-ATPase enzyme to prevent the release of gastric acid into the stomach lumen.
- The prostaglandin misoprostol inhibits gastric acid secretion (antisecretory effect) and increases bicarbonate and mucus production (cytoprotective effect).
- The cytoprotective agent sucralfate acts locally, binding to the ulcer site and forming a physical protective barrier.
- Management strategies include discontinuation of smoking, as well as reduction and discontinuation of NSAIDs.
- The primary determination of pharmacotherapeutic effectiveness is in the healing of peptic ulcers and a reduction in hyperacidity. Drug effectiveness is demonstrated by the relief of gastric pain and irritation, and ulcer healing.

BIBLIOGRAPHY

Abramowicz, M. (Ed.). (1997). Drugs for treatment of peptic ulcers. *The Medical Letter on Drugs and Therapeutics,* 39(991), 1–4.

Abramowicz, M. (Ed.). (1996). *Medical letter handbook of adverse drug reactions.* New Rochelle, NY: The Medical Letter.

Brooks, W. (1992). Short and long term management of peptic ulcer disease: Current role of H_2 antagonists. *Hepatogastroenterology,* 39(Suppl 1), 47–52.

Clearfield, H. (1992). Management of NSAID-induced ulcer disease. *American Family Physician,* 45(1), 255–258.

Freston, M., and Freston, J. (1990). Peptic ulcer in the elderly: Unique features and management. *Geriatrics,* 45(1), 39–42.

Forbes, G., Glaser, M., and Cullen, D. (1994). Duodenal ulcer treated with *Helicobacter pylori* eradication: Seven year follow-up. *Lancet,* 343(8892), 258–291.

Goroll, A., May, L., and Mulley, A. (1995). *Primary care medicine: Office evaluation and management of the adult patient.* Philadelphia: J.B. Lippincott Company.

Gugler, R., and Allgayer, H. (1990). Effects of antacids on the clinical pharmacokinetics of drugs: An update. *Clinical Pharmacokinetics,* 18, 210–219.

Hentschel, E. (1993). Effect of ranitidine and amoxicillin plus metronidazole on the eradication of *Helicobacter pylori* and the recurrence of duodenal ulcer. *New England Journal of Medicine,* 328(5), 308–312.

Hixon, L., Kelley, C., and Jones, W. (1992). Current trends in the pharmacotherapy of peptic ulcer disease. *Archives of Internal Medicine,* 152(4), 726–732.

Holland, E., and Taylor, A. (1991). Practical management of stress-related gastric ulcers. *Journal of Family Practice,* 33(6), 625–632.

Hosking, S., Lang, T., and Chung, S. (1994). Duodenal ulcer healing by eradication of *Helicobacter pylori* without antacid treatment: Randomized controlled trial. *Lancet,* 343(8896), 508–510.

Hui, W., Lam, S., and Lok, A. (1992). Maintenance therapy for duodenal ulcer: A randomized controlled comparison of seven forms of treatment. *American Journal of Medicine,* 92, 265–274.

Jess, K. (1993). Acute abdominal pain: Revealing the source. *Nursing '93,* 23(9), 34–41.

Karim, A. Rozek, L., Smith, M., et al. (1989). Effects of food and antacid on oral absorption of misoprostol, a synthetic prostaglandin E-1 analog. *Journal of Clinical Pharmacology,* 29(5), 439–443.

Katz, K., and Hollander, D. (1992). Practical pharmacology and cost-effective management for peptic ulcer disease. *American Journal of Surgery,* 163(3), 349–359.

Labaenz, J., Gyenes, E., and Ruhl, G. (1993). Omeprazole plus amoxicillin: Efficiency of various treatment regimens to eradicate *Helicobacter pylori. American Journal of Gastroenterology,* 88(4), 491–495.

Langman, M., Weil, J., and Wainwright, T. (1994). Risks of bleeding in peptic ulcers associated with individual non-steroidal anti-inflammatory drugs. *Lancet,* 343(8905), 1075–1079.

McCarthy, D. (1991). Acid peptic disease in the elderly. *Clinical Geriatric Medicine,* 7(2), 231–254.

McCarthy, D. (1991). Sucralfate. *New England Journal of Medicine,* 325(14), 1017–1025.

McQuaid, K., and Isenberg, J. (1992). Medical therapy of peptic ulcer disease. *Surgical Clinics of North America,* 72(2), 285–316.

Morley, J. (1990). Anorexia in older patients: Its meaning and management. *Geriatrics,* 45(12), 59–62.

Tierney, L, McPhee, S., and Papadakis, M. (Eds.). (1997). *Current medical diagnosis and treatment* (36th ed.). Stamford, CT: Appleton and Lange.

Tryba, M. (1991). Sucralfate versus antacids H_2 antagonists for stress ulcer prophylaxis: A meta-analysis of efficacy and pneumonia rate. *Critical Care Medicine,* 19, 942–949.

Walsh, J., and Preston, W., (1995). The treatment of *Helicobacter pylori* infection in the management of peptic ulcer disease. *New England Journal of Medicine,* 333, 984–991.

43 Laxatives and Antidiarrheal Drugs

Normal physiologic functions of the lower gastrointestinal (GI) tract include motility, absorption, and secretion. Alterations in one or more of these functions result in constipation or diarrhea. Although various drugs can be used for symptomatic relief, drug therapy does not correct the underlying cause and, in some cases, may contribute to the problem. This chapter focuses on drugs used to prevent or alleviate constipation and diarrhea.

BOWEL FUNCTION

The primary function of the colon is to absorb water, sodium, and other minerals. By removing 90 percent of the fluid, the colon converts 1000 to 2000 mL of isotonic chyme from the ileum to about 150 g of semisolid stool each day. In general, the first remnants of a meal reach the hepatic flexure in 6 hours, the splenic flexure in 9 hours, and the pelvic colon in 12 hours. Transport is much slower from the pelvic colon to the anus. As much as 25 percent of the meal's residue may still be in the rectum 72 hours later.

CONSTIPATION

Epidemiology and Etiology

Constipation is defined as infrequent defecation, a hardening or reduced caliber of stool, a sensation of incomplete evacuation, and the need to strain with bowel movements. Defecation less than three times a week is a commonly accepted criterion for the diagnosis of constipation. In bowel-conscious America, the amount of misinformation and inordinate apprehension about constipation probably exceeds that of any other health concern. Approximately four million people in the United States have constipation on a frequent basis. This figure corresponds to a prevalence of 2 percent, making constipation the most frequent GI problem seen in ambulatory care settings. The prevalence is highest in the southern United States and is reported more often by patients over age 65. In this age group, the problem is more often a result of physical inactivity rather than intrinsic bowel changes related to aging.

Constipation is three times more common in women than in men. Nonwhite patients report constipation 1.3 times more often than white patients. Patients from low income families report constipation more often than patients from higher income families. Furthermore, it is estimated that 900 people die each year in the United States from diseases associated with constipation.

Constipation of recent onset is usually related to changes in life-style or health status. Inadequate fluids or fiber in the diet is the most common cause of chronic constipation. Dietary changes such as restrictive weight loss diets, dietary changes related to aging, and poor dentition are other culprits. In contrast, constipation of long duration indicates a functional etiology (i.e., not responding to the urge to defecate) or chronic organic disease. Busy schedules with no established time for regular elimination contributes to constipation. Disorders that may originally present as constipation include hypothyroidism, diabetes mellitus, hypokalemia, hypercalcemia, and neurologic disorders. In some instances, constipation may result from drug-induced causes (see Drugs Likely to Cause Constipation).

Pathophysiology

The fundamental mechanism of constipation involves the decreased transit time of stool through the colon, along with increased reabsorption of fluid. Regardless of the cause of constipation, prolonged retention of stool in the rectum results in drying because of the reabsorption of water. The harder and drier the stool, the more difficult it is to expel.

Straining to have a stool (called the *Valsalva maneuver*) causes changes in intrathoracic pressure, leading to reduced coronary, cerebral, and peripheral circulation. Other potential problems with straining include the development of hernias and worsening symptoms of gastroesophageal reflux. Transient ischemic attacks and syncopal episodes have been noted in patients with cerebrovascular disease or deficient baroreceptor reflexes.

PHARMACOTHERAPEUTIC OPTIONS

Drugs used for the symptomatic relief of constipation are often classified as laxatives, cathartics, or purgatives. The terms are frequently used interchangeably, although not necessarily accurately. *Laxatives* loosen the bowel contents and encourage evacuation of soft stool. *Cathartics* and *purgatives* promote intense elimination activity and loss of water. The same drug can produce any of the three effects depending on the dosage and the patient's sensitivity to the drug.

Stimulant Laxatives

- ❒ Bisacodyl (DULCAGEN, DULCOLAX, FLEET LAXATIVE)
- ❒ Castor oil (NEOLOID)
- ❒ Cascara sagrada
- ❒ Casanthranol
- ❒ Phenolphthalein (ALOPHEN PILLS, ESPOTABS, EVAC-U-GEN, EVAL-U-LAX, EX-LAX, FEEN-A-MINT, MEDILAX, MODANE, PHENOLAX)
- ❒ Senna (BLACK-DRAUGHT, FLETCHER'S CASTORIA, SENEXON, SENOKOT, SENOLAX)

DRUGS LIKELY TO CAUSE CONSTIPATION

Analgesics (opioids and NSAIDs)
Aluminum-containing antacids
Anticholinergic drugs
Antidiarrheal drugs
Antiparkinson drugs
Atropine
Barium sulfate
Beta blockers
Calcium channel blockers
Cation exchange resins
Cimetidine
Clonidine
Diuretics
Ganglionic blocking drugs
Heavy metals (especially lead)
Iron supplements
MAO inhibitor antidepressants
Muscle relaxants
Osmotic laxatives (habitual use)
Stimulant laxatives (habitual use)
Phenothiazines
Phenylephrine
Phenylpropanolamine
Pseudoephedrine
Ranitidine
Sucralfate
Terbutaline
Trazodone
Tricyclic antidepressants

MAO, Monoamine oxidase; NSAIDs, nonsteroidal anti-inflammatory drugs.

Indications

Stimulant laxatives are used in the treatment of constipation associated with prolonged bedrest, constipating drugs, slowed transit times, and irritable bowel syndrome. They can also be used to evacuate the bowel before radiologic studies or surgery. Stimulants are included as part of a bowel regimen for patients with spinal cord injuries or neurologic disorders. Castor oil is not used as often today as in the past owing to its many adverse effects.

Pharmacodynamics

Stimulant laxatives are obtained from the roots, bark, and seed pods of a number of plants. They act on the intestinal wall of the small bowel and colon to increase the amount of fluid and electrolytes within the intestinal lumen. Additionally, they cause the release of prostaglandins and produce an increase in cyclic adenosine monophosphate (cAMP) concentration. This increase in cAMP concentration, in turn, increases the secretion of electrolytes and contributes to the cathartic effect.

Specifically, bisacodyl, phenolphthalein, cascara, and senna stimulate the submucosal and mesenteric plexus to produce semisoft or soft formed stool. Castor oil combines with lipase in the small bowel to produce ricinoleic acid (the active component of castor oil), which, in turn, stimulates the smooth muscle of the small bowel. Castor oil also draws more water into the bowel, producing a more watery stool. Cascara produces propulsive movements of the colon by direct chemical irritation.

Adverse Effects and Contraindications

The most common adverse effects of stimulant laxatives include mild cramping, nausea, vomiting, diarrhea, and even dehydration in susceptible individuals. Continued use of these laxatives produces irritable bowel syndrome–like diarrhea that can be severe enough to cause fluid and electrolyte imbalances. Stimulant laxatives can cause proctitis in males. Hypokalemia, tetany, and protein-losing enteropathy also occur with long-term use of stimulant laxatives. Phenolphthalein can cause a mild to severe skin rash or a severe systemic allergic reaction in susceptible individuals.

Stimulant laxatives are contraindicated in patients with hypersensitivity, abdominal pain of unknown cause (especially when associated with fever), rectal fissures, and ulcerated hemorrhoids. Castor oil is contraindicated in the presence of infestation of fat-soluble worms, during pregnancy, and in breastfeeding mothers. The aromatic fluid extract formulation of cascara sagrada contains alcohol and should be avoided in patients with known intolerance to alcohol. Excessive or prolonged use of stimulant laxatives may lead to dependence.

Pharmacokinetics

The pharmacokinetics of stimulant laxatives are identified in Table 43–1. Their onset times vary from less than 15 minutes for bisacodyl suppositories to more than 24 hours for senna preparations. Bisacodyl is minimally absorbed (less than 5 percent) following oral administration. Small amounts of bisacodyl metabolites are found in breast milk. Biotransformation takes place in the liver. The half-life of bisacodyl is unknown, although evacuation takes place in 6 to 12 hours.

Cascara is minimally absorbed when it is taken orally. It is converted to an active metabolite in the colon. Cascara circulates throughout the body to be eliminated in the bile, urine, saliva, colonic mucosa, and in breast milk. Evacuation of the bowel occurs in 6 to 10 hours.

Fifteen percent of phenolphthalein is absorbed with an onset of action in 6 to 10 hours. It is secreted in the bile, with a duration of action of 3 to 4 days. Phenolphthalein produces semisoft stools in 6 to 12 hours.

Senna is also minimally absorbed following oral administration. Its distribution, biotransformation, elimination, and half-life are unknown. It produces soft, formed stools in 1 to 3 days.

Drug-Drug Interactions

Stimulant laxatives decrease the absorption of other orally administered drugs because of increased motility and decreased transit times (Table 43–2). The enteric coating of bisacodyl and phenolphthalein is prematurely removed if it is taken concurrently with antacids or within 1 hour of consuming dairy products.

Cascara is compounded with magnesium oxide (to make it less bitter), flavoring agents, sweeteners, and alcohol (18 percent). Patients who are taking disulfiram for control of al-

TABLE 43–1 PHARMACOKINETICS OF SELECTED LAXATIVES

Drug	Route	Onset	Evacuation	Site	Stool Type
Stimulant Laxatives					
Bisacodyl	po	6–10 hr	6–12 hr	C	SS
	PR	15–60 min	15–60 min	C	SS
Castor oil	po	2–6 hr	2–3 hr	SB	W
Cascara sagrada	po	6–10 hr	6–10 hr	C	SS
Phenolphthalein	po	6–10 hr	6–12 hr	C	SS
Senna	po	6–24 hr	1–3 days	SB-C	SF
Stool Softeners					
Docusate calcium	po	24 hr–5 days	3–5 days	SB-C	SF
Docusate potassium	po	24–72 hr	3–5 days	SB-C	SF
Docusate sodium	po	24–72 hr	3–5 days	SB-C	SF
	PR	2–15 min	Hours	C	SF
Bulk-Forming Laxatives					
Psyllium	po	12 hr	2–3 days	SB-C	SF
Polycarbophil	po	12 hr	2–3 days	SB-C	SF
Methylcellulose	po	12 hr	2–3 days	SB-C	SF
Osmotic Laxatives					
Magnesium sulfate	po	3–6 hr	3–6 hr	SB-C	W
Magnesium hydroxide	po	0.5–3 hr	3–6 hr	SB-C	W
Magnesium citrate	po	0.5–3 hr	3–6 hr	SB-C	W
Sodium phosphate and	po	0.5–3 hr	3–6 hr	C	W
sodium biphosphate	PR	2–15 min	<60 min	C	W
Polyethylene glycol electrolyte solution	po	30–60 min	60 min	SB-C	W
Lubricant Laxatives					
Mineral oil	po/PR	6–8 hr	6–8 hr	C	SS
Miscellaneous Laxatives					
Glycerine	PR	0.25–5 hr	15–30 min	C	SF
Lactulose	po	24–48 hr	1–3 days	C	SF

PR, Per rectum (i.e., suppository); SB, small bowel; C, colon; SS, semisoft stool in 6–12 hr; W, watery stool in 2–6 hr; SF, soft formed stool in 1–3 days; UK, unknown.

coholism should not use cascara because of the risk of a disulfiram-like reaction.

Dosage Regimen

The dosage regimen for stimulant laxatives varies with the specific drug formulation, but in general, they are administered at bedtime for evacuation 6 to 12 hours later (see Table 43–3). For more rapid results, oral formulations may be administered on an empty stomach with a full glass of water. Suppository formulations may cause proctitis and rectal burning. If castor oil is prescribed, it should be taken early in the day and mixed with a carbonated beverage or fruit juice to increase palatability.

Stool Softeners

- ❒ Docusate calcium (PRO-CAL-SOF, SURFAK)
- ❒ Docusate potassium (DIOCTO-K)
- ❒ Docusate sodium (COLACE, CORRECTOL EXTRA GENTLE, DIALOSE, MODANE, many others)

Indications

Orally administered stool softeners are used to prevent constipation in patients who should avoid straining such as patients with a myocardial infarction or those who have had rectal surgery. When administered as an enema, they help soften fecal impactions.

Pharmacodynamics

Stool softeners incorporate water and lipids into the stool, producing an emollient action that reduces surface tension. The drugs act primarily in the jejunum and colon. By incorporating water into the stool, a softer fecal mass results (Fig. 43–1).

Adverse Effects and Contraindications

The adverse effects of orally administered stool softeners include throat irritation, mild cramps, and rashes. Diarrhea is certainly a possibility with excessive use.

Stool softeners are contraindicated in patients with hypersensitivity, abdominal pain, nausea or vomiting, especially if the constipation is associated with fever or other signs of an acute abdomen. Excessive or prolonged use of stool softeners may lead to dependency. Stool softeners are not used if prompt results are desired.

Pharmacokinetics

Small amounts of docusate may be absorbed from the small bowel following oral administration. The extent of absorption from the rectum is unknown. The onset time of

TABLE 43–2 DRUG-DRUG INTERACTIONS OF SELECTED LAXATIVES AND ANTIDIARRHEAL DRUGS

Drug	Interactive Drugs	Interaction
Stimulant/Contact Laxatives		
Bisacodyl	Antacids	Removes enteric coating of bisacodyl
Phenolphthalein		
Cascara	Disulfiram	Disulfiram-like reaction
Bulk-Forming Laxatives		
Psyllium	Cardiac glycosides	Absorption of interactive drug may be decreased
Polycarbophil	Salicylates	
	Tetracycline	
	Warfarin	
Osmotic Laxatives		
Magnesium salts	Neuromuscular blockers	Potentiates the effects of interactive drug
	Fluoroquinolone antibiotics	May decrease absorption of interactive drug
Opioid Antidiarrheals		
Diphenoxylate	Alcohol	Additive CNS depression
Difenoxin	Antihistamines	
Loperamide	Opioids	
	Sedative-hypnotics	
	Anticholinergics	Additive anticholinergic properties
	Disopyramide	
	Tricyclic antidepressants	
	MAO inhibitors	May result in hypertensive crisis
Absorbent Antidiarrheals		
Attapulgite	Aspirin	Potentiate salicylate toxicity
Bismuth subsalicylate	Tetracycline	Decreases the absorption of interactive drug
	Enoxacin	
	Heparin	Large doses may increase risk of bleeding
	Thrombolytics	
	Warfarin	

CNS, Central nervous system; MAO, monoamine oxidase

drug action varies from 2 to 15 minutes for the rectal formulation to 24 to 72 hours for the orally administered tablets or capsules (see Table 43–1). One to two days or more may be needed before a softened fecal bolus reaches the rectum and evacuation occurs.

Drug-Drug Interactions

There are no significant drug-drug interactions with docusate laxatives. However, docusate sodium should not be taken concurrently with mineral oil.

Dosage Regimen

The dosage regimen for stool softeners varies with the specific drug, although they are usually administered only once daily (Table 43–3). The drug is administered until bowel movements return to normal. Drug effectiveness is assessed after 3 days and the dosage increased as needed (maximum of 500 mg daily for docusate sodium, 300 mg daily for docusate potassium).

Bulk-Forming Laxatives

❒ Psyllium (EFFER-SYLLIUM, METAMUCIL, MODANE BULK, PERDIEM, many others); (♣) METAMUCIL, others
❒ Polycarbophil (FIBERALL, FIBERCON, FIBER-LAX, MITROLAN)
❒ Methylcellulose (CITRUCEL)

Indications

Bulk-forming laxatives such as psyllium and methylcellulose may be safely used for the long-term management of simple, chronic constipation, particularly when the disorder is related to a low-fiber diet. They are useful in situations in which straining should be avoided (e.g., myocardial infarction, rectal surgery) and are useful in the management of chronic watery diarrhea. Polycarbophil is used in the management of constipation or diarrhea associated with diverticulosis or irritable bowel syndrome.

These laxatives are the least harmful of the various types of laxatives. They do not hinder the absorption of nutrients and are less likely to be habit forming than other laxative types. Compared with stimulant laxatives that empty the entire bowel, bulk-forming laxatives have a longer onset of drug action, and because they evacuate only the descending, sigmoid colon, and rectum, the potential for dependency on bulk-forming laxatives is reduced.

Pharmacodynamics

Bulk-forming laxatives are natural and semisynthetic polysaccharides and cellulose derivatives. They combine

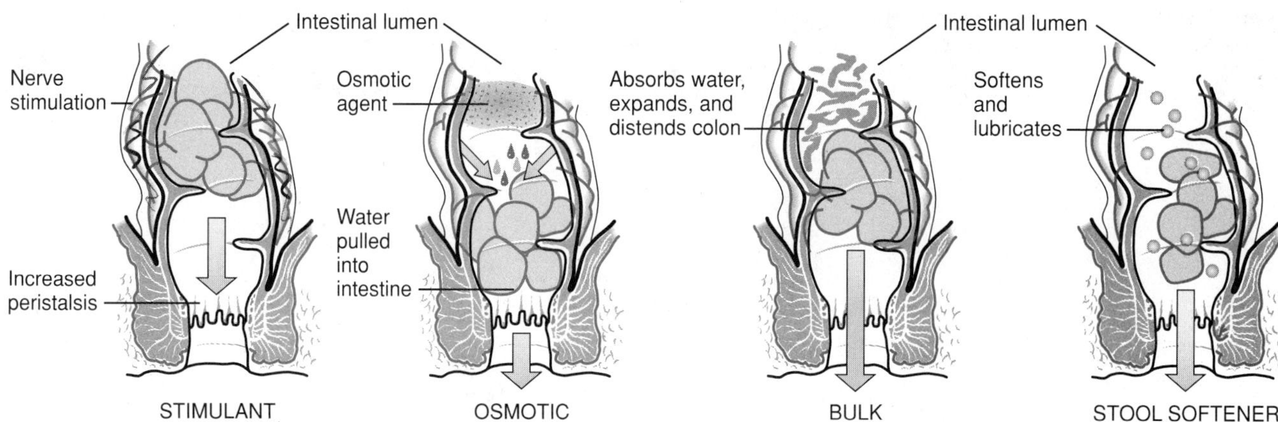

Figure 43–1 Mechanism of action of four types of laxatives. Stimulant laxatives act on the intestinal wall of the small bowel or colon to increase the amount of fluid and electrolytes within the intestinal lumen. Osmotic laxatives act by drawing water into the intestinal lumen and causing peristalsis. The greater the concentration of solutes, the greater the osmotic activity. Bulk-forming laxatives combine with water in the intestine to form an emollient gel or viscous solution. The result is an increase in peristalsis. Stool softeners produce an emollient action that reduces surface tension and thus facilitates penetration of water and lipids into the stool.

with water in the intestine to form an emollient gel or viscous solution. The result is an increase in peristalsis and a reduced transit time. Bulk-forming laxatives produce the same action as 6 to 10 g/day of dietary fiber. Antidiarrheal activity occurs because the drug takes on water within the intestinal lumen.

Adverse Effects and Contraindications

Bloating and flatulence are common undesirable adverse effects of bulk-forming laxatives. Bowel obstruction can occur if fluid intake is inadequate. In addition, allergic reactions such as urticaria, dermatitis, rhinitis, and bronchospasm can result from inhaling the powder. Esophageal obstruction has occurred in patients who have dysphagia or esophageal strictures. These laxatives are not recommended for patients with conditions that cause the esophageal or intestinal lumen to be narrowed.

Pharmacokinetics

Bulk-forming laxatives are indigestible and are not absorbed from the GI tract. The onset of action occurs in approximately 12 hours. No distribution occurs and they are eliminated in the stool. The half-life of these drugs is unknown (see Table 43–1). Bulk-forming laxatives produce a soft, formed stool in 2 to 3 days.

Drug-Drug Interactions

Bulk-forming laxatives decrease the absorption of warfarin, salicylates, and cardiac glycosides (see Table 43–2). Polycarbophil may decrease the absorption of tetracycline when the two drugs are taken concurrently. There are no known direct drug-drug interactions with methylcellulose.

Dosage Regimen

The usual adult dose of psyllium is 1 to 2 teaspoons, packets, or wafers (3 to 6 g) in a full glass of liquid two to three times daily (see Table 43–3). The packets are not standardized for volume, but each contains 3 to 3.5 g of psyllium. Up to 30 g can be taken daily in divided doses. Children older than 6 years of age receive 1 teaspoon, packet, or wafer (1.5 to 3 g) in one-half to one glass of liquid two to three times daily. The maximum pediatric dose is 15 g daily in divided doses.

Polycarbophil is given as 1 g one to four times daily or as needed. Dosage should not exceed 6 g/24 hours. For children age 2 to 6 years, 500 mg orally once or twice daily can be given. The dosage should not exceed 1.5 g/24 hours. Children ages 6 to 12 years can take 500 mg orally once to three times daily as needed, but the dosage should not exceed 3 g/24 hours. For adults and children alike, the dosage may be repeated every 30 minutes for severe diarrhea.

The dose of methylcellulose is 4 to 6 g daily. For children older than 6 years of age, 1 to 3 g can be given daily.

Laboratory Considerations

Bulk-forming laxatives may cause elevated blood glucose levels with prolonged use of formulations containing sugar.

Osmotic Laxatives

- ❒ Magnesium sulfate (Epsom Salts)
- ❒ Magnesium hydroxide (Phillips' Milk of Magnesia [MOM])
- ❒ Magnesium citrate (Citrate of Magnesia); (🍁) Citro-Mag
- ❒ Polystyrene glycol electrolyte solution (Colovage, Colyte, GoLytely, NuLytely, OCL, Peglyte); (🍁) Klean-Prep
- ❒ Sodium phosphate/biphosphate (Phospho-Soda, Fleet Enema)

Indications

Osmotic laxatives are often used to cleanse the entire intestinal tract for diagnostic purposes, to flush poisons from the system, or to remove parasites. These laxatives are useful in treating parasitic infestations because they produce a liquid stool but do not rupture the egg capsules of the parasites.

TABLE 43–3 DOSAGE REGIMEN FOR SELECTED LAXATIVES AND ANTIDIARRHEAL DRUGS

Drug	Use(s)	Dosage	Implications
Stimulant Laxatives			
Bisacodyl	Constipation related to immobility, drugs, slowed transit times, irritable bowel syndrome, spinal cord injuries, neurologic disorders	*Adult:* 5–15 mg po *or* 10 mg PR single HS dose. Maximum dose: 30 mg/day *Child younger than age 2 yr:* 5 mg PR single HS dose *Child older than age 6 yr:* 5–10 mg po single HS dose *Child age 2–12 yr:* 5–10 mg PR single HS dose	Encourage patient to retain enema or suppository 15–30 minutes before evacuating. Give oral formulations early in the day with a full glass of water
Castor oil		*Adult:* 15–60 mL po as single HS dose *Child:* 5–15 mL po as single HS dose	
Cascara sagrada		*Adults:* 0.5–1.5 mL of fluid extract (200–400 mg) as single HS dose	
Phenolphthalein		*Adult:* 30–270 mg po a single HS dose *Child age 2–5 yr:* 15–30 mg po as single HS dose or divided doses *Child age 6–11 yr:* 30–60 mg po as single HS dose or divided doses	Available as tablets, chewable tablets, wafers, and gum formulations
Senna		*Adults:* Dosage varies with formulation *Child over age 5 yr:* 50% of adult dose	Available as tablets, granules, liquid concentrate, and syrup
Stool Softeners			
Docusate calcium	Constipation in patients who should not strain	*Adult:* 240 mg po once daily *Child over age 6 yr:* 50–150 mg po once daily	Docusate calcium and potassium available as capsules; sodium formulation available as tablets, capsules, syrup, liquid, solutions, or enema
Docusate potassium		*Adult:* 100–300 mg po once daily Maximum dose: 300 mg daily *Child older than age 6 yr:* 100 mg po once daily	
Docusate sodium		*Adult:* 50–500 mg po QD *or* 50–100 mg PR once daily. Maximum dose: 500 mg daily *Child younger than 3 yr:*10–40 mg po once daily *Child 3–6 yr:* 20–60 mg po once daily *Child 6–12 yr:* 40–120 mg po once daily	
Bulk-Forming Drugs			
Psyllium	Long-term management of simple, chronic, atonic, or spastic constipation, particularly related to low-fiber diets. Chronic watery diarrhea	*Adults:* 1–2 tsp, packets, or wafers (3–6 g) po in a full glass of liquid 2–3 times daily. Not to exceed 30 g daily *Child older than age 6 yr:* 1 tsp, packet, or water (1.5–3 g) po in 1/2–1 glass of liquid 2–3 times daily. Not to exceed 15 g daily in divided doses	Must be followed by 8 ounces liquid. Not to be taken at HS to prevent obstruction
Polycarbophil	Diverticulosis, irritable bowel syndrome	*Adult:* 1–4 g po daily PRN. Not to exceed 6 g/24 hr *Child age 2–6 yr:* 500 mg po QD PRN. Not to exceed 1.5 g/24 hr *Child age 6–12 yr:* 500 mg po QD–TID PRN. Not to exceed 3 g/24 hr	For severe diarrhea, may repeat every 30 minutes. Follow with 8 ounces of liquid. Can be given throughout the day to minimize abdominal fullness.
Methylcellulose	Management of simple, chronic constipation	*Adult:* 4–6 g po daily *Child over 6 yrs:* 1–3 g po daily	Follow with 8 ounces of liquid
Osmotic Laxatives			
Magnesium sulfate	Evacuate bowel in preparation for radiographic or surgical procedures. May be used intermittently in treatment of chronic constipation	*Adult:* 10–15 g po as single dose *Child 6–11:* 5–10 g po as single dose	Best if chilled, mixed with cold fruit juice or ice. 9.9% magnesium; 8.1 mEq magnesium/g
Magnesium hydroxide		*Adult:* 30–60 mL po as single dose or in divided doses *or* 10–20 mL of concentrate *Child age 6–11 yr:* 15–30 mL as single dose or divided doses	41.7% magnesium; 34.3 mEq magnesium/g

TABLE 43-3 DOSAGE REGIMEN FOR SELECTED LAXATIVES AND ANTIDIARRHEAL DRUGS *Continued*

Drug	Use(s)	Dosage	Implications
Osmotic Laxatives *Continued*			
Magnesium citrate		*Adult:* 240 mL po as single dose *Child age 2–6 yr:* 4–12 mL po single dose *Child age 6–12 yr:* 50–100 mL po single dose	Best if chilled, mixed with cold fruit juice or ice. 16.2% magnesium; 4.4 mEq magnesium/g
Sodium phosphate/ biphosphate		*Adult:* 20–30 mL po as single dose *or* 120 mL of enema formulation *Child over age 2 yr:* 50% of adult dose PR *Child age 5–9 yr:* 2.5–10 mL po single dose *Child age 10–11 yr:* 5–10 mL po single dose	Each 20 mL of oral solution contains 96.4 mEq of sodium. Enema contains 4.4 g sodium/118 mL. Do not administer near bedtime
Polyethylene glycol electrolyte solution		*Adult:* 240 mL of solution q10 min up to 4 L until fecal discharge appears clear and has no solid material *Child:* 25–40 mL/kg/hr until fecal discharge is close and has no solid material	Patient should fast for 3–4 hours before administration and should avoid solid food within 2 hours of administration. May be given through NG tube
Lubricants			
Mineral oil	Management of constipation related to impaction, fissures, hemorrhoids	*Adult and child older than age 12 yr:* 5–45 mL as single or divided doses *or* 60–150 mL PR as single dose *Child age 2–11 yr:* 30–60 mL PR as single dose *Child age 6–12 yr:* 5–20 mL po as single or divided doses	Do not administer within 2 hours of meals, to patients in a reclining position, or to patients taking vitamin supplements or stool softeners. Moisten suppositories with water rather than lubricant because lubricants may interfere with action of the suppository
Miscellaneous Laxatives			
Glycerine	Constipation secondary to reduced gastrocolic reflex activity	*Adult:* 2–3 g PR as suppository *or* 5–15 mL as enema *Child younger than age 6 yr:* 1–1.7 g as suppository *or* 2–5 mL as enema	Usually causes evacuation of colon in 15–30 minutes
Lactulose	Treatment of chronic constipation	*Adults:* 15–30 mL/day po up to 60 mL/day	Mix with 240 mL of fruit juice, water, milk, or carbonated citrus beverage to improve flavor. May be given on an empty stomach for more rapid results
Opioid Antidiarrheals			
Diphenoxylate with atropine	Adjunct treatment for diarrhea	*Adult:* 5–20 mg/day *Child age 2–12 yr:* 0.075–0.1 mg/kg QID as liquid dosage form initially. Decrease dosage as soon as symptoms permit	Doses are based on diphenoxylate/ atropine content. One tablet or 5 mL of liquid contains 2.5 mg diphenoxylate with 0.025 mg of atropine
Difenoxin with atropine		*Adult:* Two tablets initially, then one tablet after each loose stool or every 3–4 hr PRN. Not to exceed eight tablets/day *Child:* Not recommended for use in children	Dosage based on difenoxin content. One tablet contains 1 mg difenoxin with 0.025 mg atropine
Anticholinergic			
Loperamide	Adjunct treatment of acute diarrhea. Chronic diarrhea associated with IBD. Decrease volume of ileostomy drainage	*Adult:* 4 mg initially, then 2 mg after each loose stool. Maintenance: 4–8 mg po per day. Not to exceed 8 mg/ day if OTC; 16 mg/day if prescription *Child age 6–8 yr or 24–30 kg:* 1 mg initially, then 1 mg with each loose stool. Not to exceed 4 mg/24 hr *Child age 9–11 yr or 30–47 kg:* 2 mg initially, then 1 mg with each loose stool. Not to exceed 6 mg/24 hr	OTC use in children should not exceed 2 days. Administer with clear fluids to help prevent the dehydration that accompanies diarrhea

Table continued on following page

TABLE 43–3 DOSAGE REGIMEN FOR SELECTED LAXATIVES AND ANTIDIARRHEAL DRUGS *Continued*

Drug	Use(s)	Dosage	Implications
Absorbent Antidiarrheals *Continued*			
Activated attapulgite	Adjunct in symptomatic management of mild-to-moderate acute diarrhea	*Adult:* 1.2–1.5 g after each loose stool. Not to exceed 9 g/24 hr *Child age 3–6 yr:* 300 mg after each loose stool. Not to exceed 2.1 g/24 hr *Child age 6–12:* 600 mg after each loose stool. Not to exceed 4.2 g/24 hr	Increased risk of dehydration if used in children younger than age 3 or elderly patients
Bismuth subsalicylate	Adjunct treatment of mild-to-moderate diarrhea. Traveler's diarrhea (not FDA approved for this use)	*Adult:* Two tablets q30 minutes or 30 mL q30–60 min up to eight doses/24 hr *Child age 3–6 yr:* 1/3 tablet or 5 mL q30–60 min up to eight doses/24 hr *Child age 6–9 yr:* 2/3 tablet or 10 mL q30–60 min up to eight doses/24 hr *Child age 9–12 yr:* 1 tablet or 15 mL q30–60 min up to eight doses/24 hr	Contains aspirin. The Centers for Disease Control and Prevention warns against giving drug to children or teenagers during or after recovery from chickenpox (varicella) or flulike illness because of the possible association with Reye's syndrome. It contains salicylate. Available as 262 mg tablets, or as suspension in 262 mg/5 mL or 525 mg/5 mL

FDA, Food and Drug Administration; NG, nasogastric; OTC, over the counter.

Pharmacodynamics

Osmotic laxatives produce their effects by drawing water into the intestinal lumen and causing peristalsis. The greater the concentration of solutes, the greater the osmotic activity. Hypertonic solutions cause diffusion of fluid from the plasma into the intestine to dilute the solution to an isotonic state. Magnesium salts cause an increase in the secretion of cholecystokinin from the duodenum. This activity is thought to increase the secretion and motility of the small bowel and colon, contributing to the cathartic effect.

Adverse Effects and Contraindications

The most common adverse effect of osmotic laxatives is diarrhea. However, the greater the concentration of solutes the more likely these laxatives may cause nausea. Drowsiness, bradycardia, arrhythmias, hypotension, flushing, sweating, and hypothermia are most likely to occur with parenteral administration of magnesium salts (i.e., treatment and prevention of hypomagnesemia, pregnancy-induced hypertension).

All osmotic laxatives are contraindicated in patients with nausea and vomiting of unknown origin, abdominal pain, impaction, and intestinal obstruction. Magnesium salts are contraindicated in renal disease because magnesium ions may be retained. They should be given cautiously to patients with renal disease because of their sodium content. Patients who are receiving central nervous system (CNS) depressants for seizure activity may experience a significant drop in serum calcium levels that could precipitate additional seizure activity.

Pharmacokinetics

The onset of osmotic laxatives when taken by mouth vary from 30 minutes to 6 hours depending on the preparation (see Table 43–2). Most osmotic laxatives produce a watery stool in 3 to 6 hours.

Drug-Drug Interactions

Magnesium salts potentiate the action of neuromuscular blocking drugs (see Table 43–2). The absorption of fluoroquinolone antibiotics is reduced in the presence of magnesium salts. Polyethylene glycol electrolyte solutions interfere with the absorption of orally administered drugs by decreasing transit time through the bowel. Oral drugs should not be given within 1 hour of starting laxative therapy.

Dosage Regimen

The dosages of osmotic laxatives vary with the specific drug, but most are given as a single dose (see Table 43–3). Because the greater the concentration of solutes, the more likely the patient is to become nauseated, it is important that all preparations be accompanied by at least 8 ounces of water. The water also assists the laxative to leave the stomach.

Magnesium citrate is not very soluble; therefore, large doses are needed. It is more palatable when chilled. Sodium phosphate and monophosphate has a more agreeable taste than the other compounds. It is usually given at least 2 hours before the radiologic procedure.

Polyethylene glycol electrolyte solution is given orally over 3 hours (240 mL every 10 minutes) approximately 4 to 5 hours before the procedure. It can be given by nasogastric tube if necessary at a rate of 20 to 30 mL/minute.

Lubricant Laxatives

❒ Mineral oil (AGORAL, FLEET MINERAL OIL ENEMA, others); (♣) KONDREMUL PLAIN, LANSOŸL

Indications

Mineral oil is the only lubricant laxative in use today. It is used to soften impacted stool in the management of constipation.

Pharmacodynamics

Mineral oil coats the surface of the stool and intestine with a film and retards water reabsorption to allow passage of the stool through the intestine. It does not stimulate intestinal peristalsis.

Adverse Effects and Contraindications

The adverse effects of mineral oil are few; however, anorexia, nausea, vomiting, and nutritional deficiencies can occur. Anal irritation can occur with rectal administration. Lipid pneumonia has been documented in patients who have aspirated the drug. Chronic use may decrease the absorption of fat-soluble vitamins (A, D, E, K), food, and bile salts. However, there is some evidence to suggest that only the precursor of vitamin A (carotene) is affected and that natural vitamin A is absorbed in the intestine in the presence of mineral oil.

Mineral oil is contraindicated in hypersensitivity. The rectal route is contraindicated in children younger than 2 years of age and the oral route in children is contraindicated if the child is younger than 6 years of age. Mineral oil should be used cautiously in older adults or debilitated patients because of the increased risk of lipid pneumonia. It should be used cautiously in pregnancy because it decreases the absorption of fat-soluble vitamins and can cause hypoprothrombinemia in the newborn.

Pharmacokinetics

Mineral oil is minimally absorbed following oral administration. Distribution is to the liver, spleen, mesenteric lymph nodes, and the intestinal mucosa. It produces a semisoft stool in 6 to 8 hours (see Table 43–1).

Drug-Drug Interactions

The absorption of fat-soluble vitamins is decreased in the presence of mineral oil (see Table 43–2). Similarly, concurrent use of mineral oil with stool softeners may increase the absorption of mineral oil.

Dosage Regimen

As with most other laxatives, a single dose of 5 to 45 mL is administered usually at bedtime (see Table 43–3). Routine use is discouraged. The usual dose is 60 to 150 mL if the rectal route is chosen. Children's doses vary with the age of the child and the route of administration.

Miscellaneous Laxatives

- ❐ Glycerine (FLEET BABYLAX, SANI-SUPP)
- ❐ Lactulose (CEPHULAC, CHOLAC, CHRONULAC, others); (🍁) LACTULAX

GLYCERINE

Glycerine is used for those conditions in which the rectum is filled with stool but the defecation reflex is not triggered or transit time is severely delayed. Glycerine acts by drawing water from the extravascular spaces into the lumen of the colon. Diarrhea is the most common adverse effect, although nausea, vomiting, and dehydration have also occurred. Two to three grams as a suppository or 5 to 15 mL as an enema is usually administered 30 minutes after a meal to take full advantage of the gastrocolic reflex. In children, 1 to 1.7 g as a suppository or 2 to 5 mL as an enema is given after meals.

LACTULOSE

Lactulose is a semisynthetic, hyperosmotic disaccharide that is used in the treatment of chronic constipation in adults and older adults. Its superiority to conventional laxatives has not been established. It is also used to restore regular bowel movements in patients who have had a hemorrhoidectomy, but it is not approved for such use. Lactulose is also used in the management of hepatic encephalopathy (see Chapter 45) because it lowers the pH of the colon, which, in turn, inhibits diffusion of ammonia across colonic membranes.

The most common adverse effects of lactulose include cramps, distention, flatulence, belching, and diarrhea. Lactulose is contraindicated in patients with hypersensitivity and in those who are on a low-galactose diet. Hyperglycemia has been noted in patients who have diabetes mellitus; therefore, it should be used with caution in these patients, as well as in older adults or debilitated patients. Lactulose carries a pregnancy category C designation. It is not known if lactulose is distributed to breast milk.

Less than 3 percent of lactulose is absorbed from the small intestine following oral administration. In the colon, resident bacteria biotransform the drug to lactic acid and small amounts of acetic and formic acid. The acids exert mild osmotic actions and produce soft-formed stools in 1 to 3 days. The effects of lactulose are decreased in the presence of antimicrobial drugs. The usual oral adult dose of lactulose for the management of constipation is 15 to 60 mL/day.

Critical Thinking Process

Assessment

History of Present Illness

A careful description of the patient's usual and current elimination patterns should be elicited during the health history including information about the frequency, consistency, size, and color of the stools. The health care provider should ask about any related symptoms such as abdominal pain, flatulence, or a sensation of incomplete evacuation, as well as the onset and duration of the elimination problem and any precipitating, aggravating, or mitigating factors. It is also helpful to inquire about the patient's perception of normal bowel patterns, because many patients describe themselves as constipated if they do not have a daily bowel movement. When questioning the patient about drug use, it is important to include over-the-counter drugs, especially laxatives and enemas.

Past Health History

Query the patient about past health history. Does the patient have a history of colorectal disease, hemorrhoids, or rectal fissures that may be causing discomfort? Neurologic diseases and spinal cord lesions that disrupt colon and abdominal motor nerves may provide insight into the cause of constipation. Chronic laxative or enema use can cause megacolon (dilation and hypertrophy of the colon). A history of intermittent or partially obstructing bowel lesions or metabolic disorders such as diabetes mellitus, hypothyroidism, hypokalemia, hypercalcemia, and uremia contribute to constipation.

Physical Exam Findings

Signs of constipation that may be found during the physical exam include abdominal masses with palpable tenderness. Silent or abnormal bowel sounds may be auscultated in the abdomen of the patient with constipation. A rectal exam may reveal painful areas indicating external hemorrhoids, strictures, anal tears, or abrasions. The presence of a rectal mass indicates impaction or obstructing lesion. Anal sphincter tone is increased in patients with functional problems and strictures but is decreased in constipation caused by neurologic diseases. The diameter of the rectal ampulla is markedly increased in megacolon, and bowel sounds may be reduced. Abdominal radiographs may demonstrate stool in the colon. Guaiac-positive stools may help identify an underlying cause of the constipation.

Diagnostic Testing

Diagnostic testing is not usually required in acute constipation. However, cases resistant to treatment may require some testing to establish the cause of the problem. Fecal occult blood testing provides information about ulcerative or cancerous lesions. Although it carries a 50- to 90-percent sensitivity rate, this procedure is an inexpensive method of screening for bleeding lesions that may be contributing to constipation. Occult testing is not indicated if the patient has hemorrhoids or fissures because the lesions may cause misleading positive results.

Hypokalemia evidenced in serum potassium levels may manifest as constipation. Thyroid function testing may detect hypothyroidism as a possible cause of constipation. Serum calcium levels may eliminate hypercalcemia as a cause of constipation.

Developmental Considerations

Perinatal Constipation during pregnancy is not uncommon. The effects of progesterone on smooth muscle relaxation cause decreased gastric emptying time and intestinal motility, which contribute to constipation. Constipation is also caused by mechanical compression of the bowel by the enlarging uterus and the effects of iron supplements. The increase in electrolyte and water absorption during pregnancy adds to the problem. Constipation may increase the likelihood of developing hemorrhoids.

Pediatric Stool patterns of children vary widely. Normally, neonates pass more than four stools daily during the first week of life. The frequency declines to one or two stools daily by the age of 4 years. Factors such as emotional distress, family conflict, dietary changes, febrile illness, or recent travel can alter the child's bowel habits.

A significant number of children have chronic functional constipation that often begins in infancy and tends to be self-perpetuating. Large, hard stools are retained because elimination is difficult. Chronic distention of the rectum and colon gradually decrease a child's awareness of the need to defecate. This problem results in more retention, more water reabsorption, and hardening of the stool. As the rectum becomes dilated, liquid stool oozes around the hard mass as involuntary soiling.

Geriatric Although intestinal motility decreases with age, constipation is not necessarily a problem in the older age group. Inactivity, poor appetite, tooth loss, and poor-fitting dentures contribute to the risk of constipation. Furthermore, many older adults habitually use laxatives to produce bowel movements. Chronic laxative use causes the mesenteric plexus to be less sensitive to stimulation.

Psychosocial Considerations

Pertinent life-style factors to assess in the patient with constipation include their usual activities, occupation, type and frequency of exercise, dietary and elimination habits. Could the patient be depressed or socially isolated and thus less active? Furthermore, some cultures and patients believe that autointoxication occurs if bowel movements do not occur on a regular basis (see Case Study—Constipation).

Analysis and Management

Treatment Objectives

The primary treatment objective for patients with constipation is to re-establish a normal bowel pattern and to effect comfortable stooling. The objective includes using the least number of drugs in the lowest dosages for the shortest duration of time. Correction of existing underlying conditions that may be contributing to constipation is the first step in treatment.

Treatment for constipation covers three main areas: correction of any underlying conditions that may be causing the constipation, patient education, and nondrug therapies. Prevention is the best overall treatment objective.

Treatment Options

Although there are valid indications for the use of laxatives, constipation can generally be resolved by increasing fluids and fiber in the diet, increasing exercise, and the use of appropriate bowel training. Drug therapy should be used in cases of constipation that are resistant to simple treatment measures.

Drug Variables

The initial drug of choice for constipation depends on the type and severity of constipation, the effect desired, and the underlying cause of the condition. In cases of drug-induced constipation, correction is accomplished by adjusting the drug dosage or by using alternative drugs before resorting to concurrent laxative use.

All stimulant laxatives are equally effective and less expensive than lactulose when a rapid response is desired. Some health care providers advocate the use of senna instead of the other stimulants, claiming that it is the mildest and most physiologic of all the nonfiber laxatives. There are no good studies to confirm or deny this claim, however. Stimulants should be used only for short-term treatment. Other drugs are safer and more effective for long-term management of constipation. The decision about which stimulant laxative to use can thus be based in part on availability and cost.

The osmotic laxatives are equally effective and have adverse effects similar to those of stimulant laxatives. The choice between drugs in this group and stimulant laxatives should be based on patient preference, availability, and cost. Magnesium hydroxide is usually preferred over magnesium citrate or magnesium sulfate because of its milder action.

Bulk-forming laxatives may be an appropriate choice for patients in whom a rapid response is not necessary. Bulk-forming laxatives are usually effective in 2 or 3 days, are safe for long-term use, and are least likely to cause laxative dependency. The choice of the product depends on the patient's acceptance of texture and taste (e.g., orange flavored, minty, tasteless) and its other ingredients (e.g., low sodium, sugar free), and cost. If bulk-forming laxatives are ineffective after 3 days of use, magnesium hydroxide or a stimulant laxative can be given.

Lactulose may be considered if bulk-forming laxatives are contraindicated, ineffective, or not tolerated. It can also be used for long-term management of chronic constipation, whereas magnesium hydroxide, stimulant laxatives, and stool softeners are for short-term use.

There is little therapeutic difference in the docusate stool softeners. They are primarily suitable for short-term use. Laboratory evidence suggests that docusate can be hepatotoxic and may increase the absorption of hepatobiliary toxins. They can be used if lactulose is ineffective or not tolerated.

The drug of choice for radiologic bowel preps is most often polyethylene glycol electrolyte solution because it is as effective as, or better than, cathartics, standard hydration, and enema regimens. It causes the best and most complete evacuation of the GI tract of all the available laxatives. Ordinarily, patients prefer this osmotic laxative over enema or cathartic drugs because it is more convenient (5 hours versus 3 days of drug administration), acts more quickly, and causes less discomfort. Sodium phosphate and sodium biphosphate enema in combination with bisacodyl can be used if polyethylene glycol electrolyte solution cannot be tolerated.

Patient Variables

Drug therapy may be warranted if constipation has not been relieved after 2 to 4 weeks of nondrug therapies. Patient fears of autointoxication by retained fecal matter are unfounded as long as hepatic function is normal.

For pregnant women, the drugs of choice are usually bulk-forming laxatives or stool softeners. Castor oil is not recommended during pregnancy because it may cause uterine contractions. Mineral oil is also not recommended because it interferes with the absorption of fat-soluble vitamins.

Bulk-forming laxatives are recommended for use by older adults as supplements to dietary fiber. Stool softeners may be used on a short-term basis. Osmotic and stimulant laxatives should be used sparingly because of the significant fluid and electrolyte loss produced. Use of lubricants in this age group is also discouraged. The danger of aspiration and lipid pneumonia exists with the use of mineral oil, and castor oil is too harsh for use in the older adult.

Intervention

Administration

Enteric-coated laxatives (e.g., bisacodyl, phenolphthalein) should not be taken within 1 hour of drinking milk or taking an antacid. Other laxatives (e.g., cascara sagrada, docusate potassium) should not be taken by patients who abuse alcohol.

All laxatives should be taken with a full glass of water. Psyllium formulations should be diluted at the bedside with 8 ounces of water, milk, or juice. The mixture should be taken immediately after mixing because it will congeal in a few minutes. Psyllium granules should not be chewed, taken at bedtime, or given to patients who are unable to sit upright because they may cause esophageal or intestinal obstruction.

Mineral oil should not be given to bedridden patients or children because it can cause lipid pneumonia should the patient aspirate. It should not be administered to patients in a reclining position or within 2 hours of stool softeners. Suppositories containing mineral oil should not be lubricated before administration because the lubricant may interfere with the action of the suppository. Moisten the suppository with water.

Education

Patients should be advised that laxatives are temporary measures; they are not intended for long-term treatment of constipation. Misconceptions about bowel function should be corrected. Inform the patient that autointoxication does not occur when bowel movements are less frequent. Encourage the patient to use nondrug therapies, including increased bulk in the diet, increased fluid intake, and increased activity, for bowel regulation as much as possible. Patients with abdominal pain, nausea, vomiting, or fever should be advised not to use laxatives without first consulting with their health care provider.

Anthraquinone laxatives (i.e., phenolphthalein) are eliminated in the urine. For this reason, the patient should be advised that the drug may tint acid urine a yellow-brown color and alkaline urine a pinkish red color.

Psyllium should not be taken at bedtime to minimize the possibility of intestinal obstruction. Additionally, some dosage forms of psyllium contain sugar, aspartame, or excessive sodium and should be avoided in patients on restricted diets. Bulk-forming laxatives should be taken 1 hour before or 2 hours after other drugs to promote absorption.

Evaluation

Normal bowel patterns are individually determined and may vary from three times a day to three times a week. Clinical response to treatment can be demonstrated by the passage of a soft, formed bowel movement, usually within 12 to 24 hours. In some cases, 3 days of therapy may be required to produce results. Evidence suggests that 50 percent of patients who regularly use laxatives re-establish normal bowel habits once laxative administration is discontinued.

DIARRHEA

Epidemiology and Etiology

Diarrhea is not a disease but a symptom experienced by most people at some point in their lifetime. A common definition of *diarrhea* is the occurrence of more than three stools daily. However, because the frequency of bowel movements varies with the individual, diarrhea cannot be quantified by the number of stools per day. Ordinarily, diarrhea is characterized by an increase in the frequency of profuse, watery,

Case Study Constipation

Patient History

History of Present Illness	SB is a 26-year-old female who reports to the OB clinic today with complaints of constipation. She states that she is 28 weeks pregnant. She reports her last BM was 3 days ago, and it was hard and dry. She ordinarily has one soft, formed bowel movement a day. She acknowledges not drinking enough fluids and eating primarily carbohydrates, "fast-food stuff. It's quick and easy to fix." Her activity level has declined since it started snowing. She reports that she is afraid she will fall, so she has given up her daily walk. She states that she has been faithful about taking her prenatal vitamin with iron but is taking no other medications. Thinks the iron in her vitamins is contributing to her constipation and adds to her hemorrhoidal discomfort.
Past Health History	SB's past health history is unremarkable. She had an appendectomy at age 13 and an episode of mononucleosis at age 18.
Physical Exam	VS WNL. Skin pink and warm. Mucous membranes dry. Abdominal exam reveals 28-week pregnancy. Rectal exam reveals several small, external hemorrhoids.
Diagnostic Testing	Stool guaiac is negative. Serum electrolytes, hemoglobin and hematocrit, and thyroid function tests WNL.
Developmental Considerations	Constipation in SB is related to a combination of intestinal smooth muscle relaxation associated with progesterone secretion, mechanical compression of the bowel by an enlarging uterus, and the effects of iron supplements.
Psychosocial Considerations	SB has become less active with the approach of winter and increasing gestation. SB reports that her husband is excited about the pregnancy but is worried about SB's increasing constipation.
Economic Factors	SB and her husband carry health insurance that covers perinatal care and pharmacy needs.

Variables Influencing Decision

Treatment Objectives	• Re-establish regular, comfortable stooling that empties rectum, using the least number of drugs in in the lowest dosage possible for the shortest duration of time.

Drug Variables	*Drug Summary*	*Patient Variables*
Indications	Bulk-forming laxatives and stool softeners are acceptable in the treatment of constipation during pregnancy. Castor oil can cause uterine contractions, and mineral oil interferes with absorption of nutrients.	SB is 28 weeks pregnant with decreased activity, and inadequate fiber and fluid in diet. This will become a decision point.
Pharmacodynamics	Stool softeners produce an emollient action. Bulk-forming laxatives combine with water in the intestine to form an emollient gel or viscous solution.	There are no pharmacodynamic considerations for SB.
Adverse Effects/ Contraindications	The most common adverse effect of stool softeners is diarrhea. Bulk-forming laxatives may offset potential for diarrhea and do not hinder absorption of nutrients. This will be a decision point.	There are no absolute contraindications to the use of stool softeners or bulk-producing laxatives for SB.

Drug Variables	*Drug Summary*	*Patient Variables*
Pharmacokinetics	Stool softeners and bulk-forming laxatives produce stool in 1–3 days.	There is no absolute urgency to treat SB's constipation. Fiber, fluids, and exercise are important primary modalities.
Dosage Regimen	Dosage decision based on manufacturer's recommendation.	Once- to twice-daily dosing preferred by SB. This will become a decision point.
Lab Considerations	There are no laboratory considerations related to the short-term use of either of these two laxative drug groups.	This will not be a decision point for SB treatment.
Cost Index*	Metamucil: 1 Colace: 1 Surfak: 1	These drugs are inexpensive preparations if SB chooses to purchase them OTC. Pharmacy coverage will also cover the cost.

Summary of Decision Points

- SB's constipation primarily related to 28-week pregnancy, inactivity, and lack of fiber and fluids in the diet. She will need to increase her activity and fluid intake regardless of the drug therapy used.
- There is no absolute urgency to treat SB's constipation.

DRUGS TO BE USED

- Docusate calcium 240 mg po once daily × 10 days.
- Psyllium hydrophilic muciloid 2 teaspoons in a full glass of water BID.

*Cost Index:

1 $ < 30/mo.
2 $ 30–40/mo.
3 $ 40–50/mo.
4 $ 50–60/mo.
5 $ > 60/mo.

AWP of 30, 240 mg capsules of docusate calcium is approximately $7.
AWP of 30, 50 mg capsules of docusate sodium is approximately $7.
AWP of 390 g of orange-flavored psyllium hydrophilic muciloid is approximately $7.

loose stools during a limited time period. Diarrhea is considered chronic if it persists for at least 2 weeks, produces over 300 g of stool daily, or when it subsides and returns more than 2 to 4 weeks after the initial episode.

In the last 10 years, 40,000 cases of diarrhea have been reported, resulting in 500 deaths and costing of over $50,000,000. Diarrhea is the leading cause of death in developing countries, where daily over 10,000 children younger than 5 years of age are affected. In the United States, diarrhea accounts for over 250,000 hospitalizations per year and 7.9 million office visits. Forty-eight million diarrheal episodes lasting over 48 hours occur annually.

Pathophysiology

In essence, diarrhea is caused by any factor that decreases fluid absorption in the small or large bowel, increases fluid secretion (e.g., deranged electrolyte transport), alters bowel motility, or is associated with mucosal injury. Diarrhea can be acute or chronic. Acute diarrhea is usually of bacterial or viral origin. It can be caused by bacterial overgrowth because of antimicrobial suppression of normal flora. It can also be an undesired adverse response to drug therapy in susceptible people (see Drugs Likely to Cause Diarrhea). Diarrhea that accompanies food poisoning results from consuming food or fluids that were contaminated during preparation, serving, or storage. Traveler's diarrhea occurs in persons who travel to countries where enteric pathogens are prevalent.

Although avoiding laxatives in the presence of diarrhea seems all too obvious, concealed abuse of stimulant laxatives is a surprisingly frequent cause of chronic diarrhea of unknown origin. Other common causes of chronic diarrhea include malabsorption, irritable bowel disease, and surgical procedures that shorten the intestinal tract (i.e., short-gut syndrome) or cause rapid emptying of the stomach (i.e., dumping syndrome).

Systemic manifestations of acute diarrhea include fever, nausea, vomiting, and malaise. Leukocytes, blood, and mucus may be present in the stool depending on the cause of

DRUGS LIKELY TO CAUSE DIARRHEA

Antimicrobials
Antineoplastics
Bile acids
Cardiac glycosides
Cholinergic drugs
Cholinesterase inhibitors
Guanethidine
Magnesium-containing antacids
Methyldopa
Osmotic laxatives
Quinidine
Reserpine
Stimulant laxatives

the diarrhea. *Tenesmus,* a spasmodic contraction of the anal sphincter with pain and persistent desire to defecate and cramping abdominal pain are often present with acute diarrhea. Symptoms continue until the irritant or causative agent is eliminated. The epithelial lining of the GI tract regenerates following the inflammatory response. Dehydration, electrolyte disturbances, malabsorption, and malnutrition are sequelae of chronic diarrhea.

PHARMACOTHERAPEUTIC OPTIONS

Opioid Antidiarrheals

- Difenoxin with atropine sulfate (MOTOFEN)
- Diphenoxylate with atropine sulfate (LOMOTIL, LOFENE, LOGEN, LONOX)
- Loperamide (IMODIUM, IMODIUM A-D, KAOPECTATE II CAPLETS, MAALOX ANTI-DIARRHEAL CAPLETS, PEPTO DIARRHEA CONTROL)

Indications

Opioids, as systemic antidiarrheal drugs, are the most effective antidiarrheal drugs. Although hydroalcoholic solutions of opium powder (e.g., camphorated tincture of opium, opium tincture) have long been used to treat diarrhea, synthetic opioids are now preferred. The systemic antidiarrheals are much more effective than the local preparations (e.g., absorbents, intestinal flora modifiers) in treating and controlling diarrhea. Atropine, an anticholinergic drug (see Chapter 13), is combined with diphenoxylate and difenoxin in subtherapeutic doses to discourage abuse of the preparation.

Pharmacodynamics

Opioids such as diphenoxylate and difenoxin act at the mu (μ) and possibly delta (δ) receptors to decrease intestinal motility, thereby slowing transit time. The prolonged transit time facilitates absorption of fluid, electrolytes, and solutes throughout the intestinal tract. In addition, stimulation of the opioid receptors also decrease secretion of fluid into the small intestine. Rectal sphincter tone is also increased. As a result of these actions, the fluidity, volume of stools, and frequency of defecation are reduced.

Loperamide inhibits peristalsis and prolongs transit time through direct effect on nerves in the intestinal muscle wall. It reduces fecal volume and increases viscosity and bulk while diminishing loss of fluid and electrolytes. Loperamide reduces the volume of discharge from an ileostomy and can be used in the treatment of traveler's diarrhea and chronic diarrhea associated with inflammatory bowel disease, and provides symptomatic relief of acute nonspecific diarrhea.

Adverse Effects and Contraindications

Diphenoxylate's adverse effects are caused by both mu (μ) agonist activity and nonselective muscarinic antagonism. The most common adverse effects include constipation and dizziness. Blurred vision, dry mouth and dry eyes, tachycardia, epigastric distress, nausea and vomiting, ileus, drowsiness, headache, insomnia, nervousness, and confusion are also possible. Urinary retention and flushing may occur.

Although difenoxin and diphenoxylate are effective in the treatment of mild to moderate diarrhea, they should not be used in patients with chronic ulcerative colitis or acute bacillary or amebic dysentery. When the drugs are used in patients with these conditions, it appears that they potentiate ulcerating processes in the colon and provoke the development of toxic megacolon. Opioids are also contraindicated in patients with hypersensitivity, severe liver disease, infectious diarrhea (due to *Escherichia coli, Salmonella,* or *Shigella*), and in diarrhea associated with pseudomembranous colitis *(Clostridium difficile)*. Patients who are dehydrated, or who have narrow-angle glaucoma, children younger than 2 years of age, and those with alcohol intolerance should avoid diphenoxylate preparations.

The adverse effects of loperamide are fewer than those of diphenoxylate with atropine. Drowsiness and constipation are the most common, but dizziness, nausea, and dry mouth also occur. Loperamide is contraindicated in patients with hypersensitivity, in whom constipation must be avoided, abdominal pain of unknown cause (especially if associated with fever), and alcohol intolerance. Loperamide should be used with caution in patients who have liver disease, in children younger than 2 years of age, during pregnancy and lactation, and in the older adult.

Opioids should be used cautiously in patients with inflammatory bowel disease, prostatic hypertrophy, during pregnancy, and in children. Difenoxin is not recommended for children younger than 12 years of age.

Pharmacokinetics

Diphenoxylate is well absorbed from the GI tract. Its distribution is unknown. Most of the drug is biotransformed in the liver, with some conversion to an active antidiarrheal metabolite difenoxin. Difenoxin, in turn, is biotransformed in the liver to an inactive metabolite to be eliminated. Difenoxin's half-life is about 12 hours (Table 43–4).

Loperamide is slowly and incompletely absorbed following oral administration. It apparently crosses the blood-brain barrier relatively slowly because administering doses greatly in excess of those recommended for treatment of diarrhea produce only modest effects on the CNS. Loperamide is 97-percent protein bound, undergoing enterohepatic recirculation. It is biotransformed in the liver. Thirty percent

TABLE 43–4 PHARMACOKINETICS OF SELECTED ANTIDIARRHEAL DRUGS

Drug	Route	Onset	Peak	Duration	PB (%)	$t_{1/2}$	BioA (%)
Opioids							
Diphenoxylate with atropine	po	45–60 min	2 hr	3–4 hr	UA	2.5 hr	UA
Difenoxin with atropine	po	45–60 min	2 hr	3–4 hr	UA	UA	UA
Anticholinergic							
Loperamide	po	60 min	2.5–5 hr	10 hr	97	10.8 hr	UA
Absorbent							
Activated attapulgite	po	UK	UK	UK	UK	UK	UK
Bismuth subsalicylate	po	<24 hr	UK	UK	UA	2–3 hr; 15–30 hr*	UA

*Half-life of salicylate component of bismuth subsalicylate for low doses; it is longer for higher doses
PB, Protein binding; $t_{1/2}$, elimination half-life; NA, not applicable; UA, unavailable; UK, unknown; BioA, bioavailability.

of the drug is eliminated in the stool, with minimal elimination in the urine. Its half-life is 10.8 hours.

Drug-Drug Interactions

Table 43–2 lists the drug-drug interactions with opioid antidiarrheal drugs. The interactions are not unlike those found when the opioid is used for analgesia (see Chapter 14).

Dosage Regimen

Doses of diphenoxylate with atropine are stated in terms of the diphenoxylate content. Each tablet of diphenoxylate with atropine contains 2.5 mg diphenoxylate and 0.025 mg of atropine. The usual dose of diphenoxylate is 5 mg/day, or 1 tablet after each loose stool up to a total of 20 mg (see Table 43–3). For children ages 2 to 12 years, the initial dose is usually 0.075 mg/kg four times daily. The dosage may be decreased as symptoms improve. A calibrated measuring device should be used for liquid preparations. Diphenoxylate is a Schedule V controlled drug.

Difenoxin with atropine is also dosed on the basis of its difenoxin content. Each tablet contains 1 mg of difenoxin with 0.025 mg atropine. The initial dose is two tablets, followed by one tablet after each loose stool or every 3 or 4 hours as needed. The dosage should not exceed eight tablets per day (8 mg). Difenoxin is not recommended for use in children. Difenoxin is a Schedule IV controlled drug.

The oral adult dose of loperamide for the treatment of diarrhea is 4 mg initially, then 2 mg after each loose stool up to 8 mg/day if the formulation is obtained over the counter, and 16 mg if the drug is obtained via prescription. Children's dosages initially range from 1 to 2 mg orally, followed by 1-mg tablets with each loose stool. Depending on the child's age, the dosage should not exceed 4 to 6 mg.

Laboratory Considerations

Liver function tests should be evaluated periodically during prolonged therapy with antidiarrheal drugs. Diphenoxylate with atropine may cause increased serum amylase concentrations. There are no other significant laboratory testing considerations.

Absorbents

- ❒ Activated attapulgite (KAOPECTATE, PAREPECTOLIN, DIAR-AID, DIASORB)
- ❒ Bismuth subsalicylate (PEPTO-BISMOL, BISMATROL, PINK BISMUTH)

Indications

Bismuth subsalicylate is used in the adjunctive treatment of diarrhea. It has also been used in the treatment of enterotoxigenic *E. coli* (traveler's diarrhea), although it is not approved by the Food and Drug Administration (FDA) for this use. Bismuth subsalicylate has also been added to the armamentarium in the treatment of gastritis and peptic ulcer disease associated with *Helicobacter pylori* and is sometimes used as a local protectant for the skin. The availability of this relatively inexpensive drug promotes its overuse and increases the potential for toxicity to both the salicylate and bismuth components.

Attapulgite is a nonspecific antidiarrheal drug. Although this absorbent clay produces stools with a more normal appearance, fluid loss may remain unchanged and electrolyte losses may actually increase. The claim that attapulgite facilitates removal of bacterial toxins has not been supported.

Pharmacodynamics

Bismuth subsalicylate is a relatively insoluble compound with absorbent, demulcent, astringent, and weak antacid characteristics. Although the mechanism of action is poorly understood, it is thought that the local anti-inflammatory actions of salicylate is primarily involved, decreasing the synthesis of intestinal prostaglandins. Antibacterial actions of bismuth may also be involved, especially in the prevention of traveler's diarrhea.

Attapulgite is thought to act by absorbing bacteria and toxins and decreasing water loss. The therapeutic effects are thus decreased number and water content of stools.

Adverse Effects and Contraindications

The adverse effects of bismuth subsalicylate include constipation, impaction, and gray-black tongue and stools. It is contraindicated in older adult patients who may suffer from impacted stool and in patients who are hypersensitive to aspirin. The Centers for Disease Control and Prevention recommend that bismuth subsalicylate not be used in children or teenagers during or after recovery from chickenpox (varicella) or flulike illnesses because of the association of salicylate with Reye's syndrome. Cautious use is warranted in infants, older adults, and debilitated patients because impaction is possible. Because bismuth is radiopaque, it is generally not used in patients who will be undergoing radiologic examination of the GI tract. Safe use during pregnancy and lactation has not been established. Cautious use is also warranted in patients who have diabetes mellitus or gout.

The adverse effects of attapulgite are few. It may increase the fecal elimination of sodium and potassium, but the most common adverse effect is constipation.

Pharmacokinetics

Bismuth is not absorbed; however, the salicylate is hydrolyzed from the parent compound and is 90-percent absorbed from the small bowel. The onset of action is within 24 hours. Peak and duration of action is unknown (see Table 43–4). Salicylates are highly bound to plasma proteins with bismuth subsalicylate distributed to the placenta. It also enters breast milk. The salicylate component undergoes significant hepatic biotransformation. The half-life of the salicylate component is 2 to 3 hours at low doses, and 15 to 30 hours for larger doses.

Attapulgite acts locally. The pharmacokinetics of distribution, biotransformation, and elimination routes are unknown.

Drug-Drug Interactions

If bismuth subsalicylate is taken with aspirin, it may potentiate salicylate toxicity. It decreases the absorption of tetracycline antibiotics or enoxacin (chewable tablets only). Large doses may increase the risk of bleeding in the presence of thrombolytics, warfarin, or heparin. For example, a 2-ounce dose of bismuth salts can produce the same salicylate blood level as one 5-grain tablet of aspirin. Large doses can also increase the risk of hypoglycemia from insulin or oral hypoglycemics and may decrease the effectiveness of probenecid. There is a cross-allergenicity with nonsteroidal anti-inflammatory drugs and oil of wintergreen.

Much like bismuth subsalicylate, attapulgite may decrease the GI absorption of concurrently administered drugs. Other drugs should be administered 2 to 3 hours before or 2 to 4 hours after taking attapulgite.

Dosage Regimen

A bismuth subsalicylate regimen of eight doses of 524 mg (30 mL or 2 tablets) taken every 30 minutes provides relief from the symptoms of mild diarrhea. Four 524-mg doses per day is effective for the prevention of traveler's diarrhea. The regimen should be used when one is in an endemic area, and it should be continued for 1 to 2 days after returning home. The treatment period should not exceed 3 weeks.

The adult dosage regimen for attapulgite is 1.2 to 1.5 g after each loose stool. The dosage should not exceed 9 g in 24 hours. For children, the dosage ranges from 300 mg after each loose stool for children ages 3 to 6 years, to 600 mg for children ages 6 to 12 years. Dosages should not exceed 2.1 g and 4.2 g, respectively, in 24 hours.

Laboratory Considerations

Bismuth subsalicylate causes a variety of laboratory test alterations. For example, chronic high doses may cause false-positive urine glucose tests (using copper sulfate methods), false-negative test results with enzymatic glucose tests, and falsely increased uric acid levels. It can also cause alterations in vanillylmandelic acid concentrations and liver function tests. It produces decreased serum potassium and T_3 and T_4 concentrations, and elevated prothrombin times.

Miscellaneous Antidiarrheal Drugs

- ❒ Belladonna alkaloids (DONNAGEL)
- ❒ Cholestyramine (QUESTRAN)
- ❒ Kaolin and pectin (KAOPECTATE)
- ❒ *Lactobacillus acidophilus* (LACTINEX, BACID)
- ❒ Opium tincture
- ❒ Camphorated tincture of opium (paregoric)
- ❒ Octreotide (SANDOSTATIN)

BELLADONNA ALKALOIDS

Many traditional remedies have little or no value in the treatment of acute diarrhea. These remedies include kaolin and pectin, lactobacilli, and anticholinergic preparations (muscarinic antagonists). *Belladonna alkaloids* are classified as anticholinergic drugs and include atropine, hyoscine, and hyoscyamine. However, there is no conclusive evidence that drugs in this class are effective in the treatment of diarrhea. They do, however, prevent the spasms and cramping frequently associated with acute or chronic diarrhea when given in a sufficient dose.

A single 30-mL dose of a belladonna alkaloid formulation contains a combination of kaolin and pectin, atropine, hyoscyamine, scopolamine hydrobromide, and alcohol. Because of the multiple ingredients in these products, the patient is at risk for combined adverse effects and added expense. Single-ingredient drugs are recommended to control specific symptoms. Belladonna is contraindicated in patients with narrow-angle glaucoma and intestinal obstruction because of the addition of atropine and hyoscyamine. It is given cautiously in patients with urinary tract obstruction because of its ability to cause obstruction uropathy. Patients with respiratory or cardiac disease may experience tachycardia.

CHOLESTYRAMINE

Cholestyramine, an antihyperlipidemic drug, has a direct affinity for acidic materials such as bile salts and the toxin produced by *C. difficile*. It is thought to relieve diarrhea caused by excessive bile salts and may be effective for antibiotic-induced pseudomembranous colitis, although it is not approved by the FDA for such use. Cholestyramine is described in more detail in Chapter 35.

KAOLIN AND PECTIN

Kaolin is a natural aluminum silicate clay that has been used for hundreds of years to treat diarrhea. It is most often mixed with *pectin,* a purified carbohydrate obtained from the peel of citrus fruits or from apple pulp. When pectin is cooked with sugar at the proper pH, a gel forms. The combination of the two drugs may add bulk to the stool but rarely reduce stool fluid or frequency, although they are thought to act as an absorbent and demulcent. Kaolin and pectin must be given in large doses after each bowel movement. As a result, constipation often occurs. Kaolin and pectin is not presently recognized by the FDA as effective.

LACTOBACILLUS ACIDOPHILUS

Lactobacillus acidophilus and *Lactobacillus bulgaricus* are over-the-counter preparations that are thought to promote the growth of normal intestinal flora, particularly *E. coli*. There is also the notion that increased dietary intake of products containing lactobacillus as well as lactose and dextrose (e.g., milk, buttermilk, yogurt) are all equally effective in recolonizing the intestine. However, recent research has suggested that diet therapy may be more effective than actual ingestion of the lactobacillus organism.

OPIUM TINCTURE AND CAMPHORATED TINCTURE OF OPIUM

Opium tincture and camphorated tincture of opium (paregoric) are systemic drugs that have antispasmodic and antiperistaltic actions. Although both drugs are used less often today, camphorated tincture of opium has been especially useful in the management of diarrhea associated with human immunodeficiency virus infection. Opium tincture may be added to enteral feedings to help minimize the diarrhea typically caused by such feedings. In addition, the preparation (in dilute form) may be given to suppress symptoms of withdrawal in opioid-dependent neonates.

The antidiarrheal activity of the drugs is related to the morphine content and thus are available only by prescription. Camphorated tincture of opium is a Schedule III drug that contains 0.04 percent morphine (0.4 mg/mL), 45 percent alcohol, camphor, anise oil, and benzoic acid. Opium tincture is an alcohol-based, Schedule II solution that contains 10 percent opium by weight. It is 25 times more concentrated than camphorated tincture of opium and carries a high potential for abuse.

Euphoria, analgesia, or dependence are unlikely with opium tincture or camphorated tincture of opium when using the recommended doses for short periods of time. Large doses can cause dizziness, drowsiness, fainting, flushing, and CNS depression. Adverse effects are typically dose related and include nausea, vomiting, dysphoria, constipation, and increased biliary tract pressure. Anaphylaxis is rare. Patients older than 60 years of age tend to be more sensitive to the drugs than younger patients.

Opium tincture and camphorated tincture of opium are contraindicated in patients with hypersensitivity and in those who have pseudomembranous colitis or severe ulcerative colitis (toxic megacolon may develop). The drugs should be used with caution in patients with liver disease, severe prostatic hypertrophy, and during pregnancy (Category B), as well as in patients who may be prone to opioid dependency.

Both drugs are quickly absorbed from the GI tract, with distribution to parenchymal tissues including the kidneys, lungs, liver, and spleen. Both drugs have an onset time of less than 60 minutes, with peak concentrations reached in 2 to 3 hours. Their duration of action is approximately 4 hours. Biotransformation occurs in the liver, with approximately 90 percent of the metabolites eliminated through the kidneys. The remainder is eliminated in the stool.

An average adult dose of opium tincture is 0.3 to 1 mL orally four times daily but should not exceed 6 mL/day. The average dose of camphorated tincture of opium is 5 to 10 mL once to four times daily. A child's dose is 0.25 to 0.5 mL/kg once to four times daily. Treatment of diarrhea using these agents should not exceed 48 hours. Both drugs are available in liquid form with 2 mg morphine equivalent per 5 mL.

OCTREOTIDE

Octreotide is identical to the natural hormone somatostatin (see Chapter 51) but also acts to increase absorption of fluid and electrolytes from the GI tract and increase the transit time. It has been used as an investigational drug to control severe, refractory diarrhea. Refractory diarrhea may occur with dumping syndrome, severe enterotoxic infections, short-gut syndrome, graft-versus-host disease, acquired immunodeficiency syndrome, and carcinoid tumors and vasoactive intestinal peptid tumors (vipomas). It is described as a universal inhibitor of secretory cells.

Common adverse effects of octreotide include transient nausea, diarrhea, abdominal cramping, and fat malabsorption. Headache, drowsiness, dizziness, fatigue, and weakness have been reported. Palpitations and orthostatic hypotension is possible. Gallstones may form because octreotide decreases the emptying of the gallbladder. It also alters the secretion of insulin and glucagon, leading to hyperglycemia or hypoglycemia. Because it is available only for subcutaneous or intravenous use, the patient may experience discomfort at the injection site.

Critical Thinking Process

Assessment

History of Present Illness

Much like the patient with constipation, the patient with diarrhea should be asked about usual and current elimination patterns including information about the frequency, consistency, size, and color of the stools. The health care provider should also ask about any related symptoms such as abdominal pain and flatulence, as well as onset and duration of the problem and any precipitating, aggravating, or mitigating factors. It should be determined whether there has been an increase in the consumption of laxative-like foods such as bran, lactose, sorbitol, fructose, brassica vegetables, coffee, or tea. Has the patient experienced an unexplained weight loss or been exposed to possible carriers of enteric infection? Has the patient consumed potentially contaminated food or water or traveled in foreign countries?

The patient should be asked about his or her perception of normal defecation patterns. Some patients describe themselves as having diarrhea if they have more than one stool per day regardless of the consistency. Alternating periods of constipation and diarrhea are characteristic of irritable bowel syndrome.

When questioning the patient about drug use, it is important to ask about the use of laxatives, magnesium-containing antacids, excess alcohol, caffeine-containing beverages, and herbal teas. It should also be noted whether the patient has recently taken antibiotics, digitalis, quinidine, loop diuretics, antihypertensive drugs, or ingested excessive amounts of sugar-free gums and mints that contain sorbitol.

Past Health History

A number of groups are at high risk for infectious diarrhea. Patients with a recent travel history (e.g., Peace Corps workers) and campers. Often there is a history of eating raw seafood or shellfish. Patients may also report eating in restaurants or fast-food restaurants, recently attending a picnic or banquet, or having been in close contact with children or ill family members.

Physical Exam Findings

Vital signs must be checked for postural changes, which is a reflection of significant volume depletion. Any elevation in temperature or weight loss needs to be noted. The skin is examined for rashes and lymph node enlargement. Auscultation of the abdomen often reveals hyperactive bowel sounds, and palpation may reveal tenderness, guarding, rebound, organomegaly, or masses. A rectal exam completes the physical exam.

Diagnostic Testing

Laboratory workup should be individualized. Stool examination should include size, shape, consistency, color, and odor, as well as the presence or absence of blood, mucus, pus, tissue fragments, food residues, bacteria, or parasites. The gross appearance of the stool should be assessed before administration of barium or antidiarrheal drugs.

Diarrhea stool that is mixed with mucus and red blood cells is associated with typhus, typhoid, cholera, amebiasis, and large bowel cancers. Likewise, diarrhea mixed with mucus and white blood cells is associated with ulcerative colitis, regional enteritis, shigellosis, salmonellosis, and intestinal tuberculosis. A pasty stool is associated with a high-fat content and may be indicative of a malabsorption disorder. Alterations in the size or shape of the stool indicate altered motility or abnormalities in the colonic wall.

To detect ova and parasites, stools should be sent to the laboratory while warm. The ova and parasites will not live in an environment below body temperature. Stool specimens for ova and parasites should not be refrigerated. The presence of urine in the stool specimen will destroy parasites.

A quick and simple test to detect suspected laxative abuse is to alkalinize the stool. If the stool specimen contains phenolphthalein (a common ingredient in many over-the-counter laxatives), it will turn pink.

Developmental Considerations

Perinatal Intestinal disorders in pregnancy mirror the range of GI disease in the normal population. Common etiologies include antibiotic-induced diarrhea (related to overgrowth of *C. difficile* after antibiotic therapy), functional bowel disorders, infectious gastroenteritis (bacterial, parasitic, and viral), and inflammatory bowel disorders (regional enteritis and ulcerative colitis). Acute-onset diarrhea is usually associated with a viral or bacterial infection, and although it is problematic, it is not usually voluminous in nature. Ordinarily, gastroenteritis in pregnancy does not pose significant risk to the fetus if maternal hydration is maintained. Most infections tend to be localized to the bowel mucosa and do not present a risk for infection of the fetus. Most cases of infectious diarrhea resolve without antibiotic therapy in several days, although antibiotic therapy should be considered for severe infections. The detrimental perinatal effects of GI diseases generally result from their impact on maternal nutrition.

Pediatric It is estimated that over 500 million children worldwide suffer from diarrhea each year. Acute diarrhea is the leading cause of illness in children younger than 5 years of age. The dehydration, electrolyte disturbances, and malnutrition that diarrhea causes is fatal for approximately 400 of these children a year in the United States. As a general rule, the younger the child, the greater the susceptibility and the more severe the diarrhea. Diarrhea occurs more often during infancy, is a lesser threat in early childhood, and usually constitutes only a minor problem in older children. Malnourished or debilitated children are more susceptible and tend to have more severe diarrhea.

The frequency of diarrhea in infancy is closely related to the ingestion of contaminated milk. There is a lower incidence of diarrhea in breastfed infants. Diarrhea occurs more often when there is overcrowding, substandard sanitation, inadequate facilities for preparation and refrigeration of food, and generally inadequate health care education.

Most cases of diarrhea in children are caused by bacterial, viral, and parasitic pathogens. Metabolic acidosis may be present with severe diarrhea and dehydration. Malnutrition may contribute to the severity of the condition and may be a consequence of diarrheal disease due to reduced dietary intake, malabsorption, and the catabolic response to infection. Because a child's metabolic rate is higher than that of an adult, the child is predisposed to a more rapid depletion of nutritional reserves.

Fluid replacement is important when diarrhea develops in infants and toddlers, because it can lead to life-threatening dehydration. However, antidiarrheal drugs have limited value in this age group and there is a concern about possible toxicity. Although pediatric dosages are identified for diphenoxylate with atropine and loperamide, the World Health Organization does not recommend giving either of these drugs to children. The Centers for Disease Control and Prevention and the American Academy of Pediatrics recommend that the use of oral fluid and electrolyte replacement therapy be used as the treatment of choice for most cases of dehydration caused by diarrhea.

Geriatric The causes of diarrhea in the older adult are not unlike those of others. Fifteen percent of diarrhea in the older adult is related to an infectious source, with 19 percent of the cases caused by bacterial infection, 68 percent caused by viral infections, and 3 percent caused by parasitic infections. Fecal impaction is mistaken for diarrhea because liquid stool comes around the impaction and is eliminated frequently. Fecal impaction accounts for 16 percent of diarrhea, antibiotic use in 11 percent, laxative abuse in 6 percent, and inflammatory bowel disease in 4 percent. Dietary indiscretions (e.g., too much fruit, especially bananas) and hyperosmolar tube feedings, protein-calorie malnutrition (see Chapter 59), and anxiety are also culprits. Diarrhea can be a serious problem, with associated mortality increasing dramatically in patients older than 74 years of age.

Psychosocial Considerations

American culture is very bathroom oriented. Status, and even assessed valuation of a house for tax purposes, are determined by the number of bathrooms a house has. However, persons from foreign countries may have totally different experiences with bathroom facilities. Toileting is a private activity for most people, taking place behind closed doors. During illness or hospitalization, this formerly private activity suddenly may be exposed for all to discuss, possibly view, and perhaps even worse, for others to smell.

Pertinent life-style factors to assess for the patient with diarrhea include usual activities, occupation, type and frequency of exercise, dietary and elimination habits. What is the patient's stress level? Could the stress be manifesting in part as diarrhea? Further, a sexual history is important when the patient complains of diarrhea because it may be a manifestation of gay bowel syndrome in male homosexuals.

Analysis and Management

Treatment Objectives

The excessive loss of fluid and electrolytes as well as stool that characterizes diarrhea is an important aspect of many infectious and noninfectious GI disorders. Although acute-onset diarrhea is most often of infectious origin, it is usually self-limiting and specific drug therapy is seldom warranted (unless there is evidence of GI erosion or systemic disease). Therefore, treatment objectives include the maintenance of adequate hydration and skin integrity, and the limited use of select antidiarrheal drugs.

Treatment objectives for chronic diarrhea include re-establishing bowel habits to a pattern that is normal for the patient. In order to do so, treating the underlying cause of the diarrhea is important.

Treatment Options

Drug Variables

Although an otherwise healthy adult may not be harmed by dietary abstinence during an episode of mild to moderate diarrhea, the ingestion of soft, easily digested foods and noncarbonated beverages is suggested. The oral administration of solutions containing electrolytes, glucose, and amino acids usually suffices. However, parenteral fluids may be warranted in some cases to help the patient achieve adequate hydration.

To date, there is no absolute clinical evidence that documents the therapeutic effect of antidiarrheal drugs in curing the underlying cause of the diarrhea. However, these drugs do reduce the interference with daily activities that diarrhea causes. The mainstay of nonspecific drug therapy for diarrhea continues to be the opioids. These drugs reduce the amount of fluid present in the colon, primarily by slowing transit time and thus promoting reabsorption of water and electrolytes. Opioids do not eliminate the need for fluids and electrolytes, however, and should be avoided in patients with high fever, dysentery, and antibiotic-associated pseudomembranous colitis (see Controversy—Pepto-Bismol, Loperamide, and Diarrhea).

An effective over-the-counter drug for diarrhea is bismuth subsalicylate. It can provide substantial relief in mild to moderate diarrhea and is useful in the prophylaxis of traveler's diarrhea caused by a variety of infectious agents.

Controversy

Pepto-Bismol, Loperamide, and Diarrhea

JONATHAN J. WOLFE

Diarrhea presents with compelling sequela that no patient can ignore. The definition may vary among patients. In some, it is represented by a greater than normal number of bowel movements, and in others, it may be the passage of ill-formed or liquid stools. Close definition may not matter much because diarrhea is usually self-limiting. Because the problem is acute and understandable, the patient is likely to manage it without medical consultation.

Not all diarrhea, however, is benign. In some cases, it is caused by overuse of laxatives. Many patients express concern if a daily evacuation does not occur. But, reliance on stimulant laxatives to promote daily regularity may prove harmful, particularly in an older, inactive patient with small dietary intake. Diarrhea also may be a symptom of disease. If it does not subside shortly but persists, use of antidiarrheals is inappropriate. Over-the-counter products are intended to treat only uncomplicated minor disorders. Finally, diarrhea in both the very young and the very old may have severe consequences. Dehydration and loss of electrolytes may quickly progress to life-threatening levels.

Many over-the-counter antidiarrheals are available. The simplest are adsorbent products like pectin. These agents take up excess water in the lumen of the large intestine, minimizing watery stools. Bismuth salts are very popular for both indigestion and diarrhea but not for prolonged use. Finally, opioid derivatives such as loperamide may be used. Their temporary effect on opioid receptors in the bowel wall is effective, but again these agents are proper only for short-term administration. The choice of an antidiarrheal is too often made on the basis of trade name or price. Even trade names are not foolproof. For instance, loperamide is represented in IMODIUM A-D CAPLETS, KAOPECTATE II CAPLETS, and MAALOX ANTIDIARRHEAL CAPLETS, as well as in the liquid PEPTO DIARRHEA CONTROL. The customer accustomed to these trade names may well think that he or she is purchasing a known and relatively innocuous over-the-counter product, when in fact loperamide is the active ingredient.

Critical Thinking Discussion

- What groups of patients are at risk and need to be evaluated promptly when diarrhea occurs?
- Do you experience personal difficulties when discussing diarrhea with a patient? Does this problem vary when the patient is younger than yourself, older, or of a different race?
- How may a patient characterize a present episode of diarrhea? What important factors may she not tell you at first?
- Why is persistent diarrhea in an elderly patient who is taking digoxin a critical matter?
- What concerns would you have if a patient on intravenous total parenteral nutrition reports a sudden occurrence of diarrhea? What if the flow is from an ileostomy rather than from the rectum?
- What concerns would you have if a patient being treated with gentamicin experienced a sudden onset of profuse watery diarrhea flecked with matter that looks like mucosa?

Patient Variables

Young and middle-age adults who are generally in good health can safely use antidiarrheal drugs on a short-term basis. Dehydration is less likely to occur in this age group than in young children and older adults. Diarrhea in infants, young children, and older adults can easily lead to serious fluid volume deficit. Furthermore, because glaucoma and prostatic hypertrophy are both common in older adults, combination drugs such as diphenoxylate with atropine must be used with caution.

Antidiarrheal drugs have limited value in pediatric patients, and there are concerns about possible toxicity. Although pediatric dosages for diphenoxylate with atropine and for loperamide are suggested, the World Health Organization does not recommend their use in children.

If diarrhea develops during pregnancy, it should be managed without drugs when possible. Use of opioids, which cause CNS depression, is particularly undesirable. In addition, bismuth subsalicylate should be avoided because of the salicylate component and the potential for bleeding.

Intervention

Administration

The frequency and consistency of stools and bowel sounds should be assessed before and periodically throughout the course of therapy. The risk of dependence on opioid antidiarrheal drugs increases with high-dose, long-term use. As discussed previously, subtherapeutic doses of atropine has been added to some agents to discourage abuse.

Opioid antidiarrheal drugs may be administered with food if GI upset occurs. The tablets may be crushed and administered with the patient's choice of food or fluids. If a liquid formulation is required, a calibrated measuring device should be used.

The patient can minimize the dry mouth that is associated with the atropine component of opioid antidiarrheal drugs by frequent mouth rinses, good oral hygiene, and the use of sugarless gum or candy.

Education

Because most acute diarrhea is self-limiting, the patient with no evidence of serious underlying disorders can be reassured and advised to concentrate on maintaining hydration. Sugar and electrolyte preparations are easy to take and should be encouraged. Many people think that taking fluids will worsen their diarrhea; therefore, they request opiates. The proper role of these agents should be discussed. In addition, the patient should be instructed as to the role of antibiotics and the emergence of resistant bacterial strains, the potential complications of antibiotic use, and the efficacy of antidiarrheal preparations.

Patients using opioid antidiarrheal drugs should be cautioned to take the drug exactly as directed and to avoid using alcohol or taking other CNS depressants concurrently with these drugs. Patients should not take more than the prescribed amount because of the habit-forming potential and the risk of overdose in children. If the patient is on a scheduled dosing regimen, missed doses should be taken as soon as possible unless it is almost time for the next dose. Double doses should not be taken. Patients should be advised to avoid driving or other activities that require alertness until his or her response to the drug is known. Patients should also be instructed to notify their health care provider if diarrhea persists or if fever, abdominal pain, or distention occurs.

Much can be done to relieve the perianal discomfort associated with diarrhea. Washing with warm water on absorbent cotton after each stool is helpful in lieu of using toilet paper, which can be irritating. Avoiding soap is important in order to prevent perianal irritation. A short course of hydrocortisone cream may be useful when there is considerable perianal irritation. Some patients report that cleansing gently with cotton pads soaked in witch hazel (TUCKS) provide considerable relief. The patient should be advised that ointments containing topical anesthetics should be avoided because they can be irritating in themselves.

After the diarrhea is relieved, it is usually best to have the patient avoid milk and dairy products for another 7 to 10 days because mild lactose intolerance commonly accompanies many cases of diarrhea. The best foods to consume are those that are easily digested, such as high-carbohydrate substances including rice, baked potato, toast, and applesauce. Continued replacement of fluid is important. Furthermore, once the underlying cause of the diarrhea has been identified, the patient should be advised to avoid the causative activity.

Evaluation

The therapeutic outcome of antidiarrheal treatment is relief of diarrhea. Treatment effectiveness is noted by the absence of abdominal cramping, flatulence, and other discomforts associated with diarrhea. However, if symptoms of acute diarrhea continue, fever persists, or blood or mucus appears in the stool, antidiarrheals should be discontinued and the patient re-evaluated. Patients who are unable to maintain oral hydration and who become significantly volume depleted (as evidenced by postural hypotension) require serious consideration for hospital admission and parenteral fluid replacement.

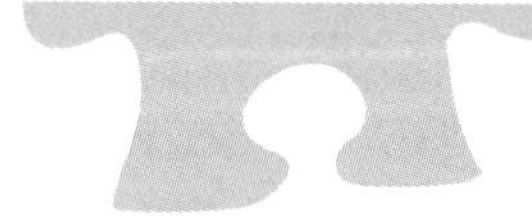

SUMMARY

- Constipation is the most frequent GI problem encountered in ambulatory care settings.
- Constipation is caused by factors such as inadequate fluid and fiber intake, lack of exercise, busy schedules with no established elimination patterns, excessive use of laxatives, and specific drugs.
- The fundamental mechanism of constipation involves the decreased transit time of stool through the colon, along with increased reabsorption of fluid.
- Patient assessment should include information about the patient's usual elimination patterns, activity levels, concomitant disease, and drug use.
- The primary treatment goal for constipation is to re-establish a normal pattern of bowel functioning and to effect comfortable elimination of the stool using the least number of drugs in the lowest dosages for the shortest duration of time.
- Treatment modalities include correction of underlying conditions that may be causing constipation, patient education, and nondrug therapies.
- When drugs are required to treat or manage constipation, they may fall into one or more of the following categories: stimulants, stool softeners, bulk-forming agents, osmotics, lubricants, and a few miscellaneous agents.

- Enteric-coated laxatives should not be taken within 1 hour of drinking milk or taking antacids. Other laxatives should not be taken by patients who abuse alcohol.
- All laxatives should be taken with a full glass of water to promote emptying of the laxative from the stomach, to promote elimination, and to reduce the potential for impaction.
- Oil-based laxatives should not be given to bedridden patients or children because of the possibility of lipid pneumonia should the patient aspirate.
- Patients should be advised that most laxatives are for short-term use only.
- Clinical response to treatment can be demonstrated by the passage of a soft, formed bowel movement, usually within 12 to 24 hours. However, normal bowel patterns are individually determined and may vary from three times a day to three times weekly.
- Diarrhea is a symptom of an underlying disorder and affects most people at some point during their lifetime. It can be caused by bacterial, viral infection, or parasitic infestation. An important cause of diarrhea is the concealed use of stimulant laxatives.
- Diarrhea results from any factor that decreases fluid absorption in the bowel, increases fluid secretion, alters bowel motility, or is associated with mucosal injury.
- The primary treatment goal for diarrhea is to re-establish a normal pattern of bowel functioning using the least number of drugs in the lowest dosages for the shortest duration of time.
- The mainstay of nonspecific drug therapy for diarrhea continues to be opioids. Bismuth subsalicylate has been used to treat traveler's diarrhea with some success.
- Miscellaneous remedies for diarrhea include anticholinergics, cholestyramine, kaolin and pectin formulations, *Lactobacillus acidophilus,* and tincture of opium, although these drugs are not generally considered first-line agents.
- The risk of dependency on opioids increases with high-dose, long-term use. Subtherapeutic doses of atropine have been added to some formulations to discourage abuse.
- Patients should be advised to take the drug exactly as directed and to avoid concurrent use of alcohol and other CNS depressants.
- Care of the patient with diarrhea is also directed toward relieving fluid and electrolyte imbalances, perianal irritation, and re-occurrence of the diarrhea.
- Treatment effectiveness of antidiarrheal drugs is noted by the absence of abdominal cramping, flatulence, and other discomforts associated with diarrhea.

BIBLIOGRAPHY

Alpers, D., Greenburg, J., and Sodeman, W. (1990). Gastroenteritis treatment tips. *Patient Care,* 24(6), 18–31.

Evans, K. (1990). Pediatric management problems: Chronic constipation. *Pediatric Nursing,* 16(6), 590–591.

Fluoire, B., Briet, F., and Florent, C. (1993). Can diarrhea induced by lactulose be reduced by prolonged ingestion of lactulose? *American Journal of Clinical Nutrition,* 58(3), 369–375.

Goroll, A., May, L., and Mulley, A. (1995). *Primary care medicine* (3rd ed.). Philadelphia: J.B. Lippincott.

Harori, D., Gurivity, J., Avorn, J., et al. (1994). Constipation: Assessment and management in an institutional elderly population. *Journal of the American Geriatrics Society,* 42(9), 947–952.

Heather, D., Howell, L., Montana, M., et al. (1991). Effect of bulk forming cathartic on diarrhea in tube-fed patients. *Heart and Lung,* 20(4), 409–413.

Montaner, J. S. (1995). Octreotide therapy in AIDS-related, refractory diarrhea: Results of a multicenter Canadian-European study. *AIDS,* 9(2), 209–210.

Murtagh, J. (1992). Diarrhea. *Australian Family Physician,* 21(5), 668–673.

Pon, D., and Dong, B. (1990). Octreotide use in AIDS. *DICP: The Annals of Pharmacotherapy,* 24(10), 951–952.

Shafik, A. (1991). Editorial: Constipation—some provocative thoughts. *Journal of Clinical Gastroenterology,* 13(3), 259–267.

Siegel, D., Edelstein, P., and Nachamkin, I. (1990). Inappropriate testing for diarrheal diseases in the hospital. *Journal of the American Medical Association,* 263(7), 979–982.

Steffan, R. (1990). Worldwide efficacy of bismuth subsalicylate in the treatment of traveler's diarrhea. *Reviews of Infectious Diseases,* 12(Suppl 1), S80–S86.

Stein, J. (1994). *Internal medicine* (4th ed.). St. Louis: Mosby–Year Book, Inc.

Talley, N., Weaver, A., Zinmeister, A., et al. (1993). Functional constipation and outlet delay: A population based study. *Gastroenterology,* 105(3), 781–790.

Tierney, L., McPhee, S., and Papadakis, M. (1997). *Current medical diagnosis and treatment* (36th ed.). Norwalk, CN: Appleton-Lange.

Turnbull, G., and Ritvo, P. (1992). Anal sphincter biofeedback relaxation treatment for women with intractable constipation syndromes. *Diseases of the Colon and Rectum,* 35(6), 530–535.

Wadle, K. (1990). Diarrhea. *Nursing Clinics of North America,* 25(4), 901–908.

Williams, S., and DiPalma, J. (1990). Constipation in the long-term care facility. *Gastroenterology Nursing,* 12(3), 179–182.

Yakabowich, M. (1990). Prescribe with care: The role of laxatives in the treatment of constipation. *Journal of Gerontological Nursing,* 16(7), 4–11.

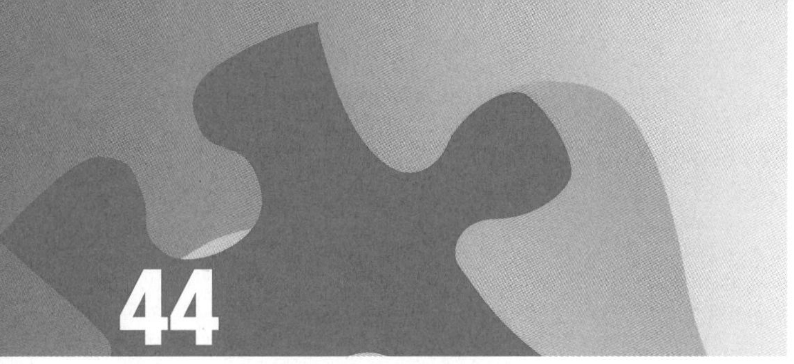

44 Antiemetic Drugs

Vomiting, often accompanied by the sensation of nausea, is the most commonly experienced phenomena related to disordered gastric motility. Nausea and vomiting are symptoms of a great many stimuli that range from overindulgence in rich and abundant food to drugs, toxins, inflammation or infection, vestibular disorders, psychogenic causes, and metabolic derangements. Treatment goals associated with the use of antiemetics include preventing or relieving the symptoms associated with the emetogenic event. Use of medication also seeks to avoid potentially life-threatening complications such as electrolyte imbalances, dehydration, and malnutrition.

NAUSEA AND VOMITING

Epidemiology and Etiology

Nausea and vomiting are common and may accompany almost any illness or stressful situation. *Nausea* is defined as an unpleasant sensation of impending vomiting. *Vomiting* is defined as the forceful expulsion of stomach contents. Sporadic cases of nausea and vomiting are fairly common, but epidemic occurrences suggest environmental exposure to viral or bacterial infections or food poisoning (e.g., staphylococcal enterotoxin).

Nausea and vomiting are also the most common adverse reactions to drug therapy. Although nausea and vomiting may occur with most drugs it is especially associated with alcohol, aspirin, opioids, antibiotics, cardiac glycosides, antineoplastic therapy, and theophylline drugs. Table 44–1 provides an overview of the most common causes of nausea and vomiting.

Pathophysiology

Vomiting is a reflex under central nervous system (CNS) control. It occurs when pathologic processes stimulate the vomiting center located in the medulla (Fig. 44–1). The vomiting center receives input from the sympathetic nervous system and cerebral cortex, the limbic system, vestibular system, and the chemoreceptor trigger zone (CTZ). Distention of the stomach, duodenum, colon, or biliary ducts from motility disorders or obstruction sends impulses to the vomiting center via the peripheral afferent of the vagus nerve. Irritation, inflammation, or cardiac, pericardial, or gastrointestinal (GI) tract ischemia can stimulate the vomiting center. Vestibular dysfunction sends impulses to the vomiting center by way of vestibular nerve connections.

The CTZ, located on the floor of the 4th ventricle, is rich in dopamine, opiate, and serotonin receptors. It is stimulated by metabolic derangements (electrolyte disorders, diabetic ketoacidosis, uremia), drugs (glycosides, antineoplastics, opiates), and toxins circulating in the blood and cerebral spinal fluid. When it is stimulated, the vomiting center initiates efferent impulses that cause a sequence of events. The glottis closes, and there is contraction of the diaphragm and abdominal muscles. The gastroesophageal sphincter relaxes and reverse peristalsis moves stomach contents upward toward the mouth for expulsion.

PHARMACOTHERAPEUTIC OPTIONS

Drugs used in the management of nausea and vomiting fall into several different drug classifications, including antihistamines, phenothiazines, prokinetic drugs, cannabinoids, serotonin antagonists, and a variety of miscellaneous agents. Benzodiazepines and corticosteroids are also used in the management of nausea and vomiting. Most of the antiemetics produce anticholinergic and antidopaminergic effects.

Antihistamines

- ❒ Cyclizine
- ❒ Dimenhydrinate (DRAMAMINE)
- ❒ Diphenhydramine (BENADRYL)
- ❒ Hydroxyzine (VISTARIL, ATARAX)
- ❒ Meclizine (ANTIVERT, ANTRIZINE, RU-VERT-M, BONINE); (🍁) BONAMINE, ANTIVERT

Indications

Antihistamines are used most often in the management of nausea and vomiting associated with motion sickness. Some antihistamines, such as diphenhydramine, are used in the management of insomnia, Parkinson-like reactions, and some nonallergic conditions. The use of antihistamines for symptom relief associated with allergies, including rhinitis, urticaria, and angioedema, is discussed in Chapter 47.

Pharmacodynamics

The ability of antihistamines to suppress nausea and vomiting is related to their ability to block the action of acetylcholine in the brain. Thus, they are also classified as anticholinergics (see Chapter 13). Not all antihistamines are effective as antiemetics, however. There is no correlation between their ability to prevent motion sickness and their potency as antihistamines or anticholinergics. Nevertheless, the mechanism by which they suppress motion sickness is unclear.

Adverse Effects and Contraindications

The most significant adverse effect of antihistamines is sedation. In addition, these drugs produce typical anticholinergic effects such as dry mouth, blurred vision, and urinary retention.

Antihistamines are contraindicated in hypersensitivity, narrow-angle glaucoma, and premature or newborn infants. Older adults are more susceptible to the anticholinergic ef-

TABLE 44–1 DISORDERS ASSOCIATED WITH NAUSEA AND VOMITING

Category	Disorders	
Gastrointestinal tract inflammation or infection	Appendicitis	Cholecystitis
	Cholelithiasis	Hepatitis
	Pancreatitis	Peptic ulcer disease
	Reye's syndrome	Postgastrectomy states
	Pyelonephritis	
Motility disorders	Gastroduodenal motor dysfunction	
	Gastroparesis (autonomic neuropathy)	
	Postvagotomy states	
Gastrointestinal obstruction	Achalasia	Gastric outlet obstruction
	Incarcerated hernia	Small bowel obstruction
	Volvulus	
Vestibular disorders	Labyrinthitis	Ménière's disease
	Motion sickness	
Increased intracranial pressure	Meningitis	
	Space-occupying lesions	
Metabolic derangements	Adrenal insufficiency	Diabetic ketoacidosis
	Thyrotoxicosis	Uremia
	Electrolyte imbalances	
Psychogenic vomiting	Eating disorders	Physical or sexual abuse
	Post-traumatic stress disorder	
Toxins	Staphylococcal enterotoxin	
Drugs	Aspirin, NSAIDs	Bromocriptine
	Cisplatin	Cyclophosphamide
	Carboplatin	Dacarbazine
	Digoxin	Doxorubicin
	Erythromycin	Ifosfamide
	Levodopa	Lithium
	NSAIDs	Nitrofurantoin
	Opioids	Phenytoin
	Tetracycline	Theophylline
	Quinidine	
Others	Motion sickness	Pain
	Unpleasant sights, sounds	

NSAIDs, Nonsteroidal anti-inflammatory drugs.

fects of antihistamines. These drugs should also be used cautiously in patients with pyloric obstruction, prostatic hypertrophy, hyperthyroidism, cardiovascular disease, or severe liver disease. Cautious use in pregnancy is advised.

Pharmacokinetics

Table 44–2 illustrates the pharmacokinetics of the various GI-related antihistamines. The antihistamines are well absorbed when they are taken orally and distributed throughout body fluids and tissues. The majority are taken orally with onset times of 15 to 60 minutes. Peak activity occurs in 1 to 4 hours with a 3- to 8-hour duration. The protein binding of the majority of the drugs is unavailable. The half-lives vary from 2 to 7 hours. The drugs are biotransformed in the liver and eliminated in the urine.

Drug-Drug Interactions

There are several drug-drug interactions possible with antihistamines (Table 44–3). Additive sedation is possible when they are used with other CNS depressants, including alcohol, antidepressants, opioid analgesics, and sedative-hypnotics. Monoamine oxidase inhibitors prolong and intensify the anticholinergic effects of antihistamines. Erythromycin, clarithromycin, ketoconazole, and itraconazole increase the risk of serious arrhythmias, particularly with astemizole and terfenadine.

Dosage Regimen

The dosage regimens for antihistamines when they are used for nausea and vomiting are identified in Table 44–4. Because most are used in the management of motion sickness, a single dose is often all that is required. Occasionally, dosing three to four times a day may be appropriate. When used for prophylaxis of motion sickness, they should be administered at least 30 minutes and preferably 1 to 2 hours before exposure to conditions that precipitate the nausea and vomiting.

Laboratory Considerations

Dimenhydrinate and meclizine cause false-negative skin tests in the presence of antihistamines. Dimenhydrinate should be discontinued 72 hours before any skin testing, whereas diphenhydramine would need to be discontinued 4 days before testing.

Phenothiazines

- ❐ Chlorpromazine (THORAZINE); (✱) CHLORPROMANYL, LARGACTIL, NOVO-CHLORPROMAZINE
- ❐ Perphenazine (TRILAFON)
- ❐ Prochlorperazine (COMPAZINE)
- ❐ Promethazine (ANERGAN, PENTAZINE, PHENAZINE, PHENCEN-50, PHENERGAN, PROREX, PROTHAZINE
- ❐ Thiethylperazine (TORECAN)

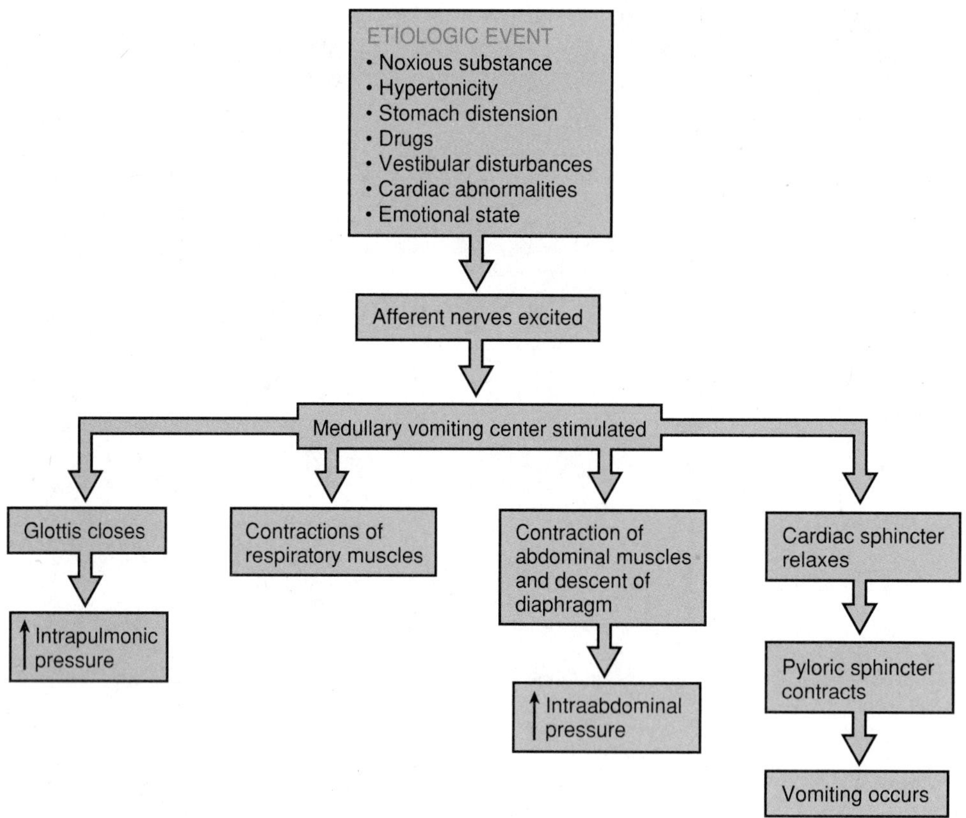

Figure 44–1 The vomiting center receives input from the sympathetic nervous system and cerebral cortex, the limbic system, vestibular system, and the chemoreceptor trigger zone (CTZ). Distention of the stomach, duodenum, colon, or biliary ducts from motility disorders or obstruction sends impulses to the vomiting center via the peripheral afferent of the vagus nerve.

Indications

Phenothiazines are used most often to suppress nausea and vomiting associated with antineoplastic therapy, radiation therapy, and toxins. The basic discussion of phenothiazines is found in Chapter 19. Promethazine is the most effective drug for motion sickness prophylaxis. Unfortunately, the sedating effect of the drug limits its usefulness.

Pharmacodynamics

The phenothiazines suppress nausea and vomiting by blockade of dopamine receptors in the CTZ. To varying degrees, these drugs also produce blockade of acetylcholine (muscarinic), histamine, and norepinephrine receptors. There is little question that blockade of these receptors is responsible for the major adverse effects of the phenothiazines.

Adverse Effects and Contraindications

Phenothiazines produce a variety of serious adverse effects. These include extrapyramidal reactions such as pseudoparkinsonism, dystonia, akathisia, and tardive dyskinesia. Other adverse effects include those related to anticholinergic actions, hypotension, and sedation. Further, phenothiazines may mask diagnostic symptoms of acute surgical conditions or neurologic syndromes. Opacities of the lens may develop with extended use of chlorpromazine. Agranulocytosis occurs 4 to 10 weeks after initiation of therapy, with recovery occurring 1 to 2 weeks following discontinuation. However, agranulocytosis may reappear if chlorpromazine therapy is restarted. Liver function abnormalities may warrant discontinuation of therapy. Chronic therapy with promethazine requires periodic evaluation of the complete blood count because blood dyscrasias may occur.

Pharmacokinetics

The pharmacokinetics of phenothiazines are identified in Table 44–2. In the majority of cases, onset occurs 30 minutes to 1 hour when the drugs are taken by mouth, with more rapid action noted when they are taken by other routes. Most phenothiazines are over 90-percent protein bound. Peak action times are unknown.

Drug-Drug Interactions

Drug-drug interactions of phenothiazines with other drugs are numerous and are identified in Table 44–3. For the most part, drug-drug interactions are of a wide variety, with each interacting drug producing somewhat distinct effects.

Dosage Regimen

The dosage regimens for selected phenothiazines when used as antiemetics are identified in Table 44–4. When comparing dosage requirements, potency is compared with that of 100 mg of chlorpromazine. Overall, low-potency phenothiazines (e.g., chlorpromazine) are more likely to pro-

TABLE 44–2 PHARMACOKINETICS OF SELECTED ANTIEMETIC DRUGS

Drug	Route	Onset	Peak	Duration	PB (%)	$t_{1/2}$
Antihistamines						
Cyclizine	po	UK	UK	4–6 hr	UK	UK
Dimenhydrinate	po	15–60 min	1–2 hr	3–6 hr	UA	UK
	po ER	UK	UK	To 12 hr		
	IM	20–30 min	1–2 hr	3–6 hr		
	IV	Rapid	UK	3–6 hr		
Diphenhydramine	po	15–60 min	1–4 hr	4–8 hr	98–99	2.4–7 hr
	IM	20–30 min	1–4 hr	4–8 hr		
	IM	Rapid	UK	4–8 hr		
Hydroxyzine	po	15–30 min	2–4 hr	4–6 hr	UA	3 hr
	IM	15–30 min	2–4 hr	4–6 hr		
Meclizine	po	60 min	UK	8–24 hr	UA	6 hr
Phenothiazines						
Chlorpromazine	po	30–60 min	UK	4–6 hr	>90	30 hr
	ER po	30–60 min	UK	10–12 hr		
	PR	1–2 hr	UK	3–4 hr		
	IM	UK	UK	4–8 hr		
	IV	Rapid	UK	UK		
Fluphenazine	po	60 min	UK	6–8 hr	> 90	Varies*
	IM	1 hr; 24–72 hr†	1.5–2 hr; UK	6–8 hr; 1–4 wk		
Perphenazine	po/IM	2–6 hr	UK	6–12 hr	>90	UK
	IV	Rapid	UK	UK		
Prochlorperazine	ER po	30–40 min	UK	10–12 hr	>90	UK
	PR	60 min	UK	3–4 hr		
	IM	10–20 min	10–30 min	3–4 hr		
	IV	Rapid	10–30 min	3–4 hr		
Promethazine	po PR, IM	10 min	UK	12 hr	65–90	UK
	IV	3–5 min	UK	12 hr		
Thiethylperazine	po	30 min	UK	UK	UA	UK
	IM/PR	UK	UK	UK	UA	UA
Prokinetic Drugs						
Cisapride	po	30–60 min	70 min	UK	97.5	8–10 hr
Metoclopramide	po	30–60 min	UK	1–2 hr	30	2.5–5 hr
	IM	10–15 min	UK	1–2 hr		
	IV	1–3 min	Immed	1–2 hr		
Cannabinoids						
Dronabinol	po	UK	2 hr	4–6 hr	97–99	25–36 hr
Nabilone	po	UK	2 hr	4–6 hr		
Serotonin Antagonists						
Granisetron	po	Rapid	60 min	To 12 hr	UA	0.9–31.1 hr‡
	IV	Rapid	30 min	To 24 hr		
Ondansetron	po/IV	Rapid	15–30 min	4 hr	70–76	3.5–5.5 hr
Miscellaneous						
Benzquinamide	IM	15 min	30 min	3–4 min	58	30–40 min
	IV	15 min	UK	3–4 hr		
Diphenidol	po	15 min	1.5–3 hr	3–4 hr	UA	4 hr
Droperidol	IM/IV	3–10 min	30 min	2–4 hr §	UA	2.2 hr
Trimethobenzamide	po	30–50 min	UA	3–4 hr	UA	UA
	PR	10–40 min	UK	3–4 hr		
	IM	15–35 min	UK	2–3 hr		
Scopolamine	po/IM/SC	30 min	60 min	4–6 hr	Low	8 hr
	Patch	4 hr	UK	72 hr		
	IV	10 min	1 hr	2–4 hr		
Corticosteroid						
Dexamethasone	po	UK	1–2 hr	2.75 days	65–71	3–4.5 hr
Dexamethasone phosphate	IM/IV	Rapid	UK	2.75 days		
Dexamethasone acetate	IM	UK	8 hr	6 days		

*The half-life of fluphenazine varies with the formulation: The half-life of fluphenazine HCl is 4.7 to 15.3 hours; fluphenazine enanthate, 3.7 days; and fluphenazine decanoate, 6.8 to 9.6 days.

†Onset and duration times for fluphenazine also vary with the specific formulation.

‡The half-life of granisetron in patients with cancer is 8 to 9 hours, with range of 0.9 to 31.1 hours; in healthy individuals, the half-life is 4.9 hours, with a range of 0.9 to 15.2 hours; in geriatric patients, the half-life is 7.7 hours, with a range of 2.6 to 17.7 hours.

§Droperidol listed as duration of tranquilization effects; alterations in consciousness may last up to 12 hours.

PB, Protein binding; $t_{1/2}$, elimination half-life; NA, not applicable; UA, unavailable; UK, unknown.

TABLE 44–3 DRUG-DRUG INTERATIONS OF SELECTED ANTIEMETIC DRUGS

Drug	Interactive Drugs	Interaction
Antihistamines		
Dimenhydrinate	Alcohol	Additive CNS depression
Diphenhydramine	Antihistamines	
Hydroxyzine	Opioids	
	Sedative-hypnotics	
Phenothiazines		
Chlorpromazine	Alcohol	Additive hypotension
Perphenazine	Antihypertensives	
Prochlorperazine	Nitrates	
Thiethylperazine	CNS depressants	Additive CNS depression
Trifluoperazine	Phenobarbital	Decreased effectiveness of chlorpromazine
	Lithium	Increased risk of lithium toxicity
	Absorbent antidiarrheals	Decreased absorption of chlorpromazine
	Antacids	
	Antithyroid drugs	Increased risk of agranulocytosis
	Bromocriptine	Decreased antiparkinson activity
	Levodopa	
	Epinephrine	Decreased vasomotor response
	Norepinephrine	
	Guanethidine	Decreased antihypertensive effects
	Beta blockers	Increased response to chlorpromazine
	Antihistamines	Increased anticholinergic effects
	Disopyramide	
	Quinidine	
	Tricyclic antidepressants	
Prokinetic Drugs		
Cisapride	Anticholinergics	Decreased effects of cisapride
	Alcohol	Accelerates sedative effects
	Benzodiazepines	
	Warfarin	Increased effects of warfarin
	Cimetidine	Increased plasma levels of cisapride
		Accelerated absorption of interactive drugs
	Ranitidine	
	Itraconazole	Increased blood levels and risk of arrhythmias
	Ketoconazole	
Metoclopramide	Alcohol	Additive CNS depression
	Antidepressants	
	Antihistamines	
	General anesthetics	
	Opioids	
	Sedative-hypnotics	
	Insulin	Diabetics may require insulin adjustment
	Haloperidol	Increased risk of extrapyramidal effects
	Phenothiazines	
	Anticholinergics	May antagonize GI effects of metoclopramide
	Opioids	
	Cyclosporine	Increased risk of toxicity to cyclosporine
	MAO inhibitors	Causes catecholamine release
	Succinylcholine	Increased risk of neuromuscular blockade
Cannabinoids		
Dronabinol	Alcohol	Additive CNS depression
Nabilone	Antihistamines	
	Opioids	
	Tricyclic antidepressants	
	Sedative-hypnotics	
	Amphetamines	Increased risk of tachycardia
	Cocaine	
	Sympathomimetics	
	Anticholinergics	
	Antihistamines	
	Tricyclic antidepressants	
Serotonin Antagonists		
Granisetron	Phenothiazines and other drugs causing extrapyramidal reactions	Increased risk of extrapyramidal reactions
Miscellaneous		
Benzquinamide	Alcohol	Additive CNS depression
Diphenidol	Antihistamines	

TABLE 44–3 DRUG-DRUG INTERATIONS OF SELECTED ANTIEMETIC DRUGS *Continued*

Drug	Interactive Drugs	Interaction
Miscellaneous *Continued*		
	Opioids	
	Sedative-hypnotics	
	Epinephrine	May cause hypertension
	Vasopressors	
Droperidol	Antihypertensives	Additive hypotension
	Nitrates	
	Alcohol	Additive CNS depression
	Antihistamines	
	Antidepressants	
	Opioids	
	Sedative-hypnotics	
Trimethobenzamide	Alcohol	Additive CNS depression
Scopolamine	Antihistamines	
	Antidepressants	
	Opioids	
	Sedative-hypnotics	
Scopolamine	Antihistamines	Additive anticholinergic effects
	Antidepressants	
	Disopyramide	
	Quinidine	

CNS, Central nervous system; GI, gastrointestinal; MAO, monoamine oxidase.

duce sedative and orthostatic hypotension and less likely to produce early extrapyramidal effects. Medium-potency phenothiazines (e.g., perphenazine) vary in their ability to produce sedation and extrapyramidal effects. High-potency phenothiazines are most likely to produce extrapyramidal effects and least likely to cause sedation and orthostatic hypotension.

Laboratory Considerations

There are several laboratory considerations with phenothiazines. Complete blood count, liver function tests, and ocular exams should be performed periodically throughout the course of therapy. Lens opacities may develop with extended use of chlorpromazine.

Chlorpromazine causes decreased hematocrit, hemoglobin, leukocytes, granulocytes, and platelet values. It may cause elevated bilirubin, alanine aminotransferase (ALT; serum glutamic-pyruvic transaminase [SGPT]), aspartate aminotransferase (AST; serum glutamic-oxaloacetic transaminase [SGOT]), and alkaline phosphatase values. Phenothiazines may also cause false-positive or false-negative pregnancy tests and false-positive urine bilirubin test results.

Thiethylperazine may cause false-positive or false-negative pregnancy tests. It also causes increased prolactin levels and interferes with gonadorelin test results.

Prokinetic Drugs

❒ Cisapride (PROPULSID)
❒ Metoclopramide (REGLAN); (✽) MAXERAN

Indications

Prokinetic drugs are helpful in treating motility disorders such as gastroparesis associated with diabetic autonomic neuropathy and postvagotomy states. They are also indicated in the management of esophageal reflux and in the treatment and prevention of postoperative nausea and vomiting when nasogastric suctioning is undesirable.

Metoclopramide is the drug of choice for suppressing nausea and vomiting related to highly emetic antineoplastic drugs (e.g., cisplatin, dacarbazine). It has also been used in the treatment of hiccoughs with some success, although it has not been approved by the Food and Drug Administration (FDA) for such use.

Cisapride is effective in treating GI reflux and gastroparesis. In addition, it is useful in the treatment of patients with chronic idiopathic constipation or with colonic hypomotility due to spinal cord injury.

Pharmacodynamics

Metoclopramide blocks dopamine receptors in the CTZ, thereby suppressing nausea and vomiting and increasing upper GI motility by enhancing the actions of acetylcholine. Although it is structurally related to procainamide (see Chapter 33), an antiarrhythmic drug, metoclopramide lacks significant local anesthetic or antiarrhythmic actions. In the GI tract it enhances motility of smooth muscle from the esophagus through the proximal small bowel, and accelerates gastric emptying and the transit of intestinal contents from the duodenum to the ileocecal valve.

Like metoclopramide, cisapride appears to enhance the release of acetylcholine at the nerve endings in the myenteric plexus. However, unlike metoclopramide, cisapride has no dopamine antagonist properties and, therefore, fewer adverse effects. However, because it increases colonic motility, it can cause diarrhea.

Adverse Effects and Contraindications

Sedation and diarrhea are common with high doses of metoclopramide. Although metoclopramide does not have useful antipsychotic effects, it can cause significant extrapyramidal symptoms, especially at high doses and espe-

TABLE 44–4 DOSAGE REGIMEN FOR SELECTED ANTIEMETIC DRUGS

Drug	Use(s)	Dosage	Implications
Antihistamines			
Cyclizine	Motion sickness, prophylaxis postoperative vomiting	*Adult:* for motion sickness, 50 mg po q4–6 hr PRN. Not to exceed 200 mg/day. For postoperative vomiting, 50 mg IM 30 min before termination of surgery, then q4–6 hr PRN	Administer IM in deep well-developed muscle. Avoid inadvertent IV administration
Dimenhydrinate	Motion sickness	*Adult:* 50 mg po/IM/IV q4hr starting 1–2 hr before departure *or* 25 mg extended release capsules po q12 hr *or* 50–100 mg PR q6–8 hr PRN. Dosage not to exceed 400 mg/day *Child 6–12 yr:* 25–50 mg po q6–8hr. Not to exceed 150 mg/day *Child:* 6–8 yr: 12.5–25 mg PR q8–12hr PRN *Child 8–12 yr:* 25–50 mg PR q8–12hr PRN *Child > 12 yr:* 50 mg PR q8–12hr PRN	Use calibrated measuring device when administering liquid dose. Administer at least 30 minutes before and preferably 1 to 2 hours before exposure to conditions that may precipitate motion sickness
Diphenhydramine	Motion sickness	*Adult:* 25–50 mg po q4–6hr *or* 10–50 mg IM/IV q2–3hr PRN. May need up to 100 mg but doses should not exceed 400 mg/day. *Child:* 1–1.5 mg/kg po q4–6hr PRN. Not to exceed 300 mg/day *or* 1.25 mg/kg (37.5 mg/m^2) IM/IV 4 times daily. Not to exceed 300 mg/day	Administer at least 30 minutes before and preferably 1–2 hours before exposure to conditions that may precipitate motion sickness. Administer IM injections into well-developed muscle. Avoid SC injections
Hydroxyzine	Antiemetic	*Adult:* 25–100 mg po/IM TID–QID. *Child:* 0.5 mg/kg (15 mg/m^2) po q6hr PRN *or* 1 mg/kg (30 mg/m^2) IM *Child < 6 yr:* 12.5 mg po q6hr PRN *Child age 6–12 yr:* 12.5–25 mg q6hr PRN	Administer IM injections into well-developed muscle using Z-track technique. Do not use deltoid site. Tissue damage may occur from SC or intra-arterial injections
Meclizine	Motion sickness	*Adults:* 25–50 mg po 60 min before exposure. May repeat in 24 hours	May cause drowsiness. Avoid concurrent use of alcohol or other CNS depressants
Phenothiazines			
Chlorpromazine	Antiemetic	*Adults:* 10–25 mg po q4h PRN *or* 50–100 mg PR q6–8 hr PRN *or* 25 mg IM initially, then 25–50 mg IM q3–4 hr PRN *or* up to 25 mg IV *Child > 6 mo:* 0.55 mg/kg (15 mg/m^2) po q4–6hr PRN *or* 1 mg/kg PR q6–8 hr PRN	Keep patient recumbent for at least 30 minutes following parenteral administration to minimize hypotensive effects
Perphenazine	Antiemetic	*Adults:* 8–16 mg/day po in divided doses. Not to exceed 24 mg/day *or* 5 mg IM initially, may be increased to 10 mg if needed *or* 1 mg IV at 1–2 min intervals to a total of 5 mg *or* as an infusion at a rate not to exceed 1 mg/min	Dilute concentrate before administration in water, milk, carbonated bevereage, soup, or tomato or fruit juice. Do not mix with beverages containing caffeine, tannics, or pectinates. Inject deep IM into well-developed muscle
Prochlorperazine	Antiemetic	*Adults & child > 12 yr:* 5–10 mg po TID–QID. May be increased q2–3 days up to 40 mg/day *or* 5–10 mg IM q3–4 hr PRN *or* 25 mg PR BID *Child 9–13 kg:* 2.5 mg po/PR QD–BID, not to exceed 7.5 mg/day *Child 14–17 kg:* 2.5 mg po BID–TID, not to exceed 10 mg/day *or* 2.5 mg PR BID–TID not to exceed 10 mg/day *Child 18–39 kg:* 2.5 mg po/PR TID *or* 5 mg BID not to exceed 15 mg/day	Administer with full glass of water to minimize gastric irritation. Inject deep IM into well-developed muscle. Dilute syrup in citrus or chocolate-flavored drinks
Promethazine	Motion sickness; treatment and prevention of nausea and vomiting	*Adult:* 25 mg po 30–60 min prior to departure for motion sickness. May be repeated in 8–12 hours. For antiemetic effects, 10–25 mg po/PR/IM/IV q4hr PRN. Initial po dose should be 25 mg *Child > 2 yrs:* 10–25 mg (0.5 mg/kg) 30–60 min before departure for motion sickness. May be given BID. For antiemetic effects, 0.25–0.5 mg/kg (7.5–15 mg/m^2) q4–6 hr *or* 12.5–25 mg po/PR/IM q4–6 hr	Administer with food or milk to minimize GI irritation. Tablets may be crushed and mixed with food or fluids for patients with difficulty swallowing. IM routes should be given into well-developed muscles. SC administration can cause tissue necrosis. Rapid IV administration can cause transient hypotension
Thiethylperazine	Antiemetic	*Adults:* 10 mg po/PR/IM QD–TID	Inject deep IM into well-developed muscle. Keep patient recumbent for at least 60 minutes following injection to minimize hypotensive effects. May cause severe hypotension if inadvertently given IV

TABLE 44–4 DOSAGE REGIMEN FOR SELECTED ANTIEMETIC DRUGS *Continued*

Drug	Use(s)	Dosage	Implications
Prokinetic Drugs			
Cisapride	Diabetic autonomic neuropathy, pseudo-obstruction	*Adults:* 10 mg QID 15 min ac and HS. May be increased to 20 mg QID. Other regimens include 5 mg TID, 10 mg BID, *or* 20 mg at HS	Instruct patient to take cisapride as directed even if feeling better.
Metoclopramide	Antineoplastic-induced nausea and vomiting	*Adults:* 1–2 mg/kg IV 30 min before treatment. Additional doses of 1–2 mg/kg may be given q2hr × 2 doses, then q3hr for 3 additional doses *Child:* 0.1–0.2 mg/kg/dose 30 min before meals and HS	IV doses should be given slowly over 1–2 minutes. Rapid infusion causes transient but intense anxiety and restlessness followed by drowsiness
	Diabetic autonomic neuropathy	*Adults:* 10 mg po 30 minutes ac and HS *or* 25 mg PR 30–60 min ac and HS.	Suppositories may be made by the pharmacist
	Postoperative nausea and vomiting	*Adults:* 10–20 mg IM	Administer near the end of surgery
Cannabinoids			
Dronabinol	Antineoplastic-induced nausea and vomiting	*Adults & Child:* 5–7.5 mg/m^2 po 1–3 hr before treatment then q2–4hr after treatment with 4–6 daily doses. Not to exceed 15 mg/m^2	Dronabinol capsules should be kept refrigerated but not frozen. Do not double doses
	Appetite stimulate in patients with AIDS	*Adults:* 2.5 mg po BID before lunch and dinner to maximum of 20 mg in divided doses	Once-daily dosing is recommended if patient is intolerant to BID regimen
Nabilone	Recalcitrant antineoplastic-induced nausea and vomiting	*Adults:* 1–2 mg po TID–QID PRN	Patients on cannabinoid therapy should be monitored closely for adverse effects because drug effects vary with each patient
Serotonin Antagonists			
Granisetron	Antineoplastic-induced nausea and vomiting	*Adults:* 1 mg po BID. First dose given at least 60 minutes prior to treatment and second dose 12 hours after the first *Adults & Children 2–16 years:* 10 mcg IV within 30 minutes of treatment	Administered only on days antineoplastic treatment is given. Single dose provides 24 hour antiemetic effects in most cases
Ondansetron		*Adults and child > 12 years:* 8 mg po 30 minutes before treatment and repeated 8 hours later then 8 mg q12 hr × 1–2 days PRN *or* 0.15 mg/kg IV 15–30 minutes prior to treatment, and q4hr × 2 doses *or* until N/V subside *or* 32 mg single dose 30 minutes before treatment *Child > 3 years:* 0.15 mg/kg IV 15–30 minutes before treatment, repeated 4 and 8 hours later *Child 4–11 years:* 4 mg po 30 minutes prior to treatment, and repeated 4 and 8 hours later—4 mg po q8hr may be given for 1–2 days following treatment	First dose should be administered before emetogenic event. Administer each dose as IV infusion over 15 minutes. Administer direct IV over 2–5 minutes
	Prophylactic postoperative nausea and vomiting	*Adults:* 4 mg IV before induction of anesthesia or postoperative	
Miscellaneous			
Benzquinamide	Prevention and treatment of nausea and vomiting associated with anesthesia and surgery	*Adults:* 50 mg (0.5–1.0 mg/kg) IM *or* 0.2–0.4 mg/kg IV. May repeat dose in 1 hour. Dosages may be repeated every 3–4 hours as needed	May be administered prophylactically at least 15 minutes before emergency from anesthesia. IM route is preferred due to arrhythmias resulting from IV use
Diphenidol	Nausea and vomiting	*Adults:* 25–50 mg po q4hr PRN *Child > 23 kg.:* 25 mg po q4hr PRN. Not to exceed 5.5 mg/kg/day	To be used only under close supervision. Observe for confusion, hallucinations
Droperidol	Postoperative and postprocedure nausea and vomiting (not FDA approved)	*Adults:* 0.5–1 mg IV q4hr PRN	Monitor BP and pulse frequently throughout course of therapy. Observe for extrapyramidal symptoms
Trimethobenzamide	Management of mild to moderate nausea and vomiting	*Adults:* 250 mg po TID–QID *or* 200 mg PR TID–QID *or* 200 mg IM TID–QID *Child 30–90 lbs:* 100–200 mg po TID–QID *or* 100–200 mg PR TID–QID *Child < 30 lbs:* 100 mg PR TID–QID	IM injections may cause pain, stinging, burning, redness, and swelling at site of injection. Give IM in gluteal region using Z-track technique. Avoid use in children who may have a viral illness (Reye's syndrome)

Table continued on following page

TABLE 44–4 DOSAGE REGIMEN FOR SELECTED ANTIEMETIC DRUGS *Continued*

Drug	Use(s)	Dosage	Implications
Miscellaneous *Continued*			
Scopolamine	Motion sickness	*Adults:* 0.5 mg Transderm-Scop system patch 4 hours before antiemetic effect is desired. 1.5 mg Transderm-V system patch is administered 12 hours before travel. For antiemetic/anticholinergic effects: 0.3–0.65 mg IM/IV/SC 3–4 times daily	Transderm-Scop patch delivers 0.5 mg over 72 hours. The Transderm-V patch delivers 1 mg over 72 hours
Corticosteroids			
Dexamethasone	Adjunct with antiemetics	10 mg po/IV 30 minutes before treatment. Follow with 4 mg po q8hr starting 4 hr after treatment	

cially in children. The extrapyramidal effects can be controlled by giving diphenhydramine, a drug with prominent anticholinergic actions. Because of its ability to increase GI motility, metoclopramide is contraindicated in the presence of obstruction, hemorrhage, and perforation of the GI tract.

Pharmacokinetics

Metoclopramide is well absorbed from the GI tract and from rectal mucosa and intramuscular (IM) tissue sites. It is widely distributed to body tissues and fluids crossing the blood-brain barrier and placenta. It enters breast milk in concentrations greater than plasma. The onset of drug action varies from minutes for the intravenous (IV) formulation to 30 to 60 minutes for the oral form (see Table 44–2). Peak action time is unknown, but the duration of action is 1 to 2 hours. There is 30-percent protein binding and a half-life of 2.5 to 5 hours. Metoclopramide is partially biotransformed in the liver, with 25 percent eliminated unchanged in the urine.

Cisapride is also rapidly and well absorbed from the GI tract, although bioavailability is low (35 to 40 percent). It enters in breast milk in small concentrations and is 97.5-percent protein bound. Cisapride is extensively biotransformed by the liver (over 90 percent), with a half-life of 8 to 10 hours.

Drug-Drug Interactions

Drug-drug interactions with prokinetic drugs are rather extensive and vary with the specific drug (see Table 44–3). Although metoclopramide can accelerate the absorption of many drugs, the decreased transit time may decrease the bioavailability of others, most notably digoxin. In addition, the delivery of food to the intestine may be altered to such an extent in patients with diabetes that an insulin dosage adjustment may be required.

Dosage Regimen

The dosage regimen for metoclopramide varies with the use of the drug (see Table 44–4). When it is used for the prevention of antineoplastic-induced nausea and vomiting, the dose is 1 to 2 mg/kg IV 30 minutes before the treatment. Additional doses of 1 to 2 mg/kg may be given every 2 hours for two doses, then every 3 hours for three additional doses.

Cisapride is dosed as 10 mg four times daily, 15 minutes before meals and at bedtime. The dosage may be increased to 20 mg four times daily. Other dosage regimens include 5 mg three times daily, 10 mg twice daily, or 20 mg at bedtime.

Laboratory Considerations

Metoclopramide may alter liver function test results and may cause increased serum prolactin and aldosterone concentrations. Cisapride has no known laboratory test interferences.

Cannabinoids

❐ Dronabinol (MARINOL)
❐ Nabilone (CESAMET)

Indications

Dronabinol and nabilone are the two cannabinoid antiemetics that are FDA approved for nausea and vomiting associated with antineoplastic therapy. Dronabinol (delta-9-tetrahydrocannabinol, THC) is the primary active ingredient in marijuana. Nabilone is a synthetic derivative of cannabinoid (not THC) and is associated with fewer CNS euphoric effects than dronabinol. They are generally used only if other treatments such as metoclopramide and ondansetron (see later) have failed. For some patients, these drugs are superior to conventional antiemetics (e.g., prochlorperazine, metoclopramide) but are generally not useful once vomiting has begun. The use of these drugs has declined somewhat since ondansetron became available.

Dronabinol was also recently approved as an appetite stimulant. The goal is to reduce anorexia and to prevent or reverse weight loss in patients with acquired immunodeficiency syndrome.

Pharmacodynamics

The mechanism by which cannabinoids suppress nausea and vomiting is unknown. It is thought that they inhibit the vomiting center in the medulla.

Adverse Effects and Contraindications

Cannabinoids produce subjective effects similar to those evoked by marijuana. Patients experience dysphoria, detachment, depersonalization, and temporal deterioration. Generally, younger patients tolerate and respond better to these drugs than older patients do. In addition to the subjective effects, cannabinoids cause tachycardia and hypotension and, therefore, must be used cautiously in patients with cardiovascular disease. Because of their CNS effects, cannabinoids are contraindicated in patients with psychiatric disorders. They are also contraindicated in patients with hypersensitivities to dronabinol, marijuana, or sesame oil; nausea and vomiting due to other causes; and during lactation. Dronabinol and nabilone are Schedule II drugs. Chronic use may lead to withdrawal syndrome on discontinuation. Safety in children under the age of 18 has not been established.

Pharmacokinetics

Cannabinoids are extensively biotransformed following absorption, resulting in a bioavailability of 10 to 20 percent. The onset time is unknown, but drug effects appear to peak in 2 hours, with a duration of action of 4 hours (see Table 44–2). Nabilone remains in the body for up to 24 hours. Cannabinoids are highly lipid soluble, entering breast milk in high concentrations. They are extensively biotransformed, with 50 percent of the drugs eliminated through biliary routes. At least one of the metabolites of the cannabinoids has psychoactive characteristics. Dronabinol is 97-percent protein bound.

Drug-Drug Interactions

Drug-drug interactions are identified in Table 44–3. Cannabinoids produce additive CNS depression if they are used concurrently with alcohol, antihistamines, opioids, tricyclic antidepressants, and sedative-hypnotics. They cause an increased risk of tachycardia when they are combined with amphetamines, cocaine, sympathomimetics, anticholinergics, antihistamines, and tricyclic antidepressants.

Dosage Regimen

The dosages of the cannabinoids are identified in Table 44–4. When dronabinol is administered orally, the dosage is 5 to 7.5 mg/m^2 taken 1 to 3 hours before the antineoplastic treatment, then every 2 to 4 hours after treatment for 4 to 6 daily doses. The dosage should not exceed 15 mg/m^2/day. When dronabinol is used as an appetite stimulate in patients with autoimmune deficiency syndrome, 2.5 mg is given orally before lunch and dinner to a maximum of 20 mg. Once-daily dosing is recommended if the patient is intolerant to a twice-daily regimen.

Nabilone is given as 1 to 2 mg orally three to four times daily. It is used most often for recalcitrant nausea and vomiting associated with antineoplastic therapy.

Serotonin Antagonists

- ❐ Ondansetron (ZOFRAN)
- ❐ Granisetron (KYTRIL)

Indications

Although ondansetron is expensive, it reduces the frequency and severity of nausea and vomiting in patients receiving highly emetogenic antineoplastic drugs (e.g., cisplatin). It is well tolerated by most patients and is even more effective when it is combined with dexamethasone. Studies have shown that ondansetron is more effective than metoclopramide in relieving nausea and vomiting.

Granisetron, the newest FDA-approved serotonin antagonist, is also used for the prevention of nausea and vomiting associated with antineoplastic drugs.

Pharmacodynamics

Serotonin receptors (5-HT_3) are located in the endings of the vagus nerve in the GI tract. It is believed that antineoplastics cause the release of serotonin from the enterochromaffin cells of the GI tract, where it is stored. These terminals send signals to serotonin receptors in the CTZ to cause nausea and vomiting. When ondansetron or granisetron is present, the released serotonin cannot bind with the receptors.

Adverse Effects and Contraindications

Granisetron's most common adverse effect is headache, although weakness, somnolence, agitation, anxiety, and CNS stimulation have also occurred. Hypertension, diarrhea, constipation, taste disorders, fever, and anaphylactoid reactions have been documented. Granisetron is contraindicated in patients with hypersensitivity and should be used with caution during pregnancy (Category B) and in children.

Ondansetron's most common adverse effects are headache and diarrhea. Dizziness, weakness, constipation, dry mouth, and abdominal pain have also been documented. Because ondansetron does not block dopamine receptors, it does not produce the extrapyramidal effects characteristic of some other antiemetics. Ondansetron is contraindicated in patients with hypersensitivity and should be used with caution during pregnancy (Category B) and in children.

Pharmacokinetics

The pharmacokinetics of ondansetron and granisetron are included in Table 44–2. The onset of drug action of both drugs is rapid when taken orally or IV, with onset times of 30 to 60 minutes. Peak drug actions are reached in 15 to 60 minutes, with a duration of drug action of 4 to 24 hours. Ondansetron is 70- to 76-percent protein bound, with a half-life of 4 hours. The protein binding of granisetron is unavailable. Both drugs are biotransformed by the cytochrome P_{450} enzyme system; therefore, inhibitors or inducers of this enzyme system may affect drug clearance. The half-lives of these drugs vary depending with the specific patient.

Drug-Drug Interactions

Concurrent use of granisetron with other drugs that cause extrapyramidal reactions may increase the risk of such reactions from granisetron (Table 44–3). There are no significant drug-drug interactions with ondansetron.

Dosage Regimen

The usual dose of granisetron is 1 mg twice daily, with the first dose given at least 60 minutes before antineoplastic treatment and the second dose given 12 hours later (Table 44–4). Granisetron is administered only on days the patient receives antineoplastic drugs. For adults and children older than 12 years of age, 10 mcg/kg is administered IV within 30 minutes of the antineoplastic treatment.

The usual dose of ondansetron is 8 mg (0.15 mg/kg) orally 30 minutes before antineoplastic therapy. The drug is given IV in the same dose if the patient is already vomiting. The dose can be repeated 4 to 8 hours later, if necessary.

Laboratory Considerations

Granisetron may cause elevated AST (SGOT) and ALT (SGPT) levels. Ondansetron may cause transient elevations in bilirubin in addition to alterations in AST (SGOT) and ALT (SGPT) levels.

Miscellaneous Drugs

- ❒ Benzquinamide
- ❒ Diphenidol (VONTROL)
- ❒ Droperidol (INAPSINE)
- ❒ Trimethobenzamide (TIGAN)
- ❒ Scopolamine (TRANSDERM SCOP)

BENZQUINAMIDE

Benzquinamide is an antiemetic used for the prevention and treatment of nausea associated with anesthesia and surgery. It acts by depressing the CTZ in the CNS. The most common adverse effect is drowsiness, although insomnia, restlessness, tremors, hypotension, and hypertension have been documented. It should be used cautiously in patients with a history of cardiovascular disease. Older adults or debilitated patients are prone to the adverse CNS effects of benzquinamide and thus require lower doses. Safety during lactation and in children has not been established.

Drug-drug interactions are many, just as with other antiemetics. Additive CNS depression can occur when benzquinamide is taken concurrently with other CNS depressants. Hypertension can develop in patients concurrently receiving vasopressors or epinephrine.

Benzquinamide is dosed as 50 mg (0.5 to 1.0 mg/kg) IM but may be repeated in 1 hour, if necessary. Dosages may be repeated every 3 to 4 hours as needed. The IV dose is 25 mg (0.2 to 0.4 mg/kg), although the IM route is preferred because of the risk of arrhythmias resulting from IV administration. It should be administered prophylactically at least 15 minutes before emergence from anesthesia. Onset occurs within 15 minutes by either route, with a duration of action of 3 to 4 hours.

DIPHENIDOL

Diphenidol is a trihexyphenidyl derivative that acts as a dopamine antagonist at the CTZ to inhibit nausea and vomiting. It is also used to prevent and control the nausea and vomiting associated with vertigo related to Ménière's disease, labyrinthitis, middle or inner ear surgery, and motion sickness.

Diphenidol produces adverse effects such as fatigue, drowsiness, disorientation, confusion, insomnia and sleep disturbances, visual hallucinations, headache, stimulation, and restlessness. It is contraindicated in patients with hypersensitivity, psychosis, or anuria. Cautious use is warranted in children; in patients with prostatic hyperplasia, glaucoma, or pyloric or duodenal stenosis; older adults; and during pregnancy and lactation.

Diphenidol is dosed in an adult at 25 to 50 mg orally every 4 hours as needed. In children who weigh over 23 kg, the oral dose is 25 mg every 4 hours as needed. The dose should not exceed 5.5 mg/kg/day.

DROPERIDOL

Droperidol is an butyrophenone antiemetic used postoperatively or after a procedure for nausea and vomiting, although it has not been FDA approved for such use. (FDA approval is for tranquilization and as an adjunct to general and regional anesthesia.) It is also useful for the nausea and vomiting associated with antineoplastic or radiation therapy and toxins. Like the phenothiazines, this butyrophenone suppresses emesis by blocking dopamine receptors in the CTZ.

The potential adverse effects are similar to those of the phenothiazines, including extrapyramidal reactions, sedation, and hypotension. It is contraindicated in patients with hypersensitivity, narrow-angle glaucoma, bone marrow depression, CNS depression, severe liver or cardiac disease, and known intolerance. It should be used cautiously in older adults and in debilitated or severely ill patients. Cautious use is also warranted in patients with diabetes, respiratory insufficiency, prostatic hyperplasia, CNS tumors, intestinal obstruction, and seizures (may lower seizure threshold), and during pregnancy or lactation. Safe use has not been established in children younger 2 years of age, although droperidol has been used during cesarean section without respiratory depression in the newborn. The usual dose of IV droperidol for nausea and vomiting is 0.5 to 1 mg every 4 hours, as needed.

TRIMETHOBENZAMIDE

Trimethobenzamide is also used in the management of mild to moderate nausea and vomiting. It is classified simply as a miscellaneous antiemetic. Although its mechanism of action is obscure, the relatively weak antiemetic effects appear to result from dopamine blockade. Trimethobenzamide is not as effective as the phenothiazines or metoclopramide but can be given IM to treat nausea and vomiting associated with antineoplastic drugs with mild to moderate emetogenic potential.

Adverse effects other than pain at the injection site include drowsiness, dizziness, allergy-type skin eruptions, extrapyramidal symptoms, and seizures. These adverse effects are uncommon, however. It is contraindicated in patients with hypersensitivity or hypersensitivity to benzocaine suppositories and in premature or newborn infants. It should be used cautiously in children who have a viral illness because it increases the risk of Reye's syndrome. Safety during pregnancy and lactation has not been established.

The usual adult oral dose of trimethobenzamide is 250 mg or a 200-mg rectal suppository three to four times daily. For children weighing 15 to 45 kg, a 100- to 200-mg dose three to four times daily as needed or 15 mg/kg/day in three to four divided doses is recommended. The dosage is the same for rectal suppositories. Children weighing less than 15 kg should receive 100 mg by suppository three to four times daily, as needed.

Drug-drug interactions with trimethobenzamide include additive CNS depression with the use of other CNS depressants such as alcohol, antidepressants, antihistamines, opioids, and sedative-hypnotics.

SCOPOLAMINE

Scopolamine is an anticholinergic (muscarinic antagonist) that is moderately effective for prophylaxis and treatment of motion sickness (see also Chapter 13). Scopolamine inhibits the muscarinic activity of acetylcholine. Thus, it corrects the imbalance of acetylcholine and norepinephrine in the CNS, which may be responsible for motion sickness.

The most common adverse effects include dry mouth, blurred vision, drowsiness, and urinary retention. It is contraindicated in patients who are hypersensitive or who are hypersensitive to bromides (injection formulation only) and those who have narrow-angle glaucoma, acute hemorrhage, or tachycardia secondary to cardiac insufficiency or thyrotoxicosis. It should be used cautiously in patients with suspected intestinal obstruction, prostatic hyperplasia, chronic renal, hepatic, pulmonary, or cardiac disease. Safe use during pregnancy and lactation has not been established.

It is well absorbed following IM, subcutaneous, and transdermal administration. It crosses placental membranes and the blood-brain barrier. Protein binding is low, with a half-life of 8 hours. Scopolamine is mostly biotransformed and eliminated through the liver.

A 1.5-mg TRANSDERM-SCOP system is applied behind the ear approximately 4 hours before antiemetic effects are desired. It delivers 0.5 mg over 72 hours. The TRANSDERM-V system delivers 1 mg over 72 hours and should be applied 12 hours before travel. Use of scopolamine is not recommended in children. The patient should be aware that he or she may have a dilated pupil on the side where the patch is worn. Prolonged use contributes to tolerance.

Benzodiazepines

Benzodiazepines such as diazepam (VALIUM) and lorazepam (ATIVAN) are also used to alleviate the nausea and vomiting associated with antineoplastic therapy. The beneficial effect of diazepam is primarily related to its reduction of anxiety. Lorazepam may be useful because of its ability to produce antegrade amnesia. It is often combined with metoclopramide and dexamethasone. The benzodiazepines are discussed in Chapter 17.

Corticosteroids

Corticosteroids confer a positive benefit when they are added to antiemetic therapy. Although many health care providers use dexamethasone, other corticosteroids such as methylprednisolone are likely to also be useful. They may be used alone, in combination with other antiemetics, or when ondansetron cannot be used. Corticosteroids tend to make patients feel better overall. The mechanism by which corticosteroids suppress vomiting is unknown.

When it is used, 10 mg of dexamethasone is taken 30 minutes before antineoplastic therapy. It is given IV in the same dose if the patient is already vomiting. The pretreatment dose is followed by 4 mg orally every 8 hours, beginning 4 hours after the antineoplastic treatment. Optimal doses have not been determined. Corticosteroids are discussed further in Chapter 52.

Critical Thinking Process

Assessment

History of Present Illness

The patient should be interviewed regarding the frequency, duration, and precipitating causes of nausea and vomiting. Accompanying symptoms and any measures that relieve the episode of nausea and vomiting should be elicited. A patient's previous experiences with nausea and vomiting may help explain the severity of the present episode. A distinction should be made between vomiting and regurgitation. Regurgitation is the passage of food into the esophagus and frequently into the mouth as well, without nausea or vomiting.

Acute-onset nausea and vomiting lasting less than 72 hours in a previously healthy person is usually caused by viral gastroenteritis or toxin exposure. Nausea and vomiting lasting over 24 hours (especially if associated with weight loss and impaired nutrition) is most often caused by GI obstruction or motility dysfunction. Further, nausea and vomiting are early manifestations of toxicity of antineoplastic therapy.

Vomiting in the early morning before eating is characteristic of the first 12 to 14 weeks of a normal pregnancy. Early morning vomiting also occurs frequently in patients with increased intracranial pressure (e.g., meningitis and space-occupying lesions of the CNS).

Nausea and vomiting without a clear relationship to meals can result from any cause but is most likely related to metabolic or vestibular disorders, drugs, or toxins. Nausea and vomiting occurring more than 2 hours after eating (especially if recurrent and not associated with significant abdominal pain) suggests gastric outlet syndrome, especially if the emesis contains food material that was eaten several hours earlier. Vomiting 2 hours after eating may also occur with motility disorders (gastroparesis associated with diabetic autonomic neuropathy and postvagotomy states), or esophageal disorders such as Zenker's diverticulum and achalasia, in which the emesis is typically undigested food. Gastroparesis is characterized by bloating, early satiety, and intractable nausea and vomiting.

Repetitive vomiting during or soon after a meal suggests different causes in children versus adults. In children, a feeding disorder associated with overfeeding or too-rapid feeding is possible. In adults, the problem is psychoneurotic vomiting, especially when there is no history of dysphagia, and vomiting can be suppressed long enough to make it to the toilet.

Past Health History

The patient should be questioned about his or her previous history of nausea and vomiting. A number of conditions and states have been associated with nausea and vomiting (see Table 44–1).

Physical Exam Findings

The physical exam is unremarkable in many cases of nausea and vomiting that stem from some of the more common causes or from motility disorders, metabolic disorders, drugs, or toxins. However, physical exam findings associated with recurrent episodes of nausea or vomiting can include an unexplained increase in tooth decay and gum disease, and evidence of dehydration or fluid and electrolyte imbalances. The physical exam in patients with gastroparesis or gastric outlet obstruction may reveal a succession splash. Patients with either acute or chronic symptoms should undergo a neurologic exam.

Diagnostic Testing

Laboratory testing should be directed by the history and physical exam. Many of the causes of nausea and vomiting have nonspecific physical findings. There are a number of tests that may be performed initially for the patient with significant nausea and vomiting, especially if the condition is accompanied by abdominal pain. These tests include serum electrolytes to evaluate for hydration, derangements, and evidence of metabolic disorders. A blood urea nitrogen and creatinine can be used in the search for evidence of renal failure or the possibility of toxicity secondary to drugs. Complete blood counts may provide evidence of infection or blood loss. Liver function tests can be used to evaluate the possibility of hepatitis, pancreaticobiliary disease, or Reye's syndrome. In patients with acute vomiting, flat and upright abdominal radiographs are obtained. Gastroparesis is confirmed by nuclear scintigraphic studies, which show delayed gastric emptying. Endoscopy or barium upper GI studies may reflect obstruction. CNS symptoms should be investigated by brain scan or magnetic resonance imaging.

Developmental Considerations

Perinatal Nausea and vomiting is common during the first trimester of pregnancy. It usually is self-limited and intermittent, beginning at about 6 weeks' and disappearing by about 12 weeks' gestation. It is commonly worse in the morning. If it is severe (hyperemesis gravidarum), acid-base and electrolyte imbalances, dehydration, or starvation may occur.

Pediatric Vomiting in infants and children may be associated with acute gastroenteritis or an acute illness (e.g., urinary tract infection, otitis media, asthma), feeding disorders, hypertrophic pyloric stenosis, or intussusception. If there is no fever, no weight loss, and no abdominal distention and the child does not appear sick, the cause may be a feeding disorder.

Geriatric Older adults are at risk for fluid volume depletion and electrolyte disturbances with vomiting, as well as a potential for injury related to drowsiness. Changes of aging may contribute to the potential for nausea and vomiting. Esophageal motility is decreased, and the distal end becomes slightly dilated. Esophageal emptying is slower, and gastric motility and emptying is reduced.

Psychosocial Considerations

Anticipatory nausea and vomiting may occur at any time after initial antineoplastic therapy. It is seen more commonly in patients who previously received drugs with high emetogenic potential. Patients younger than 50 years of age who report four or more of the following experiences may be at risk for anticipatory nausea and vomiting: susceptibility to motion sickness, or nausea or vomiting, feeling flushed or hot, or diaphoretic after their previous treatment session. Anticipatory nausea and vomiting can develop rapidly, often appearing after only one infusion and escalating in severity during subsequent treatments. Many patients find their first treatment to be much easier than they expected. However, as treatment continues, patients begin to notice the anticipatory adverse effects. With repeated treatments, the problem becomes worse.

Psychogenic vomiting can be associated with a physical syndrome, sexual abuse, post-traumatic stress, and eating disorders. Formal psychiatric assessment and psychological testing (e.g., Minnesota Multiphasic Personality Inventory) may be helpful in patients in whom psychogenic vomiting is suspected.

The expense associated with antiemetic therapy is closely related to the cause of the nausea. When the nausea and vomiting is self-limited, the expense is relatively small. However, for patients receiving antineoplastic therapies, the cost of antiemetic regimens can be rather high (see Case Study—Motion Sickness).

Analysis and Management

Treatment Objectives

Treatment goals include preventing or relieving the distressing symptoms associated with nausea and vomiting. The potentially life-threatening complications such as electrolyte imbalances, dehydration, and malnutrition should also be avoided. Additionally, treatment goals for the patient with inexorable nausea and vomiting associated with antineoplastic therapy include preventing or reducing the nausea and vomiting, thus allowing completion of effective antineoplastic regimens.

Treatment Options

The treatment of vomiting should be directed primarily at finding and correcting the underlying cause. Most causes of acute vomiting are self-limited and require no special treatment. Patients should take clear liquids (i.e., broths, tea, soups, carbonated beverages) and small quantities of dry foods (e.g., soda crackers). Hospitalization may be required for more acute vomiting. Owing to the inability to eat and loss of gastric fluids, patients can become dehydrated and develop hypokalemia and metabolic alkalosis. IV fluids and nasogastric suctioning may be needed to maintain hydration and to allow for gastric decompression.

Drug Variables

The choice of antiemetic is usually directed at symptomatic relief but depends primarily on the cause of the nausea and vomiting. Antiemetics are generally more effective for prophylaxis than for treatment. Given the complexity of the various pathways that control and stimulate vomiting, it is not surprising that no single drug is effective in all patients.

Combinations of drugs from different classes may provide better symptom control with less toxicity in some patients. Combination strategies take advantage of the synergistic mechanisms afforded to each drug. This makes possible more complete and extended prophylaxis, use of lower doses of individual drugs, and thus fewer adverse effects. For example, treatment of a patient with anticipatory, acute, or delayed forms of emesis might include a benzodiazepine (e.g., lorazepam), a serotonin antagonist (e.g., ondansetron), and a corticosteroid (e.g., dexamethasone). The decision as to the specific drug to use is thus based, in part, on potential adverse effects, because no one drug has proved to be more effective than any other drug.

Antihistamines have weak antiemetic properties but are useful in the prevention of vomiting due to motion sickness. Dimenhydrinate can be used for mild to moderate motion sickness caused by travel by automobile, air, or sea, especially if sedation is desired. For rough seas and extended journeys, transdermal scopolamine can be applied every 3 days and is more convenient than the phenothiazine promethazine or dimenhydrinate. Meclizine is almost as convenient as scopolamine, can be given once daily, and is less expensive. The decision to use dimenhydrinate and a phenothiazine such as promethazine should be based on cost. Dimenhydrinate causes less sedation than either of the other two drugs but has a high incidence of anticholinergic effects.

The incidence of nausea and vomiting associated with anesthesia is about 30 percent; thus, prophylaxis or treatment can often be useful. Postoperative nausea requires treatment in only about 5 percent of patients. Routine prophylaxis after surgery is discouraged. Further, some drugs used for the treatment of postoperative nausea and vomiting can cause hypotension and movement disorders. Patients who are at high risk for aspiration (e.g., patients with wired jaws, or patients with a history of moderate to severe postoperative vomiting) should receive prophylactic therapy. Treatment is warranted for patients with prolonged nausea (longer than 30 minutes) or repeated episodes of vomiting unrelieved by decreased vestibular stimulation (head movement). Droperidol is the drug of choice to control postoperative vomiting prophylactically owing to its effectiveness and long duration of action. However, it produces dysphoria in some patients, delays awakening, and prolongs discharge from the postanesthetic care unit. Phenothiazines, because of their relatively high incidence and severity of adverse effects, are indicated only when other antiemetics are ineffective or when only a few doses are required.

Benzodiazepines may be helpful for patients with psychogenic and anticipatory nausea and vomiting. Corticosteroids are used in combination with other agents in the treatment of antineoplastic-induced vomiting.

As a general rule, antiemetics are contraindicated when their use prevents or delays diagnosis, when signs and symptoms of drug toxicity may be masked (e.g., during digoxin therapy), and for routine use to prevent postoperative vomiting. If appropriate diagnostic tests have been obtained and no specific diagnosis has been made, a therapeutic trial of a prokinetic drug may be justified.

Patient Variables

For ambulatory patients, drugs causing minimal sedation are generally preferred. Some sedation, however, does occur even with therapeutic doses. Drugs with anticholinergic and antihistaminic properties are preferred for motion sickness. Unless sedation is desired, dimenhydrinate should be chosen instead of diphenhydramine because it is more effective for motion sickness and produces less sedation. Prophylactic treatment with scopolamine or promethazine is effective in 90 percent of patients who are susceptible to motion sickness. A note of caution, however. Diphenhydramine is often a drug that abusers seek; therefore, the quantities that are prescribed should be controlled.

Prophylactic treatment of nausea and vomiting for patients receiving antineoplastic drugs is imperative, because nausea and vomiting can curtail effective treatment. Patients receiving antineoplastic drugs with low emetogenic potential (e.g., bleomycin, chlorambucil, etoposide, fluorouracil, hydroxyurea, methotrexate, mitomycin C, vinblastine, vincristine, vindesine) who have experienced nausea or vomiting on a previous course of the drugs should receive prophylaxis. Prophylaxis should also be used when the antineoplastic drug has either a moderate or high emetogenic potential. Drugs with moderate emetogenic potential include carboplatin, carmustine, cytarabine, daunorubicin, doxorubicin, lomustine, and procarbazine. Drugs with high emetogenic potential include cisplatin, cyclophosphamide, dacarbazine, dactinomycin, mechlorethamine, and streptozocin. Because nausea and vomiting usually worsen with each treatment cycle, up to 30 percent of patients refuse further treatment. However, adequate prophylaxis and treatment can eliminate symptoms in up to 82 percent of patients.

The cost of ondansetron notwithstanding, it is often chosen for use with antineoplastic drugs that have high emetogenic potential. It is the most efficacious drug available for prophylaxis. The expense of ondansetron should be correlated with the cost of preparing the three or four parenteral drug regimens and the cost of related antiemetic rescue drugs. Further, ondansetron is well tolerated by most patients. Ondansetron in combination with dexamethasone is more effective than ondansetron alone, and it often makes patients feel better.

The nausea and vomiting that occurs during pregnancy is usually self-limited and intermittent. Therefore, routine prophylaxis or treatment is not recommended (owing to the potential for teratogenic effects). Treatment may be warranted if hyperemesis gravidarum or protracted vomiting occurs, or if nondrug measures, such as ingesting crackers and tea before morning rising, taking small, light, appetizing meals, and keeping head movement to a minimum, have failed. The usefulness of pyridoxine (vitamin B_6) as an antiemetic has not been confirmed, but it is the least likely drug to be toxic. Meclizine may be considered if pyridoxine is ineffective.

Phenothiazines are more likely to cause dystonias and other neuromuscular reactions in children than in adults. Further, most antiemetics cause drowsiness, especially in older adults and, therefore, should be used cautiously. Efforts should be made to prevent nausea and vomiting when possible.

Intervention

Administration

Most antiemetic drugs are available in oral, parenteral, and rectal dosage forms. As a general rule, oral dosage forms are preferred for prophylaxis, and rectal or parenteral forms are preferred for therapeutic use. Parenteral antiemetics should not be mixed in a syringe with other drugs. An exception is promethazine, which is often mixed with meperidine and atropine sulfate for preanesthetic medication. IM injections should be given deeply into a large muscle mass to decrease tissue irritation.

For prophylaxis, administration should be planned so that peak drug effects correspond to the time of anticipated nausea. For example, antiemetics used in the prevention of motion sickness are usually administered at least 30 minutes before travel, and preferably 1 to 2 hours before exposure. This allows time for drug dissolution and absorption. Some preparations can then be used every 3 to 4 hours as needed thereafter.

Administration of antiemetics for antineoplastic-induced nausea and vomiting should take place 5 minutes before the treatment for dexamethasone and for up to 6 to 24 hours.

Case Study Motion Sickness

Patient History

History of Present Illness

CM is a 52-year-old male who reports to the office today for a required annual employment physical. He is also requesting a prescription for motion sickness. He reports he will once again be crossing "the treacherous Drake Passage by ship" on his way to Antarctica and is worried he will not be able to perform his job as engineer should he experience motion sickness. Reports Drake Passage takes 3 days to cross. He has made the trip three times previously and reports having persistent nausea and vomiting while aboard ship. Reports he has tried OTC Benadryl and other "motion sickness pills" but found them to be less than effective.

Past Health History

CM's medical history is unremarkable except for an early benign prostatic hypertrophy that causes occasional urinary hesitancy, and "hay fever." He is scheduled to undergo skin testing upon arrival in Antarctica. He had an intermedullary rod inserted in his right femur without sequelae after an MVA at age 25. He reports taking no OTC or prescription drugs.

Physical Exam

CM's physical exam is unremarkable. Cardiac: RRR. Breath sounds clear bilaterally. CN II–XII intact. Strength bilateral upper and lower extremities equal. Bowel sounds present all four quadrants. Prostate enlarged upon palpation. Negative hernia exam.

Diagnostic Testing

Laboratory test results reveal CBC, electrolytes, UA, and EKG within normal limits. Drug screen negative.

Developmental Considerations

CM is single and feels he must remain so due to the extended periods of time he is away from home in the United States.

Psychosocial Considerations

CM reports no history of psychiatric disorders. Denies smoking, use of tobacco or alcohol since the MVA at age 25. He enjoys playing basketball and playing cards with fellow employees, occasionally dates a fellow employee.

Economic Factors

The cost of CM's annual physical exam is covered by his employer. Prescription costs are covered by employer using an in-house formulary if drug required in order for employee to function. Special permission is required if a nonformulary drug is required.

Variables Influencing Decision

Treatment Objectives

- To prevent or relieve distressing symptoms associated with nausea and vomiting.
- To prevent complications such as electrolyte imbalances, dehydration, and malnutrition.

Drug Variables	*Drug Summary*	*Patient Variables*
Indications	Meclizine and scopolamine are possible drug options because both manage motion sickness effectively in most individuals.	CM's history reveals multiple episodes of motion sickness requiring prophylaxis.
Pharmacodynamics	Meclizine has central anticholinergic, CNS depressant, and antihistaminic properties. Scopolamine inhibits muscarinic activity of acetylcholine, thus correcting imbalance of acetylcholine and norepinephrine in CNS.	There are no patient variables that affect pharmacodynamics except those related to anticholinergic adverse effects. This will become a decision point.
Adverse Effects/ Contraindications	Antihistamines used prophylactically for motion sickness may cause sedation, blurred vision, and dry mouth. Scopolamine may cause urinary hesitancy as well as above-mentioned effects.	CM reports that drowsiness is not acceptable because of his job reponsibilities while aboard ship. CM has history of early BPH. This will become a decision point.

Case Study Motion Sickness—cont'd

Drug Variables	Drug Summary	Patient Variables
Pharmacokinetics	Meclizine has a duration of action of 24 hours. Scopolamine has a duration of 72 hours if transdermal formulation is used.	There are no patient variables that effect pharmacokinetics.
Dosage Regimen	Meclizine can be taken orally once daily and repeated in 24 hours. Transdermal scopolamine can be taken once daily and the patch replaced in 48–72 hours.	CM is requesting a drug that requires no more than once-daily dosing, if possible.
Lab Considerations	Short-term use of either meclizine or scopolamine does not require laboratory monitoring. Meclizine can cause false-negative skin test results using allergen extracts.	CM is to have allergy testing done upon arrival in Antarctica. This will become a decision point.
Cost Index*	Meclizine: 1 Transdermal scopolamine: 1	Prescription costs within formulary covered by employer.

Summary of Decision Points

- Drowsiness is not acceptable because of job responsibilities while aboard ship. CM has history of early BPH.
- Scopolamine reportedly has fewer anticholinergic adverse effects than meclizine does.
- CM is to have allergy testing performed upon arrival in Antarctica. Meclizine can cause false-negative skin test results.
- Although transdermal scopolamine is more expensive than meclizine, it is best option given CM's history of BPH, upcoming allergy testing, and formulary choices.

DRUG TO BE USED

- Transderm-Scop (scopolamine) patch, one 1.5 mg patch placed behind the ear at least 4 hours before travel (will release 0.5 mg scopolamine over 72 hours). Dispense package of 4.

*Cost Index:

1 = $ <30/mo.
2 = $ 30–40/mo.
3 = $ 40–50/mo.
4 = $ 50–60/mo.
5 = $ >60/mo.

AWP of 10, 25-mg tablets of meclizine is approximately $ .80.
AWP of 4, 0.5-mg/hr patches of transdermal scopolamine is approximately $16.

Table 44–5 provides an overview of the route and administration times for selected combination treatment regimens.

Excessive sedation may occur with usual therapeutic doses of antiemetics and is more likely to occur with high doses. The sedation may be minimized by avoiding high doses when possible and assessing the patient for responsiveness before each dose. The drug may need to be reduced in dosage or frequency of administration. Also, a change in drugs may reduce adverse effects in a particular patient. Doses of phenothiazines are much smaller for antiemetic effects than for antipsychotic effects. The health care provider should be notified if the patient appears excessively drowsy or is hypotensive.

Anticholinergic effects are common to many antiemetic drugs and are more likely to occur with large doses. Hypotension, including orthostatic hypotension, may occur with any of the drugs but is most likely to occur with phenothiazines and droperidol. Therefore, the patient's blood pressure should be checked before administration.

With cannabinoids, the patient should be observed for alterations in mood, cognition, and perception of reality. According to the manufacturer, these adverse effects are well tolerated, particularly by young individuals. If necessary, tachycardia associated with the use of cannabinoids can be prevented with a beta-blocking drug such as propranolol.

Education

To help minimize nausea and vomiting, patients are advised to sip clear liquids slowly and to consume foods served cool or at room temperature. Bland foods, very sweet,

TABLE 44–5 COMBINATION ANTIEMETIC REGIMENS FOR ANTINEOPLASTIC-INDUCED NAUSEA AND VOMITING

Drugs with Low Emetogenic Potential	Drugs with Moderate Emetogenic Potential*	Drugs with High Emetogenic Potential*
Bleomycin Chlorambucil Etoposide Fluorouracil Hydroxyurea Methotrexate Mitomycin C Vinblastine Vincristine Vindesine	Carboplatin Carmustine Cytarabine Daunorubicin Doxorubicin Ifosfamide Lomustine Procarbazine	Cisplatin Cyclophosphamide Dacarbazine Dactinomycin Mechlorethamine Streptozocin

Combination Antiemetic Regimens for Patients Receiving Drugs with Low to Moderate Emetogenic Potential

Oral dronabinol every 6 hours starting 24 hours before treatment
Oral prochlorperazine every 6 hours starting 24 hours before treatment (continue combination until 24 hours after last treatment).

Oral prochlorperazine spansules twice daily on day 1 and days 3–6
IV dexamethasone daily × 5 days *or* po twice daily on days 1–5 (tapered dose)
Oral diphenhydramine 1 hour before treatment
Oral lorazepam 1 hour before treatment
IV metoclopramide 1 hour before treatment
IM droperidol 15 minutes before and every 6 hours, as needed

IV lorazepam or IV diphenhydramine 45 minutes before treatment
IV metoclopramide 30 minutes before and 90 minutes after treatment
IV dexamethasone 30 minutes before and 90 minutes after treatment

Combination Antiemetic Regimens for Patients Receiving Drugs with Moderate Emetogenic Potential

IV metoclopramide 20 minutes before and 90 minutes after treatment
IV dexamethasone 20 minutes before treatment
IV diphenhydramine 30 minutes before treatment

IV metoclopramide 20 minutes before and 90 minutes after treatment
IV dexamethasone 40 minutes before treatment
IV lorazepam 35 minutes before treatment

Combination Antiemetic Regimens for Patients Receiving Drugs with High Emetogenic Potential

IV granisetron immediately before treatment
IV dexamethasone 5 minutes before treatment
IV ondansetron 30 minutes before treatment and every 4 hours with 3 doses after treatment
IV dexamethasone 5 minutes before treatment

IV metoclopramide 20 minutes before and 90 minutes after treatment
IV dexamethasone 20 minutes before treatment
IV lorazepam 30 minutes before treatment

IV metoclopramide 30 minutes before and 90 minutes after treatment
IV diphenhydramine 45 minutes before treatment
IV dexamethasone 45 minutes before treatment

IV ondansetron 30 minutes before treatment
IV dexamethasone 30 minutes before treatment
Oral prochlorperazine SR at bedtime
Oral lorazepam at bedtime
Oral diphenhydramine at bedtime

*Emetogenic potential of some drugs is dose dependent.

fatty, salty, and spicy foods should be avoided. Some patients receiving antineoplastic therapy are unable to tolerate plain water or red meat. Visual, auditory, and olfactory stimulation should be minimized, and noxious stimuli should be removed from the environment. Avoid or decrease activity during episodes of nausea.

Good oral hygiene and frequent rinsing of the mouth with water may help relieve the bad taste and corrosion of tooth enamel by gastric acid. To relieve mouth dryness caused by the anticholinergic effects of some antiemetics, frequent rinsing and sugarless gum or candy may be used. A cool wet washcloth to the face and neck may help the patient feel more comfortable. Because pain may cause nausea and vomiting in some individuals, administration of analgesics before the event can help.

Patients should be informed that drowsiness may occur with use of antiemetics, and that driving and other activities requiring alertness should be avoided until response to the drug is known. They should also taught to take the drug as ordered and cautioned to avoid concurrent use of alcohol or other CNS depressants. Teach the patient who is taking a cannabinoid to take the drug only when he or she can be supervised by a responsible adult because of its tendency to cause mood changes. Other drugs should not be taken without the knowledge and consent of the health care provider. The patient should be advised to change positions slowly to minimize orthostatic hypotension.

Evaluation

Therapeutic effects can be observed through verbal reports of decreased nausea and a decreased frequency of or absence of vomiting. Note the patient's ability to maintain adequate intake of food and fluids, comparing his or her current weight with a baseline weight. Determine whether the dosage and administration times of the antiemetic drugs are the most effective for the individual patient.

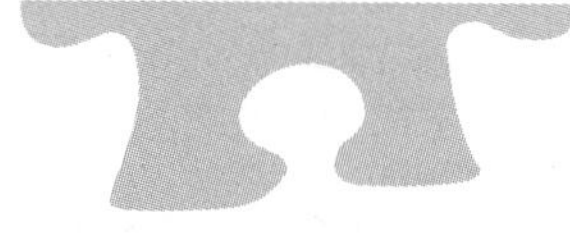

SUMMARY

- Nausea and vomiting are common and may accompany almost any illness or stressful situation and are the most common adverse response to drug therapy, particularly antineoplastic drugs.
- Conditions or states associated with nausea and vomiting include GI inflammation, infection, or obstruction; motility disorders; vestibular or intracranial disorders; metabolic derangements; toxins; and psychogenic causes.
- Nausea and vomiting occur when pathologic processes stimulate the vomiting center, which is located in the medulla. The vomiting center initiates efferent impulses, the glottis closes, there is contraction of the diaphragm and abdominal muscles, the gastroesophageal sphincter relaxes, and reverse peristalsis moves stomach contents upward toward the mouth for expulsion.
- Interview the patient regarding the frequency, duration, and precipitating causes of nausea and vomiting, including accompanying signs and symptoms, characteristics of vomitus, and measures that exacerbate or relieve nausea and vomiting.
- Note physical exam findings that suggest dehydration or fluid and electrolyte imbalance.
- Treatment goals include preventing or relieving the distressing symptoms associated with nausea and vomiting. Potentially life-threatening complications such as electrolyte imbalances, dehydration, and malnutrition should be avoided.
- The treatment of vomiting should be directed primarily at finding and correcting the underlying cause. Most causes of acute vomiting are self-limited and require no special treatment.
- The choice of an antiemetic depends primarily on the cause of the nausea and vomiting and the patient's condition, and is usually administered to relieve symptoms. Antiemetics are generally more effective for prophylaxis than for treatment.
- Treatment options include antihistamines, phenothiazines, prokinetics, cannabinoids, serotonin antagonists, and a number of miscellaneous agents. Benzodiazepines and corticosteroids have also be used as adjuncts in the treatment of nausea and vomiting.
- Combinations of drugs from different classes may provide better symptom control with less toxicity and take advantage of the synergistic mechanisms afforded each drug.
- For prophylaxis, administration times should be planned so that the peak effect corresponds to the time of anticipated nausea.
- Excessive sedation may occur with usual therapeutic doses of antiemetics and is more likely to occur with high doses. The health care provider should be notified if the patient appears excessively drowsy or is hypotensive.
- Patients should be instructed as to nondrug means of preventing and managing nausea and vomiting. They should be instructed to change positions slowly and to use caution operating machinery until drug effects are known.
- Therapeutic effects can be observed through verbal reports of decreased nausea and a decreased frequency of or absence of vomiting.

BIBLIOGRAPHY

Allan, G. (1993). The 5HT3 antagonists: New generation antiemetics. *Current Therapeutics,* 34(7), 15.

Allan, G. (1992). Antiemetics. *Gastroenterology Clinics of North America,* 21(3), 597–611.

Alpers, D. (1992). Approach to the patient with nausea and vomiting. In W. Kelly (Ed.), *Textbook of internal medicine* (2nd ed.). Philadelphia: J.B. Lippincott.

Burnett, P., and Perking, J. (1992). Parenteral ondansetron for the treatment of chemotherapy- and radiation-induced nausea and vomiting. *Pharmacotherapy,* 12(2), 120–131.

Chaffee, B., and Tankanow, R. (1991). Ondansetron: The first of a new class of antiemetic agents. *Clinical Pharmacology,* 10(6), 430–446.

Chevallier, B. (1993). The control of acute cisplatin-induced emesis: A comparative study of granisetron and a combination regimen of high-dose metoclopramide and dexamethasone. *British Journal of Cancer,* 68(1), 176–180.

Cunningham, D., and Gore, M. (1993). The real costs of emesis: An economic analysis of ondansetron as metoclopramide in controlling emesis in patients receiving chemotherapy for cancer. *European Journal of Cancer,* 29(3), 303–306.

Dershwitz, M. (1995). Advances in antiemetic therapy. *Anesthesia Clinics of North America,* 12(1), 119–132.

DiStasio, S. (1993). Zofran makes chemo bearable. *RN,* 56(5), 56–59.

Gralla, R. (1992). Antiemetic drugs for chemotherapy support: Current treatment and rationale for development of newer agents. *Cancer,* 15(Suppl 4), 1003–1006.

Grunberg, S., and Hesketh, P. (1993). Control of chemotherapy-induced emesis. *New England Journal of Medicine,* 329(24), 1790–1796.

Hockenberry-Eaton, M., and Benner, A. (1990). Patterns of nausea and vomiting in children: Nursing assessment and intervention. *Oncology Nursing Forum,* 17, 575–584.

Keller, V. (1995). Management of nausea and vomiting in children. *Journal of Pediatric Nursing,* 10(5), 280–286.

Koda-Kimble, M., and Young, L. (1995). *Applied therapeutics: The clinical use of drugs.* Vancouver, WA: Applied Therapeutics.

Mitchelson, F. (1992). Pharmacological agents affecting emesis: A review part I. *Drugs.* 43(3):295–315.

Mitchelson, F. (1992). Pharmacological agents affecting emesis: A review part II. *Drugs.* 43(4):443–463.

National Center for Health Statistics. (1991). *Current estimates from the national health interview survey, 1990.* DHHS Publication No. (PHS) 92–1509, U.S. Government.

Richardson, A. (1991). Theories of self care: Their relevance to chemotherapy-induced nausea and vomiting. *Journal of Advanced Nursing.* 16(6):671–676.

Schmitt, R., Keppler, G., Kroecker, G., et al. (1990). Controlling nausea and vomiting in outpatients. *Oncology Nursing Forum.* 17(2), 277.

45

Cation-Exchange Resins and Ammonia-Detoxifying Drugs

Toxic reactions are often perceived to be caused by stimuli external to the body. However, many endogenous substances can trigger toxicity at cellular and systemic levels. This chapter considers the drugs used to counteract two dangerous imbalances: increased levels of potassium and excess ammonia.

Maintenance of serum potassium levels within a normal range is vital to body function. Potassium is the major intracellular ion, and along with other electrolytes, sodium, chloride, calcium, and magnesium, it is closely involved in the regulation of body fluids. Elevation of serum potassium is rare in people with normal kidney function but often occurs during acute renal failure. Elevated potassium levels must be corrected because dangerously high serum potassium levels can cause cardiac, gastrointestinal, renal, and neurologic system involvement.

Ammonia is formed in the body as part of several cellular processes. Under normal conditions, it is removed quickly from the blood, converted into urea, and eliminated in the urine. However, if the liver is damaged or seriously diseased, ammonia accumulates in the blood with severe toxic consequences.

HYPERKALEMIA

Epidemiology and Etiology

A serum potassium level exceeding 5.5 mEq/L is considered *hyperkalemia*. Hyperkalemia is caused by the movement of potassium out of the cells, an increased intake of potassium, and the decreased excretion of potassium. The movement of potassium out of the cells occurs whenever severe tissue damage is present, as in crushing injuries, sepsis, fever, or surgery. The movement also occurs with metabolic acidosis and hyperglycemia or insulin deficiency. Shock also promotes hyperkalemia as a result of reduced renal function.

Elevated serum potassium levels can also occur with the concurrent use of potassium-sparing diuretics and potassium supplements, renal failure, or adrenal insufficiency. Patients with untreated adrenal insufficiency have increased potassium levels because of an aldosterone deficiency.

Excess intake of potassium can occur with dietary intake that exceeds the kidneys' ability to eliminate it and with excessive parenteral administration. Administration of stored blood further contributes to elevated potassium levels.

A sudden rise of only 1 to 3 mEq/L of potassium can be fatal. On the other hand, patients with renal failure develop severe hyperkalemia slowly and seem to adjust to the excess with few symptoms.

Pathophysiology

Potassium is the major intracellular *cation,* which is a positively charged ion important to maintenance of the balance between intracellular and extracellular fluid compartments. During *anabolism* (tissue build-up) or when glucose is converted to glycogen, potassium enters the cell. With *catabolism* (tissue breakdown or injury) potassium leaves the cell. The body conserves potassium less effectively than it conserves sodium, and the kidneys excrete potassium even when the body needs it. Normally, about 5 percent of total body potassium is eliminated each day. Serum potassium levels do not necessarily reflect total body potassium levels because most of the body's potassium is intracellular.

The active transport system for sodium and potassium is found in all cells. This pump system uses adenosine triphosphate (ATP) to move sodium out of the cell and potassium into the cell. The transporter protein is the enzyme ATPase. Approximately 60 to 70 percent of the ATP synthesized by cells, particularly muscle and nerve cells, is used to maintain the transport system. Excitable tissues (e.g., muscle, nerves, kidneys, salivary glands) have a high concentration of sodium, potassium, and ATPase. For every ATP molecule hydrolyzed, three molecules of sodium are transported out of the cell, whereas only two molecules of potassium move into the cell. This leads to an electrical membrane potential, with the inside of the cell more negative than the outside of the cell (Fig. 45–1).

Membrane potentials are decreased, and the cells become more excitable in the presence of hyperkalemia. Patients develop muscle irritability, numbness, and tingling because of overstimulation by nerve impulses. Skeletal muscle spasms, nausea, colic, and diarrhea are common. Muscles become weak as potassium is lost from the cells and because the overstimulation causes lactic acid to accumulate.

Overstimulation of the myocardium also occurs if hyperkalemia is not controlled. Electrocardiographic (ECG) tracing reflects peaked, symmetric, or tented T waves with short QT segments. The QRS complex continues to widen, and atrial arrest occurs as potassium levels continue to increase.

Intracellular potassium also shifts to extracellular fluid in patients with metabolic acidosis. Serum potassium levels rise about 0.2 to 1.7 mEq/L for every 0.1-unit fall in pH. Potassium movement out of cells occurs primarily in metabolic acidosis because of the accumulation of minerals (e.g., ammonium chloride) or hydrochloric acid. The inability of the chloride anion to permeate the cell membrane results in the transcellular exchange of hydrogen for potassium. Metabolic acidosis caused by organic acids (ketoacids and lactic acids) does not induce hyperkalemia. Acidosis associated with diabetes is due to a combination of the hyperosmolality of glucose and deficiencies of insulin, catecholamines, and aldosterone. In the absence of acidosis, serum potassium levels rise about 1 mEq/L when there is a total body potassium in excess of 50 to 200 mEq/L. However, the higher the serum potassium concentration, the smaller the excess necessary to raise the potassium levels further.

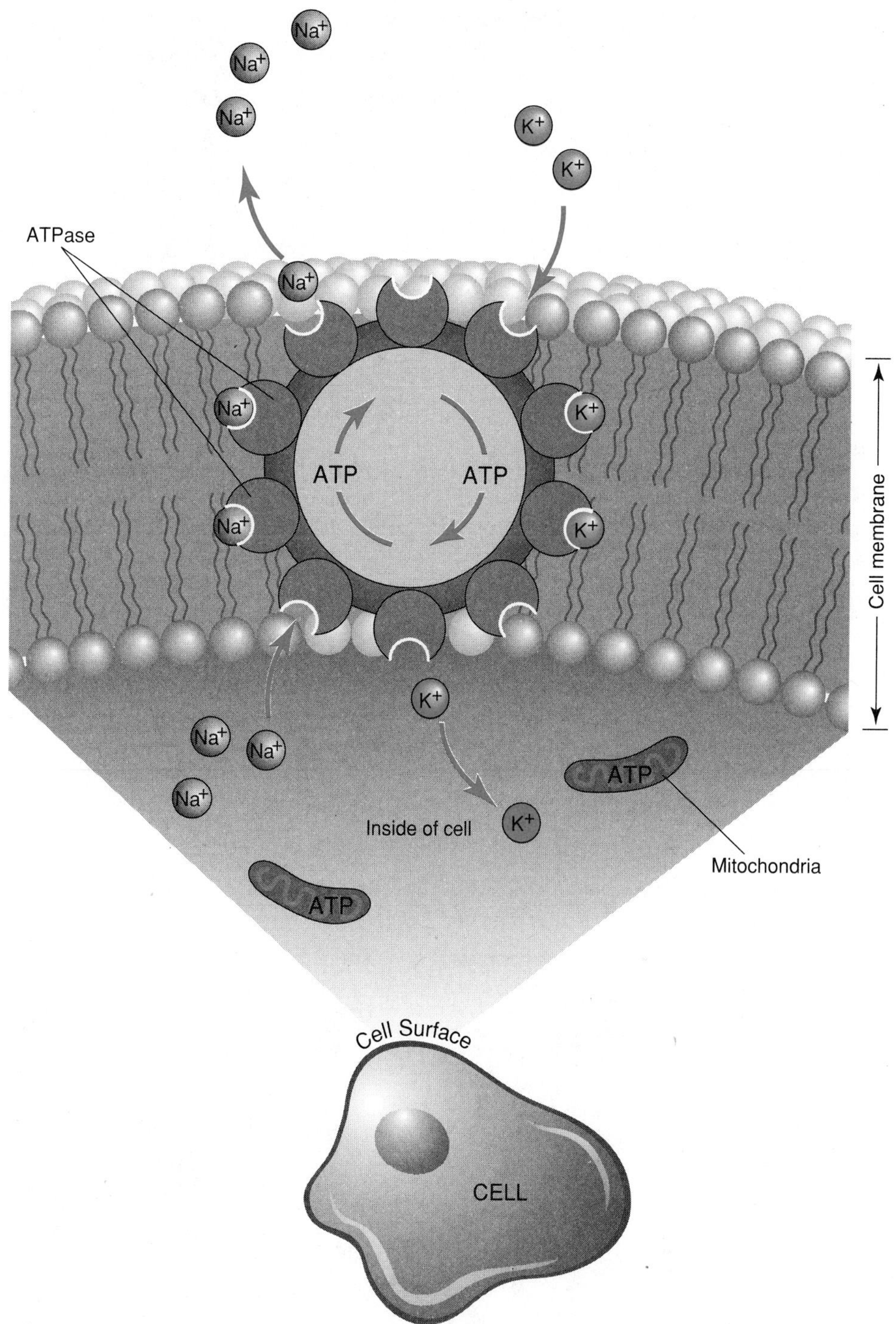

Figure 45–1 Sodium-potassium exchange system. Three sodium ions are exchanged for two potassium ions using adenosine triphosphate (ATP) to pump sodium out of the cell and potassium into the cell against a steep electrochemical gradient. An energy-containing ATP molecule, produced by the mitochondria, binds to the transporter protein, Na^+-K^+-ATPase.

PHARMACOTHERAPEUTIC OPTIONS

Cation-Exchange Resins

❒ Sodium polystyrene sulfonate (KAYEXALATE, SPS)

Indications

Sodium polystyrene sulfonate is used for the treatment of mild to moderate hyperkalemia (potassium level over 6 to 8 mEq/L). It aids in the removal of excess potassium from the body but is considered an adjunct to other measures such as restriction of potassium intake, control of acidosis, and a high-calorie diet.

Pharmacodynamics

Following oral administration, sodium is released from the resin in exchange for hydrogen ions in stomach acid. As the resin passes through the gastrointestinal (GI) tract, hydrogen ions exchange with those ions in greater concentrations. The modified resin is then eliminated in the feces. Because there is a higher concentration of potassium in the

TABLE 45–1 PHARMACOKINETICS OF CATION-EXCHANGE RESINS AND AMMONIA-DETOXIFYING DRUGS

Drug	Route	Onset	Peak	Duration	PB (%)	$t_{1/2}$
Cation-Exchange Resin						
Sodium polystyrene sulfonate	po	2–12 hr	UK	6–24 hr	NA	UK
	PR	2–12 hr	UK	4–6 hr	NA	UK
Ammonia-Detoxifying Drugs						
Lactulose	po	24–48 hr	UK	UK	UK	UK
Neomycin	po	Rapid	1–4 hr	4–6 hr	UK	2–3 hr

NA, Not applicable; PB, protein binding; PR, per rectum; $t_{1/2}$, elimination half-life; UK, unknown.

intestine, conversion of the resin to the potassium form occurs principally at this site.

Following rectal administration of sodium polystyrene sulfonate, sodium ions are partially released from the resin in exchange for other cations. Clinically, much of the exchange capacity is used for cations other than potassium such as calcium, magnesium, iron, organic cations, lipids, steroids, and proteins. Although 1 g of the resin has an in vitro exchange capacity of about 3.1 mEq of potassium, an in vivo exchange capacity greater than 1 mEq of potassium per gram of resin is unlikely.

Adverse Effects and Contraindications

The adverse effects of orally administered sodium polystyrene sulfonate include some degree of gastric irritation. Anorexia, nausea, vomiting, and constipation may occur, especially with large doses. Large oral doses can cause fecal impaction, especially in older adults. Occasionally, the resin causes diarrhea. Extensive intestinal necrosis is a rare occurrence but has been noted in patients with chronic renal failure or a kidney transplant. In all cases, the patients were azotemic, with the necrosis usually developing about 36 hours after therapy was started. Thus, the use of sodium polystyrene sulfonate is contraindicated in patients with azotemia or those who have had a kidney transplant.

Hypokalemia and clinically significant sodium retention is possible. Because the cation-exchange action of the resin is not selective for potassium, increased elimination of other cations occur also. Hypocalcemia and other electrolyte disturbances may appear.

Because sodium polystyrene sulfonate may provide a clinically significant sodium load, it should be administered cautiously to patients whose sodium intake must be restricted (e.g., those with heart failure, severe hypertension,

TABLE 45–2 DRUG-DRUG INTERACTONS OF CATION-EXCHANGE RESINS AND AMMONIA-DETOXIFYING DRUGS

Drug	Interactive Drugs	Interaction
Cation-Exchange Resin		
Sodium polystyrene sulfonate	Calcium- or magnesium-containing antacids	Decreases resin-exchanging ability; increases risk of systemic alkalosis
	Digoxin Digitoxin	Hypokalemia enhances risk of toxicity with interactive drug
Ammonia-Detoxifying Drugs		
Lactulose	Antimicrobial drugs	Prevents acidification of colon contents
	Antacids	Inhibits desired decrease in fecal pH in the colon
Neomycin	Ether Cyclopropane Halothane Nitrous oxide Tubocurarine Succinylcholine Decamethonium	Increased risk of respiratory paralysis
	Ethacrynic acid Furosemide	Increased risk of ototoxicity
	Cisplatin Methoxyflurane Carbenicillin Ticarcillin Azlocillin Mezlocillin Piperacillin	Increased risk of nephrotoxicity

and marked edema). In these patients compensatory restriction of sodium intake from other sources may be indicated.

Pharmacokinetics

The onset of orally administered sodium polystyrene sulfonate is between 2 to 12 hours, with peak drug action unknown (Table 45–1). It is distributed throughout the intestine but is not absorbed. It is eliminated in the feces in 6 to 24 hours. The duration of action of the drug when it is given rectally is 4 to 6 hours.

Drug-Drug Interactions

Concurrent use of magnesium- or calcium-containing antacids decrease the resin-exchanging ability of sodium polystyrene sulfonate. Concurrent use also increases the risk of metabolic alkalosis (Table 45–2). Hypokalemia also increases the risk of toxicity to cardiac glycosides (e.g., digoxin).

Dosage Regimen

When taken orally, sodium polystyrene sulfonate is dosed as 15 g in water or sorbitol one to four times daily (see Table 45–4). The maximum dose is 40 g four times daily. When given by rectum, 25 to 100 g of the drug is mixed with 100 mL of 0.9% sodium chloride, sorbitol, or water and given as a retention enema every 6 hours as needed. For children, the dose is 1 g per kilogram of body weight per day. Resin cookie or candy recipes are available from a pharmacist or dietician.

Laboratory Considerations

Serum potassium levels should be monitored at least daily during therapy. The duration of treatment is individually determined based on the patient's response. Intracellular potassium deficiency is not always reflected by serum potassium levels or ECG, so the clinical condition of the patient should be closely monitored.

Critical Thinking Process

Assessment

History of Present Illness

Patients with hyperkalemia should be asked if they have experienced palpitations, skipped heartbeats, or other cardiac irregularities. Information about the presence of muscle twitching, and numbness and tingling in the hands, feet, or around the mouth should be obtained. Muscle weakness ascends from the distal to proximal areas and affects the muscles of the arms and the legs. Trunk, head, and respiratory muscles are not affected until serum potassium levels reach fatal levels.

Recent changes in bowel habits, especially diarrhea, colic, and explosive bowel movements should be noted. Questions about recent medical or surgical interventions should be asked. The patient should also be questioned about urinary output, including frequency and amount of voiding. Specific information about the intake of potassium-containing foods (especially those eaten raw) and salt substitutes should be elicited because many of the substitutes contain potassium salts.

Past Health History

Information regarding a past history of diabetes mellitus and renal or adrenal insufficiency should be noted. A drug history remains vital with attention to drugs that contribute, from whatever means, to potassium retention. For example, patients taking trimethoprim, a potassium-sparing diuretic (combined with sulfamethoxazole or dapsone), have potassium levels that rise progressively. Over 25 percent of these patients have potassium levels over 5 mEq/L, and 10 percent experience life-threatening hyperkalemia. Potassium levels return to normal after the drug has been discontinued.

Physical Exam Findings

Physical exam findings of the patient with hyperkalemia includes a slow, weak pulse rate; a low blood pressure; and evidence of weakness and flaccid paralysis. Bowel sounds are hyperactive, with frequent audible rushes and gurgles. Abdominal distention and frequent, explosive, watery diarrhea may be noted. Behavioral changes are not usually seen with hyperkalemia because cardiac abnormalities cause the patient to seek help before serum potassium levels become high enough to produce neurologic manifestations.

Diagnostic Testing

A normal serum potassium level ranges between 3.5 to 5.5 mEq/L. If hyperkalemia results from dehydration, levels of other serum electrolytes may be elevated, as are hematocrit and hemoglobin levels. Hyperkalemia associated with renal failure is usually accompanied by elevations of serum creatinine and blood urea nitrogen levels, a decreased blood pH, and normal or low hematocrit and hemoglobin levels.

The common practice of repeatedly clenching and unclenching the fist during venipuncture may raise serum potassium levels by 1 to 2 mEq/L because the movement causes local release of potassium from forearm muscles.

An ECG is an insensitive method for detecting hyperkalemia. This is because 60 percent of patients with a serum potassium level greater than 6.5 mEq/L will not manifest ECG changes.

Developmental Considerations

Perinatal Hyperkalemia is relatively uncommon during pregnancy, although it is possible in the presence of renal or adrenal insufficiency, or diabetes mellitus. The normal changes of pregnancy should be considered when evaluating the pregnant woman's renal status.

Pediatric Numerous childhood illnesses cause fluid and electrolyte imbalances. However, the great majority of disturbances in hydration and electrolyte imbalance occur secondary to vomiting and diarrhea. Because plasma potassium levels can increase 0.2 to 1.7 mEq/L for each 0.1-unit fall in blood pH in such situations, immediate attention and constant surveillance is warranted.

Geriatric The older adult is susceptible to electrolyte imbalances because of the increased intake of drugs and poor intake of fluids, although hypokalemia is more common in the older adult than hyperkalemia. A common cause of hyperkalemia in the older adult is the concurrent use of potassium-sparing diuretics with potassium supplements. Other electrolyte imbalances do not have an age-frequency distribution.

Electrolyte imbalances such as hyperkalemia in the older adult may present as depression, confusion, lethargy, impaired mental functioning, anorexia, and weakness. A thorough assessment of the patient should be conducted because some of the symptoms of dehydration and electrolyte imbalance may be erroneously attributed to old age.

Psychosocial Considerations

The psychosocial needs of the patient with hyperkalemia are assessed in terms of risk factors, established support systems, previous and current coping patterns, and stability of any chronic disease. Patients with a newly diagnosed chronic illness may require counseling before acceptance and participation in self-care can begin. Even patients with long-term chronic disease cannot be assumed to require less psychosocial support.

Compliance is a major psychosocial issue for patients with hyperkalemia resulting from chronic illness. Assessment of the understanding on the part of patient and family members of the potential positive outcomes of good compliance and the negative effects of noncompliance should be noted. It must be stressed that the patient's quality of life depends on the degree of compliance with the treatment regimen.

Analysis and Management

Treatment Objectives

The treatment objectives for hyperkalemia is to normalize serum potassium levels and to prevent complications. In addition, the patient with chronic hyperkalemia will be able to prepare and administer the resin and maintain normal bowel function with neither diarrhea nor constipation.

Treatment Options

Drug Variables

Before treatment of hyperkalemia is started, the cause of the hyperkalemia should be determined and eliminated, if possible. Hyperkalemia can be anticipated and prevented in persons who have a significant decrease in urinary output for any reason, especially if they are receiving oral or intravenous potassium. Because the action of the resin is slow, treatments that shift potassium into the cells (e.g., sodium bicarbonate or dextrose, with or without insulin) or other treatments (e.g., calcium salts) are warranted. These other treatments are specifically indicated if the hyperkalemia is manifest by conduction defects (widening of the QRS complex) or arrhythmias (Table 45–3).

Sodium bicarbonate promotes the movement of potassium into the cells by increasing extracellular pH and also through direct action of the bicarbonate ion itself. Dextrose increases the release of endogenous insulin, promoting intracellular uptake of potassium. Insulin is often administered with dextrose to promote the effect of endogenous insulin. Insulin alone may be given to the hyperglycemic patient. Calcium chloride changes the relationship between membrane potential and threshold potential, restoring normal myocardial conduction. Calcium chloride does not lower serum potassium levels in any way, and, because it is short acting, it must be repeated if symptoms recur until serum potassium levels are lowered.

Patient Variables

Patients whose sodium intake must be restricted (e.g., those with heart failure, severe hypertension, or marked edema) may not be candidates for cation-exchange therapy. In these patients, compensatory restriction of sodium intake from other sources may be indicated. Cation-exchange therapy is most useful when hyperkalemia is not life-threatening and when other interventions have reduced the dangers of

TABLE 45–3 ADJUNCT TREATMENT MODALITIES FOR HYPERKALEMIA

Drug	Dosage	Mechanism	Expected Results
Sodium polystyrene sulfonate	15–60 g po or rectally	Exchanges sodium ions for potassium ions	Increases elimination of potassium via feces
Sodium bicarbonate	50–100 mEq IV over 2–5 minutes	Increases serum pH	Redistributes potassium into the cell
Dextrose 50%	25 g (50 mL) IV over 5 minutes	Increases insulin release	
Regular insulin	1 unit/3–5 g dextrose SC	Intracellular uptake of potassium	
Albuterol	10–20 mg in 4 mL 0.9% sodium chloride via nebulizer, inhaled over 10 minutes	$Beta_2$ adrenergic stimulation	
Calcium chloride	1 g (13.5 mEq) IV over 5–10 minutes	Raises threshold potential and re-establishes cardiac excitability	Reverses myocardial abnormalities
Furosemide	40–160 mg po or IV with or without sodium bicarbonate 0.5–3 mEq/kg QD	Removes potassium from the plasma	Increases elimination of potassium
Hemodialysis	Blood flow over 200–300 mL/minute (dialysate $[K^+] = 0$)	Extracorporeal potassium removal	
Peritoneal dialysis	Fast exchange over 3–4 hours	Removes potassium from peritoneal cavity	

hyperkalemia. Furthermore, use of the resin may make peritoneal or hemodialysis unnecessary.

Intervention

Administration

An osmotic laxative (i.e., sorbitol) is usually mixed with oral sodium polystyrene sulfonate to prevent constipation. It can be added to the resin powder, or a commercially prepared product may be used. Magnesium-containing laxatives should not be used, however. The powdered resin should not be mixed with foods or liquids that contain large amounts of potassium (e.g., bananas, orange juice, prune juice, apricot nectar, or milk).

When sodium polystyrene sulfonate is administered as a retention enema, each dose of the powdered resin is mixed with 100 to 200 mL of an aqueous vehicle (e.g., 25-percent sorbitol, 1-percent methylcellulose, 10-percent dextrose, or water) that has been warmed to body temperature. Alternatively, 120 to 180 mL of a commercially available suspension can be used. After an initial cleansing enema, a soft, large (French 28) rubber tube is inserted about 20 cm into the rectum, with the tip well into the sigmoid colon and secured in place. The suspension is then instilled into the rectum by gravity. After the drug is administered, the tube is flushed with 50 to 100 mL of fluid, clamped, and left in place. If leakage occurs, the hips can be elevated on pillows or the patient placed in a knee-chest position. The resin is retained in the colon for at least 30 to 60 minutes. The colon is then irrigated with a non–sodium-containing solution at body temperature to remove the resin. Approximately 2 L of solution may be needed to flush out the resin sufficiently. A Y connector with tubing may be attached to the rectal tube and the cleansing solution administered through one port of the Y and allowed to drain by gravity through the other port.

The patient should be monitored at least once daily for signs and symptoms of hypokalemia, including irritability, confusion, muscle weakness, and cardiac arrhythmias. The patient with hypertension, heart failure, or edema should be watched for evidence of sodium and fluid overload. Serum potassium and sodium levels should be monitored at least once daily during treatment.

Education

Education is the key factor in the prevention of hyperkalemia. The patient should be informed of the signs and symptoms of hyperkalemia and which findings should be reported to the health care provider. When drug therapy is necessary, the patient should be informed as to the purpose and method of drug administration and that frequent laboratory tests will be needed to monitor the effectiveness of the drug. The patient or family member should be shown how to prepare and use the resin correctly should they be self-administering the drug.

The patient should also be informed about the constipating effects of the resin and strategies to use that help prevent or reduce constipation. A high-fiber diet and 8 to 12 glasses of fluids per day will help. The health care provider should be contacted if constipation occurs or persists. Taking the drug early in the day will help prevent problems with diarrhea at night.

Diet education includes avoidance of potassium-laden foods and instruction about which foods are permissible. The patient should be taught how to determine the potassium content when reading labels. Also, it is important to teach the person doing the shopping or who prepares the meals, as well as the patient, whenever possible. Additionally, high-sodium foods, such as processed foods and lunch meats, snack foods that are high in sodium, and salt substitutes should be avoided. Many of the salt substitutes contain potassium.

Patients taking a cardiac glycoside (e.g., digoxin) should be re-educated about the signs and symptoms of toxicity because hypokalemia enhances the risk of toxicity to the glycoside drug. The patient should be taught how to take a pulse accurately and to determine its regularity and quality. The patient should also be advised to avoid calcium or magnesium antacids because they reduce the effectiveness of the resin.

Evaluation

Evaluation of drug effectiveness can be demonstrated by the normalization of serum potassium levels without adverse effects. The patient with chronic hyperkalemia is able to demonstrate how to prepare and administer the resin. He or she should maintain normal bowel function during therapy with neither constipation nor diarrhea.

HEPATIC ENCEPHALOPATHY

Epidemiology and Etiology

Hepatic encephalopathy is a state of disordered central nervous system function. Also called portal-systemic encephalopathy, it is one of the major complications of cirrhosis. It results from failure of the liver to detoxify noxious substances of GI origin because of hepatocellular dysfunction or portal-systemic shunting. Ammonia is the most readily identified toxin but is not solely responsible for the patient's disturbed mental status.

Pathophysiology

Ammonia is formed in the body in several ways: by the liver during deamination of amino acids, by epithelial cells of the proximal and distal tubules and collecting duct of the nephron, as part of the regulation of hydrogen ions, and by bacteria of the GI tract acting on urea or dietary protein. A normally functioning liver converts the absorbed ammonia to urea, a less toxic substance. Urea is then eliminated in the urine.

Damage to the liver or shunting of blood flow around the liver inhibits the conversion of ammonia to urea. The elevated serum ammonia level that results leads to hepatic encephalopathy with decreasing levels of consciousness, impaired neuromuscular functioning, and in some cases, death.

There are several conditions that can result in or contribute to hepatic encephalopathy including cirrhosis, high-protein intake, old blood in the bowel from GI bleeding, or alkalosis secondary to hyperventilation or hypokalemia, constipation, and infection. Patients with cirrhosis have a higher rate of urea breakdown in the GI tract than healthy persons. Dietary protein acts as a substrate for bacterial production of ammonia or other nitrogenous toxins. Serious GI bleeding decreases perfusion to the liver, brain, and kidneys but also contributes 15 to 20 g of protein/100 mL as ammonia substrate.

Alkalosis leads to diffusion of unionized ammonia across the blood-brain barrier to cause lethargy, confusion, and irritability. Hypokalemia is a major precipitating metabolic factor. As serum levels decrease, potassium shifts from intracellular compartment in exchange for sodium and hydrogen. The shift of hydrogen ions into the intracellular compartment increases the acid level in that compartment, decreasing pH, increasing the base in the extracellular compartment, and increasing pH. The extracellular alkalosis liberates hydrogen from ammonium (NH_4^+) and from ammonia (NH_3^+). Ammonia is gaseous and readily crosses into cells, where it accumulates and exerts toxic effects. Increased accumulation of base in the extracellular compartment from other causes can precipitate the same type of response.

Constipation allows for increased production and absorption of ammonia due to the longer contact time for bacteria and substrates. Constipation may also provoke Valsalva's maneuver while stooling and thus precipitate bleeding from esophageal varices or hemorrhoids. Infection leads to increased tissue catabolism, which also contributes to a higher nitrogen load.

PHARMACOTHERAPEUTIC OPTIONS

Ammonia-Detoxifying Drugs

- ❐ Lactulose (CEPHULAC, CHOLAC, CHRONULAC, CONSTILAC, CONSTULOSE, DUPHALAC, ENULOSE); (✱) LUCULAX
- ❐ Neomycin (MYCIFRADIN SULFATE)

Indications

Lactulose is used as an adjunct to protein restriction and supportive therapy for the prevention and treatment of hepatic encephalopathy. Lactulose has been useful in the management of hepatic encephalopathy resulting from surgical portacaval shunts or from chronic hepatic diseases such as cirrhosis. Lactulose reduces blood ammonia concentrations with improvement in the mental state of the patient.

Lactulose is also useful for the treatment of chronic constipation in adults and older adults, although its superiority to conventional laxatives has not been established. Lactulose has also been used to restore regular bowel movements in patients who have had a hemorrhoidectomy, but it is presently not approved by the Food and Drug Administration for such use.

Lactulose is not useful in the management of drug-induced encephalopathy or for encephalopathy caused by inborn errors of metabolism and electrolyte disturbances. It is not effective in the treatment of coma associated with hepatitis or other acute liver disorders.

Neomycin, an aminoglycoside antibiotic (see Chapter 24), is also used in the management of hepatic encephalopathy to decrease the population of ammonia-producing bacteria. It has been used to decrease the bacterial count in the GI tract in preparation for surgery.

Pharmacodynamics

Lactulose is a semisynthetic disaccharide that decreases blood ammonia concentrations. Although the mechanism of action is not clearly understood, the decrease in ammonia levels appears to be associated with the biotransformation of the sugar in the lower GI tract. The breakdown of lactulose to organic acids (i.e., lactic acid, formic acid, and acetic acids) causes a drop in the pH of colon contents from 7 to 5. It also inhibits the diffusion of ammonia from the colon into the blood. In addition, because the contents of the colon are more acidic than blood, ammonia (NH_3^+) is converted to ammonium ions (NH_4^+), thereby preventing its absorption. The cathartic action of lactulose is probably caused by the osmotic effect of the drug's organic acid metabolites. The metabolites expel trapped ammonium ions and other nitrogenous substances from the colon. The osmotic effect of the metabolites causes an increase in the water content of the stool and subsequent softening. The cathartic effect may not be seen for 24 to 48 hours after administration of the drug.

Neomycin acts by inhibiting protein synthesis in enteral bacteria at the level of the 30S ribosome. As a result, bactericidal effects are produced because the protein synthesis required for maintaining the structure and metabolic activity of the bacterial cell is inhibited.

Adverse Effects and Contraindications

The adverse effects of lactulose primarily affect the GI tract. During the first few days of therapy, anorexia, nausea, vomiting, and abdominal cramping are common. These effects usually subside with continued therapy, although dosage reduction may be required in some cases. Diarrhea, flatulence, distention, and belching have been noted.

Lactulose is contraindicated in hypersensitivity and for patients on a low-galactose diet. It should be used with caution in patients with diabetes mellitus, older adults, and in debilitated patients. Lactulose carries a category C rating and thus is generally avoided during pregnancy. It is not known whether lactulose is distributed to breast milk.

The primary adverse effects of neomycin are ototoxicity and nephrotoxicity, although the drug can enhance neuromuscular blockade when it is used parenterally. Hypersensitivity reactions are always possible. Neomycin is contraindicated in patients with pre-existing ototoxicity or nephrotoxicity, in patients with cross-allergenicity to aminoglycosides, and in patients with renal impairment.

Pharmacokinetics

Less than 3 percent of a dose of lactulose is absorbed from the small intestine following oral administration. The onset of action for lactulose varies with the route of administration and the patient's condition. The duration of action of a single dose may range from 6 to 8 hours. Lactulose is eliminated unchanged in the urine within 24 hours. Any unabsorbed lactulose reaches the colon unchanged, where it is transformed by bacteria to lactic acid and small amounts of acetic and formic acids. The bacteria normally present in the colon that act on lactulose include *Lactobacilli, Bacteroides, Escherichia coli,* and *Clostridia.* Neomycin is also minimally absorbed (less than 3 percent) following oral administration. Its distribution is unknown, and the onset of drug action

TABLE 45–4 DOSAGE REGIMEN FOR CATION-EXCHANGE RESINS AND AMMONIA-DETOXIFYING DRUGS

Drug	Use(s)	Dosage	Implications
Cation-Exchange Resin			
Sodium polystyrene sulfonate	Mild to moderate hyperkalemia	*Adult:* 15 g po QD–QID in water or sorbitol *or* 25–100 g/100 mL sorbitol q6hr as retention enema. Increase to 40 g po QID. *Child:* 1 g/kg/dose po or PR	Each gram contains 4.1 mEq sodium. Exchanges 1 g of sodium ions for 0.5–1 mEq potassium ions
Ammonia-Detoxifying Drugs			
Lactulose	Portal-systemic encephalopathy, chronic constipation	*Adult:* 20–30 g (30–45 mL) po TID–QID till stools are soft *or* 30–45 mL/100 mL of 0.9% NaCl *or* water per rectum q4–6hr. Retain for 30–60 minutes. Titrate dose to 2–3 stools/day	Syrup: 10 g lactulose/15 mL. Decreases blood ammonia concentrations by 25–50%. Start dose at 50 mL/hr until catharsis occurs
Neomycin	Portal-systemic encephalopathy	*Adult:* 500 mg po QID. Increase to 4–12 g po in divided doses QD. *Child:* 40–100 mg/kg/day in divided doses q4–6hr	Contraindicated in patients with renal dysfunction

varies. Peak plasma concentration from the absorbed portion of neomycin may occur 1 to 4 hours after oral or rectal administration. Orally administered neomycin is eliminated unchanged in the feces in about 4 to 6 hours. The amounts that are systemically absorbed are eliminated unchanged through the kidneys (see Table 45–1).

Drug-Drug Interactions

Theoretically, the effects of lactulose are decreased in the presence of neomycin and other oral antimicrobial drugs (see Table 45–2). It is thought that the antibiotics eliminate colonic bacteria that are necessary to transform lactulose and thereby prevent acidification of colon contents.

Neomycin interacts with a number of drugs. Respiratory paralysis can occur with concurrent use of neomycin and inhalation anesthetics or neuromuscular blockers. There is an increased risk of ototoxicity with loop diuretics and nephrotoxicity with nephrotoxic drugs.

Dosage Regimen

When given by mouth, the dose of lactulose is 20 to 30 g (30 to 45 mL) three to four times a day until the stools are soft. The dosage is then titrated to maintain two to three stools/day (Table 45–4). When lactulose is administered as a retention enema, 30 to 45 mL in 100 mL of fluid is used.

The optimal dosing of neomycin is not known. An oral starting dose of 500 mg four times daily is recommended. The dosage may be increased to 4 to 12 g/day as necessary. A child's dose of neomycin is 40 to 100 mg/kg/day in divided doses.

Laboratory Considerations

Lactulose decreases ammonia levels by 25 to 50 percent. Blood and urine electrolytes should be closely monitored when lactulose is used repeatedly.

When neomycin is used in the treatment, laboratory monitoring should include urinalysis, specific gravity, blood urea nitrogen, creatinine, and creatinine clearance before and throughout therapy. There are no known laboratory test interferences due to either lactulose or neomycin.

Critical Thinking Process

Assessment

History of Present Illness

The patient with hepatic encephalopathy usually presents with a history of failing health including reports of anorexia, nausea, vomiting, indigestion, flatulence, and constipation. Reports of vague, dull, mild or steady, wavelike abdominal pain may be noted. The pain is usually in the right upper quadrant. The patient is usually fatigued and does not tolerate activity well.

Past Health History

Encephalopathy is often a complication of loss of liver function. The patient usually has a history of Laennec's cirrhosis (secondary to alcohol abuse); therefore, information about the frequency and quantity of alcohol consumed should be elicited. Cirrhosis can also be secondary to viral hepatitis, biliary tract obstruction, right-sided heart failure, and metabolic derangement. Therefore, a history of these disorders warrants attention because as much as three-fourths of the liver can be destroyed before physiologic function is altered.

Physical Exam Findings

Manifestations of hepatic encephalopathy vary and may occur rapidly or gradually over the course of a few days. Assessment findings reflect alterations in the level of consciousness, in intellectual function, behavior and personality, and in neuromuscular function (see Stages and Symptoms of Hepatic Encephalopathy). Weight loss masked by water retention can also be seen.

Diagnostic Testing

Patients with hepatic encephalopathy have a number of abnormal laboratory tests including increased levels of total, unconjugated, and conjugated bilirubin; increased urine bilirubin and urobilinogen; and elevated liver enzymes, alanine aminotransferase (ALT; serum glutamic-pyruvic transaminase [SGPT]), aspartate aminotransferase (AST; serum glutamic-

STAGES AND SYMPTOMS OF HEPATIC ENCEPHALOPATHY

Stage 1—Prodromal Period
- Changes in sleep patterns
- Slowed responses
- Shortened attention span
- Depressed or euphoric mood
- Irritability
- Tremors
- Incoordination
- Impaired ability to write

Step 2—Impending
- Disorientation to time
- Lethargy
- Impaired calculation ability
- Decreased inhibition
- Anxiety or apathy
- Inappropriate behaviors
- Slurred speech
- Decreased reflexes
- Ataxia and asterixis

Stage 3—Stuporous
- Disorientation to place
- Confused, somnolent
- Stuporous but capable of being aroused
- Anger, rage, paranoia
- Hyperreflexia
- Clonus
- Presence of Babinski's sign
- Asterixis

Stage 4—Coma
- No intellectual functioning
- Unconscious
- Loss of deep tendon reflexes
- Responsive only to deep pain
- Hyperventilation
- Fetor hepaticus
- Increased body temperature
- Increased pulse rate

oxaloacetic transaminase [SGOT]) LDH, and alkaline phosphatase. Increased prothrombin time, decreased platelets, decreased leukocyte count, decreased red blood cell count, decreased serum albumin and serum glucose levels, hypokalemia and hyponatremia may also be noted.

Developmental Considerations

Perinatal A woman with a history of alcohol abuse has a reduced chance of conceiving due to increased potential for infertility. However, when pregnancy does occur, alcohol use places both the mother and the fetus at risk. Maternal complications of alcohol use during pregnancy include an increased risk of spontaneous abortion, stillbirth, and abruptio placentae.

Alcohol is the most common teratogen. Approximately 7 to 10 percent of child-bearing women are heavy drinkers, consuming five to six drinks on occasion and at least 45 drinks per month. In the United States, 65 percent of fetuses are exposed to alcohol. Alcohol use during pregnancy interferes with the absorption of many nutrients, overall cell growth and cell division, causes abnormal migration of neural and non-neural brain cells, inhibits DNA synthesis and interferes with amino acid availability to the fetus, and directly suppresses fetal breathing. The teratogenic manifestations of alcohol abuse can range from no effect to fetal alcohol syndrome depending on factors such as genetic sensitivity, time of exposure, and dose. Hepatic encephalopathy only compounds the potential for fetal harm.

Pediatric Common causes of cirrhosis and potential hepatic encephalopathy in infancy, childhood, and adolescence are cystic fibrosis, alpha$_1$-antitrypsin deficiency, biliary atresia, and hepatitis. The adolescent population is at particular risk for cirrhosis because hepatitis B becomes more widespread among teenage illicit parenteral drug users. The child's prognosis depends on the cause of the cirrhosis and the severity of the hepatic damage.

Geriatric Cirrhosis or other liver disease superimposed on the physical changes of the aging hepatic system increases the risk of hepatic encephalopathy. Approximately 8 to 10 percent of Americans older than 65 years of age are alcoholics. Although older adults consume less alcohol than their younger counterparts, the physical changes of aging cause it to be metabolized more slowly.

Also compounding cirrhosis is the potential for fluid and electrolyte imbalance secondary to co-morbid diseases the patient may have. Additionally, only about 3 percent of older adults meet 100 percent of the recommended daily allowances for protein, vitamins A and C, thiamine, riboflavin, and iron. Differentiation between the mental status changes due to fluid and electrolyte imbalance, or nutritional deficiencies, and the signs and symptoms of hepatic encephalopathy can be difficult to discern. Thus, a thorough patient history is vital.

Psychosocial Considerations

The patient with hepatic encephalopathy secondary to cirrhosis may experience changes in body appearance and in role relationships. Assessment of the patient's self-esteem, body image, and role relationships is important to successful treatment outcomes. If the patient is not helped to reestablish or maintain positive self-esteem, it can add to the problem of alcohol abuse and its complications (see Case Study—Hepatic Encephalopathy).

Analysis and Management

Treatment Objectives

The treatment goal for hepatic encephalopathy is an overall increase in the patient's cognitive ability from baseline status. If the patient was comatose, a return to consciousness is the goal.

Treatment Options

Many patients tolerate increased dietary protein during lactulose therapy. The drug does not, however, alter the course of the underlying liver disease. Therefore, use of lactulose in the treatment of hepatic encephalopathy does not obviate treatment of the underlying disease, nor does it preclude the use of other treatment measures.

A good clinical response has been achieved in 75 to 85 percent of patients. Because lactulose is relatively nontoxic, it is a valuable alternative to neomycin, especially when prolonged therapy is required, or when neomycin is contraindicated. Patients who previously failed to respond to

Case Study Hepatic Encephalopathy

Patient History

History of Present Illness	MM's wife accompanies her 59-year-old husband to this appointment with a 3-day history of increasing confusion, lethargy, restlessness, and irritability. She also notes that his writing has been impaired; he has involuntary muscle tremors, especially in the hands; his speech is slurred, and he has "bad breath–like a diaper pail." She reports a consumption history of a pint of whiskey a day for 15 years. She reports he has not eaten much for the last 3 days but she generally sees that he follows a high-calorie, low-protein diet. His last drink was 3 days ago.
Past Health History	MM has a history of Laennec's cirrhosis with three previous hospitalizations for GI bleeding. His last bleed was 1 year ago. He is taking no other drugs at this time but has a history of noncompliance with treatment regimens.
Physical Exam	Height: 5′9″. Weight: 167 lbs. (up 9 pounds from previous visit). BP 139/88. VSS. Spider angiomas are noted over nose and cheeks, and dilated vessels are seen over upper body and lower extremities. Multiple ecchymotic areas noted over extremities with 1+ edema of lower extremities. Bowel sounds diminished all four quadrants; liver is not palpable. General body odor of urine.
Diagnostic Testing	Electrolytes low normal. Urine bilirubin and urobilinogen, total and conjugated bilirubin, ALT (SGPT), AST (SGOT), LDH, and alkaline phosphatase are elevated. Serum ammonia elevated.
Developmental Considerations	No specific age-related changes of aging; however, because of history of cirrhosis has loss of liver function. MM's ability to progress through ages and stages of growth and development impaired due to alcohol intake.
Psychosocial Considerations	MM has been a confectionery worker for a national bakery for 24 years. He was recently relieved of his duties. MM's wife reports he has consistently lost time from work due to his alcohol intake and hospitalizations. He has attempted several times to participate in the corporation-sponsored rehabilitation program but with little success. He acknowledges that the alcohol abuse started when he began accompanying fellow employees to the local saloon after work. He has been married 37 years to the same woman who oversees his health care needs and drug regimens.
Economic Factors	MM receives financial assistance from the confectionery industry and union. Health care insurance is available through the union but he has no supplementary insurance coverage or pharmacy program eligibility.

Variables Influencing Decision

Treatment Objectives

- Decrease blood ammonia levels by 25% to 50%.
- Facilitate overall increase in the cognitive ability of the patient from baseline status.

Drug Variables	*Drug Summary*	*Patient Variables*
Indications	Neomycin: Acute treatment of portal-systemic encephalopathy (PSE) Lactulose: Chronic long-term treatment of PSE	MM has acute PSE at this time.
Pharmacodynamics	Neomycin: Inhibits bacterial protein synthesis, producing bactericidal effects. Lactulose: Inhibits nonionic diffusion of ammonia from colon into the blood stream.	MM has no pharmacodynamic variables that will affect drug decision.
Adverse Effects/ Contraindications	Neomycin: Cautious use in patients with renal insufficiency. Lactulose: Possible GI distress, improves with continued use.	MM has no history of renal insufficiency but has history of noncompliance.

Case Study continued on following page

Case Study Hepatic Encephalopathy—cont'd

Drug Variables	*Drug Summary*	*Patient Variables*
Pharmacokinetics	Neomycin: Has rapid onset but relatively short duration of action. Lactulose: Slow onset with unknown duration of action.	MM needs rapid onset of action due to acute illness but will also need long-term chronic therapy. This will become a decision point.
Dosage Regimen	Dosage of both drugs titrated to patient response.	MM unable to problem solve safely at this time so caregiver will monitor drug therapy. Also has history of noncompliance. This will become a decision point.
Lab Considerations	Serum ammonia levels checked periodically during therapy. BUN, creatinine, and creatinine clearance required before and throughout prolonged therapy with neomycin. No specific lab tests required when using lactulose.	MM's signs and symptoms more reliable for treatment success than ammonia levels. This will be a decision point.
Cost Index*	Neomycin: 1 Lactulose: 1	Cost of drugs relatively inexpensive but may become a decision point should additional drug therapies be required for MM. This may become a decision point in the future.

Summary of Decision Points

- MM has acute PSE at this time.
- MM needs rapid onset of action due to acute illness but will also require long-term chronic therapy.
- MM unable to problem solve safely at this time, so caregiver will need to monitor drug therapy. MM also has a history of noncompliance.
- Cost of drugs relatively inexpensive but may become a decision point should additional drug therapies be required for MM.
- MM's signs and symptoms more reliable for treatment success than ammonia levels.

DRUGS TO BE USED

- Neomycin 500 mg po QID until symptoms improve, then discontinue and start
- Lactulose 30–45 mL po TID–QID titrated to 2–3 stools daily

*Cost Index:

1	$ <30/mo.
2	$ 30–40/mo.
3	$ 40–50/mo.
4	$ 50–60/mo.
5	$ >60/mo.

AWP of 960 mL of lactulose (10 g/15 mL) syrup is approximately $ 30.
AWP of 100, 500 mg tablets of neomycin is approximately $ 20.

neomycin and dietary protein restriction may respond to lactulose and vice versa.

Because neomycin destroys bacteria and lactulose requires bacterial degradation to be effective, concomitant therapy with these drugs is theoretically counterproductive. It appears, however, that lactulose remains active when it is administered with neomycin, and there is some evidence that concomitant therapy may be more effective than the use of either drug alone. Some health care providers recommend neomycin for acute episodes of hepatic encephalopathy and lactulose for long-term management of chronic disease.

Intervention

Administration

Lactulose should be administered with 8 ounces of fruit juice, water, or milk to increase its palatability. Rapid results can be achieved when lactulose is given on an empty stomach. Fluids should be increased to 2 L/day. When lactulose is administered as an enema, a rectal balloon catheter should be used. The enema is retained for 30 to 60 minutes. If inadvertent evacuation occurs, the enema may be repeated.

Neomycin is ordinarily used in conjunction with erythromycin, a low-residue diet, and a laxative or enema for a preoperative bowel prep. Instruct the patient to take the neomycin as directed for the full course of therapy. Neomycin can be taken without regard to meals, but caution the patient that neomycin can cause nausea, vomiting, or diarrhea. The patient should be well hydrated (1500 to 2000 mL) during therapy.

Education

Teach the patient taking lactulose to dilute it to counteract the sweet taste and to take it on an empty stomach, thereby promoting drug action. It should be stored in a cool environment but not where the drug may freeze. The patient should report any change in bowel habits, particularly diarrhea, because diarrhea may indicate an overdose. The importance of consistent use and titration to the number of stools should be emphasized.

Instruct the patient taking neomycin to report any signs of hypersensitivity, tinnitus, vertigo, rash, dizziness, or difficulty urinating. Advise him or her of the importance of drinking plenty of fluids.

Evaluation

A patient's clearing of confusion, lethargy, restlessness, and irritability demonstrates effective treatment of hepatic encephalopathy with lactulose. Passage of soft, formed stool usually occurs within 24 to 48 hours. Improvement may occur within two hours following rectal administration and 24 to 48 hours following oral administration of lactulose. Improved neurologic status should be noted with effective neomycin therapy.

SUMMARY

- Hyperkalemia is a serum potassium level exceeding 5.5 mEq/L.
- Hyperkalemia may be caused by crushing injuries, sepsis, fever, surgery, metabolic acidosis, hyperglycemia or insulin deficiency, or shock.
- Hyperkalemia increases membrane potentials, and cells become more excitable. The cardiovascular system, the central nervous system, and the gastrointestinal tract are most often affected.
- Patients are assessed for history of palpitations, skipped beats, and other cardiac irregularities. Recent changes in bowel habits, colic, and explosive bowel movements should be noted.
- A history of diabetes mellitus, renal or adrenal insufficiency remains vital because potassium levels can be increased in their presence. Patients who are concurrently taking potassium-sparing diuretics and potassium supplements are at risk for hyperkalemia.
- The treatment objectives for the patient with hyperkalemia are to normalize serum potassium levels and to prevent complications.
- The cause of hyperkalemia should be determined before treatment is started.
- If time permits, serum potassium levels can be reduced by administering sodium polystyrene sulfonate, which is a cation-exchange resin. If potassium levels must be dropped quickly due to conduction defects or arrhythmias, treatment options include sodium bicarbonate, dextrose and insulin, and calcium chloride.
- Patient teaching includes the purpose for and method of drug administration, the potential for constipation, and the importance of adequate fluid intake.
- Evaluation of drug effectiveness includes normalization of serum potassium levels without adverse effects.
- Hepatic encephalopathy can be precipitated by increased ammonia from GI bleeding (often secondary to alcohol abuse), increased protein in the diet, hypokalemia and alkalosis, and depressed central nervous system states such as hypoxia and sedation.
- Damage to the liver or shunting of blood around the liver inhibits the conversion of ammonia to urea. Resulting elevated serum ammonia levels lead to hepatic encephalopathy, with decreased level of consciousness, impaired neuromuscular functioning, and in some cases, death.
- Patients with hepatic encephalopathy usually present with a history of failing health including reports of anorexia, nausea, vomiting, indigestion, flatulence, and constipation. Also, they often have a long history of alcohol abuse. Mental status changes are due to the build-up of ammonia in the central nervous system.
- The treatment objective for hepatic encephalopathy is to produce an overall increase in the cognitive ability of the patient from baseline status. If the patient is comatose, a return to consciousness is the goal.
- Hepatic encephalopathy is treated with a low-protein diet, lactulose, and neomycin.
- The importance of consistent use of the drug with titration to the number of stools should be emphasized.
- Effective treatment with lactulose will manifest as a clearing of confusion, lethargy, restlessness, and irritability. Improvement usually occurs within 2 hours following rectal administration and 24 to 48 hours following oral administration.

BIBLIOGRAPHY

Blanc, P., Daures, J., and Rauillon, J. (1992). Lactilol or lactulose in the treatment of chronic hepatic encephalopathy: Results of a meta-analysis. *Hepatology,* 15(2), 222–228.

Conn, H. (1995). Portal-systemic shunting and portal-systemic encephalopathy: A predictable relationship. *Hepatology,* 22(1), 365–367.

Eiam-ong, S., Kurtzman, N., and Sabatini, S. (1996). Studies on the mechanism of trimethoprim-induced hyperkalemia. *Kidney International,* 49(5), 1372–1378.

Greenberg, S., Reiser, I., and Chou, S. (1993). Trimethoprim-sulfamethoxazole induces reversible hyperkalemia. *Annals of Internal Medicine,* 119(4), 291–295.

Maddison, J. E. (1992). Neurochemical studies of hepatic encephalopathy. *Drug and Alcohol Review,* 11(4), 393–398.

McDonald, R. A. (1995). Disorders of potassium balance. *Pediatric Annals,* 24(1), 31–37.

Perazella, M. A. (1996). Hyperkalemia in the elderly: A group at high risk. *Connecticut Medicine,* 60(4), 195–198.

Perez, A. (1995). Electrolytes: Restoring the balance—hyperkalemia. *RN,* 58(11), 33–36.

Perlmutter, E. P., Sweeney, D., Herskovits, G., et al. (1996). Case report: Severe hyperkalemia in a geriatric patient receiving standard doses of trimethoprim-sulfamethoxazole. *American Journal of Medical Science,* 311(2), 84–85.

Rutecki, G. W., and Whittier, F. C. (1996). Hyperkalemia: How to identify—and correct—the underlying cause. *Consultant,* 36(3), 564–566, 569–573.

Velazquez, H., Perazella, M. A., Wright, F. S., et al. (1993). Renal mechanism of trimethoprim-induced hyperkalemia. *Annals of Internal Medicine,* 119(4), 296–301.

Unit IX

Drugs Influencing the Respiratory System

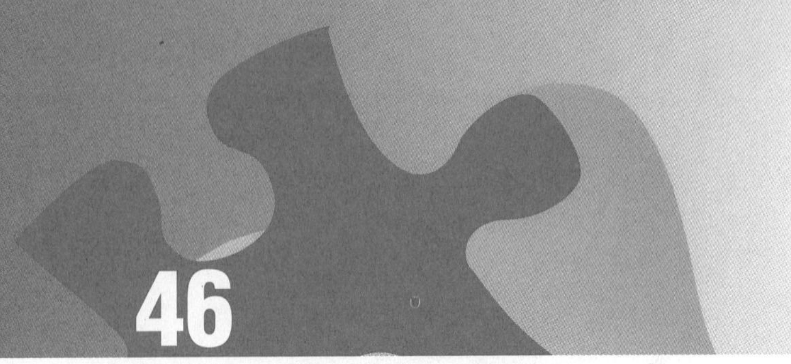

46 Antiasthmatic and Bronchodilator Drugs

Bronchodilator and antiasthmatic drugs are used in the treatment of respiratory disorders that are characterized by inflammation, bronchospasm or bronchoconstriction, mucosal edema, and excessive mucus production. Hyperactivity of the airways in response to various physical, chemical, environmental, or pharmacologic stimuli is the hallmark of asthma. Treatment is directed at preventing attacks when possible and normalizing the patient's life-style. Treatment must involve both nondrug and drug measures. As a general rule, drug therapy for hypersensitive airway disorders is more effective in relieving symptoms than in curing the underlying disorder. The health care provider generally can manage the spectrum of symptoms, but when conservative methods fall short, referral to an allergist or respiratory specialist is appropriate. Because inflammation plays such a central role in the airway dysfunction of asthma, it is not surprising that national and international guidelines for asthma management have selected this aspect of the disease as a specific therapeutic target.

ASTHMA

Epidemiology and Etiology

Asthma is defined as a chronic inflammatory disorder of the airways. It is a reversible obstructive disorder that begins at any age but most often appears in childhood. An estimated 12 million people in the United States are affected. The prevalence of asthma has increased more than 60 percent in the last 10 to 12 years. Morbidity associated with asthma is dramatic. It affects physical activity, school attendance, occupational choices, and many other aspects of daily living. Furthermore, the mortality rate related to asthma has doubled since the late 1970s. The asthma death rate for blacks ages 15 to 44 is at least five times higher than that of whites. The higher mortality rate may be associated with inaccurate assessment of disease severity, an increase in environmental allergens, inadequate medical treatment, a delay in seeking help, limited access to health care, and noncompliance with the prescribed treatment plan.

Asthma commonly has a familial predisposition. The majority of childhood cases begin between the ages of 3 and 6 years. The onset is often associated with a respiratory infection. Most patients with childhood-onset asthma improve when they reach puberty. Adult-onset asthma is more common in women than in men. Remission occurs less often in adults than in children.

Asthma can be categorized by etiology. *Intrinsic asthma* (most often seen in adults) is provoked or worsened by infection, exertion, emotion, and nonspecific environmental factors. Intrinsic asthma is not related to allergen exposure. The majority of patients with *extrinsic asthma* are *atopic,* that is, they have a hereditary predisposition to allergy. They have symptoms related to environmental allergens. The remaining patients who have the nonatopic form of the condition have extrinsic asthma related to occupational factors.

There are a number of triggers leading to asthma attacks (see Triggers of Acute Asthma Attacks). Exposure to tobacco smoke is a major precipitant of asthma symptoms in children. It increases the need for drug therapy and reduces lung function. Increased air pollution levels of respirable particulates precipitate symptoms and increase emergency room visits and hospitalization. Other factors that contribute to asthma severity include rhinitis and sinusitis, gastroesophageal reflux, viral respiratory infections, and some drugs. Approximately 5 percent of the estimated 12 million asthmatics in the United States are sensitive to sulfite-containing foods (shrimp, processed foods, avocados, acidic juices, wine, and beer; see Appendix C).

Asthma severity is classified as *mild intermittent, mild persistent, moderate persistent,* and *severe persistent.* These classifications more accurately reflect clinical manifestations of the disease. Patients at any level of severity can have mild, moderate, or severe exacerbations. Exposure of sensitive patients to allergens increases airway inflammation, hyperresponsiveness, symptoms, the need for drug therapy, and the risk of death. Substantially reducing exposure reduces these outcomes. Underdiagnosis and inadequate management are major contributors to morbidity and mortality.

Pathophysiology

Although asthma was once regarded largely as a disease of airway smooth muscle, it is now known to be a chronic inflammatory disease complicated by periodic exacerbations. Even patients with mild asymptomatic asthma have obvious, although microscopic, inflammatory changes in their airways. The changes are distinguished by infiltration of the mucosa and epithelium by activated T cells, mast cells, and eosinophils. T cells and mast cells secrete an array of chemicals in asthma, the functions of which are to direct eosinophil growth and maturation and to prevent B lymphocytes from switching from IgM to IgE, providing an explanation for the inflammatory response of asthma. The aftermath of this response is increased capillary permeability, stimulation of local and central neural reflexes, epithelial disruption and stimulation of mucus-secreting glands, smooth muscle hypertrophy, and airway wall remodeling (Fig. 46–1).

In recent years, an increased understanding of the pathophysiology of asthma has exposed a complex network of interactions among a variety of inflammatory cells and the mediators they secrete. The *leukotriene* (LT) family includes metabolites of arachidonic acid, an essential fatty acid that cannot be synthesized by animal tissues. Arachidonic acid must be obtained in the diet. Specific LTs are

TRIGGERS OF ACUTE ASTHMA ATTACKS

Environmental Factors
- Air pollutants (e.g., aerosol sprays, cigarette smoke, exhaust fumes, oxidants, perfumes, sulfur dioxides)
- Animal dander (dogs, cats, rodents, horses)
- Environmental changes (e.g., moving to new house, starting a new school)
- House-dust mite
- Pollens, spores, and mold (trees, grasses, shrubs, weeds)

Occupational Exposure
- Industrial chemicals and plastics
- Metal salts
- Pharmaceuticals
- Wood and vegetable dusts

Foods and Food Additives
- Sulfites, bisulfites, and metasulfites
- Nuts
- Milk and dairy products

Drugs
- Antibiotics
- Aspirin
- Nonsteroidal anti-inflammatory drugs (e.g., indomethacin)
- Beta blockers (e.g., propranolol)

Diseases/Conditions
- Menses
- Paranasal sinusitis
- Pregnancy
- Thyroid disease
- Viral upper respiratory infections

Other Triggers
- Exercise and cold, dry air
- Gastroesophageal reflux
- History of nasal polyps
- Strong emotions (e.g., fear, anger, laughing, crying)
- Tracheoesophageal fistula

produced by the activity of 5-lipoxygenase. Arachidonic acid is presented to the 5-lipoxygenase enzyme by 5-lipoxygenase–activating protein, a co-factor present in the nuclear membrane. The interaction leads to the formation of LTA_4, an unstable intermediate LT (Fig. 46–2). Depending on the cell type, further conversion of LTA_4 may occur by the actions of enzymes that are widespread in the tissues and circulation. LTs induce numerous biologic effects including augmentation of neutrophil and eosinophil migration, monocyte aggregation, leukocyte adhesion, increased capillary permeability, and smooth muscle contraction. These effects contribute to inflammation, edema, mucus secretion, and bronchoconstriction of the airways of asthmatic patients.

It has been shown that allergen- or anti-immunoglobulin E (IgE)–induced bronchial constriction is entirely mediated by a specific group of LTs, together with a minor histamine-dependent component. An antigen-IgE antibody complex is formed causing the release of chemical mediators in the lower respiratory tract. Histamine plays a minor role in this response. The slow-reacting substance of anaphylaxis is a more potent mediator that causes long-term contraction of bronchial smooth muscle.

For many years, it has been known that in 5 to 10 percent of patients with asthma, cyclooxygenase inhibitors (e.g., aspirin) produce profound bronchoconstriction. This is particularly true in patients with late-onset intrinsic asthma. It is now known that patients with aspirin-sensitive asthma produce greater amounts of LTs and have increased airway sensitivity when challenged by these agents.

Timing of symptoms varies greatly among patients. Bronchoconstriction can have an immediate, histamine-type pattern, or a late response with airway hypersensitivity lasting for days, weeks, or months. A second wave of symptoms sometimes appears 6 to 8 hours after initial antigen exposure. The classic manifestations of asthma are dyspnea, wheezing, and coughing in the absence of respiratory infection, especially at night.

Drugs used in the management of asthma include inhaled and systemic corticosteroids; antiallergy drugs; beta agonists; LT antagonists, the newest class of drugs; anticholinergics; and xanthines.

PHARMACOTHERAPEUTIC OPTIONS

Inhaled Corticosteroids

- ❒ Beclomethasone (BECLOVENT, BECONASE, VANCERIL, VANCENASE); (🍁) BECLODISK, BECLOFORTE
- ❒ Budesonide (RHINOCORT)
- ❒ Dexamethasone (DECADRON)
- ❒ Flunisolide (AEROBID, NASALIDE); (🍁) BRONALIDE, RHINALAR
- ❒ Fluticasone (FLOVENT, FLONASE)
- ❒ Triamcinolone (AZMACORT, NASACORT)

Indications

Inhaled corticosteroids were developed in an attempt to achieve the advantages of chronic corticosteroid therapy without the systemic adverse effects. They are useful for both acute and chronic respiratory disorders. Inhaled formulations are used in the long-term management of asthma. Corticosteroid inhalers are not indicated for relief of asthma that can be controlled by bronchodilators and other nonsteroidal drugs, in patients who require systemic corticosteroid treatment infrequently, and in the treatment of nonasthmatic bronchitis. Systemic corticosteroids are used to gain prompt control of the disease and also to manage moderate to severe persistent asthma. Hydrocortisone, prednisone, and methylprednisolone are systemic drugs (see Chapter 52) given to patients who do not respond adequately to bronchodilator therapy.

Pharmacodynamics

Corticosteroids have potent anti-inflammatory effects that reduce mucus secretion. The precise mechanism of drug action in the lung is unknown. Corticosteroids are also thought to increase the number and sensitivity of adrenergic receptors, which restores or increases the effectiveness of beta agonists.

Adverse Effects and Contraindications

The most frequent adverse effects associated with inhaled corticosteroids include headache (worse with triamcinolone

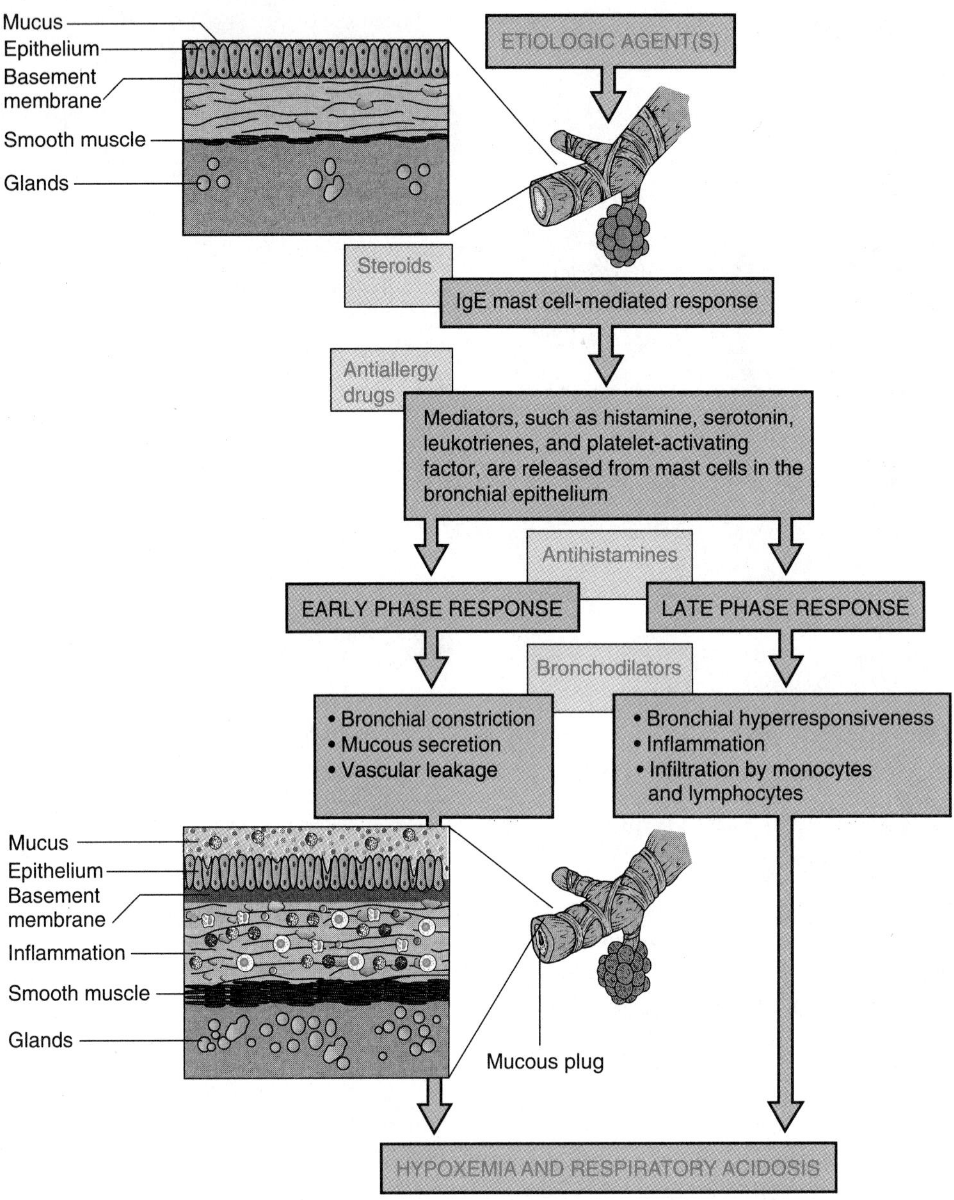

Figure 46–1 Pathophysiology of bronchial inflammation and airway hyperresponsiveness.

than others), throat itching (with budesonide), and wheezing, bronchospasm, and cough. Localized infections with *Candida albicans* or *Aspergillus niger* may be present in the mouth and pharynx. Candidiasis occurs in the larynx in 75 percent of patients using inhaled corticosteroids, although the incidence of clinically apparent infection is considerably lower. These infections may require treatment with appropriate antifungal drugs, or corticosteroid inhaler use may need to be discontinued.

A few patients complain of hoarseness and dry mouth with use of an inhaled corticosteroid. Rare cases of immediate and delayed hypersensitivity reactions, including urticaria, angioedema, rash, and bronchospasm have been reported following oral inhalation of corticosteroids.

Suppression of the hypothalamic-pituitary-adrenal (HPA) axis can occur with high doses of inhaled corticosteroids used for long periods. HPA axis suppression has been reported in adult patients who receive 32 puffs/day (approximately 1600 mcg) for over 1 month. Patients have also exhibited signs of adrenal insufficiency when they were exposed to trauma, surgery, or infections (particularly gastroenteritis) while using inhaled corticosteroids. Although inhaled steroids provide control of asthmatic symptoms, they do not provide the quantity of systemic steroid necessary to cope with these stressors. Furthermore, deaths have occurred due to adrenal insufficiency during and after transfer from systemic corticosteroids to topical drugs. A number of months are required for recovery of HPA axis function.

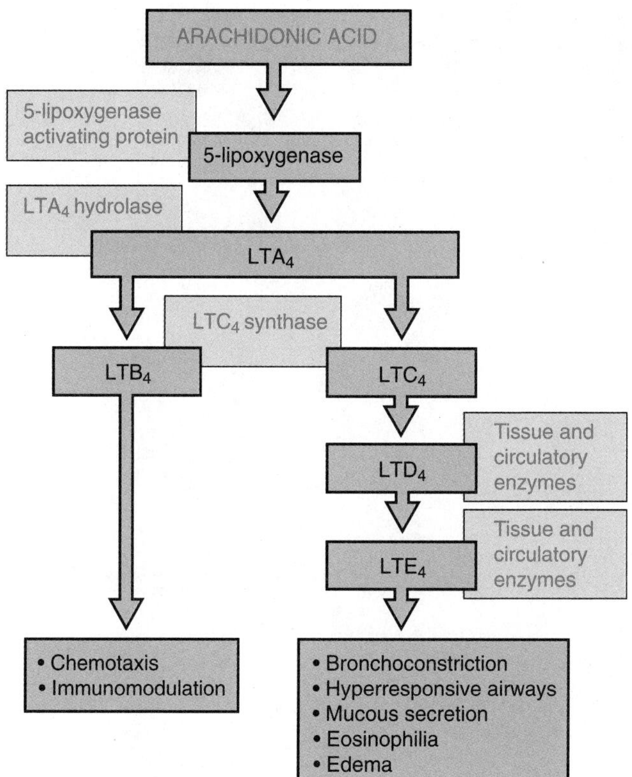

Figure 46–2 Leukotriene synthesis and activity. Five types of leukotrienes (slow-reacting substances of anaphylaxis [SRS-A]) are generated from a lipid, arachidonic acid, that is released from mast cell membranes by an intracellular phospholipase that acts on membrane phospholipids (LTA_4, LTB_4, LTC_4, LTD_4, and LTE_4). Leukotrienes are acidic, sulfur-containing lipids that produce effects similar to those of histamine. LTB_4 is a chemotactic agent that causes aggregation of leukocytes. LTC_4, LTD_4, and LTE_4 all cause contraction of smooth muscle, bronchospasm, and increased vascular permeability.

Corticosteroids are contraindicated in the primary treatment of status asthmaticus or other acute episodes of asthma in which intensive measures are required. Some inhaled corticosteroids contain fluorocarbon propellants, alcohol, propylene, or polyethylene glycol, and they should be avoided in patients with known hypersensitivity or intolerance. Corticosteroids should be used with caution in patients with peptic ulcer disease, inflammatory bowel disease, hypertension, heart failure, and thromboembolic disorders.

Pharmacokinetics

Absorption of corticosteroids occurs rapidly from all respiratory tissues. Beclomethasone and flunisolide are rapidly absorbed from the lungs, whereas triamcinolone is absorbed more slowly. Systemic absorption of inhaled corticosteroids is minimal at recommended doses. Both the relative bioavailability (systemic availability) and relative potency of inhaled corticosteroids determine the potential for systemic activity (Table 46–1).

The onset time of most inhaled corticosteroids is a few days. Peak action may not occur for up to 4 weeks in some cases. Nearly all of an inhaled corticosteroid dose delivered to the lungs is bioavailable. Approximately 80 percent of the dose from a metered-dose inhaler (MDI; without a spacer or holding chamber) is swallowed. Oral bioavailability can decrease either with the use of a spacer or holding chamber or when a drug with a high first-pass effect is used. Thus, safety is enhanced. The bioavailability of inhaled corticosteroids is as follows: beclomethasone, 20 percent; flunisolide, 20 percent; triamcinolone, 10.6 percent; budesonide, 11 percent; and fluticasone, 1 percent.

Beclomethasone is converted to an active metabolite, which adds to its potency. Flunisolide and triamcinolone are rapidly and extensively biotransformed by the liver following absorption from the lungs. The small quantities of drug that are absorbed systemically are biotransformed in the liver before elimination. The duration of drug action is unknown, although the half-life of inhaled corticosteroids varies from 1 to 15 hours.

Drug-Drug Interactions

There are no clinically significant drug-drug interactions when recommended dosages of inhaled corticosteroids are used. However, for patients who must take oral corticosteroids, attention should be paid to possible interactions. For example, corticosteroid effects can be reduced in the presence of barbiturates, rifampin, and phenytoin. There is an increased risk of gastrointestinal bleeding from systemic corticosteroids in the presence of indomethacin or salicylates. Corticosteroids also reduce salicylate levels. An increased risk of hypokalemia is possible when corticosteroids are taken concurrently with amphotericin, digitalis, or potassium-losing diuretics.

Dosage Regimen

Corticosteroids may be administered via oral inhalation using MDIs, breath-actuated MDIs, dry-powder inhalers, or using a nebulizer. One puff of corticosteroid taken two to four times daily is suggested. For children 6 to 12 years of age, one puff three to four times daily is recommended, with the maximum dose 10 puffs daily. Twice-daily regimens are nearly as effective as four administrations and are helpful in maximizing compliance. Systemic dosing of corticosteroids is discussed in Chapter 52.

After maximum response is achieved in 1 to 2 weeks, the dosage should be reduced to the lowest level that maintains control. In many cases, continued use of a corticosteroid inhaler for more than 30 days is inappropriate. Furthermore, there is no evidence that asthma control can be achieved by administration of inhaled corticosteroids in amounts exceeding the recommended dosages.

Laboratory Considerations

Inhaled corticosteroids may cause elevated serum and urine glucose levels if significant absorption has occurred. Additionally, periodic adrenal function tests for patients on chronic therapy may be necessary to assess for HPA suppression.

Antiallergy Drugs

❒ Cromolyn; (🍁) NALCROM, RYNACROM, VISTACROM
❒ Nedocromil (TILADE)

Indications

Antiallergy drugs (previously known as mast cell stabilizers) are indicated only for asthma prophylaxis. These drugs are effective for patients with chronic asthma, including allergic asthma and asthma induced by exercise, cold air, and

TABLE 46–1 PHARMACOKINETICS OF SELECTED ANTIASTHMATIC AND BRONCHODILATOR DRUGS

Drugs	Route	Onset	Peak	Duration	PB (%)	$t_{1/2}$	BioA (%)
Inhaled Corticosteroids							
Beclomethasone	INH/po	Rapid	Up to 4 wk	3.25 days	91	3–15 hr	20
Budesonide	INH	24 hr	3–7 days	UK	91	2 hr	11
Flunisolide	INH	Rapid	UA	UA	91	1–2 hr	20
Fluticasone	INH	Few days	1–2 weeks	UK	91	UA	1
Triamcinolone	INH	Few days	3–4 days	UK	91	4 hr	10.6
Anitallergy Drugs (Mast Cell Stabilizers)							
Cromolyn	INH	15 min	2–4 weeks	4–6 hr	UA	80 min	2½–3
Nedocromil	INH	2 weeks	20–40 min	4–6 hr	89	1.5–2.3 hr	2½–3
Beta Agonists							
Albuterol	po	30 min	2–2½ hr	4–8 hr	UK	2–4 hr	UA
	INH	5 min	1½–2 hr	3–8 hr			
Bitolterol	INH	3–4 min	30–120 min	5–8 hr	UK	3 hr	UA
Metaproterenol	po	15–30 min	60 min	4 hr	UK	UK	UA
	INH	1–4 min	60 min	3–4 hr			
Pirbuterol	INH	5 min	1–5 hr	6–8 hr	UK	2 hr	UA
Salmeterol	INH	10–25 min	3–4 hr	8–12 hr	UK	UK	UA
Terbutaline	po	60–120 min	2–3 hr	4–8 hr	UK	UK	30–50
	INH	5–30 min	1–2 hr	3–6 hr			
Leukotriene Antagonists							
Montelukast	po	UA	3–4 hr	UA	99	2.7–5.5 hr	63–73
Zafirlukast	po	UA	3 hr	UA	UA	10 hr	40
Zileuton	po	1.7 hr	2 hr	UA	93	1.5 hr	UA
Xanthine Derivatives							
Aminophylline	po	1–6 hr*	4–6 hr	6–8 hr	UA	3–15 hr	UA
	IV	Immediate	30 min	4–8 hr			100
Dyphylline	po	60 min*	60 min	6 hr	UA	1.8–2.1 hr	75
	IM	30–45 min	UK				
Oxtriphylline	po	15–60 min*	5 hr	6–8 hr	UA	3–15 hr	UA
	po/ER	UK	4–7 hr	12 hr			
Theophylline	po	Varies	1–2 hr	6 hr	60; 36; 35†	4–5 hr; 3–15 hr‡	UA
	po/ER	Delayed	4–8 hr	8–24 hr		3–13 hr	UA
	IV	Rapid	End of inf	6–8 hr			100
Anticholinergic							
Ipratropium	INH	5–15 min	1–2 hr	3–6 hr	UA	2 hr	

*Provided a loading dose of methylxanthine drug has been given and steady state serum levels exist.
†Protein binding of theophylline in healthy adults, neonates, and patients with cirrhosis, respectively.
‡Half-life of theophylline in patients who smoke and nonsmokers, respectively.
PB, Protein binding; $t_{1/2}$, serum half-life; UA, unavailable; UK, unknown; ER, extended-release formulation; IV, intravenous; INH, inhalation; BioA, bioavailability.

sulfur dioxide. They are mild to moderate anti-inflammatory drugs that are used as initial drug of choice for long-term therapy in children. The use of antiallergy drugs allows for reduced dosage of corticosteroids and bronchodilators. Antiallergy drugs are not effective for acute bronchospasm or status asthmaticus.

Pharmacodynamics

Cromolyn and nedocromil stabilize mast cells to inhibit activation and release of chemical mediators from eosinophils and epithelial cells. They block early and late reactions to allergens and interfere with chloride channel functions. These drugs have no direct bronchodilation characteristics.

Adverse Effects and Contraindications

Headache is common in patients on antiallergy drugs regardless of the administration route. Irritation of the trachea, cough, and bronchospasm have occurred with inhalation drugs. Although the incidence of adverse effects is relatively low, arrhythmias, hypotension, chest pain, restlessness, dizziness, central nervous system depression, seizures, anorexia, nausea, and vomiting have been noted. Fifteen to twenty percent of patients complain of an unpleasant taste from inhaled nedocromil. Sedation and coma occur with overdose. Arrhythmias are thought to be caused by the propellants used in aerosol formulations. Furthermore, it has been suggested that the propellants in aerosols may aggravate coronary artery disease.

Antiallergy drugs are contraindicated in patients with hypersensitivity to the drug. They are not used for acute episodes of asthma because they do not relieve, and may even worsen, bronchospasm when given by inhalation. They should be used with caution in patients who have impaired liver or kidney function. Safe use during pregnancy and lactation has not been established. The safety of nedocromil in children younger than 12 years of age also has not been determined.

Pharmacokinetics

Small amounts of cromolyn may reach systemic circulation after inhalation. Ninety percent of an inhaled dose of nedocromil is swallowed, with 2½ to 3 percent of the swallowed drug absorbed. Antiallergy drugs do not cross biologic membranes; hence, drug action is primarily local. The onset time of antiallergy drugs varies from 1 to 2 weeks, with peak activity ordinarily noted at 2 to 3 weeks (see Table 46–1). The duration of action of antiallergy drugs is 4 to 6 hours. The small amounts that are absorbed are eliminated unchanged in the bile and urine.

Dosage Regimen

Cromolyn is available as a capsule for use in a spinhaler and as a solution for inhalation. For adults, 20 mg (one spray) is inhaled via a nebulizer four times daily (Table 46–2). The adult dosage is used for children older than 5 years of age who use capsules and children older than 2 years of age who are using the nebulizer. Nebulizer delivery (20 mg/ampule) may be preferred for some patients. Nedocromil is administered as two inhalations four times daily for both adults and children older than 12 years of age.

Antiallergy drugs should be discontinued if a therapeutic response is not obtained with 4 weeks of therapy. Pretreatment with a bronchodilating drug may be required before use of an antiallergy drug. Pretreatment is recommended in order to increase delivery of the antiallergy drug.

Beta Agonists

- ❒ Albuterol (AIRET, PROVENTIL, VENTOLIN, others); (🍁) GEN-SALBUTAMOL, NOVO-SALMOL
- ❒ Bitolterol (TORNALATE)
- ❒ Metaproterenol (ALUPENT)
- ❒ Pirbuterol (MAXAIR)
- ❒ Salbuterol (SALBUVENT)
- ❒ Salmeterol (SEREVENT)
- ❒ Terbutaline (BRETHAIRE, BRETHINE, BRICANYL)

Indications

Short-acting beta agonists (e.g., albuterol, bitolterol, metaproterenol, pirbuterol, and terbutaline) are used for the short-term relief of bronchoconstriction and are the treatment of choice for acute exacerbations of asthma. They are effective when used prophylactically for exercise-induced bronchospasm.

The long-acting beta agonists (e.g., salbuterol, salmeterol) are used concomitantly with anti-inflammatory drugs for long-term control of symptoms, especially nocturnal symptoms. Salmeterol may provide more effective symptom control when added to standard doses of inhaled corticosteroids rather than increasing the corticosteroid dose. A more thorough discussion of beta agonists is found in Chapter 11.

Pharmacodynamics

Beta agonists act to cause airway smooth muscle relaxation by activating adenylate cyclase and increasing cyclic adenosine monophosphate (cAMP). The action produces a functional antagonism of bronchoconstriction. In addition to increasing cAMP, beta agonists inhibit release of mast cell mediators, decrease vascular permeability, and increase mucociliary clearance. They do not inhibit either the late phase inflammatory response or the subsequent bronchial hyperresponsiveness. All short-acting beta agonists are $beta_2$ specific except metaproterenol.

Adverse Effects and Contraindications

Adverse effects of short-acting beta agonists include headache, tachycardia, hypokalemia, hyperglycemia, skeletal muscle tremors, and increased lactic acid. In general, the inhaled route causes a few systemic adverse effects. Patients with pre-existing cardiovascular disease, especially the older adult, may experience adverse cardiovascular effects with inhaled therapy.

Adverse effects of long-acting beta agonists include tachycardia, hypokalemia, and prolongation of the QT interval with overdose. A diminished bronchoprotective effect may occur within 1 week of chronic therapy. The clinical significance of this effect has not been established, however. The potential significance of developing tolerance is uncertain because studies show that symptom control and bronchodilation are maintained.

Pharmacokinetics

The onset of drug action of short-acting beta agonists occurs in 5 to 30 minutes, depending on the specific drug (see Table 46–1). Peak effects are reached in 30 minutes to 2 hours, with a duration of action of 3 to 8 hours for most drugs. Compared with short-acting beta agonists, salmeterol has slower onset of action (15 to 30 minutes) but a longer duration of action (8 to 12 hours). Systemic absorption of beta agonists is minimal. Terbutaline rapidly undergoes first-pass metabolism when it is taken by mouth but has minimal absorption following inhalation. Distribution of inhaled drugs is essentially limited to the respiratory tract, although most drugs appear in breast milk in small amounts. The protein binding of beta agonists is unknown.

Biotransformation and elimination of beta agonists vary with the drug. Albuterol and metaproterenol are extensively biotransformed by the liver and other tissues. Bitolterol is converted in the lungs to colterol, the active compound. Pirbuterol and terbutaline are biotransformed by the liver and eliminated through the kidneys. The half-life of the drugs generally varies from 2 to 4 hours.

Drug-Drug Interactions

Drug-drug interactions of beta agonists are relative few but significant (Table 46–3). The additive effects of beta agonists when they are used concurrently with other adrenergic drugs or monoamine oxidase inhibitors may lead to hypertensive crisis. When they are used with beta-blocking drugs, the therapeutic effects of the beta agonist may be negated.

Dosage Regimen

The dosage of beta agonists is individualized based on patient response. In many cases, two puffs or inhalations of the short-acting drugs twice to four times daily is required.

TABLE 46–2 DOSAGE REGIMEN FOR SELECTED ANTIASTHMATIC AND BRONCHODILATOR DRUGS

Drug	Uses	Dosage	Implications*
Inhaled Corticosteroids			
Beclomethasone	Chronic steroid dependent asthma; reduces need for oral corticosteroid	*Adults and child older than 12 yr:* *Low dose:* 168–504 mcg QD is equivalent to 4–12 puffs of 42 mcg/puff MDI *or* 2–6 puffs of 84 mcg/puff MDI. *Medium dose:* 504–840 mcg QD is equivalent to 12–20 puffs of 42 mcg/puff MDI *or* 6–10 puffs of 84 mcg/puff MDI. *High dose:* Over 840 mcg QD is equivalent to > 20 puffs of 42 mcg/puff MDI *or* > 10 puffs of 84 mcg/puff MDI *Child age 6–12 yr:* *Low dose:* 84–336 mcg QD is equivalent to 2–8 puffs of 42 mcg/puff MDI *or* 1–4 puffs of 84 mcg/puff MDI *Medium dose:* 336–672 mcg QD is equivalent to 8–16 puffs of 42 mcg/puff MDI *or* 4–8 puffs of 84 mcg/puff MDI. *High dose:* > 672 mcg QD is equivalent to > 16 puffs of 42 mcg/puff MDI *or* > 8 puffs of 84 mcg/puff MDI	A 16.8-g canister of beclomethasone contains approximately 200 puffs. Advise patients using inhalation formulations and a bronchodilator concurrently to allow 5 minutes to elapse before administering the corticosteroid, unless otherwise directed by the health care provider. Instruct the patient in the correct use of the MDI. Advise the patient that corticosteroid inhalers should not be used to treat an acute asthma attack but should be continued even if other inhalation drugs are used. Patients using inhalation corticosteroids may require systemic agents for acute attacks. Advise patient to use peak flow monitoring to determine respiratory status. Rinse mouth with water immediately after inhalation to prevent mouth and throat dryness and fungal infections of mouth
Budesonide	Chronic steroid dependent asthma; reduces need for oral corticosteroid	*Adults:* *Low dose:* 200–400 mcg QD is equivalent to 1–2 inh *Medium dose:* 400–600 mcg QD is equivalent to 2–3 inh *High dose:* > 600 mcg QD is equivalent to > 3 inh *Child:* *Low dose:* 100–200 mcg QD is equivalent to 1 inh *Medium dose:* 200–400 mcg QD is equivalent to 1–2 inh *High dose:* > 400 mcg QD is equivalent to > 2 inh	Each Turbuhaler delivers 200 mcg/dose. See also implications under beclomethasone. Rinse mouth with water immediately after inhalation to prevent mouth and throat dryness and fungal infections of mouth
Flunisolide	Chronic steroid dependent asthma; reduces need for oral corticosteroid	*Adults and child older than 6 yr:* *Low dose:* 500–1000 mcg QD is equivalent to 2–4 puffs of a 250 mcg/puff MDI *Medium dose:* 1000–2000 mcg QD is equivalent to 4–8 puffs of a 250 mcg/puff MDI *High dose:* 2000 mcg QD is equivalent to > 8 puffs of a 250 mcg/puff MDI *Child:* *Low dose:* 500–750 mcg QD is equivalent to 2–3 puffs of a 250 mcg/puff MDI *Medium dose:* 1000–1250 mcg QD is equivalent to 4–5 puffs of a 250 mcg/puff MDI *High dose:* 1250 mcg QD is equivalent to > 5 puffs of a 250 mcg/puff MDI	Each 7-g canister delivers approximately 100, 250 mcg/puffs. See also implications under beclomethasone. Rinse mouth with water immediately after inhalation to prevent mouth and throat dryness and fungal infections of mouth
Dexamethasone	Chronic steroid dependent asthma; reduces need for oral corticosteroid	*Adults:* Three metered sprays via inhalation aerosol three to four times daily. Not to exceed 12 metered sprays/day *Child:* Two metered sprays via inhalation aerosol three to four times daily. Not to exceed eight metered sprays/day.	Each 12.6-g canister contains approximately 170, 84-mcg metered sprays. See also implications under beclomethasone. Rinse mouth with water immediately after inhalation to prevent mouth and throat dryness and fungal infections of mouth
Fluticasone	Chronic steroid dependent asthma; reduces need for oral corticosteroid	*Adults:* *Low dose:* 88–264 mcg QD is equivalent to 2–6 puffs of a 44 mcg/puff MDI, 2 puffs of a 110 mcg/puff MDI, *or* 2–6 inh of 50 mcg/inh DPI *Medium dose:* 264–660 mcg QD is equivalent to 2–6 puffs of a 110 mcg/puff MDI *or* 3–6 inh of a 100 mcg/inh DPI *High dose:* > 660 mcg QD is equivalent to > 6 puffs of a 110 mcg/puff MDI, > 3 puffs of a 220 mcg/puff MDI, > 6 inh of a 100 mcg/inh DPI, *or* > 2 inh of a 250 mcg/inh DPI. *Child:* *Low dose:* 88–176 mcg QD is equivalent to 2–4 puffs of a 44 mcg/puff MDI *Medium dose:* 176–440 mcg QD is equivalent to 4–10 puffs of a 44 mcg/puff MDI, 2–4 puffs of a 110 mcg/puff MDI, *or* 2–4 inh of a 100 mcg/inh DPI	Initial dosage based on prior asthma drugs. Do not change dose schedule or stop taking the drug. Teach proper use of inhaler. See also implications under beclomethasone. Rinse mouth with water immediately after inhalation to prevent mouth and throat dryness and fungal infections of mouth

TABLE 46–2 DOSAGE REGIMEN FOR SELECTED ANTIASTHMATIC AND BRONCHODILATOR DRUGS *Continued*

Drug	Uses	Dosage	Implications*
Inhaled Corticosteroids ***Continued***			
Fluticasone	Chronic steroid dependent asthma; reduces need for oral corticosteroid	*High dose:* > 440 mcg QD is equivalent to > 4 puffs of a 110-mcg/puff MDI, > 2 puffs of a 220-mcg/puff MDI, > 4 inh of a 100-mcg/inh DPI, *or* > 2 inh of a 250-mcg/inh DPI	
Triamcinolone	Chronic steroid dependent asthma; reduces need for oral corticosteroid	*Adults and child older than 12 yr:* *Low dose:* 400–1000 mcg QD is equivalent to 4–10 puffs of a 100 mcg/puff MDI. *Medium dose:* 1000–2000 mcg QD is equivalent to 10–20 puffs of a 100 mcg/puff MDI. *High dose:* > 2000 mcg QD is equivalent to > 20 puffs of a 100 mcg/puff MDI *Child:* *Low dose:* 400–800 mcg QD is equivalent to 4–8 puffs of a 100 mcg/puff MDI *Medium dose:* 800–1200 mcg QD is equivalent to 8–12 puffs of 100 mcg/puff MDI *High dose:* > 1200 mcg QD is equivalent to > 12 puffs of a 100 mcg/puff MDI	A 20-g canister contains approximately 240 puffs. See also implications under beclomethasone. Rinse mouth with water immediately after inhalation to prevent mouth and throat dryness and fungal infections of mouth
Antiallergy Drugs (Mast Cell Stabilizers)			
Cromolyn	Asthma prophylaxis	*Adults:* 2–4 puffs TID–QID via MDI *or* 1 ampule TID–QID via nebulizer *Child:* 1–2 puffs TID–QID via MDI *or* 1 ampule TID–QID	*MDI:* 1 mg/puff. *Nebulizer:* 20-mg/ampule. One dose before exercise or allergen exposure provides effective prophylaxis for 1–2 hours.
Nedocromil		*Adults:* 2–4 puffs BID–QID *Child:* 1–2 puffs BID–QID	
Beta Agonists†			
Albuterol	Reversible airway disease due to asthma or COPD	*Adults and child older than 14 yr:* 2–6 mg po TID–QID. Not to exceed 32 mg/day *or* 4–8 mg of an ER formulation BID *or* 2 puffs q4–6hr *or* 2 puffs 15–20 minutes before exercise *or* 1.25–5 mg TID via nebulizer *or* 1–2 capsules (200–400 mcg) q4–6hr via Rotahaler. Take 15 minutes before exercise *Child 6–14 yr:* 2 mg po TID–QID. Not to exceed 24 mg/day *or* 1 capsule q4–6 hr PRN via Rotahaler *Child 2–6 yr:* 0.1 mg/kg po TID. Not to exceed 2 mg TID initially. May increase to 0.2 mg/kg TID. Not to exceed 4 mg TID.	A 17-g MDI canister contains approximately 200, 90–100 mcg puffs. To use drug in a nebulizer dilute 5 mg/mL solution of drug with 2–5 mL or more of 0.9% sodium chloride or sterile water. Albuterol is compatible with cromolyn and ipratropium in nebulizer.
Bitolterol	Reversible airway disease due to asthma or COPD	*Adults and child older than 12 yr:* 2 inhalations 1–3 minutes apart, followed by additional inhalations, if needed. Not to exceed 2 inhalations q4hr *or* 3 INH q6hr. Prophylaxis: 2 inhalations q8hr.	A 6-g MDI canister contains approximately 300, 200-mcg puffs. Do not mix bitolterol with other nebulizer solutions
Metaproterenol	Reversible airway disease due to asthma or COPD	*Adults and child older than 9 yr and 27 kg.:* 20 mg po TID–QID *or* 2–3 inhalations q3–4hr. Not to exceed 12 inhalations/day *or* 5–15 inhalations of undiluted 5% solution TID–QID via nebulizer. Not to exceed q4hr use *or* 0.2–0.3 mL of a 5% solution *or* 2.5 mL of a 0.4–0.6% solution TID–QID via IPPB. Not to exceed q4hr	Metaproterenol is a nonselective drug affecting both $beta_1$ and $beta_2$ receptors A 14-g MDI canister contains approximately 200, 650-mcg puffs An aerosol solution container holds 5 mL or 100, 650- to 750-mcg inhalations. When used via IPPB, dilute each dose in 2.5 mL of 0.9% sodium chloride
Pirbuterol	Reversible airway disease due to asthma or COPD	*Adults:* 1–2 puffs q4–6 hr. Not to exceed 12 inhalations/day	A 14-g autoinhaler canister contains approximately 300, 200-mcg puffs. A 25.6-g autoinhaler canister contains approximately 400, 200-mcg puffs.
Salmeterol	Long-term prevention of symptoms (not for acute attacks or exercise-induced bronchospasm)	*Adults:* 2 puffs by MDI *or* one blister BID 12 hr apart.	A 13-g MDI canister contains approximately 120, 21-mcg puffs. MDI canister should be primed or tested before first use. Long-acting agent. If symptoms occur before next dose is due, use a rapid-acting inhaled bronchodilator to treat symptoms.

Table continued on following page

TABLE 46–2 DOSAGE REGIMEN FOR SELECTED ANTIASTHMATIC AND BRONCHODILATOR DRUGS *Continued*

Drug	Uses	Dosage	Implications*
Beta Agonists† *Continued*			
Terbutaline	Management of reversible airway disease	*Adults and child older than 12 yr:* 2.5–5 mg po q8hr to maximum of 15 mg/24 hr *or* 0.25 mg SC. May repeat once in 15–30 minutes. Not to exceed 0.50 mg/4 hr *or* 2 puffs separated by 1 minute, then q4–6 hr *Child younger than 12 yr:* 1–2 puffs q4–6 hr *or* 0.05 mg/kg/dose po q8hr. Gradually increase to 0.15 mg/kg/dose to maximum of 5 mg *or* 0.005–0.01 mg/kg/dose to maximum of 0.4 mg/kg/dose q15–20 minutes × 2 doses	Give SC injection in lateral deltoid. No proven advantage of systemic therapy over aerosol
Leukotriene Antagonists			
Montelukast	Prophylaxis and chronic long-term treatment of asthma	*Adults and child older than 15 yr:* 10 mg po daily at qHS. *Child 6–14 yr:* 5-mg chewable tablet daily at HS.	Take on an empty stomach. There is no evidence of improved efficacy with morning versus evening dosing.
Zafirlukast		*Adults:* 40 mg po BID	Take on an empty stomach. Bioavailability decreased when taken with food.
Zileuton		*Adults:* 300 mg po QID. Not to exceed 2400 mg daily	Monitor liver enzymes.
Xanthine Derivatives‡			
Aminophylline	Management of reversible airway disease due to asthma or CAL, especially nocturnal symptoms	*Adults:* Loading dose: 5 mg/kg po. Maintenance dose is 300 mg/day in divided doses q6–8 hr. May increase after 3 days to 400 mg/day and again after 3 more days to 600 mg in divided doses *Child younger than 16 yr:* Loading dose: 5 mg/kg. Maintenance dose varies based on lean body weight	Anhydrous aminophylline is 86% theophylline. Dihydrate aminophylline is 79% theophylline. Dosage determined through serum drug levels. Therapeutic range: 10–20 mcg/mL. Narrow therapeutic index. Serum levels over 20 mcg/mL associated with toxicity. Healthy adults or young smokers may require q6hr dosing. Give ER formulation q12–24 hr.
Dyphylline		*Adults:* 15 mg/kg po q6hr *or* 250–500 mg IM q6hr. Not to exceed 15 mg/kg/dose	Not a salt of theophylline. It is about 1/10 as potent as theophylline. Standard theophylline assays do not measure dyphylline concentration.
Oxtriphylline		*Adults:* 4.7 mg/kg po q8hr *or* 400–600 mg po ER formulation q12 hr *Child age 9–16 yr:* 4.7 mg/kg po q6hr *Child age 1–9 yr:* 6.2 mg/kg po q6hr	64% theophylline = 156 mg equivalent dose
Anticholinergic			
Ipratropium	Asthma maintenance therapy	*Adults:* 1–2 puffs TID–QID. Not to exceed 12 puffs/24 hr or more often than q4hr *or* 250–500 mcg TID–QID via nebulizer given	Not indicated for acute bronchospasm Can use hard candy, frequent drinks, sugarless gum to relieve dry mouth

*Metered-dose inhalers are expressed as the *actuator dose,* the amount of drug leaving the actuator and delivered to the patient. This is a labeling requirement in the United States. The actuator dose is different from the dosage expressed as the *valve dose,* the amount of drug leaving the valve, all of which is not available to the patient. The valve dose is commonly used in many European countries and in some scientific literature. Dry-powder inhaler (e.g., Turbuhaler) dosages are expressed as the amount of drug in the inhaler following activation.

†Differences in potency among and between beta agonists exist so all short-acting inhaled $beta_2$ agonists are essentially equipotent on a per puff basis.

‡Doses of xanthines are expressed in theophylline equivalents. Because of differing theophylline content, the various salts and derivatives of theophylline are equivalent on a weight basis.

MDI, Metered-dose inhaler; DPI, dry-powder inhaler; IPPB, intermittent positive-pressure breathing. CAL, chronic airway limitation.

Salmeterol is administered twice daily, 12 hours apart (see Table 46–2).

Laboratory Considerations

Beta agonists may cause a transient decrease in serum potassium concentrations when they are administered via nebulizer or in higher than recommended doses. Salmeterol may cause increased serum glucose levels. Increased serum glucose levels are rare but are more pronounced with frequent, high-dose use of salmeterol.

Leukotriene Antagonists

- ❒ Montelukast (SINGULAIR)
- ❒ Zafirlukast (ACCOLATE)
- ❒ Zileuton (ZYFLO)

Indications

Zafirlukast and zileuton are indicated for the prophylaxis and chronic treatment of asthma in adults. Zafirlukast and zileuton may be considered alternative therapy to low doses of inhaled corticosteroids or antiallergy drugs in mild persis-

TABLE 46–3 DRUG-DRUG INTERACTIONS OF SELECTED ANTIASTHMATIC AND BRONCHODILATOR DRUGS*

Drug	Interactive Drugs		Interaction
Beta Agonists			
Albuterol	Other adrenergic drugs		Additive effects may lead to hypertensive crisis
Bitolterol	MAO inhibitors		
Metaproterenol	Beta blockers		May negate therapeutic effect of adrenergic agonist
Pirbuterol			
Salmeterol			
Terbutaline			
Leukotriene Antagonists			
Zafirlukast	Warfarin	Cyclosporine	Increased risk of bleeding
Zileuton	Astemizole	Dihydropyridine CCBs	Inhibits biotransformation of interactive drugs
	Carbamazepine	Tolbutamide	
	Cisapride	Phenytoin	
	Corticosteroids	Erythromycin	Decreased effectiveness of leukotriene antagonist
		Theophylline	
		Aspirin	Increased plasma levels of zafirlukast
Xanthine Derivatives			
Aminophylline	Adrenergic agonists		Additive cardiovascular and CNS adverse effects
Dyphylline	Lithium		Decreased therapeutic effects of interactive drug
Oxtriphylline	Adrenergics	Nicotine (gum, patches, cigarettes)	May increase metabolism and decrease effectiveness of xanthine
Theophylline	Barbiturates	Phenytoin	
	Ketoconazole	Rifampin	
	Allopurinol	Disulfiram	May decrease metabolism and lead to toxicity
	Beta blockers	Interferon	
	Cimetidine	Mexiletine	
	Macrolides	Thiabendazole	
	Fluoroquinolones	Ticlopidine	
	Influenza vaccine		
	Halothane		Increased risk of arrhythmias
	Carbamazepine	Loop diuretics	Increased or decreased levels of theophylline
	Isoniazid		
Anticholinergic			
Ipratropium	Inhaled bronchodilators that contain fluorocarbon propellent		Potential additive fluorocarbon toxicity if used concurrently

*There are no significant drug-drug interactions with inhaled corticosteroids or antiallergy drugs.
CCBs, calcium channel blockers; MAO, monoamine oxidase.

tent asthma in patients older than 12 years of age. Zafirlukast and zileuton therapy can be continued during acute exacerbations of asthma but are not indicated for acute episodes. Montelukast is indicated for the prophylaxis and chronic treatment of asthma in adults and pediatric patients 6 years of age and older. These drugs are not appropriate for acute asthma attacks, including status asthmaticus. They are not bronchodilators.

Pharmacodynamics

Zileuton is a specific, orally active inhibitor of 5-lipoxygenase, the enzyme that catalyzes the formation of LTs (LTB_4, LTC_4, LTD_4, LTE_4) from arachidonic acid.

Zafirlukast is a potent competitive cysteinyl LT antagonist. By inhibiting the action of LTC_4, further conversion to other LTs is prevented and the characteristic symptoms of asthma are reduced. It is more effective in the early phase of allergen-induced airway response, with lesser effects on the late response. Neither of these drugs directly produces bronchodilation.

Montelukast is an orally active compound that binds with high affinity and selectivity to the cysteinyl LT_1 receptor (in preference to other pharmacologically important airway receptors such as the prostanoid, cholinergic, or beta receptors). It acts to inhibit physiologic actions of LTD_4 at the cysteinyl LT_1 receptor without any agonist activity.

Adverse Effects and Contraindications

The main adverse effects of LT antagonists to date include headache, dry mouth, and somnolence. Unspecified pain, abdominal pain, dyspepsia, nausea, asthenia, and myalgias have also occurred. Less common adverse effects include arthralgia, chest pain, conjunctivitis, constipation, dizziness, fever, flatulence, hypertonia, insomnia, lymphadenopathy, malaise, neck pain and rigidity, nervousness, pruritus, urinary tract infection, vaginitis, and vomiting.

LT antagonists are contraindicated in patients with hypersensitivity to the drug or to any of its inactive ingredients. Additionally, zileuton is contraindicated in patients with active liver disease and should be used with caution in patients who consume substantial quantities of alcohol or who have a past history of liver disease.

Pharmacokinetics

Zileuton is well absorbed following oral administration, with a mean peak plasma level of 1.7 hours (see Table

46–1). The absolute bioavailability of zileuton is unknown. Plasma concentrations are proportional to dose, and steady-state levels are predictable from single-dose pharmacokinetics. Zileuton is highly bound to plasma albumin, with minor binding to alpha$_1$-glycoprotein. Elimination of zileuton is predominantly via the liver with a half-life of 2½ hours. The drug is eliminated through the urine and feces.

Zafirlukast is rapidly absorbed from the gastrointestinal tract, reaching peak serum concentrations in about 3 hours. Taking the drug with food reduces its bioavailability by 40 percent. Zafirlukast is biotransformed in the liver and eliminated primarily in the feces with a half-life of about 10 hours. The half-life may be twice as long in older adults.

Montelukast is rapidly absorbed following oral administration, with peak drug activity noted in 3 to 4 hours. The mean oral bioavailability is 64 to 73 percent. It is highly bound (99 percent) to plasma proteins. It is extensively biotransformed in the liver, with elimination exclusively through the bile. The mean plasma half-life of montelukast is 2.7 to 5.5 hours in healthy young adults. With once-daily dosing, there is little accumulation of the parent drug.

Drug-Drug Interactions

Concurrent use of zafirlukast with warfarin increases the serum concentrations of warfarin and the prothrombin time. This is presumably because zafirlukast inhibits specific enzymes in the cytochrome P_{450} enzyme system. Zafirlukast also inhibits an enzyme that catalyzes the biotransformation of corticosteroids. Concurrent use with erythromycin or theophylline also lowered serum concentrations of zafirlukast, whereas concurrent use with aspirin increased serum concentrations. Table 46–3 lists other drugs that interact with zafirlukast. Phenobarbital and rifampin, which induces hepatic biotransformation, decrease the effectiveness of montelukast.

Dosage Regimen

The recommended oral dosage of zileuton for the symptomatic treatment of patients with asthma is 600 mg four times daily for a total dose of 2400 mg. For ease of administration, zileuton may be taken with meals and at bedtime (see Table 46–2).

The recommended oral dose of zafirlukast is 20 mg twice daily. It should be taken 1 hour before or 2 hours after meals.

The usual dose for adults and adolescents older than 15 years of age is 10 mg daily to be taken in the evening. One 5 mg tablet of montelukast may be given to pediatric patients 6 to 14 years of age. No dosage adjustments are thought to be necessary in this age group. The drug's safety and efficacy in children younger than 6 years of age have not been established.

Laboratory Considerations

Alanine aminotransferase (ALT; serum glutamic-pyruvic transaminase [SGPT]) and aspartate aminotransferase (AST; serum glutamic-oxaloacetic transaminase [SGOT]) elevations have been noted in patients taking LT antagonists. Transaminase elevations greater than or equal to three times the upper limit of normal have been noted. The elevations returned to normal on discontinuation of therapy. Urinary LTE_4 elimination is a marker for whole-body synthesis of LTs, and this marker can be used to monitor the bioavailability and efficacy of LT synthesis antagonists.

Xanthine Derivatives

- ❒ Aminophylline (PHYLLOCONTIN)
- ❒ Dyphylline (DILOR, LUFYLLIN)
- ❒ Oxtriphylline (CHOLEDYL)
- ❒ Theophylline (ELIXOPHYLLIN, SLO-PHYLLINE, THEO-DUR, THEOLAIR, THEOSPAN, THEOSTAT, THEOVENT, UNIPHYL, many others)

Indications

Xanthine derivatives such as theophylline are mild to moderate bronchodilator drugs. Although they are less effective than beta agonists as bronchodilators, they are principally used as adjuvants to inhaled corticosteroids for the prevention of nocturnal asthma symptoms. They also may have mild anti-inflammatory effects.

Pharmacodynamics

Xanthine derivatives produce bronchial smooth muscle relaxation by inhibiting phosphodiesterase and possibly adenosine antagonism. Only minimal bronchodilation occurs at therapeutic theophylline concentrations. Xanthines may affect eosinophilic infiltration into bronchial mucosa as well as decrease the numbers of epithelial T cells. Diaphragmatic contractility and mucociliary clearance are increased. Theophylline alleviates the early phase of asthma attacks and the bronchoconstrictive portion of the late-phase response. It has no effect on bronchial hyperresponsiveness.

Adverse Effects and Contraindications

The primary problems with xanthines are related to the relatively high incidence of adverse effects. The adverse effects are dose related, but even at therapeutic dosages, effects include headache, insomnia, gastric upset, aggravation of ulcer or gastroesophageal reflux, difficulty urinating (in older males with prostatism), and hyperactivity in some children. Hyperglycemia, hypokalemia, tachyarrhythmias (supraventricular tachycardia), and seizures have also been noted.

Pharmacokinetics

Aminophylline is well absorbed from oral dosage forms, with absorption from extended-release forms being slow but complete. Seventy-five percent of dyphylline is absorbed following oral administration. Absorption of oxtriphylline is good following oral administration. Absorption of enteric-coated and sustained-release formulations may be delayed and unreliable. Both aminophylline and oxtriphylline release theophylline following administration.

Aminophylline and oxtriphylline are widely distributed to body tissues, crossing the placental membranes. Breast milk concentrations are 70 percent those of plasma levels. Dyphylline reaches high concentrations in breast milk. The drugs are not distributed to adipose tissue.

The onset time of xanthine drug action varies from 15 to 60 minutes depending on the route of administration (see Table 46–1). Extended-release formulations of theophylline have a delayed onset time. Peak effects are noted in 1 to 7 hours, with a duration of action of 6 to 12 hours.

Aminophylline and oxtriphylline are converted to theophylline in the liver. Ninety percent of theophylline is biotransformed to caffeine, which may accumulate in neonates. Theophylline metabolites are eliminated via the kidneys. Eighty-five percent of dyphylline is eliminated unchanged by the kidneys. The half-life of theophylline varies from 3 to 13 hours depending on co-morbid diseases. Febrile illness (e.g., influenza), hypoxia, cor pulmonale, decompensated heart failure, cirrhosis, and renal disease decrease biotransformation. Smoking increases biotransformation of theophylline, thus decreasing its serum concentration.

Drug-Drug Interactions

Drug-drug interactions with xanthines are many (see Table 46–3). They produce additive cardiovascular and central nervous system effects when they are used concurrently with adrenergic drugs. Decreased effectiveness of the xanthine is seen in the presence of nicotine, barbiturates, phenytoin, ketoconazole, and rifampin. Decreased metabolism of xanthines is noted with concurrent use of erythromycin, beta blockers, cimetidine, influenza vaccine, oral contraceptives, glucocorticoids, and a number of other drugs. Theophylline levels may increase or decrease in the presence of isoniazid, carbamazepine, and loop diuretics.

Drug-Food Interactions

Regular but excessive intake of charcoal-broiled foods may decrease the effectiveness of xanthines. Excessive intake of xanthine-containing foods or beverages (e.g., colas, coffee, chocolate) increases the risk of cardiovascular and central nervous system effects. Fatty foods increase the absorption rate of xanthines. A diet high in protein increases biotransformation, leading to decreased theophylline concentrations. Conversely, a diet high in carbohydrates decreases biotransformation and increases theophylline concentrations.

Dosage Regimen

The dosage regimen for xanthine derivatives is expressed in theophylline equivalents and varies with the specific drug, patient body weight (mg/kg), route of administration, and serum drug levels. Dosages are calculated on the basis of lean body weight since theophylline does not distribute to body fat. Regardless of the theophylline salt used, dosages should be equivalent based on anhydrous theophylline content.

Individualize patient dosing. With immediate release formulations, dosing every 6 hours is generally required, especially in children. Intervals of up to 8 hours may be satisfactory in adults (see Table 46–2). Use dosage intervals to produce minimal fluctuations between peak and trough serum levels. When converting from an intermediate release to a sustained-release formulation, the total daily dose should remain the same, and only the dosing interval should be adjusted. To achieve rapid effects, an initial loading dose is required. The orally administered dose is 5 mg/kg of lean body weight. The loading dose should be reduced or eliminated if a theophylline preparation has been used in the preceding 24 hours.

Laboratory Considerations

Arterial blood gases, and fluid and electrolyte balance should be monitored in patients receiving parenteral xanthine therapy. Serum drug levels are monitored regularly for evidence of toxicity.

Anticholinergic Drug

❒ Ipratropium (ATROVENT)

Indications

The anticholinergic ipratropium is used as a bronchodilator in maintenance therapy of reversible airway obstruction due to asthma. It is not designed for use in acute bronchospasm.

Pharmacodynamics

Airway diameter is predominantly controlled by the parasympathetic nervous system. The effects of acetylcholine, the neurohormone, are increased mucus secretion and smooth muscle contraction, resulting in bronchoconstriction. Anticholinergic drugs (e.g., ipratropium) inhibit only the component of bronchoconstriction mediated by the parasympathetic nervous system. Cholinergic receptor activity in bronchial smooth muscle is inhibited, resulting in decreased concentrations of cyclic guanosine monophosphate (cGMP). Decreased levels of cGMP produce local bronchodilation. The end result is bronchodilation without systemic anticholinergic adverse effects. Ipratropium produces most bronchodilation in larger airways in contrast to beta agonists that act primarily in smaller airways. Anticholinergic drugs are discussed in more depth in Chapter 13.

Adverse Effects and Contraindications

Systemic adverse effects of ipratropium are uncommon because it is poorly absorbed. However, when it is present, the adverse effects can include nervousness, dizziness, and headache. Ipratropium is contraindicated in hypersensitive patients, and in those with allergy to atropine, belladonna alkaloids, bromide, or fluorocarbons. Its use should be avoided during acute bronchospasm. Ipratropium should be used with caution in patients who have bladder neck obstruction, glaucoma, or urinary retention. Safe use during pregnancy, lactation, or in children has not been established.

Pharmacokinetics

The onset of ipratropium's drug action occurs 5 to 15 minutes after inhalation, reaching a peak in 1 to 2 hours. Drug action may last as long as 6 hours. There is minimal systemic absorption. Small amounts are biotransformed in the liver. The half-life of ipratropium is about 2 hours.

Dosage Regimen

The usual adult dose of ipratropium is one to two inhalations via MDI three to four times daily. The dosage should not exceed 12 inhalations in 24 hours, and the drug should not be used more often than every 4 hours. When ipratropium solution is used in a nebulizer, 250 to 500 mcg is given 3 to 4 times daily. The nebulizer route is used for children with drug doses of 125 to 250 mcg given three to four times daily.

Critical Thinking Process

Assessment

History of Present Illness

Patient history is the most important component in the evaluation of a patient with suspected or confirmed asthma. The patient should be asked if he had sudden severe episodes or recurrent episodes of coughing, wheezing, or shortness of breath in the last 12 months. Has the patient had colds that settle in the chest or take more than 10 days to resolve? Does the coughing, wheezing, or shortness of breath occur during a particular season or time of the year? Does it occur in certain places or when the person is exposed to certain things (e.g., animals, tobacco smoke, perfumes)? Have the symptoms occurred during the night, early morning, or after moderate exercise, running, or other physical activity?

Determine the frequency and severity of attacks, as well as precipitating and alleviating factors. Ask if the patient uses any drugs that help him to breathe better and how often the drugs are used. Ascertain if the drugs are taken regularly or occasionally. Elicit information about allergies and the patient's status between attacks (e.g., restrictions in activities of daily living). Ask what the highest and lowest peak flow reading has been since the patient's last visit and what was done with the information.

A careful search of environmental factors should be conducted. The patient should be questioned in detail about the home environment: location, type of heating (e.g., wood burning stove or fireplace), type and quality of construction, type of insulation, humidity, nature of furnishings, presence of plants, draperies and bedding, pets and their habits, house cleaning methods, cigarette smoking, and so on. Variations in symptoms with seasons and with changes in location should be carefully recorded. Also ask about the work environment, for exposure to chemical irritants or sensitizers, physical demands, and job stressors. Does the patient cough or wheeze during the week but not on weekends when he or she is away from the workplace? Do the patient's eyes and nasal passages get irritated soon after arriving at work? The patient's clothing and dietary history should not be overlooked, especially in children, because fabrics and foods are potential allergens.

A drug history is important, especially any prescription or over-the-counter drug used to treat present or past symptoms. Determine what drugs the patient is taking, how much, and how often. Ask how many puffs of an inhaler the patient is using daily. How many inhalers has the patient used in the last month? For some patients, it is important to ask them to demonstrate their technique for using the inhaler. Information regarding the use of inhaled cocaine or nasal decongestants and antihistamines should be carefully noted.

Past Health History

When interviewing the patient, the health care provider should take pains to identify any previous allergic problems in the patient and also any allergies in close family members. This information is particularly helpful in providing support for the diagnosis of an atopic disease. The onset of symptoms in childhood is typical of allergic disease, but the onset of symptoms during adulthood does not rule out atopy.

Physical Exam Findings

A general respiratory exam includes assessment of the rate and character of respirations and skin color. For the patient with asthma, percussion of the chest may reveal hyperresonance. On auscultation, breath sounds are coarse and loud with sonorous crackles throughout the lung fields. Expiration is prolonged. Course rhonchi may be heard, along with generalized inspiratory and expiratory wheezing. The wheezing becomes high pitched as obstruction progresses. If the lungs sound clear, auscultate during forced expiration, which may bring out asthmatic wheezing.

Abnormal breathing patterns (e.g., rate below 12 or above 24, dyspnea, cough, orthopnea, wheezing, stridor) suggest respiration distress. Severe respiratory distress is characterized by tachypnea, dyspnea, use of accessory muscles of respiration, and hypoxia. Early signs of hypoxia include restlessness, confusion, anxiety, increased blood pressure, and tachycardia. Late signs of hypoxia include cyanosis and decreased blood pressure and pulse. Hypoxemia is confirmed when arterial blood gas analyses reflect decreased partial pressure of oxygen (PaO_2).

The nose is often overlooked during a physical exam or is given only a cursory inspection. The nasal mucosa is inspected for erythema, pallor, atrophy, edema, crusting, and discharge. The presence of polyps (not to be confused with turbinates), erosions, and septal perforations or deviations should be noted. A pale, boggy appearance to the mucosa is allegedly a classic sign of allergic disease, but erythema sometimes occurs in allergy and a boggy appearance certainly does not rule out sinusitis. Sinusitis may be present at the time of the exam. Mucopurulent discharge from the nares or seen in the posterior pharynx raises the possibility of sinusitis.

A child with atopy may have dark circles under the eyes (allergic shiners) and have a transverse crease above the tip of the nose from frequent upward nose rubbing (allergic salute). Erythematous conjunctiva, tearing, photophobia, and papillary edema of the lids provide supportive evidence of an allergic mechanism. Transillumination and palpation of the sinuses, a pharyngeal exam for erythema and discharge, checking the ears for evidence of otitis, and cervical node exam for adenopathy are included in the exam.

Diagnostic Testing

Few general laboratory procedures are appropriate for the patient with asthma. Pulmonary function tests provide an objective and reproducible means of evaluating the presence and severity of lung disease, as well as the response to therapy. A key measurement is *peak expiratory flow rate* (PEFR), or the greatest flow velocity that can be obtained during a forced expiration. PEFRs place the disease into physiologic categories: red, yellow, and green zones. (Fig. 46–3). In general, spirometry testing can be reliably per-

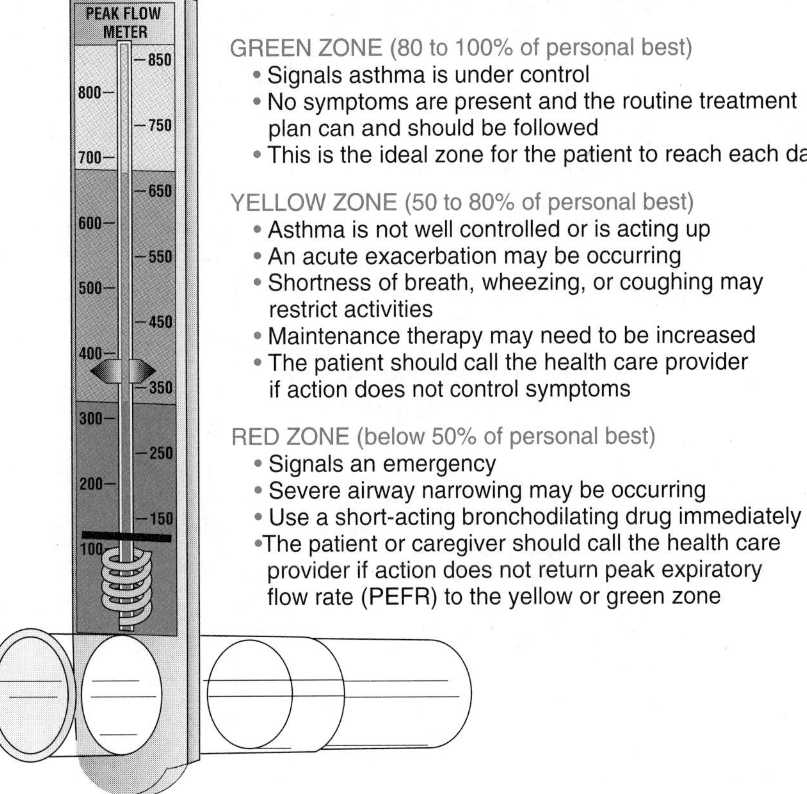

Figure 46–3 Interpreting peak expiratory flow rates. A baseline reading is required for accurate interpretation of the expiratory flow rate zones because expiration measurements are based on the patient's personal best effort rather than set levels of expiration.

formed by adults as well as children by the age of five or six. In addition, skin testing is specifically recommended for patients with persistent asthma who are exposed to perennial indoor allergens.

Developmental Considerations

Perinatal During pregnancy, a number of changes take place in the respiratory tract that are mediated by the mechanical effects of the enlarging uterus, increased oxygen demands, and the respiratory stimulant effect of progesterone. Estrogen causes hyperemia of nasopharyngeal mucosa with edema and increased production of mucus. This leads to a feeling of stuffiness and an increased tendency for epistaxis. Pregnant women should be warned of this normal change and advised against using over-the-counter drugs and nasal sprays in hope of alleviating the symptoms. A normal saline spray may be helpful in reducing some of the discomfort and should be encouraged in women who find the stuffy feeling uncomfortable.

Dyspnea is a complaint in 60 to 70 percent of normal pregnant women. The fact that it generally begins in the late first or early second trimester eliminates compression from the growing uterus as a likely cause. The sensation of dyspnea is probably due to hyperventilation and reduced $PaCO_2$ levels and an increased sensitivity to carbon dioxide by the respiratory center.

Although studies show that about 4 percent of pregnancies are complicated by asthma, the true prevalence may be much higher. Asthma may occur at any time during pregnancy. If it is diagnosed before pregnancy, it may be worsened by the pregnancy. About one-third of pregnant women with asthma are adversely affected, one-third remain the same, and one-third improve. Women with asthma usually have a return to their prepregnancy level of the disease by about 3 months postpartum.

Maternal and fetal morbidity and mortality are increased if asthma is uncontrolled during pregnancy. Maternal complications include pre-eclampsia, gestational hypertension, hyperemesis gravidarum, vaginal hemorrhage, and complications of labor. Fetal complications include increased risk of perinatal mortality, intrauterine growth retardation, preterm birth, low birth weight, and neonatal hypoxia. If asthma is controlled, the woman can maintain a normal pregnancy, with little or no increased risk to herself or the fetus.

Pediatric A strong relationship exists between viral infections and the induction of asthma in infants. Allergens play a less important role in this age group because it takes time for allergic sensitivity to develop. In children, however, allergy influences the persistence and severity of the disease (see Triggers of Acute Asthma Attacks).

Assessment of symptoms in the child is much like that of the adult but also includes a feeding history for a very young child with attention to cow's milk, eggs, and wheat. The stability of family members' relationships and stress level in the home should not be overlooked. Information about the child's toys, bedroom, and other rooms of the house where the child spends waking hours should be noted. The child's exposure level to babysitters, relatives, day care, and school environments is included. The presence or absence of symptoms in all of these areas should be noted. The source of present and past health information (often the parents) is important because valid recall of times and events associated with symptoms is critical in providing clues to the causal

Case Study Moderate Persistent Asthma

Patient History

History of Present Illness	RL is a 25-year-old Native American female who has had bronchial asthma since age 7, resulting in recurrent episodes of acute attacks. RL has been treated in the emergency room or hospitalized for asthma attacks once a month for the last 10 months. Today's attack began when she awoke this morning, although she reports wheezing during the night and having a headache. Symptoms of a URI had been present for the past 48 hours. RL has a 10-pack year history of smoking. Current drugs include cromolyn sodium four times daily and metaproterenol MDI PRN. Her wheezing this morning was not relieved by her metaproterenol MDI. She reports using up two 14-gram MDI canisters this month alone in an attempt to control her asthma.
Past Health History	RL was hospitalized at age 17 for severe respiratory distress and since then has used intermittent steroid therapy to maintain control. Her family history reveals that both parents are diabetics, as well as three of her five siblings. Her mother has a 40-year history of asthma and eczema.
Physical Exam	VS: BP 120/80, temp 97.2°F, pulse 90 and regular, and respirations 24. Height: 5'2". Weight: 190 lbs. Audible wheezes on inspiration and expiration over bilateral lung fields. Altered ratio of inspiration to expiration. Heart sounds not audible because of the wheezes. Skin pink and diaphoretic.
Diagnostic Testing	Spirometry reveals an FEV_1 of 74% of predicted with a variable PEF that exceeds 30%.
Developmental Considerations	RL is in Erikson's stage of intimacy versus isolation. She is attempting to establish intimate bonds of love and friendship, although her attempts have been hindered by her asthma.
Psychosocial Considerations	RL was married at age 20, was divorced a year later, and has one child, a daughter now age 4. She is presently in college full-time and living with her parents until she completes her education.
Economic Factors	RL has no income of her own. Her parents are supporting RL and their grandchild while RL is in school. Health care needs are covered through her parents' insurance coverage.

Variables Influencing Decision

Treatment Objectives

- Prevent chronic, troublesome symptoms (e.g., coughing or nocturnal shortness of breath, in the early morning, or after exercise)
- Maintain near-normal pulmonary function exercise and other physical activities

Drug Variables	*Drug Summary*	*Patient Variables*
Indications	Cromolyn: antiallergy drug used for asthma prophylaxis when used regularly. Beclomethasone: corticosteroids are the most effective anti-inflammatory drugs available for the treatment of asthma. Salmeterol: long-term relief of bronchoconstriction, more effective symptom control when added to standard doses of inhaled corticosteroids rather than increasing the corticosteroid dose. Effective for nighttime symptoms. All of these indications will become decision points.	RL is diagnosed with moderate persistent asthma. She has not been using the cromolyn correctly, relying on her short-acting beta agonist. These factors will become decision points.
Pharmacodynamics	Cromolyn: stabilizes mast cells. Corticosteroids: produce potent anti-inflammatory effects that also reduce mucus secretion and increase the number and sensitivity of adrenergic receptors. Salmeterol: relaxes airway smooth muscle and plays a role in increasing mucociliary clearance.	There are no pharmacodynamic considerations for RL. Cromolyn may have been effective if RL used it correctly.

Drug Variables	*Drug Summary*	*Patient Variables*
Adverse Effects/ Contraindications	Cromolyn: headache, tracheal irritation, cough, bronchospasm. Corticosteroids: headache (worse with triamcinolone than others), throat itching (with budesonide), wheezing, bronchospasm, cough, oral candidiasis. Salmeterol: headache, tachycardia, nervousness, hypertension, paradoxical bronchospasm, cough	RL's headache was relieved with acetaminophen. She believes that the headache is related to stress rather than drugs. RL is not hypertensive. She attributes her intermittent use of the cromolyn to the tracheal irritation it produces. This factor may become a decision point.
Pharmacokinetics	Cromolyn: peak activity takes 2 to 3 weeks to be observed. Corticosteroids: well absorbed from respiratory tract, although peak drug action may not be noted for up to 4 weeks. Beclomethasone has the highest bioavailablity of the available agents. Salmeterol: is a long-acting beta agonist with a slower onset than some other beta agonists.	RL needs relief from present episode of bronchospasm but also long-term relief. This factor will become a decision point.
Dosage Regimen	Cromolyn: 2 inhalations four times daily. Beclomethasone 1–2 inhalations BID via MDI with 5 minutes between puffs. Salmeterol: 2 inhalations BID at 12-hour intervals before using beclomethasone	The fewer doses RL must administer, the more likely she is to be compliant with her treatment regimen. Salmeterol will provide coverage for RL's nighttime symptoms. These factors will become decision points.
Lab Considerations	RL will need periodic spirometry testing.	There are no laboratory considerations for RL except for periodic spirometry testing.
Cost Index*	Beclomethasone MDI: 5 Salmeterol MDI: 3 Prednisone: 1	RL has pharmacy insurance through her parents' insurance policy. May need to switch to a less expensive beta agonist if cost becomes an issue

Summary of Decision Points

- Corticosteroids are all topically active, equally effective, and have few systemic adverse effects at therapeutic dosages
- There is a possibility the cromolyn is causing tracheal irritation. It may also not be effective because of RL's intermittent use.
- RL needs relief from present episode of bronchospasm as well as long-term control of symptoms.
- Salmeterol, as a long-acting beta agonist, will also provide coverage for RL's nighttime symptoms.

DRUGS TO BE USED

- Stop cromolyn sodium today
- Salmeterol 2 inhalations (50 mcg/INH) BID at 12-hour intervals before using beclomethasone MDI.
- Beclomethasone MDI 2–4 inhalations (0.0.084 mcg/INH) BID. Reduce inhalations to 1–2 BID after the first 4 weeks of therapy.
- Start oral prednisone burst regimen.

*Cost Index:
1 = $ < 30/mo.
2 = $ 30–40/mo.
3 = $ 40–50/mo.
4 = $ 50–60/mo.
5 = $ > 60/mo.

AWP of a 13-gram MDI canister (with adapter) of salmeterol is approximately $59.
AWP of a 12.2-gram MDI canister (with adapter) of beclomethasone is approximately $48.
AWP of 25 10-mg tablets of prednisone is approximately $3.

antigen. Poorly controlled asthma may delay growth in children. In general, children with asthma tend to have longer periods of reduced growth rates before puberty, males more so than females.

Geriatric Commonly, older adults who develop asthma late in life have intrinsic asthma, which does not have allergic or environmental triggers. Common estimates of the incidence of new-onset asthma after age 65 vary from 1 to 3 percent. Some health care providers indicate, however, that asthma developed in almost half of the patient population who were older than age 65. Neither IgE nor skin testing is useful in the older adult, probably because of the decrease in allergic response associated with aging. Unfortunately, treatable airway disorders in older adults often go undiagnosed, perhaps because of the high prevalence of other forms of respiratory disease and cardiac failure that may have similar clinical presentations. Some older adults may not be able to perform spirometry testing reliably. Additional tests, such as symptom scores and distance walked without dyspnea and wheezing, can be used to evaluate the patient.

Psychosocial Considerations

Many of the drugs used in the treatment of allergies and asthma are purchased by consumers over the counter. They are easily accessible to almost all persons, are easy to use, and in many cases, are generally effective. For these reasons, many patients with asthma have not been diagnosed or adequately treated. Family and societal health care beliefs and norms may keep the patient from seeking help (see Case Study—Moderate Persistent Asthma).

Analysis and Management

Treatment Objectives

Active partnership with patients remains the cornerstone of asthma management because there are many goals of asthma therapy. These goals are all-important in managing asthma effectively. The goals include

- Preventing chronic, troublesome symptoms (e.g., coughing or nocturnal shortness of breath, in the early morning, or after exercise)
- Maintaining normal or near-normal pulmonary function
- Maintaining exercise and other physical activities
- Preventing recurrent exacerbations and minimizing the need for acute care interventions
- Providing optimal drug therapy with minimal or no adverse effects
- Meeting patient and family's expectations of satisfaction with asthma care

Treatment Options

Asthma is clearly not a one-drug disease. Thus, multidrug therapy is generally the rule rather than the exception. A stepwise approach is recommended with the type and amount of drug dictated by the severity of the asthma (Fig. 46–4). Drug regimens are organized so as to gain long-term control of persistent asthma, and to treat symptoms and exacerbations with quick-relief drugs.

Two documents set the standards for the diagnosis and treatment of asthma: *Guidelines for the Diagnosis and Management of Asthma* (1991, 1997) and the *International Consensus Report on Diagnosis and Treatment of Asthma* (1992). According to these documents, chronic asthma therapy should be started when avoidance of bronchospasm-triggering factors does not control symptoms or when beta agonists are required more than twice daily for 1 week. Prophylactic therapy should be instituted before exercise in all patients with demonstrated exercise-induced asthma and in all patients who have seasonal asthma (ideally before the season for the known allergen). Corticosteroids, antiallergy drugs, LT antagonists, long-acting beta agonists, and xanthine derivatives are used for long-term control of asthma. Short-acting beta agonists and anticholinergics are used for acute asthma attacks.

Drug Variables

Inhaled Corticosteroids Because inflammation is considered an early and persistent component of asthma, therapy must be directed toward long-term suppression of the inflammation. In line with national and international guidelines, earlier and more widespread use of inhaled corticosteroids is recommended. Corticosteroids are the most effective anti-inflammatory drugs available for the treatment of asthma. Early intervention with corticosteroids improves asthma control and normalizes lung function. Early corticosteroid use may also prevent irreversible airway damage. The principal corticosteroids are topically active, equally effective, and have few systemic adverse effects at therapeutic dosages. In many countries of the world, inhaled corticosteroids have become the first-line treatment, with inhaled $beta_2$ agonists used as needed. The potential, but small, risk of adverse effects of corticosteroids is offset by their efficacy.

Still, a number of concerns remain. There is a rising trend in the prevalence, morbidity, severity, and mortality rates for asthma. Despite the well-recognized efficacy and safety of inhaled corticosteroids, many patients still have poorly controlled asthma and a poor quality of life. In addition, there are concerns about the long-term safety of inhaled corticosteroids (especially in high doses and at the extremes of age). Poor compliance with the treatment plan and poor administration technique (especially for inhaled formulations) contribute to the risk of exacerbations and adverse drug effects.

The effects of the various corticosteroids in reducing symptoms and improving PEFRs have been compared. Beclomethasone and budesonide by MDI produce comparable effects on a microgram-to-microgram basis. Beclomethasone achieves effects similar to twice the dose of triamcinolone on a microgram basis. Because the majority of patients with asthma require low corticosteroid dosages (300 to 400 mcg/day), beclomethasone is the most convenient and cost-effective preparation. Beclomethasone in high dosage (i.e., 2000 mcg/day) increases the output of urinary hydroxyproline. The increased output of this amino acid (that is produced in the digestion of hydrolytic decomposition of proteins, especially of collagens) reflects an increase in bone resorption, whereas budesonide does not cause this.

Budesonide has the highest inhaled-to-systemic ratio of the drugs available at present; however, it is less bioavailable than beclomethasone. In low dosages (i.e., less than 1000 mcg/day), the impact of differences in bioavailability between budesonide and beclomethasone is probably not significant. Budesonide administered via Turbuhaler achieved effects similar to twice the dose delivered by MDI. This sug-

Stepwise Approach for Managing Asthma in Adults and Children Over 5 Years Old

Goals of Asthma Treatment

- Prevent chronic and troublesome symptoms (e.g., coughing or breathlessness in the night, in the early morning, or after exertion)
- Maintain (near) "normal" pulmonary function
- Maintain normal activity levels (including exercise and other physical activity)
- Prevent recurrent exacerbations of asthma and minimize the need for emergency department visits or hospitalizations
- Provide optimal pharmacotherapy with minimal or no adverse effects
- Meet patients' and families' expectation of and satisfaction with asthma care

Classification of Severity: Clinical Features Before Treatment*

	*Symptoms***	*Nighttime Symptoms*	*Lung Function*
STEP 4 **Severe Persistent**	■ Continual symptoms ■ Limited physical activity ■ Frequent exacerbations	Frequent	■ FEV_1 or PEF ≤ 60% predicted ■ PEF variability > 30%
STEP 3 **Moderate Persistent**	■ Daily symptoms ■ Daily use of inhaled short-acting $beta_2$-agonist ■ Exacerbations affect activity ■ Exacerbations ≥ 2 times a week; may last days	> 1 time a week	■ FEV_1 or PEF > 60% ≤ 80% predicted ■ PEF variability > 30%
STEP 2 **Mild Persistent**	■ Symptoms > 2 times a week but < 1 time a day ■ Exacerbations may affect activity	> 2 times a month	■ FEV_1 or PEF ≥ 80% predicted ■ PEF variability 20-30%
STEP 1 **Mild Intermittent**	■ Symptoms ≤ 2 times a week ■ Asymptomatic and normal PEF between exacerbations ■ Exacerbations brief (from a few hours to a few days); intensity may vary	≤ 2 times a month	■ FEV_1 or PEF ≥ 80% predicted ■ PEF variability < 20%

* The presence of one of the features of severity is sufficient to place a patient in that category. An individual should be assigned to the most severe grade in which any feature occurs. The characteristics noted in this figure are general and may overlap because asthma is highly variable. Furthermore, an individual's classification may change over time.

** Patients at any level of severity can have mild, moderate, or severe exacerbations. Some patients with intermittent asthma experience severe and life-threatening exacerbations separated by long periods of normal lung function and no symptoms.

Illustration continued on following page

Figure 46–4 Stepwise approach for managing asthma in adults and children over 5 years old. (From the National Institutes of Health, National Heart, Lung, and Blood Institute. (1997). *Highlights of the Expert Panel Report 2: Guidelines for the Diagnosis and Management of Asthma* (Pub. No. 97-4051A). Bethesda, MD: U.S. Department of Health and Human Services.

Stepwise Approach for Managing Asthma in Adults and Children Over 5 Years Old: Treatment

Preferred treatments are in bold print.	Long-Term Control	Quick Relief	Education
STEP 4 Severe Persistent	Daily medications: ■ **Anti-inflammatory: inhaled corticosteroid (high dose)** and ■ Long-acting bronchodilator: either long-acting inhaled beta$_2$-agonist, sustained-release theophylline, or long-acting beta$_2$-agonist tablets AND ■ Corticosteroid tablets or syrup long term (2 mg/kg/day, generally do not exceed 60 mg per day).	■ Short-acting bronchodilator: **inhaled beta$_2$-agonists** as needed for symptoms. ■ Intensity of treatment will depend on severity of exacerbation; see "Managing Exacerbations of Asthma." ■ Use of short-acting inhaled beta$_2$-agonists on a daily basis, or increasing use, indicates the need for additional long-term-control therapy.	Steps 2 and 3 actions plus: ■ Refer to individual education/counseling
STEP 3 Moderate Persistent	Daily medication: ■ Either – **Anti-inflammatory: inhaled corticosteroid** (medium dose) OR – Inhaled corticosteroid (low-medium dose) and add a long-acting bronchodilator, especially for nighttime symptoms: either **long-acting inhaled beta$_2$-agonist**, sustained-release theophylline, or long-acting beta$_2$-agonist tablets. ■ If needed – Anti-inflammatory: inhaled corticosteroids (medium-high dose) AND – Long-acting bronchodilator, especially for nighttime symptoms; either **long-acting inhaled beta$_2$-agonist**, sustained-release theophylline, or long-acting beta$_2$-agonist tablets.	■ Short-acting bronchodilator: **inhaled beta$_2$-agonists** as needed for symptoms. ■ Intensity of treatment will depend on severity of exacerbation; see "Managing Exacerbations of Asthma." ■ Use of short-acting inhaled beta$_2$-agonists on a daily basis, or increasing use, indicates the need for additional long-term-control therapy.	Step 1 actions plus: ■ Teach self-monitoring ■ Refer to group education if available ■ Review and update self-management plan

Figure 46–4 *Continued*

Stepwise Approach for Managing Asthma in Adults and Children Over 5 Years Old: Treatment (continued)

Preferred treatments are in bold print.	Long-Term Control	Quick Relief	Education
STEP 2 Mild Persistent	Daily medication: ■ **Anti-inflammatory:** either **inhaled corticosteroid** (low doses) or **cromolyn or nedocromil** (children usually begin with a trial of cromolyn or nedocromil). ■ Sustained-release theophylline to serum concentration of 5-15 mcg/mL is an alternative. Zafirlukast or zileuton may also be considered for patients ≥ 12 years of age, although their position in therapy is not fully established.	■ Short-acting bronchodilator: **inhaled beta$_2$-agonists** as needed for symptoms. ■ Intensity of treatment will depend on severity of exacerbation; see "Managing Exacerbations of Asthma." ■ Use of short-acting inhaled beta$_2$-agonists on a daily basis, or increasing use, indicates the need for additional long-term-control therapy.	Step 1 actions plus: ■ Teach self-monitoring ■ Refer to group education if available ■ Review and update self-management plan
STEP 1 Mild Intermittent	■ No daily medication needed.	■ Short-acting bronchodilator: **inhaled beta$_2$-agonists** as needed for symptoms. ■ Intensity of treatment will depend on severity of exacerbation; see "Managing Exacerbations of Asthma." ■ Use of short-acting inhaled beta$_2$-agonists more than 2 times a week may indicate the need to initiate long-term-control therapy.	■ Teach basic facts about asthma ■ Teach inhaler/spacer/ holding chamber technique ■ Discuss roles of medications ■ Develop self-management plan ■ Develop action plan for when and how to take rescue actions ■ Discuss appropriate environmental control measures to avoid exposure to known allergens and irritants. (See component 4.)

↓ **Step down**
Review treatment every 1 to 6 months; a gradual stepwise reduction in treatment may be possible.

↑ **Step up**
If control is not maintained, consider step up. First, review patient medication technique, adherence, and environmental control (avoidance of allergens or other factors that contribute to asthma severity).

Notes:
- **The stepwise approach presents general guidelines to assist clinical decisionmaking; it is not intended to be a specific prescription.** Asthma is highly variable; clinicians **should tailor specific medication plans to the needs and circumstances of individual patients.**
- Gain control as quickly as possible; then decrease treatment to the least medication necessary to maintain control. Gaining control may be accomplished either by starting treatment at the step most appropriate to the initial severity of their condition or by starting at a higher level of therapy (e.g., a course of systemic corticosteroids or higher dose of inhaled corticosteroids).
- A rescue course of systemic corticosteroid may be needed at any time and at any step.
- Some patients with intermittent asthma experience severe and life-threatening exacerbations separated by long periods of normal lung function and no symptoms. This may be especially common with exacerbations provoked by respiratory infections. A short course of systemic corticosteroids is recommended.
- At each step, patients should control their environment to avoid or control factors that make their asthma worse (e.g., allergens, irritants); this requires specific diagnosis and education.

Figure 46–4 *Continued*

gests the efficacy of the drug is influenced by the delivery device. Thus, the decision to use budesonide or beclomethasone should be based on cost and the patient's preference.

Fluticasone achieves effects similar to two times the dose of beclomethasone and budesonide via MDI on a microgram basis. Fluticasone has a significant first-pass effect and, therefore, a better efficacy-to-safety relationship. The health care provider is reminded that individual patients may respond differently to different drugs.

Inhaled corticosteroids should be added to therapy if more than two inhalations of beta agonist are required on a daily basis or when symptoms are not completely reversed. Corticosteroids should be added to the treatment regimen if the PEFR or FEV_1 falls to 85 percent or less of the predicted value or best-known results. Inhaled corticosteroids are favored over oral drugs because systemic absorption is minimal at usual doses, virtually eliminating the risk of corticosteroid-induced adverse effects. High-dose therapy (i.e., 20 puffs or more per day) has been recommended for refractory cases of asthma as an alternative to systemic corticosteroids. It appears that inhaled corticosteroids are more effective than alternate-day systemic therapy with its associated complications such as cataract development, skin changes, and HPA suppression.

Orally administered prednisone therapy should be initiated if significant improvement in acute symptoms (return to at least 80 percent of normal lung function) does not occur within 30 minutes of maximum beta agonist therapy. The anti-inflammatory effect of corticosteroids is delayed at least 4 hours; therefore, intravenous (IV) administration provides little if any time advantage. Further, IV administration is significantly more expensive than using the oral route and appears to be no more effective. Parenteral hydrocortisone can be used in patients who are nauseated or who have difficulty absorbing oral drugs.

Treating children who have persistent asthma with medium-potency inhaled corticosteroids may be associated with a possible, but not predictable, adverse effect on linear bone growth. However, it appears that adverse effects are dose dependent. Use of high-dose inhaled corticosteroids in children with severe persistent asthma has significantly less potential for affecting linear growth than prolonged use of high-dose systemic corticosteroids. Systemic corticosteroids should be used in short-term (i.e., 3 to 10 days) therapy to treat moderate to severe exacerbations of asthma.

To reduce the adverse effects associated with long-term use of corticosteroids, a number of measures are recommended. Inhaled corticosteroids should be administered using spacers or holding chambers. Use the lowest dose possible to maintain control. Consider using a long-acting beta agonist with a low to medium dose of inhaled corticosteroid rather than using a higher dose of the inhaled corticosteroid. Consider adjunct use of calcium (1000 to 1500 mg/day) and vitamin D (400 units/day) supplements for postmenopausal women. Estrogen replacement therapy when appropriate may be considered for patients on doses exceeding 1000 mcg of inhaled corticosteroid per day. Growth rates in children should be monitored.

Antiallergy Drugs The chief advantage of antiallergy drugs lies in the low incidence of adverse effects, thus making them relatively safe drugs for use in children. When they are given on a daily basis, antiallergy drugs are effective in controlling persistent asthma symptoms. Furthermore, because viral infections are a common trigger for asthma in children, antiallergy drugs may prevent the inflammation associated with these illnesses.

Beta Agonists The morbidity and mortality associated with asthma have increased despite advancements in drug therapy. The increased rates may be due to a false sense of security with beta agonists that cause the patient to delay seeking medical assistance. However, beta agonists are by far the most effective bronchodilators available. They relax airway smooth muscle from the trachea to the terminal bronchioles and play a role in increasing mucociliary clearance. However, they do not inhibit either the late-phase response or the subsequent bronchial hyperresponsiveness. Orally administered beta agonists are less useful because of the increased incidence of adverse effects. Excessive use of beta agonists may cause hypokalemia. These drugs may be useful for nocturnal asthma or severe asthma.

Regularly scheduled daily use of a short-acting beta agonist is generally not recommended. However, increasing the use of beta agonists or the use of more than one canister per month indicates inadequate control of asthma and the need for initiating or intensifying corticosteroid therapy. Inhaled long-acting beta agonists are preferred over systemic drugs (when possible) because of their long duration of action and because they have fewer adverse effects than oral sustained-release drugs. Salmeterol should not be used on a regular basis in the absence of symptoms. Continuous use of beta agonists leads to a greater decline in forced expiratory volume (FEV_1) than does intermittent use.

Leukotriene Antagonists LT antagonists may be used as alternatives to low-dose inhaled corticosteroids or antiallergy drugs in patients with mild, persistent asthma over age 12. Six hundred milligrams of zileuton four times daily produces a sustained 20-percent increase in FEV_1 for up to 13 weeks. Zafirlukast appears to be modestly effective for maintenance treatment of mild to moderate asthma, but taking the drug with food markedly decreases its bioavailability. Concurrent use with many other drugs may prove troublesome.

Unlike theophylline, there is no need to monitor LT antagonist drug concentrations. Asthma symptoms are reduced by one-third, and use of inhaled corticosteroids and beta agonists fall one-fourth to one-third. However, the relative low potency and short half-lives of LT antagonists mean that dosing four times a day is required.

Xanthines Xanthines may be added as a third-line drug to the treatment regimen for patients with acute asthma, although they provide little additional benefit when used concurrently with optimal doses of inhaled beta agonists. Nevertheless, there is benefit to be gained when xanthines are used as adjuncts to inhaled corticosteroids for prevention of nocturnal asthma symptoms. Theophylline should be used only if the patient fails to improve after the first 12 hours of treatment with beta agonists, ipratropium, and prednisone. Theophylline use may also be considered for patients who cannot tolerate beta agonist therapy and whose heart rate is less than 120 beats per minute (bpm).

Initial loading doses of theophylline are needed for most patients. Steady state serum theophylline concentrations ordinarily range from 10 to 20 mcg/mL. Some patients may require slightly higher concentrations. Routine monitoring of serum drug levels is essential due to the significant toxicities, narrow therapeutic range, and individual differences in metabolic clearance. Drug absorption and biotransformation are affected by numerous factors. Each of the factors can produce significant changes in steady-state drug concentration.

Anticholinergics Anticholinergic drugs are less effective than beta agonists and are ordinarily used in combination with other bronchodilators. They may be alternative bronchodilators for patients with severe asthma or for those patients who do not tolerate inhaled beta agonists. Anticholinergics should be added to the treatment regimen for chronic asthma only after the progression from high-dose corticosteroids and beta agonists fails to control symptoms. They should not be used before beta agonist therapy because there is some concern that initially they may cause bronchoconstriction.

Anticholinergics may provide the additional benefit of bronchodilation, and they can be started along with the first dose of a beta agonist in patients with severe disease. Although they provide an additional small increase in PEFR when they are used with submaximum doses of beta agonists, anticholinergics have not been shown to reduce other variables (e.g., the need for admission to a hospital, shorter length of stay).

Patient Variables

In cases of acute bronchoconstriction and anaphylaxis, systemic corticosteroids are used for approximately 1 week in addition to other agents. For some patients, an initial continuous IV infusion of corticosteroid may be required followed by oral therapy. The patient's asthma should be reasonably stable before switching to inhaled corticosteroids. Once past the acute episode of bronchoconstriction, the patient may use an aerosol along with the patient's usual maintenance doses of systemic corticosteroid. After approximately 1 week, gradual withdrawal of the systemic steroid is started by reducing the daily or alternate-day dose. The next dosage reduction is usually made after an interval of 1 to 2 weeks, depending on the response of the patient. Generally, these decrements should not exceed 2.5 mg of prednisone or its equivalent. A slow rate of withdrawal cannot be overemphasized. The patient should be monitored closely during the transfer from systemic steroid therapy to inhaled corticosteroids. The transition may unmask allergic conditions that were previously suppressed by the systemic steroids (e.g., conjunctivitis, rhinitis, eczema).

Concerns have been voiced about whether the use of inhaled corticosteroids predisposes the patient to osteoporosis. However, because it appears that use of inhaled corticosteroids reduces the need for, and dosage of, systemic drugs, the likelihood of osteoporosis is reduced.

It appears that the risks of uncontrolled asthma are of more concern than the risks of using drugs to treat asthma. The pregnant woman with asthma should be counseled about the importance of this factor. Women using inhaled bronchodilators or corticosteroids in asthma appear to have no greater risks of congenital anomalies or adverse perinatal outcomes than the general population. The use of theophylline and cromolyn in pregnancy is also considered safe. The theophylline dosage may need to be reduced during the third trimester because of a decrease in drug clearance.

Metaproterenol by inhalation and subcutaneous terbutaline have been used extensively in pregnant women. If no satisfactory response results from initial bronchodilators, IV aminophylline should be given for the patient with an acute attack. Theophylline serum levels are closely followed. Corticosteroids should be used with severe exacerbations or for patients who do not respond to the aforementioned therapy. Methylprednisolone may be given during an acute episode. An oral prednisone taper should follow IV corticosteroid therapy.

Symptoms of asthma rarely increase during labor. Asthma drugs used in the prenatal period should be continued. Women on corticosteroid therapy before labor should receive additional corticosteroids during labor.

In managing the care of an adolescent with asthma, it should be noted that pulmonary function testing should use appropriate reference populations. Adolescents compare most closely to childhood predicted norms rather than those of an adult. A trial with cromolyn is often used when initiating anti-inflammatory therapy in an adolescent. A written treatment plan should be prepared for the student's school, including plans to ensure reliable, prompt access to drugs.

A key point to remember in managing asthma in an older patient is that chronic bronchitis or emphysema may coexist with asthma. A trial of systemic corticosteroids will determine the extent of reversibility and therapeutic benefit. Furthermore, many older adults have co-morbid conditions (e.g., arthritis, heart disease, hypertension) that are being treated with drug therapy (e.g., aspirin, beta blockers). Asthma drugs may aggravate co-existing conditions; therefore, adjustments in the drug regimen may need to be made. Be aware of the increased potential for drug-drug interactions.

Although inhaled steroids provide control of asthmatic symptoms, they do not provide the quantity of systemic steroid necessary to cope with the stressors of gastroenteritis, trauma, surgery, or infections. Furthermore, deaths have occurred due to adrenal insufficiency during and after transfer from systemic corticosteroids to topical drugs. A number of months are required for recovery of HPA axis function.

Patients should receive a written care plan based on signs and symptoms and PEFRs. PEFRs guide therapeutic decisions. Drug therapy should be increased when the PEFR is below 80 percent of the patient's personal best.

There are several aerosol delivery devices: MDI, breath-actuated MDI, dry-power inhalers, and nebulizers. Each has advantages and disadvantages. The decision for a particular delivery device should be matched with patient needs and likelihood of compliance. The technique, advantages, and disadvantages are outlined in Table 46–4.

Intervention

Administration

The technique of drug administration varies with the specific aerosol delivery device and whether or not a spacer or holding chamber device is used. However, there are several problems encountered with the use of MDIs. Many patients are unable to coordinate activation with inhalation or activate the MDI in the mouth while breathing through their nose. Some patients do not have adequate strength to activate an MDI or are unable to hold their breath for the re-

TABLE 46–4 COMPARISON OF AEROSOL DELIVERY DEVICES

Advantage(s)	Disadvantage(s)
Metered-Dose Inhaler (MDI): Actuated during slow,* deep inhalation, followed by 10-second breath holding	
• Mouth rinsing may reduce systemic absorption	Slow inhalation is difficult for some patients. May have difficulty coordinating actuation with inhalation. Patients may incorrectly stop inhalation at actuation 80% of drug is deposited in oropharynx
Breath-Actuated MDI: Slow, deep inhalation, followed by 10-second breath holding	
• Helpful for patients who are unable to coordinate actuation with inhalation	Slow inhalation difficult for some patients Patients may incorrectly stop inhalation at actuation Requires more rapid inspiration to activate than is optimal for deposition Cannot be used with currently available spacer or holding devices
Dry-Powder Inhaler (DPI): Rapid, deep inhalation with mouth closed tightly around the mouthpiece	
• Delivery may be greater than MDI depending on device and technique. • Can be used in children younger than 4 years • Most appear to have similar delivery efficacy as MDI with or without spacer or holding device • Mouth rinsing is effective in reducing systemic absorption	Dose is lost if patient exhales through device. Some devices have delivery that exceeds that of an MDI
Nebulizer: Slow tidal breathing with occasional deep breaths. Tightly fitting face mask if unable to use mouthpiece.	
• Less dependent on patient coordination or cooperation • Delivery method of choice for cromolyn in children • Delivery method of choice for high-dose $beta_2$ agonists and anticholinergics in moderate to severe exacerbations in all patients	Expensive, time-consuming Bulky; output is device dependent Significant internebulizer and intranebulizer output variances
Spacer or Holding Device: Slow inhalation or tidal breathing immediately after actuation. One actuation into device per inhalation. If face mask is used, 3–5 inhalations per actuation.	
• Easier to use than MDI alone • With face mask, allows MDI to be used with small children • Large volume devices (> 600 mL) may increase lung delivery over MDI alone in patients with poor MDI technique • Decrease oropharyngeal deposition of drug and reduces potential systemic absorption of inhaled corticosteroids that have higher oral bioavailability • Recommended for patients on medium to high doses of inhaled corticosteroids • May be as effective as nebulizer in delivering high doses of $beta_2$ agonists during severe exacerbations	Does not obviate need for coordinating actuation with inhalation Bulky; output may be reduced in some devices after cleaning Output from MDI with spacer/holding device is dependent on both MDI and spacer type

*Slow inhalation means 30 L/minute for a period of 3 to 5 seconds. Rapid inhalation means 60 L/minute for a period of 1 to 2 seconds.
Adapted from the National Institutes of Health, National Heart, Lung, and Blood Institute. (1997). *Highlights of the Expert Panel Report 2: Guidelines for the diagnosis and management of asthma* (Pub. No. 97-4051A). Bethesda, MD: U.S. Department of Health and Human Services.

quired length of time after use. Some patients inhale more than one puff with each inspiration or do not wait a sufficient amount of time between each puff (1 to 5 minutes is recommended). Not shaking the MDI before use, or holding the MDI upside down or sideways contributes to ineffective use. Not tilting the head back and opening the mouth causes the drug to bounce off the teeth, tongue, or palate, thus limiting the amount of drug reaching the patient's airways.

Some patients use both a bronchodilator inhaler and a corticosteroid inhaler. They should be advised to use the bronchodilator drug before the corticosteroid to enhance penetration of the corticosteroid into the bronchial tree. Further, several minutes should elapse after use of the bronchodilator before the corticosteroid inhaler is used. Also, by waiting, the potential toxicity from inhaled chlorofluorocarbon propellants is reduced. Some newer aerosols (e.g., PROVENTIL HFA) are formulated using hydrofluoroalkane rather than chlorofluorocarbons. Even though chlorofluorocarbons are safe for human use, it has been found that they are damaging the ozone layer of the atmosphere.

The mouth should be rinsed with water or mouthwash after each use of an inhaler to minimize dry mouth and hoarseness. Rinsing the mouth after use of inhaled corticosteroids is advised to reduce the frequent but mild candidiasis that may occur. When it is present, candidiasis responds well to antifungal drugs such as nystatin mouthwash or clotrimazole troches. The inhalation device should be washed at least daily in warm running water.

Corticosteroid preparations are not absolutely interchangeable on a microgram or per-puff basis. New delivery devices may provide greater delivery of drug to the airways, which may affect dose. Cromolyn capsules for inhalation are to be used with the Spinhaler or Halermatic device only. Patients using the antiallergy capsule and Spinhaler formulation should be instructed as to the use of the capsule and turbohaler. The capsule is placed in the turbohaler that, in turn, punctures the capsule. When the patient places the turbohaler in the mouth and inhales, the capsule spins and vibrates, causing the micronized powder to be released. The solution formulation is used with a power-operated nebulizer. Hand-operated nebulizers are unsuitable.

Dosage adjustments of theophylline preparations are based on clinical response and improvement in pulmonary function with careful monitoring of serum concentrations. If the level is too low (i.e., 5 to 10 mcg/mL), the dosage should be increased by about 25 percent at 3-day intervals until either the desired clinical response or serum concentration is achieved. The total daily dose may need to be given at more frequent intervals if asthma symptoms repeatedly occur at the end of a dosing interval. If the serum theophylline level is within the desired range (i.e., 10 to 20 mcg/mL), the present dosage level should be maintained and the serum level checked at 6- to 12-month intervals. Finer adjustments in dosage may be needed for some patients. Theophylline dosage should be decreased by 10 percent if levels are between 20 and 25 mcg/mL and the level should be rechecked in 3 days. If the level is between 25 and 30 mcg/mL, the next scheduled dose should be skipped and subsequent doses decreased by about 25 percent. Serum levels are rechecked in 3 days. When serum levels exceed 30 mcg/mL, the next two doses should be skipped and subsequent doses decreased by 50 percent. Again, the serum levels should be rechecked in 3 days. Once the patient is stabilized on a dosage, serum levels tend to remain constant.

Education Patient and family education should begin at the time of asthma diagnosis and be integrated into each step of care. Education about self-management should be tailored to the needs of each patient, maintaining a sensitivity to cultural beliefs and practices.

Because asthma is clearly not a one-drug disease, the patient must be familiar with a variety of drugs and treatment regimens. Combination therapy is generally the rule rather than the exception. Patients using inhaled corticosteroids should be taught to observe for hoarseness, cough, throat irritation, and fungal infection of the mouth and throat. Patients on immunosuppressant doses of corticosteroids should be warned to avoid exposure to chickenpox or measles. How the dose, route, and duration of corticosteroid administration affect the risk of developing disseminated infection is not known. The contribution of the underlying disease and prior corticosteroid treatment to the increased risk of infection is also not known. Patients should be told that medical advice should be sought if they are exposed to infection.

During periods of stress or a severe asthma attack, patients who have been withdrawn from systemic corticosteroids should be instructed to resume taking the drug immediately (in large doses) and to contact their health care provider for further instructions. These patients should also be instructed to carry Medic-alert identification indicating that they may need supplemental systemic steroids during periods of stress or a severe asthma attack. During withdrawal from corticosteroids, some patients experience withdrawal symptoms (e.g., lassitude, joint or muscular pain, depression) despite maintenance or even improvement in respiratory function. Patients should be encouraged to continue using the inhaler but should be carefully monitored for objective signs of adrenal insufficiency (e.g., hypotension, weight loss). If evidence of adrenal insufficiency occurs, the systemic steroid dose should be boosted temporarily and further withdrawal continued more slowly.

Monitoring of disease activity is accomplished by measuring PEFRs and keeping symptom diaries. When these interventions are properly used, they allow for early recognition of symptoms and prompt initiation or modification of therapy. Patients who experience severe and prolonged bronchospasm or other symptoms should be instructed to go to the emergency room for assistance.

Patients should be encouraged to take influenza vaccine annually and one inoculation with pneumococcal vaccine if they have chronic lung disease or other chronic conditions. Adult patients with severe persistent asthma, nasal polyps, or a history of sensitivity to aspirin or nonsteroidal anti-inflammatory drugs should be counseled regarding the risk of severe and even fatal exacerbations from using these drugs. Patients should also be encouraged to be treated for rhinitis, sinusitis, and gastroesophageal reflux, if present. Patients with asthma should all be counseled to avoid aspirin use. Routine use of chemicals to kill house-dust mites and denature the antigen is no longer recommended as a control measure.

Patients with asthma should be advised to avoid sulfite-containing and other foods to which they are sensitive (see Appendix C). The occurrence of sulfite reactions depends on the nature of the food, the level of residual sulfite, the sensitivity of the individual, and perhaps the form of residual sulfite and the mechanism of the reaction.

When bronchospasm is triggered by exercise, prophylaxis through prior inhalation of bronchodilating or antiallergy drugs is better than avoiding exercise all together, especially in children. Furthermore, the patient and family should be taught correct techniques for coughing, deep breathing, percussion, and postural drainage, when appropriate.

Evaluation

New emphasis has been placed on evaluating treatment outcomes in terms of patient perception of improvement, quality of life, and the ability to engage in activities of daily living. Effectiveness of beta agonists can be demonstrated by prevention or relief of bronchospasm and a reduction in the frequency of acute asthma attacks in patients with chronic asthma. Exercise-induced bronchospasm is prevented or reduced. Chronic asthma symptoms are relieved with corticosteroids or antiallergy drugs. Patients with asthma should strive for normal exercise tolerance, and sleep should not be interrupted by coughing or wheezing. PEFRs should be performed when symptoms appear, when there has been a change in therapy, and every 1 to 2 years thereafter. PEFRs are usually measured on wakening, and before bedtime and before and after administration of a beta agonist. That is, a minimum of twice daily and the best of three measurements on each occasion. Patients are often instructed to double the dose of inhaled corticosteroid if their PEFR is less than 75 percent of the best value, start a short course of oral corticosteroids if the PEFR is less than 50 percent of the best value, and call the health care provider if the PEFR is less than 25 percent of personal best.

Pulmonary function tests can be used to assess the effectiveness of long-term therapy. However, some patients given bronchodilators do not have a demonstrable effect on pulmonary function test results but become improved clinically. Clinical improvement is demonstrated by an increase in the distance the patient can walk, decreases in the use of as-needed drugs, and fewer reports of shortness of breath, chest tightness, and wheezing. Patients started on either oral or inhaled corticosteroids should have these drugs continued only if a positive measurable response is seen.

Thirty to fifty percent of children with chronic asthma markedly improve or become symptom free by early adulthood. Patients with less frequent attacks and normal pulmonary function test results during the initial assessment also have increased rates of remission. However, remissions are less frequent in older patients. The first drugs to discontinue in a patient with controlled asthma should be oral corticosteroids, then theophylline and ipratropium. Therapy should be continued for the duration of allergen exposure in patients with seasonal asthma.

Although the health care provider manages a wide range of asthma-related problems, when conservative methods fail to control symptoms, one must consider referral to an appropriate allergist or respiratory specialist. The FEV_1 should be assessed once to determine the reversibility of bronchoconstriction. Reversibility is indicated by an increase of 15 to 20 percent in FEV_1 after administration of a bronchodilator. Measure arterial blood gases if the patient's PEFR is less than 40 percent of predicted, the FEV_1 is less than 1.2 L, or the patient is not responding to treatment. Hospitalization should be considered for patients with an acute attack of asthma who manifest any one of the following:

- Subjective report of severe difficulty breathing
- Failure to respond fully and promptly to inhaled beta agonist therapy that was followed promptly by full doses of prednisone
- Use of accessory muscles of respiration
- A pulsus paradoxus in excess of 10 mmHg
- An FEV_1 less than 1 L/second
- Arterial pCO_2 inappropriately high for respiratory rate
- Presence of an underlying cardiac condition
- Inadequate home situation or a history of poor compliance

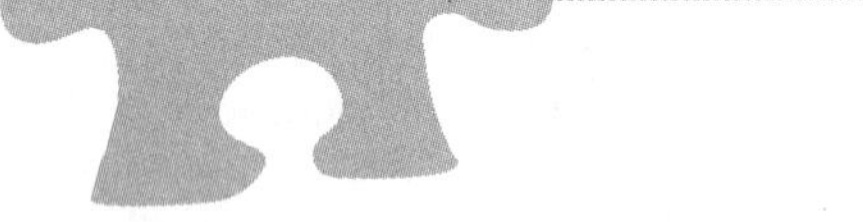

SUMMARY

- Asthma is defined as a chronic, reversible, inflammatory disorder of the airways.
- Hyperactivity of the airways to various physical, chemical, environmental, or pharmacologic stimuli is the hallmark of asthma.
- Asthma is categorized by etiology: intrinsic asthma is provoked or worsened by infection, exertion, emotion, and nonspecific environmental factors; extrinsic asthma is related to a hereditary predisposition to allergy with symptoms caused by environmental allergens.
- The severity of asthma is classified as mild intermittent, mild persistent, moderate persistent, and severe persistent.
- Inflammatory changes associated with asthma are distinguished by infiltration of mucosa and epithelium by activated T cells, mast cells, and eosinophils.
- Asthma is not a one-drug disease; thus, combination therapy is generally the rule rather than the exception.
- Drug classifications used in the management of acute and chronic asthma include beta agonists, LT antagonists, xanthine derivatives, anticholinergics, inhaled (and systemic) corticosteroids, and antiallergy drugs.
- *Guidelines for the Diagnosis and Management of Asthma* and the *International Consensus Report on Diagnosis and Treatment of Asthma* set the standards for the diagnosis and treatment of asthma.
- Short-acting beta agonists are used to relieve acute asthma symptoms. Long-acting beta agonists are used concomitantly with anti-inflammatory drugs for long-term control of symptoms, especially nocturnal symptoms.
- LT antagonists are indicated for the prophylaxis and chronic treatment of asthma in adults.
- Xanthine derivatives are mild to moderate bronchodilator drugs used principally as adjuvant to inhaled corticosteroids for the prevention of nocturnal asthma symptoms.
- Anticholinergics are used as a bronchodilator in maintenance therapy of reversible airway obstruction due to asthma.
- Inhaled corticosteroids permit chronic corticosteroid therapy without the systemic adverse effects.
- Antiallergy drugs (previously known as mast cell stabilizers) are indicated only for prophylaxis of acute asthma attacks.
- There are advantages and disadvantages to each of the drug classifications used to treat asthma. The treatment plan is individualized based on patient assessment.
- Treatment objectives include prevention of chronic, troublesome symptoms, maintaining normal pulmonary function, maintaining exercise and other physical activities, preventing recurrent exacerbations and minimizing the need for acute care interventions, providing optimal drug therapy with minimal or no adverse effects, meeting patient and family's expectations of satisfaction with asthma care.
- Peak expiratory flow rates (PEFRs) guide therapeutic decisions.
- Patients must understand the nature of their disease and how to prevent and treat its symptoms. Treatment should start with education on preventative behaviors.
- New emphasis has been placed on evaluating treatment outcomes in terms of patient perception of improvement, quality of life, and the ability to engage in activities of daily living.
- Hospitalization should be considered for patients with an acute attack of asthma that is refractory to initial treatment and in whom specific signs and symptoms exist.

BIBLIOGRAPHY

Abramowicz, M. (1996). Zafirlukast for asthma. *The Medical Letters on Drugs and Therapeutics,* 38(990), 111–112.

Adkins, J., and Brogden, R. (1998). Zafirlukast: A review of its pharmacology and therapeutic potential in the management of asthma. *Drugs,* 55(1), 121–144.

Balani, S., Xu, X., Pratha, V., et al. (1998). Metabolic profiles of montelukast sodium (Singulair), a potent cysteinyl leukotriene-1 antagonist in human plasma and bile. *Drug Metabolism and Disposition,* 25(1), 1282–1287.

Centers for Disease Control and Prevention. (1995). Asthma—United States, 1989–1992. *Mortality and Morbidity Weekly Report,* 43, 952–955.

Chanarin, J., and Johnson, S. (1994). Leukotrienes as a target in asthma therapy. *Drugs,* 47, 12–24.

Cockcroft, D. (1991). Therapy for airway inflammation in asthma. *Journal of Allergy Clinics and Immunology,* 87(5), 914–919.

Geddes, D. (1992). Inhaled corticosteroids: Benefits and risks. *Thorax,* 47, 404–407.

Harris, R., Carter, G., Bell, R., et al. (1995). Clinical activity of leukotriene inhibitors. *International Journal of Immunopharmacology,* 17(2), 147–156.

Holgate, S., Bradding, P., and Sampson, A. (1996). Leukotriene antagonists and synthesis inhibitors: New directions in asthma therapy. *The Journal of Allergy and Clinical Immunology,* 98(1), 1–13.

Imbruce, R., and Selevan, J. (1997). Pharmacoeconomics and the quality of life in the diagnosis and management of asthma—what is your FEEVY? *Journal of Care Management,* 3(3, Suppl), 1–9.

Kelloway, J. (1997). Zafirlukast: The first leukotriene-receptor antagonist approved for the treatment of asthma. *Annals of Pharmacotherapy,* 31(9), 1012–1021.

Long, D. (1997). Guidelines and realities of asthma management: The Philadelphia story. *Archives of Internal Medicine,* 157(11), 1193–1200.

Mabry, R. (1992). Corticosteroids in the management of upper respiratory allergy: The emerging role of steroid nasal sprays. *Otolaryngology: Head & Neck Surgery,* 107(6 Part 2), 855–859.

McFadden, E. R., Jr. (1994). Evolving concepts in the pathogenesis and management of asthma. *Advances in Internal Medicine,* 39, 357–394.

McFadden, E. R., Jr., and Gilbert, I. A. (1992). Asthma. *New England Journal of Medicine,* 327, 1928–1937.

National Institutes of Health. (1992). International consensus report on the diagnosis and treatment of asthma (Pub. No. 92-3091). Bethesda, MD: U.S. Department of Health and Human Services.

National Institutes of Health, National Heart, Lung, and Blood Institute. (1991). *Guidelines for the Diagnosis and Management of Asthma* (Pub. No. 91-3042). Bethesda, MD: U.S. Department of Health and Human Services.

National Institutes of Health, National Heart, Lung, and Blood Institute and World Health Organization. (1995). *Global Initiative for Asthma* (Pub. No. 95-3659). Bethesda, MD: U.S. Department of Health and Human Services.

National Institutes of Health, National Heart, Lung, and Blood Institute. (1997). *Highlights of the Expert Panel Report 2: Guidelines for the Diagnosis and Management of Asthma* (Pub. No. 97-4051A). Bethesda, MD: U.S. Department of Health and Human Services.

Spector, S. (1995). Leukotriene inhibitors and antagonists in asthma. *Annals of Allergy, Asthma, and Immunology,* 75(6 part 1), 463–474.

Sullivan S., and Weiss, K. (1993). Assessing cost-effectiveness in asthma care: Building an economic model to study the impact of alternative intervention strategies. *Allergy,* 48(17 Suppl), 146–152.

Weiss, K. (1994). The impact of pharmacologic therapy on the costs of asthma. *Allergy Proceedings,* 15(4), 189–192.

Weiss, K., Gergen, P., and Hodgson, T. (1992). An economic evaluation of asthma in the United States. *New England Journal of Medicine,* 327(8), 571–572.

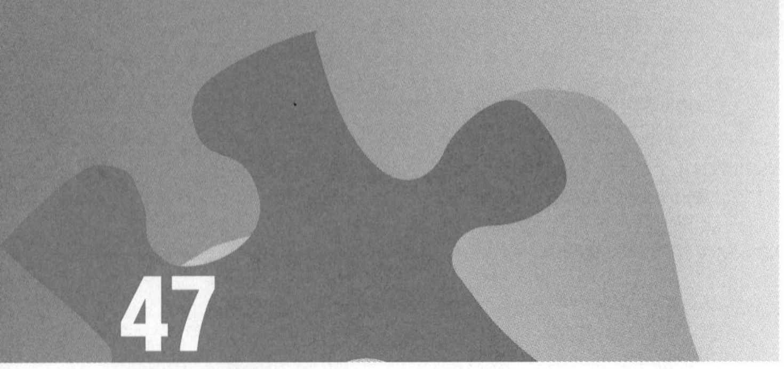

47

Antihistamines and Related Drugs

Scientific development and treatment options for allergy have exploded during the last 20 years. Health care providers are deluged with new information daily, and this new information is allowing providers to diagnose and treat allergic conditions more successfully.

ALLERGY

Epidemiology and Etiology

It is estimated that 15 to 20 percent of the North American population suffer from chronic or recurrent allergies. The allergies manifest as various types of rhinitis, urticaria, asthma, and in some cases, anaphylaxis. Asthma was discussed in Chapter 46.

There are several types of *rhinitis,* which is an acute or chronic inflammation of the mucous membranes of the nose. Rhinitis is found in 8 to 10 percent of the population younger than 20 years of age. Its etiology involves an interplay of allergens, viruses, and bacteria. *Allergic rhinitis* (i.e., hay fever) accounts for the majority of cases. It occurs most often in families with *atopy,* a hereditary predisposition for allergy. The interaction of an antigen-IgE complex on the surface of mast cells produces the symptoms associated with allergic rhinitis. Fluid rapidly moves into the tissues of the nose, causing edema of nasal mucosa. In certain individuals, antihistamines can help prevent the edematous reaction if the drug is taken before antigen exposure.

Acute episodes of allergic rhinitis tend to be seasonal, that is, symptoms disappear after a few weeks only to recur at the same time the following year. In North America, seasonal allergies are triggered by tree pollens in the spring, grasses in midsummer, and weeds in the fall, a period that typically lasts from August 15 until the first frost.

Chronic or *perennial allergic rhinitis* presents intermittently or continuously when the patient is exposed to allergens such as animal dander, wool, or certain foods. Exposure to dust mites and mold in upholstered furniture, mattresses, and pillows causes symptoms that are worse in the morning. Perennial allergic rhinitis occurs half as often as seasonal rhinitis.

Nonallergic rhinitis produces symptoms similar to those of perennial allergic rhinitis. It does not respond to allergy skin testing. *Vasomotor rhinitis* is a form of nonallergic rhinitis. It affects a substantial number of patients with chronic rhinitis with rhinorrhea. Exacerbation of symptoms results from changes in temperature and humidity, exposure to hot or cold foods, anxiety, or the ingestion of vasoactive substances in food or drinks. Many patients may simply be intolerant of the normal production of nasal mucus.

Nonallergic rhinitis with eosinophilia is an entity of chronic rhinitis and nasal eosinophilia without evidence of atopy. Nasal polyps are found more often in patients with nonallergic rhinitis with eosinophilia than in the general population, but symptoms are more difficult to treat.

Rhinitis can also develop as a result of nasal inhalation of cocaine or overuse use of topical nasal vasoconstricting sprays or drops. A rebound effect *(rhinitis medicamentosa)* occurs after several days of use, resulting in a vicious circle and more frequent use of the offending drug. Patients soon sense a dependence on the drug and characteristically have a great deal of difficulty abandoning its use.

Regardless of the cause, rhinitis results in much discomfort, absenteeism, and expense. The treatment of allergic and nonallergic rhinitis is directed toward control of symptoms. A concomitant bacterial infection, especially sinusitis, is a frequent sequelae to rhinitis.

Urticaria is a vascular reaction of the skin marked by transient appearance of wheals that are redder or paler than the surrounding skin. It is often accompanied by itching. Twenty percent of the population has experienced acute urticaria at least once, occurring without regard to genetics, age, or gender. However, at any given time, the prevalence is little more than one in 1000. Of these patients, about two-thirds have chronic urticaria. The majority of cases are acute and self-limited. Cases that persist for longer than 6 weeks are referred to as chronic urticaria. By far the most common causes of urticaria are drug reactions, stinging insect venoms, and allergenic extracts used in immunotherapy. Only persons with atopic allergy who are extremely sensitive are likely to react to ingested foods or to contact with allergens through unbroken skin. Urticaria caused by an inhaled allergen is extremely rare.

Drug allergies characterized by urticaria can develop in susceptible individuals who have shown no previous adverse response to the first dose of a drug. However, a second or subsequent exposure to even a small amount of the drug elicits an exaggerated antigen-IgE response either locally or systemically. IgE-mediated responses may occur in the skin or in the respiratory tract, causing bronchial constriction. In some patients, even limited contact with the allergen can produce fatal systemic anaphylaxis. Drugs known for producing allergic responses include aspirin, phenacetin, chloramphenicol, penicillin, streptomycin, and sulfonamides. Radiographic contrast media, polymyxin antibiotics, tubocurarine, and opiates can produce toxic-idiosyncratic reactions. Contact urticaria can be a toxic effect of formaldehyde or dimethyl sulfoxide (DMSO), a penetrating solvent used to hasten absorption of drugs through the skin. Shellfish and certain foods (e.g., strawberries) may produce the so-called urticaria of gluttony when they are eaten in large amounts. Coffee and alcohol can aggravate urticaria on a nonallergic basis.

Anaphylaxis is a life-threatening response to injected, inhaled, or ingested allergens. It can be caused by insect venoms, allergenic extracts used for immunotherapy, drugs (es-

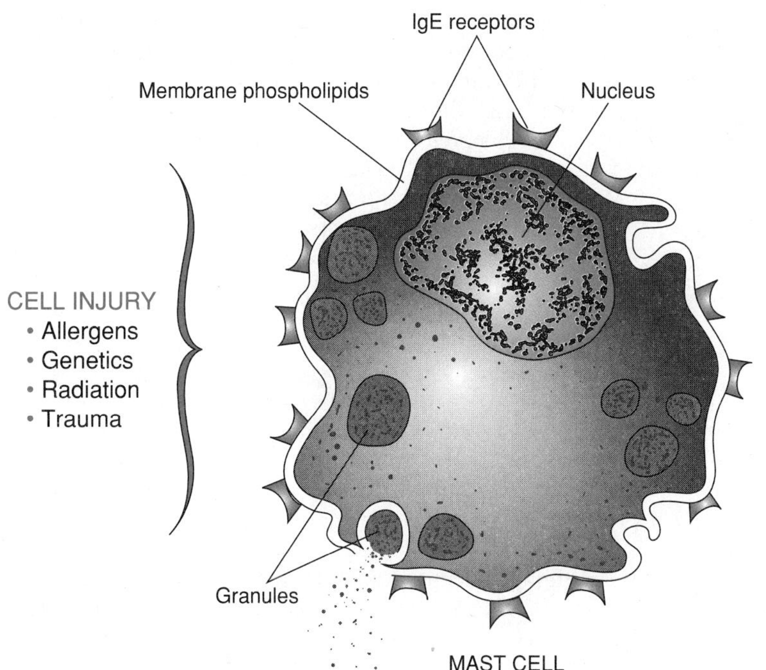

Figure 47–1 Mast cell degranulation releases chemicals that mediate the signs and symptoms of allergy. The released histamines, prostaglandins, interleukins, and leukotrienes cause local vasodilation and increased capillary permeability, hypotension, urticaria, and bronchoconstriction.

pecially injected enzymes or horse antisera, and oral or injected penicillin, contrast media), and certain foods (e.g., shellfish, nuts, legumes, eggs). In recent years, an increasing number of *anaphylactoid* reactions (those lacking evidence for allergy) have been reported that were related to exercise. Some had no identifiable cause. Any allergen that produces urticaria can produce systemic reactions if the dose, rate of administration, or reactivity of the patient is great enough. The major recognizable cause of death due to anaphylaxis is asphyxiation.

Pathophysiology

Histamine plays a central role in hypersensitivity responses. Hypersensitivity is a disorder resulting from a specific antigen-antibody reaction or a specific antigen-lymphocyte interaction. Although four different hypersensitivity responses (see Chapter 5, Table 5–2) have been identified and differ in their clinical signs and symptoms, the underlying pathophysiology is similar within each type. The reaction is initiated when the antigen-IgE complex becomes fixed to mast cells throughout the body (Fig. 47–1). There are approximately 500,000 IgE receptors on each mast cell surface. Mast cell degranulation releases chemicals that mediate the signs and symptoms of allergy and anaphylaxis. Histamine and other chemicals (i.e., prostaglandins, interleukins, and leukotrienes) that are released cause increased capillary permeability, vasodilation, hypotension, urticaria, and bronchoconstriction. Type I reactions include anaphylaxis to a bee sting, asthma, seasonal allergic rhinitis, allergies, and eczema.

Histamine binds to both H_1 and H_2 receptors. Histamine binding to H_1 receptors is responsible for increased capillary permeability, vasodilation, urticaria, bronchial constriction with wheezing and coughing, and increased gut permeability. The histamine that binds to H_2 receptors in the gut counteracts the action of H_1 receptors by decreasing overall degranulation, increasing lymphocyte activation, and decreasing neutrophil chemotaxis and enzyme release.

Direct contact with an allergen results in an antigen-IgE response with rapid release of histamine and other inflammatory mediators into body tissues. Local vasodilation is responsible for the flare, and increased capillary permeability is responsible for tissue swelling. The swellings are often referred to as hives. When the swellings are enormous, they are referred to as *angioedema*. Antihistamines taken before exposure to the antigen usually prevent urticaria.

PHARMACOTHERAPEUTIC OPTIONS

Antihistamines

Drugs used in the management of histamine-mediated disorders are synonymously referred to by several names: histamine receptor antagonists, histamine antagonists, and histamine blockers. The term antihistamine is used frequently when referring to H_1 receptor antagonists. Antihistamines were the classic first-generation drugs used for allergy.

There are six subclasses of H_1 antihistamines: ethanolamines, alkylamines, phenothiazines, piperidines, ethylenediamines, and piperazines (see First-Generation and Second-Generation Antihistamines). A second generation of H_1 antihistamines has also been developed in recent years. The second generation of H_1 drugs are actually derivatives of the piperidine subclass. In general, all subclasses of antihista-

FIRST-GENERATION AND SECOND-GENERATION ANTIHISTAMINES

First-Generation Antihistamines

Alkylamines

- Brompheniramine (BROMPHEN, DEHIST, DIAMINE, others)
- Chlorpheniramine (ALLER-CHLOR, CHLORATE, CHLOR-TRIMETON, others); (🍁) CHLORPROMANYL, LARGACTIL, NOVO-CHLORPROMAZINE
- Dexchlorpheniramine maleate (DEXCHLOR, POLADEX, POLARAMINE)
- Triprolidine hydrochloride (ACTIDIL, MYIDIL)

Ethanolamines

- Carbinoxamine maleate/pseudoephedrine
- Clemastine fumarate (TAVIST, CONTACT)
- Dimenhydrinate (DRAMAMINE, others); (🍁) APO-DIMENHYDRINATE, GRAVOL, TRAVEL TABS
- Diphenhydramine (BENADRYL, others); (🍁) ALLERDYL

Ethylenediamines

- Tripelennamine hydrochloride (PBZ, PELAMINE, TRIPELENNAMINE)

Phenothiazines

- Promethazine (PENAZINE, PHENERGAN, PHENERZINE, others); (🍁) HISTANIL

Piperazines

- Cyclizine (MAREZINE); (🍁) MARZINE
- Meclizine (ANTIVERT, BONINE)

Piperidines

- Azatadine (OPTIMINE)
- Cyproheptadine (PERIACTIN)
- Phenindamine (NOLAHIST)

Miscellaneous Antihistamine

- Hydroxyzine (VISTARIL, ATARAX)

Second-Generation Antihistamines

- Acrivastine
- Astemizole (HISMANAL)
- Azatadine (OPTIMINE)
- Azelastine (ASTELIN)
- Cetirizine (ZYRTEC; (🍁) REACTINE)
- Fexofenadine (ALLEGRA)

mines can be discussed together because for the most part they all have similar actions.

Indications

All of the H_1 antihistamines are used to treat allergic disorders. They reduce symptoms in 75 to 95 percent of patients with seasonal allergic rhinitis (hay fever). They relieve itching of the eyes, nose, and throat, and reduce rhinorrhea and sneezing. The redness, itching, and edema of acute urticaria is reduced. They are less effective in the treatment of chronic forms of urticaria.

Antihistamines can be used to treat contact dermatitis, atopic dermatitis, drug-induced skin eruptions, pruritus ani, and pruritus vulvae. Additionally, antihistamines can be used to reduce urticaria associated with mild transfusion reactions and contrast media. However, because mild allergic reactions are mediated by other substances as well as histamine, relief of symptoms may be incomplete.

Some antihistamines are used for nonallergic disorders such as motion sickness (e.g., dimenhydrinate, meclizine), nausea and vomiting (e.g., hydroxyzine, promethazine), and insomnia (e.g., diphenhydramine). The central nervous system (CNS) depressant nature of first-generation antihistamines makes these drugs useful for sedation and insomnia. Many of the over-the-counter (OTC) sleep aids contain diphenhydramine as its active ingredient. However, the dosages recommended in OTC formulations are usually too small to be effective as hypnotics.

The effectiveness of first-generation or second-generation antihistamines in treating upper respiratory infections and otitis media remains controversial. These drugs neither prevent upper respiratory infections and otitis media nor shorten the duration of symptoms. Moreover, because histamine does not mediate cold symptoms, H_1 blockade will not provide even symptomatic relief. The only benefit antihistamines have in treating upper respiratory infections is to reduce rhinorrhea.

Although antihistamines are helpful in treating urticaria and pruritus associated with anaphylaxis, they are less effective in managing the major symptoms (hypotension, bronchospasm, laryngeal edema). These symptoms are caused by chemical mediators other than histamine. Thus, antihistamines are of minimal benefit, although they can be used as adjuncts. Epinephrine (see Chapter 11) is the drug of choice for treating anaphylaxis and other serious allergic reactions.

Pharmacodynamics

H_1 antihistamines bind selectively to receptors to block the action of histamine. They do not prevent histamine release, nor do they reduce the amount of histamine released from basophils or mast cells. Some antihistamines also block the release and actions of other inflammatory mediators. Antihistamines also block the nonhistamine, muscarinic receptors of the parasympathetic nervous system. Blockade of muscarinic receptors underlies the anticholinergic adverse effects of antihistamines.

Adverse Effects and Contraindications

The adverse effects of antihistamines are often more of a nuisance than a source of serious discomfort or danger. CNS depression is characterized by slowed reaction times, diminished alertness, and drowsiness in about 20 percent of patients. Drowsiness is more common with first-generation antihistamines than with second-generation drugs. Impaired performance occurs whether or not the patient feels drowsy. Fortunately, tolerance to the sedative effect of antihistamines often develops within a few days or weeks. Second-generation antihistamines are less likely to cause CNS depression because they do not cross the blood-brain barrier. However, there are rare cases, and occasionally, the health care provider will encounter patients complaining of sedation. When the manufacturer's recommended dosages of second-generation drugs is exceeded, the likelihood of sedation increases.

In some patients (particularly children, older adults, and patients with liver disease), antihistamines can cause paradoxical excitement, nervousness, tremors, and even seizures. Impaired cognitive function, confusion, dizziness, and tinnitus have also occurred in older adults. Toxic encephalopathy has been reported after topical application of an H_1 drug such as diphenhydramine. Patients with skin breakdown are particularly susceptible because the drugs are better absorbed through skin surfaces that are not intact.

Adverse effects of H_1 antihistamines on the GI tract are common. The adverse effects include anorexia, nausea, vomiting, and diarrhea or constipation. In addition, many patients complain about the anticholinergic effects because first-generation antihistamines possess weak atropine-like properties. Cholinergic blockade results in dry mouth, nasal passages, and throat. Urinary hesitancy and palpitations have been noted. Second-generation antihistamines are least likely to produce anticholinergic adverse effects.

Adverse cardiovascular effects, including tachycardia, arrhythmias, and occasionally myocardial depression refractory to vasopressor support, have been reported with second-generation antihistamines. This is particularly true with astemizole. The arrhythmias usually occur with excessive dosages but have been reported with concurrent use of macrolide antibiotics (i.e., erythromycin, clarithromycin), imidazole antifungals (i.e., itraconazole, ketoconazole), and other drugs that inhibit the cytochrome P_{450} system. Patients with severe hepatic disease are also at risk for arrhythmias. Accordingly, these drugs are contraindicated for patients with liver disease or those who may be receiving macrolide antibiotics or imidazole antifungal drugs. In some cases, syncope preceded the development of arrhythmias.

Contraindications to the use of antihistamines include hypersensitivity, narrow-angle glaucoma, prostatic hypertrophy, stenosing peptic ulcers, bladder neck obstruction, and pregnancy. Safe use during pregnancy has not been established, although some formulations have been moved from pregnancy category C to category B in recent years. Piperazine antihistamines are teratogenic.

Pharmacokinetics

Antihistamines are generally well absorbed following oral administration. The onset of drug effects occurs within 15 to

TABLE 47–1 PHARMACOKINETICS OF SELECTED ANTIHISTAMINES AND RELATED DRUGS

Drug	Route	Onset	Peak	Duration	PB (%)	$t_{1/2}$
First-Generation Antihistamines						
Brompheniramine	po	15–30 min	1–2 hr	6–8 hr; 8–12 hr	UA	12–35 hr
Carbinoxamine/ pseudoephedrine	po	15–30 min	UA	6 hr	UA	10–20 hr
Chlorpheniramine	po	15–30 min	6 hr	4–12 hr; 8–24 hr	72	14–25 hr
Clemastine	po	15–60 min	1–2 hr	12 hr	UA	UK
Cyproheptadine	po	15–60 min	1–2 hr	8 hr	UA	UK
Dexchlorpheniramine	po	15–30 min	3 hr	3–6 hr	UA	12–15 hr
Diphenhydramine	po	15–60 min	1–4 hr	4–8 hr	98–99	2.4–7 hr
Hydroxyzine	po/IM	15–30 min	2–4 hr	4–6 hr	UA	3 hr
Promethazine	po/IM	15–30 min	UK	4–25 hr	65–90	10–14 hr
Tripelennamine	po	15–30 min	1–2 hr	4–6 hr	UA	UK
Triprolidine	po	15–60 min	1–2 hr	6–8 hr	UA	5 hr
Second-Generation Antihistamines						
Astemizole	po	1–3 days	9–12 hr	Weeks	96	100 hr; 12–19 days*
Azatadine	po	15–60 min	4 hr	12 hr	UA	9–12 hr
Azelastine	NS/po	UA	2–3 hr	UA	88; 97†	22 hr; 54 hr‡
Cetirizine	po	1–3 hr	1 hr	UA	UA	6.6–10.6; 7.0; 4.9§
Fexofenadine	po	Rapid	2.6 hr	UA	60–70	14.4 hr
Loratadine	po	1–3 hr	8–12 hr	> 24 hr	97; 73–77	8–11 hr; 20 hr‖
Corticosteroids						
Beclomethasone	INH/NS	UK	Up to 4 wks	UK	NA	15hr
Budesonide	NS	24 hr	3–7 days			2 hr
Dexamethasone	NS	Few days	UK			190 min
	INH	UK	Up to 4 wks			
Flunisolide	INH/NS	Few days	Up to 3 wks			1–2 hr
Fluticasone	NS	Few days	UK			UA
Triamcinolone	INH/NS	UK	Up to 4 wks			4 hr
Antiallergy Drugs						
Cromolyn	po	15 min	2–4 wks	4–6 hr	NA	80 min
	INH	15 min	2–4 wks			
	NS	<1 week	2–4 wks			
Lodoxamide	OPTH	1 week	UK			8.5 hr in urine
Nedocromil	INH	2 weeks	20–40 min	4–6 hr	89	1.5–2.3 hr

*Astemizole's half-life is 100 hours. The half-life of its metabolite desmethylastemizole is 12 to 19 days.

†Azelastine's plasma protein binding for the drug and its metabolite desmethylazelastine, respectively.

‡Azelastine's half-life for nasal sprays and oral formulations, respectively.

§Cetirizine's half-life for adults, school-age children, and children younger than 4 years of age, respectively.

‖Loratadine's half-life is 7.8 to 11 hours, with 97-percent protein binding; descarboethoxyloratadine, the metabolite, has a half-life of 20 hours, with 73- to 77-percent protein binding.

PB, Protein binding; $t_{1/2}$, elimination half-life; NA, not applicable; UA, unavailable; UK, unknown; NS, nasal spray; OPTH, ophthalmic; INH, inhalation.

60 minutes, with drug action lasting 4 to 6 hours (Table 47–1). Drug effects of enteric-coated or sustained-release formulations last 8 to 12 hours; however, the longer acting drugs may be less effective owing to inadequate dissolution and absorption. All first-generation antihistamines and most of the second-generation antihistamines are biotransformed by the hepatic enzyme system. They are eliminated through the urine and stool.

The half-lives and clearance rates of antihistamines are extremely variable. Children experience shorter drug elimination half-lives than that of adults. Half-life values generally increase with increasing age and in the presence of severe hepatic dysfunction.

Compared with other antihistamines, cetirizine has unique pharmacokinetic properties. Biotransformation by the hepatic enzyme system is minimal. Sixty percent of a single dose appears as unchanged drug in the urine within 24 hours. Cetirizine has a mean elimination half-life of 6.6 to 10.6 hours in adults, 7 hours in school-age children, and 4.9 hours in children younger than 4 years of age.

Drug-Drug Interactions

First-generation antihistamines enhance the adverse effects of ethanol, diazepam, and other CNS active drugs (Table 47–2). In recommended dosages, second-generation antihistamines do not potentiate CNS effects.

Dosage Regimen

Table 47–3 includes dosage regimens for selected first-generation and second-generation antihistamines. The manufacturers' dosage recommendations should be followed carefully because of the potential for misuse and overdose. The dosages for drugs used in motion sickness, nausea and vomiting are identified in Chapter 44.

Laboratory Considerations

Antihistamines can produce false-negative results in allergy skin testing; thus, they should be discontinued 72 to 96 hours before testing. Serum amylase and prolactin concentrations increase with the concurrent use of cyproheptadine and thyrotropin-releasing hormone. Promethazine can cause false-positive or false-negative pregnancy tests.

Corticosteroids

Topical corticosteroids are used in a variety of inflammatory and allergic conditions. Inhaled corticosteroids are

TABLE 47–2 DRUG-DRUG INTERACTIONS OF SELECTED ANTIHISTAMINES AND RELATED DRUGS

Drug	Interactive Drugs	Interaction
First-Generation Antihistamines		
Alkylamines Ethanolamines Ethylenediamines Phenothiazines Piperazines	Alcohol Antianxiety drugs Antipsychotic drugs Opioid analgesics Sedative-hypnotics	Additive CNS depression
	MAO inhibitors Tricyclic antidepressants	Increased duration of action of antihistamine; increased anticholinergic adverse effects
	Atropine Disopyramide Haloperidol Phenothiazines Quinidine Scopolamine	Increased anticholinergic activity and effects
Second-Generation Antihistamines		
Astemizole Fexofenadine Loratadine*	Cimetadine Clarithromycin Erythromycin Itraconazole Ketoconazole Troleandomycin	Potentially lethal arrhythmias
Azatadine	Heparin Warfarin	Decreased effect of interacting agent
	MAO inhibitors	Increased effects of azatadine
	Alcohol Barbiturates Opioids Sedative-hypnotics Tricyclic antidepressants	Increased CNS depression with higher than recommended dosages

*Although life-threatening arrhythmias have not been reported with loratadine, or the newer macrolide antibiotics, the drugs are similar and may interact in a similar manner.

CNS, Central nervous system; MAO, monoamine.

TABLE 47–3 DOSAGE REGIMEN FOR SELECTED ANTIHISTAMINES AND RELATED DRUGS

Drug	Uses	Dosage	Implications
First-Generation Antihistamines			
Brompheniramine	Nasal allergies; allergic dermatoses; adjunct in anaphylaxis; transfusion reactions	*Adults:* 4–8 mg po TID–QID *or* 8–12 mg BID of SR formulation *or* 10 mg SC/IM/IV q6–12 hr. Maximum dose: 40 mg *Child 6–12 yr:* one-half of the adult dose po *or* 0.5 mg/kg/day *or* 15 mg/m^2/day SC/IM/IV divided doses *Child younger than 6 yr:* 0.5 mg/kg/day po *or* 15 mg/m^2/day in divided doses	Administer oral doses with food or milk to decrease GI irritation. Extended-release tablets should be swallowed whole—do not crush, break, or chew
Carbinoxamine/ pseudoephedrine	Perennial and seasonal allergic rhinitis; vasomotor rhinitis; allergic conjunctivitis; common cold; allergic and nonallergic pruritus symptoms, urticaria and angioedema	*Adults:* 4–8 mg po TID–QID *Child:* 0.2–0.4 mg/kg/day	Available in combination with pseudoephedrine with or without dextromethorphan
Chlorpheniramine	Nasal allergies; allergic dermatoses; adjunct in anaphylaxis; transfusion reactions	*Adults:* 2–4 mg po TID–QID *or* 8–12 mg po QD–TID of SR formulation *or* 5–40 mg SC/IM/IV *Child 6–12 yr:* 0.35 mg/kg/day po/SC in 4 divided doses *Child older than 7 yr:* 8 mg po q12hr of SR formulation. Not recommended for children under 6 years	Administer oral doses with food or milk to decrease GI irritation. Extended-release tablets should be swallowed whole—do not crush, break, or chew
Clemastine	Perennial and seasonal allergic rhinitis; urticaria	*Adults:* 1.34–2.68 mg po BID–TID. Not to exceed 8.04 mg	Monitor for thrombocytopenia, agranulocytosis, hemolytic anemia
Cyproheptadine	Nasal allergies; allergic dermatoses; cold urticaria; appetite stimulant (unlabeled use)	*Adults:* 4 mg po q8hr. Range 4–20 mg/day in three divided doses Maximum dose: 32 mg/day *Child 6–14 yr:* 2–4 mg po q8–12 hr. Not to exceed 16 mg/day *Child 2–6 yr:* 2 mg po q8–12 hr. Not to exceed 12 mg/day	Administer with food or water to minimize GI irritation
Dexchlorpheniramine	Nasal allergies; uncomplicated urticaria; transfusion reactions; dermatographism; adjunct in anaphylaxis	*Adult and Child >12 yr:* 2 mg po q4–6 hr, *or* 4–6 mg po SR formulation at HS or q8–10 hr during the day *Child age 6–11 yr:* 1 mg po q4–6 hr *or* 4 mg sustained release formulation at HS *Child age 2–5 yr:* 0.5 mg po q4–6 hr	Do not use sustained-release formulations in children younger than 6 years of age
Diphenhydramine	Nasal allergies; allergic dermatoses	*Adults:* 25–50 mg po q4–6 hr *or* 10–50 mg IM/IV q2–3 hr PRN. (May need up to 100 mg dose, not to exceed 400 mg/day) *Adults and Child older than 12 yr:* 2% cream, gel, or stick TID–QID *Child more than 9.1 kg:* 12.5–25 mg po q4–6 hr PRN *Child weighing less than 9.1 kg:* 6.25–12.5 mg po q4–6 hr PRN *Child age 6–12 yr:* 1% cream, gel, or spray TID–QID	Use topical formulation with caution due to increased systemic absorption through abraded skin
Hydroxyzine	Pruritus	*Adults:* 25–100 mg po TID–QID. *Child:* 0.5 mg/kg po (15 mg/m^2) q6hr *Child 6–12 yr:* 12.5–25 mg po q6hr PRN *Child younger than 6 yr:* 12.5 mg po q6hr PRN	Tablets may be crushed and capsules opened and administered with food for patients who have difficulty swallowing
Promethazine	Allergic conditions	*Adults:* 25 mg po HS *or* 10–12.5 mg QID *or* 25 mg IM/IV/SUPP and may repeat in 2 hr *Child older than 2 yr:* 0.5 mg/kg po HS *or* 5–12.5 mg po TID *or* 0.125 mg/kg (3.75 mg/m^2) po q4–6 hr *or* 0.5 mg SUPP (15 mg/m^2) at HS *or* 0.125 mg/kg (3.75 mg/m^2) SUPP q4–6 hr *or* 6.25–12.5 mg SUPP TID *or* 25 mg SUPP at HS	Assess allergy symptoms before and periodically throughout the course of therapy. Tablets may be crushed and mixed with food or fluids for patients with difficulty swallowing

Table continued on following page

TABLE 47–3 DOSAGE REGIMEN FOR SELECTED ANTIHISTAMINES AND RELATED DRUGS *Continued*

Drug	Uses	Dosage	Implications
First-Generation Antihistamines *Continued*			
Tripelennamine		*Adults:* 25–50 mg po q4–6 hr up to 600 mg/day. *or* 100 mg po SR formulation q12 hr, 100 mg po q8hr may be needed *Child:* 5 mg/kg po per day *or* 150 mg/m²/day in four to six doses. Not to exceed 300 mg/day	Do not use sustained-release formulations with children. Do not crush or chew sustained-release formulations
Triprolidine		*Adults and Child > 12 yr:* 2.5 mg po q4–6 hr. Do not exceed four doses/24 hr *Child age 6–12 yr:* 1.25 mg po q4–6 hr. Do not exceed four doses/24 hr	Do not crush or chew sustained-release formulations
Second-Generation Antihistamines			
Acrivastine	Cold symptoms	*Adults:* 1 capsule q4–6 hr PRN	Combined with ephedrine, a decongestant
Azatadine	Allergy symptoms, rhinitis, chronic urticaria	*Adults:* 1–2 mg po BID. Not to exceed 4 mg/day	Not recommended for use in children
Azelastine	Seasonal allergic rhinitis	*Adults and Child older than 12 yr:* 2 sprays in each nostril BID	Reprime the pump unit and delivery system with 2 sprays or until a fine mist appears if more than 3 days have elapsed since the last use
Aztemizole	Allergic rhinitis, urticaria	*Adults and Child older than 12 yr:* 10 mg po once daily *Child 6–12 yr:* 5 mg po once daily (unlabeled) *Child < 6 yr:* 2 mg/10 kg once daily (unlabeled)	Instruct patient to take drug at least 1 hour before or 2 hours after meals since food decreases drug absorption
Cetirizine	Allergic rhinitis, chronic urticaria	*Adults:* 10 mg po once daily	Arrange for use of humidifier if thickening of secretions, nasal dryness become bothersome
Fexofenadine	Seasonal allergic rhinitis	*Adults and Child older than 12 yr:* 60 mg po BID.	Once-daily dosing is recommended for patients with impaired renal function
Loratadine	Seasonal allergic rhinitis	*Adults and Child older than 12 yrs:* 10 mg po once daily	Avoid use of alcohol, serious sedation can occur. Take on an empty stomach
Corticosteroids			
Beclomethasone	Chronic, steroid-dependent asthma; allergic rhinitis, chronic nasal inflammatory conditions	*Adults and Child older than 12 yr:* One oral INH BID–QID. Maximum dose: 168–336 mcg/day *or* one nasal spray in each nostril BID–QID daily *Child 6–12 yr:* One oral INH TID–QID. Maximum dose: 10 INH/day	Formulation: 42–50 mcg/metered spray. (200 metered sprays/16.8 g canister)
Budesonide		*Adults:* 2 sprays in each nostril BID *or* 4 sprays QD each morning	Formulation: 32 mcg/metered spray. (200 metered sprays/7 g canister)
Dexamethasone		*Adults:* 3 INH TID–QID. Maximum dose: 12 INH daily *Adults and Child older than 12 yr:* 2 sprays in each nostril BID–TID. Not to exceed 12 sprays daily *Child 6–12 yr:* 2 INH TID–QID *or* 1–2 sprays in each nostril BID. Maximum dose: 8 INH or sprays daily	Formulation: 84 mcg/metered spray. (170 metered sprays/ 12.6 g canister). Continued use past 30 days is inappropriate
Flunisolide		*Adults:* 2 INH BID. Not to exceed 8 INH *or* 2 sprays in each nostril BID–TID Maximum dose: 16 sprays daily *Child 6–14 yr:* 1 spray in each nostril BID. Not to exceed 8 sprays/day *Child younger than 6 yr:* Not recommended	Formulation: 250 mcg/metered spray (100 metered sprays/7 g canisters); 25 mcg/solution spray (200 metered sprays/25 mL bottle)
Fluticasone		*Adults:* 2 sprays in each nostril QD *or* one spray in each nostril BID after several days. Decrease to one spray in each nostril once daily. Not to exceed 4 metered sprays/day *Child older than 12 yr:* 1–2 sprays each nostril QD initially. Not to exceed 4 sprays/day	Formulation: 50 mcg/metered spray (120 metered sprays/9 g bottle)

TABLE 47–3 DOSAGE REGIMEN FOR SELECTED ANTIHISTAMINES AND RELATED DRUGS *Continued*

Drug	Uses	Dosage	Implications
Corticosteroids *Continued*			
Triamcinolone		*Adults and Child older than 12 yr:* 3 sprays TID–QID. May be given in divided doses. Not to exceed 16 sprays/day *Child 6–12 yr:* 1–2 sprays TID–QID. May be given in two divided doses. Maximum dose: 12 sprays/day	Formulation: 100 mcg/metered aerosol spray. (240 metered sprays/20 g canister); 55 mcg metered/nasal spray. (100 metered sprays/15 g canister)
Antiallergy Drugs			
Cromolyn	Prophylaxis acute asthma attack in patients with chronic asthma including allergic and exercise-induced forms	*Adults and Child older than 5 yr:* 20 mg inhaler capsule or nebulizer solution *or* 2 sprays as inhaled aerosol QID. For prophylaxis bronchospasm: 2 aerosol sprays 10–15 minutes before exposure *or* 1 spray in each nostril TID–QID up to six times daily	Formulation: 20 mg/20 mL solution; 800 mcg/aerosol spray (112 sprays/8.1 g or 200 sprays/14.2 g containers); 5.2 mg/spray (100 sprays/13 mL or 200 sprays /26 mL)
Lodoxamide		*Adults and Child older than 2 yr:* 1–2 drops in affected eye or eyes four times daily for up to 3 months	Formulation: 0.1% in 10-mL solution
Nedocromil		*Adults and Child older than 12 yr:* 2 INH QID	Formulation: 1.75 mg/spray (112 INH/16.2 g canister)

SUPP, Suppository; INH, inhalation

used in the management of reversible airway disease (see Chapter 46). Intranasal and ophthalmic corticosteroids are used in the management of allergic rhinitis and conjunctivitis (e.g., beclomethasone, budesonide, dexamethasone, flunisolide, fluticasone, and triamcinolone). Corticosteroids control symptoms; they do not cure the underlying disorder. Dermal formulations of corticosteroids have been used to treat contact dermatitis, insect stings, and some drug-induced allergies (see Chaper 64). However, because drug action and patient response does not occur immediately, these drugs are of little value in acute therapy. For mild allergic disease, inhaled, intranasal, and ophthalmic corticosteroid formulations are usually adequate. Systemic corticosteroids are reserved for severe urticaria and angioedema.

The benefit of corticosteroid use in allergic disorders stems from the ability of the drug to suppress immune response and inflammation. Corticosteroids interrupt inflammation by inhibiting the synthesis of chemical mediators (i.e., histamine, leukotrienes, and prostaglandins). Redness, warmth, edema, and discomfort are reduced. Phagocytic infiltration is suppressed, and damage from lysosomal enzyme release is averted. Furthermore, corticosteroids suppress lymphocyte proliferation to lessen the immune component of inflammation. Corticosteroids as a primary drug category are discussed further in Chapter 52.

The most common dosage of corticosteroid nasal sprays is one to two sprays in each nostril two to three times daily. The maximal daily dose should not exceed four sprays per nostril. Inhaled dosages of corticosteroids range from one to two inhalations once to four times daily (depending on the specific drug). Most of the nasal sprays and inhalation formulations are available in canisters containing 120 to 240 metered sprays.

Antiallergy Drugs

Antiallergy drugs (e.g., cromolyn, nedocromil) were originally discussed in Chapter 46 as management options for asthma. However, they are also effective in preventing seasonal and perennial allergic rhinitis, allergic conjunctivitis (although not approved by the Food and Drug Administration for such use at this time), prevention of food allergy, and prevention of acute bronchospasm.

Antiallergy drugs stabilize cell membranes; thus, histamine and the slow-reacting substance of anaphylaxis (SRS-A) from sensitized mast cells are not released. It also alters the migration of eosinophils to the inflammatory site and decreases the number of end products of inflammation. Drug action is localized.

Minimal oral absorption of the antiallergy drugs takes place following all routes of administration. Small amounts of drug may reach the circulation after inhalation, even less from other routes. Distribution of these drugs is unknown. The small amounts of drug that are absorbed are eliminated unchanged in urine and feces. Nedocromil sodium is chemically unrelated to cromolyn sodium but has similar mechanism of action and pharmacokinetic characteristics. It is effective in the management of seasonal and perennial allergic rhinitis and exercise-induced asthma but is not useful in relieving acute asthma attacks. Like cromolyn and lodoxamide, the best outcomes result from prophylactic use.

Antiallergy drugs are generally the safest drugs available for the treatment of allergy. Significant adverse effects occur in fewer than one patient of every 10,000. The most common adverse effects associated with nasal sprays include nasal stinging and congestion, throat irritation, unpleasant bitter taste, and cough. Burning eyes have been reported with ophthalmic formulations. Hoarseness has been noted with inhaled formulations.

Critical Thinking Process

Assessment

History of Present Illness

Patient history is the most important component in the evaluation of a patient with a suspected or confirmed allergy. Determine the frequency and severity of attacks, precipitating or alleviating factors, drugs used, and whether they are taken regularly or intermittently. Elicit allergies and the patient's status between attacks and any restrictions in the activities of daily living.

Patients with seasonal allergic rhinitis experience sneezing, nasal or ocular pruritus, bilateral clear watery or mucoid nasal secretions, and nasal congestion. Patients may also complain of pruritus of the upper palate and ears, and dry, scratchy, and erythematous conjunctiva. These symptoms are related to elevations of specific pollen counts. Symptoms of dust and mold allergies are less distinct because nasal congestion and clear drainage frequently occur without sneezing or pruritus. The response to mold allergies vary significantly throughout the year.

A careful search of environmental factors should be conducted. The patient should be questioned in detail about the home environment including its location, type of heating, type and quality of construction, type of insulation, and humidity. The nature of furnishings (upholstered furniture), presence of plants, draperies and bedding, pets and their habits, housecleaning methods, and cigarette smoking should also be noted. Variations in symptoms with changes in seasons and with changes in location should be carefully recorded. Ask also about the work environment and note exposure to chemical irritants or sensitizers, physical demands, and job stressors. Information about the type of clothing worn and dietary history should not be overlooked. Clothing and food are potential antigens, particularly in children. Smokers have increased symptoms of nasal congestion and thick postnasal drainage, and may be predisposed to sinusitis.

A history of pruritic wheals lasting several hours is typical of urticaria. A history of a swollen tongue or lips and epigastric discomfort may indicate GI involvement. The presence of wheezing or pharyngeal swelling suggests an anaphylactoid reaction.

It is important to record the patient's drug history, especially any prescription or OTC drug used to treat present or past symptoms. Information regarding the use of inhaled cocaine or nasal decongestants should be carefully noted. These drugs have been associated with allergy as well as rhinitis medicamentosa.

Past Health History

When interviewing the patient, the health care provider should take time to identify previous allergic problems the patient has had and any allergies in close family members. This information is particularly helpful in providing support for the diagnosis of an atopic disease. The onset of symptoms in childhood is typical of allergic disease. The onset of symptoms during adulthood, however, does not rule out atopy.

Physical Exam Findings

Examine the conjunctiva for erythema and the eyes for tearing and photophobia. Edema of the lids provides supportive evidence of an allergic mechanism. Transillumination and palpation of the sinuses, a pharyngeal exam for erythema and discharge, the ears for evidence of otitis, and palpitation of cervical nodes for adenopathy is included in the exam.

The nose is often overlooked or is given only a cursory examination. Nasal mucosa should be inspected for evidence of erythema, pallor, atrophy, edema, crusting, and discharge. The presence of polyps (not to be confused with the turbinates), erosions, and septal perforations or deviations should be noted. A pale, boggy appearance to the mucosa is allegedly a classic sign of allergic disease, but erythema sometimes occurs in allergy, and its presence certainly does not rule out sinusitis. Sinusitis may be present at the time of the exam. Mucopurulent discharge from the nares or seen in the posterior pharynx raises the possibility of sinusitis. Tenderness of the maxillary, ethmoid, or frontal sinus regions on palpation helps support a diagnosis of sinusitis.

A general respiratory exam includes assessment of the rate and character of respirations and skin color. The lungs should be examined during forced expiration, which may bring out asthmatic wheezing. Abnormal breathing patterns (e.g., rate below 12 or above 24, dyspnea, cough, orthopnea, wheezing, stridor) indicate respiratory distress. Severe respiratory distress is characterized by tachypnea, dyspnea, use of accessory muscles, and hypoxia. Early signs of hypoxia include restlessness, confusion, anxiety, increased blood pressure, and pulse. Late signs include cyanosis and decreased blood pressure and pulse. Hypoxemia is confirmed when arterial blood gas analyses demonstrate decreased partial pressure of oxygen (PaO_2).

A description and location of any skin lesions should be recorded. Urticarial lesions range in size from 0.5-cm papules to 20-cm plaques. The lesions can be circular, annular, or serpiginous in shape. Central clearing is common, and any area of the body can be involved. Urticarial lesions, if present, should be outlined in ink to aid in determining whether they are evanescent or persistent.

Diagnostic Testing

Few general laboratory tests are appropriate for the patient with an allergic disorder. A nasal or sputum smear may be examined for the presence of eosinophils. Blood eosinophilia is helpful if it is present, but its absence does not exclude allergic disease. The measurement of total serum IgE is costly and generally of limited value. In some cases, laboratory testing may include arterial blood gases, pulse oximetry, and pulmonary function testing.

Allergy testing can be helpful in patients who have significant symptoms. RAST (radioallergosorbent test) is a serum test that determines the amount of IgG immunoglobulin present against a specific allergen or allergen group. Prick or scratch testing measures clinical response to inoculation with various allergens mediated by the release of histamine and other chemicals. Intradermal testing is more sensitive but poses a higher risk of anaphylaxis. It is performed when the results of prick testing are negative or not diagnostic.

Skin testing should be selective based on clues provided by the patient's history whenever possible. In adults, testing is limited to pollens, house dust, feathers, animal danders, and mold spores. If the patient's history warrants it, skin tests to some foods may also be performed. Food testing is more useful in young children than in adults.

Developmental Considerations

Perinatal A number of changes take place in the respiratory tract during pregnancy. The changes are mediated by the enlarging uterus, increased oxygen demands, and the respiratory stimulant effect of progesterone. There is also an estrogen-induced hyperemia of the nasopharynx mucosa with concurrent edema and increased production of mucus. These changes lead to a feeling of stuffiness and an increased tendency for epistaxis. Pregnant women should be warned of this normal change and advised against using OTC nasal sprays hoping to alleviate the symptoms. However, normal saline nasal spray may be helpful in reducing some of the discomfort.

Pediatric Assessment of symptoms in the child is much like that in the adult but also includes a feeding history for a very young child, with attention to the intake of cow's milk, eggs, and wheat. The stability of family relationships and the stress level in the home should not be overlooked. Information about the child's toys, bedroom, and other rooms where the child spends waking hours should be noted. The child's exposure level to babysitters, relatives, day care, and school environments is included. The presence or absence of symptoms in all areas should be noted. The source of present and past health information (often the parents) is important. Valid recall of times and events associated with symptoms is critical in providing clues to the antigen and to establish or confirm a diagnosis. A child with atopy may have dark circles under the eyes (allergic shiners) and have a transverse crease above the tip of the nose from frequent upward nose rubbing (allergic salute).

Geriatric It is difficult to determine whether losses in somesthetic sensitivity can be attributed to changes of aging itself or to disease states that occur with greater frequency in older age. Local sinus and respiratory tract factors and comorbid diseases probably play a larger role in the allergic response than age-related changes in immunity. Clinically, older adults are more susceptible to respiratory tract and other infections, and are also likely to purchase OTC agents for self-treatment. Antihistamines such as diphenhydramine may cause dizziness, sedation, syncope, confusion, paradoxical CNS stimulation, and hypotension in older adults. Older men who have prostatic hypertrophy may have difficulty voiding while taking antihistamines because they tend to cause spasm of the urethra.

Psychosocial Considerations

Many of the drugs used in the treatment of allergies and asthma are purchased OTC by consumers. They are easily accessible to almost all persons, easy to use, and in many cases generally effective. By using OTC drugs to treat allergies, patients save a trip to the health care provider and the associated costs of a visit (see Case Study—Seasonal Rhinitis).

Analysis and Management

Treatment Objectives

Treatment objectives for the patient with an allergy primarily centers around relief of symptoms. Minimizing exposure to external trigger factors and ensuring compliance with treatment plans are also important objectives.

Treatment Options

Drug Variables

Treatment for hypersensitivity reactions involves drug management with a variety of agents, each acting on a different aspect of the response. Drug groups that can be used include antihistamines, beta agonists, and antiallergy drugs. In some cases, anticholinergics and corticosteroids may be required. Antihistamines (e.g., diphenhydramine) moderate the effects of histamine. This action reduces capillary permeability and bronchoconstriction. Beta agonists (e.g., albuterol, metaproterenol) decrease bronchoconstriction and bronchospasm. Antiallergy drugs (e.g., cromolyn) stabilize mast cell membranes. Corticosteroids (e.g., beclomethasone, prednisone) decrease inflammation. Anticholinergics block the parasympathetic response and indirectly create bronchodilation. Most of the drugs in these categories provide only symptomatic relief. No one drug is likely to abolish symptoms completely.

The choice of antihistamine depends on the goal of treatment, desired outcomes, the drug's duration of action, and adverse effects. In general, drugs are more effective for allergic rather than nonallergic forms of rhinitis, and acute allergies usually respond more favorably than chronic allergies. Long-acting formulations provide consistent symptom relief for patients with chronic allergic symptoms. A rapid-acting drug is preferred for patients with an acute reaction.

First-generation antihistamines are effective in relieving nasopharyngeal itching, sneezing, water rhinorrhea, and ocular manifestations of allergy such as itching, tearing, and erythema. However, they are not as effective for nasal congestion. Furthermore, they are sedating to various degrees and their anticholinergic effects include visual disturbances, urinary retention, and even arrhythmias in some patients.

Alkylamines (e.g., brompheniramine, chlorpheniramine) are useful in comparably low dosages and are suitable for daytime use; however, individual responses to these drugs vary and drowsiness or stimulation can result. Ethanolamines (e.g., clemastine, dimenhydrinate, diphenhydramine) are strong CNS depressants, producing a high incidence of drowsiness. In contrast, ethylenediamines (e.g., tripelennamine hydrochloride) are weak CNS depressants and therefore are less likely to cause drowsiness. However, they often cause GI distress. Piperazines (e.g., buclizine, meclizine) provide prolonged antihistaminic activity with a relatively low incidence of drowsiness. Regardless, attentiveness is decreased and operation of machinery may be unsafe. Table 47–4 provides a comparison of the various antihistamines in terms of symptom relief.

Long-term use of first-generation antihistamines has been associated with a decrease in drug efficacy in some patients. This phenomenon has been ascribed to autoinduction of hepatic biotransformation and increased clearance of the drug with successive lower serum and presumably lower tissue concentrations of the drug.

Second-generation antihistamines are more lipophobic and highly protein bound than their predecessors. They are less likely to cross the blood-brain barrier, and their sedating and anticholinergic adverse effects are minimized. Also, second-generation drugs have dose-related bronchodilating effects and provide protection against bronchospasm caused by histamine, allergens, exercise, hyperventilation, and cold, dry air.

Case Study Seasonal Rhinitis with Secondary Sinusitis

Patient History

History of Present Illness	AR is a 54-year-old female who presents to the outpatient clinic with complaints of headache, nasal congestion and sneezing, bilateral eye pain, sore throat, and a dry cough. With each episode, she stopped taking her medicine because she started to feel better, hoping to save the remaining medicine in the event she was ill in the future. Bending forward to tie her shoes makes the frontal pain more intense. She tried self-treatment with saline gargles that "helped a little," aspirin for headache, and using cold compresses over her forehead for the discomfort. She reports using previously prescribed cromolyn sodium but without much relief.
Past Health History	AR has a family history of atopy, with two sisters and a brother who have hay fever. All three have asthma of varying severity. AR denies a history of asthma or other respiratory disorders, hypertension, heart disease, or difficulty urinating. Except for hay fever she is otherwise healthy. Denies use of prescription or OTC drugs, food or drug allergy.
Physical Exam	BP 124/72. Temp: 99.4°F, pulse 76, respirations 20. TMs clean. Nasal mucosa is erythematous and edematous, with crusting, and mucopurulent discharge. Palpable sinus tenderness over frontal, ethmoid, and maxillary sinuses. Oropharynx without redness but mucopurulent, stringy drainage is noted in posterior pharynx. Breath sounds clear to auscultation bilaterally.
Diagnostic Testing	No diagnostic testing indicated for AR at this time.
Developmental Considerations	AR is a 3rd grade elementary schoolteacher.
Psychosocial Considerations	AR is a single parent with four teenage sons at home. Acknowledges that she is on a very tight budget.
Economic Factors	AR has limited resources. Is requesting to use OTC treatment regimen, if possible. Has health insurance but no pharmacy coverage.

Variables Influencing Decision

Treatment Objectives	• Promote compliance with treatment regimen and provide relief of symptoms • Promote clearing of sinus infection

Drug Variables	*Drug Summary*	*Patient Variables*
Indications	First-generation antihistamines: remain first-line drugs for treatment of allergic symptoms. Decongestants: appropriate for short-term use in nasal congestion. Antiallergy drug: appropriate for prophylaxis of allergic symptoms. Antibiotics: appropriate because sinusitis is present	AR diagnosed with seasonal rhinitis and sinusitis. Sinusitis probably secondary to viral infection. Appropriate use of antiallergy for prophylaxis would have minimized some of patient symptoms. These will become decision points.
Pharmacodynamics	Antihistamines block effects of histamine, thus decreasing symptoms. Decongestants relieve nasal congestion by constricting arterioles. Antiallergy drugs stabilize mast cells. Antibiotics appropriate for sinusitis.	AR's allergic symptoms may have been less severe if she had used the cromolyn before allergen exposure.
Adverse Effects/ Contraindications	Antihistamines: First-generation agents are sedating but remain first-line drugs. Second-generation agents less sedating. Decongestants: possibility to abuse nasal formulations. Antiallergy drug: little to no adverse effects to antiallergy drug. Antibiotic: possibility of allergic response to antibiotic.	There are no contraindications to the use of antihistamines, or decongestants, antiallergy or antibiotics for AR. Suspect chronic sinusitis with drug-resistant organism based on patient history. This is a decision point.

Drug Variables	*Drug Summary*	*Patient Variables*
Pharmacokinetics	Antihistamines: First-generation or second-generation agents have rapid onset of action. Extended-release formulations have long duration of action. Decongestants: rapid acting with long duration if extended-release formulation used. Antiallergy: slow to onset but effective if used prophylactically. Antibiotic: rapid onset with high efficacy.	There are no significant pharmacokinetic factors that would influence a drug decision. Increased moisture in nasal passages may make AR more comfortable and foster expulsion of mucus.
Dosage Regimen	Regimen of antihistamines and decongestant can be accomplished with combination, extended-release formulations. PRN prophylactic use of antiallergy agent. BID dosing regimen for antibiotic will help promote compliance. These will become decision points.	AR is more likely to be compliant with less frequent dosing of all medications, including those used for prophylaxis. This will become a decision point.
Lab Considerations	There are no significant lab considerations with the use of antihistamines and decongestants.	There is no patient-specific lab testing needed at this time.
Cost Index*	Dimetapp Extentabs: 1 Cephalosporin antibiotic: 1 Nasalcrom: 1	AR would prefer to use OTC drugs if possible rather than use prescription agents. This will become a decision point.

Summary of Decision Points

- Dimetapp Extentabs, saline nasal spray, and Nasalcrom are OTC. Only prescription would be for antibiotic.
- Could change antihistamine from first- to second-generation agent if drowsiness interferes with ADLs.
- Suspect a chronic sinusitis with possible drug-resistant organism, based on patient history.
- AR's symptoms may have been less severe if she had used the cromolyn before allergen exposure.
- Antihistamine-decongestant and antibiotic would be less expensive than brand name drugs.

DRUGS TO BE USED

- Nasalcrom 1 spray in each nostril three to six times per day at regular intervals before exposure of allergens rather than after symptoms appear.
- Brompheniramine maleate 12 mg/phenylpropanolamine HCL 75 mg (OTC as DIMETAPP EXTENTABS) tab 1 po BID PRN for antihistamine and decongestant effects
- Cephalexin 500 mg po q12 hr × 10 days

*Cost Index:
1 = $ < 30/mo.
2 = $ 30–40/mo.
3 = $ 40–50/mo.
4 = $ 50–60/mo.
5 = $ > 60/mo.

AWP of 24, 12 mg DIMETAPP EXTENTABS tablets is approximately $8.
AWP of 20, 500 mg cephalexin capsules is approximately $21.
AWP of 13 mL, 5.2 mg/inhalation sodium cromolyn (NASALCROM) container is approximately $22.
AWP of 45 mL OCEAN saline nasal spray is approximately $3; homemade nasal irrigation solution is approximately 30¢.

Topical alpha-adrenergic drugs (e.g., ephedrine, oxymetazoline, phenylpropanolamine, pseudoephedrine) have been used to alleviate nasal congestion and obstruction. The efficacy of topical drugs is limited because of rebound effects and systemic responses such as insomnia, irritability, and hypertension. The latter responses are more often seen with oral agents.

Antiallergy drugs are essentially without adverse effects. Furthermore, they are the only available drugs used for prophylaxis. Intranasal corticosteroids (e.g., beclomethasone or flunisolide) are the most potent drugs available for the relief of most forms of rhinitis. Their efficacy is comparable to those of orally administered corticosteroids but with substantially reduced adverse effects. For patients who do not adequately benefit from a full dosage of a second-generation antihistamine and a maintenance dose of an antiallergy drug, a topical corticosteroid may be used for a short period.

It should be noted that not all patients respond to drugs in the same fashion. If one drug is not effective in relieving symptoms or if excessive sedation or GI distress results, another drug from a different class may be tried.

Identifying factors that cause urticaria and strategies for elimination or avoidance of those factors provides the most satisfactory treatment regimen. First-generation antihistamines, especially cyproheptadine, hydroxyzine, and combinations of H_1 and H_2 agents, are believed to be beneficial in treating symptoms. These drugs seem to be more effective than other antihistamines, although they have a slower onset of action and have been associated with severe adverse effects. Topically applied corticosteroids are of no benefit in the treatment of urticaria, but oral formulations have been helpful in some patients.

Patient Variables

Approaches to cost containment in the treatment of rhinitis consists of a first-generation antihistamine and switching to a nonsedating preparation only if daytime sedation becomes a problem. (Daytime sedation occurs in only 10 to 25 percent of patients.) Tolerance to sedative effects is common. Substituting an inexpensive, sedating drug for the nighttime dose of a twice-daily preparation may help. It is important to keep in mind that some degree of psychomotor impairment may occur with daytime use of a first-generation drug even without noticeable sedation. Second-generation antihistamines (except for azatadine) are 15 to 30 times more expensive than many first-generation preparations (although not all first-generation drugs are inexpensive). Inhaled cromolyn and aerosol solutions are generally more expensive than nedocromil. Corticosteroids, whether for nasal use or inhalation, are generally consistent in price with antiallergy drugs.

Drug use in pregnancy should be limited. Antihistamines contained in OTC preparations (with the exception of brompheniramine) have not been shown to have deleterious effects in pregnancy or in the fetus. As with any drug, however, antihistamines should be used only when they are absolutely necessary.

Intervention

Administration

Antihistamines can prevent nasal congestion but do not relieve existing congestion. Decongestants shrink engorgement of nasal mucous membranes (see Chapter 48). Thus, they are more effective if they are taken before symptoms occur. Antihistamines should be used regularly by sensitive patients just before and during the seasonal exposures, even

TABLE 47–4 COMPARISON OF ANTIHISTAMINE AND ANTIASTHMA DRUG EFFECTS

Parameters	H_1 Receptor Specificity	Anticholinergic Effects	Performance Impairment	Relieves Sneezing	Relieves Nasal Congestion	Relieves Rhinorrhea	Relieves Ocular Symptoms	Rapid Allergy Relief
Single-Entity First-Generation Antihistamines								
Alkylamines	Effective	Moderate	Mild	Yes	No	Yes	Yes	Yes
Ethanolamines	Moderate	Significant	Marked					
Ethylenediamines	Effective	Variable–mild	Variable					
Phenothiazines	Potent	Marked	Marked					
Piperidines	Effective	Moderate	Slight					
Single-Entity Second-Generation Antihistamines								
Astemizole	Moderate to high	Little or none	Little or none	Yes	Yes	Yes	Yes	Yes
Cetirizine	Moderate	Little or none	Little or none					
Fexofenadine	Moderate to high	Little or none	Little or none					
Loratadine	Moderate to high	Little or none	Little or none					
Combination Antihistamine and Decongestant								
First generation	Moderate to potent	Mild to marked	Yes	Yes	Yes	Yes	Yes	Yes
Second generation	Moderate to high	Mild to marked	Yes	Yes	Yes	Yes	Yes	Yes
Related Drugs								
Antiallergy drugs	Moderate	NA	No	No	No	No	No	No
Topical nasal corticosteroids	No antihistamine action	No	No	Yes	Yes	Yes	No	No

when symptoms are absent. Furthermore, because these drugs may thicken respiratory tract secretions, making them more difficult to expel, the patient should be encouraged to drink 2000 to 3000 mL of fluids daily (if it is not contraindicated).

With the exception of astemizole, oral antihistamines are given with meals to minimize GI distress. The absorption of astemizole is reduced by 60 percent when it is taken with meals; therefore, it should be taken on an empty stomach (i.e., 1 hour before or 2 hours after a meal).

Patients taking first-generation antihistamines should be monitored for excessive drowsiness during the first few days of therapy. Concurrent use of sedating antihistamines with other CNS depressant drugs should be avoided. If a drug with a long half-life is used, daytime sedation can be minimized by administering the entire daily dose at bedtime.

Education

The most important aspect of allergy care is patient education. Patients must understand the nature of their disease and how to prevent and treat symptoms. Avoiding allergens has important clinical significance in limiting the severity of the disease. Patients should be told to stop smoking and to avoid other irritants or precipitating factors. This aspect is often overlooked when teaching patients who have mild allergies.

Appropriate avoidance procedures relate to the responsible allergens and differ for seasonal and perennial disease. For seasonal allergic rhinitis, patients should be advised to refrain from long walks in the woods during pollination periods. Remaining indoors with the windows closed when symptoms are severe and the pollen count is high (e.g., hot, windy, sunny days) helps reduce exposure to allergens. Some patients find air conditioners helpful, but the filter does little to remove pollen from the air. Air conditioning only makes staying indoors with the windows closed on a hot day more tolerable. The outside air intake on the conditioner should be kept closed to avoid bringing in more pollinated air. If ragweed is a problem, daisies, dahlias, and chrysanthemums should not be kept indoors because these flowers are cousins to ragweed. Minimizing dust accumulation in the bedroom and avoiding irritants such as tobacco smoke, chemical vapors, and strong perfumes lessens symptoms.

Control of perennial allergic rhinitis demands specific attention to allergens in the home. Housecleaning with a damp mop two to three times a week reduces dust. Dacron or polyester pillows should replace feather pillows. Mattresses should be covered. Areas where mold can collect (e.g., damp basements and furniture) should be cleaned thoroughly. Furnishings made of synthetic fabrics are preferable to cotton and wool and minimize dust collection. Humidification reduces dust. Patients with allergies to mold should not keep African violets or geraniums indoors. Pets may need to be removed from the home in some cases if allergic symptoms become disabling. Merely keeping the pet out of the home does not sufficiently reduce dander in the air.

Patients are instructed to take antihistamines only as prescribed or as instructed on the patient package insert contained in OTC preparations. Alcohol and other drugs should not be used without first contacting the health care provider because drugs with CNS depressant effects can cause excessive respiratory depression and death. Patients should be advised to avoid driving or operating machinery until the sedative effects of the drugs are known or the period of drowsiness has worn off. As with all drugs, antihistamines should be stored out of the reach of small children to avoid accidental ingestion.

The patient should be instructed as to the correct technique for using nasal sprays and inhalers. They should also be warned that some drugs may cause temporary stinging. In addition, teach the patient that drug canisters should be stored with the valve pointed downward and to replace the canister every 3 months, even if it is not completely empty. Patients keep inhalers in their purse or jacket pockets for extended periods, many times long after the drug has expired. By replacing the inhaler every 3 months, the patient is assured that active drug will be available when it is needed. Additionally, the delivery device of inhaled formulations should be cleaned after its use to minimize unnecessary repeated exposure to bacteria that may collect in the device. Proper cleaning also helps maintain patency of the device.

The anticholinergic properties of some antihistamines limit their use in patients with prostatic hypertrophy, those with a predisposition to urinary retention, or those who have narrow-angle glaucoma. Individuals with these disorders should be told to contact their health care provider before using an antihistamine.

Patients should be taught to consume 2000 to 3000 mL of fluids daily to help thin secretions and make them easier to remove. They should also be advised to maintain dental hygiene by brushing and flossing. The diminished salivary flow that results from the anticholinergic effects of many antihistamines contributes to dental caries and gum disease. Regular dental check-ups should be advised. Mouth dryness can be minimized by using ice, sugarless gum, or hard candy.

Patients should be advised not to drink alcohol or take other drugs without the health care provider's knowledge and consent. They should be advised that an antihistamine is often included in prescription and OTC combination products for the common cold. However, they do not relieve cold symptoms any better than a placebo. Moreover, their use exposes the patient to adverse effects without therapeutic advantage.

Patients who are using a corticosteroid concurrently with a decongestant nasal spray should be taught to use the decongestant 5 to 15 minutes before the corticosteroid. Using the decongestant first causes shrinkage of mucous membranes, whereby the corticosteroid can better reach deeper nasal passages. The patient should be taught to blow the nose in advance of nasal drug administration so as to not place the drug on the surface of secretions. The patient should also be advised to contact the health care provider if allergic symptoms do not improve within 1 month or if nasal discharge becomes purulent.

Evaluation

The principal outcomes of antihistaminic therapy are based on the reason the drugs were used. Effectiveness of treatment is demonstrated most often through patients' verbal statements. If the antihistamine was used for seasonal or perennial allergic symptoms, symptoms are relieved. If it was specifically used for its sedative characteristics, drowsiness or sleep resulted.

In patients who respond to inhaled corticosteroids, improvement in pulmonary function is usually apparent within 1 to 4 weeks after the start of treatment. Relief from allergic symptoms (e.g., rhinitis) are prevented with the use of antiallergy drugs. When conservative methods fail to control allergic symptoms the patient should be referred to an allergist. An allergist can help when an allergic etiology cannot be distinguished from vasomotor rhinitis and when the antigen or antigens must be identified for management purposes. Referral to an ear, nose, and throat specialist is warranted for symptoms related to polyps or foreign bodies, tumors, a necrotizing inflammatory condition, or atrophic rhinitis.

Patients on long-term nasal corticosteroids should have periodic otolaryngologic exams to monitor nasal mucosa and passages for infection or ulceration. Patients changing from systemic corticosteroids to inhaled formulations should be monitored for signs of adrenal insufficiency (anorexia, nausea, weakness, fatigue, hypotension, hypoglycemia) during initial therapy. Pulmonary function tests may be assessed periodically during and for several months following transfer from systemic to inhaled corticosteroids.

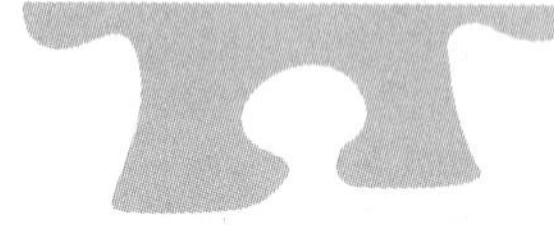

SUMMARY

- An estimated 15 to 20 percent of the population suffer from chronic or recurrent allergies, which are frequently manifested as rhinitis, urticaria, asthma, and in some cases, anaphylaxis.
- Hyperactivity of the airways to various physical, chemical, environmental, or pharmacologic stimuli is the hallmark of allergy and asthma.
- H_1 receptors play a role in allergic disorders; H_2 receptors play a role in gastric acid secretion, immune system downregulation, and feedback control of histamine release. H_3 receptors modulate cholinergic neurotransmission in the airways, in the CNS, and in the feedback control of histamine synthesis and release.
- Patient history is the most important component in the evaluation of a suspected or confirmed allergic disorder. A careful search of home, workplace, and environmental factors should be conducted.
- Allergy testing should be selective and based on clues provided by the patient's history whenever possible.
- Hyperemia of the mucosa of the nasopharynx with concurrent edema and increased production of mucus is caused by increased levels of estrogen during pregnancy. This condition leads to a feeling of nasal congestion.
- Assessment of symptoms in the child is much like that of the adult but also includes a feeding history for a very young child, with attention to the intake of cow's milk, eggs, and wheat.
- The treatment objective for the use of antihistamines, corticosteroids, and antiallergy drugs is primarily symptom relief. No one drug completely abolishes symptoms.
- There are six different categories of first-generation antihistamines, each with their own benefits and disadvantages. All are sedating to various degrees. Second-generation antihistamines are considered to be nonsedating.
- Antihistamines are more effective for allergic rather than nonallergic forms of rhinitis. Acute forms respond more favorably to drug therapy than chronic rhinitis.
- First-generation antihistamines are effective in relieving nasopharyngeal itching, sneezing, water rhinorrhea, and ocular manifestations of allergy such as itching, tearing, and erythema. However, they are less effective for nasal congestion.
- First-generation antihistamines are sedating to various degrees, and their anticholinergic effects include visual disturbances, urinary retention, and even arrhythmias in some patients.
- Second-generation antihistamines produce less sedation and anticholinergic adverse effects. These drugs have dose-related bronchodilating effects and provide protection against bronchospasm caused by histamine, allergens, exercise, hyperventilation, and cold, dry air–induced.
- Antiallergy drugs are essentially without adverse effects and are the only interventions of a prophylactic nature.
- First-generation antihistamines (cyproheptadine, hydroxyzine, and combinations of H_1 and H_2 drugs, astemizole) are believed to be beneficial in treating symptoms of urticaria.
- Antihistamines are not first-line drugs for asthma or anaphylaxis. An inhaled beta$_2$ agonist or subcutaneous epinephrine is the initial drug of choice for acute attacks of bronchospasm.
- Antihistamines can prevent nasal congestion but do not relieve existing congestion. Thus, they are more effective taken before symptoms occur.
- Patient education should include the correct use of inhalers, nebulizers, and nasal sprays and drops.
- The efficacy of drug therapy includes evidence of reduced inflammation, dilation of airways, and stabilization of mast cells. Treatment effectiveness can be demonstrated through the patient's verbal statements of symptom relief.
- When conservative methods fail to control symptoms, the health care provider should refer the patient to an appropriate allergist.

BIBLIOGRAPHY

Abramowicz, M. (1994). Intranasal budesonide for allergic rhinitis. *The Medical Letter on Drugs and Therapeutics,* 36, 63–64.

Badhwar, A., and Druce, H. (1992). Allergic rhinitis. *Medical Clinics of North America,* 76(4), 789–803.

Campoli-Richards, D., Buckley, M., and Fitton, A. (1990). Cetirizine: A review of its pharmacological properties and clinical potential in allergic rhinitis, pollen-induced asthma, and chronic urticaria. *Drugs,* 40(5), 762–781.

Corey, J. P. (1993). Advances in the pharmacotherapy of allergic rhinitis: Second generation H1-receptor antagonists. *Otolaryngology: Head & Neck Surgery,* 109(3, Part 2), 584–592.

Federal Food and Drug Administration. (1993). Reports of dangerous cardiac arrhythmias prompt new contraindications for the drug hismanal. *FDA Medical Bulletin,* 12(1), 2.

Hendeles, L. (1993). Efficacy and safety of antihistamines and expectorants in nonprescription cough and cold preparations. *Pharmacotherapy,* 13(2), 154–158.

Lang, D., Sherman, M., Polansky, M. (1997). Guidelines and realities of asthma management: The Philadelphia Story. *Archives of Internal Medicine,* 157(11), 1193–1200.

Mabry, R. (1995). Pharmacotherapy of allergic rhinitis: Corticosteroids. Otolaryngology: Head & Neck Surgery, 113(1), 120–125.

Mabry, R. (1994). Allergic and infective rhinosinusitis: Differential diagnosis and interrelationship. *Otolaryngology: Head & Neck Surgery,* 113(3, Part 2), 335–359.

Mabry, R. (1993). Therapeutic agents in the medical management of sinusitis. *Otolaryngologic Clinics of North America,* 26(4), 561–570.

Mabry, R. (1993). Topical pharmacotherapy for allergic rhinitis: Nedocromil. *American Journal of Otolaryngology,* 14(6), 379–381.

Mabry, R. (1993). Intranasal corticosteroids and cromolyn. *American Journal of Otolaryngology,* 14(5), 295–300.

Mabry, R. (1992). Topical pharmacotherapy for allergic rhinitis: New agents. *Southern Medical Journal,* 85(2), 149–154.

Mabry, R. (1992). Corticosteroids in the management of upper respiratory allergy: The emerging role of steroid nasal sprays. *Otolaryngology: Head & Neck Surgery,* 107(6, Part 2), 855–859.

Meltzer, E., Tyrell, R., and Wood, C. (1995). A pharmacologic continuum in the treatment of rhinorrhea: The clinician as economist. *Journal of Allergy and Clinical Immunology,* 95(5), 1147–1148.

National Heart, Lung, and Blood Institute, National Asthma Education Program, Expert Panel Report. (1991). *Guidelines for the Diagnosis and Management of Asthma.* Pub. No. 91–3042. Bethesda, MD: United States Department of Health and Human Services.

Ratner, P., Paull, B., Findlay, S., et al. (1992). Fluticasone propionate given once daily is as effective for seasonal allergic rhinitis as beclomethasone dipropionate given twice daily. *Journal of Allergy and Clinical Immunology,* 90(3, Part I), 285–291.

Rhinorrhea: New indications and dose forms of nasal sprays. (1996). *Modern Medicine,* 64(2), 37.

Rihoux, J., and Mariz, S. (1993). Cetirizine: An updated review of its pharmacological properties and therapeutic efficacy. *Clinical Review in Allergy,* 11(1), 65–88.

Simons, F. (1994). H_1-receptor antagonists: Comparative tolerability and safety. *Drug Safety,* 10(5), 350–380.

Simons, F., and Simons, K. (1994). The pharmacology and use of H_1 receptor antagonist drugs. *New England Journal of Medicine,* 330(23), 1663–1670.

Simons, F., and Simons, K. (1991). Second generation H_1 receptor antagonists. *Annals of Allergy,* 66(1), 5–19.

Spencer, C., Faulds, D., and Peters, D. (1993). Cetirizine: A reappraisal of its pharmacological properties and therapeutic use in selected allergic disorders. *Drugs,* 46(6), 1055–1080.

White, M. V., and Kaliner, M. A. (1992). Mediators of allergic rhinitis. *Journal of Allergy and Clinical Immunology,* 90(4, Part 2), 699–704.

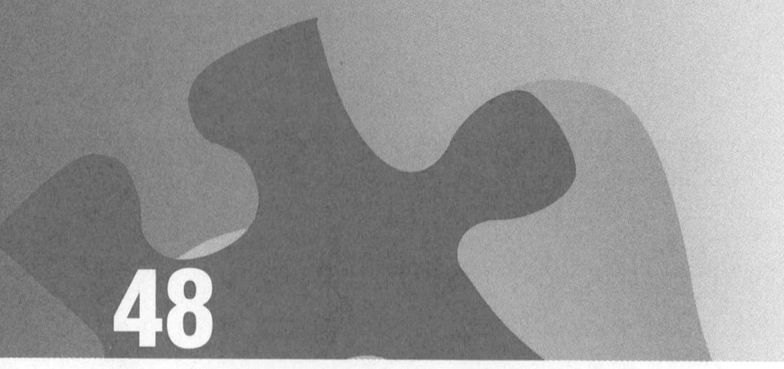

48

Expectorants, Antitussives, Decongestants, and Mucolytics

Upper respiratory disorders are generally treated with expectorants, antitussives, decongestants, and mucolytic drugs. Because most of these drugs are available over the counter (OTC), they are frequently self-prescribed. Additionally, they are widely prescribed by health care providers for a variety of upper respiratory problems, including the common cold, allergic rhinitis, idiopathic rhinitis, cough, and cystic fibrosis because of their palliative effects.

Nasal inflammation, excessive or thickened mucus, and cough add to an array of uncomfortable symptoms that may be caused by viral, bacterial, or environmental agents as well as congenital anomalies and genetic diseases. The underlying causes are often self-limiting or without cure. Expectorants and antitussives, sometimes in combination, thin mucus and relieve cough, allowing patients to perform their normal daily tasks. Decongestants shrink swollen mucous membranes and deter excessive secretions. Mucolytics alter the viscosity of mucus at the molecular level. When they are applied carefully, these drugs help the body's protective mucociliary physiology to function appropriately.

UPPER RESPIRATORY DISORDERS

Epidemiology and Etiology

Common Colds

Acute upper respiratory infections (URIs, common colds) are the most common acute infections in human beings, accounting for 10 percent (100 million) office visits annually in the United States. Health care providers see fewer of these infections because patients treat their symptoms at home using nonprescription OTC drugs or simply allow their illness to run its course. The cost of medical treatment of URIs is substantial, exceeding $10 billion per year, with over $500 million spent on OTC preparations.

Most adults average two to four colds a year, with the incidence increasing in the fall, peaking in winter, and then slowly decreasing each spring. Adult women are affected more often than men. Colds occur more commonly in families with children 2 to 7 years of age. The *coryza* syndrome is an infectious process that can be caused by 80 to 100 different viruses. Etiologic agents associated with the common cold include rhinovirus (90 percent), influenza, parainfluenza, respiratory syncytial virus, corona virus, adenovirus, echovirus, and coxsackievirus.

Rhinitis

Rhinitis is discussed in Chapter 47. In many cases, it is an allergic response to inhaled (or ingested) antigens and is the most common primary cause of nasal congestion. It is estimated that 15 to 20 percent of the population suffer from chronic or recurrent nasal congestion, although rhinitis is uncommon before the age of 3 years and rarely occurs after age 50. The highest incidence is between the ages of 30 and 40. The incidence among patients with one allergic parent is 25 percent, rising to 60 percent if both parents have atopic symptoms.

Rhinitis may be seasonal or perennial, depending on the type of allergen involved. The seasonal type is most often caused by pollens from trees (spring), grasses (summer), or weeds (fall). The perennial type is most often caused by nonseasonal allergens such as house dust and animal dander. The fecal material of the house-dust mite is the most important indoor allergen. Unfortunately, house-dust mite is present in every home regardless of how clean it is. The saliva of the cockroach is another significant allergen, especially in inner cities, but the allergens from pets, particularly cats, are also of major importance. Patients with seasonal allergic rhinitis outnumber those with perennial allergic rhinitis by about 10 to 1.

The onset of *idiopathic rhinitis,* rhinorrhea due to increased secretion of mucus from the nasal mucosa, occurs in the third to fifth decades. The disease is a chronic vasomotor disorder, with periods of exacerbation and remission unrelated to specific allergens. It is aggravated by a dry atmosphere or changes in temperature.

Atrophic rhinitis usually appears at puberty and is more common in females than in males. Hispanics, Asians, and blacks are relatively more susceptible than whites. The incidence is low in natives of equatorial Africa. Bacterial infection is thought to play an etiologic role, but the exact cause is unknown.

Cough

Although almost all people experience an acute episode of coughing at some time in their lives, most studies report a prevalence of chronic cough in only 8 to 14 percent of the population. Viral infections that produce cough are especially pronounced during the winter months, occurring more frequently in children than in adults. The most common causative organisms include influenza, parainfluenza, adenovirus, respiratory syncytial virus, rhinovirus, and coronavirus. Common etiologic agents for bacterial infections include *Streptococcus pneumoniae, Mycoplasma pneumoniae, Staphylococcus aureus, Haemophilus influenzae,* and mixed anaerobic bacteria.

Cigarette smoke is a common cause of cough. Furthermore, nonsmokers exposed to a smoke-filled room frequently develop a cough. Cough rates in smokers increase with the number of cigarettes smoked. Twenty-five percent of people who smoke one-half pack per day, 50 percent of patients who smoke one pack per day, and the majority of people who smoke two packs per day report a daily cough. Common air pollutants such as sulfur dioxide, nitrogen oxide, ammonia, ozone, and dust may also produce cough. Furthermore, cough is a frequent manifestation of asthma and other respiratory disorders, and may be an initial, predominant manifestation.

Pathophysiology

Common Cold

The virus of the common cold is transmitted by direct inoculation of the mucous membranes of the nose and eyes, usually from contaminated hands. Viral replication in the nasopharynx produces complaints of "being all stuffed up and having a runny nose." The acute catarrhal response is associated with varying degrees of nasotracheal inflammation. It results from dilation of the blood vessels in the nasal mucosa. The dilation causes engorgement of mucous membranes and an increase in mucus secretion. Characteristically, the copious nasal discharge progresses from being clear and watery to thick and sticky within 24 hours. A scratchy throat, nonproductive cough, loss of taste and smell, and sneezing are other common complaints. One of the key diagnostic findings is the absence of systemic symptoms.

Rhinitis

Allergic rhinitis is a type I hypersensitivity reaction to inhaled or ingested allergens. The antigen (e.g., pollen, dust, mold, animal dander) initially stimulates production of immunoglobulin E (IgE) antibodies that attach to receptors on mast cells and basophils in the nasal mucosa. Repeated exposure to the antigen causes release of several mediator substances, including histamine. The result is vasodilation, increased capillary permeability, smooth muscle contraction, and eosinophilia.

Idiopathic rhinitis is thought to be related to an abnormal autonomic responsiveness that results in intermittent vascular engorgement of the nasal mucosa. The signs and symptoms may be related to an allergic response or neurovascular imbalance.

With atrophic rhinitis, the mucosa changes from ciliated pseudostratified columnar epithelium to stratified squamous cell epithelium. The lamina propria is reduced in amount and vascularity.

Cough

In general, the mechanisms associated with a cough are mechanical, inflammatory, or chemical in nature. The etiologic agent stimulates afferent fibers in the vagus (cranial nerve [CN] X), trigeminal (CN V), glossopharyngeal (CN IX), or phrenic nerves. These nerves convey information to the cough center in the medulla. Efferent fibers from the cough center, in turn, carry motor impulses to the larynx and muscles of the diaphragm, chest wall, and abdomen. A cough results. In patients with excessive sputum production, increased secretions stimulate coughing.

PHARMACOTHERAPEUTIC OPTIONS

Expectorants

- ❒ Guaifenesin (HALOTUSSIN, HUMIBID, ROBITUSSIN)
- ❒ Dornase alpha (PULMOZYME, DNASE)

Indications

A variety of compounds have been promoted for their expectorant actions, but in almost all cases, efficacy is doubtful. However, there are two exceptions—guaifenesin (formerly called glyceryl guaiacolate) and dornase alpha. Guaifenesin is the only expectorant recognized by the Food and Drug Administration as safe and effective. It is the only expectorant for which scientific evidence has been found to support efficacy in decreasing the viscosity of sputum. Guaifenesin is used for the symptomatic management of cough associated with the common cold, laryngitis, bronchitis, pharyngitis, pertussis, influenza, and measles. It is also used for coughs provoked by chronic paranasal sinusitis in patients unresponsive to increased fluid intake. Guaifenesin may be found in combination with analgesics and antipyretics, antihistamines, and decongestants.

Dornase alpha helps reduce the incidence of respiratory infections and improve pulmonary function in patients with cystic fibrosis. Dornase alpha is not a replacement for other components of therapy for cystic fibrosis (e.g., antibiotics, bronchodilators, daily physical exercise).

Ammonium chloride, beechwood creosote, potassium guaiacolsulfonate, syrup of ipecac, and terpin hydrate have also been used as expectorants. The efficacy of these drugs has not been proved.

Pharmacodynamics

Guaifenesin renders a cough more productive by stimulating the flow of respiratory tract secretions. The loosened secretions are moved upward toward the pharynx by ciliary movement and by coughing. A common misconception with the use of guaifenesin is that it relieves irritated mucous membranes by preventing dryness. Evidence does not support this belief (Fig. 48–1).

Dornase alpha is a genetically engineered enzyme (recombinant human deoxyribonuclease) that hydrolyzes DNA in the sputum. It reduces the viscid elasticity of the sputum.

Adverse Effects and Contraindications

Adverse effects associated with guaifenesin include gastrointestinal (GI) distress such as nausea, vomiting, diarrhea, and abdominal pain. Dizziness, headache, rashes, and urticaria have also been noted. Guaifenesin is contraindicated in patients with hypersensitivity. Some guaifenesin preparations contain alcohol and should be avoided in patients with known intolerance to alcohol or who are taking anticoagulants. Guaifenesin inhibits platelet function.

In general, expectorants should not be used for a persistent cough associated with smoking, asthma, or emphysema, or if the cough is accompanied by excessive secretions. Safe use of expectorates during pregnancy has not been established, although guaifenesin has been used without adverse effects.

The adverse effects of dornase alpha are uncommon but voice alteration, pharyngitis, rash, chest pain, and allergic reactions may occur. There are no known contraindications or drug-drug interactions to dornase alpha.

Pharmacokinetics

The pharmacokinetics of expectorants are listed in Table 48–1. Guaifenesin is well absorbed from the GI tract after oral

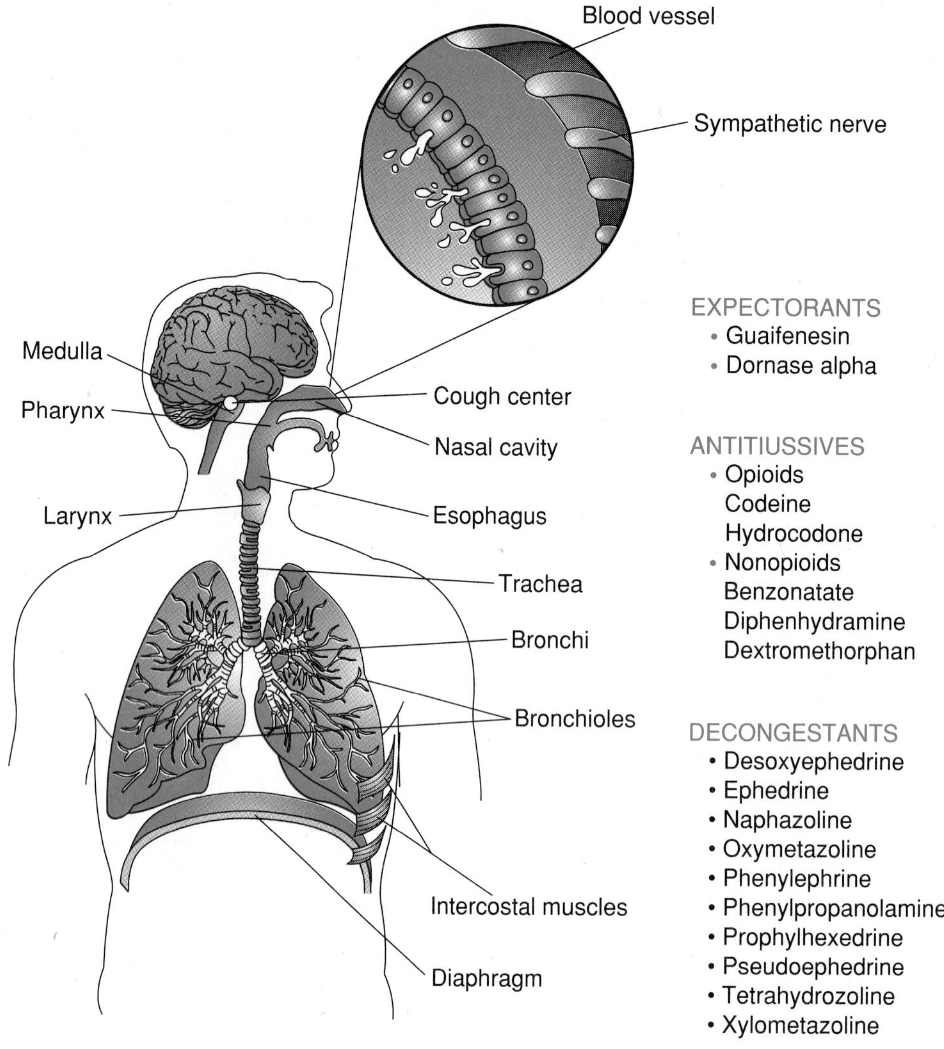

Figure 48–1 Sites of drug action for upper respiratory disorders. Drugs used to manage upper respiratory disorders fall into four classes: expectorants, antitussives, decongestants, and mucolytic drugs. Antitussive drugs act centrally in the cough center or peripherally at the site of irritation to suppress coughing. Expectorants stimulate the flow of respiratory tract secretions. Decongestants stimulate alpha receptors, causing vasoconstriction, reduced blood flow, reduced fluid exudation, and shrinkage of edematous membranes. Mucolytic drugs reduce sputum viscosity. These drugs do not eliminate the source of infection, rather they act in a palliative manner to control the symptoms and help the patient feel better.

administration. Distribution sites are unknown but its metabolites are biotransformed and eliminated through the kidneys.

The onset of the effects of dornase alpha occur within 15 minutes of nebulized administration. There is minimal systemic absorption after inhalation. Peak effects are not noted for 3 days, and the duration of drug action is unknown. It is unknown whether dornase alpha crosses the placenta or is distributed in breast milk.

Dosage Regimen

The dosage of guaifenesin depends on the specific formulation used (Table 48–2). The usual dosage is 200 to 400 mg (10 to 20 mL) four times daily. The dosage of extended release formulations is larger than for syrups, oral solutions, capsules, or tablets. Administer each dose with a full glass of water to decrease viscosity of secretions. Sustained-release formulations should be taken whole. Do not open, crush, break, or chew.

The usual dose of dornase alpha is 2.5 mg (1 ampule) once daily via aerosol mist using a compressed-air nebulizer system. Treatment should last 10 to 15 minutes. Twice-daily dosing may be beneficial for some patients.

Antitussives

NONOPIOIDS

- ❐ Benzonatate (TESSALON PERLES); (🍁) TESSALON
- ❐ Diphenhydramine (BENADRYL, COMPOZ, SOMINEX, NYTOL MAXIMUM STRENGTH, many others); (🍁) ALLERDRYL, BENADRYL
- ❐ Dextromethorphan (BENYLIN DM, ROBITUSSIN COUGH CALMERS, SUCRETS COUGH CONTROL, ST. JOSEPH COUGH SUPPRESSANT, VICKS FORMULA 44, many others); (🍁) BALMINIL DM, KOFFEX, many others

TABLE 48–1 PHARMACOKINETICS OF SELECTED EXPECTORANTS, ANTITUSSIVES, DECONGESTANTS, AND MUCOLYTICS

Drug	Route	Onset	Peak	Duration	PB (%)	$t_{1/2}$
Expectorants						
Guaifenesin	po	30 min	UA	4–6 hr	UA	UA
Dornase alpha	IV	15 min	3 days	UA	UA	UA
Antitussives						
Benzonatate	po	15–20 min	UA	3–8 hr	UA	UA
Codeine	po	< 30 min	60–90 min	4–6 hr	30–35	3 hr
Dextromethorphan	po	15–30 min	UA	3–6 hr	UA	UA
Diphenhydramine HCL	po	15–60 min	1–2 hr	4–8 hr	80–85	2.4–9.3 hr
Hydrocodone	po	Rapid	30–90 min	4–8 hr	30–35	4 hr
Decongestants						
Ephedrine	IN	1–2 min	1 hr	3 hr	UA	UA
Naphazoline	IN	< 10 min	UK	2–6 hr	UK	UK
Oxymetazoline	IN	1–2 min	5–10 min	To 12 hr	UA	UA
Phenylephrine	IN po	1–2 min	5–10 min	30 min–4 hr	UA	UA
Phenylpropanolamine	po	15–30 min	1–2 hr	3 hr*	UK	3–4 hr
Propylhexedrine	IN	0.5–5 min	UK	0.5–2 hr	UA	UA
Pseudoephedrine	po	15–30 min	30–60 min	4–6 hr 8–12 hr†	UA	UA
Tetrahydrozoline	IN	1–2 min	UK	4–8 hr	UA	UA
Xylometazoline	IN	1–2 min	5–10 min	5–6 hr	UA	UA
Mucolytics						
Acetylcysteine	Inh	Rapid	UA	Brief	UA	UA
Other Respiratory Drugs						
Alpha$_1$-proteinase inhibitor	IV	2–3 days	1–3 wks	1–2 wks	UA	4.5–5.2 days
Beractant	INT	Immed	Hr	UA	NA	UK
Colfosceril palmitrate	INT	Immed	Hr	12 hr	UA	12 hr

*Phenylpropanolamine's duration of action for extended-release formulation is 12 to 16 hours.
†Pseudoephedrine's duration of action for sustained-action formulation is 8 to 12 hours.
PB, Protein binding; $t_{1/2}$, elimination half-life; UA, unavailable; IN, intranasal formulations, usually in the form of drops or sprays; Inh, inhaled formulation; INT, intratracheal; IV, intravenous; UK, unknown.

OPIOIDS
❒ Codeine; (♣) PAVERAL
❒ Hydrocodone

Indications

Antitussives are most appropriately used to suppress dry, hacking, nonproductive coughs that keep patients awake at night. Opioids and nonopioid agents are used as antitussives. An opioid such as codeine is one of the most commonly used antitussives. Smaller doses are employed for coughs than doses used for pain relief. At low doses, the risk of dependency and undesired adverse responses are reduced.

In contrast, dextromethorphan is the most frequently used nonopioid antitussive. It is a chemical analog of codeine without its analgesic or dependency features. Nonopioid antitussives may be found in combination with antihistamines, decongestants, and expectorants in cough and cold remedies. Dextromethorphan is most effective for chronic nonproductive coughs. Diphenhydramine is the only antihistamine (see Chapter 46) with proven efficacy as an antitussive in the treatment of coughs associated with the common cold or irritants. Overall, nonopioid antitussives are thought to be as effective as opioid antitussives.

Pharmacodynamics

In general, antitussive drugs act either centrally or peripherally. Centrally acting drugs such as codeine, hydrocodone, and dextromethorphan act in the cough center in the medulla to suppress the cough. Dextromethorphan does not inhibit ciliary activity, whereas codeine does. Hydrocodone is often formulated in combination with decongestants. Dextromethorphan is a common ingredient in nonprescription cough and cold formulations.

Peripherally acting drugs such as benzonatate act at the site of the irritation that is producing the cough. Benzonatate acts as a potent local anesthetic if the integrity of the capsule is compromised.

Adverse Effects and Contraindications

Overall, opioids are limited in their usefulness because of their adverse effects (see Chapter 14). In addition they can cause dependency. The major adverse effects of opioids are apparent in the central nervous system (CNS) depression. Sedation, confusion, and hypotension may occur, especially with high doses. The most serious adverse response is respiratory depression, laryngeal edema, and anaphylaxis.

Opioids are contraindicated in patients with known hypersensitivity to the drug or to its other ingredients, and during pregnancy and lactation. Cross-sensitivity with other

TABLE 48–2 DOSAGE REGIMEN FOR SELECTED EXPECTORANTS, ANTITUSSIVES, DECONGESTANTS, AND MUCOLYTICS

Drug	Uses	Dosage	Implications
Expectorants			
Guaifenesin	Symptomatic management of cough associated with URI	*Adults:* 200–400 mg po q4hr *or* 600 mg–1.2 g po q12hr of SR formulation *Child 6–12 yrs:* 100–200 mg po q4hr *or* 600 mg po q12hrs of SR formulation. Not to exceed 1.2 g/day *Child 2–6 yrs:* 50–100 mg po q4hr. Not to exceed 600 mg/day	Administer each dose with a full glass of water to decrease viscosity of secretions. SR formulations should be taken whole. Do not open, crush, break, or chew
Dornase alpha	Cystic fibrosis	*Adults:* 2.5 mg (1 ampule) once daily via aerosol mist using a compressed-air nebulizer system	Twice-daily dosing may be beneficial for some patients
Antitussives			
Benzonatate	Nonproductive cough due to minor throat or bronchial irritation	*Adults and child older than 10 yrs:* 100 mg po TID up to 600 mg daily *Child younger than 10 yrs:* 8 mg/kg/day in 3–6 divided doses (unlabeled use)	Capsules should be swallowed whole. Release of drug from capsules may cause local anesthetic effect and choking
Codeine	Antitussive	*Adults:* 10–20 mg po q4–6hr PRN. Not to exceed 120 mg/day *Child 6–12 yrs:* 5–10 mg po q4–6hr PRN. Not to exceed 60 mg/day *Child ages 2–5 yrs:* 0.25 mg/kg po up to 4 times daily	Assess respiratory rate and pattern before and during treatment. Oral formulations may be administered with food or milk to minimize GI irritation. Narcan is the antagonist
Diphenhydramine	Allergic rhinitis Antitussive	*Adults:* 25–50 mg po q4hr PRN *Child ages 2–6 yrs:* 6.25 mg po q4hr PRN *Child ages 6–12 yrs:* 12.5 mg po q4hr PRN	Assess degree of nasal stuffiness, rhinorrhea, and sneezing before administration. Fluid intake should be maintained at 1500–2000 mL/day to decrease viscosity of bronchial secretions.
Dextromethorphan	Symptomatic relief of cough caused by minor viral URI. Chronic nonproductive coughs	*Adults and child older than 12 yrs:* 10–20 mg po q4hr *or* 30 mg po q6–8hr *or* 60 mg po q12hr of SR formulation. Not to exceed 120 mg/day *Child 6–12 yrs:* 5–10 mg po q4hr *or* 15 mg q6–8hr *or* 30 mg po q12hr of SR formulation *Child 2–6 yrs:* 2.5–7.5 mg q4hr *or* 7.5 mg q6–8hr *or* 15 mg po q12hr of SR formulation. Not to exceed 30 mg/day	15–30 mg is equivalent in cough suppression to 8–15 mg of codeine Do not immediately follow administration with fluids to prevent dilution of vehicle. Shake suspension well before administration
Hydrocodone	Antitussive	*Adults:* 5 mg po q4–6hr PRN	Assess respiratory rate and pattern prior to and during treatment. Oral formulations may be administered with food or milk to minimize GI irritation. Narcan is the antagonist
Decongestants			
Desoxyephedrine	Relief of nasal congestion that accompanies colds, allergies, or sinusitis. Adjunctive therapy of otitis media	*Adults and child older than 6 yrs:* 2 inhalations per nostril no more often than q2hr. Use not to exceed 7 days.	Emphasize need to take only as directed. Rebound congestion may occur if drug used too frequently or longer than 3–5 days. To use nasal spray: keep head upright and squeeze bottle prescribed number of times briskly while sniffing through nostril. To use nasal solution: Squeeze bulb until dropper contains correct amount of drug. Tilt head back and place 2 drops of solution into nares. Tilt head forward and toward opposite side and inhale through the nostril. Repeat with other nares. To use inhalers: warm inhaler in hand before each use. Wipe inhaler after use. Do not share drug containers with others
Ephedrine		*Adults:* 2 drops (0.5% solution) q4hr *or* 2 drops (0.25% spray)	
Naphazoline		*Adults and child older than 12 yr:* 1–2 drops/sprays (0.05% solution) no more often than q3hr	

TABLE 48–2 DOSAGE REGIMEN FOR SELECTED EXPECTORANTS, ANTITUSSIVES, DECONGESTANTS, AND MUCOLYTICS *Continued*

Drug	Uses	Dosage	Implications
Decongestants *Continued*			
Oxymetazoline		*Adults and child older than 6 yrs:* 2–3 sprays or drops (0.05% solution) BID *Child ages 2–5 yrs:* 2–3 drops (0.025% solution) BID	
Phenylephrine		*Adults and child over 12 yrs:* 2–3 sprays in each nostril q3–4hr	
Phenylpropanolamine		*Adults and child older than 12 yrs:* 25 mg po q4hr *Adults:* 75 mg po q12hr of SR formulation *Child 2–6 yrs:* 6.25 mg po q4hr *Child 6–12 yrs:* 12.5 mg po q4hr	
Propylhexedrine		*Adults and child older than 6 yrs:* 1–2 inhalations in each nostril no more than q2hr	
Pseudoephedrine		*Adults and child older than 12 yrs:* 60 mg po q4–6hr *Adults:* 120 mg po q12hr of SR formulation	
Tetrahydrozoline		*Adults and child older than 6 yrs:* 2 drops (0.1% solution) q3–4hr *Child 2–6 yrs:* 2–3 drops (0.05% solution) q4–6hr	
Xylometazoline		*Adults and child older than 12 yrs:* 2–3 drops or sprays (0.1% solution) q8–10hr *Child age 2–12 yrs:* 2–3 drops (0.05% solution) q8–10hr	
Mucolytics			
Acetylcysteine	Mucolytic	*Adults and child:* 1–10 mL of 20% solution or 2–20 mL of 10% solution q2–6hr via face mask *or* amount of 10–20% solution required to produce heavy mist via nebulizer *or* 1–2 mL of 10–20% solution q1–4hr by direct instillation	Instruct patient to clear airway completely before taking aerosol treatment. Encourage adequate fluid intake (2000–3000 mL) per day to decrease viscosity of secretions
	Acetaminophen overdose	*Adults and child:* 140 mg/kg initially followed by 70 mg/kg q4hr × 17 doses	Initial plasma acetaminophen levels are drawn at least 4 hours after ingestion of acetaminophen. Drug reacts with rubber, metals (iron, nickel, and copper). Avoid contact with these substances
Other Respiratory Drugs			
$Alpha_1$-proteinase inhibitor	Panacinar emphysema	*Adults:* 60 mg/kg IV once weekly	IV infusion rate is at least 0.08 mL/kg/minute. Should be immunized for hepatitis B before beginning therapy
Beractant	Prophylaxis and rescue of infants at high risk for IRDS or hyaline membrane disease	*Infants:* 4 mg/kg intratracheal. May repeat dose no sooner than 6 hours after preceding dose	Beractant is frozen and must be warmed before administration. Give through #5 French catheter placed with tip just beyond end of endotracheal tube above the carina. Do not instill the drug into mainstream bronchus. Quarter doses are administered, with infant placed in various positions. After each quarter-dose, the infant is ventilated with positive pressure
Colfosceril palmitate	Prophylaxis for infants at risk for IRDS	*Infants:* 2.5 mg/kg intratracheal ×2 doses. Repeat in 12 hours in all infants remaining on ventilator	Administer through sideport adapter of endotracheal tube. The infant must be in the supine midline position for the first half of the dose. Turn the infant 45 degrees to the right for 20 seconds, return to the midline position, give the second half of the dose, and then turn 45 degrees to the left for 30 seconds

IRDS, Infant respiratory distress syndrome; SR, sustained release.

nonsteroidal anti-inflammatory drugs may exist for aspirin. Aspirin-containing products should be avoided in patients with thrombocytopenia or bleeding disorders. Products containing alcohol, aspartame, saccharine, sugar, or tartrazine (FDC yellow dye #5) should be avoided in patients with hypersensitivity to these compounds. Cautious use is warranted in patients with head trauma, increased intracranial pressure, severe hepatic, renal, or pulmonary disease, hypothyroidism, adrenal insufficiency, and alcoholism. Older adults and debilitated patients are at greater risk for CNS depression caused by opioids.

Nonopioid antitussives vary in their adverse effects. Benzonatate can produce sedation, headache, and mild dizziness. Nasal congestion, pruritus, and skin eruptions, as well as GI upset have occurred. Benzonatate is contraindicated in patients with hypersensitivity. Cross-sensitivity with other ester-type local anesthetics (tetracaine, procaine, and others) may occur.

The adverse effects of diphenhydramine are related to its antihistaminic characteristics. Drowsiness, dry mouth, and anorexia are most common, but the patient may also note blurred vision, photosensitivity, tinnitus, a paradoxical excitement that is even greater in children, dizziness, and headache. It is generally contraindicated with acute attacks of asthma, in hypersensitivity, and in patients with known alcohol intolerance because some of the liquid formulations contain alcohol.

The adverse effects of dextromethorphan are few. Nausea has been noted and, with high doses, dizziness and sedation. Dextromethorphan is contraindicated in hypersensitivity, in patients taking monoamine oxidase inhibitors or selective serotonin reuptake inhibitors, and in patients with known alcohol intolerance because some products contain alcohol. It should be used cautiously in patients with a cough lasting more than 1 week or that is accompanied by fever, rash, or headache. Safe use of dextromethorphan during pregnancy and lactation or in children under the age of 2 years has not been established.

Pharmacokinetics

The pharmacokinetics of the various antitussives are similar overall (see Table 48–1). The onset of most of the drugs occurs in 15 to 30 minutes, reach peak action in 30 to 90 minutes, and have a duration of action of 3 to 8 hours. Codeine and hydrocodone are 30- to 35-percent protein bound. Diphenhydramine is 80- to 85-percent protein bound. The half-life of codeine and hydrocodone is 3 to 4 hours, whereas the half-life of diphenhydramine is 2.4 to 9.3 hours. The half-life of dextromethorphan is unknown.

Drug-Drug Interactions

CNS depressants, alcohol, sedative-hypnotics, and antidepressants provide additive CNS depression when they are used concurrently with opioid and nonopioid antitussives (Table 48–3). In addition, diphenhydramine produces additive CNS depression, and anticholinergic, and antihistaminic effects with other quinidines and disopyramide.

There are many drug-drug interactions with dextromethorphan. Concurrent use with monoamine oxidase inhibitors or selective serotonin reuptake inhibitors results in serotonin syndrome (e.g., excitation, confusion, hypotension, and hyperpyrexia). Additive CNS depression has been noted with concurrent use of antihistamines, alcohol, sedative-hypnotics, other antidepressants, or opioids. Quinidine may increase the blood levels and adverse effects of dextromethorphan.

Dosage Regimens

An antitussive dose, whether used for an adult or child, depends on the specific formulation (see Table 48–2). The dosage of extended-release formulations is larger than that of lozenges, syrups, oral solutions, capsules or tablets. Older adults or debilitated patients may require a dosage reduction because they are more susceptible to CNS depression, anticholinergic effects, and constipation than younger persons.

Decongestants

- ❒ Desoxyephedrine (VICKS INHALER)
- ❒ Ephedrine (KONDON'S NASAL JELLY, PRETZ-D, combinations)
- ❒ Naphazoline (PRIVINE)
- ❒ Oxymetazoline (AFRIN, ALLEREST, many others)
- ❒ Phenylephrine (NEO-SYNEPHRINE, CHERACOL NASAL SPRAY, SINEX); (🍁) NAFRINE
- ❒ Phenylpropanolamine HCL (TRIAMINIC, CONTACT)
- ❒ Propylhexedrine (BENZEDREX INHALER)
- ❒ Pseudoephedrine (SUDAFED, SUDAFED-SA, NOVAFED, DRIXORAL, AFRIN)
- ❒ Tetrahydrozoline (TYZINE)
- ❒ Xylometazoline (NEO-SYNEPHRINE II LONG-ACTING)

Indications

Decongestants are used to relieve symptoms associated with rhinitis, allergies, sinusitis, and colds. They have also been used as adjuncts for middle ear infections because they decrease congestion around the eustachian tubes. Eustachian tube dysfunction and ear pain during air travel is also responsive to decongestants.

Because of their popular use and lack of serious adverse effects, many topical preparations are available OTC. Some of the drugs approved by the Food and Drug Administration as safe and effective topical decongestants include oxymetazoline, phenylephrine, and xylometazoline. OTC oral formulations approved for use include phenylephrine, pseudoephedrine, and phenylpropanolamine.

Phenylpropanolamine has also been used along with behavior modification, diet, and exercise as a short-term adjunct in the management of exogenous obesity. It is also used to relieve nasal congestion resulting from deep sea diving and rebound congestion due to overuse of topical decongestants.

Pharmacodynamics

Nasal decongestants act by stimulating alpha receptors on the smooth muscle of nasal blood vessels. Stimulation of alpha receptors causes vasoconstriction and results in reduced blood flow, reduced fluid exudation, and shrinkage of edematous membranes. The response from topical use of decongestants is rapid and intense. The vasoconstriction is delayed and less intense with oral formulations.

TABLE 48–3 DRUG-DRUG INTERACTIONS OF SELECTED ANTITUSSIVES, DECONGESTANTS, AND MUCOLYTICS*

Drug	Interactive Drugs	Interaction
Antitussives		
Codeine	Alcohol	Additive CNS depression
Hydrocodone	Antidepressants	
Diphenhydramine	Antihistamines	
Dextromethorphan	Opioids	
	Sedative-hypnotics	
Diphenhydramine	Tricyclic antidepressants	Additive anticholinergic properties
	Quinidine	
	Disopyramide	
	MAO inhibitors	Intensify and prolong anticholinergic actions
Dextromethorphan	MAO inhibitors	Serotonin syndrome, hypotension, hyperpyrexia
	SSRIs	
	Quinidine	Increased blood levels and adverse effects of dextromethorphan
Decongestants		
Desoxyephedrine	Tricyclic antidepressants	Increase cardiovascular effects of phenylephrine
Ephedrine	Ergonovine	
Naphazoline	Oxytocin	
Oxymetazoline		
Phenylephrine		
Propylhexedrine		
Tetrahydrozoline		
Xylometazoline		
	Guanethidine	Decreased effect of interactive drug
	Phenothiazines	
	Beta blockers	Mutual inhibition
	Digoxin	Increased risk of arrhythmias
	Theophylline	
	MAO inhibitors	Increased vasopressor effects
	Methyldopa	
	Furazolidone	
Phenylpropanolamine	Adrenergic drugs	Additive sympathomimetic effects
	MAO inhibitors	Increased vasopressor effects
	General anesthetics	Increased risk of arrhythmias
	Reserpine	Increased risk of hypertension
	Tricyclic antidepressants	
	Ganglionic blocking drugs	
Mucolytics		
Acetylcysteine	Activated charcoal	May decrease effectiveness of acetylcysteine

*There are no significant drug-drug interactions with expectorants such as guaifenesin.
CNS, Central nervous system; MAO, monoamine oxidase; SSRIs, selective serotonin reuptake inhibitors.

Adverse Effects and Contraindications

Stinging, burning, and drying of nasal mucosa may occur with the use of nasal decongestant drops or sprays. Prolonged use of a topical nasal decongestant (more than 3 to 5 days) may produce chronic congestion (i.e., rhinitis medicamentosa). After more than 3 days of continuous use, response to these drugs becomes blunted *(tachyphylaxis),* leading to increased use, often on an hourly basis. Cessation results in marked rebound congestion, presumably due to marked reflex vasodilation and an erythematous mucosa. The congestion resolves in 2 or 3 weeks if topical decongestants are stopped. Alpha-adrenergic blocking drugs can aggravate existing rhinitis and cause mild nasal congestion in normal patients.

Occasionally, mild CNS stimulation occurs in the form of restlessness, nervousness, tremors, headache, and insomnia. Large doses may produce tachycardia, palpitations (particularly in patients with heart disease), lightheadedness, nausea, and vomiting. These adverse effects are most likely to occur in patients who are hypersensitive to adrenergic drugs. Acute psychotic reactions and excessive CNS stimulation has occurred in patients taking high doses of phenylpropanolamine combined with antihistamines. Rebound congestion and tachyphylaxis is not seen with pseudoephedrine.

The use of adrenergic decongestants is contraindicated in patients who are concurrently using monoamine oxidase inhibitors and in patients with known intolerance to active ingredients or its preservatives (bisulfites, thimerosal, aromatics, or chlorobutanol). They should be used with caution in patients who have heart disease, marked hypertension, advanced arteriosclerotic disease, insulin dependent diabetes mellitus, or hyperthyroidism. Overdosage in patients over 60 may result in hallucinations, CNS depression, and seizures.

Pharmacokinetics

The absorption of decongestants following intranasal administration is minimal. The onset of drug action occurs in 1 to 2 minutes via the intranasal route and 15 to 30 minutes when the drug is taken orally. Peak action time varies from 5 to 10 minutes to 1 to 2 hours. The duration of action ranges from 30 minutes for phenylephrine to 12 hours for pseudoephedrine (see Table 48–1).

Drug-Drug Interactions

There are extensive drug-drug interactions with decongestants. Table 48–3 provides an overview of specific interactions. Many of the interactions are related to drug effects on the cardiovascular or autonomic nervous systems. Concurrent use of drugs that acidify urine decreases the therapeutic effects of decongestants, whereas concurrent use of drugs that alkalinize the urine can contribute to toxicity.

Dosage Regimen

Dosages for nasal decongestants typically are one to two drops/sprays twice daily to every three to four hours. Oral formulations are taken no more often than every four to six hours (see Table 48–2).

Mucolytics

❒ Acetylcysteine (MUCOMYST)
❒ Sodium chloride nasal solution

Indications

Two compounds, sodium chloride nasal solution and acetylcysteine, are used as an adjunctive treatment for patients with abnormally thick mucous secretions. They are particularly helpful in patients with acute and chronic bronchopulmonary disease, atelectasis from mucous obstruction, and for patients with cystic fibrosis. Furthermore, acetylcysteine is believed to protect the liver from damage caused by acetaminophen overdose.

Pharmacodynamics

Acetylcysteine interrupts the DNA and glycoprotein bonds at the molecular level through the process of mucolysis. It reacts directly with mucus by splitting the disulfide bonds of mucoproteins. Thus, sputum viscosity is reduced and pulmonary secretions are easier to cough up. Liquefaction occurs within minutes after administration.

Acetylcysteine is believed to protect the liver from damage caused by acetaminophen by maintaining or restoring the hepatic concentration of glutathione, a tripeptide that serves to protect erythrocytes from oxidation and hemolysis. Glutathione is necessary for inactivation of acetaminophen metabolites.

Adverse Effects and Contraindications

Acetylcysteine can trigger bronchospasm in susceptible patients. For this reason, the drug is usually administered with or immediately after a bronchodilator. The most common adverse effects of acetylcysteine include a burning in the back of the throat, stomatitis, nausea, rhinorrhea, and epistaxis. It can also cause drowsiness, increased respiratory secretions, urticaria, fever, and chills. Because of its sulfur content, acetylcysteine has the additional disadvantage of smelling like rotten eggs. The drug may also corrode iron, metal, copper, or rubber.

There are no known adverse effects to the intranasal use of sodium chloride. The adverse effects of sodium chloride are seen primarily during oral and intravenous use.

Pharmacokinetics

Acetylcysteine is absorbed from the GI tract following oral administration. Action is local when inhalation route is used. The remainder of the drug is absorbed from the pulmonary epithelium. The distribution, protein binding, and half-life are unknown, although acetylcysteine is biotransformed by the liver (see Table 48–1).

Drug-Drug Interactions

Drug-drug interactions with acetylcysteine or sodium chloride are limited. Activated charcoal may adsorb acetylcysteine, thus decreasing its effectiveness as an antidote. It should not be mixed in the same solution as tetracycline, erythromycin, amphotericin B, or ampicillin (see Table 48–3).

Dosage Regimen

The method used for administration of acetylcysteine dictates the dosage used. For example, a dose of 1 to 10 mL of 20-percent solution, or 2 to 20 mL of 10-percent solution may be given undiluted three or four times daily by handheld nebulizer, aerosol, or intermittent positive-pressure breathing machine. The usual dose is 3 to 5 mL of 20-percent solution or 6 to 10 mL of a 10-percent solution. If a nebulizer is used with a croupette or tent, the quantity of a 10- to 20-percent solution sufficient to produce a heavy mist is used. Direct instillation to the airway through an endotracheal or tracheostomy tube requires 1 to 2 mL of a 10- to 20-percent solution every 1 to 4 hours (see Table 48–2).

Acetylcysteine, when used as an antagonist to acetaminophen overdose, is dosed based on body weight. Initially, 140 mg/kg of body weight is given, followed by a maintenance dose of 70 mg/kg. This can be repeated every 4 hours for up to 17 doses.

Antihistamines

Histamines are responsible for the inflammatory response. Mast cells and basophils contain large amounts of histamine. Antihistamines can be used as decongestants because they block the effects of histamine at various receptor sites in the body. Antihistamines are discussed in Chapter 46. They are divided into six groups: ethanolamines, ethylenediamines, alkylamines, piperazines, and phenothiazines. The newest generation of antihistamines are considered nonsedating. The groups differ in their anticholinergic, antiemetic (see Chapter 44), GI (see Chapter 42), and sedative effects, and all but the newer drugs have the same basic pharmacodynamics and the same major adverse effects.

Miscellaneous Respiratory Drugs

❒ $Alpha_1$-proteinase inhibitor (PROLASTIN)
❒ Beractant (SURVANTA)
❒ Colfosceril palmitate (EXOSURF)

ALPHA$_1$-PROTEINASE INHIBITOR

Alpha$_1$-proteinase inhibitor is used for chronic replacement therapy in patients with clinically demonstrable panacinar emphysema. Panacinar emphysema is a chronic hereditary and usually fatal disease that traditionally manifests itself in the third or fourth decade of life. An imbalance between elastase and alpha$_1$-antitrypsin inhibitor is believed to be the basis for the disorder.

The adverse effects of alpha$_1$-proteinase inhibitor include a fever that occurs approximately 12 hours after drug administration. The fever resolves spontaneously. Lightheadedness, dizziness, and transient leukocytosis have also been reported.

Absorption of the drug is essentially complete following IV administration. It achieves high concentrations in epithelial fluid of the lungs. The drug is broken down in the intravascular spaces, with a half-life of 4.5 to 5.2 days.

There are no significant contraindications to the use of the drug, although caution is warranted in patients who are at risk for circulatory overload. Although the drug is derived from pooled fresh human plasma and has been heat-treated to reduce the potential transmission of disease, safe use in children and during pregnancy has not been fully established. There are no known drug-drug interactions.

Alpha$_1$-proteinase inhibitor is administered IV in dosages of 60 mg/kg once weekly. The IV infusion rate is at least 0.08 mL/kg/minute. Patients should be immunized for hepatitis B before beginning therapy.

BERACTANT AND COLFOSCERIL

Beractant and colfosceril palmitate are surfactants. Surfactants are used to treat newborns at risk for infant respiratory distress syndrome (infants with gestational age under 32 weeks or birth weight under 1300 g, or both) and hyaline membrane disease in premature infants. A deficiency of surfactant prevents re-expansion of small alveoli in the lungs. This problem causes the larger alveoli to enlarge. The result is a decrease in lung compliance and inadequate pulmonary perfusion.

Surfactants lower the surface tension on alveolar surfaces during respiration and stabilize alveoli so they are less likely to collapse at resting transpulmonary pressures. These drugs replenish surfactant, restoring surface activity to the lungs. Oxygenation improves within minutes of drug administration. Both beractant and colfosceril are distributed and biotransformed by lung tissues.

Surfactants can cause adverse effects such as pulmonary and intracranial hemorrhage, hypotension, apnea, and barotrauma. Infants receiving surfactants have a higher incidence of patent ductus arteriosus. Transient bradycardia, oxygen desaturation, and an increased CO_2 tension has been noted with beractant. Beractant is contraindicated in infants who are at risk for circulatory overload. Nosocomial infections have been noted with beractant, although there has been no increase in mortality.

Gagging has been occasionally noted with colfosceril palmitate. Apnea, bradycardia, and tachycardia are rare. Failure to reduce peak ventilator inspiratory pressures after chest expansion and drug administration may result in overdistention of the lungs and fatal pulmonary air leak. Hyperoxia may develop, with failure to reduce transcutaneous oxygen saturation to less than 95 percent. Hypocapnia and reduced blood flow to the brain may result if there is failure to reduce arterial or transcutaneous CO_2 levels to below 30 mmHg.

These drugs must be administered by highly skilled health care providers. Although most health care providers believe that both drugs are equally effective, because of the differences in administration techniques, timing of doses, and patient responses, only one of the drugs should be used at any one time in neonatal nurseries. Table 48–2 discusses dosage and administration techniques.

Critical Thinking Process

Assessment

History of Present Illness

Attention should be given to obtaining a health history that includes environmental aspects and patient comfort. The patient's history may include nasal congestion, postnasal drip, nasal discharge, sneezing, sore throat, headache, itchy eyes, lacrimation, earache with decreased hearing, upper respiratory tract infection, or allergies. The sensation of postnasal drip is influenced more by the thickness of the drainage than the quantity. Ask the patient about the duration and extent of nasal congestion and about factors that precipitate or relieve the symptoms. Ask if there are times when symptoms are more pronounced under certain weather conditions, if they occur year round, or if they occur only in a particular season.

Malaise, pharyngitis, laryngitis, cough, headache, and substernal tightness and burning are common complaints in the patient with a common cold. There may be a history of a nonproductive cough or an overactive cough that interrupts the patient's sleep or produces muscular pain. The type, severity, and frequency of the cough should be assessed. Inquire about factors that trigger or relieve the cough.

Obtain a smoking history from the patient. Determine how long the patient has smoked and how many packs per day. If the patient does not smoke at present, ask if they have ever smoked. Information regarding the use of chewing tobacco should also be elicited.

Rhinorrhea is common with colds and occurs with allergic rhinitis and idiopathic rhinitis. In the classic presentation of allergic rhinitis, pruritus of the nose, eyes, and oropharynx are the predominant symptoms. Non-nasal allergic symptoms such as shortness of breath or GI distress may also be present. There is no sneezing with idiopathic rhinitis. Rhinorrhea associated with idiopathic rhinitis is watery, and the patient may indicate that the episodes are initiated by cold air, odors, nasal irritants, and stress.

Nasal and conjunctival itching occurs with allergic rhinitis but not with idiopathic rhinitis. A watery discharge from the eyes is common with allergic rhinitis, and a recurrent, severe epistaxis may be seen in patients with atrophic rhinitis.

Past Health History

Because many respiratory problems are associated with pollutants such as asbestos, fumes, organic dust particles, and chemicals, obtain information about the patient's occupation and geographic environment. In addition, determine whether there is a family history of allergy, prior allergy testing, or treatment of allergies.

Physical Exam Findings

Clear drainage depicts a localized process such as unilateral sinusitis, whereas bilateral drainage is due to a more general or systemic process. For the patient with a common cold, the nasal mucosa and pharynx may appear mildly swollen and erythematous. The edema may partially or totally occlude the nasal passages. A watery or thick, yellow nasal discharge and mild lymphadenopathy can be noted. Although fever is uncommon in adults with a common cold, it frequently occurs in children. Therefore, the patient's temperature should be taken.

The nasal mucosa of the patient with allergic rhinitis may appear pale, boggy, and edematous, or it may have a bluish color. The patient's sense of smell may be reduced. Sneezing is common. Allergic shiners, the bluish discoloration of the lower eyelids due to chronic nasal congestion, are a common finding. Nasal polyps may be noted, especially in patients with perennial rhinitis. The gesture that allergic children often display of repeatedly lifting the tip of the nose with an open palm (allergic salute) can cause a permanent transverse crease above the tip of the nose that may be seen in adulthood. Postnasal drip, which may be evident by strands of stringy mucus down the back of the pharynx, can cause frequent throat clearing and coughing. Cervical adenopathy may or may not be present.

In idiopathic rhinitis, the nasal mucosa varies from bright red to a bluish hue. If a nasal discharge is present, note the amount, color, and thickness. Clear drainage suggests a diagnosis of idiopathic, allergic, or nonallergic rhinitis, whereas thick and discolored (yellow, brown, green) drainage suggests bacterial or viral infection.

With atrophic rhinitis, epistaxis and nasal crusting with a foul odor may be present and the sense of smell may be disturbed. The throat is usually dry and, as a rule, contains crusts. A husky voice or hoarseness is common.

Assess the patient's breath sounds. A dry, nonproductive cough does not produce sputum and is not associated with chest congestion. A congested, nonproductive cough is related to chest congestion, and a small amount of mucus is produced. A congested, productive cough is identified with chest congestion and expectoration of mucus.

Diagnostic Testing

The patient's history and physical exam are the two most important aspects of assessing the patient with a cough. Laboratory tests are helpful in confirming or evaluating the severity of the etiology. Laboratory testing is not usually indicated for the patient with a common cold or rhinitis. However, if leukocytosis is present, it indicates a disorder other than the common cold. A nasal smear should be examined if exudate is present to identify the etiology. An eosinophil smear should be examined if the diagnosis is uncertain. In patients with idiopathic rhinitis, a nasal smear may also help rule out allergic rhinitis.

If allergy testing is warranted, methylxanthines and antihistamines must be discontinued at least 3 days before testing. Pulmonary function testing, radiographs, fiberoptic bronchoscopy, and arterial blood gases may be warranted in some patients.

Developmental Considerations

Perinatal Nasal stuffiness and epistaxis are fairly common during pregnancy. They are the result of estrogen-induced edema and vascular congestion of the nasal mucosa. Respiratory depression in the fetus is a theoretic possibility if a woman with severely impaired renal function chronically takes dextromethorphan during and up to the time of delivery.

Pediatric The common cold is the most prevalent infectious disease among children of all ages. Three annual waves of the common cold typically occur in children, with the greatest incidence occurring with the opening of school. The more severe cases with a tendency toward complications occur in midwinter. Another round of mild cases of the common cold also occurs in the spring.

Cold symptoms in a young child can pose additional problems. The obstruction of the upper airways cause difficulty in sucking, consumes energy, and increases oxygen needs. Restlessness, malaise, and anorexia result. A crankiness and an acetone breath odor appear due to secondary dehydration. Additionally, a mild degree of ketoacidosis can occur when fever is present. Viral enteritis may be present and accounts for an associated diarrhea.

Geriatric In the standard medical model of diagnosis, there is a 1:1 correspondence between clinical signs and symptoms and a pathologic process. However, it is believed that the medical model does not accurately define the presentation of many illnesses in the older adult. Older adults and people with chronic debilitating diseases are especially vulnerable to complications associated with upper respiratory disorders.

Psychosocial Considerations

Choices between ethnomedical options and interventions of Western medicine vary among ethnic groups and vary from one patient experience to another. At any given time, treatment of the common cold and other upper respiratory disorders may reflect exclusive use of traditional herbal remedies or a combination of herbs and Western medicine. In addition, it is often said that if families would familiarize themselves with herbs, their medicinal properties, and their uses, many visits to the health care provider would be saved. Herbs, no matter what their modern name and no matter how unorthodox they are said to be, continue to be the treatment of choice by those who value their effects (see Chapter 60).

Societal and pharmaceutical industries encourage approximately 90 percent of patients to treat URI symptoms at home. With adults experiencing an average of two to four colds a year and colds occurring more commonly in families with children, over $500 million is spent on OTC preparations (see Case Study—Common Cold with Rinorrhea).

Analysis and Management

Treatment Objectives

Treatment objectives for the patient with an upper respiratory disorder includes strategies that will prevent, minimize, or help correct symptoms. Treatment should be directed toward identifying a specific underlying etiology.

Treatment Options

Because the common cold is an acute URI of viral origin and because there is no cure for the cold, treatment is simply symptomatic. Because the common cold is a viral etiology, there is no justification for the routine use of antibiotics. Antibiotics are appropriate only if a bacterial infection is present. Furthermore, cough suppression is generally not needed in patients with uncomplicated viral respiratory infection.

Drug Variables

Because no one drug relieves all cold symptoms, a number of cold remedies containing a combination of cough and cold ingredients have been formulated by the pharmaceutical industry and are available without prescription. Combination formulations should be reserved for patients who have multiple symptoms. Most of the products contain an antihistamine (chlorpheniramine), a nasal decongestant (pseudoephedrine or phenylpropanolamine), and an analgesic (acetaminophen). Some products come in several formulations with different ingredients and are advertised for different purposes (Table 48–4). However, the drug chosen should contain only those components that are appropriate for the symptoms that are present. Patients who require relief of a single symptom are best treated with a single-entity formulation. Single formulations are preferred because they permit flexibility and individualization of dosage.

Expectorants, antitussives, decongestants, and mucolytic drugs relieve symptoms, but they are not curative. Decongestants may be helpful for the common cold and rhinorrhea, and have been shown to be more reliable than antihistamines (see Chapter 46). They are helpful not only in providing symptom relief but also for preventing sinus and eustachian tube obstruction that could result in sinusitis and otitis media, respectively.

Oral decongestants are generally less effective than topical ones and can cause systemic adverse effects. Because sympathomimetics cause systemic vasoconstriction, they may raise blood pressure when they are used in doses sufficient to alleviate nasal congestion. Oral pseudoephedrine produces a dramatic reduction in nasal symptoms. Oxymetazoline and phenylpropanolamine were also found to be effective.

There are no oral sympathomimetic drugs that provide selective local vasoconstriction. Nasal sprays are more effective for this purpose. However, they are associated with rebound congestion after the drug effect subsides, leading to abuse of the sprays.

Although few data support the effectiveness of expectorants or antitussives for the common cold, when the cough significantly interferes with sleeping or eating, an opioid antitussive can be used. Codeine is the drug of choice. In many cases, a dose before bedtime will suffice. Liquid and tablet formulations are equally effective. The potential for abuse and dependency of the opioid remains.

Nonopioid antitussives lack the potential for dependency but are not as effective as codeine. The most popular and effective OTC antitussive is dextromethorphan. It has a mild suppressant effect. Dextromethorphan does not relieve a cough associated with postnasal drip, however. Many of the nonopioid antitussives also contain alcohol, sympathomimetics, and antihistamines. The mucolytic effects of alcohol are relatively insignificant. The sympathomimetic component is of little value except in patients whose cough originates from chronic idiopathic rhinitis. The antihistamine component is most useful for patients with allergic upper airway disease and is a helpful adjunct for sleep when it is used before bedtime. Furthermore, some nonopioid formulations dull the peripheral sensory receptors. This is why mild, topical anesthetics are contained in many sprays, syrups, and cough lozenges. The efficacy of these anesthetics is questionable, however.

Expectorants such as guaifenesin are heavily consumed. Over 60 different preparations of guaifenesin are prescribed

TABLE 48–4 SELECTED EXAMPLES OF OVER-THE-COUNTER COLD, COUGH, AND ALLERGY REMEDIES

	Ingredients				
Brand Name	ANTIHISTAMINE	NASAL DECONGESTANT	ANTITUSSIVE	EXPECTORANT	ANALGESIC
ACTIFED	Triprolidine	Pseudoephedrine			
ALLEREST	Chlorpheniramine	Phenylpropanolamine			
CHERACOL D COUGH LIQUID			Dextromethorphan	Guaifenesin	
COMTREX MULTISYMPTOM COLD AND FLU RELIEF	Chlorpheniramine	Phenylpropanolamine	Dextromethorphan		Acetaminophen
CONTACT	Chlorpheniramine	Phenylpropanolamine			
CORICIDIN	Chlorpheniramine				Acetaminophen
CORICIDIN D	Chlorpheniramine	Phenylpropanolamine			Acetaminophen
TYLENOL COLD, MULTISYMPTOM	Chlorpheniramine	Pseudoephedrine	Dextromethorphan		Acetaminophen
TYLENOL LIQUID, CHILDREN'S	Chlorpheniramine	Phenylpropanolamine			Acetaminophen
DIMETAPP ELIXIR/TABLETS/EXTENTABS	Brompheniramine	Phenylpropanolamine			
DRISTAN	Chlorpheniramine	Phenylephrine			Acetaminophen
DRIXORAL COUGH AND CONGESTION LIQUID CAPS	Dexbrompheniramine	Pseudoephedrine			
NOVAHISTINE ELIXIR	Chlorpheniramine	Phenylephedrine			
NOVAHISTINE DMX		Pseudoephedrine	Dextromethorphan	Guaifenesin	
ROBITUSSIN CF		Phenylpropanolamine	Dextromethorphan	Guaifenesin	
ROBITUSSIN DM			Dextromethorphan	Guaifenesin	
ROBITUSSIN PE		Pseudoephedrine		Guaifenesin	
SINE-OFF SINUS MEDICINE	Chlorpheniramine	Phenylpropanolamine			Aspirin
SINUTAB	Chlorpheniramine	Pseudoephedrine			Acetaminophen
SINUTAB WITHOUT DROWSINESS		Pseudoephedrine			Acetaminophen

Case Study Common Cold with Rhinorrhea

Patient History

History of Present Illness	JE is a 27-year-old female who presents today with complaints of a "stuffy head," and a dry, hacking cough that is keeping her and her partner awake at night. She reports that she has had these symptoms for 3 days and that they are interfering with her work performance. She is requesting a diagnosis so that she purchases the "right medicine at the drug store." She reports that fellow workers have been sick also with "head colds," and in her work at a day care center, 12 children have been absent because of coughs and colds. She denies using other drugs at this time.
Past Health History	JE has a history of seasonal allergic rhinitis, which she was treating by avoiding suspected allergens as much as possible. She self-treats with OTC antihistamines only if the sneezing becomes uncontrollable. She denies history of cardiovascular disease, hypertension, hyperthyroidism, or diabetes mellitus. Denies drug or food allergies, or the use of home remedies.
Physical Exam	BP 116/72. Temp: 99.2° F, pulse 88, respirations 24. Tympanic membranes without bulging or retraction, landmarks visible. Nasal passages with presence of clear, discharge. Oropharynx slightly reddened with mucus present. No palpable cervical adenopathy. Breath sounds are clear bilaterally.
Diagnostic Testing	Diagnostic testing is not indicated for patients with common cold or rhinitis.
Developmental Considerations	JE believes that she finally has a position in a stable company that will maximize her contributions and also provide her with long-lasting career opportunities.
Psychosocial Considerations	She expresses concern that the infection will progress to another bout of sinusitis and cost her time away from work. She chooses to treat with OTC cough and cold remedies as much as possible to keep costs down
Economic Factors	JE does not carry health insurance because of her recent change in employment. She will pay entire cost of treatment regimen.

Variables Influencing Decision

Treatment Objectives	• Prevent, minimize, and relief of uncomfortable symptoms.

Drug Variables	*Drug Summary*	*Patient Variables*
Indications	OTC cough and cold remedies indicated for symptomatic management of uncomplicated coughs and colds.	JE diagnosed with nasopharyngitis with rhinitis. Wrong season for seasonal rhinitis. This will be a decision point.
Pharmacodynamics	Sedating cough formulation can be used for HS suppression. Daytime hours JE could use a combination of dextromethorphan and guaifenesin.	JE will only take drugs that are nonsedating owing to concerns about performance at work but wants something to help her sleep at night. This will become a decison point.
Adverse Effects and Contraindications	OTC cough and cold preparations should generally be used with caution or contraindicated in patients with a history of cardiovascular disease, hypertension, hyperthyroidism, or diabetes.	JE's history is negative for these conditions. This will not be a decison point.
Pharmacokinetics	Pharmacokinetics of majority of cold and cold remedies not a major decision point for JE.	There are no patient considerations at this time for JE regarding the pharmacokinetics of drug options. This will not be a decision point.

Case Study Common Cold with Rhinorrhea—cont'd

Drug Variables	*Drug Summary*	*Patient Variables*
Dosage Regimen	Many cough and cold remedies can be taken once daily. This simplifies the treatment regimen and promotes patient compliance.	JE is motivated toward symptom relief yet prefers treatment regimen that will minimize interference with her work performance.
Lab Considerations	Diagnostic testing is not indicated for patients with a common cold or rhinitis.	There are no patient considerations affecting the decision for treatment.
Cost Index*	Guaifenesin cough formula: 1 Dextromethorphan and guaifenesin: 1 Codeine sulfate elixir: 1	JE believes that she is able to purchase necessary OTC preparations without hardship.

Summary of Decision Points

- JE is diagnosed with nasopharyngitis with rhinitis (wrong season for seasonal rhinitis).
- JE will only take drugs that are nonsedating owing to concerns about performance at work but wants something to help her sleep at night.
- JE is motivated toward symptom relief yet prefers regimen that will minimize interference with work performance.

DRUGS TO BE USED

- Combination guaifenesin and dextromethorphan (10 mg/100 mg) 1–2 teaspoons po q4hr PRN for daytime cough suppression
- Codeine sulfate cough syrup 1–2 teaspoons po HS cough suppression
- Phenylpropanolamine 75 mg caps 1 (extended-release formulation) po q12hr for nasal congestion

*Cost index:
1 = $ < 30/mo.
2 = $ 30–40/mo.
3 = $ 40–50/mo.
4 = $ 50–60/mo.
5 = $ > 60/mo.

AWP of 15, 75-mg extended release capsules of phenylpropanolamine is approximately $.50.
AWP of 120 mL of dextromethorphan 10 mg with 100 mg guaifenesin combination oral solution is approximately $2.
AWP of 120 mL of 10 mg/5 mL codeine cough syrup is approximately $4.

when the patient insists on taking something for the cough but when clear indications for cough suppression is lacking. However, the expectorants are often combined with an effective cough suppressant. As such, they seem to provide beneficial effects, but by themselves they have no proven effect and represent unnecessary expense to the patient.

Treatment of allergic and nonallergic rhinitis is directed toward the control of symptoms. Allergic rhinitis generally responds to combined oral decongestant and antihistamine, but these agents are not usually first-line drugs. A preparation containing the least sedating or a nonsedating antihistamine should be tried first (see Chapter 46). If a response does not occur, an antihistamine from another drug class may be tried. Tolerance will develop to the drug over time. An antihistamine from another class can be substituted when the patient develops symptoms while taking a particular agent.

Nonallergic rhinitis is better treated with a decongestant only. For tenacious mucus, the use of mucolytics and expectorants can be helpful. Both allergic rhinitis and nonallergic conditions may benefit from intranasal steroid sprays, and allergic rhinitis also may be improved with topical cromolyn sodium.

Patient Variables

An enormous number of OTC preparations are available for the common cold, but only a few have been carefully studied. There is no good evidence that OTC drugs are effective in preschool children. In this age group, serious toxicity from OTC drugs are noted, especially with combination formulations. If OTC drugs are used, single-ingredient preparations are recommended.

If antitussives are used in young children, it must be done with caution because they can depress the cough reflex, leading to aspiration. Caution should also be used with combination cough and cold products because many contain aspirin because of the well-known relationship of influenza viral infection and Reye's syndrome. It is worth noting that many patients expect to receive a syrup formulation for cough suppression. Thus, prescribing the drug as a syrup may provide some psychological benefit. However, coughs that last longer than 1 week or that are accompanied by fever, rash, or headache require cautious evaluation. Furthermore, many of the preparations contain sugar and should be used carefully in patients with diabetes.

Pharmacotherapy is warranted in patients with allergic rhinitis who find avoidance of allergens impractical or ineffective. Idiopathic rhinitis is difficult to treat, but therapy must also include avoidance of precipitating factors. Immunotherapy and steroids are of no proven benefit for the patient with idiopathic rhinitis. Patients bothered by severe nasal obstruction may benefit from cryosurgery of the inferior and middle turbinates. However, surgical approaches to the treatment of nasal congestion should be reserved for patients seriously impaired by the condition. Referral to an ear, nose, and throat specialist may be indicated in some cases.

Decongestants should be used with caution in patients with heart disease, marked hypertension, advanced arteriosclerotic disease, insulin-dependent diabetes mellitus, or hyperthyroidism. Antitussives containing alcohol should be avoided in patients with a known alcohol intolerance.

Half-strength vasoconstrictive decongestant nose drops such as pseudoephedrine or phenylephrine are available for children with a common cold who are older than 3 months of age. In younger infants, sterile saline nose drops are used because a sympathomimetic decongestant can cause irritability and tachycardia. The addition of corticosteroids and antibiotics has not proved effective. Antihistamines are largely ineffective for treating the common cold. However, some health care providers have noted efficacy in relieving nasal congestion in children with acute nasopharyngitis.

Decongestant sprays can be used by older children but only with adult supervision. Orally administered decongestants are also widely used in older children to shrink engorged nasal mucosa.

Intervention

Administration

Administer cough syrups undiluted. Fluids should be withheld for up to 30 minutes after administration. Part of the therapeutic benefit of cough syrups stems from their soothing effects on pharyngeal mucosa. Capsule formulations (e.g., benzonatate perles) should not be opened or chewed. When opened or chewed, the local anesthetic effects numb oral mucosa.

The characteristics of the patient's cough (frequency, severity, productive, sputum volume, viscosity, and difficulty raising sputum) should be assessed before administration of an antitussive or mucolytic drug. The patient should be monitored for adverse reactions and hypersensitivity responses.

The patient in whom an opioid antitussive is being used should have his or her cough and sputum checked to ensure that the secretions have not inspissated (thickened). Although the dosage of an opioid antitussive is less than that used for pain, the patient's level of consciousness and respiratory depth and rate should be checked before administration. The patient should also be observed during treatment for the development of constipation.

To prevent drug-induced irritation of oral and pharyngeal membranes, the patient taking acetylcysteine should rinse the mouth after treatment. When 25 percent of the drug remains in the nebulizer, it should be diluted with an equal amount of normal saline solution to minimize reconcentration. A suction apparatus should be available for patients with an ineffective cough. A bronchodilator should be provided before the administration of acetylcysteine. Adequate patient hydration helps decrease the viscosity of the sputum.

The patient's history should be checked for possible contraindications to the use of decongestants. Decongestants can be administered as drops, nasal sprays, or oral inhalation, or they may be taken orally. Topical formulations should not be used for more than 3 to 5 days because of the high risk of rebound phenomenon.

Intranasal formulations are usually dilute, aqueous solutions prepared specifically for intranasal use. Some drugs (e.g., phenylephrine) are available also as ophthalmic solutions. The two types of solutions cannot be used interchangeably. Be sure to use the drug concentration that has been ordered. Some drug formulations are available in several concentrations. For example, phenylephrine preparations may contain 0.125, 0.25, 0.5, or 1 percent of the drug.

To minimize systemic absorption of topical decongestants, the nasal spray should be used with the patient in an upright position, squeezing the drug into each nostril. Nasal drops are administered with the head tilted back over the edge of a bed or chair. Do not touch the dropper to the nares. The recommended number of drops are instilled into each nostril with the patient breathing through the mouth. The head should remain tilted backward for 3 to 5 minutes. Give nasal decongestants to infants 20 to 30 minutes before feeding.

Adjunct therapies such as self-care measures, hydration, and humidification are also recommended.

Education

The best preventive measure to avoid catching a cold are to avoid exposure to others who are ill, engage in good handwashing, and keep the hands away from the face. A proactive approach to avoidance of coughs and colds is to send educational materials to patients at the beginning of the URI season. Pamphlets and other informational materials are usually appreciated by patients and can help cut down on unnecessary visits and telephone calls. The informational materials should include self-care hints and information about when to seek medical attention (e.g., high fever, marked pain or tenderness in an ear or sinus, increasingly purulent sputum, dyspnea, and pleuritic chest pain). In addition, the role of antibiotics in the treatment of a viral URI should be reviewed (i.e., only for complications such as otitis or sinusitis) as well as the risks of unnecessary antibiotic therapy (allergic reactions, alteration of bacterial flora, emergence of resistant strains). Unnecessary office visits and telephone calls have been reduced by as much as 30 to 40 percent through well-designed educational efforts.

Because many patients self-treat coughs, colds, and rhinitis, it is important to discuss the dangers of indiscriminate use of OTC expectorants, antitussives, and decongestants. Patients should be helped to understand which symptoms may be relieved with self-treatment and those for which self-treatment is ill-advised (see Controversy—Effectiveness of Over-the-Counter Drugs for Coughs and Congestion). Patients taking prescription drugs should be advised to contact their health care provider before taking OTC drugs.

Controversy

Effectiveness of Over-the-Counter Drugs for Coughs and Congestion
JONATHAN J. WOLFE

Coughs and congestion bring many patients to the clinic for diagnosis and treatment. The symptoms may have already led the patient to a display of over-the-counter (OTC) preparations for coughs and colds. Drugs may not be needed because the best agent for reducing viscosity of mucus is water. Water is the chief constituent of healthy secretions. Secretions are thickened by dust and cellular debris, but the presence of microorganisms change the picture. Thick, clinging mucus hinders breathing. People with asthma and other obstructive processes quickly become acutely ill in the presence of mucous plugs within their airways.

Patients often take cough products based on guaifenesin, which is widely available without prescription, incorrectly. They swallow a dose of 5 to 10 mL, but then do not drink any liquid for awhile. This is thought to allow the medicine to coat the throat, but it is the wrong way to take cough syrup. The high concentration of sugar in the syrup draws water to itself and dilutes the dose rather than providing a protective coating. Guaifenesin, indeed, is effective in oral solid form, acting to moisten the mucosa systemically.

Other OTC preparations contain a variety of active ingredients. Some may include antihistamines that dry the respiratory tree further. Patients with diabetes or glaucoma face hazards from such drugs. Other drugs contain codeine, a useful antitussive that supresses the cough center. However, after 48 hours or so, the antitussive effect of codeine falls off drastically. Dextromethorphan, a nonopioid antitussive, is a preferable agent, but continued use of either product is counterproductive. Patients also may overlook the sugar and alcohol content of cough medications. Diabetic patients are at particular risk here.

A vaporizer may be a better answer than many OTC preparations. Cool mist vaporizers are inexpensive and effective. Perhaps more effective and convenient is simply running a tub or shower with the bathroom door shut. Rapid humidification of air in a small space may bring faster relief and reduce anxiety.

Critical Thinking Discussion

- What caution would you offer to a patient with thickened secretions who is constantly blowing her nose?
- What product or products would you recommend to the patient whose nostrils are reddened and cracked from discharge and blowing?
- What method of removing thickened secretions from the nares of an infant would you recommend to parents?
- What other benefits will a patient with congestion and a low-grade fever derive by increased hydration of the mucosa?
- What characteristics of sputum or sinus discharge indicate that the patient requires evaluation by the health care provider and therapy with antibiotics?
- What inequities do you see if a poor patient spends money for OTC remedies in an attempt to avoid the cost of medical care and prescription drugs?

Relief from cold symptoms and avoidance of complications are facilitated by rest, fluids, analgesia, and perhaps inhalation of steam. Vitamin C has no proven role in the prevention or alleviation of symptoms of the common cold. Recommend that at least eight glasses or more (1500 to 2000 mL) of liquids be taken per day. Talk with the patient about the benefits of a balanced diet. They should be advised about the need for additional rest and sleep during periods of illness. The patients should be advised to stop smoking. Limiting talking, maintaining adequate environmental humidity, and chewing sugarless gum or sucking on hard candy help alleviate the discomfort caused by a chronic nonproductive cough. Instruct the patient to contact the health care provider if a cough persists for more than 1 week or if it is accompanied by fever, rash, persistent headache, or sore throat.

The patient should be instructed on the correct administration and use of nasal sprays or drops. They should be advised that nasal decongestants used for more than 7 days or in excessive amounts may produce rebound nasal congestion. Teach the patient to blow the nose gently before instilling nasal solutions or sprays. Advise patients to avoid contamination of nasal droppers or spray tips. Administration devices should be rinsed in hot water after use and allowed to dry.

Patients should be instructed in proper cough techniques. Patients with a dry, hacking cough are encouraged to take fluids freely to promote thin, easily raised sputum. Although small, opioid antitussives carry a risk of habituation and dependency. Teach the patient that recommended dosages should not be exceeded. Increasing the dose does not appreciably increase antitussive efficacy. The potential for abuse, however, is increased with an increase in dosage. Further, opioid adverse effects (i.e., respiratory depression) are potentiated by concurrent use of barbiturates or alcohol. The alcohol content of some antitussives can be as high as 40 percent. Opioids also tend to cause constipation. Thus, patients should be taught measures that help prevent constipation.

Patients should be advised to minimize caffeine intake because it may cause increased nervousness, tremors, or insomnia in the presence of decongestants. The patient should discontinue the drug and contact the health care provider if headache, nausea, vomiting, irregular pulse, extreme nervousness or restlessness, confusion, delirium, or muscle tremors occur. Drowsiness is a common adverse effect of many cough and cold preparations. The patient should be advised to use caution when driving or operating machinery.

Evaluation

The effectiveness of expectorants is demonstrated by an ability of the patient to effect a productive cough with increased sputum clearance. Antitussives should produce cough suppression, a decrease in the frequency and duration of coughing spells, and improvement in the patient's ability to sleep.

The effectiveness of topical nasal decongestants is dramatic, with efficacy noted within minutes. The patient often reports that he or she can breath easier, postnasal drip is relieved, and nasal discharge and sneezing are reduced. Oral decongestants are usually effective within 1 hour. The effectiveness of a mucolytic drug is demonstrated by decreased sputum viscosity and increased productivity.

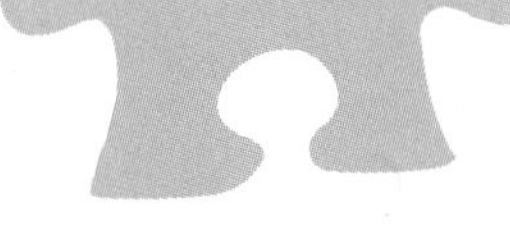

SUMMARY

- Acute URIs (common cold) are the most common acute infections in human beings, accounting for 10 percent of office visits annually in the United States. It is estimated that 15 to 20 percent of the population suffer from chronic or recurrent nasal congestion.
- Most adults average two to four colds a year, with the incidence increasing in the fall, peaking in winter, and then slowly decreasing each spring. Adult women are affected more often than men.
- Etiologic agents associated with the common cold include rhinovirus, influenza, parainfluenza, respiratory syncytial virus, coronavirus, adenovirus, echovirus, and coxsackievirus.
- Almost all people experience an acute episode of coughing at some time in their lives. A chronic cough is present in only 8 to 14 percent of the population.
- The virus of the common cold is transmitted by direct inoculation of the mucous membranes of the nose and eyes, usually from contaminated hands.
- The mechanisms associated with a cough are mechanical, inflammatory, or chemical in nature.
- Assess the patient's history for possible contraindications to the use of expectorants, antitussives, decongestants, or mucolytics. Note the character of the patient's cough, sputum characteristics, and self-treatment modalities.
- Treatment objectives include strategies that prevent, minimize, or help correct symptoms associated with upper respiratory disorders.
- Expectorants stimulate the flow and reduce the viscosity of respiratory tract secretions.
- Opioid and nonopioid antitussives act centrally or peripherally to suppress cough, reducing the frequency and intensity of the cough.
- Nasal decongestants are sympathomimetics that shrink mucous membranes, thus reducing congestion and improving nasal drainage.
- Mucolytics can be used to decrease the viscosity of secretions in patients with pulmonary diseases and cystic fibrosis. When they are taken orally, they protect the liver from acetaminophen overdose.
- Adequate hydration should be maintained throughout therapy.
- The effectiveness of expectorants is demonstrated by an ability of the patient to effect a productive cough with increased sputum clearance.
- Antitussives should produce cough suppression, a decrease in the frequency and duration of coughing spells, and improvement in the patient's ability to sleep.
- The effectiveness of topical nasal decongestants is demonstrated by the patient's report that he or she can breath easier, postnasal drip is relieved, and nasal discharge and sneezing are reduced.
- The effectiveness of a mucolytic drug is demonstrated by decreased sputum viscosity and increased productivity.

BIBLIOGRAPHY

Abramowicz, M. (Ed.). (1994). Intranasal budesonide for allergic rhinitis. *The Medical Letter of Drugs and Therapeutics,* 36(926), 63–64.

American Hospital Formulary Service. (1996). *Drug information.* Bethesda, Maryland: Author.

Benninger, M., Anon, J., and Mabry, R. (1997). The medical management of rhinosinusitis. *Otolaryngology, Head and Neck Surgery,* 117(3 Part 2), S41–49.

Benninger, M. S. (1992). Rhinitis, sinusitis, and their relationship to allergies. *American Journal of Rhinolaryngology,* 6(2), 37–39.

Creticos, P., Toglas, A., and Zimmer, P. (1992). A diagnostic dilemma: Distinguishing between colds, flu, and allergies. *The National Nurse Practitioner Symposium 13th Annual Scientific & Clinical Sessions,* August 22.

Engle, J. (1992). Topical nasal decongestants. *American Pharmacy,* 32(5), 33–37.

Fried, L., Storer, D., King, D., et al. (1991). Diagnosis of illness presentation in the elderly. *Journal of the American Geriatric Society,* 39(2), 117–123.

Gadomskin, A., and Horton, L. (1992). The need for rationale therapeutics in the use of cough and cold medicine in children. *Pediatrics,* 89(4, part 2), 774–776.

Goroll, A., May, L., and Mulley, A. (1995). *Primary care medicine: Office evaluation and management of the adult patient* (3rd ed.). Philadelphia: J.B. Lippincott.

Hendeles, L. (1993). Efficacy and safety of antihistamines and expectorants in nonprescription cough and cold preparations. *Pharmacotherapy,* 13(2), 154–158.

Hutton, N., Wilson, M., Mellits, E., et al. (1991). Effectiveness of an antihistamine-decongestant combination for young children with the common cold: A randomized, controlled clinical trial. *Journal of Pediatrics,* 118(1), 125–130.

Smith, M., and Feldman, W. (1993). Over the counter cold medications: A critical review of clinical trials between 1950 and 1991. *Journal of the American Medical Association,* 269(17), 2258–2263.

Stergachis, A., Newmann, W., Williams, K., et al. (1990). The effect of self-care minimal intervention for colds and flu on the use of medical services. *Journal of General Internal Medicine,* 5(1), 23–28.

Swartz, R. (1994). The diagnosis and management of sinusitis. *Nurse Practitioner,* 19(12), 58–63.

Ziering, R., and Klein, G. (1992). Allergic rhinitis: Measures to control the misery. *Postgraduate Medicine,* 91(1), 225–227, 231–232.

Unit X

Drugs Influencing the Endocrine System

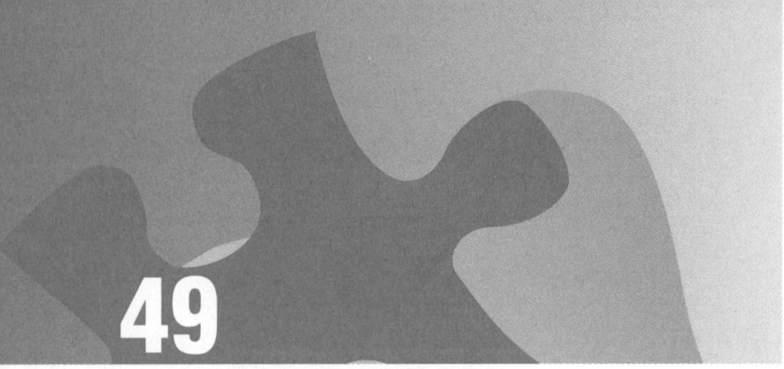

49 Pancreatic Drugs

Pancreatic drugs are used to treat hyperglycemia associated with diabetes mellitus and other forms of glucose intolerance. Plasma glucose values below 200 mg/dL usually eliminate the common signs and symptoms of diabetes. Maintaining plasma glucose values between 150 and 165 mg/dL promotes the patient's sense of well-being and good health. Furthermore, recent studies have shown that maintaining normoglycemia (80 to 120 mg/dL) prevents or minimizes the microvascular and macrovascular complications associated with diabetes mellitus.

The term *diabetes mellitus* includes four classifications: (1) insulin-dependent, or type 1, diabetes; (2) noninsulin-dependent, or type 2, diabetes; (3) secondary diabetes; and (4) diabetes associated with malnutrition. Two other types of diabetes have also been identified: impaired glucose tolerance (IGT) and gestational diabetes mellitus (GDM). This classification system was developed by the National Diabetes Data Group of the National Institutes of Health with input from the World Health Organization.

Although the classic symptoms of diabetes mellitus are similar in each classification, the two main types are different in nature. A number of different drugs are available for the management of diabetes, although the more common ones include sulfonylureas and insulin. A basic knowledge of the physiology and pathophysiology of diabetes is necessary in order to have an understanding of pharmacotherapy and the optimal goals of treatment.

DIABETES MELLITUS

Epidemiology and Etiology

Approximately 14 million people in the United States have diabetes. Of these, an estimated 6 million undiagnosed cases exist among adults. The economic costs of diabetes exceed $105 billion, approximately one-sixth of total health care costs in 1995.

Diabetes (and its complications) is the third leading cause of death from disease in the United States. It is considered the leading cause of new blindness in adults ages 20 to 74, and is the single greatest contributor to end-stage renal failure and nontraumatic amputations in adults. The incidence of amputation may be even higher for those individuals living at poverty levels. Diabetes is also a risk factor in coronary artery disease and stroke.

Type 1 Diabetes Mellitus

Type 1 diabetes mellitus accounts for approximately 10 percent of all diabetes in the United States. The annual incidence is 12 to 14 cases per 100,000 people younger than 20 years of age, with a prevalence of 1 case per 500 people younger than 16 years. Type 1 diabetes is one of the most common childhood diseases, being three to four times more common than chronic childhood diseases such as cystic fibrosis, juvenile rheumatoid arthritis, or leukemia. It is 10 times more common than nephrotic syndrome or muscular dystrophy. Approximately 40 percent of diabetic children younger than the age of 2 years present to the health care system in a coma. Of these, approximately 5 percent die.

Women are affected twice as often as men. Predisposition to type 1 diabetes is inherited as a heterogenous trait. There is a 25 to 50 percent risk of diabetes in identical twins, whereas siblings have a 6 percent risk and offspring have a 5 percent risk. Despite the strong familial influence, 90 percent of patients in whom type 1 diabetes develops do not have a first-degree relative with the disorder.

Type 2 Diabetes Mellitus

Type 2 diabetes is much more common than type 1. Type 2 diabetes is found in approximately 85 to 90 percent of all patients with diabetes in the United States. For every known case in the United States, there is one that is undiagnosed. Most often diagnosed in individuals over the age of 40, it has a relatively slow onset. The prevalence varies by ethnic group; however, the condition is markedly increased in Native Americans, blacks, and Hispanics. Prevalence also varies by geographic environment. A gene-environment interaction appears to be responsible for the condition.

There is some thought that type 2 diabetes may be an autosomal recessive trait, with a transmission rate from parent to child of 80 to 90 percent. GDM, the delivery of babies weighing more than nine pounds, having a previously identified glucose intolerance, hypertension, or significant hyperlipidemia are identifiable risk factors. Obesity and subsequent insulin resistance is a factor for 60 to 80 percent of patients with type 2 diabetes.

Secondary Diabetes

The incidence of secondary diabetes is small, but the disease is most often related to pancreatic disease or removal of pancreatic tissue, defects of insulin receptors, Cushing's syndrome, pancreatic tumors, the administration of drugs that impair insulin action, or the administration of hormones that cause hyperglycemia. The incidence will probably increase as the number of people with pancreatic disease and endocrinopathies survive longer and because more people are receiving drugs that contribute to elevated blood sugar levels.

Gestational Diabetes

GDM occurs in approximately 4 percent of pregnant women and is associated with increased fetal morbidity and mortality. Although GDM usually appears during the second or third trimesters, it usually resolves after parturition. However, women with a history of GDM have a 50- to 60-percent chance of developing IGT or type 2 diabetes within 5 to 15 years of parturition.

GDM is classified according to the age at which it was diagnosed, the length of time the disease has been present, and the degree of vascular changes that have occurred. The classification provides prognostic indicators for neonatal outcomes.

Risk factors for developing GDM include previous GDM, previous delivery of baby weighing 9 pounds or more, obesity, pregnancy after age 30, and a history of polyhydramnios or recurrent monilial vaginitis.

Pathophysiology

In the healthy individual, insulin acts to decrease the breakdown of glycogen *(glycogenolysis)* in the liver, and stimulates the formation of new glucose from fatty acids and amino acids *(glyconeogenesis)* and the formation of ketone bodies *(ketogenesis)*. At the same time, it increases the synthesis and storage of glycogen and fatty acids. In adipose tissue, insulin acts to decrease the breakdown of fat *(lipolysis)*, and to increase the production of glycerol and fatty acids. In muscle tissue, it decreases protein breakdown and amino acid output, and increases amino acid uptake, protein synthesis, and glycogen synthesis.

Insulin release from the beta cells of the islets of Langerhans occurs in response to food-related stimuli. Insulin released by the beta cells enters the portal circulation, traveling directly to the liver, where about 50 percent is used or degraded (Fig. 49–1). Insulin is secreted in a pulsatile fashion. Serum insulin levels begin to rise within minutes after a meal, reach a peak in about 3 to 5 minutes, and then return to baseline levels within 2 to 3 hours.

The body maintains a system of counter-regulatory hormones that counteract hypoglycemia-producing situations, and ensure brain function and survival. The counter-regulatory hormones include glucagon, catecholamines, growth hormone, and glucocorticoids. Alpha cells in the islet of Langerhans secrete glucagon. Glucagon maintains blood glucose by increasing the release of glucose from the liver into the blood.

Type 1 Diabetes Mellitus

Type 1 diabetes mellitus is characterized by an absolute insulin deficit related to a pancreatic beta-cell loss in the islet of Langerhans and increased insulin resistance. The result is hyperglycemia and other metabolic disturbances. Although the cause of initial islet cell injury remains unknown, it is generally thought to be associated with an autoimmune phenomena with specific human leukocyte antigens (HLA).

Type 1 diabetes can be divided into five developmental stages: genetic predisposition, environmental trigger, active autoimmunity, progressive beta-cell destruction, and overt diabetes. Islet cell antibodies (HLA-DR2, HLA-DR3, HLA-DR4) appear years before the appearance of symptoms and provide strong evidence for an autoimmune origin. These immune markers precede evidence of beta-cell deficiency and are found in 70 to 80 percent of patients with type 1 diabetes at the time of diagnosis. The risk of developing type 1 diabetes increases five to eight times when one of the immune markers is present.

The HLA-DR4 antigen is strongly associated with the cell-mediated destruction of beta cells found in type 1 diabetes. Type 1_A diabetes usually occurs before the age of 30 and is associated with a sudden onset of symptoms that require prompt treatment. The risk of heterogenous patients (HLA-DR3 and HLA-DR4) developing type 1 diabetes is 20 to 40 times higher than that of the general population. On the other hand, the HLA-DR2 antigen is associated with an unusually low risk of developing type 1 diabetes.

Type 1_B is an uncommon primary disorder associated with other autoimmune disorders such as myasthenia gravis, Hashimoto's disease, Graves' disease, and pernicious anemia. Type 1_B diabetes is associated with the HLA-DR3 antigen and occurs later in life, typically between the ages of 30 and 50.

The precise mechanism of antibody migration or attachment of immune cells to the pancreatic islet cells has not been determined. Environmental factors are thought to play a role in their destruction by producing direct toxicity, increasing the susceptibility of the beta cells to another mechanism, or triggering a beta-cell autoimmune response. Controversy remains over whether beta-cell destruction always progresses to type 1 diabetes or if it can remit. The initiating events of beta-cell destruction may be different from those of the final event that precipitate signs and symptoms.

Despite the cause, both alpha-cell and beta-cell functions are abnormal, with a lack of insulin and a relative excess of glucagon. The hyperglycemia and hyperketonemia associated with type 1 diabetes are not possible as a result of insulin deficiency alone. Glucagon must be present in relative excess. Thus, the full syndrome of diabetes is related to both hormones, a finding that may ultimately provide for new therapeutic approaches in the management of type 1 diabetes. The ratio of insulin to glucagon in the portal vein controls the metabolism of glucose and fat in the liver.

Clinical symptoms of type 1 diabetes generally appear with the destruction of approximately 80 percent of the insulin-secreting beta cells. The classic symptoms of diabetes commonly include hyperglycemia, *polydipsia* (excessive thirst), *polyphagia* (excessive hunger), and *polyuria* (frequent urination). Additionally, weight loss, blurred vision, and recurrent infections may be noted. The disease, however, may be asymptomatic in its early stages. Because of the insulin deficiency, patients are dependent on exogenous insulin to sustain metabolic functions and life.

It should be noted that the use of exogenous insulin does not distinguish type 1 diabetes from type 2 diabetes. Patients with type 2 diabetes are not prone to ketosis and are not insulin dependent but may require insulin. Table 49–1 provides a visual comparison of type 1 and type 2 diabetes based on common features.

Type 2 Diabetes Mellitus

Type 2 diabetes is characterized by decreased insulin production, decreased peripheral utilization of insulin, and insulin resistance. The factors most often associated with type 2 diabetes are the aging process, heredity, and obesity. The most powerful risk factor according to the World Health Organization is obesity. The risk increases 10 times with severe obesity. In the obese individual, insulin has a decreased ability to influence glucose uptake and metabolism in the liver, skeletal muscles, and adipose tissues. B cells that are chronically exposed to hyperglycemia become gradually less

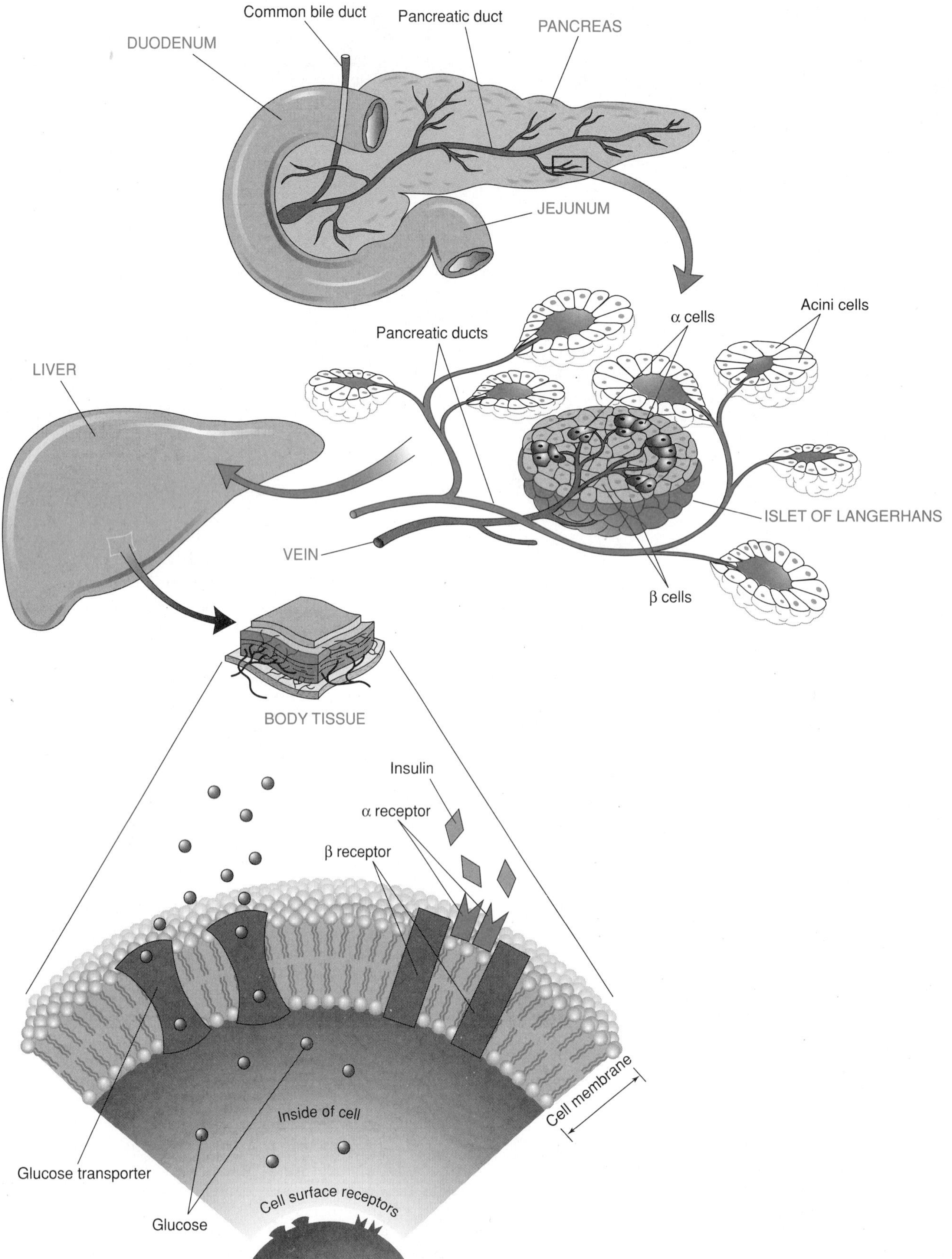

Figure 49–1 Insulin-glucose balance. Insulin is released in a pulsatile fashion by the beta cells and enters the portal circulation, where it travels directly to the liver. About 50 percent of the insulin is either used or degraded. Alpha cells in the islets of Langerhans secrete glucagon. Glucagon maintains blood glucose by increasing the release of glucose from the liver into the blood.

TABLE 49–1 COMPARISON OF TYPE 1 AND TYPE 2 DIABETES MELLITUS

Feature	Type 1	Type 2
Etiology	HLA-DR3, HLA-DR4 antigens	Strong genetic predispostion
Incidence	10% of population	85–90% of population
Age at onset	Usually under age 30 but may occur at any age	Usually over age 40
Onset of symptoms	Sudden, symptomatic	Insidious, usually asymptomatic
Manifestations	Polyuria, polyphagia, polydipsia, fatigue	Frequently none
Endogenous insulin	Absolute deficit	Relative deficit
Insulin resistance	No	Yes
Insulin receptors	Normal	Defective or decreased
Body weight at diagnosis	Nonobese	Obese in 85% of patients
Prone to ketoacidosis	Yes (DKA)	Usually resistant (HHNS)
Susceptible to infection	Yes	Yes
Poor wound healing	Yes	Yes
Drug management	Yes, Insulin	Yes, oral agents*
Dietary regimen	Yes, Essential	Yes, Essential
Weight loss program	No, in most cases	Yes, in many cases
Exercise program	Yes	Yes

*Insulin may be required in 20–30% of patients with type 2 diabetes if diet, weight loss, and exercise are ineffective.

DKA, Diabetic ketoacidosis; HHNS, hyperglycemic, hyperosmolar nonketotic syndrome.

responsive to further glucose elevations *(desensitization)*. This phenomenon is reversible with normalization of glucose levels. The ratio of proinsulin (a precursor to insulin) to insulin secreted also increases.

Patients with type 2 diabetes also have resistance to the biologic activity of insulin in both the liver and peripheral tissues *(insulin resistance)*. The decreased glucose sensitivity results in continued hepatic glucose production, even with high plasma glucose levels. This is coupled with an inability of the muscle and fat tissues to increase their glucose uptake. The mechanism causing peripheral resistance is unclear. It appears to occur after insulin binds to a receptor in the cell surface.

Multiple theories have been presented to explain the phenomenon of insulin resistance. One theory suggests that a reduced number of insulin receptors causes decreased insulin binding. Another theory holds that overeating leads to hyperinsulinemia, necessitating the development of peripheral insulin resistance to protect against hypoglycemia. In any case, the mechanism responsible for binding insulin to receptors or postreceptor activity may be reversed through weight loss.

A decrease in beta cells may be the result of progressive deterioration over time. To obscure the issue further, the ratio of alpha cells to beta cells may be completely normal in the patient with type 2 diabetes. Most patients have plasma and pancreatic insulin levels that are not decreased.

The fasting hyperglycemia and glucose intolerance associated with type 2 diabetes are usually corrected by weight loss, improvement in dietary patterns, and exercise. If the hyperglycemia is not corrected by diet and exercise, oral hypoglycemic drugs may be used to stimulate the insulin production by the pancreas and to decrease insulin resistance. When oral hypoglycemic drugs do not sufficiently correct the hyperglycemia, exogenous insulin must be used.

The clinical manifestations of type 2 diabetes are often nonspecific. The patient is often overweight and has hyperlipidemia. He or she may display some of the classic signs of diabetes, but more often have nonspecific symptoms such as fatigue, pruritus, recurrent infections and delayed wound healing, visual changes, and paresthesias.

Unlike type 1 diabetes in which the patient may develop diabetic ketoacidosis (DKA), hyperosmolar hyperglycemic nonketotic syndrome (HHNS) occurs when blood glucose levels rise. In DKA, plasma glucose are elevated above 600 mg/dL. Plasma ketones are present, and bicarbonate levels average 10 mEq/L. Sodium and potassium levels may be low, normal, or high during this time. Blood urea nitrogen (BUN) and creatinine may be elevated owing to decreased renal blood flow. HHNS presents much the same as DKA, except that glucose levels are much higher (over 1000 mg/dL), serum osmolality is approximately 360 mOsm, and ketosis is absent.

Gestational Diabetes

Changes in estrogen and progesterone levels during pregnancy stimulate hyperplasia of pancreatic beta cells. As insulin secretion increases, the utilization of peripheral glucose is also enhanced, leading to decreased fasting blood glucose levels during the first trimester. During the first half of pregnancy the elevated insulin levels divert surplus maternal calories to lipid stores and tissue glycogen.

During the second and third trimesters, progesterone, human placental lactogen hormone, and cortisol, the hormones of pregnancy, antagonize the effectiveness of insulin at the cellular level and mobilize glucose from storage sites. In addition, insulinase, a placental enzyme, accelerates degradation of insulin. The net effect is decreased insulin effectiveness, reduced peripheral uptake of glucose, and thereby, decreased amounts of glucose available to the fetus for growth.

Signs and symptoms of GDM include glucosuria on two successive office visits, recurrent monilial vaginitis, macrosomia of the fetus on ultrasound and polyhydramnios. In patients with known diabetes, symptoms vary from trimester to trimester. For most women, the diabetic state does not deteriorate because of the pregnancy itself. In fact, most women have better glycemic control than when they are not pregnant. Despite the antagonistic forces of hormones, glycemic control is often better because of the closer observation of blood glucose levels.

Impaired Glucose Tolerance

IGT occurs in patients who have higher than normal fasting glucose levels (over 200 mg/dL) but who do not fit the criteria for type 1 or type 2 diabetes. The insulin levels of these patients may be in the low-normal or high-normal range, yet they indicate a delay in insulin release. The delay in insulin release causes reactive hypoglycemia. Ten to seventy percent of patients with IGT eventually convert to type 2 diabetes. IGT almost invariably converts to normal glucose tolerance with weight reduction and exercise.

PHARMACOTHERAPEUTIC OPTIONS

Insulins

Indications

Insulin preparations are used in the treatment of type 1 diabetes. Insulin is necessary for normal carbohydrate, protein, and fat metabolism. Insulin preparations are also used in patients with type 2 diabetes who are unable to maintain control of their symptoms either by diet and exercise alone or with the addition of an oral antidiabetic drug. In addition, insulin is critical for the management of DKA. It has an important role in the treatment of HHNS, and is used in the perioperative management of both type 1 and type 2 diabetes.

Pharmacodynamics

Carbohydrates are broken down into molecules of glucose, proteins into molecules of amino acids, and fats into lipid molecules. These molecules enter the cells and are either used immediately as energy or stored for later use.

Insulin acts by binding to insulin receptor sites on cells to allow molecular transport of glucose into the cells. Cells having insulin-specific binding sites are located primarily in liver, adipose tissue, and muscle cells. They are also found in placental cells, fibroblasts, and white blood cells.

Insulin influences carbohydrate metabolism by increasing glucose uptake, increasing glucose oxidation, and increasing glucose storage. It also increases glycogen synthesis but decreases glycogenolysis. Gluconeogenesis is also decreased because of decreased delivery of fatty acids and amino acids to the liver.

Insulin facilitates the transport of amino acids into cells and increases the synthesis of protein within the cells. Insulin also potentiates the action of growth hormone. Lack of insulin can cause the protein to be broken down into amino acids, which, in turn, are transported to the liver for use in gluconeogenesis. When insulin is deficient for long periods of time, protein wasting occurs, resulting in abnormal functioning of many organs, severe weakness, and weight loss.

Insulin also promotes fat metabolism and storage. When glucose enters fat cells, it is broken down into alpha-glycerophosphate, which combines with fatty acids to form triglycerides, thereby promoting fat storage. Without insulin, fat is not stored but is released into the blood stream as free fatty acids. Other lipids (such as cholesterol and phospholipids) are also increased if insulin is lacking. The high concentration of lipids is thought to contribute to the development of atherosclerosis, appearing more frequently and developing more rapidly in people with diabetes. If excessive amounts of free fatty acids are released, and the body cannot use them as fuel; they are converted to ketone bodies that can cause acidosis and death.

Insulins are classified according to their duration of action (ultra-short acting, short-acting, intermediate-acting, long-acting), by their species of origin (human, porcine, bovine, or a mixture of bovine and porcine), and by their concentration. Human insulin is not derived from the human pancreas but is widely available as a result of recombinant DNA technologies. In theory, human insulin is slightly less immunogenic than purified porcine insulin, which, in turn, is less immunogenic than bovine insulin. When highly purified, porcine, bovine, and bovine-porcine mixtures have a relatively low, but measurable, capacity to stimulate the immune response. Beef insulin is more antigenic than pork insulin.

Adverse Effects and Contraindications

The major adverse effect of insulin is hypoglycemia. It is most often caused by too much insulin, not enough food, or excessive physical activity. When glucose levels fall gradually, symptoms are primarily limited to those of central nervous system origin (i.e., headache, confusion, drowsiness, fatigue). When glucose levels fall rapidly, the sympathetic nervous system is activated, resulting in tachycardia, palpitations, diaphoresis, and nervousness.

In some patients, hypoglycemia occurs without producing the symptoms noted earlier. As a result, the patient is unaware of the hypoglycemia until the blood sugar levels become dangerously low. Hypoglycemia unawareness is of particular concern in patients practicing tight glucose control. If hypoglycemia becomes severe, seizures, coma, and death may follow. Hypoglycemia is most likely to occur when the hypoglycemic effects of insulin peak (Fig. 49–2). For example, a short-acting insulin peaks 2 to 4 hours after administration. So, if the insulin was given at 8 AM, the risk of hypoglycemia occurs between 10 AM and 12 noon. Some intermediate-acting insulins peak 6 to 12 hours after administration. If the intermediate-acting insulin was given at 8 AM, the likelihood of hypoglycemia increases between 2 PM and 8 PM.

Dawn phenomenon may occur in some patients taking insulin, with glucose levels remaining normal until approximately 3 AM, when the nocturnal effect of growth hormone elevates blood glucose levels. In contrast, a *Somogyi phenomenon* also occurs during the night, but there is an insulin-induced hypoglycemic reaction with a rebound elevation in glucose levels. Compensatory mechanisms such as increased secretion of epinephrine, cortisol, and growth hormone are activated in the body's attempt to oppose the excessive insulin.

Cutaneous adverse effects of insulin *(lipodystrophies)* are a complication of insulin administration, characterized by changes in subcutaneous fat at the site of injection. With *lipoatrophy,* the subcutaneous fat appears to have melted away, leaving a saucer-like depression in the skin surface.

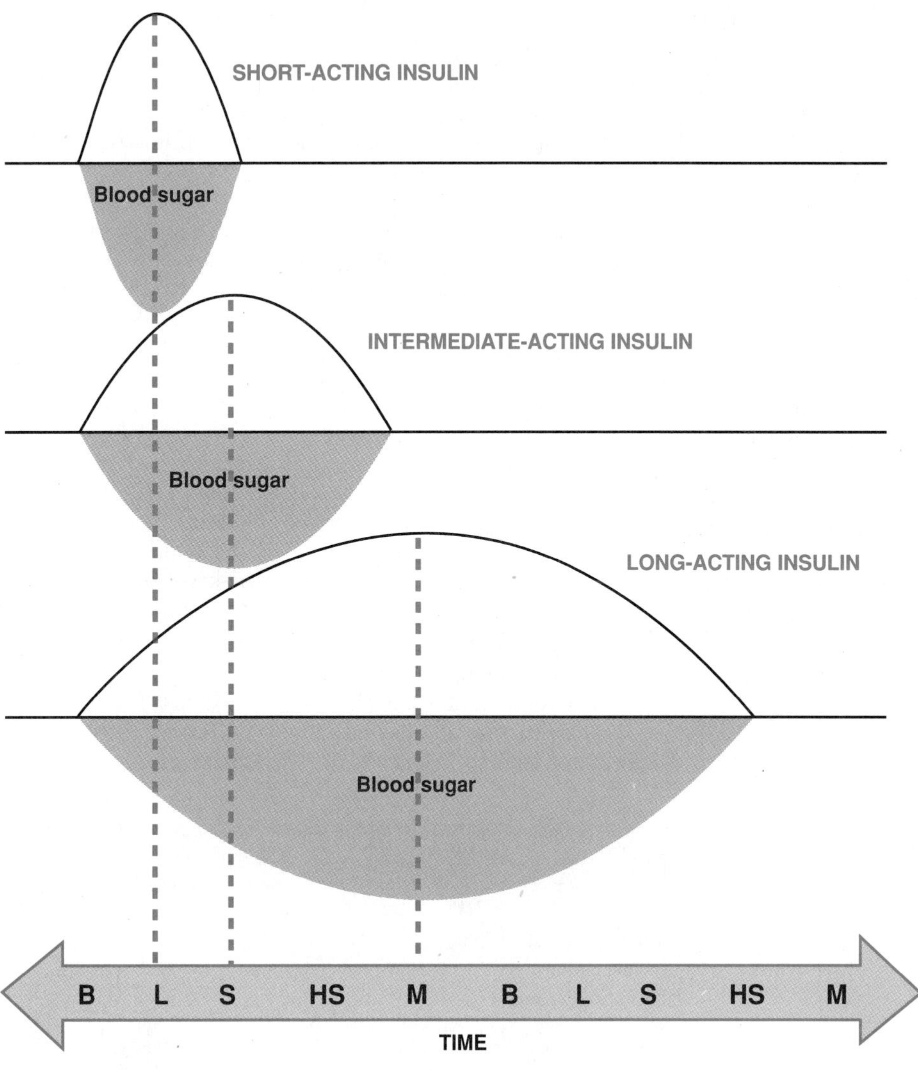

Figure 49–2 Duration of insulin action varies with the regimen prescribed. Hypoglycemia is most likely to occur when the hypoglycemic effects of insulin peak. The upward insulin curve from baseline essentially mirrors the downward blood glucose curve. For example, a short-acting insulin peaks 2 to 4 hours after administration. So, if the short-acting insulin was given at 8 AM, the risk of hypoglycemia is greatest between 10 AM and 12 noon.

The cause appears to be immunologic. Accordingly, lipoatrophy is most likely to occur with the use of insulin preparations that have a high concentration of antigenic contaminants. Because the insulin preparations today are purer than those used in the past, lipoatrophy is less of a problem. In some cases, the subcutaneous fat can be restored by injecting a highly purified insulin preparation (e.g. purified pork insulin or human insulin) directly into the site of lipoatrophy. Improvement can be seen in about 4 weeks, but full improvement can take 3 to 6 months.

Lipohypertrophy appears as a spongy, localized area at the injection site. Fat accumulates at the site because insulin stimulates fat synthesis. When use of the injection site is discontinued, the excess fat eventually is lost. Lipohypertrophy can be minimized by systematic rotation of injection sites.

Insulin allergies are caused by immunologic reactions to insulin. They are seen more commonly with animal source insulins. The most frequent allergic manifestations include immunoglobulin E (IgE)–mediated local cutaneous reactions (which include soreness, erythema, or induration at the injection site 2 hours after the injection). Localized allergic reactions occur in response to a contaminant in the insulin preparation and not to the insulin itself. Because the insulins used today are highly purified, local reactions are infrequent. On rare occasions, patients may develop life-threatening systemic responses. Systemic allergic reactions have a rapid onset and are characterized by the widespread appearance of red and intensely itchy urticaria. Systemic reactions occur in response to the insulin itself, not to a contaminant. Beef insulin, which differs from human insulin by three amino acids, is the most frequent cause of systemic reactions. Generalized reactions are least likely to occur with pork and human insulins.

Insulin resistance is a problem experienced by most individuals with diabetes at some point in the illness. With insulin resistance the insulin requirement necessary to control hyperglycemia and prevent ketosis exceeds 200 units/day. Typically, it results from a profound/complete insulin deficit in patients with type 1 diabetes and in obese patients with type 2 diabetes. Insulin resistance is characterized by one of the following anomalies: The insulin is abnormal or insulin antibodies are present, the number of insulin receptors are decreased or insulin binding to the receptors is diminished, or the receptors are not appropriately activated by the insulin.

Pharmacokinetics

Insulin is rapidly absorbed from subcutaneous administration sites. The absorption rate is determined by the type of insulin, the injection site, the injection volume, and other factors (Table 49–2). About 50 percent of insulin is biotransformed in the liver and secondarily in the kidneys (25 percent), muscles, and other tissues.

Insulin is available in ultra short-acting, short-acting, intermediate-acting, long-acting, and ultra long-acting preparations. Ultra short-acting HUMALOG (human insulin lispro) is nearly identical to that of natural insulin, but the onset of its effects occurs in about 15 minutes, with peak drug action noted in 1 hour. Because HUMALOG works so quickly, hypoglycemia can develop rapidly if adequate calories are not consumed immediately after the injection. It is the only insulin approved, at this time, for insulin infusion pump use.

Short-acting insulins are simply solutions of regular, crystalline zinc insulin dissolved in a buffer at neutral pH. The onset of effects of these preparations occur 30 minutes after subcutaneous (SC) injection, peak in 2 to 4 hours, and last 6 to 8 hours. Regular insulin is the only insulin preparation that may also be administered intravenously (IV). After IV administration, there is a rapid fall in the blood glucose concentration, usually reaching a nadir in 20 to 30 minutes. In the absence of a sustained IV infusion, insulin is rapidly cleared and glucose levels return to baseline in about 2 to 3 hours.

Intermediate-acting and long-acting insulins are formulated so that they dissolve more gradually when administered SC. They are modified by adding protamine (a large, insoluble protein), zinc, or both to slow absorption and prolong drug action. NPH insulin is a suspension of insulin in a complex with zinc and protamine in a phosphate buffer. ILETIN insulin is a mixture of crystallized and amorphous insulins in an acetate buffer, which minimizes the solubility of insulin. Intermediate-acting insulins have similar pharmacokinetic profiles. The onset of its effects occurs in 1 to 2 hours, peak in 6 to 12 hours, and have a duration of action of 18 to 26 hours.

The long-acting insulins are zinc suspensions with onset times of 1 to 3 hours. They peak in 16 to 12 hours and have a duration of action of 18 to 26 hours. The ultra long-acting insulin is an extended zinc suspension with an onset of drug action 4 to 6 hours after administration. HUMULIN U peaks in 8 to 20 hours, with a duration of action of 24 to 48 hours. The half-life of long-acting and ultra long-acting insulins makes it difficult to determine the optimal dosage, because several days of treatment are required before a steady-state concentration of circulating insulin is achieved.

Drug-Drug Interactions

The effects of insulin are potentiated in the presence of salicylates, beta blockers, monoamine oxidase inhibitors,

TABLE 49–2 PHARMACOKINETICS OF INSULINS

Drug	Species	Route	Onset*	Peak	Duration†
Ultra Short-Acting Insulin					
HUMALOG	Human	SC, IP	15 min	1 hr	3.5–4.5 hr
Short-Acting Insulins					
HUMULIN R	Human (prb)	SC, IV	30 min	2–4 hr	6–8 hr
ILETIN I REGULAR	Pork and beef	SC, IV	30 min	2–4 hr	6–8 hr
ILETIN II REGULAR	Pork	SC, IV	30 min	2–4 hr	6–8 hr
NOVOLIN R	Human (pry)	SC, IV	30 min	2.5–5 hr	8 hr
PURIFIED PORK REGULAR	Pork	SC, IV	30 min	2.5–5 hr	8 hr
VELOSULIN BR	Human (emp)	SC, IV	30 min	1–3 hr	8 hr
Intermediate-Acting Insulins					
HUMULIN N	Human (prb)	SC	1–2 hr	6–12 hr	18–24 hr
ILETIN I NPH	Pork and beef	SC	1–2 hr	6–12 hr	18–26 hr
ILETIN II NPH	Pork	SC	1–2 hr	6–12 hr	18–26 hr
NOVOLIN N	Human (pry)	SC	1.5 hr	4–12 hr	24 hr
PURIFIED PORK NPH	Pork	SC	1.5 hr	4–12 hr	24 hr
Long-Acting Insulins					
HUMULIN L	Human (prb)	SC	1–3 hr	6–12 hr	18–24 hr
ILETIN I LENTE	Pork and beef	SC	1–3 hr	6–12 hr	18–26 hr
ILETIN II LENTE	Pork	SC	1–3 hr	6–12 hr	18–26 hr
NOVOLIN L	Human (pry)	SC	2.5 hr	7–15 hr	22 hr
PURIFIED PORK LENTE	Pork	SC	2.5 hr	7–15 hr	22 hr
Ultra Long-Acting Insulins					
HUMULIN U	Human (prb)	SC	4–6 hr	8–20 hr	24–48 hr
Combination Preparations					
HUMULIN 70/30	Human (prb)	SC	30 min	2–12 hr	24 hr
HUMULIN 50/50	Human (prb)	SC	30 min	3–5 hr	24 hr
NOVOLIN 70/30	Human (pry)	SC	30 min	2–12 hr	24 hr

*Onset is for the subcutaneous route. All times are approximate.

†Maximum effects occur when insulin drug action peaks, however, actual duration of action may last longer.

prb, Produced from proinsulin synthesized by bacteria using recombinant DNA technology; emp, produced by enzymatic modification of pork insulin; pry, produced by bakers' yeast using recombinant DNA technology; IP, infusion pump; SC, subcutaneous; IV, intravenous.

sulfonamides, some angiotensin-converting enzyme inhibitors, and drugs that inhibit pancreatic function (e.g., octreotide). Beta-blocking drugs disguise the signs and symptoms of hypoglycemia. Insulin activity is antagonized in the presence of thiazide diuretics, acute alcohol ingestion, glucocorticoids, thyroid preparations, estrogens, smoking, phenothiazines, sympathomimetics, and isoniazid, and rifampin may increase insulin requirements (Table 49–3).

Dosage Regimens

Dosages and concentrations of insulin are expressed in units. This practice dates to a time when insulin preparations were impure, making it necessary to standardize them through bioassay. One unit of insulin is equal to the amount required to reduce the blood glucose concentration in a fasting rabbit to 45 mg/dL. The current international standard is a mixture of bovine and porcine insulins containing 24 units/mg. Homogeneous preparations of human insulin contain between 25 and 30 units/mg. Drug regimens are highly individualized based on the degree of glycemic response desired.

Insulin dosages for long-term therapy are usually determined by trial and error. One method involves the use of an intermediate-acting agent, such as NPH, given 30 to 60 minutes before breakfast, in an initial dose of 10 to 26 units daily. The dose may be increased by 2 to 10 units (approximately 10 percent) at daily to weekly intervals, depending on blood glucose levels. Once hyperglycemia is relatively well controlled, additional changes are usually small, 1 to 2 units at a time, and made no more often than every 2 to 3 days.

A second method for calculating dosage involves the use of a short-acting insulin. Five to 10 units are given SC 15 to 30 minutes before meals, and the dosage gradually increased based on blood glucose levels. Once hyperglycemia is controlled, an intermediate-acting insulin is substituted. With this method, the insulin is usually given once daily, just before breakfast. The initial dose of the intermediate-acting insulin is approximately two-thirds the daily dose previously established for regular insulin.

TABLE 49–3 DRUG-DRUG INTERACTIONS OF INSULINS

Interactive Drug	Interaction
Beta blockers Salicylates Monoamine oxidase inhibitors Sulfonamides Selected ACE inhibitors Octreotide	Interactive drugs potentiate effects of insulin
Acute alcohol ingestion Estrogens Glucocorticoids Isoniazid Phenothiazines Rifampin Smoking Sympathomimetics Thiazide diuretics Thyroid preparations	Interactive drugs antagonize insulin activity
Beta blockers	Masks hypoglycemia, delayed recovery from hypoglycemia

A *split dose* (twice daily) insulin regimen may be preferred because it permits a higher degree of glycemic control. Daily insulin therapy usually consists of administering two-thirds of the total daily intermediate-acting insulin in the morning, with the remaining dose given in the evening. A rapid-acting insulin might be added to either or both doses, or a combination preparation may be used.

Another method for calculating insulin dosage is based on body weight. In otherwise healthy patients with type 1 diabetes, dosing usually starts at 0.5 to 1.0 unit/kg/day. The dosage can be given as a single injection using intermediate-acting or combination preparations, or it can be divided into several daily injections. When insulin is required by patients with type 2 diabetes who exhibit insulin resistance, the insulin requirement is usually higher. Dosing for the individual with insulin resistance may start at 0.3 to 1.2 units/kg/day. Doses may be given from one to several times a day depending on the patient and the degree of glycemic control desired.

The decision to divide the insulin into multiple daily injections is made if the patient experiences midafternoon hypoglycemia and early morning hyperglycemia. Multiple daily injections may also be used if the individual is having difficulty maintaining normoglycemia or if the patient simply desires greater flexibility in life-style. Decisions to divide the insulin dosage and administer it in doses proportionate to individual needs are based on laboratory data and self-monitoring of blood glucose levels.

Insulin may also be given along with sulfonylureas (combination therapy) in type 2 diabetes. It is thought that combination therapy in type 2 diabetes is beneficial in decreasing insulin resistance.

The pregnant woman with diabetes has her insulin dosage individualized and calculated based on gestation. Ordinarily, the first indication for increased insulin occurs between 10 to 14 weeks' gestation, with the second increase occurring at approximately 28 to 32 weeks. Insulin requirements gradually increase until delivery. Table 49–4 provides only one method for the calculation of 24-hour insulin dosage over the course of three trimesters.

Insulin is available in concentrations of 100 or 500 U/mL (U-100 or U-500). U-100 is used most commonly. U-500 should be used only in cases of severe insulin resistance when the patient requires extremely large doses of insulin. REGULAR ILETIN II (concentrate) pork insulin in a concentration of 500 units/mL is available by prescription from Eli Lilly and Company for insulin-resistant patients who are hospitalized or under close medical supervision. U-500 is the only insulin that requires a prescription. Care should be taken that the patient purchases insulin syringes that correlate with the concentration of insulin used.

There are combination insulin preparations available, such as HUMULIN 70/30, which is 70 percent NPH and 30 percent regular insulin. A 50/50 combination (50 percent NPH and 50 percent regular) is also available. Premixed insulins are preferred to extemporaneous mixing by the patient, if the insulin ratio is appropriate, so as to avoid technique errors in mixing and incorrect dosing.

Laboratory Considerations

Insulin levels can be measured, but the process is costly and not usually indicated. Serum glucose levels and $HbA1_c$

TABLE 49–4 INITIATING AN INSULIN REGIMEN FOR A PREGNANT PATIENT WITH DIABETES MELLITUS

Fingerstick Blood Glucose Value	Dose of Insulin to be Administered
Step I:	
Perform fingersticks before meals and at bedtime. Administer insulin based on results using sliding scale	
<150 mg/dL	No insulin
150–200 mg/dL	8 units regular insulin
200–250 mg/dL	12 units regular insulin
250–300 mg/dL	16 units regular insulin
>300 mg/dL	20 units regular insulin
Step II:	
Recommendation if blood glucose out of desired range using protocol identified below*†	
7 AM	Adjust afternoon dose of NPH insulin
12 PM	Adjust morning dose of regular insulin
5 PM	Adjust morning dose of NPH insulin
9 PM	Adjust afternoon dose of regular insulin
3 AM	Adjust afternoon dose of NPH insulin
If blood glucose value: • Less than 60 mg/dL decrease appropriate dose by 2 units • Between 60–120 mg/dL no insulin adjustment needed • Between 120–150 mg/dL increase appropriate dose by 2 units • Between 150–180 mg/dl increase appropriate dose by 4 units • Over 180 mg/dL increase appropriate dose by 6 units † Guidelines may be liberalized if hypoglycemia frequently occurs.	
Step III:	
When glucose levels have stabilized, the daily insulin requirement is totaled and split into 2 injections with 2/3 of the total daily dose given in the morning and 1/3 given in the evening.	
Step IV:	
The morning and evening doses can then be split into 3/4 NPH and 1/4 regular insulin.	

values are sufficient to measure the effectiveness of treatment. Insulin may cause serum inorganic phosphate, magnesium, and potassium levels to decrease.

Sulfonylureas

FIRST-GENERATION DRUGS

- ❒ Acetohexamide (DYMELOR); (✱) DIMELOR
- ❒ Chlorpropamide (DIABINESE); (✱) APO-CHLORPROPAMIDE, NOVO-PROPAMIDE
- ❒ Tolazamide (TOLINASE)
- ❒ Tolbutamide (ORINASE); (✱) APO-TOLBUTAMIDE, NOVO-BUTAMIDE

SECOND-GENERATION SULFONYLUREAS

- ❒ Glipizide (GLUCATROL, GLUCATROL XL)
- ❒ Glyburide (DIABETA, GLYNASE PRESTABS, MICRONASE); (✱) APO-GLYBURIDE, EUGLUCON, GEN-GLYBE, NOVO-GLYBURIDE
- ❒ Glimepiride (AMARYL)

Indications

As a class of oral hypoglycemic drugs, sulfonylureas are used to control hyperglycemia in patients with uncomplicated, type 2 diabetes who cannot achieve appropriate control with changes in diet alone. Approximately 60 to 70 percent of patients with type 2 diabetes initially respond to sulfonylurea therapy. Sulfonylureas are ineffective in treating patients who have severely impaired function or total loss of beta cells. First-generation sulfonylureas were discovered before 1970. These compounds were found after an observation that some of the sulfonamide antibiotics produced hypoglycemic effects. Second-generation sulfonylureas were discovered after 1970. Although they are classified as second-generation drugs, there are no differences in therapeutic effectiveness compared with the first-generation drugs.

Pharmacodynamics

Sulfonylureas are effective only with type 2 diabetes, patients with a functioning pancreas. Sulfonylureas are of no value to insulin-dependent diabetics. Because type 2 diabetes is associated with a decrease in insulin secretion and impaired insulin action, sulfonylureas have been very successful in stimulating beta-cell release of insulin. In addition, sulfonylureas decrease glycogenolysis and gluconeogenesis, and at least partially reverse the postreceptor defects, increasing the number of receptor sites.

Adverse Effects and Contraindications

Adverse effects of the sulfonylureas are infrequent, occurring in about 4 percent of patients taking first-generation drugs and slightly less often in those receiving second-generation agents. The primary adverse effect is hypoglycemia because of the increase in insulin production and decrease in hepatic glucose release. Chlorpropamide has the greatest risk for severe hypoglycemia related to its extensive duration of action. Impaired renal or hepatic function can increase the risk of hypoglycemia in all sulfonylureas. Although hypoglycemia is usually mild, fatalities have occurred. Hypoglycemia is sometimes persistent, requiring infusion of dextrose for several days. Hypoglycemic reactions are most likely to develop in patients with kidney or liver dysfunction because of drug accumulation.

All first-generation sulfonylureas have a diuretic effect, with the exception of chlorpropamide, which has an antidiuretic effect. With chlorpropamide only, the patient is at risk for fluid volume excess and altered cardiac output related to the drug's antidiuretic effect. Fluid volume excess many be evidenced by weight gain, difficulty breathing, oliguria, and edema of the face, hands, and feet. Hyponatremia is less commonly seen. Chlorpropamide also exhibits disulfiram properties (alcohol flushing) and should be used cautiously in those patients who consume alcohol.

Other adverse effects of sulfonylureas include gastrointestinal (GI) distress (nausea, vomiting, cholestasis), hematologic effects (thrombocytopenia, leukopenia, hemolytic anemia, aplastic anemia), skin reactions (rash, pruritus), and an increased risk for hypothyroidism. The adverse effects are usually corrected with the cessation of therapy.

Sulfonylurea use should be avoided in patients with a history of severe reaction to a structurally related drug, such as sulfonamide antibiotics. Caution should also be taken when using the sulfonylureas in the older adult, those with impaired hepatic, thyroid, or renal function, and patients with congestive heart failure. Alterations in physiologic function caused by these disorders affect the pharmacodynamic activities of the sulfonylurea.

Use of sulfonylurea therapy is contraindicated during pregnancy. The patient should be started on insulin in order to achieve glycemic control throughout the pregnancy and counseled as to the appropriate diet and exercise program. Sulfonylureas should not be used during lactation because they pass into breast milk. In addition, sulfonylureas are contraindicated in patients with uncontrolled infection, serious burns, or trauma.

Pharmacokinetics

Sulfonylureas are well tolerated when they are taken by mouth. They are readily absorbed (over 80 percent) by the GI tract and are highly protein bound (Table 49–5). They are all biotransformed in the liver and eliminated in the urine. Patients with hepatic or renal impairment may require lower dosages or may require insulin, because the drugs and their metabolites may accumulate in the blood and increase the risk of severe and prolonged hypoglycemia.

Drug-Drug Interactions

There are many drugs that potentiate the effect of the sulfonylureas, and many that antagonize its effects (Table 49–6). A concomitant treatment plan should be carefully evaluated before starting sulfonylureas so as not to cause adverse reactions.

There are many drugs that antagonize the effects of sulfonylureas. Hormones such as glucagon, growth hormone, epinephrine, glucocorticoids, thyroid preparations, and oral contraceptives may cause hyperglycemia by decreasing insulin action. Diuretics, especially thiazide preparations, raise blood glucose levels presumably by acting to decrease potassium levels. Diazoxide is a nonthiazide diuretic that significantly elevates blood glucose levels by decreasing islet cell insulin release and stimulating the release of endogenous catecholamines. Beta blockers elevate blood glucose levels by increasing hepatic glycogenolysis that is mediated by alpha receptors. The beta blockers also mask symptoms of hypoglycemia and are not recommended for patients on hypoglycemic therapy.

Phenytoin and phenobarbital elevate plasma glucose levels. Phenytoin inhibits islet cell release of insulin. Phenobarbital acts to increase hepatic biotransformation of sulfonylureas, leading to increased drug clearance and elevated blood glucose. Nicotinic acid, a drug used in the treatment of hyperlipidemia, elevates blood glucose levels, possibly by increasing insulin resistance, but this is not completely clear. Other drugs that may cause hyperglycemia include pentamidine, cyclophosphamide, and L-asparaginase.

There are also nonprescription medications that can cause hyperglycemia. Nonsteroidal anti-inflammatory drugs may cause slight elevations in glucose levels. Cough and cold remedies often contain sugar, and this factor must be considered before using these agents. Sugar-free products are available. Nicotine from smoking may cause elevations in glucose levels. Caffeine, in large doses, has been shown to elevate blood glucose levels.

Dosage Regimen

The first-generation sulfonylureas are not as potent as the second-generation sulfonylureas and therefore require greater milligram dosages to be effective (Table 49–7). Dosages should be started low and adjusted every 4 to 7 days as needed until the desired glucose control is achieved, or until the maximum dose has been reached. If the maximum dose has not achieved a desired glucose range, changing to a more potent sulfonylurea may beneficial.

Laboratory Considerations

Oral hypoglycemic drugs may cause an increase in aspartate aminotransferase (AST; serum glutamic-oxaloacetic

TABLE 49–5 PHARMACOKINETICS OF SELECTED ORAL HYPOGLYCEMIC DRUGS

Drug	Route	Onset	Peak	Duration	PB (%)	$t_{1/2}$
First-Generation Sulfonylureas						
Acetohexamide	po	30–60 min	2–4 hr	12–18 hr	UA	30 min; 5 hr*
Chlorpropamide	po	60 min	3–6 hr	24–72 hr	High	36 hr
Tolazemide	po	4–6 hr	4–10 hr	12–24 hr	95	7 hr
Tolbutamide	po	30–60 min	3–5 hr	6–12 hr	95	7 hr
Second-Generation Sulfonylureas						
Glipizide	po	30–90 min	1–3 hr	12–24 hr	92–99	4 hr
Glyburide	po	2–4 hr	6 hr	16–24 hr	99	4–10 hr
Glimepiride	po	60 min	2–3 hr	24 hr	>99.5	5–9.2 hr
Biguanides						
Metformin	po	Days	2–2.5 wks	UK	UA	1.5–5 hr; 9–17 hr†
Alpha Glucosidase Inhibitors						
Acarbose	po	UK	1 hr	UK	UA	2 hr
Miglitol	po	Rapid	<60 min	UK	<4	2 hr
Thiazolidinedione						
Troglitazone	po	UK	UK	UK	>99	16–34 hr
Antihypoglycemia Drugs						
Glucagon	SC, IV	5–20 min	20–30 min	1–2 hr	UA	3–10 min
Diazoxide	po	60 min	8 hr	UA	90	36–60 hr
	IV	30–60 min	5 min	2–12 hr	90	36–60 hr

*Half life of acetohexamide and its metabolite, respectively.
†Half life and terminal half-life of metformin, respectively.
PB, Protein binding; $t_{1/2}$, half life; UA, unavailable; UK, unknown.

TABLE 49–6 DRUG-DRUG INTERACTIONS OF SELECTED ORAL HYPOGLYCEMIC DRUGS

Drug	Interactive Drug		Interaction
Sulfonylureas			
Sulfonylureas	Caffeine	Nicotine (smoking)	Increased risk of hyperglycemia
	Cyclophosphamide	Nicotinic acid	
	Diazoxide	NSAIDs	
	Epinephrine	Pentamidine	
	Glucagon	Rifampin	
	Glucocorticoids	Thiazide diuretics	
	Growth hormone	Thyroid hormones	
	L-asparaginase	Oral contraceptives	
	Oral anticoagulants		Hypoglycemia, increased effects of interactive drug
	Alcohol	MAO inhibitors	Effects of sulfonylurea potentiated in presence of interactive drug
	Allopurinol	Oral anticoagulants	
	Anabolic steroids	Phenobarbitone	
	Beta blockers	Phenylbutazone	
	Chloramphenicol	Probenecid	
	Clofibrate	Salicylates	
	Gemfibrozil	Sulfonamides	
	Beta blockers	Clonidine	Masks hypoglycemia, may cause delayed recovery
	Corticosteroids	Sympathomimetics	Hyperglycemia
	Dextrothyroxine	Thiazide diuretics	
	Rifampin		
Biguanide			
Metformin	Cimetidine	Nifedipine	Increased effects of metformin
	Furosemide		
	Amiloride	Quinidine	Compete for elimination pathways with metformin
	Calcium channel blockers	Ranitidine	
	Digoxin	Triamterene	
	Morphine	Trimethoprim	
	Procainamide	Vancomycin	
	Alcohol		Increased risk of lactic acidosis
	Glucocorticosteroids		
	Iodinated contrast media		
Alpha Glucosidase Inhibitors			
Acarbose	Calcium channel blockers	Oral contraceptives	May increase glucose levels and lead to loss of control of blood sugar
		Phenothiazines	
	Estrogens	Phenytoin	
	Isoniazid	Sympathomimetic	
	Loop diuretics	Thyroid hormones	
	Thiazide diuretics		
	Nicotinic acid		
	Amylase	Pancreatin	Effects of alpha glucosidase inhibitors are decreased
	Sulfonylureas		Acarbose potentiates effects of sulfonylureas
Miglitol	Activated charcoal	Pancreatin	Decreased effects of miglitol
	Amylase		
	Propranolol	Ranitidine	May decrease absorption of interactive drug
Thiazolidinedione			
Troglitazone	Cholestyramine		Significantly decreased absorption of troglitazone
	Cyclosporin		May decrease effectiveness of interactive drug
	HMG-CoA reductase inhibitors		
	Oral contraceptives		
	Tacrolimus		

MAO, Monoamine oxidase, NSAIDs, nonsteroidal anti-inflammatory drugs.

TABLE 49–7 DOSAGE REGIMEN OF ORAL HYPOGLYCEMIC DRUGS

Drug	Use(s)	Dosage	Implications
First-Generation Sulfonylurea Drugs			
Acetohexamide	Type 2 diabetes	*Adult:* 250 mg po QD. Maximum: 1500 mg Maintenance dose not to exceed 1.5 g/daily	Administer with caution to patient with impaired renal or hepatic function
Chlorpropamide	Type 2 diabetes	Adult: 250 mg po QD Maintenance dose 100–250 mg po up to 500 mg/daily. Maximum dose 750 mg/daily	Antabuse reaction. Antidiuretic effect. Administer with caution to patient with impaired renal or hepatic function. Start with lower dose in elderly
Tolbutamide	Type 2 diabetes	*Adult:* 0.25–3 g po single morning or divided doses. Maintenance dose over 2 g/day seldom required. Maximum dose, 3 g/daily	Contraindicated as sole treatment of type 1 diabetes. Administer with caution to patient with impaired renal or hepatic function. Start with lower dose in elderly
Tolazamide	Type 2 diabetes	*Adult:* 100 mg po QD if FBS less than 200 mg/dL, 250 mg po QD if FBS > 200 mg/dL. Adjust dosage according to FBS value. Maintenance dose not to exceed 1 g/daily QD Maximum dose 1 g/day	Mild diuretic effect. Administer with caution to patient with impaired renal or hepatic function. Start with lower dose in elderly patient and gradually increase dose as needed
Second-Generation Sulfonylurea Drugs			
Glipizide	Type 2 diabetes	*Adult:* 5 mg po QD before breakfast. Range: 2.5–40 mg/day. Doses over 15 mg/day should be given as two divided doses	Should be taken 30 minutes before meals. At least several days should elapse between titration steps.
Glyburide (DIABETA, MICRONASE)	Type 2 diabetes	*Adult:* 2.5–5 mg po QD with breakfast. Range: 1.25–20 mg/day. Increase in increments of no more than 1.5 mg/wk.	Slight diuretic effect. Base dosage increase in blood glucose values.
Glyburide (GLYNASE)	Type 2 diabetes	*Adult:* 1.5–3 mg po initially. Range: 0.75–12 mg/day. Doses over 6 mg/day should be given as divided doses. Increase in increments of no more than 1.5 mg/wk.	Doses may be divided. Retitrate if changing from nonmicronized to micronized form of drug.
Glimepiride	Type 2 diabetes	*Adult:* 1–2 mg po once daily initially. May increase every 1–2 weeks up to 8 mg/day. Usual dose 1–4 mg/day.	Cross-sensitivity with other sulfonylureas. May be administered once daily with the morning meal.
Biguanide			
Metformin	Type 2 diabetes	*Adult:* 500 mg po in divided doses up to 2 g/day. Maximum dose should not exceed 2.5 g/day.	Dose should be titrated based on patient response and blood glucose level. Safety and efficacy in children has not been established.
Alpha Glucosidase Drugs			
Acarbose	Type 2 diabetes in obese patient	*Adult:* 25 mg po 3 times daily at the start of each meal. Increase dosage at 4–8 week intervals as needed. Maximum dose 50 mg TID for patients under 60 kg, 100 mg po TID for patients over 60 kg.	Dosage increase based on postprandial blood glucose determinations. Glucose rather than sucrose must be used for hypoglycemia because sucrose will not be absorbed.
Miglitol	Type 2 diabetes	*Adult:* 25 mg po TID with meals. May increase to 100 mg TID if necessary.	May start with 25 mg QD if GI intolerance occurs. Take with first bite of the meal.
Antihyperglycemic Drug			
Troglitazone	Type 2 diabetes	*Adult:* Monotherapy: 400–600 mg po once daily. Increase dose to 600 mg after 6–8 weeks. Adjunct to sulfonylurea: 200 mg po daily. Increase at 2–4 week intervals to maximum of 600 mg/day. Adjunct to insulin: 200 mg po daily. Increase at 2–4 week intervals to maximum of 600 mg	If there is an inadequate response to monotherapy alternative therapeutic options should be pursued. The dosage of sulfonylurea may need to be decreased to optimize therapy. Insulin dosage should be decreased by 10–25% when fasting glucose levels decrease to less than 120 mg/dL
Antihypoglycemic Drugs			
Glucagon	Hypoglycemia related to insulin overdose	*Adult:* 0.5–1 mg IV/SC. May repeat if necessary in 20 minutes. *Child:* 25 mcg/kg IV/SC up to 1 mg. May repeat dosage if necessary in 20 minutes	Arousal response should occur in 20 minutes
Diazoxide	Hypoglycemia related to hyperinsulinism inoperable pancreatic islet cell adenoma, malignancy; islet cell hyperplasia	*Adult:* 3 mg/kg po QD in 2–3 divided doses q8hr. Maintenance dose 3–8 mg/kg po QD in 2–3 divided doses q8–12 hr *Child:* 3–8 mg/kg po QD in 2–3 divided doses q8–12 hr.	Check urine and blood glucose and ketone daily. Have insulin and tolbutamide on standby in case hyperglycemic reaction occurs. Have dopamine, norepinephrine on standby in case hypotensive reaction occurs

transaminase [SGOT]) lactate dehydrogenase (LDH), BUN, and creatinine levels. Serum sodium levels and plasma osmolality should be monitored periodically throughout therapy in patients taking chlorpropamide. Serum potassium levels should also be monitored.

Although serum levels of sulfonylureas are not routinely measured, blood glucose and $HbA1_c$ levels should be closely monitored during sulfonylurea use. Desired blood glucose levels vary with individual patients, but fasting plasma glucose values should not exceed 120 mg/dL. The complete blood count should be also monitored periodically throughout therapy, and the health care provider should be notified if a decrease in blood counts occurs.

Biguanides

❒ Metformin (GLUCOPHAGE); (🍁) NOVO-METFORMIN

Indications

Biguanides were introduced shortly after the introduction of sulfonylureas 40 years ago. The primary biguanide drug, phenformin, was withdrawn from the United States marketplace in 1977 because of a high incidence of lactic acidosis. However, metformin, a newer biguanide, is now used as adjunctive therapy in the management of type 2 diabetes. It may be used alone or in combination with a sulfonylurea in patients who have not responded adequately to a program of diet modification and exercise.

Pharmacodynamics

Metformin decreases the hepatic production of glucose, decreases intestinal absorption of glucose, and increases insulin sensitivity. When metformin is used in combination with a sulfonylurea, the combination lowers blood sugar levels more effectively than either drug used alone. This outcome is to be expected because metformin and sulfonylureas act by different mechanisms.

Adverse Effects and Contraindications

The most common adverse effects of metformin include nausea, vomiting, diarrhea, abdominal bloating, and an occasionally unpleasant metallic taste. The GI disturbances are transient and usually resolve spontaneously during therapy. Decreased vitamin B_{12} levels have been noted.

Lactic acidosis rarely occurs (0.03 cases/1000 patients) but is the most serious adverse effect of metformin (50-percent mortality rate) and the reason phenformin was removed from the market. Lactic acidosis is characterized by an increase in blood lactate levels (over 5 mmol/L), a decrease in blood pH, and electrolyte disturbances. Symptoms of lactic acidosis include unexplained hyperventilation, myalgia, malaise, and somnolence. Lactic acidosis may advance to cardiovascular collapse, acute heart failure, acute myocardial infarction, and prerenal azotemia (see Controversy—Metformin and Lactic Acidosis).

Metformin is contraindicated in patients with hypersensitivity, metabolic acidosis from any cause, underlying renal dysfunction (serum creatinine levels above 1.5 mg/dL in men or above 1.4 mg/dL in women), conditions associated with hypoxemia (e.g., heart failure), and in patients with hepatic impairment. Metformin should be used with caution in older adults and debilitated patients, patients under stress from infection or surgical procedures, hypoxic patients, or patients with pituitary deficiency or hyperthyroidism. Safe use during pregnancy and lactation has not been established.

Pharmacokinetics

Fifty to sixty percent of metformin is absorbed from the small intestine following oral administration. Food delays or decreases the extent of absorption. Metformin is distributed primarily to intestinal mucosa and salivary glands. The onset of hypoglycemic drug action takes several days, with peak effects noted in 2 to 4 weeks. The duration of drug action is unknown. Metformin is almost entirely eliminated unchanged by the kidneys and has a biphasic half-life.

Controversy

Metformin and Lactic Acidosis

JONATHAN J. WOLFE

The appearance of second-generation sulfonylurea drugs (e.g., glipizide, glyburide) was a welcome improvement in diabetes management. These drugs have been associated with higher potency and lower levels of adverse effects than their precursors. They are also perceived as safer and more efficacious than previous oral antidiabetic agents such as phenformin, because the occurrence of lactic acidosis was clearly associated with its use. Accordingly, the introduction of metformin as an oral antidiabetic stirred negative memories of lactic acidosis and death among many health care providers.

Metformin is chemically related to phenformin. However, the risk of lactic acidosis with this drug is reported to be about 0.03 cases/1000 patient-years of use. Nevertheless, in approving marketing metformin the Food and Drug Administration required that a boxed warning about lactic acidosis be included. This seems a reasonable response to an adverse effect, which is approximately 50-percent fatal. It is also a complication requiring immediate treatment in an emergency department setting with personnel familiar with the disorder.

Much of the warning indicates that people with renal disease are more prone to lactic acidosis. This suggests prudent steps in patient selection. Similarly, patients who are unable to control their intake of alcohol are poor candidates for metformin. Finally, recommendations about discontinuing the drug in the face of stressors such as surgery go far toward protecting the patient. Most of all, it is critical for patients taking this drug to understand prodromal signs of lactic acidosis. It is precisely here that patient education and periodic review of cautions about lactic acidosis may prove maximally effective.

Critical Thinking Discussion

- What three signs, although nonspecific, may indicate the onset of lactic acidosis?
- What advantages does metformin offer as a single agent for antidiabetic therapy in the patient who has been able to control the disease solely by diet?
- What dosage level of metformin and sulfonylureas are ideal when the two products are used in combination to treat diabetes? Does such a combination increase the likelihood of lactic acidosis?
- Why might a patient insist on a lengthy trial of metformin and a second oral drug rather than changing to therapy with subcutaneous insulin?
- Does metformin appear to pose as great a hazard to the patient as does uncontrolled diabetes mellitus?

Drug-Drug Interactions

There are many drug-drug interactions with metformin. A number of drugs compete with metformin for elimination pathways, and thus, altered drug responses may occur. Cimetidine, furosemide, and nifedipine increase the effects of metformin. Iodinated contrast materials alter renal function, and thus, the elimination of metformin is delayed, increasing the risk of lactic acidosis.

Dosage Regimen

Initially, a 500-mg tablet of metformin is taken by mouth with morning and evening meals. The dosage may be increased in 500-mg increments at weekly intervals up to 2 g/day. Dosages exceeding 2 g/day should be administered as 1000 mg with morning and evening meals. If dosages of more than 2.5 g are needed, the dose should be taken three times daily with meals. The maximum daily dose should not exceed 2.5 g/day.

If 850-mg tablets of metformin are used, the initial dose is 850 mg is taken with the morning meal. The dosage may be increased in 850-mg increments every other week in divided doses. Maintenance therapy is 850-mg twice daily with morning and evening meals. The maximum dose should not exceed 850 mg three times daily.

Laboratory Considerations

Metformin may cause a decrease in serum vitamin B_{12} levels without producing clinical manifestations. It rarely causes anemia but anemia is reversible with discontinuation of metformin or supplementation with vitamin B_{12}. Serum glucose and $HbA1_c$ values should be monitored periodically throughout therapy. Metformin may decrease serum potassium levels.

Alpha-Glucosidase Inhibitors

❒ Acarbose (PRECOSE)
❒ Miglitol (GLYSET)

Indications

Acarbose and miglitol are used in the management of type 2 diabetes in conjunction with dietary therapy. Both drugs may be used concurrently with sulfonylurea drugs.

Pharmacodynamics

Acarbose and miglitol lower blood sugar levels by inhibiting the enzyme alpha glucosidase in the GI tract. The inhibition of this enzyme results in delayed glucose absorption and digestion of carbohydrates, which, in turn, reduces postprandial hyperglycemia. For this reason, this group of drugs is popularly known as starch blockers. They tend to cause weight loss. Alpha glucosidase inhibitors may be of value to the obese diabetic patient, but they are not indicated for patients with normal weight because of its effect on nutrition.

Adverse Effects and Contraindications

The most common adverse effects of acarbose include abdominal pain, diarrhea, and flatulence. Elevated transaminases have been noted in some patients taking acarbose. Low serum iron levels have been noted with miglitol. A rash has also been reported with miglitol.

Pharmacokinetics

Less than 2 percent of acarbose is absorbed systemically. The minimal amounts that are absorbed are eliminated by the kidneys with a half-life of 2 hours. Drug action peaks in 1 hour, but the duration of drug action is unknown.

Miglitol is completely absorbed at lower doses (25 mg). Fifty to seventy percent is absorbed at 100-mg doses. Miglitol is primarily distributed into extracellular fluid, with small amounts entering breast milk. It is not biotransformed. The small amounts that are absorbed are eliminated essentially unchanged in the urine.

Drug-Drug Interactions

There are many drug-drug interactions with acarbose and miglitol. A number of drugs may increase glucose levels in diabetic patients and lead to loss of glycemic control. The effects of alpha glucosidase inhibitors are decreased with the concurrent use of intestinal absorbents; thus, concurrent use should be avoided. Both acarbose and miglitol potentiates the effects of sulfonylurea drugs.

Dosage Regimen

Acarbose is taken three times daily at the beginning of each meal. The dosage may be increased at 4- to 8-week intervals as needed and tolerated. The usual dosage range is 50 to 100 mg three times daily. Dosage should not exceed 50 mg three times daily in patients weighing less than 60 kg or 100 mg three times daily in patients weighing more than 60 kg.

Twenty-five milligrams of miglitol are taken by mouth three times daily with meals. The dosage may be increased up to 100 mg three times daily, if necessary. If GI intolerance occurs, therapy should be started at 25 mg once daily.

Laboratory Considerations

Serum glucose, $HbA1_c$, AST (SGOT), and ALT (SGPT) should be monitored periodically throughout alpha glucosidase inhibitor therapy. Elevation of liver function test results may require dosage reduction or discontinuation of acarbose therapy.

Thiazolidinedione

❒ Troglitazone (REZULIN)

Indications

Troglitazone is indicated as an adjunct to diet and exercise in patients with type 2 diabetes. It should not be used as monotherapy in patients who had been previously well-controlled on sulfonylureas. Troglitazone may be added as an adjunct to a sulfonylurea but should be added to, not substituted for, the sulfonylurea. It may also be used as an adjunct for patients taking insulin; however, secondary causes of poor glycemic control should be investigated and treated before starting troglitazone therapy.

Pharmacodynamics

Troglitazone lowers glucose by improving target cell response to insulin. It has a unique mechanism of action that is dependent on the presence of insulin for activity. Troglitazone decreases hepatic glucose output and increases insulin-dependent glucose disposal in skeletal muscle. The mechanism of action is thought to involve binding to nuclear receptors that regulate the transcription of a number of insulin responsive genes critical for the control of glucose and lipid metabolism. It does not stimulate insulin secretion. Plasma lactate and ketone body formation are also decreased with troglitazone. Unlike the sulfonylureas, troglitazone is not an insulin secretagogue.

Adverse Effects and Contraindications

Patients receiving troglitazone in combination with insulin or oral hypoglycemic drugs may be at risk for hypoglycemia. Hypoglycemia has not been observed when troglitazone is used as monotherapy and would not be expected given the mechanism of action.

Troglitazone therapy in anovulatory, premenopausal women with insulin resistance may result in resumption of ovulation. These patients are at risk for contraception.

Hemoglobin and white blood cell counts have decreased in patients taking troglitazone. These changes occurred within the first 4 to 8 weeks of therapy. These changes may be due to the dilutional effects of increased plasma volume and have not been associated with any significant adverse hematologic effects.

Severe idiosyncratic hepatocellular injury has been reported but is rare. The hepatic injury is usually reversible but hepatic failure and death have been reported. Hepatic injury has occurred after both short-term and long-term troglitazone therapy. Anorexia, nausea, vomiting, abdominal pain, fatigue, and dark urine is suggestive of hepatic involvement.

Troglitazone is contraindicated in patients with known hypersensitivity to the drug or any of its components. The drug should not be used in patients with type 1 diabetes because troglitazone enhances the effects of circulating insulin. It does not lower glucose levels in patients who lack endogenous insulin. It should be used with caution in patients with hepatic disease.

Dosage Regimen

When troglitazone is used as monotherapy, the usual dosage is 400 to 600 mg once daily. If necessary, the dosage is increased to 600 mg after 6 to 8 weeks.

If troglitazone is used as an adjunct to sulfonylurea, the usual daily dosage is 200 mg. The dosage is increased at 2- to 4-week intervals to a maximum of 600 mg/day.

Used as an adjunct to insulin, the usual dose of troglitazone is 200 mg daily. The dosage is increased at 2- to 4-week intervals to a maximum of 600 mg. The insulin dose should be decreased by 10 to 25 percent when fasting glucose levels decrease to less than 120 mg/dL. Further adjustments should be individualized based on patient response.

Laboratory Considerations

There is no specific laboratory testing required for patients taking troglitazone. However, because of the risk of hepatic injury, liver function testing should be performed before the start of therapy, again within the first 1 to 2 months of therapy, and then every 3 months during the first year of therapy. Liver function testing should be performed periodically thereafter and at the first symptoms suggestive of liver dysfunction. Troglitazone should be discontinued if the patient develops jaundice or ALT (SGPT) levels three times the upper limit of normal.

Newer Antidiabetic Drug

Repaglinide (PRANDIN) is the first benzoic acid derivative to be used as an antidiabetic drug. Repaglinide is taken at a dose of 0.5 to 4.0 mg three times daily before meals. It augments the early insulin response associated with food intake and decreases the excess prandial and postprandial glucose excursions in the patient with type 2 diabetes. Because repaglinide is rapidly eliminated, little or no hypoglycemia is seen. This new drug also improves glycemic control when it is added to metformin therapy in patients whose diabetes is poorly controlled on metformin alone.

Antihypoglycemic Drugs

- ❒ Glucagon
- ❒ Glucose (INSTA-GLUCOSE, GLUTOSE)
- ❒ Diazoxide (HYPERSTAT)

GLUCAGON

Glucagon is indicated for the treatment of severe hypoglycemia in patients with diabetes. It can be used to treat hypoglycemia that results from insulin overdosage. It is useful though only if liver glycogen is available for use; thus, it is ineffective in chronic states of hypoglycemia or starvation and adrenal insufficiency. Glucagon is also used as an adjunct to barium in upper GI studies. It relaxes the esophagus, stomach, duodenum, small bowel, and colon to decrease peristalsis, thus improving outcomes of the exam.

Glucagon is a natural polypeptide hormone secreted by the alpha cells of the pancreas in response to hypoglycemia. It maintains plasma levels of glucose by stimulating hepatic glycogenolysis and gluconeogenesis. Glucagon effects carbohydrate metabolism in a manner exactly opposite that of insulin. It promotes the breakdown of glycogen, reduces glycogen synthesis, and stimulates the biosynthesis of glucose. Whereas insulin acts to lower plasma glucose concentrations, glucagon causes glucose levels to rise.

Adverse effects of glucagon, such as nausea and vomiting, are rare. A rash, dizziness, and respiratory distress have been documented but are infrequent. Glucagon is contraindicated in patients with hypersensitivity to beef or pork protein. The diluent contains glycerine and phenol and thus glucagon should be avoided in patients with hypersensitivity to these ingredients. It should be used with caution in patients with a history of insulinoma or pheochromocytoma.

Glucagon is usually given IV or SC, with an onset time of 5 to 20 minutes. Peak drug action is noted in 30 minutes, with a duration of drug action of 1 to 2 hours. It is extensively biotransformed by the liver and kidneys.

Large doses of glucagon may enhance the effects of warfarin. It negates the response to insulin and oral hypoglycemic drugs. Hyperglycemia effects are intensified and prolonged in the presence of epinephrine.

The dosage of glucagon when used to treat hypoglycemia is 0.5 to 1 mg IV or SC. If there is no response, the dosage may be repeated in 20 minutes. Once consciousness has been restored, oral carbohydrates should be given. The carbohydrates will help prevent recurrence of hypoglycemia and help restore hepatic glycogen content. For children, the dose is 25 mcg/kg IV or SC and the dosage repeated in 20 minutes if there is no response.

GLUCOSE

Glucose is used to treat or manage hypoglycemia. It is a monosaccharide that is absorbed from the intestine and then either used or stored by the body. The only adverse effect reported is nausea. No clinically significant drug-drug interactions have been noted.

Approximately 10 to 20 g are administered orally. Because glucose is not absorbed from the oral cavity, it must be swallowed to produce an effect. The dosage may be repeated in 10 minutes, if necessary. Use in children should be under the supervision of the health care provider.

DIAZOXIDE

Diazoxide is an oral glucose–elevating drug that acts by decreasing insulin release. It is used in the management of hypoglycemia due to hyperinsulinism in infants and children, inoperable pancreatic islet cell adenoma or malignancy, extrahepatic malignancy, and islet cell hyperplasia. It is not indicated for the treatment of functional hypoglycemia. It is also used for the short-term treatment of malignant and nonmalignant hypertension in hospitalized patients.

The most commonly reported adverse effects include a decrease in urine output, resulting in edema of the hands, feet or lower extremities, weight gain, and possibly congestive heart failure in susceptible individuals. Other adverse effects include taste alterations, anorexia, nausea, vomiting, abdominal pain, and constipation. With chronic use, it may cause increased hair growth on the arms, legs, back, and forehead. Tachycardia and thrombocytopenia have also been reported. Hyperglycemia or ketoacidosis are noted with diazoxide overdose.

Diazoxide is rapidly absorbed when it is taken orally, with an onset of drug action in less than 1 hour. The duration of drug action is less than 8 hours. Diazoxide is over 90-percent bound to albumin, biotransformed in the liver, and eliminated in the urine.

The initial adult dose is diazoxide is 1 mg/kg every 8 hours. The maintenance dose is 3 to 8 mg/kg divided into 2 to 3 doses and administered every 8 to 12 hours. The maximum dose is usually 15 mg/kg/day.

DRUGS INFLUENCING BLOOD GLUCOSE LEVELS

Drugs That Elevate Blood Glucose Levels	*Drugs That Decrease Blood Glucose Levels*
Allopurinol	Alcohol
Adrenocorticotropic hormone	Allopurinol*
Amphetamines	Anabolic steroids
Asparaginase	Beta blockers
Beta blockers	Clofibrate*
Carbonic anhydrase inhibitors	Chloramphenicol*
Caffeine (in large quantities)	Fenfluramine
Calcium channel blockers	Guanethidine
Cyclophosphamide	Histamine-2 antagonists
Decongestants	Insulin
Diazoxide	Isoniazid
Epinephrine	Monoamine oxidase inhibitors
Estrogens	Oral anticoagulants*
Furosemide	Oxyphenbutazone*
Glucagon	Oxytetracycline
Glucose gel/tablets	Pentamidine
Glucocorticoids	Phenylbutazone*
Growth hormone	Probenecid
Lithium	Salicylates*
Marijuana	Sulfonamides*
Morphine	
Nicotine (smoking)	
Nicotinic acid	
Oral contraceptives	
Phenytoin	
Pentamidine	
Thiazide diuretics	
Thyroid hormones	

*Interact with sulfonylurea drugs only.

Critical Thinking Process

Assessment

History of Present Illness

On the patient's arrival at the office or acute care setting, information must be obtained related to the reason for the visit. If there is a history of diagnosed diabetes, the patient should be questioned as to the type and how long it has been since the original diagnosis was made. The patient should be queried as to specific symptoms and how long they have been present. Subjective information to be sought would include level of fatigue, polyuria, polydipsia, polyphagia, blurry vision, and dry or itching skin. Information regarding recent stressors, life changes, and any other precipitating factors should be elicited. Dietary restrictions, the degree to which self-blood glucose monitoring is done, activity levels, and the extent of patient education regarding diabetes should also be ascertained. Information sought would also include data about other drugs taken that may affect blood glucose levels (see Drugs Influencing Blood Glucose Levels) and identification of risk factors for atherosclerosis, such as smoking, hypertension, obesity, hyperlipidemia, and family history.

Questions that may guide the health care provider in assessing complications of diabetes include the following: Does the patient experience intermittent claudication (leg pain) when walking or exercising? Has there been a noticeable change in color, temperature, tingling or pain in the extremities? Has the patient experienced blurred or double vision, blind spots, or floaters within the field of vision? When eating, are there feelings of fullness, followed by bloating and flatus? Has there been difficulty voiding? It should be remembered that in an attempt to establish a diabetes-related database, general assessment data should not be overlooked.

Past Health History

Obtaining a complete past health history is important in assessing the patient with diabetes. History of major illnesses, childhood illnesses, surgical operations, social habits, and immunizations should be obtained.

Of particular importance to the person with diabetes is obtaining information about the family history of diabetes, heart disease, stroke, and the patient's history of obesity. For female patients, a gestational history should be obtained, including information about hyperglycemia, delivery of an infant weighing more than 9 pounds, toxemia, stillbirth, polyhydramnios, or other complications of pregnancy. Smoking, excessive alcohol intake, fatigue, emotional upset, and some over-the-counter drugs may exacerbate hyperglycemia.

The frequency, severity, and cause of acute complications, such as ketoacidosis and hypoglycemia, as well as precipitating factors such as accompanying illness or infection, should be included in the history. Prior infections, particularly of the skin, foot, dental, and genitourinary tracts, can put the patient at risk for future problems and should be noted. Symptoms and treatment of chronic complications associated with diabetes such as eye, heart, kidney, nerve, and sexual function, and peripheral vascular and cerebrovascular disease should be included when obtaining past history.

Physical Exam Findings

A complete physical exam should be performed with an initial or interim evaluation. Because patients with diabetes are at greater risk for eye, kidney, nerve, cardiac, and vascular complications, a head-to-toe assessment should be performed. The complications of diabetes include signs of retinopathy, neuropathy, and decreased peripheral circulation. Clinical manifestations of retinopathy include tortuosity or beading of the retinal blood vessels, pinpoint hemorrhages, or exudates on the retinal surface. Retinopathy may lead to blindness. Manifestations of neuropathy include decreased sensation, decreased reflexes, and positional blood pressure changes. These manifestations are assessed by evaluating reflexes, vibratory senses, and response to sharp and dull sensations. Decreased peripheral circulation is manifest as decreased skin temperature and weak posterior tibial or dorsalis pedis pulses. Neuropathy may lead to amputations. For the patient with type 1 diabetes, insulin injection sites should also be assessed. Skin turgor should also be assessed to determine the state of dehydration. In children, growth and maturity may be delayed.

The presence of fruity odor on the breath may be detected if the patient is experiencing ketoacidosis. The level of consciousness is determined by the patient's orientation and response to stimulation. Vital signs, including blood pressure, should be noted.

Diagnostic Test Findings

Each patient should undergo laboratory testing appropriate for the condition. Laboratory tests may include determination of blood glucose levels, electrolyte studies, BUN, serum creatinine, microalbuminuria, and glycosylated hemoglobin levels, pH and CO_2 levels. Tests are conducted to establish a diagnosis of diabetes, determine glycemic control and to determine the extent of associated complications and risk factors.

Connecting peptide (C-peptide) can be measured to diagnose type 1 diabetes. C-peptide is formed during the conversion of proinsulin to insulin in the beta cells of the pancreas. Because C-peptide and insulin are formed in equal amounts, this test indicates the amount of endogenous insulin production. Normally, a strong correlation exists between levels of insulin and C-peptide, except possibly in obese persons and in the presence of islet cell tumors. Patients with type 1 diabetes usually have no or low concentrations of C-peptide, whereas patients with type 2 diabetes tend to have normal or elevated levels.

A fasting glucose level should be obtained, if possible, to determine the patient's level of control, or to confirm the diagnosis of diabetes. If the patient is receiving an IV dextrose solution, the results of the test must be analyzed with that variable in mind. Critical values in adults are readings less than 60 mg/dL or more than 500 mg/dL.

Two-hour postprandial blood glucose readings reflect the efficiency of insulin-mediated glucose uptake by peripheral tissues. Normally, blood glucose levels return to fasting levels within 2 hours. Smoking and caffeine can lead to falsely elevated values at 2 hours, whereas strenuous exercise can lead to falsely decreased values.

Glycosylated hemoglobin (HbA_{1c}) levels help determine the amount of so-called sugar-coated hemoglobin A (glycohemoglobin) and identifies the average blood glucose level for the previous 3-month period. Most simply, glycohemoglobin is blood glucose bound to hemoglobin. The test provides evidence as to the adequacy of dietary or insulin therapy, determines the duration of hyperglycemia in new cases of juvenile onset diabetes with acute ketoacidosis, and provides a sensitive estimate of glucose imbalance in mild cases of diabetes. In addition, it may be used as a mechanism for determining the effectiveness of old and new forms of therapy, such as oral hypoglycemia drugs, single or multiple insulin injections, and beta cell transplantation. Test results are not affected by time of day, meal intake, exercise, recently administered diabetic drugs, emotional stress, or patient cooperation.

The amount of glycosylated hemoglobin found and stored by the red blood cell depends on the amount of glucose available to it over the cell's 120 day life-span. A normal range for the nondiabetic is 4.0 to 7.0 percent. Values are increased in patients who are poorly controlled and in those patients with newly diagnosed diabetes. In these instances, HbA_{1c} levels comprise 8 to 12 percent of the total hemoglobin. With optimal insulin control, HbA_{1c} levels return toward normal.

A fasting lipid profile (total cholesterol, high-density lipoprotein cholesterol, low-density lipoprotein, and triglycerides) help determine the risk for cardiovascular complications. These results should be taken into consideration when conducting dietary counseling. BUN and serum creatinine levels should be measured in all adults, or when proteinuria is present, to determine the degree of renal dysfunction or damage. Microalbuminuria may be used to detect early renal damage. Alterations in these exams should be taken into account when prescribing medications, because many drugs are eliminated by the kidney. Urinalysis should include ketones, glucose, and protein, and a culture should be obtained if microscopic findings are abnormal or if symptoms are present.

In addition, thyroid function tests should be included because diabetes is associated with thyroid disease. Retinal photographs provide an effective means to document retinal status and are performed when a diagnosis of type 2 diabetes is made, or 5 years after a diagnosis of type 1 diabetes. Nerve conduction tests may be performed when abnormalities such as tingling, numbness, or pain are noted.

Developmental Considerations

Perinatal Pregnancy-related morbidity and mortality in patients with diabetes has been significantly reduced over the past decade. However, the mortality risk remains higher in the diabetic population than in the nondiabetic population. Intensive antepartum surveillance of diabetic pregnancies is crucial.

The stress of pregnancy may also affect the previously nondiabetic woman. Increased demands on the pancreas can cause elevated glucose levels, which are associated with macrosomia, neonatal hypoglycemia, hypocalcemia, polycythemia, and hyperbilirubinemia. All women should be screened for GDM between the 24th and 28th week of gestation. If it is suspected that a glucose intolerance exists, full diagnostic glucose tolerance testing should be performed.

If the woman is diagnosed with GDM, she should be counseled regarding diet, exercise, and home glucose monitoring. If unable to control glucose levels with diet and exercise alone, insulin is necessary to control blood glucose levels. Women with GDM cannot take oral hypoglycemic agents because they cross placental membranes. GDM usually resolves after delivery, but the woman has a greater risk for developing type 2 diabetes and should be evaluated at the first postpartum visit and regularly thereafter.

Pediatric Insulin is almost always required with a diagnosis of pediatric diabetes, the aim being to closely simulate the plasma insulin levels seen in the nondiabetic individual. Insulin dosage can be difficult to regulate in pediatric and adolescent patients because calorie intake, activity levels, and hormonal levels fluctuate. The adolescent with diabetes must contend with peer pressure, teenage dietary practices, and growth spurts. As a general rule, the earlier the onset of diabetes, the more years there are for complications to develop.

Geriatric Most older adults have type 2 diabetes associated with age-related impairment of both pancreatic beta cells and insulin action. The older patient is more likely to be overweight and have lower activity levels that, in turn, lead to insulin resistance. In addition, factors that predispose the older adult to diabetes may exist, including co-morbid illnesses and the use of hyperglycemia-inducing drugs.

Psychosocial Considerations

Although patients with diabetes are not at greater risk for developing psychological problems, they are at risk for psychosocial complications related to their illness. Women with type 1 diabetes are at higher risk for developing eating disorders such as anorexia nervosa and bulimia, and patients with long-standing diabetes have an increased risk for developing depression and anxiety. A diagnosis of diabetes can be very frightening to those who have preconceived ideas about the disease. Compliance may be dependent on the person's ability to make necessary changes in life-style.

Stress is thought to play a major role in the management of diabetes. Not only does stress cause a change in eating or exercise behaviors, but the physiologic response to stress has a direct relationship to blood glucose levels. Inquiries about stressful events should be a routine part of an evaluation.

For many people, the thought of injections can be overwhelming and frightening. Many devices are available to assist patients in self-administering injections while minimizing the sense of pain. Family members may be helpful in assisting with injections. Special consideration may need to be given to those who fear needles. Compliance may be minimal if the patient cannot overcome the fear.

Many people with diabetes find it difficult to comply with recommended meal plans. Because eating is such a social activity, many people lack the support they may need to persist in a regimented manner. Ethnic and cultural variations of meal patterns may also influence the treatment plan. Evaluation of the patient's educational level is vital if patient teaching and treatment regimens are to be successful (see Case Study—Insulin-Dependent Type 2 Diabetes).

Analysis and Management

Treatment Objectives

The primary goal in managing the diabetic patient is to control blood glucose at levels that minimize symptoms of hyperglycemia and avoid hypoglycemia. To the extent that complications of diabetes may be related to hyperglycemia, the goal of treatment should be normalization of both fasting and postprandial blood glucose concentrations. Treatment regimens aimed at lowering blood glucose levels to or near normal levels in all patients is mandated by the following proven benefits:

- The risk of DKA and HHNC with their accompanying morbidity and mortality is markedly reduced
- Polyphagia, polydipsia, weight loss, fatigue, and vaginitis or balanitis may be decreased
- The development or progression of diabetic retinopathy, nephropathy, and neuropathy are greatly reduced
- Near-normalization of blood glucose levels is associated with a less atherogenic lipid profile

Individual treatment objectives should take into account the patient's ability to understand and carry out the treatment regimen, his or her risk for severe hypoglycemia, and other factors that may increase risk or decrease benefit (e.g., very young, older adults, end-stage renal disease, advanced cardiovascular or cerebrovascular disease, or other co-morbid disorders that materially shorten the life-span).

Treatment Options

Pharmacotherapeutic options vary based on the type of diabetes. Patients with type 1 diabetes are dependent on insulin and would not benefit from the oral hypoglycemic drugs. Insulin is also indicated for patients with acute decompensated diabetes, as in DKA. Persons with GDM may require insulin to protect the fetus. Primary or secondary failure of oral hypoglycemic drugs may also lead to the need for supplemental insulin. Patients with type 2 diabetes may take oral hypoglycemics.

Case Study Insulin-Dependent Type 2 Diabetes Mellitus

Patient History

History of Present Illness	VH is a 72-year-old black female who presents to the clinic today for 3-month follow-up of her type 2 diabetes mellitus. She reports having periods of hyperglycemia several times a week for last 3 months but thought she was just tired. She reports following an 1800-calorie ADA diet as learned in diabetic education class. Reports no signs or symptoms of UTI, skin breakdown, or recent vision changes.
Past Health History	VH has history of hemoglobinopathy, congestive heart failure, hypertension, and previous transmetatarsal amputation left foot. Last eye exam: 3 months ago. Retinopathy present. Present meds: digoxin 0.25 mg po QD; gemfibrozil 600 mg po BID; metoprolol 50 mg po BID; naproxen 500 mg po BID; glipizide 10 XL mg. po QD.
Physical Exam	VS: BP 170/96, pulse 88, respirations 16. Weight: 143 (up from 135 3 months ago). Height: 5'2". Skin warm, dry. Mucous membranes dry. Thyroid nonpalpable. S_3 heart sound present. Bilateral pulses 2+. No evidence skin breakdown bilateral lower legs or feet. Old transmetatarsal incision evident.
Diagnostic Testing	Current labs: UA for C&S negative. UA shows trace protein, 250 mg/dL glucose. HbA_{1c} 9% (hemoglobinopathy underestimates HbA_{1c}). Cholesterol 193 mg/dL. Triglyceride 724 mg/dL. FBS 268 mg/dL. SBGM report indicates AM blood sugar readings consistently ranging from 200–220 mg/dL. before meals and at bedtime.
Developmental Considerations	Husband attended diabetic classes with VH. Reports that he does all the shopping and cooking, followed prescribed dietary regimen. Are retired floral shop owners.
Psychosocial Considerations	Have 3 children who live out of state but are in contact about once a month. Active in church women's group. Wears special orthotic shoes to accommodate transmetatarsal amputation.
Economic Factors	Both husband and wife are on Social Security disability with military health care and pharmacy coverage. Husband reports that he is unsure of accuracy of glucose monitoring device currently in use. It is 5 years old.

Variables Influencing Decision

Treatment Objectives

- Control blood glucose at levels that will help minimize symptoms of hyperglycemia and yet avoid hypoglycemia.
- Prevent, postpone, reverse complications associated with long-term history of dibetes mellitus.

Drug Variables	*Drug Summary*	*Patient Variables*
Indications	Oral hypoglycemic drugs most often used in the management of type II diabetes. Long-acting insulin may cover glucose levels since VH no longer responsive to oral drugs. This will become a decision point.	VH blood glucose levels remain elevated each AM in spite of maximum dose of sulfonylurea. This will become a decsion point.
Pharmacodynamics	Insulin acts by binding to insulin receptor sites on cells to allow transport of glucose into cell. Glipizide XL stimulate beta cell release of insulin. VH's pancreas is no longer as functional as before.	Insulin will reduce blood glucose levels to target range and minimize continued risk of complications.
Adverse Effects/ Contraindications	Potential for hypoglycemia exists for both insulin and oral drugs.	VH is aware of signs and symptoms of hypoglycemia and the interventions required. This will remain a decision point because she will require update of information.

Drug Variables	*Drug Summary*	*Patient Variables*
Pharmacokinetics	Peak action and duration relative to specific drug. BIDS regimen will act to better stabilize blood sugar over a longer period of time than glipizide XL.	There are no patient variables at this time that directly influence pharmacokinetics. Patient routinely eats three meals/day and has HS snack
Dosage Regimen	Insulin dosages are individualized based on patient blood glucose readings. VH afraid of self-administration of insulin. Husband willing to provide injections. This will become a decision point. BIDS regimen recommended.	Patient faithfully monitors blood glucose. Is able to follow dosage regimen with sufficient instructions.
Lab Considerations	Change in dosage regimen requires weekly monitoring until status stabilizes. This will become a decision point.	Transportation to military health care facility for lab work provided by church group. This is not a decision point.
Cost Index*	Glipizide XL: 4 Ultralente insulin: 1 Syringes: 1 Alcohol wipes: 1 One-Step glucose monitor device and strips (kit): 5	Insulin supplies and glucose monitoring equipment provided by military health care system. This is not a decision point. Glipizide XL formulary drug at military facility.

Summary of Decision Points

- Long-acting insulin may cover glucose levels since VH no longer responsive to oral drugs.
- BIDS regimen will act to better stabilize blood sugar over a longer period of time than glipizide XL.
- VH aware of signs and symptoms of hypoglycemia and interventions required.
- Transportation to military health care facility for lab work provided by church group.
- VH afraid of self-administration of insulin. Husband willing to provide injections.
- Insulin supplies and glucose monitoring equipment provided by military health care system.

DRUGS TO BE USED

- Continue glipizide XL 10 mg po QD each AM
- Start Ultralente insulin, 10 units at bedtime
- Replace glucose monitoring device and strips

*Cost Index:
1 $ < 30/mo.
2 $ 30–40/mo.
3 $ 40–50/mo.
4 $ 50–60/mo.
5 $ > 60/mo.

AWP of 100, 10 mg tablets of glipizide XL is approximately $64.
AWP of one 10 mL vial of U-100 Ultralente Insulin is approximately $25.
AWP of 100, 28 gauge, 1/2", 1 mL syringes is approximately $25.
AWP of One-Step II glucose monitor with strips (Kit) is approximately $150.

Drug Variables

Insulins Human insulin is the preferred choice in pregnant women and in women with diabetes who are considering pregnancy. Additionally, it is recommended for those with allergies or immune responses to animal source insulin, those initiating insulin therapy, and those who will be using insulin only intermittently.

Attempts should be made to identify the underlying cause of any hypersensitivity responses to insulin by measuring insulin-specific IgG and IgE antibodies. If patients have allergic reactions to mixed porcine-bovine insulin, human insulin should be used. If the allergy is severe, treatment involves the use of systemic glucocorticoids. If allergy persists, desensitization may be attempted and is successful in about 50 percent of patients.

Dawn phenomenon may be corrected by changing the time of the evening dose of intermediate acting insulin to bedtime instead of dinner time. The Somogyi phenomenon may be corrected by decreasing the evening dose of intermediate acting insulin or eating a more substantial bedtime snack. The lipodystrophies can be minimized by proper rotation of injection sites. Insulin allergies may be corrected by a change to the less antigenic human insulin. Insulin resistance is treated by changing the insulin to a purer preparation or by changing from an animal source to human insulin.

When recommending treatment schedules for patients with odd work or sleep schedules, it is important to keep in mind the type of insulin and dosage administration times so as not to coincide with high activity times or times when it would be unrealistic to comply. If a prescribed regimen does not fit with the patient's schedule, compliance with the treatment plan will be difficult and the patient may be set up to fail. Education is necessary to learn how to incorporate daily routines and special occasions into the treatment regimen.

Human insulin preparations, although less antigenic, are more expensive than animal preparations. There are many blood glucose testing products available that are compact, easy to use, and reasonably priced. The strips for these products are costly and should be taken into consideration when putting a testing plan in place for the patient. The patient's financial situation should be assessed before providing a treatment plan. Supplies to maintain tight diabetes control can be costly. Support groups and organizations may also be able to provide financial assistance or resources for those who may not be able to afford the high cost of diabetes supplies.

Oral Hypoglycemic Drugs Oral hypoglycemic agents are used when type 2 diabetes cannot be controlled by alterations in diet, weight loss, and exercise. Sulfonylureas should be used only after a 4- to 6-week trial of diet and exercise. Unfortunately, many health care providers find it easier to prescribe a drug than to educate the patient on the benefits of weight-reducing diets and exercise. Dietary management should be maintained after beginning oral medication for diabetes.

All sulfonylureas appear to be equally efficacious. Concentrations of glucose are often lowered sufficiently to relieve symptoms of hyperglycemia, but they may not reach normal levels. If the patient does not respond, it is called primary failure. When glycemic control is initially achieved but then lost, as occurs in 5 to 10 percent of patients per year, secondary failure takes place. Secondary failure may result from noncompliance with diet and exercise programs, disease progression, a stressful event or condition, or misdiagnosis of a patient with a slow-onset type 1 diabetes. Failure of sulfonylureas is an indication for insulin therapy. Sulfonylureas are not likely to be effective for a patient on a dietary regimen who still has a fasting glucose level above 250 mg/dL.

First-generation sulfonylureas are chemically and pharmacologically similar. Tolbutamide is the least potent form, and chlorpropamide the most potent form. Second-generation drugs are more potent than first-generation oral hypoglycemics on a per-milligram basis and, therefore, are given in smaller dosages. They appear to have fewer adverse effects and drug-drug interactions compared with first generation drugs. Patients are still at risk, however, for hypoglycemia because the actions of the medications are essentially the same. Acetohexamide has uricosuric properties and is the preferred sulfonylurea for patients with gout.

Although oral hypoglycemic drugs are sometimes referred to as oral insulins, they are completely different from insulin. True insulins cannot be given by mouth because it is a protein that is destroyed by proteolytic enzymes in the GI tract. Insulin is given only by the parenteral route.

Consideration should be given to the half-life and duration of the sulfonylurea agent. A long-acting sulfonylurea is more likely to place the patient at risk for severe, prolonged hypoglycemia, especially if the patient is older, has poor nutrition, or renal, cardiovascular, or hepatic disease.

Generally speaking, if two sulfonylureas have failed to give adequate control, the patient may be a candidate for insulin therapy. There are no indications for the concomitant use of two oral hypoglycemic agents.

Patient Variables

In formulating a treatment plan for the patient with diabetes, consideration should be given to the patient's age, school or work schedule and conditions, physical activity, eating patterns, social situation and personality, cultural variables, and the presence of complications of diabetes or other co-morbid conditions. Implementation of the management plan requires that each aspect be understood, reasonable, and agreed on by the patient and the health care provider.

A patient's perception of the illness and the strength of her health care beliefs and convictions significantly influence the success of management regimens. The risk of experiencing unpleasant adverse drug effects such as hypoglycemia may alter a patient's compliance and should be considered when developing a plan of care. The patient, as well as family members, when appropriate, should be instructed on the importance of continued medical management and follow-up. Referral to a diabetes management team provides for improved, individualized and comprehensive instruction, and facilitates more effective follow-up and compliance.

The pharmacotherapeutic regimen is individualized and based in part on the type of diabetes and the motivation level of the patient. Tighter control of blood glucose levels require the patient to perform home blood glucose monitoring several times per day, to take his or her prescribed medications faithfully, exercise, and regularly visit the health team. This type of management program is not recommended for everyone, especially for the patient with autonomic neuropathy who may not recognize a hypoglycemic event, or for the patient with ischemic heart disease in whom hypoglycemia may precipitate a dangerous arrhythmia.

Intervention

Administration

Insulins Insulin is available in different types and strengths and is taken from different species. Check the type, species, dose, and expiration date before administration. The various types of insulins should not be interchanged without first contacting the health care provider. Use only insulin syringes to draw up the required dose. The unit markings on the insulin syringe must match the insulin's units per milliliter. Special syringes are available for doses less than 50 units.

Injection Technique For the patient who requires insulin, it is important to demonstrate correct dosage preparation and injection technique. Insulin is most often given by the SC route. In emergency situations, regular insulin may be given IV. Insulin cannot be taken orally because it is a protein that would be destroyed by proteolytic enzymes in the stomach.

Insulin may be injected into SC tissue of the upper arm, abdomen, anterior and lateral aspects of the thigh, and the buttocks (see Appendix F). Most patients are taught to inject insulin at a 90-degree angle. Those with less subcutaneous tissue may need to inject at a 45-degree angle to avoid intramuscular injection. Aspiration is not necessary. The insulin should be at room temperature, and injection sites should be rotated to minimize disfiguring lipodystrophies that slow insulin absorption.

There is considerable variation in absorption rates among various areas of the body. Therefore, rotation within one area at a time is recommended (e.g., rotating systemically across and over the abdomen only) rather than rotating to different areas with each injection. The abdomen has the fastest rate of absorption, followed by the arms, thighs, and buttocks. Exercise increases the rate of absorption from injection sites and should be taken into consideration when choosing a site.

Delivery Systems There are a variety of insulin delivery systems on the market. Jet injectors are available for those who are afraid of needles or for those who are unable to use syringes. These devices deliver insulin in a fine pressurized stream through the skin without the use of a needle. Absorption and peak insulin levels may be altered by the injector, necessitating caution by the patient. Typically, onset and peak action of the insulin occur earlier when these devices are used. The injectors are expensive and may traumatize the skin if they are used incorrectly.

Penlike devices are available that have insulin-containing cartridges inserted into a penlike holder. After the attachment of a disposable needle, the insulin is injected by selecting a dose and depressing a button once for each 1- to 2-unit increment desired, or once for the entire selected dosage. Although needles are used for the injection, there is no need for insulin to be drawn from multidose vials, adding to the convenience and accuracy of administration. The penlike devices may be helpful for patients who need multiple daily injections and for those who are visually or neurologically impaired.

Subcutaneous insulin pumps are available as an alternative to conventional injection therapy and can provide excellent glucose control, but they require strong motivation on the part of the patient. The pumps deliver a constant basal rate of insulin throughout the day and night, with the capability of delivering a bolus of insulin at mealtime. The needle, attached to a syringe via a long strip of plastic tubing, remains indwelling in the subcutaneous tissue of the abdomen. Patients program the pump to deliver the optimal amount of insulin, based on self-monitoring of blood glucose levels. Patients must be alert to tenderness and erythema at the insertion site, which indicate abscess or staphylococcal infection.

In the acute setting, during periods of illness or stress, a continuous IV infusion of regular insulin may be required. If more rapid onset but reduced duration of action is required, intramuscular injection may be performed but is not recommended for routine injections.

Insulin Handling and Storage Insulin deteriorates when it is exposed to excessive heat, light, or agitation. Constant refrigeration is not needed for the newer preparations, although patients should be instructed to refrigerate, not freeze, extra bottles until needed. Extra vials of insulin should be kept on hand in case of breakage. Vials in current use should be kept at room temperature to minimize irritation at the injection site caused by cold insulin. Insulin may lose its potency after it has been in use for over 30 days, especially when it is kept at room temperature. Insulin vials should always be inspected for clumping before each use.

Short-acting and intermediate-acting insulins may be mixed in the same syringe and used immediately or stored for later use. ILETIN insulins can be mixed together. However, because of the binding to zinc, ILETIN insulins should not be mixed with regular insulin. To do so may cause a delay in the onset of the action of regular insulin.

Intermediate-acting and long-acting insulin multidose vials must be gently but thoroughly rolled between the palms to mix the suspension before withdrawing the required dose. The bottle should not be shaken vigorously because the protein molecules become denatured by the whipping action. Frothing or foaming of the solution indicates the start of protein breakdown.

Equipment Disposal The patient should be taught proper syringe disposal, which varies from state to state. Unless the syringe is to be reused, it should be placed in a puncture-resistant container or needle clipping device. The syringe is less likely to be reused by another individual if the plunger is removed from the syringe before disposal.

Syringe manufacturers cannot guarantee sterility of needles that are reused. However, insulin contains bacteriostatic additives that inhibit the growth of bacteria commonly found on skin. For some patients syringe reuse is not only safe but economical. Immunosuppressed patients may be more at risk for infection than others and syringe reuse is not appropriate for these individuals. In addition, needles become dull when used several times, causing injections to become painful. Cleansing needles that are to be reused with alcohol should be avoided because the alcohol removes protective oils and contributes to quicker development of dull needles.

Oral Hypoglycemic Drugs Oral hypoglycemic drugs may be administered once in the morning or divided into two doses. The drug should be taken with meals to ensure best diabetic control and minimize gastric irritation. The drug should not be taken after the last meal of the day in order to avoid hypoglycemia episodes during the night. Tablets may be crushed and taken with fluids, applesauce, or pudding if the patient has difficulty swallowing.

Gradual dosage adjustment is not necessary when converting patients from other oral hypoglycemic drugs or insulin dosages of less than 20 units/day to sulfonylureas. Patients taking 20 to 40 units/day should convert gradually by receiving tolbutamide and a 25- to 50-percent reduction in insulin dose the first day, with gradual insulin dosage reduction as tolerated. Patients taking glyburide may discontinue insulin immediately. Patients taking more than 40 units/day should have a 29- to 50-percent reduction in insulin dose the first day, with a gradual insulin dosage adjustment as tolerated. Blood glucose levels should be monitored three times daily during the conversion period.

When transferring patients from oral hypoglycemic drugs (other than chlorpropamide) to metformin, no transition period is necessary. When transferring the patient from chlorpropamide, care should be exercised during the first 2 weeks of therapy (due to the prolonged retention of chlorpropamide) because overlapping drug effects make hypoglycemia possible. If there is an inadequate response to maximum dose of metformin within 4 weeks, an oral sulfonylurea drug may be added while continuing metformin at the maximum dosage.

Education

The most important part of diabetes management, in addition to compliance with the treatment plan, is patient education. Compliance is enhanced when the patient understands and can use the information provided. Except during periods of acute illness, the teaching needs of the patient with diabetes should be given high priority. Comprehensive diabetic education is beyond the scope of this text except as it relates to pharmacotherapy. As always, the use of teaching-learning principles must be applied to the teaching plan.

Educational materials should be written or adapted to the patient's learning ability, life-style, and sociocultural variables. In most instances, the use of printed materials encourages the patient to review the information or procedures at a later date. Family members or other support systems should be included in the educational plan so they can act as a resource and to help the patient gain compliance.

Support groups are also helpful as a learning resource and help with the development of realistic expectations. In rural communities where support groups may not be available, regional or national organizations are usually accessible for resource information and support. In addition, specialists such as diabetes nurse educators, dietitians, physical therapists, and behaviorists are good resources when educating a patient regarding diabetes. In relation to diabetic control in general, the patient with diabetes must be taught blood glucose monitoring techniques, the importance of meal planning, exercise, the signs and symptoms of insulin excess and deficiency, how to cope with sick days and insulin reactions, and when to seek professional attention.

Glucose Monitoring Urine or blood glucose monitoring is recommended for patients with type 1 and type 2 diabetes. Patients should be taught to test blood glucose levels before each meal and at bedtime. The more closely blood glucose levels approach normal, the less likely complications are to develop (although strict control does not always ensure that complications will not occur). The development of blood glucose meters has made urine testing for glucose obsolete for most patients. Further, urine glucose testing can be affected by fluid intake and by many drugs. Testing, however, is irrelevant if the patient does not know what to do with the results.

As with any pharmacotherapeutic regimen, the patient's knowledge base and ability to carry out the prescribed plan of care should be assessed. For the patient who is or will be receiving insulin, the patient's cognitive and physical ability to perform skills (i.e., adequate vision, fine motor skills) and the ability to prepare or obtain regularly scheduled meals and snacks should be taken into consideration. If the patient is unable to perform these tasks, it could increase their risk for severe hypoglycemia or severe hyperglycemia. Family members and home health professionals can be trained to assist with these tasks and can be helpful in preventing acute complications. If resources are not available to assist the patient, the desire to use insulin therapy should be reconsidered in view of patient safety.

Hypoglycemia The patient should be instructed on signs, symptoms, and proper treatment of hypoglycemia and when to notify his or her health care provider. As discussed in the section on diagnostic test findings, the characteristic symptoms of hypoglycemia depend on whether the hypoglycemia came on slowly or rather suddenly. Most hypoglycemic episodes can be prevented by adhering to regularly scheduled meal times and snacks, the careful timing of exercise, and proper dosing of insulin. Patients should be instructed to carry at least 15 g of fast-acting carbohydrate to treat hypoglycemia. Fifteen grams of fast-acting carbohydrate is contained, for example, in the following foods:

- Four to six ounces of fruit juice (without added sugar)
- One-half cup of regular (not diet) carbonated beverage
- Six Life Savers
- Two or three squares of graham crackers
- Four teaspoons of granulated sugar
- One cup of milk
- Six sugar cubes
- One-half cup of regular gelatin (not diet)

When the reaction is severe and the patient cannot swallow, a glucagon injection should be administered. Family members, roommates, and co-workers should be instructed in the use of glucagon for situations when the individual cannot be treated orally. All patients should be instructed to carry medical identification to alert others of the diabetes in case of emergency.

Meal Planning Exogenous insulin acts whether there is food present or not. Therefore, meal planning is one of the most important steps in diabetes management. Advise the patient that having diabetes does not mean they will have to give up all of the foods that they now enjoy. However, meal planning must become a big part of their treatment. Nutritional recommendations for patients with diabetes are similar to the recommendations of the American Heart Association, the National Cancer Institute, the Nutritional Committee for Recommendations for Children with Diabetes of the American Academy of Pediatrics, and the U.S. Dietary Guidelines. However, the patient should have an individualized meal plan, including three meals and three snacks, and be shown how to make daily meal choices. Calorie levels are individualized as to the patient's weight, desired weight, and activity level. The meal plan should be realistic and provide as much flexibility as possible to allow for integration into the individual's life-style. Low-fat meal principles should be enforced and alternative cooking methods should be used. Sugar substitutes should be offered. High-fiber diets should be encouraged because fiber slows the absorption of glucose from the GI tract and lowers total cholesterol and low-density lipoprotein cholesterol. The patient should be followed at regular intervals to ensure that changes in life-style are noted and appropriate adjustments are made to the nutritional program. Patients with weight loss goals may need more frequent follow-up.

Exercise Regular exercise is recommended for all persons with diabetes. Patients should be counseled as to benefits of exercise, an exercise plan, and precautions to take while exercising. The benefits of exercise include better glycemic control, improved cardiovascular health, weight loss, decreased anxiety, improved self-image, and disease prevention. An exercise plan should always include a low-intensity warm up and a postexercise cool down. Aerobic exercise is the most beneficial type of exercise to achieve glycemic and cardiovascular benefits. The patient should be taught first to discuss the intensity, duration, and frequency of exercise with the health care provider, and the exercise regimens individualized should be based on the patient's ability and health. The patient should be instructed as to protective footwear and other protective equipment, and his or her feet should be inspected daily and after exercise by the patient or other sighted individual. Exercise in extreme heat or cold should be avoided. It is important that the patient understand that exercise during periods of poor metabolic control should be avoided and to carry at least 15 g of fast-acting carbohydrate at all times to treat hypoglycemia should it occur. If the patient takes insulin, blood glucose levels should be monitored before, during, and after exercise. An exercise regimen that is carried out at a convenient time and location helps improve compliance with the exercise program.

Stress management is important in the proper management of blood glucose levels. Any physical or emotional stress affects glycemic control, and the patient may require an increased dosage during this time. The patient may find it helpful to visit with a behaviorist to counteract any emotional stress that may be having an effect on the individual's health. Family members should be included, as appropriate.

The patient with diabetes who travels must take their antidiabetic agents and related equipment with them. The patient should be taught to take extra insulin and syringes in separate carry-on baggage should their luggage be misplaced while in route. Specially designed containers for insulin and syringes are commercially available.

Sick Day Behaviors The patient should be instructed on what to do when illness interferes with the management plan. Blood sugar levels should be checked at least every 4 hours to detect hyperglycemia. The patient should continue taking his or her medication as directed, even if he or she is unable to follow the meal plan. If the patient is unable to take foods, fluids, or required medications, he should contact the health care provider because insulin may be required during this time. Ten to fifteen grams of carbohydrate should be consumed every hour. Liquids such as regular soda, popsicles, and jello (sweetened) are examples of sick day foods that provide the needed carbohydrates. Eight ounces of water should be consumed per hour to avoid dehydration. The health care provider should be notified if blood glucose levels exceed 250 mg/dL or there is fever exceeding 101.1° F for more than 24 hours, the patient is unable to take in fluids, breathing becomes shallow, or there is chest pain. It is important that the patient and family understand sick day guidelines because proper management can avoid hospitalization.

Evaluation

Effectiveness of pharmacotherapeutics for the patient with diabetes is demonstrated by control of blood glucose levels without the appearance of hypoglycemia or hyperglycemic episodes. In patients receiving combination drug therapy treatment, effectiveness is demonstrated by a reduction in insulin requirements.

SUMMARY

- Diabetes mellitus is a disorder of carbohydrate, protein, and fat metabolism.
- Approximately 14 million people in the United States have diabetes. Of these, an estimated 6 million undiagnosed cases exist among adults.
- Diabetes (and its complications) is the third leading cause of death from disease in the United States. It is considered to be the leading cause of new blindness in adults and is the single greatest contributor to end-stage renal failure and nontraumatic amputations in adults.
- Type 1 diabetes mellitus accounts for approximately 10 percent of all diabetes in the United States. Type 2 diabetes accounts for approximately 85 to 95 percent of all diabetes.
- Secondary diabetes is most often related to pancreatic disease or removal of pancreatic tissue, defects of insulin receptors, Cushing's syndrome, pancreatic tumors, the administration of drugs that impair insulin action, or the administration of hormones that cause hyperglycemia.
- GDM occurs in approximately 4 percent of pregnant women and is associated with increased fetal morbidity and mortality.
- The patient with type 1 diabetes has an absolute insulin deficit with hyperglycemia. This patient depends on insulin for survival.
- The patient with type 2 diabetes has a relative insulin deficit and insulin resistance. This patient may be treated by weight loss, diet, and exercise alone, or he or she may require oral hypoglycemic drug therapy.
- Subjective information to be sought for the patient history includes the level of fatigue, complaints of polyuria, polyphagia, polydipsia, blurry vision, and dry or itchy skin.
- Because patients with diabetes are at greater risk for eye, kidney, nerve, and cardiovascular complications, a head-to-toe assessment should be conducted.
- The primary goal in managing the diabetic patient is to control blood glucose at levels that reduce glucose levels to normal and avoid hypoglycemia.
- Drugs used to treat type 2 diabetes include oral hypoglycemic drugs such as sulfonylureas, biguanides, alpha glucosidase inhibitors, and antihyperglycemic thiazolidinedione drugs.
- Oral hypoglycemic drugs act by encouraging the release of insulin from the pancreas, decrease glycogenolysis and gluconeogenesis, and increase the sensitivity of the body tissues to insulin.
- Insulin is used in the management of type 1 diabetes. It acts by binding to insulin receptor sites on cells to allow molecular transport of glucose into the cells.
- Treatment schedules for patients with odd work, school, or sleep schedules should be kept in mind when planning the type of insulin and dosage administration times so as not to coincide

with high activity levels or times when it would be unrealistic to comply.

- Teaching needs of the patient on insulin include injection techniques, delivery systems, insulin handling and storage, equipment disposal, self–blood glucose monitoring, adverse effects, sick day behaviors, and the importance of balancing diet and exercise.
- The evaluation of insulin or oral hypoglycemic drug therapy can be demonstrated by control of blood glucose levels without the appearance of hypoglycemic or hyperglycemic episodes.

BIBLIOGRAPHY

Abramowicz, M. (Ed.). (1995). Metformin for non-insulin-dependent diabetes mellitus. *The Medical Letter of Drugs and Therapeutics,* 37(948), 41–42.

Abramowicz, M. (Ed.). (1996). Acarbose for diabetes mellitus. *The Medical Letter of Drugs and Therapeutics,* 38(967), 9–10.

American College of Obstetricians and Gynecologists. (1991). *Classification of diabetes in pregnancy* (Technical Bulletin No. 92). Washington, DC: Author.

American Diabetes Association. (1998). Clinical practice recommendations. Standards of medical care for patients with diabetes mellitus. *Diabetes Care,* 21(1), 1–26.

American Diabetes Association. (1994). Nutrition recommendations and principles for people with diabetes mellitus. *Journal of the American Dietetic Association,* 94(5), 504–506.

Bailey, C. J. (1993). Metformin—An Update. *General Pharmacology,* 24(6), 1299–1309.

Barnett, A. (1994). Diabetes mellitus, hypertension, ACE inhibitors: A significant risk. *Nursing Times,* 990(2), 62–64.

Bloomgarden, Z. (1998). Troglitazone: An agent for reducing insulin resistance. *A Special Report: Managing Type 2 Diabetes: New Science and New Strategies,* March, 33–39.

Coniff, R., Shapiro, J., and Bray, G. (1995). Multicenter placebo-controlled trial comparing acarbose with placebo, tolbutamide plus acarbose in non-insulin dependent diabetes mellitus. *American Journal of Medicine,* 98(5), 443–463.

Dagogo, J. S., and Santiago, J. (1998). The natural history of type 2 diabetes. *A Special Report: Managing Type 2 Diabetes: New Science and New Strategies.* March, 7–12.

Diabetes Control and Complications Trial (DCCT) Group. (1993). The effect of intensive treatment of diabetes on the development and progression of long-term complications in insulin dependent diabetes mellitus. *New England Journal of Medicine,* 329(14), 977–986.

Ertel, N. (1998). Newer therapeutic agents for type 2 diabetes. *A Special Report: Managing Type 2 Diabetes: New Science and New Strategies.* March, 25–32.

Gan, S., Barr, J., and Arieff, A. (1992). Biguanide-associated lactic acidosis: Case report and review of literature. *Archives of Internal Medicine,* 152(11), 2333–2338.

Garrison, M., and Campbell, K. (1993). Identifying and treating common and uncommon infections in the patient with diabetes. *The Diabetes Educator,* 19(6), 522–531.

Genuth, S. (1998). Diabetic retinopathy, nephropathy, and neuropathy: The importance of controlling glycemia. *A Special Report: Managing Type 2 Diabetes: New Science and New Strategies.* March, 19–24.

Harley, J. (1993). Preventing diabetic foot disease. *Nurse Practitioner,* 18(10), 37–44.

Heppard, M., and Garite, T. (1992). *Acute obstetrics: A practical guide.* St. Louis: Mosby–Year Book.

Kerr, C. (1995). Improving outcomes in diabetes: A review of the outpatient care of NIDDM patients. *Journal of Family Practice,* 40(1), 63–75.

LeMone, P. (1994). Responses of the older adult to the effects and management of diabetes mellitus. *MEDSURG Nursing,* 3(2), 122–127.

Moses, R. G., Slobodnuik, R., Donnelly, T., et al. (1997). Additional treatment with repaglinide provides significant improvement in glycemic control in NIDDM patients poorly controlled on metformin. (Abstract.) *Diabetes,* 46(Suppl 1), 93A.

Schmidt, L., Post, K., McGill, J., et al. (1994). The relationship between eating patterns and metabolic control in patients with non-insulin dependent diabetes mellitus (NIDDM). *The Diabetes Educator,* 20(4), 317–321.

Spollett, G. (1993). Intensive insulin therapy in insulin dependent diabetes and combination therapy. *Nurse Practitioner,* 18(7), 27–38.

Tierney, L., McPhee, S., and Papadakis, M. (1997). *Current medical diagnosis and treatment* (36th ed.). Norwalk, CN: Appleton & Lange.

Tinker, L., Heins, J., and Holler, H. (1994). Commentary and translation: 1994 recommendations for diabetes. *Journal of the American Dietetic Association,* 94(5), 507–511.

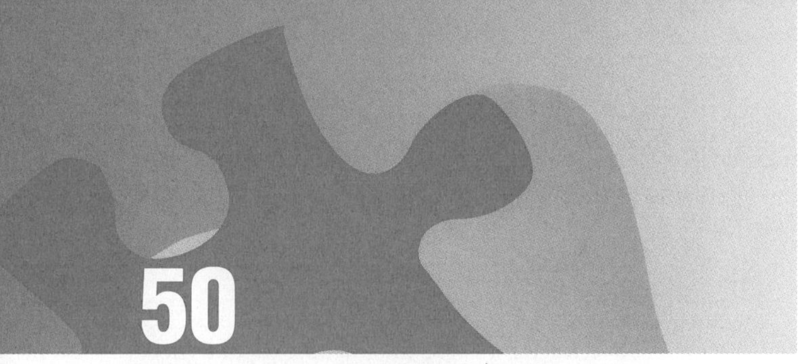

50

Thyroid and Parathyroid Drugs

The function of the thyroid gland is to take iodine from the circulation, combine it with the amino acid tyrosine, and convert it to triiodothyronine (T_3) and thyroxin (T_4) (Fig. 50–1). The thyroid gland stores T_3 and T_4 while waiting for release into the circulation under influence of thyroid-stimulating hormone (TSH). Thyroid hormones not bound to circulating plasma proteins provide the true determinate of thyroid status for the patient.

Alteration of thyroid gland function produces some of the most common endocrine disorders. *Thyrotoxicosis* (hyperthyroidism) is a result of excessive production of thyroid hormones. *Hypothyroidism* is caused by a deficiency of thyroid hormones.

The function of the parathyroid gland is to secrete parathyroid hormone (PTH), whose main function is the control of the level of ionized calcium in extracellular fluid and to defend the body against hypocalcemia. PTH stimulates osteolysis by osteoclasts that release calcium and phosphate into extracellular fluid. It increases the renal tubular reabsorption of calcium (and magnesium). PTH decreases the renal tubular reabsorption of phosphate and of bicarbonate, enhancing their urinary loss. It also increases the synthesis of the active form of vitamin D, called calcitriol, from its precursor through activation of a specific enzyme in the kidney. It directly enhances absorption of calcium in the intestines.

Alteration of parathyroid gland functioning thus produces hyperparathyroidism (i.e., hypercalcemia) or hypoparathyroidism (i.e., hypocalcemia). Although they are not as common as thyroid disorders, parathyroid disorders can be life-threatening depending on their severity.

HYPERTHYROIDISM

Epidemiology and Etiology

Hyperthyroidism, one of the most common endocrine disorders, commonly affects women between the ages of 20 and 40. The incidence appears to peak between the ages of 50 and 60 and is seven times greater in people over age 65. Hyperthyroidism is four times more prevalent in women than in men, with approximately 1 percent of the women in the United States developing hyperthyroidism in their lifetime. Later in life, it affects men and women equally. Relapse after treatment and remission is most likely to occur during a postpartum period.

The incidence of hyperthyroidism in pregnancy is extremely low, affecting approximately 1 in every 500 to 2000 pregnancies. Its presence is associated with a significant increase in neonatal mortality. Untreated hyperthyroidism results in premature labor, congenital abnormalities, and low birth weight.

The most common cause of hyperthyroidism despite age or gender is Graves' disease (toxic diffuse goiter). Graves' disease accounts for about 85 percent of cases of hyperthyroidism. Further, about 15 percent of patients with this autoimmune disorder have a first-degree relative with the same disorder, and about half of the relatives have circulating thyroid autoantibodies. Another form of hyperthyroidism, toxic multinodular goiter (TMNG), is usually noted after the age of 50 and is more common in women than in men. Other causes of hyperthyroidism include thyroid adenoma, radiation-induced thyroiditis, thyroid carcinoma, trophoblastic tumors, and dermoid-secreting tumors of the ovary.

Pathophysiology

Hyperthyroidism produces a state of hypermetabolism with increased sympathetic nervous system activity. Many of the signs and symptoms result from the action of certain IgG immunoglobulins (long-acting thyroid-stimulating hormones [LATS]) on the thyroid gland. TMNG has one or more autonomous hyperfunctioning thyroid nodules. A toxic adenoma, the least common cause of hyperthyroidism, is produced when one or more of the adenomas function without TSH or other thyroid stimulation.

Excessive thyroid hormones affect carbohydrate, protein, and fat metabolism. There is an increased absorption of glucose and diminished sensitivity to exogenous insulin. Protein breakdown exceeds protein synthesis, resulting in a negative nitrogen balance. Synthesis, mobilization, and breakdown of fats are increased. The net effect is lipid depletion and a chronic state of protein-energy malnutrition (PEM). Excess thyroid hormones increase the excretion of cholesterol in the feces, with an increase in transformation of cholesterol to bile salts. Additionally, the conversion of B vitamins to their respective coenzymes is impaired.

Thyroid hormones increase the number of beta receptor sites in the heart. Excess thyroid hormones increase heart rate and stroke volume, thus increasing cardiac output and peripheral blood flow. Systolic blood pressure is also elevated.

Hyperactivity of thyroid hormones also produces hypercalcemia and decreases the secretion of PTH hormones. Alterations in the menstrual cycle can be related to hypothalamic or pituitary disturbances. An increase in sex hormone–binding globulins may also produce symptoms such as oligomenorrhea or amenorrhea. The hyperdynamic state also affects the skin, hair, nails, and eyes (Table 50–1).

Drug-induced or spontaneous remissions may occur with hyperthyroidism. The rate of remission is greater for patients diagnosed early in their disease, who have mild hyperthyroidism, or small goiters. The rate is also greater in those treated for extended periods with antithyroid drugs.

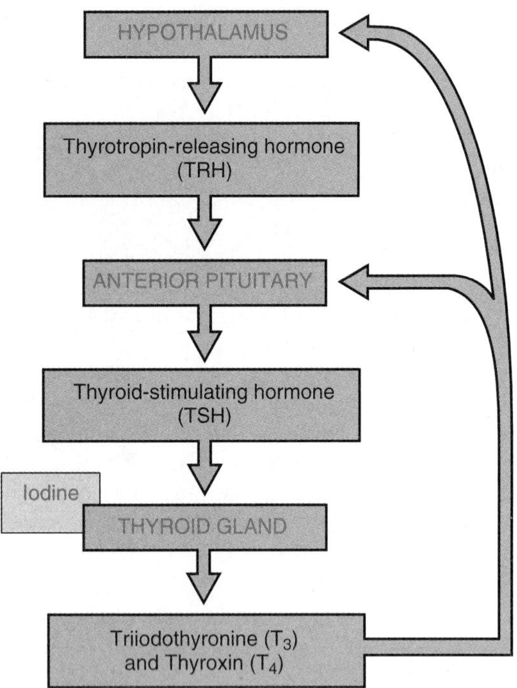

Figure 50–1 Thyroid hormone secretion is regulated through a negative feedback loop involving the hypothalamus, the anterior pituitary, and the thyroid gland.

PHARMACOTHERAPEUTIC OPTIONS

Antithyroid Drugs

❐ Propylthiouracil (PTU); (✱) PROPYL-THYRACIL
❐ Methimazole (TAPAZOLE)

Indications

The thioureylene drugs PTU and methimazole are used in almost all patients to manage manifestations of hyperthyroidism. They are first-line drugs used in the treatment of thyrotoxicosis, helping maintain normal metabolism until the natural course of the disease produces a spontaneous remission.

Pharmacodynamics

By inhibiting the synthesis of thyroid hormones, PTU and methimazole reduce the signs and symptoms of hyperthyroidism. In addition to blocking the synthesis of thyroid hormones, PTU also reduces the peripheral conversion of T_4 to the more potent T_3. In contrast, methimazole does not have this effect. In fact, methimazole can antagonize the inhibition caused by PTU if they are taken together. A *euthyroid* state is usually restored within 4 to 8 weeks. Remission usually occurs with 3 to 6 months of therapy.

PTU and methimazole also reduce serum concentrations of thyroid-stimulating immunoglobulins (TSIs) and increase suppressor T-cell activity. This finding suggests that the drugs have immunosuppressive actions.

Adverse Effects and Contraindications

The adverse effects of antithyroid drugs are notorious, but they are no different or more frequent than those of other commonly used drugs. The incidence of adverse effects of PTU and methimazole is small, varying from 3 to 7 percent. A rash, either a mild papular rash or urticaria, fever, arthralgias, and arthritis are all apparently dose related. Purpura and pruritus are occasionally seen. Skin reactions often subside spontaneously, whether or not the drug is withdrawn. Nausea and vomiting and nasal stuffiness are also common.

Benign transient leukopenia (i.e., white blood cell count less than 4000/mm^3) develops in about 12 percent of adult patients. However, leukopenia is not an antecedent to agranulocytosis, and its presence does not require stopping the drug. The likelihood of cross-allergenicity between PTU and methimazole is approximately 50 percent. So, although the appearance of adverse effects to one drug may suggest that a substitution of the other thioamide is warranted, undesirable sequelae may occur.

TABLE 50–1 COMPARISON OF HYPERTHYROIDISM AND HYPOTHYROIDISM

Signs and Symptoms of Hyperthyroidism	Signs and Symptoms of Hypothyroidism
Goiter	Weakness
Dyspnea on exertion	Dry, course skin
Tiredness	Lethargy, slow speech
Hot hands	Eyelid, facial, or peripheral edema
Palpitations	Cold intolerance
Heat intolerance	Thick tongue
Sweaty palms	Coarseness of hair
Diaphoresis	Cardiac enlargement
Pulse rate over 90 bpm	Pallor of skin
Fine tremors of fingers	Memory impairment
Lid lag	Constipation
Nervousness, anxiety	Hair loss
Weight loss but increased appetite	Anorexia but weight gain
Exophthalmos	Dyspnea
Constipation, diarrhea	Hoarseness
Scanty menses	Menorrhagia
Free thyroxine (FT_4) levels elevated	Free thyroxine (FT_4) levels decreased
Free triiodothyronine (FT_3) levels elevated	Free triiodothyronine (FT_3) levels decreased
Thyroid-stimulating hormone (TSH) levels decreased	Thyroid-stimulating hormone (TSH) levels elevated

Agranulocytosis is the most feared adverse reaction to thioureylenes, occurring in 0.2 percent of patients. It usually develops within 90 days of starting therapy and is characterized by high fever, bacterial pharyngitis, and an absolute granulocyte count below 250/mm^3. Fortunately, the patient's white blood cell count normalizes in 7 to 10 days once the drug has been stopped. Fatalities related to antithyroid drug use are rare.

Antithyroid drugs readily cross the placenta to inhibit fetal thyroid hormone secretion. Suppression of thyroid function in the fetus leads to fetal goiter and hypothyroidism. Administering thyroid hormones to the mother does not reverse the effects of the drugs on the fetus because T_3 and T_4 hormones do not cross the placenta. Furthermore, the long-term consequences of neonatal hypothyroidism are not clear. There is approximately a 30-percent probability of mental retardation.

Pharmacokinetics

Both PTU and methimazole are well absorbed from the GI tract, concentrating in the thyroid gland. PTU and methimazole have similar onset times, peak, and duration of action (Table 50–2). The onset of the effects of PTU occurs in 10 to 21 days compared with 1 week for methimazole. It should be noted that previously synthesized body stores of thyroid hormones must be depleted before a clinical response is noted.

Methimazole peaks in 4 to 10 weeks in contrast to PTU, which takes 6 to 10 weeks to peak. Both drugs have a duration of action of several weeks, but the duration varies with the dosage and the half-life. Elimination of the drugs and their metabolites is primarily through the kidneys.

PTU and methimazole are transported across placental membranes. Only about one fourth of the serum concentration of PTU crosses the placenta compared with that of methimazole. PTU is present in breast milk in one tenth the concentration of methimazole.

Drug-Drug Interactions

There are several clinically significant drug-drug interactions with antithyroid drugs (Table 50–3). There is an increased risk of bleeding when antithyroid drugs are taken with oral anticoagulants. Increased therapeutic effects and toxicity of theophylline, metoprolol, propranolol, and cardiac glycosides may be noted as the patient moves from a hyperthyroid state to a euthyroid state.

Dosage Regimen

The dosage of antithyroid drugs is adjusted to achieve and maintain T_3, T_4, and TSH levels in the normal range. The initial recommended dose of PTU is 300 mg every 8 hours, with a daily maximum of 900 mg (see Table 50–4). PTU generally cannot be given as a single daily dose owing to its short duration of action. Once a euthyroid state has been achieved, the disorder can often be maintained with smaller doses. Once-a-day to twice-a-day dosing is also possible. The maintenance dose of PTU is usually 100 to 150 mg daily.

TABLE 50–2 PHARMACOKINETICS OF SELECTED THYROID AND PARATHYROID DRUGS

Drugs	Route	Onset	Peak	Duration	PB (%)	$t_{1/2}$	BioA (%)
Selected Antithyroid Drugs							
Propylthiouracil	po	10–21 days	6–10 weeks	weeks	75–80	1–2 hrs	80–95
Methimazole	po	1 wk	4–10 wks	weeks	0	6–13 hrs	80–95
Sodium iodide^{131}	po	3–6 days	UK	56 days	0	8 days	100
Selected Thyroid Hormones							
Levothyroxine (T_4)	po	48 hrs	1–3 wks	1–3 wks	99	7 days	48–79
Liothyronine (T_3)	po	48 hrs	24–72 hrs	72 hrs	99	1–2 days	95
Liotrix (T_3, T_4)	po	UK	T_3: 24–72 hrs T_4: 1–3 wks	T_3: 72 hrs T_4: 1–3 wks	99	T_3: 1–2 days T_4:7 days	48–95
Selected Hypocalcemic Drugs							
Pamidronate	IV	24 hrs	7 days	300 days	UK	1.6 hrs/ 27.2 hrs*	100
Etidronate	IV	24 hrs	3 days	11 days	UK	5–7 hrs	100
Calcitonin salmon	IM SQ	15 min	2–4 hrs	6–8 hrs	UK	70–90 min	UK
Gallium nitrate	IV	24 hrs	5 days	7.5 days	UK	24 hr	100
Plicamycin	IV	24–48 hr	72 hr	7–10 days	UA	UA	100
Selected Hypercalcemic Drugs							
Calcium	po	UK	UK	UK	>90	UK	66
	IV	Immediate	Immediate	0.5–2 hr	45	UK	100
Selected Vitamin D Analogs							
Calcitriol	po	2–6 hr	2–6 hr	3–5 days	UK	3–8 hr	UA
Dihydrotachysterol	po	10–24 hr	2 wks	2 wks†	UK	UK	UK
Ergocalciferol	po	12–24 hrs†	4 wks	2 mo‡	UK	UK	UK

*Pamidronate's first and second phase half-life
†Therapeutic effects of ergocalciferol may take 10–14 days
‡Duration of hypercalcemic effects for vitamin D analogs
PB, Protein binding; $t_{1/2}$, elimination half-life; NA, not applicable; BioA, bioavailability; UA, unavailable; UK, unknown.

TABLE 50–3 DRUG-DRUG INTERACTIONS OF SELECTED THYROID AND PARATHYROID DRUGS

Drug	Interactive Drugs	Interaction
Selected Antithyroid Drugs		
Propylthiouracil	Oral anticoagulants	Increased risk of bleeding
Methimazole	Theophylline Metoprolol Propranolol Digitalis glycosides	Increased risk of toxicity of interacting drug as patient moves from hyperthyroid to euthyroid state
Thyroid Hormones		
Levothyroxine Liothyronine	Cholestyramine Colestipol	Impaired absorption of thyroid hormones
Liotrix Thyroid	Epinephrine	Increased risk of coronary events
	Insulin Oral hypoglycemics	Increased blood sugar levels with desiccated thyroid
Selected Hypocalcemic Drugs		
Etidronate Pamidronate	Calcium supplements Antacids Iron	Decreased absorption of etidronate
	Cardiac glycosides Neurotoxic drugs	Increased risk of glycoside toxicity
Calcitonin	Calcium supplements Vitamin D	Antagonize calcium-lowering effect of calcitonin
Selected Hypercalcemic Drugs		
Calcium preparations	Digitalis glycosides	Increased inotropic and toxic effects of interacting drug
	Magnesium antacids	Competes with interacting drug for absorption
	Tetracycline Fluoroquinolones Iron salts Phenytoin Verapamil Calcium channel blockers	Decreased effects of orally interacting drugs
	Atenolol	Decreased effectiveness of interactive drug
	Thiazide diuretics	Concurrent use may result in hypercalcemia
	Sodium polystyrene sulfonate	Reduced ability of interacting drug to decrease serum potassium levels
Vitamin D Analogs		
Vitamin D analogs	Cholestyramine Colestipol Mineral oil	Decreased absorption of analog
	Thiazide diuretics	Concurrent use in patients with hypoparathyroidism may result in hypercalcemia
	Glucocorticoids	Decreased effectiveness of vitamin D analogs
	Cardiac glycosides	Increased risk of arrhythmias
	Barbiturates Hydantoin anticonvulsants Primidone Sucralfate	Increased vitamin D requirements

In contrast, methimazole can be given as a single daily dose. Because it is 10 to 50 times as strong as PTU, initial doses of methimazole are 15 mg/day for mild disease, 30–40 mg/day for moderate disease, and 60 mg/day every 8 hours for severe disease.

Laboratory Considerations

Owing to the potential for blood dyscrasias with thioureylenes, periodic monitoring of the complete blood count, liver function tests, protein, creatine phosphokinase (CPK), and TSH levels should be done.

Radioiodine

❒ Sodium Iodide[131] (IODOTOPE THERAPEUTIC)

Indications

Sodium iodide[131] (^{131}I) has its widest use in the treatment of hyperthyroidism in the older adult and in the diagnosis of thyroid disorders. It is clearly suggested for patients with a history of heart disease, although its use is contraindicated in patients with a recent myocardial infarction.

Pharmacodynamics

The destructive beta rays of ^{131}I act almost exclusively on the parenchymal cells of the thyroid to reduce hormone synthesis. There is little or no damage to surrounding tissues.

Adverse Effects and Contraindications

The major adverse effect of ^{131}I is iatrogenic hypothyroidism. The development of hypothyroidism is so characteristic that it is considered a consequence of therapy rather than a true adverse effect. Radiation thyroiditis and parotiditis are possible and may cause dryness and irritation of the mouth and throat. The most common adverse effects include nausea, vomiting, and diarrhea.

Hypothyroidism develops in at least 50 percent of patients within the first year of ^{131}I therapy, with an annual increase of 2 to 3 percent each year. Consequently, within 10 to 20 years, nearly all patients will become hypothyroid. For this reason, it is mandatory that the patient receive close, life-long, follow-up care.

Pharmacokinetics

^{131}I is readily absorbed from the gastointestinal (GI) tract and taken up by the thyroid gland. The onset of drug action occurs in 3 to 6 days, and the isotope has a half-life of 8 days. Over 99 percent of its radiant energy is expended within 56 days (see Table 50–2).

Drug-Drug Interactions

Propranolol and antithyroid drugs hasten the control of hyperthyroidism while awaiting the full effects of ^{131}I (see Table 50–3).

Dosage Regimen

The effective dose of ^{131}I differs among patients based primarily on the size of the thyroid, the iodine uptake of the gland, and the rate of release of radioactive iodine from the gland. The usual total dose is 4 to 10 mCi (Table 50–4). Depending to some extent on the dosage adopted, 50 to 60 percent of patients are cured by a single dose; 20 to 30 percent require two doses. The remainder of patients require three or more doses before the disorder is controlled.

Critical Thinking Process

Assessment

History of Present Illness

The patient with hyperthyroidism most often reports anxiety, diaphoresis, fatigue, hypersensitivity to heat, nervousness, and palpitations. The patient may also voice confusion about losing weight in spite of an increased appetite. Anorexia and constipation are infrequent. Often, there are reports of problems with the eyes such as difficulty focusing. The patient may also note peripheral edema, diarrhea, and oligomenorrhea or amenorrhea.

Past Health History

The patient with hyperthyroidism may have a history of atrial fibrillation, angina, or heart failure. Sufficient information about the patient's past history should be obtained to help distinguish hyperthyroidism from anxiety neurosis (especially at menopause) or other diseases associated with hypermetabolic states (e.g., pheochromocytoma, acromegaly). Myasthenia gravis causes some of the same ophthalmoplegic signs as that of hyperthyroidism. Orbital tumors can cause exophthalmos.

Physical Exam Findings

Generally, the patient with hyperthyroidism is nervous and thin. Muscle wasting may be evident. Vital signs reflect tachycardia, irregular pulse, and a widened pulse pressure. The skin is moist and velvety, and may show increased pigmentation or *vitiligo.* Hair is often fine and thin. Spider angiomas and gynecomastia may be evident also. Lid lag may be present with a lack of accommodation on exam. Exophthalmos may also be evident, and the patient may appear to stare. In severe cases, the patient may be unable to close the eyelids and must have the lids taped shut to protect the eyes.

An exam of the neck reveals an enlarged thyroid gland that is either smooth or nodular and symmetric or asymmetric. A thyroid bruit may be noted on auscultation, although absence of a bruit or of changes in the appearance of the neck does not rule out hyperthyroidism. Exam of the chest may reveal evidence of paroxysmal atrial fibrillation, a harsh pulmonary systolic murmur, and the presence of an S_3 heart sound.

Deep tendon reflexes are hyperactive and fine tremors of the fingers and tongue may be present. Mental status changes range from mild exhilaration to delirium. In the elderly patient, however, apathy, lethargy, and depression may be evident.

Diagnostic Testing

Laboratory diagnosis of hyperthyroidism is generally straightforward. All forms of hyperthyroidism (except that caused by a rare pituitary TSH-secreting tumor) are associated with low or undetectable serum TSH concentrations. With the widespread availability of sensitive TSH assays, the thyroid-releasing hormone (TRH) test has become obsolete. In addition, most patients have elevated circulating levels of T_3, T_4, and free T_4. The 24-hour radioiodine uptake test is neither sensitive nor specific for hyperthyroidism. It is, however, useful in distinguishing hyperthyroidism that may develop during the postpartum period from postpartum thyroiditis and in confirming the diagnosis of subacute thyroiditis.

If the patient has only one or two characteristic signs and symptoms of hyperthyroidism, the pretest probability of this condition is low, and no testing is required. However, if the health care provider is compelled to test, the free T_4 level is a better reflection of the patient's true hormonal status. If the patient exhibits five or more characteristic signs and symptoms, the ultrasensitive TSH is probably the best indicator of patient thyroid status because of its higher sensitivity.

Developmental Considerations

Perinatal Minor changes in thyroid function occur during pregnancy. High estrogen levels during pregnancy stimulate the liver to increase its production of thyroxine-binding globulins. Increased globulin levels result in the elevation of T_3 and T_4, with elevated T_4 levels lasting 6 to 12

TABLE 50–4 DOSAGE REGIMEN FOR THYROID AND PARATHYROID DRUGS

Drug	Use(s)	Dosage	Implications
Selected Antithyroid Drugs			
Propylthiouracil	Hyperthyroidism	*Adult:* 300–400 mg po QD in divided doses. Maintenance: 100–150 mg po QD. Maximum dose 900 mg/day *Neonate:* 10 mg/kg/day po in divided doses *Child ages 6–10:* 50–150 mg po QD *Child over age 10 yr:* 150–300 mg po QD Maintenance dose based on patient response	May administer in two to four divided doses. Pharmacist will compound into enema or suppository if needed. Cannot be given as single dose because of short duration of action. Maintenance dose usually ½–⅔ of the initial dose once patient is euthyroid
Methimazole	Hyperthyroidism	*Adult:* mild disease: 15 mg.po daily. Moderately severe disease: 30–40 mg po daily. Severe disease: 60 mg po q8 hr. Maintenance: 5–15 mg po QD *Child:* 0.4 mg/kg every 8 hours in divided doses. Maintenance dose is 1/2 initial dose.	Continue initial dosage until euthyroid state achieved. May be given as single dose because of long half-life
Sodium iodide^{131}	Hyperthyroidism	*Adult:* 4–10 mCi po x1 based on serum thyroxine level and thyroid size	50–60% of patients are cured by single dose. 20–30% require second dose
	Thyroid cancer	*Adult:* 50–150 mCi po	May repeat dosage in 6–12 months depending on clinical status
Selected Thyroid Hormones			
Desiccated thyroid	Hypothyroidism	*Adult and child:* 30 mg po QD. Increase by 15 mg po every 20 days till desired response reached. Maintenance: 65–120 mg po QD	Dosage increases made at 2-week intervals. Maintenance doses may be higher in growing child than in adult
	Myxedema	*Child:* 16 mg po QD for 2 weeks; 32 mg po QD for 2 weeks. Maintenance: 50–120 mg po QD	Increase daily dosage at monthly or greater intervals on basis of lab tests
Levothyroxine*	Hypothyroidism	*Adult:* 0.05 mg po QD. Increase by 0.025 mg po every 2–3 wks. Maintenance: 0.075–0.125 mg po QD	Slower onset but longer duration of action than T_3
	Myxedemic coma	*Adult:* 200–500 mcg IV. If no response in 24 hr, may give additional 100–300 mcg Maintenance: 50–100 mcg/day	
	Congenital hypothyroidism	*Child age 0–6 mo:* 0.025–0.05 mg po QD *Child age 6–12 mo:* 0.05–0.75 mg po QD *Child age 1–5 yrs:* 0.075–0.1 mg po QD *Child age 6–12 yrs:* 0.1–0.15 mg po QD *Child over 12 yrs:* 0.15 mg po QD	
Liothyronine	Hypothyroidism	*Adult:* .25 mcg po QD. Increase by 12.5–25 mcg every 1–2 weeks till desired response. Maintenance: 25–75 mcg po QD *Child, elderly, patients with CAD:* 5 mcg/day	Possess actions similar to that of T_4—onset more rapid, but shorter duration of action—allows quicker dosage adjustment
	Simple goiter	*Adult:* 5 mcg po QD. Increase by 5–10 mcg po every 1–2 weeks; after 25 mcg reached may increase by 12.5–25 mcg at 1 week intervals till desired response achieved. Usual dose: 75 mcg/day	
	Myxedema	*Adult:* 5 mcg/day initially. Increase by 5–10 mcg/day every 1–2 weeks until 25 mg is reached then increase by 12.5–50 mcg every 1–2 weeks. Usual maintenance dose: 50–100 mcg/day	
	Congenital hypothyroidism	*Child under 3 yrs:* 5 mg po QD *Child over 3 yrs:* 5 mcg po QD. Increase by 5 mcg po every 3–4 days till desired response achieved. Approximately 20 mcg/day may be sufficient in infants	
Liotrix	Hypothyroidism	*Adult:* 50 mcg levothyroxine/12.5 mcg liothyronine. Increase by 50 mcg levothyroxine/12.5 mcg liothyronine every month until desired response achieved. Maintenance: 50–100 mcg levothyroxine/12.5–25 mcg liothyronine daily *Geriatric:* 12.5–25 mcg levothyroxine/3.1–6.2 mcg liothyronine daily. Increase by 12.5–25 mcg levothyroxine/3.1–6.2 mcg liothyronine q6–8wk until desired response achieved	A constant fixed ratio of T_3 and T_4 by weight. Represents thyroid hormone equivalents (e.g., 60 mg desiccated thyroid = 0.1 mg T_4 = 25 mcg T_3)
Selected Hypocalcemic Drugs			
Pamidronate	Hyperparathyroidism	*Adult:* 60–90 mg IV over 24 hours	Do not mix with calcium-containing infusions, such as Ringers. Current saline hydration should be undertaken
Etidronate	Hyperthyroidism	*Adult:* 7.5 mg/kg/day IV × 3 days then switch to 20 mg/kg/day po	

TABLE 50–4 DOSAGE REGIMEN FOR THYROID AND PARATHYROID DRUGS *Continued*

Drug	Use(s)	Dosage	Implications
Selected Hypocalcemic Drugs *Continued*			
Calcitonin-salmon	Hyperthyroidism	*Adult:* 4 IU/kg SQ/IM every 12 hours. Increase to 8 IU/kg SQ/IM every 6 hours	Intradermal skin test should precede therapy with calcitonin salmon. Watch for anaphylaxis
Gallium nitrate	Hyperparathyroidism	*Adult:* 100–200 mg/m^2 daily × 5 days IV	Allow a 3–4 week rest period between courses of therapy
Plicamycin	Hypercalcemia	15–25 mcg/kg IV once daily for 3–4 days. May be repeated after 7 days or 1–3 times weekly	
Selected Hypercalcemic Drugs			
Calcium	Hypoparathyroidism	*Adult:* 500 mg po BID–QID 1–2 hours after meals	Chewable tablets preferred to standard tablets due to more consistent bioavailability. Calcium salts differ in their percentage of elemental calcium
	Hypocalcemic tetany	*Adult:* 4.5–16 mEq IV. Repeat until symptoms are controlled *Child:* 0.5–0.7 mEq/kg IV three to four times daily until tetany is controlled	Transient increases in BP occurs with IV administration, especially in older adults or patients with hypertension. Extravasation can cause cellulitis, necrosis, and sloughing of tissues. Check IV site for patency.
	Emergency treatment hypocalcemia	*Adult:* 7–14 mEq IV. Dose may be repeated every 1–3 days based on patient response *Child:* 1–7 mEq IV *Infant:* Less than 1 mEq	
Selected Vitamin D and Vitamin D Analogs			
Calcitriol	Hypoparathyroidism	*Adult:* 0.25–2.7 mcg po QD. Maintenance dose 0.5–2.7 mcg po daily *Child:* 0.04–0.08 mcg/kg/day po	Dosage adjusted as necessary to maintain serum calcium levels. May be administered without regard to meals. May be mixed with juice, cereal, or food, or dropped directly into the mouth. Serum calcium levels should be maintained at 8–10 mg/dL
Dihydrotachysterol	Hypocalcemic tetany	*Adult:* 0.25–2.5 mg po QD × 3 days. Maintenance: 0.25–1.0 mg po QD	
	Hypoparathyroidism Pseudohypopara-thyroidism	*Adult:* 0.75–2.5 mg/day × several days then 0.2–1 mg/day up to 1.5 mg/day. *Child:* 1–5 mg/day × 4 days then 0.5–1.5 mg/day.	
Ergocalciferol	Vitamin D deficiency	*Adult:* 1000–2000 units/day po initially then 400 units/day maintenance *Child:* 1000–4000 units/day po initially then 400 units/day maintenance	
	Hypoparathyroidism	*Adult:* 50,000–150,000 units/day po *Child:* 50,000–200,000 units/day	

*Product	T_3/T_4 (mcg)	Thyroid Equiv. (mg)
Thyrolar 1/4	4.1/12.5	15
Thyrolar 1/2	6.25/25	30
Thyrolar 1	2.5/50	60
Thyrolar 2	25/100	120
Thyrolar 3	37.5/150	180

weeks postpartum. Serum concentrations of free T_3 and T_4 are essentially unchanged. Serum levels of TSH are normal to slightly low during pregnancy. Human chorionic gonadotropin (hCG) produced by the placenta has weak thyroid-stimulating activity.

Pediatric Neonatal hyperthyroidism results from the transfer of maternal TSIs to the fetus. It is usually transient, lasting only 1 to 3 months. This is because the half-life of neonatal TSIs is approximately 2 weeks. TSIs stimulate the fetal thyroid to produce thyroid hormones, causing fetal or neonatal hyperthyroidism. Neonatal hyperthyroidism depends on maternal TSIs and not on the mother's thyroid status. Therefore, infants of euthyroid women with a previous history of hyperthyroidism are also at risk. Measurement of maternal TSI levels is useful to predict the likelihood of neonatal hyperthyroidism.

Geriatric Hyperthyroidism frequently goes undetected in older persons. There are several reasons for this problem. The patient has fewer diagnostic signs and symptoms, coexisting diseases may mask symptoms, and the symptoms that are commonly present in the younger population may be absent in older adults. Confirmation of hyperthyroidism, therefore, relies heavily on laboratory test results.

Symptoms of hyperthyroidism in the older adult are often atypical. Only about 25 percent of older adults have the classic hyperactivity, restlessness, and nervous appearance. The older adult may or may not have tachycardia or moist, flushed skin. Classic eye manifestations are rare. The most frequent patient reports relate to anorexia and a loss of ambition. Weight loss is the most frequent objective finding. An enlarged thyroid is present in 80 percent of those affected. More than 75 percent

Case Study Hyperthyroidism

Patient History

History of Present Illness	JC is a 35-year-old part-time secretary and mother who arrived at the clinic accompanied by her husband. She complains of nervousness, insomnia, an inability to focus on her daily activities, and heat intolerance. JC also reports that she is losing weight although she is eating constantly. She has had difficulty swallowing and a noticeable change in the frequency and consistency of her bowel movements. Her menstrual flow and its frequency have decreased over the last 3 months. In addition, JC states her neighbor thinks she is on "some kind of uppers" because of the nervousness.
Past Health History	JC denies a history of previous thyroid disorders but reports that her mother developed an "overactive thyroid" at age 33. She denies a history of surgery or neurologic, musculoskeletal, or other hormonal disorders.
Physical Exam	Height: 5'7". Present weight: 113 pounds (10–15 pounds below her usual weight). VS: BP 146/72 (BP 1 year ago 120/70), apical pulse 112 and irregular, respirations 24. Temperature 98.8 F. Bruits are noted over the thyroid gland on auscultation. Exophthalmos is evident. JC is unable to close her eyelids completely, and her visual fields are impaired. Her hair is fine, soft, and silky, and her skin is moist and smooth. JC has hyperactive DTRs and fine tremors. Her decreased attention span is evident.
Diagnostic Testing	JC's diagnostic workup reflects an elevated T_3RIA, T_4, and free T_3 and T_4 levels. The serum TSH concentration is low. Antithyroglobulin and antimicrosomal antibody values are elevated. Her TSI is positive. An ECG reflects tachycardia and atrial fibrillation. A pregnancy test reveals that JC is not pregnant.
Developmental Considerations	JC's husband reports that she thinks she may be pregnant because her periods are less frequent and decreased in amount.
Psychosocial Considerations	JC's husband describes his wife as a normally quiet, well-organized individual, who finishes projects she starts, one who coordinates family activities very well. Over the last 3 months he reports she has become unorganized, and doesn't finish projects or activities she has started. He also reports that she does not like to take medicine of any kind. JC's husband also reports that she eats large quantities at mealtimes and snacks between meals. He has noticed her wearing lightweight blouses and shorts, although it is fall and the weather is cool. They have been arguing recently because she wants the windows open. He gets cold and wants them closed.
Economic Factors	JC's husband is a bank executive. He reports that the family enrolled in a health plan that covers clinic visits and hospitalizations. The prescription drug plan requires a co-payment for prescription drugs. He believes that the insurance premiums are reasonable and the plan supports their health care needs.

Variables Influencing Decision

Treatment Objectives

- Restore a euthyroid state by returning plasma TSH levels to the low normal range.
- Symptom relief while waiting for therapeutic effectiveness of drug to be achieved.

Drug Variables	*Drug Summary*	*Patient Variables*
Indications	Either PTU or methimazole may be used in the treatment of hyperthyroidism.	JC has been diagnosed with hyperthyroidism so this is a decision point.
Pharmacodynamics	The quantitative significance of decreased peripheral conversion by PTU has not been established. It would, however, provide a theoretical explanation for the choice of PTU over methimazole.	No patient-related variable to affect decision.

Case Study Hyperthyroidism—cont'd

Drug Variables	*Drug Summary*	*Patient Variables*
Adverse Effects/ Contraindications	Contraindicated in pregnancy and during lactation. Adverse effects are those related to hypothyroidism.	JC is neither pregnant nor lactating, so this is generally not a major decision point.
Pharmacokinetics	Although the onset time of methimazole is sooner than that of PTU, a clinical response may be seen sooner with PTU.	JC and her husband wish her to return to euthyroid state as soon as reasonable, so this is a decision point.
Dosage Regimen	Both PTU and methimazole are initially administered every 8 hours.	Once-a-day dosing would likely foster better compliance; therefore, this becomes a decision point.
Lab Considerations	Requires monitoring of lab values periodically throughout therapy.	TSH low and T_4 levels high. TSI is elevated, so this is a decision point for treatment.
Cost Index*	Propylthiouracil: 3 Methimazole: 1	JC feels health plan supports her medical needs so this is not a decision point.

Summary of Decision Points

- The quantitative significance of decreased peripheral conversion by PTU provides a theoretical explanation for the choice of PTU over methimazole.
- If compliance is good, methimazole is effective when administered once daily, whereas PTU is less effective.
- Even at minimal recommended dosages, the cost of a 30-day supply of PTU is approximately 2 times that of methimazole.

DRUG TO BE USED

- Methimazole 10 mg po QD initially. Dosage to be adjusted based on patient response after 2 or 3 weeks.

*Cost Index:

1 $ < 30/mo.
2 $ 30–40/mo.
3 $ 40–50/mo.
4 $ 50–60/mo.
5 $ > 60/mo.

AWP of 100, 10 mg tablets of methimazole is approximately $ 23.
AWP of 100, 50 mg tablets of propylthiouracil (PTU) is approximately $ 46.

of patients have cardiovascular symptoms such as palpitations, heart failure, atrial fibrillation, and angina pectoris.

Laboratory reports indicate there is an age-related decrease in T_3 levels in healthy older adults. Male T_3 levels decrease by age 60. Female levels do not show a consistent decrease until age 70 or 80 years. The normal decrease in T_3 levels makes the diagnosis of mild hyperthyroidism difficult. Circulating T_4 levels also decrease modestly with age. The reduction may be due to reduced metabolism of the aging thyroid gland, where most of T_4 is produced. There is also an age-related increase in TSH levels.

Psychosocial Considerations

The wide variation in the signs and symptoms of hyperthyroidism may affect the patient's activities of daily living. Workplace relationships may be affected because of the hyperactive state of the patient. Mood swings, irritability, decreased attention span, and manic behavior may be experienced. Although the patient may not be aware of some of the mood changes, fellow employees and family members can usually note the changes (see Case Study—Hyperthyroidism).

Analysis and Management

Treatment Objectives

The treatment objective for hyperthyroidism is to reduce the levels of circulating thyroid hormones in anticipation of a spontaneous remission. Reducing the uncomfortable signs and symptoms is also important.

Treatment Options

Historically, surgery was the first-line treatment for hyperthyroidism. It is not used as frequently today but may be appropriate for children, adolescents, pregnant women unable to tolerate PTU, and adults who are unresponsive to antithyroid drugs and who refuse radioiodine. Antithyroid drugs and radioiodine have replaced surgery as the treatments of choice. Although these drugs are generally safe and effective, none of them are perfect. They do, however, provide satisfactory outcomes for most patients.

Drug Variables

The primary drugs used in the treatment of hyperthyroidism include the thioureylenes PTU or methimazole. The advantage of using antithyroid drugs is that they provide an opportunity for the patient to have a spontaneous remission, and thus, life-long drug treatment regimens are avoided. On the other hand, however, the disadvantage is that permanent remissions occur in only about 30 percent of patients. Continuous and repeated therapy is usually required.

The indications and adverse effects of both PTU and methimazole are essentially the same. However, for bothersome symptoms, long-acting beta-blocking drugs (propranolol, metoprolol, atenolol, nadolol) (see Chapter 11) are usually given as adjunctive therapy until the thioureylene restores the patient to a euthyroid state. The long-acting form of propranolol is preferred to propranolol itself, which has a short duration of action.

PTU is the drug of choice for pregnant hyperthyroid women because of its limited placental transfer and low potency. Another reason PTU is the drug of choice during pregnancy is the reported development of scalp defects in fetuses exposed to methimazole in utero. Both PTU and methimazole are pregnancy category D agents. Antithyroid drugs are not teratogenic; however, neonatal thyroid function can be affected.

Serum T_3 and T_4 levels decrease more rapidly in patients treated with methimazole. Although the differences in PTU and methimazole serum levels are insignificant, moderate doses of methimazole pose a lower risk of agranulocytosis.

Should a remission occur, life-long follow-up is indicated. If a remission is not achieved, the patient may require a second course of antithyroid therapy or radioiodine.

^{131}I is concentrated only in areas of the thyroid that are functional. Suppressed perinodular areas are spared radiation exposure. Therefore, hypothyroidism, although it can occur, is less of a problem. There are several advantages to using ^{131}I. First, no other body tissues are exposed to detectable amounts of ionizing radiation. Because ^{131}I is taken by mouth, it is easy to administer. The health care provider should administer ^{131}I only after stopping any other antithyroid agents.

Patient Variables

Because hyperthyroidism usually remits during pregnancy, it is usually controlled with low doses of an antithyroid drug. It may even be possible to stop antithyroid drug therapy. On the other hand, the disease may worsen or relapse after delivery.

The economic factor alone makes PTU less desirable than methimazole. Even at minimal recommended dosages, the cost of a 30-day supply of PTU is approximately three times that of methimazole.

Intervention

Administration

Antithyroid drugs should be administered at the same time each day in three equally divided doses. If a dose is missed, the patient should be instructed to take it when it is remembered. If it is almost time for the next dose, both doses should be taken. The health care provider should be contacted if more than one dose is missed.

Education

The patient and family should be taught about the therapeutic and adverse effects of thyroid hormones and antithyroid drugs on the body. Signs and symptoms of imbalance should also be discussed. Insufficient drug prolongs the period of thyrotoxicity, whereas too much may cause hypothyroidism. An interruption in therapy may result in symptoms reappearing. Lack of compliance also reduces the likelihood of a permanent remission. After the initial treatment period, manifestations of imbalance should be reported so that dosages can be changed.

When radioiodine therapy is used, teach the patient to increase fluid intake to 3 to 4 L/day for 48 hours. Sufficient fluid intake helps remove ^{131}I from the body. The patient should also be instructed to void frequently so as to not expose the gonads to radiation. The patient should report redness, swelling, sore throat, or the development of mouth lesions. The patient need not restrict contact with other people because the dosage of ^{131}I is relatively small. There is no need to restrict the use of the public restrooms.

The patient should be instructed to stop the antithyroid drug and notify the health care provider if symptoms of infection occur. Sore throat, enlarged lymph nodes, GI upsets, fever, rash, and jaundice are particularly important. The importance of periodic blood tests and medical follow-up should be stressed.

Further, the patient should be cautioned against taking over-the-counter (OTC) drugs. OTC drugs, such as decongestants, contain vasopressor compounds that are poorly tolerated by patients with hyperthyroidism. Antidiarrheal drugs containing kaolin will absorb an antithyroid drug, thereby reducing its absorption. Further, the health care provider should be contacted before taking any drugs containing iodine.

Because a positive clinical response to antithyroid drugs cannot be expected for days to weeks, immediate interventions are sometimes required that help reduce symptoms of hyperthyroidism. The patient should be encouraged to continue wearing lightweight clothing and to use lightweight bed linens. The environment should be kept cool with high humidity.

Rest is important to conserve energy and reduce fatigue. However, because of the patient's high metabolic rate, it is often difficult to achieve. The patient should be taught that control of environmental temperature, lighting, and noise levels minimizes unnecessary stimuli. All possible strategies should be used to help induce sleep. Additionally, persons working with, or around a patient with hyperthyroidism should maintain a calm but efficient manner because patients are unnecessarily stimulated by hustle and bustle. On the other hand, the patient may become impatient with slow responses.

The patient should be informed that they will begin to feel better after the initial few weeks of treatment. Because antithyroid drug therapy is lengthy, the patient needs encouragement to maintain compliance.

Because hyperthyroidism affects young women, the patient should be advised to contact the health care provider should they become pregnant. The treatment regimen may need to be changed to protect the unborn child.

The patient should be taught to consume a diet high in vitamins, minerals, and protein, and to include sufficient calories to prevent weight loss. More frequent meals or snacks are usually needed. Foods to avoid include those high in residue or those with laxative effects. Stimulants such as coffee, tea, cola drinks, chocolate, and foods containing caffeine should also be avoided. Body weight should be monitored two to three times weekly. Calorie intake should be gradually reduced as symptoms of hyperthyroidism subside. A reduction in calories should not be difficult because the patients appetite will decrease with treatment. The intake of vitamins, minerals, and dietary nutrients, however, should be maintained, although calories are reduced.

The patient should be advised to carry Medic-Alert identification describing the treatment regimen. Dentists should be informed of the treatment regimen before treatment is provided so as to minimize potentially adverse effects of any anesthetics used.

Evaluation

Antithyroid drugs induce a permanent remission in about 30 percent of patients with hyperthyroidism. Treatment effectiveness for hyperthyroidism can be demonstrated by a decrease in the severity of signs and symptoms (e.g., lowered pulse rate and weight gain). Thyroid function test results return to normal levels, and the patient should reflect a euthyroid state rather than a hypothyroid state secondary to drug therapy. Reduced TSI levels generally suggest a remission has taken place and that therapy can be modified or withdrawn.

If a remission is not achieved, the patient may require a second course of antithyroid therapy, or radioiodine. Approximately 20 percent of patients with a remission develop spontaneous hypothyroidism with antithyroid drug therapy alone. The need for life-long follow-up remains.

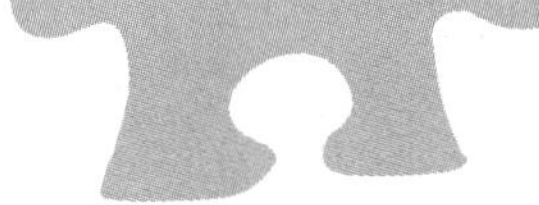

HYPOTHYROIDISM

Epidemiology and Etiology

Hypothyroidism is the result of inadequate peripheral thyroid hormone levels. Although the typical patient with hypothyroidism is a female over age 50 years, the disease can occur at any age and in either gender. Most cases occur between the ages of 30 and 60 years. Hypothyroidism is at least twice as prevalent as hyperthyroidism.

More than 90 percent of patients with hypothyroidism have primary thyroid atrophy. In North America, Hashimoto's thyroiditis (chronic lymphocytic thyroiditis, autoimmune thyroiditis) is the most common cause. Prior treatment with radioiodine or thyroidectomy are the next most common causes of hypothyroidism. Hypothyroidism may also co-exist with other autoimmune disorders such as rheumatoid arthritis, systemic lupus erythematosus, or pernicious anemia.

Fewer than 6 percent of hypothyroidism cases are related to secondary or central causes. Secondary hypothyroidism is most often caused by failure of the pituitary to synthesize sufficient quantities of TSH. Postpartum pituitary necrosis (Sheehan's syndrome) and a pituitary tumor are the most frequent causes of secondary hypothyroidism. A recently recognized cause of hypothyroidism is cancer therapy with interleukin-2 (IL-2), alpha-interferon, or granulocyte macrophage–colony stimulating factor (GMCSF).

Commonly used drugs such as lithium, iodine, amiodarone, and para-aminosalicylic acid may also cause secondary hypothyroidism. Lithium interferes with the biosynthesis and release of thyroid hormone and may cause elevated serum TSH levels a few weeks after therapy is started. Iodine blocks the release of thyroid hormone. Amiodarone, a commonly used antiarrhythmic agent, is rich in iodine and is fat soluble. It remains in the body many weeks after therapy is stopped. Additionally, patients who take health tonics or eat kelp may be receiving too much iodine. Other goitrogenic (thyroid stimulants) food substances include turnips, cabbage, spinach, soybeans, and seafood.

Pathophysiology

In primary hypothyroidism, the production of thyroid hormones is inadequate. The thyroid gland enlarges in an attempt to compensate for the inadequacy and a goiter is formed. Insufficient quantities of thyroid hormones result in an overall decrease in the basal metabolic rate and a variety of system manifestations. There is decreased cerebral blood flow, leading to hypoxia and mental status changes. A reduction in stroke volume and heart rate cause lowered cardiac output. Peripheral vascular resistance increases to maintain systolic blood pressure. A variety of electrocardiographic changes are noted (e.g., bradycardia, prolonged PR interval, depressed P waves, low-amplitude).

Hemodynamic alterations associated with reduced blood flow caused decreased renal elimination of water, an increase in total body water, and dilutional hyponatremia. There is also a reduction in the production of erythropoietin. A decrease in red cell mass leads to anemias. Vitamin B_{12}, iron, and folate deficiencies may also occur.

There is a general slowing of GI system functioning. Decreased appetite, constipation, weight gain, and fluid retention develop. Decreased protein metabolism leads to delayed skeletal and soft tissue growth and produces a slightly positive nitrogen balance. Abnormalities in lipid metabolism cause an increase in cholesterol and triglyceride levels. This increase is associated with the development of atherosclerosis and subsequent heart disease.

The metabolism of estrogens and androgens is altered. The patient experiences increased sensitivity to exogenous insulin and decreased absorption of glucose. Reduced secretions from sweat and sebaceous glands result in dry, flaky skin. Head and body hair become brittle. Nails are slow growing, and there is delayed wound healing. The accumulation of hyaluronic acid in interstitial spaces cause the characteristic puffy appearance *(myxedema)* seen in hypothyroidism. The reason for the accumulation of this hydrophilic proteoglycan is unknown.

Myxedematous changes in respiratory muscles lead to hypoventilation and carbon dioxide retention. Pleural effusions associated with dyspnea are possible, although the effusions may be asymptomatic.

There is a decreased rate of muscle contraction and relaxation, and increased bone density that contributes to muscle aching and joint stiffness. Deep tendon reflexes are decreased.

PHARMACOTHERAPEUTIC OPTIONS

Thyroid Hormones

- ❒ Desiccated thyroid USP (ARMOUR THYROID)
- ❒ Levothyroxine (LEVOTHROID, SYNTHROID, T_4); (🍁) ELTROXIN, PMS-SODIUM
- ❒ Liothyronine (CYTOMEL, T_3)
- ❒ Liotrix (THYROLAR, T_3/T_4)
- ❒ Thyroglobulin

Indications

Inasmuch as hypothyroidism, myxedema, simple goiter, and cretinism result from hypofunction of the thyroid gland, the use of thyroid agents represent true replacement therapy. Levothyroxine is the drug of choice for replacement therapy in patients with diminished or absent thyroid functioning. Thyroid hormones include both natural and synthetic derivatives. Natural products are derived from beef and pork.

Pharmacodynamics

Thyroid hormones act to increase the metabolic rate of body tissues. They promote gluconeogenesis, thus increasing the utilization and mobilization of glycogen stores. The drugs also stimulate protein synthesis, cell growth and differentiation, and aid in the development of the central nervous system (CNS).

Adverse Effects and Contraindications

There are few adverse effects of levothyroxine or liothyronine other than those indicating overdosage. The most common adverse effects include irritability, insomnia, nervousness, headache, weight loss, and tachycardia. The adverse effects are essentially those of hyperthyroidism.

A few patients may be allergic to the tartrazine dye used in the yellow (100 mcg) or green (300 mcg) levothyroxine tablets. Although the incidence of tartrazine sensitivity in the general population is low, it is frequently found in patients who have aspirin hypersensitivity. Levothyroxine rarely results in clinical toxicity. The most life-threatening adverse effect is cardiovascular collapse.

Pharmacokinetics

When it is given by mouth, levothyroxine is variably absorbed (48 to 79 percent) from the GI tract. When it is taken on an empty stomach, preferably before breakfast, absorption is increased. It is well distributed to body tissues undergoing enterohepatic recirculation. The onset time is 48 hours, with peak effects observed in 1 to 3 weeks (see Table 50–2). The duration of action is 1 to 3 weeks. Biotransformation takes place in the liver, with excretion through the feces. Because of strong binding to plasma proteins (99 percent) levothyroxine has a serum half-life of about 7 days, making serum levels stable with once daily dosing.

Liothyronine is almost completely absorbed following oral administration. It is distributed to many body tissues. The onset time is 48 hours, with peak effects noted in 24 to 72 hours. Biotransformation takes place in the liver and other body tissues. The duration of action is 72 hours. The half-life of the drug is less than 1 to 2 days, making it less desirable for long-term therapy.

Drug-Drug Interactions

Drugs that lower cholesterol such as cholestyramine impair the absorption of thyroid hormones (see Table 50–3). Several hours should separate administration of these drugs. The use of epinephrine with levothyroxine increases the risk of coronary events in patients with coronary artery disease. Desiccated thyroid has been shown to increase insulin or oral hypoglycemic requirements in patients with diabetes.

Dosage Regimen

The dosage of thyroid hormones is individualized to approximate the patient's deficit of thyroid hormone. A reasonable drug regimen is a daily dose of 50 mcg of levothyroxine for 2 weeks, followed by a daily dose of 100 mcg for the subsequent 2 weeks (see Table 50–4). With this regimen, a clinical response can be established and plasma TSH concentrations returned to a normal range.

The optimal daily dose is usually between 100 and 150 mcg. Some patients may require a little as 50 mcg daily, whereas others need as much as 400 mcg. Serum TSH levels should be checked 6 to 8 weeks after therapy is started and the dosage adjusted, if necessary.

Laboratory Considerations

Periodic monitoring of TSH and T_4 levels is warranted during thyroid hormone therapy. The concurrent use of thyroid hormones in patients with elevated biliary tract pressure may cause increases in plasma amylase and lipase. Further, the determination of these levels may be unreliable for 24 hours after administration of opioids.

Critical Thinking Process

Assessment

History of Present Illness

The patient with hypothyroidism most often complains of cold intolerance; coarse, dry skin; decreased sweating; swelling of the eye lids; and lethargy. Frequent complaints also include anorexia, constipation, hair loss, hoarseness or aphonia, swelling of the legs or face, and memory impairment.

Past Health History

When obtaining a health history, the health care provider elicits information related to congenital anomalies, stress, trauma, infection, and radiation exposure. Furthermore, information about co-morbid diseases such as rheumatoid arthritis, systemic lupus erythematosus, and pernicious anemia should be elicited. Pre-existing conditions presently treated with thyroid hormones must be included. A family history that is positive for thyroid abnormalities is important to note.

Physical Exam Findings

The physical exam should include an assessment of vital signs, height and weight, cardiac rhythm and regularity, skin color, temperature and texture, and the texture of hair and nails. With hypothyroidism, there may be a notable loss of the outer third of the eyebrow. Vision, deep tendon reflexes, and mental status should also be examined.

Assessment of other body systems should include the presence or absence of tremor, pain, and proximal muscle weakness, as well as the presence of periorbital or peripheral edema, slow speech, and hoarseness.

Diagnostic Testing

T_3 and T_4 levels may remain within a broad range of normal, even when the patient has true, but mild, hypothyroidism. A slight elevation of TSH assay is also present. The serum TSH value, however, may be misleading in patients who have pituitary or hypothalamic hypothyroidism.

The T_4 level should not be relied on to define the patient's thyroid status. Although the values may fall within the normal range, individually it is abnormal. There are many drugs and other disorders that produce falsely low T_4 values. Falsely low values may occur as the result of reduced serum thyroxine–binding globulins (e.g., nephrotic syndrome, protein loss by the gut, glucocorticoids), or displacement of T_4 from binding proteins (e.g., high-dose salicylates, the use of furosemide in renal failure, phenytoin).

Antimicrosomal antibodies are present in the sera of 90 percent of middle age patients but may be negative in young patients. Antithyroglobulin antibodies are noted a few years after the antibodies are found. The elevation presumably represents a response to antigens leaking from the damaged thyroid.

Developmental Considerations

Perinatal Pregnant women and newborns should be monitored for potential thyroid abnormalities as a basic standard of care, although hypothyroidism is uncommon in pregnancy. However, if the condition is left untreated, it may cause a higher rate of stillbirths, abortions, and congenital abnormalities. Fetal thyroid hormone production starts at 12 weeks' gestation. Low T_4 levels in the mother during the first trimester may result in impairment of fetal brain development.

Fetal thyroid state can be monitored by measuring thyroid hormones in amniotic fluid. Neonatal hypothyroidism occurs independently of maternal thyroid disease and is routinely screened via TSH testing 5 to 7 days after birth. If breastfeeding is desired by mothers who are on thyroid hormones, infant thyroid hormone levels should be monitored.

Pediatric Thyroid disease may be congenital, with onset occurring from birth to 2 years. If the condtion is left untreated, it affects growth and development, causing mental retardation. The incidence of congenital hypothyroidism is approximately 1:4000, with a 1- to 3-percent prevalence reported in school children. Untreated hypothyroidism results in a syndrome called *cretinism*. Cretinism, hypothyroidism of infancy, is caused by thyroid hormone deficiency during fetal or early neonatal life. It may be related to maternal iodine deprivation or congenital thyroid abnormalities.

Acquired hypothyroidism may be due to unknown causes, thyroiditis, secondary to pituitary deficiency, or operative removal of the thyroid gland. Hypothyroidism occurring after 18 months of age is associated with reversible mental slowness. Between the ages of 1 and 5 years of age, the cause of hypothyroidism is usually maldeveloped or ectopic thyroid tissue.

Prompt diagnosis and treatment of hypothyroidism in children is necessary to prevent developmental retardation. Ossification of the epiphyses and brain growth and development are particularly affected. A delay of only 3 months in treatment of neonatal hypothyroidism causes irreversible mental retardation.

Thyroid disease is the most common endocrine disorder of adolescence. During adolescence, the prognosis of thyroid disease is usually good with appropriate therapy.

Geriatric The clinical manifestations of hypothyroidism in the older adult is often subtle and can mistakenly be attributed to normal changes of aging. Hypothyroidism can present as carpal tunnel syndrome, dementia, pernicious anemia, or elevated cholesterol in addition to the common signs and symptoms previously discussed. Because clinical symptoms of thyroid disease are unreliable in this age group, routine laboratory screening is recommended.

Psychosocial Considerations

The patient's psychological response to thyroid disease is influenced by the perceived state of health and the severity of the symptoms. Access to health care and the ability to obtain appropriate drugs helps alleviate concerns about potential disability. Daily activities can be affected if symptoms persist untreated.

Analysis and Management

Treatment Objectives

The primary objective in the management of hypothyroidism is to restore the patient to a euthyroid state and to maintain plasma TSH levels in the low-normal range. Symptomatic relief of the symptoms of hypothyroidism is also a treatment objective. Management includes the gradual replacement of thyroid hormones and a low-calorie diet to promote weight loss. Life-long therapy should be expected.

Treatment Options

Drug Variables

Thyroid hormone replacement is the only treatment available for hypothyroidism. Levothyroxine provides standardized, predictable effects, thereby preventing the wide variety of symptomatic and metabolic disturbances associated with insufficient thyroid production. However, the patient's response is greatly affected by age, the cause and duration of the goiter, and the degree of nodularity.

Although thyroid hormone preparations are economical, standardization of iodine content or bioassay is inexact. Synthetic derivatives are generally preferred over natural hormones because their composition is known and constant. A combination of T_3 and T_4 (liotrix) is available but is not recommended because transient hyperthyroidism could precipitate angina or arrhythmias.

Levothyroxine use has a number of advantages over other thyroid hormones (e.g., desiccated thyroid) including a uniform potency, relatively low cost, and lack of foreign protein antigenicity. It has been suggested that liothyronine (T_3) is safer than levothyroxine because it is more potent and has a shorter half-life (2 to 3 days). Serum levels fall more rapidly when the drug is stopped; however, the advantages of liothyronine are offset by difficulties in dosage regulation. The difficulties can result in more frequent cardiovascular problems and symptoms of hyperthyroidism. Liothyronine is seldom used because of undesirable characteristics that cause short, alternating periods of hyperthyroidism and hypothyroidism. In addition, more frequent dosing is required, making it less desirable for prolonged therapy than the pure T_4 preparations. Other disadvantages include altered thyroid function tests and a higher cost.

Furthermore, small dosage tablets facilitate the titration of thyroid status. At present, the cost of brand name levothyroxine differs little from that of generic formulations. Most care providers avoid prescribing generic levothyroxine primarily because of concerns about quality control (see Guidelines for the Initial Use of Levothyroxine).

Patient Variables

In patients with signs and symptoms of hypothyroidism, TSH levels greater than 15 mU/L, and T_4 levels below normal values can be effectively treated with thyroid hormone replacement. Patients with mild or no symptoms of hypothyroidism, moderately elevated TSH levels (6 to 15 mU/L), and T_4 levels within normal limits should be treated early rather than later for subclinical hypothyroidism. Thyroid hormone replacement is not required in patients with TSH levels that are within the normal limits and T_4 levels that are low or low normal.

Patients who have been on thyroid hormone replacement for many years but for whom an initial diagnosis is not well documented are often encountered. In such patients, determine whether or not replacement therapy is still warranted by decreasing the dose by 50 percent and check the TSH level in 4 to 6 weeks. If the TSH remains normal, the dose can be decreased by another 50 percent for 4 to 6 weeks and then discontinued entirely. The TSH is used as a guide to the patient's thyroid status.

Intervention

Administration

Blood pressure and apical pulse should be assessed before and periodically during therapy. Overdosage is manifested as hyperthyroidism with similar signs and symptoms (tachycardia, chest pain, nervousness, insomnia, diaphoresis, tremors, weight loss). If tachyarrhythmias or chest pain develop, the usual intervention is to withhold the thyroid hormone for 2 to 6 days. Acute overdose is treated by induction of emesis or gastric lavage.

A levothyroxine suspension is readily available for patients who cannot or will not swallow whole tablets. It can be given by spoon or dropper. A crushed tablet may be sprinkled over a small amount of cooked cereal or applesauce.

GUIDELINES FOR INITIAL LEVOTHYROXINE THERAPY IN ADULTS

Rapid: Full Estimated Replacement Dose
- Begin at 0.1 mg daily for 6 to 8 weeks; may be adjusted based on TSH and T_4 levels
- Healthy young patients with mild hypothyroidism
- Most patients when hypothyroidism occurs shortly after surgery or radioiodine treatment of hyperthyroidism, unless known cardiac disease is present

Routine: Subreplacement Dose
- Begin at 0.075 to 0.1 mg daily for first 4 to 6 weeks; may be increased in increments of 0.025 to 0.05 mg every 4 to 6 weeks if tolerated
- Most healthy patients younger than 45 or 50 years

Cautious Use:
- Begin at 0.05 mg daily for first 4 weeks; may be increased in increments of 0.025 to 0.05 mg every 4 to 6 weeks if tolerated
- Patients over the age of 45 or 50 years
- Young patients with multiple risk factors for coronary artery disease
- Younger patients with severe or long-standing hypothyroidism

Extremely Cautious Use:
- Begin at 0.025 mg or less daily for first 4 weeks; may be increased in increments of 0.025 to 0.05 mg or less every 4–6 weeks, if tolerated
- Patients with angina and arrhythmias, and elderly patients
- Patients over the age of 45 or 50 years with multiple risk factors for coronary artery disease
- Older patients with severe or long-standing hypothyroidism

*The clinical assessment of the patient must take precedence over arbitrary guidelines. Data from Chopra, J. (1998). Hypothyroidism. In R. Rakel (Ed.). *Conn's current therapy 1998*. (pp. 644–649). Philadelphia: W. B. Saunders. Used with permission.

Education

The patient should receive an explanation of the disorder and the fact that treatment for hypothyroidism is life-long. Response to treatment usually takes several weeks to manifest. The patient should be advised that maximal response may not be seen for several months.

Patients should be instructed to take levothyroxine exactly as directed, on an empty stomach, and at the same time each day. Administration before breakfast helps prevent insomnia. If a dose is missed, it should be taken as soon as it is remembered. The health care provider should be notified if more than two or three doses are missed. However, because of levothyroxine's long half-life, in some cases, the forgotten doses may be taken all at once. The drug should not be discontinued without first talking with the health care provider.

Because the bioavailability of levothyroxine may differ between preparations, the patient should be cautioned not to change brands of levothyroxine with prescription refills. The concurrent use of other OTC drugs should be avoided unless otherwise instructed. Additive CNS and cardiac stimulation may occur with decongestants.

The patient and family should be taught how to take a pulse. A resting pulse rate over 100 bpm may indicate overdose. Thus, the drug should be withheld and the health care provider notified.

The importance of follow-up should be stressed. Thyroid function tests should be performed regularly during the initial phase of treatment, and at least yearly during therapy.

Evaluation

The patient's clinical response to levothyroxine can be evaluated by resolution of signs and symptoms of hypothyroidism. The expected response includes weight loss, an increased sense of well-being, and greater energy levels. The texture and characteristics of hair, skin, and nails should normalize, and constipation should be corrected.

Serum T_4 levels can be used to monitor the effectiveness of therapy. If serum T_4 levels are low but the TSH is normal, measurement of free T_4 levels is warranted. Persistent clinical and laboratory evidence of hypothyroidism in spite of adequate replacement indicates poor patient compliance, poor absorption, excessive fecal loss, or inactivity of the formulation. Intracellular resistance to thyroid hormones is rare.

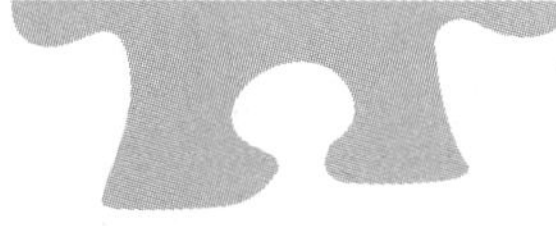

HYPERPARATHYROIDISM

Epidemiology and Etiology

Hyperparathyroidism (HPT), an increasingly recognized disorder, is defined as hypercalcemia secondary to excessive production of PTH. A relatively common disorder that affects 1:500 to 1:1000 people, it occurs two to four times more often in postmenopausal women than in men. It is rare before puberty but the incidence increases dramatically after age 50. It is the third most common endocrine disorder following diabetes mellitus and thyroid disease.

The etiology of primary HPT is unknown, but a single parathyroid adenoma accounts for 80 to 85 percent of cases. The adenoma is often clonal in nature, implying a defect in the gene that regulates PTH. Carcinoma of the parathyroid gland is rare, occurring in less than 2 percent of cases.

Risk factors in the development of primary HPT include a childhood history of radiation therapy to the neck or use of the drug lithium. Although in most cases HPT occurs sporadically, it also appears in assorted patterns as a familial disorder.

Secondary HPT is a response to vitamin D deficiency or the hypocalcemia of chronic renal disease. Hyperplasia of the parathyroid gland is found in 10 to 15 percent of cases. Eventually, the hyperplastic glands develop autonomous function and no longer respond to the normal feedback mechanisms (Fig. 50–2).

Pathophysiology

Regardless of etiology, the pathogenesis of primary HPT is related to the development of hypercalcemia. Patients with HPT are said to have difficulty with "bones, stones, abdominal groans, psychic moans, and fatigue overtones."

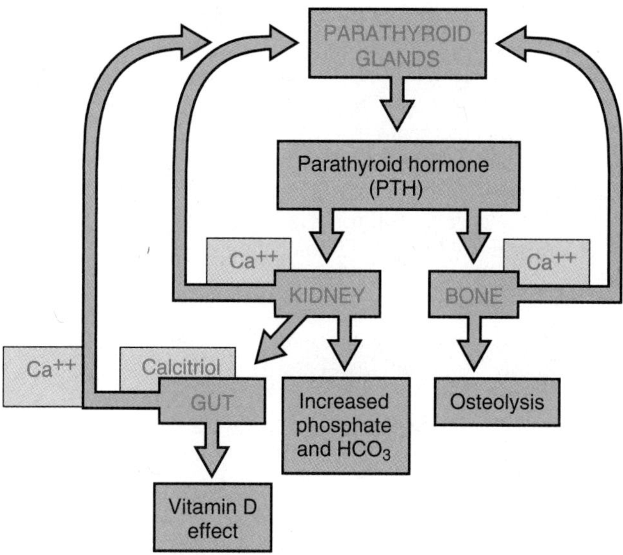

Figure 50–2 Parathyroid hormone secretion is regulated through a negative feedback loop involving the kidneys, bones, and intestine.

Increased quantities of PTH act directly on the kidneys. Calcium resorption (not reabsorption) and phosphate elimination increases in the renal tubules. Under ordinary circumstances, serum calcium levels are maintained within a narrow range despite large swings in calcium absorption during the day. These variations contribute to elevated serum calcium levels and low phosphorus levels.

In patients with a parathyroid adenoma, PTH secretion is excessive for a given serum calcium level. Elevated serum calcium levels are secondary to the loss of negative feedback. In contrast, patients with feedback control of PTH secretion but who have an increased number of parathyroid cells cause oversecretion of PTH. In some cases, production of a PTH-like substance from nonparathyroid tissue keeps the parathyroid glands from responding to the increased calcium levels.

Increased bicarbonate elimination and decreased acid elimination produce metabolic acidosis, urinary alkalosis, and hypokalemia. Stones containing calcium oxalate or phosphate may develop as a consequence of hypercalciuria. In addition, the glomerular filtration rate increases and renal tubular acidosis (RTA) occurs.

Hypertension may be noted in acute hypercalcemia, most likely as a result of vasoconstriction. In contrast, with a chronic hypercalcemic state, the development of hypertension is due to renal damage.

Increased levels of PTH lead to increased absorption of calcium by the intestines. It does so in the presence of increased vitamin D production by the kidneys.

In severe cases of HPT, thirst, anorexia, nausea, and vomiting are outstanding symptoms. There may also be anemia, asthenia, weight loss, and constipation. Hypercalcemia leads to increased secretion of gastrin and pepsin, resulting in peptic ulcer disease. An increase in pancreatitis is also noted.

Hypersecretion of PTH from any cause can lead to a bone disorder known as *osteitis fibrosa cystica generalisata.* Excessive PTH increases osteoclastic activity and decreases osteoblastic activity. This results in the release of calcium and phosphorus into the circulation and decalcification of bone. However, only 33 percent of HPT cases show minor degrees of decalcification. Another 33 percent display obvious skeletal abnormalities. The remaining 33 percent display advanced bone changes.

When the normal solubility of serum calcium is exceeded, calcium deposits in soft tissue. Tissue deposits can occur in the cornea, conjunctiva, myocardium, and kidneys. The deposits are most likely to occur with long-standing hypercalcemia.

PHARMACOTHERAPEUTIC OPTIONS

Hypocalcemic Drugs

- Etidronate (DIDRONEL)
- Pamidronate (AREDIA)
- Calcitonin salmon (CALCIMAR, MIACALCIN, SALMONINE, OSTEOCALCIN)
- Calcitonin human

Indications

Etidronate and pamidronate are hypocalcemic drugs. Pamidronate is a potent inhibitor of bone resorption and may be used for treatment of hypercalcemia due to HPT or malignancy. The drug is under study for use in the management of postmenopausal osteoporosis and Paget's disease. These two drugs may also be used in the treatment and prophylactic management of heterotopic calcification associated with total hip replacement or spinal cord injury. They have also been used successfully to relieve bone pain in patients with metastatic prostate and breast cancer.

Calcitonin salmon is also a hypocalcemic drug found to be useful for most forms of acute, severe hypercalcemia associated with increased bone resorption. It has been safely used to decrease the rate of bone turnover and to lower serum calcium levels. Any loss of efficacy may be due to calcitonin-induced reduction of serum phosphate levels. However, unidentified factors may also be involved. Calcitonin has also been used in the treatment of osteogenesis imperfecta but is not approved by the Food and Drug Administration (FDA) for that use at this time. It is approved by the FDA for treatment of symptomatic Paget's disease and osteoporosis.

Pharmacodynamics

Hypocalcemic drugs prevent bone resorption by attaching to bone mineral to be absorbed into newly formed bone matrix. They may also inhibit the activity of the bone-wasting osteoclasts.

Much like the other hypocalcemic agents, calcitonin salmon decreases serum calcium levels through directly inhibiting bone resorption. It also promotes the renal excretion of calcium, but its effectiveness varies.

Adverse Effects and Contraindications

Common adverse effects of hypocalcemic drugs include fatigue, anorexia, nausea, vomiting, constipation, and abdominal pain. A metallic taste or loss of taste is also possible. Bone pain and generalized discomfort is relatively common. Local irritation at an intravenous (IV) injection site may occur if the drug is given parenterally. Fluid and electrolyte imbalance is more likely with pamidronate than with etidronate.

Calcitonin is generally devoid of serious adverse effects. However, anaphylaxis is more common with the salmon source of the drug. Nausea, vomiting, a strange taste in the mouth, and facial flushing have been known to occur.

Pharmacokinetics

IV pamidronate is 100-percent absorbed, resulting in complete bioavailability. It is rapidly distributed, with 50 percent of a dose retained by bone. It reaches high concentrations in the liver, spleen, teeth, and tracheal cartilage. The onset of the drug action of pamidronate is 24 hours, with peak activity noted in 7 days. The half-life is biphasic. The first phase lasts 1.6 hours, and the second phase lasts 27.2 hours. The elimination half-life from the bone, however, is 300 days. The duration of action of pamidronate is unknown. Pamidronate causes a gradual decline in serum calcium levels over several days that tends to last for weeks to months.

When used IV to treat hypercalcemia, etidronate is completely absorbed. Only 1 to 6 percent of the drug is absorbed following oral administration. Interestingly, its onset time is 24 hours (as measured by decreased urinary calcium excretion). It takes 3 days to reach peak drug action, and it has a duration of action of 11 days. Fifty percent of the absorbed dose is eliminated unchanged in the urine. Unabsorbed drug is eliminated through the feces. The half-life of etidronate is 5 to 7 hours.

There are two sources of calcitonin, salmon and human. The salmon source of calcitonin is more potent than human sources on a weight basis. It also has a longer duration of action. Because calcitonin is destroyed in the GI tract, calcitonin salmon requires parenteral administration. It is completely absorbed using subcutaneous (SC) or intramuscular (IM) routes, with an onset time of 15 minutes. The distribution of calcitonin is unknown, but it does not appear to cross the placenta. Peak effects are reached in 2 to 4 hours. It is rapidly biotransformed in the kidneys, blood, and tissues. The half-life is 70 to 90 minutes, with a duration of action of 8 to 24 hours (see Table 50–2).

Drug-Drug Interactions

There are few drug-drug interactions with hypocalcemic drugs. Vitamin D and calcium supplements antagonize the calcium-lowering effect of calcitonin (see Table 50–3).

Dosage Regimen

Two of the hypocalcemic agents are available in parenteral form for IV use. An oral dose of pamidronate is soon to be approved. Pamidronate is administered IV over a 24-hour period, with a dosage range of 30 to 90 mg. Patients with severe hypercalcemia should be started at the 90-mg dose (see Table 50–4).

Etidronate is administered IV as 7.5 mg/kg/day for 3 days. The patient may then be switched to 20 mg/kg/day by mouth. Concurrent saline hydration should be undertaken with pamidronate or etidronate therapy.

Calcitonin salmon is administered with an initial dose of 4 IU/kg SC or IM every 12 hours. The dose may be increased to 8 IU/kg every 6 hours, as needed. An intradermal skin test should precede therapy with calcitonin salmon. The patient should be closely watched for anaphylaxis with the initial injection.

Laboratory Considerations

Patients taking pamidronate should have electrolytes (including calcium, phosphorus, and magnesium), hemoglobin, and creatinine closely monitored. A complete blood count (CBC) and platelet count should be monitored during the first 2 weeks of hypocalcemic therapy. Monitor the blood urea nitrogen (BUN) and creatinine before and periodically throughout therapy. Stable or reversible increases in BUN and creatinine may occur in patients with hypercalcemia.

Etidronate interferes with bone uptake of technetium in diagnostic scans. Decreased urinary elimination of hydroxyproline and serum alkaline phosphatase are often the first clinical signs of treatment effectiveness in patients with Paget's disease.

Miscellaneous Hypocalcemic Drugs

- ❐ Gallium nitrate (GANITE)
- ❐ Plicamycin (MITHRACIN)

GALLIUM NITRATE

Gallium nitrate is now being used more often because it has even fewer adverse effects than plicamycin. Gallium nitrate inhibits calcium resorption from bone. The most common adverse effects include renal toxicity and hypophosphatemia. Hearing loss, optic neuritis, visual impairment, and hypocalcemia have been noted.

The drug is contraindicated in patients with severe renal impairment (serum creatinine exceeding 2.5 mg/dL) and should be used with caution in patients with renal impairment. Safe use during pregnancy and lactation has not been established.

Gallium nitrate is administered IV with complete bioavailability. It is eliminated unchanged by the kidneys, with a half-life of 24 hours. The half-life increases to 72 to 115 hours with prolonged infusions. Peak action is reached in 5 days, with a duration of action of 7.5 days.

The usual dose of gallium nitrate is 100 to 200 mg/m^2 daily for 5 days. A 3- to 4-day rest period is recommended between courses of therapy. Serum calcium and phosphate levels should be monitored twice weekly to determine treatment effectiveness. Oral phosphate therapy may be needed should hypophosphatemia develop. Serum albumin levels should also be monitored before and periodically throughout therapy.

PLICAMYCIN

Plicamycin is an antineoplastic agent that is very effective in lowering serum calcium levels. Plicamycin antagonizes the action of vitamin D and inhibits the action of parathyroid hormone on osteoclasts. The most common adverse effects include hypocalcemia and thrombocytopenia. CNS irritability or depression and GI upset have been noted, as well as fluid and electrolyte imbalances.

The drug should be used with caution in patients with hypersensitivity, bleeding disorders, depressed bone marrow reserve, hypocalcemia, and severe renal or liver disease. It should be used with caution in patients of child-bearing age, active infections, chronic debilitating illnesses, and renal or hepatic impairment. Safe use in children has not been established.

The onset of the hypocalcemic effect of plicamycin occurs in 24 to 48 hours when it is administered IV, with peak activity seen after 24 hours. The duration of action is 1 to 2 weeks.

The dosage of plicamycin is about one tenth that used for antineoplastic therapy, and thus, the adverse effects are proportionately lower. The usual dose to treat hypercalcemia is 15 to 25 mcg/kg once daily for 3 to 4 days. The dosage may be repeated after 7 days or one to three times weekly.

Monitor the CBC with differential, platelet count, prothrombin time, and bleeding times, and electrolytes before and periodically throughout therapy. Plicamycin may cause thrombocytopenia, leukemia, anemia, hypocalcemia, hypokalemia, and hypophosphatemia. Notify the health care provider if the platelet count drops below 150,000/mm^3, prothrombin time is elevated four or more seconds above the control, or the leukocyte count is less than 4000/mm^3.

Critical Thinking Process

Assessment

History of Present Illness

The patient with hyperparathyroidism may report problems related to the musculoskeletal system that include simple back pain, joint pains, painful shins, or muscle spasms. Depression or anxiety, arthralgias, and nausea and vomiting may also be noted. Complaints of constipation, abdominal pain, ulcers, muscle weakness, and fatigue are also frequent.

Past Health History

When interviewing the patient, the examiner should include questions about a history of calcium oxalate or calcium phosphate renal calculi, thyroid disease or surgery, neck dissection, renal failure, or adrenal insufficiency (Addison's disease). The patient may also note a personal history of sarcoidosis, milk-alkali syndrome, multiple myeloma, cancer with metastasis, or seizures that required therapy.

Physical Exam Findings

The physical exam should include vital signs, height and weight, and skin color and texture. The eyes should be examined for corneal changes related to precipitation of calcium in the corneas (band keratopathy), conjunctivitis, papilledema, blepharospasm, and photophobia.

Intense pruritus may accompany severe hypercalcemia with evidence of broken skin surfaces. In hyperparathyroidism associated with renal failure, calcium also precipitates in the soft tissues, especially around the joints. Bony tenderness may be noted on palpation.

Diagnostic Testing

The hallmarks of primary hypercalcemia are elevated ionized or total serum calcium levels and elevated PTH levels. PTH-C (C-terminal fragments) levels are also elevated. The

C assays tend to have higher values and are more widely accepted as indicators of hyperparathyroidism. Sodium phosphorus levels tend to be low. The results are then correlated with the patient's clinical picture.

Most patients with primary hypercalcemia show no evidence of bone disease. However, with untreated, longstanding hyperparathyroidism, extensive bone erosion results. The bone resorption is readily demonstrated in the cortex of the phalanges. In a small number of patients who have significant osteitis, serum alkaline phosphatase levels are also elevated. The elevation reflects osteoblastic activity.

Because of the effects of PTH, bicarbonate levels are reduced and serum chloride levels are elevated. The concentration of cyclic adenosine monophosphate (cAMP) in the urine is also increased. Urinary calcium levels may be normal or elevated. Its measurement is used in the diagnosis of familial benign hypercalcemia. However, marked hypercalciuria may suggest a non–PTH-related hypercalcemia. Other causes of hypercalcemia can be readily identified by other clinical manifestations or by laboratory studies.

Developmental Considerations

Perinatal Hypercalcemia in pregnancy is rare. Only about 80 cases have been described in the medical literature. More pregnant patients are diagnosed with symptomatic hypercalcemia than nonpregnant patients. This probably reflects the lack of routine screening of calcium levels rather than an increased severity of the disease. Intact PTH levels are not altered by pregnancy, and therefore, the evaluation of hypercalcemia during pregnancy is similar to that of nonpregnant patients.

The treatment of choice for primary hypercalcemia during pregnancy is parathyroidectomy. Surgery is usually performed during the second trimester, when fetal body systems are developed, but before the third trimester, when a greater chance of premature labor exists. When parathyroidectomy is contraindicated, oral phosphate therapy may be appropriate for some patients. Treatment with hormones or biphosphates is contraindicated.

Pediatric Parathyroid hormone excess manifested by hypercalcemia is very rare in children. When it is present, the clinical manifestations include renal colic, bone pain and bone masses, and osteoporosis.

Geriatric Older adults may exhibit signs of hypercalcemia such as progressive hypertension, lethargy, drowsiness, depression, and GI discomfort. Radiation therapy to the neck or chest may precipitate the disorder, as well as a history of lithium use.

Psychosocial Considerations

The notion that the patient with hypercalcemia has difficulty with "bones, stones, abdominal groan, psychic moans, and fatigue overtones" is well known. These problems impact the patient's ability to carry out activities of daily living. The variety of signs and symptoms cause the patient to seek medical attention numerous times over the course of the disease.

Analysis and Management

Treatment Objectives

The primary treatment objective for hypercalcemia is to control the underlying disease. Management is aimed at reducing serum calcium levels.

Treatment Options

Drug Variables

There is no totally acceptable medical treatment regimen for hypercalcemia. Surgical removal of the abnormal parathyroid gland has been the treatment of choice in symptomatic patients. Symptomatic patients are usually dehydrated; therefore, hydration with isotonic saline is the first step in treatment. In addition, calcium intake is restricted and electrolyte deficits (i.e., potassium and magnesium) are corrected. When expansion of plasma volume has been accomplished, a loop diuretic such as furosemide is given to promote urinary elimination of calcium. If it is used too early in treatment, however, furosemide may further dehydrate the patient and worsen the hypercalcemia. Therefore, it should be used only after circulatory volume has been restored. Thiazide diuretics should not be used because they decrease the elimination of calcium and worsen the hypercalcemia.

Hypocalcemic drugs such as etidronate, pamidronate, and calcitonin salmon have been used with some success in the management of mild hypercalcemia. Because of the adverse GI effects and possibility of bone pain, neither etidronate and pamidronate are drugs of choice for the treatment of hypercalcemia. Calcitonin salmon has fewer GI adverse effects and may be more desirable. Calcitonin may also be given SC or by nasal spray and would be appropriate in patients with low weight and small body frame.

Glucocorticoids have been effective for hypercalcemia associated with sarcoidosis and hypervitaminosis D. They are not useful for hypercalcemia that occurs with hyperparathyroidism or with production of a PTH-related hormone. At present, no PTH-inhibiting drug is available.

Hypercalcemic states have also been reduced with the administration of phosphate. Phosphate promotes the deposition of calcium in the bone and soft tissues. Phosphate use is discouraged, however, because of the risk of fatal calcifications in the lungs, kidney, and other soft tissues.

Patient Variables

Patients receiving cardiac glycosides should be given hypocalcemia therapy with caution because of an increased risk for cardiac glycoside toxicity.

Conjugated estrogen has been used in some patients to reduce bone resorption and serum calcium levels. In many patients, estrogen therapy helps stabilize the disease. However, a history of estrogen-receptor–positive breast cancer contraindicates this therapy option. In addition, for patients who refuse surgery or who are not candidates, drugs that suppress PTH-mediated bone turnover may be useful.

Intervention

Administration

Etidronate should be administered on an empty stomach at least 2 hours before or after a meal. Intravenous etidronate is diluted in normal saline and administered over 2 hours. The patient should be monitored for bone pain and reports of GI adverse effects. Serum phosphate levels usually return to normal 2 to 4 weeks after therapy. With long-term therapy (over 3 months), the risk of fractures increases. Etidronate may cause systemic reactions including tetany.

Allergy testing is usually done before initiating calcitonin salmon therapy. If the skin test produces a wheel, the drug should not be given. If more than 2 mL of calcitonin salmon is to be administered, an IM route is preferred. To minimize the flushing effect of the drug, it should be given at bedtime. Injection sites should be rotated.

The patient should follow-up with the health care provider to monitor serum calcium, phosphorus, alkaline phosphatase, and PTH levels. The levels should normalize within a few months of the start of therapy. Periodic monitoring of urine for casts should also be performed.

Vigorous saline hydration, maintaining a urine output of 2000 mL/24 hours, should be undertaken concurrently with pamidronate therapy but should be initiated cautiously in patients with underlying congestive heart failure. Advise the patient to notify the health care provider of pain at the infusion site or if bone pain becomes severe or persistent.

Education

Patients should be advised to take the hypocalcemia drug as directed. If a dose is missed but remembered within 2 hours of the next dose, it should be taken. Patients should be taught to not double dose. Patients should be advised that calcium supplements, antacids, and iron may decrease the absorption of etidronate, antagonizing the drugs beneficial effects. The correct technique for SC injection should be included in patient teaching. The patient should be reassured that the flushing and warm sensation following injection is transient and usually lasts about 1 hour. Nausea following injection tends to decrease with continued therapy.

The patient should be taught to watch for signs of hypocalcemic tetany with the first several doses of hypocalcemic drugs. Nervousness, irritability, paresthesia, and muscle twitching should be immediately brought to the attention of the health care provider. Signs of hypercalcemic relapse (bone or flank pain, renal calculi, anorexia, nausea, vomiting, thirst, lethargy) should be promptly reported.

Evaluation

The effectiveness of drug therapy will be evidenced by lowered serum calcium levels and fewer complaints of bone pain and fractures.

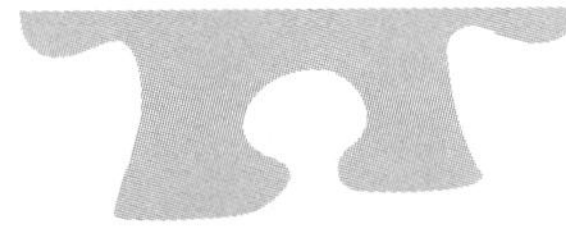

HYPOPARATHYROIDISM

Epidemiology and Etiology

Hypoparathyroidism is defined according to its two primary causes. The most common, insufficient amounts of PTH (true hypoparathyroidism), is caused by surgical removal of the gland. It is uncommon following a simple thyroid lobectomy, but the incidence of hypoparathyroidism following total thyroidectomy is 3 to 5 percent. The average age of onset for idiopathic hypoparathyroidism is 16 years. Pseudohypoparathyroidism is inherited, affecting females twice as often as males. The average age of onset for pseudohypoparathyroidism is 8.5 years. Familial occurrences of idiopathic hypoparathyroidism are rare. Secondary disease may occur after surgery.

Pseudohypoparathyroidism is a rare familial disorder characterized by target tissue resistance to PTH. The idiopathic form is associated with absent or decreased PTH secretion from hypoplastic or damaged parathyroid glands. Functional hypoparathyroidism may also occur as the result of magnesium deficiency. Magnesium deficiency, most often caused by malabsorption and alcoholism, prevents the secretion of PTH.

Prolonged administration of anticonvulsant drugs such as phenytoin and phenobarbital, the antimicrobial drug rifampin, glutethimide, and other enzyme-inducing drugs may induce hypocalcemia.

Pathophysiology

Deficiency of PTH secretion leads to hypocalcemia and hyperphosphatemia. PTH release occurs in response to low serum calcium levels, and secretion is suppressed by the elevated levels. Calcium reabsorption in the intestines is decreased. When there is insufficient calcium to meet metabolic needs, calcium stores in the bones are reduced. Chronic calcium insufficiency can result in bone demineralization. Low levels of PTH also cause decreased renal clearance of phosphorus, thereby enhancing its tubular reabsorption.

There are several factors that depress calcium transport across the small intestine. For example, phytate, oxalate, and probably phosphate in the bowel promote the formation of a complex that is not absorbed from the wall of the gut. Because calcium is responsible for neuromuscular integrity, the clinical manifestations of hypocalcemia become evident. Tetany refers to the involuntary muscle spasms that affect muscles of the upper and lower extremities. Carpopedal spasms, paresthesias of the lips and hands, and occasionally laryngeal stridor may occur. When respiratory muscles are involved, respiratory distress may result.

PHARMACOTHERAPEUTIC OPTIONS

Hypercalcemic Drugs

- ❒ Calcium carbonate (OS-CAL, TITRALAC, TUMS); (🍁) APO-CAL, CALCITE, CALGLYCINE, CALSAN, MYLANTA LOZENGES, NU-CAL
- ❒ Calcium gluconate
- ❒ Calcium lactate, acetate, chloride

Indications

Oral calcium preparations are used in the treatment and management of mild hypocalcemia associated with hypoparathyroidism, pseudohypoparathyroidism, achlorhydria, chronic diarrhea, pancreatitis, vitamin D deficiency, and hyperphosphatemia. Calcium carbonate has also been used as an antacid (see Chapter 40). It is used as an adjunct in the prevention of postmenopausal osteoporosis. Calcium acetate is used to control hyperphosphatemia in end-stage renal failure (see Chapter 41).

Pharmacodynamics

Calcium is rapidly distributed to extracellular fluids to restore calcium levels and re-establish homeostasis. Its action is especially important in the functioning of the nervous, cardiovascular, and skeletal systems. In the nervous system, calcium helps regulate excitability and transmitter release. For the cardiovascular system, calcium plays a role in myocardial contraction and the coagulation of blood. Calcium is also required for the structural integrity of the skeletal system. It acts as a sedative on the body; therefore, decreased excitability of the neuromuscular system takes place.

Adverse Effects and Contraindications

The most common adverse effects of calcium salts include constipation, nausea, and vomiting. Calcium has been known to cause gastrointestinal distress from increased gas production. The most severe adverse effects include arrhythmias and cardiac arrest.

Prolonged use of high doses of calcium produces other symptoms such as hypercalcemia with alkalosis, hypomagnesemia and hypophosphatemia, mood and mental changes, GI hemorrhage, and milk-alkali syndrome.

Calcium preparations are contraindicated in patients with hypercalcemia, renal calculi, and ventricular fibrillation. They should be used cautiously in patients who are taking cardiac glycosides or in those who have severe respiratory insufficiency or renal disease.

Pharmacokinetics

Orally administered calcium requires vitamin D for absorption to take place in the duodenum and proximal jejunum. Calcium absorption is facilitated by the presence of PTH and a pH of 5 to 7. Absorption also depends on dietary factors, such as calcium binding to fiber, phytic, oxalic, and fatty acids (see Appendix C). When calcium is taken with large amounts of foods containing these acids, calcium absorption is impaired. When calcium is bound, calcium salts form insoluble soaps.

Calcium readily enters extracellular fluid to be distributed to the bone. It crosses the placenta and enters breast milk. It is eliminated primarily in the stool, with a small amount (20 percent) eliminated in the urine.

Drug-Drug Interactions

All of the calcium salts enhance inotropic and toxic effects of cardiac glycoside preparations. Calcium competes with magnesium for GI absorption and decreases the absorption of tetracycline and the fluoroquinolones. It is also an antagonist to the effects of verapamil and other calcium channel blockers. Cholestyramine, colestipol, and mineral oil may decrease the absorption of vitamin D (see Table 50–3).

Dosage Regimen

The various calcium salts differ in their percentage of elemental calcium (see Table 50–4). These differences must be accounted for when determining dosage. For example, if 1 g of elemental calcium from either calcium carbonate or calcium lactate is desired, 2.5 g of calcium carbonate or nearly 7 g of calcium lactate is required to provide the calcium ordered.

Laboratory Considerations

Intravenous calcium may cause a false decrease in serum and urine magnesium (Titan yellow method) and transient elevations of plasma II-OHCS levels by the Glenn-Nelson technique. Values normalize after 1 hour. Urinary steroid values (17-OHCS) may be decreased.

Vitamin D and Vitamin D Analogs

- ❒ Calcitriol (1,25-dihydroxycholecalciferol, CALCIJEX, ROCALTROL)
- ❒ Dihydrotachysterol (DHT, HYTAKEROL)
- ❒ Ergocalciferol (CALCIFEROL, DRISDOL)

Indications

Calcitrol is used in the management of hypocalcemia related to chronic renal failure and hypoparathyroidism or pseudohypoparathyroidism. Dihydrotachysterol is used for the treatment of hypophosphatemia and hypocalcemia, as well as for the prevention and treatment of rickets, vitamin D deficiency, and postoperative and idiopathic tetany. Ergocalciferol is used for prophylaxis and treatment of vitamin D deficiency, hypophosphatemia, and hypocalcemia, as well as for the treatment of osteodystrophy, osteomalacia secondary to chronic convulsant therapy, and rickets.

Pharmacodynamics

Vitamin D and vitamin D analogs are necessary for adequate absorption of calcium and phosphorus from the intestine, for regulating renal excretion, and for proper disposition of calcium in the bone. It regulates calcium homeostasis in conjunction with parathyroid hormone and calcitonin.

Dietary vitamin D is primarily cholecalciferol or ergocalciferol. Cholecalciferol is formed from 7-dehydrocholesterol in skin exposed to ultraviolet light. Dihydrotachysterol and ergocalciferol are inactive forms of vitamin D and may be thought of as precursors to the more active forms.

Adverse Effects and Contraindications

The adverse effects of vitamin D and its analogs are primarily manifestations of toxicity (hypercalcemia). Weakness, headache, somnolence, photophobia, nausea, vomiting, dry mouth, constipation, metallic taste, polydipsia, anorexia, and weight loss have been noted. Hypertension and arrhythmias, hypercalcemia, muscle pain, and bone pain are possible.

Vitamin D and its analogs are contraindicated in patients with hypersensitivity, hypercalcemia, and vitamin D toxicity. Large doses of vitamin D should be avoided during pregnancy. The drugs should be used with caution in patients with hyperparathyroidism, sarcoidosis, and in patients taking cardiac glycosides. Safe use during pregnancy has not been established. Chronic excessive vitamin D intake in children may lead to mental and physical retardation and suppression of linear growth.

Pharmacokinetics

Vitamin D and its analogs are readily absorbed from the GI tract. Dihydrotachysterol and ergocalciferol are well absorbed but in an inactive form. It is distributed to breast milk, lymph, liver, skin, brain, spleen, and bones. The peak activity of calcitriol given orally occurs in 2 to 6 hours. The duration of action of vitamin D ranges from 3 to 5 days for calcitriol taken orally to 6 months or more for ergocalciferol.

Dihydrotachysterol and ergocalciferol are biotransformed to active metabolites by sunlight, the liver, and the kidneys. The half-lives of vitamin D preparations is 3 to 8 hours, with 50 percent eliminated in bile, feces, or urine. The remainder is stored for months in body tissues, especially the liver and bones.

Drug-Drug Interactions

Cardiac glycosides may be more likely to cause arrhythmias in patients who are also receiving vitamin D analogs. Thiazide diuretics may trigger hypercalcemia in patients with hypoparathyroidism who are taking vitamin D. A number of other drug-drug interactions are identified in Table 50–3.

Dosage Regimen

The dosage of vitamin D analogs varies with the specific drug. Calcitriol is administered initially as 0.25 to 2.7 mcg daily. The dosage is adjusted as necessary to maintain normal serum calcium concentrations.

When it is used for hypoparathyroidism or pseudohypoparathyroidism, dihydrotachysterol is administered initially as 0.75 to 2.5 mg daily. Maintenance doses are usually 0.2 to 1.0 mg daily but should not exceed 1.5 mg/daily.

When it is used for hypoparathyroidism or pseudohypoparathyroidism in adults, ergocalciferol is dosed at 50,000 to 150,000 units po daily. Children's dosages range upward to 200,000 units daily.

Laboratory Considerations

Serum ionized calcium concentrations should be drawn weekly during initial therapy. BUN, serum creatinine, alkaline phosphatase, PTH levels, urinary calcium/creatinine ratio, and 24-hour urinary calcium levels should be measured periodically throughout therapy. A fall in alkaline phosphatase levels may signal the onset of hypercalcemia. Overdosage of vitamin D compounds is associated with a serum calcium level times phosphate (Ca x P) level of greater than 70 and an elevated BUN, alanine aminotransferase (ALT; serum glutamic-pyruvic transaminase [SGPT]) and aspartate aminotransferase (AST; serum glutamic-oxaloacetic transaminase [SGOT]). Vitamin D analogs may cause a false increase in serum cholesterol values.

Critical Thinking Process

Assessment

History of Present Illness

Patients with acute hypocalcemia may report muscle cramps, tingling of the circumoral area, hands, and feet. Symptoms of chronic hypoparathyroidism include blurring of vision, personality changes, and anxiety.

Past Health History

The patient's past history should elicit information regarding pancreatitis, osteomalacia, renal failure, malabsorption syndrome, low calcium levels, or a history of neck surgery.

Physical Exam Findings

Acute hypoparathyroidism causes tetany, with muscle cramps, irritability, carpopedal spasm, and seizures. In most cases, the neuromuscular irritability caused by low calcium levels may be demonstrated by tapping over the facial nerve just in front of the ear. A unilateral contraction of facial muscles occurs *(Chvostek's sign)*. Carpopedal spasms may be induced by placing a blood pressure cuff on the arm and inflating it above systolic pressure *(Trousseau's test)* for a period of 3 minutes. Deep tendon reflexes may be hyperactive.

Slit-lamp examination of the eyes may show early posterior lenticular cataract formation. Papilledema may be noted. Chronically low levels of calcium may be associated with dental abnormalities (pitting or delayed eruptions) or subcutaneous calcifications. Prolonged hypocalcemia causes changes in the skin, hair, and nails, as well as the teeth and lens of the eye. If the condition is left untreated, cataracts may develop within a few years. The skin becomes coarse, dry, and scaly. Alopecia may develop with patchy or absent eyelashes and eyebrows. The nails become thin and brittle with transverse grooves. Dentition may be delayed and hypoplastic.

Diagnostic Testing

True hypoparathyroidism is associated with low levels of intact PTH in light of low total and ionized calcium concentrations. Serum and urinary calcium levels are low, with high serum and urinary phosphate levels. Alkaline phosphatase levels are normal.

Serum calcium is largely bound to serum albumin. Therefore, the serum calcium level should be corrected for serum albumin level using the following formula:

$$\text{Corrected serum calcium} = \text{serum calcium mg/dL} + (0.8 \times [4.0 - \text{albumin g/dL}])$$

An electrocardiogram (ECG) may be needed to evaluate the heart rhythm and the QT interval. Radiographic tests may be used to determine the presence of renal calculi, fractures, bony tumors, osteoporosis, or tuberculosis.

Developmental Considerations

Perinatal Hypoparathyroidism in pregnancy is relatively uncommon. However, more pregnant patients are diagnosed with symptomatic hypoparathyroidism than nonpregnant patients. This finding probably reflects the lack of routine screening of calcium levels rather than an increased severity of the disease. Intact PTH levels are not altered by pregnancy, and therefore, diagnosis of hypoparathyroidism during pregnancy is similar to that of nonpregnant patients.

Neonates may have hypoparathyroidism secondary to maternal hypercalcemia, with 25 percent of the cases resulting in fetal death, 50 percent resulting in tetany, and 2 percent having a congenital absence of parathyroid glands and thymus. The congenital absence of these structures may cause early death.

Pediatric Clinical manifestations of hypoparathyroidism in children are secondary to hypocalcemia. The signs and symptoms include tetany; generalized tonic-clonic, absence, and simple partial seizures; carpopedal spasms; muscle cramps or twitching; paresthesias; and respiratory stridor.

Case Study Hypoparathyroidism

Patient History

History of Present Illness	SM is a 47-year-old divorced man who has returned to the surgical clinic after having a total thyroidectomy 3 days ago at the ambulatory surgery center. He is complaining of lethargy, irritability, muscle cramps, and circumoral tingling.
Past Health History	SM has 10 year history of alcohol abuse, consuming one to two six-packs of beer daily. He has had no alcohol in the last 8 months since joining Alcoholic's Anonymous. Because of his alcohol abuse, he developed chronic gastroenteritis. He has curtailed his intake of calcium because it contributes to diarrhea and admits that he does not follow a balanced diet. He has no allergies and takes no medications.
Physical Exam Findings	Height: 5'9". Present weight: 155 pounds. VS: BP 136/88, apical pulse 88, respirations 24. Temperature: 98.6°F. Incision does not show redness, edema, or exudate. Wound edges are approximated, and staples remain in place. Breath sounds clear on auscultation. Chvostek's test is positive, and Trousseau's sign is present. DTRs are hyperactive. Skin is warm, dry, and scaly.
Diagnostic Testing	Total serum calcium level is low at 7.8 mg/dL. (Norm: 8.8–10.0 mg/dL.) Ionized calcium value is 4.0 mg/dL. (Norm: 4.4–5.4 mEq/L.) Total plasma proteins (albumin and globulins) are also low at 5 g/dL. (Norm: 6–8 g/dL.) Serum phosphorous level: 5.0 mg/dL. (Norm: 2.7–4.5 mg/dL.) Serum magnesium 1.0 mEq/L. (Norm: 1.3–2.1 mEq/L.) BUN, creatinine, and electrolytes WNL.
Developmental Considerations	No specific developmental considerations for SM at this time.
Psychosocial Considerations	SM is a civil engineer who travels a great deal. He pays child support for two young children.
Economic Factors	SM carries health insurance through his employer but no pharmacy coverage

Variables Influencing Decision

Treatment Objectives	• Maintain serum calcium levels in a slightly low but asymptomatic range. • Prevent long-term complications such as renal stones and ectopic calcifications.

Drug Variables	*Drug Summary*	*Patient Variables*
Indications	Calcium preparations appropriate in the treatment of hypocalcemia related to hypoparathyroidism.	This will become a decision point because SM is diagnosed with hypoparathyroidism secondary to parathyroidectomy.
Pharmacodynamics	Calcium salts in combination with vitamin D analog enhance the intestinal absorption of calcium, so this becomes a decision point.	No patient-related variables that would affect the decision.
Adverse Effects/ Contraindications	Nausea, vomiting, and constipation are the most common adverse effects.	This will become a decision point because of SM's history of gastroenteritis secondary to alcohol abuse.
Pharmacokinetics	No significant pharmacokinetic implications at this time.	No patient related variables that would affect the decision.
Dosage Regimen	A daily calcium intake of 2000–4000 mg is required. Chewable tablets preferred formulation. Will need concurrent vitamin D analog.	Patient agreeable to taking chewable tablets, so this is not a decision point.

Case Study Hypoparathyroidism—cont'd

Drug Variables	Drug Summary	Patient Variables
Lab Considerations	Serum calcium, phosphorus, and albumin levels to be monitored before start of therapy and periodically throughout.	Patient willing to return for follow-up lab work.
Cost Index*	Calcium carbonate: 1 Vitamin D: 1	Patient has no pharmacy insurance.

Summary of Decision Points

- Calcium salts in combination with vitamin D analog enhance the intestinal absorption of calcium.
- Calcium carbonate is the drug of choice in the treatment of chronic hypocalcemia related to hypoparathyroidism.
- Patient history of gastroenteritis may complicate plan to use calcium.

DRUGS TO BE USED

- Calcium carbonate 600 mg with vitamin D 250 IU po BID 1–2 hours after meals

*Cost Index:

1 $ < 30.mo.
2 $30–40/mo.
3 $40–50/mo.
4 $50–60/mo.
5 $ > 60/mo.

AWP of 60, 600 mg tablets of calcium carbonate with vitamin D 250 IU is approximately $3.

The skin can be dry and coarse. Maculopapular skin eruptions and eczematous dermatitis can occur. The hair is often brittle with areas of alopecia. Nails are thin and brittle, and there is dental and enamel hypoplasia.

Children with pseudohypoparathyroidism are short and have round facies with short, thick necks. The fingers and toes are stubby, with dimpled skin over the knuckles. Calcium deposits in subcutaneous soft tissue is common. Mental retardation is a more prominent feature of pseudohypoparathyroidism than of the idiopathic form. Mood swings, memory loss, depression, and confusion can occur.

Candidiasis of the nails and mouth occurs with the idiopathic form but seldom with pseudohypoparathyroidism. Furthermore, papilledema, thought to be related to increased intracranial pressure, may occur in the idiopathic form but is rare in pseudohypoparathyroidism.

Geriatric Older adults may be susceptible to hypoparathyroidism because of dietary deficiencies of calcium and vitamin D, or because of decreased activity and lack of exposure to sunshine. Secondary causes of hypoparathyroidism that may occur more often in older adults include cancer of the prostate, pancreatitis, and liver or renal disease. Elderly patients are more susceptible to osteoporosis with the potential for spontaneous fractures.

Psychosocial Considerations

Prolonged hypocalcemia may produce changes in the skin, hair, muscle coordination, and pain from ulcers or pancreatitis. These problems adversely affect the patient's self-esteem and ability to perform the activities of daily living (see Case Study—Hypoparathyroidism).

Analysis and Management

Treatment Objectives

Regardless of the cause of hypoparathyroidism, the primary objectives are twofold. Maintain serum calcium levels in a slightly low but asymptomatic range. In keeping calcium levels on the low side of normal, long-term complications such as renal stones and ectopic calcifications are avoided.

Treatment Options

Drug Variables

Calcium carbonate is the most efficient form of calcium available and is the drug of choice in the treatment of chronic hypocalcemia related to hypoparathyroidism. It is also less expensive than other formulations. Calcium carbonate is also a weak phosphate binder that is helpful in controlling the serum phosphate levels associated with renal failure.

Therapy with vitamin D should be started as soon as oral calcium is begun. The vitamin D drug of choice for chronic hypoparathyroidism is ergocalciferol (vitamin D_2). With proper dosages the patient's serum calcium levels can be maintained within normal limits. It provides a more stable serum calcium level than do the shorter acting vitamin D preparations. Dihydrotachysterol has a shorter duration of action than ergocalciferol and is more effective in the mobilization of calcium from bone.

Patient Variables

Calcium formulations are useful in patients who avoid dairy products and admit to having a poor diet. Alcohol use or abuse may contribute to magnesium deficiency. In addition, the parathyroid glands may have been inadvertently removed during a thyroidectomy. Replacement hormone therapy is indicated when calcium levels are below normal and the patient is symptomatic. Some literature suggests that once-daily dosing of calcium supplements is better absorbed when taken at bedtime.

The treatment of choice for hypoparathyroidism during pregnancy consists of calcium and vitamin D. It should be noted that if hypoparathyroidism during pregnancy remains untreated, a high maternal and fetal mortality ensues. Further neonatal hyperparathyroidism may develop in response to the hypocalcemia. Breast-feeding may cause hypervitaminosis D in the infant because vitamin D is eliminated in the breast milk.

Calcium is given to neonates to treat tetany, to overcome cardiac toxicity of hyperkalemia, for cardiopulmonary resuscitation, and to treat the acute symptoms of lead colic. As in the management of the adult, the pharmacotherapeutic management of either form of hypoparathyroidism in a child is the maintenance of normal serum calcium levels. Some children may be treated with oral calcium salts alone. Others may also require supplemental vitamin D. Close follow-up is crucial to the well-being of the child. Serum calcium and phosphorus levels are checked twice weekly during initial therapy and then monthly thereafter.

Intervention

Administration

Oral calcium preparations should be taken 2 to 3 hours after eating. Calcium tablets should be chewed well before swallowing and followed by a full glass of water.

Intravenous calcium must be administered slowly into a large vein to avoid local trauma and cardiac arrhythmias. Undiluted calcium should be given at a rate of 0.5 to 1.0 mL/minute. It should be diluted in normal saline and given slowly at the rate of 1 L per 12 to 24 hours. The IV site should be closely monitored for extravasation, necrosis, or sloughing. Thromboses of peripheral veins also may occur with IV calcium. The patient's blood pressure should be checked periodically during the administration of IV calcium. ECG monitoring is essential to detect QT changes and inverted T-wave abnormalities.

Monitoring of serum calcium levels at regular intervals, at least every 3 months, is important. Urine calcium levels with spot urine determinations should also be monitored and kept below 30 mg/dL, if possible.

Education

The patient taking hypocalcemic drugs should be taught to avoid taking enteric-coated drugs within 1 hour of calcium carbonate. Doing so will result in premature dissolution of the tablets.

Calcium carbonate should not be taken concurrently with foods containing large amounts of oxalic acid (e.g., spinach, Swiss chard, rhubarb, beets) or phytic acid (e.g., brans, whole grain cereals). The concurrent administration of dairy products (phosphorus) may produce a milk-alkali syndrome that is manifested as headache, confusion, nausea, and vomiting.

The patient should also be taught that calcium preparations may cause constipation; thus, they should be encouraged to increase bulk and fluid in the diet and to increase mobility. Severe constipation may indicate toxicity, necessitating contact with the health care provider.

Evaluation

The effectiveness of drug therapy for hypoparathyroidism will be evidenced as resolution of hypoparathyroid symptoms and an increase in serum calcium levels to a more normal range.

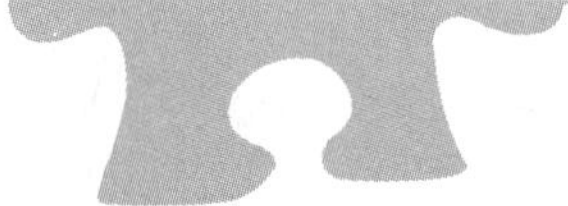

SUMMARY

- Hyperthyroidism occurs as a result of excessive secretion of thyroid hormones and is four times more common in females under the age of 40 than in males.
- The incidence of hyperthyroidism peaks between the ages of 50 and 60, and is seven times more common over the age of 65. Men and women are equally affected.
- Thyroid-stimulating immunoglobulins cause enlargement of the thyroid gland and cause excessive secretion of thyroid hormones. A state of hypermetabolism is produced that affects all body systems.
- Assessment of the patient includes history of present illness, past health history, physical exam findings, diagnostic testing, developmental, and psychosocial considerations.
- Management of hyperthyroidism is aimed at reducing the levels of circulating thyroid hormones and alleviating symptoms.
- Treatment options for hyperthyroidism include the antithyroid drugs propylthiouracil or methimazole. Beta blocking drugs may also be used as adjunctive therapy.
- Propylthiouracil is the drug of choice for pregnant hyperthyroid women because of its limited placental transfer and low potency.
- Stress the importance of compliance with the drug regimen but caution patients to stop the antithyroid drug and notify the health care provider if symptoms of infection occur.
- Manage signs and symptoms with environmental controls and appropriate interventions while waiting for therapeutic effectiveness to be achieved.
- Therapeutic effectiveness of antithyroid drugs is demonstrated by a decreased pulse rate and weight gain. Thyroid hormone levels should return to normal and the patient reflect a clinically euthyroid state.
- More than 90% of the patients with hypothyroidism have primary thyroid atrophy. Hashimoto's thyroiditis is the most common cause.
- T_3 and T_4 levels may remain within a normal range even when the patient has a true mild hypothyroidism.

- Antimicrosomal and antithyroglobulin antibodies are often found in the sera of patients.
- Hypothyroidism is the result of inadequate peripheral thyroid hormone levels.
- Insufficient thyroid hormones result in an overall decrease in the basal metabolic rate producing multisystem manifestations.
- Assessment of the patient includes history of present illness, past health history, physical exam findings, diagnostic testing, developmental and psychosocial considerations.
- The findings of the assessment will be consistent with the diagnosis of hypothyroidism.
- The primary aim of treatment is to restore a euthyroid state and alleviate symptoms.
- Pharmacotherapeutic options include levothyroxine and methimazole.
- Teach the patient and family the effects of thyroid hormones on the body.
- There are few adverse effects associated with thyroid hormone use except those that indicate overdosage.
- Monitor vital signs prior to and periodically throughout thyroid hormone therapy to alert the health care provider of possible overdosage.
- Development of chest pain and tachyarrhythmias signals overdosage.
- Teach the patient that therapy for hypothyroidism is lifelong and to avoid changing brands of thyroid hormones with prescription refills.
- Therapeutic effectiveness of thyroid hormone therapy is determined by the presence of weight loss, greater energy levels, and an increased sense of well-being. Serum TSH and T_4 levels return to normal range.
- Primary hyperparathyroidism is defined as hypercalcemia secondary to the excessive production of parathyroid hormone (PTH). Secondary hyperparathyroidism is a response to the hypocalcemia of chronic renal disease or vitamin D deficiency.
- Hyperparathyroidism is a relatively common disorder affecting postmenopausal women two to four times more often than men. It is the third most common endocrine disorder.
- A single parathyroid adenoma accounts for 80 to 85 percent of the cases of primary HPT.
- The hallmarks of primary hyperparathyroidism are elevated total serum and ionized calcium levels with an elevated intact PTH.
- Assessment of the patient includes history of present illness, past health history, physical exam findings, diagnostic testing, developmental, and psychosocial considerations.
- The pharmacotherapeutic objective of treatment of hyperparathyroidism is to control the underlying disease and to restore calcium levels to a normal range.
- Pamidronate, etidronate, and calcitonin are possible drug options used in the treatment of hyperparathyroidism.
- Allergy testing is done prior to initiating calcitonin therapy. Monitor for anaphylaxis.
- Patients should be monitored for development of bone pain and complaints of adverse GI effects.
- Therapeutic effectiveness of hypercalcemic drugs is demonstrated by lowered serum calcium levels and fewer complaints of bone pain and the absence of fractures.
- Hypoparathyroidism is related to an insufficient amount of PTH (true hypoparathyroidism) and is most often caused by surgical removal of the gland.
- Pseudohypoparathyroidism is a rare familial disorder characterized by target tissue resistance to PTH. The idiopathic form is associated with absent or decreased PTH secretion from hypoplastic or damaged glands.
- Deficiency of PTH secretion leads to hypocalcemia and hyperphosphatemia.
- Assessment of the patient includes history of present illness, past health history, physical exam findings, diagnostic testing, developmental and psychosocial considerations.
- Neuromuscular irritability caused by hypocalcemia affects muscles of the upper and lower extremities. Carpopedal spasms, paresthesias of the lips and hands, and occasionally laryngeal stridor may occur. When respiratory muscles are involved, respiratory distress may result.
- The primary objective of hypoparathyroidism is to maintain serum calcium levels in a slightly low, but asymptomatic range. In so doing, long-term complications are avoided.
- Calcium salts such as calcium carbonate and vitamin D preparations are the drugs of choice in the treatment of hypocalcemia.
- Therapeutic effectiveness of hypocalcemic therapy is noted with resolution of hypocalcemic symptoms and an increase in serum calcium levels to normal range.

BIBLIOGRAPHY

American Society of Hospital Pharmacists. (1990). *Hospital formulary service.* Author.

Bemben, D., Winn, P., Hamm, R., et al. (1994). Thyroid disease in the elderly: Part I: Prevalence of undiagnosed hypothyroidism. *Journal of Family Practice,* 38(6), 583–588.

Berg, G., Michanek, A., Holmberg, E., et al. (1996). Iodine-131 treatment of hyperthyroidism: Significance of effective half-life measurements. *The Journal of Nuclear Medicine,* 37(2), 228–232.

Berg, G., Michanek, A., Holmberg E., et al. (1996). Clinical outcome of radioiodine treatment of hyperthyroidism: A follow-up study. *Journal of Internal Medicine,* 239(2), 165–171.

Bishnoi, A., and Sachmechi, I. (1996). Thyroid disease during pregnancy. *American Family Physician,* 53(1), 215–220.

Braverman, L., and Utiger, R. (Eds.). (1991). *Werner and Ingbar's the thyroid: A fundamental and clinical text.* Philadelphia: J.B. Lippincott.

Burrow, G., Fisher, D., and Larsen, P. (1994). Maternal and fetal thyroid function. *The New England Journal of Medicine,* 331(6), 1972–1078.

Catz, B. (1990). Hypothyroidism. In S. Falk (Ed.), *Thyroid disease, endocrine surgery, nuclear medicine, and radiotherapy.* New York: Raven.

Cushing, G. (1993). Subclinical hypothyroidism. *Postgraduate Medicine,* 94(1), 95–107.

DeGroot, L., and Larsen, P. (1994). *The thyroid and its diseases* (5th ed.). New York: Wiley.

Foley, T. (1993). Goiter in adolescents. *Adolescent Endocrinology,* 22, 593–604.

Franklyn, J. (1994). The management of hyperthyroidism. *New England Journal of Medicine,* 330(24), 1731–1738.

Geffner, D., and Hershman, J. (1992). β-adrenergic blockade for the treatment of hyperthyroidism. *American Journal of Medicine,* 93, 61–65.

Heitman, B., and Irizarry, A. (1995). Hypothyroidism: Common complaints, perplexing diagnosis. *The Nurse Practitioner,* 20(3), 54–60.

Hurley, D. and Gharib, H. (1995). Detection and treatment of hypothyroidism and Graves' disease. *Geriatrics,* 50(4), 41–44.

Isley, W. (1993). Thyroid dysfunction in the severely ill and elderly: Forget the classic signs and symptoms. *Postgraduate Medicine,* 94(3), 111–128.

Johnson J., and Felicetta, J. (1992). Hyperthyroidism: A comprehensive review. *Journal of American Academy of Nurse Practitioners,* 4(1), 8–14.

Johnson, J., and Felicetta, J. (1992). Hypothyroidism: A comprehensive review. *Journal of American Academy of Nurse Practitioners,* 4(4), 131–138.

Kennedy, J., and Caro, J. (1996). The ABC's of managing hyperthyroidism in the older patient. *Geriatrics,* 51(5), 22–24.

Lazarus, J. (1991). Thyroid disease in relation to pregnancy. *Clinical Endocrinology,* 34, 91–98.

Lazarus, J. (1996). Investigation and treatment of hypothyroidism. *Clinical Endocrinology,* 44(2), 129–131.

Liang, B., Feld, S., and Smith, L. (1996). Outcomes and the patient: A case-based review of the AACE clinical practice guidelines for the management of thyroid disease. *Hospital Physician,* 32(10), 26.

Mandel, S., Brent, G., and Larsen, P. (1993). Levothyroxine therapy in patients with thyroid disease. *Annals of Internal Medicine,* 119, 492–502.

Martinez, M., Derksen, D., and Kapsner, P. (1993). Making sense of hypothyroidism: An approach to testing and treatment. *Postgraduate Medicine,* 93, 135–145.

Mokshagundam, S., and Barzel, U. (1993). Thyroid disease in the elderly. *American Geriatrics Society,* 41, 1361–1367.

Murakami, Y., Takamatsu, J., Sakane, S., et al. (1996). Changes in thyroid volume in response to radioactive iodine for Graves' hyperthyroidism correlated with activity of thyroid-stimulating antibody and treatment outcome. *The Journal of Clinical Endocrinology and Metabolism,* 81(9), 3257–3260.

Nicolini, U., Venegoni, E., Acaia, B., et al. (1996). Prenatal treatment of fetal hypothyroidism: Is there more than one option? *Prenatal Diagnosis,* 16(5), 443–448.

Singer, P., Cooper, D., Levy, E., et al. (1995). Treatment guidelines for patients with hyperthyroidism and hypothyroidism. Standards of Care Committee, American Thyroid Association. *The Journal of the American Medical Association,* 273(10), 808–812.

Streff, M., and Pachucki-Hyde, L. (1996). Management of the patient with thyroid disease. *The Nursing Clinics of North America,* 31(4), 779–796.

Surks, M., Chopra, I., and Mariash, C. (1990). American Thyroid Association Guidelines for Use of Laboratory Tests in Thyroid Disorders. *Journal of the American Medical Association,* 263(11), 529–532.

Torring, O., Tallstedt, L., Wallin, G., et al. (1996). Graves' hyperthyroidism: Treatment with antithyroid drugs, surgery, or radioiodine-A prospective, randomized study. Thyroid Study Group. *The Journal of Clinical Endocrinology and Metabolism,* 81(8), 2986–2993.

Wartofsky, L. (1996). Treatment options for hyperthyroidism. *Hospital Practice,* 31(9), 69–73.

Wolf, P., Meek, J. (1992). Practical approach to the treatment of hypothyroidism. *American Family Physician,* 45, 722–731.

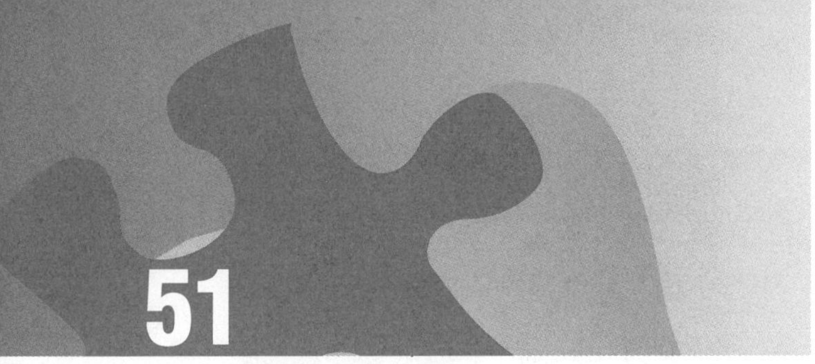

51 Pituitary Drugs

Pituitary disorders are characterized by an excess or deficit of pituitary-secreted hormones. Hormonal excess or deficit can be caused by malfunctioning of the pituitary gland or by extrapituitary factors. Pituitary tumors are the major cause of hormone excess. Other causes of hormone excess can be related to ectopic hormone–secreting sites or the presence of substances, such as drugs, that enhance hormone secretion. In contrast, hormone deficit is usually related to pituitary defects.

PITUITARY FUNCTION

The pituitary gland weighs about 0.5 g and is located beneath the hypothalamus in a small fossa of the sphenoid bone called the sella turcica. The gland is composed of three distinct lobes: anterior, intermediate, and posterior.

The anterior pituitary has multiple functions, and because of its ability to regulate other endocrine gland function, it is known as the master gland. The anterior lobe (adenohypophysis) of the pituitary contains five cell types that synthesize six different polypeptide and glycoprotein hormones. The polypeptide hormones include prolactin (PRL), adrenocorticotropin (ACTH, corticotropin), and growth hormone (GH). PRL is responsible for stimulating the production of breast milk in the mammary glands. ACTH stimulates the secretion of corticosteroids, and GH enhances systemic body growth. Synthesis of pituitary hormones occurs in response to the secretion of releasing factors and inhibiting factors from the hypothalamus (Table 51–1).

The glycoproteins that are synthesized include thyrotropin (thyroid-stimulating hormone [TSH]), luteinizing hormone (LH), and follicle-stimulating hormone (FSH). TSH stimulates the growth of the thyroid gland and the secretion of thyroid hormones. LH stimulates the maturation of the corpus luteum and production of progesterone after ovulation. In males, it stimulates the production of testosterone. FSH is responsible for development of ovarian follicles and estrogen secretion in females and spermatogenesis in males.

The posterior pituitary (neurohypophysis) secretes two peptide hormones, antidiuretic hormone (ADH, vasopressin) and oxytocin. The two hormones and their carrier proteins are synthesized in the cell bodies of these neurons. ADH is synthesized in the hypothalamus and stored in the posterior pituitary. Oxytocin is responsible for uterine activity during pregnancy and contributes to the release of breast milk. There is no known function for this peptide hormone in men.

These glands, like all endocrine glands, do not operate in isolation. They are part of classic feedback systems in which their responses to signals from body tissues are regulated to maintain a stable level of activity. The pituitary and hypothalamus also respond to physiologic states, including, for example, core and skin temperature and plasma osmolarity changes as well as to internal circadian rhythms. The circadian rhythms impart a daily pattern to the rates of hypothalamic activity and endocrine secretion.

PITUITARY DYSFUNCTION

Epidemiology and Etiology

In general, pituitary disorders are rare, affecting only a few per 100,000 persons per year. Benign tumors (adenomas) of the pituitary gland are the most common causes (15 percent) of pituitary disorders and can arise from any of the cells of the pituitary gland. Microadenomas (tumors under 10 mm in diameter) usually lead to oversecretion of pituitary hormones. This is because most pituitary tumors retain the capacity to secrete hormones or hormone fragments. A few secrete multiple hormones: GH and PRL are the most frequent combination (7 percent). Further, because the pituitary gland is enclosed in a small fossa, macroadenomas (equal to or greater than 10 mm in diameter) lead to the compression or destruction of the pituitary tissue, which leads to decreased pituitary hormone secretion.

Several processes, such as a pituitary tumor, vascular thrombosis leading to pituitary necrosis, infiltrative granulomatous diseases, and idiopathic or perhaps autoimmune destruction of pituitary cells, may result in pituitary insufficiency. Occasionally, a patient exhibits isolated pituitary hormone failure. Under these circumstances, the cause of the deficiency is likely to be in the hypothalamus and involve the corresponding releasing hormone.

Pathophysiology of Anterior Pituitary Disorders

Polypeptide Hormones

PRL is a pituitary hormone whose principal action is to stimulate the synthesis and release of breast milk in the mammary glands. It has a molecular structure similar to that of GH, and some of the biologic characteristics of both hormones overlap. The release of PRL is inhibited by hypothalamic pituitary-inhibiting factor and dopamine, a neurotransmitter. In their absence, increased PRL secretion and lactation occur. Prolactinomas are the most common pituitary disorder. About 30 percent of all pituitary adenomas secrete enough PRL to cause hyperprolactinemia, and about 25 percent of those secrete both PRL and GH. Suppression of gonadal function is the major clinical indication of hyperprolactinemia in both males and females. Hypersecretion induces galactorrhea if other hormonal requirements (i.e., insulin, estrogen, and GH) are met. Men experience infertility and impotence. Women have an increased risk of osteoporosis and occasionally develop hirsutism, menstrual disturbances (amenorrhea), vaginal dryness, and dyspareunia. Hyposecretion of PRL is associated with lower lactation in women.

TABLE 51–1 PHYSIOLOGIC EFFECTS OF PITUITARY HORMONES

Hormone	Releasing Hormone	Target Organ	Effect(s)
Anterior Pituitary Hormones			
Growth hormone (GH, somatotropin)	GHRH (somatotropin)	All tissues	Enhances systemic body growth
Prolactin (PRL)	PRH	Mammary glands	Stimulates the production of breast milk in mammary glands
Thyroid-stimulating hormone (TSH, thyrotropin)	TRH	Thyroid gland	Stimulates the growth of the thyroid gland and the secretion of thyroid hormones
Adrenocorticotropic hormone (ACTH, corticotropin)	CRH	Adrenal cortex	Stimulates the production of corticosteroids
Follicle-stimulating hormone (FSH)	GnRH	Ovaries, testes	Stimulates ovarian follicles in females, estrogen secretion, and spermatogenesis in males
Luteinizing hormone (LH)	GnRH	Ovaries, testes	Stimulates the maturation of the corpus luteum and production of progesterone after ovulation in females. In males, it stimulates the production of testosterone
Posterior Pituitary Hormones			
Antidiuretic hormone (ADH)	—	Renal tubules and glomerulus	Facilitates water reabsorption in renal tubules and induces vasoconstriction at the glomerular level
Oxytocin	—	Uterine and other smooth muscles	Initiates uterine contraction

Releasing hormones: GHRH, growth hormone–releasing hormone; GnRH, gonadotropin-releasing hormone; TRH, thyroxin-releasing hormone; CRH, corticotropin-releasing hormone.

GH is the principal hormonal regulator of somatic growth. It has no specific target organ but rather influences carbohydrate, protein, and fat metabolism throughout the body. The effects of GH include stimulating growth of skin, muscle, visceral tissues, bone, and cartilage. GH also induces insulin resistance and lipolysis. For GH to be released, the person must have at least 2 hours of sleep daily. Secretion of GH is also increased during exercise, hypoglycemia, stress, and neurogenic stimulation. Secretion is decreased in hyperglycemia, in obesity, in hypothyroidism, and with emotional deprivation.

Excessive GH secretion is almost always caused by a pituitary tumor. Oversecretion of GH produces different effects in children and adults. In children, excess GH leads to increased proportional growth (giantism). On the other hand, adults with excessive GH production exhibit disproportional growth (acromegaly). Hyposecretion of GH results in dwarfism.

ACTH regulates the release of glucocorticoids from the adrenal cortex (and to a lesser degree mineralocorticoids). Corticotropic adenomas are less common and result in excessive secretion of ACTH. Excessive ACTH secretion, in turn, leads to hypersecretion of glucocorticoids, a condition known as Cushing's syndrome (Fig. 51–1). Cortisol, the principal glucocorticoid, has primarily catabolic effects in most tissues. Clinical manifestations of androgen or mineralocorticoid excess may also be present depending on the etiology of the syndrome. Cushing's syndrome is a serious condition, with a 5-year mortality of 50 percent if left untreated.

Hyposecretion of ACTH is the predominant cause of primary adrenal insufficiency (see Chapter 52). The widespread changes that develop when the pituitary is damaged or surgically removed are predictable in terms of the known hormonal functions of the gland. Levels of plasma ACTH may be undetectable in normal individuals when they are obtained under basal conditions. Therefore, demonstration of deficiency requires the use of stimulatory testing.

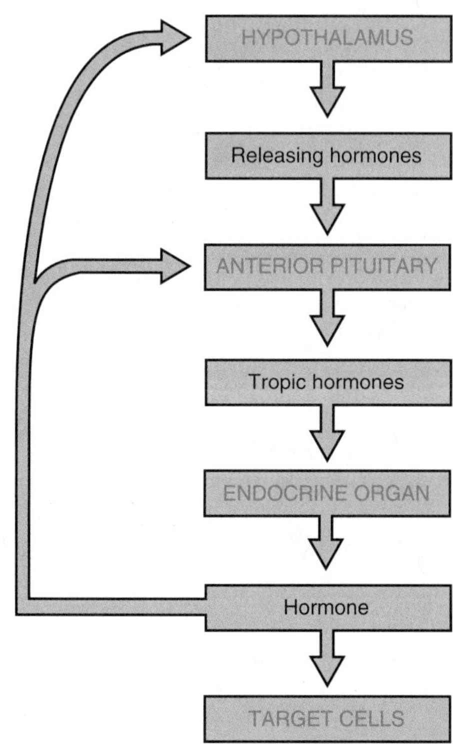

Figure 51–1 The hypothalamic-pituitary control of hormone levels, with negative feedback loops identified.

Glycoprotein Hormones

TSH regulates the growth and secretion of the thyroid gland as well as secretory activity of thyroid hormones. Hyposecretion results in hyperthyroidism, whereas hypersecretion results in thyroid hormone deficiency and hypothyroidism (see Chapter 50). Thyrotropic adenomas cause increased production of TSH. Excessive TSH leads to hyperactivity of the thyroid gland and the development of goiter. Hyperthyroidism is also referred to as thyrotoxicosis, toxic goiter, and Graves' disease. TSH deficiency is associated with hypoactivity of the thyroid gland and decreased plasma levels of thyroid hormones.

LH and FSH are responsible for regulating development of primary and secondary sex characteristics and secretion of male and female hormones from ovaries and testes. In females, LH stimulates the maturation of the corpus luteum and the production of progesterone after ovulation. In males, it stimulates the production of androgens. Hypersecretion of LH results in primary gonadal failure (see Chapter 53). FSH stimulates ovarian follicles in females and spermatogenesis in males. Deficiency of FSH results in anovulation or aspermatogenesis. Hypersecretion results in primary gonadal failure.

Gonadotrophic adenomas are associated with increased FSH or LH. Increased plasma levels of FSH and LH result in impaired sex organ functioning such as amenorrhea, impotence, and infertility. FSH and LH deficiencies result in sexual malfunctioning in men and women.

Pathophysiology of Posterior Disorders

Hormones secreted by the posterior pituitary gland (neurohypophysis) are produced by nerve cells in the hypothalamus. The two hormones that are produced, ADH (vasopressin) and oxytocin, are stored in the pituitary. ADH controls water balance in the body by increasing the permeability of the cells of the distal tubules in the kidney to water, thus decreasing the formation of urine. Osmolality, thirst, and blood volume regulate the secretion of ADH. An increase in osmotic pressure or a decrease in volume increases ADH secretion. Excessive ADH, in turn, causes a condition known as syndrome of inappropriate ADH secretion that causes severe water retention. ADH deficiency is referred to as diabetes insipidus. Patients with diabetes insipidus are unable to control the amount of water lost in urine, leading to polyuria.

Oxytocin stimulates the musculature of the uterus and also causes ejection of milk from the alveoli of the breasts (see Chapter 55). The uterus of a nonpregnant woman does not respond to normal concentrations of oxytocin. The uterus of a pregnant woman is more sensitive. Oxytocin is secreted in greater amounts during parturition and during breastfeeding. It is similar to ADH in respect to water homeostasis, response to secretory stimuli, and renal action.

PHARMACOTHERAPEUTIC OPTIONS

Drug therapies that use pituitary hormones are limited and primarily include replacement and suppressive therapies; and diagnostic testing also uses pituitary hormones. All pituitary hormones are proteins (with the exception of dopamine). This makes them expensive and difficult to obtain in amounts sufficient to use therapeutically. In addition, protein increases the risk of allergic reactions. These problems make replacement therapy with target organ hormones safer and more economical. Their therapeutic effects as well as adverse effects are the same as those found with naturally existing hormones.

Anterior Pituitary Hormone Replacement Drugs

- ❒ Corticotropin (ACTH, ACTHAR, HP ACTHAR GEL)
- ❒ Cosyntropin (CORTROSYN)
- ❒ Somatrem (PROTROPIN)
- ❒ Somatropin (HUMATROPE, NUTROPIN)

Indications

Corticotropin and cosyntropin are given diagnostically to stimulate the synthesis of hormones by the adrenal cortex (i.e., glucocorticoids, mineralocorticoids, androgens). They are not effective unless the adrenal cortex can respond. A corticotropin stimulation test is used to differentiate primary from secondary adrenocortical insufficiency. After injection of corticotropin, plasma cortisol levels rise in patients with secondary insufficiency. Corticotropin can also be used as an anti-inflammatory or immunosuppressant agent when conventional glucocorticoid therapy fails, and it is sometimes used to help manage adrenal crisis.

Somatrem and somatropin are two forms of GH synthesized by recombinant DNA technology. They are therapeutically equivalent to endogenous GH. The drugs are used to increase growth in children with growth failure or who have delayed physiologic development due to insufficient endogenous GH secretion. The drugs are ineffective when impaired growth results from other causes or if they are used after puberty when the epiphyses of long bones have closed.

Pharmacodynamics

The pharmacodynamics of hormone replacement drugs are similar to those of naturally occurring hormones. Corticotropin functions in an enzymatic manner to stimulate the adrenal cortex to release cortisol, corticosterone, several weakly androgenic steroids, and a small amount of aldosterone. The physiologic effects are seen in the relief of symptoms of insufficient cortisol, including increased energy levels, and stabilized fluid and electrolyte balance.

Somatrem and somatropin stimulate growth via their effects on most body tissues and especially on epiphyseal plates. Somatropin has the same amino acid sequence as for the endogenous pituitary hormone, whereas somatrem has one additional amino acid. The use of these GHs lead to increased cellular size and increased growth rate. Specifically, they facilitate transport of amino acids across cell membranes. This movement increases nitrogen balance and decreases urea production. GH also decreases the transport of glucose into the cells and decreases its utilization, causing what is known as a diabetogenic effect. They facilitate the release of free fatty acids from adipose tissues, leading to increased fat storage in the liver and increased availability of fatty acids for energy. This effect is referred to as the ketogenic or lipolytic effect because it results from fat lipolysis and leads to the conversion of fatty acids to ketone bodies.

Many of these actions are mediated by substances called somatomedins, which are synthesized in the liver and other tissues. Under the regulation of GH, they promote growth of cartilage and bone. In children, GH is essential to stimulate linear bone growth.

When somatrem or somatropin is given to adults with adult-onset pituitary insufficiency, a marked increase in serum lipoprotein concentration occurs. Specifically, studies have shown that high-density lipoproteins increase and low-density lipoproteins remain unchanged.

Adverse Effects and Contraindications

Corticotropin's adverse effects predominantly appear with chronic use of dosages exceeding 40 units/day. The most common adverse effects include depression, nausea, petechiae, hypokalemia, sodium retention, and adrenal suppression. Effects on the central nervous system include seizures, vertigo, headache, personality changes, and mental disturbances such as euphoria, mood swings, and psychosis. Impaired wound healing, thinning of the skin, petechiae, ecchymosis, facial erythema, increased diaphoresis, and hyperpigmentation may occur. Hypertension, congestive heart failure, necrotizing angiitis, fluid volume overload, hypocalcemia, hypokalemia, alkalosis, and negative nitrogen balance have also occurred. Long-term use suppresses pituitary release of corticotropin, which, in turn, may cause adrenocortical hyperplasia, decreased glucose tolerance, suppression of growth in children, steroid myopathy, and muscle weakness. Patients who are sensitive to porcine products may experience an allergic response from corticotropin. The adverse effect associated with cosyntropin is hypersensitivity, including anaphylaxis.

Corticotropin is contraindicated in patients with Cushing's syndrome. Because it exacerbates symptoms, it is also contraindicated in patients with diabetes and psychotic or psychopathic disorders. Use in patients with active tuberculosis or acquired immunodeficiency syndrome (AIDS) should be avoided because it decreases immunity and increases the risk of gastrointestinal (GI) perforation and hemorrhage. Cautious use is warranted in patients with hypertension or heart failure because of sodium and water retention. It should also be used with caution in patients who have myasthenia gravis because it causes muscle weakness.

Locally, somatrem and somatropin cause pain and swelling at the injection site. Furthermore, approximately 30 to 40 percent of all somatrem-treated patients and 7 to 20 percent of children develop antibodies to the drug. Resistance to treatment is rare and frequently can be overcome by increasing the dose of the hormone. In addition, somatrem depresses thyroid function and insulin production. Other adverse affects include hypothyroidism and slipped femoral epiphyses. Patients with a familial history of diabetes should be monitored carefully when receiving GH replacements because these drugs may precipitate a hyperglycemic episode in susceptible individuals. Furthermore, untreated hypothyroidism may interfere with the growth response to GH. It is not known if the drug is eliminated in breast milk, and animal reproduction studies have not been conducted with GH drugs (pregnancy category C).

Pharmacokinetics

Because corticotropin is a protein substance, it is destroyed by proteolytic enzymes in the digestive tract if taken by mouth. Therefore, it must be given parenterally. The onset times for the intravenous (IM) and intravenous (IV) formulations is 5 minutes (Table 51–2). The gelatin repository formulation peaks in 3 to 12 hours, with a 10- to 25-hour duration. The IV formulation peaks in 1 hour, and its duration of action is unknown. Its plasma half-life is 20 minutes. Although the precise distribution of corticotropin is unknown, it is thought that the hormone does not cross the placenta.

Somatrem and somatropin are given by the subcutaneous (SC) or IM route. Serum GH levels are greater after an SC abdominal injection than after an SC thigh injection. Individual absorption rates vary widely. In circulation, the drugs are extensively bound to plasma protein, thus extending their half-life. The elimination half-life ranges from 20 minutes for somatropin to 5 hours for somatrem, depending on the route of administration. Ninety percent of the drugs is biotransformed in the liver and eliminated by the kidneys. Biotransformation and elimination are more rapid in adults than in children.

Drug-Drug Interactions

Table 51–3 lists the drug-drug interactions of selected pituitary drugs. Enzyme-inducing drugs (e.g., barbiturates, phenytoin, rifampin) increase the biotransformation of glucocorticoids when taken concurrently with corticotropin or cosyntropin.

Somatrem and somatropin taken concurrently with either glucocorticoids or corticotropin decrease the growth response. Anabolic steroids increase the growth response.

Dosage Regimens

In general, the dosages of pituitary hormone replacement drugs are highly individualized and adjusted frequently according to patient response (Table 51–4). Although dose-response curves for somatrem and somatropin have been proposed, the optimal schedule for treatment has not been established. Although SC and IM routes are equally effective, SC injections are preferred because they are less painful. SC injections may lead to local lipoatrophy, however.

Laboratory Considerations

Corticotropin and cosyntropin have significant impact on blood glucose and plasma cortisol levels. When corticotropin is used to diagnose adrenal insufficiency, plasma cortisol concentrations and urine 17-ketosteroids and 17-hydroxycorticosteroids are measured before and after drug administration. Therapeutic response is equated with a rise in the plasma and urine steroid concentrations. Corticotropin decreases white blood cell counts and serum potassium and calcium levels and suppresses reactions to allergy skin tests. It causes an increase in blood sugar levels, especially in patients with diabetes, and increases serum sodium, cholesterol, and lipid values. Serum protein-bound iodine and thyroxine concentrations decrease.

Somatrem reduces glucose tolerance, total protein, and thyroid function test results (thyroxine-binding capacity and radioactive iodine uptake).

TABLE 51–2 PHARMACOKINETICS OF SELECTED PITUITARY DRUGS

Drugs	Route	Onset	Peak	Duration	PB (%)	$t_{1/2}$	BioA (%)
Hormone-Suppressant Drugs							
Bromocriptine	Oral	2 hr; 1–2 hr*	8 hr; 4–8 wk*	24 hr; 4–8 hr*	93–96	4–4.5 hr; 45–50 hr†	3–6
Octreotide	SC	Rapid	30 min	12 hr	65	1.5 hr	UK
Anterior Pituitary Replacement Drugs							
Corticotropin	IM	5 min	3–12 hr	10–25 hr	UA	20 min	UA
	IV		1 hr	UK			100
Cosyntropin	IM	UK	45–60 min	UK	UA	15 min	UA
	IV						100
Somatrem	SC	3 months	2–6 hr	12–48 hr	20–25	3–5 hr	UA
	IM						
	IV					20–30 min	100
Somatropin	SC	3 months	2–4 hr	36 hr	UA	20–25 min	UA
	IM						
Posterior Pituitary Replacement Drugs							
Desmopressin	Nasal	30 min	1–5 hr	8–20 hr	UA	7.8 min; 75.5 min‡	UA
Lypressin	Nasal	60 min	30–120 min	3–8 hr	UA	15 min	UA
Vasopressin	IM	60 min	2–4 hr	2–8 hr	UA	10–20 min	UA
	SC						
Vasopressin tannate in oil	IM	60 min	2–4 hr	48 hr§	UA	UA	UA

* Effect on serum prolactin levels and effects on growth hormone levels, respectively.
†The half-life of bromocriptine is biphasic. The initial phase is about 4.5 hours in duration and the terminal phase, 45–50 hours.
‡The half-life of desmopressin is biphasic. The initial phase is 7.8 minutes in duration and the terminal phase, 75.5 minutes.
§The duration of action of vasopressin tannate in oil (PTO) for any given dose depends on how well the PTO is resuspended and can vary substantially.
BioA, Bioavailability; PB, protein binding; $t^1/_2$, elimination half-life; UA, unavailable; UK, unknown.

Posterior Pituitary Hormone Replacement Drugs

❐ Desmopressin acetate (DDAVP, STIMATE)
❐ Lypressin (DIAPID)
❐ Vasopressin (PITRESSIN); (🍁) PRESSYN

Indications

Vasopressin (ADH), in either natural or synthetic form, is used primarily to control hypothalamic diabetes insipidus. It is not effective in treating nephrogenic diabetes insipidus, a condition in which the kidneys are unable to respond appropriately to this hormone. It is also used as an IV or intraarterial infusion in the emergency management of massive GI bleeding. It is also used to relieve postoperative intestinal gaseous distention and to dispel gas appearing before abdominal radiography.

Desmopressin acetate and lypressin are synthetic analogs of ADH. The therapeutic uses of both drugs are the same as those for ADH. Additionally, because of its dose-dependent increase in plasma factor VIII (antihemophilic factor), desmopressin is used to treat hemophilia A and B and von Willebrand's disease. In recent years, desmopressin has also been used in the management of primary nocturnal enuresis that is unresponsive to other treatment modalities.

Pharmacodynamics

Prepared from bovine and porcine pituitaries, vasopressin has pressor as well as antidiuretic activity. As analogs of vasopressin, desmopressin and lypressin act in the distal tubules and collecting ducts of the kidneys to increase cellular permeability to water. Thus, the amount of water reabsorbed increases and urine output decreases. It is important to note that the amount of vasopressin necessary to promote water conservation is seldom high enough to produce widespread pressor activity. In large doses, desmopressin and lypressin stimulate smooth muscle contraction, especially of arterioles. The vasoconstriction, in turn, decreases blood flow to the splenic, coronary, GI, pancreatic, skin, and muscular systems. Direct administration of vasopressin into the superior mesenteric artery constricts the gastroduodenal, superior mesenteric, and splenic arteries, thus decreasing portal blood pressure and reducing blood loss.

Also in large doses, desmopressin and lypressin increase peristalsis of the large bowel and contraction of the smooth muscle of the gallbladder and urinary bladder. Some oxytocic activity may also occur, causing uterine contractions.

Adverse Effects and Contraindications

The adverse effects of vasopressin are usually mild in small dosages. The most common adverse effects include circumoral pallor, abdominal cramps, nausea, sweating,

TABLE 51–3 DRUG-DRUG INTERACTIONS OF SELECTED PITUITARY DRUGS

Drug	Interactive Drugs	Interaction(s)
Hormone Suppressants		
Bromocriptine	Alcohol Antihistamines Opioid analgesics Sedative-hypnotics	Increased CNS depression
	Levodopa	Additive neurologic effects of bromocriptine
	Haloperidol Imipramine Methyldopa Reserpine Phenothiazines Tricyclic antidepressants	Increase prolactin levels and decrease effectiveness of bromocriptine
	Antihypertensive drugs	Increased hypotensive effects
Octreotide	Cyclosporine	Reduced blood levels of interactive drug
	Chlorpropamide Carbamazepine Insulin	May alter requirements for interactive drug
Anterior Pituitary Hormone Replacement Drugs		
Corticotropin	Barbiturates Phenytoin Rifampin	Increased glucocorticoid metabolism
	Insulin Oral hypoglycemic drugs	May increase requirements for interactive drug
	Estrogens Oral contraceptives	May block metabolism of corticotropin
	Salicylates	Increased risk for GI bleeding
	Amphotericin B Diuretics Furosemide Mezlocillin Piperacillin Ticarcillin	Additive hypokalemia
Cosyntropin	Blood or whole plasma	May inactivate cosyntropin
Somatrem Somatropin	Adrenocorticoids Glucocorticoids Corticotropin	Growth response inhibited
	Anabolic steroids Estrogens Thyroid hormones	Epiphyseal closure accelerated
Posterior Pituitary Hormone Replacement Drugs		
Lypressin Desmopressin Vasopressin	Carbamazepine Chlorpropamide Clofibrate Fludrocortisone	Increased antidiuretic effects
	Alcohol Demeclocycline Heparin Lithium Norepinephrine	Decreased antidiuretic effects
	Ganglionic-blocking drugs	Increased vasopressor effects
	Barbiturates Cyclopropane	Synergistic effects

CNS, Central nervous system; GI, gastrointestinal.

tremor, and a pounding headache. Uterine cramping and diarrhea may occur because of the oxytocic and smooth muscle–stimulant effects of vasopressin. Shifts in fluid volumes occur with initial therapy. Patients who may have difficulty tolerating the fluid shifts (e.g., heart failure) should be cautiously treated.

Large doses of vasopressin produce cardiovascular effects such as blood pressure elevations, anginal pain, and arrhythmias. Myocardial infarction has occurred. The pressor effects of vasopressin are not usually evident with the amounts used to manage polyuria. However, in patients with coronary artery disease, even small doses have been found to precipitate angina, especially in the older adult.

The adverse effects of desmopressin acetate and lypressin are usually infrequent and mild. The most common are

TABLE 51–4 DOSAGE REGIMENS FOR SELECTED PITUITARY DRUGS

Drug	Uses	Dosage	Implications
Hormone-Suppressant Drugs			
Bromocriptine	Hyperprolactinemia	*Adult:* 1.25–2.5 mg po QD. Increase every 3–7 days up to 2.5 mg BID–TID	Dosages for children not yet established. Other uses may require different dosages
	Acromegaly	*Adult:* 1.25–2.5 mg po QD × 3 days. Increase by 1.25–2.5 mg po q3–7 days until optimal response obtained. Range: 10–30 mg po QD up to 100 mg	
	Pituitary prolactinoma (unlabeled use)	*Adult:* 5–7.5 mg po QD. Range 1.25–20 mg po QD	
Octreotide	Acromegaly associated with pituitary tumor (unlabeled use)	*Adult:* 100–200 mcg SC TID	Dosage should not exceed 750 mg daily
Anterior Pituitary Hormone Replacement Drugs			
Corticotropin	ACTH replacement; treatment purposes	*Adult:* 20 units SC/IM QID *or* 40–80 units of gel formulation q25–72 hr	Refrigerate repository form and administer with 22-gauge needle
	Diagnosis of ACTH deficiency	*Adult:* 10–25 units zinc formulation in 500 mL D5W by IV infusion over 8 hr *or* 20 units SC/IM	Direct IV infusion should be given over 2 minutes
Cosyntropin	Diagnosis of ACTH deficiency	*Adult:* 0.25–0.75 mg SC/IM × 1 *or* 0.25 mg in D5W *or* NSS IV at 0.04 mg/hr *Child under 2 yr:* 0.125 mg IM × 1	Direct IV infusion should be given over 2 minutes
Somatrem	GH deficiency	*Child:* 0.06–0.1 mg/kg SC/IM three times weekly *or* 0.26 IU/kg SC/IM 3 times weekly	Dosages are titrated based on patient response. Dosage of somatropin differs for each specific brand name product
Somatropin		*Child:* 0.18–0.3 mg/kg SC/IM weekly	
Posterior Pituitary Hormone Replacement Drugs			
Desmopressin	Neurogenic diabetes insipidus	*Adult:* 10 mcg intranasally at HS *or* 2–4 mcg SC/IV in two divided doses. Increase by 2.5-mcg increments until satisfactory response occurs. Maintenance: 10–40 mcg SC as single or divided doses QD–TID *Child:* 5 mcg intranasally at HS. Increase by 2.5-mcg increments. Maintenance: 2–4 mcg/kg/day (5–30 mcg) as single dose or in two divided doses	Maintenance doses are given in single or divided doses. An extra morning dose of 5 mcg may be needed by pediatric patients, 10 mcg by adult patients
	GI bleeding	*Adults and child over 3 mo:* 0.3 mcg/kg repeated as needed *Adults and child >50 kg:* 1 spray (150 mcg) in each nostril *Adults and child <50 kg:* 1 spray (150 mcg) in one nostril	
Lypressin	Hypothalamic diabetes insipidus	*Adult:* 1–2 sprays intranasally QID	Intranasal forms 0.185 mg/mL
Vasopressin	Hypothalamic diabetes insipidus	*Adult:* 5–10 units SC/IM BID–TID *or* 2.5–5 units SC/IM q2–3 days (oil formulation) *Child:* 2.5–10 units SC/IM TID–QID *or* 1.25–2.5 units SC/IM q2–3 days (oil formulation)	Give with 1–2 glasses of water at time of SC/IM administration to minimize GI effects

ACTH, Adrenocorticotropic hormone; GH, growth hormone; GI, gastrointestinal.

rhinitis, local irritation of nasal passages, and heartburn. Headache, conjunctivitis, rhinorrhea, and nasal congestion have also occurred.

Pharmacokinetics

Vasopressin, whether in its natural or synthetic form, is a protein and is destroyed by enzyme activity when it is taken orally. Therefore, these drugs must be administered parenterally or by inhalation. The onset time for vasopressin and its analogs ranges from 30 to 60 minutes, with peak activity occurring 30 minutes to 4 hours later (see Table 51–2). The duration of action and half-lives also vary a great deal. Desmopressin has a biphasic half-life, with the first phase occurring in 7.8 minutes and the terminal phase in 75.5 minutes.

Drug-Drug Interactions

There are several drug-drug interactions associated with vasopressin and its analogs. In general, antidiuretic effects may be increased or decreased by the concurrent administration of alcohol, heparin, carbamazepine, or lithium (see Table 51–3).

Dosage Regimen

As with many other endocrine system drugs, the dosages of vasopressin and its analogs are determined according to patient response. Vasopressin is administered in units ranging from 5 to 10 two to three times daily. For vasopressin tannate in oil, a longer acting formulation, the usual dose is 2.5 to 5 units SC or IM every two to three days. Children's dosages are individualized in the range of 2.5 to 10 units SC or IM three to four times daily. The dosage for the long-acting formulation is 1.25 to 2.5 units SC or IM every 2 or 3 days.

Desmopressin therapy is initiated in a stepwise fashion. After a nightly dose to control nocturia is established, a larger morning dose or two divided doses are used during the day. Desmopressin is usually taken intranasally using an insufflator but can also be given intravaginally and is available in a parenteral form. The desmopressin dosage ranges from 2 to 4 mcg/kg/day (0.1 to 0.4 mL by insufflation) for pediatric patients and up to 10 mcg for adults. The average adult maintenance dose is 10 to 40 mcg, given as a single dose or in one to three divided doses. Chronic intranasal use may cause tolerance, or tachyphylaxis may develop if IV desmopressin is given more frequently than every 24 to 48 hours. IV desmopressin has 10 times the antidiuretic effect of intranasal desmopressin.

When desmopressin is used for its antihemorrhagic effects, the IV dosage is 0.3 mcg/kg in adults and children to one spray (150 mcg) in each nostril.

Lypressin used for hypothalamic diabetes insipidus is dosed as one to two nasal sprays (0.185 mg/mL/spray) four times daily. An extra dose may be administered at bedtime if needed.

Laboratory Considerations

Patients receiving vasopressin should have urine specific gravity and urine volume as well as serum electrolytes monitored throughout therapy. Plasma factor VIII concentrations and bleeding times should be measured when the drug is used in hemophilia A and B and von Willebrand's disease.

Hormone Suppressant Drugs

- ❒ Bromocriptine (PARLODEL)
- ❒ Octreotide (SANDOSTATIN)

Indications

Bromocriptine is a direct-acting dopamine receptor agonist that is used clinically for the treatment of hyperprolactinemia (galactorrhea/amenorrhea) of various causes and acromegaly. It decreases lactation and produces shrinkage of a prolactinoma. It is also used in the treatment of pituitary adenomas (prolactinomas) and in the management of male infertility due to PRL-dependent hypogonadism, although it is not approved by the Food and Drug Administration for these purposes.

Octreotide is used primarily to treat excess GH production associated with acromegaly. It also helps control symptoms in patients with carcinoid tumors and vasoactive intestinal peptide tumors (VIPomas), reducing the volume of secretions produced by the stomach and intestine. It has also been used in the management of diarrhea associated with AIDS, although it has not been approved by the Food and Drug Administation for such use.

Pharmacodynamics

Bromocriptine decreases PRL secretion through direct action on the pituitary gland. It also promotes ovulation and ovarian activity in patients with amenorrhea, thus restoring fertility. Bromocriptine is also known to decrease GH levels in acromegalic patients, but its mechanism remains unclear.

Octreotide is identical to the natural GH somatropin. It suppresses the secretion of serotonin, gastrin, glucagon, insulin, vasoactive intestinal peptide, and GH. Compared with somatostatin (GH-inhibiting hormone), octreotide is very powerful. Octreotide has 45 times the potency of somatostatin in inhibiting the effects of GH. Somatostatin is not used clinically owing to its short half-life (1 to 3 minutes).

Adverse Effects and Contraindications

The response and tolerance to bromocriptine vary among patients. The adverse effects are generally related to its activity as a dopaminergic agonist. The adverse effects are classified into two groups—those related to initial therapy and those associated with long-term use. Initial effects include nausea, vomiting, and postural hypotension. There is a first-dose phenomenon that can be evidenced by sudden cardiovascular collapse. Long-term effects include constipation, confusion, vivid dreams, delusions, hallucinations, dyskinesia, alcohol intolerance, and digital vasospasm. All adverse effects can be reduced by decreasing the dose or discontinuing the drug. When the dose of bromocriptine is increased gradually, the incidence of nausea decreases. Other adverse effects include nasal congestion, tinnitus, rash, and depression. Pleural effusions may occur with long-term therapy.

Bromocriptine is contraindicated in patients with hepatic and renal dysfunction and in patients with hypersensitivity to the drug, to ergot alkaloids, or to bisulfites (capsules only). Because bromocriptine results in lowered lactation, it should not be used by breastfeeding mothers or in those under the age of 15. It should be cautiously used in pregnant patients and in patients with cardiac disease and mental disturbances. It may restore fertility; thus, additional contraception may be required if pregnancy is undesirable.

There are many adverse effects with octreotide, but they are usually of short duration. GI adverse effects of octreotide are milder than those seen with bromocriptine. Nausea, abdominal cramps, bloating, and moderate diarrhea are frequently noted, as well as circumoral pallor, sweating, tremors, and a pounding headache. Octreotide should be used cautiously in patients with gallbladder disease owing to the increased tendency toward gallstones. Dosage reduction may be required in patients with renal failure. Hyperglycemia or hypoglycemia can occur, and malabsorption of fat may be aggravated. The impact of bromocriptine and octreotide on pregnancy are not yet clear (category B).

Pharmacokinetics

Bromocriptine is partially absorbed from the GI tract, with the onset time varying depending on whether the drug is used for its effects on serum PRL levels or on GH (see Table 51–2). Over 90 percent of the plasma bromocriptine is bound to albumin. It is completely biotransformed in the liver by first-pass kinetics. The majority is eliminated via bile, with less than 5 percent eliminated in the urine. The half-life of bromocriptine is biphasic. The initial phase takes 4 to 4.5 hours, with a terminal phase of 45 to 50 hours.

Octreotide is rapidly absorbed after SC administration, reaching peak plasma levels in 30 minutes. The half-life of octreotide is about 1.5 hours, with a duration of action of up to 12 hours. About one third of the dose is eliminated unchanged in the urine.

Drug-Drug Interactions

Table 51–3 lists drug-drug interactions of bromocriptine and octreotide. Drugs that cause increased PRL secretion (e.g., haloperidol, imipramine) reduce the effectiveness of bromocriptine. Octreotide alters the requirements for insulin or oral hypoglycemic drugs and reduces the blood levels of cyclosporine.

Dosage Regimens

The dosage of bromocriptine is adjusted every 3 to 7 days based on patient need and response (see Table 51–4). Octreotide is administered SC three times daily. Dosages for children have not yet been established. Taking one to two glasses of water at the same time the SC injection is given minimizes the GI distress associated with octreotide.

Laboratory Considerations

Because of their impact on GH, bromocriptine and octreotide have a significant impact on plasma glucose levels. Patients taking either drug should receive close monitoring of plasma glucose levels.

Bromocriptine can cause an elevated BUN and serum alanine aminotransferase (ALT; serum glutamic-pyruvic transaminase [SGPT]), aspartate aminotransferase (AST; serum glutamic-oxaloacetic transaminase [SGOT]), creatine kinase, alkaline phosphatase, and uric acid levels. The elevations are usually transient and are not clinically significant.

Octreotide can cause a slight increase in liver enzymes and decreased serum thyroxine concentrations. Seventy-two–hour fecal fat and serum carotene determinations should be performed periodically to monitor for possible drug-induced aggravation of fat malabsorption.

Critical Thinking Process

Assessment

History of Present Illness

When eliciting the patient's history of present illness, be alert to the time of onset, sequences of events, changes in complaints, and description of symptoms (e.g., polyuria, polydipsia, polyphagia, weight gain, and visual difficulties). Symptoms need to be recorded regarding location, severity, tempo, quality, and what relieves or aggravates them.

Past Health History

Asking about previous illnesses cues the patient to recall past events of medical-surgical, psychiatric, or obstetric significance. The patient should be queried about previous hospitalizations, childhood and adult illnesses, surgical procedures, head injuries and trauma. A history of head trauma or visual changes is valuable in evaluating pituitary causes of polyuria. A menstrual and fertility history should also be noted. Patients should be asked about sexual growth and development (axillary and pubic hair growth, genital development), menstrual patterns, and fertility status. The patient should be questioned about hypersensitivity to any corticosteroids or porcine products.

Inquire about family members' illnesses, state of health or cause of death, and age. Identify any disorders occurring in family members that may relate to the patient's reports of symptoms (e.g., diabetes, thyroid disease, anemia, epilepsy, headaches, strokes, kidney disease, mental illness, and other conditions).

Physical Exam Findings

In general, a complete physical exam should be completed for the patient with pituitary disorders. Pay special attention to the status of the patient's renal, cardiovascular, and respiratory systems. A thorough neurologic exam should be performed. The patient's blood pressure should be checked with the patient lying and standing. An accurate intake and output recording should be kept, and the patient should be monitored for edema. The patient's height, weight, and stature should be noted and compared with growth charts in the case of children, or to standardized tables for adults. The patient with suspected growth abnormalities should also have his or her ring size, heel pad thickness, and soft tissue volume noted.

Diagnostic Testing

Laboratory testing of the patient with a pituitary disorder may include any of a number of tests. Tests that might be used to diagnose or monitor pituitary disorders include measurements of urine specific gravity and osmolarity, urine for FSH and LH, 17-ketosteroids, and 17-hydroxycorticosteroids. Serum electrolytes, blood sugar, and hormonal testing, such as ADH, cortisol, GH, PRL, somatomedin-C, and thyroid function tests, may also be performed. Vasopressin (cortisol stimulation) may be included. Computed tomography or magnetic resonance imaging scans can be used for visualization of anatomic structures.

Developmental Considerations

Perinatal Because of the lack of controlled human studies, the risks associated with pituitary hormone suppressant and replacement drugs are not well established. However, the risk-benefit analysis for the use of a particular drug should be evaluated on individual basis.

Use of corticotropin in pregnancy has demonstrated no adverse fetal effects. However, corticosteroids have been suspected of causing malformations. Because corticotropin stimulates the release of endogenous corticosteroids, this relationship should be considered if prescribing the drug to women during child-bearing years.

A threefold increase in circulating levels of endogenous vasopressin has been reported during the last trimester of pregnancy and in labor compared with the nonpregnant state. Although such occurrences are infrequent, the induc-

Case Study Diabetes Insipidus

Patient History

History of Present Illness	JS is a 53-year-old white male who presents to the outpatient clinic today with complaints of increased thirst (particularly for ice cold water) for the past 2 to 3 weeks and increased urination that keeps him up at night. He adds that epigastric fullness and anorexia is a problem. He states he has had an unintentional weight loss of 15 pounds over the last 2 to 3 weeks.
Past Health History	JS's past health history is positive for broken nose with obstructed right naris. He denies a history of brain tumor, head trauma, TIA, stroke, or granulomatous disease. He has no known drug or food allergies and denies use of prescription or OTC drugs. JS states he has frequent, severe episodes of allergic rhinitis secondary to hay fever.
Physical Exam Findings	JS appears mildly dehydrated and restless. Skin warm and dry with poor skin turgor. BP 104/62, pulse 100, respiration 20.
Diagnostic Testing	Urine specific gravity 1.001 with an osmolality of 175 mOsm/kg. Total 24-hour urinary output is 10.4 L. Serum sodium is 129 mEq/L. Serum osmolality is 350 mOsm/kg. BUN: 20 mg/dL. Creatinine: 1.5 mg/dL. MRI is unremarkable.
Developmental Considerations	JS has no significant age-related changes in hepatic, renal, or cardiac functioning.
Psychosocial Considerations	JS is a high school teacher. He is married and has three grown children. He is planning to retire within the next 10 years and is concerned that his diagnosis will prevent the couple from traveling in Europe.
Economic Factors	JS is covered by a private health insurance that includes pharmacy coverage with a $10 co-pay; however, philosophically he believes drugs are generally too expensive.

Variables Influencing Decision

Treatment Objectives	• Restore renal function and prevent dehydration and hyponatremia

Drug Variables	*Drug Summary*	*Patient Variables*
Indications	Diagnosis and treatment of diabetes insipidus.	JS has been diagnosed with hypothalamic diabetes insipidus.
Pharmacodynamics	The three drugs mimic the action of endogenous ADH.	The three drugs have similar actions. This variable is not a decision point.
Adverse Effects/ Contraindications	Vasopressin, lypressin, and desmopressin: Water intoxication, rhinitis, hypernatremia, hypertension, and abdominal cramps.	JS has frequent, severe episodes of rhinitis. Intranasal routes of drug administration should be avoided. This will become a decision point.
Pharmacokinetics	Lypressin and vasopressin have a shorter duration than desmopressin.	There is no direct pharmacokinetic variable affecting the decision.
Dosage Regimen	Lypressin is given nasally. Desmopressin is given nasally and parenterally. Vasopressin is given parenterally. Desmopressin: 2–4 mcg/day in two doses SC or IV. Vasopressin: 5–10 units two to three times a day SC or IM as needed. Vasopressin tannate in oil: 2.5–5 units q2–3 days IM.	Desmopressin is preferred over vasopressin because it requires fewer doses per day; however, this benefit may be offset by the cost of the drug. Further, vasopressin tannate in oil is dosed even less frequently than vasopressin; therefore, this becomes a decision point.

Drug Variables	*Drug Summary*	*Patient Variables*
Lab Considerations	Urine osmolarity, urine specific gravity, serum electrolytes, BUN, creatinine before and periodically throughout therapy.	This is not a decision factor, although JS should be taught the importance of follow-up lab testing.
Cost Index*	Desmopressin: 5 Lypressin: 5 Vasopressin: 5 Vasopressin tannate in oil: 5	Although these drugs are expensive, cost is not a major decision factor for JS because his insurance covers all but the $10 co-pay.
Summary of Decision Points	• JS has been diagnosed with hypothalamic diabetes insipidus. • JS has frequent episodes of severe rhinitis and a history of broken nose obstruction, thus contraindicating the use of the intranasal route for replacement therapy. • In general, desmopressin is preferred over vasopressin on basis of dosage frequency; however, owing to the cost of desmopressin, vasopressin may be used with similar efficacy. The Pitressin tannate in oil (PTO) formulation is dosed every 2–3 days.	
DRUG TO BE USED	• Vasopressin tannate in oil, 1 mg IM when previous dose has worn off (every 1–3 days). Dosage to be increased based on patient response.	

*Cost Index:
1 $<30/mo
2 $ 30–40/mo.
3 $ 40–50/mo.
4 $ 50–60/mo.
5 $>60/mo.

AWP of a multidose vial of vasopressin (20 units/mL) is approximately $150.
AWP of a multidose vial of vasopressin tannate in oil (20 units/mL) is approximately $90.
AWP of a multidose vial of desmopressin acetate (4 mcg/mL) for injection is approximately $245.
AWP of an 8-mL vial of lypressin (0.185 mg/mL) nasal spray is approximately $48.

tion of uterine activity has been reported after IM or intranasal vasopressin. The IV use of desmopressin, which is most often given intranasally, has also been reported to cause uterine contractions. Vasopressin has not been shown to produce tonic uterine contractions that could be deleterious to the fetus or threaten a pregnancy. However, it is classified as a category C drug and should be used during pregnancy only when clearly indicated.

Bromocriptine, used for the treatment of infertility due to hyperprolactinemia or pituitary tumors, including acromegaly, is usually discontinued as soon as pregnancy is diagnosed.

Pediatric The use of pituitary drugs in children older than 6 months of age has been fairly safe. Because of the immaturity of the negative feedback mechanisms in children, the plasma levels of exogenous pituitary hormones might be difficult to regulate. Caution is needed in evaluating the efficiency of any of the pituitary drugs. Because children are more susceptible to fluid volume disturbance, drug therapies should be carefully chosen.

Geriatric Owing to the age-related decline in hepatic and renal functioning, older adults are at higher risk for drug overdose. Older adults taking pituitary drugs should have routine monitoring of hepatic and renal functioning.

Psychosocial Considerations

In general, pituitary disorders do not, in and of themselves, produce significant psychosocial dysfunctions. However, the disorders treated by pituitary drugs are mostly observable and might cause the patients some degree of social discomfort. Treatment is more likely to alleviate the social discomfort associated with pituitary-related illnesses than add to it (see Case Study—Diabetes Insipidus).

Analysis and Management

Treatment Objectives

Owing to the rarity of pituitary disorders and the rapidly advancing concepts of their management, endocrine consultation is usually indicated. However, the overall goal of treatment is to bring the plasma levels of the affected hormone or hormones to within a normal range. With hormone excess, the relevant goal is to suppress the production of that hormone. With hormone deficits, the goal is to replace the deficient hormone and maintain or improve existing system functioning.

Treatment Options

Most drug therapy is used to replace or supplement naturally occurring hormones in situations involving inadequate function of the pituitary gland. Conditions resulting from excessive amounts of pituitary hormones are more often treated with surgery or radiation therapy.

Drug Variables

Because of the limited choice of drugs available for treating pituitary disorders, it is difficult to establish the criteria for selecting one drug over another. Even when more than one drug is available to treat the same disorder, they are likely to have comparable pharmacokinetics and pharmacodynamics. For example, even though drug manufacturers recommend corticotropin for treatment of diseases that respond to glucocorticoids, corticotropin is less predictable and less convenient than glucocorticoids and has no apparent advantages.

Patient Variables

The use of pituitary drugs should be decided on an individual basis. Dosages of any pituitary hormone must be individualized because responsiveness of affected tissues varies. Extra caution is needed when pituitary drugs are used in children and older adults, because they lack the ability to regulate drug activity. If drugs are to be used during pregnancy, the mother and the fetus should be monitored very closely.

GH has great potential for misuse, primarily because of its real and perceived effects on body size and composition. Enhanced athletic performance is the most commonly desired result. GH is useless for stimulating linear growth in adults because of the closure of epiphyseal plates. Yet adult athletes often seek GH to increase muscle mass and decrease body fat in a manner that is undetectable by current drug testing programs.

Intervention

Administration

The drug should be administered as directed, and the patient should be monitored for allergic reactions and undesired clinical responses. With a few exceptions, most pituitary drugs are available for parenteral use only. Most of the drugs have a very short half-life, so it is important to ensure that the patient is compliant with medication administration. And finally, because pituitary drugs are very potent, extra care is needed when preparing the drugs for use to prevent drug overdose.

Anterior Pituitary Hormones Patients allergic to porcine products should receive an intradermal test dose before receiving therapeutic or diagnostic dosages of corticotropin. Hypersensitivity reactions (i.e., wheezing, rash or hives, bradycardia, irritability, seizures, nausea and vomiting) are more likely to occur with the SC route or prolonged therapy. Additionally, patients on prolonged corticotropin therapy should routinely have hematologic values, electrolytes, and serum and urine glucose values examined. Blood or urine glucose levels should be monitored periodically throughout therapy for patients on somatrem or somatropin.

GH drugs must be refrigerated before and after reconstitution with bacteriostatic water for injection. The solution should be clear after reconstitution. Reconstituted vials should be used within 14 days of reconstitution. The patient's height and weight, thyroid function, and glucose tolerance should be checked at regular intervals. Somatropin injections should be given at least 48 hours apart.

Posterior Pituitary Drugs The ampule of vasopressin tannate in oil should be shaken vigorously to disperse the ingredients uniformly. One to two glasses of water should be taken when the injection is given to minimize adverse GI effects. The health care provider should be alert for signs of water toxicity. In the case of toxicity, the drug should be withdrawn and the patient's fluid intake restricted until the urine specific gravity is at least 1.015.

Desmopressin acetate is administered through a flexible nasal catheter used to measure the liquid. Once the drug is drawn into the catheter, one end is placed in the patient's nose and the other end in the patient's mouth. The patient then blows into the catheter to deposit the drug in the nasal passageways.

Lypressin should be administered by holding the bottle upright, with the patient in a vertical position with the head upright. No more than three sprays should be taken at any one time. The two drugs should not be inhaled.

Hormone-Suppressant Drugs Bromocriptine should be administered with food or milk to minimize gastric distress. Tablets may be crushed if the patient has difficulty swallowing. Taking it at bedtime may help reduce the nausea. Blood pressure should be monitored before and frequently during drug therapy. The patient should be advised to remain supine during and for several hours after the first dose because severe hypotension may occur. Ambulation and transfer during initial dosing should be supervised to prevent injury from the hypotension.

The preferred injection sites for octreotide are the hip, thigh, and abdomen. The injection sites should be rotated, and multiple injections to one site within a short time period should be avoided. The drug should be allowed to reach room temperature before administration to minimize local reactions at the injection site. The injections should be administered between meals and at bedtime.

Education

Proper planning is important for the patient receiving hormonal therapy. The amount of teaching can vary based on the treatment plan. For example, when the patient is a child, make sure that the family has a responsible caregiver who will ensure compliance with the plan of treatment. The caregiver and the patient may need to learn how to administer injections. In addition to teaching injection techniques, orient the patient and caregivers to how and where to get the drugs and the supplies for giving injections. It is important to teach the patients and caregivers what to expect from the treatment and what kind of changes should be reported to the health care provider. Routine monitoring of drug and hormone levels should be stressed.

Teaching plans must include information about consequences of abruptly discontinuing treatment, physical changes to expect, and physical changes that must be brought to the attention of the health care provider. The patient should be advised to wear or carry Medic-Alert identification. He or she should be taught to avoid the use of over-the-counter drugs and to consult with the health care provider before adding any other drug to the treatment regimen.

The patient taking corticotropin should be advised to avoid immunizations that use live vaccines because use of corticotropin decreases immunity. The patient should be instructed to notify the health care provider if fever, sore throat, muscle weakness, sudden weight gain, or edema develops. A dietitian can provide instructions about sodium-restricted diets that are high in vitamin D, protein, and potassium.

Patients taking drugs that may cause drowsiness should use caution when driving or engaging in activities requiring alertness until the drug response is known. Caution the patient to avoid concurrent alcohol and over-the-counter drug use during the course of treatment without first checking with the health care provider.

Evaluation

Evaluation of treatment outcomes is important and can be accomplished in a number of different ways. If the goal is to bring the hormone level to the normal range, then routine monitoring of the plasma level of the drug and the affected hormone or hormones is sufficient. But if the goal of the treatment is to produce some organ change, then specific organ monitoring is needed. For example, if synthetic ADH is given for the treatment of diabetes insipidus, then close monitoring of urine osmolarity and volume is vital. Finally, because of the integration of the endocrine system, it is important to evaluate the functioning of the other endocrine glands, for example, by monitoring blood glucose levels.

A patient's clinical response to GH can be evaluated by the child's attainment of adult height. The patient should be monitored for development of neutralizing antibodies if the growth rate does not exceed 2.5 cm in 6 months.

With vasopressin and its analogs, the effectiveness of treatment can be evaluated by observing for decreased urinary output, increased urine specific gravity, decreased signs of dehydration, and decreased thirst. The patient should, however, be monitored for evidence of water intoxication (e.g., drowsiness, listlessness, headache).

To monitor the effectiveness of treatment for hyperprolactinemia, serum PRL concentrations should be measured monthly during initial therapy and twice yearly thereafter. Serum GH levels and insulin-like growth factor concentrations should be monitored periodically during therapy. The effectiveness of therapy can be demonstrated by a decrease in galactorrhea in 6 to 8 weeks and decreased serum levels of GH in patients with acromegaly.

The effectiveness of treatment with octreotide can be demonstrated by a relief of symptoms and suppressed tumor growth in patients with pituitary tumors associated with acromegaly.

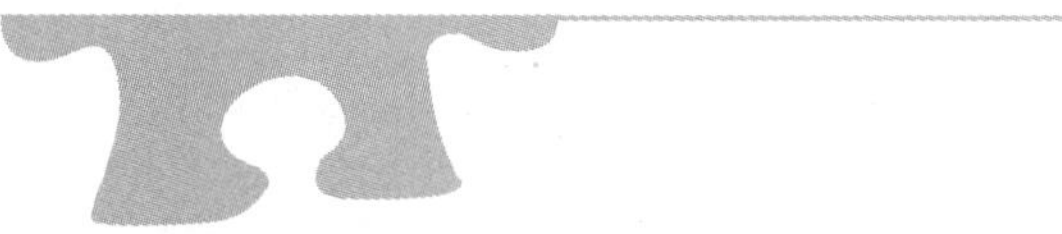

SUMMARY

- The pituitary gland has two distinct areas responsible for the secretion of eight different hormones—the anterior and posterior pituitary.
- The anterior pituitary (adenohypophysis) secretes polypeptide hormones (GH, ACTH, PRL) and glycoprotein hormones (LH, FSH, TSH).
- The posterior pituitary (neurohypophysis) is responsible for storing and releasing vasopressin (ADH) and oxytocin, which are produced by the hypothalamus.
- Pituitary disorders can be classified as those with excessive hormone production and disorders with deficient hormone production.
- Excessive pituitary hormones exert their effects on the target organs, causing hyperactivity of those organs. Hormone excess is associated with manifestations such as giantism, acromegaly, and galactorrhea/amenorrhea
- Hormone deficits are associated with disorders such as diabetes insipidus and dwarfism.
- For a patient with hormone excess, the goal is to suppress the production of the hormone and keep plasma levels within normal limits.
- In the case of hormone deficiency, the goal is to replace the hormone using an exogenous synthetic form of the hormone.
- Pituitary hormone replacement drugs include corticotropin and cosyntropin (ACTH preparations), somatrem and somatropin (GH preparations), and desmopressin, lypressin, and vasopressin (ADH preparations).
- Preparations of ACTH such as corticotropin and cosyntropin are used primarily for the diagnosis of adrenocorticoid function and for the treatment of conditions responsive to glucocorticoid therapy.
- Somatrem and somatropin produce increased growth and metabolic activity in children who lack GH.
- Vasopressin and its analogs (desmopressin and lypressin) reduce urine formation, thus conserving water. Vasopressin is also a potent vasoconstrictor that may be used in the management of GI bleeding.
- Pituitary hormone–suppressant drugs include bromocriptine and octreotide.
- Suppressant drugs are used to manage hypersecretion of anterior pituitary hormones that cause hyperprolactinemia and acromegaly.
- Patients or their caregivers may need to learn how to administer injections or be taught how to use the drugs using an intranasal route.
- Because of the potency of the pituitary drugs, extra care should be used when preparing these drugs for administration.
- Close monitoring for adverse effects as well as therapeutic effects is required.
- Drug effectiveness can be evaluated through monitoring of plasma levels of hormones.
- Desired and undesired changes in organ functioning, brought about by the agent, should be evaluated on routine basis.

BIBLIOGRAPHY

Allen, D., Blizzard, R., and Rosenfeld, R. (1995). The use—and misuse—of growth hormone. *Patient Care,* January 30, 41–57.

Blackwell, R. (1992). Hyperprolactinemia: Evaluation and management. *Endocrinology and Metabolic Clinics of North America, 21*(1), 105–124.

Bullock, B. (Ed.). (1996). *Pathophysiology: Adaptations and alterations in function* (4th ed.). Philadelphia: J.B. Lippincott.

Chong, B., Newton, T., (1993). Hypothalamic and pituitary pathology. *Radiologic Clinics of North America, 31*(5), 1147–1153.

Greenspan, F. (Ed.) (1991). *Basic and clinical endocrinology* (3rd ed.). Norwalk, CT: Appleton & Lange.

Hughes, J., Ellisworth, C., and Harris, B. (1995). Clinical case seminar: A 33-year-old woman with a pituitary mass and panhypopituitarism. *Journal of Clinical Endocrinology and Metabolism, 80*(5), 1521–1525.

Jenkins, D., and Stewart P. (1993). Advances in medical therapy for pituitary disease: Treating patients with growth hormone excess and deficiency. *Journal of Clinical Pharmacy and Therapeutics, 18,* 155–163.

Klibanski, A., and Zervas, N. (1991). Diagnosis and management of hormone secreting pituitary adenomas. *New England Journal of Medicine, 324*(12), 822–831.

Kumar, V., Cotran, R., and Robbins, S. (1992). *Basic pathology* (5th ed.). Philadelphia: W.B. Saunders.

Lee, L., and Gumomski, J. (1992). Adrenocortical insufficiency: A medical emergency. *AACN Clinical Issues in Critical Care Nursing,* 3, 319–330.

Malakey, W. (1993). Prolactomas. *Advances in Endocrinology and Metabolism,* 4, 197–217.

Morley, T., and Korenman, S. (Eds.). (1992). *Endocrinology and Metabolism in the elderly.* Boston: Blackwell Scientific Publications.

Panidis, D., Russo, D., Skiadopoulos, S., et al. (1994). Hypothalamic-pituitary deficiency after Weil's syndrome: A case report. *Fertility and Sterility, 62*(5), 1077–1079.

Reasner, C. (1990). Anterior pituitary disease. *Critical Care Nursing Quarterly, 13*(3), 62–66.

Robinson, A., and Fitzsimmons, M. (1994). Diabetes insipidus. *Advances in Endocrinology and Metabolism, 5,* 261–296.

Schlechte, J., and Iverson, R. (1990). Pituitary tumors. *Advances in Endocrinology and Metabolism, 1,* 261–181.

Sikes, P. (1992). Endocrine responses to the stress of critical illness. *AACN Clinical Issues in Critical Care Nursing, 3,* 379–391.

Vance, M. (1992). Growth hormone: Non-growth promoting uses in humans. *Advances in Endocrinology and Metabolism, 3,* 259–269.

Vance, M. (1994). Hypopituitarism. *New England Journal of Medicine, 330*(23), 1651–1662.

Wardhaugh, B. (1992). Evaluating growth hormone treatment. *Nursing Standards, 6*(48), 33–36.

Wilson, D., and Rosenfeld, R. (1990). New directions in the diagnosis and treatment of growth failure. *Advances in Endocrinology and Metabolism, 1,* 95–128.

Wilson, J. (Ed.) (1991). *Harrison's principles of internal medicine* (12th ed.). New York: McGraw-Hill.

Wise, B., and Case, B. (1994). Recombinant human growth hormone. *ANNA Journal, 21*(1), 87–89.

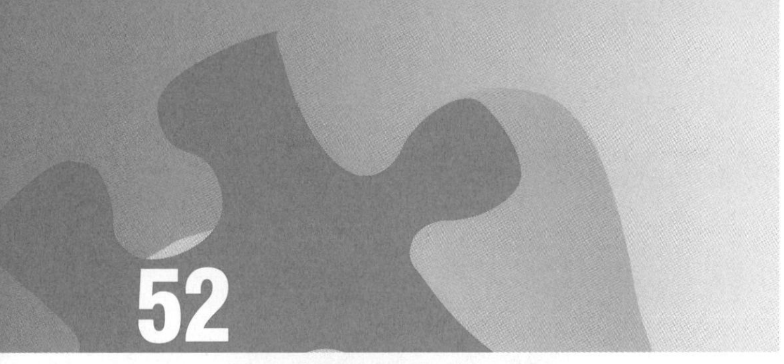

52 Adrenal Cortex Drugs and Inhibitors

Exogenously administered adrenal cortex hormones (e.g., prednisone) or steroids have assumed a major role in the management of various diseases since the 1940s (Clinical Indications for the Use of Adrenal Corticosteroids). Although complication rates associated with the administration of exogenous hormones are high, many lives are saved or improved with corticosteroid use.

The adrenal cortex produces two classes of hormones: corticosteroids and androgenic steroids. Androgenic steroids are discussed in Chapter 53. The corticosteroids are further divided into glucocorticoid and mineralocorticoid steroids. Corticosteroids primarily affect carbohydrate metabolism, whereas mineralocorticoids (aldosterone) regulate sodium balance. When adrenal cortex function is compromised, synthetic compounds can replace naturally produced substances to maintain normal bodily function. In addition, supraphysiologic doses of glucocorticoids lessen the immune response and sometimes decrease the negative consequences associated with inflammation.

In rare cases, adrenal hormones are produced by the body in levels beyond its requirements. When appropriate, drug therapy can suppress the release of adrenal hormones.

This chapter reviews pathologic processes that are treated or ameliorated with the use of adrenal cortex hormones. The consequences associated with high levels of steroids, either naturally occurring or iatrogenically produced, are described. Information about conditions causing overproduction of glucocorticoids is reviewed, along with drug treatments suppressing adrenal hormone production. Finally, an overview of various drug administration options is included.

ADRENAL INSUFFICIENCY

Epidemiology and Etiology

Adrenal insufficiency results in decreased levels of adrenal cortex hormones—glucocorticoids (cortisol, corticosterone, and cortisone), mineralocorticoids (aldosterone), and androgens (testosterone). In recent years, the incidence of adrenal insufficiency has increased as a result of improved diagnostic techniques, the use of newer drugs that may have cytotoxic action, and the increased use of high-dose glucocorticoids. Nonetheless, adrenal insufficiency is still considered to be a rare disorder. In the United States, most cases of adrenal insufficiency are due to an autoimmune destruction of the adrenal gland, with a 2 to 3 times greater incidence in females than in males.

Hyposecretion of adrenal hormones occurs either because of direct damage to the adrenal cortex (primary adrenal insufficiency) or because a pathologic process has impinged on the production or secretion of adrenal cortex hormones (secondary adrenal insufficiency). In either case, secretion of adrenal hormones is insufficient (chronically or acutely) to support normal body functions.

Primary Adrenal Insufficiency

Dysfunction of the adrenal glands results in primary adrenal insufficiency (Addison's disease). It is frequently due to chronic destructive disease and results in loss of the major adrenal hormones cortisol and aldosterone. Idiopathic (probably autoimmune) insufficiency is now ranked as the leading cause of Addison's disease, followed by tuberculosis, infiltrative processes such as fungal lesions and metastatic carcinoma, traumatic or hemorrhagic injury to both adrenal glands, or gram-negative sepsis (Waterhouse-Friderichsen syndrome). Exogenous causes of adrenal insufficiency include abdominal radiation therapy, the use of adrenal toxic drugs such as mitotane, and adrenalectomy.

Secondary Adrenal Insufficiency

Pathologic conditions of the hypothalamic-pituitary-adrenocortical (HPA) axis cause decreased cortisol and adrenal androgen production with continued but sometimes decreased aldosterone secretion. Hypothalamic or pituitary tumors, postpartum necrosis of the pituitary gland (Sheehan's syndrome), high-dose radiation therapy of the pituitary or other intracranial lesions, and hypophysectomy are all contributing causes. In addition to pathologic hyposecretion of hypothalamic or pituitary hormones, when administered in supraphysiologic levels, glucocorticoids (e.g., prednisone) cause a suppression of the HPA axis via the negative feedback system.

Pathophysiology

Insufficient adrenal hormones cause defects associated with the loss of glucocorticoid (cortisol) and mineralocorticoid (aldosterone) action. The action of the releasing factors from the hypothalamus (e.g., corticotropin-releasing hormone [CRH]) and stimulating hormones from the pituitary gland (i.e., adrenocorticotropic hormone [ACTH]) is essentially quelled (Fig. 52–1). Impaired secretion of cortisol results in decreased formation of glycogen (gluconeogenesis) from noncarbohydrate sources (e.g., amino acids or fatty acids). There is also depletion of liver and muscle glycogen and, thus, hypoglycemia.

Decreased gastric acid production and a decreased glomerular filtration rate also occur. Anorexia, weight loss, and a reduced excretion of urea nitrogen results. Reduced aldosterone secretion causes alterations in the clearance of sodium, water, and potassium by the kidneys. Because of the alterations in water and electrolyte excretion, hypokalemia, hyponatremia, and hypovolemia result. Potassium retention also promotes the reabsorption of hydrogen ions, thus ultimately leading to metabolic acidosis.

Low androgen levels may result in the loss of body, axillary, and pubic hair. The hair loss is especially noticeable in

CLINICAL INDICATIONS FOR THE USE OF ADRENAL CORTICOSTEROIDS	
Acute Spinal Cord Injury	
Adrenal Insufficiency	
Primary	Secondary
Allergic Reactions	
Food and drug reactions	Angioedema
Contact dermatitis	
Neurologic Problems	
Cerebral edema	Postcraniotomy
Closed head injury	Exacerbation of multiple sclerosis
Collagen Diseases	
Systemic lupus erythematosus	Giant cell arteritis
Polymyalgia rheumatica	
Congenital Adrenal Hyperplasia	
Dermatologic Problems	
Severe seborrheic, contact, and atopic dermatitis	Angioedema or urticaria
Severe psoriasis	Severe erythema multiforme
Gastrointestinal Disorders	
Regional enteritis	Inflammatory bowel disease
Ulcerative colitis	
Hematologic Disorders	
Hemolytic anemia	Idiopathic thrombocytopenic purpura
Leukemia	Multiple myeloma
Hypercalcemia with Neoplasms	
Sarcoidosis	Carcinoma
Musculoskeletal Inflammation	
Arthritis—degenerative	Synovitis
Acute gouty arthritis	Tendinitis
Ankylosing spondylitis	Bursitis
Myasthenia Gravis	
Neoplastic Conditions	
Nephrotic Syndrome	
Ophthalmologic Disorders	
Uveitis	Allergic conjunctivitis
Optic neuritis	
Organ Transplant	
Respiratory Diseases	
Asthma	Allergic rhinitis
Aspiration pneumonia	Chronic airway limitation, especially with bronchospasm
Rheumatic Disorders	
Rheumatoid arthritis	
Septic Shock	
Thyroiditis	

females, in whom the adrenals are responsible for the major production of androgens. It is important to note that the severity of symptoms is related to the degree of hormone deficiency.

Acute insufficiency (addisonian crisis) is life-threatening. The patient's physiologic requirement for glucocorticoids and mineralocorticoids exceeds the available supply. In most cases, the crisis is precipitated by a stressful event (e.g., severe infection, surgery, or trauma). It also occurs when there is a pre-existing deficiency of adrenal hormones. The pathophysiology of acute insufficiency is similar to that for chronic insufficiency. The one exception is a patient who presents with bilateral adrenal hemorrhage. These patients may have normal sodium and potassium levels because the time frame from the initial event may be too short for a noticeable change to occur. Without prompt intervention, sodium and potassium levels fall quickly. Intravascular volume depletion occurs secondary to the loss of mineralocorticoid, leading to more severe hypotension.

CONGENITAL ADRENAL HYPERPLASIA

Epidemiology and Etiology

Congenital adrenal hyperplasia (CAH) is transmitted as an autosomal recessive trait. The frequency varies throughout the world. In the United States, the incidence of CAH is

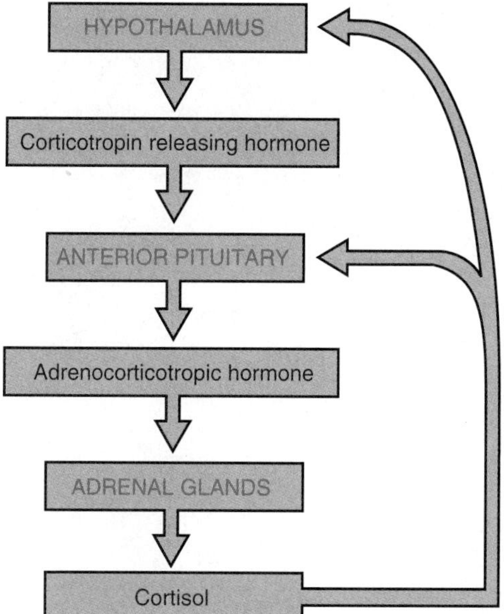

Figure 52–1 The hypothalamic-pituitary-adrenal axis shows that cortisol production is dependent on an intact hypothalamus, pituitary gland, and adrenal gland. It operates as a negative feedback system.

1 in approximately 80,000 to 100,000 live births. The most common form of CAH is due to a 21-hydroxylase deficiency.

Pathophysiology

Congenital enzyme deficiencies in the metabolic pathways of the glucocorticoids lead to low adrenal corticosteroid levels. Low adrenal corticosteroid levels, in turn, signal the pituitary gland to release more ACTH for adrenal stimulation. High levels of ACTH lead to hyperplasia of adrenal tissue as a compensatory mechanism to increase hormone production. Unfortunately, the adrenal cortex is still unable to synthesize the needed hormones. In contrast, androgens also stimulated by ACTH are produced in excessive quantities.

Clinical manifestations of CAH are virilization of the female fetus and adrenal corticosteroid insufficiency in both the male and female. Sodium and water depletion leading to hypovolemia, dehydration, and shock are evident at times.

PHARMACOTHERAPEUTIC OPTIONS

Glucocorticoids

- ❒ Cortisone (CORTONE)
- ❒ Hydrocortisone (CORTEF, HYDROCORTONE); (🍁) HYCORT
- ❒ Methylprednisolone (DEPO-MEDROL, MEDROL, SOLU-MEDROL)
- ❒ Prednisolone (DELTA-CORTEF, DUEPRED, HYDELTRA)
- ❒ Prednisone (DELTASONE, METICORTEN); (🍁) WINPRED

Indications

Glucocorticoids are used to treat many different disorders. Corticosteroid drugs that are applied topically in ophthalmic, otic, and dermatologic disorders are discussed in Chapters 62, 63, and 64, respectively.

Corticosteroid drug therapy is indicated in the treatment of adrenal insufficiency and CAH when naturally occurring adrenal hormones are not present in sufficient quantities to sustain life. Of particular importance are disorders characterized by the lack of cortisol. Glucocorticoids are given to replace or substitute for the natural hormones (both glucocorticoids and mineralocorticoids) in cases of insufficiency and to suppress corticotropin when excess secretion causes adrenal hyperplasia.

Glucocorticoids are clearly indicated for shock resulting from adrenal insufficiency. Maximal levels of glucocorticoids are already produced in hemorrhagic or cardiogenic shock and in other forms of severe stress. Administering exogenous glucocorticoids probably has little therapeutic effect in these conditions. On the other hand, anaphylactic shock resulting from an allergic response may be effectively treated with glucocorticoids because they increase or restore cardiovascular responsiveness to adrenergic drugs.

Pharmacodynamics

The adrenal hormone cortisol produces many physiologic effects. At the cellular level, cortisol accounts for 95 percent of glucocorticoid activity as a group, with about 15 to 25 mg secreted daily. Corticosterone has a small degree of activity, with about 1.5 to 4 mg secreted daily. Cortisone itself has little activity and is secreted in minute quantities. Endogenous glucocorticoids are cyclically secreted, with the largest amount produced in the morning and the smallest amount during the evening hours (in people on a normal day-night schedule). Whether of endogenous or exogenous origin, glucocorticoids affect carbohydrate, protein, and fat metabolism. They also produce effects on inflammatory and immune responses; on the nervous, musculoskeletal, respiratory, and gastrointestinal systems; and on fluid and electrolyte balance.

It is important to distinguish between the physiologic effects of glucocorticoids and pharmacologic effects. Physiologic effects occur at low levels (i.e., the levels produced by the release of glucocorticoids from healthy adrenals, or by the administration of low-dose exogenous glucocorticoids). Pharmacologic effects occur at supraphysiologic doses. These effects are achieved when glucocorticoids are required to treat disorders unrelated to adrenocortical function (e.g., allergic reactions, asthma, and inflammation).

Carbohydrate, Protein, and Fat Metabolism

Glucocorticoids stimulate the formation of glucose (*gluconeogenesis*) by causing the breakdown of protein to amino acids. The amino acids are transported to the liver, where they are converted to glucose through enzymatic action. The glucose is then returned to the circulation for use by body tissues, or is stored in the liver as glycogen. There is a moderate decrease in the cell's use of glucose by an unknown mechanism (anti-insulin effects). Additionally, there is increased production but decreased use of glucose. Higher blood levels of glucose thus promote a diabetic-like state. These actions also increase the amount of glucose stored as glycogen in the liver, skeletal muscles, and other tissues.

The effects of glucocorticoids on protein metabolism include an increased breakdown of protein to amino acids. The rate at which amino acids are transported to the liver and converted to glucose is increased. There is also a decreased rate at which new proteins are formed (antianabolic effects) from dietary and other amino acids. The combination of increased breakdown of cell protein and decreased protein synthesis produces protein depletion in almost all body cells except those of the liver. Thus, glycogen stores are increased, whereas protein stores are decreased.

Fatty acids are mobilized from adipose tissue, resulting in increased fatty acid concentration in the plasma. The oxidation of fatty acids within body cells is also stimulated.

Central Nervous System

Glucocorticoids affect mood and central nervous system excitability. Physiologic levels help maintain normal nerve excitability. Increased or pharmacologic amounts decrease nerve excitability, slow activity in the cerebral cortex, and alter brain wave patterns. Secretion of CRH by the hypothalamus and of corticotropin by the anterior pituitary gland is decreased. There is further suppression of glucocorticoid secretion by the adrenal cortex.

Musculoskeletal Actions

Muscle strength is maintained when glucocorticoids are present in physiologic amounts. Glucocorticoids support functioning of striated muscle, primarily by maintaining circulatory competence. Muscle atrophy (from protein breakdown) occurs when glucocorticoids are used in supraphysiologic doses. In addition, they inhibit bone formation and growth, and increase bone breakdown. They decrease the intestinal absorption and increase the renal excretion of calcium. These two actions contribute to bone demineralization (osteoporosis) in adults and to decreased linear growth in children.

Respiratory System Actions

Although glucocorticoids do not have bronchodilating action, it is thought they play a role in maintaining the bronchodilating responsiveness to endogenous catecholamines (e.g., epinephrine). Glucocorticoids stabilize mast cells as well as other cells to inhibit the release of bronchoconstrictive and inflammatory chemicals (e.g., histamine).

Gastrointestinal System Actions

Glucocorticoids decrease the viscosity of gastric mucus. The decreased protective properties of the mucus is thought by some to contribute to the development of peptic ulcer disease.

Fluid and Electrolyte Actions

Glucocorticoids cause the retention of sodium and therefore water, and increase the excretion of calcium and potassium.

Stress Protection

Glucocorticoids have a permissive effect on the action of catecholamines, thereby supporting blood pressure during times of stress. Working together, the catecholamines and glucocorticoids maintain blood pressure and plasma glucose content. If corticosteroid levels are insufficient, as they are in adrenal insufficiency, circulatory collapse and death can follow.

ADVERSE EFFECTS OF SUPRAPHYSIOLOGIC DOSES OF CORTICOSTEROIDS

Cushingoid Features and Musculoskeletal Changes

Facial rounding—Moon face
Dorsal hump—Buffalo hump
Supraclavicular fossa fullness
Central obesity
Osteoporosis
Muscle wasting
Myopathy
Weakness

Nervous System Changes

Headache	Restlessness
Vertigo	Seizures
Insomnia	Pseudotumor cerebri

Mood Changes

Depression	Psychosis
Euphoria	Suicidal gestures

Fluid and Electrolyte Imbalances

Hypernatremia	Fluid retention
Hypokalemia	Hypertension
Hypocalcemia	Peripheral edema
Metabolic alkalosis	Congestive heart failure

Skin Changes

Striae	Hirsutism
Fragile skin	Acne
Impaired wound healing	Ecchymosis

Ophthalmologic Complications

Cataracts	Glaucoma

Miscellaneous

Increased susceptibility to infection
Gastrointestinal irritation
Glucose intolerance and diabetes mellitus
Decreased growth in children

Adverse Effects and Contraindications

Glucocorticoids are naturally occurring substances, and at normal physiologic levels, they have no adverse effects or contraindications. Adverse effects occur when the dosage is greater than the body's requirements for the hormones (Adverse Effects of Supraphysiologic Doses of Corticosteroids).

No contraindications exist when glucocorticoids are given for replacement therapy in adrenal insufficiency. However, they are contraindicated in patients with systemic fungal infections and in those who are hypersensitive to the drug formulations. Glucocorticoids should be used with caution in patients at risk for infections because they may decrease the immune response. In patients with existing infections they may mask signs and symptoms so that infections become more severe before being recognized and treated. They should also be used with caution in patients with diabetes mellitus, peptic ulcer disease, inflammatory bowel disorders, hypertension, congestive heart failure, and renal insufficiency.

Glucocorticoids cross into breast milk. Exogenous formulations ingested by the infant from breast milk suppress the HPA axis. Therefore, mothers who exceed normal corticosteroid levels are advised not to breastfeed their infants.

Pharmacokinetics

The rate of absorption for glucocorticoids depends on the route of administration and the specific glucocorticoid. When they are taken orally, glucocorticoids are readily absorbed in the upper jejunum. Following intramuscular (IM) injection, absorption is rapid with two types of glucocorticoid esters (i.e., sodium phosphates and sodium succinates) and relatively slow with other derivatives (e.g., acetates, acetonides, tebutates). Absorption from local sites of injection (e.g., intra-articular, intrasynovial) is slower than from IM sites. Corticosteroid preparations are classified according to their therapeutic effects as short acting, intermediate acting, and long acting. Peak plasma levels are achieved within 30 to 100 minutes (Table 52–1).

The duration of action of glucocorticoids is a function of dosage, route of administration, and solubility. Glucocorticoids are highly bound to the plasma proteins, transcortin, and albumin. For those drugs that are administered orally or by intravenous routes, the duration of action is determined largely by the biologic half-life. With IM administration, the duration of action is a function of water solubility. Highly soluble formulations have a duration that is shorter than that of less soluble formulations. For locally administered glucocorticoids, the duration of action is a function of solubility as well as of the specific site of administration.

Glucocorticoids are biotransformed by microsomal enzymes in the liver. Commercially prepared drugs, such as prednisone and cortisone, require hepatic conversion to prednisolone or cortisol, respectively, to achieve glucocorticoid effects. Further biotransformation by the liver conjugates the glucocorticoids with glucuronic acid to permit excretion by the kidneys.

Drug-Drug Interactions

Various drug-drug interactions are possible among glucocorticoids and other drugs (Table 52–2), especially when the dosage exceeds the physiologic norm. Drugs that induce microsomal enzymes (e.g., barbiturates, phenytoin, rifampin, and other glucocorticoids) increase adrenal hormone biotransformation and may require increased dosages of glucocorticoids. Conversely, drugs that inhibit microsomal enzymes (e.g., erythromycin and oral contraceptives) decrease biotransformation and may require a decreased corticosteroid dosage to achieve similar effects.

Glucocorticoids cause sodium and fluid retention and potassium excretion. Hence, diuretic therapy may be compromised. Additionally, thiazide diuretics, furosemide, and amphotericin B potentiate the potassium-depleting effects of glucocorticoids, leading to severe hypokalemia.

TABLE 52–1 PHARMACOKINETICS OF SELECTED ADRENAL CORTEX DRUGS AND INHIBITORS

Drug	Route	Onset	Peak	Duration	PB (%)	$t_{1/2}$	BioA (%)
Short-Acting Corticosteroids							
Cortisone	po	Rapid	2 hr	1.25–1.5 days	Very high	30 min	UA
	IM	slow	20–48 hr		Very high		100
Hydrocortisone	po	6 hr	1 hr		High		UA
	IM	rapid	4–8 hr		High		UA
	IV	rapid	1 hr		High		100
Intermediate-Acting Corticosteroids							
Methylprednisolone	po	UA	1–2 hr	1.25–1.5 days	High	>3.5 hr	UA
	IV	Rapid	UA			UA	100
Prednisolone	po	1 hr	1–2 hr			2.1–3.8 hr	UA
	IV	rapid	1 hr			2.1–3.8 hr	100
Prednisone	po	1 hr	1–2 hr		High to very high	1 hr	UA
Triamcinolone	po	UA	1–2 hr	2.25 days	High	2–5 hr	UA
Long-Acting Corticosteroids							
Dexamethasone	po	UA	1–2 hr	2.75 days	High	5 hr	UA
	IM	UA	8 hr	6 days	High	3–4.5 hr	UA
Betamethasone	po	UA	1–2 hr	3.25 days	High	3–5 hr	UA
	IM	1–3 hr	UA	7 days	High	3–5 hr	UA
Mineralocorticoids							
Fludrocortisone	po	UA	1.7 hr	1–2 days	High	3.5 hr*	UA
Desoxycorticosterone	IM	UA	UA	UA	High	1.2 hr	UA
Adrenal Hormone Inhibitors†							
Aminoglutethimide	po	3–5 days	1.5 hr	1.5–3 days	Low	11–16 hr; 5–9 days‡	UA
Metyrapone	po	24 hr	1 hr	4 hr	UA	1–2.5 hr	UA
Mitotane	po	2–3 days	3–5 hr	UA	UA	18–159 days	UA

*Fludrocortisone remains therapeutically active for 24–48 hours.

†Time of onset of adrenal suppression with adrenal hormone inhibitors (e.g., corticosteroid excretion in urine).

‡During aminoglutethimide therapy, the half-life increases with prolonged therapy (1 year of therapy). Inital $t_{1/2}$ of aminoglutethimide is 11–16 hours, followed by 5–9 days.

BioA, Bioavailability; IM, intramuscular; IV, intravenous; PB, protein binding; $t_{1/2}$, elimination half-life; UA, unavailable.

TABLE 52–2 SELECTED DRUG-DRUG INTERACTIONS OF ADRENAL CORTEX DRUGS AND INHIBITORS

Drug	Interactive Drug	Interaction
Corticosteroids		
Betamethasone	Aminoglutethimide	Induces microsomal enzymes, decreases effects of corticosteroid
Cortisone	Carbamazepine	
Dexamethasone	Phenobarbital	
Hydrocortisone	Phenytoin	
Methylprednisolone	Rifampicin	
Prednisolone	Erythromycin	Decreases biotransformation of corticosteroid
Prednisone	Troleandomycin	
	Antacids	Decreases absorption of corticosteroid
	Anticoagulants	Increases or decreases in clotting
	Antihypertensives	Loss of some antihypertensive effectiveness due to mineralocorticoid effects of corticosteroids
	Oral contraceptives	Decreases renal clearance of corticosteroids; decreases metabolism of corticosteroids
	Estrogens	
	Salicylic acid	Increases biotransformation of salicylic acid
	NSAIDs	Additive GI irritation
	Thiazide diuretics	Potentiates potassium depleting effects of glucocorticoid—possible severe hypokalemia
	Furosemide	
	Amphotericin B	
	Skin-testing agents	Decreases reactivity of the skin test—false-negative reactions
	Isoniazid	Decreases renal clearance of corticosteroid
	Ketoconazole	
	Insulin	Decreases effectiveness of interactive drug
	Oral hypoglycemics	
Mineralocorticoids		
Fludrocortisone	Aminoglutethimide	Induces microsomal enzymes
	Carbamazepine	
	Phenobarbital	
	Phenytoin	
	Rifampicin	
	Diuretics	Decreases effectiveness of diuretics; significant potassium depletion with non–potassium-sparing diuretics
	Potassium supplements	
Adrenal Hormone Inhibitors		
Aminoglutethimide	Dexamethasone hydrocortisone	Increases biotransformation of aminoglutethimide
	Oral anticoagulants	Increases biotransformation of interacting drug; decreases effectiveness of interacting drug
	Medroxyprogesterone	Decreases steady state concentration of interacting drug
	Theophylline	
	Digoxin	
	Alcohol	May potentiate action of adrenal hormone–inhibiting drug
Metyrapone	Phenytoin	Increases biotransformation of metyrapone–inaccurate test results
	Estrogens	Subtherapeutic response to metyrapone—inaccurate test results
Trilostane	Thiazide diuretics, loop diuretics	Decreases potassium loss

NSAIDs, Nonsteroidal anti-inflammatory drugs.

High doses of glucocorticoids increase serum glucose levels. Therefore, insulin and oral hypoglycemics may appear ineffective. Increased dosages of the antidiabetic drugs may be required.

Higher than normal doses of glucocorticoids may increase the biotransformation and renal clearance of salicylates. Therefore, therapeutic dosages of salicylates are more difficult to achieve and rapid cessation of glucocorticoid therapy may result in salicylate toxicity.

Dosage Regimens

Dosage regimens of glucocorticoids are highly individualized. For a given patient with any disease, the dosage is determined empirically (by trial and error). For patients whose disease is not an immediate threat to life, the dosage should be low initially and then increased gradually until symptoms are under control. In the event of a life-threatening situation, a large initial dose should be used, and if a response does not occur rapidly, the dose should be doubled or tripled.

When glucocorticoids are used for prolonged periods, the dosage should be reduced (after the patient is stabilized) to be the smallest effective dose possible. Prolonged treatment with supraphysiologic doses should be provided only if the disorder is life-threatening or if it has the potential to cause permanent disability. Increased dosages may be needed at times of stress (unless the dosage is high to begin with).

The adult adrenal glands secrete an average of 20 mg of cortisol per day. Therefore, 15 to 25 mg per day of hydrocortisone (or its equivalent) is recommended for adrenal insufficiency (Tables 52–3 and 52–4).

TABLE 52–3 DOSAGE REGIMEN FOR SELECTED ADRENAL HORMONES AND INHIBITORS

Drug	Use(s)	Dosage*	Implications
Corticosteroids			
Betamethasone Betamethasone sodium phosphate	Inflammation and immunosuppression	*Adult:* 2.4–4.8 mg po QD *or* 0.5–9 mg/day parenterally	Long-acting glucocorticoid. Suppresses HPA at doses of 0.6 mg/day. Contraindicated in the presence of infection
	Local anti-inflammatory effects	*Adult:* 6–15 mg q2–7 days by local injection	Absorption slow but complete. After acute episode of inflammation doses are decreased or tapered off when possible
Cortisone Cortisone acetate	Adrenal insufficiency; congenital adrenal hyperplasia	*Adult:* 10–37 mg po QD in divided doses *or* 20–330 mg IM QD. Maintenance: Reduce dose in small increments until lowest dose that maintains satisfactory clinical response is reached. *Child:* 0.1–0.2 mg po QD	Short-acting glucocorticoid. Suppresses HPA axis at doses > 20 mg/day. Carefully monitor growth and development in infants and children on prolonged therapy. Taper doses when discontinuing high-dose or long-term therapy
	Inflammation and immunosuppression	*Adult:* 25–300 mg po QD *or* 0.2–1.25 mg/kg/day parenterally	
	Local anti-inflammatory effects	*Adult:* 5–75 mg by local injection	Dosage depends on degree of inflammation, location, and size of area
Dexamethasone Dexamethasone acetate Dexamethasone sodium phosphate	Inflammation and immunosuppression	*Adult:* 0.5–9 mg po QD in three to four divided doses *or* 0.5–24 mg/day IM/IV (phosphate) *or* 6–16 mg/day (acetate) *Child:* 0.024–0.34 mg/kg/day po *or* 6–40 mcg/kg/day parenterally	IM acetate salt is long acting. Suppresses HPA axis at chronic doses of 0.75 mg/day. Adrenal suppression lasts 2.75 days
	Local anti-inflammatory effects	*Adult:* 0.8–16 mg by local injection	Dosage depends on degree of inflammation, location, and size of area
	Local anti-inflammatory effects on lungs	*Adult:* 300 mcg (three puffs) TID–QID. Maximum dose 1200 mcg/day *Child:* 200 mcg TID–QID. Maximum dose 800 mcg/day	Chronic high-dose use may lead to systemic absorption
Flunisolide	Local anti-inflammatory effects on lungs	*Adult:* 500 mcg (two puffs) BID. Maximum dose 2000 mcg/day	250 mcg/puff. Not recommended for children under 6 years
Hydrocortisone	Adrenal insufficiency; congenital adrenal hyperplasia	*Adult:* 15–25 mg po QD in divided doses *Child:* 0.5–0.75 mg/kg/day	For adults, give ⅔ of dose in morning and ⅓ of dose in evening. May increase doses during periods of physical or emotional stress
Hydrocortisone sodium succinate	Inflammation and immunosuppression	*Adult:* 10–320 mg po QD *or* 15–250 mg QD parenterally *Child:* 2–32 mg/kg/day po *or* 0.16–1 mg/kg/day parenterally	Suppresses adrenal function with chronic use at doses >20 mg/day
Methylprednisolone Methylprednisolone sodium succinate Methylprednisolone acetate Methylprednisolone sodium phosphate	Inflammation and immunosuppression	*Adult:* 8–240 mg po QD *or* 10–1000 mg/day *or* 10–240 mg q4hr parenterally *Child:* 0.117–1.66 mg/kg/day po *or* 0.2–2.0 mg/kg/day parenterally	Suppresses adrenal function at chronic doses of 4 mg/day. Practically devoid of mineralocorticoid activity
Prednisone Prednisone sodium phosphate	Adrenal insufficiency; congenital adrenal hyperplasia	*Adult:* 5–60 mg po QD Individualized dosage *Child:* 4–5 mg/m² po in equal divided doses q12hr	Reduce dose in small increments at intervals until lowest dose that maintains satisfactory clinical response is reached
	Inflammation and immunosuppression	*Adult:* 5–60 mg po QD *or* 4–60 mg/day parenterally *Child:* 0.14–2 mg/kg/day po; 0.05–0.25 mg/kg/day parenterally	Suppresses adrenal function at chronic doses of 5 mg/day. Has minimal mineralocorticoid activity
	Local anti-inflammatory effects	*Adult:* 2–30 mg q3days to q3 weeks by local injection	Dosage depends on degree of inflammation, location, and size of area

Table continued on following page

TABLE 52–3 DOSAGE REGIMEN FOR SELECTED ADRENAL HORMONES AND INHIBITORS *Continued*

Drug	Use(s)	Dosage*	Implications
Corticosteroids *Continued*			
Triamcinolone	Inflammation and immunosuppression	*Adult:* 4–48 mg po QD *Child:* 0.117–1.66 mg/kg/day	Suppresses adrenal function at chronic doses of 4 mg/day. Suppression lasts 2.25 days
	Local anti-inflammatory effects on lungs	*Adult:* 200 mcg (two puffs) TID–QID. Maximum dose 1600 mcg/day *Child age 6–12 yrs:* 100–200 mcg TID–QID	100 mg/puff. Not recommended for children younger than 6 years of age
Mineralocorticoid			
Fludrocortisone	Adrenal insufficiency	*Adult:* 0.1 mg po three times a week to 0.2 mg po QD *Child:* 0.1–0.2 mg po QD	Dosages are adjusted to maintain water and sodium balance. Use with cortisone or hydrocortisone
Corticosteroid Inhibitors			
Aminoglutethimide	Cushing's syndrome; ectopic ACTH-producing tumors; adrenal enzyme inhibition	*Adult:* 250 mg po BID–TID × 14 days. Increase until desired effects are achieved to a maximum of 2 g/day. Maintenance: 250 mg po QID	Dosages are decreased or discontinued if signs and symptoms of adrenal insufficiency appear
Mitotane	Cushing's syndrome	*Adult:* 500–1000 mg po QD in divided doses. Increase every 2–4 weeks until desired effects achieved. Maximum of 4 g/day Maintenance: 500–2000 mg po QD in divided doses	Larger dose given in the evening to lessen discomfort associated with therapy. Dosages are decreased or discontinued if signs and symptoms of adrenal insufficiency appear
Trilostane	Cushing's syndrome, especially pituitary-dependent forms; adrenal enzyme inhibition; ectopic ACTH-producing tumors	*Adult:* 30 mg po QID × 3 days. Increase in 3–4 day intervals until desired effects are achieved. Maximum dosage 480 mg/day. Maintenance: 120–360 mg po QD in divided doses	Pediatric dosage has not been established. Dosages are decreased or discontinued if signs and symptoms of adrenal insufficiency appear
Metyrapone	Testing of HPA axis function; adrenal enzyme inhibition	*Adult:* 750 mg po q4hr × 6 doses, 4 days after administration of ACTH *Child:* 15 mg/kg q4hr × 6 doses	Used in conjunction with ACTH suppression test Corticosteroids are discontinued before testing

*All anti-inflammatory and immunosuppressive doses are given as a typical range. Doses much higher than those indicated are used during emergency situations. Initial therapy may include multiple divided doses. With long-term therapy, early morning administration and alternate-day therapy is recommended.

The replacement dosage for glucocorticoids in children is 12 mg/m^2. The glucocorticoid is administered in two doses, two thirds in the early morning and the other one third in the late afternoon. During periods of stress additional amounts of the selected glucocorticosteroid is required.

Laboratory Considerations

Testing of blood cortisol levels is possible but not practical for drug therapy monitoring. Normally, cortisol levels vary greatly throughout the day, with peak levels occurring around 6 to 8 AM, about half peak levels at 4 to 5 PM, and

TABLE 52–4 DOSE EQUIVALENCIES AND RELATIVE CORTICOSTEROID EFFECTS

Drug	Equivalent Dose (mg)*	Relative Glucocorticoid Effect (Anti-inflammatory)	Relative Mineralocorticoid Effect (Sodium Retaining)
Betamethasone	0.6	25	0
Cortisone	25	1	1
Dexamethasone	0.75	25	0
Hydrocortisone	20	0.8	0.8
Methylprednisolone	4	5	0.5
Paramethasone	2	10	0
Prednisolone	5	4	0.8
Prednisone	5	4	0.8
Triamcinolone	4	5	0

Note: These values refer to drug doses given systemically. This information does not apply to locally administered therapy.

*Approximate oral or IV dose needed to produce equivalent anti-inflammatory effects.

lowest levels at midnight. Serum cortisol levels can be drawn at different times but with knowledge of expected variations. The normal range at 8 AM is 7 to 25 mcg/dL, and at 8 PM, it should be less than 10 mcg/dL. However, the clinical presentation of the patient is a more reliable indicator of drug effectiveness.

Mineralocorticoids

- ❒ Fludrocortisone (FLORINEF)
- ❒ Desoxycorticosterone acetate injection (DOCA)

Indications

Mineralocorticoids are used primarily as replacement therapy for patients with adrenal insufficiency or with salt-losing forms of CAH. Fludrocortisone is the drug of choice for chronic mineralocorticoid replacement. It is potent, possessing significant glucocorticoid activity. In most cases, however, concomitant therapy with a glucocorticoid such as cortisone or hydrocortisone is required. In some cases of adrenal insufficiency, a glucocorticoid with a more potent mineralocorticoid effect is used alone when sodium and blood pressure levels remain normal.

Desoxycorticosterone (DOCA) is rarely used in chronic therapy because the most effective route of administration is intramuscular. Fludrocortisone, administered orally, has the potent sodium-retaining effect of a mineralocorticosteroid, as well as some glucocorticosteroid effects.

Pharmacodynamics

Mineralocorticoids affect the distal renal tubules, causing reabsorption of sodium and water and the excretion of potassium and hydrogen ions.

Adverse Effects and Contraindications

Mineralocorticoids are naturally occurring substances and, at normal physiologic levels, have no adverse effects or contraindications. Adverse effects are a direct consequence of fludrocortisone's mineralocorticoid activity. When the dosage is too high, sodium and water are retained, whereas potassium is lost. These effects on water and sodium can result in expansion of blood volume, hypertension, edema, cardiac enlargement, and hypokalemia. Cases of hypertensive encephalopathy and permanent brain damage have been described with the use of DOCA injection.

In children, treatment with mineralocorticoids can cause suppression of the HPA axis, leading to decreased secretion of growth hormone. Treatment is aimed at administering the lowest dosage possible to maintain growth within the 50th percentile for children of the same age.

Pharmacokinetics

Fludrocortisone is readily absorbed when given orally. DOCA requires sublingual, subcutaneous implantation, or IM injection to avoid first-pass biotransformation by the liver. Once they are absorbed, mineralocorticoids are highly bound to plasma proteins. Peak levels are reached in 1.7 hours (see Table 52–1). The plasma half-life of fludrocortisone is 3.5 hours, but the drug remains therapeutically active for 24 to 48 hours. Biotransformation occurs primarily in the liver, and the metabolites are excreted by the kidneys.

Drug-Drug Interactions

Drugs that induce microsomal enzymes increase the biotransformation of mineralocorticoids (see Table 52–2). Mineralocorticoids increase potassium excretion. When they are taken concurrently, non–potassium-sparing diuretics may cause severe hypokalemia. Patients who need supplemental potassium require greater than normal doses.

Drug-Food Interactions

Sodium content in the diet is monitored and adjusted based on clinical presentation of the patient. When mineralocorticoid dosage levels are relatively low, additional sodium may be necessary to maintain normal fluid and electrolyte balance. On the other hand, sodium restrictions are necessary when adrenal hormone levels are relatively high. Given the tendency toward hypokalemia, patients are not placed on a potassium-restricted diet.

Dosage Regimen

The adult dose of fludrocortisone varies widely from 0.1 mg two times weekly to 0.2 mg daily (see Table 52–3). The usual daily dosage is 0.1 mg. The pediatric dosage range is between 0.1 and 0.2 mg daily. Dosage adjustments are required to meet individual needs. If hypertension or fluid retention occur, the dosage is reduced.

Dosage must be reduced if hypoalbuminemia is present. Normally, mineralocorticoids are highly bound to plasma proteins, especially albumin. With hypoalbuminemia, more drug is free in the circulation and is pharmacologically active. This increases the incidence and severity of adverse effects if the dosage is not reduced.

For patients who are receiving chronic therapy, the dosage must be increased during periods of stress. Although what is stressful to one patient may not be so to another, some common stressors exist. Surgery and anesthesia, infections, anxiety, and temperature extremes may require an increased dosage of mineralocorticoid drug.

Many forms of synthetic adrenal hormones are available. The formulations vary with respect to pharmacokinetic properties (particularly biotransformation), duration of action, and mineralocorticoid and glucocorticoid effects. The oral route is preferred when mineralocorticoids must be given systemically. Parenteral administration is indicated for patients who are seriously ill or who are unable to take oral formulations.

Laboratory Considerations

Laboratory testing of serum drug levels is not considered practical. Drug efficacy is best determined by clinical presentation.

Critical Thinking Process

Assessment

The patient may present with signs and symptoms that are consistent with either adrenal insufficiency or excessive glucocorticoid levels. Therefore, the health care provider is watchful for a wide spectrum of abnormal findings indicating the need to maintain, reduce, or increase the dosage of the adrenal hormone. Glucocorticoid dosing varies from person to person and changes even for the same individual from time to time. A thorough assessment allows for more informed decisions to be made about the dosage required.

History of Present Illness

For the patient with adrenal insufficiency, the health care provider asks questions about changes in activity levels because lethargy, fatigue, and muscle weakness are often present. Gastrointestinal problems such as anorexia, nausea, vomiting, weight loss, diarrhea, and abdominal pain are also of interest. Salt craving is discussed because it is often a symptom of adrenal hypofunction. Female patients may report menstrual changes related to weight loss, and males may note impotence.

Past Health History

A past medical history aids in identifying potential etiologic factors in the development of adrenal insufficiency. The health care provider should inquire whether the patient has had intracranial surgery, or radiation therapy to the head or abdomen. Significant medical problems such as tuberculosis, diabetes, congestive heart failure, or peptic ulcer disease should be noted because these conditions may develop from or be exacerbated by administration of glucocorticoids. All past and current drugs are recorded, specifically the use of anticoagulants, cytotoxic drugs, or glucocorticoids.

Determining what the patient perceives to be a stressful situation and how that patient reacts under stressful conditions is also important. During periods of increased stress, the body requires additional amounts of adrenal hormones to achieve the same physiologic effects.

Physical Exam Findings

The clinical manifestations of adrenal insufficiency vary from patient to patient, and the severity of signs is related to the degree of hormone deficiency. Thorough assessment of the skin, mucous membranes, knuckles on the hand, areolae, and surgical scars is essential. Increased pigmentation, especially over skin folds and pressure areas, is a classic sign of insufficiency. With primary adrenal insufficiency, areas of decreased pigmentation may be noted because of the autoimmune destruction of the melanocytes. In secondary disease, there is no change in skin pigmentation.

Signs of hypoglycemia may be noted because of impaired gluconeogenesis. The patient should be assessed for diaphoresis, tachycardia, and tremors. With primary insufficiency, cortisol and aldosterone deficiencies result in volume depletion; therefore, the patient should be examined for evidence of dehydration. A deficiency of aldosterone may present as hyperkalemia with arrhythmias.

Diagnostic Testing

With adrenal insufficiency, laboratory findings may include a low serum cortisol, decreased fasting blood sugar, low serum sodium levels, and elevated potassium, and blood urea nitrogen (BUN) levels. Plasma ACTH and melanocyte-stimulating hormone levels are elevated because of the loss of the HPA feedback system.

Plasma cortisol levels are drawn at various times throughout the day and evening to determine whether the normal diurnal pattern of a rise in the early morning (peaking around 8 AM to 7 to 25 mcg/dL) and a fall in the evening (less than 10 mcg/dL) to almost undetectable levels near midnight is evident. Levels lower than expected suggest some form of adrenal insufficiency. Cortisol levels of less than 5 mcg/dL at 8 AM are considered diagnostic. Care providers should be familiar with the sleep patterns of the patient because the expected diurnal pattern changes when the person habitually works throughout the night and sleeps in the daytime.

It is important to note that although basal cortisol and ACTH levels may be helpful, definitive stimulation testing is required to confirm a diagnosis of adrenal insufficiency. Cortisol samples are drawn at baseline and again 45 minutes after the IM injection of cosyntropin. A diagnosis of adrenal insufficiency is likely if levels fail to rise at least 10 mcg/dL. Plasma ACTH levels are higher than normal with primary adrenal insufficiency.

Free cortisol and metabolites of adrenal hormones (17-hydroxycorticosteroids and 17-ketosteroids) are eliminated with the urine. Levels are reduced with adrenal insufficiency. On initiation of drug therapy, metabolite excretion returns to normal levels.

An electrocardiogram can indicate an elevated potassium level. Signs characteristic of hyperkalemia include peaked T waves, a widening QRS complex, and an increase in the PR interval.

Developmental Considerations

Perinatal Couples with a history of adrenal hormone disorders who are thinking about conception must consider the potential consequences to both the mother and fetus. Glucocorticoids taken for physiologic replacement therapy should not affect the pregnant woman or the fetus. However, maintaining exact physiologic drug requirements during pregnancy is virtually impossible given the increased stress and the physical changes of pregnancy (see Chapter 6). Glucocorticoids given in higher than normal doses may cause problems to either the mother or fetus. Relative overdosage with glucocorticoids causes sodium and water retention, resulting in elevated blood pressure and edema for some women. Possible blood pressure elevations and peripheral edema associated with pregnancy may be worsened.

Glucocorticoids are teratogenic in laboratory animals. However, no clinical studies on humans exist that demonstrate an association between congenital malformations and the therapeutic use of adrenal hormones.

Infants born to mothers receiving large doses of glucocorticoids are monitored closely for signs and symptoms of adrenal insufficiency immediately after birth. Supplemental doses of steroids may be required temporarily by the newborn. The health care provider determines whether the infant's adrenal glands can be stimulated naturally with the gradual withdrawal of exogenous steroids.

Pediatric Managing corticosteroid replacement therapy is difficult for younger patients because of age and need for physical growth. With suppression of the HPA axis, growth hormone is also suppressed. A delicate balance must be maintained between growth and delivery of adequate glucocorticoid replacement.

The most significant problem associated with glucocorticoid replacement therapy in children is the suppression of growth hormone (GH), resulting in failure of the child's growth to normal adult stature. When given as replacement therapy for adrenal insufficiency or CAH, the dosage is adjusted to approximate minimal levels necessary for body functioning. Although regulation of GH arises from alternate mechanisms, GH release is decreased with HPA suppression. Health care providers closely monitor the growth of the child, attempting to maintain the child's growth in the 50th percentile for similar age groups. Supplemental doses of GH are controversial but may be used during predicted high-growth periods to stimulate normal development.

Geriatric Administration of glucocorticoids to older patients pose many challenges. Although the pharmacodynamics of glucocorticoids are similar for both young and old adults, normal physiologic changes and pathophysiologic changes that are common with aging make monitoring for overdosing or underdosing difficult. Normal changes of aging such as weakness, fatigue, anorexia, and sparse hair are also seen in adrenal insufficiency. Slight-to-moderate immunosuppression, development of cataracts, redistribution of body mass, changes in vessel compliance, decreased glucose tolerance, alterations in gastrointestinal functioning, and thinning of the skin are also associated with normal changes of aging and may be difficult to distinguish from the signs and symptoms of adrenal insufficiency. Additionally, many older patients have pre-existing fluid and sodium retention associated with hypertension and heart failure. The added burden of glucocorticoids increases fluid and sodium retention, leading to further pathology. When used in the elderly, the corticosteroid dose is usually reduced because of the decreased muscle mass, plasma volume, hepatic biotransformation, and renal elimination.

Psychosocial Considerations

Depending on the degree of insufficiency, the patient may appear lethargic, apathetic, depressed, confused, or psychotic. The health care provider should monitor the patient for orientation to time, place, and person. Families may report that the patient has decreased energy levels, and is emotionally labile and forgetful. Such changes place serious stressors on family relationships (see Case Study—Adrenal Insufficiency).

Analysis and Management

Treatment Objectives

The objective of treatment for adrenal insufficiency is to reduce patient symptoms to a tolerable level. Reasonable goals for drug therapy should be set in collaboration with the patient.

Drug Variables

Adrenal insufficiency, whether caused by Addison's disease, adrenalectomy, or inadequate CRH secretion, requires replacement of both glucocorticoids and mineralocorticoids. Hydrocortisone and cortisone are usually the drugs of choice because they have greater mineralocorticoid activity compared with other glucocorticoids. If additional mineralocorticoid activity is required, fludrocortisone is most convenient because it can be given by mouth.

Androgens normally produced in the adrenal cortex are also limited with adrenal insufficiency, but generally are not replaced unless clinically indicated (see Chapter 53).

Treatment of CAH requires either adrenalectomy to halt androgen overproduction or corticosteroid therapy to suppress the HPA axis. Thus, the release of androgens from the adrenal glands is decreased and the missing hormones are replaced.

Treatment of secondary adrenal insufficiency includes the administration of either the hypothalamic-releasing factor (i.e., CRH) or pituitary-stimulating hormone (i.e., ACTH) that signals the release of adrenal cortex hormones. However, hypothalamic and pituitary hormones drugs are expensive and must be administered parenterally.

Patient Variables

Adult patients are maintained on fairly consistent daily drug doses once clinical signs and symptoms of adrenal insufficiency are stabilized. Periods of stress (physical and/or emotional) require increased drug therapy to sustain the metabolic functions of adrenal hormones. Patients with certain pre-existing medical conditions such as diabetes and hypertension may find regulation of both their adrenal insufficiency and other chronic conditions more difficult.

Children require frequent drug dosage changes as they grow. With long-term use, glucocorticoids impair growth and development by their action on protein and bone metabolism. Permanent stunting is unusual. Regulation of adrenal insufficiency and adrenal hormone replacement requires very close monitoring.

There are several guidelines for corticosteroid dosage during stress. For patients with upper respiratory infections (e.g., viral), any febrile illness, strenuous exercise, gastroenteritis with vomiting and diarrhea, or minor surgery, doubling the daily maintenance dose is usually sufficient. Once the stressful period is over, the dosage may be reduced.

If infection occurs during long-term glucocorticoid therapy, appropriate antibiotics are again indicated. Additionally, increased doses of glucocorticoids are often indicated to cope with the added stress of the infection.

If the patient must undergo anesthesia and surgery, even greater doses of glucocorticoids may be given for several days. For example, a patient undergoing abdominal surgery may require 300 to 400 mg of hydrocortisone on the day of surgery. The dose can be gradually reduced to the usual maintenance dose within about 5 days if postoperative recovery is uncomplicated. As a general rule, it is astute to administer excessive doses temporarily rather than to risk inadequate doses and adrenal insufficiency. Specific regimens will vary, however, according to the type of anesthesia, surgical procedure, health care provider preference, and patient condition.

Further, additional glucocorticoids may be given in other stressful situations as well. One extra dose of hydrocortisone (e.g., 100 mg) may be adequate for a short-term stress situation, such as after a traumatic injury, angiogram, pneumoencephalogram, or other invasive diagnostic test.

Intervention

Administration

Glucocorticoids, when they are used for adrenal insufficiency, are administered orally in the early morning and late afternoon to simulate natural glucocorticoid diurnal rhythms. Ideally, the drug is taken between 6 and 9 AM, with the second dose given between 4 and 6 PM. Patients who

Case Study Adrenal Insufficiency

Patient History

History of Present Illness	PK is a 4-year-old boy accompanied to the clinic by his parents. He is complaining of tummy ache, muscle weakness, diarrhea, irritability, and lack of ability to keep up with his 5-year-old brother in play. He has not been eating well for several weeks, and his mother believes that he has lost weight. For the last week, PK frequently asks to lie down and refuses to play outside with his brother. He complains of headache and, his mother states that he is frequently sweaty. The parents have seen no evidence of seizure activity.
Past Health History	PK has been well and developing normally until approximately 1 week ago. Other than insignificant acute illnesses, PK has been seen only for regularly scheduled well-child examinations. He has no known allergies to medications, foods, or environmental elements. Family history is noncontributory.
Physical Exam	PK is irritable but cooperates with examination. Vital signs are all well within normal limits for age except blood pressure, which is slightly lower than expected for age. Weight is down 2 pounds since last visit 2 months ago. Skin is smooth, warm, pale, and moist with elastic turgor with no evidence of infection or purpura. Normal male pattern hair distribution with no flaking noted. Lungs are clear to auscultation. Normal sinus rhythm with no murmur. Abdomen is slightly distended and tender to deep palpation in all four quadrants. Pupils are equal, round, and reactive to light and accommodation. No nuchal rigidity elicited wtih Kernig's or Brudzinski's signs. Gait is symmetric and equal with no ataxia.
Diagnostic Testing	Serum Na, 134 mEq/L; serum K, 5.0 mEq/L; Serum Ca, 12 mg/dL; BUN, 19 mg/dL; FBS, 62 mg/dL. CBC shows moderate neutropenia, lymphocytosis, and hemoconcentration.
Developmental Considerations	PK is more susceptible to suppression of the HPA axis and decreased secretion of growth hormone with treatment. The lowest possible dosage of glucocorticosteroid is used in an attempt to maintain PK's growth within the 50th percentile of children his own age.
Psychosocial Considerations	Because PK is not yet in school and stays at home with his mother during the day, adapting his schedule to allow for his increased appetite, nutritional needs, needs for rest, and administration of medication is not problematic.
Economic Factors	PK and his 5-year-old brother live with both parents in a middle-class neighborhood. The father works full time, and the mother is able to stay home with the boys. All family members are covered by an HMO through the father's employment. All prescription drugs are $5.00 per prescription, regardless of the drug cost.

Variables Influencing Decision

Treatment Objectives	• Replace adrenal hormones to prevent life-threatening consequences associated with the lack of naturally occurring corticosteroids.

Drug Variables	*Drug Summary*	*Patient Variables*
Indications	Glucocorticoids (GCS): Short-acting glucocorticoids are used in the treatment of adrenal insufficiency. Mineralocorticoids (MCS): Adjunctive therapy for adrenal insufficiency with glucocorticoids to avoid excessive water and sodium loss.	PK has been diagnosed with congenital adrenal hyperplasia.
Pharmacodynamics	Replacement hormones act similarly to naturally occurring hormones.	All GCS have similar pharmacodynamics; the only decision point arises if PK does not improve with one preparation; in that case, another will be tried. Fludrocortisone is the only orally administered MCS for chronic use.

Drug Variables	*Drug Summary*	*Patient Variables*
Adverse Effects Contraindications	Adverse effects of GCS and MCS occur with relative overdose. Adverse effects are lessened by keeping dosages at the lowest dose possible and administering early in the morning.	PK requires replacement therapy to maintain normal metabolic functions. If adverse effects occur, dosages may be decreased or other drugs used. Will be a decision point with signs of overdosage; may consider halting MCS. PK is more susceptible to infections.
Pharmacokinetics	All short-acting GCS have similar pharmacokinetics. Fludrocortisone is the only preparation available.	Because similar drug categories have similar pharmacokinetics, this is not a decision point with chronic therapy.
Dosage Regimen	As a replacement drug, GCS and MCS are given early in the morning and at 4 PM (if evening dose is indicated) to simulate the natural diurnal release of adrenal hormones.	GCS dosing is highly individualized. A decision point occurs with need to increase or decrease dosage. Dosages are increased as PK grows, during periods of emotional upset, with infection, or if surgery is necessary. Dosages are decreased with signs of relative overtreatment. Dosing with MCS is a decision point.
Lab Considerations	GCS and MCS affect the levels of sodium, calcium, potassium, nitrogen, and glucose. Serum drug levels are not a practical measurement of therapeutic effects. Baseline measurements and weekly monitoring is continued until pathologic signs and symptoms are resolved.	PK has normal hepatic and renal function and should have no problems with laboratory data as long as therapy is maintained at the appropriate level. This is not a decision point.
Cost Index*	Prednisone: 1 Fludrocortisone: 3	Since PK's medications are covered by an HMO, cost is not a decision point.

Summary of Decision Points

- Short-acting GCS are preferred in the treatment of adrenal insufficiency.
- Pharmacodynamics in general is not a major consideration. However, use of an MCS may not be necessary if fluid and electrolyte balances are maintained well with only GCS therapy.
- Determining the appropriate dosage of GCS is difficult when administered to a growing child.

DRUGS TO BE USED

- Prednisone 4–5 mg/m^2 po QD in divided doses q12hr
- Fludrocortisone 0.1 mg po QD

*Cost Index:
1 = $ <30 mo
2 = $ 30–40 mo
3 = $ 40–50 mo
4 = $ 50–60 mo
5 = $ >60 mo

AWP of 100, 25-mg tablets of cortisone acetate is approximately $47.
AWP of 100, 0.25-mg tablets of dexamethasone is approximately $5.
AWP of 100, 20-mg tablets of hydrocortisone is approximately $8.
AWP of 100, 4-mg tablets of methylprednisolone is approximately $45.
AWP of 100, 5-mg tablets of prednisone is approximately $4.
AWP of 100, 4-mg tablets of triamcinolone is approximately $9.
GCS = Glucocorticosteroids
MCS = Mineralocorticosteroids

routinely work during the night may need to make scheduling adjustments.

Education

Educational needs for the patient taking glucocorticoids are extensive. Patients must be aware that hormone replacement is a life-long need. In addition, a diagnosis of adrenal insufficiency requires significant participation by the patient in the treatment plan. By identifying potential emotional and environmental stressors, and discussing possible interventions the health care provider can help minimize crises. Careful attention by the health care provider to patient and family education may alleviate the anxiety that often surrounds chronic illness.

Patients and families are instructed as to the clinical manifestations and the possibility of overtreatment and undertreatment, as well as the occasional need to temporarily increase drug dosages during times of stress. They should also be taught about the need to avoid stressful situations where possible and to practice stress-reducing techniques.

Patients are instructed to avoid becoming fatigued, even if steroid therapy has resulted in increased energy levels. A normal exercise regimen is required to prevent excessive muscle wasting and to help maintain bone mass; however, it should be interspersed with adequate rest periods.

Patients with adrenal insufficiency are more prone to infections and are taught to avoid crowds and people with known infections. Treatment for even minor infections is initiated quickly.

Dietary needs are discussed, including the need for a high-carbohydrate, high-protein diet. Generally, potassium and sodium are not restricted. Dietary sodium intake should remain constant after the requirements for mineralocorticoid replacement have been determined. A shift of sodium intake in either direction would necessitate a concomitant change in the dosage of mineralocorticoid replacement. Abrupt decreases in sodium intake can precipitate an adrenal crisis. In climates where there is great variation in temperatures, mineralocorticoid dosage may need to be adjusted.

Patients should be taught that when drug levels are maintained at near-normal physiologic levels, no dietary alterations are necessary. However, should drug dosages exceed physiologic levels, patients may need to limit foods high in sodium to prevent fluid retention, edema, and hypertension. In contrast, patients with adrenal insufficiency who do not have adequate hormone levels may require additional sodium to maintain homeostatic fluid balance. Dietary adjustments are made based on the clinical presentation of the patient. Additionally, patients need to avoid foods that cause gastric irritation because the condition may be worsened by glucocorticoid therapy.

Occasionally, a female patient with primary adrenal insufficiency may experience muscle weakness or decreased libido. These symptoms are most often due to the loss of adrenal androgens. It can be treated with IM injections of small amounts of testosterone.

Patients should be instructed on the need to wear a Medic-Alert identification bracelet or necklace.

Evaluation

With adequate treatment, blood pressure and other vital signs stabilize; fluid, electrolyte, and blood sugar levels return to normal; appetite and physical strength improve; and weight is regained. Likewise, the patient has minimal to no signs and symptoms of overtreatment.

Patients are knowledgeable about the disease, appropriate treatment plans, and potential for complications. Finally, the patient is aware of the potential need to make dosage adjustments in drug therapy.

SUPPRESSION OF IMMUNE AND INFLAMMATORY RESPONSES

Epidemiology and Etiology

Autoimmune and Inflammatory Disorders

Pathologic conditions activate the immune system as part of the natural healing process. Activation of the immune system triggers the inflammatory response as a means of protecting the body and initiating healing. Unfortunately, at times, the inflammatory response can overwhelm the body, leading to direct tissue damage. Furthermore, the immune system can be activated inappropriately, as in the case of an autoimmune disorder. In autoimmune disorders, the body no longer recognizes itself. Thus, the immune system initiates autodestruction and elimination of its own tissue through various inflammatory processes.

Many pathologic conditions are associated with widespread inflammation or autodestruction. Inflammation usually has the most detrimental consequences. Among autoimmune disorders are asthma, chronic respiratory diseases, rheumatoid and collagen diseases, nephrotic syndrome, and dermatologic disorders.

Organ and Tissue Transplant

Medical therapy now allows for the replacement of defective body tissue or organs with healthy compatible donor tissue. The introduction of foreign tissue requires matching between the host and donor blood and tissue types. Unfortunately, except in special ideal matchings (i.e., identical twins and auto-transplantation), some incompatibilities always exist between the host and donor tissue. Incompatibilities initiate the immune response and destruction of the transplanted tissue.

Pathophysiology

Regardless of the cause or location of inflammation, signs and symptoms include localized or widespread edema, erythema, heat, pain, and exudate. Each symptom can be explained as a process necessary for restoration of the affected tissue to normal function. When the symptoms are prolonged or impinge on normal tissue and organ function, the inflammatory process becomes a pathologic consequence (i.e., severe pain, limitations in activities, altered functional ability) rather than the means to repair tissue.

Any time a foreign material is introduced into the body, an inflammatory response occurs as the natural means of destroying the foreign substance. Briefly, a large amount of plasma-like fluid leaks out of capillaries into the damaged area and becomes clotted. Leukocytes migrate to the area followed by tissue healing, largely by growth of fibrous scar tissue.

With organ or tissue transplantation, the body reacts to rid the system of the foreign tissues. The host body is unable to differentiate between therapeutic and pathologic invasion. Thus, the immune system reacts to defend the body against intrusion even if that means rejecting a vital organ.

PHARMACOTHERAPEUTIC OPTIONS

Glucocorticoids

- ❒ Betamethasone (CELESTONE, SELESTOJECT) (✽) BETNESOL, SELESTOJECT
- ❒ Cortisone (CORTONE); (✽) CORTONE
- ❒ Dexamethasone (DECADRON, DEXASONE, HEXADROL, others); (✽) DEXASONE
- ❒ Flunisolide (AEROBID)
- ❒ Hydrocortisone (CORTEF, HYDROCORTONE); (✽) HYCORT
- ❒ Methylprednisolone (A-METHAPRED, DEPO-MEDROL, MEDROL, SOLU-MEDROL, others)
- ❒ Paramethasone
- ❒ Prednisolone (DELTA-CORTEF)
- ❒ Prednisone (DELTASONE, ORASONE, STERAPRED, others)
- ❒ Triamcinolone (ARISTOCORT, KENACORT, AZMACORT, KENALOG, TRILONE, others)

Indications

Glucocorticoids are used for their anti-inflammatory or immunosuppressive properties to prevent, alleviate, or palliate the detrimental effects of the immune response and inflammation. Corticosteroid therapy is effective in the treatment of autoimmune disorders, prevention of transplant rejection, suppression of hypersensitivity reactions, alleviation of cerebral edema, and in many other disorders. For patients who have had a transplant, drug therapy is continued as long as the transplanted tissue is in place (usually life-long).

Corticosteroid selection is based on the desired effects of therapy. The specific type of corticosteroid therapy is determined by the disease occurrence and location of the body system most influenced, the route of administration, and the potential duration of therapy.

Pharmacodynamics

Glucocorticoids act through several mechanisms to interrupt inflammatory and immune responses. These drugs can inhibit the synthesis of chemical mediators (i.e., prostaglandins, leukotrienes, and histamine) and thereby reduce swelling, warmth, redness, and pain. In addition, glucocorticoids suppress the infiltration of phagocytes; therefore, damage from the release of lysosomal enzymes is averted. Last, glucocorticoids suppress proliferation of lymphocytes, reducing the immune component of inflammation. A decrease in the number of eosinophils and lymphocytes as well as a decreased production of antibodies result in immunosuppressive effects.

It should be noted, however, that the mechanisms by which glucocorticoids suppress inflammation are broader in scope than those of nonsteroidal anti-inflammatory drugs (see Chapter 15). The anti-inflammatory effects of glucocorticoids are also related to the synthesis of specific regulatory proteins. Glucocorticoids penetrate cell membranes to bind to intracellular receptors. The receptor-steroid complex binds to chromatin in the DNA of the cell's nucleus. The interaction with chromatin triggers the transcription of messenger RNA molecules that, in turn, code for regulatory proteins, thereby increasing the synthesis of such proteins.

Normally, physiologic doses of glucocorticoids probably do not significantly affect inflammation and healing; however, large amounts inhibit all stages of the inflammatory and immune responses.

In patients with asthma, glucocorticoids increase the number of beta receptors and increase or restore the responsiveness of the receptors to beta-adrenergic bronchodilating drugs. In asthma, chronic airway limitation, and rhinitis, the drugs decrease inflammation and mucus secretion.

Adverse Effects and Contraindications

Pharmacologic doses of glucocorticoids produce effects similar to normal activities of cortisol. Unfortunately, when given in supraphysiologic doses, in addition to the desired effects, unwanted responses are frequently seen. Many of the adverse effects associated with steroid therapy are natural consequences of high levels of the hormone. For example, signs and symptoms of Cushing's syndrome are similar to the clinical problems faced by people who take glucocorticoids for suppression of immune and inflammatory responses.

Suppression of the immune system with pharmacologic doses of glucocorticoids allows for overgrowth of infecting organisms. Subclinical infections may become clinically significant after the initiation of steroid therapy. Use of steroid therapy for patients with systemic fungal infections and herpes simplex is contraindicated. Use of corticosteroid therapy must be avoided in patients with known bacterial infections unless concurrent antibiotic therapy is initiated. Immunosuppression from glucocorticoid therapy in the patient with a fungal or herpes infection can lead to a fulminating systemic infection.

Use of topically administered glucocorticoids on an open wound must be avoided. Loss of skin integrity allows for systemic absorption and possible systemic adverse effects.

Glucocorticoids should be used with caution in patients at risk for infections and in patients with infections. They should also be used cautiously in patients with diabetes mellitus (they cause or worsen hyperglycemia), peptic ulcer disease, inflammatory bowel disorders, hypertension, congestive heart failure, and renal insufficiency.

Corticosteroid therapy is frequently associated with an increased prevalence of peptic ulcers. However, controlled studies show no clinically significant difference between patients treated with glucocorticoids and a control group treated without drug therapy. Perhaps the ulcerogenic potential of glucocorticoids is due to changes in the gastric lining, which thereby allows other factors such as foods and other drugs to cause damage. Therefore, foods known to cause irritation and pain for the patient must be avoided, especially during steroid therapy.

Glucocorticoids cross into breast milk. Exogenous glucocorticoids ingested by the infant from breast milk suppress the HPA axis. Therefore, mothers who are undergoing drug therapy are advised not to nurse.

Pharmacokinetics

When they are taken orally, glucocorticoids are readily absorbed in the upper jejunum. Peak plasma levels are achieved within 30 to 100 minutes. Parenterally administered doses are also rapidly absorbed, with peak plasma levels achieved quickly. Other routes of administration are not intended for systemic absorption; however, some systemic absorption occurs with any route. The onset of action after oral or parenteral administration is rapid, although resolution of inflammation may take 1 to several days to become clinically evident.

Glucocorticoids are highly bound to the plasma proteins transcortin and albumin. Only the unbound portion is active. Plasma half-life varies with different preparations and is classified according to therapeutic effects as short, intermediate, or long acting (see Table 52–1). Additionally, the biologic or therapeutic effects of these drugs last much longer than their half-life and are of greater importance when determining which preparation to use.

Glucocorticoids are biotransformed by microsomal enzymes in the liver. Commercially prepared drugs, such as prednisone and cortisone, require hepatic conversion to prednisolone or cortisol, respectively, to achieve glucocorticoid effects. Further, biotransformation by the liver conjugates the glucocorticoids with glucuronic acid and allows elimination by the kidneys.

Drug-Drug Interactions

Various interactions are possible among glucocorticoids and other drug therapies (see Table 52–2), especially when the dosage exceeds the physiologic normal range. Drug-drug interactions are discussed under the section on pharmacotherapeutic options for adrenal insufficiency.

Drug-Food Interactions

Patients receiving glucocorticoid therapy may be required to limit their intake of foods high in sodium to prevent fluid retention, edema, and hypertension. Dietary adjustments are made based on the clinical presentation of the patient. Additionally, patients must avoid foods causing gastric irritation to prevent the possibility of ulcer formation.

Dosage Regimen

The specific preparation used is determined by the disorder being treated, the route of administration, the projected length of therapy, the patient's response, and the personal experience of the health care provider. Different preparations are administered via various routes (Table 52–5). The dosage regimen for glucocorticoids necessary to achieve suppression of immunity and inflammation are included on Table 52–3. Occasionally, certain patients respond more favorably to one preparation than another. Thus, changes in the particular therapy may be necessary. Dose equivalencies were described in Table 52–4.

Pharmacologic doses, given orally, include amounts higher than the normal physiologic range and include a wide variety of dosages. Dosage must be determined on an individual basis from one patient to another. However, as a rule of thumb, the dosage administered must be high enough and given for a sufficient period to control symptoms. In general, therapeutic effects are achieved with 1 mg/kg/day of prednisone (or the equivalent) given in one to three divided doses. Owing to rapid absorption from the gastrointestinal (GI) tract, oral and parenteral dosages are equivalent. Dosage regimens include low dosages (e.g., prednisone 5 to 15 mg/day), moderate dosages (e.g., prednisone 0.5 mg/kg/day), high dosages (e.g., prednisone 1 to 3 mg/kg/day), and massive dosages (e.g., prednisone 15 to 30 mg/kg/day).

TABLE 52–5 ADMINISTRATION ROUTES FOR SELECTED CORTICOSTEROIDS

Agent	Routes of Administration
Beclomethasone	INH
Betamethasone	PO, IV, IM, IA, IB, ID, IS, TOP
Cortisone	PO, IM
Dexamethasone	PO, IV, IM, INH, IA, IB, IS, TOP
Flunisolide	INH
Hydrocortisone	PO, IV, IM, SC, IA, IB, IL, IS, TOP
Methylprednisolone	PO, IV, IM, IA, IB, IS, TOP
Prednisolone	PO, IV, IM, IA, IB, IS
Prednisone	PO
Triamcinolone	PO, IM, INH, IA, IB, ID, IS, TOP

IA, Intra-articular; IB, intrabursal; ID, intradermal; IL, intralesional; IM, intramuscular; INH, oral/nasal inhalation; IS, intrasynovial; IV, intravenous; PO, oral; SC, subcutaneous; TOP, topical.

Recommended dosing frequencies vary from regular daily doses (usually low dosage) of the drug of choice to intermittent dosing (moderate to high dosages). Many of the primary disorders treated with glucocorticoids lend themselves to intermittent therapy during periods of symptom exacerbation. Some patients may need drug therapy for a limited time. Treatment regimens are referred to as a "burst" or "pulse" of steroids. The patient is given a large dose initially and then slowly weaned off the drug. The burst can last from 7 to 10 days. A sample burst schedule is included in Table 52–6.

Laboratory Considerations

No particular laboratory test is available to monitor the therapeutic drug levels of glucocorticoids in suppressing inflammation. Clinical presentation is the best way of determining the efficacy of therapy. Laboratory testing to follow the progress of particular pathologies is appropriate in verifying the control of the primary disorder.

An in-depth discussion of ACTH stimulation testing is beyond the scope of this chapter. However, the test can determine if the adrenal cortex is able to resume normal functioning after a prolonged period of suppression and possible disuse atrophy. When evidence of HPA axis suppression is present, drug therapy continues, is when appropriate, the patient is weaned off therapy much more gradually.

Critical Thinking Process

Assessment

History of Present Illness

When adrenal hormone therapy is used in the treatment of inflammatory disorders or to prevent transplant rejection, the patient is questioned about the recurrence of symptoms associated with the primary disorder or rejection. The focus

TABLE 52–6 BURST SCHEDULES

Hydrocortisone Therapy—Used When Short-Term, High-Dose Therapy Is Needed, Followed by Tapering and Discontinuance

	SUN DAY 1	MON DAY 2	TUES DAY 3	WED DAY 4	THURS DAY 5	FRI DAY 6	SAT DAY 7
Morning	40 mg	40 mg	40 mg	40 mg	40 mg	20 mg	None
Noon	40 mg	20 mg	None	None	None	None	None
Evening	40 mg	40 mg	40 mg	20 mg	None	None	None

Methylprednisolone Therapy—Used When Changing to Alternate-Day Therapy

	SUN DAY 1	MON DAY 2	TUES DAY 3	WED DAY 4	THURS DAY 5	FRI DAY 6	SAT DAY 7
Morning	32 mg	32 mg	32 mg	16 mg	16 mg	16 mg	16 mg
Evening	32 mg	32 mg	32 mg	16 mg	16 mg	16 mg	None
	SUN DAY 8	MON DAY 9	TUES DAY 10	WED DAY 11	THURS DAY 12	FRI DAY 13	SAT DAY 14
Morning	16 mg	16 mg	8 mg	8 mg	8 mg	None	8 mg
Evening	None	None	None	None	None	None	None
	SUN DAY 15	MON DAY 16	TUES DAY 17	WED DAY 18	THURS DAY 19	FRI DAY 20	SAT DAY 21
Morning	None	8 mg	None	8 mg	None	8 mg	None
Evening	None	None	None	None	None	None	None

of specific questions to be asked is guided by knowledge of the signs and symptoms of normal versus abnormal function of the body system being treated. Judgments about the potential consequences of the glucocorticoids versus an exacerbation of the inflammatory disorder are made only after careful review of the patient's history.

Past Health History

Past health history, including allergies, drug history, concomitant disease, and activities to reduce mental stress, is important to elicit. Although glucocorticoids are given to treat allergic reactions, individuals can develop allergic reactions to synthetic steroid preparations. Determination of concurrent or recent drug therapy is important because many drugs use metabolic pathways in the liver similar to glucocorticoids.

Significant medical problems such as tuberculosis, diabetes, heart failure, and peptic ulcer disease should be noted because these conditions may develop from or be exacerbated by administration of glucocorticoids. All past and current drugs are recorded, especially the use of anticoagulants, cytotoxic drugs, or glucocorticoids.

Determining what the patient perceives to be a stressful situation and how the patient reacts under stressful condition is also important. During periods of increased stress, the body requires additional amounts of the adrenal hormone to achieve the same physiologic effects.

Physical Exam Findings

The health care provider is aware that any patient taking glucocorticoids may experience physical signs consistent with iatrogenic Cushing's syndrome but may also experience secondary adrenal insufficiency. Therefore, the care provider must be watchful of a wide spectrum of abnormal findings that may indicate the need to maintain, reduce, or increase the dosage of the adrenal hormone.

The physical exam focuses on abnormalities associated with the particular primary disease causing inflammation. Additionally, the physical includes an assessment of vital signs with special attention to blood pressure elevations or orthostatic changes in pressure. Measures indicating fluid balance status are also assessed, including neck vein distention, peripheral edema, lung sounds, mucous membranes, and skin turgor. Evaluation of eyes and vision for glaucoma or cataracts is performed for early detection and treatment.

Thorough assessment of the skin and musculoskeletal system is essential for anyone taking high doses of glucocorticoids. Physical changes resulting from glucocorticoid therapy include muscle wasting and weakness, redistribution of fatty tissue to central areas of the body (moon face, buffalo hump, truncal obesity), striae, thin and fragile skin that bruises easily, acneiform eruptions, hirsutism, and poor wound healing.

Diagnostic Testing

Patients receiving glucocorticoids for the anti-inflammatory or immunosuppressive properties will no longer exhibit the normal diurnal pattern of cortisol secretion. Thus, serum cortisol levels are not helpful in estimating the therapeutic benefits of synthetic steroids in suppressing inflammatory reactions.

Free cortisol as well as metabolites of adrenal hormones (17-hydroxycorticosteroids and 17-ketosteroids) are eliminated in the urine. Metabolites are elevated in 24-hour urinalysis when glucocorticoids are used for immune and inflammation suppression.

An ACTH stimulation test diagnoses HPA axis suppression after initiation and weaning of glucocorticoid therapy, and suggests an iatrogenic adrenal insufficiency. In addition to diagnosing hormonal disorders, laboratory and radiographic findings are used to assess the impact of the use of glucocorticoids on body systems. Glucocorticoids have a profound effect on electrolyte levels. Therefore, monitoring serum sodium, potassium, and calcium levels is essential. While receiving high doses of glucocorticoids, patients tend to retain sodium and lose potassium and calcium. Hyperglycemia occurs frequently, along with increased white blood cell and lymphocyte counts.

Bone density studies reveal the amount of bony matrix loss for patients receiving long-term therapeutic corticosteroid therapy. Upper and lower GI imaging aids in the assessment for potential ulcerations in the mucosal lining.

Developmental Considerations

Perinatal Adequate reproductive studies have not been completed with glucocorticoids to show an effect on female fertility. Increases or decreases in the motility and number of spermatozoa have been reported in some men taking glucocorticoids.

Use of glucocorticoids in pregnant women and women of child-bearing age requires weighing the potential benefits to the mother against potential hazards to both the mother and fetus. Glucocorticoids are teratogenic in laboratory animals. However, no clinical studies on humans exist that demonstrate an association between congenital malformations and therapeutic use of adrenal hormones.

Use of glucocorticoids in average and large doses causes water and sodium retention, resulting in an elevation of blood pressure and edema for some patients. For women with pre-existing elevated blood pressure or peripheral edema, the addition of a corticosteroid may potentiate the problem.

Infants born to mothers receiving large doses of glucocorticoids are monitored closely for signs and symptoms of adrenal insufficiency. The newborn may temporarily require supplemental doses of steroids. Efforts are made to determine whether the infant's adrenal glands can be naturally stimulated with the gradual withdrawal of exogenous steroids.

Pediatric When high doses of glucocorticoids are necessary to treat pathologic conditions in children, diminished growth is a concern due to HPA suppression. The result is failure of the child to grow to normal adult stature. Although regulation of GH comes from other mechanisms, GH release is decreased with HPA suppression. Health care providers closely monitor the growth of the child, attempting to maintain the child's growth within the 50th percentile for similar age groups. Supplemental doses of GH are controversial but may be used during predicted high growth periods to stimulate normal development. Dosing of glucocorticoids is maintained at the lowest possible levels, given on alternate days, and tapered off as quickly as possible. Children and adolescents experience body image problems associated with Cushingoid features and short stature.

Geriatric Administration of glucocorticoids in older patients poses many challenging problems. Although the pharmacodynamics of adrenal steroids is similar for both young and old adults, normal physiologic changes of aging and pathologic disorders commonly associated with aging make the use of glucocorticoids worse for older adults.

Psychosocial Considerations

Health care providers should question the patient about past experiences with glucocorticoid therapy to determine adverse as well as beneficial effects of the drug therapy. Questions such as did the patient feel better while under treatment, what therapeutic and adverse effects occurred, how did the patient feel emotionally, and what happened when the patient was weaned off the drug are all important in determining the patient's experience with glucocorticoids. If the health care provider suspects that the patient will not comply with the prescribed treatment plan, the issue is discussed with the patient and alternate measures for treatment also explored.

Analysis and Management

Treatment Objectives

Special care is taken to determine the risks and benefits of initiating glucocorticoid therapy in supraphysiologic dosages. Anti-inflammatory and immunosuppressive therapy is aimed at maintaining the lowest glucocorticoid dosage possible without the recurrence of symptoms of the original disorder.

Treatment Options

Drug Variables

The classic corticosteroid used for its anti-inflammatory effects is hydrocortisone (cortisol). A variety of other preparations are available with differing durations of action and potency. All have equal anti-inflammatory effects when they are given in equivalent dosages. Selecting a specific drug to use is based on the relative anti-inflammatory and mineralocorticoid (sodium-retaining) potency, as well as the plasma and half-life of the drug. When drug therapy is aimed at anti-inflammation and immunosuppression, agents with relatively less mineralocorticoid potency are desirable.

Patient Variables

Initiation of glucocorticoids in doses higher than the normal physiologic levels begins only after carefully weighing the potential benefits with the potential adverse effects. Patients with severe pathologic signs and symptoms associated with a disease process causing inflammation or overactivation of the immune response may require corticosteroid therapy to preserve life or functional ability. Perinatal, pediatric, and geriatric variations are considered before the initiation of therapy.

Intervention

Administration

Adverse drug effects are lessened by keeping the dosage of the glucocorticoid at the lowest level possible. Giving the drug early in the morning or using an alternate-day therapy (ADT) regimen is helpful in minimizing adverse effects.

Acute disorders requiring systemic glucocorticoids respond best to high quantities of drug given in divided daily doses, usually over 4 to 10 days. Once the desired response is achieved or the acute situation is resolved, the patient begins to reduce the dose. The first alteration is a change from divided daily doses to once-a-day dosing, usually taken early in the morning. If symptoms do not recur, the dosage amount is decreased further over a period of approximately 1 week, then corticosteroid therapy ceases.

Patients receiving single morning doses of glucocorticoids over a relatively short period of time (less than 14 days) can generally have the drug discontinued without weaning. If the patient experiences signs and symptoms of adrenal insufficiency, drug therapy may be reinitiated and weaning slowly continued over a longer period.

For patients requiring long-term corticosteroid therapy, ADT is the preferred choice of therapy. Only short-acting glucocorticoids (e.g., prednisone, prednisolone, methylprednisolone) are used for ADT. ADT lessens HPA axis suppression. Weaning to ADT is accomplished in a variety of ways. One weaning method suggests a once-a-day schedule. A dosage equivalent to 2½ to 3 times the minimal daily dosage is given on an every-other-day basis. Surprisingly, administration of higher dosages of glucocorticoids given on alternate days leads to fewer adverse effects than lower dosages given daily. When the patient demonstrates a tolerance for the ADT regimen, the dosage is gradually decreased while the patient is monitored for signs and symptoms of recurrence of the original disease.

When the glucocorticoid is injected into a joint or soft tissue, the patient is advised to limit activities involving the injected joint or tissue for 1 to several days. Limiting activities may be somewhat difficult for the patient because after injection, the affected area begins to feel better and the patient is tempted to return to his or her regular activities, causing additional stress on the tissue or joint.

Education

Educational needs for the patient taking adrenal hormones is extensive and not unlike that of the patient taking them for adrenal insufficiency. Patients are made aware of clinical manifestations for both iatrogenic Cushing's syndrome and adrenal insufficiency. In addition, the health care provider advises the patient of the possible psychological responses that he or she may experience during both the therapy period and the period of drug tapering. Some patients enjoy the benefits of therapy with minimal adverse effects, whereas others find the adverse effects an uncomfortable substitute for the signs and symptoms of the original disorder.

Patients receiving supraphysiologic doses of glucocorticoids for inflammation or immunosuppression commonly experience adverse effects consistent with iatrogenic Cushing's syndrome. The patient should be made aware that taking steroids may lead to some degree of HPA axis suppression.

Often patients regulate their own corticosteroid dosage based on personal responses and daily activities or stress levels. Patients are advised to maintain dosages at the lowest possible levels to achieve therapeutic effects. The health care provider should discuss the palliative nature of glucocorticoid therapy. Other treatment modalities used in the cure or direct treatment of the primary disease must not be discontinued because of improvement in physical abilities due to steroid therapy.

Evaluation

The best way to determine the effectiveness of corticosteroid therapy for suppression of the immune and inflammatory responses is by evaluation of clinical presentation of the patient. When treatment is effective, pathologic signs and symptoms of the primary disease are resolved to an acceptable level. Given the multitude of adverse effects of high-dose glucocorticoid therapy, an evaluation of the effectiveness of treatment is not complete until the patient has been assessed for the presence and extent of the less desirable effects of treatment. With proper therapy, dosages kept at lowest level, oral agents taken early in the morning, ADT when possible, and local administration versus systemic administration when appropriate, patients generally display fewer problems associated with therapy. Close monitoring for potentially dangerous adverse effects includes examination of skin integrity, bone mass studies to monitor density, laboratory analysis for early signs of infection, eye and vision checks for early detection of glaucoma and cataracts, and assessment of vital signs and fluid balance status.

CUSHING'S SYNDROME

Epidemiology and Etiology

Cushing's syndrome, or hypercortisolism, is a relatively rare condition characterized by the overproduction of cortisol, whether secreted by the adrenal cortex (endogenous) or administered as therapy for another clinical disorder (exogenous, iatrogenic). The condition affects predominantly women in an 8:1 ratio compared with men. The average age of onset of Cushing's syndrome is between ages 20 and 40, but it may occur up to the age of 60.

Excessive endogenous secretion may be caused by increased production of ACTH by pituitary adenomas (Cushing's disease); ectopic production of ACTH by a tumor in the GI tract, pancreas, or lung; or production by an autonomously functional adrenal tumor. Adrenal tumors are usually unilateral and are responsible for approximately 25 percent of all cases of Cushing's syndrome. In adults, approximately 50 percent of these tumors are malignant. The remainder of the cases are due to bilateral adrenal hyperplasia that is caused by pituitary or nonendocrine tumors that produce excessive ACTH.

Hypersecretion by the adrenal cortex also leads to hyperaldosteronism and excessive amounts of androgens. Hypersecretion by the adrenal medulla results in excessive secretion of catecholamines, of which 80 percent is epinephrine and the remainder norepinephrine.

Pathophysiology

Cushing's syndrome is characterized by an exaggeration of the normal physiologic action of glucocorticoids. Adrenocortical hyperplasia results in the loss of normal diurnal rhythms; a decreased responsiveness to prolactin, thyrotropin, and gonadotropin to their respective releasing hormones; and abnormal sleeping patterns. Although some of the changes are due to excessive amounts of glucocorticoids, others are linked to a yet unidentified hypothalamic abnormality.

Patients with Cushing's syndrome have a *cushingoid* appearance as a result of alterations in nitrogen, carbohydrate, and mineral metabolism. An increase in total body fat results from a decreased turnover of plasma fatty acids, and a redistribution of bulk to a more truncal pattern. Moderate to marked increases in the breakdown of tissue protein and a marked increase in urinary nitrogen levels occur. These changes result in decreased muscle mass with a proximal myopathy, atrophic skin, decreased bone matrix, and a loss of total skeletal calcium. High levels of glucocorticoids kill lymphocytes within organs that contain these cells, such as the liver, spleen, and lymph nodes. Thus, the immune response is reduced. In most cases, there is evidence of increased androgen production with acne, hirsutism, and in rare instances, clitoral hypertrophy. Increased androgen production also interrupts the normal pituitary-ovarian axis, thereby decreasing production of estrogens and progesterone from the ovary, causing oligomenorrhea.

PHARMACOTHERAPEUTIC OPTIONS

Adrenal Corticosteroid Inhibitors

- Aminoglutethimide (CYTADREN)
- Metyrapone
- Mitotane (LYSODREN)
- Trilostane

Indications

Although adrenal corticosteroid inhibitors relieve hypercortisolism in some patients, drugs are seldom the preferred form of therapy. However, several drugs are available to block the synthesis of adrenal hormones and are used for testing the function of the HPA axis.

Aminoglutethimide is used as a temporary means of decreasing excessive corticosteroid production in patients awaiting more definitive therapy (e.g., surgery). In patients with adrenal adenomas and carcinomas, or ectopic ACTH-secreting tumors, morning plasma cortisol levels are reduced by about 50 percent. The drug does not influence the underlying disease process. Therefore, once therapy is discontinued, excessive production of glucocorticoids will resume.

Aminoglutethimide has also been used to produce a so-called medical adrenalectomy in patients with advanced breast cancer and in patients with metastatic cancer of the prostate.

Pharmacodynamics

Corticosteroid inhibitors act primarily by inhibiting enzyme activity in the adrenal cortex and preventing the conversion of cholesterol to pregnenolone. In turn, the synthesis of all adrenal steroids is inhibited.

Adverse Effects and Contraindications

Adverse effects of corticosteroid inhibitors are common. Patients complain of nausea with abdominal distress, headaches, drowsiness, dizziness, and a morbilliform (measles-like) skin rash. Additional adverse effects include hematologic abnormalities, hypothyroidism, muscle pain, and fever. Masculinization may occur in females, and precocious sexual development may occur in males.

Pharmacokinetics

Because there is limited use of corticosteroid inhibitors, little is known of their pharmacokinetic properties. They are absorbed when they are taken orally and generally have a half-life of between 8 and 13 hours. Mitotane is the exception, with a half-life of 18 to 159 days (see Table 52–1). Biotransformation occurs in the liver, with metabolites eliminated by the kidneys.

Drug-Drug Interactions

Adrenal corticosteroid inhibitors can inhibit or promote the biotransformation of synthetic adrenal hormones (see Table 52–2).

Dosage Regimens

The dosage varies depending on the drug used (see Table 52–3). Patients are generally started on smaller doses and gradually increased as signs and symptoms such as abdominal pain lessen. Doses are increased until clinical evidence of Cushing's syndrome is lessened. The drugs are administered in divided doses throughout the day, usually every 4 to 6 hours.

Laboratory Considerations

No laboratory tests for drug effectiveness are available. Urine sampling helps validate the effects of therapy. Analysis of 24-hour urine samples for 17-hydroxyglucocorticoids and 17-ketogenic steroids reveals increased urinary elimination of corticosteroid byproducts.

Critical Thinking Process

Assessment

History of Present Illness

Patients with hypercortisolism present with a variety of complaints. The health care provider should ask about changes in activity or sleep patterns, changes in body appearance or skin integrity, or if they have fatigue and muscle weakness. Because osteoporosis is a common occurrence in hypercortisolism, patients are asked if they have bone pain or a history of fractures. A history of frequent infections or frequent bruising may also be noted. Female patients may report a cessation of menses, and men may report impotence. Mental symptoms such as emotional lability, irritation, confusion, and depression may be present and identified by a family member.

Past Health History

Past health history includes assessment of drug and alcohol intake. Excessive alcohol intake can produce clinical features similar to Cushing's syndrome. A history of chronic conditions (e.g., diabetes, hypertension, and renal insufficiency) may impact the disease process and drug therapy. Current drug therapy is important to note because of potential drug-drug interactions.

Physical Exam Findings

Physical changes associated with hypercortisolism can be extensive, necessitating an extensive exam of all body systems. The many physical changes can be disturbing for the patient. The most striking changes are the redistribution of fat to the center of the body (truncal obesity), the appearance of a buffalo hump, and a moon face. The trunk is large with thin legs and arms and the presence of generalized muscle wasting and weakness.

Characteristic skin changes include increased blood vessel fragility that leads to bruises, thin translucent skin, and delayed wound healing. Reddish purple striae are often present on the upper thighs and abdomen. A fine coating of hair over the face and body and the appearance of acne are also common. Coarse, thin body hair and balding in the temporal area may be noted, as well as hirsutism and clitoral hypertrophy (rare). In addition, hypertension is a common finding in patients with hypercortisolism.

Diagnostic Testing

Various diagnostic tests are used to identify the etiology of Cushing's syndrome, including radiographic studies, magnetic resonance imaging, and dexamethasone suppression test. Additionally, hypercortisolism has many metabolic consequences that may be identified through blood and urine testing. Plasma ACTH levels vary depending on the etiology of hypercortisolism. In Cushing's syndrome, ACTH levels are low to unmeasurable. In ectopic syndromes, the ACTH level is elevated.

In hypercortisolism, basal levels of urinary free cortisol, 17-ketosteroids, and 17-hydroxyglucocorticoids are all elevated. Urinary calcium, potassium, and glucose levels are also elevated.

Dexamethasone testing serves as an initial screening method for Cushing's syndrome. Plasma cortisol levels are measured the morning following a midnight oral dose of dexamethasone. Normally, plasma cortisol levels are less than 5 mg/dL. Further definitive testing for Cushing's syndrome is required if plasma levels are higher than 5 mg/dL.

The metyrapone test is used to assess HPA axis feedback responses. Metyrapone lowers serum cortisol levels and, therefore, stimulates ACTH secretion. A normal response is an increase in ACTH and 11-deoxycortisol levels.

Developmental Considerations

Perinatal Little information about the safety of adrenal hormone inhibitors and pregnancy exists. Women with Cushing's syndrome are less likely to conceive. If the disorder occurs during pregnancy, the fetus also receives higher than normal cortisol levels, resulting in potential negative consequences on fetal growth and development. Interestingly, treatment with metyrapone during the second and third trimesters may block enzyme activity, leading to adrenal insufficiency for the fetus.

Pediatric Cushing's syndrome has an effect on the growth and development of children. The physical changes associated with high levels of cortisol are particularly devastating for children and adolescents concerned with appearance. Little is known about treatment of children with adrenal hormone inhibitors and the safety of pharmaceutical agents is not well established.

Geriatric Skin changes associated with Cushing's syndrome are exaggerated in older patients. Excessive skin thinning, blood vessel fragility, and fat redistribution occur as a natural part of aging and worsen with high levels of cortisol. Older patients are also more likely to have other chronic conditions complicating disease progression and treatment.

Psychosocial Considerations

Hypercortisolism can result in emotional lability. The health care provider should question the patient about recent mood swings, irritability, confusion, or depression. Patients can become neurotic or psychotic as a result of changes in cortisol levels. Because the patient experiences a change in physical appearance, the health care provider should attempt to identify which changes are particularly troubling to the patient.

Patients with hypercortisolism experience extreme fatigue and require frequent rest periods. They may have trouble performing normal activities of daily living, thereby contributing to the potential for dysfunctional family relationships.

Analysis and Management

Treatment Objectives

The primary treatment objective for the patient with hypercortisolism is to control excessive amounts of cortisol and the pathologic consequences.

Treatment Options

Drug Variables

Drug therapy is used primarily for identification of the etiology and palliative treatment. Although all corticosteroid inhibitors have similar pharmacodynamic properties, the effectiveness of drug therapy can be erratic and less than satisfactory. Corticosteroid inhibitors can potentially produce signs and symptoms associated with adrenal insufficiency.

Patient Variables

Patients with concurrent chronic diseases such as diabetes and hypertension have fluid and electrolyte imbalances with and without drug therapy. The presence of comorbid disorders needs to be taken into consideration when planning therapy. In addition, patients may experience additional anxiety when the etiology of their signs and symptoms is difficult to pinpoint or when treatment options are limited. Treatment of children is extremely difficult given that the Food and Drug Administration has no established dosages for adrenal corticosteroid inhibitors.

Intervention

Administration

Adrenal hormone inhibitor therapy requires multiple daily dosing. Patients are started on smaller doses with increases to achieve desired effects. All preparations are administered orally, and dosages are decreased with the appearance of signs and symptoms of adrenal insufficiency.

Education

Patients are taught the signs and symptoms of adrenal insufficiency. Unfortunately, many of the clinical indicators of adrenal insufficiency are not specific, nor are they very different from those of Cushing's syndrome. Patients are warned of the sometimes erratic nature of drug therapy effectiveness and the possibility of recurrence in physical problems of Cushing's syndrome.

Evaluation

Therapy is considered to be effective when signs and symptoms of Cushing's syndrome are lessened without complications of adrenal insufficiency. Vital signs stabilize, serum electrolytes including glucose levels return to normal, and emotional changes are less disruptive. Often, surgical removal of the adrenal glands is necessary, but this approach, in turn, results in acute adrenal insufficiency. Adequate treatment of the adrenal insufficiency is required thereafter.

SUMMARY

- Adrenal insufficiency results in decreased levels of adrenal cortex hormones: glucocorticoids (cortisol and cortisone), mineralocorticoids (aldosterone), and androgens (testosterone).
- Pathologic conditions of the HPA axis lead to secondary adrenal insufficiency.
- Dysfunction of the adrenal glands results in primary adrenal insufficiency.
- Congenital enzyme deficiencies in the metabolic pathways of glucocorticoids lead to low hormone levels and CAH.
- Sodium and water depletion leading to hypovolemia, dehydration, and shock may become evident.
- Physiologic symptoms of adrenal insufficiency include weakness, fluid and electrolyte imbalances, hypoglycemia, hypotension, weight loss, nausea, vomiting, anorexia, abdominal pain, and mental status changes.
- Clinical manifestations of CAH are virilization of the female fetus and adrenal corticosteroid insufficiency in both the male and female.
- Glucocorticoid replacement is required to prevent life-threatening consequences associated with the lack of naturally occurring adrenal hormones.
- Allow for changes in dosages to reflect changes in stress levels of the patient.
- Treatment of primary adrenal insufficiency requires replacement of glucocorticoids and mineralocorticoids in some instances.
- Treatment for CAH requires either adrenalectomy to suppress the HPA axis or the administration of replacement hormones as needed.
- Extensive teaching about the medications and the importance of taking the drug daily at the prescribed times is required.
- Patients are knowledgeable about the disease, appropriate treatment plans, and potential for complications.
- Allow for changes in dosage to meet special physical and emotional needs such as stress, surgical procedures, trauma, and physical growth.
- Note any signs and symptoms associated with relative overdosing and underdosing of the medications.
- Autoimmune and inflammatory disorders activate the immune system as part of the natural healing process. The inflammatory response can overwhelm the body and lead to direct tissue damage.
- In autoimmune disorders the immune system initiates autodestruction and elimination of its own tissue through various inflammatory processes.
- Examples of inflammatory and autoimmune disorders include asthma, chronic respiratory diseases, rheumatoid diseases, collagen diseases, nephrotic syndrome, and dermatologic problems.
- The immune system is unable to differentiate between therapeutic (transplantation of a healthy organ) and pathologic invasion, and reacts to defend the body against intrusion even if that means rejecting a vital organ.
- Treatment objectives are to suppress the detrimental effects of inflammation and the immune response, and to lessen but not cure the primary pathologic process.
- Supraphysiologic doses of glucocorticoids are often needed.
- Local versus systemic administration of glucocorticoids are preferred when possible.
- After the initiation of therapy, the health care provider assesses the signs and symptoms of the primary disorder and also looks for physical and emotional changes associated with glucocorticosteroid therapy.
- Drug therapy is initiated in dosages high enough to cause suppression of signs and symptoms of inflammation.
- When possible, drug therapy is tapered and stopped when clinical effects are achieved for the particular inflammatory disorder.
- When long-term therapy is required, attempts are made to maintain the dosage at the smallest level possible, give the dose early in the morning, and administer on an ADT schedule.
- Clinical outcomes are noted to be successful when the signs and symptoms of inflammation are resolved.
- Cushing's syndrome, or hypercortisolism, is characterized by overproduction of the adrenal hormone cortisol.
- Etiologic factors include cortisol-secreting adrenal tumors and increased ACTH production from either the pituitary gland or an ectopic source.
- The most common form is iatrogenic Cushing's syndrome caused by excessive amounts of exogenous adrenal hormones.
- The physical appearance of patients with Cushing's syndrome is classified as cushingoid.
- Drug therapy is palliative to maintain fluid and electrolyte balance.
- Adrenal corticosteroid inhibitors are administered in increasing dosages until signs and symptoms of hypercortisolism are diminished.
- Therapy is effective when signs and symptoms of Cushing's syndrome are lessened without complications of adrenal insufficiency. Vital signs, electrolytes, and glucose levels return to normal, and emotional changes are less disruptive.

REFERENCES

Derendorf, H., Hochhaus, G., Mollmann, H., et al. (1993). Receptor-based pharmacokinetic-pharmacodynamic analysis of corticosteroids. *Journal of Clinical Pharmacology,* 33(2), 115–123.

Dyer, J. (1993). Drug watch. *American Journal of Nursing,* 93(10), 56–57.

Edwards, C., and Walker, B. (1993). Cortisol and hypertension: What was not so apparent about "apparent mineralocorticoid excess." *Journal of Laboratory and Clinical Medicine,* 122(6), 632–634.

Elsasser, W., and von Eickstedt, K. (1992). Corticotropins and corticosteroids. In M. N. G. Dukes (Ed.), *Meyer's side effects of drugs* (12th ed.). Amsterdam: Elsevier Science.

Hadden, J., and Smith, D. (1992). Immunopharmacology: Immunomodulation and immunotherapy. *Journal of the American Medical Association,* 268(20), 2964–2969.

Handerhan, B. (1992). Recognizing adrenal crisis: How to respond to severe steroid withdrawal. *Nursing,* 22(4), 33.

Hansten, P., and Horn, J. (1991). The top 40 drug interactions. *Drug Interactions Newsletter,* 11(1), 483–487.

Henriques, H., and Lebovic, D. (1995). Defining and focusing perioperative steroid supplementation. *American Surgeon,* 61(9), 809–813.

Holland, E., and Taylor, T. (1991). Glucocorticoids in clinical practice. *The Journal of Family Practice,* 32(5), 512–519.

Ismail, K., and Wessely, S. (1995). Psychiatric complications of corticosteroid therapy. *British Journal of Hospital Medicine,* 53(10), 495–499.

Lake, K., and Kilkenny, J. (1992). The pharmacokinetics and pharmacodynamics of immunosuppressive agents. *Critical Care Nursing Clinics of North America,* 4(2), 205–221.

Lepoittevin, J., Drieghe, J., and Dooms-Goossens, A. (1995). Studies in patients with corticosteroid contact allergy. *Archives of Dermatology,* 131(1), 31–37.

Marx, J. (1995). How the glucocorticoids suppress immunity. *Science,* 270(5234), 286–290.

McEvoy, G. (Ed.). (1995). *American hospital formulary service drug information.* Bethesda, Md: American Society of Hospital Pharmacists.

Milgrom, H., and Bender, B. (1995). Behavioral side effects of medications used to treat asthma and allergic rhinitis. *Pediatrics in Review,* 16(9), 333–335.

Payne, J. (1992). Immune modification and complications of immunosuppression. *Critical Care Nursing Clinics of North America,* 4(1), 43–61.

United States Pharmacopeial Convention. (1996). *Drug information for the health care professional* (16th ed.). Rockville, Md: Author.

van Burren, M., Boer, P., and Koomans, H. (1993). Effects of acute mineralocorticoid and glucocorticoid receptor blockade on the excretion of an acute potassium load in healthy humans. *Journal of Clinical Endocrinology and Metabolism,* 77(4), 902–909.

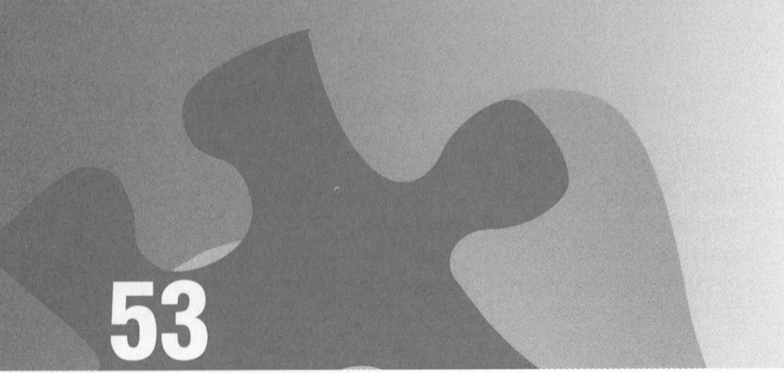

53 Androgens and Anabolic Steroids

Knowledge of androgens and their effect on male reproductive disorders increased significantly during the 1930s. Androgenic substances were extracted from urine, testosterone was isolated from the testes, and its synthesis was accomplished. Additional study of the androgens noted two distinct actions, virilizing activity and protein anabolic activity. Current knowledge indicates an overlap in the actions of androgens and anabolic steroids; each drug group possesses some properties of the other group.

HYPOGONADISM

Epidemiology and Etiology

Hypogonadism is caused by deficient secretion of testosterone by the testes. Hypogonadism, whether a result of chromosomal, pituitary, or testicular disorders, involves the nondevelopment or regression of secondary male characteristics along with a fragile libido and waning potency. It may be classified as disease in the testes themselves (primary hypogonadism) or as insufficient gonadotropin secretion by the pituitary (secondary hypogonadism). The distinction and differential diagnosis between the two disorders are essential to the choice of drug therapy.

Both primary and secondary hypogonadism may occur in the prepubertal or postpubertal male. Hypogonadism is commonly seen in primary care. It generally has significant effects on the psychosocial as well as the physical well-being of the male patient.

Pathophysiology

The testes are composed of two functional parts. The interstitium contains Leydig's cells, which synthesize and secrete testosterone, the principal hormone of the testis. The seminiferous tubules contain Sertoli's cells, which surround the germ cells that produce mature sperm. Testicular function is primarily controlled by the gonadotropin hormone, luteinizing hormone, and follicle-stimulating hormone, which are secreted by the anterior pituitary gland (Fig. 53–1). Luteinizing hormone binds to receptors on Leydig's cells to stimulate testosterone production. Follicle-stimulating hormone binds to receptors on Sertoli's cells and is important in the initiation and quantitative maintenance of spermatogenesis.

Gonadotropin secretion by the pituitary depends on stimulation by gonadotropin-releasing hormone, a protein produced by the hypothalamus that stimulates secretion of both luteinizing hormone and follicle-stimulating hormone. Pulsatile secretion of gonadotropin-releasing hormone and stimulation of the pituitary are necessary for normal gonadotropin secretion. Central nervous system activation and maintenance of hypothalamic secretion of gonadotropin-releasing hormone stimulate gonadotropin.

Prepubertal Hypogonadism

In prepubertal hypogonadism, more commonly known as delayed puberty, androgenic stimulation of undifferentiated embryonic tissues is deficient or absent. Lack of stimulation results in undeveloped and immature male sex accessory organs.

Prepubertal hypogonadism can be caused by deficient production of testicular steroids (congenital and acquired), insensitivity syndrome of target organs (e.g., receptor defects, 5α-reductase deficiency), deficient secretion of pituitary gonadotropin, deficient hypothalamic secretion of gonadotropin-releasing hormone, hyperprolactinemia, or other unknown factors. Onset of normal pubertal development is delayed. Male secondary sexual characteristics and behavior, accelerated growth, and the initiation of spermatogenesis do not occur.

Postpubertal Hypogonadism

Postpubertal hypogonadism is classified as either hypergonadotropic primary or hypogonadotropic secondary hypogonadism. Hypergonadotropic hypogonadism occurs as a result of testicular destruction (i.e., castration, radiation, mumps orchitis). Defects in testicular response to gonadotropin release lead to decreased secretion of testosterone and, as a result of normal feedback mechanisms, high levels of circulating gonadotropins. In the absence of adequate testosterone levels, spermatogenesis is impaired.

Hypogonadotropic testicular failure secondary to hypopituitarism in the adult is usually associated with complete destruction or removal of the pituitary gland. In this situation, gonadotropin levels are low because of feedback inhibition. In the absence of adequate gonadotropin secretion, Leydig's cells are not stimulated to secrete testosterone, and sperm maturation is not promoted in Sertoli's cells. Spermatogenesis depends not only on appropriate stimulation by gonadotropins but also on an appropriate response by the testes.

PHARMACOTHERAPEUTIC OPTIONS

Androgens

- ❒ Fluoxymesterone (HALOTESTIN, ANDROID-F)
- ❒ Methyltestosterone (ANDROID, ORETON METHYL, TESTRED, VIRILON); (🍁) METANDREN
- ❒ Testosterone base (ANDRO, HISTERONE, TESAMONE, TESTAQUA, TESTOJECT); (🍁) MALOGEN
- ❒ Testosterone cypionate (ANDRO-CYP, ANDRONATE, DEPOTEST, DEPO-TESTOSTERONE); (🍁) DEPO-TESTOSTERONE CYPIONATE
- ❒ Testosterone enanthate (DELATEST, EVERONE, TESTONE LA, ANDRO L.A.)

❒ Testosterone propionate injection (TESTEX); (🍁) MALOGEN
❒ Transdermal testosterone (TESTODERM)

Indications

The primary use of the androgen testosterone is in replacement therapy. In both prepubertal and postpubertal primary and secondary hypogonadism, for which the treatment goal is the initiation and maintenance of spermatogenesis, other drugs are given along with the androgen therapy.

Another therapeutic use of testosterone is in secondary or tertiary hormonal treatment for palliation of advanced inoperable breast cancer in women who are 1 to 5 years past menopause. Less common uses for testosterone and the 17α-alkylated androgens (fluoxymesterone and methyltestosterone) are based on their ability to stimulate erythropoiesis by enhancing renal and extrarenal production of erythropoietin. In the past, androgen therapy has been used in the treatment of various anemias (e.g., aplastic anemia, the anemia associated with chronic renal failure, myelofibrosis, and myelodysplastic syndromes). The advent of recombinant erythropoietin (see Chapter 41) has eliminated the need for androgen therapy in anemias.

The use of testosterone for idiopathic thrombocytopenic purpura, autoimmune thrombocytopenia in systemic lupus erythematosus, and classic hemophilia is controversial. Further, although androgens have been used in the past to prevent postpartum breast engorgement, to manage the symptoms of osteoporosis, and to enhance athletic performance, these uses are not recommended.

Pharmacodynamics

Testosterone produces both androgenic and anabolic effects by binding to androgen receptors in skeletal muscle, the prostate gland, and bone marrow. The binding of testosterone with its receptors promotes the synthesis of specific messenger RNA molecules. In some tissues, testosterone is initially converted to dihydrotestosterone in order to permit binding with the androgen receptors. Further, the hormone-receptor pairs serve as models for production of specific proteins. The effects of testosterone are evidenced through these proteins.

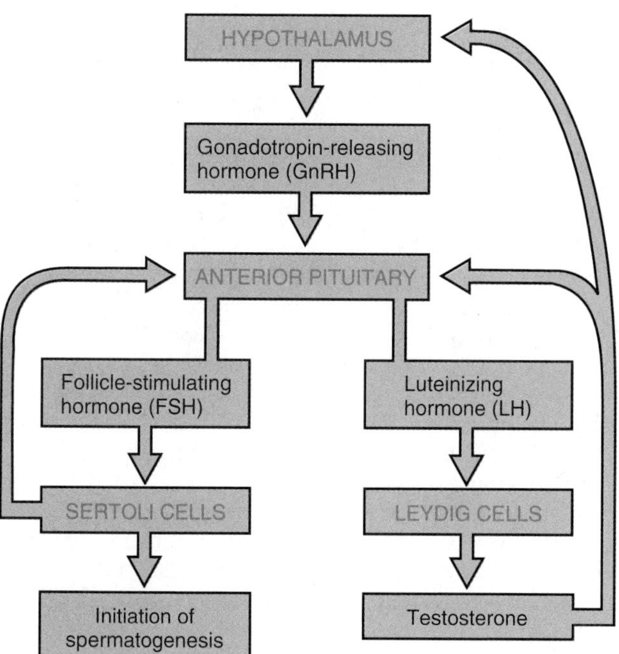

Figure 53–1 Testosterone production is dependent on an intact hypothalamus, pituitary gland, and Leydig's cells in the testis. Spermatogenesis requires both an intact pituitary gland and Sertoli cell function. The two feedback loops influence continuous hormone production.

Adverse Effects and Contraindications

Testosterone has many adverse effects. The central nervous system effects are headache, anxiety, depression, sleeplessness, and excitement. Adverse cardiovascular effects include edema (with fluoxymesterone and methyltestosterone), polycythemia, and suppression of clotting factors II, V, VII, and X (with testosterone and fluoxymesterone). Bladder irritability, vaginitis, nausea, vomiting, gastric irritation, diarrhea, jaundice, hepatotoxicity, peliosis hepatis, hepatic neoplasm, and cholestatic hepatitis (with methyltestosterone) have been documented. In prepubertal males, priapism (abnormal, continued, painful erection) and phallic enlargement have been seen. Premature epiphyseal closure, paresthesias, and acne may be noted in prepubertal males as well. Genitourinary adverse effects in postpubertal males include testicular atrophy, oligospermia, decreased ejaculatory volume, urinary hesitancy, epididymitis, impotence, and gynecomastia.

In females, clitoral enlargement may be noted. Alterations in metabolic and endocrine functioning include the development of hypercalcemia and, in females, facial hair growth, libido changes, a deepening of the voice, and menstrual irregularities.

The adverse effects of androgens are often related to dosage and duration of administration. Male patients who are receiving androgens for replacement therapy are usually minimally affected. However, female patients need to be monitored closely owing to the possibility of irreversible virilization.

These drugs are contraindicated in females during pregnancy (Category X), in patients with serious cardiac, hepatic, or renal diseases, and in those with hypersensitivity to the drugs. Men with cancer of the breast or prostate and patients with sensitivity or allergy to mercury compounds should also avoid androgenic therapy. It is not known whether androgens are excreted in breast milk. However, androgens would rarely be used by lactating women.

Pharmacokinetics

The pharmacokinetics of androgenic hormones vary with the individual drug. However, the onset of action of most intramuscular (IM) formulations is slow, and their duration of action ranges from 1 to 3 days to 2 to 4 weeks (Table 53–1). Testosterone is 99 percent protein bound. The formulations are biotransformed in the liver, and most have a half-life of 10 to 100 minutes, although fluoxymesterone's half-life is 9.2 hours. The cypionate formulation has a half-life of up to 8 days. Androgens are eliminated through the urine and feces.

Drug-Drug Interactions

The action of anticoagulants may be increased when they are given in combination with androgens. The synthetic oral

TABLE 53–1 PHARMACOKINETICS OF SELECTED ANDROGENS AND ANABOLIC STEROIDS

Drug	Route	Onset	Peak	Duration	PB (%)	t½	BioA (%)
Androgen							
Testosterone	po	Slow	UK	1–3 days	98	10–100 min	UA
	TD	Rapid	2–4 hr	22–24 hr	98	10–100 min	UA
Testosterone cypionate (LA)	IM	Slow	UK	2–4 wk	98	8 days	UA
Testosterone enanthate (LA)	IM	Slow	UK	2–4 wk	98	10–100 min	UA
Testosterone propionate (SA)	IM	Slow	UK	1–3 days	98	10–100 min	UA
Methyltestosterone	po	Rapid	2 hr	UA	98	2.5–3.5 hr	UA
	Buccal	Rapid	1 hr	UA	98	UA	UA
Fluoxymesterone	po	Rapid	2 hr	UA	98	9–10 hr	UA
Anabolic Steroids							
Stanozolol	po	Rapid	UA	UA	98	UK	UA
Oxymetholone	po	Rapid	UA	UA	98	9 hr	UA
Danazol	po	2 hr	6–8 wk	3–6 mo	98	4.5 hr	UA
Oxandrolone	po	Slow	UA	UA	98	0.5 hr; 9 hr*	UA
Nandrolone phenpropionate	IM	Slow	1–2 days	UA	98	UA	UA
Nandrolone decanoate	IM	Slow	3–6 days	UA	98	UK	UA
Anabolic Hormone Inhibitor							
Finasteride	po	30 min	1–2 hr; 8 hr; 6 mo†	2 wk	90	6 hr	UA
Antiandrogens							
Bicalutamide	po	UK	31.3 hr	UK	UA	5.8 days	UA
Cyproterone	po	UK	UK	UK	UK	UK	UA
Flutamide	po	UK	UK	UK	92–96	UK	UA

*First-phase and second-phase half-lives, respectively.

†Peak blood levels of finasteride, effect on 5α-dihydrotestosterone, and effect on prostatic symptoms, respectively.

LA, Long-acting formulation; SA, short-acting formulation; UA, unavailable; UK, unknown; t½, elimination, half-life; PB, protein binding; BioA, bioavailability.

androgens produce stronger reactions than testosterone (Table 53–2). Administration of imipramine with methyltestosterone may produce paranoia.

Dosage Regimen

The propionate, cypionate, and enanthate esters of testosterone should not be confused and are not interchangeable drugs. Their durations of action differ somewhat. The adverse effects of androgens cannot be quickly reversed by discontinuing these drugs, because of their long duration of action. The usual dose of testosterone enanthate or testosterone cypionate is 50 to 400 mg IM every 2 to 4 weeks. (Table 53–3). The preparation is oil based and is given deep in the gluteal area. Transdermal formulations (10 mg/40 cm^2 or 15 mg/60 cm^2) are available. Fluoxymesterone therapy is continued for 1 month to achieve a subjective response and for 2 to 3 months for objective effects.

Laboratory Considerations

Androgen replacement therapy should provide normal physiologic serum testosterone levels (300 to 900 mcg/dL or 10 to 30 nmol/L) as well as correction of the clinical manifestations of hypogonadism. Testosterone levels should be in the midnormal range 1 week after the first testosterone injection and should exceed the lower limit of the normal range immediately before the next injection.

Because of androgens' potential for severe hepatic damage, periodic liver function tests are recommended. In patients taking high doses of androgens, hemoglobin and hematocrit levels should be regularly checked to monitor for polycythemia. Serum cholesterol levels may increase during androgen therapy, particularly in patients with a history of coronary artery disease or myocardial infarction. Blood glucose and total serum thyroxine levels may be decreased. Free thyroid hormone levels remain unchanged. Increased creatinine and creatinine clearance values may last for 2 weeks after therapy is initiated.

In females with breast cancer receiving palliative androgen therapy, urine and serum calcium levels should be checked frequently, because androgens may induce hypercalcemia. Care should be taken, however, to note whether a serum and/or urine calcium elevation is due to androgen therapy or to bony metastases.

TABLE 53–2 DRUG-DRUG INTERACTIONS OF SELECTED ANDROGENS AND ANABOLIC STEROIDS

Drug	Interactive Drugs	Interaction(s)
Androgens		
Testosterone	Anticoagulants	Increased action of anticoagulants
Methyltestosterone	Imipramine	Paranoid response
Androgens	Oxyphenbutazone	Increased serum levels of interactive agent
	Oral hypoglycemic agents	Increased hypoglycemic response
	Insulin	
Anabolic Steroids		
Anabolic steroids	Anticoagulants	Increased action of anticoagulants
	Sulfonylureas	Increased hypoglycemic effects
	Adrenal corticosteroid	Increased edema formation
	ACTH	
Anabolic Hormone Inhibitor		
Finasteride	Theophylline	Decreased theophylline clearance
Antiandrogens		
Flutamide	Leuprolide	Synergism
Bicalutamide	Warfarin	Possible increased effectiveness of interactive drug

Newer Androgens

Subcutaneously implanted testosterone pellets are available in the United States but have not been used extensively. The pellets are more commonly used in other countries. Two to 6 pellets containing 150 to 450 mg of testosterone are implanted, with the intent that testosterone levels will be within a normal range in 4 to 6 months. The need for a minor surgical procedure to implant the pellets and the large number of pellets to be implanted have contributed to the unpopularity of this formulation. The rare possibility of pellet extrusion and the risk of local hematoma formation, inflammation, infection, and fibrosis have also contributed to its lack of use.

A longer-acting 17-beta-hydroxyl testosterone ester, testosterone buciclate (20-Aet-1), has been developed and is in clinical trials. Two testosterone transdermal systems are available. The matrix type involves the application of one 6-mg dosage patch to the clean, dry, and hairless skin of the scrotum every 22 to 24 hours. The reservoir type consists of a patch that may be applied to clean, dry skin of the back, abdomen, upper arms, or thighs every 22 to 24 hours. Patches are available in 2.5- and 5-mg.

Critical Thinking Process

Assessment

History of Present Illness

A principal aim in assessment of the patient with hypogonadism is determining the patient's perception of the illness or health problem. It is important to understand what concerns or symptoms caused the patient to seek health care. Eliciting from the patient the symptoms, their onset, and their duration is critical.

The adult male with primary hypogonadism may present to the health care provider with a history of infertility, reduced libido and potency, alterations in behavior (e.g., loss of motivation or irritability), and perhaps, some loss of secondary sexual characteristics. He may have noted decreases in axillary and pubic hair, muscle mass, and testicular and penile size, as well as changes in body shape that reflect a more "female-like" fat distribution.

Past Health History

A thorough health history is needed, because some chronic diseases and conditions may prohibit the use of androgens. For example, androgens are contraindicated in males with a past history of cancer of the breast or prostate. A history of hepatic, cardiac, and renal disease may also preclude the use of these drugs. Additionally, a history of prostatic hypertrophy and hypercalcemia may eliminate their use.

Information concerning current medication usage should be obtained, because androgens alter the effectiveness of certain drugs. Allergy or sensitivity to mercury compounds contraindicates the use of testosterone as well.

Physical Exam Findings

Physical exam findings of primary hypogonadism in an adult male may include feminization in physical appearance and atrophy of external genitalia. Reduced muscle mass and decreased axillary and pubic hair may also be evident.

Diagnostic Testing

Diagnostic endocrine studies are used to determine whether the suspected hypogonadal state exists because of a testicular, pituitary, or hypothalamic dysfunction. Evaluation and monitoring of hypogonadism consists of serum testosterone measurements. Testosterone levels fluctuate, generally being higher in the morning, so more than one assay may be necessary for careful evaluation. A low serum testosterone level is further evaluated in light of serum levels of luteinizing hormone and follicle-stimulating hormone. Luteinizing hormone and follicle-stimulating hormone levels tend to be high in patients with primary hypogonadism but low or inappropriately normal in men with hypogonadotropic hypogonadism. Patients with low gonadotropin

TABLE 53–3 DOSAGE REGIMENS FOR SELECTED ANDROGENS AND ANABOLIC STEROIDS

Drug	Use(s)	Dosage	Implications
Androgens			
Testosterone propionate	Androgen replacement	*Adult:* 25–50 mg IM 2–3 times weekly	Do not confuse testosterone propionate, cypionate, and enanthate; each has a different duration of action
	Delayed puberty	*Child:* 100 mg IM monthly for limited duration	
	Palliation of breast cancer in females	*Adult:* 50–100 mg IM 3 times weekly	
Testosterone cypionate	Androgen replacement	*Adult:* 50–400 mg IM q2–4 wk	Side effects cannot be quickly reversed by discontinuing drug, owing to its long duration
	Delayed puberty	*Child:* 50–200 mg IM q2–4 wk	For limited duration in delayed puberty
	Palliation of brease cancer in females	*Adult:* 200–400 mg IM q2–4 wk	
Testosterone enanthate	Androgen replacement	*Adult:* 50–400 mg IM q2–4 wk	Side effects cannot be quickly reversed by discontinuing drug, owing to its long duration
	Delayed puberty	*Child:* 100 mg IM monthly for 4–6 mo	Maximum dose 100 mg monthly
	Palliation of breast cancer in females	*Adult:* 200–400 mg q2–4 wk	Side effects cannot be quickly reversed by discontinuing drug, owing to its long duration
Testosterone transdermal	Androgen replacement	*Adult:* 1 patch daily (4–6 mg)	Discontinue after 6–8 wk if no results For proper dosing, a morning serum testosterone level should be used Potential for transfer of testosterone from scrotal patch to the female sexual partner, resulting in mild virilization
Methyltestosterone	Hypogonadism; male climacteric and impotence	*Adult:* 10–50 mg po QD	
	Postpubertal cryptorchidism	*Adult:* 30 mg po QD	
	Palliation of breast cancer in females	*Adult:* 50–200 mg po QD; 25–100 mg buccal QD	
Fluoxymesterone	Hypogonadism	*Adult:* 5–20 mg po QD	Monitor geriatric patients for evidence of prostatic hypertrophy and carcinoma
	Inoperable breast cancer in females	*Adult:* 10–40 mg po QD in divided doses	Continue for 1 mo for subjective response; 2–3 mo for objective response
Anabolic Steroids			
Danazol	Hereditary angioedema	*Adult:* 400–600 mg po QD initially. Maintenance: 100–600 mg po QD or QOD	Titration to lowest dose possible to prevent long-term adverse effects For maintenance, alternate-day dosing, or regimen of several days with drug followed by several days without
	Endometriosis	*Adult:* 100–200 mg po BID for mild cases; 400 mg po BID for moderate to severe cases	Treatment duration 3–6 mo
	Fibrocystic breast disease	*Adult:* 100–400 mg po QD in two divided doses	Treatment duration 2–6 mo
Stanozolol	Prophylactic use to decrease frequency and severity of attacks of hereditary angioedema	*Adult:* 2 mg po TID. Maintenance: 2 mg po QD or QOD *Child:* 1–2 mg po QD	Maintenance dose based on patient response Prophylactic therapy is not recommended in children, but drug may be used in acute attack
Oxymetholone	Anemias caused by deficient red blood cell production; acquired or congenital anemias; myelofibrosis; hypoplastic anemias due to myelotoxic drugs	*Adult:* 1–5 mg/kg po QD	Treatment trial period 3–6 mo Response not often immediate Continuous maintenance usually necessary with congenital aplastic anemia
Oxandrolone	Promote weight gain in medically related weight loss	*Adult:* 2.5 mg po BID–QID. Increase as needed to 20 mg po QD	A course of 2–4 wk is usually adequate
Nandrolone decanoate	Management of anemia in renal insufficiency	*Adult:* 50–100 mg IM weekly at 1–4 wk intervals for females; 50–200 mg IM weekly at 1–4 wk intervals for males *Child age 2–13 yrs:* 25–50 mg IM q3–4 wk	If possible, therapy should be intermittent

TABLE 53–3 DOSAGE REGIMENS FOR SELECTED ANDROGENS AND ANABOLIC STEROIDS *Continued*

Drug	Use(s)	Dosage	Implications
Anabolic Steroids *Continued*			
Nandrolone phenpropionate	Palliation of metastatic breast cancer in females	*Adult:* 25–100 mg IM weekly	If possible, therapy should be intermittent Therapy may continue up to 12 wk The required dose may be 2–3 times the amount needed for androgen replacement
Anabolic Hormone Inhibitor			
Finasteride	Benign prostatic hypertrophy	*Adult:* 5 mg po QD	A 6-mo regimen may be required before clinical response is noted
Antiandrogens			
Flutamide	Prostate cancer	*Adult:* 250 mg po q8hr	Given in combination with luteinizing hormone–releasing hormone analog therapy
Bicalutamide		*Adult:* 50 mg po QD	

levels may undergo further evaluation for other pituitary abnormalities, such as hyperprolactinemia. The hemoglobin and hematocrit values may be slightly below the normal male range owing to hypogonadism. The laboratory workup should include both urine and blood tests. Additionally, spermatogenesis may be impaired.

Developmental Considerations

Perinatal Androgens and anabolic steroids are not used during pregnancy because of the teratogenic risk.

Pediatric Hypogonadism in the adolescent male is usually not diagnosed until the patient reaches 16 or 17 years of age, when delayed puberty can be ascertained. At that time, diagnostic testing would consist of an endocrine evaluation to determine the specific cause of the dysfunction.

The adolescent male can benefit from androgen therapy; however, caution must be exercised, as androgens accelerate epiphyseal closure and may affect linear growth. X-ray studies of the epiphyseal area of the hand and wrist area should be performed on a regular basis, usually every 6 months, during androgen therapy.

Generally, in the prepubertal male with delayed onset of puberty, androgen therapy with testosterone is likely to be only one part of the drug regimen. Other drugs that may be used are luteinizing hormone–releasing hormone, human chorionic gonadotropin, and gonadotropin-releasing hormone.

Geriatric Administration of androgens increases the risk of prostatic hypertrophy and prostate cancer in elderly males. Additionally, chronic disease is more common in the geriatric population. Hence, the elderly patient with a history of liver, cardiac, or renal disease should be given androgen therapy with caution.

Psychosocial Considerations

Conditions that necessitate androgen therapy require a sexual history for an accurate diagnosis. The patient may be reluctant to verbalize such intimate concerns. A teenage male with diminished secondary sex characteristics may be embarrassed to share such information. Further, adolescents in general are striving for their own identity separate from that of their parents at a time when hypogonadism may increase parental involvement in their lives. Similarly, an adult male with decreased libido and impotence may have trouble expressing concerns, because the changes hypogonadism produces may be thought of as "normal" with increasing age.

During androgen therapy, virilizing and masculinizing effects are seen in both males and females. The changes in body image may be unwanted and may lead to lowered self-esteem and possible noncompliance with drug therapy. However, some of the adverse effects are reversible if the drug dosage can be reduced. (see Case Study—Primary Hypogonadism).

Analysis and Management

Treatment Objectives

The treatment objective for the adult male with primary hypogonadism due to testicular dysfunction is to restore sexual function, normalize behavior, and promote virilization. In prepubertal males who are androgen deficient, treatment interventions are directed at re-establishing and maintaining masculine characteristics and functions.

Treatment Options

Drug Variables

The oral androgens (methyltestosterone and fluoxymesterone) generally have weaker therapeutic effects than the injectable testosterone esters. Part of the reason for their lower efficacy is their biotransformation in the liver. Additionally, oral, sublingual, and buccal formulations cost more than intramuscular (IM) forms and carry a greater risk for adverse effects. The buccal and sublingual preparations have a bitter taste as well.

Injectable testosterone comes as short-acting aqueous solutions or long-acting solutions in oil. The short-acting solutions require more frequent administration—two to three times a week—and generally are not as readily available for use. The formulation of choice is usually a long-acting solution, which is administered once or twice a month. The drug of choice for the hypogonadal adult male is either testosterone enanthate or testosterone cypionate because of these agents' greater efficacy, lower cost, and longer duration of action.

Patient Variables

The major patient variable influencing androgenic therapy is compliance. The masculinizing and virilizing effects of the androgens may be an issue affecting compliance. However, if IM injections of testosterone are chosen instead of the oral synthetic androgens, compliance becomes less of an issue. (see controversy—Androgens and Anabolic Steroids: Not Just for Pro Sports).

Case Study Primary Hypogonadism

Patient History

History of Present Illness	AB is a 62-year-old male with vague complaints of decreased motivation and an inability to perform sexually for the last several months. He believes that his scrotum and penis have gotten smaller. He thinks this may be due to his age but wants verification.
Past Health History	AB denies history of cardiac, renal, hepatic, or prostate disease or carcinoma. No recent weight loss or gain. He exercises sporadically and takes no prescription or over-the-counter medications. States he does not like taking drugs in general.
Physical Examination	VSS. Decreased muscle mass relative to visit of 5 years ago. Relative atrophy of genitalia with loss of pubic and axillary hair. Prostate exam reveals 25–30 g bilobular organ. Other systems exam unremarkable.
Diagnostic Testing	Electrolytes, liver function values, blood urea nitrogen, creatinine, lipid panel, hemoglobin within normal limits. Serum calcium levels 8.5 mg/dL. Testosterone level 220 mcg/mL (normal, 300–900 mcg/mL). Twenty-four–hour urine for LH, 25 IU/24 hr (normal, 5–20 IU/24 hr). Twenty-four–hour urine for FSH, 30 IU/24 hr (normal, 1–20 IU/24 hr).
Developmental Considerations	Married male who may be at risk for benign prostatic hypertrophy. Adult children live in the same community.
Psychosocial Considerations	Concerned about what he describes as symptoms of "aging." Reluctant to verbalize specific concerns about sexual performance, but states he feels like "less of a man."
Economic Factors	AB belongs to an HMO with pharmacy privileges. Income derived from job in construction.

Variables Influencing Decision

Treatment Objectives	• Restore sexual function, normalize behavior, and promote virilization.

Drug Variables	*Drug Summary*	*Patient Variables*
Indications	Hormone replacement for primary hypogonadism.	AB's diagnosis based on clinical symptoms and laboratory studies. Low testosterone and elevated LH and FSH levels make this a decision point.
Pharmacodynamics	Drugs under consideration have similar pharmacodynamics.	Not a decision point, since patient variables have no direct relationship to pharmacodynamics.
Adverse Effects/ Contraindications	Synthetic oral testosterone preparations have a greater tendency to cause adverse effects.	Good practice to use drug with the least potential for adverse effects. This is a decision point.
Pharmacokinetics	Oral drugs have shorter duration of action than IM formulations.	AB will benefit from drug with a longer duration of action.
Dosage Regimen	Oral drugs need to be taken 2–3 times a day compared with IM formulations that are taken 1–2 times a month.	AB would prefer no drugs be used; however, IM route interferes less with life-style than po formulations; therefore, this also is a decision point.
Laboratory Considerations	Baseline complete blood count and liver function, and lipid measurements recommended; may be repeated in 3–6 months. Both IM and oral drugs may affect liver function, blood count, and lipid levels.	Not a decision point, but AB will need laboratory monitoring prior to starting therapy and then periodically throughout.

Case Study Primary Hypogonadism—cont'd

Drug Variables	*Drug Summary*	*Patient Variables*
Cost Index*	Oral androgens: 5 IM androgens: 1	Cost is a decision point. Oral androgens are much more expensive than IM formulations.
Summary of Decision Points	• Low testosterone and elevated LH and FSH levels confirmed diagnosis of primary hypogonadism. • IM androgens have a much longer duration and cost considerably less than oral formulations. • IM androgens are effective in treating primary hypogonadism with less chance of adverse effects.	
DRUG TO BE USED	• Testosterone enanthate 300 mg IM every 3 weeks until therapeutic response noted.	

*Cost Index:

1 = $< 30/mo.
2 = $ 30–40/mo.
3 = $ 40–50/mo.
4 = $ 50–60/mo.
5 = $> 60/mo.

AWP of 100, 10-mg tablets of methyltestosterone is approximately $25.
AWP of 100, 10-mg tablets of fluoxymesterone is approximately $111.
AWP of 10mL of 100 mg/mL injectable testosterone cypionate is approximately $15.
AWP of 10mL of 100 mg/mL injectable testosterone enanthate is approximately $15.

Intervention

Administration

Oral androgen preparations should be administered with food to decrease the possibility of gastric distress. IM injections of androgens should be given deep into the gluteal muscle using a Z-track technique.

The transdermal formulation of testosterone should be worn on a shaved area of the scrotum for 22 hours a day. Chemical depilatories should not be used to remove hair from the scrotal surface before application of the transdermal patch. A new patch is applied daily. There is a potential for transfer of testosterone from the scrotal patch to a female sexual partner, who may be affected by mild virilization.

Education

Owing to the virilizing and masculinizing effects of androgens, patients need a full understanding of the potential changes in secondary sex characteristics that may accompany therapy. Health care providers should be sensitive to the emotional responses of both male and female patients to therapy. The patient should be instructed to discuss his/her emotional responses to a changing body image with the health care provider. The changes that do occur should be monitored, because some changes may necessitate a reduction in dosage or discontinuation of the drug.

Patients should be made aware of the importance of follow-up supervision by the health care provider. Laboratory tests must be performed periodically to monitor response to therapy.

Patient teaching should also include information about the possibility of fluid retention with both oral and IM testosterone formulations. The fluid retention requires the patient to monitor body weight on a regular basis. A weight gain of more than 2 lb per week should be reported to the health care provider. The patient may need instruction regarding dietary sodium restriction and/or the use of diuretics. Patients also must be taught that if a dose of an orally administered androgen is missed, the next dose should not be doubled to correct the omission.

Evaluation

The efficacy of androgen replacement therapy is assessed primarily by monitoring the patient's clinical response. Although there is variability in response, most men experience an awakening of libido, resumption of sexual activity, and improved sense of well-being 1 to 2 months after androgen therapy is started. Whether therapy continues depends on the patient's symptoms.

HEREDITARY ANGIOEDEMA

In 1882, Sir William Osler described the features of hereditary angioedema (HAE) that occurred in five generations of a family. Osler had observed abdominal pain and both cutaneous and laryngeal edema in one family. Concluding that the symptoms were all one disorder, he com-

Controversy

Androgens and Anabolic Steroids: Not Just in Pro-Sports
JONATHAN J. WOLFE

The emergence of abuse patterns has led many states to classify steroids as controlled substances. This is a reasonable response to a class of drugs whose role in therapy is limited, but whose potential for abuse is high. It is a sad fact that those who divert androgens and anabolic steroids reap monstrous profits from willing users desirous of enhancing athletic prowess. Even more appalling is the choice by some coaches, who have been entrusted to develop athletic skill among adolescents and young adults, to suggest using these products as adjuncts to strength training. The scandal attached to such practices in former Soviet Block countries related to their development of Olympic athletes seems to have lost its ability to chasten current athletes and trainers worldwide.

Body builders and sculptors of both sexes are also susceptible to the temptation to use androgens and steroids. Human growth hormone has also sparked the interest of those seeking larger and more impressive stature. It seems an unproductive quest to challenge such trends in a society that reveres physique and an advertising industry that links physical attributes to the promotion of every sort of consumable product.

However, health care practitioners increasingly see the regrettable effects of these bad choices. The human skeleton was not designed to carry the mass of a 340-pound (155 kg) lineman. Knees and hips racked by arthritis are poor 30th birthday presents. The cardiac damage brought on by bulk-up diets and the fluid retention attributable to steroid use shortens life and diminishes its quality. Concentration on physical development toward unattainable and artificial standards curses those who abuse this class of drugs as well as others who fast and purge to attain an unrealistically slender body. The abuse of physical conditioning with or without steroids is a public health issue.

Critical Thinking Discussion

- Your local high school football team regularly fields junior and senior defensive linemen weighing over 240 pounds. You have known these boys as normal-sized junior high school students. What techniques may they be using under proper supervision to achieve such mass? Are these players likely to resist using anabolic steroids if a trainer or older student role model offers them?
- Androgenic steroids produce gynecomastia and testicular atrophy in a significant number of abusers. What further history should you elicit when examining a 17-year-old athlete before fall football camp, when you note that this 220-pound young man was normomastic a year ago but now presents with obvious gynecomastia? He denies using marijuana.
- You have been asked to make a presentation about the hazards of steroid abuse to a 7th grade class at your local junior high school. Your information includes coverage of the drugs banned by the International Olympic Committee. One young man challenges you, asserting that he intends to become a professional ball player, adding: "You can't make it for college scholarships or in the pros if you aren't man enough to do whatever it takes to be the strongest and the fastest!"

mented on its hereditary nature. It was determined in 1917 that HAE is inherited as an autosomal dominant trait.

Not until 1962 was more definitive work performed on this disorder. It was determined at that time that HAE results from a deficiency in the inhibition of complement. The causative factor, a low level of C1 esterase inhibitor (C1 INH), was discovered in 1963.

Epidemiology and Etiology

HAE accounts for only 2 percent of clinical angioedema. It is estimated that HAE occurs in 1:50,000 to 1:150,000 individuals. One-half of those affected have had significant symptomatology by age 7 years, and two-thirds by adolescence.

Pathophysiology

As an immune response is initiated, reactions are triggered that enhance or expand the patient's original response to an antigen. The complement system consists of a group of sequentially acting proteins, C1 through C9, in the globulin portion of serum. Two activating systems, called the classic and alternative pathways, lead to a final common pathway that operates in cell lysis and stimulates the release of inflammatory mediators. The classic pathway is usually activated by antigen-antibody complexes, but C1, its first component, can also be activated by a variety of serum proteins.

C1 esterase inhibitor (C1 INH) is one of a group of serum protease inhibitors from the serpin family. Other examples of this group are antithrombin III, alpha$_1$-antitrypsin, and angiotensinogen. The proteins react with and inactivate their target proteases. Activated C1 esterase is the target for which C1 INH is named. The primary function of the inhibitor is to act as a regulatory brake on the complement activation process. C1 INH is the initial mediator in the classic complement pathway and is a major inhibitor of several steps of the formation of bradykinin as well.

An autosomal dominant disorder, HAE results from a genetic deficiency of functional C1 esterase inhibitor. C1 INH deficiency allows unopposed activation of the first component of complement, with the subsequent breakdown of its two substrates, C2 and C4. With this deficiency, there is a local release of vasoactive peptides and greater vascular permeability.

Two types of HAE exist, but they have essentially the same phenotype. In the predominant type I form—accounting for about 80 percent of all cases—there is a lack of production of C1 INH synthesis because of the faulty gene, with low serum levels. Twenty percent of individuals have type II HAE, which manifests as normal production of nonfunctional C1 INH. The gene for C1 INH has been mapped on chromosome 11 in the q13 region.

PHARMACOTHERAPEUTIC OPTIONS

Anabolic Steroids

- ❒ Danazol (DANOCRINE); (🍁) CYCLOMEN
- ❒ Nandrolone phenpropionate injection (DURABOLIN, NANDROBOLIC, HYBOLIN IMPROVED)
- ❒ Nandrolone decanoate (DECA-DURABOLIN, HYBOLIN DECANOATE, NEO-DURABOLIC, ANDROLONE-D, KABOLIN)
- ❒ Oxandrolone (OXANDRIN); (🍁) ANAPOLON
- ❒ Oxymetholone (ANADROL-50)
- ❒ Stanozolol (WINSTROL)

Indications

There are several indications for the use of anabolic steroids (attenuated androgens), including HAE, endometriosis, and fibrocystic breast disease. Less commonly, these agents are used in palliation of metastatic breast cancer (without hypercalcemia) and for treatment of anemias caused by deficiencies in red blood cell production. Anabolic steroids are unacceptable for use in patients with osteoporosis or alcoholic hepatitis.

Pharmacodynamics

Anabolic steroids, which resemble testosterone, promote anabolic (rather than catabolic) activity by blocking cortisol uptake in muscle and liver cells. Cortisol normally acts as a catabolic agent, but by blocking cortisol uptake in muscle cells, anabolic steroids reduce muscle breakdown and increase muscle mass. When cortisol uptake is blocked in liver cells, the action of cortisol on the body's stress response is affected. Additionally, these drugs decrease plasma protein synthesis in the liver and enhance their effects by increasing the amount of free drug in the plasma. The mechanism of action of the anabolic steroids in HAE is still unclear, but they appear to raise C1 inhibitor activity and C4 serum concentrations by increasing the hepatic synthesis of C1 INH.

Adverse Effects and Contraindications

Like the androgens, anabolic steroids have a number of adverse effects. Excitement, insomnia, habituation, and depression are manifestations of central nervous system involvement. Gastrointestinal and genitourinary adverse effects are nausea, vomiting, diarrhea, cholestatic jaundice, hepatic necrosis, hepatocellular neoplasms, peliosis hepatis (with long-term therapy), and death. Endocrine effects in prepubertal males include phallic enlargement and greater frequency of erections; in the postpubertal male, acne, inhibition of testicular function with oligospermia, gynecomastia, testicular atrophy, chronic priapism, epididymitis, bladder irritability, change in libido, and impotence may occur. In females, hirsutism, acne, hoarseness or a deepening of the voice, clitoral enlargement, changes in libido, menstrual irregularities, and male-pattern baldness have been noted. Other adverse effects of anabolic steroids are fluid retention and edema. Patients with seizure disorders may note increased activity.

Use of anabolic steroids in all pregnant (Category X) and lactating females and in male patients with hormone-dependent cancers (breast or prostatic) is contraindicated. Other contraindications are any use that is intended to enhance physical appearance or athletic performance, the presence of nephrosis or the nephrotic phase of nephritis, and in females with cancer of the breast who have accompanying hypercalcemia. Anabolic steroids are controlled substances, listed under Schedule III of the Controlled Substances Act. Although nonprescription sale of the drugs is illegal, they are readily available.

Pharmacokinetics

Anabolic steroids vary in onset from slow to rapid (see Table 53–1). Their peak and duration of action are unknown, as are the half-life and percentage of protein binding. It is known that these drugs are widely distributed, are biotransformed in the liver, and are eliminated in the urine.

Drug-Drug Interactions

The concurrent use of anticoagulants and anabolic steroids may potentiate anticoagulant activity (see Table 53–2). The hypoglycemic action of sulfonylureas may increase when they are taken in conjunction with anabolic steroids. Administration of the anabolic steroids with an adrenal steroid or adrenocorticotropic hormone may exacerbate edema.

Dosage Regimen

Dosage regimens for patients taking anabolic steroids for therapeutic reasons vary with the specific use (see Table 53–3). In most cases, intermittent therapy is desirable. Titration to the lowest possible dose helps prevent long-term adverse effects. Response to recommended regimens is slow; it is often weeks to months before therapeutic efficacy is noted.

Laboratory Considerations

Anabolic steroids may influence the results of laboratory tests. Laboratory values that may rise in the presence of anabolic steroids are Bromsulphalein test results and aspartate transaminase (serum glutamic-oxaloacetic transaminase), alanine transaminase (serum glutamate pyruvate transaminase), serum bilirubin, and alkaline phosphatase measurements. Cholesterol levels and prothrombin times may increase because of suppression of clotting factors II, V, VII, and X. Low-density lipoprotein levels and resin uptake of triiodothyronine and thyroxine also increase.

Laboratory values that may decrease in the presence of anabolic steroids are serum high-density lipoprotein and protein-bound iodine levels, thyroxine-binding capacity, and radioactive iodine uptake. Free thyroxine levels remain normal.

Other laboratory tests whose results are altered by anabolic steroid therapy are the metyrapone test (serum, plasma, or urine cortisol) and glucose tolerance test. Creatinine and creatine excretion may also increase.

Critical Thinking Process

Assessment

History of Present Illness

Patients with HAE may report swelling of the face and extremities lasting 2 to 3 days with no known precipitating factor. Occasionally, patients present with crampy abdominal pain accompanied by watery diarrhea and, in extreme cases, partial to complete airway obstruction.

Past Health History

The clinical history of the patient with HAE varies greatly, making a diagnosis difficult. Diagnosis of HAE is suspected if there is a positive family history of the disease. Other support for the diagnosis includes a history of attacks of swelling and unexplained abdominal colic. A patient's age at the time of the initial attack is of little help in making the diagnosis. In most patients, the initial episode occurred in early childhood; however, a few patients with HAE have their first attack between the ages of 50 and 70 years. Some patients have weekly attacks, whereas others have occasional attacks spread over several decades.

Case Study Hereditary Angioedema

Patient History

History of Present Illness	JK, a 30-year-old female, reports swelling of her extremities, lips, and periorbital area. This attack of swelling has lasted 2 days. Several months ago, she had a similar episode that lasted for "several" days and included abdominal cramping and diarrhea.
Past Health History	Unremarkable. JK reports that she remembers her maternal aunts having occasional swelling of the face. Takes no medication at present time but has documented history of compliance with medications.
Physical Exam	VSS. Physical exam unremarkable except for obvious edema of periorbital region and arms, with mild swelling in lower extremities.
Diagnostic Testing	Routine blood work within normal limits. hCG negative. C4 complement level 8 mg/dL (normal, 10–30 mg/dL). C1 INH level 4 mg/dL (normal 8–24 mg/dL).
Developmental Considerations	JK never married but is raising her sister's children.
Psychosocial Considerations	Patient expresses normal concern about the unknown.
Economic Factors	JK's income is "satisfactory for my needs," although she does not have pharmacy insurance through her employer.

Variables Influencing Decision

Treatment Objectives	• To decrease the frequency and severity of attacks of hereditary angioedema (HAE).

Drug Variables	*Drug Summary*	*Patient Variables*
Indications	To decrease the frequency and severity of attacks of HAE.	JK diagnosed with type I HAE on basis of clinical symptoms and lab work. This will become a decision point.
Pharmacodynamics	All anabolic steroids under consideration have similar pharmacodynamics. Stanozolol has lower androgen:anabolic ratio than danazol.	JK has no variables that become a decision point.
Adverse Effects/ Contraindications	All anabolic steroids have similar adverse effects; however, stanozolol demonstrates less androgenic action.	Will be a decision point, because JK wants to minimize the masculinizing effects of treatment.
Pharmacokinetics	Similar for all anabolic steroids.	Not a decision point for JK.
Dosage Regimen	Drugs available in oral and IM formulations. This is a decision point.	JK is a responsible, working female. Noncompliance is not an anticipated problem. Long-term therapy may or may not be indicated.
Laboratory Considerations	Baseline complete blood count and measurements of liver function and lipids recommended; may be repeated in 3–6 months.	This is not a decision point. All anabolic steroids require periodic follow-up lab work during treatment. JK has history of keeping appointments.
Cost Index*	Stanozolol: 1 Danazol: 5	Cost is a decision point. JK does not have pharmacy insurance.

Summary of Decision Points	• JK diagnosed with type I HAE. • JK wants to minimize masculinizing effects of treatment. • Decision regarding use of oral versus IM formulation. • Stanozolol demonstrates less androgenic effect than danazol, owing to its lower androgen:anabolic ratio. This is particularly important in females. • Stanozolol is significantly less expensive than danazol.
DRUG TO BE USED	• Stanozolol 2 mg po TID for 5 days initially. If response favorable, decrease dosage over 2–3 months to 2 mg daily.

*Cost Index:
1 = $<30/mo.
2 = $ 30–40/mo.
3 = $ 40–50/mo.
4 = $ 50–60/mo.
5 = $>60/mo.

AWP of 100, 2-mg tablets of stanozolol is approximately $66.
AWP of 100, 50-mg tablets of danazol is approximately $189.

Physical Exam Findings

During an acute attack, the patient exhibits facial and/or extremity swelling. Occasionally, abdominal palpation reveals a tender abdomen with crampy pain.

Diagnostic Testing

Associated abnormal laboratory findings pertain to the complement system and include a low level of C4 in the presence of normal C1 and C3 levels, and a low level of C1 INH in about 80 to 85 percent of patients with HAE. It is usually recommended that a C4 evaluation be performed as a simple screening test for HAE, and the diagnosis confirmed by measurement of C1 INH levels. In 20 percent of patients, this inhibitor protein may be present in normal or even increased amounts, but its function is abnormal (type II HAE). A functional or qualitative C1 INH assay is imperative before type II HAE can be ruled out. The C4 level is decreased in both types of HAE.

Developmental Considerations

Perinatal Anabolic steroids are not used during pregnancy because of the teratogenic risk. Clitoral hypertrophy and fused labia have been noted in fetuses exposed to danazol.

Danazol was originally developed as a drug for the treatment of endometriosis. Pregnancy has a suppressive effect on endometriosis, however, so it is unlikely that a pregnant woman would be taking danazol for this indication. Furthermore, when the drug is administered, ovulation is usually suppressed. Because danazol may be effective in the treatment of immune thrombocytopenic purpura, classic hemophilia, and alpha$_1$-antitrypsin deficiency, it is conceivable that health care providers will encounter more patients who began taking this drug while unknowingly pregnant.

Pediatric The adverse effects of giving anabolic steroids to young children are not fully understood. The risk-to-benefit ratio needs to be evaluated carefully before anabolic steroids are prescribed. In children, anabolic steroids may accelerate epiphyseal maturation more quickly than linear growth, thus compromising adult height. The drug effects may continue for up to 6 months after the drug has been discontinued.

Geriatric Older adults often have hypertension and other cardiovascular disorders that may be aggravated by the sodium and water retention associated with anabolic steroids. In men, the drugs may increase prostate size and interfere with urination, raise the risk of prostate cancer, and cause excessive sexual stimulation and priapism.

Psychosocial

Some patients may be concerned about taking anabolic steroids because of an awareness of their reputation for abuse. The health care provider must be sensitive to the patient's concerns and explain the different uses of the drugs. (see Case Study—Hereditary Angioedema).

Analysis and Management

Treatment Objectives

The primary treatment objective in HAE is to decrease the frequency and severity of attacks. Further, the patient must avoid overuse and/or abuse of these drugs because of their "body-building" effects.

Treatment Options

Drug Variables

Anabolic steroids are accepted as useful for long-term prevention of HAE. Two oral anabolic steroids, stanozolol and danazol, are widely prescribed for preventive therapy of HAE. Both are highly effective and have been reported to control symptoms in more than 90 percent of cases. The drugs have similar pharmacodynamics, pharmacokinetics, and adverse effects. However, stanozolol is the drug of choice because of its lower cost per dose and, more important, because of its lower anabolic:androgenic ratio. The lower ratio reduces the masculinizing effects, particularly in the female patient.

Patient Variables

The biggest variables involve the past and present health history of the patient. A past medical history of cardiac, renal, or hepatic disease should signify the use of much caution in prescribing anabolic steroids. The risk-to-benefit ratio needs to be heavily weighed. Patients with diabetes who are receiving anabolic steroids may find that their blood glucose levels are decreased, thereby necessitating a reduction in their insulin or oral hypoglycemic dose, or a change in diet.

Similarly, in children for whom anabolic steroid therapy is being considered for the management of HAE, the risk-to-benefit ratio must be thoroughly scrutinized. The potential therapeutic benefit of anabolic steroids should offset the risk of premature epiphyseal closure. Further, the safety and efficacy of stanozolol in children with HAE have not been established.

Adherence to a drug regimen is important in prevention or control of any disease process. In anabolic steroid therapy, the presence of masculinizing and virilizing adverse effects could lead to noncompliance with the drug regimen. Although these adverse effects would be more tolerable for males, females might discontinue the drug if such effects occur. Thus, it is important for the health care provider to consider use of stanozolol, which has the least potential for such effects.

The ease of administration, availability, and cost make stanozolol compatible with any acute care, ambulatory care, long-term care, or home care environment. The minimal effective dose of anabolic steroids should be used because of their potential adverse effects. To calculate the minimal effective dosage, the patient's clinical response, and not strictly the levels of C4 and C1 INH, should be considered. At times, a patient's C4 and C1 INH levels are below normal, but the patient remains asymptomatic.

Intervention

Administration

The anabolic steroids are available in tablets for oral use or in solution for deep IM injection into gluteal muscle. The oral tablet formulations should be taken with food or milk to decrease the risk of gastrointestinal disturbances.

Education

Regular medical supervision is essential for patients taking anabolic steroids. Periodic laboratory tests to monitor liver function, lipids, hemoglobin, and hematocrit are needed. Because anabolic steroids cause sodium, chloride, water, potassium, phosphate, and calcium imbalances, electrolytes should be closely monitored. Ankle swelling or a weight gain of more than 2 lb per week should be reported to the health care provider. Restriction of dietary sodium and/or the use of diuretics may be indicated.

Because of the potential virilizing and masculinizing effects of the androgens and anabolic steroids, patients must be fully informed of the potential for changes in secondary sex characteristics. The changes that do occur should be monitored, because certain changes require a reduction in dosage or discontinuation of the drug. Health care providers should be sensitive to the possible emotional responses of both male and female patients to changes in body image. Patients must also be taught that if they miss a dose, they should not double up on the next dose, but should continue with the original dosage.

Evaluation

The effectiveness of anabolic steroids in the management of HAE is evidenced by reductions in frequency and severity of attacks. Comparing the frequency of attacks before and after a trial period of anabolic steroids is necessary. The minimal dosage should be given, and the dose should be titrated according to the clinical response of the patient, not the serum levels of C1 INH and C4.

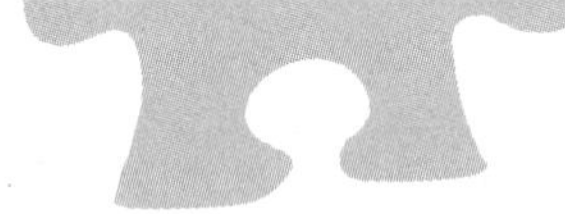

ANABOLIC HORMONE INHIBITOR

The anabolic hormone inhibitor finasteride (PROSCAR) is used in the symptomatic management of benign prostatic hypertrophy. It is a synthetic compound that competitively inhibits the steroid 5-alpha-reductase, an intracellular enzyme that normally converts testosterone to the potent androgen 5-alpha-dihydrotestosterone. The development of the prostate gland depends on levels of dihydrotestosterone. Thus, inhibiting dihydrotestosterone production reduces prostatic tissue and diminishes the symptoms of benign prostatic hypertrophy. However, it may be necessary to give finasteride for 6 months before a satisfactory patient response is achieved.

The adverse effects associated with finasteride include impotence, decreased libido, and smaller volume of ejaculate. The drug should be used with caution in patients with liver disease. Further, the male patient should not expose a female sex partner to a crushed tablet of finasteride, because of the potential for teratogenic effects in a male fetus.

Finasteride is well absorbed by mouth, with an onset time of 30 minutes. Peak blood levels are reached in 1 to 2 hours, but the effects on dihydrotestosterone are not seen for 8 hours. The drug is 90 percent protein bound and is biotransformed in the liver. Thirty-nine percent of the compound is eliminated in the urine, and 57 percent in the feces.

Finasteride decreases the clearance of theophylline. Additionally, serum concentrations of prostate-specific antigen are decreased in a patient taking finasteride, even in the presence of prostate cancer.

ANTIANDROGENS

- ❒ Cyproterone (ANDROCUR); (🍁) BERLEX
- ❒ Flutamide (EULEXIN)
- ❒ Bicalutamide (CASODEX)

The antiandrogens interfere with androgens at the androgenic target tissues of the prostate gland, bone marrow, and skeletal muscle. Drugs in this category are cyproterone, flutamide, and bicalutamide.

Cyproterone

Cyproterone, a pure antiandrogen, is used for severe hirsutism. It interferes with the binding of androgen to the nuclei receptor. Although this agent is widely used in Europe, it is considered an orphan drug in the United States and is not currently approved by the U.S. Food and Drug Administration for general use.

Flutamide

Flutamide is a nonsteroidal antiandrogen used in combination with leuprolide, a synthetic luteinizing hormone–releasing hormone, for the treatment of prostate carcinoma. It acts by interfering with testosterone uptake in the nucleus or with testosterone activity in target tissues. It arrests tumor growth in androgen-sensitive tissues (i.e., prostate).

The most common adverse effects of flutamide are hot flashes, decreased libido, impotence, gynecomastia, diarrhea, nausea, and vomiting. Although there are other adverse effects, the most serious is a drug-induced hepatitis. Use of flutamide is contraindicated in patients with hypersensitivity and during pregnancy.

Flutamide is rapidly and completely absorbed when taken by mouth and is eliminated in the urine and feces as metabolites. The half-life is 6 to 8 hours, with a 94 percent plasma protein binding. Alanine aminotransferase (ALT; serum glutamic-pruvic transaminase [SGPT]) aspartate aminotransferase (AST; serum glutamic-oxaloacetic transminase [SGOT]), and alkaline phosphatase may be elevated in the presence of flutamide.

The usual oral dose of flutamide is 250 mg every 8 hours.

Bicalutamide

Like flutamide, bicalutamide is a nonsteroidal antiandrogen agent. It is also used in the treatment of prostate cancer in combination with leuprolide. It acts by binding to cytosol androgen in target tissue, thereby competitively inhibiting the action of androgens.

The most common adverse effects of bicalutamide are similar to those of flutamide. Bicalutamide is contraindicated in patients with hypersensitivity and during pregnancy. It should be used with caution in patients with a history of renal or hepatic disease, in the older adult, and during lactation.

Bicalutamide is well absorbed taken by mouth, is metabolized in the liver, and is eliminated in the urine and feces. It should be used with caution in patients also receiving anticoagulant therapy, because bicalutamide displaces the anticoagulant from its binding sites. Blood urea nitrogen, creatinine, bilirubin, ALT (SGPT), and AST (SGOT) may be elevated in the presence of bicalutamide.

The usual oral dose of bicalutamide is 50 mg taken every day.

SUMMARY

- Hypogonadism is caused by a deficiency of testosterone secretion by the testes, whether a result of chromosomal, pituitary, or testicular disorders.
- It involves nondevelopment or regression of the secondary male characteristics along with a fragile libido and waning potency.
- Hypogonadism may occur in prepubertal or postpubertal males.
- Hypogonadism may have significant effects on the psychosocial and physical well-being of affected males.
- Hypogonadism may be classified as primary (due to a disease in the testes) or secondary (due to insufficient gonadotropin secretion by the pituitary gland).
- With delayed puberty, androgenic stimulation of undifferentiated embryonic tissues is absent or deficient. Lack of stimulation results in underdeveloped and immature male sexual organs.
- Hypergonadotropic hypogonadism occurs as a result of destruction of the testes (i.e., by castration, radiation, mumps, orchitis) and causes alterations in virilization, impotence, and/or libido.
- The treatment objectives for the adult male with primary hypogonadism are to restore sexual function, normal behavior, and virilization.
- In prepubertal males who are androgen deficient, treatment interventions are directed at re-establishing and maintaining masculine characteristics and functions.
- Options for the treatment of the prepubertal and postpubertal male with an androgen deficiency include using oral androgens (fluoxymesterone or methyltestosterone) or the IM solutions of testosterone enanthate and testosterone cypionate.
- Physical exam may reveal decreased secondary sexual characteristics such as reductions in axillary and pubic hair and muscle mass, loss of testicular and penile size, and changes in body shape to reflect a more "female-like" fat distribution.
- The patient may describe a history of reduced libido and potency, irritability, and loss of motivation.
- Care of the patient with hypogonadism requires regular medical supervision and periodic laboratory serum evaluation.
- Patient compliance may be an issue because of the masculinizing and virilizing effects of androgens. Patients need full knowledge about the possible effects and instructions on how to respond to the outcomes.
- Evaluation of the efficacy of androgen replacement is primarily based on the patient's clinical response and not strictly on serum testosterone levels.
- HAE accounts for only 2 percent of cases of clinical angioedema.
- One-half of those affected will have had an "attack" by age 7 years, and two-thirds by adolescence.
- HAE is an autosomal dominant disorder that results from a genetic deficiency of functional C1 esterase inhibitor (C1 INH).
- In type I HAE (80 percent of all cases), there is a lack of C1 INH. In type II HAE (the remaining 20 percent), C1 INH is present but nonfunctional.
- C1 INH deficiency or dysfunction allows unopposed activation of the first component of the complement cascade, with the consequent breakdown of C2 and C4, allowing for local release of vasoactive peptides and greater vascular permeability.
- The objective of treatment for HAE is to decrease the frequency and severity of attacks.

- Anabolic steroids are widely accepted in the long-term prevention of HAE attacks. Two oral drugs, stanozolol and danazol, are widely prescribed for prophylaxis.
- During an acute attack, patients report swelling of the face and extremities lasting 2 to 3 days with no known precipitating factor(s).
- Occasional patients may have crampy abdominal pain with watery diarrhea.
- A medical emergency exists in patients with laryngeal edema that causes airway obstruction.
- Definitive diagnosis is made on the basis of laboratory measurements of C1 INH and C4 and clinical symptoms.
- Patients may require long-term therapy with anabolic steroids to decrease the symptoms of HAE.
- Patient compliance may be an issue in anabolic steroid therapy because of the drugs' masculinizing and virilizing effects, particularly in females.
- The effectiveness of anabolic steroids in HAE is evidenced by fewer and less severe attacks.
- Anabolic hormone inhibitors such as finasteride are used in the symptomatic management of benign prostatic hypertrophy.
- Finasteride is a synthetic compound that competitively inhibits the steroid 5-alpha-reductase; thus, inhibition of dihydrotestosterone production diminishes prostatic tissue as well as the symptoms of benign prostatic hypertrophy.
- Six months of finasteride treatment may be necessary before a satisfactory patient response is achieved.
- Flutamide and bicalutamide are used with a luteinizing hormone–releasing hormone analog, such as leuprolide, for the treatment of prostate cancer.

BIBLIOGRAPHY

Barakat, A., and Castaldo, A. (1993). Hereditary angioedema: Danazol therapy in a 5-year-old child. *The Pediatric Forum,* 147, 931–932.

Drug facts and comparisons. (1996). St. Louis: Author.

Elnicki, D. (1992). Hereditary angioedema. *Southern Medical Journal,* 85(11), 1084–1090.

Gooren, L. (1994). A ten-year study of the oral androgen testosterone undecanoate. *Journal of Andrology,* 15(3), 212–215.

Matsumoto, A. (1994). Hormonal therapy of male hypógonadism. *Endocrinology and Metabolism Clinics of North America,* 23(4), 857–875.

Morales, A., Johnston, B., Heaton, J., et al. (1994). Oral androgens in the treatment of hypogonadal impotent men. *The Journal of Urology,* 152, 1115–1118.

Osterman, J. (1994). Androgen replacement therapy. *Current Therapy in Endocrinology and Metabolism,* 5, 286–291.

Schwartz, F., and Miller, R. (1994). Androgens and anabolic steroids. In Craig, C., and Stizel, R. (Eds.). *Modern pharmacology* (4th ed.). Boston: Little, Brown.

Sim, T., and Grant, J. (1990). Hereditary angioedema: Its diagnostic and management perspectives. *The American Journal of Medicine,* 88, 656–664.

Talavera, A., Larraona, J., Ramos, J., et al. (1995). Hereditary angioedema: An infrequent cause of abdominal pain with ascites. *The American Journal of Gastroenterology,* 90(3), 471–473.

U.S. Pharmacopeial Convention, Inc. (1998). *Drug information for the health professional* (18th ed.). Taunton, MA: Rand McNally.

Wang, C., and Swerdloff, R. (1995). Androgens. In Smith, C., and Reynard, A. (Eds.). *Essentials of pharmacology.* Philadelphia: W.B. Saunders.

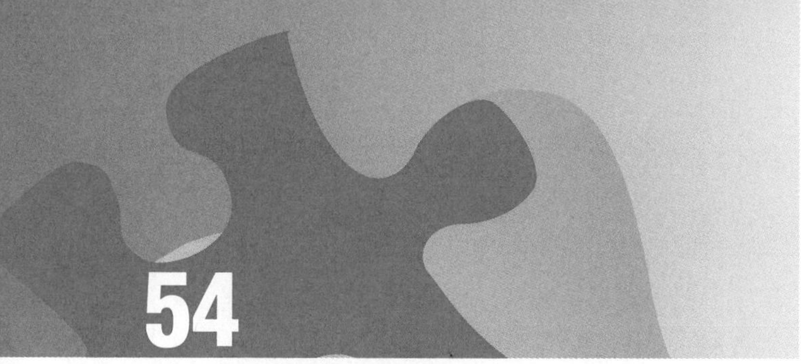

54 Hormonal Contraceptives and Related Drugs

Only in the last half of the 20th century has it become acceptable to discuss issues related to the female reproductive cycle, such as conception and contraception, abnormal bleeding, and menopause. As knowledge of physiologic and pathophysiologic conditions has grown, so has the availability of treatment and management options. The treatment and management choices can become quite confusing, however, and require an understanding of the normal reproductive cycle as well as variations from normal.

Female hormones are administered in the clinical setting for both contraceptive and noncontraceptive purposes. Noncontraceptive uses of estrogens are for the management of menopausal symptoms, osteoporosis, prostatic cancer, and, in some patients, carcinoma of the breast. Noncontraceptive uses of progestins include the treatment of amenorrhea, dysfunctional uterine bleeding, endometrial carcinoma, and endometriosis. Combinations of estrogens and progestins are used to prevent conception.

MENSTRUAL CYCLE

The primary female reproductive organs, the ovaries, have two main functions. They secrete female sex hormones, and they develop and release ova. At birth, a female infant has 1 to 2 million egg cells. By puberty, approximately 300,000 to 400,000 inactive eggs remain. The process of ovulation begins after puberty, when the hypothalamic-pituitary-ovarian axis is fully developed. During a woman's reproductive years, approximately 300 to 400 mature ova are released. The remainder fail to ovulate, and degenerate. The menstrual cycle occurs at two levels, the ovary and the endometrium.

Ovulatory Response

The ovulatory cycle is divided into three phases: the menstrual phase, the follicular phase, and the luteal phase (Fig. 54–1). The first day of menstrual bleeding is day 1 of the cycle. During the first 4 to 5 days, a large group of ovarian follicles begin to grow. The hypothalamus responds to low levels of estrogen and progesterone from the end of the previous cycle by producing *gonadotropin-releasing hormone* (GnRH). GnRH is released in a pulsatile manner, every 1 to 3 hours. Regular pulses of GnRH are important for regular cycling. Many menstrual disorders are related to abnormal GnRH pulsatility. GnRH travels to the anterior pituitary to stimulate the release of *follicle-stimulating hormone* (FSH). As a result, the group of follicles continue to develop. One follicle becomes dominant as it matures over the next 8 to 12 days.

Granulosa cells in the dominant *graafian follicle* produce more estrogen and have more FSH and *luteinizing hormone* (LH) receptors than other follicles in the group. Through a negative feedback mechanism, estrogen reduces secretion of FSH from the anterior pituitary (Fig. 54–2).

The granulosa cells also produce *inhibin,* which suppresses FSH stimulation of other follicles. As a result, follicles with fewer FSH receptors fail to develop and die. The dominant follicle also has theca cells that produce androgens in response to LH secretion from the pituitary.

By days 13 to 15 of the cycle, 1 or 2 days before ovulation, higher levels of estrogen stimulate LH release from the anterior pituitary, causing a sudden rise in LH. There are smaller increases in progesterone and inhibin at this time. The LH surge triggers the remaining events necessary for ovulation. Completion of the first meiotic division, along with production of prostaglandins and proteolytic enzymes, allows for rupture of the follicle and release of the ovum. The LH surge occurs approximately 34 to 36 hours before ovulation and lasts about 48 hours. As LH production peaks, estrogen levels drop.

Following ovulation, the ruptured ovarian follicle acquires additional LH receptors and becomes the *corpus luteum.* If fertilization occurs, the corpus luteum continues to produce large amounts of progesterone and lesser amounts of estrogen and androgens. If the ovum is not fertilized, the corpus luteum degenerates after approximately 14 days, and menstrual bleeding occurs. FSH levels again start to rise about 2 days before the menses begin, in response to decreased levels of progesterone and inhibin. Follicular development for the next cycle begins.

Estrogen is produced primarily in the ovaries and in lesser amounts by the adrenal cortex. The major estrogen produced by the ovaries is *estradiol.* During pregnancy, large quantities of estrogens are produced by the placenta. Some of the estradiol is converted to estrone and estriol in the periphery. These estrogens are less potent than estradiol itself. Estradiol is synthesized from cholesterol or acetyl coenzyme A in the ovaries.

In the male, small amounts of testosterone are converted to estradiol and estrone by the testes. Additional estrogen is produced through enzymatic conversion of testosterone in peripheral tissues such as the liver, fat, and skeletal muscle.

Progesterone, the principal endogenous hormone, prepares the uterus for implantation of a fertilized ovum. Progesterone is produced largely by the corpus luteum (and in smaller amounts by the adrenal cortex) and is regulated by LH secretion from the anterior pituitary. If implantation takes place, the developing trophoblast produces its own luteotropic hormone *(human chorionic gonadotropin),* which acts on the corpus luteum to promote continued progesterone secretion. Secretion of progesterone by the placenta during pregnancy is necessary for maintenance of the pregnancy and preparation of the endometrium for labor.

Endometrial Response

As the ovarian events are taking place (*i.e.,* the development of a mature follicle), the endometrial lining of the

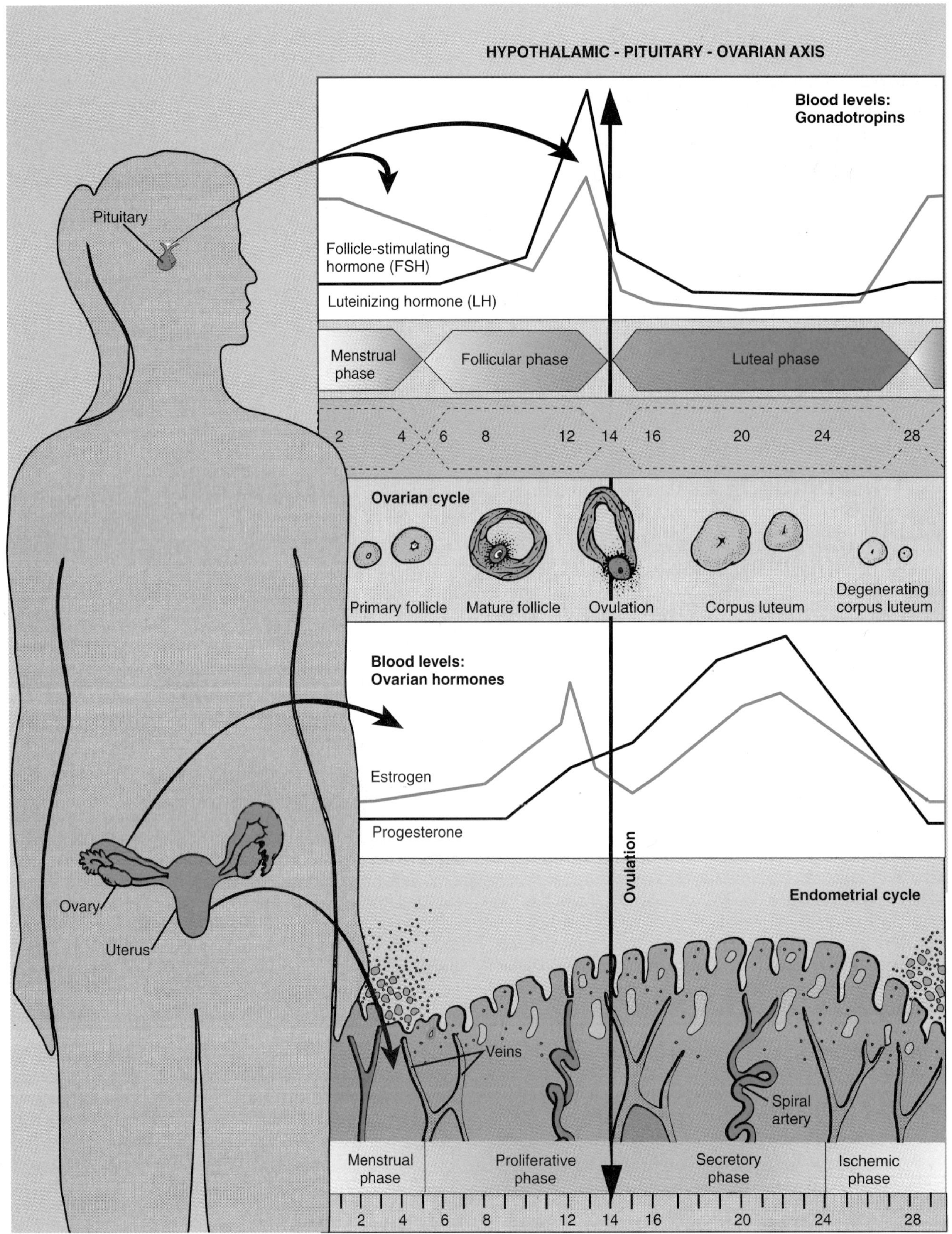

Figure 54–1 Hormonal events during menstrual cycle. The female menstrual cycle is composed of an ovulatory response and an endometrial response, which is composed of a menstrual phase, a follicular phase, and a luteal phase. (Adapted from Nichols, F. H., and Zwelling, E. [1997]. *Maternal-newborn nursing: Theory and practice* [p. 193]. Philadelphia: W. B. Saunders. Used with permission; data from Speroff, L., Glass, R., and Kase, N. [1994]. *Clinical gynecologic endocrinology and infertility* [5th ed.]. Baltimore: Williams & Wilkins.)

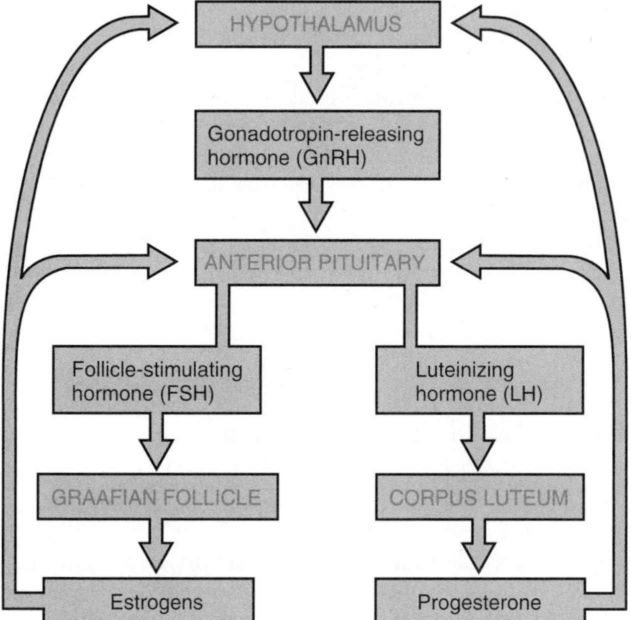

Figure 54–2 The Hypothalamic-pituitary-ovarian (HPO) axis illustrates the pathways to the production of estrogen and progesterone with the feedback pathways identified.

uterus is also undergoing cyclic changes. During the *follicular* phase, estrogen produced by the developing follicle causes the endometrium to grow rapidly. Following ovulation, progesterone produced by the corpus luteum stimulates the endometrium to increase in thickness and vascularity in preparation for implantation of a fertilized ovum. If implantation does not occur, the corpus luteum degenerates, and there is spasm of vessels in the endometrium. As a result, the endometrium becomes necrotic and starts to shed approximately 14 days after ovulation. The menstrual cycle thus begins anew.

Changes at Puberty

Beginning in fetal life, the ovaries secrete low levels of estrogen. Estrogen secretion increases between the ages of 9 and 12 years, triggering sexual maturation. Puberty is complete with the first menstrual cycle, when the female is capable of sexual reproduction. As puberty begins, hypothalamic production of GnRH increases, as does secretion of LH and FSH from the anterior pituitary. As a result, the ovaries produce higher levels of the sex hormones, estrogen, progesterone, and androgen.

Genitalia and secondary sex characteristics develop, such as the breasts and pubic and axillary hair. The sex hormones also stimulate the ovaries to release mature ova, leading to menstruation. Estrogens are responsible for the brisk growth of long bones during puberty. They also guide epiphyseal closure, thereby bringing linear growth to a halt.

Changes at Menopause

Menopause, defined as the absence of menstruation for a period of 6 to 12 months, is reached by most women between the ages of 40 and 58 years, with an average age of 51 years. Changes leading to menopause occur over several years before menses actually cease. Menopause occurs when the ovaries can no longer perform the function of ovulation and estrogen production. Because estrogen secretion stops, the woman's body undergoes physiologic changes.

During the period before menses completely cease, the woman's cycles begin to change because of lower estrogen levels and higher FSH levels. An inadequate luteal phase can result in irregular cycles. Although the likelihood of fertility is reduced, a woman may still become pregnant during this *perimenopausal* period. FSH and LH levels both rise until a few years after menopause, when they gradually decline.

Some estrogen is still produced in the postmenopausal woman from sources other than the ovary. *Androstenedione,* produced primarily by the adrenal cortex, is converted to estrone. The conversion of androgens to estrogen is variable. Body weight and age affect the amount of circulating estrogen in the postmenopausal woman. In early menopause, estrogen production is adequate to sustain estrogen-dependent tissues such as breasts, urethra, vagina, and vulva. Symptoms of estrogen loss include atrophic organ changes, vasomotor instability ("hot flashes"), vaginal dryness, and stress incontinence or urinary frequency. Atrophic changes, in addition to other normal changes of aging, and the effects of child-bearing may lead to cystocele formation and uterine prolapse. Symptoms of vaginitis, dyspareunia, stenosis, and urethritis are common. Postmenopausal women are also at higher risk for osteoporosis and cardiovascular disease.

The hot flash is a common experience of postmenopausal women. Forty to 70 percent of women experience hot flashes, and 25 to 49 percent have episodes of sweating during menopause. Many women report intense heat, with or without perspiration, over the upper body. It lasts a relatively short time but can be most disturbing at night, waking the patient from sleep. However, not all hot flashes are caused by estrogen deficiency, and verification should be obtained by an FSH measurement. The origin of hot flashes is poorly understood, but they seem to originate in the hypothalamus. At the same time that a hot flash begins, there is a surge in LH and an increase in GnRH secretion.

Loss of bone density affects approximately 25 million Americans and causes more than 1 million fractures each year. During the first 20 years following the onset of menopause, white women experience a 50 percent loss in trabecular bone and a 30 percent loss in cortical bone. Osteoporosis is uncommon in black women. Vertebral bone is commonly affected, accounting for the dorsal kyphosis seen in older women. In addition to estrogen loss, smoking and the use of caffeine, alcohol, and steroids also increases the risk of osteoporosis. Weight-bearing exercise and calcium supplementation reduce this risk.

Cardiovascular disease, primarily from atherosclerosis, is the principal cause of death in the United States. During reproductive years, women have three and one-half times lower risk of developing coronary artery disease than men. This is because younger women have higher levels of high-density lipoproteins (HDLs) and lower levels of low-density lipoproteins (LDLs). The level of HDL is affected by estrogen; as a result, the risk of cardiovascular disease doubles after menopause, and postmenopausal women are more likely to die after a heart attack. High concentrations of LDLs and low levels of HDLs are correlated with a greater incidence of atherosclerosis.

PATHOPHYSIOLOGIC DISRUPTIONS

Amenorrhea

Amenorrhea is the absence of menses. It is usually divided into primary and secondary amenorrhea. Primary amenorrhea is either an absence of menses by age 14 years without development of secondary sex characteristics, or the absence of menses by age 16 years with or without development of secondary sex characteristics. Primary amenorrhea may be caused by underdevelopment or malformation of the reproductive organs or by endocrine disturbances, genetic disorders (e.g., Turner's syndrome, ovarian dysgenesis with dwarfism), or central nervous system disorders.

Secondary amenorrhea is defined as the absence of menses for at least three cycles *(oligomenorrhea)* or for 6 months in a woman who has previously menstruated. Possible causes of secondary amenorrhea are many and include pregnancy, lactation, menopause, stress, disease, endocrine imbalances, tumors, weight abnormalities, excessive exercise, certain drugs, anatomic abnormalities, genetic factors, and previous surgery.

Polycystic ovarian syndrome is a common cause of secondary amenorrhea. Also known as Stein-Leventhal syndrome, this disorder occurs when follicular cysts continue to grow as a result of chronic androgen imbalance. As a result, these patients do not ovulate, or when they do, their menses are irregular, heavy, and prolonged. Normal elimination of FSH and 17-ketosteroid is found, but infertility is usually persistent. Polycystic ovarian syndrome may be asymptomatic, or the patient may report infertility, excess body hair, acne, or weight gain.

Dysmenorrhea

Dysmenorrhea is painful menstruation with lower abdominal cramping before and/or during menses. It affects a large number of women of child-bearing age and may be primary or secondary.

Primary dysmenorrhea usually begins shortly after menarche, is associated with ovulatory cycles, and occurs in the absence of pelvic disease. Excessive prostaglandin is produced in the endometrium, causing intense uterine contractions. In addition, other smooth muscles contract (e.g., in the gastrointestinal system), resulting in the symptoms of nausea, vomiting, and diarrhea. The pain may radiate to the back, sacrum, and/or inner thighs.

Secondary dysmenorrhea usually is painful menstruation owing to an identifiable pathologic cause. Possible causes of secondary dysmenorrhea are extrauterine, intrauterine, and intramural (i.e., within the uterine wall) diseases. The pain is progressive and occurs as a result of inflammation, ischemia, overdistention, hemorrhage, or perforation. Signs and symptoms include gastrointestinal distress, urinary tract complaints, backache, and/or heavy menstrual bleeding.

Premenstrual Syndrome

Premenstrual syndrome is the presence of symptoms in the period before menstruation or in the early days of the menstrual period. It is also referred to as premenstrual tension. The definition and diagnosis of premenstrual syndrome depend on the timing and the cyclic nature of symptoms rather than on specific clinical manifestations. Symptoms may begin at the time of ovulation and increase until the menses, or they may appear at ovulation, abate, and then reappear and increase until menses. A combination of physical, psychological, and behavioral symptoms occurs in a cyclic fashion. Typically, they appear during the late luteal phase and subside 1 to 2 days after the onset of menses. Etiologies include many physical and psychological factors. No one single cause accounts for all the symptoms. In true premenstrual syndrome, the symptoms cease with the onset of menses or last no more than a few days into the cycle.

Dysfunctional Uterine Bleeding

Dysfunctional uterine bleeding (DUB) is defined as menstrual cycles that are excessive in frequency, duration, or amount of flow. DUB is more commonly seen at both ends of the reproductive life-span. For up to 2 years during adolescence, menstrual cycles may be anovulatory as the hypothalamic-pituitary-ovarian axis matures. As ovarian function declines during the perimenopausal period, menstruation may become irregular. Approximately 10 to 15 percent of cases of DUB related to ovulatory cycles have an anatomic rather than hormonal origin.

Normal ovarian function usually cycles an average of every 28 days. Abnormal frequency consists of cycles that occur more often than every 24 days or less often than every 35 days. The duration of menstrual periods varies among individuals but in general is 5 to 7 days. Although it is difficult to measure blood loss during menses, excessively heavy flow should be considered abnormal. The average menstrual blood flow ranges from 35 to 105 mL. The amount of blood loss is based on the patient's perception, an estimate of the number of pads or tampons used, and the impact on the woman's usual functioning. Some patients with DUB report excessive bleeding with a normal cycle interval *(hypermenorrhea or menorrhagia)*. Others report irregular, frequent bleeding *(polymenorrhea, metrorrhagia)*.

Potential causes of DUB may be complications of pregnancy and reproductive tract diseases, such as polyps, infection, endometriosis, fibroids, malignancies, and functional cysts. Systemic illness, such as thrombophlebitis, liver disease, obesity, diabetes, hypertension, and adrenal disorders, may secondarily result in DUB. The use of hormonal contraceptives or intrauterine devices can also cause abnormal menstrual bleeding.

PHARMACOTHERAPEUTIC OPTIONS

Estrogens

- ❒ Conjugated estrogens (PREMARIN)
- ❒ Diethylstilbestrol (DES), (STILPHOSTROL)
- ❒ Ethinyl estradiol (ESTINYL)
- ❒ Esterified estrogens (ESTRATAB, MENEST)
- ❒ Estradiol (ALORA, CLIMARA, ESTRACE, ESTRADERM, ESTRING, VIVELLE)
- ❒ Estradiol cypionate (DEPGYNOGEN, DEPO-ESTRADIOL, DEPOGEN)

- ❐ Estradiol valerate (DELESTROGEN, DIOVAL, DURAGEN, ESTRADIOL LA, ESTRA-L, VALERGEN)
- ❐ Estrone (AQUEST, ESTRONE 5)
- ❐ Estropipate (OGEN, ORTHO-EST)

Indications

Estrogens are used in the management of menopausal symptoms as well as for prophylaxis of osteoporosis and treatment of prostatic cancer, and female hypogonadism. Estrogens are also used to treat DUB, although progestins are ordinarily preferred for this disorder. In selected cases, estrogens have been used in the management of female acne in doses designed to suppress gonadotropins and in selected women with estrogen-receptive breast cancer.

Menopausal Symptoms

When used in the management of menopausal symptoms, low-dose oral estrogen provides effective relief of vasomotor symptoms. Ordinarily, conjugated estrogens are preferred for vasomotor symptoms and are taken on a cyclic schedule. Atrophic vaginitis is also responsive to estrogen therapy and can be treated with oral or vaginal estrogen formulations. The role of estrogen in relieving other symptoms of menopause (e.g., muscle cramps, arthralgia, anxiety, palpitations, dizziness) has not been determined.

A great deal of evidence is available to show that estrogen replacement lowers the frequency of arm and hip fractures secondary to osteoporosis. The prophylactic effect of estrogen appears to be greatest when estrogens are taken before significant osteoporosis occurs. Additional calcium in the diet also causes the rate of vertebral fractures to decline by as much as 80 percent. However, because only 35 percent of postmenopausal women develop significant osteoporosis, and because weight-bearing exercise and increased calcium intake are also effective, the routine prophylactic use of estrogen may be hard to justify in some instances.

Protection against cardiovascular disease is a major benefit of estrogens for the postmenopausal patient. Estrogen has inhibitory effects on the development of atherosclerosis, decreasing levels of LDL and increasing levels of HDL. Estrogen has also been shown to protect arterial walls from the accumulation of lipoproteins, and to exhibit vasodilating and antiplatelet actions. Other possible benefits of estrogen therapy on cardiovascular disease are a direct inotropic effect on the heart and improvement in utilization of peripheral glucose. Postmenopausal women who are taking estrogen have been shown to have lower levels of circulating insulin.

Ovarian Failure

Ovarian failure occurs when a woman younger than 35 years is depleted of estrogen-producing follicles. Such failure is often idiopathic. There may be an accelerated loss of follicles because of genetics, autoimmune disease, infection, or iatrogenic trauma. When used to manage primary ovarian failure, estrogen replacement replicates the events of puberty, when given at the appropriate time. Genital structures grow to normal size, breasts develop, axillary and pubic hair grows, and the body assumes a feminine contour. Estrogen does not however, affect growth spurts or produce changes in the ovary.

Breast and Prostate Cancer

Estrogen provides palliation and prolongation of life in postmenopausal women who have estrogen-receptive breast cancer. It should be noted, however, that estrogens are not the preferred treatment. These drugs should be used only if surgical resection of the breast and radiation therapy have been ruled out. Breast cancer survivors considered for estrogen therapy should be at least 5 years past menopause, because use of estrogens before this time may promote cancer growth rather than impede it. Biopsy should demonstrate the presence of estrogen receptors. Cancers that lack estrogen receptors are unlikely to respond to estrogen therapy. Diethylstilbestrol (DES) is the estrogen most often used for cancer therapy.

Estrogens can be of value in treating prostate cancer, because they suppress androgen production. They are reserved for patients in whom the prostatic cancer is well advanced. In these patients, estrogen may induce histologic remission as well as regression of the metastasis.

Pharmacodynamics

The precise mechanism by which estrogens produce their effects is unknown. They circulate briefly in the blood stream before reaching target cells. They passively enter target cells and combine with receptor proteins in the cell cytoplasm. The estrogen-receptor complex then interacts with DNA to produce RNA and new DNA. Once stimulated, these substances stimulate cell production and production of various proteins. The receptors are found in the estrogen-receptive female reproductive tract, breast, pituitary gland, and hypothalamus.

Adverse Effects and Contraindications

The most common adverse effect of estrogen is nausea. Fortunately, nausea diminishes with continued use and is rarely so severe as to require stopping therapy. Large doses may cause anorexia, vomiting, and diarrhea.

Prolonged estrogen therapy unopposed by progesterone (i.e., without the concurrent use of progestins) increases abnormal growth of the endometrium. This can result in hyperplasia, atypia, and a 4- to 14-fold increase in the risk of endometrial cancer. The abnormalities occur whether estrogen is given continuously or cyclically. As dosage and duration of treatment increase, the risk of endometrial cancer also rises. Approximately 10 percent of women with endometrial hyperplasia and a larger percentage with atypia develop cancer.

The effect of estrogen on development of breast cancer is still under investigation. Estrogens are not thought to be carcinogenic, nor do they cause breast cancer. However, they can promote the growth of estrogen-receptive tumors. Estrogen-dependent breast cancer should be ruled out before estrogen therapy is started. Further, estrogen should be used cautiously in the patient with a strong family history of breast cancer or a personal history of breast nodules, fibrocystic disease, or abnormal mammogram. The use of estrogens in the treatment of breast cancer or bony metastasis can lead to severe hypercalcemia.

The incidence of gallbladder disease is higher in women taking estrogen. Estrogens can cause jaundice in patients with pre-existing liver disease (cholestatic jaundice). Other adverse effects are headache, dizziness, and depression.

Estrogen should not be used during pregnancy. Females who were exposed in utero to diethylstilbestrol have a higher risk of developing a rare form of cervical or vaginal cancer later in life. Diethylstilbestrol was used in years past to prevent miscarriage. The cancer appears most commonly around the age of 19 years. After age 30, the chance of developing either vaginal or cervical cancer declines to a very low level. The incidence is estimated to be 0.01 to 0.1 percent. Although diethylstilbestrol has been associated with these two types of cancer, there is reason to believe that other estrogen preparations may present a similar risk. Other reports of the use of diethylstilbestrol during pregnancy have suggested a relationship with congenital heart defects and limb reductions. Testicular hypoplasia has been noted in males exposed in utero to DES.

Pharmacokinetics

In general, exogenous estrogens are readily absorbed via the gastrointestinal tract, skin, and mucous membranes. When applied topically, enough drug is absorbed to produce systemic effects. The depot formulations are absorbed over a period of days. Natural estrogens circulate by binding to sex hormone–binding globulin and albumin. They are 50 to 80 percent bound to plasma proteins.

The limited effectiveness of orally administered natural estrogens is due not to poor absorption but to active biotransformation in the liver. A proportion of some estrogens are eliminated in the bile and undergo enterohepatic circulation. Degradation occurs through conversion to less active products (e.g., estriol) through oxidation to nonestrogenic substances, and by conjugation with sulfuric and gluconic acids. Nonsteroidal estrogens are also rapidly biotransformed and thus require daily dosing to be effective. Elimination is primarily renal and varies at different times of the menstrual cycle, and during the female's life-span.

Drug-Drug Interactions

The simultaneous use of estrogen with other drugs can diminish or enhance their effects (Table 54–1). Several antibiotics (e.g., tetracyclines, ampicillin, rifampin, griseofulvin) and anticonvulsant drugs (e.g., phenobarbital, phenytoin, primidone) can accelerate the elimination of estrogens. The effects of estrogen may be enhanced in the presence of ascorbic acid.

The action of clotting factors is increased by estrogen, thus diminishing the effects of oral anticoagulants. Additionally, glucose tolerance is reduced, thus decreasing the effectiveness of antidiabetic drugs.

The effects of other drugs are increased by estrogen. Anti-inflammatory effects of hydrocortisone are enhanced, as is the pain-relieving effect of meperidine. The effects of tricyclic antidepressants are also enhanced.

TABLE 54–1 DRUG-DRUG INTERACTIONS OF SELECTED HORMONAL CONTRACEPTIVES AND RELATED DRUGS

Drug	Interactive Drug(s)	Interaction
Estrogens		
Estrogens	Barbiturates	Decreased effects of interactive drugs
	Carbamazepine	
	Chloramphenicol	
	Alcohol	
	Dihydroergotamine	
	Ethosuximide	
	Glucocorticoids (systemic)	
	Mineral oil	
	Oral neomycin	
	Phenylbutazone	
	Phenytoin	
	Primidone	
	Ampicillin	Accelerated elimination of hormone, thus reducing its effectiveness
	Griseofulvin	
	Rifampin	
	Sulfonamides	
	Tetracyclines	
	Antidiabetic drugs	Decreased effectiveness of interactive drug
	Oral anticoagulants	
	Dantrolene	Increased risk of hepatic toxicity to interactive drug
	Nicotine	Increased risk of thromboembolic phenomena
	Ascorbic acid	Increased effects of estrogen
	Hydrocortisone	Enhanced anti-inflammatory effects
	Imipramine	Increased effectiveness of interactive drug
	Meperidine	
	Theophylline	
	Tricyclic antidepressants	
Progestins		
Progesterone	Rifampin	Reduced plasma levels of progesterone
	Bromocriptine	Decreased effects of interactive drug
Medroxyprogesterone	Aminoglutethimide	Decreased contraceptive effectiveness
Hydroxyprogesterone	Bromocriptine	Decreased effects of interactive drug

Dosage Regimens

The dosage and route of estrogen administration should be individually determined according to the indication and patient circumstances. Exogenous estrogen can be administered orally, parenterally, transdermally, or intravaginally (Table 54–2).

When estrogens are used for replacement therapy, either cyclic or continuous administration can be employed. The purpose of a *cyclic regimen* is to simulate estrogen secretion during the normal menstrual cycle. With cyclic regimens, estrogen is taken daily for 21 days and then stopped for 1 week. The sequence is then repeated as long as treatment is indicated. The addition of a progestin during the last 10 days of the cycle promotes endometrial breakdown, thus diminishing the risk of endometrial cancer. The addition of progestin is essential for the woman who has a uterus. If withdrawal bleeding occurs, it will begin toward the end of the week of no treatment, and the estrogen can be resumed before the induced menstrual period ceases. The estrogens should be used in the lowest effective dose and for the shortest possible time.

Estrogen dosage for the treatment of cancer is substantially higher than that used for other indications. Daily administration regimens may be used rather than cyclic regimens. Because cyclic regimens are not involved, a long-acting intramuscular formulation (e.g., estradiol cypionate, estradiol valerate) may be used rather than an oral formulation.

Laboratory Considerations

Estrogens have favorable effects on cholesterol levels. Levels of LDL are reduced, whereas levels of HDL are elevated. There is conjecture, but no proof, that these effects on cholesterol metabolism may explain the lower incidence of myocardial infarction observed in premenopausal women. Lipid values should be monitored in patients with a personal or family history of hyperlipidemia who are taking estrogen.

Measuring estradiol blood levels in patients receiving estrogen is difficult, owing to the differences in tests available and inconsistencies among individual patients. However, measurement of estradiol blood levels may be useful in the patient already on estrogen therapy who continues to complain of symptoms. Adequacy of therapy cannot be determined by measuring FSH levels.

Estrogens may raise levels of serum glucose, sodium, triglyceride, phospholipid, cortisol, prothrombin, and coagulation factors VII, VIII, IX, and X. They can also decrease serum folate, pyridoxine, and antithrombin III values. False interpretations of thyroid function values, false elevations in norepinephrine platelet-induced aggregation, and false decreases in metyrapone have been noted with estrogen therapy.

Progestins

- ❒ Hydroxyprogesterone caproate (HYLUTIN)
- ❒ Medroxyprogesterone acetate (PROVERA, AMEN, CURRETAB, CYCRIN)
- ❒ Megestrol acetate (MEGACE)
- ❒ Norethindrone (MICRONOR, NOR Q.D.)
- ❒ Norethindrone acetate (AYGESTIN)
- ❒ Progesterone (CRINONE, FEMOTRONE, GESTEROL, PROGESTAJECT, PROMETRIUM)

Indications

Progestins, as a class of hormones, have been used in the management of menopause, dysfunctional uterine bleeding, amenorrhea, endometriosis, threatened or habitual abortion, and premenstrual syndrome, and as a palliative measure in recurrent or metastatic endometrial cancer. Progestins have also been used in the management of hypoventilation secondary to extreme obesity and chronic airway limitation disorders. The primary use of progestins in contraception is discussed later in this chapter.

Menopausal Symptoms

Progestin is added to estrogen regimens in the postmenopausal patient to prevent endometrial overgrowth and cancer. The addition of a progestin for a postmenopausal woman who still has a uterus is required. The beneficial effects of estrogen in the prevention of osteoporosis are not reduced by the addition of progesterone.

Dysfunctional Uterine Bleeding

DUB is characterized by irregular cycles and episodes of prolonged bleeding. It usually results from continuous action of estrogen on the endometrium, combined with an insufficient amount and poor cycling of progesterone. Progesterone causes abnormal bleeding to cease and helps re-establish a regular monthly cycle.

Amenorrhea

Progesterone has been used in the assessment of the amenorrheic patient after exclusion of pregnancy and the measurement of TSH and prolactin. The progestational challenge evaluates the amount of endogenous estrogen and the patency of the uterus and vagina. If endogenous estrogen levels are adequate, treatment with a progestin for 5 to 10 days is followed by withdrawal bleeding when the progestin is discontinued. If estrogen levels are low, it may be necessary to induce endometrial proliferation with an estrogen before giving progestin. Cyclic therapy can be used to promote regular monthly flow. An anovulatory woman is treated monthly (or, in some cases, every 2 to 3 months) with a progesterone regimen in order to prevent overexposure of the endometrium to estrogen.

Endometriosis

Endometriosis is a disorder in which endometrial tissue is transplanted to an abnormal location (e.g., uterine wall, ovary, abdominal cavity). This disorder is painful and a common cause of infertility and spontaneous abortion. Treatment of endometriosis with progestins is directed at engendering regression of the ectopic endometrial growths. Prolonged treatment, designed to prevent menstruation for many months, also prevents bleeding of endometrial tissues into the peritoneal cavity. Favorable effects have been achieved with continuous use of estrogen, but better results are derived from the continuous use of oral progestins. Although the use of progesterone relieves symptoms of endometriosis, it is not effective in increasing the pregnancy rate in affected patients. Danazol, an androgenic hormone (see Chapter 53), is also used in the management of endometriosis.

TABLE 54–2 DOSAGE REGIMEN FOR SELECTED HORMONAL CONTRACEPTIVES AND RELATED DRUGS

Drug	Use(s)	Dosage
Estrogen and Estrogen Derivatives		
Conjugated estrogen	Menopausal symptoms	0.3–1.25 mg po QD
	Dysfunctional uterine bleeding	
	Dysfunctional uterine bleeding	25 mg po IM/IV; may repeat one in 6–12 hours
	Primary ovarian failure	1.25 mg/day po cyclically
	Primary hypogonadism	2.5–7.5 mg/day in divided doses × 20 days, off 10 days
	Atrophic vaginitis	1–2 g vaginal cream daily for 1–2 weeks, then 1–2×/week
	Postcoital contraception	15 mg po BID × 5 days *or* 50 mg IV on 2 consecutive days
	Osteoporosis prophylaxis	0.625 mg po QD, cyclically
Estrone	Female hypogonadism	0.1–1.0 mg IM per week in single or divided doses
	Primary ovarian failure	
	Vasomotor symptoms	0.1–0.5 mg IM 2–3 times per week
	Atrophic vaginitis	
	Osteoporosis prophylaxis	1.25 mg po QD
	Inoperable prostate cancer	2–4 mg IM 2–3 times per week
Estropipate	Vasomotor symptoms	0.625 mg po QD × 3 weeks, 7–10 days off, repeat
	Female hypogonadism	1.25–7.5 mg po QD × 3 weeks, 7–10 days off, repeat
	Primary ovarian failure	
	Osteoporosis prophylaxis	0.625 mg/day po (25 days of a 31-day cycle/month)
	Atrophic vaginitis	2–4 g QD intravaginally, cyclically
Esterified estrogens	Female hypogonadism	2.5–7.5 mg po QD in divided doses × 3 weeks, 7–10 days off
	Vasomotor symptoms	0.3–1.25 mg po QD × 3 weeks, 7–10 days off, repeat
	Atrophic vaginitis	
	Inoperable breast cancer	10 mg po TID × 3 months
	Inoperable prostate cancer	1.25–2.5 mg po TID
	Primary ovarian failure	2.5–7.5 mg po QD estrogen in divided doses × 3 weeks, with oral progestin given the last 5 days of estrogen therapy
Estradiol	Menopausal symptoms	0.05–2.0 mg po QD × 3 weeks, 7–10 days off, repeat sequence; or QD Monday–Friday, none on Saturday or Sunday
	Female hypogonadism	
	Vasomotor symptoms	1–2 mg po QD cyclically or 2–4 g vaginally for 12 weeks, reduce dosage by 50% over 1–2 weeks or 0.05 mg/24 hr topically 2 × week cyclically or 12.5 cm^2 patch once weekly
	Atrophic vaginitis	
	Female hypogonadism	
	Primary ovarian failure	
	Osteoporosis prophylaxis	0.5 mg po QD × 3 weeks, 7–10 days off
	Breast cancer	10 mg po TID
	Prostate cancer	1–2 mg po TID
Estradiol valerate	Vasomotor symptoms	10–20 mg IM q4 weeks
	Atrophic vaginitis	
	Female hypogonadism	
	Primary ovarian failure	
	Prostate cancer	30 mg or more IM q1–2 weeks
Estradiol cypionate	Vasomotor symptoms	1–5 mg IM q3–4 weeks
	Female hypogonadism	1.5–2.0 mg IM every month
Ethinyl estradiol	Vasomotor symptoms	0.02–0.15 mg po QD × 3 weeks, 7–10 days off, repeat
	Osteoporosis prophylaxis	0.01 mg po QD
	Female hypogonadism	0.05 mg po TID during first 2 weeks of menstrual cycle followed by 2 weeks of progesterone; continue for 3–6 months, then 2 months off
	Postcoital contraception	2.5 mg po BID × 5 days
	Breast cancer	1 mg po TID
	Prostate cancer	0.15–2.0 mg po QD
Diethylstilbestrol	Postcoital contraception	25 mg po BID × 5 days
	Breast cancer	15 mg po QD
	Prostate cancer	1–3 mg po QD; maintenance: 1 mg/day
Combination Estrogens and Progestins		
Conjugated estrogen and medroxyprogesterone acetate	Menopausal symptoms	0.625 mg estrogen/2.5 mg progesterone or 0.625 mg estrogen/5 mg progesterone po, 21 days on and 7 days off
	Primary ovarian failure	1.25 mg po QD, cyclically
Esterified estrogen and methyltestosterone	Menopausal symptoms not relieved by estrogen alone	0.625 mg estrogen/1.25 mg testosterone po QD or 1.25 mg estrogen/ 2.5 mg testosterone po QD
Ethinyl estradiol and levonorgestrel	Menopausal symptoms	50 mcg to 0.5 mg po QD × 21 days or 28 days
	Female hypogonadism	
	Postcoital contraception	2 tablets po q 12 hr × 2 doses
Progesterone Preparations		
Hydroxyprogesterone caproate	Amenorrhea	250–375 mg IM q4 weeks; may be followed by cyclic estrogen therapy
	Dysfunctional uterine bleeding	
	Endometrial cancer	1-g doses given 1–7 days/week
Medroxyprogesterone acetate	Secondary amenorrhea	5–10 mg po QD for 5–10 days; start at any time in cycle
	Dysfunctional uterine bleeding	
	Endometriosis	150 mg IM every 3 months
	Endometrial cancer	
	Vasomotor symptoms	10 mg po daily

TABLE 54–2 DOSAGE REGIMEN FOR SELECTED HORMONAL CONTRACEPTIVES AND RELATED DRUGS *Continued*

Drug	Use(s)	Dosage
Progesterone Preparations ***Continued***		
Megestrol acetate	Breast cancer	40 mg po QID
	Endometrial cancer	40–320 mg po in divided doses
Norethindrone	Amenorrhea Dysfunctional uterine bleeding	5–20 mg po on days 5–25 of menstrual cycle
	Endometriosis	10 mg po QD initially, then 30 mg QD po for maintenance
Norethindrone acetate	Amenorrhea Dysfunctional uterine bleeding	2.5–10 mg po QD on days 5–25 of menstrual cycle
	Endometriosis	5 mg po QD × 2 weeks. Increase in increments of 2.5 mg/day every 2 weeks until 15 mg/day is reached
Progesterone	Amenorrhea	5–10 mg IM QD × 6–8 days, 8–10 days before menstrual period
	Dysfunctional uterine bleeding	5–10 mg IM for 6 days; begin progesterone therapy after 2 weeks of estrogen therapy

Threatened and Habitual Abortion

The corpus luteum produces the majority of the progesterone necessary to maintain a pregnancy until about 10 to 12 weeks of gestation. Exogenous administration of high-dose progestins (e.g., medroxyprogesterone, norethindrone) via suppository has been used extensively in an attempt to prevent recurrent pregnancy loss. However, there is no evidence that treatment with progestins is effective in the majority of patients. High-dose progestins pose a risk to the fetus for abnormalities such as limb reductions, heart defects, and masculinization of the female fetus.

Progestins have also been used after assisted reproductive technology to promote a successful pregnancy, particularly if the woman is known to have a low level of endogenous progesterone. Progestin doses should remain low, and the drug should be discontinued when placental production of progestins becomes sufficient to support the pregnancy (approximately 12 weeks of gestation).

Premenstrual Syndrome

Progesterone suppositories have been used for years in an attempt to relieve symptoms of premenstrual syndrome. Progesterone is thought to produce a more favorable hormonal balance. However, little therapeutic effect has been demonstrated.

Endometrial Cancer

Progestins (e.g., medroxyprogesterone acetate, megestrol acetate) may be used as palliatives in the management of recurrent or metastatic endometrial cancer. They are thought to cause regression of the tumor and remission of the cancer. Several months of therapy may be needed before a clinical response is seen. Megestrol acetate may also provide palliation for women with breast cancer.

Pharmacodynamics

Progesterone is secreted by the corpus luteum during the last half of the menstrual cycle, after ovulation. It continues the changes in the endometrium begun by estrogens during the first half of the menstrual cycle. Progesterone secreted during the second half of the menstrual cycle converts the endometrium from a proliferative state to a secretory state. Progesterone also acts on the endocervical glands, causing their secretions to become scant and viscous. This action is opposite that of estrogen, which promotes the flow of profuse, watery secretions.

Progesterone generally has opposite effects on the metabolism of lipids from those of estrogen. Progesterone decreases HDLs and increases LDLs, thereby raising the risk of cardiovascular disease.

The potent antiestrogenic effects of progestins explain their effects on the endometrium. They are responsible for the conversion of estradiol to estrone sulfate in a form that is quickly eliminated from the cell. This occurs by stimulating 17-beta-hydroxysteroid dehydrogenase (which catalyzes the oxidation of estradiol to the less potent estrone) and estrogen sulfotransferase (which catalyzes the sulfation and inactivation of estrogens). In addition, progestins inhibit the proliferation of estrogen receptors that normally occurs with estrogen action. Thus, estrogen effects on target cells are decreased.

Progestins also suppress the transcription of oncogenes by estrogen. The therapeutic effects of progestins include prevention of hyperplasia, inhibition of endometrial growth following ovulation, and the prevention of atrophy during pregnancy and use of oral contraceptives.

Adverse Effects and Contraindications

Progestins are sometimes poorly tolerated, leading the patient to discontinue therapy. Because of progestin's action on the endometrium, patients may complain of breakthrough bleeding, spotting, and amenorrhea. Other complaints are breast tenderness, bloating, and depression. Jaundice, edema, lethargy, photosensitivity, nausea, and exacerbation of acute intermittent porphyria have also been reported.

Administration of high-dose progestins during the first 4 months of pregnancy has been associated with masculinization of the female fetus, limb reductions, and heart defects. Women who become pregnant while taking progestins should be advised of the potential risks to the fetus. Contraindications to the use of progestins are similar to those for estrogen.

Pharmacokinetics

Regardless of the route of administration, daily administration of progestins is necessary because of their extensive first pass effect. The first-past effect also renders orally administered progestins relatively ineffective. Although progestins formulated in an oil base are rapidly absorbed and biotransformed quickly, they are relatively effective if given in sufficient daily doses.

In addition to biotransformation in the liver, progestins are biotransformed in the endometrium and the myometrium. Small amounts of progestins are stored in fat tissue, and the remainder are highly protein bound. The half-life of progesterone in the circulation is a few minutes. Progestin is eliminated primarily by the kidneys, with a small portion eliminated via the bile and feces.

Drug-Drug Interactions

Plasma levels of progesterone are reduced in the presence of rifampin because of greater biotransformation of the drug (see Table 54–1). Progesterone may also decrease the effectiveness of bromocriptine when the two drugs are used concurrently for galactorrhea or amenorrhea.

Dosage Regimens

Many orally active and parenteral formulations of progestins are available. It is not feasible to compare the relative clinical effectiveness of progestin formulations, because comparisons are limited in number and because different responses have been noted. The relative potencies of the progestins are not the same. Some progestins possess more or less estrogenic and androgenic activities than others (see Table 54–2).

Cyclic therapy is employed in DUB to establish a regular monthly cycle. Doses of 5 to 10 mg of norethindrone taken every 4 to 6 hours are usually effective in stopping DUB in 24 hours. To permit a respite from bleeding 5 mg can be given twice daily for 1 to 2 weeks. Withdrawal bleeding at the end of the treatment regimen can be likened to a normal menstrual flow. It is usually accompanied by menstrual cramps. However, the cramps are self limiting. Other progestins can be used, but those without inherent estrogenic activity are more effective when combined with an estrogen.

To prevent a recurrence of bleeding, cyclic therapy is required. Oral progestin is started 5 days after the onset of each menstrual period and continued for the next 20 days. This cycle promotes a repeating pattern of endometrial proliferation following endometrial breakdown and menstruation. Aqueous suspensions of progesterone are particularly painful when given intramuscularly and are less frequently used.

Norethindrone acetate may be used in the management of endometriosis. Oral doses of 5 mg daily are used for 2 weeks, after which the dose is increased in increments of 2.5 mg per day every 2 weeks until 15 mg per day is reached. Therapy may be continued for 6 to 9 months. Symptomatic relief is seen in about 80 percent of patients, and fertility returns in about 50 percent of patients.

Medroxyprogesterone acetate 10 mg daily may be used alone to treat vasomotor symptoms in the patient who has had breast cancer. The addition of 1000 mg of calcium daily supplies protection against osteoporosis. However, atrophic symptoms of menopause, such as vaginal dryness and dyspareunia, may worsen.

Laboratory Considerations

The effect of progestins on lipoproteins appears to be dose related. A physiologic dose of progestins appears to not alter the favorable effects of estrogen on lipoproteins. Either a decrease or no significant change in HDL cholesterol may be seen with low doses of progesterone. Progestins also have been shown to raise serum glucose and insulin levels and cause a relative insulin sensitivity.

Short-Acting Oral Contraceptives

Typically called the "the pill," a combined estrogen-progesterone oral contraceptive (Table 54–3) has been on the market for more than 35 years. These agents are among the most widely used drugs requiring a prescription. They are also the most popular form of reversible birth control in the United States. Currently, 10 million women in the United States and 60 million worldwide are estimated to take oral contraceptives. Conception can be averted by interfering with the reproductive process at any step from the development of the female ovum to implantation of the fertilized ovum.

Indications

The most common oral contraceptive is a combination of an estrogen and a progestin. Single-hormone formulations are also available. A progestin-only formulation has come to be called the "minipill." Minipills were developed to eliminate the estrogen component, the drug thought to be responsible for most of the adverse effects of the contraceptive. However, the minipill has become less popular because of the irregular menstrual cycles it produces as well as its lower efficacy rate. Estrogen-only formulations are known as postcoital, or "morning after," pills. However, combination pills have a contraceptive efficacy rate of 98 to 99 percent, whereas the progestin-only formulation has a reported efficacy of 97 to 98 percent. Thus, the minipill has fallen from favor with most women. It is used postpartum by breast-feeding women until they wean their babies, however, without problematic adverse effects.

Combination estrogen-progestin oral contraceptives (OCs) are an effective, reversible form of birth control. Although the primary purpose of oral contraceptives is to control fertility, several noncontraceptive uses have been identified. "The pill" can make menstrual periods more regular. It also has a protective effect against pelvic inflammatory disease, an infection of the fallopian tubes or uterus that is a major cause of infertility.

Progestin-only minipills are useful contraceptives for women who are lactating, who are older than 40 years, or for whom estrogen-containing preparations are contraindicated.

Postcoital contraception may be necessary for the following situations: (1) another form of contraception has been forgotten, (2) another form of contraception has failed (e.g., condom breakage, dislodging of a diaphragm), (3) rape, or (4) ambivalence following intercourse. Large doses of combination pills are used when such one-time protection is needed.

Treatment of DUB can be accomplished with oral contraceptives that have high estrogenic activity. Dysmenorrhea due to excessive prostaglandin production should be treated with antiprostaglandin agents. However, for dysmenorrhea occurring with irregular bleeding or endometriosis, OCs

TABLE 54–3 COMPARISON OF SELECTED CONTRACEPTIVE FORMULATIONS

	Combination						
Trade Name	ESTROGEN COMPONENT	PROGESTIN COMPONENT	**Estrogen Activity**	**Progesterone Activity**	**Androgen Activity**	**Endometrial Activity**	**Spotting and Breakthrough Bleeding(%)***
High-Dose Combination Monophasics							
OVRAL	0.05 mg ethinyl estradiol	0.5 mg norgestrel	Hi	Hi	Hi	Int	4.5
NORINYL 1 + 35	0.05 mg mestranol	1 mg norethindrone	Lo–Int	Int	Lo	Int–Hi	10.6
ORTHO-NOVUM 1/50	0.05 mg mestranol	1 mg norethindrone	Lo–Int	Int	Lo	Int–Hi	10.6
OVCON-50	0.05 mg ethinyl estradiol	1 mg norethindrone	Hi	Int	Int	Int	11.9
DEMULEN 1/50	0.05 mg ethinyl estradiol	1 mg ethynodiol diacetate	Lo	Hi	Lo	Int	13.9
Low-Dose Combination Monophasics							
LO-OVRAL	0.03 mg ethinyl estradiol	0.3 mg norgestrel	Lo–Int	Lo–Int	Int	Lo–Int	9.6
OVCON-35	0.035 mg ethinyl estradiol	0.4 mg norethindrone	Int–Hi	Lo	Lo	Int	11.0
DESOGEN	0.03 mg ethinyl estradiol	0.15 mg desogestrel	Int	Int–Hi	Lo	Lo–Int	9.9
ORTHO-CEPT	0.03 mg ethinyl estradiol	0.15 mg desogestrel	Int	Int–Hi	Lo	Lo–Int	9.9
LEVLEN, NORDETTE	0.03 mg ethinyl estradiol	0.15 mg levonorgestrel	Lo–Int	Lo–Int	Int	Int	14.0
ORTHO-CYCLEN	0.035 mg ethinyl estradiol	0.25 mg norgestimate	Int–Hi	Lo	Lo	Lo–Int	14.3
NORINYL 1 + 50	0.035 mg ethinyl estradiol	1 mg norethindrone	Int–Hi	Int	Int	Int	14.7
ORTHO-NOVUM 1/35	0.035 mg ethinyl estradiol	1 mg norethindrone	Int–Hi	Int	Int	Int	14.7
MODICON	0.035 mg ethinyl estradiol	0.5 mg norethindrone	Int–Hi	Lo	Lo	Int	14.6
BREVICON	0.035 mg ethinyl estradiol	0.5 mg norethindrone	Int–Hi	Lo	Lo	Int	14.6
LOESTRIN FE 1.5/30	0.03 mg ethinyl estradiol	1.5 mg norethindrone acetate	Lo	Hi	Hi	Int	25.2
LOESTRIN 1.5/30	0.03 mg ethinyl estradiol	1.5 mg norethindrone acetate	Lo	Hi	Hi	Int	25.2
LOESTRIN FE 1/20	0.03 mg ethinyl estradiol	1.5 mg norethindrone acetate	Lo	Hi	Hi	Int	25.2
LOESTRIN 1/20	0.02 mg ethinyl estradiol	1 mg norethindrone acetate	Lo	Int–Hi	Int–Hi	Int	29.7
DEMULEN 1/35	0.035 mg ethinyl estradiol	1 mg ethynodiol diacetate	Int	Hi	Int	Hi	37.4
ALESSE	0.02 mg ethinyl estradiol	0.1 mg levonorgestrel	Int	Lo	Int	Int	UA
Combination Biphasics							
ORTHO-NOVUM 10/11	0.035 mg ethinyl estradiol	10 days 0.5 mg norethindrone	Int–Hi	Lo–Int	Int	Int	19.6
	0.035 mg ethinyl estradiol	11 days 1 mg norethindrone					
JENEST-28	0.035 mg ethinyl estradiol	7 days 0.5 mg norethindrone	Int–Hi	Lo	Int	Int	14.1
	0.035 mg ethinyl estradiol	14 days 1.0 mg norethindrone					
Combination Triphasics							
ORTHO-NOVUM 7/7/7	0.035 mg ethinyl estradiol	7 days 0.5 mg norethindrone	Hi	Lo–Int	Int	Int	12.2
	0.035 mg ethinyl estradiol	7 days 0.75 mg norethindrone					
	0.035 mg ethinyl estradiol	7 days 1 mg norethindrone					
TRI-LEVLEN, TRIPHASIL	0.03 mg ethinyl estradiol	6 days 0.05 mg levonorgestrel	Int	Lo	Int	Int	15.1
	0.04 mg ethinyl estradiol	5 days 0.075 mg levonorgestrel					
	0.03 mg ethinyl estradiol	10 days 0.125 mg levonorgestrel					
ORTHO TRI-CYCLEN	0.035 mg ethinyl estradiol	7 days 0.18 mg norgestimate	Int–Hi	Lo	Lo	Int	17.5
	0.035 mg ethinyl estradiol	7 days 0.215 mg norgestimate					
	0.035 mg ethinyl estradiol	7 days 0.25 norgestimate					
TRI-NORINYL	0.035 mg ethinyl estradiol	7 days 0.5 mg norethindrone	Int–Hi	Int	Int	Int	14.7
	0.035 mg ethinyl estradiol	9 days 1 mg norethindrone					
	0.035 mg ethinyl estradiol	5 days 0.5 mg norethindrone					
Combination Estrophasic							
ESTROSTEP 21 and ESTROSTEP FE	0.02 mg ethinyl estradiol	5 days 1 mg norethindrone acetate	Lo–Int	Int–Hi	Int	Int	UA
	0.03 mg ethinyl estradiol	7 days 1 mg norethindrone acetate					
	0.035 mg ethinyl estradiol	9 days 1 mg norethindrone acetate					
Progestin-Only Minipills							
OVRETTE	None	0.075 mg norgestrel	None	Lo	Lo	Hi	34.9
MICRONOR	None	0.35 mg norethindrone	VL	Lo	Lo	Hi	42.3
NOR-Q.D.	None	0.35 mg norethindrone	VL	Lo	Lo	Hi	42.3

Hi, high; Int, intermediate; Lo, low; VL, very low; UA, unavailable.

*Reported prevalence of spotting and breakthrough bleeding during third cycle of use. Information should not be precisely compared.

Data from Dickey, R. (1994). *Managing contraceptive pill patients* (8th ed.). Durant, OK: Essential Medical Information Systems; *Nurse Practitioner Prescribing Reference*. (1998). New York: Prescribing Reference, Inc.

with a high progestin component are beneficial. Standard low-dose pills are useful for teens with DUB or dysmenorrhea.

Oral contraceptives suppress excessive androgen production and may be useful in the treatment of polycystic ovarian syndrome. A relatively high estrogen dose with progestin may be required to adequately suppress ovarian function.

When it is important to retain fertility in the patient with endometriosis, a low-dose estrogen/high-dose progestin OC may be used. Blocking ovulation reduces the severity of endometriosis and lengthens the time of remission.

Although danazol is more effective in treating the symptoms of fibrocystic breast disease, OCs are useful when effective contraception is also desired. A pill with a low dose of estrogen is required.

Because estrogen replacement therapy (ERT) has been shown to favorably affect bone resorption in postmenopausal women, it would be reasonable to expect that OCs containing estrogen would have a similar effect. Evidence has been conflicting, however. Although some women have a gain in bone mass, others have shown none.

There are some data to suggest that the incidence of pelvic inflammatory disease caused by some but not all organisms may be reduced in users of oral contraceptives. Several theories may account for this finding. Thickened cervical mucus may reduce the ascent of organisms. In addition, there is a less favorable environment for bacterial growth with the decreased menstrual bleeding seen with use of these agents. Rates of *Chlamydia,* gonorrhea, and human immunodeficiency virus infections, however, are not lower in users of OCs.

The risk of venous thrombosis and/or myocardial infarction was a concern with the older OC formulations that contained high doses of estrogen. With newer formulations containing 35 mcg of estrogen or less, the rates of thromboembolism in users of oral contraceptives are similar to those in other women of similar age who are not taking hormones. It is now clear that habitual smoking and oral contraceptive use, not age, are the primary risk factors for myocardial infarction in women.

Pharmacodynamics

Estrogen and progestin interfere with fertility in a number of ways. It is clear that as currently used, the combination inhibits ovulation by suppressing FSH and LH. Estrogen inhibits the secretion of FSH, and the action of progestin inhibits the release of LH. In addition, estrogen and progestin alter the development of endometrium, thus making implantation of a fertilized ovum unlikely. Further, a thick tenacious mucus is secreted under the influence of progestin, creating a hostile environment for, or even a barrier to, the passage of sperm.

Adverse Effects and Contraindications

Breakthrough bleeding occurs when estrogen stimulation is not sufficient to maintain the endometrium. It most commonly occurs within the first few cycles of OC use. Inadequate estrogen or progesterone may also result in amenorrhea following a pill cycle.

The estrogen component of OCs has been linked to complaints of nausea, vomiting, and breast tenderness and enlargement. Oral contraceptives containing more than 0.05 mg of estrogen are associated with higher risks of cardiovascular disorders, including thromboembolism, myocardial infarction, cerebrovascular accidents, and hypertension. The potential for complications increases with the dosages of estrogen and progestin, duration of OC use, age of the patient, and cigarette smoking.

Both the estrogen and progestin components can cause fluid retention and weight gain. The progestins used in oral contraceptives exert some androgenic activity, depending on the type and dose. As a result, the patient may experience hair growth and acne. Irregular bleeding is more common with the progestin-only minipill. Absolute and relative contraindications to oral contraceptives are listed in Table 54–4. Cholestatic jaundice is the most severe adverse effect of oral contraceptives.

Contraindications to the use of oral contraceptives include reproductive cancer, thrombophlebitis, myocardial infarction, hepatic tumors, coronary artery disease, cerebrovascular accidents, and age greater than 40 years. Cautious use of OCs is warranted in patients with depression, hypertension, renal disease, seizure activity, rheumatic disease (including systemic lupus erythematosus), migraine headaches, amenorrhea, irregular menses, fibrocystic breast disease, gallbladder disease, acute mononucleosis, and sickle cell disease, as well as in heavy smokers.

Pharmacokinetics

Hormonal contraceptives are well absorbed following oral administration. They are slowly absorbed when given via injection or implantation. Their distribution and half-life are unknown. The onset and peak action of oral contraceptives are approximately 1 month. Their duration of action is 1 month for oral formulations, 3 months for injectable formulations, and as much as 5 years for implants.

Drug Drug Interactions

Synergistic or antagonistic effects may occur when OCs are used concomitantly with other drugs. Oral contraceptives may be less effective when taken concurrently with a variety of antimicrobials, anticonvulsants, rifampin, analgesics, antihistamines, chenodiol, and griseofulvin. When OCs are used along with tricyclic antidepressants, the adverse effects of the antidepressants may become evident at lower dosages. Intermenstrual bleeding may be the first sign of a drug-drug interaction and reduced efficacy of the oral contraceptive.

Dosage Regimens

Oral contraceptives are available in monophasic, biphasic, and triphasic regimens. With monophasic regimens, the daily estrogen and progestin dosage remains constant throughout the cycle. In a biphasic regimen, the estrogen dosage remains constant, but the progestin dosage is increased during the last half of the cycle. The dosages of both estrogen and progestin change in triphasic regimens.

Oral contraceptive therapy is usually started with a formulation whose estrogen content is equivalent to or less than 0.035 mg. Most OCs currently available are taken sequentially for 21 days, followed by 7 days on which either no pill is taken or an inert or iron-containing pill is taken.

TABLE 54–4 CONTRAINDICATIONS TO THE USE OF CONTRACEPTIVES

	Absolute Contraindications	Relative Contraindications
Short-acting contraceptives	History of deep vein thrombosis or pulmonary embolus Antiphospholipid antibody syndrome Protein C deficiency Protein S deficiency Antithrombin III deficiency Estrogen-dependent breast cancer History of heart disease, cerebrovascular accident, uncontrolled hypertension Smoking in patient older than 35 years Pregnancy Active liver disease Intestinal malabsorption syndrome Concurrent use of rifampin	Migraine headaches Severe depression Oligomenorrhea/amenorrhea Diabetes mellitus with retinopathy or nephropathy Symptomatic mitral valve prolapse History of jaundice or pruritus of pregnancy Family history of thromboembolic disease Family history of elevated triglycerides Epilepsy Sickle cell disease Gallbladder disease Elective surgery
Long-acting contraceptives	Active thrombophlebitis Thromboembolic disease Undiagnosed genital bleeding Benign or malignant liver tumors Known or suspected breast cancer Active liver disease	Smoking (> 15 daily) in patient older than 35 years History of ectopic pregnancy Diabetes mellitus Hypercholesterolemia Severe acne Hypertension History of cardiovascular disease Gallbladder disease Severe vascular or migraine headaches Severe depression Compromised immune system Concomitant use of phenytoin, phenobarbital, carbamazepine, rifampin

The sequence is started 5 days after the onset of menses and is repeated as long as indicated. Day 1 is the first day of the period. The cycle is repeated every 28 days, regardless of whether breakthrough bleeding or spotting occurs. The pills should be taken at the same time each day. An additional form of birth control (e.g., condom, diaphragm) is recommended during the first week of OC use. Oral contraceptives can be started approximately 1½ to 2 weeks postpartum owing to the increased clotting risk, as long as breastfeeding is not desired.

Hormonal contraceptives are also available as progestin-only minipills. Unlike combination OCs, they are started on day 1 of the menstrual cycle and are taken continuously thereafter. There is no break between cycles.

Laboratory Considerations

Oral contraceptives may increase levels of clotting factors VII, VIII, IX, and X, thyroxin-binding globulin, protein-bound iodine, thyroxine, platelet aggregation, and results of Bromsulphalein, bilirubin, and liver function tests (alanine transaminase, aspartate transaminase). The estrogen component in OCs increases HDL levels and decreases LDL levels. Total cholesterol and LDL are increased by progestins, whereas levels of triglycerides and HDL are decreased. The newer generation of progestins (desogestrel and norgestimate) have been shown to raise levels of HDL while leaving LDL essentially unchanged. In the past, high-dose contraceptives caused a slight increase in glucose and insulin levels.

Long-Acting Contraceptives

- ❒ Depot medroxyprogesterone acetate (DEPO-PROVERA)
- ❒ Implantable levonorgestrel (NORPLANT, NORPLANT II)
- ❒ Intrauterine devices (PARAGARD COPPER-T 380A, PROGESTASERT PROGESTERONE T)

Three types of long-acting contraceptives are currently available in the United States: the subdermal implant system levonorgestrel, the depot formulation of medroxyprogesterone acetate, and the hormone-releasing intrauterine device (IUD). These systems use forms of progestin. The long-acting contraceptives are useful for women who are sexually active and desire effective contraception with relative ease of use. They are also indicated for women who have experienced estrogen-related adverse effects from oral contraceptives, who have difficulty remembering to take pills regularly, or who have heavy menstrual periods resulting in anemia. Women with hypertension or a history of vascular thrombosis are also candidates for these contraceptive methods.

INJECTABLE PROGESTINS

Depot medroxyprogesterone acetate (DMPA) may be helpful with DUB that occurs during perimenopause, in addition to providing contraception. DEPO-PROVERA is also useful for mentally retarded patients, for whom compliance with a drug requiring daily administration may be an issue. The quantity of breast milk has increased in women using DEPO-PROVERA, but the amount of drug found in the breast milk is small. Other beneficial effects of this agent are reduced anemia due to smaller menstrual blood loss, decreased incidence of candidal vulvovaginitis and pelvic inflammatory disease, and a lower risk of endometrial cancer.

Much like other progesterone systems, DMPA prevents pregnancy in three ways: It inhibits ovulation, changes the cervical mucus to help prevent sperm from reaching the egg, and changes the lining of the uterus to prevent the fertilized egg from implanting in the endometrium. It is a crystalline substance that deposits in tissue and reabsorbs slowly. Plasma levels adequate to achieve contraception are obtained within 24 hours of injection and are maintained for at least 14 weeks. DMPA carries no estrogenic or androgenic effects.

The most common problems with DMPA are irregular bleeding, mastalgia, weight gain, and depression. Most women become amenorrheic after 6 to 12 months of use. Serious weight gain and depression require discontinuation of the drug and may not be relieved for 6 to 8 months following discontinuation. Bone density also is decreased more often with the long-term use of medroxyprogesterone than with other forms of contraception.

The usual dosage of DMPA is 150 mg administered intramuscularly within the first 5 days of the menstrual cycle. A back-up contraceptive method should be used for the first 2 weeks after initial administration. An average of 12 months, and as much as 2½ years, may be required for the return of fertility.

IMPLANTABLE PROGESTINS

The subdermal system of implantable levonorgestrel consists of Silastic rods containing 36 mg of levonorgestrel. The matchstick rods are surgically implanted in the inner aspect of the upper arm, where they slowly and continuously release levonorgestrel. The system acts much like the progestin-only OCs, in that the cervical mucus becomes thick and tenacious, creating a barrier to sperm migration. Ovulation and endometrial growth are suppressed, and implantation is discouraged. The six-rod NORPLANT implant provides contraceptive protection for up to 5 years (or until the rods are removed). The two-rod NORPLANT II system contains 70 mg of levonorgestrel and protects from conception for up to 3 years; it is quicker, easier, and less painful to insert than the original NORPLANT system.

NORPLANT should be inserted during the first 7 days after menstruation, parturition, or abortion or miscarriage. The sticks should be removed at the end of their effective period and replaced if contraception is still desired. NORPLANT has been successfully used in lactating patients when implanted 6 weeks after delivery. In the first months following implantation, approximately 0.085 mg of hormone is released each day. By 9 months, the dosage decreases to about 0.35 mg per day, and by 18 months, to about 0.3 mg per day. The drug is slowly biotransformed by the liver. Blood levels of levonorgestrel become undetectable 10 to 14 days after removal of the system.

The most common adverse effects of NORPLANT systems are related to menstrual irregularities. Prolonged bleeding occurs in approximately 28 percent of women, spotting in 17 percent, amenorrhea in 9.4 percent, and irregular onset of bleeding in about 7.6 percent. More frequent bleeding occurs in 7 percent of women. Most irregular bleeding cycles become more regular within 6 to 12 months of implantation. Galactorrhea, cervicitis, vaginitis, abdominal pain, leukorrhea, and musculoskeletal pain have been noted in 5 percent of patients. Other, minor side effects are acne, weight gain or loss, hirsutism, depression and other mood changes, anxiety, and nervousness. A small percentage of patients have had difficulty with removal of the implants owing to the formation of adhesions. Infection at the implantation site and expulsion of the implants are rare.

Because FSH continues to be released at a level about half of normal, the incidence of ovarian cysts is increased in NORPLANT users. Fertility is rare in users of this system, but when conception does occur, it is more likely to be ectopic than in patients experiencing normal menstrual cycles.

INTRAUTERINE DEVICES

An IUD is a T-shaped contraceptive device inserted into the uterus. Two types of IUDs are available in the United States. The PARAGARD COPPER-T 380A and the PROGESTASERT PROGESTERONE T. The PARAGARD IUD can remain in place for 10 years, but the PROGESTASERT IUD must be replaced every year. The IUD is effective and well tolerated in women who have had children.

It is not entirely clear how IUDs prevent pregnancy. They seem to prevent fertilization either by immobilizing the sperm on their way to the fallopian tubes or by changing the endometrium so a fertilized ovum cannot implant. There is a slow, continuous release of 0.65 mg per day from an IUD, an amount too small to elevate systemic progesterone levels.

The most common adverse effects of IUD use are increased menstrual bleeding and dysmenorrhea during the first few months of use. Serious complications from IUDs are rare, although IUD users may be at higher risk of developing pelvic inflammatory disease. Other complications are uterine perforation, abnormal bleeding, and cramps. These complications occur most often during and immediately after insertion of the IUD. Some women report increased vaginal discharge.

Intrauterine devices are contraindicated in the patient who is at risk for sexually transmitted diseases or has a history of pelvic inflammatory disease. Therefore, it is preferred that the candidate be in a mutually monogamous relationship. Because of the possibility of infection, the IUD is not recommended for women who have not had children or who are at greater risk for subacute bacterial endocarditis. Other relative contraindications for IUD use are a history of ectopic pregnancy, anatomic variations that make insertion difficult, and a history of impaired fertility.

New and Future Hormonal Contraceptives

Newer forms of progestins available for oral contraceptive use include desogestrel, norgestimate, and gestodene. Desogestrel and norgestimate are biologically similar. They have several beneficial effects.

Desogestrel strongly suppresses ovarian function and follicular development. The incidence of breakthrough and irregular bleeding is reduced owing to the excellent cycle control. Desogestrel has a lower affinity for androgen receptors than levonorgestrel or gestodene, and so has fewer androgenic adverse effects (e.g., acne). Desogestrel also causes less weight gain, has less influence on blood pressure, and interferes little or not at all with the positive effect of estrogen on lipid metabolism.

Capronor contains biodegradable capsules of levonorgestrel that are placed under the skin. Insertion and removal are easier than with NORPLANT, because a fibrous sheath does not form around the capsules. They provide contraception for 12 to 18 months and are still being tested in the United States. Capronor's adverse effects are similar to those of NORPLANT.

Implanon is a single, subdermal implant that contains progestin 3-ketodesogestrel. It is expected to provide contraception for 2 to 3 years. The irregular bleeding patterns seen with Implanon are similar to those seen with NORPLANT and capronor, but because Implanon contains a less androgenic form of progesterone, there is less acne and weight gain.

Biodegradable, subdermal pellets containing norethindrone are being tested to determine the number and size of pellets required to provide contraception. They appear to provide protection for 12 to 18 months and to completely degrade within 24 months of insertion. Current research centers on determining the size, number of pellets, and hormone preparation necessary for contraception. Adverse effects of the pellets include abnormal bleeding for the first few months, which usually returns to normal. Insertion of the pellets is simple, but they sometimes fracture during removal.

A vaginal Silastic ring containing the progestin-only levonorgestrel is also available for contraception. It is placed like a diaphragm, high in the vagina. Progesterone is released gradually and absorbed through the vagina. Irritation of the vaginal mucosa has been a problem in clinical trials. Contraception is provided for 6 months.

Combination estrogen and progestin vaginal rings containing 50 mg ethinyl estradiol and 100 mg levonorgestrel release small amounts of hormone with each menstrual cycle. Such a ring is placed in the vagina on day 7 of the menstrual cycle and removed after 21 days to allow withdrawal bleeding. Expulsion of the ring and interference with intercourse are common problems.

GnRH agonists and antagonists are being formulated as biodegradable microcapsules or Silastic implants. They suppress ovarian function, leading to a hypoestrogenic state. Complications of insufficient estrogen are common. These drugs are being investigated for use in men also. Hormonal contraception in men is difficult, because sperm production is continuous, not cyclic as in women. Methods such as implants, injections, and pills that inhibit spermatogenesis to a low enough level to provide contraceptive benefits are being investigated.

Critical Thinking Process

Assessment

History of Present Illness

The first step in assessing the patient who presents with disorders of the menstrual cycle or for contraceptive counseling is to obtain the reason for the visit. Information should be obtained as to age, drugs or contraceptives used, and a description of complaints. A complete menstrual history, including age at menarche, and usual interval and duration of menses, should be obtained. Questions about the presence or absence of premenstrual symptoms, such as breast tenderness, bloating, or abdominal pain that occurs midway between menstrual periods *(mittelschmerz)*, should be included. Signs and symptoms, such as the amount and duration of abnormal bleeding, pain associated with bleeding or intercourse, headaches, presence or absence of abdominal pain, hirsutism, vasomotor symptoms, vaginal dryness, mastalgia and breast discharge, and infertility, should all be explored. If the patient reports heavy menses, the health care provider should determine whether it is associated with periods of dizziness, fainting, or lightheadedness. The extent to which the menstrual disorder is interfering with the woman's activities of daily living should also be established.

Past Health History

In addition to a menstrual history, information is gathered regarding past illnesses, hospitalizations, and surgeries. Any chronic diseases, particularly thyroid, hepatic, renal, or other endocrine disorders, should be noted. The health care provider should ask about a history of coagulopathies, excessive bruising, varicose veins, or thrombophlebitis. Previous gynecologic surgery or treatment for gynecologic disorders, such as abnormal Papanicolaou smear, endometriosis, or leiomyoma, is important to note.

An obstetric history—details of past pregnancies, ectopic pregnancy, abortions (spontaneous or therapeutic)—should be obtained. Postpartum hemorrhage or infection should be asked about.

Drugs the patient is currently taking or has recently taken may affect the diagnosis and/or management of menstrual cycle disorders or contraceptive choices. The use of tobacco, alcohol, antibiotics, or illicit drugs should be explored. Other life-style habits that may be important to elicit are recent or extreme weight loss or gain, exercise, stress, and sexual practices.

Physical Exam Findings

After a thorough history is obtained, a complete head-to-toe physical examination should be performed. While performing the exam, the health care provider should note general body habitus, development of secondary sexual characteristics, distribution of body fat, distribution and texture of hair, any bruises, and color of mucous membranes. Baseline vital signs, including height and weight, should be evaluated.

The presence of hirsutism, acne, and exophthalmos as well as the color of the sclera should be noted. Extraocular eye movements and the patient's visual field should be tested. The thyroid should be examined for nodules or enlargement, and any lymphadenopathy noted. The breasts should be examined for dimpling or retraction of tissue, masses, and discharge. The health care provider should use this opportunity to counsel the patient concerning breast self-examination.

The external genitalia should be examined for lesions, erythema, and any obstruction, such as an imperforate hymen or septum. Clitoromegaly, and the presence of vaginal discharge, erythema, or vaginal or cervical lesions or polyps should be noted. The color of mucous membranes of the vagina and signs of estrogen deficiency, such as absence of rugae or atrophy, should be included. A bimanual exam should be performed to determine uterine size and any tenderness. The adnexa should be palpated for masses or tenderness. The abdomen should be examined for any masses, organomegaly, hernias, or tenderness.

Diagnostic Testing

Women of child-bearing age who present with abnormal menstrual bleeding or for contraception should have a pregnancy test. Urine testing for pregnancy is usually sufficient. A Papanicolaou smear and complete blood count are basic tests that will be helpful in evaluating any female patient. Thyroid function tests (thyroxine and thyroid-stimulating hormone) are useful in evaluating amenorrhea. If the patient's history or exam findings suggest, liver function tests, coagulation tests, progesterone level, and cervical cultures for *Chlamydia* and gonorrhea may be ordered. If a pituitary tumor is suspected, a prolactin measurement is recommended. If the prolactin level is high, computed tomography or magnetic resonance imaging will be needed to rule out pituitary adenoma.

Transvaginal ultrasonography may be useful in evaluating the patient who presents with a complaint of pelvic pain. This procedure can provide evidence of uterine size, endometrial thickening, presence of ovarian cysts, presence of leiomyoma, and the suspicion or likelihood of an ectopic pregnancy.

In the perimenopausal or menopausal patient presenting with intermenstrual bleeding, an FSH level higher than 40 IU/mL indicates ovarian failure (5 to 20 IU/mL is normal). An endometrial biopsy evaluates for uterine proliferation or hyperplasia. Office hysteroscopy is practical to visualize the endometrium and obtain directed sampling in the patient who is not actively bleeding. Dilatation and curettage may be required if an adequate sample cannot be obtained by biopsy or hysteroscopy, or if treatment is unsuccessful.

Developmental Considerations

Perinatal In the patient of child-bearing age who presents with menstrual cycle or gynecologic disorders, the past gynecologic and obstetric history and plans for future childbearing are crucial to diagnosis. The possibility of pregnancy as a source of the complaints should always be pursued. The health care provider's first encounter with patients of this age group is often for pregnancy care or for contraception. Women usually do not appreciate meeting their health care provider for the first time when they have already been asked to change to an examining gown and to place their legs in the stirrups for a pelvic exam. It may be helpful to elicit the chief complaint, history of present illness, and medical history prior to having the patient change into a gown.

Pediatric Examination of the pediatric patient must be adapted to the individual developmental needs. The usual dorsal lithotomy examination position is not always appropriate. Very young children may be examined in the frog-leg position, or in their mother's arms. Adequate visualization of the prepubertal female genitalia can usually be accomplished by gently retracting the labia majora and applying traction downward on the vagina. Pelvic anatomy can be palpated through the rectum. If the use of invasive instruments is required, they must be small.

Foreign bodies inserted into the vagina are common sources of bleeding, discharge, or odor in the pediatric patient. Other gynecologic problems in pediatric patients may be the result of abuse or molestation, or trauma.

It takes approximately 2 years for the hypothalamic-pituitary-ovarian axis to fully mature. As a result, an adolescent's menstrual cycles are frequently anovulatory. Irregular menstrual bleeding and dysmenorrhea are common complaints of the adolescent female seeking care. In obtaining the sexual history of such a patient, it is important to ask about the onset of secondary sexual characteristics and about sexual activity, including the number of partners and use of condoms. Unless bleeding is heavy, a bimanual exam and/or ultrasound is usually sufficient to adequately assess the patient. A Papanicolaou smear should be obtained if the patient is sexually active. Management depends on the signs and symptoms, history, physical exam, and need for contraception.

Adolescents are undergoing a number of physical and emotional changes that are confusing for many. The health care provider is in an excellent position to offer support during this time. Confidentiality is important to the adolescent patient.

Geriatric Management of patients during perimenopause or menopause depends on symptoms and individual needs. Past and current medical history is essential. After pathologic causes of abnormal bleeding or pain are eliminated, the patient can be managed with various drugs, depending on the patient's life-style, medical condition, and personal preferences. At this time, the patient should be assessed for the likelihood of age-related complications, such as osteoporosis, urogenital atrophy, cancer of the genital tract, and cardiovascular disease.

Psychosocial Considerations

Human sexuality is a complex phenomenon encompassing biologic, psychological, and sociocultural aspects. Biologic aspects are the anatomy and physiology of sexual development and sexual activities, and psychological aspects consist of gender identity, sexual self-concept, and valuing oneself as a male or female. Sociocultural aspects include sexual orientation learned from the value systems of the family, peers, and community. All of these aspects are interrelated and interdependent.

Changing social norms have made discussion of menstrual cycle concerns more acceptable. However, some patients continue to feel extremely uncomfortable discussing issues of menstrual function. For these reasons, the health care provider should be prepared to deal with this aspect of care. He or she should become knowledgeable about sexuality and sexual norms, and should use this knowledge to understand the patient's behavior and reactions to sexuality in health and illness. The health care provider must be aware of differences in cultural and individual attitudes and perspectives regarding sexuality and the menstrual cycle. He or she should pay attention to the attitudes and words used by the patient to describe the symptoms. In some cases, it may be well to begin the interview with discussion of other subjects, such as physical or family questions, and then move to questions about menarche, age of onset of sexual development, and so on. The discussion should focus on the patient's general knowledge and expectations of the visit before moving to specific concerns.

Assessment information includes the patient's knowledge about hormonal therapies. Compliance with hormonal therapy involves the willingness to take the drugs as prescribed, to have breast and pelvic exams, and to arrange for blood pressure measurements every 6 to 12 months. (See Case Study—Postmenopausal Bleeding.)

Case Study Postmenopausal Bleeding

Patient History

History of Present Illness	AD is a 59-year-old white female with a history of no menses for 8 years, until the onset 2 months ago of irregular vaginal bleeding. Other symptoms are dyspareunia, hot flushes, and stress incontinence. She believes that she is a little shorter than she used to be.
Past Health History	AD is allergic to sulfa. She denies tobacco or alcohol use. She takes no drugs, other than Tylenol or Motrin for occasional aches and pains, a multivitamin, and daily calcium supplement. She has no history of cardiovascular disease or bone fractures, and has never had hormonal replacement therapy. She has had three vaginal deliveries, but no gynecologic surgery. Her last Papanicolaou smear was 2 years ago. The lipid profile done at that time was normal.
Physical Exam Findings	BP 106/60; height 5′4″; weight 150 lb. Small degree of kyphosis. Pelvic exam: labia atrophic; vagina pink, no rugae; first-degree cystocele; uterus small, nontender, no adnexal mass or tenderness.
Diagnostic Testing	Pap smear normal. Endometrial biopsy reveals atrophic endometrium. Thyroid profiles normal. Cholesterol level 239 mg/dL; HDL 30 mg/dL.
Developmental Considerations	AD is in the normal menopausal age range and is at risk for complications of postmenopausal syndrome.
Psychosocial Considerations	AD has not been concerned about the risks/benefits of hormonal replacement therapy, because she has not experienced any symptoms in the past. She is married and is sexually active.
Economic Factors	AD has insurance coverage with her husband's health plan and pharmacy plan.

Variables Influencing Decision

Treatment Objectives	• Relieve patient's symptoms and minimize complications of menopausal syndrome. • Initiate treatment plan with the least risks and greatest benefits for the patient.

Drug Variables	*Drug Summary*	*Patient Variables*
Indications	Symptoms of menopausal syndrome: irregular bleeding, urogenital atrophy, stress incontinence, kyphosis.	AD has no evidence of endometrial hyperplasia or neoplasia; does have menopausal syndrome.
Pharmacodynamics	Estrogen: Endogenous estrogen is produced by the ovaries and adrenals; converted from androgens; responsible for normal menses; regulated through negative and positive feedback mechanisms through the anterior pituitary and hypothalamus. Progestin: Antiestrogenic effect; inhibits proliferation of estrogen receptors, decreasing estrogen's effect on target cells. Therapeutic effects: prevents hyperplasia, inhibits endometrial growth following ovulation.	AD still has her uterus. In a patient with a uterus, both hormones are required to prevent overgrowth of the endometrium. This will become a decision point.
Adverse Effects/ Contraindications	Estrogen: Increased incidence of thromboembolic disease, hypotension, altered carbohydrate metabolism, gallbladder disease; endometrial cancer if unopposed; contraindicated in patients with history of breast cancer. Progestin: Breast tenderness, bloating, depression; contraindications same as estrogen.	This will be a decision point owing to signs/ symptoms of menopausal syndrome.

Case Study continued on following page

Drug Variables	*Drug Summary*	*Patient Variables*
Pharmacokinetics	Estrogen: Produces same response as endogenous hormone; natural estrogens rapidly biotransformed in liver; nonsteroidal estrogens require daily dosing; parenteral administration suspensions are absorbed over several days; well absorbed through skin and mucous membranes; great interindividual and intraindividual variability; elimination primarily renal. Progestin: Rapidly biotransformed in liver; requires daily dosing; biotransformed in the endometrium and the myometrium; small amounts stored in fat; elimination primarily renal.	AD has normal renal and kidney function, so this will not become a major decision point.
Dosage Regimen	Oral: Daily continuous and sequential method: estrogen, days 1–25 each month; progesterone, first 14 days or last 10 days of estrogen use. Transdermal: 0.05–0.1 mg 1–2×/wk. Intravaginal: 0.3–1.25 mg intravaginally q HS for 1 month, followed by 2–3×/wk.	Because AD has symptoms of urogenital atrophy, the method and route of administration will be a decision point. Initial therapy with intravaginal cream may be helpful. She will eventually need combination hormonal replacement therapy. Daily dosing should be adequate to prevent osteoporosis.
Laboratory Considerations	Estrogen: Favorable effect on lipid profile; tendency of oral estrogen to lower fasting insulin levels; clotting factors not altered with postmenopausal doses. Progestin: Effect on lipid profile dose related; not significant with low doses; may increase serum glucose and insulin levels.	AD has had a slightly abnormal lipid profile within past 2 years. No history of thromboembolic disease, family history of cardiovascular disease, or diabetes. Routine assessment of lipoproteins is recommended every 5 years for women in the postmenopausal age group.
Cost Index*	Oral estrogen: 1 Transdermal estrogen: 5 Intravaginal estrogen: 1 Progestin: 1	AD is able to obtain medication through her husband's insurance plan with a minimal co-pay.

Summary of Decision Points

- AD is a candidate for hormonal replacement therapy for her menopausal symptoms.
- Estrogen not contraindicated owing to normal endometrial biopsy.
- Addition of progestin required because AD still has her uterus.
- After a careful explanation of the risks and benefits of hormonal replacement therapy, the patient must decide whether to proceed with treatment.
- Route of administration variable, depending on AD's symptoms and preference.
- Intravaginal cream indicated as initial therapy owing to symptoms of atrophic vaginal bleeding.
- Daily oral progestin administration effective for prevention of endometrial hyperplasia.

DRUGS TO BE USED

- Initial treatment with PREMARIN 0.625 mg/g intravaginal cream q HS for 1 month. Patient to be reevaluated for treatment efficacy. At that time, she will be started on PREMARIN 0.625 mg po daily on days 1–25 each month, with PROVERA 10 mg po daily on days 16–25.

*Cost Index:

1 = $< 30/mo.
2 = $ 30–40/mo.
3 = $ 40–50/mo.
4 = $ 50–60/mo.
5 = $> 60/mo.

AWP of Premarin vaginal cream, 0.625 mg/g in a 42.5-g tube, is approximately $34.
AWP of 60, 0.625-mg tablets of PREMARIN is approximately $24.
AWP of 60, 10-mg tablets of PROVERA is approximately $28.
AWP of 8 transdermal estrogen (ESTRADERM) 0.05-mg patches/24 hrs is approximately $18.

Analysis and Management

Treatment Objectives

Treatment objectives for the patient presenting with complaints of menstrual cycle disorders consist of accurate diagnosis followed by amelioration or elimination, when possible, of the symptoms. A primary management goal should be to choose the method that carries the fewest risks and adverse effects, is the least invasive, and is appropriate for the patient's age and circumstances.

For the patient seeking contraception, the goals are similar to those noted previously. The patient should be provided with effective and reversible contraception that carries a minimum risk for adverse effects.

For the perimenopausal woman, the goals are relief of menopausal symptoms and reduction of the risks for cardiovascular disease and osteoporosis.

Treatment Options

Drug Variables

The choice of drug is largely determined by the cost and convenience to the patient. Oral therapy is usually preferred: the action begins promptly and the treatment can be terminated at will. The specific drug used may need to be changed to account for diminished efficacy of some orally administered drugs.

The choice of estrogen formulations depends on the reason for use and the desired route of administration. Conjugated estrogens are routinely used and are associated with fewer liver problems than other preparations. Diethylstilbestrol is the only estrogen approved for use as a postcoital contraceptive. Such use is recommended for females who are victims of rape or incest or whose physical or mental health is threatened by pregnancy. To be effective, the drug should be started within 24 hours of the unprotected intercourse, if possible, and no later than 72 hours.

Dysfunctional Uterine Bleeding Pharmacotherapeutic options for treatment of amenorrhea include use of combination OCs or progesterone. Low-dose combination drugs are preferred in the patient who is sexually active, a nonsmoker, and younger than 35 years. Combination OCs are also the drugs of choice for the patient with DUB who desires contraception as well. If the patient does not need contraception, or pregnancy is not desired, oral medroxyprogesterone acetate is indicated. If the patient is experiencing heavy bleeding, estrogen may need to be added to the progestin regimen.

Dysmenorrhea For patients with complaints of dysmenorrhea, prostaglandin inhibitors are the preferred drug. Most nonsteroidal anti-inflammatory drugs are effective in relieving primary dysmenorrhea in 70 to 90 percent of cases. These agents work enzymatically, inhibiting prostaglandin production without affecting endometrial development. They can be started with the onset of menstrual flow and rarely need to be used for more than 72 hours. Examples are ibuprofen, naproxen, mefenamic acid, diflunisal, and ketoprofen.

If the patient also desires contraception, low-dose OCs are indicated. These drugs, which suppress both menstrual fluid volume and prostaglandin release (but not synthesis) by causing endometrial hypoplasia, are effective in preventing dysmenorrhea in 60 to 80 percent of patients. Oral contraceptives should be used only in patients requiring both contraception and relief of dysmenorrhea. If there is no improvement with OCs used for 3 months, a nonsteroidal anti-inflammatory drug should be added for the next 3 months. If this combination provides no relief after 6 months, a laparoscopy should be considered.

Premenstrual Syndrome Treatment of premenstrual syndrome is controversial. The first-line management options are not hormonal; they consist of vitamin and mineral supplements and symptomatic relief with prostaglandin inhibitors, spironolactone, clonidine, or GnRH agonists. Depression may be treated with tryptophan or selective serotonin reuptake inhibitors. After other options have been tried without results, micronized progesterone may be used. (Micronized progesterone is made by breaking the drug up into very small pieces.) Its use, however, has not been shown to be superior to that of a placebo.

Menopausal Symptoms Estrogen therapy for menopause must begin early, before the osteoporotic process has begun. Estrogen replacement therapy does not reverse bone loss that has already occurred, although it appears to be effective in preventing further bone loss once it is started. In addition, if estrogen therapy is discontinued, bone loss will resume. Other possible effects of estrogen therapy on cardiovascular disease are a direct inotropic action on the heart and improved peripheral glucose metabolism, affecting insulin production. Hyperinsulinemia exerts an atherogenic effect on blood vessels. Postmenopausal women on estrogen therapy have been shown to have lower levels of circulating insulin.

Because long-term use of estrogen during menopause has been associated with endometrial cancer, the benefits of long-term therapy must be weighed against potential risks. Vasomotor symptoms decline spontaneously over time, however, so long-term use of estrogen may not be necessary.

Contraception Many methods of contraception are available for the patient who is sexually active and desires to delay fertility. Nonpharmacologic options are barrier methods, such as the diaphragm, cervical cap, spermicides, and condom. Nonhormonal IUDs are available and prevent implantation of the fertilized ovum. Pharmacologic options include combination OCs in various doses, progestin-only pills, progesterone-releasing IUDs, injectable progesterone, and progesterone subdermal implants. The proper choice should be individualized and depends on the patient's preferences, life-style, and health. Table 54–5 contains a quick overview of current contraceptive methods, their estimated effectiveness, and their availability.

Combination oral contraceptives contain one of two estrogens, predominantly ethinyl estradiol. They also contain one of eight progestins, which differ significantly in progestational and androgenic effects and also in the extent of biotransformation to estrogenic substances. The effects of a given combination drug are a result of the specific combination of estrogen and progestin. The effects of estrogen in combination formulations are similar when they are prescribed in equipotent doses, but progestins differ in progestogenic, estrogenic, antiestrogenic, and androgenic activity. Consequently, their adverse effects differ to some extent. The patient may tolerate one formulation better than another.

Currently available low-dose pills have fewer associated risks than earlier versions. Women who smoke, however, es-

TABLE 54–5 ESTIMATED EFFECTIVENESS OF CONTRACEPTIVE METHODS

Contraceptive Method	Estimated Effectiveness (%)	Availability
Male condom	88*	OTC
Female condom	79	OTC
Diaphragm with spermicide	82	Rx
Cervical cap with spermicide	64–82†	Rx
Spermicide alone	79	OTC
Combined oral contraceptive	>99	Rx
Progestin-only oral contraceptive ("minipill")	>99‡	Rx
Injection (DEPO-PROVERA)	>99	Rx
Implant (NORPLANT)	>99	Rx
Intrauterine device	98–99	Rx
Periodic abstinence	Approx. 80§	Patient teaching
Surgical sterilization, male or female	Over 99	Surgery required

OTC, over the counter; Rx, prescription.
*Effectiveness rate for polyurethane condoms has not been established.
†Less effective for women who have had a baby because the birth process stretches the vagina and cervix making it more difficult to achieve a proper fit.
‡Based on perfect use, when the woman takes the pill every day as prescribed.
§Efficacy varies based on specific method used.

pecially those older than 35 years, and women with certain medical conditions, such as a history of blood clots or breast or endometrial cancer, may be advised against taking "the pill." Oral contraceptives can contribute to cardiovascular disease, including high blood pressure, blood clots, and blockage of the arteries.

One of the biggest questions has been whether OCs increase the risk of breast cancer in past and present pill users. Research has suggested than a woman's risk of breast cancer 10 years after discontinuing birth control pills is no higher than that of women who never have used them. During and for the first 10 years after discontinuing the use of OCs, a woman's risk is only slightly higher than the risk for a woman who has never used them.

Early oral contraceptive formulations contained larger amounts of estrogen and produced a relatively high incidence of potentially serious adverse effects. Currently available formulations contain smaller amounts of estrogen, and adverse effects are expected to decrease, although their long-term effects remain unknown. Despite the lower estrogen dosage, oral contraceptives may still be safest when given to nonsmoking women younger than 35 years who do not have a history of migraine headaches, hypertension, thromboembolic problems, or diabetes mellitus.

All multiphasic OC formulations are rational first choices in most women, because they contain less progestin than monophasic formulations and they mirror the normal menstrual cycle. Further, multiphasic formulations are believed to have less effect on carbohydrate and lipid metabolism, and are as effective for contraception as monophasics. The advantages of multiphasic formulations, however, may not offset the disadvantages—confusion concerning the distinctly colored tablets, less flexibility in regard to missed doses, and a higher incidence of benign ovarian cysts.

In contrast, monophasic combinations with less estrogenic activity may be the drug of choice. These formulations provide a steady blend of estrogenic, progestational, and androgenic activity with a permissible rate of breakthrough bleeding. Compared with multiphasic formulations, the monophasic types are associated with a lower incidence of ovarian cysts.

If one OC formulation results in spotting or breakthrough bleeding (signs of estrogen deficiency), an OC with a higher estrogen content can be substituted. Likewise, if nausea, edema, or breast discomfort becomes evident (signs of estrogen excess), an OC with a lower estrogen dosage may be chosen. Progestin dosage can also be adjusted to accommodate symptoms of deficiency or excess. Changes in OC preparations can be made at the beginning of any new cycle.

Minipills can decrease menstrual bleeding and cramps, as well as the risk of endometrial and ovarian cancer and pelvic inflammatory disease. Because they contain no estrogen, minipills do not carry the risk of blood clots that is associated with estrogen in combined pills. They are a good option for women who cannot take estrogen because they are breastfeeding or because they have severe headache or high blood pressure with estrogen-containing products.

NORPLANT failures are rare, but the rate is higher with increased body weight. IUDs have one of the lowest failure rates of any contraceptive method. In the population in which the IUD is appropriate—women in a mutually monogamous, stable relationship who are not at high risk for infection—the IUD is a very safe and effective contraceptive method. (See Controversy—Hormonal Contraceptives.)

Patient Variables

Personal preference is a major factor in determining the best hormonal regimen. Even the best form of hormonal therapy is ineffective if improperly used. The health care provider should spend the time necessary to educate the patient about the available options. The choice of method is then made on the basis of informed consent.

In determining the patient's need or desire for hormonal therapy, many other factors must also be taken into account. They are the patient's specific complaints, age (developmental and physical), life-style, physical assessment findings, and laboratory data. Therapy may require continuous use for a long time, and compliance may be an issue, especially

Controversy

Hormonal Contraceptives

JONATHAN J. WOLFE

No pharmaceutical agent has had as profound an impact on society during the past 30 years as hormonal contraceptives. The abilities to treat most infections, alter lipid metabolism, regulate cardiac function, and influence the course of mental illness, which are provided by other, concurrently developed agents, are remarkable in themselves. They pale, however, in comparison with the almost flawless control over reproductive function that hormonal contraceptives confer. Worldwide population trends clearly show the effect of access to these sophisticated medications. In some cases, abortion rates testify to a willingness to substitute far riskier means of birth control in nations where contraceptives are either not available or unacceptable.

Oral contraceptives are often viewed by patients as benign products. Certainly, the risks of pregnancy and delivery are far greater than the risk of using hormonal contraceptives, especially the newer low-dose drug combinations. However, many patients stand at substantial risk; and indeed, the acceptance of any drug therapy is a matter for sober reflection. Patients who have either a personal history of clotting disorders, or a family history of certain malignancies, and patients who smoke have higher risk profiles. Many of them require careful counseling before hormonal contraceptives are chosen over other methods.

Critical Thinking Discussion

- What counseling should you offer a minor, 15 years of age, who requests an examination and prescription for oral contraceptives without the knowledge of her parents?
- Why are oral contraceptives more acceptable to American patients than contraceptive implants (e.g., NORPLANT)?
- The privacy associated with oral contraceptives makes them highly desirable. What aspects of these products are least desirable for individual patients?
- Name the three most important interactions between hormonal contraceptives and other drugs. What is the best source for information about these potentially grave drug-drug interactions?
- Is it fair for public health authorities to have access to hormonal contraceptives at prices far below those that community pharmacies must pay for the same drugs? Is it good public policy to subsidize access to these drugs for some citizens?

if adverse effects are particularly annoying. Other physical conditions, especially those that involve other drug therapies, are also important to consider in order to avoid drug-drug interactions.

Menopausal Symptoms Alternatives to hormonal replacement therapy can be useful for a woman who is reluctant to use hormones or has a contraindication to or intolerance of either estrogen or progestin. Estrogen is intolerable for about 10 percent of women. Alternative therapies, such as herbal remedies, are generally not well studied and may not be as efficacious as hormonal therapy. This said, the decision to accept hormonal replacement therapy should be made with knowledge about possible options and their associated benefits and risks. The patient should understand that although a decision to use a specific management modality has been made, the choice is not life-long. The decision can always be re-evaluated as the woman's thinking and circumstances change. Table 54–6 provides an overview of hormonal replacement regimens.

For women who are experiencing severe menopausal symptoms but dislike the idea of taking a drug to get rid of them, life-style changes and alternative and complementary treatment modalities may be appropriate (see Chapter 60). Likewise, for women who are having few symptoms, life-style changes may be the only treatment needed. Because taking hormones to prevent cardiovascular disease and osteoporosis is a different issue from taking them to treat symptoms, the patient's decision is made more difficult, and the values surrounding the issue may be different. Helping the patient to explore family history and the overall impact of her longevity on the potential for these disorders will assist in making an appropriate decision. What effect would life-style changes, such as diet, exercise, weight loss, stress reduction, and quitting smoking, have on these same diseases?

The critical question is when to start estrogen or hormonal therapy. Although the current trend is to start all women on hormones at menopause and have them taking hormones for life, it is not the only choice. Because the greatest effect on decreasing mortality from heart disease seems to be in those women currently taking hormones, it may make sense to wait until the patient is in her 60s or 70s to start therapy. If it turns out that hormones work because they dilate blood vessels, then the patient would want to have been taking hormones when a myocardial infarction occurs. On the other hand, there are data suggesting that estrogen should be started right at menopause to prevent the bone loss of osteoporosis. There are no absolute answers to these issues at this time, rendering decision-making that much more difficult.

Contraception Factors that should be noted when selecting an OC include the patient's goals for family planning, age, frequency of intercourse, and motivation and ability to comply with a treatment plan. For a woman who frequently engages in intercourse, OCs or a progestin implant may be appropriate. Likewise, for a patient for whom sexual activity is infrequent, a condom, diaphragm, or spermicide may offer the necessary protection against pregnancy and can offer protection against sexually transmitted diseases. These combinations may be especially beneficial for the woman who has multiple sexual partners. If compliance is an issue, as it can be with the use of OCs, condoms, or a diaphragm, an IUD, or a progestin implant can be a reasonable choice. For couples whose family planning goals have already been met, sterilization of either partner may be a desirable alternative to drug therapy.

Women who have had a contraceptive failure while correctly taking a low-estrogen OC should receive a higher-estrogen formulation. Further, women who are taking other drugs that reduce the efficacy of the OCs (e.g., phenobarbital, phenytoin, carbamazepine, rifampin) should also be started on a higher-estrogen formulation.

Patients with acne, lipid abnormalities, cardiovascular risks, or metabolic abnormalities may benefit from an OC with reduced androgenic activity. These products have fewer cardiovascular and metabolic adverse effects. However, a patient can be started on a multiphasic product and re-evaluated after a few months to determine whether these conditions have worsened or improved.

The contraceptive implants provide an effective means of contraception, although the efficacy of the formulation may be weight dependent, and the adverse effects are similar to those of progestin-only oral formulations. Further, surgery is

TABLE 54–6 EXAMPLES OF HORMONAL REPLACEMENT REGIMENS

Regimen	Component	Administration	Drug Options
Continuous combined	Estrogen	Daily	0.625 mg conjugated estrogen 0.625 mg estrone 1 mg micronized estradiol*
	Progesterone	Daily	2.5 mg medroxyprogesterone acetate 0.35 mg norethindrone Micronized progesterone†
Continuous sequential	Estrogen	Daily	0.625 mg conjugated estrogen 0.625 mg estrone 1 mg micronized estradiol*
	Progesterone	Days 1–14	5 mg medroxyprogesterone acetate Micronized progesterone†
Cyclical sequential	Estrogen	Days 1–25	0.625 mg conjugated estrogen 1 mg micronized estradiol*
	Progesterone	Days 1–14 or Days 13–25	5 mg medroxyprogesterone acetate Micronized progesterone†
Cyclical combined	Estrogen	Days 1–25	0.625 mg conjugated estrogen
	Progesterone	Days 1–25	2.5 mg medroxyprogesterone acetate 0.35 mg norethindrone acetate Micronized progesterone†
Continuous‡	Estrogen	Days 1–30	0.625 mg conjugated estrogen

*Micronized estradiol (ESTRACE).
†Dose and route of micronized progesterone (CRINONE, PROMETRIUM) vary from patient to patient.
‡Estrogen-only dosage regimen for women who no longer have a uterus.

required for their insertion and removal, and they are rather costly.

Progestin-only minipills may be an appropriate choice in women with absolute contraindications to estrogens. Although minipills are less effective than the combination OCs (2 to 3 percent versus 0.3 to 1.2 percent failure rate, respectively), their use may be considered whenever contraception is desired for women who cannot tolerate estrogen at all, or for those women who are breastfeeding. The use of progestin-only formulations should be contemplated whenever contraception is desired in women who cannot take estrogen (e.g., because of systemic lupus erythematosus, varicose veins, or estrogen-induced hypertension).

Breakthrough bleeding is the most common reason for switching formulations. For most healthy young women, spotting is not an ominous sign and is ordinarily managed with a watch-and-wait approach for several months. In general, many cases of breakthrough bleeding can be managed by switching to a different formulation, regardless of the estrogen or progestin activity. If the breakthrough bleeding continues to occur during the first 10 days of use (usually indicating estrogen deficiency), switching to a formulation with higher estrogenic activity is appropriate. If, however, the breakthrough bleeding occurs after the tenth day (usually indicating a progestin deficiency), switching to a formulation with higher progestin activity is warranted.

For women who report the development or worsening of acne, hair growth, or hypertension, switching to a formulation with a lower androgenic activity is appropriate. Scanty periods or amenorrhea is common with long-term use of oral contraceptives. If the amenorrhea is not due to pregnancy, the addition of 0.2 mg of ethinyl estradiol or 0.625 mg of conjugated estrogen for the first 7 days of the next two or three cycles often results in a return of withdrawal bleeding.

Healthy nonsmoking women can continue to use oral contraceptives without increased risk until the age of 50 years. Oral formulations should not be used in women older than 35 years who smoke, because of their markedly increased risk of cardiovascular disease. When pregnancy is wanted, the contraceptive should be stopped approximately 3 months ahead of conception to allow for accurate dating of the pregnancy. There does not appear to be a higher risk of birth defects if conception occurs within the first month after the contraceptive agent is discontinued.

Oral contraceptives should be restarted approximately 4 to 6 weeks postpartum. This period allows coagulation to return to normal levels and permits lactation to become established. Nevertheless, in women who may be sexually active during the early postpartum period and who will not use alternative methods of birth control, oral contraceptives can be restarted immediately. Although it is generally considered safe for a woman to use oral contraceptives while breastfeeding if she is otherwise healthy and lactation is established, the practice remains controversial.

Intervention

Administration

Contraceptives and other hormones may be administered by many routes. Each patient's circumstances must be considered in determining the most appropriate route. The packaging of many hormonal products is designed so that the products are taken only on a certain day in the cycle. To prevent confusion regarding when to start therapy, the package design should be taken into account. Oral contraceptives are available in 21-day or 28-day packs. The last seven pills of a 28-day pack are placebos only. This packaging provides the convenience of taking a pill every day without needing to count days off.

In general, multiphasic OCs are started on day 1 of the menses to ensure first-cycle inhibition of ovulation. Monophasic OCs are started on day 5 or 6 of the menses. Ovulation is inhibited as long as the OC is started on one of these days.

Alternative dosing schedules have been effectively used by some patients. For example, if the timing of the menstrual flow is problematic, such as for honeymoon, holidays, or athletics, skipping a period is possible. To cause a change in cycle, a new 21-day package is started as soon as the previous one has been completed. The patient should be advised that breakthrough bleeding may occur with this regimen. For other women who are taking a triphasic formulation with a significant increase in the progestin component, a new package may be started from front to back. This regimen minimizes the chance of spotting as a result of a relative fall in progesterone levels. For the patient taking monophasic products who experiences headaches or migraines the week she is off contraceptives, consideration should be given to changing to a different oral contraceptive.

Education

For many women, a gynecologic exam is the most likely time to seek medical care. Therefore, it is a valuable time to educate such a patient about her body and its function, as well as illness prevention and health maintenance. The woman should be taught about the benefits of regular check-ups, accompanied by an annual Papanicolaou smear and breast exam, as well as the value of regular breast self-examinations in between. The important roles that diet and exercise play in her current and future health, including prevention of osteoporosis and cardiovascular disease, should be emphasized.

When a patient presents with a medical condition, whether it be natural, such as menopause, or a disruption of a natural physiologic mechanism, she should be given information concerning the treatment options available. This information should be provided at the appropriate age and educational level for her understanding.

If drug treatment is advised, information should include appropriate indications, benefits, and potential adverse effects. Package inserts may be given to the patient to furnish complete information. In addition, specific instructions may be needed, depending on the indication and/or treatment chosen. Noncompliance and discontinuation of the drug may be avoided by proper counseling at the start of therapy.

Hormonal Replacement Therapy The perimenopausal or menopausal patient should be assured that her condition is a natural occurrence. However, she should also be advised that the loss of ovarian function may result in physical changes that can be ameliorated or avoided by the use of hormonal replacement therapy. She should be counseled about the risks of osteoporosis, cardiovascular changes, and urogenital atrophy. Information should be provided concerning the risks and benefits of hormonal replacement therapy, allowing the woman to make an informed choice among the treatment options. She should also be encouraged to incorporate exercise and dietary changes into her life, and to stop smoking. The menopausal or perimenopausal patient should also be given information appropriate to her age range as to early recognition of disorders such as cardiovascular disease and diabetes. She should be taught to perform monthly breast self-examination and to have a pelvic exam and Papanicolaou smear yearly.

At the start of hormonal replacement therapy, the patient should be counseled to keep records of the onset, duration, and amount of any uterine bleeding. She should be also advised of the importance of keeping follow-up appointments.

Contraception The patient should be advised that oral contraceptives, IUDs, subdermal implants, and contraceptive injections do not provide protection against the human immunodeficiency virus or sexually transmitted diseases. Any patient using hormonal contraceptives should be counseled about the risks of smoking and development of deep vein thrombosis.

The patient should be informed that for maximal effectiveness, OCs should be taken at approximately the same time each day. Information should be provided concerning what to do in the event of missed pills, for the occurrence of diarrhea or vomiting, or about concomitant use of drugs that may interfere with the pill's effectiveness. The most appropriate action in any of these circumstances is to use a back-up contraceptive method until the next menstrual period.

Generally speaking, if one dose of an OC is missed, it should be taken as soon as it is remembered. If two doses are missed, the patient should take two tablets of the OC for the next 2 days, and should use a supplemental birth control method also for the rest of the pill cycle while continuing to take the OC. If more than two consecutive doses are missed, contraception for that cycle is questionable, and a new package of pills should be started after pregnancy has been ruled out and the menses begins.

For postcoital contraception, the general rule is two tablets of OVRAL immediately and two tablets again in 12 hours. If LO/OVRAL, NORDITTE, LEVLEN, TRIPHASIL or TRI-LEVLEN, are used, four tablets should be taken immediately, and four additional tablets taken 12 hours later. This procedure is often used in emergency rooms for victims of rape. This regimen applies if the drug is taken within 3 days of the unprotected intercourse. Nausea is common with this dosage, and eating a snack with the pills may be helpful. Warning signs of estrogen excess—severe leg pain, severe abdominal pain, chest pain or shortness of breath, severe headaches or dizziness, blurred or loss of vision, and jaundice—should be described. The woman should be told that her next menstrual period may not occur at the usual time, and to return for a pregnancy test if menses does not occur within 4 weeks. She should also receive counseling about appropriate forms of birth control for regular use.

When using either of the NORPLANT subdermal systems, the patient should be informed that the implants become effective within 24 hours of insertion and that effectiveness lasts for about 3 to 5 years (depending on the formulation used), at which time they should be replaced. The patient should be counseled concerning signs of infection and told to return to the health care provider if symptoms occur. She should be informed that irregular bleeding is common for the first few months to 1 year after insertion of the implants. Follow-up care is important if bleeding becomes heavy.

The woman using an IUD birth control method should be taught to check for the presence of the IUD strings in the vagina after each period, because the IUD can be expelled during menstruation without the patient's being aware of it. She should also be counseled to return to the health care provider if signs of infection appear, such as fever, pelvic pain, severe cramping, or increased bleeding. If she misses a period, she should contact the health care provider immediately to evaluate for the possibility of pregnancy.

Evaluation

The female patient should be seen by a health care provider annually for routine gynecologic follow-up, regardless of whether she receives drug treatment. The first return visit should be scheduled for after completion of three cycles of hormone treatment. A history of the menstrual cycle should be obtained at each visit.

If a woman receiving estrogens develops persistent or recurrent vaginal bleeding, an evaluation should be conducted for endometrial cancer. All patients on estrogen therapy should have endometrial biopsy every 2 to 3 years. Additional follow-up depends on the particular condition and treatment regimen chosen. For example, it is reasonable to have a patient who is taking OCs or hormones to treat DUB, amenorrhea, or dysmenorrhea return for evaluation of the effectiveness of the treatment and adverse effects.

The postmenopausal patient who is started on estrogen replacement or hormonal replacement therapy also needs to be re-evaluated in 3 months. This length of time is sufficient for the occurrence of improvement in atrophy of the vagina and other menopausal symptoms, as well as drug adverse effects.

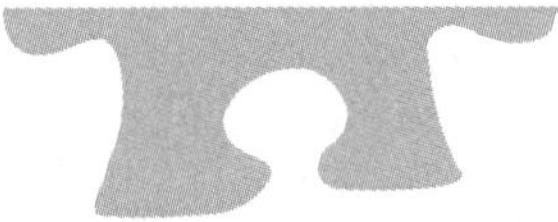

SUMMARY

- The ovarian cycle can be divided into three phases: follicular phase, ovulatory phase, and luteal phase. The endometrium cycle prepares the endometrium for implantation by an ovum.
- Gonadotropin-releasing hormone from the hypothalamus stimulates release of FSH from the anterior pituitary gland.
- LH is released from the anterior pituitary in response to elevated levels of estrogen.
- Estrogen secretion increases between ages 9 and 12 years, triggering sexual maturation, and begins to decline as the woman enters the perimenopausal period at about 40 years.
- Disruptions of the normal menstrual cycle may occur; they include amenorrhea, dysmenorrhea, premenstrual syndrome, DUB, and polycystic ovarian syndrome.
- A complete history and physical exam must be performed in order to determine the probable etiology of the patient's complaint or to identify appropriate therapy for menopause or contraception.
- The patient who presents with a disorder of the menstrual cycle or who requests contraceptive counseling should have a complete history and physical exam.
- Attention should be given to menstrual cycle history, pregnancy history, thyroid, cardiovascular, renal, and endocrine irregularities, malignancies, and thromboembolic phenomena.
- Laboratory testing may consist of pregnancy testing, Papanicolaou smear, complete blood count, and measurements of thyroid and liver function, FSH, and LH.
- Whether the patient is seeking treatment of a pathologic condition, contraception, or prevention of menopausal symptoms, the option that has the lowest dosage and fewest side effects, while providing the desired therapeutic effects, should be chosen.
- Estrogen and progestin preparations are available for the treatment of menopausal symptoms. If the patient still has her uterus, progestin should be given concomitantly to avoid endometrial hyperplasia.
- Many forms of hormonal preparations are available as contraceptives, including oral estrogen-progesterone combinations, oral progestin-only pills, intramuscular progesterone, subdermal implants, and progesterone-releasing IUDs.
- The patient should be advised that oral contraceptives, IUDs, subdermal implants, and contraceptive injections do not provide protection against the human immunodeficiency virus or sexually transmitted diseases.
- In general, multiphasic OCs are started on day 1 of the menses to ensure first-cycle inhibition of ovulation. Monophasic OCs are started by day 5 or 6 of the menses. Ovulation is inhibited as long as the OC is started on one of these days.
- If one dose of an OC is missed, it should be taken as soon as it is remembered. If two doses are missed, two tablets of the OC should be taken for the next 2 days and a supplemental birth control method also used. If more than two consecutive doses are missed, contraception for that cycle is questionable, and a new package of pills should be started after pregnancy has been ruled out and the menses begins.
- For postcoital contraception, the general rule is two tablets immediately and two more tablets in 12 hours. This regimen applies if the drug is taken within 3 days of the unprotected intercourse.
- Initiation of hormonal therapy necessitates a follow-up visit in 3 months to evaluate its efficacy and adverse effects. This length of time is sufficient for the occurrence of improvement in atrophy of the vagina and other menopausal symptoms, as well as the drug's adverse effects.

BIBLIOGRAPHY

American College of Obstetricians and Gynecologists. (1996). *Guidelines for women's health care.* Washington, DC: Author.

Ali, N., and Twibell, K. (1994). Barriers to osteoporosis prevention in perimenopausal and elderly women. *Geriatric Nurse,* 15, 201–205.

Archer, D. (1994). Clinical and metabolic features of desogestrel: A new oral contraceptive preparation. *American Journal of Obstetrics and Gynecology,* 170(5), 1550–1555.

Archer, D. (1995). Management of bleeding in women using subdermal implants. *Contemporary Obstetrics and Gynecology,* 40(7), 11–25.

Burkman, R. (1994). Noncontraceptive effects of hormonal contraceptives: Bone mass, sexually transmitted disease and pelvic inflammatory disease, cardiovascular disease, menstrual function, and future fertility. *American Journal of Obstetrics and Gynecology,* 170(5), 1569–1574.

Chuong, C., Pearsall-Otey, L., and Rosenfeld, B. (1995). A practical guide to relieving PMS. *Contemporary Nurse Practitioner,* 1(5), 31–37.

Darney, P. (1994). Hormonal implants: Contraception for a new century. *American Journal of Obstetrics and Gynecology,* 170(5), 1536–1542.

Dickey, R. (1994). *Managing contraceptive pill patients* (8th ed.). Durant, OK: Essential Medical Information Systems.

Glass, R. (1993). *Office gynecology* (4th ed.). Baltimore: Williams & Wilkins.

Goldzieher, J. (1994). Menopause: A deficiency state. *Advances in Obstetrics and Gynecology,* 1, 159–173.

Hatcher, R., Trussell, J., Stewart, F., et al. (1994). *Contraceptive technology* (16th ed.). New York: Irvington Publishers.

Kaunitz, A. (1994). Long-acting injectable contraception with depot medroxyprogesterone acetate. *American Journal of Obstetrics and Gynecology,* 170(5), 1543–1549.

Love, S. (1997). *Dr. Susan Love's hormone book: Making informed decisions about menopause.* New York: Random House.

McKeon, V. (1994). Hormone replacement therapy: Evaluating the risks and benefits. *Journal of Obstetric, Gynecologic, and Neonatal Nursing,* 23(8), 647–657.

Moore, A., and Noonan, M. (1996). A nurse's guide to hormone replacement therapy. *Journal of Obstetric, Gynecologic, and Neonatal Nursing,* 25(1), 24–31.

Rayburn, W., and Carey, J. (1996). *Obstetrics and gynecology.* Baltimore: Williams & Wilkins.

Rosenfeld, J. (1997). *Women's health in primary care.* Baltimore: Williams & Wilkins.

Seltzer, V., and Pearse, W. (1995). *Women's primary health care: Office practice and procedures.* New York: McGraw-Hill.

Speroff, L., Glass, R., and Kase, N. (1994). *Clinical gynecologic endocrinology and infertility* (5th ed.). Baltimore: Williams & Wilkins.

Thorneycroft, I. (1993). Contraception in women older than 40 years of age. *Obstetrics and Gynecology Clinics of North America,* 20(2), 273–278.

Youngkin, E., and Davis, M. (1994). *Women's health: A primary care clinical guide.* Norwalk, CT: Appleton & Lange.

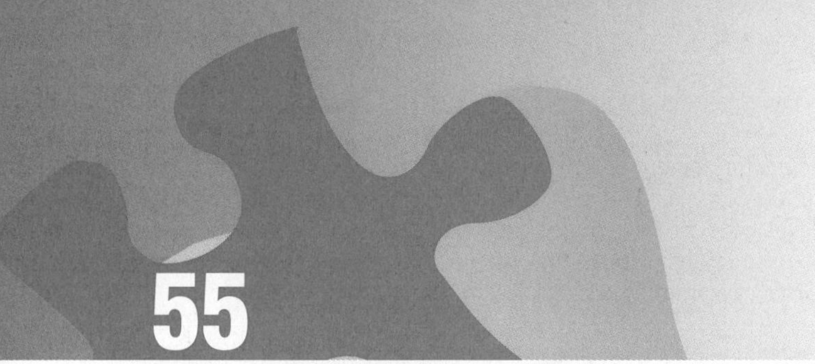

55 Uterine Motility Drugs

Pregnancy is a dynamic state. From the start of pregnancy, the fate of the fetus is directly related to that of its mother. Any substances ingested, inhaled, or otherwise received by the mother may pass through the placenta to the fetus unless it is destroyed or changed on its passage. Substances that cross placental membranes usually reach concentrations of 50 to 100 percent of the initial amount to which the mother was exposed. The resulting biochemical reactions can affect the growing fetus as well as the mother and gestation.

There are three groups of drugs available to stimulate uterine activity. The principal use of *uterine stimulants* such as oxytocin is for the induction of labor. *Prostaglandins* are used principally for abortion, whereas ergot alkaloids are used in control of postpartum bleeding. *Tocolytic* drugs have only one use: suppression of preterm labor (PTL).

Whenever drug therapy is indicated during pregnancy, it is vital to consider the benefit versus the risk of its use on the fetus. Few drugs are considered safe for use during pregnancy, and drug use is generally contraindicated. Despite the general principle that drug use should be avoided, the pregnant woman may require drug therapy for a variety of problems, including treatment of PTL or induction of labor.

PHYSIOLOGY OF LABOR

Causes of Labor

The etiology for the initiation of labor is not understood. Research has provided a number of theories based on observable biochemical factors (Fig. 55–1). It is known that there is a dramatic drop in progesterone and a surge of estrogen just before the onset of labor. In humans, progesterone withdrawal does not occur till after delivery of the fetus. Estrogen levels have been shown to increase markedly during the last 2 or 3 weeks of pregnancy. The estrogen domination is credited with the increased myometrial excitability noted 2 to 3 weeks before labor. Estrogen is also credited for the increase in the number of oxytocin receptors in the myometrium.

Oxytocin is a naturally occurring stimulant of uterine contractions. The oxytocin theory is based on evidence that the number of oxytocin receptors in the myometrial tissue of the uterus increases dramatically toward the end of gestation. Oxytocin is also thought to interact with the endometrial (decidual) tissue of the uterus to release prostaglandins. A direct link between oxytocin and the initiation of labor has been difficult to establish because labor will ensue in the complete absence of oxytocin. This occurrence does not eliminate the importance of oxytocins in the process of labor but merely questions their role in the onset of labor.

There is increasing evidence that prostaglandins play an important role in the onset of labor. The decidua, myometrium, and fetal membranes are known to produce prostaglandins, and prostaglandins are known to cause uterine contractions. During labor, prostaglandin levels in blood, urine, and amniotic fluid rise dramatically. Prostaglandins can induce labor at any point in gestation whether they are given orally, intravenously (IV), intramuscularly (IM), or instilled into the amniotic fluid. Prostaglandin inhibitors are known to prolong gestation and lengthen labor.

The fetal-maternal communication theory is presently considered the most viable theory. The premise is that there are two arms to the initiation of labor—the paracrine (fetal) and the endocrine. The paracrine system is the interaction between the fetal membranes and the decidua. This system is held responsible for maintaining the pregnancy. The hypothesis is that diminishing support of the fetal paracrine system stimulates a decidual response. The decidual response, in turn, is theorized to initiate labor. Conversely, this theory states that it is the fetus that maintains the pregnancy by preventing decidual activation.

Stages and Progression of Labor

Labor is separated into three distinct stages. Many health care providers refer to the first few hours after delivery of the placenta as the fourth stage of labor. The first stage begins with uterine contractions that cause progressive cervical change and is complete when the cervix is dilated to 10 cm. Today, the evaluation and management of labor is fundamentally based on the Friedman curve. Friedman divided labor into two phases—latent and active. The latent phase is defined as the time period from the onset of cervical change until 3 cm of dilatation is achieved. During the active phase, the cervix continues to dilate approximately 1 to 2 cm/hour. This speed of progress of cervical dilatation exists from 3 to 8 cm of dilation but then may slow down from 8 to 10 cm.

The second stage begins when dilation of the cervix is complete and ends with the delivery of the infant. The normal time frame for this stage is a few minutes to 2 hours. If surveillance indicates that the fetus is in good health and is continuing its decent, many health care providers will allow the second stage to continue past 2 hours.

The third stage begins with the delivery of the infant and ends with the delivery of the placenta. The mean length of the third stage is 6 minutes after delivery, with the majority of placentas delivered in 30 minutes.

During the fourth stage of labor, the mother and infant are closely observed. This is a time of transition for the infant and recovery for the mother. The beginning of the family relationship and bonding also occurs during this stage.

INDUCTION OF LABOR

Most births occur without the need for obstetric intervention. In some cases, however, pharmacotherapeutic in-

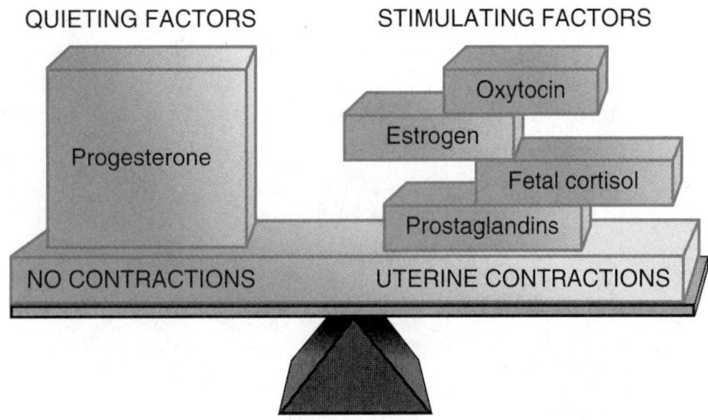

Figure 55–1 Initiating labor. A delicate balance exists between the biochemical factors related to gestation. Those factors identified on the right side of the fulcrum provide stimulus for uterine contractions and the initiation of labor. Progesterone on the left exerts a quieting effect on uterine contractions. Labor begins when the balance of these factors changes. (Adapted from Olds, S. B., London, M. L., and Ladewig, P. W. [1996]. *Maternal-newborn nursing: A family-centered approach* [5th ed., p. 573]. Menlo-Park, CA: Addison-Wesley. Copyright © 1996 by Addison-Wesley Nursing. Reprinted by permission.)

tervention is necessary to maintain the safety of the woman and the fetus. Induction of labor is the attempt to initiate uterine contractions before their spontaneous onset. The use of a uterine stimulant for either inducing or augmenting labor varies from hospital to hospital, city to city, and county to county. Their use ranges from 5 to 40 percent.

There are many reasons for the induction of labor. Maternal indications include pre-eclampsia or maternal conditions such as renal disease. Fetal indications comprise postmaturity syndrome, oligohydramnios, macrosomia (large baby), intrauterine growth restriction, or fetal death. Labor induction is accomplished through the use of cervical ripening drugs, and drugs that cause contractions.

Augmentation of labor is any attempt to stimulate uterine contractions when labor has already begun but the uterine contractions are found to be inadequate. Augmentation is begun when the cervix is not dilating, the fetus is not descending, or the contractions have proved to be weak via measurement by an intrauterine pressure catheter.

If labor must be initiated, the biophysical preparation for labor that normally takes place during the third trimester may not have occurred. Therefore, the initial drug-induced uterine contractions must promote these activities by causing a myometrial cell inflammatory response that frees arachidonic acid so it is converted to prostaglandins. As the level of synthesized prostaglandins increases, myometrial gap junctions form so that the uterus can respond in a coordinated fashion and the active phase of labor begins.

PHARMACOTHERAPEUTIC OPTIONS

Oxytocin

❒ Oxytocin (OXYTOCIN INJECTION, PITOCIN, SYNTOCINON, SYNTOCINON NASAL SPRAY)

Indications

Oxytocin is used for initial induction of labor in patients with a favorable cervix (Bishop's score of 5 or less) or in patients of gravida three or more (Table 55–1). It may also be used to augment labor, to control uterine bleeding after delivery, and to induce abortions. An oxytocin nasal spray promotes the letdown of breast milk. Oxytocin is also used during antepartum testing to assess fetal well-being.

Pharmacodynamics

Oxytocin produces contractions characteristic of contractions that occur during labor and delivery; however, the cervix must be inducible (ripe) for the drug to be effective. Topical prostaglandin (PGE_2) has been found to be helpful in ripening the cervix when it is applied the night before the induction. During the last trimester of pregnancy, it is known that the number of oxytocin receptors in the myometrium of the uterus dramatically increases. Oxytocin is known to increase the force and frequency of contractions but is less effective before the build up of oxytocin receptors in the myometrium.

In the breast, the myoepithelium, a type of smooth muscle, will contract in response to oxytocin. Milk is forced by these contractions into large sinuses, where it is readily available to the sucking infant.

Adverse Effects and Contraindications

Maternal adverse effects include both those caused by the drug and those caused by contractions. Excessive contractions, or increased strength of the contractions, can possibly cause increased blood loss, uterine rupture, and pelvic hematoma. Rare but severe reactions include fatal afibrinogenemia, anaphylaxis, cardiac arrhythmias (e.g., premature

TABLE 55–1 BISHOP'S SCORE

	Number of Points			
Criteria	0	1	2	3
Cervical dilation (cm)	0	1–2	3–4	>5
Cervical effacement (%)	0–30	40–50	60–70	>80
Cervical consistency	Firm	Moderate	Soft	—
Cervical position	Posterior	Central	Anterior	—
Fetal station	−3	−2	−1	+1, +2

Adapted from Bishop, E. (1964). Pelvic scoring for elective induction. *Obstetrics and Gynecology,* 24, 266. Reprinted with permission from the American College of Obstetricians and Gynecologists.

ventricular contractions), subarachnoid hemorrhage, coma, and death. Less severe reactions may include hypertension or hypotension, nausea, and vomiting. Oxytocin is known to cause water intoxication and death with prolonged use.

Adverse fetal reactions are often associated with excessive contractions or high uterine resting tone. Potential fetal reactions to oxytocin include abruptio placentae, bradycardia, arrhythmias, fetal trauma, brain damage, and fetal death secondary to asphyxia.

Contraindications to the use of oxytocin include hypersensitivity to the drug, abnormal fetal presentation, pronounced cephalopelvic disproportion, placenta previa, fetal distress, and other conditions in which vaginal delivery is not indicated.

Pharmacokinetics

Oxytocin is readily absorbed from the oral mucosa and when given parenterally. The nasal passages are a less efficient route of delivery. Oxytocin is not administered orally because it will be destroyed by chymotrypsin in the gastrointestinal (GI) tract. The half-life of oxytocin is 1 to 5 minutes (Table 55–2). Biotransformation occurs in the liver with elimination by the kidneys. Oxytocinase, a circulating enzyme produced in early pregnancy, is also capable of inactivating the drug.

Drug-Drug Interactions

A number of drug-drug interactions are associated with oxytocin. Vasoconstrictors given concurrently with oxytocin have been linked to severe hypertension (Table 55–3). Cyclopropane anesthesia is known to create tachycardia and hypotension or bradycardia with atrioventricular rhythms. Similarly, thiopental given with oxytocin has been associated with a delay in anesthesia induction. Norepinephrine, prochlorperazine, and warfarin sodium have also been cited as causing drug interactions.

Dosage Regimen

Controversy is prevalent when discussing the dosage and administration of oxytocin for induction or augmentation of labor. There are proponents of low-dose oxytocin and others believe in using high doses. Most pharmacology references recommend beginning with 0.5 to 2 mU/minute by IV infusion pump. The dosage may be increased by 1 to 2 mU/minute at 15- to 30-minute intervals until adequate uterine contraction pattern is established. The Association of Women's Health, Obstetrics, and Neonatal Nursing and the American College of Obstetrics and Gynecology guidelines recommend 0.5 to 1 mU/minute, increasing 1 mU/minute every 30 to 60 minutes. High-dose oxytocin, starting at 6 mU and increasing by 6 mU/minute every 20 to 40 minutes has also been recommended, without an increase in morbidity or mortality. The desired cervical dilation rate of 1 cm/hour can be used as a guide for increasing oxytocin infusion rates. An infusion rate of 2 to 8 mU/minute is usually sufficient to achieve a cervical dilation rate of 1 cm/hour. A dosage of more than 20 mU/minute at term is rarely needed (Table 55–4).

TABLE 55–2 PHARMACOKINETICS OF SELECTED UTERINE MOTILITY DRUGS

Drug	Route	Onset	Peak	Duration	PB (%)	$t_{1/2}$	BioA (%)
Oxytocin							
Oxytocin	IV	Immed	UK	1 hour	UA	3–5 min	100
	IM	3–5 min	UK	30–60 min	UA	3–5 min	UA
	Spr	Few min	UK	20 min	UA	< 10 min	UA
Prostaglandins							
Dinoprostone*	IC	Rapid	30–45 min	UK	NA	UK	NA
Carboprost	IM	15 min	30 min	2 hr	NA	UK	NA
Misoprostol	Vag	UA	UA	UA	UA	UA	UA
Ergot Alkaloids							
Ergonovine maleate	IV	1 min	UK	45 min	UA	UK	100
	IM	2–5 min	UK	3 hr	UA	UK	UA
	po	5–15 min	UK	3 hr	UA	UK	UA
Methylergonovine	IV	Immed	UK	45 min–3 hr	UA	30–120 min	100
	IM	2–5 min	0.5 hr	3 hr	UA		78
	po	5–10 min	UK	3 hr	UA		60
Beta$_2$ Agonists							
Ritodrine	IV	Immed	30–60 min	UK	32	6 min; 1.5–2.5 hr†	100
	po	Rapid	30–60 min	UK	32		30
Terbutaline sulfate	IV	6–15 min	15–30 min	1.5–4 hr	UA	3–4 hr	100
	SQ						
	po	30 min	1–2 hr	4–8 hr	UA	UA	30–50
Magnesium sulfate	IV	Immed	UA	30 min	UA	UA	100
	IM	1 hr	UA	3–4 hr	UA	UA	UA

*Dinoprostone: time of onset for cervical ripening. Time to abortion via suppository is 10 minutes, with a peak of 12–24 hours and a 2- to 3-hour duration of action.

†Ritodrine: distribution half-life 6 minutes; second phase is 1.5–2.5 hours with an elimination half-life of over 10 hours.

PB, Protein binding; $t_{1/2}$, elimination half-life; NA, not applicable; UA, unavailable; UK, unknown; IC, intracervical, per vagina, BioA, bioavailability.

TABLE 55–3 DRUG-DRUG INTERACTIONS FOR SELECTED UTERINE MOTILITY DRUGS

Drug	Interaction Drug	Interaction
Uterine Stimulants		
Oxytocin	Vasopressors	Severe hypertension
	Cyclopropane anesthesia	Excessive hypotension
Prostaglandins		
Dinoprostone	Oxytocins	Augments effects of interacting drug
Carboprost		
Misoprostol	Magnesium-containing antacids	Increased risk of diarrhea
Ergot Alkaloids		
Ergonovine maleate	Vasopressors	Excessive vasoconstriction
Methylergonovine maleate	Dopamine	
	Nicotine	
$Beta_2$ Agonists		
Ritodrine	Sympathomimetics	Increased adrenergic effects
Terbutaline	Decongestants	
	Vasopressors	
	Beta blockers	Decreased therapeutic effects of beta agonist
	Corticosteroid	Fatal pulmonary edema
	MAO inhibitors	Hypertensive crisis

MAO, Monoamine oxidase

Oxytocin used for postpartum bleeding is administered as 10 mU intramuscularly (IM) after delivery of the placenta or as an IV drip of 10 to 40 mU per 1000 mL of IV fluids. The IV drip rate is 10 titrated at a rate that will control uterine atony.

The nasal spray formulation is used to promote milk letdown. One spray into one or both nostrils 2 to 3 minutes before nursing or pumping breasts is recommended.

Laboratory Considerations

Owing to its short-term use, therapeutic serum levels of oxytocin are not determined. Instead, the response of the uterus to stimulation is used to titrate the drug. Oxytocin is not known to interfere with other laboratory tests.

Prostaglandins

- Dinoprostone (CERVIDIL, PROSTIN E_2); (✱) Prepidil Gel
- Carboprost tromethamine (HEMABATE); (✱) Prostin/15M
- Misoprostol (CYTOTEC)

Indications

The primary obstetric use of prostaglandins at this time is for termination of pregnancy between the gestational ages of 12 and 20 weeks, or a uterus of less than 20 weeks in size (an abortifacient). It may also be used in the management of a missed abortion of up to 28 weeks' gestation. During the second and third trimesters, prostaglandins can induce contractions of sufficient strength to cause complete evacuation of uterine contents. Misoprostol, in combination with mifepristone (RU486), a morning-after contraceptive drug (see Chapter 54), has been shown to be effective for termination of early pregnancies. Prostaglandins are promoters of uterine contraction, spontaneous labor, and delivery.

More recently, dinoprostone and misoprostol have been used to ripen an unfavorable cervix (Bishop's score of 5 or less) in pregnancy at or near term when induction of labor is indicated.

Carboprost is used to promote uterine contractions and involution to limit the amount of blood loss during a postpartum hemorrhage. However, it is reserved for bleeding that is refractory to more conventional drug therapies (e.g., oxytocin, ergot alkaloids). It can also be used to initiate ripening of the cervix before the induction of labor. Prostaglandins are also used to maintain the patency of the ductus arteriosus in neonates with certain types of heart disease.

Pharmacodynamics

PGE_2 and $PGF_{2\alpha}$ are bioactive metabolites of arachidonic acid, derivatives of fatty acids. The amnion and chorion are responsible for the majority of PGE_2 production, whereas PGF_2 is preferentially produced in the decidua and myometrium. Unlike true hormones, however, prostaglandins do not travel to distant sites to produce effects. They act on the very tissues in which they are made. Degradation of prostaglandins is so rapid that these substances rarely escape their tissue of origin intact.

Exogenous prostaglandins are thought to stimulate the smooth muscle of the myometrium directly to cause uterine contraction during a second-trimester abortion. Because uterine contractions begin slowly, about 18 hours may pass before expulsion of the fetus takes place. Unlike other abortifacients, however, prostaglandins are not feticidal. Hence, an aborted fetus may show transient signs of life.

The exact mechanism of action of prostaglandins, however, is unknown. It is theorized that intracellular concentrations of cyclic 3′,5′-adenosine monophosphate (cAMP), or the regulation of cellular membrane calcium transport may be involved. There are several assertions that hint at the pharmacodynamic actions of prostaglandins. First, exoge-

TABLE 55–4 DOSAGE REGIMEN FOR SELECTED UTERINE MOTILITY DRUGS

Drug	Uses	Dosage	Implications
Oxytocics			
Oxytocin	Induction or augmentation of labor	0.5–2 mU/min IV via infusion pump. Increase by 1 mU/min q30–60min IV. Maintenance: Titrate to minimum of three contractions in 10 minutes	Uterine response should start within 3–5 minutes and persist for 2–3 hours
	Control postpartum bleeding	10 mU after delivery of placenta. IV drip: 10–40 mU/1000 IV solution titrated to control uterine atony	Not recommended for IV push administration
SYNTOCINON NASAL SPRAY	Promote milk letdown	1–2 sprays to each naris 2–3 min before breastfeeding or pumping.	Hold bottle upright and squeeze into nostrils while sitting up, not lying down
Prostaglandins			
Dinoprostone	Cervical ripening	25 mg vaginal suppository q2–4 hr, remove when active labor. Maximum: 240 mg. Gel: 0.5–5 mg q4–6 hr × 1–2 doses	May start oxytocin 60 minutes after last dose
Carboprost	Postpartum hemorrhage	250 mcg deep IM; may repeat q15–90 min × 2 doses	Not for IV use. Must be refrigerated
	Pregnancy termination	250 mcg IM q1.5–3.5 hr based on patient response. Maximum: 12 mg in 48 hours	
Misoprostol	Pregnancy termination (unlabeled)	100–200 mcg q12 hrs intravaginally	
Ergot Alkaloids			
Ergonovine maleate	Postpartum hemorrhage	0.2–0.4 mg IM q6–12hr. Not to exceed 1 mg total	Usual course of treatment 48 hours. Total dosage should not exceed five doses
Methylergonovine	Postpartum hemorrhage	0.2–0.4 mg IM q6–12hr. Not to exceed 1 mg total	
Beta$_2$ Agonists			
Ritodrine	Tocolysis	0.1 mg per IV infusion pump. 10 mg po 30 minutes before stopping IV therapy, then 10 mg po × 2 hr × 24 hr. Increase by 0.05 mg q10–15 min based on patient response. Maintenance: 0.15–0.35 mg/min × 12 hr; 10–20 mg po q4–6 hr. Total dose not to exceed 120 mg/day. Oral: 10 mg q2hr × 24 hr then q4–6 hr	Use of an IV infusion pump is recommended
Terbutaline sulfate	Tocolysis (unlabeled)	IV start at 5 mcg/min. Increase by 5 mcg q10–15 min to max of 60–80 mcg/min *or* 0.25 mg SC q3–4 hr *or* 5 mg po q2–6 hr	Use of an IV infusion pump is recommended

nous prostaglandins induce uterine contractions that are comparable in frequency and duration to those occurring naturally. The prostaglandin content of the amniotic fluid, umbilical cord blood, and maternal blood increases at term and during labor. Furthermore, the ability of the uterus to synthesize prostaglandins increases at term. Last, it has been noted that labor is delayed and prolonged by drugs that inhibit prostaglandin synthesis.

Prostaglandins mimic the process by which natural cervical ripening occurs. A local application of prostaglandin results from breakdown of collagen. Cervical ripening is not dependent on uterine stimulation.

Adverse Effects and Contraindications

GI adverse effects are very common. Nausea, vomiting, and diarrhea occur in up to 60 percent of patients as a result of prostaglandin stimulation of GI smooth muscle. These responses can be minimized by pretreatment with antiemetic and antidiarrheal drugs.

The adverse effects of prostaglandins depend in part on their formulation as well as their dosage. The endocervical gels most often cause a warm feeling in the vagina, back pain, fever, and uterine contraction abnormalities. Patients receiving the suppository formulation most often complain of headache and chills. Up to 70 percent of patients receiving dinoprostone in 20-mg doses have fevers as high as 101°F. The fevers may continue for approximately 6 hours after dosing and are resistant to aspirin. Hypotension is more common than hypertension.

Intense uterine contractions can result in uterine rupture, cervical trauma, cervical lacerations, painful chemical cervicitis, and retained placenta. Anaphylaxis is possible.

Vascular symptoms including hot flashes, flushing, headaches, lightheadedness, fainting sensations, a diastolic blood pressure drop of 20 mmHg, cardiac arrhythmias, and death have been reported. Respiratory symptoms including wheezing, dyspnea, bronchospasm, coughing, tightness of chest, and chest pain have accompanied the administration of these drugs. Underlying cardiac disease and asthma are relative contraindications for prostaglandin administration.

Pharmacokinetics

Intravaginal dinoprostone is well absorbed through vaginal mucosa, with the onset of contractions noted in as little as 10 minutes after insertion. The effects last for 2 to 3 hours. This drug has been administered orally, IV, intra-amniotically, and extra-amniotically. The intra-amniotic and extra-amniotic routes are not recommended because of unacceptably high incidence of adverse affects. Dinoprostone is biotransformed in the kidneys, lungs, spleen, and other bodily tissues. The drug and its metabolites are principally eliminated by the kidney. Small amounts are eliminated in feces. The half-life of dinoprostone is unknown (see Table 55–2).

Carboprost is absorbed slowly by the IM route, with an onset time of drug action of 15 minutes, and peak action is reached in 2 hours. Biotransformation takes place by the action of tissue enzymes. The pharmacokinetics of vaginal use of misoprostol are not available.

Dosage Regimens

Dinoprostone suppositories are used to terminate pregnancies in which the uterine size is equivalent to 20 weeks or less. A 20-mg dinoprostone intravaginal suppository is placed every 3 to 5 hours until delivery of uterine contents. The dosage should not exceed a total of 240 mg. If it is appropriate, IV oxytocin can be used concurrently at doses of 10 to 100 mU/hour (see Table 55–4). The oxytocin can be started as soon as 1 hour after the first dose of dinoprostone. It is recommended that oxytocin be added to the regimen if delivery has not occurred 24 to 36 hours after induction.

Induction of cervical ripening has been achieved with 0.5 mg to 5.0 mg doses of dinoprostone gel. The gel is placed in close proximity to the cervix at 4- to 6-hour intervals, followed by IV oxytocin administration 4 to 6 hours after the last gel administration. A diaphragm may be used to hold the gel next to the cervix. One or two doses are usually administered, although up to four doses have been used for some patients. The patient should remain in a supine position for at least 30 minutes after drug administration.

Carboprost is also used for termination of pregnancy during the second trimester (13 to 20 weeks). An IM dose of 250 mcg is given initially, followed by 250 mcg every 1.5 to 3.5 hours as needed. It should be used no longer than 48 hours, and a total dose of 12 mg IV is contraindicated due to the severe complications of bronchospasm, vomiting, hypertension, and anaphylaxis.

Carboprost is also used for postpartum hemorrhage as a single IM injection of 250 mcg. In some cases, multiple doses at 15- to 90-minute intervals may be used. The total dosage should not exceed 2 mg (eight doses).

Although misoprostol is not approved by the FDA for abortifacient use at this time, it is administered as a 100- to 200-mcg tablet, placed in the posterior fornix every 12 hours. *Laminaria digitata,* a species of kelp or seaweed, may be used concurrently for second-trimester terminations. When it is dried, *Laminaria* has the ability to absorb water and expand with substantial force. It has been used to dilate the cervical canal in induced abortion.

Misoprostol used for cervical ripening is administered in doses of 25- to 50-mg tablets placed in the posterior fornix every 2 to 4 hours. Oxytocin may be started 1 to 2 hours after the last dose of misoprostol.

Ergot Alkaloids

- ❒ Ergonovine maleate (ERGOTRATE MALEATE)
- ❒ Methylergonovine (METHERGINE)

Indications

The effects of ergot alkaloids have been recognized for over 2000 years. The first documented use of these drugs was noted 400 years ago. Midwives used ergot to augment labor and to stop postpartum bleeding long before physicians started using it. The first documentation of use by a physician to hasten childbirth was in 1818. However, by 1824, a dramatic rise in stillbirths was noted and it was recommended to limit the use to controlling hemorrhage only.

Ergonovine and methylergonovine are used to increase the strength, duration, and frequency of uterine contractions in uterine atony, and decrease postpartum and postabortion bleeding. Their ability to induce sustained uterine contraction makes them particularly suited for these purposes. Ergot alkaloids are not used for induction of labor but are used to slow bleeding after birth.

Ergonovine has also been used in the management of migraine headache, especially of the use of ergotamine, which is generally more effective, has been accompanied by paresthesias. Its unlabeled uses include diagnostic testing for Prinzmetal's angina, and to provoke coronary artery spasm during coronary arteriography.

Pharmacodynamics

Ergot is a naturally occurring fungus found on rye plants. Spores of this fungus are spread by the wind or flying insects and carried to the ovaries of young grains. A growth of tissue forms and hardens. These hard purple growths are a major source of commercial ergot. Ergonovine has proved to be the most effective uterine stimulant. Methylergonovine is a derivative of ergonovine and produces effects similar to those of the natural alkaloid.

The mechanism of action for all the ergot alkaloids apparently is the result of their actions as partial antagonists or agonists at the tryptaminergic, adrenergic, and dopaminergic receptors. The uterine-stimulating effects of ergot alkaloids appear to be involved with the interactions of receptors for biogenic amines. The prolactin-inhibiting effects are accomplished by direct action on the pituitary and hypothalamus, causing the release of prolactin-inhibiting factor via the dopamine receptors.

Ergot alkaloids can cause vasoconstriction of arterioles and veins. This action is the basis for using certain alkaloids in the treatment of migraine headaches.

Adverse Effects and Contraindications

Nausea, vomiting, dizziness, and a headache are the most common adverse effects of ergot alkaloids. Other adverse effects include tinnitus, *ergotism* (a constellation of signs and symptoms that include blood pressure changes, weak pulse, dyspnea, chest pain, numbness and coldness of the extremities), confusion, excitement, delirium, hallucinations, convulsions, and coma.

Hypertension is also known to occur, especially in women with pre-eclampsia or underlying hypertension. In these patients, the use of ergot alkaloids is contraindicated due to instances of cerebrovascular accidents, seizures, and severe arrhythmias. They should also be used cautiously in patients with hepatic or renal impairment.

Pharmacokinetics

Oral and parenterally administered ergonovine maleate and methylergonovine maleate are rapidly absorbed by either route. IV usage is limited to life-threatening situations only. The GI tract absorbs approximately 60 percent of methylergonovine. The onset of uterine contractions is noted 2 to 5 minutes after IM administration, continuing for approximately 45 minutes. Following oral administration, the onset of uterine contractions occurs in 5 to 15 minutes, with drug action lasting 3 hours or longer. Peak serum levels are attained within 30 minutes to 3 hours via the oral route (see Table 55–2).

Only very small amounts of ergot alkaloids are eliminated in urine. It is believed that ergonovine maleate and methylergonovine are eliminated through nonrenal mechanisms with elimination in the feces.

Drug-Drug Interactions

Ergot alkaloids can produce excessive vasoconstriction when they are used with other vasopressors, such as dopamine or nicotine (see Table 55–3).

Dosage Regimen

Dosages for methylergonovine and ergonovine are exactly the same. When they are used as an oxytocic, the usual oral or sublingual dose is 0.2 to 0.4 mg. The dose can be repeated every 6 to 12 hours. Oral doses are given till heavy bleeding slows or up to 7 days of continued administration. The usual course, however, is 48 hours. The IM or IV dosage routes are usually 0.2 mg every 2 to 4 hours, up to 5 doses. A change to an oral formulation should then be made. Total dosage should not exceed 1 mg or five IM administrations. Administration is usually held until after passage of the placenta (see Table 55–4).

PRETERM LABOR

The largest cause of infant morbidity and mortality is a preterm birth. PTL is defined as the onset of labor with cervical change before completion of the 37th week of pregnancy. In the majority of patients with PTL, the exact etiology of the condition is unknown.

Certain conditions are known to predispose women to PTL. It has been postulated that up to one-third of preterm deliveries are due to infection. Chorioamnionitis, an infection of the membranes that cover the fetus, is implicated in the majority of these cases. Closely associated with infection and PTL is premature rupture of membranes (PROM). In the patient with PROM, onset of labor often occurs shortly after the rupture, especially when infection is the cause. The period of time between membrane rupture and delivery is known as the latency period. If infection is not the cause of PROM, this latency period may last from a few days to weeks. An overdistended uterus, due to either multiple gestation or polyhydramnios, is known to increase the chance of PTL. Fetal anomalies, especially chromosomal abnormalities, and death of the fetus are known to precipitate labor. Cervical incompetence and certain uterine anomalies will predispose women to preterm deliveries. Placenta problems (e.g., placenta previa or abruptio placentae) may cause PTL in a percentage of patients with these problems. The true cause of PTL is found in only a small percentage of patients. The majority of cases are classified as cause unknown.

PHARMACOTHERAPEUTIC OPTIONS

Alcohol was the first drug to be used to stop labor. It is rarely if ever used for that purpose today since the discovery of other drugs with tocolytic properties (see Controversy—Uterine Motility Drugs). All of the drugs currently used for tocolysis were originally created for the treatment of other diseases. The drugs covered in this chapter are discussed for their therapeutic use as tocolytics only.

Beta$_2$ Agonists

- ❒ Ritodrine (YUTOPAR)
- ❒ Terbutaline (BRICANYL, BRETHINE)

Indications

Beta$_2$ agonists are commonly used drugs for the treatment of PTL. Terbutaline is more commonly used because it is less expensive. Ritodrine is the only drug approved for tocolytic use by the FDA. In general, ritodrine is reserved for pregnancies in which the gestational age is greater than 20 weeks and less than 34 or 36 weeks. The desire to use a tocolytic drug (i.e., to prolong intrauterine development) should be balanced against the risks of early delivery to both the mother and fetus.

Pharmacodynamics

Beta$_2$ agonists are believed to stimulate the production of cyclic cAMP by the activation of the enzyme adenyl cyclase. The increase in cAMP appears to increase the uptake and sequestration of intracellular calcium. This lack of available calcium prevents activation of the contractile proteins of smooth muscle cell, creating uterine smooth muscle relaxation. A decrease in the intensity and duration of contractions results.

Adverse Effects and Contraindications

As might be expected, the administration of beta$_2$ agonists produces a number of cardiovascular and metabolic adverse effects in the mother. Cardiac adverse effects include tachycardia, widening pulse pressure, chest pain or tightening, heart murmur, palpitations, and cardiac arrest. ST-T wave depression and T-wave inversion have been reported with terbutaline administration. Although there are few changes in the mean arterial pressure, a dose-related tachycardia and increase in cardiac output occur. The response is

Controversy

Uterine Motility Drugs
JONATHAN J. WOLFE

Therapy in response to inappropriately early labor has advanced radically in the past 3 decades. Formerly, obstetric care in the face of premature labor largely involved use of bedrest. In acute settings, the principal therapeutic intervention involved use of intravenous ethanol. Neither treatment offered great expectations of good outcomes. Complete bedrest in advanced pregnancy predictably enhanced the chance of clotting disorders, pneumonia, and the other sequelae one expects with inactivity. Alcohol infusion (in combination with dextrose) was not appropriate for long-term use.

In the 1970s, a new product for management of preterm labor was introduced. Ritodrine, a beta-receptor agonist, offered important improvement in responding to the condition. The good this drug may accomplish is clear, because prematurely delivered children suffer disproportionately from a variety of severe disorders. The premature neonate also is far more likely to die than the full-term child. Within the limits of maternal tolerance, ritodrine allows continuous and effective ablation of inappropriate labor.

Controversy involving the use of this drug is twofold. The first relates to the mother's exposure to potential harm. A trade-off is required in the case of a pregnant patient with diabetes mellitus, steroid-treated asthma, and a variety of cardiac ailments. Severe pulmonary complications, sometimes manifested postpartum, are also associated with the drug. The second dilemma stems from commercial use of ritodrine. Home care using labor monitoring devices is available in many markets. These devices can provide data over telephone links to prompt administration of tocolytics, such as ritodrine. However, in a managed care setting, it is difficult to establish the cost-benefit ratio of outpatient tocolysis.

Critical Thinking Discussion

- In choosing to use monitoring and tocolytic interventions, what level of hazard to the neonate is acceptable in the case of a mother who is otherwise healthy and has had an uneventful pregnancy?
- What alternative use could be made of the money spent on monitoring for premature labor and providing home intravenous therapy?
- Imagine that a marketing representative from a home care company has met with you in your office to explain the labor monitoring and intravenous drug therapy available from his company. What ethical concerns would you, as a practitioner, have about recommending this provider to one of your patients?
- What harm might come to a patient as the result of choosing either to use or not to use tocolytic therapy?
- In an acute care setting, what additional monitoring would be appropriate for meeting the outcomes of tocolytic therapy?

probably the result of a reflex response to the lowered diastolic pressure and direct action on $beta_1$ receptors in the heart.

Adverse effects commonly associated with beta agonist use include tremors, restlessness, jitteriness, nervousness, emotional upset, and anxiety. Headache, nausea, vomiting, erythema, malaise, and lethargy have also been reported.

There is decreased renal elimination of sodium, potassium, and water. This is presumably due to the enhanced secretion of renin. If hydration during $beta_2$ agonist therapy is overly vigorous, pulmonary edema may result, with or without evidence of myocardial failure. Evidence of cardiac disease is a contraindication to the use of $beta_2$ agonists. Patients complaining or showing signs of severe cardiac symptoms should be worked up for occult cardiac disease.

Ritodrine and similar drugs can cause marked hyperglycemia. Although treatment is not usually required, persistent hyperglycemia may result in fetal tachycardia, hyperinsulinemia, and reactive hypoglycemia in the fetus should parturition proceed. The use of beta agonists in patients with diabetes is hazardous and is usually contraindicated.

Hypokalemia is another consequence of ritodrine administration. This state reflects a movement of potassium into the intracellular compartment. Total body stores are not reduced, and treatment is not usually indicated.

Pharmacokinetics

The bioavailability of oral ritodrine is approximately 30 percent with peak plasma levels attained in 30 to 60 minutes. IV ritodrine has an immediate onset, with peak drug action noted in 30 to 60 minutes. Ritodrine is 100 percent bioavailable, with a half-life of 6 minutes. Elimination of both terbutaline and ritodrine is partially achieved through biotransformation in the liver to inactive conjugates. The majority of the drugs and the inactive conjugates are eliminated in urine (see Table 55–2).

Drug-Drug Interactions

Beta-blocking drugs antagonize the effects of ritodrine and terbutaline; therefore, concurrent use should be avoided. Simultaneous use with other sympathomimetic drugs is not recommended due to the possible additive effect. Use with potent anesthetic agents, meperidine, and diazoxide may also cause hypotension and cardiac arrhythmias. Hypertension will be caused by concomitant use of anticholinergic agents. Concurrent use with tricyclic antidepressants or monoamine oxidase inhibitors may potentiate the vascular system effects (see Table 55–3).

Intravenous use of a $beta_2$ agonist increases the woman's risk for pulmonary edema. Additional use of corticosteroid to promote fetal lung maturity increases the chance of pulmonary edema even further; therefore, the patient should be monitored for signs and symptoms of pulmonary edema. Concomitant use of IV magnesium sulfate and a subcutaneous $beta_2$ agonist is contraindicated except during emergency transport because of a significant risk of pulmonary edema, hypotension, and cardiac arrhythmias.

Dosage Regimen

The dosage of ritodrine is individualized by balancing uterine response and unwanted effects. Intravenous administration is initially started at 0.1 mg/minute and increased by 0.05 mg/minute every 10 to 15 minutes until the desired effects are attained. The usual effective dosage is between 0.15 and 0.35 mg/minute and is continued for at least 12 hours after uterine contractions cease.

Oral ritodrine therapy is started at 10 mg approximately 30 minutes before terminating IV therapy. The usual dosage for the first 24 hours is 10 mg every 2 hours. The dosage is then decreased to 10 to 20 mg every 4 to 6 hours. The total oral dosage should not exceed 120 mg/day.

Intravenous doses of terbutaline sulfate are titrated until contractions cease. The administration of IV terbutaline requires the use of an infusion pump for the safety of the patient. The patient is started on 5 mcg/minute. The dosage is increased by 5 mcg approximately every 10 to 15 minutes to a maximum dose of 60 to 80 mcg/minute. Maternal and fetal heart rates are monitored and the infusion is decreased if the heart rates exceed 130 and 170, respectively. The lowest effective dose is then continued for at least 12 hours before discontinuing IV administration and starting the patient on subcutaneous terbutaline.

The recommended subcutaneous dose of terbutaline is 0.25 mg every 2 to 6 hours. The average administration frequency after IV therapy is every 3 to 4 hours. Subcutaneous terbutaline is often used as a first-line drug when patients present with PTL and minimal cervical dilatation. The drug is administered via infusion pump at 50 mcg/hour, with boluses of 250 mcg as needed. The usual oral maintenance dose of terbutaline can be 5 mg by mouth every 4 to 6 hours until term, but it can be titrated to patient response (see Table 55–4).

Laboratory Considerations

Serum glucose levels should be monitored in patients with diabetes. Serum electrolytes including sodium and potassium levels should be monitored in patients on concurrent potassium depleting drugs. Therapeutic drug levels of beta$_2$ agonists are not usually performed because the drug is titrated to uterine activity.

Other Tocolytic Drugs

MAGNESIUM SULFATE

The primary indication for magnesium sulfate is the treatment of seizures associated with pre-eclampsia. It was subsequently found to have tocolytic effects. Magnesium sulfate causes uterine relaxation through a direct effect on uterine smooth muscle. Both the frequency and the force of contractions are reduced. Labor is arrested at magnesium levels ranging from 6 to 8 mEq/L. Because magnesium does not sensitize the heart to catecholamines or promote hyperglycemia, it may be preferred to beta$_2$ agonists in women with hyperthyroidism or diabetes. Prolonging the pregnancy for at least 48 hours allows time to stimulate fetal surfactant production in the fetus using other drugs.

Intravenous magnesium sulfate is started with a bolus of 4 to 6 g, then the infusion is continued at 1 to 4 g/hour. The IV infusion is continued for 24 to 48 hours when the patient is started on subcutaneous (SC) terbutaline or oral magnesium. Prolonged infusions are not recommended but have been employed with careful monitoring. The recommended oral therapy is 1 g of magnesium gluconate every 2 to 4 hours. However, oral therapy is not often used because of the adverse effect of diarrhea.

With serum magnesium levels of 4 mEq/L and above, patients may experience hot flashes, flushing, sweating, nausea, vomiting, headache, and depression of reflexes. At serum levels of 8 to 10 mEq/L, patients may complain of blurred vision, double vision, and lethargy. The deep tendon reflexes are depressed or absent. Respiratory arrest, flaccid paralysis, and severe central nervous system depression may occur at serum levels above 13 to 15 mEq/L. Serum levels equal to or greater than 25 mEq/L will produce cardiac arrest and circulatory collapse. Neonatal central nervous system depression may occur in infants born to mothers who are taking magnesium. An attendant, preferably a neonatal nurse practitioner or neonatologist, who is familiar with neonatal resuscitation should be attending the delivery.

CALCIUM CHANNEL BLOCKER

Nifedipine, a calcium channel blocker (see Chapter 32), may also be used to treat PTL although it is not FDA approved for such use. Nifedipine works to inhibit the transmembranous influx of calcium ions. This factor inhibits the contractile process of uterine smooth muscle.

NONSTEROIDAL ANTI-INFLAMMATORY DRUGS

Nonsteroidal anti-inflammatory drugs (i.e., prostaglandin inhibitors) such as indomethacin and sulindac have been used to prolong gestation in both term and preterm pregnancies. The overall experience with indomethacin is limited; however, it may be the drug of choice in the management of PTL if IV access is not possible (such as during transfer to high-risk care centers) or if polyhydramnios (excessive amniotic fluid) is present.

The use of indomethacin in the management of PTL has the potential for adverse effects in the fetus. Nonsteroidal anti-inflammatory drugs should not be used in gestations greater than 34 weeks and use should be limited to 48 hours. Of particular importance is the possibility of premature closure of the ductus arteriosus and the production of pulmonary hypertension. However, fetal echocardiography can detect early signs of constriction of the ductus and its use may allow for continued administration of indomethacin or related drugs in those instances in which evidence of ductal constriction is absent. Indomethacin also causes a dose-dependent oligohydramnios owing to decreased fetal urinary output. Oligohydramnios is reversible on discontinuation of the drug.

Drugs that Improve Neonatal Outcome

Corticosteroids have been given to the mother in PTL to prepare the infant for survival when a preterm birth is anticipated. Corticosteroids are used to induce fetal surfactant production.

It is believed that fetal lungs produce surfactant in response to a cascade of hormonal signals. Fetal corticosteroids are postulated to be involved in this process, although the exact mechanism of action is unknown. There is evidence that corticosteroids reduce the incidence of fetal respiratory distress syndrome (RDS), necrotizing enterocolitis, electrolyte imbalances, and patent ductus arteriosus in premature infants who are treated prenatally.

Critical Thinking Process

Assessment

History of Present Illness

The assessment of the patient requiring drugs to induce, augment, or stop labor begins with a detailed nursing history and physical. The plan of care is created from the information obtained. Eliciting the patient's perception of what brought her to the hospital is the focus of the questions asked. It is exceedingly important to determine the gestational age of the fetus, because the type of drug therapy may differ considerably based on this information. Questions to ask include whether the last menstrual period was normal, the length of her cycles, whether an ultrasound was done early in the pregnancy, if the ultrasound results changed her due dates, and if the health care provider ever questioned the dates. If the patient is experiencing contractions, the assessment includes time of onset, duration, frequency, and the perceived strength of the contraction. Has the patient noted leaking of vaginal fluid? If the answer is yes, it is important to ascertain the quantity, color, and odor of the fluid.

Recent sexual intercourse, due to the release of prostaglandins from the cervix and prostaglandins in the semen, may cause the onset of contractions. Therefore, a patient in PTL should be asked about recent sexual intercourse.

A complete assessment of the current pregnancy includes reviewing the first, second, and third trimester of the pregnancy for any problems or complications. It is important to determine whether the mother has had previous contractions or bleeding episodes. If the answer is yes, query the patient as to what treatment was initiated and if it was effective. Reviewing the prenatal records, when available, is an essential part of assessing the current pregnancy. The fetus is also a patient; therefore, questions should be asked about fetal movement.

Past Health History

Important information is gained through the assessment of the past medical and surgical history. As part of the drug history, allergies to both food and drugs, including physiologic responses, need to be documented. Document current and previous drug use including prescription drugs, over-the-counter drugs, illicit drugs, and alcohol intake.

The patient's past obstetric history can often be insightful. The outcome of all previous pregnancies should be identified. This includes information about any abortions (spontaneous or elective), and previous term or preterm deliveries. The length of labor, type of delivery, the gestational age at delivery, weight of the infant, and any complications are important to ascertain. The past use of drugs to prevent delivery or to induce delivery is important to note.

Physical Exam Findings

The physical exam should include the evaluation of vital signs, along with the assessment of fetal heart tones. A sterile vaginal exam or sterile speculum exam is performed depending on the status of the fetal membranes and gestational age of the fetus. Before the 37th week or if it must be determined whether the patient is leaking amniotic fluid, a sterile speculum exam should be done in place of the sterile vaginal exam. The speculum exam eliminates cervical stimulation, which can cause the release of prostaglandins, thus initiating contractions. The speculum exam also decreases the chance of vertical transmission of bacteria that can occur with a vaginal exam. Deep tendon reflexes should be evaluated on all patients.

Diagnostic Testing

An initial external fetal monitor strip evaluation yields a wealth of information. The baseline fetal heart rate, the variability, and the presence of periodic changes are evaluated. The monitor strip also informs the health care provider of the timing and duration of uterine contractions. The strength of contractions cannot be truly assessed without an internal uterine pressure catheter.

The patient's urine should be assessed for evidence of dehydration, urinary tract infection, and pre-eclampsia. The urine should also be checked for ketones, nitrates, leucocyte esterase, and protein.

Routine blood work for a laboring patient is a complete blood count (CBC) and blood drawn and placed on hold in the event the patient needs a transfusion. The patient with PTL is evaluated for infection through blood work and amniocentesis.

Developmental Considerations

Pregnancy is a developmental challenge and a pivot point in life that is accompanied by stress and anxiety, whether the pregnancy is desired or not. Pregnancy can be viewed as a developmental stage, with its own distinct developmental tasks. If a pregnancy terminates in the birth of a child, the couple enters a new stage of life together. However, the couple must face the realities of labor and birth before parenthood can be achieved.

Assessment of how the woman's pregnancy alters her body image and necessitates a reordering of social relationships and role change should be determined. There may be ambivalence, acceptance, introversion, and mood swings as the woman undertakes to maintain her soundness and that of her family, and at the same time, incorporate new life into the family system. The partner is often viewed as a bystander or observer of the pregnancy. Evaluation of the partner's perception of the pregnancy should be performed. Continued re-evaluation will need to be accomplished as the pregnancy progresses.

Psychosocial Considerations

Assessing the patient and her partner's views of labor, induction, and use of drugs is an important factor. Couples may have prepared a birth plan. Reading this plan may provide some insight into their views about the laboring and delivery process. Some women perceive the use of any drug during labor as a failure, others are terrified at the thought of labor without some type of pain relief drug or anesthesia. Previous sexual abuse or rape can affect the course of the labor and the amount of discomfort the patient experiences during vaginal exams and subsequent labor.

Society as a whole tends to view labor as a natural process. "Women have been dropping babies in the fields for years" is a persuasive attitude that has been quoted many times. Therefore, women who require induction of labor or PTL may believe that they have failed or their body has failed them. Added to this problem is anxiety and fear the patient and family have about the survival of the infant. Parents often experience tremendous apprehension about the survival and quality of life of their unborn child. Compounding this issue is the persuasive feeling of powerlessness the patient and partner often experience. In America's multicultural society, understanding the patient's cultural views of the labor experience influences how the health care provider perceives the patient's attitudes and influences the plan of care (see Case Study—Preterm Labor).

Case Study Preterm Labor

Patient History

History of Present Illness	AD is an 18-year-old white female G_1P_0 at 30 weeks' gestation. AD complains of awakening at 0300 with an intermittent backache that continued to worsen and at 0530 the pains were 7 minutes apart. She called her doctor, who told her to go to the hospital. Denies leaking or bleeding. Denies recent sexual intercourse. Pregnancy has been uncomplicated until backache began. AD received terbutaline but the drug was ineffective in relieving her preterm labor.
Past Health History	AD denies allergies to food or medications. She denies other health problems or hospitalizations. She smoked 1ppd until she discovered she was pregnant, then she quit. Occasional alcohol use when not pregnant. Denies use of street drugs. At present, she is taking prenatal vitamins 1 each day.
Physical Exam Findings	VS: BP 120/60, pulse 80, respiration 22, temperature 99°F. Sterile vaginal exam reveals cervix is 2 cm dilated, 80% effaced, and fetal head is at a −1 station. Patient is breathing heavily through the contractions. Remainder of exam unremarkable.
Diagnostic Testing	Gestation confirmed by a first trimester ultrasound. FHTs: 160 and reassuring. Uterine contractions every 5–7 minutes for a full minute. CBC, CRP, and clot to hold are sent to the lab. An amniocentesis is performed, and fluid sent to lab to r/o infection and assess status of fetal lung maturity.
Psychosocial Considerations	Family out of state. Partner present and supportive. Have started Lamaze classes.
Economic Factors	AD and her partner have no health insurance or pharmacy coverage. Are concerned about cost of prenatal care, potential for extended hospitalization, and aftercare.

Variables Influencing Decision

Treatment Objectives

- Arrest preterm labor
- Deliver if infection present
- Promote fetal induction of surfactant and preventative therapy (if required)

Drug Variables	*Drug Summary*	*Patient Variables*
Indications	Ritodrine reserved for pregnancies greater than 20 weeks but less than 34–36 weeks. This will become a decision point. Prostaglandin not required for cervical ripening.	AD and husband desire pregnancy to go to term, if possible. This will become a decision point. Cervix dilated to 2 cm.
Pharmacodynamics	Uterine smooth muscle relaxation. A decrease in intensity and duration of contractions results.	AD is in preterm labor. She takes no other drugs with which there would be a drug-drug interaction.
Adverse Effects/ Contraindications	$Beta_2$ agonists produce cardiovascular and metabolic adverse effects in the mother.	Benefit of tocolysis outweights risk at this time. AD will be taught what to expect.
Pharmacokinetics	IV ritodrine onsets immediately with peak effects reached in 30–60 minutes. This becomes a decision point.	There is time for ritodrine therapy to reach peak effects.
Dosage Regimen	Initial dose 50 mcg to be titrated based on balance of patient response and unwanted effects.	There is no patient variable here, so this is not a decision point.
Lab Considerations	Electrolytes to be monitored. Serum drug levels not required.	No specific lab work required due to AD variables.

Case Study continued on following page

Drug Variables	*Drug Summary*	*Patient Variables*
Cost Index*	IV ritodrine: 5 po ritodrine: 5 IV oxytocin: 1	Premature delivery of a 30-week fetus will entail neonatal intensive care and the potential for complication due to prematurity. This will become a decision point.

Summary of Decision Points

- Ritodrine reserved for pregnancies greater than 20 weeks but less than 34–36 weeks.
- Premature delivery of a 30-week fetus will entail neonatal intensive care and the potential for complications due to prematurity.
- Delivery may be necessary if an infection is causing the preterm labor because fetal antibiotic therapy is needed, which can not be accomplished through the mother.
- IV ritodrine onsets immediately with peak effects reached in 30–60 minutes.

DRUGS TO BE USED

- Ritodrine hydrochloride 50 mcg IV per infusion pump initially, titrate to response. Increase every 10–15 minutes as response warrants.
- Ritodrine hydrochloride 10 mg po q4–6 hr once removed from IV formulation
- Oxytocin for induction if infection present and delivery is required

*Cost index:

1 $ < 30/mo
2 $ 30–40/mo
3 $ 40–50/mo
4 $ 50–60/mo
5 $ > 60/mo

AWP of 30mg/100 mL, 5% ritodrine/dextrose premixed solution is approximately $125.
AWP of 60, 10-mg tablets of ritodrine hydrochloride is approximately $150.
AWP of 10 mL, 10 IU/mL multidose via 1 oxytocin for injection is approximately $7.

Cultural assessment is an important aspect of history taking. The health care provider should identify the primary beliefs, values, and behaviors that relate to pregnancy and child-bearing. This includes information about ethnicity, degree of affiliation with the ethnic group, patterns of decision-making, religious preferences, language and communication styles, and common etiquette practices. An exploration of the couple's expectation of the health care system should also be noted. The degree to which these variables are in concert with the woman's personal values, beliefs, and behaviors is important when planning care. Discrepancies should be considered and a determination made as to whether the patient's system is supportive, neutral, or harmful in relation to possible interventions. The health care provider then faces two considerations: identifying ways of persuading the patient to accept the proposed therapy, or accepting her rationale for refusing therapy if she is not willing to change her belief system.

Analysis and Management

Treatment Objectives

The goal of treatment with a uterine stimulant is to establish regular contractions that occur every 3 to 5 minutes and last for 60 to 90 seconds. To effect cervical effacement and dilation, a rate that mimics normal spontaneous labor (approximately 1 cm/hour) is desired to deliver a fetus vaginally without increasing the risk to the mother or the fetus. The goal in abortifacient treatment is to cause evaluation of uterine contents with increasing maternal risk for complications.

The treatment goal in tocolysis is to stop uterine contractions, and to prevent progression of cervical effacement and dilation. Additionally, it is desired to delay delivery of the fetus long enough (24 to 48 hours) to permit acceleration of fetal lung maturity if the gestation is less than 32 weeks.

Treatment Options

Uterine Stimulants Augmentation of labor may be indicated when nondrug measures such as amniotomy (artificial rupture of membranes) and nipple stimulation are unsuccessful. It may also be appropriate in cases in which prolongation of pregnancy is dangerous to the mother (e.g., hypertension, diabetes) or the fetus. Oxytocin is considered the initial treatment if Bishop's score is 5 or more patients who are gravida one or two. However, induction of labor without cervical softening has a high failure rate. Oxytocin should not be used to induce labor for any reason other than medical necessity. The convenience of the health care provider or patient is an unacceptable reason for induction.

The use of prostaglandins produces effective preinduction cervical ripening. When prostaglandins are administered locally, they decrease the duration of labor, shorten the induction to delivery period, decrease the dosage of oxytocin, and reduce the overall failure of induction. Further, uterine response to oxytocin is enhanced in the presence of PGE_2. However, the time to induction and duration of labor are longer with prostaglandin gel, although patient acceptance is greater.

Selection of a uterine stimulant to be used as an abortifacient depends on gestational age. During weeks 1 to 12, suction dilatation and curettage is the procedure of choice. Mifepristone (RU486) may also be used in some instances. Other drugs are generally ineffective during this time. During weeks 13 to 20, dilation plus evacuation is generally preferred. Oxytocin is less effective during this time but may be used as an adjunct, if necessary. Hypertonic solutions (e.g., saline, urea) behave as poisons to the placenta and fetus, thus acting as an abortifacient.

Mifepristone is employed in combination with prostaglandins (i.e., misoprostol) for termination of early pregnancy. It is given first, and the prostaglandin is administered 48 hours later. The combination of the two drugs stimulates uterine contractions and the expulsion of uterine contents. The oral formulations of both drugs make the procedure more convenient and less expensive than IM prostaglandins.

Tocolytics Tocolytics stop contractions for 24 to 48 hours but there is debate about whether they improve perinatal outcomes or reduce the overall rate of preterm birth. There is a trend that suggests tocolytics decrease infant mortality in gestations of 24 to 27 weeks only. Because perinatal morbidity and mortality are not altered, the indication for tocolysis is to delay delivery long enough to administer corticosteroids to the mother. The corticosteroids hasten fetal lung maturity and reduce the incidence of respiratory distress in the premature newborn.

In general, tocolysis is indicated if the onset of labor is between 24 and 32 weeks' gestation, with documented cervical dilatation and uterine contractions that occur every 7 to 10 minutes and lasting 30 seconds. Therapy is used only if there are no contraindications to stopping PTL; when major maternal illness cannot be controlled; in the presence of pre-eclampsia, abruptio placentae, chorioamnionitis, and severe fetal anomalies that are incompatible with life; or in the case of fetal demise.

When the decision to use a tocolytic drug is made, treatment is likely to be successful if cervical dilatation is less than 4 cm and cervical effacement is less than 80 percent. Tocolysis is usually not attempted if the membranes have ruptured because there is a risk of infection. Subcutaneous terbutaline is the drug of choice if the cervix is less than 3 cm dilated. Intravenous magnesium sulfate or a $beta_2$ agonist is used for women with cervical dilation over 3 cm. After 48 hours, indomethacin, a nonsteroidal anti-inflammatory drug, may be added if IV tocolysis is not slowing uterine contractions.

Intervention

Administration

Uterine Stimulants Fetal maturity, presentation, and pelvic adequacy should be assessed before administration of oxytocin. Further, the character, frequency, and duration of uterine contractions, resting uterine tone, and fetal heart rate should be monitored during therapy. A Y connection should be used when preparing the IV infusion so that the oxytocin solution can be discontinued if necessary while access to a vein is maintained. Oxytocin should not be administered by more than one route simultaneously, and infusion should be stopped if any of the following conditions exist:

- Contractions are less than 2 minutes apart
- Contractions are stronger than 50 to 65 mmHg on the uterine pressure monitor
- Resting uterine pressure is greater than 15 to 20 mmHg
- Contractions that last longer than 60 to 90 seconds
- A significant change in fetal heart rate occurs

Should any of these conditions occur, the oxytocin should be discontinued, the patient turned onto the left side (to prevent fetal anoxia), and given oxygen, and the health care provider notified immediately. Terbutaline 0.125 to 0.25 mg IV push can be used for fetal distress. Magnesium sulfate should be available if excessive stimulation of the myometrium occurs and the patient has a known cardiac defect. Additionally, the patient should be monitored for signs and symptoms of water intoxication (drowsiness, listlessness, confusion, headache, anuria). The health care provider should be notified if the patient's condition suggests intoxication.

As with oxytocin use, the frequency, duration, force of contractions, and uterine resting tone should be monitored during prostaglandin therapy. Dinoprostone-induced adverse effects can be minimized by pretreatment with an antidiarrheal, antiemetic, and antipyretic (e.g., acetaminophen) drug before the use of high-dose prostaglandin.

For cervical ripening, the degree of effacement should be determined before the insertion of the prostaglandin. The health care provider should use caution to prevent contact of the prostaglandin with the skin. The patient should be in a dorsal recumbent position, and the cervix should be visualized by the examiner. Sterile technique is used when inserting the prostaglandin gel or suppository. The patient should remain supine for 15 to 30 minutes to minimize leakage from the cervical canal. During low-dose prostaglandin use, the fetus should be monitored for 2 hours after the medication is administered. Patients with hypertension should not receive an ergot alkaloid.

Tocolytics Before administration of a tocolytic drug, the patient's blood pressure, heart rate, blood glucose levels, and fluid status should be evaluated, as well as the fetal heart rate. The patient should be placed on the left side to minimize blood pressure changes during the infusion. IV administration of a $beta_2$ agonist or magnesium sulfate should be accomplished with the use of an infusion pump in order to accomplish titration better. The use of sodium chloride for infusion should be avoided due to the risk of pulmonary edema. Ritodrine is incompatible with any other drug in solution or in the syringe.

Magnesium sulfate infusions should always be administered via IV pumps due to the serious consequences of extremely high magnesium levels. The patient's respiratory rate and patellar reflex should be monitored before and throughout therapy. Patient reports of symptoms that reflect excessive dosage should be managed by decreasing or shutting off the IV infusion and closely observing the patient until lab results are available. Calcium gluconate, the reversal agent for magnesium sulfate, should be on hand. Serum magnesium levels and renal function should be monitored periodically throughout administration of parenteral magnesium sulfate.

There are many drug-drug interactions associated with parenteral administration of magnesium. A drug interaction reference should be consulted before mixing magnesium sulfate in either Y connectors, piggyback containers, or syringes.

Education

Uterine Stimulants Patients receiving oxytocin infusions should be advised to expect contractions that are similar to menstrual cramps after administration has begun. They should be advised of the goal of therapy and informed that the infusion rate will be adjusted based on their response. Women receiving prostaglandins at high doses should be forewarned of the side effects of nausea, vomiting, diarrhea, and high temperatures that often occur and that you will be premedicating them to lessen these effects.

Inform the patient who is to receive a prostaglandin that she may note a warm feeling in her vagina during drug administration. When a prostaglandin is used as an abortifacient, the patient should be advised to notify the health care provider if fever, chills, foul-smelling vaginal discharge, lower abdominal pain, or increased bleeding occurs. Once expulsion of uterine contents and placenta has occurred, the patient should be thoroughly examined for trauma (cervical or uterine lacerations).

Tocolytics Educational needs of the patient at risk for PTL include reinforcement of preterm birth prevention principles and warning signs of early labor. The patient receiving oral tocolytic therapy should be advised that contractions may resume even with therapy. Instruct the patient to contact her health care provider for reinstitution of IV therapy if signs of labor reappear. Women who are receiving $beta_2$ agonists should be advised regarding the drugs' common adverse effects.

Patients on magnesium sulfate should be informed that this drug may cause nausea and vomiting, especially with the loading dose. Other important information to include in patient teaching includes a flushed feeling, burning at the IV site, lethargy, blurred vision, and dry mouth.

Patients at risk for preterm delivery should be educated about the drugs that may be used to promote fetal lung maturity and the reasons for their use. Emotional support is vital during therapy.

Evaluation

The effectiveness of uterine stimulants such as oxytocin can be demonstrated by the onset of effective contractions and an increase in uterine tone without indications of fluid volume excess. The effectiveness of prostaglandins can be demonstrated by the presence of cervical ripening and the induction of labor. If therapy is not successful in 10 or 12 hours, oxytocin should be discontinued and the patient allowed to rest. The infusion may be restarted the following day.

The effectiveness of tocolysis is demonstrated by the discontinuation of uterine contractions and no further progression of cervical effacement and dilation. Additionally, tocolysis is considered a success if delivery of the fetus has been delayed long enough (24 to 48 hours) to permit acceleration of fetal lung maturity.

SUMMARY

- The etiology for the initiation of labor is unknown, but several theories have been proposed.
- Labor is separated into three distinct stages: progressive cervical change, dilation of cervix and delivery of infant, and delivery of placenta.
- Pharmacotherapeutic interventions may be necessary to maintain the safety of the woman and the fetus.
- Induction or augmentation of labor is accomplished through the use of cervical ripening drugs and drugs that cause contractions.
- PTL is defined as the onset of labor with cervical change before completion of the 37th week of gestation. The etiology of PTL is often unknown.
- Complete assessment of the pregnant woman includes reviewing past and present history, including an obstetric and drug history.
- The couple's expectations, values, beliefs, and behaviors around the perinatal experience are important to assess and include in the plan of care.
- The goal of treatment with a uterine stimulant is to establish regular contractions that occur every 3 to 5 minutes and last 60 to 90 seconds.
- The treatment goal in tocolysis is to stop uterine contractions and to prevent the progression of cervical effacement and dilation.
- Oxytocins are used for the initial induction of labor in patients with favorable cervix or in patients who are gravida three or greater.
- The primary use of prostaglandins is for the termination of pregnancy. They are also used to ripen an unfavorable cervix.
- Ergot alkaloids have been used to decrease postpartum bleeding secondary to uterine atony.
- $Beta_2$ agonists, magnesium sulfate, calcium channel blockers, and nonsteroidal anti-inflammatory drugs are used in the treatment of PTL.
- Drug dosage and administration are titrated to patient response.
- Fetal maturity, presentation, pelvic adequacy, maternal vital signs, and fetal heart rate should be assessed before the start of therapy and periodically thereafter.
- The effectiveness of uterine stimulants can be demonstrated by the onset of effective contractions and an increase in uterine tone without indications of fluid volume excess.
- The effectiveness of tocolysis is demonstrated by the discontinuation of uterine contractions, and progression of cervical effacement and dilatation.

BIBLIOGRAPHY

Akoury, H. A., MacDonald, F. J., Brodie, G., et al. (1991). Oxytocin augmentation of labor and perinatal outcome in nulliparas. *Obstetrics and Gynecology,* 78(2), 227–230

American College of Obstetricians and Gynecologists. (1991). Induction and augmentation of labor. *ACOG Technical Bulletin.* No. 157. Washington D.C.: Author.

Brodsky, P., and Pelzar, E. (1991). Rationale for oxytocin administration protocols. *Journal of Gynecology, Obstetrics, Neonatal Nursing,* 20(6), 440–444.

Bugalho, A., Bique, C., Machungo, F., et al. (1994). Induction of labor with intravaginal misoprostol on intrauterine fetal death. *American Journal of Obstetrics and Gynecology,* 171(2),538–541.

Carlan, S., O'Brien, W., Jones, M., et al. (1995). Outpatient oral sulindac to prevent recurrence of preterm labor. *Obstetrics and Gynecology,* 85(1), 769–773.

Carlan, S., O'Brien, W., O'Leary, T., et al. (1992). Randomized comparative trial of indomethacin and sulindac for the treatment of refractory preterm labor. *Obstetrics and Gynecology,* 79(2), 223–228.

Creasy, R., and Resnik, R. (1989). *Maternal fetal medicine: Principles and practice.* (2nd ed.). Philadelphia: W. B. Saunders.

Cunningham, F., MacDonald, P., Leveno, K., et al. (1993). *William's obstetrics* (19th ed.). Norwalk, CT: Appleton & Lange.

Day, M., and Snell B. (1993). Use of prostaglandins for induction of labor. *Journal of Nurse-Midwifery,* 38(2), 42S–48S.

Fletcher, H., Mitchell, S., Frederick, J., et al. (1994). Intravaginal misoprostol versus dinoprostone as cervical ripening and labor-inducing agents. *Obstetrics and Gynecology,* 83(2), 244–247.

Gilman, A., Rall, T., Nies, A., et al. (1990). *The pharmacological basis of therapeutics* (8th ed). New York: Pergamon Press.

Hales, K., Rayburn, W., Turnbull, G., et al. (1994). Double-blind comparison of intracervical and intravaginal prostaglandin E_2 for cervical ripening and induction of labor. *American Journal of Obstetrics and Gynecology,* 171(4), 1087–1091.

Heyborn, K., Burke, S., and Porreco, R. (1990). Prolongation of premature gestation in women with hemolysis, elevated liver enzymes, and low platelets. *Journal of Reproductive Medicine,* 35(1), 53–57.

Higby, K., Xenakis, E., and Pauerstien, C. (1993). Do tocolytic agents stop preterm labor? A critical and comprehensive review of efficacy and safety. *American Journal of Obstetrics and Gynecology,* 168(4), 1247–1259.

Husstein, P. (1991). Use of prostaglandins for induction of labor. *Seminars in Perinatology,* 15, 173–181.

Johnson, P. (1993). Suppression of preterm labour. *Drugs,* 45(5), 684–692.

Knuppel, R., and Drukker, J. (1993). *High risk pregnancy: A team approach* (2nd ed.). Philadelphia: W. B. Saunders.

Lacy, C., Armstrong, L., Lipsy, R., et al. (1993). *Drug information handbook.* Houston: Lexi-Comp, Inc.

Magann, E., Bass, D., Chauhan, S., et al. (1994). Antepartum corticosteroids: Disease stabilization in patients with the syndrome of hemolysis, elevated liver enzymes, and low platelets (HELLP). *American Journal of Obstetrics and Gynecology,* 171(4), 1148–1153.

McEvoy, G. (1993). *American hospital formulary service drug information.* Bethesda, MD: American Society of Hospital Pharmacists.

Miller, F., Chibbar, R., and Michell, A. (1993). Synthesis of oxytocin in amnion, chorion, and decidua: A potential paracrine role for oxytocin in the onset of human parturition. *Regulatory Peptides,* 45(1993), 247–251.

Satin, A., Leveno, K., Sherman, L., et al. (1994). High-dose oxytocin: 20- versus 40-minute dosage interval. *Obstetrics and Gynecology,* 83(2), 234–238.

Sawai, S., O'Brien, W., Mastrogiannis, D., et al. (1992). NSAIDs: Maternal and fetal considerations. *American Journal of Reproductive Immunology,* 28(3-4), 141–147.

Thorp, J., Parriott, J., Ferrette-Smith, D., et al. (1994). Antepartum vitamin K and phenobarbital for preventing intraventricular hemorrhage in the premature newborn: A randomized, double-blind, placebo-controlled trial. *Obstetrics and Gynecology,* 83(1), 70–76.

Travis, B., and McCullough, J. (1993). Pharmacotherapy of preterm labor. *Pharmacotherapy,* 13(1), 28–36.

Wing, D., Rahall, A., Jones, M., et al. (1995). A comparison of misoprostol and prostaglandin E_2 gel for preinduction cervical ripening and labor induction. *American Journal of Obstetrics and Gynecology,* 172(6), 1804–1810.

Wing, D., Rahall, A., Jones, M., et al. (1995). Misoprostol: An effective agent for cervical ripening and labor induction. *American Journal of Obstetrics and Gynecology,* 172(6), 1811–1816.

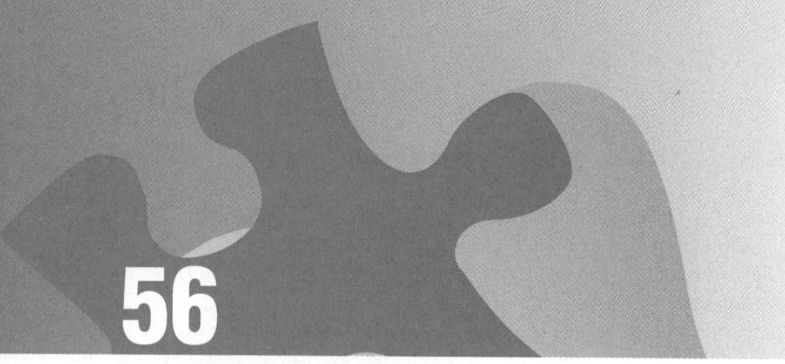

56 Fertility Drugs

In the United States, it is estimated that one to two million couples of child-bearing age (15 to 44 years old) are unsuccessful in their attempts to achieve pregnancy. The last 10 years have brought a tremendous increase in the knowledge of the human reproductive system and a simultaneous expansion in medical interventions for the treatment of infertility. Still, only 50 to 60 percent of couples with diagnosed infertility can expect to achieve pregnancy and carry the fetus to term with the expert diagnosis and interventions available today.

Infertility is defined as an inability to conceive after 1 year of unprotected coitus or an inability to carry a fetus to term. Primary infertility occurs in couples with no history of pregnancy with either partner. Secondary infertility occurs when there has been a previous pregnancy, regardless of the outcome. In general, infertility rates increase with age and are more prevalent in certain populations. Blacks have a 1.5-percent greater incidence of infertility than whites. Many couples have several reasons for their infertility. It is estimated that 40 percent of infertility is due to male factors, 40 percent due to female factors, and 20 percent due to both. Therefore, it is essential to conduct a thorough evaluation of both partners in the diagnostic phase of treatment.

The physiologic events of normal fertility are discussed in Chapter 54. It is important to review the information on the menstrual cycle and the physiologic and pharmacologic effects of estrogens and progestins. Information on testosterone from Chapter 53 should also be reviewed. In particular, the roles of luteinizing hormone (LH) and follicle-stimulating hormone (FSH) in male and female reproduction should be noted. Finally, consideration should be given to the pulsatile nature of gonadotropin-releasing hormone (GnRH), the hormone that controls the release of LH and FSH and is essential to normal reproductive function.

FEMALE FERTILITY DISORDERS

Female fertility disorders include problems related to follicular maturation, ovulation, pituitary disorders, or luteal phase defects. Fertilization, implantation, and growth and development of the ovum may also be a problem. Uterine, tubal, and pelvic disorders also contribute to infertility (Table 56–1).

Ovulation Disorders

Disorders of ovulation are due to hypothalamic, pituitary, or ovarian dysfunction. Ovulatory dysfunction accounts for approximately 25 percent of female infertility. The hormonal system that sends feedback from the hypothalamus to the pituitary to the ovaries and then back can malfunction at any point.

Hypothalamic dysfunction produces a hypogonadotropic state. The inactivity of GnRH results in decreased secretion of gonadotropins, primarily LH, producing amenorrhea. Amenorrhea may be caused by disruption of estrogen production, which, in turn, impacts hypothalamic function. It has been shown that GnRH is inhibited by the feedback effects of ovarian steroids on the endogenous opiate system of the hypothalamus. Chronic stimulation of brain opioid activity is implicated as a cause of amenorrhea.

Prolactin levels are increased when gonadotropin levels are decreased. Opiate antagonists have been found to be effective in these women for increasing the LH pulse frequency suppressed by the excess opiates they produce.

Kallman's syndrome, a type of hypogonadotropic hypogonadism, is a rare congenital defect caused by a deficiency of GnRH. This syndrome appears to be genetically heterogeneous. Karyotyping reveals a normal female. Agenesis or hypoplasia of the olfactory lobes is associated with decreased luteinizing hormone–releasing factor (LRF). Patients present with primary amenorrhea, decreased gonadotropin levels, and a lack of sexual development, as well as an inability to perceive odors. Although the ovaries are responsive to administered gonadotropins, ovulation cannot be induced.

Amenorrhea following the discontinuation of oral contraceptives is rare. It is possible that the woman had a history of undiagnosed abnormalities of the hypothalamic-pituitary-ovarian (HPO) axis before pill use or developed it during therapy. Because most women resume menstruation within 6 months, a definitive diagnosis should be delayed until that time.

If the exact cause of amenorrhea is unknown, it is termed idiopathic hypothalamic dysfunction. Clinically, these patients have normal gonadotropin levels and exhibit withdrawal bleeding following progesterone challenge. GnRH levels are low or GnRH is released improperly; however, most patients with this disorder ovulate with pharmacotherapy.

Pituitary Disorders

Examples of pituitary disorders affecting fertility include hyperprolactinemia and prolactin-secreting adenomas. Prolactin acts at the level of the gonads, the pituitary, or the hypothalamus to inhibit gonadotropin secretion. When prolactin secretion is low, LH and estrogen levels may also be low. Hyperprolactinemia in women is associated with amenorrhea.

Many drugs can cause an excess amount of circulating prolactin, as can stress and pituitary adenomas. In the postpartum period, the ovary is resistant to exogenous gonadotropin stimulation due to the hyperprolactinemic state induced by nipple stimulation. This often results in anovulation and is the basis for the belief that breastfeeding is a form of contraception. However, breastfeeding alone as a postpartum contraceptive has proved to be unreliable.

Hypopituitarism, or Sheehan's syndrome, occurs as a result of acute necrosis of the anterior pituitary. During preg-

TABLE 56–1 DISORDERS OF FERTILITY

Female Disorders of Fertility	Male Disorders of Fertility
Ovulation Disorders	**Pretesticular Disorders**
Hypothalamic amenorrhea	Hypogonadotropic hypogonadism
Kallman's syndrome	Isolated gonadotropin deficiency
Birth control pills	Pituitary failure
Idiopathic hypothalamic dysfunction	Hyperprolactinemia
Stress, weight loss, anorexia	Chronic disease
	Kallman's syndrome
Pituitary Disorders	**Testicular Disorders**
Hyperprolactinemia	Dysfunctional spermatogenesis
Sheehan's syndrome	Toxins
Hypogonadotropic hypogonadism	Infection
	Varicocele
	Klinefelter's syndrome
Ovarian Disorders	**Post-Testicular Disorders**
Gonadotropin-resistant ovary syndrome	Absence of vas deferens
Polycystic ovary syndrome	Obstructions
Premature ovarian failure	Vasectomy
Luteinized unruptured follicle syndrome	Retrograde ejaculation
Disorders of sexual development	Physiologic/psychogenic dysfunction
	Spinal cord injury
	Sperm autoimmunity
	Hypospadias
Uterine, Tubal, and Pelvic Disorders	
Structural anomalies	
Tubal damage	
Endometriosis or endometritis	
Uterine leiomyomas	
Asherman's syndrome	
Unfavorable cervical mucus	
Luteal Phase Defects	
Other Disorders	
Heat	
Radiation	
Chemicals	
Endocrine disorders	
Complications of pregnancy (abortion, cesarean section, postpartum infection, ectopic pregnancy)	

nancy, the anterior pituitary enlarges, increasing the oxygen demand and blood flow to the gland. In cases of postpartum hemorrhage and shock, the pituitary is particularly vulnerable to damage from ischemia. Prompt diagnosis and volume replacement is essential for survival. The degree of hypopituitarism is highly variable, and the pituitary response to GnRH may be normal, diminished, or absent. Subsequent pregnancy has been reported after spontaneous, complete, or partial recovery.

Hypogonadotropic hypogonadism is associated with an insufficient secretion of GnRH and subsequent deficiency of gonadotropins. The appearance of secondary sex characteristics is dependent on sex steroids, which are lacking in these patients. The syndrome often goes undetected until puberty, at which point patients present with persistent sexual infantilism. A genetic or developmental defect, it is found in both males and females. Females have primary amenorrhea and immature ovaries that readily respond to gonadotropin.

Ovarian Dysfunction

Gonadotropin-resistant ovary syndrome is found in patients with both primary and secondary amenorrhea. In the presence of elevated gonadotropins, particularly FSH, the follicles fail to respond. Estrogen levels are low or low normal, whereas FSH and LH levels are found to be normal or high. The etiology, then, is thought to be the presence of ovarian antigonadotropin-receptor antibodies, which may indicate autoimmune disease. Ovarian biopsy is necessary to make a definitive diagnosis. These patients do not respond to gonadotropin administration and therefore pregnancy is virtually impossible.

In polycystic ovary syndrome (PCO), virtually all androgenic hormones are found to be elevated. Patients with this condition frequently present with anovulation, hirsutism, hyperprolactinemia, and obesity. However, the combination of these symptoms and infertility is not unique to PCO. It is important to assess the patient for other endocrinopathies. Elevated LH and low or normal FSH levels are secondary to decreased levels of GnRH. The follicular cysts in the ovaries do not mature fully. Chronic anovulation causes a lack in the negative feedback system that keeps estrogen levels in balance, further suppressing FSH. The administration of FSH to the patient with PCO elevates estrogen levels and decreases androstenedione and testosterone. The result is ovulation.

Premature ovarian failure affects a group of patients with a history of menstrual infrequency or irregularity, who have ceased menstruating before the age of 40, and who have no apparent genetic abnormalities. Their symptoms usually include amenorrhea, elevated gonadotropins, and decreased estrogens. Varying profiles of gonadotropins and steroid hormones are found, many of which are typical of postmenopausal women. It is thought that oocytes are prematurely depleted, a deficient number were developed prenatally, or excessive gonadotropic stimulation has occurred. Autoimmune response to gonadotropins or their receptors is also suspect. Hormone replacement therapy is often prescribed, and in some cases, ovulation induction has been successful.

The condition of regular menses without the normal release of an ovum has been described as luteinized unruptured follicle syndrome. This syndrome has been found in women with normal cycles. It is considered to be a sporadic and infrequent cause of infertility, probably a result of occasional desynchronized mechanisms of ovulation.

There are many instances of developmental aberrations that inhibit or preclude fertility. Many go undetected until the etiology of infertility or recurrent abortion is sought. Structural anomalies of the uterus, vagina, and cervix may be detected by manual exam, during delivery or surgery, or by sonogram or radiographic imaging. Examples include uterine didelphia (so-called double uterus), bicornate uterus, and septate uterus. Uterine and cervical defects can be the result of developmental defects of unknown etiology or the effects of exposure to teratogenic substances during pregnancy.

Gonadal dysgenesis occurs as a result of an embryonic developmental defect. Examples of chromosomal anomalies that adversely affect fertility are Turner's syndrome, Klinefelter's syndrome, and pseudohermaphroditism or true hermaphroditism. Fertility is rarely possible in patients with disorders of sexual development.

Luteal Phase Defects

Approximately 3 to 4 percent of infertile women are diagnosed as having luteal phase defects. In women who have a history of habitual abortion, the incidence may be higher. An inadequate luteal phase is the result of a deficient secretion of progesterone by the corpus luteum after normal, spontaneous ovulation. This results in an inadequate stimulation of the endometrium and inability to conceive or maintain the pregnancy. Inadequate luteal function is often only a natural consequence of similarly inadequate folliculogenesis. Luteal phase deficiency consistently accompanies follicular phase FSH deficiency.

Uterine, Tubal, and Pelvic Disorders

A history of pelvic inflammatory disease, septic abortion, intrauterine device use, ruptured appendix, or ectopic pregnancy should alert the health care provider to the possibility of tubal damage. The fallopian tubes consist of three muscular layers and are lined with ciliated cells that wave in the direction of the uterus. Their secretory and contractile functions are vital to the transport of both the sperm and ovum, and ultimately, the delivery of the embryo to the uterus after fertilization.

The secretory activity of the fallopian tubes, which is mainly under the influence of estrogen, varies in response to the hormonal fluctuations of the menstrual cycle. As ovulation approaches and estrogen production increases, secretions accumulate in the tubal lumen to assist in sperm transport. After fertilization, owing to the effects of progesterone, the secretions decrease and the fluid becomes clear. This allows the cilia to move the embryo through the tubes to the uterus. If the cilia are destroyed or the tubes are twisted, scarred, or blocked, this transport process is impaired.

Endometriosis is one of the most common gynecologic disorders. It is defined as the presence of hormonally responsive endometrial tissue found implanted outside the endometrial cavity. Although the etiology and pathogenesis are not clear, it is postulated that during menstruation, endometrial cells reflux through the tubes and attach to the pelvic structures. Endometrial fragments are most commonly found in dependent pelvic structures but may also be carried by the lymph and vasculature to distant sites.

Ectopic endometrial tissue contains receptors for estrogen, progesterone, and androgens. They respond to the fluctuating serum levels of these hormones much the same as normal endometrium, with monthly bleeding that results in inflammation and peritoneal scarring. When the ovaries and tubes are involved, ovum transport is often obstructed by adhesions and the distortion of the anatomic structures in relation to each other.

Endometriosis is indicated when there are complaints of dysmenorrhea, dyspareunia, and infertility. Symptoms, however, vary greatly and, by themselves, cannot be used to measure the severity of the disease. Laparoscopy should be used to confirm the diagnosis. Treatment options include surgery, medical therapy, or a combination of medical and surgical treatment.

Acquired uterine defects are commonly seen in cases of infertility. Uterine leiomyomas, or fibroids, are benign pelvic tumors affecting approximately 20 percent of American women. Interference with the proliferation of the endometrium may prevent normal expansion of the uterus as pregnancy progresses. Fibroids may cause habitual abortion or abnormalities of implantation, predisposing the pregnancy to placenta previa and premature labor. They occur more often in later reproductive years and are three to nine times more prevalent in blacks than in whites.

A woman who has been exposed to diethylstilbestrol can present with a wide range of aberrations of fertility from cervical incompetencies to uterine cavity anomalies. Many of these problems are surgically repairable, and a nearly normal pregnancy may ensue. Others, however, require assisted reproductive techniques (ART) and have a marginal success rate.

Intrauterine adhesions, or Asherman's syndrome, cause the destruction of a large area of the endometrium, usually as a result of postpartum curettage, curettage after missed abortion, or infection. Amenorrhea or recurrent abortions may ensue due to an insufficient amount of tissue left to provide for proper implantation. Hysteroscopy allows direct visualization of adhesions and a means by which lysis can be performed. High-dose estrogen-progestin treatment is added for 2 to 3 months to promote re-epithelialization of the endometrium.

Cervical factors also contribute to infertility. Inspection of the cervical mucus allows the health care provider to directly observe the effects and timing of hormonal activity. Further study of the chemical properties as well as the contents of the mucus provides more detailed information that may be helpful in the diagnosis and treatment. In some cases, there is a lack of cervical mucus or cervical stenosis. These conditions can be seen in women who were exposed to diethylstilbestrol in utero and women whose cervical glands have been destroyed by cervical cautery or conization.

MALE FERTILITY DISORDERS

Infertility in men accounts for 40 to 60 percent of problems of conception. Disorders can be classified as pretesticular, testicular, and post-testicular (see Table 56–1).

Pretesticular Disorders

Pretesticular disorders include hypothalamic and pituitary disorders such as hypogonadotropic hypogonadism (Kallman's syndrome and isolated gonadotropin deficiency), pituitary failure, delayed or premature sexual development, and congenital adrenal hyperplasia. This category of patients has defects of the hypothalamic-pituitary axis that are either acquired or hereditary.

In most of these patients, hypothalamic dysfunction results in decreased or absent release of GnRH. Testicular biopsy reveals immature testes with underdeveloped Leydig's cells that are unable to produce testosterone. Both sexual development and spermatogenesis are dependent on the quantity of gonadotropins secreted. Treatment with various hormones usually promotes sexual maturation and, hence, the restoration of fertility.

Prolactin plays a role in male fertility, much as it does in females. Many studies have suggested that prolactin synergizes with LH and testosterone to increase reproductive function in the male. Almost all males with prolactin-producing pituitary tumors are impotent, regardless of their testosterone level. Suppression of prolactin with the administration of bromocriptine or removal of the tumor restores sexual function.

Chronic disease can be another source of pretesticular infertility. Diabetes mellitus can cause a lack of emission or retrograde ejaculation. Cystic fibrosis or recurrent upper respiratory infections may cause abnormalities of the seminal vesicles, vas deferens, and epididymis, or cause immotile cilia syndrome that interferes with the transport of sperm through the ductal system.

Testicular Disorders

Testicular disorders include dysfunctional spermatogenesis due to genetic or abnormal development or causes such as varicocele; exposure to toxins, drugs, and radiation; or infections. Examination of the cellular development of germ cells during various stages of spermatogenesis is necessary to classify disorders of sperm maturation. Semen studies are used for this purpose. Drugs that affect spermatogenesis include alcohol, amebicides, anabolic steroids, cimetidine, homogenated hydrocarbons, nicotine, nitrofurantoin, sulfonamide drugs, and sulfasalazine.

Infection may cause epididymitis, orchitis, or epididymo-orchitis (a combination of the two). Common causative organisms include *Escherichia coli,* streptococci, staphylococci, *Neisseria gonorrhoeae,* and *Chlamydia.* Infertility may occur as a result of a recurrent or chronic infection that causes mechanical obstruction from scarring.

The mumps virus can cause acute orchitis and, in pubertal or adult males, may result in damage to the seminiferous tubules and Leydig's cells, creating testosterone deficiency, hypogonadism, and infertility.

In some cases, the etiology of infertility is reversible with surgical intervention. Varicocele is an abnormal dilatation or varicosity of the veins that drain the testicle. Varicoceles are found in up to 15 percent of the male population. Of those, approximately 50 percent have poor semen quality. Some studies have shown improved pregnancy rates in partners of men who have undergone surgery.

Post-Testicular Disorders

Post-testicular causes of infertility include a congenital absence of the vas deferens, obstructive problems, vasectomy, retrograde ejaculation, and sexual dysfunction related to physiologic and psychogenic problems, or spinal cord injuries. New technologies are aimed at improving vasectomy resections. Electroejaculation implants may be used for voluntary nerve innervation in patients with spinal cord injuries. Improvement of semen processing for therapeutic insemination may also promote fertility.

Sperm autoimmunity can occur in men if their immune system identifies the spermatozoa as foreign when they first appear at puberty. If this problem occurs, there is a decrease in sperm motility and viability due to agglutination or clumping and immobilization. Current treatments have inconclusive efficacy, but in the case of idiopathic infertility, sperm agglutination tests may be indicated.

PHARMACOTHERAPEUTIC OPTIONS

Many advances in the treatment of infertility have been made in the last few decades. Ovulatory dysfunction, once a hopeless situation for achieving pregnancy, now constitutes one of the most successful areas of new technology. If the infertility problems are due solely to problems of ovulation, current drug preparations can increase the couple's chances of conceiving to near that of the general population. Before beginning treatment for ovulation induction, other endocrinopathies must first be eliminated. ART also uses these principal drugs, but protocols for their use can vary.

Bromocriptine (PARLODEL)

Indications

Bromocriptine is indicated for patients with infertility associated with hyperprolactinemia, pituitary adenomas, and galactorrhea. It is also used for the restoration of menstrual function in patients who so desire it or for those in whom restoration of ovarian function is necessary for the prevention of bone loss.

Oligospermia, if caused by elevated prolactin levels, may also be treated with bromocriptine. Males show an increased sperm count when elevated prolactin levels are corrected.

Pharmacodynamics

Bromocriptine resembles the neurotransmitter dopamine in structure and is able to bind to dopamine receptors in the pituitary gland. Prolactin secretion from the pituitary gland is then inhibited, reducing prolactin levels. By substantially reducing elevated prolactin levels, bromocriptine can restore ovulation and ovarian function in amenorrheic women. This appears to be accomplished by direct suppression of pituitary secretion or by stimulating dopamine receptors in the hypothalamus to release prolactin-inhibiting factor. It may also act on dopaminergic receptors in the ovary to restore ovulation. There is evidence that it may stimulate ovulation in women whose prolactin level is not elevated and does not decrease with use, indicating it may have an effect on hypothalamic release of LH-releasing hormone.

Bromocriptine also suppresses galactorrhea and prolactin levels in men. In most patients with hyperprolactinemia, if bromocriptine is discontinued, prolactin returns to pretreatment levels within 1 to 6 weeks. Amenorrhea returns in 4 to 24 weeks, and galactorrhea returns in 2 to 12 weeks.

Adverse Effects and Contraindications

The most frequently experienced adverse effects of bromocriptine are nausea and vomiting related to gastrointestinal (GI) intolerance. These symptoms usually resolve spontaneously within a few days and may be avoided by a slow increase of the dosage to achieve the desired effects. Some patients experience severe postural hypotension and syncope on initiation of therapy. Hypertension, although rare, occurs usually after about 2 weeks of therapy. Treatment should be discontinued if hypertension; severe, progressive, or unremitting headache; or signs of central nervous system toxicity are present.

Patients wishing to breastfeed should not take bromocriptine owing to its suppressive effects on lactation. Prolactin levels in the fetus of pregnant women treated with bromocriptine were found to be decreased in utero but returned to normal after birth. Bromocriptine is routinely discontinued when conception is verified.

Pharmacokinetics

Bromocriptine is rapidly and completely absorbed in the GI tract. A single dose has been found to decrease serum prolactin levels within 2 hours, with maximal suppression occurring within 8 hours (Table 56–2). The most therapeutic effects in hyperprolactinemic patients are seen after 4 weeks of therapy. Approximately 90 to 96 percent is bound to serum albumin. The half-life of a 2.5-mg dose in the first phase is 3 to 4.5 hours, whereas the terminal phase is 45 to 50 hours. Bromocriptine is biotransformed in the liver and eliminated in the feces through biliary elimination. A small percent is eliminated in the urine.

Drug-Drug Interactions

The effectiveness of bromocriptine in decreasing prolactin levels may be antagonized by drugs known to elevate prolactin such as amitriptyline, imipramine, phenothiazines, and methyldopa (Table 56–3). Additive neurologic effects may occur with levodopa as well as additive hypotensive effects when the drug is used with antihypertensives. Severe hypertension may occur when bromocriptine is given concomitantly with certain ergot alkaloids, which may lead to severe cardiovascular and central nervous system complications.

Drug-Food Interactions

Sulfites contained in some commercial food preparations may cause an allergic reaction in susceptible patients. The use of alcohol is contraindicated.

Dosage Regimen

For the treatment of hyperprolactinemic causes of amenorrhea, hypogonadism, and infertility, the usual dose is 1.25 to 2.5 mg/day, with the goal of 2.5 mg twice daily (Table 56–4). Tablets may be split to be given throughout the day or may be administered at bedtime. If the initial 2.5-mg daily dose is well tolerated during the first week of treatment, a second 2.5-mg dose can be added. Prolactin levels

TABLE 56–2 PHARMACOKINETICS OF SELECTED FERTILITY DRUGS

Drug	Rte	Onset	Peak	Duration	PB (%)	$t_{½}$	BioA (%)
Bromocriptine	po	30–90 min	1–2 hr	8–12 hr*	90–96	3–4.5; 45–50 hr†	UA
Clomiphene citrate	po	5–14 days	UK	UK	UA	5 days	UA
Human menopausal gonadotropin	IM	UK	Fe:18 hr; M:4 mo	UK	UA	LH: 4 hr; FSH: 70 hr	UA
Human chorionic gonadotropin	IM	2 hr	6 hr	36–72 hr	UA	23 hr	UA
Gonadorelin acetate	IV/SC	Rapid to slow	2–6 hr	3–5 hr	UA	2–8 min	100
Leuprolide acetate	SC	1–2 wks‡	2–4 hr	3–4 wk	7–15	3 hr	94
FSH	IM	UK	6–18 hr	UA	UA	2.9 hr	UK
Testosterone	IM	UK	UK	1–3 days; 2–4 wk§	98	10–100 min; 8 days‖	UK

*The most therapeutic effects of bromocriptine when used in hyperprolactinemia are seen after 4 weeks of therapy.
†First-phase half-life of bromocriptine is 3 to 4.5 hours, whereas terminal phase is 45 to 50 hours.
‡Onset of leuprolide action follows a transient increase during the first week of therapy; depot formulation.
§Duration of action of testosterone is 1 to 3 days for base and propionate formulations; 2 to 4 weeks for cypionate and enanthate formulations.
‖Half-life of testosterone base is 10 to 100 minutes; 8 days for testosterone cypionate.
$t_{½}$, Elimination half-life; BioA, bioavailability; FSH, follicle-stimulating hormone; PB, protein binding; SC, subcutaneously; UA, unavailable; UK, unknown.

TABLE 56–3 DRUG-DRUG INTERACTIONS OF SELECTED FERTILITY DRUGS

Drug(s)	Interactive Drug(s)	Interaction
Bromocriptine	Amitriptyline Imipramine Phenothiazines Methyldopa Progesterone	Reduced effectiveness of bromocriptine to reduce prolactin levels
	Levodopa	Additive neurologic effects
	Antihypertensives	Additive hypotensive effects
	Ergot alkaloids	Severe hypertension
Leuprolide	Antiandrogens Megestrol Flutamide	Additive antineoplastic effects

should be rechecked, and if adequate suppression has not occurred, the dosage may be increased to 7.5 mg/day.

If oral administration is not possible, some have found perivaginal administration to be equally effective while reducing symptoms. Current research has developed both a delayed-release oral preparation and an injectable form of bromocriptine that may soon be more readily available.

Laboratory Considerations

Prolactin levels should be assessed to obtain the desired effect at the lowest possible dose. Bromocriptine has been associated with transient elevations in plasma concentrations of alanine aminotransferase (ALT; serum glutamic-pyruvic transaminase [SGPT]), aspartate aminotransferase (AST; serum glutamic-oxaloacetic transaminase [SGOT]), alkaline phosphatase, uric acid, and blood urea nitrogen (BUN). Transient increases in g-glutamyl transferase and creatine kinase were also found.

Clomiphene Citrate

❒ Clomiphene citrate (CLOMID, MILOPHENE, SEROPHENE)

Indications

Use of clomiphene citrate is indicated in the treatment of ovulatory failure. These patients respond to a progesterone

TABLE 56–4 DOSAGE REGIMEN FOR SELECTED FERTILITY DRUGS

Drug	Use(s)	Dosage	Implications
Bromocriptine	Hyperprolactinemia	*Female:* 2.5–7.5 mg po QD. Begin ½ tablet QD and add one to two tablets QD over 2 wk	If extremely sensitive, may give intranasally. Check PRL levels after 4 wk, then PRN
Clomiphene citrate	Oligospermia, anovulation, polycystic ovary syndrome	*Female:* 50 mg po × 5 days, repeat in 30 days; 100 mg po × 5 days. Increase to 150 mg QD if still unresponsive *Male:* 25 mg QD with 5-day rest period and repeat *or* 100 mg on MWF	First-line drug for primary infertility. Gonadotropin surge expected 5–10 days after last dose. May be repeated up to six cycles before considered "failed." Check BBT and U/S by day 5
Follicle-stimulating hormone	Failed clomiphene therapy; PCO with elevated LH/FSH	*Female:* 75 IU IM QD for 7–12 days, followed by 5000–10,000 units hCG 1 day after last dose of FSH. If evidence of ovulation but no pregnancy, repeat regimen × 2 cycles before increasing dose to 150 IU QD × 7–12 days followed by hCG. May repeat × two more courses	Individualize dose. Ovarian hyperstimulation usually occurs during 2 wk post-treatment period. Instruct to have intercourse daily beginning day before hCG until ovulation. If ovaries overly enlarged, hold hCG. Larger doses not recommended. Multiple births possible. Very expensive
Human chorionic gonadotropin	Anovulatory women pretreated with menotropins. Hypogonadotropic hypogonadism secondary to pituitary deficiency	*Female:* 5000–10,000 units IM 1 day after last dose of hMG *Male:* 500–1000 units 3×/wk × 3 wk then 2×/wk for 3 wk; *or* 4000 units 3×/wk × 6–9 mo, then decrease to 2000 units 3×/wk × 3 mo	Closely monitor ovary size during stimulation treatment. Do not administer hCG if abnormally enlarged to avoid OHSS. Warn couple about the possibility of multiple births
Human menopausal gonadotropin	Follicle stimulation for ART. Ovulation dysfunction, luteal phase deficiency, idiopathic and male factor infertility	*Female:* 150 IU (75 IU FSH and 75 IU LH) IM QD × 6–12 days, starting on day 2–3. Repeat × 3 cycles before doubling dose (300 IU) *Male:* Pretreat with hCG until secondary sex characteristics appear approximately 4–6 mo, then 150 IU IM 3×/wk with 2000 units hCG 2×/wk for 4 mo to detect sperm in ejaculate. May increase to 300 IU hMG	See warnings under FSH and hCG about OHSS and multiple births. Treatment very expensive ($45 or more per 150 IU ampule: $1000/cycle)
Leuprolide acetate	Controlled ovulation induction for ART	*Female:* Begin midluteal phase of previous cycle. Give 1 mg SC QD for about 2 wk, decrease to 0.5 mg SC QD when hMG or FSH is started	Not FDA approved for this use. Adds to cost but may find cost savings due to fewer canceled cycles due to decreased frequency of OHSS

ART, Assisted reproductive techniques; BBT, basal body temperature; FDA, Food and Drug Administration; FSH, follicle-stimulating hormone; hCG, human chorionic gonadotropin; hMG, human menopausal gonadotropin; LH, luteinizing hormone; MWF, Monday, Wednesday, and Friday; OHSS, ovarian hyperstimulation syndrome; PCO, polycystic ovary syndrome; PRL, prolactin; PRN, polyradiculoneuropathy; U/S, ultrasound.

challenge test by bleeding, meaning that they have normal or nearly normal levels of endogenous estrogen. They may have a history of regular cycles without ovulation or they may have oligomenorrhea, but ovulatory dysfunction must be demonstrated. Patients with PCO may benefit from treatment with clomiphene because the drug competes for the estrone-binding sites and inhibits negative feedback. If the high levels of estrogen are not inhibited, gonadotropin secretion continues to be inhibited, suppressing ovulation.

Clomiphene has been used in a limited number of patients for menstrual disorders, endometrial anaplasia or hyperplasia, persistent lactation, oligospermia, and fibrocystic breast disease. However, it is not approved for these purposes. It is also used for the treatment of male infertility.

Pharmacodynamics

Clomiphene's precise mechanism of action is unknown. It appears to compete with estradiol for estrogen binding sites in the hypothalamus, where it increases the release of GnRH to stimulate the pituitary to increase FSH and LH secretion. Clomiphene stimulates the events of the normal cycle that lead to ovulation.

Clomiphene has no progestational, androgenic, corticotropic, or antiandrogenic effects. It does not appear to interfere with normal adrenal or thyroid function.

Adverse Effects and Contraindications

The most common adverse effects of clomiphene citrate are menopause-like hot flashes. The hot flashes are related to the antiestrogenic properties of the medication, which causes vasomotor flushing. Abdominal bloating, distention, and discomfort have also been reported, as well as breast tenderness, nausea and vomiting, headache, and visual disturbances. Other side effects include hair loss or dryness, urinary frequency, increased appetite, weight gain, skin rash, tension, fatigue, insomnia, dizziness, and mood swings.

Clomiphene is contraindicated in women with preexisting ovarian cysts and those with persistent ovarian enlargement after treatment has begun. The ovary may increase in size for several days after the drug is discontinued. Normally, the enlargement spontaneously subsides without any intervention or sequela. If ovarian enlargement does occur, the treatment should be stopped and the dosage of the next cycle decreased.

Some patients with PCO are unusually sensitive to the gonadotropin levels induced by normal doses of clomiphene and may have an exaggerated response. Again, discontinuation of the medication is recommended and the condition is expected to resolve spontaneously.

Clomiphene citrate is contraindicated in patients who are hypersensitive to gonadotropins, patients with liver disease or with a history of liver dysfunction, and in women with abnormal uterine bleeding of unknown etiology. It is also contraindicated in those with pituitary tumors and thyroid and adrenal dysfunction. The patient and her partner should be warned about the risk of multiple gestation, especially with higher doses, and about the risks inherent in a multiple gestation pregnancy.

Pharmacokinetics

Clomiphene citrate is taken orally and is readily absorbed in the GI tract. Its half-life is about 5 days, but traces have been found in feces for up to 6 weeks. The biotransformation appears to take place in the liver, and it is eliminated in feces. There is evidence that some of the drug may be stored in body fat or undergo enterohepatic circulation to be slowly released from the body.

Dosage Regimen

Following a negative pregnancy test, clomiphene therapy is started on day 5 of the cycle. The initial dosage of clomiphene is 50 mg/day for 5 days. If this regimen is unsuccessful, 100 mg may be administered in the same manner, also beginning day 5. If ovulation or a normal luteal cycle is still not achieved, the dosage may be increased by 50 mg/cycle, up to 150 mg. Dosages higher than 150 mg/day are unlikely to induce ovulation. In the absence of adverse effects, this high dose may be repeated for 3 to 4 months, after which time clomiphene citrate therapy is considered ineffective.

The practice of beginning the treatment on day 5 correlates with the day when the dominant follicle is being selected. Beginning the clomiphene earlier results in multiple gestation more frequently. Earlier administration may be used in the recruitment of oocytes for ART such as in vitro fertilization, in which the goal is to mature a number of ova for retrieval in one cycle.

The gonadotropin surge is expected from 5 to 10 days after the last dose of clomiphene. The patient is instructed that for optimal results to be achieved, coitus should occur every day for 1 week beginning 5 days after the last dose of medication. The majority of patients ovulate after the first course of treatment. Those with prolonged amenorrhea may be less responsive, but up to 80 percent can be expected to ovulate and approximately 40 percent will become pregnant. The pregnancy rate in those without other causes of infertility approaches that of the general population, approximately 80 to 90 percent. The greater the number of cycles in which the drug is administered, regardless of the number of ovulations induced, the lower the pregnancy rate. Positive results seem to diminish if pregnancy is not achieved within six cycles unless other causes of infertility are discovered and corrected.

When the patient is unresponsive and the basal body temperature chart (used to detect progesterone levels from the corpus luteum) is inconclusive, human chorionic gonadotropin (hCG) may be added to the regimen (Fig. 56–1). This method is used to improve the midcycle LH surge but requires more accurate timing. If this supplemental treatment also fails to produce pregnancy, progesterone may be added or treatment with human menopausal gonadotropin (hMG) begun. In some practices, clomiphene is also used to regulate ovulation in patients receiving artificial insemination.

Laboratory Considerations

No clinically important hematologic or renal abnormalities have been reported with clomiphene citrate. Rarely, alteration in liver function tests and cholesterol synthesis may occur. It may cause increases in serum thyroxine and thyroid-binding globulin levels.

Close monitoring of follicle development and determination of ovulation can be evaluated with urine or serum estrogen levels. During cycles in which ovulation was assisted

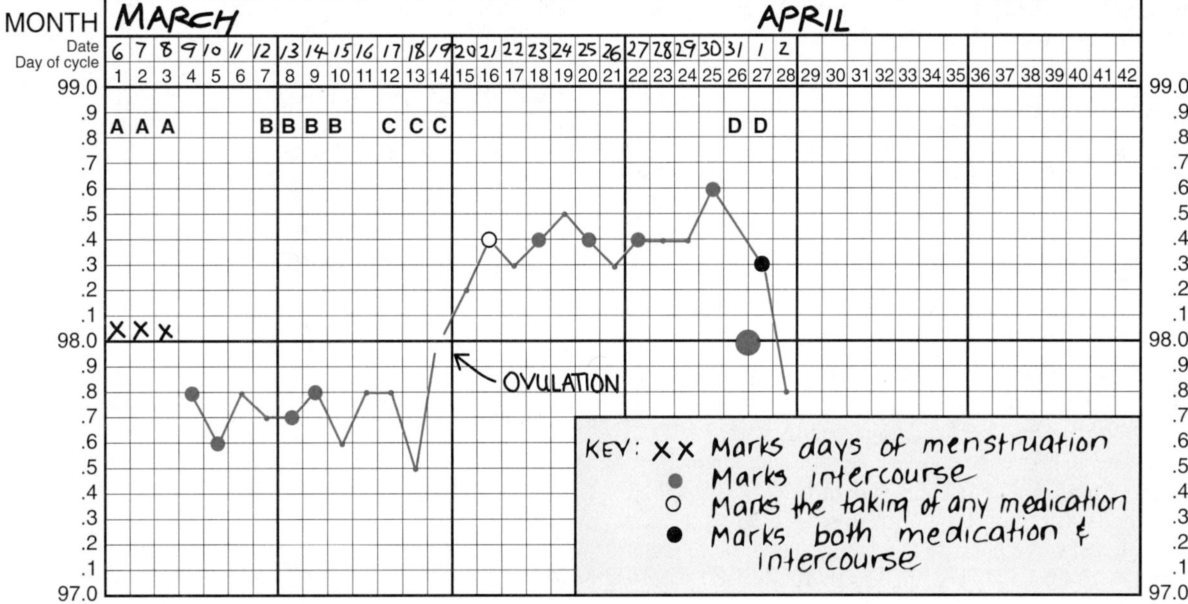

Figure 56–1 Basal body temperature graph. A basal body temperature graph identifies infertility testing intervals. Testing intervals are represented by *A*, semen analysis; *B*, hysterosalpingography; *C*, postcoital test; and *D*, endometrial biopsy. (Reprinted with permission from Garner, C. [1991]. An overview of infertility. In Garner C. [Ed.], *Principles of infertility nursing* [p. 4] Boca Raton, FL: CRC Press, copyright CRC Press, Boca Raton, Florida.)

by hCG, endometrial growth was inhibited by the antiestrogenic activity of clomiphene. Endometrial thickness can be monitored by ultrasound and optimally should be 6 mm or more for successful implantation.

Human Menopausal Gonadotropin

❒ Human menopausal gonadotropin (menotropins, hMG, PERGONAL)

Indications

Clinical indications for the use of hMG include ovulatory dysfunction, luteal phase defects, and idiopathic infertility. Demonstration of ovarian competence and tubal patency is necessary for fertilization and implantation to take place. Male factor infertility and ART candidates are also treated with hMG. In women in whom ART is indicated, hMG is also used to induce a large number of eggs to mature in one cycle for retrieval and in vitro fertilization.

Use of hMG is indicated in patients with hypothalamic pituitary failure, but who have ovarian function with normal gonadotropin levels or who respond to the progesterone challenge with bleeding. Women for whom the clomiphene citrate/hCG therapy is ineffective are candidates, as are those on clomiphene citrate with abnormal cervical mucus.

Pharmacodynamics

The FSH and LH in hMG, which is directly administered, bypass the hypothalamus and pituitary gland and bind to the ovarian granulosa and thecal cells, respectively. This process leads to follicular proliferation and maturation, followed by development of the corpus luteum. To induce ovulation of the mature ovum, a single large dose of hCG, having LH activity, is administered.

In males, LH stimulates spermatogenesis. Men who have had adequate virilization with hCG treatment require 3 months of concomitant hMG treatment to promote spermatogenesis.

Adverse Effects and Contraindications

The likelihood of ovulation is dose related, as are the complications. Hot flashes are a common side effect. Ovarian enlargement may be mild to moderate with the same complaints as that of clomiphene, but the incidence of the severe ovarian hyperstimulation syndrome (OHSS) is greater.

OHSS develops in approximately 1 percent of patients and can be life-threatening. As the ovaries are hyperstimulated, mild enlargement can progress to a critical condition with ascites, pleural effusion, hypovolemia, hypotension, oliguria, and electrolyte imbalance. The ovaries are at risk for rupture due to their excessive size from the development of multiple follicular cysts, corpora lutea, and stromal edema. Increased coagulability and decreased renal perfusion are the major complications. Hemoconcentration occurs, while renal hypoperfusion leads to hyperkalemia, and azotemia.

hMG is contraindicated in women with primary ovarian failure, thyroid or adrenal dysfunction, intracranial lesions, pituitary insufficiency, or genital bleeding of unknown etiology. In men, contraindications include normal pituitary function, primary testicular failure, or infertility due to causes other than hypogonadotropic hypogonadism.

Pharmacokinetics

hMG is destroyed in the GI tract and, therefore, must be administered by intramuscular (IM) injection. Its biotransformation is not fully understood. Like other gonadotropins, glomerular filtration with further breakdown in the proximal tubule is followed by completed clearance in the reticuloendothelial system of the liver. Blood levels have been found to decrease in a biphasic manner (see Table 56–2).

Following one IM dose of hMG, approximately 8 percent is found unchanged when eliminated in the urine.

Dosage Regimen

hMG is a purified preparation of the gonadotropins LH and FSH extracted from the urine of postmenopausal women. The commercial preparation contains a 1:1 ratio of FSH (75 IU) and LH (75 IU). It is an expensive therapeutic agent, and because of its greater complication rate, it should be used only with careful evaluation and by a qualified reproductive technology specialist.

The dosage of hMG is individually determined to produce follicular maturation. To minimize the risk of ovarian hyperstimulation with hMG/hCG therapy, the lowest dose possible should be used. The dosage begins with 75 IU of both FSH and LH for 9 to 12 days, until follicular maturation has occurred. Then, a single dose of hCG is given IM 1 day after the last dose of hMG. This dose of hCG stimulates the midcycle LH surge because the dose of LH in hMG is not high enough to do so. The couple is then advised to have coitus the day of the hCG injection and the 2 days after. If there is evidence of ovarian hyperstimulation, owing to the fragility of the stimulated ovary, further coitus and strenuous exercise should be avoided.

If pregnancy does not occur but there is evidence of ovulation, this regimen may be repeated at least two more times. If ovulation did not occur, the dose of hMG can be increased to 150 IU each for both LH and FSH. The regimen may be repeated twice more. There may be some advantage to adding purified FSH to the treatment regimen.

In order to prevent ovarian hyperstimulation, estrogen measurements and ultrasound determination of follicular size are necessary to determine the best moment to administer the ovulatory dose of hCG. At least by day 7 of hMG therapy, urine or blood estrogen levels are measured and drug dosage is adjusted for the rest of the cycle. Observation of cervical mucus changes is also used.

To stimulate spermatogenesis with hMG, full masculinization, as evidenced by the presence of secondary sex characteristics, must first be achieved. Pretreatment with hCG is necessary in the case of primary or secondary hypogonadotropic hypogonadism. Once pretreatment is complete, concomitant use of hCG and hMG can begin. The initial dose is 75 IU each of LH and FSH, three times weekly, with 2000 USP units of hCG two times weekly. Spermatozoa should then be evident in the ejaculate. If they are not, the dosages of hMG can be increased and the regimen repeated.

Laboratory Considerations

Serum estradiol levels are determined beginning on day 7 of hMG administration and are repeated every 1 to 3 days. Depending on the estradiol level, the subsequent dose of hMG is then individualized for the rest of the cycle. Midcycle estradiol levels, which are taken early in the morning after an evening dose of hMG is given, should be between 1000 and 1500 pg/mL for best results. From 1500 to 2000 pg/mL, the risk of hyperstimulation is great, and above 2000 pg/mL, hCG is generally withheld.

In addition, ultrasound monitoring of follicular size is used. In a normal cycle, when the follicle reaches 20 to 24 mm it is mature. In cycles induced by hMG, clomiphene citrate, and FSH, follicles may be considered ready for the dose of hCG when they are slightly smaller (16 to 18 mm). By the time of actual rupture of the follicles, they will have increased in size. Measurement of endometrial thickness by ultrasound is also used to determine the optimal time for administration of hCG. Pregnancy success rates are greatest when endometrial thickness is greater than 6 mm.

Human Chorionic Gonadotropin

❒ Human chorionic gonadotropin (hCG) A.P.L., CHOREX, CHORIGON, CHORON, CORGONJECT, FOLLUTEIN, GLUKOR, GONIC, PREGNYL)

Indications

In women whose cause of infertility is not primary ovarian failure, hCG is used in conjunction with hMG and FSH to stimulate ovulation. It is also used in combination with hMG to stimulate spermatogenesis in males who have primary or secondary hypogonadotropic hypogonadism.

Pharmacodynamics

hCG is a polypeptide hormone produced by the placenta and obtained from the urine of pregnant women. It is composed of alpha and beta subunits, with the alpha subunit being identical to that found in the gonadotropins FSH and LH. The beta subunits differ in their amino acid chain.

The action of hCG is identical to that of LH in that it stimulates the production of gonadal steroid hormones by inducing the production of androgen by the Leydig's cells of the testes and progesterone by the corpus luteum of the ovary. In this way, androgens in the male cause the development of secondary sex characteristics and testicular descent. Its use promotes the development of delayed secondary sex characteristics and, when it is given with hMG, stimulates spermatogenesis. In the female, FSH stimulation in the ovary causes maturation of the follicle, whereas the LH surge promotes ovulation. hCG can substitute for LH in this capacity.

Adverse Effects and Contraindications

Occasional headaches are reported, as well as fatigue, irritability, depression, pain at the injection site, and edema. Some investigators have suggested that owing to its profound effect on the ovaries, there is a higher incidence of OHSS in cycles during which hCG is used as the ovulation stimulant.

Contraindications are similar to those of hMG. Androgen secretion induced by hCG may cause fluid retention. It should be used with caution in patients with asthma, seizure disorders, migraines, and cardiac or renal problems. Safe use during pregnancy has not been established, and hCG may cause fetal toxicity.

Pharmacokinetics

hCG is destroyed in the GI tract and, therefore, is administered parenterally. Following IM injection, an increase in serum levels can be found within 2 hours. Peak concentrations occur in 6 hours and last for 36 to 72 hours. Serum levels begin to decline after 48 hours and are almost undetectable within 72 hours.

The distribution is mainly to the testes in males and to the ovaries in females. A small amount may also be found in the proximal tubules of the kidneys. Elimination is via the kidneys, with approximately 10 percent eliminated within the first 24 hours, whereas the remainder may be detected for up to 3 to 4 days.

Dosage Regimen

The dosage of hCG is dependent on the particular use and the individual patient. When it is used concomitantly with hMG and FSH, a single IM injection is administered 24 hours after the last dose of hMG or FSH is given. The dose of hCG recommended for ovulation induction is 5000 to 10,000 USP units. Ovulation is expected 24 to 40 hours later. Treatment regimens for the male patient are discussed in the section on hMG.

Laboratory Considerations

To avoid OHSS, hCG should not be given if estradiol levels are too high or follicle growth is excessive, particularly if the number of large follicles exceeds 5.

hCG may interfere with the results of radioimmunoassays for gonadotropins, especially LH. The laboratory should be informed of the therapy when levels are requested. Because hCG is the same hormone used to diagnose pregnancy, patients should be alerted that a false-positive test may result for up to 14 days after administration.

Follicle-Stimulating Hormone

❒ Follicle-stimulating hormone (urofollitropin, METRODIN)

Indications

Similar to hMG, clinical indications for the use of FSH include ovulatory dysfunction, luteal phase defects, idiopathic infertility, male factor infertility, and ART. Women in whom pregnancy is desired as soon as possible due to advanced maternal age are also considered candidates.

In women who have elevated LH levels, as in PCO, the additional LH found in hMG (which contains equal amounts of FSH and LH) may stimulate premature ovulation. Some studies have indicated that the use of purified forms of FSH may decrease this complication and consequently produce a higher pregnancy rate. Other studies indicate that FSH, when used in addition to hMG, enhances the pregnancy rate, especially for hyporesponders.

Pharmacodynamics

In women who do not have primary ovarian failure, FSH stimulates the maturation of a cohort of follicles by causing an elevation of the endogenous FSH level. Unlike menotropins, there is a less pronounced elevation of LH. In the normal menstrual cycle, as the follicular phase progresses, one follicle matures more rapidly and becomes the dominant follicle. When the FSH level begins to fall off during the mid- to late follicular phase, the less mature follicles begin to atrophy, whereas the dominant follicle continues to mature in spite of decreasing levels of FSH. When exogenous FSH is administered, the nondominant follicles receive the additional stimulation they need to continue to mature; thus, a larger cohort of mature follicles are recruited per ovulation cycle, increasing the fertilization potential.

Like hMG, FSH is extracted from the urine of postmenopausal women. In women who have demonstrated normal ovarian function, its follicle-stimulating effects override the single follicular development of the normal cycle. Unlike hMG, it lacks LH, and, therefore, only endogenous LH is present. If the endogenous LH level is insufficient to induce rupture of the follicles, treatment with hCG is usually required.

Adverse Effects and Contraindications

Adverse reactions to FSH are similar to those found with hMG use, the most prominent being OHSS. The course of action and teaching should be carried out the same as with hMG. Other adverse reactions occur infrequently and include ovarian cysts, ovarian enlargement, pelvic or abdominal discomfort, headache, pain or swelling at the injection site, and breast tenderness. As with all gonadotropins, the risk of multiple births is associated with FSH use.

FSH is contraindicated in women with primary ovarian failure, ovarian cysts, or enlargement unrelated to PCO; abnormal uterine bleeding; uncontrolled thyroid or adrenal dysfunction; or pituitary tumor.

Pharmacokinetics

Like other gonadotropins, FSH is only bioactive when it is given IM. Its half-life is about 2.9 hours. Biotransformation takes place in the proximal tubules of the kidneys and the hepatic reticuloendothelial system.

Dosage Regimen

The recommendation for initial dose of FSH is 75 IU/day IM for 7 to 12 days, followed by 5000 to 10,000 units of hCG 1 day after the last dose. The dosage may need to be individualized. The couple should be instructed to have daily coitus beginning the day before the dose of hCG is administered. When ultrasound measurement and estrogen levels indicate that adequate follicular growth is not achieved, treatment may continue after 12 days. If ovulation does not occur or ovulation occurs but does not result in pregnancy, this regimen may be repeated for two to three more cycles. If the treatment is still unsuccessful, some health care providers may increase the dose in subsequent cycles to 150 IU per day.

When FSH is used for in vitro fertilization, therapy is started on day 2 or 3 of the menstrual cycle. The dose is 150 mg/day until adequate follicular size is achieved but should not exceed 10 to 12 days. If the ovaries are enlarged on day 12, hCG is withheld in that cycle to avoid OHSS.

Laboratory Considerations

See discussion under hMG for information regarding monitoring follicular growth, endometrial thickness, and timing of administration of hCG.

Leuprolide Acetate

❒ Leuprolide acetate (LUPRON DEPO-PED, LUPRON, LUPRON DEPOT)

Indications

Leuprolide acetate is a GnRH agonist and is often used during ART to help control the secretion of endogenous LH and FSH. Use of leuprolide acetate is indicated in those patients with elevated baseline levels of these gonadotropins. In many reproductive practices, it is used routinely for improved control in ART cycles.

Depending on the desired effect, leuprolide can be used in short-term and long-term regimens. Short cycles are beginning to gain popularity as ovulation inducers, being used much the same way as hCG. Research is being conducted to determine the benefits to its use. Compared with ovulation induction with hMG and hCG, it is believed to cause fewer cases of OHSS.

Long-term regimens started on day 3, early in the follicular phase of the preceding cycle or on day 21, in the midluteal phase, are instituted when there is concern about controlling the maturation process of the follicles in ART. Premature luteinization can occur when the endogenous LH level interferes with the rate of follicle maturation. The use of leuprolide to suppress the endogenous hormone may help control the stimulation process.

Pharmacodynamics

Leuprolide has an affinity for pituitary GnRH receptor sites. Initially, it has a stimulating effect, causing a rise in the LH and FSH levels. With longer use, approximately 2 to 4 weeks, it has the opposite effect, causing a suppression of the secretion of gonadotropin-releasing hormone and, hence, decreased LH and FSH.

During ART, endogenous hormones may interfere with stimulation and maturation of the ovum. Excess FSH may influence follicular response, resulting in suboptimal follicular development and inadequate estrogen production. When LH levels are abnormally elevated, the exact moment of the LH surge and subsequent rupture of mature follicles becomes more difficult to predict. Because timing of ovum retrieval is crucial to the success of ART procedures, a premature LH surge can result in canceled cycles. Studies estimate that approximately 15 to 30 percent of ART cycles must be canceled owing to unsatisfactory response to hormonal stimulation. This contributes to the loss of precious time and financial resources. It is generally believed that the addition of GnRH agonist to the ART cycle assists with scheduling and decreases cancellation rates.

Adverse Effects and Contraindications

Hot flashes and sweats, as well as mild headache, may be caused by leuprolide. Irritation, pain, or reaction at the injection site may also occur.

Pharmacokinetics

Leuprolide is administered subcutaneously. The plasma half-life is approximately 3 hours. The biotransformation, distribution, and elimination is unknown.

Dosage Regimen

When started in the previous cycle, some health care providers teach patients to self-administer 1.0 mg subcutaneously per day. Then, when gonadotropin therapy is begun, the daily dose of leuprolide is decreased to 0.5 mg/day. For use in place of hCG, a single subcutaneous dose of 500 mcg of leuprolide has been given with a success rate similar to that of hCG.

Laboratory Considerations

When leuprolide is used to induce ovulation in place of hCG, it may be useful to monitor LH levels as well as estradiol. Again, ultrasound is also used to determine follicular growth and leuprolide is administered when two or more follicles have reached adequate size.

Gonadal function tests may be abnormal for up to 12 weeks following treatment. Elevated AST (SGOT), lactate dehydrogenase (LDH), alkaline phosphatase, triglyceride, low-density lipoprotein, and cholesterol levels may be found as well as decreased white cells and high-density lipoproteins.

Gonadorelin Acetate

❐ Gonadorelin acetate (GnRH, FACTREL, LUTREPULSE)

Indications

Gonadorelin acetate (GnRH) is useful in treating infertility caused by absent or dysfunctional secretion of endogenous GnRH from the hypothalamus. Women with hypothalamic amenorrhea who have a deficiency of endogenous GnRH are the best candidates for this type of treatment. Multiple pregnancy is also possible. Some women with PCO respond favorably to this treatment, but owing to their hypersensitivity, lower doses must be used and the advantages are not as great. Hyperprolactinemic patients who cannot tolerate bromocriptine have also been treated successfully with gonadorelin.

Pharmacodynamics

Endogenous GnRH is released in a pulsatile fashion from the hypothalamus in order to properly stimulate the release of gonadotropins from the pituitary. The frequency and amplitude of the pulses are critical to the stimulatory effects of GnRH. Before this knowledge, single-dose injections of gonadorelin were effective for the first 2 to 4 weeks of therapy, elevating the plasma level of gonadotropins. At that point, however, gonadorelin began to desensitize the receptor sites on the pituitary and suppressed the secretions of gonadotropins.

Pulsatile administration of synthetic gonadorelin binds to pituitary receptor sites and simulates the natural secretion pattern, stimulating FSH and LH secretion. In turn, the natural sequence of maturation of one follicle and ovulation occurs.

Adverse Effects and Contraindications

One of the advantages to gonadorelin treatment is a decreased incidence of OHSS. Although this is still a precaution and monitoring of ovarian stimulation is necessary, there have been fewer reported cases than in women treated with hMG. Local infection at the site of injection is also a problem. Use of the subcutaneous route may eliminate this problem. Gonadorelin should not be administered in conjunction with ovulation stimulators.

Pharmacokinetics

Gonadorelin is poorly absorbed by the GI tract and, therefore, must be administered subcutaneously or intravenously. It is supplied for use in the LUTREPULSE pump to be given continuously over 24 hours in preprogrammed doses at a set frequency. It is widely distributed in the extracellular space and has a half-life of about 2 to 8 minutes (see Table 56–2). It is mainly biotransformed and eliminated by the kidneys. Some individuals with prolonged hypogonadism may be resistant to initial treatment and require priming with gonadorelin for several days before they respond with increased gonadotropin levels.

Dosage Regimen

Gonadorelin is formulated as a hydrochloride (FACTREL) or acetate (LUTREPULSE). The dosage of the hydrochloride formulation is 100 mcg subcutaneously or intravenously. The acetate formulation is administered via the LUTREPULSE pump. A 5-mcg dose is given every 90 minutes in doses from 1 to 20 mg. Observation of the ovaries by ultrasound and estradiol levels is initiated after about 4 days and repeated every 3 to 4 days. The patient requires between 10 and 20 days of therapy for ovulation to occur. Some health care providers continue treatment for 2 more weeks to maintain the corpus luteum. Others add hCG or progesterone for luteal phase support. For gonadorelin-resistant patients, priming with repeated doses for several days may be required.

Laboratory Considerations

As with all ovulation inducers, it is necessary to monitor the development of the follicle. Ultrasound and regular assessment of estradiol levels, as well as cervical mucus evaluation, are commonly used. Although it is less common, close observation for OHSS is advised.

Testosterone

❒ Testosterone

Testosterone is used mainly for replacement of endogenous hormone when there is deficient endocrine function of the testes (see Chapter 52). Because the therapeutic efficacy of testosterone use in the infertile male has not been established, the risks associated with synthetic androgens may outweigh the benefits. Permanent azoospermia can result with high doses when the drug is used to induce rebound increases in sperm count. Misuse of androgens by athletes and body builders has occurred due to their anabolic and androgenic effects. Nonmedical use is believed to be common.

Adverse reactions to testosterone include acne, flushing, gynecomastia, habituation, changes in libido, and edema. IM testosterone may cause local irritation and the rate of absorption to vary. With prolonged therapy, or in excessive doses, oligospermia and decreased ejaculatory volume may occur. Case reports suggest that adverse effects include increased aggression, antisocial behavior, and psychotic manifestations. There is a long list of potential physical damage to heart, liver, and bone formation, as well as other associated adverse effects, making testosterone a potentially dangerous drug.

ADJUNCTIVE AND EXPERIMENTAL DRUGS USED TO TREAT INFERTILITY

Approximately 25 percent of male infertility is due to unknown causes. Various treatment regimens have produced somewhat inconclusive results and often prove to be very expensive. Tamoxifen citrate is an oral antiestrogen that has been used in the treatment of idiopathic male infertility. It is structurally similar to clomiphene citrate and has also been used to stimulate ovulation. The precise mechanism of action is not known. Antiestrogens are thought to block estrogen receptors in the hypothalamus, resulting in a decrease in the inhibition of GnRH. This allows an increase in the GnRH with a subsequent increase in the secretion of LH and FSH. Elevated gonadotropins stimulate the production of testosterone in the testes, leading to enhanced spermatogenesis. Tamoxifen may be used in conjunction with clomiphene citrate. The course of treatment should be at least 3 months, which is the length of one spermatogenic cycle.

Testolactone is an antineoplastic agent with antiestrogenic effects. It prevents the conversion of androgens to estrogens. When testolactone is used with GnRH in men with hypothalamic GnRH deficiency, it enhances the release of LH and FSH and stimulates testicular maturation and spermatogenesis.

Men with high sperm antibody titers may benefit from treatment with immunosuppressive therapy. The most common drugs of choice are glucocorticoids, but evidence of their efficacy is inconclusive. Treatment for antisperm antibodies may be more successful if intrauterine insemination procedures are employed. Patients with elevated circulating androgens and hirsutism are hyporesponders to ovulation inducers. Dexamethasone inhibits corticotropin release and decreases adrenal androgen level in the ovarian follicle. It is given in oral doses of 0.5 to 0.75 mg every evening and is continued until pregnancy is achieved.

Dexamethasone is also being used as an adjunct for treatment in women with high circulating androgen levels. Excess androgens cause elevated LH and FSH levels, which interfere with normal gonadotropin feedback mechanisms. A complete medical workup for evaluation of symptoms associated with increased androgens, such as hirsutism, oily skin or acne, weight gain, and irregular menses should be performed. The usual dose of dexamethasone is 0.5 to 0.75 mg po at bedtime. It may be used with clomiphene, hMG, or FSH during induction of ovulation.

Progesterone is used for luteal phase support in patients with luteal phase defects. Supplemental progesterone enhances endometrial development. Progesterone is usually given as vaginal suppositories in 25-mg doses twice daily, 50-mg doses every evening, or 100-mg capsules three times daily.

Critical Thinking Process

Assessment

Assessment of the couple desiring treatment for infertility requires a thorough assessment of both the female and the male partner. A primary assessment, including a comprehensive history and physical exam should be performed before an expensive, time-consuming, and emotionally arduous investigation is initiated.

History of Present Illness

Pretreatment assessment is essential before starting treatment for infertility and should include a thorough history that will identify potential medical or drug-induced causes. Patients usually report an inability to conceive after an extended period of time of unprotected sexual relations. In other cases, an inability to carry a fetus to term is the chief complaint. A thorough sexual history is obtained from both partners, and it is essential to begin formation of a database. The sexual history should include information on the frequency as well as the timing of coitus and the use of drugs that may decrease fertility. The use of lubricants, positions used, and douching practices should also be noted.

The health care provider should elicit information regarding the male partner's history of groin injury, mumps after adolescence, and acute viral illnesses in the past 3 months. A surgical history should be noted, including hernia repair, vasectomy, reversal of a vasectomy, or varicocele repair.

Past Health History

The female patient's database should include a complete reproductive and menstrual history, including specific information related to premenstrual syndrome, mittelschmerz (midcycle ovulation pain), dysmenorrhea, amenorrhea, or intermenstrual spotting. History of pelvic disease, ovarian cysts, endometriosis, hormone-dependent tumors, sexually transmitted diseases (STDs), and pelvic inflammatory disease (PID) should be noted. Prior radiation exposure or diethylstilbestrol, the use of contraceptives, and a history of the patient's smoking and alcohol use should be noted. The use of contraceptive measures in the past (type, duration, and complications of use) and when they were used should be elicited.

Exposure to potentially toxic substances, sitting for extended hours, strenuous exercise, and the use of hot baths after exercise should be noted, particularly in the case of the male partner. Further, a genetic history, history of birth defects, and reproductive problems in family members should be included in the database.

Physical Exam Findings

The infertile female should have a baseline pelvic exam. Attention should be paid to the size, shape, position, and mobility of the uterus; the presence of congenital anomalies; and endometriosis. Evaluation of the adnexa, ovary size, fixations, and tumors should be noted. A rectovaginal exam should be performed noting the presence of retroflexed or retroverted uterus, or a rectouterine pouch mass.

The male exam should note the presence or absence of phimosis, location of the urethral meatus, and size and consistency of each testis, vas deferens, and epididymis. The presence of a varicocele should be noted. The rectal exam is used to identify the size and consistency of the seminal vesicles and prostate, with microscopic evaluation of prostatic fluid used to gather evidence of infection.

Vital signs including blood pressure, temperature, height, and weight should be noted in both partners. The female patient should also be examined for evidence of thyroid dysfunction (e.g., exophthalmos, lid lag, tremor, palpable gland).

Diagnostic Testing

All patients with infertility problems need a thorough workup prior to pharmacotherapy. Basal body temperature charts are used to assess for biphasic elevations and evidence of ovulation. A semen analysis is also performed during early diagnostic testing. Routine lab tests include LH, FSH, and estradiol levels; thyroid studies (T_3, T_4, T_7, and TSH); and prolactin levels. Other evaluation methods include cervical mucus studies, hysterosalpingogram, laparoscopy, laparotomy, endometrial biopsy, and postcoital semen analysis. For the male partner, assessment includes an evaluation of endocrine functioning and semen analysis.

Developmental Considerations

For many couples, treatment for infertility represents a final chance to have biologic children before resorting to adoption. A waiting period of up to 7 years is not uncommon for couples attempting to adopt a child. Couples who choose to remain childless need as much support for their decision as does the couple who chooses to accept fertility treatment. Answers to questions that address the couple's self-image, guilt and blame, and sexuality are important data to obtain.

Psychosocial Considerations

Fertility treatment is often complicated, expensive, and emotionally as well as physically draining. Receiving the diagnosis of infertility is often a life-altering event. Patients may demonstrate an array of reactions ranging from denial to anger and grief. They may experience repercussions, such as low self-esteem, marital discord, divorce, and parenting difficulties when the treatment is successful. Ethical and religious issues often further complicate the course of treatment. Counseling, referrals, and individualized support as well as follow up are important aspects of the care provided by the fertility specialists and perinatal team.

When a multiple pregnancy is the outcome of treatment for infertility, the cost of prolonged hospital bedrest is enormous. When the multiple pregnancy culminates in premature delivery, with the potential for a neonatal demise, the daily costs increase exponentially.

Pharmacotherapeutic treatment of infertility is a very costly endeavor with relatively few guarantees of success. Routine laboratory and ultrasound monitoring before and during treatment need to be considered, as do other diagnostic tests and procedures. The cost throughout the rest of the pregnancy are variable and highly unpredictable.

Clomiphene citrate is usually the first drug used in patients requiring ovulation induction. It is relatively inexpensive and requires fewer office visits and interventions when compared with other drugs used for this purpose.

hMG is significantly more expensive than clomiphene citrate. An ampule is estimated to cost approximately $45, and, therefore, the cost of treatment can run up to $1000 for one cycle of the medication alone. FSH is as expensive as hMG. The average cost of one dose of hCG is approximately $50. Leuprolide and progesterone, commonly used adjuvant treatments, add to the expense. Their use requires consider-

Case Study Infertility

Patient History

History of Present Illness	DJ is a 35-year-old nullipara who complains of failure to become pregnant after 5 years of unprotected intercourse. She visits today, accompanied by partner, for follow up and treatment of infertility secondary to obstructive pathology.
Past Health History	DJ's history is benign for contributing factors to infertility. Her menses started at age 12 with 28–29 day cycles, lasting 4–5 days. She reports no unusual discomfort, bleeding, or symptoms of PMS. History is negative for STDs and PID. No family history of infertility. Mother had four spontaneous term pregnancies without complications.
Physical Exam	VSS. Height: 5′7″. Weight: 130 lbs. Manual exam reveals slightly retroverted uterus with ovaries of normal size and location. Speculum exam reveals nulliparous cervix with no unusual findings. Remainder of physical unremarkable.
Diagnostic Testing	LH, FSH, estradiol, thyroid function studies, prolactin levels, cervical mucus, hysterosalpingogram, and laparoscopy are WNL.
Developmental Considerations	DJ is considered to be of advanced maternal age. In light of diagnosis is immediate candidate for ART. Possibility of multiple embryo development would satisfy the couple's desire for family in one pregnancy.
Psychosocial Considerations	DJ and partner have experienced a wide range of emotions from denial to anger and grief. They have experienced low self-esteem and marital discord for a time. Counseling provided needed support while waiting for diagnosis. Relationship now stable and supportive. Couple willing and capable of doing whatever is necessary for DJ to conceive, including IVF.
Economic Factors	DJ and partner are gainfully employed and have financial stability and a large savings account from which they can draw funds if required to pay for one cycle of ovulation induction (approximately $10,000) and IVF procedure. Cost of laboratory and ultrasound monitoring covered by health insurance.

Variables Influencing Decision

Treatment Objectives	• Foster follicle stimulation for ART. • Achieve and maintain pregnancy.

Drug Variables	*Drug Summary*	*Patient Variables*
Indications	Leuprolide, FSH, hCG support luteal phase and maintain pregnancy through its first trimester.	DJ diagnosed with infertility secondary to obstructive pathology.
Pharmacodynamics	Leuprolide to suppress endogenous LH and FSH to control stimulation process better. Will induce maturation of multiple follicles. hCG will cause LH surge, leading to final maturation of ova so eggs can be retrieved for IVF.	DJ and husband aware of potential for multiple pregnancies which are acceptable to them. This is not a decision point.
Adverse Effects/ Contraindications	Caution must be used to avoid OHSS.	Couple knowledgeable of risk factors and adverse effects of ART.
Pharmacokinetics	Varies with individual drug and patient. This will not become a decision point.	DJ's medical history negative for renal or hepatic disorders that would affect pharmacokinetics of drugs.

Case Study continued on following page

Drug Variables	Drug Summary	Patient Variables
Dosage Regimen	Fertility treatment regimens complicated. Regimens require close attention by couple. This will become a decision point.	Couple motivated and capable of compliance with complicated drug regimen. This will not become a decision point.
Laboratory Considerations	Thyroid and lipid panel, pregnancy test before treatment.	Pregnancy test negative.
Cost Index*	Leuprolide acetate: 5 hCG: 5 FSH: 5	Financially secure couple willing to absorb cost of treatment. This will not be a decision point.

Summary of Decision Points

- Couple knowledgeable of risk factors and adverse effects of ART.
- Complicated dosage regimen requiring close attention by couple.
- Expensive treatment regimen but financially secure couple willing to absorb cost of treatment.

DRUGS TO BE USED

- Step 1: Leuprolide acetate 0.5 mg SC BID initially, to start in midluteal phase of prevous cycle until FSH started, then single 0.5 mg doses SC daily.
- Step 2: Follicle-stimulating hormone 150 IU IM QD for 7–12 days to start on day 3 of cycle.
- Step 3: Human chorionic gonadotropin (hCG) 10,000 units IM 24 hours after last dose of leuprolide acetate and FSH.

*Cost Index:
1 = $ < 30/mo.
2 = $ 30–40/mo.
3 = $ 40–50/mo.
4 = $ 50–60/mo.
5 = $ > 60/mo.

AWP of a 2-week supply of 5-mg/mL leuprolide acetate kit is approximately $300.
AWP of 10,000 units/dose human chorionic gonadotropin powder for injection with diluent is approximately $32.
AWP of 150 IU of follicle-stimulating hormone is approximately $48.

ation of the motivation and willingness of the participants in this type of intervention.

Before beginning the treatments, the couple must be made fully aware of the costs, the amounts they can expect to be reimbursed by their insurance if they are covered, and the expense that can be incurred if complications ensue. In other words they need to understand the economic implications of multiple birth. Hospitalization costs for the antepartum woman and the potential cost of multiple premature infants can be devastating. (see Case Study—Infertility).

Analysis and Management

Treatment Objectives

The general objective in the treatment of infertility is to determine the cause of the infertility and to correct, if possible, endocrinopathies, infections, anatomic aberrations, and hormonal imbalances or deficiencies. The use of ART is very common in the field of infertility.

The goal of pregnancy, with minimal adverse reactions, takes skill and timing to achieve. Studies have shown that up to 90 percent of patients taking hMG ovulate, whereas 50 to 70 percent will achieve pregnancy after an average of three treatment cycles. Some have noted improved cervical mucus with hMG that may be therapeutic in itself, making coitus more natural and efficient. Multiple pregnancy rates range from 10 to 30 percent and mostly result in twins, with five percent of the pregnancies resulting in three or more fetuses. The spontaneous abortion rate is 20 to 25 percent, which is slightly higher than the general norm (see Controversy—The Ethics of Using Fertility Drugs).

Treatment Options

Drug Variables

Although clomiphene is a first-line agent, in the case of an anatomic abnormality such as nonpatent fallopian tubes, ovulation induction followed by coitus and normal fertilization, conception, and implantation is not an option. In this case, the health care provider moves straight to ART with drugs such as hMG, FSH, and hCG. The particular regimen is largely based on the preference of the health care provider.

Controversy

The Ethics of Using Fertility Drugs
JONATHAN J. WOLFE

Reproductive health presents the thorniest moral questions faced by health care providers. The topic of promoting fertility by drug administration may produce less ardent political arguments than does abortion, but it contains clear conflicts and difficult choices.

Couples who want children but cannot conceive them experience a unique type of emotional suffering. They live in a world where abortion is easily available, the adoption process is difficult and lengthy, and abuse of children is the fodder of daily news. Every new tale of child abuse appears an affront to justice, particularly to couples who find a bitter sting in their continued infertility. Surely one can argue that they deserve relief.

Other participants in the area of fertility promotion may hold complementary if differing viewpoints. The issue of justice is easy to assert. However, how many pregnancies come to disaster because prenatal care is lacking? How much prenatal care could be purchased for the price of a single in vitro fertilization or artificial insemination? Do numbers win out, or does the claim of the individual person?

The hazard of fertility treatments also demands a hearing. Preparation for harvesting ova requires painful and lengthy hormonal treatment. Aside from cost and short-term adverse effects, are long-term health effects also possible? The use of ovulation-stimulating drugs can produce showers of ova, contributing to multiple births that may be complicated by prematurity. Do parents have the right to demand neonatal intensive care for quadruplets in order to overcome infertility? Is it ethical to advocate abortion for some fetuses in a multiple pregnancy in order to improve the odds for one or two others? The entire issue of fertility treatment remains morally unacceptable when one's beliefs forbid any intervention in conception.

Critical Thinking Discussion

- What alternatives should be available to a couple who cannot conceive children?
- What increases in insurance premiums in your own plan are acceptable to ensure that all infertile participants have access to fertility treatment?
- Does a single woman who desires to bear children have the same right to treatment of infertility as a married couple?
- Is surrogacy a proper resource for an infertile couple when the woman cannot carry a pregnancy to successful termination?
- What considerations would you have a patient reflect on before consenting to infertility treatment?

Different providers routinely use drugs they are most familiar with and in which they have the most confidence to bring about the best results.

Patient Variables

Compliance with the complex regimen of fertility treatment requires a firm understanding of the plan of care, with attention to timing of drug administration and coital activities. An understanding of the couple's relationship and commitment to a treatment regimen is vital to treatment success.

Intervention

Administration

Clomiphene citrate should be taken exactly as directed at the same time each day. Missed doses should be taken as soon as they are remembered. The dose should be doubled if it is not remembered until the next dose is due. The health care provider should be notified if more than one dose is missed.

hCG is destroyed in the GI tract, necessitating a painful IM injection. The IM formulation requires reconstitution using normal saline provided by the manufacturer. Steps should be taken to relieve the discomfort of the IM injection as much as possible. The reconstituted drug is stable for 90 days when it is refrigerated.

Leuprolide acetate is only for IM injection. The patient should be instructed to store the drug at room temperature. When hMG is used, the reconstituted formulation should be used immediately and any unused portion discarded.

Education

When treatment is initiated, the couple should be taught to self-administer the subcutaneous injections. Information on aseptic technique and what to watch for infection at the injection site should be included. Warnings about the importance of compliance should be provided. The patient should be instructed to report signs and symptoms of ovarian hyperstimulation to the health care provider as soon as possible. The correct procedure for monitoring basal body temperature should be included in the teaching. The importance of follow-up meetings with the health care provider should be emphasized.

Evaluation

The effectiveness of bromocriptine therapy can be demonstrated by the resumption of normal ovulatory menstrual cycles and restoration of fertility. Clomiphene citrate effectiveness is demonstrated by the occurrence of ovulation, as measured by estrogen elimination, biphasic body temperature elevations, and endometrial histologic changes. If conception is not achieved after three to four treatment cycles, the original diagnosis should be re-evaluated.

hMG effectiveness is evaluated by the maturation of follicles. hMG therapy is followed by hCG, which, in turn, should lead to ovulation. If ovulation does not occur after three to six menstrual cycles, therapy may be discontinued. For the male, effectiveness is evident by increased spermatogenesis after 4 months of therapy. Treatment effectiveness of hCG can be noted by an increase in spermatogenesis in males.

Although the couple may believe that the only successful outcome of treatment is a pregnancy, that outcome cannot and should not be guaranteed. However, when pregnancy has been detected and the embryonic sac and heart rate can be detected by ultrasound, treatment with fertility drugs is considered successful.

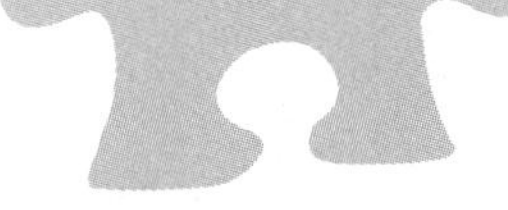

SUMMARY

- In the United States, there are an estimated 1 to 2 million couples of child-bearing age who are unsuccessful in their attempts to conceive.

- Infertility is defined as an inability to conceive after 1 year of unprotected coitus or an inability to carry a fetus to term.
- Alterations in the HPO axis are responsible for a large proportion of female infertility.
- Female fertility disorders include problems related to follicular maturation, ovulation, pituitary disorders, luteal phase defects, and uterine, tubal, and pelvic disorders.
- Male fertility problems include a variety of dysfunctions that can be classified as pretesticular, testicular, and post-testicular disorders.
- Assessment of the couple desiring treatment for infertility requires a thorough assessment of both the female and male partner.
- A primary assessment, including a comprehensive history and physical exam should be performed before an expensive, time-consuming, and emotionally arduous investigation is initiated.
- The primary objectives in the treatment of infertility are induction of ovulation, the control of interference with hormonal response, and the restoration of spermatogenesis.
- Drug therapy can modify the HPO axis that controls GnRH, FSH, and LH secretion.
- Drug options include bromocriptine, clomiphene citrate, FSH, GnRH, hCG, leuprolide acetate, menotropins, and urofollitropin.
- Treatment regimens often use a combination of drugs, and, therefore, therapy should be carried out by a specialist in infertility.
- The patient should be referred to specialists and support groups as needed (i.e., an endocrinologist, a urogenital surgeon, infertile family support groups).
- Special attention should be paid to patient teaching regarding self-administration of drugs, complications, adverse effects, and the importance of follow up.
- Treatment regimens require that the couple be highly educated about the drug therapy, appropriate timing of drug therapy in relation to coitus, and the importance of follow-up monitoring.
- The couple should be supported around decisions to remain childless or to proceed with adoption.
- When pregnancy has been detected and the embryonic sac and heart rate can be detected by ultrasound, treatment with fertility drugs is considered successful.
- Although the couple may believe that the only successful outcome of treatment is a pregnancy, that outcome cannot and should not be guaranteed.

BIBLIOGRAPHY

Bernstein, J., Potts, N., and Mattor, J. (1985). Assessment of psychological dysfunction associated with infertility. *Journal of Obstetric, Gynecologic, and Neonatal Nursing,* 14(6 Suppl), 63S–66S.

Blenner, J. (1990). Attaining self-care in infertility treatment. *Applied Nursing Research,* 3(3), 98–104.

Castelbaum, A., and Lessey, B. (1995). Insights into the evaluation of the luteal phase. *Infertility and Reproductive Medicine Clinics of North America,* 6(1), 199–213.

Dobbs, K., Dumesic, D., Dumesic, J., et al. (1994). Differences in serum follicle-stimulating hormone uptake after intramuscular and subcutaneous human menopausal gonadotropin injection. *Fertility and Sterility,* 62(5), 978–983.

Fanchin, R., de Zeigler, D., Castracane, V., et al. (1995). Physiopathology of premature progesterone elevation. *Fertility and Sterility,* 64(4), 796–801.

Filicori, M., Flamigni, C., Cognigni, G., et al. (1996). Different gonadotropin and leuprorelin ovulation induction regimens markedly affect follicular fluid hormone levels and folliculogenesis. *Fertility and Sterility,* 65(2), 387–393.

Garner, C. (1991). *Principles of infertility nursing.* Boca Raton, FL: CRC Press.

Gerris, J., De Vits, A., Joostens, M., et al. (1995). Triggering of ovulation in human menopausal gonadotrophin-stimulated cycles: Comparison between intravenously administered gonadotrophin-releasing hormone (100 and 500 μg), GnRH agonist (buserelin, 500 μg) and human chorionic gonadotropin (10,000 IU). *Human Reproduction,* 10(1), 56–62.

Gilman, A., Rall, T., and Nies, A. (1990). *Goodman and Gilman's The pharmacological basis of therapeutics* (8th ed.). New York: Pergamon Press.

Ginsburg, K., Yeko, T., Heiner, J., et al. (1995). Adjunctive agents in ovulation induction. *American Journal of Obstetrics and Gynecology,* 172(2), 782–785.

Greenblatt, E., Meriano, J., and Casper, R. (1995). Type of stimulation protocol affects oocyte maturity, fertilization rate, and cleavage rate after intracytoplasmic sperm injection. *Fertility and Sterility,* 64(3), 557–563.

Isaacs, J., Wells, C., Williams, D., et al. (1996). Endometrial thickness is a valid monitoring parameter in cycles of ovulation induction with menotropins alone. *Fertility and Sterility,* 65(2), 262–266.

Jinno, M., Ubukata, Y., Satou, M., et al. (1996). An improvement in the embryo quality and pregnancy rate by the pulsatile administration of human menopausal gonadotropin in patients with previous unsuccessful in vitro fertilization attempts. *Fertility and Sterility,* 65(2), 382–386.

Lobo, R. (1993). Unexplained infertility. *Journal of Reproductive Medicine,* 38(4), 241–249.

Lolis, D., Tsolas, O., and Messinis, I. (1995). The follicle-stimulating hormone threshold level for follicle maturation in superovulated cycles. *Fertility and Sterility,* 63(6), 1272–1277.

Neumann, P., Gharib, S., and Weinstein, M. (1994). The cost of a successful delivery with in-vitro fertilization. *The New England Journal of Medicine,* 331(4), 239–243.

O'Shea, D., Kettel, M., Isaacs, J., et al. (1995). Ovulation induction in the poor responder or hyperresponder. *American Journal of Obstetrics and Gynecology,* 172(2), 788–791.

Olive, D. (1995). The role of gonadotropins in ovulation induction. *American Journal of Obstetrics and Gynecology,* 172(2), 759–765.

Paulson, R. (1993). In-vitro fertilization and other assisted reproductive techniques. *Journal of Reproduction Medicine,* 38(4), 261–268.

Remohi, J., Gutierrez, A., Vidal, A., et al. (1994). The use of gonadotrophin-releasing hormone analogues in women receiving oocyte donation does not affect implantation rates. *Human Reproduction,* 9(9), 1761–1764.

San Roman, G., Long, C., Reshef, E., et al. (1995). Monitoring the ovulation induction cycle. *American Journal of Obstetrics and Gynecology,* 172(2), 785–787.

Schlaff, W., Yazigi, R., Olive, D., et al. (1995). The empiric use of gonadotropin therapy and intrauterine insemination. *American Journal of Obstetrics and Gynecology,* 172(2), 778–781.

Scott, R., Bailey, S., Kost, E., et al. (1994). Comparison of leuprolide acetate and human chorionic gonadotropin for the induction of ovulation in clomiphene citrate-stimulated cycles. *Fertility and Sterility,* 61(5), 872–879.

Scott, R., Leonardi, G., Hofmann, G., et al. (1993). A prospective evaluation of clomiphene citrate challenge test screening of the general population. *Obstetrics and Gynecology,* 82(4), 539–544.

Sengoku, K., Tamate, K., Takaoka, Y., et al. (1994). A randomized prospective study of gonadotrophin with or without gonadotrophin-releasing hormone agonist for treatment of unexplained infertility. *Human Reproduction,* 9(6), 1043–1047.

Seppala, M., and Hamberger, L. (1991). *Frontiers in human reproduction.* New York: The New York Academy of Science.

Shoham, Z., Zosmer, A., and Insler, V. (1991). Early miscarriage and fetal malformations after induction of ovulation (by clomiphene citrate and/or human menotropins), in-vitro fertilization, and gamete intrafallopian transfer. *Fertility and Sterility,* 55(1), 1–11.

Strickler, R., Radwanska, E., and Williams, D. (1995). Controlled ovarian hyperstimulation regimens in assisted reproductive technologies. *American Journal of Obstetrics and Gynecology,* 172(2), 766–772.

Toback, B. (1992). Recent advances in female infertility care. *NAACOG's Clinical Issues,* 3(2), 313–319.

Wysowski, D. (1993). Use of fertility drugs in the United States, 1973 through 1991. *Fertility and Sterility,* 60(6), 1096–1098.

Yen, S., and Jaffe, R. (1986). *Reproductive endocrinology, physiology, pathophysiology, and clinical management* (2nd ed.). Philadelphia: W. B. Saunders.

Youngkin, E. (1994). *Women's health: A primary care clinical guide.* East Norwalk, CT: Appleton and Lange.

Drugs Influencing Nutritional Balance

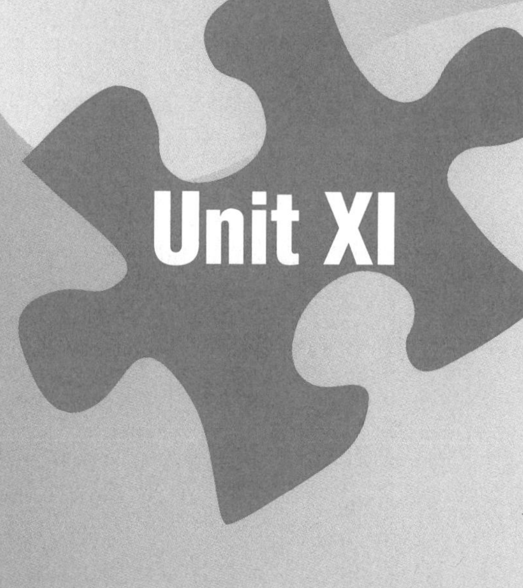

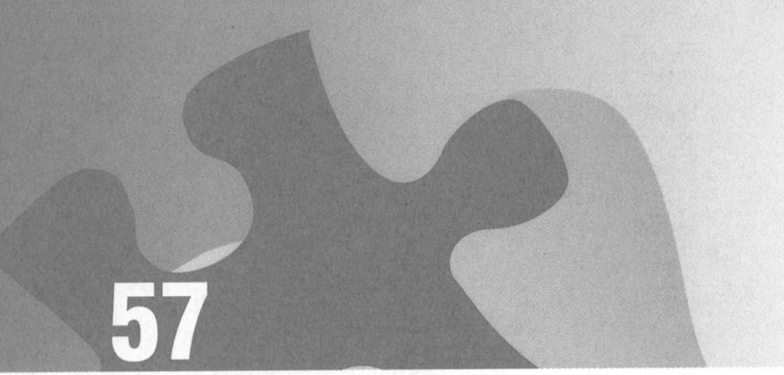

57 Intravenous Therapy

Intravenous (IV) therapy is used extensively today to maintain fluid and electrolyte balance as well as for nutritional support, the infusion of blood and blood components, and drug administration. Although the technology and expertise needed to deliver IV therapy has evolved over five centuries, the major breakthroughs occurred during the 20th century. Between 1900 and 1930, the discovery of pyrogens, blood groups, antigens, and components necessary for nutritional support led to more extensive and successful treatment modalities. Technologic improvements included more effective sterilization procedures, flexible plastic peripheral and central catheters, implantable ports, blood preservatives, and recovery procedures. Parenteral nutrition and fat emulsion therapy were also important to improved patient care.

The purpose of this chapter is to discuss the role of IV therapy in relation to the biochemical processes that ensure a continuous state of equilibrium within the body. Optimal IV therapy requires an understanding of basic physiologic needs for fluids, electrolytes, acid-base balance, and nutrients within the body, as well as the pathophysiology of imbalances. The role played by the homeostatic organs in the body must also be considered when delivering IV fluids. Frequently, if the cause of the imbalance can be identified and reversed through early aggressive intervention, the need for long-term therapy can be avoided.

PHYSIOLOGY AND PATHOPHYSIOLOGY

All body systems are dependent on fluids, electrolytes, acid-base balance, and nutrients for maintenance of a healthy state. Homeostasis is maintained primarily through fluid intake and output, the distribution of fluids and electrolytes, intake and utilization of daily nutrient requirements, and regulation of renal, cardiovascular, pulmonary, and endocrine systems. Deficiencies in any of the mechanisms results in imbalances affecting the entire body.

Homeostatic requirements are easily met by a healthy adult. However, in the presence of acute or chronic illness, age extremes in either direction, altered mental status, or immobility, it may be impossible for a person to maintain a state of equilibrium. The results may be an imbalance in the form of excesses or deficits in fluids, electrolytes, acid-base components, or nutrients. When equilibrium is no longer present, the resulting imbalances may be life threatening.

Origins of Imbalance

Fluids

Body fluids function in the maintenance of blood volume, transportation of substances to and from cells, regulation of temperature, provision for a medium for cellular metabolism, removal of waste by-products from the body, and performance of hydrolysis for digestive purposes. In a healthy adult, approximately 60 percent of the total body weight is made up of fluids and electrolytes. The amount and distribution varies with body fat, age, and gender. Fat tissue has less fluid content than lean tissue, resulting in a lower percentage of body water in obese adults. As adult weight increases, the proportion of water weight decreases.

Body fluids are distributed into two distinct compartments. The intracellular fluid (ICF) compartment accounts for approximately 40 percent of adult weight (average adult weighs 70 kg). The extracellular fluid (ECF) compartment accounts for another 20 percent of the weight. The extracellular volume is primarily made up of plasma in the vascular system and interstitial fluid occupying the space between cells in tissues. Plasma is responsible for approximately 5 percent of the total body weight, while the interstitial fluid accounts for the other 15 percent. The fluid that occupies the pleural, peritoneal, subarachnoid, gastric, and synovial spaces is also ECF.

These compartments constantly exchange contents. Four mechanisms move particles through cell membranes and from the intravascular space to the interstitial space. Osmosis, diffusion, and filtration are passive processes, in contrast to the active transport that occurs when ions move from an area of low concentration to an area of higher concentration. Active transport requires energy in the form of adenosine triphosphate (ATP) for ion transport to occur. ATP is released by the cell and provides the energy necessary for substances to pass through cell membranes. The movement of sodium from the ICF to the ECF uses the sodium-potassium pump and is an example of active transport.

Electrolytes

Electrolytes are elements or compounds that dissociate in water or other solvents and whose concentrations are expressed in milliequivalents per liter (mEq/L). Ions characteristically have the ability to conduct electrical current and to actively unite as well as to dissolve in fluids. They are either positively charged (cations) or negatively charged (anions). The major electrolytes found in the body include the cations sodium, potassium, calcium, and magnesium. The anions include chloride, phosphate, bicarbonate, and sulfate. Each fluid compartment in the body contains electrolytes in varying concentrations. Alterations in the normal concentration of electrolytes result in serious, if not life-threatening, complications for the patient.

Acid-Base Balance

Acid-base balance within the body requires maintenance of arterial pH within the narrow range of 7.35 to 7.45. The pH reflects actual hydrogen ion concentration of the blood. There is an inverse relationship between hydrogen ions and pH. As hydrogen ion concentration goes up or down, the pH moves in the opposite direction. High concentrations of hydrogen ions result in a low pH (acid), whereas a decrease in hydrogen ions results in an elevated pH (alkaline). Any arterial pH below 6.80 or above 7.80 is incompatible with life.

Acid-base balance is dependent on a balanced relationship between acids that give up hydrogen ions and buffers that accept ions. Acids are constantly produced through metabolic processes. The normal ratio of acid to base necessary to maintain a neutral pH is one part acid (mainly carbonic acid) to 20 parts base (mainly bicarbonate) (Fig. 57–1). Bicarbonate is the buffer that takes on hydrogen ions, preventing the concentration from increasing.

The normal pH of blood is maintained by buffering systems, as well as by the lungs and the kidneys. The primary buffering system is the bicarbonate-carbonic acid system. Phosphates and proteins also buffer, assisting in the maintenance of a neutral pH. These mechanisms are responsible for most of the hydrogen ion buffering that occurs in the body.

Homeostatic Organs

The major organs involved in fluid and electrolyte balance include the heart and blood vessels, kidneys, lungs, hypothalamus, endocrine glands (adrenal, parathyroids, and pituitary glands), and gastrointestinal (GI) tract. Each of these organs plays a significant role in maintaining the delicate balance of fluids and solutes within the body.

Heart and Blood Vessels

Renal perfusion is essential for homeostasis and is dependent on receiving at least 25 percent of the normal cardiac output. The cardiovascular system maintains renal perfusion through cardiac output, coupled with total peripheral resistance. These two mechanisms provide the kidney with the necessary blood flow to maintain a normal glomerular filtration rate. When the cardiac output or systemic resistance is diminished, renal function is impaired and alterations in homeostasis result.

Kidneys

The kidneys' role in fluid, electrolyte, and nonelectrolyte balance is fundamental to homeostasis. The kidneys perform critical functions, including

- Selective elimination and reabsorption
- Production of bicarbonate ions
- Elimination of foreign substances, chemical wastes, and metabolic by-products
- Secretion of renin for maintenance of blood pressure and extracellular volume
- Promotion of calcium absorption through the activation of vitamin D
- Production of erythropoietin to stimulate red blood cell production

Renal insufficiency (see Chapter 41) results in imbalances affecting virtually all of the electrolytes, as well as fluids, pH, and other parameters.

Lungs

The lungs help maintain acid-base balance through regulation of oxygen and carbon dioxide levels in the blood. Tachypnea increases the elimination of carbon dioxide, resulting in an alkalotic state. Conversely, retention of carbon

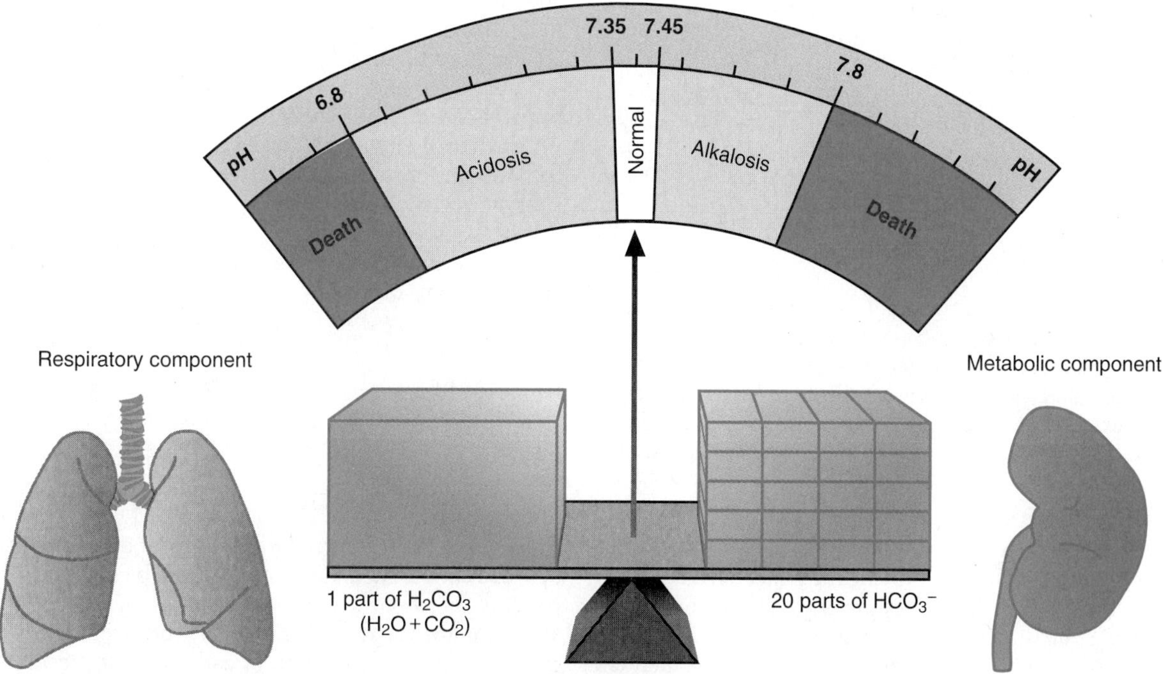

Figure 57–1 Relation of bicarbonate to carbonic acid. (From Black, J. M., and Matassarin-Jacobs, E. [1997]. *Medical-surgical nursing: Clinical management for continuity of care* [5th ed., p. 332]. Philadelphia: W. B. Saunders. Used with permission.)

dioxide, as in hypoventilation, results in an acidotic state. The lungs also play a role in insensible fluid loss through respiration, with approximately 500 mL of water leaving the lungs of a normal adult every 24 hours.

Hypothalamus

The hypothalamus, together with the pituitary gland, assists in regulation of fluid volume. Receptors in the hypothalamus respond to changes in the osmolality of ECF by regulating the sensation of thirst and changing the production rate or secretion of antidiuretic hormone (ADH). ADH is produced by the hypothalamus and stored in the posterior lobe of the pituitary. In the presence of increased blood osmolality, thirst is triggered, and ADH is secreted. ADH acts on the kidneys to increase water absorption in the tubules, thereby lowering the osmolality of ECF. Thus, the urine is more concentrated, and the blood is less concentrated.

Endocrine Glands

In addition to the pituitary gland, two other endocrine glands play a role in homeostasis of fluid and electrolytes. The adrenal cortex produces the mineralocorticoid aldosterone that acts on the kidneys to increase the absorption of sodium and water while increasing the elimination of potassium. The adrenal medulla produces epinephrine and norepinephrine, which play a role in the maintenance of blood pressure and therefore renal perfusion. The parathyroid glands regulate the serum calcium concentrations required for normal neuromuscular excitability, blood clotting, and permeability of cell membranes.

Gastrointestinal Tract

Healthy functioning of the GI tract is necessary for fluid and electrolyte balance, as well as for a well-nourished state. Absorption of nutrients and the absorption and reabsorption of water take place in the gut. GI disorders can result in a state of dehydration, electrolyte imbalance, and malnourishment. IV therapy or total parenteral nutrition (TPN) is required when the GI tract is not able to maintain a well-nourished and homeostatic state.

Nutrition

Nutritional status is dependent on the ability to ingest, absorb, digest, assimilate, and eliminate the nutrients necessary to maintain proper body structure and function. A balance in fluid and electrolytes, as well as of carbohydrates, proteins, lipids, vitamins, and minerals, is required. All of these nutrients produce an optimal state of health and well-being.

Carbohydrates

Carbohydrates in the diet provide the major source of energy for all body functions. They are particularly important for normal brain functioning. In addition to energy, they spare protein catabolism, prevent ketosis, and also play a role in the biotransformation of other nutrients. Inadequate carbohydrate intake results in many symptoms, including depression, fatigue, protein wasting, and electrolyte imbalances.

Proteins

Proteins are nitrogenous compounds composed of essential and nonessential amino acids. They contain a variety of other elements including sulfur, phosphorus, iron, iodine, and other essential constituents of living cells. Protein in the diet is the major building material in the body and is the major building block of muscles, blood, integument, nails, hair, and the internal organs. Protein also is necessary for the production of hormones, enzymes, antibodies, and energy as well as waste elimination. Inadequate protein intake results in abnormal growth and development, lethargy and weakness, decreased stamina, depression, poor resistance to infection, poor wound healing, and chronic illness. Protein intake that exceeds dietary requirements can contribute to fluid volume imbalances.

Lipids

Lipids include any of the free fatty acids in the blood. They include cholesterol, triglycerides, fatty acids, phospholipids, lipoproteins, and neutral fats. The lipids are stored in the body and used as necessary for reserve energy. Blood lipid elevation can result from and also can cause disorders such as atherosclerosis. High blood lipid levels may be associated with excessive intake of dietary lipids. Inadequate fat intake is rarely a problem because the average American diet has an abundant supply of fat. The body can also synthesize fats from sources other than actual fat intake. Persons who cannot ingest any food need parenteral replacement of lipids.

Vitamins and Minerals

Vitamins (organic compounds) and minerals (inorganic compounds) are present in the tissue and fluids of the body and are necessary for normal metabolic and physiologic functioning. Extensive coverage of all of vitamins and minerals is beyond the scope of this text, but they are discussed in Chapter 58 and in any nutrition textbook. Vitamins and minerals are essential nutritional components for all ages. An inadequate intake or an inability to use one or more of the vitamins or minerals results in a need for replacement. A consistent deficiency in any of the essential vitamins and minerals results in a variety of signs and symptoms. Excessive intake of certain vitamins and minerals can lead to signs and symptoms of toxicity.

Imbalances

Acidosis

Acidosis can be metabolic or respiratory in origin. Excessive loss of fluids with an alkaline pH or high concentrations of bicarbonate ions (intestinal, bile, and pancreatic fluids) result in an increase in chloride ions and a drop in blood pH. Inability of the kidneys to produce bicarbonate can also result in metabolic acidosis.

Respiratory acidosis is caused by the retention of carbon dioxide and the production of carbonic acid, resulting in a pH below 7.35. Acidosis results in increasing weakness and progresses to coma if it is not corrected. IV treatment of acidosis requires parenteral fluids that increase pH, such as sodium lactate or sodium bicarbonate.

Alkalosis

The cause of alkalosis, like acidosis, can be metabolic or respiratory in origin. Gastric juices have an acidic pH, and when they are lost over a period of time, the result is metabolic alkalosis. The alkalosis is due to the loss of chloride ions and the retention of bicarbonate ions. Tachypnea or hyperventilation results in blowing off carbon dioxide, thereby lowering carbonic acid. In the presence of an abnormally high pH, the body is incapable of ionizing calcium, resulting in muscular hyperirritability and tetany. Metabolic alkalosis requires replacement of chloride ions with an infusion of solutions such as sodium chloride, potassium chloride, or, if replacement of chloride without sodium is indicated, ammonium chloride. Respiratory alkalosis may require therapy directed at rebreathing the exhaled carbon dioxide.

Excesses

Excesses can occur in fluid volume as well as electrolyte concentration. Excesses of fluid volume may be due to an increase in the total body fluid or an alteration in the distribution between fluid compartments. Fluid excess in general follows an increase in sodium and remains isotonic. The most frequent cause of fluid volume excess is cardiac insufficiency. The insufficiency results in decreased renal perfusion, diminished glomerular filtration rate, increased renin secretion, and excessive aldosterone, causing sodium and water retention. Renal failure due to other insults can also result in fluid volume excesses. Table 57–1 provides a comparison of assessment findings for patients who have a fluid volume excess versus a deficit.

Protein deficiencies lead to fluid volume excess in interstitial fluid and ICF, resulting in a deficit of intravascular volume. Fluid replacement therapy can also be the source of iatrogenic fluid volume excess.

Excesses in electrolyte concentration include hyperkalemia, hypernatremia, hypercalcemia, hypermagnesemia, acidosis (excess hydrogen ions), and alkalosis (excess bicarbonate ions). These excesses are seen most frequently in patients with chronic renal disease but can result from dysfunctions of other homeostatic mechanisms. Excesses in serum electrolytes can also result from excessive oral intake or from parenteral replacement therapy. Electrolytes are found in a variety of commonly used over-the-counter drugs that need to be monitored in patients prone to electrolyte excesses.

Nutrients are required in specific amounts. Nutritional excesses occur when the intake of the nutrient exceeds the

TABLE 57–1 COMPARISON OF FLUID VOLUME EXCESS AND DEFICITS

Assessment Parameter	Fluid Volume Excess	Fluid Volume Deficit
General survey	Confusion, irritability Weight gain Bounding pulse Increased blood pressure Venous distention Growth and development delay	Lethargy Weight loss Weak or thready pulse Decreased blood pressure and pulse pressure Tachycardia Orthostatic hypotension Temperature low (depends on etiology) Growth and developmental delay Decreased activity*
Integumentary	Warm, moist, supple skin Tight, shiny skin Edema with possible pitting	Dry skin Decreased skin turgor Possible tenting of skin
Head, face, neck	Taut fontanelles* Increased head circumference*	Sunken fontanelles* Dry, cracked lips Furrowed tongue Lack of tears* Dry mucous membranes
Respiratory	Inspiratory crackles Increased respiratory rate Shortness of breath Dyspnea on exertion Paroxysmal nocturnal dyspnea Pulmonary edema	Normal breath sounds Dry mucous membranes and thick secretions
Cardiovascular	Elevated central venous pressure Chest pain in cardiac patients	Decreased central venous pressure Decreased cardiac output Decreased tissue perfusion Cardiac arrhythmias
Elimination	Intake exceeds output Urine has low specific gravity	Decreased output Urine has high specific gravity
Neuromuscular	Decreased level of consciousness Seizure activity Irritability	Lethargy, disorientation Seizure activity Confusion
Laboratory data	Hemoglobin and hematocrit normal or low Electrolytes values decreased	Hemoglobin and hematocrit elevated Electrolyte values increased

*Pediatric findings

body requirements. Excesses can lead to a variety of symptoms depending on the nutrient involved. Sustained excessive intake of carbohydrates and lipids results in obesity and may lead to various disease processes. Hypervitaminosis can result from excessive intake of vitamins that occasionally reach toxic levels.

Deficits

Intravascular fluid (IVF) volume deficits may result from an actual loss of fluid from the body or a shift from the vascular to the interstitial space, where it accumulates. Actual loss of intravascular fluid is most frequently caused by a primary GI abnormality, vomiting and diarrhea secondary to a systemic problem, protracted high fever, or nasogastric suction. Other potential causes are dysfunction of any of the previously discussed homeostatic mechanisms. Renal, endocrine, and neurologic dysfunction can result in excessive urinary output, leading to fluid volume deficit.

Fluid volume deficits from the loss of water alone result in hypovolemia, and if the deficits are uncorrected, the condition may lead to dehydration. In dehydration, the deficit is hypertonic, fluid is lost without solutes or electrolytes, and both the ECF and the ICF volumes decrease. In a hypotonic dehydrated state (loss of fluid that has relatively more salt than water), fluid leaves the ECF and moves into the ICF. Replacement therapy is determined by the type of dehydration.

Electrolyte deficiencies occur when ions are lost faster than they are replaced. Electrolytes leave the body as solutes in urine, stool, gastric secretions, or any other bodily fluid. Common electrolyte deficits include hypokalemia, hyponatremia, hypocalcemia, hypomagnesemia, acidosis, and alkalosis. Electrolyte deficiencies can also occur when parenteral or diuretic therapy does not include replacement of affected electrolytes.

Nutritional deficits occur when there is an inability to ingest and use any of the required nutrients. Deficits may be specific to one nutrient, vitamin, or mineral, or may be global due to GI dysfunction or other severe illnesses. Nutritional deficiencies affect all body tissues and make recovery from illness more difficult. Interventions are directed at the specific deficit, etiology of the deficit, and the severity of the problem. Interventions range from conservative oral replacement therapy to total parenteral nutrition via a centrally placed venous access device.

PHARMACOTHERAPEUTIC OPTIONS

IV therapy is one of the most frequently used treatment modalities in acute and chronic health care. It is initiated after careful patient assessment, interpretation of laboratory findings, and consideration of the many treatment options. There are literally hundreds of IV therapy solutions on the market. In order to provide quality care, it is necessary to understand the basic concepts underlying therapy as well as the specific actions and uses of the different fluids. Complete coverage of all the available formulas is beyond the scope of this book but is available in books devoted to that purpose. The knowledge necessary for initiation and management of patients receiving common IV fluids to maintain balance, restore losses, and meet nutritional requirements is the focus of this chapter.

The choice of solutions requires knowledge of daily water needs, tonicity of body and IV fluids, electrolyte requirements, pH of blood and IV fluids, and calorie and other nutrient requirements. IV fluids may be classified as crystalloids (solutions composed mainly of water with dissolved electrolytes or dextrose) or colloids (solutions composed of water, proteins, and small amounts of carbohydrates and lipids). The solutions may also be categorized based on:

- Content (water, sugar, sodium, other electrolytes, and nutrients)
- Osmolality or tonicity (hypertonic, isotonic, or hypotonic)
- Ionic particles (acidic, alkaline, electrolytes, balanced)
- Indications for use (hydrating, replacing, balancing, and nutrition)

In this chapter, IV fluids are categorized as *crystalloids,* which include saline solutions, dextrose solutions, and multiple-electrolyte solutions. In reality, these categories overlap. For example, solutions are available that contain both saline and dextrose, or dextrose with multiple electrolytes. The mechanism of action of the various solutes is not different whether they are isolated or are in solution with other nutrients. For this reason, they can be discussed independently, keeping in mind that they are frequently used in combination.

Colloids include albumin and plasma protein fraction, dextran, and hetastarch (HES). Other IV fluids include acid-base correction solutions, parenteral nutrition solutions, and fat emulsions.

Crystalloids

SALINE SOLUTIONS

- ❒ Saline solutions
- ❒ Dextrose solutions
- ❒ Multiple-electrolyte solutions

Indications

Saline solutions are frequently the fluid of choice for fluid replacement, but they vary in the amount of sodium chloride (0.225, 0.33, 0.45, 0.9, 3, and 5 percent) in the solution. Differences in the osmolality determine the mechanism of action and, therefore, use of the solution. The therapeutic effects of saline solutions are partially dependent on the tonicity of the solution (Fig. 57–2). Isotonic saline (0.9 percent NaCl) is used primarily for simple hydration and to replace ECF lost in situations such as GI suctioning, in which the loss resulted in a loss of chloride at an equal or greater rate than sodium. The chloride in saline is also helpful in compensating for the increase in bicarbonate ions in metabolic alkalosis accompanying fluid loss. Isotonic saline is also used clinically in fluid challenges to test kidney function. Fluid challenges may precede implementation of therapies that require good renal function.

Isotonic saline is also the only IV fluid used when transfusing blood products. It does not hemolyze blood cells. It is used before and after a transfusion to prime and clear the IV line. It is also useful in thinning blood products if they are running slowly owing to their high viscosity.

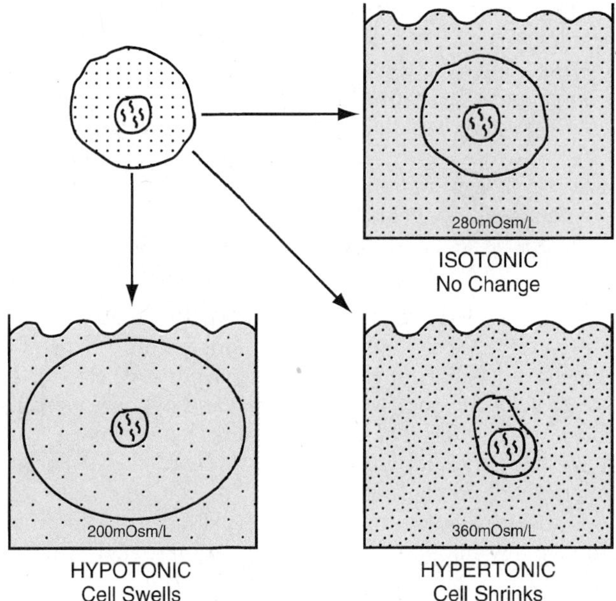

Figure 57–2 Comparison of tonicity of intravenous fluids. Hypotonic solutions move from the vascular system into dehydrated cells. Isotonic solutions remain within the vascular system. Hypertonic solutions pull free water from edematous cells into the circulation. (From Guyton, A. C., and Hall, J. E. [1996]. *Textbook of medical physiology* [9th ed., p. 304]. Philadelphia: W. B. Saunders. Used with permission.)

Hypotonic solutions (e.g., 0.225, 0.33, and 0.45 percent NaCl) are often used in the management of hypernatremia and insensible water losses, as well as to hydrate patients who are dehydrated but not hyponatremic.

Hypertonic solutions (e.g., 3 and 5 percent NaCl) are used cautiously in the management of water intoxication. They are also used in the treatment of cerebral edema, treatment of shock due to addisonian crisis, and hyponatremia. Inappropriate use of these hypertonic solutions has led to fatalities.

Pharmacodynamics

The major pharmacodynamic effects of saline solutions are dependent on the tonicity of the solution. Saline solutions, as well as other IV fluids, are described as isotonic, hypotonic, or hypertonic.

Isotonic solutions (those whose osmotic pressures are approximately equal to that of normal plasma—310 mEq/L) trigger the least movement of water from the IVF compartment into or out of the ICF or interstitial compartments. Isotonic saline replaces sodium, chloride, and water without altering the osmolality of normal plasma.

Hypotonic solutions (those whose osmotic pressures are less than that of plasma [less than 250 mEq/L]) cause water to leave the IVF compartment and successively to enter the interstitial and ICF compartments. Hypotonic saline provides water in excess of that needed to eliminate the salt. After osmotic equilibrium is achieved, the ICF and the ECF have the same osmolality. Total body water is increased by the amount of fluid infused.

Hypertonic solutions (those whose osmotic pressures exceed that of plasma [greater than 375 mEq/L]) draw water from the interstitial and ICF compartments into the IVF compartment. They dilute the ECF compartment with an increase in total body water. When the fluid osmolality exceeds that of plasma, hypertonic saline works well in keeping sodium in the IVF compartment. It pulls fluid from the ICF compartment and interstitial spaces. When saline is given in hypertonic concentrations, it may result in spilling potassium into the urine.

Adverse Effects and Contraindications

Hypertonic and hypotonic solutions may injure tissue cells. Hypertonic solutions shrink cells, whereas hypotonic solutions cause swelling and lysis of cells. The cells most often affected in practice are the red blood cells (RBCs). If such solutions are administered by clysis, or if they infiltrate from an IV line, tissue necrosis and sloughing may result.

Rapid infusion of IV fluids can produce toxicity from excesses of any or all of the constituent components. Fluid excesses produce circulatory overload and hypertension. Saline solutions have the potential to cause hypernatremia and, as a result, hypokalemia. The end result of the imbalances may be peripheral, pulmonary, and cerebral edema, as well as congestive heart failure. Excess chloride results in loss of bicarbonate ions and can cause acidosis in patients receiving continuous saline infusions and in those with precarious acid-base balances.

Water intoxication is a serious potential complication of excessive hypotonic fluid administration. In contrast, administration of hypertonic saline solutions contributes to dehydration. Fluid volume excess is of particular concern in high-risk populations such as the elderly and those with cardiac, renal, or hepatic disease.

Pharmacokinetics

IV saline solutions are rapidly and widely distributed by osmosis and diffusion throughout body systems. The distribution pattern is dependent on the tonicity of body and IV fluids. Saline solutions are eliminated primarily through the kidneys.

Drug-Drug Interactions

The role of sodium in maintenance of blood pressure may result in an antagonism of the effects of antihypertensive drugs. The severity of the effect is dependent on the amount of sodium in the solution. Sodium chloride is incompatible with amphotericin B, levarterenol, mannitol, and other water-soluble drugs.

Dosage Regimen

Isotonic and hypotonic saline solutions are given by continuous IV infusion at a rate dependent on age, weight, laboratory values, and patient condition. The usual adult dosage is 1 to 2 L in a 24-hour period, with frequent monitoring of signs, symptoms, and laboratory values. In an average adult the daily sodium requirements are more than met with the 154 mEq of sodium and chloride that are contained in 1 L of normal saline. The patient must be assessed for signs of sodium retention.

The dosage of hypertonic saline depends on the clinical situation. It is given based on the severity of hyponatremia and the patient's overall condition. It is generally administered at a rate not to exceed 100 mL/hour, with continual monitoring of signs, symptoms, and laboratory values. Hypertonic saline should be administered only with constant monitoring and a delivery system that prevents excessive or rapid delivery.

DEXTROSE SOLUTIONS

Dextrose in the form of glucose is commonly used in IV solutions because it is the best available carbohydrate, is well utilized by tissues, and provides readily available energy for cellular activity. Dextrose solutions are used to meet the caloric requirements of the patient.

Dextrose is available in concentrations of 2.5, 5, 10, 20, 25, 30, 40, 50, 60, and 70 percent in water, which determines the tonicity of the fluid. Dextrose solutions, like saline solutions, are hypotonic (e.g. 2.5 percent dextrose), isotonic (e.g., 5 and 10 percent dextrose) and hypertonic (e.g., 20 and 50 percent dextrose). The percentage of dextrose determines the clinical use. Dextrose is available for specialty use in combination with alcohol, HES, dextran, and sodium chloride, potassium, and other electrolytes.

Dextrose is frequently used in saline solutions. IV fluids that have a combination of the two (e.g., 0.9 percent NaCl and 0.2 percent dextrose, 0.45 percent NaCl and 5 percent dextrose, 0.9 percent NaCl and 5 percent dextrose) are used to provide electrolytes, calories, and optimal osmolality.

Indications

Dextrose and water in lower concentrations (less than 10% dextrose) are used for the purposes of peripheral hydration, providing calories, and assessing of kidney function in patients with no need for electrolyte replacement. If electrolyte replacement is indicated, it may be added to dextrose solutions. The calories provided by dextrose solutions decrease utilization of body protein stores and lower excess ketone production. Proteins are spared when 400 cal/day of dextrose are administered.

Higher concentrations of dextrose are used for reversing hypoglycemia and provide calories for nourishment when less fluid is indicated. Dextrose is used in conjunction with amino acids for total parenteral nutrition.

Pharmacodynamics

Five percent dextrose solutions are approximately isotonic compared with blood. As the percentage of carbohydrate increases above 5 percent, they become hypertonic. The water in a dextrose solution provides immediate hydration for the patient. The dextrose in the solution is rapidly metabolized, leaving water in the intravascular space. The result is a change in osmotic pressure that makes the water available for cellular and interstitial tissue rehydration.

Dextrose provides immediate calories for the metabolic requirements of the body. Carbohydrate solutions use natural sugars such as dextrose and fructose. Fructose, however, has some disadvantages. Fructose may increase serum levels of lactate and urate if it is administered rapidly, and it is considerably more expensive than dextrose. Glucose is converted to glycogen in the liver, preventing unnecessary use of protein for energy and preventing ketosis by decreasing the burning of fat. Dextrose transfusions in the presence of insulin additives result in a shift of potassium from ECF to ICF.

The monosaccharide form of sugar provides 3.4 cal/g, meaning that 1 L of 5 percent dextrose yields 170 cal, whereas 10 percent dextrose provides 340 cal/L, 20 percent dextrose provides 680 cal/L, and 50 percent dextrose contains 1700 cal/L. A seriously ill patient who receives 3 L of 5 percent dextrose in water solutions receives less than 600 cal/day. Without additional calorie intake, protein catabolism and metabolic acidosis soon develop. Additional calorie intake can be achieved through the use of TPN.

Adverse Effects and Contraindications

Adverse effects of glucose solutions include hyperglycemia, fluid overload, hyperosmolar syndrome, electrolyte disturbances, rebound hypoglycemia, and hypoglycemic alkalosis or acidosis. The hyperglycemia, hyperosmolar syndrome and rebound hypoglycemia are more likely to occur with the concentrated solutions.

All dextrose solutions are acidic (pH 3.5 to 5) and may produce thrombophlebitis at peripheral sites. High concentrations are best given using a centrally placed IV line.

Dextrose solutions must be used cautiously in patients with glucose intolerance. Caution is necessary in patients at risk of fluid volume overload.

Pharmacokinetics

Dextrose and water are rapidly distributed. The water is eliminated by the kidneys if it is not needed in the body. If the dextrose level in the blood exceeds the renal threshold, it also will be eliminated by the kidney.

Drug-Drug Interactions

Dextrose solutions given IV increase insulin and oral hypoglycemic requirements for patients with diabetes. Dextrose solutions are incompatible with vitamin B_{12}, kanamycin, phenytoin, sodium bicarbonate, warfarin, and many other drugs. Dextrose solutions cause hemolysis of whole blood when mixed in the same IV line.

Dosage Regimen

The recommended dosage of dextrose solutions depends on the patient's age, weight, health status, and dextrose concentration. When isotonic or hypotonic solutions are used for fluid replacement in adults, 1 to 3 L are given over a 24-hour period, with ongoing assessments for fluid volume overload. In children, the dosage and rate is dependent on size. When treating children, a pediatric-specific reference must be consulted.

The dosage for 5 percent dextrose and water for adults and children is usually 0.5 to 0.8 g/kg/hr. This rate is used when hydrating the patient rapidly and, in the absence of other pathology, does not result in marked glycosuria.

Hypertonic dextrose (e.g., 50 percent dextrose) is used in adults with hypoglycemic emergencies. It is usually given as a 50 mL bolus (or less if sufficient). The dosage may be repeated if insulin-induced hypoglycemia persists. Less concentrated dextrose solutions are also used to treat hypoglycemia and nutritional deficits. Hypoglycemia in neonates and infants is reversible with lower concentrations of dextrose (10 to 15 percent dextrose) delivered at a slower rate, dependent on blood sugar and rapidity of response.

MULTIPLE-ELECTROLYTE SOLUTIONS

A number of multiple-electrolyte solutions that are commercially available have varying concentrations of electrolytes. As with other solutions, the use of multiple electrolyte solutions is based on the patient's diagnosis, physical assessment, and laboratory values. Some are for maintenance of homeostasis, whereas others are for the purpose of replacing specific fluids. The contents of specific solutions are available from the label on each container, or through pharmacy reference books produced for that specific purpose. Of these solutions, lactated Ringer's is the most commonly used and is referred to by the same name regardless of the manufacturer. Other than lactated Ringer's, multiple-electrolyte solutions are declining in clinical use.

Indications

Multiple-electrolyte solutions are used for the purpose of maintaining body fluids and electrolytes within the normal range. When body fluids are being lost at a rapid rate (e.g., hemorrhage, burns, vomiting, fistulas, GI suction), multiple-electrolyte solution fluids are used for rapid replacement because they approximate the plasma contents. Multiple-electrolyte solutions are also useful in daily maintenance of homeostasis when the patient is not able to obtain maintenance requirements enterally.

Lactated Ringer's is a good multipurpose solution and is considered to be almost physiologic. It is most often used to correct isotonic fluid volume deficits. It is used in hypovolemia due to third space fluid shifts following major surgery or trauma.

Pharmacodynamics

The major actions of multiple-electrolyte solutions result from their electrolytes and the water. Dextrose, when included, is for energy. The mechanism of action of the electrolytes is partially dependent on the tonicity of the solution. Commonly used multiple-electrolyte solutions are slightly hypotonic or isotonic in osmolality and have some combination of sodium, chloride, calcium, lactate, phosphate, potassium, magnesium, and sometimes dextrose.

Lactated Ringer's has concentrations of 130 mEq/L of sodium, 4 mEq/L of potassium, 3 mEq/L of calcium, 28 mEq/L of lactate, and 109 mEq/L of chloride. The combination results in a balanced solution that has 137 mEq/L of anions and of cations for a total concentration or 274 mEq/L. Other electrolyte solutions have different concentrations of electrolytes based on the replacement needs of the patient.

Potassium is an electrolyte that is easily and frequently lost from the body and must be added at higher concentrations in some clinical situations. A higher concentration is available in premixed solutions or can be added to the solution before the infusion is started.

Hypertonic multiple-electrolyte solutions are available. They are hypertonic as a result of the 5 percent dextrose that is added to increase the electrolyte contents. The dextrose is added for the purpose of sparing protein, and it changes the tonicity of the fluid.

Adverse Effects and Contraindications

The risk of fluid volume overload must always be considered when infusing isotonic, hypotonic, or hypertonic IV fluids. Adverse effects include overtransfusion of fluid or electrolytes. Excessive parenteral fluids may also result in the wasting of electrolytes if replacement is not sufficient. When electrolyte solutions are used in concentrations greater than plasma concentrations, there is a potential for electrolyte excesses that can be life threatening.

Lactated Ringer's should not be used in patients with an inability to metabolize the lactate in the solution. Patients at high risk for impaired lactate metabolism include those with liver disease, Addison's disease, severe pH imbalances, shock, or cardiac failure.

Pharmacokinetics

The multiple-electrolyte solutions are rapidly and widely distributed throughout the IVF compartment and made available to the ICF and interstitial spaces. Distribution within these spaces is dependent on diffusion and osmosis, as well as active transport. The lactate in lactated Ringer's is quickly biotransformed to bicarbonate, making it useful in the treatment or prevention of metabolic acidosis. The fluid and electrolytes are eliminated in the urine and stool, with a small amount eliminated through insensible losses. The ultrafiltration of electrolytes that takes place in the kidneys depends on the level of electrolytes in the plasma.

Drug-Drug Interactions

Interactions depend on the electrolytes present and their concentration in the solution. When infusing electrolyte solutions, it is important to consult the pharmacist or a desk reference as to the potential interactions of the electrolytes with other treatment modalities or drugs. Each electrolyte has a potential interaction with a variety of substances and should be looked up individually.

Dosage Regimen

Dosage and administration are determined by the solution contents and the patient's age, weight, and overall condition—especially renal function. In patients with renal impairment, the dosage and rate of administration must be altered accordingly. Electrolyte replacement is based on average daily requirements, coupled with current and ongoing losses.

Colloids

- ❒ Albumin and plasma protien fraction
- ❒ Dextran (DEXTRAN 40, 10 percent LMD)
- ❒ Hetastarch (HESPAN, hydroxyethyl starch [HES])
- ❒ Whole blood
- ❒ Plasma

Volume expanders increase the total volume of body fluid. When plasma volume is reduced as the result of simple fluid and electrolyte loss, the deficit may be corrected in many patients by the simple replacement of saline. However, when the initial losses are of a more complex and critical nature, a plasma volume expander (volume extender, plasma substitutes) may be indicated.

The IV solutions previously discussed have been crystalloids. Volume expanders are colloids, osmotically active, and draw fluid into the IVF space from the ECF space. Volume expanders are available as plasma derivatives like albumin and plasma protein fraction (PPF) or in synthetic form such as dextran (low molecular weight [LMW], dextran 40; high molecular weight [HMW], dextran 70/75) and HES.

ALBUMIN AND PLASMA PROTEIN FRACTION

Albumin and PPF are used to provide volume expansion in situations in which crystalloid solutions are not adequate (such as plasma exchange, shock, and massive hemorrhage). They are also used in the treatment of acute liver failure, burns, and hemolytic disease of the newborn.

Albumin is composed of 96 percent albumin, 4 percent globulin, and traces of other proteins extracted from plasma. It is available as a 5 percent solution that is osmotically equivalent to plasma and also as a concentrated (hypertonic) 25 percent solution.

PPF, on the other hand, is made up of 83 percent albumin and 17 percent globulins extracted from plasma. It is less pure than albumin and contains a higher degree of other plasma proteins. It is available only as a 5 percent solution.

There are no ABO blood group antibodies present with albumin and PPF. Therefore, compatibility is not a factor. Albumin and PPF solutions cannot transmit hepatitis or the human immunodeficiency virus. The pasteurization process used to prepare the products destroys the viruses. Chapter 38 discusses blood and blood products in more depth.

DEXTRAN

Dextran is similar to human albumin in that it expands plasma volume by drawing fluid from the interstitial space to the IVF space. Dextran 40 is an LMW polysaccharide that is used as a volume expander but also as prophylaxis for thrombosis and embolism. LMW dextran not only corrects hypovolemia but also appears to improve microcirculation independent of simple volume expansion. It minimizes the sludging of blood that accompanies shock. In a patient who has whole blood or plasma loss, a single infusion of dextran increases circulating blood volume and improves the hemodynamic status for over 24 hours. On the other hand, dextran 70 or 75 (depending on the pharmaceutical preparation) is an HMW polysaccharide that is used primarily to expand plasma volume in impending or hypovolemic shock.

Dextran is formed by the action of a bacterium. It has osmotic properties but no oxygen-carrying capacity. The LMW molecules are eliminated by the kidneys. The remainder slowly cross capillary membranes to be oxidized over a period of weeks. The persistence of dextran and its metabolic disposal are desirable features.

The incidence of adverse reactions in otherwise healthy patients is less than 10 percent. However, dextran is a potent antigen, stimulating histamine release and anaphylaxis. Therefore, conditions such as asthma contraindicate the use of dextran. Other contraindications to the use of dextran include renal failure, severe dehydration, pregnancy, and heart failure. Slight bleeding tendencies have been reported after Dextran administration.

HETASTARCH (HESPAN [HES])

HES, like dextran, is used for its osmotic properties but has no oxygen-carrying capacity. In the management of shock and in postoperative cardiac patients, HES has the same efficacy as albumin. HES is less likely to cause an allergic reaction than dextran.

HES is made from hydroxyethyl starch, a cornstarch. A 6 percent solution approximates the colloidal osmotic pressure of albumin. When it is given IV, HES expands blood volume by 1 to 2 times the amount infused. About 40 percent of an LMW dose is readily eliminated in 24 hours. The HMW preparation is slowly biotransformed, with only about 1 percent of a dose present after 2 weeks.

However, HES does produce a mild bleeding tendency, nausea, vomiting, myalgia, and swelling of the parotid gland.

WHOLE BLOOD

Whole blood, although it is not considered a true volume expander, is composed of red blood cells that contain plasma proteins (e.g., globulins, antibodies), stable clotting factors, an anticoagulant, and a preservative. It is used to treat acute, massive blood loss requiring the oxygen-carrying properties of red blood cells along with the volume expansion provided by plasma. When it is used, whole blood should resolve the symptoms of hypovolemic shock and anemia.

However, acute loss of as much as one third of a patient's total blood volume can often be managed with crystalloid or colloid solutions. Signs and symptoms that indicate whole blood may be appropriate include acute blood loss with hypotension, tachycardia, shortness of breath, and pallor. If a patient is actively bleeding, the hematocrit and hemoglobin values may fluctuate due to rapid fluid shifts. In a nonbleeding patient, one unit (500 mL) of whole blood should increase the hematocrit by 3 percent and hemoglobin by 1 g/dL. In spite of the benefits of whole blood, advances in the use of blood components have made whole blood transfusions rarely required and often medically inappropriate.

PLASMA

Plasma is the cell-free portion of blood and constitutes 60 percent of total blood volume. Two types of plasma are available for transfusion—fresh or fresh frozen. Fresh frozen plasma (FFP) contains 91 percent water, 7 percent proteins (i.e., albumin, globulins, antibodies, and clotting factors), and 2 percent carbohydrates. Both types contain all of the clotting factors except platelets. Clotting Factor V is stable for about 10 days. Factor VIII is stable for 2 days but then decreases by 30 percent over time. Factors VII, IX, X, XI, and XII and fibrinogen remain fairly stable.

FFP may be a useful adjunct in massive transfusion to prevent dilutional hypocoagulability and in patients with severe liver disease who have limited synthesis of plasma clotting factors. FFP transfusions are rarely indicated if the prothrombin time and partial thromboplastin time are less than 1.5 times normal.

Fresh plasma can be stored for 35 to 40 days. Frozen plasma can be stored for up to 1 year. FFP is separated within 4 hours of donation and is frozen within 6 hours. It takes approximately 45 minutes to thaw and must be used within 24 hours. Storage in a liquid state after 24 hours of thawing results in the loss of labile clotting Factors V and VIII.

Plasma, as a product of human origin, carries the risk of transmitting hepatitis B, hepatitis C, or human immunodeficiency virus but not cytomegalovirus. For units of plasma derived from a single donor, the risk is no greater than that for a single transfusion of whole blood. Pooled plasma preparations are heated during processing to minimize the risk of viral transmission. Plasma contains no red blood cells and crossmatching is not required, although ABO compatible plasma should be used.

Adverse effects and hazards include chills and fever, allergic reactions, and circulatory overload. Circulatory overload can be avoided with the use of specific coagulation concentrates when high levels of clotting factors are required. When large volumes are used, citrate toxicity and hypothermia may occur.

The amount (dosage) administered depends on the clinical situation and may be determined by serial laboratory assays of coagulation. One unit for an adult usually contains 225 to 275 mL of anticoagulated plasma, with 200 to 400 mg of fibrinogen, 200 units of Factor VIII, and 200 units of Factor IX, as well as the other stable and labile clotting factors. For pediatric patients and in other special circumstances, smaller volumes with proportionally smaller coagulation factors may be available.

Parenteral Nutrition Solutions

Parenteral nutrition has been commercially available since 1969 and has dramatically improved the management of patients who, for a variety of reasons, do not take in enough food to meet the nutritional needs of the body. Parenteral nutrition is used to promote protein synthesis (anabolism), decrease protein breakdown (catabolism), maintain a positive nitrogen balance, and promote fluid and electrolyte homeostasis in patients with a variety of conditions. The three major choices of parenteral support include:

- Peripheral protein-sparing solutions that are composed of water, amino acids, and sometimes dextrose, vitamins, or electrolytes
- Peripheral parenteral nutrition (PPN) solutions that are hypotonic or isotonic and that are composed of dextrose, amino acids, lipid emulsions, electrolytes, vitamins, and trace elements
- Central-line TPN solutions that are hypertonic and that provide complete nutrition. TPN is composed of dextrose, amino acids, electrolytes, vitamins, minerals, trace elements, and lipid emulsion

Indications

The goal in using TPN is to keep the patient in a positive nitrogen balance while allowing for growth of new body tissue (see Conditions Warranting Parenteral Nutrition).

The minimal energy needs for a normal resting adult are between 1400 and 1800 kcal/day. Patients who have had surgical procedures may require a minimum of 3000 kcal/day. For patients who are severely septic, traumatized, or burned, 5000 to 10,000 kcal/day may be required. An IV solution of 5 percent dextrose in water supplies only 170 cal/L. Thus, ordinary IV therapy does not provide sufficient calories or protein to support the patient's nutritional needs.

CONDITIONS WARRANTING PARENTERAL NUTRITION

- Inability to use the alimentary tract for enteral feedings
- Intolerance of long-term enteral feedings or inability to provide sufficient nutrition by enteral feeding alone
- Illness that is sustained and debilitating
- Impaired absorption of protein from the GI tract
- Long-term wound infection, abscess, or fistula resulting in extreme nitrogen loss
- Bowel rest required for longer than 1 week secondary to GI surgery, injury, or inflammatory GI disorders
- Hypoproteinemia due to loss of protein or substantial increase in protein requirements
- Chronic diarrhea or vomiting
- Persistent weight loss in excess of 10 percent of body weight
- Liver and renal failure resulting in altered amino acid requirements

TPN provides complete nutritional support for patients with long-term needs. In contrast, PPN is used to meet a patient's nutritional needs when those needs are short term, when calorie requirements do not exceed 2500 kcal/day, or when the patient is not a candidate for TPN due to inaccessibility of a central vein. PPN is not sufficient for patients who have greater nutritional requirements or for those requiring long-term complete nutritional support.

Pharmacodynamics

Parenteral nutrition preparations vary in tonicity. PPN solutions are hypotonic or isotonic, whereas centrally delivered TPN is hypertonic. Carbohydrates (primarily dextrose) and lipids provide calories necessary for biotransformation, prevent the use of protein for energy, and prevent or correct nitrogen imbalances. Amino acids provide calories, promote anabolism, and prevent or decrease the catabolism of protein. Thus, wound healing is promoted and tissue wasting is prevented. Trace elements, vitamins, and minerals are added to the solutions for the purpose of meeting the daily patient requirements and to replace excessive losses as they occur. The absence of these components results in a variety of specific signs and symptoms depending on the nutrient, trace element, and electrolyte involved.

Adverse Effects and Contraindications

Metabolic abnormalities related to the infusion of large amounts of glucose, including hyperglycemia and hypoglycemia, are common. Excessive amounts of dextrose may result in steatosis (fatty liver) and, unless appropriate action is taken, may prove fatal. If liver function tests are elevated, the health care provider should be notified for appropriate adjustments.

An abrupt termination of hypertonic dextrose solutions (which stimulates insulin secretion) results in rebound hypoglycemia. The usual procedure is to reduce the infusion rate by 50 percent for ½ to 1 hour before discontinuation of TPN unless patients are receiving enteral feedings. The rate of peripheral solutions does not need to be tapered.

The use of amino acids, when they are given without carbohydrates, as in protein-sparing peripheral therapy, may result in ketosis. Most major electrolyte imbalances occur in patients ill enough to be on parenteral nutrition.

The most common electrolyte imbalances associated with parenteral nutrition include excesses and deficits in serum levels of potassium, sodium, phosphate, calcium, and magnesium. Another complication that can occur is hypersensitivity to any of the components. An alteration in the composition of the solution may be required.

Sepsis is the most frequent complication of TPN therapy. The use of strict aseptic technique in the preparation and storage of the infusion is essential to prevent bacterial contamination. One of the first signs of sepsis is glucose intolerance (provided that it was not a pre-existing condition).

Pharmacokinetics

PPN and central-line parenteral nutrition solutions are widely distributed. Biotransformation occurs, as with other forms of nutrition, through the anabolic process with elimination of metabolites in the urine and feces.

Drug-Drug Interactions

Many drugs are incompatible with parenteral nutrition solutions, and a pharmacist should be consulted before any drugs are added to parenteral nutrition products. In general, TPN is not a proper vehicle for drug administration. Patients receiving TPN should receive all other therapies through venous access not used for TPN. As administration systems and solutions change, so do the drugs that can be safely administered with TPN solutions.

Insulin requirements typically increase while the patient is receiving parenteral nutrition. Glucocorticoids, diuretics, or tetracycline may inhibit the protein-sparing effects of the amino acids and exaggerate negative nitrogen balance.

Dosage Regimen

Commercially prepared TPN base solutions are available for both central and peripheral use (Table 57–2). These solutions contain dextrose and nitrogen in the form of amino acids or protein hydrolysates. They may also contain minimal amounts of electrolytes and vitamins. Additional electrolytes (e.g., sodium, potassium, chloride, calcium, magnesium, and phosphate), as well as vitamins and trace elements, may be required.

Calories are supplied primarily by 20 or 50 percent dextrose. The administration of 100 to 150 g of dextrose daily has a protein-sparing effect. Because most patients who receive TPN have a nutritional deficit, their daily calorie needs are well above average. These patients must receive a minimum of 2000 cal/day. A formula for estimating calories in parenteral solutions is contained in Appendix E.

A healthy person requires about 56 g of protein daily. In a patient with nutritional deficits, nitrogen requirements may exceed 150 g/day. This quantity ensures a positive nitrogen balance. Standard base solutions of TPN provide approximately 5 to 6 g of nitrogen or about 128 to 140 cal/L.

Base solutions often contain small amounts of electrolytes. Additional amounts may be added to meet normal daily requirements. The following are considered normal daily electrolyte requirements:

- Sodium: 60 to 200 mEq
- Potassium: 50 to 160 mEq
- Chloride: 100 to 200 mEq
- Magnesium: 20–30 mEq
- Phosphate: 30 to 100 mmol

Vitamins are usually added to TPN solutions to meet body needs. If a multivitamin is used, the requirement for vitamin B_{12} is met without the need for supplemental injections. Vitamin K and folic acid are usually ordered separately based on patient needs.

The trace elements zinc, copper, manganese, cobalt, and iodine are added to the TPN solution according to patient needs. Zinc levels are closely monitored because zinc stores may be depleted within a week or two of starting TPN. Additional amounts of zinc and selenium are added as necessary.

Fat Emulsions

Indications

Parenteral fat emulsions, commonly referred to as lipids, can be used in conjunction with parenteral nutrition solutions to prevent endogenous fatty acid deficiencies. Fat emulsions have a low tonicity and provide more than twice as much energy as TPN solutions.

Fat emulsions are required when TPN continues for more than 2 to 3 weeks to prevent nutritional deficiencies. The use of fat emulsions enhances protein repletion, improves glucose tolerance, and reduces fluid retention. They are especially recommended for patients with diabetes mellitus (for better glucose control and lower insulin requirements) and respiratory failure (less carbon dioxide produced from oxidation of fats).

Pharmacodynamics

The onset, peak, and duration of action of fat emulsions are unknown. Fat emulsions are isotonic and can be used to offset the high osmolality of the TPN solution. Fat emulsions contain 1.2 percent egg yolk phospholipids as an emulsifier and glycerol to adjust tonicity.

The major fatty acids contained in fat emulsions include oleic, palmitic, stearic, and linolenic acid. These fatty acids provide a concentrated source of energy, spare protein, and offer a high satiety value. Because they slow gastric secretions and retard gastric emptying, they delay the rapid development of hunger.

Linoleic acid, as a polyunsaturated fatty acid is a presursor to linolenic acid. It is the only required dietary fat that cannot be synthesized by the body. If it is not furnished in the diet, deficiency symptoms result. Food sources of linoleic acid include safflower, sunflower, and corn oils, with lesser amounts present in soybean and canola oil. It is also present in small amounts in green leafy vegetables, seaweed, and meat fats. Palmitic and stearic acids, the most prevalent fatty acids, are found in animal fats, cheese, butter, coconut oil, and chocolate. The most abundant monounsaturated fatty acid is oleic acid, which is found in olive, peanut, and canola oils.

Adverse Effects and Contraindications

Adverse effects of fat emulsions are usually observed with excessive doses. Acute reactions include fever, chills, vomiting, headache, a feeling of pressure over the eyes, and

TABLE 57–2 PARENTERAL NUTRITION FORMULATIONS

TPN Solutions	Manufacturer	Amino Acid Concentration (%)	Composition
Aminess	ClinTec Nutrition	5.2	EAA, acetate, histidine
Aminosyn	Abbott Laboratories	3	EAA, acetate, sodium
		5, 7, 10	EAA, acetate, potassium
Aminosyn M	Abbott Laboratories	3.5	EAA, acetate, chloride, magnesium, phospate, potassium, sodium
Aminosyn/Dextrose	Abbott Laboratories	3	EAA, acetate, dextrose (5%–25%), potassium
		4.5	EAA, acetate, chloride, dextrose (25%), potassium
Aminosyn/Lytes	Abbott Laboratories	7, 8.5	EAA, acetate, chloride, magnesium, phosphate, potassium, sodium
Aminosyn-RF	Abbott Laboratories	5.2	Only EAA with acetate, arginine, histidine, potassium
BranchAmin	ClinTec Nutrition	4	Contains only isoleucine, leucine, valine with phosphate
Freamine HBC	McGaw, Inc.	6.9	EAA/NEAA (including 4% high BCAA), acetate, chloride, sodium
Freamine III	McGaw, Inc.	8.5, 10	EAA, acetate, chloride, potassium, sodium
Freamine III/Lytes	McGaw, Inc.	3	EAA, acetate, chloride, magnesium, phosphate, potassium, sodium
Hepatamine	McGaw, Inc.	8	EAA/NEAA (inc. BCAA, dec. AAA and methionine), acetate, chloride, sodium
Nephramine	McGaw, Inc.	5.4	Only EAA, acetate, chloride, cysteine, histidine, sodium
Novamine	ClinTech Nutrition	8.5, 11	EAA, acetate
ProCalAmine	McGaw, Inc.	3	EAA, NEAA, acetate, calcium, chloride, 3% glycerine, magnesium, phosphate, potassium, sodium, taurine*
RenAmin	ClinTech Nutrition	6.5	EAA/NEAA, acetate, chloride
Travasol		5.5, 8.5, 10	EAA, acetate, chloride
Travasol/Lytes		5.5, 8.5	EAA, acetate, chloride, magnesium, phosphate, sodium
TrophAmine	McGaw, Inc.	6	EAA, NEAA, taurine*
Fat Emulsions†	**Manufacturer**	**Amino Acid Concentration (%)**	**Composition**
Intralipid	ClinTech Nutrition	10, 20	Soybean oil
Liposyn	Abbott	10, 20	
Liposyn II	Abbott	10, 20	50% Soybean and 50% safflower oil
Liposyn III	Abbott	10, 20	Soybean oil
Nutrilipid	Kendell-McGaw	10, 20	Soybean oil
Soyacal		10, 20	
Travamulsion		10, 20	

*Amino acid required by neonates.
†Each solution contains 1.2 percent egg phopholipids.
EAA, Essential amino acids; NEAA, nonessential amino acids; BCAA, branched chain amino acids; AAA, aromatic amino acids.

pain in the chest or back. They usually occur during the initial transfusion. Milder reactions are pruritus and urticaria. Signs of thrombophlebitis at the injection site can also occur.

Chronic administration of fat emulsions results in the deposition of fat pigment in Kupffer's cells of the liver and a decrease in hemoglobin concentration. The effects are reversible when the emulsion is discontinued. Fat overload syndrome is characterized by hyperlipidemia, fever, focal seizures, leukocytosis, hepatomegaly, splenomegaly, spontaneous bleeding, and shock.

A capillary fatty embolism may also occur. Fat emulsions require complex processes to keep the fat particles emulsified in an aqueous system. The stabilizer is egg yolk phospholipids. When fat particles aggregate, the particle size increases, with larger particles rising to the surface. This process is known as creaming. Discard creamed solution. Agitation cannot possibly render fat emulsions safe after creaming has occurred. If, however, the process continues, the aggregates combine, placing the patient at risk for an capillary fat embolism. In addition, solutions in which the emulsion appears to have separated or is oily should not be used. Lipid emulsions must be administered only with IV sets containing a 1.2 micron filter. This filter will retain fat particles if the emulsion cracks. This is a crucial patient safety matter—there are no exceptions.

Fat emulsions are administered with caution in patients at risk for fat embolism, such as those with long bone fractures, and in patients with severe hepatic damage, anemia, or coagulation disorders. Reports have indicated that infants have decreased lipid clearance with increased serum levels of fatty acids after infusion. Therefore, the fat emulsions should be administered with extreme caution to premature and low birth weight infants.

Fat emulsions are contraindicated in patients with hyperlipidemias, lipoid nephrosis, and pancreatitis that is accompanied by lipemia. Because egg yolk phospholipids are used to stabilize the solution a history of severe egg allergy prohibits their use. Safe use in pregnancy has not been established. Fat emulsions are identified as pregnancy category C drugs.

Pharmacokinetics

It is believed that fat emulsions are managed by the body in the same manner that ingested fats are metabolized. The protein in the blood serves as an emulsifier, forming lipid-protein complexes. The complexes are carried to the liver, adipose tissue, muscle, and other cells, where they are converted to free fatty acids and glycerol. Free fatty acids are then transported to tissues, where they are oxidized for an energy source or resynthesized and stored as triglycerides. When they are needed for energy, triglycerides are mobilized and oxidized.

Drug-Drug Interactions

Heparin is the only drug that may be added to fat emulsions. It helps speed clearance of the lipids from the plasma.

Dosage Regimen

Several fat emulsions are available in the United States (see Table 57–2). They are prepared from either soybean oil, safflower oil, or a combination of both and provide a mixture of neutral triglycerides and unsaturated fatty acids. They are administered either peripherally or through a central IV line.

Of the total daily calories required, 4 to 8 percent need to be endogenous fatty acids to prevent fatty acid deficiency. Twenty to 40 percent of the total daily calories should be fat, with the remaining calories supplied by TPN solutions. Minimal fat requirements can be met by administering 500 mL of a 10 percent solution two to three times weekly. A 10 percent solution provides 1.1 kcal/mL, with a 20 percent solution providing 2 kcal/mL. It is recommended that the daily adult dose of fat emulsion not exceed 2 to 3 g/kg/day.

A 10 percent solution should be administered at 1 mL/minute for the initial 15 to 30 minutes, then increased to 85 to 125 mL/hour. The infusion rate should not exceed 500 mL on the first day. The dosage may be increased on the second day. A 20 percent solution should be administered at 0.1 mL/minute for the initial 10 to 15 minutes, then increased to 1 g/kg over 4 hours. The rate should not exceed 100 mL/hour.

Fat emulsions can be added piggyback into the TPN solutions. Because of a lower specific gravity, the fat emulsion solution must be hung higher than the TPN solution to prevent the emulsion from backing up into the TPN line. Special 1.2-micron filters are always used during the administration of fat emulsion solutions.

Critical Thinking Process

Assessment

History of Present Illness

The history of present illness describes in detail the presenting signs and symptoms. The description should include the symptoms that led the patient to seek care. The reason for initiating fluid, electrolyte, or nutritional infusion therapy will become of foremost importance. Why did the present illness result in the need for IV fluids? Will the objective be to prevent potential complications, alleviate an acute symptom, or palliate an ongoing chronic problem?

Past Health History

In the case of ongoing medical problems, access to previous charts or data is helpful in planning individualized interventions. A past history of renal, pulmonary, cardiovascular, or endocrine disorders is of special interest in patients who are beginning IV therapy due to the higher risk of complications in these individuals.

Physical Exam Findings

A head-to-toe physical exam should be completed and documented before the initiation of therapy if the patient's condition permits. Critical assessments of fluid, electrolyte, or nutritional imbalances include general appearance and mental status, vital signs, accurate daily weights, and intake and output. The skin turgor and temperature, as well as the condition of the mucous membranes, the lips, the hair, and the nails, should be noted. In infants, head circumference and the integrity of the fontanelles should be noted. Jugular venous distention, the presence of crackles or wheezes, edema, and dysrhythmias give the health care provider a sense of cardiovascular integrity. Involuntary neuromuscular activity, altered deep tendon reflexes, or changes in sensation may suggest electrolyte imbalances as well. Table 57–1 provides an overview of physical exam findings related to fluid volume excess or deficits.

Diagnostic Testing

Laboratory data play an important part in the assessment of a patient who receives IV therapy. The rapidity with which lab values can change magnifies the need for careful monitoring. Baseline studies that are appropriate before and throughout IV therapy may include a complete blood count, electrolytes, platelet count, prothrombin time, and blood urea nitrogen (BUN), as well as carbon dioxide, glucose, creatinine, total protein, uric acid, liver function studies, cholesterol, and triglyceride levels.

Daily monitoring of laboratory data varies based on the solution used. After the patient is stabilized, less frequent routine monitoring is appropriate. With all parenteral nutrition, daily, if not more frequent, monitoring of glucose, in addition to intake, output, and weight, is indicated. Liver function, electrolytes, BUN, and creatinine are checked two to three times weekly. Periodic evaluation of all baseline studies, as well as nitrogen balance, iron, trace elements, and total lymphocyte count, is recommended.

Common diagnostic tests may include an electrocardiogram, which provides information about the electrolytes that affect cardiac muscle. Chest radiographs assess for pulmonary edema and cardiomegaly. These tests may be routinely ordered for high-risk patients or as needed on any patient receiving parenteral nutrition.

Developmental Considerations

Perinatal Physiologic changes during pregnancy affect the fluid, electrolyte, and nutritional balance in women (see Chapter 6). In the first trimester, human chorionic gonadotropin secretion can cause nausea and vomiting, alter carbohydrate biotransformation, and result in changes in smell and taste. IV therapy may be required if *hyperemesis gravidarum* (severe vomiting in early pregnancy) occurs. In rare but severe cases, TPN may be required until vomiting subsides.

Pediatric As discussed in Chapter 7, infants and small children have a proportionately higher percentage of total body water than adults. The distribution of fluid is also different in infants. The relative percentage of ECF in neonates is higher. ECF leaves the body through the lungs, GI tract, and kidneys. For this reason and the fact that an infant's daily water turnover is greater than that of adults, infants are more susceptible to fluid volume deficits than older children and adults.

The smaller the child, the higher the risk for fluid volume overload by virtue of size alone. IV therapy in infants and children should be delivered with small drop factor tubing, small containers, and infusion pumps. Caution must be taken to prevent the older child from tampering with the delivery system. Tamper-proof systems and close monitoring decreases the likelihood of IV fluid volume overload. Records of intake and output with a parenteral fluid record and urine specific gravities should be maintained at the child's bedside.

IV therapy in children results in anxiety and feelings of threat. Time spent gaining the child's and parent's trust, and allowing the parents to remain with the child, will improve the experience. Psychosocial implications vary depending on the child's age, personality, and developmental stage. Observation of the child and interviews with the parents before starting therapy assists in planning the appropriate interventions for the child. Infants who require long-term therapy with TPN should be included in stimulation programs to minimize developmental delays.

Geriatric The normal aging process is accompanied by a decrease in the efficiency of the body's compensatory mechanisms. This results in a narrow margin of safety and a longer recovery time once homeostasis has been interrupted. Fluid, electrolyte, and nutritional imbalances are common problems among the ill elderly. Imbalances often increase the frequency and length of hospital stay and may threaten the patient's ability to return to an independent lifestyle.

Physical changes of aging predispose the patient to iatrogenic fluid and electrolyte imbalances (see Chapter 8). Rapid infusion of IV fluids has dramatic implications due to the inability of homeostatic mechanisms to respond to rapid changes in fluid volume. Geriatric patients with a history of renal or heart disease require the same precautions as pediatric patients.

Psychosocial Considerations

An awareness of the patient's cultural, ethnic, and religious background may be important when considering IV therapy. The patient and family should be made aware of what the procedure involves and what solution is being used. If the patient or family has concerns about the procedure or fluid used, it is necessary to address those concerns before initiating therapy. The use of blood and blood products is more likely to be of concern in some patients than the use of synthetic products. If the patient's religious beliefs preclude the use of blood products, the appropriate health care provider should be notified and the information documented in the patient's record. Alternative IV solutions may be available for this patient, or a court order may be obtained if a blood transfusion is the only proper therapy.

Analysis and Management

Treatment Objectives

The major objectives of IV therapy include maintenance of daily requirements, replacement of existing deficits, and restoration of ongoing or concurrent losses. Management of the patient receiving IV therapy for actual or potential fluid, electrolyte, or nutritional imbalances is focused on the prevention of complications in patients at risk. Treatment is directed at regulating fluid volume and osmolality, avoiding acid-base disturbances, avoiding electrolyte imbalances, and preventing malnourishment or severe catabolism. The selection of fluid for therapy is based on the assessment findings, laboratory results, and underlying pathology.

Treatment Options

The cost of IV therapy, whether for replacement or expansion of fluid volume or for nutritional support, varies with the solutions used, the duration of treatment, and the patient monitoring that is required.

A thorough investigation of alternatives is warranted before a decision is made to use TPN. The cost of TPN in the United States varies from one hospital to another, as well as from one geographic region to another. The estimated daily cost of inpatient TPN therapy varies from $75 to $500, with a median cost of approximately $200 daily. Outpatient costs exceed $50,000/year. On the other hand, implementation of TPN is cost effective compared with the cost of malnutrition. For example, the cost of healing a single decubitus ulcer, which is one complication of malnutrition, ranges from $5000 to $40,000 and may take several months.

The fat emulsions are relatively expensive compared with the cost of dextrose solutions and, therefore, may not be used routinely in adults on short-term (less than 3 weeks) parenteral therapy. They are less expensive than TPN solutions. Again, the cost of combined TPN and fat emulsion therapy remains less than the cost of managing complications of nutritional deficiencies. Comparative costs of IV fluids can be obtained from the pharmacy or purchasing department.

The expenses incurred during IV therapy include not only the cost of the solutions but also the cost of the access devices, tubing, and infusion pumps. The requirement for sterility and frequent equipment changes increases the expense. It is important to be conscious of cost and to select the least expensive means to achieve management goals. Each time a decision is made to change IV fluids before a hanging bag is completed and each time a bag is changed prematurely, the cost to the patient increases. Furthermore, an infusion pump is necessary for patients with compromised renal, cardiac, or neurologic function, or if the specific solution infused warrants a pump for safety. Other significant supplemental costs include pharmacy compounding fees, physician fees for therapeutic monitoring, and fees for laboratory studies.

Intervention

Administration

How fluids are administered is an important part of IV therapy. Administration decisions include not only what solution to use but also which venous access device is appropriate and what delivery system is indicated. Venous access devices are selected based on the quality of the patient's veins, age, clinical condition, anticipated duration of treatment, and the solution type and amount to be delivered. Peripherally inserted needles or catheters work well for most forms of IV therapy. Small sizes are usually sufficient unless large amounts of fluid must be given rapidly or if the fluid is viscous. Centrally placed catheters, implanted infusion ports, and peripherally inserted central catheters are indicated for patients who require long-term therapy. These access devices have greater longevity and also make it possible to deliver solutions that are irritating to smaller veins. IV therapy should be discontinued as early as possible to prevent infusion-related complications.

Although the use of an infusion pump results in an additional charge to the patient, in many clinical situations, it is a necessary piece of safety equipment. Parenteral nutrition and lipids also require the use of an infusion pump. An accurate infusion rate is extremely important for patients with selected renal, cardiovascular, endocrine, or neurologic disorders. In addition, an infusion pump must always be used for fluids with additives such as heparin, aminophylline, insulin, and large doses of potassium.

Determining intake and output, as well as planning for future fluid needs, is vital to successful therapy. Documentation that is easily interpreted is important when providing IV therapy. Recording the infusion site and condition and the amount of fluid started, infused, and discarded is important. Encouraging the conscious patient to report any change in the way he or she feels is important. With sustained IV therapy, regular monitoring of serum sodium, potassium, chloride, and bicarbonate levels is indicated, as well as periodic measurements of acid-base balance.

Dextrose solutions require monitoring of the blood glucose level at a frequency based on the patient's condition and the concentration of solution. The hypotonic and isotonic solutions have little effect on blood glucose levels of patients who are not glucose intolerant. Hypertonic glucose solutions require frequent monitoring of blood glucose levels in all patients.

Monitoring serum electrolytes is indicated when using multiple electrolyte solutions. In potassium replacement therapy, cardiac monitoring or an ECG may be indicated. This is especially true of patients receiving cardiac drugs or patients with a history of cardiac disease. It is a good idea to administer a fluid challenge to test renal function before starting aggressive electrolyte replacement. Ongoing monitoring of BUN and creatinine levels is indicated with continuous therapy.

The laboratory should be notified if the patient has received volume expanders because the lab values of some common tests may be altered by the expanders. Dextran, for example, results in a false elevation of blood glucose, urinary protein, alanine aminotransferase (ALT; serum glutamic-pyruvic transaminase [SGPT]), aspartate aminotransferase (AST; serum glutamic-oxaloacetic transaminase [SGOT]), and bilirubin levels.

Total Parenteral Nutrition Solutions Total parenteral nutrition solutions for adults are usually started at a rate of 40 to 50 mL/hour. Rates are determined based on age, weight, lab values, and heart and renal function. A slow infusion rate allows for microsomal proteins within the body to use the TPN products. Additionally, the pancreas is slowly stimulated, thereby increasing its release of insulin. The infusion rate is increased over a 24-hour period until the desired maximum rate is reached.

Once the patient is stabilized on TPN, the infusion may be interrupted for a short period (e.g., 2 hours) each day. The period that TPN is interrupted may be gradually increased to 8 hours. A 5 to 10 percent dextrose solution may be hung during the 2-hour period. It is thought that periodic interruption of TPN infusions promotes better use of nutrients and fats that have accumulated in the liver.

Patients receiving TPN solutions with high concentrations of glucose must be monitored for hyperglycemia. Supplemental administration of insulin may be required. TPN solutions containing less than 25 percent dextrose generally do not require supplemental insulin after the first day or two. Experience has shown that a sliding scale insulin dose is used for a day or two to learn daily requirements, then regular insulin is added to the TPN bag with sliding scale insulin used as a backup. Regardless of the regimen that is used, patients with diabetes are carefully monitored throughout TPN therapy, and insulin adjustments are made accordingly.

Hypoglycemic reactions may occur should a TPN solution with greater than 20 percent glucose be suddenly discontinued. A 10 percent glucose in water solution should be hung and run at the same rate as the previous solution until the TPN can be restarted. Any TPN solution that has been interrupted must be discarded.

To avoid the possibility of contamination and degradation of additives (e.g., vitamins), TPN solution containers should be changed every 24 hours. TPN tubing is also changed every 24 to 72 hours, depending on local policy. TPN bags, tubing, and filters are changed daily without exception. Filters prevent problems (e.g., phlebitis) due to particulate contaminants. They are also life saving in cases of precipitates. The 1.2-micron filter is life saving in case of a cracked lipid emulsion. It is thought that the filters assist in preventing infection, although their effectiveness has not been substantiated. Blood, drugs, and other IV fluids are administered through a separate IV line to avoid contamination of the TPN catheter.

Fat Emulsions In general, fat emulsions are administered over an 8- to 12-hour period. The initial infusion rate is 30 mL/hour. Adverse effects usually appear within the first

30 minutes of the infusion, although late reactions are possible. The fat emulsion tubing may be piggybacked into the Y connector on the primary tubing closest to the IV insertion site. By piggybacking the emulsion at this site, the length of time the emulsion is in contact with TPN solution is reduced. Because fat emulsion particles are very large, a 1.2-micron in-line filter is used.

Blood, some drugs, and other IV fluids are administered through a separate IV line to avoid contamination of the fat emulsion. Routine blood work should be delayed until 2 to 6 hours after the infusion of a fat emulsion, so that the extra fat in the blood stream will not distort results. In addition, as much as possible, the patient should not be transported anywhere, because this will cause agitation of the bottle.

Education

Education of the patient who is to receive IV therapy is determined by the patient's needs and the delivery setting. An awareness of the patient's cultural, ethnic, and religious background may be important when considering IV therapy. IV therapy is especially threatening to those who have not experienced it before. The patient and family should be told what the procedure involves and what solution is being used. If there are concerns about the procedure or the fluid being administered, it is important to address those concerns before starting the infusion. The use of blood products is more likely to be of concern than the use of synthetic IV solutions. The patient's religious beliefs may preclude the use of blood products. The patient's beliefs should be noted on the patient's records and appropriate health care providers notified.

In acute care settings with extremely ill patients, in which IV therapy orders may change rapidly, information is given in small amounts and at a very basic level. However, IV therapy is often administered in settings in which a health care provider is not present. In this situation, education of the patient and any other home-based caregivers is important.

First, the patient or caregivers need to understand why the IV therapy is required and how the infusion delivery system works. They need to learn techniques for assessment and care of the access site. They also need basic information about the fluid being administered and any storage precautions, potential complications, or side effects. Finally, they must know what information needs to be documented and how to get professional help when needed.

Providing the information in an organized manner, both verbally and in written form with demonstration and return demonstrations, is effective in increasing the retention of information. Video tapes can be used to educate patients and families involved in long-term home IV therapy.

Fluid and electrolyte imbalances may cause mental status changes, restlessness, and irritability in the patient. Confused patients may play with the IV tubing, change the rate, or dislodge the venous access device. Caregivers should be instructed how to manage the infusion in such a situation. Repeated explanations, as well as protection from injury during the infusion, is important.

Home Intravenous Therapy A patient's desire to stay at home, control care, and minimize the cost of care, coupled with reimbursement concerns focused on shorter lengths of hospital stay, make home IV therapy an increasingly popular option. Patients suitable for home IV therapy include those requiring hydration, TPN, IV drugs for pain control, antibiotics, or cancer chemotherapy. Home IV therapy presents some concerns and implications that are unique. The most significant concern is that of educating the patient and caregivers. The assessment, plan, and interventions for IV therapy are not different in the home, but the need for education of the recipient far exceeds that required for an inpatient setting. Perinatal, pediatric, and geriatric patients in particular, may require more intensive assessment, education, and care depending on their physical, mental, and emotional status. Safe home care therapy can be achieved only through impeccable assessment and education.

Many aspects of education are necessary for home IV therapy. The education content includes:

- Signs and symptoms of excesses and deficits
- Aseptic technique and signs and symptoms of infection
- Mechanics of IV therapy and troubleshooting infusion pumps
- Infusion schedule and rate
- Documentation of response to therapy and for reimbursement
- Emergency care and contacts

Providing education in verbal and written form with clear, concise, and specific guidelines makes IV therapy in the home a safe, viable option. It should be noted that pharmacists cannot dispense home IV drugs without written documentation of proper education of the patient or caregiver.

Coordination of home care services is also a consideration in home IV therapy. Certainly, coordination requires communication with the patient and caregiver, but it also requires communication with pharmacists, health care providers, and equipment companies as well. In order to efficiently and cost effectively provide home therapy, the services must be coordinated to prevent home therapy from becoming fragmented, duplicated, or unsafe.

Home IV therapy poses unique economic problems due to different insurance and other payor requirements. The home care nurse, social worker, and discharge planner play central roles in the process because they know the rules and regulations governing home care and can provide answers to questions regarding reimbursement for home care services.

Evaluation

During the evaluation phase, the health care provider evaluates the effectiveness of IV therapy. The evaluation is based on indicators developed in relation to the pharmacotherapeutic objectives. If the original purpose of therapy was to correct an existing fluid imbalance or nutritional problem, evaluation determines whether the problem has been corrected or alleviated. Skin turgor, the presence or absence of thirst, the presence of absence of edema, growth (in infants), changes in body weight and urine characteristics, and the conditions of mucous membranes (i.e., dry, moist, pink) indicate changes in hydration levels. In situations in which therapy was started as a maintenance or preventive procedure, evaluation ensures that maintenance has been achieved without an excess or deficit occurring.

The health care provider should evaluate the laboratory tests used when monitoring IV therapy. Evaluation of complete blood count, electrolytes, platelet count, prothrombin time, BUN, and liver function studies, as well as carbon dioxide, glucose, creatinine, total protein, uric acid, cholesterol, and triglyceride levels should be undertaken.

Because IV therapy is invasive, the potential for infection and sepsis increases. The insertion site, as well as laboratory tests, should be monitored for signs and symptoms of infection. If infection at the insertion site is suspected, all lines should be removed and the TPN solution and catheter tips should be cultured. Peripheral blood culture is also needed. The culture usually indicates the presence of *Staphlococcus epidermis,* which is most likely caused by poor technique. If the patient receiving TPN complains of sudden chills, fever, or chest or back pain, suspect that the patient has septicemia. Other sources of infection should also be ruled out.

The patient's psychological response to IV therapy should also be evaluated. Did the patient accept the therapy? Because meal times are generally considered a social activity, not eating can have major psychological effects on some patients, even to the point of hallucinating about food. If long-term therapy is required, how is the patient coping with not eating ordinary meals? Are the patient and caregivers able to cope with the prescribed therapy? For the patient receiving TPN therapy, reassurance should be provided that his or her appetite will return to normal when this form of feeding is discontinued.

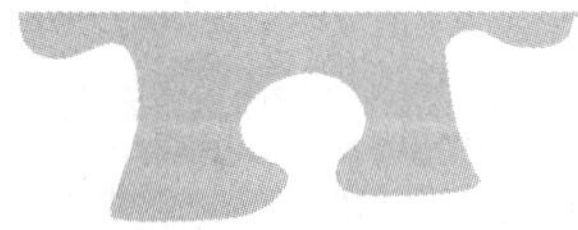

SUMMARY

- IV therapy is an extensively used treatment modality for the purpose of fluid and electrolyte maintenance or replacement, nutritional support, blood and blood component replacement, and drug administration.
- IV therapy requires an understanding of fluids, electrolytes, acid-base balance, and nutrients within the body, as well as the pathophysiology of imbalances.
- Homeostatic organs involved in balance or imbalances include heart and blood vessels, kidneys, lungs, hypothalamus, endocrine glands, and GI tract.
- Fluid and electrolyte balance is also dependent on sufficient carbohydrates, proteins, lipids, vitamins, and minerals.
- Imbalances that occur may result in acidosis or alkalosis or in excesses or deficits of fluids, electrolytes, and nutrients.
- A past history of renal, pulmonary, cardiovascular, or endocrine disorders places the patient at higher risk of complications related to IV therapy.
- The objectives of IV therapy include maintenance of daily requirements, replacement of existing deficits, and restoration of ongoing or concurrent losses.
- Management of a patient receiving IV fluids requires that the health care provider understand the effect of the various solutions on the body and the potential side effects for the patient.
- Solutions that may be used include saline solutions, dextrose solutions, multiple-electrolyte solutions, volume expanders, and parenteral nutrition formulas.
- IV solutions provide nutrients for energy and anabolism, electrolytes for normal physiologic functions, fluids for maintenance of normal levels of ICF and ECF, and ions for acid-base balance.
- Isotonic solutions expand the ICF and ECF compartments equally, while not altering vascular osmolality.
- Hypotonic solutions transcend all membranes from vascular spaces to tissues and cause cells to swell.
- Hypertonic solutions pull fluid from the ICF and interstitial fluid spaces, causing cells to shrink.
- Saline solutions are used to replace fluid losses. Glucose solutions provide calories and hydration for patients who do not need electrolyte replacement. Multiple-electrolyte solutions are used to replace fluids and electrolytes.
- Volume expanders increase the total volume of body fluid. Blood and blood products are used to replace volume, the oxygen-carrying properties of blood, clotting factors, and other components.
- Parenteral nutrition is used to promote protein synthesis, decrease protein breakdown, maintain a positive nitrogen balance, and promote fluid and electrolyte balance.
- Total parenteral nutrition is used to keep the patient in a positive nitrogen balance, provides nutritional support for patients with long-term needs, and promotes growth of new body tissue.
- Fat emulsions are used as an adjunct with TPN to prevent essential fatty acid deficiencies. Fat emulsions have a low tonicity and provide more than twice as much energy as TPN solutions.
- Extensive education of the patient and caregivers is required for safe IV therapy.
- No two patients respond exactly the same to IV therapy. The patient's response depends on many individualized factors, including age, height, weight, general physical condition, and drug and other therapies.
- The more extensive and lengthy the use of IV solutions, the greater the likelihood of complications.
- Complications include fluid overload, infiltration, thrombophlebitis and thromboembolism, pain at the administration site, infection and sepsis, electrolyte imbalance, acid-base imbalance, and reactions to specific IV fluids.

BIBLIOGRAPHY

Armstrong, C., Mayhall, C., and Miller, K. (1990). Clinical predictors of infection of central venous catheters used for total parenteral nutrition. *Infection Control and Hospital Epidemiology,* 11(2), 71–78.

Charnow, J., Fandek, N., and Johnson, P. (Eds.). (1993). *Medication administration & I.V. therapy manual* (2nd ed.). Philadelphia: Springhouse Corporation.

Drug facts and comparisons. (1997). St. Louis: Facts and Comparisons.

Hennessy, K., Orr, M., and Curtas, C. (1990). Nutrition support nursing: A specialty practice: Historical development. *Clinical Nurse Specialist,* 4(2), 67–70.

Horne, M., Heitz, U., and Swearingen, P. (1991). *Fluid, electrolyte and acid-base balance.* St. Louis: Mosby–Year Book.

LaRocca, J. (1994). *Handbook of home care IV therapy.* St. Louis: Mosby.

Lin, E. (1991). Nutrition support: Making the difficult decision. *Cancer Nursing,* 14(5), 261–269.

Marrelli, T. (1994). *Home health standards and documentation guidelines for reimbursement* (2nd ed.). Chicago: Mosby.

McCance, K., and Huether, S. (1998). *Pathophysiology: The biologic basis for disease in adults and children.* St. Louis: Mosby.

Metheny, N. (1996). *Fluid and electrolyte balance: Nursing considerations.* Philadelphia: J. B. Lippincott Company.

National Blood Resource Education Program, Nursing Education Working Group. (1990). *Transfusion therapy guidelines for nurses.* Washington, D.C.: U.S. Department of Health and Human Services.

Perry, S., Pillar, B., and Radany, M. (1990). The appropriate use of high-cost, high-risk technologies: The case of total parenteral nutrition. *Quality Review Bulletin,* 16(6), 214–217.

Phillips, L., and Kuhn, M. (1996). *Manual of I.V. therapeutics.* Philadelphia: F.A. Davis.

Vallerand, A., and Deglin, J. (1995). *Davis's guide for IV medications.* Philadelphia: F. A. Davis.

Weinstein, S. (1996). *Plumer's principles & practices of intravenous therapy* (5th ed.). Philadelphia: J. B. Lippincott.

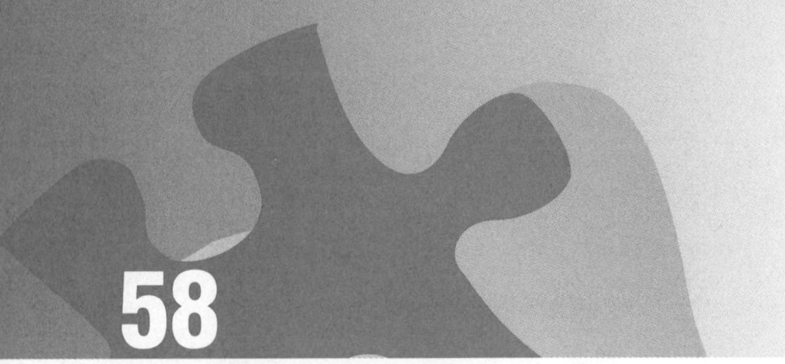

58 Vitamins and Minerals

Consumers are continually seeking ways to stay healthy. And an individual's health may be at risk if the myth that essential vitamins and minerals are obtained if the correct foods are consumed in the appropriate quantities is believed. For decades, this has been the position of the United States Food and Drug Administration (FDA) as well as the health care and food industries. Many of the chronic diseases seen today can be linked to unhealthy life-styles, especially on a nutritional level. Further, more than 30 percent of all patients admitted to acute care facilities demonstrate some degree of malnutrition. Additionally, the nutritional status of patients often deteriorates when hospitalization exceeds 2 weeks.

There are approximately 50 known essential nutrients, including vitamins, minerals, essential fatty acids, and amino acids. These nutrients must be acquired from the diet or from supplements in order to maintain minimal health and to prevent specific deficiency diseases such as pellagra, beriberi, and scurvy. Deficiency diseases, however, are not the common health problems faced in America and other industrialized nations. Modern problems are degenerative diseases, and nutrients play an important role in preventing these conditions.

From a historical perspective, the leading causes of death in the United States have followed three epidemiologic trends. Typhoid, typhus, and yellow fever contributed to high infectious disease mortality rates until the late 1800s. Beginning in 1900, three of the four leading causes of death were infectious diseases. At the start of the new millennium, the epidemiologic trend will be characterized by degenerative and man-made disease. The prevention and therapeutic uses of vitamins and minerals target these conditions.

CURRENT HEALTH ISSUES

Since the 1960s, attention has increasingly focused on the relationship of nutrition to degenerative disease. Although this interest is driven to some degree by the rapid increase in number and longevity of older adults, it is also prompted by the desire to prevent premature deaths from cancer and cardiovascular disease.

Approximately two-thirds of deaths in the United States are caused by degenerative disease. Of the 10 leading causes of death, four are associated with diet (heart disease, stroke, diabetes, and some kinds of cancer) and two with excessive alcohol consumption (accidents and suicide). Further, skipping meals, dieting, and relying on processed and fast foods contribute to nutrient deficiency and the risk of disease later in life. High-risk groups for nutritional deficits include adolescents, women who are pregnant or lactating, and older adults. The consumption of both sugar and caffeine has increased, and only 20 percent of adults consume the recommended five servings of fruits and vegetables daily. In light of these findings, health care providers have started to recognize that individuals suffering from diseases, injury, or other medical conditions have nutrient needs higher than the recommended dietary allowances. Some health care providers recommend that additional nutritional supplements be taken because it is almost impossible to consume the caloric intake needed to provide the required vitamins and minerals. Vitamins and minerals are essential to life and good health, and yet less than 10 percent of Americans meet even the recommended dietary allowances (RDAs).

Recommended Dietary Allowances

The basic American standard for nutrition is the RDA. The RDA specifies the levels of essential nutrients judged to be adequate by the Food and Nutrition Board of the National Academy of Sciences for the daily needs of most healthy adults. These standards are updated periodically to reflect current knowledge. The levels are intended to be met by consuming a wide variety of foods. However, nutrient requirements vary greatly from one person to another. For this reason, the RDAs for most nutrients are designed to exceed average requirements and to ensure that the needs of almost everyone are met. Nutrient intakes falling below those specified by RDAs are not necessarily inadequate, but the risk of deficiency increases the more the intake falls below recommended levels. An overwhelming majority of men and women consume less than 65 percent of the RDA for at least one nutrient.

The RDAs are intended to be applied to the needs of population groups; however, they can reasonably be used to estimate the risk of nutrient deficiency if intakes are averaged over a sufficient period of time. It would be a mistake to assume that individuals whose diets do not meet the RDAs are necessarily malnourished because the RDAs include a margin of safety to allow for individual variations. For this reason, arbitrary cutoff points (e.g., two-thirds of the RDA, 70 percent of the RDA) are frequently used as the levels below which there is a significant risk of nutrient inadequacy. It is equally erroneous to assume that because the average nutrient intakes for a population group meet the RDAs, no malnutrition exists in individuals within that group. Notwithstanding, it has been proposed that the RDAs provide four reference points for each nutrient: (1) a deficient level of intake, (2) average requirements, (3) RDA, and (4) upper safe level of intake. Interactions among nutrients and the potential roles of nutrients and other food constituents in reducing the risk of chronic disease should also be examined.

Nutritional Supplements

The FDA establishes safe standards for the manufacture of both prescription and over-the-counter (OTC) drugs in order to ensure consumer protection. However, vitamin and mineral supplements are not classified as drugs and thus are not controlled by the FDA. The labels on these products rarely inform the consumer about use, safe dosage, or adverse effects.

In 1994, the Dietary Supplement Health and Education Act was signed, giving the FDA more authority to regulate the marketing of dietary supplements. In spite of this law, manufacturers of vitamins, minerals, herbs, botanicals, amino acids, and other dietary supplements do not have to establish the safety of their products before they are sent to market. Instead, the government must prove that a supplement or an ingredient contained in a supplement is unsafe before the product can be taken off the shelves.

VITAMINS

Vitamins are compounds that indirectly assist other nutrients through the processes of digestion, absorption, biotransformation, and elimination. Thirteen vitamins are needed by the body to maintain health. Vitamins are divided into two classes: fat-soluble and water-soluble (see Classification of Vitamins and Minerals).

Each fat-soluble vitamin has a distinct and separate physiologic role. For the most part, these vitamins are absorbed along with other lipids. Efficient absorption requires the presence of bile and pancreatic juice. Then the vitamins are transported to the liver via the lymph system as a part of lipoproteins and stored in various body tissues. Vitamins are not normally eliminated in the urine.

Most water-soluble vitamins are ingredients of essential enzyme systems. Many support energy biotransformation. Water-soluble vitamins are not stored in appreciable amounts and are normally eliminated in small quantities in the urine. Thus, a daily supply is desirable to avoid depletion and interruption of normal physiologic functions.

CLASSIFICATION OF VITAMINS AND MINERALS

Fat-Soluble Vitamins	*Water-Soluble Vitamins*	*Macrominerals*	*Microminerals*
Vitamin A	Vitamin B complex	Sodium	Chromium
Vitamin D	Thiamin (vitamin B_1)	Potassium	Manganese
Vitamin E	Riboflavin (vitamin B_2)	Chloride	Selenium
Vitamin K	Niacin (vitamin B_3)	Calcium	Silicon
	Pantothenic acid	Phosphorus	Vanadium
	Pyridoxine (vitamin B_6)	Magnesium	
	Cyanocobalamin (vitamin B_{12})	Iron	
	Biotin	Zinc	
	Folic acid	Copper	
	Vitamin C	Iodine	

Fat-Soluble Vitamins

VITAMIN A

❒ Vitamin A (AQUASOL A)

Functions

Vitamin A has been named *retinol* in reference to its specific function in the retina of the eye. It is a component of the visual pigments (rhodopsin, iodopsin) and, as such, is essential to the integrity of photoreception in the rods and cones of the retina. Vitamin A also plays an important role in growth and development of skeletal and soft tissues. It is necessary for the development of bone through the effect on protein synthesis and bone cell differentiation and the enamel-forming epithelial cells in the development of teeth. Vitamin A also has a role in maintaining normal epithelial structures by promoting mucin production. It is necessary in the differentiation of basal cells into mucus epithelial cells.

Vitamin A may also play a part in cell membrane regulation as an enzyme co-factor in steroid and mucopolysaccharide synthesis, which is essential in growth and reproduction. It enhances resistance to carcinogenesis, possibly by destabilizing lysosomes or enhancing antitumor immunity, or through direct cytotoxic action on abnormal cells.

Pharmacokinetics

Beta-carotene is responsible for the deep orange and yellow colors in many fruits and vegetables. These provitamin *carotenoids* are converted to vitamin A with varying degrees of efficiency. They are described in terms of *beta-carotene.* Beta-carotene is split in the cytoplasm of the intestinal mucosal cells into retinyl esters. Retinyl esters are transported via the lymph system to the circulation and then to the liver as a part of chylomicrons and lipoproteins. Retinol-binding protein combines with retinol at the time of mobilization from the liver. The esters are removed from the circulation by the kidneys.

Approximately 90 percent of vitamin A is stored in the liver, with the remainder deposited in fat, the lungs, and kidneys. Gradual accumulations of vitamin A in the liver peak in adult life. Hepatic storage of vitamin A allows a temporary reduced intake of vitamin A to take place without a significant impact on body functioning.

The effects of beta-carotene are somewhat different from that of vitamin A. Beta-carotene inactivates single oxygen molecules, which is what make it an *antioxidant.* It is believed that the protective antioxidant function is performed by the intact beta-carotene molecule rather than its vitamin A.

Dietary Sources

Dietary sources of vitamin A are many. Preformed vitamin A occurs only in foods of animal origin, either in storage areas such as the liver or associated with the fat of milk and eggs. It is also found in dark green leafy vegetables, and red-yellow-orange fruits and vegetables. Deeper colors are associated with higher levels of carotenoids. The top 10 provitamin A sources in the American diet include carrots, vegetable soups, sweet potatoes, beef stew, mixed vegetables, and cantaloupe. Vitamin A also appears in fish oils (e.g., cod liver oil, halibut liver oil).

Deficiency States

Vitamin A deficiency is generally associated with malnutrition and infectious disease. In almost every infectious disease, vitamin A deficiency is known to occur in greater frequency and severity, and with an increased incidence of mortality. Vitamin A deficiency results in night blindness, xerophthalmia (abnormal dryness of the conjunctiva and cornea), loss of corneal substance, and scarring.

Vitamin A deficiency produces characteristic changes in skin texture in which blockage of the hair follicles with plugs of keratin causes the skin to become dry, scaly, and rough goose flesh. The changes are first noted on the forearms and thighs, but in advanced states, the whole body can be involved.

There is a shrinking, hardening, and progessive deterioration of epithelial tissues and reduced resistance to invasion by bacteria, viruses, or parasites. Without vitamin A, the protective barrier of mucous membranes is lost. The number of circulating T cells as well as their response is reduced.

An overgrowth of bone with resultant nerve lesions and growth retardation can occur. The growth retardation is characterized by osteoplastosis, impaired protein synthesis, and loss of appetite. The patient may complain of dry, rough skin and vague apathy. An increased risk of lung and gastrointestinal (GI) infections in children can lead to an increased death rate.

Dosage Regimen

The requirement for vitamin A was originally defined in terms of international units (IU), which continue to be in wide use. However, the preferred measurement now expresses vitamin A activity in terms of micrograms (mcg) of retinol, beta-carotene, or other mixed carotenoids. The RDA for vitamin A is identified in Table 58–1. Specific recommendations vary with age, gender, and the patient's reproductive status.

Excess States

Excess vitamin A is stored in the liver, which creates the potential for toxic effects ranging from anorexia and irritability to hepatomegaly and seizures. The earliest signs of *hypervitaminosis A* have been reported in patients with liver disease, children, and pregnant women. Excess retinol causes changes in biologic membranes when the amount ingested exceeds the binding capacity of retinol-binding proteins. Beta-carotene intake that exceeds 300 mg results in orange discoloration of skin, weakness, low blood pressure, weight loss, and low white cell count. Unlike jaundice, in *hypercarotenodermia,* the sclera of the eye is clear. When excess intake of carotene is discontinued, the skin normally clears in a short time.

A single dose of retinol of more than 660,000 IU (200 mg) in adults or 330,000 IU (100 mg) in children can cause hypervitaminosis A. Symptoms include headache, fatigue, weakness, anorexia, nausea, and vomiting. A bulging fontanelle may be seen in children.

Chronic hypervitaminosis A is usually a reflection of intake exceeding 10 times the RDA or 14,000 IU (4.2 mg of retinol) for infants or 33,000 IU (10 mg of retinol) for an adult. Vitamin A consumption that exceeds 10,000 IU/day causes significantly lower plasma glucose and insulin responses to oral glucose than those in individuals taking less than 8000 IU/day. The greater the intake of vitamin A, the more effective insulin is in stimulating glucose disposal. Patient responses to chronic hypervitaminosis A are highly variable. Symptoms disappear in weeks or months when the supplement is discontinued. Vitamin A is also teratogenic, and congenital malformations are likely to develop in fetuses exposed to high levels.

VITAMIN D

- ❒ Calcitriol (vitamin D_3) (CALCIJEX, ROCALTROL)
- ❒ Dihydrotachysterol (DHT) (HYTAKEROL)
- ❒ Ergocalciferol (vitamin D_2) (CALCIFEROL, DRISDOL); (🍁) OSTOFORTE, RADIOSTOL

Functions

Vitamin D plays a role in immmunity, reproduction, insulin secretion, and the differentiation of keratocytes. It is a constituent of the calcium-controlling hormone calcitriol, which promotes the intestinal absorption of calcium and phosphorus. It also stimulates the renal reabsorption of phosphate and stimulates the release of calcium from bone tissue.

Pharmacokinetics

Ingested forms of vitamin D are absorbed from the intestine along with lipids. Vitamin D is bound to vitamin D–plasma–binding protein for transport to storage sites in the liver, skin, brain, bone, and other tissues (Fig. 58–1).

Cholecalciferol (vitamin D_3) is formed in the skin through the action of ultraviolet light on 7-dehydrocholesterol. Cholecalciferol is converted in the liver to the active metabolite, 25-hydroxycholecalciferol (25 OHD_3). 25 OHD_3 is five times as potent as cholecalciferol. The most active form of vitamin D, calcitriol, also known as 1,25-dehydroxycholecalciferol-1,25$(OH)_2D_3$, is produced in the kidneys and is 10 times more potent than cholecalciferol.

Calcitriol increases the uptake of calcium and phosphate from the intestine and on the bone to increase their mobilization. Calcitriol synthesis is regulated by serum levels of calcium and phosphorus. Parathyroid hormone is released in response to low serum calcium levels and appears to stimulate renal production of 1,25$(OH)_2D_3$.

Dietary Sources

Cholecalciferol, formed from 7-dehydrocholesterol, is naturally found in animal foods (e.g., herring [225 IU], salmon [142 IU], sardines [85 IU], chicken liver [45 IU], canned shrimp [30 IU]). It is found in small and highly variable amounts in butter, cream, egg yolks, and liver. The best food sources of vitamin D are fish liver oils. Approximately 98 percent of all milk is fortified with 10 mcg/quart (400 IU/quart) of irradiated ergosterol (vitamin D_2). Most powdered milk and evaporated milk are also fortified, as well as some margarines, butter, certain cereals, and infant formulas. Milk used to make cheese or yogurt is not ordinarily fortified.

Deficiency States

Vitamin D deficiency causes inadequate absorption of calcium and phosphorus. This deficiency, in turn, leads to low levels of serum calcium and stimulation of parathyroid hormone secretion. The elevated parathyroid hormone secretion raises serum calcium levels by moving calcium from

TABLE 58–1 DOSAGE REGIMEN OF SELECTED VITAMINS

Vitamin	Primary Prevention*	Maximum Dosage for Correction of Deficiencies	Implications
Fat-Soluble Vitamins			
Vitamin A	420–1800 mcg po daily (1400–6000 IU)	300 mcg po daily as a single dose (100,000 IU)	1 IU = 0.3 mcg retinol
Vitamin D	10 mcg po daily (400 IU)	Malabsorption: 50,000 IU Uncomplicated deficiency: 1000 IU	1 IU = 0.025 mcg pure crystalline vitamin D
Vitamin E	3–4 mg α-TE po daily (4–15 IU)	100 mg po daily	1 IU = 1 mg α-TE
Vitamin K	1 mcg/kg,† *TPN:* 2–10 mg IM/IV weekly. *Hemorrhagic disease of newborn:* 0.5–1 mg SC/IM/IV within 1 hr of birth	2.5–10 mg po/SC/IM/IV. May repeat in 12–48 hr if necessary or in 6–8 hr after parenteral dose. Maximum: 25–50 mg	There is no standardized unit of measurement
Water-Soluble Vitamins			
Thiamin (B_1)	0.5 mg/1000 kcal with a minimum of 1 mg/day regardless of total intake	*Adults:* 5–10 mg po TID *or* 5–100 mg IM/IV TID *Child:* 10–50 mg po in divided doses *or* 10–25 mg/day IM/IV	Sensitivity reactions and death from IV administration have occurred. An intradermal test dose is recommended in patients with suspected sensitivity
Riboflavin (B_2)	0.4–1.8 mg daily po	*Adult:* 5–30 mg po daily in divided doses for several days, then 1–4 mg/day *Child over 12 yr:* 3–10 mg/day for several days, then 0.6 mg/1000 calories ingested	Patients self-administering should be cautioned not to exceed the RDA
Niacin (B_3)	10–20 mg daily po	*Adults:* Up to 500 mg po daily *or* 50–100 mg IM/SC 5 or more times daily *or* 25–100 mg IV 2 or more times daily *Child:* Up to 300 mg po daily in divided doses	Niacin activity expressed in niacin equivalents (NE) 1 mg of niacin or 60 mg of tryptophan = 1 NE. Patients self-administering should be cautioned not to exceed the RDA
Pantothenic acid (B_5)	4–7 mg	No recommendation available	
Pyridoxine (B_6)	2–10 mg daily	*Drug-induced deficiency:* 50–200 mg daily po/IM/IV for 3 weeks, then 25–100 mg/day *Chronic alcoholism:* 50 mg po daily for 2–4 weeks. May be continued indefinitely *Pyridoxine-dependency syndrome:* 30–600 mg/day IM/IV initially, then 50 mg/day po for life *Isoniazid overdose (over 10 g):* Amount in mg equal to amount of isoniazid ingested given as 4 g IV, then 1 g IM q30 min	A pyridoxine dose of 0.016 mg parallels the intake of 6 g of protein. Dosages vary depending on specific use
Cyanocobalamin (B_{12})	2.5–3 mg daily po	*Adults:* 1–25 mcg/day po to 100 mcg daily. *or* 30 mcg/day IM/SC for 6–7 days, then 100–200 mcg/month. Doses up to 1000 mcg have been used	Hydroxocobalamin is better absorbed than cyanocobalamin since absorption from GI tract requires intrinsic factor and calcium
Folic acid	35–200 mcg daily po Pregnancy: 400 mcg daily Lactation: 280 mcg daily	1000 mcg daily	Patients self-administering should be cautioned not to exceed the RDA.
Ascorbic acid	50–100 mg	*Adults:* 100–250 mg po/IV/IM/SC one to three times daily *Child:* 100–300 mg/day po/IV/IM/SC in divided doses	100 mg for smokers is recommended for smokers under primary prevention

*Specific recommendations vary with age, gender, and reproductive status.

†There are no specific recommendations for vitamin K when used for primary prevention. Dosage is an estimated minimum daily requirement. Dosage is also given for prevention of hypoprothrombinemia for patients on total parenteral nutrition.

TPN, Total parenteral nutrition; α-TE, alpha-tocopherol equivalent.

the bone into serum. In adults, this movement manifests as *osteomalacia,* a condition characterized by decreased bone density and strength. Osteomalacia is more likely to occur during times of increased need for calcium, such as during pregnancy and lactation. In children, this sequence of events produces inadequate mineralization of bones, a condition known as rickets. Rachitic bones are unable to withstand ordinary stresses and strains, resulting in the appearance of bowlegs, knock knees, pigeon breasts, and frontal bossing of the skull. Because of vitamin D fortification of foods, rickets is now rare in the United States.

Dosage Regimen

The normal adult is assumed to obtain sufficient vitamin D from sunlight exposure and the incidental ingestion of small amounts in foods. However, dark-skinned persons may have only 5 percent of ultraviolet light penetrate the

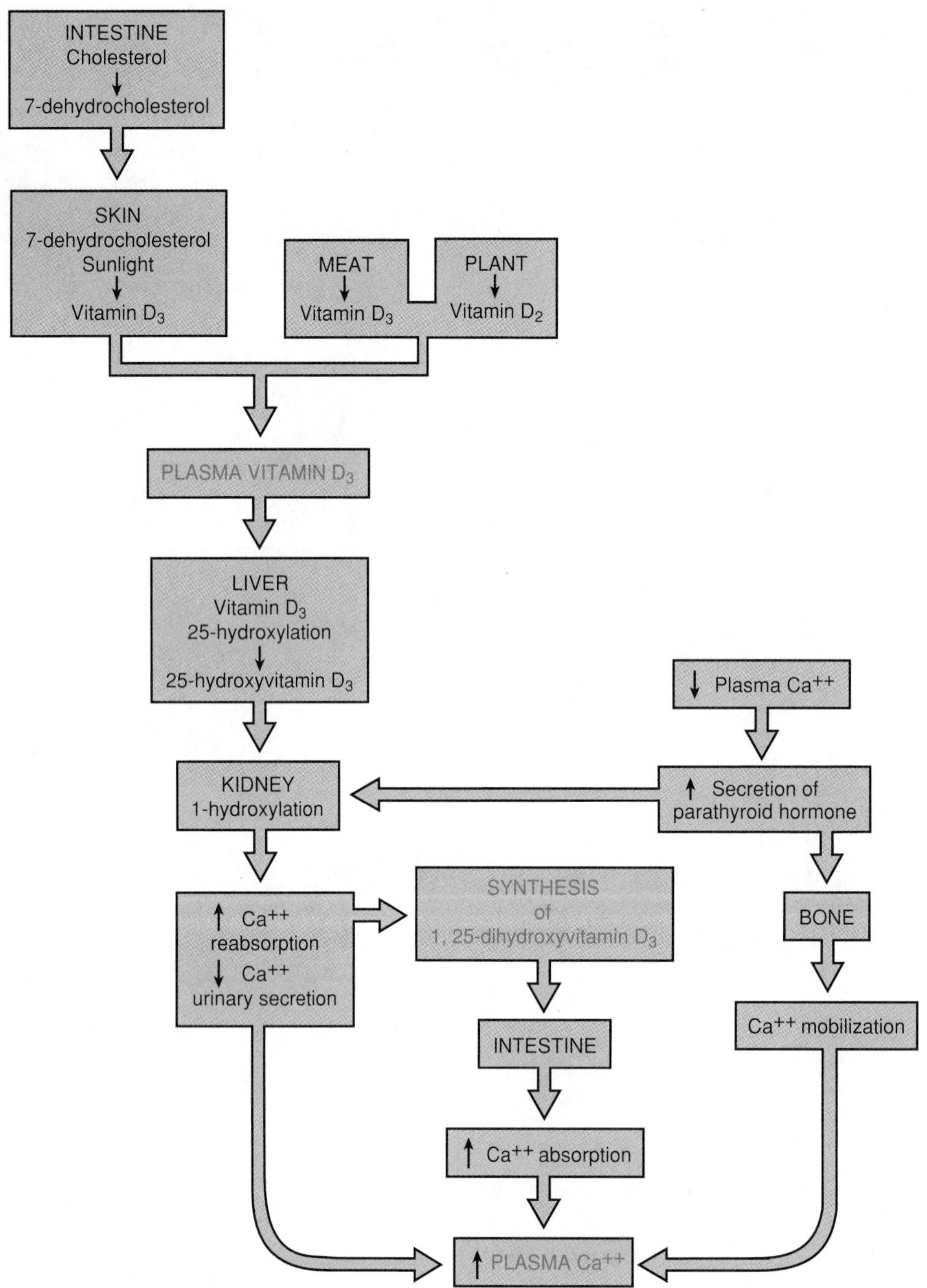

Figure 58–1 Vitamin D and calcium interaction. Vitamin D is converted to 25-hydroxyvitamin D_3 (25[OH]D_3) in the liver and to 1,25-dihydroxyvitamin D_3 in the kidneys. Regulation of plasma calcium concentration is controlled by vitamin D and parathyroid hormone (PTH). Vitamin D and PTH regulate plasma calcium concentration by acting on the intestines, kidneys, and bone. (Adapted from Page, C. P., Curtis, M. J., Sutter, M. C., et al. (1997). *Integrated pharmacology* [pp. 496–497]. St. Louis: Mosby. Used with permission.)

deeper layers of the skin, where vitamin D is synthesized. Pigementation is limiting only if exposure periods to ultraviolet light are short. With longer exposure and a higher intensity of exposure, the same circulating concentration of cholecalciferol can be obtained.

Supplemental vitamin D is not required except for persons who are chronically shielded from sunlight. These may be persons who are homebound, living in sunless areas with high atrmospheric pollution, those who wear clothing that completely covers the body, or those working at night and staying indoors during the day. Circumstances that require long submarine voyages and living in the Antarctic require a small daily supplement of vitamin D.

Excess States

Acute *hypervitaminosis D* results from high dosage (over 70,000 IU) or prolonged administration of vitamin D. It develops with dosages 12 times the RDA. Chronic toxicity can occur with ingestion of 10,000 IU. Hypervitaminosis D produces signs and symptoms of hypercalcemia. The signs and symptoms of hypercalcemia include weakness, fatigue, lassitude, headache, nausea, vomiting, diarrhea, renal impairment, and hypertension. Calcification of soft tissues tends to develop. This calcification is most dangerous in the kidneys. High serum calcium is the most serious complication in patients with heart failure who are taking cardiac glycosides because calcium excess tends to increase the risk of toxicity to these drugs. The first step in the treatment of vitamin D excess is to stop the intake.

Vitamin D excess may also cause cessation of growth for up to 6 months, and permanent stunting of stature may result. Persons who have had hypervitaminosis D may retain permanent hypersensitivity to normal doses of the vitamin.

VITAMIN E

❒ Vitamin E (alpha tocopherol; AQUASOL E, E-200, E-400, E-1000, E-COMPLEX-600, E-VITAMIN, VITA-PLUS E); (🍁) WEBBER VITAMIN E

Functions

Vitamin E has both antioxidant properties and immune integrity properties. It both enhances and protects the immune system. Vitamin E appears to prevent cellular and subcellular membranes from deterioration by scavenging oxygen-containing free radicals. The scavenging prevents free radicals from catalyzing peroxidation of the polyunsaturated fatty acids (PUFAs) that constitute the structural components of cells. The destruction leads to abnormal cellular structure and compromised cellular function. The ability of vitamin E to circumvent such destruction has led to the notion that it may be useful in preventing conditions associated with free radical destruction (e.g., aging, the effects of environmental toxins, some forms of carcinogenesis).

Some health care providers believe that vitamin E helps reduce menopausal symptoms such as hot flashes, feminine dryness, and shrinkage. The antioxidant properties of vitamin E have been associated with the healing of chronic resistant dermatitis of the hands.

Vitamin E can antagonize vitamin K and should not be used by patients undergoing treatment for blood clotting disorders.

Pharmacokinetics

Vitamin E activity in foods is contributed by the *tocopherols* (α, β, τ, Δ) and the tocotrienols. It acts to prevent peroxidation of PUFAs. Vitamin E resides inside low-density lipoprotein particles to prevent renal elimination of vitamin molecules and disarms the free radicals from within. This activity explains its important characteristic as an antioxidant. The absorption of vitamin E is inefficient, ranging between 20 and 80 percent. Vitamin E is stored in the liver and to a larger extent in fatty tissues. It is biotransformed in the liver, entering the enterohepatic circulation. The metabolites are eventually eliminated in both the urine and feces.

Dietary Sources

Since vitamin E is fat soluble, the richest sources are high-fat foods like vegetable oils. Seed oils (e.g., wheat germ oil, corn oil, soybean oil, sunflower oil) are the richest source of vitamin E. Smaller amounts are present in fruits, vegetables, and animal fats. Peanut, olive, coconut, and fish oils are poor sources of vitamin E.

Deficiency States

Vitamin E deficiencies are uncommon. When they are present, they are usually related to malabsorption or lipid transport abnormalities (e.g., abetalipoproteinemia). Deficiency of vitamin E is associated with symptoms of peripheral neuropathy. A deficiency of vitamin E lowers host resistance by depressing the proliferation of lymphocytes, lowering the antibody response to pathogens, and lowering delayed hypersensitivity reactions. These responses have an impact on the immunologic response to cancers, helminthic infestations, and chronic infections.

Newborns have low tissue concentrations of vitamin E because little vitamin E is transferred across placental membranes. Breast milk contains a sufficient amount of vitamin E to meet the needs of a breastfeeding infant.

Dosage Regimen

An exact dosage recommendation for vitamin E is not possible because the consumption of PUFAs varies significantly among individuals. There is no evidence that vitamin E deficiency exists in the United States; thus, the RDA is based on the amount consumed in the average American diet.

Vitamin E activity is expressed in milligrams of alpha tocopherol equivalents (α-TE). The average American's intake of α-TE is estimated to be 7.4 to 9 mg α-TE/day. The average intake of PUFA is 21 g/day. This is equivalent to an α-TE:PUFA ratio of 0.4.

Excess States

The risk of vitamin E toxicity is relatively low, even at relatively high levels. Toxicity occurs with more than 4000 IU of vitamin E per day. Some health care providers have noted signs and symptoms of toxicity with an intake as low as 2000 IU/day. Signs and symptoms of excess include headache, fatigue, blurred vision, and diarrhea. Vitamin E toxicity in preterm infants is characterized by respiratory distress, renal failure, liver disease, ascites, and thrombocytopenia.

VITAMIN K

❒ Phytonadione (AQUAMEPHYTON, MEPHYTON)

Functions

Vitamin K functions as a lipid co-factor for membrane-bound peptide carboxylase. The co-factor is essential for the formation of prothrombin (factor II), proconvertin (factor VII), plasma thromboplastin component (factor IX), and Stuart factor (factor X) in the liver. The cascade theory of blood coagulation is noted in Figure 36–1 in Chapter 36. Vitamin K may also participate in oxidative phosphorylation in the tissues.

Pharmacokinetics

Vitamin K occurs naturally in two forms: phylloquinone (vitamin K_1), which is found in green plant foods, and menaquinone (vitamin K_2), which is formed as the result of bacterial action in the intestinal tract. Phylloquinone and menaquinone are also available in water-soluble formulations. The fat-soluble synthetic formulation menadione (vitamin K_3) is twice as potent as primary food sources for vitamin K_3.

Vitamin K is primarily absorbed from the upper intestine in the presence of bile and dietary fats. It is incorporated into chylomicrons and lipoproteins, and carried to the liver. None of the forms of vitamin K are stored in large quantities in the body. Vitamin K is biotransformed in the liver and eliminated in the urine and feces.

Dietary Sources

Dietary sources of large quantities of vitamin K include green, leafy vegetables, particularly kale, turnip greens, spinach, broccoli, cabbage, and lettuce. Other vegetables (cauliflower, tomatoes), fruits, cereals (wheat bran), dairy products (cheese, egg yolks) and meat (liver) contain smaller amounts. An average mixed diet contains 300 to 500 mcg/day of vitamin K. Significant amounts are formed by the bacterial flora in the GI tract.

Deficiency States

Vitamin K deficiency is usually associated with inadequate intake or absorption. Deficiency is common in newborns owing to the lack of dietary intake of vitamin K and the lack of intestinal synthesis of the vitamin during the first week of life. After infancy, deficiency usually results from diseases that interfere with absorption (biliary tract and GI disorders) or use of vitamin K (cirrhosis, hepatitis). In persons who consume large quantities of alcohol, deficiency is related to decreased intake and impaired use. Drug-induced deficiency develops with use of oral anticoagulants or other drugs that act as vitamin K antagonists. Deficiency is also possible with the use of antibiotics because they reduce the synthesis of bacteria in the intestine. Deficiency caused by antibiotic use is rare, however.

The signs and symptoms of vitamin K deficiency include petechiae, ecchymosis, bleeding into the joints or muscles, hematemesis, hematuria, GI bleeding, asthenia, and hypovolemic shock.

Dosage Regimen

The dosage regimen of vitamin K is usually expressed in micrograms, although no standard unit of measurement has been identified. The RDA for vitamin K is 65 to 70 mcg daily. Half of this amount is supplied by the intestinal synthesis by bacteria and the remainder by dietary intake of vitamin K–containing foods.

Excess States

An excess of vitamin K is unlikely to occur from dietary intake. It may occur when vitamin K is used as an antagonist to oral anticoagulants, although clinical manifestations rarely develop. When vitamin K is given to a patient who is receiving oral anticoagulants, the patient will be resistant to the drug for a period of 2 to 3 weeks. Elevated plasma levels of vitamin K are seen in patients with hypertriglyceridemia. Excessive doses of synthetic vitamin K have produced kernicterus in an infant. The water-miscible forms of vitamin K have a much wider margin of safety.

Water-Soluble Vitamins

THIAMINE

❒ Thiamine (BIAMINE); (🍁) BETAXIN, BEWON

Functions

Thiamine (vitamin B_1), in either its pyrophosphate or triphosphate form, functions as a coenzyme vital in Krebs' cycle. Although thiamine is essential for biotransformation of fats, proteins, and nucleic acids, it is most strongly associated with the oxidative decarboxylation of pyruvate, which is concerned only with carbohydrate biotransformation, to acetyl coenzyme A. Without thiamine triphosphate, pyruvate cannot enter Krebs' cycle and energy deprivation results. In addition, the triphosphate form is also involved in the oxidative decarboxylation of alpha keto acids derived from the amino acids methionine, threonine, leucine, isoleucine, and valine. Thiamine triphosphate also functions as an alternate pathway for glucose oxidation. It plays a role in the transmission of impulses on nerve membranes, possibly by promoting sodium influx.

Pharmacokinetics

Thiamine is well absorbed from the GI tract and widely distributed to body tissues. It crosses the intestinal membranes by active transport systems in specific areas of the small intestine. Plasma protein binding is minimal. Thiamine is stored in variable degrees in the liver and eliminated through the kidneys.

Dietary Sources

Dietary sources of thiamine include meat, poultry, fish, egg yolk, dried beans, whole grain cereal products, and peanuts.

Deficiency States

Thiamine deficiencies are no longer common in the United States, but when it does occur, it is usually related to the overconsumption of refined foods (e.g. white flour, sugar). These foods displace nutrient-rich whole foods in the diet. Alcohol-related thiamine deficiency (Wernicke-Korsakoff syndrome) is the third most common cause of dementia in the United States. A deficiency of thiamine also leads to a reduced production of antibodies and increases the risk for infection.

Signs and symptoms of thiamine deficiency (*beriberi*) include confusion, tachycardia, and an enlarged heart. So-called dry beriberi is associated with muscular wasting, energy deprivation, inactivity, and peripheral neuropathy with paralysis of the lower extremities. So-called wet beriberi is precipitated by a high carbohydrate intake, along with strenuous physical exertion. It is characterized by peripheral edema due to biventricular heart failure with pulmonary edema.

Infantile beriberi, although rare, has been identified in infants fed unusual formulas without adequate thiamine supplementation. Deterioration of the infant occurs suddenly with cardiac failure and cyanosis.

Dosage Regimen

Because of the close relationship between thiamine and energy biotransformation, the RDA is based on energy intake. The RDA for children, adolescents, and adults is 0.5 mg/1000 kcal, with a minimum of 1 mg/day regardless of total intake. An additional 0.4 mg/day is recommended for pregnant women and 0.5 mg/day during lactation to allow for increased energy needs and the elimination of thiamine in breast milk.

Excess States

There are no known toxic effects from thiamine.

RIBOFLAVIN

❒ Riboflavin

Functions

Riboflavin (vitamin B_2) is a constituent of two coenzymes: flavin mononucleotide and flavin adenine dinucleotide. It is essential for the completion of several reactions in the energy cycle that produces adenosine triphosphate (ATP). It is also a component of amino acid oxidases and xanthine oxidase that are involved in the oxidation of amino acids and hydroxy acids to alpha keto acids and the oxidation of a number of purines. It may also function in the production of corticosteroids and red blood cells, as well as in gluconeogenesis.

Pharmacokinetics

Riboflavin is well absorbed from the proximal small intestine in the presence of food. Plasma protein binding is minimal. Although riboflavin is stored in small amounts in the liver and kidney, the quantities stored are not sufficient to meet all of the body's needs. Thus, riboflavin must be regularly supplied in the diet. Riboflavin is biotransformed in the liver to variable degrees and eliminated in the urine depending on the intake and relative need of the tissues for the vitamin.

Dietary Sources

The best dietary sources of riboflavin are milk (fresh, canned, or powdered), cheddar cheese, and cottage cheese. Organ meats (e.g., beef liver) contain appreciable amounts of riboflavin. Other lean meats, eggs, and green, leafy vegetables are also important sources of riboflavin. Riboflavin is synthesized by intestinal bacteria but not in appreciable amounts. Sixty percent of riboflavin is lost when flour is milled; thus, most breads and cereals are enriched with riboflavin.

Deficiency States

Riboflavin deficiencies usually occur in combination with deficiencies of other water-soluble vitamins. The deficiency must exist for several months for signs and symptoms of riboflavin deficiency to appear. Early signs of *ariboflavinosis* include photophobia, lacrimation, burning and itching of the eyes, capillary overgrowth around the cornea, glossitis, angular stomatitis (cracks in the corners of the mouth), and cheilosis (fissuring of the lips). Eye disorders such as burning, itching, lacrimation, photophobia, and vascularization of the cornea are possible. Seborrheic dermatitis, a greasy eruption of the skin in the nasolabial folds, scrotum, or vulva, may appear.

Dosage Regimen

Riboflavin requirements are based on the amount required to maintain tissue reserves, as well as on urinary elimination, red blood cell riboflavin levels, and erythrocyte glutathione reductase activity. The RDA for riboflavin in an average healthy adult is 1.7 mg/day. Requirements are increased during pregnancy and lactation (1.3 mg/day).

Excess States

There are no known toxic effects for riboflavin.

NIACIN

❒ Niacin (NIA-BID, NIACOR, NICO-400, NICOBID, NICOLAR, NICOTINEX, SLO-NIACIN); (🍁) NOVO-NIACIN

❒ Niacinamide (nicotinamide)

Functions

Niacin (vitamin B_3) is the generic term for nicotinamide (niacinamide) and nicotinic acid. It is obtained from food and the endogenous synthesis from tryptophan. It is essential for glycolysis, fat synthesis and tissue respiration. It functions as a coenzyme in many metabolic processes after being converted to nicotinamide, the physiologically active form. Large doses of niacin decrease lipoprotein and triglyceride synthesis by inhibiting the release of free fatty acids from adipose tissue and decreasing hepatic lipoprotein synthesis. It lowers total cholesterol and raises high-density lipoprotein levels (see also Chapter 35). Because niacin is easily converted to niacinamide, it is frequently used therapeutically in that form to avoid the vasodilating effect of nicotinic acid.

The timed-release form of niacin helps reduce hypoglycemic symptoms, especially during withdrawal from sugar. It can also lower blood pressure and improve circulation by dilating blood vessels. Because of this action, some individuals experience flushing of the skin similar to that produced by an allergic reaction. This flushing is not harmful and usually disappears within 15 to 20 minutes. However, timed-release niacin must be used with caution because it can sometimes cause elevation of liver enzymes, and on rare occasions, it can cause hepatitis in sensitive individuals. Another form of niacin is inositol hexaniacinate, which causes no flushing, liver problems, uric acid elevations, or histamine-induced gastric acid release. It has the same cholesterol-lowering capacity as regular niacin. Niacin has been found to reduce migraine headaches, reduce dizziness found in Ménière's disease, and reduce the symptoms of Raynaud's phenomenon.

Pharmacokinetics

The absorption of niacin takes place in the small intestine. Only a small amount of niacin is stored in the body. Excess niacin is eliminated through the kidneys in the urine.

Dietary Sources

The richest sources of niacin are organ meats, brewer's yeast, and peanuts and peanut butter. Lean meats, poultry, and fish are also rich sources of niacin. These foods are rich in both niacin and tryptophan. Most foods rich in animal protein are also rich in tryptophan. Although milk and eggs contain small amounts of niacin, they are excellent sources of tryptophan. To lesser degrees, beans, peas and other legumes, most nuts, and whole grains or enriched cereals also contain niacin and tryptophan. Intestinal bacteria synthesize some niacin.

Deficiency States

Niacin deficiency is most common in persons who have severely inadequate diets with very little protein. Early niacin deficiency manifests as muscular weakness, anorexia, indigestion, and skin eruptions. Severe niacin deficiency leads to *pellagra,* which is characterized by skin eruptions, dementia, diarrhea, tremors, and sore tongue. The skin is cracked and pigmented, and scaly dermatitis is present in the areas that are exposed to sunlight. Lesions of the central nervous system (CNS) lead to confusion, hallucinations, disorientation, and impairment of peripheral motor and sensory nerves. Inflammation of the mucous membranes of the GI tract causes digestive abnormalities.

Dosage Regimen

Niacin activity is expressed in niacin equivalents (NEs). One milligram of niacin or 60 mg of tryptophan equals 1 NE. Niacin dosages range from 5 to 20 mg daily for primary prevention to as much as 600 mg daily to correct severe nutritional deficiency. Nicotinamide is the preferred drug because it does not cause the unpleasant flushing and burning sensations that accompany nicotinic acid therapy. Patient response to nicotinamide becomes observable within 24 hours, with cessation of diarrhea and less redness of the tongue. In some cases, the CNS manifestations of pellagra may never respond, most likely because of a previous prolonged state of malnutrition.

Excess States

The large doses of niacin (2 to 6 g daily) that are used to treat hyperlipidemia (types I and II) result in transient flushing, headache, cramps, and nausea and vomiting, as well as increased blood sugar and uric acid levels. Liver function tests reflect hepatic response to excess niacin.

PANTOTHENIC ACID

Functions

Pantothenic acid (B_5) is needed to restore normal adrenal function, which can become depleted in times of stress. As a vital constituent of acetyl coenzyme A, it is involved in the release of energy from carbohydrates and in the degradation and biotransformation of fatty acids. In addition to functioning in the citric acid cycle, it is involved in the synthesis of cholesterol, phospholipids, steroid hormones, and orphyrin for hemoglobin and choline.

Pharmacokinetics

Pantothenic acid is readily absorbed from the GI tract. It is distributed to all tissues. Pantothenic acid is apparently not degraded in the body because the intake and elimination of the vitamin are approximately equal. Approximately 70 percent of the absorbed pantothenic acid is eliminated in the urine.

Dietary Sources

Pantothenic acid is present in all plant and animal tissues. Primary sources of pantothenic acid include egg yolk, kidney, liver, and yeast. Broccoli, lean beef, skim milk, sweet potatoes, and molasses are also fair sources of pantothenic acid. Much of the pantothenate in meat is lost during thawing and cooking. Approximately half of the pantothenic acid contained in flour is lost in the milling process.

Deficiency States

No deficiency state has been identified with pantothenic acid, although a deficiency can lead to depression, fatigue, and insomnia.

Dosage Regimen

A daily intake of 4 to 7 mg of pantothenic acid is most likely sufficient for adults. A higher intake may be needed in pregnant or lactating women. The average intake of pantothenic acid in the American diet ranges from 5 to 20 mg/day.

Excess States

No serious toxic effects of pantothenic acid are known. However, ingestion of large amounts may cause diarrhea.

PYRIDOXINE

❒ Pyridoxine (NESTREX, RODEX); (🍁) HEXA-BETALIN

Functions

Pyridoxine (vitamin B_6) has three interchangeable forms (pyridoxine, pyridoxal, and pyridoxamine) that are coenzymes serving a role in many metabolic functions. These three forms convert to the coenzyme pyridoxal phospate (PLP). The functions of pyridoxine include decarboxylation, transamination, transulfuration, and the conversion of tryptophan to niacin. It is required for glycogenolysis, the synthesis of hemoglobin, and the formation of antibodies. The formation of sphingolipids involved in the development of the myelin sheath surrounding nerve cells is also pyridoxine-dependent. Pyridoxine may also be required for the conversion of linoleic acid to arachidonic acid, as well as for the formation and regulation of neurotransmitters such as epinephrine, norepinephrine, tyramine, dopamine, serotonin, and gamma-aminobutyric acid.

Pharmacokinetics

All three forms of pyridoxine are absorbed by the mucosal cells of the upper small intestine. They are phosphorylated here to form pyridoxal phosphate and pyridoxamine phosphate. Pyridoxal phosphate is distributed bound to plasma albumin. Some pyridoxine is stored in the body, but a large percentage is eliminated in the urine. Fifty percent of the total body content of pyridoxine is stored in muscle.

Dietary Sources

Dietary sources of pyridoxine include yeast, wheat germ, pork, glandular meats (particularly liver), whole grain cereals, legumes, potatoes, bananas, and oatmeal. Milk, eggs, vegetables, and fruit contain small amounts.

Deficiency States

Pyridoxine deficiency occurs as the result of inadequate intake or impaired absorption, although it is relatively rare. There are many drugs, however, that interfere with the biotransformation or performance of pyridoxine, particularly cycloserine, isoniazid, hydralazine, and penicillamine (see Appendix C). Signs and symptoms of pyridoxine deficiency include skin and mucous membrane lesions, malaise, depression, and glucose intolerance. Extreme deficiency leads to CNS abnormalities in infants whose formulas do not contain pyridoxine. A deficiency syndrome has been noted in mentally retarded children with an inborn error of pyridoxine biotransformation. The inborn error manifests as uncontrollable seizures. Pyrixodine supplementation must be started in the neonatal period to prevent irreversible mental retardation.

Dosage Regimen

The RDA for pyridoxine is noted in Table 58–1. Pyridoxine requirements increase as protein intake increases. Pyridoxine intake appears adequate when the vitamin is taken in a ratio of 0.016 mg/1 g of protein. The RDA is two times the daily RDA for protein. Additional protein intake during pregnancy and lactation parallel the increase needed in pyridoxine. Pyridoxine levels in breast milk correlate with the adequate intake in the maternal diet. Infants to age 6 months should have 0.3 mg/day, and 0.6 mg/day should be given to older infants. The RDAs for children and adolescents are based on average protein intake.

Although the approach is considered to be controversial, up to 500 mg of pyridoxine has been shown to be effective in the treatment of premenstrual syndrome, and dosages as high as 250 mg have been used for the treatment of carpal tunnel syndrome.

Excess States

The risk of toxicity to pyridoxine is low; however, prolonged ingestion of high doses has resulted in severe ataxia and sensory neuropathy. Discontinuation of the drug has resulted in complete recovery within 6 months.

COBOLAMIN

- ❒ Cyanocobalamin (CRYSTAMINE, CRYSTI 1000, CYANOJECT, CYOMIN); (🍁) ANACOBIN, RUBION
- ❒ Hydroxocobalamin (HYDROBEXAN, HYDRO COBEX, HYDRO-CRYSTI 12, LA-12)

Functions

Cobalamin (B_{12}) is essential to biotransformation of all cells, particularly those of the GI tract, bone marrow, and CNS. It is also required for normal red blood cells, growth, and the biotransformation of carbohydrate, proteins, and fats. Along with folic acid, choline, and methionine, cobalamin participates in the synthesis of nucleic acids, purine, and pyrimidines. It is also vital to DNA synthesis, and it affects myelin formation.

Pharmacokinetics

Hydrochloric acid in the stomach releases cobalamin from its peptide bonds. In the presence of intrinsic factor from the stomach, cobalamin is absorbed in the intestinal tract. The cobalamin/intrinsic factor complex is absorbed in the membranes of the ileum. Calcium is necessary for the transfer to occur to pinocytotic vesicles. Once it is absorbed, cobalamin circulates bound to plasma proteins. The highest concentrations of cobalamin are found in the liver and, to some extent, in the kidney. Enterohepatic circulation recycles cobalamin from bile and other intestinal secretions; thus, it may take 5 or 6 years for a cobalamin deficiency to manifest. Excess cobalamin is eliminated in the urine.

Dietary Sources

The richest dietary sources of cobalamin are liver, kidney, milk, eggs, fish, cheese, and muscle meats. Some cooked sea vegetables contain cobalamin in the same concentration as beef liver. Well over half of the cobalamin (40 to 90 percent) is lost during pasteurization and evaporation. Vegetables contain cobalamin only through contamination or bacterial synthesis. The small amount of cobalamin that is synthesized in humans is not absorbed because the synthesis takes place in the colon beyond the terminal ileum.

Deficiency States

Cobalamin deficiency produces megaloblastic or pernicious anemia. *Megaloblastic anemia* is associated with glossitis, hypospermia, GI disorders, decreased numbers of but abnormally large red blood cells, fatigue, and dyspnea. With severe deficiency, leukopenia, thrombocytopenia, cardiac arrhythmias, heart failure, and infections may occur. Megaloblastic anemia precedes neurologic changes in the majority of patients. Subacute degeneration of cerebral white matter in the brain, optic nerves, spinal cord, and peripheral nerves has been noted. Symptoms include numbness, tingling, and burning of the feet, as well as stiffness and generalized weakness of the legs.

Cobalamin deficiency presenting in the older adult manifests as yellow skin tones resulting from concurrent anemia and jaundice due to ineffective erythropoiesis; a smooth, beefy red tongue; and neurologic disorders. Impaired mentation and depression may also be present, although these findings may also be related to elevated homocysteine levels.

Dosage Regimen

Vitamin B_{12} deficiencies can be corrected by administering cyanocobalamin, a purified, crystalline form of vitamin B_{12}, either parenterally or orally through a nutritional supplement if malabsorption is not the primary problem. Parenterally, cyanocobalamin can be administered by intramuscular (IM) or deep subcutaneous injection. It should never be given IV. After the condition is corrected, 100 mcg will be required to maintain life-long health. Normal RDAs of cyanobalamin range from 0.3 mcg/day for infants to 3 mcg/day for adults. This amount provides for substantial body stores in view of the increasing prevalence of achlorhydria, atrophic gastritis, and pernicious anemia in persons older than 60 years of age. Additional cyanocobalamin is recommended during pregnancy and lactation. By increasing a man's vitamin B_{12} to 1000 mcg/day, sperm production can increase to over 100 million.

Excess States

No toxic effects of cobalamin are known. Dosages as high as 100 mcg/day have been taken without apparent harm.

FOLIC ACID

❐ Folic acid (folate); (🍁) APO-FOLIC, NOVO-FOLACID

Functions

Folic acid is also known as folacin, folate, and pteroylglutamic acid. It forms coenzymes known as tetrahydrofolates involved in one-carbon transfers in biotransformation. Folic acid is essential for the synthesis of the purines guanine and adenine and of the pyrimidine thymine, compounds necessary to DNA and RNA synthesis. Folic acid and cobalamin regulate the formation of red blood cells in the bone marrow. It serves as a single carbon carrier in the formation of heme.

Folic acid may be important in the protection against cervical cancer. For example, folic acid can reverse cervical dysplasia, which prevents cervical cancer, and it is also helpful in the prevention of lung cancer. Other uses of folic acid include the prevention and treatment of gum disease and gout.

Pharmacokinetics

Folic acid is broken down to a monoglutamate form by enzymes from the pancreas and the intestinal mucosa. It is then absorbed by carrier-mediated active transport. A small percentage of folic acid is absorbed by pH-sensitive passive diffusion. During or after absorption, the monoglutamate form of folic acid is changed to methyltetrahydrofolic acid and is stored.

Dietary Sources

The best sources of folic acid are liver, kidney beans, lima beans, and fresh, dark green, leafy vegetables, particularly broccoli, asparagus, and spinach. Orange juice, white bread, dried beans, green salads, and ready-to-eat cereals are the major food sources of folic acid, contributing about one-third of the total daily intake. Only small quantities of folic acid are contained in milk, eggs, fruits (except oranges), root vegetables, and most meats. Only 25 to 50 percent of dietary folic acid is nutritionally available, but intestinal bacteria synthesize large amounts, which add to the daily intake.

Deficiency States

Folate deficiency may be the most common vitamin deficiency in humans. Deficiency results in poor growth, megaloblastic anemia and other blood disorders, elevated blood levels of homocysteine (a blood chemical linked to the clogging of arteries), glossitis, and GI tract disturbances. Low plasma folate and cobalamin levels have been associated with elevated plasma homocysteine levels and an increased risk of heart disease. Some health care providers believe that folic acid deficiency is an independent risk factor for heart disease, unrelated to cholesterol levels, hypertension, or diabetes.

Conditions that enhance the body's need for folic acid such as pregnancy, hemolytic anemia, leukemia, Hodgkin's disease, the use of certain drugs (e.g., oral contraceptives, sulfasalazine, diphenylhydantoin, barbiturates), and protein malnutrition impair the utilization of folic acid. Excessive alcohol intake impairs the absorption of folic acid or increases its elimination. Neural tube defects (e.g., spina bifida, anencephaly) have been associated with folic acid deficiency. Low red blood cell folate levels have also been found to enhance the other risk factors for cancer and human papillomavirus infection.

Dosage Regimen

The RDA for folic acid has been established at 3 mcg/kg/day, which is equivalent to the average intake of the United States and Canadian populations. It has been estimated that 75 percent of abnormalities related to neural tube defects could be prevented by the use of folic acid supplements.

Excess States

There are no known toxic effects to folic acid, although dosages of 15 mg have been reported to cause abdominal distention, loss of appetite, nausea, sleep disturbances, and interference with zinc absorption. Excess folic acid may also prevent the recognition of vitamin B_{12} deficiency.

BIOTIN

Functions

Biotin assists in the transfer of carbon dioxide from one compound to another, thus playing an important role in carbohydrate, fat, and protein biotransformation. Biotin is not produced in the body but is synthesized in the lower GI tract by bacteria. Biotin is a constituent of a coenzyme for carboxylation and deamination reactions. It is required in the synthesis of fatty acids, generation of the tricarboxylic acid cycle, and the formation of purines. Biotin is metabolically related to folic acid, pantothenic acid, and cobalamin.

Pharmacokinetics

Biocytin, the natural fragment released by degradation, is readily absorbed. Biotin is released during hydrolysis of biocytin and taken up by the muscle, liver, and kidneys. It is protein bound in most natural foods. A vegetarian diet may alter the normal flora of the bowel to enhance synthesis of biotin or promote its absorption, or both.

Dietary Sources

Biotin is synthesized in considerable amounts by intestinal bacteria but may also be obtained from liver, kidneys, egg yolk, soybeans, and yeast. Moderately good sources of biotin are milk, fish, nuts, and oatmeal. Fruits, vegetables, and meat are poor sources of biotin.

Deficiency States

The signs and symptoms of biotin deficiency in adults include dermatitis, glossitis, lassitude, depression, hyperesthesia, pallor, anorexia, loss of sleep, depression, muscle pains, and hypercholesterolemia. In infants younger than 6 months of age, biotin deficiency appears as seborrheic dermatitis and alopecia. Biotin deficiency is a common disorder in patients receiving total parenteral nutrition, although there is an inherited form of biotin deficiency (i.e., biotin-dependent multiple carboxylase deficiency syndrome). The anticonvulsant drugs primidone and carbamazepine inhibit biotin transport in the intestine, leading to deficiency.

Dosage Regimen

The RDA for biotin has not been established because of the lack of knowledge regarding its bioavailability in foods. The RDA has been provisionally set at 30 to 100 mcg/day, which appears to meet the needs of most healthy adults.

Excess States

No known toxic effects are produced by biotin.

ASCORBIC ACID

❐ Ascorbic acid (sodium ascorbate; ASCORBICAP, CEBID, CECON, CEMILL, CENOLATE, CETANE, CEVALIN, CEVI-BID, CE-VI-SOL, FLAVORCEE, SUNKIST VITAMIN C); (🍁) APO-C, KAMU-JAY

Functions

Ascorbic acid (vitamin C) is the most commonly used dietary supplement in the United States. It is essential as either a coenzyme or co-factor for collagen formation and, thus, is required for wound healing and tissue repair. These collagen tissues include connective tissue, cartilage, bone matrix, tooth dentin, skin, and tendons. It has been associated with the healing of fractures, bruises, pinpoint hemorrhages, and bleeding gums.

Ascorbic acid plays a part in the biotransformation of iron and folic acid, as well as in the synthesis of fats and proteins, the preservation of blood vessel integrity, and resistance to infection. It blocks the degradation of ferritin to hemosiderin, from which iron is poorly mobilized, thus ensuring a more available supply in the form of ferritin. Ascorbic acid is essential in the oxidation of phenylalanine and tyrosine, the conversion of folic acid to tetrahydrofolic acid, and the formation of serotonin and norepinephrine.

The value of ascorbic acid as an antioxidant is under investigation. There is evidence to suggest that ascorbic acid, as well as vitamin A (particularly beta-carotene and other carotenoids), pyridoxine, and folic acid, protects the body by supporting antioxidant activity. The free radical theory demonstrates why it is important to protect the body with dietary supplements, specifically ascorbic acid, vitamin E, and beta-carotene. Keep in mind that there are both unstable and stable oxygen molecules shooting about in the body. The stable oxygen molecule is essential to life. There are also some unstable oxygen molecules (free radicals) that enable the body to successfully fight inflammation, kill bacteria, and control the smooth muscle tone, which regulates the working of internal organs and blood vessels. However, too many free radicals may be generated by exposure to air pollution, cigarette smoke, ultraviolet light, pesticides, and contamination in food, and even from too much exercise. Although the healthy body can more or less control its own production of free radicals, too many free radicals create a problem. They begin to run wild, successfully attacking healthy as well as unhealthy tissues and sometimes resulting in heart disease, various cancers, and many other diseases (see Conditions Mediated by Free Radical Damage).

CONDITIONS MEDIATED BY FREE RADICAL DAMAGE

Arteriosclerosis	Liver cirrhosis
Autoimmune diseases	Myocardial infarction
Cancer	Nephrotoxicity
Cataracts associated with diabetes	Nutrient deficiencies
Chronic airway limitation	Parkinson's disease
Contact dermatitis	Premature aging
Drug toxicity	Premature retimopathy
Emphysema	Senile dementia and neurologic degeneration
Hypertensive cerebrovascular injury	Thermal injuries
Immune deficiency of aging	Viral infection (including autoimmune deficiency syndrome)
Inflammatory bowel disease	
Iron overload disease	

Adapted from Joseph Pizzorno, from the book *Total Wellness*, Prima Publishing, Rocklin, CA. Copyright © 1996 by Joseph Pizzorno. Buy or order at better bookstores or call (800) 632-8676. www.primapublishing.com. Used with permission.

Pharmacokinetics

Ascorbic acid is readily absorbed from the small intestine by an active mechanism and diffusion. Ninety percent of ascorbic acid from foods is bioavailable to the body when taken in quantities between 20 and 120 mg. At very high dosages, bioavailability falls to only 16 percent. Diets high in zinc and pectin may decrease absorption, whereas absorption may be increased in the presence of natural citrus extract.

Ascorbic acid is readily taken up by the tissues of the adrenal glands, the kidneys, liver, and spleen, appearing in equilibrium with serum levels. Amounts in excess of those needed by the body are eliminated in the urine as oxalic acid or ascorbic acid, or are exhaled as carbon dioxide.

Dietary Sources

Evidence suggests that naturally occurring ascorbic acid and supplemental products are equally bioavailable. The best dietary sources of ascorbic acid are acidic, fresh citrus fruits and raw, leafy vegetables, as well as tomatoes. Strawberries, cantaloupe, cabbage, green peppers, and properly prepared potatoes are also good sources of ascorbic acid.

The ascorbic acid content of fruits and vegetables varies with the conditions under which they are grown and the degree of ripeness when harvested. Refrigeration and quick freezing help retain the vitamin.

Deficiency States

The occurrence of frank *scurvy* is rare, although marginal deficiencies may occur in people whose diets are devoid of fruits and vegetables, people who consume excess quantities of alcohol, older adults with very limited diets, critically ill people under chronic stress, and infants fed exclusively cow's milk.

Mild deficiency of ascorbic acid is reflected as irritability, malaise, arthralgia, and an increased tendency to bleed. More severe deficiencies involve most body tissues. The effects include gingivitis; bleeding of the gums, anosmia, skin, joints and other areas; disturbances of bone growth; anemia; loosening of the teeth; follicular hyperkeratosis; loss of hair; and dry, itchy skin. Because of defects in collagen synthesis, wounds fail to heal and scars of previous wounds may break down. Secondary infections develop in the site of altered skin and mucous membrane integrity. Neurotic disturbances that include hypochondriasis, hysteria, and depression, followed by decreased psychomotor performance, are common. Coma and death may occur if scurvy is not treated.

The elimination of ascorbic acid is increased when the patient is under stress and when the patient has received adrenocorticotrophic hormone by injection. This loss is due to high adrenocortical hormone activity. The immunologic activity of leukocytes, the production of interferon, the inflammatory response, and the integrity of the mucous membranes all contribute to resistance to infection. The value of ascorbic acid in the prevention and treatment of the common cold has not been supported.

Dosage Regimen

The minimum RDA of ascorbic acid needed to prevent scurvy is approximately 10 mg daily. However, this dosage does not provide for acceptable reserves. The RDA of 60 mg prevents the onset of scorbutic symptoms for 4 weeks and provides a margin of safety. Regular intake of supplemental vitamin has had a strong impact on serum levels of the vitamin independent of other variables affecting nutritional status. Additional ascorbic acid is necessary for persons under emotional or environmental stress, such as fever, infection, trauma, or in hot environments. Persons who smoke have lower serum concentrations of ascorbic acid. It is suggested that smokers increase their intake of ascorbic acid to at least 100 mg/day.

Excess States

Excessive intake of ascorbic acid may result in diarrhea from the osmotic effect of the unabsorbed vitamin passing through the intestinal tract. Megadoses of ascorbic acid may produce excessive amounts of oxalate and urate in the urine and subsequent renal calculi. Excessive ascorbic acid may also cause retention of iron stores, particularly in blacks who are sensitive to iron.

Antioxidants in foods have been shown to combat the effects of harmful free radicals in physiologic amounts. However, ascorbic acid and other antioxidants taken in excess of physiologic needs may act as pro-oxidants in some populations. Rebound scurvy may be seen when massive doses of ascorbic acid are taken and then suddenly discontinued. For this reason, high-dose ascorbic acid therapy should be withdrawn slowly.

MINERALS AND TRACE ELEMENTS

Minerals, which are found in body fluids, serve a structural function in the body. There are 16 essential minerals are required to maintain health. Supplements of minerals and trace elements are determined by the amount needed to maintain body tissues. *Minerals* (macrominerals) are defined as those requiring a dosage of 100 mg/day. The macrominerals are primarily electrolytes and include calcium, magnesium, potassium, sodium, phosphorus, chloride, and sulfur. If less than 100 mg/day is required by the body, the substance is called a *trace mineral* or micromineral. Microminerals include chromium, cobalt, copper, fluoride, iodine, iron, manganese, molybdenum, selenium, silicon, zinc, and vanadium.

Sodium, Potassium, and Chloride

Sodium, potassium, and chloride are briefly discussed in Chapter 57. Because they are so closely related in the body, it is convenient to discuss them together. Sodium makes up 2 percent of the total mineral content of the body; potassium, 5 percent; and chloride, 3 percent. Although they are distributed throughout the body, sodium and chloride are predominantly extracellular ions, and potassium is predominantly the intracellular ion.

These three ions maintain four important physiologic functions in the body: (1) water balance and distribution, (2) osmotic equilibrium, (3) acid-base balance, and (4) muscular irritability. The sodium-potassium-ATPase pump is important in volume regulation, maintenance of membrane potential (along with calcium), glucose transport, and transport of amino acids such as alanine, proline, tyrosine, and tryptophan.

Sodium assists in regulating osmotic pressure, water balance, conduction of electrical impulses in nerves and muscles, and electrolyte and acid-base balance. It influences the permeability of cell membranes, assists in the movement of substances across cell membranes, and participates in many intracellular chemical reactions. It is found in large quantities in saliva, gastric secretions, bile, and pancreatic and intestinal secretions. Sodium is present in most foods. Proteins contain relatively large amounts, vegetables and cereals contain moderate to small amounts, and fruit contains little to no sodium. The major source of sodium in the diet is table salt that is added to food during cooking, processing, and seasoning. One teaspoon of salt contains 2.3 g of sodium.

Potassium is present in all body fluids. As an intracellular ion, potassium helps maintain osmotic pressure, fluid and electrolyte balance, and acid-base balance. Along with sodium in extracellular fluid, potassium helps regulate neuromuscular irritability. Potassium is required for conduction of nerve impulses and contraction of skeletal and smooth muscle. It is especially important in activity of the myocardium. Potassium also participates in carbohydrate and protein biotransformation. It helps transport glucose into cells and is required for glycogen formation and storage. Potassium is also required for the synthesis of muscle proteins from amino acids and other components. Potassium is present in most foods, including meat, whole grain breads or cereals, bananas, citrus fruits, tomatoes, and broccoli.

Chloride is an ionized form of the element chlorine and is the main anion of extracellular fluid. With sodium, chloride functions to maintain osmotic pressure and water balance. It forms hydrochloric acid in gastric mucosal cells and helps regulate electrolyte and acid-base balance by competing with bicarbonate ions for sodium. Chloride also participates as a homeostatic buffering mechanism in which chloride shifts in and out of red blood cells in exchange for bicarbonate. Most of dietary chloride is ingested as sodium chloride. Foods high in sodium are also high in chloride.

Sodium, potassium, and chloride are readily absorbed from the GI tract and are eliminated through the kidneys in the urine, feces, and sweat.

Sulfur

Sulfur is present in the body as a component of three amino acids: cystine, cysteine, and methionine; as such, it is present in all proteins. It is an essential component of three vitamins: thiamine, biotin, and pantothenic acid. It is most prevalent in insulin and in the keratin of hair, skin, and nails. Excess inorganic sulfur is eliminated in the urine. Food sources of sulfur include meat, poultry, fish, eggs, dried beans, broccoli, and cauliflower.

Calcium

❒ Calcium acetate (PHOSLO)
❒ Calcium carbonate (BIOCAL, CAL CARB-HD, CALTRATE, CHOOZ, OS-CAL, OYSCO, OYST-CAL, OYSTER CALCIUM, TITRILAC, TUMS, many others); (🍁) APO-CAL, CALCITE, CALGLYCINE, CALSAN, MEGA-CAL, NU-CAL

Functions

Calcium is the most abundant mineral in the body, making up 39 percent of the total body minerals and 1.5 to 2 percent of body weight. Ninety-nine percent is found in the bones and teeth. The remaining 1 percent is in the intravascular fluids and within soft tissues. Approximately half of that contained in intravascular fluids is bound to protein, mostly albumin, and the remaining half is free, ionized calcium. Therefore, the total plasma calcium level does not reflect the exact amount of free, active calcium in the body.

Calcium is required in the transmission of nerve impulses and in the regulation of heartbeat. The proper balance of calcium, sodium, potassium, and magnesium ions maintains muscle tone and controls nerve irritability.

Calcium initiates the formation of a blood clot by stimulating the release of thromboplastin from platelets. It is also a vital co-factor in the conversion of prothrombin to thrombin and in the conversion of fibrinogen to fibrin. Calcium is also essential in the regulation of blood pressure and may help protect against colon cancer.

Pharmacokinetics

Calcium is primarily absorbed in the part of the duodenum where an acid medium prevails. Absorption is greatly reduced in the lower part of the GI tract, where the contents are alkaline. Ordinarily, only about 20 to 30 percent of calcium taken by mouth, either as foods or supplements, is absorbed. Calcium is absorbed through the action of calcitriol ($1,25[OH]_2D_3$). Calcitriol increases calcium uptake at the brush border of the intestinal mucosa by stimulating production of a calcium-binding protein. Calcitriol also stimulates the activity of intestinal enzymes such as alkaline phosphatase.

Three distinct fractions of calcium make up total serum calcium: ionized calcium, anion-complexed calcium (bound with phosphate), and protein-bound calcium (bound primarily with albumin or globulin). Ionized calcium equilibrates rapidly with protein-bound calcium. Plasma-ionized calcium is controlled primarily by parathyroid hormone, calcitonin, and vitamin D. Total protein levels change along with changes in plasma protein levels, although the ionized fraction usually remains within normal limits.

Dietary Sources

Dietary sources of calcium include dark green leafy vegetables, such as kale, collard greens, turnip greens, mustard greens, and broccoli, and seafood, such as sardines, clams, oysters, and canned salmon. Soybeans are rich in calcium, which is absorbed in a manner similar to that of calcium contained in milk. Oxalic acid limits the availability of calcium in some plant foods. Oxalic acid is contained in rhubarb, spinach, chard, and beet greens. Fortified orange juice contains as much calcium as milk.

Deficiency States

Clinical conditions that can cause calcium deficiency are many and include changes in dietary habits, GI function, calcium-binding, medical disorders, and many drugs. Dietary changes that can cause calcium deficiency include inadequate dietary intake or vitamin D deficiency, or both, or an excess intake of phosphorus, which combines with calcium so that neither mineral is absorbed. Malabsorption of fat in the intestine or diarrhea can also cause a calcium deficiency. There is less ionized calcium available in metabolic alkalosis. Patients receiving multiple transfusions of stored blood are at risk for calcium deficiency because the calcium is combined with citrate for storage.

Patients with renal failure are at risk for calcium deficiency. Pancreatitis causes the release of lipases into soft tissue spaces so that the free fatty acids that are formed bind with calcium. Burns, Cushing's disease, hypoparathyroidism, inadvertent removal of the parathyroid glands, wounds, alcoholism, tumor lysis syndrome, and liver disease may contribute to calcium deficiency.

A number of drugs can cause hypocalcemia. Magnesium sulfate, colchicine, and neomycin inhibit parathyroid hormone secretion. Aspirin, anticonvulsants, and estrogen alter the biotransformation of vitamin D. Phosphate preparations decrease serum calcium levels, and steroids decrease calcium mobilization. Loop diuretics reduce calcium absorption from the renal tubules, and antacids and laxatives decrease calcium absorption (see also Appendix C).

Calcium deficiency results in *tetany* (twitching around the mouth, tingling and numbness of the fingers, carpopedal spasms, facial spasm, laryngospasm, seizures, death). Peristalsis is increased with resultant diarrhea. Arrhythmias, palpitations, weak pulse, and hypotension result from the increase in cell irritability. Decreased myocardial contraction leads to decreased cardiac output. Pathologic fractures occur secondary to calcium loss from the bone. Patients are also at risk for bleeding because the intrinsic pathway for blood coagulation is inhibited. Other signs of calcium deficiency include brittle nails, depression, insomnia, and periodontal disease.

Dosage Regimen

The RDA of calcium for adults is based on estimates of obligatory loss and an absorption rate of 30 to 40 percent. The dosage for infants from 6 to 12 months of age is 400 mg; for infants 6 months to 1 year of age, the RDA is 600 mg. Children ages 1 to 10 years should have 800 to 1200 mg, and children ages 11 to 14 years should have 1200 to 1500 mg daily. Women age 25 to 35 should have 1000 mg daily, and postmenopausal women should have 1000 to

1500 mg daily. Additional amounts of calcium are recommended to meet the needs of pregnancy and lactation. Postmenopausal women who are not on estrogen replacement therapy should consume 1200 mg of elemental calcium daily (Table 58–2). Bone loss in calcium-supplemented postmenopausal women can be further decreased by increasing the intake of zinc, copper, and manganese. Adult men should consume a minimum of 800 mg daily. There is some evidence to suggest that increasing the calcium intake to approximately 1300 mg/day from diet and providing a calcium citrate malate supplement for 18 months significantly increases the total body and spinal bone density of adolescent girls. This group has an additional 1.3 percent of skeletal mass added per year. The increased bone mass may provide additional protection against osteoporosis in the future.

Excess States

Excessive calcium intake can cause anorexia, nausea, vomiting, decreased peristalsis, distention, and constipation. The increased calcium level enhances hydrochloric acid, gastrin, and pancreatic enzyme release, and slows GI transit time. Mild to moderate neurologic depression may occur and manifest as weakness, fatigue, depression, and difficulty concentrating. With severe excess, there is extreme lethargy, depressed sensorium, confusion, and coma.

Arrhythmias, heart block, and cardiac arrest are likely to be due to a shortened repolarization time. Digoxin toxicity

TABLE 58–2 DOSAGE REGIMEN FOR SELECTED MINERALS

Mineral	Primary Prevention	Dosage Required to Correct Deficiencies	Implications
Calcium	800–1200 mg po daily	*Adult:* 1–2 g po daily *Child:* 45–65 mg/kg/day po	Total serum calcium levels: 7.6–11 mg/dL depending on age. Use caution with calcium preparations: dosages may be expressed in milligrams, grams, or milliequivalents of calcium
Phosphorus	800–1200 mg po daily	Varies with reason for use	The average calcium to phosphorus ratio should be 1:1.6. Serum phosphorus levels: 2.7–4.5 mg/dL
Magnesium	*Adults:* Chloride formulation: 5 mg magnesium/kg/day. Hydroxide formulation: 5 mg magnesium/kg/day. Oxide formulation: 5 mg/ magnesium/kg/day *Child:* Chloride formulation: 100 mg/magnesium/day. Hydroxide formulation: 100 mg magnesium/day. Oxide formulation: 100 mg magnesium/day	*Adults:* Chloride formulation: 200–400 mg magnesium/day in three to four divided doses. Hydroxide formulation: 200–400 magnesium/day in three to four divided doses. Oxide formulation: 200–400 mg magnesium/day in three to four divided doses *Child age 6–11 yr:* Chloride formulation: 3–6 mg magnesium/kg/day in three to four divided doses Hydroxide formulation: 3–6 mg magnesium/kg/ day in three to four divided doses. Oxide formulation: 3–6 mg magnesium/kg/day in three to four divided doses	The average calcium to magnesium ratio should be 4:1. Serum magnesium levels: 1.5–2.5 mEq/L. Magnesium chloride is 12% magnesium or 9.8 mEq magnesium/g. Magnesium hydroxide is 41.7% magnesium or 34.4 mEq magnesium/g. Magnesium oxide is 60.3% magnesium or 49.6 mEq magnesium/g
Iron	*Adults:* Fumarate: 200 mg/day po. Gluconate: 325 mg/day po. Sulfate: 300–325 mg/day po. Elemental iron: 50–100 mg TID *Child:* Fumarate: 3 mg/kg/day po. Sulfate: 5 mg/kg/day po. Elemental iron: 4–6 mg/kg/day in three divided doses	*Adults:* Fumarate: 200 mg po TID–QID. Controlled-release form may be given BID. Gluconate: 325–650 mg po QID. Sustained-release capsules may be given BID. Sulfate: 300 mg po BID–QID. Timed-release tablets may be given twice daily. *Child:* Fumarate: 3–6 mg/kg TID. Sulfate: 10 mg/kg po TID	RDA is set at 10 mg/day. Iron absorption is decreased by one-third to one-half with concurrent administration of food. Vitamin C may slightly increase the absorption of oral iron preparations. Use oral formulations cautiously in patients with peptic ulcer disease and ulcerative colitis, and in patients with allergies to tartrazine. Indiscriminate use may lead to iron overload
Zinc	10–15 mg/day; 25–30 mg for pregnant and lactating women	*Adults:* 2.5–4 mg/day IN, additional 2 mg/day in acute catabolic states *Child younger than 5 yr:* 100 mcg/kg/day IV	Doses expressed in mg of elemental zinc. Zinc sulfate contains 23% zinc Serum copper levels: 114 ± 14 mcg/100 mL
Copper	*Adults:* 0.5–3 mg po daily *Child:* 0.7–2 mg/day *Child 6 mo–1 yr:* 0.6–0.7 mg/day *Infants to 6 mo:* 0.4–0.6 mg/day	Individualized based on patient needs	
Iodine	40–200 mcg daily	*Adult:* Lugol solution: 0.1–0.3 mL po TID. SSKI: 0.3–0.6 mL po TID–QID (equal to 300 mg K1)	Dilute iodine solutions and administer orally. SSKI contains 1 g potassium iodide/mL. Lugol solution contains 50 mg iodine/mL plus 100 g of potassium iodide/mL
Chromium	50–200 mg	Unknown	—
Manganese	0.5–5 mg daily	Unknown	Estimated safe and effective daily intake
Selenium	0.01–0.02 mg daily	Unknown	Estimated safe and effective daily intake

contributes to the arrhythmias. Kidney stones are possible because of calcium precipitates. Polyuria occurs because of osmotic diuresis and volume depletion. The kidney's ability to concentrate urine results in polyuria.

Phosphorus

Functions

Phosphorus aids in bone growth and mineralization of teeth. It is a component of molecules such as ATP and cyclic adenosine monophosphate (cAMP), which are essential for energy biotransformation while maintaining the structural integrity of cells. It also plays a part in cellular immunity. Phosphorus is needed for phosphorylation and dephosphorylation, which are important steps in the activation and deactivation of many enzymes by cellular phosphatases and kinases. Phosphate is also a buffer in intracellular fluids and the kidneys, where it acts in the elimination of hydrogen ions. Phosphate reacts with hydrogen, releasing sodium in the process. Sodium is then reabsorbed under the influence of aldosterone.

Approximately 80 percent of phosphorus contained in the body is in the form of calcium phosphate crystals ($CaPO_4$). Phosphorus is the second most abundant mineral in the body, second only to calcium. Most of the inorganic phosphorus is contained in two forms: H_2PO_4 and HPO_4.

Pharmacokinetics

Regardless of the form, most phosphorus is absorbed as inorganic phosphate. Phosphorus is hydrolyzed in the intestinal lumen by alkaline phosphatase and released as inorganic phosphate. The acidic environment of the proximal duodenum maintains the solubility of phosphorus and thus the bioavailability.

Phosphorus is eliminated through the kidneys. Phosphate elimination is reduced in the presence of increased plasma insulin, thyroid-stimulating hormone, growth hormone, and glucagon levels; in metabolic or respiratory alkalosis; and with contraction of the extracellular fluid.

Dietary Sources

As a rule of thumb, good sources of protein are also good sources of phosphorus. Good sources of both include milk, meat, poultry, fish, and eggs. Other food sources of phosphorus include dairy products, nuts, legumes, cereals, and grains. A small amount is contained in fruits and juices, soft drinks, coffee, and tea. These foods contain about 3 percent of the RDA for phosphorus.

Deficiency States

Phosphorus deficiency is unlikely because the element is widely available in a variety of foods. Clinical hypophosphatemia most often results from the long-term administration of IV glucose or total parenteral nutrition without added phosphorus, excessive use of phosphate-binding drugs (see Chapter 41), hyperparathyroidism, the treatment of diabetic ketoacidosis, and alcoholism with or without decompensated liver disease. Premature infants can also develop clinical hypophosphatemia if they are fed unfortified human milk.

The signs and symptoms of hypophosphatemia include muscular weakness, encephalopathy, cardiomyopathy with congestion, hemolytic anemia, ventilatory collapse, and GI and skin hemorrhages.

Dosage Regimen

The RDA for phosphorus approximates that of calcium for all age groups—800 to 1200 mg daily (see Table 58–2).

Excess States

Phosphorus excess is rare, but when it is present, it may cause tachycardia, nausea and diarrhea, abdominal cramps, muscle weakness, and hyperreflexia.

Magnesium

❒ Magnesium chloride (SLO-MAG)
❒ Magnesium citrate (CITROMA); (🍁) CITRO-MAG
❒ Magnesium oxide (MAG-OX 400, MAOX 420, URO-MAG)
❒ Magnesium sulfate (Epsom salt)

Functions

Magnesium is second only to potassium in concentration in intracellular fluid. Fifty percent of the body's magnesium is stored in bone, 49 percent is contained in intracellular fluid, and 1 one percent in the plasma.

Calcium and magnesium have complementary roles. Calcium gives bones their strength, whereas magnesium helps them maintain their elasticity to prevent injury. More than half of the body's magnesium is found in bones. Along with calcium, magnesium moderates the transmission of impulses to nerves and the contraction of skeletal, smooth, and cardiac muscle. It accomplishes this process through effects on more than 300 enzyme systems. Magnesium is responsible for transportation of sodium and potassium across the cell membrane and the synthesis and release of parathyroid hormone. Magnesium is necessary for the conversion of ATP to ADP and thus the release of energy. It influences the utilization of sodium, potassium, calcium, and phosphate, and activates enzymes necessary for the biotransformation of carbohydrates, proteins, fats, and cyanocobalamin. Magnesium also promotes vasodilation of peripheral arteries and arterioles.

Pharmacokinetics

Magnesium is absorbed from the small intestine at the same site as calcium, although the rate of absorption varies from 35 to 45 percent. Most absorption occurs in the jejunum through simple and facilitated diffusion. The efficiency of absorption varies with the composition of the diet as a whole, the magnesium status of the individual, and the amount consumed in the diet. Vitamin D has no effect on the absorption of magnesium.

Magnesium is carried in the plasma as free ions or as a complex with phosphate, citrate, or protein. Maintenance of serum levels depends on absorption, elimination, and transmembranous cation flux rather than on hormonal regulation, as are calcium and phosphorus. The kidneys conserve magnesium (especially when intake is low). Reabsorption tends to vary inversely with that of calcium.

Dietary Sources

Magnesium is abundant in foods. The best food sources of magnesium include seeds, nuts, legumes, and unmilled cereal grains and dark green vegetables. Diets high in refined foods, meat, and dairy products are usually lower in magnesium than diets rich in vegetables and unrefined grains. Magnesium is lost during refining of foods such as flour, rice, and sugar, and is not added during processing.

Deficiency States

Magnesium status is difficult to determine because serum levels remain constant over a wide range of intake levels. However, magnesium deficiency may be precipitated by any condition in which there is decreased intake, increased loss, or a shift in electrolyte balance. Increased calcium or phosphorus intake can decrease magnesium absorption from the intestines. Magnesium deficiency is possible in patients with renal disease, on diuretic therapy, and who have malabsorption syndrome, hyperthyroidism, pancreatitis, kwashiorkor, diabetes, parathyroid gland disorders, postsurgical stress, and vitamin D–resistant rickets.

Many drugs increase the risk of magnesium deficiency. Excessive amounts of phosphorus (from overuse of antacids) inhibits the intake of magnesium from the intestine. Diuretics and antibiotics interfere with renal handling of magnesium as either a primary action or an adverse effect. Loop, osmotic, and thiazide diuretics; aminoglycoside antibiotics; carbenicillin; amphotericin B; cisplatin; corticosteroids; and cardiac glycosides are the usual offenders. The neurologic trauma associated with cocaine abuse has also been linked to magnesium deficiency.

Deficiency of magnesium results in muscle spasm, personality changes, anorexia, nausea, and vomiting. Tetany, myoclonic jerks, athetoid movements, seizures, and coma have also been reported. If the magnesium deficiency continues, parathyroid hormone, calcium and potassium levels drop and sodium is retained. Neuromuscular changes appear along with other signs.

Dosage Regimen

The RDA for magnesium is 50 to 450 mg daily, although specific recommendations vary with age, gender, and reproductive status (see Table 58–2).

Excess States

The signs and symptoms of hypermagnesemia include flaccid paralysis, CNS depression, anesthesia, and even paralysis, especially in patients with renal insufficiency. Cardiac arrest in diastole is possible. There may also be an increased incidence of congenital defects in exposed embryos.

Iron

- ❐ Ferrous fumarate (FEMIRON, FEOSTAT, FUMASORB, FUMERIN, HEMOCYTE, IRCON, PALMIRON); (🍁) NOVO-FUMAR, PALAFER
- ❐ Ferrous gluconate (FERGON, FERRALET, SIMRON); (🍁) APO-FERROUS GLUCONATE, FERTINIC, NOVO-FERROGLUC
- ❐ Ferrous sulfate (FEOSOL, FER-IN-SOL, FER-IRON, FERO-GRADUMET, FEROSPACE, FERRALYN, FERRA-TD, MOL-IRON, SLOW FE); (🍁) APO-FERROUS SULFATE, FERO-GRAD, NOVO-FERROSULFA
- ❐ Iron dextran (INFED); (🍁) IMFERON

Functions

Nearly three-fourths of body iron is in hemoglobin in red blood cells. Hemoglobin is required for transport and use of oxygen by body cells. About one-fourth is stored in the liver, bone marrow, and spleen as ferritin and hemosiderin. Ferritin is a complex of ferric hydroxide and a protein, apoferritin, which originates in the reticuloendothelial system. Ferritin reflects the body iron stores and is a good indication of iron storage status. Hemosiderin is similar to ferritin but contains more iron and is very insoluble. The remaining small amount is in myoglobin and enzymes or bound to transferrin in the plasma. Transferrin is a transport protein and with beta-globulin regulates iron absorption. Myoglobin aids oxygen transport and use by the muscles. Enzymes are important in cellular respiration. Iron also appears to be involved in immune function. High levels of ferritin are required for proper function of the immune system. Iron is also critical for normal brain development and function at all ages. It is also involved in the function and synthesis of neurotransmitters and possibly myelin.

Pharmacokinetics

The absorption of iron from food varies considerably and is estimated to be about 10 percent under normal circumstances. Absorption is influenced by several factors. Iron absorption is increased in the presence of dietary ascorbic acid. The acidity of gastric fluids increases the solubility of dietary iron. Calcium combines with phosphate, oxalate, and phytate. If this reaction does not occur, iron combines with these substances and produces nonabsorbable compounds. Physiologic states that increase iron absorption include periods of increased blood formation such as pregnancy and growth.

Normal iron elimination is less than 1 mg/day, being eliminated in the urine, sweat, bile, and feces, and from the skin in desquamated cells. The average women loses another 0.5 mg of iron daily and 15 mg monthly during menses.

Dietary Sources

The average diet supplies the body with about 12 to 15 mg/day of iron, of which only 5 to 10 percent is absorbed (0.6 to 1.5 mg). The best dietary sources of iron are liver, oysters, shellfish, kidney, heart, lean meat, poultry, and fish. Dried beans and vegetables are the best plant sources of iron. Other foods that contain iron are egg yolks, dried fruits, dark molasses, whole grain and enriched breads, wines, and cereals. Milk and milk products are almost devoid of iron. Iron-fortified cereal is a substantial source of iron for children up to 12 months of age.

Deficiency States

Iron deficiency is the most common nutritional deficiency and the most common cause of anemia among women and children worldwide. Groups considered at most risk for iron deficiency include infants younger than 2 years of age, adolescents (particularly girls), pregnant women, and older adults.

Iron deficiency is most often caused by chronic blood loss but can also be aggravated by a diet insufficient in iron, protein, folic acid and vitamin B_{12}, pyridoxine, and ascorbic acid. Menstruation is the most common cause of iron deficiency in women.

Anemia may also develop as a result of faulty iron absorption. Factors that decrease the absorption of iron include the lack of hydrochloric acid in the stomach and the use of antacids, which produce an alkaline environment. Combining iron with phosphates, oxalates, or phytates in the intestine results in insoluble and nonabsorbable compounds. Increased intestinal motility decreases the absorption of iron by decreasing the contact time with intestinal mucosa. Steatorrhea and other malabsorption disorders also decrease the absorption of iron.

Iron deficiency as well as iron overload can alter the immune response and result in an infection. The infection is likely to occur because iron is required by bacteria for growth and reproduction. T-cell and natural killer-cell concentrations are reduced with iron deficiency, and mitogenic response is muted. Transferrin and lactoferrin, two iron-binding proteins, seem to protect against infection by withholding iron from the organisms that need it for proliferation.

Dosage Regimen

Supplemental iron is usually administered to increase the available iron in the blood. Dosage is calculated in terms of elemental iron. Iron preparations vary greatly in the amount of elemental iron they contain. Ferrous sulfate, for example, contains 20 percent iron. Thus, each 300-mg tablet provides about 60 mg of elemental iron. With the usual dosage regimen of one tablet three times daily, the daily dose of elemental iron is 180 mg.

The RDA for a normal term infant is based on an average need of 1.5 mg/kg/day during the first year of life. Thereafter, the RDA is set at 10 mg/day and continues until adolescence (see Table 58–2). Males' need for iron declines after the adolescent growth spurt, but female needs continue to be high until after menopause. There is an increased need for iron during pregnancy.

Excess States

Iron overload can be caused by hereditary hemochromatosis and transfusion overload. Iron overload in blacks may be linked to a combination of dietary iron intake and the presence of a predisposing gene that is separate from any HLA-linked gene.

Zinc

❒ Zinc sulfate (ORAZINC, VERAZINC, ZINC-220, ZINCATE, ZINKAPS); (🍁) PMS-EGOZINC

Functions

Zinc helps maintain the health of the eyes, skin, hair, and joints; stabilizes cell membranes against free-radical damage, thereby improving our immune system; improves reproduction success by increasing the sperm count in males; reduces menopause-associated depression; and helps prevent excessive menstrual flow (when taken with choline). Zinc is also an essential component of many enzymes (e.g., alcohol dehydrogenase, DNA polymerase, retinol dehydrogenase). It may help protect the heart from cardiomyopathy and angiopathy. Zinc is also a constituent of the hormone insulin. Zinc supplements help with burn and wound healing, as well as in the treatment of acne and skin disorders. It is one of the several nutrients that is helpful in macular degeneration. Zinc has also been used in high doses to treat prostate enlargement.

Pharmacokinetics

Zinc is poorly absorbed from the GI tract (20 to 30 percent), although the mechanism is not well understood. A protein-rich meal promotes zinc absorption by forming zinc–amino acid chelates that present zinc in a more absorbable form. It is taken up first by the liver before it is redistributed to other tissues. It is widely distributed and concentrates in muscle, bone, skin, kidney, liver, pancreas, retina, prostate, red blood cells, and white blood cells. It is highly bound to plasma albumin, although some zinc is transported by transferrin and by alpha$_2$ macroglobulin. Plasma zinc levels drop by 50 percent in the acute-phase response to injury, probably from sequestration by the liver. Ninety percent of the mineral is eliminated in the feces, with the remainder lost in urine and sweat.

Dietary Sources

Dietary sources of zinc include meat, fish, poultry, milk, and milk products, providing 80 percent of the total dietary zinc. Oysters, shellfish, liver, cheese, whole grain cereal, dry beans, and nuts are also sources of zinc. The zinc density of the American diet appears to be 5.6 to 5.7 mg/1000 calories.

Deficiency States

Zinc deficiency is most often caused by a diet high in unrefined cereal and unleavened bread. Acquired zinc deficiency may develop as the result of malabsorption, starvation, or increased loss through urinary, pancreatic, or other exocrine secretions. Patients abusing alcohol and those receiving total parenteral nutrition have developed signs of clinical zinc deficiency because of the underlying disease process.

The first indication of a zinc deficiency is often hypogeusia (decreased taste acuity). Prolonged zinc deficiency may result in hypogonadism, growth retardation, mental disturbances, anemia, lethargy, diverse forms of skin lesions, delayed wound healing, alopecia, and susceptibility to frequent infections. Testicular function may be adversely affected by a low level of zinc. Mental depression as well as other mental disorders such as neurotic and compulsive states have been corrected by the administration of 15 to 150 mg of zinc per day.

Dosage Regimen

A positive zinc balance is attained with intakes of 112.5 mg/day from a mixed diet, based on a 20 percent efficacy of absorption. The RDA is 10 to 15 mg/day. Oral contraceptives may alter zinc distribution; however, there is no evidence available showing that these changes alter the dietary requirement.

Excess States

Excess oral ingestion of zinc to the point of toxicity is rare. However, continued supplementation in excess of the RDA will interfere with copper absorption. The most serious form of zinc toxicity is seen in patients with renal failure who are on hemodialysis. The signs and symptoms of overdose include nausea, vomiting, and diarrhea.

Copper

Functions

Copper is necessary for the function of the antioxidant enzyme superoxide dismutase as well as connective tissue maintenance and immune function. Copper is also vital for production of red blood cells, apparently by regulating storage and release of iron for hemoglobin. It also works with vitamin C in the production of collagen and elastin. Copper is essential for correct functioning of the central nervous, cardiovascular, and skeletal systems.

Pharmacokinetics

Copper is absorbed from the stomach, but maximal absorption takes place in the small intestine. It is transported bound to plasma albumin. Some copper is stored in the liver, with elimination via the bile into the intestine and feces. Small amounts of copper are present in urine, sweat, and menstrual blood.

Dietary Sources

Copper is widely distributed in foods. The average daily intake of copper is 1.0 to 1.5 mg, which is lower than the 2 to 3 mg that is recommended to be safe and adequate. Foods high in copper are oysters, liver, kidneys, chocolate, nuts, dried legumes, cereals, dried fruits, poultry, and shellfish.

Deficiency States

Copper deficiency is manifested in adults as microcytic hemochromic anemia, followed by neutropenia and leukopenia. Neutropenia and leukopenia are the best early indicators of copper deficiency. Because copper is stored in the liver, copper deficiency is not readily apparent. Bone changes include osteoporosis, metaphyseal spur formation, and soft tissue calcification noted in infants on prolonged total parenteral nutrition. Subperiosteal hemorrhages develop, and hair and skin depigmentation appears. There is defective elastin formation. Cerebral and cerebellar degeneration develops, which finally leads to death.

Copper deficiency is also possible as a result of a sex-linked recessive defect called Menkes' disease. Affected infants experience growth retardation, defective keratinization and pigmentation of the hair, hypothermia, degenerative changes in aortic elastin, abnormalities of the metaphyses of long bones, and progressive mental deterioration.

Dosage Regimen

The RDA for copper has not been established; rather, the recommendation is 1.5 to 3 mg/day for adolescents and adults. The dosage is estimated to be safe and adequate for daily intake (see Table 58–2).

Excess States

Copper toxicity damages the liver, kidneys, and other organs. Ceruloplasmin, the alpha$_2$ globulin that transports copper, increases during pregnancy and with the use of oral contraceptives. Serum concentrations of copper in pregnant women are approximately twice those in nonpregnant women. Increased serum copper concentrations can also be found in patients with pellagra, acute and chronic infections, and liver disease. The meaning of these elevations is unknown. Bile contains substantial amounts of copper; thus, copper excesses are possible with any form of chronic liver disease. Wilson's disease, a rare progressive autosomal recessive disorder, is associated with a defect in copper biotransformation and accumulation of copper in the liver. This mineral is suspected of being both mutagenic and carcinogenic.

Iodine

- ❒ Saturated solution of potassium iodide (PIMA, SSKI, THYRO-BLOCK)
- ❒ Strong iodine solution (LUGOL SOLUTION)

Functions

The body normally contains 20 to 30 mg of iodine, with more than 75 percent concentrated in the thyroid gland. The remainder is distributed throughout the body, particularly in the lactating mammary gland, gastric mucosa, and blood. Iodine, part of the hormone thyroxine, regulates growth and development, basal metabolic rate, and body temperature. Iodine is used as a supplement during long-term parenteral nutrition and as an adjunct with other antithyroid drugs in the preparation for thyroidectomy (see also Chapter 50).

Pharmacokinetics

Iodine is readily absorbed in the form of iodide. It circulates free and in a protein-bound state. Iodine is stored in the thyroid, where it is used to synthesize two hormones: triiodotyrosine (T_3) and thyroxine (T_4). When the hormones are broken down, iodine is conserved if needed and stored in the liver. Selenium is important in iodine biotransformation. Elimination of iodine is primarily through the kidneys in urine, although small amounts are eliminated in the feces.

Dietary Sources

Seafood (clams, lobster, oysters, sardines, other saltwater fish) is the best source of iodine. Saltwater fish contains 300 to 3000 mcg/kg of iodine, whereas fresh water fish contains only 20 to 40 mcg/kg of iodine. Iodine content in vegetables varies with the amount of iodine in the soil where they are grown. The iodine content of milk and eggs depends on the amount present in animal feed. Milk produced in the United States contains 5 to 10 times as much iodine as is found in the milk of many European countries. Iodized salt remains an important food source of iodine. Iodized salt helps prevent goiter.

Deficiency States

Iodine deficiency is generally associated with the development of simple goiter, which is an enlargement of the thyroid gland. The deficiency may be absolute, particularly in geographic regions where there is suboptimal iodine intake. Iodine deficiency is a preventable cause of mental deficiency *(cretinism)*, especially during pregnancy. Signs and symptoms of iodine deficiency include sluggishness and weight gain.

Dosage Regimen

The RDA for iodine is 150 mg for adults. Larger amounts are needed for children and pregnant or lactating women.

Excess States

Iodism, or iodine excess, like iodine deficiency, inhibits thyroid function. Enlargement of the thyroid may develop in response to this effect. Acute poisoning by iodine solutions causes severe damage to the exposed tissues of the GI tract. Chronic iodism is characterized by increased secretions of the respiratory tract, a brassy taste, soreness of oropharyngeal tissues, eye irritations, and GI irritation. Signs and symptoms include soreness of the teeth and gums, coryza, sneezing, eyelid swelling, enlargement and tenderness of the parotid and submaxillary glands, bloody diarrhea, fever, anorexia, and depression. Iodism is unlikely with dietary intake but may occur with excessive intake of drugs containing iodine.

Other Minerals

CHROMIUM

Chromium potentiates insulin action and, as such, influences carbohydrate, protein, and fat biotransformation. It is a part of glucose tolerance factor, a biologically active substance manufactured in the body that regulates sugar biotransformation. Glucose tolerance factor is a hormone-like compound that helps insulin move glucose out of the blood and into cells.

It is believed that chromium deficiency has something to do with the high incidence of diabetes in older adults, although research has not substantiated this claim to date. Chromium deficiency may result in insulin resistance, so that elevated insulin levels are required to maintain insulin-dependent functions as well as an impaired function in the presence of normal hormone concentrations. Insulin resistance is recognized as a major independent risk factor for cardiovascular disease.

Dietary intake is a factor in the amount of chromium needed. The recommended supplementary range is 50 to 200 mcg/day. Consuming large quantities of foods high in refined sugar requires more insulin and, therefore, more chromium. To reach the recommended range of 50 mcg of chromium, one would have to eat 3000 calories per day. The precise assessment of chromium in foods is difficult because biologically available chromium and inorganic chromium cannot be distinguished from one another. Brewer's yeast, oysters, liver, and potatoes are high in chromium. Seafoods, whole grains, cheeses, chicken, meats, and bran also contain fair amounts of chromium. Dairy products, fruits, and vegetables have little chromium.

Ninety percent of diets are deficient in chromium owing to modern agricultural techniques and the consumption of refined foods. Signs and symptoms of deficiency include anxiety, fatigue, elevated serum cholesterol and triglyceride concentrations, an increased incidence of aortic plaque, corneal lesions, decreased fertility and sperm counts, and glucose intolerance. Supplemental trivalent chromium is believed to improve these symptoms significantly.

MANGANESE

Manganese is a component of enzymes (e.g., pyruvate carboxylase, glutamine synthetase). It plays a role in oxidative phosphorylation, fatty acid biotransformation, and mucopolysaccharide synthesis. Manganese is required for the formation of connective and body tissues, growth and reproduction, and carbohydrate and lipid biotransformation.

Manganese is absorbed throughout the small intestine. Iron and cobalt compete for the same binding sites as magnesium for absorption. Men absorb less manganese than women. The difference in genders may be related to iron status. In young women, heme iron has no influence on manganese status. Manganese is bound to a macroglobulin, transferrin, and transmanganin for transport. Elimination occurs primarily through the feces.

Dietary sources of manganese include whole grains, legumes, nuts, tea, fruits, and vegetables. Animal sources, dairy products, and seafood are poor sources of manganese. Substantial amounts are present in instant coffee and tea.

Deficiency of manganese appears to affect sterility in both genders. Striking skeletal abnormalities and ataxia characterize the children of deficient mothers. Manganese excess occurs as a result of absorption through the respiratory tract. Excess manganese accumulates in the liver and CNS, producing parkinsonian symptoms.

SELENIUM

This nonmetallic chemical element forms part of the structure of the antioxidant enzyme glutathione peroxidase. It appears to protect the body from toxic effects of mercury and cadmium. Selenium combines with tocopherol to protect cell membranes and organelle membranes from free-radical lipid peroxidase damage. It facilitates the union between oxygen and hydrogen at the end of the metabolic chain, transfers ions across cell membranes, and aids in immunoglobulin and ubiquinone (coenzyme Q) synthesis. Adequate intake of selenium reduces menopause-related hot flashes, stimulates the immune response, protects the liver, detoxifies environmental carcinogens and mutagens, and helps cells breathe. Selenium also helps reduce the incidence of heart disease and decreases the risk of cancer, including colon and breast cancer, with its antioxidant effect. It also helps displace mercury, a toxic heavy metal from the tissues. The absorption of selenium occurs in the upper segment of the small intestine. It is transported via albumin and alpha$_2$ globulin.

Food sources of selenium include Brazil nuts, seafood, kidney, liver, meat, and poultry. Fruits and vegetables are low in selenium. Grains vary in selenium content depending on where they were grown and the selenium content of the soil and water.

Despite a wide range of intake, selenium deficiency is rare in humans. Cardiomyopathy in patients on long-term total parenteral nutrition has been associated with selenium deficiency. Selenium deficiency, combined with other factors, causes Keshan disease, a cardiomyopathy that is not related to coronary heart disease but that affects children. Selenium deficiencies have also been linked to reduced male fertility, increased spontaneous abortions, epidemics of viruses that are normally harmless, and reduced growth rates. A deficiency of selenium reduces glutathione peroxidase activity, causing jaundice in neonates. Deficiency of selenium can also lead to seborrheic dermatitis, dandruff, macular degeneration, low thryoid function, inflammation of the heart muscle, high cholesterol levels, and pancreatic insufficiency. Although animal studies have suggested that high selenium intake can protect against some cancers, in some cases, selenium may be toxic and actually may stimulate tumor growth. The dietary intake at which selenium intake becomes toxic has not been identified.

SILICON

Silicon has been recognized in the last 2 decades as an essential trace mineral. Chemically, it is similar to carbon, forming organosilicon compounds that are larger than previous compounds and that have different properties. Silicon apparently affects macromolecules such as glycosaminoglycan, collagen, and elastin. Thus, it is involved in the initiation and rate of calcification of bone as well as the composition of cartilage. This latter role suggests that inadequate silicon may be associated with the development of some joint disorders. Silicon may be important during times of stress associated with low dietary calcium, high dietary aluminum, and inadequate thyroid function. The role silicon plays in the development of atherosclerosis, osteoarthritis, and hypertension cannot be substantiated at this time.

Deficiency of silicon in animals has resulted in structural abnormalities of the skull, depressed collagen content of bone, and long bone abnormalities. Dietary intake of silicon varies with the quantity of unrefined grains with high fiber content, cereal products, and root vegetables consumed. Plant foods, particularly unrefined grains, contain large amounts of silicon, with the most concentrated source of silicon being beer. It is thought that the RDA for silicon may be in the range of 2 to 5 mg/day.

VANADIUM

Vanadium acts to inhibit enzymes that hydrolyze phosphate ester bonds (e.g., sodium/potassium/adenosine triphosphatase, ribonucleases, phosphatases). It appears to produce insulin-like effects and has been shown to stimulate glycogen synthesis, activate glycolysis, and inhibit glucose-6-phosphatase activity. In addition, vanadium may affect thyroid and iodine function.

Dietary sources of vanadium include grains and grain products and cereals. Meat, fish, and poultry contain moderate amounts of vanadium.

FLUORIDE

Fluoride is a component of tooth enamel, conferring maximal resistance to dental caries. It strengthens bones, probably by promoting calcium retention. Adequate intake before the age of 50 or 60 years may decrease the risk of osteoporosis and subsequent fractures in later years.

Fluoride is present in water, soil, plants, and animals in small amounts. It is often added to community drinking water supplies. Dietary sources of fluoride include drinking water and processed foods that have been prepared or reconstituted with fluoridated water. Small amounts of fluoride are contained in fruits and vegetables. Fluoride is contained in tea leaves, and the amount can be important depending on the strength and the extent of tea consumption. Soups and stews made with fish and meat bones also provide fluoride. Mechanically deboned meat and poultry, as well as seafood, and beef liver are high in fluoride.

Fluoride deficiency is indicated by the presence of dental caries and a greater increase in the severity of osteoporosis. Excessive quantities of fluoride result in mottling of teeth and osteosclerosis. Mild fluorosis can appear with as much as 0.1 mg/kg/day. The mottling of teeth associated with excessive fluoride is not usually visible and has no negative effects.

COBALT

Cobalt is a component of vitamin B_{12}. It is required for normal function of all body cells and for the maturation of red blood cells. Most of the body's cobalt is stored in the liver, with lesser quantities stored in the spleen, kidneys, and pancreas. It is eliminated primarily in the urine, with small amounts found in feces and sweat.

In humans, a vitamin B_{12} deficiency produces pernicious anemia. The effect of excess quantities of cobalt has not been established, although it appears that it may produce polycythemia, bone marrow hyperplasia, and increased blood volume.

Critical Thinking Process

Assessment

History of Present Illness

Nutritional assessment should be conducted for all patients in a health care system. Information obtained in a nutritional assessment is usually used as the basis for designing the nutritional care plan. Assessment of the healthy patient includes information about current weight; usual weight; and if weight has been gained or lost in the past month, 6 months, last year, and over the last 2 years. Ask if there has been a change in appetite, if the patient takes vitamin and mineral supplements, and if a special diet is followed at home. Have there been changes in taste and smell (see Appendix C)? Ask about any anorexia, *ageusia* (absence or impairment of the sense of taste), *dysgeusia* (distortion of the sense of taste), *anosmia* (absence of the sense of smell), chewing or swallowing problems, frequent meals away from home, an inability to eat for more than 7 to 10 days, and maintenance of IV fluids for more than 5 days. Inquire if the patient has problems with heartburn, bloating, flatus, diarrhea, constipation, or abdominal distention. Determine the frequency of the problem and if home remedies are used to treat the complaint.

Past Health History

Inquire about the patient's past history of alcohol use and recent major surgery of the GI tract. Determine if the patient has chronic health problems and how they are managed. Determine if a dietary modification is required for the chronic illness, and identify any drugs used in its treatment.

Physical Exam Findings

Physical signs and symptoms of poor nutrition provide vital supporting evidence for a diagnosis of a nutritional problem. The physical exam can also identify chronic medical conditions that may be related to nutritional deficiencies.

Anthropometry, including measurements of height, weight, certain body circumferences (e.g., calf measurement, midarm), and skin-fold thickness, are useful because body growth is related to nutrition. A body mass index should be calculated based on height and weight measurements. If the patient is in a balanced state of nutrition, height, weight, skin-fold thickness, and body circumferences should fall within normal limits on standardized tables.

Because dental caries are preventable to some extent and are partially caused by poor nutritional practices, a dental exam for dental caries and gum condition should be a part of the total assessment. This factor is particularly true with elderly clients, who may eat poorly because of loosely fitting dentures or missing teeth.

Table 58–3 provides an overview of the signs and causes of malnutrition. Findings of concern that indicate the need for an in-depth assessment to determine a nutritional versus other causes include

- Sudden or unexplained weight loss of 10 percent or more of body weight
- Rapid weight loss of more than 2 pounds per week
- Significant change in weight after age 25
- Height for age is above the 10th percentile, but weight for height is less than the 5th percentile in children
- Excess weight for height (greater than the 95th percentile) in children)

Diagnostic Testing

Many biochemical tests are the most objective measures of nutritional status, but not all are appropriate, nor is a single test diagnostic of a nutritional status. Laboratory tests can be helpful in detecting subclinical or marginal deficiencies, such as anemia, when clinical signs are not yet evident. They are also helpful in confirming a suspicion of a deficiency based on dietary or clinical evaluation. However, caution must be used in interpreting results, because they can be dependent on the disease state and the various treatment modalities. The most common laboratory testing performed includes hemoglobin and hematocrit, complete blood count with differential, serum albumin, total protein, serum glucose, folate levels, and urinalysis; this group of tests is recommended as a minimum evaluation data set.

Developmental Considerations

Perinatal During pregnancy, there should be an increase in all nutrients to meet the physiologic demands of maternal changes and fetal growth. The amount of increase in essential nutrients depends on a number of factors. These factors include the woman's general nutritional status before pregnancy, current health status, age and parity, amount of time between pregnancies, height and bone structure, weight, and

TABLE 58–3 PHYSICAL SIGNS AND CAUSES OF MALNUTRITION

Body Part	Signs of Malnutrition	Deficient Nutrient
Hair	Lacks natural shine, dull, sparse, straight, color changes, easily plucked	Multiple nutrient deficiencies
Face	Malar and supraorbital pigmentation, nasolabial seborrhea, moon face	Riboflavin, niacin, pyridoxine
Eyes	Pale conjunctiva, conjunctiva and corneal xerosis, keratomalacia, redness and fissuring of eyelid corners	Vitamin A, iron
Lips	Cheilosis, angular fissure and scars	Niacin, riboflavin
Tongue	Glossitis	Folic acid, niacin, cyanocobalamin, pyridoxine
	Magenta color	Riboflavin
	Pale, atrophic	Iron
	Filiform papillary atrophy	Niacin, folic acid, cyanocobalamin, iron
Teeth	Mottled enamel	Excess fluoride
Gingiva	Spongy, bleeding, receding	Ascorbic acid
Glands	Thyroid enlargement (goiter)	Iodine
Skin	Follicular hyperkeratosis, xerosis with flaking	Vitamin A, insufficient unsaturated and essential fatty acids
	Hyperpigmentation	Folic acid, niacin, cyanocobalamin
	Petechiae	Ascorbic acid
	Pellagrous dermatitis	Niacin
	Scrotal and vulval dermatosis	Riboflavin
Nails	Koilonychia (spoon nails), brittle, ridged	Iron
Musculoskeletal system	Frontal and parietal bossing, epiphyseal swelling, craniotabes (soft, thin skull bones in infants), persistently open anterior fontanelle, knock knees or bowlegs, beading of ribs (rachitic rosary)	Vitamin D
Gastrointestinal system	Hepatomegaly	Multiple deficiencies
Nervous system	Mental confusion and irritability	Thiamine, niacin
	Sensory loss, motor weakness, loss of position sense, loss of vibratory sense, loss of ankle and knee jerks, calf tenderness	Thiamine
Cardiac	Cardiac enlargement, tachycardia	Thiamine

activity level. If the woman's nutritional status is poor before she becomes pregnant, the additional demands of pregnancy on her body may further compromise her nutritional status.

Adolescent pregnancies have been associated with low birthweight, short gestational periods, and perinatal mortality. High parity or conceptions that occur more often than 12 months apart deplete the woman's nutritional reserves. Low pre-pregnancy weight and insufficient weight gain during pregnancy may result in low-birthweight infants and other complications of pregnancy.

Pediatric Nutrients likely to be low or deficient in children's diets include calcium, iron, zinc, pyridoxine, magnesium, and vitamin A. Clinical signs of malnutrition in American children, however, are rare. Children at nutritional risk include those from deprived families; those from the inner city; homeless children; children with anorexia, poor appetite, and poor eating habits; children with chronic disease (e.g., cystic fibrosis) or liver disease; and those on dietary programs for obesity or who are vegetarians.

Weight is a more sensitive measure of growth and an earlier clue to nutritional inadequacy than length or height. Head circumference for an infant is not useful as a nutritional screening tool. Head size increases so slowly after age 3 that malnutrition has little effect on it. Head circumference is useful primarily as an indicator of non-nutritional abnormalities. Check the fontanelle in children.

Geriatric Lack of transportation, loss of functional ability, immobility, limited income, and living alone may lead to social isolation. Older adults living alone may be deprived of stimulating interaction with others and thus lack incentive to cook and eat meals. Depression frequently accompanies social isolation and the sense of loss experienced with the death of a spouse or friends, retirement, changes in body appearance, impaired vision, and poor physical fitness. Lack of interest in eating and anorexia, common symptoms of depression, result in limited food intake and increased risk of nutrient deficiency. There is growing concern that the elderly are particularly deficient in vitamin B_{12}, vitamin B_6, and folate.

Psychosocial Considerations

Some patients and their families have an inadequate income. Poor dietary intake is associated with low income status. Limited access to food and food choices plus inadequate facilities for food storage and preparation has a significant impact on both the quantity and quality of food intake. Inquire as to who does the shopping and cooking.

Analysis and Management

Treatment Objectives

Many people take vitamin and mineral supplements in an effort to promote health and prevent deficiencies. Treatment objectives should center on ingesting appropriate amounts and sources of dietary vitamins and minerals, avoiding megadoses of vitamin supplements and minerals unless recommended by the health care provider, and avoiding symptoms of vitamin or mineral deficiency or excess. The need for vitamin and mineral supplementation is based on the following considerations:

- Daily requirements of the nutrient for healthy individuals
- The nature of the deficiency, disease, or injury
- Body storage of the specific nutrient
- Normal and abnormal losses of the nutrient through the skin, urinary tract, and GI tract
- Possible nutrient-drug interactions

Treatment Options

Vitamin and Mineral Variables

Vitamins prescribed by health care providers to prevent or treat deficiencies exert the same physiologic effects as those obtained from foods. Synthetic vitamins have the same structure and function as natural vitamins derived from animal and plant sources. There is no evidence to suggest that natural vitamins are superior to synthetic vitamins. Further natural vitamins are usually more expensive. Vitamin formulations available OTC cannot and should not be used interchangeably or indiscriminately without concern for safety.

For deficiency states, oral vitamin preparations are preferred when possible. They are usually effective, safe, and convenient to administer and relatively inexpensive. If the deficiency involves a single vitamin, that vitamin alone should be taken rather than using a mutivitamin. However, a multivitamin product may be used because one vitamin deficiency usually does not occur in isolation. Dosages should be titrated as near as possible to the amount needed by the body.

Many OTC products promoted for use as dietary supplements contain 50 percent of the RDA. In patients who consume a reasonably well-balanced diet, nutrient needs may be exceeded if these supplements are used. Products used for the treatment of deficiencies may contain as much as 300 to 500 percent above the RDA. These products should not contain more than the recommended amounts of vitamin A, vitamin D, and folic acid. Further, combination products (i.e., multivitamins) often contain minerals as well, although the quantities are ordinarily much smaller than those recommended for the average adult's daily needs.

Multivitamins for treating deficiencies should be used only for therapeutic purposes and for limited periods. When fat-soluble vitamins are given to correct deficiency, there is a risk of producing excess states. When water-soluble vitamins are used, excesses are less likely but may still occur with large doses (see Controversy—Dietary Supplements—Some Real Issues).

Patient Variables

There are many vitamin supplements available OTC, varying in number, type, and specific ingredients. Some contain a single vitamin, whereas others are combinations of different vitamins. Some persons believe that megadoses of vitamins promote health and provide other beneficial effects. There is no evidence to suggest, however, that dosages exceeding those needed for normal body functioning are beneficial and, in fact, can be harmful in some cases.

Health care providers do not agree on the use of vitamin and mineral supplements in pregnancy. Some believe that if the woman has a well-balanced diet, supplementation other than iron and folic acid is usually unnecessary. However, accepted practice in antepartum care today is the routine prescription of prenatal vitamins. In general, the pregnant women needs additional folic acid, pyridoxine, ascorbic

Controversy

Dietary Supplements—Some Real Issues
JONATHAN J. WOLFE

A patient asks you about a canned dietary product advertised on television. He had internalized the message that older people are healthier if they drink this product as part of their diet. However, his only income is a fixed pension and you know that he lives in relative poverty. Buying this dietary product will force him to buy less of other types of food, wash his clothes less often, and keep his three-room home colder in winter.

Patients come to their practitioners constantly seeking answers about health issues. Sometimes they are actually asking for an interpretation of what is important and what is specious. Such requests frequently involve dietary supplementation. Patients are bombarded by recommendations—usually with no scientific grounding, but based in anecdote—that they should take a particular vitamin supplement or add a particular food to their diets. Often, the recommendation comes from a source with an economic interest in their decision.

Vitamin supplementation is relatively inexpensive and hardly controversial. A multivitamin taken on a daily basis is probably not needed but is not likely to cause harm. The issue with some supplements is not certain. Some are suggested without a known established minimum daily requirement. Some are not standardized or are prepared from materials that are not assayed. Their worth may be impossible to establish. Even toxicity may be unknown. Some supplements are actually harmful in superphysiologic doses. This is true particularly of fat-soluble vitamins and nutrients containing metallic elements.

Health care providers are challenged daily to give guidance in dietary supplementation. The basic guideline that no one needs vitamins who eats a balanced diet often fails the test. Patients may have unusual dietary habits, perhaps derived from traditions we do not understand.

Critical Thinking Discussion

- What collaboration can you suggest between yourself and dietitians to act as a bridge to cover uncertain areas about diet supplements?
- What community resources can you find to educate yourself about issues related to dietary supplements?
- Do you perceive sellers of natural products and dietary supplements as adversaries or potential allies?
- What reference should you use to look up interactions between vitamin and other nutritional supplements and your patient's drugs?

acid, vitamins A, D, and E, calcium, phosphorus, iron, zinc, copper, magnesium, and iodine. These nutrients may be supplied with a prenatal vitamin.

Premature infants require the same vitamins and minerals as full-term infants. Poor body stores, physiologic immaturity, illness, and rapid growth increase the need for supplementation. The American Academy of Pediatrics does not support routine use of vitamin and mineral supplements for normal, healthy children. The exception is fluoride in unfluoridated areas. Parents who desire to give a vitamin and mineral supplement need not be concerned. The quantities of vitamins and minerals contained in supplements do not exceed those of the RDA; however, megadoses should be avoided.

Adolescents incorporate two times the amount of calcium, iron, zinc, and magnesium during growth spurts. Forty-five percent of bone growth occurs during these growth spurts. Adolescents, thus, are in need of additional supplementation. Their need for vitamins A and E, ascorbic acid, pyridoxine, and folic acid are the same as for an adult, but they need additional thiamine, riboflavin, niacin, vitamin B complex, and vitamin D.

As lean body mass declines with age, perhaps so does the need for trace elements needed for muscle metabolism. Glucose intolerance associated with aging may indicate the need for additional chromium. Increased calcium is needed owing to bone loss from osteoporosis, hypochlorhydria, and decreased intestinal absorption of calcium. Zinc requirements decline in the older adult, but these patients are in need of additional beta carotene, vitamin D, vitamin E, ascorbic acid, and cyanocobalamin owing to loss of intrinsic factor. Pyridoxine, cyanocobalamin, and folic acid confer protection against elevated homocysteine levels, an independent factor for cardiovascular disease, and certain neurologic deficits.

The RDA needed for wound healing includes additional ascorbic acid and vitamin A. For patients receiving tube feedings, the RDA for vitamins and minerals depends on the specific volume of feeding taken and the specific needs of the patient.

Intervention

Administration

Most vitamin and mineral supplements are taken on a once-daily basis. Oral vitamin products should not be taken at the same time as mineral oil because the oil absorbs vitamins and thus prevents their systemic absorption. Orally administered supplements should be taken with a full glass of water. Oral niacin preparations (except for timed-release forms) should be taken with or after meals or at bedtime. The patient should be instructed to sit or lie down for about 30 minutes after administration to reduce the risk of falls secondary to vasodilation, dizziness, and hypotension caused by the drug. The vasodilation occurs within a few minutes but may last up to 1 hour. IM or intravenous (IV) administration should be reserved for patients in whom oral administration is not feasible.

Parenterally administered vitamins should be given with care to avoid tissue damage. Manufacturers' instructions should be reviewed before administering the drug. Careful aspiration of IM or subcutaneous injections should be done to avoid inadvertent IV administration. Because sensitivity reactions have occurred with thiamine, an intradermal test dose is recommended. Z-track technique may be used for IM injections of cyanocobalamin, thiamine, and phytonadione. Gentle pressure should be applied to the site after administration.

Education

Patients should be taught that taking a vitamin and mineral supplement each day does not preclude the importance of eating a well-balanced diet, because vitamins in their natural form are often better than those synthesized in the laboratory. It is important to counsel the patient about the advisability of taking megadoses of vitamins and minerals. All vitamins and minerals should be kept out of the reach of young children and should never be referred to as candy. No known benefit to health results from ingesting more mineral nutrients than the body needs. Some vitamins and minerals are toxic if they are taken in more than the recommended doses.

Advise patients that although hemoglobin levels return to normal after about 2 months of iron therapy, an additional 6 months of therapy is recommended to restore the body's iron stores. Tell the patient taking liquid iron preparations to dilute and sip the formula through a straw to avoid staining the teeth. Patients should be aware that iron preparations turn the stools dark green or black.

Evaluation

Treatment effectiveness can be demonstrated through resolution of symptoms of deficiency with no evidence of overdosage.

SUMMARY

- RDAs for vitamins are established by the Food and Nutrition Board of the National Academy of Sciences. RDAs represent 100 percent of vitamin intake considered necessary to avoid deficiency.
- Vitamins prescribed by health care providers to prevent or treat deficiencies exert the same physiologic effects as those obtained from foods.
- Vitamins are compounds that indirectly assist other nutrients through the processes of digestion, absorption, biotransformation, and elimination.
- Vitamins are divided into two groups: fat-soluble and water-soluble. Fat-soluble vitamins include vitamins A, D, E, and K. Water-soluble vitamins include thiamine, riboflavin, niacin, pyridoxine, pantothenic acid, biotin, cyanocobalamin, and folic acid.
- Vitamin A is required for normal vision, growth, bone development, skin, and mucous membranes.
- Vitamin D is plays an important role in the regulation of calcium and phosphorus biotransformation.
- Vitamin E acts as an antioxidant in preventing destruction of certain fats, including the lipid portion of cell membranes. It may also increase absorption, hepatic storage, and use of vitamin A.
- Vitamin K is essential for blood clotting. It activates precursor proteins found in the liver into clotting factors: prothrombin, proconvertin, plasma thromboplastin component, and the Stuart factor.
- Thiamine acts as a coenzyme in carbohydrate biotransformation and is essential for energy production.
- Riboflavin serves as a coenzyme in biotransformation and is necessary for growth. It may function in the production of corticosteroids and red blood cells, and in gluconeogenesis.
- Niacin is essential for glycolysis, fat synthesis, and tissue respiration. After conversion to nicotinamide, the physiologically active form, it functions as a coenzyme in many metabolic processes
- Pyridoxine serves as a coenzyme in many metabolic processes and functions in the biotransformation of carbohydrates, proteins, and fats. It is a part of the enzyme phosphorylase, which helps release glycogen from the liver and muscle tissue
- Pantothenic acid is a component of acetyl coenzyme A and is essential for cellular biotransformation of carbohydrates, proteins, and fats and for synthesis of cholesterol, steroid hormones, phospholipids, and porphyrin.
- Folic acid is essential for the normal biotransformation of all body cells, for normal red blood cells, and for growth.
- Cyanocobalamin is essential for biotransformation of all body cells, particularly those of the bone marrow, nervous tissue, and GI tract; normal red blood cells; growth; and biotransformation of carbohydrates, proteins, and fats.
- Biotin is essential to carbohydrate and fat biotransformation.
- Ascorbic acid is essential as a coenzyme or co-factor for collagen formation and thus is required for wound healing and tissue repair. It has been associated with the healing of fractures, bruises, pinpoint hemorrhages, and bleeding gums.
- Minerals, which are found in body fluids, serve as structural functions in the body. There are 16 essential minerals required by our body to maintain health.
- Calcium is required in the transmission of nerve impulses and in the regulation of heartbeat, maintenance of muscle tone, and formation of a blood clot.
- Calcium and magnesium have complementary roles. Calcium gives bones their strength, whereas magnesium helps them maintain their elasticity to prevent injury.
- Phosphorus aids in bone growth and mineralization of teeth. It is a component of ATP and cAMP, which are essential for energy biotransformation, maintenance of cellular integrity, and immune response.
- Nearly three-fourths of body iron is in hemoglobin in red blood cells. Hemoglobin is required for transport and use of oxygen by body cells.
- Zinc is a component of many enzyme systems and is necessary for normal cell growth, synthesis of nucleic acids, and the synthesis of carbohydrates and proteins. It may be essential for the use of vitamin A.
- Copper is necessary for the function of the antioxidant enzyme superoxide dismutase as well as connective tissue maintenance and immune function.
- Iodine, part of the hormone thyroxine, regulates growth and development, basal metabolic rate, and body temperature.
- Chromium aids glucose by increasing the effectiveness of insulin and facilitating the transport of glucose across cell membranes.
- Manganese plays a role in oxidative phosphorylation, fatty acid biotransformation, and mucopolysaccharide synthesis. Manganese is required for the formation of connective and body tissues, growth and reproduction, and carbohydrate and lipid biotransformation.
- Selenium partners with tocopherol to protect cell membranes and organelle membranes from free-radical lipid peroxidase damage.
- Silicon affects macromolecules such as glycosaminoglycan, collagen, and elastin. Thus, it is involved in the initiation and rate of calcification of bone as well as the composition of cartilage.
- Vanadium inhibits enzymes that hydrolyze phosphate ester bonds. It appears to produce insulin-like effects and has been shown to stimulate glycogen synthesis, activate glycolysis, and inhibit glucose-6-phosphatase activity.
- Cobalt is a component of vitamin B_{12}. It is required for normal function of all body cells and for the maturation of red blood cells.
- Information obtained in a nutritional assessment is usually used as the basis for designing the nutritional care plan.
- Treatment objectives center on ingestion of appropriate amounts and sources of dietary vitamins and minerals, avoiding

megadoses of vitamin supplements and minerals unless recommended by the health care provider and avoiding symptoms of vitamin or mineral deficiency or excess.

- There is no evidence to suggest, however, that dosages exceeding those needed for normal body functioning are beneficial, and in fact, they may be harmful in some cases.
- Treatment effectiveness can be demonstrated through resolution of symptoms of deficiency with no evidence of over-dosage.

BIBLIOGRAPHY

Beaton, G. (1996). Statistical approaches to establish mineral element recommendations. *The Journal of Nutrition,* 126, 2320S–2329S.

Bhanot, D., Thompson, K., and McNeil, J. (1994). Essential trace elements of potential importance in nutritional management of diabetes mellitus. *Nutrition Research,* 14, 593–604.

Blumberg, J. (1994). To take antioxidant pills or not? The debate heats up. *Tufts University Diet and Nutrition Letter,* 12, 3–6.

Borek, C. (1995). *Maximize your health-span with antioxidants: The babyboomer's guide.* New Canaan, CN: Keats Publishing Company.

Dickinson, V. A., Block, G., and Russek-Cohen, E. (1994). Supplement use, other dietary and demographic variables, and serum vitamin C in NHANES II. *Journal of the American College of Nutrition,* 13(1), 22–32.

Facchini, F., Coulston, A., and Reaven, G. (1996). Relation between dietary vitamin intake and resistance to insulin-mediated glucose disposal in healthy volunteers. *American Journal of Clinical Nutrition,* 63, 946–950.

Frishman, R. (1996). Aging alters mineral needs. *Hardvard Health Letter,* 21, 6–8.

Gormley, J. (1996). Minerals top the list of nutrients women need for health and energy. *Better Nutrition,* 58, 28–30.

Grodner, M., Anderson, S., and DeYoung, S. (1996). *Foundations and clinical applications of nutrition: A nursing approach.* St. Louis: Mosby.

Harvey, C., and Hoffman, I. (1996). AHF launches nutritional intervention study to combat prostate cancer. *Primary Care and Cancer,* 16, 33–34.

Hennekens, C., During, J., Manson, J. et al. (1996). Lack of effects of long-term supplementation with beta carotene on the incidence of malignant neoplasms and cardiovascular disease. *The New England Journal of Medicine,* 334, 1145–1149.

Janson, M. (1996). *The vitamin revolution in health care.* Greenville, NH: Arcadia Press.

Johnson, P. (1996). New approaches to establish mineral element requirements and recommendations: An introduction. *The Journal of Nutrition,* 126, 2309S–2312S.

Kolasa, K., Lackey, C., and Poehlman, G. (1996). When patients ask about vitamin-mineral supplements. *Patient Care,* 30, 85–99.

Kushi, L., Folsom, A., Prineas, R., et al. (1996). Dietary antioxidant vitamins and death from coronary artery disease in postmenopausal women. *The New England Journal of Medicine,* 334 (18), 1156–1162.

LaChance, P. (1998). Overview of key nutrients: Micronutrient aspects. *Nutrition Review,* 56(4 Pt 2), S34–S39.

Lukasi, H., and Penland, J. (1996). Functional changes appropriate for determining mineral element requirements. *The Journal of Nutrition,* 126(9 Suppl), 2354S–2365S.

Mahan, L., and Escott-Stump, S. (1996). *Krause's food, nutrition, & diet therapy* (9th ed.). Philadelphia: W.B. Saunders Company.

Meyers, D., Maloley, P., and Weeks, D. (1996). Safety of antioxidant vitamins. *Archives in Internal Medicine,* 156(9), 925–935.

Nielson, F. (1996). How should dietary guidance be given for mineral elements with beneficial actions or suspected of being essential? *The Journal of Nutrition,* 126, 2377S–2386S.

O'Dell, B. (1996). Endpoints for determining mineral element requirements: An introduction. *The Journal of Nutrition,* 126, 2342S–2345S.

Olson, P., Torp, E. C., Mahon, R. T., et al. (1994). Oral vitamin E for refractory hand dermatitis. *Lancet,* 343(8898), 672–673.

Omenn, G., Goodman, G., Thomquist, M., et al. (1996). Effects of a combination of beta carotene and vitamin A on lung cancer and cardiovascular disease. *The New England Journal of Medicine,* 334(18), 1150–1155.

Pennington, J. (1996). Intakes of minerals from diets and foods: Is there a need for concern? *The Journal of Nutrition,* 126, 2304S–2309S.

Pennington, C. (1998). Disease-associated mulnutrition in the year 2000. *Journal of Postgraduate Medicine,* 74(868), 65–71.

Pennington, J., and Schoen, S. (1996). Total diet study: Estimated dietary intakes of nutritional elements: 1982–1991. *International Journal of Vitamin and Nutritional Research,* 66(4), 350–362.

Pizzorno, J. (1996). *Total wellness.* Rocklin, CA: Prima Publishing.

Rayman, M. (1997). Dietary selenium: Time to act. *British Medical Journal,* 314, 387–389.

Smith, S. (1996). Sorting through vitamins, minerals in a pill: What you need to know. Part 2. *Environmental Nutrition,* 19, 1–3.

Stephens, N., Parsons, A., Schofield, P., et al. (1996). Randomixed controlled trial of vitamin E in patients with coronary disease: Cambridge Head Antioxidant Study (CHAOS). *Lancet,* 347, 781–786.

Tucker, K. (1996). The use of epidemiologic approaches and meta-analysis to determine mineral element requirements. *The Journal of Nutrition,* 126, 2365S–2373S.

Webb, D. (1995). Vitamins, minerals, potions, and pills: Which supplements for you? *American Health,* 14, 48–55.

Wein, D. (1994). Five less-celebrated minerals your body can't do without. *Environmental Nutrition,* 17, 1–3.

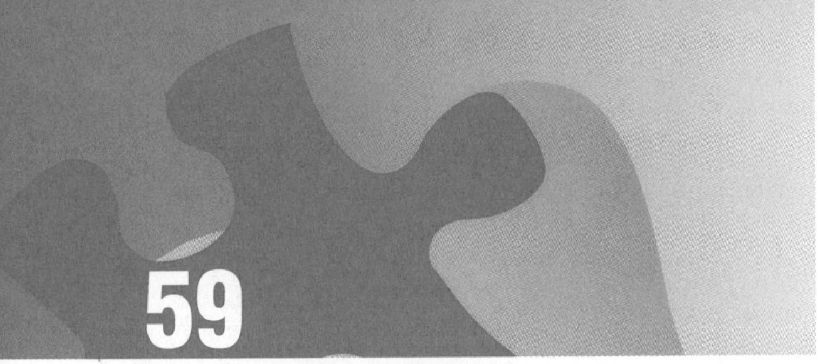

59

Enteral Products

Malnutrition can be defined as a deficiency, imbalance, or excess of nutrients. Nutritional deficiencies result in a deficit of the nutrients required to support body processes and an attendant lack of energy. *Overnutrition,* on the other hand, may result in an excess of one or more nutrients, which can lead to nutritional imbalances. People in the United States frequently consume excessive calories; however, their diets may still lack specific nutrients in amounts adequate to meet their body's needs during strenuous exercise, times of stress, trauma, illness, or surgery. Serious nutritional deficiencies, as evidenced by weight loss, pressure sores, dehydration, hepatic failure, and chronic infections, are observed in 10 to 65 percent of older adults in long-term care settings and 25 to 45 percent of all admissions to acute care facilities.

Vitamin and mineral deficiencies lead to specific problems discussed in Chapter 58. These nutrient deficiency conditions are compounded when they occur concurrently with protein or calorie deficiencies. For example, depressed vitamin C and protein levels result in poor wound healing. Indeed, deficiencies of several nutrients are more prevalent than an isolated nutrient deficiency.

Clinically, *protein-energy malnutrition* (PEM) is more common than vitamin or mineral deficiencies. PEM includes three disorders: marasmus, kwashiorkor, and marasmic-kwashiorkor. These disorders are caused by protein and energy deficiencies and may be exacerbated by patient age, disease or infection, environmental stress, and other nutritional deficits. PEM is a consequence of long-term nutritional deficiency rather than the result of not eating properly for 1 day. As such, it is most often seen in children living in extreme poverty and in patients with chronic illness.

MALNUTRITION

Epidemiology and Etiology

Although poverty is still the major cause of malnutrition, the condition is by no means confined to the underdeveloped parts of the world. Anyone can become undernourished if there is a serious neglect of diet. Further, with increasing numbers of homeless people, immigrants, and migrant workers, along with the implementation of managed care, malnutrition has become prevalent in the community as well as acute care settings.

Individuals may become *malnourished* (unintended loss of over 10 percent of usual body weight) in the hospital as a result of an inability to absorb nutrients or refusal to eat foods provided. Illness, stress, and trauma have catabolic effects that increase nutritional requirements in situations in which oral intake is minimal. Conditions such as cancer, acquired immunodeficiency syndrome, gastrointestinal (GI) disorders, heart failure, chronic pulmonary disease, renal and hepatic failure, alcoholism, and conditions with high metabolic needs (i.e., hyperthyroidism, trauma) are more frequently associated with malnutrition. Additionally, a number of institutional practices affect the nutritional health of hospitalized patients (see Undesirable Practices Affecting the Nutritional Health of Hospital Patients).

Malnourishment in the community may be a result of difficulty in purchasing and preparing food, financial constraints, or poor cooking facilities. Ignorance of the basic principles of nutrition is almost as great a cause of malnourishment as poverty. Misplaced faith in vitamins as a substitute for food can contribute to malnourishment if carried to an extreme. An overreliance on excessively processed foods can also lead to malnourishment. Modern methods of processing and refining foods sometimes cause a loss of valuable nutrients. However, this danger is recognized by both the manufacturers and the government, who try to retain and restore the nutritional value of many foods. Alcoholism, which often leads a person to rely on alcohol at the expense of food, is another cause of malnutrition. People who want to lose or gain weight, have food allergies, or consciously avoid certain foods may endanger their health by consuming a diet that lacks essential nutrients.

Pathophysiology

In malnourished states, endogenous energy stores are used to maintain body functions. For example, glucose is the obligatory fuel for brain cells and red blood cells. Glycogen stores are depleted in 12 to 24 hours during fasting. With starvation, the body is unable to convert significant amounts of fatty acids to glucose, and glycogen becomes the predominant fuel. With continued starvation, hepatic gluconeogenesis is enhanced.

Because the body does not maintain reserve protein stores, the protein contained in visceral organs is vital. Visceral protein is used when exogenous protein is unavailable. Protein from lean muscle mass and, to some extent, visceral proteins are used to maintain basic maintenance needs. Even mild protein loss impairs normal metabolic processes and immune responses. However, with prolonged starvation, the body adapts to conserve vital proteins.

Normal fat stores represent the largest energy resource, providing more than 150,000 calories. The basal metabolic rate drops as the body attempts to conserve available fuel. Ketones, a by-product of fat metabolism, are used for energy instead of glucose, thereby decreasing the rate of protein catabolism. Use of fat as fuel results in less protein and nitrogen loss. In addition, decreased insulin secretion promotes lipolysis.

When a patient's intake is inadequate over an extended period of time in meeting physiologic requirements, the body is virtually starved. The degree of starvation and stress determine the extent and type of malnutrition.

Even well-nourished patients may develop PEM in a little as 2 weeks. PEM affects the whole body, especially metabolic

UNDESIRABLE PRACTICES AFFECTING THE NUTRITIONAL HEALTH OF HOSPITAL PATIENTS

1. Failure to record height and weight.
2. Rotation of staff at frequent intervals.
3. Diffusion of responsibility for patient care.
4. Prolonged use of glucose and saline intravenous feedings.
5. Failure to observe patients' food intake.
6. Withholding meals because of diagnostic tests.
7. Use of tube feedings in inadequate amounts, of uncertain composition, and under unsanitary conditions.
8. Ignorance of the composition of vitamin mixtures and other nutritional products.
9. Failure to recognize increased nutritional needs due to injury or illness.
10. Performance of surgical procedures without first making certain that the patient is optimally nourished, and failure to give the body nutritional support after surgery.
11. Failure to appreciate the role of nutrition in the prevention of and recovery from infection; unwarranted reliance on antibiotics.
12. Lack of communication and interaction between physician and dietitian. As staff professionals, dietitians should be concerned with the nutritional health of *every* hospital patient.
13. Delay of nutrition support until the patient is in an advanced state of depletion, which is sometimes irreversible.
14. Limited availability of laboratory tests to assess nutritional status; failure to use those that are available.

From Butterworth, C. E. (1974). The skeleton in the hospital closet. *Nutrition Today,* 9(2), 4–8. Used with permission.

systems, in which it causes reduced synthesis of enzymes and plasma proteins, increased susceptibility to infection, poor wound healing, and mental weariness. PEM involves two distinct deficiency states: marasmus and kwashiorkor. A combination of protein and calorie deficiency is called marasmic-kwashiorkor. Physical changes associated with PEM are identified in Table 59–1.

Marasmus and kwashiorkor are actually two different disorders, although the diets implicated in each are not significantly different. Marasmus seems to be a normal adaptation to starvation, whereas kwashiorkor develops when the body can no longer adapt to the starvation because of a co-morbid condition or infection. The maladaptation may be responsible for the clinical and biochemical differences in the disorders.

Marasmus

Marasmus, or energy deficiency, is a chronic condition of protein and calorie undernutrition that varies in severity. Marasmus may occur secondary to tuberculosis, malabsorption disorders, chronic infections, anorexia nervosa, and alcohol abuse. Isolated or hospitalized older adults are also at risk. Marasmus is characterized by gradual wasting that leads to severe cachexia.

When caloric intake is inadequate, available fat stores and, to some extent, muscle proteins are depleted. Weight loss is due to loss of muscle and fat. Muscle wasting, which is evident primarily in the extremities and trunk, also occurs in the intestines, heart, and other organs. Visceral protein measurements (serum albumin and transferrin) may be within normal limits or slightly decreased (usually not below 2.8 g/dL). Thus, immunocompetence and wound healing are reasonably good.

Although marasmus is not particularly life-threatening, nutritional support should be initiated to prevent the development of hypoalbuminemia in the event that stress or trauma occurs. Response and cure are slow. Appropriate planning is vital to ensure long-term changes in eating patterns and improvement in nutritional status.

Kwashiorkor

Kwashiorkor (hypoalbuminemia) is a syndrome of severe protein deficiency caused by an inadequate intake of good quality protein, although total protein intake may or may not be adequate. In the United States, kwashiorkor most of-

TABLE 59–1 COMPARISON OF MARASMUS AND KWASHIORKOR

Parameters	Marasmus	Kwashiorkor
Nutrient intake	Decreased protein and calorie intake	Decreased protein intake
Course	Months to years	Weeks
Appearance	Wasted appearance Weight $<$ 80% of standard Triceps skinfold $<$ 3 mm Midarm muscle circumference $<$ 15 cm	Well-nourished appearance Easy hair pluckability Moon face, edema Wasted muscles in upper extremity
Laboratory results	Serum albumin within normal limits Transferrin within normal limits	Serum albumin $<$ 2.8 g/dL TIBC $<$ 200 mcg/dL WBC $<$ 1500 mm^3 Anergy
Clinical course	Response to short-term stressors reasonably preserved	Infections Poor wound healing Pressure sores Skin breakdown
Mortality rate	Low unless due to co-morbid disease	High

TIBC, Total iron-binding capacity; WBC, white blood cell.

Adapted from Heimburger D.C., and Weinsier, R.L. (1997). *Handbook of clinical nutrition* (3rd ed., p. 171). St. Louis: Mosby. Used with permission.

ten occurs secondary to malabsorption disorders, cancer and cancer therapies, certain kidney diseases, iatrogenic causes, and hypermetabolic illnesses.

Stress-induced hypoalbuminemia increases the length of hospitalization by 29 percent, mortality fourfold, and development of nosocomial infection and sepsis almost 2.5 times above that seen with marasmic PEM. Typical cases are patients under acute stress who have been on standard intravenous (IV) dextrose solutions for an extended period of time (2 weeks or more). The continuous carbohydrate supply from IV dextrose solutions interferes with normal physiologic adaptive functions of starvation, whereby increased amounts of fats are catabolized for energy. Additionally, elevated levels of epinephrine, glucagon, and cortisol cause hyperglycemia. Also, the tissues are insulin resistant.

Signs and symptoms that may indicate kwashiorkor include edema and bloating related to the low serum albumin levels. Visceral organ functions are impaired, as evidenced by low total lymphocyte counts and low protein levels (prealbumin, albumin, and transferrin). Weight loss may not be apparent because of the edema. Muscular wasting; depigmentation of hair and skin; scaly, flaky skin; mental apathy, and retarded growth and maturation are also evident. Anthropometric indices may remain stable because somatic proteins are relatively stable.

Compared with the relatively normal laboratory findings of marasmus, kwashiorkor can be principally diagnosed using laboratory results. Protein levels gradually decrease as a result of inadequate hepatic synthesis. In some cases, classic symptoms of kwashiorkor (i.e., skin breakdown, poor wound healing, edema, and easily pluckable hair) are present. A fatty liver may develop, although serum cholesterol and triglyceride levels remain low.

Marasmic-Kwashiorkor

Marasmic-kwashiorkor combines the symptoms of both deficiency states. The loss of subcutaneous fat becomes very apparent when the edema is reduced in the early stages of treatment. Acute stress, in addition to chronic starvation, results in marasmic-kwashiorkor or PEM. Decreased body weight, muscle mass, skinfold thickness, and immune incompetence are evident. It is an extremely serious, life-threatening disorder in which vigorous nutritional therapy is essential and requires close monitoring.

PHARMACOTHERAPEUTIC OPTIONS

Enteral Formulas

Several types of formulas are available to meet the nutritional needs of different disease states and conditions. The Food and Drug Admininstration defines *formulas* as medical foods formulated to be consumed or administered for the specific dietary management of a disease or condition for which distinctive nutritional requirements have been established.

With more than 50 medical food products available, the formulations differ in osmolality, digestibility, caloric density, protein, fat, lactose, carbohydrate content, viscosity, and the presence of other nutrients. Changes are constantly made to the composition of old formulas, and new formulas are developed as a result of new knowledge. The nutrient contents of different types of formulas are noted in Table 59–2.

Polymeric formulas are composed usually of high molecular weight molecules that are formed by a combination of simpler molecules (monomers). They are the most widely used formulas and meet the needs of approximately 90 percent of patients without major organ failure. Specialized polymeric formulas and elemental formulas are used when regular polymeric formulas do not meet patient needs.

Polymeric Formulas

Polymeric formulas contain adequate amounts of protein to promote anabolism in catabolic or malnourished patients. They include fiber for long-term feedings to help regulate bowel function, may be blended to use normal foods, and are concentrated for conditions requiring fluid restriction. Polymeric formulas provide intact nutrients (whole proteins and long-chain triglycerides) but require a fully functional intestinal tract. Use of the gut is physiologically natural, and nutrients are used efficiently. Nutrients are digested and absorbed in the same fashion as regular foods. Following absorption of nutrients, they are metabolized in the same fashion as nutrients from foods.

Because of the prevalence of lactose intolerance, most commercially prepared formulas are lactose free. Some polymeric formulas are flavored, thus increasing their acceptance as oral supplements. Oral supplemental feedings may be used any time nutrient requirements exceed the amount of nutrients the patient is able to ingest. Most polymeric formulas contain 1 cal/mL but may contain up to 2 cal/mL.

Polymeric formulas are available as a powder to be mixed with milk or water and in ready-to-use liquid forms. The sources of carbohydrates, proteins, and fats vary. The recommended daily intake (RDIs) for vitamins and minerals are met when the patient is given 1000 to 2000 mL of formula.

Although RDIs are used as a standard, these amounts may not be adequate for many hospitalized patients. Many provide fiber, which is believed to help maintain gut integrity and bowel function, especially when formulas are the sole source of nutrition support. In addition to their convenience, commercially prepared formulas are microbiologically safe and are consistent in their nutrient content and osmolality.

Specialized Polymeric Formulas

Specialized polymeric formulations are designed for patients with a normally functioning GI tract but who also have metabolic problems. Increasing numbers of special formulations are available in response to growing knowledge and interest in the nutritional requirements in certain disease states (e.g., renal and liver disorders, respiratory failure, immune incompetence, diabetes, and conditions causing hypermetabolism). Many products have been formulated for oral consumption.

Hypermetabolic States

Specialty polymeric formulas have been designed to meet the nutritional requirements for patients who are in a hypercatabolic state (trauma, burns, sepsis). Hypercatabolic conditions elicit a hormonal response that promotes increased proteolysis and hydrolysis of branched-chain amino acids

TABLE 59–2 NUTRIENT CONTENT OF DIFFERENT TYPES OF FORMULAS

Nutritional Element	Blended	Polymeric	Elemental
Protein	Meat Milk Eggs Soy	Soy isolates Caseinates Lactalbumin	Hydrolyzed whey Casein Soy Lactalbumin hydrolysate
Carbohydrate	Vegetables Milk Cereals Starch	Glucose polymers Maltodextrins Corn syrup	Maltodextrin starch Sucrose Tapioca starch Modified cornstarch Fructose Oligosaccharides
Fat	Meat Whole milk Egg	Corn oil Safflower oil Soy oil Fish oils	MCT oil Sunflower oil Lecithin Soy oil Soy lecithin
Fiber	Fruits Vegetables Soy polysaccharides	Lignin Cellulose Hemicellulose Pectin	NA
Examples	COMPLEAT MODIFIED COMPLEAT REGULAR	CRITICARE HN ENRICH ENSURE ENSURE HN ISOCAL ISOCAL HN JEVITY RESOURCE SUSTACAL TRAUMACAL ULTRACAL	FIBERSOURCE FIBERSOURCE HN HEPATIC-AID II ISOSOURCE ISOSOURCE HN LIPISORB OSMOLITE OSMOLITE HN PEPTAMEN TRAVASORB HEPATIC TRAVASORB RENAL

NA, Not applicable.

(BCAA) (leucine, isoleucine, and valine) in skeletal muscle. Skeletal muscle uses BCAAs for energy, and along with other amino acids, BCAAs are used for gluconeogenesis, enzyme synthesis, wound healing, and immunocompetence. Because serum BCAA levels are decreased in hypercatabolic states, the elemental formulas are BCAA enriched. Specialized formulas (e.g., CRITICARE HN, TRAUMACAL, REPLETE) containing 40 to 50 percent BCAA are available, whereas standard polymeric formulas contain 25 to 33 percent BCAAs. If the patient can tolerate high protein intake (1.5 to 2 g/kg/day), BCAA-enriched formulas should not be necessary. They may be used in situations in which positive nitrogen balance has not been achieved within a reasonable period of time after the patient has received standard feeding or formulas supplying adequate protein and energy.

Pulmonary Insufficiency

Several conditions involving the respiratory system affect nutritional status, including chronic airway limitation (chronic bronchitis and emphysema), sleep apnea, and adult respiratory distress syndrome. Patients with chronic bronchitis are often overweight and hypercapnic. Patients with emphysema tend to be underweight and hypoxemic. Additionally, patients with emphysema tend to have deterioration of lung parenchyma that corresponds to the degree of nutritional depletion. Formulas designed for patients with pulmonary insufficiency help maintain nutritional status and prevent muscle atrophy, especially of intercostal and diaphragmatic muscles. Because of their nutrient composition, specialty formulas enhance the ability to wean patients from ventilator support.

High-carbohydrate feedings and overfeeding increase carbon dioxide production, oxygen consumption, and ventilatory requirements. Fat oxidation produces less carbon dioxide per calorie. Therefore, these specialized polymeric formulas (e.g., PULMOCARE, NUTRIVENT) decrease ventilatory requirements by decreasing carbon dioxide production and oxygen consumption. Carbohydrate-to-fat ratios are more important for hypercapnic patients, so the type of formula needed should be individually determined.

For severely compromised patients, specialized enteral formulas with a high-fat (66 to 68 percent) and low-carbohydrate (32 to 34 percent) content may be beneficial. The product provides more than 1.5 to 2 cal/mL because there is an increased tendency to retain fluid. Carbohydrate-to-fat ratios are more important for hypercapnic patients. Initially, only 80 to 90 percent of maintenance calories are provided by formulas. Formulas that provide more than 60 percent of the calories from carbohydrate should be avoided.

Hepatic Disease

Because nutrient intake of patients with hepatic disease is usually poor, malnutrition becomes a characteristic feature of liver disease. Hepatic diseases alter the use of carbohydrates, proteins, and fats. Triglycerides, ammonia levels, and blood levels of aromatic amino acids are elevated, whereas BCAA levels are low, and alterations in glucose tolerance are demonstrated.

It appears that BCAA-enriched formulas are effective in the resolution of encephalopathy and in the improvement of nutritional status, thereby improving survival. Although protein is desperately needed, protein intake must be altered in patients with advanced hepatic failure and impending encephalopathy. BCAA-enriched formulas are designed to promote protein use, stimulate liver protein synthesis, and prevent encephalopathy. By modifying amino acid mixtures and providing increased amounts of protein, hepatocyte regeneration is stimulated.

Specialized formulas used for hepatic disease (HEPATIC-AID II, TRAVASORB HEPATIC) contain high quantities (50 percent) of BCAAs and low quantities of the aromatic amino acids and methionine. Protein allowance is determined by monitoring blood urea nitrogen and serum ammonia levels and mental status.

Diabetes Mellitus

Diabetic patients with frequent hypoglycemic episodes may exhibit slow gastric emptying. Contributing factors relating to gastroparesis include secretory abnormalities, peptic ulcer disease, high-fat or hyperosmolar formulas, gastric mucosal alterations, and increased antibody production. A low-carbohydrate formula may help stabilize blood glucose levels. The use of monounsaturated fats promotes normal levels of lipoproteins. Intermittent feedings may also improve metabolic control in diabetic patients. Simulation of a normal meal pattern may result in increased nutrient absorption and glucose use.

The carbohydrate content of the formula may have a significant effect on glycemic response. Commercial formulas such as GLUCERNA and CHOICE DM are specifically designed for patients with diabetes. Carbohydrates are restricted to 33 percent, and soluble fiber is added. Fat content is 50 percent of the calories with a large portion of the fat monounsaturated. Because of the formula's high cost and the variability among patient responses, it may be advantageous to start diabetic patients (especially if they are non-insulin dependent) on a regular formula, with a normal distribution of energy nutrients. Blood glucose levels should be monitored closely, especially initially. The formula is changed if the blood glucose levels are exceptionally high.

When continuous feedings are necessary in the critically ill patient, insulin may be provided via continuous peripheral IV infusion or subcutaneously through use of a sliding scale. Use of an IV insulin drip is rather treacherous, however, especially if the enteral feeding stops but the insulin drip continues to run. This practice is not advisable unless constant monitoring is available.

Renal Failure

Supplementation of essential amino acids may be required in patients with uremia. Specialty formulas (e.g., AMIN-AID, NEPRO, SUPLENA, TRAVASORB RENAL) are frequently recommended, not only because the total protein of the diet is limited in renal failure but also because the amino acid patterns are specially designed to meet patient needs. Renal formulations may also be used when dialysis must be avoided or to decrease dialysis requirements. Maintenance of adequate calories has been associated with improvement in blood urea nitrogen, serum phosphorus, and potassium levels, as well as survival rates.

The specialized formulas contain essential amino acids as the nitrogen source. By supplying only essential amino acids, urea production decreases by recycling the nitrogen into the synthesis of nonessential amino acids (NEAAs). They promote a positive nitrogen balance in renal patients who cannot tolerate much protein. Research has shown that these products are not superior to formulas containing a mixture of essential and nonessential amino acids.

Immune Suppression

Immune function is affected by PEM and a variety of disease states. Certain components of traditional enteral formulas adversely affect immune function. For example, omega-6 polyunsaturated fatty acids (PUFAs), the traditional lipids contained in enteral formulations, affect the lipid composition of the cell membrane and are ultimately metabolized to prostaglandin E_2. High concentrations of prostaglandin E_2 are immunosuppressive and inhibit T-cell mitogenesis, the production of lymphokines, and the generation of cytotoxic cells. Therefore, many formulas have been introduced to modulate immune response using a variety of specific nutrients.

Manipulation of the amount and type of lipids may affect the patient's response to disease, injury, and infection. The amino acid arginine, omega-3 fatty acids, and ribonucleic acid (RNA) have drawn attention for their role in immunostimulatory effects. Omega-3 PUFAs are metabolized to 3-series prostanoids and 5-series leukotrienes that are less immunosuppressive. Limiting the fat of patients who are immunosuppressed may be beneficial. During periods of stress, lipids may be the preferred fuel, and in several formulations, the omega-6 PUFAs are replaced with the less immunosuppressive omega-3 PUFAs.

Arginine is an amino acid necessary for collagen synthesis and normal tissue growth. It has important effects on host defense mechanisms. Supplemental amounts of arginine have been shown to promote wound healing, enhance T-cell function, enhance lymphocyte blastogenesis, and increase the percentage of T-helper lymphocytes in postoperative cancer patients. Use of supplemental arginine for only 3 days has been shown to increase the amounts of circulating natural killer and leukocyte-activated killer cells, and their respective cytotoxicities in women with breast cancer.

Broad application of these products cannot be fully endorsed. Although the substances contained in the formulas are normally considered to be nutrients, when used to stimulate the immune system, they are more appropriately considered pharmacologic drugs.

Blended Formulas

Regular foods may be blended to a liquid consistency for use in tube feeding. Baby foods can be used with the addition of some liquid. Because the proportions of carbohydrate, protein, and fat are similar to those in a regular diet, the feeding is well tolerated by patients with a normally functioning GI tract. Some patients prefer blended foods because they provide a better variety at a reduced cost.

Bacterial contamination and inconsistency of nutrient composition with homemade formulas are potential problems. The feeding tube may become clogged if the particle size is too large or the mixture too thick.

Blended products are also commercially available. These products contain natural foodstuffs plus additional vitamins and minerals, as well as moderate amounts of fiber.

Elemental Formulas

There are two types of elemental formulas on the market. Semielemental formulas contain proteins that have been enzymatically hydrolyzed back into peptide fragments and free amino acids. The protein is a balanced mixture of essential and nonessential amino acids. Strictly elemental formulas contain pure amino acids.

Older elemental formulas are powders that are mixed with water to form hypertonic solutions. Some newer products include ready-to-use liquids. Newer products have a lower osmolality than those containing solely amino acids. The carbohydrate sources are oligosaccharides and disaccharides. Older formulas contain very little fat. Several newer products contain medium-chain triglyceride oils. Electrolytes, minerals, and trace elements are also present.

If the patient has a normally functioning intestinal tract, there is no evidence that elemental formulas are superior to polymeric formulas. They are sometimes given indiscriminately, even though a less expensive polymeric formula would be more appropriate. When the GI tract is not wholly functional (as in short bowel syndrome), or when fecal residue should be minimal (as before an operation), elemental formulas may be needed. Because of their amino acid and peptide content, elemental formulas are not very palatable and are usually administered by feeding tube.

Hydrolyzed protein formulas promote healing and improved health. Elemental formulas may enhance gut recovery after prolonged total parenteral nutrition or bowel rest. Elemental formulas require minimal digestion and do not significantly stimulate pancreatic, biliary, and intestinal secretions. They are rapidly absorbed in the proximal small intestine and are adequately absorbed, even in some patients with of short bowel syndrome.

Critical Thinking Process

Assessment

History of Present Illness

How long a patient can withstand inadequate nutritional intake is influenced by many factors that include age, previous state of health and nutrition, and the presence of sepsis. A well-nourished adult in a moderately catabolic state can usually tolerate up to 14 days of starvation without encountering significant problems. However, if the patient is between 60 and 70 years of age, tolerance of starvation is no more than 10 days. For a patient older than 70, tolerance drops to no more than 7 days.

Past Health History

A thorough dietary history reveals significant information that is necessary for determining the optimal route of administration, type of formula, and other factors related to a nutritional support regimen (see Dietary History). Subjec-

DIETARY HISTORY

Fluid Balance

Usual fluid intake amount
- Recent changes in amount (increased, decreased, or unchanged)
- Beverage preferences
- Frequency of intake
- Beverages not tolerated

Nutritional Status

Teeth and mouth
- Condition of teeth
- Dentures
- Difficulties in chewing
- Soreness in mouth
- Difficulty swallowing
- Problems with choking
- Recent changes in taste

Recent weight changes showing either gain or loss

Appetite and food preferences
- Recent appetite changes (increased, decreased, or unchanged)
- Food likes and dislikes
- Foods not tolerated and why
- Food allergies
- Where meals are taken
- Who purchases and prepares the food
- Snacking habits
- Number of feedings daily
- Vitamin or mineral supplements used
- Budgeting problems
- Alcohol intake (type, frequency, amount)
- Personal or religious restrictions (e.g., kosher or vegetarian)
- Dietary concerns

Nutrient adequacy—Use of these techniques for determining actual and habitual dietary intake provides rough estimates that can be compared with established standards (RDI, Food Guide Pyramid, Dietary Guidelines for Americans)
- Dietary recall—a recollection of all foods and amounts eaten by the person on the previous day
- Food diary—maintained by the person for 3 to 7 days and consisting of a record of foods eaten, the amounts, method of preparation, where the food is eaten, and time of intake
- Food frequency form—food checklist to determine the number of times per day, week, or month specific foods or categories of food are eaten

Gastrointestinal Problems
- Excessive belching or heartburn
- Indigestion
- Nausea
- Vomiting

Elimination
- Constipation or diarrhea
- Recent changes in bowel movements
- Frequency of bowel movements
- Use of laxatives or enemas, or other practices
- Difficulty with urination
- Recent changes in urinary elimination patterns (increased, decreased, or unchanged)

Current Prescribed and Over-the-Counter Drug Use

Adapted from Davis, J., and Sherer, K. (1994). *Applied nutrition and diet therapy for nurses* (2nd ed., p. 287). Philadelphia: W. B. Saunders. Used with permission.

tive information gathered in a diet history can help determine nutritional adequacy of the patient's usual intake. Other factors influencing intake, such as other family members or significant others, economic status, and social and recreational activities, are important in understanding overall dietary intake. Mobility, independence, and transportation indicate the patient's ability to obtain and prepare an enteral feeding. For instance, patients who need to receive feedings at home must have muscle strength and dexterity to open a can. Knowledge of the patient's occupation and daily activities can indicate general energy level.

Screening intake for food group consumption can provide meaningful information about the nutrient quality of food intake. This information can be collected by interview (recall) or by a record the patient maintains. A nutrient intake record is used to provide a rough estimate of actual nutrient intake that can be compared with standards. Frequently, only key nutrients, which include calories, protein, fat, dietary fiber, calcium, and vitamins A and C, are used to assess overall nutrient intake. A dietary history minimizes the time and expense involved in more tedious nutritional assessments.

Other data that must be assessed include concurrent diseases or conditions (especially gastroesophageal reflux) and drugs, or genetic factors that may modify a patient's nutrient requirements, absorption, use, or elimination of nutrients. A good dietary history should disclose information regarding inadequate food and fluid intake, as well as abnormal fluid losses. When previous food intake or accelerated catabolism result in weight loss and less-than-normal body stores, nutrition support should be implemented as early as possible. Recent weight changes may be caused by increased nutrient losses and requirements. Food allergies or intolerances may influence the type of formula that is appropriate. Emotional factors should not be ignored.

In most acute care facilities, nursing staff records the amount of each food consumed for evaluation by the dietitian. All foods eaten within the designated time period should be documented, including snacks and foods provided by family and friends.

Physical Exam Findings

Physical exam findings can reveal existing nutritional deficiencies, especially in the skin, eyes, mouth, skeleton, and nervous system (Table 59–3). However, signs of malnutrition are often nonspecific. Different problems may produce the same specific clinical finding. For this reason, clinical findings must correlate with other assessment parameters, laboratory data, and diet history.

TABLE 59–3 CLINICAL FINDINGS ASSOCIATED WITH NUTRIENT DEFICIENCIES

Anatomic Feature	Physical Findings	Possible Nutrient Deficiency
Hair	Alopecia	Protein, biotin, zinc
	Dyspigmentation	Protein, biotin
	Flag sign	Protein
	Easily plucked hair	Protein
Nails	Transverse ridging	Protein
	Koilonychia	Iron
Skin	Dryness	Vitamin A, essential fatty acids, zinc
	Follicular hyperkeratosis	Vitamins A and C, essential fatty acids
	Perifollicular petechiae	Vitamins A and C
	Purpura	Vitamins C and K
	Dermatitis	Niacin
	Nasolabial seborrhea	Niacin, riboflavin, vitamin B_6
	Pigmentation, desquamation of sun-exposed areas	Niacin
Eyes	Night blindness	Vitamin A
	Bitot's spot	
	Xerophthalmia	Riboflavin
	Angular blepharitis	
Perioral	Cheilosis	Vitamin B_6, riboflavin, niacin
	Angular stomatitis	Riboflavin, niacin, vitamin B_6
Oral	Bleeding, swollen gums	Vitamin C
	Magenta tongue	Riboflavin
	Atrophic papillae	Iron, niacin, folate, vitamins B_{12}, C, and E
	Glossitis	Riboflavin, niacin, folate, iron, and vitamins B_6 and B_{12}
	Hypogeusia	Zinc
Subcutaneous tissue	Edema	Protein, thiamin
	Wasting	Energy
Musculoskeletal system	Muscle wasting	Protein
	Bowlegs	Vitamin D, calcium
	Beading of ribs	Vitamin D, protein
	Tenderness	Vitamin C
Neurological	Dementia	Niacin, vitamin B_{12}
	Confabulation, disorientation	
	Peripheral neuropathy	Thiamin, vitamins B_6 and B_{12}
	Tetany	Calcium, magnesium
Other	Parotid enlargement	Protein
	Heart failure	Thiamin, phophorus
	Poor wound healing, decubitus ulcers	Protein, vitamin C, zinc

Height and Weight Body weight is a nonspecific measure of all body components, including fat, proteins, and fluid balance. It is one of the most expedient and helpful indicators of nutritional status.

Information regarding the patient's weight and height can be obtained from the patient or family if direct measurements are impossible, but these measurements are seldom accurate. A fixed measuring guide attached to a vertical flat surface, such as a wall, is a more accurate measurement of height than the measuring rod on platform scales. The measurement may be accomplished by having the patient stand as straight and tall as possible.

Because of its significance in assessing nutritional status, care must be taken to obtain accurate weight. The patient's weight is compared with standards to determine if the patient is overweight, of normal weight, or underweight. In a clinic setting, clothing should be minimal and shoes should not be worn. Patients in the hospital should be weighed at the same time of day, preferably before breakfast and after voiding. The same scale should be used, and the patient should have on similar clothing at each weighing.

All scales should be professionally calibrated at least semiannually, in addition to adjustment of the zero balance on the horizontal beam of the scale before each use. Use of scales that are appropriate for the patient's mobility status is important. Wheelchair scales are used if the patient is able to sit, especially if the patient is weighed daily. Bed scales are necessary for bedridden patients.

A simple method of estimating desirable weight has been used. For women, estimated desirable weight is calculated using 100 pounds for the first 60 inches (5 feet) in height with an additional 5 pounds added for each additional inch in height over 60 inches. For men, the estimated desirable weight is calculated using 106 pounds for the first 60 inches with an additional 6 pounds added for each additional inch in height. An additional 10 percent is added or subtracted for a large or small frame, respectively. For patients with paraplegia, 5 to 10 percent is subtracted, and for those with quadriplegia, 10 to 15 percent is subtracted. Again, these are unscientific measures and can provide only an estimate of appropriate weight.

Height-weight tables developed by life insurance companies are widely used. The charts were developed to predict mortality on the basis of weight and are not predictive of medical conditions associated with weight. Judgments about nutritional status based solely on height and weight are limited in their reliability and do not reflect body fat or hydration status. Deviations from ideal body weight (IBW) indicate the degree of depletion or overweight. Evaluation of the significance of weight change can be a useful tool (see Evaluation of Weight Change).

EVALUATION OF WEIGHT CHANGE

Use equation

$$\text{Percent weight change} = \frac{\text{usual weight} - \text{actual weight}}{\text{usual weight} \times 100}$$

And compare to standard

Time Period	Significant Weight Loss (%)	Severe Weight Loss (%)
1 week	1–2	>2
1 month	5	>5
3 months	7.5	>7.5
6 months	10	>10

Since weight is directly related to bone structure, frame size is another aspect that must be considered when determining appropriate weight. The simplest technique for determining frame size are wrist measurements (see Determination of Frame Size).

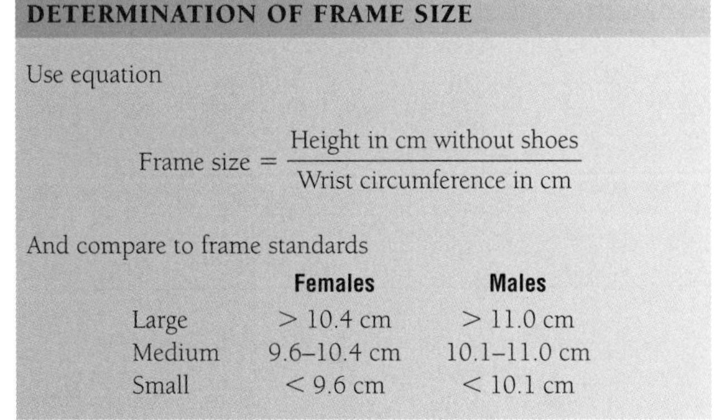

DETERMINATION OF FRAME SIZE

Use equation

$$\text{Frame size} = \frac{\text{Height in cm without shoes}}{\text{Wrist circumference in cm}}$$

And compare to frame standards

	Females	Males
Large	> 10.4 cm	> 11.0 cm
Medium	9.6–10.4 cm	10.1–11.0 cm
Small	< 9.6 cm	< 10.1 cm

Weight loss can be an ominous sign, indicating use of lean body mass (muscle and organ tissue) for energy. If fluid loss is not significant, weight loss is a better indicator of current nutritional status. It reflects loss of vital protein stores (muscle and organ tissue) for energy. This occurs rapidly with significantly inadequate caloric intake. During a high-stress condition, and especially if IV dextrose solutions are being administered, protein stores are catabolized. Weight status may be maintained, falsely indicating adequate nutrition, because water and collagen replace the fat and muscle tissue being catabolized. This common finding in PEM is particularly apparent in obese patients.

The rate of weight loss is also important. Daily weight fluctuations of 2.2 pounds reflect body fluid changes of 1 L. Examinination of trends over a period of time is more helpful for indicating nutritional status.

Triceps Skinfold Anthropometric measurements are used to identify adequacy of nutritional status or malnutrition and to detect loss or gain of body components relative to previous measurements. Anthropometric measurements such as triceps skinfold, subscapular skinfold, and midarm muscle circumference measurements may be used to identify the status of somatic protein and fat stores (Fig. 59–1). Anthropometric measurements help confirm or discredit visual appraisals. Since 50 percent of fat stores are subcutaneous, skinfold thickness indicates energy reserves. The amount of body fat, indirectly measured by skinfold measurements, is also an indirect indicator of previous caloric balance (intake versus requirements). Special skinfold calipers are required for this technique. Although body fat increases with age, the sum of skinfold measurements remains constant, indicating that fat accumulates in locations other than subcutaneous sites.

Body Mass Index Body mass index (BMI), which is body weight divided by the height squared, estimates total

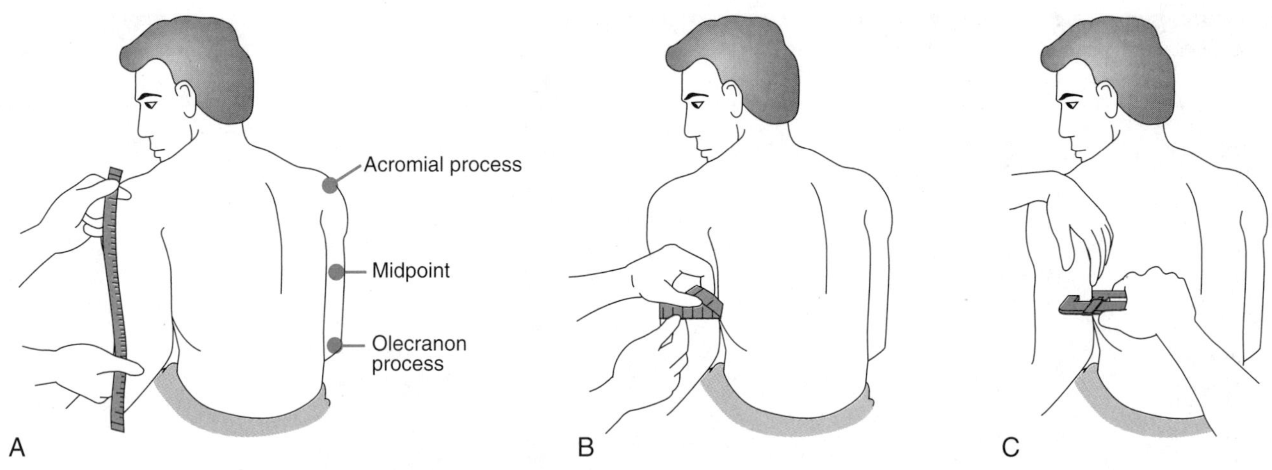

D

MEASUREMENT		STANDARD	90%	60%
Midarm circumference (MAC)	Men	29.3 cm	26.4 cm	17.6 cm
	Women	28.5 cm	25.7 cm	17.1 cm
Triceps skinfold (TSF)	Men	12.5 mm	11.3 mm	7.5 mm
	Women	16.5 mm	14.9 mm	9.9 mm
Midarm muscle circumference (MAMC)	Men	25.3 cm	22.8 cm	15.2 cm
	Women	23.2 cm	20.9 cm	13.9 cm

Calculate the midarm muscle circumference (MAMC) using the following formula:
MAMC (in cm) = [MAC in cm] – [(0.314) × (TSF in mm)]

Figure 59–1 Tricep skinfold measurement. *A,* Measure and mark the midpoint of the upper arm. *B,* Measure the circumference of mid–upper arm. *C,* Measure skin-fold thickness of triceps using special calipers. (From Black, J. M., and Matassarin-Jacobs, E. [1997]. *Medical-surgical nursing: Clinical management for continuity of care* (5th ed., p. 240). Philadelphia: W. B. Saunders. Used with permission.)

body mass. BMI has the highest correlation with actual body fat (Table 59–4). BMI minimizes the effect of height and is useful for descriptive and comparison purposes. Patients with BMI calculations of less than 19 are classified as underweight and are at risk for disorders such as respiratory disease, tuberculosis, digestive disease, and some cancers. The major weakness in the use of a BMI is the lack of distinction between heaviness resulting from adiposity and heaviness related to muscularity or edema. Classifications ranging from morbid obesity to severe PEM can be made based on BMI (see Body Mass Index Classifications). The reader is referred to a nutrition textbook for additional information on anthropometric measurements and body mass index calculations.

Diagnostic Testing

Laboratory testing provides objective information about nutritional status and is warranted when other parameters suggest possible malnutrition. Use of laboratory testing requires knowledge of the purpose of each test, awareness of normal values, and knowledge of factors that may cause alterations in the results. In some cases, marginal nutritional deficiencies can be detected before overt clinical signs appear. In general, clinical and dietary assessments can be confirmed from laboratory data by confirming suspicions or indicating possible causes.

Urine is routinely checked for specific gravity, protein, pH, and acetone. Urinary values of these parameters generally fluctuate more than serum levels of the same parameters, reflecting recent rather than usual intake. Hemoglobin, hematocrit, total protein, serum albumin or prealbumin, and total lymphocyte counts collectively reflect protein nutriture. Determinations of sodium and potassium, glucose,

BODY MASS INDEX CLASSIFICATIONS

Classification	Body Mass Index
Severe or morbid obesity	>40
Moderate obesity	30–40
Mild obesity	27.5–30
Obesity	>27.5
Appropriate weight (+65 years)	24–29
Appropriate weight (55–64 years)	23–28
Appropriate weight (45–54 years)	22–27
Appropriate weight (35–44 years)	21–26
Appropriate weight (25–34 years)	20–25
Appropriate weight (19–24 years)	19–24
Mild PEM	17.0–18.4
Moderate PEM	16.0–16.9
Severe PEM	<16

PEM, Protein-energy malnutrition.

Data from James, W. P., Ferro-Luzzi, S., and Waterlow, J.C. (1988). Definition of chronic energy deficiency in adults. Report of a working party of the International Dietary Energy Consultation Group. *European Journal of Clinical Nutrition,* 42, 969–981; and Bray, G. A., and Gray, D. S. (1988). Obesity. Part 1: Pathogenesis. *Western Journal of Medicine,* 149, 429–441.

TABLE 59–4 BODY WEIGHTS IN POUNDS ACCORDING TO HEIGHT AND BODY MASS INDEX*†

	Body Mass Index, kg/m²													
Height, in	19.0	20.0	21.0	22.0	23.0	24.0	25.0	26.0	27.0	28.0	29.0	30.0	35.0	40.0
	Body Weight, lb													
58.0	90.7	95.5	100.3	105.0	109.8	114.6	119.4	124.1	128.9	133.7	138.5	143.2	167.1	191.0
59.0	93.9	98.8	103.8	108.7	113.6	118.6	123.5	128.5	133.4	138.3	143.3	148.2	172.9	197.6
60.0	97.1	102.2	107.3	112.4	117.5	122.6	127.7	132.9	138.0	143.1	148.2	153.3	178.8	204.4
61.0	100.3	105.6	110.9	116.2	121.5	126.8	132.0	137.3	142.6	147.9	153.2	158.4	184.8	211.3
62.0	103.7	109.1	114.6	120.0	125.5	130.9	136.4	141.9	147.3	152.8	158.2	163.7	191.0	218.2
63.0	107.0	112.7	118.3	123.9	129.6	135.2	140.8	146.5	152.1	157.7	163.4	169.0	197.2	225.3
64.0	110.5	116.3	122.1	127.9	133.7	139.5	145.3	151.2	157.0	162.8	168.6	174.4	203.5	232.5
65.0	113.9	119.9	125.9	131.9	137.9	143.9	149.9	155.9	161.9	167.9	173.9	179.9	209.9	239.9
66.0	117.5	123.7	129.8	136.0	142.2	148.4	154.6	160.8	166.9	173.1	179.3	185.5	216.4	247.3
67.0	121.1	127.4	133.8	140.2	146.5	152.9	159.3	165.7	172.0	178.4	184.8	191.1	223.0	254.9
68.0	124.7	131.3	137.8	144.4	151.0	157.5	164.1	170.6	177.2	183.8	190.3	196.9	229.7	262.5
69.0	128.4	135.2	141.9	148.7	155.4	162.2	168.9	175.7	182.5	189.2	196.0	202.7	236.5	270.3
70.0	132.1	139.1	146.1	153.0	160.0	166.9	173.9	180.8	187.8	194.7	201.7	208.6	243.4	278.2
71.0	135.9	143.1	150.3	157.4	164.6	171.7	178.9	186.0	193.2	200.3	207.5	214.6	250.4	286.2
72.0	139.8	147.2	154.5	161.9	169.2	176.6	183.9	191.3	198.7	206.0	213.4	220.7	257.5	294.3
73.0	143.7	151.3	158.8	166.4	174.0	181.5	189.1	196.7	204.2	211.8	219.3	226.9	264.7	302.5
74.0	147.7	155.4	153.2	171.0	178.8	186.5	194.3	202.1	209.9	217.6	225.4	233.2	272.0	310.9
75.0	151.7	159.7	167.7	175.6	183.6	191.6	199.6	207.6	215.6	223.5	231.5	239.5	279.4	319.4
76.0	155.8	164.0	172.2	180.4	188.6	196.8	205.0	213.2	221.4	229.5	237.7	245.9	286.9	327.9

*Each entry gives the body weight in pounds (lb) for a person of a given height and body mass index.
†Desirable body mass index range in relation to age
From Bray, G. A, and Gray, D. S. (1988). Obesity. Part 1. Pathogenesis. *Western Journal of Medicine*, 149, 431. Used with permission.

and cholesterol and triglyceride levels are indicative of electrolyte balance and carbohydrate and lipid metabolism.

Vitamin Levels Although some mineral (calcium, chloride, phosphorus, magnesium) levels are easy to determine, elaborate testing techniques are required to assess most vitamin levels. These tests are expensive, and many agencies are not equipped to perform the tests on a routine basis. Examples of tests for vitamin levels include urinary thiamine, riboflavin, vitamin B_{12}, *N*-methylnicotinamide (niacin), and serum levels for carotene and vitamins A and C. Dietary deficiency of a vitamin results in decreased elimination (or conservation) before laboratory changes or physical signs of deficiency are evident. Early detection of vitamin deficiency may prevent more serious complications (see discussion in Chapter 58).

Protein Levels Laboratory evaluation of protein status can be determined by several tests: serum albumin, transferrin, prealbumin, and 24-hour urine urea nitrogen. Plasma proteins are affected by stress and renal and hepatic disease.

Albumin, which is synthesized in the liver, transports small molecules (including many drugs, hormones, and vitamins) and provides 70 percent of the colloidal osmotic pressure of plasma. When colloid osmotic pressure decreases, peripheral edema may develop. This process leads to decreased absorption of nutrients and diarrhea from intestinal villi. Albumin levels correlate with changes in midarm muscle circumference. In some cases, low serum levels indicate reduced synthesis (liver dysfunction), catabolism, loss to interstitial fluids, and abnormal external loss. In addition to malnutrition, serum albumin levels decrease in the presence of fluid volume excess and bedrest. Serum albumin levels are good indicators of long-term nutritional status if there is no current illness or condition.

Transferrin, an iron-carrying protein, has a shorter half-life than albumin, and its measurement is more sensitive to current status. Low levels indicate protein deficiency, which is accompanied by increased risks of *anergy* (lack of energy), sepsis, and mortality. Although low levels of albumin place the patient at increased risk, physiologic stress, such as infection or surgery, may also cause low albumin and transferrin levels. Although malnutrition is not evident, patients need adequate nutrition support to prevent further decreases.

Prealbumin is a more sensitive test for recent nutritional problems and correlates better with nitrogen balance than albumin or transferrin. Thus, a prealbumin level is a better indicator of visceral protein anabolism. Assessment of visceral proteins is identified in Table 59–5.

Urea is the major waste product of protein catabolism. A 24-hour urine urea nitrogen clearance test can be used to determine the extent of protein catabolism and adequacy of protein intake. In catabolic patients, protein breakdown is much more rapid than synthesis. Approximately three-fourths of ingested nitrogen is excreted.

To determine the adequacy of protein and caloric intake, an estimate of protein intake (over the previous 2 or 3 days) is necessary. A 3-day average, using the formula for estimated nitrogen balance found in Appendix C, should be positive by more than 0.04 g of nitrogen/kg/day to ensure positive nitrogen balance. If the value obtained is a negative number, more protein is needed.

Immunologic Testing Immune status is reflected in the total lymphocyte count (TLC). A differential white blood cell count alone has limited value; it must always be interpreted in light of the TLC. A depressed lymphocyte count predisposes a patient to infection. TLCs are calculated by multi-

TABLE 59–5 ASSESSMENT OF VISCERAL PROTEINS

Protein	Functions	Half-Life	Normal	Degree of Malnutrition: Mild	Moderate	Severe
Albumin (g/dL)	Carrier protein; maintains colloid osmotic pressure	21 days	> 3.5	3–3.5	2.5–3	< 2.5
Transferrin (mg/dL)	Transports iron	8–10 days	> 200	180–200	160–180	< 160
Prealbumin (mg/dL)	Transports thyroxin and retinol-binding protein	2–3 days	> 15	10–15	5–10	< 5
Total lymphocyte count/mm^3	Reflects immune status	NA	> 1500	1200–1500	800–1200	< 800

NA, Not applicable.

From Davis, J. R., and Sherer, K. (1994). *Applied nutrition and diet therapy for nurses* (2nd ed., p. 299). Philadelphia: W. B. Saunders. Used with permission.

plying the white blood cell count by the percentage of lymphocytes (using a decimal figure). Moderate nutritional problems are characterized by a TLC between 800 and 1200/mm^3. Patients whose values fall below are considered to be severely malnourished and anergic. The TLC is affected by many medical conditions and fluctuates significantly.

Developmental Considerations

Perinatal Most indications for nutritional supplements in the general patient population also apply to pregnant women. Prevention of malnutrition during the second and third trimesters, when maternal and fetal components are expanding rapidly, results in a favorable outcome. Extensive nutritional deficits in the last half of pregnancy have a significant effect on the infant's birth weight. Hyperemesis gravidarum is a potential indication for enteral support.

Pediatric Preterm infants are likely candidates for enteral feedings because of a weak or absent suck reflex. Additionally, the GI tract of the infant is immature, with inadequate lower esophageal sphincter pressure, delayed gastric emptying because of decreased secretion of gastric acid and increased production of gastrin, impaired GI motility, and limited GI enzyme and hormone secretion. Because of inadequate nutrient stores, preterm infants should be provided with sufficient nutrients to allow for a growth rate comparable to the intrauterine growth rate.

Geriatric Assessment of the hydration status in an older adult is essential because signs of dehydration are similar to many of the physical changes seen with aging. Because the changes of aging occur at varying rates, older adults differ from one another more than any individuals in other age group. The nutritional status of older adults may be poor because of oral or dental health problems, inadequate alterations in taste and smell, financial status, an inability to shop and prepare food, or polypharmacy.

In general, aging results in changes in body composition. There is a decline in lean body mass and total body water, and relatively higher amounts of adipose tissue. Weight begins to decrease after age 70, but rapid weight changes should be noted to avoid overlooking changes that may indicate a disease process. The older adult may experience decreased thirst and reduced renal concentration, which increases the risk of dehydration.

Psychosocial Considerations

Psychosocial adjustments to malnutrition and enteral feeding states may be difficult because of the numerous psychological and varied social meanings of food. Enteral nutrition reduces feedings to the bare essentials of nourishment. By its very nature, tube feedings dramatically bypass the sensory pleasures that normally accompany eating. Deprivation of the gustatory experiences related to tasting, chewing, and swallowing food; drinking liquids; and appetites for favorite foods are associated with enteral feedings. Regardless of whether the impairment is temporary or permanent, patients mourn the loss of oral gratifications and pleasures they experienced from eating.

Television and magazine advertisements constantly exhort consumers to eat or drink. Family life and social activities are frequently focused around eating. Enteral feedings become stressful and uncomfortable for the patient and family rather than being a uniting force. The patient may retreat to another room or eat or drink only small amounts.

Additionally, enteral feedings disrupt the normal biosensory cues that stimulate appetite and signal satiety. Patients and caretakers should be reassured that they are receiving adequate nutrition, even if they are experiencing hunger pangs. Positive signs, such as weight gain and increased stamina, can be emphasized.

Sadness, depression, or anger are common responses to changes in life-style or inability to perform activities of daily living. Leisure and social activities are important to the patient. Assessment of the patient's body image helps determine the ideal route of administration and method of delivery for the enteral feeding. Many patients who require nasoenteric feeding tubes do not wish to go out in public.

Changes in life-style can be minimized by carefully assessing the patient's needs and determining the best formula and method of delivery to control GI symptoms such as flatus, diarrhea, constipation, nausea, borborygmus, or fullness.

Many times the patients have become cachectic, unattractive, weak, and unable to ambulate before implementation of enteral feedings. Their bodies may be repulsive to them. Some patients welcome the initiation of enteral feedings that help them regain weight and restore strength. However, the presence of a nasal feeding tube or gastrostomy may compound patients' perception of disfigurement. Acceptance of the feeding tube may be just as difficult as acceptance of a temporary or permanent ileostomy or colostomy. The health care provider helps in this adjustment by allowing patients an opportunity to ventilate their feelings.

Patients requiring enteral feedings for more than a couple of months are more likely to become depressed than one whose therapy is short term. About 80 percent of patients experience depression during the first 3 to 6 months of enteral feedings at home. Episodes of sadness, social withdrawal, and feelings of hopelessness may be experienced. Symptoms of depression can be very similar to those of severe malnutrition: apathy, decreased energy, loss of interest in the environment, severe asthenia, anorexia, nausea, a variety of somatic complaints, crying, headaches, and social withdrawal. If depression is not diagnosed, poor compliance with feedings is likely to occur, with resultant metabolic abnormalities and dehydration.

Patients and families are unique in their ability to support one another in their needs. Personality characteristics and behavioral patterns of the patient and family shape psychological responses to this treatment. The addition of an enteral feeding with other care needs can further compound psychological reactions. Compliance with the nutritional regimen can be increased by individualizing care plans congruent with level of physical health and personality styles.

A determination of what was normal for this family unit before the illness is important. An assessment would include whether the family previously dealt openly with such issues, the closeness and stability of the family unit, and whether the patient was an active or passive member of the family. Families may be reluctant for the patient to return to established roles within the family. The family may experience additional strain because the person who is ill may be the primary force in establishing family cohesion and stability or was the primary breadwinner.

An assessment will also determine availability of nonfamily resources, as well as willingness of family members to become involved with the patient's treatment and to assume responsibility for changing roles and activities. Long-term dependence on a single caregiver can lead to feelings of anger and resentment on the part of the caregiver and feelings of guilt in the patient. Even in a loving relationship, the caregiver may experience burnout.

Ethical Concerns Nutrients provided through tube feedings can be perceived as heroic, optional medical treatment similar to other life-sustaining medical treatment decisions. In contrast, however, enteral feedings may be viewed as a unique life support system that provides food and is an essential part of humane care. Therefore, ethical issues are often of concern, especially for terminally ill or comatose patients.

Clinical decisions as to whether to forgo enteral feedings can be complex. Values such as respect for patient autonomy and performance of professional beneficence may be contradictory. The American Nurses' Association views patient advocacy as a responsibility of all health care professionals. Each patient is to be treated with dignity and respect. Factors that must be assessed include the patient's diagnosis, prognosis, and function rather than age. Ethical issues such as quality of life and life expectancy are other variables. Unfortunately, economics can also become a factor in determining treatment modalities.

Informed consent means that the patient must be competent to make an informed decision about the proposed treatment, must have adequate information about the possible risks and benefits of the treatment, and must make the decision voluntarily in accordance with personal values and goals. If the patient is unable to express his or her desire in this matter, the wishes of the family or legal representative should prevail. Occasionally, a health care provider's moral conflicts with a patient's decision to forgo nutrition support complicates the plan of care.

It is frequently impossible to predict who will benefit from enteral feedings. Thus, the decision to withdraw enteral feedings should be continually reassessed. If the therapeutic plan proves futile, it may be in the best interest of the patient to withdraw the feedings.

Analysis and Management

Treatment Objectives

The primary treatment objectives for the patient with malnutrition are to (1) decrease weight loss, (2) restore anabolism by furnishing nutrients that meet increased demands, (3) replace tissue protein losses, and (4) alleviate the clinical manifestations of the condition. A variety of feeding modalities can be used to help meet these objectives, but the cardinal guideline is to use the gut if it is working rather than parenteral nutrition modalities.

Treatment Options

Increasing oral intake is the ideal method for nutritional support. It is the least expensive and invasive and the most enjoyable. Oral feedings consist of using regular foods, frequent feedings, or foods modified in texture or flavor. The calorie and protein content of foods provided, and the overall intake, can be improved by following the guidelines in Table 59–6. If adequate intake is not achieved, oral supplements of nutritionally complete formulas can be added to the diet, or nutrient-dense foods can be provided. When nutritional support is initiated, calories and protein are gradually increased to allow for readaptation of metabolic and intestinal functions. In some cases, enteral and parenteral feedings may be required to provide nutrients and to restore metabolic balance better. Repletion of nutrients that is excessively aggressive can result in metabolic imbalances such as hypophosphatemia and cardiorespiratory failure.

Enteral feeding is appropriate for patients who have been without nutrition for 5 to 7 days, for patients whose duration of illness is anticipated to be more than 10 days, and for the patient who is malnourished. To implement an enteral feeding, the patient must have a functional GI tract.

The advantages of feedings that use the gut are obvious. They are physiologically more natural, less expensive, and nutritionally more complete than common parenteral solutions. Further, nutrients administered via the gut are used efficiently and metabolic upsets are less likely to occur. Bowel rest for any reason (for example, starvation, GI tract dysfunction) leads to atrophy in the small and large bowel. It is not

TABLE 59–6 DETERMINATION OF CALORIES, PROTEIN, AND FLUID REQUIREMENTS

Calories Per Day

Status	Adults cal/kg IBW	Infants and Children	cal/kg
Basal energy needs	25–30	Preterm infants	100–120
Ambulatory, maintain weight	30–35	0–6 months	105
Malnutrition, mild stress	40	1–3 years	100
Severe injuries and sepsis	50–60	4–6 years	85
Extensive burns	80	7–10 years	86
Pregnancy (2nd and 3rd trimester)	Add 300 cal	11–14, boys	60
		11–14, girls	48
Lactation	Add 500 cal	15–18, boys	42
		15–18, girls	38

Protein Per Day

Status	Adult Estimated Requirements (g/kg/day)
Normal adult	0.8–1.0
Moderately stressed (infection, fracture, surgery)	1.0–2.0
Severely stressed (burns, multiple fractures)	2.0–2.5
Pregnancy/lactation	Add 10–15 g to above calculations

Infants and Children	Normal (g/kg/day)	Sressed (g/kg/day)
Preterm	3.5–4.0	—
0.0–6 months	2.2	2.2–3.0
6 months–1 year	2.0	1.6–3.0
1–3 years	1.8	1.2–3.0
4–6 years	1.5	1.1–3.0
7–10 years	1.2	1.0–2.5
11–14 years	1.0	1.0–2.5
15–18 years	0.85	1.0–2.5

Fluid Requirements Per Day

Adults	ml/kg
18–64 years	30–35
55–65 years	30
>65 years	25
Infants and Children	**ml/kg**
Preterm (<1000 g)	150
Preterm (>1000 g)	100–150
Infants and child 1–10 kg	100
Child 11–20 kg	1000 mL + 50 mL/kg for each kg > 10 kg
Child > 20 kg	1500 mL + 20 mL/kg for each kg > 20 kg

certain whether enteral feedings maintain GI integrity by promoting anatomic (villous structure) or immune functions, but bacterial translocation is decreased. However, endotoxins from translocation of bacteria can trigger a hypermetabolic response and a septic state, ultimately resulting in multiple system organ failure. Enteral feedings also foster more normal substrate distribution. Early initiation of enteral feeding is associated with maintenance or a more rapid establishment of positive nitrogen balance, lessened hypermetabolic response, prevention of paralytic ileus, and reduced cost.

During anabolism, adequate nonprotein calories (carbohydrates and fats) must be supplied for energy in order to use protein for tissue rebuilding. Normal energy requirements are in the range of 25 to 35 cal/kg/day.

Protein can be synthesized only if energy (i.e., calorie) requirements are met. Normal protein requirements are 0.8 to 1.0 g/kg daily. A patient with an illness has increased requirements for healing and optimal immune response. If protein intake is inadequate, as much as 1 pound of tissue protein can be catabolized daily. Additional protein is needed in the presence of sepsis, fever, infection, trauma, exudates, or hemorrhaging. Protein and energy requirements can be calculated as shown in Table 59–6.

Provision of adequate amounts of fluids to replace normal fluid losses and losses from exudates, hemorrhage, vomiting, diuresis, and fever is essential. However, most enteral feedings do not provide adequate fluid. Eighty percent of a 1-calorie/mL formula is available as fluid for the body. Fiber-containing formulas may cause constipa-tion and even impaction without additional fluids. Additional fluids are also necessary in patients receiving large protein and electrolyte loads, those receiving additional fiber, those with hyperthermia, those with decreased renal concentrating ability, or those with extensive tissue breakdown. Fluid requirements are also shown in Table 59–6. Severe shifts in fluid balance and in the metabolism of phosphorus, potassium, glucose, and magnesium caused by malnutrition should be corrected before implementing feedings.

Formula Variables

Once the daily calories, protein, and fluid needs of the patient are determined, the appropriate formula is selected.

The route of administration must be known at this point because this can affect the type of formula chosen and the method of delivery.

Route Enteral nutrition can be administered by a number of routes. The route chosen depends on anticipated duration of feeding, condition of the GI tract, and potential for aspiration. Small, soft-bore tubes made of polyurethane or silicone elastomers are available in several sizes and come with stylets to facilitate their placement.

The most common route for short-term feedings is a nasogastric tube inserted into the stomach. Longer, more flexible weighted tubes can also be passed to the duodenum (nasoduodenal) and the jejunum (nasojejunal) (Fig. 59–2). Permanent feeding tube placement (gastrostomy, esophagostomy, or jejunostomy) is indicated for long-term enteral feeding. The tube is surgically inserted at the appropriate location and sutured in place. The placement of a percutaneous endoscopic gastrostomy (PEG) tube can be performed at the bedside with minimal sedation. If necessary, a gastrostomy can be used as an access to the jejunum to minimize reflux and aspiration. A jejunostomy tube can be placed during a laparotomy, especially for preoperative malnutrition, major upper abdominal operations, and the postoperative anticipated need for antineoplastic drugs or radiation therapy.

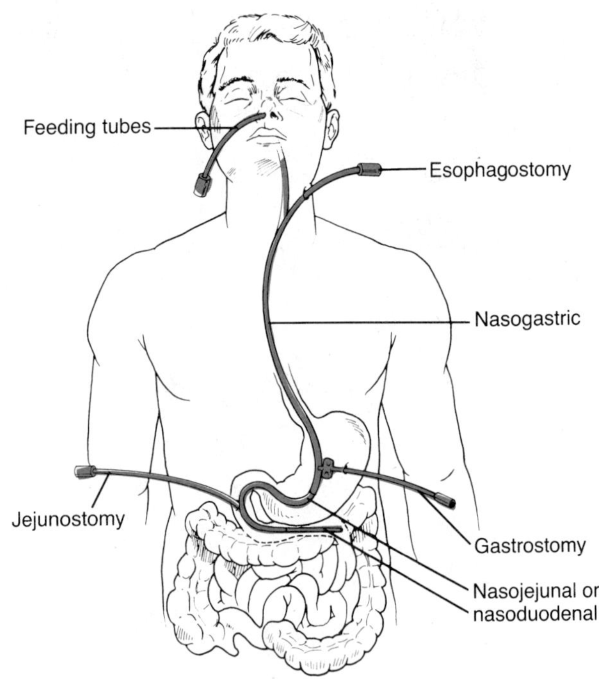

Figure 59–2 Enteral feeding tube placement. The most common route for short-term feedings is a nasogastric (NG) tube inserted into the stomach. Longer, more flexible weighted tubes can also be passed to the duodenum (nasoduodenal) and the jejunum (nasojejunal). Permanent feeding tube placement (gastrostomy, esophagostomy, or jejunostomy) is indicated for long-term enternal feeding. (From Mahan, L. K., and Escott-Stump, S. [1996]. *Krause's food, nutrition, & diet therapy* (9th ed., p. 429). Philadelphia: W. B. Saunders. Used with permission.)

Tube placement beyond the stomach requires notification of the pharmacist because placement of the tube in the duodenum or jejunum alters delivery and absorption of some drugs. For example, a tube in the jejunum affects absorption of a drug designed to be administered into the stomach because of the lack of an acidic medium and the time the drug would normally be in the stomach.

Method Formulas can be administered intermittently using bolus feedings, continuously, or by cyclic infusion. The best administration method for a patient depends on many factors, including the patient's medical condition, tolerance, and preference. Facility policies and staffing are also important in determining method of delivery.

Bolus feedings are more appropriate to supplement oral intake by ambulatory patients. Bolus feedings can be delivered only to the stomach. Tolerance of bolus feedings is dependent on the functional ability of the GI tract. Rapid administration of 300 to 400 mL of formula through a syringe in a short period of time (e.g. 10 minutes) is generally not recommended. Bolus feedings are associated with a high risk of gastric retention, aspiration, nausea, vomiting, diarrhea, distention, and cramps.

Intermittent feedings are administered over a 30- to 60-minute period, delivering approximately 300 to 400 mL every 3 to 6 hours. The feeding is better tolerated if the administration rate is 6 to 12 mL/min. The equipment required for bolus feedings is minimal—only an enteral feeding bag. Gravity feeding systems must be more closely monitored than those using a mechanical pump. Intermittent feedings are a practical and inexpensive method for enteral feedings at home. They are frequently used for diabetic patients because the pseudonormal meal feeding patterns result in improved metabolic control.

Continuous feedings are recommended if all of the patient's nutrition is provided via enteral feeding, for critically ill patients, or for patients receiving feedings into the small bowel. These feedings are infused over a 24 hour period. In an acute care setting, continuous feedings are advantageous because the nutrients are used more efficiently and permit quicker achievement of the caloric goal (see Controversy Box).

Cyclic feedings are infused over 8 to 16 hours, either during the day or night. If patients are able to eat, nighttime cyclic feedings are preferred. Nighttime feedings allow more freedom during the day. Conversely, patients who are at risk of aspirating or tube dislodgment may need daytime feedings.

A mechanical pump is necessary for feedings administered into the distal duodenum or proximal jejunum, when elemental formulas are used, for patients who have limited absorptive area, or for patients who are at high risk for aspiration. The mechanical pump is more dependable than the gravity drip method, which is subject to an uneven flow rate. To ensure the patient's mobility, a portable pump can be used. Continuous infusions reduce the risk of abdominal distention. Precise flow rates are important and are checked for accuracy every one to 2 hours.

Formula The formula to be used should provide adequate calories, protein, and 100 percent of the RDI of vitamins and minerals. Additional water is usually necessary to maintain a satisfactory urinary output. If the formula chosen provides less fluid than the patient's requirement, additional water should be provided. This approach is particularly important to prevent dehydration, especially in infants, children, and older adults.

Once the method of administration (bolus, intermittent, continuous, or cyclic) has been determined, divide the total

Controversy

Drug Dosing Issues in Continuous Versus Bolus Feedings
JONATHAN J. WOLFE

The placement of a feeding tube exposes a patient to various hazards. Nasogastric intubation carries risks of aspiration during placement. It can also cause esophageal perforation. The percutaneous endoscopic gastrostomy tube avoids these risks but involves surgical intervention and produces a permanent breach in skin integrity. Either tube requires continuous attention to skin care and patency. Both tubes make it possible to overfeed a patient inadvertently or to introduce products of high osmolality. Errors in feeding can produce sequelae ranging from diarrhea to metabolic imbalances.

Another set of problems with the use of enteral tubes is their possible wrong use for drug dosing. It is fairly well established that bolus feeding through tubes is preferable in most cases. The cycle of fullness and emptying stimulates physiologic patterns familiar to the patient who can feed independently. However, feeding with elemental and other specialized products may best be accomplished with a continual infusion. In either case, it is possible to dose incorrectly.

Many drugs are not commercially available as oral liquids. Administering tablets and capsules presents many difficulties. Some drugs may suspend nicely in liquids, but others are insoluble. Some, indeed, cannot be crushed because they are timed-release formulations. Crushing or dissolving a timed-release formulation may expose a patient to a toxic overdose if the dose is released all at once. Crushed tablets may obstruct a feeding tube. Tablet coatings and the inert talc and other excipients can coagulate in the tube. Even oral liquids may not be suitable for use in a feeding tube. Many contain high-sugar syrups that can cause osmotic diarrhea.

Finally, drugs may prove physically incompatible with tube feeding products. Some drugs may need to be given on an empty stomach. This means dosing between boluses or stopping the infusion. In any case, drug administration through enteral tubes requires flushing with water before and after the dose. All of these precautions make feeding and dosing regimens complex and confusing.

Critical Thinking Discussion

- What teaching is appropriate for the adult patient who is to have a feeding tube placed?
- Should the required drugs be mixed with the enteral feeding or given separately from the feeding? Why or why not?
- Under what circumstances may a patient validly refuse to have a tube placed?
- How might an interdisciplinary patient care team deal with the problems of combining drug dosing with enteral feeding?

volume of formula by the number of hours or feedings the formula is providing. Additional fluid volume should be equally distributed throughout the day and can be used to flush the tube before, during, and after feedings and drug administration.

Cost The cost of enteral formulas varies from one location to another, with prices influenced by market competition. Standard polymeric formulas (1 kcal/mL) usually cost less than $15/day. Elemental formulas are three to four times more expensive than polymeric formulas. Specialized formulas may be more expensive than routine polymeric formulas (specialized polymeric formulas can cost as much as $100/day or more), but the cost may not be significant depending on the specific formula.

Enteral feedings using a standard polymeric formula are 10 to 20 percent as costly as parenteral feedings. In contrast, the cost of total parenteral nutrition in acute care settings ranges from $100 to over $500 per liter, depending on the ingredients. A more important factor to be considered is the formula's availability. Hospitals and supply outlets cannot maintain supplies of all types of formulas. Costs for tubes and pumps range from $6 to $150 per day.

One fact to be noted is that the cost for 1 month of enteral feedings taken by mouth costs less than 1 day in the hospital. Furthermore, when considering the cost of enteral feedings, the cost of malnutrition should also be acknowledged. The expense of healing pressure sores, only one complication of malnutrition, is estimated to be over $50,000 per patient.

Patient Variables

Pediatric Nutrients that are easily digested and absorbed (i.e., human milk or formula that replaces some of the fat and lactose with medium chain triglyceride [MCT] oil and glucose polymers) should be provided to the preterm infant. The use of human milk is advantageous because of its immunologic protective effects, growth factors, and other constituents. Because of the slower growth rate of preterm infants fed human milk, fortification of human milk with protein, sodium, calcium, and phosphorus, as provided in SIMILAC NATURAL CARE and ENFAMIL HUMAN MILK FORTIFIER, may be needed. Most commercial formulas for infants provide 24 cal/oz. Standard infant formulas are not recommended for preterm infants. Specially developed infant formulas are available for preterm infants.

Full-term infants have more mature organ systems than preterm infants do (see also Chapter 6). Compared with adults, however, their ability to digest starch and absorb fat is less efficient.

Implementation of enteral feedings for children at risk should be initiated as soon as possible. Pediatric patients have low reserves but high metabolic demands. All nutrients should be provided in adequate amounts to promote normal growth for the patient's age and sex. Adult formulas are not ideal for the pediatric patient because of a high renal solute load and insufficient vitamin and mineral levels. One commercial formula furnishes 1 cal/mL and provides an energy and nutrient profile designed to meet the needs of this age group. All infants must be carefully monitored to prevent dehydration.

Geriatric Older adults receiving a hyperosmolar formula are especially prone to hypernatremia and fluid volume deficit, because the formula promotes loss of water into the bowel.

Intervention

Administration

Feedings administered directly into the duodenum or jejunum should be isotonic (about 300 mOsm/L). Patients receiving high osmolality formulas often have difficulty tolerating the feeding. High solute loads can be managed by controlling the rate of infusion rather than diluting the formula. If the patient has had food in the GI tract in the previous 24 hours, a full-strength isotonic or slightly hypertonic formula (300 to 500 mOsm) given at a rate of 50 to 75 mL/hour is appropriate. If nourishment has been withheld longer than 7 days or if enteral nutrition is necessary because of inadequate oral intake or compromised GI function and a hyperosmolar formula is to be used, the feeding should be started at a rate of 30 to 50 mL/hour. The infusion rate may be advanced 15 to 25 mL/hour every 8 to 12 hours until the optimal caloric goal is reached.

The infusion rate is increased as tolerated to achieve adequate nutrient, fluid, and electrolyte requirements but as soon as possible. Three to five days may be required for the patient to adapt to the feeding and the formula. Too rapid an increase in the infusion rate causes abdominal cramping, nausea, and diarrhea and may require starting the adaptive process over again. Even if feeding falls behind schedule, increasing the rate is not advisable. Advancing the rate and the strength of the formula simultaneously is not recommended.

Most formulas can be safely hung for 8 hours. Prefilled, ready-to-use containers offer a decreased risk of contamination during handling, preparation, and formula transfer. To prevent unacceptable contamination levels, delivery sets should be changed every 24 hours.

Underfeeding and Overfeeding Failure to administer adequate formula volume is most often attributed to interruptions for diagnostic tests, physical and respiratory therapy, and tube obstruction. Because as many as 30 to 50 percent of hospitalized patients are malnourished, interruptions in feedings may retard recovery. If enteral feedings are the only nutrition modality used, the total energy level provided must be adequate to prevent malnutrition but yet not be excessive to avoid complications of overfeeding. Complications associated with overfeeding include excessive carbon dioxide production and subsequent acidosis, cholestasis, hyperglycemia, pulmonary edema, lipogenesis, and hepatic complications.

Gastric residuals should be checked before each bolus feeding to prevent overfilling. (Gastric residuals are not checked for tubes placed in the duodenum or jejunum.) Patients should also be questioned regarding fullness and examined for abdominal distention for overfilling, which can lead to nausea, vomiting, and aspiration. The usual rule of thumb is to withhold the feeding and recheck the residual in 1 hour if the residual exceeds 100 to 150 mL or if more than half of the volume previously infused is aspirated. To reduce loss of gastric secretions and electrolytes, the aspirate should be reinstilled immediately after measuring residuals. After 1 hour, if the residual is less than 100 mL or less than half of the previous volume, the feeding may be administered. If excessive residual (over 300 mL) persists, the reason for slowed gastric emptying should be determined and the problem resolved. With many narrow-bore, pliable feeding tubes, residuals may be unreliable.

With continuous or cyclic feedings, residuals are checked every 2 to 4 hours. If the residual is two to three times the hourly rate, the health care provider should be notified for appropriate changes in infusion rate.

Tube Obstruction Obstructed feeding tubes cause havoc for patients and interrupt feedings until the tube is cleared or replaced. There are several common reasons for feeding tube obstruction. A 1.5- to 2-kcal/mL formula, a very thick formula, or another highly viscous product may obstruct a feeding tube by coagulating in the stomach's acidic environment. When it is aspirated, the coagulated formula may stick to the lumen, further contributing to obstruction. The smaller the lumen of the feeding tube, the greater the risk of obstruction. Feeding rates of less than 50 mL/hour may also contribute to an obstructed feeding tube. Flushing feeding tubes with 50 to 100 mL of water every 4 hours, before and after drug administration, and before and after feedings reduces the risk of obstruction.

Action should be taken as soon as possible to clear an obstructed tube. Several methods have been effective in opening an obstructed tube. The head of the bed should first be elevated or the patient positioned upright. The tube is then flushed with room temperature water, cranberry juice, or sugar-free, caffeine-free, chocolate-free carbonated beverage such as Diet Sprite or 7-UP. Pancrelipase, a pancreatic enzyme, or 1 teaspoon of meat tenderizer in 4 ounces of water may be administered and the tube clamped for 15 minutes to 1 hour. When attempting to declog a tube, aspirate as much liquid as possible so the agent comes into contact with the obstruction. A lumen that cannot be unclogged requires tube replacement, thus contributing to the cost of enteral feedings and patient discomfort. Avoid forcing a tube open. High pressure can rupture viscera and require emergency surgery.

Drug-Formula Interactions A frequently overlooked source of problems for patients receiving enteral formulas is drug-formula interactions. When and how to administer drugs when enteral feedings are necessary is dependent on the method of administering the feeding and the specific drug to be used (see Controversy—Drug Dosing Issues in Continuous Versus Bolus Feedings). In general, mixing drugs with feeding formulas should be avoided. Optimal absorption is obtained if the drugs are administered 2 hours before or after a feeding. Further, highly acidic (pH less than 4) drugs such as potassium chloride and pseudoephedrine can coagulate the enteral formula. Carbamazepine suspension adheres to polyvinyl chloride feeding tubes. Bulk-forming laxatives (e.g., hydrophilic psyllium mucilloid [METAMUCIL]) congeal and occlude the tube. Small fragments of drugs may adhere to the tube, trapping subsequent fragments that build up with time. As much as possible, only liquid drug forms should be used. Feeding tubes should be flushed with water before and after drug administration. Five to ten milliliters of water should be given between drugs when multiple drugs must be administered.

Serum concentrations of phenytoin, theophylline, carbamazepine, and methyldopa are decreased in patients receiving enteral formulas. Therefore, it is recommended that enteral feedings be stopped 1 hour before and 2 hours after administration of these drugs.

Warfarin resistance has been reported in patients receiving enteral feedings. The interaction was first attributed to the unrecognized presence of vitamin K in the formula. Recent evidence indicates that the binding of warfarin to the components of the feeding formula (e.g., soy proteins or proteinaceous caseinate salts) may contribute to this phenomenon. Despite decreases in the vitamin K content of formulas, the problem still persists.

Diarrhea Diarrhea occurs in 5 to 30 percent of patients who receive enteral feedings, with the incidence reaching 68 percent in patients in intensive care units. However, contrary to popular opinion, in most cases, the diarrhea is not caused by the formula itself. In 60 percent of cases, drugs are responsible for diarrhea, the formula is responsible in 30 percent of cases, and in 10 percent, *Clostridium difficile* organisms are responsible for the diarrhea. Daily stool output of more than 250 g/day is classified as diarrhea.

Most oral drug solutions have an osmolality of more than 1000 mOsm/mL. Diarrhea is likely to develop if the hyperosmolar solutions are not diluted. Also, liquid drugs frequently contain sorbitol as a sweetener, increasing the risk of an osmotic diarrhea. Potassium chloride, if it is not sufficiently diluted, or other diarrhea-inducing drugs (especially magnesium-containing antacids) may also be culprits.

Intragastric drug administration may delay gastric emptying or result in dumping of gastric contents into the small bowel. Diluting the drug with 10 to 30 mL of tap water and flushing the tube before and after administering each drug can decrease the viscosity of the drug. Thus, passage through the tube is facilitated, preventing osmotic diarrhea.

The risk of diarrhea from bacterial contamination of formulas is affected by such variables as initial contamination, composition of solution (which affects the rate of bacterial growth), presence of preservatives, number of manipulations involved in the preparation of the formula, and the mode and duration of administration (hang time of the formula). Life-threatening sepsis can result from contaminated enteral solutions; therefore, care must be taken in their preparation and administration to prevent contamination and excessive bacterial growth.

Malnutrition may affect formula tolerance in several ways. Anatomic changes in the GI tract (blunted villi height) may result in fewer intestinal disaccharidases and, consequently, formula intolerance accompanied by diarrhea. Serum albumin levels of less than 3 g/dL correlate significantly with increased risk of diarrhea in patients receiving enteral feedings.

Antibiotic use or infections frequently lead to a *Clostridium difficile*–induced colitis. Diarrhea associated with antibiotic use can often be alleviated by administering oral vancomycin and IV or oral metronidazole. The organism *Lactobacillus acidophilus* (LACTINEX) has been used to restore the normal GI flora. Opioid antidiarrheal drugs should not be used for pathogen-induced diarrhea. GI motility is reduced, thereby prolonging exposure to pathogens and increasing the risk of sepsis. Decreased GI tract motility or the use of histamine-2 blockers can also cause diarrhea secondary to bacterial overgrowth.

Treatment with kaolin pectate antidiarrheal drugs has been effective in retarding diarrhea having no organic cause. A fiber-containing formula may also be helpful because the fiber normally absorbs water and electrolytes.

Education

In today's health care environment, many patients receive enteral feedings at home. Home feedings require that patients and families obtain the required instruction before discharge from the acute care setting with careful follow-up in the home. An interdisciplinary effort involving a health care provider, dietitian, psychiatrist, social worker, pharmacist, and discharge planner should be included in the management of the patient.

The patient and preferably at least one other individual should be taught and allowed to assume full responsibility for feedings before discharge from the hospital. Clear, concise written instructions provided before discharge contribute to the patient's confidence and ease the transition to home. Skills that must be learned and demonstrated include (1) preparation and administration of formula, including techniques for storage, preparation, infusion, and manipulation; (2) tube and site care; and (3) recognition and appropriate response to complications, equipment maintenance, and malfunctions. Patients must learn where to obtain the necessary feeding supplies and how to access financial resources that may be available. Full attention with regard for patient and family needs, including emotional, psychological, social, and financial needs, as well as the patient's medical and nutritional condition, contribute to a successful home enteral program.

Although sanitary techniques are important and should be discussed, procedures used at home do not have to be as closely followed as in the hospital. Infusion bags and tubings used for bolus or cyclic feedings can be carefully rinsed daily with either soapy water or diluted vinegar and rinsed in tap water. The bag can be reused for up to 7 days without significant bacterial contamination.

Ordinarily, nasogastric tubes are not used for home enteral feedings, but they are occasionally necessary. Patients should be taught how to check proper placement of the tubing by aspirating stomach contents. If the patient belches when pushing air into the tube, the formula should not be infused. Changes in the length of tube outside the nose may mean that the tube has moved out of position and should not be used until the proper position has been verified.

The social aspects of mealtime should be maintained as much as possible, encouraging mealtimes in the usual manner to minimize patient isolation. If it is allowed, the patient may chew gum at this time. Other adjustments that need to be considered are social and festive occasions and vacations, in which food plays a major role.

Evaluation

Enteral feedings should result in the improvement of nutritional parameters, including anthropometric measurements and laboratory values. Patients should be receiving adequate calories and protein to maintain body weight. When evaluating weight changes, weight loss can be masked by sodium and water retention. If the patient needed to gain weight and received adequate and appropriate nutritional supplements, nutritional support was successful.

Serum proteins, especially prealbumin, should be monitored at least weekly. It is imperative to monitor electrolytes during enteral feedings and to correct deficiencies, or to compensate for increases in serum concentrations when appropriate.

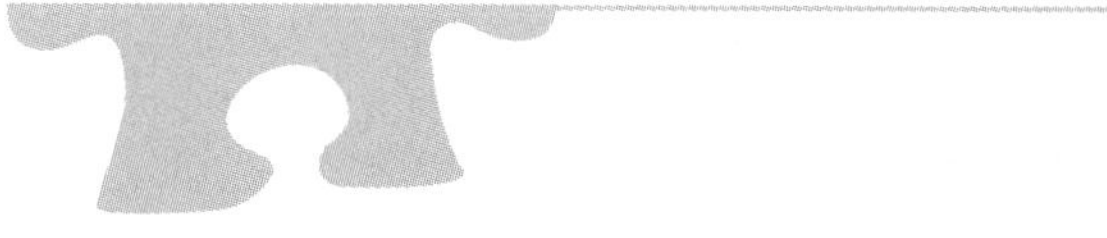

SUMMARY

- Physical problems interfering with the normal ability to consume food orally necessitates a plan for nutrition support.
- PEM can be described as a continuum between marasmus and kwashiorkor. In marasmus, fat stores are used for energy. When

stress occurs, if energy and protein requirements are unmet, kwashiorkor develops.

- Kwashiorkor is life-threatening because of delayed wound healing and impaired resistance to infection. Certain vitamin and mineral deficiencies frequently accompany PEM and should be evaluated.
- The general rule of nutritional support programs is to use the gut if it works.
- Enteral feedings that use the GI tract are the physiologically natural method of feeding and permit more efficient use of nutrients. The method of nutrition support should be the least invasive, most natural, most cost-effective method that can be adapted to the patient's life-style.
- Polymeric formulas are made from intact nutrients (carbohydrate, protein, and fat). These require normal digestive and absorptive capacity of the GI tract.
- Polymeric formulas have a high nitrogen content for use with catabolic or malnourished patients, include fiber for long-term feedings to help regulate bowel function, may be blenderized to use normal foods, and are concentrated for conditions requiring fluid restriction.
- Specialized polymeric formulas are available for patients with hypermetabolic disorders, renal or pulmonary conditions, glucose intolerance, gastrointestinal or pancreatic disease, and immune dysfunction.
- Elemental formulas contain nutrients that have been enzymatically hydrolyzed to free amino acids or smaller peptide fragments.
- Elemental formulas are appropriate for patients with minimal digestive capacity, limited absorptive surface of GI tract (short bowel syndrome, celiac sprue), or protein-losing enteropathy (e.g., inflammatory bowel disease, radiation enteritis), or when fecal residue should be minimal.
- Assessment of food intake; a medical history; simple, inexpensive anthropometric measurements (at least weight and height); and routine basic laboratory findings are used to evaluate the patient's nutritional status and progress during therapy.
- Formula selection should be based on the patient's nutritional status, nutrient use, the status of major organ function, GI absorption, and fluid balance.
- With sufficient energy intake, both polymeric and elemental formulas provide 100 percent of the RDIs of vitamins and minerals.
- Enteral feeding tubes can deliver nutrients into the stomach, the duodenum, or the jejunum. Feedings into the stomach use the whole GI tract.
- Feeding methods may be bolus, continuous, or cyclic, depending on the needs of the patient and the environment. Feedings into the duodenum or jejunum require continuous or cyclic feedings.
- Evaluation of patient response must be maintained to determine the effectiveness of the formula and the patient's tolerance to prevent serious side effects that may occur.

BIBLIOGRAPHY

Alexander, J. (1990). Nutrition and translocation. *Journal of Parenteral and Enteral Nutrition,* 14, 170S–174S.

Benya R., and Mobarhan S. (1991). Enteral alimentation: Administration and complications. *Journal of American College of Nutrition,* 10, 209–219.

Bockus, S. (1991). Trouble shooting your tube feedings. *American Journal of Nursing,* 19(5), 24–30.

Bower, R. (1990). Nutritional and metabolic support of critically ill patients. *Journal of Parenteral and Enteral Nutrition,* 14, 257S–259S.

Bowers, D. (1992). The logistics of enteral nutrition support: Current practice for the initiation and progression of tube feeding. In K. Kudsk and G. Zaloga (Eds.), *Enteral nutrition support of the 1990s: Innovations in nutrition, technology, and techniques* (pp. 33–34). Report of the Twelfth Ross Roundtable on Medication Issues. Columbus, OH: Ross Laboratory, Inc.

Brackenridge, B., and Campbell, R. (1990). Enteral nutritional support and supplementation in diabetes. *Diabetes Educator,* 16(6), 463–465.

Bray, G., and Gray, D., (1988). Obesity. Part I: Pathogenesis. *Western Journal of Medicine,* 149, 429–441.

Brittenden, J., Park, K., Hayes, P., et al. (1992). Effect of arginine on natural cytotoxicity in cancer patients and healthy volunteers. *British Journal of Surgery,* 79, A442.

Brown, R. (1992). Pharmacology in the ICU: Drugs and enteral nutrition. In K. Kudsk and G. Zaloga (Eds.), *Enteral nutrition support of the 1990s: Innovations in nutrition, technology, and techniques* (pp. 35–39). Report of the Twelfth Ross Roundtable on Medication Issues. Columbus, OH: Ross Laboratory, Inc.

Butterworth, C. E., Jr. (1974). The skeleton in the hospital closet. *Nutrition Today,* 9(2), 4–8.

Charland, S., Bartlett, D., and Torosian, M. (1994). Effect of protein-calorie malnutrition on methotrexate pharmacokinetics. *Journal of Parenteral and Enteral Nutrition,* 18, 45–49.

Constans, T., Bacq, Y., Bréchot, J. F., et al. (1992). Protein-energy malnutrition in elderly medical patients. *Journal of the American Geriatrics Society,* 40, 263–268.

Cummins, A. (1995). Malabsorption and villous atrophy in patients receiving enteral feeding. *Journal of Parenteral and Enteral Nutrition,* 19(3), 193–198.

Davis, J. R., and Sherer, K. (1994). *Applied nutrition and diet therapy for nurses* (2nd ed.). Philadelphia: W. B. Saunders.

DeChiccio, R., and Matarese, L. (1992). Selection of nutrition support regimens. *Nutrition in Clinical Practice,* 7, 239–245.

Fischer, J. (1990). Branched-chain-enriched amino acid solutions in patients with liver failure: An early example of nutrition pharmacology. *Journal of Parenteral and Enteral Nutrition,* 14, 249S–256S.

Fleisher D., Sheth, N., and Kou, J. H. (1990). Phenytoin interactions with enteral feedings administered through nasogastric tubes. *Journal of Parenteral and Enteral Nutrition,* 14(5), 513–516.

Frankel, W., Choi, D., Zhang, W., et al. (1994). Soy fiber delays disease onset and prolongs survival in experimental *Clostridium difficile* ileocecitis. *Journal of Parenteral and Enteral Nutrition,* 18, 55–61.

Frankenfield, D., and Beyer, P. (1991). Dietary fiber and bowel function in tube-fed patients. *Journal of American Dietetic Association,* 91(5), 591–599.

Heimburger, D. C., and Weinsier, R. L. (1997). *Handbook of clinical nutrition* (3rd ed.). St. Louis: Mosby.

James, W. P., Ferro-Luzzi, S., and Waterlow, J. C. (1988). Definition of chronic energy deficiencies in adults. Report of a working party of International Dietary Energy Consultation Group. *European Journal of Clinical Nutrition,* 42, 969–981.

Kerstetter, J., Holthauser, B., and Fitz, P. (1992). Malnutrition in the institutionalized older adult. *Journal of the American Dietetic Association,* 92(9), 1109–1116.

Kohn, C. (1991). The relationship between enteral formula contamination and length of enteral delivery. *Journal of Parenteral and Enteral Nutrition,* 15(2), 567–571.

McClave, S., Mitoraj, T., Thielmeier, K., et al. (1992). Differentiating subtypes (hypoalbuminemic versus marasmic) of protein-calorie malnutrition incidence and clinical significance in a university hospital setting. *Journal of Parenteral and Enteral Nutrition,* 16(4), 337–342.

Mears, E. (1994). Prealbumin and nutrition assessment. *Dietetic Currents,* 21(1), 1–4.

Melnik, G. (1990). Pharmacologic aspects of enteral nutrition. In J. Rombeau and M. Caldwell (Eds.), *Clinical nutrition: Enteral and tube feeding* (2nd ed, pp. 472–509). Philadelphia: W .B. Saunders.

Mendenhall, C. L., Moritz, T. E., Roselle, G. A., et al. (1995). Protein energy malnutrition in severe alcoholic hepatitis: Diagnosis and response to treatment. *Journal of Parenteral and Enteral Nutrition,* 19(4), 258–265.

Metheny, N. A., Clouse, R. E., Clark, J. M., et al. (1994). pH testing of feeding-tube aspirates to determine placement. *Nutrition in Clinical Practice,* 9(5), 185–190.

Mobarhan S., and Trumbore L. (1991). Enteral tube feeding: A clinical perspective on recent advances. *Nutrition Reviews,* 49(5), 129–140.

Mukau, L., Talamini, M., and Sitzmann, J. (1994). Elemental diets may accelerate recovery from total parenteral nutrition induced gut atrophy. *Journal of Parenteral and Enteral Nutrition,* 18, 75–78.

Patterson, M. L., Dominguez, J. M., Lyman, B., et al. (1990). Enteral feeding in the hypoalbuminemic patient. *Journal of Parenteral and Enteral Nutrition,* 14(4), 362–365.

Perry, S., Pillar, B., Radary, M. H., et al. (1990) The appropriate use of high-cost, high-risk technologies: The case of total parenteral nutrition. *Quality Review Bulletin,* 16(6), 214–217.

Peters, A., and Davidson, M. (1992). Effects of various enteral feeding products on postprandial blood glucose response in patients with Type I diabetes. *Journal of Parenteral and Enteral Nutrition,* 16(1), 69–74.

Rolandelli, R. H., DePaula, J. A., Guenter, P., et al. (1990). Critical illness and sepsis. In J. L. Rombeau and M. Caldwell (Eds.), *Clinical nutrition: Enteral and tube feeding* (2nd ed., pp. 288–305). Philadelphia: W. B. Saunders.

Rowland, M. (1990). Self-reported weight and height. *American Journal of Clinical Nutrition,* 52(6), 1125–1133.

Shankardass, K., Churchman, S., Chelswick, K., et al. (1990). Bowel function of long-term tube-fed patients consuming formulae with and without dietary fiber. *Journal of Parenteral and Enteral Nutrition,* 14(5), 508–512.

Silk, D., and Payne-James, J. (1990). Complications of enteral nutrition. In J. Rombeau and M. Caldwell (Eds.), *Clinical nutrition: Enteral and tube feeding* (2nd ed.). Philadelphia: W. B. Saunders.

Skeie, B., Kvetan, V., Gil, K. M., et al. (1990). Branch-chain amino acids: Their metabolism and clinical utility. *Critical Care Medicine,* 18(5), 549–571.

Smith, C. E., Marien, L., Brogdon, C., et al. (1990). Diarrhea associated with tube feeding in mechanically ventilated critically ill patients. *Nursing Research,* 39(3), 148–152.

Talbot, J. (1991). Guidelines for the scientific review of enteral food products for special medical purposes. *Journal of Parenteral and Enteral Nutrition,* 15, 99S–173S.

Webber-Jones, J., Sweeney, K., Winterbottom, A., et al. (1992). How to declog a feeding tube. *Nursing '92,* 22, 62–64.

Weddle, D. O, Schmeisser, D., Barnish, M., et al. (1991). Inpatient and post-discharge course of the malnourished patient. *Journal of the American Dietetic Association* 91(3):307–311.

Welch, S. K., Hanlon, M. D., Waits, M., et al. (1994). Comparison of four bedside indicators used to predict duodenal feeding tube placement with radiography. *Journal of Parenteral and Enteral Nutrition,* 18(6), 525–530.

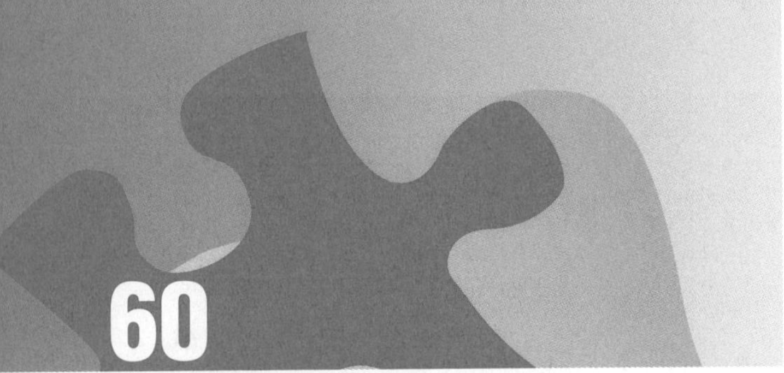

60 Complementary and Adjunctive Therapies

Modern complementary and adjunctive therapies being used to enhance conventional Western medical practice are really not new. Their roots can be traced to early Greek and Chinese treatments. These therapies include naturopathy, homeopathy, acupuncture, and phytotherapy.

Phytotherapy, the use of plant-based medicine, has become increasingly popular in Europe and the United States. It uses plants—the leaves, flowers, stems, and roots—to treat illness. Plants applied medicinally are technically called *botanicals,* but the terms *herb* and *botanical* are often interchanged. This chapter explains the active constituents, mechanisms of action, system application, and adjunctive use of selected herbs. Adverse effects and contraindications are examined, as well as any botanical-drug interactions. The issue of toxic herbs and precautions regarding their use are addressed in the Critical Thinking section of this chapter.

HOLISTIC HEALTH CARE

Complementary and adjunctive therapies are considered holistic. *Holism,* derived from the Greek word *holos,* meaning a whole, is based on the notion that health is a vital dynamic state, which reflects a profound will and wisdom to maintain wellness rather than simply the absence of disease. *Vis mediatrix naturae,* the healing force of nature, is the underlying precept of holism. It maintains that all living things can self-heal; human organisms are believed to encompass inherent self-defense mechanisms against illness. When they are properly stimulated, these mechanisms will heal.

Although natural therapies are often described as cutting edge, they are actually much older than conventional Western interventions. Experts estimate that herbal remedies and Ayurveda, the traditional medicine of India, are over 5000 years old. Egyptians used fragrant oils in what may have been an early version of aromatherapy. Hydrotherapy was routine in ancient Greece and Rome. And homeopathy, one of the newest adjunctive therapies, is only 200 years old.

Allopathic medicine, marked by drug development and surgery, is a recent development. The American attitude that health can be found in the medicine chest is a product of the 20th century and the advent of antibiotics. This period has heralded life-saving discoveries such as penicillin and the Salk polio vaccine. It seems only reasonable that investigators may develop similar drugs to eradicate cancer, heart disease, and other dreaded diseases. But disease and the development of pharmaceuticals are extraordinarily complex biochemical problems, and solutions often create new challenges, as evidenced in severe side effects of some medications and growing drug resistance of many antibiotics. Thus, patients search for alternatives to prescription drugs. Complementary and adjunctive therapies, like herbal drugs, are appealing because they have few adverse effects.

The use of complementary and adjunctive therapies for health problems has been increasing since the 1960s. It is now widespread in the United States, and more health care providers are including some forms of alternative and complementary therapies in their practice. In 1990, a national survey conducted by physicians at Harvard Medical School found that one in three Americans visited providers of complementary therapies. In fact, in recent years, more Americans visited health care providers who use complementary and adjunctive therapies than primary care physicians (425 million visits versus 388 million visits). Nursing schools and medical schools across the nation are beginning to include these therapies in their curricula. Additionally, a number of health maintenance organizations and insurance companies are reimbursing for holistic therapies.

Rising health care costs also may be a factor in the recent surge of interest. People want to control their health care destinies, and insurance companies look for the best care results for the lowest cost. In addition, Americans affected by newly discovered chronic diseases such as acquired immunodeficiency and chronic fatigue syndromes, conditions that contemporary health care modalities cannot cure, are seeking alternative treatments. Many patients are also attracted to the health care provider who uses complementary and alternative treatment modalities because they treat the whole person—body, mind, and spirit. Patients find the individualized approach particularly appealing in an age of managed care and impersonal group practices.

As a result of the increased interest in complementary and adjunctive therapies, increasing health care costs, and loss of individualized care, the Office of Alternative Medicine of the National Institutes of Health was created to evaluate the efficacy of these modalities. The office has since grown considerably with an original 1992 budget of $2 million increasing to $12 million in 1997. The mandate of this federally funded agency is to investigate and evaluate alternative therapies and their effectiveness in relieving suffering, illness, and disease. Although the Office of Alternative Medicine does not operate as a referral service, it does serve as an public information clearinghouse as well as a research training program. Table 60–1 provides an overview of the categories of complementary and alternative therapies.

Naturopathy

The first precept of *naturopathy,* one of the disciplines of holistic medicine, is based on the concept of the healing force of nature. This intervention emphasizes the prevention of disease and the maintenance of health. A second principle of naturopathy is derived from the Hippocratic oath: First do no harm. Practitioners of naturopathy avoid therapies that weaken the body's innate ability to self-heal or take over a function of the body. Naturopathic practice also empha-

TABLE 60–1 CATEGORIES OF COMPLEMENTARY AND ALTERNATIVE MEDICAL PRACTICE

Mind-Body Interventions	
Art therapy	Biofeedback
Dance therapy	Guided imagery
Humor	Hypnotherapy
Meditation	Music therapy
Prayer therapy	Psychotherapy
Relaxation	Support groups
Yoga	
Alternative Systems of Practice	
Acupuncture	Ayurveda
Community-based practices	Environmental medicine
Homeopathic medicine	Latin American rural practices
Native American practices	Naturopathic medicine
Past life therapy	Shamanism
Tibetan medicine	Traditional Asian medicine
Manual Healing	
Acupressure	Alexander technique
Biofield therapeutics	Chiropractic medicine
Feldenkrais method	Massage therapy
Osteopathy	Reflexology
Rolfing	Therapeutic touch
Trager method	
Herbal Medicine	
Various herbs	
Diet, Nutrition, Life-Style Changes	
Changes in life-style	Diet
Gerson therapy	Macrobiotics
Megavitamins	Nutritional supplements
Bioelectromagnetic Applications	
Bluelight treatment/artificial lighting	
Electroacupuncture	
Electromagnetic fields	
Electromagnetic and neuromagnetic stimulation	
Magnetoresonance spectroscopy	
Pharmacologic and Biologic Treatments	
Antioxidizing and oxidizing agents	
Cell treatment	
Chelation treatment	
Metabolic therapy	

From a pamphlet produced by the Office of Alternative Medicine, National Institutes of Health, Bethesda, MD.

sizes the concepts of wellness, prevention, and the health care provider as teacher.

As defined by the Department of Labor, naturopathic physicians diagnose and treat patients with treatments based on natural laws. Naturopaths are trained to diagnose and treat on the primary care level and may prescribe some drugs and do minor surgery. Their modalities include phytotherapy, electrotherapy, minor orofacial surgery, mechanotherapy, and naturopathic corrections and manipulations. Other treatments used by naturopathic doctors include nutrition, with an emphasis on whole foods, and vitamin supplements. Naturopathic health care providers do not perform major surgery, use x-rays or radium therapeutically, or prescribe conventional pharmaceutical drugs.

Training for a degree in naturopathic medicine is conducted in 4-year, postgraduate institutions. The naturopathic curriculum includes courses in medical pathology, microbiology, histology, physical and clinical diagnosis, and pharmacognosy. Clinical training in botanical medicine, pharmacognosy, hydrotherapy and physiotherapy, therapeutic nutrition, and homeopathy is also required.

States with naturopathic licensure laws (doctor of naturopathy, N.D.) require a pre-med residency in naturopathic medicine consisting of at least 4 years of didactic work and 4100 hours of study obtained in a college or university recognized by the state examining board. Naturopathic health care providers are considered the general practitioners of the natural healing world. States that license naturopathic health care providers include Alaska, Arizona, Connecticut, Hawaii, Maine, Montana, New Hampshire, Oregon, Utah, Vermont, and Washington.

Homeopathy

The root words of *homeopathy* come from the Greek *homoios,* meaning like, and *pathos,* meaning suffering. Homeopathy is a medical system that endeavors to help the body heal itself by treating like with like. The law of similars or like cures like is based on the theory that if a large amount of the substance causes symptoms in a healthy volunteer, a smaller amount of the same substance can be used to treat an ill patient. Although considered controversial by contemporary medical science, homeopathy is not a new idea. The Greek physician Hippocrates noted that things that caused illness (e.g., poisons) could be used to treat the illnesses they caused.

Dr. Samuel Hahnemann, an 18th-century German physician, is essentially credited with founding homeopathy. Dr. Hahnemann considered the medical practices of the time barbaric because patients were regularly bled, leeched, and blistered to purge them of fluids believed to cause their illness. He became convinced that there were three systems of medicine: (1) prevention, in which the causes of illness, such as poor hygiene, are removed and illness prevented; (2) *contraria contraris,* in which treatment produces conditions antagonistic to the illness (allopathy); and (3) *similia similibus curentur,* meaning like cures like, in which a substance that causes symptoms in a healthy person will cure similar symptoms (when given in a much smaller dose) in an ill person. An example of such a substance is quinine. Spurred by a report that quinine could relieve the symptoms of malaria but doubting that this was achieved by an astringent quality, Dr. Hahnemann experimented with quinine and found that it caused malaria-like symptoms in himself and other healthy individuals. *Similia similibus curentur* became the first law on which homeopathy is based, the law of similars.

The second premise of homeopathy was to give the smallest dose possible. Hanhemann also believed that if more than one remedy was given at a time, the combination might have a different effect on the body and it would be more difficult to pinpoint which remedy was having which effect. Thus, the most important principle of homeopathy is to prescribe to each individual.

Many people believe it is the tiny size of the dose that makes a remedy homeopathic because these remedies are sold over the counter (OTC) in minute doses. This is not the case. The healing power of the remedy is ascribed to the transfer of its vibrational pattern into a substrate of water, alcohol, or lactose. A tincture is made directly from source material. One drop of the tincture is then mixed with 99 drops of water or alcohol to make the first potency. The mixture is vigorously shaken over 100 times, a process called succussion. One drop of the succussion mixture is combined with 99 drops of water or alcohol, and the process is repeated. Succussion makes the remedy more potent. Potentized remedies are used to make pills and creams or may be taken as a tincture.

Homeopathic practitioners emphasize that assessment of all aspects of the physical, mental, and emotional life of a patient is central to the prescription of appropriate remedies. The goals of homeopathy are to select a remedy that will bring about a sense of well being on all levels, both physical and emotional; to alleviate physical symptoms; and to restore a patient to a state of creative energy. Worldwide, homeopathy is commonly practiced in India, Mexico, and Russia. According to the National Center for Homeopathy, about four in every 10 people in France and one in three people in England use homeopathy.

Clinical evidence on the efficacy of homeopathy is highly contradictory, and yet it appears to be superior to conventional medicine for many patients. However, definite conclusions on the effectiveness of homeopathy cannot yet be made. It appears that homeopathic treatments, used in conjunction with oral rehydration therapy, shortened the course of diarrhea in a clinical trial with pediatric patients in Nicaragua. However, homeopathic remedies have not been found to be effective in relieving pain or inflammation.

Overall, homeopathic remedies are considered relatively safe. Reports to the U.S. Food and Drug Administration (FDA) on illness caused by homeopathic remedies have been discounted. However, homeopathic remedies are reported by health care providers to potentiate the effects of pharmaceutical drugs. Anecdotal reports suggest that patients may experience a reduced need for pharmaceutical drugs when they are taken in conjunction with homeopathic remedies.

Homeopathy is practiced by a wide range of health care providers, including medical doctors, naturopathic physicians, nurses, and dentists. Certificate programs in homeopathic medicine are offered by universities that educate natural healers as well as homeopathic healers. Homeopathic health care providers include physicians (MDs) or osteopathic physicians (DOs) who have completed additional work in homeotherapeutics. These individuals may use the initials DHt (Diplomate of Homeotherapeutics) after they pass an exam consisting of a presentation of 10 cases treated with homeopathic medicine with 3 years of follow-up. They also must successfully complete a written exam, an oral exam, and a casetaking. Their work is supervised by a panel of physicians.

Traditional Chinese Medicine

Traditional Chinese medicine is based on the concept that energy, also termed *Chi* (*qi*) or life force energy, is the center of body functions. Chi is the intangible force that animates life and enlivens all activity. Wellness is a function of a balanced and harmonious flow of chi, whereas illness or disease results from disturbances in its flow. Wellness also requires preserving an equilibrium between the contrasting states of yin and yang (the dual nature of all things). The underlying principle of traditional Chinese medicine is preventive in nature, and the body is viewed as a reflection of the natural world.

Traditional Chinese medicine has been practiced in China for at least 3000 years. It relies on a variety of treatment modalities, including acupuncture and moxibustion. Herbal therapy is used to prevent as well as treat illness and to balance or harmonize bodily processes. *Chi Kung* (or qi gong) contains elements of meditation, relaxation training, visualization, movement, posturing, and breathing exercises. It is practiced as a form of exercise for physical fitness and as a self-healing tool. Massage and manipulation promote the flow of chi and remove blockages.

Four substances, blood, *jing* (essence or substance of all life), *shen* (spirit), and fluids (bodily fluids other than blood) constitute the fundamentals of Chinese medicine. The nutritional modality of Chinese medicine comprises several components: food used as a means of obtaining nutrition, food used as a tonic or medicine, and the abstention from food. Foods are classified according to taste (sour, bitter, sweet, spicy, and salty) and property (cool, cold, warm, hot, and plain) in order to regulate yin, yang, chi, and blood. *Gui-Jin* links the functions of various foods to corresponding internal organs, channels, and various parts of the body for the purpose of interpreting the functional mechanisms of foods. In other words, foods are consumed in order to improve the functions of the corresponding organs.

Within the framework of traditional Chinese medicine, meridians form channels that carry blood and chi throughout the body, forming the web of life. These are not literal channels, but rather 14 invisible vertical networks that unify all parts of the body and connect the inner and the outer body. In traditional Chinese medicine, organs are viewed not as anatomic concepts but as energy fields.

Acupuncture is the insertion of thin needles into points on the meridians to stimulate the body's chi or vital energy (Fig. 60–1). This therapy is used to treat disharmony in the body that leads to disease. Disharmony, or loss of balance, is caused by a weakening of the ying force in the body, which preserves and nurtures life, and the yang force, which generates and activates life. Related to the concept of acupuncture is the use of moxibustion, or the application of heat, and acupressure, or pressure, along meridian acupuncture points to bring balance to body substances.

Acupuncture has been applied to produce regional anesthesia. Its method of action appears to be through needle stimulation triggering the release of opioids, natural morphine-like substances, into the body. In 1997, a National Institutes of Health panel endorsed acupuncture as clearly effective for postoperative pain from dental surgery, as well as nausea and vomiting from chemotherapy and anesthesia. Additionally, the panel judged that acupuncture may also be effective for migraine headaches, arthritis, menstrual cramps, low-back pain, and tennis elbow.

The use of Chinese herbs is integral to the practice of Oriental medicine. The Chinese pharmacopoeias were published as early as the third century BC and contain herbs and minerals as well as animal products. Typically, a Chinese medicinal formula incorporates three to five different substances.

Phytotherapy

In botany, an herb is a green plant without a woody stem. In medicine, the term is extended to include any plant, or part

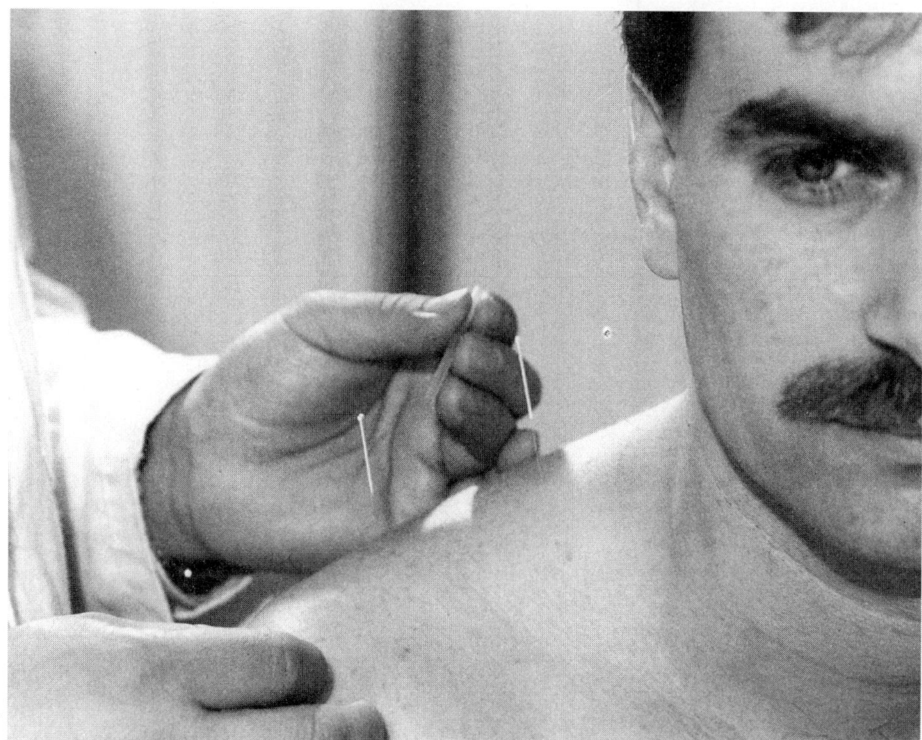

Figure 60–1 Acupuncture site on the shoulder. Acupuncture does no harm and has virtually no adverse effects. Although its method of action is not understood, acupuncture's ability to produce measurable change in the areas of the brain that perceive pain has been documented. (Photo courtesy of The New Center College, Syosset, New York 11791.)

of a plant, that can be used to make a remedy. Thus, the term herb embraces seaweed, ferns, flowers, roots, bulbs, barks, seeds and leaves, and includes cooking herbs, spices, as well as many fruits and vegetables. Phytotherapy (from the Greek *phyto* for plant) is the science of using plant-based medicines to treat illness. *Phytomedicines* have a significant history of research and use in clinical settings, most notably in Europe.

Phytomedicines occupy the middle ground between drugs and food. At one end of the herbal spectrum are strong remedies that have been used as the source of modern drugs (e.g., poppies used for opium and deadly nightshade for atropine). At the other end of the spectrum are nourishing remedies such as bladderwrack and horsetail, rich sources of vitamins and essential trace minerals. For many phytomedicines, the active ingredients and their mechanism of action have been defined. The scientific basis of phytomedicine is investigated using the same scientific tools, such as double-blind, placebo-controlled clinical trials, as other drugs.

More than 80 percent of the population worldwide uses botanical preparations as medicine (Fig. 60–2). In most industrialized countries, herbalism is experiencing an unprecedented renaissance. Every third American is thought to use some form of alternative therapy, and use of alternative therapies is more common among well-educated, upper income, white Americans in the 25- to 49-year-old age range. Although Germany leads the market with approximately $3 billion in annual sales, the United States is second in line with $1.5 billion in annual sales. The United States is followed by Italy, the United Kingdom, Spain, the Netherlands, and Belgium. Echinacea, ginseng, ginkgo, saw palmetto, and cranberry account for a large portion of these sales.

Research information on phytotherapy as a modality of complementary medicine is exploding. Medline, the National Institutes of Health's database on health sciences topics, listed over 3700 peer-reviewed journal articles in the category of medicinal plants in the database for 1990 to 1997. Virtually all contemporary health care providers examine patients who routinely use complementary or adjunctive therapies. Yet only three in 10 of these patients discuss complementary or adjunctive therapies with their health care provider.

PHYTOMEDICINAL OPTIONS

Bilberry

Bilberry *(Vaccinium myrtillus)* is a relative of the blueberry and cranberry. This shrub produces small, sweet blackberries. It was used by British pilots during World War II to improve night vision.

Indications

Bilberry may be useful for simple diarrhea. There are preliminary indications that it may be useful in preventing and treating eye conditions such as diabetic retinopathy and night blindness, macular degeneration, glaucoma, and cataracts. It may also be effective for varicose veins and hemorrhoids.

Pharmacodynamics

The active constituents in bilberry are anthocyanosides, bioflavonoids that act as antioxidants. Bilberry is also thought to contain pectin. Pectin is a soluble fiber that counteracts diarrhea by acting as an antioxidant and preventing damage to small blood vessels. It acts by keeping capillary walls strong and flexible. It also helps maintain the flexibility of the walls of red blood cells and allows them to pass through the capil-

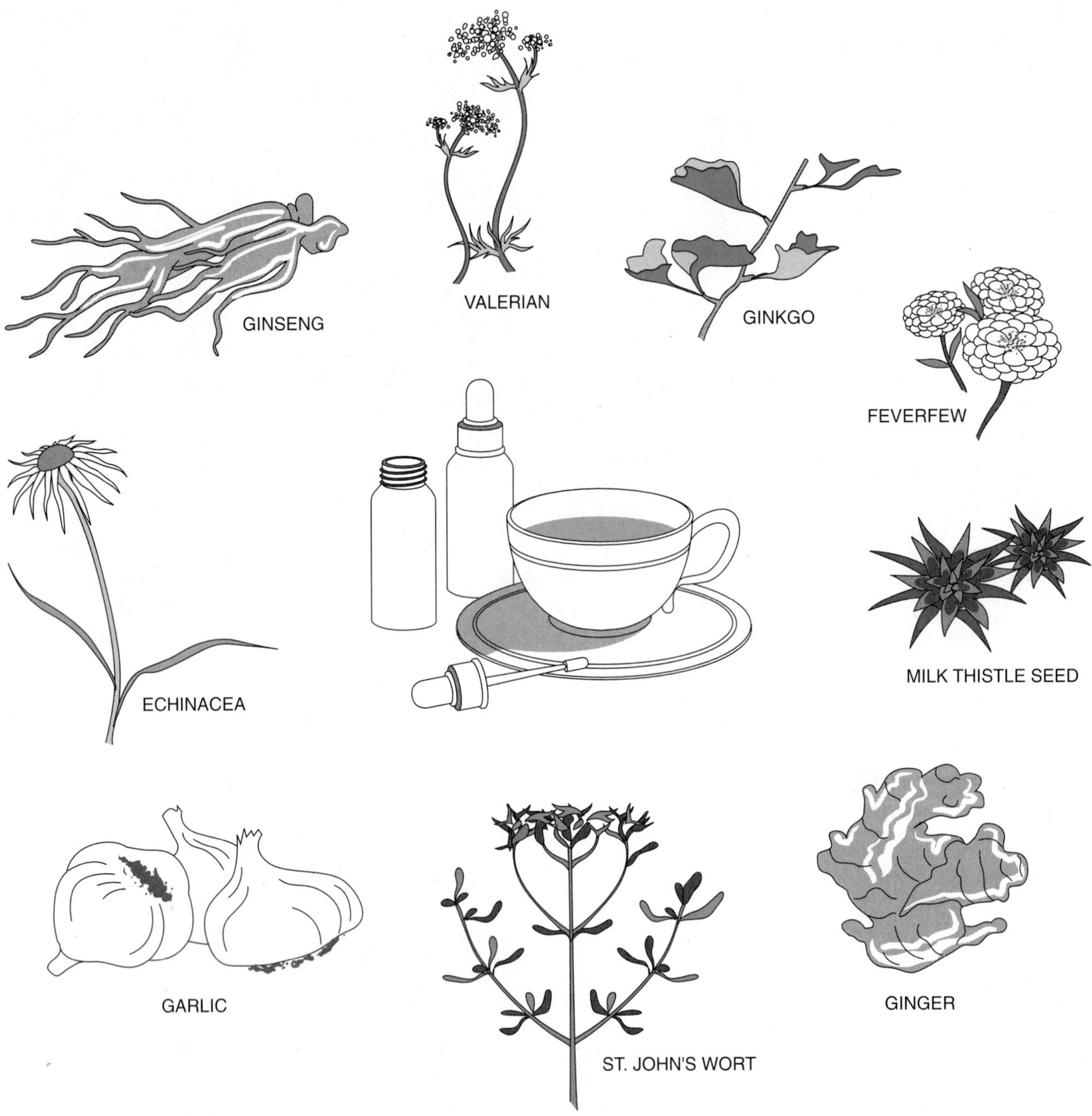

Figure 60–2 Components of selected phytomedicinals. Phytomedicines are made from flowers, seeds, stems, bark, and roots, and their extracts are commonly used in a variety of phytomedicinals, including tea, capsules, and ointments.

laries better. In addition, this herb supports and strengthens collagen structures, inhibits the growth of bacteria, acts as an anti-inflammatory agent, and is thought to have antiaging and anticancer effects. The fresh berries have a laxative effect. Bilberry may prolong blood coagulation.

Adverse Effects and Contraindications

The adverse effects of bilberry appear to be few.

Drug-Drug Interactions

Bilberry may prolong coagulation time. Thus, it should be used with caution in patients who are concurrently taking aspirin, anticoagulants, vitamin E, fish oils, garlic, or ginger. Bilberry interferes with iron absorption when taken internally.

Dosage Regimen

The usual dose of bilberry in tablets or capsules is 240 to 480 mg of dried berry extract taken in two divided doses (Table 60–2). The extract is standardized to at least 25 percent anthocyanosides.

Black Cohosh

Black cohosh (*Cimicifuga racemosa*) is a showy plant native to North American forests. It is also known as black snakeroot, rattleweed, rattleroot, squawroot, and cimicifuga. The drug was introduced by Native Americans, who valued it for a wide variety of conditions ranging from rheumatism to sore throat and diseases of women. It was also used to stimulate menstrual flow.

Indications

Black cohosh is now used primarily for premenstrual syndrome and menopausal symptoms such as hot flashes. Herbalists also recommended black cohosh for dysmenorrhea and rheumatism, and as an antispasmodic, astringent, diuretic, expectorant, and sedative. There is evidence that it

TABLE 60–2 DOSAGE REGIMEN FOR SELECTED HERBAL REMEDIES*

Agent	Uses	Dosage	Implications
Bilberry	Simple diarrhea	*Adult:* 240–480 mg of dried berry extract taken in two to three divided doses daily	Extract is standardized to at least 25% anthocyanosides
Black cohash	Menopausal symptoms, PMS	*Adult:* 40 mg daily	Use no more than 6 months continuously. Allow several weeks between uses
Echinacea	Nonspecific immune system stimulant	*Adult:* 15 to 30 drops of hydroalcoholic formulation taken two to five times daily. Dried root: 1 to 2 g. Tincture: 0.75 to 1 teaspoon. Fluid extract: 0.25 to 0.5 teaspoon. Solid (dry powdered) 3.5% extract: 300 mg	Cycled use (8 weeks followed by 1 week rest) is recommended because of the possibility of weakened effects with continued use
Feverfew	Migraine headaches, menstrual pain, asthma, dermatitis, and arthritis	*Adult:* 250 mcg po daily	Continuous use for at least four to 6 weeks is recommended
Garlic	Mild hypertension, anticoagulation antibacterial, antiviral, antifungal agent, . reduction of total serum cholesterol and triglyceride levels, prophylaxis for stroke	*Adult:* Chew one clove daily	Formulation should deliver a minimum of 10 mg of alliin or a total allicin potential of 5000 mcg
Ginger	Dyspepsia, diuretic, dizziness	*Adult:* 2–4 g po in divided doses/day *or* two cups of tea using 1 tsp fresh root *or* 1½ tsp powdered root/cup *or* eat two 1-inch squares of candied ginger. Repeat in 4 hr, if necessary	May aggravate gallstones. Do not use for postoperative nausea since it can prolong bleeding, or use concurrently with bilberry. Dosage should not exceed 1 g/day during pregnancy
	Nausea and vomiting. hyperemesis gravidarum	*Adult:* 1–2 g po in two divided doses/day	
	Motion sickness	*Adult:* 1000 mg po taken 30 minutes before planned trip and then 500–1000 mg every 4 hr if symptoms return.	
Ginkgo biloba extract	Age-related decline in mental function	*Adult:* 120 to 160 mg po daily	Solid and liquid form are available with each tablet and capsule containing 40 mg of *Gingko biloba* extract
Ginseng	Immune system stimulant, erogenic aid	*Adult:* 100 mg of 4–7% Chinese ginseng po once or twice daily *or* 2–4 mL of 33% fluid extract Siberian ginseng taken po one to three times daily	Cycled use in 2 to 3 week intervals with a 1 to 2 week rest period is advised for Chinese ginseng and 5 to 7 weeks' rest for Siberian ginseng
Hawthorn	Hypertension, atherosclerosis, angina, early-stage congestive heart failure	*Adult:* 160 mg of the dried berries, leaves, and flower po daily *or* 20–40 drops of standardized tincture three times daily	Use only under the direction of health care provider. Use product standardized to 18.75% oligomeric procyanidins and 2.2% flavonoids
Milk thistle	Hepatoprotectant	*Adult:* 140 mg of standardized seed extract is taken po three times daily	Capsules contain 200 mg of concentrated seed extract representing 140 mg of silybin
Saw palmetto	Benign prostatic hyperplasia	*Adult:* 160 mg of the standardized liposterolic extract is taken po twice daily	Six to eight weeks of continuous use is recommended before assessing efficacy
St. John's wort	Mild to moderate depression	*Adult:* 300 mg of the herb standardized to 0.3 percent hypericin taken by mouth three times daily *or* 40–80 drops of tincture three times daily *or* 1–2 heaping teaspoons of dried herb per cup of water taken twice daily	Avoid concurrent use with opioids, amphetamines, over-the-counter cold and flu preparations. Several weeks may pass before improvement is noted
Valerian root	Insomnia, anxiety	*Adult:* Insomnia: 300 to 400 mg (50 to 100 drops) of standardized valerian root extract, 1 hour before bedtime *or* 1 teaspoon of dried root per cup of water used as a tea. The dosage may be repeated two to three times if needed. Anxiety: 200–300 mg each morning	Standardized root extracts should contain at least 0.5 percent valerenic acid

*Patients should be advised that herbs are not regulated in the United States at this time. Because there are no standards in the United States, formulations vary widely in potency and recommended dosages. When discrepancies exist in the above-mentioned dosages, the dosage instructions on the product label should be followed.

will promote labor in the pregnant women. Popular lay press claims suggest that it may also be useful for lowering blood pressure and cholesterol levels, as well as for reducing mucus production. It has also been suggested that black cohosh may be helpful for poisonous snake bites.

Pharmacodynamics

The pharmacodynamic studies of black cohosh have been conducted primarily in Europe. The active ingredients include triterpenoid glycosides, isoflavones, and aglycones, which include acteine, cimicifugin, isoflerulic acid, oleic acid, palmitic acid, pantothenic acid, phosphorus, racemosin, tannins, and vitamin A. A methanol extract of black cohosh has been noted to contain substances that bind to estrogen receptors. The extract also appears to suppress luteinizing hormone but not follicle-stimulating hormone. These findings have been interpreted to mean that black cohosh possesses some degree of estrogen-like activity.

Adverse Effects and Contraindications

Large doses of black cohosh cause dizziness, headaches, nausea, stiffness, and trembling. It should not be used during pregnancy until birth is imminent or in the presence of chronic disease.

Drug-Drug Interactions

There are no known drug-drug interactions with black cohosh, although the herb should not be used in patients taking antihypertensive drugs.

Dosage Regimen

The safe dosage regimen for black cohosh is yet to be established. The therapeutic dose approved by the German regulatory agency is 40 mg/day. It has been noted that 8 mg/day taken for 8 weeks has suppressed luteinizing hormone activity, suggesting that this dose may stimulate synthesis of estrogen.

Echinacea

Echinacea *(Echinacea purpurea)*, also known as snakeroot, purple coneflower, Sampson root, or hedgehog, is a member of the daisy family native to the central United States. It was the most commonly used herb of the Plains Indians. Nine species of echinacea grow in the United States. In addition to *E. purpurea* there is also *E. pallida* and *E. angustifolia.*

Echinacea was first introduced in about 1871 as a blood purifier to counteract blood poisoning. It was later used for problems ranging from bee stings, rattlesnake bites, and chronic nasal congestion to toothache and leg ulcers.

Indications

At present, the most common adjunctive use of echinacea is to prevent or moderate symptoms of colds and flu. Echinacea also acts as a nonspecific immune system stimulant. Either the drug is taken internally to increase the body's resistance to various infections or it is applied locally for its wound-healing action. It has been approved by the German Commission C to enhance resistance to upper respiratory infections. Topically, echinacea may provide antioxidant protection against ultraviolet A and ultraviolet B light rays. It is also used topically more often in Germany to treat hard-to-heal wounds, eczema, burns, psoriasis, and herpes simplex.

Pharmacodynamics

The active ingredients of echinacea have been identified as high-molecular-weight polysaccharides. Other constituents of echinacea include flavonoids, caffeic acid derivatives (e.g., echinacoside), essential oils, polyacetylenes, alkylamides, and miscellaneous chemicals including resins, glycoproteins, sterols, minerals, and fatty acids. The polysaccharides have been targeted in echinacea as the immune-enhancing agents.

Several mechanisms may account for the immune-boosting properties of echinacea. It is thought to stimulate phagocytosis, increase the motility of leukocytes, and increase the number of T cells. Arabinogalactan, one of the plant's polysaccharides, has been shown to activate macrophages to produce tumor necrosis factor and other immune potentiators such as interferon. Echinacea has been shown to help protect the body from infection by stabilizing hyaluronic acid, one component of the ground substance in connective tissue. Hyaluronic acid, a mucopolysaccharide, protects cells and connective tissue from invasion by microorganisms. Further, echinacea's inhibitory action on lipoxygenase suggests anti-inflammatory activity and justifies its use for infection.

Adverse Effects and Contraindications

Echinacea has been identified as essentially nontoxic when it is taken orally, and it is apparently safe for women who are pregnant or lactating, although allergies are possible. This herb should not be used by persons with systemic autoimmune illnesses, including tuberculosis, acquired immunodeficiency syndrome, collagen diseases such as lupus erythematosus, multiple sclerosis and other autoimmune diseases, or allergies to the sunflower family.

Drug-Drug Interactions

There are no known drug-drug interactions with echinacea.

Dosage Regimen

The dosage of echinacea depends on the potency of the particular formulation. Commercially available products are usually 380-mg capsules. Standardized preparations should contain 3.5 percent echinacoside. One to three capsules are taken three times daily with water at mealtime. The dosage of a hydroalcoholic formulation (22 percent alcohol) is 15 to 30 drops taken two to five times daily. Other dosage forms of echinacea include dried root (1 to 2 g), tincture (0.75 to 1 teaspoon), fluid extract (0.25 to 0.5 teaspoon). Cycled use (8 weeks of use, followed by 1 week rest) of echinacea is recommended because of the possibility of weakened effects with continued use.

Feverfew

Feverfew *(Tanacetum parthenium)* is a short, bushy, perennial, a member of the daisy family. Its yellow flowers and yellow-green leaves resemble those of chamomile. Its name is simply a corruption of the Latin term *febrifugia,* or fever reducer. Historically, the plant was used as an antipyretic.

Indications

Today, feverfew has become a popular prophylaxis for migraine headaches and is also used to relieve menstrual pain, asthma, dermatitis, and arthritis. In Canada, feverfew is sanctioned as a preventive therapy for migraine headache.

Pharmacodynamics

The principal active constituent of feverfew is parthenoid, a sesquiterpene lactone. Feverfew also contains essential oils (0.02 to 0.07 percent). Feverfew may act by reducing the inflammatory process and inhibiting the release of serotonin, which has been implicated in migraine headaches.

Adverse Effects and Contraindications

Long-term studies on the adverse effects of feverfew have not been conducted. Other problems that may be associated with feverfew include palpitations, a slightly heavier menstrual flow, and colicky abdominal pain. Feverfew is a potential allergen for those who are sensitive to ragweed. The most common adverse effect reported with feverfew has been mouth ulcerations and an inflamed tongue, in individuals who chew the dried leaves. Feverfew is contraindicated in pregnant and lactating women, and is not recommended for children younger than 2 years of age.

Drug-Drug Interactions

No drug-drug interactions have been noted with feverfew at this time.

Dosage Regimen

The average daily dose for migraines is 125 mg of dried feverfew leaf standardized to 0.2% parthenolide.

Garlic

Garlic, consisting of the bulb *Allium sativum,* is a member of the botanical family *Lilliaceace* and belongs to the same genus as the onion *(A. cepa),* leek *(A. ampeloprasum),* and shallot *(A. ascalonicum).* As a medicinal herb, garlic has been used since the earliest days of recorded history. It grows wild almost everywhere in the world, and every culture has recognized its enormous healing powers. To the Greek physician Galen (AD 130–200), it was known as the great panacea. To the gangs who worked on the great pyramids of Egypt, it was a daily ration given to them to maintain their strength and prevent disease. Because of its supremacy in strengthening immunity, cleansing the blood, and driving out infection, it was championed by the people of central Europe as one of the weapons of choice to combat the depredations of the legendary blood-drinking vampires.

Indications

Garlic is a popular herbal product marketed in the United States whose effects are supported by scientific and clinical evidence. One thousand papers on the therapeutic effects of garlic have been published in the last 20 years. Garlic is used to treat mild hypertension and for blood clotting disorders. It may be used as an antibacterial, antiviral, and antifungal agent, and it is believed to have some anticancer properties. The most effective use of garlic is in the reduction of total serum cholesterol and triglyceride levels, and it has been shown to have a modest effect in lowering blood pressure. It may also provide some protection against stroke. Popular lay press claims suggest that garlic may be used also as an anthelmintic, antispasmodic, diuretic, carminative and digestant, and expectorant.

Pharmacodynamics

Garlic bulbs contain an odorless, sulfur-containing amino acid derivative known as alliin. When the bulb is crushed or bruised, alliin comes into contact with alliinase and is converted to allicin, the active ingredient in garlic. The parent substance alliin has no antibacterial properties; however, allicin has potent antibacterial activity against numerous gram-positive and gram-negative organisms. Allicin carries a strong garlic odor and is also extremely unstable. In order to obtain the volatile oil from garlic, the bulbs are subjected to steam distillation. The compounds yielded include diallyldisulfide, diallyltrisulfide, methylallylsulfides, dimethylsulfides, dithiins, and ajoenes, all garlic-smelling compounds.

Ajoene is the compound in garlic that has been proposed to act as an antithrombotic agent. Ajoene also increases fibrinolysis, the breakdown of fibrin, which slows blood coagulation. The antithrombotic and fibrinolytic actions of garlic have been shown to be at least as potent as aspirin in slowing the blood clotting mechanism.

Garlic has also been shown to hinder the metabolism of cholesterol, prevent the oxidation of low density lipoproteins, and increase bile acid secretion. It may also exert a mild antihypertensive activity. Allicin is the probable agent in garlic that promotes these actions.

Dried garlic preparations contain neither allicin, the antibacterial component, or ajoene, the anticoagulant agent. Allicin and ajoene may be present in garlic that has been dried at a relatively low temperature, but it is unstable in the presence of acids. Thus, when dried garlic is consumed, the enzyme is destroyed by stomach acid, and little conversion to active ingredients takes place. Therefore, dried garlic preparations are most effective if they are enteric coated. The enteric-coated formulations should be more effective (theoretically) than even fresh garlic, in which alliinase is destroyed in the stomach. Fresh garlic releases its active components primarily in the mouth during chewing, not later in the stomach. Germany' Commission E recommends that fresh garlic be used.

Adverse Effects and Contraindications

Consumption of moderate quantities of garlic on a daily basis should not pose any risk for healthy persons. However, larger doses required for therapeutic efficacy (over 5 cloves/day) can cause heartburn, flatulence, garlic taste or odor, and related gastrointestinal problems. There are no reported allergic reactions or known contraindications to the use of garlic during pregnancy or lactation. Garlic is not suitable for children younger than 3 years of age.

Drug-Drug Interactions

Because garlic reduces coagulation, persons taking aspirin or other anticoagulant drugs should avoid eating large amounts of the herb.

Dosage Regimen

Recommended doses of garlic in a commercial preparation should deliver a minimum of 10 mg of alliin or a total allicin potential of 5000 mcg. The recommended dosage of raw garlic is to chew one clove daily. Odor-controlled, enteric-coated garlic powder supplements can be used for those who are hesitant about the odor.

Ginger

Ginger *(Zingiber officinale)* is a rhizome (underground stem) native to the orient. It is also known as Jamaica ginger, African ginger, Cochin ginger, black ginger, and race ginger. The plant has a green-purple flower and resembles an orchid. It continues to be valued throughout the world as a spice.

Indications

It is used as a digestive aid, stimulant, diuretic, antiemetic, and treatment for dizziness. Ginger has also shown efficacy in the treatment of hyperemesis gravidarum (excessive vomiting during pregnancy), although long-term use during pregnancy is not recommended. Ginger is used in Germany as a remedy for dyspepsia and as prophylaxis for motion sickness. Owing to its anti-inflammatory actions, other applications of ginger include arthritis, both rheumatoid and osteoarthritis, and muscular pain.

Pharmacodynamics

The active constituent in ginger includes a volatile oil (1 to 4 percent) that contains sesquiterpene hydrocarbons, zingiberene, and bisabolene. Pungent oleoresin components of the plant include shogaols and gingerols. These pungent components are thought to be the most pharmacologically active. The antiemetic activity of ginger is primarily situated in the gastrointestinal tract. Although it appears the shogaols and gingerols may also act on the vestibular impulses to the autonomic centers of the brain. Ginger has not been shown to influence the inner ear or the oculomotor system.

Ginger exerts anticoagulant effects by inhibiting thromboxane production. The sesquiterpene gingerol is responsible for the blood thinning action of ginger. Ginger has mild anti-inflammatory and analgesic effects due to the inhibition of leukotrienes and prostaglandins.

Adverse Effects and Contraindications

There are no reports at this time of severe ginger toxicity. However, it has been suggested that severe overdoses of ginger carry the potential for central nervous system depression and arrhythmias. Ginger is generally contraindicated in patients with a history of gallstones and should be used by these patients only after consultation with the health care provider.

Drug-Drug Interactions

Ginger should not be taken concurrently with anticoagulants, aspirin, or bilberry because the risk of bleeding is increased.

Dosage Regimen

Ginger is usually taken in the form of capsules, each containing 500 mg of powdered ginger. When it is used as an antiemetic, 1 to 2 g of ginger are taken in two divided doses. For maximum effect on motion sickness, ginger should be used several days before travel, with continuous usage for duration of the trip. Ginger may also be consumed as a tea or in the form of candied ginger. Dosages of more than 6 g have been shown to increase exfoliation of gastric epithelial cells. Ingestion of these amounts of ginger may result in gastric distress and potential ulcer formation.

Ginkgo

Ginkgo *(Ginkgo biloba)* is the oldest living species of tree. It can be traced back more than 200 million years to the fossils of the Permian period. It was used medically in China for hundreds of years and is now a popular ornamental tree in parks and gardens throughout the world. The ginkgo tree is hardy, thriving along heavily trafficked streets of major cities.

Indications

Because of gingko's numerous pharmacologic actions, it is used to treat varicosities, post-thrombotic syndrome, obliterative arterial disease of the lower limbs, and intermittent claudication. Gingko has been found to be useful for treating age-related decline in mental function (short-term memory loss, poor concentration, possibly dementia), cognitive disorders secondary to depression, tinnitus, and vertigo. Gingko has also been shown to be effective in alleviating depression in older adults, especially in patients with chronic cerebrovascular insufficiency who are not responding to standard drug therapy. Early-stage senility of the Alzheimer's type may also be improved by gingko.

Pharmacodynamics

The herbal extract of gingko (GBE) is derived from green-picked GBE leaves that have been specifically developed for pharmaceutical purposes. The leaves are extracted with an acetone-water mixture, the organic solvent is removed, and the extract is processed, dried, and standardized. Standardized preparations of GBE typically contain 24 percent ginkgo, flavone glycosides, flavonoids (including the bioflavonoids quercetin, kaempferol, and isorhammnetin), and six percent terpene lactones (ginkgolides and bilobalide).

The flavonoids are primarily responsible for GBE's antioxidant activity, particularly damage to the lipid layer of the cell membrane, and the ability to inhibit platelet aggregation. The flavone glycosides also mildly inhibit platelet aggregation.

The ginkgolides act as platelet-activating factor antagonists. Platelet-activating factor not only promotes aggregation of blood platelets but also is involved in many of the effects of allergic response. Allergic responses include bronchoconstriction, cutaneous vasodilation, hypotension, and release of inflammatory compounds from phagocytes. It is suggested that GBE and the ginkgolides attach to platelet-activating factor binding sites to reduce these effects. Bilobalide, in action with the ginkgolides, has been shown to increase blood flow in the brain and protect brain tissue from the effects of hypoxia.

Adverse Effects and Contraindications

The adverse effects of GBE are few. Very large doses of GBE may cause restlessness, headache, nausea, vomiting, diarrhea, and allergic skin reactions. GBE should be used with caution in patients taking anticoagulants or bilberry because of an increased risk of bleeding.

Unprocessed gingko leaves in any form should be avoided. They contain several potent allergens known as ginkgolic acids. These compounds, which are removed during the processing of GBE, are closely related to urushiol, the chemical that puts the itch in poison ivy. No contraindications to the use of GBE during pregnancy or lactation have been noted.

Drug-Drug Interactions

GBE may interact with anticoagulants, aspirin, and perhaps bilberry, thus increasing the risk of bleeding.

Dosage Regimen

Ginkgo leaves are used in the form of concentrated, standardized GBE. The product is marketed in both solid and liquid form, with each tablet and capsule containing 40 mg of GBE. The normal adult dose of GBE is 120 to 160 mg daily. The recommended dosage for cerebrovascular insufficiency and early-stage Alzheimer's disease is 240 mg daily. Six to eight weeks of therapy may be needed before therapeutic efficacy is noted.

Ginseng

Ginseng is a yellowish, radish-like herb that has a rich history in Eastern medicine. It is used as a culinary root vegetable in China, particularly in making soup. In China, ginseng has been in continuous use for over 4000 years and has a broad range of medicinal uses. It is expensive and not widely available in the United States.

There are numerous varieties of ginseng, and almost all are cultivated. The most common are *Panax ginseng,* also called Korean, Chinese, or Asian ginseng, and *Eleutherococcus senticosus.* These two types of ginseng are considered the most important species because of the frequency of their use and the amount of research that has been dedicated to them.

There are also four closely related species. The American variety of ginseng is *P. quinquefolius.* It grows wild more or less commonly in wooded areas from Quebec, Canada, to Minnesota and south to Georgia and Oklahoma. Because it has been intensively sought in the United States, it has been declared an endangered species. Ginseng is a slow-growing and exacting plant that takes at least 6 years to produce a marketable root.

Japanese ginseng is *P. japonicum* and Himalayan ginseng is *P. pseudoginseng. Eleutherococcus senticosus,* or Siberian ginseng, is a related species of the ginseng family but contains different active constituents from the *Panax* species.

Reference to colors of ginseng indicate the herb process. Red ginseng refers to the ginseng root that has been sterilized and preserved through steam treatment, thus turning it red. White ginseng is the dried root. There is no chemical difference between the red and white varieties.

Indications

Ginseng has been used to stimulate the immune system and has been used as an ergogenic aid (i.e., an aphrodisiac) in healthy men and women. It has also been used to relieve fatigue and stress, to enhance mental performance and cardiovascular function, and to regulate plasma glucose levels in persons with type II diabetes. It is analogous to the ubiquitous vitamin tablets. Perhaps the most widely cited reason for using ginseng is its purported ability to help the body compensate for physical and mental fatigue. Athletes use it to increase physical endurance. It enhances cardiovascular response both during and after strenuous physical activity and enables the body to make better use of its energy stores. Students use ginseng to avoid physical fatigue and improve cognitive function. Students taking ginseng may demonstrate significant improvement in arithmetic and deductive reasoning skills.

Pharmacodynamics

Ginseng species differ primarily in their composition and mechanism of action. *P. ginseng* is the most complex, with 13 identified ginsenosides. The interaction of the ginsenosides contributes to ginseng's attribution as an adaptogen. Adaptogens, by definition, must be innocuous and cause minimal disruption of physiologic functioning, and they must have nonspecific activity irrespective of the direction of the pathologic state. Increased vitality and resistance to either physical, chemical, or biologic stress are characteristic of adaptogens. Triterpenoid saponin glycosides are the principal active constituents in ginseng. Other components of ginseng are volatile oils, β-sitosterol, phytohormones, and panaxin, a volatile oil. Standardized extracts of the herb contain 4 to 7 percent ginsenosides.

Because of the interaction of the ginsenosides, which are all contained in small amounts in the root of the plant, the whole root is used in herbal preparations. For example, the actions of two ginsenosides in ginseng, Rb_1 and Rg_1, exert different yet harmonizing influences on the body. Rb_1 has a hypoactive effect on blood pressure and a mildly sedative effect, whereas Rg_1 is believed to exert a mildly stimulatory action on the central nervous system.

Ginseng has been documented to increase levels of T cells and natural killer cells, and to stimulate production of white blood cells in cancer patients undergoing antineoplastic therapy. The effect of ginseng on type II diabetes has been investigated. It appears that ginseng improves the mood, improves physical performance, and reduces fasting blood glucose and body weight. Improvements in glycosylated hemoglobin (HbA1c), aminoterminalpropeptide (PIIINP) concentration, and physical activity have been noted.

Ginseng also appears to have a modulating effect on the hypothalamic-pituitary-adrenal axis. By inducing secretion of adrenocorticotropic hormone, ginseng assists in the production and secretion of certain adrenal hormones. Ginseng has an analogous relationship with many of the body's homeostatic control mechanisms and several secondary actions on metabolic activity of the body in times of stress. Ginseng has also shown promise in combating age-related disorders by increasing the life-span of cells. It is also thought to stimulate nerve growth factor, which normally becomes deficient with increasing age.

Adverse Effects and Contraindications

Mild adverse effects of ginseng, such as headache, insomnia, anxiety, skin rashes, and diarrhea, are usually the result of inappropriate dosage levels. Long-term consumption of ginseng is reported to cause hypertension, nervousness, insomnia, and episodes of morning diarrhea, otherwise known as the ginseng abuse syndrome. Ginseng abuse syndrome, however, is rare.

Ginseng is contraindicated in patients with known hypertension, asthma, emphysema, fibrocystic breast disease, clotting disorders, or arrhythmias. The safety of ginseng use by pregnant or lactating women has not been determined.

Drug-Drug Interactions

Ginseng has no reported drug-drug interactions. Caffeine used concurrently with ginseng may cause overstimulation and gastrointestinal distress.

Dosage Regimen

A great variation exists in both dosing quantities of ginseng and the interval time between doses. The species and strengths of the dose can be tailored to match the appropriate treatment. Notwithstanding, ginseng in concentrations of 4 to 7 percent is generally regarded as safe in dosages of 100 mg once or twice daily. Cycled use of Chinese ginseng in 2- to 3-week intervals with a rest period of 1 to 2 weeks is advised.

For Siberian ginseng, the acceptable safe dosage for the 33 percent fluid extract is 2 to 4 mL taken one to three times daily. For the dry extract of the root, 2 to3 g daily in two or three divided doses is recommended. The dosage of concentrated solid extract is 300 to 400 mg daily. The most important aspect of dosing and the only universally accepted practice is to space the regimens apart. With long-term use, a 1- to 2-week drug holiday is recommended every 5 to 7 weeks if Siberian ginseng is used.

Hawthorn

Hawthorn *(Crataegus oxyacantha)* is a small to medium-sized tree that is native to Europe. Other species of hawthorn include *C. monogyna* and *C. pentagyna*. The leaves, blossoms, and fruits of the plant are used in modern standardized extracts. Much research has been conducted on hawthorn using proprietary extracts that are not available in the United States. Only leaf and blossom formulations are approved for use in Germany.

Indications

Hawthorn has applications for the cardiovascular system. It may be used in the management of hypertension, atherosclerosis, angina, and possibly early-stage congestive heart failure. It should not be used, however, for acute angina because drug action is slow.

Pharmacodynamics

The chemical composition of hawthorn leaves, berries, and blossoms contains oligomeric procyanidins and a mixture of flavonoids. Flavonoid constituents of hawthorn include vitexin, quercetin and rutin, and oligomeric procyanidins. The oligomeric procyanidins and the flavonoids are the active constituents of the herb. Cardiotonic amines, choline and acetylcholine, purine derivatives, amygdalin, triterpene acids, and pectins are other chemical constituents of hawthorn.

Drug actions of hawthorn are related to the high concentrations of flavonoids and oligomeric procyanidins. Flavonoids have been shown to inhibit lipid peroxidation by their action as free radical scavengers. The flavonoid quercetin limits oxidation of low-density lipoproteins.

The cardiovascular activity of hawthorn extract has been demonstrated. Hawthorn preferentially dilates coronary blood vessels and reduces peripheral vascular resistance, thus lowering blood pressure and the risk of angina. It improves the metabolic processes of the heart through its inotropic (strength of the contraction) and chronotropic (heart rate) effects. The high concentration of flavonoids in hawthorn also exert antioxidant action, mitigating free radical damage to the cardiovascular system by increasing the levels of intracellular vitamin C. In addition, hawthorn inhibits angiotensin-converting enzyme (ACE), which converts angiotensin I to angiotensin II, a powerful blood vessel constrictor.

Adverse Effects and Contraindications

Long-term use of hawthorn appears to be safe. Safe use of hawthorn extract during pregnancy or lactation has not been established. Persons with cardiovascular disease should consult a qualified health care provider for information on the appropriate use of hawthorn.

Drug-Drug Interactions

No drug-drug interactions have been noted with hawthorn and commonly available prescription drugs.

Dosage Regimen

A typical daily dosage of hawthorn is 160 mg of the dried berries, leaves, and flowers taken as two divided doses. Higher doses should be used only under the direction of a health care provider. Hawthorn may also be taken as 20 to 40 drops of tincture three times daily. Products standardized to oligomeric procyanidins (18.75 percent) and flavonoids (2.2 percent), usually measured as vitexin, give more predictable results.

Milk Thistle

Milk thistle *(Silybum marianum)* is a tall plant with prickly leaves and a milky sap. It is a member of the daisy family that is also known as St. Mary's thistle, blessed thistle, and Our Lady's thistle. It is native to the Mediterranean region but is naturalized to the eastern United States, California, and other parts of North America. Milk thistle has been used since the 16th century to enhance liver function.

Indications

Milk thistle is known as the liver herb because of its hepatoprotective characteristics. It has been used to reduce hepatotoxicity caused by the use of psychoactive drugs such as phenothiazines and in the treatment of overdose of the death cap mushroom *(Amanita phalloides)*. Milk thistle may also be used as an adjunctive therapeutic tool for inflammatory liver damage due to cirrhosis, hepatitis, and fatty infiltration caused by alcohol or other toxins.

Pharmacodynamics

The active constituent of milk thistle is silymarin, which is found in highest concentrations in the seeds of the plant. Silymarin consists of flavonolignins, unique forms of flavonoids. The flavonolignins include silybinin, silydianin, and silychristine. Silybinin is considered the most important component of silymarin.

Silymarin specifically supports the liver by protecting hepatocytes from toxins and increasing the ability of liver cells to regenerate by stimulating protein synthesis. A strong inhibitory effect of silymarin on leukotriene B_4 by the Kupffer cells partially accounts for the hepatoprotective effects. In addition, silybin is thought to both inhibit the peroxidase process and stimulate ribonucleic acid synthesis in hepatocytes.

Dramatic evidence of silymarin's protection of liver cells is its action on the death cap mushroom. One of the death cap mushroom contains phalloidine, one of the quickest and most toxic liver poisons. Phalloidine acts to destroy the outer membrane of liver cells, and it can lead to death within 3 to 7 days of eating the mushroom. Silymarin binds to sites on liver cell membranes to make sites unavailable to phalloidine, and the cell membrane is protected from phalloidine damage. Silymarin reverses the organ failure and encephalopathy associated with ingestion of the mushroom.

Silymarin has also been shown to regenerate hepatocytes that have been damaged due to chronic viral hepatitis B or alcohol use if the liver cells have not been irreversibly damaged. It appears to reverse liver cell damage (evidenced on biopsy), increase blood protein levels, and decrease liver enzyme levels. Abdominal discomfort, decreased appetite, and fatigue are also improved with silymarin treatment.

Silybinin, one of the compounds on silymarin, has been shown to stabilize the membranes of the hepatocytes by decreasing the turnover rate of membrane phospholipids. As an antioxidant, silymarin stimulates glutathione production. Glutathione is a powerful endogenous antioxidant, ten times greater than vitamin E.

Adverse Effects and Contraindications

There are no known contraindications to the use of milk thistle extract at recommended doses. In rare cases, milk thistle may cause loose stools and diarrhea. No reports of toxicity with long-term use of silymarin have been reported. Patients with decompensated cirrhosis should avoid alcohol-based milk thistle extract. Patients with allergies to ragweed should avoid milk thistle. Safe use during pregnancy and lactation has not been established.

Drug-Drug Interactions

There are no known drug-drug interactions with milk thistle.

Dosage Regimen

Standardized extracts of milk thistle containing at least 70 percent silymarin should be used. The most widely accepted dosage regimen for milk thistle is 140 mg taken three times daily. Capsules of milk thistle contain 200 mg of concentrated seed extract representing 140 mg of silymarin.

Silymarins is very poorly soluble in water; thus, the herb is not very effective taken in the form of tea.

Saw Palmetto

Saw palmetto *(Serenoa repens, Sabal serrulata),* also known as sabal, is a shrublike palm tree that is native to the southeastern portion of the United States. It is found in Florida, Georgia, Louisiana, and South Carolina but is also found in the West Indies. Its fruits were used during the early 1900s as a mild diuretic and for chronic cystitis and an enlarged prostate.

Indications

Saw palmetto acts to reduce symptoms of benign prostatic hyperplasia (BPH). Its use in the treatment of BPH has been substantiated through research. BPH is a nonmalignant abnormal growth of the prostate gland. This condition affects 50 to 60 percent of men between the ages of 40 and 60, and over 90 percent of men older than 80 years of age. BPH has a significant impact on life-style owing to its irritative symptoms and obstruction to urinary flow.

Saw palmetto extract has been found to compare favorably with the pharmaceutical drug finasteride in the management of BPH. The saw palmetto extract, however, has fewer adverse effects, including impotence and decreased libido, than finasteride. Saw palmetto helps initiate urine flow, and to decrease urinary frequency, residual volumes, nocturia, and dysuria. Saw palmetto reduces the symptoms of BPH; it does not reduce the size of the prostate. There are also claims by the popular lay press that it is beneficial in the treatment of asthma and bronchitis, as well as breast enlargement in women.

Pharmacodynamics

The active constituents of saw palmetto are derived from the red-brown-black berries that contain free fatty acids and sterols. The berries contain approximately 1.5 percent of an oil (betasitosterol) that contains saturated (80 to 95 percent) and unsaturated fatty acids and sterols. A purified liposterolic extract of the berries is used medicinally.

As a phytomedicine, saw palmetto acts as a weak antiandrogen to reduce the action of 5α-reductase. The 5α-reductase enzyme converts testosterone to dihydrotestosterone (DHT). As men age, 5α-reductase activity is increased. DHT fosters changes in prostatic cell growth by binding to androgen receptor sites in prostate cells to increase cell growth and division. The lipophilic extract of saw palmetto is said to block the action of the enzyme and inhibit binding of DHT to prostate cells, limiting overproduction of cells and prostatic enlargement. Saw palmetto may reverse atrophy of the testes and mammary glands and may increase sperm production. Saw palmetto is also thought to have anti-inflammatory activity, specifically for the prostate.

Adverse Effects and Contraindications

No significant adverse effects of saw palmetto extract have been reported. Large amounts of saw palmetto may cause diarrhea. There is no evidence that saw palmetto alters prostate-specific antigen (PSA) values.

Drug-Drug Interactions

There are no known drug-drug interactions with saw palmetto.

Dosage Regimen

For mild (stage I) or moderate (stage II) BPH, a dosage of 160 mg of the standardized liposterolic extract is taken twice daily. Six to eight weeks of continuous use is recommended before assessing efficacy. Long-term use of saw palmetto extract to reduce symptoms of BPH is generally needed. Tea made with saw palmetto is of little value because few of the active ingredients are water soluble.

St. John's Wort

St. John's wort *(Hypericum perforatum),* an aromatic perennial herb, has gained much popular attention as an antidepressive. St. John's wort is also known as amber, goat week, Johnswort, and Klamath weed. The plant's name is derived from the yellow flower it produces at St. John's Tide (the summer solstice), June 24th, the day traditionally celebrated as the birthday of John the Baptist. The small black dots containing red pigment and the translucent spots on the leaves provide the plant's signature appearance. Mystical properties were attributed to St. John's wort in the Middle Ages, prompting people to place it under their pillows to ward off death. The herb was known to Dioscorides and Hippocrates. The plant is native to Europe but is found throughout the United States.

Indications

St. John's wort is used as an antidepressant and has applications for mild to moderate depression. It is not appropriate for patients experiencing suicidal ideations, psychotic behaviors, or severe depression. The efficacy of St. John's wort as an antidepressant is comparable to that of imipramine.

Pharmacodynamics

The active ingredient in St. John's wort is thought to be hypericin, which is contained in the red pigment of the leaves. Other ingredients include pseudohypericin, flavonoids, xanthones, tannin (10 percent), and essential oils (1 percent). When the leaves of the plant are rubbed, a red stain is produced. This stain is hypericin, a photosensitizing substance of the plant.

The exact mechanism of action of St. John's wort is unclear. Some health care providers suggest that drug action may be a combination of low-grade monoamine oxidase inhibition and blockade of the reuptake of norepinephrine and serotonin. Other mechanisms have also been proposed. St. John's wort is also thought to possess antibacterial, antiviral, and wound healing activity.

Adverse Effects and Contraindications

The reported adverse effects of St. John's wort include gastrointestinal distress, emotional vulnerability, fatigue, pruritus, and weight gain. Although the adverse effects of St. John's wort are reported to be milder and with fewer incidences than with prescription drugs, patients taking St. John's wort may experience adverse effects in the first 2 to 4 weeks of use. Photosensitivity is possible, particularly in patients with fair skin; thus bright sunlight should be avoided. Inflammation of mucous membranes and dermatitis has occurred with large dosages or prolonged use.

American herbal experts advise that St. John's wort should not be used by pregnant or lactating women.

Drug-Drug Interactions

There are no known drug-drug interactions with St. John's wort, although concomitant use of prescription antidepressants, including fluoxetine and monoamine oxidase inhibitors, such as phenelzine and tranylcypromine, is not advised. Other drugs that should not be taken concurrently with St. John's wort include opioids, amphetamines, OTC cold and flu preparations.

Dosage Regimen

The recommended dose of St. John's wort is 300 mg of the herb, standardized to 0.3 percent hypericin taken by mouth three times daily. Forty to eighty drops of tincture may be used three times daily or one to two cups of tea taken each morning and evening. The tea is made with 1 to 2 heaping teaspoons of dried herb per cup. Several weeks may pass before improvement is noted.

Valerian Root

Valerian root *(Valeriana officinalis)* is a tall perennial herb whose hollow stem bears leaves with white or reddish flowers. Valerian consists of the dried rhizome and roots, which continue to be used after more than 1000 years as a valued tranquilizer and sleep aid. Valerian is also known as wild valerian and garden heliotrope. According to the legend, the Pied Piper enticed rats from the village of Hamelin with valerian. The vertical rhizome and its numerous rootlets are harvested in the autumn of the second year of growth. It is these parts that possess the volatile essential oil that contains the distinctive and, to some, disagreeable odor. The odor is said to be attractive to rats.

Indications

Valerian is used as a sedative and sleep aid. Valerian seems to improve the quality of sleep, reduces the time it takes getting to sleep (even in older persons and poor or irregular sleepers), but it produces no morning hangover. Valerian has also been used to reduce anxiety and may be effective in relieving muscle spasms.

Valerian in combination with lemon balm (*Melissa officinalis*) appears to be comparable to the benzodiazepines (e.g., triazolam) in shortening sleep latency and increasing sleep quality. Patients treated with a valerian–lemon balm combination experience no daytime sedation or loss of concentration. Valerian has also been used as adjunctive therapy for benzodiazepine (e.g., diazepam, lorazepam) withdrawal.

Pharmacodynamics

At the present time, the identity of the ingredients responsible for the sedative effects of valerian remain unknown. The identified components include volatile essential oils and the sesquiterpene derivatives valerenic acid and valeranone. Most of the major European pharmaceutical companies producing valerian root extracts have chosen to remove the one active ingredient valepotriate in the finished product. This action was taken because of the uncertainty regarding possible carcinogenic effects. The valepotriates demonstrate alkylating activity in vitro because of their epoxide structure. These compounds may inhibit thymidine incorporation into DNA, leading to impaired mitochondrial function. The valepotriate-free extracts now being used have the same potential for sedation and the same antianxiety action as the natural root.

The mechanism of action of valerian root appears to be similar to that of benzodiazepines, but valerian root is not addicting. Valerian binds to gamma-aminobutyric acid–A receptor sites to depress central nervous system activity. With weak binding of these receptor sites, sedation is caused without adverse effects, addiction, or dependence.

Adverse Effects and Contraindications

Although valerian may cause a headache or mild, temporary stomach upset, at recommended dosages, the herb has no known serious adverse effects. Too much of the herb may cause a severe headache, nausea, morning headache, and blurred vision. Alcohol use does not increase valerian's sedative properties, and valerian can be used safely while operating a car or other machinery.

Valerian and VALIUM (diazepam) are sometimes confused because of the similarity in spelling of the names and because both drugs have antianxiety actions. Valerian, however, is a much milder antianxiety drug.

Drug-Drug Interactions

Valerian should not be used concurrently with other sedative-hypnotic, antianxiety, or antidepressant drugs.

Dosage Regimen

Valerian root is administered in the form of a tea, tincture, or extract. It can also be added to bath water for external application to treat insomnia. Standardized root extracts should contain at least 0.5 percent valerenic acid. The recommended dosage of valerian for treatment of insomnia is 300 to 400 mg (50 to 100 drops) of standardized valerian root extract given 1 hour before bedtime. A tea may be prepared using 1 teaspoon of dried root per cup of water. The dosage may be repeated two to three times if needed. For anxiety, an added morning dose of 200 to 300 mg is suggested.

Critical Thinking Process

Assessment

A directed history that includes questions to determine the use of phytomedicines or other complementary modalities, including naturopathic treatment, homeopathic remedies, Chinese herbs, or acupuncture, is an important assessment tool for health care providers. The health care provider should query patients who seek advice on the use of herbal remedies about the following: Why are you interested in taking this product? What allergies, if any, do you have to plant materials? Are you now pregnant or breastfeeding? What prescription or OTC drugs are you currently taking?

If the patient reports a symptom, it is important to identify the specific herbal preparation he or she is using. Many people are not sure what they are using, in part because many OTC preparations are combinations of plant products. Many foreign preparations include herbs about which little is known, particularly Asian and Indian herbs.

HERBS FREQUENTLY ASSOCIATED WITH ALLERGIC REACTIONS

Angelica	Dandelion	Milk thistle	Rosewood
Arnica	Feverfew	Hops	Royal jelly
Camphor	Gravel root	Hydrangea	Yarrow
Chamomile	Jasmine	Motherwort	Yohimbine
Cowslip	Lavender	Parsley	

Patients should be asked about the existence of comorbid diseases or conditions and allergies (see Herbs Frequently Associated with Allergic Reactions). At a minimum, the physical exam should include height and weight, blood pressure, pulse, and breath sounds. Further examination will most likely be system focused, based on the patient's reports. Depending on the herbal remedy used, liver function and kidney function tests should be performed before and throughout therapy. Allergy skin testing may have to be performed for some patients before the use of herbal remedies.

Factors that influence choices of cures are bound to cultural beliefs about the causes of illness. Herbal remedies are important aspects of the treatment process for many persons of color. Contemporary medical practices neither assimilate or stamp out folk practices. Health care providers, therefore, must learn an effective diplomacy in order to understand and deal responsibly with the cultural beliefs and practices of their patients.

Many people have turned away from conventional therapies because they believe that natural substances such as herbs are safer than synthetic substances. Patients may not realize the pharmacotherapeutic properties of herbal remedies. The slogan all natural may lead them to believe that all herbal products are safe because they do not think of them as drugs.

Analysis and Management

Treatment Objectives

Regardless of the system or type of therapy used, virtually all complementary and adjunctive therapies share four basic components. They empower the patient to play an integral role in recovering their health and wellness, as well as in maintaining it. They encourage a balanced life-style, with appropriate rest, sleep, exercise, nutrition, and emotional tranquility. The interventions are directed at the individual rather than at the symptoms. And lastly, complementary and adjunctive therapies recognize that good health is dependent on balance or harmony of all aspects of our lives.

Treatment Options

Drug Variables

Herbs are usually chosen to work in unison with the inherent healing powers of the body. Despite obvious conflicts, herbalism and conventional medicine are not at odds with each other. What one does well, the other tends to do poorly, and vice versa. For example, contemporary medicine treats diseases using drugs that contain isolated compounds.

The isolated compounds work well but are often potent and have serious adverse effects. However, for acute conditions, there is no substitute. On the other hand, traditional phytotherapy uses the whole herb. Whole herbs contain hundreds of compounds that may work in concert for a better overall effect than one compound alone could deliver and yet they are gentler and safer than isolated drug compounds.

Whatever the approach, phytotherapy or conventional medicine, self-treatment with herbs is appropriate only for minor, self-limiting conditions. For example, fevers are treated with herbs such as feverfew to bring down the temperature by encouraging the body to sweat. Recurrent infections may be treated with echinacea, which stimulates the immune system to help the body fight off infection. In addition, many herbs strengthen a particular organ or body part. Hawthorn strengthens the heart, and milk thistle is thought to protect the liver. Tonics such as ginger help relieve motion sickness and the nausea associated with pregnancy.

The vast majority of botanical producers are unlicensed and are not required to demonstrate efficacy, safety, or quality. Even though they are often promoted as harmless, herbal remedies are by no means free from adverse effects. Thus, every effort should be made to obtain the highest quality product available.

Patient Variables

Pregnant women generally like herbs for their relative safety and lack of adverse effects, although no herbal remedy should be taken during pregnancy without first consulting the health care provider. Herbs contraindicated during pregnancy include angelica, Chinese angelica, comfrey, dang gui, devil's claw, ginseng, lady's mantle, licorice, motherwort, peppermint, sage, thyme, uva ursi, vervain, wild yam, and yarrow. Pregnant women should also avoid any herbal laxative except dandelion and yellow dock and any worming herbs except garlic. When a woman is breastfeeding, herbs that the infant should avoid should also be avoided by the mother. Lactating women should also avoid sage, which tends to dry up breast milk.

Children respond very well to herbal remedies, but children's illnesses can develop very quickly. An accurate diagnosis from the health care provider should be obtained before beginning an herbal remedy (see Controversy—Unconventional Answers to Illness).

Controversy

Unconventional Answers to Illness

JONATHAN J. WOLFE

Patients and their caregivers are increasingly interested in unconventional approaches to health promotion and disease treatment. Americans in particular, schooled to be careful consumers and armed with wide stores of uncensored information, often ask whether nontraditional treatments may be tried in their own cases. Some want to avoid painful procedures. Some want a last resort after traditional medicine has failed to produce a satisfactory result.

Mainstream health care providers have begun to accept that treatments other than surgery and drugs may offer real value. This is abundantly clear in the treatment of pain, in which behavioral therapies conclusively offer benefit with minimal cost or adverse effects. Rehabilitation therapy has also advanced rapidly. At present, interest in massage and acupuncture seem to provide evidence of a broader acceptance that adjunctive treatment has value. It seems that the process by which modern Western science–based medicine overcame its rivals may have relegated useful treatments to an obscurity that is now being overcome.

Patients are increasingly demanding these modalities. A fine balance will be required between a request based on some compelling but unreliable anecdote in unrefereed literature and a choice based on experience in controlled conditions.

Critical Thinking Questions

- A 36-year-old man with intractable pain following a lumbar injury and four attempts at surgical restoration tells you that he has received real benefit from drinking six cups of tea made from a natural herb that his wife buys at the local health food store. What is an appropriate response to this statement? What information should you document about the tea, its preparation, and its use? How do you measure this when following his progress?
- A 77-year-old woman has moderate pain from her incurable breast cancer, which has metastasized to her ribs and thoracic spine. She reacts negatively to your suggestion to use a transcutaneous electrical nerve stimulator (TENS) unit and imaging as means to reduce her suffering and limit adverse effects from opioid drugs. What answer is appropriate to her statement, "You are only suggesting this because I am old and poor—and my insurance company doesn't want to spend more on drugs for me!" Will you be able to offer this option to her later? What change in her condition could make such adjunctive treatments proper to offer?
- An orthopedic surgeon in your clinic has become interested in acupuncture and has taken several courses in its use at West Coast hospitals and colleges. Your assistance is requested for a procedure. The surgeon wants you to prep and drape the patient's back, then using aseptic technique, hand her 65 needles that she will insert into points marked on the patient's torso. Is this request proper? Under state law, may you assist in this procedure? What personal reservations do you have about taking an active part in this unconventional treatment? What further information do you need?

Intervention

Administration

Herbal remedies should be taken exactly as identified on the package label. The adage that if a little is good, more is better is not correct. For some herbal remedies, a fine line exists between safe dosages and toxicity. There are a number of ways herbs can be used. The formulation chosen depends on the herb to be used, the purpose for its use, and to some degree, personal preference.

Bulk herbs are sold loose to be used as teas; however, bulk herbs rapidly loose their potency. Herbs should have a vibrant color and a strong aroma. Leaves and flowers purchased should be as close as possible to whole. Herbs that have been shielded from light and stored in opaque containers to preserve their potency are preferred. The active ingredients of the herb must be water soluble to be effective in a tea formulation.

Extracts are made by pressing herbs with a heavy hydraulic press and soaking them in alcohol or water. The excess alcohol or water is allowed to evaporate, yielding a concentrated extract. Extracts are the most effective form of herbs, particularly for people with severe illnesses or malabsorption syndromes. Alcohol-free extracts, if available, are best. Herbal extracts are generally diluted in a small amount of water before being ingested.

Tinctures are liquid extracts of plants, often in an alcohol base. Tinctures are used internally or externally in gargles, douches, compresses, liniments, mouthwashes, and baths. These formulations are stable, convenient, and easy to take and digest. Tinctures are taken by the dropperful in a small amount of juice or water. Glycerine-based tinctures are available for those who want or need to avoid alcohol.

Capsules and tablets contain powdered or freeze-dried herbs or extracts. Freeze-drying preserves potency better than powdering, which exposes the herb to heat and oxygen. Both powdered and freeze-dried formulations may contain binders and fillers, and thus may not be fully absorbed. Capsules and tablet formulations are an option for herbs that have an unpleasant taste.

Water-based extractions include teas and decoctions, which can be used as skin washes, gargles, compresses, and lotions, or diluted as eye baths, douches, and baths. *Teas* are made using 1 ounce (25 g) of a dried herb or 2 ounces (50 g) of fresh herb and 500 mL of boiling water. The herb is placed in a pot, the boiling water is poured over the herb, and the pot is covered. The herb should be brewed for 1 to 3 minutes if flowers are used, 2 to 4 minutes if the herb's leaves are used, and 4 to 10 minutes if the bark, roots, or hard seeds of the herb are used. *Decoctions* are brewed from seeds, bark, and roots using the same quantities as for a tea. The herb is placed in a pan, covered with water, and covered with a tight lid. The mixture is allowed to come to a boil and then simmered for 20 to 30 minutes. The mixture is then strained and water added to make 500 mL. Syrups are made from decoctions and reduced slowly over low heat to one-third the original amount. Cane sugar or honey is added (2.2 pounds or 1 kilogram) for every 500 mL of decoction. The syrup is then poured into a clean, dark-glass bottle; labeled; and stored in a cool place.

An herbal compress is made using a cloth soaked in a warm or cool standard tea solution and applied directly to an injured area. It is used cold for inflammations; warm for spasms, cramps, and muscle tension; and hot for joints and swellings. Abscesses are treated by alternating hot with cold compresses.

Ointments are formulated from an extract, tea, pressed juice, or powdered form of an herb. The herbal substance is added to a salve that is applied to an affected area. A *poultice* is a hot, soft, moist mass of ground or granulated herbs spread on muslin or other loosely woven cloth and applied for up to 24 hours on a sore or inflamed area of the body to relieve pain and inflammation. The cloth is changed when it cools.

Education

Patients should be advised that herbs are not regulated in the United States at this time. Because there are no standards

TABLE 60–3 POTENTIAL ADVERSE EFFECTS OF HERBAL EXTRACTS

Herbal Remedy	Adverse Effects
Black cohosh	Nausea, vomiting
Caraway	Nausea, vomiting, CNS depression
Cardamon	Nausea, vomiting, diarrhea
Castor bean	Nausea, vomiting, bleeding, protoplasmic toxin, phytotoxin
Chomper	Digitalis toxicity
Cinnamon	Local skin and eye irritation; vomiting, GU irritation
Coconut	Diarrhea
Cola nut	Insomnia, anxiety, tachycardia, worsening PUD
Darniana	GU irritation; may exacerbate pre-existing UTI
Dandelion	Vomiting
Foxglove	Vomiting, bradycardia, dysrhythmia
Gentian	Nausea, vomiting
Goldenseal	Paresthesia, hypertension, CNS stimulation, respiratory failure
Grindelia	Drowsiness, bradycardia, mydriasis, increased blood pressure, nephrotoxicity, cardiotoxicity
Hellebore	Vomiting, hypotension, bradycardia
Hops	Possibility of hemolysis
Hydrangea	Dizziness, nausea, vomiting, chest pain
Jalap	Volume depletion, excessive catharsis, watery diarrhea
Jimsonweed	Hallucinations, anticholinergic syndrome, contact dermatitis
Kava-kava	Hallucinations, yellowish skin, drowsiness
Lobelia	Headache, nausea, vomiting, seizures, coma, hepatotoxicity possible
Maté	Hallucinations, diaphoresis, caffeinism, venous peripheral vascular disease
Mormon tea	Hypertension, tachycardia, nervousness, anxiety
Morning glory	Hallucinations, confusion, nausea, diarrhea, coma
Nutmeg, mace	Nausea, vomiting, hypothermia, chest pain, dizziness, headache
Oleander	Vomiting, diarrhea
Pennyroyal oil	Hepatotoxicity, seizures, GI bleeding
Periwinkle	Hallucinations, dry mouth, drowsiness, nausea, ataxia, hepatotoxicity, seizures, decreased bowel sounds, alopecia
Royal jelly	Severe bronchospasm
Scotch broom	Vomiting
Snakeroot	Bradycardia, diarrhea, dizziness, hypotension, miosis, nasal congestion, coma
Tobacco	Nicotine syndrome
Valerian	Vomiting, drowsiness
Wormwood	Seizures, coma
Yohimbe bark	Abdominal distress, fatigue, weakness, paralysis, elevated blood pressure, hallucinations

CNS, Central nervous system; GU, genitourinary; PUD, peptic ulcer disease; UTI, urinary tract infection.

in the United States, formulations vary widely in potency and recommended dosages. Although most herbs are nontoxic when they are used at recommended dosages, there are herbs with identified toxic ingredients (Table 60–3). These herbs include for example, arnica, belladonna, hemlock, lily of the valley, and sassafras. Patients should also be told of the resources that are available to them regarding herbal remedies.

Herbs contained in commercial herbal tea products are considered safe when consumed in moderate amounts and rarely cause problems even for heavy users. Some individuals, however, may experience adverse reactions with some ingredients of herbal tea preparations when they are consumed in very large amounts.

Self-treatment with herbs is appropriate only for minor self-limiting conditions. When the decision is made to use an herbal remedy, a few cautionary tips should be taught. The patient should be taught to learn about the therapy before engaging in its use. The more that is known about the efficacy of the remedy, the quality of the herb, and its adverse effects, the safer the remedy may be. Herbs should not be taken casually. Herbs should be used only when the body has a specific need. They should not be used on a regular basis. Patients should be helped to understand that herbs take longer to work than conventional pharmaceuticals.

The patient should be taught to buy from companies he or she trusts. If possible, ask how and where the herbs are grown and processed. The answer to this question provides the patient with a sense of the quality control used. Only standardized herbal remedies are recommended.

Start with a single herb with less than the recommended dose, and carefully monitor the response. This is particularly important if the patient is an older adult or below average weight for height. Herbs should be avoided entirely if the patient is pregnant or lactating.

Information about potential drug-drug interactions or drug-food interactions should be obtained. The herbal remedy should be stopped immediately if the patient experiences adverse effects.

Evaluation

The therapeutic effectiveness of complementary and adjunctive therapies has been determined by patient self-reports and careful research. However, to date only a handful of herbs have been approved by the FDA for selected applications, so that any lay press book or article touting the benefits of an herbal remedy must be considered in light of the scientific literature on safety. The Office of Alternative Medicine was established to support the studies of complementary and adjunctive therapies.

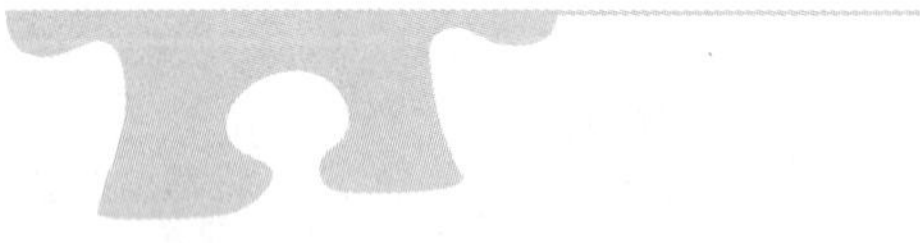

SUMMARY

- Holistic therapies emphasize the healing force of nature and the body's ability to heal itself.
- Naturopathy uses natural methods of healing. Practitioners are trained in naturopathic medical schools, which are similar to conventional medical schools. Modalities of naturopathy include phytomedicines, nutrition, and the use of nutritional supplements.
- Homeopathy is based on the law of similars, the minimum dose, and the single remedy. Many contemporary health care providers practice homeopathy, using remedies that are nontoxic.
- Balancing chi (energy), acupuncture uses needles inserted along energy lines of the body called meridians. Therapeutic applications of acupuncture include regional anesthesia and reduction of postoperative nausea and vomiting.
- Phytotherapy is the science of using plant-based medicines to treat illness. Use of herbal remedies is becoming more widespread among health care providers and the public alike.
- Assessment techniques, particularly directed histories, should incorporate questions to determine use of complementary medical therapies, herbal medicines, or homeopathic remedies.
- Commonly used herbal remedies include black cohosh, bilberry, echinacea, feverfew, garlic, ginger, GBE, ginseng, hawthorn, milk thistle, saw palmetto, St. John's wort, and valerian.
- Bilberry is an herbal remedy that may be used to treat simple diarrhea and may prevent eye irritations such as glaucoma and macular degeneration.
- Black cohosh may relieve symptoms associated with menopause and PMS. This herbal remedy suppresses luteinizing hormone and has estrogen-like activity.
- Echinacea is used to strengthen the immune system and as an adjunctive treatment to reduce the duration and severity of symptoms of colds and influenza.
- Feverfew relieves migraine headache by relaxing smooth muscle and reducing platelet aggregation.
- Garlic acts on the cardiovascular system and lowers hyperlipoproteinemia. The antithrombotic and fibrinolytic actions of garlic are at least as potent as those of aspirin.
- Ginger has been used as an antiemetic. One therapeutic application of ginger has been for the reduction of nausea and vomiting after surgery.
- Constituents of GBE act as platelet-activating factor antagonists. GBE has been used as an adjunctive treatment for cerebral insufficiency and dementia.
- Ginseng is termed an adaptogen and has a normalizing effect, is nonspecific (affects the whole organism in a positive way), and is nontoxic. Ginseng has been studied for therapeutic use in diabetes and to alleviate stress and fatigue.
- Hawthorn has a concentration of flavonoids, particularly oligomeric procyanidins. The cardiovascular system is affected by hawthorn. Therapeutic applications for hawthorn are conditions associated with early-stage congestive heart disease.
- Silymarin is the principal active constituent of milk thistle. Milk thistle is used as a hepatoprotective agent in patients with inflammatory liver conditions and cirrhosis.
- The berries of the saw palmetto plant are the source of the active constituents in the phytomedicine. Saw palmetto is used as an adjunctive treatment for benign prostatic hyperplasia.
- St. John's wort is used as an antidepressant, with applications for mild to moderate depression. St. John's wort has been shown to be as efficacious as imipramine in the treatment of mild to moderate depression.
- Valerian has been used as a sleep aid and acts to weakly bind the same central nervous system receptor sites as that of benzodiazepines. Valerian has no addictive or physical dependence-producing properties.

- There are a number of ways herbs can be used. The formulation chosen depends on the herb to be used, the purpose for its use, and, to some degree, personal preference.

BIBLIOGRAPHY

al Sadi, M., Newman, B., and Julious, S. (1997). Acupuncture in the prevention of post operative nausea and vomiting. *Anaesthesia,* 52(7), 658–661.

Bastyr University, Natural Product Research Consultants. (1996). *Phytotherapy: Herbal medicine meets clinical science.* Seattle: Bastyr University Continuing Professional Education Program.

Bastyr University, Natural Product Research Consultants. (1996). *Herbal medicine: An introduction for pharmacists.* Seattle: Bastyr University Continuing Professional Education Program.

Bone, M., and Wilson, D. (1990). Ginger root, a new antiemetic: The effect of ginger root on postoperative nausea and vomiting after major gynecological surgery. *Anaesthesia,* 45, 669–671.

Brown, D. (1993, 1994, 1995, 1996). *Quarterly Review of Natural Medicine.* Seattle: Natural Product Research Consultants.

Brown, D. (1995). *Herbal prescriptions for better health.* Rocklin, CA: Prima Publishing.

Brown, D., Austin, S., and Reichert R. (1997). *Early-stage congestive heart failure.* Condition Specific Monograph Series. Seattle: Natural Product Research Consultants.

Brown, D. (1995). *Phytofact sheets.* Seattle: Natural Product Research Consultants.

Burton Goldberg Group. (1994). *Alternative medicine: The definitive guide.* Washington: Future Medicine Publishing Inc.

Cardinale, V. (1997). Alternative pharmacy: Natural therapies gaining acceptance. *Drug Topics,* July, 61–62.

Carraro J., Raynaud J., Koch G., et al. (1996). Comparison of the phytotherapy (Permixon) with finasteride in the treatment of benign prostate hyperplasia: A randomized international study of 1098 patients. *The Prostate,* 29, 231–240.

Centers for Disease Control and Prevention. (1995). Self-treatment with herbal and other plant-derived remedies in rural Mississippi. MMWR *Morbidity and Mortality Weekly Report,* 11(44), 204–207.

Collinge, W. (Ed.) (1996). *The American holistic health association complete guide to alternative medicine.* New York: Warner Books.

De Schepper, L. (1998). *The people's repertory: Your guide to safe, effective homeopathic remedies.* Santa Fe, NM: Full of Life Publishing.

de Weerdt, J., Bootsma, H., Hendricks, H. (1996). Herbal medicines in migraine prevention: Randomized, double-blind, placebo-controlled crossover trial of feverfew preparation. *Phytomedicine,* 3(3), 225–230.

Dressing H., Riemann D., Low, M., et al. (1992). Insomnia: Are valerian/lemon balm combinations of equal value to benzodiazepine? *Therapiewoche,* 42, 726–736.

Eisenberg, D., Kessler, R., Foster, C., et al. (1993). Unconventional medicine in the US: Prevalence, costs, and patterns of use. *New England Journal of Medicine,* 328, 246–252.

Ernst, E. (1998). Harmless herbs: A review of the recent literature. *The American Journal of Medicine,* 104(2), 170–178.

Ernst, E., and Kaptchuk, T. (1996). Homeopathy revisited. *Archives of Internal Medicine,* 19, 2612–2615.

FDA Warns against dietary supplement product, "Chomper." *FDA Medical Bulletin,* 27(2), 1–2.

FDA Consumer (1996). Homeopathy: Real medicine or empty promises? 30(10), 15–20.

Harrar, G., and Sommer, H. (1994). Treatment of mild to moderate depressions with hypericum. *Phytomedicine,* 1, 3–8.

Hung O., Shih, R., Chiang, W., et al. (1997). Herbal preparation use among urban emergency department patients. *Academic Emergency Medicine,* 4, 209–213.

Klausner, A. (1998). EN's herbal medicine cabinet: Top 10 herbs you can trust. *Environmental Nutrition,* 21(5), 1, 4–6.

Keller, E., and Bzdek, V. (1986). Effects of therapeutic touch on tension headache pain. *Nursing Research,* 35(2), 101–106.

Kleijnen, J., and Knipschild, P. (1992). Ginkgo biloba. *Lancet,* 340(8828), 1136–1139.

Lokken P., Straumsheim P., Tveiten, D., et al. (1995) Effect of homeopathy on pain and other events after acute trauma: Placebo-controlled trial with bilateral oral surgery. *British Medical Journal,* 310(6992), 1439–1445.

McCaleb, R. (1992). Food ingredient safety evaluation. *Food and Drug Law Journal,* 47, 657–663.

Mowrey, D. B., and Clayson, D. E. (1982). Motion sickness, ginger, and psychophysics. *Lancet,* 1(8273), 655–657.

Muller, J., and Clauson, R. (1997). Pharmaceutical considerations of common herbal medicine. *The American Journal of Managed Care,* 3(11), 1753–1770.

Murphy, J. J., Heptinstall, S., and Mitchell, J. R. (1988). Randomised double-blind placebo-controlled trial of feverfew in migraine prevention. *Lancet,* 2(8604), 189–192.

Murray M. (1995). *The healing power of herbs* (2nd ed.) Rocklin, CA: Prima Publishing.

Niebyl, J. (1992). Drug therapy during pregnancy. *Current Opinion in Obstetrics and Gynecology,* 4(1), 43–47.

Pachter, L. (1994). Culture and clinical care: Folk illness beliefs and behaviors and their implications for health care delivery. *Journal of the American Medical Association,* 271(9), 690–694.

Peterson J. (1996). Acupuncture in the 1990s. *Archives of Family Medicine,* 5, 237–240.

Phillips, S., Ruggier, R., and Hutchinson, S. (1993). *Zingiber officinale* (ginger): An antiemetic for day case surgery. *Anaesthesia,* 48(8), 715–717.

Pizzorno, J., and Murray, M. (1991). *Encyclopedia of natural medicine.* Rocklin, CA: Prima Publishing.

Schoenberger, D. (1992). The influence of immune-stimulating effects of pressed juice from *Echinacea purpurea* on the course and severity of colds. *Forum Immunologie,* 8, 2–12.

Sotaniemi, E., Haapakoski, E., and Rautio, A. (1995). Ginseng therapy in non-insulin-dependent diabetic patients. *Diabetes Care,* 8 (10), 1373–1375.

Sullivan, K. (Ed.). (1997). *The complete family guide to natural home remedies.* New York: Barnes and Noble Books.

Tyler, V., and Foster, S. (1996). Herbs and phytomedicinal plants. In T. Covington (Ed.), *Handbook of nonprescription drugs* (11th ed.). Washington, DC: American Pharmaceutical Association.

Tyler, V. (1994). *Herbs of choice: The therapeutic use of phytomedicinals.* New York: Haworth Press.

Tyler, V. (1993). *The honest herbal: A sensible guide to the use of herbs and related remedies* (3rd ed.). New York: Haworth Press.

Vorbach, E., Hubner, W., and Arnoldt, K. (1994). Effectiveness and tolerance of the Hypericum Extract LI 160 in comparison with imipramine: Randomized double-blind study with 135 outpatients. *Journal of Geriatric Psychiatry and Neurology,* 7(1 suppl), S19.

Youngkin, E., and Israel, D. (1996). A review and critique of common herbal alternative therapies. *Nurse Practitioner,* 21(10), 39–62.

Warshafsky, S., Kamer, R., and Sivak, S. (1993). Effect of garlic on total serum cholesterol. A metaanalysis. *Annals of Internal Medicine.* 119:599–605.

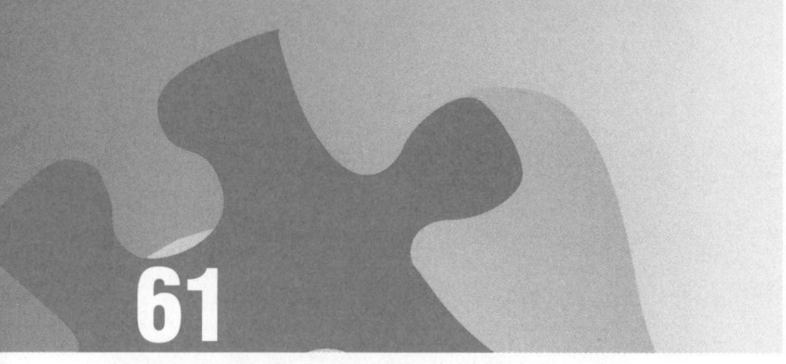

61

Alkalinizing and Acidifying Drugs

The basis for all acid-base relationships is *pH,* the hydrogen ion concentration of body fluids. The normal pH range of blood is 7.35 to 7.45. Even a slight deviation in the hydrogen ion concentration causes profound changes in the rate of chemical reactions. An increase in hydrogen ions makes body fluids more acidic, and a decrease makes them more alkaline. Despite the day-to-day reliability of the body's pH-regulating processes, alkalinizing or acidifying drugs are sometimes needed to correct imbalances. To understand the use of alkalinizing and acidifying drugs in treating acid-base imbalance, an overview of normal regulatory mechanisms is needed.

ACID-BASE BALANCE AND IMBALANCE

To maintain acid-base balance, the body has three major lines of defense: the bicarbonate-carbonic acid buffer system, the respiratory system, and the renal system. The bicarbonate-carbonic acid buffer system can be conceptualized as a sponge. Depending on the specific situation, the sponge either soaks up surplus hydrogen ions or releases them. It acts within seconds to prevent excessive changes in hydrogen ion concentrations. The respiratory system influences pH through control of carbon dioxide exhalation. If a sudden change in pH occurs, the respiratory system, working alone, readjusts the concentration of hydrogen ions within 1 to 3 minutes. The kidneys help regulate pH through regulation of bicarbonate elimination. Although the kidneys are the most powerful of the control mechanisms, when they work alone, several hours to a day or more is needed to restore balance. The hemoglobin and phosphate system also help maintain the body's acid-base balance. Each of these mechanisms shares the responsibility for maintaining normal hydrogen ion concentration.

Balance Mechanisms

Bicarbonate-Carbonic Acid Buffer System

The primary buffer system of the body consists of a combination of carbonic acid and sodium bicarbonate in the same solution. Carbonic acid is a very weak acid, its ability to dissociate into hydrogen ions and bicarbonate ions being less powerful than that of other acids. Most carbonic acid in solution dissociates to carbon dioxide and water, with a net result of high concentrations of dissolved carbon dioxide but only a weak concentration of acid. Hydrolysis of bicarbonate in solution yields the hydroxyl ion and thus increases the alkalinity of the solution. Normally, to maintain acid-base balance (pH of 7.35 to 7.45), the ratio of carbonic acid to base bicarbonate must be 1:20. There are also small amounts of other buffers such as potassium bicarbonate, calcium bicarbonate, and magnesium bicarbonate in the body.

Respiratory System

Carbon dioxide is continuously formed in the body by different metabolic processes. For example, the carbon in foods is oxidized to carbon dioxide. Carbon dioxide diffuses out of the cells into the interstitial fluids and then into intravascular fluids. It is transported to the lungs, where it diffuses into the alveoli to be exhaled. If the metabolic rate is increased, the concentration of carbon dioxide in extracellular fluids is also increased. If the respiratory rate increases, the expiration of carbon dioxide increases, lowering the amount of carbon dioxide in extracellular fluids.

The respiratory system, through a feedback mechanism, acts to control hydrogen ion concentration through the direct action of hydrogen ions on the respiratory center in the medulla. Additionally, changes in ventilation rate and depth alter hydrogen ion concentration of body fluids. When the hydrogen ion concentration of the extracellular fluid increases, the rate and depth of respirations increase and more carbon dioxide is exhaled. Carbon dioxide concentration in the extracellular fluid thus decreases, leading to a drop in hydrogen ion concentration and an increase in pH.

Renal System

Because the kidneys eliminate varying amounts of acid or base, they play a vital role in the control of pH. The renal mechanism involves events occurring in the renal tubules, including hydrogen ion secretion, sodium reabsorption, bicarbonate elimination into the urine, and ammonia secretion into the tubules. Bicarbonate entering the renal tubules changes in proportion to the extracellular bicarbonate concentration. When bicarbonate concentrations in the extracellular fluid remain normal, hydrogen secretion and the filtration of bicarbonate normally balance and neutralize each other. Although the renal mechanism is slow to act, it differs from the respiratory mechanism in that it continues to respond until the extracellular pH reaches normal.

An inability of the body to maintain acid-base balance results in respiratory or metabolic alkalosis, respiratory or metabolic acidosis, or a combination of imbalances (Table 61–1). Furthermore, these imbalances can occur as three forms: primary, mixed, and compensated.

Primary imbalances originate from an acute condition such as respiratory alkalosis resulting from hyperventilation. *Mixed imbalances* occur when one disorder results in acidosis and the other disorder results in alkalosis, when both disturbances are acidotic, or when both are alkalotic. *Compensated imbalances* involve the body's attempt to bring the pH back to normal after a primary imbalance has occurred. The body compensates for a primary imbalance by initiating the opposite imbalance. Compensated imbalances are usually found with chronic disorders (e.g., chronic airway limitation). In essence, respiratory imbalances are compensated for by the

TABLE 61–1 OVERVIEW OF ACID-BASE BALANCE

Condition	Possible Etiology	Imbalance Mechanism
Respiratory Acidosis		
Reduced elimination of hydrogen ions	Respiratory depression related to Anesthetics, drugs (especially opioids) Poisons Electrolyte imbalances Trauma and spinal cord injury Cerebral edema Guillain-Barré syndrome Poliomyelitis Myasthenia gravis Airway obstruction Alveolar-capillary obstruction related to Vascular occlusive disease Pneumonia Pulmonary edema Tuberculosis Cystic fibrosis Atelectasis Adult respiratory distress syndrome Emphysema Lung cancer Inadequate chest expansion Muscle weakness Skeletal deformities	*Acute Acidosis:* Increases in carbon dioxide cause carbonic acid and hydrogen content to increase and the pH to decrease *Chronic Acidosis:* Renal response to increase in carbon dioxide. Hydrogen ions eliminated. Reabsorption of sodium bicarbonate helps restore pH
Respiratory Alkalosis		
Excessive loss of carbon dioxide	Hyperventilation related to Fear Anxiety Mechanical ventilation CNS stimulation related to Catecholamine Progesterone Salicylates Hypoxemia related to Asphyxiation Asthma High altitudes Pneumonia Pulmonary emboli Shock	*Acute alkalosis:* Carbon dioxide blown off causing a base excess and pH increases *Chronic alkalosis:* Renal response to decreased carbon dioxide. More bicarbonate excreted. Chloride retained to restore pH
Metabolic Acidosis		
Overproduction of hydrogen ions	Excessive oxidation fatty acids related to Diabetic ketoacidosis Starvation Hypermetabolism related to Heavy exercise Seizure activity Fever Hypoxia, ischemia Excessive ingestion acids related to Salicylate intoxication Methanol ingestion Ethanol intoxication	Addition of large amounts of fixed acids in blood results in loss of bicarbonate and decreased pH. Immediate respiratory response results in decreased carbon dioxide levels but not sufficient to correct imbalance
Reduced elimination of hydrogen ions	Renal failure	
Reduced production of bicarbonate	Renal failure Liver failure Pancreatitis	
Increased elimination of bicarbonate	Dehydration Diarrhea Buffering of organic acids	
Metabolic Alkalosis		
Increased base components	Administration parenteral base related to Blood transfusion Parenteral nutrition Sodium bicarbonate	Loss of acid or retention of base results in elevated pH and bicarbonate. Minimal respiratory response results in normal or elevated carbon dioxide levels. Bicarbonate-carbonic acid buffer system activated and respirations become slow and shallow. Kidneys retain more hydrogen and excrete more bicarbonate
Increased base components	Excessive ingestion of base related to Antacids Milk-alkali syndrome Cushing's syndrome	
Decreased acid components	Gastric suctioning Hyperaldosteronism Prolonged vomiting Thiazide diuretics	

CNS, Central nervous system.

renal system; metabolic imbalances are compensated for by the respiratory system.

Hemoglobin System

Hemoglobin in red blood cells uses a process called the *chloride shift* to help maintain acid-base balance. The shift is regulated by the level of oxygen in blood plasma. There is a reciprocal exchange of chloride ions for bicarbonate ions.

Phosphate System

The phosphate buffer system acts in the same manner as the bicarbonate-carbonic acid system to regulate acid-base balance. Strong acids are neutralized to form a weak acid of sodium diphosphate and sodium chloride, resulting in a slight change in pH. When a strong base is added to the system, it is neutralized to form a weak base and water. The result changes the pH slightly toward the alkaline side. The total buffering power of this system is less than that of the bicarbonate-carbonic acid system. However, the role of the bicarbonate-carbonic acid system in the kidney tubules does increase the buffering power of the phosphate system.

Pathophysiology

Because alkalosis and acidosis are manifestations of many conditions rather than a separate disease state, their actual incidence is unknown. However, the most common disorder is respiratory alkalosis, followed by respiratory acidosis, metabolic alkalosis, and metabolic acidosis. Mixed imbalances are also possible.

Alkalosis

Alkalosis is defined as a decrease in hydrogen concentration of the blood and is reflected by an arterial pH above 7.45. It is not a disease as such but a consequence of a pathogenic process. Alkalosis results from an actual or relative increase in the concentration or strength of base in the blood.

In an actual base excess, the concentration of base components is proportionately higher than normal compared with the concentration of acid components. There is either an overproduction of base or reduced elimination of bases, usually bicarbonate.

In a relative base excess, the concentration of acid components is decreased. The base excess results from either increased elimination of acids (as hydrogen ions) or reduced production of acids.

Alkalosis causes disturbances in metabolism and pulmonary respiration with serious and potentially life-threatening results. The most common manifestations of alkalosis include stimulation of the central nervous system (CNS), neuromuscular, and cardiovascular systems.

Respiratory Alkalosis

Respiratory alkalosis, occurring as a result of alveolar hyperventilation, results in decreased serum carbon dioxide levels (hypocapnia). Excessive exhalation of carbon dioxide causes decreased serum carbon dioxide levels and decreased carbonic acid production. In turn, the arterial pH increases.

The body attempts to compensate by increasing renal elimination of bicarbonate. In compensating for the respiratory alkalosis, both carbonic acid and base bicarbonate levels are decreased. The most common causes of respiratory alkalosis include hypoxia, pulmonary disease, and drugs (particularly aspirin and other salicylates).

Metabolic Alkalosis

Metabolic alkalosis results from excessive accumulation of fixed bases or excessive loss of fixed acids in body fluids. A major cause of metabolic alkalosis is loss of fixed acids, such as hydrochloric acid (HCl), from the stomach, either through gastric suctioning or excessive vomiting. The loss of acid increases pH. Carbonic acid dissociates and bicarbonate concentration increases through renal absorption. This results in increased renal elimination of hydrogen, potassium, and chloride. Chloride competes with bicarbonate for combination with sodium. Thus, when chloride levels fall, bicarbonate levels rise. As pH increases, calcium binding increases and serum calcium levels decrease, creating hypocalcemia. Serum potassium levels also decrease as a result of the body's attempt to maintain electrical neutrality. Most of the serious manifestations of alkalosis are attributed to the accompanying hypocalcemia.

The body attempts to compensate for metabolic alkalosis through hypoventilation. Stimulation of chemoreceptors is decreased, slowing the respiratory rate and conserving carbon dioxide, thus elevating pH. The most common causes of metabolic alkalosis include vomiting or suctioning and the administration of alkalinizing salts (e.g., sodium bicarbonate).

Acidosis

Acidosis is defined is an arterial blood pH below 7.35. Like alkalosis, acidosis is not a specific disease but rather a symptom of a disease or pathologic process. Acidosis results from an actual or relative increase in the concentration of acids.

In actual acidosis, the concentration of acid components does not increase. Instead, the concentration of base components is decreased (base deficit), which makes the fluid more acid than alkaline. An actual base deficit results from processes that cause either increased elimination of base (usually bicarbonate) or reduced production.

Acidosis causes significant changes in physiologic functions. Many of the early signs and symptoms of acidosis manifest as depression of the CNS, neuromuscular, cardiovascular, and respiratory systems.

Respiratory Acidosis

Respiratory acidosis is a primary acid-base imbalance resulting from retention of carbon dioxide secondary to hypoventilation. Abnormally slow or shallow respirations, or poor alveolar ventilation resulting in inadequate gas exchange causes carbon dioxide to accumulate in the lungs and the serum, increasing carbonic acid levels circulating in the blood and lowering pH. Low arterial pH and elevated serum carbon dioxide levels (hypercapnia) constitute respiratory acidosis. It can be acute, as in sudden ventilatory failure, or chronic, as in emphysema. The body attempts to compensate by increasing the renal reabsorption of bicarbonate.

Metabolic Acidosis

Metabolic acidosis results from excessive accumulation of acids or loss of base in body fluids. Fixed acids, such as

HCl, are produced by metabolism or ingested foods. Chloride, a component of HCl, competes with bicarbonate for combination with sodium. Excessive chloride retention or ingestion increases the production of fixed acids. The inability of the kidneys to retain sufficient bicarbonate results in excessive hydrogen and eventually metabolic acidosis. Metabolic acidosis never results from a respiratory problem, with the exception of lactic acidosis from anaerobic metabolism.

Increased levels of circulating hydrogen results in rapid stimulation of peripheral chemoreceptors and, within minutes, increases the respiratory rate and the onset of acidosis. The body attempts to compensate for metabolic acidosis through hyperventilation, which results in reduced carbon dioxide levels.

PHARMACOTHERAPEUTIC OPTIONS

Alkalinizing Drugs

- ❒ Acetazolamide (DIAMOX)
- ❒ Sodium acetate
- ❒ Sodium bicarbonate (NEUT)
- ❒ Sodium citrate/citric acid (SHOHL SOLUTION, BICITRA, ORACIT)
- ❒ Sodium lactate
- ❒ Tromethamine (THAM)

Indications

Alkalinizing drugs such as sodium bicarbonate, acetate, citrate, lactate, and tromethamine are used to increase blood pH and, thus, correct metabolic acidosis.

Sodium bicarbonate is also used to increase urinary pH in patients with barbiturate, lithium, or salicylate toxicities in an attempt to enhance elimination of these drugs. Sodium bicarbonate may be used as an adjunct to other therapy for the treatment of hyperkalemia to promote the reuptake of potassium into the cells.

Tromethamine is also used on a short-term basis to correct acidosis associated with cardiac disease, bypass surgery, or after cardiac arrest. Because it is sodium free, it can be used to prevent or correct acidosis in patients for whom sodium retention would be hazardous.

Acetazolamide is used to facilitate removal of phenobarbital or lithium after overdose. It is not recommended for use with salicylate overdose because both drugs can cause metabolic acidosis. It has also been used to offset the cerebral edema encountered with exposure to high altitudes.

Pharmacodynamics

Sodium bicarbonate dissociates in the blood to increase bicarbonate and decrease hydrogen concentration. As the hydrogen ions are eliminated in the urine, urinary pH rises. Sodium acetate, lactate, and citrate must first be converted to bicarbonate and then act in the same fashion as sodium bicarbonate.

Tromethamine combines with hydrogen ions from carbonic acid to form bicarbonate and a cationic buffer. It also acts as an osmotic diuretic to increase urine flow and urine pH, and to eliminate fixed acids, carbon dioxide, and electrolytes.

Acetazolamide, a carbonic anhydrase inhibitor (see Chapter 39), raises urinary pH but paradoxically lowers blood pH by promoting the elimination of sodium, potassium, bicarbonate, and water. The bicarbonate ion alkalinizes the urine and, by reducing bicarbonate levels, also acidifies the blood.

Adverse Effects and Contraindications

The adverse effects associated with alkalinizing drugs are usually associated with large dosages. Excessive sodium bicarbonate causes metabolic alkalosis that manifests as hyperirritability, tetany, or both. When administered too rapidly to correct diabetic ketoacidosis, tissue hypoxia, cerebral dysfunction, and lactic acidosis can result. The high sodium content (276 mg of sodium bicarbonate) causes water retention and edema in some patients. Thus, sodium bicarbonate should be used cautiously in patients with congestive heart failure, renal failure, or other disorders of fluid balance. Sodium bicarbonate is contraindicated in patients with chloride losses or hypocalcemia. Oral administration of sodium bicarbonate produces gastric distention and flatus when it combines with HCL in the stomach and releases carbon dioxide.

Sodium citrate produces fewer adverse effects than sodium bicarbonate, but in excess, it can also cause metabolic alkalosis or tetany, or may aggravate existing cardiovascular disease by increasing calcium levels. Orally administered sodium citrate produces a laxative-like effect.

Sodium lactate also produces fewer adverse effects than sodium bicarbonate but in excess can cause metabolic acidosis (rather than alkalosis). Because the sodium content is high (204 mg/g), water retention and edema may develop. Furthermore, it should not be used with an acute disorder or in patients with hepatic impairment because the conversion of lactate to bicarbonate occurs in the liver.

The adverse effects of tromethamine range from irritation at the IV injection site to hypoglycemia, respiratory depression, and hyperkalemia. Tromethamine can accumulate to toxic levels in patients with impaired liver function. The drug is contraindicated in pregnant women and in patients with uremia or chronic respiratory acidosis. Respiratory depression can occur in patients who chronically hypoventilate and in those receiving drugs that depress respirations. Tromethamine is contraindicated in patients with hyperphosphatemia and hypocalcemia.

Acetazolamide produces a wide range of adverse effects. CNS reactions include headache, sedation, confusion, and paresthesias. In a patient with severe liver disease, acetazolamide can raise the blood sugar, decrease uric acid elimination, produce metabolic acidosis, and precipitate hepatic coma. Hypersensitivity reactions and bone marrow depression can lead to aplastic anemia.

Pharmacokinetics

Sodium bicarbonate is 100 percent bioavailable when administered intravenously (IV). The drug has an immediate onset, with peak drug action reached in 15 minutes (Table 61–2). It is widely distributed to extracellular fluid. Sodium bicarbonate is eliminated in the urine with an unknown half-life.

At a pH of 7.4, 30 percent of tromethamine is nonionized and, therefore, is capable of reaching equilibrium with body

TABLE 61–2 PHARMACOKINETICS OF SELECTED ALKALINIZING AND ACIDIFYING DRUGS*

	Route	Onset	Peak	Duration	PB (%)	$t_{1/2}$	BioA (%)
Alkalinizing Drugs							
Sodium bicarbonate	IV	Immed	15 min	1–2 hr	UA	UA	100
Tromethamine	IV	UK	UK	UK	UK	UK	100
Acidifying Drugs							
Ascorbic acid	po	2 days–3 wks	UK	UK	UK	UK	UA
	SC						
	IV	Immed					100
Ammonium chloride	IV	UA	1–3 hr	UA	UK	UK	100
Arginine hydrochloride	IV	Immed	20–30 min	1 hr	UK	UK	100

*As noted in intracellular fluids.
PB, Protein binding; t½, elimination half-life; UK, unknown; UA, unavailable; BioA, bioavailability.

water. The drug penetrates cells and neutralizes acidic anions of intracellular fluid. Elevation in pH has been noted 1 hour after administration. Tromethamine is biotransformed in the liver and eliminated in the urine.

Drug-Drug Interactions

Drug-drug interactions for alkalinizing drugs are identified in Table 61–3. The most common interactions are related to their ability to increase the reabsorption or to facilitate elimination of interacting drugs.

Dosage Regimen

The dose of a specific alkalinizing drug is individualized based on laboratory calculations of bicarbonate levels needed. Sodium bicarbonate is initially administered as 1 mEq/kg of body weight, to be followed by 0.5 mEq/kg every 10 minutes. The dosage is then based on the formula identified in Table 61–4. The dosages for sodium citrate and lactate are also individualized.

The usual dosage range for tromethamine is 1 to 5 mmol/kg of body weight, administered in acute situations over 5 to 15 minutes. The need for additional tromethamine is determined by serial measurements of serum bicarbonate concentrations and calculation of the base deficit. It should not be given for more than 24 hours except in life-threatening situations.

Laboratory Considerations

Serum sodium, potassium, calcium, bicarbonate, and osmolality levels should be monitored before and throughout

TABLE 61–3 DRUG-DRUG INTERACTIONS OF SELECTED ALKALINIZING AND ACIDIFYING DRUGS

Drug	Interactive Drugs	Interaction
Alkalinizing Drugs		
Sodium bicarbonate	Amphetamines Ephedrine Flecainide Mecamylamine Methadone Pseudoephedrine Quinidine Quinine	Increases reabsorbtion of interactive drugs
	Aspirin Chlorpropamide Salicylates Lithium Phenobarbital Tetracycline	Increased elimination of interactive drug
	Glucocorticoids	Excessive sodium retention
Acidifying Drugs		
Arginine hydrochloride	Estrogens Progestin	May elevate growth hormone response
	Glucagon Insulin Sulfonylureas	Reduced response to interactive drug.
	Potassium-sparing diuretics	Increases risk of hyperkalemia.

TABLE 61–4 DOSAGE REGIMEN FOR SELECTED ALKALINIZING AND ACIDIFYING DRUGS

Drug	Uses	Dosage	Implications
Alkalinizing Drugs			
Acetazolamide	Alkalinize urine in phenobarbital or lithium overdose	Individualized dosage based on the overdosed drug	Check urinary pH frequently
Sodium bicarbonate	Metabolic acidosis in cardiac arrest	1 mEq/kg IV to be followed by 0.5 mEq/kg every 10 min as needed	Step 1: Base deficit = desired bicarbonate level − patient's bicarbonate level. Step 2: Bicarbonate dosage (mEq) = 0.4 × kg body weight × base deficit
	Less severe metabolic acidosis	2–5 mEq/kg IV over 4–8 hr	
	Chronic renal failure	20–36 mEq/kg po QD in divided doses	Dosage necessary to achieve serum bicarbonate level of 18–20 mEq/L
	Alkalinizing urine	48 mEq po followed by 12–24 mEq po q4hr	Check urinary pH frequently.
Sodium citrate and citric acid	Metabolic acidosis	*Adult:* Up to 5 mL/min IV of dilute solution based on patient's chloride deficit. 10–30 mL po after QID and HS *Child:* 5–15 mL po QID and HS	1 mL of solution = 1 mmol of sodium bicarbonate
	Alkalinize urine in drug overdose	4–12 g po QD in divided doses q4–6hr	Check urinary pH frequently
Sodium lactate	Metabolic acidosis for patients who cannot tolerate oral product	Dosage (mL of 1/6 molar solution) = 0.8 × body weight (lb) × (60 −plasma CO_2 value)	Converts to sodium bicarbonate in the liver
	Alkalinize urine in drug overdose	30 mL/kg IV of a 1/6 molar solution *or* po in divided doses over 24 hr	
Tromethamine	Metabolic acidosis associated with CABG, cardiac arrest, or cardiac disease	Dosage (mL of 0.3 molar solution) = body weight (kg) × (normal HCO_3^- − patient HCO_3^- in mEq/L). Infuse IV over 1 hr or more to a maximum of 24 hr. *Cardiac arrest:* Range: 3.5–6 mL/kg of a 0.3 molar solution	Not to be used longer than 24 hours to avoid serious adverse effects.
Acidifying Drugs			
Ammonium chloride	Metabolic alkalosis	Based on patient chloride deficit but usually 100–200 mEq in 500–1000 mL IV solution. Dosage (mEq) = chloride deficit in mEq/L × 0.2 × kg body weight. Dilute solution not to exceed 5 mL/minute	Available as IV solution of 5.35 g/20 mL. Each gram of ammonium chloride reduces the carbon dioxide–combining power of a 70-kg adult by about 1.1 volume % or 16 mg/kg will lower the carbon dioxide–combining power by 1 volume %
	Acidify urine	4–12 g po in divided doses q4–6hr *Child:* 75 mg/kg/day in four divided doses	
Arginine monohydrochloride	Metabolic alkalosis related to chloride loss (unlabeled)	Arginine dosage (g) = patient's base deficit × body weight (kg) divided by 9.6	Should be administered via indwelling needle or IV catheter into antecubital vein
Ascorbic acid	Acidify urine in drug overdose	4–12 g po QD in divided doses	
Hydrochloric acid	Severe metabolic alkalosis unresponsive to fluid and electrolytes; decompensated CHF or renal failure with oliguria	Dose HCl (mEq) = (0.2 L/kg × kg body weight) × (103 − observed serum chloride) 0.1–0.2 molar solution IV at 0.2 mEq/kg/hr or less - Additional doses based on q4hr arterial blood gases	Give through central venous IV line
Sodium chloride	Metabolic alkalosis	250, 500, 1000 mL IV infused over 8–24 hr	Monitor serum sodium levels

CABG, Coronary artery bypass graft

therapy. Renal function and pH testing should also be performed. In emergency situations, arterial blood gases should be monitored frequently. Urinary pH should be monitored every 4 hours when these drugs are used for urinary alkalinization in drug overdose.

Sodium bicarbonate antagonizes the effects of pentagastrin and histamine during testing of gastric acid secretion. Administration of sodium bicarbonate should be avoided in the 24 hours preceding the test.

Acidifying Drugs

- ❒ Ammonium chloride
- ❒ Arginine hydrochloride
- ❒ Ascorbic acid (ASCORBICAP)
- ❒ Hydrochloric acid (HCl)

Indications

Three acidifying drugs are used to correct metabolic alkalosis: ammonium chloride, arginine hydrochloride, and HCl. Ammonium chloride is specifically useful in correcting acidosis when sodium chloride is contraindicated (e.g., patient with a fluid overload). Ammonium chloride and ascorbic acid may serve as urine-acidifying drugs. These two drugs can be used to increase the effectiveness of certain urinary antibacterial drugs (see Chapter 40) and to enhance drug elimination in drug overdose.

The Food and Drug Administration has approved arginine hydrochloride only for evaluation of pituitary function. Therefore, use of this product to treat metabolic alkalosis is considered investigational.

The patient in metabolic acidosis may need chloride ions as well. Thus, patients can receive both the hydrogen ions and chloride ions by receiving an infusion of HCl. However, it is exacting to prepare and administer. Overdose results in severe adverse effects. For this reason, ammonium chloride is often used because it provides both hydrogen and chloride ions using parenteral or oral doses.

Pharmacodynamics

Ammonium chloride, which has a fixed anion, is an acidifying salt that is converted to urea in the liver. Hydrogen and chloride ions are liberated, thus lowering blood pH. It lowers urinary pH by producing an acid urine and changing the elimination rate of many drugs and drug metabolites.

Arginine provides hydrogen ions via biotransformation to HCL. In turn, it directly lowers blood pH by providing the blood with hydrogen ions. Arginine also stimulates the pituitary release of growth hormone and prolactin, and the pancreatic release of glucagon and insulin. The exact mechanism of action is unclear, but these actions appear to be independent of adrenergic control and changes in blood glucose concentrations. Arginine also elevates serum gastrin levels.

Ascorbic acid directly acidifies the urine by producing hydrogen ions and lowering urinary pH.

Adverse Effects and Contraindications

The adverse effects of acidifying drugs are usually mild. Ammonium chloride can cause anorexia, nausea, vomiting, and thirst when taken orally. Using enteric-coated tablets may minimize adverse gastrointestinal (GI) effects; however, absorption of this dosage form is unpredictable.

Large doses of ammonium chloride can cause metabolic acidosis secondary to hyperchloremia, especially in patients with impaired renal function. Other adverse effects of large doses of ammonium chloride include rash, headache, hyperventilation, bradycardia, progressive drowsiness, confusion, and excitement alternating with coma. Calcium-deficient tetany, hyperglycemia, glucosuria, twitching, hyperreflexia, and electroencephalogram changes have also been reported. Most of these adverse effects are related to ammonia toxicity resulting from inability of the liver to convert ammonium ions to urea. Because the acidifying action of ammonium chloride depends on hepatic conversion to urea, the drug is contraindicated in patients with liver disease. Safe use in perinatal and pediatric populations has not been established.

Arginine hydrochloride has a low incidence of adverse effects; however, rapid IV infusion may produce flushing, nausea, vomiting, numbness, headache, and local venous irritation. Extravasation from an IV site causes superficial phlebitis and necrosis. Nasal obstruction and discharge, choking, sweating, and tachycardia have also been reported during IV administration of arginine. These effects may represent an allergic response to the drug. Abdominal pain and bloating have been reported following oral administration.

High doses of ascorbic acid can produce nausea, vomiting, diarrhea, abdominal cramps, flushing, headache, and insomnia. In patients with glucose-6-phosphate dehydrogenase deficiency, hemolytic anemia can develop after the administration of high doses of ascorbic acid.

Pharmacokinetics

Ammonium chloride taken orally is completely absorbed in 3 to 6 hours. Drug action peaks 1 to 3 hours after IV administration (see Table 61–2). Ammonium chloride is biotransformed to HCl and urea, which is then eliminated via the kidneys, and HCl.

Arginine has an immediate onset when it is given IV, with peak drug action noted in 20 to 30 minutes. The duration of action of arginine is 1 hour. Arginine is incorporated into many biochemical pathways in the liver, filtered at the glomerulus, and almost completely reabsorbed by the renal tubules.

Drug-Drug Interactions

Drug-drug interactions of acidifying drugs are identified in Table 61–3. Estrogens and estrogen-progestin combination drugs may elevate growth hormone response and reduce the glucagon and insulin response to arginine. Severe, potentially fatal hyperkalemia has occurred following arginine therapy. The patients affected were those with hepatic disease who had taken spironolactone 2 or 3 days before receiving arginine. The combined use of potassium-sparing diuretics and arginine should thus be avoided.

Dosage Regimen

The dosage regimen of acidifying drugs is individualized. The dosage of ammonium chloride is calculated based on the patient's chloride deficit. The dosage of arginine is calculated based on the base deficit (see Table 61–4). To acidify urine in the treatment of drug overdose, ascorbic acid is dosed daily in 4 to 12 g orally in divided doses.

Laboratory Considerations

The patient's acid-base and electrolyte balance should be monitored before and throughout treatment with acidifying drugs. Blood urea nitrogen (BUN) and creatinine measurements should be taken before arginine is used because the drug contains large amounts of metabolizable nitrogen, which causes a temporary elevation in nitrogen levels. Liver function tests should also be monitored.

Critical Thinking Process

Assessment

History of Present Illness

Whether the origin of alkalosis is respiratory or metabolic, the patient's symptoms are the result of the body's attempt to compensate for the imbalance. Many of the symptoms are also related to the hypocalcemia and hypokalemia that usually accompany alkalosis.

In alkalosis, stimulation of the CNS appears in the patient's reports of lightheadedness, vertigo, agitation, and confusion. One of the earliest symptoms of alkalosis is a tingling sensation in the fingers and toes or around the mouth. Palpitations and dry mouth may also be noted.

Early complaints associated with acidosis include general malaise and headache. The patient may also report nausea, vomiting, and abdominal pain. As the acidosis worsens, the patient becomes drowsy, confused, and finally, unconscious. Alkalosis is manifested as CNS depression. Patient complaints also include symptoms related to hypocalcemia and hypokalemia. Numbness and tingling of the hands, toes, and lips, irritation, and anxiety are noted in mild hypocalcemia. The patient with hypokalemia may complain of anorexia, muscle weakness, shortness of breath, fatigue, irritability, and excessive urination.

Past Health History

Determine whether the patient has a recent history of vomiting or diarrhea; a history of heart or renal failure, cirrhosis, diabetes mellitus, or chronic airway limitation; or recent surgery. A drug history is important to elicit because drugs cause or contribute to acid-base imbalance. Family members should be used as a source of information because some alterations in acid-base balance cause changes in the patient's cognitive function or emotional status.

It is important to gather detailed dietary history in order to determine caloric intake as well as the appropriate proportions of carbohydrates, fats, and proteins. The patient should be asked specifically if he or she has been fasting or following a strict diet during the preceding week. Knowledge about dietary intake can be vital in evaluating metabolic imbalances.

Physical Exam Findings

Clinical manifestations of alkalosis are the result of hypocalcemia or hypokalemia. The presence of Trousseau's sign and Chvostek's sign may be noted with hypocalcemia. In addition, carpopedal spasms, tetany, hyperactive deep tendon reflexes, skeletal muscle weakness, and muscle cramping and twitching are evident. Syncopal episodes, seizures, and coma are possible. Although skeletal muscles contract as a result of overstimulation, the muscles themselves become weaker because of the alkalosis and hypokalemia. Hand-grasp strength is reduced, and the patient may be unable to support body weight or walk. Respiratory efforts become less effective as the skeletal muscles of respiration become weaker. Because alkalosis produces increased myocardial irritability, especially in the presence of an accompanying hypokalemia, the heart rate increases and the pulse becomes thready. The blood pressure may be normal or low.

Clinical manifestations of acidosis are similar whether the cause is respiratory or metabolic. Depressed CNS function is common in patients with acidosis and may be manifested as lethargy progressing to confusion, especially in the older adult. The patient becomes stuporous as acidosis worsens or if it is accompanied by hyperkalemia. The acidotic state and accompanying hyperkalemia cause a decrease in muscle tone and deep tendon reflexes. The muscle weakness is bilateral and can progress to flaccid paralysis.

If the acidosis is of respiratory origin, breathing effectiveness is greatly diminished, with respirations rapid but shallow. If the acidosis has a metabolic origin, the rate and depth of respirations increase in proportion to the increase in hydrogen ion concentration. The respirations are rapid, deep, and regular and are not under voluntary control (*Kussmaul's respirations*). The skin and mucous membranes are pale to cyanotic in color because respirations are ineffective.

However, in metabolic acidosis, in which respirations are essentially unaffected and the rate increased, the patient's skin is pink, warm, and dry. Cardiovascular manifestations of acidosis include tachycardia. As acidosis worsens or is accompanied by hyperkalemia, electrical activity through the heart is reduced and bradycardia results. As a result of changes in heart activity, peripheral pulses can be difficult to locate and are easily obliterated with light pressure. Hypotension is the result of vasodilation.

Diagnostic Testing

The most common laboratory tests for the diagnosis and monitoring of acid-base balance are the pH, carbon dioxide, bicarbonate, and electrolyte levels of the blood.

A pH greater than 7.45 indicates alkalosis. Because the clinical manifestations of metabolic alkalosis are similar to those of respiratory alkalosis, it is important to monitor arterial blood gas values and serum electrolytes as well as patient signs and symptoms to determine the cause (Table 61–5).

The presence of acidosis is also detected by checking arterial blood gases, as well as evaluating potassium and chloride levels. When arterial pH falls below 7.35, acidosis is present. The patient with acidosis should have one or more electrocardiographic evaluations, primarily to detect changes associated with hyperkalemia. The changes associated with hyperkalemia include peaked T waves, a wide QRS complex, and a prolonged PR interval. Ventricular arrhythmias are common.

Developmental Considerations

Perinatal Because pregnancy increases cell numbers and additional oxygen is required, hormonal and anatomic changes are directed at facilitating oxygen availability. Progesterone stimulates the respiratory rate. Additionally, pregnancy induces a small degree of hyperventilation as tidal volume (amount of air breathed with ordinary respiration) decreases steadily throughout pregnancy. In the process, excess carbon dioxide is blown off. The resulting decrease in carbonic acid creates a pH difference in pregnancy. Although the normal pH range is still between 7.35 to 7.45, in pregnancy, the pH tends toward the upper range of 7.42 to 7.45. Thus, there may be a slight degree of respiratory alkalosis throughout pregnancy.

TABLE 61–5 LABORATORY FINDINGS IN ACID-BASE IMBALANCES

		Gas Parameters*			Electrolytes†		
Imbalance	Compensation	pH	$PaCO_2$	HCO_3	K^+	Ca^{++}	Cl^-
Respiratory alkalosis	Uncompensated	↑ 7.45	↓ 35	N			
	Partially compensated	↑ 7.45	↓ 35	↓ 22			
	Compensated	N	↓ 35	↓ 22	↓	↓	↑
Respiratory acidosis	Uncompensated	↓ 7.35	↑ 46	N			
	Partially compensated	↓ 7.35	↑ 46	↑ 26			
	Compensated	N	↑ 46	↑ 26	↑	N	↑↓
Metabolic alkalosis	Uncompensated	↑ 7.45	N	↑ 26			
	Partially compensated	↑ 7.45	↑ 26	↑ 26			
	Compensated	N	↑ 46	↑ 26	↓	↓	↓
Metabolic acidosis	Uncompensated	↓ 7.35	N	↓ 22			
	Partially compensated	N or ↓ 7.35	↓ 35	↓ 22			
	Compensated	N	↓ 35	↓ 22	↑	N	↑

*Arterial blood gas values at sea level:
pH 7.35–7.45
$PaCO_2$ 35–46 mmHg
HCO_3 22–26 mEq/L

†Electrolyte levels relative to sodium values. Normal electrolyte values:
Potassium 3.5–5.0 mEq/L
Chloride 98–106 mmol/L
Calcium 8.8–10.0 mg/dL

↑Lab values above normal range; ↓Lab values below normal range; N, normal.

Pediatric Acid-base buffering systems are less well developed in infants and children than in adults, and they tend to develop acid-base imbalances more easily. Common conditions that predispose an infant to acid-base imbalances include fevers, upper respiratory infections, vomiting, and diarrhea. Furthermore, infants and small children are less able to describe symptoms such as thirst or changes in sensation (e.g., paresthesias). Therefore, a careful evaluation of early changes in acid-base balance should be performed.

Geriatric Age is an important variable in assessing the patient with an acid-base imbalance because the geriatric patient is more vulnerable to conditions that cause acid-base imbalance. Conditions that contribute to acidosis or alkalosis include cardiac, renal, and pulmonary impairments; diabetes mellitus; persistent diarrhea; pancreatitis; and fever.

Alkalosis causes the myocardium to be more sensitive to digitalis derivatives, resulting in an increased risk for digitalis toxicity. Because many older adults take one or more cardiac drugs or diuretics, information about prescribed or over-the-counter drugs should be noted. Many of these drugs alter acid-base, fluid, or electrolyte balance.

Because of decreased chest wall compliance, elasticity of lung tissues, number of alveoli, and respiratory muscle strength, the older adult cannot eliminate carbon dioxide as readily. This limits the patient's ability to compensate for metabolic alterations and predisposes the patient to respiratory acidosis.

The physical changes of aging also result in a decrease in nephrons. The older adult may take 18 to 48 hours to achieve acid-base balance after an upset, whereas a younger adult may need only 6 to 10 hours. By returning some substances to body fluids and eliminating others, the kidneys compensate (in several hours) for even large deviations from normal. However, as aging continues, compensatory abilities decline.

Psychosocial Considerations

A complete psychosocial assessment is important because behavioral changes resulting from CNS irritability or depression may be the first observable clinical manifestation of an acid-base imbalance. The health care provider should observe and objectively document the patient's presenting behaviors.

Analysis and Management

Treatment Objectives

Treatment goals for alkalosis are directed at increasing the level of hydrogen ions; preventing further hydrogen, potassium, calcium, and chloride losses; and restoring fluid balance. Treatment goals for acidosis are directed at correcting the underlying cause of the acidosis and normalizing acid-base balance. It should be evident that overtreating one type of imbalance may upset the balance in the opposite direction. Thus, caution should be used when determining specific treatment modalities.

Treatment Options

Respiratory Alkalosis Because alkalosis is a manifestation of other abnormal processes, treatment is most effective when it is first directed at the underlying abnormality. Mild asymptomatic alkalosis requires no specific treatment. With hysterical hyperventilation, symptoms are alleviated by having the patient rebreathe a mixture of carbon dioxide and oxygen from a large paper bag or by giving inhalations of 5 percent carbon dioxide at intervals.

If a patient is to be exposed to high altitudes, 2 days of pretreatment with acetazolamide (250 mg twice daily) produces a mild metabolic acidosis. The mild acidosis offsets the initial respiratory alkalosis on exposure to high altitude and thus minimizes symptoms due to hyperventilation.

Respiratory Acidosis The only practical treatment for respiratory acidosis involves improvement of the basic underlying cause of the hypoventilation. The possibility of drug abuse should be considered in otherwise healthy individuals who suddenly develop acute respiratory depression. Naloxone, an opioid antagonist (see Chapter 14), should be considered for use in all comatose patients in whom no apparent cause of respiratory depression can be identified.

If the underlying cause of respiratory acidosis is pneumonia, appropriate antimicrobial therapy should be started. It should be noted that oxygen therapy in patients with chronic hypercapnia should be given with extreme caution and in the lowest possible concentration to avoid serious tissue hypoxia. Hypoxemia may be the primary stimulus to respiration in this situation. Sudden increases in arterial carbon dioxide values produced by oxygen administration may result in cessation of respirations. Administering alkalinizing salts has no place in the management of chronic respiratory acidosis. In severe respiratory acidosis, particularly in asthmatic patients, it may be essential to correct the pH derangement directly by infusing sodium bicarbonate solution.

Metabolic Alkalosis Treatment that is effective for metabolic alkalosis is different from treatment that is effective for respiratory alkalosis. Therefore, the health care provider must be able to distinguish between metabolic and respiratory alkalosis in order to prevent and manage the condition.

In most cases, acute metabolic alkalosis can be corrected by the IV administration of adequate amounts of sodium chloride solution. The ability of a neutral salt to correct an acid-base imbalance is based on physiologic rather than chemical mechanisms. For example, in alkalosis due to vomiting, the body is depleted of water, hydrogen, chloride, and to a lesser degree, sodium. Once an adequate extracellular volume is re-established, normal renal mechanisms become effective and sodium, along with bicarbonate, is eliminated in the urine.

In severe cases of metabolic alkalosis, the severity of symptoms can be corrected with an acidifying salt such as ammonium chloride because, in the presence of normal hepatic function, the alkalosis can be corrected without waiting for renal mechanisms to come into play. Ammonium chloride is used when it is desirable to lower the systemic pH promptly and directly without reliance on either renal or hepatic mechanisms. The infused acid is immediately buffered by circulating blood, although mild hemolysis may occur. This procedure should be considered as a heroic measure to be used only when more conventional therapy has failed. Because of its high chloride content, arginine hydrochloride has been recommended by some health care providers as a systemic acidifier for the management of extreme metabolic alkalosis. However, use of the drug should not preclude the use of IV sodium chloride and potassium chloride.

In some cases, the primary purpose of therapy for metabolic alkalosis is to change the pH of the urine. When renal function is normal, this is readily accomplished by using either alkalinizing or acidifying salts. Their use produces a modest distortion in systemic acid-base balance. However, in edema-forming states, when the renal reabsorption of sodium is inappropriately high, alkalinizing salts are poorly eliminated. Furthermore, in the presence of renal insufficiency, the capacity of the kidney to compensate for acidosis is diminished, and acidifying salts may have harmful systemic effects.

Metabolic Acidosis In most cases, the treatment for metabolic acidosis is aimed at the underlying cause. Certain general principles serve as useful guidelines for treatment. Disorders characterized by failure of bicarbonate regeneration or reduced elimination of inorganic acids represent acidosis. Thus, the treatment of these disorders requires administering relatively modest amounts of bicarbonate. For example, in chronic renal failure, alkali therapy is generally not required unless plasma bicarbonate levels fall below 16 to 18 mEq/L. If the acidosis is more severe, bicarbonate supplementation in the form of SHOHL SOLUTION can be used.

Treatment of patients with metabolic acidosis due to external bicarbonate loss varies with the nature of the disorder. For example, in acute acidosis due to GI losses, sodium bicarbonate can be given cautiously to raise the plasma bicarbonate concentration to 16 mEq/L over a 12- to 24-hour period rather than to repair the entire bicarbonate deficit. The use of bicarbonate in this manner is valid only if there are no further GI losses.

If the underlying cause is diabetic ketoacidosis, the usual treatment includes fluids and insulin. Insulin promotes glucose utilization by the cells and thus completes oxidation of ketoacids. Simultaneously, ketogenesis is reduced. Therefore, alkali therapy is ordinarily not necessary. Additionally, because the hyperventilatory response to acidosis in some diabetic patients is governed by arterial rather than central medullary chemoreceptors, IV sodium bicarbonate may result in arterial alkalinization and a fall in the ventilation rate. In severe ketoacidosis, IV sodium bicarbonate may be necessary to increase serum bicarbonate levels and neutralize nonvolatile acid accumulation.

Sodium bicarbonate is seldom used alone for the treatment of metabolic acidosis. If hypokalemia is present, it should be corrected with potassium replacement before the administration of sodium bicarbonate. If sodium bicarbonate is given in the presence of hypokalemia, the acidosis may be corrected, using potassium to shift back into the cells, but the resulting severe hypokalemia may culminate in cardiac arrest.

In the case of alcoholic ketoacidosis, IV sodium chloride and glucose are usually ordered. Because blood insulin values are generally decreased in alcoholic ketoacidosis–associated hypoglycemia, insulin is contraindicated. It may induce a life-threatening hypoglycemia. Alkali therapy should not be used unless the metabolic acidosis is in the lethal range. The same considerations apply to starvation ketosis.

Intervention

Administration

Laboratory monitoring is required for initial dosage calculations and future adjustments. Thus, arterial blood gases should be drawn using the correct technique and immediately delivered to the laboratory for analysis. The health care provider is responsible for minimizing errors in arterial

TABLE 61–6 POTENTIAL ABG SAMPLING ERRORS

Sampling Error	Effects: pH	Effects: $PaCO_2$	Effects: PaO_2	Implications
Air bubbles in syringe	↑	↓	↑	Immediately expell all air bubbles. Do not agitate or use sample that appears frothy
Inadvertent venous sample or venous contamination of arterial sample	↓	↑	↓	Avoid use of femoral artery. Use needle with short bevel. Do not overshoot artery and then withdraw to catch it. Watch for autofilling of syringe with arterial puncture. Verify questionable results with new sample
Alteration of pH due to presence of anticoagulant	↓	–	–	Use lithium heparin, if possible. Use 1:1000 units/mL concentration. Use minimum 2-mL discard sample with arterial line aspiration
Dilution of sample due to presence of anticoagulant	↑	↓	↓	Use syringe with minimum dead space. Use dried heparin if available
Effects of metabolism on white blood cells in sample	↓	↑	↓	Place sample on ice immediately after drawing with analysis occurring within 20 minutes. Have sample analyzed immediately if patient has leukocytosis

Data from Malley, W.J. (1990). *Clinical blood gases: Application and noninvasive alternatives.* Philadelphia: W.B. Saunders Company.
↑Lab values above normal range. ↓Lab values below normal range.

blood gas analysis (ABG) due to faulty specimen collection. Potential sampling errors and their implications are identified in Table 61–6.

Interventions for the patient with alkalosis or acidosis are directed toward maintaining and monitoring existing system functioning as well as correcting the acid-base imbalance. Thus, the patient's history of a pre-existing condition that may contraindicate the use of an alkalinizing or acidifying drug, or warrant their cautious use, should be reviewed.

IV alkalinizing and acidifying drugs should be given in a patent, free-flowing IV line. To prevent incompatibilities, the IV line should be flushed before and after drug administration. Syringe, Y connector compatibilities, additive compatibilities, and potential drug-drug interactions should also be noted. Infusion rates should be carefully monitored.

Attention should be paid to the IV site for evidence of extravasation, phlebitis, or irritation. Extravasation of alkalinizing drugs should be treated by elevating the extremity, applying warm compresses, and administering hyaluronidase, lidocaine, or both, as indicated to minimize tissue damage.

Orally administered drugs should be taken as ordered with a full glass of water. A missed dose should be taken as soon as remembered unless it is almost time for the next dose. Doses should not be doubled if missed.

Sodium bicarbonate should not be taken concurrently with milk products. Renal calculi or hypercalcemia may result. Sodium citrate/citric acid is more palatable when diluted with 60 to 90 mL of water and refrigerated before use. It should be administered 30 minutes after meals or bedtime snack to minimize its saline laxative effects. Tromethamine should not be used for more than 24 hours to help minimize severe adverse effects.

The patient should be closely monitored for signs and symptoms of overdosage of the alkalinizing or acidifying drug. Respiratory rate, volume, patterns, breath sounds, and ABGs should be monitored. The patient should be observed and attended to as necessary to ensure safety. Restraints may be needed in some cases. Skin color, temperature, peripheral pulses, and capillary refill should be assessed.

If signs of overdosage appear (CNS irritability or depression), the drug should be witheld and the health care provider notified. The patient may need to be switched to a different drug or the drug may need to be discontinued.

Education

Patients should be advised of the importance of regular follow-up examinations to monitor serum electrolyte levels and acid-base balance. As with any other drug, the patient and family should be taught the name of the drug, its purpose, dosage and frequency, and possible adverse effects. The patient taking sodium bicarbonate on a prolonged basis may develop GI distress and flatulence. Because GI distress contributes to noncompliance and subsequent acute acidosis, a different alkalinizing drug may be required. Patients and families should be taught how to prepare and administer the drug and to avoid certain activities if the alkalinizing drug is one that may cause drowsiness (e.g., acetazolamide).

The patient should be taught to recognize signs of fluid retention such as rings that have gotten tighter, ankles that are swelling, or a weight gain of 2 to 3 pounds in a few days. The patient should be advised to report these signs promptly.

The patient should be cautioned to avoid activities that require alertness if drowsiness is a problem or if a sedative-hypnotic drug is employed for insomnia. The patient with diabetes should be instructed to monitor his or her blood glucose values because certain alkalinizing and acidifying drugs can cause hypoglycemia and hyperglycemia, respectively.

Evaluation

Serum electrolyte values are monitored at least daily or every other day until a return to normal occurs and then less frequently. Resolution of the signs and symptoms of the acid-base imbalances should occur without the appearance of the opposite disorder.

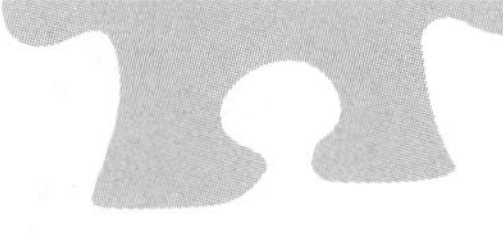

SUMMARY

- The body uses three primary defense mechanisms to maintain acid-base balance: the bicarbonate-carbonic acid buffer system, the respiratory system, and the renal system.
- Respiratory alkalosis occurs when alveolar hyperventilation results in excessive loss of carbon dioxide. Respiratory acidosis results primarily from decreased alveolar ventilation, leading to retention of carbon dioxide.
- Metabolic alkalosis results from the loss of hydrogen ions or the accumulation of base components such as bicarbonate. Metabolic acidosis results from a decrease in base components, or through increased hydrogen ion levels.
- Determine whether the patient has a history of heart or renal disease, cirrhosis, diabetes mellitus, chronic obstructive pulmonary disease, or recent surgery or other risk factors for acid-base imbalance.
- Patients should be monitored for evidence of CNS stimulation or depression representative of alkalosis or acidosis, respectively.
- When appropriate, acidosis is corrected with sodium bicarbonate or another alkaline product such as tromethamine. The underlying cause of acidosis must always be treated. Alkalosis may be corrected with ammonium chloride.
- Care must be taken when correcting either imbalance not to overtreat and produce the opposite imbalance.
- IV alkalinizing and acidifying drugs should be given in a patent, free-flowing IV line. The IV line should be flushed before and after administration of the drugs to prevent incompatibilities.
- The patient should be monitored for signs and symptoms of overdosage of the alkalinizing or acidifying drug.
- Patients should be advised of the importance of regular follow-up examinations to monitor serum electrolyte levels and acid-base balance and to monitor progress.
- Resolution of the signs and symptoms of the acid-base imbalances should occur without the appearance of the opposite disorder.

BIBLIOGRAPHY

American Society of Hospital Pharmacists. (1996). *AHFS Drug Information '96*. Bethesda, MD: Author.

Boweby, H., and Elanjian, S. (1992). Necrosis caused by extravasation of arginine hydrochloride. *Annals of Pharmacotherapy, 26*(2), 263–264.

Cullen, L. (1992). Interventions related to fluid and electrolyte balance. *Nursing Clinics of North America, 27*(2), 569–597.

Faria, S., Taylor, L. (1997). Interpretation of arterial blood gases by nurses. *Journal of Vascular Nursing, 15*(4), 128–130.

Feeney-Stewart, F. (1990). The sodium bicarbonate controversy. *Dimensions of Critical Care Nursing, 9*(1), 22–28.

Hardman, J., Limbird, L. Molinoff, P., et al. (1996). *Goodman and Gilman's the pharmacological basis of therapeutics*. (9th ed.). New York: McGraw-Hill.

Malley, W. (1990). *Clinical blood gases: application and noninvasive alternatives*. Philadelphia: W.B. Saunders.

Marik, P., Kussman, B., Lipman, J., et al. (1991). Acetazolamide in the treatment of metabolic alkalosis in critically ill patients. *Heart and Lung, 20*(5 Part 1), 455–459.

Narins, R. (Ed.) (1994). *Maxwell and Kleeman's clinical disorders of fluid and electrolyte metabolism*. (5th ed.). New York: McGraw-Hill.

Nasimi, A., Cardona, J., Berthier, M., et al. (1996). Hydrochloric acid infusion for treatment of severe metabolic alkalosis in a neonate. *Clinical Pediatrics, 35*(5), 271–272.

Rose, B. (1994). *Clinical physiology of acid-base and electrolyte disorders* (4th ed.). New York: McGraw-Hill.

Rutecki, G., and Whittier, F. (1991). Acid-base interpretation: Five rules, and how they help in everyday cases. *Consultant, 31*(11), 44–46, 55, 59.

Sica, D. (1992). Renal disease, electrolyte abnormalities, and acid-base imbalance in the elderly. *Clinics in Geriatric Medicine, 10*(1), 197–211.

Sing, R., Brancas, C., and Sing, R. (1995). Bicarbonate therapy in the treatment of lactic acidosis: Medicine or toxin? *Journal of the American Osteopathic Association, 95*(1), 52–55.

Unit XII

Drugs Influencing Sensory Perception

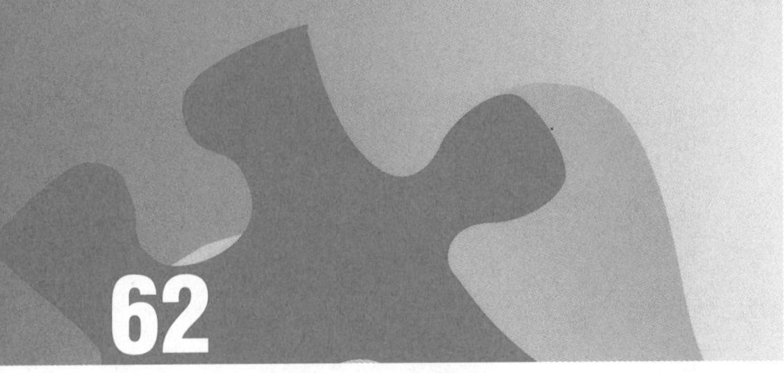

62

Ophthalmic Drugs

Visual disorders are a peril to patients, largely because vision is one of the most cherished of senses. Although many eye disorders are correctable with eyeglasses or contact lenses, others require drugs to control or treat the problem.

OPHTHALMIC DISORDERS

Eye disorders can occur at any age. The disorders may be due to a wide variety of causes, but the majority can be categorized as refractive disorders, infections or inflammatory conditions, and glaucoma.

Glaucoma

Epidemiology and Etiology

Five to ten million people in the United States are estimated to have elevated intraocular pressure (IOP). Another 2 million have glaucoma, although 50 percent are unaware of its presence. In addition, an estimated 80,000 Americans are blind as a result of the disease. The incidence of blindness is about 1.5 percent; however, in blacks ages 45 to 65, the prevalence is at least five times that of whites in the same age group.

Glaucoma is generally divided into two types based on the angle of the anterior chamber: open angle (i.e., wide angle) and closed angle (i.e., narrow angle). Glaucoma is further divided into primary and secondary forms. Primary glaucoma is precipitated by intrinsic pathologic change within the eye. Secondary forms are associated with other eye disorders, such as lens displacement, anterior chamber hemorrhage, lacerations, or contusions. Secondary glaucoma is also associated with systemic disease or the use of certain drugs.

Primary open-angle glaucoma is the most prevalent form and is thought to be genetically determined. It is a multifactorial, insidious, slowly progressing disorder that is usually asymptomatic until extensive, irreversible loss of visual field has occurred. Primary open-angle glaucoma is most common in people over 40. As many as one third of patients with primary open-angle glaucoma have an IOP that exceeds 22 mmHg on a single measurement (normal range 15 ± 2.5 mmHg). The risk that patients with ocular hypertension will develop visual field loss ranges from 0.5 percent to 1 percent per year. The most common cause of chronic open-angle glaucoma is degenerative changes in the trabecular meshwork, resulting in decreased outflow of aqueous humor.

Primary closed-angle glaucoma affects one out of every 1000 people over the age of 40. Women are affected more often than men. The female-to-male ratio is 4:1 in whites and Eskimos. Many cases are precipitated by emotional upset, low-level illumination, or use of drugs that dilate the pupil (e.g., adrenergics, antianxiety drugs, antihistamines, antiparkinson drugs, antispasmodics, benzodiazepines, cold preparations, phenothiazines, and tricyclic antidepressants). Other drugs such as central nervous system stimulants, appetite suppressants, and bronchodilators produce minimal pupillary dilation and have no proven adverse influence on IOP in either normal eyes or eyes with open-angle glaucoma.

The potential to develop glaucoma increases almost exponentially with escalating IOP. However, not all patients with ocular hypertension develop glaucoma. Modest elevations in IOP can sometimes be tolerated without injury to the optic nerve. In contrast, some patients with glaucoma have an IOP in the normal range. Risk factors for glaucoma include heredity, black race, diabetes mellitus, myopia, systemic vascular disease, and advancing age.

Pathophysiology

Glaucoma results from interference with the drainage of aqueous humor from the anterior chamber. Aqueous humor is secreted by ciliary epithelium and transported to the posterior chamber, where it passes through the pupil to the anterior chamber (Fig. 62–1). About 80 percent of the total outflow passes through the trabecular meshwork in the anterior chamber angle, enters the canal of Schlemm, and then appears in the ocular venous circulation. The remaining 20 percent flows through the uveoscleral pathway to the ciliary body into the suprachoroidal space. It drains into venous circulation in the ciliary body, choroid, and sclera. IOP is the balance among the rate of humor produced by the ciliary body, the resistance to outflow, and the level of episcleral venous pressure.

In normotensive glaucoma, the IOP falls in or below the normal range of 15 ± 2.5 mmHg and is sometimes accompanied by a wide diurnal and postural fluctuation. The anterior chamber angle is normal, the optic nerves are cupped, and visual fields show characteristic peripheral defects. The etiology of normotensive glaucoma is unknown. Patients with this stable form of glaucoma do not require treatment but should have co-morbid diseases (e.g., anemia, arrhythmias, heart failure) treated to prevent ischemia of the optic nerve.

Secondary glaucoma disrupts the flow pattern of aqueous humor. Edematous tissues may inhibit the outflow of the humor through the trabecular meshwork. Delayed healing of corneal wounds may result in epithelial cell growth into the anterior chamber. Secondary glaucoma is less common than the primary form and is typically found on diagnosis or treatment of a co-morbid disease.

Inflammation and Infection

Epidemiology and Etiology

The red eye is a physical manifestation of inflammation caused by vasodilation of the conjunctival, episcleral, and scleral vessels. The common diagnoses associated with red eye include bacterial, viral, fungal, allergic, and irritative

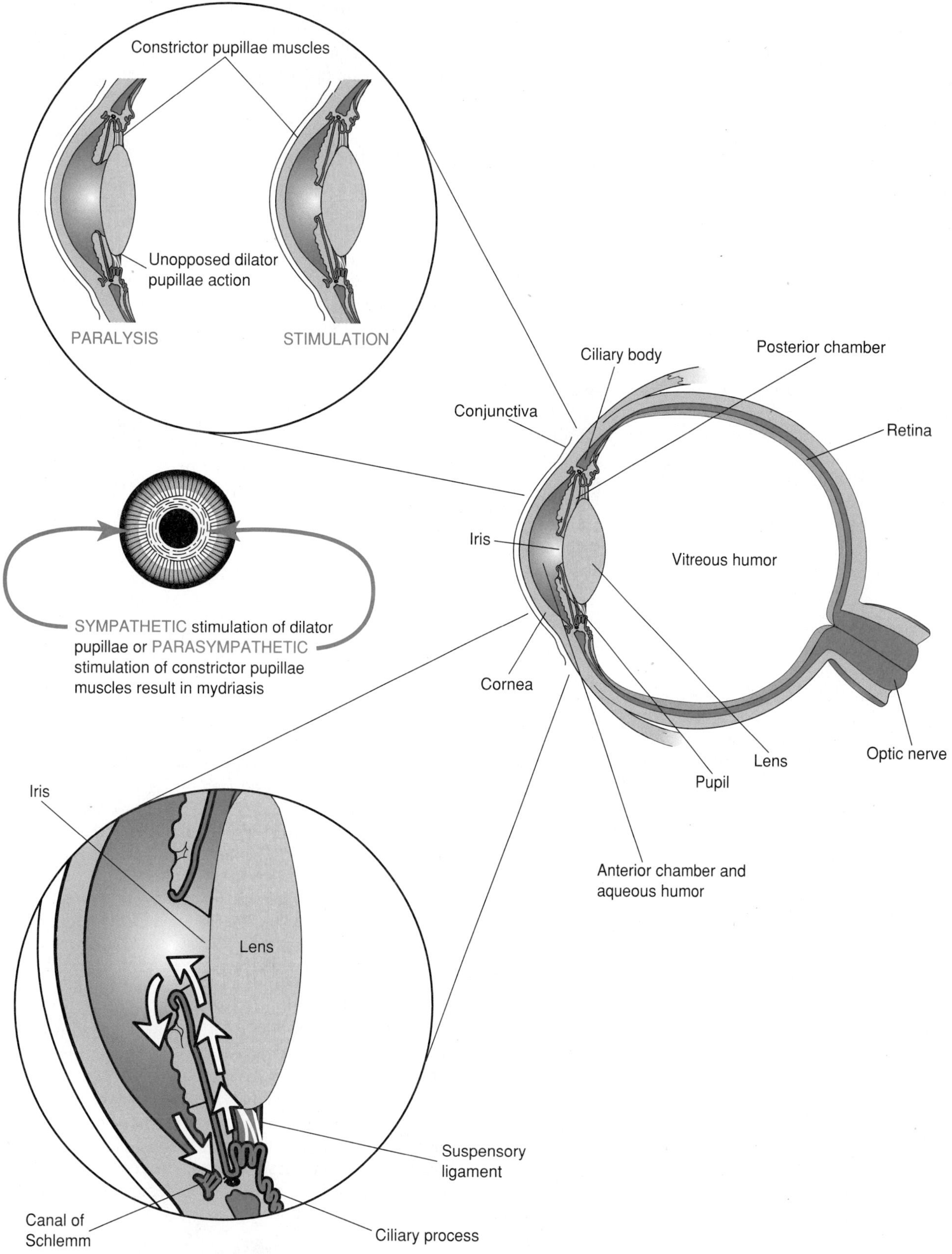

Figure 62–1 Ophthalmic drug action. Cholinergic miotics (e.g., pilocarpine) cause miosis by contracting the iridic sphincter and dilating vessels and the collection channels to increase outflow. They contract ciliary muscles, leading to a deeper anterior chamber, a wider angle, and increased outflow of aqueous humor. Anticholinesterase miotics (e.g., isoflurophate) increase the amount of acetylcholine available near ciliary muscles and the iridic sphincters, causing them to contract and the pupil to dilate. Adrenergics (e.g., epinephrine) stimulate beta$_2$ receptors in the outflow channels to increase the outflow of aqueous humor. Anticholinergic drugs (e.g., tropicamide) paralyze ciliary muscles and relax the iris, causing pupillary dilation and cycloplegia.

conjunctivitis; corneal abrasions and foreign bodies; subconjunctival hemorrhage; episcleritis or scleritis; keratitis; iritis; and acute closed-angle glaucoma.

Two to three percent of all ambulatory patients present with symptoms of one of the above-mentioned ocular disorders. Viral conjunctivitis and allergic reactions are more common than bacterial conjunctivitis. Viral conjunctivitis occurs in epidemics and is most common in young adults. On the other hand, bacterial conjunctivitis is seen in patients of all ages at any time of the year. It may occur in an epidemic form known as *pink eye*. Allergic conjunctivitis is sporadic and seasonal, occurring frequently in patients with a history of allergies during times of high pollen counts. Irritative conjunctivitis is most often caused by exposure to dust or smoke.

Corneal abrasions and foreign bodies occur most often in patients who spend time out of doors or in environments such as metal shops or lumber mills. Subconjunctival hemorrhage can occur as a result of trauma or as a result of recurrent Valsalva maneuvers such as coughing or during labor and delivery. Episcleritis and scleritis occur in patients with systemic autoimmune and connective tissue disorders. Immunocompromised patients may also be at risk for keratitis. Approximately 50 percent of patients with iritis are positive for the HLA-type B27 antigen, suggesting there is a genetic predisposition to the disorder.

Pathophysiology

The classic description of acute inflammation includes *rubor* (redness), *tumor* (edema), *calor* (warmth), and *dolor* (pain, discomfort). The manifestations can be divided into two categories—vascular and cellular responses. (See Chapter 15 for more thorough explanation of inflammation.)

The vascular response begins almost immediately after injury or exposure to microorganisms. A momentary period of vasoconstriction is followed immediately by vasodilation of the arterioles and venules that supply the area. As a result, the area becomes congested, red, and warm. An increase in capillary permeability allows fluid to escape into tissues to cause edema. Pain follows as the result of tissue swelling and the release of chemical mediators.

The cellular response is marked by the movement of white blood cells into the area of injury. As fluid leaves the capillaries, blood viscosity increases, and white blood cells move to the periphery of the vessel. They migrate into tissue spaces, where they wander guided by microorganisms and cellular debris. The white cells engulf and degrade the organisms and cellular debris from the area of inflammation.

PHARMACOTHERAPEUTIC OPTIONS

The major approach to the management of glaucoma is pharmacotherapy. Antiglaucoma drugs fall primarily into the following categories: cholinergic miotics, (direct-acting agents), anticholinesterase miotics (indirect-acting agents), ocular beta blockers, adrenergics, anticholinergics, carbonic anhydrase inhibitors, and osmotics.

Another grouping of ocular drugs produces *mydriasis* (pupillary dilation) and *cycloplegia* (paralysis of accommodation). A third grouping includes the anti-inflammatory and antimicrobial drugs. This third group is composed of antibiotics, antifungals, antivirals, antiseptics, and corticosteroids. Other ophthalmic drugs include anesthetics, antiallergy agents, enzyme preparations, artificial tears, irrigating solutions, and contact lens products.

Antiglaucoma Drugs

CHOLINERGIC MIOTICS

❒ Carbachol (CARBOPTIC, ISOPTO CARBACHOL); (✱) MIOSTAT

❒ Pilocarpine (ADSORBOCARPINE, AKARPINE, ISOPTO CARPINE, OCUSERT PILO, PILAGAN, PILOCAR, PILOPINE HS, PILOPTIC, PILOPTO-CARPINE, PILOMIOTIN, PILOSTAT); (✱) MINIMS PILOCARPINE, MIOCARPINE

Indications

Cholinergic miotics are indicated for the management of glaucoma. Pilocarpine has long been the drug of choice for primary open-angle glaucoma and many other chronic glaucomas. It is also used (in 0.5 to 1 percent concentrations) for emergency management of acute closed-angle glaucoma. Pilocarpine is used for long-term therapy when the IOP remains elevated after laser or conventional surgery, or if a patent iridotomy does not relieve the angle closure. In patients with tonic pupils (Adie's syndrome), a weak concentration of pilocarpine is useful for identifying denervation supersensitivity and the possibility of long-term treatment.

Cholinergic miotics are also used in the treatment of strabismus (an inward deviation of one eye relative to the other [accommodative esotropia]).

Pharmacodynamics

Cholinergic miotics are direct-acting drugs that produce effects similar to those produced by acetylcholine (ACh), the parasympathetic nervous system neurohormone. ACh action is stopped by hydrolysis of cholinesterase, resulting in contraction of the iridic sphincter and miosis. Vasodilation of blood vessels and of collection channels peripheral to the canal of Schlemm increases the outflow of aqueous humor. Contraction of the ciliary muscle and a deepening of the anterior chamber improves the filtration angle, also increasing the outflow of aqueous humor. Ciliary muscle action leaves the eye in accommodation of near vision. Although hydrolysis occurs at various rates, once it is complete, the pupil returns to the premedicated state. Pilocarpine does not appear to have a clinically significant effect on aqueous humor production.

Although such cases are rare, cholinergic miotics (especially potent agents) may close rather than open the angle of the canal of Schlemm and worsen angle closure. This paradoxical effect results from a miosis-induced pupillary blockade or a forward movement of the lens associated with ciliary muscle contraction.

Adverse Effects and Contraindications

Pilocarpine is ordinarily better tolerated than other miotics. Nevertheless, adverse effects commonly associated with cholinergic miotics include irritation, conjunctivitis, and blepharitis. Allergic reactions and systemic effects are uncommon, although retinal detachment, obstruction of the lacrimal apparatus, synechiae (adhesion of the iris to the lens and cornea), iridic cysts, and cataracts have been noted with prolonged use. Tolerance and resistance have also been noted.

Unusual hypersensitivity or overdose produces systemic manifestations such as headache, salivation, diaphoresis, abdominal discomfort, diarrhea, respiratory distress, bradycardia, arrhythmias, and a drop in the blood pressure. Cholinergic miotics should be used with caution in patients with a history of asthma, heart failure, peptic ulcer disease, Parkinson's disease, epilepsy, or hyperthyroidism.

Pharmacokinetics

Carbachol's onset time to miosis (rather than onset of drug action) is 2 to 5 minutes, with reduction in IOP reached in about 6 hours. Miotic drug effects and the reduction in IOP persist for about 4 hours (Table 62–1).

Pilocarpine, on the other hand, produces miosis in 10 to 30 minutes. Maximal reduction of IOP occurs in 1 to 1.5 hours, which correlates with the maximal decrease in outflow resistance. The duration of pilocarpine's miotic action is 4 to 8 hours, with IOP reduction lasting 4 to 14 hours. Melanin in the iris is a binding site for pilocarpine; thus, reduction in IOP may be decreased in heavily pigmented eyes.

Drug-Drug Interactions

Carbachol and pilocarpine may be ineffective in reducing IOP when they are used concurrently with flurbiprofen (Table 62–2). Flurbiprofen is a nonsteroidal anti-inflammatory miotic inhibitor.

Dosage Regimen

Carbachol and pilocarpine are given in dosages that are sufficient to maintain the IOP at a level that prevents further damage to the optic disc and progressive loss of visual field (Table 62–3). Variations in IOP at different times of day should be taken into account.

ANTICHOLINESTERASE MIOTICS

- ❒ Demecarium (HUMORSOL)
- ❒ Echothiophate (PHOSPHOLINE IODIDE)
- ❒ Isoflurophate
- ❒ Physostigmine (ESERINE SULFATE)

Indications

Anticholinesterase miotics (i.e., cholinesterase inhibitors) are also used in the treatment of glaucoma in patients who have *aphakia* (absence of a lens). Demecarium, isoflurophate, and echothiophate are long-acting, potent drugs and have been associated with cataract formation. Thus, they are reserved for patients refractory to short-acting miotics, ocular beta-blocking drugs, epinephrine, and carbonic anhydrase inhibitors. Laser trabeculoplasty or filtering surgery (i.e. trephination, thermal sclerostomy, or sclerectomy) may be preferred to the long-acting miotics, especially if the lens is present. In the absence of a lens or when there is no sign of an imminent retinal detachment, strong miotics can be used to treat chronic glaucoma. The short-acting drug physostigmine is not well tolerated by patients and is seldom used today for prolonged treatment.

In addition to their use in glaucoma, anticholinesterase miotics have been used to diagnose and treat strabismus. By inducing accommodation peripherally, these drugs decrease accommodative effort and reduce convergence.

Pharmacodynamics

Anticholinesterase miotics are indirect-acting drugs that are subclassified into two groups, those producing reversible activity and those with irreversible activity. Both groups reduce enzymatic destruction of ACh by inactivating cholinesterase. Thus, ACh accumulates. The additional ACh acts on ciliary muscles and iridic sphincters to cause pupillary constriction and ciliary muscle contraction.

The reversible drugs demecarium and physostigmine act on plasma cholinesterase to halt its activity. In contrast, echothiophate and isoflurophate decrease both plasma and red blood cell cholinesterase. Complexes are formed at the site of enzyme action, irreversibly impairing the destructive function of cholinesterase. Destruction of ACh then depends on the synthesis of new enzyme. The effects of irreversible drugs may last several days or weeks, whereas reversible drug effects last 12 to 36 hours.

Adverse Effects and Contraindications

Anticholinesterase miotics produce a variety of adverse effects as a result of their local effects on ocular structures. Accommodative myopia can be problematic in young patients, and pupillary constriction may interfere with vision, especially in patients with central lens opacities. Other common local effects include eyelid twitching, browache, headache, eye pain, ciliary and conjunctival congestion, and lacrimation. Anticholinesterase drugs may cause eyelid spasm, which is annoying to the patient. Conjunctivitis and contact dermatitis may develop with localized allergy. Allergic responses were more prevalent when physostigmine solutions were used but are less common today. Long-term use of strong miotics can cause conjunctival thickening and obstruction of the nasolacrimal canals.

Cataract development may be hastened with the use of anticholinesterase miotics, particularly in patients over age 60. Echothiophate is particularly a problem. In addition, pupillary blockade, local vascular congestion, and occasional forward movement of the lens may cause a sudden or, more often, an insidious angle closure and an increase in IOP (even in eyes with only moderately narrow angles). Patients with advanced cataracts may be particularly at risk.

Pharmacokinetics

The onset of miosis for anticholinesterase miotics varies from 10 minutes to 4 hours (see Table 62–1). IOP is reduced in approximately 24 hours, with a duration of miotic action lasting 3 to 10 days for reversible agents and days to weeks for irreversible agents. Pressure reduction can last as little as 12 hours or as much as several weeks depending on the specific drug.

Drug-Drug Interactions

Concurrent use of anticholinesterase miotics with organophosphate insecticides or pesticides can result in cardiovascular and respiratory arrest. Carbamate, succinylcholine, and systemic anticholinesterase inhibitors also increase the risk of cardiovascular and respiratory arrest if they

TABLE 62–1 PHARMACOKINETICS OF SELECTED OPHTHALMIC DRUGS

Drug	Onset of Drug Action	Onset of Miosis	Peak Miosis; IOP Reduction	Duration of Miotic Action; IOP Reduction	Onset of Mydriasis; Cycloplegia	Maximal Mydriasis; Cycloplegia	Duration of Mydriasis; Cycloplegia	Effect on Aqueous Outflow
Cholinergic Miotics								
Carbachol	10–20 min	2–5 min	UA; 6 hr	4–8 hr; 4 hr	NA	NA	NA	Inc
Pilocarpine	1.5–2 hr	10–30 min	30 min; 1–1.5 hr	4–8 hr; 4–14 hr*	NA	NA	NA	Inc
Anticholinesterase Miotics								
Demecarium	15–60 min	2–4 hr	2 hr; 24 hr	3–10 days; 24–48 hr†	NA	NA	NA	Inc
Echothiophate	5–10 min	10–30 min	2 hr; 24 hr	1–4 wk; days-weeks†	NA	NA	NA	Inc
Isoflurophate	10–30 min	10–30 min	2 hr; 24 hr	1–4 wk; 1 week†	NA	NA	NA	Inc
Physostigmine	10–15 min	10–15 min	UA; 2–6 hr	UA; 12–36 hr	NA	NA	NA	Inc
Beta Blockers								
Betaxolol	30–60 min	30–60 min	2 hr	12 hr	NA	NA	NA	Dec
Carteolol	UA	UA	12 hr	UA	NA	NA	NA	Dec
Levobunolol	< 60 min	< 60 min	2–6 hr	UA; 24 hr	NA	NA	NA	Dec
Metipranolol	< 30 min	< 30 min	UA	12–24 hr	NA	NA	NA	Dec
Timolol	30 min	30 min	1–2 hr	12–24 hr	NA	NA	NA	Dec
Adrenergics								
Apraclonidine	NA	NA	NA; 3–5 hr	NA; UA	60 min; NA	3–5 hr; NA	12 hr; NA	Dec
Dipivefrin	30 min	NA	NA; 60 min	NA; 12 hr	Minutes	UA	UA	Dec
Epinephrine	5 min	NA	NA; 4 hr	24 hr; NA	Minutes	30 min; NA	1–3 hr; NA	Dec
Phenylephrine	NA	NA	NA	NA	0–60 min; NA	15–60 min	3–7 hr; NA	Dec
Carbonic Anhydrase Inhibitors								
Acetazolamide	2 hr	30 min–2 hr	NA; 18–24 hr	2–4 hr; 8–12 hr	NA	NA	NA	NA
Dichlorphenamide	30–60 min	NA	NA; 2–4 hr	6–12 hr	NA	NA	NA	NA
Methazolamide	2–4 hr	NA	NA; 10–18 hr	NA; 10–18 hr	NA	NA	NA	NA
Osmotics								
Glycerine (po)	10–30 min	NA	NA; 1–1.5 hr	NA; 4–8 hr	NA	NA	NA	Inc
Isosorbide (po)	10–30 min	NA	NA; 1–1.5 hr	NA: 5–6 hr	NA	NA	NA	Inc
Mannitol (IV)	30–60 min	NA	NA; 60 min	NA; 6–8 hr	NA	NA	NA	Inc
Urea (IV)	30–45 min	NA	NA; 60 min	1–2 hr; 3–10 hr	NA	NA	NA	Inc
Anticholinergic Mydriatics and Cycloplegics								
Atropine	NA	NA	NA	NA	30–40 min; 1–3 hr	30–40 min; 1–3 hr	7–12 days; 6–14 days	Dec
Cyclopentolate	NA	NA	NA	NA	30–60 min; 15–60 min	30–60 min; 25–75 min	24 hr; 0.25–1 day‡	Dec
Homatropine	NA	NA	NA	NA	10–30 min; 30–90 min	10–30 min; 30–90 min	6 hr–3 days; 10–48 hr	Dec
Scopolamine	NA	NA	NA	NA	20–30 min; 30–60 min	20–30 min; 30–60 min	3–7 days; 3–7 days	Dec
Tropicamide	NA	NA	NA	NA	20–40 min; 20–35 min	20–40 min; 20–40 min	6–7 hr; 1–6 hr	Dec

*Pilocarpine duration of IOP action depends on concentration.
† Duration of decrease in IOP for demecarium, echothiophate, and isoflurophate may last up to one month.
‡Cyclopentolate: recovery of accomodation; recovery from mydriasis may take several days.
Dec, Decrease; Inc, increase; IOP, intraocular pressure; NA, not applicable; UA, unavailable.

TABLE 62–2 DRUG-DRUG INTERACTIONS OF SELECTED OPHTHALMIC DRUGS

Drug	Interactive Drugs	Interaction
Cholinergic Miotics		
Carbachol	Flurbiprofen	Decreases effects of carbachol
Anticholinesterase Miotics		
Demecarium	Carbamate	Cardiovascular and respiratory arrest if used concurrently
Echothiophate	Organophosphate insecticides	
Isoflurophate	Organophosphate pesticides	
Physostigmine	Succinylcholine	
	Systemic anticholinesterase inhibitors	
Isoflurophate	Chymotrypsin	Inhibits isoflurophate activity
Beta Blockers		
Timolol	Calcium channel blockers	Additive mydriasis
	Carbonic anhydrase inhibitors	
	Cholinergic miotics	
	Dipivefrin	
	Echothiophate	
	Epinephrine	
	Pilocarpine	Synergistic
	Oral beta blockers	Additive bradycardia
	Quinidine	
	Verapamil (oral formulation)	Bradycardia and asystole
	Reserpine	Decreased capacity for "flight or fight"
Adrenergics		
Epinephrine	Atropine	Increased risk of hypertension and tachycardia
	Indomethacin	Inhibits ocular hypotensive action
Phenylephrine	Atropine	Pressor effects of phenylephrine enhanced
	Guanethidine	
	MAO inhibitors	
	Methyldopa	
	Reserpine	
	Tricyclic antidepressants	
Carbonic Anhydrase Inhibitors		
Acetazolamide	Methenamine	Decreases the excretion of interactive drug
	Procainamide	
	Quinidine	
	Diflunisol	Increases therapeutic and toxic effects of carbonic anhydrase inhibitor
Osmotics		
Glycerine	Diuretics	Increases IOP-lowering effects of glycerin

MAO, Monoamine oxidase.

are used concurrently with the anticholinesterase miotics (see Table 62–2). Chymotrypsin inhibits isoflurophate activity.

Dosage Regimen

Anticholinesterase miotics are strong and should be applied topically using the lowest effective dosage. Because these drugs come in a variety of concentrations and formulations, caution should be used to administer the correct drug (see Table 62–3).

BETA BLOCKERS

- ❒ Betaxolol (BETOPTIC, BETOPTIC S)
- ❒ Carteolol (OCUPRESS)
- ❒ Levobunolol (BETAGAN LIQUIFILM)
- ❒ Metipranolol (OPTIPRANOLOL)
- ❒ Timolol (TIMOPTIC, TIMOPTIC-XE); (🍁) APO-TIMOP

Indications

Glaucoma treatment has been greatly influenced by topically administered beta blockers. They are used in the management of primary and chronic open-angle glaucoma, aphakic glaucoma, and some secondary glaucomas. They may also be useful in the emergency treatment of acute closed-angle glaucoma when given with systemic ocular hypotensive drugs and pilocarpine. They are useful for some childhood glaucomas. Timolol accounts for 70 percent of all glaucoma drugs used and has become the standard for all ocular beta blockers.

Either topical or systemic administration is effective. Oral agents may be especially helpful when there are additional indications for beta blockers (e.g., angina pectoris or systemic hypertension).

Pharmacodynamics

Although the exact mechanism of action is unknown, all ocular beta blockers antagonize the effect of circulating catecholamines on beta$_2$ receptors in ciliary epithelium, thus causing a fall in aqueous humor production. IOP is reduced by both selective and nonselective beta blockers. The ocular beta blockers differ in their affinity for cardiac (beta$_1$) and noncardiac (beta$_2$) receptors. Betaxolol is selective for the beta$_1$ receptor. In concentrations of 0.125 to 0.5 percent, it has been shown to ef-

TABLE 62–3 DOSAGE REGIMEN FOR SELECTED OPHTHALMIC DRUGS

Drug	Use(s)	Dosage	Nursing Implications
Cholinergic Miotics			
Carbachol	Primary open-angle glaucoma; chronic glaucoma; seconday glaucoma	*Adults:* 1–2 gtts each eye initially q6–8 hr	Drug concentration and dosage frequency adjusted to maintain IOP in desired range. Available in 0.75%–3% concentrations. Check label carefully
Pilocarpine		*Adults:* 1–2 gtts each eye up to 6×/ day *or* 0.5 inch ribbon to lower conjunctival sac	Drug concentration and dosage frequency adjusted to maintain IOP in desired range. 1%–6% concentration solutions available in combination with 1% epinephrine bitartrate and 2% concentration in combination with physostigmine. Check labels carefully for correct drug and concentration
Pilocarpine ocular system		*Adults:* One 20 mcg *or* 40 mcg ocular system placed into lower conjuntival sac each week	Ocular system is gently moved to upper conjunctival sac by pressure through closed eyelids. Each system releases 20 or 40 mcg of drug per hour for 1 week
Anticholinesterase Miotics			
Demecarium	Primary open-angle glaucoma, chronic glaucoma, refractory glaucoma, strabismus	*Adults:* 1 gtt each eye BID to 2×/ week based on patient response	0.125%–0.25% solutions available. Check labels carefully for correct concentration.
Echothiophate		*Adults:* 1 gtt each eye q12–48 hr	Available in 0.03%, 0.06%, 0.125%, and 0.25% concentrations. Check labels carefully for correct concentration
Isoflurophate		*Adults:* ¼th inch in lower conjunctival sac each eye q12–72 hr	Available as 0.025% ointment only
Physostigmine	Primary open-angle glaucoma only	*Adults:* 1–2 gtts each eye QID	Available as 0.25% ointment or 0.25%–0.5% solution. Check label carefully for correct concentration
Ocular Beta Blockers			
Betaxolol	Chronic open-angle glaucoma; aphakic glaucoma; some seconday glaucoma	*Adults:* 1 gtt solution BID	Available as 0.25%–0.5% solution. Check label carefully
Carteolol		*Adults:* 1 gtt solution BID	Available as 1% solution only
Levobunolol		*Adults:* 1 gtt solution QD–BID	Available as 0.25%–0.5% solution. Check label carefully
Metipranolol		*Adults:* 1 gtt solution QD–BID	Available as 0.3% solution only
Timolol		*Adults:* 1 drop of 0.25% solution BID. May be increased to one drop of 0.5% solution BID if response unsatisfactory. Gel formulaiton: 0.5% once daily	May produce fewer local adverse effects than miotics and are better tolerated by patients with active accommodation or cataracts
Adrenergics			
Apraclonidine	Primary open-angle glaucoma, seconday glaucoma, ocular exams, uveitis, eye irritation	*Adults:* one gtt in affected eye 1 hr before procedure	Use cautiously in patients with history of cardiovascular disease
Dipivefrine		*Adults:* 1 gtt q12 hr	If miotic agent is ordered concurrently, administer miotic first. If dipivefrin is only antiglaucoma drug used, to switch from epinephrine, administer dipivefrin when next epinephrine dose is due. To switch from other antiglaucoma drugs, continue other drug for the 1st day of dipivefrin therapy. Available as 0.1% solution
Epinephrine		*Adults: Glaucoma:* 1–2 gtts solution to affected eye QD–BID. *Mydriasis:* 1–2 gtts into the eye; may repeat once PRN.	Available as 0.1% solution. May be given as infrequently as every 3 days. When used with miotics, instill miotic first. Safe use in children has not been established
Phenylephrine		*Adults: Mydriasis:* 1 gtt of 2.5% *or* 10% solution on upper limbus. May be repeated in 1 hour. *Uveitis:* 1 gtt of 2.5% *or* 10% solution on surface of cornea with atropine *Glaucoma:* 1 gtt of 10% solution repeated as often as necessary. May use in conjunction with miotics. *Intraocular surgery:* 2.5% *or* 10% solution 30–60 min before procedure. *Refraction:* 1 gtt of cycloplegic drug followed in 5 minutes by 1 gtt of 2.5% solution and in 10 minutes by another drop of cycloplegic drug. *Fundoscopic exam:* 1 gtt of 2.5% solution each eye. *Eye irritation:* 1–2 gtts of 0.12% solution to affected eye	Precede instillation with local anesthetic to prevent tearing and dilution of solution. Available as 0.8–0.12% and 10% solutions. Check labels carefully

TABLE 62–3 DOSAGE REGIMEN FOR SELECTED OPHTHALMIC DRUGS *Continued*

Drug	Use(s)	Dosage	Nursing Implications
Anticholinergics			
Atropine	Refraction, diagnostic purposes, uveitis, keratitis, secondary glaucoma, intraoperative and postoperative mydriasis and cycloplegia	*Adults:* 1–2 gtts QD–QID *Child:* 1–2 gtts QD–TID	Adult dosage available as 0.5%–3% solution or 0.5%–1% ointment. Check labels carefully. Child dosage available as 0.5% solution
Cyclopentolate		*Adults: Refraction:* 1–3 gtts of solution once; *Before ophthalmoscopy:* one gtt of solution once	Available as 0.55%, 1%, and 2% solution. Check label carefully
Homatropine		*Adults: Refraction:* 1–2 gtts 5% solution every 5 minutes × 2–3 doses *or* 1–2 drops of 2% solution every 10–15 minutes × 5 doses; *Uveitis:* one drop of 2%–5% solution BID–TID	Available as 2%–5% solutions. Check label carefully
Scopolamine		*Adults:* 1–2 gtts in affected eyes one hour before exam	Available as 0.25% solution
Tropicamide		*Adults:* 1–2 gtts of solution repeated in 5 minutes; then every 20–30 minutes PRN to maintain mydriasis	Available as 0.5%–1% solutions. Check label carefully
Carbonic Anhydrase Inhibitors			
Acetazolamide	Glaucoma, preoperative and postoperative eye surgery	*Adults:* 62.5–250 mg tablets po BID–QID *or* 500 mg capsules QD–BID *or* 500 mg IV/IM and repeated PRN in 2–4 hours *Child:* 8–30 mg/kg (300–900 mg/m^2) po daily in divided doses *or* 5–10 mg/kg IV/IM q6 hr	The prolonged release preparation given once daily is better tolerated by some patients
Dichlorphenamide		*Adults:* 100–200 mg po q12 hr initially, then maintenance dose of 25–50 mg QD–TID	No recommended dosages for children. Take oral formulations with food to minimize GI irritation. Long-acting capsules may be opened and sprinkled on soft food, but do not crush, chew, or swallow contents dry
Dorzolamide		*Adults:* 1 gtt in affected eye TID	
Methazolamide		*Adults:* 25–50 mg po BID–TID	
Osmotics			
Glycerine	Short-term reduction of IOP and vitreous volume, acute closed-angle glaucoma, preoperative and postoperative chronic glaucoma, retinal detachment, cataract extraction, keratoplasty, secondary glaucoma	*Adults:* 1–1.8 g/kg po of a 50%–75% solution. May be given more than once daily if necessary necessary	Usually given 1–1.5 hr preoperatively. Ocular penetration poor
Isosorbide		*Adults:* 1.5 g/kg po initially then QID if necessary	Dosage range 1–3 g/kg. Ocular penetration good
Mannitol		*Adults & Child:* 0.5–2 g/kg of a 20% solution infused IV over a 30–60 minute period	Ocular penetration very poor
Urea		*Adults:* 0.5–2 g/kg of a 30% solution administered IV at a rate of 60 drops/minute. The usual dose is 1 g/kg *Child:* 0.5–1.5 g/kg of a 30% solution infused over a 30-minute period	Ocular penetration good

GI, Gastrointestinal; IOP, intraocular pressure.

fectively reduce IOP as much as 35 percent from baseline. Metipranolol and carteolol are both nonselective drugs and are comparable to timolol in reducing IOP. Some beta blockers also have local anesthetic and partial agonist activity.

Adverse Effects and Contraindications

Although ocular beta blockers are customarily well tolerated, some adverse effects have been reported. They may cause mild ocular irritation, conjunctival hyperemia, eye pain, headache, decreased corneal sensitivity, transient dry eye syndrome, local hypersensitivity reactions, superficial punctate keratitis, blepharoptosis, and blurring of central vision. Refractive changes due to withdrawal of miotics may be responsible for some reports of blurred vision.

Timolol can be systemically absorbed to produce adverse effects related to blockade of cardiac and noncardiac beta receptors. It should be used with caution in patients with uncontrolled heart failure or atrioventricular conduction disturbances. Sudden death has occasionally occurred, although a cause-and-effect relationship has not been established.

Gentle eyelid closure or light pressure over the inner canthus of the eye following drug application reduces the likelihood of systemic reactions and increases ocular contact time. The adverse effects of beta blockers are most noticeable the first 2 weeks of therapy.

Timolol also reduces forced expiratory volume (FEV_1) in patients with chronic airway limitation and may precipitate bronchospasm. Like other nonselective beta blockers, it should not be used in patients with a history of asthma or chronic airway disease. Although such cases are rare, this drug has produced vasomotor rhinitis. Both cardiac and pulmonary adverse effects may be additive to those of the anticholinesterase miotics. Cardiac sympathetic tone and the strength of myocardial contraction are reduced by timolol, even when plasma levels are undetectable.

Timolol has been shown to decrease libido in both genders and lead to impotence and reduced ejaculation volume in men. Because ocular timolol is one of the most commonly used drugs in the United States, all patients complaining of sexual dysfunction should be asked if they are using this drug.

On occasion, ocular beta blockers increase the frequency of hypoglycemic episodes and mask the symptoms of hypoglycemia in type I diabetic patients. And although such cases are rare, timolol has caused hyperkalemia in some patients. Timolol is transmitted in breast milk and thus should be used with caution in nursing mothers.

Pharmacokinetics

All ocular beta blockers relieve IOP for at least 12 hours. The ocular hypotensive action of betaxolol lasts about 12 hours. The hypotensive effects of levobunolol, timolol, and metipranolol may persist for 24 hours or more (see Table 62–1).

Drug-Drug Interactions

When used alone, ocular beta blockers do not dilate the pupil. However, the mydriatic effect of epinephrine is enhanced in the presence of beta blockers (see Table 62–2). Thus, combined therapy may be dangerous in patients with narrow filtration angles. Timolol also has additive effects with calcium channel blockers. Bradycardia has been associated with the concurrent use of timolol eyedrops and oral quinidine.

Although indomethacin, a nonsteroidal anti-inflammatory drug (NSAID), may attenuate the antihypertensive effect of oral beta blockers, it does not affect the ocular hypotensive action of timolol. Close observation is needed when administering a beta blocker concurrently with catecholamine-depleting drugs such as reserpine.

Dosage Regimen

Ocular beta blockers come in a variety of concentrations. The concentration and dosage frequency are adjusted based on patient response (see Table 62–3). Timolol 0.5 percent gel once daily, or timolol 0.5 percent solution twice daily, have been found equally effective in lowering IOP. Carteolol 1 percent and timolol 0.25 percent twice daily were also effective. Metipranolol in concentrations ranging from 0.1 to 0.6 percent is comparable to timolol 0.25 to 0.5 percent in reducing IOP. Betaxolol 0.125 and 0.5 percent, and timolol 0.5 percent administered twice daily were effective in decreasing IOP, with similar adverse effect profiles.

ADRENERGIC AGONISTS

- ❐ Apraclonidine (IOPIDINE)
- ❐ Brimonidine tartrate (ALPHAGAN)
- ❐ Dipivefrin (PROPINE); (🍁) OPHTHO-DIPIVEFRIN
- ❐ Epinephrine (EPIFRIN, GLAUCON, EPINAL, EPPY/N)
- ❐ Phenylephrine (AK-DILATE, AK-NEFRIN, MYDFRIN, NEOSYNEPHRINE, PHENOPTIC, PREFRIN LIQUIFILM, RELIEF); (🍁) MINIMS PHENYLEPHRINE

Indications

Epinephrine and its analogs are used in the management of primary open-angle glaucoma and other chronic glaucomas. In addition, they are used to dilate the pupil for funduscopic exams, to prevent hemorrhage of small ocular vessels, and as an ocular decongestant during allergic reactions. They may be administered alone for initial treatment, especially when beta blockers are ineffective or not tolerated. Epinephrine is also used to supplement miotics or carbonic anhydrase inhibitors.

Apraclonidine is used to prevent the elevation of IOP following argon laser trabeculoplasty, iridotomy and capsulotomy, and cataract surgery. Dipivefrin is an effective ocular hypotensive drug for patients with open-angle glaucoma.

Phenylephrine is generally reserved for the short-term pupillary dilation needed for eye exams. Nonprescription concentrations are used as a topical decongestant (vasoconstrictor), but even at low concentrations, these drugs may dilate the pupil if enough drug penetrates the corneal epithelium.

Brimonidine tartrate is the newest topical agent for the treatment of elevated IOP associated with primary open-angle glaucoma or ocular hypertension. The drug is a second-generation alpha agonist.

Pharmacodynamics

The data are conflicting regarding the mechanisms involved in the adrenergic control of aqueous humor dynamics. Current evidence suggests that aqueous humor production and outflow is mediated primarily by beta mechanisms. Although the sphincter and ciliary muscles are largely under parasympathetic control, adrenergic receptors have also been found in these tissues. Beta receptors are primarily found in the ciliary muscles. Both alpha and beta receptors are found in the sphincter muscle of the iris. Activation of $beta_2$ receptors in the canal of Schlemm increases outflow, an action that may involve stimulation of prostaglandin synthesis and, hence, uveoscleral drainage. Activation of beta receptors in the ciliary bodies produces a slight, transient, clinically unimportant increase in aqueous production, whereas blockade of receptors decreases production. When it is used alone, epinephrine produces a 30 to 35 percent decrease in the rate of aqueous humor production. Concurrent use of adrenergics with carbonic anhydrase inhibitors may produce a 65 to 70 percent decrease in aqueous humor production.

Dipivefrin is a prodrug form of epinephrine. It penetrates the cornea more readily than epinephrine because it is highly lipid soluble. Once in the eye, it is converted to its active form by ocular enzymes.

Brimonidine tartrate works to reduce production of aqueous humor in the eye and to increase its outflow.

Adverse Effects and Contraindications

Epinephrine produces browache, headache, blurred vision, eye irritation, and excessive tearing in some patients. Systemic effects such as tachycardia, hypertension, and faintness rarely occur with epinephrine, but rebound miosis can occur, especially in patients older than 50 years of age. The ocular and systemic adverse effects of dipivefrin are the same as for epinephrine but are generally less common and less severe.

Topical epinephrine and its analogs can cause pupillary dilation, even when used with miotics. They are contraindicated before iridectomy in closed-angle glaucoma because they may precipitate an acute attack. Although such cases are rare, epinephrine may cause a temporary elevation of IOP when it is used without miotics in patients with open-angle glaucoma. This phenomenon may be related to the release of pigment particles from the iris into the aqueous humor.

The most common systemic adverse effects of apraclonidine is a sensation of dry mouth or nose. It occurs more often in patients treated with the 1-percent solution than with the 0.25- or 0.125-percent solutions.

The most important and common adverse effect of chronic phenylephrine use is rebound congestion of the conjunctiva, in which the vessels become progressively more dilated. Patients with rebound effects should be referred for professional eye care for differential diagnosis and management. Further, because a patient can use phenylephrine indiscriminately to quiet an irritated eye, the drug can induce pupillary dilation and may precipitate closed-angle glaucoma in susceptible patients. This adverse effect is more likely to occur if the cornea is damaged or diseased, allowing increased corneal drug penetration.

Phenylephrine should be used with caution in patients who have a history of cardiovascular disease or diabetes mellitus and in patients taking interactive drugs. Phenylephrine should not be used as an ocular irrigant due to its potential adverse effects.

Pharmacokinetics

The onset of action of adrenergic ocular drugs ranges from 5 minutes for epinephrine to 30 minutes for dipivefrin. Peak decrease in IOP occurs in 1 to 5 hours with a duration of drug action of 12 to 24 hours (see Table 62–1).

Drug-Drug Interactions

Concurrent use of ocular adrenergics is discouraged in patients taking atropine preparations because of the risk of hypertension and tachycardia (see Table 62–2). The ocular hypotensive effect of epinephrine is partially inhibited with concurrent use of indomethacin. The pressor effects of phenylephrine may be enhanced in patients taking atropine, tricyclic antidepressants, monoamine oxidase inhibitors, reserpine, guanethidine, or methyldopa.

Dosage Regimen

Only 2.5-percent adrenergic solutions are recommended for routine use, especially for infants and older adults (see Table 62–3). The risks of adverse effects are greatly increased with the use of 10-percent solutions. Epinephrine and dipivefrin solutions cause discoloration of soft contact lenses. The lenses should be removed before administration and left out for approximately 30 minutes.

CARBONIC ANHYDRASE INHIBITORS

- ❒ Acetazolamide (DIAMOX)
- ❒ Dichlorphenamide (DARANIDE)
- ❒ Dorzolamide (TRUSOPT)
- ❒ Methazolamide (NEPTAZANE)

Indications

Carbonic anhydrase inhibitors are used in the long-term treatment of open-angle glaucoma and other chronic glaucomas refractory to cholinergic miotics, beta blockers, and epinephrine. They are considered ocular hypotensives and are used also to decrease IOP for preoperative and postoperative eye surgery patients. In addition, they are used along with miotics, ocular beta blockers, and osmotics for the emergency treatment of acute closed-angle glaucoma. Patients younger than 40 years of age tolerate these drugs better than older patients.

Acetazolamide is the most common carbonic anhydrase inhibitor and is used for all types of glaucoma. It is usually considered a second-line drug and is used after other treatment regimens (e.g., cholinergic miotics, beta blockers, adrenergics) alone or in combination have failed to control IOP. Because of its diverse actions, acetazolamide is also used for other purposes (see Chapter 39).

Pharmacodynamics

Carbonic anhydrase inhibitors block ocular carbonic anhydrase in the ciliary epithelium, thus lowering IOP. Carbonic anhydrase catalyzes the reversible action that is involved in the hydration of carbon dioxide and dehydration of carbonic acid. The systemic acidosis that is produced enhances the ocular hypotensive effects. With maximal dosages, these drugs reduce aqueous humor production by about 40 percent.

By reducing aqueous humor formation, carbonic anhydrase inhibitors decrease IOP, usually resulting in pupillary miosis and opening of the anterior chamber angle. These drugs should be used only for short-term treatment before iridectomy because the lowered IOP may mask the fact that the angle is still partly closed. Permanent closure of the angle can result.

Adverse Effects and Contraindications

The most common adverse effects of carbonic anhydrase inhibitors include alteration in taste, anorexia, gastrointestinal distress (nausea, vomiting, diarrhea), malaise, fatigue, weakness, nervousness, and loss of libido. Lethargy and depression are common but often go unnoticed until the drug is discontinued and the patient notices a sudden improvement in his or her emotional state. Many patients cannot tolerate carbonic anhydrase inhibitors for prolonged periods because of the malaise syndrome. Transient myopia has been reported and may result from changes in hydration or a forward movement of the lens. Confusion, ataxia, tremor, and tinnitis are rare. Although such cases are rare, patients taking these drugs may develop dermatitis, myopia, agranulocytosis, and aplastic anemia.

Carbonic anhydrase inhibitors cause alkalinization of the urine and may complicate therapy with drugs that are dependent on urine pH for elimination or reabsorption. Methazolamide has the same actions as acetazolamide but is safer for patients with renal calculi or chronic airway limitation because it alters acid-base balance to a smaller degree.

Carbonic anhydrase inhibitors are contraindicated in patients with low serum sodium or potassium levels, hepatic or renal disease, suprarenal gland failure, or hyperchloremic acidosis. Further, because carbonic anhydrase inhibitors have teratogenic potential, these drugs should be avoided during the first trimester of pregnancy.

Pharmacokinetics

Most body tissues contain carbonic anhydrase in amounts greater than those needed for physiologic functioning. Almost 99 percent of carbonic anhydrase must be inhibited to significantly reduce aqueous humor formation. The onset of drug action is 30 minutes to 4 hours after administration, with peak effects noted in 10 to 24 hours. The duration of drug action varies with the specific agent but ranges from 8 to 18 hours. The duration of action of sustained-release formulations is usually 18 to 24 hours.

Different brands of acetazolamide vary in bioavailability, and some products have been found to have significant lot-to-lot variations. For this reason, bioequivalence requirements have been proposed for all carbonic anhydrase inhibitors. Acetazolamide is 93-percent protein bound and does not undergo biotransformation. Seventy percent of a dose is recovered in the urine within 24 hours. Its half-life is 5 hours.

Methazolamide is well absorbed, is only 55 percent protein bound, and diffuses into tissues more readily than acetazolamide. Only 25 percent of the dose is eliminated unchanged in the urine. There is no information available about its metabolites.

Dichlorphenamide appears to be well absorbed, with maximal effects observed 2 to 4 hours after administration. Extensive studies of its pharmacokinetic properties have not been conducted.

Drug-Drug Interactions

Acetazolamide decreases the elimination of methenamine, procainamide, and quinidine, and it increases the elimination of lithium. The NSAID diflunisal competes with acetazolamide for plasma protein binding sites, thereby increasing both the therapeutic and toxic effects of acetazolamide.

Dosage Regimen

Although carbonic anhydrase inhibitors are usually given by mouth, the sodium salt of acetazolamide can also be given intravenously or intramuscularly, if necessary. Taking the drug with meals, lowering the dosage, supplementing with sodium bicarbonate, or substituting one carbonic anhydrase inhibitor for another may alleviate some of the gastrointestinal adverse effects associated with their use.

Laboratory Considerations

Diuresis causes serum potassium levels to fall during the first few weeks of treatment with carbonic anhydrase inhibitors. It usually returns to near normal levels unless a potassium-wasting diuretic is also taken. Although the hypokalemia that results is clinically insignificant, potassium levels should still be monitored.

Carbonic anhydrase inhibitors reduce uric acid elimination, thus increasing blood uric acid levels. The hyperuricemia is usually asymptomatic and rarely leads to exacerbation of gout.

Adverse hematopoietic reactions most often appear within the first 6 months of treatment. The mortality rate in patients who develop aplastic anemia from carbonic anhydrase inhibitors is about 50 percent. The value of routine blood monitoring has been questioned, but patients should be instructed to promptly report the development of symptoms such as sore throat, fever, fatigue, pallor, easy bruising, epistaxis, purpura, or jaundice.

OSMOTICS

- ❒ Glycerine (OPHTHALGAN, ADSORBONAC SOLUTION, MURO 128, AK-NaCL)
- ❒ Isosorbide (ISMOTIC)
- ❒ Mannitol (OSMITROL)
- ❒ Urea (UREAPHIL)

Indications

Osmotics are used for the short-term reduction of IOP and vitreous volume in patients with glaucoma, corneal edema, and corneoscleral lacerations. They are also used for preoperative and postoperative surgical repair of a detached retina, cataract extraction, and keratoplasty. Osmotic drugs cause an immediate and marked fall in IOP and reduction of vitreous humor volume and are generally effective even in patients who do not respond to miotics or carbonic anhydrase inhibitors.

Pharmacodynamics

Osmotic drugs cause the plasma to be hypertonic compared with intraocular fluid. By increasing osmolarity, osmotics cause fluid to be drawn from the corneal epithelium to the tear film to be eliminated from the eye through the trabecular meshwork. Osmotics also decrease aqueous humor production by their action on hypothalamic osmoreceptors. They also aid in opening the angle by reducing the fluid volume in the posterior segment of the eye, temporarily reducing pressure behind the iris. If a miotic is then effective in opening the angle, the pressure may remain normal even after osmotic effects have dissipated.

Adverse Effects and Contraindications

Osmotics commonly produce headache, nausea, and vomiting. Diarrhea occasionally occurs. Glycerine may cause hyperglycemia and glycosuria and should be used with caution in patients with diabetes mellitus. Confusion and amnesia may occur in older patients, but frank hyperosmolar nonketotic coma is a rare event. Osmotics decrease the volume of cerebrospinal fluid and can lead to severe pounding headaches. Also, the shift in body fluids may increase the workload on the heart and precipitate heart failure.

Isosorbide produces effects similar to that of glycerin, although it does not adversely effect blood glucose levels and is preferred for patients with diabetes. It may also cause less nausea and vomiting than glycerin.

Mannitol's adverse effects are similar to those of glycerin and isosorbide, but in addition, chills, dizziness, and chest pain have been reported. The drug has occasionally caused agitation, disorientation, seizures, and anaphylactoid reactions. An acute increase in intravascular volume with subsequent fluid overload may result in pulmonary edema or intracranial hemorrhage. Fatalities have been reported.

Urea is irritating to the tissues, causing pain at the site of infusion. Necrosis may result if extravasation occurs. Superficial and deep thrombosis may develop if urea is infused into the veins of the lower extremities. This drug is contraindicated in patients with severely impaired renal or hepatic functioning.

Pharmacokinetics

Glycerine is well absorbed following oral administration, remaining in the intravascular space. It is 80-percent biotransformed in the liver, with the remaining 10 to 20 percent transformed in the kidneys. Its half-life is 30 to 45 minutes. Reduction of IOP begins within 10 minutes and peaks in 60 to 90 minutes. Its duration of action is approximately 5 hours. When glycerin is used to reduce corneal swelling, its duration of action is 3 to 5 hours. The onset and peak are unknown.

The onset of isosorbide occurs 10 to 30 minutes after oral administration, peaks in 60 to 90 minutes, and has a duration of action of 5 to 6 hours. It is biotransformed in the liver and has a half-life of 5 to 9.5 hours. It is eliminated in the urine. Isosorbide is often used for patients with diabetes because it does not biotransform to provide calories.

Mannitol is completely bioavailable when it is administered intravenously. It is confined to the extracellular spaces and does not usually cross the blood-brain barrier or eye membranes. Mannitol is eliminated through the kidneys, with minimal biotransformation by the liver. Its half-life is 100 minutes. Mannitol has an onset time of 30 to 60 minutes, a peak of 1 hour, and a duration of action of 6 to 8 hours.

Urea has an onset time of 30 to 45 minutes, with peak action seen in 60 minutes. The duration of action is 5 to 6 hours. Biotransformation and half-life of urea is unknown.

Drug-Drug Interactions

Glycerine may cause slightly elevated serum and urine glucose concentrations. Diuretics enhance the IOP-lowering effects of glycerin. Hypokalemia increases the risk of cardiac glycoside toxicity.

Dosage Regimen

Glycerine is administered orally as 1 to 1.5 g/kg of a 50- to 75-percent solution. The drug may be given more than once daily, if needed. Lemon juice or instant coffee may be added to unflavored preparations to increase palatability. Palatability is also enhanced by pouring the solution over crushed ice and drinking it through a straw. Patients should not be permitted to drink additional water.

Isosorbide is given orally as 1.5 g/kg initially. It may be given up to four times daily, if necessary. Palatability is increased when the drug is poured over cracked ice.

Mannitol is dosed in both adults and children as 0.5 to 2 g/kg of a 20-percent solution infused intravenously over a 30- to 60-minute period. It may be discontinued when the desired effect has been obtained, even if the full dose has not been given. A total dose of 1 g/kg is usually sufficient, but small doses are sometimes effective. (Note: Mannitol should not be confused with mannitol hexanitrate, an antianginal drug.)

In adults, urea is administered intravenously as 0.5 to 2 g/kg of a 30-percent solution given at a rate of 60 drops per minute. The usual dose is 1 g/kg. For children, the usual dose is 0.5 to 1.5 g/kg of a 30-percent solution infused over a 30-minute period.

Osmotics should not be administered through the same intravenous line as blood or blood products.

Antimicrobial Drugs

As with other body structures, there are three categories of organisms that can cause eye infections: bacteria, viruses, and fungi. And also as with other body parts an appropriate antimicrobial should be used to treat the infection. A culture and sensitivity of ocular fluid, exudate, or tissue can be performed to identify the specific organism, but this procedure is seldom done. Ordinarily, treatment is started before culture results are known.

ANTIBIOTICS

- ❒ Chloramphenicol (CHLOROPTIC)
- ❒ Ciprofloxacin (CILOXAN)
- ❒ Gentamicin (GENTACIDIN, GENOPTIC, GARAMYCIN)
- ❒ Norfloxacin (CHIBROXIN)
- ❒ Ofloxacin (OCUFLOX)
- ❒ Polymixin B sulfate
- ❒ Polymixin B sulfate with bacitracin zinc and neomycin sulfate (NEOSPORIN)
- ❒ Polymixin B sulfate with trimethoprim (POLYTRIM)
- ❒ Sulfacetamide sodium (AK-SULF, BLEPH-10, ISOPTO CETAMIDE, OCUSULF-10, SODIUM SULAMYD, SULF-10, SULF-15); (✱) SULFEX
- ❒ Tobramycin (TOBREX)

Antibiotics can be administered topically or systemically to treat bacterial eye infections. They are used to treat problems such as corneal ulcerations, blepharitis, endophthalmitis, trachoma, and retinitis due to human immune deficiency syndrome. Systemic antibiotics are discussed in Chapter 24.

Bacitracin, cephalosporins, chloramphenicol, and gentamicin act to inhibit the growth of (bacteriostasis), or directly kill (bacteriocidal), bacteria by inhibiting protein synthesis in susceptible organisms. Bacitracin is effective against gram-positive organisms. Chloramphenicol, cephalosporins, and gentamicin are used to treat gram-positive and gram-negative infections. Sulfacetamide prevents the uptake of para-aminobenzoic acid, a metabolite of bacterial folic acid synthesis, and is also effective in eradicating gram-positive and gram-negative bacterial infections. Most ophthalmologists recommend the use of a broad-spectrum antibacterial drug until sensitivity has been determined. Broad-spectrum drugs provide complete coverage and minimize hypersensitivity reactions.

Bacitracin and chloramphenicol penetrate the cornea and conjunctiva. In addition, chloramphenicol also penetrates aqueous humor. Gentamicin penetrates poorly through an intact cornea but penetrates well through corneal abrasions. The intraocular penetration of sulfacetamide varies. Bacitracin, chloramphenicol, and gentamicin are eliminated via the nasolacrimal system. The elimination route of the other drugs is unknown. The onset and duration of action vary according to the patient's disorder and response to treatment.

ANTIVIRALS

- ❒ Idoxuridine
- ❒ Trifluridine (VIROPTIC)
- ❒ Vidarabine (VIRA-A OPHTHALMIC OINTMENT)

A number of ocular antiviral drugs have emerged in recent years for the treatment of viral infections. Idoxuridine, vidarabine, and trifluridine are the three standard agents used in the treatment of cytomegalovirus retinitis, but they are also useful for human immunodeficiency virus–induced iridocyclitis and anterior uveitis. Other antiviral drugs are discussed in Chapter 25.

Idoxuridine is poorly absorbed intraocularly. Vidarabine and trifluridine are found in trace amounts in the aqueous humor after application to a cornea that has an epithelial defect or inflammation. Neither drug displays significant systemic absorption.

Idoxuridine, vidarabine, and trifluridine interfere with DNA synthesis in susceptible organisms. Idoxuridine, the first ocular antiviral drug developed, is invaluable in treating herpes simplex of the cornea because it prevents the virus from feeding off the cells of the corneal epithelium.

To prevent recurrence of herpes, antiviral drugs should continue to be administered for 5 to 7 days after healing has occurred. Improvement usually occurs in 7 to 8 days and may continue for as long as 21 days.

ANTIFUNGALS

- ❒ Natamycin (NATACYN)

Antifungal drugs are used to treat infections such as fungal keratitis and endophthalmitis, which occur frequently after an eye injury or eye surgery. Further, the frequency of fungal corneal ulcers has increased in recent years, most likely associated with the increased used of corticosteroids and their depression of the immune system. Additionally, the use of broad-spectrum antibiotics has contributed to the incidence. Because ocular antifungal drugs are poorly absorbed by the eyes, ocular infections are a challenge to treat. Other antifungal drugs are discussed in Chapter 25.

Natamycin is the only ocular antifungal drug available in the United States. It is considered the drug of choice for the initial treatment of fungal keratitis because of its broad spectrum. It is also effective in treatment of blepharitis and conjunctivitis. Natamycin does not reach measurable levels in the deeper corneal layers (unless a defect in the epithelium is present), and thus it may not reach deep corneal mycoses. The 5-percent suspension acts by increasing the permeability of the fungal cell membrane.

Anti-Inflammatory Drugs

Corticosteroids and NSAIDs constitute the two drug groups used to counter ocular inflammation. They suppress the immune system, causing signs and symptoms to be reduced or disappear.

CORTICOSTEROIDS

- ❒ Dexamethasone (DECADRON, MAXIDEX)
- ❒ Fluorometholone (FLAREX, FML)
- ❒ Medrysone (HMS)
- ❒ Prednisolone acetate (PRED MILD, INFLAMASE FORTE)

Corticosteroids have been used in the treatment of ocular inflammation since the 1950s and include dexamethasone, fluorometholone, medrysone, and prednisolone. They vary in their ability to decrease corneal inflammation from 23 to 52 percent, and they protect the eye from scarring and neovascularization. The salt formulation affects the ability of the drug to penetrate the cornea. Biphasic salts penetrate an intact cornea better than water-soluble salts. However, the ability to penetrate the cornea does not suggest therapeutic effectiveness. Corticosteroids are more effective for acute than chronic disorders but are contraindicated in the presence of infection because they are not bacteriocidal and tend to mask infections. Corticosteroid preparations are available in combination with antimicrobial agents.

Corticosteroids are available in combination with antimicrobial drugs or antihistamines. For example, prednisolone is available in combination with gentamicin (PRED-G), with neomycin and polymixin B sulfate (POLY-PRED), or with SULFACETAMIDE (Isopto Cetapred). Hydrocortisone acetate is available in combination with chloramphenicol and polymixin B sulfate. Dexamethazone is combined with polymixin B sulfate and neomycin (MAXITROL)

Orally administered corticosteroids have been associated with lowered resistance to infection and modification of the inflammatory response. The drugs can mask serious ocular disease if they are not closely monitored. Additionally, corticosteroid use has been associated with the development of posterior subcapsular cataract (PSC) formation. This is particularly true in patients who are using 10 to 16 mg/day of oral prednisone or its equivalent for 1 year or more. There is a 70-percent incidence of PSC in patients treated with dosages exceeding 16 mg/day over the same time period. Patients receiving less than 10 mg/day or the equivalent are less likely to develop PSC, although patient sensitivity varies. Any patient receiving long-term oral corticosteroids should have routine eye exams and be instructed not to rub the eyes because ocular corticosteroids increase bruisability of the delicate eye tissues. There are no significant interactions between ocular corticosteroids and other drugs.

NONSTEROIDAL ANTI-INFLAMMATORY DRUGS

- ❒ Diclofenac (VOLTAREN EYE DROPS)
- ❒ Flurbiprofen (OCUFEN)
- ❒ Ketoralac (ACULAR)
- ❒ Rimexolone (VEXOL)
- ❒ Suprofen (PROFENAL)

Ocular NSAIDs have a variety of uses, including inhibition of intraoperative miosis, postoperative cataract surgery, prevention or treatment of cystoid macular edema, iritis, iridocyclitis, episcleritis, seasonal allergic conjunctivitis, contact lens-associated conjunctivitis, and vernal conjunctivitis.

Ocular NSAIDs inhibit prostaglandin synthesis and reduce prostaglandin-mediated effects (i.e., miosis, increased vascular permeability, conjunctival hyperemia, and changes in IOP). Ocular NSAIDs are well tolerated but do produce transient burning and stinging when they are administered. Dendritic keratitis is also possible. Assess for abnormal bleeding because excessive systemic absorption may interfere with platelet aggregation.

OCULAR ANTIHISTAMINES

- ❒ Cromolyn sodium (CROLOM)
- ❒ Levocabastine (LIVOSTIN)
- ❒ Lodoxamide tromethamine (ALOMIDE)
- ❒ Olopatadine (PATANOL)
- ❒ Sodium cromoglycate

Ocular antihistamines are used in the management of seasonal allergic conjunctivitis. Sodium cromoglycate may be effective as an alternative to those who fail to respond to more conservative antiallergy measures. However, this drug has been in short supply and solutions must be compounded for ophthalmic use. Lodoxamide tromethamine is a mast cell–stabilizing drug that is thought to be at least as effective as sodium cromoglycate in treating allergic ocular disorders including vernal keratoconjunctivitis. Ocular antihistamines block histamine receptors in the eye. The most common adverse effects include headache, burning, and stinging.

Miscellaneous Ophthalmic Drugs

OCULAR ANTICHOLINERGICS

- ❒ Atropine (ISOPTO ATROPINE)
- ❒ Cyclopentolate (CYCLOGYL)
- ❒ Homatropine (ISOPTO HOMATROPINE)
- ❒ Scopolamine (ISOPTO HYOSCINE)
- ❒ Tropicamide (MYDRIACYL)

Indications

Ocular anticholinergic drugs (also commonly known as mydriatics and cycloplegics) are used to produce mydriasis for refraction and other diagnostic purposes. They can be used in the treatment of anterior uveitis and keratitis, as well as for some secondary forms of glaucoma. They also facilitate mydriasis during ocular surgery and decrease postoperative complications. Atropine and scopolamine were discussed in Chapter 13, along with other muscarinic antagonists; thus, only ocular considerations are discussed here.

Pharmacodynamics

Ocular anticholinergics block the action of parasympathetic nervous system stimulation. There is paralysis of ciliary muscles and relaxation of the muscles of the iris resulting in pupil dilation and loss of accommodation (*cycloplegia*). A cycloplegic drug dilates the pupil and paralyzes accommodation, whereas a mydriatic drug dilates the pupil without affecting accommodation.

Adverse Effects and Contraindications

Adverse effects, including toxic reactions, can occur with systemic absorption of an ocular anticholinergic through the nasolacrimal ducts and episcleral blood vessels. Ocular responses include blurred vision, photophobia, and precipitation of closed-angle glaucoma. Systemic effects may include dry mouth, constipation, fever, tachycardia, and central nervous system effects.

Pharmacokinetics

The majority of ocular anticholinergics reach maximal mydriasis and cycloplegia 15 to 60 minutes after administration depending on the specific drug (see Table 62–1). Their duration of action varies. Mydriatic effects can last from 6 hours to 12 days, whereas cycloplegic effects can last from 6 hours to 7 days.

Dosage Regimen

The dosage of ocular anticholinergic drug depends on the purpose for its use. For refraction and use preoperatively and postoperatively, the dosage is usually 1 drop administered once daily in the affected eye (see Table 62–3). Caution should be used to check the specific labels carefully because the drugs come in a variety of concentrations.

OCULAR DECONGESTANTS

- ❒ Naphazoline (AK-CON, ALBALON, ALLEREST EYE DROPS, NAPHCON, NAPHCON FORTE, PRIVING, others)

Ocular decongestants stimulate alpha receptors in vascular smooth muscle of the eye, resulting in local vasoconstriction. These drugs are typically used for the short-term treatment of superficial corneal vascularity (i.e., congestion, itching, minor irritation, and hyperemia). The most common adverse effects include headache, nervousness, dizziness, weakness, hypertension, and arrhythmias with systemic absorption. Other adverse effects are transient burning, stinging, dryness, blurred vision, mydriasis, and increased or decreased IOP. Rebound congestion and eye redness may occur if the drug is overused.

The onset of the drug's effects occurs in 10 minutes, with a duration of action of 2 to 6 hours. Some systemic absorption does occur. The usual dose is 1 drop placed in the conjunctival sac every 3 to 4 hours. Naphazoline should not be used for more than 3 to 5 days unless the individual is under the direction of a health care provider.

DIAGNOSTIC AIDS

- ❒ Rose bengal
- ❒ Fluorescein (AK-FLUOR, FLUORESCITE, FLUOR-I-STRIP, others)
- ❒ Fluoracaine
- ❒ Fluorexon

Several drugs are available for diagnostic purposes: rose bengal, fluorescein sodium, and fluorexon. Rose bengal is a dye used for ordinary ocular examinations or when superficial corneal or conjunctival tissue changes are suspected. Rose bengal is available from several manufacturers in a 1-percent solution or as 1.3-mg strips.

Fluorescein sodium is a nontoxic water-soluble dye that is applied to the cornea or conjunctiva of the eye to identify denuded areas of epithelium, or foreign bodies. However, because fluorescein is easily contaminated with *Pseudomonas aeruginosa*, the dye is impregnated on strips of filter paper. The dry filter paper is moistened with a sterile solution and then gently brought into contact with eye tissues, allowing the dye to disperse. The dye stains denuded areas of epithelium a bright green color, and a green ring will surround a foreign body. Conjunctival loss is stained a yellow color. The staining of the eye disappears in about 30 minutes. Staining of the skin can be washed off with mild soap and water. Fluorescein is available in concentrations that vary from 2- to 25-percent solutions. Strips are available as 0.6-mg, 1-mg, and 9-mg formulations.

Fluorescein is also used in fitting hard contact lens, to test the patency of the nasolacrimal system, and to identify defects in retinal pigment. Fluorexon is used to fit soft contact lenses because it has less than 55 percent water content and does not stain soft lenses. The lenses are flushed with saline after exposure to fluorexon (0.35-percent solution). If the nasolacrimal system is patent, the dye will appear in nasal secretions. Fluoracaine is administered intravenously as an aid in retinal angiography to identify retinal defects.

Fluoracaine, a combination of fluorescein and a local anesthetic, is used to facilitate removal of foreign bodies from the eye. One drop of a 0.25-percent solution is used.

OCULAR ANESTHETICS

- ❒ Proparacaine (ALCAINE, OPHTHETIC); (🍁) DIOCAINE
- ❒ Tetracaine (PONTOCAINE); (🍁) MINIMS TETRACAINE

Because the cornea and conjunctiva contain delicate sensory nerves, surgery and some diagnostic procedures involving the eye would be impossible without anesthetics. Local anesthetics are particularly helpful when general anesthesia is considered unnecessary or unduly risky. Ocular anesthetics are also used for foreign body and suture removal, for conjunctival or corneal scraping, and for lacrimal canal manipulation. Ocular drugs anesthetize the corneal surface so that tonometry measurements can be taken. The usual dose is one to two drops into the conjunctival sac every hour during the day, and every 2 hours at night as needed (see Chapter 16 for information about other local anesthetics).

Proparacaine and tetracaine act by stabilizing neurons so they are less permeable to ions, thus interfering with cell activity. Additional drops may be required to anesthetize an inflamed eye because the vasculature carries the anesthetic away. Systemic adverse effects can occur if the ocular anesthetic is absorbed through the nasolacrimal system.

The ocular anesthetics can cause transient eye pain and redness. Prolonged use can cause loss of visual acuity, keratitis, scarring, corneal opacities, and delayed corneal healing. They should be used with caution and the patient told not to rub the eyes, explaining that corneal abrasion may occur because the usual signal for pain is absent. A protective eye patch should be worn while the eye is anesthetized.

The only significant drug-drug interaction involves tetracaine. Because it interferes with the antibacterial action of sulfonamides, it should be administered 30 minutes apart from the tetracaine.

LUBRICANTS

- ❒ Sodium chloride (ADSORBONAC, MURO 128)
- ❒ Polyvinyl alcohol (HYPOTEARS)
- ❒ Petrolatum and mineral oil (LACRI-LUBE)
- ❒ Petrolatum, mineral oil, and lanolin (DURATEARS NATURALE)

The availability of synthetic chemicals appropriate for topical ocular use has resulted in the development of various solutions that help alleviate dry eyes. The use of water-soluble polymer solutions and bland, nonmedicated ointments remains the primary therapy. Because almost all of these products are available without a prescription, the health care provider and pharmacist often carry the primary responsibility to assist and counsel the patient regarding their selection and proper use. Although the purpose of ocular lubricants is to increase the viscosity of existing tears, it must be noted that high viscosity alone does not necessarily provide relief for all dry eye conditions.

Perhaps the most important property of the cellulose ethers in artificial tear formulations is that they stabilize the tear film and prevent tear evaporation. Beneficial effects generally occur without irritation or toxicity to ocular tissues. Clinical results and patient acceptance remain the final criteria for determining efficacy of treatment of dry eyes. It must be emphasized that no single formulation has yet been identified that will universally improve clinical signs and symptoms while maintaining patient comfort and acceptance.

IRRIGANTS

Extraocular irrigating solutions (e.g., physiologic saline) are used to clear away unwanted materials or debris from the ocular surface while maintaining moisture. One of the most useful applications of extraocular irrigants is in ocular lavage following chemical injuries to the eyes. Penetrating chemicals, such as alkalis, must be washed out immediately. Although the ideal irrigating solution for this purpose is physiologic saline, water may be the only available, practical solution, and it can be used when no commercial ocular irrigant is available. In emergency situations involving alkali or acid burns, prompt professional evaluation and treatment by an ophthalmologist is required.

Ocular irrigants are used on a short-term basis only. They are not to be used for open wounds in or near the eyes. All ophthalmic irrigating solutions are available without a prescription and can be used by patients and health care providers alike.

Ocular irrigants should not be administered with a contact lens in place because the solutions tend to cause contact lens irritation by reducing the mucin component of the tear film or, in the case of rigid gas permeable lenses, by reducing the hydrophilicity of the lens surface. Further, absorption of the preservatives contained in the irrigant by a soft contact lens can have an adverse effect on the corneal epithelium. Although irrigating solutions may be used to wash out the eyes after contact lens wear, they have no particular value as contact lens wetting, cleansing, or cushioning solutions.

CONTACT LENS PRODUCTS

Annual sales of contact lens care products exceed $400 million in pharmacies and $900 million overall. More than 200 nonprescription contact lens care products are available. Product selection depends on products' compatibility with each other as well as with the specific contact lens (i.e., conventional hard lenses, soft contact lenses, or rigid gas permeable lenses).

The basic considerations for a well-formulated contact lens solution include pH, viscosity, isotonicity with tears, stability, sterility, and provision for maintenance of sterility (bacteriocidal action). The pH comfort range is not well defined because the pH of tears varies. The normal pH of the eye is 7.4. It is best to have a weakly buffered solution that can readily adjust to any tear pH because highly buffered solutions cause significant discomfort and, in some cases, ocular damage. However, stability of the solution components takes precedence over comfort.

The potential for bacterial contamination of contact lens solution is great because of the daily use of the solution. Depending on the specific lens care procedure, a single container of solution may last for a month or more. Therefore, the solution must contain a bacteriocidal agent that is both effective over the long term and nonirritating with daily use. Commonly used antibacterial agents include benzalkonium chloride, thimerosal, and sorbic acid, all of which cause irritation, depending on the concentration and patient sensitivity.

Many adverse effects have been reported when a patient who wears contact lens ingests or topically applies certain drugs (Table 62–4). The pharmacologic effects of certain topically administered drugs may be enhanced when soft lenses are in place. The soft lens absorbs the drug and releases it over time, thus creating a sustained-release dosage form. Drug effects may be decreased because the lens absorbs the drug and binds it so that it is released into the eye. Further, contact time of the drug with the eye is increased regardless of the type of contact lens. Finally, increased drug absorption may occur secondary to compromised corneal epithelium that is present during contact lens wear. Further, the preservatives, vehicles, tonicity, and pH of the solution could alter the lenses. For example, hypertonic solutions such as 10 percent sodium sulfacetamide or 8 percent pilocarpine may cause soft lens dehydration and lens disfigurement.

Drugs with an acidic pH promote lens dehydration and steepening, whereas alkaline drugs promote hydration and flattening. Topical suspensions can cause a buildup of particulate matter, leading to discomfort and lens intolerance. Gel and oil formulations alter the relationship between the contact lens and the surface of the cornea. Finally, the active ingredient of certain topical products such as epinephrine may discolor lenses.

Some systemic drugs are secreted into the tears and may interact with contact lenses. For example, the antimicrobial drug rifampin stains the lenses and tears orange. Gold salts are secreted into the tears and may cause ocular irritation. Other drugs may affect tear production, the refractive properties of the eye, the shape of the cornea, or the actual lens of the eye.

In general, patients should be advised to avoid any ocular solution or ointment when contact lenses are in place. The only exceptions to this rule are products that are specifically formulated to be used with contact lenses.

TABLE 62–4 DRUG-CONTACT LENS INTERACTIONS

Drug/Drug Group	Effect on Contact Lens
Anticholinergics Antihistamines Diuretics Timolol Tricyclic antidepressants	Tear volume decreased
Cholinergics Reserpine	Tear volume increased
Diagnostic dyes Phenothiazines Epinephrine (topical) Phenylephrine Fluorescein (topical) Rifampin Nicotine Nitrofurantoin Sulfasalazine Phenazopyridine Tetracycline Tetrahydrozoline (topical)	Color changes in lens
Pilocarpine (8%) Sulfacetamide (10%)	Changes in tonicity of lens
Chlorthalidone Oral contraceptives Clomiphene Primodone	Lid or corneal edema
Gold salts Isotretinoin Salicylates	Ocular inflammation/irritation
Acetazolamide Sulfadizine Sulfamethizole Sulfosoxazole	Induction of myopia
Digoxin (increased glare) Ribavarin (cloudy lens)	Miscellaneous

Adapted from Engle, J. (1990). Contact lens care. *American Druggist*, January, 54–65. Used with permission.

Critical Thinking Process

Assessment

History of Present Illness

The most common chief eye complaint is often a change or loss of vision, but the effects may also be less specific, such as headache or eyestrain. Symptoms can often be divided into problems that affect appearance, vision, and sensation. Furthermore, it is not unusual for the patient to be unable to verbalize a specific complaint. Therefore, elicit information regarding the onset, location, duration, and characteristics (such as frequency and severity) of the symptoms. Determine whether there have been abnormal sensations such as itching, burning, or pain noted. The circumstances surrounding the onset of symptoms are important, as well as the patient's response to any treatment.

The drug history should include the current use of any drugs because many systemically administered drugs affect the eyes (Table 62–5). Ask if the patient uses eye drops or ointments, and note the name, dose, and dosage frequency. Determine whether over-the-counter eye preparations are used that may dry the eyes (e.g., antihistamines, decongestants). Determine whether the patient has ever had an allergic reaction to eye drugs or other reactions that affected the eyes.

TABLE 62–5 SYSTEMIC DRUGS PRODUCING OCULAR ADVERSE EFFECTS

Drug Category	Drug	Effect(s)
Adrenergics	Nasal decongestants	Reduced visual acuity, mydriasis, miosis, ocular palsies
	Reserpine	
Analgesics	Ibuprofen	Reduced visual acuity (rare), miosis
	Opioids (including pentazocine)	Miosis. With opioid withdrawal, irregular pupils, diplopia, paresis of accommodation, tearing
Antiarrhythmics	Amiodarone	Cataracts, keratopathy, optic neuritis, reduced visual acuity
	Quinidine	
Anticholinergics	Atropine	Cycloplegia, decreased accommodation, mydriasis, photophobia
	Idiclyclomine	
	Glycopyrrolate	
	Propantheline	
	Scopolamine	
	Trihexyphenidyl	
Anticoagulants	Heparin	Retinal hemorrhage
	Warfarin	
Anticonvulsants	Carbamazepine	Blurred vision, diplopia
	Phenytoin	Cataracts, nystagmus
	Trimethadione	Visual glare
Anesthetics	Propofol	Inability to open eyes
Antidepressants	Tricyclic antidepressants	Cycloplegia, mydriasis (most common)
	Fluoxetine	Eye tics (paroxysmal contractions of lateral eye muscles)
Antidiabetic drugs	Chlorpropamide	Mydriasis, optic neuritis, diplopia, conjuntivitis
Antihistamines	Chlorpheniramine	Blurred vision, decreased lacrimal secretions, mydriasis
Antihypertensives	Clonidine	Dry, itchy eyes, miosis
	Diazoxide	Lacrimation
	Guanethidine	Blurred vision, miosis, conjunctivitis, ptosis
	Reserpine	Conjunctivitis, miosis
Anti-inflammatory drugs	Gold salts	Corneal deposits, conjunctivitis, conjunctival deposits, nystagmus
	Indomethacin	Reduced visual acuity, oculogyric crisis, color vision disturbances, change in tear quality
	Phenylbutazone	Conjunctivitis, reduced visual acuity, retinal hemorrhage, optic neuritis, corneal erosions
	Salicylates	Retinal hemorrhages, mydriasis, conjunctivitis, optic neuritis, nystagmus
	Chloroquine	Ptosis, pigment changes, optic atrophy
Antilipemic drugs	Lovastatin	Cataracts
Antimicrobial drugs	Amantadine	Corneal lesions
	Chloramphenicol	Optic neuritis, changes in visual acuity
	Chloroquine	Corneal deposits, macular degeneration
	Ethambutol	Retrobulbar neuritis
	Gentamicin	Pseudotumor cerebri (rare)
	Isoniazid	Optic neuritis
	Nalidixic acid	Brightly colored appearance of objects
	Sulfonamides	Conjunctivitis, myopia, optic neuritis, nystagmus, photosensitivity
	Streptomycin	Optic neuritis
	Quinine	Diplopia
	Piperazine	Reduced visual acuity
	Ethionamide	Optic neuritis
	Tetracyclines	Myopia (rare, transient), papilledema
Antineoplastic drugs	Busulfan	Cataracts
	Carmustine	Arterial narrowing Intraretinal hemorrhages Nerve fiber layer infarcts
	Cytarabine	Blurred vision, keratoconjunctivitis, ocular burning, photophobia
	Doxorubicin	Conjunctivitis, excessive tearing
	Fluorouracil	Lacrimation, ocular irritation
	Tamoxifen	Corneal opacities, reduced visual acuity, retinopathy
	Vinca alkaloids	Extraocular muscle paresis, ptosis
Antiparkinson drugs	Levodopa	Mydriasis
Barbiturates	All	Ptosis, mydriasis, nystagmus, diplopia, conjunctivitis
Biologic response modifiers	Interlukin-2	Diplopia, palinopsia, scotomata
Benzodiazepines	Diazepam	Reduced visual acuity, nystagmus, diplopia
Calcium channel blockers	All	Blurred vision, transient blindness
Cardiac glycosides	Digitalis	Altered color vision, acuity
Cholinergics	Neostigmine	Ptosis, nystagmus
CNS depressants	Cannabis	Vision changes, diplopia
CNS stimulants	Amphetamines	Vision changes, mydriasis, oculogyric crises
Diuretics	Carbonic anhydrase inhibitors	Myopia
	Thiazides	

TABLE 62–5 SYSTEMIC DRUGS PRODUCING OCULAR ADVERSE EFFECTS *Continued*

Drug Category	Drug	Effect(s)
Hormones	ACTH	Papilledema
	Clomiphene	Blurred vision, mydriasis, visual field changes, visual sensations
	Oral contraceptives	Optic neuritis, pseudotumor cerebri, retrobulbar neuritis
Phenothiazines	Chlorpromazine	Lens deposits, retinal pigment deposits
	Prochlorperazine	Vision changes, oculogyric crises
	Thioridazine	Pigmentary retinopathy
Sedative Hypnotics	Chloral hydrate	Diplopia, conjunctivitis
	Ethchlorvynol	Optic neuritis, nystagmus
	Haloperidol	Vision changes, mydriasis, oculogyric crises
	Trilafon	Oculogyric crisis, optic neuritis
	Thioridazine	Vision changes, mydriasis
	Mellaril	
Uricosurics	Allopurinol	Cataracts; macular lesions (rare)
Others	Vitamin A	Nystagmus, diplopia, ocular palsies, papilledema, exophthalmia
	Vitamin D	Calcium deposits
	Nicotinic acid	Optic neuritis
	Chlorambucil	Papilledema
	Antihistamines	Miosis, vision changes, photophobia, reduced lacrimation

ACTH, Adrenocorticotropic hormone; CNS, central nervous system.

The most common ocular disorder is a red eye. It may be caused by minor irritation, inflammatory disorders or infection, allergy, vascular congestion, subconjunctival hemorrhage, and trauma. Changes in the external appearance may include abnormal positioning, lesions, redness, and edema.

Visual changes may be related to eye abnormalities and problems along the visual pathway. Patient complaints often include glare or halos resulting from scratches on the lens of glasses, uncorrected refractive errors, dilated pupils, corneal edema, or cataracts. "Floaters" in the field of vision may represent inflammatory cells, blood cells, pigment, or strands in the vitreous. The patient may complain of double vision in one or both eyes that may be due to refractive errors, muscle imbalance, or neuromuscular disorders.

Patient descriptions of abnormal sensations include eyestrain, pressure, or fullness; a pulling; or generalized headache. The location of the abnormal sensation may be described as behind the eye (retrobulbar), within the eye, or surrounding the eye (periocular). Deep internal aching may suggest inflammation or infection, muscle spasm, or glaucoma. Spasm of the ciliary muscle and the sphincter of the iris appears with inflammation and results in browache and photophobia or miosis. Itching is ordinarily a sign of allergy. Dryness, burning, or a sensation of a foreign object in the eye can occur with mild corneal irrigation or dry eyes. Tearing can be due to irritation or an abnormality of the lacrimal ducts. Infections, noninfectious irritations, and allergic reactions may manifest as complaints of increased ocular secretions.

Past Health History

The past health history focuses on the patient's general state of health. Ask specifically about chronic, systemic disorders that are commonly associated with eye disorders (e.g., diabetes, arthritis, hypertension, thyroid disease). Inquire about childhood illnesses and immunizations, particularly about rubella (measles).

If glasses or contact lenses are currently worn, ask when the last eye exam was performed and when the prescription was last changed. Determine whether the patient has had eye (e.g. laser treatments) or brain surgery.

Many eye disorders have a familial predisposition; thus, it is important to inquire specifically about *myopia* (nearsightedness, near vision better than distant vision), *hyperopia* (farsightedness, far vision better than near vision), glaucoma, and strabismus. Other common familial disorders affecting the eyes include macular degeneration, migraines, sickle cell anemia, retinitis pigmentosa, and retinoblastoma.

Physical Exam Findings

Assess the patient with an eye disorder for redness, swelling, tearing, discharge, and decreased visual acuity. The external exam includes the eyebrows, lashes, lids, lacrimal apparatus, anterior portion of the eyes, pupils, sclera, conjunctiva, cornea, and irises. Symmetry and alignment should be noted. Hair loss over the lateral aspects of the eyebrows occurs with aging and is considered normal. Also, in the older adult, a thin, white ring around the edge of the cornea may be seen *(arcus senilis)* and is also considered a normal change of aging.

Tests for ocular motility, corneal light reflex (Hirschberg's test), cover-uncover test, visual acuity, and visual fields should be completed. It is important to remember that while an abnormal acuity suggests an uncorrected refractive error or pathologic process, normal acuity does not exclude disease or disorder of the visual system. Further, patients who wear contact lenses may not respond to the corneal reflex test to the same degree as patients who do not wear them because they become somewhat insensitive to the stimulus. Internal eye structures are visible only through direct and indirect funduscopic exams.

The patient's physical features should be observed for age and any obvious deformities. For example, hand deformities and abnormal gait may provide a clue to the diagnosis of associated eye disorders such as *Sjögren's syndrome* (i.e., rheumatoid arthritis, xerostomia, and keratoconjunctivitis sicca).

Diagnostic Testing

For the patient with glaucoma, a tonometry reading reflects increased IOP. Aqueous humor maintains the shape of the eye with a relatively uniform pressure within the globe. As pressure increases, the eye becomes firmer and a greater force is required to cause the same amount of indentation with the tonometer. Normal pressure is considered to be 15 ± 2.5 mmHg. The IOP should be measured at different times of day, because variations of as much as 10 mmHg or more may occur over a 24-hour period. The use of fluorescein staining and special lighting (Wood's lamp) can help identify corneal or conjunctival damage or the presence of a foreign body.

Developmental Considerations

Perinatal Just as with a nonpregnant individual, pregnant women may have visual disorders that require pharmacotherapy. The normal changes of pregnancy may alter visual acuity in some cases. Systemic absorption of ocular drugs should be considered when assessing the patient's signs and symptoms. The woman should be questioned about visual blurring or changes, or scotomata. The results of the funduscopic exam should be recorded on the patient's record.

The elevated blood sugar levels that accompany gestational diabetes may cause alterations in vision. The woman's blood sugar should be checked at the appropriate time during the three gestational periods. A hypertensive crisis can also alter vision; thus, the woman's blood pressure should be monitored regularly and a record maintained.

Pediatric Few studies of ophthalmic drug use in children have been reported. Further, the conditions for which adults need therapy (e.g., glaucoma, cataracts) rarely occur in children. However, glaucoma may be present at birth, even though 50 percent of affected infants have symptoms that may not be readily apparent. Symptoms usually develop during the first year of life. In about 40 percent of cases, the IOP is elevated in the fetus, and the infant is born with ocular enlargement. Both eyes are affected in about 75 percent of the infants, but the severity of the disorder varies.

Geriatric The incidence of cataracts, dry eye, retinal detachment, glaucoma, *entropion,* and *ectropion* increases with age. *Ptosis* may also occur with aging but also results from edema, disorders of the third cranial nerve, and neuromuscular disorders. Older adults are at risk for ocular disorders, especially glaucoma and cataracts. They are also more likely to have cardiovascular disorders that can be aggravated by systemic absorption of topical eye drugs. The principles of drug therapy are the same as those for young adults, however.

Psychosocial Considerations

When assessing the patient with an eye disorder, factors that influence ocular health should be noted as well as health management behaviors. Questions about the nature of the patient's work include information about exposure to irritating fumes, smoke, or airborne particles. The use of safety goggles or protective eyewear when engaging in sports activities (e.g., racquetball, baseball, contact sports), a problem of sufficient lighting, or glare in the workplace should be noted. If contact lenses are worn, are the lenses cared for correctly and regularly, and are they stored as recommended? If the patient has a chronic disease, does the patient actively manage the disease?

Because the level of independence varies with the individual eye disorder, information supplied by the patient or family helps to determine how much help may be needed with the activities of daily living. Referrals to home health care or social services for assistance with rehabilitation or finances may be needed in some cases. Planning for housekeeping and meal preparation, safety in the home environment (because of altered vision), transportation, and assistance with the eyes should be explored and documented.

It is important to note how the patient is coping with chronic alterations in vision. Although people adapt differently, patients usually experience stages of grief and loss and may be at any stage of the process. Loneliness may be a significant finding. Patients may be understandably anxious during physical exams because improvement has not occurred, or it may be found that vision loss has progressed (see Case Study—Glaucoma).

Analysis and Management

Treatment Objectives

The primary goal in the treatment of glaucoma is to facilitate the outflow of aqueous humor through the outflow channels, thus preventing damage to the ganglion cells and optic nerve fibers, and loss of visual field. The main treatment goals in the management of infection and inflammation are to reduce symptoms and to prevent recurrence of the disorder while minimizing adverse effects.

Treatment Options

Drug Variables

Ocular solutions are sterile, easily administered, and usually do not interfere with vision. The disadvantage is that the solutions are in contact with the eye for a short time. Ointments, on the other hand, are comfortable on administration and stay in contact with the eye for longer periods. The problem with ointments is that a film or haze tends to form over the eye that interferes with vision. They may also cause a higher incidence of contact dermatitis than solutions, and the majority are not sterile formulations. Ocular gels and ocuserts, the newer delivery systems, were developed to overcome the problems associated with conventional eye drops and ointments. The advantage to using ocuserts is their longer duration of action, which, in turn, increases patient compliance. Ocusert use also avoids the peak-and-valley responses that have been associated with solutions and ointments.

Treatment of glaucoma varies with the type of glaucoma and the presence of co-morbid conditions. Most patients are treated first with ocular beta blockers, then with epinephrine, pilocarpine, and anticholinesterase miotics, and finally with carbonic anhydrase inhibitors. However, drug selection for the patient with primary open-angle glaucoma largely depends on how well the patient tolerates adverse effects. If the first topical drug fails to reduce pressure sufficiently and noncompliance has been ruled out as a cause of treatment failure, substitution of another drug is recommended before proceeding to combination therapy. Laser trabeculoplasty is usually reserved for patients whose IOP has not been suffi-

Case Study Glaucoma

Patient History

History of Present Illness	LH is a 65-year-old black man who reports to the ophthalmologist today on referral from his primary care nurse practitioner. He has been complaining of eye pain; reduced visual acuity, particularly peripheral vision; and persistent headaches. He denies inflammation, itching, or discharge. He reports that the vision changes started about 6 weeks ago and have gotten progressively worse. He reports taking an OTC nonsteroidal anti-inflammatory drug for occasional arthritis pain and has no known drug allergies.
Past Health History	LH's history is unremarkable for cardiovascular, respiratory, or renal disease. His last eye exam was about 6 months ago when he had his last eyeglass prescription filled.
Physical Exam	Physical exam reveals white sclera, pink conjunctiva, without inflammation or discharge noted. Visual acuity 20/80 (large Snellen). Funduscopic exam unremarkable at this time—no AV nicking, papilledema, exudates.
Diagnostic Testing	Schiøtz tonometry value 21 mmHg (normal: 15 ± 2.5).
Developmental Considerations	Although a widower, LH is active in his church, driving the van for church activities.
Psychosocial Considerations	LH states he is "one of the luckies" who does not have a problem with systemic hypertension but participates in his community to increase awareness in his culture. "My vision just can't go now. I have too much to do."
Economic Factors	LH receives a small retirement check and is covered by both Medicare and FHP insurance. He wants his care to be cost effective and yet therapeutic without "draining the insurance."

Variables Influencing Decision

Treatment Objectives

- Facilitate outflow of aqueous humor, thus preventing damage to optic nerve and loss of visual field
- Reduce eye discomfort and headache

Drug Variables	*Drug Summary*	*Patient Variables*
Indications	Cholinergic miotics, anticholinesterase miotics, anticholinergics, adrenergics, carbonic anhydrase inhibitors, and osmotics are all appropriate for use with primary open-angle glaucoma. Beta blockers are efficacious, most commonly used, and usually considered standard of care.	LH's diagnosis is an early stage of primary open-angle glaucoma. This will become a decision point.
Pharmacodynamics	Ocular beta blockers decrease production of aqueous humor, thus decreasing volume	There is no patient variable that influences pharmacodynamics at this time.
Adverse Effects/ Contraindications	Ocular beta blockers produce fewer adverse effects than miotics and are better tolerated by patients in most cases. They can precipitate cardiorespiratory distress in susceptible individuals.	LH's cardiorespiratory history is negative. Although he has eye pain at this time and a headache, his condition may improve with the use of a beta blocker and reduction in pressure.
Pharmacokinetics	Ocular beta blockers relieve IOP for at least 12 hours. Timolol's effects persist for up to 24 hours.	There is no patient variable that influences pharmacokinetics at this time.

Case Study continued on following page

Case Study Glaucoma—cont'd

Drug Variables	*Drug Summary*	*Patient Variables*
Dosage Regimen	Timolol is dosed as one drop of 0.25% solution BID, as are most other ocular beta blockers, or as a once daily instillation of 1/4th inch 0.5% gel.	Consider once-daily gel formulation to promote compliance, reduce blurring, and maintain nocturnal IOP. BID treatment regimen may also meet treatment objectives but reduces likelihood of compliance.
Lab Considerations	Regular tonometry readings should be performed during treatment.	LH expresses willingness to keep follow-up appointments for tonometry measurements.
Cost Index*	Timolol: 2 Betaxolol: 3 Metipranolol: 1	Although metipranolol is the least expensive, LH wishes to the use most cost-effective drug.

Summary of Decision Points

- LH has been given a diagnosis of an early stage of primary open-angle glaucoma.
- Ocular beta blockers such as timolol are the standard of care in 70% of patients with this form of glaucoma.
- Consider once-daily gel formulation at HS to promote compliance, reduced blurring, and maintain nocturnal IOP within normal limits. BID treatment regimen may reduce likelihood of compliance.
- LH has no pre-existing cardiovascular condition and is not taking other drugs that may interact with timolol.
- LH wishes to be cost effective as well as therapeutic in his care

DRUGS TO BE USED

- Timolol 0.25% ointment, 1/4 inch to lower conjunctival sac at HS

*Cost Index:
1 = $ < 30/mo.
2 = $ 30–40/mo.
3 = $ 40–50/mo.
4 = $ 50–60/mo.
5 = $ > 60/mo.

AWP of 3, 5-mL containers of 0.25% timolol ointment to the affected eye twice daily for 3 months is approximately $31.
AWP of 2, 5-mL bottles of 0.25% betaxolol solution to affected eye twice daily for a 3 month regimen is approximately $40.
AWP of 2, 5-mL bottles of 0.3% metipranolol solution to affected eye twice daily for a 3 month regimen is approximately $25.

ciently lowered despite maximally tolerated therapy with an ocular miotic, beta blocker, epinephrine, and orally administered carbonic anhydrase inhibitor.

There is no rationale for combining drugs with similar pharmacologic action (e.g., a cholinergic miotic and an adrenergic). Further, it is thought that such combinations are likely to increase adverse effects.

Cholinergic Miotics and Anticholinesterase Miotics A cholinergic miotic historically has been the principal and initial drug used for chronic open-angle glaucoma; however, beta blockers are now preferred for initial therapy. Miotics should be avoided when iritis is present because they may aggravate the inflammatory process. Although miotics are beneficial in many forms of noninflammatory secondary glaucoma, they are not as effective when obstruction of the outflow channels is due to particulate matter (e.g., red blood cells, tumor cells, inflammatory cells).

If control of IOP is not achieved with optimal use of a cholinergic miotic such as pilocarpine, anticholinesterase drugs are usually prescribed as second-line therapy. However, these drugs have been associated with the formation of iris cysts. These may be prevented by the use of phenylephrine in combination with the anticholinesterase miotic.

Ocular Beta Blockers Timolol appears to be as effective as pilocarpine or epinephrine in lowering IOP in open-angle glaucoma, may be more efficacious in nocturnal control of IOP, and is often better tolerated. An abrupt rise in IOP may occur when timolol replaces other antiglaucoma drugs. Ocular hypotensive effects and the incidence of adverse effects are similar for both timolol and levobunolol. However, levobunolol is more expensive than timolol whether it is administered once or twice daily. The efficacy of betaxolol in decreasing IOP has been demonstrated, but the magnitude of the decrease may not be as great as with timolol. Betaxolol

(1 percent) has been shown to produce fewer cardiovascular adverse effects than 0.5 percent timolol. It is also better tolerated than timolol in patients with chronic airway limitation. It should be considered for use when topical beta blockers are indicated. Topical metipranolol appears to offer no advantage over timolol or levobunolol in the treatment of glaucoma, but like timolol, metipranolol reportedly produces corneal anesthesia. Metipranolol has been cited as the most cost-effective agent in treating primary open-angle glaucoma; however, the increased frequency of burning and stinging, as well as granulomatous anterior uveitis, may limit its use.

Metipranolol has been associated with a greater incidence of stinging or burning on administration than other ocular beta blockers, and it has also been associated with the development of granulomatous anterior uveitis. Significantly fewer patients report stinging and burning with carteolol than with timolol.

Adrenergics Dipivefrin's effect on IOP is slightly less than that of 2 percent epinephrine, but its mydriatic effect is comparable. Pharmacologically, timolol and epinephrine should be antagonistic. However, there appears to be evidence that there is a small additive effect when timolol and epinephrine are given concurrently. The small additive effect is probably a result of the secondary alpha effect of epinephrine on outflow after the beta receptors in the ciliary bodies have been blocked. Still, the partial additive effects of epinephrine and timolol may be worthwhile for some patients. In contrast to timolol, the outflow effects of adrenergic drugs appears to be preserved when they are used in combination with betaxolol.

Carbonic Anhydrase Inhibitors The adverse effects of carbonic anhydrase inhibitors have led to their withdrawal in more than 50 percent of patients. Thus, the development of topical formulations that would be effective in lower doses and cause fewer reactions is desirable. The investigational drugs MK-417 (sezolamide), and MK-927 (dorlazemide) are based on modifications of an ethoxzolamide-like structure. Dorlazemide is specific for carbonic anhydrase isoenzyme II, the isoenzyme present in ciliary processes. It is the most potent carbonic anhydrase inhibitor developed thus far. It is more active in lowering IOP in primary open-angle glaucoma and ocular hypertension, and it may be somewhat better tolerated than sezolamide. Dorzolamide is somewhat more active than sezolamide, with a peak mean IOP reduction of 26.2 percent and 22.5 percent for sezolamide. Because of the short duration of action of these compounds, topical application three times daily is recommended. Oral acetazolamide may have a more consistent pressure-lowering effect than methazolamide.

Osmotics Glycerine is probably safer than intravenously administered agents such as mannitol and urea, but it has a slower onset of action. Mannitol and urea are equally effective in reducing IOP and vitreous volume, but mannitol is more convenient to administer and less toxic. Orally administered glycerine and isosorbide are not as rapidly effective as intravenous agents but often are preferred because of their safety and convenience.

The systemic effects of dehydration that occur with the use of the intravenous osmotic drugs are less likely with glycerin than with the others. Isosorbide produces a more significant diuresis than glycerin, and catheterization may be necessary. Mannitol may be less likely than urea to penetrate ocular fluids in the presence of inflammation and, in this situation, would be more effective than urea.

Patient Variables

Special consideration should be given to treatment of open-angle glaucoma in patients with cataracts. A beta blocker or the adrenergic dipivefrin is usually preferred because miotics may further impair vision. In addition, the long-acting miotics may exacerbate cataracts and increase the risk of complications during or after cataract surgery. Furthermore, the prolonged use of miotics may lead to permanent miosis and thus interfere with the evaluation of the optic disc and macula.

Cholinergic Miotics Stronger concentrations of pilocarpine may be required in patients with dark irides, because topical miotics are less effective in heavily pigmented eyes. In patients older than 50 years of age who do not have cataracts, pilocarpine is better tolerated than other available miotics. Carbachol is sometimes substituted when resistance or tolerance develops to pilocarpine or when a slightly longer acting drug is needed.

Laser iridotomy or conventional iridotomy is the definitive treatment for primary closed-angle glaucoma. The IOP is usually lowered with drugs before these procedures. A combination of two or more agents, including osmotics, carbonic anhydrase inhibitor, ocular beta blockers, and adrenergics, is often used preoperatively. After surgery, any residual glaucoma is managed in a stepwise fashion with drug therapy, laser trabeculoplasty, and filtering surgery, as indicated.

Anticholinesterase Miotics The development of cataracts after long-term administration of anticholinesterase miotics has limited the usefulness of these drugs in glaucoma therapy. Although cataract formation has not been observed in children or young adults, the usefulness of these drugs in young patients with strabismus must be balanced against the possible risk that cataract development will be hastened later in life.

Ocular Beta Blockers Betaxolol may cause more local eye irritation than timolol. Although it is safer than a nonselective beta blocker, β_1 selectivity is not absolute and bronchospasm has occasionally occurred in patients with chronic airway limitation. Bradycardia, syncope, and sinus arrest are rare. Other adverse effects are similar to timolol.

The ability of metipranolol to reduce IOP is comparable to that of 0.5 percent timolol and 0.5 to 1 percent levobunolol. In combination therapy, metipranolol 0.1 and 2-percent pilocarpine produces a greater reduction in IOP in patients with open-angle glaucoma than either drug alone. In one study, the combination of pilocarpine and metipranolol stabilized IOP in up to 95 percent of patients whose glaucoma was inadequately controlled by previous antiglaucoma drugs.

Intervention

Administration

Assess for redness, swelling or other irritation, and systemic effects that were not present before treatment was started. Because drug containers of otic and ocular drugs are similar in appearance in many cases, only ocular formulations should be used. Otic and dermatologic drug formulations should not be used in the eye. Eye drops that have changed color or become cloudy should be discarded. Further, the use of eye cups is discouraged because of the potential for contamination and risk of spreading disease.

The normal healthy eye holds about 10 microliters of fluid. The average eye dropper delivers 25 to 50 microliters per drop. Thus, more than a capful is not useful. When more than one drop is to be administered, it is best to wait 5 minutes between drops. The wait ensures that the original drop is not rinsed away by the second or that the second drop is not diluted by the first.

Wash the hands thoroughly before administering ocular drugs. The patient should be instructed to tilt the head backward or to be in a lying position with the eye gazing upward. The lower lid is gently pulled down, and holding the dropper above the eye, the drop is placed inside the lower lid. The lid is released slowly. The patient should be instructed not to blink or rub the eye for approximately 30 seconds.

For adults with a strong blink reflex or for pediatric patients, the closed-eye technique can be used to administer eye drops. Have the patient lie down, place the drop on the inner canthus of the eyelid. Opening the lid causes the drops to fall into the eye by gravity.

Systemic absorption of eye drops can cause adverse reactions. Nasolacrimal occlusion is effective in decreasing drug loss through the nasolacrimal system into the posterior nasopharynx. The occlusion is accomplished by placing a finger over the inner canthus for a period of 3 to 5 minutes. This permits maximal drug effects while using lower concentrations and less frequent administrations.

When ointments are used for the first time, the first one-fourth inch should be squeezed out and discarded. To facilitate ointment flow, warm the container for a few minutes by holding it in the hand. Gently pull down the lower lid and place one-fourth to one-half inch of ointment inside the lower lid by gently squeezing the tube. Instruct the patient to close the eye for 1 to 2 minutes and roll the eye in all directions. The patient should be advised that temporary blurring may occur with the use of ointments. Remove excess ointment around the eye or ointment tube with tissue. Wait at least 5 minutes for drops and 10 minutes before using another drug if the patient is using more than one ocular agent.

Cholinergic Miotics and Anticholinesterase Miotics Cholinergic and anticholinesterase miotic solutions and ointment forms require frequent instillation. Frequent instillation decreases patient compliance. When possible, miotic solutions should be administered at bedtime to minimize blurring and interference with vision. The adverse effects of cholinergics are less severe, however, and occur less often than those produced by anticholinesterase drugs.

Carbonic Anhydrase Inhibitors When oral liquid acetazolamide is needed, crush the tablets and mix them with a highly flavored carbohydrate syrup such as raspberry, cherry, or chocolate. Tablets can also be softened in hot water and added to honey or syrup. Sustained-release capsules should not be opened or crushed.

Osmotics Topical osmotic solutions such as glycerin may cause pain and eye irritation. A topical local anesthetic is usually instilled shortly before administration of the topical osmotic. Do not give the patient hypotonic fluids following administration of an osmotic solution, because these fluids will cancel the osmotic effect of the osmotic.

Education

The patient with eye conditions (particularly glaucoma) associated with possible blindness often has high levels of anxiety. As a result, they may be unable to comprehend simple verbal administration instructions. Written instructions are helpful to ensure compliance. Patients should be encouraged to continue regular use of their drugs for effective treatment of glaucoma. Because chronic glaucoma is a silent disease, much like hypertension, there is little positive reinforcement to continue therapy. The only noticeable effects are the drug's adverse effects.

The patient who requires ocular drugs should be taught how to store and administer the preparation properly (see Appendix F). The label should be checked to be sure that the correct drug and concentration is used. Solutions that become cloudy or darkened should be discarded. Eye drugs should be stored as noted on the label. Some require refrigeration. Most preparations have a 3-month shelf-life once they are opened or to the end of the current illness. If the drug is stored past these times, it may become contaminated.

The patient should be taught to maintain the sterility of the drug as well as the dropper. The tube tip or dropper should not come in contact with anything else, including the skin. A dropper should be held with the tip pointing downward to prevent the drug from flowing into the dropper bulb. The container should be closed when it is not in use.

The patient should also be taught what adverse effects indicate a worsening of the condition as well as the signs of improvement. Specific instructions about what to do and whom to contact should be provided if adverse effects appear. Patients should be instructed when to contact the health care provider for follow-up and to avoid sharing their eye drugs with others. Other individuals requiring eye drugs should have their own supply. Ocular drugs should not be stopped without the knowledge of the health care provider.

Cholinergic Miotics and Anticholinesterase Miotics Patients taking cholinergic miotics or anticholinesterase miotics should be advised that they may have difficulty adjusting to changes in lighting. This problem can be particularly serious for the older adult patient because their adaptation abilities and visual acuity are often reduced. Nighttime can be especially dangerous. Advise the patient to use the drug at bedtime to minimize interference caused by blurring.

Because blurring and difficulty in focusing may occur, instruct the patient to avoid hazardous activities (e.g., driving, operating machinery). Anticholinesterase miotics can cause spasm of the blink reflex, which can be particularly annoying to some patients.

Ocular Beta Blockers A fall in blood pressure and pulse can occur due to concomitant blockade of beta receptors in the heart and vascular system. Therefore, all other beta-blocking drugs should be discontinued before using an ocular beta blocker, such as timolol. Frequent checks of blood pressure and pulse during the initial phase of therapy and later during maintenance are usually necessary. Further, a tendency toward tolerance has been noted with long-term beta-blocker therapy; therefore, periodic measurements of IOP are warranted.

Adrenergics The patient should also be advised to remove soft contact lenses before administering a miotic drug because of the possibility of staining.

Evaluation

When evaluating the effectiveness of IOP-lowering drugs, the IOP should be measured at different times during the day, because variations of as much as 10 mmHg or more may occur over a 24-hour period. In addition, the condition of the optic nerve and visual field status must be determined at least twice a year, or more frequently when indicated. The close monitoring is necessary to ensure that there is no further progressive damage from insufficient lowering of pressure, intermittent noncompliance, or other causes.

A reduction in inflammation, discharge, and discomfort should be noted. In some cases, the use of the drug (e.g., ocular antivirals) may need to continue for 5 to 7 days to prevent recurrence of the infection.

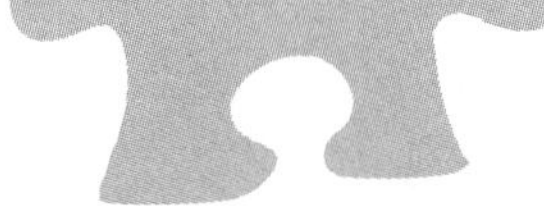

SUMMARY

- Eye disorders can occur at any age and can be due to a wide variety of causes. They are most often categorized as refractive disorders, infections or inflammatory conditions, and glaucoma.
- Five to ten million people in the United States have an elevated IOP, and at least 2 million have glaucoma. Fifty percent of those with glaucoma are unaware of its presence.
- Two to three percent of all ambulatory patients present with conjunctivitis, corneal abrasions and foreign bodies, subconjunctival hemorrhage, episcleritis or scleritis, keratitis, iritis, and acute closed-angle glaucoma.
- Viral conjunctivitis and allergic reactions are more common than bacterial conjunctivitis, which occurs in epidemics, most often in young adults.
- Bacterial conjunctivitis is seen in patients of all ages at any time of the year. It may also occur in an epidemic form known as "pink eye." Allergic conjunctivitis is sporadic and seasonal, occurring frequently in patients with a history of allergies during times of high pollen counts. Irritative conjunctivitis is most often caused by exposure to dust or smoke.
- Primary glaucomas are precipitated by intrinsic pathologic changes within the eye. Secondary forms are associated with other eye or systemic diseases.
- All forms of glaucoma result from interference with the outflow of aqueous humor from the anterior chamber.
- A drug history should include any medications in current use because many drugs affect the eyes.
- If glasses or contact lenses are currently worn, ask when the last eye exam was performed and when the prescription was last changed.
- Assess the patient with an eye disorder for redness, swelling, tearing, discharge, and decreased visual acuity. The external exam includes the eyebrows, lashes, lids, lacrimal apparatus, anterior portion of the eyes, pupils, sclera, conjunctiva, cornea, and irises. For the patient with glaucoma, a tonometry reading will reflect increased IOP.
- Older adults are at risk for ocular disorders, especially glaucoma and cataracts. They are also more likely to have cardiovascular disorders that can be aggravated by systemic absorption of topical eye drugs. The principles of drug therapy are the same as for young adults, however.
- The primary goal in the treatment of glaucoma is to facilitate the outflow of aqueous humor through the outflow channels, thus preventing loss of visual field.
- Treatment goals in the management of infection and inflammation are to reduce symptoms and to prevent recurrence of the disorder while minimizing adverse effects.
- Drugs that reduce IOP include adrenergics, carbonic anhydrase inhibitors, and osmotics. Drugs that constrict the pupil and reduce IOP in glaucoma and ocular hypertension include cholinergic miotics, anticholinesterase miotics, and ocular beta blockers.
- Mydriatics and cycloplegics are used primarily for intraocular exam and refractions. Some mydriatics are also used to treat open-angle glaucoma.
- Corticosteroids and NSAIDs reduce ocular edema, redness, and scarring.
- Antimicrobial drugs reduce infection caused by bacteria, viruses, and fungal organisms.
- Lubricants are used in the treatment of dry eye.
- Ocular drugs available for diagnostic purposes include rose bengal, fluorescein sodium, and fluorexon.
- Local anesthetics are especially helpful when general anesthesia is considered unnecessary or unduly risky, for use in foreign body and suture removal, for conjunctival or corneal scraping, and for lacrimal canal manipulation.
- The availability of lubricants for topical ocular use has resulted in alleviation of dry eyes. The use of water-soluble polymer solutions and bland, nonmedicated ointments remains the primary therapy.
- Extraocular irrigating solutions are used to clear away unwanted materials or debris from the ocular surface while maintaining their moisture. One of the most useful applications of extraocular irrigants is in ocular lavage following chemical injuries to the eyes.
- A variety of over-the-counter contact lens solutions and products exist. Product selection depends on the products' compatibility with each other as well as with the specific contact lens.
- The health care provider should teach the patient and family how to administer the prescribed ocular drug. Written instructions are helpful to ensure compliance with the treatment regimen.

BIBLIOGRAPHY

Ball, S., and Scheider, E. (1992). Cost of beta adrenergic receptor blocking agents for ocular hypertension. *Archives of Ophthalmology,* 110(5), 654–657.

Brooks, A., and Gilles, W. (1992). Ocular beta blockers in glaucoma management. *Drugs in Aging,* 2, 208–221.

Dabezies, O. (Ed.) (1992). *Contact lenses: The CLAO guide to basic science and clinical practice* (2nd ed.) Boston: Little, Brown.

Goa, K., and Chrisp, P. (1992). Ocular diclofenac: A review of its pharmacology and clinical use in cataract surgery, and potential in other inflammatory ocular conditions. *Drugs in Aging,* 2(6), 473–486.

Hurvitz, L., Kaufman, P., and Robin, A. (1991). New developments in the drug treatment of glaucoma. *Drugs,* 41(4), 514–532.

Katz, J., and Tielsch, J. (1996). Visual function and visual acuity in an urban adult population. *Journal of Visual Impairment and Blindness,* 90(5), 367.

Leibowitz, H., Ryan, W., and Kupferman, A. (1992). Comparative antiinflammatory efficacy of topical corticosteroids with low glaucoma-inducing potential. *Archives in Ophthalmology,* 110(1), 118–120.

Lembach, R. (1990). Rigid gas permeable contact lenses. *Journal of CLAO,* 16(2), 129–134.

Lippa, E., Schuman, J., and Higginbotham, E. (1991). MK-507 versus sezolamide: Comparative efficacy of two topically active carbonic anhydrase inhibitors. *Ophthalmology,* 98(3), 308–312.

Singh, K., and Zimmerman, T. (1995). Update on the status of topical beta blockers in the treatment of glaucoma. *Ophthalmology Clinics of North America,* 8(2), 295.

The Glaucoma Laser Trial Research Group. (1990). The glaucoma laser trial (GLT):2. Results of argon laser trabeculoplasty versus topical medicines. *Ophthalmology,* 97, 1403–1413.

Shedden, A. (1993). Multiclinic, double-masked study of 0.5% Timoptic XE once daily versus 0.5% Timoptic twice daily. *Ophthalmology,* 100, 111.

Sherwood, M. (1991). New topical treatments for glaucoma. *Ophthalmology Clinics of North America,* 4(4), 803.

Tielsch, J., Sommer, A., and Katz, J. (1991). Racial variations in the prevalence of primary open-angle glaucoma: The Baltimore Eye Survey. *Journal of the American Medical Association,* 266(3), 369–374.

Urtti, A., Rouhiainen, H., Kaila, T., et al. (1994). Controlled ocular timolol delivery: Systemic absorption and intraocular pressure effects in humans. *Pharmaceutical Research,* 11(9), 1278–1282.

Urtti, A., and Salminen, L. (1993). Drug delivery approaches to minimize systemic concentration of ocularly administered drugs. *Surveys in Ophthalmology,* 37(6), 435–456.

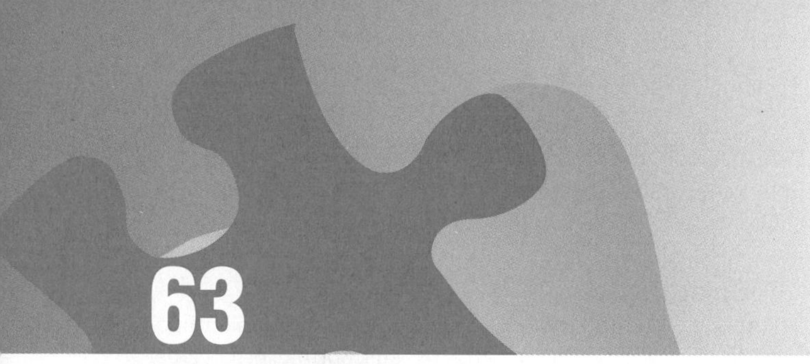

63

Otic Drugs

Treatment of middle and inner ear disease often requires oral or parenteral medications. External ear pathologies, however, depend on topical otic drugs administered locally to prevent or treat disorders. Otic drugs instilled directly into the external meatus of the ear include antibiotics, anti-infective agents, anti-inflammatory agents, anesthetics, drying drugs, and cerumen solvents. These drugs are used exclusively for their local actions, and direct administration allows distribution to all surface areas of the external canal. Many otic drugs are combinations of two or more agents and are primarily used to treat external ear infections, inflammation, pain, and the removal of excessive or impacted cerumen.

INFECTION

Epidemiology and Etiology

Infection of the external ear *(otitis externa)* is common when the integrity of the external canal is compromised, allowing invasion of pathogenic organisms into the tissue. Patients whose ears are frequently exposed to water due to swimming, bathing, or environmental factors are at greatest risk for alterations in the integrity of the skin tissue of the external ear. Additionally, patients who traumatize the skin with cotton swabs or other foreign objects inserted into the canal are at risk for development of an external ear infection. Pathogens causing external otitis include *Pseudomonas aeruginosa, Staphylococcus aureus, Escherichia coli, Proteus species,* and anaerobes.

Pathophysiology

Infection results in inflammation and pain. External canal structures become red, edematous and painful to even slight touch. Extensive swelling leads to a conductive type hearing loss due to obstruction of the canal. Fever, malaise, anorexia, and fatigue reflect signs of systemic involvement and require systemic therapy rather than topical preparations. Acute otitis media and infections of the inner ear require systemic antibiotic therapy to combat the organism effectively.

PHARMACOTHERAPEUTIC OPTIONS

Antibiotics

❒ Chloramphenicol otic (CHLOROMYCETIN OTIC); (🍁) Sopamycetin

Indications

Otic antibiotics are used in the treatment of external otitis, a superficial infection of the ear. Chloramphenicol otic is the prototype otic antibiotic that is most commonly used in the United States. In addition, otic antibiotics are sometimes prescribed in the treatment of chronic suppurative otitis media and otorrhea following tympanotomy tube insertion. Systemic antibiotics are used when the infection is extensive or resistant to antibiotic therapy. Relief of symptoms of external otitis occurs within a week of the initial use of topical antibiotics. Pain associated with external otitis is generally severe enough to ensure compliance with the therapeutic regimen. However, untreated external otitis can progress to necrotizing external otitis, resulting in an increase in both morbidity and mortality.

Pharmacodynamics

Otic antibiotics work via direct contact with the microorganism on the skin. They are not designed for systemic absorption. As a broad-spectrum antibiotic, chloramphenicol otic acts on both gram-negative and gram-positive organisms such as *S. aureus, E. coli, Haemophilus influenzae, P. aeruginosa, Aerobacter aerogenes, Klebsiella pneumoniae,* and *Proteus* species. It produces primarily bacteriostatic effects by inhibiting protein synthesis.

Adverse Effects and Contraindications

Contact dermatitis is the most common adverse effect of chloramphenicol otic. Itching, burning, angioneurotic edema (e.g., local wheals accompanied by swelling of subcutaneous tissue), urticaria, vesicular lesions, and maculopapular dermatitis are associated with contact dermatitis. Prolonged use can lead to an overgrowth of nonsusceptible organisms including fungi. Otic antibiotics are contraindicated in patients with a perforated tympanic membrane. Chloramphenicol otic is ototoxic if it enters the inner ear and round window.

Cautious use of otic antibiotics is warranted in pregnant or lactating women because otic antibiotics have not been studied in this group. They are probably safe because systemic absorption is negligible. Patients with known adverse reactions to kanamycin, paromomycin, streptomycin, or gentamicin should use chloramphenicol with caution.

Allergies to preservatives such as benzethonium chloride, sulfites, and thiomersal need to be considered because many otic preparations contain these products.

Pharmacokinetics

Typical pharmacokinetic properties do not apply to topical otic antibiotics. These drugs are not designed to be absorbed, biotransformed, or eliminated systemically. Absorption of otic antibiotics occurs only superficially through the otic tissue. The otic antibiotic must remain in direct contact with the infected otic tissue long enough to be effective. If

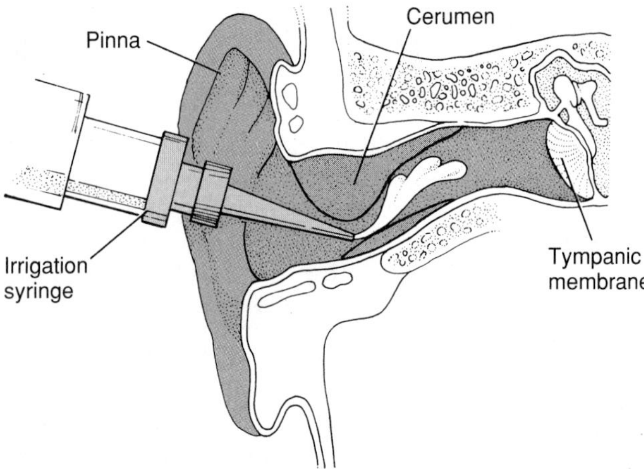

Figure 63–1 Irrigation of the external canal. A stream of warm water is directed above or below the blockage. This allows back pressure to push out cerumen and other debris rather than further impact the external canal. (From Ignatavicius, D. D., Workman, M. L., and Mishler, M. S. [1995]. *Medical-surgical nursing: A nursing process approach* [2nd ed., p. 1370]. Philadelphia: W. B. Saunders. Used with permission.)

possible, before administration of the otic antibiotic, all exudate, cerumen, debris, and other secretions should be removed from the canal via warm water irrigation (Fig. 63–1). Elimination is via evaporation, normal physiologic ear cleaning, and water irrigation.

Drug-Drug Interactions

Given the topical nature of otic preparations, the likelihood of drug-drug interactions are rare. On the contrary, topical otic anti-inflammatory and otic analgesic drugs are often used concurrently to alleviate ear discomfort. No known drug-drug interactions exist with chloramphenicol otic.

Dosage Regimen

The dosage for chloramphenicol otic is 2 to 3 drops administered to the effected ear three times daily (Table 63–1). Chloramphenicol should not be used for longer than 10 days.

Laboratory Considerations

The effectiveness of chloramphenicol is well documented, rarely requiring that exudate from the ear be cultured before administration. When otic therapy is ineffective and signs and symptoms of external ear infection continue, cultures and sensitivities may be taken to determine the infecting organism and the best drug for treatment.

Audiology testing with tympanometry may be performed to assess hearing and to determine movement potential of the tympanic membrane. It is most often performed with persistent infection or when the infection is thought to have affected the patient's hearing.

Antibacterial and Drying Agents

- ❐ Acetic acid (VOSOL)
- ❐ Acetic acid and Burow solution (OTIC DOMEBORO)
- ❐ Acetic acid and hydrocortisone (VOSOL HC)
- ❐ Boric acid and isopropyl alcohol (DRI/EAR, EAR-DRY, SWIM-EAR)

Indications

Antibacterial otic drops are used to treat superficial infections of the external ear caused by susceptible organisms. Drying drugs suppress the growth of organisms and help prevent recurrent ear canal infection. Drying drugs are used frequently by swimmers who have repeated ear infections.

Pharmacodynamics

Antibacterial and drying otic drugs contain either acetic or boric acid, astringents, weak antimicrobials (both antibacterial and antifungal), and isopropyl alcohol as a drying agent. The antibacterial drugs eliminate and prevent susceptible organisms from accumulating in the external ear canal via weak antimicrobial action and drying of the external ear canal tissue.

Adverse Effects and Contraindications

Adverse reactions include local irritation and contact dermatitis with burning, stinging, pruritus, tenderness, erythema, rash, urticaria, and edema. The external ear canal is observed closely for signs of local irritation or worsening of the pretreatment symptoms. Patients are instructed to discontinue use if irritation occurs and to call their health care provider. Antibacterial and drying drugs are not used when the tympanic membrane has been perforated. Allergies to preservatives such as benzethonium chloride, sulfites, and thiomersal need to be considered because many otic preparations contain these products.

Pharmacokinetics

Antibacterial and drying drugs are designed to be effective through direct contact with external ear canal tissue. Normal pharmacokinetics do not apply to otic antibacterial and drying drugs because they are not designed for absorption, distribution, or biotransformation. Drug elimination is through evaporation, normal physiologic ear cleaning, or water irrigation.

Dosage Regimen

Four to six drops of the antibacterial and drying solution are instilled into the external canal one to four times daily as needed (see Table 63–1).

INFLAMMATION AND PAIN

Epidemiology and Etiology

Structures of the external ear become inflamed for a variety of reasons including allergic reactions, trauma, and infection. Patients living in areas of high humidity or who engage in water activities are more likely to have problems with otic inflammation.

Pathophysiology

With inflammation, blood flow to the area increases, capillary permeability increases, and fluid flows into the effected tissues, producing edema and erythematous coloring.

TABLE 63–1 DOSAGE REGIMEN FOR SELECTED OTIC DRUGS

Drug	Use(s)	Dosage	Implications
Antibiotics			
Chloramphenicol 0.5% otic solution	For superficial external ear canal infections.	*Adult and child:* 2–3 drops TID	Do not use for more than 10 days. Consider supplementing with systemic antibiotics in all but superficial infections
Antibacterial and Drying Drugs			
Acetic acid 2% and Burow's solution	For superficial infections of the external ear canal.	*Adult and child:* 4–6 drops q2–3 hr as needed	Not to be used for extended periods
Boric acid and isopropyl alcohol	Suppression of growth of organisms to prevent recurrent ear canal irritation.	*Adult and child:* 5 drops TID–QID	
Acetic acid Acetic acid and hydrocortisone		*Adult and child:* 5 drops TID–QID	Clean ear prior to use. May substitute saturated cotton wick for 1st 24 hours
Steroids			
Desonide and acetic acid	Inflammation of external ear canal caused by infection or trauma.	*Adult and child:* 2–3 drops TID	Treatment period not to exceed 4 days
Dexamethasone sodium phosphate 0.1%	Steroid responsive inflammation of external canal	*Adult and child:* 3–4 drops BID–TID	May substitute saturated cotton wick moistened as needed. Replace in 12–24 hrs
Steroid-Antibiotic Combinations			
Hydrocortisone and neomycin sulfate-polymixin B	Infections of external auditory canal	*Adults:* 4 drops TID–QID *Child:* 3 drops TID–QID	Clean ear prior to use. Not to be used longer than 10 days. Reevaluate if no improvement in 7 days. Ototoxicity with prolonged use
Hydrocortisone-polymixin B	Infections of external auditory canal, fenestration cavities, mastoidectomy		
Hydrocortisone-neomycin sulfate	Susceptible infections of external auditory canal, fenestration cavities, mastoidectomy		
Otic Anesthetics			
Benzocaine	Analgesia in acute otitis media.	*Adult and child:* Fill ear canal	Use with caution if history of allergy to local anesthetics
Benzocaine and antipyrine	Analgesia in acute otitis media. Adjunct in cerumen removal	*Adult and child:* Fill ear canal. May repeat q1–2 hr PRN. Insert moistened cotton plug.	Treat infection with systemic antibiotics. Discard 6 months after dropper is put into solution.
Benzocaine, antipyrine, and phenylephrine	Analgesia in acute otitis media	*Adult and child:* Fill ear canal.	
Ceruminolytics			
Triethanolamine-polypeptide oleate-dondensate 10%	Cerumen removal	*Adult and child:* Fill the ear canal and let remain for 15–30 minutes. May repeat × 1 PRN	Irrigate repeatedly with warm water.
Carbamide peroxide 6.5%	Cerumen removal	*Adult and child:* 5–10 drops. May repeat 2 × daily for up to 4 days.	May irrigate with warm water.

As a sensory organ, the ear contains many sensory nerve fibers that, when inflamed, produce significant pain. Thus, drug therapy is designed to alleviate pain through either the reduction of inflammation or direct anesthetic effects.

PHARMACOTHERAPEUTIC OPTIONS

Steroid and Steroid-Antibiotic Combinations

- ❒ Desonide and acetic acid (TRIDESILON)
- ❒ Dexamethasone sodium phosphate (DECADRON)
- ❒ Hydrocortisone and neomycin sulfate (✽) COLY-MYCIN SOTIC
- ❒ Hydrocortisone, neomycin sulfate, and polymyxin B (CORTISPORIN OTIC, DROTIC, EAR-EZE, LAZERSPORIN-C, OTOMYCIN-HPN, OTOSPORIN); (✽) CORTISPORIN
- ❒ Hydrocortisone and polymyxin B (OTOBIOTIC OTIC)

Indications

Inflammation of the external canal caused by infection or trauma leads to severe pain. Corticosteroids are given to reduce inflammation and control pain, either alone or in combination with an otic antibiotic and otic anesthetic. Hydrocortisone and dexamethasone are the most common corticosteroids used as otic drugs. The broad-spectrum antibiotic neomycin sulfate is used in combination with corticosteroids because of its bactericidal effect. Combinations of corticosteroids and antibiotics are used to treat superficial infections causing pain and inflammation. The corticosteroid helps alleviate discomfort, whereas the antibiotic treats the infection.

Pharmacodynamics

Steroid and steroid-antibiotic combinations are given to reduce dermal reactions to inflammation, edema, pruritus, and pain. Similar to other topical steroids, the exact mechanism of action is not fully understood. Topical steroids most likely act to decrease inflammation by suppressing the immune response. They require direct contact with the skin and are given for their local topical effect.

Adverse Effects and Contraindications

The most common adverse effects of steroid and steroid-antibiotic combinations are overgrowth of organisms, delayed healing, and contact dermatitis. Limiting the length of treatment to no more than 4 days helps prevent problems. Steroid and steroid-antibiotic combinations are contraindicated in patients with a perforated tympanic membrane, herpes simplex, vaccinia, and varicella. Cautious use of steroids and steroid-antibiotic combinations is warranted in pregnant or lactating women because neither type has been studied in this group.

Once again, allergies to preservatives such as benzethonium chloride, sulfites, and thiomersal need to be considered because many otic preparations contain these products.

Pharmacokinetics

Normal pharmacokinetics do not apply to steroids and steroid-antibiotic combinations because they are not designed for absorption, distribution, or biotransformation. Some drug may be absorbed unintentionally through the skin depending on the dosage, integrity of the skin, the length of use, and whether an occlusive dressing was used. The drugs are eliminated via evaporation, normal physiologic ear cleaning, and water irrigation. Little fear of interactions among otic steroids and other drugs exists unless the otic steroid is systemically absorbed.

Dosage Regimen

Two to three drops of solution are instilled into the external canal of the affected ear (see Table 63–1).

Laboratory Considerations

Rarely is the exudate from the ear cultured before administration of otic corticosteroids. When therapy is ineffective and signs and symptoms of external ear infection continue, cultures and sensitivities are taken to determine the infecting organism and the best drug for treatment.

Otic Anesthetics

- ❒ Benzocaine (AMERICAINE OTIC, OTOCAIN)
- ❒ Benzocaine-antipyrine (ALLERGEN EAR DROPS, AURALGAN OTIC, AUROTO OTIC, OTOCALM EAR); (🍁) AURALGAN
- ❒ Benzocaine, antipyrine, and phenylephrine (TYMPAGESIC)

Indications

Otic anesthetics contain benzocaine and are used for the relief of pain and pruritus associated with the acute congestion of serous otitis and external otitis. Otic anesthetics have no effect on microorganisms or inflammation.

Pharmacodynamics

Otic anesthetics temporarily stabilize the neuronal membranes to decrease membrane permeability to sodium ions. Depolarization of the neuronal membrane is inhibited, thereby blocking the initiation and conduction of nerve impulses and sensitivity to pain.

Adverse Effects and Contraindications

Otic anesthetics tend not to blanch the tympanic membrane or mask the otoscopic landmarks; however, benzocaine may mask the symptoms of fulminating infection of the middle ear if it is used indiscriminately. Rarely, methemoglobinemia may result from the use of otic benzocaine. Methemoglobinemia causes respiratory distress and cyanosis requiring treatment with intravenous methylene blue.

As with other otic drugs, anesthetics are not used in patients with a perforated tympanic membrane. No teratogenic studies have been conducted with pregnant women; hence, safety in pregnancy has not been established. Allergies to preservatives such as benzethonium chloride, sulfites, and thiomersal need to be considered because many otic drugs contain these products.

Pharmacokinetics

Much like the other otic drugs, to be effective, topical anesthetics must come in direct contact with ear tissue. Normal pharmacokinetics do not apply to cerumen solvents because they are not designed for absorption, distribution, or biotransformation.

Drug-Drug Interactions

Benzocaine antagonizes the antibacterial activity of sulfonamides and should not be administered together. When both benzocaine and sulfonamides must be used, the potential drug interaction is avoided if benzocaine preparations are instilled in the ear first to achieve anesthesia. The pooled benzocaine is then removed before the administration of the sulfonamide.

Dosage Regimen

Four to five drops are instilled into the external canal. The dosage may be repeated every 1 to 2 hours while severe pain persists (see Table 63–1).

CERUMEN IMPACTION

Epidemiology and Etiology

Cerumen, or ear wax, is a normal sebaceous gland secretion functioning to protect and lubricate the canal. The primary action of cerumen is to gather bacteria and debris for removal. Normally, when the external ear canal gets wet and drains, cerumen is eliminated. Various factors lead to decreased elimination of cerumen compared with production. When elimination is decreased, the cerumen may become impacted in the canal. The incidence of cerumen impaction is greater in the geriatric population.

Pathophysiology

Patients with cerumen impaction may have no symptoms or may complain of a sensation of fullness in the ear, with or without associated conductive hearing loss. Complaints of pain, itching, or bleeding from the ear may also be associated. Treatment requires removal of the impacted cerumen via warm water irrigation. If the impaction is resistant to irrigation, commercially prepared ceruminolytics can be used to soften the cerumen for ease of removal.

PHARMACOTHERAPEUTIC OPTIONS

Ceruminolytics

- Carbamide peroxide (AURO EAR DROPS, DEBROX ear drops, E-R-O EAR DROPS, MURINE EAR DROPS)
- Triethanolamine, polypeptide oleate, and condensate (CERUMENEX ear drops)

Indications

Ceruminolytic drugs help soften cerumen for removal. They are used for easy removal of cerumen without painful instrumentation with a metal curette. Cerumen removal is necessary for otoscopic examination, audiometry, and tympanometry and when the patient experiences discomfort or hearing loss from excessive or dry cerumen. Additionally, cerumen solvents provide antiseptic protection.

Pharmacodynamics

Ceruminolytics contain glycerin to soften cerumen and carbamide peroxide to loosen debris by effervescence of oxygen. They act to emulsify and disperse excess or impacted cerumen.

Adverse Effects and Contraindications

Ceruminolytics are irritating and may cause a severe eczematoid allergic reaction, especially with prolonged exposure. If the patient experiences excessive irritation, adequate softening of cerumen may often be achieved with plain anhydrous glycerin followed by flushing with plain warm water. The friability of older skin, especially of the external canal, may contribute to a greater incidence of contact dermatitis when used in the geriatric population.

Ceruminolytics are not used in patients with a perforated tympanic membrane. No teratogenic studies have been conducted with pregnant woman; hence, their safety in pregnancy has not been established. Allergies to preservatives such as benzethonium chloride, sulfites, and thiomersal need to be considered because many otic drugs contain these products.

Pharmacokinetics

Normal pharmacokinetics do not apply to cerumen solvents because they are not designed for absorption, distribution, or biotransformation. The drug is placed directly on the effected tissue and is then mechanically eliminated using warm water irrigation.

Dosage Regimen

Correct dosage requires filling of the ear canal with the drug while the patient's head is tilted at a 45-degree angle. Patients may use the ceruminolytic over a 2- to 3-day period to soften the cerumen (see Table 63–1). The drug is then used once every week or two to prevent recurrence.

OTOTOXICITY

When inner ear structures or the auditory nerve (cranial nerve VIII) are damaged by drug therapies, the drugs are considered *ototoxic*. Two areas of the inner ear are commonly affected by toxic substances, the cochlea and the vestibular system. Damage occurs as different structures are affected. A variety of mechanisms, including toxic levels of drugs in the perilymphatic fluid, may damage the hair cells in the organ of Corti. Additionally, drug therapy can change enzymatic activity in the inner ear, causing damage.

Topical and systemic drugs can be toxic, with ototoxicity resulting at therapeutic drug levels. The ototoxicity of topical otic drugs is primarily related to the drug coming into direct contact with the inner ear structures. Therefore, consequences of ototoxicity are lessened if the tympanic membrane is intact, thus preventing direct contact with the inner ear. Some controversy exists regarding the use of otic drugs in the treatment of chronic otitis media when the patient has a tympanic perforation.

Different categories of drugs that are known to be ototoxic include the aminoglycosides and other antibiotics, loop diuretics, antimalarial, nonsteroidal anti-inflammatory drugs, and some antineoplastic drugs. Specific substances and the area most commonly effected are found in Table 63–2. Unfortunately, neomycin, a highly ototoxic agent, is commonly found in topical otic drugs. Assessment for an intact tympanic membrane is essential before the administration of any otic preparation containing neomycin.

Symptoms of ototoxicity depend on the inner ear structure that is most effected. Tinnitus and sensorineural hearing loss are present with damage to the cochlea. Damage to the vestibular apparatus produces vertigo, ataxia, lightheadedness, headache, giddiness, inability to focus or fixate on images, nausea, vomiting, and cold sweats. Factors such as dosage, renal function, concomitant use of other ototoxic chemicals, inherent susceptibility, age, and exposure to high-intensity noise impact the ototoxic effects of different drugs.

Effects on hearing loss secondary to ototoxic drugs can be transient or permanent, unilateral or bilateral, and dose related or non–dose related. In addition to auditory function tests, monitoring of renal function is essential in patients who are being treated with ototoxic drugs. Renal function tests are indicators of drug and drug-by-product clearance. Ototoxicity is increased with decreased renal function. Older patients are especially prone to developing ototoxicity because of a normal age-related decline in renal function.

TABLE 63–2 IMPACT OF OTOTOXIC SUBSTANCES ON AUDITORY AND VESTIBULAR FUNCTION

Drug	Auditory Problems	Vestibular Problems
Antibiotics		
Amikacin	++	+
Chloramphenicol	+to++	+
Erythromycin	+to++	+
Gentamicin	++	+
Kanamycin	++	+
Neomycin	++	+
Streptomycin	++	+
Tobramycin	++	+
Vancomycin	++	+
Diuretics		
Acetazolamide	+	+
Ethacrynic acid	++	+
Furosemide	++	+
Nonsteroidal Anti-Inflammatory Agents		
Ibuprofen	+	
Indomethacin	+	+
Naproxen	+	
Salicylates	++	
Other Drugs		
Alcohol		++
Cisplatine	+	+
Nitrogen mustard	+	+
Quinine	+	++
Quinidine	+	++

+, Slight; ++, significant.

Adapted from Ignatavicius, D. D., Workman, M. L., and Mishler, M. S. (1995). Medical-surgical nursing: A nursing process approach (2nd ed., p. 1356). Philadelphia: W. B. Saunders. Used with permission.

Critical Thinking Process

Assessment

Assessment of past and current health history with a physical examination is necessary before the administration of otic drugs. Follow-up assessments are performed to determine the effectiveness of the drugs administered.

History of Present Illness

Patients with ear disorders require a comprehensive nursing history to determine problems, goals, and interventions that are appropriate for treatment. The health care provider queries the patient for a review of the present illness, including bathing and swimming behaviors, recent trauma to the ear or head, and any changes in hygiene activities, or products used in or around the ears. In addition, the health care provider specifically inquires about the use of over-the-counter or prescription drugs the patient is currently taking. Complaints of malaise, anorexia, and fatigue are noted.

Past Health History

A past health history summarizing the patient's overall health should be completed. The health care provider determines whether the female patient is pregnant or lactating. Few of the otic preparations have been studied in this population and are used only with caution. In addition, the dates and results of any audiometric or tympanography testing are documented.

Substances causing irritation to the skin are discussed with the patient. Allergies to drugs, foods, preservatives (e.g., benzethonium chloride, thimerosal, and sulfites), and hygiene products used in or near the ear should be elicited from the patient.

Concomitant diseases such as upper respiratory tract infections, head injury, and neurologic disorders should be identified. Otic disorders and cerumen impaction may cause hearing loss, dizziness, and ataxia similar to those caused by some severe neurologic disorders.

Physical Exam Findings

The ear exam begins with an inspection and palpation of the external ear and mastoid, followed by an otoscopic visualization. Finally, signs of systemic infection such as fever are noted. Cerumen impaction is evident when the entire length of the external canal and the tympanic membrane cannot be visualized.

Diagnostic Testing

Discharge from the external ear is rarely cultured. However, a culture and sensitivity test is performed in cases in which the initial therapy fails to produce a response. Additionally, audiometry testing with tympanometry is performed to assess hearing and to determine movement potential of the tympanic membrane.

Should the health care provider suspect that inflammation and pain is associated with a systemic disorder, laboratory testing may include a complete blood count and sedimentation rate. Allergy testing is used to determine substances that are irritating to particular patients.

Developmental Considerations

Perinatal As a general rule, the incidence of otic disorders in the pregnant woman are no greater than that of the general population. However, systemic antibiotics should be used with caution because some of the drugs are teratogenic in nature. For example, chloramphenicol readily crosses the placental membranes and may produce gray baby syndrome (i.e., fetal abdominal distention, drowsiness, low body temperature, cyanosis, hypotension, and respiratory distress). Any otic drug that is absorbed systemically has teratogenic potential, although otic drugs are not appreciably absorbed systemically.

Pediatric Children are more susceptible to disorders of the middle ear than to external otitis because of their relatively straight and short eustachian tube. The eustachian tube can easily be blocked by the adenoid tissue in the nasopharynx, especially in conjunction with upper respiratory tract infections. The straight, short external canal of childhood makes children less susceptible to cerumen impaction than adults.

Generally, children who are diagnosed with otitis media are treated with systemic antibiotics. Most otic preparations are not recommended for use in infants younger than 1 year of age because of the danger of potential systemic absorption. Systemic absorption may hinder the normal development of infants.

In addition, infants who feed from a bottle while lying down are more likely to have pooling of fluids in their nasopharynx and eustachian tubes, resulting in a greater risk of serous otitis and otitis media. The most common use of otic drops in infants and children with serous otitis and otitis media is for the treatment of ear pain. Systemic antibiotic drugs are necessary to treat the otitis media.

Geriatric The friability of older skin, especially of the ear canal, may contribute to a greater incidence of contact dermatitis and systemic absorption of otic drugs. A stiffening of the cilia of the ear, combined with a higher keratin content of cerumen, causes cerumen to impact easily, decreasing the ability to hear. In addition, physiologic changes of aging may alter the presentation of an otic disorder, causing the disorder to be overlooked. The older patient should be monitored for adverse effects more frequently.

Psychosocial Considerations

Sleeping patterns are often disrupted by ear disorders. Further, patients living in humid environments are more susceptible to ear infections. Prior diagnoses of an external otitis increase the risk of recurrence. Cerumen is naturally removed when the ear canal is washed out during showering. People who shower or wash their hair infrequently are more prone to cerumen impaction. Appropriate use of otic preparations just before bedtime may relieve discomfort and enhance sleeping patterns.

Handwashing and proper disposal of contaminated ear drainage may prevent spread to others. If the patient wears some form of ear device for employment (e.g., telephone ear piece or ear plugs), the devices should be kept clean and free of debris. Ear devices should not be shared with other workers.

Analysis and Management

Treatment Objectives

Treatment objectives include relieving ear pain, and reducing infection and inflammation. To prevent further episodes of external otitis, the use of otic drying drugs keep the external canal dry and less likely to support organism growth. When cerumen is the problem, the treatment objective is to soften and remove excessive cerumen from the external canal, decrease conductive hearing loss, and improve comfort.

Treatment Options

Drug Variables

The Federal Food and Drug Administration does not recommend the use of otic preparations in patients with a perforated tympanic membrane.

Only one otic antibiotic is available for otic use. All otic antibacterial and drying drugs, and steroid and steroid-antibiotic combinations have similar pharmacokinetics and pharmacodynamics. Steroids and anesthetics are used primarily for pain control and relief of inflammation. Patients with minimal to no pain do not require steroids or anesthetic otic drugs. When they are used, treatment is provided for only a limited time.

Patients who are noncompliant should not be given otic anesthetics, or they are given a very limited quantity. Prolonged use of anesthetics may mask the signs and symptoms of fulminating infection.

Several commercial preparations are available to soften cerumen. Anhydrous glycerine is very inexpensive and when used over several days can be as effective as other ceruminolytic products. The cost of different products varies but all are relatively inexpensive.

Patient Variables

Patients known to have skin sensitivity to any topical preparation should use ceruminolytics with caution to avoid possible skin irritation. Thorough teaching about alternate methods for cerumen removal and ways to prevent impaction is important.

Intervention

Administration

Otic drugs are instilled directly into the external canal. In cases in which the external auditory canal is obstructed with edema, an ear wick is devised from a small piece of gauze and inserted beyond the edematous portion of the canal toward the tympanic membrane (Fig. 63–2). Otic drops are applied to the outside portion of the gauze wick to be absorbed along the gauze into the depths of the canal. Because of the discomfort involved with insertion of an ear wick, the gauze need only be changed every 2 days. Generally, at the end of 2 days, edema in the canal has subsided and the otic drug is administered directly to the ear canal. Following administration, a cotton pledget is inserted into the canal to keep the solution from draining out.

Antibacterial and drying drugs are instilled in the external canal in a manner similar to that used for other otic drugs. Following use of these drugs, the ear canal is carefully dried with compressed air or a hair dryer on the cool or low-heat setting. The canal is not dried with a cotton swab. If cerumen has accumulated in the external canal, the cerumen debris is removed before the use of the antibacterial solution.

Dosages of ceruminolytics are measured in drops. The ear canal is liberally filled and the solution allowed to remain in

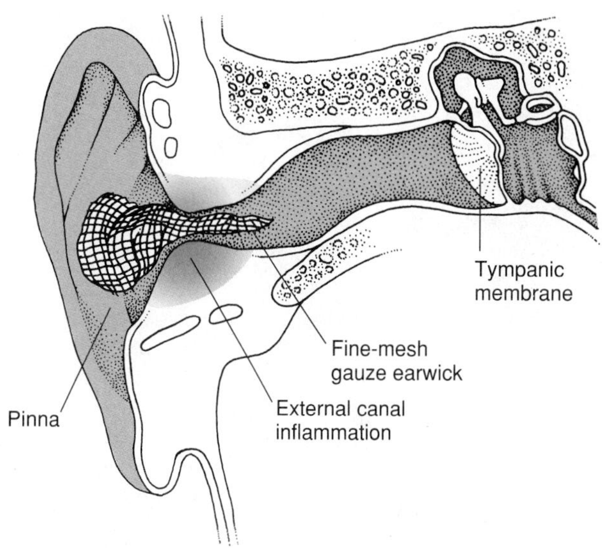

Figure 63–2 Earwick for instillation of antibiotics into the external canal. Otic solutions are placed on the external portion of the earwick to be absorbed through the canal. This is particularly helpful when the canal is blocked by edema. (From Ignatavicius, D. D., Workman, M. L., and Mishler, M. S. [1995]. *Medical-surgical nursing: A nursing process approach* [2nd ed., p. 1369]. Philadelphia: W. B. Saunders. Used with permission.)

Case Study External Otitis

Patient History

History of Present Illness	CC is an 8-year-old Hispanic female who is accompanied to the clinic by her mother. Approximately 3 days ago, CC began complaining of purulent green-yellow ear drainage from her right ear with associated pain and a feeling that her ear was "clogged up and itchy." Her mother has been giving her acetaminophen 325 mg BID for the persistent right ear pain, but there was no improvement. In addition, her mother has been filling the right ear with cotton to capture the drainage. At home her temperature has been 98.6° F orally. She denies complaints of anorexia, fatigue, and malaise. Her mother denies trauma to the ear, hearing loss, dizziness, and ataxia.
Past Health History	CC and her mother deny any prevous history of ear problems. She does not wear a hearing aid or any other device in her ears. CC's audiogram and tympanogram, performed last year in school, are reported as normal. CC is essentially well, with no known respiratory, skin irritation, or neurologic problems. She has no known allergies to medications, foods, preservatives, or hygiene products. CC takes no medications on a regular basis. Family history is noncontributory. She denies past problems with herpes simplex and vaccinia, and reports varicella at age 4.
Physical Exam	No complaints of pain with manipulation of the left pinna; right pinna manipulation elicits pain response. No tenderness over mastoid processes bilaterally. Left ear canal clean and clear. Right ear canal edematous and erythematous, with moderate amount of wet yellowish drainage. Otoscopic exam reveals left TM intact, pearly gray with no perforation. Right tympanic membrane unable to visualize entirety due to external ear canal swelling and tenderness. Portion of tympanic membrane visualized appears intact and noninflamed.
Diagnostic Testing	Will treat and have CC return to clinic for culture and sensitivities if nonresponsive after 3 days. Will consider audiometric and tympanometry only if problem persists.
Developmental Considerations	CC is in 2nd grade. Will need assistance with administration of otic drug. She and her mother will also need education regarding administration, care of items contaminated with otic discharge, and appropriate handwashing. School has a full-time school nurse.
Psychosocial Considerations	CC has been swimming daily at the local swimming pool. She uses a mild baby shampoo daily. No new shampoos or hair products have been used. Mother explains that CC has not been sleeping well the last few nights and was complaining of ear pain. Mother reports no special precautions taken with soiled ear materials and sporadic handwashing.
Economic Factors	CC and her mother live alone in a small house near the clinic. Ms. C. works full-time and has health insurance for CC. Ms. C. does not have a car and relies on walking for her transportation. The nearest discount pharmacy is about 2 miles away.

Variables Influencing Decision

Treatment Objectives	• Alleviate ear pain by reducing inflammation and providing direct anesthetic effect. • Prevent further episodes of external otitis through use of otic drying agents to keep external ear canal dry and less likely to support organism growth.

Drug Variables	*Drug Summary*	*Patient Variables*
Indications	Antibiotics: For treatment of superficial infections of external ear. Steroid/Steroid-Antibiotic: Inflammation of external canal caused by infection or trauma. Antibacterial/drying drug: Suppression of organism growth and prevention of recurrent external canal irritation. Anesthetics: For relief of pain and pruritus.	CC has edema and erythema right external canal with purulent drainage. She has a 3-day period of itching and pain.

Drug Variables	*Drug Summary*	*Patient Variables*
Adverse Effects/ Contraindications	Contact dermatitis with urticaria and burning (vesicular lesions, maculopapular lesions). Rarely, angioneurotic edema with local wheals, swelling of subcutaneous tissue. Ototoxic if enters inner ear. Contraindicated with perforated membrane.	CC has no known skin disorders, no known allergies. TM appears to be intact but not visible due to edema. She has no indication of middle ear infection, herpes simplex, vaccinia, or varicella. Mother denies use of OTC preparations.
Pharmacodynamics	Effects produced through direct contact with skin. Various otic agents work to treat and/or prevent different problems. Use of a single antibiotic agent versus a steroid-antibiotic combination agent is a decision point. Drugs within the same class have similar pharmacodynamics, and therefore, determining the particular drug within a class is not a decision point.	CC has edema and erythema in the right external canal with purulent drainage and a 3-day period of itching and pain. The decision is to use several otic agents to alleviate pain and inflammation, treat the infection, and prevent recurrence of the infection.
Dosage Regimen	Dosage regimen is based on health care provider information and recommended dosage for CC's size. Drying agents are administered in the morning and before bedtime. Use of anesthetic based on patient level of discomfort.	Mother will administer otic drops in the morning and evening. School nurse will administer midday dose if CC brings them to school. Mother and school nurse are reliable. No problems with compliance are expected. CC needs to remember to take ear drops to school and bring them home each day. Preferably, both mother and school nurse could have the otic agents. However, this may not be cost effective. This could be a decision point.
Lab Considerations	Rarely is exudate from the ear cultured before therapy. If signs and symptoms persist after treatment, culture and sensitivities may be performed to determine the infecting organism and the best agent for treatment. Audiometry testing with tympanometry may be performed to assess hearing and movement potential of TM with infection that persists.	This may be a decision point if CC's infection persists after her initial course of treatment.
Cost Index*	Hydrocortisone/neomycin/polymixin B: 1 Benzocaine: 1 Boric acid/isopropyl alcohol: 1	No one agent is more effective than another. Mother will purchase least expensive preparation.

Summary of Decision Points

- Dosage regimen may require two bottles of each otic agent used (one for home and one for school). If one is used, will have to rely on 8 year old to transport back and forth to school.
- Otic anesthetics are only used while otic pain exists.
- Cultures and sensitivities on otic drainage are only indicated in persistent cases that are not respondent to treatment.

DRUGS TO BE USED

- Hydrocortisone-neomycin sulfate-polymyxin B: 3 drops affected ear TID
- Benzocaine otic solution: Fill ear canal PRN for pain
- Boric acid/isopropyl alcohol 5 drops to affected ear TID

*Cost Index:
1 = $ < 30/mo.
2 = $ 30–40/mo.
3 = $ 40–50/mo.
4 = $ 50–60/mo.
5 = $ > 60/mo.

AWP of hydrocortisone/neomycin/polymixin otic drops is approximately $10 for a 10-mL bottle.
AWP of benzocaine otic solution is approximately $14 for a 10-mL bottle.
AWP of boric acid/isopropyl alcohol solution is approximately $10 for a 10-mL bottle.

Case Study Cerumen Impaction

Patient History

History of Present Illness	KZ is a 73-year-old Italian-American male. Complains of itching in the ears, feeling of fullness, and partial loss of hearing in both ears for the last month. No complaints of bleeding from the ear canals. Denies using any over-the-counter otic preparations.
Past Health History	Throughout his life, KZ has had recurrent problems with excessive and dry cerumen. Previously has had ear irrigations by his physician but no irrigations for approximately 2 years. Denies history of otitis media and tympanic membrane perforation. Denies history of skin irritation or eczema. No known allergies to food preservatives. Medications include hydrochlorothiazide for hypertension.
Physical Exam	Bilaterally pinna of equal size and appearance. Elongated lobes bilaterally. No tenderness with manipulation of the pinna nor compression of the tragus bilaterally. Unable to visualize either tympanic membranes due to excessive yellow-brown cerumen. No drainage noted in external canal opening. Decreased hearing demonstrated bilaterally by inability to hear whispered words from 1 to 2 feet away. Weber tuning fork test reveals lateralization to left ear.
Diagnostic Testing	None
Developmental Considerations	KZ may need assistance with administration of otic agents.
Psychosocial Considerations	KZ showers daily in the morning but avoids getting water in his ears. Denies swimming and resides in a very dry climate. KZ appears reliable and willing to comply with therapy recommendations. KZ is married, and his wife is willing to assist him as necessary.
Economic Factors	KZ is living on his retirement income and feels able to purchase over-the-counter otic agents. He owns and drives his own car for transportation.

Variables Influencing Decision

Treatment Objectives

- Soften and remove excessive cerumen from the external canal, decrease conductive hearing loss, and improve comfort level.

Drug Variables	*Drug Summary*	*Patient Variables*
Indications	For softening and removal of cerumen from the external ear canal.	KZ has bilateral excessive dry cerumen obstructing his external canals.
Pharmacodynamics	All ceruminolytics contain glycerin to soften cerumen and carbamide peroxide to loosen cerumen debris via the effervescence of oxygen release.	Because all ceruminolytics are similar in action, and one is no more efficacious than another, this is not a decision point.
Adverse Effects/ Contraindications	Can be irritating to the external canal and surrounding tissue; may cause a severe eczematoid allergic reaction with prolonged exposure.	Will be a decision point because unable to visualize KZs tympanic membrane bilaterally; however, he is not complaining of increased temperature, pain, nor experiencing ear drainage commonly associated with TM perforation. Will also be a decision point in regard to skin irritation. KZ has no history of skin irritation nor eczema.
Pharmacokinetics	Normal pharmacokinetics do not apply to ceruminolytics as the drug is not designed for absorption, distribution, or metabolism. All ceruminolytics help eliminate cerumen mechanically followed by warm water irrigations.	Because all ceruminolytics have similar pharmacokinetics, this is not a decision point.

Drug Variables	*Drug Summary*	*Patient Variables*
Dosage Regimen	Fill the external canal with the ceruminolytic and allow the drug to remain in place for 15–30 minutes. Follow with warm water irrigation. Ceruminolytics may be repeated daily until the ear canal is free of cerumen.	Because KZ is reliable and will have his wife help with ceruminolytic administration and warm water irrigation, dosage regimen and compliance will not be a problem to be used as a decision point.
Lab Considerations	None	None
Cost Index*	Trolamine-polypeptide oleate-condensate: 1 Carbamide peroxide: 1	Since KZ's otic agents are relatively inexpensive, cost is not a major decision point. Patients are instructed to purchase the least expensive over-the-counter preparation.

Summary of Decision Points

- The adverse effects of ceruminolytics require attention to possible skin irritation.
- Ceruminolytics are contraindicated with perforated tympanic membranes.
- Because all ceruminolytics are similar, specific choices should be the least expensive.

DRUGS TO BE USED

- Trolamine-polypeptide oleate-condensate to affected ear daily

*Cost Index: 1 = $ < 30/mo.
2 = $ 30–40/mo.
3 = $ 40–50/mo.
4 = $ 50–60/mo.
5 = $ > 60/mo.

AWP of 15 ml of a 6.5% trolamine-polypeptide oleate-condensate solution is approximately $6.
AWP of 15 mL of 6.5% carbamide peroxide is approximately $5.

place for 15 to 30 minutes. The patient then repeatedly irrigates the external canal with warm water using an ear syringe (see Fig. 63–1). The irrigation displaces and evacuates the cerumen from the external canal. The whole procedure can be repeated daily until the canal is cleared of cerumen. In cases in which cerumen is resistant to removal, the ceruminolytic agent is instilled in the evening and a cotton pledget is inserted, allowing the medication to remain in place overnight. The ear is then irrigated the next morning as stated earlier. After clearing the impaction, patients may repeat the procedure weekly to remove loose cerumen and prevent development of future impaction.

Education

Patients are taught the general principles of otic drug storage and administration. Solutions are kept tightly closed and stored at 59° to 86° F. Administration of cold otic drugs causes nausea, vomiting, and ataxia. The patient is instructed to warm the ear drop container to body temperature passively by holding it in the hands for 5 to 10 minutes. Ear drops should never be warmed in a microwave oven.

Administration of ear drops requires special positioning of the patient. The person administering the ear drops should wash his or her hands thoroughly. If the patient must administer the ear drops alone, have the patient sit in front of a mirror and tilt the head so the affected ear is up. The patient carefully drops the warmed solution into the ear without the dropper touching the ear or putting the dropper down. The patient is cautioned to avoid contact with the tip of the dropper to prevent contamination of the entire bottle of solution.

Otic drugs are more easily administered by someone other than the patient. Family members or friends can be instructed on the administration of otic drugs. In children, the external pinna should be displaced down and back to open the canal, whereas in adults, the pinna should be displaced up and back. Hold this position for 2 to 5 minutes, allowing the drug to disperse into the canal. Repeat to the opposite ear if indicated. If the dropper accidentally touches the ear, the dropper is wiped clean with a tissue before replacing it back in the bottle. When administering otic antibiotics, a cotton pledget is inserted in the external canal to prevent the drug from leaking out. To prevent cross-contamination and infection, patients are cautioned not to share otic drugs with other persons. Handwashing and proper disposal of contaminated ear drainage and soiled cotton pledget prevents spread to others. Special instructions are given, and the patient is cautioned not to use otic drops in the eyes.

Special teaching needs with regard to steroid and steroid-antibiotic combinations, and anesthetics include teaching the patient to limit the use of pain-controlling drugs to only when ear pain is present. Further, patients are also cautioned against keeping drugs from previous illnesses and self-medicating for recurrent ear problems. Patients are instructed that a change in the treatment regimen may be required if pain continues after 2 or 3 days of use.

Patients having cerumen problems are taught about the normal production, function, and elimination of cerumen. They are also taught nonpharmacologic means for the removal of cerumen from the canal. Allowing warm water from a shower to run in the ear and using a clean towel to wipe out the larger ear structures daily is effective. Finally, patients are told of the potential for hearing loss with impaction. If there has been a recent change in hearing associated with the impaction, the patient can expect hearing to markedly improve with removal of the impacted cerumen. If hearing does not return, the patient is instructed to contact a health care provider to have additional hearing testing and tympanometry conducted.

Otic discomfort often disrupts sleeping patterns. Appropriate use of otic drugs before retiring for the night may enhance sleeping patterns. Significant improvement is noted after 1 or 2 days of antibiotic therapy. Patients are taught to monitor symptoms and to contact the health care provider if symptoms persist or worsen.

Patients should be instructed to avoid activities that might dilute or wash out an otic drug from the ear. Such activities include showering without proper ear protection and swimming with the head exposed to water. Ideally, antibacterial and drying drugs are used upon rising, at bedtime, and after bathing, swimming, or circumstances when the ear has been exposed to added moisture. If an ear device (e.g., hearing aid, telephone ear piece, or ear plugs) is worn, it should be kept clean and free of debris. Ear devices should not be shared with others.

Evaluation

Evaluation involves determining the efficacy of the otic preparation. When the drugs are effective, the patient no longer complains of pain, edema, itching, or sensorial or perceptual alterations. Effectiveness of antibacterial and drying drugs is noted when external otitis does not recur.

When hearing loss persists after other signs and symptoms are resolved, audiology testing with tympanometry may be performed. Decreased movement of the tympanic membrane indicates conductive hearing loss, which requires additional diagnosis and corrective measures to restore hearing.

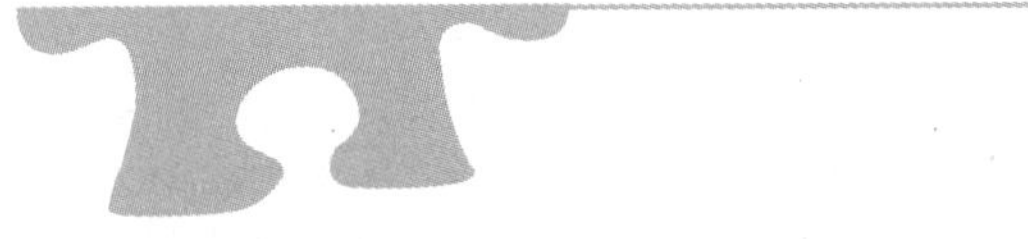

SUMMARY

- Treatment of otic disorders may require the use of topical otic drugs as well as systemic drugs.
- External ear canal infections are common for people whose ears are frequently exposed to moisture due to swimming, bathing, or high humidity environments.
- Usual pathogens causing external ear infections include *P. aeruginosa*, *S. aureus*, *E. coli*, and *Proteus* species, and anaerobes.
- External otic infection causes local inflammation and pain. Symptoms of fever, malaise, anorexia, and fatigue reflect systemic involvement. Moist environments and humidity facilitate the growth of microorganisms.
- Local inflammation and swelling cause external ear canal obstruction, leading to conductive hearing loss.
- Structures of the ear become inflamed for a variety of reasons, including allergic reactions, trauma, and infection.
- With inflammation, blood flow to the area increases, capillary permeability is increased, and fluid flows into the effected tissue producing edema and erythematous coloring.
- As a sensory organ, the ear canal contains many sensory nerve fibers that produce significant pain.
- Cerumen impaction is more common in the geriatric population.
- Cerumen is a normal sebaceous gland secretion of the ear, functioning to protect and lubricate the external canal. Normally, cerumen is eliminated when the ear canals get wet.
- When cerumen is not eliminated properly, the external canal may become impacted with cerumen.
- Damage to inner ear structures can be caused by certain chemicals or ototoxic drugs.
- Categories of drugs known to be ototoxic include aminoglycosides and other antibiotics, loop diuretics, antimalarials, nonsteroidal anti-inflammatory drugs, and some antineoplastic drugs.
- Tinnitus and sensorineural hearing loss are present with damage to the cochlea.
- Damage to the vestibular apparatus produces vertigo, lightheadedness, headache, giddiness, inability to focus or fixate on images, nausea, vomiting, and cold sweats.
- Factors such as dosage, renal function, concomitant use of other ototoxic agent, inherent susceptibility, age, and exposure to high-intensity noise impact the ototoxic effects.
- Treatment objectives for otic infection are aimed at eliminating the infection relieving inflammation and pain. Treatment objectives for pain associated with inflammation are accomplished by decreasing local edema, blocking local sensation of pain, and treating the etiology of the inflammation.
- Treatment objectives for cerumen impaction are to soften and remove excessive cerumen from the external canal, decrease conductive hearing loss, and improve comfort level.
- Inflammation associated with infection, trauma, or allergic reaction is quickly resolved with antibiotics, antibacterial and drying drugs, steroid or steroid-antibiotic combinations.
- Pain subsides quickly when the ear is treated with otic anesthetics.
- In children, the external pinna should be displaced down and back to open the canal, whereas in adults, the pinna should be displaced up and back to administer otic drugs.
- Administer otic ceruminolytics, and then irrigate the ear with warm water.
- If conductive hearing loss is associated with the infection, hearing returns to normal with resolution of the infection.
- Hearing loss associated with cerumen impaction is resolved with clearing of cerumen.

BIBLIOGRAPHY

Andaz, C., and Whittet, H. (1993). An in vitro study to determine efficacy of different wax-dispersing agents. *Journal of Otorhinolaryngology,* 55(2), 97–99.

Barlow, D., Duckert, L., Kreig, C., et al. (1995). Ototoxicity of topical otomicrobial agents. *Acta Otolaryngologica* 115(2), 231–235.

Drug Facts and Comparisons. (1998). St. Louis: A Walters Kluwer Co.

Hanger, H., and Mulligen, G. (1992). Cerumen: Its fascination and clinical importance: A review. *Journal of the Royal Society of Medicine,* 85(6), 346–349.

Hayback, P. (1993). Tuning into ototoxicity. *Nursing,* 23(6), 34–41.

Jung, T., Rhee, C., Lee, C., et al. (1993). Ototoxicity of salicylate, nonsteroidal anti-inflammatory drugs, and quinine. *Otolaryngologic Clinics of North America,* 26(5), 791–810.

Mahoney, D. (1993). Cerumen impaction: Prevalence and detection in nursing homes. *Journal of Gerontological Nursing,* 19(4), 23–29.

Malkiewicz, J., and Hull, R. (1998). Ear assessment. In D. Ignatavicius, L. Workman, M. Mishler (Eds.), *Medical-surgical Nursing: A nursing process approach* (3rd ed.) Philadelphia: W. B. Saunders.

Martin, J. (1998). Interventions for ear and hearing disorders. In D. Ignatavicius, L. Workman, M. Mishler (Eds.), *Medical-surgical Nursing: A nursing process approach* (3rd ed.). Philadelphia: W. B. Saunders.

Meyer, M. (1993). *Coping with medications.* San Diego: Singular Publishing Group.

Rohn, G., Meyerhoff, W., and Wright, C. (1993). Ototoxicity of topical agents. *Otolaryngologic Clinics of North America,* 26(5), 747–758.

Welling, D., Forrest, L., and Goll, F. (1995). Safety of ototopical antibiotics. *Laryngoscope,* 105(5), 471–474.

Winslow, E. (1994). Hearing loss? Check for impacted cerumen. *American Journal of Nursing,* 94(10), 55.

Wintermeyer, S. (1994). Chronic suppurative otitis media. *Annals of Pharmacotherapy,* 28(9), 1089–1099.

Zivic, R., and King, S. (1993). Cerumen-impaction management for clients of all ages. *Nurse Practitioner: American Journal of Primary Health Care,* 18(3), 33–34, 36.

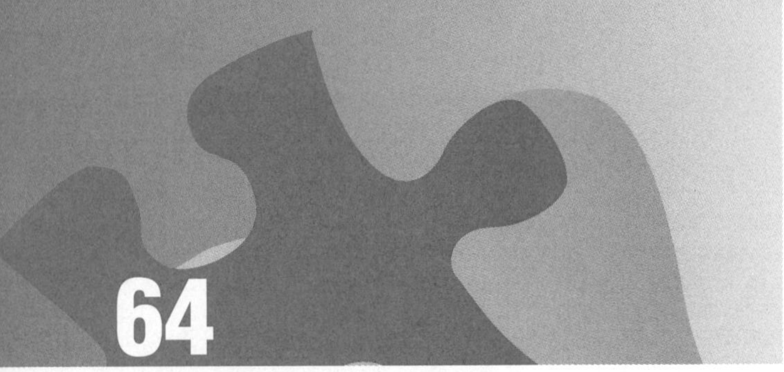

64

Dermatologic Drugs

The skin has been described as the largest organ in the body. It covers the body's surface and acts as a shield from the environment. Skin diseases are one of the most common concerns that arise in the health care setting. Almost all health care providers see patients with dermatologic problems during the course of their career. Because skin disease can be a devastating experience, history is rich with accounts of humanity's attempt to minister to the skin.

For most diseases, drugs are administered at a site that is distant from the target organ; however, in dermatology, drugs can be directly applied to the site. Topical therapy can be used to restore skin hydration, alleviate symptoms, reduce inflammation, protect the skin, reduce scales and callus, cleanse and débride, and eradicate microorganisms. Some skin problems, such as burns and decubitus ulcers, take extensive, aggressive intervention to resolve. In rare cases, the skin ailment may be so difficult to diagnose that only hypotheses of treatment are possible.

STRUCTURE AND FUNCTION OF THE SKIN

The skin is composed of three distinct layers: the epidermis, the dermis, and subcutaneous tissue. These layers as well as other features of the skin are depicted in Figure 64–1. Skin appendages such as the hair and nails make up a fourth component.

Epidermis

The *epidermis,* the outer layer of the skin, is composed almost entirely of closely packed cells. Its primary function is to retard the loss of fluids from the inner body to the outside environment. It also acts as a barrier against the entry of foreign substances.

Four distinct cellular layers make up the epidermis: the basal layer, stratum spinosum, stratum granulosum, and the stratum corneum. Cell division occurs in the *basal layer,* the deepest layer and the only epidermal cells that are mitotically active. All cells of the epidermis arise from this layer. The epidermis has no direct blood supply of its own, relying on diffusion for its nutrition. It normally takes 3 to 4 weeks for the epidermis to produce new cells and push older cells outward. During the ascent upward through the epidermal layers, the *keratinocytes* (the cells of the epidermis that synthesizes keratin) become smaller and flatter. As they near the skin surface, they die. Their cytoplasm becomes *keratin,* a hard, fibrous, proteinaceous material. The keratin provides the outer layer of the epidermis with flexibility and elasticity. This outer layer is referred to as the *stratum corneum.*

Above the basal layer is the *stratum spinosum.* This cellular layer is called spinous because of the delicate spinelike processes projecting from its surfaces. The stratum spinosum absorbs water. Water absorption is readily seen when the skin of the palms and the soles become white and swollen during bathing.

In the granular cell layer, the *stratum granulosum,* cells acquire additional keratin and become more flattened. The degradative enzymes found in granular cells are responsible for the destruction of internal cellular components. Enzymatic function is necessary for the differentiation of keratinocytes to cornified cells.

Cells of the *stratum corneum,* the fourth layer, are large, flattened, polyhedral-shaped cells that are filled with keratin. They are stacked vertically, producing a tightly packed, semi-impermeable layer that is the major physical barrier of the skin. Through a process that is not completely understood, the stratum corneum undergoes continuous exfoliation (i.e., shedding). The shedding completes the growth cycle of the epidermis.

The skin has the lowest water permeability of any biologic membrane. This property, combined with the complex protein keratin in the stratum corneum, allows the skin to function as a barrier that does not hinder drug absorption. Because the skin is not an absolute barrier, transdermal absorption occurs.

Three other important cell types are located in the epidermis: melanocytes, Langerhans cells, and Merkel cells. *Melanocytes* are found primarily in the basal layer. They produce melanin, transferring it to keratinocytes, which, in turn, is deposited over the surface of the nucleus on the side facing the sun. The difference in skin pigmentation depends mostly on the activity level of the melanocytes rather than on the number, size, and dispersion of the cells in the skin.

Langerhans cells serve as the first-line immunologic defense, protecting against environmental antigens. They function as antigen-presenting cells migrating to lymph nodes. They contribute to the uptake, processing, and presentation of a foreign substance to T lymphocytes.

Merkel cells are considered touch receptors. They are thought to detect mechanical deformities of the epidermis and to regulate epithelial proliferation. Unlike melanocytes and Langerhans cells, Merkel cells do not shed under normal circumstances. This characteristic raises the question, however, as to how they maintain their positions against the upward movement of keratinocytes.

Dermis

The *dermis* lies beneath the epidermis, is composed largely of collagen, and is approximately 40 times thicker than the epidermis. Collagen fibers, the most abundant protein in the body, constitute about 70 percent of the dry weight of the dermis. Most importantly, it contributes to the support and nourishment of the epidermis. The basement membrane is the linkage that integrates epidermis to dermis. The basement membrane along with elastic and reticular fibers comprise the dermal matrix. Reticular fibers are overabundant in certain pathologic conditions such as granulomas and tumors.

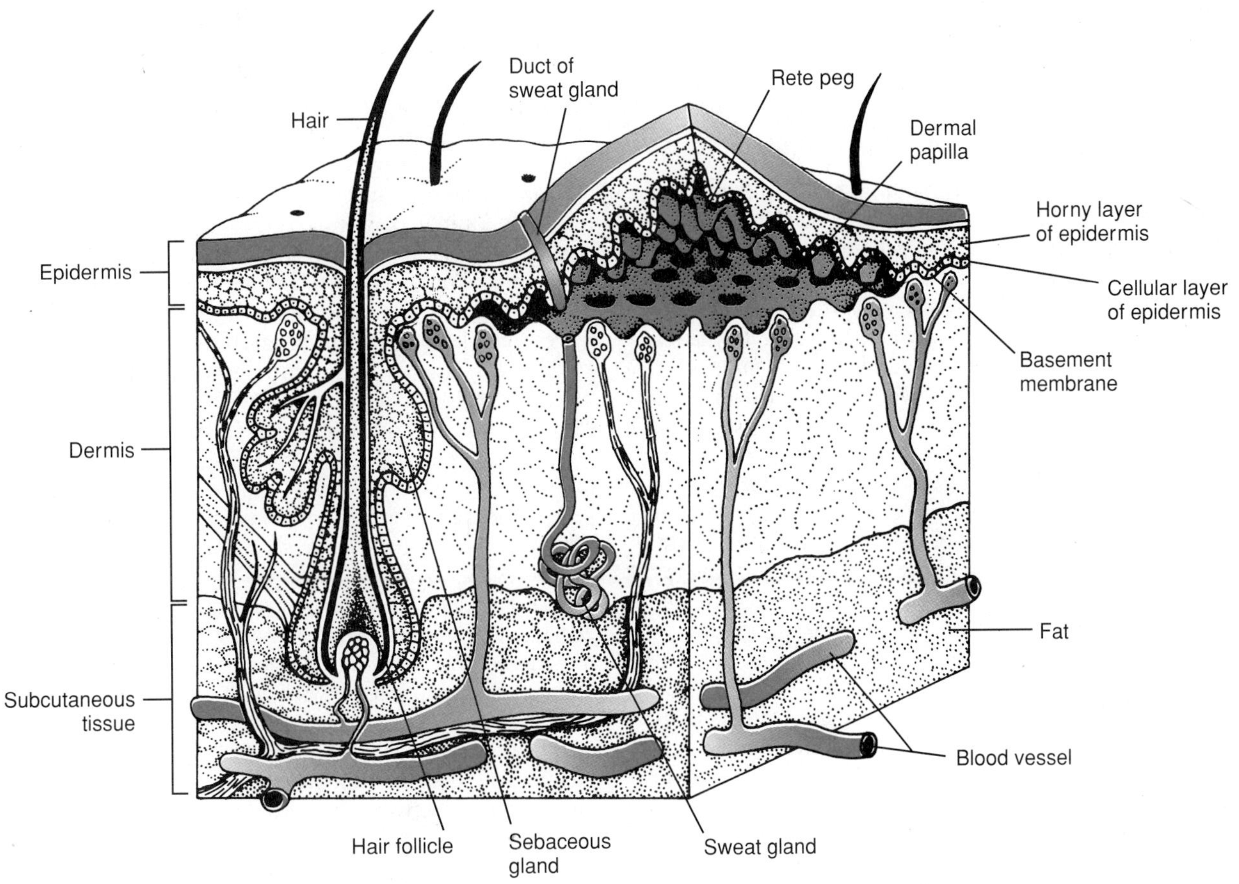

Figure 64–1 The anatomy of the skin includes the three growth layers of the epidermis and other stuctures. (From Ignatavicius, D., Workman, M., and Miehler, M. [1995]. *Medical-surgical nursing: A nursing process approach.* [2nd ed, p. 1910]. Philadelphia: W. B. Saunders. Used with permission.)

Three groups of mesodermal cells make up the dermis. Of these, the reticulohistiocytic group, consisting of histiocytes and mast cells, are linked to many skin diseases such as atopic and contact dermatitis, and lichen planus. The myeloid group of cells are the origin of various dermatoses, especially those with an allergic etiology. The cells of the lymphoid group contribute to inflammatory lesions of the skin. Myeloid and lymphoid groups of cells also exist in specific neoplasms of the skin.

Other structures found in the dermis include nerves and blood vessels, the sebaceous glands and hair follicles (pilosebaceous apparatus), and eccrine and apocrine glands. Apocrine glands open into hair follicles and are found in the axillae, breast areas, and genital organs. Bacteria grow on their secretions and yield characteristic body odors. Eccrine glands (sweat glands) are widely distributed over much of the body but are found predominantly on the palms of the hands and the soles of the feet. The eccrine glands help regulate body temperature and protect against excessive dryness.

Sebaceous glands are large fat-containing cells that produce sebum. The *sebum,* an oily substance, lubricates and protects the skin so the skin is not only water repellent but also antiseptic. Normal skin pH is 4.5 to 5.5. This acid pH provides a protective mechanism because microorganisms grow best at a pH of 6 to 7.5. Fungal infections are the most common disorders of the pilosebaceous apparatus. Furthermore, stimulation of the sebaceous follicle by a surge of androgenic hormones is a contributing factor in the development of acne.

Sensory nerves integrate tactile sensations such as heat, touch, pressure, and pain between the skin and the brain. Motor nerves, part of the involuntary sympathetic nervous system, control the sweat glands, smooth muscles of the skin, and arterioles.

The arterioles help control temperature and provide nutrition to the skin. Temperature regulation is achieved via pathways located in the papillary dermis. By conducting heat from internal structures to the skin surface, heat is removed from the body. Arteriolar circulation carries nutrients to the skin.

Subcutaneous Tissue

A layer of *subcutaneous tissue* lies beneath the dermis. It is largely made up of fat. It insulates the body from cold, cushions deep tissues from trauma, and serves as a reserve source of calories.

SKIN DISORDERS

Skin disorders are classified in several ways. They can be classified as noninfectious inflammatory diseases, infectious inflammatory diseases (caused by bacteria, fungi, or viruses), skin conditions caused by sunlight or pressure, and malignant tumors of the skin.

Noninfectious Inflammatory Dermatoses

Dermatitis and eczema are noninfectious inflammatory dermatoses. *Dermatitis* is a general term that denotes an inflammation of the skin caused by exogenous irritants, allergens, or trauma. The term *eczema* is often used as a synonym for endogenous dermatitis. Regardless of the cause, dermatitis is usually characterized by erythema, vesicle formation, edema, oozing, excoriation, crusting, and scaling. With chronic scratching, the tissues become thickened *(lichenification)*.

Atopic dermatitis, also called atopic eczema, is a pruritic dermatosis. People with atopy tend to develop pruritus under stress. Forty to sixty-five percent of patients with this disease have a family history of hay fever or asthma with a hereditary predisposition to a lowered cutaneous threshold to pruritus. Most react to common food and inhaled allergens by producing immunoglobulin E (IgE) antibodies. In adults, the dermatitis may be a response to harsh chemicals or scratching, with lesions most often noted on the forehead, wrists, feet, and sides of the neck. There may be lichenification on flexor surfaces with continued scratching and rubbing. Lesions in infants and children are found primarily on the cheeks and extensor surfaces of the antecubital or popliteal surfaces. Infantile atopic dermatitis can start as early as 4 to 6 months of age, disappearing by about ages 3 to 5. Sometimes it continues as childhood atopic dermatitis, beginning at age 2 to 4 and disappearing around age 10. In some cases, it continues into adulthood.

Contact dermatitis is a rash resulting from contact between an allergen and the skin. It is a form of allergic exogenous dermatitis and may be caused by chemicals or mechanical irritation. Common substances that produce contact dermatitis include plants (e.g., poison ivy), jewelry containing nickel, adhesive tape, shoe leather, elastic, rubber, cosmetics, and perfumes. Contact dermatitis has clinical features that include red, thick, crusty, fissured, suppurating areas in various stages. The affected areas are those that have been in direct contact with the offending substance.

Seborrheic dermatitis affects hairy areas, often appearing on the scalp, eyebrows, ears, or sternum. The skin becomes red, scaly, and greasy looking, and often itches. Untreated patients may excoriate the skin by scratching, thus allowing a secondary infection to develop. In babies, scalp seborrhea is called "cradle cap." In the adult, mild seborrhea may appear as dandruff. Patients with acquired immunodeficiency syndrome or parkinsonism may develop especially prominent seborrhea.

Urticaria (hives) is an IgE-mediated allergic response to external agents (e.g., insect bites) or to internal allergens (i.e., food allergies) that reach the skin through the blood stream. The characteristic lesion of urticaria is itchy and edematous, and has an erythematous wheal with a pallid center. The lesions typically blanch with pressure. Urticaria occurs in about 15 to 20 percent of the population. It is usually self-limiting but may also become chronic. Chronic urticaria appears as a large hive without the sensation of itching. It is often accompanied by angioedema.

Psoriasis is a chronic, papulosquamous disorder that alters the appearance of the epidermis by increasing its thickness. It follows an erratic course. The primary defect is an accelerated maturation of the epidermis. Instead of epidermal turnover taking 26 to 28 days, epidermal cells complete their growth cycle in less than 7 days. Symmetric patches appear on extensor surfaces, knees, elbows, buttocks, or on the scalp. Initial papules coalesce into red plaques. Both papules and plaques are covered with silvery scales that may be pruritic. The nails often become thick, irregular, and exhibit pits of 1 mm or less. Removal of the scales frequently leaves fine bleeding points called *Auspitz's sign.*

Pityriasis rosea is also a papulosquamous disease but is self-limited. It initially presents with a single oval salmon-colored patch (herald patch) that is covered with scales 2 to 10 cm in diameter. The major patches appear on the trunk, following the cleavage lines of the skin. Smaller patches appear on peripheral areas. It occurs predominantly in females ages 10 to 35. Seasonal onset is typical during fall and spring.

Lichen planus, another papulosquamous disease, produces lesions that are 2 to 8 mm in size and are flat and purple, the borders of which are polygonal. The surface of the lesions are criss-crossed with white or silver lines called *Wickham's striae.* The lesions first appear on flexor surfaces of the wrists and forearm, the legs above the ankles, the sacral area, penis, or mucous membranes. The onset of the disease occurs between the ages of 30 and 70.

Infectious Inflammatory Dermatoses

Bacterial Infections

Bacterial infections of the skin are most often caused by *Streptococci* or *Staphylococci* invasion of the skin where the barrier function has been compromised by damage or inflammation. Organisms may be introduced below the epidermis by trauma or by disturbances in normal anatomy (hair follicle, hangnail). Virulence of the organisms and host immune factors combine to determine whether the infection will occur and the extent of the infection.

Cellulitis is characterized by tenderness, edema, and erythema that spreads to subcutaneous tissues. *Erysipelas* is a form of cellulitis caused by group A *Streptococcus pyogenes.* The visible signs include round or oval patches on the skin that promptly enlarge and spread, becoming swollen, tender, and red. The affected skin is hot to the touch, and occasionally, the adjacent skin blisters. Systemic manifestations such as headache, malaise, fever, chills, vomiting, and complete prostration can occur.

Folliculitis is an infection of hair follicles. It most often occurs on the scalp or bearded areas of the face.

Furuncles (boils) and *carbuncles* (a cluster of boils) are usually caused by *Staphylococci aureus.* They are often a symptom of poor health. Furuncles tend to recur, resulting from infection of hair follicles. They usually appear on the neck, face, axillae, buttocks, thighs, and perineum. Carbuncles involve multiple hair follicles with pustules. Like furuncles, carbuncles are caused by pus-forming bacteria. Systemic manifestations may develop and include malaise, fever, leukocytosis, and bacteremia. Scar tissue is formed with healing.

Impetigo is a superficial skin infection that is highly contagious and usually found on exposed skin surfaces in children. It is caused by group A *Streptococcus pyogenes, Staphylococcus aureus,* or both. It is not uncommon to find the disease in adolescents who are involved in wrestling activities at school because the microorganisms seem to harbor on the wrestling mats. The lesions are rapidly crusting clear vesicles, 2 to 3 mm to 2 cm in diameter. The honey-colored crusts are moist and oozing. If the crusts are removed, the base is red and eroded.

Fungal Infections

Fungal infections of the hair, skin, and nails are a major source of morbidity throughout the world. It has been estimated that fungal infections account for 5 percent of new outpatient referrals to dermatologists in temperate climates and as much as 20 percent in tropical climates. Most of the infections are caused by either dermatophytes or by yeasts, most commonly the Candida species.

Tinea (ringworm) is a superficial infection in which the fungus lives on the dead horny layer of the skin. It causes the skin to scale and disintegrate, the nails to crumble, and hair to break off. Lesions often appear as scaly, erythematous, circular lesions. *Tinea pedis* refers to fungal infection of the feet (athlete's foot). It is transmitted through shared bathing facilities where warm, moist feet enhance fungal growth. Men are more commonly affected than women.

Tinea unguium (onychomycosis) is a fungal infection of toenails often seen in persons who have long-standing tinea pedis. The affected nails appear dull and thick. The distal edge becomes separated from the nail bed (onycholysis) causing a misshapen appearance. Fingernails may also become infected.

Tinea capitis is ringworm of the scalp. It is common in the pediatric age group and is highly contagious. A consistent sign is the broken-off hair "stub" that leads to patches of partial baldness.

Tinea cruris is a fungal infection of the groin; *tinea corporis,* infection of the body, *tinea barbae,* the beard; and *tinea manus* the hand. *Tinea versicolor* appears as a brown discoloration.

Candidiasis is a yeast infection caused by *Candida albicans.* Predisposition to candidiasis occurs in people treated with antibiotics, women taking oral contraceptives, those who are on corticosteroid or antineoplastic therapies, babies and adults in diapers, and in people who are immunosuppressed (e.g., diabetes mellitus, acquired immunodeficiency syndrome). Candida has a predilection for warm, moist sites; thus, intertriginous sites (skin folds), the mouth, and vagina are common sites for infection. With candidal growth, the skin may be denuded, leaving a raw, glistening base. Red papules (satellite lesions) are scattered away from the margins of the raw areas. The presence of the scattered papules is useful in distinguishing candidiasis from tinea. The most prominent symptom of vaginal candidiasis is severe itching.

Viral Infections

Skin lesions are common in viral infections. They may be caused by replication of the virus in the skin, by immune responses of the host, or both. Viral infections of the skin include herpes simplex, herpes zoster, varicella (chickenpox), verrucae, and other dermatoses.

Herpes simplex lesions appear as vesicles with an inflamed base. Primary infections have an incubation period of up to 2 weeks. Type I herpes infections involve the skin and oral cavity. Type II herpes infections most often involve the skin of neonates, which can lead to encephalitis. The genital mucosa is a common site for herpes infections. Herpes infections can also spread to the lungs and brain in immunocompromised individuals. Recurrent infection is due to either a reactivation of an older infection or new infection.

Herpes zoster (shingles) is caused by reactivation of the chickenpox virus, varicella. The virus survives in a latent form in dorsal root ganglia. Certain stimuli allow the virus to traverse down the axon to the skin, where vesicles appear in a dermatome distribution pattern. Pain, itching, or irritation precede the skin eruption by 48 to 72 hours. The lesions begin with a red base, on which appears a small but enlarging clear vesicle. The vesicle becomes white and then yellow before rupturing. Fluid oozes to form a crust that may require 7 to 10 days to heal. Systemic symptoms may be present.

Verrucae (warts) are of various types. Verruca vulgaris is a viral infection of the hands and fingers. Verruca plantaris (plantar wart) is an inward growth on the sole of the foot. It may be covered by a callus or hyperkeratosis. Verrucae plana are flat warts located on the dorsum of the hands and face. *Condylomata acuminatum* are cauliflower-like growths in the anogenital area (genital warts). They, too, are often associated with hyperkeratosis.

Acne Vulgaris

Acne vulgaris is a skin disorder commonly found in 30 to 85 percent of adolescents and young adults. The lesions usually appear on the face, neck, chest, shoulders, and back. Open *comedones* are the most common lesions of mild acne. A comedo forms when sebum combines with keratin to form a plug within a skin pore. Oxidation causes the exposed surface of the sebum plug to turn black, hence the term blackhead. Closed comedones, known often as whiteheads, develop when pores fill below the skin surface with sebum and scales. In its most severe form, acne is characterized by abscesses and inflammatory cysts.

Acne is stimulated by the increased production of androgens during adolescence. Under their influence, sebum production and the turnover of follicular epithelial cells increase, leading to plugging of the pores. Symptoms are exacerbated by the activity of *Propionibacterium acnes,* an organism that converts sebum into irritating fatty acids. The bacterium releases chemotactic factors that promote inflammation. Oily skin, hormonal changes, and a genetic predisposition are additional contributing factors.

Acne vulgaris is classified as follows: Grade I acne includes primarily sparse comedones. Grade II acne is characterized by comedones, papules, and occasional pustules. In grade III acne, there is a predominance of papules and pustules with small cysts. With grade IV acne, there are overt signs of cystic acne. Treatment regimens vary with the grade.

Trauma

Trauma can contribute to an infection when physical injury disrupts the integrity of the skin surface. Common wounds include lacerations (cuts or tears), abrasions (shearing or scraping of the skin), puncture wounds, surgical avulsions, traumatic amputations, incisions, and burns.

Burns are classified according to the depth of destruction. Superficial partial-thickness burns (first-degree) involve only the epidermis, are painful, and appear red or pink and dry. There are no blisters. An example of a superficial, partial-thickness burn is a mild sunburn.

Deeper partial-thickness (second-degree) burns involve the epidermis and parts of the dermis. These burns are red, moist, blistered, and painful. Mottling, with pink or red to waxy white areas with blisters and edema are often present. The entire epidermal and dermal layers are affected in a deep second-degree or partial-thickness burn. Sweat glands and hair follicles remain intact.

Full-thickness (third-degree) burn injuries are painless because nerve fibers are destroyed. The burns may vary in color with much edema noted. The eschar is hard, dry, and leathery, but the wound leaks fluid absorbed from the underlying tissues.

A blackened, depressed, full-thickness burn involving muscle, fascia, and bone is classified as a fourth-degree burn. Exposure of bones and ligaments is common. When bone is involved, the wound appears dull and dry.

Drug Reactions

Drug reactions take on many forms and are caused by a variety of mechanisms. A rather common form is a fine, reddish papular rash over the trunk (or any part of the body). Five percent of patients have an extended hospital stay as the result of adverse drug reactions, with 10 percent of hospitalized patients experiencing at least one adverse drug reaction. Allergic manifestations to drugs may or may not result in specific antibody formation or sensitized lymphocytes. For this reason, the recognition of clinical manifestations of a drug reaction is of utmost importance. Adverse drug reactions to dermatologic preparations are noted in Table 64–1.

Infestations and Bites

The bites of bees, wasps, hornets, and yellow jackets are potential causes of skin lesions, and they are responsible for approximately 50 to 100 reported deaths a year. Most victims are younger than age 20. Males are twice as likely to be affected, possibly because they are involved in outdoor work. Reactions are more frequent when stings occur around the head and neck, but reactions can occur from bites in other areas as well. Severe edema of the pharynx, epiglottis, and trachea is the major cause of death in sensitive people. Reactions may range in severity from transient redness, edema, and pain to acute anaphylactic shock (usually within 15 minutes). The peak reaction usually appears within 48 to 72 hours and lasts up to 7 days. Neurologic, vascular reactions, or immune-complex disease may also be seen.

Ulcerations

An ulceration of the skin and subcutaneous tissue over or near a bony prominence is referred to as a *decubitus ulcer* (bedsore). Decubitus ulcers are caused by sustained pressure or friction of a body part resting against an external object. Other factors such as poor nutritional status, inadequate hydration, and a compromised immune response increases the risk of ulcer formation.

A decubitus ulcer reflects several pathophysiologic tissue changes. Obstruction of capillary blood flow by externally applied pressure causes tissue hypoxia (lack of oxygen to the tissue). An early sign of pressure is blanching erythema, an area of redness to the skin that turns white when pressed with a finger. Nonblanching erythema is a more serious sign of impaired blood supply to the tissues. Deeper, irreversible tissue damage is likely when hyperemia persists. Muscle damage can occur if ischemia persists for long periods. A cycle of cellular death and release of metabolic wastes into the surrounding tissues accompanies ischemia. Edema encroaches on interstitial spaces, slowing tissue perfusion and increasing hypoxia.

Decubitus ulcers are categorized by stages. A stage I ulcer involves the superficial layer of skin. There is visible erythema that does not resolve within 30 minutes of pressure relief. Stage II ulcers involve loss of epidermis with possible penetration into, but not through, the dermis. The wound base is moist, pink, and painful. A stage III ulcer involves subcutaneous tissue, making a shallow crater. Deep tissue destruction extends through subcutaneous tissue to fascia, muscle layers, joints, or bone. Eschar, necrotic tissue, tunneling, exudate, and infection appears with stage III ulcers, but there is usually no pain. Stasis dermatitis often precedes a venous stasis ulcer and is found on the lower legs. There is a brown, eczematous appearance. Stasis ulcerations are often secondary to poor vasculature and venous stasis but may be confused with viral rashes.

PHARMACOTHERAPEUTIC OPTIONS

Antiseptics

- ❒ Ethanols (isopropyl alcohol)
- ❒ Oxidizing antiseptics (hydrogen peroxide, benzoyl peroxide)
- ❒ Biguanides (chlorhexidine gluconate, HIBICLENS)
- ❒ Iodines (povidone-iodine, BETADINE)
- ❒ Chlorine preparations (DAKIN'S SOLUTIONS)
- ❒ Metallics (silver nitrate, silver sulfadiazine, zinc oxide)
- ❒ Phenol derivatives (hexachlorophene, PHISOHEX, resorcinol)
- ❒ Acetic acid
- ❒ Gentian violet
- ❒ Sulfur

Indications

Antiseptics are organic or inorganic preparations that kill or inhibit the growth of bacteria, fungi, and viruses; however, antiseptics are used primarily to prevent infections rather than to treat them. Different organisms are sensitive to different antiseptics. Most antiseptics differ in spectrum and effectiveness, and are not interchangeable. Vegetative forms of bacteria are most sensitive to antiseptics, followed by fungi, lipophilic viruses, tubercle bacilli, and hydrophilic viruses. Bacterial and fungal spores are resistant to most antiseptics. The therapeutic index of an antiseptic is a crucial

TABLE 64–1 ADVERSE DRUG REACTIONS WITH TOPICAL DERMATOLOGIC PREPARATIONS

Common Drug-Induced Dermatologic Reactions

ACNEIFORM REACTIONS		URTICARIA		ALOPECIA	
ACTH	Iodides	ACTH	Mercurials	Alkylating drugs	Levodopa
Androgenic hormones	Isoniazid	Amitriptyline	Nitrofurantoin	Allopurinol	Norethindrone acetate
Bromides	Lithium	Barbiturates	Opioids	Anticoagulants	Oral contraceptives
Corticosteroids	Oral contraceptives	Bromides	Penicillin	Antimetabolites	Propranolol
Cyanocobalamin	Trimethadione	Chloramphenicol	Penicillinase	Antithyroid drugs	Retinoids
Ethambutol	Phenytoin	Dextran	Pentazocine	Colchicine	Trimethadione
Ethionamide	Phenobarbital	Enzymes	Phenothiazines	Heavy metals	Vitamin A
Hydantoins		Erythromycin	Salicylates	Indomethacin	
		Griseofulvin	Serums		
		Hydantoins	Streptomycin		
		Insulins	Sulfonamides		
		Iodides	Tetracyclines		
		Meperidine	Thiouracil		
		Meprobamate			

PHOTOSENSITIVE REACTIONS		PURPURA		CONTACT DERMATITIS	
Acetohexamide	Oral contraceptives	ACTH	Gold salts	Bacitracin	Meprobamate
Amitriptyline	Phenytoin	Allopurinol	Griseofulvin	Benzocaine	Neomycin
Antimalarials	Phenothiazines	Amitriptyline	Iodides	Benzoyl peroxide	Nitrofurazone
Barbiturates	Salicylates	Anticoagulants	Meprobamate	Chloramphenicol	PABA
Carbamazepine	Sulfonamides	Barbiturates	Penicillin	Chlorpromazine	Penicillin
Citrus fruits	Sulfonylureas	Chloral hydrate	Phenylbutazone	Ephedrine	Phenol
Doxycycline	Tetracyclines	Chlorpropamide	Quinidine	Formaldehyde	Streptomycin
Gold salts	Thiazides	Chlorpromazine	Rifampin	Iodine	Sulfonamides
Griseofluvin	Topical corticosteroids	Corticosteroids	Sulfonamides	Isoniazid	Thiamine
Haloperidol	Tricyclic antidepressants	Digitalis	Thiazides	Lanolin	Thimerosal
Nortriptyline			Trifluoperazine		

Life-Threatening Drug-Induced Skin Eruptions

STEVENS-JOHNSON SYNDROME (ERYTHEMA MULTIFORME)		EXFOLIATIVE DERMATITIS		LUPUS ERYTHEMATOSUS	
Ampicillin	Oxyphenylbutazone	PAS	Isoniazid	Aminosalicylic acid	Oral contraceptives
Barbiturates	Penicillin	Barbiturates	Isosorbide	Chlorpromazine	Penicillamine
Carbamazepine	Pentazocine	Carbamazepine	Measles vaccine	Chlortetracycline	Penicillin
Chloramphenicol	Phenobarbital	Chlorpropamide	Nitroglycerine	Corticosteroid withdrawal	Phenobarbital
Chlorpropamide	Phenytoin	Demeclocycline	Oral hypoglycemics	Digitalis	Phenothiazines
Clindamycin	Procaine penicillin	Diphtheria vaccine	Oxyphenylbutazone	Ethosuximide	Primidone
Codeine	Sulfonamides	Furosemide	Penicillin	Gold compounds	Propylthiouracil
Novobiocin	Tetracyclines	Gold	Phenothiazines	Griseofulvin	Rifampin
		Griseofulvin	Phenytoin	Hydantoins	Streptomycin
		Tetracyclines	Sulfonamides	Hydralazine	Sulfonamides
			Tetracyclines	Isoniazid	Tetracyclines
				Methyldopa	Thiazides
				Methysergide	Trimethadione

ACTH, Adrenocorticotropic hormone; PABA, para-aminobenzoic acid; PAS, aminosalicylic acid.

consideration because the agent must be considerably more toxic to surface pathogens than to adjacent living tissues. There are a variety of antiseptics including ethanols, oxidizing agents, biguanides, iodines, chlorine preparations, metallic antiseptics, phenol derivatives, and miscellaneous agents (e.g., acetic acid, gentian violet, sulfur).

Adverse effects of antiseptics vary with the specific drug; however, most are irritating to skin surfaces. In some cases, they interfere with the body's natural healing processes. Further, most antiseptics are drying to the skin.

Ethanols may be used for cleansing intact skin before injections or surgical incisions. They are bactericidal to common bacteria but are less effective against viruses and fungi. When applied to the skin, alcohols kill approximately 90 percent of bacteria within 2 minutes, if the area is kept moist for that period. When applied as a single swipe and left to evaporate, about 75 percent of bacteria are killed. Ethanols, however, are irritating to denuded skin and open wounds, causing a burning type of pain. Furthermore, tissue injury is increased in the presence of ethanols, and proteins coagulate to form a mass under which bacteria proliferate. Ethanols are also drying to healthy skin.

Oxidizing antiseptics are used for wound cleansing, cleansing of tracheostomy tubes, to remove cerumen from the external ear, as a mouthwash diluted with equal parts of water, saline, or commercial mouthwash, and in the treatment of acne vulgaris. Hydrogen peroxides act through oxidation-reduction processes to alter surface tension, thus increasing the permeability of the organism's cell wall and leakage of cell contents. These agents liberate oxygen when in contact with pus or organic substances. Hydrogen peroxide is more effective as a débriding and cleansing agent than as an antiseptic. It is of doubtful value on intact skin. Benzoyl peroxide is bactericidal for anaerobic bacteria (e.g., *Corynebacterium*) and is often used in the treatment of acne vulgaris.

Biguanides are generally effective against both gram-positive and gram-negative organisms. Some gram-negative organisms are resistant to this type of antiseptic; however, little, if any, absorption occurs through the skin of adults. The degree of absorption in children is unknown. Biguanides are used primarily as a skin cleanser to prevent the spread of microorganisms.

Iodines are used in the prevention and treatment of infections of the skin, scalp, and mucous membranes of the mouth and vagina. They are bactericidal to most bacteria, fungi, and viruses, but antiseptic activity depends on the concentration of iodine. When applied to the skin, a 1-percent solution kills approximately 90 percent of bacteria within 90 seconds.

Chlorine preparations are used for infected wounds when other agents or methods are not effective or available. They exert bactericidal action dissolving necrotic materials and blood clots. They also delay blood clotting, which may, in turn, interfere with wound healing.

Metallics are most often used in the treatment of burn wounds and for cauterizing warts or wounds. Silver sulfadiazine is widely used in the treatment of burns. It penetrates burn eschar to exert antibacterial action against *Pseudomonas* and many other organisms. Zinc preparations may be used in the treatment of eczema, impetigo, tinea infections, venous stasis ulcers, pruritus, psoriasis, and seborrhea. In fact, zinc pyrithione is a common ingredient in over-the-counter (OTC) dandruff shampoos.

Phenol derivatives are used most often for handwashing and preoperative skin cleansing. Hexachlorophene is bacteriostatic against gram-positive bacteria but is relatively ineffective against gram-negative bacteria and fungi. Fungal and gram-negative organisms may actually increase in number with the chronic use of hexachlorophene preparations. Furthermore, it has been shown to be systemically absorbed, especially after repeated applications. In some cases, resorcinol is used in the treatment of acne, tinea infections, dermatitis, psoriasis, and other cutaneous lesions.

The American Medical Association recommends that hexachlorophene not be used routinely to bathe infants. It is heavily absorbed through broken skin or when applied excessively and has been shown to cause neurotoxicity.

Acetic acid, gentian violet, and sulfur also have antiseptic actions. Acetic acid has been used for wound, bladder, vaginal, and otic irrigations and in dressing surgical wounds. In a 5-percent concentration it is bactericidal to many organisms including *Pseudomonas*. In concentrations of less than 5 percent, it is bacteriostatic.

Gentian violet, a dye derived from coal tar, is used therapeutically as a topical antimicrobial. It is effective against gram-positive bacteria and many fungi but is ineffective against gram-negative and acid-fast organisms. It may be used for oral and vaginal fungal infections.

Sulfur has fungicidal and keratolytic properties, and it may be used alone or in combination with other keratolytic agents (e.g., coal tar, resorcinol, salicylic acid). It is widely used in dermatology for the treatment of psoriasis, seborrhea, and dermatitis.

Soaps and detergents are not antiseptics because they do not kill or inhibit organisms but instead facilitate mechanical cleansing of the skin. Although sometimes referred to as disinfectants, they are usually too strong for application to skin or mucous membranes. The term disinfectant is generally used in reference to sterilizing inanimate objects.

Astringents

Astringents are substances that result in vasoconstriction when used topically. The principal ingredients in astringents are the salts of metals such as lead, iron, zinc, permanganates, and tannic acid. They act by coagulating proteins on a cell surface and decreasing sensitivity. The adverse effects of astringents are related to the degree of vasoconstriction produced by the preparation and their frequency of use.

Emollients and Lubricants

Emollients and lubricants are oily or fatty substances that are used to keep the skin soft and to prevent water evaporation. They lubricate psoriatic plaques, for example, thereby easing the removal of scales and reducing formation of fissures in intertriginous areas. Mineral oil, lanolin, or petrolatum, for example, are used to relieve pruritus and skin dryness.

The adverse effects of emollients and lubricants are related specifically to the active ingredient in the preparation. The most common is excessive greasiness of the skin and an increased incidence of acne.

Antimicrobial Drugs

Antimicrobial drugs change the nature of protein structure in the pathogen, causing coagulation of proteins, inhibition of cell wall synthesis, and disturbance of enzymatic processes. Antimicrobial drugs are either bactericidal or bacteriostatic to bacteria, fungi, and viruses. They may be administered locally or systemically to treat dermatologic disorders. In many severe, chronic, deep, or generalized bacterial infections, systemic antibiotics are preferred over topicals. Generally, topical antibiotics have limited clinical use for acute, superficial, and relatively localized infections. When antibacterial drugs are needed, the less absorbable antibiotics such as bacitracin, polymixin B, and neomycin are generally used. Several combinations of these products are available for use.

Topical antifungal and antiviral drugs are also generally effective. There are four classes of topical antifungal drugs currently available (see Chapter 25). Claims of unique efficacy are made by each new topical antifungal drug that appears. All have a cure rate of approximately 85 percent for acute infections and much less for chronic ones. Systemic therapy may be warranted if the patient is immunocompromised and refractory to topical therapies. Antimicrobial drugs are discussed extensively in Chapters 24 through 27.

The most common adverse effects of topical antimicrobials include local irritation, pruritus, burning sensations, and vesicular and maculopapular dermatitis. Topical neomycin in particular has been associated with toxicity. The risk is greater in patients with decreased renal function and increased drug absorption. In general, antimicrobials are safe, but long-term use may encourage the emergence of resistant organisms.

Anti-Inflammatory Drugs

Many skin conditions respond to topical or intralesional administration of adrenal corticosteroids. Although most often applied topically, they may also be administered systemically for severe disorders. Fluorinated topical corticosteroids are used in the treatment of disorders such as psoriasis because of their anti-inflammatory, antipruritic, and vasoconstrictive actions. They also have an ability to decrease cellular proliferation. When high-potency topical corticosteroids are used, the patient should be switched to less potent agents before treatment is stopped to minimize the risk of rebound flare of the disease.

The potent halogenated corticosteroids are the most likely to cause atrophy, telangiectasia, purpura, striae, and acneiform eruptions. Thin-skinned areas are particularly susceptible to the development of atrophy. Purpura is seen on the dorsal aspect of the forearms and hands with long-term use of potent corticosteroids. Allergic contact dermatitis, burning sensations, dryness, itching, hypopigmentation, facial hirsutism, folliculitis, moon facies, and alopecia (usually of the scalp) are also possible. Other adverse effects include overgrowth of bacteria, fungi, and virus, and immunosuppression. Fluorinated steroids may cause rosacea if they are used on the face. Infants may have more severe symptoms of rosacea because of a relative increase in body surface area.

Proteolytic Enzymes

❒ Proteolytic enzymes (ELASE)

Proteolytic enzymes are used to chemically débride burn wounds, decubitus ulcers, and venous stasis ulcers. Enzymatic débridement removes sloughing tissue and helps facilitate granulation of the wound. To avoid delayed healing, the proteolytic enzyme should be discontinued when the wound is clean with healthy, pink, granulation tissue present. Surgical débridement may be required if a decubitus ulcer is very serious or if complications, such as osteomyelitis, are present. Surgical skin closure or grafting may be required after chemical débridement has taken place.

Adverse effects of proteolytic enzymes consist of a mild, transient pain, paresthesias, bleeding, and transient dermatitis. Even with high concentrations, adverse effects are minimal, primarily consisting of local hyperemia. Adverse effects severe enough to warrant discontinuation of therapy have occasionally occurred. No systemic toxicity has been observed as a result of topical application of proteolytic enzymes.

Keratolytics

Keratolytic drugs such as salicylic acid soften scales and loosen the horny layer of skin. They are used in the treatment of warts, corns, calluses, and other keratin-containing skin lesions.

Hypersensitivity and damage to renal tubules has been reported, thus limiting the usefulness of some keratolytics (e.g., ammoniated mercury). They should not be used on reddened, irritated skin or an any area that is infected, if the patient has diabetes mellitus, or poor peripheral circulation.

Melanizing and Demelanizing Drugs

❒ Trioxsalen (TRISORALEN)
❒ Methoxsalen (OXSORALEN)
❒ Hydroquinone (PORCELANA, ESOTÉRICA)
❒ Monobenzone

Melanizing drugs are used to stimulate deposition of melanin in vitiligo, a disorder characterized by a loss of pigmentation. Two closely related drugs of the psoralen family, trioxsalen and methoxsalen, are the major melanizing drugs. Exposure to ultraviolet light is an integral part of the treatment protocol because the psoralens are effective in stimulating melanocytes only after photoactivation.

Demelanizing preparations include hydroquinone and monobenzone, which are occasionally used to bleach blemishes such as freckles, old-age spots, and the melasma of pregnancy or oral contraception. Some preparations of hydroquinone are formulated in an opaque base that shields ultraviolet light. Protecting the effected area from ultraviolet light significantly hastens the response. Hydroquinone is contraindicated in patients with miliaria, sunburn, skin irritation, or when depilatory agents are used.

Adverse effects associated with melanizing drugs are minimal, but some patients experience nausea, GI irritation, protoporphyria, and an exacerbation of lupus erythematosus. The only adverse effect of demelanizing drugs is a skin rash.

Sunscreens

Sunscreens protect the skin from excessive sunlight, thereby preventing sunburn and reducing the potential for wrinkles and skin cancer. It has been projected that use of a sun protection factor (SPF) 15 from age 6 months through 18 years results in a 78 percent reduction in the incidence of skin cancer over a person's lifetime. However, sunscreens can be toxic if products with high SPF values are used on infants. Sunscreens are capable of causing contact dermatitis and photosensitivity reactions in some patients.

Pharmacokinetics

There are several factors that influence transdermal absorption of drugs. Drug penetration and absorption are increased as much as 10 percent with hydration of the stratum corneum. Hydration causes the cells to swell, decreasing their density and thereby decreasing their resistance to diffusion. High ambient humidity increases hydration of the skin, as do certain drug formulations. Occlusion under impermeable plastic film enhances drug absorption by preventing transepidermal water loss and increasing epidermal hydration. Further, the more occlusive the formulation (e.g., emulsions, ointments) the greater the permeability. The low solubility of some formulations limits drug concentration and reduces the rate of absorption.

Because absorption of topical drugs occurs by passive diffusion, higher drug concentrations increase the amount of drug absorbed. Absorption from abraded or damaged skin surfaces is also much greater than that from intact skin and when drugs are left in place for prolonged periods.

Mucous membranes, facial skin, and intertriginous areas are sites of enhanced drug penetration, and often toxicity, because of the thinness of the stratum corneum. In addition, hair follicles and sweat ducts provide epidermal fenestrations that provide limited but low-resistance pathways for drug penetration.

Topical absorption from areas with thick skin (e.g., the palms of the hand and the soles of the feet) is relatively slow. Peak rates are not achieved for 12 to 24 hours. However, large fluctuations in plasma concentrations and increased first-pass effects commonly seen with some orally administered drugs can sometimes be avoided with transdermal administration. The use of topical rather than systemic drugs also may improve the therapeutic index of many compounds and enhance patient compliance.

Most topically administered dermatologic drugs have limited distribution. However, the skin functions as a reservoir for some drugs. For example, a topical corticosteroid under occlusion for 24 hours establishes a drug reservoir in the stratum corneum that can persist for as long as 2 weeks. Most drugs that pass through the stratum corneum to the epidermis are biotransformed there. Drugs that are not biotransformed in the epidermis pass unchanged into the systemic circulation. Drugs reaching the systemic circulation are eliminated through the kidneys, much like orally administered agents.

Critical Thinking Process

Assessment

History of Present Illness

Initial questions to be elicited from a patient with a dermatologic complaint should include when and where the disorder began. Establishing the time of onset helps determine whether the problem is acute or chronic or whether relapse has occurred. Knowledge about the site of the initial lesion and if there is pruritus may also be helpful. The distribution and development of individual lesions is often characteristic; therefore, information regarding any changes in the lesions should be elicited. Determining whether the patient has had any other symptoms helps distinguish systemic from localized problems. Information about what has been done to treat the disorder should be noted because many types of lesions are altered by therapies, some for the better, some for the worse.

The patient should also be asked about the effect of sunlight on the disorder because several disorders may result from photosensitivity. Questions about possible exposure to others with a similar skin condition helps elicit information about contagious illness. Asking the patient what he or she thinks may be causing the problem may provide some insight into the cause. Often however, the patient guesses incorrectly.

Other factors to be considered are the patient's profession, home, and workplace environments. It is important to understand what the patient comes in contact with and to what extent. For example, does the patient work around chemicals? What is the home environment like? Are there pets, plants, or flowers in the home or workplace? Patient-determined or health care provider–prescribed factors that may have alleviated the condition and the patient's psychological response to the problem should also be noted. A travel history can also be helpful, particularly if the travel included hiking or exposure to a variety of outdoor plants, shrubs, and trees. Does the patient engage in recreational activities that involve prolonged exposure to the sun or unusual cold. Inquire about the use of tanning salons. More than one million persons per day use tanning salons, and very limited federal regulation has been provided regarding safe use.

Ask also about the patient's self-care habits. Determine the frequency with which soaps, lotions, abrasives, and cosmetics are used. Record the brand names of any products used. Ask if there have been recent changes in bedding or clothing, or how these items are cleaned. Inquire about exercise and sleep patterns because these factors affect circulation, nourishment, and wound healing.

Past Health History

Patients should be asked if they have had a similar problem in the past. This question may help reveal a recurrent condition. They should also be asked about the presence of other types of skin lesions or rashes and other illnesses they now have or had in the past.

It is important to gather a thorough family history—genetically transmitted dermatologic conditions include alopecia (loss of patches of hair), ichthyosis, atopic dermatitis, and psoriasis—with particular attention to eczema, asthma, hay fever, and allergies. Systemic diseases with dermatologic manifestations include diabetes, blood dyscrasias, and connective tissue diseases such as lupus erythematosus. The background check helps the health care provider find clues that contribute to the dermatologic condition and the patient's response to treatment. Knowledge of these disorders would be of assistance, for example, in managing patients with atopic dermatitis.

A thorough drug history should also be gathered because a vast number of dermatologic reactions to drugs is possible. Use of products obtained from health food stores should also be elicited. Some products may even be life-threatening. The most common drugs involved in life-threatening drug-induced skin eruptions are identified in Table 64–1.

Physical Exam Findings

A differential diagnosis of a dermatologic problem is based on one feature—the appearance of the skin lesion. Therefore, inspection and palpation are essential when evaluating skin lesions. Examination should be accomplished by comparing the left side of the body to the right using a good light source.

Lesions should be inspected for the following variables: color, size, shape, margin characteristics, location and distribution (localized or generalized), texture, temperature, and odor. The arrangement (clustered, linear, annular, or dermatomal), whether the lesions are primary or secondary (Fig. 64–2), and if there is evidence of healing should also be noted. Descriptions of the lesions need to be specific, using the metric system for measurement.

Palpation of lesions is important, particularly for patients with dark skin. For example, erythema may not be noticeable, but warmth and edema of the involved area can be identified through palpation. The effect of pressure and any pulsatility should also be identified.

The use of the Norton Scale, or the Braden Scale for Predicting Pressure Sore Risk can help identify patients and the specific factors that place them at risk for decubitus ulcers. All patients at risk should undergo a systematic skin inspec-

PRIMARY LESIONS (Original Appearance)

NONPALPABLE

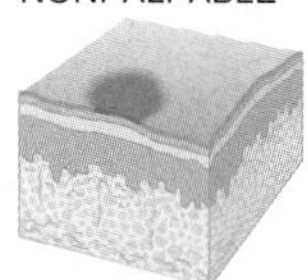

Macule: A spot, circumscribed, up to 1 cm; not palpable; not elevated above or depressed below surrounding skin surface; hypopigmented, hyperpigmented, or erythematous. **Example:** freckles. Referred to as **patch** if greater than 1 cm. **Examples:** café au lait spots, mongolian spots.

PALPABLE, SOLID

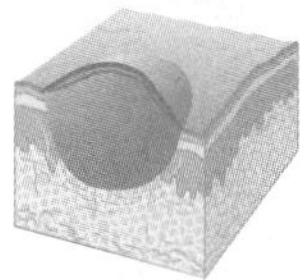

Papule: A bump, palpable and circumscribed, elevated and less than 5 mm in diameter; may be pigmented, erythematous, or flesh-toned. **Example:** elevated nevus (mole).

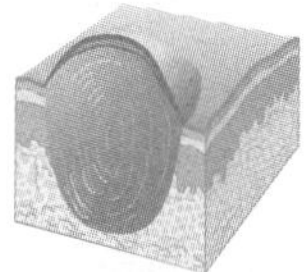

Nodule: A lesion similar to a papule, with a diameter of 5 mm to 2 cm; may have a significant palpable dermal component. **Examples:** fibroma, xanthoma, intradermal nevi.

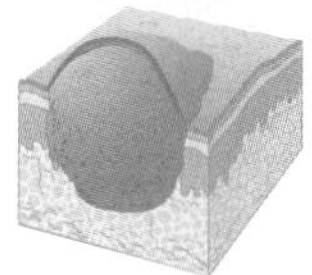

Tumor: Any mass lesion; generally larger than a nodule; may be either malignant or benign. **Example:** lipoma.

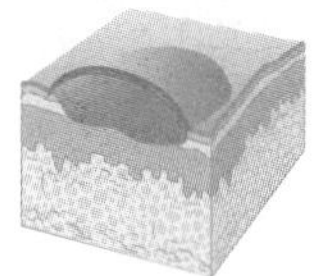

Plaque: Usually well-circumscribed lesion with large surface area and slight elevation.
Examples: psoriasis, lichen planus.

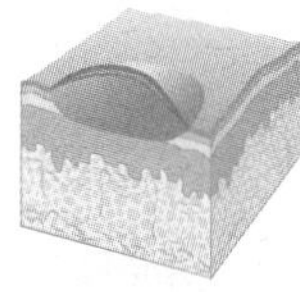

Wheal: An elevation in the skin, with a smooth surface, sloping borders, and (usually) light pink color; caused by acute areas of edema in the skin; may appear, disappear, or change form abruptly within minutes or hours; size ranges from 3 mm to 20 cm.
Example: mosquito bite.

PALPABLE, FLUID-FILLED

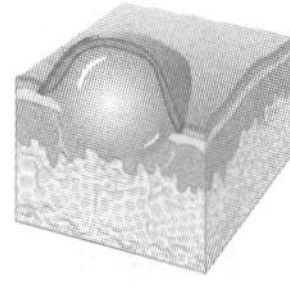

Vesicle: A small blister (up to 5 mm in diameter); fluid collection may be subcorneal, intraepidermal, or subepidermal.
Example: herpes simplex (early stages).

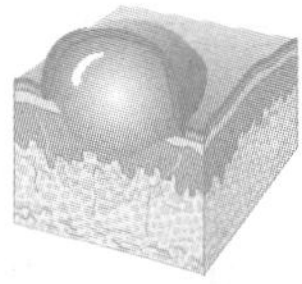

Bulla: A blister larger than 5 mm; fluid may be located at various levels. **Examples:** pemphigus, pemphigoid.

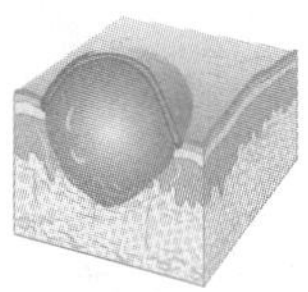

Pustule: An elevated, well-circumscribed lesion containing purulent exudate.
Example: acne vulgaris.

Figure 64–2 Skin lesions are assessed as primary or secondary. Primary lesions are recognizable structural changes in the skin. Secondary lesions are primary lesions that have changed because of the natural progression of the lesion or because of scratching, irritation, or secondary infection. (From Copstead, L. C. [1995]. *Perspectives on pathophysiology* [pp. 1048–1049]. Philadelphia: W. B. Saunders. Used with permission.)

Illustration continued on following page

tion at least once a day. Particular attention is paid to bony prominences.

Primary lesions develop without any preceding skin changes. In many cases, primary lesions are not seen and one must depend on the patient to describe how the lesion looked when it first appeared. Primary lesions include macules, papules, patches, plaques, nodules, wheals, vesicles, bullae, and pustules. Dermatologic diagnoses rely heavily on these primary lesions.

Secondary lesions result from changes in primary lesions and are influenced by scratching or infection. These changes may be brought about by the patient or the patient's environment and often occur in the epidermal layer of skin. Secondary lesions include scales, crusts, lichenification, keloids, scars, excoriations, atrophy, ulcers, and fissures.

Diagnostic Testing

Skin testing is conducted for three major reasons: to detect a person's sensitivity to allergens such as dust or pollen, to determine sensitivity to organisms believed to cause disease, and to determine if cell-mediated immune functioning is normal.

There are three types of skin tests: scratch tests, patch tests, and intradermal testing. Other special tests are important in the field of dermatology such as fungus examinations, biopsies, and cytodiagnosis. For scratch tests, extremely small quantities of allergens are introduced into small scratches made on the patient's back or forearm. A positive reaction is swelling or redness at the site within 30 minutes. Intradermal testing is performed by injecting the substance within the layers of the skin (e.g., Mantoux test for tuberculosis). Urticaria and atopic dermatitis are also tested using these methods. With a patch test, a small gauze square is impregnated with the substance in question and applied to the skin of the forearm. A positive reaction is swollen or reddened skin at the site of the patch after a given period of time.

Fungal cultures are performed to identify the specific type of fungus. Examinations are accomplished by scraping the diseased skin or mucous membrane and viewing it under microscopy. Potassium hydroxide testing determines the presence of mycelial fragments, arthrospores, and budding yeast cells. The use of a Wood's lamp helps determine the presence of a fungus. When potassium hydroxide is used in a darkened room, infected hair will fluoresce a bright yellow-green.

Biopsies are an important tool in ruling out malignancies of skin nodules when the etiology is unknown. A small sample of skin tissue is excised from the patient, stained, and examined under the microscope.

The Tzank test is the microscopic assessment of fluids and cells from vesicles and bullae. A smear of cells is col-

SECONDARY LESIONS (Modification of Original Appearance)

DAMAGED OR DIMINISHED SKIN SURFACE

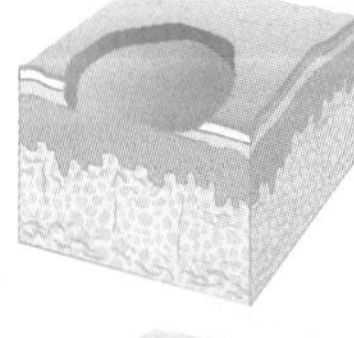

Erosion: Loss of epidermis that does not extend into dermis. **Example:** ruptured chicken pox vesicle.

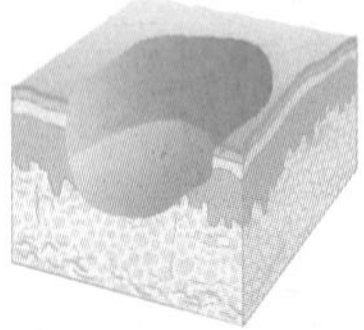

Ulcer: Loss of skin through the epidermis; healing results in scar formation. **Example:** stasis ulcer.

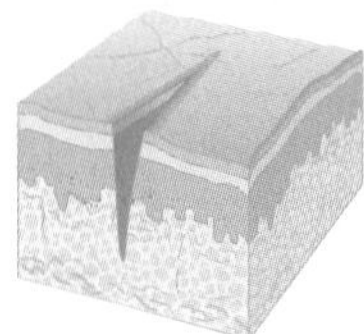

Fissure: A split in all epidermal layers of skin **Example:** athlete's foot.

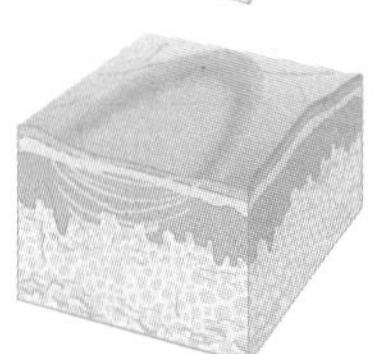

Atrophy : Diminution of epidermal surface; skin looks thinner and more translucent than normal; atrophy of the dermal layers may result in wasting or depression of the skin surface. **Example:** arterial insufficiency.

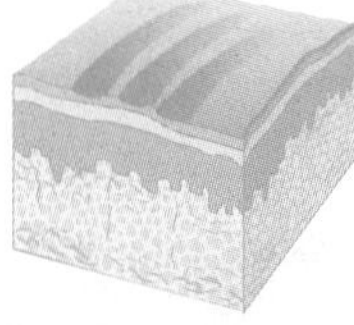

Excoriation: Loss of outer skin layers from scratching or rubbing. **Example:** scratched insect bite.

AUGMENTED OR INCREASED SKIN SURFACE

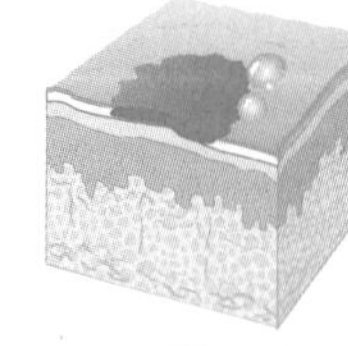

Crust: A collection of serous exudate and debris on the surface of damaged or absent outer skin layers. **Example:** impetigo.

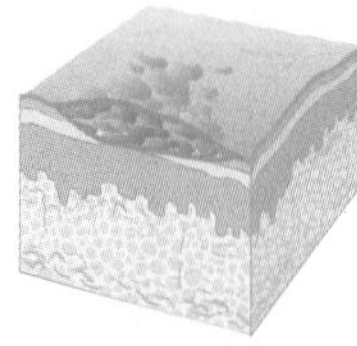

Scale: A compact portion of desquamating stratum corneum; may vary in size, thickness, and consistency. **Examples:** psoriasis scale (compact and thick), pityriasis rosea scale (thin and small).

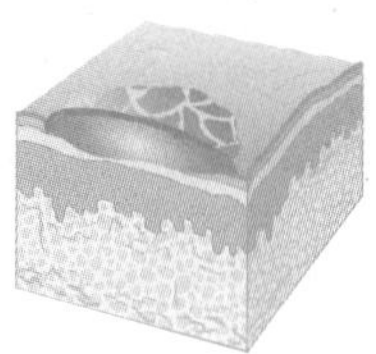

Lichenification: Epidermal thickening and roughening of the skin with increased visibility of skin surface furrows. **Example:** chronic atopic dermatitis.

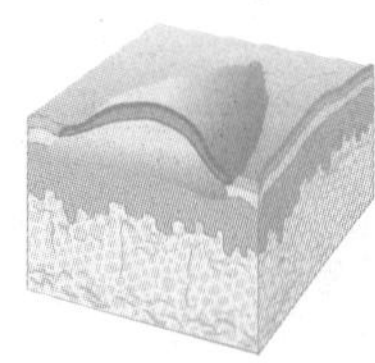

Scar : A collection of fibrous tissue that forms to replace lost epidermal and dermal tissue. **Examples:** surgical scar, acne scar.

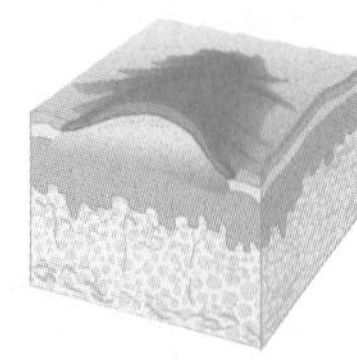

Keloid: Augmentation of scar tissue, creating a significant elevation on the skin surface after healing. **Examples:** postsurgical scar, post-acne scar.

Figure 64–2 *Continued*

lected from the affected area and prepared for microscopic observation. A cytologic assessment is then performed. Tzank testing is useful in testing bullous diseases, vesicular virus eruptions, and basal cell epitheliomas.

X-ray studies and blood and urine tests are sometimes helpful in dermatology patients who may have a systemic disease. For example, an antinuclear antibody test should be ordered in a patient with the skin lesions of systemic lupus erythematosus. A serology test is performed for a patient with a skin rash of suspected syphilis. Furthermore, a complete blood count and differential are always helpful in gauging the severity of infection and hematologic response. Wound cultures are indicated in patients who have open, weeping wounds in unusual areas such as the perineum.

Developmental Considerations

Perinatal Alterations in hormonal balance, mechanical stretching of tissues, and stress are responsible for melasma (chloasma), the mask of pregnancy. It is caused by increased melanin and appears as a blotchy, brownish tone to the skin over the jaw and the forehead of some women. *Striae gravidarum* (stretch marks) may also appear. Vascular abnormalities can cause spider angiomas and palmar erythema. Oily skin, hirsutism, and fingernail changes are other skin abnormalities seen during pregnancy.

Pediatric Providing drug therapy for children presents a unique set of challenges. Children undergo profound physiologic changes, and failure to understand these changes and their effects can lead to underestimation or overestimation of drug dosage. The potential for failure of therapy, severe adverse reactions, or fatal toxicity must be considered when treating children.

Children have an increased risk of systemic toxicity from topically applied drugs for two reasons. First, because of their greater surface area-to-weight ratio, a given amount of applied drug represents a greater dose (in milligrams per kilograms) compared with that of adults. Secondly, at least in preterm neonates, the permeability of the skin is increased (see Chapter 7).

The most common skin disease of the adolescent is acne, which can be devastating. The development of acne and the associated hormonal changes in adolescents are accompanied by feelings of self-doubt and a normal self-consciousness. When dealing with an adolescent with skin problems, body image considerations become a basic part of the treatment care plan.

Geriatric Physiologic changes of aging affect the skin. Progressive impairment of the peripheral vascular circulation alters the cutaneous response to physical trauma, cold, and infection. In contrast to pediatric patients, the skin of older adults is less permeable to drugs, perhaps because of the altered lipid content and loss of subcutaneous tissue (see Chapter 8). Changes in the central nervous system modify the perception of itching and pain, and atrophy of the reticuloendothelial system may impair the immune response. Also, emotional factors are certainly important and may prolong or exacerbate a skin disorder.

Psychosocial Considerations

Skin diseases are visible and therefore have a profound psychological effect on the person who may have to go through life with a perceived abnormality. Visually or physically disabling chronic skin disorders have been associated with chronic unemployment, poor mental health, and even suicide. Furthermore, there are a variety of cultural attitudes toward illness. In light of this, it is best not to assume, based on someone's ethnicity, that a certain idea or belief is held about their own dermatologic illness. Stereotyping inhibits an effective patient–health care provider relationship. It is better to ask patients how they feel about the condition and to individualize care.

Diet is influenced by culture. Some diets, especially those that are high in fat and calories (particularly non-nutritious calories) contribute to skin disorders. For example, there is a large list of foods that can cause urticaria (see Appendix C) in susceptible individuals. It is important to know the patient's normal eating habits when evaluating a skin disease.

Socioeconomic considerations cannot be ignored. Compliance with a treatment plan and return for follow-up care are influenced by social expectations or financial ability to pay for desired medications and treatments. Many topical therapies are expensive and cost is a factor that influences patient compliance with the treatment plan.

At every pharmacy, the cost to the patient is calculated using a specific formula. Usually, a pharmacy charge is added to the result. One large prescription is usually less costly (although not necessarily inexpensive) than the same amount of drug given using refills because the pharmacy charge is added to each refill. This may be particularly true with inexpensive drugs, when the pharmacy charge composes most of the patient cost. (see Case Study—Contact Dermatitis).

Analysis and Management

Treatment Objectives

Prevention is a key objective in the control of dermatologic disorders. General treatment objectives, however, for the patient with a skin disorder includes identifying and removing the cause (when possible). Additional objectives include restoring, protecting, and maintaining normal structure and function of the skin, reducing inflammation, reducing scales and calluses, cleansing and débriding, eradicating microorganisms, and providing symptom relief.

Treatment Options

In general, when choosing between conclusions suggested by the patient's history and observations made by the health care provider, the findings of the physical examination should take precedence. Collaborating with the patient regarding the formulation to be used may help improve compliance with the treatment regimen.

There are many dermatologic agents and formulations that can be used to prevent or manage many skin problems. The decision as to which agents to use include whether the lesion is dry or moist, pruritic, inflammatory, whether or not there is an infectious agent, and the location and spread of the lesion. In general, it is better for the health care provider to be thoroughly familiar with a few dermatologic drugs and treatment methods than to attempt to use many forms. Naturally, the course of some endogenous skin diseases cannot be altered. However, steps can be taken to prevent their occurrence and to minimize their effects.

Case Study Contact Dermatitis

Case Study

History of Present Illness	SM is a 66-year-old retired horticulturist who presents to the health care provider with complaints of periorbital redness, itching, and weeping. He denies exposure to known environmental irritants, ophthalmic medications, or the use of new skin care products. He acknowledges that he rubbed his face and eyes 2 days ago while he had his work gloves on. Had one other episode with similar characteristics about 2 months ago that "went away on its own" while he was on vacation. Character of lesions and distribution have not changed. Current medications are hydrochlorothiazide 25 mg po QD for mild hypertension.
Past Health History	SM denies history of drug or food allergies but has a family history of asthma. He has mild "seasonal hay fever."
Physical Exam	Diffuse, erythematous, vesicular lesions over forehead, periorbital region, and cheeks. Eyelids are edematous but without vesicular lesions. No evidence of secondary lesions at this time. Afebrile. No evidence of systemic involvement.
Diagnostic Testing	Patch test of 2 years ago evidences contact allergy to common herbicide used at nursery.
Developmental Considerations	SM spends Sunday afternoons leading children's tours of the local botanical gardens.
Psychosocial Considerations	SM is a widower who retired as a horticulturist 2 years ago. He works occasionally during busy seasonal periods and fills in when other employees are on vacation. He enjoys woodworking in his shop at home, making and refinishing furniture.
Economic Factors	SM lives on a fixed retirement income. He is enrolled in Medicare parts A and B and carries a secondary insurance that covers any additional charges and pharmacy needs.

Variables Influencing Decision

Treatment Objectives

- Remove or avoid underlying allergen.
- Reduce severity of pruritus.
- Reduce inflammatory process.

Drug Variables	*Drug Summary*	*Patient Variables*
Indications	Topical steroids used for the relief of inflammatory and pruritic manifestations of corticosteroid-responsive dermatoses.	SM's dermatitis is confined to periorbital region. High-potency formulations should be avoided. This will become a decision point.
Pharmacodynamics	Exert anti-inflammatory, and antipruritic effects. Concomitant use of moisturizer hydrates epidermis, thereby enhancing healing.	May take 2 to 3 weeks for full resolution of dermatitis.
Adverse Effects/ Contraindications	Suppression of HPA axis with large dose, large surface areas, or with use of occlusive dressings. Avoid contact with eyes.	Anticipate low-dose corticosteroid for short-term use, no dressing, and facial surface is a relatively small area. This becomes a decision point.
Pharmacokinetics	Steroid creams are well absorbed through hydrated skin. Retained in stratum corneum producing long duration of action.	Long duration of action related to storage site permits once to twice a day dosing.

Drug Variables	*Drug Summary*	*Patient Variables*
Dosage Regimen	Applied 2 to 4 times daily. 30 g is an appropriate quantity for face.	SM would prefer to keep the dosage regimen simple. This is a decision point.
Lab Considerations	There are no definitive laboratory considerations applicable to short-term, low-dose topical steroid use. However, if HPA suppression suspected, urinary free cortisol test and ACTH stimulation tests helpful in evaluating status.	There are no significant laboratory considerations, so this will not be a decision point in SM's treatment.
Cost Index*	Triamcinolone acetonide cream: 1 Hydrocortisone butyrate cream: 1	Triamcinolone acetonide is the least expensive of the two products, although both products fall into same cost index. This becomes a decision point.

Summary of Decision Points

- High-potency steroids should not be used on the face.
- Nongreasy cream formulation cosmetically acceptable and easy to use on face.
- Low-dose corticosteroid is acceptable for short-term use, without dressings, and on small surface area.
- Long duration of action permits once-daily to twice-daily dosing.
- Triamcinolone is least expensive compared with hydrocortisone butyrate.
- Appropriate to use moisturizer concomitantly to promote hydration and healing.

DRUG TO BE USED

- Triamcinolone acetonide (ARISTOCORT, KENALOG) 0.025% cream. Apply thin layer to affected area twice daily for 10 to 14 days. Dispense 15 g.
- Concomitant use of moisturizer.

*Cost Index: 1 = $ < 30/mo.
2 = $ 30–40/mo.
3 = $ 40–50/mo.
4 = $ 50–60/mo.
5 = $ > 60/mo.

AWP of 15 g triamcinolone acetonide is approximately $7
AWP of 15 g hydrocortisone butyrate cream 0.1% is approximately $18

Drug Variables

Because there are a vast number of preparations and formulations available in the United States and Canada, it would be impossible to discuss them all. Further, not all generic topical drugs are equivalent to their brand name counterparts, either in potency or in the presence of ingredients that may cause irritation or allergy. When in doubt about the proper method of treatment, it is generally considered prudent to undertreat rather than overtreat the disorder.

Many patients use OTC skin care products, such as moisturizers, cleansers, and sunscreens. Sometimes these products are optimal for the patient's skin type and are compatible with topical drugs. However, many times this is not the case. For example, oily moisturizers used by patients with acne are likely to undermine the beneficial effect that would be obtained from drying agents. Although the effectiveness of the drying agent could still be achieved without taking this factor into consideration, a better effect can be achieved when the use of both products are coordinated with the patient's skin type.

Further, the most effective results are obtained when the degree of moisturizing or drying associated with a specific drug is tailored to the patient's skin type. The most effective topical drug is the one that produces just enough moisture or dryness to meet the patient's needs. Figure 64–3 provides an overview of the continuum of topical bases and demonstrates the range of OTC products on the market today. The formulation used for the base affects potency and cosmetic acceptability. A description of the various vehicles and formulations can be found in Table 64–2.

Management of the patient with a dermatologic disorder may require monitoring of systemic parameters as well as monitoring of skin lesions. Complete blood counts,

Moisturizing ←			Neutral	→ Drying	
Oleaginous Bases	Water-in-Oil Emulsions	Oil-in-Water Emulsions	Oil-Free Emulsions with Emollient Esters	Strictly Oil-Free Emulsions	Alcohol Solutions
–	–	–	–	–	–
–	–	–	–	Gels	–
–	–	–	–	–	–
Water-Free Products	Oil-Based Products	Water-Based Products	Glycerin/ P.Glycol Bases	– Water Solutions	Other Volatile Solutions

Figure 64–3 Continuum of topical bases. Products to the left in this model become increasingly moisturizing. Products toward the right of the model are increasingly drying. The more moisturizing the product, the greasier it becomes and the less acceptable it is to patients. The ideal product is one that is neither too moisturizing or too drying. (From Scheman, A. J., and Severson, D. L. [1997]. *Pocket guide to medications used in dermatology* [5th ed., p. 6]. Baltimore: Williams & Wilkins. Used with permission.)

and liver function and renal function testing may be required for drugs that have a potential for systemic absorption.

Antibacterial Drugs There is little definitive evidence on which to base antibiotic selection for bacterial skin infections. The high prevalence of *Streptococci,* the sensitivity of some community-acquired *Staphylococci* to penicillin, and low cost make it a reasonable choice. If after 24 to 48 hours the patient is still febrile or not improving, a penicillinase-resistant drug can be substituted. Antibiotic therapy should continue for 10 to 14 days, depending on the rate of clinical resolution.

Antifungal Drugs Because the primary effect of most antifungal drugs is to prevent colonization of new organisms, any drug should be used for a minimum of 4 weeks to eradicate the infection. For example, scalp infections begin at the root, which is 3 to 4 mm below the skin surface. Because scalp hair grows about 1 mm per week, treatment should be continued for 4 to 6 weeks. Many fungal infections of the nails begin in the matrix, and thus, cure consists of eradication of the organism from that protected site. Treatment can take 6 to 12 months for fingernails and 12 to 24 months for toenails. However, the success rate is probably less than 60 percent.

Anti-Inflammatory Agents A correlation exists between the potency and the therapeutic efficacy of corticosteroids (Table 64–3). Application frequency depends on the site, response to the drug, and the application technique. Less potent formulations should be used on areas such as the face, the dorsum of the hands, groin, scrotum, and axillae because of the risk of striae with more potent preparations. Highest potency corticosteroids are restricted to no more than 45 g/week and should be used no longer than 2 weeks. Retention of the drug in the stratum corneum makes one to two applications per day sufficient. For children, preparations in the low or mildly potent category of preparations are recommended.

Acne Vulgaris The Food and Drug Administration has published a monograph on topical acne drugs, based on recommendations of the Advisory Panel on OTC Antimicrobial (II) Drug Products. Benzoyl peroxide, sulfur, and resorcinol with sulfur are considered to be safe and effective for the treatment of acne. Salicylic acid in concentrations of 0.5 to 2.0 percent is also safe and effective. Data are insufficient to determine the safety of concentrations over 2 percent.

Antiseptics, which are available in many formulations, are classified as unsafe or ineffective. Astringents (aluminum and zinc salts), which promote drying through vasoconstriction, are generally classified as ineffective. The antimicrobial povidone-iodine is considered safe, but data are insufficient to permit its final classification as effective. (see Controversy—Dermatologic Drugs).

Decubitus Ulcers Treatment regimens for decubitus ulcers vary a great deal from agency to agency, health care provider to health care provider, and patient to patient. Treatment depends on the stage of the ulcer and the condi-

Controversy

Dermatologic Drugs

JONATHAN J. WOLFE

Drugs used in dermatology are usually unexceptionable. Local anesthetic agents in small doses make minor surgery acceptable. Doses of epinephrine too small for systemic actions enhance the effect of those anesthetics. And topical drugs, even those containing potent steroids, represent a low risk when used correctly. Not many systemic medications are regularly used for dermatologic effect. However, the decision to use this last group of drugs demands careful thought and monitoring.

The classic systemic drug taken for dermatologic effect is surely tetracycline. The antibiotic is used at a low dose over a long time for acne treatment. It seems innocuous but may not be so. The female patient taking this drug may also be sexually active and taking oral contraceptives. Many women have become pregnant because of the interaction between oral contraceptives and tetracycline (or other oral antibiotic preparations). Later, the child may also have discolored teeth because of the presence of this common drug during gestation.

Isotretinoin, an antiacne agent derived from vitamin A poses a special risk. Again, it is women and neonates who bear most of the risk. Isotretinoin is a known teratogenic agent. Its use in pregnancy is associated with grave birth defects. Only a trust-based relationship with one's patient can permit the candid history needed for prescribing this drug. The sexually active woman who takes this class of drug must not, under any circumstances, become pregnant. The prohibition extends after the drug is stopped until it is fully eliminated (which is a lengthy matter with a lipid-soluble vitamin).

Critical Thinking Discussion

- An 18-year-old female patient suffers from disfiguring cystic acne. She has been taking isotretinoin since she was 17 years old. She now is planning her wedding, but needs to remain on the drug for another 6 months. Her liver tests have remained normal, and her progress is good. She tells you that her fiancé's religion does not permit contraception or abortion. What choices do you have as her caregiver?
- A 15-year-old boy takes 250 mg of tetracycline once daily for moderate to severe acne. He presents with a rash that disappears when the drug is discontinued. What alternatives can you suggest for oral antiacne therapy?
- A 22-year-old woman is planning her honeymoon in the Bahamas. She takes 250 mg of tetracycline daily for her moderate acne. She has been sexually active for the past four years. You have worked with her to meet her outcome of effective contraception. How can you help assure her that her stay in the tropics will be a happy memory under this regimen?

TABLE 64–2 VEHICLES AND FORMULATIONS

Vehicle/Formulation	Physical Characteristics	Advantages and Disadvantages	Examples
Ointments	Up to 10% of active ingredients in a fatty base such as petrolatum or lanolin, or in nongreasy bases	*Advantages:* Very moisturizing due to thick barrier that prevents water loss. Best reserved for thick, scaling, or keratotic lesions. Prolonged, protective action when applied at night. *Disadvantages:* Greasier than creams. Not suitable for use on hairy areas or on oozing surfaces	Betamethasone dipropionate (DIPROLENE), acyclovir (ZOVIRAX), combination antibiotics (NEOSPORIN, BACITRACIN)
Emollients	Base preparations of fixed oils such as olive oil, cotton seed, or flaxseed	*Advantages:* Keep skin soft. Prevent evaporation of water and development of dryness. *Disadvantages:* Avoid lanolin-based agents if there is an allergy to wool	Lanolin, petrolatum, vitamin A and D creams and ointments, vitamin E oil, cream, liquid, ointment (AQUACARE, NUTRAPLUS, LUBRIDERM, NIVEA SKIN CARE)
Creams (solid emulsions)	Active ingredients incorporated into emulsion-type hydrophobic base that vanishes when rubbed in.	*Advantages:* Good for daytime use, particularly with potent active ingredients that are effective when rubbed into oozing, denuded surfaces	Hydrocortisone cream (ASPERCREME, MYOFLEX CREME)
Lotions (liquid emulsions)	Powder suspended in oil or water with active ingredients. Requires shaking to disperse ingredients.	*Advantages:* Best suited for hairy areas or for lesions that are wet and oozing. Protects and cools acutely inflamed areas on face and on hairy body surfaces. *Disadvatages:* Are more drying than creams	Calamine lotion (CALADRYL)
Aqueous solutions	Active ingredients incorporated into a liquid that contains water as the solvent.	*Advantages:* Only mildly drying due to a slow evaporation of water. *Disadvantages:* Alcohol solutions are very drying because ethanol and other low-molecular-weight alcohols are volatile and rapidly evaporate.	Aluminum acetate (BUROW SOLUTION), potassium permanganate, zinc stearate, boric acid, DAKIN SOLUTION
Pastes	Ointments into which powders are mixed (e.g. zinc oxide, starch, talc, small amounts of tars, salicylic acid)	*Advantages:* Prolonged protective and occlusive action. Porous enough to permit heat to escape from the skin. *Disadvantages:* Not suited for hairy surfaces or on oozing areas.	Zinc oxide paste, anthralin paste
Paints	Liquids used to touch up small localized areas or intertriginous surfaces	*Advantages:* Desirable drying effect on moist areas where two skin surfaces meet *Disadvantages:* Sometimes stain and are messy	Gentian violet, salicylic acid; CASTELLANI PAINT
Powders	Materials in fine particles for dusting on surfaces	*Advantages:* Absorb moisture and reduce friction from large areas. Exert cooling or protective effects. *Disadvantages:* May cause irritation of respiratory tract in susceptible individuals and small children	PEDI-DRI FOOT POWDER, talcum powder, ZEASORB POWDER
Gels	Semisolid oil-based product of precipitated or coagulated colloid. Contains large amounts of water. Deposits film of active ingredients on skin	*Advantages:* Used in hairy areas as well as on smooth skin *Disadvantages:* Are somewhat drying when used on nonhairy areas	Betamethasone dipropionate (DIPROLENE GEL), coal tar gel (PSORIGEL), SEA BREEZE FACIAL CLEANSING GEL
Rubs and liniments	Have higher proportions of oil than ordinary lotions. Include counterirritants such as methyl salicylate, camphor, oil of cloves, capsaicin	*Advantages:* Used for pain relief on intact skin. May include antiseptic, analgesic, anesthetic additives. Can be formulated as gel, cream, lotions, or ointment *Disadvantages:* Ingredients are irritating to abraded skin. Some preparations are greasy	VICKS VAPORUB, MYOFLEX CREME BEN-GAY, ZOSTRIX

Table continued on following page

TABLE 64–2 VEHICLES AND FORMULATIONS *Continued*

Vehicle/Formulation	Physical Characteristics	Advantages & Disadvantages	Examples
Colloidal and emollient baths	Decrease the drying effect of water	*Advantages:* Soothing to irritated skin and help relieve itching *Disadvantages:* May cause bath tub to be slippery increasing the risk for falls	ALPHA KERI BATH OIL, AVEENO REGULAR BATH, AVEENO OILATED BATH
Soaps	Sodium salts palmitic, oleic, and stearic fatty acids. Prepared by saponifying fats or oils with alkalies. Consistency depends on the acid and alkali used	*Advantages:* Some contain antiseptics but only work to the degree that they mechanically clean the skin *Disadvantages:* Dry and irritating if used excessively	YARDLEY ALOE-VERA SOAP, BORAXO POWDERED HAND SOAP
Cleansers	Contain an emollient substance with the pH adjusted to be neutral or slightly acidic	*Advantages:* Recommended for persons with sensitive, dry, or irritated skin, or those who may have had a previous reaction to a soap product *Disadvantages:* May contain soaps	AVEENO CLEANSING BAR, PHISODERN, LOWILA CAKE
Hydrocolloid dressings	Composed of hydrophilic granules embedded in a polymer base. Absorbs water from wound to form protective gel	*Advantages:* Stimulates tissue granulation. Excludes bacteria. Waterproof. Easy application. Reduces pain	DUODERM, RESTORE, ULTEC
Transparent dressings	Thin, polyurethane adhesive dressings. Permeable to vapor and gas. Supports cellular regeneration	*Advantages:* Wound is visible. Waterproof. Good adhesion. Cost effective *Disadvantages:* Nonabsorbent. Difficult to apply. Limited to superficial lesions	TEGADERM, OPSITE

tion of the wound bed. Recommended treatment protocols for stage I or II decubitus ulcers consist of silicon sprays and the use of transparent (TEGADERM, OPSITE) or hydrocolloidal dressings (DUODERM). Treatment regimens for stage III decubitus ulcers include the use of wet to dry dressings, proteolytic enzyme débridement, and hydrocolloidal dressing. Wet-to-dry dressings and enzymatic or surgical débridement has been suggested for stage IV decubitus ulcers. Because of pre-existing multiple pathogens, wound cultures of decubiti are not recommended.

Patient Variables

The quantity of drug needed for a planned treatment regimen is an important factor when ordering a topical agent. For example, a 10- to 14-day course of a topical drug that is applied two to three times daily requires 30 g for the face, 45 g for the hands or feet, 60 g for arms or legs, and 60 to 90 g for the trunk. Coverage for the entire body requires 120 to 150 g or more.

Intervention

Administration

Standard precautions are recommended when handling a patient with skin disease. Prudent handwashing prevents self-inoculation of other body parts and minimizes the possibility of spreading the condition to others.

Manufacturers' instructions for application should be followed. Applying one drug on top of another should be avoided unless otherwise indicated. Before applying antiseptics, ensure that dirt, soil, organic matter, or other contaminants are removed from the skin surface. Such materials not only harbor organisms but provide a physical barrier that restricts access of the antiseptic and may chemically inactivate specific antiseptics.

Emollients are greasier than creams and thus are best reserved for thick, scaling, or keratotic lesions. They are very moisturizing owing to a thick barrier that prevents water loss and exerts prolonged, protective action when applied at night. When using emollients, application should begin at the midline and follow long, even strokes outward and downward in the direction of hair growth. This technique reduces the risk of follicle irritation and skin inflammation. Patients with an allergy to wool should avoid the use of emollients, however.

Lotions are best suited for hairy areas or for wet, oozing lesions. They are more drying than creams. Creams are good for daytime use and should be rubbed in until they disappear. They are particularly effective when rubbed into oozing, denuded areas.

Ointments and pastes are not suited for hairy areas or on oozing surfaces. Pastes are applied with a tongue blade and are porous enough to permit heat to escape from the skin. They are, however, not suitable for hairy surfaces or on oozing lesions. To remove the paste, a cloth soaked with mineral oil or vegetable oil is used.

Paints have a drying effect on moist areas where two skin surfaces are in contact. They sometimes stain the skin and clothing and are messy to use.

Before applying topical proteolytic enzymes, the wound should be thoroughly cleansed with water or saline. Antiseptics such as hexachlorophene, heavy metal compounds, benzalkonium chloride, nitrofurazone, and iodides should

TABLE 64–3 EXAMPLES OF TOPICAL CORTICOSTEROID PREPARATIONS*

Group Potency	Preparation	Formulation
Group I (highest)	Augmented betamethasone dipropionate 0.05% (DIPROLENE, DIPROSONE, VALISONE, others)	Cream, ointment, lotion
	Clobetasol propionate 0.05% (TEMOVATE); [🍁] DERMOVATE	Cream ointment, solution
	Halobetasol propionate 0.05% (ULTRAVATE)	Cream, ointment
	Diflorasone diacetate 0.05% (PSORCON)	Cream, ointment
Group II (high)	Amcinonide 0.1% (CYCLOCORT)	Ointment
	Betamethasone dipropionate 0.05% (DIPROSONE)	Ointment
	Desoximetasone 0.25% (TOPICORT)	Cream, ointment
	Fluocinonide 0.05% (LIDEX); [🍁] LIDEMOL, LYDERM	Cream, gel, liniment, solution
	Halcinonide 0.1% (HALOG)	Cream, ointment
Group III (medium-high)	Amcinonide 0.1% (CYCLOCORT)	Cream
	Betamethasone dipropionate 0.05% (DIPROSONE, MAXIVATE)	Cream
	Diflorasone diacetate 0.05% (FLORONE, MAXIFLOR, PSORCON)	Cream, ointment
Group IV (medium)	Desoximetasone 0.05% (TOPICORT LP)	Cream
	Flurandrenolide 0.05% (CORDRAN); [🍁] DRENISON	Ointment
	Hydrocortisone butyrate 0.1% (LOCOID)	Ointment
	Hydrocortisone valerate 0.2% (WESTCORT)	Ointment
	Mometasone furoate 0.1% (ELOCON); [🍁] ELOCOM	Cream, ointment
	Triamcinolone acetonide 0.1% (ARISTOCORT, KENALOG)	Ointment
Group V (low)	Alclometasone dipropionate 0.05% (ACLOVATE)	Cream
	Betamethasone valerate 0.1% (VALISONE)	Cream
	Flurandrenolide 0.05% (CORDRAN)	Cream
	Fluocinolone acetonide 0.025% (SYNALAR, SYNEMOL, FLUONID)	Cream
	Hydrocortisone butyrate 0.1% (LOCOID)	Cream
	Hydrocortisone valerate 0.2% (WESTCORT)	Cream
	Triamcinolone acetonide 0.1% (ARISTOCORT, KENALOG, KENONEL); [🍁] TRIADERM	Cream, lotion
Group VI (mild)	Desonide 0.05% (DESOWEN, TRIDESILON)	Cream
	Fluocinolone acetonide 0.01% (FLUOCET, FLUONID, SYNALAR) [🍁] FLUODERM, FLUONID	Solution
Group VII (lowest)	Dexamethasone 0.1% (DECADRON)	Gel, ointment
	Hydrocortisone 0.5%, 1%, 2.5% (HYTONE, SYNACORT)	Cream, ointment, lotion

*It is recommended that one become familiar with and use one agent from each category, making the selection on the basis of cost, cosmetic acceptability, and efficacy.

Adapted from Goroll, A., May, L., and Mulley, A. (1995). *Primary care medicine: Office evaluation and management of the adult patient* (p. 907). Philadelphia: J. B. Lippincott. Used with permission.

not be used before or during the use of proteolytic enzymes because they have the potential for inactivating the enzyme. Any ointment previously applied should be removed before fresh application of the enzyme. Ointment is applied directly to the wound tissue and then covered with a thin layer of moist gauze or other nonadhering dressing. Enzyme activity depends on adequate moisture; therefore, the dressings are kept moist at all times and changed one to three times daily. Care should be taken not to allow the enzyme to contact healthy skin.

Keratolytics are for external use only. They should not be applied over moles, birthmarks, warts with hair growing from them, or warts on the face or mucous membranes. They should be kept away from fire or flames.

Occlusive dressings should be applied over small surface areas only. The use of occlusive dressings increases the risk of adverse systemic effects. Large body areas should not be wrapped.

Education

It is vital for the patient to understand the importance of handwashing each time the affected skin area is touched. Good hygiene of the unaffected areas of the body should be maintained and the affected area cleansed only in the prescribed fashion. The patient should avoiding touching the affected areas as much as possible and to dress in a manner that will minimize contact with the involved area.

Teach patients that soaps, cleansers, and detergents should be used only in the axillae and groin, and on the feet by persons with dry or irritated skin. Unless the patient's occupation exposes him or her to excessive soiling, most patients need not use soap on all body surfaces. When informed, most patients often comply with this restriction rather than to a total ban on soap. Baths containing a small amount of bath oil may be used but are less effective than application of oils to the skin after bathing.

The patient should be taught how to apply the prescribed drug and to continue its use for the recommended time period, even if results are not immediate or the symptoms are slow in subsiding. They should be informed that acute skin disorders do not clear up in 3 to 4 days. In some cases, it can take several weeks or months before significant improvement is noted. However, if the condition worsens, the patient should contact the health care provider.

Burns Burns can be avoided by using common-sense techniques. Patients should be taught to keep matches out of the reach of children, and they should be taught the dangers of fire. Handles on pots and pans should be turned inward toward the wall. A fire extinguisher should be close at hand, and a smoke alarm should be installed in the home.

Sunburns are potentially dangerous and can lead to extensive skin damage. Skin damage is caused by excessive exposure to the sun's ultraviolet rays. Damage can be minimized by avoiding long periods of time in the sun; wearing loose, light clothing that covers exposed body parts; and using a sunscreen.

Sunscreen products are labeled in terms of SPF. The higher the SPF value, the greater the protection. Preparations with high SPF values are recommended for people with fair skin who sunburn easily and those who are allergic to sunlight. Sunscreens with low SPF values may be used by those who tan without experiencing a sunburn. In addition, the health care provider should make sure that patients understand the need for a sunscreen when photosensitizing drugs (e.g., tetracycline) are used and should aid in the selection of an appropriate agent.

The best way to choose a sunscreen is by skin type, the length of time spent in the sun, the usual intensity of the sun in the patient's geographic area, and the formulation preferred. The intensity of sunlight at 5000 feet is about 20 percent greater than that at sea level and is at its highest between the hours of 10 AM and 2 PM in most areas. Fresh snow and white sand are effective reflectors that intensify the brilliance of sunlight.

The recommended SPF values for various skin types are as follows:

- SPF 8 or higher: usually very fair complexion with red or blonde hair and freckles; always burns, never tans
- SPF 6 to 7: usually fair skinned; burns easily, minimal tanning
- SPF 4 to 5: sometimes burns but gradually tans
- SPF 2 to 3: minimal burning, always tans
- SPF 2: rarely ever burns, always tans
- No sunscreen: never burns, tans darkly

Sunscreens should be applied 30 minutes to 1 hour before sun exposure to allow absorption into the skin. It should be reapplied every 2 hours, and after swimming or sweating. Even sunscreens that are labeled waterproof or water resistant are removed by toweling and perspiration.

Decubitus Ulcers The most effective way to treat a decubitus ulcer is to prevent it in the first place. Skin care should be individualized but at minimum should be cleansed at the time of soiling and at routine intervals. The patient should be taught about environmental factors that lead to skin drying, such as low humidity and exposure to cold. Massage over bony prominences should be avoided. Exposure to moisture due to incontinence, perspiration, or wound drainage should also be avoided. The use of proper positioning, transferring, and turning techniques minimizes skin injury due to friction and shearing forces. Adequate protein and calorie intake are necessary to promote tissue integrity and healing. Nutritional supplements or support should be available as required. Rehabilitation efforts should be instituted as early as possible in the treatment regimen.

Evaluation

Acute skin lesions should decrease in size and eventually disappear when treatment has been successful. It should be noted, however, that acute skin lesions do not resolve in 3 to 4 days. They require time and frequent observation. Chronic skin conditions, some decubitus ulcers, and severe burns may take weeks to months or even years to heal. Recorded changes help determine progress toward achieving the desired outcome or resolution of the skin disorder. Furthermore, because the affected area is visible, drug therapy can be directly and continuously monitored, although not always quantitatively.

SUMMARY

- The primary function of the epidermis is to retard the loss of fluids from the inner body to the outside environment. The dermis contributes to the support and nourishment of the epidermis. The subcutaneous tissues insulate the body from cold, cushion deep tissues from trauma, and serve as a reserve source of calories.
- Noninfectious, inflammatory dermatoses include atopic dermatitis, contact dermatitis, seborrheic dermatitis, urticaria, psoriasis, pityriasis rosea, and lichen planus.
- Infectious, inflammatory dermatoses include bacterial, fungal, and viral infections.
- Acne vulgaris is a common adolescent skin disorder that is characterized by open and closed comedones, and in some cases, abscesses and inflammatory cysts.
- Skin trauma can cause infection when physical injury disrupts skin integrity.
- Drug reactions can manifest as a variety of skin disorders including local and diffuse lesions as well as life-threatening systemic reactions.
- Infestations and insect bites are potential causes of skin lesions with reactions that range from redness and itching to anaphylaxis.
- Decubitus and stasis ulcers are breaches in skin integrity and increase the risk for infection and delayed healing.
- Topical drug classifications that may be used in the management of dermatologic disorders include antiseptics, astringents, emollients and lubricants, antimicrobials, anti-inflammatory agents, proteolytic enzymes, keratolytics, melanizing/demelanizing agents, and sunscreens.
- Adverse effects of topical agents range from local drying, pruritus, urticaria, erythema, blistering and peeling to systemic effects such as Stevens-Johnson syndrome and anaphylaxis.
- Factors that influence the absorption of topical dermatologic drugs include the degree of skin hydration and humidity, occlusion, drug concentration, and the site of administration.
- Management of the patient with a dermatologic disorder may require monitoring of systemic laboratory parameters as well as monitoring of the lesions.
- General treatment objectives for the patient with a skin disorder include prevention, identifying and removing the cause, restor-

ing and maintaining normal structure and function of the skin, and providing symptom relief.

- In general, it is better for the health care provider to be thoroughly familiar with a few dermatologic drugs and treatment methods than to attempt to use many.
- Patients and their families should be educated as to the cause of the skin disorder and how to minimize its recurrence and spread to other body surfaces or other persons.
- Clear instructions regarding application of the topical dermatologic agent should be provided. Compliance with the plan of care will improve with documented patient understanding of the regimen.
- Subacute skin lesions should decrease in size and eventually disappear when treatment has been successful. Chronic skin conditions, some decubitus ulcers, and severe burns may take weeks to months or even years to heal.

BIBLIOGRAPHY

Abram, S. (1995). *Control of communicable diseases in man.* Washington, D.C.: American Public Health Association.

American Medical Association. (1995). *Drug evaluation annual.* Milwaukee: Author.

Barnett, J. (1995). Topical antibiotics. *Topics in Emergency Medicine,* 1(17), 40–42.

Braden, B. (1989). Clinical utility of the Braden Scale for predicting pressure sore risk. *Decubitus,* 2(3), 44–46, 50–51.

Bryant R. (1992). *Acute and chronic wounds: Nursing management.* St. Louis: Mosby.

Greenberger, N., and Hinthorn, D. (1993). *History taking and physical examination: Essentials and clinical correlates.* St. Louis: Mosby–Year Book.

Habif, T. (1996). *Clinical dermatology: A color guide to diagnosis and therapy.* (3rd ed.). St. Louis: Mosby.

Ives, T. (1992). Benzoyl peroxide. *American Pharmacy,* 32, 33–38.

Keyser, J. (1992). Foot wounds in diabetic patients. *Postgraduate Medicine,* 91, 98–109.

Jarvis, C. (1996). *Physical examination and health assessment* (2nd ed.). Philadelphia: W. B. Saunders.

Lesher, J., Levine, N., and Treadwell, P. (1994). Fungal infections of the skin. *Patient Care,* 28, 16–44.

Lowe, N. (1993). *Practical psoriasis therapy* (2nd ed.). St. Louis: Mosby–Year Book.

Mandell, G., Bennett, J., and Dolin, R. (1995). *Principles and practice of infectious diseases* (4th ed.). New York: Churchill Livingstone.

Nicol, N., and Huether, S. (1998). Alteration in the integument in children. In K. McCance and S. Huether (Ed.), *Pathophysiology: The biologic basis for disease in adults and children* (3rd ed.). St. Louis: Mosby–Year Book. pp. 1555–1569.

Nguyen, Q., Alyssa, K., and Schwartz, R. (1994). Management of acne vulgaris. *American Family Physician,* 50(1), 89–96.

Panel on the Prediction and Prevention of Pressure Ulcers in Adults. (May 1992). *Pressure ulcers in adults: Prediction and prevention. Quick reference guide for clinicians.* AHCPR Publication No. 92–0050. Rockville, MD: Agency for Health Care Policy and Research. Public Health Service, U.S. Department of Health and Human Services.

Scheman, A. and Severson, D. (1997). *Pocket guide to medications used in dermatology* (5th ed.). Baltimore: Williams & Wilkins.

United States Pharmacopeial Convention. (1994). *USP DI: Drug information for the health care professional* (14th ed.). Rockville, MD: Author.

Yarkony, G. (1994). Pressure ulcers: A review. *Archives of Physical Medicine and Rehabilitation,* 75(8), 908–917.

Unit XIII

Appendices

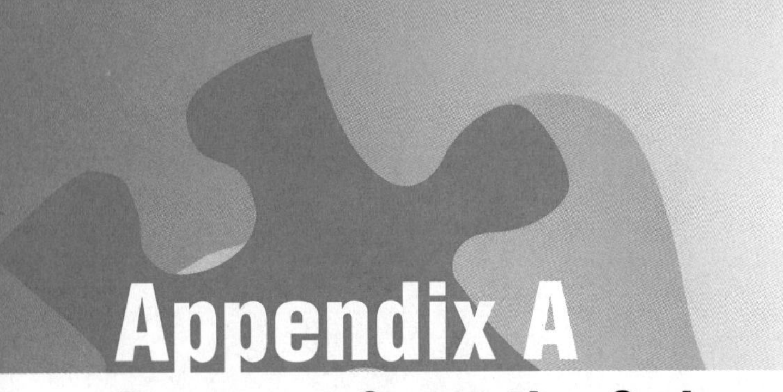

Appendix A

Resources Supporting Orphan Drug Development

National Information Center for Orphan Drugs and Rare Diseases (NICODARD)
Federal Food and Drug Administration Office of Orphan Product Development
5600 Fishers Lane HF-35 Room 8-73
Rockville, MD 20857
800-300-7469
http://www.fda.gov/orphan/about/progovn.htm

The Office of Orphan Product Development (OOPD) is located in the office of the Commissioner of the Food and Drug Administration. OOPD administers the orphan drug products development program.

National Organization for Rare Disorders (NORD)
Fairwood Professional Building
100 Route 37, P.O. Box 8923
New Fairfield, CT 06812-8923
800-999-6673
203-746-6518
203-746-6481 (FAX/TDD)
Online: http://www.healthy.net/pan/cso/cioi/NORD.HTM

NORD serves as a clearinghouse for information on rare diseases, offers networking programs linking patients and family members, and administers several drug assistance programs for indigent patients. Reports available on over 3000 orphan diseases.

Pharmaceutical Research Manufacturers Association (PhRMA)
1100 15th Street NW
Washington, DC 20005
202-835-3400
202-835-3429 (FAX)
http://www.phrma.org

Membership in PhRMA represents approximately 100 United States companies that have a primary commitment to pharmaceutical research.

National Institutes of Health (NIH)
9000 Rockville Pike
Building 10
Bethesda, MD 20892
301-496-4000
http://www.nih.gov

NIH is one of the world's foremost biomedical research centers and the federal focal point for biomedical research in the United States. The goal of NIH research is to acquire new knowledge that will help prevent, detect, diagnose, and treat disease and disability from the rarest genetic disorder to the common cold.

Centers for Disease Control and Prevention (CDCP)
1600 Clifton Road, NE
Atlanta, GA 30333
404-639-3311
404-639-3286
http://www.cdc.gov

A major agency of the Department of Health and Human Services, CDCP is concerned with all phases of control of communicable, vector-borne, and occupational diseases and with the prevention of disease, injury, and disability. The CDCP's responsibilities include epidemiology, surveillance, detection, laboratory science, ecological investigations, training, disease control methods, chronic disease prevention, health promotion, and injury prevention and control.

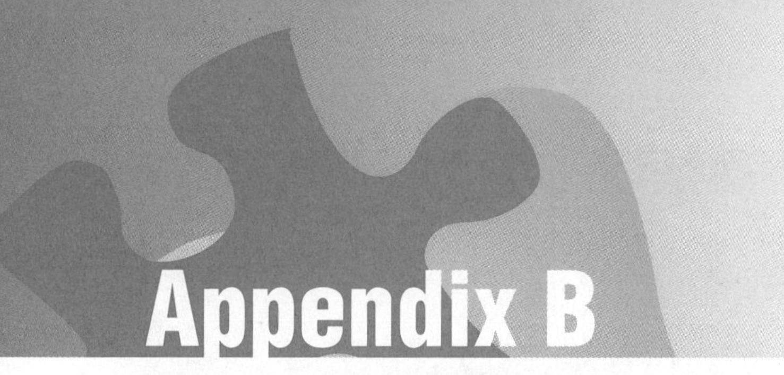

Appendix B

Selected Internet-Accessible Information Databases*†

Resource	Internet Address
Medical Subject Directories	
Achoo: The Internet Health Directory	http://www.achoo.com
Directory of Internet-accessible medical resources. Arranged into human life, medical practice, and business of health with scope notes on the contents. Includes a search feature of the entire directory	
Diseases, Disorders and Related Topics	http://www.mic.ki.se/diseases/index.html
Arranged by mesh (Medical Subject Headings: U.S. National Library of Medicine's controlled vocabulary) subject headings. Links to extensive disease information	
Martindale's The Reference Desk	http://www.sci.lib.uci.edu/HSG/Ref.html
Links to materials primarily created by teaching hospitals for the health care provider. Medical collection includes dental center, veterinary center, pharmacy center, nursing center, public health center, nutrition center, clinic—primary care, and others	
Health World	http://www.healthy.net
Most material here is alternative medicine, both original materials and links or other alternative medicine sources	
MedWeb: Biomedical Internet Resources	http://www.cc.emory.edu/WHSCL/medweb.html
Thorough, divided into content areas with subsections on consumer health, disabilities, documents, electronic publications, guides, health sciences societies and associations, and lists of Internet resources	
Primary Care Internet Guide	http://www.uib.no/isf/guide/guide.html
Information for the primary care provider. Includes links to catalogs, libraries, and search engines, including medical journals, miscellaneous medicine, family practice, family medicine, general practice, public health, nursing, occupational and environmental medicine, medical history, medical education, and medical students	
Clinical Resources	
Agency for Health Care Policy and Research (AHCPR)–Supported Guidelines	http://text.nlm.nih.gov/ftrs/dbaccess/ahcpr
Each guideline is available in three versions: a clinical practice guideline, quick reference guideline, and consumer guideline. Topics include acute pain management, urinary incontinence, pressure ulcer in adults, cataract in adults, depression in primary care, sickle cell disease, evaluation and management of early HIV infection, benign prostatic hyperplasia, management of cancer pain, unstable angina, heart failure, otitis media with effusion in young children, quality determinants of mammography, acute low back problems in adults, poststroke rehabilitation, and cardiac rehabilitation	
Centers for Disease Control and Prevention (CDCP) Guidelines	http://wwwonder/cdc/gov/wonder/prevguid/prevguid.html
Office guidelines and recommendations published by the U.S. Centers for Disease Control and Prevention for the prevention of diseases, injuries, and disabilities	
United States Food and Drug Administration	http://www.fda.gov
Access to information related to drugs and drug regulation	
University of Iowa Family Practice Handbook	http://vh.radiology.uiowa.edu/Providers/ClinRef/FPHandbook/FPHomepage.html
Intended for health care providers, focuses on diagnosis and treatment of common illnesses	
University of Iowa Virtual Hospital	http://vh.radiology.uiowa.edu/Welcome/Welcome.html
Offers online materials for patient education and the health care provider	
National Jewish Center for Immunology and Respiratory Medicine	http://www.njc.org
Extensive patient education information relating to asthma, allergy, and respiratory immunology with links to other sites	
Clinician's Handbook of Preventive Services	http://indy.radiology.uiowa.edu/Providers/ClinGuide/PreventionPractice/TableOfContents.html
Sections on screening, immunization, prophylaxis, and counseling for children, adolescents, adults, and older adults	
Consumer and Patient Education	
American Family Physician Patient Information	http://vh.radiology.uiowa.edu:80/Providers/Publications/AmericanFamily/AFPHomePage.html
Online versions of consumer health information originally published in the journal *American Family Physician*	

Resource	Internet Address
Resources for Primary Care Physicians Links to patient education materials by topic	http://www.coolware.com/health/pcp/pateduc.html
The Herb Resource Foundation Offers monographs on individual herbs for a fee	http://www.herbs.org http://sunsite.unc.edu/hrf/
The American Botanical Council Nonprofit. Produces a quarterly journal, *Herbalgram* (by subscription, in conjunction with the Herb Research Foundation), and offers herb information packets for a fee and mail-order books	http://www.herbalgram.org.
Medicinal Plants of North America Information on medicinal plants of North America	http://probe.nalusda.gov:/8300/cgi_bin/browse/mpnadb
Drugs	
Antibiotics Guideline Sections on history, action mechanisms, resistance, host-antibiotic-microbe interactions, isolation of specific organisms in the laboratory, determination of antibiotic susceptibilities, and descriptions of specific antibiotic classes	http://aisr.lib.tju.edu/CWIS/OAC/antibiotics_guide/intro.html
Antibiotics Usage Guidelines Guide formulated for use at Medical College of Wisconsin. Specific treatment recommendations for common infections by drug name, drug class, organism, empiric therapy by site, and antimicrobial therapy in HIV-infected patient	http://www.intmed.mcw.edu/AntibioticGuide.html
Center Watch Information about clinical trials worldwide. Also has information about newly approved drugs	http://www.centerwatch.com/
Clinical Pharmacology Database searchable by trade or generic name. Information includes description, mechanism of action, pharmacokinetics, chemical diagram, picture of drug, indications, dosage, contraindications/precautions, drug interactions, adverse reactions, patient information, and product identification and classification	http://www.gsm.com/clinphrm/monographs.html
Doctor's Guide to New Drugs or Indications Information about new drugs or new indications in the United States and worldwide	http://www.pslgroup.com/NEWDRUGS.HTM
Drug InfoNet Information about drugs, diseases, questions to experts, and links to other sites; names, addresses, and phone numbers for many pharmaceutical manufacturers	http://www.druginfonet.com/
Farmaweb Information about drugs in English and Spanish	http://www.farmaweb.com/
Glaxo Wellcome Pharmacology Guide Quick reference guide to most of the important terms and concepts of pharmacology	http://www.glaxowellcome.co.uk/netscape/science/phguide/index.htmlh/
HealthTouchOnLine Drug Information Searchable database of drugs with information on drug uses, precautions, and side effects	http://www.healthtouch.com/level1/p dri.html
PharmInfoNet Drug Database Browsable database of drugs by trade or generic name. Links to online articles about the drug from several sources, including company press releases, *Medical Sciences Bulletin,* Internet FAQs, *Internet Mental Health Monograph,* and other sources	http://pharminfo.com
Pharmacology Glossary: Boston University School of Medicine Information on symbols and terms used in pharmacology	http://med-amsa.bu.edu/Pharmacology/Programmed/glossary.html
Pharmacokinetics Learning module on pharmacokinetics from Thomas Jefferson University	http://jeffline.tju.edu/CWIS/OAC/pharmacology/pharm guide/menu.html

Resources provided in this table should not be used in lieu of contact with health care providers. Inclusion in this list does not constitute endorsement.

*This listing presents only a small sampling of the resources available online. Use the medical subject indices to locate additional resources. Addresses on the World Wide Web are case sensitive; use of both upper and lower combinations is necessary.

†To determine if the online Web offering is reliable, ask the following questions:

- Who maintains the site?
- Is there an editorial board or listing of names and credentials of those responsible for preparing and reviewing the contents of the site?
- Does the site link to other sources of medical information?
- When was the site last updated?
- Are graphics and multimedia files, such as video or audio clips, available?
- Does the site charge an access fee?

Domain names:

.edu = educational institutions
.org = nonprofit organizations
.gov = government (nonmilitary)
.mil = military
.com = commercial
.net = network organizations

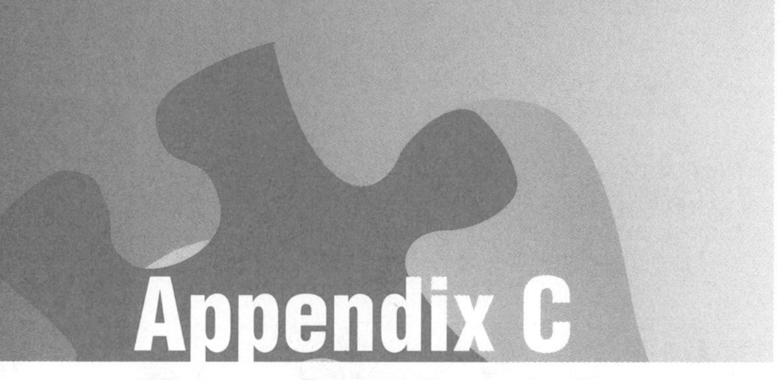

Appendix C

Dietary Considerations

FORMULAS RELATED TO DIET AND WEIGHT

Calculation of Ideal Body Weight

$$\% \text{ IBW} = \text{actual weight} \times 100$$

Midarm Muscle Circumference (MAMC)

$$\text{MAMC (cm)} = \text{MAC (cm)} - 3.14 \text{ (TSF) (cm)}$$

Estimated Nitrogen Balance (ENB)

$$\text{ENB} = \frac{\text{protein input (g)}}{6.25} - (24 \text{ hr UUN [g]} + 4)$$

FOODS THAT ACIDIFY THE URINE

Breads
Cereals
Cheeses
Cranberries
Eggs
Fish
Meats
Plums
Poultry
Prunes
Tomatoes
Tomato sauce

FOODS THAT ALKALINIZE THE URINE

All fruits (except cranberries, plums, and prunes)
All vegetables (except corn and lentils)
Buttermilk
Chestnuts
Coconuts
Cream
Milk

FOODS HIGH IN DOPAMINE

Broad (fava) beans

FOODS HIGH IN FOLIC ACID

Cantaloupe
Dark green leafy vegetables
Liver
Navy beans
Nuts
Oranges
Whole wheat products
Yeast

FOODS HIGH IN OXALIC ACID

Beets
Chard
Cranberries
Gooseberries
Rhubarb
Spinach

FOODS HIGH IN PURINES

Anchovies
Broth
Consommé
Mincemeat
Organ meats
Roe
Sardines
Scallops

FOODS HIGH IN CALCIUM

Blackstrap molasses
Bok choy
Broccoli
Clams
Canned salmon/sardines
Cream soups
Milk and dairy products
Oysters
Spinach
Tofu

FOODS HIGH IN IRON

Cereals
Dried beans/peas
Dried fruit
Leafy green vegetables
Lean red meats
Organ meats

FOODS HIGH IN VITAMIN D

Breads
Cereals
Fish
Fish liver oils
Fortified milk

FOODS HIGH IN POTASSIUM

Apricots
Artichokes
Avocado
Bananas
Broccoli
Brussel sprouts
Cantaloupe
Carrots
Chard
Chicken
Dried fruit
Garbanzo beans
Grapefruit
Honeydew melon
Ketchup
Kidney beans
Lima beans
Navy beans
Pears
Pinto beans
Potatoes
Prunes
Prune juice
Pumpkin
Oranges
Orange juice
Rhubarb
Spinach
Soy beans
Tomatoes
Tomato/vegetable juice
Turkey
Watermelon
Whole milk

FOODS HIGH IN PHYTATES

Brans
Whole grain cereals

FOODS CONTAINING SULFITES

Acidic juices
Avocados
Beer
Dried fruits
Dried vegetables
Instant potatoes
Processed foods
Shrimp
Wine

FOODS HIGH IN SODIUM

Baking mixes
Barbecue sauce
Butter/margarine
Buttermilk
Canned soup
Canned seafood
Canned/bottled spaghetti sauce
Canned chili
Ketchup
Cold cuts
Cured meats
Dried soup mixes
Fast foods
Ham
Macaroni and cheese
Most Chinese food
Olives
Parmesan cheese
Pickles
Potato chips
Potato salad
Pretzels
Relish
Salted nuts
Sauerkraut
Soy sauce

FOODS HIGH IN VITAMIN K

Asparagus spears
Avocado
Broccoli, raw and cooked
Canola, salad, soybean oil
Coleslaw
Collard greens
Dill pickles
Dry soybeans
Green cooked peas
Head, Bibb, red leaf lettuce
Margarine
Mayonnaise
Olive oil
Raw bean pods
Raw cucumber peel
Raw endive
Raw green scallion
Raw leaf kale
Raw parsley
Raw red cabbage
Sauerkraut

CAFFEINE SOURCES

Coffee (150 mL)

Brewed coffee (115 mg)
Brewed decaffeinated coffee (3 mg)
Instant coffee (65 mg)
Instant decaffeinated coffee (2 mg)
Percolated coffee (80 mg)

Tea (150 mL)

Brewed, U.S. brand (40 mg)
Brewed, imported (60 mg)
Iced tea (35 mg)
Instant tea (30 mg)

Carbonated Beverages (360 mL)

Citrus drinks (0–54 mg)
Coca-cola (45 mg)
Diet Pepsi (38 mg)
Dr. Pepper (40 mg)
Ginger ale (0 mg)
Mellow Yellow (40 mg)
Mountain Dew (53 mg)
Mr Pibb (54 mg)
Orange drinks (0 mg)
Other soft drinks (0–43 mg)
Pepsi-Cola (41 mg)
Root beer (0 mg)
Soda, seltzer (0 mg)
Tab (47 mg)

Foods

Baker's chocolate (26 mg/30 mL)
Chocolate milk (5 mg/240 mL)
Cocoa (4 mg/150 mL)
Dark, semisweet chocolate (20 mg/30 mL)
Chocolate syrup (4 mg/30 mL)
Chocolate cake/frosting (15.8 mg/one-twelfth of cake)
Milk chocolate (6 mg/1 oz)

TYRAMINE-RESTRICTED DIETS

General Information

- Tyramine-restricted diets are designed for patients taking monoamine oxidase (MAO) inhibitors, drugs that have been reported to cause hypertensive crisis when taken concurrently with tyramine-rich foods. These include foods in which aging, protein breakdown, and putrefaction are used to increase flavor. As little as 5–6 mg of tyramine can produce a response, and 25 mg is a dangerous amount.
- Food sources of other pressor amines, such as histamine, dihydroxyphenylalanine, and hydroxytyramine, are also avoided.
- Avoid over-the-counter drugs such as decongestants, cold remedies, and antihistamines.

Foods To Be Avoided

Cheeses: New York State Cheddar, Gruyere, Stilton, Emmentaler, Brie, Camembert, processed American

Other Aged Cheeses: Blue, Boursault, brick, cheddars, Gouda, mozzarella, Parmesan, Romano, Roquefort

Wines, Beers, and Ales: All tap beer, Chianti, domestic nonalcoholic beer, Riesling, sauterne, sherry, vermouth

Yeast and Yeast Products: Homemade bread, yeast extracts such as soup cubes, canned meats, and marmite

Meat: Aged game, beef and chicken liver, canned meats with yeast extracts, any meats marinated over 24 hours

Fish (salted dried): Cod, herring, pickled herring

Other: Anchovies, broad bean pods, chocolate, cream (especially sour), dates, dried figs, eggplant, nuts, overripe fruit, raisins, salad dressing, sauerkraut, soy sauce, vanilla, yogurt

Foods Containing Tyramine that Should Be Cautiously Consumed by Persons Taking MAO Inhibitors

Avocado (fresh)—maximum 1 per day
Aspartame-containing foods and beverages—not more than 3 servings per day
Chocolate candy—up to 4 oz per day
Cottage cheese or cream cheese, fresh—up to 4 oz per day of each
Monosodium glutamate in prepared foods, snack foods, Chinese foods—minimize use
Processed American cheese, fresh—up to 2 oz per day
Raspberries—not more than 1½ oz per day
Sour cream—up to 4 oz per day
Soybean paste or tofu—not more than ½ oz per day
Yogurt—8 oz fresh, refrigerated, or frozen

TABLE C–1. EFFECT OF FOODS ON DRUG ABSORPTION

Drug Absorption Reduced or Delayed		Drug Absorption Enhanced
Acetaminophen	Hydrocortisone	Carbamazepine
Alcohol	Hydrochlorothiazide	Chlorothiazide
Amoxicillin	Ibuprofen	Diazepam
Ampicillin	Isoniazid	Dicumarol
Aspirin	Levodopa	Diftalone
Atenolol	Nafcillin	Erythromycin estolate, ethylsuccinate
Cefaclor	Oxacillin	Griseofulvin
Cephalexin	Oxytetracycline	Hydralazine
Diclofenac	Penicillin G, VK	Labetalol
Digoxin	Phenobarbital	Metoprolol
Doxycycline	Propantheline	Nitrofurantoin
Erythromycin stearate	Rifampin	Phenytoin
	Sotalol	Propranolol
Tetracycline	Sulfonamides	Spironolactone

TABLE C–2. SELECTED LISTING OF DRUGS CAUSING PRIMARY NUTRIENT MALABSORPTION

Drug	Use(s)	Nutrient	Mechanism
Antacids	Hyperacidity	Calcium, iron, magnesium, zinc	Raises gastric pH and chelates the minerals
Aspirin	Analgesia, antipyretic	Calcium, iron	Damages gastric villi and microvilli; inhibits brush border enzymes and intestinal transport systems for nutrients
Cimetidine	Hyperacidity	Vitamin B_{12}	Reduces cleavage from its dietary sources, reduces secretion of intrinsic factor
Cholestyramine	Hypercholesterolemia	Fat, iron, vitamins A, E, K, B_{12}	Binding agent for bile salts, nutrients
Colchicine	Gout	Fat, vitamin B_{12}, sodium, potassium, carotene, lactose	Enzyme damage, inhibits cell division
Coumarin	Anticoagulation	Vitamin K	Antagonizes vitamin K activity
Cephalosporins	Antibiotic	Vitamin K	Depletes vitamin K
Cisplatin	Antineoplastic	Magnesium	Depletes magnesium
Diuretics	Diuresis	Sodium, potassium, magnesium, zinc	Increases elimination of nutrient
D-Penicillamine	Disease-modifying antirheumatic drug	Pyridoxine (vitamin B_6), zinc	Interferes with pyridoxine metabolism, chelates heavy metals
Ethylenediaminetetraacetate	Heavy metal poisoning	Zinc	Chelates heavy metal
Furosemide	Diuresis	Calcium	Reduces calcium absorption
Hydralazine	Hypertension	Pyridoxine (B_6)	Interferes with pyridoxine metabolism
Isoniazid, cycloserine	Tuberculosis	Pyridoxine (B_6)	Interferes with pyridoxine metabolism
Levodopa	Parkinson's disease	Pyridoxine (B_6)	Interferes with pyridoxine metabolism
Methyldopa	Hypertension	Vitamin B_{12}, folic acid, iron	Unclear, possible autoimmune action
Methotrexate	Disease-modifying antirheumatic, antineoplastic	Folate	Inhibits synthesis of specific enzymes by competing with vitamin or vitamin metabolites
Mineral oil	Laxative	Vitamins D, K, beta-carotene	Nutrients dissolve in oil; excreted in stool
Neomycin	Antibacterial	Fat, vitamin B_{12}, sodium, potassium, iron, calcium, lactose, sucrose	Binds bile salts, lowers pancreatic lipase
Para-aminosalicylic acid	Antimycobacterial	Vitamin B_{12}	Enzyme damage, inhibits cell division
Phenolphthalein	Laxative	Vitamins D, K, calcium	Rapid intestinal transit, decreased absorption
Potassium chloride	Potassium replacement	Vitamin B_{12}	Lowers ileal pH
Pyrimethamine	Malaria Ocular toxoplasmosis	Folate	Inhibits synthesis of specific enzymes by competing with vitamin or vitamin metabolites
Sulfasalazine	Ulcerative colitis	Folic acid	Blocks mucosal uptake of folic acid
Trimethoprim	Antibacterial	Folic acid	Competitive inhibitor of folate transport mechanisms

TABLE C–3. SELECTED LISTING OF DRUGS AFFECTING TASTE AND SMELL

Drug Class	Drugs
Amebicides, antihelmintics	Metronidazole, niridazole
Analgesics	Codeine, hydromorphone, morphine
Anesthetics (local)	Amylocaine, benzocaine, enzocaine, cocaine, procaine, tetracaine
Anticoagulants	Phenindione
Anticonvulsants	Phenytoin
Antifungal drugs	Griseofulvin
Antihistamines	Chlorpheniramine, cycloheptadine
Antihypertensives	Captopril
Antilipemic	Clofibrate
Antimicrobial drugs	Methicillin
Antineoplastic drugs	5-Fluorouracil
Antiparkinson drugs	Baclofen, chlormezanone, levodopa
Antithyroid drugs	Methimazole, thiouracil, methylthiouracil, propylthiouracil
Central nervous system stimulants	Amphetamines (bitter taste), psilocybin
Corticosteroids	Cortisone, prednisone
Diuretics	Diazide, diazoxide, furosemide (peculiar sweet taste)
Hypoglycemia drugs	Glipizide, phenformin (metallic taste)
Immunosuppressive drugs	D-Penicillamine, doxorubicin, methotrexate, azathioprine
Analgesics, antipyretics, anti-inflammatory drugs; disease-modifying drugs	Allopurinol, colchicine, gold, levamisole, phenylbutazone, 5-thiopyridoxine
Psychoactive drugs	Amitriptyline, carbamazepine, chlordiazepoxide, chlorpromazine, meprobamate, diazepam, flurazepam, lithium carbonate (metallic taste), phenytoin, triazolam, trifluoperazine
Skeletal muscle relaxants	Baclofen, chlormezanone, levodopa
Toothpaste ingredients	Sodium lauryl sulfate

TABLE C–4. SELECTED DRUG-FOOD INTERACTIONS

Class	Drug	Foods	Interaction
Antibiotics	Erythromycin Penicillin	Acidic fruit juices, carbonated beverages	Decreases drug's effect
	Tetracycline	Dairy products, iron	Impairs absorption
Anticoagulants	Warfarin sodium	Fatty fish; foods high in vitamin K; avocado; green leafy vegetables; broccoli	Potential bleeding; can reverse or reduce drug's effects
Anticonvulsants	Phenytoin	Foods high in folic acid; supplements high in calcium	Decreases seizure threshold
Antidepressants	Amitriptyline	Crackers, cookies, Brazil nuts, walnuts, eggs, pasta, meat, fowl, fish, cheese, cranberries, bread, plums, prunes, corn, lentils, peanuts	Interferes with benefits of drug
	MAO inhibitors	Foods containing tyramine or dopamine; alcoholic beverages; large amounts of caffeine	Hypertensive crisis
	Lithium	Large amounts of caffeine	Decreases drug's effects
	Phenelzine	Foods containing tyramine or dopamine	Hypertensive crisis; agitation
Antihistamines	SUDAFED PROCARDIA HISMANAL	Alkaline foods, grapefruit juice	Increases adverse effects
Cardiac glycosides	Digoxin	Bran	Decreases drug's effects
Diuretics	Furosemide Bumetanide Ethacrynic acid	High-sodium foods or antacids	Increases body fluid and blood pressure; alters electrolyte balance
	Triamterene Spironolactone Amiloride	Potassium-rich foods	Hyperkalemia
Bronchodilators	Theophylline	Charcoal-broiled beef Caffeine	Reduces effectiveness Increases adverse effects
Antihypertensives	Felodipine	Grapefruit juice	Increases serum level
	Hydralazine	Nutritional supplements such as ENSURE, SUSTACAL, MERITENE	Decreases effectiveness
Acne drugs	Isotretinoin	Fats, vitamin A supplements	Increases triglycerides; toxicity; adverse effects
Antiparkinson drugs	Levodopa, SINEMET	Vitamin B_6, meat or meat extracts; liquid nutritional supplements	Reduces effectiveness

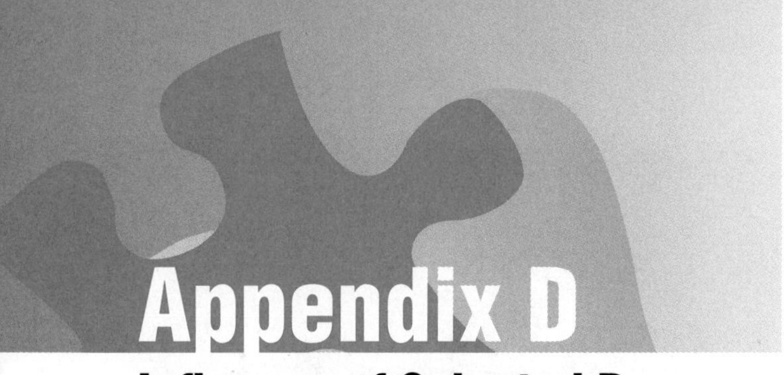

Appendix D

Influence of Selected Drugs on Laboratory Values

Drug	Increase in Values/False Positive	Decrease in Values/False Negative
Sympathetic Nervous System Drugs		
Epinephrine	Blood glucose Serum lactic acid	
Isoproterenol		Serum potassium
Reserpine	Serum prolactin Urinary catecholamine Urinary VMA	
Parasympathetic Nervous System Drugs		
Bethanechol	Amylase AST (SGOT) Lipase	
Propantheline	ANA	
Glycopyrrolate	Uric acid	
Opioid Analgesics and Related Drugs		
Opioids in general	Amylase, lipase	
Propoxyphene	AST (SGOT), ALT (SGPT) Alkaline phosphatase LDH Bilirubin	
Dezocin	Alkaline phosphatase AST (SGOT)	Hemoglobin
Anti-Inflammatory, Disease-Modifying Antirheumatic Drugs		
Salicylates in general	Urinary glucose (copper sulfate method) Uric acid VMA TSH 5-HIAA	Urinary glucose (enzymatic test method) Serum potassium Cholesterol
Propionic acid derivatives in general (may alter urine albumin, bilirubin, 17-ketosteroids, 17-hydroxycorticosteroid determinations)	BUN Creatinine Potassium Alkaline phosphatase LDH AST (SGOT), ALT (SGPT)	Urinary electrolytes Blood glucose Hemoglobin Hematocrit Leukocyte Platelet Creatinine clearance
Acetic acid derivatives in general (blood glucose values may be altered)	Alkaline phosphatase LDH AST (SGOT), ALT (SGPT) BUN Creatinine Potassium	Urinary electrolytes Hemoglobin Hematocrit Leukocyte Platelet Creatinine clearance
Diclofenac	BUN Creatinine Electrolytes Urinary uric acid	Urine electrolyte Serum uric acid
Anthranilic acids and enolic acids in general	Alkaline phosphatase LDH AST (SGOT), ALT (SGPT)	Hemoglobin Hematocrit Leukocyte Platelet

Drug	Increase in Values/False Positive	Decrease in Values/False Negative
Anti-Inflammatory, Disease-Modifying Antirheumatic Drugs *Continued*		
	BUN, creatinine Serum electrolytes	Urinary electrolytes
Gold products in general	AST (SGOT), ALT (SGPT) LDH	
Azathioprine		Serum uric acid Urinary uric acid Albumin
Cyclophosphamide (may suppress positive reactions to skin tests for *Candida,* mumps, tuberculin PPD)	Pap smear	
Methotrexate	Serum uric acid	
Allopurinol	Alkaline phosphatase Bilirubin AST (SGOT), ALT (SGPT)	Blood glucose
Colchicine (may interfere with urinary 17-hydroxy-corticosteroid concentration)	AST (SGOT) Alkaline phosphatase Urine hemoglobin	
Probenecid	Urinary glucose (using copper sulfate method)	
Antianxiety and Sedative-Hypnotic Drugs		
Clonazepam	Bilirubin AST (SGOT), ALT (SGPT)	
Oxazepam		Uptake of ^{131}I and ^{123}I
Chlordiazepoxide	Bilirubin	Metyrapone tests
Clorazepate (may alter results of 17-ketosteroids and 17-ketogenic steroids)	AST (SGOT), ALT (SGPT)	Uptake of ^{131}I and ^{123}I
Butabarbital	Urine glucose (using copper sulfate method)	Urine glucose (using enzymatic method)
Meprobamate	Urinary steroids	
Antidepressant and Antimania Drugs		
Amitriptyline	Bilirubin	Metyrapone
Doxepine (may alter blood glucose levels)	Alkaline phosphatase	
Imipramine		
Nortriptyline (may alter blood glucose values)		
Sertraline	AST (SGOT), ALT (SGPT) Cholesterol Triglycerides	
Amoxapine (may alter blood glucose values)	Serum prolactin	
Antipsychotic Drugs		
Acetophenazine	Pregnancy tests PBI (increase in PBI not attributable to an increase in thyroxine)	
Chlorpromazine Fluphenazine Mesoridazine Thioridazine Trifluoperazine (all may cause false positive or false negative pregnancy tests)	Bilirubin AST (SGOT) ALT (SGPT) Alkaline phosphatase Urine bilirubin	Allergy skin tests Hematocrit Hemoglobin Leukocytes Granulocytes Platelets
Risperidone Thioridazine Trifluoperazine	Serum prolactin	
Risperidone	AST (SGOT), ALT (SGPT)	
Central Nervous System Drugs		
Amphetamine Dextroamphetamine (both may interfere with urinary steroid determinations)	Plasma corticosteroid	
Pemoline	LDH Alkaline phosphatase AST (SGOT), ALT (SGPT)	
Skeletal Muscle Relaxants		
Baclofen	Blood glucose Alkaline phosphatase AST (SGOT), ALT (SGPT)	

Drug	Increase in Values/False Positive	Decrease in Values/False Negative
Skeletal Muscle Relaxants *Continued*		
Metoxalone	Blood glucose Bilirubin Calcium Cholesterol Creatinine LDL Triglycerides Uric acid	Magnesium Potassium Urinary sodium Urinary calcium PBI
Methocarbamol	Urinary 5-HIAA Urinary VMA	
Anticonvulsants		
Phenobarbital		Bilirubin (values altered in neonates, epileptics, and people with hyperbilirubinemia)
Primidone		Bilirubin
Clonazepam		Uptake of ^{131}I, ^{123}I
Clorazepate	Bilirubin AST (SGOT), ALT (SGPT)	Uptake of ^{131}I, ^{123}I
Phenytoin	Alkaline phosphatase GTT Blood glucose	
Valproates	Urinary ketones	
Gabapentin	Urinary proteins (using dipstick method)	
Acetazolamide	Chloride Urine glucose Urine protein 17-Hydroxycorticosteroids Blood ammonia Uric acid Urine urobilinogen Urine calcium	Potassium Bicarbonate Leukocytes Red blood cells
Carbamazepine		Pregnancy (using hCG method)
Antiparkinson and Myasthenia Gravis Drugs		
Carbidopa/levodopa	BUN AST (SGOT), ALT (SGPT) Alkaline phosphatase Bilirubin Coombs' test LDH PBI Urine ketone (using dipstick method) Urine glucose (using copper sulfate method)	Urine glucose (using enzymatic methods)
Bromocriptine	BUN AST (SGOT), ALT (SGPT) Alkaline phosphatase Uric acid	
Antibacterial Drugs		
Sulfadiazine Sulfamethizole Sulfamethoxazole Sulfasalazine Sulfisoxazole	Urinary glucose (using copper sulfate method)	
Sulfisoxazole	Urinary protein (using sulfosalicylic acid method and Urobilistix methods)	
Penicillins in general	Urine glucose (using copper sulfate method) Direct Coombs' test AST (SGOT), ALT (SGPT) LDH Alkaline phosphatase	
Carbenicillin	AST (SGOT), ALT (SGPT)	
Mezlocillin	Urine protein	Potassium
Piperacillin	Creatinine AST (SGOT), ALT (SGPT) Bilirubin Alkaline phosphatase Sodium Direct Coombs' test	

Drug	Increase in Values/False Positive	Decrease in Values/False Negative
Antibacterial Drugs *Continued*		
Cephalosporins in general	Coombs' test	
	AST (SGOT), ALT (SGPT)	
	Alkaline phosphatase	
	Bilirubin	
	LDH	
	BUN	
	Creatinine	
Cefaclor	Urine glucose (using copper sulfate method)	
Cefamandole		
Cefotetan		
Cefoxitin		
Cefuroxime		
Cephazolin		
Cephalexin		
Cephalothin		
Cephapirin		
Cephradine		
Cefotetan	Urine creatinine	
Cefoxitin	Serum creatinine	
Cefamandole	Urine protein	
Tetracyclines in general	AST (SGOT), ALT (SGPT)	
	Alkaline phosphatase	
	Bilirubin	
	Amylase	
	BUN (except for doxycycline)	
	Urinary catecholamines	
Aminoglycosides in general	BUN	Calcium
	AST (SGOT), ALT (SGPT)	Magnesium
	Alkaline phosphatase	Potassium
	Bilirubin	Sodium
	Creatinine	
	LDH	
Macrolides in general	Bilirubin	Leukocytes
	AST (SGOT), ALT (SGPT)	Platelets
	LDH	
	GTT	
	Alkaline phosphatase	
	CK	
	Potassium	
	Prothrombin time	
	BUN	
	Creatinine	
	Blood glucose	
Fluoroquinolones in general	AST (SGOT), ALT (SGPT)	
	LDH	
	Bilirubin	
	Alkaline phosphatase	
Ofloxacin (may alter blood glucose levels)		Leukocytes
Ciprofloxacin	BUN	
Norfloxacin	Creatinine	
Aztreonam	AST (SGOT), ALT (SGPT)	
	Alkaline phosphatase	
	LDH	
	Creatinine	
	Prothrombin	
	Partial thromboplastin time	
	Eosinophils	
	Coombs' test	
Clindamycin	Alkaline phosphatase	Leukocytes
	Bilirubin	Eosinophils
	Creatine kinase	Platelets
	AST (SGOT), ALT (SGPT)	
Chloramphenicol	Urinary glucose (using copper sulfate method)	
Imipenem/cilastatin	BUN	
	AST (SGOT), ALT (SGPT)	
	Alkaline phosphatase	
	Bilirubin	
	Creatinine	
Vancomycin	BUN	

Drug	Increase in Values/False Positive	Decrease in Values/False Negative
Antiviral and Antifungal Drugs		
Didanosine	AST (SGOT), ALT (SGPT)	
	Alkaline phosphatase	
	Bilirubin	
	Uric acid	
	Amylase	
	Lipase	
	Triglycerides	
Lamivudine	Amylase	
Stavudine	Amylase	
	Lipase	
	AST (SGOT), ALT (SGPT)	
	Alkaline phosphatase	
Zalcitabine	AST (SGOT), ALT (SGPT)	
	Alkaline phosphatase	
Foscarnet (may cause abnormal A-G ratios)	AST (SGOT), ALT (SGPT)	
Antitubercular and Antileprotic Drugs		
Isoniazid	Urine glucose (using copper sulfate method)	
Rifampin	BUN	
	AST (SGOT), ALT (SGPT)	
	Alkaline phosphatase	
	Bilirubin	
	Uric acid	
	Coombs' test	
Pyrazinamide (may interfere with urine ketone determinations)		
Streptomycin	BUN	Calcium
	AST (SGOT), ALT (SGPT)	Magnesium
	Alkaline phosphatase	Potassium
	Bilirubin	Sodium
	Creatinine	
	LDH	
Antihelmintic, Antimalarial, and Antiparasitic Drugs		
Mebendazole	BUN	Hemoglobin
	AST (SGOT), ALT (SGPT)	
	Alkaline phosphatase	
Quinine (interferes with 17-hydroxycorticosteroid determinations)	17-ketogenic steroids (using Zimmerman method)	
Antineoplastic Drugs		
Busulfan	Uric acid	
	Cytology results	
Thiotepa	AST (SGOT), ALT (SGPT)	
	LDH	
	Bilirubin	
	Uric acid	
	Creatinine	
	BUN	
Cyclophosphamide	Pap smears	
Chlorambucil	ALT (SGPT)	
Ifosfamide	Bilirubin	
Topotecan	AST (SGOT), ALT (SGPT)	
Mechlorethamine	Serum uric acid	
	Urine uric acid	
Melphalan	Serum uric acid	
	5-HIAA	
Carboplatin	Bilirubin	Potassium
	Alkaline phosphatase	Calcium
	AST (SGOT)	Magnesium
		Sodium
Cisplatin	BUN	Potassium
	Creatinine	Calcium
		Magnesium
		Phosphate
		Sodium
Carmustine	AST (SGOT)	
	Bilirubin	
	Alkaline phosphatase	
Cladribine	Uric acid	

Drug	Increase in Values/False Positive	Decrease in Values/False Negative
Antineoplastic Drugs *Continued*		
Cytarabine	Uric acid	
Doxorubicin		
Etoposide		
Lomustine		
Methotrexate		
Mitoxantrone		
Teniposide		
Vinblastine		
Vincristine		
Vinorelbine		
Dacarbazine	AST (SGOT), ALT (SGPT)	
	Uric acid	
	BUN	
Fludarabine	AST (SGOT)	
	Alkaline phosphatase	
Mercaptopurine	Blood glucose	
	Uric acid (when sequential multiple analyzer is used to determine values of either test)	
Pentostatin	AST (SGOT), ALT (SGPT)	
	LDH	
Thioguanine	AST (SGOT), ALT (SGPT)	
	LDH	
	Bilirubin	
	Alkaline phosphatase	
Fluorouracil	5-HIAA	
Daunorubicin	AST (SGOT)	
Idarubicin	ALT (SGPT)	
	LDH	
	Bilirubin	
	Alkaline phosphatase	
Paclitaxel	Triglycerides	
Irinotecan	Alkaline phosphatase	
	AST (SGOT)	
Hydroxyurea	BUN	
	Creatinine	
	Uric acid	
L-Asparaginase (may interfere with thyroid function tests)	Urine uric acid	Calcium
	Serum uric acid	
Mitotane		
		Uric acid
		PBI
Pegaspargase	BUN	Calcium
	Creatinine	
	Blood glucose	
Inotropic		
Amrinone		Potassium
Anticoagulants and Antiplatelet Drugs		
Ticlopidine	Cholesterol	
	Triglycerides	
	AST (SGOT), ALT (SGPT)	
	Alkaline phosphatase	
Heparin	Plasma free fatty acids	Triglycerides
	AST (SGOT), ALT (SGPT)	Cholesterol
Enoxaparin	AST (SGOT), ALT (SGPT)	
Antianginal Drugs		
Nitroglycerine	Urinary catecholamines	
	Urinary VMA concentration	
Isosorbide		Cholesterol
Antiarrhythmic Drugs		
Procainamide	AST (SGOT), ALT (SGPT)	
	Alkaline phosphatase	
	LDH	
	Bilirubin	
	Coombs' test	
Mexilitine	ANA	
	AST (SGOT)	
Phenytoin	Alkaline phosphatase	
	GTT	
	Blood glucose	

Drug	Increase in Values/False Positive	Decrease in Values/False Negative
Anticoagulants and Antiplatelet Drugs ***Continued***		
Quinidine	CK	
Lidocaine		
Mexiletine		
Flecainide		
Propafenone		
Disopyramide	AST (SGOT), ALT (SGPT)	Hematocrit
		Hemoglobin
	Bilirubin	Glucose
Phenytoin	Alkaline phosphatase	Dexamethasone, metyrapone test, PBI
	Glucose	Urinary steroids
Flecainide	CK	
Propafenone		
Acebutolol		
Esmolol (both may interfere with glucose/insulin tolerance tests)		
Propranolol	Serum K	Glucose
	Uric acid	
	AST (SGOT), ALT (SGPT)	
	Alkaline phosphatase	
	LDH	
Verapamil	Liver function tests	
Bretylium		Urinary epinephrine, norepinephrine, VMA, epinephrine
Antihypertensive Drugs		
ACE inhibitors in general	AST (SGOT), ALT (SGPT)	
	Alkaline phosphatase	
	Bilirubin	
	Uric acid	
	Blood glucose	
	Positive ANA	
Acebutolol	Alkaline phosphatase	
Metoprolol	LDH	
	AST (SGOT), ALT (SGPT)	
Amiodarone	AST (SGOT), ALT (SGPT)	
	Alkaline phosphatase	
	ANA	
Captopril	Urinary ketones	
Nifedipine	ANA	
	Direct Coombs' test	
Nimodipine		Platelets
Nonselective beta blockers in general	BUN	
	Lipoproteins	
	Potassium	
	Triglycerides	
	Uric acid	
Selective beta blockers in general	ANA	
	Blood glucose	
Propafenone	ANA	
Antilipemic Drugs		
Probucol	Bilirubin	Hemoglobin
	Blood glucose	Hematocrit
	BUN	Eosinophils
	CK	
	AST (SGOT), ALT (SGPT)	
	Alkaline phosphatase	
	Uric acid	
Cholestyramine	AST (SGOT), ALT (SGPT)	Calcium
	Alkaline phosphatase	Sodium
	Phosphorus	Potassium
	Chloride	
	Prothrombin time	
Gemfibrozil	Blood glucose	Hemoglobin
		Hematocrit
		Leukocyte
		Potassium

Drug	Increase in Values/False Positive	Decrease in Values/False Negative
Antilipemic Drugs *Continued*		
HMG-CoA reductase inhibitors in general (may cause thyroid function abnormalities)	Alkaline phosphatase Bilirubin	
Diuretic Drugs		
Carbonic anhydrase inhibitors in general	Urinary proteins 17-Hydroxycorticosteroids	
Bumetanide	Urinary phosphates	
Torsemide	Cholesterol Lipids	
Thiazide diuretics in general	Blood glucose Urine glucose Bilirubin Calcium Creatinine Uric acid Cholesterol LDL Triglycerides	Magnesium Potassium Sodium Urinary calcium PBI
Spironolactone	Plasma cortisol concentrations	
Urinary Antimicrobial and Related Drugs		
Nitrofurantoin	Blood glucose Bilirubin Alkaline phosphatase BUN Creatinine Urine glucose (using copper sulfate method)	
Peptic Ulcer and Hyperacidity Drugs		
Aluminum hydroxide	Serum gastrin	Serum phosphate
Histamine-2 antagonists in general	AST (SGOT), ALT (SGPT) Creatinine Prolactin	Parathyroid hormone
Nizatidine	Urobilinogen Alkaline phosphatase	
Ranitidine	Urine protein (using sulfosalicylic acid method)	
Omeprazole	AST (SGOT), ALT (SGPT)	Thyroxine (T_4)
Lansoprazole (may alter RBC, WBC, platelet levels)	Creatinine Gastrin levels Cholesterol Triglycerides Electrolytes	Electrolytes Creatinine
Metoclopramide	Prolactin Aldosterone	
Laxatives and Antidiarrheal Drugs		
Bismuth subsalicylate		Serum potassium T_3 and T_4
Diphenoxylate/atropine	Amylase	
Cascara	Blood glucose	Potassium
Psyllium	Blood glucose	
Lactulose	Blood glucose	
Antiemetics		
Hydroxyzine		Allergen skin tests
Meclizine		
Ondansetron	Bilirubin AST (SGOT), ALT (SGPT)	
Droperidol	Amylase Lipase	
Antiasthmatic and Bronchodilating Drugs		
Epinephrine	Blood glucose Serum lactic acid	
Salmeterol	Blood glucose Serum potassium	
Inhaled glucocorticoids in general (if significant absorption occurs)	Blood glucose Urine glucose	
Zafirlukast	ALT (SGPT)	

Drug	Increase in Values/False Positive	Decrease in Values/False Negative
Antihistamines and Related Drugs		
Astemizole Azatadine Brompheniramine Chlorpheniramine Triprolidine Clemastine Dimenhydrinate Diphenhydramine		Allergy skin testing
Pancreatic Drugs		
Insulin		Inorganic phosphate Magnesium Potassium
Oral hypoglycemics	AST (SGOT) LDH BUN Creatinine	
Thyroid and Parathyroid Drugs		
Levothyroxine Liothyronine Liotrix	TSH	AST (SGOT), ALT (SGPT) LDH Protime CK PBI Blood glucose Bilirubin
Propylthiouracil Methimazole	AST (SGOT) ALT (SGPT) LDH Alkaline phosphatase Bilirubin Prothrombin time	
Adrenal Cortex Drugs and Inhibitors		
Corticosteroids in general	Cholesterol Lipids Sodium Blood glucose	Uptake of ^{131}I and ^{123}I Potassium Calcium Leukocytes
Fludrocortisone		Potassium
Androgens and Anabolic Steroids		
Testosterone	17-Ketosteroid concentrations Chloride Potassium Phosphate Sodium	FSH LH
Hormonal Contraceptives and Related Drugs		
Estrogens	HDL Triglycerides Blood glucose Sodium Phospholipid Cortisol Prolactin Prothrombin Factors VII, VIII, IX, X	LDL Folate Pyridoxine Antithrombin III Pregnanediol

ANA, antinuclear antibodies; ALT (SGPT), alanine transaminase (serum glutamic-pyruvic transaminase); AST (SGOT), aspartate transaminase (serum glutamic-oxaloacetic transaminase); CK, creatine kinase; FSH, follicle-stimulating hormone; GTT, glutamyltransferase; hCG, human chorionic gonadotropin; 5-HIAA, 5-hydroxyindoleacetic acid; LDH, lactate dehydrogenase; LDL, low-density lipoproteins; LH, luteinizing hormone; PBI, protein-bound iodine; T_3, triiodothyroinine; T_4, thyroxine; TSH, thyroid-stimulating hormone; VMA, vanillylmandelic acid.

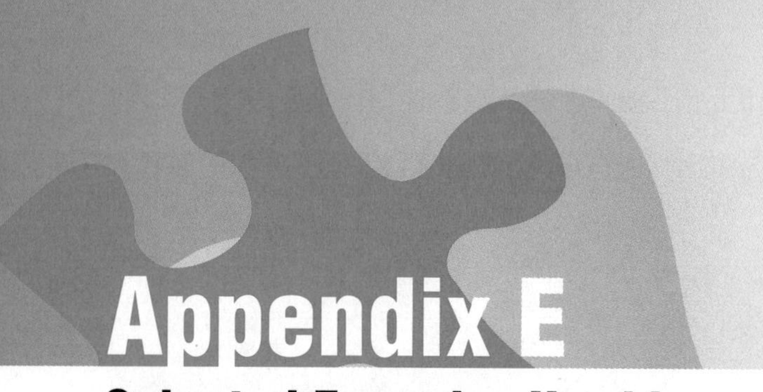

Appendix E

Selected Formulas Used in Pharmacotherapeutics

FORMULA METHOD FOR DOSAGE

Number of tablets, capsules, liquid needed

$$= \frac{\text{Dose ordered (what you want)}}{\text{Dose available (what you have on hand)}} \times \text{Vehicle}$$

RATIO METHOD FOR DOSAGE

$$\frac{\text{Dose ordered}}{\text{Amount to give } (X)} \times \frac{\text{Available unit}}{1}$$

Proportion Method

Dose ordered : 1 :: Amount to give (X) : Available unit

DIMENSIONAL ANALYSIS METHOD FOR DOSAGE

Number of tablets or capsules to be given

$$= \text{Order in mg} \times \frac{\text{1 tablet or capsule}}{\text{What 1 tablet or capsule is in mg}}$$

If amounts are in different units of measurement:

Number of tablets or capsules to be given = Order in mg

$$\times \frac{\text{1 tablet or capsule}}{\text{What 1 tablet or capsule is in grams}} \times \frac{1}{\text{1000 mg}}$$

CALCULATION OF INTRAVENOUS FLOW RATE

mL/hr

$$= \frac{\text{Amount to be infused in mL} \times \text{drop factor (gtt/mL)}}{\text{Desired administration time in minutes}}$$

$$\text{Drops/minute} = \frac{\text{mL/hour}}{4}$$

CALCULATING THE STRENGTH OF A SOLUTION

Solution strength   Desired solution strength

$$\frac{X}{100} = \frac{\text{Amount of drug}}{\text{Amount of finished solution (mL)}}$$

CALCULATION OF APPROPRIATE DILUENT VOLUMES

$$V_{(\text{final})} = V_{(\text{initial})} \times \frac{\text{mOsm}_{(\text{initial})}}{\text{mOsm}_{(\text{desired})}}$$

Example: To determine the degree of product dilution required, the initial product volume, $V_{(\text{initial})}$, is multiplied by the factor required to reduce initial osmolality to the point of tolerability. The difference between initial and final volume, $V_{(\text{final})}$, should be the volume of diluent added, $V_{(\text{diluent})}$. For instance, 10 mL of a product with an initial osmolality of 2000 mOsm requires 30 mL of sterile water to reduce osmolality to 500 mOsm.

$$V_{(\text{final})} = 10 \text{ mL} \times \frac{2000 \text{ mOsm}}{500 \text{ mOsm}}$$

CALCULATION OF BODY SURFACE AREA (BSA)

$$\text{BSA (m}^2) + \sqrt{\frac{\text{height (cm)} \times \text{wt (kg)}}{3600}}$$

CALCULATION OF IDEAL BODY WEIGHT (IBW)

$$\% \text{ IBW} = \text{actual weight} \times 100$$

DRUG DOSING IN RENAL FAILURE

$$V_d = \frac{\text{Total amount of drug administered}}{\text{Concentration of drug in plasma}}$$

$$\text{Dose} = V_d \times \text{blood level desired}$$

$$\text{Blood level} = \frac{\text{Dose}}{V_d}$$

CROCKCROFT AND GAULT EQUATION FOR CALCULATION OF CREATININE CLEARANCE

$$\text{CrCl}_{(\text{males})} = \frac{(140 - \text{age}) \times (\text{Weight kg})}{(72) \times \text{serum creatinine in mg/100 mL}}$$

$$\text{CrCl}_{(\text{females})} = \frac{(140 - \text{age}) \times (\text{Weight kg}) \times 0.85}{(72) \times \text{serum creatinine in mg/100 mL}}$$

CALCULATION OF IRON DEXTRAN DOSE FOR IRON DEFICIENCY ANEMIA

mg of iron =

$$\frac{0.3 \times \text{weight in pounds} \times (100 - [\text{Hgb in g\%}] \times 100)}{14.8}$$

(Note: Base dosage of iron dextran on hematologic response with frequent hemoglobin determinations. For patients weighing less than 14 kg [30 pounds], give 80% of the calculated dose.)

CALCULATION OF IRON DEXTRAN DOSE FOR BLOOD LOSS

Replacement iron (in mg) = blood loss (in mL) × Hct

CORRECTED SERUM CALCIUM

"Corrected" Serum Ca
= Serum Ca (mg/dL) + {0.8 × [4.0 − albumin g/dL]}

CONVERSION FROM LONG-ACTING TO IMMEDIATE-RELEASE DOSAGE FORMS

1. Calculate the total daily dose for the long-acting preparation.
2. Determine an appropriate dosing interval for the immediate-release form by selecting a value between 1 and 2 times the drug's half-life.
3. Divide the value from step 2 into 24: This will provide the number of doses to be given per day.
4. Determine the new dose by dividing the total daily dose by the number of doses given per day (step 3).

To illustrate, a patient is taking a long-acting theophylline preparation at a dose of 400 mg twice a day via a feeding tube. Changing to 200 mg of the immediate-release form every 6 hours offers a convenient dose and schedule and provides a relatively smooth drug plasma profile that approximates that of the previous long-acting formulation.

Example: Theophylline SR 400 mg po BID
Theophylline $t_{1/2}$ = 4–5 hours

400 mg × 2 doses per day = 800 mg

1.5 × 4 hours ($t_{1/2}$) = 6 hours

$$\frac{24}{6} = 4 \text{ doses per day}$$

$$\frac{800 \text{ mg}}{4 \text{ doses/day}} = 200 \text{ mg/dose}$$

CALCULATING AVERAGE ADULT DOSE OF CRYOPRECIPITATE

The following steps may be used in determining the appropriate number of units of cryoprecipitate:

1. Blood volume (mL) = kg of body weight × 70 mL/kg
2. Plasma volume (mL) = blood volume (mL) × (1.0 − hematocrit)
3. Units of factor VIII required = patient's plasma volume (mL) × (desired factor VIII level units/mL − initial factor VIII level units/mL)
4. Bags of cryoprecipitate = units of factor VIII/100

For example, to raise the factor VIII level to 0.5 unit/mL in a 70-kg adult with a hematocrit of 40% and an initial factor VIII level of 0 units/mL,

1. kg × 70 mL/kg = 4900 mL
2. 4900 mL × (1.0 − 0.4) = 2940 mL
3. 2940 mL × (0.5 − 0) − 1470 units
4. 1470 units/100 = 14.7 bags of cryoprecipitate

To achieve the desired therapeutic level, this dose may need to be repeated in 8 to 12 hours.

ESTIMATING KILOCALORIES IN PARENTERAL SOLUTIONS

Glucose in amino acid solutions:

Concentration of solution × g of glucose in solution
= physiologic amino acid infused × fuel factor

Example: To determine the number of kcal/g in 3000 mL of D5W,

$$\frac{3000 \text{ mL} \times 5 \text{ mg glucose}}{100 \text{ mL}} = \frac{150 \text{ g glucose} \times 3.4 \text{ kcal}}{1 \text{ g}}$$
$$= 510 \text{ kcal}$$

To determine the amount of protein in 2000 mL of 3.5% amino acid solution,

$$\frac{2000 \text{ mL} \times 3.5 \text{ g amino acid}}{1000 \text{ mL}} = 70 \text{ g amino acids/protein}$$

FAT EMULSIONS

1 mL of 10% fat emulsion = 1.1 kcal/mL;
number of mL × 1.1 = kcal

1 mL of 20% fat emulsion = 2.0 kcal/mL;
number of mL × 2 = kcal

Example: 500 mL of a 20% fat emulsion = 500 mL × 2 kcal/mL = 1000 kcal

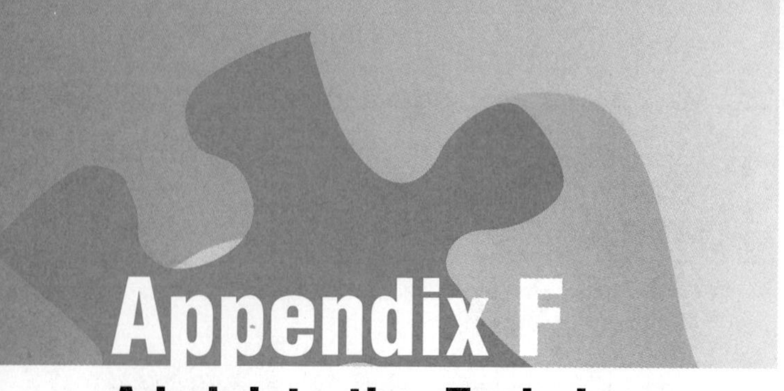

Appendix F
Administration Techniques

Elizabeth Kissell

ADMINISTERING OPHTHALMIC DRUGS

1. Ask the patient to look upward.
2. Gently retract the lower lid with your thumb or index finger against the cheek bone to expose the lower conjunctival sac (Fig. F–1).
3. Rest your hand holding the dropper or tube of ointment on the patient's forehead. Without touching the dropper to the eye structures, instill the prescribed number of drops into the conjunctival sac. If you are using an ointment, apply it in a thin stream evenly along inside the edge of the entire lower eyelid from the inner to the outer canthus (Fig. F–2).
4. Have the patient close the eyes gently. Using a clean tissue, gently wipe away excess medication, moving from the inner to outer canthus.

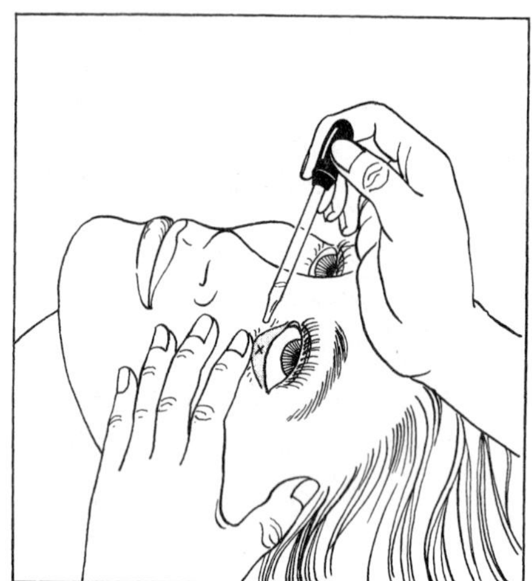

Figure F–1.

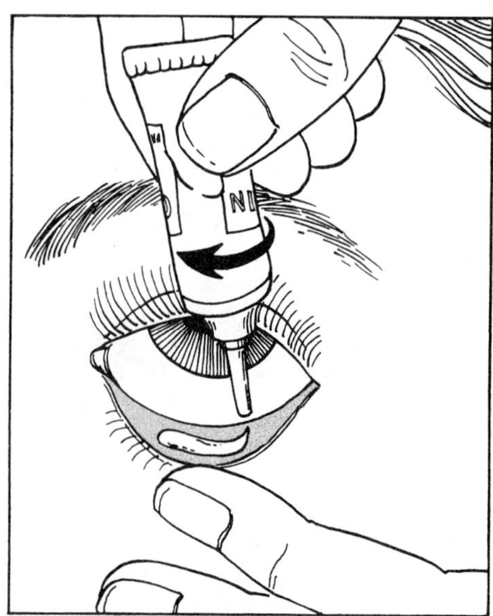

Figure F–2.

ADMINISTERING OTIC DRUGS

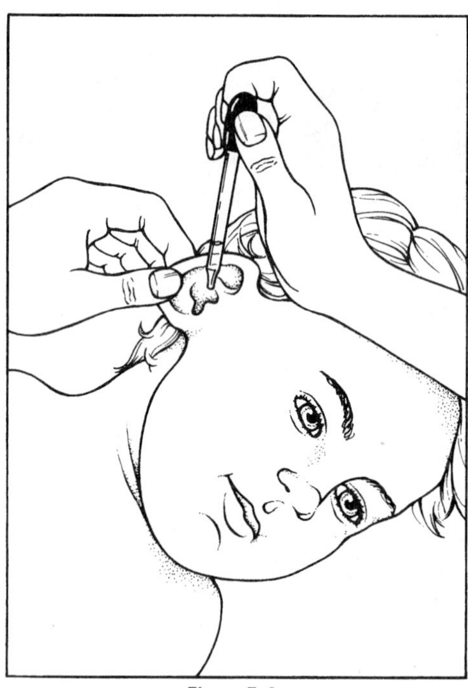

Figure F–3.

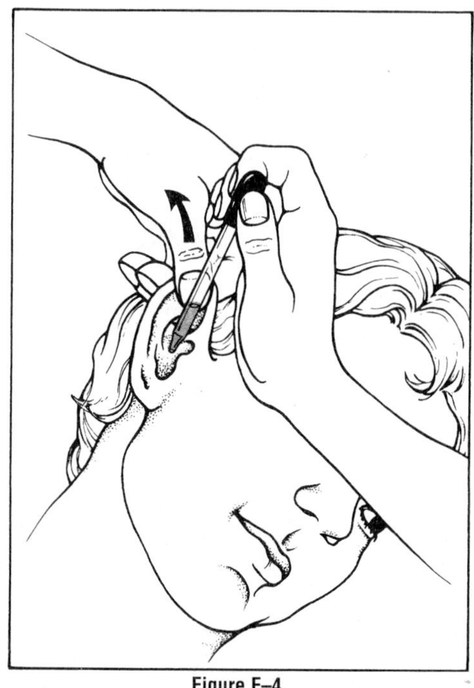

Figure F–4.

1. Using one hand, straighten the ear canal by gently pulling the auricle down and back for children under 3 years of age (Fig. F–3), or upward and outward for children over 3 years and adults (Fig. F–4).
2. Rest your hand holding the medication dropper 1 cm (½ inch) above the ear canal.
3. Instill drops on the side of the auditory canal, allowing them to flow in without falling directly on the tympanic membrane.
4. Ask the patient to maintain a side-lying position for 2 to 3 minutes. Apply gentle pressure on the tragus, or gently massage the tragus with your finger.
5. If drops are ordered for the other ear as well, wait 5 minutes and repeat this procedure.

ADMINISTERING NASAL DROPS AND SPRAYS

1. Ask the patient to lie supine and assist in positioning the head properly. When using drops, see the positions for the ethmoid and sphenoid sinuses (Fig. F–5) or the nasal passageways and frontal and maxillary sinuses (Fig. F–6). When using spray for young children, keep the head in an upright position; for older children and adults, tilt the head backward and support it with your free hand.

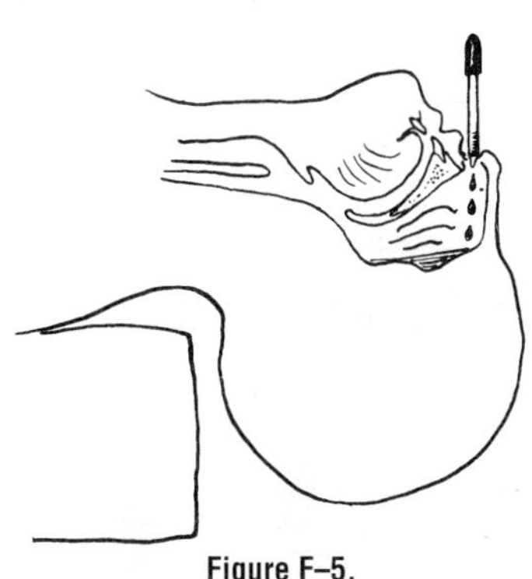

Figure F–5.

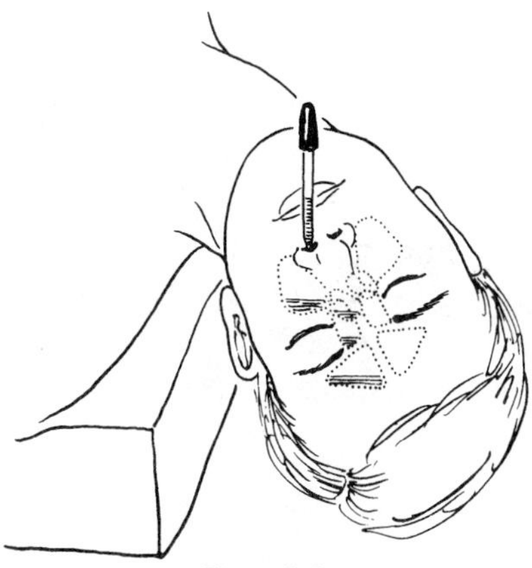

Figure F–6.

2. Hold the medicine dropper 1 cm (½ inch) above the naris with its tip pointing toward the upper membrane of the nasal cavity, and instill the prescribed number of drops. Have the patient remain in the supine position for 5 minutes. When a spray is used, occlude the opposite naris and administer the spray. Ask the patient to inhale as the spray enters the nasal passages.
3. Caution the patient against blowing the nose for several minutes. However, patients may blot a runny nose.

MIXING INSULIN IN ONE SYRINGE

1. Determine the total units of insulin to be administered from the medication vial (Fig. F–7).

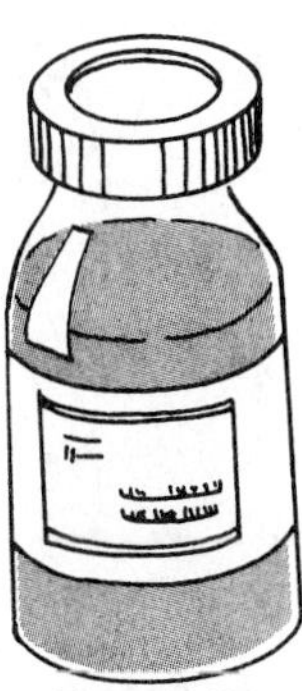

Figure F–7.

2. Rotate each vial between your hands for at least 1 minute.
3. Cleanse the rubber stoppers of both vials with alcohol.

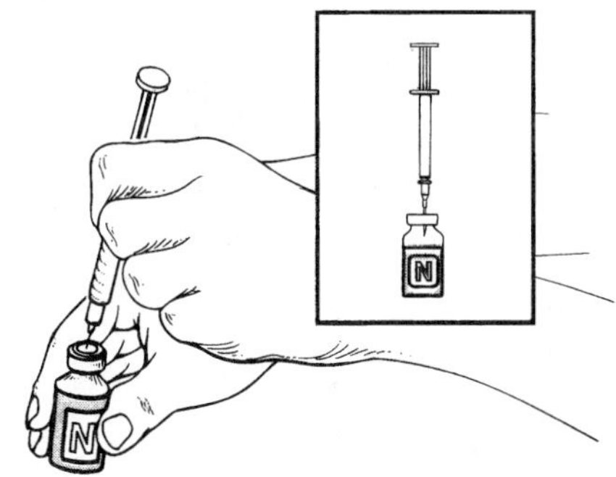

Step A: Inject air into longer-acting (cloudy) insulin
Figure F–8.

4. Inject air into the vial equal to the amount of modified (cloudy) insulin to be administered (Fig. F–8).
5. Remove the insulin syringe and needle from the modified (cloudy) insulin vial.

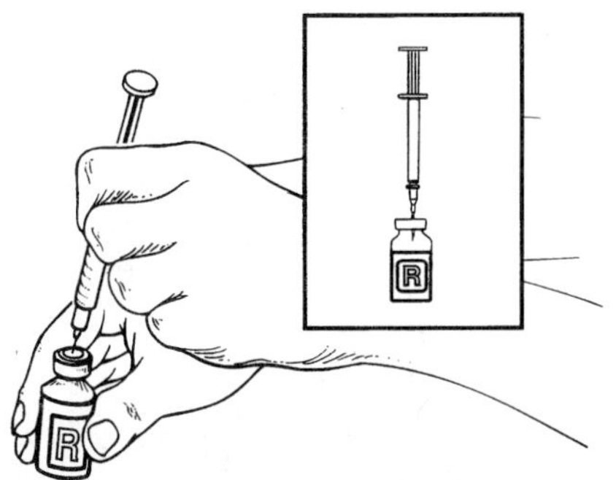

Step B: Inject air into short-acting (clear) insulin
Figure F–9.

6. Inject air into the vial equal to the amount of regular (clear) insulin to be administered (Fig. F–9).

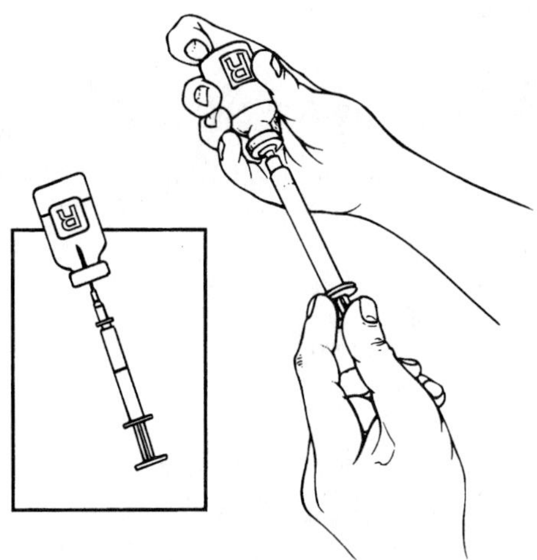

Step C: Withdraw prescribed amount of short-acting (clear) insulin

Figure F–10.

7. Withdraw the exact amount of regular (clear) insulin. Verify the amount of regular (clear) insulin with another RN (Fig. F–10).
8. Cleanse the rubber seal of the modified (cloudy) insulin again and insert needle.

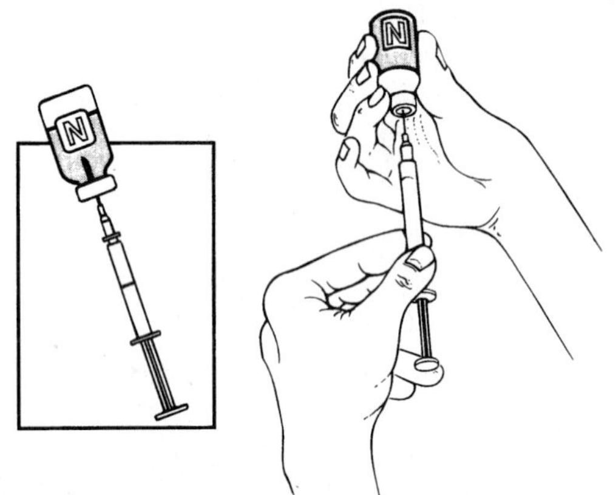

Step D: Withdraw prescribed amount of longer-acting (cloudy) insulin

Figure F–11.

9. Withdraw the exact amount of modified (cloudy) insulin, ensuring that the total amount of medication in the syringe now equals the total units of insulin to be administered. Check total units with another RN (Fig. F–11).
10. Insulin is to be administered within 5 minutes of drawing up medication.

LOADING A PREFILLED SYRINGE SYSTEM

1. Three steps (*A* through *C*) illustrate the loading of a prefilled cartridge system (Fig. F–12).

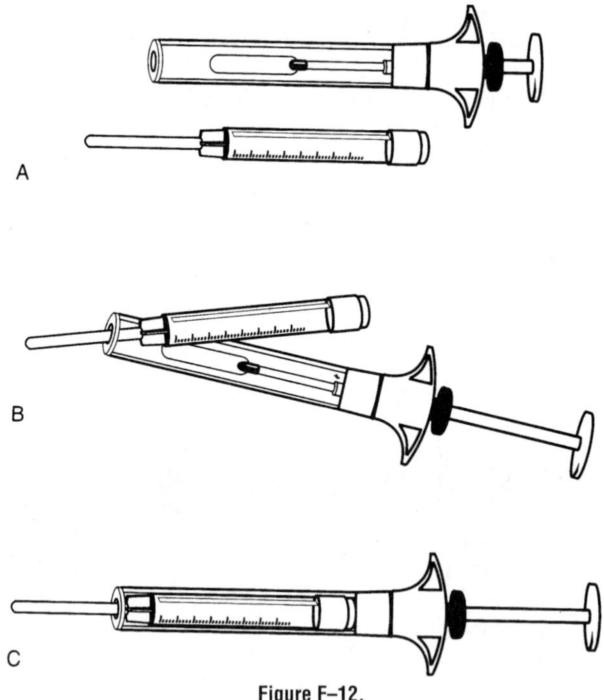

Figure F–12.

2. A closed system devised for medication administration includes a barrel *(left)* and a medication cartridge *(right)* (Fig. F–13).

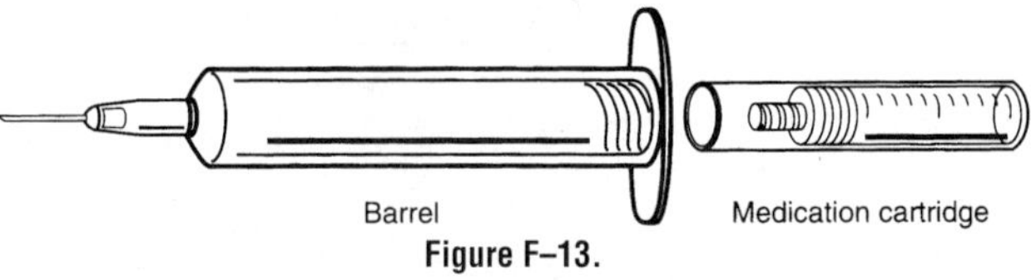

Figure F–13.

LOCATING PARENTERAL INJECTION SITES*

Adults

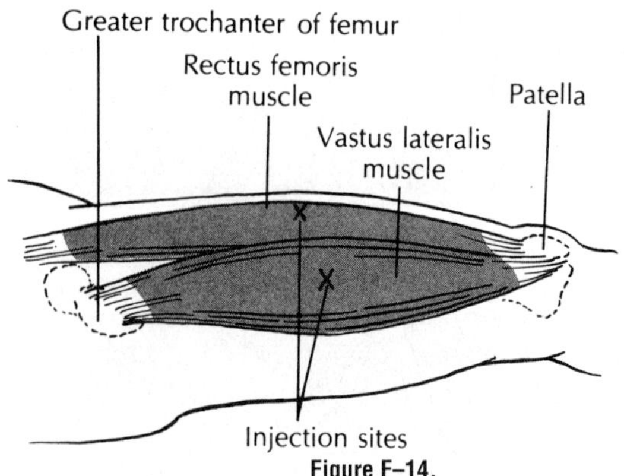

Figure F–14.

1. Vastus lateralis site—The injection site is located on the lateral aspect of the area formed by one hand breadth above the upper border of the patella and one hand breadth below the greater trochanter (Fig. F–14).

Sites are in order of preference.

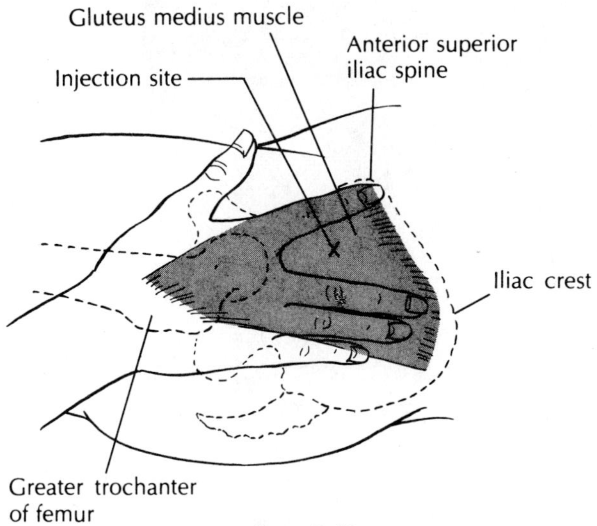

Figure F–15.

2. Ventrogluteal site—To locate the right ventrogluteal site, place your left hand with the palm over the right greater trochanter and your index finger on the right anterior superior iliac spine. Point your thumb toward the umbilicus. Spread your third finger away, and point it toward the top of the iliac crest. The injection site is in the center of the "V" formed between your index and third fingers. Use your right hand in the same manner to locate the left ventrogluteal site (Fig. F–15).

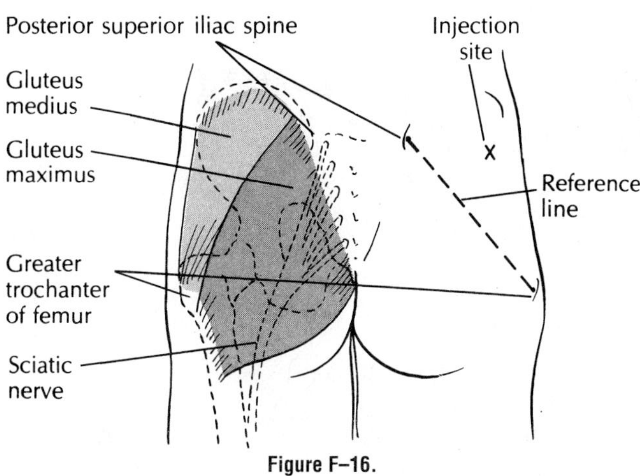

Figure F–16.

3. Dorsogluteal site—Have the patient lie prone with the toes turned medially or in a side-lying position, with the upper leg flexed. Palpate the greater trochanter and posterior superior iliac spine. Draw an imaginary line between these two points. The injection site is above and lateral to the line (Fig. F–16).

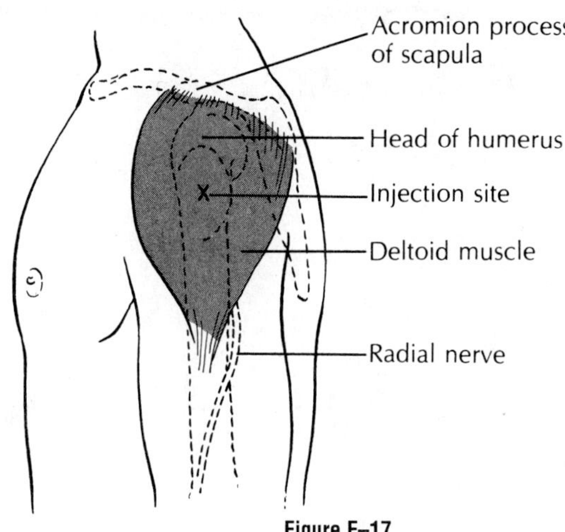

Figure F–17.

4. Deltoid site—Fully expose the patient's upper arm. Locate the acromion process. The injection site is 2 to 3 fingerbreadths below the acromion process on the lateral aspect of the upper arm (Fig. F–17).

Infants

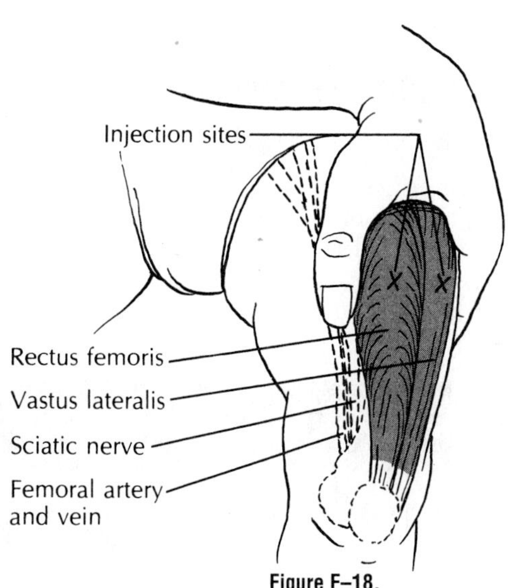

Figure F–18.

1. Rectus femoris site—Draw an imaginary line from the patella to the greater trochanter. Locate the medial outer aspect of the area that is ⅓ the distance from the patella to the greater trochanter. Standing at the infant's head, place your thumb on the inside of the muscles of the infant's left leg and your index finger on the outside, creating the U-shaped area of the injection site (Fig. F–18).

Children

1. Rectus femoris site—Use the same technique as in infants.
2. Vastus lateralis site—Locate the knee and greater trochanter. The site is in the medial outer aspect of the

TABLE F–1. APPROPRIATE VOLUME FOR VARIOUS PARENTERAL INJECTION SITES

Injection Site	Adult	Child	Infant
Vastus lateralis	≤3 mL	≤2 mL	Do not use
Ventrogluteal	≤2.5 mL	Age 3 to preschoolers ≤1 mL Preschoolers ≤1.5 mL School age ≤2 mL Older children ≤2.5 mL	Do not use
Dorsogluteal	≤2 to 3 mL	Age 3 to 6 years ≤1.5 mL Age 6 to 15 years ≤2 mL Over age 15 years ≤2 to 3 mL	Do not use
Deltoid	≤0.5 to 2 mL	Do not use	Do not use
Rectus femoris	NA	≤0.5 to 1 mL; needle size ≤1 inch	≤0.5 to 1 mL; needle size ≤1 inch

NA, not applicable.

middle ⅓ of the area between the knee and greater trochanter. This site is appropriate for school-age children to those 18 years of age.

3. Ventrogluteal site—Do not use this site for children younger than 3 years of age. This site (described in #2 under adults) may be used after age 3, if the child has been walking for at least 1 year.
4. Dorsogluteal site—Do not use this site for children younger than 3 years of age. This site (described in #3 under adults) may be used in children after age 3.

ADMINISTERING INTRAMUSCULAR (IM) DRUGS

1. Inspect areas for skin integrity. Palpate the area for tenderness, masses, or inflammation.
2. Locate the site and cleanse.
3. Administer the drug using the Z-track method with the needle held at a 90-degree angle.
4. After waiting 10 seconds, withdraw the needle steadily. Apply gentle pressure to the site using an alcohol swab or sterile gauze.

The Z-track technique for an IM injection helps prevent leakage of medication back into the subcutaneous tissue and should be used when the medication to be administered is irritating to the tissue. *A,* Normal tissue before the injection; *B,* altered tissue during the injection; *C,* normal tissue after the injection (Fig. F–19).

ADMINISTERING SUBCUTANEOUS (SC) DRUGS

1. Inspect areas for skin integrity. Palpate the area for tenderness, masses, or inflammation.
2. Locate the site and cleanse. Rotate sites.
3. Administer the drug with the needle held at a 45- to 90-degree angle. Do not aspirate when administering heparin (Fig. F–20).

TABLE F–2. EQUIPMENT NEEDED FOR AN INTRAMUSCULAR INJECTION

Equipment	Adult	Child	Infant
Syringe	2 to 3 mL	1 to 2 mL	1 mL
Needle	19 to 23 gauge, 1 to 1½ inch	25 to 27 gauge, ½ to 1 inch	25 to 27 gauge, ⅝ inch

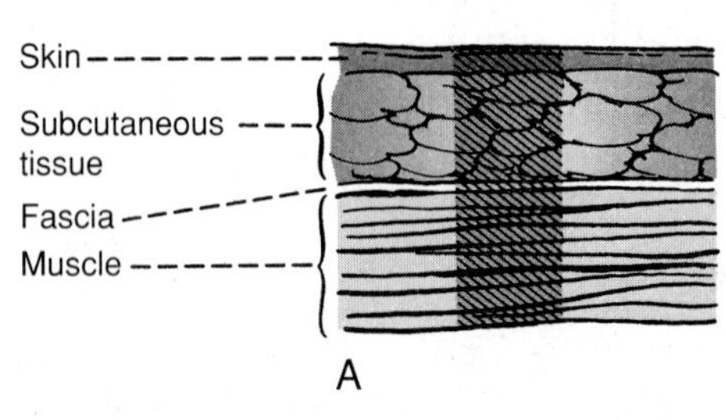

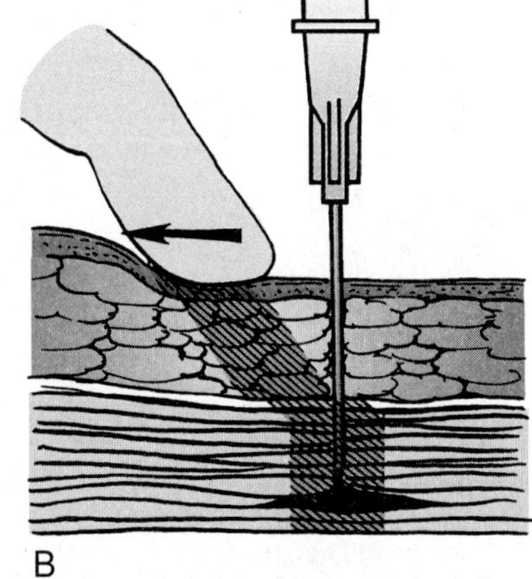
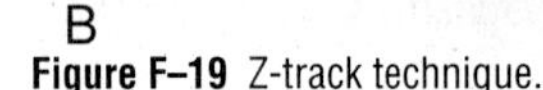

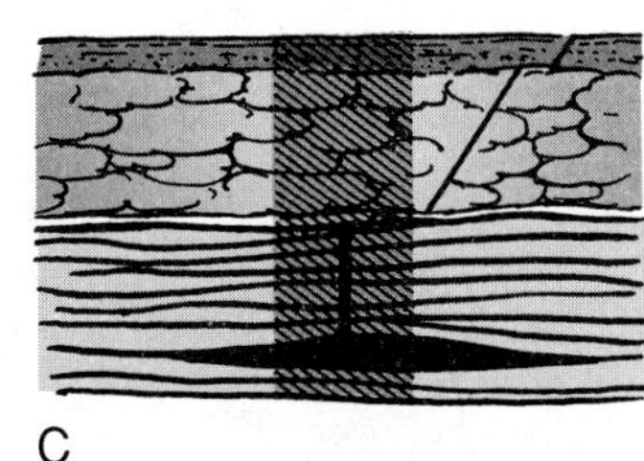

Figure F–19 Z-track technique.

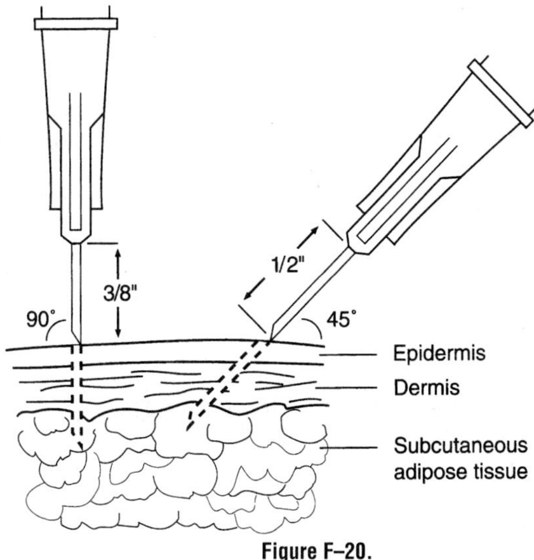

Figure F–20.

4. Wait 10 seconds before withdrawing the needle.
5. Apply gentle pressure to the site using an alcohol swab or sterile gauze, but do not massage.

ADMINISTERING INTRADERMAL (ID) DRUGS

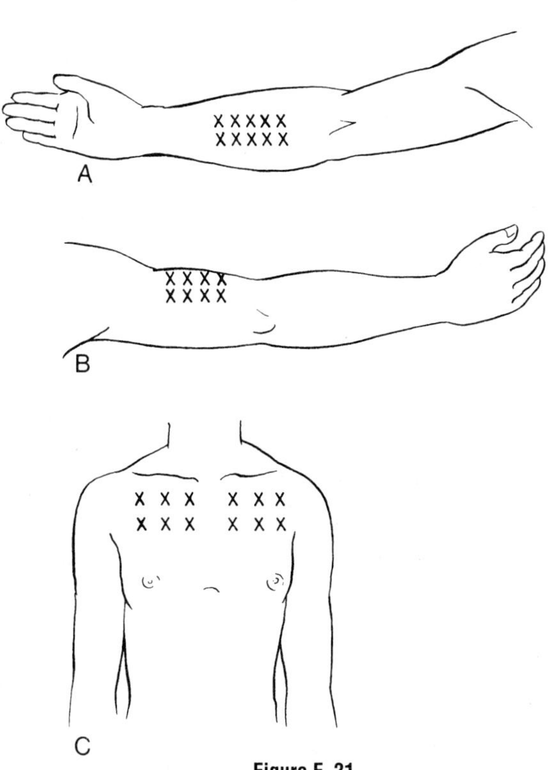

Figure F–21.

1. Determine the site to be used for ID injection (Fig. F–21).
2. Insert the needle slowly with the bevel up at a 10- to 15-angle under the outer layer of skin. When resistance is felt, advance the needle approximately 3 mm

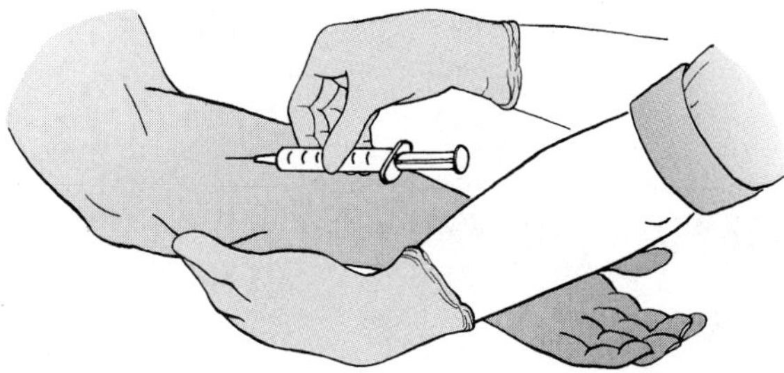

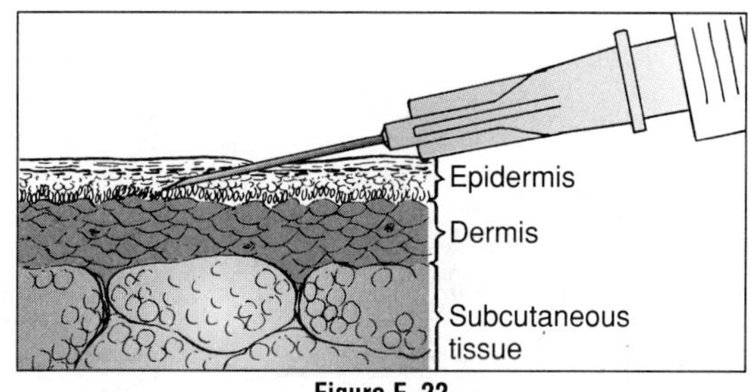

Figure F–22.

(⅛ inch) below the skin surface. The tip of the needle can be seen under the skin (Fig. F–22).
3. Slowly inject the drug. Observe the development of a small bleb.
4. Withdraw the needle. Do not massage the injection site.

ADMINISTERING INTRAVENOUS (IV) PUSH DRUGS THROUGH AN EXISTING LINE

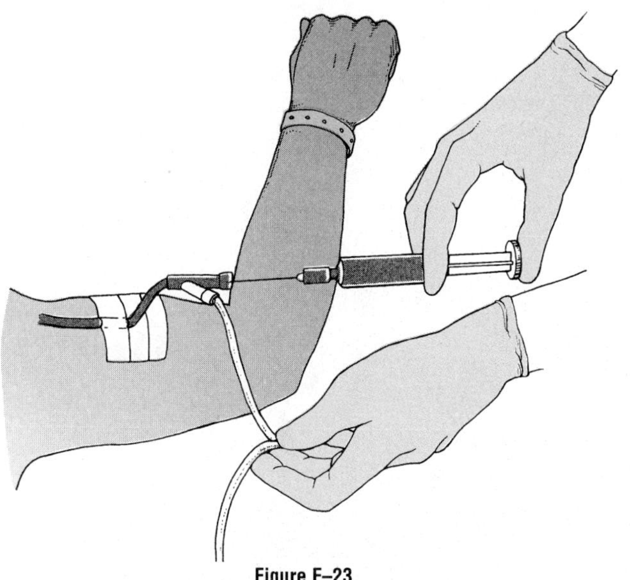

Figure F–23.

1. Connect the needle and syringe or the syringe directly to the port. Pinch the tubing above the injection port to occlude the IV line (Fig. F–23).
2. Pull back on the plunger to note blood return.

3. Administer the drug over the prescribed rate.
4. After the drug is administered, re-establish the primary infusion line.

ADMINISTERING INTRAVENOUS (IV) PUSH DRUGS THROUGH AN INTERMITTENT INFUSION DEVICE

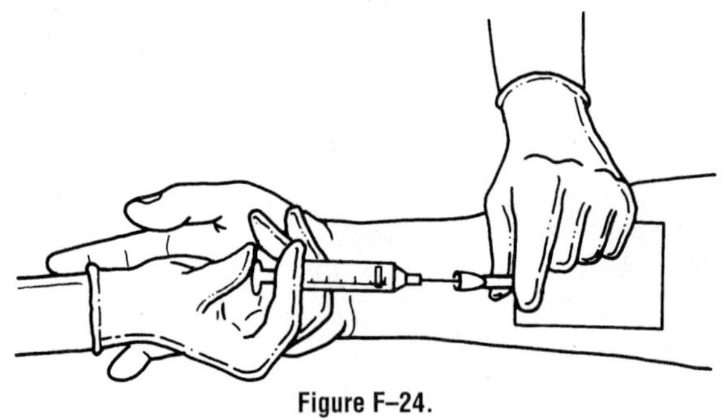

Figure F–24.

1. Prepare and administer flush solution or solutions according to the agency's policy.
2. Connect the needle and syringe or the syringe directly to the intermittent infusion device (Fig. F–24).
3. Administer the drug over the prescribed rate.
4. After the drug is administered, follow the agency's policy on flushing.

ADMINISTERING VAGINAL MEDICATIONS

1. Ask the patient to lie in the dorsal recumbent or Sims' position.
2. Remove the suppository from its foil wrapper. Apply a water-soluble lubricant to the rounded end of the suppository and to your index finger. If you are using an applicator, follow the manufacturer's directions on the package insert.

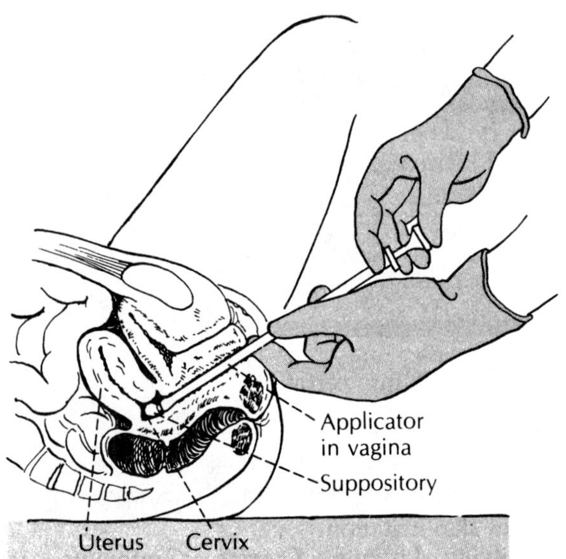

Figure F–25.

3. Using your other hand, gently spread the patient's labial folds.
4. Using your index finger, insert the rounded end of the suppository into the vagina, directing it along the posterior wall for the entire length of your index finger. If you are using an applicator, insert it into the vagina for 5 to 7 cm (2 to 3 inches). Depress the plunger to release the drug into the vagina (Fig. F–25).
5. Withdraw your index finger or the applicator.
6. Ask the patient to remain on her back for at least 10 minutes.

ADMINISTERING RECTAL SUPPOSITORIES

1. Ask the patient to lie in the Sims' or left lateral position with the upper leg flexed.
2. Remove the suppository from its foil wrapper. Apply a water-soluble lubricant to the rounded end of the suppository and your index finger.
3. Separate the patient's buttocks with your other hand. Ask the patient to breathe slowly through the mouth.

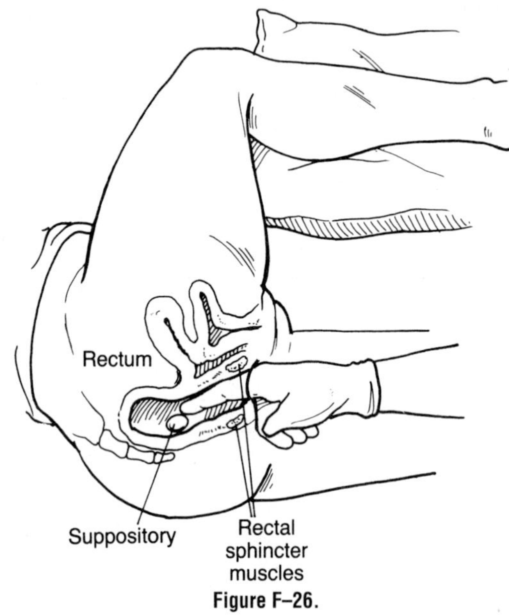

Figure F–26.

4. Using your index finger, insert the suppository through the anus beyond the internal sphincter: 10 cm (4 inches) in adults and 5 cm (2 inches) in children (Fig. F–26).
5. Withdraw your index finger and gently wipe the perianal area clean.
6. Ask the patient to remain lying flat or on the side for 5 to 15 minutes.

The illustrations in this Appendix come from the following sources and are used with permission: Figures F–2, 3, 4, 7, 8, 9, 10, 11, 12, 13, 14, 16, 20, 21, 23, 24, and 26 from Lammon, C. B., Foote, A. W., Leli, P. G., et al. (1995). *Clinical nursing skills* (pp. 578, 581, 589, 605, 606, 612, 619, 622, 625, 630). Philadelphia: W. B. Saunders. Figures F–1, 15, 17, 18, 19, 22, and 26 from Bolander, V. B. (1994). *Sorensen and Luckmann's basic nursing: A psychophysiologic approach* (3rd ed., pp. 1276, 1277, 1294, 1302). Philadelphia: W. B. Saunders. Figures F–5, 6, and 25 from deWit, S. C. (1994). *Rambo's nursing skills for clinical practice* (4th ed., pp. 909 and 994). Philadelphia: W. B. Saunders.

Appendix G

Effects of Selected Maternal Drug Ingestion on the Fetus or Neonate

Drugs	Cat*	Significance	Trimester/Term
Analgesics/Anti-Inflammatory Drugs			
Acetaminophen	B	No reported adverse effects; analgesic of choice during pregnancy	1st
Fentanyl	B/D	No reported adverse effects; may produce loss of fetal heart rate variability without causing fetal hypoxia	Term
Hydrocodone	B	No reported adverse effects; neonatal withdrawal is possible in infants exposed in utero to prolonged maternal ingestion	Term
Meperidine HCL	B	Loss of beat-to-beat variability; decreased neonatal respirations; late depression effects in newborn	Term
Morphine	B	SGA; depressed newborn; neonatal death	Neonatal
Nalorphine	D	Statistically significant reduction in neonatal depression has not been demonstrated, may increase neonatal depression if an improper opioid-to-opioid antagonist ratio is used	Term
Naloxone	B	Significant increases in number, duration, and amplitude of fetal heart rate accelerations may occur; significant increases in number of fetal body movements and percentage of time spent breathing may occur	Term
NSAIDs	B	No documented teratogenicity; may prolong pregnancy and inhibit labor; maintenance of PDA questionable, resulting in PPHN; blood clotting and hyperbilirubinemia reported in neonates	L&D
Oxycodone	B/D	No reported adverse effects	Term
Pentazocine	B	Withdrawal	Term
Propoxyphene	C	Neonatal withdrawal	Term
Salicylates	C	Neonatal bleeding; coagulation defects; premature closing of ductus arteriosus; diminished factor XII; toxicity with excessive maternal ingestion; may prolong pregnancy; may cause slight increased risk of cardiac defects	Term
Anesthetic Drugs			
Cyclopropane	—	Infant depression from narcosis	Term
Halothane	—	Infant depression from narcosis; spontaneous abortion	Term
Nitrous oxide	—	Questionable fetal anomalies; spontaneous abortion	Early
Bupivicaine HCL	—	Bradycardia; stillborn with PCB	Labor
Chloroprocaine	—	Possible bradycardia with PCB; little transfer to fetus; probably safest anesthetic for fetus; possible maternal neurologic effects	Labor
Lidocaine	B	Fetal bradycardia; may cause CNS depression in newborn	Labor-neonatal
Mepivacaine HCL	—	Fetal bradycardia; stillborn with PCB; substandard motor nerve response and poor muscle tone in fetus	Labor-neonatal
Prilocaine HCL	—	Less bradycardia than with lidocaine or mepivacaine, but metabolite causes methemoglobinemia	Labor
Procaine, tetracaine	—	May depress fetus by direct effect or via maternal hypotension	L&D
Anticoagulants			
Heparin	C	No reported congenital defects; drug does not cross placental membranes	Entire
Warfarin sodium	D	Embryopathy (fetal warfarin syndrome), CNS defects, spontaneous abortion, stillbirth, prematurity, hemorrhage; mental retardation, blindness, spasticity, seizures, deafness, scoliosis, growth failure, death	1st
Antidiabetic Drugs			
Insulin	B	Possible caudal regression syndrome	1st
Tolbutamide	D	Possibly teratogenic; neonatal hypoglycemia; neonatal thrombocytopenia	Entire
Antimicrobial Drugs			
Acyclovir	C	No documented fetal effects; at high dosage may cause chromosomal breakage	Entire

Drugs	Cat*	Significance	Trimester/Term
Antimicrobial Drugs *Continued*			
Amphotericin B	B	No documented fetal effects	—
Ampicillin	B	No known adverse effects; may not reach therapeutic levels in utero	—
Cephalosporins	B	No reported adverse effects; high dosage may be required to achieve therapeutic effects in fetus	—
Chloramphenicol	C	Fetal levels equal maternal levels; gray baby syndrome	Near term
Chloroquine	D	Fetal CNS damage, particularly to auditory nerve; possibly abnormal retinal pigmentation; congenital deafness	Entire
Clindamycin	B	Concentrates in fetal liver; no adverse effects on fetus yet reported	—
Erythromycin	B	Crosses placenta only at high maternal dosages; fetal level 25% of maternal; no adverse effects demonstrated	—
Gentamicin sulfate	C	Possible ototoxicity; fetal levels well below toxic adult levels; if maternal levels therapeutic, probably adequate for bacterial control in fetus	—
Isotretinoin	X	CNS, cardiac, facial anomalies	Entire
Kanamycin sulfate	D	Fetal concentration 40% of maternal, probably ototoxic	Entire
Metronidazole	C	Not recommended in 1st trimester; mutagenic in bacteria; questionably embryotoxic	1st
Neomycin	D	No reported adverse effects	—
Nitrofurantoin	B	Hemolytic anemia in mother or fetus with G6PD deficiency	Near term
Nystatin	A/UK	Safe for *Candida* infections of skin, mucous membranes, intestinal tract. Use has not been associated with teratogenesis	—
Penicillin	B	Fetal levels 20–50% of maternal; no adverse effects reported	—
Ribavarin	X	Teratogenic and/or embryolethal in all animal species	Entire
Phenazopyridine	B	No teratogenicity studies have been done. Relatively contraindicated because other drugs are preferable	
Streptomycin	D	8th cranial nerve damage; micromelia; slight danger of multiple skeletal anomalies	Entire
Sulfonamides	B	Hyperbilirubinemia; kernicterus; thrombocytopenia; possibility of hemolysis in G6PD deficiency (category D if near term)	Near term
Tetracycline	D	Inhibition of bone growth; discoloration of teeth; possible micromelia; syndactyly, hypospadias, and inguinal hernia; maternal fatty liver may result in stillbirth	Entire
Tobramycin sulfate	C	No increased incidence of malformation; possibly ototoxic. More study needed	—
Trimethoprim-sulfamethoxazole	C	Teratogenic in animals—primarily cleft palate; may cause fetal resorption. No documented teratogenesis in humans	1st
Zidovudine	C	No documented fetal effects	—
Antihistamine			
Brompheniramine	B	Statistically increased risk of teratogenicity	1st
Antithyroid Drugs			
Methimazole	D	Goiter; approximately 30% probability of mental retardation	Week 14 on
Potassium iodide	X	Fetal goiter; mental retardation	Week 14 on
Propylthiouracil	D	Goiter; approximately 30% probability of mental retardation	Week 14 on
Radioiodine	X	Congenital hypothyroidism; cretinism	Week 14 on
Asthmatic Drugs			
Albuterol	C	Does not cause birth defects; adverse effects related to metabolic and cardiovascular drug effects	Near term
Aminophylline	C	No increase in abnormalities; tachycardia, vomiting, jitteriness in fetus after drug given to mother	Near term
Cromolyn sodium	C	No increase in fetal anomalies reported; high doses may cause fetal growth retardation and stillbirth in animals	Entire
Terbutaline	B	Does not cause birth defects; adverse effects similar to those of albuterol	Near term
Theophylline	C	No documented birth defects; transient tachycardia, irritability, vomiting may occur in newborns	Near term
Cardiovascular Drugs			
ACE inhibitors such as captopril	C	Decreased uterine blood flow; increased fetal morbidity and mortality; may cause oligohydramnios	2nd and 3rd
Methyldopa	C	Decrease of intracranial volume after 1st trimester exposure	After 1st
Beta blockers	C	Possible association with teratogenesis; neonatal hypoglycemia; IUGR; neonatal bradycardia and respiratory depression	1st; near term
Digoxin	B	Equilibration between mother and fetus after one week of treatment; lack of documented effects on fetus	?
Heparin	C	Probably little fetal effect since does not cross placenta; maternal osteoporosis and thrombocytopenia	Entire
Nifedipine	C	Possible fetal hypoxemia and acidosis	Entire
Quinidine	C	May cause neonatal thrombocytopenia	Entire
Verapamil	C	May cause a decrease in uterine blood flow and cause fetal hypoxia and bradycardia	Entire
Warfarin sodium	D	Hemorrhagic death in utero; numerous fetal deformities reported	Entire

Drugs	Cat*	Significance	Trimester/Term
Central Nervous System Drugs			
Alcohol	D	Fetal alcohol syndrome (FAS); IUGR, maxillary hypoplasia; narrow palpebral fissures, microcephaly, mental retardation	Entire
Amphetamines	D	Transposition of the great vessels; biliary atresia; cleft palate; generalized arthritis, learning disabilities, poor motor coordination, IUGR	4th through 12 wk
Caffeine (>600 mg/day)	C	Spontaneous abortion, IUGR, increased incidence of cleft palate, other anomalies suspected	Entire
Cocaine		Learning disabilities, poor state organization, decreased interactive behavior, CNS anomalies, cardiac anomalies, GU anomalies, SIDS	
Dextroamphetamine	C	Congenital heart defects, hyperbilirubinemia	Entire
Diethylpropion	B	No reports linking drug to congenital defects	—
Methylphenidate	C	No reports linking drug to congenital defects	—
Nicotine (½–1 PPD)		Increased rate of spontaneous abortion; increased incidence of abruptio placentae; SGA; small head circumference, decreased length, SIDS	
Barbiturates	B	All drugs cross placenta; are stored in fetal liver, brain, and placenta; fetal concentration greater than maternal; fetus may be addicted; hyperreflexia; hyperactivity; vasomotor instability; neonatal bleeding, coagulation defects, thrombocytopenia; possible congenital malformation; enzyme inducers	Entire
Carbamazepine	C	Fetal carbamazepine syndrome; craniofacial, CNS and cardiovascular malformations	1st
Chlordiazepoxide	D	Possible increased incidence of congenital anomalies if taken during first 42 days of pregnancy	First 42 days
Diazepam	D	Possible increased incidence of congenital anomalies, including cleft palate Cord level approximately equal to maternal blood level; hypotonia, hypothermia, impaired cold response; possible withdrawal symptoms, decreased beat-to-beat variability in neonatal heart rate; thrombocytopenia; withdrawal syndrome may last up to 10 days	First 42 days; near term
Diphenhydramine	C	Thrombocytopenia; possible association with cleft palate	Near term; 1st
Fluoxetine	B	No documented adverse fetal effects	—
Heroin	B/D	Withdrawal symptoms; convulsions; death; IUGR; respiratory alkalosis; hyperbilirubinemia	Entire
Lithium carbonate	D	Possible alteration in cardiac rhythm; altered thyroid function tests in fetus; possible goiter; jaundice; electrolyte imbalance; neonatal hypotonia; CNS depression; congenital anomalies; lethargy and cyanosis in newborn	Near term
Methadone	B/D	Fetal distress, meconium aspiration, hyperbilirubinemia, severe withdrawal symptoms with abrupt termination of drug; neonatal death	Neonatal
Phenothiazines	UK	Withdrawal, extrapyramidal dysfunction; delayed respiratory onset; hyperbilirubinemia; hypotonia or hyperactivity; decreased platelet count	
Phenytoin sodium	D	High incidence of anomalies (abnormal genitalia; cleft lip/palate; hypoplasia of distal phalanges, diaphragmatic hernia; fetal hydantoin syndrome, microcephaly, mental retardation); associations documented only with chronic exposure	1st, 2nd
Trimethadione	D	Mental retardation; facial dysmorphogenesis, cardiovascular hemorrhage, depletion of vitamin K–dependent clotting factors, IUGR	Entire
Valproic acid	D	Possible association with microcephaly; possible fetal hydantoin syndrome; spina bifida; facial dysmorphogenesis, perinatal distress, behavioral abnormalities	Entire
Diuretics			
Acetazolamide	C	Limb defects	1st
Ammonium chloride	B	Fetal acidosis	Near term
Furosemide	C	Increased fetal urine output without circulatory disturbance; possible electrolyte imbalance	Near term
Thiazide diuretics	D	Bone marrow depression; thrombocytopenia; neonatal death; ascites; possible chronic hypokalemia, hypoglycemia	Near term
Gastrointestinal Drugs			
Cimetidine, ranitidine	B	Possible transient liver impairment in newborn	Near term
Metoclopramide	B	No documented fetal effects	—
Hormonal Drugs			
Androgens	—	Masculinization of female fetus	—
Bromocriptine	X	No evidence of teratogenicity exists; should be stopped with pregnancy	—
Corticosteroids	B	Cleft palate in early pregnancy; newborn adrenal failure, placental insufficiency, and possible acceleration of fetal lung maturity in late pregnancy	See note
Diethylstilbestrol	X	Anomalies of female reproductive tract; uterine and vaginal adenosis, epididymal cysts, hypotrophic testes, infertility	Early
Estrogens	D	Possible masculinization of female fetus; may be embryotoxic	Entire
Oral contraceptives	D	Possible limb reduction defects; possible cardiac anomalies; questionable Pierre Robin syndrome	Early
Immunizing Drugs			
Hepatitis B	B	No reported adverse effects	—

Drugs	Cat*	Significance	Trimester/Term
Immunizing Drugs *Continued*			
Measles virus	C	Infected fetus; may increase abortion rate	Entire
Mumps	C	Infected fetus with uncertain effects on fetal development	Entire
Pertussis	C	Maternal febrile response may lead to abortion; no fetal anomalies reported	Early
Poliovirus	C	Probably safe during pregnancy	—
Rubella vaccine	C	Rubella syndrome	—
Tetanus immune globulin	B	No reported adverse effects	—
Tetanus/diphtheria toxoid	C	Probably safe during pregnancy	—
Psychoactive Drugs			
Phencyclidine (PCP, "angel dust")	X	Flaccid appearance; poor head control; impaired neurologic development	Entire
Lysergic acid diethylamide (LSD)	C	Chromosomal breakage	Entire
Marijuana	C	IUGR; potentially impaired immunologic mechanisms	Entire
Vitamins and Minerals			
Ascorbic acid	A	MDR has no adverse effects; deficiency may lead to abortion and premature delivery	Entire
Ferrous fumarate, gluconate, sulfate	A	Safe and accepted supplementation during pregnancy and lactation	Entire
Folic acid	A	Deficiency has severe effects on developing embryo; possible neural tube defects	Early
Pyridoxine HCl (vitamin B_6)	A	MDR dosage has no known adverse fetal effects; deficiency has questionable association with nausea and vomiting of pregnancy; possible maternal neurologic problems with high doses	Entire
Riboflavin (vitamin B_2)	A	MDR has no known adverse fetal effects; deficiency may be related to prematurity and abortion	Early
Thiamine (vitamin B_1)	A	MDR has no known adverse effects; deficiency may lead to abortion	Early
Vitamin A	A	Intracranial hypertension; growth retardation	Entire
Vitamin D	A	Mental retardation; hypercalcemia	Entire
Vitamin K	C	Excess may lead to hyperbilirubinemia; deficiency may cause fetal hemorrhage	Near term

*Risk factor if used for prolonged periods or in high doses at term

ACE, Angiotensin-converting enzyme; Cat, FDA pregnancy category; GU, genitourinary; SGA, small for gestational age; PPHN, persistent pulmonary hypertension of the newborn; PCB, paracervical block; CNS, central nervous system; G6PD, glucose 6-phosphate dehydrogenase; IUGR, intrauterine growth retardation; RDS, respiratory distress syndrome; MDR, minimal daily requirement; Near term, time period near labor and delivery as well as neonatal period.

Appendix H

Product Information for Selected Nutritional Supplements and Enteral Formulas*

Product (Manufacturer)	cal/mL	mOsm/kg	CHO, g (% cal)	Pro, g (% cal)	Fat, g (% cal)	Fiber, g	Vol for 100% RDA	Comments
1.0 Cal/mL POLYMERIC FORMULAS FOR TUBE FEEDING OR NUTRITIONAL SUPPLEMENT†								
BOOST (Mead Johnson)	1.06		164 (68)	10 (17)	4 (15)	—	1180	Flavored; not intended for tube feeding; low in fat; increased amounts of antioxidants
ENSURE (Ross)	1.06	470	145 (55)	37 (14)	37 (32)	—	1887	Flavored
ENSURE HN (Ross)	1.06	470	141 (53)	44 (17)	36 (30)	—	1321	Flavored; nutrient dense, high nitrogen
NUTREN 1.0 (Clintec)	1.00	300–390§	127 (51)	40 (16)	38 (33)	—	1500	Available in flavors and with fiber (14 g/1000 mL)
PROMOTE (Ross)	1.0	350	130 (52)	62 (25)	26 (23)	—	1250	Flavored; high nitrogen, nutrient dense, fat blend recommended by AHA, contains omega-3 fatty acids, fortified with ultratrace minerals,‡ carnitine, and taurine
RESOURCE (Sandoz)	1.06	430	140 (54)	37 (14)	37 (32)	—	1890	Flavored
SUSTACAL LIQUID (Mead Johnson)	1.0	650	140 (55)	61 (24)	23 (21)	—	1080	High nitrogen, flavored
SUSTACAL WITH FIBER (Mead Johnson)	1.06	480	140 (53)	46 (17)	35 (30)	6	1420	Flavored
SUSTACAL 8.8 (Mead Johnson)	1.06	500	148 (56)	37 (14)	35 (30)	—	1890	Nutrient dense, flavored

Product (Manufacturer)	cal/mL	mOsm/kg	CHO, g (% cal)	Pro, g (% cal)	Fat, g (% cal)	Fiber, g	Vol (mL) for 100% RDA	Comments
1.0 cal/mL POLYMERIC FORMULAS PRIMARILY FOR TUBE FEEDINGS								
COMPLEAT MODIFIED (Sandoz)	1.07	300	140 (53)	43 (16)	37 (31)	4.2	1500	Blenderized from natural foods; contains ultratrace minerals‡
COMPLEAT REGULAR (Sandoz)	1.07	450	130 (48)	43 (16)	43 (36)	4.2	1500	Blenderized from natural foods; contains lactose and ultratrace minerals‡
ENTRITION (Clintec)	1.0	300	136 (55)	35 (14)	35 (32)	—	2000	—
ENTRITION HN (Clintec)	1.0	300	114 (46)	44 (18)	41 (37)	—	1300	High nitrogen
ENTRITION WITH FIBER (Clintec)	1.0	300	127 (51)	40 (16)	38 (33)	14	1500	Contains ultratrace minerals‡
FIBERSOURCE (Sandoz)	1.2	390	170 (56)	43 (14)	41 (30)	10	1500	Contains ultratrace minerals‡ and 50% of fat from MCTs

Table continued on following page

1.0 cal/mL POLYMERIC FORMULAS PRIMARILY FOR TUBE FEEDINGS *Continued*								
Product (Manufacturer)	**cal/mL**	**mOsm/kg**	**CHO, g (% cal)**	**Pro, g (% cal)**	**Fat, g (% cal)**	**Fiber, g**	**Vol (mL) for 100% RDA**	**Comments**
FIBERSOURCE HN (Sandoz)	1.2	390	160 (52)	53 (18)	41 (30)	6.8	1500	High nitrogen; contains ultratrace minerals,‡ and 50% of fat from MCTs
ISOCAL (Mead Johnson)	1.06	270	135 (50)	34 (13)	44 (37)	—	1890	—
ISOCAL HN (Mead Johnson)	1.06	270	123 (46)	44 (17)	45 (37)	—	1250	Nutrient dense, high nitrogen
ISOSOURCE (Sandoz)	1.2	360	170 (56)	43 (14)	41 (30)	—	1500	Contains ultratrace minerals;‡ 50% of fat from MCTs
ISOSOURCE HN (Sandoz)	1.2	330	160 (52)	53 (18)	41 (30)	—	1500	High nitrogen; contains ultratrace minerals,‡ taurine. and carnitine; 50% of fat from MCTs
ISOTEIN HN (Sandoz)	1.2	300	160 (52)	68 (23)	34 (25)	—	1770	Powder; high nitrogen; contains ultratrace minerals‡
JEVITY (Ross)	1.06	310	152 (53)	44 (17)	37 (30)	14	1320	Fortified with ultratrace minerals,‡ taurine and carnitine; 50% fat from MCTs
OSMOLITE (Ross)	1.06	300	145 (55)	37 (14)	39 (31)	—	1887	50% of fats from MCTs; fortified with ultratrace minerals‡
OSMOLITE HN (Ross)	1.06	300	141 (53)	44 (17)	37 (30)	—	1321	50% of fats from MCTs; fortified with ultratrace minerals‡
REPLETE (Clintec)	1.0	350	113 (45)	63 (25)	33 (30)	—	1500	Flavored; high nitrogen; available with fiber
ULTRACAL (Mead Johnson)	1.06	310	123 (46)	44 (17)	45 (37)	14	1180	High nitrogen, nutrient dense, flavored

1.5 cal/mL AND ABOVE FORMULAS FOR TUBE FEEDINGS OR NUTRITIONAL SUPPLEMENT								
Product (Manufacturer)	**cal/mL**	**mOsm/kg**	**CHO, g (% cal)**	**Pro, g (% cal)**	**Fat, g (% cal)**	**Fiber, g**	**Vol (mL) for 100% RDA**	**Comments**
ENSURE Plus (Ross)	1.5	690	200 (53)	55 (15)	53 (32)	—	1420	High calorie, flavored
ENSURE Plus HN (Ross)	1.5	690	200 (53)	63 (17)	50 (30)	—	947	High calorie, high nitrogen; flavored
ISOCAL HCN (Mead Johnson)	2.0	640	200 (40)	75 (15)	102 (45)	—	1000	High calorie and nitrogen, fortified with ultratrace minerals‡
NUTREN 1.5 (Clintec)	1.5	410–590§	170 (45)	60 (16)	68 (39)	—	1000	Flavored; less sweet taste; 50% of fat from MCTs
NUTREN 2.0 (Clintec)	2.0	710	196 (39)	80 (16)	106 (45)	—	750	Flavored; less sweet taste
RESOURCE PLUS (Sandoz)	1.5	600	200 (53)	55 (15)	53 (32)	—	1600	Flavored
TWO CAL HN (Ross)	2	690	217 (43)	84 (17)	91 (40)	—	947	High nitrogen, fortified with ultratrace minerals;‡ designed for stressed patients

FORMULAS FOR SPECIFIC CONDITIONS								
Product (Manufacturer)	**cal/mL**	**mOsm/kg**	**CHO, g (% cal)**	**Pro, g (% cal)**	**Fat, g (% cal)**	**Fiber, g**	**Vol for 100% RDA**	**Comments**
Metabolically Stressed								
CRITICARE HN (Mead Johnson)	1.06	650	220 (82)	38 (14)	5 (5)	—	1890	Equal percentage of free amino acids and small peptides; fortified with additional amounts of vitamin C and B-complex vitamins

FORMULAS FOR SPECIFIC CONDITIONS								
Product (Manufacturer)	**cal/mL**	**mOsm/kg**	**CHO, g (% cal)**	**Pro, g (% cal)**	**Fat, g (% cal)**	**Fiber, g**	**Vol for 100% RDA**	**Comments**
Metabolically Stressed								
IMPACT (Sandoz)	1.0	375	132 (53)	56 (22)	28 (25)	—	1500	High protein (intact), enriched with arginine, RNA, and omega-3 fatty acids; contains ultratrace minerals;‡ available with fiber (10 g/1000 mL)
PERATIVE (Ross)	1.3	425	177 (55)	67 (21)	37 (25)	—	1155	Small peptides (elemental); enriched with arginine, carnitine, taurine, and ultratrace minerals‡
REABILAN HN (O'Brien)	1.33	490	158 (48)	58 (18)	52 (35)	—	1875	High nitrogen, small peptides
REPLETE (Clintec)	1.0	290–350	113 (45)	63 (25)	33 (30)	—	1000	Flavored and unflavored without or with fiber (10 g of fiber/1000 mL); fortified with vitamins A and C, zinc, and glutamine to promote healing
STRESSTEIN (Sandoz)	1.2	910	170 (57)	70 (23)	28 (20)	—	2000	Powder; BCAA enriched; contains MCTs and ultratrace minerals‡
TRAUMACAL (Mead Johnson)	1.5	490	145 (38)	83 (22)	68 (40)	—	3000	High calorie, high nitrogen, moderate CHO; increased amounts of nutrients needed for wound healing
Impaired GI Function								
ACCUPEP HPF (Sherwood)	1.0	490	188 (76)	40 (16)	10 (9)	—	1600	Powder, hydrolyzed protein (elemental), 50% of fat from MCTs
ADVERA (Ross)	1.3	504	215 (66)	60 (19)	23 (16)	9	1500	Flavored; fortified with beta-carotene and omega-3 fatty acids; increased levels of vitamins E, C, B_6, B_{12}, and folic acid
ALITRAQ (Ross)	1.0	575	165 (66)	53 (21)	16 (13)	—	1500	Powdered; flavored; peptides and free amino acids (elemental), supplemented with glutamine and arginine; fortified with ultratrace minerals,‡ taurine, and carnitine; designed for metabolically stressed patients with impaired GI function
LIPISORB (Mead Johnson)	1.0	320	116 (46)	35 (14)	48 (40)	—	1970	Powdered; flavored; unique MCT formulation for fat malabsorption
PEPTAMEN (Clintec)	1.0	270	127 (51)	40 (16)	39 (33)	—	1500	Flavored; peptides and free amino acids (elemental); supplemented with glutamine, arginine, ultratrace minerals,‡ taurine, and carnitine; 70% of fat from MCTs; designed for metabolically stressed patient with impaired GI function
REABILAN (O'Brien)	1	350	131 (53)	31 (13)	39 (35)	—	2250	Short-chain peptides
TOLEREX (Sandoz)	1.0	550	230 (91)	21 (8)	2 (1)	—	3160	Powder; free amino acids (elemental)
TRAVASORB HN (Clintec)	1.0	560	175 (70)	45 (18)	14 (12)	—	2000	Powder; peptide (elemental); 60% of fat from MCTs
VITAL HN (Ross)	1.0	500	185 (74)	42 (17)	11 (9)	—	1500	Powder; free amino acids (elemental); high nitrogen; enriched with ultratrace minerals‡
VIVONEX T.E.N. (Sandoz)	1.0	630	206 (82)	38 (15)	3 (3)	—	2000	Powder; free amino acids; BCAA enriched with glutamine and arginine
Glucose Intolerance								
CHOICE DM (Mead Johnson)	1.0	440	106 (40)	45 (17)	51 (43)	14	1000	Enriched with antioxidants and ultratrace minerals‡
GLUCERNA (Ross)	1.0	375	94 (33)	42 (17)	56 (50)	14	1422	Fat blend high in monounsaturated fatty acids; enriched with ultratrace minerals‡

FORMULAS FOR SPECIFIC CONDITIONS *Continued*

Product (Manufacturer)	cal/mL	mOsm/kg	CHO, g (% cal)	Pro, g (% cal)	Fat, g (% cal)	Fiber, g	Vol for 100% RDA	Comments
Renal Disorders								
NEPRO (Ross)	2	635	215 (43)	70 (14)	96 (43)	—	950‖	Flavored; high calorie, moderate protein, low electrolytes, low fluid, designed for patients with chronic or acute renal failure on dialysis
SUPLENA (Ross)	2	600	255 (51)	30 (6)	96 (43)	—	950‖	High calorie, low protein, low electrolyte, low fluid, contains carnitine and taurine; designed for nondialyzed renal patients; flavored
TRAVASORB RENAL (Clintec)	1.35	590	270 (81)	23 (7)	18 (12)	—	N/A	Nutritionally incomplete (only water-soluble vitamins present); EAA, contains histidine and arginine; 70% fat from MCTs
Hepatic Conditions								
HEPATIC-AID II (Kendall-McGaw)	1.17	560	168 (57)	44 (15)	36 (28)	—	N/A	Nutritionally incomplete; powder; amino acids; BCAA enriched; low aromatic amino acids and methionine; contains arginine
Pulmonary Conditions								
NUTRIVENT (Clintec)	1.5	450	100 (27)	68 (18)	94 (55)	—	1000	High fat with MCTs
PULMOCARE (Ross)	1.5	520	106 (28)	63 (17)	92 (55)	—	950	Flavored; high fat, low CHO; fortified with ultratrace minerals‡

*All formulas are liquid, ready to use, lactose free, and nutritionally adequate when the amount indicated is provided unless otherwise noted.
†Formulas are frequently flavored, making them suitable for oral or tube feedings.
‡CHOICE DM ultratrace minerals including selenium, chromium, and molybdenum.
§Varies owing to added flavors.
‖Except phosphorus, magnesium, and vitamins A and D, which are limited on renal diets.
BCAA, branched-chain amino acids; CHO, carbohydrates; GI, gastrointestinal; MCT, medium-chain triglycerides; N/A, not available; Pro, protein; RDA, recommended daily allowance.
Adapted from Davis, J., and Sherer, K. (1994). *Applied nutrition and diet therapy for nurses* (2nd ed, pp. 1050–1055). Philadelphia: W. B. Saunders. Used with permission.

Index

Note: Page numbers in *italics* refer to illustrations; page numbers followed by t refer to tables, and those followed by b refer to boxed material.

A

B

C

D

F

G

H

I

J

K

L

M

N

O

P

Q

R

S

T

U

V

W

X

Y

Z

Pharmacotherapeutic Terms and Phrases in English and Spanish

BASIC GREETINGS AND QUESTIONS

SALUDOS Y PREGUNTAS BASICAS

English	Spanish
Hello	Hola
Good morning, good afternoon, good evening.	Buenos días, buenas tardes, buenas noches.
What is your name? How old are you?	¿Cómo se llama usted? ¿Cúantos años tiene?
What is your phone number?	¿Cuál es su número de teléfono?
What is your address?	¿Cuál es su dirección?
How are you? How are you doing?	¿Cómo est usted? ¿Cómo le va?
How many . . ., What . . ., Where . . ., Who . . ., Why . . ., How . . .	Cúantos (as)..., Qué..., Dónde..., Quién..., Por qué..., Cómo...

TERMS FOR HEALTH HISTORY

EXPRESIONES PARA LA HISTORIA CLINICA

How do you feel? Good, bad, tired, dizzy.	¿Cómo se siente? Bien, mal, cansado(a), mareado(a).
Are you constipated? Do you have diarrhea?	¿Está estreñido(a)? ¿Tiene diarrea?
Do you have nausea?	¿Tiene náuseas?
Do you have a fever?	¿Tiene usted fiebre?
Is this affecting your daily activities?	¿Le afecta esto sus actividades diarias?
Have you had these symptoms before? For how long? Minutes, hours, days, months, more than six months?	¿Ha tenido estos síntomas antes? ¿Por cuánto tiempo? ¿Minutos, horas, días, meses, más de seis meses?
Are you taking any medications now? What color is the medicine? Green, yellow, clear, white, dark, brown?	¿Está tomando alguna medicina ahora? ¿De qué color es la medicina? ¿Verde, amarilla, transparente, blanca, oscura, marrón/café?
Do you have the medicine with you now?	¿Tiene la medicina en este momento?
Show me, please. How many pills do you take? One, two, three, four, five, six, seven, eight, nine, ten?	Enséñemela, por favor. ¿Cúantas pastillas? ¿Una, dos, tres, cuatro, cinco, seis, siete, ocho, nueve, diez?
Are you allergic to any medicines? Are you allergic to any foods?	¿Tiene alergias a algunas medicinas? ¿Tiene alergias de algunas comidas?
Do you have pain? Where is the pain?	¿Tiene algún dolor? ¿Dónde le duele?
Annoying, bothering; brief; burning; cold; constant; doesn't let me rest; crushing; cramping; discomfort; dull; excruciating; heavy; hot; itching; periodic, comes and goes; strong/severe; throbbing	Un dolor molesto; breve; que quema, que arde, / "como que le quema;" frío; constante, "que no le deja descansar;" aplastastante, / "como que lo están moliendo"; como calambre; incómodo; no agudo; agudisimo; pesado, / "como que tiene un gran peso encima;" caliente; de picázon; no constante, "que va y viene;" fuerte; "como que le palpita"
What color is your urine?	¿De qué color es la orina?
Do you drink alcohol? Do you smoke?	¿Toma alcohol? ¿Fuma?

TERMS FOR PHYSICAL EXAM

EXPRESIONES PARA EL EXAMEN FISICO

Are you ready? Can you feel this? Left, right. Let me feel your pulse; . . . blood pressure. Let me see your abdomen, chest, ears, eye, forehead, heart, lungs, mouth, nose, skin, stomach, throat, tongue . . .	¿Está lísto(a)? ¿Puede sentir esto? A la izquierda, a la derecha. Permítame tomarle el pulso; ... la presión arterial. Permítame examinarle el vientre, el pecho, las orejas, el ojo, la frente, el corazón, los pulmones, la boca, la nariz, la piel, el estómago, la garganta, la lengua...
Cough. Take a deep breath. Cough again.	Tosa. Respire profundo. Tosa otra vez.